MOSBY'S
MEDICAL & NURSING
DICTIONARY

MOSBY'S
MEDICAL & NURSING
DICTIONARY

Illustrated

Thirty-two page full-color anatomy atlas

Laurence Urdang
Editor in Chief

Helen Harding Swallow
Managing Editor

THE C. V. MOSBY COMPANY

ST. LOUIS • TORONTO • LONDON 1983

MOSBY

A TRADITION OF PUBLISHING EXCELLENCE

Publisher: Thomas Allen Manning
Assistant editor: Nancy L. Mullins
Designer: Diane Beasley
Production: Jeanne Bush

The C.V. Mosby Company
11830 Westline Industrial Drive, St. Louis, Missouri 63141

Library of Congress Cataloging in Publication Data

Main entry under title:

Mosby's medical and nursing dictionary.

1. Medicine—Dictionaries. 2. Nursing—
Dictionaries. I. Urdang, Laurence. II. Swallow,
Helen Harding. III. C. V. Mosby Company.
R121.M89   610'.3'21   82-6450
ISBN 0-8016-5194-8   AACR2

AT/D/D 9 8 7 6 5 4 3 2 1   02/B/277

CONSULTING CONTRIBUTORS

Violet A. Breckbill, R.N., Ph.D.
Case Western Reserve University
University Hospitals of Cleveland
Cleveland, Ohio

Joyce E. Dains, R.N., M.S.N.
University of Texas
Houston, Texas

Donna Diers, R.N., M.S.N.
Yale University
New Haven, Connecticut

Claire M. Fagin, R.N., Ph.D.
University of Pennsylvania
Philadelphia, Pennsylvania

Marilyn E. Flood, R.N., Ph.D.
University of California Hospital
San Francisco, California

Jane Hirsch, R.N., M.S.
University of California
San Francisco, California

Eugene Johnson, Ph.D.
Washington University
St. Louis, Missouri

Judith B. Krauss, M.S.N.
Yale University
New Haven, Connecticut

Jannetta MacPhail, R.N., Ph.D., F.A.A.N.
Case Western Reserve University
University Hospitals of Cleveland
Cleveland, Ohio

Susan Molde, R.N., M.S.N.
Yale University
Yale New Haven Hospital
New Haven, Connecticut

Mary N. Moore, R.N., M.S.N.
University of Pennsylvania
Philadelphia, Pennsylvania

Helen K. Mussallem, O.C., B.N., M.A.,
Ed.D., O.St.J., LL.D., D.Sc., F.R.C.N.
Past Executive Director
Canadian Nurses Association
Ottawa, Ontario, Canada

Marie L. O'Koren, R.N., Ed.D., F.A.A.N.
University of Alabama
Birmingham, Alabama

Ginette Rodger, M.N.Adm.
Executive Director
Canadian Nurses Association
Ottawa, Ontario, Canada

Margretta M. Styles, R.N., Ed.D., F.A.A.N.
University of California
San Francisco, California

June D. Thompson, R.N., M.S.
University of Texas
Houston, Texas

STAFF

Editor in Chief:
Laurence Urdang

Managing Editor:
Helen Harding Swallow, B.A., R.N., M.S.N., CNM

Chief Writers:
Barbara Guidos, B.A., M.A.
John Bernard Landry, B.A.
Elsie Rosner, B.S., M.A.

Writers:
Janice M. Bohall, R.N. • Lawrence S. Carlton, M.D., F.A.C.P., Senior Attending Physician in Medicine, Physician Coordinator Nurse Practitioner Program, Hartford Hospital, Hartford, Connecticut • Mary Lee Evans, R.N., M.S.N., Assistant Professor, College of Nursing, University of Rhode Island, Kingston, Rhode Island • Janet I. Hirsch, R.N., M.S., Ed.D., Associate Professor of Nursing, University of Rhode Island, Kingston, Rhode Island • John Hoover, B.S., Pharmacist • Aaron Klein, B.A., M.S. • Leslie L. Lewis, L.L.B., AMWA, life fellow, associated with Rush-Presbyterian-St. Luke's Medical Center, Chicago, Illinois • Willard J. Morse, Jr., M.D., F.A.C.O.G., Attending Obstetrician-Gynecologist, Women's and Infant's Hospital, Providence, Rhode Island; Medical Director, New Beginnings Birth Center, Warwick, Rhode Island • Penelope Steiner, B.A., B.S., M.Ph., Instructor, State University of New York, Downstate Medical Center, Brooklyn, New York • Roberta E. Weisbrod, Ph.D.

Pronunciation Editor:
Antoinette Baicich d'Oronzio, B.A., M.A.

Editorial Assistants:
Elsie P. Chapman, A.S.
John J. Czepiel, B.A.
Joyce P. Donovan, B.A.
Jesse White-Fresé, A.S.C.

Typographic and systems design by:
Laurence Urdang

Programming and composition by:
Alexander Typesetting, Inc.

EDITOR'S FOREWORD

The second half of the twentieth century has seen an information explosion many times greater than that which characterized the sixteenth and seventeenth centuries in Europe. The enormous number of professionals and specialists in virtually every field of activity has contributed to new ideas, and new ideas breed new language. Communication among professionals of all persuasions and between professionals and the lay public cannot take place without language, and it is specifically in the lexicon—the word stock—of language that the communication of new ideas is documented.

Some people think that dictionaries represent the judgment of editors as to what the words of a language ought to mean. But that notion is erroneous: the meanings of words are established by the convention of their users. It is the lexicographer's profession to interpret those conventions, to examine the ways the language is used, and to describe the meanings of the words and expressions in keeping with those ways. It is an ancillary, though customary function of the compiler and editor of dictionaries to define the terms, occasionally—depending on the kind of dictionary being prepared—to show how they are pronounced, where they originated, how and under what circumstances they are used, and to give other information about them. The technique of defining, or of describing what a term means by interpreting its various senses in language that is simpler than the term being defined, is one of the chief functions of the lexicographer. The writing of definitions is, essentially, an art, not a science. To be sure, there are certain conventions that may be followed and certain structures (and strictures) to be observed, but in the final analysis, it must be the user of the dictionary who decides the success of the work.

Mosby's Medical and Nursing Dictionary is an entirely new work, not based on a long line of dictionaries published over the last decades. Such a project presents certain difficulties to its compilers and editors; on the other hand, it provides the opportunity to take a fresh look at the style of defining, unhampered by a style established dozens of years earlier that is probably inappropriate to the needs of users today. The concept of an encyclopedic format suggests thorough coverage—that is, tending toward explanatory presentation of information rather than toward dry, brief, terse definitions such as those found in ordinary dictionaries. In this sense, definitions in this dictionary usually include more information than do general dictionaries, whose users are most often satisfied with relatively succinct definitions of technical terms, understanding that if they want fuller information, they must go to specialized works.

We believe that in *Mosby's Medical and Nursing Dictionary* we have compiled, written, and edited a reference book of consummate usefulness to nurses as well as to other health professionals. Its definitions are full; the breadth of coverage is as complete as is practical while retaining a convenient size and affordable price. Every effort has been made to present the most up-to-date information in understandable English, using full sentences, without recourse to a skimpy, telegraphic style that may create ambiguity and interfere with clarity. The illustrations, tables, and appendices supplement the text.

Many, many people have been involved in the various states of preparing the dictionary, but none more important to its successful culmination than Thomas A. Manning, Publisher of the Mosby Press and special products division, The C.V. Mosby Company. We are grateful to him and to Nancy Mullins, Assistant Editor, not only for all their help but for their forbearance during some of the more difficult periods of compilation.

Laurence Urdang

FEATURES AND BENEFITS

DEFINITIONS

The definitions are written in encyclopedic style rather than in the brief, terse format found in ordinary dictionaries. The definitions usually contain more information than those in other dictionaries. This was done to be comprehensive enough to be useful, although for more in-depth information, the reader must consult more specialized textbooks and references.

VOCABULARY

Particular attention was given to selecting the most up-to-date, current terminology, such as "nursing diagnosis," "humanistic nursing model," "maternal-infant bonding," and "nursing process."

ABBREVIATIONS

Standard abbreviations for entries are included and cross-referenced to their full definitions.

ARRANGEMENT

The basic arrangement of the information in the dictionary is alphabetical, but a few words of explanation may prove helpful.

All words and phrases have been alphabetized letter-by-letter—that is, in word-by-word alphabetization, sequences are arranged in this order:

in vitro	hip replacement
in vivo	Hippocrates
inactive colon	
inanimate	

in letter-by-letter alphabetization, these sequences are arranged thus:

inactive colon	Hippocrates
inanimate	hip replacement
in vitro	
in vivo	

Entry words and phrases containing Arabic or Roman numerals follow those that are identical except for the numeral and precede those that have an alphabetic character in place of the numeral. Where there is more than one such entry, they are given in numerical order. For example:

s,	Mobitz I heart block,
S,	Mobitz II heart block,
S_1,	type I hypersensitivity,
S_2,	type II hypersensitivity,
S_3,	type III hypersensitivity,

A few chemical formulas appear as entries; these follow the same rule. For example:

CNS syndrome,	NMR,
CO,	N_2O,
CO_2,	nobelium,

For entry words that are changed drastically in spelling to form plurals or that have more than one plural, the plural or plurals are shown for spelling. The first form shown is the more common except when plurals are of more or less equal frequency. For example:

carcinoma, *pl.* **carcinomas, carcinomata.**
cortex, *pl.* **cortices.**
lentigo, *pl.* **lentigenes.**
diplococcus, *pl.* **diplococci.**

Sometimes the plural of a word is more often encountered than its singular. Such an entry is shown in its plural form, followed by the singular. For example:

bacteria, *sing.* **bacterium.**

At the ends of many entries appear other forms in which the word appears; that is, if the entry word is a noun, the adjective form is often given, if an adjective, the noun or verb form is shown. For example:

agitated, . . . **—agitate,** *v.,* **agitation,** *n.*
physiology, . . . **—physiologic, physiological,** *adj.*
therapy, . . . **—therapeutic,** *adj.,* **therapist,** *n.*

Some entries contain information about other sub-entries within their text because understanding of the subentry was felt to be clearer in the context of the main entry. In such cases, there is always a main entry listing for the subentry, with a cross reference showing where it is to be found. For example:

equine encephalitis, an arbovirus infection, characterized by inflammation of the nerve tissues of the brain and spinal cord, with high fever, headache, nausea, vomiting, myalgia and neurologic symptoms, as visual disturbances, tremor, lethargy, and disorientation. The virus is transmitted by the bite of an infected mosquito. Horses are the primary host of the particular viruses that cause the infection; man is a secondary host. **Eastern equine encephalitis (EEE)** is a severe form of the infection. It occurs along the eastern seaboard of the United States and lasts longer and causes more deaths and residual morbidity than **Western equine encephalitis (WEE),** which occurs throughout the United States and results in a mild, brief illness, as does **Venezuelan equine encephalitis (VEE),** which is common in Central and South America, Florida, and Texas.

• • •

Western equine encephalitis. See **equine encephalitis.**

Abbreviations are almost always referred to their full forms, where they are defined. In those cases when a subentry has its own abbreviation, its full form is given followed by a reference showing where its definition can be found. For example:

I.V., abbreviation for **intravenous.**
WEE, abbreviation for Western equine encephalitis. See **equine encephalitis.**

In general, the arrangement of information is straightforward, self-evident, and simple to follow.

PRONUNCIATION

Many of the words encountered in medicine and nursing are common English terms that any person can pronounce: *head, heart, stomach, vein, artery,* etc. Therefore, pronunciations are given only for those words and phrases that might present difficulty because they are unfamiliar, because their pronunciations cannot be derived from their spellings, or both.

An attempt has been made to respell such entries in a simplified system that is unambiguous. The following table equates the respelling symbols with common English words.

a	*as in*	alms, father, hurrah
æ	*as in*	at, bat
ai	*as in*	I, fight, sly
au	*as in*	out, bout, now
b	*as in*	book, robber, rub
ch	*as in*	charge, catcher, watch
d	*as in*	dog, ladder, lad
e	*as in*	elf, shelf
ei	*as in*	ate, bait, bay, care
f	*as in*	fat, offer, off
g	*as in*	good, dagger, dog
h	*as in*	happy, mohair
i	*as in*	eat, beat, bee
I	*as in*	it, bit
j	*as in*	June, major, judge
k	*as in*	keep, skip, maker, make
l	*as in*	lad, slip, silly, kill
m	*as in*	make, smart, summer, sum
n	*as in*	need, snip, dinner, din
ng	*as in*	sing
o	*as in*	cot, ox, doff
ɔ	*as in*	awful, dawn, straw
oi	*as in*	oil, coil, boy
ou	*as in*	oat, boat, go
p	*as in*	pot, spot, dipper, dip
r	*as in*	rub, bring, merry, hair
s	*as in*	set, messy, mess
sh	*as in*	sharp, cashier, mash
t	*as in*	tone, stone, better, bet
th	*as in*	thin, moth
th	*as in*	this, mother, smooth
u	*as in*	ooze, boot, too, sure
U	*as in*	cook
v	*as in*	very, river, save
w	*as in*	wait, beware
y	*as in*	year, use (yuz)
z	*as in*	zoo, razor, jazz
zh	*as in*	azure, rouge
ə	*as in*	*the unstressed vowel sound in* above, fluent, qualify, melody, locust *and as in the stressed vowel sound in* earn, fern, fir, come, cup, burn

Foreign Sounds

A   *as in French* pâté
ã   *as in French* en
æ̃   *as in French* fin
œ   *as in French* oeuf, *German* König
œ̃   *as in French* un
R   *as in any foreign r-sound, as French* roulade, *German* reisen, *Spanish* pero, perro, *Italian* caro, carro
χ   *as in German* ich, ach, *Scottish* loch
Y   *as in French* pur, *German* für

PLURALS

When a plural of a word is not a native English formation, only the spelling of the plural is shown in the headword. The following list of pronunciations of these plurals may be useful.

Endings	Example	Pronunciation
-a (ə)	**inoculum,** *pl.* **inocula.**	Inok′yUlə
-ae (i)	**vertebra,** *pl.* **vertebrae.**	vər′təbri
-ata (ətə)	**hematoma,** *pl.* **hematomata.**	hi′mətou′mətə
-des (diz)	**epulis,** *pl.* **epulides.**	Ipyu′lIdiz
-en (ən)	**Gestalt,** *pl.* **Gestalten.**	geŝhtal′tən
-es (iz)	**psychosis,** *pl.* **psychoses.**	saikou′siz
-i (ai)	**calculus,** *pl.* **calculi.**	kæl′kyUlai
-ones (ou′niz)	**comedo,** *pl.* **comedones.**	kom′Idou′niz

ILLUSTRATIONS

Nearly 400 illustrations visually supplement the definitions. A 32-page full-color anatomy atlas precedes a complete anatomy table.

APPENDIX

Complete, detailed information you can USE is found in the appendix. Extensive tables and charts on conversion rules, units of measurements, normal laboratory values, health history, RDA's, Washington Development and Denver Screening Guides, drug interaction and trade drug names cross-referenced to generic names, DSM III's directories of nursing associations in the United States and Canada, burn centers, a complete patient education section, and a unique table of communicable and infectious diseases.

CREDITS

Appreciation is expressed to the following Mosby authors whose titles provided a valuable resource toward the compilation of this dictionary:

Anthony, C.P., and Thibodeau, G.A.: Textbook of anatomy and physiology, ed. 9, 1979. • Barber, J.M., and Budassi, S.A.: Mosby's manual of emergency care: practices and procedures, 1979. • Barnard, K.E., and Erickson, M.L.: Teaching children with developmental problems: a family care approach, ed. 2, 1976. • Beck, E.W.: Mosby's atlas of functional human anatomy, 1982. • Bower, F.L., and Bevis, E.O.: Fundamentals of nursing practice: concepts, roles, and functions, 1979. • Brooks, S.M., and Paynton-Brooks, N.: The human body: structure and function in health and disease, ed. 2, 1980. • Conover, M.B.: Understanding electrocardiography: physiological and interpretive concepts, ed. 3, 1980. • Fogel, C.I., and Woods, N.F.: Health care of women: a nursing perspective, 1981. • Goth, A.: Medical pharmacology: principles and concepts, ed. 10, 1981. • Groer, M.W., and Shekleton, M.E.: Basic pathophysiology: a conceptual approach, 1979. • Hahn, A.B., Barkin, R.L., and Oestreich, S.J.K.: Pharmacology in nursing, ed. 15, 1982. • Hilt, N.E., and Cogburn, S.B.: Manual of orthopedics, 1980. • Iorio, J.: Childbirth: family centered nursing, ed. 3, 1975. • Jensen, M.D., Benson, R.C., and Bobak, I.M.: Maternity care: the nurse and the family, ed. 2, 1981. • Malasanos, L., et al.: Health assessment, ed. 2, 1981. • McClintic, J.R.: Human anatomy, 1982. • Parcel, G.S.: Basic emergency care of the sick and injured, ed. 2, 1982. • Pasquali, E.A., et al.: Mental health nursing: a bio-psycho-cultural approach, 1981. • Phibbs, B.: The human heart: a consumer's guide to cardiac care, 1982. • Phipps, W.D., Long, B.C., and Woods, N.F.: Medical-surgical nursing: concepts and clinical practice, 1979. • Schottelius, B.A., and Schottelius, D.D.: Textbook of physiology, ed. 18, 1978. • Smith, A.L.: Microbiology and pathology, ed. 12, 1980. • Tucker, S.M., et al.: Patient care standards, ed. 2; 1980. • U.C.S.F.: Mosby's manual of clinical nursing procedures, 1981. • Whaley, L.F., and Wong, D.L.: Nursing care of infants and children, 1979. • Williams, S.R.: Nutrition and diet therapy, ed. 4, 1981. • Young, C.G., and Austrin, M.G.: Learning medical terminology step by step, ed. 4, 1979.

We acknowledge the following additional sources of information and material used:

American Burn Association: Burn care services in the United States, Rockville, Md. Department of Health and Human Services. • American Cancer Society: Cancer facts and figures (1982), 1982, New York, The Society. • American Heart Association: Heart facts, Dallas, Texas, 1982, The Association. Reprinted with permission, American Heart Association. • The American Hospital Association: A patient's bill of rights, 1975, Chicago, The Association. • American Nurses Association: State and territorial boards of nursing, Kansas City, Mo., The Association. • American Psychiatric Association: DMS III classification axes I and II categories and codes, Washington, D.C., The Association. • American Society for Psychoprophylaxis in Obstetrics of Los Angeles, Inc.: The A.S.P.O. Lamaze review sheet, Pacific Palisades, California. • Canadian Nurses Association: Directory of professional nursing associations, The Canadian Nurse, Ottawa, Canada. • Canadian Pharmaceutical Association: Poison control centers in Canada; in Compendium of pharmaceuticals and specialties, ed. 16, Ontario, Canada, 1981, The Association. • Church, C.F., and Church, H.N.: Bowes and Church's food values of portions commonly used, ed. 12, Philadelphia, J.B. Lippincott Co. • National Clearinghouse for Poison Control Centers: Poison control centers in the United States and territories, Rockville, Maryland, U.S. Department of Health and Human Services. • Nursing '81 Career Directory: Nursing '81, Springhouse, Pennsylvania, 1981, Intermed Communications, Inc. Reprinted with permission from Nursing '81 Career Directory Nursing 1981. Copyright 1981 Intermed Communications, Inc. All rights reserved. • Teasdale, G. and Jennette, B.: Assessment of coma and impaired consciousness: a practical scale, Lancet 2:81-84, 1974. • Vaughan, V.C. and McKay, R.J.: Nelson's textbook of pediatrics, ed. 10, Philadelphia, 1979, W.B. Saunders Co.

CONTENTS

MOSBY'S
MEDICAL & NURSING
DICTIONARY

A

a, symbol for **arterial blood.**

A, symbol for **alveolar gas.**

a-, a combining form meaning 'without, not': *abacterial, abaptiston, abasia.*

AA, **1.** abbreviation for **Alcoholics Anonymous. 2.** abbreviation for **achievement age.**

AACCN, abbreviation for **American Association of Critical Care Nurses.**

AACN, abbreviation for **American Association of Colleges of Nursing.**

AAIN, abbreviation for **American Association of Industrial Nurses.**

AAMC, abbreviation for **American Association of Medical Colleges.**

AAN, abbreviation for **American Academy of Nursing.**

AANA, abbreviation for **American Association of Nurse Anesthetists.**

AANN, abbreviation for **American Association of Neurological Nurses.**

AANNT, abbreviation for **American Association of Nephrology Nurses and Technicians,** an organization of nurses and technicians working in the fields of dialysis and renal disease.

AAPA, abbreviation for **American Academy of Physicians' Assistants.**

A.A.P.B., abbreviation for **American Association of Pathologists and Bacteriologists.**

A.A.P.M.R., abbreviation for **American Academy of Physical Medicine and Rehabilitation.**

AART, abbreviation for **American Association for Respiratory Therapy.**

AAUP, abbreviation for **American Association of University Professors.**

AAV, abbreviation for **adenoassociated virus.**

ab-, a combining form meaning 'from, off, away from': *abarthrosis, abarticulation, abaxial.* Also **abs-.**

abalienation (æbeil′yənei′ʃən), **1.** a state of physical deterioration or mental decay. **2.** a state of insanity. — **abalienate,** *v.,* **abalienated,** *adj.*

abandonment of care, (in law) wrongful cessation of the provision of care to a patient, usually by a physician.

abarthrosis (æb′arθrou′sıs). See **diarthrosis.**

abarticular (æb′artık′yulər), **1.** of or pertaining to a condition that does not affect a joint. **2.** of or pertaining to a site or structure remote from a joint.

abasia (əbei′ʒhə), the inability to walk, as in paralytic abasia which paralyzes the leg muscles. — **abasic, abatic,** *adj.*

abaxial (æbæk′sıəl), **1.** of or pertaining to a position outside the axis of a body or structure. **2.** of or pertaining to a position at the opposite extremity of a structure.

Abbokinase, a trade name for a plasminogen activator (urokinase).

Abbot pump (æb′ət), a small portable pump that can be adjusted and finely calibrated to deliver precise amounts of medication in solution through an intravenous infusion set. It is similar to a Harvard pump, but the flow rate may be increased or decreased by smaller increments.

ABC, abbreviation for **aspiration biopsy cytology.**

abdomen (æb′dəmən, æbdou′mən), the portion of the body between the thorax and the pelvis. The abdominal cavity contains the lower portion of the esophagus, the stomach, the intestines, the liver, the spleen, and the pancreas. The walls of the abdominal cavity are lined with the parietal layer of the peritoneum, a serous membrane. The covering, or outermost layer of each organ, is formed by the visceral layer of the peritoneum. A small amount of serous fluid in the space between the membranous layers allows the organs to slide freely, as in the normal process of digestion, evacuation, and breathing. Also called *Informal.* **belly.** — **abdominal,** *adj.*

abdominal actinomycosis. See **actinomycosis.**

abdominal aorta, the portion of the descending aorta that passes from the aortic hiatus of the diaphragm into the abdomen, descending ventral to the vertebral column, and ending at the fourth lumbar vertebra where it divides into the two common iliac arteries. It supplies many different parts of the body, as the testes, ovaries, kidneys, and stomach. Its branches are the celiac, superior mesenteric, inferior mesenteric, middle suprarenals, renals, testicular, ovarian, inferior phrenics, lumbars, middle sacral, and common iliacs. See also **descending aorta.** Compare **thoracic aorta.**

abdominal aponeurosis, the conjoined tendons of the oblique and transverse muscles of the abdomen.

abdominal bandage, a broad supportive bandage commonly used after abdominal surgery.

abdominal binder, a bandage or elasticized wrap that is applied around the lower part of the torso to support the abdomen. An abdominal binder is sometimes applied after abdominal surgery to decrease discomfort, thereby increasing a patient's ability to begin ambulatory activities and accelerate convalescence. A kind of abdominal binder is **scultetus binder.**

abdominal delivery, the delivery of a child through a surgical incision in the abdomen. The procedure performed may be any of the several kinds of Caesarean section.

abdominal fistula, an abnormal passage from an abdominal organ to the surface of the body. In a colostomy, a passage from the bowel to an opening on the surface of the abdomen is created surgically.

abdominal hernia, a hernia in which a loop of bowel protrudes through the abdominal musculature, often through the site of an old surgical scar. Also called **ventral hernia.** See also **hernia.**

abdominal pain, acute or chronic localized or diffuse pain in the abdominal cavity. Abdominal pain is a significant complaint because its cause may require immediate surgical or medical intervention. The most common causes of severe abdominal pain are inflammation, perforation of an intra-abdominal structure, circulatory obstruction, intestinal or ureteral obstruction, or rupture of an organ located within the abdomen. Specific conditions include appendicitis, perforated gastric ulcer, strangulated hernia, superior mesenteric arterial thrombosis, and small and large bowel obstruction. The differential diagnosis of the cause of acute abdominal pain requires localization and characterization of the pain by means of light and deep percussion, auscultation and palpation and by abdominal, rectal, or pelvic examination. Direct physical examination may be supplemented by various laboratory and radiologic examinations. Aspiration of peritoneal fluid for bacteriological and chemical evaluation is sometimes indicated. Conditions producing acute abdominal pain that may require surgery include appendicitis, acute or severe and chronic diverticulitis, acute and chronic cholecystitis, cholelithiasis, acute pancreatitis, perforation of a peptic ulcer, carious intestinal obstructions, abdominal aortic aneurysms, and trauma affecting any of the abdominal organs. Gynecological causes of acute abdominal pain that may require surgery include: acute pelvic inflammatory disease, ruptured ovarian cyst, and ectopic pregnancy. Abdominal pain associated with pregnancy may be caused by the weight of the enlarged uterus; rotation, stretching or compression of the round ligament; or squeezing or displacement of the bowel. In addition, uterine contractions associated with premature labor may produce severe abdominal pain. Chronic recurrent abdominal pain may be psychosomatic in origin or simply the result of overeating or aerophagia. When the symptoms are recurrent, an organic cause is considered. Organic sources of abdominal pain include peptic ulcer, hiatus hernia, gastritis, chronic cholecystitis and cholelithiasis, chronic pancreatitis, pancreatic carcinoma, chronic diverticulitis, intermittent low-grade intestinal obstruction and functional indigestion. Some systemic conditions may be responsible for abdominal pain. Examples of these include systemic lupus erythematosus, lead poisoning, hypercalcemia, sickle cell anemia, diabetic acidosis, porphyria, tabes dorsalis, and black widow spider poisoning.

abdominal pregnancy, an extrauterine pregnancy in which the conceptus develops in the abdominal cavity after being extruded from the fimbriated end of the Fallopian tube or through a defect in the tube or uterus. The placenta may implant on the abdominal or visceral peritoneum. Abdominal pregnancy may be suspected when the abdomen has enlarged but the uterus has remained small for the length of gestation. Abdominal pregnancies constitute approximately 2 per cent of ectopic pregnancies and approximately .01 per cent of all pregnancies. The condition results in perinatal death of the fetus in approximately 90 per cent of cases, maternal death in approximately 6 per cent. Because of its rarity, the condition may be unsuspected, and diagnosis is often delayed. Ultrasound or x-ray visualization showing gas in the maternal bowel below the fetus is diagnostic of the condition. Surgical removal of the placenta, sac, and embryo or fetus is necessary, but the procedure is often complicated by massive bleeding, and, as the placenta tends to adhere firmly to the peritoneum and to the bowel, complete removal is seldom possible. Postoperative sequelae may include necrotization of retained placental tissue, infection, continued bleeding, and sterility.

abdominal pulse, the pulse of the abdominal aorta.

abdominal reflex, a superficial neurological reflex obtained by firmly stroking the skin of the abdomen, normally resulting in a brisk contraction of abdominal muscles in which the umbilicus moves toward the site of the stimulus. This reflex is lost in diseases of the pyramidal tract. See also **superficial reflex.**

abdominal surgery, any operation which involves an incision into the abdomen, usually performed under general anesthesia. Before surgery a complete blood count, a type and cross-match of the blood, and a urinalysis are done. Often, an enema is given. The skin is shaved and cleansed from the nipple line to the pubis. A barbiturate is often given at bedtime; food and fluids by mouth are forbidden after midnight. Shortly before surgery a barbiturate or tranquilizer and a narcotic are usually given, along with an anticholinergic agent, as atropine. Postoperatively, the nurse ensures that the airway is open, checks tubes and catheters, connects drainage tubes to collection containers, and checks the dressing for excessive bleeding or drainage. Close observation of vital signs is essential. A careful record is kept of fluid intake and output. The patient is turned and is helped to cough and breathe deeply every hour. Medication is given as needed for relief from pain. Some kinds of abdominal surgery are **appendectomy, cholecystectomy, colostomy, gastrectomy, laparotomy.** See also **acute abdomen.**

abdominal tenaculum. See **tenaculum.**

abdomino-, a combining form meaning 'pertaining to the abdomen': *abdominocentesis, abdominoscopy, abdominothoracic.*

abdominocentesis (æbdom'ınousenti'sıs). See **paracentesis.**

abdominocyesis (æbdom'ınousaii'sıs), an abdominal pregnancy.

abdominoscopy (æbdom'ınos'kəpi), a procedure for examining the contents of the peritoneum in which an electrically illuminated tubular device is passed through a trocar into the abdominal cavity. See also **laparoscopy.**

abducens nerve, the sixth cranial nerve which originates in the pons in the brainstem. It is a motor nerve controlling the movement of the lateral rectus muscle of the eye.

abducent nerve, either of a pair of cranial nerves essential for lateral eye movements. They branch to the rectus lateralis and pass through a notch below the posterior clinoid process, connecting to two areas in the brain. Also called **nervus abducens, sixth nerve.**

abduction, movement of a limb away from the body. Compare **adduction.**

abduction boots, a pair of orthopedic casts for the lower extremities, available in both short-leg and long-leg configurations, with a bar incorporated at ankle-level to provide hip abduction. Abduction boots are used for postoperative positioning and immobilization after hip adductor releases and to promote proper positioning during healing after surgery to repair structures in the lower extremities.

abductor (æbdək'tər), a structure that draws another part away from the midline of the body, as a muscle that abducts. Compare **adductor.**

Abernethy's sarcoma (æb'ərni'thiz), a malignant neoplasm of fat cells, usually occurring on the trunk.

aberrant (æber'ənt), **1.** of or pertaining to a wandering from the usual or expected course, as various ducts, nerves, and vessels in the body. **2.** (in botany and zoology) of or pertaining to an abnormal individual, as certain atypical members of a species.

aberrant ductule, a rudimentary structure in the male, situated near the epididymis, that consists of vestigial remains of the caudal part of the embryonic mesonephric tubules. A similar vestigial structure, the paroophoron, is found in the female. See also **appendix epididymis, paradidymis.**

aberrant goiter, an enlargement of a supernumerary or ectopic thyroid gland.

abetalipoproteinemia (əbei'təlaip'ouprou'tini'miə), a rare inherited disorder of fat metabolism, characterized by acanthocytosis, low or absent serum betalipoproteins, and hypocholesterolemia. In severe cases steatorrhea, ataxia, nystagmus, motor incoordination, and retinitis pigmentosa occur.

abient (æb'iənt), characterized by a tendency to move away from stimuli. Compare **adient.** – **abience,** *n.*

abiogenesis, spontaneous generation; the theory that organic life can originate from inanimate matter. Compare **biogenesis.** – **abiogenetic,** *adj.*

abiosis (æb'iou'sis), a nonviable condition or a situation that is incompatible with life. – **abiotic,** *adj.*

abiotrophy (æb'iot'rəfi), a premature depletion of vitality or the deterioration of certain cells and tissues, especially those involved in genetic degenerative diseases. – **abiotrophic,** (æb'iətrou'fık) *adj.*

ablation (æblei'shən), an amputation, an excision of any part of the body, or a removal of a growth or harmful substance.

ablatio placentae. See **abruptio placenta.**

ablepsia (əblep'siə), the condition of being blind. Also called **ablepsy.**

abnerval current, an electric current that passes from a nerve to and through muscle.

abnormal behavior, maladaptive acts or activities detrimental to the individual and to society. The acts range from the transitory inability to cope with a stressful situation to persistent bizarre or destructive behavior or total disorientation and withdrawal from the realities of everyday life. See also **behavior disorder.**

abnormal psychology, (in psychology) the study of mental disorders and maladaptive behavior, including neuroses and psychoses, and of normal phenomena that are not completely understood, like dreams and altered states of consciousness.

ABO blood groups, the most important of several systems for classifying human blood based on the antigenic components of the red blood cell. The ABO blood group is identified by the presence or absence of two different antigens, A or B, on the surface of the erythrocyte. The four blood types in this grouping, A, B, AB, and O, are determined by and named for these antigens. Type AB indicates the presence of both antigens; type O the absence of both. Corresponding antibodies, anti-A, and anti-B agglutinins, can be found in the plasma of type O blood. The plasma components of type A and type B blood are, respectively, devoid of anti-A and anti-B agglutinins; both agglutinins are absent from type AB blood plasma. In addition to its significant role in blood banks and transfusion therapy, the ABO blood grouping contributes to forensic medicine, genetics, and, together with the less important blood groups, to anthropology and legal medicine. See also **Rh factor, transfusion.**

aboiement (ʌbwamã'), an involuntary making of abnormal sounds.

aborted systole, a contraction of the heart that is usually premature and is not associated with a peripheral pulse.

abortient (əbɔrˈs̆hənt). See **abortifacient.**

abortifacient (əbɔrˈtɪfeiˈs̆hənt), **1.** producing abortion. **2.** an agent that effects abortion.

abortion, spontaneous or induced termination of pregnancy before the fetus has developed enough to be expected to live if born. See also **incomplete abortion, induced abortion, spontaneous abortion, therapeutic abortion.**

abortion-on-demand, a concept promoted by pro-choice health advocates that it is the right of a pregnant woman to have an abortion performed at her request. That right may be limited by time of gestation, or it may pertain to any period of gestation.

abortus fever, a form of brucellosis, the only one endemic to North America. It is caused by *Brucella abortus,* an organism so named because it causes abortion in cows. Infection in humans results from the ingestion of contaminated milk from cows infected with *B. abortus,* from handling infected meat, or from skin contact with the excreta of living infected animals. Streptomycin and tetracycline are usually prescribed together as treatment. Also called **Rio Grande fever.** See also **brucellosis.**

abouchement (æbus̆hmañˈ), the junction of a small blood vessel with a large blood vessel.

aboulia. See **abulia.**

abrachia (əbreiˈkiə), the absence of arms. — **abrachial,** *adj.*

abrasion, a scraping, or rubbing away of a surface by friction. Abrasion may be the result of trauma, as a skinned knee; of therapy, as in dermabrasion of the skin for removal of scar tissue; or of normal function, as the wearing down of a tooth by mastication. Compare **laceration.** See also **friction burn.** — **abrade,** *v.,* **abrasive,** *adj.*

abreaction (æbˈriækˈs̆hən), an emotional release resulting from mentally reliving or from bringing into consciousness, through the process of catharsis, a long-repressed, painful experience. See also **catharsis.**

abrosia (əbrouˈz̆hə), the act of fasting or abstaining from food.

abruptio placenta, separation of the placenta implanted in normal position in a pregnancy of twenty weeks or more or during labor prior to delivery of the fetus. It occurs approximately once in two hundred births, and, because it often results in severe hemorrhage, it is a significant cause of maternal and fetal mortality. Hypertension and pre-eclampsia are associated with increased rates of occurrence, but in many cases there is no explanation. Complete separation brings about immediate death of the fetus. Bleeding from the site of separation causes abdominal pain, uterine tenderness, and tetanic uterine contraction. Bleeding may be concealed within the uterus or may be evident externally, sometimes as sudden massive hemorrhage. Shock and death can come in minutes. Caesarean section must be performed immediately and rapidly. Extensive extravasation of blood within the wall of the uterus may deplete fibrinogen, prolong clotting time, bring about intractable bleeding, and, by damaging the musculature of the uterus, prevent the uterus from contracting well after delivery. Hysterectomy may be necessary to prevent exsanguination. Partial separation may occasion little bleeding and may not interfere with fetal oxygenation. If the pregnancy is near term, labor may be permitted or induced by means of amniotomy. A premature pregnancy may be allowed to continue under close observation of the mother at bed rest. The nurse must be alert to the possibility that bleeding is present but concealed internally and that if all the blood can escape, there may be little pain. Also called **ablatio placentae, accidental hemorrhage.** Compare **placenta previa.** See also **Couvelaire uterus.**

abscess, a cavity containing pus and surrounded by inflamed tissue, formed as a result of suppuration in a localized infection (characteristically, a staphylococcal infection). Healing usually occurs when an abscess drains or is incised. If an abscess is deep in tissue, drainage is effected by means of a sinus tract that connects it to the surface.

absent without leave (AWOL), (in psychiatry) describing a patient who runs away from a psychiatric facility.

absolute alcohol. See **dehydrated alcohol.**

absolute cephalopelvic disproportion. See **cephalopelvic disproportion.**

absolute growth, the total increase in size of an organism or a particular organ or part, as the limbs, head, or trunk.

absolute refractory period. See **refractory period.**

absorb, the act of engorging or taking up various substances, as the tissues of the kidneys and intestines absorb fluids.

absorbable gauze, a gauzelike material, produced from oxidized cellulose, that can be absorbed. It is applied directly to bleeding tissue for hemostasis.

absorbed dose, (in radiotherapy) the energy imparted by ionizing radiation per unit mass of irradiated material at the place of interest. The unit of absorbed dose is the rad, which equals 100 ergs per gram.

absorbent dressing, a dressing of any material applied to a wound or incision to absorb secretions.

absorbent gauze, a gauze for absorbing fluids. The form, weight, and use vary. Gauze may be a fine fabric in rolled single layers for spiral bandages, or it may be a thick, many-layered pad for a sterile pressure dressing.

absorption, **1.** the incorporation of matter by other matter through chemical, molecular, or physical action, as the dissolving of a gas in a liquid or the taking up of a liquid by a porous solid. **2.** (in physiology) the passage of substances across and into tissues, as the passage of digested food molecules into intestinal cells or the passage of liquids into kidney tubules. Kinds of absorption in physiology are **agglutinin absorption, cutaneous absorption, external absorption, interstitial absorption, intestinal absorption, parenteral absorption, pathologic absorption. 3.** (in radiology) the absorption of radiant energy by living or nonliving matter with which the radiation reacts.

absorption fever. *Obsolete.* See **puerperal fever.**

abstinence, voluntary avoidance of any substance or the performance of any act for which the person has an appetite.

abstract, a condensed scientific article, literary piece, or address.

abstract thinking, the final stage in the development of the cognitive thought processes in the child. During this phase thought is characterized by adaptability, flexibility, and the use of abstractions and generalizations. Problem solving is accomplished by drawing logical conclusions from a set of observations, as making hypotheses and testing them. This type of thinking appears from about 12 to 15 years of age, usually after some degree of education. Compare **concrete thinking, syncretic thinking.**

abulia, aboulia (əbu'liə), a loss of the ability or a reduced capacity to function voluntarily or to make decisions.

abuse, improper use of equipment, a substance, or a service, as a drug or program, either intentionally or unintentionally. See also **drug abuse.**

abuse of process, (in law) a civil action for damages in which it is alleged that the legal process has been used in a manner not contemplated by law. This action might be brought by a health practitioner attempting to countersue a patient or by a psychiatric patient attempting to demonstrate wrongful confinement.

a.c. (in prescriptions) abbreviation for *ante cibum,* a Latin phrase meaning 'before meals.' The times of administration are commonly 7 A.M., 11 A.M., and 5 P.M.

Ac, symbol for **actinium.**

AC, abbreviation for **alternating current.**

ac-. See **ad-.**

academic ladder, the hierarchy of faculty appointments in a university through which a faculty member must advance from instructor, to assistant professor, associate professor, and, finally, to professor.

acampsia (əkæmp'siə), a condition in which a joint becomes rigid. See also **ankylosis.**

acantha (əkæn'thə), a spine or a spinous projection. – **acanthoid,** *adj.*

acantho-, a combining form meaning 'thorny or spiky': *acanthesthesia, acanthoid, acantholysis.*

acanthocyte (əkæn'thəsait), an abnormal red blood cell

with spurlike projections giving it a thorny appearance. Large numbers are present in abetalipoproteinemia; fewer occur in cirrhosis and in certain malabsorption syndromes. Compare **burr cell.** See also **abetalipoproteinemia, acanthocytosis.**

acanthocytosis (əkæn'thousaitou'sis), the abnormal presence of acanthocytes in the circulating blood system, most commonly associated with abetalipoproteinemia in which as many as 80 per cent of the erythrocytes are acanthocytes. Also called **Bassen-Kornzweig syndrome.** See also **abetalipoproteinemia.**

acanthoma (æk'ænthou'mə), any benign or malignant tumor arising from the prickle cell layer of the epidermis.

acanthoma adenoides cysticum. See **trichoepithelioma.**

acanthoma verrucosa seborrheica. See **seborrheic keratosis.**

acanthosis (æk'ənthou'sis), an abnormal thickening of the prickle cell layer of the skin, as in eczema and psoriasis. See also **acanthosis nigricans, epidermis.** – **acanthotic,** *adj.*

acanthosis nigricans, a skin disease characterized by hyperpigmented, warty lesions of the axillae and other body folds. There are benign and malignant forms, the latter associated with cancers of the gastrointestinal tract. See also **acanthosis.**

acardia (eikar'diə), a rare congenital anomaly in which the heart is absent. It is sometimes seen in a conjoined twin whose survival until birth depended upon the circulatory system of its twin. – **acardiac,** *adj.*

acardius (ækar'diəs), **acardiacus** (æk'ardai'əkəs), an acardiac fetus. Kinds of acardius include **acardius acephalus, acardius acormus, acardius amorphus.** Also called **fetus acardiacus.**

acardius acephalus, an acardiac fetus that lacks a head and most of the upper part of the body.

acardius acormus, an acardiac fetus that has a grossly defective trunk.

acardius amorphus, an acardiac fetus with a rudimentary body that does not resemble the normal form. Also called **acardius anceps.**

acariasis (æk'ərai'əsis), any disease caused by an acarid, as scrub typhus, which is caused by trombiculid mites.

acarid (æk'ərid), one of the many mites that are members of the order Acarina which includes a great number of parasitic and free-living organisms. Most are yet undescribed, but several types are of medical interest because they infect humans. The kinds associated with disease are those acting as intermediate hosts of pathogenic agents, those that directly cause skin or tissue damage, and those that cause loss of blood or tissue fluids. Important as vectors of scrub typhus and other rickettsial agents are the six-legged larvae of trombiculid mites, which are parasitic of humans, many other mammals, and birds.

acaro-, a combining form meaning 'pertaining to mites': *acarodermatitis, acaroid, acarophobia.*

accelerated hypertension. See **malignant hypertension.**

acceleration, an increase in the speed or velocity of an object or reaction. Compare **deceleration.** —**accelerator,** *n.*

acceleration phase, (in obstetrics) the first period of active labor, characterized by an increased rate of dilatation of the cervical os as charted on a Friedman curve.

acceptable daily intake (ADI), the maximum amount of any substance that can be safely ingested by a human. Ingestion of amounts in excess of the ADI may cause toxic effects.

acceptor, 1. an organism that receives from another person or organism living tissue, as transfused blood or a transplanted organ. 2. a substance or compound that combines with a part of another substance or compound. Compare **donor.**

accessory, 1. a supplement employed chiefly for convenience or for safety, as the electric elevator mechanisms for hospital beds. 2. (in anatomy) a structure that serves one of the main anatomical systems, as the accessory sex organs in men and women or the accessory organs of the skin, as the hair, the nails, and the skin glands.

accessory chromosome, an unpaired X or Y sex chromosome. See also **monosome.**

accessory muscle, a relatively rare anatomic duplication of a muscle which may appear anywhere in the muscular system. The most common sign associated with an accessory muscle is the appearance of a soft tissue mass. Differential diagnosis without surgical intervention and exploration is difficult because of the similar appearance of some tumors or soft tissue masses, as ganglia. The appearance of the soft tissue mass associated with an accessory muscle may be transient or it may be constant, depending on the location of the accessory muscle in relation to motion. In many individuals with accessory muscles, specific treatment is not indicated unless the accessory muscle interferes with normal function.

accessory nerve, either of a pair of cranial nerves essential for speech, swallowing, and certain movements of the head and shoulders. Each nerve has a cranial and a spinal portion, communicates with certain cervical nerves, and connects to the nucleus ambiguus of the brain. Also called **eleventh nerve, nervus accessorius, spinal accessory nerve.**

accessory pancreatic duct, a small duct opening into the pancreatic duct or duodenum near the mouth of the common bile duct.

accessory phrenic nerve, the nerve that joins the phrenic nerve at the root of the neck or in the thorax, forming a loop around the subclavian vein. It may arise from the nerve to the subclavius or from the fifth cervical nerve. Resection of the phrenic nerve to immobilize the diaphragm may be only partially successful if the accessory phrenic nerve is not also resected. Compare **phrenic nerve.**

accessory sinus of the nose. See **nasal sinus.**

ACCH, abbreviation for **Association for the Care of Children's Health.**

accidental hemorrhage. See **abruptio placentae.**

acclimate (əklaɪ′mɪt, æk′lɪmeɪt), **acclimatize** (əklaɪ′-mətaɪz), the process of adjusting physiologically to a different climate, especially to changes in altitude and in temperature. —**acclimation, acclimatization,** *n.*

accommodation, 1. the state or process of adapting or adjusting one thing or set of things to another. 2. the continuous process or effort of the individual to adapt or adjust to his surroundings in order to maintain a state of homeostasis, both physiologically and psychologically. 3. (in sociology) the reciprocal reconciliation of conflicts between individuals or groups concerning habits and customs, usually through a process of compromise, arbitration, or negotiation. Also called **adjustment.** Compare **adaptation.**

accommodation reflex, an adjustment of the eyes for near vision, consisting of pupillary constriction, convergence of the eyes, and increased convexity of the lens. Also called **ciliary reflex.** See also **pupillary reflex.**

accomplishment quotient, a numerical evaluation of a person's achievement age compared to mental age, expressed as a ratio multiplied by 100. See also **achievement quotient, intelligence quotient.**

accouchement (əkuʃ′mant), *Archaic.* childbirth; obstetric delivery.

accouchement forcé (fɔrseɪ′), a dangerous, out-of-date obstetric operation in which the fetus is rapidly delivered through a forcibly dilated cervix.

accreditation, a process whereby a professional association or nongovernmental agency grants recognition to a school or institution for demonstrated ability in a special area of practice or training, as the accreditation of hospitals by the Joint Commission of Accreditation for Hospitals or of nursing schools by the National League for Nursing. Compare **certification, licensure.**

accrementition (æk′rɪmentɪʃ′ən), growth or increase of size by the addition of similar tissue or material, as in cellular division, simple fission, budding, or germination.

accretio cordis (əkri′ʃiou), an abnormal condition in which there is an adhesion of the pericardium to a structure around the heart.

accretion (əkri′ʃən), 1. growth or increase by the addition of material of the same nature that is already present. 2. the adherence or growing together of parts that are normally separated. 3. the accumulation of foreign material, especially within a cavity. —**accrete,** *v.,* **accretive,** *adj.*

accretionary growth, an increase in size resulting from the accumulation of new tissue through the process of mitosis or the addition of material similar to that which is already present.

acecarbromal (æs'əkarbrou'məl), a sedative-hypnotic.
■ INDICATION: It is prescribed in the treatment of anxiety.
■ CONTRAINDICATIONS: Known hypersensitivity to this drug or to other bromides prohibits its use.
■ ADVERSE EFFECTS: Among the more serious adverse reactions are bromism, dizziness, skin rash, and gastrointestinal disturbances.

acedia (əsi'diə), a condition of listlessness and a form of melancholy, marked by indifference and sluggish mental processes.

acelius (eisil'iəs), an individual without a body cavity.

acentric (eisen'trik), 1. the characteristic of having no center. 2. (in genetics) describing a chromosome fragment that has no centromere.

-aceous, a combining form meaning 'pertaining to or of the nature of' something specified: *coriaceous, foliaceous, testaceous.*

acephalo-, a combining form meaning 'having no head': *acephalobrachia, acephalus, acephaly.*

acephalobrachia (æsef'əloubrei'kiə), a congenital anomaly in which a fetus lacks both arms and a head.

acephalus (æsef'ələs), a fetus lacking a properly developed head. — **acephalous,** *adj.*

acephaly, acephalia, acephalism, a congenital defect in which the head is absent or not properly developed. — **acephalic,** *adj.*

acet-, a combining form meaning 'vinegar': *acetify, acetoin, acetyl.*

acetabulum (æs'ıtæb'yələm), *pl.* **acetabula.** the large, cup-shaped, articular cavity at the juncture of the ilium, the ischium, and the pubis, containing the ball-shaped head of the femur.

acetaminophen (əset'əmin'əfin), an analgesic and antipyretic containing no aspirin.
■ INDICATIONS: It is often prescribed for mild to moderate pain and fever.
■ CONTRAINDICATION: Known hypersensitivity to acetaminophen prohibits its use.
■ ADVERSE EFFECTS: Among the most serious adverse reactions are anaphylaxis and hemolytic anemia. Overdosage can result in fatal hepatic necrosis.

acetate kinase, an enzyme that catalyzes the transfer of a phosphate group from adenosine triphosphate to acetate. Also called **acetokinase.**

acetazolamide (æs'ıtəzou'ləmaɪd), a carbonic anhydrase inhibitor.
■ INDICATIONS: It is prescribed for edema, glaucoma, and epilepsy (primarily petit mal).
■ CONTRAINDICATIONS: Hyponatremia, hypocalemia, se-

vere liver or kidney disease or dysfunction, Addison's disease, or known hypersensitivity to this drug prohibits its use.
■ ADVERSE EFFECTS: Among the most serious adverse reactions are anorexia, acidosis, hyperuricemia and crystalluria. Gastrointestinal disturbances and lethargy are common.

Acetest (æs'ətest'), a trademark for a product used to test for the presence of abnormal quantities of acetone in the urine of patients with diabetes mellitus or other metabolic disorders. A large quantity of acetone causes a rapid change in the color of the Acetest tablet. See also **acidosis, ketone bodies.**

acetic acid (əsi'tık, əset'ık), a clear, colorless, pungent liquid that is miscible with water, alcohol, glycerin, and ether and that constitutes 3 to 5 per cent of vinegar. Acetic acid is produced commercially by the destructive distillation of wood or from methyl alcohol, or it may be converted from ethyl alcohol by the action of many aerobic bacteria. Various concentrations of acetic acid are used in the manufacture of plastics, dyes, insecticides, cellulose acetate, photographic chemicals, and pharmaceutical preparations, including vaginal jellies and antimicrobial solutions for the treatment of superficial infections of the external auditory canal. Also called **ethanoic acid.**

acetic fermentation, the production of acetic acid or vinegar from a weak alcoholic solution.

acetoacetic acid (æs'ıtouəsi'tık, əsi'touəsi'tık), a colorless, oily compound produced in the body by the metabolism of lipids and pyruvates. It is excreted in trace amounts in normal urine and in elevated levels in diabetes mellitus, especially in ketoacidosis. Acetoacetic acid, a ketone body, is also increased during starvation owing to incomplete oxidation of fatty acids. Soluble in water, alcohol, and ether, acetoacetic acid decomposes at temperatures below 100°C to acetone and carbon dioxide. Also called **acetone carboxylic acid, acetylacetic acid, diacetic acid.**

acetohexamide, a sulfanylurea oral antidiabetic.
■ INDICATION: It is prescribed in the treatment of adult onset diabetes mellitis.
■ CONTRAINDICATIONS: Unstable diabetes, severe liver or kidney dysfunction, or known hypersensitivity to this drug or to other sulfanylureas prohibits its use.
■ ADVERSE EFFECTS: Among the most serious adverse reactions are blood dyscrasias, hypoglycemia, and allergic reactions. Gastrointestinal disturbances are common.

acetokinase (æs'ıtoukai'neis, əsi'toukai'neis). See **acetate kinase.**

acetol kinase, an enzyme that catalyzes the transfer of a phosphate group from adenosine triphosphate to hydroxyacetone.

acetone (æs'ıtoun), a colorless, aromatic, volatile liquid found in small amounts in normal urine and in larger quantities in the urine of diabetics. Commercially prepared acetone is used to clean the skin before injections, but prolonged exposure to the compound can be irritating. It also has many varied industrial uses.

acetone bodies. See **ketone bodies.**

acetone carboxylic acid (kar'boksıl'ık). See **acetoacetic acid.**

acetophenazine maleate, a phenothiazine tranquilizer.
- INDICATION: It is prescribed in the treatment of psychotic disorders.
- CONTRAINDICATIONS: Parkinson's disease, the concurrent administration of central nervous system depressants, liver or renal dysfunction, severe hypotension, or known hypersensitivity to any phenothiazine prohibits its use.
- ADVERSE EFFECTS: Among the more serious adverse effects are hypotension, liver toxicity, a variety of extrapyramidal reactions, blood dyscrasias, and hypersensitivity reactions.

acetophenetidin. See **phenacetin.**

acetylacetic acid (əsi'tıləsi'tık, æs'ıtıləsi'tık). See **acetoacetic acid.**

acetylcarbromal. See **acecarbromal.**

acetylcholine chloride, a miotic.
- INDICATIONS: It is prescribed to cause rapid miosis during ocular surgery and to reverse the effects of cycloplegic and mydriatic medications.
- CONTRAINDICATIONS: There are no known contraindications.
- ADVERSE EFFECTS: Systemic effects of acetylcholine may occur and opacities of the lens of the eye may be caused by a hypertonic solution of the drug.

acetylcoenzyme A (acetyl-CoA) (əsi'tılkouen'zaim, æs'ıtılkouen'zaim), a molecule that is formed in the course of several important metabolic processes. The formation of acetylcoenzyme A is the critical intermediate step between anaerobic glycolysis and the Krebs' citric acid cycle.

acetylsalicylic acid (əsi'təlsæl'ısıl'ık). See **aspirin.**

ACh, abbreviation for **acetylcholine.**

achalasia (æk'əlei'ẑhə), an abnormal condition characterized by the inability of a muscle to relax, particularly the cardiac sphincter of the stomach.

Achard-Thiers syndrome (æẑh'artirz'), a hormonal disorder seen in postmenopausal women with diabetes, characterized by growth of body hair in a masculine distribution. Treatment includes mechanical removal or bleaching of excess hair and hormonal therapy to correct endocrine imbalances related to systemic disease. See also **hirsutism, hypertrichosis.**

ache, 1. a pain characterized by persistence, dullness, and, usually, moderate intensity. An ache may be localized, as in a stomach ache, headache, or bone ache, or general, as the myalgia that accompanies a viral infection or a persistent fever. 2. to suffer from a dull, persistent pain of moderate intensity.

achievement age, the level of a person's educational development as measured by an achievement test and compared with the normal score for chronological age. Compare **mental age.** See also **development age.**

achievement motivation, an intrapsychic drive that initiates behavior directed toward the attainment of a particular goal. Compare **physiological motivation, social motivation.**

achievement quotient (AQ), a numerical expression of a person's achievement age, determined by various achievement tests, divided by the chronological age and expressed as a multiple of 100. Compare **intelligence quotient.** See also **accomplishment quotient.**

achievement test, a standardized test for the measurement and comparison of knowledge or proficiency in various fields of vocational or academic study. Compare **aptitude test, intelligence test, personality test, psychological test.**

Achilles tendon (əkıl'iz). See **tendo calcaneus.**

Achilles tendon reflex, a deep tendon reflex consisting of plantar flexion of the foot when a sharp tap is given directly to the tendon of the gastrocnemius muscle at the back of the ankle. This reflex is often absent in diabetics and people with peripheral neuropathies. A sluggish return of the flexed foot may be seen in patients with hypothyroidism. A hyperactive reflex may be due to hyperthyroidism or to pyramidal tract disease. Also called **ankle reflex, calcaneal tendon reflex.** See also **deep tendon reflex.**

achlorhydria (ei'klɔrhai'driə), an abnormal condition characterized by the absence of hydrochloric acid in the gastric juice. The ability to produce gastric juice with a pH of less than 6 is tested when the subject is stimulated with an intramuscular injection of pentagastrin. Achlorhydria occurs most commonly in atrophy of the gastric mucosa, pernicious anemia, and gastric carcinoma; it is also found in severe iron-deficiency anemia. Achlorhydria in a patient with symptoms of gastric ulcer almost always indicates that the lesion is malignant. Protein digestion is severely impaired in patients with achlorhydria, but overall digestion in the alimentary tract is relatively normal, since trypsin and other enzymes of the pancreas and small intestine are not affected. See also **pernicious anemia.** – **achlorhydric,** *adj.*

achondroplasia (eikon'drouplei'ẑhə), 1. See **rickets.** a skeletal condition involving disordered growth of cartilage, often due to nutritional deficiency. 2. a familial disorder of the growth of cartilage in the epiphyses of the long bones and skull that results in premature ossification, permanent limitation of skeletal development, and dwarfism typified by protruding forehead, and short, thick arms and legs on a normal trunk. Familial achondroplasia is inherited as a Mendelian dominant; the chance is 50 per cent that an offspring of an affected parent will be affected. The majority of affected individuals die during gestation or the first year of life. The minority that survive have relatively normal longevity. There is no treatment. Antenatal diagnosis is possible. Also called **chondrodystrophy.**

achondroplastic dwarf, the most common type of dwarf, characterized by disproportionately short limbs, a normal-sized trunk, large head with a depressed nasal bridge and small face, stubby trident hands, and lordosis. The condition results from an inherited defect in bone-forming tissue and is often associated with other defects or abnormalities, although there is usually no involvement of the central nervous system and intelligence is normal. See also **achondroplasia.**

achromatocyte (ei'kroumæt'əsait). See **achromocyte.**

achromocyte (eikrou'məsait), a sickle-shaped, hypochromic erythrocyte, perhaps the result of a ruptured red blood cell which lost hemoglobin. Also called **achromatocyte.**

Achromycin V, a trade name for an antibiotic (tetracycline hydrochloride).

achylia (eikai'liə), an absence or severe deficiency of hydrochloric acid and pepsinogen in the stomach. This condition may also occur in the pancreas, when the exocrine portion of that gland fails to produce digestive enzymes. Also called **achylosis.** See also **achlorhydria.** — **achylous,** adj.

achylous (əkai'ləs), 1. of or pertaining to a lack of gastric juice or other digestive secretions. 2. of or pertaining to a lack of chyle.

acicular (əsik'yulər), needle-shaped, as certain leaves and crystals.

acid, 1. a compound that yields hydrogen ions when dissociated in solution. Acids turn blue litmus red, have a sour taste, and react with bases to form salts. Acids have chemical properties essentially opposite to those of bases. See also **alkali.** 2. Slang. lysergic acid diethylamide. See **lysergide.**

acid-, a combining form meaning 'sour, acid': *acidemia, acidophil, aciduric.*

-acid, 1. a combining form meaning an 'acid': *diacid, monacid, sulfacid.* 2. a combining form meaning 'pertaining to acid': *subacid, semiacid, superacid.*

acid-base balance, a condition existing when the net rate at which the body produces acids or bases equals the net rate at which acids or bases are excreted. The result of acid-base balance is a stable concentration of hydrogen ions in body fluids. See also **acid, base.**

acid-base metabolism, the metabolic processes that maintain the balance of acids and bases essential in regulating the composition of body fluids. Acids release hydrogen ions and bases accept them; the number of hydro-

gen ions present in a solution governs whether it is acid, alkali, or neutral. Hydrogen ions are measured on a pH scale of one to fourteen, with a reading of seven being neutral. Above seven, the solution is alkaline; below seven, it is acid. Blood is slightly alkaline, ranging from 7.35 to 7.45. Metabolic buffer systems within the body maintain this ratio, and, when it is upset, either acidosis or alkalosis results. Acidosis may be caused by diarrhea, vomiting, uremia, diabetes mellitus, and the action of certain drugs. Alkalosis may be caused by over-ingestion of alkaline drugs, loss of chloride in gastric vomitus, and the action of certain diuretic drugs. See also **acid-base balance, acidosis, alkalosis, pH.**

acid bath, a bath taken in water containing a mineral acid to help reduce excessive sweating.

acid burn, damage to tissue caused by exposure to a strong acid. The severity of the burn is determined by the kind of acid and the duration and extent of exposure. Emergency treatment includes washing the affected area with large amounts of water and neutralizing the causative agent with a dilute solution of sodium bicarbonate.

acid dust, an accumulation of highly acidic particles of dust. Such substances accumulate in the atmosphere and account for much of the smog hanging over large metropolitan areas. Many respiratory illnesses, as lung cancer and asthma, may be aggravated or caused by such dust.

-acidemia, a combining form meaning an 'increased hydrogen-ion concentration in the blood': *lactacidemia, lipacedemia, oxybutyricacidemia.*

acid-fast stain, a method of staining used in bacteriology in which a smear on a slide is flooded with carbolfuchsin stain, decolorized with acid alcohol, and counterstained with mythylene blue. Acid-fast organisms resist decolorization and appear red against a blue background when viewed under a microscope. The stain may be performed on any clinical specimen but is most commonly used in examining sputum for *Mycobacterium tuberculosis,* an acid fast bacillus. A kind of acid-fast stain is the **Ziehl-Neelsen stain.**

acid flush, a runoff of precipitation with a high acid content, as may occur during thaws in various parts of the world. Acid flushes may pollute rivers and reservoirs, killing fish and endangering the health of adjacent populations.

acidify, 1. to make a substance acid, as through the addition of an acid. 2. to become acid. Compare **alkalize.**

acid mist, mist containing a high concentration of acid or particles of any toxic chemical, as carbon tetrachloride or silicon tetrachloride. Such chemicals are often used by industry and stored in tanks that may leak their contents into residential areas, becoming especially dangerous if the toxic substance mixes with fog. Inhalation of acid mists may irritate the mucous membranes, the eyes, and the respiratory tract and seriously upset the chemistry of the body.

acidophil (æs′ɪdoufɪl, əsɪd′əfɪl), **1.** a cell or cell constituent with an affinity for acid dyes. **2.** an organism that thrives in an acid medium. —**acidophilic,** *adj.*

acidophilic adenoma, a tumor of the pituitary gland, characterized by cells that can be stained red with an acid dye. Gigantism and acromegaly are caused by an acidophilic adenoma. Also called **eosinophilic adenoma.**

acidophilus milk (æs′ɪdof′ələs), milk inoculated with cultures of *Lactobacillus acidophilus,* used in various enteric disorders to change the bacterial flora of the gastrointestinal tract.

acidosis, an abnormal increase in hydrogen ion concentration in the body owing to an accumulation of an acid or the loss of a base. The various forms of acidosis are named for the cause of the condition, as respiratory acidosis results from respiratory retention of CO_2, and diabetic acidosis results from an accumulation of ketones associated with poorly controlled diabetes mellitus. Treatment depends on diagnosis of the underlying pathology and concurrent correction of the acid-base imbalance. Compare **alkalosis.**

acid perfusion test, a test to demonstrate sensitivity of the esophagus to acid, a condition suggestive of reflux esophagitis. 0.1 normal hydrochloric acid and normal saline are dripped alternately into the esophagus via a nasal-esophageal tube without telling the patient which solution is being infused. A positive response is pain with acid but not with saline. An alternative method is to compare acid barium swallows with neutral barium swallows. If acid sensitivity is present, diffuse spasm of the esophagus may be seen by fluoroscopy when acid barium is infused and no spasm with neutral barium. Also called **Bernstein test.**

acid phosphatase, an enzyme that synthesizes phosphate esters of carbohydrates in an acid medium. See also **phosphatase.**

acid poisoning, a toxic condition caused by the ingestion of a toxic acid agent such as hydrochloric, nitric, phosphoric, or sulfuric acids, some of which are ingredients in cleaning compounds. Emergency treatment includes giving copious amounts of water or milk to dilute the acid. Vomiting is not induced and mild solutions of alkali are not given. The victim is transported immediately to the hospital for observation of any corrosive damage to the esophagus, for metabolic abnormality, and for mechanical removal of the acid by gastric intubation and lavage. Compare **alkali poisoning.**

acid precipitation, the precipitation of moisture, as rain or snow, with high acidity caused by release into the atmosphere of pollutants from industry, motor vehicle exhausts, and other sources. Acid precipitation with a pH of 5.6 or less is blamed by various authorities for numerous human health problems, fish kills, and the destruction of timber. Also called **acid rain, acid snow.**

acid therapy, a method for removing warts, which employs plaster patches impregnated with acid, as 40 per cent salicylic acid, or with acid drops, as 5 to 16.7 per cent salicylic and lactic acids in flexible collodion. The application is made every 12 to 24 hours for 2 to 4 weeks. Acid therapy is not usually recommended for body areas that perspire heavily or that are likely to become wet or for exposed body parts where the patches would detract from the patient's appearance.

Acidulin, a trade name for a gastric acidifier (glutamic acid hydrochloride).

acinar adenocarcinoma. See **acinic cell adenocarcinoma.**

Acinetobacter (æs′ɪni′təbæk′tər), a genus of nonmotile, aerobic bacteria of the family Neisseriaceae which often occurs in clinical specimens. The *Acinetobacter* contains gram-negative or gram-variable cocci and does not produce spores. This bacterium grows on regular media without serum and is oxidase-negative and catalase-positive.

acinic cell adenocarcinoma, an uncommon, low-grade malignant neoplasm that develops in the secreting cells of racemose glands, especially the salivary glands. The tumor consists of cells with clear or slightly granular cytoplasm and small eccentric dark nuclei. Also called **acinar adenocarcinoma, acinous adenocarcinoma.**

acinitis (æs′ənai′tɪs), any inflammation of the tiny, grape-shaped portions of certain glands.

acinous adenocarcinoma (æs′ɪnəs). See **acinic cell adenocarcinoma.**

acinus (æs′ɪnəs), *pl.* **acini. 1.** any small saclike structure in the body. Also called **alveolus. 2.** a subdivision of the lung consisting of the tissue distal to a terminal bronchiole.

ACMC, abbreviation for **Association of Canadian Medical Colleges.**

acmesthesia (æk′mɪsθi′źhə), a sensation of a pinprick or of a sharp point touching the skin.

acne, an inflammatory, papulo-pustular skin eruption, occurring usually on the face, neck, shoulders, and upper back. Its cause is unknown but involves bacterial breakdown of sebum into fatty substances irritating to surrounding subcutaneous tissue. Treatment includes topical and oral antibiotics, topical vitamin A derivatives, benzyl benzoate, and dermabrasion. Kinds of acne include **acne conglobata, acne vulgaris, chloracne, rosacea.** See also **comedo.** —**acneiform,** *adj.*

acne artificialis, an eruption in the skin caused by an external irritant.

acne cachecticorum, an eruption or irritation of the skin that may occur in patients who are very weak and debilitated. It is characterized by soft, mildly infiltrated pustular lesions.

acne conglobata (koŋ'gloubeɪ'tə), a severe form of acne with abscess, cyst, scar, and keloid formation. Acne conglobata may affect the lower back, buttocks, and thighs as well as the face and chest. Also called **cystic acne.**

acneform (æk'nifɔrm), resembling acne.

acneform drug eruption, any one of various skin reactions to a drug, characterized by papules and pustules erupting in acne, with or without comedones.

acnegenic (æk'nɪjen'ɪk), causing or producing acne.

acne indurata, a pathological skin condition characterized by extensive papular lesions that often produce severe scars.

acne keratosa, a skin condition characterized by hard conical plugs which usually appear at the corners of the mouth and inflame surrounding tissue.

acne necrotica miliaris, a rare, chronic type of folliculitis of the scalp, occurring mostly in adults and characterized by tiny pustules.

acne neonatorum, a skin condition of infants caused by sebaceous gland hyperplasia and characterized by the formation of comedones, nodules, and cysts on the nose, cheeks, and forehead.

acne papulosa, a common pathological skin condition that develops papular lesions. It is considered a papular form of acne vulgaris.

acne rosacea. See **rosacea.**

acne vulgaris, a common form of acne seen predominantly in adolescents and young adults. Acne vulgaris is probably an effect of androgenic hormones, (which stimulate the production of sebum), and *Corynebacterium acnes* in the piliary canal.

ACNM, abbreviation for **American College of Nurse-Midwives.**

ACOG, abbreviation for **American College of Obstetricians and Gynecologists.**

acognosia (æk'əgnou'žhə), a knowledge of remedies.

aconeus, one of seven superficial muscles of the posterior forearm. A small triangular muscle, it originates on the dorsal surface of the lateral condyle and inserts in the olecranon process of the ulna. It is innervated by a branch of the radial nerve, which contains fibers from the seventh and eighth cervical nerves, and it functions to extend the forearm.

acoria (ækɔr'iə), a condition characterized by constant hunger, even when the appetite is small.

acorn-tipped catheter, a flexible catheter with an acorn-shaped tip, used in various diagnostic procedures, especially in urology.

acou-, acu-, a combining form meaning 'pertaining to hearing': *acouesthesia, acoulalian, acouophonia.*

-acousia, -acusia, a combining form meaning a '(specified) condition of the hearing': *amblyacousia, bradyacousia, dysacousia.* Also **-acusis, -akusis.**

acousma (əkuz'mə), *pl.* **acousmas, acousmata.** a hallucinatory impression of strange sounds.

acoustic, acoustical, of or pertaining to sound or hearing.

-acoustic, 1. a combining form meaning 'pertaining to the hearing organs': *entacoustic, otacoustic.* 2. a combining form meaning 'pertaining to amplified sound waves': *micracoustic, microcoustic, stethacoustic.* Also **-acoustical.**

acoustic microscope, a microscope in which the object being viewed is scanned with sound waves and its image reconstructed with light waves. Acoustic microscopes produce excellent resolution of the objects being studied and allow very close examination of cells and tissues without staining or damaging the specimen.

acoustic nerve, either of a pair of cranial nerves essential to the sense of hearing, having two distinct sets of fibers called the cochlear nerves and the vestibular nerves, and connecting to three areas in the brain. Also called **eighth nerve.**

acoustic neurilemoma. See **acoustic neuroma.**

acoustic neurinoma. See **acoustic neuroma.**

acoustic neurofibroma. See **acoustic neuroma.**

acoustic neuroma, a benign tumor that develops from the eighth cranial (acoustic) nerve and grows within the auditory canal. Depending on the location and size of the lesion, tinnitus, increasing deafness, headache, facial numbness, papilledema, dizziness, and an unsteady gait may result. Paresis and difficulty in speaking and swallowing may occur in the later stage. It may be unilateral or bilateral. Also called **acoustic neurilemoma, acoustic neurinoma, acoustic neurofibroma.**

acoustic trauma, a gradual loss of hearing caused by exposure to loud noise over an extended period of time or a sudden loss of hearing, partial or complete, caused by an explosion, a severe blow to the head, or other accident. Hearing loss may be temporary or permanent.

acousto-optics (əkus'touop'tɪks), a field of physics that studies the generation of light waves by ultrahigh-frequency sound waves. Knowledge gained by such study is applied chiefly in the transmission of information by acousto-optic devices.

ACP, 1. abbreviation for **American College of Pathologists.** 2. abbreviation for **American College of Physicians.**

acquired, (in genetics) of or pertaining to a characteristic, condition, or disease originating after birth and caused not by hereditary or developmental factors but by a reaction to environmental influences outside of the organism. Compare **congenital, familial, hereditary.**

acquired immunity, any form of immunity that is not innate and is obtained during life. It may be natural or artificial and actively or passively induced. **Naturally acquired immunity** is obtained by the development of antibodies resulting from an attack of infectious disease or by the transmission of antibodies from the mother through the placenta to the fetus or to the infant through the colostrum. **Artificially acquired immunity** is obtained by vaccination or by the injection of antiserum. Compare **natural immunity**. See also **active immunity, passive immunity**.

acquired reflex. See **conditioned reflex**.

ACR, abbreviation for **American College of Radiologists**.

acrid, sharp or pungent, bitter and unpleasant to the smell or taste.

acridine (æk'rɪdin), a benzopyridine compound used in the synthesis of dyes and drugs. Its derivatives include fluorescent yellow dyes and the antiseptic agents acriflavine hydrochloride, acriflavine base, and proflavine.

acro-, a combining form meaning 'pertaining to the extremities': *acro-agnosis, acro-ataxia, acrocyanosis*.

acrocentric (æk'rousen'trɪk), pertaining to a chromosome in which the centromere is located near one of the ends so that the arms of the chromatids are extremely uneven. Compare **metacentric, submetacentric, telocentric**.

acrocephalosyndactylism (æk'rousef'əlousɪndæk'təlɪz'-əm). See **Apert's syndrome**.

acrocephaly (æk'rousef'əli). See **oxycephaly**.

acrochordon (æk'roukɔr'don), a benign, pedunculated skin tag commonly occurring on the eyelids or neck or in the axilla or groin.

acrocyanosis (æk'rousai'ənou'sɪs), a condition characterized by cyanotic discoloration, coldness, and sweating of the extremities, especially the hands, caused by arterial spasm that is usually precipitated by cold or by emotional stress. Warming induces vasodilation, and the blue discoloration becomes mottled with red. Abnormal sympathetic nerve activity or overreaction to certain stimuli may be responsible for the vasospasm that typically occurs in Raynaud's disease and is also seen in rheumatoid arthritis, in scleroderma, and in workers who operate pneumatic air hammers. Acrocyanosis may be treated with sympatholytic drugs, and attacks may be prevented by not smoking and by avoiding exposure to cold. A kind of acrocyanosis is **peripheral acrocyanosis of the newborn**. Also called **Raynaud's sign**.

acrodermatitis, an eruption of the skin caused by a parasitic mite, which is a member of the order Acarina.

acrodermatitis enteropathica (en'təroupæth'ɪkə), a rare, chronic disease of infants characterized by vesicles and bullae of the skin and mucous membranes, alopecia, diarrhea, and failure to thrive. It may be lethal if not treated. Diiodohydroxyquin is usually prescribed.

acromegalic eunuchoidism, a rare disorder characterized by genital atrophy and the development of female secondary sex characteristics, occurring in men with advanced acromegaly caused by a chromophil adenoma in the anterior pituitary gland. Initially, the gonadal function of the anterior lobe may be stimulated, but with the growth of the tumor, the patient may become impotent,

lose facial, axillary, and pubic hair, develop a soft skin and a feminine distribution of fat. Also called **retrograde infantilism**.

acromegaly (æk'rəmeg'əli), **acromegalia,** a chronic metabolic condition characterized by a gradual, marked enlargement and elongation of the bones of the face, jaw, and extremities. The condition, which afflicts middle-aged persons, is caused by the overproduction of growth hormone and is treated by x ray or surgery, often involving partial resection of the pituitary gland. Compare **gigantism**. See also **adenohypophysis, growth hormone**. — **acromegalic,** *adj.*

acromioclavicular articulation, the gliding joint between the acromial end of the clavicle and the medial margin of the acromion of the scapula. The joint has six ligaments.

acromion (əkrou'miən), the lateral extension of the spine of the scapula, forming the highest point of the shoulder and connecting with the clavicle at a small oval surface in the middle of the spine. It gives attachment to the deltoideus and trapezius. Also called **acromion process**. Compare **coracoid process**. — **acromial,** *adj.*

acronym, a word formed by the initial letters or syllables of other words as *CAT*, which is the acronym for *C*omputerized *A*xial *T*omography. Most acronyms are composed of the initial capital letters of their full forms and differ from abbreviations in that they are pronounced and treated as words grammatically. — **acronymic,** *adj.*

acroparesthesia (æk'roupær'ɪsfhi'ʒə), **1.** an extreme sensitivity at the tips of the extremities of the body, caused by compression of the nerves in the affected area or by polyneuritis. **2.** a disease characterized by tingling, numbness, and stiffness in the extremities, especially in the fingers, the hands, and the forearms. It sometimes produces pain, skin pallor, or mild cyanosis. The disease occurs in a simple form, which may produce acrocyanosis, and in an angiospastic form, which may produce gangrene.

acrophobia, a pathological fear or dread of high places that results in extreme anxiety. The obsessive phenomenon is most frequently seen in persons who are overconscientious, shy, pedantic, punctilious, or painstakingly addicted to orderliness and symmetry. In many cases the cause can be traced to some repressed, fear-producing experience involved with heights, usually occurring in childhood. Therapy is planned to attempt to overcome or eliminate the phobic reaction. See also **obsession, phobia**.

acrosomal cap. See **acrosome**.

acrosomal head cap. See **acrosome**.

acrosomal reaction, the pattern of various chemical changes that occur in the anterior of the head of the spermatozoon in response to contact with the ovum and that lead to the penetration by the sperm and fertilization of the ovum.

acrosome, the caplike structure surrounding the anterior end of the nucleus of a spermatozoon. It is derived from the Golgi apparatus within the cytoplasm and contains enzymes that function in the penetration of the ovum during fertilization. Also called **acrosomal cap, acrosomal head cap.** See also **acrosomal reaction.** — acrosomal, *adj.*

acrotic (əkrot'ık), 1. of or pertaining to the surface or to the skin glands. 2. of or pertaining to the absence or the weakness of a pulse.

ACSM, abbreviation for the **American College of Sports Medicine.**

act-. a combining form meaning 'to do, drive, act': *action, activate, actor.*

ACTH, abbreviation for **adrenocorticotropic hormone.**

Acthar, a trade name for adrenocorticotropic hormone (corticotropin).

Actidil, a trade name for an antihistamine (triprolidine hydrochloride), used for the symptomatic relief of allergic conditions.

Actifed, a trade name for a fixed-combination drug containing an adrenergic bronchodilator and vasoconstrictor (pseudoephedrine hydrochloride) and an antihistamine (triprolidine hydrochloride).

actigraph (æk'tıgræf), any instrument that records changes in the activity of a substance or an organism and produces a graphic record of the process, as an electrocardiograph machine, which produces a record of cardiac activity.

actin, a protein found in muscle fibers that acts with myosin to bring about contraction and relaxation. See also **myosin.**

actin-. See **actino-.**

acting out, the expression of intrapsychic conflict or painful emotion through overt behavior that is usually neurotic, defensive, and unconscious and that may be destructive or dangerous. In controlled situations, like psychodrama, Gestalt therapy, or play therapy, such behavior may be therapeutic in itself and may also serve to reveal to the patient the underlying conflict governing his behavior. See also **transference.**

actinic (æktın'ık), of or pertaining to radiation, as sunlight or x rays.

actinic dermatitis, a skin inflammation or rash resulting from exposure to sunlight, x ray, or atomic particle radiation. Chronic or recurrent actinic dermatitis can predispose to skin cancer. See also **actinic keratosis.**

actinic keratosis, a slowly developing, localized thickening of the outer layers of the skin as a result of chronic, excessive exposure to the sun. Treatment of this potentially malignant lesion includes surgical excision, cryotherapy, and topical chemotherapy. Also called **senile keratosis.**

actinin (æktın'ın), a protein that forms part of the complex of actin and myosin in a muscle fiber. The precise function of actinin is not known, but some researchers believe it may help to maintain the regular architecture of the myofibrils.

actinium (Ac), a rare, radioactive metallic element. Its atomic number is 89; its atomic weight is 227. It occurs in some ores of uranium.

actino-, actin-, a combining form meaning 'pertaining to a ray or to radiation': *actinocardiogram, actinocutitis, actinogen.*

Actinomyces (æk'tınoumai'siz), a genus of anaerobic, gram-positive bacteria. The species that may cause disease in man, *Actinomyces israelii,* is normally present in the mouth and throat. See also **actinomycosis.**

actinomycin D. See **dactinomycin.**

actinomycosis (æk'tınoumaikou'sıs), a chronic, systemic disease characterized by deep, lumpy abscesses that extrude a thin, granular pus through multiple sinuses. The disease occurs worldwide but is seen most frequently in those who live in rural areas. It is not spread from person to person or from animal to humans. The various species of *Actinomyces* are species specific. The causative organism in humans is *A. israelii,* a normal inhabitant of the bowel and mouth. Disease occurs following tissue damage, usually in the presence of another infectious organism. It is diagnosed by microscopic identification of sulfur granules, pathognomic of *Actinomyces,* in the exudate. There are three principal forms of actinomycosis. **Cervicofacial actinomycosis** occurs with the spread of the bacterium into the subcutaneous tissues of the mouth, throat, and neck, secondary to dental or tonsillar infection. The process begins with a hard swelling over the angle of the lower jaw and neck. The swelling becomes indurated, and sinus tracts form, draining the pus to the skin. Remarkably little pain accompanies these abscesses, even when they are so deep as to involve the bone of the jaw. **Thoracic actinomycosis** may represent proliferation of the organism from cervicofacial abscesses into the esophagus, or it may result from inhalation of the bacterium into the bronchi. The infection may spread through the lungs, reaching the pleura, or through the esophagus into the mediastinum. Ribs, heart, and the great vessels may then be affected. Fever, cough, draining sinuses, weight loss, night sweats, and, rarely, pleural effusion are characteristic of this form of the disease. **Abdominal actinomycosis** usually follows an acute inflammatory process in the stomach or intestines, as appendicitis, diverticulum of the large bowel, or a perforation of the stomach. A large mass may be palpated, and sinus tracts may be found in the groin or other area that drains exudate from abscesses deep in the abdomen. Rarely, a pelvic form of abdominal actinomycosis occurs following insertion of an intrauterine contraceptive device. All forms of actinomycosis are treated with at least six weeks of daily injections of penicillin in large doses. Surgical excision or incision and drainage of deep or large abscesses may be necessary. Abdominal actinomycosis can be cured in 40 per cent of cases, thoracic actinomycosis in 80 per cent, and cervicofacial actinomycosis in 90 per cent.

action alternatives, (in nursing) any of several possible actions or courses of action chosen by a nurse as part of a goal-oriented nursing care plan and performed to resolve a problem or to modify the effects a particular problem has on a patient.

action current, a current produced in a cell membrane of a nerve or muscle by the electrical activity in the tissue. This current serves to depolarize adjacent membrane areas and thereby initiates a repetition of the action potential along the nerve fiber.

action level, the level of concentration at which an undesirable or toxic component of a food is considered dangerous enough to public health to warrant government prohibition of the sale of that food. The United States Food and Drug Administration tests foods for action levels.

action potential, an electrical impulse consisting of a self-propagating series of polarizations and depolarizations, transmitted across the cell membranes of a nerve fiber during the transmission of a nerve impulse and across the cell membranes of a muscle cell during contraction or other activity of the cell.

activated charcoal, a general-purpose antidote and a powerful pharmaceutic adsorbent.

■ INDICATIONS: It is prescribed in the treatment of acute poisoning and to control flatulence.

■ CONTRAINDICATIONS: There are no known contraindications, but activated charcoal is ineffective in poisoning caused by a strong acid or alkali or by cyanide.

■ ADVERSE EFFECTS: There are no known adverse effects.

activated 7-dehydrocholesterol. See **vitamin D₃.**

activation factor. See **factor XII.**

activator, 1. a substance, force, or device that stimulates activity in another substance or structure, especially a substance that activates an enzyme. 2. a substance that stimulates the development of an anatomical structure in the embryo. 3. an internal secretion of the pancreas. 4. an apparatus for making substances radioactive, as a cyclotron or neutron generator.

active algolagnia. See **sadism.**

active assisted exercise, the movement of the body or any of its parts primarily through the individual's own efforts but accompanied by the aid of a therapist or some other device, as an exercise machine. See also **exercise, passive exercise.**

active euthanasia, the killing of an individual suffering from an incurable illness or an irreparable injury, especially by administering a lethal drug. Also called **mercy killing, positive euthanasia.** Compare **passive euthanasia.**

active exercise, repetitive movement of a part of the body as a result of voluntary contraction and relaxation of the controlling muscles. Compare **passive exercise.** See also **aerobic exercise, anaerobic exercise.**

active immunity, a form of acquired immunity that results from the production of antibodies in the cells. Antibodies develop naturally after infection or artificially after vaccination.

active movement, muscular action at a joint owing to voluntary effort without outside help. Compare **passive movement.**

active play, any activity from which one derives amusement, entertainment, enjoyment, or satisfaction by taking a participatory rather than a passive role. Children of all age groups engage in various forms of active play, from the exploration of objects and toys by the infant and toddler to the formal games, sports, and hobbies of the older child. Compare **passive play.**

active resistance exercise, the movement or exertion of the body or any of its parts performed totally through the individual's own efforts against a resisting force. See also **progressive resistance exercise.**

active site, the place on the surface of an enzyme where its catalytic action occurs.

active transport, the movement of materials across the membrane of a cell by means of chemical activity that allows the cell to admit larger molecules than would otherwise be able to enter. Expediting active transport are carrier molecules within the cell that bind themselves to incoming molecules, rotate around them, and disconnect, setting the incoming molecule free inside the cell wall. The entry of large molecules in the process of active transport disturbs the equilibrium of the internal environment of the cell, which compensates for the imbalance by releasing materials through its membrane. Active transport is the means by which the cell absorbs glucose and other substances needed to sustain life and health. Certain enzymes play a role in active transport, providing a chemical "pump" that helps move substances through the cell membrane. Compare **osmosis, passive transport.**

active treatment. See **treatment.**

activities of daily living (ADL), the activities usually performed in the course of a normal day in the client's life, as eating, dressing, washing, or brushing the teeth. The ability to perform the activities of daily living may be compromised by a variety of causes, including chronic illnesses and accidents. The limitation imposed may be temporary or permanent; rehabilitation may involve relearning the skills or learning new ways to accomplish an activity. Nursing has a significant role in helping a client to maintain or regain his ability to perform the necessary activities of daily living, thus remaining independent to the greatest degree possible. An ADL check-list is often used before discharge from the hospital. If any activities cannot be adequately performed, arrangements are made with an outside agency, as a visiting nurse service, or with family members to provide the necessary assistance to the client. Follow-up with physical therapy on an outpatient basis may be useful in maintaining or increasing the client's ability to perform the activities.

actual cautery, the application of heat, rather than a chemical substance, in the destruction of tissue.

actual charge, the amount actually charged or billed by a medical practitioner for a service. The actual charge may not be the same as that paid for the service by an insurance plan.

actual damages. See **damages.**

actualize, the act of fulfilling a potential, as by a person who may develop capabilities through experience and education.

acu-, **1.** a combining form meaning 'pertaining to a needle': *acuclosure, aculeate, acupressure.* **2.** a combining form meaning 'pertaining to hearing': *acuesthesia.* Also **acou-.**

acuminate wart. See **condylomatum acuminatum.**

acupressure (æk′yəpreśh′ər), a therapeutic technique of applying digital pressure in a specified way on designated points on the body to relieve pain, produce anesthesia, or regulate a bodily function.

acupuncture (æk′yəpərŋk′ćhər), a method of producing analgesia or altering the function of a system of the body by inserting fine, wire-thin needles into the skin at specific sites on the body along a series of lines, or channels, called meridians. The needles are twirled or energized electrically or warmed. Acupuncture originated in the Far East and has gained increasing attention in the West since the early 1970s. Research seeks to determine the usefulness of acupuncture and to understand the mechanisms by which it produces analgesia or alters sensory function. Some studies indicate that the analgesic effect of this technique is reversed by naloxone, suggesting that the release of enkephalin is significantly involved. See also **moxibustion.** – **acupuncturist,** *n.*

acupuncture point, one of many discrete points on the skin along the several meridians, or chains of points of the body. Stimulation of any of the various points may induce an increase or decrease in function or sensation in an area or system of the body. The meridians are named and the points numbered to allow specific location of the points to be stimulated in acupuncture, acupressure, or moxibustion.

-acusis. See **-acousia.**

acute, **1.** (of a disease or disease symptoms) beginning abruptly with marked intensity or sharpness, then subsiding after a relatively short period of time. **2.** sharp or severe. Compare **chronic.**

acute abdomen, an abnormal condition characterized by the acute onset of severe pain within the abdominal cavity. An acute abdomen requires immediate evaluation and diagnosis, as it may indicate a condition that requires surgical intervention. Information about the onset, duration, character, location, and symptoms associated with the pain is critical in making an accurate diagnosis. The patient is asked what decreases or increases the pain; constant, increasing pain is associated with appendicitis and diverticulitis, whereas intermittent pain is more likely indicative of a bowel obstruction, ureteral calculi, or gallstones. Appendicitis may often be differentiated from a perforated ulcer by the slower development of pain. Although sometimes misleading because of referral, radiation, or reflection of pain, the patient's report of the location of the pain may serve to identify a specific organ or system. Factors in the patient's history that are useful in the diagnosis and management of an acute abdomen include changes in bowel habits, weight loss, bloody stool, diarrhea, and clay-colored stool. Also called **surgical abdomen.** See also **abdominal pain.**

acute alcoholism, drunkenness or intoxication resulting from excessive consumption of alcoholic beverages. The syndrome is temporary and is characterized by depression of the higher nervous centers causing impaired motor control, stupor, lack of coordination, and often nausea, dehydration, headache, and other physical symptoms. Compare **chronic alcoholism.**

acute (angle-closure) glaucoma. See **glaucoma.**

acute bacterial arthritis. See **septic arthritis.**

acute care, a pattern of health care in which a patient is treated for an acute episode of illness, for the sequelae of an accident or other trauma, or during recovery from surgery. Acute care is usually given in a hospital by specialized personnel using complex and sophisticated technical equipment and materials, and it may involve intensive care. This pattern of care is often necessary for only a short time, unlike chronic care.

acute cervicitis. See **cervicitis.**

acute childhood leukemia, a progressive, malignant disease of the blood-forming tissues that is characterized by the uncontrolled proliferation of immature leukocytes and their precursors, particularly in the bone marrow, spleen, and lymph nodes. It is the most frequent cancer in children, with a peak onset occurring between the ages of two and five years.

■ OBSERVATIONS: Acute leukemia is classified according to cell type: **acute lymphoid leukemia (ALL)** includes lymphatic, lymphocytic, lymphoblastic, and lymphoblastoid types; **acute nonlymphoid leukemia** includes granulocytic, myelocytic, monocytic, myelogenous, monoblastic, and monomyeloblastic types (the myelocytic and monocytic series are abbreviated AML). ALL is predominantly a disease of childhood, whereas AML occurs in all age groups. The traditional classification of leukemia into chronic and acute types is based on duration or expected course of the illness and the relative maturity of the leukemic cells. Although this classification is still used, particularly to differentiate the childhood, or acute, from the adult, or chronic, forms of the disease, it is no longer valid as a prognostic indication. The exact etiology of the disease is unknown, although various factors are implicated, including genetic defects, immune deficiency, viruses, and carcinogenic environmental factors, primarily ionizing radiation. In acute leukemia, large immature leukocytes accumulate rapidly and infiltrate other tissues of the body, especially the reticuloendothelial system, causing decreased production of erythrocytes and platelets. Neutropenia, anemia, an increased susceptibility to infection and hemorrhage, and weakening of the bones with a tendency to fracture also occur. Initial symptoms of the disease include fever, pallor, fatigue, anorexia, secondary infections (usually of the mouth, throat, or lungs), bone and joint pain, subdermal or submucosal hemorrhage, and enlargement of the spleen, liver, and lymph nodes. Onset may be abrupt or follow a gradual, progressive course. Involvement of the central nervous system may lead to leukemic meningitis. Characteristically, a peripheral blood smear reveals many immature leukocytes. The diagnosis is confirmed by bone marrow aspiration or biopsy and examination, which show a highly elevated number of lymphoblasts with almost complete absence of erythrocytes, granulocytes, and megakaryocytes. The prognosis is poor in untreated cases and death usually occurs within six months following the onset of symptoms. Survival rates have dramatically increased in recent years with the use of antileukemic agents in combination regimens. Remission of five-years or longer occurs in 50 to 70 per cent of children with ALL, with 20 to 30 per cent achieving complete remission. For children with AML, the prognosis is poorer, and the remission rate is far less.

■ INTERVENTION: Treatment of acute leukemia consists of a three-stage process involving the use of chemotherapeutic agents and irradiation. In the first, or remission induction phase, complete destruction of all leukemic cells is achieved within a four- to six-week period using a combination drug therapy regimen. The main drugs used in ALL are the corticosteroids, usually three daily oral doses of prednisone; vincristine, administered intravenously once a week; and L-asparaginase, given intramuscularly three times a week for a total of nine doses. Allopurinol, a xanthine-oxidase inhibitor, is usually administered to inhibit uric acid production. Other drugs used in various combination regimens in sequential cycles include methotrexate, 6-mercaptopurine, cyclophosphamide, cytosine, arabinoside, hydroxyurea, daunorubicin, and adriamycin. In children with AML the primary drugs for induction remission are 6-thioguanine, daunomycin, cytosine arabinoside, 5-azacytidine, vincristine, and prednisone.

The child is usually hospitalized for part or all of the treatment because of the many side effects of the drugs and the high risk of complications, especially infection and hemorrhage. If severe hemorrhaging occurs and does not respond to local treatment, platelet transfusions may be necessary, and in cases of severe anemia, especially during induction therapy, whole blood or packed red cells may be needed to raise hemoglobin levels. The second stage of treatment involves prophylactic maintenance to prevent leukemic infiltration of the central nervous system. Therapy usually consists of daily high-dose cranial irradiation for about two weeks following induction remission and weekly or twice-weekly doses of intrathecal methotrexate, for a total of five or six injections, although in some cases only the drug is given. In small children the irradiation is limited to the cranium to prevent retardation of linear growth, but older children may receive craniospinal radiation. Therapy to maintain remission usually begins after the child is discharged from the hospital and consists of various regimens of drugs in combination. A common schedule includes daily oral doses of 6-mercaptopurine and weekly doses of oral methotrexate, intermittent short-term therapy with prednisone and vincristine, and periodic doses of intrathecal methotrexate for prophylaxis against spread to the central nervous system. Complete blood counts are done weekly or monthly, and bone marrow examinations are performed every three to four months to detect myelosuppression and drug toxicity. Maintenance therapy is discontinued after a period of two to three years if initial remission is maintained. Continuous treatment beyond three years is not advised, as the adverse affects of the medications increase with prolonged use. Relapse occurs in as many as 20 per cent of treated children. If relapse occurs, the child begins the treatment cycle again, usually with prednisone, vincristine, and a combination of other drugs not previously tried. With each relapse the prognosis becomes poorer. Other treatments for prolonging remission include immunotherapy using periodic inoculation with BCG vaccine or bone marrow transplant, which has been successful in inducing long-term remissions in about 10 to 20 per cent of the cases, especially those with AML or severe, terminal ALL.

■ NURSING CONSIDERATIONS: Nursing care for the child with acute leukemia involves intensive physical and emotional support during all phases of the disease, its diagnosis, and treatment. Foremost is the preparation of the child and parents for the various diagnostic and therapeutic procedures, including venipuncture, bone marrow aspiration or biopsy, lumbar puncture, and x-ray treatment. Specific medical and nursing management depends on the particular regimen of drug therapy, although most of the chemotherapeutic agents used in treatment cause myelosuppression that may lead to secondary complications of infection, hemorrhage, and anemia. Overwhelming infection is a major problem and one of the most frequent causes of death. Severe neutropenia indicates increased risk of infection. It may occur during immunosuppressive therapy or after prolonged antibiotic therapy. The most common infectious organisms are viruses, especially varicella, herpes zoster, herpes simplex, measles, mumps, rubella, and poliomyelitis, both gram-positive and gram-negative bacteria, including *Staphylococcus aureus, S. epidermidis, group-A beta-hemolytic Streptococcus, Pseudomonas aeruginosa, Escherichia coli, Proteus,* and *Klebsiella,* and various parasites and fungi, especially *Pneumocystis carinii* and *Candida albicans.* To prevent infection, the nurse isolates the child as much as possible, screens visitors for active infection, institutes strict aseptic procedures, monitors temperature closely, evaluates possible sites of infection (as needle punctures), encourages adequate nutrition, and helps the child to avoid exertion or fatigue, and, at discharge, teaches the child and parents the necessity for avoiding all known sources of infection, primarily the common childhood communicable diseases. Preventive measures to control infection also help to decrease the tendency toward hemorrhage. Special attention is given to skin care, oral hygiene, cleanliness of the perineal area, and restriction of activities that could result in accidental injury. A major nursing consideration is the management of the many side effects resulting from drug toxicity and irradiation, including nausea and vomiting, anorexia, oral and rectal ulceration, alopecia, hemorrhagic cystitis, and peripheral neuropathy, including weakness and numbing of the extremities and severe jaw pain. Although corticosteroid treatment usually increases the appetite and produces a euphoric sense of well-being in the child, it also causes moon face, which is reversed with cessation of the steroid therapy. During maintenance therapy, the nurse continues to provide emotional support and guidance, specifically teaching parents which side effects are normal reactions to drugs and which indicate toxicity and require medical attention. In terminal stages of the disease, relief of discomfort and pain become the primary focus. Effective measures include careful physical handling of the child, frequent position changes, avoidance of pressure on painful areas, and control of annoying environmental factors, as excessive light and noise. Nonsalicylate analgesics are used as needed, depending on the severity of pain.

acute cholecystitis. See **cholecystitis.**

acute delirium, an episode of delirium that is sudden, severe, and transient. See also **delirium.**

acute disease, a disease characterized by a relatively short duration of symptoms that are usually severe. An episode of acute disease results in recovery to a state comparable to the patient's state of health and activity prior to the disease, in passage into a chronic phase, or in death. See also **chronic.**

acute epiglottitis, epiglottiditis, a severe, rapidly progressing bacterial infection of the upper respiratory tract that occurs in young children, primarily between the ages of two and seven. It is characterized by sore throat, croupy stridor, and an inflamed epiglottis, which may cause sudden respiratory obstruction and be quickly fatal. The infection is generally caused by *Haemophilus influenzae,* type B, although streptococci may occasionally be the causative agent. Transmission occurs by infection with airborne particles or contact with infected secretions. The diagnosis is made by bacteriologic identification of *H. influenzae,* type B, in a specimen taken from the upper respiratory tract or in the blood. An x-ray film of the neck from the side shows an enlarged epiglottis and distention of the hypopharynx, which distinguishes the condition from croup. Direct visualization of the inflamed, cherry-red epiglottis by depression of the tongue or indirect laryngoscopy is also diagnostic but may produce total acute obstruction and is attempted only by trained personnel with equipment to establish an airway or to provide respiratory resuscitation, if necessary.
■ OBSERVATIONS: The onset of the infection is abrupt and it progresses rapidly. The first signs—sore throat, hoarseness, fever, and dysphagia—may be followed by an inability to swallow, drooling, varying degrees of dyspnea, inspiratory stridor, and marked irritability and apprehension. Difficulty in breathing may progress to severe respiratory distress in minutes or hours. Suprasternal, supraclavicular, intercostal, and subcostal inspiratory retractions may be visible. The hypoxic child appears frightened and anxious; the color of the skin ranges from pallor to cyanosis.
■ INTERVENTION: Establishment of an airway is urgent, either by endotrachial intubation or by tracheostomy. Humidity and oxygen are provided, and airway secretions are drained or suctioned. Intravenous fluids are usually required, and antibiotic therapy is initiated immediately, usually with penicillin, ampicillin, or chloramphenicol. Sedatives are contraindicated because of their depressant effect on the respiratory system, and steroids, antihistamines, and adrenergic drugs are not usually of any therapeutic value.
■ NURSING CONSIDERATIONS: The nurse may assist intubation or tracheostomy once the diagnosis is confirmed. Intensive nursing care is required for a child with acute epiglottitis. Frequent changing of clothing and bed linen may be necessary to prevent chilling. The most acute phase of the condition passes within 24 to 48 hours and intubation is rarely needed beyond three to four days. As the child responds to therapy, breathing becomes easier, and there is usually rapid recovery so that bed rest and quiet activity to relieve boredom become primary nursing

concerns. The infection may spread, causing such complications as otitis media, pneumonia, and bronchiolitis. Complications of the tracheostomy may also develop, including infection, atelectasis, cannula occlusion, tracheal bleeding, granulation, and stenosis, and delayed healing of the stoma.

acute febrile polyneuritis. See **Guillain-Barré syndrome.**

acute gastritis. See **gastritis.**

acute glomerulonephritis, a noninfectious disease of the glomerulus of the kidney that occurs following a streptococcal infection, most often in childhood. The symptoms are hematuria, proteinuria, decreased production of urine, and edema. Children usually recover completely; adults may develop scar tissue in the glomerulus and consequent decrease of renal function. Treatment may include limitation of dietary protein and sodium, diuretics, antihypertensives, and antibiotics. See also **chronic glomerulonephritis, subacute glomerulonephritis, uremia.**

acute hallucinatory paranoia, a form of paranoia in which hallucinations are combined with the systematized delusions. Also called **paranoia hallucinatoria.**

acute hallucinosis. See **alcoholic hallucinosis.**

acute hemorrhagic leukoencephalitis. See **acute necrotizing hemorrhagic encephalopathy.**

acute idiopathic polyneuritis. See **Guillain-Barré syndrome.**

acute idiopathic thrombocytopenic purpura. See **idiopathic thrombocytopenic purpura.**

acute interstitial nephritis. See **interstial nephritis.**

acute laryngotracheobronchitis (LTB). See **croup.**

acute lymphoblastic leukemia. See **acute lymphocytic leukemia.**

acute lymphocytic leukemia (ALL), a progressive, malignant disease characterized by large numbers of immature cells, closely resembling lymphoblasts in the bone marrow, the circulating blood, the lymph nodes, the spleen, the liver, and other organs. The number of normal blood cells is reduced. About 80 per cent of the 2,250 cases a year in the United States occur in children, with the greatest number diagnosed between the ages of two and five. The risk of the disease is greatly increased for people with Down's syndrome and for siblings of leukemia patients. The disease has a sudden onset and rapid progression marked by fever, pallor, anorexia, fatigue, anemia, hemorrhage, bone pain, splenomegaly, and recurrent infection. Blood and bone marrow studies are used for diagnosis and for determining the type of proliferating lymphocyte, which may be B cells, T cells (that usually respond poorly to therapy), or null cells (as are found in most cases). Treatment includes intensive combination chemotherapy, therapy for secondary infections and hyperuricemia, irradiation, and intrathecal methotrexate.

Frequent blood transfusions may be required, and an important aspect of care is sensitive concern for the emotional needs of the children and their families. Modern therapy results in remissions for 83 to 92 per cent of young ALL patients and five-year tumor-free survival for 50 per cent, with the best response in children between the ages of two and ten. Also called **acute lymphoblastic leukemia.** See also **acute childhood leukemia.**

acute mastitis. See **mastitis.**

acute myelocytic leukemia (AML), a malignant neoplasm of blood-forming tissues characterized by the uncontrolled proliferation of immature granular leukocytes that usually have azurophilic Auer rods in their cytoplasm. The typical symptoms, appearing abruptly or, more often, gradually, are spongy bleeding gums, anemia, fatigue, fever, dyspnea, moderate splenomegaly, joint and bone pains, and repeated infections. Chloromas (greenish granulocytic sarcomas) may develop in bone or soft tissue. AML may occur at any age, but it most frequently affects adolescents and young adults. The risk of the disease is increased among people who have been exposed to massive doses of radiation and among individuals with certain blood dyscrasias, as polycythemia vera, primary thrombocytopenia, and refractory anemia. Variants of AML, in which only one cell line proliferates, are erythroid, eosinophilic, basophilic, monocytic, and megakaryocytic leukemias. The diagnosis is based on differential blood count and bone biopsies. Chemotherapy with various combinations of drugs, including cyclophosphamide, cytosine arabinose, daunorubicin, methotrexate, prednisone, and vincristine, is the primary form of treatment. Allopurinol is frequently administered prior to chemotherapy to reduce the risk of urate crystalluria and ureteral obstruction. Repeated transfusions of red cells and platelets may be required. Radiotherapy, immunotherapy, and marrow transplantation are also used, but long remissions resulting from any form of treatment are rare, and death may be caused by an infection, a hemorrhage, or an obstruction produced by leukocytes in a blood vessel. Also called **acute nonlymphocytic leukemia, granulocytic leukemia, myelogenous leukemia, myeloid leukemia, splenomedullary leukemia, splenomyelogenous leukemia.** See also **acute childhood leukemia.**

acute necrotizing gingivitis, a fusospirochetal infection characterized by necrotic, foul-smelling ulcers of the gums and throat, fever, and enlarged lymph nodes in the neck. It is usually associated with poor oral hygiene and is most common in conditions in which there is crowding and malnutrition. Treatment includes peroxide mouth washes, antibiotics, metronidazole, and dental care. Also called **trench mouth, Vincent's angina, Vincent's infection.**

acute necrotizing hemorrhagic encephalopathy, a degenerative disease of the brain, characterized by marked edema, numerous minute hemorrhages, necrosis of blood vessel walls, especially those of small veins, demyelination of nerve fibers, and infiltration of the meninges with neutrophils, lymphocytes, and histiocytes. Typical signs are severe headache, fever, and vomiting; convulsions may occur, and the patient may rapidly lose consciousness. Treatment consists of decompression by withdrawing cerebrospinal fluid and administration of large doses of steroids, but the disease is frequently fatal in one to six days. This kind of encephalopathy is thought to be caused by an immunologic mechanism, but the disease often resembles acute bacterial meningitis or herpes simplex encephalitis. Also called **acute hemorrhagic leukoencephalitis.**

acute nonlymphocytic leukemia (ANLL). See **acute myelocytic leukemia.**

acute pain, severe pain, as may follow surgery or trauma or accompany myocardial infarction or other conditions and diseases. Acute pain occurring in the first 24 to 48 hours after surgery is often difficult to relieve, even with drugs. Some studies show that patients over age 50 need less analgesia to relieve acute pain than do younger patients. Another study indicates that 23 percent of surgical patients, except for orthopedic patients, do not require analgesia. Acute pain in individuals with orthopedic problems originates from the periosteum, the joint surfaces, and the arterial walls. Muscle pain associated with bone surgery results from muscle ischemia rather than muscle tension. Acute abdominal pain often causes the individual involved to lie on one side and draw up the legs in the fetal position. Compare **chronic pain.** See also **pain intervention.**

acute paranoid disorder, a psychopathological condition characterized by a persecutory delusional system of rapid onset, quick development, and short duration, usually lasting less than six months. The disorder, which rarely becomes chronic, is most commonly seen in persons who have experienced drastic changes in their environment, such as immigrants, refugees, prisoners, military inductees, and, in a less severe form, those leaving home for the first time.

acute promyelocytic leukemia, a malignancy of the blood-forming tissues, characterized by severe bleeding, scattered bruises, a low fibrinogen level and platelet count, and the proliferation in bone marrow of promyelocytes and blast cells with distinctive Auer rods. Management of the disease requires replacement of coagulation factors and the administration of cytotoxic antileukemia drugs.

acute psychosis, one of a group of disorders in which the ability to process information is diminished and disordered. The cause of the particular disorder may be a known physiologic abnormality. In other cases the physiologic abnormality may not be recognized, but the defect in function is clearly present. Delirium and acute

brain syndrome are associated with known pathophysiology in the brain and are characterized by disorientation, disturbance of memory, and lapses in consciousness. Acute functional psychosis is associated with unknown pathophysiology and varying signs and symptoms that progress from insomnia and agitation to paranoid or grandiose delusions, mania, emotional lability, and hallucinations. An acute psychosis of any kind requires prompt diagnosis and treatment. The impaired judgment, confusion, and turmoil suffered has disastrous effects on all aspects of the patient's life. Antipsychotic medication and psychotherapy often bring about remission.

acute pyelonephritis. See **pyelonephritis.**

acute pyogenic arthritis, an acute bacterial infection affecting one or more joints, caused by trauma or a penetrating wound and occurring most frequently in children. Typical signs are pain, redness, and swelling in the affected joint, muscular spasms in the area, chills, fever, diaphoresis, and leukocytosis. Treatment consists of immobilization of the joint, the intravenous administration of an antibiotic, analgesia, and sedation. If required, the joint may be irrigated with normal saline and antibiotic. Hospitalization is usually required.

acute radial nerve palsy, a type of mononeuropathy characterized by damage to the radial nerve and consequent weakening of the muscles of the forearm. It may be caused by excessive compression of the radial nerve against a hard surface in individuals insensitized by the intake of alcohol or sedatives. It may also be caused by the repeated compression of the nerve by various weights, as the weight of the head of a bed partner. Time and the withdrawal of causative compression usually assure full recovery.

acute radiation exposure, exposure of short duration to intense ionizing radiation, usually occurring as the result of an accident in an industrial installation, a nuclear power plant, or a vehicle transporting radioactive material or from proximity to a detonated atom bomb. Exposure of the whole body to approximately 10,000 rads causes neurological and cardiovascular breakdown and is fatal within 24 hours. A dose between 500 and 1,200 rads destroys gastrointestinal mucosa, produces bloody diarrhea, and may cause death in several days. Death may occur weeks after exposure to a dose of 200 to 500 rads because of the destructive effect on blood-forming organs, but 600 rads is generally considered the fatal dose. See also **radiation exposure.**

acute respiratory distress syndrome (ARDS), a respiratory emergency characterized by respiratory insufficiency and failure usually following aspiration of a foreign body, cardiopulmonary bypass surgery, gram-negative sepsis, multiple blood transfusions, oxygen toxicity, trauma, pneumonia or other respiratory infection. It may also occur in such diseases as Guillain-Barré syndrome, muscular dystrophy, myasthenia gravis, emphysema, asthma, or poliomyelitis. Also called **shock lung, wet lung.**

■ OBSERVATIONS: The symptoms and signs of ARDS include shortness of breath, rapid breathing, flail chest, inadequate oxygenation of the arterial blood, increase in arterial PCO_2 and a decrease in the arterial pH. The changes that occur within the lungs include damage to the membranes of the capillaries, hemorrhage, capillary leaking, interstitial edema, impairment in gas exchange, and ventilation-perfusion abnormalities. These sequellae lead to decreased compliance and increased dyspnea.

■ INTERVENTION: The patient with ARDS usually requires mechanical ventilation, usually using positive-end-expiratory-pressure (PEEP). Treatment is directed toward establishing an airway, administering oxygen, improving the underlying condition, and removing the cause. Particular care in administrating oxygen is necessary in patients with chronic obstructive lung disease who have elevated levels of PCO_2, as a sudden or marked decrease in the PCO_2 may result in decreased respiratory effort. These patients also receive intermittent-positive-pressure breathing (IPPB) therapy every few hours, modified to administer low-flow oxygen to aid in ventilation and to reduce CO_2 levels. Also used in management are suctioning of the respiratory passages as necessary, and ultrasonic mist therapy, postural drainage, and cupping and vibration. When ventilation cannot be maintained and there is evidence of a rising PCO_2, mechanical ventilation with a respirator is necessary. Positive-end-expiratory-pressure is widely used in the treatment of ARDS. Sedatives are given with caution because they depress respiration.

■ NURSING CONSIDERATIONS: The patient with ARDS requires constant and meticulous nursing care, reassurance, and observation for changes in respiratory function and adequacy including signs of hypercapnia, especially confusion, skin flushing, and behavior changes that include aggressiveness. Increasing hypoxia may be recognized by tachycardia, elevated blood pressure, and increased peripheral resistance; fulminant respiratory failure is accompanied by falling blood pressure and cyanosis. If PEEP is being used, the nurse is careful to see that there is not a sudden disappearance of breath sounds accompanied by signs of respiratory distress—an indication that pneumothorax is present. Care is taken when weaning patients from the ventilator, and intermittent mandatory ventilation (IMV) may be used. Adequate humidification, respiratory therapy, sterile suction techniques, hourly hyperinflation and position changes are continued as necessary. Weight is taken frequently, x-ray films of the chest are taken and evaluated, and bacteriologic cultures of secretions are performed in the laboratory. Throughout treatment, ventilation is carefully monitored using blood gas studies and spirometry.

acute rheumatic arthritis, arthritis that occurs during the acute phase of rheumatic fever.

acute rhinitis. See **coryza.**

acute rickets. See **infantile scurvy.**

acute schizophrenia, a form of schizophrenia that is characterized by the sudden onset of personality disorganization with symptoms that include confusion, emotional turmoil, fear, depression, dreamlike dissociation, and bizarre behavior. Episodes appear suddenly in persons whose previous behavior has been relatively normal and are usually of short duration. Recurrent episodes are common, and in some instances a more chronic type of the disorder may develop. Also called **undifferentiated schizophrenia.** See also **schizophrenia, schizophreniform disorder.**

acute transverse myelitis, an abnormal condition characterized by inflammation of the entire thickness of the spinal cord, affecting both the sensory and the motor nerves. It is the most destructive form of myelitis and can develop rapidly, accompanied by necrosis and neurologic disorder that commonly persist after recovery. Patients who develop spastic reflexes soon after the onset of this disease are more likely to recover. This disorder may develop from a variety of causes, as acute multiple sclerosis, measles, pneumonia, and the ingestion of certain toxic agents, as carbon monoxide, lead, and arsenic. Such poisonous substances can destroy the entire circumference of the spinal cord, including the myelin sheaths, the axis cylinders, and the neurons, and can also cause hemorrhage and necrosis.

■ OBSERVATIONS: Acute transverse myelitis starts very quickly with sensory and motor dysfunctions below the level of the spinal cord damage. Within two days of onset, one or both legs of the affected patients may suffer flaccid paralysis following the advent of pain and sensory loss. Resulting severe spinal cord damage may cause shock with associated hypotension and hypothermia. Sphincter function and reflex losses are also common signs. Diagnosis is commonly based on the rapid onset of paraplegia, but it must rule out spinal cord tumor and identify any associated underlying infection.

■ INTERVENTION: There is no effective treatment and the prognosis for complete recovery is poor. Any underlying infection is identified and treated accordingly. Some patients with myelitis induced by multiple sclerosis or by various infections have received steroid treatments, but the results of such therapy are inconclusive.

■ NURSING CONSIDERATIONS: Proper nursing care of the patient with acute transverse myelitis involves frequent assessment of vital signs and constant vigilance for any signs of spinal shock, as hypotension and profuse sweating. Foley catheters must be meticulously maintained to avoid urinary tract infections, and proper skin care is needed to prevent infections and decubitus ulcers. To prevent contractures nurses commonly assist the patient with range-of-motion exercises and assure that the patient is properly aligned. Also important, especially for the patients who develop paraplegia, are physical therapy, bowel and bladder training, and consistent instruction and encouragement throughout the rehabilitation period.

ACVD, abbreviation for *atherosclerotic cardiovascular disease.*

-acy, a combining form meaning a 'state or quality of': *anthropocracy, lunacy, physiocracy.*

acyesis (æ′sāii′sıs), **1.** the absence of pregnancy. **2.** a condition of sterility in women.

ad-, a combining form meaning 'to, toward, addition to, or intensification': *adneural, adoral, adrenal.* Also **ac-, af-, ag-, ap-, as-, at-.**

-ad, a combining form meaning 'toward (a specified terminus)': *anteriad, iniad, obeliad.*

A/D, abbreviation for **analog-to-digital.**

ADA, 1. abbreviation for **American Dental Association, 2.** abreviation for **American Diabetes Association, 3.** abbreviation for **American Dietetic Association.**

adactyly (eidæk′tıli), a congenital defect in which one or more digits of the hand or foot are missing.

adamantinoma (æd′əmæn′tınou′mə). See **ameloblastoma.**

adamantoblastoma (æd′əmæn′toublæstou′mə). See **ameloblastoma.**

Adam's apple, *Informal.* the bulge at the front of the neck produced by the thyroid cartilage of the larynx. Also called **laryngeal prominence.**

Adams-Stokes syndrome, a condition characterized by sudden recurrent episodes of loss of consciousness owing to incomplete heart block. Seizures may accompany the episodes. Also called **Stokes-Adams syndrome.**

adaptation, a change or response to stress of any kind, as inflammation of the nasal mucosa in infectious rhinitis or an increase in crying in a frightened child. Adaptation may be normal, self-protective, and developmental, as a child learning to talk; it may be all encompassing, creating further stress, as polycythemia, naturally occurring at high altitudes, which provides more oxygen-carrying red blood cells but which may also lead to thrombosis, venous congestion, or edema. The degree and nature of adaptation shown by a patient is evaluated regularly by the nurse. It is a measure of the effectiveness of nursing care, the course of the disease, and the ability of the patient to cope with stress. See also **stress.**

adaptation model, (in nursing) a conceptual framework that focuses on the patient as an adaptive system, one in which nursing intervention is required when a deficit develops in the patient's ability to cope with the internal and external demands of the environment. These demands are classified in four groups: physiologic needs, the need for a positive self-concept, the need to perform so-

cial roles, and the need to balance dependence and independence. The nurse assesses the patient's maladaptive response and identifies the kind of demand that is causing the problem. Nursing care is planned to promote adaptive responses in order to cope successfully with the current stress on the patient's well-being. This model is frequently used as a conceptual framework for programs of nursing education.

adaptation syndrome. See **general adaptation syndrome.**

adaptor RNA. See **transfer RNA.**

Addams, Jane (1860–1935), an American social reformer. In 1889 she founded Hull House in Chicago, one of the first social settlements in the United States, where volunteers from many disciplines, including nursing, lived and continued working in their professions. She was at the center of most of the social reforms of her time and was an inspiration to those in the nursing profession who were striving to establish high educational standards and better working conditions. She was co-recipient of the Nobel peace prize in 1931.

addiction, compulsive, uncontrollable dependence on a substance, habit, or practice to such a degree that cessation causes severe emotional, mental, or physiological reactions. Compare **habituation.**

Addis count (æd′ıs), a method for counting red blood cells, white blood cells, epithelial cells, casts, and protein content in a sedimented 12-hour urine sample. Results are expressed as the number of each formed element excreted per 24 hours. The count is useful for diagnosing and managing kidney disease, as there should be none or nearly none of these components in the urine.

Addisonian anemia. See **pernicious anemia.**

Addisonian crisis. See **adrenal crisis.**

Addison's crisis (æd′ısənz). See **adrenal crisis.**

Addison's disease, a life-threatening condition caused by partial or complete failure of adrenocortical function, often owing to autoimmune processes, infection (especially tubercular or fungal), neoplasm, or hemorrhage in the gland. All three general functions of the adrenal cortex are lost: glucocorticoid, mineralocorticoid, and androgenic. Also called **Addisonism, Addison's syndrome.** See also **adrenal crisis, hypoadrenalism.**

■ OBSERVATIONS: The disease is characterized by weakness, decreased endurance, increased pigmentation of the skin and mucous membranes, anorexia, dehydration, weight loss, gastrointestinal disturbances, anxiety, depression and other emotional distress and decreased tolerance to cold. The onset is usually gradual, occurring over a period of weeks or months. Laboratory tests show abnormally low blood concentrations of sodium and glucose, a greater than normal level of serum potassium, and a decreased urinary output of certain steroids. The diagnosis is established if, after stimulation with adrenocorticosteroids, the amount of cortisol in the plasma and steroid in the urine fails to increase.

■ INTERVENTION: Treatment includes replacement therapy with glucocorticoid and mineralocorticoid drugs, an adequate intake of fluids, control of sodium and potassium balance, and a diet high in carbohydrate and protein. The person's requirements for glucocorticoid, mineralocorticoid, and salt are increased by stress, as in infection, trauma, and surgical procedures. Follow-up care includes frequent monitoring of sugar in the blood or urine, urinary acetone, and continued administration of corticoid drugs.

■ NURSING CONSIDERATIONS: The complications of Addison's disease include high fever, psychotic behavior, and adrenal crisis (Addisonian crisis). Under careful management, the patient's resistance to infection, capacity for work, and general well-being may be maintained. Nurses administer steroid and other drugs, observe the patient for signs of abnormal sodium and potassium levels, monitor body weight and fluid intake and output, and encourage an adequate intake of nutrients. The patient needs protection against stress while in the hospital and instruction in the importance of avoiding stress at home. The significance of emotional distress, the value of wearing a medical-alert bracelet or tag, the signs of impending crisis, the use of a prepared kit for emergencies, and the importance of scrupulous attention to drug and diet regimens are emphasized before discharge. Discharge teaching also emphasizes the need to take cortisone after meals or with milk to avoid gastric irritation and the development of ulcers.

Addison's keloid, a firm, white or pinkish patch of connective tissue on the skin, sometimes surrounded by a purplish areola. The lesion may involute, leaving a scar. Also called **circumscribed scleroderma, localized scleroderma, morphea.**

Addison's syndrome. See **Addison's disease.**

adduction, movement of a limb toward the body. Compare **abduction.**

adductor (ədək′tər), a muscle that acts to cause adduction. Compare **abductor, tensor.**

adductor brevis, a somewhat triangular muscle in the thigh and one of the five medial femoral muscles. Arising from the inferior ramus of the pubis, between the gracilis and the obturator externus, it passes downward, backward, and to the side to insert into the line leading from the lesser trochanter to the linea aspera of the femur. It is innervated by a branch of the obturator nerve, which contains fibers from the third and fourth lumbar nerves, and it acts to adduct and rotate the thigh medially and to flex the leg. Compare **adductor longus, adductor magnus, gracilis, pectineus.**

adductor canal, a triangular channel beneath the sartorius muscle and between the adductor longus and vastus medialis through which the femoral vessels and the saphenous nerve pass. Also called **Hunter's canal.**

adductor longus, the most superficial of the three adductor muscles of the thigh and one of five medial femoral muscles. A triangular muscle that arises from the anterior surface of the pubis, it spreads to form a broad fleshy belly, passing downward, backward, and to the side to insert into the linea aspera of the femur, between the vastus medialis and the adductor magnus. It is innervated by a branch of the obturator nerve, which contains fibers from the third and fourth lumbar nerves, and it functions to adduct and flex the thigh. Compare **adductor brevis, adductor magnus, gracilis, pectineus.**

adductor magnus, the long, heavy triangular muscle of the medial aspect of the thigh. It arises from the inferior rami of the ischium and pubis and the inferior margin of the ischial tuberosity. The fibers of the muscle insert into the rough surface of the greater trochanter, into the linea aspera via a broad aponeurosis, and into the distal third of the femur via a rounded, thick tendon. The muscle is innervated by the obturator nerve, which contains fibers of the third and fourth lumbar nerves, and by a branch of the sciatic nerve. The adductor magnus acts to adduct the thigh. The proximal portion acts to rotate the thigh medially and to flex it on the hip; the distal portion acts to extend the thigh and rotate it laterally.

aden-. See **adeno-.**

adenalgia (æd′ənæl′jə), a condition characterized by pain in any of the glands. Also called **adenodynia.**

adenectomy (æd′ənek′təmi), the surgical removal of any gland.

Aden fever (ei′dın). See **dengue.**

-adenia, a combining form meaning '(condition of the) glands': *anadenia, heteradenia, poradenia.*

adenine arabinoside (æd′ənin ær′əbın′əsaid). See **vidarabine.**

adenine-D-ribose. See **adenosine.**

adenitis (æd′ənai′tıs), an inflammatory condition of a lymph node or gland. Acute adenitis of the cervical lymph nodes manifests itself as a sore throat and stiff neck, simulating mumps if severe. It is usually a sign of secondary infection related to an oral, pharyngeal, or ear infection. Scarlet fever may cause an acute suppurative cervical adenitis as may infectious mononucleosis. Swelling of the lymph nodes in the back of the neck is often the result of a scalp infection, insect bite, or infestation by head lice. Inflammation of the lymph nodes of the mesenteric portion of the peritoneum often produces pain and other symptoms similar to those of appendicitis. Mesenteric adenitis may be mistaken for appendicitis, but, characteristically, mesenteric adenitis is preceded by a respiratory infection, the pain is less localized and less constant than in appendicitis, and it does not increase in severity. Generalized adenitis is a secondary symptom of syphilis.

Therapy requires treatment of the primary infection by the administration of antimicrobial agents, application of warm compresses and, in rare cases, incision and drainage. Compare **acinitis.**

adeno-, aden-, a combining form meaning 'pertaining to a gland': *adenocarcinoma, adenocellulitis, adenofibrosis.*

adenoacanthoma (æd'ɪnɔuæk'ænθou'mə), a malignant neoplasm derived from glandular tissue with squamous differentiation shown by some of the cells.

adenoameloblastoma (æd'ɪnɔuæm'əloublæstou'mə), *pl.* **adenoameloblastomas, adenoameloblastomata.** a benign tumor of the maxilla composed of ducts lined with columnar or cuboidal epithelial cells. It develops in tissue that normally gives rise to the teeth, and it is most often seen in young people.

adenoassociated virus (AAV) (æd'ɪnɔuəsou'sieitɪd), a defective virus that can reproduce only in the presence of adenoviruses. It is not yet known what role, if any, these organisms have in causing disease.

adenocarcinoma (æd'ɪnɔukarsɪnou'mə), *pl.* **adenocarcinomas, adenocarcinomata.** any one of a large group of malignant, epithelial cell tumors of the glands. Specific tumors are diagnosed and named by cytologic identification of the tissue affected, as an adenocarcinoma of the uterine cervix is characterized by tumor cells resembling the glandular epithelium of the cervix. — **adenocarcinomatous,** *adj.*

adenocarcinoma in situ, a localized growth of abnormal glandular tissue that may become malignant. It is most common in the endometrium and in the large intestine.

adenocarcinoma of the kidney. See **renal cell carcinoma.**

adenocele (æd'ɪnɔusil'), a cystic, glandular tumor.

adenochondroma (æd'ənɔukondrou'mə), *pl.* **adenochondromas, adenochondromata.** a neoplasm of cells derived from glandular and cartilaginous tissues, as a mixed tumor of the salivary glands. Also called **chondroadenoma.**

adenocyst (æd'ənəsɪst), **adenocystoma** (æd'ənɔusɪstou'mə), *pl.* **adenocystomas, adenocystomata.** a benign epithelial tumor in which the cells form glandular structures and cysts. A kind of adenocystoma is **papillary adenocystoma lymphomatosum.**

adenocystic carcinoma, a malignant neoplasm composed of cords of uniform small epithelial cells arranged in a sievelike pattern around cystic spaces which often contain mucus. The tumor occurs most frequently in the salivary glands, breast, mucous glands of the upper and lower respiratory tract, and, occasionally, in vestibular glands of the vulva. Although it grows slowly, it is malignant and tends to spread along the nerves, causing neurologic damage. Facial paralysis often results from adenocystic carcinoma of the salivary gland. Blood-borne metastases in bones and in the liver have been reported.

Also called **adenoid cystic carcinoma, adenomyoepithelioma, cribriform carcinoma, cylindroma, cylindromatous carcinoma.**

adenodynia (æd'ənɔudɪn'iə). See **adenalgia.**

adenoepithelioma (æd'ɪnɔuep'ɪθhi'liou'mə), *pl.* **adenoepitheliomas, adenoepitheliomata.** a neoplasm consisting of glandular and epithelial components.

adenofibroma (æd'ɪnɔufaibrou'mə), *pl.* **adenofibromas, adenofibromata.** a tumor of the connective tissues that contains glandular elements. A kind of adenofibroma is **adenofibroma edematodes.**

adenofibroma edematodes, a neoplasm consisting of glandular elements and connective tissue in which there is marked edema, as in a nasal polyp.

adenohypophysis (æd'ɪnɔuhæipof'ɪsɪs), the anterior lobe of the pituitary gland. It secretes growth hormone, thyrotropin, adrenocorticotropic hormone, melanin stimulating hormone, follicle stimulating hormone, luteinizing hormone, prolactin, beta lipotropin, and endorphins. Releasing hormones from the hypothalamus regulate secretion by the anterior pituitary. Adenohypophyseal hormones control activities of the thyroid, gonads, adrenal cortex, breast, and other endocrine glands. Also called **anterior pituitary.**

adenoid (æd'ɪnoid). See **pharyngeal tonsil.** — **adenoidal,** *adj.*

adenoidal speech, an abnormal manner of speaking caused by hypertrophy of the adenoidal tissue that normally exists in the nasopharynx of children. It is often characterized by a muted, nasal quality and may be corrected by a natural reduction of the swollen tissues or by surgical excision of the adenoids.

adenoid cystic carcinoma. See **adenocystic carcinoma.**

adenoidectomy (æd'ɪnoidek'təmi), removal of the lymphoid tissue in the nasopharynx. The surgical procedure may be performed because the adenoids are enlarged, causing obstruction, or chronically infected, and normal adenoids may be excised as a prophylactic measure during tonsillectomy. Preoperative procedures include a partial thromboplastin time test and for black patients a sickle cell preparation test. The operation is performed under general anesthesia in children, but local anesthesia may be used in adults. After removal of the adenoids, bleeding is stemmed with pressure; in some cases vessels may be ligated with sutures or an electrocoagulation current may be used. Postoperatively, the patient is observed for signs of hemorrhage and the pulse is checked every 15 minutes for the first hour and every 30 minutes for several hours thereafter. See also **tonsillectomy.**

adenoid hyperplasia, a condition in which enlarged adenoid glands cause partial respiratory obstruction, especially in children. Enlarged adenoids, often in association with enlarged tonsils, are a frequent cause of recurrent otitis media, sinusitis, and conduction deafness. Severe nasopharyngeal obstruction can result in alveolar hypoventilation and pulmonary hypertension with congestive heart failure. Treatment is usually surgical removal of the adenoids.

adenoleiomyofibroma (æd′ɪnoʊlaɪ′oʊmaɪ′oʊfaɪbroʊ′mə), *pl.* **adenoleiomyofibromas, adenoleiomyofibromata.** a benign tumor derived from smooth muscle with connective tissue and epithelial elements.

adenolipoma (æd′ɪnoʊlɪpoʊ′mə), *pl.* **adenolipomas, adenolipomata.** a neoplasm consisting of elements of glandular and fatty tissue.

adenolipomatosis (æd′ɪnoʊlɪpoʊmətoʊ′sɪs), a condition characterized by the growth of numerous adenolipomas in the groin, axilla, and neck.

adenolymphoma (æd′ɪnoʊlɪmfoʊ′mə), *pl.* **adenolymphomas, adenolymphomata.** See **papillary adenocystoma lymphomatosum.**

adenoma (æd′ɪnoʊ′mə), *pl.* **adenomas, adenomata.** a benign tumor of glandular epithelium in which the cells of the tumor are arranged in a recognizable glandular structure. An adenoma may cause excess secretion by the affected gland, as acidophilic pituitary adenoma resulting in an excess of growth hormone. Kinds of adenomas include **acidophilic adenoma, basophilic adenoma, fibroadenoma, insulinoma.** – **adenomatous,** *adj.*

-adenoma, a combining form meaning a 'tumor composed of glandular tissue or glandlike in structure': *sarcoadenoma, splenadenoma, syringadenoma.*

adenoma sebaceum (sebeɪ′siəm), an abnormal skin condition consisting of multiple, small, yellowish-red, waxy papules on the face, composed chiefly of fibrovascular tissue. Adenoma sebaceum is part of the complex known as tuberous sclerosis.

adenomatoid (æd′ɪnoʊ′mətoɪd), resembling a glandular tumor.

adenomatosis (æd′ɪnoʊmətoʊ′sɪs), an abnormal condition in which hyperplasia or tumor development affects two or more endocrine glands, usually the thyroid, adrenals, or pituitary. Also called **multiple endocrine adenomatosis.**

adenomatous goiter, an enlargement of the thyroid gland owing to an adenoma or numerous colloid nodules.

adenomyoepithelioma (æd′ɪnoʊmaɪ′oʊep′ɪfhi′lioʊ′mə). See **adenocystic carcinoma.**

adenomyofibroma (æd′ɪnoʊmaɪ′oʊfaɪbroʊ′mə), *pl.* **adenomyofibromas, adenomyofibromata,** a fibrous tumor that contains glandular and muscular components.

adenomyoma (æd′ɪnoʊmaɪoʊ′mə), *pl.* **adenomyomas, adenomyomata.** a tumor of the endometrium of the uterus, characterized by a mass of smooth muscle containing endometrial tissue and glands. It usually causes dysmenorrhea.

adenomyomatosis (æd′ɪnoʊmaɪ′oʊmətoʊ′sɪs), an abnormal condition characterized by the formation of benign nodules resembling adenomyomas, found in the uterus or in parauterine tissue.

adenomyosarcoma (æd′ɪnoʊmaɪ′oʊsarkoʊ′mə), *pl.* **adenomyosarcomas, adenomyosarcomata.** a malignant tumor of soft tissue containing glandular elements and striated muscle. A kind of adenomyosarcoma is **Wilms' tumor.**

adenomyosis (æd′ɪnoʊmaɪoʊ′sɪs), **1.** a benign neoplastic condition characterized by tumors composed of glandular tissue and smooth muscle cells. **2.** a malignant neoplastic condition characterized by the invasive growth of uterine mucosa in the wall of the uterus or the oviducts.

adenopathy (æd′ənop′əfhi), an enlargement of any gland, especially a lymphatic gland. – **adenopathic,** *adj.*

adenosarcoma (æd′ɪnoʊsarkoʊ′mə), *pl.* **adenosarcomas, adenosarcomata.** a malignant glandular tumor of the soft tissues of the body.

adenosarcorhabdomyoma (æd′ɪnoʊsar′koʊræb′doʊmaɪoʊ′mə), *pl.* **adenosarcorhabdomyomas, adenosarcorhabdomyomata.** a tumor composed of glandular elements, embryonal connective tissue, and striated muscle.

adenosine (əden′əsin, əden′əsɪn), a compound derived from nucleic acid, composed of adenine and a sugar, D-ribose. Adenosine is the major molecular component of the nucleotides adenosine monophosphate, adenosine diphosphate, adenosine triphosphate and of the nucleic acids deoxyribonucleic acid and ribonucleic acid. Also called **adenine-D-ribose.** See also **adenosine phosphate.**

adenosine 3′:5′-cyclic phosphate. See **cyclic adenosine monophosphate.**

adenosine deaminase, an enzyme that catalyzes the conversion of adenosine to the nucleoside inosine through the removal of an amino group. See also **adenosine.**

adenosine diphosphate, a product of the hydrolysis of adenosine triphosphate.

adenosine hydrolase, an enzyme that catalyzes the conversion of adenosine into adenine and pentose.

adenosine kinase, an enzyme in the liver and kidney that catalyzes the transfer of a phosphate group from adenosine triphosphate to produce adenosine phosphate.

adenosine monophosphate (AMP), an ester, composed of adenine, D-ribose, and phosphoric acid, that affects energy release in work done by a muscle.

adenosine phosphate, a compound consisting of the nucleotide adenosine attached through its ribose group to one, two, or three phosphoric acid molecules. Kinds of adenosine phosphate, all of which are interconvertible, are **adenosine diphosphate, adenosine monophosphate, adenosine triphosphate.**

adenosine triphosphatase (ATPase), an enzyme that catalyzes the hydrolysis of adenosine triphosphate to adenosine diphosphate and inorganic phosphate. Among various enzymes in this group associated with cell membranes and intracellular structures, mitochondrial ATPase is involved in obtaining energy for cellular metabolism and myosin ATPase is involved in muscle contraction.

adenosis (æd'ənou'sıs), **1.** a disease in any gland, especially a lymphatic gland. **2.** an abnormal development or enlargement of glandular tissue.

adenovirus (æd'ınouvaï'rəs), any one of the 31 medium-sized viruses of the Adenoviridae family, pathogenic to man, that cause conjunctivitis, upper respiratory infection, or gastrointestinal infection. After the acute and symptomatic period of illness, the virus may persist in a latent stage in the tonsils, adenoids, and other lymphoid tissue. — **adenoviral,** *adj.*

adenylate (əden'ıleit), to convert a substance to adenylic acid.

adenylate kinase, an enzyme in skeletal muscle, the heart, brain, and liver that activates hexokinase to make possible the transfer of phosphate from adenosine diphosphate to fructose or glucose. Also called **myokinase.**

adenylic acid (æd'ınıl'ık). See **adenosine monophosphate.**

adequate and well-controlled studies, clinical and laboratory studies that the sponsors of a new drug are required by law to conduct to demonstrate the truth of the claims made for its effectiveness. See also **control.**

adermia (ədər'miə), a congenital or acquired skin defect or the absence of skin.

ADH, abbreviation for **antidiuretic hormone.**

adhere, the act of sticking together or becoming fastened, as two surfaces that may be fastened with or as with glue.

adherence, 1. the quality of clinging or being closely attached. **2.** the process in which a person follows rules, guidelines, or standards, especially as a patient follows the prescription and recommendations for a regimen of care.

adhesion (ædhi'ʒhən), a band of scar tissue that binds together two anatomical surfaces which are normally separate from each other. Adhesions are most commonly found in the abdomen where they form following abdominal surgery, inflammation, or injury. A loop of intestine may adhere to unhealed areas and cause an intestinal obstruction if scar tissue develops and constricts the lumen of the bowel, blocking the intestinal flow. The condition is characterized by abdominal pain, nausea and vomiting, distention, and an increase in pulse rate without a rise in temperature. Nasogastric intubation and suction may relieve the blockage. If not, surgery may be necessary to separate adhering surfaces. See also **adhesiotomy, intestinal obstruction.**

adhesiotomy (ædhi'ziot'əmi), the surgical removal of adhesions, usually performed to relieve an intestinal obstruction. See also **abdominal surgery.**

adhesive absorbent dressing, an absorbent dressing on an adhesive backing.

adhesive pericarditis, a condition characterized by adhesions between the visceral and the parietal layers of the pericardium or by adhesions between the pericardium and the mediastinum, diaphragm, or chest wall. Adhesions between the pericardial layers may completely obstruct the pericardial cavity. Adhesive pericarditis may seriously impair normal movements of the heart.

adhesive peritonitis, an inflammation of the peritoneum, characterized by adhesions between adjacent serous surfaces. This condition may be marked by exudations of serum, fibrin, cells, and pus, accompanied by abdominal pain and tenderness, vomiting, constipation, and fever.

adhesive plaster, a strong fabric material covered on one side with an adhesive. Often water-repellent, it may be used to hold bandages and dressings in place, to immobilize a part, or to exert pressure. Also called **adhesive tape.**

adhesive pleurisy, inflammation of the pleura with exudation, causing obliteration of the pleural space through the fusion of the visceral pleural layer covering the lungs and the parietal layer lining the walls of the thoracic cavity.

adhesive skin traction, one of two kinds of skin traction in which the therapeutic pull of traction weights is applied with adhesive straps that stick to the skin over the body structure involved, especially a fractured bone. Adhesive skin traction is used only when continuous traction is desired and skin care for the affected area presents no serious problem. The adhesive straps used to secure the traction system to the body area involved spread the pull over a wide plot of skin, decreasing the vulnerability of the patient to skin breakdown. Compare **nonadhesive skin traction.**

ADI, abbreviation for **acceptable daily intake.**

adiathermance (æ'daiəthər'məns), the quality of being unaffected by heat waves.

adient (æd'iənt), characterized by a tendency to move toward rather than away from stimuli. Compare **abient.** — **adience,** *n.*

Adie's pupil (ei'diz). See **Adie's syndrome.**

Adie's syndrome, a pathological condition of the pupil, characterized by abnormal pupillary accommodation. In near vision the affected pupil contracts and dilates slower than the pupil on the opposite side and does not usually react normally to direct and indirect light. Adie's syndrome is considered a pupillary muscle problem rather than a motor problem and does not indicate any neurological disease. Also called **Adie's pupil.**

adip-. See **adipo-.**

adipectomy (æd'ıpek'təmi). See **lipectomy.**

adiphenine hydrochloride (ədıf'lənin), an anticholinergic with smooth muscle relaxant properties that has been used for spastic disorders of the gastrointestinal and genitourinary tract.

adipic (ədɪpˈɪk), of or pertaining to fatty tissue.

adipo-, adip-, a combining form meaning 'pertaining to fat': *adipocele, adipogenesis, adipokinin.*

adipocele (ædˈɪpousilˈ), a hernia containing fat or fatty tissue. Also called **lipocele.**

adipofibroma (ædˈɪpoufaɪbrouˈmə), *pl.* **adipofibromas, adipofibromata.** a fibrous neoplasm of the connective tissue in which there are fatty components.

adiponecrosis (ædˈɪpounɪkrouˈsɪs), a necrosis of fatty tissue in the body. —**adiponecrotic,** *adj.*

adiponecrosis subcutanea neonatorum, an abnormal dermatolgic condition of the newborn characterized by patchy areas of hardened subcutaneous fatty tissue and a bluish-red discoloration of the overlying skin. The lesions, often a result of manipulation during delivery, spontaneously resolve within a period of days to several weeks without scarring. Also called **pseudosclerema, subcutaneous fat necrosis.**

adipose (ædˈɪpous), fatty. Adipose tissue is composed of fat cells arranged in lobules. See also **fat, fatty acid, lipoma.**

adipose tumor. See **lipoma.**

adiposogenital dystrophy (ædˈɪpouˈsoujenˈɪtəl), a disorder occurring in adolescent boys, characterized by genital hypoplasia and feminine secondary sex characteristics, including female distribution of fat. It is caused by hypothalamic malfunction or by a tumor in the anterior pituitary gland. A subnormal body temperature, low blood pressure, and reduced blood sugar are frequently associated with the disorder. Diabetes insipidus often occurs because of hyposecretion of antidiuretic hormone, and involvement of the hypothalamic satiety center may induce overeating and result in pronounced obesity. If a tumor is present, there may be drowsiness and symptoms of increased intracranial pressure. Treatment may include the administration of testosterone and a weight reduction program, excision or radiologic ablation of a tumor, and replacement of hormones, as necessary. Also called **adiposogenital syndrome, Fröhlich's syndrome.**

adiposogenital syndrome. See **adiposogenital dystrophy.**

aditus (ædˈɪtəs), an approach or an entry.

adjunct, (in health care) an additional substance, treatment, or procedure used for increasing the efficacy or safety of the primary substance, treatment, or procedure or to facilitate its performance. —**adjunctive,** *adj.*

adjunctive psychotherapy, a form of psychotherapy that concentrates on improving a person's general mental and physical outlook without trying to resolve basic emotional problems. Some kinds of adjunctive psychotherapy

are **music therapy, occupational therapy, physical therapy, recreational therapy.**

adjunct to anesthesia, one of a number of drugs of five different classes. Each class of drug has a use in anesthetic procedures, as well as a therapeutic indication in other aspects of health care. Adjuncts to anesthesia are used as premedications, as intravenous supplements to hypnotic or analgesic medications, and as neuromuscular blocking agents, analeptics, and therapeutic gases. Premedications are given to reduce anxiety, sedate the patient, reduce salivation and secretions of the respiratory passages, and prevent bradycardia. Strong analgesics, sedatives and hypnotics, phenothiazenes, anticholinergics, and antianxiety agents are also sometimes prescribed as premedications. Intravenous hypnotic and analgesic supplements, given to augment the effects of nitrous oxide, include morphine, demerol, diazepam, fentonyl, and droperidol. Neuromuscular blocking agents are given to produce and sustain relaxation of the skeletal muscles during the surgical procedure. These agents are of two kinds: depolarizing or nondepolarizing. Depolarizing agents (including succinylcholine), act by depolarizing the postsynaptic membranes, rendering them refractory to stimulation and producing muscle paralysis. Nondepolarizing agents, including tubocurarine, methocurine, gallamine, and pancuronium, act by competing with acetylcholine for receptor sites on the postjunctional receptor sites, producing paralysis of the muscles. The use of these agents usually requires assisted or controlled respiration by an anesthetist or anesthesiologist and a careful evaluation of the recovery of neuromuscular transmission in the postoperative period. Analeptics may be administered to stimulate the function of the central nervous system in ventilatory insufficiency owing to drug overdose, drowning, electric shock, carbon monoxide poisoning, or other condition resulting in hypoxemia. The effects of these agents are transitory and may paradoxically result in further depression; therefore, they are not usually recommended. Therapeutic gases include carbon dioxide and oxygen and various general anesthetics. Carbon dioxide and oxygen are given to maintain normal respiratory metabolism and function and as vehicles to carry anesthetic gases.

adjusted death rate. See **standardized death rate.**

adjustment. See **accommodation.**

adjustment reaction, a temporary disorder of varying severity that occurs as an acute reaction to overwhelming stress in persons of any age who have no apparent underlying mental disorders. Symptoms include anxiety, withdrawal, depression, brooding, temper outbursts, crying spells, attention-getting behavior, enuresis, loss of appetite, aches, pains, and muscle spasms. It can result from such situations as separation of an infant from its mother, the birth of a sibling, loss or change of a job, death of a loved one, or forced retirement. Symptoms usually recede and eventually disappear as stress diminishes. See also **psychoneurotic disorder.**

adjuvant therapy (æd'jəvənt), the treatment of a disease with substances that enhance the action of drugs, especially drugs that promote the production of antibodies.

ADL, abbreviation for **activities of daily living.**

administration of parenteral fluids, the intravenous infusion of various solutions to maintain adequate hydration, restore blood volume, reestablish lost electrolytes, or provide partial nutrition.

■ METHOD: Fluid is administered parenterally through a closed system consisting of a bottle of sterile solution, a catheter, and an attached intracatheter or scalp vein needle that is inserted into a peripheral vein and securely taped to the patient's arm or leg. The fluid is infused slowly. Five per cent dextrose in distilled water may be used to maintain volume or restore blood volume; ascorbic acid and vitamin B are often added to the solution. Five per cent dextrose in saline solution plus potassium chloride may be infused to reestablish electrolyte balance, but potassium is contraindicated in renal failure and untreated adrenal insufficiency. A one sixth molar lactate solution may be administered if sodium is deficient, and an ammonium chloride solution may be administered when replacement of chloride is required. Distilled water containing 10 to 20 per cent glucose or fructose may be used to supply carbohydrate, but, since these solutions are hypertonic, additional hydration is needed for proper excretion. Low molecular weight dextran is frequently used as a plasma volume expander in treating shock, but it increases bleeding time and is contraindicated in pregnancy and severe renal disease. During parenteral fluid administration, the venipuncture site is observed every one to two hours for signs of redness, swelling, warmth, and leakage; for the security and comfort of the tape; and for the position of the patient's extremity. The flow rate, the level, color, and clarity of the fluid, the label, and the patency of the tubing are checked, and the patient is monitored for signs of dehydration, fever, and signs of circulatory overload, as headache, tachycardia, elevated blood pressure, dyspnea, engorged neck veins, and pulmonary edema.

■ NURSING ORDERS: Depending on the service, the nurse may select the necessary equipment, prepare the venipuncture site, check the labels of fluid bottles for content, and perform the venipuncture. During the administration of fluid, the nurse keeps the system closed, watches the flow rate, records the amount of solution given, and observes the venipuncture site and the patient's general condition. If there are any signs of increased blood volume, the nurse reduces the flow of the infusion until further orders are obtained. The nurse changes the dressing daily

and ensures that the patient understands the importance of keeping the extremity still, of not disturbing the tubing, and of reporting pain or swelling.

■ OUTCOME CRITERIA: Parenteral fluid therapy is usually uneventful but infants, elderly patients with circulatory or renal impairment, and burn patients, whose plasma may shift suddenly from interstitial tissue, causing increased blood volume, require special attention.

adnexa, *sing.* **adnexus.** tissue or structures in the body that are next to or near another, related structure. The ovaries and the uterine tubes are adnexa of the uterus. – **adnexal,** *adj.*

adolescence, 1. the period in development between the onset of puberty and adulthood. It usually begins between the ages of 11 and 13, with the appearance of secondary sex characteristics, and spans the teen years, terminating at 18 to 20 years of age with the acquisition of completely developed adult form. During this period the individual undergoes extensive physical, psychological, emotional, and personality changes. 2. the state or quality of being adolescent or youthful. See also **postpuberty, prepuberty, psychosexual development, psychosocial development, pubarche.**

adolescent, 1. of, pertaining to, or characteristic of adolescence. 2. one in the state or process of adolescence; a teenager.

adolescent vertebral epiphysitis (ɪpɪf'ɪsai'tɪs). See **Scheuermann's disease.**

ADP, abbreviation for **adenosine diphosphate.**

adrenal cortex, the greater portion of the adrenal or suprarenal gland, fused with the gland's medulla and producing mineral corticoids, androgens, and glucocorticoids, hormones essential to homeostasis. The outer cortex is normally a deep-yellow color; the inner part, dark-red or brown. It is recognizable in the embryo during the sixth week as a groove in the coelom at the base of the mesentery near the cranial end of the mesonephros.

adrenal cortical carcinoma, a malignant neoplasm of the adrenal cortex that may cause adrenogenital syndrome or Cushing's syndrome. Such tumors vary in size, occur at any age, and are more common in females than in males. Metastases frequently develop in the lungs, liver, and other organs. See also **adrenogenital syndrome, Cushing's syndrome.**

adrenal crisis, an acute, life-threatening state of profound adrenocortical insufficiency in which immediate therapy is required. It is characterized by glucocorticoid deficiency, a drop in extracellular fluid volume, and hyperkalemia. Also called **Addisonian crisis.** See also **Addison's disease, adrenal cortex.**

■ OBSERVATIONS: Typically, the patient appears to be in shock or coma with a low blood pressure, severe prostration, and loss of vasomotor tone. The person's medical history may include Addison's disease or reveal symptoms indicating its presence. Laboratory tests show hyperkalemia and hyponatremia.

■ INTERVENTION: An intravenous isotonic solution of sodium chloride containing a water-soluble glucocorticoid is administered rapidly. Vasopressor agents may be necessary to combat hypotension. If the patient is vomiting, a nasogastric tube is usually inserted. Total bed rest and the monitoring of blood pressure, temperature, and other vital signs are mandatory. After the first critical hours the patient is followed as for Addison's disease and steroid dosage is tapered to maintenance levels. In all cases the precipitating cause is sought. Infection and a failure to increase the maintenance dose is a common cause of crisis in people who have Addison's disease.

■ NURSING CONSIDERATIONS: Nursing care during adrenal crisis includes eliminating all forms of stimuli, especially loud noises or bright lights. The patient is not moved unless absolutely necessary and is not allowed to perform self-care activities. If the condition is identified and treated promptly, the prognosis is good. Discharge instructions include a reminder to the patient to seek medical attention in any stressful situation, whether physiologic or psychologic, in order to prevent a recurrence of the crisis.

adrenalectomy (ədri'nəlek'təmi), the surgical removal of one or both adrenal glands or the resection of a portion of one or both glands, performed to reduce the excessive secretion of adrenal hormones when an adrenal tumor or a malignancy of the breast or prostate is present. The incision is made under the 12th rib in the rear flank area, under a general anesthetia. Preoperative laboratory tests include electrolytes, fasting blood sugar, and glucose tolerance. Corticosteroid drugs are given, and frequent blood-pressure measurements are recorded. Before surgery, a nasogastric tube is inserted and a venous cutdown is done. Postoperative care focuses on monitoring vital signs and maintaining blood pressure with an I.V. solution containing a vasopressor and corticosteroids. An abrupt drop in blood pressure, increasing weakness, and a rise in temperature are signs of acute corticosteroid insufficiency. Blood electrolyte levels are checked frequently, and fluid intake and output are carefully recorded. Steroids are given by mouth a few days after surgery. When oral steroids can be tolerated the dosage is tapered to a maintenance level; if both glands were removed, the maintenance dosage continues for life. Stress and fatigue must be avoided. See also **Addison's disease, Cushing's syndrome.**

adrenal gland, either of two secretory organs perched atop the kidneys. Each consists of two parts having independent functions: the cortex and the medulla. The adrenal cortex, in response to adrenocorticotropic hormone secreted by the anterior pituitary, secretes cortisol and androgens. Adrenal androgens serve as precursors that are converted by the liver to testosterone and estrogens. Renin from the kidney controls adrenal cortical production of aldosterone. The adrenal medulla manufactures the catecholamines epinephrine and norepinephrine.

Adrenalin, a trade name for an adrenergic (epinephrine).

adrenaline (ədren'əlin, ədren'əlin). See **epinephrine.**

adrenalize (ədri'nəlaiz), to stimulate or excite.

adrenal virilism, the development in a female of male secondary sexual characteristics resulting from excessive production of androgenic hormones or to tumors of the ovary, as arrhenoblastoma, hilus cell tumor, or gynandroblastoma. Also called **masculinization, virilization.**

adrenarche (æd'rɪnar'ki), the intensified activity in the adrenal cortex that occurs at about eight years of age and increases the elaboration of various hormones, especially androgens.

adrenergic (æd'rɪnər'jɪk), 1. of or pertaining to sympathetic nerve fibers of the autonomic nervous system. 2. of or pertaining to drugs or hormones that mimic the effects of sympathetic stimulation. 3. an adrenergic drug. Compare **cholinergic.**

adrenergic blocking agent. See **antiadrenergic.**

adrenergic drug. See **adrenergic.**

adrenergic fibers, nerve fibers of the autonomic nervous system that release the neurotransmitter norepinephrine. Most postganglionic sympathetic fibers are of this type.

adrenergic receptor, a site in a sympathetic effector cell that reacts to adrenergic stimulation. Two types of adrenergic receptors are recognized: alpha-adrenergic receptors and beta-adrenergic receptors. In general, stimulation of alpha receptors is excitatory of the function of the host organ or tissue, and stimulation of the beta-receptors is inhibitory.

-adrenia, a combining form meaning '(degree or condition of) adrenal activity': *anadrenia, dysadrenia, hypadrenia.*

adrenocorticotropic (ədri'noukər'tɪkoutrop'ɪk), **adrenocorticotrophic** (ədri'noukər'tɪkoutrof'ɪk), of or pertaining to stimulation of the adrenal cortex.

adrenocorticotropic hormone, adrenocorticotrophic hormone (ACTH), a hormone of the anterior pituitary gland that stimulates the growth of the adrenal gland and the secretion of corticosteroids. ACTH secretion, regulated by corticotropin releasing factor (CRF) from the hypothalamus, increases in response to a low level of circulating cortisol and to stress, fever, acute hypoglycemia, and major surgery. Under normal conditions there is a diurnal rhythm in ACTH secretion with an increase beginning after the first few hours of sleep and reaching a peak at the time a person awakens. ACTH stimulates the formation of cyclic adenosine monophosphate (AMP), which is thought to activate the enzyme system that catalyzes the conversion of cholesterol to pregnenolone, the precursor of all steroidal hormones. A purified preparation of ACTH in gelatin is widely used in the treatment of rheumatoid arthritis, acquired hemolytic anemia, intractable allergic states, various dermatologic diseases, and many other disorders. Also called **corticotropin.**

adrenodoxin (ədri'noudok'sın), a protein, produced by the adrenal glands, that participates in the transfer of electrons within animal cells.

adrenogenitalism (ədri'noujen'ıtəlız'əm), a condition characterized by hypersecretion of adrenocortical androgens, resulting in somatic masculinization. Excessive production of the hormone may be caused by a virilizing adrenal tumor, congenital adrenal hyperplasia, or an inborn deficiency of enzymes required to transform endogenous androgenic steroids to glucocorticoids. Girls born with adrenogenitalism may be pseudohermaphroditic with clitoral enlargement and labial fusion in infancy and later hirsutism, low vocal pitch, acne, amenorrhea, and masculine distribution of hair and development of muscles. Boys with congenital adrenogenitalism show precocious development of the penis and prostate and of pubic and axillary hair, but their testes remain small and immature because negative feedback from the high level of adrenal androgens prevents the normal pubertal increase in pituitary gonadotropin. Children with the disorder are unusually tall, but their epiphyses close prematurely and as adults they are abnormally short. Virilizing tumors are more common or more frequently diagnosed in women. They usually occur between the ages of 30 and 40 but may arise later, after the menopause. Signs of the tumor in women include hirsutism, amenorrhea, oily skin, ovarian changes, muscular hypertrophy, and atrophy of the uterus and breasts. Treatment may involve tumor resection, administration of cortisol, and plastic surgical procedures. Electrolytic epilation may be indicated. See also **pseudohermaphrodism.**

adrenogenital syndrome (ædri'noujen'ıtəl), an endocrine disorder resulting from abnormal activity of the adrenal cortex. Less than normal amounts of cortisol and more than normal amounts of androgen are produced, causing precocious puberty in boys and masculinization of the external genitalia in girls (pseudohermaphrodism). Most often congenital, the condition may be acquired in adulthood as a result of medication or a tumor that suppresses or stimulates the adrenal glands. In female infants the syndrome usually is obvious at birth, and is characterized by enlargement of the labia and clitoris. In males the diagnosis is often not made until the age of four or older when precocious development of the phallus and underdevelopment of the testes are seen. Treatment to restore hormonal balance is often achieved with a corticosteroid. Early reconstructive surgery of the female genitalia may be necessary to achieve normal development. Also called

congenital adrenal hyperplasia. See also **adrenal virilism, pseudohermaphrodism.**

Adriamycin. See **doxorubicin hydrochloride.**

adromia (ədrou'miə), the absence of the conductive capacity of any nerve that normally innervates a muscle.

adult, 1. one who is fully developed and matured and who has attained the intellectual capacity and the emotional and psychological stability characteristic of a mature person. **2.** a person who has reached full legal age. Compare **child.**

adult celiac disease. See **celiac disease.**

adulteration, the debasement or dilution of the purity of any substance, process, or activity by the addition of extraneous material.

adult hemoglobin. See **hemoglobin A.**

adulthood, the phase of development characterized by physical and mental maturity.

adult polycystic disease (ADP). See **polycystic kidney disease.**

adult respiratory distress syndrome (ARDS), a set of symptoms including decreased compliance of lung tissue, pulmonary edema, and acute hypoxemia. It may be caused by shock, chest trauma, aspiration, fat embolism, or massive viral pneumonia and is often characterized by the development of a uniform hyaline membrane covering the alveolar epithelium. The membrane interferes with the production of pulmonary surfactant and impedes the exchange of oxygen and carbon dioxide. The condition is similar to respiratory distress syndrome of the newborn. Treatment may include oxygen therapy by positive and expiratory pressure, fluid restriction, diuretics, and corticosteroids. Complications of this condition are oxygen toxicity and pulmonary sepsis. See also **congestive atelectasis, shock lung, wet lung.**

adult celiac disease. See **celiac disease.**

adult rickets, a disease affecting adults that resembles rickets. See also **osteomalacia, rickets.**

advanced life support (ALS). See **Emergency Medical Technician-Advanced Life Support.**

adventitious (æd'ventıʃ'əs), of or pertaining to an accidental condition or an arbitrary action.

adventitious bursa, an abnormal bursa that develops as a response to friction or pressure.

adverse drug effect, a harmful, unintended reaction to a drug administered at normal dosage.

adynamia (æd'ınei'miə), lack of physical and emotional drive owing to psychodynamic weakness. A kind of adynamia is **adynamia episodica hereditaria.** See also **asthenia.** —**adynamic,** *adj.*

adynamia episodica hereditaria, a condition seen in infancy, characterized by muscle weakness and episodes of flaccid paralysis. It is inherited as an autosomal dominant trait. Also called **hyperkalemic periodic paralysis.**

adynamic fever, an elevated temperature with a feeble pulse, nervous depression, and a cool, moist skin. Also called **asthenic fever.**

adynamic ileus. See **ileus.**

Aedes (eii′diz), a genus of mosquito, prevalent in tropical and subtropical regions. Several species are capable of transmitting pathogenic organisms to man, including dengue and yellow fever.

aer-. See **aero-.**

aerate (eir′eit), the act of charging a substance or a structure with air, carbon dioxide, or oxygen.

aero-, aer-, a combining form meaning 'pertaining to air or to gas': *aerobe, aerocystography, aerodontalgia.*

Aerobacter aerogenes (er′oubæk′tər eroj′miz). See *Enterobacter cloacae.*

aerobe (eir′oub), a microorganism that lives and grows in the presence of free oxygen. Kinds of aerobe are **facultative aerobe, obligate aerobe.** Compare **anaerobe.** – **aerobic,** *adj.*

aerobic exercise, mild to moderate muscular exertion below the level that produces metabolic acidosis. Compare **anaerobic exercise.** See also **active exercise, passive exercise.**

aerobic glycolysis. See **glycolysis.**

aerobics. See **aerobic exercise.**

aerodontalgia (er′oudontæl′jə), a painful sensation in the teeth owing to decreased atmospheric pressure, as may occur at high altitudes.

aeroembolism (eir′ouem′bəlız′əm). See **embolism.**

aerophagy (eirof′əji), **aerophagia** (eir′oufei′jə), the swallowing of air, usually followed by belching, gastric distress, and flatulence.

aerosinusitis (eir′ousai′nəsai′tıs), inflammation, edema, or hemorrhage of the frontal sinuses, caused by expansion of air within the sinuses when barometric pressure is decreased, as in aircraft at high altitudes. Also called **barosinusitis.**

aerosol, 1. nebulized particles suspended in a gas or air. **2.** a pressurized gas containing a finely nebulized medication for inhalation therapy. **3.** a pressurized gas containing a nebulized chemical agent for sterilizing the air of a room.

aerotitis (eir′ətai′tıs), an inflammation of the ear caused by changes in atmospheric pressure. Also called **barotitis.**

aerotitis media, inflammation or bleeding in the middle ear owing to a difference between the air pressure in the middle ear and that of the atmosphere, as occurs in sudden changes in altitude, in diving, or in hyperbaric chambers. Symptoms are pain, tinnitus, diminished hearing, and vertigo. Also called **barotitis media.**

Æsculapius (es′kyʊlei′piəs), the ancient Greek god of medicine. According to legend, Æsculapius, the son of Apollo, was trained by the centaur Chiron in the art of healing, becoming so proficient that he not only cured sick patients but also brought the dead back to life. Because Zeus feared that Æsculapius could help humans escape death altogether, he killed the healer with a bolt of lightning. Later, Æsculapius was raised to the stature of a god and was worshiped also by the Romans, who believed he could prevent pestilence. Serpents were regarded as sacred by Æsculapius, and he is symbolized in modern medicine by a staff with a serpent entwined about it.

-aesthesia, -esthesia, a combining form meaning '(condition of) feeling, perception, or sensation': *allaesthesia, cinaesthesia, hypercrysaesthesia.*

-aesthetic. See **-esthetic.**

af-. See **ad-.**

afebrile (eifi′brəl, eifeb′rəl), without fever.

affect, an outward manifestation of a person's feelings or emotions. – **affective,** *adj.*

affective disorder. See **major affective disorder.**

affective melancholia, *Obsolete.* the depressive phase of bipolar disorder. See also **depression.**

affect memory, a particular emotional feeling that recurs whenever a significant experience is recalled.

afferent (æf′ərənt), proceeding toward a center, as applied to arteries, veins, lymphatics, and nerves. Compare **efferent.**

affidavit, a written statement that is sworn to before a notary public or an officer of the court.

affiliated hospital, a hospital that is associated to some degree with a medical school or health program.

affirmative defense, (in law) a denial of guilt or wrongdoing based on new evidence rather than on simple denial of a charge, as a plea of immunity according to a good samaritan law. The defendant bears the burden of proof in an affirmative defense.

afibrinogenemia (æfai′brınoujıni′miə), a rare, hematologic disorder characterized by a relative lack or absence of fibrinogen in the blood. It may be the result of a primary, congenital blood dyscrasia, or it may be acquired, as in disseminated intravascular coagulation.

African lymphoma. See **Burkitt's lymphoma.**

African sleeping sickness. See **African trypanosomiasis.**

African tick fever. See **relapsing fever.**

African trypanosomiasis, a disease caused by the parasites *Trypanosoma brucei gambiense* or *Trypanosoma brucei rhodesiense,* transmitted to man by the bite of the tsetse fly. African trypanosomiasis occurs only in the tropical areas of Africa, where tsetse flies are found. The disease progresses through three phases: localized, at the site of invasion of the organism; systemic, marked by fever, chills, headache, anemia, edema of the hands and feet, and enlargement of the lymph glands; and neurologic, marked by symptoms of central nervous system involvement, including lethargy, sleepiness, headache, convulsions, and coma. The disease is fatal unless treated, though it may be years before the patient reaches the neurologic phase. Antimicrobial medication specific for the treatment of trypanosomiasis is available in the United States only from the Center for Disease Control. Kinds of African trypanosomiasis are **Gambian trypanosomiasis, Rhodesian trypanosomiasis.** Also called **African sleeping sickness, sleeping sickness.** See also **trypanosomiasis, tsetse fly.**

Afrin, a trade name for an adrenergic vasoconstrictor (oxymetazoline hydrochloride), used as a decongestant.

afterbirth. the tissue, fluid, and blood expelled from the uterus after childbirth, including the placenta, the amnion and the chorion, and some amniotic fluid, blood, and bloodclots.

afterloading, (in radiotherapy) a technique in which an unloaded applicator or needle is placed within the patient at the time of an operative procedure and subsequently loaded with the radioactive source under controlled conditions in which health care personnel are protected against exposure to radiation. A kind of afterloading is **remote afterloading.**

afterpains, contractions of the uterus common during the first days postpartum. They tend to be strongest in nursing mothers and multiparas, resolve spontaneously, and rarely require analgesia. The nurse may reassure the mother that afterpains are normal and prove that the uterus is contracting as it should.

Ag, symbol for **silver.**

ag-. See **ad-.**

AGA, abbreviation for **appropriate-for-gestational-age.**

agamete (eɪgæm′ɪt), **1.** any of the unicellular organisms that reproduce asexually by multiple fission, such as bacteria and protozoa. **2.** any asexual reproductive cell, as a spore or merozoite, that forms a new organism without fusion with another cell.

agametic (eɪ′gəmi′tɪk), **agamous,** asexual; without recognizable sex organs or gametes.

agamic, reproducing asexually, without the union of gametes; asexual.

agammaglobulinemia (ægæm′əglob′yulɪni′miə), a rare disorder characterized by the absence of the serum immunoglobulin, gamma globulin, associated with an increased susceptibility to infection. The condition may be transient, congenital, or acquired. The transient form is common in infancy before six weeks of age when the infant becomes able to synthesize the immunoglobulin. The congenital form is rare, sex-linked, and results in decreased production of antibodies. The acquired form usually occurs in association with a malignant disease like leukemia, myeloma, or lymphoma. See also **Bruton's agammaglobulinemia, gamma globulin, immune globulin.**

agamocytogeny (əgæm′ousaitoj′əni). See **agamogenesis.** – **agamocytogenic,** adj.

agamogenesis (əgæm′oujen′əsɪs), asexual reproduction,

as by budding or simple fission of cells; parthenogenesis. Also called **agamocytogeny, agamogony.** – **agamogenetic, agamogenic,** adj.

agamogony (æg′əmog′əni). See **agamogenesis.** – **agamogonic,** adj.

agamont (æg′əmont). See **schizont.**

agamous (æg′əməs). See **agametic.**

agar-agar (a′gara′gar), a dried hydrophilic, colloidal product obtained from certain species of red algae. Because it is unaffected by bacterial enzymes, it is widely used as the basic ingredient in solid culture media in bacteriology. Agar-agar is also used as a suspending medium, as an emulsifying agent, and as a bulk laxative. Also called **agar.**

agency, (in law) a relationship between two parties in which one authorizes the other to act in his behalf as his agent. It usually implies a contractual arrangement between two parties managed by a third party, the agent.

agenesia corticalis, the failure of the cortical cells of the brain, especially the pyramidal cells, to develop in the embryo, resulting in infantile cerebral paralysis and severe mental retardation.

agenesis (eijen′ɪsɪs), **agenesia** (ei′jɪni′žə), **1.** congenital absence of an organ or part, usually caused by a lack of primordial tissue and failure of development in the embryo. **2.** impotence or sterility. Compare **dysgenesis.** – **agenic,** adj.

agenetic fracture, a spontaneous fracture owing to an imperfect osteogenesis.

ageniocephaly (eijen′iousef′əli), **ageniocephalia** (eijen′-iousifeil′yə), a form of otocephaly in which the brain, cranial vault, and sense organs are intact but the lower jaw is malformed. – **ageniocephalic, ageniocephalous,** adj.

agenitalism (eijen′ɪtəlɪz′əm), a symptom complex owing to the lack of the secretion of the sex hormones, caused by the absence or malfunction of the ovaries or testes.

agenosomia (əjen′əsou′miə), a congenital malformation characterized by the absence or defective formation of the genitals and protusion of the intestines through an incompletely developed abdominal wall.

agenosomus (əjen′əsou′məs), a fetus with agenosomia.

agent, (in law) a party authorized to act on behalf of another and to give the other an account of such actions. – **agency,** n.

age of majority, the age at which a person is considered to be an adult in the eyes of the law.

agglutination (əglu′tɪnei′šən), the aggregation or clumping together of insoluble particles as a result of their interaction with specific antibodies called agglutinins, commonly used in blood typing and in identifying or estimating the strength of immunoglobulins or immune sera. See also **agglutinin, blood typing, precipitin.**

agglutination inhibition test, a serologic technique useful in testing for certain unknown soluble antigens. The unknown antigen is mixed with a known agglutinin. If there is a reaction, the agglutinin can no longer agglutinate the cells or particles that carry its corresponding antigen, and the unknown antigen is thus identified. One type of pregnancy test is based on agglutination inhibition.

agglutinin (əglu′tɪnɪn), a specific kind of antibody whose interaction with antigens is manifested as agglutination. Usually multivalent, agglutinins act on insoluble antigens in stable suspension to form a cross-linking lattice that may clump or precipitate. Compare **precipitin.** See also **agglutination, blood typing, hemagglutination.**

agglutinin absorption, the removal from immune serum of antibody by treatment with homologous antigen, followed by centrifugation and separation of the antigen-antibody complex.

agglutinogen (æg′lutɪn′əjɪn), any antigenic substance that causes agglutination by the production of agglutinin.

aggregate anaphylaxis, an exaggerated reaction of hypersensitivity rapidly induced by the injection of an antigen that forms a soluble antigen-antibody complex.

aggression, a forceful, self-assertive action or attitude that is expressed physically, verbally, or symbolically. It may arise from innate drives or occur as a defensive mechanism and is manifested by either constructive or destructive acts directed toward oneself or against others. Kinds of aggression are **constructive aggression, destructive aggression, inward aggression.**

aggressive personality, a personality with behavior patterns characterized by irritability, tantrums, destructiveness, or violence in response to frustration.

aging, the process of growing old, owing in part to a failure of body cells to function normally or to produce new body cells to replace those that are dead or malfunctioning. Normal cell function may be lost through infectious disease, malnutrition, exposure to environmental hazards, or genetic influences. Among body cells that exhibit early signs of aging are those that normally cease dividing after reaching maturity. See also **senile.**

agitated, describing a condition of psychomotor excitement characterized by purposeless, restless activity. Pacing, crying, and laughing without apparent cause are often seen and may serve to release nervous tension associated with anxiety, fear, or other mental stress. – **agitate,** v., **agitation,** n.

agitated depression, a form of depression characterized by severe anxiety accompanied by continuous physical restlessness. See also **depression.**

agitographia (æj′ɪtougræf′iə), a condition characterized by abnormally rapid writing in which words or parts of words are unconsciously omitted. The condition is commonly associated with agitophasia.

agitolalia (æj′ɪtoulei′liə). See **agitophasia.**

agitophasia (æj′ɪtoufei′źhə), a condition characterized by abnormally rapid speech in which words, sounds, or syllables are unconsciously omitted, slurred, or distorted. The condition is commonly associated with agitographia. Also called **agitolalia.**

agnathia (ægnæth′iə), **agnathy** (æg′nəthi), a developmental defect characterized by total or partial absence of the lower jaw. It is usually accompanied by the union or approximation of the ears. Compare **synotia.** See also **otocephaly.** – **agnathous,** adj.

agnathocephalus (ægnæth′əsef′ələs), a fetus with agnathocephaly.

agnathocephaly (ægnæth′əsef′əli), **agnathocephalia** (ægnæth′ousɪfeil′yə), a congenital malformation characterized by the absence of the lower jaw, defective formation of the mouth, and placement of the eyes low on the face with fusion or approximation of the zygomas and the ears. See also **otocephaly.** – **agnathocephalic, agnathocephalous,** adj.

agnathus (ægnæth′əs), a fetus with agnathia.

agnogenic myeloid metaplasia. See **myeloid metaplasia.**

agnosia (ægnou′źhə), total or partial loss of the ability to recognize familiar objects or persons through sensory stimuli as a result of organic brain damage. The condition may affect any of the senses and is classified accordingly as auditory, visual, olfactory, gustatory, or tactile agnosia. Also called **agnosis.** See also **autotopagnosia.**

-agnosia, a combining form meaning '(condition of the) loss of the faculty to perceive': *autotopagnosia, fingeragnosia, paragnosia.* Also **-agnosis.**

-agogue, -agog, a combining form meaning an 'agent promoting the expulsion of a (specified) substance': *lymphagogue, succagogue, uragogue.*

agonal thrombus (æg′ənəl), an aggregation of blood platelets, fibrin, clotting factors, and cellular elements that forms in the heart in the process of dying.

agonist (æg′ənɪst), **1.** a contracting muscle whose contraction is opposed by another muscle (an antagonist). **2.** a drug or other substance having a specific cellular affinity that produces a predictable response.

agoraphobia (æg′ərəfou′biə), an anxiety disorder characterized by a fear of being in an open, crowded, or public place, as a field, tunnel, bridge, congested street, or busy department store, where escape may be difficult or help not available in case of sudden incapacitation. The obsessive phenomenon is observed more often in women than in men and generally can be traced to some sudden loss or separation occurring in childhood. Treatment consists of psychotherapy to uncover the cause of the phobic reaction followed by behavior therapy, specifically the systemic desensitization and flooding techniques for reducing the anxiety and altering the behavioral response. If untreated, fear and avoidance behavior dominate life, and the person refuses to leave home. See also **phobia**.

-agra, a combining form meaning a 'pain or painful seizure': *cardiagra, podagra, trachelagra*.

agranular endoplasmic reticulum. See **endoplasmic reticulum**.

agranulocyte (eigræn′yʊlousait′), any leukocyte that does not contain cytoplasmic granules, as a monocyte or lymphocyte. Compare **granulocyte**. See also **leukocyte**.

agranulocytosis (ægræn′yʊlousaitou′sis), an abnormal condition of the blood, characterized by a severe reduction in the number of granulocytes (basophils, eosinophils, and neutrophils), resulting in fever, prostration, and bleeding ulcers of the rectum, mouth, and vagina. It is an acute disease and may be an adverse reaction to a medication or the result of radiation therapy.

agraphia (eigræf′iə), an abnormal neurologic condition characterized by loss of the ability to write, resulting from injury to the language center in the cerebral cortex. – **agraphic**, *adj*.

agrypnia (agrip′niə). See **insomnia**.

agrypnotic (æg′ripnot′ik), **1.** insomniac. **2.** a drug or other substance that prevents sleep.

AHA, abbreviation for **American Hospital Association.**

"aha" reaction, (in psychology) a sudden realization or inspiration, experienced especially during creative thinking. Some psychologists associate great scientific discoveries and artistic inspirations with this reaction, which is not necessarily related to intelligence. The term has apparently replaced **aha experience,** formerly used by psychologists, especially those of the Gestalt school, to label experiences in which an individual utters "Aha!" during a moment of revelation.

AHF, abbreviation for **antihemophilic factor.**

AHH, abbreviation for **aryl hydrocarbon hydroxylase.**

AI, abbreviation for **artificial intelligence.**

AID, abbreviation for **artificial insemination donor.**

AIH, abbreviation for **artificial insemination husband.**

air, the colorless, odorless gaseous mixture constituting the earth's atmosphere. It consists of 78 per cent nitrogen, 21 per cent oxygen, almost 1 per cent argon, small amounts of carbon dioxide, hydrogen, and ozone, traces of helium, krypton, neon, and xenon, and varying amounts of water vapor.

air bath, the exposure of the naked body to warm air for therapeutic purposes. Also called **balneum pneumaticum**.

air cells of the nose. See **nasal sinus**.

air conditioner lung. See **humidifier lung**.

air embolism, the abnormal presence of air in the cardiovascular system, resulting in obstruction of the flow of blood through the vessel. Air may be inadvertently introduced by injection, during intravenous therapy or surgery, or traumatically, as by a puncture wound. See also **decompression sickness, embolus, gas embolism**.

air encephalography. See **encephalography**.

airplane splint, a splint used for immobilizing a fractured humerus during healing. The splint holds the arm in an abducted position at shoulder level, with the elbow bent. It extends to the waist and may be made of wire or leather, or it may be supported by a plaster body.

air pump, a pump that forces air in or out of a cavity or chamber.

air sickness. See **motion sickness**.

air thermometer, a thermometer using air as its expansible medium. See also **thermometer**.

airway clearance, ineffective, a nursing diagnosis accepted by the Fourth National Conference on the Classification of Nursing Diagnoses. The etiology of the problem is decreased energy or fatigue, infection, obstruction, or secretions of the tracheobronchial tree, perceptual or cognitive impairment, or trauma. The defining characteristics of the condition include abnormal breath sounds, change in the rate or depth of respiration, tachypnea, cough, cyanosis, and dyspnea. See also **nursing diagnosis**.

airway obstruction, an abnormal condition of the respiratory system characterized by a mechanical impediment to the delivery or to the absorption of oxygen in the lungs, as in broncheospasm, choking, croup, laryngospasm, chronic obstructive lung disease, goiter, tumor, or pneumothorax.

■ OBSERVATIONS: If the obstruction is minor, as in sinusitis or pharyngitis, the person is able to breathe, but not normally. If the obstruction is acute, the person may grasp the neck, gasp, become cyanotic, and lose consciousness.

■ INTERVENTION: Acute airway obstruction requires rapid intervention to save the person's life. A bolus of food, a collection of mucus, or a foreign body may be removed manually, by suction, or with the Heimlich maneuver. Obstruction of the airway owing to inflammatory or allergic reaction may be treated with bronchodilating drugs, corticosteroids, intubation, and the administration of oxygen. An emergency tracheotomy may be required if the obstruction cannot be mechanically removed or pharmacologically reduced within a few minutes.

■ NURSING CONSIDERATIONS: The patient is usually very apprehensive and may physically resist assistance. The cause of the obstruction is identified, if possible. Medical assistance is summoned, and the most highly trained person available begins emergency care, including removing the obstruction, if possible; administering oxygen; and performing cardiopulmonary resuscitation, if necessary. See also **aspiration, cardiopulmonary resuscitation, Heimlich maneuver.** *(See next page for illustration)*

FIRST-DEGREE OBSTRUCTION

Obstruction allows passage of air in both directions

SECOND-DEGREE OBSTRUCTION

Inhalation

Air able to move past the obstruction in one direction only. Air passages enlarge during inspiration and diminish during expiration.

Expiration

COMPLETE OBSTRUCTION

Air unable to move in either direction. FB and edematous mucosa obliterate passage.

AIRWAY OBSTRUCTION

Nasopharynx
Soft tissue
Oropharynx
Tongue
Larynx
Esophagus
Trachea

AIRWAY OBSTRUCTION BY TONGUE

akathisia (æk′əthi′źhə),   an abnormal condition characterized by restlessness and agitation, as seen in tardive dyskinesia.   –**akathisiac**, *adj.*

akinesia (ei′kıni′źhə, ei′kaıni′źhə),   an abnormal state of motor and psychic hypoactivity or muscular paralysis. –**akinetic**, *adj.*

akinetic apraxia,   the inability to perform a spontaneous movement. See also **apraxia.**

akinetic mutism,   a state in which a person is unable or refuses to move or to make sounds, resulting from neurological or psychological disturbance.

Akineton,   a trade name for an anticholinergic (biperiden hydrochloride or biperiden lactate), used as an antiparkinsonian.

-akusis.   See **-acousia.**

Al,   symbol for **aluminum.**

-al¹, -ale,   a combining form meaning 'pertaining to or characterized by': *appendiceal, calcyeal, meningeal.*

-al²,   a combining form designating a compound containing a member of the aldehyde group: *benzal, chloral, ethanal.*

ala (ei′lə), *pl.* **alae.**   **1.** any winglike structure. **2.** the axilla.

ala auris,   the auricle of the ear.

ala cerebelli (ser′əbel′ai),   the ala of the central lobule of the cerebellum.

ala cinerea (sınir′iə),   the triangular area on the floor of the fourth ventricle of the brain from which the autonomic fibers of the vagus nerve arise.

ala nasi (nei′sai),   the outer flaring cartilaginous wall of each nostril.

Al-Anon,   an international organization that offers guidance and counseling for the relatives, friends, and associates of alcoholics. See also **Alcoholics Anonymous.**

ala of the ethmoid,   a small projection on each side of the crista galli of the ethmoid bone. Each ala fits into a corresponding depression of the frontal bone.

ala of the ilium,   the upper flaring portion of the iliac bone.

ala of the sacrum, the flat extension of bone on each side of the sacrum.

alar ligament, one of a pair of ligaments that connects the axis to the occipital bone and limits rotation of the cranium. Also called **check ligament, odontoid ligament.** Compare **membrana tectoria.**

alarm reaction, the first stage of the general adaptation syndrome, characterized by the mobilization of the various defense mechanisms of the body or the mind to cope with a stressful situation of a physical or emotional nature. See also **stress.**

alastrim (æl′əstrɪm), a mild form of smallpox, thought to be caused by a weak strain of *Poxvirus variolae.* Unlike smallpox, alastrim is rarely fatal. Also called **Cuban itch, milkpox, variola minor.** See also **smallpox.**

Alateen, an international organization that offers guidance and counseling for the children of alcoholics. See also **Alcoholics Anonymous.**

ala vomeris (vou′mərɪs), an extension of bone on each side of the upper border of the vomer.

alb-, a combining form meaning 'white': *albedo, albugo, albumen.*

alba (æl′bə), *Latin.* 'white,' as in linea alba.

Albers-Schönberg disease (al′bersšhœn′berg). See **osteopetrosis.**

albinism (æl′bɪnɪz′əm), an abnormal congenital condition characterized by partial or total lack of melanin pigment in the body. Total albinos have pale skin which does not tan, white hair, pink eyes, nystagmus, astigmatism, and photophobia. Albinos are prone to severe sunburn, actinic dermatitis, and skin cancer.

Albright's syndrome (ɔl′braits), a disorder characterized by fibrous dysplasia of bone, isolated brown macules on the skin, and endocrine dysfunction. It causes precocious puberty in girls but not in boys. The osseous lesions are reddish-gray, gritty fibromas containing areas of coarse fiber that may be confined to one bone or occur in several, frequently causing deformities. Hyperthyroidism is present in some cases. Treatment may involve osteotomy, curettage, and bone grafts. Also called **Albright-McCune-Sternberg syndrome, osteitis fibrosa disseminata.**

albumin (ælbyu′mɪn), a water-soluble, heat-coagulable protein containing carbon, hydrogen, oxygen, nitrogen, and sulfur. Various albumins are found in practically all animal tissues and in many plant tissues. Determination of the levels and kinds of albumin in urine, blood, and other body tissues is the basis of a number of laboratory diagnostic tests.

albumin A, a blood serum constituent that gathers in cancer cells but is deficient in circulation in cancer patients.

albumin (human), a plasma-volume expander.
- INDICATIONS: It is prescribed in the treatment of hy-

poproteinemia, hyperbilirubinemia, and hypovolemic shock.
- CONTRAINDICATIONS: Severe anemia or cardiac failure prohibits its use.
- ADVERSE EFFECTS: Among the most serious adverse reactions are chills, hypotension, fever, and urticaria.

albuminuria (ælbyu′mɪnyur′iə). See **proteinuria.**

-albuminuria, a combining form meaning a '(specified) condition characterized by excess serum proteins in the urine': *noctalbuminuria, nyctalbuminuria, pseudalbuminuria.*

Alcaine, a trade name for a local anesthetic agent (proparacaine).

Alcock's canal (æl′koks), a canal formed by the obturator internus muscle and the obturator fascia through which the pudendal vessels and nerve pass. Also called **pudendal canal.**

alcohol, **1.** (U.S.P.) a preparation containing at least 92.3 per cent and not more than 93.8 per cent by weight of ethyl alcohol, used as a topical antiseptic and solvent. **2.** a clear, colorless, volatile liquid that is miscible with water, chloroform, or ether, obtained by the fermentation of carbohydrates with yeast. **3.** a compound derived from a hydrocarbon by replacing one or more hydrogen atoms with an equal number of hydroxyl (OH) groups. Depending on the number of hydroxyl radicals, alcohols are classified as monohydric, dihydric, trihydric. Some kinds of alcohol are **rubbing alcohol, sugar alcohol, unsaturated alcohol.**

alcohol bath, a procedure for decreasing an elevated body temperature. A tepid solution of 25 to 50 per cent alcohol in water is sponged lightly on each limb, then on the trunk, turning the person only once from supine to prone position and then back again. Some sources recommend the placement of a hot-water bottle at the feet and a cold compress on the head to accelerate heat loss through vasodilation, to promote the comfort of the patient during the procedure, and to reduce the temperature of the circulation to the brain. As the alcohol evaporates quickly, the bed is less likely to get wet, the patient does not need to be dried, and, for an equal result, the solution does not need to be as cold as a plain bath with cold water.

alcoholic cirrhosis. See **cirrhosis.**

alcoholic fermentation, the conversion of carbohydrates to ethyl alcohol.

alcoholic hallucinosis, a form of alcoholic psychosis characterized primarily by auditory hallucinations, abject fear, and delusions of persecution. The condition develops in acute alcoholism shortly after stopping or reducing the intake of alcohol. Also called **acute hallucinosis.** See also **alcoholic psychosis, hallucination.**

alcoholic-nutritional cerebellar degeneration, a sudden, severe incoordination in the lower extremity, characteristic of poorly nourished alcoholics. The patient walks, if at all, with an ataxic or wide-based gait. It is important to distinguish between this condition and cerebellar tumors, multiple sclerosis, and other neurologic disorders which have similar motor impairments. Treatment consists of improved nutrition, abstinence from alcohol, and physical therapy. Also called **cerebellar cortical degeneration.** See also **alcoholism.**

alcoholic paranoia, paranoia associated with chronic alcoholism.

alcoholic psychosis, any of a group of severe mental disorders, such as pathological intoxication, delirium tremens, Korsakoff's psychosis, and acute hallucinosis, characterized by brain damage or dysfunction that results from the excessive use of alcohol.

Alcoholics Anonymous (AA), an international nonprofit organization, founded in 1935, consisting of abstinent alcoholics whose purpose is to help alcoholics stop drinking and maintain sobriety through group support, shared experiences, and faith in a power greater than themselves. The A.A. program, which emphasizes both medical and religious resources for help in overcoming alcoholism, consists of attending meetings and coping with abstinence "one day at a time." Meetings are held at convenient times in factories, schools, churches, hospitals, and many other institutions and community buildings. Similar groups who work with the children, relatives, friends, and associates of alcoholics are Al-Anon and Alateen.

alcoholic trance, a state of automatism resulting from intoxication.

alcoholism, the extreme dependence on excessive amounts of alcohol, associated with a cumulative pattern of deviant behaviors. Alcoholism is a chronic illness with a slow, insidious onset, which may occur at any age. The etiology is unknown, but cultural and psychosocial factors are suspect, and families of alcoholics have a higher incidence of alcoholism. Frequent intoxication has cumulative destructive effects on an individual's family and social life, working life, and physical health. The most frequent medical consequences of alcoholism are central nervous system depression and cirrhosis of the liver. The severity of each of these is increased in the absence of food intake. Alcoholic patients also may suffer from alcoholic gastritis, peripheral neuropathies, auditory hallucinations, and cardiac problems. Abrupt withdrawal of alcohol in addiction causes weakness, sweating, and hyperreflexia. The severe form of alcohol withdrawal is called delirium tremens. Extreme caution should be used in administering drugs to the alcoholic patient because of the possibility of additive central nervous system depression. The treatment of alcoholism consists of psychotherapy (especially group therapy, by organizations like Alcoholics Anonymous), electroshock treatments, or drugs

that cause an aversion to alcohol. See also **delirium tremens.**

alcohol poisoning, poisoning caused by the ingestion of any of several alcohols, of which ethyl, isopropyl, and methyl are the most common. Ethyl alcohol (grain alcohol) is found in whiskies, brandy, gin, and other beverages. Ordinarily, it is lethal only if large quantities are ingested in a brief period. Isopropyl alcohol is more toxic: ingestion of eight ounces may result in respiratory or circulatory failure. Methyl alcohol (wood alcohol) is extremely poisonous: in addition to nausea, vomiting, and abdominal pain, it may cause blindness, and death may follow the consumption of only two ounces. Treatment for alcohol poisoning includes gastric lavage, intravenous administration of sodium bicarbonate and dextrose, bedrest, the oral or intravenous administration of ethanol oxygen, and, if necessary, hemodialysis.

Aldactazide, a trade name for a fixed-combination drug containing two diuretics (hydrochlorothiazide and spironolactone).

Aldactone, a trade name for a diuretic (spironolactone).

Aldase, a trade name for an enzyme (hyaluronidase), used as an adjunct to anesthesia.

aldolase (æl′dəleıs), an enzyme found in muscle tissue that catalyzes the step in anaerobic glycolysis involving the breakdown of fructose 1,6-diphosphate to glyceraldehyde 3-phosphate. The enzyme can also catalyze the reverse reaction. See also **glycolysis.**

Aldomet, a trade name for an antihypertensive (methyldopa).

Aldoril, a trade name for a fixed-combination drug containing a diuretic (hydrochlorothiazide) and an antihypertensive (methyldopa).

aldosterone (æl′doustɪroun′, ældos′tɪroun), a steroid hormone produced by the adrenal cortex that regulates sodium and potassium balance in the blood.

aldosteronism (æl′doustɪrou′nızəm, ældos′tɪrənɪz′əm), a condition characterized by hypersecretion of aldosterone, occurring as a primary disease of the adrenal cortex or, more often, as a secondary disorder in response to various extra-adrenal pathologic processes. Primary aldosteronism may be caused by adrenal hyperplasia or by an aldosterone-secreting tumor, as in Conn's syndrome. Secondary aldosteronism is associated with increased plasma renin activity and may be induced by the nephrotic syndrome, hepatic cirrhosis, idiopathic edema, congestive heart failure, trauma, burns, or other kinds of stress. Hypersecretion of aldosterone promotes sodium retention and potassium excretion, leading to increased blood volume and blood pressure, alkalosis, muscular weakness, tetany, paresthesias, nephropathy, ventricular arrhythmias, and other cardiac abnormalities. The electrolyte imbalance in aldosteronism usually causes polydipsia and polyuria. Treatment of primary aldosteronism caused by a tumor may include surgical resection and chemotherapy with the adrenal cytotoxic agent mitotane. Spironolactone, an aldosterone antagonist, is frequently used to treat symptoms of aldosteronism. Also called **hyperaldosteronism.**

aldosteronoma (æl'dɔustɪr'ənou'mə), *pl.* **aldosteronomas, aldosteronomata.** an aldosterone-secreting adenoma of the adrenal cortex that is usually small and occurs more frequently in the left than the right adrenal gland, causing hyperaldosteronism with salt retention, expansion of the extracellular fluid volume, and increased blood pressure.

Aleppo boil (əlep'ou). See **oriental sore.**

aleukemic leukemia, a type of leukemia in which the total leukocyte count remains within normal limits and few abnormal forms appear in the peripheral blood. Diagnosis requires tissue examination, usually of the bone marrow. Also called **subleukemic leukemia.** See also **leukemia.**

aleukemic myelosis. See **myeloid metaplasia.**

aleukia (eilu'kiə), a marked reduction in or the complete absence of white blood cells or blood platelets. Compare **leukopenia, thrombocytopenia.** See also **aplastic anemia.**

aleukocythemic leukemia. See **subleukemic leukemia.**

alexia (əlek'siə), an abnormal neurologic condition characterized by an inability to comprehend written words. Compare **dyslexia.** – **alexic,** *adj.*

alg-. See **algesi-.**

alga (æl'gə), *pl.* **algae** (æl'ji). any of a large group of nonmotile, or motile, marine plants containing chlorophyll. Many genera and species of algae are found worldwide; all belong to the phylum Thallophyta. – **algal,** *adj.*

alge-. See **algesi-.**

algesi-, alg-, alge-, algo-, a combining form meaning 'pertaining to pain': *algesia, algesiogenic, algesthenia.*

-algesia, a combining form meaning '(condition of) sensitivity to pain': *asphalgesia, haphalgesia, hyperthermalgesia.*

-algesic, a combining form meaning 'pertaining to sensitivity to pain': *analgesic, hypalgesic, paralgesic.*

-algia, a combining form meaning 'pain, painful condition': *epigastralgia, sacralgia, uteralgia.* Also **-algy.**

-algic, a combining form meaning 'related to pain': *cardialgic, ophthalmalgic, tibialgic.*

algid malaria, a form of malaria caused by the protozoan *Plasmodium falciparum,* characterized by coldness of the skin, profound weakness, and severe diarrhea. See also **falciparum malaria, malaria.**

algo-. See **algesi-.**

algolagnia (æl'goulæg'niə), a form of sexual perversion characterized by sadism or masochism.

algolagniac (æl'gəlæg'niæk). See **sadomasochism.**

algophobia (æl'goufou'biə), an anxiety disorder characterized by an abnormal, pervasive fear of experiencing pain or of witnessing pain in others. See also **phobia.**

alienation, 1. the act or state of being estranged or iso-lated. 2. *Obsolete.* insanity or mental derangement, now generally restricted to medical jurisprudence or forensic psychiatry. See also **depersonalization.**

alienist, *Obsolete.* a psychiatrist, especially one who specializes in giving legal evidence concerning the mental competence of persons appearing before a court of law.

alimentary bolus. See **bolus,** def 1.

alimentary canal. See **digestive tube.**

alimentation (æl'ɪmentei'ʃən), nourishment. See also **feeding.**

aliphatic acid (æl'ɪfæt'ɪk), an acid of a nonaromatic hydrocarbon characterized by an open carbon chain.

-alis, a combining form meaning 'pertaining to' something specified: *corticalis, rhomboidalis, vesicalis.*

alkali (æl'kəlai), a compound with the chemical characteristics of a base. Alkalis combine with fatty acids to form soaps, turn red litmus blue, and enter into reactions that form water-soluble carbonates. See also **acid, base.** – **alkaline,** *adj.* **alkalinity,** *n.*

alkali burn, tissue damage caused by exposure to an alkaline compound like lye. Treatment includes washing the area with copious amounts of water to remove the chemical and applying vinegar or other mildly acidic substance diluted with water to neutralize any remaining acid and to decrease the discomfort. The victim should be immediately taken to a medical facility if the tissue damage is more than slight and superficial. Compare **acid burn.**

-alkaline, a combining form meaning 'of or referring to alkali': *silicoalkaline, subalkaline, vegetoalkaline.*

alkaline-ash, residue in the urine having a pH of higher than 7.

alkaline-ash producing foods, foods that may be ingested in order to produce an alkaline pH in the urine, thereby reducing the incidence of acidic urinary calculi, or that may be avoided in order to reduce the incidence of alkaline calculi. Some of the foods that result in alkaline ash are milk, cream, buttermilk, fruit (except prunes, plums, and cranberries), vegetables (except corn and lentils), almonds, chestnuts, coconuts, and olives.

alkaline bath, a bath taken in water containing sodium bicarbonate, used especially for skin disorders.

alkaline phosphatase, an enzyme, involved in bone mineralization, that hydrolyzes phosphoric esters and functions optimally at 9.3 pH. Most alkaline phosphatase in normal serum is derived from bone, but the enzyme is produced also in the liver, intestinal mucosa, placenta, breast, and other tissues. Plasma levels of alkaline phosphatase rise rapidly in the first month of life, fall slowly after the third month, increase again during bone growth in preadolescence; levels decrease in senility, anemia, and malnutrition. Increased concentrations of the enzyme in serum, reflecting increased proliferation or activity of osteoblasts, are found in skeletal disorders, as rickets, osteomalacia, and Paget's disease; elevated levels occurring in liver disorders, biliary obstruction, or intrahepatic cholestasis reflect impaired hepatic excretory function. Serum alkaline phosphatase is also increased in hyperparathyroidism and in hereditary hyperphosphatasia, characterized by thickness of the calvaria, large areas of increased density at the base of the skull, and deformities of the shafts and epiphyses of long and short bones.

alkalinize (æl'kəlɪnaɪz), **alkalize** (æl'kəlaɪz), **1.** to make a substance alkaline, as through the addition of a base. **2.** to become alkaline. Compare **acidify.**

alkali poisoning, a toxic condition caused by the ingestion of an alkaline agent like liquid ammonia, lye and some detergent powders. Emergency treatment includes giving copious amounts of water or milk to dilute the alkali. Vomiting is not induced and mild acids are not administered. The victim is transported immediately to the hospital for observation of any corrosive damage to the esophagus or of any metabolic abnormality and for mechanical removal of the alkali by gastric intubation and lavage. Compare **acid poisoning.**

alkalosis (æl'kəlou'sɪs), an abnormal condition of body fluids, characterized by a tendency toward an increased pH, as from an excess of alkaline bicarbonate or a deficiency of acid. Respiratory alkalosis may be caused by hyperventilation, resulting in an excess loss of carbon dioxide and a carbonic acid deficit. Metabolic acidosis may result from an excess intake or retention of bicarbonate, loss of gastric acid in vomiting, potassium depletion, or any stimulus that increases the rate of sodium-hydrogen exchange. Alkalosis is said to be compensated if an adaptive mechanism, as a buffer system, carbon dioxide retention, or bicarbonate excretion, prevents a shift in pH. Treatment of uncompensated alkalosis involves correction of dehydration and various ionic deficits to restore the normal acid-base balance in which the ratio of carbonic acid to bicarbonate is twenty to one. Compare **acidosis.**

alkaptonuria (ælkæp'tounyʊr'iə), a rare inherited disorder resulting from the incomplete metabolism of tyrosine, an amino acid, in which abnormal amounts of homogentisic acid are excreted, staining the urine dark. In this disorder, which is transmitted by an autosomal recessive gene, a key metabolic enzyme is absent from the body. Usually, the condition does not cause symptoms until middle age, at which point ochronosis, a type of arthritis, may develop. — **alkaptonuric,** *adj.*

Alkeran, a trade name for an antineoplastic (melphalan).

alkylating agent, a substance that promotes alkylation.

ALL, abbreviation for **acute lymphocytic leukemia.** See also **acute childhood leukemia.**

all-. See **allo-.**

allanto-, a combining form meaning 'pertaining to a sausage or to the allartois': *allantochorion, allantoid, allantotoxicon.*

allantoidoangiopagus (æl'antoɪd'ouæn'jiop'əgəs), conjoined twin fetuses of unequal size that are united by the vessels of the umbilical cord. Also called **omphaloangiopagus.** See also **omphalosite.** — **allantoidoangiopagous,** *adj.*

allantois (əlæn'toʊɪs), a tubular extension of the yolk sac endoderm that extends with the allantoic vessels into the body stalk of the embryo. In human embryos, allantoic vessels become the umbilical vessels and the chorionic villi. See also **body stalk, umbilical cord.** — **allantoic,** *adj.*

allele (əlil'), **1.** one of two or more alternative forms of a gene that occupy corresponding loci on homologous chromosomes. **2.** Also called **allelomorph.** one of two or more contrasting characteristics transmitted by alternative genes.

allelo-, a combining form meaning 'pertaining to another': *allelocatalysis, allelomorph, allelotaxis.*

allelomorph (əli'ləmɔrf). See **allele.**

allergen (æl'ərjɪn), a substance that can produce a hypersensitive reaction in the body but is not necessarily intrinsically harmful. Some common allergens are pollen, animal dander, house dust, feathers, and various foods. Some studies indicate that one of every six Americans is hypersensitive to one or more allergens. The bodies of normal individuals develop a natural or acquired immunity to allergens, but in less fortunate individuals the immune system may be overly sensitive to foreign substances and to others produced naturally by the body. The body normally protects itself against allergens or antigens by the complex chemical reactions of the humoral immune and the cell-mediated immune systems. Methods to identify specific allergens affecting individuals continue to improve. The most common method involves a skin test in which several allergens can be examined simultaneously. — **allergenic,** *adj.*

allergenic (æl'ərjen'ɪk), of or pertaining to a substance that tends to cause hypersensitivity reactions in certain individuals.

allergic, **1.** of or pertaining to allergy. **2.** having an allergy.

allergic alveolitis. See **diffuse hypersensitivity pneumonia.**

allergic asthma, a form of asthma caused by the exposure of the bronchial mucosa to an inhaled airborne antigen. This allergen causes the production of antibodies that bind to mast cells in the bronchial tree. The mast cells then release histamine which stimulates contraction of bronchial smooth muscle and causes mucosal edema. Psychological factors may provoke asthma attacks in bronchi already sensitized by allergens. Hyposensitization treatments are more effective for pollen sensitivity than for house dust, animal hair, molds, and insects. Often, a diurnal pattern of histamine release is seen, causing variable degrees of bronchospasm at different times of the day. Also called **extrinsic asthma.** Compare **intrinsic asthma.** See also **asthma, asthma in children, status asthmaticus.**

allergic bronchopulmonary aspergillosis, a form of aspergillosis that occurs in asthmatics when the fungus *Aspergillus fumigatus,* growing within the bronchial lumen, causes a Type I or Type III hypersensitivity reaction. The characteristics of the condition are similar to those of asthma, including dyspnea and wheezing. Chest examination and pulmonary function tests may reveal airway obstruction. Serologic tests usually reveal precipitating antibodies to *A. fumigatus.* Bacteriologic and microscopic examination of sputum may reveal *A. fumigatus* in addition to Charcot-Leyden crystals. Eosinophilia is usually also present. Compare **aspergillosis.**

allergic conjunctivitis, an abnormal condition characterized by hyperemia of the conjunctiva owing to an allergy. Common allergens that cause this condition are pollen, grass, topical medications, air pollutants, occupational irritants, and smoke. It is bilateral and usually starts before puberty and lasts about 10 years, commonly recurring in a seasonal pattern.

■ OBSERVATIONS: The common signs of allergic conjunctivitis are tearing and pain, accompanied by discharge and conjunctival hyperemia. Eosinophils predominate in stained blood smears, and diagnosis is commonly based on cultures and sensitivity tests to identify the causative allergen.

■ INTERVENTION: Treatment of allergic conjunctivitis commonly includes the administration of vasoconstrictor eyedrops, as epinephrine, cold compresses to relieve itching, and the administration of oral histamines.

■ NURSING CONSIDERATIONS: Warm compresses and ointments or eyedrops may be administered.

allergic coryza, acute rhinitis caused by exposure to any allergen to which the person is hypersensitive.

allergic cutaneous angiitis. See **allergic vasculitis.**

allergic interstitial pneumonitis. See **bagassosis.**

allergic reaction, a hypersensitive response to an allergen to which an organism has previously been exposed and to which the organism has developed antibodies. Subsequent exposure causes the release of histamine and a variety of symptoms including urticaria, eczema, dyspnea, bronchospasm, diarrhea, rhinitis, sinusitis, laryngospasm and anaphylaxis. Eosinophilia is usually present, revealed in a differential white blood-cell count.

allergic rhinitis, inflammation of the nasal passages, usually associated with watery nasal discharge and itching of the nose and eyes, owing to a localized sensitivity reaction to house dust, animal dander, or an antigen, commonly pollen. The condition may be seasonal, as in hay fever, or perennial, as in allergy to dust or animals. Treatment includes the local, systemic, or topical administration of antihistamines, avoidance of the antigen, and hyposensitization by injections of diluted antigen in gradually increasing amounts.

allergic vasculitis, an inflammatory condition of the blood vessels that is induced by an allergen. Disseminated intravascular inflammation sometimes occurs in patients treated with iodides, penicillin, sulfonamides, and thioureas. Allergic cutaneous vasculitis is characterized by itching, malaise, a slight fever, and by the presence of papules, vesicles, urticarial wheals, or small ulcers on the skin.

allergy, a hypersensitive reaction to intrinsically harmless antigens, most of which are environmental. Studies show that one of every six Americans has a severe allergy and that more than 20 million Americans have allergic reactions to airborne or inhaled allergens, as cigarette smoke, house dust, and pollens. Allergic rhinitis, which is associated with airborne allergens, affects predominantly young children and adolescents but occurs in all age groups. Allergies are classified according to Types I, II, III, and IV hypersensitivity. Types I, II, and III involve different immunoglobulin antibodies and their interaction with different antigens. Type IV allergy is associated with contact dermatitis and T-cells which react directly with the antigen and cause local inflammation. Allergies are divided into those that produce immediate or antibody-mediated reactions and those that produce delayed or cell-mediated reactions. Immediate allergic reactions involve Types I, II, and III hypersensitivity and antigen-antibody reactions that activate certain enzymes, creating an imbalance between these enzymes and their inhibitors. Immediate allergic reactions also release certain substances into the circulation, as histamine, bradykinin, acetylcholine, gamma globulin G, and leukotaxine. Delayed allergic reactions are caused by antigens but do not seem to depend on antibodies. Depending on the type of hypersensitivity involved, some common symptoms of allergy are bronchial congestion, conjunctivitis, edema, fever, urticaria, and vomiting. Severe allergic reactions, as anaphylaxis, can cause systemic shock and death. Symptoms of limited duration, as those associated with hay fever, serum sickness, bee stings, and urticaria, can be suppressed by glucocorticoids administered as supplements to primary therapy. The effect of such steroids may be considerably delayed. Severe allergic reactions, as anaphylaxis and angioneurotic edema of the glottis, commonly require immediate therapy with epinephrine administered subcutaneously. When allergic reactions are life-threatening, steroids, as dexamethasone sodium phosphate, may be administered intravenously. For milder diseases, as serum sickness and hay fever, antihistamines are usually administered. See also **allergy testing.**

allergy testing, any one of the various procedures used in identifying the specific allergens that afflict the patients involved. Such tests are helpful in prescribing treatment to prevent allergic reactions or to reduce their severity. Skin testing is the most common kind of procedure for allergy testing and commonly exposes the patient to small quantities of the suspected allergens. Positive reactions usually occur within 20 minutes and are commonly manifested as varying degrees of erythema. Factors considered in performing allergy tests include the medical history of the patient, the allergy history, the environment, and the diet. Individuals to be tested are usually instructed to discontinue the use of any antihistamines at least 24 hours before the test, as these drugs can interfere with normal test responses. The most common kinds of allergy testing include the intradermal, scratch, patch, conjunctival, and use tests.

allied health personnel. See **paramedical personnel.**

alligator forceps, 1. a forceps with heavy teeth and a double clamp, employed in orthopedic surgery. 2. a forceps with long, thin, angular handles and interlocking teeth.

allo-, all-, a combining form meaning 'differing from the normal, reversal, or referring to another': *allobiosis, allochezia, allopathy.*

allodiploid (æl′oudɪp′lɔid), **allodiploidic,** 1. of or pertaining to an individual, organism, strain, or cell that has two genetically distinct sets of chromosomes derived from different ancestral species, as occurs in hybridization. 2. such an individual, organism, strain, or cell.

allodiploidy (æl′oudɪp′lɔidi), the state or condition of having two genetically distinct sets of chromosomes derived from different ancestral species.

alloeroticism (æl′ourot′ɪsɪzəm), **alloerotism** (æl′ouer′-ɪtɪz′əm). See **heteroeroticism.**

allogamy (əlog′əmi). See **cross fertilization.** – **allogamous,** *adj.*

allohexaploid (æl′ouhek′səploid), **allohexaploidic.** See **allopolyploid.**

allometric growth, the increase in size of different organs or parts of an organism at various rates. Also called **heterauxesis.** Compare **isometric growth.** See also **allometry.**

allometron, a quantitative change in the proportional relationship of the parts of an organism as a result of the evolutionary process.

allometry (əlom′ɪtri), the measurement and study of the changes in proportions of the various parts of an organism in relation to the growth of the whole or within a series of related organisms. – **allometric** (æl′əme′trɪk), *adj.*

allopathic physician, a physician who treats disease and injury with active interventions, as medical and surgical treatment, intended to bring about effects opposite from those produced by the disease or injury. Almost all practicing physicians in the United States are allopathic. Compare **chiropractic, homeopathy.**

allopathy (əlop′əthi), a system of medical therapy in which a disease or an abnormal condition is treated by creating an environment that is antagonistic to the disease or condition, as an antibiotic toxic to a pathogenic organism is given in an infection or an iron supplement may be given to increase the synthesis of hemoglobin in iron deficiency anemia.

allopentaploid (æl′əpen′təploid), **allopentaploidic.** See **allopolyploid.**

alloplastic maneuver, (in psychology) a process that is part of adaptation, involving an adjustment or change in the external environment. Compare **autoplastic maneuver.**

alloploid (æl′əploid), **alloploidic.** See **allodiploid, allopolyploid.**

alloploidy (æl′əplɔi′di). See **allodiploidy, allopolyploidy.**

allopolyploid (æl′əpol′ɪploid), **allopolyploidic,** 1. of or pertaining to an individual, organism, strain, or cell that has more than two genetically distinct sets of chromosomes derived from two or more different ancestral species, as occurs in hybridization. They are referred to as allotriploid, allotetraploid, allopentraploid, allohexaploid, and so on, depending on the number of multiples of haploid sets of chromosomes they contain. 2. such an individual, organism, strain, or cell. Compare **autopolyploid.**

allopolyploidy (æl′əpol′ɪplɔi′di), the state or condition of having more than two genetically distinct sets of chromosomes from two or more ancestral species. Compare **autopolyploidy.**

allopurinol (æl′əpyur′ənol), a xanthine oxidase inhibitor.

■ INDICATIONS: It is prescribed in the treatment of gout and other hyperuricemic conditions.

■ CONTRAINDICATIONS: It is not prescribed for children (except those with hyperuricemia secondary to malignancy), for lactating mothers, or for people suffering an acute attack of gout. Known hypersensitivity to this drug prohibits its use.

■ ADVERSE EFFECTS: Among the most serious adverse reactions to this drug are blood dyscrasias and severe rashes and other allergic reactions. Gastrointestinal disturbances also may occur.

all or none law, the principle that the heart muscle, under any stimulus above the threshold level, regardless of the intensity, will either contract to the maximum extent or not at all. The principle also applies to single strands of muscle and nerve fibers, although the degree of response when an entire muscle or nerve trunk is stimulated depends on the number of fibers stimulated. Also called **Bowditch's law.**

allotetraploid (æl′outet′rəploid), **allotetraploidic.** See **allopolyploid.**

allotrio-, a combining form meaning 'strange or foreign': *allotriodontia, allotriogeustia, allotriophagy.*

allotriploid (əlot'rıpɔid), **allotriploidic.** See **allopolyploid.**

allowable charge, the maximum amount that a third party, usually an insurance company, will pay to reimburse a provider for a specific service.

allowable costs, components of an institution's costs that are reimbursable as determined by a payment formula. In general, costs of services not considered to be reasonable or necessary to the proper delivery of health services are excluded from allowable costs.

alloy (æl'ɔi), a mixture of two or more metals or of substances with metallic properties. Most alloys are formed by mixing molten metals that dissolve in each other. A number of alloys have medical applications, as those used for prostheses and in dental amalgams. See also **amalgam.**

aloe (æl'ou), the inspissated juice of various species of *Aloe* trees, formerly used as a cathartic but generally discontinued because it often causes severe intestinal cramps.

alopecia (æl'əpi'shiə), partial or complete lack of hair resulting from normal aging, endocrine disorder, drug reaction, anticancer medication, or skin disease. Also called **baldness.** Kinds of alopecia include **alopecia areata, alopecia totalis, alopecia universalis.**

alopecia areata, a disease of unknown cause in which there are well-defined bald patches on the head and other hairy parts of the body. The condition is usually self-limited and clears completely within 6 to 12 months without treatment. Recurrences are common.

alopecia totalis, an uncommon condition characterized by the loss of all the hair on the scalp. The cause in unknown, and the baldness is usually permanent. No treatment is known. Compare **alopecia areata, alopecia universalis.**

alopecia universalis, a lack of hair on all parts of the body, occasionally an extension of alopecia areata. Compare **alopecia totalis.**

alpha, the first letter of the Greek alphabet, often used in chemical nomenclature to distinguish one variation in a chemical compound from others.

alpha-adrenergic blocking agent. See **antiadrenergic.**

alpha-adrenergic receptor. See **alpha receptor.**

alpha-aminoisovalerianic acid. See **valine.**

Alphadrol, a trade name for a glucocorticoid (fluprednisolone).

alpha fetoprotein (AFP), a protein normally synthesized by the liver, yolk sac, and gastrointestinal tract of a human fetus, but which may be found elevated in the sera of adults having certain malignancies. AFP measurements in amniotic fluid are used for early diagnosis of fetal neural defects, as spina bifida and anencephaly. Elevated serum levels may be present in ataxia telangiectasia, hereditary tyrosinemia, cirrhosis, alcoholic hepatitis, and viral hepatitis. Although not a specific marker for malignancies, AFP may be used to monitor effectiveness of surgical and chemotherapeutic management of hepatomas and germ cell neoplasms.

alpha-galactosidase, a form of the enzyme that catalyzes the conversion of alpha-D-galactoside to D-galactose.

alpha hemolysis, the development of a greenish zone around a bacterial colony growing on blood-agar medium, characteristic of pneumococci and certain streptococci and caused by the partial decomposition of hemoglobin. Compare **beta hemolysis.**

alpha-hydroxypropionic acid. See **lactic acid.**

Alphalin, a trade name for vitamin A.

alpha-methyldopa. See **methyldopa.**

alpha receptor, any one of the postulated adrenergic components of receptor tissues that responds to norepinephrine and to various blocking agents. The activation of the alpha receptors causes such physiological responses as increased peripheral vascular resistance, dilation of the pupils, and contraction of pilomotor muscles. Also called **alpha-adrenergic receptor.** Compare **beta receptor.**

alpha rhythm. See **alpha wave.**

alpha state, a condition of relaxed, peaceful wakefulness devoid of concentration and sensory stimulation. It is characterized by the alpha rhythm of brain wave activity, as recorded by an electroencephalograph, and is accompanied by feelings of tranquillity and a lack of tension and anxiety. Biofeedback training and meditation techniques are used as means of achieving the state.

Alpha Tau Delta (æl'fə tɑu' del'tə), a national fraternity for professional nurses.

alpha tocopheryl. See **vitamin E.**

alpha wave, one of the four types of brain waves, characterized by a relatively high voltage or amplitude and a frequency of 8 to 13 Hz. Alpha waves are the "relaxed waves" of the brain and constitute the majority of waves recorded by electroencephalograms registering the activity of the parietal and the occipital lobes and the posterior parts of the temporal lobes when the individual is awake but nonattentive and relaxed, with the eyes closed. Opening and closing the eyes affects the patterns of the alpha waves and the beta waves. Also called **alpha rhythm.** Compare **beta wave, delta wave, theta wave.**

ALS, 1. abbreviation for **antilymphocyte serum.** 2. abbreviation for **advanced life support.** See **Emergency Medical Technician-Advanced Life Support.** 3. abbreviation for **amyotrophic lateral sclerosis.**

altered state of consciousness (ASC), any state of awareness that differs from the normal awareness of a conscious person. Altered states of consciousness have been achieved, especially in Eastern cultures, by many individuals using various techniques, as long fasting, deep breathing, whirling, and chanting. Researchers now recognize that such practices can affect the chemistry of the body and help to induce the desired state. Experiments suggest that telepathy, mystical experiences, clairvoyance, and other altered states of consciousness may be subconscious capabilities in most individuals and can be used to improve health and help fight disease.

alternate generation, alternation of generations, a type of reproduction in which a sexual generation alternates with one or more asexual generations, as in many plants and lower animals.

alternating current (AC), an electrical current that reverses direction and changes in magnitude, according to a consistent sinusoidal pattern. Compare **direct current.**

alternating pulse, a regular, steady pulse in which a strong beat is followed by a weak one. It is characteristic of left-ventricular failure. Also called **pulsus alternans.**

alternative inheritance, the acquisition of all genetic traits and conditions from one parent, as in self-pollinating plants and self-fertilizing animals.

altitude sickness, a syndrome associated with the relatively low concentrations of oxygen in the atmosphere at altitudes encountered during mountain climbing or travel in unpressurized aircraft. The acute symptoms may include dizziness, headache, irritability, breathlessness, and euphoria. Older people and those affected by pulmonary or cardiac disorders may suffer pulmonary edema, heart failure, or prostration, requiring emergency treatment and removal to lower altitudes. A chronic form of altitude sickness is characterized by an increased production of red blood cells, resulting in blood that is thick and difficult to move through the circulatory system. See also **polycythemia.**

alum, a topical astringent, used primarily in lotions and douches. Alum is applied topically as a 0.5-5 per cent solution. It is not to be confused with caustic pencils made from silver nitrate.

alum bath, a bath taken in water containing alum, used primarily for skin disorders.

aluminum (Al), a widely used metallic element and the third most abundant of all the elements. Its atomic number is 13; its atomic weight is 26.97. It occurs in the ores feldspar, mica, and kaolin but most abundantly in bauxite. Aluminum is commonly obtained by purifying bauxite to produce alumina, which is reduced to aluminum. It is light and durable and used extensively in the manufacture of aircraft components, prosthetic devices, and dental appliances. It is also a component of many antacids, antiseptics, astringents, and styptics. Aluminum salts, as aluminum hydroxychloride, can cause allergic reactions in susceptible individuals. Aluminum hydroxy-

chloride is the most commonly used agent in antiperspirants and is also effective as a deodorant.

aluminum acetate solution.   See **Burow's solution.**

Alupent, a trade name for a beta-adrenergic bronchodilator (metaproterenol sulfate).

alve-, a combining form meaning 'trough, channel, cavity': *alvei, alveolate, alveolus.*

alveolar adenocarcinoma, a neoplasm in which the tumor cells form alveoli.

alveolar canal, any of the canals of the maxilla through which the posterior superior alveolar blood vessels and the nerves to the upper teeth pass. Also called **dental canal.**

alveolar cell carcinoma, a malignant pulmonary neoplasm that arises in a bronchiole and spreads along alveolar surfaces. The tumor consists of cuboidal or nonciliated columnar epithelial cells with abundant eosinophilic cytoplasm that may contain droplets of mucus. This form of lung cancer, which occurs less frequently than bronchogenic squamous cell carcinoma or oat cell carcinoma, is characterized clinically by a severe cough and copious sputum. Also called **bronchiolar carcinoma.**

alveolar duct, the terminal segment of a respiratory bronchiole in the lung.

alveolar fistula.   See **dental fistula.**

alveolar soft part sarcoma, a tumor in subcutaneous or fibromuscular tissue, consisting of numerous large round or polygonal cells in a netlike matrix of connective tissue.

alveolitis (æl'viəlai'tıs), an allergic pulmonary reaction to the inhalation of antigenic substances characterized by acute episodes of dyspnea, cough, sweating, fever, weakness, and pain in the joints and muscles lasting from 12 to 18 hours. Recurrent episodes may lead to chronic obstructive lung disease with weight loss, increasing exertional dyspnea, and interstitial fibrosis. X rays of the lungs may show cellular thickening of alveolar septa and ill-defined generalized infiltrates. Kinds of alveolitis include **bagassosis, farmer's lung, pigeon breeder's disease.**

alveolo-, a combining form meaning 'pertaining to an alveolus': *alveoloclasia, alveolodontal, alveoloplasty.*

alveolus (ælvi'ələs), a small saclike structure. See also **dental alveolus, pulmonary alveolus.** – **alveolar,** *adj.*

alymphocytosis (ælım'fousaitou'sıs), an abnormal reduction in the total number of lymphocytes circulating in the blood. It is similar to lymphocytopenia but usually implies a more severe reduction. Compare **aplastic anemia, lymphocytopenia.** See also **leukocyte, lymphocyte.**

Alysine, a trade name for an analgesic (sodium salicylate).

Alzheimer's disease (alts'haimərz), presenile dementia, characterized by confusion, restlessness, agnosia, speech disturbances, inability to carry out purposeful movements, and hallucinosis. The patient may become hypomanic, refuse food, and lose sphincter control without local impairment. The disease usually begins in later middle life with slight defects in memory and behavior and occurs with equal frequency in men and women. Typical pathologic features are miliary plaques in the cortex and fibrillary degeneration within pyramidal ganglion cells. Treatment can only be palliative, but maintaining proper nutrition may delay the progression of the disease.

Am, symbol for **americium.**

A.M.A., abbreviation for **American Medical Association.**

amalgam (əmæl′gəm), **1.** a mixture or combination. **2.** an alloy of mercury and another metal or metals.

Amanita, a genus of mushrooms. Some species, as *Amanita phalloides,* are poisonous, causing hallucinations, gastrointestinal upset, and pain that may be followed by liver, kidney, and central nervous system damage.

amantadine hydrochloride (əmæn′tədin), an antiviral and antiparkinsonian drug.

■ INDICATIONS: It is prescribed in the prophylaxis and early treatment of influenza virus A$_2$, and for symptomatic treatment of parkinsonian symptoms.

■ CONTRAINDICATIONS: It is used with caution in patients with congestive heart failure and during pregnancy and lactation. Known hypersensitivity to this drug prohibits its use.

■ ADVERSE EFFECTS: Among the most serious adverse reactions are central nervous system effects and livedo reticularis. Nervousness, blurred vision, and slurred speech also may occur.

amasesis (æm′əsi′sis), the inability to chew food, caused by paralysis of the muscles of mastication, impaired teeth, poorly fitted dentures, or a psychiatric problem.

amastia (əmæs′tiə), absence of the breasts in women caused by a congenital defect, an endocrine disorder resulting in faulty development, lack of development of secondary sex characteristics, or a bilateral mastectomy. Also called **amazia.**

amaurosis (æm′ɔrou′sis), blindness, especially lack of vision resulting from an extraocular cause, as disease of the optic nerve or brain, diabetes, renal disease, or systemic poisoning produced by excessive use of alcohol or tobacco. Unilateral or, more rarely, bilateral amaurosis may follow an emotional shock and may continue for days or months. Amaurosis may accompany an attack of acute gastritis. One kind of congenital amaurosis is transmitted as an autosomal recessive trait. —**amaurotic** (əm′ərot′ik), *adj.*

amaurosis congenita of Leber. See **Leber's congenital amaurosis.**

amaurosis fugax (fu′gæks), transient episodic blindness. Compare **amaurosis.**

amaurosis partialis fugax (fu′gæks), transitory partial blindness, usually caused by vascular insufficiency of the retina or optic nerve as a result of carotid artery disease.

amaurotic familial idiocy. See **Tay-Sachs disease.**

amazia (əmei′ziə). See **amastia.**

amb-. See **ambo-.**

ambenonium chloride (æm′bınou′niəm), a cholinergic.

■ INDICATION: It is prescribed in the treatment of myasthenia gravis.

■ CONTRAINDICATIONS: Intestinal and urinary obstructions or known hypersensitivity to this drug prohibits its use.

■ ADVERSE EFFECTS: Among the more serious adverse reactions are increased bronchial secretions, muscle cramps, and nausea.

Ambenyl, a trade name for a fixed-combination drug containing a narcotic analgesic-antitussive (codeine sulfate), two antihistamines (bromodiphenhydramine hydrochloride and diphenhydramine hydrochloride), an expectorant (potassium guaiacolsulfonate) and ammonium chloride.

amber mutation, (in molecular genetics) a genetic alteration in which a polypeptide chain terminates prematurely, because the triplet of nucleotides that normally code for the next amino acid in the chain becomes UAG, the uracil-adenine-guanine sequence that signals the end of the chain. Also called **nonsense mutation, ochre mutation.**

ambi-, a combining form meaning 'on both sides': *ambidexterity, ambilateral, ambiversion.*

ambient air standard, the maximum tolerable concentration of any air pollutant, as lead, nitrogen dioxide, sodium hydroxide, or sulfuric dioxide. Federal authorities in the United States have indicated that only Los Angeles, Chicago, Salt Lake City, and Metropolitan New York may not meet the ambient air standard for nitrogen dioxide and that those cities and many others throughout the world have an atmosphere polluted by various toxic chemicals that are dangerous to breathe. Research and medical evidence show the strong correlation between many diseases and toxic chemicals, but little is known about the precise effects and movement of airborne pollutants.

ambiguous genitalia, external genitalia that are not normal and morphologically typical of either sex, as occurs in pseudohermaphroditism.

ambilhar. See **niridazole.**

ambivalence (æmbɪv′ələns), **1.** a state in which a person experiences conflicting feelings, attitudes, drives, desires, or emotions, as love and hate, tenderness and cruelty, pleasure and pain. To some degree, ambivalence is normal. Treatment in severe, debilitating cases consists of psychotherapy appropriate to the underlying cause. **2.** uncertainty and fluctuation owing to an inability to make a choice between opposites. **3.** a continuous oscillation or fluctuation. —**ambivalent** (æmbɪv′ələnt), *adj.*

ambivert (æm′bɪvərt′), a person who possesses some of the characteristics of both introversion and extroversion.

amblyopia (æm′blɪou′piə), reduced vision in an eye that appears to be structurally normal when examined with an ophthalmoscope. Kinds of amblyopia are **suppression amblyopia, toxic amblyopia.**

ambo-, amb-, a combining form meaning 'both or on both sides': *ambosexual.*

Ambodryl, a trade name for an antihistamine (bromodiphenhydramine hydrochloride).

ambulance, an emergency vehicle usually used for the transport of patients to a medical facility in cases of accident, trauma, or sudden, severe illness.

ambulatory, able to walk, hence describing a patient who is not confined to bed, or designating a health service for people who are not hospitalized.

ambulatory automatism, aimless wandering or moving about or performance of mechanical acts without conscious awareness of the behavior. See also **fugue, poriomania.**

ambulatory care, all health services provided on an outpatient basis to those who visit a hospital or other health care facility and depart after treatment on the same day.

amcinonide, a topical corticosteroid.
- INDICATION: It is used as an anti-inflammatory agent.
- CONTRAINDICATIONS: Viral and fungal diseases of the skin, circulation impairment, or known hypersensitivity to steroids prohibits its use.
- ADVERSE REACTIONS: Among the most serious adverse reactions are various skin reactions. Systemic side effects may occur from prolonged or excessive application.

ameba, amoeba, a microscopic, single-celled, parasitic organism. Several species may infect man, including *Entamoeba histolytica* and *E. coli.* See also **amebiasis.** — **amebic,** *adj.*

-ameba, -amoeba, a combining form meaning a '(specified) protozoan': *caudameba, Dientameba, Entameba.*

amebiasis, amoebiasis (æm′ibaɪ′əsɪs), an infection of the intestine or liver by species of pathogenic amebae, particularly *Entamoeba histolytica,* acquired by ingesting food or water contaminated with infected feces. Mild amebiasis may be asymptomatic; severe infection may cause profuse diarrhea, acute abdominal pain, jaundice, anorexia, and weight loss. It is most serious in infants, the elderly, and debilitated people. Metronidazole is usually effective in curing the infection. See also **ameba, amebic abscess, amebic dysentery, hepatic amebiasis.**

amebic abscess, a collection of pus formed by disintegrated tissue in a cavity, usually in the liver, caused by the protozoan parasite *Entameba histolytica.* Cysts of the organism, ingested in fecally contaminated food or water, pass through the digestive tract into the intestine, where active trophozoites of the parasite are released. The trophozoites enter the intestinal mucosa, causing ulceration, nausea, vomiting, abdominal pain, and severe diarrhea, and they may invade the liver and produce an abscess. Oral metronidazole and chloroquine hydrochloride administered orally or intramuscularly are used in treating hepatic amebic abscesses.

amebic dysentery, an inflammation of the intestine caused by infestation with *Entamoeba histolytica* and characterized by frequent, loose stools flecked with blood and mucus. Intestinal amebiasis is often accompanied by symptoms of liver involvement. Also called **intestinal amebiasis.** See also **amebiasis,** *Entamoeba histolytica,* **hepatic amebiasis.**

amelanotic (æm′ɪlənot′ɪk), of or pertaining to tissue that is unpigmented because it lacks melanin.

amelia (əmi′liə), **1.** a birth defect, marked by the absence of one or more limbs. The term may be modified to indicate the number of legs or arms missing at birth, as **tetramelia** for the absence of all four limbs. **2.** a psychological trait of apathy or indifference associated with certain forms of psychosis.

amelification (əmel′ɪfɪkeɪ′ʃhən), the differentiation of ameloblasts, or enamel cells, into the enamel of the teeth.

ameloblast (æm′ɪloublæst′), an epithelial cell from which the enamel of the teeth is formed. — **ameloblastic,** *adj.*

ameloblastic fibroma, an odontogenic neoplasm in which there is a simultaneous proliferation of mesenchymal and epithelial tissues but no development of dentin or enamel.

ameloblastic hemangioma, a highly vascular tumor of cells covering the dental papilla. See also **hemangioma.**

ameloblastic sarcoma, a malignant odontogenic tumor, characterized by the proliferation of epithelial and mesenchymal tissue without the formation of dentin or enamel.

ameloblastoma (æm′əloublæstou′mə), a highly destructive, malignant, rapid growing tumor of the jaw.

amelodentinal (æm′ələouden′tɪnəl), pertaining to both the enamel and dentin of the teeth.

amelogenesis (æm′ələoujen′ɪsɪs), the formation of the enamel of the teeth. — **amelogenic,** *adj.*

amelogenesis imperfecta, a hereditary dental defect characterized by a brown coloration of the teeth and resulting from either severe hypocalcification or hypoplasia of the enamel. The condition, which is inherited as an autosomal dominant trait, is classified according to severity as agenesis, in which there is complete lack of enamel; enamel hypoplasia, in which defective matrix formation causes the enamel to be normal in quality of hardness but deficient in quantity; or enamel hypocalcification, in which defective maturation of the ameloblasts results in the normal quantity of enamel, though it is soft and undercalcified in context. Also called **hereditary brown enamel, hereditary enamel hypoplasia.** Compare **denti-**

nogenesis imperfecta. See also **enamel hypocalcification, enamel hypoplasia.**

amenorrhea (ei'menəri'ə), the absence of menstruation. Amenorrhea is normal prior to sexual maturity, during pregnancy, after menopause, and during the intermenstrual phase of the monthly hormonal cycle but is otherwise caused by dysfunction of the hypothalamus, pituitary gland, ovary, or uterus, by the congenital absence or surgical removal of both ovaries or the uterus, or by medication. **Primary amenorrhea** is the failure of menstrual cycles to begin. **Secondary amenorrhea** is the cessation of menstrual cycles once established. See also **hypothalamic amenorrhea, post-pill amenorrhea.** —**amenorrheic.** *adj.*

amentia (eimen'shə), **1.** *Obsolete. See* **mental retardation. 2.** a state of mind characterized by apathy and disorientation, bordering on stupor, as in Stearns' alcoholic amentia. Also called **confusional insanity.**

Americaine, a trade name for a local anesthetic (benzocaine).

American Academy of Nursing (AAN), the honorary organization of the American Nurses' Association, created to recognize superior achievement in nursing in order to promote advances and excellence in nursing practice and education. A person who is elected to membership is given the title of Fellow of the American Academy of Nursing and may use the abbreviation FAAN as an honorific.

American Academy of Physical Medicine and Rehabilitation (A.A.P.M.R.), a national association of professional health-care workers concerned with the diagnosis of physical impairment and the development of therapies and devices to improve physical function.

American Academy of Physicians' Assistants (AAPA), a national organization of physicians' assistants or associates.

American Association for Respiratory Therapy (AART), a national organization of nurses and other health workers in the field of respiratory therapy.

American Association of Colleges of Nursing (AACN), an organization of baccalaureate and graduate schools of nursing that was established to deal with various issues of nursing education.

American Association of Critical Care Nurses (AACCN), a national organization of nurses who work in critical care units.

American Association of Industrial Nurses (AAIN), a national professional association of nurses working in industry and concerned with issues in occupational health.

American Association of Medical Colleges (AAMC), a national organization of faculty members and deans of medical schools.

American Association of Neurological Nurses (AANN), a national organization of nurses working in the field of neurology.

American Association of Nurse Anesthetists (AANA), a professional association of certified registered nurse anesthetists. The AANA is the accrediting agency for schools of nurse anesthetists. See also **nurse anesthesist.**

American Association of Pathologists and Bacteriologists (A.A.P.B.), a national professional organization of specialists in pathology and bacteriology.

American Association of University Professors (AAUP), a national organization of faculty members of institutions of higher learning. The AAUP represents faculty in matters of academic freedom, appointment policies, and procedures and serves as the bargaining agent for the faculties of some universities.

American College of Obstetricians and Gynecologists (ACOG), the national organization of obstetricians and gynecologists. It is concerned with the education of physicians in the specialty standards of practice, the continued education and well-being of its members, and the board certification of eligible members as fellows of the organization.

American College of Pathologists (ACP), a national professional organization of physicians who specialize in pathology.

American College of Physicians (ACP), a national professional organization of physicians.

American College of Radiologists (ACR), a national professional organization of physicians who specialize in radiology.

American Journal of Nursing, the professional journal of the American Nurses' Association (ANA). It contains articles and papers of general and specialized clinical interest to nurses and is the principal resource regarding the profession and employment in the profession in the United States. It is one of five magazines published by the American Journal of Nursing Company of which ANA is the sole owner.

American leishmaniasis, a group of mucocutaneous infections caused by various species of *Leishmania,* characterized by disfiguring ulcerative lesions of the nose, mouth, and throat. These infections are most prevalent in southern Mexico and in Central and South America. Illness may be prolonged, rendering patients susceptible to serious secondary infections. Kinds of American leishmaniasis are **chiclero's ulcer, espundia, forest yaws, uta.** Also called **mucocutaneous leishmaniasis, New World leishmaniasis.** See also **leishmaniasis.**

American Medical Association (A.M.A.), a professional association whose membership is made up of approximately half of the total licensed physicians in the United States, including practitioners in all recognized medical specialties as well as general primary care physicians. The A.M.A. is governed by a Board of Trustees and House of Delegates who represent various state and local medical associations as well as government agencies such as the Public Health Service and medical departments of the Army, Navy, and Air Force. The A.M.A. maintains directories of all qualified physicians (including nonmembers) in the United States, including graduates of foreign medical colleges, evaluates prescription and nonprescription drugs, advises congressional and state legislators regarding proposed health-care laws, and publishes a variety of journals that report on scientific and socioeconomic developments in the field of medicine. See also **British Medical Association.**

American mountain fever. See **Colorado tick fever.**

American Nurses' Association (ANA), the national professional association of registered nurses in the United States. It was founded in 1896 to improve standards of health and the availability of health care given in order to foster high standards for nursing, to promote the professional development of nurses, and to advance the economic and general welfare of nurses. The ANA is made up of 53 constituent associations from 50 states, the District of Columbia, Guam, and the Virgin Islands, representing more than 900 district associations. National conventions are held biennially in even-numbered years. Members may join one or more of the five Divisions on Nursing Practice: Community Health; Gerontological; Maternal and Child Health; Medical-Surgical; and Psychiatric and Mental Health Nursing. These Divisions are coordinated by the Congress for Nursing Practice. The Congress evaluates changes in the scope of practice, monitors scientific and educational developments, encourages research, and develops statements that describe ANA policies regarding legislation affecting nursing practice. Other commissions within the Association include the Commission on Nursing Education, the Commission on Nursing Services, the Commission on Nursing Research, and the Economic and General Welfare Commission (E and GW), which functions at the local, state, and national level. The programs of the E and GW Commission are intended to ensure fair compensation for nurses, working conditions that are conducive to high quality nursing care, and a pool of qualified nurses adequate for the health-care needs of the country. In addition, the ANA is politically active on the federal level in all issues relevant to nursing. Statistical services enable the Association to fulfill its role as the most authoritative source of data on nursing in the United States. The publications of the ANA include the *American Nurse,* a newspaper, the *Publications List,* and *The American Journal of Nursing,* the professional journal of the Association.

American Psychiatric Association (APA), a national professional psychiatric society concerned with the development of standards for psychiatric facilities, the formulation of mental health programs, the dissemination of data, and the promotion of psychiatric education and research. It publishes the *Diagnostic and Statistical Manual of Mental Disorders.*

American Red Cross, one of more than 120 national organizations that seek to reduce human suffering through various health, safety, and disaster relief programs in affiliation with the International Committee of the Red Cross. The Committee and all Red Cross organizations evolved from the Geneva Convention of 1864, following the example and urging of Swiss humanitarian Jean Henri Dunant, who aided wounded French and Austrian soldiers at the Battle of Solferino in 1859. The American Red Cross has more than 130 million members in about 3,100 chapters throughout the United States. Volunteers comprise the entire staffs of about 1,700 chapters. Other chapters maintain small paid staffs and some professionals but depend largely on volunteers. The American Red Cross blood program collects and distributes more blood than any other single agency in the United States and coordinates distribution of blood and blood products to the U.S. Defense Department on request or during national emergencies. The organization annually collects about four million blood donations and gives blood to more than 4,000 hospitals. American Red Cross nursing and health programs include courses in the home on parenthood, prenatal and postnatal care, hygiene, and venereal disease. Nursing students are enrolled for service in American Red Cross community programs and during disasters. Four area offices at Alexandria, Virginia, Atlanta, Georgia, St. Louis, Missouri, and San Francisco, California, supervise and assist 70 divisions of the American Red Cross and direct field staff members assigned to military installations. National headquarters of the organization is at 17th and D Streets, NW, Washington, D.C. 20006. The President of the United States is honorary chairman of the organization, for which a 50-member board of governors, all volunteers, develops policy. The symbol of the American Red Cross, like that of most other Red Cross societies throughout the world, is a red cross on a field of white; in Switzerland it is a white cross on a red field, in Muslim countries, a red crescent, in Israel, a red star of David, and, in Iran, a red lion and sun.

American Society of Radiologic Technologists (ASRT), a national professional organization of technicians specialized in radiology.

American trypanosomiasis. See **Chagas' disease.**

American Type Culture Collection (ATCC), a nonprofit, nongovernmental organization that is concerned with the preservation of specimens of cellular and microbiological cultures and with the distribution of the cultures to research centers and laboratories in the academic, scientific, and medical communities.

americium (Am), a manmade radioactive element of the actinide group. Its atomic number is 95; its atomic weight is 243.

Ameslan (æm'ıslæn), acronym for American Sign Language, a method of communication with the deaf that relies primarily on the position, shape, and motion of the hands and fingers for the transmission of concepts and messages.

amethopterin. See **methotrexate.**

ametropia (æm'ıtrou'piə), a condition characterized by an optical defect involving an error of refraction, as astigmatism, hyperopia, myopia. – **ametropic,** *adj.*

Amicar, a trade name for a hemostatic (aminocaproic acid).

amide-compound local anesthetic, any of more than two dozen compounds that are safe, versatile, and effective local anesthetics. If hypersensitivity to a drug in this group precludes its use, one of the ester-compound local anesthetics may provide analgesia without adverse effect. Some kinds of amide-compound local anesthetics are **bupivacaine, dibucaine, etiodocaine, lidocaine, mepivacaine, prilocaine.**

amido-, a combining form meaning 'the presence of the radical NH_2 along with the radical CO': *amido-acetal, amidobenzene, amidopyrine.*

amidobenzene (əmi'douben'zin, æm'ıdouben'zin). See **aniline.**

Amigen, a trade name for a nutritional replacement or supplement (protein hydrolysate injection), used in parenteral alimentation.

amikacin sulfate, an aminoglycoside antibiotic.

■ INDICATION: It is prescribed in the treatment of various severe infections that are resistant to other antibiotics.

■ CONTRAINDICATIONS. Concurrent use of certain diuretics or known hypersensitivity to this or other aminoglycosides prohibits its use. The drug is used with caution in patients who have impaired renal function or myasthenia gravis.

■ ADVERSE EFFECTS: Among the more serious adverse reactions are nephrotoxicity, auditory and vestibular ototoxicity, and neuromuscular blockade. Gastrointestinal disturbances, pain at the site of injection, and hypersensitivity reactions may occur.

Amikin, a trade name for an antibacterial (amikacin sulfate).

amine (æm'ın, əmin'), (in chemistry) any organic compound that contains nitrogen.

amine pump, *Informal.* an active transport system in the presynaptic nerve endings that takes up released amine neurotransmitters. Adverse reactions to some drugs, notably tricyclic antidepressants, block this function, resulting in a high concentration of norepinephrine in cardiac tissue and resultant tachycardia and arrhythmia. See also **monoamine oxidase inhibitor.**

aminoacetic acid (əmi'nouəsi'tık, æm'ınouəsi'tık), a nonessential amino acid occurring as a natural ingredient of many proteins; as a synthetic compound, it is used as a dietary supplement and a gastric antacid. Also called **glycine, glycocoll.**

amino acid, an organic chemical compound composed of one or more basic amino groups and one or more acidic carboxyl groups. Twenty of the more than 100 amino acids that occur in nature are the building blocks of peptides, polypeptides, and proteins. See also **essential amino acid.**

aminoaciduria (æmi'nouæs'ıdyur'iə), the abnormal presence of amino acids in the urine that usually indicates an inborn metabolic defect, as in cystinuria.

aminobenzene (əmi'nouben'zin, æm'ınouben'zin). See **aniline.**

aminobenzoic acid, a metabolic product of the catabolism of the amino acid tryptophan. Also called **anthralinic acid.**

aminocaproic acid (əmi'noukəprou'ık, æm'ınoukəprou'ık), a hemostatic.

■ INDICATION: It is prescribed to stop excessive bleeding that results from hyperfibrinolysis.

■ CONTRAINDICATION: Active intravascular coagulation prohibits its use.

■ ADVERSE EFFECTS: Among the most serious adverse reactions are thrombosis and hypotension. Inhibition of ejaculation, nasal congestion, diarrhea, and various allergic reactions also may occur.

Aminodur, a trade name for a muscle relaxant and respiratory stimulant (aminophylline).

aminoglycoside antibiotic. See **antibiotic.**

amino oxidase. See **monoamine oxidase.**

aminophylline (æm'ənoufıl'ın, æm'ənoufıl'in), a bronchodilator.

■ INDICATIONS: It is prescribed in the treatment of bronchial asthma, emphysema, and bronchitis.

■ CONTRAINDICATIONS: Known hypersensitivity to this drug or other xanthine medication prohibits its use. It is used with caution in patients who have peptic ulcer and those in whom cardiac stimulation would be harmful.

■ ADVERSE EFFECTS: Among the more serious adverse reactions are gastrointestinal disturbances, central nervous system stimulation, palpitations, tachycardia, and nervousness.

aminosalicylic acid, a tuberculostatic antibacterial.

■ INDICATIONS: It is prescribed in the treatment of pulmonary and extrapulmonary tuberculosis.

■ CONTRAINDICATION: Known hypersensitivity to this drug prohibits its use.

■ ADVERSE EFFECTS: Among the most serious adverse reactions are hypersensitivity reactions, including drug fever. Gastrointestinal disturbances are common.

aminosuccinic acid (əmi'nousəksɪn'ɪk, æm'-ɪnousəksɪn'ɪk).   See **aspartic acid.**

aminotransferase.   See **transaminase.**

amitosis (æm'ətou'sɪs),   direct cell division in which there is simple fission of the nucleus and cytoplasm. It does not involve the complex stages of chromatin separation of the chromosomes that occur in mitosis. – **amitotic,** *adj.*

amitriptyline,   a tricyclic antidepressant.

■ INDICATION: It is prescribed in the treatment of depression.

■ CONTRAINDICATIONS: Concomitant administration of monoamine oxidase inhibitors, recent myocardial infarction, or known hypersensitivity to this drug or to other tricyclic medication prohibits its use. It is used with caution in patients having a seizure disorder or in those with cardiovascular disease.

■ ADVERSE EFFECTS: Among the more serious adverse reactions are sedation and a variety of gastrointestinal, cardiovascular, and neurologic reactions. This drug interacts with many other drugs.

AML,   abbreviation for **acute myelocytic leukemia.**

ammonia,   a colorless aromatic gas consisting of nitrogen and hydrogen, produced by the decomposition of nitrogenous organic matter. Some of its many uses are as an aromatic stimulant, a detergent, and an emulsifier.

ammoniacal fermentation,   the production of ammonia and carbon dioxide from urea by the enzyme urease.

ammoni-,   a combining form meaning 'pertaining to ammonium': *ammoniemia, ammonirrhea, ammoniuria.*

amnesia,   a loss of memory owing to brain damage or to severe emotional trauma. Kinds of amnesia are **anterograde amnesia, hysterical amnesia, post-traumatic amnesia, retrograde amnesia.**

amnestic apraxia,   the inability to carry out a movement in response to a request owing to a lack of ability to remember the request rather than to a loss of motor function. See also **apraxia.**

amnio-,   a combining form meaning 'pertaining to the amnion': *amniogenesis, amnioma, amniorrhexis.*

amniocentesis (æm'niousenti'sɪs),   an obstetric procedure in which a small amount of amniotic fluid is removed for laboratory analysis. It is usually performed between the sixteenth and twentieth weeks of gestation to aid in the diagnosis of fetal abnormalities.

■ METHOD: Using ultrasound scanning techniques the position of the fetus and the location of the placenta are determined. The skin on the mother's abdomen is aseptically prepared and a local anesthetic is usually injected. A needle attached to a syringe is introduced into a part of the uterus where there is the least chance of perforating the placenta or scratching the fetus. Between 20 and 25 ml of amniotic fluid are aspirated. Amniocentesis is performed to diagnose various genetic defects, including chromosomal abnormalities, neural tube defects, and Tay-

Sachs disease. It is also performed to discover the sex of the fetus if certain sex-linked genetic defects are suspected. Later in pregnancy amniocentesis may be performed to assess fetal maturity by testing the lecithin-sphingomyelin (L/S) ratio in the laboratory prior to therapeutic termination of pregnancy. The fluid may be tested for the concentration of creatinine, another indicator of fetal maturity. When postmaturity is suspected, amniocentesis is performed to examine the amniotic fluid for meconium.

■ NURSING ORDERS: Proof of informed consent is required to be signed by the woman prior to amniocentesis. Specifically stated in the consent form are the reason for performing the procedure and the facts that fluid is to be removed after needle puncture of the uterus, that ultrasound imaging techniques are usual adjuncts, that the procedure may fail to give the results intended, and that spontaneous abortion, nausea, abdominal pain, or fetal injury may occur. The woman is reassured that complications and failure are rare; she is given emotional support before, during, and after the procedure. In testing for genetic abnormalities three or more weeks are usually necessary for tissue culture before a diagnosis may be made; this waiting period is extremely stressful for the mother. The woman is warned to report any signs of infection or of the onset of labor. Rh immune globulin is often given to pregnant women who are Rh negative.

■ OUTCOME CRITERIA: Spontaneous abortion occurs in approximately one per cent of women undergoing amniocentesis. Perforation of the placenta or a blood vessel in the umbilical cord or placenta may cause hemorrhage or isoimmunization and hemolytic disease of the fetus, possibly leading to fetal death. Maternal and fetal infection with attendant morbidity or mortality may occur, but it is rare. Premature rupture of the membranes, premature labor or trauma to the fetus or umbilical cord may occur. The procedure is not usually performed for genetic diagnosis unless the mother plans to terminate the pregnancy if the procedure indicates the presence of a genetic disease or abnormality.

amnion (æm'nion),   a membrane, continuous with and covering the fetal side of the placenta, that forms the outer surface of the umbilical cord and becomes the outermost layer of the skin of the developing fetus. Compare **chorion.**

amniotic fluid,   a liquid produced by the fetal membranes and the fetus. It surrounds the fetus throughout pregnancy, usually totaling about 1,000 ml at term. In addition to providing the fetus with physical protection, the amniotic fluid is a medium of active chemical exchange. It is secreted and resorbed by cells lining the amniotic sac at a rate of 500 ml/hr at term, and is swallowed, metabolized, and excreted as fetal urine at a rate of 50 ml/hr. Its chemical constituents are those of maternal and fetal plasma in different concentrations. Its pH is close to neutral. Amniotic fluid itself is clear, though desquamated fetal cells and lipids give it a cloudy appearance.

amniotic sac, a thin-walled bag that contains the fetus and amniotic fluid during pregnancy, having a capacity of 4 to 5 liters at term. The wall of the sac extends from the margin of the placenta. The amnion, chorion, and decidua that make up the wall are each a few cell layers thick. They are closely applied – though not fused – to each other and to the wall of the uterus. The intact sac and its fluid provide for the equilibration of hydrostatic pressure within the uterus, and, during labor, effect the uniform transmission of the force of uterine contractions to the cervix for dilatation. See also **amnion, chorion, decidua.**

amobarbital, a barbiturate sedative-hypnotic.
- INDICATIONS: It is prescribed for the relief of anxiety and insomnia and as an anti-convulsant.
- CONTRAINDICATIONS: Porphyria or known hypersensitivity to barbiturates prohibits its use.
- ADVERSE EFFECTS: Among the most serious adverse reactions are respiratory and circulatory depression, drug hangover, and various allergic reactions. It is also involved in many drug interactions.

amoeba. See **ameba.**

-amoeba. See **-ameba.**

amoebiasis (æm'ibai'əsis). See **amebiasis.**

amoebic dysentery. See **amebic dysentery.**

amorph (ei'mɔrf, əmɔrf'), an inactive gene; a mutant allele that has little or no effect on the expression of a trait. Compare **antimorph, hypermorph, hypomorph.**

amorphic, (in genetics) of or pertaining to a gene that is inactive or nearly inactive so that it has no determinable effect.

amoxapine, an antidepressant similar to the tricyclics.
- INDICATION: It is prescribed in the treatment of mental depression.
- CONTRAINDICATIONS: It is used with caution in conditions where anticholinergics are contraindicated, in seizure disorders, and in patients with cardiovascular disorders. Concomitant administration of monoamine oxidase inhibitors, recent myocardial infarction, or known hypersensitivity to this drug prohibits its use.
- ADVERSE EFFECTS: Among the most serious adverse reactions are sedation and anticholinergic side effects. A variety of gastrointestinal, cardiovascular, and neurological reactions may also occur. It is involved in many potential drug interactions.

amoxicillin, a semisynthetic oral penicillin similar to ampicillin.
- INDICATIONS: It is prescribed in the treatment of several infections that are caused by a susceptible gram-negative or gram-positive organism.

- CONTRAINDICATION: Known hypersensitivity to any penicillin prohibits its use.
- ADVERSE EFFECTS: Among the most serious adverse reactions are anaphylaxis, nausea, and diarrhea. Various allergic reactions and rashes are common.

Amoxil, a trade name for an antibiotic (amoxicillin).

AMP, abbreviation for **adenosine monophosphate.**

ampere (æm'pir), a unit of measurement of the amount of electrical current. An ampere, according to the meter-kilogram-second (MKS) system, is the amount of current passed through a resistance of one ohm by an electrical potential of one volt. The standard international ampere is the amount of current which deposits 0.001118 gm of silver per second when passed, according to certain specifications, through a silver nitrate solution. See also **ohm, volt.**

amph-. See **amphi-.**

amphetamine, a central nervous system stimulant used in treating narcolepsy, as part of a program for the management of children with attention deficit disorder, and as an adjunct to diet in treating exogenous obesity. Amphetamine increases systolic and diastolic blood pressures and acts as a weak bronchodilator and respiratory stimulant; it has a high potential for abuse, resulting in tolerance, psychological dependence, and severe social disability. Overdosage of the drug may cause nausea, vomiting, diarrhea, abdominal cramps, cardiac arrhythmias, restlessness, tremor, hyperreflexia, tachypnea, confusion, assaultiveness, hallucinations, and panic states. Also called *Slang.* **speed.**

amphi-, amph-, a combining form meaning 'on both sides': *amphiarthrosis, amphiaster, amphibious.*

amphiarthrosis (æm'fiarfhrou'sis). See **cartilaginous joint.**

amphigenesis (æm'fijen'isis). See **amphigony.**

amphigenetic (æm'fijinet'ik), **1.** produced by the union of gametes from both sexes. **2.** bisexual; having both testicular and ovarian tissue.

amphigonadism (æm'figou'nədiz'əm), true hermaphroditism; having both testicular and ovarian tissue. — **amphigonadic,** *adj.*

amphigonous inheritance, the acquisition of genetic traits and conditions from both parents. Also called **biparental inheritance, duplex inheritance.**

amphigony (æmfig'əni), sexual reproduction. Also called **amphigenesis.** — **amphigonic,** (əm'figon'ik) *adj.*

amphikaryon (æm'fikær'ion), a nucleus containing the diploid number of chromosomes. — **amphikaryotic,** *adj.*

amphimixis (æm'fimik'sis), **1.** the union of germ cells in reproduction so that both maternal and paternal hereditary characteristics are derived; interbreeding. **2.** (in psychoanalysis) the union and integration of oral, anal, and genital libidinal impulses in the development of sexuality.

ampho-, a combining form meaning 'both': *amphochromophil, amphodiplopia, amphogenic.*

amphoric breath sound, an abnormal, hollow blowing sound heard with a stethoscope. It indicates a cavity opening into the bronchus, or a pneumothorax.

amphotericin B (æm'fətǝr'ǝsɪn), an antifungal medication.
■ INDICATION: It is prescribed for topical or systemic use in the treatment of fungal infections.
■ CONTRAINDICATION: Known hypersensitivity to this drug prohibits its use.
■ ADVERSE EFFECTS: Among the most serious adverse reactions, when used systemically, are thrombophlebitis, blood dyscrasias, nephrotoxicity, nausea and fever. When used topically, local hypersensitivity reactions are the most common adverse reactions.

ampicillin, a semi-synthetic penicillin.
■ INDICATION: It is prescribed in the treatment of a variety of infections caused by a broad spectrum of sensitive gram-negative and gram-positive organisms.
■ CONTRAINDICATION: Known hypersensitivity to any penicillin prohibits its use.
■ ADVERSE EFFECTS: Among the most serious adverse reactions are anaphylaxis, nausea, and diarrhea. Fever, rashes, other allergic reactions, and suprainfection also may occur.

amplification, (in molecular genetics) **1.** a process in which the amount of plasmid DNA is increased in proportion to the amount of bacterial DNA by treatment with certain substances, including chloramphenicol. **2.** the replication in bulk of an entire gene library. — **amplify,** *v.*

amplitude, width or breadth of range or extent, as amplitude of accommodation or amplitude of convergence.

amplitude of accommodation, the total accommodative power of the eye, determined by the difference between the refractive power for farthest vision and that for nearest vision.

amplitude of convergence, the difference in the power needed to turn the eyes from their far point to their near point of convergence.

ampule, ampoule (æm'pyul), a small, sterile glass or plastic container that usually contains a single dose of a solution to be administered parenterally.

ampullary tubal pregnancy, a kind of tubal pregnancy in which implantation occurs in the ampulla of one of the Fallopian tubes. See also **tubal pregnancy.**

amputation, the surgical removal of a part of the body or a limb or part of a limb, performed to treat recurrent infections or gangrene in peripheral vascular disease, to remove malignant tumors, and in severe trauma. Under general anesthesia the part is removed and a shaped flap is cut from muscular and cutaneous tissue to cover the end of the bone, with a section left open for drainage if infection is present. Preoperative care includes an assessment of circulation in the affected limb and the shaving and cleansing of the area. Postoperatively, the stump is elevated on a pillow, and, if necessary, protected with plastic from urinary and fecal contamination. Vital signs are monitored carefully. If a soft dressing is used, it is watched for excessive bleeding. If the dressing is rigid (a cast) it must remain in place for 8 to 14 days. Should the cast come off inadvertently, the stump must be wrapped tightly at once with elastic compresssion bandage, and plans are made to replace the cast. With the cast on, the patient can stand briefly after 24 hours and bear some weight on a prosthesis. The stump is moved frequently to prevent circulatory complications and tissue necrosis. Medication may relieve incisional and phantom limb pain. Kinds of amputation include **closed amputation, open amputation, primary amputation, secondary amputation.**

amputation neuroma, a form of traumatic neuroma that may develop near the stump after the amputation of an extremity.

amputee, a person who has had one or more extremities traumatically, congenitally, or surgically removed. See also **congenital amputation.**

Amsler grid (æms'lǝr), a checkerboard grid of intersecting dark horizontal and vertical lines with one dark spot in the middle. To discover a visual field defect, the person simply covers or closes one eye, and looks at the spot with the other. A visual field defect is perceived as a defect, distortion, blank, or other fault in the grid. The person may record the defects directly on a paper copy of the grid that may be kept as a permanent record.

Amsterdam dwarf, a person affected with de Lange's syndrome, in which short stature and severe mental retardation are associated with many other abnormalities.

amyelinic neuroma, a tumor that contains only nonmyelinated nerve fibers.

amyl-. See **amylo-.**

amyl alcohol, a colorless, oily liquid that is only slightly soluble in water but can be mixed with ethyl alcohol, chloroform, or ether.

amyl alcohol tertiary. See **amylene hydrate.**

amylase (æm'ɪleɪs), an enzyme that catalyzes the hydrolysis of starch into smaller carbohydrate molecules. Alpha-amylase, found in saliva, pancreatic juice, malt, certain bacteria, and molds, catalyzes the hydrolysis of starches to dextrins, maltose, and maltotriose. Beta-amylase, found in grains, vegetables, and malt, is involved in the hydrolysis of starch to maltose. See also **enzyme.**

amylene hydrate, a clear, colorless liquid with a camphorlike odor, miscible with alcohol, chloroform, ether, or glycerin and used as a solvent and a hypnotic.

amylic fermentation, the formation of amyl alcohol from sugar.

amyl nitrite, a vasodilator.
- INDICATION: It is prescribed to relieve the vasospasm of angina pectoris.
- CONTRAINDICATIONS: Known hypersensitivity to this drug or to other nitrites prohibits its use.
- ADVERSE EFFECTS: Among the more serious adverse reactions are hypotension, allergic reactions, nausea, headache, and dizziness.

amylo-, amyl-, a combining form meaning 'pertaining to starch': *amyloclast, amylodextrin, amyloid.*

amyloidosis (æm'ılɔidɑu'sıs), a disease in which a waxy, starchlike, glycoprotein (amyloid) accumulates in tissues and organs, impairing their function. There are two major forms of the condition. **Primary amyloidosis** usually occurs with multiple myeloma. Patients with **secondary amyloidosis** usually suffer from another chronic infectious or inflammatory disease, as tuberculosis, osteomyelitis, rheumatoid arthritis, or Crohn's disease. The cause of both types of amyloidosis is unknown. Almost all organs are affected, most often the heart, lungs, tongue, and intestines in primary amyloidosis, and the kidneys, liver, and spleen in the secondary type. Diagnosis is made through biopsy of the suspected organ. There is no known cure for amyloidosis, and treatment in the secondary type is aimed at alleviating the underlying chronic disease. Patients with renal amyloidosis are frequently candidates for kidney dialysis and transplantation.

amylopectinosis (æm'ıloupek'tınou'sıs). See **Andersen's disease.**

amyotonia (ei'maiɑtou'niɑ), an abnormal condition of skeletal muscle, characterized by a lack of tone, weakness, and wasting, usually the result of motor neuron disease. – **amyotonic,** *adj.*

amyotonia congenita. See **Oppenheim's disease.**

amyotrophic lateral sclerosis (ALS) (ei'maiɔutrof'ık), a degenerative disease of the motor neurons, characterized by atrophy of the muscles of the hands, forearms, and legs spreading to involve most of the body. It results from degeneration of the motor neurons of the anterior horns and cortico spinal tracts, beginning in middle age and progressing rapidly, causing death within two to five years. There is no known treatment. Also called **Lou Gehrig's disease.** See also **Aran-Duchenne muscular atrophy.**

Amytal, a trade name for a sedative (amobarbital).

an-, 1. a combining form meaning 'upward, backward, excessive, or again': *anelectrotonic, anion, anode.* 2. a combining form meaning 'not': *anaerogenic, analgesia, anaphia.* Also **ana-.**

ANA, abbreviation for **American Nurses' Association.**

ana-. See **an¹.**

anabolic steroid, any one of several compounds derived from testosterone or prepared synthetically to promote general body growth, to oppose the effects of endogenous estrogen, or to promote masculinizing effects. All such compounds cause a mixed androgenic-anabolic effect. Anabolic steroids are prescribed in the treatment of aplastic anemia, red-cell aplasia, and hemolytic anemia and in anemias associated with renal failure, myeloid metaplasia, and leukemia. Some common compounds used in such therapies are calusterone, methandriol, and nandrolone. Anabolic steroids used in the palliation of carcinoma of the breast in women carry the risk of causing masculinization. The earliest symptoms of such undesirable effects are acne, the growth of facial hair, and the hoarsening or deepening of the voice. Continued use of these compounds in women may also produce prominent musculature, excessive body hair, and hypertrophy of the clitoris.

anabolism (ɑnæb'ɑliz'ɑm), constructive metabolism characterized by the conversion of simple substances into the more complex compounds of living matter. Compare **catabolism.** – **anabolic,** *adj.*

anaclisis (æn'ɑklai'sıs), 1. a condition, normal in childhood but pathologic in adulthood, in which a person is emotionally dependent on other people. 2. a condition in which a person consciously or unconsciously chooses a love object because of a resemblance to the mother, father, or other person who was an important source of comfort and protection in infancy. – **anaclitic,** *adj.*

anaclitic depression, a syndrome occurring in infants, usually following sudden separation from the mothering person. Symptoms include apprehension, withdrawal, incessant crying, refusal to eat, sleep disturbances, and, eventually, stupor leading to severe impairment of the infant's physical, social, and intellectual development. If the mothering figure or a substitute is made available within one to three months, the infant recovers quickly with no long-term effects. See also **hospitalism.**

anacrotic pulse (æn'ɑkrot'ık), (on a sphygmographic tracing) a pulse characterized by one transient drop in amplitude on the curve of the primary elevation. It is seen in valvular aortic stenosis.

anadicrotic pulse (æn'ɑdaikrot'ık), (on a sphygmographic tracing) a pulse characterized by two transient drops in amplitude on the curve of primary elevation.

anadidymus, conjoined twins that are united in the upper portion of the body but are separated in the lower half.

anadipsia (æn'ɑdıp'siɑ), extreme thirst, often occurring in the manic phase of manic-depressive psychosis. The condition is the result of dehydration owing to the excessive perspiration, continuous urination, and relentless physical activity produced by the intense excitement characteristic of the manic phase.

Anadrol, a trade name for an androgen (oxymetholone), used as an anabolic agent.

anaerobe (æneir'oub), a microorganism that grows and lives in the complete or almost complete absence of oxygen. Anaerobes are widely distributed in nature and in the body. Some kinds of anaerobes are **facultative anaerobe, obligate anaerobe.** Compare **aerobe.** See also **anaerobic infection.** —**anaerobic,** *adj.*

anaerobic (æn'ərou'bık), **1.** pertaining to the absence of air or oxygen. **2.** able to grow and function without air or oxygen.

anaerobic exercise, muscular exertion sufficient to result in metabolic acidosis owing to accumulation of lactic acid as a product of muscle metabolism. Compare **aerobic exercise.** See also **active exercise, passive exercise.**

anaerobic glycolysis. See **glycolysis.**

anaerobic infection, an infection caused by an anaerobic organism, usually occurring in deep puncture wounds that exclude air or in tissue that has diminished oxygen-reduction potential as a result of trauma, necrosis, or overgrowth of bacteria. Kinds of anaerobic infection are **gangrene, tetanus.** See also *Clostridium.*

anaerobic myositis. See **gas gangrene.**

anakatadidymus, conjoined twins that are united in the middle but separated at both the upper and lower parts of the body.

anal (ei'nəl), of or pertaining to the anus.

anal agenesis. See **imperforate anus.**

anal canal, the final portion of the alimentary tract, about 4 cm long, between the rectal ampulla and the anus.

anal character, (in psychoanalysis) a kind of personality exhibiting patterns of behavior originating in the anal phase of infancy, characterized by extreme orderliness, obstinacy, perfectionism, cleanliness, punctuality, and miserliness, or their extreme opposites. See also **anal stage, psychosexual development.**

anal crypt, the depression between rectal columns that encloses networks of veins which, when inflamed and swollen, are called hemorrhoids.

analeptic (æn'əlep'tık). See **central nervous system stimulant.**

anal eroticism, anal erotism, (in psychoanalysis) libidinal fixation at or regression to the anal stage of psychosexual development, often reflected in such personality traits as miserliness, stubbornness, and overscrupulousness. Compare **oral eroticism.** See also **anal character.**

anal fissure, a linear ulceration or laceration of the skin of the anus.

anal fistula, an abnormal opening on the cutaneous surface near the anus, usually resulting from a local crypt abscess and also common in Crohn's disease. A perianal fistula may or may not communicate with the rectum. Also called **fistula in ano.**

analgesia (æn'əlji'ziə), a lack of pain without loss of consciousness.

analgesia algera (æl'jerə). See **anesthesia dolorosa.**

analgesic (æn'əlji'zık), **1.** relieving pain. **2.** a drug that relieves pain.

analgesic cocktail, *Informal.* an individualized mixture of drugs used for pain relief in specific syndromes. See also **lytic cocktail.**

anal membrane. See **cloacal membrane.**

anal membrane atresia. See **imperforate anus.**

analog, analogue, **1.** a substance, tissue, or organ that is similar in appearance or function to another but differing in origin or development, as the eye of a fly and the eye of a human. **2.** a drug or other chemical compound that resembles another in structure or constituents but has different effects. Compare **homolog.**

anal reflex, a superficial neurological reflex obtained by stroking the skin or mucosa of the region around the anus, which normally results in a contraction of the external anal sphincter. This reflex may be lost in disease of the pyramidal tract above the upper lumbar spine level. See also **superficial reflex.**

anal sadism, (in psychoanalysis) a sadistic form of anal eroticism, manifested by such behavior as aggressiveness and selfishness. Compare **oral sadism.**

anal stage, (in psychoanalysis) the pregenital period in psychosexual development, occurring between the ages of one and three years, when preoccupation with the function of the bowel and the sensations associated with the anus are the predominant source of pleasurable stimulation. It is regarded as an important determinant of ultimate personality type. Adult patterns of behavior associated with fixation on this stage include either extreme neatness, orderliness, cleanliness, perfectionism, and punctuality, or their extreme opposites. See also **anal character, psychosexual development.**

anal stenosis. See **imperforate anus.**

analysand (ənæl'ısænd), a person undergoing psychoanalysis.

analysis, **1.** the separation of substances into their constituent parts and the determination of the nature, properties, and composition of compounds. **2.** (in chemistry) **qualitative analysis** is the determination of the elements present in a substance; **quantitative analysis** is the determination of how much of each element is present in a substance. **3.** *Informal,* psychoanalysis. —**analytic,** *adj.* **analyze,** *v.*

analysis of variance (ANOVA), a series of statistical procedures for determining the differences, attributable to chance alone, among two or more groups of scores.

analyst, **1.** a psychoanalyst. **2.** a person who analyzes the chemical, physical, or other properties of a substance or product.

analytic psychology, **1.** the system in which phenomena, such as sensations and feelings, are analyzed and classified by introspective rather than by experimental methods. Compare **experimental psychology.** **2.** a system of analyzing the psyche according to the concepts developed by Carl Gustav Jung. It differs from the psychoanalysis of Sigmund Freud in stressing a racial or collective unconscious and a mystical, religious factor in the development of the personal unconscious and in minimizing the importance of sexual influence on early emotional and psychological development. Also called **Jungian psychology.**

analyzing, (in five-step nursing process) a category of nursing behavior in which the health care needs of the client are identified and the goals of care are selected. The nurse interprets data, identifies problems involving the client, the client's family, and significant others, establishes priorities among goals, integrates the information, and projects the expected outcomes of nursing activities. Although analyzing follows assessing and precedes planning in the five steps of the nursing process, in practice, analyzing is integral to effective nursing practice at all steps of the process. See also **evaluating, implementing.**

anamnesis (æn'æmni'sɪs), **1.** remembrance of the past. **2.** the accumulated data concerning a medical or psychiatric patient and the patient's background, including family, previous environment, experiences, and particularly, recollections, for use in analyzing his condition. Compare **catamnesis.**

anaphase (æn'əfeiz), the third of four stages of nuclear division in mitosis and in each of the two divisions of meiosis. In mitosis and the second meiotic division the centromeres divide and the two chromatids, which are arranged along the equatorial plane of the spindle, separate and move to the opposite poles of the cell, forming daughter chromosomes. In the first meiotic division the pairs of homologous chromosomes separate from each other and move intact to the opposite poles of the spindle. See also **interphase, meiosis, metaphase, mitosis, prophase, telophase.**

anaphylactic hypersensitivity, an IgE or IgG dependent, immediate-acting humoral hypersensitivity response to an exogenous antigen. An intradermal skin test produces a wheal and flare reaction and edema within 30 minutes. Histamine, kinins, and other substances are released from mast cells, causing vasodilation and muscle contraction. Systemic anaphylaxis, atopic allergies, hayfever, and insect-sting reactions are all anaphylactic hypersensitivity reactions. Also called **type I hypersensitivity.** Compare **cell-mediated hypersensitivity, cytotoxic hypersensitivity, immune complex hypersensitivity.** See also **anaphylactic shock.**

anaphylactic shock, a severe and sometimes fatal systemic hypersensitivity reaction to a sensitizing substance, as a drug, vaccine, certain food, serum, allergen extract, insect venom, or chemical. This condition may occur within seconds from the time of exposure to the sensitizing factor and is commonly marked by respiratory distress and vascular collapse. The more quickly any systemic atopic reaction occurs in the individual after exposure, the more severe the associated shock is likely to be. The involved allergen enters the systemic circulation and triggers an incomplete humoral response that allows the allergen to combine with IgE and cause the release of histamine. Also entering into the reaction are IgG and IgM, which cause the release of complement fractions, further stimulating histamine action.

■ OBSERVATIONS: Anaphylactic shock can occur within seconds or minutes after exposure to an allergen. The first symptoms are intense anxiety, weakness, sweating and shortness of breath. Other symptoms may include hypotension, shock, cardiac dysrhythmia, respiratory congestion, laryngeal edema, nausea, and diarrhea.

■ INTERVENTION: If the patient is conscious and normotensive, treatment requires the immediate injection of epinephrine intramuscularly or subcutaneously with vigorous massage of the injection site to assure faster distribution of the drug. If the patient is unconscious, epinephrine is administered intravenously. The airway is maintained and the patient is carefully monitored for signs of laryngeal edema, which may require the insertion of an endotracheal tube or a tracheotomy and oxygen therapy. The signs of laryngeal edema include stridor, hoarseness, and dyspnea. Cardiopulmonary resuscitation may be required for cardiac arrest; it often involves closed-chest heart massage, assisted ventilation, and the administration of sodium bicarbonate.

■ NURSING CONSIDERATIONS: Nursing care of patients experiencing anaphylactic shock requires the performance of appropriate emergency treatment and the close monitoring of the patient for hypotension and decreased circulatory volume; volume expanders, as plasma, saline, and albumin, are often ordered. After the emergency, other medications, as subcutaneous epinephrine, corticosteroids, and diphenhydramine I.V. are administered as prescribed; blood pressure, central venous pressure, and urinary output are monitored. Patients with food allergies that produce anaphylactic shock are instructed to avoid offending allergens; patients with insect sting allergies are instructed to carry emergency anaphylactic kits when outdoors. Such kits contain epinephrine, antihistamine, and tourniquets.

anaphylactoid purpura. See **Henoch-Schönlein purpura.**

anaphylaxis (æn'əfəlæk'sɪs), an exaggerated hypersensitivity reaction to a previously encountered antigen. The response, which is mediated by antibodies of the IgE class of immunoglobulins, causes the release of histamine, kinin, and substances that affect smooth muscle. The reaction may be a localized wheal and flare of generalized itching, hyperemia, angioedema, and, in severe cases, vascular collapse, bronchospasm, and shock. The severity of symptoms depends on the original sensitizing dose of the antigen, the amount and distribution of antibodies, and the route of entry and size of the dose of antigen producing anaphylaxis. Insect stings, contrast media containing iodide, aspirin, antitoxins prepared with animal serum, and allergens used in testing and desensitizing patients who are hypersensitive produce anaphylaxis in some individuals. Penicillin injection is the most common cause of anaphylactic shock. Kinds of anaphylaxis are **aggregate anaphylaxis, antiserum anaphylaxis, cutaneous anaphylaxis, cytotoxic anaphylaxis, indirect anaphylaxis, inverse anaphylaxis. – anaphylactic, anaphylactoid,** *adj.*

anaplasia (æn'əplei'źhə), a change in the structure of cells and in their orientation to each other characterized by a loss of differentiation and reversion to a more primitive form. Anaplasia is characteristic of malignancy. Compare **metastasis. – anaplastic,** *adj.*

anaplastic astrocytoma. See **glioblastoma multiforme.**

anasarca (æn'əsar'kə), generalized, massive edema. Anasarca is often observed in edema associated with renal disease when fluid retention continues for an extended period of time. See also **edema. – anasarcous,** *adj.*

anastomosis (ənæs'təmou'sɪs), *pl.* **anastomoses.** a surgical joining of two ducts or blood vessels to allow flow from one to the other. It may be performed to bypass an aneurysm or a vascular or arterial occlusion. Under general anesthesia a section of the patient's saphenous vein or a synthetic prosthesis of Dacron, Teflon, or Orlon is grafted to the prepared vessels. Postoperative nursing care includes preventing tissue injury and wound infection by the use of a bed cradle over the incision, and padded rails. An adequate airway is maintained, oxygen is given if necessary, and vital signs are closely monitored. The systolic blood pressure is kept at about 20 mm of mercury above normal to maintain blood flow through the graft. Lack of blood flow may allow the graft to close, a major complication that requires exploratory surgery, and sometimes, amputation. Distal pulses on both legs are evaluated and their locations marked. Capillary filling time and the color and temperature of the skin are checked. Prophylactic antibiotic therapy may be started. Urinary output is monitored to be certain it is more than 30 cc for two consecutive hours. The patient is turned and frequently encouraged to cough and breathe deeply. Kinds of anastomoses are **end-to-end anastomosis, side-to-side anastomosis.** See also **aneurysm, bypass.**

anastomosis at elbow joint, a convergence of blood vessels at the elbow joint, consisting of various veins and portions of the brachial and deep brachial arteries and their branches.

anatomical dead space, an area in the trachea, bronchi, and air passages containing air that does not reach the alveoli during respiration. As a general rule, the volume of air in the anatomical dead space in milliliters is approximately equal to the weight in pounds of the involved individual. Certain lung disorders, as emphysema,

increase the amount of anatomical dead space. Compare **physiological dead space.**

anatomical position, a position of the body in which a person stands erect, facing directly forward, feet pointed forward slightly apart, arms hanging down at the sides with palms facing forward. This is the standard neutral position of reference used to describe sites or motions of various parts of the body. See also **body position.**

anatomical snuffbox, a small, cuplike depression on the back of the hand near the wrist, formed by the tendons reaching toward the thumb and index finger as the thumb is abducted, the wrist flexed, and the digits extended.

anatomic curve, the curvature of the different segments of the vertebral column. In the lateral contour of the back, the cervical curve appears concave, the thoracic curve appears convex, and the lumbar curve appears concave.

anatomic impotence. See **impotence.**

anatomy, 1. the study, classification, and description of structures and organs of the body. Kinds of anatomy are **applied anatomy, comparative anatomy, descriptive anatomy, gross anatomy, microscopic anatomy, morbid anatomy, surface anatomy.** 2. the structure of an organism. 3. a text on anatomy. 4. *Archaic.* dissection of a body.

Anavar, a trade name for an androgen (oxandrolone), used as an anabolic agent.

-ance. See **-ency.**

Ancobon, a trade name for an antifungal (flucytosine).

ancrod (æn'krod), the venom of the Malayan pit viper, used to remove fibrinogen from the circulation, thus preventing clotting of the blood.

-ancy. See **-ency.**

ancylo-, anchylo-, ankylo-, a combining form meaning 'bent or in the form of a loop': *ancylostomatic, ancylostomiasis, ancylostomo-anemia.*

Ancylostoma (ærŋ'kɪlos'təmə), a genus of nematode that includes *Necator americanus,* the most common North American hookworm.

ancylostomiasis (æn'səlos'təmæi'əsɪs), hookworm disease, more specifically that caused by *Ancylostoma duodenale, A. braziliensis,* or *A. canium.* Infection by *A. duodenale* is generally more harmful and less responsive to treatment than that by *Necator americanis,* which is the hookworm most often found in the southern United States. Clinical manifestations and treatment are similar for all types of hookworms. Infection may be prevented by eliminating fecal pollution of soil and by wearing shoes. See also **hookworm.**

Andersen's disease, a rare glycogen-storage disease characterized by a genetic deficiency of branching enzyme (amylo-1:4, 1:6 transglucosisase), causing the deposition in tissues of abnormal glycogen with long inner and outer chains. Infants with the disease are normal at birth but fail to thrive and soon show hepatomegaly, splenomegaly, and hypotonic muscles, associated with the progressive development of liver cirrhosis or heart failure of unknown mechanisms. Diagnosis is by enzyme assays of white blood cells and fibroblasts. There is no specific therapy for the disease, which is usually fatal in the first few years of life. Also called **amylopectinosis, Cori's disease, glycogen storage disease Type IV.**

andr-. See **andro-.**

andreioma (æn'driou'mə). See **arrhenoblastoma.**

andreoblastoma (æn'drioublæstou'mə). See **arrhenoblastoma.**

andro-, andr-, a combining form meaning 'pertaining to man or to the male': *androcyte, androgen, androgone.*

androgamone (æn'drougæm'oun), a gamone secreted by the male gamete.

androgen (æn'drəjin), a drug that increases male characteristics. Natural hormones, as testosterone and its esters and analogs, are primarily used as substitutional therapy during the male climacteric. Androgens may be administered orally or parenterally. See also **anabolism.** — **androgenic,** *adj.*

androgynous (ændroj'inəs), **1.** (of a man or woman) having some characteristics of both sexes. Social role, behavior, personality, and appearance are reflections of individuality and are not determined by gender. **2.** hermaphroditic. Compare **gynandrous.** — **androgyny,** *n.*

android pelvis, a type of pelvis in which the structure is characteristic of the male. It is not uncommon in women. The bones are thick and heavy and the inlet is heart-shaped. The sacrum inclines anteriorly, the side walls are convergent, and the pubic arch is small. The diameters of the midplane and the outlet are smaller than in the normal gynecoid pelvis, and vaginal delivery is likely to be difficult unless the overall pelvis is large and the fetus small.

androma (ændrou'mə). See **arrhenoblastoma.**

androsterone (ændros'təroun), originally believed to be the principal male sex hormone, it is used less frequently since the discovery of testosterone. The greater potency of several other male sex hormones has relegated androsterone largely to historical biochemical interest. See also **testosterone.**

-ane, a combining form designating hydrocarbons of the paraffin series: *butane, lindane, xylane.*

Anectine, a trade name for a depolarizing agent (succinylcholine chloride), used as an adjunct to anesthesia.

anemia, a disorder characterized by a decrease in hemoglobin in the blood to levels below the normal range. According to the pathophysiological classification, anemia is a reflection of any one (or more) of three basic processes: decreased hemoglobin or red cell production, increased red cell destruction, or blood loss. A separate and distinct morphological classification system describes anemia by the hemoglobin content of the red cells (normochromic or hypochromic) and by differences in red cell size (macrocytic, normocytic, or microcytic).

■ OBSERVATIONS: Depending on its severity, anemia may be accompanied by some or all of a number of clinical findings that stem directly from the diminished oxygen carrying capacity of the blood. These include fatigue, exertional dyspnea, dizziness, headache, insomnia, and pallor, especially of the mucous membranes. Anorexia and dyspepsia, palpitations, tachycardia, cardiac dilatation and systolic murmurs also occur. Understanding the pathophysiology of the anemia is a prerequisite for rational therapy, including the recognition that iron deficiency is, by far, the most common causative factor. Specific tests are first directed at this kind of anemia. Additional laboratory studies may be required to establish the presence of the less common forms.

■ INTERVENTION: The therapeutic response to anemia is highly variable and depends on the specific causative factors involved. Moderate to severe anemia, with hemoglobin levels that are below 7 to 8 gm/100ml, may call for transfusion of one or more units of blood, especially if the condition is acute and accompanied by specific clinical signs. Depending on the kind of anemia, treatment aims at providing supplements of the deficient component, eliminating the cause of the blood loss, or alleviating the hemolytic component. The latter may involve the administration of adrenal corticosteroids or, possibly, splenectomy. Appropriate laboratory tests and other examinations are usually repeated at intervals to monitor the response, the need for continued therapy, and the extent of return to normal levels.

■ NURSING CONSIDERATIONS: The nurse emphasizes to the patient the importance of adequate diet to supply blood building components. The patient's need for rest is stressed, especially in the face of cardiac and respiratory symptoms. The time needed for recovery and the need for repeated blood tests to evaluate the progress of therapy are outlined. The patient is also cautioned, where applicable, to be alert for signs of increasing anemia or resumption of blood loss. When transfusions are given, the nurse is alert for indications of a transfusion reaction.

-anemia, -anaemia, a combining form meaning '(condition of) red blood cell deficiency or its remedy': *achylanemia, melanemia, sulfanemia.* Also **-nemia.**

anemia of pregnancy, a condition of pregnancy characterized by a reduction in the concentration of hemoglobin in the blood. It may be physiologic or pathologic. In physiologic anemia of pregnancy, the reduction in concentration results from dilution because the plasma volume expands more than the red blood cell volume. The hematocrit in pregnancy normally drops several points below the level it was before pregnancy. In pathologic anemia of pregnancy, the oxygen-carrying capacity of the blood is deficient owing to disordered erythrocyte production or excessive loss of erythrocytes through destruction or bleeding. Pathologic anemia is a common complication of pregnancy occurring in approximately one half of all pregnancies. Disordered production of erythrocytes may result from nutritional deficiency of iron, folic acid, or vitamine B_{12}, or from chronic disease, malignancy, chronic malnutrition, or exposure to toxins. Destruction of erythrocytes may result from inflammation, chronic infection, sepsis, autoimmune disorders, microangiopath, or a hematologic disease in which the red cells are abnormal. Excessive loss of erythrocytes through bleeding may result from abortion, bleeding hemorrhoids, intestinal parasites, as hook worm, placental abnormalities, as placenta previa and premature separation, or postpartum uterine atony.

anemic anoxia, a condition characterized by a deficiency of oxygen in body tissues, resulting from a decrease in the number of erythrocytes in the blood or in the amount of hemoglobin.

anemo-, a combining form meaning 'pertaining to the wind': *anemopathy, anemophobia, anemotropism.*

anencephaly (æn'ensef'əli), congenital absence of the brain and spinal cord in which the cranium does not close and the vertebral canal remains a groove. Transmitted genetically, anencephaly is not compatible with life. It can be detected early in gestation by amniotic fluid tap and analysis or by ultrasonography. See also **neural tube defect.**

anergic stupor, a kind of dementia characterized by quietness, listlessness, and nonresistance.

anergy, 1. lack of activity. 2. an immunodeficient condition characterized by a lack of or diminished reaction to an antigen or group of antigens. This state may be seen in advanced tuberculosis and other serious infections and in some malignancies. – **anergic,** *adj.*

aneroid (æn'əroid), not containing a liquid, used especially to describe a device in contrast to one performing a similar function that does contain liquid, as aneroid sphygmomanometer, which does not contain a column of liquid mercury.

Anestacon, a trade name for an endourethral local anesthetic solution (2% lidocaine hydrochloride).

anesthesia, the absence of normal sensation, especially sensitivity to pain, as induced by an anesthetic substance or by hypnosis or as occurs with traumatic or pathophysiologic damage to nerve tissue. Anesthesia induced for medical or surgical purposes may be topical, local, regional, or general and is named for the anesthetic agent used, the method or procedure followed, the area or organ anesthetized, or the age or class of patient served. See also specific anesthetic agents and forms of anesthesia.

anesthesia dolorosa (dou'lərou'sə), a severe, spontaneous, paradoxical pain in an anesthetized area. Also called **analgesia algera.**

anesthesia machine, an apparatus for administering inhalant anesthetic agents. Although there are many different models, all have the following features: an accommodation for a source of gas; a meter to measure the flow of gas; vessels for volatilizing and mixing the anesthetic agents and the carrier gases; and a system for delivery of the gas to the patient.

anesthesia patients, classification of, the system by which the American Society of Anesthesiologists classifies anesthesia patients in 5 categories by anesthetic risk factors. Class I includes patients who are generally healthy, without serious organic, physiologic, biochemical, or psychiatric problems, and for whom anesthesia is required only for a local condition, as an inguinal hernia or fibroid uterus. Class II includes patients who have mild to moderate systemic problems, whether involving or extraneous to the condition requiring anesthesia, as anemia, mild diabetes, essential hypertension, extreme obesity, or chronic bronchitis. Class III includes patients who have severe systemic disturbances or disease, whether or not related to the procedure requiring surgical anesthesia. Class IV includes patients who are suffering from a life-threatening, but not necessarily terminal, condition that may or may not be related to the intended surgical procedure. Class V includes the moribund patient who has little chance of survival, as a person in shock with a burst abdominal aneurysm or a massive pulmonary embolus. The letter E is added to the roman numeral to indicate an emergency procedure, as a patient scheduled for an elective herniorrhaphy who becomes an emergency case when his hernia becomes an obstruction.

anesthesia screen, a metal inverted U-shaped frame that attaches to the sides of an operating table, 12 to 18 inches above a patient's upper chest. It is covered with a sheet to prevent contamination of an operative site on the chest or abdomen by airborne infection from the patient or the anesthetist and to provide a wide sterile field for the surgeon.

anesthesiologist, a physician trained in the administration of anesthetics and in the provision of respiratory and cardiovascular support during anesthetic procedures. Compare **nurse-anesthetist.**

anesthesiology (æn'əsfhi'ziol'əji), the branch of medicine that is concerned with the relief of pain and with the administration of medication to relieve pain during surgery. It is a specialty requiring competency in general medicine, a broad understanding of surgical procedures, a wide knowledge of clinical pharmacology, biochemistry, cardiology, and respiratory physiology. See also **anesthesiologist, nurse anesthetist.**

anesthetist (ənes'fhətist), 1. a person who administers anesthesia. 2. an anesthesiologist. See also **nurse anesthetist.**

anetoderma (æn'ɪtɒuder'mə), an idiopathic, patchy atrophy and looseness of skin for which there is no known effective treatment.

aneuploid (æn'yʊploid), **aneuploidic,** **1.** of or pertaining to an individual, organism, strain, or cell that has a chromosome number that is not an exact multiple of the normal, basic haploid number characteristic of the species. Variation occurs through individual chromosomes rather than an entire set so that there are more or less than the normal diploid number found in the somatic cell. **2.** such an individual, organism, strain, or cell. Compare **euploid.** See also **monosomy, trisomy.**

aneuploidy (æn'yʊploi'di), any variation in chromosome number that involves individual chromosomes rather than entire sets. There may be fewer chromosomes, as in Turner's syndrome, or more chromosomes, as in Down's syndrome. Such individuals have various abnormal physiological and morphological traits. Compare **euploidy.** See also **monosomy, trisomy.**

aneurysm (æn'yʊrɪz'əm), a localized dilatation of the wall of a blood vessel, usually caused by atherosclerosis and hypertension, or, less frequently, by trauma, infection, or a congenital weakness in the vessel wall. Aneurysms are most prominent and significant in the aorta but also occur in peripheral vessels and are fairly common in the lower extremities of older people, especially in the popliteal arteries. An arterial aneurysm may be a saccular distention affecting only part of the circumference of the vessel, it may be a fusiform or cylindroid dilatation of a section of the vessel, or it may be a longitudinal dissection between layers of the vascular wall. A sign of an arterial aneurysm is a pulsating swelling that produces a blowing murmur on auscultation with a stethoscope. An aneurysm may rupture, causing hemorrhage, or thrombi may form in the dilated pouch and give rise to emboli that may obstruct smaller vessels. Kinds of aneurysms include **aortic aneurysm, berry aneurysm, cerebral aneurysm, compound aneurysm, dissecting aneurysm, mycotic aneurysm, racemose aneurysm, Rasmussen's aneurysm, ventricular aneurysm.** – **aneurysmal,** *adj.*

aneurysm needle, a needle equipped with a handle, used to ligate aneurysms.

ANF, abbreviation for **American Nurses' Foundation.**

angi-. See **angio-.**

angiitis (æn'jiaɪ'tɪs), an inflammatory condition of a vessel, chiefly a blood or lymph vessel. A kind of angiitis is **consecutive angiitis.** See also **vasculitis.**

angina (ænjaɪ'nə, æn'jɪnə), **1.** a spasmodic, cramplike choking feeling. **2.** a term now used primarily to denote the paroxysmal thoracic pain and choking feeling caused by anoxia of the myocardium (angina pectoris). **3.** a descriptive feature of various diseases characterized by a feeling of choking, suffocation, or crushing pressure and pain. Kinds of angina are **intestinal angina, Ludwig's an-**gina, Prinzmetal's angina, streptococcal angina. – **anginal,** *adj.*

-angina, a combining form meaning 'severe ulceration, usually of the mouth or throat': *herpangina, juxtangina, monocytangina.*

angina decubitus, a condition characterized by periodic attacks of angina pectoris that occur when the person is lying down.

angina dyspeptica, a painful condition caused by gaseous distention of the stomach that mimics angina pectoris.

angina epiglottidea, a painful condition caused by inflammation of the epiglottis.

angina pectoris, a paroxysmal thoracic pain caused most often by myocardial anoxia owing to atherosclerosis of the coronary arteries. The pain radiates down the inner aspect of the left arm and is frequently accompanied by a feeling of suffocation and impending death. Attacks of angina pectoris are often related to exertion, emotional stress, and exposure to intense cold. The pain may be relieved by rest and vasodilation of the coronary arteries by medication, as with nitroglycerin.

angina sine dolore, a painless episode of coronary insufficiency.

angina trachealis. See **croup.**

angio-, angei-, angi-, a combining form meaning 'pertaining to a vessel, usually a blood vessel': *angioblastic, angiochondroma, angioglioma.*

angioblastic meningioma (æn'jiɒublæs'tɪk), a tumor of the blood vessels of the meninges covering the spinal cord or the brain.

angioblastoma (æn'jiɒublæstou'mə), *pl.* **angioblastomas, angioblastomata.** a tumor of blood vessels in the brain. Kinds of angioblastomas are **angioblastic meningioma, cerebellar angioblastoma.**

angiocardiogram (æn'jiɒukar'diəgræm'), a radiograph of the heart and the vessels of the heart. A radiopaque substance is injected forcibly into a vein in the

ANGIOCATHETER SECURING METHOD

antecubital space and x rays are taken as the radiopaque contrast medium passes through the heart and its vessels. Nausea and vomiting are common untoward reactions; urticaria, shortness of breath, or anaphylaxis may also occur. An antihistimine and oxygen are kept close at hand during the procedure. Angiocardiograms are performed by a member of the radiology department.

angiochondroma (æn'jiɔukondrou'mə), *pl.* **angiochondromas, angiochondromata.** a cartilaginous tumor characterized by an excessive formation of blood vessels.

angioedema (æn'jiɔuidi'mə). See **angioneurotic edema.**

angioendothelioma (æn'jiɔuen'douthi'liou'mə). See **hemangioendothelioma.**

angiofibroma (æn'jiɔufaibrou'mə), *pl.* **angiofibromas, angiofibromata.** an angioma containing fibrous tissue. Also called **fibroangioma.**

angioglioma (æn'jiɔugliou'mə), *pl.* **angiogliomas, angiogliomatas.** a highly vascular tumor composed of neuroglia.

angiography (æn'jiog'rəfi), the x-ray visualization of the internal anatomy of the heart and blood vessels following the intravascular introduction of radiopaque contrast medium. The procedure is used as a diagnostic aid in myocardial infarction, vascular occlusion, calcified atherosclerotic plaques, cerebrovascular accident, portal hypertension, renal neoplasms, renal artery stenosis as a causative factor in hypertension, pulmonary emboli, and congenital and acquired lesions of pulmonary vessels. The contrast medium may be injected into an artery or vein or introduced into a catheter inserted in a peripheral artery and threaded through the vessel to a visceral site. Since the iodine in the contrast medium may cause a marked allergic reaction in some patients, testing for hypersensitivity is indicated before the radiopaque substance is used. Following the procedure the patient is monitored for signs of bleeding, and bed rest for a number of hours is indicated. —**angiographic,** *adj.*

angiohemophilia (æn'jiɔuhi'məfi'liə, æn'jiɔuhem'əfi'liə). See **Von Willebrand's disease.**

angiokeratoma (æn'jiɔuker'ətou'mə), *pl.* **angiokeratomas, angiokeratomata.** a vascular, horny neoplasm on the skin, characterized by clumps of dilated blood vessels, clusters of warts, and thickening of the epidermis, especially the scrotum and the dorsal aspect of the fingers and toes.

angiokeratoma circumscriptum, a rare skin disorder characterized by discrete papules and nodules in small patches on the legs or on the trunk.

angiokeratoma corporis diffusum, an uncommon familial disease in which phospholipids are stored in many parts of the body, especially the blood vessels, causing vasomotor, urinary, and cutaneous disorders, and, in some cases, muscular abnormalities. Characteristic signs of the disease are edema, hypertension, and cardiomegaly,

especially enlargement of the left ventricle; diffuse nodularity of the skin; albumin, erythrocytes, leukocytes, and casts in the urine; and vacuoles in muscle bundles. Also called **Fabry's disease, Fabry's syndrome.**

angiolipoma (æn'jiɔulipou'mə), *pl.* **angiolipomas, angiolipomata.** a benign neoplasm containing blood vessels and tissue. Also called **lipoma cavernosum, telangiectatic lipoma.**

angioma (æn'jiou'mə), *pl.* **angiomas, angiomata.** any benign tumor made up primarily of blood vessels (hemangioma) or lymph vessels (lymphangioma). Most angiomas are congenital; some, like cavernous hemangiomas, disappear spontaneously.

-angioma, a combining form meaning a 'tumor composed chiefly of blood and lymph vessels': *fibroangioma, glomangioma, telangioma.*

angioma arteriale racemosum, a vascular neoplasm characterized initially by the intertwining of many small, newly formed, dilated blood vessels. Subsequently, normal blood vessels become affected.

angioma cavernosum. See **cavernous hemangioma.**

angioma cutis, a nevus composed of a network of dilated blood vessels.

angioma lymphaticum. See **lymphangioma.**

angioma serpiginosum, a cutaneous disease characterized by rings of tiny vascular points resembling grains of pepper. Also called **Hutchinson's disease.**

angiomatosis (æn'jioumətou'sis), a condition characterized by the presence of numerous vascular tumors. A kind of angiomatosis is **hemorrhagic familial angiomatosis.**

angiomyoma, *pl.* **angiomyomas, angiomyomata.** a tumor composed of vascular and muscular tissue elements.

angiomyoneuroma (æn'jioumai'ounurou'mə), *pl.* **angiomyoneuromas, angiomyoneuromata.** See **glomangioma.**

angiomyosarcoma (æn'jioumai'ousarkou'mə), *pl.* **angiomyosarcomas, angiomyosarcomata.** a tumor containing vascular, muscular, and connective tissue elements.

angioneuroma (æn'jiounurou'mə), *pl.* **angioneuromas, angioneuromata.** See **glomangioma.**

angioneurotic anuria, an abnormal condition characterized by an almost complete absence of urination caused by destruction of tissue in the renal cortex. See also **anuria.**

angioneurotic edema (æn'jiounurot'ik), an acute, painless, dermal, subcutaneous, or submucosal swelling of short duration involving the face, neck, lips, larynx, hands, feet, genitalia, or viscera. It may result from food or drug allergy, infection, or emotional stress or it may be hereditary. Treatment depends upon the cause. For severe forms, subcutaneous injections of epinephrine, intubation, or tracheotomy may be necessary to prevent respiratory obstruction. Prevention depends on the identification and avoidance of etiologic factors. Also called **angioedema.** See also **anaphylaxis, hives, serum sickness, urticaria.**

angiosarcoma (æn′jiousarkou′mə), a rare, malignant tumor consisting of endothelial and fibroblastic tissue. Also called **hemangiosarcoma.** Compare **angioma.**

angiotensin (æn′jiouten′sın), a polypeptide occurring in the blood causing vasoconstriction, increased blood pressure, and the release of aldosterone from the adrenal cortex. Angiotensin is formed by the action of renin on angiotensinogen, an alpha-2-globulin that is produced in the liver and constantly circulates in the blood. Renin, elaborated by juxtaglomerular cells in the kidney in response to decreased blood volume and serum sodium, acts as an enzyme in the conversion of angiotensinogen to angiotensin I, which is rapidly hydrolyzed to form the active compound angiotensin II. The vasoconstrictive action of angiotensin II decreases the glomerular filtration rate and the concomitant action of aldosterone promotes sodium retention, with the result that blood volume and sodium reabsorption increase. Plasma angiotensin increases during the luteal phase of the menstrual cycle and is probably responsible for an elevated level of aldosterone during that period. Angiotensin is inactivated by peptidases, called angiotensinases, in plasma and tissues.

angle, 1. the space or the shape formed at the intersection of two lines, planes, or borders. The divergence of the lines, planes, or borders may be measured in degrees of a circle. 2. (in anatomy and physiology) the geometric relationships between the surfaces of body structures and the positions affected by movement.

angstrom (æŋ′strəm), **angstrom unit,** a unit of measure of length equal to 0.1 millimicron (1/10,000,000 meter).

angular movement, one of the four basic kinds of movement allowed by the various joints of the skeleton in which the angle between two adjoining bones is decreased, as in flexion, or increased, as in extension. Compare **circumduction, gliding, rotation.**

angular vein, one of a pair of veins of the face, formed by the junction of the frontal and the supraorbital veins. At the root of the nose each angular vein receives the flow of venous blood from the infraorbital, the superior palpebral, the inferior palpebral, and the external nasal veins becoming the first part of one of the two facial veins.

angulated fracture, a fracture in which the fragments of bone are angulated.

anhedonia (æn′hidou′niə), the inability to feel pleasure or happiness from experiences that are ordinarily pleasurable. Compare **analgesia.** – **anhedonic,** *adj.*

anhidrosis (æn′hıdrou′sıs, æn′haidrou′sıs), an abnormal condition characterized by inadequate perspiration. – **anhidrotic,** *adj.*

anhidrotic (æn′hıdrot′ık, æn′haidrot′ık), 1. of or pertaining to anhidrosis. 2. an agent that reduces or suppresses sweating.

Anhydron, a trade name for a diuretic and antihypertensive (cyclothiazide).

-an, -ian, a combining form meaning 'belonging to, characteristic of, similar to': *amphibian, protozoan salpingian.*

anicteric hepatitis (æn′ıkter′ık), a mild form of hepatitis in which there is no jaundice (icterus), usually seen in infants and young children. Symptoms include anorexia, gastrointestinal disturbances, and slight fever. SGOT and SGPT are elevated. The infection may be mistaken for flu or go unnoticed. Compare **hepatitis.** See also **icterus, jaundice.**

anidean (ænıd′iən), **anidian, anidous** (æn′ıdəs), formless; shapeless; denoting an undifferentiated mass, as an anideus.

anideus (ænıd′iəs), an anomalous, rudimentary conceptus consisting of a simple rounded mass with little indication of the body parts. A kind of anideus is **embryonic anideus.** Also called **fetus anideus.**

aniline (æn′ılin), an oily, colorless poisonous liquid with a strong odor and burning taste, formerly extracted from the indigo plant and now made synthetically using nitrobenzene in the manufacture of aniline dyes. Industrial workers exposed to aniline are at risk of developing methemoglobinemia and bone marrow depression. Also called **amidobenzene, aminobenzene.**

anilinparasulfonic acid (æn′ılınpær′əsəlfon′ık). See **sulfanilic acid.**

anima (æn′ımə), 1. the soul or life. 2. the active ingredient in a drug. 3. (in Jungian psychology) a person's true, inner, unconscious being or personality, as distinguished from overt personality, or persona. 4. (in analytic psychology) the female component of the male personality. Compare **animus.**

animal pole, the active, formative part of the ovum protoplasm that contains the nucleus and bulk of the cytoplasm and where the polar bodies form. In mammals it is also the site where the inner cell mass gives rise to the ectoderm. Also called **germinal pole.** Compare **vegetal pole.**

animal starch. See **glycogen.**

animus (æn′ıməs), 1. the active or rational soul; the animating principle of life. 2. the male component of the female personality. 3. (in psychiatry) a deep-seated antagonism that is usually controlled but may erupt with virulence under stress. Compare **anima.**

anion (æn′ai′ən), 1. a negatively charged ion which is attracted to the positive electrode (anode) in electrolysis. 2. a negatively charged atom, molecule, or radical. Compare **cation.**

anion exchange resin, any one of the simple organic polymers with high molecular weights that exchange anions with other ions in solution. Anion exchange resins are used as antacids in treating ulcers. Compare **cation exchange resin.**

anion gap, the difference between the concentrations of serum cations and anions, determined by measuring the concentrations of sodium cations and chloride and bicarbonate anions. It is helpful in the diagnosis and treatment of acidosis, and it is estimated by subtracting the sum of sodium and bicarbonate concentrations in the plasma from that of sodium. It is normally about 8 to 14 mEq/liter and represents the negative charges contributed to plasma by unmeasured ions or ions other than those of chloride and bicarbonate, mainly phosphate, sulfate, organic acids, and plasma proteins. Anions other than chloride and bicarbonate normally constitute about 12 mEq/liter of the total anion concentration in plasma. Acidosis can develop with or without an associated anion increase. An increase in the anion gap often suggests diabetic ketoacidosis, drug poisoning, renal failure, or lactic acidosis and usually warrants further laboratory tests.

anise (æn′ɪs), the fruit of the *Pimpinella anisum* plant. Extract of anise is used in the preparation of carminatives and expectorants.

aniseikonia (æn′aisaikou′niə), an abnormal ocular condition in which each eye perceives the same image as being of a different size.

aniso-, a combining form meaning 'unequal or dissimilar': *anisochromia, anisodont, anisognathous.*

anisocytosis (ænai′sousaitou′sɪs), an abnormal condition of the blood characterized by red blood cells of variable and abnormal size. Compare **poikilocytosis.** See also **macrocytosis, microcytosis.**

anisogamete, a gamete that differs considerably in size and structure from the one with which it unites, as the macrogamete and microgamete of certain sporozoa. Compare **heterogamete, isogamete.** – **anisogametic,** *adj.*

anisogamy, sexual conjugation of gametes that are of unequal size and structure, as in certain thallophytes and sporozoa. Compare **heterogamy, isogamy.** – **anisogamous,** *adj.*

anisokaryosis (ænai′soukær′iou′sɪs), significant variation in the size of the nucleus of cells of the same general type. – **anisokaryotic,** *adj.*

anisometropia (ænai′səmətrou′piə), an abnormal ocular condition characterized by a difference in the refractive powers of the eyes.

anisopoikilocytosis (ænai′soupoi′kilousaitou′sɪs), an abnormal condition of the blood characterized by red blood cells of variable and abnormal size and shape. See also **anisocytosis, erythrocyte, morphology, poikilocytosis.**

ankle, 1. the joint of the tibia, the talus, and the malleoli. 2. the part of the leg where this joint is located.

ankle bandage, a figure-of-eight bandage looped under the sole of the foot and around the ankle. The heel may be covered or left exposed, although covering is preferable as it prevents "window edema."

ankle bone. See **talus.**

ankle reflex. See **Achilles tendon reflex.**

ankylo-. See **ancylo-.**

ankylosing spondylitis (ærɳ′kilou′sɪɳ), a chronic inflammatory disease of unknown etiology, first affecting the spine and adjacent structures, and commonly progressing to eventual fusion (ankylosis) of the involved joints. In extreme cases the patient develops a forward flexion of the spine, called a "poker spine" or "bamboo spine." The disease affects primarily males under the age of 30, and generally burns itself out after a course of 20 years. There is a strong hereditary tendency. In addition to the spine, the joints of the hip, shoulder, neck, ribs, and jaw are often involved. When the costovertebral joints are involved, the patient may have difficulty in expanding the rib cage while breathing. Ankylosing spondylitis is a systemic disease, often affecting the eyes and the heart. Many patients with the disease also have inflammatory bowel disease. The aim of treatment is to reduce pain and inflammation in the involved joints, usually with nonsteroidal anti-inflammatory drugs. Physical therapy aids in keeping the spine as erect as possible to prevent flexion contractures. In advanced cases surgery may be performed to straighten a badly deformed spine. Compare **rheumatoid arthritis.** See also **ankylosis, Marie-Strumpell disease.**

ankylosis (ærɳ′kilou′sɪs), 1. fixation of a joint, often in an abnormal position, usually resulting from destruction of articular cartilage and subchondral bone, as occurs in rheumatoid arthritis. 2. Also called **arthrodesis, fusion.** surgically induced fixation of a joint to relieve pain or provide support.

anlage, (in embryology) the undifferentialed layer of cells from which a particular organ, tissue, or structure develops; primordium rudiment. See also **blastema.**

ANLL. abbreviation for **acute nonlymphocytic leukemia.** See **acute myelocytic leukemia.**

Annals, *Informal. Annals of Internal Medicine,* a professional journal in internal medicine.

annular (æn′yulər), describing a ring-shaped lesion surrounding a clear, normal, unaffected disk of skin.

annular ligament, a ligament that encircles the head of the radius and holds it in the radial notch of the ulna. Distal to the notch, the annular ligament forms a complete fibrous ring.

anodmia (ænod′miə). See **anosmia.** – **anodmatic, anodmic,** *adj.*

anodontia (æn′oudon′chə), a congenital defect in which some or all of the teeth are missing.

anodyne (æn′ədɑin), a drug that relieves or lessens pain. Compare **analgesic.**

anomalo-, a combining form meaning 'uneven or irregular': *anomalopia, anomaloscope, anomalotrophy.*

anomaly (ənom'əli), **1.** deviation from what is regarded as normal. **2.** congenital malformation, as the absence of a limb or the presence of an extra finger. — **anomalous,** *adj.*

anomia (ənou'miə), a form of aphasia characterized by the inability to name objects, caused by a lesion in the temporal lobe of the brain.

anomie, anomy (æn'əmi), a state of apathy, alienation, anxiety, personal disorientation, and distress, resulting from the loss of social norms and goals previously valued.

anoopsia (æn'ouop'siə), a strabismus in which one or both eyes are deviated upward.

Anopheles (ənof'əliz'), a genus of mosquito, many species of which transmit malaria-causing parasites to man. See also **malaria.**

anopia (ænou'piə), blindness resulting from a defect in or the absence of one or both eyes.

-anopia, -anopsia, 1. a combining form meaning '(condition involving) nonuse or arrested development of the eye': *hemianopia, hesperanopia, duadrantopia.* **2.** a combining form meaning '(condition of) defective color vision': *cyanopia, deuteranopia, tritanopia.* Also **-anopsia.**

anorchia, anorchism, congenital absence of one or both testes.

anorectal (æn'ourek'təl, ei'nourek'təl), of or pertaining to the anal and rectal portions of the large intestine.

anorectic (æn'ərek'tɪk), **1.** of or pertaining to anorexia. **2.** lacking appetite. **3.** causing a loss of appetite, as anorexiant drug. — **anorectous, anorexiant,** *adj.*

anorexia (æn'ərek'siə), lack or loss of appetite, resulting in the inability to eat. The condition may result from poorly prepared or unattractive food or surroundings, unfavorable company, or various psychological causes. Compare **pseudoanorexia.** See also **anorexia nervosa.** — **anorexic,** *adj.*

anorexia nervosa (nərvou'sə), a psychoneurotic disorder characterized by a prolonged refusal to eat, resulting in emaciation, amenorrhea, emotional disturbance concerning body image, and an abnormal fear of becoming obese. The condition is seen primarily in adolescents, predominantly in girls, and is usually associated with emotional stress or conflict, such as anxiety, irritation, anger, and fear, which may accompany a major change in the person's life. Treatment consists of measures to improve nourishment, followed by therapy to overcome the underlying emotional conflicts.

anosmia (ænoz'miə), loss or impairment of the sense of smell, commonly occurring as a temporary condition resulting from a head cold or respiratory infection or when intranasal swelling or other obstruction prevents odors from reaching the olfactory region. It becomes a permanent condition when the olfactory neuroepithelium or any part of the olfactory nerve is destroyed as a result of intracranial trauma, neoplasms, or disease, as atrophic rhinitis or the chronic rhinitis associated with the granulomatous diseases. In some instances, the condition may be caused by psychological factors, as a phobia or fear associated with a particular smell. Kinds of anosmia are **anosmia gustatoria, preferential anosmia.** Also called **anodmia, anosphrasia, olfactory anesthesia.** — **anosmatic, anosmic,** *adj.*

anosmia gustatoria, the inability to smell foods.

anosognosia (æn'əsognou'Źhə), an abnormal condition characterized by a real or feigned inability to perceive a defect, especially paralysis, on one side of the body, possibly attributable to a lesion in the right parietal lobe of the brain.

anosphrasia (æn'əsfrei'Źhə), **anosphresia** (æn'əsfri'Źhə). See **anosmia.**

ANOVA, abbreviation for **analysis of variance.**

anovulation (æn'ovyʊlei'Śhən), failure of the ovaries to produce, mature, or release eggs, owing to ovarian immaturity or postmaturity; to altered ovarian function, as in pregnancy and lactation; to primary ovarian dysfunction, as in ovarian dysgenesis; or to disturbance of the interaction of the hypothalamus, pituitary gland, and ovary, caused by stress or disease. Hormonal contraceptives prevent conception by suppressing ovulation. Anovulation may be an adverse side effect of other medications prescribed in the treatment of other disorders. — **anovulatory** (ænov'yʊlətor'i), *adj.*

anoxia (ænok'siə), an abnormal condition characterized by a relative or a total lack of oxygen. Anoxia may be local or systemic and may be the result of an inadequate supply of oxygen to the respiratory system or of an inability of the blood to carry oxygen to the tissues, as in anemic anoxia, or of the tissues to absorb the oxygen from the circulation, as in histiocytic anoxia. Kinds of anoxia include **cerebral anoxia, stagnant anoxia.** — **anoxic,** *adj.*

-ans, a combining form meaning '-ing': *aberrans, penetrans, proliferans.*

ansa (æn'sə), *pl.* **ansae.** (in anatomy) a looplike structure resembling a curved handle of a vase.

ansa cervicalis (sər'vɪkæl'ɪs), one of three loops of nerves in the cervical plexus, branches of which innervate the infrahyoid muscles. It has a superior root, which connects with the hypoglossal nerve and contains fibers of the first and the second cervical nerves, and an inferior root, which connects with the second and the third cervical nerves. Also called **ansa hypoglossi.**

ansa hypoglossi. See **ansa cervicalis.**

answer, (in law) the response of a defendant to the complaint of a plaintiff. The answer contains a denial of the plaintiff's allegations and may also contain an affirmative defense or a counterclaim. It is the principal pleading on the part of the defense and is prepared in writing, usually by the defense attorney, and submitted to the court.

ant-. See **anti-.**

Antabuse, a trade name for an alcohol deterrent (disulfiram).

antacid, 1. opposing acidity. 2. a drug or dietary substance that buffers, neutralizes, or absorbs hydrochloric acid in the stomach. Most antacids are not absorbed systemically. Antacids containing aluminum and calcium are constipating; those containing magnesium have a laxative effect.

antagonist, 1. one who contends with or is opposed to another. 2. (in physiology) any agent, such as a drug or muscle, that exerts an opposite action to that of another. Kinds of antagonists include **associated antagonist, competitive antagonist, direct antagonist.** Compare **agonist.** 3. (in dentistry) a tooth in the upper jaw that articulates during mastication or occlusion with a tooth in the lower jaw. — **antagonistic,** *adj.,* **antagonize,** *v.*

antagonist drug, a drug that opposes the action of another drug by neutralization, by receptor-site blockade, or by other means. See also **narcotic antagonist.**

ante-, a combining form meaning 'before in time or in place': *anteflexion, antenatal, antepartal.*

anteflexion, an abnormal position of an organ in which the organ is tilted acutely forward, folded over on itself.

antenatal. See **prenatal.**

antenatal diagnosis. See **prenatal diagnosis.**

Antepar (æn'tɪpar), a trade name for an anthelmintic (piperazine citrate).

antepartal care, care of a pregnant woman during the time in the maternity cycle that begins with conception and ends with the onset of labor. See also **intrapartal care, prenatal nutrition, postpartal care.**

■ METHOD: A medical, surgical, gynecologic, obstetric, social, and family history is taken with particular emphasis

Commonly used antacids

Trade name	Drug composition	Comments
Maalox	Magnesium and aluminum hydroxide	Preferred antacid Good buffering effect Good taste Nonconstipating Low sodium content Can cause hypermagnesemia in patients with renal failure
Maalox Plus	Magnesium and aluminum hydroxide Simethicone	Same as above Antiflatus
Mylanta	Magnesium and aluminum hydroxide Simethicone	Same as Maalox Plus
Amphojel	Aluminum hydroxide gel	Constipating Can interfere with absorption of anticholinergic drugs Contains sodium Decreases absorption of phosphate Good antacid effect Give with water so that medication reaches stomach Can be given by continuous drip (1 part Amphojel to 2 or 3 parts water)
Gelusil	Magnesium trisilicate Magnesium and aluminum hydroxide	Slower buffering effect Gelatin effect in stomach to coat and protect the ulcer Nonconstipating
Riopan	Magaldrate (chemical combination of magnesium and aluminum hydroxide)	Rapid antacid action High acid-buffering effect No acid rebound Nonconstipating Low sodium content Can cause hypermagnesemia in patients with renal failure
Marblen	Magnesium and calcium carbonate Aluminum hydroxide Magnesium trisilicate	Neutralizes more acid than other antacids Nonconstipating Low sodium content
Alka-2	Calcium carbonate	Rapid neutralization of acid Constipating May cause hypercalcemia May cause acid rebound Not suitable for long-term therapy

on the discovery of familial or transmissable diseases. A physical examination is performed, including observation and evaluation of the skin, thyroid gland, heart, breasts, abdomen, lungs, and pelvic organs. The vaginal part of the pelvic examination includes a pap smear and tests for *Neisseria gonorrhea, Candida albicans,* and *Trichomonas vaginalis.* Blood pressure, weight, urinalysis for sugar and protein, measurement of the hAeight of the fundus and auscultation of the fetal heart are routinely performed at monthly intervals or even more frequently. Laboratory tests are performed to determine blood type and Rh factor, hematocrit, and hemoglobin. A serologic test for syphilis is performed and various diagnostic studies may be done to discover viral infections. Amniocentesis may be performed if certain fetal abnormalities are suspected.

■ NURSING CONSIDERATIONS: The parents are encouraged to discuss their concerns about the pregnancy, to understand the physiological processes, to report decreased fetal activity, to take a preparation-for-labor class, and to plan for the infant's needs.

■ OUTCOME CRITERIA: The basic goal of prenatal care is a healthy mother, who is ready emotionally and physically to give birth to a healthy baby. Increasingly, that goal has come to include the mother's and father's satisfaction with the birth itself and a minimal use of obstetric intervention. Information, emotional support, good nutrition, and careful observation help most mothers to achieve healthy, happy intrapartal and postpartal periods of the maternity cycle.

anterior, 1. the front of a structure. 2. of or pertaining to a surface or part situated toward the front or facing forward. Also called **ventral.** Compare **posterior.**

anterior asynclitism. See **asynclitism.**

anterior atlantoaxial ligament, one of five ligaments connecting the atlas to the axis. It is fixed to the inferior border of the anterior arch of the atlas and to the ventral surface of the body of the axis. Compare **posterior atlantoaxial ligament.**

anterior atlanto-occipital membrane, one of two broad, densely woven fibrous sheets that form part of the atlanto-occipital joint between the atlas and the occipital bone. It is continuous with two articular capsules and strengthened ventrally by a strong, rounded cord connecting the base of the occipital bone to the anterior arch of the atlas. Also called **anterior atlanto-occipital ligament.** Compare **posterior atlanto-occipital membrane.**

anterior cardiac vein, one of several small vessels that return deoxygenated blood from the ventral portion of the myocardium of the right ventricle to the right atrium. In some individuals, the right marginal vein opens into the right atrium, and, in those instances, is regarded as one of the anterior cardiac veins. See also **coronary sinus.**

anterior common ligament. See **anterior longitudinal ligament.**

anterior crural nerve. See **femoral nerve.**

anterior cutaneous nerve, one of a pair of cutaneous branches of the cervical plexus. It arises from the second and the third cervical nerves, bends around the middle of the sternocleidomastoideus, crosses the muscle obliquely, passes beneath the platysma, and divides into the ascending and the descending branches. The ascending branches pass upward, pierce the platysma, and are distributed to the cranial, the ventral, and the lateral parts of the neck. The descending branches are distributed to the skin of the ventral and the lateral parts of the neck as far down as the sternum.

anterior fontanel. See **fontanel.**

anterior longitudinal ligament, the broad, strong ligament attached to the ventral surfaces of the vertebral bodies. It extends from the occipital bone and the anterior tubercle of the atlas to the sacrum. Also called **anterior common ligament.** Compare **posterior longitudinal ligament.**

anterior mediastinal node, a node in one of the three groups of thoracic visceral nodes of the lymphatic system that drains lymph from the nodes of the thymus, pericardium, and sternum. They are located ventral to the brachiocephalic veins and to the arterial trunks from the aortic arch. The efferents of the nodes form the right and the left bronchomediastinal trunks. Compare **posterior mediastinal node.** See also **lymph, lymphatic system, lymph node.**

anterior mediastinum, a caudal portion of the mediastinum in the middle of the thorax, bounded ventrally by the body of the sternum and parts of the fourth through the seventh ribs and dorsally by the parietal pericardium, extending downward as far as the diaphragm. It contains a few lymph nodes and a few vessels and a thin layer of subserous fascia, which is separated from the endothoracic fascia by a fascial cleft. Compare **middle mediastinum, posterior mediastinum, superior mediastinum.**

anterior nares, the ends of the nostrils that open anteriorly into the nasal cavity and allow the inhalation and the exhalation of air. Each is an oval opening that measures about 1.5 cm anterioposteriorly and about one cm in diameter. The anterior nares connect with the nasal fossae. Also called **nostrils.** Compare **posterior nares.**

anterior neuropore, the opening of the embryonic neural tube in the anterior portion of the forebrain. It closes at the 20 somite stage, which indicates the end of horizon XI in the numerical anatomical charting of human embryonic development. Compare **posterior neuropore.** See also **horizon.**

anterior pituitary. See **adenohypophysis.**

anterior tibial artery, one of the two divisions of the popliteal artery, arising in back of the knee, dividing into six branches, and supplying various muscles of the leg and foot. Its six branches are the posterior tibial recurrent, fibular, anterior tibial recurrent, muscular, anterior medial malleolar, and anterior lateral malleolar. Compare **posterior tibial artery.**

anterior tibial node, one of the small lymph glands of the lower limb, lying on the interosseous membrane near the proximal portion of the anterior tibial vessels. Compare **inguinal node, popliteal node.**

anterograde amnesia, the inability to recall events of long ago with normal recall of recent events. Compare **anterograde memory.**

anterograde memory, the ability to recall events of long ago but not those of recent occurrence. Compare **anterograde amnesia.** Also called **senile memory.**

anteroposterior (æn′tɪroupostir′ɪər), from the front to the back of the body, commonly associated with the direction of the roentgenographic beam.

anteversion, an abnormal position of an organ in which the organ is tilted forward on its axis, away from the midline.

anthelmintic (ænt′helmɪn′tɪk), **1.** of or pertaining to a substance that destroys or prevents the development of parasitic worms, as filariae, flukes, hookworms, pinworms, roundworms, schistosomes, tapeworms, trichinae, and whipworms. **2.** an anthelmintic drug. An anthelmintic may interfere with the parasites' carbohydrate metabolism, inhibit their respiratory enzymes, block their neuromuscular action, or render them susceptible to destruction by the host's macrophages. Among a number of drugs used in treating specific helmintic infections are piperazine, pyrantel pamoate, pyrvinium pamoate, mebandazole, niclosamide, hexylresorcinol, diethylcarbamazine, and theabendazole.

-anthema, a combining form meaning a '(specified) type of eruption, rash': *eisanthema, enanthema, exanthema.*

anthraco-, a combining form meaning 'pertaining to a carbuncle or to carbon dioxide': *anthracoid, anthraconecrosis, anthracosis.*

anthracosis (æn′fhrəkou′sɪs), a chronic lung disease occurring in coal miners, characterized by the deposit of coal dust in the lungs and the formation of black nodules on the bronchioles and resulting in focal emphysema. The condition is aggravated by cigarette smoking. There is no specific treatment; most cases are asymptomatic and the progress of the condition may be halted by the prevention of further exposure to coal dust. Also called **black lung, coalworker's pneumoconiosis, miner's pneumoconiosis.** See also **inorganic dust.**

anthracosis linguae. See **parasitic glossitis.**

anthralin (æn′fhrəlɪn), a topical antipsoriatic.

■ INDICATIONS: It is prescribed in the treatment of psoriasis and chronic dermatitis.

■ CONTRAINDICATIONS: Renal dysfunction or known hypersensitivity to this drug prohibits its use. It is not applied to acute psoriatic eruptions or near the eyes.

■ ADVERSE EFFECTS: The most serious adverse reaction is nephrotoxicity resulting from systemic absorption.

anthralinic acid. See **aminobenzoic acid.**

anthrax (æn′fhræks), a disease affecting primarily farm animals (cattle, goats, pigs, sheep, and horses), caused by the bacterium *Bacillus anthracis.* Anthrax in animals is usually fatal. Humans most often acquire it when a break in the skin comes into direct contact with infected animals and their hides, but they may also contract a pulmonary form of anthrax by inhaling the spores of the bacterium. The cutaneous form begins with a reddish-brown lesion which ulcerates and then forms a dark scab. The signs and symptoms that follow include internal hemorrhage, muscle pain, headache, fever, nausea, and vomiting. The pulmonary form, called woolsorter's disease, is often fatal unless treated early. Treatment for both forms is penicillin G or tetracycline. A vaccine is available for veterinarians and for others for whom anthrax is an occupational hazard. Also called **malignant pustule.**

anthropo-, a combining form meaning 'pertaining to man or to a human being': *anthropocentric, anthropocracy, anthropoid.*

anthropoid pelvis, a type of pelvis in which the inlet is oval; the anteroposterior diameter is much greater than the transverse and, owing to the posterior inclination of the sacrum, the posterior portion of the space in the true pelvis is much greater than the anterior portion. The side walls are somewhat convergent and the ischial spines are prominent. If the pelvis is large, vaginal delivery is not compromised, but the occiput posterior position of the fetus is favored. This type of pelvis is present in 40 per cent of nonwhite women and in more than 25 per cent of white women.

anti-, ant-, a combining form meaning 'against or over against': *antialexin, antibiosis, antichlorotic.*

antiadrenergic (æn′tɪæd′rənər′jɪk), **1.** of or pertaining to the blocking of the effects of impulses transmitted by the adrenergic postganglionic fibers of the sympathetic nervous system. **2.** an antiadrenergic agent. Drugs that block the response to norepinephrine by alpha-adrenergic receptors reduce the tone of smooth muscle in peripheral blood vessels, causing increased peripheral circulation and decreased blood pressure. Alpha-blocking agents include ergotamine derivatives, used in treating migraine; phenoxybenzamine and phentolamine, administered for Raynaud's disease, pheochromocytoma, and diabetic gangrene; and tolazoline hydrochloride, administered to patients with spastic vascular disease. Agents that block beta-adrenergic receptors decrease the rate and force of heart contractions among other effects. Propranolol and its congeners are beta-blocking agents. Also called **sympatholytic.** Compare **adrenergic.**

antiadrenergic drug. See **antiadrenergic.**

antianemic, 1. of or pertaining to a substance or procedure that counteracts or prevents a deficiency of erythrocytes. 2. an agent used to treat or to prevent anemia. Whole blood is transfused in the treatment of anemia resulting from acute blood loss, and packed red cells are usually administered when the deficiency is caused by chronic blood loss. Transfusions of blood components are used in the treatment of aplastic anemia. Iron-deficiency anemia, the most common form of anemia, is usually treated with oral preparations of ferrous sulfate, fumerate, or gluconate, but a parenteral preparation is indicated for people who are unable to absorb iron from the gastrointestinal tract or for those who develop nausea and diarrhea when taking iron orally. Cyanocobalamin is administered parenterally in the treatment of pernicious anemia. Folic acid is prescribed to correct a deficiency of that vitamin in the anemias accompanying general malnutrition or alcoholic cirrhosis and to treat the common anemia of infants who are on a milk diet exclusively. A combination of folic acid and vitamin B_{12} is prescribed for people who are anemic owing to an inadequate dietary intake of both vitamins.

antiantibody, an immunoglobulin formed as the result of the administration of an antibody that acts as an immunogen. The antiantibody then interacts with the antibody. See also **antibody, immune globulin.**

antianxiety agent. See **sedative-hypnotic.**

antiarrhythmic, 1. of or pertaining to a procedure or substance that prevents, alleviates, or corrects an abnormal cardiac rhythm. 2. an agent used to treat a cardiac arrhythmia. A defibrillator that delivers a precordial electric shock is often used to restore a normal rhythm to rapid, irregular atrial or ventricular contractions. A pacemaker may be implanted in a patient with an extremely slow heart rate or other arrhythmia. The electrode catheter of an external pacemaker may be threaded through a vein to the heart in cases of ventricular standstill or complete heart block. Two of the major antiarrhythmic drugs are lidocaine, which increases the threshhold of electrical stimulation in the ventricles during diastole, and a combination of disopyramide, procainamide, and quinidine, which decrease the excitability of the myocardium and prolong the refractory period. The beta-adrenergic blocking agent propranolol may be used in treating arrhythmias. Isoproterenol is indicated for complete heart block and ventricular arrhythmias requiring an increased force of cardiac contractions to establish a normal rhythm. Atropine may be used in the treatment of bradycardia, a sedative in the treatment of tachycardia, and digitalis in the treatment of atrial fibrillation. See also **arrhythmia.**

antibacterial (æn′tıbæktir′iəl), 1. of or pertaining to a substance that kills bacteria or inhibits their growth or replication. 2. an antibacterial agent. Antibiotics synthesized chemically or derived from various microorganisms exert their bactericidal or bacteriostatic effect by interfering with the production of the bacterial cell wall, by interfering with protein synthesis, nucleic acid synthesis, or cell membrane integrity, or by inhibiting critical biosynthetic pathways in the bacteria.

antiberiberi factor. See **thiamine.**

antibiotic, 1. of or pertaining to the ability to destroy or interfere with the development of a living organism. 2. an antimicrobial agent, derived from cultures of a microorganism or produced semisynthetically, used to treat infections. The penicillins, derived from species of the fungus *Penicillium* or manufactured semisynthetically, consist of a thiazolidine ring fused to a beta-lactam ring connected to side chains; these agents exert their action by inhibiting mucopeptide synthesis in bacterial cell walls during multiplication of the organisms. Penicillin G and V are widely used in treating many gram-positive coccal infections but are inactivated by the enzyme penicillinase produced by strains of staphylococci; cloxacillin, dicloxacillin, methicillin, nafcillin, and oxacillin are penicillinase-resistant penicillins. Broad-spectrum penicillins effective against gram-negative organisms are ampicillin, carbenicillin, and hetacillin. Hypersensitivity reactions, as rash, fever, bronchospasm, vasculitis, and anaphylaxis are relatively common side effects of penicillin therapy. Aminoglycoside antibiotics, composed of amino sugars in glycoside linkage, interfere with the synthesis of bacterial proteins and are used primarily for the treatment of infections caused by gram-negative organisms. The aminoglycosides include gentamicin derived from *Micromonospora,* semisynthetic amikacin, kanamycin, neomycin, streptomycin, and tobramycin. These agents commonly cause nephrotoxic and ototoxic reactions as well as gastrointestinal disturbances. Macrolide antibiotics, consisting of a large lactone ring and deoxamino sugar, interfere in protein synthesis of susceptible bacteria during multiplication without affecting nucleic acid synthesis. Oleandomycin, which is added to feed to improve the growth of poultry and swine, and broad-spectrum erythromycin, used to treat various gram-positive and gram-negative infections and intestinal amebiasis, are macrolides derived from species of *Streptomyces.* Erythromycin may cause mild allergic reactions and gastrointestinal discomfort, but nausea, vomiting, and diarrhea occur infrequently with the usual oral dose. Polypeptide antibiotics derived from species of Streptomyces or certain soil bacilli vary in their spectra; most of these agents are nephrotoxic and ototoxic. Bacitracin and vancomycin are polypeptides used to treat severe staphylococcal infections; capreomycin and vancomycin are antituberculosis agents; and gramicidin is included in ointments for topical infections. Among polypeptide antibiotics effective against gram-negative organisms, colistin and neomycin are administered for diarrhea caused by enteropathogenic *Escherichia coli;*

polymixin B, although neurotoxic, is the drug of choice for acute *Pseudomonas* infections. Antifungals, including amphotericin B and nystatin, apparently bind to sterols in fungus cell membranes and change their permeability; griseofulvin grossly distorts terminal hyphae of fungi. Amphotericin B is effective against many kinds of fungi; it may cause fever, vomiting, diarrhea, generalized pains, anemia, renal dysfunction, and other adverse effects when administered intravenously. Oral griseofulvin is used to treat various fungal infections of the skin and nails and may cause hypersensitivity reactions, gastrointestinal disturbances, fatigue, and insomnia. Nystatin is applied locally for the treatment of oral and vaginal candidiasis; candicidin is also used for vaginal candidiasis. The tetracyclines, including the prototype derived from *Streptomyces,* chlortetracycline, demeclocycline, doxycycline, minocycline, and oxytetracycline, are active against a wide range of gram-positive and gram-negative organisms and some rickettsiae. Antibiotics in this group are primarily bacteriostatic and are thought to exert their effect by inhibiting protein synthesis in the organisms. Tetracycline therapy may cause gastrointestinal irritation, photosensitivity, renal toxicity, and hepatic toxicity, and administration of a drug of this group during the last half of pregnancy, during infancy, or before the age of eight may result in permanent discoloration of the teeth. The cephalosporins, derived from the soil fungus *Cephalosporium* or produced semisynthetically, inhibit bacterial cell wall synthesis, resist the action of penicillinase and are used in treating infections of the respiratory tract, urinary tract, middle ear, and bones, as well as septicemia caused by a wide range of gram-positive and gram-negative organisms. The group includes cefadroxil, cefamandole, cefazolin, cephalexin, cephaloglycin, cephaloridine, cephalothin, cephapirin, and cephradine. Treatment with a cephalosporin may cause nausea, vomiting, diarrhea, enterocolitis, or an allergic reaction, as rash, angioedema, or exfoliative dermatitis; use of antibiotics in this group is contraindicated in patients who have shown hypersensitivity to a penicillin. Chloramphenicol, a broad-spectrum antibiotic initially derived from *Streptomyces venezuelae,* inhibits protein synthesis in bacteria by interfering with the transfer of activated amino acids from soluble RNA to ribosomes. Since the drug may cause life-threatening blood dyscrasias, its use is reserved for the treatment of acute typhoid fever, serious gram-negative infections (including *Hemophilus influenzae* meningitis,) and rickettsial diseases.

antibiotic sensitivity tests, a laboratory method for determining the susceptibility of bacterial infections to therapy with antibiotics. After the infecting organism has been recovered from a clinical specimen, it is cultured and tested against several antibiotic drugs, often in two groups, gram-positive and gram-negative. If the growth of the organism is inhibited by the action of the drug, it is reported as sensitive to that antibiotic. If the organism is not susceptible to the antibiotic in question, it is reported as resistant to that drug. See also **Gram's stain.**

antibody, an immunoglobulin, essential to the immune system, produced by lymphoid tissue in response to bacteria, viruses, or other antigenic substances. An antibody is specific to an antigen. Each class of antibody is named for its action. Among the many antibodies are agglutinins, bacteriolysins, opsonins, precipitin. See also **epitope, plasma protein, T cell.**

antibody instructive theory, a theory that each antigenic contact in the life of an individual develops a new antibody, as when an immunoglobulin-covered B cell comes in contact with an antigen and subsequently produces plasma cells and memory cells. The theory maintains that the random contact of B cells with antigens induces the reticuloendothelial system to instruct memory cells to produce antibodies against antigens at any time. Compare **antibody specific theory.**

antibody specific theory, a theory maintaining that the body develops antibody patterns before or shortly after birth and can recognize any antigen and increase antibodies specific to that antigen at any time. The theory holds that the body contains an enormous number of diverse clones of cells, each genetically programmed to synthesize a different antibody. This theory further maintains that any antigen entering the body selects the specific clone programmed to synthesize the antibody for that antigen and stimulates the cells of the clone to proliferate and produce more of the same antibody. Also called **clonal selection theory.** Compare **antibody instructive theory.**

antibromic. See **deodorant.**

anticholinergic, 1. of or pertaining to a blockade of acetylcholine receptors which results in the inhibition of the transmission of parasympathetic nerve impulses. 2. an anticholinergic agent that functions by competing with the neurotransmitter acetylcholine for its receptor sites at synaptic junctions. Anticholinergic drugs reduce spasms of smooth muscle in the bladder, bronchi, and intestine; relax the iris sphincter; decrease gastric, bronchial, and salivary secretions; decrease perspiration; and accelerate impulse conduction through the myocardium by blocking vagal impulses. Many anticholinergic agents reduce parkinsonian symptoms; atropine in large doses stimulates the central nervous system and in small doses acts as a depressant. Among numerous cholinergic blocking agents are anisotropine methylbromide, belladonna, glycopyrrolate, hyoscyamine sulfate, methixene hydrochloride, and scopolamine. Various members of the group are used to treat spastic disorders of the gastrointestinal tract, to reduce salivary and bronchial secretions preoperatively, or to dilate the pupil. Also called **parasympatholytic.** Compare **cholinergic.**

anticholinergic agent. See **anticholinergic.**

anticholinesterase (æn'tıkol'ənes'təreis), a drug that inhibits or inactivates the action of acetylcholinesterase. Drugs of this class cause acetylcholine to accumulate at the junctions of various cholinergic nerve fibers and their effector sites or organs, allowing potentially continuous stimulation of cholinergic fibers throughout the central and peripheral nervous systems. Anticholinesterase drugs include neostigmine, edrophonium, and pyridostigmine. Neostigmine and pyridostigmine are prescribed in the treatment of myasthenia gravis; edrophonium in the diagnosis of myasthenia gravis and the treatment of overdosage of curariform drugs. Many agricultural insecticides have been developed from anticholinesterases; these are the highly toxic chemicals called organophosphates. Nerve gases developed as potential chemical-warfare agents contain potent, irreversible forms of anticholinesterase.

anticipatory guidance, the psychological preparation of a patient to help relieve fear and anxiety of an event expected to be stressful, as the preparation of a child for surgery by explaining what will happen and what it will feel like and the showing of equipment or the part of the hospital where the child will be.

anticoagulant, 1. of or pertaining to a substance that prevents or delays coagulation of the blood. 2. an anticoagulant drug. Heparin, obtained from the liver and lungs of domestic animals, is a potent anticoagulant that interferes with the formation of thromboplastin, with the conversion of prothrombin to thrombin, and with the formation of fibrin from fibrinogen. Synthetic coumarin and phenindione derivatives administered orally are vitamin K antagonists that prevent coagulation by inhibiting the formation of certain clotting factors.

anticodon (æn'tıkou'don), (in genetics) a sequence of three nucleotides in transfer RNA that pairs complementarily with a specific codon of messenger RNA during protein synthesis to specify a particular amino acid in the polypeptide chain. See also **genetic code, transcription, translation.**

anticonvulsant, 1. of or pertaining to a substance or procedure that prevents or reduces the severity of epileptic or other convulsive seizures. 2. an anticonvulsant drug. Hydantoin derivatives, especially sodium diphenylhydantoin, apparently exert their anticonvulsant effect by stabilizing the cell membrane and decreasing intracellular sodium, with the result that the excitability of the epileptogenic focus is reduced. Diphenylhydantoin prevents the spread of excessive discharges in cerebral motor areas and suppresses dysrhythmias originating in the thalamus, frontal lobes, and other brain areas. Phenacemide and primidone are also used in treating grand mal epilepsy, and succinic acid derivatives, valproic acid, paramethadione, and various barbiturates are among the drugs prescribed to limit or prevent petit mal seizures. Many of these agents have a potential for producing fetal malformations when administered to pregnant women.

antidepressant, 1. of or pertaining to a substance or a measure that prevents or relieves depression. 2. an antidepressant agent. Tricyclic antidepressant agents, as amitryptyline and imipramine hydrochloride, block re-uptake of amine neurotransmitters, but the exact mechanism of the antidepressant action of these drugs is unknown. Monoamine oxidase (MAO) inhibitors, as isocarboxazid, pargyline hydrochloride, phenelzine sulfate, and tranylcypromine, increase the concentration of epinephrine, norepinephrine, and serotonin in storage sites in the nervous system, and it is theorized that this increased level of

Anticonvulsants used to prevent seizures

Drug	Use related to seizure type	Average daily dose	Toxic effects
Phenytoin sodium (Dilantin)	Grand mal, focal, psychomotor	0.4 to 0.6 g (divided dose)	Ataxia, vomiting, nystagmus, drowsiness, rash, fever, gum hypertrophy, lymphadenopathy
Phenobarbital (Luminal)	Grand mal, focal, psychomotor (adjunctive)	0.1 to 0.4 g (divided dose)	Drowsiness, rash
Primidone (Mysoline)	Grand mal, focal, psychomotor	0.5 to 2.0 g	Drowsiness, ataxia
Mephenytoin (Mesantoin)	Grand mal, focal, psychomotor	0.3 to 0.5 g	Ataxia, nystagmus, pancytopenia, rash
Ethosuximide (Zarontin)	Petit mal, psychomotor, myoclonic, akinetic	750 to 1500 mg	Drowsiness, nausea, agranulocytosis
Trimethadione (Tridione)	Petit mal	0.3 to 2.0 g (divided dose)	Rash, photophobia, agranulocytosis, nephrosis
Diazepam (Valium)	Status epilepticus, mixed	8 to 30 mg	Drowsiness, ataxia
Carbamazepine (Tegretol)	Grand mal, psychomotor	0.3 to 2.0 g	Rash, drowsiness, ataxia

monoamines in the brain stem is responsible for the drugs' antidepressant effect. MAO inhibitors also have antihypertensive action.

antidiuretic, 1. of or pertaining to the suppression of urine formation. 2. an antidiuretic agent. Antidiuretic hormone (vasopressin), produced in hypothalamic nuclei and stored in the posterior lobe of the pituitary gland, suppresses urine formation by stimulating the resorption of water in distal tubules and collecting ducts in the kidneys. —**antidiuresis,** n.

antidiuretic hormone (ADH), a hormone that decreases the production of urine by increasing the reabsorption of water by the renal tubules. ADH is secreted by cells of the hypothalamus and stored in the posterior lobe of the pituitary gland. It is released in response to a decrease in blood volume, an increased concentration of sodium or other substances in plasma, or by pain, stress, or the action of certain drugs. ADH can cause contraction of smooth muscle in the gastrointestinal tract and blood vessels, especially capillaries, arterioles, and venules. Acetylcholine, methacoline, nicotine, large doses of barbiturates, anesthetics, epinephrine, and norepinephrine stimulate ADH release; ethanol and phenytoin inhibit production of the hormone. Synthetic ADH is used in the treatment of diabetes insipidus. Also called **vasopressin.**

antidote (æn′tɪdout), a drug or other substance that opposes the action of a poison. An antidote may be mechanical, acting to coat the stomach and prevent absorption; or chemical, acting to make the toxin inert; or physiologic, acting to oppose the action of the poison, as a sedative given to a person who has ingested a large amount of a stimulant.

antidromic conduction (æn′tɪdrom′ɪk), the conduction of a neural impulse backward from a receptor in the midportion of an axon. As synaptic junctions allow conduction in one direction only, any backward, antidromic impulses that occur fail to pass the synapse, dying at that point. Compare **orthodromic conduction.**

antiembolism hose, elasticized stockings worn to prevent the formation of emboli and thrombi, especially in patients after surgery or those restricted to bed. Return flow of the venous circulation is promoted, preventing venous stasis and dilation of the veins, conditions that predispose to thromboembolic disorders.

antiemetic, 1. of or pertaining to a substance or procedure that prevents or alleviates nausea and vomiting. 2. an antiemetic drug or agent. Belladonna derivatives, bromides, barbiturates and other sedatives, and substances that protect the stomach lining, as lime water or mild gastric astringents, have weak antiemetic properties. Chlorpromazine and other phenothiazines are the most effective antiemetic agents. In motion sickness scopolamine and antihistamines provide relief. Marijuana may alleviate the nausea induced by certain antineoplastic drugs in cancer patients.

antiepileptic (æn′tɪepɪlep′tɪk). See **anticonvulsant.**

antifebrile. See **antipyretic.**

antifungal, 1. of or pertaining to a substance that kills fungi or inhibits their growth or reproduction. 2. an antifungal, antibiotic drug. Amphotericin B, effective against a broad spectrum of fungi, probably acts by binding to sterols in the fungal cell membrane and changing the membrane's permeability. Griseofulvin, another broad-spectrum antifungal agent, binds to the host's new keratin and renders it resistant to further fungal invasion. Miconazole inhibits the growth of common dermatophytes, including yeastlike *Candida albicans,* and nystatin is effective against yeast and yeastlike fungi.

antigen (æn′tɪjən), a substance, usually a protein, that causes the formation of an antibody and reacts specifically with that antibody.

antigen-antibody reaction, a process of the immune system in which immunoglobulin coated B cells recognize an intruder or antigen and stimulate antibody production to protect the body against infection. The T cells of the body assist in the antigen-antibody reaction, but the B cells play the key role. Antigen-antibody reactions activate the complement system of the body, amplifying the humoral immunity response of the B cells and causing lysis of the antigenic cells. Antigen-antibody reactions involve the binding of antigens to antibodies to form antigen-antibody complexes that may render the toxic antigen harmless, agglutinize antigens on the surface of microorganisms, or activate the complement system by exposing the complement-binding sites on the antibody molecule. Complement protein immediately binds to these sites and triggers the activity of the other complement proteins to produce cytolysis of the antigen cells. The antigen-antibody reaction may start immediately with antigen contact, or it may start 48 hours later. Antigen-antibody reactions are essential to the immune response of the body and are precipitated by contact of antigenic protein molecules with antibody protein molecules. The antigen-antibody reactions occur and antigen-antibody complexes are formed when unique areas on the surfaces of antigen molecules fit precisely into appropriate concave combining sites on the surfaces of antibody molecules. Various amounts of IgM, IgG, IgA, IgE, and IgD are normally present during any antigenic challenge. Antigenic-antibody reactions normally produce immunity, but they can also produce allergy, autoimmunity, and fetomaternal hematologic incompatibility. In immediate allergic reactions, antigens provoke the production of specific antibodies that may circulate freely in the serum or may become attached to specific cells. Antigen-antibody reaction in the immediate allergic response activates certain enzymes and causes an imbalance between these enzymes and their inhibitors. Simultaneously released into the circulation are certain pharmacologically active substances, as acetylcholine, bradykinin, histamine, gamma globulin G, and leukotaxine. Autoimmunity makes it impossible for the immune system to distinguish between self and a foreign substance. There are several theories, that seek to explain why the body reacts to autoimmune diseases by producing antibodies that attack not only the invading organisms but the cells of the body as well. They are the forbidden clone theory, the sequestered antigens theory, and the immune complex activity theory. The antigen-antibody reactions associated with autoimmunity are still not well understood. In erythroblastosis fetalis, an antigen-antibody reaction stems from the incompatibility of the fetal and the maternal blood and produces a maternal antibody that acts against fetal red cells. ABO incompatibility involves the antigen-antibody reaction between maternal antibodies and fetal blood cells when maternal and fetal blood groups differ.

antigen determinant, a small area on the surface of an antigen molecule that fits a combining site of an antibody molecule and binds the antigen in the formation of an antigen-antibody complex. Antigen determinants commonly consist of a sequence of amino acids which decrees the shape of these reactive areas. Also called **epitope.**

antigenicity (æn'tɪjənɪs'əti), the quality of causing the production of antibodies. The degree of antigenicity depends on the kind and amount of the particular substance, the condition of the host, and the degree to which the host is sensitive to the antigen and able to produce antibodies.

antigerminal pole. See **vegetal pole.**

antiglobulin (æn'tɪglob'yulɪn), an antibody against human globulin, occurring naturally or prepared in laboratory animals. Specific antiglobulins are used in the detection of specific antibodies, as in blood typing. See also **antiglobulin test, Coomb's test, precipitin.**

antiglobulin test, a test for the presence of antibodies that coat and damage red blood cells as a result of any of several diseases or conditions. The test can detect Rh antibodies in maternal blood and is used to anticipate hemolytic disease of the newborn. It is also used to diagnose and screen for autoimmune hemolytic anemias and to determine the compatibility of blood types. When exposed to a sample of the patient's serum, the antiglobulin serum will cause agglutination if human globulin antibody or its complement is present. Also called **Coombs' test.** See also **autoimmune disease, erythroblastosis fetalis.**

antihemophilic C factor. See **plasma thromboplastin antecedent.**

antihemophilic factor (AHF), blood factor VIII, a systemic hemostatic.

■ INDICATION: It is prescribed in the treatment of hemophilia A, a deficiency of Factor VIII.

■ CONTRAINDICATIONS: There are no known contraindications.

■ ADVERSE EFFECTS: The most serious adverse reaction is hepatitis, because the factor is obtained from pools of human plasma. Various allergic reactions may also occur.

antihistamine (æn'tɪhɪs'təmɪn, æn'tɪhɪs'təmin), any substance capable of reducing the physiological and pharmacological effects of histamine, including a wide variety of drugs that block histamine receptors. Many such drugs are readily available as nonprescriptive medicines for the management of allergies. Toxicity resulting from the overuse of antihistamines and their accidental ingestion by children is common and sometimes fatal. These substances do not stop the release of histamine, and the ways in which they act on the central nervous system (CNS) are not completely understood. The antihistamines are divided into H_1 and H_2 blockers depending on the responses to histamine they prevent. The H_1 blocking drugs, as the alkylamines, ethanolamines, ethylenediamines, and piperazines, are effective in the symptomatic treatment of acute exudative allergies, as pollinosis and urticaria. The H_2 blocking drugs, as cimetidine, are effective in the control of gastric secretions and are often used in the treatment of duodenal ulcers. Antihistamines can both stimulate and depress the CNS. The side effects of H_1 blockers may include sedation, nausea, constipation, and dryness of the throat and respiratory tract. About 25 per cent of the individuals who use antihistamines experience some bothersome reaction. —**antihistaminic,** *adj.*

antihypertensive, 1. of or pertaining to a substance or procedure that reduces high blood pressure. 2. an antihypertensive agent. Various drugs achieve their antihypertensive effect by depleting tissue stores of catecholamines in peripheral sites, by stimulating pressor receptors in the carotid sinus and heart, by blocking autonomic nerve impulses that constrict blood vessels, by stimulating central inhibitory alpha-adrenergic receptors, or by direct vasodilation. Thiazides and other diuretic agents reduce blood pressure by decreasing blood volume. Among the numerous drugs used to treat hypertension are rauwolfia and veratrum alkaloids, diazoxide, guanethidine, methyldopa, pargyline hydrochloride, and trimethaphan camsylate.

anti-infection vitamin. See **vitamin A.**

anti-inflammatory, 1. of or pertaining to a substance or procedure that counteracts or reduces inflammation. 2. an anti-inflammatory drug or agent. Betamethasone, prednisolone, prednisone, and other synthetic glucocorticoids are used extensively in treating inflammation. The basis of the anti-inflammatory effect of salicylates and nonsteroidal anti-inflammatory agents, as phenylsutazone, indomethacin, appears to involve inhibition of prostaglandin biosynthesis.

antilipidemic (æn'tɪlɪp'ɪdi'mɪk), **1.** of or pertaining to a regimen, diet, or agent that reduces the amount of lipids in the serum. **2.** a drug used to reduce the amount of lipids in the serum. Antilipidemic diets and drugs are prescribed to reduce the risk of atherosclerotic cardiovascular disease (ACVD) based on two facts: atheromatous plaques contain free cholesterol, and lower serum cholesterol levels and less coronary heart disease are found in populations consuming a low-fat diet than in those on a high-fat diet. Although it has not been proven that food intake affects the development of ACVD, a prudent low-fat diet with polyunsaturates replacing saturated fats is considered a valuable preventive measure by many cardiologists. A number of pharmacologic agents are used to reduce serum lipids, but it is not established whether drug-induced lowering of serum cholesterol or triglyceride levels has a beneficial effect, no effect, or a detrimental effect on ACVD morbidity or mortality. Clofibrate reduces very low density lipoproteins in serum; the drug may reduce the risk of a second, non-fatal myocardial infarction but it increases the risk of cholelithiasis, cardiac arrhythmias, intermittent claudication, and thromboembolism. Cholestyramine exerts its antilipidemic action by combining with bile acids in the intestine to form an insoluble complex which is excreted in the feces; it may reduce serum cholesterol markedly but it prevents the absorption of essential fat soluble vitamins and may be associated with several serious side effects. Colestipol also binds and removes bile acids from the intestine; sitosterol may interfere with intestinal absorption of cholesterol, but the exact mechanism of its action and that of antilipidemic probucol are unknown. Dextrothyroxine lowers serum lipid levels by stimulating hepatic catabolism and excretion of cholesterol and its metabolites. See also **hyperlipidemia.**

Antilirium, a trade name for a narcotic antagonist (physostigmine salicylate), used as an adjunct to anesthesia.

antilymphocyte serum (ALS), a serum prescribed as an immunosuppressive agent for the reduction of rejection reactions in organ transplant and as an adjunct in chemotherapy for malignant neoplasms. Its effects have been promising in some cases of leukemia and in kidney transplant. It is associated with some adverse effects, as serious serum sickness, generalized infection, anaphylaxis, and antigen-antibody-induced glomerulonephritis.

antimalarial (æn'tɪməleɪr'iəl), **1.** of or pertaining to a substance that destroys or suppresses the development of malaria plasmodia or to a procedure that exterminates the mosquito vectors of the disease, as spraying insecticides or draining swamps. **2.** an antimalarial drug that destroys or prevents the development of plasmodia in human hosts. Chloroquine hydrochloride and hydroxychloroquine sulfate are effective against *Plasmodium vivax, P.*

malariae, and certain strains of *P. falciparum.* Chloroguanide is effective against *P. falciparum* infections.

antimetabolite (æn'tɪmɪtæb'əlaɪt), a drug or other substance that resembles a normal human metabolite and interferes with its function in the body, usually by competing for the metabolite's receptors or enzymes. Among the antimetabolites used as antineoplastic agents are the folic acid analog methotrexate and the pyrimidine analogs fluorouracil and floxuridine. Antineoplastic mercaptopurine, an analog of the nucleotide adenine and the purine base hypoxanthine, is a metabolic antagonist of both compounds. Thioguanine, another member of a large series of purine analogs, interferes with nucleic acid synthesis. Cytarbine, used in the treatment of acute myelocytic leukemia, is a synthetic nucleoside that resembles cytidine and kills cells actively synthesizing DNA, apparently by inhibiting the enzyme DNA polymerase.

antimicrobial (æn'timaɪkrou'biəl). See **antibacterial.**

Antiminth, a trade name for an anthelmintic (pyrantel pamoate).

antimitochondrial antibody (æn'timaɪ'toukon'driəl, æn-'timɪt'oukon'driəl), an antibody that acts specifically against mitochondria. These antibodies are not normally present in the blood of healthy people. A laboratory test for the presence of the antibodies in the blood is a valuable diagnostic aid in liver disease, as a biopsy of the liver may not yield affected tissue. Low titers may occur in chronic hepatitis, drug-induced hepatotoxicity, and various other diseases. High titers are virtually diagnostic of primary biliary cirrhosis.

antimony, a bluish, crystalline metallic element occurring in nature, both free and as salts. Various antimony compounds are used in the treatment of filariasis, leishmaniasis, lymphogranuloma, schistosomiasis, and trypanosomiasis and as an emetic. See also **tartar emetic.**

antimony poisoning, poisoning caused by the ingestion or inhalation of antimony or antimony compounds, characterized by vomiting, sweating, diarrhea, and a metallic taste in the mouth. Irritation of the skin or mucous membrane may result from external exposure. Severe poisoning resembles arsenic poisoning. British anti-lewisite is used for chelation. Antimony and antimony compounds are common ingredients of many substances used in medicine and industry.

antimony potassium tartrate, an antischistosomal.

■ INDICATION: It is prescribed in the treatment of infection caused by *Schistosoma japonicum.*

■ CONTRAINDICATIONS: Anemia, severe hepatic, renal, or cardiac insufficiency, or known hypersensitivity to this drug prohibits its use.

■ ADVERSE EFFECTS: Among the most serious adverse reactions are circulatory collapse from too rapid injection and coughing and vomiting during and after injection.

Potentially serious allergic reactions and blood dyscrasias are occasionally observed.

antimorph, a mutant gene that inhibits or antagonizes the normal influence of its allele in the expression of a trait. Compare **amorph, hypermorph, hypomorph.**

antimuscarinic (æn'tımǝs'kǝrın'ık), inhibiting the stimulation of the postganglionic parasympathetic recepter.

antimutagen (æn'tımyu'tǝjın), 1. any substance that reduces the rate of spontaneous mutations or counteracts or reverses the action of a mutagen. 2. any technique that protects cells against the effects of mutagenic agents. – **antimutagenic,** adj.

antineoplastic (æn'tıni'ouplæs'tık), 1. of or pertaining to a substance, procedure, or measure that prevents the proliferation of malignant cells. 2. a chemotherapeutic agent that controls or kills cancer cells. Drugs used in the treatment of cancer are cytotoxic but are generally more damaging to dividing cells than to resting cells. Cycle-specific antineoplastic agents are more effective in killing proliferating cells than in killing resting cells, and phase-specific agents are most active during a specific phase of the cell cycle. Most anticancer drugs prevent the proliferation of cells by inhibiting the synthesis of DNA by various mechanisms. Alkylating agents, as nitrogen mustard derivatives, ethylenimine derivatives, and alkyl sulfonates, interfere with DNA replication by causing cross-linking of DNA strands and abnormal pairing of nucleotides. Antimetabolites exert their action by interfering with the formation of compounds required for cell division. The folic acid analog and 5-fluorouracil, a pyrimidine analog, inhibit enzymes required for the formation of the essential DNA constituent thymidine. Hypoxanthine analog 6-mercaptopurine and 6-thioguanine, an analog of guanine, interfere with the biosynthesis of purine. Vinblastine and vincristine, alkaloids derived from the periwinkle plant, disrupt cell division by interfering with the formation of the mitotic spindle. Antineoplastic antibiotics, as adramycin, daunomycin, and mitomycin, block or inhibit DNA synthesis, while actinomycin-D and mithramycin interfere with RNA synthesis. Cytotoxic chemotherapeutic agents may be administered orally, intravenously, or by infusion. All have untoward and unpleasant side effects and are potentially immunosuppresive and dangerous. Estrogens and androgens, although not considered antineoplastic agents, frequently cause tumor regression when administered in high doses to patients with hormone-dependent cancers. See also **alkylating agent, antimetabolite.**

antineoplastic antibiotic, a chemical substance derived from a microorganism or a synthetic analog of the substance, used in cancer chemotherapy. Actinomycin-D, employed in the treatment of Wilms' tumor, testicular carcinoma, choriocarcinoma, rhabdomyosarcoma, and some other sarcomas, exerts its antineoplastic effect by interfering with RNA synthesis. Mithramycin, with a similar mechanism of action, is also administered for testicular cancer and for trophoblastic neoplasms. Adriamycin, a broad spectrum agent that is especially useful in treating breast carcinoma, lymphomas, sarcomas, and acute leukemia, and closely related daunomycin, which is also effective in acute leukemias, block the biosynthesis of RNA. Mitomycin-C, prescribed for gastric, breast, cervical, and head and neck carcinomas, cross links strands of DNA. Bleomycin, used in the treatment of squamous cell carcinomas of the head and neck, testicular carcinoma, and lymphomas, damages DNA and prevents its repair. Antineoplastic antibiotics depress bone marrow and usually cause nausea and vomiting; several cause alopecia. Adriamycin and daunomycin may be cardiotoxic, and mitomycin and bleomycin may produce pulmonary changes.

antineoplastic hormone, a chemical substance produced by an endocrine gland or a synthetic analog of the naturally occurring compound, used to control certain disseminated cancers. Hormonal therapy is designed to counteract the effect of an endogenous hormone required for the growth of the tumor. The estrogens diethylstilbestrol (DES) and ethinyl estradiol are employed in palliative treatment of a prostatic carcinoma that is nonresectable or unresponsive to radiotherapy. An androgen, as testosterone propionate, testolactone, or fluoxymesterone, may be administered postoperatively to control disseminated breast cancer in women whose tumors are estrogen dependent. The antiestrogen tamoxifen produces responses in many patients with advanced estrogen-dependent breast cancer. Parodoxically, large doses of estrogen, frequently used to control disseminated breast cancer in postmenopausal women, apparently check the growth of tumors by inhibiting the secretion of estrogen by the adrenal gland. Some progestins produce a favorable response in women with disseminated endometrial carcinoma and, occasionally, in patients with prostatic or renal cancers. These progestins include megestrol acetate, medroxyprogesterone acetate, and 17-alpha-hydroxyprogesterone caproate.

antineuritic vitamin. See **thiamine.**

antinuclear antibody, an antibody directed at components of cellular nuclei, as DNA, found in patients with various diseases, as systemic lupus erythematosus.

antiparallel, (in molecular genetics) the condition in which molecules, as strands of DNA, are parallel but point in opposite directions.

antiparasitic, 1. of or pertaining to a substance or procedure that kills parasites or inhibits their growth or reproduction. 2. an antiparasitic drug including amebicides, anthelmintics, antimalarials, schistosomicides, trichomonacides, and trypanosomicides.

antiparkinsonian (æn'tıpar'kınsou'niǝn), of or pertaining to a substance or procedure used to treat parkinsonism. Drugs for this neurological disorder are of two kinds: those that compensate for the lack of dopamine in the corpus striatum of parkinsonism patients, and anticholinergic agents that counteract the activity of the abundant acetylcholine in the striatum. Synthetic levodopa, a dopamine precursor that crosses the blood-brain barrier, is administered to patients to reduce the rigidity, sluggishness, dysphagia, drooling, and instability characteristic of the disease, but the drug does not alter the relentless course of the disorder. Centrally active cholinergic blockers, notably benztropine, biperiden, procyclidine, and trihexyphenidyl, may relieve tremors and rigidity and improve mobility. The antiviral agent amantadine is often effective in the treatment of parkinsonism; the mechanism of its action is not established, but it apparently causes an increased release of dopamine in the brain. Therapeutic approaches to the relief of the symptoms of parkinsonism include alcohol injection, cautery, cryosurgery, and surgical excision performed to destroy the globus pallidus (reducing rigidity) and parts of the thalamus (reducing tremor). Extrapyramidal symptoms similar to idiopathic parkinsonism are frequently induced by antipsychotic drugs. See also **tardive dyskinesia.**

antiperistaltic (æn′tıper′ıstɔl′tık, æn′tıper′ıstæl′tık), **1.** of or pertaining to a substance that inhibits or diminishes peristalsis. **2.** an antiperistaltic agent. Narcotics, as paregoric, diphenoxylate, and loperamide hydrochloride, are antiperistaltic agents used to provide symptomatic relief in diarrhea. Anticholinergic (parasympatholytic) drugs reduce spasms of intestinal smooth muscle and are frequently prescribed to decrease excessive gastrointestinal motility.

antipernicious anemia factor.   See **cyanocobalamin.**

antipruritic, 1. of or pertaining to a substance or procedure that tends to relieve or prevent itching. **2.** an antipruritic drug. Topical anesthetics, corticosteroids, and antihistamines are used as antipruritic agents.

antipsychotic (æn′tısaıkot′ık), **1.** of or pertaining to a substance or procedure that counteracts or diminishes symptoms of a psychosis. **2.** an antipsychotic drug. Phenothiazine derivatives are the most frequently prescribed antipsychotics for use in the treatment of schizophrenia and other major affective disorders. They apparently act by enhancing the filtering mechanisms of the reticular formation in the brain stem. Common side effects of phenothiazines are a dry mouth, blurred vision, and extrapyramidal reactions requiring treatment with antiparkinsonian agents. See also **antidepressant, neuroleptic, tranquilizer.**

antipyretic, 1. of or pertaining to a substance or procedure that reduces fever. **2.** an antipyretic agent. Such drugs usually lower the thermodetection set point of the hypothalamic heat regulatory center, with resulting vasodilation and sweating. Widely used antipyretic agents are acetaminophen, administered orally or through rectal suppositories, aspirin, and other salicylates. A tepid alcohol sponge bath or lukewarm tub bath may decrease an elevated temperature, and hypothermia produced by a cooling blanket is sometimes used for patients with a prolonged, high fever. Also called **antifebrile, antithermic, febrifuge.**

antipyretic bath, a bath in which tepid water is used to reduce the temperature of the body.

antiscorbutic vitamin.   See **ascorbic acid.**

antisense, (in molecular genetics) a strand of DNA containing the same sequence of nucleotides as messenger RNA (mRNA).

antisepsis (æn′tısep′sıs), destruction of microorganisms to prevent infection. — **antiseptic,** *adj.*

antiseptic (æn′tısep′tık), **1.** tending to inhibit the growth and reproduction of microorganisms. **2.** a substance that tends to inhibit the growth and reproduction of microorganisms.

antiseptic dressing, a dressing treated with an antiseptic, germicide, or bacteriostat, applied to a wound or an incision to prevent or treat infection.

antiseptic gauze, gauze permeated with an antiseptic solution, sometimes packaged in individual, sealed packets.

antiserum (æn′tısır′əm), *pl.* **antisera, antiserums.** serum of an animal or human containing antibodies against a specific disease, used to confer passive immunity to that disease. Antisera do not provoke the production of antibodies. There are two types of antiserum. Antitoxin is an antiserum that neutralizes the toxin produced by specific bacteria, but it does not kill the bacteria. Antimicrobial serum acts to destroy bacteria by making them more susceptible to the leukocytic action. Polyvalent antiserum acts on more than one strain of bacteria; univalent antiserum acts on only one strain. Antibiotic drugs have largely replaced antimicrobial antisera. Caution is always to be used in giving antiserum of any kind, as hepatitis or hypersensitivity reactions can occur. Also called **immune serum.** Compare **vaccine.**

antiserum anaphylaxis, an exaggerated reaction of hypersensitivity in a normal person caused by the injection of serum from a sensitized individual. Also called **passive anaphylaxis.**

antisocial personality, a person who exhibits attitudes and overt behavior contrary to the customs, standards, and moral principles accepted by society. Also called **psychopathic personality, sociopathic personality.** See also **antisocial personality disorder.**

antisocial personality disorder, a condition characterized by repetitive behavioral patterns that lack moral and ethical standards and bring a person into continuous conflict with society. Symptoms include aggressiveness, callousness, impulsiveness, irresponsibility, hostility, a low frustration level, a marked emotional immaturity, and poor judgment. A person who has this disorder neglects the rights of others, is incapable of loyalty to others or to social values, is unable to feel guilt or to learn from experience, is impervious to punishment, and tends to rationalize his behavior or to blame it on others. The disorder is usually recognized before adulthood and often persists throughout life. Adverse environmental influences, biological deficiencies, and unconscious conflicts resulting from aberrant family relationships may contribute to the development of the disorder. Most individuals with this condition manage to function in society despite frequent bouts with authorities, but many are referred by courts to prisons. Also called **antisocial reaction.** See also **psychopath, sociopath.**

antisocial reaction. See **antisocial personality disorder.**

antistreptolysin-O test (ASOT, ASLT) (æn'tıstrɛp'-təlaı'sınou'), a streptococcal antibody test for finding and measuring serum antibodies to streptolysin-O, an exotoxin produced by most group A and some group C and G streptococci. The test is often used as an aid in the diagnosis of rheumatic fever. A low titer of anti-streptolysin-O antibody is present in most people, since streptococcal infection is common. Elevated or increasing titers indicate a recent infection. See also **Lancefield's classification.**

antithermic. See **antipyretic.**

antithyroid drug, any one of several preparations that can inhibit the synthesis of thyroid hormones and are commonly used in the treatment of hyperthyroidism. The major antithyroid drugs are thioamides, as propyl-thiouracil, methimazole, and carbimazole. In the body such substances interfere with the incorporation of iodine into the tyrosyl residues of thyroglobulin required for the production of the hormones thyroxine and triiodothyronine. These drugs are often used to control hyperthyroidism during an anticipated remission and before a thyroidectomy. Such substances cross the placenta, can cause fetal hypothyroidism and goiter, and are contraindicated for mothers who breastfeed their children.

antitoxin (æn'tıtok'sın), a subgroup of antisera usually prepared from the serum of horses immunized against a particular toxin-producing organism, as botulism antitoxin given therapeutically in botulism and tetanus and diptheria antitoxin given prophylactically to prevent those infections.

antitrust, (in law) against the operation, establishment, or maintenance of a monopoly in the manufacture, production, or sale of a commodity, providing of a service, or practice of a profession.

antitussive (æn'tıtəs'ıv), **1.** against a cough. **2.** any of a large group of narcotic and nonnarcotic drugs that act on the central and peripheral nervous systems to suppress the cough reflex. Because the cough reflex is necessary for clearing the upper respiratory tract of obstructive secretions, antitussives should not be used with a productive cough. Codeine and hydrocodone are potent narcotic antitussives. Dextromethorphan is an equally effective antitussive with no dependence liability. Antitussives are administered orally, usually in a syrup with a mucolytic or expectorant and alcohol, or, sometimes, in a capsule with an antihistaminic and a mild analgesic.

antivenin (æn'tıven'ın), a suspension of venom-neutralizing antibodies prepared from the serum of immunized horses. Antivenin confers passive immunity and is given as a part of emergency first aid for various snake and insect bites.

Antivert, a trade name for an antiemetic (meclizine hydrochloride).

antiviral (æn'tıvaı'rəl), destructive to viruses.

antivitamin, a substance that inactivates a vitamin.

antixerophthalmic vitamin. See **vitamin A.**

antr-. See **antro-.**

antral gastritis, an abnormal narrowing of the antrum, or distal portion of the stomach. The narrowing is not a true gastritis, but a radiographic finding which may represent gastric ulcer or tumor. Compare **gastritis.**

antro-, antr, a combining form meaning 'pertaining to an antrum or sinus': *antrocele, antrodynia, antrophore.*

antrum cardiacum (æn'trəm), a constricted passage from the esophagus to the stomach, lying just inside the opening formed by the cardiac sphincter.

Anturane, a trade name for a uricosuric (sulfinpyrazone).

anuresis (æn'yuri'sıs). See **anuria.** – **anuretic,** *adj.*

anuria (ənur'ıə), the inability to urinate, the cessation of urine production, or a urinary output of less than 100 to 250 ml per day. Anuria may be caused by kidney failure or dysfunction, a decline in blood pressure below that required to maintain filtration pressure in the kidney, or an obstruction in the urinary passages. A rapid decline in urinary output, leading ultimately to anuria and uremia, occurs in acute renal failure. Although patients can live up to two weeks with anuria, death may occur within 24 hours of the total loss of urinary function. Uremia develops in anuria as the amount of waste products and potassium in the bloodstream increases because the kidneys cannot excrete them. The failure of the kidney to excrete hydrogen ions leads to acidosis, and the cells of the body then tend to release more potassium than usual. Fever, trauma, and infection, to which the uremic patient is particularly susceptible, tend to cause rapid catabolism of body tissue that further increases serum potassium levels. Symptoms of high potassium levels include extreme muscle weakness, numbness, and cardiac arrhythmia. Heart failure may suddenly occur. Management of anuria includes limitation of potassium and protein intake, medication to increase the rectal excretion of potassium, dialysis, regulation of fluid intake, and careful monitoring of blood chemistry and fluid balance. Protection of the patient from infection and from injury is critical. Kinds of anuria include **angioneurotic anuria, calculus anuria, obstructive anuria, postrenal anuria, prerenal anuria, renal anuria.** Also called **anuresis.** – **anuric,** *adj.*

anus (ei′nəs), the opening at the end of the anal canal.

anxietas (ærɡzaiʹɪtæs), a state of anxiety, nervous restlessness, or apprehension, often accompanied by a feeling of oppression in the epigastrium. Kinds of anxietas are **anxietas presenilis, anxietas tibiarum.**

anxietas presenilis, a state of extreme anxiety caused by approaching senility.

anxietas tibiarum. See **restless legs syndrome.**

anxiety, a state or feeling of apprehension, uneasiness, agitation, uncertainty, and fear resulting from the antici-

---

Signs of anxiety

Appearance
↑ Muscle tension (rigidity)
Skin blanches, pales
↑ Perspiration, clammy skin
Fatigue
↑ Small motor activity (e.g., restlessness, tremor)

Behavior
↓ Attention span
↓ Ability to follow directions
↑ Acting out
↑ Somatizing
↑ Immobility

Conversation
↑ Number of questions
Constant seeking of reassurance
Frequent shifting of topics of conversation
Describes fears with sense of helplessness
Avoids focusing on feelings
Focuses on equipment or procedures

Physiological signs mediated through autonomic nervous system
↑ Heart rate
↑ Rate or depth of respirations
Rapid extreme shifts in body temperature, blood pressure, menstrual flow
Diarrhea
Urinary urgency
Dryness of mouth
↓ Appetite
↑ Perspiration
Dilation of pupils

Signs of anxiety are dependent on the degree of anxiety. Mild anxiety heightens the use of capacities, whereas severe and panic states severely paralyze or overwork capacities.

---

pation of some threat or danger, usually of intrapsychic rather than external origin, whose source is generally unknown or unrecognized. The condition may result as a rational response to a certain situation that produces tension, like taking an examination or applying for a job, or from a general concern about the uncertainties of life. It is a pathologic condition if it is not based in reality and if it is so severe that it results in the inability to function in the everyday activities of life. Kinds of anxiety include **castration anxiety, free-floating anxiety, separation anxiety, situational anxiety.**

anxiety attack, an acute, psychobiological reaction manifested by intense anxiety and panic. Symptoms vary according to the intensity of the attack but typically include palpitations, shortness of breath, dizziness, faintness, profuse sweating, pallor of the face and extremities, gastrointestinal discomfort, and a vague feeling of imminent death. Attacks usually occur suddenly, last from a few seconds to an hour or longer, and vary in frequency from several times a day to once a month. Treatment consists of reassurance, administration of a sedative, if necessary, and appropriate psychotherapy to identify the stresses perceived as threatening. See also **anxiety, anxiety neurosis.**

anxiety complex. See **castration anxiety.**

anxiety neurosis, a neurotic disorder characterized by persistent anxiety. The symptoms range from mild, chronic tenseness, with feelings of timidity, fatigue, apprehension, and indecisiveness, to more intense states of restlessness and irritability that may lead to aggressive acts or indecisiveness. In extreme cases, the overwhelming emotional discomfort is accompanied by physical reactions, including tremor, sustained muscle tension, tachycardia, dyspnea, hypertension, increased respiration, and profuse perspiration. Other physical signs include changes in skin color, nausea, vomiting, diarrhea, restlessness, immobilization, insomnia, and changes in appetite, all occurring without underlying organic cause. The symptoms of anxiety may be controlled with medication, such as tranquilizers, but psychotherapy is the preferred treatment and sometimes cures the neurosis. Also called **anxiety reaction, anxiety state.** See also **anxiety, anxiety attack.**

anxiety reaction. See **anxiety neurosis.**

AORN, abbreviation for **Association of Operating Room Nurses.**

aorta (eiɔr′tə), the main trunk of the systemic arterial circulation, comprised of four parts: the ascending aorta, the arch of the aorta, the thoracic portion of the descending aorta, and the abdominal portion of the descending aorta. It starts at the aortic opening of the left ventricle, where it has a diameter of about 3 cm, rises a short distance toward the neck, bends to the left and dorsally over the root of the left lung, descends within the thorax on the left side of the vertebral column, and passes through the aortic hiatus of the diaphragm into the abdominal cavity. Opposite the caudal border of the fourth lumbar vertebra, it narrows to about 1.75 cm in diameter and branches into the two common iliac arteries.

aortic aneurysm, a localized dilatation of the wall of the aorta caused by atherosclerosis, hypertension, or, less frequently, by syphilis. The lesion may be a saccular distention, a fusiform or cylindroid swelling of a length of the vessel, or a longitudinal dissection between the outer and middle layers of the vessel wall. Syphilitic aneurysms almost always occur in the thoracic aorta and usually involve the aortic arch, while more common atherosclerotic aneurysms are usually in the abdominal section of the great vessel below the renal arteries and above the bifurcation of the aorta. These lesions often contain atheromatous ulcers covered by thrombi that may discharge emboli, causing obstruction of smaller vessels. A bulging abdominal aortic aneurysm may impinge on a ureter, vertebra, or other adjacent structure, causing pain. A pulsatile mass may be detected in a routine examination, but in many cases the first sign is life-threatening hemorrhage, resulting from rupture of the lesion. A diagnosis of an unruptured aneurysm may be made using x rays of the abdomen, which show a ring of calcification around the dilatation, or with an angiogram. Treatment of small chronic aneurysms includes the use of antihypertensive drugs to reduce pressure on the weak area of the vessel, analgesics to relieve pain, and agents to reduce the force of cardiac contraction. Acute or large aneurysms are resected, and the segment of the aorta is replaced with synthetic prostheses. Cardiopulmonary bypass is required during surgical repair of an aneurysm of the ascending, transverse, or descending aorta but not for an abdominal aneurysm. Common postoperative complications are renal failure and ileus. See also **dissecting aneurysm.**

aortic arch. See **arch of the aorta.**

aortic arch syndrome, any of a group of occlusive conditions of the aortic arch producing a variety of symptoms related to obstruction of the large branch arteries, including the innominate, left common carotid, or left subclavian. Such conditions as atherosclerosis, Takayasu's disease, and syphilis may cause aortic arch syndrome. The symptoms include syncope, temporary blindness, hemiplegia, aphasia, or memory loss.

aortic body reflex, a normal chemical reflex initiated by a decrease in oxygen concentration in the blood and, to a lesser degree, by increased carbon dioxide and hydrogen ion concentrations that act on chemoreceptors in the wall of the arch of the aorta and result in nerve impulses that cause the respiratory center in the medulla to increase respiratory activity. See also **carotid body reflex.**

aortic stenosis, a cardiac anomaly characterized by a narrowing or stricture of the aortic valve owing to congenital malformation or to fusion of the cusps, as may result from rheumatic fever. Aortic stenosis obstructs the flow of blood from the left ventricle into the aorta, causing decreased cardiac output and pulmonary vascular congestion. Clinical manifestations include faint peripheral pulses, exercise intolerance, anginal pain, and a systolic murmur. Diagnosis is confirmed by cardiac catheterization and echocardiography. Surgical repair is usually indicated, followed by frequent examinations, since recurrence of the stenosis and bacterial endocarditis are relatively common sequelae. Children with aortic stenosis are usually restricted from strenuous, competitive sports activities. See also **congenital cardiac anomaly.**

aortic valve, a tricuspid valve in the heart between the left ventricle and the aorta. It is composed of three semilunar cusps that close in diastole to prevent blood from flowing back into the left ventricle from the aorta. The three cusps are separated by sinuses which resemble tiny buckets when they are filled with blood. These cup-shaped flaps grow from the lining of the aorta and, in systole, open to allow oxygenated blood to flow from the left ventricle into the aorta and on to the peripheral circulation. The right coronary artery arises from the sinus between the right posterior cusp of the valve and the aortic wall; the left coronary artery arises from the sinus of the left posterior cusp. The anterior cusp is the third flap of the valve. Compare **mitral valve, pulmonary valve.**

aortitis (ei′ɔrtai′tis), an inflammatory condition of the aorta, occurring most frequently in tertiary syphilis and occasionally in rheumatic fever. Kinds of aortitis are **rheumatic aortitis, syphilitic aortitis.**

aortography (ei′ɔrtog′rəfi), a radiographic process in which the aorta and its branches are injected with any of various contrast media for visualization. —**aortographic,** *adj.*

aortopulmonary fenestration, a congenital anomaly characterized by an abnormal fenestration in the ascending aorta and the pulmonary artery cephalad to the semilunar valve, allowing oxygenated and unoxygenated blood to mix, resulting in a decrease in the oxygen available in the peripheral circulation.

aosmic, anosmic.

ap, 1. Also **apo-.** a combining form meaning 'separation or derivation from': *apeidosis, apentric.* **2.** See **ad-.**

APA, abbreviation for **American Psychiatric Association.**

apathy (æp′əthi), an absence or suppression of emotion, feeling, concern, or passion; an indifference to things generally found to be exciting or moving. The condition is commonly seen in patients with neurasthenic neurosis and schizophrenia. —**apathetic,** *adj.*

APC, abbreviation for **aspirin, phenacetin, caffeine.**

APD, abbreviation for **adult polycystic disease.** See **polycystic kidney disease.**

apepsia nervosa (əpep′siə nərvou′sə). See **anorexia nervosa.**

aperient (əpir′iənt). See **aperitive.**

aperitive (əper′ɪtɪv), **1.** a mild laxative. **2.** acting as a mild laxative. Also called **aperient.**

Apert's syndrome (ʌperz′), a rare condition characterized by an abnormal craniofacial appearance in combination with partial or complete syndactyly of the hands and the feet. The specific cause of Apert's syndrome is not known, but the condition appears to be the result of a primary germplasm defect. Characteristic features of this condition include premature synostosis of the cranial bones, with resultant growth disturbances. Some signs of Apert's syndrome are a peaked and vertically elongated head, widespread and bulging eyes, and a high, arched posterior palate with bony defects of the maxilla and the mandible. The degree of syndactyly varies greatly and may be complete, with the apparent fusion of all the digits externally. The treatment of Apert's syndrome usually includes an osteotomy of the cranial bones to prevent increased intracranial pressure. The syndactyly may be surgically corrected, the specific procedure depending on the severity of the deformity. Also called **acrocephalosyndactylism.**

aperture, an opening or hole in an object or anatomical structure. See specific apertures.

aperture of frontal sinus, an external opening of the frontal sinus into the nasal cavity.

aperture of glottis, an opening between the true vocal cords and the arytenoid cartilages.

aperture of larynx, an opening between the pharynx and larynx.

aperture of sphenoid sinus, a round opening between the sphenoid sinus and nasal cavity, situated just above the superior nasal concha.

apex (ei′peks), pl. **apices** (ei′pɪsiz). the top, the end, or the tip of a structure, as the apex of the heart, the apices of the teeth.

apex beat, a pulsation of the left ventricle of the heart, palpable and sometimes visible at the fifth intercostal space, approximately 9 cm to the left of the midline.

apexcardiogram (ei′pekskar′diəgræm′), a graphic representation of the pulsations of the chest over the heart in the region of the cardiac apex.

apex cordis (kɔr′dis), the pointed lower border of the heart. It is directed downward, forward, to the left, and is usually located at the level of the fifth intercostal space.

apex pulmonis (pəlmou′nis), the rounded upper border of each lung, projecting above the clavicle into the root of the neck.

Apgar score (æp′gar), the evaluation of an infant's physical condition, usually performed one minute and five minutes after birth, based on a rating of five factors that reflect the infant's ability to adjust to extrauterine life. A pediatrician, Virginia Apgar, M.D. developed the system for the rapid identification of infants requiring immediate intervention or transfer to an intensive-care nursery.

■ METHOD: The infant's heart rate, respiratory effort, muscle tone, reflex irritability, and color are scored from a low value of zero to a normal value of two. The five scores are combined, and the totals at one minute and five minutes are noted; for example, Apgar 9/10 is a score of 9 at one minute and 10 at five minutes. See table **Apgar Score.**

■ OUTCOME CRITERIA: A score of 0 to 3 represents severe distress, a score of 4 to 7 indicates moderate distress, and a score of 7 to 10 indicates an absence of difficulty in adjusting to extrauterine life. The five-minute score is normally higher than the one-minute score. As a normal, vigorous, healthy newborn almost always has bluish hands and feet at one minute, the first score will include a "1" rather than a perfect "2"; but at five minutes the blueness may have passed and a score of "2" may be given. A five-minute score of 0 to 1 correlates with a 50 per cent neonatal mortality rate; infants that survive exhibit three times as many neurologic abnormalities at one year of age as do children with a five-minute score of 7 or more.

■ NURSING ORDERS: A low one-minute score requires immediate intervention, including giving oxygen, clearing the nasopharynx, and, usually transfer to an intensive care nursery. A baby with a low score that persists at five minutes requires expert care, which may include assisted ventilation, umbilical catheterization, cardiac massage, blood gas evaluation, medication to correct acid-base deficit, or medication to reverse the effects of maternal medication.

Infant evaluation at birth—Apgar scoring system

	0	1	2
Heart rate	Absent	Slow (below 100 beats/minute)	Over 100 beats/minute
Respiratory effort	Absent	Slow or irregular	Good crying
Muscle tone	Limp	Some flexion of extremities	Active motion
Response to catheter in nostril (tested after oropharynx is clear)	No response	Grimace	Cough or sneeze
Color	Blue or pale	Body pink, extremities blue	Completely pink

APHA, abbreviation for **American Public Health Association.**

aphagia (æfei'jə), a condition characterized by the loss of the ability to swallow owing either to organic or to psychological causes. A kind of aphagia is **aphagia algera.** See also **dysphagia.**

aphagia algera, a condition characterized by the refusal to eat or swallow because doing so causes pain.

aphakia (əfei'kiə), **aphacia** (əfei'shə), (in ophthalmology) a condition in which part or all of the crystalline lens of the eye has been surgically removed, usually in the treatment of cataracts. — **aphakic, aphacic,** adj.

aphasia (əfei'zhə), an abnormal neurologic condition in which language function is defective or absent owing to an injury to certain areas of the cerebral cortex. The deficiency may be sensory or receptive, in which language is not understood, or expressive or motor, in which words cannot be formed or expressed. Sensory aphasia may be complete or partial, affecting specific language functions, as in dyslexia or alexia. Expressive aphasia may be complete, as in dysphasia, in which speech is impaired or as in agraphia, in which writing is affected or it may be partial, diminishing either or both functions. Most commonly, the condition is a mixture of incomplete expressive and receptive aphasia. It may occur following severe head trauma, prolonged hypoxia, or cardiovascular accident. It is sometimes transient, as when the swelling in the brain that follows a stroke or injury subsides and language returns. Intensive speech therapy and effort by the patient and the patient's family have many times been successful in restoring language function. See also **Broca's area.**

-aphia, a combining form meaning a 'condition of the sense of touch': *araphia, hyperaphia, paraphia.* Also **-haphia.**

aphonia (eifou'niə), a condition characterized by loss of the ability to produce normal speech sounds owing to overuse of the vocal cords, organic disease, or psychological causes, such as hysteria. Kinds of aphonia include **aphonia clericorum, aphonia paralytica, aphonia paranoica, spastic aphonia.** See also **speech dysfunction.** — **aphonic, aphonous,** adj.

aphonia clericorum (kler'ɪkɔr'əm), a condition characterized by a loss of the voice from overuse.

aphonia paralytica (pær'əlɪt'ɪkə), a condition characterized by a loss of the voice owing to paralysis or disease of the laryngeal nerves.

aphonia paranoica (pær'ənɔi'kə), an inability to speak that lacks an organic basis and that is characteristic of some forms of mental illness.

aphonic speech (eifon'ɪk), abnormal speech in which vocalizations are whispered.

-aphrodisia, a combining form meaning a '(specified) condition of sexual arousal': *anaphrodisia, hypaphrodisia.*

aphronia (əfrou'niə), (in psychiatry) a condition characterized by an impaired ability to make common-sense decisions. — **aphronic,** n., adj.

aphthous fever, an acute, extremely contagious, rhinovirus infection of cloven-hooved animals. It is characterized by the development of ulcers on the skin around the mouth, on the mucous membrane in the mouth, and on the udders. Horses are immune. Uncommonly, the virus is transmitted to man by direct contact with infected animals or their secretions or with contaminated milk. Also called **foot-and-mouth disease.**

aphthous stomatitis, a recurring condition characterized by the eruption of painful ulcers (commonly called canker sores) on the mucous membranes of the mouth. The cause is unknown, but there is evidence to suggest that aphthous stomatitis is an immune reaction. See also **canker sore.**

APIC, abbreviation for American **Association for Practitioners of Infection Control.**

apical dental ligament, a ligament connecting the axis to the occipital bone. It extends from the process of the axis to the anterior margin of the foramen magnum and lies between the two alar ligaments, blending with the anterior atlanto-occipital membrane. It is considered a rudimentary intervertebral disc and contains traces of the embryonic notochord.

APKD, abbreviation for **adult polycystic disease.** See **polycystic kidney disease.**

aplasia (əplei'zhə), **1.** a developmental failure resulting in the absence of an organ or tissue. **2.** in hematology, a failure of the normal process of cell generation and development. See also **aplastic anemia, hyperplasia.** — **aplastic,** adj.

aplasia cutis congenita, the congenital absence of a localized area of skin. The defect occurs predominantly on the scalp, less frequently on the limbs and trunk, and is usually covered by a thin, translucent membrane or scar tissue, or it may be raw and ulcerated. The conditon is genetically transmitted, although the mode of inheritance is not known.

aplastic, **1.** pertaining to the absence or defective development of a tissue or organ. **2.** failure of a tissue to produce normal daughter cells by mitosis. See also **aplastic anemia.** — **aplasia,** n.

aplastic anemia, a deficiency of all of the formed elements of the blood, representing a failure of the cell-generating capacity of the bone marrow. It may be caused by neoplastic disease of the bone marrow, or, more commonly, by destruction of the bone marrow by exposure to toxic chemicals, ionizing radiation, or some antibiotics or other medications. Rarely, an idiopathic form of the disease occurs.

apnea (æpni'ə, æp'niə), an absence of spontaneous respiration. Kinds of apnea include **cardiac apnea, deglutition**

apnea, periodic apnea of the newborn, primary apnea, reflex apnea, secondary apnea. —apneic, *adj.*

apo-, ap-, a combining form meaning 'separation or derivation from': *apobiosis, apocarteresis, aponeurosis.*

apocrine gland, one of the large, deep exocrine glands located in the axillary, anal, genital, and mammary areas of the body. The apocrine glands secrete sweat that has a strong, characteristic odor. Compare eccrine gland. See also exocrine gland.

apodial symmelia. See sirenomelia.

apomorphine hydrochloride, an emetic.

■ INDICATION: It is prescribed to induce vomiting.

■ CONTRAINDICATIONS: Impending shock, narcosis, extreme inebriation from drugs or alcohol, or known hypersensitivity to this drug or other morphine derivatives prohibits its use. The drug is used with caution in debilitated patients or in those having cardiac decompensation.

■ ADVERSE EFFECTS: Among the more serious reactions are central nervous system depression, respiratory depression, and circulatory failure. Euphoria and tremors may occur.

aponeurosis (æp′ounurou′sis), *pl.* aponeuroses. a strong sheet of fibrous connective tissue that serves as a tendon to attach muscles to bone or as fascia to bind muscles together.

aponeurosis of the obliquus externus abdominis, the strong membrane that covers the entire ventral surface of the abdomen and lies superficial to the rectus abdominis. Fibers from both sides of the aponeurosis interlace in the midline to form the linea alba. The upper part of the aponeurosis serves as the inferior origin of the pectoralis major; the lower part ends in the inguinal ligament.

apophyseal fracture (æp′əfiz′iəl), a fracture that separates an apophysis of a bone from the main osseous tissue at a point of strong tendinous attachment.

apophysitis (epof′əsai′tis), a condition characterized by the inflammation of an outgrowth or swelling, especially a bony outgrowth that is not separated from the bone. Apophysitis occurs most frequently as a disorder of the foot caused by disease of the epiphysis of the quadrangular bone at the back of the tarsus.

apoplexy (æp′əplek′si), 1. *Obsolete.* a cerebrovascular accident, resulting in paralysis. 2. a hemorrhage within an organ. —apoplectic, *adj.*

apothecaries' measure, a system of graduated liquid volumes originally based on the minim, formerly equal to one drop of water but now standardized to 0.06 ml. 60 minims equal one fluid dram, 8 fluid drams equal one fluid ounce, 16 fluid ounces equal one pint, 2 pints equal one quart, 4 quarts equal one gallon. See also apothecaries' weight, metric system.

apothecaries' weight, a system of graduated amounts arranged in order of heaviness and based upon the grain, formerly equal to the weight of a plump grain of wheat but now standardized to 65 mg. 20 grains equal one scruple, 3 scruples equal one dram, 8 drams equal one ounce, 12 ounces equal one pound. Compare avoirdupois weight. See also apothecaries' measure, metric system.

apparent death. See death.

appellant (əpel′ənt), (in law) a party that brings an appeal to an appellate court. Having lost the case in a lower court, the appellant requests the court to reconsider the case.

appellate court, a court of law that has the power to review the decision of a lower court. It does not make a new determination of the facts of the case; it reviews only the way in which the law was applied in the case.

appellee (æp′əli′), (in law) a party in an appeal that won the case in a lower court. The appellee argues that the decision of the lower court should not be modified by the appellate court.

appendage, an accessory structure attached to another part or organ. Also called appendix.

appendectomy (æp′əndek′təmi), the surgical removal of the vermiform appendix through an incision in the right lower quadrant of the abdomen. The operation is performed in acute appendicitis to remove an inflamed appendix before it ruptures and prophylactically at the time of other abdominal surgery. Unless the appendix has burst and peritonitis is present or suspected, postoperative care and nursing considerations are the same as for any other abdominal operation. If the appendix has burst, a drain may be left in the incision, dressing changes are more frequent, and appropriate antibiotics are prescribed; ileus may be present and pain may be acute. Intravenous fluids, electrolytes, sedatives, and narcotic analgesics are usually given. See also abdominal surgery, peritonitis.

appendiceal, appendicial (æp′endish′əl), appendical (əpen′dikəl), of or pertaining to the vermiform appendix.

appendicitis (əpen′disai′tis), inflammation of the vermiform appendix, usually acute, which if undiagnosed leads rapidly to perforation and peritonitis. The most common symptom is constant pain in the right lower quadrant of the abdomen around McBurney's point, which the patient describes as having begun as intermittent pain in midabdomen. To decrease the pain, the patient keeps his knees bent to avoid tension of abdominal muscles. Appendicitis is characterized by vomiting, a low-grade fever of 99 to 102°, an elevated white blood count, rebound tenderness, a rigid abdomen, and decreased or absent bowel sounds. The inflammation is caused by an obstruction as a hard mass of feces or a foreign body, in the lumen of the appendix, fibrous disease of the bowel wall, an adhesion, or a parasitic infestation. Treatment is appendectomy, within 24 to 48 hours of the first symptoms, because delay usually results in rupture and peritonitis as fecal matter is released into the peritoneal cavity. The fever rises sharply once peritonitis begins, and the patient may have sudden relief from pain followed by increased, diffuse pain. The nurse is alert to the other indications of peritonitis: increasing abdominal distention, tachycardia, rapid shallow breathing, and restlessness. If peritonitis is suspected, intravenous antibiotic therapy, fluids, and electrolytes are given. Appendicitis is most apt to occur in teenagers and young adults and is more frequent in males. See also **appendectomy, appendix, McBurney's point, perforate, peritonitis.**

appendix, *pl.* **appendixes, appendices. 1.** Also called **appendage.** an accessory part of a main structure. **2.** See **vermiform appendix.**

appendix dyspepsia, an abnormal condition characterized by the impairment of the digestive function associated with chronic appendicitis. See also **dyspepsia.**

appendix epididymidis, a cystic structure sometimes found on the head of the epididymis. It represents a remnant of the mesonephros.

appendix epiploica, *pl.* **appendices epiploicae.** one of the fat pads, 2 to 10 cm long, scattered through the peritoneum along the colon and the upper part of the rectum, especially along the transverse and the sigmoid parts of the colon.

appendix vermiformis (vər'mɪfɔɪ'mɪs). See **vermiform appendix.**

apperception (æp'ərsep'shən), **1.** mental perception or recognition. **2.** (in psychology) a conscious process of understanding or perceiving in terms of a person's previous knowledge, experiences, emotions, and memories. — **apperceptive,** *adj.*

applied anatomy, the study of the structure and morphology of the organs of the body as it relates to the diagnosis and treatment of disease. Also called **practical anatomy.** Kinds of applied anatomy are **pathological anatomy, radiological anatomy, surgical anatomy.**

applied chemistry, the application of the study of chemical elements and compounds to industry and the arts.

applied psychology, 1. the interpretation of historical, literary, medical or other data according to psychological principles. **2.** any branch of psychology that emphasizes practical rather than theoretical approaches and objectives, as clinical psychology, child psychology, industrial psychology, educational psychology.

applied science. See **science.**

appositional growth, an increase in size by the addition of new tissue or similar material at the periphery of a particular part or structure, as in the addition of new layers in bone and tooth formation. Compare **interstitial growth.**

approach-approach conflict, a conflict resulting from the simultaneous presence of two or more incompatible impulses, desires, or goals, each of which is desirable. Also called **double-approach conflict.** See also **conflict.**

approach-avoidance conflict, a conflict resulting from the presence of a single goal or desire that is both desirable and undesirable. See also **conflict.**

appropriate-for-gestational-age (AGA) infant, a newborn infant whose size, growth, and maturation is normal for gestational age, whether delivered prematurely, at term, or later than term. Such infants, if born at term, fall within the average range of size and weight on intrauterine growth curves, measuring from 48 to 53 cm in length and weighing between 2,700 and 4,000 gm.

apractognosia (eipræk'tognou'ziə). See **constructional apraxia.**

apraxia (əpræk'siə), an impairment in the ability to perform purposeful acts or to manipulate objects. The condition is primarily neurologic but occurs in several forms. **Sensory apraxia** is characterized by impairment caused by a loss of the perception of the use of an object. **Motor apraxia** is characterized by an inability to use an object or perform a task without any loss of perception of the use of the object or the goal of the task. **Amnestic apraxia** is characterized by an inability to perform the function owing to an inability to remember the command to perform it. — **apraxic,** *adj.*

Apresoline Hydrochloride, a trade name for an antihypertensive (hydralazine hydrochloride).

aptitude, a natural ability, tendency, talent, or capability to learn, understand, or acquire a particular skill; mental alertness.

aptitude test, any of a variety of standardized tests for measuring an individual's ability to learn certain skills. Compare **achievement test, intelligence test, personality test, psychological test.**

AQ, abbreviation for **achievement quotient.**

aqua amnii. See **amniotic fluid.**

Aquamephyton, a trade name for vitamin K (phytonadione).

aqueduct of Sylvius. See **cerebral aqueduct.**

aqueous (ei'kwiəs, æk'wiəs), **1.** watery or waterlike. **2.** a medication prepared with water. See also **aqueous humor.**

aqueous humor, the clear, watery fluid circulating in the anterior and posterior chambers of the eye. It is produced by the ciliary processes and is reabsorbed into the venous system at the iridocorneal angle by means of the sinus venosus, or canal of Schlemm.

AR, abbreviation for **assisted respiration.**

Ar, symbol for **argon.**

Ara-A. See **vidarabine.**

arabinosylcytosine (ær'əbɪn'ousɪlsæi'təsin). See **cytarabine.**

arachidonic acid (ær'əkɪdon'ɪk), an essential fatty acid that is a component of lecithin and a basic material for the biosynthesis of some prostaglandins.

arachn-. See **arachno-.**

arachno-, arachn-, a combining form meaning 'pertaining to the arachnoid membrane or to a spider': *arachnoidal, arachnoidea, arachnolysin.*

arachnodactyly (əræk′noudæk′təli), a congenital condition of having long, thin, spiderlike fingers and toes. See **Marfan's syndrome.**

arachnoid (əræk′nɔid), a delicate, fibrous structure resembling a cobweb or spiderweb, as the arachnoid membrane that forms the middle of three protective layers of meninges surrounding the brain and spinal cord. – **arachnoidal,** *adj.*

arachnoidea encephali (ær′æknɔi′diə ensef′əli). See **arachnoid membrane.**

arachnoid membrane, a thin, delicate membrane enclosing the brain and the spinal cord, interposed between the pia mater and the dura mater. The subarachnoid space lies between the arachnoid membrane and the pia, and the subdural space lies between the arachnoid membrane and the dura. Also called **arachnoid.**

arachnoid of the spinal cord, a membrane surrounding the spinal cord.

Aramine, a trade name for an adrenergic (metaraminol bitartrate).

Aran-Duchenne muscular atrophy (æræn′dushen′), a form of amyotrophic lateral sclerosis affecting the hands, arms, shoulders, and legs at the onset before becoming more generalized.

arbitrator (ar′bitrei′tər), an impartial person appointed to resolve a dispute between parties. The arbiter listens to the evidence as presented by the parties in an informal hearing and attempts to arrive at a resolution acceptable to both parties. – **arbitration,** *n.*

arbovirus (ar′bouvai′rəs), any one of more than 300 arthropod-borne viruses that cause infections characterized by a combination of two or more of the following: fever, rash, encephalitis, and bleeding into the viscera or skin. Dengue, yellow fever, and equine encephalitis are three common arboviral infections. Treatment is symptomatic for all arbovirus infections. Vaccines have been developed to prevent infection from some arboviruses.

arch-. See **archi-.**

arche-. See **archi-.**

archenteric canal (ar′kənter′ik). See **neurenteric canal.**

archenteron, *pl.* **archentera.** the primitive digestive cavity formed by the invagination of the blastula in the embryonic development of many animals. It corresponds to the tubular cavity in the vertebrates that connects the amniotic cavity with the yolk sac. Also called **archigaster, coelenteron, gastrocoele, primitive gut.** See also **gastrula.** – **archenteric,** *adj.*

archetype (ar′kitaip′), **1.** an original model or pattern from which a thing or group of things is made or evolves. **2.** (in analytic psychology) an inherited primordial idea or mode of thought derived from the experiences of the human race and present in the unconscious of the individual in the form of drives, moods, and concepts. See also **anima.** – **archetypal, archetypic, archetypical,** *adj.*

archi- arch-, arche-, a combining form meaning 'first, beginning, or original': *archiblastoma, archenteron, archicyte.*

archiblastoma (ar′kiblæstou′mə), *pl.* **archiblastomas, archiblastomata.** a tumor composed of cells derived from the layer of tissue surrounding the germinal vesicle.

archigaster (ar′kigæs′tər). See **archenteron.**

archinephric canal (ar′kinef′rik). See **pronephric duct.**

archinephric duct. See **pronephric duct.**

archinephron, *pl.* **archinephra.** See **pronephros.** – **archinephric,** *adj.*

archistome (ar′kistoum′). See **blastopore.**

archo-, a combining form meaning 'pertaining to the rectum or anus': *archocele, archoptoma, archostenosis.*

arch of the aorta, one of the four portions of the aorta, giving rise to three arterial branches called the brachiocephalic, left common carotid, and the left subclavian arteries. The arch rises at the level of the cranial border of the second sternocostal articulation of the right side, passes to the left in front of the trachea, bends dorsally, and becomes part of the descending aorta. Also called **aortic arch.**

arcing spring contraceptive diaphragm, a kind of contraceptive diaphragm in which the flexible metal spring that forms the rim is a combination of a flexible coil spring and a flat, band spring made of stainless steel. The rubber dome is approximately 1½ inches deep, and the diameter of the rubber-covered rim is between 5½ and 10 cm. Ten sizes, in increments of 0.5 cm, allow the clinician to fit the diaphragm to each individual woman. The kind of spring and the size of the rim in millimeters are stamped on the rim, as, for example, 75 mm arcing spring. This kind of diaphragm is prescribed for a woman whose vaginal musculature is relaxed and does not afford strong support, as in first degree cystocele, rectocele, or uterine prolapse; if the uterus is in an abnormal position, the arcing spring may offer better protection than the coil or flat spring, being stronger and better able to prevent the diaphragm from slipping out of the fornices of the vagina, thereby leaving the cervix exposed. Many women who have had a vaginal delivery are fitted with an arcing spring diaphragm, as some loss of vaginal muscle tone commonly occurs. An unusually long or short vagina or a vagina of unusual contour may often be well fitted with an arcing spring diaphragm. It is the most commonly prescribed kind of diaphragm, and, while heavier than the other kinds, is usually found to be comfortable to use. Compare **coil spring contraceptive diaphragm, flat spring contraceptive diaphragm.** See also **contraceptive diaphragm fitting.**

ARDS. 1. abbreviation for **adult respiratory distress syndrome.** 2. abbreviation for **acute respiratory distress syndrome.**

area, (in anatomy) a limited anatomical space that contains a specific structure of the body or within which certain physiologic functions predominate, as the aortic area and the association areas of the cerebral cortex.

arenavirus (ær'ınəvai'rəs), any one of a group of viruses usually transmitted to man by oral or cutaneous contact with the excreta of wild rodents. Individual arenaviruses are identified with specific geographical areas, as **Bolivian hemorrhagic fever,** in one river valley in Bolivia, **Lassa fever,** in Nigeria, Liberia, and Sierra Leone, and **Argentine hemorrhagic fever,** in two agricultural provinces in Argentina. Arenavirus infections are characterized by slow onset, fever, muscle pain, rash, petechiae, hemorrhage, delirium, hypotension, and ulcers of the mouth. Treatment is supportive; there is no specific antimicrobial agent or vaccine. Fluid and electrolyte balance, rest, and adequate nutrition are the goals of treatment.

areola (æri'oulə), pl. **areolae.** 1. a small space or a cavity within a tissue. 2. a circular area of a different color surrounding a central feature, as the discoloration about a pustule or vesicle. 3. the part of the iris around the pupil.

areola mammae (mæm'i), the pigmented, circular area surrounding the nipple of each breast. Also called **areola papillaris.**

areola papillaris (pæp'ılar'ıs). See **areola mammae.**

areolar gland (əri'ələr), one of the large sebaceous glands in the areolae encircling the nipples on the breasts of women. The areolar glands secrete a lipoid fluid that lubricates and protects the nipple during nursing, and contain smooth muscle bundles that cause the nipples to become erect when stimulated. Also called **gland of Montgomery.**

areolar tissue, a kind of connective tissue having little tensile strength and consisting of loosely woven fibers and areolae. Also called **fibroareolar tissue.** Compare **fibrous tissue.**

Arfonad, a trade name for a ganglion blocking agent antihypertensive (trimethaphan camsylate).

argentaffin cell, a cell containing serotonin-secreting granules that stain readily with silver and chromium parts. Such cells occur in most regions of the gastrointestinal tract and are especially abundant in the crypts of Lieberkühn. Also called **enterochromaffin cell, Kulchitsky's cell.** See also **carcinoid, carcinoid syndrome.**

argentaffinoma (ar'jentæf'ınou'mə), pl. **argentaffinomas, argentaffinomata.** a carcinoid tumor arising most often from argentaffin cells (Kultschitzky's cells) in epithelium of the crypts of Lieberkühn in the gastrointestinal tract. The neoplasm, which occurs chiefly in middle-aged or elderly persons, may be a nodule or plaque in the early stage and a growth encircling the bowel in the later stage.

Highly vascular tumors formed of silver-staining argentaffin cells may also develop in the bronchi.

argentaffinoma syndrome. See **carcinoid syndrome.**

Argentine hemorrhagic fever, an infectious disease caused by an arenavirus transmitted to humans by the ingestion of food contaminated by the excreta of infected rodents and by personal contact. Initially, it is characterized by chills, fever, headache, myalgia, anorexia, nausea, vomiting, and a general feeling of malaise. As the disease progresses, the patient may develop a high fever, dehydration, hypotension, flushed skin, abnormally slow heartbeat, bleeding from the gums and internal tissues, hematuria, and hematemesis. There may be involvement of the central nervous system, shock, and pulmonary edema. There is no specific treatment for the disease other than hydration, rest, warmth, and adequate nutrition. Rarely, intravenous fluids and dialysis are necessary. Usually, the prognosis is complete recovery. See also **arenavirus.**

argininemia (ar'jınını'miə), an autosomal recessive disorder characterized by an increased amount of arginine in the blood caused by a deficiency of arginase. Without arginase, ammonia cannot be metabolized into urea. Partial deficiency may result in hyperammonemia, metabolic alkalosis, convulsions, hepatomegaly, mental retardation, and growth failure; total deficiency is fatal. See also **ammonia, urea.**

argon (Ar), a colorless, odorless, chemically inactive gas and one of the six rare gases in the atmosphere. Its atomic weight is 8; its atomic number is 39.9.

Argyll Robertson pupil, a pupil that constricts on accommodation but not in response to light. It is most often seen in advanced neurosyphilis.

ariboflavinosis (ɪraɪ'boʊfleɪ'vɪnoʊ'sɪs), a condition caused by deficiency of vitamin B_2 in the diet and characterized by lesions at the corners of the mouth, on the lips, and around the nose and eyes, by seborrheic dermatitis, and by various visual disorders. See also **riboflavin.**

Aristocort, a trade name for a glucocorticoid (triamcinolone).

arithmetic mean. See **mean,** def. 2.

Arlidin, a trade name for a peripheral vasodilator (nylidrin hydrochloride).

arm, 1. a portion of the upper limb of the body between the shoulder and the elbow. The bone of the arm is the humerus. The muscles of the arm are the coracobrachialis, the biceps brachii, the brachialis, and the triceps brachii. Investing these structures is the brachial fascia. The arm is innervated by various nerves, as the ulnar nerve and the radial nerve, and is nourished by various arteries, as the brachial artery and the radial collateral artery. 2. *Nontechnical.* the arm and the forearm. See also **shoulder joint.**

arm bone. See **humerus.**

arm cylinder cast, an orthopedic device of plaster of Paris or fiberglass, used for immobilizing the upper limb from the wrist to the upper arm. It is most often applied to aid the healing of a dislocated elbow, for postoperative immobilization or positioning of the elbow, or in the correction or the maintenance of a correction of a deformity of the elbow.

armpit.   See **axilla.**

Arnold-Chiari malformation (ar′nəldkiar′i),   a congenital herniation of the brain stem and lower cerebellum through the foramen magnum into the cervical vertebral canal, often associated with hydrocephalus and spina bifida. See also **neural tube defect.**

aromatic alcohol,   a fatty alcohol in which part of the hydrogen of the alcohol radical is replaced by a phenyl hydrocarbon.

aromatic bath,   a medicated bath in which aromatic substances or essential oils are added to the water.

arrest,   to inhibit, restrain, or stop, as to arrest the course of a disease. See also **cardiac arrest.**

arrested dental caries,   dental caries in which the area of decay has stopped progressing and infection is not present but in which the demineralized area in the tooth remains as a cavity.

arrested development,   the cessation of one or more phases of the developmental process in utero before normal completion, resulting in congenital anomalies. Also called **developmental arrest.**

arrheno-,   a combining form meaning 'male': *arrhenoblastoma, arrhenogenic, arrhenoplasm.*

arrhenoblastoma (æri′nɔublæstou′mə),   an ovarian neoplasm whose cells mimic those in testicular tubules and secrete male sex hormone, causing virilization in females. Also called **andreioma, andreoblastoma, androma, Sertoli-Leydig cell tumor.**

arrhenoma (ær′ınɔu′mə).   See **arrhenoblastoma.**

arrhythmia, arrythmia (ərɪ*th*′miə, ərɪ*th*′miə,)   any deviation from the normal pattern of the heartbeat. Kinds of arrhythmias include **atrial fibrillation, atrial flutter, heart block, premature beat, sinus arrhythmia.** – **arrhythmic, arrhythmical,** *adj.*

arsenic (As),   an element that occurs throughout the earth's crust in metal arsenides, arsenious sulfides, and arsenious oxides. Its atomic number is 33; its atomic weight is 74.91. The arsenic atom occurs in the elemental form and in trivalent and pentavalent oxidation states. This element has been used for centuries as a therapeutic agent and as a poison and continues to have limited use in some trypanocidal drugs, as melarsoprol and tryparsamide. The introduction of nonarsenical trypanosomicides with less dangerous side effects in the treatment of trypanosomiasis has greatly reduced its use. Arsenic is usually not mined in raw form but recovered as a byproduct from the smelting of copper, lead, zinc, and other ores. Such processes release arsenic into the environment as does the leaching of large amounts of the element from

the soil by mineral springs and the effluent from geothermal power plants. It is a component of coal, released during combustion. The environmental distribution of arsenic assures its concentration in the food chain. Many compounds containing arsenic are used as pesticides, herbicides, and as feed additives for poultry and livestock. Fruit, vegetables, fish, and shellfish contain significant concentrations of arsenic. The average daily human consumption of this element is about 900 μg, most of which is ingested in food and water. The average concentration in the human adult is about 20 mg, an amount stored mainly in the liver, the kidney, the gastrointestinal tract, and the lungs. Small concentrations lodge in the muscles and neural tissue. Trivalent arsenicals, as inorganic arsenite, inhibit many enzymes and are poorly absorbed from the gastrointestinal tract. The mechanisms for the biotransformation of arsenicals in humans are not well understood. Most arsenicals are slowly excreted from the body, which accounts for the toxicity of the element. Most arsenic in the body is excreted in the urine and the feces. The pentavalent forms of arsenicals are rapidly excreted and cause much less toxicity than the trivalent forms. Chronic exposure to inorganic arsenicals, especially the trivalent compounds, may cause severe damage to the gastrointestinal lining, kidneys, central nervous system, bone marrow, liver, and blood system. Small doses of inorganic arsenic cause mild vasodilation; larger doses induce capillary dilation, cardiac disorders, and diminished blood volume. Various studies show a strong connection between the intensity and duration of exposure to arsenic and lung cancer in metal workers. Federal restrictions on arsenic levels in food and occupational environments have greatly reduced the incidence of both acute and chronic arsenic poisoning.

arsenic poisoning,   poisoning caused by the ingestion or inhalation of arsenic or a substance containing arsenic, an ingredient in some pesticides, herbicides, dyes, and medicinal solutions. Small amounts absorbed over a period of time may result in chronic poisoning, producing nausea, headache, coloration and scaling of the skin, hyperkeratoses, anorexia, and white lines across the fingernails. Ingestion of large amounts of arsenic results in severe gastrointestinal pain, diarrhea, vomiting, and swelling of the extremities. Renal failure and shock may occur, and death may result. Determination of the presence of arsenic in the urine, hair, or fingernails is diagnostic. Treatment includes gastric lavage with water and administration of British anti-lewisite, intravenous fluid therapy, and other supportive treatment as indicated for anemia, renal failure, or shock.

Artane,   a trade name for an anticholinergic (trihexyphenidyl hydrochloride).

arteri-.   See **arterio-.**

arteria alveolaris inferior. See **inferior alveolar artery.**

arterial, of or pertaining to an artery.

arterial blood gas, the oxygen and carbon dioxide in arterial blood, measured by various methods to assess the adequacy of ventilation and oxygenation, and the acid-base status. The oxygen content of arterial blood, normally 15 to 22 volumes per cent, is decreased in chronic obstructive lung disease, flail chest, kyphoscoliosis, neuromuscular impairment, obesity, hypoventilation, and postoperative respiratory complications. Oxygen saturation of hemoglobin is normally 95 per cent or higher. The partial pressure of oxygen (PaO_2), normally 80 to 100 mm Hg, is increased in polycythemia and hyperventilation and decreased in anemias, cardiac decompensation, chronic obstructive pulmonary disease, and certain neuromuscular disorders. The carbon dioxide content, normally 46 per cent, is increased in emphysema and aldosteronism and by severe vomiting; it is decreased in starvation, acute renal failure, diabetic acidosis, and severe diarrhea. Partial pressure of carbon dioxide, normally 38 to 42 mm Hg, may be higher in emphysema, obstructive lung disease, and reduced function of the respiratory center and lower in pregnancy and in the presence of pulmonary emboli and anxiety. The normal pH of arterial blood is 7.40.

arterial circle of Willis, the anastomosis at the base of the brain, formed by the anterior and the posterior cerebral arteries and branches of the internal carotid and the basilar arteries. The three arterial trunks supply each cerebral hemisphere, arise from the arterial circle of Willis. The trunks are the anterior, giving rise to the two anterior cerebral arteries, anterolateral, giving rise to the two middle cerebral arteries, and posterior, giving rise to the two posterior cerebral arteries.

arterial insufficiency, inadequate blood flow in arteries caused by occlusive atherosclerotic plaques or emboli, by damaged, diseased, or intrinsically weak vessels, by arteriovenous fistulas, aneurysms, hypercoagulability states, or heavy use of tobacco. Signs of arterial inadequacy include pale, cyanotic, or mottled skin over the affected area, absent or decreased sensations, tingling, diminished sense of temperature, muscle pains, as intermittent claudication in the calf following continuous exercise, reduced or absent peripheral pulses, and, in advanced disease, atrophy of muscles of the involved extremity. Arterial insufficiency may be diagnosed by checking and comparing peripheral pulses in contralateral extremities, by angiography, by ultrasound using a Doppler device, and by skin temperature tests. Normally immersion of an extremity in hot water increases the skin temperature of the opposite limb, but this usually does not occur in arterial disease; immersion of the patient's hand in ice water raises the bl ⁴ pressure about 45 mm Hg and the pulse pressure 2C while in the normal individual

the blood pressure increases only 25 mm Hg and the pulse pressure does not change. Treatment of arterial insufficiency may include a diet low in saturated fats, moderate exercise, sleeping on a firm mattress, the use of a vasodilator, and, if indicated, surgical repair of an aneurysm or arteriovenous fistula. Smoking, prolonged standing, and sitting with the knees bent are discouraged.

arterial insufficiency of lower extremities, a condition characterized by hardening, thickening, and loss of elasticity of the walls of peripheral arteries causing decreased circulation, sensation, and function. Symptoms include sharp, cramping pain during exercise or rest at night, numbness, skin changes ranging from pallor to ulceration, and loss of hair on the legs. Pedal and popliteal pulses may be diminished or absent. Laboratory studies usually show elevated plasma lipids.

arterial pressure, the stress exerted by the circulating blood on the walls of the arteries. The amount of arterial pressure in an individual is the product of the cardiac output and the systemic vascular resistance. A number of extrinsic and intrinsic factors serve to regulate and to maintain a reasonably constant arterial pressure. Extrinsic factors include neurological stimulation, catecholamines, prostaglandins and other hormones. Intrinsic factors include chemoreceptors and pressure-sensitive receptors in the arterial walls that act to cause vasoconstriction or vasodilation. Arterial blood pressure is commonly measured with a sphygmomanometer and stethoscope. Stress, hypervolemia, hypovolemia, and various drugs may alter the arterial pressure. See also **blood pressure.**

arterial wall, the fibrous enclosure of the many vessels that carry oxygenated blood from the heart to structures throughout the body, and of the pulmonary arteries that carry venous blood from the heart to the lungs. The arteries, like the veins, are cylindrical tubes enclosed by layers of different kinds of tissue. The inner layer is composed of a membrane of endothelium, a subendothelial layer of delicate connective tissue, and an internal elastic membrane. The endothelium of the inner layer is composed of a single layer of simple squamous cells and is continuous with the endothelium of the capillaries and the endocardium of the heart. The middle layer of tissue around each artery comprises most of the arterial wall and is composed of circular sheets of smooth muscle cells and elastic tissue. The outer layer consists of areolar connective tissue with a fine network of collagenous and elastic fibers. Most of the arteries in the body are of medium size, with a diameter of about four mm. The muscular coat is well developed, and nerves from the sympathetic system control the flow of blood into the areas served by the artery. The middle layer in smaller arteries is almost entirely muscular and in larger arteries is more elastic. The thickness of the outer layer varies with the location of the artery. In protected areas, as the abdominal and cranial cavities, the outer layer of associated arteries is very thin, but in more exposed locations, as in the limbs, it is much thicker. Larger arteries have a thick inner layer which in older people may contain atherosclerotic plaques of cholesterol and calcium salts or other pathological deposits.

arterio-, arteri-, a combining form meaning 'pertaining to an artery': *arteriosclerosis, arteriovenous, arteritis.*

arteriogram (artir'iəgræm'), an x ray of an artery injected with a radiopaque medium. See also **arteriography.**

arteriography (artir'iog'rəfi), a method of radiologic visualization of arteries performed after radiopaque contrast medium is introduced into the blood stream or into a specific vessel by injection or through a catheter. See also **angiography.** —**arteriographic,** *adj.*

arteriola (artir'iou'lə). See **arteriole.**

arteriole (artir'ioul), one of the blood vessels of the smallest branch of the arterial circulation. Blood flowing from the heart is pumped through the arteries to the arterioles to the capillaries into the veins and returned to the heart. The muscular wall of the arterioles constricts and dilates in response to neurochemical stimuli; thus, arterioles play a significant role in peripheral vascular resistance and in regulation of blood pressure.

arteriosclerosis, a common arterial disorder characterized by thickening, loss of elasticity, and calcification of arterial walls, resulting in a decreased blood supply, especially to the cerebrum and lower extremities. The condition often develops with aging, and in hypertension, nephrosclerosis, scleroderma, diabetes, and hyperlipidemia. Typical signs include intermittent claudication, changes in skin temperature and color, altered peripheral pulses, bruits over an involved artery, headache, dizziness, and memory defects. The use of vasodilators and exercise to stimulate collateral circulation may relieve symptoms of arteriosclerosis, but there is specific treatment for the disorder. Preventive measures include therapy of predisposing diseases, continued activity in later life, adequate rest, and avoidance of stress. Kinds of arteriosclerosis are **atherosclerosis, Mönckeberg's arteriosclerosis.**

arteriovenous (artir'iouvi'nəs), of or pertaining to arteries and veins.

arteriovenous angioma of the brain, a congenital tumor consisting of a tangle of coiled, usually dilated arteries and veins, islets of sclerosed brain tissue, and, occasionally, cartilaginous cells. The lesion, which may be distinguished by an intracranial bruit, generally arises in the vascular system of the pia mater and may grow to 8 project deeply into the brain, causing seizures and progressive hemiparesis.

arteriovenous fistula, an abnormal communication between an artery and vein occurring congenitally or resulting from trauma, infection, arterial aneurysm, or a malignancy. A continuous murmur and palpable thrill may be detected over the fistula and may be obliterated by compressing the feeding artery; this maneuver may slow the heart beat (Branham's sign). Chronic arteriovenous fistulas may give rise to varicosities, cutaneous ulcers, and cardiac enlargement. A congenital fistula may result in a cavernous hemangioma. If an arteriovenous fistula is limited in size and is in an accessible location, it can be treated by surgical excision. An arteriovenous fistula is often created surgically to provide access to the bloodstream of patients receiving hemodialysis.

arteritis (ar'tərai'tıs), an inflammatory condition of the inner layers or the outer coat of one or more arteries, occurring as a clinical entity or accompanying another disorder, as rheumatoid arthritis, rheumatic fever, polymyositis, or systemic lupus erythematosus. Kinds of arteritis include **infantile arteritis, rheumatic arteritis, Takayasu's arteritis, temporal arteritis.** See also **endarteritis, periarteritis.**

arteritis umbilicalis, a septic inflammation of the umbilical artery in newborn infants, usually by the bacteria of the species *Clostridium tetani.*

artery, one of the large blood vessels of arterial circulation carrying blood from the heart to the arterioles. The wall of an artery has three layers: the **tunica adventitia,** the outer coat; the **tunica media,** the middle coat; and the **tunica intima,** the inner coat. See also **arteriole.**

artery forceps, any forceps used for grasping, compressing, and holding the end of an artery during ligation. Generally self-locking, its handles are scissorlike. Also called **hemostatic forceps.**

arthr-, arthro-, a combining form meaning 'pertaining to a joint': *arthralgia, arthrocentesis.*

arthralgia (arfhræl'jiə), any pain that affects a joint. —**arthralgic,** *adj.*

-arthria, a combining form meaning a '(specified) condition involving the ability to articulate': *anarthria, dysarthria, pararthria.*

-arthritic, a combining form meaning 'pertaining to an arthritic condition': *antarthritic, antiarthritic, postarthritic.* Also **-arthritical.**

arthritis, any inflammatory condition of the joints, characterized by pain and swelling. See also **osteoarthritis, rheumatoid arthritis.**

arthritis deformans. See **rheumatoid arthritis.**

arthrocentesis (ar'frousıntı'sıs), the puncture of a joint with a needle and the withdrawal of fluid, performed to obtain samples of synovial fluid for diagnostic purposes. A local anesthetic is usually administered; meticulous asepsis is observed in the procedure. Normal synovial fluid is a clear, straw-colored, slightly viscous liquid that forms a white, ropy mucin clot when mixed with glacial acetic acid; but if inflammation is present, as in rheumatoid arthritis, the fluid is watery and turbid and its mixture with glacial acetic acid results in a flocculent, easily broken clot. The number of leukocytes, especially polymorphonuclear cells, and the protein content are increased and the glucose level is decreased if inflammation is present. Synovial fluid samples are also cultured and examined microscopically to diagnose a septic process, as bacterial arthritis.

arthrodesis. See **ankylosis,** def. 2.

arthrodia (arθrou′diə). See **gliding joint.**

arthrogryposis multiplex congenita, fibrous stiffness of one or more joints, present at birth, often associated with incomplete development of the muscles that move the involved joints and degenerative changes of the motor neurons that innervate those muscles. The cause of the condition, which is uncommon, is unknown. Physiotherapy to loosen the joints is the only treatment.

arthropathy (arθrop′əthi), any disease or abnormal condition affecting a joint. — **arthropathic,** adj.

arthroplasty (ar′θrəplæst′i), the surgical reconstruction or replacement of a painful, degenerated joint, to restore mobility to a joint in osteoarthritis, rheumatoid arthritis, or to correct a congenital deformity. Under general anesthesia one of two procedures is used: either the bones of the joint are reshaped and soft tissue or a metal disc is placed between the reshaped ends, or all or part of the joint is replaced with a metal or plastic prosthesis. Preoperative care includes the typing and cross-matching of blood. Postoperatively, the patient is immediately placed in traction to immobilize the affected limb. Exercise to increase muscle strength and range of motion is allowed in a slow, progressive schedule. Frequent checks of distal circulation are necessary if a cast is in place. The nurse watches for signs of surgical shock, thrombophlebitis, pulmonary embolism, or fat embolism. Antibiotics are usually given to prevent infection which is the most common cause of failure of the surgery. See also **osteoarthritis.**

arthropod (ar′θrəpod′), a member of the Arthropoda, a large phylum of animal life which includes crabs and lobsters as well as mites, ticks, spiders, and insects. Arthropods generally are distinguished by a jointed exoskeleton (shell) and paired, jointed legs; they bite, sting, cause allergic reactions, and carry viruses and other disease agents.

arthroscopy (arθros′kəpi), the examination of the interior of a joint, performed by inserting a specially designed endoscope through a small incision. The procedure, used chiefly in knee problems, permits biopsy of cartilage or synovium, the diagnosis of a torn meniscus, and, in some instances, the removal of loose bodies in the joint space. — **arthroscopic,** adj.

Arthus reaction (artus′), a rare, severe, immediate hypersensitivity reaction to a foreign substance, which is usually not irritating but, in certain individuals is antigenic. An acute local inflammatory reaction occurs at the site of injection. A sterile abscess may form that is slow to heal and that may become necrotic and secondarily infected. Also called **Arthus phenomenon.**

articul-, a combining form meaning 'pertaining to a joint': *articular, articulatio.*

articular capsule, an envelope of tissue that surrounds a freely moving joint, composed of an external layer of white fibrous tissue and an internal synovial membrane. See also **fibrous capsule.**

articular cartilage. See **cartilage.**

articular disc, the platelike end of certain bones in movable joints, developed from unabsorbed mesoderm and sometimes closely associated with surrounding muscles or with cartilage.

articular fracture, a fracture involving the articular surfaces of a joint.

articulatio cubiti (artık′yulei′shiou). See **elbow joint.**

articulatio ellipsoidea. See **condyloid joint.**

articulatio genus. See **knee joint.**

articulation. See **joint.**

articulation of the pelvis, any one of the connections between the bones of the pelvis, involving four groups of ligaments. The first group connects the sacrum and the ilium; the second, the sacrum and the ischium; the third, the sacrum and the coccyx; and the fourth, the two pubic bones.

articulatio plana. See **gliding joint.**

articulatio sellaris. See **saddle joint.**

artifact, anything extraneous or irrelevant, as a substance, structure, piece of information, etc.

artificial fever, an elevated body temperature produced by artificial means, as the injection of malarial parasites or of a vaccine known to produce fever symptoms, or by applying heat to the body. An artificial fever may be prescribed for a patient to arrest a disease that is sensitive to elevated body temperatures. Also called **fever therapy.**

artificial impregnation. See **artificial insemination.**

artificial insemination, the introduction of semen into the vagina or uterus by mechanical or instrumental means rather than by sexual intercourse. The procedure is planned to coincide with the expected time of ovulation so that fertilization can occur. Kinds of artificial insemination are **artificial insemination donor, artificial insemination husband.** Also called **artificial impregnation.** See also **menstrual cycle.**

artificial insemination donor (AID), artificial insemination in which the semen specimen is provided by an anonymous donor. The procedure is used primarily in cases where the husband is sterile. Also called **heterologous insemination.** Compare **artificial insemination husband.**

artificial insemination husband (AIH), artificial insemination in which the semen specimen is provided by the husband. The procedure is used primarily in cases of impotency or when the husband is incapable of sexual intercourse because of some physical disability. Also called **homologous insemination.** Compare **artificial insemination donor.**

artificial intelligence (AI), the capability of a device, as an industrial robot, to perform functions previously thought to require human intelligence. Computer technology produces many instruments and systems that mimic and surpass some human capabilities, as speed of counting, correlating, sensing, and deducing.

artificial kidney, a device used to rid blood, circulated outside of the body, of substances usually excreted in urine. It usually consists of a set of tubes or catheters for passing the blood between the person and a membrane unit for hemodialysis and a dialysate supply system. Also called **kidney machine.** See also **hemodialysis, peritoneal dialysis.**

artificial limb. See **prosthesis.**

artificial lung. See **Drinker respirator.**

artificially acquired immunity. See **acquired immunity.**

artificial pacemaker. See **cardiac pacemaker.**

artificial respiration, the process of maintaining respiration by manual or mechanical means when normal breathing has stopped. Effective ventilation of the lungs may fail because of bronchial obstruction by swelling, a foreign body, increased secretions, neuromuscular weakness, status asthmaticus, exhaustion, pharmacologic depression, or trauma to the chest wall. Before attempting to administer artificial respiration, the airway is tested

Position for pinching nose closed

Position for making seal around
patient's mouth

ARTIFICIAL RESPIRATION

and any obstruction removed; the pulse is palpated and the need for cardiopulmonary resuscitation is evaluated. See also **cardiopulmonary resuscitation, resuscitation, ventilator.**

artificial selection, the process by which the genotypes of successive plant and animal generations are determined through controlled breeding. Compare **natural selection.**

aryl hydrocarbon hydroxylase (AHH), an enzyme that converts carcinogenic chemicals in tobacco smoke and in polluted air into active carcinogens within the lungs. Aryl hydrocarbon hydroxylase is the subject of numerous studies to determine why some smokers develop cancer and others do not. Experimental blood tests indicate that the level of aryl hydrocarbon hydroxylase may be a factor in hereditary predisposition of a cigarette smoker to cancer.

As, symbol for **arsenic.**

as-. See **ad.**

ASA, abbreviation for **American Society of Anesthesiologists.**

asbestosis (æs′bestou′sis), a chronic lung disease caused by the inhalation of asbestos fibers that results in the development of alveolar, interstitial, and pleural fibrosis. Asbestos miners and workers are most frequently affected, but the disease sometimes occurs in other people who have been exposed to asbestos building materials. Chest x-ray films show the characteristic small linear opacities distributed throughout the lungs. The disease is progressive: shortness of breath develops, eventually, in respiratory failure. Cigarette smoking and continuous exposure to asbestos aggravate the condition. Fatal mesothelial tumors sometimes occur. There is no treatment. See also **chronic obstructive lung disease, inorganic dust.**

ASC, abbreviation for **altered state of consciousness.**

ascariasis (æs′kərai′əsis), an infection caused by a parasitic worm, *Ascaris lumbricoides,* that migrates through the lungs in its larval stage. The eggs are passed in human feces, contaminating the soil and allowing transmission to the mouths of others through hands, water, or food. After hatching in the small intestine, the larvae travel through the wall of the intestine, whence they are carried by the lymphatics and blood to the lungs. Early respiratory symptoms of coughing, wheezing, and fever are caused by the passage through the respiratory tract. The larvae are swallowed, they mature in the jejunum, where they release eggs, and the cycle is repeated. Intestinal infection may result in abdominal cramps and obstruction. In children, migration of the adult worms into the liver, gall bladder, or peritoneal cavity may cause death. The infective eggs are readily identified in the feces. Piperazine citrate, pyrantel pamoate, and mebendazole, are effective treatments. The disease can be prevented by educating people, especially children, about good sanitation habits and handwashing.

Ascaris (æs′kərıs), a genus of large parasitic intestinal roundworms, as *Ascaris lumbricoides,* a cause of ascariasis, found throughout temperate and tropical regions.

ascending aorta, one of the four main sections of the aorta, branching into the right and left coronary arteries, rising from the semilunar valve of the heart, curving to the right near the cranial border of the second right costal cartilage, and lying about 6 cm deep to the dorsal surface of the sternum. It is about 5 cm long and has three small aortic sinuses at its origin, opposite the aortic valve.

ascending colon, the segment of the colon that extends from the cecum in the lower right side of the abdomen to the transverse colon at the hepatic flexure on the right side, usually at the level of the umbilicus.

ascending current. See **centripetal current.**

ascending oblique muscle. See **obliquus internus abdominis.**

ascending pharyngeal artery, one of the smallest arteries that branch from the external carotid artery, deep in the neck, supplying various organs and muscles of the head, as the tympanic cavity, the longi capitis, and the colli. It divides into five branches, the pharyngeal, palatine, prevertebral, inferior tympanic, and posterior meningeal.

ascending urography. See **urography.**

Ascheim-Zondek (AZ) test (ash′haimtson′dek), an obsolete biologic test for pregnancy.

ascites (əsai′tiz), an abnormal intraperitoneal accumulation of a fluid containing large amounts of protein and electrolytes. Ascites may be detectable when more than 500 ml of fluid has accumulated. The condition may be accompanied by general abdominal swelling, hemodilution, edema, or a decrease in urinary output. Identification of ascites is made through auscultation, percussion, and palpation. Ascites is a complication of cirrhosis, congestive heart failure, nephrosis, malignant neoplastic disease, peritonitis, or various fungal and parasitic diseases. Ascites is treated with dietary therapy and diuretic drugs; abdominal paracentesis may be performed to relieve pain and improve respiratory and visceral function by relieving the pressure of the accumulated fluid. By lowering pressure within the portal system, paracentesis is therapeutic in ascites accompanied by bleeding. See also **paracentesis.** — **ascitic,** *adj.*

ascites adiposus. See **chylous ascites.**

ascites precox, an abnormal accumulation of fluid within the peritoneal cavity preceding the development of generalized edema associated with pericarditis. See also **ascites.**

ascorbemia (æs′korbi′miə), the presence of ascorbic acid in the blood in amounts greater than normal, usually reflecting only an excess of ascorbic acid in the diet.

ascorbic acid (əskor′bık), a water soluble, white crystalline vitamin present in citrus fruits, tomatoes, berries, potatoes, and fresh, green, leafy vegetables, such as broccoli, brussels sprouts, collards, turnip greens, parsley, sweet peppers, and cabbage. It is essential for the formation of collagen and fibrous tissue for normal intercellular matrices in teeth, bone, cartilage, connective tissue, and skin, and for the structural integrity of capillary walls. It also aids in fighting bacterial infections and interacts with other nutrients. Signs of deficiency are bleeding gums, tendency to bruising, swollen or painful joints, nosebleeds, anemia, lowered resistance to infections, and slow healing of wounds and fractures. Severe deficiency results in scurvy. An excess of ascorbic acid may cause a burning sensation during urination, diarrhea, skin rash, and nausea, and may disturb the absorption and metabolism of vitamin B_{12}. Tests for glycosuria, uric acid, and iron may be inaccurate when large amounts of the vitamin are being administered. Also called **antiscorbutic vitamin, cevitamic acid, vitamin C.** See also **ascorbemia, bioflavonoid, scurvy.**

ascorburia (æs′korbyur′iə), the presence of ascorbic acid in the urine in amounts greater than normal, usually reflecting only an excess of ascorbic acid in the diet.

ASD, abbreviation for **atrial septal defect.**

-ase, a combining form used in naming enzymes: *lipoidase, oxidase, protease.*

Asellacrin, a trade name for a growth stimulant (somatropin).

Asendin, a trade name for an antidepressant (amoxapine).

asepsis (eisep′sıs), **1.** the absence of germs. **2. medical asepsis,** the removal or destruction of disease organisms or infected material. **3. surgical asepsis,** protection against infection before, during, or following surgery by the use of sterile technique. — **aseptic,** *adj.*

aseptic fever, a fever not associated with infection. Mechanical trauma, as in a crushing injury, can cause fever even when no pathogenic microorganism is present. Although the exact mechanism is not understood, fever in such cases is believed to result from the breakdown of leukocytes or from the absorption of avascular tissue.

aseptic gauze, 1. sterile gauze prepared and packed for surgical use. **2.** any gauze that is free of microorganisms.

aseptic meningitis, an inflammation of the meninges that is caused by one of a number of viruses, including coxsackieviruses, nonparalytic polio viruses, echoviruses, and mumps. The disease is especially common in children during the late summer and early fall. In about one third of the cases no pathogen can be demonstrated, but analysis of cerebrospinal fluid reveals increased numbers of white blood cells, normal glucose concentration, and no bacteria. Symptoms vary depending upon the causative agent and may include fever, headache, stiff neck and back, nausea, and skin rash. No specific treatment is available. Supportive therapy is directed toward maintaining hydration and controlling the fever. Complete recovery, without complication or residual effect, is usual.

Asepto syringe, a trade name for a bulb-fitted, blunt-tipped syringe used primarily for irrigation of wounds.

asexual (eisek'shuəl), **1.** not sexual. **2.** of or pertaining to an organism that has no sexual organs. **3.** of or pertaining to a process that is not sexual. — **asexuality,** *n.*

asexual dwarf, an adult dwarf whose genital organs are underdeveloped.

asexual generation, any type of reproduction that occurs without the union of male and female gametes, as fission, budding, sporulation, or parthenogenesis. Also called **direct generation, nonsexual generation.**

asexualization (eisek'shuəlizei'shən), the process of making one incapable of reproduction; sterilization of an individual or animal by castration, vasectomy, removal of the ovaries, or other means.

asexual reproduction, a type of reproduction found in plants and lower animals in which new organisms are formed without the union of gametes, as occurs in budding, fission, and spore formation. Compare **sexual generation.**

Asherman syndrome (æsh'ərmən), secondary amenorrhea in a hormonally normal woman, caused by obliteration of the endometrial cavity by adhesions that form as a result of curettage or infection. It is diagnosed by hysterography and may be treated by secondary curettage (to remove adhesions), followed by placement in the uterus of a device to prevent reformation of adhesions during healing.

Asian flu. See **influenza.**

-asis, a combining form meaning an 'action, process, or result of': *basis, metabasis, oxydasis.*

ASLT, abbreviation for **antistreptolysin-O test.**

ASOT, abbreviation for **antistreptolysin-O test.**

asparaginase (æspær'əjineis), an enzyme that catalyzes the hydrolysis of asparagine to asparaginic acid and ammonia. Asparaginase is used as a chemotherapeutic agent in the treatment of acute lymphoblastic leukemia.

aspartate kinase, an enzyme that catalyzes the transfer of a phosphate group from adenosine triphosphate to aspartate to produce phosphoaspartate.

aspartate transaminase (æspar'teit), an enzyme that catalyzes the breakdown of the amino acid aspartic acid to fumaric acid and ammonia by transferring an amino group from the aspartic acid molecule to another molecule.

aspartic acid (æspar'tik), a nonessential amino acid present in sugar cane, beet molasses, and the breakdown products of many proteins. Pure aspartic acid is a water-soluble, colorless crystalline substance. In the Krebs' citric acid cycle, aspartic acid and oxaloacetic acid are interconvertible. Aspartic acid is used in culture media, dietary

supplements, detergents, fungicides, and germicides. Also called **aminosuccinic acid.**

aspergillic acid (æs'pərjil'ik), an antibiotic substance derived from *Aspergillus flavus,* an aflatoxin-producing mold found on corn, grain, and peanuts.

aspergillosis (æs'pərjilou'sis), an infection caused by a fungus of the genus *Aspergillus,* most commonly affecting the ear but capable of causing inflammatory, granulomatous lesions on or in any organ. The infection is relatively uncommon and typically occurs in a person already weakened by some other disorder. Topical fungicides can be used on the skin; amphotericin B is used to treat systemic aspergillosis, especially if it has spread to the lungs. The prognosis, as for most systemic fungal infections, is poor.

Aspergillus (æs'pərjil'əs), a genus of fungi that is a common contaminant in the laboratory and a cause of nosocomial infection. The fungus has hyphae and spores, lives in the soil, is ubiquitous, and proliferates rapidly. Inhalation of the spores of the two pathogenic species, *Aspergillus fumigatus* and *A. flavus,* is common, but infection is rare.

aspermia (eispər'miə), lack of formation or ejaculation of semen.

asphyxia (æsfik'siə), severe hypoxia leading to hypoxemia and hypercapnea, loss of consciousness, and, if not corrected, death. Some of the more common causes of asphyxia are drowning, electric shock, aspiration of vomitus, lodging of a foreign body in the respiratory tract, inhalation of toxic gas or smoke, and poisoning. Artificial ventilation and oxygen are promptly administered to avoid damage to the brain. The underlying cause is then treated. See **artificial respiration.** — **asphyxiate,** *v.,* **asphyxiated,** *adj.*

aspirating needle, a long hollow needle used to remove fluid from a cavity, vessel, or structure of the body.

aspiration (æs'pirei'shən), **1.** the act of taking a breath, inhaling. **2.** the act of withdrawing a fluid, as mucus or serum, from the body by a suction device. See also **aspiration pneumonia.** — **aspirate,** *n.*

aspiration biopsy, the removal of living tissue for microscopic examination by suction through a fine needle attached to a syringe. The procedure is used primarily to obtain cells from a lesion containing fluid or when fluid is formed in a serous cavity. See also **cytology, needle biopsy.**

aspiration biopsy cytology (ABC), a microscopic examination of cells obtained directly from living body tissue by aspiration through a fine needle. It is used primarily as a diagnostic procedure, generally as a technique for detecting nuclear and cytoplasmic changes in cancerous tissue. Compare **exfoliative cytology.**

aspiration of vomitus, the inhalation of regurgitated

gastric contents into the pulmonary system. See also **aspiration, aspiration pneumonia.**

aspiration pneumonia, an inflammatory condition of the lungs and bronchi caused by the inhalation of vomitus containing acid gastric contents. See also **pneumonia.**

■ OBSERVATIONS: Aspiration pneumonia most often occurs during anesthesia or recovery from anesthesia or during a seizure of acute alcoholic intoxication or other condition characterized by vomiting and a decreased level of consciousness.

■ INTERVENTION: Treatment requires prompt suctioning of the bronchi and the administration, under pressure, of 100 per cent oxygen. Continued artificial ventilation may be required. Corticosteroids are usually given to diminish inflammation. The sputum is cultured regularly, and any bacterial infection thus diagnosed is treated with an appropriate antibiotic. As long as oxygen is required, frequent analyses of the levels of gases in the blood are performed.

■ NURSING CONSIDERATIONS: The pulse rate and quality of respirations, level of consciousness, and the color of the skin are carefully monitored. Infection and respiratory failure are frequent complications. Aspiration pneumonia may be avoided by correctly positioning unconscious patients with the head low and turned to the side and by paying careful attention to the maintenance of an adequate airway. An oral airway is left in place until the patient can take it out, and secretions are removed by suction as necessary.

aspirator, any instrument that removes a substance from body cavities by suction, as a bulb syringe, piston pump, or hypodermic syringe.

aspirin, an analgesic, antipyretic, and antirheumatic.

■ INDICATIONS: It is prescribed to reduce fever and for the relief of pain and inflammation.

■ CONTRAINDICATIONS: Bleeding disorders, peptic ulcer, pregnancy, the concomitant use of anticoagulants, or known hypersensitivity to salicylates prohibits its use.

■ ADVERSE EFFECTS: Among the most serious adverse reactions are gastrointestinal effects (ulcers, occult bleeding); sustained treatment with large doses can cause clotting defects, liver toxicity, and renal toxicities. An asthmatic-like and other allergic reactions are occasionally seen. Dyspepsia is the most common adverse effect.

aspirin poisoning. See **salicylate poisoning.**

ASRT, abbreviation for **American Society of Radiologic Technologists.**

Assam fever (æsæm′). See **kala-azar.**

assault, 1. an unlawful act that places another person, without that persons's consent, in fear of immediate bodily harm or battery. The act must be presently possible, thus causing well-founded apprehension in the victim of the assault. 2. the act of committing an assault. 3. to threaten a person with bodily harm or injury.

assertion training. See **assertive training.**

assertive training, a technique used in behavior therapy to help individuals become more self-assertive and self-confident in interpersonal relationships. It focuses on the direct, honest statement of feelings and beliefs, both positive and negative. The technique is learned by role playing in a therapeutic setting, usually in a group, followed by practice in actual situations. Also called **assertion training.**

assessing, (in five-step nursing process) a category of nursing behavior that includes gathering, verifying, and communicating information relative to the client. The nurse collects information from verbal interactions with the client, the client's family and significant others; examines standard data sources for information; systematically checks for symptoms and signs; determines the client's ability to perform self-care activities; assesses the client's environment; and identifies reactions of the staff (including the nurse who is performing the assessment) to the client and to the client's family and significant others. To verify the data the nurse confirms the observations and perceptions by gathering additional information; discusses the orders and decisions made by other members of the staff with them, when indicated; and personally evaluates and checks the patient's condition. The nurse reports the information that has been gathered and verified. Although assessing is the first of the five steps of the nursing process, preceding analyzing, in practice assessing is integral to effective nursing practice at all steps of the process. See also **evaluating, implementing, planning.**

assessment, (in medicine and nursing) 1. an evaluation or appraisal of a condition. 2. the process of making such an evaluation. 3. (in a problem-oriented medical record) an examiner's evaluation of the disease or condition based on the patient's subjective report of the symptoms and course of the illness or condition and the examiner's objective findings, including data obtained through laboratory tests, physical examination, and medical history. See also **nursing assessment, problem-oriented medical record.** —**assess,** v.

assessment of the aging patient, an evaluation of the changes characteristic of advancing years exhibited by an elderly person.

■ METHOD: The patient is measured, weighed, examined, observed, and questioned about physical, functional, and behavioral changes; height normally diminishes 0.5 inch with aging, and weight steadily decreases in men over 65 years old but increases in women. The skin is examined for dryness, wrinkles, sagging, thinning over the back of the hands, areas of vitiligo, keratoses, warts, skin tags, senile telangiectases, and the hair for depigmentation, lack of lustre, and thinning or loss on the scalp and in the axillary and the pubic areas. Observations are made of enlargement of the nose and ears relative to face size, dryness of the eyes, discoloration of the sclera and iris, an opaque ring near the edge of the cornea (arcus senilis), decreased size of the pupil, and diminished peripheral vision. Tests are performed to determine if there is hearing loss, especially of high frequency tones, decreased tidal volume, diminished peripheral perfusion, or deviation of the trachea, especially if scoliosis is present. Examination may reveal gum recession, loss of teeth and taste perception, diminished salivation, a decreased resting heart rate and cardiac output, and an easily palpable arterial pulse. The elderly patient may show decreased muscle mass, osteoarthritic joints, Heberden's or Bouchard's nodes at finger joints, contracture of lateral fingers, osteoporosis, a broad-based stance, and slow voluntary movements. The sense of position, of smell and of touch and the sensitivity to heat and cold may be diminished, and deep tendon reflexes may be decreased. Signs of aging that may be found in women are pendulous, flaccid breasts; vaginal narrowing and shortening, and diminished lubrication, causing painful coitus; and effects of long-term estrogen therapy, as uterine bleeding, mastalgia, weight gain, fluid retention, and hypertension. Signs of aging in men include decrease in the size and firmness of the testes and in the amount and viscosity of seminal fluid, an increased diameter of the penis, and prostatic hypertrophy; libido and a sense of satisfaction usually do not diminish.

■ NURSING ORDERS: The nurse faces the patient during the evaluation, establishes eye contact, repeats questions if necessary, avoids shouting, and addresses the person by name. If the patient's visual perception and tactile sense are diminished, the nurse uses color contrasts and items of marked textural differences in the assessment.

■ OUTCOME CRITERIA: Aging does not progress at a uniform rate and its effects may vary widely from one individual to the next, but, in many cases, changes considered normal in elderly patients are disease processes that may respond to treatment. A careful assessment distinguishes the effects of pathology from those of aging and elucidates the care needed by the patient.

assimilation, 1. the process of incorporating nutritive material into living tissue; the end stage of the nutrition process, following digestion and absorption or occurring simultaneously with absorption. 2. (in psychology) Compare **apperception.** the incorporation of new experiences into a person's pattern of consciousness. 3. (in sociology) the process in which a person or a group of people of a different ethnic background become absorbed into a new culture. —**assimilate,** v.

assisted breech, an obstetrical operation in which a baby being born feet or buttocks first is permitted to deliver spontaneously as far as its umbilicus and is then extracted. Also called **partial breech extraction.** Compare **breech extraction.**

assisted ventilation. See **IPPB.**

associate degree in nursing, an academic degree awarded upon satisfactory completion of a two-year course of study, usually at a community or junior college. The recipient is eligible to take the national licensing examination to become a registered nurse. An associate degree in nursing is not available in Canada.

associate nurse, U.S. 1. (in primary nursing) a nurse who is responsible for implementing a primary nurse's care plans. 2. in some states, a registered nurse who holds a diploma from a hospital school of nursing or an associate degree from a two-year academic school of nursing.

association, 1. a connection, union, joining, or combination of things. 2. (in psychology) the connection of remembered feelings, emotions, sensations, thoughts, or perceptions with particular persons, things, or ideas. Kinds of association are **association of ideas, clang association, controlled association, dream association, free association.**

association area, any part of the cerebral cortex involved in the integration of sensory information. Also called **association cortex.**

association cortex. See **association area.**

Association for Practitioners of Infection Control (APIC), a national professional organization of nurses who work in the field of infection control.

Association for the Care of Children's Health (ACCH), an international, interdisciplinary organization concerned with the psychosocial needs of children and their families in health-care settings. A quarterly journal and a bimonthly newsletter are available to members. There are affiliate organizations throughout the United States and Canada.

Association of Canadian Medical Colleges (ACMC), a Canadian organization of the deans and faculty members of the nation's sixteen medical schools. It is concerned with all aspects of the education of physicians and acts as the liaison between the member schools and other professional organizations and governmental agencies. The official languages of the ACMC are French and English.

association of ideas, a mental connection established between similar or simultaneously occurring ideas, feelings, or perceptions.

Association of Operating Room Nurses (AORN), a national organization of operating room nurses.

association test, a technique used in psychiatric diagnosis and in educational and psychological evaluation in which a person is asked to respond to a stimulus word with the first word that comes to mind. The time taken to respond and the associations offered are compared to pretested responses and are classified and enumerated for diagnostic significance. Also called **word association test.**

associative play, a form of play in which a group of children participate in similar or identical activities without formal organization, group direction, group interaction, or a definite goal. The children may borrow or lend toys or pieces of play equipment and they may imitate others in the group, but each child acts independently, as on a playground or among a group riding tricycles or bicycles. Compare **cooperative play.** See also **parallel play, solitary play.**

astatine (At), a very unstable, radioactive element that occurs naturally in very small amounts. Its atomic number is 85; its atomic weight is 210.

-aster, a combining form meaning 'star-shaped': *cytaster, diaster, oleaster.*

astereognosis (əstir'iognou'sis), a neurologic disorder characterized by an inability to identify objects by touch.

asterixis (æs'tərik'sis), a hand-flapping tremor, often accompanying metabolic disorders. The tremor is usually induced by extending the arm and dorsiflexing the wrist. Asterixis is seen frequently in hepatic coma. Also called **flapping tremor, liver flap.**

asteroid body, an irregular star-shaped structure which develops in the giant cells in certain diseases, including sarcoidosis, actinomycosis, and nocardiosis.

asthenia (æsfhi'niə), **1.** the lack or loss of strength or energy; weakness; debility. **2.** (in psychiatry) lack of dynamic force in the personality. Kinds of asthenia include **asthenia gravis hypophyseogenea, myalgic asthenia, neurocirculatory asthenia, tropical anhidrotic asthenia.** See also **adynamia.** — **asthenic,** *adj.*

-asthenia, a combining form meaning '(condition of) depleted vitality': *gangliasthenia, neurasthenia phlebasthenia.*

asthenic fever, *Archaic.* an abnormal rise in body temperature associated with mental depression and characterized by a weak pulse and cool, moist skin.

asthenic habitus, a body structure characterized by a slender build with long limbs, an angular profile, and prominent muscles or bones.

asthenic personality, a personality characterized by low energy, lack of enthusiasm, and oversensitivity to physical and emotional strain. A person who has this kind of personality may be easily fatigued and self-pitying, and he may place the burden of his physical and emotional difficulties on others.

asthma (æz'mə), a respiratory disorder characterized by recurring episodes of paroxysmal dyspnea, wheezing on expiration, coughing, and viscous mucoid bronchial secretions. The episodes may be precipitated by inhalation of allergens or pollutants, infection, vigorous exercise, or emotional stress. Treatment includes elimination of the causative agent, hyposensitization, aerosol or oral bronchodilators, and short term use of corticosteroids. Beta-adrenergic drugs, barbiturates, and narcotics are contraindicated. Repeated attacks often result in emphy-sema and permanent obstructive lung disease. See also **allergic asthma, asthma in children, intrinsic asthma, status asthmaticus.**

-asthma, a combining form meaning '(condition of) labored breathing': *acetonasthma, cardiasthma, corasthma.*

asthma crystal. See **Charcot-Leyden crystal.**

asthma in children, an obstructive respiratory condition characterized by recurring attacks of paroxysmal dyspnea, wheezing, prolonged expiration, and an irritative cough that is a common, chronic illness in childhood. Onset usually occurs between the ages of three and eight. Asthmatic attacks are caused by constriction of the large and small airways, resulting from bronchial smooth-muscle spasm, edema or inflammation of the bronchial wall, or excessive production of mucus. It is a complex disorder involving biochemical, immunologic, infectious, endocrinologic, and psychologic factors. Asthma in children is usually extrinsic, that is, most attacks are associated with an allergenic hypersensitivity to a foreign substance, as airborne pollen, mold, house dust, certain foods, animal hair and skin, feathers, insects, smoke, and various chemicals or drugs. In infants, especially those born into a family with a history of allergic reactions, food allergy is a common precipitating factor. In some instances, episodes are triggered by nonallergenic factors, as infection or inflammation, bronchial compression from external pressure, obstruction by a foreign body, physical stress resulting from fatigue or exercise, exposure to cold air, or psychological stress. Such cases are classified as nonallergic, or intrinsic asthma. A few cases may be caused by an inherited or acquired defect of adrenergic and cholinergic control of airway diameter. There is a strong hereditary factor associated with the disease. As many as 75 per cent of children with asthma have a family history of the disorder, and the child usually has other allergic manifestations, as hay fever, eczema, or urticaria. The disease occurs twice as often in boys as in girls prior to puberty, but both boys and girls are affected equally during adolescence. Also called **bronchial asthma.**

■ OBSERVATIONS: The condition is often confused with acute middle and lower respiratory tract infections, congenital stridor, obstruction of the bronchi or trachea, bronchial or tracheal compression, and cystic fibrosis. The diagnosis is generally determined by observation during a physical examination, a medical history confirming a presence of allergic reactions and familial allergic disease, and, to a lesser degree, laboratory tests and x rays, which primarily eliminate identification of other diseases. A unique diagnostic feature is the presence of large numbers of eosinophils and their crystalloid degenerative fragments, called Charcot-Leyden crystals, in the sputum. Pulmonary function tests are valuable for assessing the degree of airway obstruction and the volume of gas exchange. Asthmatic episodes vary greatly in frequency, duration, and degree of symptoms, ranging from occasional periods of wheezing, mild coughing, and slight dypsnea to severe attacks that can lead to total airway obstruction and respiratory failure. An attack may begin gradually or abruptly and is often preceded by an upper respiratory infection. In general, episodes caused by infection have a gradual onset and are of long duration, while those resulting from allergenic factors are acute and subside quickly if the causative agent is removed. Typically, an attack begins with shortness of breath, paroxysms of wheezing, and a hacking, nonproductive cough. As secretions increase, the expiratory phase becomes prolonged, the cough gets deeper and more rattling, and a large quantity of thick, tenacious, mucoid sputum is produced as the attack subsides. The child appears apprehensive, speaks in a panting manner, and may assume a bent-over position to facilitate breathing. The prolonged expiratory phase is not as noticeable in infants and young children. In severe spasm or obstruction the respirations become shallow and irregular. A sudden increase in the rate of respiration, repeated hacking, and nonproductive coughing are indicative of lack of air movement with impending ventilatory failure and asphyxia. Children with chronic asthma develop a barrel chest from the continuous hyperventilated state and usually carry their shoulders in an elevated position to make better use of the accessory muscles of respiration.

■ INTERVENTION: An acute asthmatic attack is a medical emergency and requires immediate relief of bronchial obstruction with bronchodilating drugs, reduction of mucosal edema, and removal of excess bronchial secretions. The major drugs used to relieve bronchospasm are the beta-adrenergic agents, including epinephrine, isoproterenol, ephedrine, isoetharine, metaproterenol, terbutaline, and salbutamol; the methylxanthines, including theophylline and aminophylline; corticosteroids; expectorants; sedatives; and antibiotics for cases in which infection is the triggering mechanism. Rarely, an acute attack does not respond to any of these measures, resulting in status asthmaticus. Hospitalization is required. The child is usually in a state of dehydration and acidosis with hypoxia and hypercapnia. Management consists of intravenous fluids; humidified oxygen given by tent, face mask, or cannula; administration of sodium bicarbonate or tromethamine to keep pH at acceptable levels; and use of bronchodilators to alleviate bronchospasm and of antibiotics to reduce risk of infection. Children with mild, intermittent episodes of asthma are treated with bronchodilators in aerosol sprays, which provide quick relief and are effective in controlling an attack at the outset; oral administration is preferred for younger children. Those with persistent chronic asthma receive daily oral doses of a bronchodilator, often theophylline, usually in combination with an expectorant and corticosteroids. Broncho-

spasm induced by exercise can be treated prophylactically with cromolyn sodium, which inhibits the release of histamine in the lungs. Long-range management and treatment consist of physical training and exercises to induce physical and mental relaxation, improve posture, strengthen respiratory musculature, and develop better breathing patterns. Hyposensitization is recommended when an allergen is known and cannot be avoided. Prognosis for children with asthma varies considerably; many children lose their symptoms at puberty. Prognosis depends on the number and severity of symptoms, emotional factors, and the family history of allergy.

■ NURSING CONSIDERATIONS: The primary focus of nursing care for children with acute asthma is to relieve symptoms of respiratory distress by initiating intravenous infusion and oxygen therapy, correcting acidosis, and administering bronchodilators and corticosteroids. The nurse implements measures to promote physical comfort, induce rest, and reduce fatigue and anxiety. It is especially important to reassure the child and parents concerning procedures, equipment, and prognosis. The nurse also plays an important role in the long-term support of children with chronic asthma, primarily in teaching the child and parents about the disease and how to cope with the condition. Once an allergen is determined, the home environment may be modified to reduce contact with the causative agents. The nurse teaches the child and parents how to use prescribed medications, especially nebulizers and aerosol devices, how to detect early signs of an attack so that it can be controlled with medication, how to determine any adverse effects of the drugs, especially the dangers of overuse, and how to implement physical exercise and play activities as therapeutic measures, especially those that promote proper breathing techniques. Children with emotional problems require special attention; psychological stresses often trigger asthmatic attacks, and psychotherapy or behavior therapy is often necessary.

-asthmatic, a combining form meaning 'pertaining to asthma, its symptoms, or its treatment': *antiasthmatic, nonasthmatic, postasthmatic.*

asthmatic eosinophilia, a form of eosinophilic pneumonia, characterized by allergic bronchospasm, by expectoration of bronchial casts containing eosinophils and mycelium, and by cough and fever. The condition usually occurs in the fourth or fifth decade of life, and is twice as common in women as in men. It is a result of hypersensitivity to *Aspergillus fumigatus* or *Candida albicans.* Untreated, the condition may result in pleural effusion, pericarditis, ascites, encephalitis, hepatomegaly, and respiratory failure. Treatment is similar to that for asthma and includes administration of corticosteroids and antibiotics. Desensitization to the allergen is not usually effective. See also **allergic asthma, eosinophilic pneumonia.**

Astiban, a trade name for an investigational parasiticide (sodium stibocaptate), available only from the Center for Disease Control.

astigmatism (əstɪg′mətɪz′əm), an abnormal condition of the eye in which the light rays cannot be focused clearly in a point on the retina because the spherical curve of the cornea is not equal in all meridians. Vision is blurred and use of the eyes causes discomfort. The person cannot accommodate to correct the problem. The condition usually may be corrected with contact lenses or with eyeglasses ground to neutralize the defect.

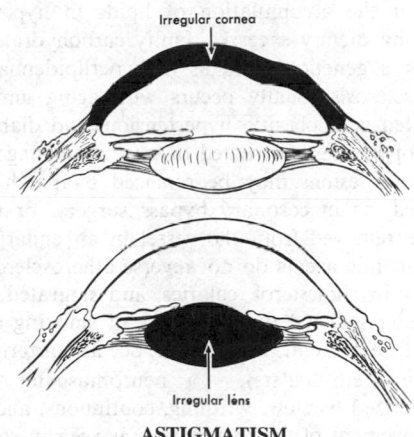

Irregular cornea

Irregular lens

ASTIGMATISM

astragalus (æstræg′ələs), *pl.* **astragali.** See **talus.**

astringent (əstrɪn′jɪnt), **1.** a substance that causes contraction of tissues upon application, usually used locally. **2.** having the quality of an astringent. — **astringency,** *n.*

astringent bath, a bath in which alum, tannic acid, or another astringent is added to the water.

astro-, a combining form meaning 'pertaining to a star, or star-shaped': *astroblastoma, astrocytoma, astrophorous.*

astroblastoma (æs′trɒublæstou′mə), *pl.* **astroblastomas, astroblastomata.** a malignant neoplasm of the brain and spinal cord. Cells of an astroblastoma lie around blood vessels or, in some cases, cluster around connective tissue septa.

astrocytic glioma (æs′trɒusaɪ′tɪk). See **astrocytoma.**

astrocytoma (æs′trɒusaɪtou′mə), *pl.* **astrocytomas, astrocytomata.** a primary tumor of the brain composed of astrocytes and characterized by slow growth, cyst formation, invasion of surrounding structures, and, often, the development of a highly malignant glioblastoma within the tumor mass. Complete surgical resection of an astrocytoma may be possible early in the development of the tumor.

astrocytosis, an increase in the number of neuroglial cells with fibrous or protoplasmic processes frequently observed in an irregular area adjacent to degenerative lesions, as abscesses, certain brain neoplasms, and encephalomalacia. Astrocytosis represents a reparative process, and in some cases it may be diffuse in a fairly large region.

asymmetrical (ei′sɪmet′rɪkəl, æsɪmet′rɪkəl), **asymmetric** (ei′sɪmet′rɪk, æs′ɪmet′rɪk), (of the body or parts of the body) unequal in size or shape; different in placement or arrangement about an axis. Compare **symmetrical.** — **asymmetry** (eisɪm′ɪtri, æsɪm′ɪtri), *n.*

asymmetric tonic neck reflex. See **tonic neck reflex.**

asynclitism (əsɪŋ′klɪtɪz′əm), presentation of a parietal aspect of the fetal head to the maternal pelvic inlet in labor, the sagittal suture being parallel to the transverse diameter of the pelvis but anterior or posterior to it. In normal labor, the fetal head usually engages with some degree of asynclitism. **Anterior asynclitism,** in which the anterior parietes present, is called Nägele's obliquity. **Posterior asynclitism** is called Litzmann's obliquity. See also **engagement, mechanism of labor.**

asynergy (eisɪn′ərji), **1.** a condition characterized by faulty coordination among groups of organs or muscles that normally function harmoniously. **2.** the state of muscle antagonism found in cerebellar disease. See also **ataxia, cerebellum.**

asyntaxia (ei′sɪntæk′siə), any interference with the orderly sequence of growth and differentiation of the fetus during embryonic development, resulting in one or more congenital anomalies. A kind of asyntaxia is **asyntaxia dorsalis.** See also **developmental anomaly.**

asyntaxia dorsalis, failure of the neural tube to close during embryonic development. See also **neural tube defect.**

asystole (eisɪs′təli, eisɪstol′ɪk), the absence of a heartbeat, as distinguished from fibrillation in which electrical activity persists but contraction ceases. Cardiotoxic asystole is characterized by a brief period of cardiac arrest caused by an acceleration in the heart rate. Asystole requires immediate cardiopulmonary resuscitation with cardiac massage and adequate ventilation. If these measures fail to initiate heart contractions a discharge with a defibrillator may be administered and, if that is ineffective, an intracardiac injection of epinephrine may be given (taking care to avoid direct myocardial injection), or 5 to 10 ml. of 1.0 per cent calcium chloride may be injected into the ventricular cavity. Also called **cardiac arrest, cardiac standstill.** — **asystolic,** *adj.*

At, symbol for **astatine.**

at-. See **ad-.**

Atabrine Hydrochloride, a trade name for an antimalarial (quinacrine hydrochloride).

Atarax, a trade name for an antianxiety, antiemetic, and anticholinergic (hydroxyzine hydrochloride).

atavism (æt′əvɪz′əm), the appearance in an individual of traits or characteristics more like those of a grandparent or earlier ancestor than of the parents. Atavistic data may offer clues to an examining physician of genetic or familial health factors. — **atavistic,** *adj.*

ataxia (ətæk'sɪə), an abnormal condition characterized by impaired ability to coordinate movement. A staggering gait and postural imbalance are caused by a lesion in the spinal cord or cerebellum, which might be the sequela of birth trauma, congenital disorder, infection, degenerative disorder, neoplasm, toxic substance, or head injury. See also **hereditary ataxia.**

ataxic aphasia (ətæk'sɪk). See **motor aphasia.**

ataxic speech, abnormal speech characterized by faulty formation of the sounds owing to neuromuscular dysfunction.

ATCC, abbreviation for **American Type Culture Collection.**

-ate[1], **1.** a combining form meaning 'acted upon or being in a (specified) state': *degenerate, disparate, enucleate.* **2.** a combining form meaning 'possessing': *caudate, cuspidate, longipedate.*

-ate[2], **1.** a combining form meaning a 'chemical compound derived from a (specified) source': *silicate, sulfate, opiate.* **2.** a combining form meaning an 'acid compound': *acetate, oxalate, phosphate.*

atelectasis (æt'ɪlek'təsɪs), an abnormal condition characterized by the collapse of lung tissue, preventing the respiratory exchange of carbon dioxide and oxygen. Symptoms include diminished breath sounds, a mediastinal shift toward the side of the collapse, fever, and increasing dyspnea. The condition may be caused by obstruction of the major airways and bronchioles, by pressure on the lung from fluid or air in the pleural space, or by pressure from a tumor outside the lung. As the remaining portions of the lung eventually hyperinflate, oxygen saturation of the blood is often nearly normal. Loss of functional lung tissue may secondarily cause increased heart rate, blood pressure, and respiratory rate. The retained secretions are rich in nutrients for the growth of bacteria, a condition often leading to stasis pneumonia in critically ill patients. See also **postoperative atelectasis, primary atelectasis.**

atelectatic rale, an abnormal intermittent crackling sound heard during auscultation of the chest. It usually disappears after the individual being examined coughs or breathes deeply several times.

ateliotic dwarf, a dwarf whose skeleton is incompletely formed, resulting from the nonunion of the epiphyses and diaphyses during bone development.

atelo-, a combining form meaning 'imperfect or incomplete': *atelocardia, ateloglossia, atelopodia.*

atheroma (æth'ɪrou'mə), *pl.* **atheromas, atheromata.** an abnormal mass of fat or lipids, as in a sebaceous cyst or in deposits in an arterial wall. — **atheromatous,** *adj.*

atheromatosis (æth'ɪroumətou'sɪs), the development of many atheromas.

atherosclerosis (æth'ərousklərou'sɪs), a common arterial disorder characterized by yellowish plaques of cholesterol, lipids, and cellular debris in the inner layers of the walls of large and medium-sized arteries. With the formation of the plaques, the vessel walls become thick, fibrotic, and calcified, and the lumen narrows, resulting in reduced circulation in organs and areas normally supplied by the artery. Atheromatous lesions are major causes of coronary heart disease, angina pectoris, myocardial infarction, and other cardiac disorders. The pathogenesis of atherosclerosis is not clear; it may be induced by injury to arterial endothelium, the proliferation of smooth muscle in vessel walls, or the accumulation of lipids in hyperlipidemia caused by dietary excesses, faulty carbohydrate metabolism, or a genetic defect, as in hyperlipidemia Type II. Atherosclerosis usually occurs with aging and is often associated with obesity, hypertension, and diabetes. Segments of arteries obstructed or severely damaged by atheromatous lesions may be replaced by patch grafts or bypassed, as in coronary bypass surgery, or the lesion may be removed from the vessel in an endarterectomy. Antilipidemic agents do not reverse atherosclerosis, but a diet low in cholesterol, calories, and saturated fats, adequate exercise, and the avoidance of smoking and stress may help to prevent the disorder. See also **arteriosclerosis.**

athetosis (æth'ɪtou'sɪs), a neuromuscular condition characterized by slow, writhing, continuous, and involuntary movement of the extremities, as seen in some forms of cerebral palsy and in motor disorders resulting from lesions in the basal ganglia.

athiaminosis (əthaɪ'əmɪnou'sɪs), a condition resulting from lack of thiamine in the diet. See also **beriberi, thiamine.**

athlete's foot. See **tinea.**

athlete's heart, the typical, enlarged heart of an athlete trained for endurance, characterized by a slow rate of contractions, an increased pumping capacity, and greater than average ability to deliver oxygen to skeletal muscles.

athletic habitus, a physique characterized by a well-proportioned, muscular body with broad shoulders, thick neck, deep chest, and flat abdomen. Compare **asthenic habitus.** See also **mesomorph.**

Athrombin-K (eɪθrom'bɪn keɪ'), a trade name for an anticoagulant (warfarin).

Ativan, a trade name for an antianxiety agent (lorazepam), used as an adjunct to anesthesia.

atlanto-occipital joint (ætlæn'touoksɪp'ɪtəl), one of a pair of condyloid joints formed by the articulation of the atlas of the vertebral column with the occipital bone of the skull. It includes two articular capsules, two membranes, and two lateral ligaments. The atlanto-occipital joint permits nodding and lateral movements of the head.

atlas, the first cervical vertebra, articulating with the occipital bone and the axis.

atmo-, a combining form meaning 'pertaining to steam or vapor': *atmocausis, atmolysis, atmotherapy.*

atmosphere, 1. the natural body of air, composed of approximately 20 per cent oxygen, 78 per cent nitrogen, and 2 per cent carbon dioxide and other gases, that covers the surface of the earth. 2. an envelope of gas, which may or may not duplicate the natural atmosphere in chemical components. 3. a unit of gas pressure that is usually defined as being equivalent to the average pressure of the earth's atmosphere at sea level, or about 14.7 pounds per square inch. —**atmospheric,** *adj.*

atmospheric pressure, the pressure exerted by the weight of the atmosphere. The atmospheric pressure at sea level is approximately 15 pounds per square inch. With increasing altitude the pressure decreases: at 30,000 feet, approximately the height of Mt. Everest, the air pressure is 4.3 pounds per square inch. Also called **barometric pressure.**

atom, 1. (in physics) the smallest division of an element that exhibits all the properties and characteristics of the element. It is comprised of neutrons, electrons, and protons. The number of protons in the nucleus of every atom of any given element is the same and is called its atomic number. 2. *Nontechnical.* the amount of any substance that is so small further division is not possible. 3. *Informal.* a minute amount of any substance. —**atomic,** *adj.*

atomic number, the number of protons in the nucleus of every atom of a particular element. The atomic number equals the number of electrons, and their number and arrangement determine the chemical characteristics of the atom, with the exception of its atomic weight and radioactivity. See also **atom, electron, proton.**

atomic weight, the relative mass of an atom based on the weight of an atom of carbon-12.

atomize. See **nebulize.**

atomizer, a device for reducing a liquid and ejecting it as a fine spray or vapor.

atonia (eitou'niə), an abnormal lack of muscle tone. —**atonic,** *adj.*

atonia constipation, constipation caused by the failure of the colon to respond to the normal stimuli for evacuation. It may occur in elderly or bedridden patients or after prolonged dependence on laxatives. To prevent impaction of fecal material in the colon and rectum, a moderately irritant oral laxative or a mild suppository may be recommended. Patients are encouraged to develop regular, unhurried bowel habits and may be given a diet rich in fruits and vegetables. If fecal impaction develops, it may be removed by means of a mild enema or manual disimpaction, with the use of anesthetic agents. Also called **colon stasis, lazy colon.** See also **fecalith, inactive colon.**

atonic, 1. weak. 2. lacking normal tone, as in the case of a muscle that is flaccid. 3. lacking vigor, as an atonic ulcer, which heals slowly. —**atony,** *n.*

atonic bladder. See **flaccid bladder.**

atonic impotence. See **impotence.**

atopic (eitop'ik), of or pertaining to a hereditary tendency to develop immediate allergic reactions, as asthma, atopic dermatitis, or vasomotor rhinitis, owing to the presence of an antibody (atopic reagin) in the skin and sometimes the bloodstream. —**atopy,** *n.*

atopic asthma. See **extrinsic asthma.**

atopic dermatitis, an intensely pruritic, often excoriated, maculo-papular inflammation commonly found on the face, antecubital and popliteal areas of allergy-prone individuals. Although it may occur at any age, it is most common in infants and clears completely in half the cases by 18 months of age. Treatment includes discovery and avoidance of allergens, topical and parenteral corticosteroids, tar ointments, antihistamines, and wet compresses of Burow's solution. Also called **atopic eczema, infantile eczema.** Compare **contact dermatitis.** See also **atopic.**

atopic eczema. See **atopic dermatitis.**

atopic reagin. See **reagin.**

atoxic (eitok'sik). See **nontoxic.**

ATP, abbreviation for **adenosine triphosphate.**

TPase, abbreviation for **adenosine triphosphatase.**

ATPD, abbreviation for *ambient temperature, ambient pressure, dry.*

ATPS, abbreviation for *ambient temperature, ambient pressure, saturated* (with water vapor).

atresia (ətri'źhə), the absence of a normal body opening, duct, or canal, as the anus, vagina, or external ear canal. —**atresic, atretic,** *adj.*

-atresia, a combining form meaning a 'condition of occlusion': *gynatresia, hedratresia, urethratresia.*

atresic teratism (ətri'sik), a congenital anomaly in which any of the normal openings of the body, as the mouth, nares, anus, or vagina, fail to form.

atreto-, a combining form meaning 'closed, or imperforate': *atretoblepharia, atretolemia, atretorrhinia.*

atrial appendix. See **auricle.**

atrial failure, an abnormal condition characterized by the failure of the atrium to fill adequately and distend the associated ventricle. The atria provide a pumping function and a reservoir function for the heart and normally contribute 15 to 20 per cent of ventricular filling. Tachycardia commonly increases this proportion. In normal individuals or in patients with mild heart disease, loss of the atrial pumping function may not change cardiac output at rest but may decrease the output during exercise. Atrial failure is commonly caused by mechanical abnormalities, fibrillation, or dysdynamic myocardial failure. Heart failure caused by atrial failure may occur with the onset of atrial fibrillation in patients who have compensated heart disease. Such individuals may develop congestive heart failure even when under treatment with digitalis to control the ventricular response rate. Atrial fibrillation very rarely produces heart failure in people with otherwise normal hearts.

atrial fibrillation, a condition characterized by rapid, random contractions of the atria, causing irregular ventricular beats at the rate of 130 to 150 a minute. The atria may discharge more than 350 impulses a minute, but some do not pass the atrioventricular junction. The ventricles cannot contract in response to all the stimuli that are received, and ventricular contractions become disordered. The arrhythmia occurs most frequently in rheumatic heart disease, mitral stenosis, and atrial infarction. The rapid pulsations result in a decreased cardiac output, and the disorganized contractions of the atria promote thrombus formation in the upper chambers. Treatment consists of the administration of digitalis or of quinidine or the use of electric shock to restore a normal sinus rhythm.

atrial gallop, an abnormal cardiac rhythm in which a low-pitched, extra sound is heard late in diastole on auscultation of the heart. It indicates increased resistance to ventricular filling and is frequently heard in hypertensive cardiovascular disease, coronary artery disease, and aortic stenosis. Also called **S4.** See also **gallop, heart sound.**

atrial myxoma, a benign, pedunculated gelatinous tumor that originates in the interatrial septum of the heart. It may cause palpitations, disseminated neuritis, nausea, weight loss, fatigue, dyspnea, fever, and, occasionally, sudden loss of consciousness owing to obstruction of the flow of blood through the heart.

atrial septal defect (ASD), a congenital cardiac anomaly characterized by an abnormal opening between the two atria. The severity of the condition depends on the size and location of the defect, which is dependent on the stage at which embryonic development was arrested. The defects are classified as ostium secundum defect, in which the aperture in the septum secundum of the fetal heart fails to close; ostium primum defect, in which there is inadequate development of the endocardial cushions; and sinus venosus defect, in which the superior portion of the atrium fails to develop. Atrial septal defects cause an increased flow of oxygenated blood into the right side of the heart which is usually well tolerated, since it is delivered under much lower pressure than in ventricular septal defect. Clinical manifestations include right atrial and ventricular enlargement, a characteristic harsh, scratchy systolic murmur, and a fixed splitting of the second heart sound, which does not vary with respiration. X rays and electrocardiograms generally show right atrial and ventricular enlargement, although definitive diagnosis is made by cardiac catheterization. Surgical closure is indicated in most cases but unless the defect is severe is usually postponed until later childhood to prevent com-

plications during early adulthood, as atrial arrhythmias, bacterial endocarditis, and congestive heart failure. Also called **atrioseptal defect.** See also **congenital cardiac anomaly.**

atrio-, a combining form meaning 'pertaining to the atrium of the heart': *atriocommisuropexy, atrionector, atrioseptopexy.*

atrioseptal defect. See **atrial septal defect.**

atrioventricular (AV) block (ei'triouventrik'yələr), the slowed conduction or stoppage of the cardiac excitatory impulse, occurring at the atrioventricular node, bundle of His, or its branches. Kinds of AV block include first-degree block, with prolonged AV conduction, second-degree block, with partial AV block, and third-degree block with complete atrioventricular block. An overdose of digitalis, degenerative or inflammatory cardiac disease, or acute myocardial infarction may precipitate the condition. AV block is a common indication for the insertion of a cardiac pacemaker.

atrioventricular bundle. See **bundle of His.**

atrioventricular (AV) node, an area of specialized cardiac muscle that receives the cardiac impulse from the sinoatrial (SA) node and conducts it to the atrioventricular bundle of His and thence to the walls of the ventricles. The AV node is located in the septal wall of the right atrium.

atrioventricular septum, a small portion of membranous septum that separates the atria from the ventricles of the heart.

atrioventricular valve, a valve in the heart through which blood flows from the atria to the ventricles. The valve between the left atrium and left ventricle is the mitral valve; the right atrioventricular valve is the tricuspid valve.

at risk, the state of an individual or population being vulnerable to a particular disease or injury. The factors determining risk may be environmental or physiological. An example of an environmental factor is exposure to harmful substances or organisms. An example of a physiological factor is genetic predisposition to a disease.

atrium (ei'triəm), *pl.* **atria.** a chamber or cavity, especially the right and left atria of the heart.

atrium of the heart, one of the two upper chambers of the heart. The right atrium receives deoxygenated blood from the superior vena cava, the interior vena cava, and the coronary sinus. The left atrium receives oxygenated blood from the pulmonary veins. Blood is emptied into the ventricles from the atria during diastole.

Atromid-S, a trade name for an antihyperlipidemic (clofibrate).

-atrophia, **1.** a combining form meaning a 'condition of malnutrition': *metatrophia, metratrophia, pantatrophia.* **2.** a combining form meaning a 'progressive decline of a body part': *dermatrophia, neuratrophia, splenatrophia.* Also -**trophy.**

atrophic arthritis. See **rheumatoid arthritis.**

atrophic catarrh, an abnormal condition characterized by inflammation and discharge from the mucous membranes of the nose, accompanied by the loss of mucosal and submucosal tissue. Compare **hypertrophic catarrh.** See also **catarrh.**

atrophic fracture, a spontaneous fracture caused by atrophy, as in the bones of an elderly person.

atrophic gastritis, a chronic inflammation of the stomach, associated with degeneration of the gastric mucosa. Seen in elderly patients and in persons with pernicious anemia, atrophic gastritis may cause epigastric pain. Even though less acid is being produced by the stomach, antacids are helpful in relieving discomfort. See also **gastritis, pernicious anemia.**

atrophy (æt'rəfi), a wasting or diminution of size or physiological activity of a part of the body owing to disease or other influences. A skeletal muscle may undergo atrophy because of lack of physical exercise or as a result of neurologic or musculoskeletal disease. Cells of the brain and central nervous system may atrophy in old age because of restricted blood flow to those areas. See also **aging.** – **atrophic,** *adj.*

atropine sulfate, an antispasmodic and anticholinergic.
■ INDICATIONS: It is prescribed in the treatment of gastrointestinal hypermotility, inflammation of the iris or the uvea, cardiac arrhythmias, parkinsonism, certain kinds of poisoning, and as an adjunct to anesthesia.
■ CONTRAINDICATIONS: Gastrointestinal obstruction, glaucoma, hepatitis, liver or kidney dysfunction, porphyria, or known hypersensitivity to this drug or other anticholinergics prohibits its use.
■ ADVERSE EFFECTS: Among the more serious adverse reactions are tachycardia, loss of taste, nausea, diarrhea, skin rash, and eye pain.

attachment, 1. the state or quality of being affixed or attached. 2. (in psychiatry) a mode of behavior in which one individual relates in an affiliative or dependent manner to another; a feeling of affection or loyalty that binds one person to another. Such relationships develop at critical periods during life and any failure to form these attachments, because of lack of the opportunity or the inability to relate, can lead to personality deviation disorders or maladaptive behavior. 3. See **bonding.** 4. (in dentistry) any device, as a retainer or artificial crown, used to secure a partial denture to a natural tooth in the mouth.

attending physician, the physician who is responsible for a particular, usually private, patient. In a university setting, an attending physician often also has teaching responsibilities and holds a faculty appointment. Also called, *Informal.* **attending.**

attention deficit disorder, a syndrome affecting children, adolescents, and, rarely, adults characterized by learning and behavior disabilities. The symptoms may be mild or severe and are associated with functional deviations of the central nervous system without signs of major neurologic or psychiatric disturbance. The people affected are usually of normal or above average intelligence. Symptoms include impairment in perception, conceptualization, language, memory, and motor skills, decreased attention span, increased impulsivity and emotional lability, and usually, but not always, hyperactivity. The condition is ten times more prevalent in boys than in girls and may result from genetic factors, biochemical irregularities, or perinatal or postnatal injury or disease. There is no known cure, and symptoms often subside or disappear with time. Medication with methylphenidate, permoline, or the dextroamphetamines is frequently prescribed for children with hyperactive symptoms, and some form of psychotherapeutic counseling is often recommended. Some treatments include abstinence from certain foods and food additives. Also called **hyperactivity, hyperkinesis, minimal brain dysfunction.** See also **learning disability.**

Attenuvax, a trade name for an active immunizing agent (live measles virus vaccine).

attic, the. See **epitympanic recess.**

attitudinal reflex, any reflex initiated by a change in position of the head or by a change in position of the head with respect to the position of the body. Kinds of attitudinal reflexes include **tonic neck reflex, tonic labyrinthine reflex.** Also called **statotonic reflex.**

attrition, the process of wearing away or wearing down by friction.

-**ature,** a noun-forming combining form: *armature, ligature, tubulature.*

Au, symbol for **gold.**

audioanalgesia, the use of music to enhance relaxation and to distract a patient's mind from pain, as during dentistry. The procedure has also been tried experimentally during labor.

audiogram (ɔ'diəgræm'), a chart showing the acuteness of hearing of an individual as indicated by the ability to hear sounds and to distinguish different speech sounds. See also **audiometry.**

audiology, a field of research devoted to the study of hearing, especially impaired hearing that cannot be corrected by medical means. – **audiologic,** *adj.*

audiometer (ɔ'diom'ətər), an electrical device for testing the hearing and for measuring bone and air conduction. Earphones are placed over the ears; the ear not being tested receives a masking noise from the machine while the ear being tested is stimulated by a series of tones, from very low to very high frequencies at various decibels of intensity. The patient signals when a tone is heard, and the results are noted on an audiogram.

audiometry (ɔ'diom'ıtri), the testing of the acuity of the sense of hearing. Various audiometric tests determine the lowest intensity of sound at which an individual can perceive an auditory stimulus (hearing threshold), hear different frequencies, and distinguish different speech sounds. Pure tone audiometry assesses the person's ability to hear frequencies, usually ranging from 125 to 8,000 hertz (Hz), and can indicate if a hearing loss is caused by a middle-ear problem or by one in the inner ear or the auditory nerve. In this test the subject sits in a soundproof booth and signals when sounds are first heard through earphones. The sound will be of a given frequency, as the operator will have been slowly increasing the decibel level. Speech audiometry tests the ability to repeat selected words. Impedance audiometry is an objective method of assessing the conductive mechanism of the middle ear by measuring muscle responses to sound with a probe inserted in the ear canal. Cortical audiometry indicates auditory acuity by measuring and averaging electrical potentials evoked from the cortex of the brain by pure tones. Localization audiometry is a method for measuring the individual's ability to locate the source of a pure tone received binaurally in a sound field. — **audiometric,** *adj.*

auditory ossicles, the incus, the malleus, and the stapes, small bones in the middle ear that articulate with each other and the tympanic membrane. Sound waves are transmitted through them as the tympanic membrane vibrates.

auditory system assessment, an evaluation of the patient's ears and hearing and an investigation of present and past diseases or conditions that may be responsible for an auditory impairment.

■ METHOD: In an interview with the patient, oral or written questions are used to determine if the individual has earaches, decreased or absent hearing in one or both ears, vertigo, a feeling of fullness, itching, or of the heart pulsating in the ears. The person is asked if there is a ringing or buzzing in the ears or a popping noise when yawning or swallowing, if the voice echoes, if the ears drain a clear, yellow, red, or dark substance, and if the person uses oils, cotton swabs, or hairpins to clean the ears. Observations are recorded of the patient's general appearance, blood pressure, pulse, temperature, and respirations, the ability to hear or to lip-read or use a hearing aid. The person's startle reflex, tolerance of loud sounds, allergies, use of medication, especially of eardrops, streptomycin, salicylates, and quinine, and the color, character, and amount of ear drainage are carefully noted. The presence of otitis media, otosclerosis, acoustic nerve tumor, labyrinthitis, Ménière's disease, diabetes mellitus, arteriosclerosis, hypertension, mastoiditis, or a cerebral tumor, head contusion, or skull fracture is investigated. It is determined if the patient previously underwent stapes mobilization, suffered from otitis media, head trauma, or syphilis, or if the person is exposed to a high decibel level on the job or to recreational ear hazards, as in swimming. Diagnostic procedures indicated by the history may include an audiogram, audiometric test, a mastoid x ray, otologic examination, Rinne and Weber tuning-fork tests, and microbiologic studies for potential pathogens in smears of ear drainage.

■ NURSING ORDERS: The nurse conducts the interview, makes the observations, and collects the pertinent background information and the results of the diagnostic procedures.

■ OUTCOME CRITERIA: A thorough assessment of the patient's auditory system is essential in establishing the diagnosis of an ear disorder.

auditory tube. See **eustachian tube.**

Auer body (au'ər). See **Auer rod.**

Auer rod, an abnormal, needle-shaped or round, pink-staining inclusion in the cytoplasm of myeloblasts and promyelocytes in acute myelogenous or myelomonocytic leukemia. These inclusions contain enzymes such as acid phosphatase, peroxidase, and esterase, and may represent abnormal derivatives of cytoplasmic granules. The finding of Auer rods in stained smears of blood may help to differentiate acute myelogenous leukemia from acute lymphoblastic leukemia. Also called **Auer body.**

aur-, a combining form meaning 'pertaining to the ear': *auralgan, auricle, auricular.*

aura (ɔr'ə), *pl.* **aurae. 1.** a sensation, as of light or warmth, that may precede an attack of migraine or an epileptic seizure. **2.** *pl.* **auras.** an emanation of light or color surrounding a person as seen in Kirlian photography and studied in current nursing research in healing techniques.

aural[1] (ɔr'əl), of or pertaining to the ear or hearing. — **aurally,** *adv.*

aural[2], of or pertaining to an aura.

aural forceps, a dressing forceps with fine, bent tips, used in aural surgery.

Aureomycin, a trade name for a tetracycline antibiotic (chlortetracycline hydrochloride).

auricle (ɔr'ıkəl), **1.** Also called **pinna.** the external ear. **2.** the left or right cardiac atrium, so named because of its earlike shape.

auricular, 1. of or pertaining to the auricle of the ear. **2.** otic.

auricularis anterior, one of three extrinsic muscles of the ear. Arising from the anterior portion of the fascia in the temporal area and inserting into a projection in front of the helix, it is innervated by the temporal branch of the facial nerve and functions to move the auricula forward and upward. Some people can voluntarily contract the auricularis anterior to move the ears. Compare **auricularis posterior, auricularis superior.**

auricularis posterior, one of three extrinsic muscles of the ear. Arising from the mastoid area of the temporal bone by short aponeurotic fibers and inserting into the lower part of the cranial surface of the concha, it is innervated by the posterior auricular branch of the facial nerve and serves to draw the auricula backward. Compare **auricularis anterior, auricularis superior.**

auricularis superior, a thin, fan-shaped muscle that is one of three extrinsic muscles of the ear. It arises in the fascia of the temporal area and converges to insert with a thin, flattened tendon into the cranial surface of the auricula. It is innervated by a temporal branch of the facial nerve and acts to draw the auricula upward. Compare **auricularis anterior, auricularis posterior.**

auriculoventriculostomy (ɔrɪk'yulouventrɪk'yulos'kəpi), a surgical procedure that directs cerebrospinal fluid into the general circulation in the treatment of hydrocephalus, usually in the newborn. In this procedure, a polyethylene tube is passed from the lateral ventricle through a burr hole in the parietal skull area under the scalp and into the jugular vein for the discharge of cerebrospinal fluid into the superior vena cava or the right atrium. The insertion of the tube into these structures that have one-way valves is to avoid reflux of the blood into the ventricles and to continue the drain of excess cerebrospinal fluid when ventricular pressure increases. This procedure is performed to correct the communicating and the obstructive forms of hydrocephalus.

auriosis (ɔr'iou'sɪs). See **chrysiasis.**

aurothioglucose (ɔr'outhai'ouglu'kous), an antiarthritic used in chrysotherapy.

■ INDICATION: It is prescribed for adjunctive treatment of adult and juvenile rheumatoid arthritis.

■ CONTRAINDICATIONS: Severe uncontrolled diabetes, renal or hepatic dysfunction, a history of infectious hepatitis, hypertension, heart failure, systemic lupus erythematosus, agranulocytosis, hemorrhagic diathesis, pregnancy, or known hypersensitivity to this drug prohibits its use.

■ ADVERSE EFFECTS:Among the most serious adverse effects are kidney and renal damage and various allergic reactions. Dermatitis and lesions of mucous membranes are common.

auscultation (ɔ'skəltei'shən), the act of listening for sounds within the body to evaluate the condition of the heart, lungs, pleura, intestines, or other organs or to detect the fetal heart sound. Auscultation may be performed directly but most commonly a stethoscope is used to determine the frequency, intensity, duration, and quality of the sounds. During auscultation of the chest, the patient usually sits upright and is instructed to breathe slowly and deeply through the mouth. The anterior and posterior surfaces of the thorax are auscultated from apex to base with comparisons made between the right and left sides; when the posterior chest is examined the patient is asked to bring the shoulders forward so that a greater surface of the lung can be auscultated. The heart and abdomen may be auscultated with the patient supine or sitting upright. – **auscultate,** v.

auscultatory percussion. See **auscultation, percussion.**

Australia antigen, hepatitis B surface antigen (HB-sAG), found in the serum of a person who has acute or chronic serum hepatitis or who is a carrier for that virus. Extremely dilute concentrations of the antigen can cause the disease. Medical personnel must take adequate precautions to avoid autoinoculation, especially in dialysis units, blood banks, and laboratories. Blood banks routinely screen for Australia antigen to avoid causing active hepatitis infection in a transfusion recipient. See also **hepatitis.**

Australian Q fever. See **Q fever.**

autacoid (ɔ'təkɔid), any of a group of substances, as hormones, that are produced in one organ and are transported via blood or lymph as a means to control a physiologic process in another part of the body.

autism, a mental disorder characterized by extreme withdrawal and an abnormal absorption in fantasy, accompanied by delusion, hallucination, and an inability to communicate verbally or to otherwise relate to people. Schizophrenic children are often autistic. See also **infantile autism.** – **autistic,** adj.

auto-, a combining form meaning 'pertaining to self': autoblast, autocatharsis, autoclasis.

autoantibody (ɔ'touæn'tɪbod'i), an immunoglobulin that reacts against a normal constituent in a person's body, as nuclear material in the patient with systemic lupus erythematosus. There are several mechanisms that may trigger the production of autoantibodies. An antigen formed during fetal development and then sequestered may be released as a result of infection or trauma and elicit the synthesis of autoantibodies, as occurs in autoimmune thyroiditis, sympathetic uveitis, and aspermia. Antibodies produced against certain streptococcal antigens during infection may cross-react with myocardial tissue, causing rheumatic heart disease, or with glomerular basement membrane, causing glomerulonephritis. Normal body proteins may be converted to autoantigens by chemicals, infectious organisms, or therapeutic drugs. Autoantibodies are found against gastric parietal cells in pernicious anemia, against platelets in autoimmune thrombocytopenia, and against antigens on the surface of erythrocytes in autoimmune hemolytic anemia.

autoantigen (ɔ'touæn'tɪjɪn), an endogenous body constituent that stimulates the production of autoantibody and a resulting autoimmune reaction against one or more tissues of the person in whom the abnormal reaction occurs. See also **autoantibody.**

autochthonous idea, an idea that originates in the unconscious and arises spontaneously in the mind, independent of the conscious train of thought.

autodiploid (ɔ'toudɪp'lɔid), **autodiploidic,** **1.** of or pertaining to an individual, organism, strain, or cell containing two genetically identical or nearly identical chromosome sets that are derived from the same ancestral species and result from the duplication of the haploid set. **2.** such an individual, organism, strain, or cell. Compare **allodiploid.** See also **autopolyploid.**

autodiploidy (ɔ'toudɪp'lɔidi), the state or condition of having two genetically identical or nearly identical chromosome sets from the same ancestral species. Such a state enables cell division to occur in a normal manner. Compare **allodiploidy.**

autoeroticism, **1.** sensual, usually sexual, gratification of the self, usually obtained through the stimulus of one's own body without the participation of another person and derived from such acts as stroking, masturbation, fantasy, or from other oral, anal, or visual sources of stimulation. **2.** sexual feeling or desire occurring without any external stimulus. **3.** (in Freudian psychoanalytic theory) an early phase of psychosexual development, occurring in the oral and the anal stages. Also called **autoerotism.** Compare **heteroeroticism. autoerotic,** *adj.*

autoerotism. See **autoeroticism.**

autoerythrocite sensitization syndrome (ɔ'touɪrɪfh'-rəsait). See **Gardener-Diamond syndrome.**

autoerythrocyte sensitization (ɔ'touərɪfh'rəsait), an unusual disorder characterized by the spontaneous appearance of painful, hemorrhagic spots on the anterior aspects of the arms and legs, resulting from hypersensitivity to the patient's own red blood cells. Autoimmune hemolytic anemia, an extreme example of hypersensitivity to antigens on the surface of the patient's erythrocytes, may cause fulminant hemolysis, fever, abdominal pain, hyperbilirubinemia, thrombosis, and shock.

autogenesis (ɔ'toujen'əsɪs), **1.** abiogenesis. **2.** self-produced; originating from within the organism. Also called **autogeny.** Compare **heterogenesis, homogenesis.** — **autogenetic,** *adj.*

autogenous (ɔtoj'ənəs), **1.** self-generating. **2.** originating from within the organism, as a toxin or vaccine.

autogeny (ɔtoj'əni). See **autogenesis.** — **autogenic,** *adj.*

autograft, surgical transplantation of any tissue from one part of the body to another location in the same individual. Autografts are commonly used to replace skin lost in severe burns.

autographism (ɔtog'rəfiz'əm). See **dermatographia.**

autohexaploid (ɔ'touhek'səploid), **autohexaploidic.** See **autopolyploid.**

autoimmune disease, one of a large group of diseases characterized by the subversion or alteration of the function of the immune system of the body. Antigens nor-mally present in the internal cells stimulate the development of antibodies, and the antibodies, unable to distinguish antigens of the internal cells from external antigens, act against the internal cell to cause localized and systemic reactions. These reactions affect the epithelial and the connective tissues of the body, causing a variety of diseases that can be divided into two general categories: the collagen diseases (including systemic lupus erythematosus, dermatomyositis, periarteritis nodosa, scleroderma, and rheumatoid arthritis) and the autoimmune hemolytic disorders (including idiopathic thrombocytopenic purpura, acquired hemolytic anemia, and autoimmune leukopenia). The precise pathophysiologic processes and the etiology of these diseases are unknown and remain under study.

■ OBSERVATIONS: The manifestations and clinical characteristics depend on the specific disease and on the organ or systems affected. See specific diseases.

■ INTERVENTION: Therapy includes corticosteroid, antiinflammatory, and immunosuppressive drugs. The symptoms are treated specifically, as a transfusion for hemorrhage, analgesics for pain, and physical therapy for the prevention of contracture. Diet may be regulated for specific needs, as iron might be increased to treat anemia in a person with thrombocytopenic purpura, or calories might be reduced in a weight-loss diet for a person with rheumatoid arthritis. Surgical treatment may be corrective or preventive, as a hip replacement in rheumatoid arthritis or a splenectomy in thrombocytopenic purpura.

■ NURSING CONSIDERATIONS: Many of these diseases are characterized by periods of crisis and periods of remission. During a crisis, the patient may be hospitalized and require extensive nursing care, with relief from pain, applications of heat or cold, range of motion exercises, or assistance in movement and ambulation. The nurse observes for signs of hemorrhage, puts side rails or a trapeze in place if necessary, protects the person from infection, and prevents chilling or overheating. As the patient is in particular need of emotional support, the nurse helps the person to verbalize feelings of anger and frustration, to recognize limitations, to focus on strengths, to set realistic goals, and to understand the disease process. It is important also to teach the patient and the family the side effects of the drugs being prescribed as well as how the drugs are to be taken.

autoimmunity, an abnormal characteristic or condition in which the body reacts against constituents of its own tissues. Some authorities believe autoimmunity indicates an inability of the immune system in the body to distinguish between autoantigens and foreign substances because of some change in the function of the cellular components of the immune system. Autoimmunity may result in hypersensitivity and autoimmune disease. It is not yet fully understood, but there are several common theories to explain autoimmunity, as the forbidden clone theory, the sequestered antigens theory, and the immune complex activity theory.

automatic behavior. See **automatism.**

automatic bladder. See **spastic bladder.**

automatic infiltration detector, a temperature-sensitive device that activates an alarm and automatically stops an intravenous infusion when infiltration of the intravenous fluid occurs. The device detects any cooling of the skin at the intravenous site, a common sign of infiltration. The detector is usually secured to the skin with tape and attaches by a small cable to the fluid monitoring circuit of an intravenous pump.

automatism (ɔtom'ətɪz'əm), **1.** (in physiology) involuntary function of an organ system independent of apparent external stimuli, as the beating of the heart, or dependent upon external stimuli but not consciously controlled, as the dilation of the pupil of the eye. **2.** (in philosophy) the theory that the body acts as a machine and that the mind, whose processes are solely dependent on brain activity, is a noncontrolling adjunct of the body. **3.** (in psychology) mechanical, repetitive, and undirected behavior that is not consciously controlled, as seen in psychomotor epilepsy, hysterical states, and such acts as sleepwalking. Kinds of automatism include **ambulatory automatism, command automatism, immediate posttraumatic automatism.** Also called **automatic behavior.**

autonomic (ɔ'tənom'ɪk), of or pertaining to the autonomic nervous system.

autonomic drug, any of a large group of drugs that mimic or modify the function of the autonomic nervous system.

autonomic dysreflexia, a dysreflexia that is the result of impaired function of the autonomic nervous system.

autonomic nervous system, the part of the nervous system that regulates involuntary vital function, including the activity of the cardiac muscle, the smooth muscle, and the glands. It has two divisions: the **sympathetic nervous system** accelerates heart rate, constricts blood vessels, and raises blood pressure; the **parasympathetic nervous system** slows heart rate, increases intestinal peristalsis and gland activity, and relaxes sphincters.

autonomic reflex, any of a large number of normal reflexes governing and regulating the functions of the viscera. Autonomic reflexes control such activities of the body as blood pressure, heart rate, peristalsis, sweating, and urination.

autonomous bladder. See **flaccid bladder.**

autonomy, the quality of having the ability or tendency to function independently. — **autonomous,** *adj.*

autopentaploid (ɔ'toupen'təploid), **autopentaploidic.** See **autopolyploid.**

autoplastic maneuver, (in psychology) a process that is part of adaptation, involving an adjustment within the self. Compare **alloplastic maneuver.**

autopolyploid (ɔ'toupol'ɪploid), **1.** Also **autopolyploidic.** of or pertaining to an individual, organism, strain, or cell that has more than two genetically identical or nearly identical sets of chromosomes that are derived from the same ancestral species. They result from the duplication of the haploid chromosome set and are referred to as autotriploid, autotetraploid, autopentaploid, autohexaploid, and so on, depending on the number of multiples of the haploid chromosomes they contain. **2.** such an individual, organism, strain, or cell. Compare **allopolyploid.** See also **allodiploid.**

autopolyploidy (ɔ'toupol'ɪploi'di), the state or condition of having more than two identical or nearly identical sets of chromosomes. Compare **allopolyploid.**

autopsy, a post-mortem examination performed to confirm or determine the cause of death. Also called **necropsy, thanotopsy.** — **autopsic, autopsical,** *adj.,* **autopsist,** *n.*

autopsy pathology, the study of disease by the examination of the body after death by a pathologist. The organs and tissues are first described by their appearance at the time of dissection, then by their appearance in the microscopic examination of small representative samples of tissue taken for their diagnostic value.

autoserous treatment (ɔ'təsir'əs), therapy of an infectious disease by inoculating the patient with the patient's own serum.

autosite (ɔ'təsäit), the larger, more normally formed member of unequal or asymmetrical, conjoined twins upon whom the other smaller fetus is dependent for various physiologic functions and for nutrition and growth. Compare **parasitic fetus.** — **autositic.** *adj.*

autosomal (ɔ'təsou'məl), **1.** pertaining to or characteristic of an autosome. **2.** pertaining to any condition transmitted by an autosome.

autosomal-dominant inheritance, a pattern of inheritance in which the transmission of a dominant gene on an autosome causes a characteristic to be manifested. Males and females are affected with equal frequency. Affected individuals have an affected parent (unless the condition is the result of a fresh mutation). Half of the children of a heterozygous affected parent are affected. All of the children of a homozygous affected parent are affected. Normal children of an affected parent do not carry the trait. Traits can be traced vertically through previous generations. A family history may be illustrated by drawing a pedigree. The first case, the propositus, appears suddenly in the pedigree, usually as a mutation. Achondroplasia, osteogenesis imperfecta, polydactyly, and Marfan's syndrome are autosomal-dominant disorders. Compare **autosomal-recessive inheritance.**

autosomal inheritance, a pattern of inheritance in

which the transmission of traits depends on the presence or absence of certain genes on the autosomes. The pattern may be dominant or recessive, and males and females are affected with equal frequency. The majority of hereditary disorders are the result of a defective gene on an autosome. See also **autosomal-dominant inheritance, autosomal-recessive inheritance.**

autosomal-recessive inheritance, a pattern of inheritance in which the transmission of a recessive gene on an autosome results in a carrier state if the person is heterozygous for the trait and in the affected state if the person is homozygous for the trait. Males and females are affected with equal frequency. Affected individuals have unaffected parents who are heterozygous for the trait. One fourth of the children of two unaffected heterozygous parents are affected. All of the children of two homozygous affected parents are affected. The children of a couple in which one parent has the trait and the other does not are all carriers who show no effect of the trait. There is usually no family history of the trait; it becomes manifest when two unaffected parents who are heterozygous for a particular recessive gene have a child who is homozygous for the trait. Cystic fibrosis, phenylketonuria, and galactosemia are examples of autosomal-recessive inheritance.

autosome (ɔ'tɜsoum), any chromosome that is not a sex chromosome and that appears as a homologous pair in the somatic cell. Man has 22 pairs of autosomes, which are involved in transmitting all genetic traits and conditions other than those that are sex-linked. Also called **euchromosome.**

autosplenectomy (ɔ'tousplɪnek'təmi), a progressive shrinking of the spleen which may occur in sickle-cell anemia. The spleen is replaced by fibrous tissue and becomes nonfunctional.

autosuggestion, an idea, thought, attitude, or belief suggested to oneself, often as a formula or incantation, as a means of controlling one's behavior. Compare **suggestion.**

autotetraploid (ɔ'toutet'rəploid), **autotetraploidic.** See **autopolyploid.**

autotopagnosia, the inability to recognize or localize the various parts of the body owing to organic brain damage. Also called **body-image agnosia.** See also **proprioception.**

autotriploid (ɔ'toutrɪp'loid), **autotriploidic.** See **autopolyploid.**

autumn fever. See **leptospirosis.**

auxanology (ɔks'ənol'əji), the scientific study of growth and development. – **auxanologic, auxanological,** adj.

auxesis (ɔksi'sɪs), pl. **auxeses.** an increase in size or volume owing to cell expansion rather than to an increase in the number of cells or tissue elements; hypertrophy. Also called **auxetic growth.** Compare **merisis.** – **auxetic,** adj., n.

auxo-, a combining form meaning 'pertaining to growth, to acceleration, or to stimulation': *auxochrome, auxocyte, auxotonic.*

AV, abbreviation for **atrioventricular.**

avantin (æv'əntɪn). See **isopropyl alcohol.**

avascular (eivæs'kyulər), **1.** (of a tissue area) not receiving a sufficient supply of blood. The reduced flow may be the result of blockage by a blood clot or the deliberate stoppage of flow during surgery or of measures taken to control a hemorrhage. **2.** (of a kind of tissue) not having blood vessels.

Aventyl Hydrochloride, a trade name for an antidepressant (nortriptyline hydrochloride).

aversion conditioning. See **aversion therapy.**

aversion therapy, a form of behavior therapy in which punishment or unpleasant or painful stimuli, like electric shock or drugs that induce nausea, are used in the suppression of undesirable behavior. The procedure is used in treating such conditions as drug abuse, alcoholism, gambling, overeating, smoking, and various sexual deviations. Also called **aversive conditioning.** See also **behavior therapy.**

aversive stimulus, a stimulus, as electric shock, that causes psychic or physical pain. See also **aversion therapy.**

Avertin, a trade name for a general anesthetic (tribromoethanol).

avitaminosis (eivai'təmɪnou'sɪs), a condition resulting from a deficiency of or the lack of absorption or utilization of one or more essential vitamins in the diet. Also called **hypovitaminosis.** Compare **hypervitaminosis.** See also specific vitamins.

Avlosulfon, a trade name for a leprostatic antibacterial (dapsone).

AV nicking, a vascular abnormality on the retina of the eye, visible on ophthalmologic examination, in which a vein is compressed by an arteriovenous crossing. The vein appears "nicked," owing to constriction or spasm. It is a sign of hypertension, arteriosclerosis, and other vascular conditions.

Avogadro's law (æv'ougad'rouz), a law in physics stating that equal volumes of all gases at a given temperature and pressure contain the identical number of molecules.

avoidance, (in psychiatry) a conscious or unconscious defense mechanism, physical or psychological in nature, by which an individual tries to avoid or escape from unpleasant stimuli, conflicts, or feelings, as anxiety, fear, pain, or danger.

avoidance-avoidance conflict, a conflict resulting from the confrontation of two or more alternative goals or desires that are equally aversive and undesirable. Also called **double-avoidant conflict.** See also **conflict.**

avoidance conditioning, the establishment of certain patterns of behavior in order to avoid unpleasant or painful stimuli.

avoirdupois weight, the English system of weights in which there are 7,000 grains, 256 drams, or 16 ounces to one pound. One ounce in this system equals 28.35 grams and one pound equals 453.59 grams. Compare **apothecaries' weight.** See also **metric system.**

avulsed teeth (əvəlst'), teeth that have been forcibly displaced from their normal position. In some cases they can be surgically reimplanted, but this procedure is not often successful. See also **avulsion.**

avulsion, the separation, by tearing, of any part of the body from the whole, as an umbilical cord torn in the process of delivering the placenta. —**avulse,** v.

avulsion fracture, a fracture caused by the tearing away of a fragment of bone where a strong ligamentous or tendinous attachment forcibly pulls the fragment away from osseous tissue.

awake anesthesia, an anesthetic procedure in which analgesia and anesthesia are accomplished without loss of consciousness and the concomitant need for life support equipment, personnel, and expertise. Dental procedures, surgery on a limb or an extremity, and certain kinds of head surgery are ordinarily performed using awake anesthesia. Awake anesthesia is not as complete as general anesthesia, and muscle relaxation may not be very deep. Various combinations of sedatives, tranquilizers, and low concentrations of anesthetic gas may be used. Also called **conscious sedation.**

AWOL, abbreviation for **absent without leave.**

ax-, a combining form meaning 'pertaining to an axis': *axial, axofugal, axon.* Also **axio-, axon-.**

axial current, the central part of the blood current.

axial gradient, 1. the variation in metabolic rate in different parts of the body. **2.** the development toward the body axis or its parts in relation to the metabolic rate in the various parts.

axial illumination. See **illumination.**

axial neuritis. See **parenchymatous neuritis.**

axilla (æksɪl'ə), pl. **axillae.** a pyramid-shaped space forming the underside of the shoulder between the upper part of the arm and the side of the chest. Also called **armpit.**

axillary anesthesia. See **brachial plexus anesthesia.**

axillary artery, one of a pair of continuations of the subclavian arteries that starts at the outer border of the first rib and ends at the distal border of the teres major, where it becomes the brachial artery. It has three parts and six branches, supplying various chest and arm muscles, as the pectorals, deltoid, and subclavius. The six branches are the highest thoracic, thoracoacromial, lateral thoracic, subscapular, posterior humeral circumflex, and the anterior humeral circumflex.

axillary nerve, one of the last two branches of the posterior cord of the brachial plexus before the posterior cord becomes the radial nerve. The axillary nerve passes over the insertion of the subscapularis, crosses the teres minor, and leaves the axilla, accompanied by the posterior humeral circumflex artery. It passes through the quadrilateral space bounded by the neck of the humerus, the two teres muscles, and the long head of the triceps and divides into a posterior branch and an anterior branch. The posterior branch innervates the teres minor, part of the deltoideus, and part of the skin overlying the deltoideus; the anterior branch winds around the neck of the humerus and innervates the deltoideus. Some fibers of the nerve also supply the capsule of the shoulder joint.

axillary node, one of the lymph glands of the axilla that help to fight infections in the chest, armpit, neck, and arm and to drain lymph from those areas. The 20 to 30 axillary nodes are divided into the lateral group, the anterior group, the posterior group, the central group, and the medial group. The lateral group is associated with lymphatic vessels that drain the whole arm; the anterior group with vessels that drain the thoracic muscles; the posterior group with vessels that drain the dorsal muscles of the neck and the muscles of the thoracic wall; the central group with vessels that drain the lymph from the nodes of the three preceding groups; the medial group with afferent vessels that drain lymph from the breast and efferent vessels that form the subclavian lymphatic trunk. See also **lymphatic system, lymph node.**

axillary vein, one of a pair of veins of the upper limb that begins at the junction of the basilic and the brachial veins near the distal border of the teres major and becomes the subclavian vein at the outer border of the first rib. It receives deoxygenated blood from the venous tributaries that correspond to the branches of the axillary artery and near its termination, from the cephalic vein. It contains a pair of valves at the distal border of the subscapularis. Compare **subclavian vein.**

axio-. See **ax-.**

axis, pl. **axes. 1.** (in anatomy) a line that passes through the center of the body, or a part of the body, as the frontal axis, binauricular axis, basifacial axis. **2.** the second cervical vertebra about which the atlas rotates, allowing the head to be turned, extended, and flexed. Also called **epistropheus, odontoid vertebra.**

axis artery, one of a pair of extensions of the subclavian arteries, running into and supplying the upper limb, continuing into the forearm as the palmar interosseous artery. Each artery is divided into subclavian, axillary, and brachial portions, developing radial and ulnar arteries from the brachial section.

axis traction, 1. the process of pulling a baby's head with obstetric forceps in a direction in line with the path of least resistance, following the curve of Carus through the mother's birth canal. **2.** *Informal.* any mechanical device attached to obstetric forceps to facilitate pulling in the proper direction.

axoaxonic synapse (æk'soʊæksonʹɪk), a type of synapse in which the axon of one neuron comes in contact with the axon of another neuron.

axodendritic synapse (æk'soʊdendrɪtʹɪk), a type of synapse in which the axon of one neuron comes in contact with the dendrites of another neuron.

axodendrosomatic synapse (æk'soʊden'droʊsoʊmætʹɪk), a type of synapse in which the axon of one neuron comes in contact with both the dendrites and the cell body of another neuron.

axon (æk'son), the cylindrical extension of a nerve cell that conducts impulses away from the neuron cell body. Axons may be bare or sheathed in myelin. Also called **axis cylinder.** Compare **dendrite.**

axon-. See ax-.

axon flare, vasodilation, reddening, and increased sensitivity of skin surrounding an injured area, caused by an axon reflex. Axon flare or reflex is considered part of a triple response in which injury or stroking of the skin results in local reddening, the release of histamine or a histaminelike substance, a surrounding flare, and wheal formation. A pin prick in the involved area causes more intense pain than a similar stimulus prior to injury.

axoplasmic flow (æk'soʊplæzʹmɪk), the continuous pulsing, undulating movement of the cytoplasm between the cell body of a neuron, where protein synthesis occurs, and the axon fiber in order to supply it with the substances vital for the maintenance of activity and for repair. The nerve fiber is totally dependent on the cell body for metabolites and any interruption in the axoplasmic flow caused by disease or trauma results in the degeneration of the unsupplied areas of the axon.

axosomatic synapse (æk'soʊsoʊmætʹɪk), a type of synapse in which the axon of one neuron comes in contact with the cell body of another neuron.

azathioprine, an immunosuppressive.

■ INDICATIONS: It is prescribed to prevent organ rejection following transplantation and in the treatment of lupus erythematosis and other systemic inflammatory diseases.

■ CONTRAINDICATION: Known hypersensitivity to this drug prohibits its use.

■ ADVERSE EFFECTS: Among the most serious adverse reactions are bone marrow depression and hepatotoxicity. Nausea and fever are common.

azo-, a combining form meaning 'containing nitrogen': *azocarmine, azoimide, azorubin.*

azoospermia (eɪzoʊ'əspərʹmiə), lack of spermatozoa in the semen. It may be caused by testicular dysfunction or by blockage of the tubules of the epididymis, or it may be induced by vasectomy. Infertility but not impotence is associated with azoospermia. Compare **oligospermia.**

azotemia (æz'oʊtiʹmiə), the retention in the blood of excessive amounts of nitrogenous compounds. This toxic condition is caused by failure of the kidneys to remove urea from the blood and is characteristic of uremia. See also **uremia.** – **azotemic,** *adj.*

AZ test. See **Ascheim-Zondek test.**

azul. See **pinta.**

azula. See **pinta.**

Azulfidine, a trade name for an antibacterial (sulfasalazine).

azygosperm. See **azygospore.**

azygospore, a spore that is produced directly from a gamete that does not undergo conjugation, as in certain algae and fungi. Also called **azygosperm.**

azygous, azygos, occurring as a single entity or part, as any unpaired anatomical structure; not part of a pair. – **azygos,** *n.*

azygous vein, one of the seven veins of the thorax. Beginning opposite the first or second lumbar vertebra, it rises through the aortic hiatus in the diaphragm and passes to the right of the vertebral column to the fourth thoracic vertebra, then arches ventrally over the root of the right lung, and ends in the superior vena cava. It receives numerous veins, as the hemiazygous veins, several esophageal veins, and the right bronchial vein. Compare **internal thoracic vein, left brachiocephalic vein, right brachiocephalic vein,**

B

B, symbol for **boron.**

Ba, symbol for **barium.**

BA, abbreviation for **Bachelor of Arts.**

Babcock's operation, the extirpation of a varicosed saphenous vein by inserting an acorn-tipped sound, tying the vein to the sound, and drawing it out.

babesiosis (bəbi'siou'sıs), an infection caused by protozoa of the genus *Babesia.* The infective organism is introduced into the host through the bite of ticks of the species *Ixodes dammini.* Symptoms include headache, fever, nausea and vomiting, myalgia, and hemolysis. Also called **babesiasis.**

Babinski's reflex (bəbın'skiz), dorsiflexion of the big toe with extension and fanning of the other toes elicited by firmly stroking the lateral aspect of the sole of the foot. The reflex is normal in newborn infants and abnormal in children and adults in whom it may indicate a lesion in the pyramidal tract. Also called **Babinski's sign.**

baby, 1. an infant or young child, especially one who is not yet able to walk or talk. 2. to treat gently or with special care.

baby talk, 1. See also **lallation.** the speech patterns and sounds of young children learning to talk, characterized by mispronunciation, imperfect syntax, repetition, and phonetic modifications, as lisping or stuttering. 2. the intentionally oversimplified manner of speech, imitative of young children learning to talk, used by adults in addressing children or pets. 3. the speech patterns characteristic of regressive stages of various mental disorders, especially schizophrenia.

bachelor of science in nursing (BSN), an academic degree awarded upon satisfactory completion of a four-year course of study in an institution of higher learning. The recipient is eligible to take the national certifying examination to become a registered nurse. A BSN degree is prerequisite to advancement in most systems and institutions that employ nurses. Compare **associate degree in nursing, diploma program in nursing.**

bacill-, a combining form meaning 'pertaining to any rod-shaped bacterium': *bacillemia, bacillicidal, bacillosis.*

Bacillaceae (bæs'əlei'sıi), a family of *Schizomycetes* of the order *Eubacteriales,* consisting of gram-positive, rod-shaped cells that can produce cylindrical, ellipsoid, or spherical endospores situated terminally, subterminally, or centrally. These cells are chemoheterotropic and mostly saprophytic, commonly appearing in soil. Some are parasitic on insects and animals and are pathogenic. The family includes the genus *Bacillus,* which is aerobic, and the genus *Clostridium,* which is facultatively anaerobic.

bacillary dysentery. See **shigellosis.**

bacille Calmette-Guérin (BCG) (kælmet'geiræ'), an attenuated strain of tubercle bacilli, used in many countries as a vaccine against tuberculosis, most often administered intradermally, using a multiple-puncture disc. It appears to prevent the more serious forms of tuberculosis and to give some protection to persons living in areas where tuberculosis is prevalent. BCG is also administered to stimulate the immune response in people who have certain kinds of malignancy. It induces a positive tuberculin reaction and may mask early, active infection by removing the diagnostic sign of conversion from the negative to the positive skin reaction. See also **tuberculin test, tuberculosis.**

bacilliform (bəsıl'ıfɔrm), rod-shaped in form, like a bacillus.

bacilluria (bæs'əlur'ıə), the presence of bacilli in the urine.

Bacillus, a genus of aerobic, gram-positive spore-producing bacteria in the family Bacillaceae, order Eubacteriales, including 33 species, three of which are pathogenic and the rest saprophytic soil forms. Many microorganisms formerly classified as *Bacillus* are now classified in other genera. See also **Bacillaceae.**

Bacillus anthracis, a species of gram-positive, facultative anaerobe that causes anthrax. The spores of this organism, if inhaled, can cause a pulmonary form of anthrax; spores can live for many years in animal products, as hides and wool, and in soil. See also **anthrax, woolsorter's disease.**

bacillus Calmette-Guérin vaccine. See **BCG vaccine.**

bacitracin (bæs'ıtrei'sın), an antibacterial.

■ INDICATION: It is prescribed for skin infections sensitive to bacitracin.

■ CONTRAINDICATION: Known hypersensitivity to this drug prohibits its use.

■ ADVERSE EFFECTS: Among the more serious adverse reactions are nephrotoxicity and skin rash.

back, the posterior portion of the trunk of the body between the neck and the pelvis. The back is divided by a middle furrow that lies over the tips of the spinous processes of the vertebrae. The upper cervical vertebrae cannot be felt in this furrow, but the seventh cervical vertebra is easily distinguished just above the more prominent first thoracic vertebra. The skeletal portion of the back includes the thoracic and the lumbar vertebrae and both scapulas, The root of the spine of the scapula is on a level in the back with the spine of the third thoracic vertebra, and the inferior angle of the scapula is on a level with the spine of the seventh thoracic vertebra. The superficial muscles of the back are large and include the trapezius, the rhomboideus major, and the latissimus. The deep muscles of the back are the erector spinae iliocostalis, interspinales, intertransversarii, longissimus, multifidi, rotatores, splenius, semispinales, spinales, transversocostal, and transversospinal. The nerves that innervate the various muscles of the back include some branches of the dorsal primary divisions of the spinal nerves, the lateral branches of the dorsal primary division of the middle and the lower cervical nerves, some branches of the primary division of the spinal nerves, and some branches of the ventral primary divisions of the spinal nerves. The back may be affected by various orthopedic diseases and disorders of the spine, as ankylosing spondylitis, hemivertebra, kyphosis, Pott's disease, scoliosis, and spasmodic torticollis. The back may also be affected by trauma, as fractures, spinal dislocations, and ruptured intervertebral discs. Lower back problems are common.

backache, pain in the lumbar, lumbosacral, or cervical regions of the back, varying in sharpness and intensity. Causes may include muscle strain or other muscular disorders or pressure on the root of a nerve, as the sciatic nerve, owing in turn to a variety of factors, including a ruptured vertebral disc. Treatment may include heat, ultrasound, and devices to provide support for the affected area while in bed or while standing or sitting, bed rest, surgical intervention, and medications to relieve pain and relax spasm of the muscle of the affected area.

backcross, (in genetics) **1.** the cross of a first filial-generation hybrid with one of the parents or with a genotype that is identical to the parental strain. **2.** the organism or strain produced by such a cross.

background radiation, naturally occurring radiation emitted by materials in the soil, ground waters, and building material, radioactive substances in the body [especially potassium -40 (^{40}K)], and cosmic rays from outer space. The average person is exposed each year to 44 millirads (mrad) of cosmic radiation, 44 mrads from external terrestrial radiation and 18 mrads from naturally occurring internal radioactive sources.

back pressure, pressure that builds in a vessel or a cavity as fluid is accumulated. The pressure increases and extends backward if the normal mechanism for egress or

passage of the fluid is not restored. See also **backward failure.**

backward failure, cardiac failure marked by elevated venous pressure and diminished arterial pressure, most commonly beginning as left ventricular failure that results in decreased output. Backward failure develops when the ventricle cannot empty and the blood backs up in the pulmonary veins and the lungs, causing pulmonary edema.

bacter-. See **bacterio-.**

bacteremia (bæk'tırı'mıə), the presence of bacteria in the blood. Undocumented bacteremias occur frequently and usually abate spontaneously. Bacteremia is demonstrated by blood culture. Antibiotic treatment, if given, is specific for the organism found and appropriate to the locus of infection. Compare **septicemia.** See also **septic shock.** – **bacteremic,** adj.

bacteremic shock. See **septic shock.**

bacteria (bæktir'iə), sing. **bacterium.** any of the small unicellular microorganisms of the class Schizomycetes. The genera vary morphologically, being spherical (cocci), rod-shaped (bacilli), spiral (spirochetes), or comma-shaped (vibrios). The nature, severity, and outcome of any infection caused by a bacterium are characteristic of that species.

-bacteria, a combining form meaning 'genus of microscopic plants forming the class Schizomycetes': *lysobacteria, nitrobacteria, streptobacteria.*

bacterial aneurysm. See **mycotic aneurysm.**

bacterial endocarditis, an acute or subacute bacterial infection of the endocardium or the heart valves or both. The condition is characterized by heart murmur, prolonged fever, bacteremia, splenomegaly, and embolism. The acute variety progresses rapidly and is usually caused by staphylococci or pneumococci. The subacute variety is usually caused by lodging of streptococcus viridans in valves of the heart damaged by rheumatic fever. Prompt treatment of both types with antibiotics, as penicillin, cephalosporin, or gentamicin given intravenously, is essential to prevent destruction of the valves and cardiac failure. See also **endocarditis, subacute bacterial endocarditis.**

bacterial food poisoning, a toxic condition resulting from the ingestion of food contaminated by certain bacteria. Acute infectious gastroenteritis caused by various species of salmonella is characterized by fever, chills, nausea, vomiting, diarrhea, and general discomfort beginning 8 to 48 hours after ingestion and continuing for several days. Similar symptoms caused by staphylococcus, usually *S. aureus,* appear much sooner and rarely last more than a few hours. Food poisoning caused by the neurotoxin of *Clostridium botulinum* is characterized by gastrointestinal symptoms, disturbances of vision, weakness or paralysis of muscles, and, in severe cases, respiratory failure. See also **botulism.**

bacterial kinase, 1. a kinase of bacterial origin. 2. a bacterial enzyme that activates plasminogen, the precursor of plasmin.

bacterial plaque, a film comprised of microorganisms that attaches to the teeth and often causes caries and infections of the gums. Mucin secreted by the salivary glands is also a component of plaque; it varies in thickness and consistency depending on individual metabolism, dental hygiene, diet, and environmental factors. Also called **dental plaque.**

bacterial protein, any protein produced by a bacterium.

bactericidal (bæktir′ɪsaɪ′dəl), destructive to bacteria. Compare **bacteriostatic.**

bactericidin, an antibody that kills bacteria in the presence of complement.

bacterio-, bacter-, a combining form meaning 'pertaining to any bacterial microorganism': *bacteriogenic, bacteriophytoma, bacteriosis.*

bacteriocidal, capable of acting to kill bacteria. Compare **bacteriostatic.**

bacteriologist, a specialist in bacteriology.

bacteriology, the scientific study of bacteria. – **bacteriologic, bacteriological,** *adj.*

bacteriolysin (bæktir′ɪəlaɪ′sɪn), an antibody that causes the breakdown of a particular species of bacterial cell. Complement is usually also necessary for this reaction. See also **bacteriolysis.**

bacteriolysis (bæktir′iol′əsɪn), the breakdown of bacteria intracellularly or extracellularly. See also **bacteriolysin.** – **bacteriolytic,** *adj.*

bacteriophage (bæktir′iəfeɪj′), any virus that causes lysis of host bacteria, including the blue-green "algae." Bacteriophages resemble other viruses in that each is composed of either ribonucleic acid or deoxyribonucleic acid. They vary in structure from simple fibrous bodies to complex forms with contractile "tails." Bacteriophages associated with temperate bacteria may be genetically intimate with the host and are named after the bacterial strain for which they are specific, as coliphage and corynebacteriophage. – **bacteriophagic,** *adj.*, **bacteriophagy,** *n.*

bacteriostatic (bæktir′iəstæt′ɪk), tending to restrain the development or the reproduction of bacteria. Compare **bacteriocidal.**

bacteriuria (bæktir′iyur′iə), the presence of bacteria in the urine. The presence of more than 100,000 pathogenic bacteria per ml of urine is usually considered significant and diagnostic of urinary tract infection. See also **urinary tract infection.**

bacteroid, bacterioid, 1. of, pertaining to, or resembling bacteria. 2. a structure that resembles a bacterium. – **bacteroidal, bacterioidal,** *adj.*

Bacteroides (bæk′təroɪ′diz), a genus of obligate anaerobic bacilli normally found in the colon, mouth, genital tract, and upper respiratory system. Severe infection may result from the invasion of the bacillus through a break in the mucous membrane into the venous circulation, where thrombosis and bacteremia may occur. Foul-smelling abcesses, gas, and putrefaction are characteristic of infection with this organism. Of the 30 species, *Bacteroides fragilis* is the most common and most virulent.

Bactrim, a trade name for a fixed-combination drug containing two antibacterials (sulfamethoxazole and trimethoprim).

BAEP, abbreviation for **brain stem auditory evoked potential.**

bag, 1. a flexible or dilatable sac or pouch designed to contain gas, fluid, or semisolid material such as crushed ice. An **Ambu bag** or **breathing bag** is used to control the flow of respiratory gases entering the lungs of a patient. Several types of bags are used in medical or surgical procedures to dilate the anus, vagina, or other body openings. 2. **bag of waters,** the membranous sac of amniotic fluid surrounding the fetus in the uterus of a pregnant woman.

bagasse (bəgæs′), the crushed fibers or the residue of sugar cane.

bagassosis (bæg′əsou′sɪs), a self-limited lung disease caused by an allergic response to bagasse, the fungi-laden, dusty debris left after the syrup has been extracted from sugar cane. It is characterized by fever, dyspnea, and malaise. Treatment may include corticosteroid drugs taken by mouth. To prevent a recurrence of the condition, the antigen should be avoided. Also called **allergic interstitial pneumonitis.** See also **organic dust.**

bagging, *Informal.* the artificial respiration performed with a ventilator or respirator bag, as an ambu-bag or Hope resuscitator. The bag is squeezed to deliver air to the patient's lungs as the mask is held over the mouth. During general anesthesia the anesthetist may also use this technique to correct the respiratory pattern of an unconscious patient.

bag of waters. See **amnion.**

Bain Breathing Circuit, a continuous-flow anesthetic system that does not require a soda-lime absorber.

Bainbridge reflex (bein′brɪj), a cardiac reflex consisting of an increased pulse rate, resulting from stimulation of stretch receptors in the wall of the left atrium. It may be produced by the infusion of large amounts of intravenous fluids.

BAL, abbreviation for **British anti-lewisite.**

balance, 1. an instrument for weighing. 2. a normal state of physiologic equilibrium. 3. a state of mental or

emotional equilibrium. **4.** to bring into equilibrium.
—**balanced,** *adj.*

balanced anesthesia, *Informal.* one of a number of variable techniques of general anesthesia in which no single anesthetic agent or preset proportion of the combination of agents is used; rather, an individualized mixture of anesthetics is prescribed according to the needs of a particular patient for a particular operation. One type of balanced anesthesia may combine a local or regional anesthetic with general anesthesic agents; another may combine a muscle relaxant, an analgesic, oxygen, an anesthetic gas, and a sedative.

balanced diet, a diet containing all of the essential nutrients that cannot be synthesized in adequate quantities by the body, in amounts adequate for growth, energy needs, nitrogen equilibrium, repair of wear, and maintenance of normal health.

balanced polymorphism, the recurrence in a population of an equalized mixture of homozygotes and heterozygotes for specific genetic traits, which are maintained from generation to generation by the forces of natural selection. Compare **genetic polymorphism.**

balanced suspension, a system of splints, ropes, slings, pulleys, and weights for suspending the lower extremities of the body, used as an aid to healing and recuperation from fractures or from surgical operations.

balanced traction, a system of balanced suspension that supplements traction in the treatment of fractures of the lower extremities or following various operations affecting the lower parts of the body.

balanced translocation, the transfer of segments between nonhomologous chromosomes in such a way that there are changes in the configuration but not in the total number of chromosomes, so that each cell or gamete contains no more or no less than the normal amount of diploid or haploid genetic material. See also **translocation.**

balanic (bəlæn′ık), of or pertaining to the glans penis or the glans clitoridis.

balanitis (bæl′ənaı′tıs), inflammation of the glans penis.

balanitis xerotica obliterans (zırot′ıkə oυblıt′əræns), a chronic skin disease of the penis, characterized by a white, indurated area surrounding the meatus. Local antibacterial and anti-inflammatory agents are used to treat it.

balano-, a combining form meaning 'pertaining to the glans penis': *balanocele, balanoplasty, balanoposthitis.*

balanoplasty (bæl′ənouplæs′ti), an operation involving plastic surgery of the glans penis.

balanoposthitis (bæl′ənouposthaı′tıs), a generalized inflammation of the glans penis and prepuce, characterized by soreness, irritation, and discharge, occurring as a complication of bacterial or fungal infection. Smear and culture can determine the causative agent—often a common venereal disease—whereupon specific antimicrobial ther-

apy can be instituted. Circumcision may be considered in severe cases. To relieve discomfort, the inflamed area can be irrigated with a warm saline solution several times a day.

balanopreputial (bæl′ənouprıpyu′ṩəl), of or pertaining to the glans penis and the prepuce.

balanorrhagia (bæl′ənoυreı′jiə), balanitis in which pus is discharged copiously from the penis.

balantidiasis (bæl′əntıdaı′əsıs), an infection caused by ingestion of cysts of the protozoan *Balantidium coli.* In some cases the organism is a harmless inhabitant of the large intestine, but infection with *B. coli* usually causes diarrhea. Infrequently the infection progresses, and the protozoan invades the intestinal wall and produces ulcers or abcesses, which may cause dysentery and death. The diagnosis is made by the identification of cysts and trophozoites in the stool or in the exudate from intestinal ulcers. Metronidazole is usually prescribed to treat the infection.

Balantidium coli (bæl′əntıd′iəm), the largest and the only ciliated protozoan species that is pathogenic to man, causing balantidiasis. The organism is seen in two life stages: the motile trophozoite and the encysted cercaria. It is a normal inhabitant of the domestic hog and is transmitted to man by the ingestion of cysts excreted by the hog.

baldness, absence of hair, especially from the scalp. See also **alopecia.**

BAL in Oil, a trade name for an antidote to arsenic, gold, and mercury poisoning (dimercaprol).

Balkan frame, an overhead, rectangular frame, attached to the bed of an orthopedic patient, for use in attaching splints, suspending or changing the position of immobilized limbs, and for continuous traction involving weights and pulleys.

ball, a relatively spherical mass, as one of the chondrin balls imbedded in hyaline cartilage.

ball-and-socket joint, a synovial joint in which the globular head of an articulating bone is received into a cuplike cavity, allowing the distal bone to move around an indefinite number of axes with a common center, as in hip and shoulder joints. Also called **enarthrosis, spheroidea.** Compare **condyloid joint, pivot joint, saddle joint.**

ballism (bæl′ızəm), an abnormal neuromuscular condition characterized by uncoordinated swinging of the limbs and jerky movements. Ballism is associated with extrapyramidal disorders, as Sydenham's chorea.

ballismus (bəlız′məs), an abnormal condition characterized by violent flailing motions of the arms and, occasionally, the head, resulting from injury to the subthalamic nucleus. **Hemiballismus** is a unilateral form of the condition. Also called **ballism.**

ballistocardiogram (bəlıs′toυkar′diəgræm′), a record of the movement of the body—toward the head and toward the feet—caused by the thrust of the heart during systolic ejection of the blood into the aorta and the pulmonary arteries. The patient is placed on a special table that is so delicately balanced that vibrations of the body can be recorded by a machine attached to the table. The ballistocardiogram is a sensitive tool that is useful in measuring cardiac output and the force of contraction of the heart.

balloon septostomy. See **Rashkind procedure.**

balloon-tip catheter, a catheter bearing a nonporous inflatable sac around its distal end. After insertion of the catheter the sac can be inflated with air or sterile water, introduced via injection into a special port at the proximal end of the catheter. The inflated sac serves to secure the catheter in the correct position. Kinds of balloon-tip catheters include **Foley catheter, Swan-Ganz catheter.**

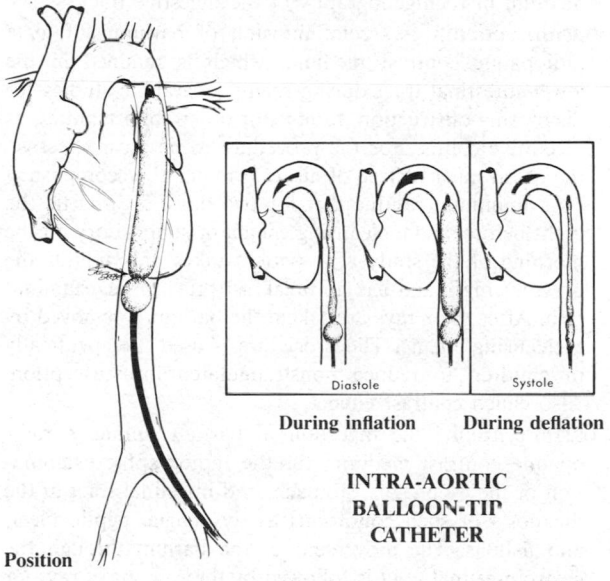

Diastole   Systole

During inflation   During deflation

**INTRA-AORTIC
BALLOON-TIP
CATHETER**

Position

ballottable head, a fetal head that has not descended and become fixed in the maternal bony pelvis.

ballottement (bəlot′mənt), a technique of palpating a floating structure by bouncing it gently and feeling it rebound. Ballottement of a fetus within a uterus is an objective sign of pregnancy. In late pregnancy, a fetal head that can be ballotted is said to be **floating** or **unengaged,** as differentiated from a fixed or an engaged head which cannot be easily dislodged from the pelvis.

ball thrombus, a relatively round, coagulated mass of blood containing platelets, fibrin, and cellular fragments, that may obstruct a blood vessel or an orifice, usually the mitral valve of the heart.

ball-valve action, the intermittent opening and closing of an orifice by a buoyant, ball-shaped mass which acts as a valve. Some kinds of objects that may act in this manner are kidney stones, gallstones, and blood clots.

balm, 1. a healing or a soothing substance, as any of various medicinal ointments. 2. an aromatic plant of the genus *Melissa* that relieves pain.

balneology, a field of medicine that deals with the chemical compositions of various mineral waters and their healing characteristics, especially in baths. — **balneologic,** *adj.*

balneotherapy (bæl′niʊfher′əpi), a use of baths in the treatment of many diseases and conditions.

balneum pneumaticum. See **air bath.**

balsam, any of a variety of resinous saps, generally from evergreens, usually containing benzoic or cinnamic acid. Balsam is sometimes used in rectal suppositories and dermatologic agents as a counterirritant.

bamboo spine, the characteristically rigid spine of advanced ankylosing spondylitis. Also called **poker spine.** See also **ankylosing spondylitis.**

band, 1. (in anatomy) a bundle of fibers, as seen in striated muscle, that encircles a structure or binds one part of the body to another. 2. (in dentistry) a strip of metal that fits around a tooth and serves as an attachment for orthodontic components. 3. Also called **stab form.** *Informal.* the immature form of a segmented granulocyte characterized by a sausage-shaped nucleus. It is the only immature leucocyte normally found in the peripheral circulation. Bands represent 3 to 5 per cent of the total white cell volume. An increase in the relative number of bands indicates bacterial infection or acute stress to the bone marrow.

bandage, 1. a strip or roll of cloth or other material that may be wound around a part of the body in a variety of ways to secure a dressing, maintain pressure over a compress, or immobilize a limb or other part of the body. 2. to apply a bandage.

bandage shears, a sturdy pair of scissors used to cut through bandages. The blades of most bandage shears are angled to the shaft of the instrument, and the lower blade has a rounded blunt protuberance to facilitate insertion under the bandage without harming the patient's skin.

band cell, any one of the developing granular leukocytes in circulating blood, characterized by a curved or indented nucleus. Band cells are intermediate leukocytic forms between metamyelocytes and adult leukocytes with segmented nuclei.

banding, (in genetics) any of several techniques of staining chromosomes with fluorescent stains or chemical dyes that produce a series of lateral light and dark areas whose intensity and position are characteristic for each chromosome. Banding patterns are identified according to the staining technique used, as C-banding, G-banding, Q-banding, and R-banding. Also called **chromosome banding.**

Bandl's ring (bæn'dəlz). See **pathologic retraction ring.**

Bangkok hemorrhagic fever. See **dengue.**

bank blood, anticoagulated, preserved blood collected from doners in units of 500 ml and stored under refrigeration for future use. Dated and identified as to blood type, it is stored for a usual maximum period of 21 days. Bank blood may be used directly after cross-matching against the recipient's blood or for the extraction and preparation of any of its components. See also **packed cells, pooled plasma, whole blood.**

Banthine, a trade name for an anticholinergic (methantheline bromide), used as an antispasmodic.

Banting treatment, a therapeutic regimen for obesity, consisting of a low-carbohydrate, high-protein diet. Also called **Banting diet.**

Banti's syndrome (bæn'tiz), a serious, progressive disorder involving several organ systems, characterized by portal hypertension, splenomegaly, anemia, leukopenia, gastrointestinal tract bleeding, and cirrhosis of the liver. Obstruction of the blood vessels that lie between the intestines and the liver leads to venous congestion, an enlarged spleen, and abnormal destruction of red and white blood cells. Early symptoms are weakness, fatigue, and anemia. Surgical removal of the spleen and creation of a portacaval shunt to improve portal circulation are sometimes necessary. Since the syndrome is often a complication of alcoholic cirrhosis of the liver, medical treatment includes prescribing improved nutrition, vitamins, abstinence from alcohol, and rest. Also called **Banti's disease.** See also **cirrhosis, portacaval shunt, portal hypertension.**

bar-. See **baro-.**

baralyme (BL) (bær'əlaim), a chemical compound used to absorb exhaled carbon dioxide in an anesthesia rebreathing system.

Bárány's syndrome. See **caloric test.**

barber's itch. See **sycosis barbae.**

barbiturate (barbich'ureit, barbich'ərit), a derivative of barbituric acid that acts as a sedative or hypnotic.

-barbituric, a combining form meaning an 'acid used medicinally for its soporific effects': *dibromobarbituric, isobarbituric, phenylethylbarbituric.*

barbiturism (barbich'əriz'əm), **1.** acute or chronic poisoning by any of the derivatives of barbituric acid. Ingestion of such preparations in excess of therapeutic quantities may be fatal or may produce physiologic, pathologic, and psychologic changes, as depressed respiration, cyanosis, disorientation, and coma. **2.** addiction to a barbiturate.

Bard-Pic syndrome (bard'pik'), a condition characterized by progressive jaundice and cachexia, associated with advanced pancreatic cancer.

Bard's sign, the increased oscillations of the eyeball in organic nystagmus when the patient tries to visually follow a target moved from side to side across the line of sight. Such oscillations usually cease during the same test if the patient has congenital nystagmus.

bar graph, a graph in which frequencies are represented by bars extending from the ordinate or the abscissa, allowing the distribution of the entire sample to be seen at once.

bariatrics, the field of medicine that focuses on the treatment and the control of obesity and diseases associated with obesity.

barium (Ba), a pale yellow, metallic element classified with the alkaline earths. Its atomic number is 56; its atomic weight is 137.36. The acid-soluble salts of barium are poisonous. Barium carbonate, formerly used in medicine, is now used to prepare the cardiac stimulant, barium chloride; fine, milky barium sulfate is used as a contrast medium in roentgenography of the digestive tract.

barium enema, a rectal infusion of barium sulfate, a radiopaque contrast medium, which is retained in the lower intestinal tract during roentgenographic studies for diagnosing obstruction, tumors, or other abnormalities, as ulcerative colitis. For the procedure to be most effective, the colon must be free of all fecal material, accomplished by a minimum residue diet for two days, a cathartic the night before, and a cleansing enema or suppository on the morning of the study. The patient takes only liquids the previous night and has no breakfast prior to the examination. After the x rays are taken, the barium is removed by a cleansing enema. The procedure is used therapeutically in children to reduce nonstrangulated intussusception. Also called **contrast enema.**

barium meal, the ingestion of barium sulfate, a radiopaque contrast medium, for the radiographic examination of the esophagus, stomach, and intestinal tract in the diagnosis of such conditions as dysphagia, peptic ulcer, and fistulas. The movement of the barium through the gastrointestinal tract is followed by fluoroscopy, x rays, or both. Prior to the test, the patient receives nothing by mouth for at least eight hours. Also called **barium swallow.** See also **G.I. series.**

barium sulfate, a radiopaque medium used as a diagnostic aid in roentgenology.

■ INDICATION: It is prescribed for x-ray examination of the gastrointestinal tract.

■ CONTRAINDICATION: Known hypersensitivity to this drug prohibits its use.

■ ADVERSE EFFECTS: Among the more serious complications is severe constipation.

barium swallow. See **barium meal.**

Barlow's disease (bar'louz). See **infantile scurvy.**

Barlow's syndrome, an abnormal cardiac condition characterized by an apical systolic murmur, a systolic click, and an electrocardiogram indicating inferior ischemia. These signs are associated with mitral regurgitation caused by prolapse of the mitral valve. Also called **electrocardiographic-auscultatory syndrome.**

baro-, bar-, a combining form meaning 'pertaining to pressure': *baresthesia, barognosis, barospirator.*

barognosis, *pl.* **barognoses.** the ability to estimate weight.

barograph, an instrument that continuously monitors barometric pressure and provides a record on paper of pressure changes.

barometer, an instrument for measuring atmospheric pressure, commonly consisting of a slender tube filled with mercury, sealed at one end, and inverted into a reservoir of mercury. At sea level the normal height of mercury in the tube is 760 mm. At higher elevations the mercury column height (barometric pressure) is less. Fluctuations in barometric pressure may occur preceding major changes in the weather, making a barometer useful in weather forecasting. — **barometric,** *adj.*

barometric pressure (bær'əmet'rɪk). See **atmospheric pressure.**

baroreceptor (bær'ourɪsep'tər), one of the pressure-sensitive nerve endings in the walls of the atria of the heart, the vena cava, the aortic arch, and the carotid sinus. Baroreceptors stimulate central reflex mechanisms that allow physiologic adjustment and adaptation to changes in blood pressure via vasodilation or vasoconstriction. Baroreceptors are essential for homeostasis.

barosinusitis (bær'ousai'nəsai'tɪs). See **aerosinusitis.**

Barosperse, a trade name for a radiopaque medium (barium sulfate).

barotitis (bær'ətai'tɪs). See **aerotitis.**

barotitis media. See **aerotitis media.**

barotrauma (bær'outrɔ'mə, bær'outrau'mə), physical injury sustained as a result of exposure to increased environmental pressure, as barotitis media, rupture of the lungs, or paranasal sinuses, as may occur among deep-sea divers or caisson workers.

Barr body. See **sex chromatin.**

barrel chest, a large, rounded thorax, considered normal in some stocky individuals and certain others who live in high-altitude areas and consequently develop increased vital capacities. Barrel chest, however, may also be a sign of pulmonary emphysema.

Barr-Epstein virus. See **Epstein-Barr virus.**

Barré's sign, the inability of a hemiplegic to maintain a flexed position on the side of the lesion when placed in a prone attitude with the lower limbs flexed at the knees: the leg on the side of the lesion extends.

Barrett's esophagus (bær'ɪts). See **Barrett's syndrome.**

Barrett's syndrome, a disorder of the lower esophagus marked by a benign ulcerlike lesion in columnar epithelium, resulting most often from chronic irritation of the esophagus by gastric reflux of acidic digestive juices. Major symptoms include dysphagia and heartburn. Symp-

toms may be relieved by eating frequent small meals, avoiding foods that produce gas, taking antacid medication, and elevating the head of the bed to prevent passive reflux when lying down.

barrier, a wall or other obstacle that can restrain or block the passage of substances. Barrier methods of contraception, as the condom or cervical diaphragm, prevent the passage of spermatazoa into the uterus. Membranes and cell walls of body tissues function as screenlike barriers to permit the movement of water or certain other molecules from one side to the other while preventing the passage of other substances. Barriers in kidney tissues adjust automatically to regulate the retention or excretion of water and other substances according to the needs of organ systems elsewhere in the body. See also **barrier nursing.**

barrier nursing, nursing care of a patient in isolation, performed to prevent the spread of infection by creating an aseptic barrier around the patient. Gown, mask, and gloves are worn by staff or visitors entering the room; the number of staff entering the room is kept to a minimum, and visitors are limited. Contaminated substances are handled according to strict protocols. Specific techniques vary with the indication for isolation. A patient with an infection may be isolated to prevent others from contracting the infection; a patient who is extremely susceptible to infection may be isolated for protection against possible infection from others.

bartholinitis (bar'təlɪnai'tɪs), an inflammatory condition of one or both Bartholin's glands, caused by bacterial infection. Usually, the causative microorganism is a species of *Streptococcus* or *Staphylococcus* or a strain of gonococci. The condition is characterized by swelling of one or both glands, pain, and the development of an abscess in the infected gland. A fistula may develop from the gland to the vagina, anus, or perineum. Treatment includes local application of heat, often by soaking in hot water, antibiotics, or, if necessary, incision of the gland and drainage of the purulent material or excision of the entire gland and its duct.

Bartholin's cyst (bar'təlɪnz), a cyst that arises from one of the vestibular glands or from its ducts, filling with clear fluid which replaces the suppurative exudate characteristic of chronic inflammation.

Bartholin's duct, the major duct of the sublingual gland.

Bartholin's gland, one of two small, mucus-secreting glands located on the posterior and lateral aspect of the vestibule of the vagina. Also called **greater vestibular glands.**

Barton, Clara (1821–1912), an American philanthropist, humanitarian, and founder of the American National Red Cross. During the Civil War, she was a volunteer nurse, often on the battlefield, and at its end she organized a bureau of records to help in the search for missing men. When the Franco-Prussian War erupted, she assisted in the organization of military hospitals in Europe in association with the International Red Cross. This experience led to her advocacy of an American Red Cross organization, of which she became the first president.

Bartonella (bar'tənel'ə), a genus of small, gram-negative flagellated pleomorphic coccobacilli. Members of the genus are intracellular parasites that infect red blood cells and the epithelial cells of the lymph nodes, liver, and spleen. They are transmitted at night by the bite of a sandfly of the genus *Phlebotomus.* The only known species of *Bartonella* is *B. bacilliformis,* the organism that causes bartonellosis. Owing to its distinctive appearance, it is easily identified on microscopic examination of a smear of blood stained with Wright's stain.

bartonellosis (bar'tənəlou'sis), an acute infection caused by *Bartonella bacilliformis,* transmitted by the bite of a sandfly. It is characterized by fever, severe anemia, bone pain, and, several weeks after the first symptoms are observed, by multiple nodular or verrucose skin lesions. The disease is endemic in the valleys of the Andes in Peru, Colombia, and Ecuador. The treatment usually includes chloramphenicol, penicillin, streptomycin, or tetracycline. Untreated, the infection is often fatal. Also called **Carrión's disease, Oroya fever, verruga peruana.**

Barton forceps (bar'tən). See **obstetric forceps.**

Barton's fracture, a fracture of the distal articular surface of the radius, which may be accompanied by the dorsal dislocation of the carpus on the radius.

Bartter's syndrome (bar'tərz), a rare hereditary disorder, characterized by hyperplasia of the juxtaglomerular apparatus and secondary hyperaldosteronism. Renin and angiotensin levels may be elevated, but blood pressure usually remains normal. Early signs in childhood are abnormal physical growth and mental retardation, often accompanied by chronic hypokalemia and alkalosis.

bary-, a combining form meaning 'heavy or difficult': *baryecoia, baryencephalia, baryphonia.*

basal, of or pertaining to the fundamental or the basic, as basal anesthesia, which produces the first stage of unconsciousness, and the basal metabolic rate, which indicates the lowest metabolic rate.

basal anesthesia, 1. a state of unconsciousness just short of complete surgical anesthesia in depth, in which the patient does not respond to words but still reacts to pinprick or other noxious stimuli. 2. narcosis produced by injection or infusion of potent sedatives alone, without added narcotics or anesthetic agents. 3. any form of anesthesia in which the patient is completely unconscious, in contrast to awake anesthesia. Also called **narcoanesthesia.**

basal body temperature, the temperature of the body taken in the morning, orally or rectally, after at least five hours of sleep and before doing anything else, including getting out of bed, smoking a cigarette, moving around, talking, eating, or drinking.

basal body temperature method of family planning, a natural method of family planning that relies on the identification of the fertile period of the menstrual cycle by noting the progesterone mediated rise in basal body temperature of 0.5° to 1.0°F that occurs with ovulation. The rate and pattern of the increase varies greatly from woman to woman, and somewhat from cycle to cycle in any one woman. Several cycles are observed and careful records are kept in which the woman takes her temperature at the same time every morning, before doing anything else. It may be taken orally or rectally but should be done the same way every day. Talking, getting up, smoking a cigarette, eating, or even moving about in bed may change the temperature. Many other factors may also change the reading, including infection, stress, a bad night's sleep, medication, or environmental temperature. If any of these are present the woman notes them on her record. The fertile period is considered to continue until the temperature is above the baseline for five days; the rise occurs slowly during all five days or increases rapidly, reaching a plateau at which it remains for three or four days. The days following that period are considered 'safe' unfertile days. Abstinence is required from six days before the earliest day that ovulation was noted to occur during the preceding six months until the fifth day after the rise in temperature in the current cycle. Another way of calculating the possible beginning of the fertile days is to subtract nineteen days from the shortest complete menstrual cycle of the preceding six months. The basal body temperature method is more effective when used with the ovulation method than is either method used alone. The combination of these methods is called the symptothermal method of family planning. Compare **calendar method of family planning, ovulation method of family planning.**

basal bone, 1. (in prosthodontics) the osseous tissue of the mandible and the maxillae, except for the rami and the processes, which provides support for artificial dentures. 2. (in orthodontics) the fixed osseous structure that limits the movement of teeth in the creation of a stable occlusion.

basal cell, any one of the cells in the base layer of stratified epithelium.

basal cell acanthoma. See **basal cell papilloma.**

basal cell carcinoma, a malignant, epithelial cell tumor that begins as a papule and enlarges peripherally, developing a central crater that erodes, crusts, and bleeds. Metastasis is rare, but local invasion destroys underlying and adjacent tissue. In 90 per cent of cases, the lesion is seen between the hairline and the upper lip. The primary cause of the cancer is excessive exposure to the sun or to x rays. Treatment is eradication of the lesion, often by electrodesiccation or cryotherapy. Also called **basal cell epithelioma, basaloma, carcinoma basocellulare, hair matrix carcinoma.** See also **rodent ulcer.**

basal cell epithelioma. See **basal cell carcinoma.**

basal cell papilloma, a benign, epidermal neoplasm characterized by multiple yellow or brown raised oval lesions that usually develop in middle age. Also called **basal cell acanthoma, seborrheic keratosis, seborrheic wart.**

basal ganglia, the islands of gray matter within each cerebral hemisphere, the most important being the caudate nucleus, the putamen, and the pallidium. The basal ganglia are surrounded by the rings of the limbic system and lie between the thalamus of the diencephalon and the white matter of the hemisphere.

basal lamina, a thin, noncellular layer of ground substance lying just under epithelial surfaces. Constituting the uppermost layer of the basement membrane, it can be examined with an electron microscope. Also called **basement lamina.**

basal layer. See **stratum basale.**

basal membrane, a sheet of tissue that forms the outer layer of the choroid and lies just under the pigmented layer of the retina. It is composed of elastic fibers and a thin homogenous layer.

basal metabolic rate (BMR), the amount of energy used in a unit of time by a fasting, resting subject to maintain vital functions. The rate, determined by the amount of oxygen utilized, is expressed in calories consumed per hour per square meter of body surface area or per kilogram of body weight.

basal metabolism, the amount of energy needed to maintain essential basic body functions, as respiration, circulation, temperature, peristalsis, and muscle tone, measured when the subject is awake and at complete rest, has not eaten for 14 to 18 hours, and is in a comfortable, warm environment. It is expressed as a basal metabolic rate, according to large calories per hour per square meter of body surface.

basaloid carcinoma, a rare, malignant neoplasm of the anal canal containing areas which resemble basal call carcinoma of the skin, though a basaloid carcinoma is the more rapidly invasive and malignant of the two. The tumor may spread to the skin of the perineum.

basaloma (bei'səlou'mə). See **basal cell carcinoma.**

basal temperature, the temperature of a healthy individual immediately after at least eight hours of relaxed sleep and a fast of 14 to 18 hours.

base, 1. Compare **alkali.** A chemical compound that combines with an acid to form a salt. **2.** a molecule or radical that takes up or accepts protons. **3.** the major ingredient of a compounded material, particularly one that is used as a medication. Petroleum jelly is frequently used as a base for ointments.

base analogue, an analogue of one of the purine or the pyrimidine bases normally found in ribonucleic acid or deoxyribonucleic acid.

Basedow's goiter (ba'sɪdouz), an enlargement of the thyroid gland, characterized by the hypersecretion of thyroid hormone following iodine therapy.

basement lamina. See **basal lamina.**

basement membrane, the fragile, noncellular layer of tissue that secures the overlying, layers of stratified epithelium. It is the deepest layer, may contain reticular fibers, and can be selectively stained with silver stains.

base of the heart, the portion of the heart opposite the apex, directed to the right side of the body. It forms the upper border of the heart, lies just below the second rib, and involves primarily the left atrium, part of the right atrium, and the proximal portions of the great vessels. Passing between the base of the heart and the bodies of the fifth to the eighth thoracic vertebrae are the descending aorta, the esophagus, and the thoracic duct.

base of the skull, the floor of the skull, containing the anterior, middle, and posterior cranial fossae and numerous foramina, as the optic foramen, foramen ovale, foramen lacerum, and foramen magnum.

base pair, a pair of nucleotides in a nucleic acid. One of the pair must be a purine, the other, a pyrimidine. Base pairing finds guanine paired with cytosine and adenine paired with thymine.

base pairing, (in molecular genetics) the association in nucleic acids of the purine bases adenine and guanine with the pyrimidine bases cytosine, thymine, and uracil. In DNA, adenine always pairs with thymine, and guanine always pairs with cytosine. In RNA, adenine invariably pairs with uracil, and guanine invariabily pairs with cytosine.

base ratio, the ratio of molar quantities of the bases in ribonucleic and deoxyribonucleic acids.

bas-fond, the bottom or fundus of any structure, especially the fundus of the urinary bladder.

basi-, basio-, a combining form meaning 'pertaining to a foundation or a base': *basicranial, basilaris, basiotribe.*

-basia, a combining form meaning 'ability to walk': *abasia, brachybasia, dysbasia.*

-basic, a combining form meaning 'relating or containing alkaline compounds': *ammonobasic, polybasic, tribasic.*

basic amino acid, an amino acid that has a positive electric charge in solution. The basic amino acids are arginine, histidine, and lysine.

basic health services, the minimum degree of health care considered to be necessary to maintain adequate health and protection from disease.

basilar, of or pertaining to a base or a basal area.

basilar artery, the single arterial trunk formed by the junction of the two vertebral arteries at the base of the skull, extending from the inferior to the superior border of the pons, dividing into the left and right cerebral arteries, and supplying the internal ear and parts of the brain through the five branches of each artery. The branches are the pontine, labyrinthine, anterior inferior cerebellar, superior cerebellar, and posterior cerebral.

basilar artery insufficiency syndrome, the composite of clinical indicators associated with insufficient blood flow through the basilar artery, a condition that may be caused by arterial occlusion. Some of the common signs of this syndrome are dizziness, blindness, numbness, depression, dysarthria, dysphagia, and weakness on one side of the body.

basilar membrane, the cellular structure that forms the floor of the cochlear duct and is supported by bony and fibrous projections from the cochlear wall. It provides a fibrous base for the spiral organ of Corti.

basilar plexus, the venous network interlaced between the layers of the dura mater over the basilar portion of the occipital bone. It connects the two petrosal sinuses and communicates with the anterior vertebral venus plexus.

basilar sulcus, the sulcus that cradles the basilar artery, in the midline of the pons.

basilic vein (bəsɪl′ɪk), one of the four superficial veins of the arm, beginning in the ulnar part of the dorsal venous network and running proximally on the posterior surface of the ulnar side of the forearm. It veers toward the anterior surface of the forearm distal to the elbow and is joined by the median cubital vein, then ascends obliquely between the biceps brachii and the pronator teres and crosses the brachial artery. It then runs proximally along the medial border of the biceps brachii, pierces the deep fascia, and ascends to join the brachial vein to form the axillary vein. Compare **dorsal digital vein, median antebrachial vein.**

basiloma (bæs′ɪlou′mə), pl. **basilomas, basilomata.** a carcinoma composed of basal cells. A kind of basiloma is **basiloma terebrans.** Also called **basaloma.**

basiloma terebrans (ter′əbrænz), a basal cell epithelioma that is invasive.

basio-. See **basi-.**

basioccipital, of or pertaining to the basilar process of the occipital bone.

basion, the midpoint on the anterior margin of the foramen magnum of the occipital bone, opposite the opisthion in the middle of the posterior margin.

basis pedunculi cerebri. See **crus cerebri.**

basophil (bei′səfɪl), a granulocytic white blood cell characterized by a segmented nucleus that contains granules that stain blue when exposed to a basic dye. Basophils represent 1 per cent or less of the total white blood cell count. The relative number of basophils increases in myeloproliferative diseases and decreases in severe allergic reactions. Compare **eosinophil, neutrophil.** See also

agranulocyte, differential white blood cell count, granulocyte, leukocyte, polymorphonuclear leukocyte.

basophilic adenoma, a tumor of the pituitary gland composed of cells that can be stained with basic dyes. Cushing's syndrome is often caused by a basophilic adenoma. Compare **acidophilic adenoma, chromophobic adenoma.**

basophilic leukemia, an acute or chronic malignant neoplasm of blood-forming tissues, characterized by large numbers of immature basophilic granulocytes in peripheral circulation and in tissues. See also **acute myelocytic leukemia.**

basophilic stippling, the abnormal presence of punctate, basophilic granules in the red blood cells, observed under the microscope on a gram-stained smear of the blood. Stippling is characteristic of lead poisoning. See also **basophil, lead poisoning.**

basosquamous cell carcinoma (bei′souskwei′məs), a malignant epidermal tumor composed of basal and squamous cells.

Bassen-Kornzweig syndrome (bæs′ənkorn′swaig). See **abetalipoproteinemia.**

bath, (in the hospital) a cleansing procedure performed daily by or for almost all patients to help prevent infection, preserve the unbroken condition of the skin, stimulate circulation, promote oxygen intake, maintain muscle tone and joint mobility, and provide comfort.
■ METHOD: The bath may be a bed or tub bath, a shower, or a partial bath, depending on the patient's condition and preference and the room temperature. The bath period may be used to instruct the patient on hygienic measures. Observations are made of the general cleanliness and odor of the patient's body, the color, dryness, turgor, and elasticity of the skin, the condition of the hair, hands, feet, fingernails and toenails. Any discoloration, abrasion, rash, discharge, perineal or rectal irritation, clubbing of the digits, hair loss, or evidence of lice is carefully noted. Mild soap and water are used for the bath and a lanolin-based lotion is used for the after-bath massage. The patient's hair is combed daily and shampooed as desired; finger- and toenails are cleaned and trimmed whenever required. Petroleum jelly or other suitable lubricant and a thin layer of cornstarch are applied to the perineal and perianal areas if indicated.
■ NURSING ORDERS: The nurse gives the bed bath in a setting that provides privacy for the patient. Firm, gentle strokes are used to wash, dry, and massage the person; vigorous rubbing is avoided. The partial bath is given with the patient seated in or on the side of the bed, or in a chair. Self-help is encouraged, and the procedure is completed as soon as possible to avoid chilling. In preparation for a tub bath, the nurse checks the safety strips in the bottom of the tub and the temperature of the water, and assists the patient into the tub. Precautions are taken

to avoid chilling, and on completion of the bath the nurse may help the patient out of the tub. In preparation for a shower, the nurse explains the operation of the dials regulating the water temperature, provides a bath mat, and cautions the patient not to become chilled.

■ OUTCOME CRITERIA: A daily bath helps to prevent decubiti, provides an opportunity to assess external signs of disease and effects of therapy, and improves the patient's sense of well-being and self-esteem.

bathesthesia (bæth'əsthi'Zhə), bathyesthesia, a deep sensibility, as that associated with organs or structures beneath the surface of the body, as muscles and joints.

bathmic evolution (bæth'mik). See **orthogenic evolution.**

batho-. See **bathy-.**

bathy-, batho-, a combining form meaning 'pertaining to depth, deep': *bathycentesis, bathypnea, bathomorphic.*

bathycardia (bæth'əkar'diə), an abnormal but nonpathological condition characterized by an unusually low position of the heart.

battered woman syndrome (BWS), repeated episodes of physical assault on a woman by the man with whom she lives, often resulting in serious physical and psychological damage to the woman. Such violence tends to follow a predictable pattern. The violent episodes usually follow verbal argument and accusation and are accompanied by verbal abuse. Almost any subject—housekeeping, money, childrearing—may begin the episode. Over time the violent episodes escalate in frequency and severity. Once a month becomes once a week; a shove becomes a punch. Most battered women report that they thought that the assaults would stop, but, unfortunately, study shows that the longer the women stay in the relationship the more likely they are to be seriously injured. Less and less provocation seems to be enough to trigger an attack once the syndrome has begun. The use of alcohol increases the severity of the assault; a man who usually shoves or slaps his partner is more likely to punch or kick her if he is drunk. Other drugs do not have this effect; the man is more likely to be abusive as the drug is wearing off. Battering occurs in cycles of violence. The first phase is characterized by the man acting increasingly irritable, edgy, and tense. Verbal abuse, insults, and criticism increase, and shoves or slaps begin. The second phase is the time of the acute, violent activity. As the tension mounts, the woman becomes unable to placate the man, and she may argue or defend herself. The man uses this as the justification for his anger and assaults her, often saying that he is 'teaching her a lesson.' The third stage is characterized by apology and remorse on the part of the man, with promises of change. The calm continues until tension builds again. The battered woman syndrome occurs at all socioeconomic levels, and one half to three quarters of female assault victims are the victims of an attack by a lover or husband. It is estimated that between one and two million women a year are beaten by their husbands. Men who grew up in homes in which the father abused the mother are more likely to beat their wives than are men who lived in nonviolent homes. Personal and cultural attitudes also affect the incidence of wife-battering. Aggressive behavior is a normal part of male socialization in most cultures; physical aggression may be condoned as a means of resolving a conflict. A personality profile obtained by psychological testing reveals the typical battered woman to be reserved, withdrawn, depressed, and anxious, with low self-esteem, a poorly integrated self-image, and a general inability to cope with life's demands. The parents of such women encouraged compliance, were not physically affectionate, and socially restricted their daughters' independence, preventing the widening of social contact that normally occurs in adolescence. Victims of the battered woman syndrome are often afraid to leave the man and the situation; change, loneliness, and the unknown are perceived as more painful than the beatings. Nurses are in an excellent position to offer assistance to battered women in several ways, as encouraging a woman to talk about the battering and the injuries may help her to admit what she may have been too embarrassed to reveal even to her parents. A realistic appraisal of the situation is then possible; the woman wants to hear that the nurse thinks the battering will not recur but the nurse can tell her only that the usual pattern is for the abuse to continue and to become more severe. The woman may be referred to the social service department or given directions for contacting special community agencies, as a battered women's shelter or a hotline to a counseling service. Caring for and counseling a battered woman often require great patience because she is usually ambivalent about her situation and may be confused to the point of believing that she deserves the assaults she has suffered. Records are maintained to document the extent of the problem, including the form of abuse reported, the injuries sustained, and a summary of similar incidents and previous admissions.

battery, 1. a complex of two or more electrolytic cells connected together to form a single source providing direct current or voltage. 2. a series or a combination of tests to determine the cause of a particular illness or the degree of proficiency in a particular skill or discipline.

Battey bacillus (bæt'i), any of a group of atypical mycobacteria, including *Mycobacteria avium* and *M. intracellulare,* that cause a chronic pulmonary disease resembling tuberculosis. These organisms are resistant to most of the common bacteriostatic and antibiotic medications. Surgical resection of involved lung tissue may be necessary and may improve the outcome in serious cases. Rest, good nutrition, and general supportive care are usually recommended. Compare **tuberculosis.**

battledore placenta (bæt'əldər'), a placenta to which the umbilical cord is attached at the periphery.

Battle's sign, a small hemorrhagic spot behind the ear that appears in cases may indicate a fracture of a bone of the lower skull.

batyl alcohol, an alcohol found in fish liver oil that is used to treat bracken poisoning in cattle.

Baudelocque's diameter (bou'dəloks'). See **external conjugate.**

Baudelocque's method, (in obstetrics) a maneuver used to convert a face presentation to a vertex presentation. The operator flexes the fetal head vaginally and applies counter pressure to the back of the head abdominally while an assistant rotates the fetus in the direction of flexion until the vertex is fixed in the pelvis.

Baynton's bandage (bein'tənz), a spiral adhesive wrap applied to the leg over a dressing, used in the treatment of indolent ulcers of the leg.

BBB, abbreviation for **blood-brain barrier.**

B cell, a type of lymphocyte that originates in the bone marrow. A precursor of the plasma cell upon suitable antigenic stimulation, it is one of the two lymphocytes that play a major role in the body's immunologic response. See also **plasma cell, T cell.**

BCG, abbreviation for **bacillus Calmette-Guérin.**

BCG vaccine, an active immunizing agent prepared from bacillus Calmette-Guérin.

■ INDICATION: It is prescribed most commonly for immunization against tuberculosis.

■ CONTRAINDICATIONS: Hypogammaglobulinemia, immunosuppression, or concomitant use of corticosteroids or isoniazid prohibits its use. It is not given following a vaccination for smallpox, nor is it given to patients with a positive tuberculin reaction or a burn.

■ ADVERSE EFFECTS: Among the most serious adverse reactions are anaphylaxis and disseminated pulmonary tuberculosis. Pain, inflammation and granuloma may develop at site of injection.

BCNU. See **carmustine.**

B complex vitamins, a large group of water soluble substances that includes **vitamin B$_1$ (thiamine), vitamin B$_2$ (riboflavin), vitamin B$_3$ (niacin), vitamin B$_6$ (pyridoxine), vitamin B$_{12}$ (cyanocobalamin), biotin, choline, carnitine, folic acid, inositol,** and **para-aminobenzoic acid.** The B complex vitamins are essential in converting carbohydrates into glucose to provide energy, for metabolism of fats and proteins, for normal functioning of the nervous system, for maintenance of muscle tone in the gastrointestinal tract, and for the health of skin, hair, eyes, mouth, and liver. They are found in brewer's yeast, liver, wholegrain cereals, nuts, eggs, meats, fish, and vegetables and are produced by the intestinal bacteria. Maintaining milk-free diets or taking antibiotics may destroy these bacteria. Symptoms of vitamin B deficiency include nervousness,

depression, insomnia, neuritis, anemia, alopecia, acne or other skin disorders, and hypercholesterolemia. See also specific vitamins.

b.d. See **b.i.d.**

Be, symbol for **beryllium.**

beaded, 1. of or having a resemblance to a row of beads. 2. of or pertaining to bacterial colonies that develop along the inoculation line in various stab cultures. 3. of or pertaining to stained bacteria that develop more deeply stained beadlike granules.

beaker cell. See **goblet cell.**

BEAM, abbreviation for **brain electrical activity map.**

bean, the pod-enclosed flattened seed of numerous leguminous plants. Beans used in pharmocological preparations are alphabetized by specific name.

Becker's muscular dystrophy, a chronic degenerative disease of the muscles, characterized by progressive weakness. It occurs in childhood between 8 and 20 years of age. It occurs less frequently, progresses more slowly, and has a better prognosis than the more common pseudohypertrophic form of muscular dystrophy. The pathophysiology of the disease is not understood; it is transmitted genetically as an autosomal recessive trait. Also called **benign pseudohypertrophic muscular dystrophy.**

Beck I operation, a surgical procedure to provide collateral circulation to the heart. The operation roughens the surface of the epicardium and the parietal lining of the pericardium, applies an irritant, as powdered asbestos, to these surfaces, partially closes the coronary sinus at its entrance to the right atrium, and grafts the parietal pericardium and the mediastinal fat to the myocardium. Compare **Beck II operation.**

Beck II operation, an operation in two stages that provides collateral circulation to the heart. In the first stage, a venous graft is placed between the aorta and the coronary sinus to shunt arterial blood. In the second stage of the procedure, executed two to three weeks after the first stage, the coronary sinus is partially closed to raise pressure within the sinus and force oxygenated blood from the aorta to flow into the coronary vessels. Compare **Beck I operation.**

Beck's triad, a combination of three symptoms that characterize cardiac compression: high venous pressure, low arterial pressure, and a small, quiet heart.

Beckwith's syndrome, an hereditary disorder of unknown etiology associated with neonatal hypoglycemia and hyperinsulinism. Clinical manifestations include gigantism, macroglossia, omphalocele or umbilical hernia, visceromegaly, hyperplasia of the kidney and pancreas, extreme enlargement of the cells of the adrenal cortex, and often various other abnormalities. Treatment consists of adequate glucose, diazoxide, and glucocorticoid therapy. Subtotal pancreatectomy is often necessary in cases of beta-cell hyperplasia, nesidioblastosis, or beta-cell tumor of the pancreas.

Beckwith-Wiedemann syndrome. See **EMG syndrome.**

beclomethasonedipropionate, a glucocorticoid.
■ INDICATION: It is prescribed in an inhaler in the treatment of bronchial asthma.
■ CONTRAINDICATIONS: Status asthmaticus, acute asthma, or known hypersensitivity to this drug prohibits its use.
■ ADVERSE EFFECTS: Among the more serious adverse reactions of systemic administration are the symptoms of adrenal insufficiency. Hoarseness, sore throat, and fungal infections of the oropharynx and larynx may occur.

bed, (in anatomy) a supporting matrix of tissue, as the nail beds of modified epidermis over which the fingernails and the toenails move as they grow.

bedbug, a blood-sucking arthropod of the species *Cimex lectularius* that feeds on humans and other animals. The bedbug can be removed after covering it with petrolatum. The bite, which causes itching, pain, and redness, can be treated with a lotion or cream containing a corticosteroid or other topical anti-inflammatory or analgesic preparation.

Bednar's aphthae (bed′narz), the small, yellowish, slightly elevated ulcerated patches that normally occur on the posterior portion of the hard palate of newborn babies. Compare **Epstein's pearls, thrush.**

bedside manner, 1. the behavior of a nurse or doctor as perceived by a patient. 2. an agreeable and satisfying professional demeanor in the eyes of a patient.

bedsore. See **decubitus ulcer.**

Bee-cell pessary. See **pessary.**

beef tapeworm. See *Taenia saginata.*

beef tapeworm infection, an infection caused by the tapeworm *Taenia saginata,* transmitted to humans when they eat contaminated beef. The adult worm can live for years in the intestine of humans without causing any symptoms. The infection is rarely found in the U.S. because beef is carefully inspected before being made available, but it is commonly found in other parts of the world. See **tapeworm infection.**

bee sting, an injury caused by the venom of bees, usually accompanied by pain and swelling. The stinger of the honeybee usually remains implanted and should be removed. Pain may be alleviated by application of an ice pack or a paste of sodium bicarbonate and water. Serious reactions may result from multiple stings, stings on some areas of the head, or the injection of venom directly into the circulatory system. In a hypersensitive person, a single bee sting may result in death owing to anaphylactic shock and bronchospasm. Hypersensitive individuals are encouraged to carry emergency treatment supplies with them when the possibility of bee sting exists. Compare **wasp.**

behavior, 1. the manner in which a person acts or performs. 2. any or all of the activities of a person, including physical actions, which are observed directly, and mental activity, which is inferred and interpreted. Kinds of behavior include **abnormal behavior, automatic behavior, invariable behavior, variable behavior.**

behavioral objective, a goal in therapy or research that concerns an act or a specific behavior or pattern of behaviors.

behavioral reflex. See **conditioned response.**

behavioral science, any of the various interrelated disciplines, as psychiatry, psychology, sociology, and anthropology, that observes and studies human activity, including psychological and emotional development, interpersonal relationships, values, and mores.

behavior disorder, any of a group of antisocial behavior patterns occurring primarily in children and adolescents, as overaggressiveness, overactivity, destructiveness, cruelty, truancy, lying, disobedience, perverse sexual activity, criminality, alcoholism, and drug addiction. The most common motivating force for such reactions is hostility, which is manifested either overtly or covertly and is precipitated by a disturbed relationship between the child and his parents, an unstable home situation, and, in some cases, by organic brain dysfunction. Behavior disorders may be symptomatic of other neuroses or psychoses, as childhood schizophrenia. Treatment may include psychotherapy, milieu therapy, medication, and family counseling. See also **antisocial personality disorder.**

behaviorism, a school of psychology founded by John B. Watson that studies and interprets behavior by observing measurable responses to stimuli without reference to consciousness, mental states, or subjective phenomena, as ideas and emotions. See also **neobehaviorism.**

behaviorist, a disciple of the school of behaviorism.

behavioristic psychology. See **behaviorism.**

behavior modification. See **behavior therapy.**

behavior systems model, a conceptual framework describing factors that may affect the stability of a person's behavior. The model examines systems of behavior, not the behavior of an individual at any particular time. In this model, behavior is defined as an integrated response to stimuli. Several subsystems of behavior form man's eight microsystems, which are: ingestion, elimination, dependency, sex, achievement, affiliation, aggression, and restoration. Each subsystem comprises several structural components called "imperatives," which are goal, set, choice, action, and support. The goal of nursing care is to attain, maintain, or restore balance of the subsystems of behavior for the stability of the patient.

behavior therapy, a kind of psychotherapy that attempts to modify observable, maladjusted patterns of behavior by the substitution of a new response or set of responses to a given stimulus. The treatment techniques involve the methods, concepts, and procedures derived from experimental psychology and include assertiveness training, aversion therapy, contingency management, flooding, modeling, operant conditioning, and systemic desensitization. Also called **behavior modification.** See also **biofeedback.**

Behçet's disease, a rare and severe illness of unknown cause, mostly affecting young males and characterized by severe uveitis and retinal vasculitis. Some other signs are optic atrophy and aphthalike lesions of the mouth and the genitals, indicating diffuse vasculitis. Also called **Behçet's syndrome.**

Behla's bodies (beɪˈlɑz). See **Plimmer's bodies.**

BEI, abbreviation for **butanol extractable iodine.**

bejel (bejˈəl), a nonvenereal form of syphilis prevalent among children in the Middle East and North Africa, caused by the spirochete *Treponema pallidum II.* It is transmitted by person-to-person contact and by the sharing of drinking and eating utensils. The primary lesion is usually on or near the mouth, appearing as a mucous patch, followed by the development of pimplelike sores on the trunk, arms, and legs. Chronic ulceration of the nose and soft palate occurs in the advanced stages of the infection. Destructive changes in the tissues of the heart, central nervous system, and mouth, often associated with the venereal form of syphilis, rarely develop. Intramuscular injection of penicillin is effective in curing the infection, but if extensive tissue destruction has occurred, scar tissue forms and may be permanently disfiguring.

Békésy audiometry (bekˈɪsi), a method of testing hearing in which the subject presses a signal button while listening to a pure tone that is progressively diminished in intensity and releases the button when the sound no longer is heard. Continuous and interrupted tones are used in the test.

bel, a unit that expresses intensity of sound. It is the logarithm (to the base 10) of the ratio of the power of any specific sound to the power of a reference sound. The most common reference sound has a power of 10^{-16} watts per cm^2, or the approximate minimum intensity of sound at 1000 cycles per second, that is perceptible to the human ear. An increase of one bel approximately doubles the intensity or loudness of most sounds.

belching. See **eructation.**

belladonna, the dried leaf and flowering or fruiting tops of *Atropa belladonna,* a common perennial called deadly nightshade, containing the alkaloids hyoscyamine and atropine.

bellows murmur, a blowing sound, as air moving in and out of a bellows.

Bell's law, an axiom stating that the ventral spinal roots are motor and the dorsal spinal roots are sensory. Also called **Bell-Magendie law, Magendie's law.**

Bell's mania, *Obsolete.* a mood disorder characterized by acute delirium. See also **delirium, mania.**

Bell's palsy, a paralysis of the facial nerve, resulting from trauma to the nerve, compression of the nerve by a tumor, or, most often, from an unknown cause. Any or all branches of the nerve may be affected. The person may not be able to open an eye or close the mouth. The condition may be unilateral or bilateral, transient or permanent. Plastic surgery may reduce the deformity.

Bell's phenomenon, a sign of peripheral facial paralysis, manifested by the upward and outward rolling of the eyeball when the affected individual tries to close the eye.

belly. See **abdomen.**

belly button. See **umbilicus.**

belonephobia (belˈənəfouˈbiə), a morbid fear of sharp-pointed objects, especially needles and pins.

Benadryl, a trade name for an antihistaminic (diphenhydramine hydrochloride).

Bence Jones protein (bens), a protein found almost exclusively in the urine of patients with multiple myeloma. The protein constitutes the light chain component of myeloma globulin; it coagulates at temperatures of 45° to 55°C and redissolves completely or partially on boiling. See also **multiple myeloma, protein.**

bench research, *Informal.* (in medicine) any research done in a controlled laboratory setting using other than human subjects.

Bendectin, a trade name for a fixed-combination drug containing an antihistamine (doxylamine succinate) and a vitamin (pyridoxine hydrochloride), used for treating nausea in pregnancy.

bending fracture, a fracture indirectly caused by the bending of an extremity, as of the foot or of the big toe.

bendroflumethiazide (benˈdroufluˈməθaiˈəzaid), a diuretic and antihypertensive.

■ INDICATIONS: It is prescribed in the treatment of hypertension and edema.

■ CONTRAINDICATIONS: Anuria or known hypersensitivity to this drug, to other thiazide medication, or to sulfonamide derivatives prohibits its use.

■ ADVERSE EFFECTS: Among the more serious adverse reactions are hypokalemia, hyperglycemia, hyperuricemia, and various hypersensitivity reactions.

bends, the. See **decompression sickness.**

Benedict's qualitative test, a test for sugar in the urine based on the reduction by glucose of cupric ions to a colored cuprous oxide precipitate when it is placed in an alkaline solution. Eight drops of urine are added to 5 ml of Benedict's solution; the mixture is boiled for one to two minutes and then cooled. Formation of an orange or red precipitate indicates more than 2 per cent sugar (called 4+), yellow indicates 1 per cent to 2 per cent sugar (called 3+), olive green indicates .5 per cent to 1 per cent sugar (called 2+), and green indicates less than .5 per cent sugar (called 1+).

Benemid, a trade name for a uricosuric (probenecid).

benign, (of a tumor) noncancerous and therefore not an immediate threat, even though treatment eventually may be required for health or cosmetic reasons. Compare **malignant.**

benign hypertension, a misnomer implying an innocent elevation of blood pressure. Since any sustained elevation of blood pressure may adversely affect health, it is incorrect to refer to the condition as 'benign.' Compare **malignant hypertension.** See also **essential hypertension.**

benign intracranial hypertension. See **pseudotumor cerebri.**

benign juvenile melanoma, a benign, pink or fuchsia raised papule with a scaly surface, usually on a cheek and occurring most commonly in children between the ages of 9 and 13 years. It may be mistaken for a malignant melanoma. Also called **compound melanocytoma, spindle cell nevus, Spitz nevus.**

benign mesenchymoma, a benign neoplasm that has two or more definitely recognizable mesenchymal elements in addition to fibrous tissue.

benign neoplasm, a tumor, characteristically localized, that has a fibrous capsule, limited potential for growth, a regular shape, and cells that are well differentiated. A benign neoplasm does not invade surrounding tissue or metastasize to distant sites. It causes harm only by pressure and does not usually recur after surgical excision. Some kinds of benign neoplasms are **adenoma, fibroma, hemangioma, lipoma.** See also **malignant neoplasm.**

benign prostatic hypertrophy, enlargement of the prostate gland, common among men by the age of 50. The condition is not malignant or inflammatory but is usually progressive and may lead to obstruction of the urethra and to interference with the flow of urine, possibly causing frequency of urination, the need to urinate during the night, pain, and urinary tract infections. Treatment consists of conservative measures: regular sexual release, hot baths, prostatic massage, avoidance of alcohol or excessive fluid intake, and voiding upon the urge to do so. Surgical resection of the enlarged prostate is sometimes necessary. Compare **prostatitis.** See also **prostatectomy.**

benign pseudohypertrophic muscular dystrophy. See **Becker's muscular dystrophy.**

benign stupor, a state of apathy or lethargy, as occurs in severe depression.

benign thrombocytosis. See **thrombocytosis.**

benign tumor, a neoplasm that does not invade other tissues or metastasize in other sites. A benign tumor is usually well encapsulated, and its cells exhibit less anaplasia than those of a malignant growth. Some benign tu-

mors must be excised to prevent damage or death, because the tumor may grow to occupy space needed by an organ or tissue.

Bennet's small corpuscle (ben'əts). See **Drysdale's corpuscle.**

Bennett's fracture, a fracture that runs obliquely through the base of the first metacarpal bone and into the carpometacarpal joint, detaching the greater part of the articular facet. Bennett's fracture may be associated with dorsal subluxation or with dislocation of the first metacarpal.

Benoquin, a trade name for a depigmenting agent (monobenzone).

benoxinate hydrochloride, a topical anesthetic.

■ INDICATIONS: It is used for ophthalmologic anesthesia in surgical procedures, in removing sutures or foreign objects from the eye, and in tonometry.

■ CONTRAINDICATION: Known hypersensitivity to this drug prohibits its use.

■ ADVERSE EFFECTS: Among the more serious adverse reactions are slight pain when first instilled, corneal damage with excessive or prolonged use, and hypersensitivity reactions.

Benoxl, a trade name for a topical antiseptic (benzoyl peroxide), used in the treatment of acne.

bent fracture, an incomplete greenstick fracture.

bentonite, colloidal, hydrated aluminum silicate, which, when added to water, swells to approximately twelve times its dry size. It is used as a bulk laxative and as a base for skin care preparations.

Bentyl, a trade name for an anticholinergic antispasmodic (dicyclomine hydrochloride).

benzalkonium chloride, a disinfectant prepared in an aqueous solution in various strengths.

benzathine penicillin G. See **penicillin G benzathine.**

Benzedrex, a trade name for an adrenergic vasoconstrictor (propylhexedrine).

Benzedrine, a trade name for a central-nervous-system stimulant (amphetamine sulfate).

benzene poisoning, a toxic condition caused by ingestion of benzene, the inhalation of benzene fumes or exposure to benzene-related products such as toluene or xylene, characterized by nausea, headache, dizziness, and incoordination. In acute cases, respiratory failure or ventricular fibrillation may cause death. Chronic exposure may result in aplastic anemia or a form of leukemia. Benzene poisoning by inhalation is treated with ventilatory assistance and oxygen; poisoning by ingestion is treated with gastric intubation, removal of the poison, and lavage. See also **nitrobenzene poisoning.**

benzethonium chloride (ben'zıfhou'nıəm), a topical anti-infective used for disinfecting the skin and for treating some infections of the eye, nose, and throat. It is also used as a preservative in some pharmaceutical preparations.

benzocaine, a local anesthetic agent derived from aminobenzoic acid, used in many over-the-counter compounds for pruritus and pain. Benzocaine has a low incidence of toxicity, but sensitization to it may occur with prolonged or frequent use. Suppositories containing benzocaine may cause methemoglobinemia in infants and small children. A minimum of 5 per cent benzocaine is required in a compound to be effective.

benzodiazepine derivative (ben'zoudaiæz'əpin), one of a group of psychotropic agents, including the tranquilizers chlordiazepoxide, diazepam, oxazepam, and chlorazepate, prescribed to alleviate anxiety and the hypnotics flurazepam and nitrazepam, prescribed in the treatment of insomnia. Some of the drugs have further clinical application: diazepam is often prescribed to relieve spasm of the muscles and to increase the seizure threshold. Tolerance and physical dependence occur with prolonged high dosage. Withdrawal symptoms, including seizures, and acute psychosis, may follow abrupt discontinuation. Adverse reactions to the benzodiazepines include drowsiness, ataxia, and a paradoxical increase in aggression and hostility; these reactions are not commonly seen in association with the usual recommended dosage.

benzoic acid (benzou'ık), a keratolytic agent, usually used with salicylic acid as an ointment in the treatment of athlete's foot and ringworm of the scalp. It has little antifungal action but makes deep infections accessible to more potent preparation. Mild irritation may occur at the site of application.

benzonatate (benzou'nəteit), a nonopiate antitussive.
■ INDICATION: It is prescribed to suppress the cough reflex.
■ CONTRAINDICATIONS: Known hypersensitivity to this drug prohibits its use.
■ ADVERSE EFFECTS: There are no known serious reactions. Vertigo, headache, constipation, and hypersensitivity reactions, usually mild, sometimes occur.

benzotropine mesylate, an anticholinergic agent.
■ INDICATION: It is prescribed in the treatment of Parkinson's disease.
■ CONTRAINDICATIONS: Narrow angle glaucoma, asthma, obstruction of the genitourinary or gastrointestinal tract, severe ulcerative colitis, or known hypersensitivity to this drug prohibits its use.
■ ADVERSE EFFECTS: Among the more serious adverse effects are blurred vision, drowsiness, central nervous system effects, tachycardia, dry mouth, decreased sweating, and hypersensitivity reactions.

benzoyl peroxide, an antibacterial, keratolytic, drying agent.
■ INDICATION: It is prescribed in the treatment of acne.
■ CONTRAINDICATION: Known hypersensitivity to this drug prohibits its use. It is not used in the eye, on inflamed skin, or on mucous membranes.
■ ADVERSE EFFECTS: Among the more serious adverse reactions are excessive drying and allergic contact sensitization.

benzphetamine hydrochloride, a sympathomimetic used as an anorexic agent.
■ INDICATION: It is prescribed to decrease the appetite in the treatment of obesity.
■ CONTRAINDICATIONS: Arteriosclerosis, cardiovascular disease, hypertension, glaucoma, hyperthyroidism, or known hypersensitivity to this or other sympathomimetic drugs prohibits its use.
■ ADVERSE EFFECTS: Among the more serious adverse reactions are restlessness, insomnia, tachycardia, increased blood pressure, and dry mouth.

benzquinamide (benzkwın'əmaid), an antiemetic.
■ INDICATIONS: It is prescribed in the treatment of postoperative nausea and vomiting.
■ CONTRAINDICATIONS: Severe hypertension, severe cardiovascular disease, or known hypersensitivity to this drug prohibits its use. It is not usually administered to children or to pregnant women.
■ ADVERSE EFFECTS: Among the most serious adverse reactions are sudden increase in blood pressure and cardiac arrhythmia. Drowsiness, chills, and shivering are commonly noted.

benzthiazide, a diuretic and antihypertensive.
■ INDICATIONS: It is prescribed in the treatment of hypertension and edema.
■ CONTRAINDICATIONS: Anuria or known hypersensitivity to this drug, to other thiazide medication, or to sulfonamide derivatives prohibits its use.
■ ADVERSE EFFECTS: Among the more serious adverse effects are hypokalemia, hyperglycemia, hyperuricemia, and hypersensitivity reactions.

benzyl alcohol, a clear, colorless, oily liquid, derived from certain balsams, used as a topical anesthetic and as a bacteriostatic agent in solutions for injection. Also called **phenyl carbinol, phenyl methanol.**

benzyl carbonol. See **phenylethyl alcohol.**

Berger rhythm (bər'gər). See **alpha wave.** Also called **Berger wave.**

Berger wave. See **Berger rhythm.**

Bergonié-Tréboneau law (beʀgɔnyei'tʀeibɔnou'), (in radiotherapy) a rule stating that the radiosensitivity of tissue depends on the number of undifferentiated cells, their mitotic activity, and the length of time they are actively proliferating.

beriberi (ber'iber'i), a disease of the peripheral nerves owing to a deficiency of or an inability to assimilate thiamine. It is frequently caused by a diet limited to polished white rice, and it occurs in endemic form in eastern and southern Asia. Rare cases in the United States are associated with stressful conditions, as hypothyroidism, infections, pregnancy, lactation, and chronic alcoholism. Symptoms are fatigue, diarrhea, appetite and weight loss, disturbed nerve function causing paralysis and wasting of limbs, edema, and heart failure. Administration of thiamine prevents and cures the disease. Also called **athiaminosis, kakke disease.** See also **thiamine.**

berkelium (Bk), an artificial radioactive transuranic element. Its atomic number is 97; its atomic weight is 247.

Berlock dermatitis (bər'lok), an abnormal skin condition, characterized by hyperpigmentation and skin lesions, caused by a unique reaction to psoralen-type photosynthesizers, commonly used in perfumes, colognes, and pomades, as oil of bergamot. This condition affects mostly women and children and may result from the use of products containing psoralens and from exposure to ultraviolet light. Although only about 5 per cent of the radiation of the sun is ultraviolet light and much of that is absorbed by oxygen and ozone, the level of ultraviolet radiation reaching the earth, especially on a sunny day, is sufficient to cause the lesion to appear.

■ OBSERVATIONS: Berlock dermatitis commonly produces an acute erythematous reaction, as that associated with sunburn. The area affected becomes hyperpigmented and surrounded by darker pigmentation. Areas of the neck where perfume containing oil of bergamot is applied often become affected by pendantlike lesions. Diagnosis is based on the appearance of such signs and on patient history that may include recent exposure to psoralens.

■ INTERVENTION: Treatment of Berlock dermatitis seeks to identify and eliminate the cause of the condition. Topical steroids may be administered to relieve discomfort.

■ NURSING CONSIDERATIONS: Patients with Berlock dermatitis benefit from advice about the complications of prolonged exposure to sunlight and ultraviolet light. They also appreciate the justifiable reassurance that the lesions will vanish within a few months.

Bernard-Soulier syndrome (bərnard'sulyei'), a coagulation disorder characterized by an absence of or a deficiency in the ability of the platelets to aggregate owing to the relative lack of an essential glycoprotein in the membranes of the platelets. On microscopic examination the platelets appear large and dispersed. The use of aspirin may provoke hemorrhage in people who have this condition. Following trauma and surgery, loss of blood may be greater than normal and transfusion may be required.

Bernoulli's law (bərnu'liz), a law of chemistry stating that the velocity of a gas or a fluid flowing through a tube is inversely proportional to the pressure it exerts against the side of the tube: the greater the velocity, the lower the pressure.

Bernoulli's principle, (in physics) a principle stating that the sum of the velocity and the kinetic energy of a fluid flowing through a tube is constant. The greater the velocity the less the lateral pressure on the wall of the tube. Thus, if an artery is narrowed by an atherosclerotic plaque, the flow of blood through the constriction increases in velocity and decreases in lateral pressure.

Bernstein test. See **acid perfusion test.**

berry aneurysm, a small, saccular dilatation of the wall of a cerebral artery, occurring most frequently at the junctures of vessels in the circle of Willis. A berry aneurysm may be the result of a congenital developmental defect and may rupture without warning, causing intracranial hemorrhage.

berylliosis (bərıl'iou'sıs), poisoning that results from the inhalation of dusts or vapors containing beryllium or beryllium compounds. It is characterized by granulomas throughout the body and by diffuse pulmonary fibrosis, resulting in a dry cough, shortness of breath, and chest pain. Symptoms may not appear for several years following exposure. See also **inorganic dust.**

beryllium (Be), a steel-gray, light-weight metallic element. Its atomic number is 4; its atomic weight is 9.012. Beryllium occurs naturally as beryl and is used in metallic alloys and in fluorescent powders. Inhalation of beryllium fumes or particles may cause the formation of granulomas in the lungs, skin, and subcutaneous tissues. See also **berylliosis.**

bestiality (bes'chiæl'ıti), **1.** a brutal or animal-like character or nature. **2.** conduct or behavior characterized by beastlike appetites or instincts. **3.** sexual relations between a human being and an animal. **4.** sodomy. Also called **zooerastia.** See also **zoophilia.**

beta (β), the second letter of the Greek alphabet, employed as a combining form with chemical names to distinguish one of two or more isomers or to indicate the position of substituted atoms in certain compounds. Compare **alpha.**

beta-adrenergic blocking agent. See **antiadrenergic.**

beta-adrenergic receptor. See **beta receptor.**

beta-adrenergic stimulating agent. See **adrenergic.**

beta-carotene, an ultraviolet screen.

■ INDICATION: It is prescribed to ameliorate photosensitivity in patients with erythropoetic protoporphyria.

■ CONTRAINDICATIONS: It is used with caution in patients with impaired renal or hepatic function. Known hypersensitivity to this drug prohibits its use.

■ ADVERSE EFFECTS: No serious adverse reactions have been observed. Diarrhea may occur.

beta cells, 1. insulin-producing cells situated in the islands of Langerhans. They contain granules that are soluble in alcohol and tend to be concentrated in the central portion of each islet. The insulin-producing function of the beta cells tends to accelerate the movement of glucose, amino acids, and fatty acids out of the blood and into the cellular cytoplasm, countering glucagon function of alpha cells. **2.** the basophilic cells of the anterior lobe of the pituitary gland.

Betadine, a trade name for a topical anti-infective (povidone-iodine).

beta fetoprotein, a protein found in fetal liver and in some adults with liver disease. It is now known to be identical with normal liver ferritin. See also **alpha fetoprotein, ferritin, fetoprotein.**

beta-galactosidase. See **lactase.**

beta hemolysis, the development of a clear zone around a bacterial colony growing on blood-agar medium, characteristic of certain pathogenic bacteria. Compare **alpha hemolysis.**

beta-hemolytic streptococci, the pyogenic streptococci of groups A, B, C, E, F, G, H, K, L, M, and O that cause hemolysis of red blood cells in blood agar in the laboratory. These organisms cause most of the acute streptococcal infections seen in humans, including rheumatic fever, scarlet fever, many cases of pneumonia and septicemia, and streptococcal sore throat. Penicillin is usually prescribed to treat these infections when they are suspected, even before the results of the bacteriologic culture are available, because it is known that these organisms as a group are sensitive to the effects of penicillin, and because the sequelae of untreated streptococcal infection may include glomerulonephritis and rheumatic fever.

beta-ketobutyric acid. See **acetoacetic acid.**

Betalin S, a trade name for vitamin B_1 (thiamine hydrochloride).

betamethasone, a glucocorticoid.
▪ INDICATIONS: It is prescribed as a topical anti-inflammatory agent.
▪ CONTRAINDICATIONS: Systemic fungal infections, dermatologic viral and fungal infections, impaired circulation, or known hypersensitivity to this drug prohibits its use.
▪ ADVERSE EFFECTS: Among the more serious adverse reactions associated with prolonged use of the drug are gastrointestinal, endocrine, neurologic, and fluid and electrolyte disturbances.

Betapar, a trade name for a glucocorticoid (meprednisone).

beta particle, an electron or positron emitted from the nucleus of an atom during radioactive decay of the atom.

beta receptor, any one of the postulated adrenergic components of receptor tissues that responds to epinephrine and such blocking agents as prepanolol. Activation of beta receptors causes various physiological reactions, as relaxation of the bronchial muscles, increased cardiac rate, and the force of cardiac contraction. Also called **beta-adrenergic receptor.** Compare **alpha receptor.**

beta rhythm. See **beta wave.**

betatron (bei′tətron), a cyclic accelerator that produces high-energy electrons by magnetic induction. The magnetic field of the betatron deflects electrons into a circular orbit, and an increasing magnetic orbital flux produces an induced circumferential electric field which accelerates the electrons.

beta wave, one of the four types of brain waves, characterized by relatively low voltage and a frequency of more than 13 Hz. Beta waves are the "busy waves" of the brain, recorded by electroencephalograph from the frontal and the central areas of the cerebrum when the patient is awake and alert with eyes open. Also called **beta rhythm.** Compare **alpha wave, delta wave, theta wave.**

bethanechol chloride (bəfhæn′əkol), a cholinergic.
▪ INDICATIONS: It is prescribed in the treatment of urinary retention and neurogenic atony of the bladder.
▪ CONTRAINDICATIONS: Uncertain strength of the bladder, obstruction of the gastrointestinal or urinary tract, hyperthyroidism, peptic ulcer, bronchial asthma, cardiovascular disease, epilepsy, Parkinson's disease, hypotension, or known hypersensitivity to this drug prohibits its use. It is not given during pregnancy.
▪ ADVERSE EFFECTS: Among the more serious adverse reactions are flushing, headache, gastrointestinal distress, diarrhea, excessive salivation, sweating, and hypotension.

bezoar (bi′zor), a hard ball of hair and vegetable fiber that may develop within the intestines of humans but more often is found in the stomachs of ruminants. In some societies it was formerly considered a useful medicine and possessed of certain magical properties. It is apparently still used as a therapeutic and mystical device by some, especially in the Far East.

B/F, a symbol for *black female,* often used in the initial identifying statement in a patient record.

B-galactosidase. See **lactase.**

bhang, bang (bæng), an Asian Indian hallucinogenic, composed of dried leaves and the young stems of uncultivated *Cannabis sativa.* It is usually ingested as a boiled mixture with milk, sugar, or water; it produces euphoria. It also may be smoked or chewed. See also **cannabis.**

bi-, **1.** See **bio-.** **2.** Also **bis-.** a combining form meaning 'twice, two': *biarticular, bicapsular, bicaudal.*

Bi, symbol for **bismuth.**

-bia, a combining form meaning 'creature possessing a mode of life': *aerobia, coenobia, Euphorbia.*

bias, **1.** an oblique or a diagonal line. **2.** a prejudiced or subjective attitude. **3.** (in statistics) the systematic distortion of a statistic caused by a particular sampling process. **4.** (in electronics) a voltage applied to an electronic device, as a vacuum tube or a transistor, to control operating limits.

bicarbonate of soda. See **sodium bicarbonate.**

biceps. See **biceps brachii.**

biceps brachii, the long fusiform muscle of the upper arm on the anterior surface of the humerus, arising in two heads from the scapula. The short head arises in a thick flat tendon from the corocoid process, the long head arises in the glenoid cavity. Both parts of the muscle converge in a flattened tendon that inserts into the radius of the forearm. The biceps brachii is innervated by branches of the musculocutaneous nerve, containing fibers from the fifth and the sixth cervical nerves. It flexes the arm and the forearm and supinates the hand. The long head draws the humerus toward the glenoid fossa, strengthening the shoulder joint. Also called **biceps, biceps flexor cubiti.** Compare **brachialis, triceps brachii.**

biceps femoris, one of the posterior femoral muscles. It has two heads at its origin. The long head arises from the tuberosity of the ischium and from the inferior part of the sacrotuberous ligament; the short head arises from the linea aspera and from the lateral intermuscular septum. The fibers passing from both heads join in a tendon that inserts into the lateral side of the fibula, and by a few fibers, into the lateral condyle of the tibia. The tendon of insertion forms the lateral hamstring. The long head of the muscle is innervated by branches of the sciatic nerve containing fibers from the first three sacral nerves. The short head is innervated by a branch of the peroneal nerve containing fibers from the fifth lumbar and first two sacral nerves. The biceps femoris flexes the leg and rotates it laterally and extends the thigh and tends to rotate it laterally. Also called **hamstring muscle.**

biceps flexor cubiti. See **biceps brachii.**

biceps reflex, a contraction of a biceps muscle produced when the tendon is tapped with a percussor in testing deep tendon reflexes.

Bickerdyke, Mary Ann (1817–1901), an American nurse who, after taking a short course in homeopathy, cared for the sick and wounded on the battlefields during the Civil War. She insisted on cleanliness, good food, and the best of medical care for her patients. At night, she searched the battlefield with a lantern looking for survivors.

biconcave, concave on both sides, especially as applied to a lens. —**biconcavity,** *n.*

biconvex, convex on both sides, especially as applied to a lens. —**biconvexity,** *n.*

bicornate, having two horns or processes.

bicuspid (baïkəs′pɪd), **1.** having two cusps or points. **2.** one of the two teeth between the molars and canines of the upper and lower jaw. Also called **premolar tooth.**

bicuspid valve. See **mitral valve.**

b.i.d., (in prescriptions) abbreviation for *bis in die,* a Latin phrase meaning 'twice a day.' The times of administration are commonly 9 A.M. and 7 P.M.

bidactyly (baïdæk′tɪli), an abnormal condition in which the second, third, and fourth digits on the same hand are missing and only the first and fifth are represented. Also called **lobster-claw deformity. bidactylous,** *adj.*

bidermoma (baï′dərmou′mə), *pl.* **bidermomas, bidermo-**

mata. a teratoid neoplasm composed of cells and tissues originating in two germ layers.

biduotertian fever, a form of malaria characterized by overlapping paroxysms of chills, fever, and other symptoms, caused by infection with two strains of *Plasmodium,* each having its own cycle of symptoms, as in quartan and tertian malaria. See also **malaria.**

bifid, split into two parts.

bifocal, **1.** of or pertaining to the characteristic of having two foci. **2.** (of a lens) having two areas of different focal lengths.

bifurcation, a splitting into two branches, as the trachea, which branches into the two bronchi at about the level of the fifth thoracic vertebra.

Bigelow's lithotrite (bɪg′əlouz), a long-jawed lithotrite, passed through the urethra, for crushing a calculus in the bladder.

bigeminal pulse, an abnormal pulse in which two beats in close succession are followed by a pause during which no pulse is felt. See also **trigeminal pulse, trigeminy.**

bigeminy (bæijem′ɪni), **1.** an association in pairs. **2.** a cardiac arrhythmia characterized by two beats in rapid succession followed by a longer interval. The arrhythmia is usually related to premature ventricular beats. —**bigeminal,** *adj.*

bilabe (baï′lɛib), a narrow forceps used to remove small calculi from the bladder.

bilaminar, of or pertaining to the characteristic of having two layers, as the basal lamina and the reticular lamina that constitute the basement membrane of the epithelium.

bilaminar blastoderm, the stage of embryonic development prior to mesoderm formation in which only the ectoderm and entoderm primary germ layers have formed. Compare **trilaminar blastoderm.**

bilateral, **1.** having two sides. **2.** occurring or appearing on two sides. A patient with bilateral hearing loss may have partial or total deafness in both ears. **3.** having two layers.

bilateral long leg spica cast, an orthopedic device of plaster of Paris, fiberglass, or other casting material that encases and immobilizes the trunk cranially as far as the nipple line and both legs caudally as far as the toes. A horizontal crossbar to improve immobilization connects the parts of the cast encasing both legs at ankle level. The bilateral long leg spica cast is used to aid the healing of fractures of the hip, the femur, the acetabulum, or the pelvis and for the correction or the maintenance of the correction of a hip deformity. Compare **one-and-a-half spica cast, unilateral long leg spica cast.**

bile, a bitter, yellow-green secretion of the liver. Stored in the gall bladder, bile receives its color from the presence of bile pigments, as bilirubin. Bile passes from the gall bladder through the common bile duct in response to the presence of a fatty meal in the duodenum. Bile emulsifies these fats, preparing them for further digestion and absorption in the small intestine. Any interference in the flow of bile will result in the presence of unabsorbed fat in the feces and in jaundice. Also called **gall.** See also **biliary obstruction, jaundice.** — **biliary,** *adj.*

bile acid, a steroid acid of the bile, produced during the metabolism of cholesterol. On hydrolysis bile acid yields glycine and cholic acid.

bile solubility test, a bacteriologic test used in the differential diagnosis of pneumococcal and streptococcal infection. A broth culture of each organism is placed into two tubes. Ox bile is added to one and salt to the other. Pneumococci dissolve in ox bile, resulting in a clear solution; streptococci do not dissolve, resulting in a cloudy solution. The tube with salt is used for comparative purposes.

Bilharzia (bɪlharʹziə). See *Schistosoma.*

bilharziasis (bɪlʹharzaiʹəsɪs). See **schistosomiasis.**

bili-, a combining form meaning 'pertaining to the bile': *biliary, bilidigestive, bilifuscin.*

biliary (bɪlʹierʹi), referring to bile or to the gall bladder and its ducts, which transport bile. These are often called the **biliary tract** or the **biliary system.** See also **bile, biliary calculus.**

biliary atresia, congenital absence or underdevelopment of one or more of the biliary structures, causing jaundice and early liver damage. As the condition worsens, the child may show retarded growth and develop portal hypertension. Surgery can correct the defective ducts in only a small percentage of cases. Most infants die in early childhood from biliary cirrhosis. It is essential for the physician to distinguish between this condition and neonatal hepatitis, which is treatable. See also **biliary cirrhosis.**

biliary calculus, a stone formed in the biliary tract, consisting of bile pigments and calcium salts. Biliary calculi may cause jaundice, right upper quadrant pain, obstruction, and inflammation of the gall bladder. If stones cannot pass spontaneously into the duodenum, intravenous cholangiography will reveal their location, and they can be surgically removed. Also called **choledocholithiasis, gallstones.** See also **cholangitis, cholecystitis, cholelithiasis.**

biliary cirrhosis, an inflammatory condition in which the flow of bile through the ductules of the liver is obstructed. Biliary cirrhosis most commonly affects women in their middle years, and its cause is unknown. It is characterized by abdominal pain, jaundice, steatorrhea, and enlargement of the liver and spleen. The disease is a slowly progressive one, and in its end stages closely resembles cirrhosis of the liver. There is no specific medical or surgical treatment. Care must be taken to rule out obstruction of the biliary structures outside the liver,

since the latter condition can be treated successfully. Compare **biliary calculus, biliary obstruction.**

biliary colic, a type of smooth-muscle or visceral pain specifically associated with the passing of stones through the bile ducts. Also called **cholecystalgia.** See also **biliary calculi.**

biliary duct, a duct through which bile passes from the liver to the duodenum.

biliary fistula, an abnormal passage from the gall bladder, a bile duct, or the liver to an internal organ or the surface of the body. Biliary fistulae opening into the colon, duodenum, hepatic duct, peritoneal cavity, pleural space, or skin are complications in cholelithiasis; a gall stone entering the duodenum may become impacted, usually in the ileocecal valve, and cause intestinal obstruction.

biliary obstruction, blockage of the common or cystic bile duct, usually caused by one or more gallstones. It impedes bile drainage and produces an inflammatory reaction. Uncommon causes of biliary obstruction include choledochal cysts, pancreatic and duodenal tumors, Crohn's disease, pancreatitis, echinococcosis, ascariasis, and sclerosing cholangitis. Stones, consisting chiefly of cholesterol, bile pigment, and calcium, may form in the gall bladder and in the hepatic duct in persons of either sex at any age but are more common in middle-aged women. Increased amounts of serum cholesterol in the blood, as occurs in obesity, diabetes, hypothyroidism, biliary stasis, and inflammation of the biliary system promote the formation of gallstones. Cholelithiasis may be asymptomatic until a stone lodges in a biliary duct, but the patient usually has a prior history of indigestion and discomfort after eating fatty foods.

■ OBSERVATIONS: Biliary obstruction is characterized by severe epigastric pain, often radiating to the back and shoulder, nausea, vomiting, and profuse diaphoresis. The dehydrated patient may have chills, fever, jaundice, clay-colored stools, dark, concentrated urine, an electrolyte imbalance, and a tendency to bleed because the absence of bile prevents the synthesis and absorption of fat-soluble vitamin K.

■ INTERVENTION: The patient is placed in bed in a semi-Fowler's position and is usually administered intermittent nasogastric suctioning, parenteral fluids with electrolytes and fat-soluble vitamins, and medication for pain. Antibiotics, anticholinergic and antispasmodic drugs, and a cholecystogram or ultrasound scan may be ordered. The blood pressure, temperature, pulse, and respirations are noted, and the patient is helped to turn, cough, and deep breathe every two to four hours. The intake and output of fluids are measured and the color and character of urine and stools are noted. When the nasogastric tube is removed, the patient initially receives a low-fat liquid diet and progresses to a soft or normal diet, as tolerated; up to 2,500 ml of fluids a day are forced, unless contraindicated. Cholecystectomy is usually the definitive treatment, but, in most cases, surgery is delayed until the patient's condition is stabilized and any prothrombin deficiency (owing to vitamin K malabsorption) is corrected.

■ NURSING CONSIDERATIONS: The patient may experience intense pain as obstruction causes biliary colic. Instruction is given on the importance of adhering to a low-fat diet and reporting recurrence of symptoms if discharge occurs prior to surgery. Cholecystectomy usually requires several days of intensive nursing care and support. See **cholecystectomy.**

biliary tract cancer, a relatively rare malignancy in an extrahepatic bile duct, occurring slightly more often in men than in women, characterized by progressive jaundice, pruritus, weight loss, and, in the later stages, by severe pain. Transhepatic cholangiography and x rays following the introduction of a contrast medium into the common bile duct and pancreatic duct are used to identify and determine the site of the lesion. Results of laboratory studies indicative of extrahepatic biliary obstruction include greater than normal levels of serum alkaline phosphatase and bilirubin in the blood. If the tumor is in the ampulla of Vater, occult blood may be found in the stool. The tumor is an adenocarcinoma; it may be papillary or flat and ulcerated. It is generally inoperable if it is located in the hepatic or common bile duct, but periampullary lesions may be treated by pancreato-duodenectomy. In cases of an inoperable tumor, various surgical procedures may be performed palliatively to improve the flow of bile. Preoperative, postoperative, and palliative irradiation are also used. With the exception of a rare remission induced by 5-fluorouracil, chemotherapy is not effective in treating these lesions.

biligulate (bailɪg′yəlɪt), having two tongues or two tonguelike structures.

bilious (bɪl′yəs), **1.** of or pertaining to bile, **2.** characterized by an excessive secretion of bile, **3.** characterized by a disorder affecting the bile.

bilirubin (bɪl′ɪru′bɪn), the orange-yellow pigment of bile, formed principally by the breakdown of hemoglobin in red blood cells after termination of their normal lifespan. Water-insoluble, unconjugated bilirubin normally travels in the bloodstream to the liver, where it is converted to a water-soluble, conjugated form and excreted into the bile. In a healthy person, about 250 mg of bilirubin are produced daily, and the majority of that is eventually excreted from the body in the stool. The characteristic yellow pallor of jaundice is caused by the accumulation of bilirubin in the blood and in the tissues of the skin. Testing for bilirubin in the blood provides valuable information for diagnosing and evaluating liver disease, biliary obstruction, and hemolytic anemia. See also **jaundice, van den Bergh test.**

biliuria (bɪl′ɪyur′iə), the presence of bile in the urine.

biliverdin (bɪl′ɪvər′dɪn), a greenish bile pigment formed in the breakdown of hemoglobin and converted to bilirubin. See also **bile, bilirubin.**

Billroth's operation I, the surgical removal of the pylorus in the treatment of gastric cancer. The proximal end of the duodenum is anastomosed to the stomach.

Billroth's operation II, the surgical removal of the pylorus and duodenum. The cut end of the stomach is anastomosed to the jejunum through the transverse mesocolon.

bilobulate, bilobular, having two lobes.

bilocular, biloculate, (in biology) **1.** divided into two cells. **2.** containing two cells.

bimanual, of or pertaining to the functioning of both hands.

binary fission, direct division of a cell or nucleus into two equal parts. It is the common form of asexual reproduction of bacteria, protozoa, and other lower forms of life. Also called **simple fission.** Compare **multiple fission.**

binaural stethoscope (bainɔr′əl), a stethoscope having two earpieces.

bind, 1. to bandage or wrap in a band. **2.** to join together with a band or with a ligature. **3.** (in chemistry) to combine or unite molecules by employing reactive groups within the molecules or by using a binding chemical. Binding is especially associated with chemical bonds that are fairly easily broken, as in the bonds between toxins and antitoxins.

Binet age (bɪnei′), the mental age of an individual, especially a child, as determined by the Binet-Simon tests, which are evaluated on the basis of tested intelligence of the normal individual at any given age. The Binet age corresponding to 'profoundly retarded' is 1 to 2 years; to 'severely retarded,' 3 to 7 years; and to 'mildly retarded,' 8 to 12 years.

binocular, 1. pertaining to both eyes, especially regarding vision. **2.** a microscope, telescope, or field glass that can accommodate viewing by both eyes.

binocular fixation, the process of having both eyes directed at the same object at the same time. This is essential to having good depth perception.

binocular ophthalmoscope, an ophthalmoscope having two eyepieces through which stereoscopic examination of the eye may be made.

binocular parallax (pær′əlæks), the difference in the angles formed by the sight lines to two objects situated at different distances from the eyes. Binocular parallax is a major factor in depth perception. Also called **stereoscopic parallax.**

binocular perception, the visual ability to judge depth or distance by virtue of having two eyes.

binomial, containing two names or terms.

binovular, developing from two distinct ova, as in dizygotic twins. Also called **diovular.** Compare **uniovular.**

binovular twins. See **dizygotic twins.**

bio-, a combining form meaning 'pertaining to life': *bioassay, biogenesis, biolysis.* Also **bi-.**

bioassay (baɪ'ouæs'ei, baɪ'ouəsei'), the laboratory determination of the concentration of a drug or other substance in a specimen by comparing its effect on an organism, an animal, or an isolated tissue with that of a standard preparation. Also called **biological assay.**

bioavailability, the degree of activity or amount of an administered drug or other substance that becomes available for activity in the target tissue.

biochemical genetics. See **molecular genetics.**

biochemistry, the chemistry of living organisms and life processes. Also called **biological chemistry, physiological chemistry.**

bioequivalent (baɪ'ouɪkwɪv'ələnt), (in pharmacology) **1.** of or pertaining to a drug that has the same effect on the body as another drug, usually one nearly identical in its chemical formulation. **2.** a bioequivalent drug. — **bioequivalence,** *n.*

biofeedback, a process providing a person with visual or auditory information about the autonomic physiological functions of his body, as blood pressure, muscle tension, and brain wave activity, usually through use of instrumentation. By trial and error, the person learns to consciously control these processes, which were previously regarded as involuntary. Biofeedback may be used clinically to treat many conditions, as hypertension, insomnia, and migraine headache.

bioflavonoid (baɪ'ouflei'vənoid), a generic term for any of a group of colored flavones found in many fruits and essential for the absorption and metabolism of ascorbic acid. The bioflavonoids are needed for the maintenance of collagen and of the capillary walls and may aid in protection against infection. The components are citrin, hesperidin, rutin, flavones, and flavonoids. Rich sources include lemons, grapes, plums, grapefruit, black currants, apricots, buckwheat, cherries, blackberries, and rose hips. Deficiency can result in a tendency to bleed or bruise easily. The bioflavonoids are completely nontoxic. Also called **vitamin P.** See also **ascorbic acid.**

biogenesis (baɪ'oujen'əsɪs), **biogeny,** **1.** the doctrine that living material can originate only from pre-existing life and not from inanimate matter. **2.** the origin of life and living organisms; ontogeny and phylogeny. — **biogenetic,** *adj.*

biogenetic law. See **recapitulation theory.**

biogenic (baɪ'oujen'ɪk), **1.** produced by the action of a living organism, as fermentation. **2.** essential to life and the maintenance of health, as food, water, proper rest.

biogenic amine, one of a large group of naturally occurring biologically active compounds most of which act as neurotransmitters. The most dominant, norepinephrine, is involved in such physiologic functions as emotional reactions, memory, sleep, and arousal from sleep. Other biochemicals of the group include three catecholamines: histamine, serotonin, and dopamine. These substances are active in regulating blood pressure, elimination, body temperature, and many other centrally mediated bodily functions.

biogenous (baɪoj'ənəs), **1.** biogenetic. **2.** biogenic.

biogeny (baɪoj'əni). See **biogenesis.**

biological, biologic, any medicinal preparation made from living organisms or the products of living organisms. Kinds of biologicals are **antigens, antitoxins, serums, vaccines.**

biological assay. See **bioassay.**

biological half-life, the time required for the body to eliminate one-half of an administered dosage of any substance by regular physiological processes. The time required is approximately the same for both the stable and radioactive isotopes of a specific element. See also **effective half-life, half-life.**

biological vector. See **vector.**

biologic psychiatry, a school of psychiatric thought that stresses the physical, chemical, and neurological causes of and treatments for mental and emotional disorders.

biology, the scientific study of plants and animals. Some branches of biology are **biometry, ecology, molecular biology,** and **paleontology.**

biome (baɪ'oum), the total group of biological communities existing in and characteristic of a given geographic region, as a desert, woodland, or marsh. A biome includes all plants, animals, and microorganisms of a particular region.

biomechanics, the study of mechanical laws and their application to living organisms, especially the human body and its locomotor system. — **biomechanical,** *adj.*

biomedical engineering, a system of techniques in which knowledge of biological processes is applied to solve practical medical problems and to answer questions in biomedical research.

bionics, the science of applying electronic principles and devices, as computers and solid-state miniaturized circuitry, to medical problems, as artificial pacemakers used to correct abnormal heart rhythms. — **bionic,** *adj.*

biophore (baɪ'əfɔr'), according to Weismannism, the basic hereditary unit contained in the germ plasm from which all living cells develop and all inherited characteristics are transmitted. Compare **gemmule.**

biopsy, **1.** the removal of a small piece of living tissue from an organ or other part of the body for microscopic examination to confirm or establish a diagnosis, estimate prognosis, or follow the course of a disease. **2.** the tissue excised for examination. **3.** *Informal.* to excise tissue for examination. Kinds of biopsy include **aspiration biopsy, needle biopsy, punch biopsy, surface biopsy.** — **bioptic,** *adj.*

biopsychic (bai′ousai′kık), of or pertaining to psychical factors as they relate to living organisms.

biopsychology. See **psychobiology.**

biopsychosocial (bai′ousai′kousou′shəl), of or pertaining to the complex of biological, psychological, and social aspects of life.

biorhythm, any cyclic, biological event or phenomenon, as the sleep cycle, the menstrual cycle, or the respiratory cycle. — **biorhythmic,** *adj.*

-biosis, a combining form meaning 'life': *macrobiosis, necrobiosis, otobiosis.*

biostatistics (bai′oustətıs′tıks), numerical data on births, deaths, diseases, injuries, and other factors affecting the general health and condition of human populations. Also called **vital statistics.**

biosynthesis, any one of thousands of chemical reactions continually occurring throughout the body in which simple molecules form complex biomolecules, especially the carbohydrates, the lipids, the proteins, the nucleotides and the nucleic acids. Biosynthetic reactions constitute the anabolism of the body. — **biosynthetic,** *adj.*

biotaxis (bai′outæk′sıs), the ability of living cells to develop into certain forms and arrangements. See also **cytoclesis.** — **biotactic,** *adj.*

biotaxy (bai′outæk′si), 1. biotaxis. 2. the systematic classification of living organisms according to their anatomical characteristics; taxonomy.

biotechnology, the study of the relationships between humans or other living organisms and machinery, as the health effects of word processor equipment on office workers or the ability of airplane pilots to perform tasks when traveling at supersonic speeds.

-biotic, 1. a combining form meaning 'pertaining to life': *anabiotic, catabiotic, microbiotic.* 2. a combining form meaning 'possessing a (specified) mode of life': *endobiotic, parabiotic, photobiotic.*

biotin (bai′ətın), a colorless, crystalline, water-soluble B complex vitamin that acts as a coenzyme in fatty acid production and in the oxidation of fatty acids and carbohydrates. It also aids in the utilization of protein, folic acid, pantothenic acid, and vitamin B_{12}. Rich sources are egg yolk, beef liver, kidney, unpolished rice, brewer's yeast, peanuts, cauliflower, and mushrooms. Since biotin is synthesized by intestinal bacteria, naturally occurring deficiency disease is unknown, although it can be induced by large quantities of raw egg whites in the diet. Symptoms include scaly dermatitis, grayish pallor, extreme lassitude, anorexia, muscle pains, insomnia, some precordial distress, and slight anemia. Also called **vitamin H.**

biotin deficiency syndrome, an abnormal condition caused by a deficiency of biotin, characterized by derma-

titis, hyperesthesia, muscle pain, anorexia, slight anemia, and changes in electrocardiographic activity of the heart. The average daily requirement of biotin for an adult is 100 to 200 μg; the average American diet provides 100 to 300 μg of the vitamin. Authorities have observed spontaneous deficiency of biotin in some individuals who have eaten raw eggs over a long period of time. Some authorities consider seborrheic dermatitis in infants a form of biotin deficiency. Some common sources of biotin are egg yolks, liver, and yeast.

biotope, a specific biological habitat or site.

biotransformation (bai′outræns′fərmei′shən), the chemical changes a substance undergoes in the body, as by the action of enzymes. See also **metabolic.**

Biot's respiration (biouz′), an abnormal respiratory pattern, characterized by irregular breathing with periods of apnea. The breathing may be slow and deep or rapid and shallow and is often accompanied by sighing. Biot's respiration is symptomatic of meningitis or increased intracranial pressure.

biparental inheritance. See **amphigonous inheritance.**

biparietal (baipərai′ətəl), of or pertaining to the two parietal bones of the head, as the biparietal diameter.

biparietal diameter, the distance between the protuberances of the two parietal bones of the skull.

bipartite, having two parts.

biped, 1. having two feet. 2. any animal with only two feet.

bipedal, capable of locomotion on two feet.

bipenniform (baipen′ıfɔrm), (of bodily structure) having the bilateral symmetry of a feather, as the pattern formed by the fasciculi that converge on both sides of a muscle tendon in the rectus femoris. Compare **multipenniform, penniform, radiate.**

biperiden hydrochloride (baiper′ədın), an anticholinergic agent.

■ INDICATIONS: It is prescribed in the treatment of Parkinsonism and drug-induced extrapyramidal disorders.

■ CONTRAINDICATIONS: Narrow angle glaucoma, asthma, obstruction of the genitourinary or gastrointestinal tract, or known hypersensitivity to this drug prohibits its use.

■ ADVERSE EFFECTS: Among the more serious adverse reactions are blurred vision, central nervous system effects, tachycardia, dry mouth, decreased sweating, and hypersensitivity reactions.

biperiden lactate, an anticholinergic agent.

■ INDICATIONS: It is prescribed in the treatment of Parkinson's disease and drug-induced extrapyramidal disorders.

■ CONTRAINDICATIONS: Narrow angle glaucoma, asthma, obstruction of the genitourinary or gastrointestinal tract, or known hypersensitivity to this drug prohibits its use.

■ ADVERSE EFFECTS: Among the more serious adverse reactions are blurred vision, central nervous system effects, tachycardia, dry mouth, decreased sweating, and hypersensitivity reactions.

biphasic (baɪfeɪ′zɪk), having two phases, parts, aspects, or stages.

Biphetamine, a trade name for a fixed-combination drug containing two central stimulants (amphetamine and dextroamphetamine), formerly prescribed as an anorexiant.

bipolar, 1. having two poles, as in certain electrotherapeutic treatments using two poles or in certain bacterial staining that affects only the two poles of the microorganism under study. 2. (of a nerve cell) having an afferent and an efferent process.

bipolar disorder, a major affective disorder characterized by episodes of mania and depression. One or the other phase may be predominant at any given time, one phase may appear alternately with the other, or elements of both phases may be present simultaneously. Characteristics of the manic phase are excessive emotional displays, excitement, euphoria, hyperactivity accompanied by elation, boisterousness, impaired ability to concentrate, decreased need for sleep, and seemingly unbounded energy, often accompanied by delusions of grandeur. In the depressive phase, marked apathy and underactivity are accompanied by feelings of profound sadness, loneliness, guilt, and lowered self-esteem. Causes of the disorder are multiple and complex, often involving biological, psychological, interpersonal, and social and cultural factors. Treatment includes antidepressants, tranquilizers and antianxiety drugs, or the use of electroconvulsive therapy for persons who present an immediate and serious risk of suicide, followed by long-term psychotherapy. Careful nursing observation is important during depression, particularly during the recovery from depression, because of the possibility of suicide.

bipolar lead, 1. an electrocardiographic conductor having two electrodes placed on different body regions, with each electrode contributing significantly to the record. 2. *Informal.* a tracing produced by such a lead on an electrocardiograph.

bipotentiality, the characteristic of acting or reacting according to either of two potentials.

bird breeder's lung. See **pigeon breeder's lung.**

bird-headed dwarf, a person affected with Seckel's syndrome, a congenital disorder characterized by a proportionate shortness of stature; a proportionately small head with hypoplasia of the jaws, large eyes, and a beaklike protrusion of the nose; mental retardation; and various other skeletal, cutaneous, and genital defects. Also called **nanocephalic dwarf.**

birth, 1. event of being born, the coming of a new person out of its mother into the world. 2. the childbearing event, the bringing forth by a mother of a baby. 3. a medical event, the delivery of a fetus by an obstetric attendant.

birth canal, *Informal.* the passage that extends from the inlet of the true pelvis to the vaginal orifice through which an infant passes during vaginal birth.

birth control, use of a drug, device, or practice to prevent or to delay pregnancy. See also **family planning.**

birth defect. See **congenital anomaly.**

birthing chair, a chair used in labor and delivery to promote the comfort of the mother and the efficiency of parturition. The chair may be specially designed, having many technical features, or it may be a simple three-legged stool with a high, slanted back and a circular seat with a large central hole in it. The newer birthing chairs allow the woman to sit straight up or to recline. The chair has a lower section that may be removed or folded out of the way. Lights, mirrors, and basins may be attached for the attendant's convenience. The upright position appears to shorten the time in labor, particularly the second or expulsive stage of labor, probably owing to gravity and increased participation of the mother. The chair is not suitable for use with anesthesia.

birth injury, trauma suffered by a baby while being born. Some kinds of birth injury are **Bell's palsy, cerebral palsy, Erb's palsy.**

birthmark, any localized skin discoloration or blemish, flat or raised, present at birth or appearing shortly thereafter. Kinds of birthmarks include **mole, nevus, strawberry mark.**

birth rate, the proportion of the number of births in a specific area during a given period to the total population of that area, usually expressed as the number of births per 1000 of population. Compare **crude birth rate, refined birth rate, true birth rate.**

birth trauma, 1. any physical injury suffered by an infant during the process of delivery. 2. the supposed psychic shock, according to some psychiatric theories, that an infant suffers during delivery.

birth weight, the measured heaviness of a baby when born, usually about 3,500 gm (7.5 lbs.) in the United States. 97 per cent of newborns weigh between 2,500 gm (5.5 lbs.) and 4,500 gm (10 lbs.). Babies weighing less than 2,500 gm at term are considered **small-for-gestational-age.** Babies weighing more than 4,500 gm are considered **large-for-gestational-age** and are often infants of diabetic mothers.

bis-, a combining form meaning 'twice, two': *bisacomial, bisaxillary, bisferious.* Also **bi-.**

bisacodyl (bɪsæk′oʊdɪl), a carthartic.

■ INDICATIONS: It is prescribed in the treatment of acute or chronic constipation, to empty the bowel pre- or postoperatively or before diagnostic radiographic procedures.

■ CONTRAINDICATIONS: Abdominal pain, nausea, vomiting, rectal fissures, ulcerated hemorrhoids, or known hypersensitivity to this drug prohibits its use.

■ ADVERSE EFFECTS: Among the more serious adverse reactions are colic, abdominal pain, and diarrhea.

bisect, to divide into two equal lengths or parts.

bisexual (bīsek′shuəl), **1.** hermaphroditic; having gonads of both sexes. **2.** possessing physical or psychological characteristics of both sexes. **3.** engaging in both heterosexual and homosexual activity. **4.** desiring sexual contact with persons of both sexes.

bisexual libido, (in psychoanalysis) the tendency in a person to seek sexual gratification with people of either sex.

bishydroxycoumarin (bɪs′hīdrok′sɪku′mərɪn). See **dicumarol.**

bismuth (Bi), a reddish, crystalline, trivalent metallic element. Its atomic number is 83; its atomic weight is 209. It is combined with various other elements, as oxygen, to produce numerous salts used in the manufacture of many pharmaceutical substances.

bite block. See **occlusion rim.**

bitegage (bīt′geij′), a prosthetic dental device that helps attain proper occlusion of the teeth rooted in the maxilla and the mandible.

bitelock (bīt′lok′), a dental device for retaining the occlusion rims in the same relation outside the mouth as inside the mouth.

bitemporal, of or pertaining to both temples or both temporal bones.

biteplate, a device used in dentistry as a diagnostic or a therapeutic aid for prosthodontics or for orthodontics. It is fabricated of wire and plastic, worn in the palate, and may also be used to correct temperomandibular joint problems or as a splint in restoring the full mouth.

bithionol (TBP) (bɪthai′ənol), a pale gray powder, soluble in acetone, alcohol, or ether, used as a local antiseptic and administered orally in the treatment of infestations of the giant liver fluke (*Fasciolasis*) and of the lung fluke (*Paragonimus westermani*) that cause parasitic hemoptysis in Asiatic countries.

Bithynia (bəthin′iə), a genus of snails, species of which act as intermediate hosts to *Opistorchis.*

biting in childhood, a natural behavior trait and reflex action in infants, acquired at about five to six months of age in response to the introduction of solid foods in the diet and the beginning of the teething process. The activity represents a significant modality in the psychosocial development of the child, since it is the first aggressive action the infant learns and through it the infant learns to control the environment. The behavior also confronts the infant with one of the first inner conflicts, because biting can produce both pleasing and displeasing results. Biting during breast feeding causes withdrawal of the nipple and anxiety in the mother, yet it also serves as a means of soothing teething discomfort. Infants continue to use biting as a mechanism for exploring their surroundings. Toddlers and older children often use biting for expressing aggression toward their parents and other children, especially during play or as a means of gaining attention. Most children normally outgrow the tendency unless severe maladaptive or emotional problems are present. See also **psychosexual development, psychosocial development.**

Bitot's spots (bitouz′), white or gray triangular deposits on the bulbar conjunctiva adjacent to the lateral margin of the cornea, a clinical sign of vitamin A deficiency.

bitrochanteric lipodystrophy, an abnormal and excessive deposition of fat on the buttocks and the outer aspect of the upper thighs, occurring most commonly in women. See also **lipodystrophy.**

bitterling test (bɪt′ərlɪŋ), a test for pregnancy in which the small, carplike bitterling fish of Japan is immersed in a quart of fresh water containing two teaspoonsful of the urine of the woman being tested. If she is pregnant the long oviduct of the bitterling grows from its belly.

biuret test, a method for detecting urea and other soluble proteins in serum. In alkaline solution, copper sulfate ions react with the peptide bonds of proteins to produce a purple color, called the biuret reaction. The amount of serum protein in a sample solution is estimated by comparing its color with that of a standard solution whose protein concentration is known.

bivalent (bīveil′ənt), **1.** (in genetics) a pair of synapsed homologous chromosomes that are attached to each other by chiasmata during the early first meiotic prophase of gametogenesis. The structure serves as the basis for the tetrads from which gametes are produced during the two meiotic divisions. Also called **divalent. 2.** (in chemistry) See **valence,** def. 1. – **bivalence,** *n.*

bivalent chromosome, a pair of synapsed homologous chromosomes during the early stages of gametogenesis. See also **bivalent.**

bivalve cast, an orthopedic cast used for immobilizing a section of the body for the healing of one or more broken bones or for correction or the maintenance of correction of an orthopedic deformity. The bivalve cast is cut in half to monitor and detect pressure under the cast, especially with a patient who has decreased sensation or who has no sensation in the portion of the body surrounded by the cast. An area of the skin that is subjected to prolonged pressure from a cast may become infected, and early signs of pressure are almost impossible to detect. The bivalve cast is cut into anterior and posterior portions to facilitate inspection of the patient's skin. If dangerous pressure areas are detected, "windows" are often cut out of the cast over the pressure areas to relieve the problem.

bizarre leiomyoma. See **epithelioid leiomyoma.**

Bk, symbol for **berkelium.**

BL, abbreviation for **baralyme.**

black damp. See **damp.**

Black Death, *Informal.* bubonic plague, especially the epidemic in the fourteenth century that killed over 25,000,000 people in Europe. See also **bubonic plague, plague,** *Yersinia pestis.*

Blackfan-Diamond syndrome, a rare congenital disorder evident in the first three months of life, characterized by severe anemia, very low reticulocyte count, but normal numbers of platelets and white cells. Also called **congenital hypoplastic anemia.** See also **anemia.**

black fever. See **kala-azar.**

black hairy tongue. See **parasitic glossitis.**

blackhead. See **comedo.**

black light. See **Wood's light.**

black lung. See **anthracosis.**

black lung disease. See **pneumoconiosis.**

blackout, *Informal.* a temporary loss of vision or consciousness resulting from cerebral ischemia.

black plague. See **bubonic plague.**

black tongue. See **parasitic glossitis.**

blackwater fever, a serious complication of chronic falciparum malaria, characterized by jaundice, hemoglobinuria, acute renal failure, and the passage of bloody dark red or black urine owing to massive intravascular hemolysis. Death occurs in 20 to 30 per cent of all cases; mortality is particularly high among Europeans. See also **falciparum malaria, malaria.**

Blackwell, Elizabeth (1821–1910), a British-born American physician, the first woman to receive a medical degree. She established the New York Infirmary, a 40-bed hospital staffed entirely by women, with which Marie Zakrzewski was associated for a time. At the infirmary, she began training nurses in a four-month course. Her influence helped others to establish nursing schools to improve patient care.

black widow spider, a poisonous insect found in many parts of the world. The venom injected with its bite causes perspiration, abdominal cramps, nausea, headaches, and dizziness of various levels of intensity. Small children, old people, or those with heart conditions are most severely affected and may require hospitalization and the administration of an antivenin.

black widow spider antivenin, a passive immunizing agent.

■ INDICATION: It is prescribed in the treatment of black widow spider bite.

■ CONTRAINDICATIONS: Known hypersensitivity to this drug or to horse serum prohibits its use.

■ ADVERSE EFFECTS: Among the more serious adverse reactions are allergic reactions.

bladder, 1. a membranous sac serving as a receptacle for secretions. 2. the urinary bladder.

bladder cancer, the most common malignancy of the urinary tract. It is characterized by a tumor or by multiple growths that tend to recur in a more aggressive form. Malignant neoplasia of the bladder occurs 2.3 times more often in men than in women, is more prevalent in urban than in rural areas, and may be increasing in incidence. The risk for developing bladder cancer is increased with cigarette smoking and exposure to carcinogens, as aniline dyes, and with the use of beta-naphthylamine, mixtures of aromatic hydrocarbons, or benzidine and its salts, used in chemical, paint, plastics, rubber, textile, petroleum, and wood industries and in medical laboratories. Other predisposing factors are chronic urinary tract infections, calculous disease, and schistosomiasis; in Egypt, where *Schistosoma haematobium* infestations are extremely common, the bladder is the most frequent site of cancer. Early symptoms of a bladder cancer include hematuria, frequent urination, dysuria, and cystitis. Urinalysis, excretory urography, cystoscopy, or transurethral biopsy are performed for diagnosis. The majority of bladder malignancies are transitional cell carcinomas; a small percentage are squamous cell carcinomas or adenocarcinomas. Superficial or multiple lesions may be treated by fulguration or open loop resection. A segmental resection is usually performed if the tumor is at the dome or in a lateral wall of the bladder, but total cystectomy may be performed for an invasive lesion of the trigone. In patients requiring cystectomy, a conduit is constructed to divert urine to the colon, to a rectal bladder, or to an abdominal stoma. External radiation may be administered preoperatively or as palliation for inoperable lesions. Internal radiation, the introduction of radioisotopes via a balloon of a catheter, or the implantation of radon seeds may be used in treating small localized tumors on the bladder wall. Medications that are often used as palliatives are 5-fluorouracil and adriamycin. See also **cystectomy.**

bladder flap, *Informal.* the vesicouterine fold of peritoneum that is incised during low cervical Caesarean section so that the bladder can be separated from the uterus to expose the lower uterine segment for incision. The flap is reapproximated with sutures during closure to cover the uterine incision. See also **Caesarean section.**

Blalock-Taussig procedure (blei′loktə′sig), surgical construction of a shunt as a temporary measure to overcome congenital pulmonary stenosis and atrial-septal defect, as in an infant born with tetralogy of Fallot. Preoperatively, a cardiac catheterization is done to identify the defect or defects and the levels of arterial blood gases are analyzed. Hypothermia anesthesia and a cardiac bypass machine are utilized. The subclavian artery is joined end-to-end with the pulmonary artery, directing blood from the systemic circulation to the lungs. Thrombosis of the shunt is the major postoperative complication. Nursing care includes giving humidified oxygen by nasotracheal tube, monitoring fluids and electrolytes, maintaining the I.V., and giving nasogastric feedings. Restlessness may signal a lack of oxygen or a low cardiac output. Permanent surgical correction is performed in early childhood. See also **heart surgery.**

blanch, **1.** causing to become pale, as a spider angiomata may be blanched using digital pressure. **2.** whitening or bleaching a surface or substance. **3.** becoming white or pale, as from vasoconstriction accompanying fear or anger.

bland, mild or having a soothing effect.

bland diet, a diet that is mechanically, chemically, physiologically, and, sometimes, thermally nonirritating. It is often prescribed in the treatment of peptic ulcer, ulcerative colitis, gall bladder disease, diverticulosis and diverticulitis, gastritis, idiopathic spastic constipation, mucous colitis, and after abdominal surgery. The diet may include eggs, meat, poultry, fish, and enriched fine cereals; milk is usually an important ingredient. A bland diet may be planned that includes or excludes any specific foods. Spicy or highly seasoned foods, carbonated beverages, raw fruits and vegetables, and rich desserts are avoided. See also **sippy diet.**

blanket bath, the procedure of wrapping the patient in a wet pack and then in blankets.

-blast, a combining form meaning an 'embryonic state of development': *leucoblast, megaloblast, osteoblast.*

blast cell, any immature cell, as an erythroblast, a lymphoblast, or a neuroblast.

-blastema, a combining form meaning a 'mass of living substance': *epiblastema, scleroblastema, scytoblastema.*

blastema (blæsti′mə), *pl.* **blastemas, blastemata.** **1.** any mass of living protoplasm capable of growth and differentiation, specifically the primordial undifferentiated cellular material from which a particular organ or tissue develops. **2.** in certain animals, a group of cells capable of regenerating a lost or damaged part or of giving rise to a complete organism in asexual reproduction. **3.** the budding or sprouting area of a plant. — **blastemal, blastematic, blastemic,** *adj.*

blastid, blastide, the site in the fertilized ovum where the pronuclei fuse and the nucleus forms.

blastin, any substance that provides nourishment for or stimulates the growth or proliferation of cells, as allantoin.

blasto-, a combining form meaning 'pertaining to an early embryonic or developing stage': *blastocele, blastocytoma, blastomatosis.*

blastocoele, blastocoel, blastocele, the fluid-filled cavity of the blastocyst in mammals and the blastula or discoblastula of lower animals. The cavity increases the surface area of the developing embryo for better absorption of nutrients and oxygen. Also called **cleavage cavity, segmentation cavity, subgerminal cavity.**

blastocyst (blæs′təsɪst), the embryonic form that follows the morula in human development. It is a spherical mass of cells having a central, fluid-filled cavity (blastocele) surrounded by two layers of cells. The outer layer (trophoblast) later forms the placenta; the inner layer (embryoblast) later forms the embryo. Implantation in the wall of the uterus usually occurs at this stage, on approximately the eighth day after fertilization.

blastocyte, an undifferentiated embryonic cell prior to germ layer formation. — **blastocytic,** *adj.*

blastocytoma (blæs′tousaɪtou′mə). See **blastoma.**

blastoderm, the layer of cells forming the wall of the blastocyst in mammals and the blastula in lower animals during the early stages of embryonic development. It is produced by the cleavage of the fertilized ovum and gives rise to the primary germ layers, the ectoderm, mesoderm, and endoderm from which the embryo and all of its membranes are derived. In animals in which the ovum contains a large amount of yolk and undergoes partial cleavage, the cells form a small caplike structure, or cellular disc, above the yolk mass. Kinds of blastoderm are **bilaminar blastoderm, embryonic blastoderm, extraembryonic blastoderm, trilaminar blastoderm.** Also called **germinal membrane.** — **blastodermal, blastodermic,** *adj.*

blastodisc, blastodisk, the disclike nonyolk area of the protoplasm surrounding the animal pole where cleavage occurs in a fertilized ovum containing a large amount of yolk, as in birds and reptiles. As cleavage continues the blastomeres form a convex structure, the blastula, which eventually develops into the embryo.

blastogenesis (blæs′toujen′əsɪs), **1.** asexual reproduction by budding. **2.** the theory of the transmission of hereditary characteristics by the germ plasm, as opposed to the theory of pangenesis. **3.** the early development of the embryo during cleavage and formation of the germ layers. **4.** the process of transforming small lymphocytes in tissue culture into large blastlike cells by exposure to phytohemagglutin or other substances, often for the purpose of inducing mitosis. — **blastogenetic,** *adj.*

blastogenic, **1.** originating in the germ plasm. **2.** initiating tissue proliferation. **3.** relating to or characterized by blastogenesis.

blastogeny (blæstoj′əni), the early stages in ontogeny; the germ plasm history of an organism or species, which traces the history of the inherited characteristics.

blastokinin (blæs′təkaɪ′nɪn), a globulin, secreted by the uterus in many mammals, that may stimulate and regulate the implantation process of the blastocyst in the uterine wall. Also called **uteroglobulin.**

blastolysis, destruction of a germ cell or blastoderm. — **blastolytic,** *adj.*

blastoma (blæstou′mə), *pl.* **blastomas, blastomata.** a neoplasm of embryonic tissue developing from the blastema of an organ or tissue. A blastoma derived from a number of scattered cells is pluricentric and one arising from a single cell or group of cells is unicentric. Also called **blastocytoma.** – **blastomatous,** *adj.*

blastomatosis (blæs'toumətou'sis), the development of many tumors derived from embryonic tissue.

blastomere (blæs'təmir), one of a pair of cells that develops in the first mitotic division of the segmentation nucleus of a fertilized ovum. The two blastomeres divide and subdivide to form the morula in the first several days of pregnancy. – **blastomeric,** *adj.*

blastomerotomy, the destruction or the separation of blastomeres, either caused naturally or induced artificially. Also called **blastotomy.** – **blastomerotomic,** *adj.*

Blastomyces (blæs'toumai'siz), a genus of yeastlike fungus, usually including the species *Blastomyces dermatitidis,* which causes North American blastomycosis, and *Paracoccidioides brasiliensis,* which causes South American blastomycosis.

blastomycosis (blæs'toumaikou'sis), an infectious disease caused by a yeastlike fungus, *Blastomyces dermatitidis,* that usually affects only the skin but may invade the lungs, kidneys, central nervous system, and bones. The disease is most common in young men living in North America, particularly the southeastern United States, but outbreaks have occurred in Africa and Latin America. Skin infections often begin as small papules on the hand, face, neck, or other exposed areas where there has been a cut, bruise, or other injury and spread gradually and irregularly into surrounding areas. When the lungs are involved, x-ray films of the chest show tumors resembling cancer. The person usually has a cough, dyspnea, chest pain, chills, and a fever with heavy sweating. Diagnosis is made by identification of the disease organism in a culture of specimens from lesions. Treatment usually involves the administration of a fungicidal antibiotic, amphotericin B. Recovery usually begins within the first week of treatment. Also called **Gilchrist's disease.** See also **fungus, mycosis.**

blastopore (blæs'təpɔr), (in embryology) the invagination into a blastula that occurs in the process of the blastula becoming a gastrula.

blastoporic canal. See **neurenteric canal.**

blastosphere. See **blastula.** – **blastospheric,** *adj.*

blastotomy (blæstot'əmi). See **blastomerotomy.** – **blastotomic,** *adj.*

-blastula, a combining form meaning an 'early embryonic stage in the development of a fertilized egg': *coeloblastula, diblastula, steroblastula.*

blastulation, the transformation of the morula into a blastocyst or blastula by the development of a central cavity, the blastocoele.

BLB mask, abbreviation for **Boothby-Lovelace-Bulbulian mask.**

bleb (bleb), an accumulation of fluid under the skin, usu-

ally associated with lesions that are smaller than normal blisters. – **blebby,** *adj.*

bleed, 1. to lose blood from the blood vessels of the body. The blood may flow externally, through an orifice or a break in the skin, or it may flow internally, into a cavity, an organ, or the spaces between the tissues. The color, quantity, and source of the blood are noted. 2. to cause blood to flow from a vein or an artery.

bleeder, 1. *Informal.* a person who has hemophilia or any other vascular or hematologic condition associated with a tendency to hemorrhage. 2. *Informal.* a bleeding blood vessel, especially one cut during a surgical procedure.

bleeding, the release of blood from the vascular system as a result of damage to or inadequacy of one or more blood vessels. See also **blood clotting.**

bleeding time, the time required for blood to stop flowing from a tiny wound. A test of bleeding time is the Ivy method, in which a blood pressure cuff on the upper arm is inflated to 40 mm of mercury and a small wound is made with a scalpel and a template on the volar surface of the arm. Prolonged bleeding times are most often the result of uremia, a disorder of platelet function or the ingestion of aspirin or other anti-inflammatory medications. Normal Ivy bleeding time is from 2 to 6 minutes. See also **hemostasis.**

blending inheritance, the apparent fusion in the offspring of distinct, dissimilar characteristics of the parents, usually of a quantitative nature, as height, with segregation of the specific traits failing to appear in successive generations. This pre-Mendelian concept of inheritance is now explained in terms of multiple pairs of genes that have a cumulative effect. See also **polygene.**

blenn-. See **blenno-.**

blenno-, blenn-, a combining form meaning 'pertaining to mucus': *blennemesis, blennostasis, blennothorax.*

blennorrhea (blen'əri'ə), 1. See also **swimming pool conjunctivitis.** excessive discharge of mucus. 2. *Obsolete.* gonorrhea. Also called **blennorrhagia.**

Blenoxane, a trade name for an antineoplastic (bleomycin sulfate).

bleomycin sulfate, an antineoplastic antibiotic.

■ INDICATION: It is prescribed in the treatment of a variety of neoplasms.

■ CONTRAINDICATION: Hypersensitivity to this drug prohibits its use.

■ ADVERSE EFFECTS: Among the most serious adverse reactions are pneumonitis, pulmonary fibrosis, and a syndrome of hyperpyrexia and circulatory collapse. Rashes and skin reactions commonly occur.

blephar-. See **blepharo-.**

blepharal, of or pertaining to the eyelids.

-blepharia, a combining form meaning '(condition of the) eyelid': *ablepharia, atretoblepharia, macroblepharia.*

blepharitis (blef'ərai'tıs), an inflammatory condition of the lash follicles and Meibomian glands of the eyelids, characterized by swelling, redness, and crusts of dried mucus on the lids. **Ulcerative blepharitis** is caused by bacterial infection. **Nonulcerative blepharitis** may be caused by psoriasis, seborrhea, or an allergic response.

MARGINAL BLEPHARITIS

blepharoadenoma (blef'ərouæd'ɪnou'mə), *pl.* **blepharoadenomas, blepharoadenomata.** a glandular epithelial tumor of the eyelid.

blepharoatheroma (blef'ərouæth'ərou'mə), *pl.* **blepharoatheromas, blepharoatheromata.** a tumor of the eyelid.

blepharo-, blephar-, a combining form meaning 'pertaining to the eyelid or eyelash': *blepharochalasis, blepharal, blepharelosis.*

blepharoncus (blef'əron'kəs), a neoplasm of the eyelid.

blepharoplegia (blef'əroupli'jə), paralysis of the eyelid.

-blepsia, a combining form meaning '(condition of) sight': *acyanoblepsia, chionablepsia, hemiablepsia.* Also **-blepsy.**

-blepsy. See **-blepsia.**

blight, any disease of plants caused by fungus.

blighted ovum, a fertilized ovum that fails to develop. On x-ray or ultrasonic visualization it appears to be a fluid-filled cyst attached to the wall of the uterus. It may be empty, or it may contain amorphous parts. Many first trimester spontaneous abortions represent the expulsion of a blighted ovum. Suction curettage may be necessary if the blighted ovum is retained.

blind fistula, an abnormal passage with only one open end; the opening may be on the body surface or on or within an internal organ or structure. Also called **incomplete fistula.**

blind intubation. See **intubation.**

blind loop, a redundant segment of intestine. Bacterial overgrowth occurs and may lead to malabsorption, obstruction, and necrosis. Blind loops may be created by surgical procedures, as side-to-side ileotransverse colostomy.

blindness, the inability to see.

blind spot, 1. a normal gap in the visual field occurring when an image is focused on the space in the retina occupied by the optic disc. 2. an abnormal gap in the visual field owing to a lesion on the retina or in the optic pathways or to hemorrhage or choroiditis, often perceived as light spots or flashes.

blister, a vesicle or bulla.

bloat, a swelling or filling with gas, as the distention of the abdomen from swallowing air or from intestinal gas.

block anesthesia. See **conduction anesthesia.**

blocking, 1. preventing the transmission of an impulse by the injection of an anesthetic. 2. interrupting an intracellular biosynthetic process, as by the injection of actinomycin D. 3. being unable to remember or involuntarily interrupting a train of thought or speech, usually owing to emotional or mental conflict. 4. repressing an idea or emotion to keep it from obtruding into the consciousness.

blocking antibody, an antibody that fails to cross link and cause agglutination. When such antibodies are present in high concentration they tend to interfere with the action of other antibodies by occupying all of the antigenic sites. See also **antigen-antibody reaction, hapten.**

blood, the liquid pumped by the heart through all of the arteries, veins, and capillaries. It consists of a clear yellow fluid, called plasma, and the formed elements, a series of different cell types, all with varying functions. The major function of the blood is to transport oxygen and nutrients to the cells and to remove from the cells carbon dioxide and other waste products for detoxification and elimination. The normal adult has a total blood volume of 7 to 8 per cent of body weight. This is approximately equivalent to 70 ml/kg of body weight for men and about 65 ml/kg for women. It moves at a speed of about 30 cm/second, with a complete circulation time of 20 seconds. Compare **lymph.** See also **blood cell, erythrocyte, leukocyte, plasma, platelet.**

blood agar, a culture medium consisting of blood and nutrient agar, used in bacteriology to cultivate certain microorganisms, including *Staphylococcus epidermidis, Diplococcus pneumoniae,* and *Clostridium perfringens.*

blood bank, an organizational unit responsible for collecting, processing, and storing blood to be used for transfusion and other purposes. It is usually a subdivision of a laboratory in a hospital and is often charged with the responsibility for all serological testing. See also **bank blood, component therapy, transfusion.**

blood-brain barrier (BBB), an anatomical-physiological feature of the brain thought to consist of walls of capillaries in the central nervous system and surrounding glial membranes. The barrier separates the parenchyma of the central nervous system from blood. The blood-brain barrier functions in preventing or slowing the passage of various chemical compounds, radioactive ions, and disease-causing organisms, as viruses from the blood into the central nervous system.

blood buffers, a system of buffers, composed primarily of dissolved carbon dioxide and bicarbonate ions, which functions in maintaining the proper pH of the blood. See also **buffer, pH.**

blood cell, any one of the formed elements of the blood, including red cells (erythrocytes), white cells (leukocytes), and platelets (thrombocytes). Together they normally constitute about 50 per cent of the total volume of the blood. See also **erythrocyte, leukocyte, platelet.**

blood clot, a semi-solid, gelatinous mass, the end result of the clotting process in blood. It ordinarily consists of red cells, white cells, and platelets enmeshed in an insoluble fibrin network. Compare **embolus, thrombus.** See also **blood clotting, fibrinogen.**

blood clotting, the conversion of blood from a free-flowing liquid to a semi-solid gel. Although it can occur within the intact blood vessel, the process usually starts with tissue damage and exposure of the blood to air. Within seconds of injury to the vessel wall, platelets clump at the site. If normal amounts of calcium, platelets, and tissue factors are present, prothrombin will be converted to thrombin. Thrombin then acts as a catalyst for the conversion of fibrinogen to a mesh of insoluble fibrin, in which all of the formed elements are immobilized. Also called **blood coagulation.** Compare **hemostasis.** See also **anticoagulant.**

blood coagulation. See **blood clotting.**

blood count, *Nontechnical.* a computation of the number of cells per cu mm of blood performed for a variety of diagnostic purposes. Approximately 4.5 and 5.0 million red cells per cu mm are considered normal for women and men, respectively. Normally, leukocytes range between 5,000 and 10,000 cells per cu mm. The relative number of the types of white cells is also important for diagnostic purposes and is reported as a percentage of the total white count. See also **anemia, differential white blood cell count, platelet.**

blood culture medium, a liquid enrichment medium for the growth of bacteria in the diagnosis of blood infections. It contains a suspension of brain tissue in meat broth with dextrose, peptone, and citrate and has a pH of 7.4.

blood donor, anyone who donates his blood to a blood bank or directly to another person. See also **blood bank, transfusion.**

blood dyscrasia, a pathologic condition in which any of the constituents of the blood are abnormal or are present in abnormal quantity, as in leukemia or hemophilia.

blood fluke, a parasitic flatworm of the class Trematoda, genus *Schistosoma,* including the species *S. haematobium, S. japonicum,* and *S. mansoni.* See also *Schistosoma,* **schistosomiasis.**

blood gas, gas dissolved in the liquid part of the blood. Blood gases include oxygen, carbon dioxide, and nitrogen. *(See next column for illustration)*

blood gas determination, an analysis of the pH of the blood and the concentration and pressure of oxygen, carbon dioxide, and hydrogen ion in the blood. It can be

	pH	CARBONIC ACID	BICARBONATE
ACIDOSIS	Low	Increase	Decrease
ALKALOSIS	High	Decrease	Increase

Acid-base balance is normally maintained by three different body systems: the respiratory system, the renal system, and the buffer system.

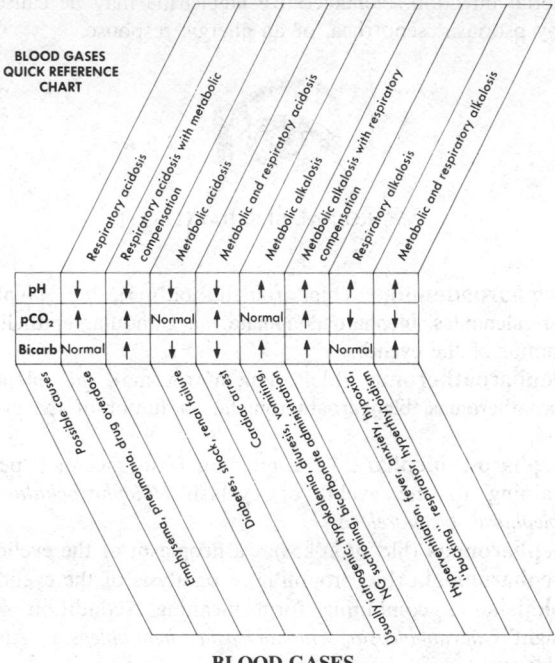

BLOOD GASES

performed rapidly as an emergency procedure to assess acid-base balance and ventilatory status. Blood gas determination is often important in the evaluation of cardiac failure, hemorrhage, kidney failure, drug overdose, shock, uncontrolled diabetes mellitus, or any other condition of severe stress. The blood for examination is drawn from a vein or artery as ordered, placed in ice, and immediately transported for analysis. See also **acid-base balance, acidosis, alkalosis, oxygenation, PCO_2, pH, PO_2.**

blood glucose. See **blood sugar.**

blood group, the classification of blood based on the presence or absence of genetically determined antigens on the surface of the red cell. More than 14 different grouping systems have been described; their relative importance depends on their clinical significance in transfusion therapy. See also **ABO blood groups.**

blood island, one of the clusters of mesodermal cells that proliferate on the outer surface of the embryonic yolk sac and give it a lumpy appearance. The outermost cells flatten into primitive endothelium; the inner cells develop primitive blood plasma and elaborate hemoglobin within their cytoplasm.

blood lavage, the removal of toxic elements from the blood by the injection of serum into the veins.

blood patch. See **epidural blood patch.**

blood plasma, the liquid portion of the blood, free of its formed elements and particles. Plasma represents approximately 50 per cent of the total volume of blood and contains glucose, proteins, amino acids, and other nutritive materials, urea and other excretory products, as well as hormones, enzymes, vitamins, and minerals. Compare **serum.** See also **blood, plasma protein, pooled plasma.**

blood poisoning. See **septicemia.**

blood pressure (BP), the pressure exerted by the circulating volume of blood on the walls of the arteries, the veins, and the chambers of the heart. Overall blood pressure is maintained by the complex interaction of the homeostatic mechanisms of the body, moderated by the volume of the blood, the lumen of the arteries and arterioles, and the force of the cardiac contraction. The pressure in the aorta and the large arteries of a healthy young adult is approximately 120 mm Hg during systole and 70 mm Hg in diastole. The pulse pressure is approximately 50 mm Hg. ■ METHOD: The blood pressure is most often measured by auscultation, using an aneroid or mercury sphygmomanometer, a stethoscope, and a blood pressure cuff. The cuff is placed around the upper arm and inflated to a pressure greater than the systolic pressure, occluding the artery. The diaphragm of the stethoscope is placed over the brachial artery in the antecubital space and the pressure in the cuff is slowly released. No sound is heard until the cuff pressure falls to less than the systolic pressure in the artery; at that point a pulse is heard. As the cuff pressure continues to fall slowly, the pulse continues; first becoming louder, then dull and muffled. These sounds, called the sounds of Korotkoff, are produced by turbulence of the blood flowing through a vessel that is partially occluded as the arterial pressure falls to the low pressure of diastole. When the cuff pressure is less than the diastolic pressure no pulse is heard. Thus the cuff pressure at which the first sound is heard is the systolic blood pressure indicative of the pressure in the large arteries during systole; the cuff pressure at which the sounds stop is the diastolic blood pressure, indicative of the pressure on the arteries during diastole. Other methods include the use of palpation in place of auscultation to determine the systolic pressure: the pressure at which a pulse is first palpated in the antecubital space is noted; using a calibrated strain gauge or a mercury manometer attached to an oscillograph, the arterial pressure may be monitored directly through a cannula placed in the artery. ■ NURSING ORDERS: The intervals at which the patient's blood pressure is to be taken are specified. The pressure in both arms is taken the first time the procedure is performed; persistent major difference between the two readings is indicative of the presence of a vascular occlusion. The blood pressure may be taken using the thigh and the popliteal space, but to obtain an accurate reading the leg should be at the level of the heart. A larger cuff is used when taking the blood pressure of an obese person and for all people when using the thigh location. ■ OUTCOME CRITERIA: Any factor that increases peripheral resistance or cardiac output affects the blood pressure. Strong emotion, for example, tends to do both; therefore, it is important to try to secure a blood pressure reading when the person is at rest. Increased peripheral resistance usually increases the diastolic pressure, and increased cardiac output tends to increase the systolic pressure. Blood pressure increases with age, owing primarily to the decreased distensibility of the veins. As a person grows older an increase in systolic pressure precedes an increase in diastolic pressure.

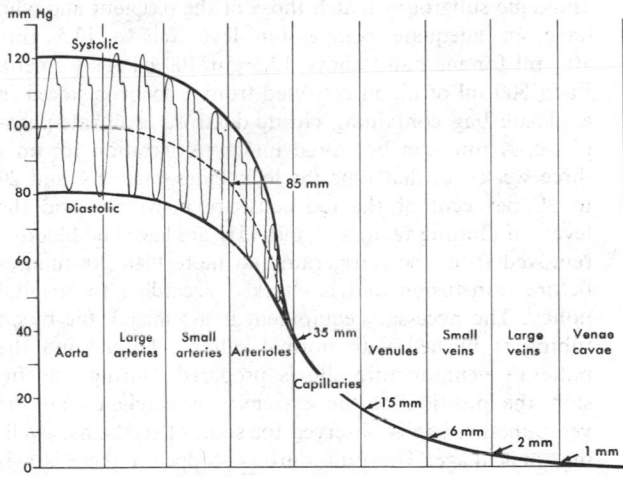

BLOOD PRESSURE GRADIENT

blood pump, 1. a pump for regulating the flow of blood into a blood vessel during transfusion. 2. See also **oxygenation.** A component of a heart-lung machine that pumps the blood through the machine for oxygenation and then through the peripheral circulatory system of the body.

blood serum. See **serum.**

blood substitute, a substance used as a replacement for circulating blood or for extending its volume. Plasma, human serum albumin, packed red cells, platelets, leukocytes, and concentrates of clotting factors are often administered in place of whole blood transfusions in the treatment of various disorders. Substances that are sometimes used in solution to expand blood volume include dextran, hetastarch, albumin solutions, or plasma protein fraction. Perfluorocarbon emulsions that are being tested as blood substitutes are able to carry oxygen to tissues, have a long shelf-life without refrigeration, and do not induce antigen-antibody reactions.

blood sugar, 1. one of a group of closely related substances, as glucose, fructose, and galactose, that are normal constituents of the blood and are essential for cellular metabolism. 2. *Nontechnical.* Also called **blood glucose.** The concentration of glucose in the blood, represented in milligrams of glucose per deciliter of blood. See also **hyperglycemia, hypoglycemia.**

blood test, 1. any test which determines something about the characteristics or properties of the blood. 2. *Informal.* a serologic test for syphilis.

blood transfusion, the administration of whole blood or a component, as packed red cells, to replace blood lost through trauma, surgery, or disease.

■ METHOD: Blood for transfusion is obtained from a healthy donor or donors whose ABO blood group and antigenic subgroups match those of the recipient and who have an adequate hemoglobin level (above 13.5 gm/100 ml for men and above 12.5 gm/100 ml for women). Each 500 ml of blood collected from a donor is stored in a plastic bag containing citrate-dextrose or citrate-phosphate. A unit can be stored under refrigeration for only three weeks; at that time the leukocytes, platelets, and 20 to 30 per cent of the red cells are nonviable, and the levels of clotting factors V and VIII are low. The blood is removed from the refrigerator no more than 30 minutes before transfusion and is checked according to hospital policy. The necessary equipment is assembled, the blood tubing is flushed with normal saline solution, and the patient's venipuncture site is prepared. During transfusion the position of the extremity is checked, and the venipuncture site is observed for signs of erythema, swelling, or leakage. The procedure is stopped if there is evidence of a systemic reaction. An acute hemolytic reaction, characterized by chills, fever, headache, back pain, decreased blood pressure, hematuria, and nausea, may occur if the recipient's and donor's blood groups are not exactly matched. Circulatory overload may cause shortness of breath, lung congestion, and frothy sputum. A pyrogenic reaction caused by bacteria or an antigen on the leukocytes or platelets of the transfused blood may result in fever, chills, and palpitations. An allergic reaction to serum protein in transfused blood may be characterized by urticaria, laryngeal edema, and asthmatic wheezing. After a transfusion has been completed, pressure is applied to the venipuncture site and a bandage or dressing is applied. The patient is observed for an hour to make certain that a reaction does not occur.

■ NURSING ORDERS: The nurse prepares the required equipment and venipuncture site, observes the patient during and after transfusion, and instructs the patient to report any symptoms associated with the procedure.

■ OUTCOME CRITERIA: All possible measures are taken to prevent the reactions which occur in an estimated 2 to 3 per cent of transfused patients. Acute hemolytic reactions can be fatal; delayed hemolysis, characterized by jaundice and anemia, may occur weeks or months after transfusion. Air embolism may occur if blood is administered under air pressure after hemorrhaging; massive replacement may cause hyperkalemia, thrombocytopenia, ammonia and citrate toxicity. Viral hepatitis and cytomegalovirus disease may be transmitted by transfused blood, but in most cases transfusion is an uneventful procedure.

blood typing, identification of genetically determined antigens on the surface of the red blood cell, used to determine a person's blood group. Usually a blood bank prodecure, it is the first step in testing donor's and recipient's blood to be used in transfusion and is followed by cross matching. See also **ABO blood groups, blood group, Rh factor, transfusion reaction.**

blood urea nitrogen (BUN), the amount of nitrogenous substance present in the blood as urea. BUN is a rough indicator of kidney function. It is elevated in kidney failure, shock, gastrointestinal bleeding, diabetes mellitus, and some tumors. BUN levels are decreased in liver disease, malnutrition, and normal pregnancy. See also **azotemia.**

blood vessel, any one of the network of tubes that carries blood. Kinds of blood vessels are **arteries, arterioles, capillaries, veins, venules.**

blood warming coil, a device constructed of coiled plastic tubing, used for warming reserve blood before massive transfusions, as those often required for patients who develop extensive gastrointestinal bleeding. Administration of cold blood in such transfusions may cause the patient to go into shock. The blood-warming coil is a prepackaged, sterile single-use device. Aseptic technique is used to remove the coil from its wrapper. The coil is immersed in water warmed to 99°F (37.6°C), and blood from the transfusion bag is allowed to flow through the coil until warm enough to administer. The coil is equipped with clamps for control of the blood flow to the primary transfusion line. During prolonged transfusions the blood-warming coil is replaced every 24 hours. Compare **electric blood warmer.**

bloody show. See **vaginal bleeding.**

blow-out fracture, a fracture of the floor of the orbit caused by a blow that suddenly increases the intraocular pressure.

blue baby, an infant born with cyanosis caused by a congenital heart lesion, as transposition of the great vessels, tetralogy of Fallot, or by incomplete expansion of the lungs (congenital atelectasis). Tetralogy of Fallot is the most common congenital cyanotic cardiac lesion and is characterized by a large ventricular septal defect, pulmonic stenosis, right ventricular hypertrophy, and overriding aorta. The effects are related to the size of the defect, but, children with the disorder often squat to relieve dyspnea. In transposition of the great vessels, the aorta arises from the right ventricle and the pulmonary artery from the left ventricle with the result that two separate, parallel paths of circulation exist and the blood is not oxygenated. Congenital cyanotic heart lesions are diagnosed by cardiac catheterization, angiography, or echocardiography and are corrected surgically, preferably in early childhood. See also **congenital cardiac anomaly, congenital heart disease, tetralogy of Fallot.**

blue bloater. See **chronic bronchitis.**

blue fever, *Informal.* Rocky Mountain spotted fever, so named for the dark cyanotic discoloration of the skin following the initial rickettsial infection. See also **rickettsiosis, Rocky Mountain spotted fever, typhus.**

blue nevus, a sharply circumscribed, usually benign, steel-blue skin nodule with a diameter between 2 and 7 mm. It is found on the face or upper extremities, grows very slowly, and persists throughout life. Nodular blue nevi found on the buttocks or in the sacrococcygeal region occasionally become malignant. Any sudden change in the size of such a lesion demands surgical attention and biopsy. The dark color is caused by large, densely packed melanocytes deep in the dermis of the nevus. Compare **melanoma.**

blue phlebitis. See **phlegmasia cerulea dolens.**

blue spot, 1. Also called **macula cerulea.** One of a number of small greyish-blue spots that may appear near the armpits or around the groins of individuals infested with lice, as in pediculosis corporis and pediculosis pubis. These spots are usually less than one cm in diameter and are caused by a substance in the saliva of lice that converts bilirubin to biliverdin. **2.** Also called **Mongolian spot.** One of a number of dark blue or mulberry-hued round or oval spots that may appear as a congenital condition in the sacral regions of certain children under four or five years of age. They usually disappear spontaneously as the affected individual matures.

blunt dissection, a dissection performed by separating tissues along natural lines of cleavage, without cutting.

blunthook, 1. a sturdy hook-shaped bar used in obstetrics for traction between the abdomen and the thigh in cases of difficult breech deliveries. **2.** a hook-shaped device with a blunt end used in embryotomy.

blush, a brief, diffuse erythema of the face and neck, commonly the result of dilatation of superficial small blood vessels in response to heat or sudden emotion.

B/M, symbol for *black male,* often used in the initial identifying statement in a patient record.

B.M.A., abbreviation for **British Medical Association.**

BMR, abbreviation for **basal metabolic rate.**

BOA, abbreviation for **born out of asepsis.**

board certification, (in medicine) a process in which an individual is tested in a medical specialty or subspecialty. Physicians are approved to practice after successfully completing requirements of specialty or subspecialty

Boards. The various medical professional organizations provide board certification examinations. Successful candidates are called "Fellows," as Fellow of the American College of Surgeons (F.A.C.S.), Fellow of the American College of Obstetrics and Gynecology (F.A.C.O.G.). Board certification is required to attain the privilege of professional practice in a hospital, including the admission of patients, the use of hospital resources, or the performance of certain diagnostic tests or surgery.

board certified, (in medicine) denoting a physician who has passed the certification examination administered by a medical specialty board and has been certified as a specialist in a particular field of medicine. The professional is then called a fellow of the specialty organization.

board eligible, (in medicine) denoting a physician who has completed the educational requirements necessary for eligibility to take the specialty board examinations. See also **board certified.**

board of health, an administrative body acting on a municipal, county, state, provincial, or national level. The functions, powers, and responsibilities of boards of health vary with the locales. Each board is generally concerned with the recognition of the health needs of the people and the coordination of projects and resources to meet and identify these needs. Among the tasks of most boards of health are prevention of disease, health education, and implementation of laws pertaining to health.

Boas' test (bou'æzɪz), **1.** Also called **resorcinol test.** A test for hydrochloric acid in the contents of the stomach, in which a glass rod dipped in a specially prepared reagent is touched to a drop of filtered stomach liquid. A scarlet streak forms along the rod in the presence of hydrochloric acid. The reagent, which is warmed before the rod is dipped, contains 5 gm of resorcinol and 5 gm of sugar dissolved in 100 ml of dilute alcohol. **2.** a test for free hydrochloric acid in the contents of the stomach in which filtered stomach fluid is boiled with a special reagent, containing five parts of resorcinol, three parts of cane sugar, and 92 parts of 94 per cent alcohol. Free hydrochloric acid produces a transient rosy mirror. **3.** a test for lactic acid in a sample of gastric juice that depends on the oxidation of the lactic acid to aldehyde and formic acid by the action of sulfuric acid and manganese. The test detects the aldehyde by the addition of Nessler's reagent or by the formation of iodoform with the addition of iodine solution. **4.** Also called **chlorophyll test.** A test for gastric motility in which a fasting patient drinks 400 ml of water which has been tinted green by the addition of 20 drops of chlorophyll solution. After 30 minutes the contents of the stomach are aspirated and the amount of tinted water that has passed through the stomach is determined.

body, 1. the whole structure of an individual with all the organs. **2.** a cadaver or a corpse. **3.** Also called **corpus,**

soma. the largest or the main part of any organ, as the body of the tibia or the body of the vastus lateralis.

body fluid, a fluid contained in the three fluid compartments of the body, the blood plasma of the circulating blood, the interstitial fluid between the cells, and the cell fluid within the cells. Blood plasma and interstitial fluid make up the extracellular fluid; the cell fluid is the intracellular fluid. The chemical constituents of the fluids vary greatly; for example, sodium is present in large amounts in both compartments of the extracellular fluid but is nearly absent in the intracellular fluid; protein is present in the blood plasma and cell fluid, but not in the interstitial fluid.

body image, a person's subjective concept of his physical appearance. The mental representation, which may be realistic or unrealistic, is constructed from self-observation, the reactions of others, and a complex interaction of attitudes, emotions, memories, fantasies, and experiences, both conscious and unconscious. A marked inability to conceptualize one's personal body characteristics may be caused by organic brain damage, as in autotopagnosia, by a physical disability, as the loss of a limb, or by psychological and emotional disturbances, as in anorexia nervosa.

body-image agnosia. See **autotopagnosia.**

body jacket, an orthopedic cast that encases the trunk of the body but does not extend over the cervical area; it may be equipped with shoulder straps. It is used to help immobilize the trunk for the healing of spinal injuries and scoliosis and for postoperative positioning and immobilization after spinal surgery.

body language, a set of nonverbal signals, including body movements, postures, gestures, spatial positions, facial expressions, and bodily adornment, that give expression to various physical, mental, and emotional states.

body mechanics, the field of physiology that studies muscular actions and the function of muscles in maintaining the posture of the body.

body movement, motion of all or part of the body, especially at a joint or joints. Some kinds of body movements are **abduction, adduction, extension, flexion, rotation.**

body odor, a fetid smell associated with stale perspiration. Freshly secreted perspiration is odorless, but after exposure to the atmosphere and bacterial activity at the surface of the skin, chemical changes occur to produce the odor. Common body odor usually can be eliminated by bathing with soap and water. Body odors also can be the result of discharges from a variety of skin conditions, including cancer, fungus, hemorrhoids, leukemia, and ulcers. See also **bromhidrosis.**

body of Retzius (ret′sias), any one of the masses of protoplasm containing pigment granules at the lower end of a hair cell of the organ of Corti in the internal ear.

body position, attitude or posture of the body. Some kinds of body position are **anatomical position, decubitus position, Fowler's position, prone position, supine position, Trendelenburg position.**

body righting reflex, any one of the neuromuscular responses to restore the body to its normal upright position when it has been displaced. The righting reflexes involve complicated mechanisms and processes associated with the structures of the internal ear, as the utricle, the saccule, the macula, and the semicircular canals. Also involved in the righting mechanism are receptors for the vestibular branch of the eighth cranial nerve. Any change in the position of the head produces a change in the pressure on the gelatinous membrane of the macula and causes tiny otoliths within the membrane to pull on hair cells, stimulating adjacent receptors of the vestibular nerve. The fibers of the nerve transmit impulses to the brain, producing a sense of position of the head by a sensation of change in the gravitational pull, activating muscles that tend to restore the body to its optimum position. Also activating righting reflexes are proprioceptors in muscles and tendons and visual nerve impulses. Interruption of the impulses associated with body-righting reflexes may disturb equilibrium and cause nausea and vomiting.

body stalk, the elongated part of the embryo that is connected to the chorion. The stalk first extends from the posterior end of the embryo to the chorion but later moves to the midventral region and forms the lengthening umbilical cord. As the embryo develops and the amnion expands, the umbilical cord comes to enclose the body stalk and the yolk sac.

body surface area (BSA). See **surface area.**

body systems model, (in nursing education) a conceptual framework in which illness is studied in relation to the functional systems of the body, as the circulatory, nervous, gastrointestinal, and reproductive. In this model, nursing care is directed toward manipulating the patient's environment in such a way that the signs and symptoms of the health problem are alleviated. As the body systems model focuses on the disease rather than the patient, current educational programs tend to integrate it with other concepts that allow the nurse to approach the patient in a more holistic framework, recognizing the complexity of the external and internal agents that contribute to illness and to health.

body temperature, the level of heat produced and sustained by the body processes. Variations and changes in body temperature are major indicators of disease and other abnormalities. Heat is generated within the body through metabolism of food and lost from the body surface through radiation, convection, and evaporation of perspiration. Heat production and loss are regulated and controlled in the hypothalamus and brain stem. Fever is usually a function of an increase in the generation of heat, but some abnormal conditions, as congestive heart failure, produce slight elevations of body temperature through impairment of the heat-loss function. Contributing to the failure to dissipate heat are reduced activity of the heart, lower rate of blood flow to the skin, and the insulating effect of edema. Diseases of the hypothalamus or interference with the other regulatory centers may produce abnormally low body temperatures. Normal adult body temperature, as measured orally, is 98.6°F. Oral temperatures ranging from 96.5°F to 99°F are consistent with good health, depending on the physical activity of the person, the ambient temperature, and the particular, normal body temperature for that person. Axillary temperature is usually 1°F lower than the oral temperature. Rectal temperatures may be 0.5° to 1.0°F higher than oral readings. Body temperature appears to vary one to two degrees throughout the day, with lows recorded early in the morning and peaks between 6 P.M. and 10 P.M. This diurnal variation may increase in range during a fever. While adult body temperature, normal and abnormal, tends to vary within a relatively narrow range, the temperatures of children respond more dramatically and rapidly to disease, changes in ambient temperature, and levels of physical activity.

Boeck's sarcoid (beks).   See **sarcoidosis.**

boil, a skin abscess. See **furuncle.**

boiling point, the temperature at which a substance passes from the liquid to the gaseous state at a particular atmospheric pressure. See also **evaporation.**

bole, any of a variety of soft, friable clays of various colors, although usually red from iron oxide. They consist of hydrous silicate of aluminum, are used as pigments, and were once commonly used as absorbents and astringents. See also **kaolin.**

Bolivian hemorrhagic fever, an infectious disease caused by an arenavirus, generally transmitted from infected rodents to humans through contamination of food by rodent urine, though direct transmission between people has also been observed. After an incubation period of from one to two weeks, the patient experiences chills, fever, headache, muscle ache, anorexia, nausea, and vomiting. As the disease progresses, hypotension, dehydration, bradycardia, pulmonary edema, and internal hemorrhages may occur. The mortality may reach 30 per cent; pulmonary edema is the most common cause of death. There is no specific therapy. Peritoneal dialysis is sometimes performed. Also called **Machupo.** See also **Argentine hemorrhagic fever, Lassa fever.**

bolus,   1. Also called **alimentary bolus.** a round mass, specifically a masticated lump of food ready to be swallowed. **2.** a large round preparation of medicinal material for oral ingestion, usually soft and not prepackaged. **3.** a dose of a medication or a contrast material, radioactive isotope, or other pharmaceutical preparation injected all at once intravenously. **4.** See **bole.**

Bombay phenotype, a rare genetic trait involving the phenotypic expression of the ABO blood groups. The gene for the H antigen, which in the usual dominant form of HH or Hh is responsible for the precursor necessary for the production of the A and B antigens, is homozygous recessive in individuals with this trait so that the expression of the A, B, and H antigens is suppressed. Cells of such individuals are phenotypically of blood type O even though they are genotype AB, and the serum contains anti-A, anti-B, and anti-H antigens. In such cases the offspring from two phenotypic O blood type parents may be blood type AB. The phenomenon is an example of the intricate interaction of linked genes in which one gene on a chromosome controls the expression or suppression of another gene that is not its allele. The trait is named for the city in which it was first reported. See also **ABO blood groups.**

bonding, the attachment process that occurs between an infant and the parents, especially the mother, and is significant in the formation of affectionate ties that later influence both the physical and psychological development of the child. The process is reciprocal and is usually initiated immediately following birth by placing the nude infant on the mother's abdomen so that both the parents and child can see and touch one another and begin to interact. The newborn is in an alert, reactive state for about 30 minutes to an hour after birth and displays such behavior as crying, sucking, clinging, grasping, and following with the eyes, which in turn stimulates the expression of the parenting instincts. Especially important in initiating bonding is eye-to-eye contact, fondling of the infant, soothing talk, and other affectionate behavior that begins to create positive emotional ties. Another essential element is the amount of contact that occurs between parents and the newborn, especially crucial with premature and high-risk infants. New concepts in normal delivery procedures, especially the trend toward more natural childbirth, allowing the father to participate and even to assist in the delivery, and the parental involvement in the care of premature and ill newborns help to facilitate stronger parent-infant relationships. Specific behavioral traits are common for each parent during the early attachment process. Mothers are more concerned with physically touching and holding the infant, while fathers are more intent on forming a sense of absorption, preoccupation, and visual interest in the child—what has been called paternal engrossment. By about the second to third week of life there is a definite reciprocal pattern of interacting behavior, involving an attention and nonattention cycle, during each encounter of parents and child. At the peak of the attention phase, the infant reaches out toward the parent and is very attentive. This is followed in a short time by deceleration of excitement in the infant and a turning away from the parent. This nonattentive phase prevents the infant from being overwhelmed by excessive stimuli, and no amount of visual or verbal attempt will regain his attention. Recognition of these cycles and especially the fact that the nonattention phase is not a form of rejection help both the mother and father to develop competence in parenting. Assessment of the attachment process is an important function of the nurse and requires skill in terms of observation and interviewing. The nurse observes the mother's reactions, especially while feeding, bathing, and comforting her infant, for potential signs of inadequate or delayed mothering. Perhaps the most important actions for forming positive parent-child attachment are eye contact in the *en face* position and embracing the infant close to the body. Many variables determine the development of attachment and parenting, including the parents' fantasies about the child, the conditions surrounding the pregnancy, what arrangements have been made concerning changes in lifestyle with the addition of a dependent family member, and what type of parenting the mother and father received as children. Since bonding is always a reciprocal process, the nurse can also instruct parents on ways of encouraging various developmental behavior, especially during the first year of life, which, in turn, enhances the responsiveness of the infant and creates a closer attachment. Parents who are aware of the child's expected level of performance promote trust and security in the child. Such awareness and especially early contact between parents and child, primarily during the neonatal period, reduce the later risk of neglect or child abuse. Although bonding is considered primarily an emotional response, it is theorized that there may be some biochemical and hormonal interaction in the mother that may stimulate the response, but studies are still inconclusive. Also called **maternal-child attachment**. See also **maternal deprivation syndrome, maternal-infant bonding**.

bone, **1.** the dense, hard, and slightly elastic connective tissue, comprising the 206 bones of the human skeleton. It is composed of compact osseous tissue surrounding spongy cancellous tissue permeated by many blood vessels and nerves and enclosed in membranous periosteum. Long bones contain yellow marrow in longitudinal cavities and red marrow in their articular ends. Red marrow also fills the cavities of the flat and the short bones, the bodies of the vertebrae, the cranial diploe, the sternum, and the ribs. Blood cells are produced in active red marrow. Osteocytes form bone tissue in concentric rings around an intricate Haversian system of interconnecting canals that accommodates blood vessels, lymphatic vessels, and nerve fibers. **2.** any single element of the skeleton, as a rib, the sternum, or the femur. See also **connective tissue**.

bone cancer, a skeletal malignancy occurring as a primary sarcomatous tumor in an area of rapid growth or, more frequently, as a metastasis from cancer elsewhere in the body. Primary bone tumors are comparatively rare, but the incidence peaks during adolescence, then decreases, and rises slowly after the age of 35. In adults bone cancer is strongly linked to exposure to ionizing radiation, especially in applying paints containing radium to watch dials. Paget's disease, hyperparathyroidism, chronic osteomyelitis, old bone infarcts, and fracture cal-

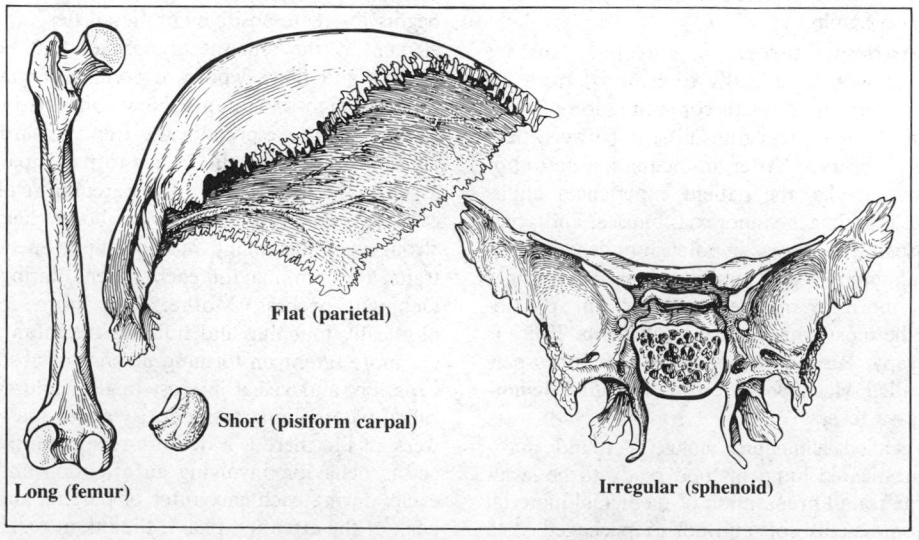

Flat (parietal)

Short (pisiform carpal)

Long (femur)

Irregular (sphenoid)

CLASSIFICATION OF BONE BY SHAPE

losities increase the risk of bone tumors, but most osseous malignancies are metastatic lesions found most often in the spine or pelvis and less often in sites away from the trunk. Bone cancers progress rapidly but are often difficult to detect; pain that increases at night may be the only symptom. X rays, radioisotopic scans, arteriography, and biopsies are diagnostic; alkaline phosphatase levels are elevated in osteoblastic tumors, and serum calcium and urinary calcium are increased in highly destructive lesions; but in other bone lesions, blood studies are often equivocal. The most common osseous malignancies are osteosarcomas, followed by chrondrosarcomas, fibrosarcomas, and Ewing's sarcoma. Surgical treatment consists of local resection of slow-growing tumors or amputation, including the joint above the tumor, if the lesion is particularly virulent and fast-growing. Radiotherapy may be administered preoperatively or as the primary form of treatment of radiosensitive tumors, as Ewing's sarcoma, reticulum cell sarcoma, and multiple myeloma. Chemotherapy, using a combination of adriamycin, cyclophosphamide, vincristine, and actinomycin D, is often effective in curing Ewing's tumors. The use of interferon and other forms of immunotherapy is experimental.

bone-cutting forceps, a kind of forceps that has long handles, single or double joints, and heavy blades.

bone marrow, specialized, soft tissue filling the spaces in cancellous bone of the epiphyses. Fatty, **yellow marrow** is found in the compact bone of most adult epiphyses. **Red marrow** is found in many bones of infants and children and in the spongy bone of the proximal epiphyses of the humerus and femur and in the sternum, ribs, and vertical bodies of adults. It is composed of myeloid tissue and is essential in the manufacture and maturation of red blood cells.

Bonine, a trade name for an antiemetic (meclizine hydrochloride).

Bonnevie-Ullrich syndrome (bon'viul'rɪk). See **Turner's syndrome**.

booster injection, the administration of an antigen, as a vaccine or toxoid, usually in a smaller amount than the original immunization, given to maintain the immune response at an appropriate level.

Boothby-Lovelace-Bulbulian (BLB) mask, an apparatus for the administration of oxygen, consisting of a mask fitted with an inspiratory-expiratory valve and a rebreathing bag.

boracic acid (boræs'ɪk). See **boric acid**.

borax bath, a medicated bath in which borax and glycerin are added to the water.

borborygmus (bor'bərɪg'məs), *pl.* **borborygmi.** an audible abdominal sound produced by hyperactive intestinal peristalsis. Borborygmi are rumbling, gurgling, and tinkling noises heard in auscultation. Although increased intestinal activity may be noted in cases of gastroenteritis and diarrhea, true borborygmi are more intense and episodic. Borborygmi accompanied by vomiting, distension, and intestinal cramps suggest a mechanical obstruction of the small intestine.

borderline schizophrenia. See **latent schizophrenia.**

Bordetella (bor'dɪtel'ə), a genus of gram-negative coccobacilli, some species of which are pathogens of the respiratory tract of man, including *Bordetella bronchiseptica, B. parapertussis,* and *B. pertussis.* See also **parapertussis, pertussis.**

boric acid (bor'ɪk), a white, odorless powder or crystalline substance used as a buffer and formerly employed as a topical antiseptic and eye wash. Also called **boracic acid, orthoboric acid.**

Bornholm disease (born'houm, born'houlm), a viral disease of epidemic potential that appears as a sudden pain in the area of the diaphragm, accompanied by malaise, nausea, headache, and intermittent fever. Also called **devil's grip, epidemic pleurodynia.**

born out of asepsis (BOA), (in a hospital) a newborn infant that was not delivered in the usual place in an obstetric unit. Depending on the policy of the institution, a BOA-designated infant may have been born on the way to the hospital, in the hospital, on the way to the delivery suite, or in a labor room.

■ OBSERVATIONS: Initial assessment on the admitting unit includes evaluation of respiration, quality of cry, skin color, apical pulse rate, muscle tone, reflexes, temperature, condition of umbilical cord or cord-stump, ability to suck, presence of meconium, congenital defect, skin eruption, or signs of sepsis, including jaundice, anorexia, vomiting, diahrrea, irritability or lethargy, high-pitched cry, and hypothermia or hyperthermia.

■ INTERVENTION: The usual steps in caring for a newborn are performed. Head and chest circumferences are measured, weight is taken, the baby is placed in a warmer until the axillary temperature is 36.5°C. Vitamin K and silver nitrate are usually given, a bath is given when the body temperature is over 36.5°C and stable. In many hospitals BOA infants are placed in a special nursery, isolated from other infants to prevent contagion should the BOA baby be infected.

■ NURSING CONSIDERATIONS: Daily care for the newborn BOA is the same as that given to other newborns, but, in addition, close observation for signs of sepsis is also made. The parents are involved in the care of the infant as soon as is possible, and the usual instructions are given for care of the baby at home after discharge.

boron (B), a nonmetallic element, similar to aluminum. Its atomic number is 5; its atomic weight is 10.8. Elemental boron occurs in the form of dark crystals and as a greenish-yellow amorphous mass. Certain concentrations of this element are toxic to plant and animal life, but plants need traces of boron for normal growth. It is the characteristic element of boric acid, which is used chiefly as a dusting powder and ointment for minor skin disorders. Boric acid in solution was formerly extensively employed as an anti-infective and eyewash, but the high incidence of toxic reactions and fatalities associated with these preparations has greatly reduced their use.

Borrelia (bərel'iə), a genus of coarse, unevenly coiled, helical spirochetes, several species of which cause tickborne and louseborne relapsing fever. The organism is spread to offspring from generation to generation. This does not occur in lice. Many animals serve as reservoirs and hosts for *Borrelia*. The spirochete may be identified by microscopic examination of a smear of blood stained with Wright's stain; it is also easily inoculated onto culture media for bacterial culture and identification.

Bostock's catarrh, *Obsolete.* See **hay fever.**

Boston exanthem, an epidemic disease characterized by scattered, pale red maculopapules on the face, chest, and back, occasionally accompanied by small ulcerations on the tonsils and soft palate. There is little or no adenopathy, and the rash disappears spontaneously in two or three weeks. It is caused by echovirus 16 and requires no treatment. Compare **herpangina.**

bottle feeding, feeding an infant or young child from a bottle with a rubber nipple on the end, sometimes called artificial feeding because it is done as a substitute for or supplement to breast feeding.

■ METHOD: The infant is held on one arm close to the body of the mother or nurse during feeding. The bottle is held at an angle to assure that the nipple is always filled with liquid so that the infant does not ingest air while feeding. For a newborn infant, rest periods may be given every several minutes. Once or twice in the course of the feeding and again at the end the infant is encouraged to burp by being held upright on the mother's or nurse's shoulder or on its stomach on the feeder's lap. Gentle rubbing or patting on the back and pressure on the stomach often helps to induce burping.

■ OUTCOME CRITERIA: Bottle feeding is used as a substitute for breast feeding when the mother is unable to breast feed or chooses not to. Bottle feeding can also be substituted for breast feeding occasionally, once lactation has been established. Bottle feeding is recommended if the mother has active tuberculosis or other active, acute contagious disease, if she has a serious chronic disease, as cancer or cardiac disease, or has recently undergone extensive surgery. Severe mastitis, narcotic addiction, or concurrent use of medication that is secreted in the breast milk usually requires the mother to bottle feed.

■ NURSING ORDERS: The formula contains protein, fats, carbohydrates, vitamins, and minerals in amounts similar to those in breast milk. The formula may be warmed before feeding by immersing the bottle in warm water for several minutes (although this is not necessary), and the

size of the nipple hole is adjusted to the needs of the infant. Smaller infants need larger nipple holes which require less sucking. Premature, or weak infants, may be fed using a special, long soft nipple through which it is very easy for the infant to feed.

bottle-mouth syndrome. See **nursing-bottle caries.**

botulism (boch'əlɪz'əm), an often fatal form of food poisoning caused by an endotoxin produced by the bacillus *Clostridium botulinum.* The toxin is ingested in food contaminated by *C. botulinum,* although it is not necessary for the live bacillus to be present if the toxin has been produced. In rare instances, the toxin may be introduced into the human body through a wound contaminated by the organism. Botulism differs from most other types of food poisoning in that it develops without gastric distress and may not occur for from 18 hours up to a week after the contaminated food has been ingested. Botulism is characterized by a period of lassitude and fatigue followed by visual disturbances, as double vision, difficulty in focusing the eyes, and loss of ability of the pupil to accommodate to light. Muscles may become weak, and the patient often develops dysphagia. Nausea and vomiting occur in less than half the cases. Hospitalization is required and antitoxins are administered. Sedatives are given, mainly to relieve anxiety. Approximately two thirds of the cases of botulism are fatal, usually as a result of respiratory complications. For those who survive, recovery is slow. Most botulism occurs after eating improperly canned or cooked foods. See also *Clostridium.*

bouba (bu'bə). See **yaws.**

Bouchard's node (busharz'), an abnormal cartilaginous or bony enlargement of a proximal interphalangeal joint of a finger, usually occurring in degenerative diseases of the joints. Compare **Heberden node.**

bougie (bu'zhi), a thin, cylindrical instrument made of rubber, waxed silk, or other flexible material for insertion into canals of the body in order to dilate, examine, or measure them.

-boulia. See **-bulia.**

boulimia. See **bulimia.**

bounding pulse, a pulse that, on palpation, feels full and springlike owing to an increased thrust of cardiac contraction or an increased volume of circulating blood within the elastic structures of the vascular system.

bouquet fever. See **dengue.**

Bourneville's disease (burn'vɪlz). See **tuberous sclerosis.**

boutonneuse fever (bu'tənuz'), an infectious disease caused by *Rickettsia conorii,* transmitted to humans through the bite of a tick. The onset of the disease is characterized by a lesion called a tache noire, or black spot, at the site of the infection, fever lasting from a few days to two weeks, and a papular erythematous rash that spreads over the body to include the skin of the palms and soles. Treatment usually involves administration of antibiotics. There is no prophylactic medication available, and prevention depends primarily upon avoiding ticks. The disease is similar to Rocky Mountain spotted fever and to other rickettsial diseases. It is prevalent in parts of Europe, Asia, Africa, and the Middle East. See also **rickettsiosis, Rocky Mountain spotted fever.**

Bowditch's law (bɑu′dĭchīz). See **all or none law.**

bowel. See **intestine.**

bowel elimination, alteration in: constipation, a nursing diagnosis accepted by the Fourth National Conference on the Classification of Nursing Diagnoses. The etiology of the condition is to be developed at a later conference. The defining characteristics include decreased activity level; decreased frequency of elimination; a hard, formed stool; a palpable rectal mass; a reported feeling of pressure or fullness in the rectum, and straining at stool. Abdominal pain, appetite impairment, back pain, headache, and interference with daily living may also be present. See also **nursing diagnosis.**

bowel elimination, alteration in: diarrhea, a nursing diagnosis accepted by the Fourth National Conference on the Classification of Nursing Diagnoses. The etiology of the condition is to be developed at a later conference. The defining characteristics include abdominal pain, cramping, increased frequency of elimination, increased frequency of bowel sounds, loose or liquid stools, and urgency of defecation. A change in the color of the feces may also be noted. See also **nursing diagnosis.**

bowel elimination, alteration in: incontinence, a nursing diagnosis accepted by the Fourth National Conference on the Classification of Nursing Diagnoses. The etiology of the condition is to be developed at a later conference. The defining characteristic of the problem is the involuntary passage of stool. See also **nursing diagnosis.**

bowel training, a method of establishing regular evacuation by reflex conditioning, used in the treatment of fecal incontinence, impaction, chronic diarrhea, and autonomic hyperreflexia. In patients with autonomic hyperreflexia, distention of the rectum and bladder causes paroxysmal hypertension, restlessness, chills, diaphoresis, headache, elevated temperature, and bradycardia.

■ METHOD: The patient's previous bowel habits are ascertained and the necessity of developing a program to induce an evacuation at the same time each day or every other day is explained. Exercises to strengthen abdominal muscles, as pushing up, bearing down, and contracting the musculature, are demonstrated. A bedside commode is provided and privacy is ensured. The patient is instructed to recognize and respond promptly to signals indicating a full bowel, as goose pimples, perspiration, piloerection on arms or legs, and to develop cues to stimulate the urge to defecate, as drinking coffee, massaging the abdomen, pressing the inner thigh, or stroking the anus. Fluids to 3,000 ml daily are encouraged; prune juice, orange juice, and coffee are included in the daily diet, and the importance of having well-balanced meals that include bulk and roughage and of avoiding constipating foods, as bananas, beans, and cabbage, is discussed. Depending on the patient and the problem, the training program may involve drinking four to ten ounces of prune juice each night or 12 hours prior to the time set for evacuation, drinking warm water, coffee, or milk 30 minutes before the set time, and inserting a lubricated glycerine suppository prior to the set time. The patient is told that no formed stools for three days, semiliquid feces, restlessness, and discomfort are signs of impending impaction and that the condition may be treated with a laxative suppository or with a tap water or oil retention enema. The importance of reporting symptoms of autonomic hyperreflexia to the physician is stressed, and the possibility that emotional stress or illness may cause accidental incontinence after the program is established is discussed.

■ NURSING ORDERS: The nurse provides instruction and encourages the patient to establish a program of regular evacuation.

■ OUTCOME CRITERIA: Reflex conditioning is often an effective method of developing regular bowel habits in incontinent patients, especially those who are highly motivated and are given good instruction and understanding support. Young persons with spinal cord lesions are able to develop automatic defecation when adequately trained, but some elderly incontinent people may not be able to learn the program.

Bowen's disease (bou′ənz). See **intraepidermal carcinoma.**

Bowen's precancerous dermatosis. See **intraepidermal carcinoma.**

bowleg (bou′leg′). See **genu varum.**

Bowman's capsule (bou′mənz), the cup-shaped end of a renal tubule containing a glomerulus. Also called **glomerular capsule.**

box bath. See **cabinet bath.**

boxer's fracture, a fracture of one or more metacarpal bones, usually the fourth or the fifth, caused by punching a hard object. Such a fracture is often distal, angulated, and impacted.

Boyle's law, (in physics) a law stating that the product of the volume and pressure of a gas compressed at a constant temperature remains constant.

BP, abbreviation for **blood pressure.**

Br, symbol for **bromine.**

brace, an orthopedic device, sometimes jointed, to support and hold any movable part of the body in the correct position to allow function, as a leg brace permits walking and standing. Compare **splint.**

brachi-, a combining form meaning 'pertaining to the arm': *brachialgia, brachiation, brachiocyllosis.*

-brachia, a combining form meaning an 'anatomical condition involving an arm': *acephalobrachia, diantebrachia, monobrachia.*

brachial (brei'kiəl), of or pertaining to the arm.

brachial artery, the principal artery of the upper arm that is the continuation of the axillary artery. It has three branches and terminates at the bifurcation of its main trunk into the radial artery and the ulnar artery.

brachialis (brei'kiæl'ɪs), a muscle of the upper arm, covering the anterior part of the elbow joint and the distal half of the humerus. It arises from the anterior surface of the humerus and inserts, by a thick tendon, into the tuberosity of the coronoid process of the ulna. It is innervated by a branch of the musculocutaneous nerve, containing fibers from the fifth and the sixth cervical nerves, and functions to flex the forearm. Compare **biceps brachii, triceps brachii.**

brachial plexus, a network of nerves in the neck, passing under the clavicle and into the axilla, originating in the fifth, sixth, seventh, and eighth cervical and first thoracic spinal nerves and innervating the muscles and skin of the chest, shoulders, and arms.

brachial plexus anesthesia, an anesthetic block of the region innervated by the anterior divisions of the last four cervical and first thoracic nerves. The plexus extends from the transverse processes to the apex of the axilla, where the terminal nerves are formed. Because of the anatomy of the area, many approaches are possible, the axillary being most common; supraclavicular and interscalene are also used. Perivascular axillary block has the least incidence of complications, it being limited to minimal extravasation of blood. Other approaches may result in Horner's syndrome, phrenic nerve palsy, pneumothorax, recurrent laryngeal paralysis, sensory deficits, paresthesias, or hematomas. See also **regional anesthesia.**

brachial plexus paralysis. See **Erb's palsy.**

brachial pulse, the pulse of the brachial artery, palpated in the antecubital space.

brachiocephalic arteritis (brei'kiousəfæl'ɪk). See **Takayasu's arteritis.**

brachiocephalic artery, one of the three arteries that branch from the arch of the aorta, running about 5 cm from the level of the cranial border of the second right costal cartilage, ascending cranially, dorsally, and obliquely to the right, and dividing into the right common carotid and the right subclavian arteries.

brachiocephalic trunk. See **brachiocephalic artery.**

brachioradialis (brei'kiourei'diæl'ɪs), the most superficial muscle on the radial side of the forearm. It arises from the lateral supracondylar ridge of the humerus and from the lateral intermuscular septum and inserts, by a flat tendon, into the styloid process of the radius. It is innervated by a branch of the radial nerve, which contains fibers from the fifth and the sixth cervical nerves, and it functions to flex the forearm.

brachioradialis reflex, a deep tendon reflex, elicited by striking the lateral surface of the forearm proximal to the distal head of the radius, characterized by normal slight elbow flexion and forearm supination. It is accentuated by disease of the pyramidal tract above the level of the fifth cervical vertebra. See also **deep tendon reflex.**

-brachium, a combining form meaning 'arm or armlike growth': *antibrachium, prebrachium, pontibrachium.*

brachy-, a combining form meaning 'short': *brachycheilia, brachygnathia, brachyskelous.*

brachycephaly (bræk'ɪsef'əli), **brachycephalia, brachycephalism,** a congenital malformation of the skull in which premature closure of the coronal suture results in excessive lateral growth of the head, giving it a short, broad appearance with a cephalic index of between 81 and 85. See also **craniostenosis.** – **brachycephalic, brachycephalous,** *adj.*

Bradford frame, a rectangular orthopedic frame made of pipes to which heavy movable straps of canvas are attached, running from side to side to support a patient in a prone or supine position. The straps can be removed to permit the patient to urinate or defecate while remaining immobile.

Bradford solid frame, a rectangular orthopedic device of metal covered with canvas to aid in immobilization, especially of children in traction. The Bradford solid frame provides support for the entire body and is especially appropriate for patients who are under five years of age, hyperactive, or mentally retarded. The main purpose of the device is to assist in maintaining proper immobilization, positioning, and alignment by controlling movement. To facilitate nursing care, the Bradford solid frame is not placed directly on a bed but elevated at both ends by plywood blocks or by other suitable devices. It is most often used with Bryant traction but never with balanced suspension traction, cervical traction, cervical tongs, or certain other kinds of traction.

Bradford split frame, a rectangular orthopedic device of metal covered with two separate pieces of canvas fastened at both ends of the frame. Used especially in pediatrics to aid in the immobilization of children in traction, it is divided in the middle by a large opening designed to accommodate the excretory functions of an incontinent patient in a hip spica cast. The division also allows for the upper and lower extremities of the patient to be elevated separately and for the maintenance of a clean and dry cast. When the purpose of the frame is to provide elevation only, the head end of the frame is elevated to help assure a clean and dry cast by the flow of excretory matter by gravity. The frame is equipped with three webbing straps to prevent the patient from sliding on the frame. Two straps are anchored at the upper end of the frame around the metal portion, one strap on each side. Both straps are then passed under the canvas cover to the opening in the middle of the frame. If the cast encasing the patient is a short leg hip spica, the straps are secured around the thigh section of the cast. If the cast extends to the toes of one or both legs, the straps are wrapped around the portion of the frame at the opening in the middle and then secured around the thigh section. The third strap is placed around the waist of the patient and around the frame. For an incontinent child, a plastic funnel leading into the bedpan is positioned below the opening in the frame.

Bradley method, a method of psychophysical preparation for childbirth developed by Robert Bradley, M.D., comprising education about the physiology of childbirth, exercise and nutrition during pregnancy, and techniques of breathing and relaxation for control and comfort during labor and delivery. The father is extensively involved in the classes and acts as the mother's "coach" during labor. The first stage of labor is divided into two parts. During the latent phase the woman is encouraged to carry on her normal activities until she feels the need to concentrate on the contractions. During the active phase the uterine cervix dilates from about 5 cm to 10 cm, the contractions occur every $1\frac{1}{2}$ to 3 minutes and last from 40 to 90 seconds, the interval between contractions tends to decrease, and the length and intensity of the contractions tend to increase. The father helps the mother to relax by repeating reminders to relax the various parts of her body, by massaging and touching her as he has learned she finds relaxing, and by arranging and rearranging pillows to support her in a 'lounge chair' position. During contractions, she breathes deeply and slowly—in through the nose and out through the mouth. Her abdominal wall lifts with each inhalation and falls with each exhalation. She may close her eyes and try to visualize the baby's head pressing against the cervix, causing it to dilate. She is encouraged by the close support of the father, the midwife or obstetrician, and the nurse. During the second stage of labor, the uterine cervix is fully dilated, the contractions are strong and expulsive, occurring every $1\frac{1}{2}$ to 2 minutes and lasting 60 to 90 seconds. The mother, feeling the urge to bear down and push, allows her knees to fall away from each other without forcibly drawing her thighs against her abdomen as in other methods. She breathes in and out deeply once or twice, waiting for the contraction to build in strength, then she bears down while holding her breath. She pushes as hard as necessary to relieve the pressure or urgency of the contraction. The father may count seconds for her so that she can push for 10 or for 15 seconds, as necessary. He also checks to see that her legs and buttocks are relaxed, and he reminds her to keep her perineum relaxed, to concentrate, and to 'let

the baby out.' As the baby is born, with the mother still in a semi-sitting position, the infant is placed on her abdomen and then nursed as soon as it wants. The mother is given a glass of orange juice and often walks back to her room with the father and the baby. Among the advantages of the method are its simplicity, the involvement of the father, and the realistic approach to the efforts and discomfort of labor. Also called **husband-coached childbirth.** Compare **Lamaze method, Read method.**

brady-, a combining form meaning 'slow, dull': *bradyacusia, bradydiastalsis, bradyphagia.*

bradycardia (brăd′ĭkar′dĭə), an abnormal circulatory condition in which the myocardium contracts steadily but at a rate of less than 60 contractions a minute. The heart normally slows during sleep, and, in some physically fit people, the pulse may be quite slow. Pathologic bradycardia may be symptomatic of a brain tumor, digitalis toxicity, or vagotonus. Cardiac output is decreased, causing faintness, dizziness, chest pain, and, eventually syncope and circulatory collapse. Treatment may include administration of atropine, implantation of a pacemaker, or reduction of digitalis dosage.

bradykinesia (brăd′ĭkĭni′źhə, brăd′ĭkăini′źhə), an abnormal condition characterized by slowness of all voluntary movement and speech, as caused by parkinsonism, other extrapyramidal disorders, and certain tranquilizers.

bradypnea (brăd′ĭpni′ə), an abnormally slow rate of breathing. Also called **oligopnea.** See also **respiratory rate.**

Braille, a system of printing for the blind consisting of raised dots or points that can be read by touch.

brain, the portion of the central nervous system contained within the cranium. It consists of the cerebrum, cerebellum, pons, medulla, and midbrain. Specialized cells in its mass of convoluted, soft, gray or white tissue coordinate and regulate the functions of the central nervous system.

brain concussion, a violent jarring, or shaking, or other blunt nonpenetrating injury to the brain caused by a sudden change in momentum of the head. Characteristically, after a mild concussion there may be a transient loss of consciousness followed, on awakening, by a headache. Severe concussion may cause prolonged unconsciousness and disruption of certain vital functions of the brain stem, as respiration and vasomotor stability. The treatment for a person recovering from a concussion consists principally of observation for signs of intracranial bleeding. Also called **concussion.**

brain death, an irreversible form of unconsciousness characterized by a complete loss of brain function while the heart continues to beat. The legal definition of this condition varies from state to state. The usual clinical criteria for brain death include the absence of reflex activity, movements, and respiration. The pupils are dilated and fixed. As hypothermia, anesthesia, poisoning, or drug intoxication may cause deep physiologic depression that resembles brain death, a diagnosis of brain death requires that the electrical activity of the brain be evaluated and shown to be absent on two electroencephalograms performed 12 to 24 hours apart. Also called **irreversible coma.** Compare **coma, sleep, stupor.**

brain electrical activity map (BEAM), a topographic map of the brain created by a computer that is able to respond to the electrical potentials evoked in the brain by a flash of light. Potentials recorded at 4-millisecond intervals are converted into a many-colored map of the brain showing them to be positive or negative. The waves may be observed traveling through the brain. If the wave is disordered, blocked, too small, or too large, there may be a tumor or other lesion causing the abnormal pattern.

brain fever, *Informal.* any inflammation of the brain or meninges. See also **encephalitis.**

brain scan, a diagnostic procedure employing radioisotope imaging techniques to localize and identify intracranial masses, lesions, tumors, or infarcts. Radioisotopes are injected intravenously to circulate to the brain where they accumulate in abnormal tissue. The radioisotopes are traced and photographed by a scintillator, or scanner, and the size and location of the abnormality are determined. The nature and rate of accumulation of radioisotopes in pathologic tissue in some cases are diagnostic of a particular lesion. A brain scan, which is painless, requires no special preparation other than injection of the isotopes and an explanation of the procedure. Compare **CAT scan.** See also **isotope, radioisotope.**

brain stem, the portion of the brain comprising the medulla oblongata, the pons, and the mesencephalon. It performs motor, sensory, and reflex functions and contains the corticospinal and the reticulospinal tracts. The 12 pairs of cranial nerves from the brain arise mostly from the brain stem. Compare **medulla oblongata, mesencephalon, pons.**

brain stem auditory evoked potential (BAEP), the most reliable evoked potential for predicting nerve damage during surgery in the auditory nerve region. A clicking sound is made and the EEG waves from the auditory area of the patient's brain are observed. Cessation or absence of electrical activity may indicate damage or destruction.

brain tumor, a neoplasm of the intracranial portion of the central nervous system that is usually invasive but does not spread beyond the cerebrospinal axis. Brain tumors, which are not rare, cause significant morbidity and mortality, but increasing numbers are successfully treated. Intracranial tumors in children are usually the result of a developmental defect. In adults 20 to 40 per cent of malignancies in the brain are metastatic lesions from cancers in the breast, lung, gastrointestinal tract, kidney, or any site of a malignant melanoma. The etiology of primary brain tumors is not known, but the risk is increased in individuals exposed to vinyl chloride, in the siblings of cancer patients, and in recipients of renal transplant being treated with immunosuppressant medication. During pregnancy a meningioma may suddenly develop or increase in size, suggesting that this tumor is stimulated by hormonal factors. Symptoms of a brain tumor are often those of increased intracranial pressure, as headache, nausea, vomiting, papilledema, lethargy, and disorientation. Various localizing signs also occur, as loss of vision in the eye on the side of an occipital neoplasm. Diagnostic measures include visual field and funduscopic examinations, skull x rays, electroencephalography, cerebral angiography, brain scanning, computerized axial tomography, and spinal fluid studies. Lumbar puncture may not be performed if increased intracranial pressure is obvious. A broad spectrum of tumors may be found in the brain, but gliomas, chiefly astrocytomas, are the most common malignancies. Rapidly growing medulloblastomas often occur in children. Benign meningiomas are the only intracranial neoplasms more common in women than in men. Craniopharyngiomas, generally found in children and young adults, are benign but impinge on critical structures and are difficult to remove. Schwannomas most often arise from the eighth cranial nerve and cause deafness; but they are generally benign. Surgery is the initial treatment for most primary tumors of the brain. Radiotherapy is indicated for inoperable lesions, medulloblastomas, tumors with multiple foci, and as postoperative treatment of residual tumor tissue. Beams of neutrons and high energy pi-mesons currently show promise in the treatment of highly malignant brain lesions. The blood-brain barrier impedes the effect of some antineoplastic agents but responses are obtained in some cases treated with procarbazine and various nitrosoureas administered alone or with vincristine. Compare **spinal cord tumor.**

bran bath, a bath in which bran has been boiled in the water, used for the relief of skin irritation.

branched chain ketoaciduria. See **maple syrup urine disease.**

branched tubular gland, one of the many multicellular glands with one excretory duct from two or more tube-shaped secretory branches as some of the gastric glands.

branchial fistula, a congenital, abnormal passage from the pharynx to the external surface of the neck, resulting from the failure of a branchial cleft to close during fetal development. Introduction of a sound into a branchial fistula may cause pallor and arrhythmic pounding of the heart. Also called **cervical fistula.**

brand name. See **trade name.**

brassfounder's ague. See **metal fume fever.**

brassy eye. See **chalkitis.**

Braun's canal (braunz). See **neurenteric canal.**

Braxton-Hicks contraction (bræk'stənhıks'), irregular tightening of the pregnant uterus that begins in the first trimester and increases in frequency, duration, and intensity as pregnancy progresses. Contractility of uterine muscle increases in pregnancy. Near term, strong Braxton-Hicks contractions are often difficult to distinguish from the contractions of true labor. See also **false labor.**

Brazilian trypanosomiasis. See **Chagas' disease.**

breach of contract, the failure to perform as promised or agreed in a contract. The breach may be complete or partial and may occur by repudiation, by failure to recognize the contract, or by prevention or hindrance of performance.

breach of duty, 1. the failure to perform an act required by law. 2. the performance of an act in an unlawful way.

breakbone fever. See **dengue.**

breast, 1. the anterior aspect of the chest. 2. a mammary gland.

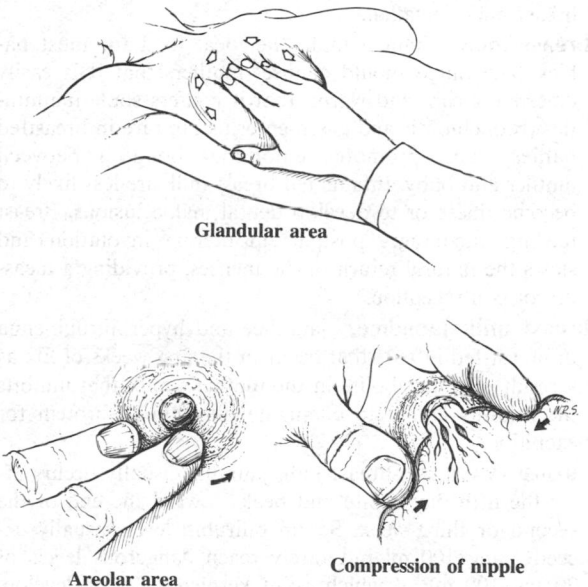

Glandular area

Areolar area

Compression of nipple

BREAST PALPATION

breast cancer, a malignant neoplastic disease of breast tissue, the most common malignancy in women in the United States. The incidence increases exponentially with age from the third to the fifth decade and reaches a second peak at age 65, suggesting that breast cancer in premenopausal women may be related to ovarian hormonal function and in postmenopausal patients to adrenal function. Based on the great prevalence of breast cancer in affluent countries, especially in high socioeconomic groups, it is thought that a high fat diet may be a causative factor, but the relationship is unproven and the etiology is unknown. Risk factors include a family history of breast cancer, nulliparity, exposure to ionizing radiation, early menarche, late menopause, obesity, diabetes, hypertension, chronic cystic disease of the breast, and, possibly, postmenopausal estrogen therapy. Women who are over 40 when they bear their first child and patients with malignancies in other body sites also have an increased risk of developing breast cancer. Initial symptoms, detected in most cases by self-examination, include a small painless lump, thick or dimpled skin, or nipple retraction. As the lesion progresses there may be nipple discharge, pain, ulceration, and enlarged axillary glands. The diagnosis may be established by a careful physical examination, mammography, and cytologic examination of tumor cells obtained by biopsy. Infiltrating ductal carcinomas are found in about 75 per cent of cases and infiltrating lobular, infiltrating medullary, colloid, comedo, or papillary carcinomas in the others. Tumors are more common in the left than in the right breast and in the upper and outer quadrant than in the other quadrants. Metastasis through the lymphatic system to axillary lymph nodes and to bone, lung, brain, and liver is common, but there is evidence that primary carcinomas of the breast may exist in multiple sites and that tumor cells may enter the blood stream directly without passing through lymph nodes. Surgical treatment, depending on the assessment of the tumor, may be a radical, modified radical, or simple mastectomy, with dissection of axillary nodes, or a lumpectomy. Postoperative radiotherapy, chemotherapy, or both are usually prescribed. Chemotherapeutic agents frequently administered in various combinations are cyclophosphamide, methotrexate, 5-fluorouracil, phenylalanine mustard (L-PAM), thio-TEPA, adriamycin, vincristine, and prednisone. The presence of estrogen receptors in breast tumors is considered an indication for ovarian ablation, adrenalectomy, or hypophysectomy or for the administration of androgens or antiestrogens in order to reduce the amount of endogenous estrogen. Implantation of a prosthesis following mastectomy is gaining currency but is painful initially and is not universally approved. Less than one per cent of breast cancers occur in men, but those with Klinefelter's syndrome are at 60 times greater risk. In men, the tumor may be successfully treated with surgical excision and with combination chemotherapy, orchiectomy, adrenalectomy, or hypophysectomy. The prognosis is generally less favorable in women. See also **lumpectomy, mastectomy.**

Visual examination

Palpation

BREAST SELF-EXAMINATION

breast examination, a process in which the breasts and their accessory structures are observed and palpated in assessing the presence of changes or abnormalities that could indicate malignant disease. See also **self-breast examination.**
■ METHOD: The breasts are observed with the patient sitting with her arms at her sides, sitting with her arms over her head, back straight, then leaning forward, and, finally, sitting upright, as she contracts the pectoral muscles. The breasts are observed for symmetry of shape and size and for surface characteristics, including moles or nevi, hyperpigmentation, retraction or dimpling, edema, abnormal distribution of hair, focal vascularity, or lesions. With the patient still sitting, the axillary nodes and the supraclavicular and subclavicular areas are palpated. With the patient lying down on her back, each breast is

shifted medially, and the glandular area in each is palpated with the flat of the fingers of a hand in concentric circles or in a pattern like the spokes of a wheel, from the periphery inward. The areolar areas, the nipples, and the tail of Spence in the upper outer quadrant extending toward the axilla are then palpated.
■ NURSING CONSIDERATIONS: The patient should be taught how to perform a self-breast examination and encouraged to do it monthly. Many women find it helpful to check their breasts every time they shower for the first few months after being taught the procedure to practice and to become very familiar with their own breasts.
■ OUTCOME CRITERIA: Early diagnosis greatly improves the rate of cure in cancer of the breast. The breast examination thoroughly performed serves as a valuable means of screening women to discover those who require further diagnostic examination by xeroradiography, mammography, biopsy, or, less frequently, by thermoradiography.

breast feeding, suckling or nursing. **1.** giving a baby milk from the breast. **2.** taking milk from the breast. See **breast milk, lactation.**

breast milk, human milk, the ideal food for most babies. The nurse should counsel mothers that it is easily digested, clean, and warm, that it confers some immunities (bronchiolitis and gastroenteritis are rare in breastfed babies), and promotes emotional bonding between mother and baby. Infants fed breast milk are less likely to become obese or to develop dental malocclusions. Breast feeding encourages postpartum uterine involution and slows the natural return of the menses, providing a measure of contraception.

breast milk jaundice, jaundice and hyperbilirubinemia in breast-fed infants that occur in the first weeks of life as a result of a metabolite in the mother's milk that inhibits the infant's ability to conjugate bilirubin to protein for excretion.
■ OBSERVATIONS: Breast milk jaundice usually occurs after the fifth day of life and peaks toward the end of the second or third week. Serum bilirubin levels usually exceed 5 mg/100 ml but rarely reach dangerous levels of 20 mg/100 ml, at which point kernicterus may develop. The infant seems normal and healthy but the skin, the whites of the eyes, and the serum are jaundiced.
■ INTERVENTION: If serum bilirubin exceeds acceptable levels, breast feeding may be interrupted until there is a decrease to the normal range, usually a period of one to three days. During this interval, the infant is bottle-fed with a supplemental formula and the mother uses a breast pump or manual devices to maintain lactation without becoming engorged. Phototherapy may be used to accelerate excretion of bilirubin through the skin.
■ NURSING CONSIDERATIONS: The primary concern of the nurse is to observe for signs of increasing jaundice, to

monitor serum bilirubin levels, and, usually, to reassure the mother that her child is well and that the jaundice resolves slowly but completely in time.

breast pump, a device for withdrawing milk from the breast.

breast self-examination (BSE). See **self-breast examination.**

breathing. See **respiration.**

breathing pattern: ineffective, a nursing diagnosis accepted by the Fourth National Conference on the Classification of Nursing Diagnoses. The etiology of the condition includes neuromuscular impairment, pain, musculoskeletal impairment, impairment of perception or cognition, anxiety, decreased energy, and fatigue. The defining characteristics of the problem include dyspnea, shortness of breath, tachypnea, fremitus, abnormal concentrations of arterial blood gases, cyanosis, cough, nasal flaring, change in depth of respiration, pursed-lip breathing or prolonged expiratory phase, increased anteroposterior diameter of the chest, use of accessory muscles of breathing, and altered excursion of the chest wall with respiration. See also **nursing diagnosis.**

breathing tube, a device inserted into the trachea through the mouth or nose to assure a patent airway for adequate respiration during artificial or assisted ventilation. See also **extubation, intubation.**

breathlessness. See **dyspnea.**

breath sound, the sound of air and carbon dioxide passing in and out of the respiratory system as heard with a stethoscope. Vesicular and tracheal breath sounds are normal. Decreased breath sounds may indicate an obstruction of an airway, collapse of a portion or all of a lung, thickening of the pleurae of the lungs, emphysema, or other chronic obstructive lung disease.

Breckinridge, Mary (1881–1965), an American nurse, who founded the Frontier Nursing Service, in Kentucky. The Service was designed to improve the obstetrical care of women living in the remote mountainous area. The nurses in the Service had training in midwifery and reached their patients on horseback and on foot, often encountering personal danger. The Service began training midwives and stimulated the increase of other midwifery schools.

breech birth, parturition in which the baby emerges feet, knees, or buttocks first. Breech birth is often hazardous: the body may deliver easily but the aftercoming head may become trapped by an incompletely dilated cervix because babies' heads are usually larger than their bodies. See also **assisted breech, version and extraction.**

breech extraction, an obstetrical operation in which a baby being born feet or buttocks first is grasped before any part of the trunk is born and delivered by traction. Compare **assisted breech.**

breech presentation, intrauterine position of the fetus in which the buttocks or feet present, occurring in approximately 3 per cent of labors. Kinds of breech presentation are **complete breech, footling breech, frank breech.** Compare **vertex presentation.** See also **breech birth.**

bregma (breg'mə), the junction of the coronal and sagittal sutures on the top of the skull. —**bregmatic,** adj.

Brenner tumor, an uncommon, benign ovarian neoplasm consisting of nests or cords of epithelial cells containing glycogen that are enclosed in fibrous connective tissue. The tumor may be solid or cystic and is sometimes difficult to distinguish from certain granulosa-theca cell neoplasms.

brepho-, a combining form meaning 'pertaining to an embryo, fetus, or newborn infant': *brephoplastic, brephopolysarcia, brephotrophic.*

Brethine, a trade name for a bronchodilator (terbutaline sulfate).

bretylium tosylate (brɪtɪl'ɪəm tou'sɪleɪt), an antiarrhythmic.

■ INDICATIONS: It is prescribed in the treatment of life-threatening ventricular arrhythmias when other measures have not been effective.

■ CONTRAINDICATION: Known hypersensitivity to this drug prohibits its use.

■ ADVERSE EFFECTS: Among the more serious adverse reactions are hypotension, nausea and vomiting, diarrhea, and nasal stuffiness.

Bretylol, a trade name for an adrenergic blocking agent (bretylium tosylate), used as an antiarrhythmic agent.

brevi-, a combining form meaning 'short': *brevicollis, breviflexor, breviradiate.*

Brevital Sodium, a trade name for a barbiturate (methohexital sodium), used as a general anesthetic.

brewer's yeast, a preparation containing the dried pulverized cells of a yeast, as *Saccharomyces cerevisiae,* that is used as a leavening agent and as a dietary supplement. It is one of the best sources of the B complex vitamins and of many minerals and is also a high grade of protein. Brewer's yeast may protect against toxicity of large doses of vitamin D, is used to prevent constipation, and is a good source of enzyme-producing agent.

Bricanyl, a trade name for a beta-adrenergic drug (terbutaline sulfate).

bridge of Varolius. See **pons.**

bridging, 1. a nursing technique of positioning a patient so that bony prominences are free of pressure on the mattress by using pads, bolsters of foam rubber, or pillows to distribute body weight over a larger surface. 2. a nursing technique for supporting a part of the body, as the testicles in treating orchitis using a Bellevue bridge made of a towel or other material.

brief psychotherapy, (in psychiatry) treatment directed toward the active resolution of personality or behavioral problems rather than toward the speculative analysis of the unconscious. It usually concentrates on a specific problem or symptom and is limited to a specified number of sessions with the therapist.

Bright's disease, *Obsolete.* a kidney disease, especially glomerulonephritis.

Brill-Symmer's disease (brɪl'sɪm'ərz). See **giant follicular lymphoma.**

Brill-Zinsser disease (brɪl'zɪn'sər), a mild form of typhus that recurs in a person who appears to have completely recovered from a severe case of the disease. Some rickettsiae remain in the body after the symptoms of the disease abate, causing the recurrence of symptoms, especially when stress, illness, or malnutrition weaken the person. Treatment with antibiotics may eradicate the organism. See also **endemic typhus, epidemic typhus, rickettsiosis, typhus.**

Briquet's syndrome (brɪkeiz'). See **somatization disorder.**

Brissaud's dwarf (brisouz'), a person affected with infantile myxedema in which short stature is associated with hypothyroidism.

Bristamin, a trade name for an antihistamine (phenyltoloxamine citrate).

British anti-lewisite (BAL), a heavy metal antagonist. Also called **dimercaprol.**

■ INDICATIONS: It is prescribed in the treatment of Wilson's disease, and in the treatment of acute arsenic, mercury, or gold poisoning, as from an overdosage with mercurial diuretics, arsenicals, or gold salts or from an accidental ingestion of mercury, gold, or arsenic.

■ CONTRAINDICATIONS: Hepatic or renal insufficiency, poisoning with cadmium, iron, or selenium, or known hypersensitivity to the drug prohibits its use.

■ ADVERSE EFFECTS: Among the most serious adverse reactions are nephrotoxicity, acidosis, convulsions, and abnormal cardiovascular functions. Mild reactions include pain at the injection site, nausea, excessive salivation, and parasthesia.

British Medical Association (B.M.A.), a national professional organization of physicians in the United Kingdom.

British Pharmacopoeia, the official British reference work setting forth standards of strength and purity of medications and containing directions for their preparation in order to ensure that the same prescription written by different doctors and filled by different pharmacists will contain exactly the same ingredients in the same proportions. The first *British Pharmacopoeia* was published in 1864 by the General Medical Council; it superseded the *London Pharmacopoeia,* which had been published since 1618. See also **British Medical Association.**

brittle bones. *Nontechnical.* See **osteogenesis imperfecta.**

brittle diabetes, a chronic, difficult to control disease of carbohydrate metabolism, characterized by inexplicable oscillations between hypoglycemia and ketoacidosis. See also **diabetes mellitus.**

broad beta disease, a familial type of hyperlipoproteinemia in which a lipoprotein, high in cholesterol and triglycerides, accumulates in the blood. The condition, which affects males in their 20s and females in their 30s and 40s, is characterized by yellowish nodules (xanthomas) on the elbows and knees, peripheral vascular disease, and elevated serum cholesterol levels. People with this disease are at risk of developing early coronary disease. Therapy includes dietary measures to reduce weight and serum lipids. See also **hyperlipidemia, hyperlipoproteinemia.**

broad ligament, a folded sheet of peritoneum draped over the uterine tubes, the uterus, and the ovaries. It extends from the sides of the uterus to the sidewalls of the pelvis, dividing the pelvis from side to side and creating the vesicouterine fossa and pouch in front of the uterus and the rectouterine fossa and pouch behind it. Also called **ligamentum latum uteri.**

Broca's area (brou'kəz), an area, involved in speech production, situated on the inferior frontal gyrus of the brain.

Brodie's abscess, a form of osteomyelitis consisting of an indolent staphylococcal infection of bone, usually in the metaphysis of a long bone of a child, characterized by a necrotic cavity surrounded by dense granulation tissue. See also **osteomyelitis.**

Brodmann's areas (brod'manz), the 47 different areas of the cerebral cortex that are associated with specific neurologic functions and distinguished by different cellular components. Compare **motor area.** See also **cerebral cortex.**

brom-, bromo-, a combining form meaning 'odor, stench': *bromacetone, bromhidrosis, bromoacetophenon.*

bromhidrosis (brou'mɪdrou'sɪs), an abnormal condition in which the apocrine sweat has an unpleasant odor. The odor is usually caused by bacterial decomposition of perspiration on the skin. Treatment includes frequent bathing, changing of socks and underclothes, and the use of deodorants, antibacterial soaps, and dusting powders. Also called **body odor.**

bromide (brou'maid), a compound in which the negative element is bromine, especially a salt of hydrobromic acid. Bromides, once widely prescribed as sedatives, are now seldom used for that purpose because they may cause serious mental disturbances as side effects.

bromine (Br), a toxic, red-brown, liquid element of the halogen group. Its atomic number is 35; its atomic weight is 79.909. Bromine is used in industry, in photography, in the manufacture of organic chemicals and fuels, and in medications. Bromine gives off a red vapor that is extremely irritating to the eyes and the respiratory tract. Liquid bromine is irritating to the skin; bromates used as neutralizers in cold wave products are toxic if ingested. Bromides are binary compounds of bromine; they have been used as sedatives, hypnotics, and analgesics and are still used in some nonprescription, over-the-counter preparations. Prolonged use of these products may cause brominism, a toxic condition characterized by acneiform eruptions, headache, loss of libido, drowsiness, and fatigue. See also **bromide.**

bromo-. See **brom-.**

bromoderma (brou'moudər'mə), an acneiform, bullous, or nodular skin rash, occurring as a hypersensitivity reaction to ingested bromides.

brompheniramine maleate (brom'fənır'əmin), an antihistamine.

■ INDICATIONS: It is prescribed in the treatment of a variety of hypersensitivity reactions, including rhinitis, skin reactions, and itching.

■ CONTRAINDICATIONS: Asthma or known hypersensitivity to this drug prohibits its use. It is not given to newborn infants, lactating mothers, or to other people for whom anticholinergic medications are contraindicated.

■ ADVERSE EFFECTS: Drowsiness, skin rash, hypersensitivity reactions, dry mouth, and tachycardia commonly occur.

Brompton's cocktail, an analgesic solution containing alcohol, morphine or heroin, cocaine, and, in some cases, a phenethiazine. The cocktail is administered in the control of pain in the terminally ill patient. Given frequently in small doses, it may relieve pain for many months. It was developed at the Brompton Hospital in England. Also called **Brompton's mixture.**

Bromsulphalein (BSP) test (bromsəl'fælin), a trade name for sulfobromophthalein, a dye prepared for use in a highly sensitive, nonspecific test that measures the ability of liver cells to remove the sulfobromophthalein from the blood. Forty-five minutes after intravenous injection, more than 95 per cent of the dye is normally cleared from the blood. The test is rarely indicated in current clinical practice because it may cause severe allergic reactions, and because it cannot indicate a specific dysfunction of the liver. See also **sulfobromophthalein.**

bronch-, a combining form meaning 'pertaining to the bronchus': *bronchiectasis, bronchiotetany, bronchodilation.*

bronchial asthma. See **asthma in children.**

bronchial breath sound, an abnormal sound heard with a stethoscope over the lungs, indicating consolidation owing to pneumonia or compression. Expiration and inspiration produce loud, high-pitched sounds of equal duration.

bronchial fremitus, a vibration that can be palpated or auscultated on the chest wall over a bronchus congested by secretions that rattle as the air passes during respiration.

bronchial hyperreactivity, an abnormal respiratory condition characterized by reflex bronchospasm in response to histamine or a cholinergic drug. It is a universal feature of asthma and is used in the differential diagnosis of asthma and heart disease. An asthmatic person experiences episodes of bronchospasm in response to the cholinergic effect of endogenous histamine and to exposure via inhalation of histamine or a cholinergic drug like methacholine in testing for asthma.

bronchial tree, an anatomical complex of the bronchi and the bronchial tubes. The bronchi branch from the trachea and the bronchial tubes branch from the bronchi. The right bronchus is wider and shorter than the left bronchus, and it diverges less abruptly from the trachea. The right bronchus branches into three subsidiary bronchi, one passing to each of the three lobes that comprise the right lung. The left bronchus is smaller in diameter but about twice as long as the right bronchus and passes inferior to the pulmonary artery before branching into the bronchi for the inferior and the superior lobes of the left lung.

bronchiectasis (brong'kiek'təsis), an abnormal condition of the bronchial tree, characterized by irreversible dilatation and destruction of the bronchial walls. The condition is sometimes congenital, but is more often a result of bronchial infection or of obstruction by a tumor or an aspirated foreign body. Symptoms of bronchiectasis include a constant cough productive of copious purulent sputum, hemoptysis, chronic sinusitis, clubbing of fingers, and persistent moist, coarse rales. Some of the complications of bronchiectasis are pneumonia, lung abscess, empyema, brain abscess, and amyloidosis. Treatment includes frequent postural drainage, antibiotics, and, rarely, surgical resection of the affected part of the lungs.

bronchiolar carcinoma. See **alveolar cell carcinoma.**

bronchiole (brong'kioul), a small airway of the respiratory system extending from the bronchi into the lobes of the lung. There are two divisions of bronchioles: the terminal bronchioles pass inspired air from the bronchi to the respiratory bronchioles and expired waste gases from the respiratory bronchioles to the bronchi. The respiratory bronchioles function similarly, allowing the exchange of air and waste gases between the alveolar ducts and the terminal bronchioles. — **bronchiolar,** *adj.*

bronchiolitis (brong'kioulai'tis), an acute viral infection of the lower respiratory tract that occurs primarily in infants aged 2 to 12 months, characterized by expiratory wheezing, respiratory distress, and obstruction at the level of the bronchioles. The most common causative agents are the respiratory syncytial viruses (RSV) and the parainfluenza viruses. *Mycoplasma pneumoniae,* the rhinoviruses, enteroviruses, and measles virus are less common etiologic agents. Transmission occurs by infection with airborne particles or by contact with infected secretions. The diagnosis consists of evidence of hyperinflation of the lungs through percussion or chest x ray.

■ OBSERVATIONS: The condition typically begins as an upper respiratory tract infection with serous nasal discharge and, often, low-grade fever. Increasing respiratory distress follows, characterized by tachypnea, tachycardia, intercostal and subcostal retractions, a paroxysmal cough, an expiratory wheeze, and, often, an elevated temperature. The chest may appear barrel-shaped; x rays show hyperinflated lungs and a depressed diaphragm. Respiration becomes more shallow, causing increased alveolar oxygen tension and leading to respiratory acidosis. Complete obstruction and absorption of trapped air may lead to atelectasis and respiratory failure. Blood-gas determinations indicate the degree of oxygen saturation and carbon dioxide retention.

■ INTERVENTION: Routine treatment includes humidity and oxygen via a mist tent, vaporizer, or Croupette, generally combined with oxygen; an adequate fluid intake, usually given intravenously because of tachypnea, weakness, and fatigue; suctioning of the airways to remove secretions, and rest. Endotracheal intubation is indicated when carbon dioxide retention occurs, when bronchial secretions do not loosen and clear, or when oxygen therapy does not alleviate hypoxia. Such medications as antibiotics, bronchodilators, corticosteroids, cough suppressants, and expectorants are not routinely used. Sedatives are contraindicated because of the suppressant effect they exert on the respiratory tract. The infection typically runs its course in seven to ten days, with good prognosis. A major complication is bacterial infection, most commonly following prolonged use of a mist tent. The disorder is often confused with asthma: a family history of allergy, the presence of other allergic manifestations, and improvement with epinephrine injection is usually indicative of asthma, not bronchiolitis. Cystic fibrosis, pertussis, the bronchopneumonias, and foreign body obstruction of the trachea are other disorders that may be confused with bronchiolitis.

■ NURSING CONSIDERATIONS: The focus of nursing care is to promote rest and to conserve the child's energy by reducing anxiety and apprehension; to increase the ease of breathing with humidity and oxygen as needed; to aid in changing position for comfort; and to induce drainage of secretions or to suction when necessary. Fever is usually controlled by the cool atmosphere of the mist tent and by administering antipyretics as needed. Frequent changing of clothing and bed linen is often necessary in a mist environment to reduce chilling. Vital signs and chest and breath sounds are continuously monitored to detect early signs of respiratory distress. Children with bacterial infections are isolated to prevent cross contamination.

bronchitis (brŏŋkaiʹtis), an acute or chronic inflammation of the mucous membranes of the tracheobronchial tree. **Acute bronchitis** is characterized by a productive cough, fever, hypertrophy of mucus-secreting structures, and back pain. Caused by the spread of upper respiratory viral infections to the bronchi, it is often observed with or following childhood infections like measles, whooping cough, diphtheria, and typhoid fever. Treatment includes bedrest, aspirin, expectorants, and appropriate antibiotic therapy. **Chronic bronchitis** is distinguished by an excessive secretion of mucus in the bronchi with a productive cough for at least 3 consecutive months in at least 2 successive years. Additional symptoms are frequent chest infections, cyanosis, hypoxemia, hypercapnia, and a marked tendency for the development of cor pulmonale and respiratory failure. Causes of chronic bronchitis include cigarette smoking, air pollution, chronic infections, and abnormal physical development of the bronchi that distorts the structures sufficiently to interfere with bronchial drainage. Most common in adults, it is often a complication of cystic fibrosis in children. Treatment includes the cessation of cigarette smoking, avoidance of airway irritants, the use of expectorants, and postural drainage. Currently, prophylactic antibiotics, steroids, and desensitization therapy are not recommended.

bronchodilator, a substance, especially a drug, that relaxes contractions of the smooth muscle of the bronchioles to improve ventilation to the lungs. Pharmacologic bronchodilators are prescribed to improve aeration in asthma, bronchiectasis, bronchitis, and emphysema. Commonly used bronchodilators include corticosteroids, ephedrine, isoproterenol, theophyllin, and various derivatives and combinations of these drugs. Beclamethasone and triamcinolone are available in aerosol form. The adverse effects vary, depending on the particular class of the bronchodilating drug. In general, bronchodilators are given with caution to people with impaired cardiac function. Nervousness, irritability, gastritis, or palpitations of the heart may occur.

bronchofibroscopy. See **fiberoptic bronchoscopy.**

bronchogenic carcinoma, one of the more than 90 per cent of malignant lung tumors that originate in bronchi. Lesions, usually the result of cigarette smoking, may cause coughing and wheezing, fatigue, chest tightness, aching joints, and in the late stages, bloody sputum, clubbing of the fingers, weight loss, and pleural effusion. Diagnosis is made by bronchoscopy, sputum cytology, lymph node biopsy, and radioisotope scanning procedures, but exploratory surgery may be required. About 45 per cent of the tumors are squamous cell or epidermoid carcinomas, 33 per cent are oat cell carcinomas, and 15 to 20 per cent are adenocarcinomas. Surgery is the most effective treatment, but approximately 50 per cent of cases are advanced and inoperable when first seen. Palliative treatment includes radiotherapy and chemotherapy.

bronchopneumonia,   an acute inflammation of the lungs and bronchioles, characterized by chills, fever, high pulse and respiratory rates, bronchial breathing, cough with purulent bloody sputum, severe chest pain, and abdominal distension. The disease is usually a result of a spread of bacterial infection from the upper respiratory tract to the lower respiratory tract, caused by *Mycoplasma pneumoniae, Staphylococcus pyogenes,* or *Streptococcus pneumoniae.* Atypical forms of bronchopneumonia may occur in viral and rickettsial infections. The most common cause in infancy is the respiratory syncytial virus. The condition results in pleural effusion, empyema, lung abscess, peripheral thrombophlebitis, respiratory failure, congestive heart failure, and jaundice. Treatment includes an antibiotic, often penicillin or ampicillin, oxygen therapy, supportive measures to keep the bronchi clear of secretions, and relief of pleural pain. Compare **aspiration pneumonia, eosinophilic pneumonia, interstitial pneumonia.**

bronchopulmonary,   of or pertaining to the bronchi and the lungs of the respiratory system.

bronchoscope (broŋ'kəskoup'),   a curved, flexible tube for visual examination of the bronchi. It contains fibers that carry light down the tube and project an enlarged image up the tube to the viewer. The bronchoscope is used to examine the bronchi, to secure a specimen for biopsy or culture, or to aspirate a foreign body from the respiratory tract. See also **fiberoptic bronchoscopy.** — **bronchoscopic,** *adj.*

bronchoscopy,   the visual examination of the tracheobronchial tree, using the standard rigid, tubular metal bronchoscope or the narrower, flexible fiberoptic bronchoscope, which has greatly expanded the diagnostic and therapeutic applications of the procedure. The patient is in a fasting state and is usually sedated prior to the examination, which is routinely performed under topical anesthesia. In addition to visualization, the procedure can be used for suctioning, for obtaining a biopsy and fluid or sputum for examination, for removal of foreign bodies, and for diagnosing such conditions as localized atelectasis, bronchial obstruction, lung abscess, and tracheal extubation. See also **bronchoscope.** — **bronchoscopic,** *adj.*

bronchospasm,   an abnormal contraction of the smooth muscle of the bronchi, resulting in an acute narrowing and obstruction of the respiratory airway. A cough with generalized wheezing usually indicates this condition. Bronchospasm is a chief characteristic of asthma and bronchitis. Treatment includes the use of active bronchodilators, catecholamines, corticosteroids, or methylxanthines, and of preventive drugs, as cromolyn sodium. See also **asthma, bronchitis.**

bronchus (broŋ'kəs), *pl.* **bronchi.** any one of several large air passages in the lungs through which pass inspired air and exhaled waste gases. Each bronchus has a wall consisting of three layers. The outermost is made of dense fibrous tissue, reinforced with cartilage. The middle layer is a network of smooth muscle. The innermost layer consists of ciliated mucous membrane. Kinds of bronchi are **lobar bronchus, primary bronchus, secondary bronchus, segmental bronchus.** See also **arteriole, bronchiole.** — **bronchial,** *adj.*

Bronkephrine,   a trade name for a sympathomimetic bronchodilator (ethylnorepinephrine hydrochloride).

Bronkosol,   a trade name for a bronchodilator (isoetharine hydrochloride), used for temporary relief of bronchial asthma, acute paroxysms, and bronchial spasms of bronchitis and emphysema.

Brown-Séquard's treatment (braun'seikardz').   See **organotherapy.**

Brown-Séquard syndrome,   a traumatic neurologic disorder resulting from compression of one side of the spinal cord, above the tenth thoracic vertebrae, characterized by spastic paralysis on the injured side of the body, loss of postural sense, and loss of the senses of pain and heat on the other side of the body.

brown spider,   a poisonous insect, also known as the brown recluse or violin spider, found in both North and South America. The venom from its bite usually creates a blister surrounded by concentric white and red circles. This so-called "bull's eye" appearance is helpful in distinguishing it from other spider bites. The wound ordinarily ulcerates and sometimes becomes infected. Pain, nausea, fever, and chills are common, but the reaction is usually self-limited. Antivenin is not available in the United States.

Brucella abortus.   See **abortus fever.**

brucellosis (bru'səlou'sis),   a disease caused by any of several species of the gram-negative coccobacillus *Brucella.* Brucellosis is most prevalent in rural areas among farmers, veterinarians, meat packers, slaughterhouse workers, and livestock producers. Primarily a disease of animals (including cattle, pigs, and goats), humans usually acquire it by ingesting contaminated milk or milk products or through a break in the skin. It is characterized by fever, chills, sweating, malaise, and weakness. The fever often comes in waves, rising in the evening and subsiding during the day, occurring at intervals separated by periods of remission. Other signs and symptoms may include anorexia and weight loss, headache, muscle and joint pain, and an enlarged spleen. In some patients, the disease is acute; more often, it is chronic, recurring over a period of months or years. Although brucellosis itself is rarely fatal, treatment is important because serious complications such as pneumonia, meningitis, and encephalitis can develop. Tetracycline plus streptomycin is the treatment of choice; bed rest is also important. Also called **Cyprus fever, Malta fever, Mediterranean fever, rock fever, undulant fever.** See also **abortus fever.**

Bruch's disease. See **Marseilles fever.**

Brudzinski's sign (brudzɪn′skiz), an involuntary flexion of the knee when the neck is passively flexed, seen in patients with meningitis.

bruise. See **ecchymosis.**

bruit (brut), an abnormal sound or murmur heard while auscultating an organ or gland, as the liver or thyroid. The specific character of the bruit, its location, and when it occurs in a cycle of other sounds are all of diagnostic importance.

Brushfield's spots, pinpoint, white or light yellow spots on the iris of a child with Down's syndrome. Occasionally, they are seen in normal infants, but their absence may help to rule out Down's syndrome.

Bruton's agammaglobulinemia, a sex-linked, inherited condition characterized by the absence of gamma globulin in the blood. Patients with this syndrome are deficient in antibodies and susceptible to repeated infections. Compare **agammaglobulinemia.** See also **gamma globulin.**

bruxism (brək′sızəm), the compulsive, unconscious grinding of the teeth, especially during sleep or as a mechanism for the release of tension during periods of extreme stress in the waking hours. Also called **bruxomania.**

bruxomania (brək′soumei′niə). See **bruxism.**

bry-, a combining form meaning 'full of life': *bryocyte, bryocytole, bryocytic.*

Bryant traction, an orthopedic mechanism used only with infants to immobilize both lower extremities in the treatment of a fractured femur or in the correction of the congenital dislocation of the hip. This mechanism consists of a traction frame supporting weights, connected by ropes that run through pulleys to traction foot plates worn by the infant involved. The traction pull elevates the lower extremities to a vertical position with the patient supine, the trunk and the lower extremities forming a right angle. The weight applied to the traction mechanism is usually less than 35 pounds. Compare **Buck's traction.**

BSA, abbreviation for **body surface area.** See **surface area.**

BSE, abbreviation for **breast self-examination.** See **self-breast examination.**

BSN, abbreviation for **bachelor of science in nursing.**

BSP, abbreviation for **Bromsulphalein.**

BTPD, abbreviation for *body temperature, ambient pressure, dry.*

BTPS, abbreviation for *body temperature, ambient pressure, saturated* (with water vapor).

buba (byu′bə, bu′bə). See **yaws.**

bubbling rale, an abnormal chest sound characteristic of moisture moving in the lungs. Compare **amphoric breath sound, atelectatic rale, dry rale.**

bubo (byu′bou), *pl.* **buboes.** a greatly enlarged, inflamed lymph node usually in the axilla or groin, associated with such diseases as chancroid, lymphogranuloma venereum, and plague. Treatment includes specific antibiotic therapy, application of moist heat, and sometimes, incision and drainage.

bubonic plague, the most common form of plague, characterized by painful buboes in the axilla, groin, or neck, fever often rising to 106°F, prostration with a rapid, thready pulse, hypotension, delirium, and bleeding into the skin from the superficial blood vessels. The symptoms are caused by an endotoxin released by a bacillus, *Yersinia pestis,* introduced into the body by the bite of a rat flea that has bitten an infected rat. Inoculation with plague vaccine confers partial immunity; infection provides lifetime immunity. Treatment includes antibiotics, supportive nursing care, surgical drainage of buboes, isolation, and stringent precautions against spread of the disease. Conditions favor a plague epidemic when a large infected rat population lives with a large nonimmune human population in a damp, warm climate. Improved sanitary conditions and the eradication of rats and rat fleas may prevent outbreaks of the disease. Killing the rats and not the fleas promotes human infection. Also called **Black Death, black plague.** Compare **pneumonic plague, septicemic plague.** See also **bubo.**

bucca-. See **bucco-.**

buccal (bək′əl), of or pertaining to the inside of the cheek, the surface of a tooth, or the gum next to the cheek.

buccal administration of medication (bək′əl), oral administration of a drug, usually in the form of a tablet, by placing it between the cheek and the teeth or gum until it dissolves.

buccal fat pad, a fat pad in the cheek under the subcutaneous layer of the skin, over the buccinator. It is particularly prominent in infants and is often called a sucking pad.

bucci-. See **bucco-.**

buccinator (bək′sınei′tər), the main muscle of the cheek, one of the 12 muscles of the mouth. It arises from the maxilla above and the mandible below, inserting in the lips; its superficial surface is covered by the buccopharyngeal fascia and the buccal fat pad. Its deep part is pierced by the duct of the parotid gland opposite the second molar tooth. The buccinator, innervated by buccal branches of the facial nerve, compresses the cheek, acting as an important accessory muscle of mastication by holding food under the teeth.

bucco-, bucca-, bucci-, a combining form meaning 'pertaining to the cheek': *buccocervical, buccodistal, buccogingival.*

buccopharyngeal (bək′oufərɪn′jiəl), of or pertaining to the cheek and the pharynx or to the mouth and the pharynx.

bucket-handle fracture, a fracture that produces a tear in a semilunar cartilage along the medial side.

bucking, *Informal.* **1.** gagging on an endotracheal tube. **2.** involuntarily resisting insufflation by a positive pressure respirator.

Buck's skin traction, an orthopedic procedure that applies traction to the lower extremity, with the hips and the knees extended. It is used to help in the treatment of hip and knee contractures, in postoperative positioning and immobilization, and in disease processes of the hip and the knee. This type of traction may be unilateral, involving one leg, or bilateral, involving both legs.

Buck's traction, one of the most common orthopedic mechanisms by which pull is exerted on the lower extremity with a system of ropes weights, and pulleys. Buck's traction, which may be unilateral or bilateral, is used to immobilize, position, and align the lower extremity in the treatment of contractures and diseases of the hip and knee. The mechanism commonly consists of a metal bar extending from a frame at the foot of the patient's bed, supporting traction weights connected by a rope passing through a pulley to a cast or a splint around the affected body structure. Compare **Bryant traction.**

Budd-Chiari syndrome (bəd′kiær′i), a disorder of hepatic circulation, marked by venous obstruction, which leads to liver enlargement, ascites, extensive development of collateral vessels, and severe portal hypertension. Also called **Chiari's syndrome, Rokitansky's disease.**

budding, a type of asexual reproduction in which the cell produces a budlike projection containing chromatin that eventually separates from the parent and develops into an independent organism. It is a common form of reproduction in the lower animals and plants, as sponges, yeasts, and molds.

Buerger's disease (bər′gərz). See **thromboangiitis obliterans.**

buffer, a substance or group of substances that absorbs hydrogen ions when a base is added to the system and that releases hydrogen ions upon the addition of an acid. Buffers minimize changes of pH in a chemical system. Among the functions carried out by buffer systems in the body are maintenance of the acid-base balance of the blood and maintenance of the proper pH in kidney tubules. See also **blood buffers, pH.**

buffy coat transfusion. See **granulocyte transfusion.**

bulbar paralysis, a degenerative neurologic condition characterized by progressive paralysis of the lips, tongue, mouth, pharynx, and larynx. The condition occurs most commonly in people over 50 years of age, in multiple sclerosis, and in amyotrophic lateral sclerosis.

bulbourethral gland, one of two small glands located on each side of the prostate, draining to the urethra. Bulbourethral glands secrete a fluid component of the seminal fluid.

bulb syringe, a blunt-tipped, flexible syringe usually made of rubber or plastic. Bulb syringes are used primarily for irrigating external orifices, as the auditory canal.

bulbus oculi (bəl′bəs). See **eye.**

-bulia, a combining form meaning '(condition of the) will': *abulia, parabulia, hyperbulia.* Also **-boulia.**

bulimia (byulɪm′iə), **boulimia,** an insatiable craving for food, often resulting in episodes of continous eating followed by periods of depression and self-deprivation. **– bulemic,** *n., adj.*

bulk. See **dietary fiber.**

bulk cathartic, a cathartic that acts by softening and increasing the mass of fecal material in the bowel. Bulk cathartics contain a hydrophilic agent like methylcellulose or psyllium seed.

bulla (bul′ə, bəl′ə), *pl.* **bullae.** a thin-walled blister of the skin or mucous membranes greater than one centimeter in diameter containing clear, serous fluid. Compare **vesicle.** **– bullous,** *adj.*

bulldog forceps, short, spring forceps for clamping an artery or vein for hemostasis. The jaws may be padded to avoid injury to vascular tissue.

bullet forceps, a kind of forceps that has thin, curved, serrated blades designed for extracting a foreign object, as a bullet, from the base of a puncture wound.

bullous myringitis, an inflammatory condition of the ear, characterized by fluid-filled vesicles on the tympanic membrane and the sudden onset of severe pain in the ear. The condition often occurs with bacterial otitis media. Treatment includes the administration of antibiotics, analgesics, and surgical draining of the vesicles. See also **otitis media.**

bulphthalmos. See **congenital glaucoma.**

Buminate, a trade name for a blood-volume expander (human albumin).

BUN, abbreviation for **blood urea nitrogen.**

-bund, a combining form meaning 'prone to' something specified: *furibund, moribund.*

bundle branch block, an abnormality in the conduction of the cardiac impulse through the fibers of the bundle of His. If many fibers are affected, the heart rate is reduced; the pacemaker function is relegated to the ventricles and peripheral perfusion is impaired. The condition may occur following myocardial infarction, in ischemic heart disease, or in certain degenerative neurological diseases. An artificial pacemaker may be used to maintain adequate cardiac function.

bundle of His (hɪs), a band of fibers in the myocardium through which the cardiac impulse is transmitted from the atrioventricular (AV) node to the ventricles. The bundle of His begins at the AV node, follows the membranous septum of the heart and divides to form the left bundle branch and the right bundle branch. The right bundle branch continues toward the apex and spreads throughout the right ventricle. The left bundle branch penetrates the fibrous septum and spreads throughout the left ventricle. The ends of both bundle branches within the ventricles are composed of Purkinje fibers. Also called **atrioventricular bundle, His bundle.**

bunion (bən′yən), an abnormal enlargement of the joint at the base of the great toe. It is caused by inflammation of the bursa, usually as a result of chronic irritation and pressure from poorly fitted shoes. It is characterized by soreness, swelling, thickening of the skin, and lateral displacement of the great toe.

Bunyamwera arbovirus, one of a group of arthropod-borne viruses that infect man, carried by mosquitoes from rodent hosts causing a mild disease characterized by headache, weakness, low-grade fever, myalgia, and a rash. Convalescence is prolonged. Outbreaks have occurred in North America, South America, Africa, and Europe.

buphthalmos (byʊfθæl′məs). See **congenital glaucoma.**

bupivacaine hydrochloride (byupɪv′əkein), a local anesthetic.

■ INDICATIONS: It is prescribed for caudal, epidural, peripheral, or sympathetic anesthetic block.

■ CONTRAINDICATIONS: Known hypersensitivity to this drug or to any of the amide class of local anesthetics prohibits its use.

■ ADVERSE EFFECTS: Among the more serious adverse reactions are central nervous system disturbances, cardiovascular depression, and hypersensitivity reactions. The adverse effects vary depending on the condition of the patient, the dosage, and the route of administration.

Burkitt's lymphoma (bər′kıts), a malignant neoplasm composed of undifferentiated lymphoreticular cells that form a large osteolytic lesion in the jaw or, in children, an abdominal mass. The tumor, which is seen chiefly in Central Africa, is characteristically a gray-white mass with a brainlike consistency, sometimes containing areas of hemorrhage and necrosis. Central nervous system involvement often occurs, and other organs may be affected. The Epstein-Barr virus (EBV), a herpesvirus, may be the cause of this lymphoma. Chemotherapy usually results in rapid shrinking of the osteolytic lesion and complete cure of the disease. Also called **African lymphoma, Burkitt's tumor.**

Burkitt's tumor. See **Burkitt's lymphoma.**

burn, any injury to tissues of the body caused by heat, electricity, chemicals, or gases in which the extent of the injury is determined by the amount of exposure of the cell to the agent and to the nature of the agent. The treatment of burns includes pain relief, careful asepsis, prevention of infection, maintenance of the balance in the body of fluids and electrolytes, and good nutrition. Severe burns of any etiology may cause shock, which is treated before the wound. See also **chemical burn, electrocution, thermal burn.**

burn center, a health care facility that is designed to care for patients who have been severely burned. A network of burn centers has been established throughout the

		Depth of burn / Detailed classification	Pain and pinprick sensitivity	Appearance	Healing time	End result of healing	Treatment
1°		Erythema only, no loss of epidermis	Hyperalgesia	Erythema		Normal skin	Allow to heal by natural processes / Protect from further injury and infection
		Superficial, no loss of dermis	Hyperalgesia or normal		6-10 days	Normal skin	
2°	Partial skin loss	Intermediate, healing from hair follicles	Normal to hypo-algesia	Erythema to opaque, white blisters are characteristic	7-14 days	Normal to slightly pitted and/or poorly pigmented	
		Deep, healing from sweat glands	Hypoalgesia to analgesia		14-21 days	Hairless and depigmented / Texture normal to pitted or flat and shiny	
3°	Whole skin loss	Deep dermal, occasionally heal from scattered epithelium	Analgesia	White opaque to charred, coagulated; subcutaneous veins may be visible	More than 21 days	Poor texture / Hypertrophic Scar frequent	Elective skin grafting may save time and give better end result
		Whole skin loss, healing from edges only			Never if area is large	Hypertrophic scar and chronic granulations unless grafted	Skin grafting mandatory
4°	Deep tissue loss	Deep structure loss	May be some algesia				

BURN CLASSIFICATION

United States and Canada that provide sophisticated advanced techniques of care for burn victims.

burnout, the condition of having no energy left to care, resulting from chronic, unrelieved job-related stress and characterized by physical and emotional exhaustion and, sometimes, by physical illness. The professional loses concern for the clients, no longer has positive feelings, sympathy, or respect for patients, and often develops cynical, dehumanized perceptions of people, labeling them in a derogatory manner. Causes of burnout peculiar to the nursing profession often include stressful, even dangerous, work environments; lack of support; lack of respectful relationships within the health care team; low pay scales, with a broadening gulf between nurse's and physician's salaries; shift changes and long work hours with overtime causing shifts to last from 12-16 hours; general understaffing of hospitals; pressure from the responsibility of providing continuous high levels of care over long periods of time; frustration and disillusionment resulting from the difference between job realities and job expectations; and sexism.

burn therapy, the management of a patient burned by flames, a hot liquid, or explosive, chemical, or electric current. Partial-thickness burns may be first degree, involving only the epidermis, or second degree, involving the epidermis and corium, while full-thickness or third degree burns involve all skin layers. Second degree burns covering more than 30 per cent of the body and third degree burns on the face and extremities, or more than 10 per cent of the body surface, are critical. In the first 48 hours of a severe burn, vascular fluid, sodium chloride, and protein rapidly pass into the affected area causing local edema, blister formation, hypovolemia, hypoproteinemia, hyponatremia, hyperkalemia, hypotension, and oliguria. The initial hypovolemic stage is followed by a shift of fluid in the opposite direction resulting in diuresis, increased blood volume, and decreased serum electrolytes. Potential complications in serious burns include circulatory collapse, renal damage, gastric atony, paralytic ileus, infections, septic shock, pneumonia, and stress ulcer (Curling's ulcer), characterized by hematemesis and peritonitis.

■ METHOD: The extent of the burn, its cause, and time of occurrence and the patient's age, weight, allergies, and any preexisting illness are recorded. If respiratory distress is present, endotracheal intubation or tracheostomy may be performed. Specimens are obtained for urinalysis, blood type, blood urea nitrogen level, hematocrit, prothrombin time, electrolyte levels, blood gases, and for cultures of nasal, throat, wound, and stool organisms. Parenteral fluids and electrolytes, antibiotics, tetanus prophylaxis, and pain medication are administered as ordered; large doses of analgesics and sedatives are avoided when possible in order to prevent depressing respiration and the masking of symptoms. An indwelling urinary catheter is inserted and a nasogastric tube and catheter for monitoring central venous pressure may be indicated. Local treatment of the burn may be by the closed method or the more frequently used open method in which the injured area is cleaned and exposed to air and the patient is kept warm by a blanket or linen over a bed cradle or by a heater or lamp. In the closed method, a germicidal or bacteriostatic cream, ointment, or solution is applied to the burn, and the wound is covered with a dressing. A porcine heterograft may be used to cover the wound temporarily; this technique prevents loss of fluid and reduces the risk of infection, but the graft dries in one or two days and may pull and cause pain. Newly developed artificial skin holds great promise for treating severe burns. During the acute stage of a burn, the patient's blood pressure, pulse, respiration, and cerebrovascular pressure are checked every 30 to 60 minutes and the rectal temperature every two to four hours. Oral hygiene, assistance in turning, coughing, and deep breathing are provided every two hours, and the patient's sensorium is evaluated hourly. If oral fluids are ordered, juices and carbonated drinks are offered but plain water and ice chips are avoided. Fluid intake and output are measured hourly; if a child excretes less than 1.0 ml/kg of urine or an adult less than 0.5 ml/kg, a diuretic or an increase in intravenous infusion of fluid may be necessary. Blood transfusions, steroid therapy, and antipyretics may be ordered; aspirin is contraindicated. Excessive chilling and exposure to upper respiratory and wound infections are carefully avoided. Burned extremities are elevated, and contractures are prevented by using firm supports to keep affected areas properly aligned, as by using a footboard to keep the feet at a 90° angle to the ankles in burns of the lower extremities or by having the patient grasp a ball when the back of the hand is burned. In burns of the arm, axilla, or chest, the arm of the affected side is supported at a 90° angle to the body slightly above shoulder height. Linear incision of the eschar on the wound may be required if the constricting crust interferes with circulation or respiration. The patient is weighed daily at the same time on the same scale, and, after the initial acute period, an adequate intake of a high-calorie, high-protein diet is encouraged; to stimulate appetite the patient is offered frequent small meals of preferred foods and beverages that are high in potassium. Vitamins may be required. Tranquilizers may be given prior to wound care, but narcotics for pain usually are not needed after the acute phase. The patient is encouraged to stand for a few minutes every hour or every second hour and is generally able to walk in seven to ten days, but convalescence may be prolonged. Burned patients often are frightened, withdrawn, and disoriented initially, but after a few days they may become angry, depressed, or rebellious and in need of emotional support to help them cooperate with their treatment and rehabilitation. Extensive plastic surgery and repeated skin grafts may be required to restore function and the physical appearance of burn patients.

■ NURSING ORDERS: The burned patient requires intensive, prolonged care to avoid complications and prevent disfiguring contractures. The nurse administers parenteral fluids, medication, and wound care, closely monitors the patient, limits physical discomfort, provides emotional support and diversion, and encourages the family to visit regularly and to become involved in the patient's care.

■ OUTCOME CRITERIA: The outcome for the severely burned patient depends greatly on the detailed, near-constant care required during the acute phase of treatment. Scarring may cause residual dysfunction and discouragement. Encouragement to participate fully in physical therapy and to continue treatments may be helpful. Although protection from infection is essential, the nurse does not isolate the patient unless necessary.

Burow's solution (byur′ouz), a liquid preparation containing aluminum sulfate, acetic acid, precipitated calcium carbonate, and water, used as a topical astringent, antiseptic, and antipyretic for a wide variety of skin disorders. Also called **aluminum acetate solution.**

burp, *Informal.* **1.** to belch or eructate. **2.** a belch, or eructation.

burr cell, one of a variety of cells or cell fragments that have spicules, or tiny projections on the surface. Compare **acanthocyte.**

burrowing flea. See *Tunga penetrans.*

bursa (bər′sə), *pl.* **bursae. 1.** a fibrous sac between certain tendons and the bones beneath them. Lined with a synovial membrane that secretes synovial fluid, the bursa acts as a small cushion that allows the tendon as it contracts and relaxes to move over the bone. See also **adventitious bursa, bursa of Achilles, olecranon bursa, prepatellar bursa. 2.** a sac or closed cavity. See also **omental bursa, pharyngeal bursa.**

bursa of Achilles, bursa separating the tendon of Achilles and the calcaneus.

bursitis (bərsai′tis), an inflammation of the bursa, the connective tissue structure surrounding a joint. Bursitis may be precipitated by arthritis, infection, injury, or excessive or traumatic exercise or effort. The chief symptom is severe pain of the affected joint, particularly on movement. The goals of treatment for bursitis include the control of pain and the maintenance of joint motion. A frequent measure used for the relief of acute pain is an intrabursal injection of an adrenocorticosteroid, followed by procaine infusion. Other commonly used treatments are analgesics, anti-inflammatory agents, cold, and immobilization of the inflamed site. After the inflammatory process has subsided, heat may be helpful. In chronic cases surgery may be required to remove calcium depos-

its. Some kinds of bursitis are **housemaid's knee, miner's elbow, weaver's bottom.** See also **rheumatism.**

bursting fracture, any fracture that disperses multiple bone fragments, usually at or near the end of a bone.

Buschke's disease (bush′kəz). See **cryptococcosis.**

busulfan, an alkylating agent.

■ INDICATION: It is prescribed in the treatment of chronic myelocytic leukemia.

■ CONTRAINDICATIONS: Radiation, depressed neutrophil or platelet counts, concurrent administration of neoplastic medication, or known hypersensitivity to this drug prohibits its use.

■ ADVERSE REACTIONS: Among the more serious adverse reactions are depression of the bone marrow and severe nausea and diarrhea. Amenorrhea commonly occurs.

butabarbital sodium (byu′təbar′bitəl), a sedative.

■ INDICATIONS: It is prescribed for the relief of anxiety, nervous tension, and insomnia.

■ CONTRAINDICATIONS: Porphyria, seizure disorders, or known hypersensitivity to this drug prohibits its use.

■ ADVERSE EFFECTS: Among the more serious adverse reactions are jaundice, skin rash, and paradoxical excitement.

butanoic acid (byu′tənou′ik). See **butyric acid.**

butanol extractable iodine (BEI) (byu′tənol), iodine in the blood that can be separated from plasma proteins by extraction with the organic solvent butanol. Measurement of BEI indicates the level of thyroid hormone in the blood.

butaperazine maleate, an antipsychotic.

■ INDICATIONS: It is prescribed in the treatment of schizophrenia and chronic brain syndrome.

■ CONTRAINDICATIONS: Bone marrow depression, the concomitant use of an antiadrenergic, or known hypersensitivity to this drug or to other phenothiazines prohibits its use. It is not given to children under 12 years of age.

■ ADVERSE EFFECTS: Among the more serious adverse reactions are skin rash, leukopenia, tardue dyskinesia, and jaundice.

Butazolidin, a trade name for an antirheumatic (phenylbutazone).

Butesin Picrate, a trade name for a local anesthetic (butamben picrate).

Butisol Sodium, a trade name for a sedative (butabarbital sodium).

butorphanol tartrate (byutor′fənol), a parenteral narcotic of the phenanthrene family, given for surgical premedication and as an analgesic component of balanced anesthesia. Because it provides almost immediate relief from pain when given intravenously and begins to take effect within 10 minutes when given intramuscularly (with peak analgesic activity within 30 to 60 minutes), it is useful for the relief of moderate to severe pain associated with surgical procedures. Butorphanol tartrate is not given to patients known to be sensitive to phenanthrenes or to persons dependent on narcotics, as it may provoke withdrawal symptoms. Toxicity may result from the use of butorphanol with other narcotics.

butterfly bandage, a narrow adhesive strip with broader winglike ends used to approximate the edges of a superficial wound and to hold the sides together as they heal. It is used in place of a suture in certain cases. Also called **butterfly.**

butterfly fracture, a bone break in which the center fragment contained by two cracks forms a triangle.

butterfly rash, an erythematous, scaling eruption of both cheeks joined by a narrow band of rash across the nose. It is seen in lupus erythematosus, rosacea, and seborrheic dermatitis.

buttermilk, **1.** the slightly sour-tasting liquid residue remaining after the solids in cream have been churned into butter. It is nearly fat free and, except for a relatively low content of vitamin A, is nutritionally comparable to whole milk. **2.** cultured milk made by the addition of certain organisms to fat-free milk.

buttock. See **nates.**

buttonhole, a small slitlike hole in the wall of a structure or a cavity of the body.

buttonhole fracture, any fracture caused by the perforation of a bone by a bullet.

button suture, a technique in suturing in which the ends of the suture material are passed through buttons on the surface of the skin and tied. It is used to prevent the suture from cutting through the skin.

butyl, a hydrocarbon radical, the compounds of which are obtained from petroleum. Butyl compounds, some of which are toxic and irritating, are used in a variety of industrial and medical applications, including anesthesia.

butyl alcohol (byu'tıl), a clear liquid derived from beet molasses.

Butyn Sulfate, a trade name for a local anesthetic agent (butacaine sulfate).

butyr-, a combining form meaning 'pertaining to butter': *butyraceous, butyric, butyrinase.*

butyric acid (byutır'ık), a fatty acid occurring in rancid butter, feces, urine, perspiration, and, in trace amounts, in the spleen and blood. Butyric acid is used in the preparation of flavorings, emulsifying agents, and pharmaceuticals. Also called **butanoic acid, propylformic acid.**

butyric fermentation, the conversion to butyric acid of carbohydrates.

butyrophenone (byu'tərufi'nōun), one of a small group of major tranquilizers used in treating psychosis, to decrease the choreic symptoms of Huntington's chorea and the tics and coprolalia of Gilles de la Tourette's syndrome, and as an adjunct in neurolept anesthesia. The two principal butyrophenones are haloperidol and droperidol. Butyrophenones are pharmacologically and clinically similar to the phenothiazines.

BWS, abbreviation for **battered woman syndrome.**

bypass, any one of various surgical procedures to divert the flow of blood or other natural fluids from normal anatomical courses. A bypass may be either temporary or permanent. Bypass surgery is commonly performed in the treatment of cardiac and gastrointestinal disorders.

byssinosis (bıs'nou'sıs), an occupational respiratory disease characterized by shortness of breath, cough, and wheezing. The condition is an allergic reaction to dust or fungi in cotton, flax, and hemp fibers. The symptoms are typically more pronounced on Mondays when the workers return after a weekend break and are reversible in the early stages. Prolonged exposure of many years results in chronic airway obstruction, bronchitis, and emphysema with fibrosis, leading to respiratory failure, pulmonary hypertension, and cor pulmonale. Treatment is symptomatic for the irreversible changes of emphysema and chronic bronchitis. Compare **black lung disease.**

C

c, symbol for **capillary blood**.

c, abbreviation for **curie**.

C, symbol for **concentration of gas in the blood**.

Ca, symbol for **calcium**.

cabinet bath, a bath in which the patient is enclosed in a cabinet, except for the head, and heated by hot air or radiant heat. Also called **box bath**.

Cabot's splint (kæb′əts), a metal splint worn behind the thigh and leg for support.

cac-. See **caco-**.

cacao, 1. cocoa. 2. the substance *Theobroma cacao*. 3. the seeds of *Theobroma cacao*.

cacesthesia (kæk′əsfhi′źhə), any morbid feeling or disordered sensibility. —**cacesthetic,** *adj.*

cachet, any lenticular edible capsule that encloses a dose of medicine.

cachexia (kəkek′siə), general ill health and malnutrition, marked by weakness and emaciation, usually associated with serious disease, as tuberculosis or cancer. Also called **cachexy.** —**cachectic,** *adj.*

cachexy (kəkek′si). See **cachexia**.

cachinnation (kæk′ənei′šhən), an excessive laughter for no apparent reason, often part of the behavioral pattern in schizophrenia. —**cachinnate,** *v.*

caco-, cac-, a combining form meaning 'ill, bad': *cacodontia, cacogeusia, cacosmia.*

cacodemonomania (kæk′oudi′mənoumei′niə), an abnormal mental condition in which the patient claims to be possessed by an evil spirit.

cacophony (kəkof′əni), *pl.* **cacophonies.** a harsh or discordant sound or a mixture of confused, different sounds. —**cacophonic, cacophonous,** *adj.*

cadaver, a dead body used for dissection and study.

cadmium (Cd), a metallic, bluish-white element that resembles tin. Its atomic number is 48; its atomic weight is 112.40. Cadmium has many uses in industry and was formerly used in medications. Such medications have been replaced by less toxic drugs. Cadmium bromide, used in engraving, lithography, and photography, can cause severe gastrointestinal symptoms if swallowed. Cadmium may also cause poisoning by inhalation of fumes from metal-plating processes or by the ingestion of acidic foods prepared and stored in cadmium-lined containers, as lemonade in certain metal cans.

cadmium poisoning, poisoning resulting from the inhalation of cadmium in fumes created by welding, smelting, or other industrial processes involving solder. The effects may include vomiting, dyspnea, headache, prostration, pulmonary edema, and, possibly, years later, cancer. Treatment for acute poisoning includes intravenous fluids and hyperbaric oxygen.

caduceus (kədu′siəs), the wand of the god Hermes or Mercury, used as the symbol for the U.S. Army Medical Corps. It is represented as a staff with two serpents coiled around it and is often confused with the staff of Æsculapius.

caenogenesis. See **cenogenesis**.

Caesarean hysterectomy, a surgical operation in which the uterus is removed at the time of Caesarean section. It is performed most often for complications of Caesarean section, usually intractable hemorrhage. Less often it is done to treat preexisting gynecologic disease, as an intraepithelial cervical neoplasia. It is rarely done electively for sterilization because the danger of hemorrhage is greater when both procedures are performed simultaneously.

Caesarean section, a surgical procedure in which the abdomen and uterus are incised and a baby is delivered transabdominally. It is performed when abnormal maternal or fetal conditions exist that are judged likely to make vaginal delivery hazardous. Approximately 15 per cent of births in the United States are by Caesarean section; the operation is performed less frequently in other countries. The maternal mortality is 0.1 to 0.2 per cent. Maternal indications for the operation include hemorrhage from placenta previa or abruptio placenta, severe preeclampsia, and dysfunctional labor. Delivery by Caesarean section at a prior parturition is no longer considered an absolute indication for repeating it in future deliveries. Caesarean birth is less traumatic for babies than difficult midforceps delivery. Fetal indications for the operation include fetal distress, cephalopelvic disproportion, and abnormal presentation, as breech and transverse lie. The incision in the skin of the abdomen may be horizontal or vertical, regardless of the kind of internal incision into the uterus. Because she must begin mothering while she is recovering from major surgery, the mother requires special care that provides for both her postoperative medical needs and her need to nurture her new baby, who may also be ill or recovering during the crucial neonatal period. See also classical Caesarean section, extraperitoneal Caesarean section, low cervical Caesarean section.

café-au-lait spot (kæf'eioulei'), a pale tan macule the color of coffee with milk. Several café-au-lait spots developing simultaneously are associated with neurofibromatosis, but occasional cafe-au-lait spots occur normally. See also **neurofibromatosis**.

Cafergot, a trade name for a fixed-combination drug containing caffeine and ergotamine, commonly administered in the treatment of migraine headaches.

caffeine, a central nervous system stimulant.
■ INDICATIONS: It is prescribed to counteract migraine, drowsiness, and mental fatigue.
■ CONTRAINDICATIONS: It is used with caution in patients with heart disease and gastric ulcer. Known hypersensitivity to this drug prohibits its use.
■ ADVERSE EFFECTS: Among the most serious adverse reactions are tachycardia and diuresis. Gastrointestinal distress, restlessness, and insomnia are common.

-caine, a combining form naming synthetic alkaloid anesthetics: *isocaine, metycaine, neurocaine.*

caisson disease (kei'son). See **decompression sickness**.

caked, formed into a compact mass or crust, as the scab of coagulated blood on a healing wound.

calabar swelling (kæl'ɔbar), an abnormal condition characterized by fugitive, swollen lumps of subcutaneous tissue caused by a parasitic, filarial worm endemic to central and west Africa. The swollen areas migrate with the worm through the body at a speed of about one cm per minute and may become as large as a small egg. At times the worm may move under the conjunctiva of the eye and may live in the anterior chamber of the eye. Treatment includes the oral administration of diethylcarbamazine, which destroys the adult worms and their offspring. Antihistamines and other medications may be given. A kind of calabar swelling is *Loa loa.* See also **loiasis**.

Caladryl, a trade name for a topical, fixed-combination drug containing a protectant (calamine) and an antihistaminic (diphenhydramine hydrochloride).

calamine (kæl'əmain), a pink, odorless, powdered concoction used as a protectant or as an astringent and sometimes prepared as a lotion. It is composed of zinc oxide with 0.5 per cent ferric oxide.

calc-, 1. a combining form meaning 'pertaining to lime or limestone': *calcarea, calcariuria, calciosis.* 2. a combining form meaning 'pertaining to the heel': *calcaneum, calcaneocavus, calcanodynia.*

calcaneal, of or pertaining to the calcaneus at the back of the tarsus.

calcaneal spurs, abnormal, often painful, bony outgrowths on the lower surface of the calcaneus, resulting from chronic traumatic pressure on the heel.

calcaneal tendon. See **Achilles tendon**.

calcaneal tendon reflex. See **Achilles tendon reflex**.

calcaneal tuberosity, a transverse elevation on the plantar surface of the calcaneus to which are attached the abductor digiti minimi, the long plantar ligament, and various other muscles, including the abductor hallucis and the flexor digitorum brevis.

calcaneodynia (kælkei'nioudin'iə), a painful condition of the heel.

calcaneum (kælkei'niəm). See **calcaneus**.

calcaneus (kælkei'niəs), the heel bone. The largest of the tarsal bones, it articulates proximally with the talus and distally with the cuboid. — **calcaneal, calcanean,** *adj.*

calcar (kæl'kar), *pl.* **calcaria.** a spur or a structure that resembles a spur.

calcareous, of or pertaining to calcium or lime.

calcarine (kæl'kərain'), 1. having the shape of a spur. 2. of or pertaining to the calcar.

calcarine fissure, a fissure between the cuneus and the lingual gyrus on the medial surface of the occipital lobe of the brain. Also called **calcarine sulcus**.

calcarine sulcus. See **calcarine fissure**.

calcifediol, a physiological form of Vitamin D.
■ INDICATION: It is prescribed in the treatment of metabolic bone disease associated with chronic renal failure.
■ CONTRAINDICATIONS: Hypercalcemia, vitamin D toxicity, or known hypersensitivity to this drug prohibits its use.
■ ADVERSE EFFECTS: Among the most serious adverse reactions are renal toxicity and those reactions associated with hypercalcemia, as soft tissue calcification and gastrointestinal and central nervous system disturbances.

calciferol (kælsif'ɔrol), a fat-soluble, crystalline, unsaturated alcohol produced by ultraviolet irradiation of ergosterol and used as a dietary supplement in the prophylaxis and treatment of rickets, osteomalacia, and other hypocalcemic disorders. It occurs naturally in milk and fishliver oils. Also called **ergocalciferol, oleovitamin D₂, vitamin D₂.** See also **rickets, viosterol**.

calcific aortic disease, an abnormal condition characterized by small deposits of calcium in the aorta.

calcification, the accumulation of calcium salts in tissues. Normally, about 99 per cent of all the calcium entering the human body is deposited in the bones and teeth; the remaining one per cent is dissolved in body fluids, as the blood. Disorders affecting the delicate balance between calcium and other minerals, parathyroid hormone, and vitamin D can result in calcium deposits in arteries, kidneys, lung alveoli, and other tissues, interfering with usual organ functions. See also **calcitonin, calcium, calculus**.

calcified fetus. See **lithopedion**.

Calcimar, a trade name for calcitonin.

calcitonin (kæl'sitou'nin), a hormone produced in parafollicular cells of the thyroid that participates in regulating the blood level of calcium and stimulates bone mineralization. A synthetic preparation of the hormone is used in the treatment of certain bone disorders. Calcitonin acts to reduce the blood level of calcium and to inhibit bone resorption, while parathyroid hormone acts to increase blood calcium and bone resorption. Calcitonin has a short-term effect in enhancing bone formation and causes transient decreases in the volume and acidity of gastric juice and in the volume of amylase and trypsin in pancreatic juice. The hormone also promotes the excretion of phosphate, sodium, and calcium by decreasing their reabsorption in kidney tubules. The secretion of calcitonin is regulated by the amount of calcium in plasma, and an infusion of calcium may increase the concentration of the circulating hormone two- to threefold. Men usually have a higher level of plasma calcitonin than women.

calcitriol, a regulator of calcium metabolism.

■ INDICATIONS: It is prescribed in the management of hypocalcemia occurring in patients undergoing chronic renal dialysis.

■ CONTRAINDICATIONS: Hypercalcemia, evidence of vitamin D toxicity, or known sensitivity to this drug prohibits its use.

■ ADVERSE EFFECTS: Among the more serious adverse reactions are renal toxicity and those associated with hypercalcemia, as soft tissue calcification, and gastrointestinal and central nervous system disturbances.

calcium (Ca), an alkaline earth metal element. Its atomic number is 12; its atomic weight is 40. Its metallic form is a white, flammable solid, somewhat harder than lead. Calcium is commonly produced by the electrolysis or by the thermal dissociation of calcium chloride. Calcium carbonate is the most common calcium compound, which, when treated with hydrochloric acid, forms calcium chloride. Calcium also occurs as a component of the natural compound gypsum, which forms plaster of Paris when heated. It is also a component of calcium cyanamid, a fertilizer and progenitor of other nitrogen compounds. Calcium is the fifth most abundant element in the human body and occurs mainly in the bone. The body requires calcium ions for the transmission of nerve impulses, muscle contraction, blood coagulation, cardiac functions, and other processes. It is a component of extracellular fluid and of the cells of soft tissue. The average daily human intake of calcium varies from 200 to 2,500 mg. In the United States dairy products are the major dietary sources of this element. The daily dietary allowances recommended by the Federal Food and Nutrition Board vary from 360 mg for infants to 1,200 mg for women 15 to 18 years of age. More than 90 per cent of the calcium in the body is stored in the skeleton, which constantly exchanges its supplies with the calcium of the interstitial fluids. The endocrine system controls the concentration of ionized calcium in the plasma. Only a fraction of this amount is ionized and diffusable; the rest is bound to proteins, especially albumin. It is the ionized, diffusable portion of calcium that figures in the physiological changes associated with hypocalcemia. About one third of the calcium ingested by humans is absorbed, primarily in the small bowel. Vitamin D, calcitonin, and parathyroid hormone are essential in the metabolism of calcium. The degree of cell permeability varies inversely with calcium ion concentration. Abnormally high levels of ionized calcium in the extracellular fluid can produce muscle weakness, lethargy, and coma. A relatively small decrease from the normal level of this element can produce tetanic seizures.

calcium chloride, a concentrated solution of the chloride salt of calcium used to replenish calcium in the blood.

■ INDICATIONS: It is prescribed for hypocalcemic tetany and as an antidote for magnesium poisoning or an overdose of magnesium sulfate.

■ CONTRAINDICATIONS: Renal insufficiency, ventricular fibrillation, hypercalcemia, or known hypersensitivity to this drug prohibits its use.

■ ADVERSE EFFECTS: Among the more serious adverse reactions is hypercalcemia.

■ CAUTION: Calcium chloride is never injected into tissue.

calcium pump, a theoretical, energy-requiring mechanism for transmitting calcium ions across a cell membrane from a region of low calcium ion concentration to one of higher concentration. Compare **sodium pump.**

calculus (kæl′kyuləs), *pl.* **calculi** (kæl′kyulӕi). a pathological stone formed of mineral salts. Calculi are usually found within hollow organs or ducts and can cause obstruction and inflammation. Kinds of calculi include **biliary calculus, renal calculus.** Also called **stone.** See also **gallstone.**

Calderol, a trade name for a calcium regulator (calcifediol).

Caldwell-Moloy pelvic classifacation (kɔl′dwelmӕloi′), a system for classifying the structure of the bony pelvis of the female. The types in this system are android, anthropoid, gynecoid, and platypelloid. The sacrum, sidewalls, sacrosciatic notch, ischial spines, pubic arch, and ischial tuberosities are the anatomic points of reference used to determine pelvic type. The classification system requires that a mixed pelvis be named for the character of its posterior section with the name of the type characterized by the anterior portion following a hyphen, as in a gynecoid-android pelvis. See also **pelvic classification.**

calefacient (kæl′əfei′shənt), **1.** making or tending to make anything warm or hot. **2.** an agent that imparts a sense of warmth when applied, as a hot-water bottle or a hot compress.

calendar method of family planning, a natural method of family planning in which the fertile period of a woman's menstrual cycle is identified by an examination of at least six menstrual cycles recorded on a calendar. If the length of the cycle varies, twelve cycles are recorded. It is assumed that ovulation occurs fourteen days before the onset of menstruation and that during the four days before the expected or usual day of ovulation, the day of ovulation, and the three days after ovulation, fertilization may occur. Abstinence is required during the fertile period. In a woman with a regular cycle this period is from the eighteenth to the eleventh days prior to the first day of the next menstrual period. However, if the cycle varies in length, the number of variance days between the shortest and longest cycles is added to the period of abstinence, allowing for the earliest and latest day of ovulation and the surrounding, 'unsafe days.' Thus, if menstruation occurs every 24 to 30 days, abstinence would be required from the sixth to the nineteenth days of the cycle. The calendar method is more effective as an adjunct to the symptothermal method of family planning than if used alone. Also called **rhythm method.** Compare **basal body temperature method of family planning, ovulation method of family planning, symptothermal method of family planning.**

calf, *pl.* **calves.** the fleshy mass at the back of the leg below the knee, composed chiefly of the gastrocnemius muscle.

calf bone. See **fibula.**

caliber, calibre, the diameter of a tube or a canal, as any of the blood vessels.

California encephalitis, a common, acute viral infection that affects the central nervous system. Epidemics occur mainly in the Midwest, on the Eastern Seaboard, and in Texas and Louisiana. The virus was first isolated in California. The infection generally follows one of two clinical courses. The mild form is characterized by headache, malaise, gastrointestinal symptoms, and a fever that may reach 104°F. The more severe form may be marked by a sudden onset of fever, vomiting, headaches, lethargy, and signs of neurologic involvement, as loss of reflexes, disorientation, seizure, loss of consciousness, and flaccid paralysis. Recovery usually begins in a week. Mortality is very low, but a significant number of patients have neurological sequelae for a year or more. Treatment usually involves administration of anticonvulsant and sedative medications. See also **arbovirus, encephalitis.**

californium (Cf), an artificial element in the actinide group. Its atomic number is 98. Californium isotopes discovered so far have atomic weights ranging from 244 to 245.

calipers, an instrument with two hinged, adjustable, curved legs, used to measure the thickness or the diameter of a convex body or solid.

caliper splint, a splint for the leg consisting of two metal rods running from the back of a band around the thigh or from a cushioned ring around the lower portion of the pelvis. The rods are attached to a metal plate under the shoe below the arch of the foot.

Calliphoridae (kæl'əfɔr'ədi), a family of medium-sized to large flies that belong to the order Diptera, serve as pathogenic vectors, and may cause myiasis in humans. These flies include the genera *Auchmeromyia, Calliphora, Cordylobia, Cochliomyia, Chrysomyia, Lucilia, Phaenicia,* and *Phormia.*

callomania, an abnormal psychological condition characterized by delusions of personal beauty.

callosal fissure, a groove following the convex aspect of the corpus callosum.

callosity (kəlos'əti). See **callus.**

calloso marginal fissure (kalou'sou), a long, irregular groove on the medial surface of a cerebral hemisphere. It divides the cingulate gyrus from the medial frontal gyrus and from the paracentral lobule. Also called **cingulate sulcus.**

callus, 1. a common, usually painless thickening of the epidermis at locations of external pressure or friction. Also called **callosity.** Compare **corn.** 2. bony deposit formed between and around the broken ends of a fractured bone during healing. — **callous,** *adj.*

calmodulin, a polypeptide protein that mediates a variety of biochemical and physiological processes, including the contraction of muscles and the release of norepinephrine. Depending on its form and function, calmodulin may act independently of, in concert with, or antagonistically to reactions involving cyclic adenosine-monophosphate.

calor (kæl'ɔr), heat, as that generated by inflammation of tissues or that from the normal metabolic processes of the body.

calor-, a combining form meaning 'pertaining to heat': *calorie, calorifacient, calorization.*

caloric, of or pertaining to heat or calories.

caloric test, a procedure for determining if the ear is diseased or normal. The test alternately irrigates the ear with hot water and cold water. If the ear is normal the hot water irrigation produces a rotatory nystagmus toward the irrigated side. Cold water irrigation produces a rotatory nystagamus away from the irrigated side. If the ear is diseased, irrigation produces no nystagmus. Also called **Barany's syndrome.**

calorie, 1. the amount of heat required to raise one gram of water one degree Celsius at atmospheric pressure. Also called **gram calorie, small calorie.** 2. a quantity of heat equal to 1,000 small calories. Also called **great calorie, kilogram calorie, large calorie.** 3. a unit, equal to the large calorie, used to denote the heat expenditure of an organism and the fuel or energy value of food. — **caloric,** *adj.*

calorific (kæl′ərɪf′ɪk), pertaining to the production of heat.

calorigenic (kəlɔr′ɪjen′ɪk), of or pertaining to a substance or process that produces heat or energy or that increases the consumption of oxygen.

calorimeter (kæl′ərɪm′ɪtər), a device used for measuring quantities of heat generated by friction, by chemical reaction, or by the human body. — **calorimetric**, *adj.*

calorimetry, the measurement of the amounts of heat radiated and the amounts of heat absorbed. Compare **direct calorimetry, indirect calorimetry.** — **calorimetric,** *adj.*

calusterone (kəlu′stəroun), an antineoplastic androgen.

■ INDICATION: It is prescribed in the treatment of cancer of the breast.

■ CONTRAINDICATIONS: Cardiac and renal disease, hypercalcemia, or known sensitivity to the drug prohibits its use. It is not given to pregnant or lactating women.

■ ADVERSE EFFECTS: Among the more severe adverse reactions are fluid retention and hypercalcemia. Masculinization with clitoral enlargement, hirsutism, acne, alopecia, and erythrocytemia also occur.

calvaria, the skull cap or superior portion of the skull, which varies greatly in shape from individual to individual. In some persons, the calvaria is relatively oval, in others it is more circular. It is traversed by the coronal suture between the frontal and the parietal bones, by the sagittal suture in the midline between the two parietal bones, and by the upper part of the lambdoidal suture between the parietal bones and the occipital bone. The inner surface of the calvaria is indented to accept the convolutions of the cerebrum and furrowed for the branches of the meningeal vessels. It also contains the superior sagittal sinus, affords attachment at its margins for the falx cerebri, and posteriorly, in some individuals it accommodates the openings of the parietal foramina. The soft spots in the skull of an infant are situated on the surface of the calvaria at the junction of the sagittal and the coronal sutures and at the junction of the sagittal and lambdoid sutures. See also **bregma.**

calvities (kælvɪsh′iiz), the condition of baldness. — **calvous,** *adj.*

calyx (kei′lɪks), *pl.* **calyces** (kæl′ɪsiz), **calyxes. 1.** a cup-shaped organ. **2.** a renal calyx. **3.** the wall of an ovarian follicle after expulsion of the ovum at ovulation. Also spelled **calix.**

cambium layer, 1. the loose, inner cellular layer of the periosteum that develops during ossification. **2.** a cellular layer that lies between the wood and the bark in plants.

camera, (in anatomy) any cavity or chamber, as those of the eye or the heart.

camphor, a colorless or white crystalline substance with a penetrating odor and pungent taste, occurring naturally in certain plants, especially *Cinnamomum camphora.* Also called **camphora, gum camphor.**

camphora (kæmfɔr′ə). See **camphor.**

camphor bath, an air bath in which the air is filled with camphor vapor.

camphor salicylate, a crystalline substance formed by the fusion of 84 parts of camphor and 65 parts of salicylic acid, used in skin ointments and administered internally for diarrhea.

camptodactyly, the permanent flexion of one or more fingers. — **campodactylic,** *adj.*

camptomelia (kæmp′təmi′liə), a congenital anomaly characterized by bending of one or more limbs causing permanent bowing or curving of the affected area. See also **camptomelic syndrome.** — **camptomelic,** *adj.*

canal, (in anatomy) a narrow tube or channel. Some kinds of canals are **adducto canal, Alcock's canal, alveolar canal.**

Canadian Association of University Schools of Nursing (CAUSN), a national Canadian organization of nursing schools affiliated with institutions of higher learning.

Canadian Association of University Teachers (CAUT), a national Canadian organization representing the interests of all who teach in the universities of the provinces and territories of Canada. The official languages of the CAUT are French and English.

Canadian crutch, a wooden or a metal device that helps a disabled patient stand or walk. It consists of two uprights with a crosspiece to accommodate the hand and a concave crosspiece that fits the armpit for support.

***Canadian Journal of Public Health* (CJPH),** the official publication of the Canadian Public Health Association.

***Canadian Medical Association Journal* (CMAJ),** the official publication of the Canadian Medical Association.

Canadian Nurses' Association (CNA), the official national organization for the professional registered nurses of Canada who are members of the ten provincial nurses' associations and the Northwest Territory's association. The CNA, a federation of these eleven associations, is supported by contributions of the 140,000 members of the regional associations. The chief objective of the CNA is to promote conditions conducive to the good health of the people and to good patient care. It is concerned with the quality and quantity of nurses available, the standards of preparation for nurses, the social and economic welfare of nurses, the advancement of competence and expertise within the profession, the promotion of unity and understanding among the members, and the representation of the organized profession of nurses nationally and internationally. A board of twenty-three elected volunteers and a permanent staff working at CNA House in Ottawa manage the affairs of the organization. Among the services provided are a research and advisory unit that studies trends in nursing and health and prepares briefs, when necessary; a library containing reference works, the archives of the CNA, and up-to-date lists of educational programs in nursing; an information service that collects and disseminates information about nursing and publishes *The Canadian Nurse* and *L'Infirmière Canadienne;* a labor relations service; a testing service; a governmental liaison service; and an international service that facilitates a working relationship with various organizations, as the World Health Organization and the Pan American Health Organization. All services are provided in the two official languages, English and French.

Canadian Nurses' Association Testing Service (CNATS), the organizational affiliate of the Canadian Nurses' Association that is concerned with testing the graduates of approved schools of nursing to qualify as registered nurses.

Canadian Nurses' Foundation (CNF), a national Canadian foundation organized to support scholarship in nursing. The CNF awards financial support to nurses undertaking graduate studies in nursing and to nurses planning research in nursing.

Canadian Nurses' Respiratory Society (CNRS), an organization of nurses working with or interested in alleviating the problems of respiratory disease. The CNRS is an affiliate of the Canadian Nurses' Association and it is a section of the Canadian Lung Association.

Canadian Orthopedic Nurses' Association (CONA), a national Canadian organization concerned with the nursing care of orthopedic patients and the continuing education of nurses working in orthopedics. Membership includes orthopedic nurses and other professionals concerned with orthopedics.

Canadian Public Health Association (CPHA), a national Canadian organization concerned with issues in public health and epidemiology. Membership is open to professionals and to others interested in these issues.

canaliculus (kæn′əlık′yuləs), *pl.* **canaliculi.** a very small tube or channel, like the tiny Haversian canaliculi throughout bone tissue.

canalization, the formation of canals or of passages through any tissue.

canal of Schlemm (shlem), a tiny vein at the angle of the anterior chamber of the eye that connects with the pectinate villi, draining the aqueous humor and funneling it into the blood stream. Also called **Schlemm's canal.**

cancellous (kæn′sıləs), (of tissue) latticelike, porous, spongy. Cancellous tissue is normally present in the interior of many bones, where the spaces are usually filled with marrow.

cancer, 1. a neoplasm characterized by the uncontrolled growth of anaplastic cells that tend to invade surrounding

tissue and to metastasize to distant body sites. **2.** any of a large group of malignant neoplastic diseases characterized by the presence of malignant cells. Each cancer is distinguished by the nature, site, or clinical course of the lesion. The basic etiology of cancer is undetermined, but many potential causes are recognized. More than 80 per cent of cases of cancer are attributed to cigarette smoking, exposure to carcinogenic chemicals, ionizing radiation, and ultraviolet rays; overexposure to the sun is the major cause of skin cancer. Many viruses induce malignant tumors in animals, and viral particles are detected in some human tumors; but there is no clear evidence that any microorganism causes human cancer. The high incidence of various kinds of cancer in certain families suggests that genetic susceptibility is an important factor. An excess rate of malignant tumors in organ transplant recipients following immunosuppressive therapy indicates that the immune system plays a major role in controlling the proliferation of anaplastic cells. The basic defect may be a biochemical anomaly that triggers abnormal cell growth and glucose metabolism and in which certain vital proteins and respiratory enzymes are reduced. The incidence of different kinds of cancer varies markedly with sex, age, ethnic group, and geographic location. The age-adjusted death rate for oral cancer is almost ten times higher in Hong Kong than in Denmark and that for prostate cancer is more than ten times greater in Sweden than in Japan, but leukemia mortality is similar throughout the world. In the United States, cancer is second only to heart disease as a cause of mortality and is the leading cause of death of children between the ages of 3 and 14. The most common sites for the development of malignant tumors are the lung, breast, colon, uterus, oral cavity, and bone marrow. Surgery remains the major form of treatment, but irradiation is widely used as preoperative, postoperative, or primary therapy; chemotherapy, with single or multiple antineoplastic agents, is often highly effective. Many malignant lesions are curable if detected in the early stage. Depending on the site, the warning signal may be a change in bowel or bladder habits, a nonhealing sore, unusual bleeding or discharge, a thickening or lump in the breast or elsewhere, indigestion or dysphagia, an obvious change in a wart or mole, or a nagging cough or persistent hoarseness. *(See next page for tables)*

cancer bodies. See **Russell's bodies.**

cancericidal (kæn′sərısai′dəl), of or pertaining to a substance or procedure capable of destroying cancer cells.

cancer in situ. See **carcinoma in situ.**

cancer of the small intestine, a neoplastic disease of the duodenum, jejunum, or ileum. Its characteristics vary, depending on the kind of tumor and the site, but may include abdominal pain, vomiting, weight loss, diarrhea, intermittent bowel obstruction, gastrointestinal bleeding, or a mass deep in the right abdomen. Diagnosis is made

Most frequent type of cancer by age (except for nonmelanoma skin cancer)

Age (yrs)	Site
0 to 10	Leukemia, cancer of the brain and kidney, lymphoma, cancer of the eye and connective tissue
10 to 20	
Males	Leukemia, Hodgkin's disease, cancer of the brain, bone, and testis
Females	Carcinoma in situ of cervix, leukemia, cancer of the brain, Hodgkin's disease, cancer of the thyroid
20 to 30	
Males	Hodgkin's disease, cancer of the testis, leukemia, melanoma of skin, cancer of the brain
Females	Cancer of the uterus, thyroid, and breast, Hodgkin's disease, melanoma of skin
30 to 40	
Males	Cancer of the lung, testis, colon and rectum, Hodgkin's disease, melanoma of skin
Females	Cancer of the uterus, breast, thyroid, ovary, and melanoma of skin
40 to 50	
Males	Cancer of the lung, colon and rectum, bladder, brain, and larynx
Females	Cancer of the breast, uterus, colon and rectum, ovary, and lung
50 to 60	
Males	Cancer of the lung, colon and rectum, prostate gland, bladder, and larynx
Females	Cancer of the breast, uterus, colon and rectum, lung, and ovary
60 to 70	
Males	Cancer of the prostate gland, lung, colon and rectum, bladder, and stomach
Females	Cancer of the breast, colon and rectum, uterus, lung, and ovary
Over 70	
Males	Cancer of the prostate gland, colon and rectum, lung, bladder, stomach
Females	Cancer of the colon and rectum, breast, uterus, stomach, and pancreas

Cancer's seven warning signals

Adults	Children
Change in bowel or bladder habit	Marked change in bowel or bladder habits; nausea and vomiting for no apparent cause
Unusual bleeding or discharge	Bloody discharge of any sort: blood in urine, spontaneous nosebleed or other type hemorrhage, failure to stop bleeding in the usual time
Thickening or lump in breast or elsewhere	Swellings, lumps, or masses anywhere in the body
Obvious change in wart or mole	Any change in the size or appearance of outward growths, such as moles or birthmarks
Nagging cough or hoarseness	Unexplained stumbling in a child
A sore that does not heal	A generally run-down condition
Indigestion or difficulty in swallowing	Pains or the persistent crying of a baby or child, for which no reason can be found

with barium x-ray examination, but such studies may be inconclusive until lesions are large. Adenocarcinomas, the most common tumors, occur more frequently in the duodenum or upper jejunum and form polypoid or constricting napkin-ring growths. Lymphomas, found most often in the lower small intestine, may impair bowel motility by invading nerves and in some cases are associated with a malabsorption syndrome. Less common tumors of the small intestine are carcinoids, usually found in the ileum, and sarcomas, usually seen in the jejunum and ileum. A leiomyosarcoma may sometimes form a large extraluminal mass but does not metastasize, unlike other cancers of the small intestine. Surgery, including a wide resection of mesenteric lymph nodes, is indicated for adenocarcinomas. Irradiation is not effective in ablation of these tumors but is recommended postoperatively for lymphomas to treat metastatic lesions in mesenteric lymph nodes, the liver, and spleen. Resection of carcinoids is advised to prevent bowel obstruction even if metastatic disease is present, and some patients with these lesions may respond to chemotherapeutic agents, as cyclophosphamide, 5-fluorouracil, methotrexate, and streptozotocin. Cancer of the small intestine, which is uncommon considering the great length and surface area of that organ, occurs slightly more often in men than in women.

cancer staging, a system for describing the extent of a malignant tumor and its metastases, used to plan appropriate treatment and predict prognosis. Staging involves a careful physical examination, diagnostic procedures, and, ultimately, surgical exploration. The standardized system developed by the American Joint Committee for Cancer Staging and End Results Reporting uses the letter T to represent the tumor, N for the regional lymph node involvement, M for distant metastases, and numerical subscripts in each category to indicate the degree of dissemination. According to this system $T_1N_0M_0$ designates a small, localized tumor; $T_2N_1M_0$ is a larger primary tumor that has extended to regional nodes and $T_4N_3M_3$ is a very large lesion involving regional nodes and distant sites. The Ann Arbor System classifies Hodgkin's disease as

Stages I to IV according to the number and location of involved lymph nodes in relation to the diaphragm and the involvement of extralymphatic organs or tissues, based on numerous diagnostic procedures and by a staging laparotomy. Other systems may be used for staging breast carcinoma, colorectal cancer, and cutaneous melanoma.

cancer-ulcer, a carcinomatous ulceration.

cancr-, chancr-, a combining form meaning 'pertaining to cancer': *cancriform, cancroid, cancrology.*

cancriform (kæng′krifɔrm), of or pertaining to a lesion resembling a cancer.

cancroid, 1. of or pertaining to a lesion resembling a cancer. 2. a moderately malignant skin cancer.

candela. See **candle.**

candicidin (kæn′dəsai′dɪn), an antifungal agent.

■ INDICATION: It is prescribed in the treatment of vaginitis caused by *Candida albicans* or by other species of *Candida.*

■ CONTRAINDICATION: Known hypersensitivity to this drug prohibits its use.

■ ADVERSE EFFECTS: Among the most serious adverse reactions are irritation of the vulvar and perivulvar area. Allergic reactions occur rarely.

Candida (kæn′dɪdə), a genus of yeastlike fungi including the common pathogen, *Candida albicans.*

Candida albicans (kæn′dɪdə æl′bəkænz), a common, budding, yeastlike, microscopic fungal organism normally present in the mucous membranes of the mouth, intestinal tract, vagina, and on the skin of healthy people. Under certain circumstances, it may cause superficial infections of the mouth or vagina and, less commonly, serious invasive systemic infection and toxic reaction. See also **candidiasis.**

candidiasis (kæn′dɪdai′əsɪs), any infection caused by a species of *Candida,* usually *Candida albicans,* characterized by pruritus, a white exudate, peeling, and easy bleeding. Diaper rash, intertrigo, vaginitis, and thrush are common topical manifestations of candidiasis. Endocarditis, other inflammatory conditions of the heart and liver, and infection of the kidney, spleen, and lungs sometimes occur in debilitated patients. Treatment includes the oral and topical administration of antifungal drugs, as nystatin, clotrimazole, and, rarely, amphotericin-B. Gentian violet, painted on the inflamed mucosa of the mouth or vagina or in intertrigo or diaper rash, on the skin, is messy but effective.

Candiru fever (kæn′dɪru′), an arbovirus infection transmitted to humans by the bite of a sandfly, characterized by an acute fever, headache, and muscle aches. Recovery occurs, without treatment, within a few days. It occurs mainly in the forests of Brazil. See also **arbovirus, sandfly fever.**

candle, (in optics) the basic unit of measurement for luminous intensity, equal to $\frac{1}{60}$ of the luminous intensity of a square centimeter of a black body heated to 1773.5°C or the solidification temperature of platinum, adopted in 1948 as the international standard of luminous intensity. Also called **candela.**

candy-striper, *Informal.* a hospital volunteer, named for the striped pink and white uniforms traditionally worn by the young people who perform this service.

cane-cutter's cramp. See **heat cramp.**

canefield fever. See **field fever.**

canine tooth, any one of the four teeth, two in each jaw, situated immediately lateral to the incisor teeth in the human dental arches. The canine teeth are larger and stronger than the incisors, and they project beyond the level of the other teeth in both arches. Their roots sink deeply into the bones, causing marked prominences on the alveolar arch. The upper canine teeth, or eye teeth, are larger and longer than the lower ones and have a distinct basal ridge. The lower canine teeth, or stomach teeth, are situated nearer the middle line than the upper ones, and their summits correspond to the intervals between the upper canines and the incisors. The crowns of the canines are very large and conical and taper to blunted points or cusps. The canines erupt as deciduous teeth about 16 to 20 months after birth. The eruption of the permanent canines occurs during the eleventh or the twelfth year of life.

canker, an ulcer or sore, especially in the mouth. Also called **aphthous stomatitis.**

canker sore, an ulcerous lesion of the mouth, characteristic of aphthous stomatitis. See also **aphthous stomatitis.**

cannabis (kæn′əbis), a psychoactive drug derived from the flowering tops of hemp plants. It has no currently acceptable clinical use in the United States but has been employed effectively as an antiemetic in some cancer patients to counter the nausea and vomiting associated with chemotherapy. Cannabis is controlled under Schedule I of the Comprehensive Drug Abuse Prevention and Control Act of 1970 and may be legally obtained for research and special medical applications authorized by the Drug Enforcement Administration of the U.S. Department of Justice. The common hemp from which cannabis is obtained is an herbaceous annual of which *Cannabis sativa* is the sole species. The two subspecies are *indica* and *americana.* All parts of the plant contain psychoactive substances or cannabinoids, the highest concentrations of which are in the flowering tops of the plant. *Cannabis sativa* grows in many parts of the world, and cannabis is used in different psychoactive ways among various populations. The cannabinoids synthesized by the hemp plant include cannabinol, cannabidiol, cannabinolic acid, cannabigerol, cannabicyclol, and several isomers of tetrahydrocannabinol (THC). THC is believed to cause the most characteristic psychological effects, which include alterations of mood, memory, motor coordination, cognitive ability, and self-perception. Most users of cannabis smoke marijuana cigarettes containing dried and chopped leaves of the hemp plant. Other users ingest the drug. The effects vary, depending on the dosage, the type of administration, and the experience of the user. In marijuana illicitly obtained and used in the United States the concentration of THC varies widely from 0.5 to 6 per cent, and its absorption into the blood stream depends on the smoking technique of the user and the destruction of cannabinoids by pyrolysis. Oral doses of 20 mg of THC or the smoking of a cigarette containing 2 per cent of THC most commonly produces euphoria in the user and changes in mood and sense of time. Oral doses of cannabis equivalent to several cigarettes impair short-term memory and the capacity to complete tasks requiring multiple steps to reach a specific goal. Low doses of cannabis seldom impair the ability to perform simple motor tasks but commonly hinder more complex actions, as driving and flying, which involve complex sensory perception, concentration, and information processing. Cannabis may also enhance the nondominant senses of touch, taste, and smell. Higher doses in some persons can produce delusions, paranoid feelings, anxiety, and panic. This drug also increases the heart rate and systolic blood pressure. Pharmacological effects of smoking marijuana occur within minutes after smoking begins and produce peak plasma concentrations of THC within 10 to 30 minutes. The effects of one cigarette rarely last more than 2 or 3 hours. Marijuana is about three times more powerful when smoked than when taken orally. The smoking of marijuana has increased throughout the world since the 1960s, and, in 1977, approximately 60 per cent of young adults polled in the United States reported some experience with the drug. The most recent studies indicate that it is used by many individuals in all socioeconomic and ethnic groups. Much of the controversy over the drug centers on the harsh penalties for possessing it and on the growing indications that heavy use of marijuana, especially by adolescents, adversely affects health, social adjustment, and productivity. Research indicates that some cannabinoids may be therapeutic as anticonvulsants and helpful in reducing intraocular pressure associated with glaucoma. Also called **bhang, ganja, grass, hashish, marijuana, pot, reefer, tea, weed.**

cannon wave, a radical 'a' wave in the jugular pulse, characteristic of a complete heart block and of premature ventricular beats of the heart. Cannon waves are caused by the contraction of the right atrium of the heart after contraction of the right ventricle has closed the tricuspid valve.

cannula (kæn′yələ), pl. **cannulas, cannulae.** a flexible tube containing a stiff, pointed trocar that may be inserted into the body, guided by the trocar. As the trocar is removed, a body fluid may be passed through the cannula to the outside. – **cannular, cannulate,** adj.

cannulation, cannulization, the insertion of a cannula into a body duct or cavity, as into the trachea, bladder, or a blood vessel. – **cannulate, cannulize,** v.

cantharis, pl. **cantharides** (kænθær′ɪdiz). the dried insects Cantharis vesicatoria containing cantharidin, formerly used as a topical vesicant. Also called **Spanish fly.**

cantho-, a combining form meaning 'pertaining to the canthus': cantholysis, canthorraphy, canthotomy.

canthus (kæn′θəs), pl. **canthi.** the angle at the medial and the lateral margins of the eyelids. The medial canthus opens into a small space containing the opening to a lacrimal duct. Also called **palpebral commissure.** – **canthic,** adj.

Cantil, a trade name for an anticholinergic antispasmodic (mepenzolate bromide).

cap, abbreviation for Latin capiat 'let him or her take,' used in medicinal prescriptions.

CAP, (in molecular genetics) an abbreviation for **catabolic activator protein.** CAP participates in initiating the transcription of RNA in organisms without a true nucleus, as bacteria.

capeline bandage (kæp′əlin), a caplike covering used for protecting the head, shoulder, or a stump. Also called **Hippocrates' bandage.**

capillaritis, an abnormal condition characterized by a progressive pigmentary disorder of the skin without inflammation but with dilation. It does not involve any systemic problems and runs a benign self-limiting course.

capillarity. See **capillary action.**

capillary (kæp′ɪler′i), one of the tiny blood vessels (about 0.008 mm in diameter) joining arterioles and venules. Through their walls, which consist of a single layer of endothelial cells, blood and tissue cells exchange various substances.

capillary action, the action involving molecular adhesion by which the surface of a liquid in a tube is either elevated or depressed, depending on the cohesiveness of the liquid molecules. The more cohesive the molecules the more elevated will be the surface of the liquid. Less cohesive liquid molecules will adhere to the surfaces of the tube in which they are contained and depress the surface of the liquid. Also called **capillarity.**

capillary angioma. See **cherry angioma.**

capillary bed, a capillary network.

capillary flames. See **telangiectatic nevus.**

capillary fracture, any thin hairlike fracture.

capillary hemangioma, a blood-filled birthmark or benign tumor consisting of closely packed, small blood vessels. Commonly found in infants, it first grows, then spontaneously disappears in early childhood without treatment. Surgical removal will not usually be attempted unless frequent trauma and bleeding are present. Also called **hemangioma simplex, strawberry mark.** Compare **cavernous hemangioma, nevus flammeus.**

capillary pulse. See **Quincke's pulse.**

capillovenous, of or pertaining to the venous capillaries.

capillus (kəpɪl′əs), *pl.* **capilli.** one of the hairs of the body, especially one of the hairs of the scalp.

capit-, a combining form meaning 'pertaining to the head': *capitate, capitopedal, capitular.*

capitate, having the shape of a head.

capitate bone, one of the largest carpal bones, located at the center of the wrist and presenting a rounded head that fits the concavity of the scaphoid and the lunate bones. Various ligaments are attached to the rough dorsal and palmar surfaces. The capitate articulates with the scaphoid and lunate proximally, the second, third, and fourth metacarpals distally, the trapezoid on the radial side, and the hamate on the ulnar side. Also called **os capitatum, os magnum.**

capitulum (kəpɪ́ch′ələm), *pl.* **capitula.** a small, rounded prominence on a bone where it articulates with another bone.

capitulum humeri, a rounded eminence at the distal end of the humerus. It articulates with the radius.

-capnia, a combining form meaning '(condition of) carbon dioxide content in the blood': *acapnia, eucapnia, hypocapnia.*

capnograph (kæp′nəgræf), an instrument used in anesthesia, respiratory physiology, and respiratory therapy to produce a tracing, or capnogram, which shows the proportion of carbon dioxide in expired air.

capric acid (kæp′rɪk), a white, crystalline substance with a rancid odor, occurring as a glyceride in natural oils. Capric acid is used in the production of perfumes, flavors, wetting agents, and food additives. Also called **decanoic acid, decoic acid.**

caps-, kaps-, a combining form meaning 'capsule or container': *capsitis, capsulation, capsuloplasty.*

capsid (kæp′sɪd), the layer of protein enveloping a virion. A capsid is composed of structural units, called capsomeres, and its symmetry may be cubic or helical.

capsula, *pl.* **capsuli.** See **capsule.**

capsular swelling test. See **quellung reaction.**

capsule, **1.** Compare **tablet.** a small, soluble container, usually made of gelatin, used for enclosing a dose of medication for swallowing. **2.** a membranous shell surrounding certain microorganisms, as the pneumococcus bacterium. **3.** a well-defined anatomical structure which encloses an organ or part, as the capsule of the adrenal gland.

capsulectomy (kæp′səlek′təmi), the surgical excision of a capsule, usually the capsule of a joint or the capsule of the lens of the eye.

capsule of Tenon. See **fascia bulbi.**

capsule of the kidney, the fatty enclosure of the kid-

ney, consisting of adipose tissue continuous at the hilus with the fat of the renal sinus. This investment of perirenal fat covers the fibrous capsule and helps to protect the organ from bumps and shocks. Compare **Bowman's capsule.**

capsule of the lens. See **lens capsule.**

capsuloma (kæp′səlou′mə), *pl.* **capsulomas, capsulomata.** a neoplasm of the renal capsule or the subcapsular area.

capsulotomy, an incision into the capsule of the eye, as in an operation to remove a cataract.

captain-of-the-ship doctrine, the medicolegal principle that the physician is ultimately responsible for all patient-care activities and thus may be held accountable and may be sued for negligence or malpractice when the act at issue is performed by an employee or other person under the physician's control, even if not ordered by the physician.

caput (kei′pət, kæp′ət), *pl.* **capita** (kæp′ɪtə). **1.** the head. **2.** the enlarged or prominent extremity of an organ or part. Some kinds of capita include **caput costae, caput epididymis, caput femoris, caput fibulae, caput humeri, caput mallei, caput mandibulae, caput ossis metacarpalis, caput phalangis, caput radii, caput stapedis, caput succedaneum.**

caput costae, the head of a rib; it articulates with a vertebral body.

caput epididymidis, the head of the epididymis.

caput femoris, the head of the femur; it fits into the acetabulum.

caput fibulae, the head of the fibula; it articulates with the lateral condyle of the tibia.

caput humeri, the head of the humerus; it fits into the glenoid cavity of the scapula.

caput mallei, the head of the malleus.

caput mandibulae, the articular process of the ramus of the mandible.

caput ossis metacarpalis, the metacarpal head; it articulates with the proximal phalanx of the same digit.

caput phalangis, the articular head at the distal end of the proximal and middle phalanges.

caput radii, the head of the radius; it articulates with the capitulum of the humerus.

caput stapedis, the head of the stapes.

caput succedaneum, a localized pitting edema in the scalp of a fetus that may overlie sutures of the skull. It is usually formed during labor as a result of the circular pressure of the cervix on the fetal occiput. On vaginal examination the swelling may be mistaken for unruptured membranes. If the caput enlarges appreciably during labor, it may give an erroneous impression of fetal descent on successive examinations. At birth the baby's head may appear markedly deformed, but the swelling begins to resolve immediately and is usually gone in a few days. Compare **cephalhematoma, molding.**

carapace (kær'əpeis'), a horny shield or shell covering the dorsal surface of an animal, as a turtle.

carate (kərat'ei). See **pinta.**

carbachol (kar'bəkɔl), a parasympathomimetic agent.

■ INDICATIONS: It is prescribed in the treatment of glaucoma, for use in ocular surgery, and to oppose the action of cycloplegic and mydriatic medication.

■ CONTRAINDICATIONS: Corneal abrasion, acute iritis, or known hypersensitivity to this drug prohibits its use.

■ ADVERSE EFFECTS: Among the more serious adverse reactions are accommodative spasm and conjunctival hyperemia.

carbamate kinase, a liver enzyme that catalyzes the transfer of a phosphate group from adenosine triphosphate, associated with ammonia and carbon dioxide, to form adenosine diphosphate and carbamoylphosphate.

carbamazepine (kar'bəmæz'əpin), an analgesic and anticonvulsant.

■ INDICATIONS: It is prescribed in the treatment of trigeminal neuralgia and certain seizure disorders.

■ CONTRAINDICATIONS: Concomitant use of monoamine oxidase inhibitors, a history of bone marrow depression, or known hypersensitivity to this drug or to any of the tricyclic antidepressants prohibits its use.

■ ADVERSE EFFECTS: Among the more serious adverse reactions are life-threatening blood dyscrasias, drowsiness, dizziness, ataxia, and nausea. Dermatologic and hypersensitivity reactions may occur.

carbamide peroxide, a topical anti-infective and cerumenolytic.

■ INDICATIONS: It is prescribed in the treatment of canker sores and other minor inflammatory conditions of the gums and mouth and to soften impacted earwax.

■ CONTRAINDICATION: Perforated eardrum prohibits its use.

■ ADVERSE EFFECTS: The most serious adverse reaction is local irritation.

carbenicillin disodium (kar'bənəsɪl'ɪn), a semisynthetic penicillin antibiotic.

■ INDICATION: It is prescribed in the treatment of certain infections.

■ CONTRAINDICATIONS: Known hypersensitivity to this drug or to other penicillins prohibits its use.

■ ADVERSE EFFECTS: Among the more serious adverse effects are hypersensitivity reactions, neurological disturbances, and clotting defects. The high sodium content (5.5-6.5 mEg/gm) may aggravate fluid and electrolyte imbalance in people affected with kidney, heart, or liver disease.

carbidopa, a DOPA decarboxylase inhibitor.

■ INDICATION: It is prescribed in combination with DOPA in the treatment of idiopathic Parkinson's disease.

■ CONTRAINDICATIONS: Glaucoma, hypertension, the use of a monoamine oxidase inhibitor within the past 14 days, or known hypersensitivity to this drug prohibits its use.

■ ADVERSE EFFECTS: Among the most serious adverse reactions are gastrointestinal bleeding, cardiac irregularity, hemolytic anemia, tardive dyskinesia, mental depression, blurred vision, and activation of malignant melanoma.

carbinoxamine maleate (kar'bənok'səmin), an antihistamine.

■ INDICATIONS: It is prescribed in the treatment of a variety of hypersensitivity reactions, including rhinitis, skin reactions, and itching.

■ CONTRAINDICATIONS: Asthma or known hypersensitivity to this drug prohibits its use. It is not administered to newborn infants or lactating mothers.

■ ADVERSE EFFECTS: Among the more serious adverse reactions are tachycardia and other side effects of anticholinergic medications. Drowsiness, skin rash, hypersensitivity reactions, and dry mouth commonly occur.

carbo-, carbon-, a combining form meaning 'carbon, charcoal': *carbonate, carboneol, carbonometry.*

Carbocaine Hydrochloride, a trade name for a local anesthetic (mepivacaine hydrochloride).

carbocyclic (kar'bousaɪ'klɪk). See **closed-chain.**

carbohydrate, any of a group of organic compounds, the most important being sugar, starch, cellulose, and gum. They are classified according to molecular structure as mono-, di-, tri-, poly-, and heterosaccharides. Carbohydrates constitute the main source of energy for all body functions and are necessary for the metabolism of other nutrients. They are synthesized by all green plants and in the body are either absorbed immediately or stored in the form of glycogen. Cereals, vegetables, fruits, rice, potatoes, legumes, and flour products are the major sources of carbohydrates. They can also be manufactured in the body from some amino acids and the glycerol component of fats. Symptoms of deficiency include fatigue, depression, breakdown of essential body protein, and electrolyte imbalance. Excessive consumption of carbohydrates may result in tooth decay, obesity, diabetes mellitus, hypertension, cardiovascular disease, anemia, cancer, and kidney dysfunction.

carbohydrate metabolism, the sum of the anabolic and catabolic processes of the body involved in the synthesis and breakdown of carbohydrates, principally galactose, fructose, and glucose. Some of the processes are glycogenesis, gluconeogenesis, and glycolysis. Energy-rich phosphate bonds are produced in many metabolic reactions requiring carbohydrates.

carbolated camphor, a mixture of 1.5 parts camphor with 1.0 parts each of alcohol and phenol, used as an antiseptic dressing for wounds.

carbol-fuchsin stain, a preparation used in the treatment of superficial fungal infections. It contains boric acid, phenol, reorcinol, fuchsin, acetone, and alcohol in water. Also called **Castellani's paint.**

carbolic acid (karbol'ik), a poisonous, colorless-to-pale-pink crystalline compound obtained from coal tar distillation and converted to a clear liquid with a strong odor and burning taste by the addition of ten per cent water. Low concentrations of carbolic acid are used in antiseptic preparations. Also called **hydroxybenzene, oxybenzene, phenic acid, phenol, phenylic acid, phenylic alcohol.**

carbolic acid poisoning. See **phenol poisoning.**

carbon (C), a nonmetallic, chiefly tetravalent element. Its atomic number is 6; its atomic weight is 12.011. Carbon occurs in pure form in diamond and graphite and is a component of all living tissue. Most of the study of organic chemistry focuses on the vast number of carbon compounds. Carbon occurs in impure form in charcoal, coke, and soot, and in the atmosphere as carbon dioxide. Carbon is essential to the chemistry of the body, participating in many metabolic processes and acting as a component of carbohydrates, amino acids, triglycerides, deoxyribonucleic and ribonucleic acids, and many other compounds. Carbon dioxide produced in glycolysis is important in the acid-base balance of the body and in controlling respiration. Carbon is a component of carbon monoxide, which can be lethal if inhaled, and of many hydrocarbons, the fumes of which can cause death from respiratory failure. Brief incidental exposures to low concentrations of solvent vapors that contain carbon, as gasoline, lighter fluids, aerosol sprays, and spot removers, may be relatively harmless, but exposures to concentrations of hydrocarbon vapors often found in the home and in manufacturing environments may be dangerous. Many occupational pulmonary diseases, as coal worker's pneumoconiosis, black lung disease, aluminosis (bauxite lung), baritosis, berylliosis, and byssinosis, are caused by chronic inhalation of dusts containing carbon compounds. See also **carbon-11, carbon-14.**

carbon-. See **carbo-.**

carbon-11, a radioisotope of carbon with a half-life of 20 minutes. It is produced by a cyclotron and emits positrons. Compare **carbon-14.**

carbon-14, a beta-emitter with a half-life of 5,600 years. It occurs naturally, arising from cosmic rays, and is used as a tracer in studying various aspects of metabolism and in dating relics which contain natural carbonaceous materials. Compare **carbon-11.**

carbon arc lamp, an electric lamp producing a strong white light of adjustable intensity from an arc of current between carbon electrodes.

carbon cycle, the steps by which carbon in the form of carbon dioxide is extracted from and returned to the atmosphere by living organisms, especially human beings. The process starts with the photosyntetic production of carbohydrates by plants, progresses through the consump-

tion of carbohydrates by animals and human beings, and ends with the exhalation of carbon dioxide by those same animals and human beings, and also with the release of carbon dioxide during the decomposition of dead plants and animals. Various chemical processes intervene between the ingestion of carbohydrates and the release of carbon dioxide. Carbohydrate metabolism starts with the movement of glucose through cell membranes and subsequently involves glycolysis, the processes of the citric acid cycle, electron transport, and oxidative phosphorylation. See also **Krebs' citric acid cycle.**

carbon damp. See **damp.**

carbon dioxide (CO_2), a colorless, odorless gas produced by the oxidation of carbon. Carbon dioxide, as a product of cell respiration, is carried by the blood to the lungs and is exhaled. The acid-base balance of body fluids and tissues is affected by the level of carbon dioxide and its carbonate compounds. Solid carbon dioxide (dry ice) is used in the treatment of some skin conditions.

carbon dioxide bath, a bath taken in water that is saturated with carbon dioxide. See also **Nauheim bath.**

carbon dioxide tension, the partial pressure of carbon dioxide gas, expressed as $PaCO_2$, which is proportional to its percentage in the blood or lungs. It is expressed quantitatively in mm Hg. Alveolar $PaCO_2$ directly reflects adequate pulmonary gas exchange in relation to blood flow. A high rate of ventilation causes a lower alveolar $PaCO_2$, a lower rate of breathing leads to higher amounts of alveolar and blood carbon dioxide. The $PaCO_2$ is measured by glass electrodes in samples of arterial blood. Normal values for arterial and alveolar carbon dioxide tension are between 37 and 43 mm Hg. Higher levels occur in conditions of slow blood flow or increased metabolic rate. Below-normal values are caused by hyperventilation, respiratory alkalosis, or rapid rates of blood flow. See also **carbon dioxide, hypercapnia, hyperventilation, hypoventilation.**

carbon monoxide, a colorless, odorless, poisonous gas produced by the combustion of carbon or organic fuels in a limited oxygen supply, as in the cylinders of an internal combustion engine. Carbon monoxide combines irreversibly with hemoglobin, preventing the formation of oxyhemoglobin and reducing the oxygen supply to the tissues. Prolonged exposure to high levels of carbon monoxide results in asphyxiation.

carbon monoxide poisoning, a toxic condition in which carbon monoxide gas has been inhaled and absorbed in the lungs, displacing oxygen from the red blood cells and decreasing the capacity of the blood to carry oxygen to the cells of the body. Characteristically, headache, dyspnea, drowsiness, confusion, cherry-pink skin, unconsciousness, and apnea occur in sequence as the level of carbon monoxide in the blood increases. The most common source of carbon monoxide in cases of poisoning is exhaust fumes from an automobile. Treatment includes removal of the victim from the toxic environment, resuscitation, and administration of oxygen.

carbon tetrachloride, a colorless, volatile, toxic liquid used as a solvent and in fire extinguishers. Ingestion of the liquid or inhalation of the fumes usually results in headaches, nausea, depression, abdominal pain, and convulsions. In poisoning by inhalation, ventilatory assistance and oxygen may be necessary. In poisoning by ingestion, removal of the poison and gastric lavage are the usual treatments. Carbon tetrachloride is particularly toxic to the kidneys and liver: permanent damage to these organs may result.

carboprost tromethamine, a prostaglandin.

■ INDICATIONS: It is prescribed to induce abortion during the second trimester.

■ CONTRAINDICATIONS: Acute pelvic inflammatory disease and known hypersensitivity to this drug prohibits its use. It is used with caution in patients who have cardiac, pulmonary, hepatic, or renal disease, asthma, jaundice, diabetes, or epilepsy, and in those who have had uterine surgery.

■ ADVERSE EFFECTS: Among the more serious adverse reactions are fever, vomiting, and diarrhea. Cervical trauma may occur.

carboxyhemoglobin (karbok'sihi'məglou'bın, karbok'si-hem'əglou'bın), a compound produced by the exposure of hemoglobin to carbon monoxide. Carbon monoxide from the environment is inhaled into the lungs, absorbed through the alveoli, and bound to hemoglobin in the blood, blocking the sites for oxygen transport. Oxygen levels decrease and, when the decrease is excessive, hypoxia and anoxia result. See also **carbon monoxide poisoning, oxyhemoglobin.**

carboxyl, a monovalent radical COOH characteristic of organic acids. The hydrogen of the radical can be replaced by metals to form salts.

carbuncle (kar'bəŋkəl), a cluster of staphylococcal abscesses or boils containing purulent matter in deep, interconnecting, subcutaneous pockets. Eventually pus discharges to the skin surface through numerous openings. Common sites for carbuncles are the back of the neck and the buttocks. Diabetes mellitus and hypogammaglobulinemia may be associated diseases. Treatment may include the use of antibiotics, hot compresses, and surgical drainage.

carbunculosis, an abnormal condition, characterized by the bacterial infection of the hair follicle resulting in the formation of deep, painful abscesses that drain through multiple openings onto the skin surface, usually around hair follicles. Carbunculosis is a form of folliculitis, most commonly caused by the coagulase-positive *Staphylococcus aureus*. The lesions caused by this condition may result in fever and malaise.

■ OBSERVATIONS: Carbunculosis commonly follows persistent *S. aureus* infection and furunculosis. Diagnosis is based on obvious skin lesions, a patient history of previous furunculosis, and *S. aureus* revealed in wound culture.

■ INTERVENTION: Treatment of carbunculosis requires the administration of systemic antibiotics. The prognosis depends on the severity of the infection and the physical condition of the patient.

■ NURSING CONSIDERATIONS: Nursing care for this disorder is mainly supportive and educative to impress the patient with the importance of meticulous personal and family hygiene. The nurse explains that reducing the intake of sugars and fats is important and cautions the patient never to squeeze a boil because it may rupture into the surrounding area. The patient is also instructed not to share towels and washcloths with other family members because this may spread the bacteria. Also stressed is the importance of boiling towels and washcloths before reusing them and the need for daily changes of boiled clothes and bedsheets. The patient is additionally encouraged to change dressings frequently and to discard them in paper bags. Since carbunculosis commonly follows furunculosis, which is often a disorder associated with diabetes, the patient should have a thorough physical examination.

carcin-, a combining form meaning 'pertaining to cancer': *carcinelcosis, carcinogen, carcinolytic.*

carcinectomy (kar'sınek'təmi), the excision of a cancer.

carcinoembryonic antigen (CEA), an antigen present in very small quantities in adult tissue. A greater than normal amount is suggestive of cancer. Tests for its presence aid in screening, in evaluating recurrent or disseminated disease, and in gauging the success of surgical ablation of malignant tumors.

carcinogen (karsın'əjın), a substance that causes the development of a cancer.

carcinogenic (kar'sınəjen'ık), of or pertaining to the ability to cause the development of a cancer. Also called **cancerigenic, cancerogenic.**

carcinogenicity (kar'sınoujınıs'ıti), of or pertaining to the ability to cause the development of a cancer.

carcinoid (kar'sınoid), a small yellow tumor derived from argentaffin cells in the gastrointestinal mucosa that secrete serotonin, other catecholamines, and similar compounds. Carcinoid tumors spread slowly locally but may later metastasize widely. Their secretions often cause systemic symptoms. Also called **argentaffinoma, Kulchitsky-cell carcinoma.** See also **argentaffin cell, carcinoid syndrome.**

carcinoid syndrome, the systemic effects of serotonin-secreting carcinoid tumors manifested by flushing, diarrhea, cramps, skin lesions resembling pellagra, labored breathing, palpitations, and valvular heart disease, especially of the pulmonary valve. Treatment includes surgical excision of the tumor, if feasible, the administration of alpha-adrenergic blocking agents to produce vasodilation, and medication to counteract bronchospasm. Also called **argentaffinoma syndrome.** See also **carcinoid.**

carcinolysis (kar'sınol'ısıs), the destruction of cancer cells, as by the action of an antineoplastic drug. — **carcinolytic,** adj.

carcinoma (kar'sınou'mə), pl. **carcinomas, carcinomata.** a malignant epithelial neoplasm that tends to invade surrounding tissue and to metastasize to distant regions of the body. It develops most frequently in the skin, large intestine, lungs, stomach, prostate gland, cervix, or breast. The tumor is characteristically firm, irregular and nodular, with a well-defined border in some places; as a result, it usually cannot be clearly dissected and excised without removing normal surrounding tissue. Macroscopically, it is whitish with diffuse, dark hemorrhagic patches, and it has yellow areas of necrosis in the center. Microscopically, the tumor cells are characterized by anaplasia, abnormal size and shape, disproportionately large nuclei, and clumps of nuclear chromatin. — **carcinomatous,** adj.

-carcinoma, a combining form meaning a 'malignant tumor composed of epithelial cells, with a tendency to metastasize': ophthalmocarcinoma, osteocarcinoma, phlebocarcinoma.

carcinoma basocellulare. See **basal cell carcinoma.**

carcinoma cutaneum. 1. See **basal cell carcinoma. 2.** See **squamous carcinoma.**

carcinoma en cuirasse, a rare neoplasm accompanying advanced breast cancer and characterized by progressive fibrosis and rigidity of the skin of the chest, neck, back, and, occasionally, the abdomen. Another type, an extraperitoneal extension of gelatinous carcinoma of the rectum, encases the abdominal cavity in a rigid shell.

carcinoma fibrosum. See **scirrhous carcinoma.**

carcinoma gigantocellulare. See **giant cell carcinoma.**

carcinoma in situ, a premalignant neoplasm that has not invaded the basement membrane but shows cytologic characteristics of invasive cancer. Such neoplastic changes in stratified squamous or glandular epithelium are frequently seen on the uterine cervix and also occur in the anus, bronchi, buccal mucosa, esophagus, eye, lip, penis, uterine endometrium, vagina, and in the lesions of senile keratosis. Cervical carcinoma in situ is treated successfully by various methods, including cryosurgery, electrocautery, and simple hysterectomy. Lesions of this kind in pregnant women sometimes regress in the months after delivery. Also called **cancer in situ, intraepithelial carcinoma, preinvasive carcinoma.** See also **erythroplasia of Queyrat.**

carcinoma lenticulare, a form of carcinoma tuberosum or scirrhous skin cancer characterized by the development of many small, relatively flat nodules that often coalesce to form larger areas resembling a fungous infection.

carcinoma medullare. See **medullary carcinoma.**

carcinoma molle. See **medullary carcinoma.**

carcinoma mucocellulare. See **Krukenberg's tumor.**

carcinoma scroti, an epithelial cell carcinoma of the scrotum.

carcinoma simplex, an undifferentiated epithelial tumor in which the stroma and neoplastic epithelial cells do not have a definite microscopic pattern.

carcinoma spongiosum, a carcinoma that is soft and spongy with small and large cavities in it. See also **medullary carcinoma.**

carcinoma telangiectaticum, a neoplasm of the capillaries of the skin causing dilatation of the vessels and red spots on the skin that blanch with pressure.

carcinomatoid (kar'sınou'mətoid), resembling a carcinoma.

carcinomatosis, an abnormal condition characterized by the extensive spread of carcinoma throughout the body.

carcinoma tuberosum. See **tuberous carcinoma.**

carcinoma villosum (vılou'səm). See **villous carcinoma.**

carcinomectomy (kar'sınoumek'təmi). See **carcinectomy.**

carcinophilia (kar'sınoufil'iə, kar'sınoufil'yə), the property in which there is an affinity for carcinomatous tissue. — **carcinophilic,** adj.

carcinosarcoma (kar'sınousarkou'mə), pl. **carcinosarcomas, carsinosarcomata.** a malignant neoplasm composed of carcinomatous and sarcomatous cells. Tumors of this type may occur in the esophagus, thyroid gland, and uterus.

carcinosis (kar'sınou'sıs), pl. **carcinoses.** a condition characterized by the development of many carcinomas throughout the body. Kinds of carcinoses are **carcinosis pleurae, miliary carcinosis, pulmonary carcinosis.** Also called **carcinomatosis.**

carcinosis pleurae, a secondary malignancy of the pleura in which nodules develop throughout the membranes.

carcinostatic (kar'sınoustæt'ık), of or pertaining to the tendency to slow or halt the growth of a carcinoma.

carcinous (kar'sınəs). carcinomatous.

card-, cardio-, a combining form meaning 'heart': cardioclasis, cardiography, cardiomegaly.

cardia, 1. the opening between the esophagus and the cardiac portion of the stomach. **2.** the portion of the stomach surrounding the esophagogastric connection, characterized by the absence of acid cells. **3.** an obsolete term formerly and vaguely used to describe the heart and the region around the heart. — **cardiac,** adj.

cardia-. See **cardio-.**

-cardia, a combining form meaning a 'type of heart action or location': araiocardia, brachycardia, miocardia.

cardiac, **1.** of or pertaining to the heart. **2.** pertaining to a person with heart disease. **3.** of or pertaining to the proximal part of the stomach.

-cardiac, **1.** a combining form meaning 'to characterize types and locations of heart ailments': *gravidocardiac, intracardiac, precardiac.* **2.** a combining form meaning 'to identify heart ailment patients': *diplocardiac, hemicardiac, phrenopericardiac.*

cardiac aneurysm. See **ventricular aneurysm.**

cardiac apnea, abnormal, temporary absence of respiration, as in Cheynes-Stokes respiration.

cardiac arrest, a sudden cessation of cardiac output and effective circulation, usually precipitated by ventricular fibrillation and, in some instances, by ventricular asystole. When cardiac arrest occurs, delivery of oxygen and removal of carbon dioxide stop, tissue cell metabolism becomes anaerobic, and metabolic and repiratory acidosis ensue. Immediate initiation of cardiopulmonary resuscitation is required to prevent heart, lung, kidney, and brain damage. Also called **cardiopulmonary arrest.** See also **cardiopulmonary resuscitation.**

cardiac arrhythmia, an abnormal rate or rhythm of atrial or ventricular myocardial contraction. The condition may be caused by a defect in the ability of the sinoatrial node to maintain its pacemaker function, or by a failure of the bundle of His, the bundle branches, or the Purkinje network to conduct the contractile impulse. Increased metabolic demand, as in exercise or fever, or altered metabolic function, as in acidosis, alkalosis, hypokalemia, or hypocalcemia, results in an arrhythmia if the capacity of the heart to adjust to the particular stress is exceeded. Kinds of arrhythmia include **bradycardia, extrasystole, heart block, premature atrial contraction, premature ventricular contraction, tachycardia.**

(See next page for table)

cardiac asthma, an attack of asthma associated with heart disease, as ventricular failure, and characterized by predominant pulmonary congestion with some bronchoconstriction.

cardiac catheter, a long, fine catheter designed to be passed into the heart through a blood vessel. Used for diagnosis, it allows the determination of blood pressure and the rate of flow in the vessels and chambers of the heart and the identification of abnormal anatomy. Medication may be instilled directly into a coronary vessel, often with visualization by tomography.

cardiac catheterization, a diagnostic procedure in which a catheter is introduced into a large vein, usually of an arm or a leg, and threaded through the venous system to the heart.

■ METHOD: A sterile radiopaque catheter 100 to 125 cm in length is passed through an incision into the vein, through the vein to the superior vena cava, and into the right atrium and other structures to be studied. The course of the catheter is followed with fluoroscopy, and radiographs may be taken. An electrocardiogram is monitored on an oscilloscope. As the catheter tip passes through the chambers and vessels of the heart the pressure of the flow of blood is monitored, and samples of the blood are taken to study the oxygen content.

■ OUTCOME CRITERIA: Formerly, only the right side of the heart could be catherterized; now, the left side may also be studied, but it requires passage through the arterial circulation into the left ventricle. Many conditions may be accurately identified and assessed using cardiac catheterization, including congenital heart disease, tricuspid stenosis, and valvular incompetence. Among the risks of the procedure are local infection, cardiac arrhythmia, and thrombophlebitis.

■ NURSING ORDERS: Cardiac catheterization takes from 1 to 3 hours and the patient has to lie still during the entire procedure. It is not painful, but, because it is anxiety producing, the patient needs explanation and emotional support. A young child may need anesthesia in order to lie still. An antiobiotic is often given the day before. The pulse on the operative side and the blood pressure on the other side of the body are monitored every 15 minutes for one hour and every half hour thereafter. The temperature may be elevated for several hours, and there may be pain at the site of the incision. The nurse observes for signs of infection, thrombophlebitis, and cardiac arrhythmia. Cardiac catheterization is often performed by a special team in a special laboratory. By offering information and counseling, a member of the team may be of great help to the patient and the nursing staff before and after the procedure.

cardiac compression. See **cardiac tamponade.**

cardiac conduction defect, any impairment of the electrical pathways and the specialized muscular fibers that conduct action impulses to contract the atria and the ventricles. Conduction defects may develop in the sinus node, the atrioventricular node, the bundle of His, the left or the right fiber bundles, or the Purkinje fibers. Defective transmission of cardiac impulses along the conduction routes may be caused by ischemic coronary disease or by an occlusion, a lesion, or other pathological factor.

cardiac cycle, the cycle of events during which an electrical impulse is conducted through special fibers over the muscle of the myocardium, from the sinoatrial (SA) node of the atrioventricular (AV) node, to the bundle of His and the bundle branches, and to the Purkinje fibers, causing contraction of the atria followed by contraction of the ventricles. Contraction occurs with depolarization of the muscle fibers; recovery requires repolarization. Deoxygenated blood enters the right atrium of the heart from the superior vena cava and is pumped through the tricuspid valve into the right ventricle. With ventricular contraction, the blood is pumped through the semilunar valve into the pulmonary artery and the lungs for oxygenation.

Comparison of cardiac arrhythmias

Pattern interpretation

Normal
Prolonged AV conduction
PAC with aberrant ventricular conduction
Premature junctional beat
PVC
PVC with retrograde concealed conduction
PVC with retrograde atrial conduction

Arrhythmia	Description	Etiology	Symptoms/consequences	Treatment
Sinus tachycardia	P waves present followed by QRS Rhythm regular Heart rate 100 to 150	Increased metabolic demands Decreased oxygen delivery; CHF, shock, hemorrhage, anemia	May produce palpitations Prolonged episodes may lead to decreased cardiac output	Treat underlying cause Occasionally sedatives

Sinus tachycardia   100-160
Sinus bradycardia   Below 60
Sinus arrhythmia   Irregular
Sinus exit block

Rate of sinus node is 110. Conduction is normal.

Originating in sinus node

Sinus bradycardia	P waves present Rhythm regular Heart rate less than 60	Physical fitness Parasympathetic stimulation (sleep) Brain lesions Digitalis excess	Very low rates may cause decreased cardiac output; light-headedness, faintness, chest pain	Atropine if cardiac output is decreased Pacemaker

Rate is 48. Rhythm is regular and conduction is normal.

Complete heart block	Atria and ventricles beat independently P waves have no relation to QRS Heart rate 20 to 40	Digitalis toxicity Infectious disease Coronary artery disease Myocardial infarction	Very low rates may cause decreased cardiac output; light-headedness, faintness, chest pain	Pacemaker Isoproterenol to increase heart rate

P waves are clearly seen and occur regularly at rate of 72. Ventricles are beating independently under control of nodal pacemaker at rate of 32.

continued.

Comparison of cardiac arrhythmias—cont'd

Arrhythmia	Description	Etiology	Symptoms/consequences	Treatment
Atrial fibrillation	Rapid, irregular waves (over 350/min) Ventricular rhythm irregularly irregular Heart rate varies, may be increased to 150 to 170/min	Rheumatic heart disease Mitral stenosis Atrial infarction	Pulse deficit Decreased cardiac output if rate is rapid Promotes thrombus formation in atria	Digitalis Quinidine Cardioversion

Disorganized electrical activity

Atrial fibrillation with controlled ventricular response and coarse fibrillatory line

Arrhythmia	Description	Etiology	Symptoms/consequences	Treatment
Premature atrial beats	Early P wave followed by normal QRS Rhythm irregular	Stress, ischemia, atrial enlargement, caffeine, nicotine	May produce palpitations Frequent episodes may decrease cardiac output Is sign of chamber irritability	Sedation Quinidine

II

Junctional premature beats

Arrhythmia	Description	Etiology	Symptoms/consequences	Treatment
Premature ventricular beats	Early wide bizarre QRS, not associated with a P wave Rhythm irregular	Stress, acidosis, ventricular enlargement Electrolyte imbalance Drug toxicity (digitalis, quinidine) Hypoxemia, hypercapnia	Same as PAB	Procainamide (Pronestyl) Lidocaine Oxygen Sodium bicarbonate Potassium Treat CHF
Ventricular fibrillation	Chaotic electrical activity No recognizable QRS complex	Myocardial infarction Electrocution Freshwater drowning Drug toxicity	No cardiac output Absent pulse or respiration Cardiac arrest	Defibrillation Epinephrine Sodium bicarbonate

Disorganized electrical activity

Chaotic ventricular activity is reflected in erratic ECG pattern.

Arrhythmia	Description	Etiology	Symptoms/consequences	Treatment
Ventricular standstill	Can only be distinguished from ventricular fibrillation by ECG P waves *may* be present No QRS "Straight line"	Myocardial infarction Chronic diseases of conducting system	Same as ventricular fibrillation	CPR Pacemaker Intracardiac epinephrine

Oxygen-rich blood is returned to the heart through the branches of the pulmonary veins to the left atrium and is then passed through the mitral valve into the left ventricle. With ventricular contraction, the blood is pumped through the aortic semilunar valve into the aorta for peripheral circulation. The contractions of the left and the right atria are nearly simultaneous; they precede the nearly simultaneous contractions of the ventricles. The atria begin to repolarize during ventricular depolarization. On electrocardiogram the cycle is shown as a series of waves, called P, Q, R, S, and T waves, that includes the QRS complex and as two segments that connect the waves, the PR segment and the ST segment. Structural, chemical, or electrical abnormalities may cause a large variety of abnormalities in electrical conduction, muscular contraction, and blood flow in the heart. The ECG may reflect these abnormalities by changes in the shape and duration of the waves and segments of the ECG that represent phases of the cardiac cycle. See also specific waves and specific segments.

cardiac impulse, the movement of the thorax, caused by the beating of the heart. It is readily palpable and easily recorded.

cardiac massage, repeated, rhythmic compression of the heart applied directly, during surgery, or through the intact chest wall in an effort to maintain circulation after cardiac arrest or ventricular fibrillation. See also **cardiopulmonary resuscitation.**

cardiac monitor, a device for the continuous observation of cardiac function. It may include electrocardiograph and oscilloscope readings, recording devices, and a visual or audible record of heart function and rhythm. An alarm system may be set to alert staff of variation from a certain rate.

cardiac monitoring, a continuous check on the functioning of the heart with an electronic instrument that provides an electrocardiographic reading on an oscilloscope. Each ventricular contraction of the heart is indicated by either a flashing light or an audible sound. The indicator is often integrated with an alarm system that is triggered by a pulse rate above or below predetermined limits. The procedure is performed most often in an intensive care unit, although devices are available for patients who are ambulatory. See also **electrocardiography.**

cardiac murmur, an abnormal sound associated with the flow of blood through the heart, which may indicate incomplete closing of one or more heart valves or may be a sign of valvular stenosis. Depending on various characteristics, as intensity, frequency, and duration, a cardiac murmur may be a benign or a pathogenic sign. Also called **heart murmur.**

cardiac muscle, a special striated muscle of the myocardium, containing dark intercalated discs at the junctions of abutting fibers. Cardiac muscle is an exception among involuntary muscles, which are characteristically smooth. Its contractile fibrillae resemble those of skeletal muscle but are only one third as large in diameter, are richer in sarcoplasm, and contain centrally located instead of peripheral nuclei. Studies with the electron microscope indicate that the intercalated discs in cardiac muscle represent cell boundaries. The connective tissue of cardiac muscle is sparser than that of skeletal muscle.

cardiac output, the volume of blood expelled by the ventricles of the heart, equal to the amount of blood ejected at each beat (the stroke output), multiplied by the number of beats in the period of time used in the computation. Cardiac output is commonly measured by the thermodilution technique in which a Swan-Ganz catheter with a thermistor electrode at the tip is inserted in the pulmonary artery, and a certain amount of a cold solution is injected through the lumen of the catheter into the right atrium. The thermistor determines the temperature of the solution when it reaches the pulmonary artery, and the output is calculated on the basis of the temperature change; the increase in the temperature of the solution is inversely related to the functioning of the heart. A normal heart in a resting adult ejects from 2.5 to 3.6 liters of blood per minute. A decreased output at rest is usually indicative of a late stage in abnormal cardiac performance; its failure to increase during exercise occurs much earlier in a malfunctioning heart.

cardiac output, alteration in: decreased, a nursing diagnosis accepted by the Fourth National Conference on the Classification of Nursing Diagnoses. The etiology of the condition is to be developed at a later conference. The defining characteristics include variations in blood pressure, arrhythmias, fatigue, jugular vein distention, color changes of the skin and mucous membranes, oliguria, decreased peripheral pulses, cold and clammy skin, rales, dyspnea, orthopnea, and restlessness. Other characteristics that frequently occur are change in mental status, shortness of breath, syncope, vertigo, edema, cough, frothy sputum, cardiac gallop, and weakness. See also **nursing diagnosis.**

cardiac pacemaker. See **pacemaker.**

cardiac plexus, one of several nerve complexes situated close to the arch of the aorta. The cardiac plexuses contain sympathetic and parasympathetic nerve fibers which leave the plexuses, accompany the right and the left coronary arteries, and enter the heart. Some of the fibers from the plexuses terminate in the sinoatrial node; others terminate in the atrioventricular node and in the atrial myocardium.

cardiac reserve, the potential capacity of the heart to function well beyond its basal level, responding to the demands of various physiological and psychological changes.

cardiac resuscitation. See **cardiopulmonary resuscitation.**

cardiac sphincter, a ring of muscle fibers at the juncture of the esophagus and stomach.

cardiac standstill, the complete cessation of contractions of the heart, resulting in circulatory failure, unconsciousness, respiratory arrest, and death. Cardiac standstill requires immediate cardiopulmonary resuscitation, open cardiac massage, or stimulation of the heart with an electric current. It may be caused by myocardial infarction, chronic disorder of the conduction system of the myocardium, systemic diseases, or metabolic disturbance. Also called **cardiac arrest, cardioplegia.**

cardiac stimulant, a pharmacologic agent which increases the action of the heart. Cardiac glycosides, as digitalis, digitoxin, digoxin, delanoside, lanatoside, acetyldigitoxin, and ouabain, increase the force of myocardial contractions and decrease the heart rate and conduction velocity, allowing more time for the ventricles to relax and become filled with blood. These glycosides, which are composed of a steroid nucleus, lactone ring, and a sugar, are used in the treatment of congestive heart failure, atrial flutter and fibrillation, paroxysmal atrial tachycardia, and cardiogenic shock. Toxic signs and symptoms, resulting from an overdose or the cumulative effect of slowly eliminated digitalis preparations, include anorexia, nausea, vomiting, diarrhea, abdominal pain, headache, muscle weakness, confusion, drowsiness, irritability, visual disturbances, bradycardia or tachycardia, ectopic heart beats, bigeminy, and a pulse deficit. Epinephrine, a potent vasopressor and cardiac stimulant, is sometimes used to restore heart rhythm in cardiac arrest but is not employed in treating heart failure or cardiogenic shock. Isoproterenol hydrochloride, which is related to epinephrine, may be used in treating heart block. Dobutamine hydrochloride and dopamine are employed in the short-term treatment of cardiac decompensation owing to depressed contractility.

cardiac tamponade, compression of the heart produced by the accumulation in the pericardial sac of fluid or of blood resulting from the rupture of a blood vessel of the myocardium, as by a penetrating wound.

■ OBSERVATIONS: Signs of cardiac tamponade may include distended neck veins, hypotension, decreased heart sounds, tachypnea, peripheral pulses that are weak or absent or that fall sharply during inspiration (pulsus paradoxus), elevated cerebrovascular pressure, reduced left atrial pressure, and a pericardial friction rub. The patient, who is usually anxious and restless, may sit upright or lean forward and the skin may be pale, dusky, or cyanotic. The electrocardiogram generally shows decreased cardiac voltage and the chest x ray may reveal an enlarged heart shadow ("water bottle" heart).

■ INTERVENTION: The patient is maintained on bed rest;

the head of the bed is elevated 45 degrees, and a defibrillator and emergency drugs are kept at the bedside. Blood pressure, respiration, apical pulse, and cerebrovascular, atrial, and pulmonary wedge pressures are checked every 15 to 30 minutes. Auscultation for pulsus paradoxus is performed and peripheral pulses are checked every 30 minutes. A 12-lead electrocardiogram is usually ordered, and, when possible, the patient is placed on a cardiac monitor and the rhythm strip is checked every hour. Cardiotonic and antiarrhythmic drugs and measures for controlling pain are administered as ordered. Aspiration of the fluid or blood in the pericardial sac (pericardiocentesis) is performed for diagnosis and for therapy. If surgery is indicated the patient is prepared for the procedure, and the bleeding vessel or vessels are ligated.

■ NURSING CONSIDERATIONS: The patient with life-threatening cardiac tamponade is usually cared for in an intensive care unit. A drain may be in place in the pericardial sac. Coughing and deep breathing are painful, and recovery may be lengthy and difficult. The patient requires extensive physical and emotional care.

cardiac valve. See **heart valve.**

Cardilate, a trade name for an antianginal (erythrityl tetranitrate).

cardinal frontal plane, the plane that divides the body into front and back portions. Also called **vertical plane.**

cardinal horizontal plane, the plane that divides the body into upper and lower portions. Also called **transverse plane.**

cardinal ligament, a sheet of subserous fascia extending across the pelvic floor as a continuation of the broad ligament. It is embedded in the adipose tissue on each side of the vagina and is formed by the fasciae of the vagina and the cervix converging at the lateral borders of these organs. The ligament forms ventral and dorsal extensions at the lateral portion of the pelvic diaphragm. The ventral extension joins the tissue supporting the bladder. The dorsal extension blends with the uterosacral ligaments. The vaginal arteries course across the pelvis in close association with the cardinal ligament. See also **broad ligament.**

cardinal movements of labor, the typical sequence of positions assumed by the fetus as it descends through the pelvis during labor and delivery, usually designated as engagement, flexion, descent, internal rotation, extension, and external rotation or restitution. The birth canal is a curved cylinder; the head must enter it in a downward, transverse direction but exit it in a more forward, anteroposterior direction. In a vertex presentation, engagement of the head in the pelvic inlet requires flexion of the head with chin on chest. Following descent, the head must undergo extension to turn forward and be born under the symphysis. The pelvic inlet is somewhat heart-shaped and the fetal head enters it facing obliquely; but the pelvic outlet is somewhat diamond-shaped and the head usually exits it facing posteriorly and must undergo internal rotation to do so. Following delivery of the head, the shoulders remain for a time in the oblique plane and the head undergoes external rotation or restitution to allow the widest diameter of the shoulders to be delivered from the longer anteroposterior diameter of the pelvic outlet.

cardinal position of gaze, (in ophthalmology) one of six positions to which the normal eye may be turned. Each position requires the function of a specific ocular muscle and a cranial nerve. The positions and the corresponding muscles and nerves are as follows:

straight nasal: medial rectus and the third cranial nerve.

up nasal: inferior oblique and the third cranial nerve.

down nasal: superior oblique and the fourth cranial nerve.

straight temporal: lateral rectus and the sixth cranial nerve.

up temporal: superior rectus and the third cranial nerve.

down temporal: inferior rectus and the third cranial nerve.

cardinal sagittal plane, the plane that divides the body into left and right portions. Also called **midsagittal plane.**

cardinal symptom. See **symptom.**

cardio-, cardia-, a combining form meaning 'pertaining to the heart': *cardiocele, cardiocirrhosis, cardiodynia.*

cardiocirculatory (kar'dioʊsɔr'kyʊlətɔr'i), of or pertaining to the heart and the circulation.

cardiogenic shock (kar'dioʊjen'ɪk), an abnormal condition often characterized by low cardiac output in association with acute myocardial infarction and congestive heart failure. This condition is difficult to diagnose because of complex hemodynamic variations in affected individuals. Although low cardiac output is a common sign of this disorder, cardiogenic shock may also occur in association with normal or higher-than-normal output. Fast determination of blood volume is important to proper therapy. Cardiogenic shock is fatal in about 80 per cent of cases, and immediate therapy is necessary to save affected individuals. Depending on the signs, therapy may include the administration of fluids, diuretics, or vasoactive drugs and the application of various devices, as pacing catheters. A variety of surgical procedures may be part of the therapy but are not usually employed.

cardiogram, an electronically recorded tracing of cardiac activity.

cardiography, the technique of graphically recording the movements of the heart by means of a cardiograph.

cardiologist, a physician specializing in the diagnosis and treatment of disorders of the heart.

cardiology, the study of the anatomy, normal functions, and disorders of the heart.

cardiolysis, an operation that separates the heart and the pericardium from the sternal periosteum in a proce-

dure to correct adhesive mediastinopericarditis. The operation resects the ribs and the sternum over the pericardium.

cardiomegaly (kar'dioʊmeg'əli), hypertrophy of the heart caused most frequently by hypertension and also occurring in arteriovenous fistula, congenital aortic stenosis, ventricular septal defect, patent ductus arteriosus, and Paget's disease. In athletes an enlarged, well functioning heart is a normal finding.

cardiomyopathy (kar'dioʊmaiop'əθhi), any disease that affects the myocardium, as alcoholic cardiomyopathy.

cardioplegia (kar'dioʊpli'jə). See **cardiac standstill.**

cardiopulmonary, of or pertaining to the heart and the lungs.

cardiopulmonary arrest. See **cardiac arrest.**

cardiopulmonary bypass, a procedure used in heart surgery in which the blood is diverted from the heart and lungs by means of a pump oxygenator and returned directly to the aorta.

cardiopulmonary resuscitation (CPR), a basic emergency procedure for life support, consisting of artificial respiration and manual external cardiac massage. It is used in cases of cardiac arrest to establish effective circulation and ventilation in order to prevent irreversible cerebral damage owing to anoxia. External cardiac massage compresses the heart between the lower sternum and the thoracic vertebral column. During compressions, blood is forced into systemic and pulmonary circulation, and venous blood refills the heart when the compression is released. Mouth-to-mouth breathing or a mechanical form of ventilation is used concomitantly with CPR in order to oxygenate the blood being pumped through the circulatory system.

▪ METHOD: Basic cardiopulmonary resuscitation requires no adjunctive equipment, although mechanical devices can be used. It can be done by one or two rescuers and involves three interrelated actions: opening the airway, restoring breathing, and restoring circulation. For an adult, the procedure is performed in the following manner:

1) The patient is placed on a hard flat surface, as a CPR board, a backboard, or, if necessary, the floor. Resuscitation efforts are not delayed while the rescuer is waiting for such a support.

2) The patient is examined closely. If unresponsive, the patient is tapped on the shoulder, or the ear is pinched. The rescuer asks loudly, "Can you hear me? Are you all right?" If there is no response, it is assumed the patient is unconscious.

3) The rescuer establishes and maintains an open airway. In the supine position, relaxed muscles allow the tongue to drop back in the throat, blocking the airway. This can be easily relieved by tilting the head. One hand is placed beneath the patient's neck and the other on the forehead,

the one lifting the neck while the other applies pressure on the forehead. This extends the neck and lifts the tongue from the back of the throat. In a case of suspected cervical spine injury, the neck is not hyperextended. Instead, the lower jaw is lifted by placing the fingers behind the angles of the patient's jaw in front of the earlobes and displacing it upward. If available, an oropharyngeal airway is inserted; if not, the head is held in position, either tilted back or with jaw lifted, throughout the resuscitation procedure.

4) The rescuer evaluates the need for artificial respiration by looking, listening, and feeling for signs of air exchange or respiratory effort. If there is no spontaneous exchange and if there is no stoma over the larynx, regular artificial respiration is begun immediately. If there is a stoma, mouth-to-stoma respiration is initiated.

5) To begin artificial respiration, the rescuer rotates the hand that has been placed on the patient's forehead and, using the thumb and index finger of this hand, pinches the nostrils closed. A tight seal is made with the rescuer's mouth around the mouth of the patient, and four breaths, each of increasing strength and volume, are given. The rescuer's mouth is removed and the patient is allowed to exhale passively. The rescuer watches the chest fall and then breathes in another series of breaths. The cycle is repeated every five seconds as long as respiratory deficiency exists. If indicated, mouth-to-nose respiration may be used. If the chest does not expand, the head is repositioned and ventilation is again attempted. A second unsuccessful attempt indicates an obstructed airway. See also **Heimlich maneuver.**

6) The rescuer takes the pulse and checks for cardiac arrest. If the pulse is absent or inadequate, the carotid artery is palpated for five seconds immediately after the four initial breaths are given. Absence or questionable pressure of the pulse at that time indicates the need to begin external cardiac compression.

7) To start external massage, the rescuer takes a position facing the side of the patient. To find the correct location for the hands (the landmark position), the chest is uncovered and the xiphoid process is identified. With the middle finger on the notch and the index finger next to it, the heel of the other hand is placed on the sternum, directly adjacent to the fingers marking the xiphoid. With the fingers extended upward and away from the ribs, the first hand is placed on top of the second and the fingers are interlocked. With arms straight, the rescuer rocks back and forth from the hip joints, exerting sufficient downward pressure with the forward swing of the body to depress the patient's sternum from $1^1/_2$ to 2 inches. It is extremely important to be positioned properly in order to avoid depressing the xiphoid process and the possibility of causing severe internal injury. After each compression, a rest is allowed for a time equal to the time of compres-

sion, but the hands are not moved from their position on the chest. The cycle is repeated using a ratio of 15 compressions to two breaths at the rate of 80 compressions a minute. The proper rhythm may be achieved by counting "one and two and three," up to 15. If two rescuers are available, CPR is performed with one rescuer giving compressions and the other giving breaths, at a five-to-one ratio at a rate of 60 compressions a minute. The proper rhythm can be determined by counting "one-one thousand, two-one thousand," up to five-one thousand. Effectiveness of CPR is checked frequently by palpating the carotid for the return of a spontaneous heartbeat and by watching for "pinking" of the skin, constriction of the pupils, and a return of respiration. If the rescuer doing compressions becomes tired, a switch may be made by changing the counting rhythm to "switch-one thousand, two-one thousand," up to five-one thousand. At the end of that cycle, the rescuer giving compressions moves the patient's head and checks the pulse. The rescuer who has been at the head, after giving a breath, moves to the patient's side, and checks the pulse for five seconds. If the pulse is absent or its pressure is inadequate, the rescuer at the head says, "No pulse. Continue CPR."

The technique for infants up to one year of age and for children up to eight years of age is like that for adults, with the following exceptions. In infants, the neck is not hyperextended because soft cartilage and neck tissues may occlude the airway if the head is tilted too far; placing a hand beneath the shoulders of an infant provides adequate tilt. The rescuer's mouth covers the infant's mouth and nose, and the infant's pulse is checked on the brachial artery. For infants, only the tops of the index and middle fingers of one hand are used to compress the sternum; for small children, the heel of one hand is used. Because the ventricles of the heart in infants and small children lie higher in the chest cavity than they do in adults, external pressure is applied midsternum and only to a depth of $^1/_2$ to 1 inch for infants and to 1 to $1^1/_2$ inches for children. The rate of cardiac compression for infants is 100 a minute, with breaths interposed as quickly as possible after each five compressions—approximately one every three seconds. The rate of compression for children is 80 a minute, with ventilations delivered once every four seconds. Less air is necessary for a child than for an adult. For an infant, only the air held in the cheeks is puffed in.

■ OUTCOME CRITERIA: To provide adequate basic life support, these rules for correct performance should be followed:

1) CPR is not interrupted for more than five seconds, except for endotracheal intubation or for moving a patient. In these cases, the interruption does not exceed 15 seconds.

2) Compressions are smooth, regular, and uninterrupted.

3) The patient is stabilized before transportation to a more convenient site.

4) The pressure on the chest is completely released after each compression, although the palm of the hand remains in contact with the chest wall.

5) The shoulders of the rescuer are placed directly above the patient's sternum in order to provide the most effective thrusts.

6) The sternum is depressed to the correct degree according to the size and age of the patient.

7) The xiphoid process is not compressed because of the danger of lacerating the liver.

8) Gastric distension is not relieved unless it becomes so severe that it interferes with ventilation.

CPR is used only in cases of sudden cardiac arrest. Even if CPR is initiated as soon as possible and all steps are performed correctly, there are some cases, as with severe emphysema or crushing chest injuries, in which it is not successful. Even properly performed, CPR may cause rib fractures in some patients. Other complications include fracture of the sternum, separation of costochondral cartilage, hepatic hematoma, lung contusions, and fat embolism. The danger of complications is minimized by correct performance. Properly performed external cardiac massage can produce a systolic blood pressure peaking at more than 100 mm Hg in the carotid arteries. With no heartbeat the diastolic pressure is 0; thus, the mean pressure with CPR is usually about 40 mm Hg and the flow of arterial blood is approximately 25 per cent to 35 per cent of the normal flow. These figures point out the need for immediate action and for continuous effort in order to effect a rescue; they also indicate that CPR can be effective and can save lives if properly given in a carefully monitored fashion. CPR is an interim measure used until advanced life support action and definitive measures can be taken. Once initiated, it is continued until one of the following occurs: spontaneous circulation and respiration are restored; resuscitation efforts are transferred to someone who can continue life-support procedures, either basic or advanced; a physician assumes responsibility for the patient; the patient is handed over to the care of a medical facility; or the rescuer is physically unable to continue.

■ NURSING ORDERS: Cardiopulmonary resuscitation is considered an emergency procedure, and knowledge of the principles, procedures, requirements, and complications of this maneuver is essential. In the hospital, there are additional tasks to perform to implement CPR. Primarily, the nurse evaluates the extent of the emergency and the indications for initiating lifesaving measures. The nurse is also prepared to undertake immediate action should it be necessary to do so before the medical team arrives. If not immediately involved in performing CPR, the nurse prepares for the initiation of definitive therapy

by readying equipment, including an electrocardiograph, a defibrillator, a tracheostomy set, oxygen, and a suction machine. Epinephrine for direct injection into the heart, sodium bicarbonate to combat acidosis, and calcium chloride to stimulate cardiac contraction are also prepared for injection and properly labeled. While resuscitation proceeds, efforts are made to start an intravenous infusion and ECG electrodes are applied to the patient. In the hospital, the decision to terminate resuscitation efforts is made by a physician.

Two-rescuer CPR position

Cardiac compression

CARDIOPULMONARY RESUSCITATION (CPR)

cardiorrhaphy, an operation in which the heart muscle is sutured.

cardioscope, an obsolete device for inspecting and manipulating the internal structures of the heart.

cardiospasm (kar′dɪoʊspæz′əm), a form of achalasia characterized by a failure of the cardia at the distal end of the esophagus to relax, causing dysphagia and regurgitation, and sometimes requiring surgical division of the muscle.

cardiotachometer, an instrument that continuously monitors and records the heartbeat.

cardiotomy, 1. an operation in which the heart is incised. **2.** an operation in which the cardiac end of the stomach or cardiac orifice is incised.

cardiotonic (kar'diouton'ik), **1.** of or pertaining to a substance that tends to increase the efficiency of contractions of the heart muscle. **2.** a pharmacologic agent that increases the force of myocardial contractions. Cardiac glycosides, derived from certain plant alkaloids, exert a tonic effect by altering the transport of electrolytes across the myocardial membrane, causing an increased influx of sodium and calcium and an increased efflux of potassium. Digitalis, digitoxin, and digoxin, widely used cardiac glycosides obtained from leaves of a species of foxglove, increase the force of myocardial contractions, extend the refractory period of the atrioventricular node, and, to a lesser degree, affect the sinoatrial node and the heart's conduction system. Other cardiac glycosides are ouabain and strophanthin, obtained from species of *Strophanthus;* scillaridin, derived from squill; and bufotalin, obtained from the skin and saliva of a European toad.

cardiotoxic, having a toxic or injurious effect on the heart.

cardiovascular (kar'diouvæs'kyular), of or pertaining to the heart and blood vessels.

cardiovascular assessment, an evaluation of the condition, function, and abnormalities of the heart and circulatory system.

■ METHOD: The patient is asked to describe the onset, duration, location, and characteristics of any pain present and the occurrence of weakness, fatigue, shortness of breath, fever, coughing, wheezing, and palpitations. Questions are asked regarding episodes of fainting, indigestion, nausea, edema of extremities, cyanosis, changes in vision, and whether the hands and feet ever feel numb or cold. The person's general appearance, color, assumed position, the rate and rhythm of arterial pulses, the presence of pulsus paradoxus or pulsus alternans, and the distention, pulsation, and pressure of neck veins are observed. The blood pressure, temperature, rate and character of respirations are checked, and the precordium is examined for the point of maximal impulse, symmetry, the cardiac border, pulsations, and evidence of lifts or bulges. Auscultation of the chest is performed to determine the intensity, pitch, duration, timbre, origin, and frequency of heart sounds and murmurs and to identify the location and character of breath sounds, including rales, rhonchi, and rubs. The color, temperature, turgor, and dryness or sweating of the skin are noted, and the appearance of the extremities, capillary filling time, nails, and lesions are described. The patient's level of consciousness, reflexes, neurologic signs, and responses to pain are recorded, along with data on concurrent hypertension, obesity, diabetes, and any pulmonary and renal conditions. Information is obtained on any previous cardiovascular surgery and illnesses, as rheumatic fever, myocardial infarction, angina, congenital heart disease, occlusive vascular disease, and lung and kidney disorders. Pertinent background data include the patient's response to stress, methods of coping, relationships, occupation, environment, sleep pattern, exercise levels, leisure activities, and use of alcohol and tobacco. Other factors considered in the evaluation are the patient's history of medication with digitalis preparations, antihypertensives, diuretics, aspirin, sleeping pills, and over-the-counter cold and influenza remedies and a family history of heart disease, hypertension, diabetes, obesity, vascular disorders, stroke, and renal disease. Diagnostic aids are an electrocardiogram, chest x ray, echocardiogram, coronary arteriogram, cardiac catheterization, arterial and pulmonary wedge pressure readings. Appropriate laboratory studies include a complete blood count, hemoglobin and hematocrit determinations, electrolyte and clotting profiles, and assays of serum cholesterol, triglycerides, serum glutamic oxaloacetic transaminase serum, creatine phosphokinase and lactic acid dehydrogenase.

■ NURSING ORDERS: The nurse usually obtains the patient's history, records the external observations, checks the blood pressure, temperature, respiration, and pulse, auscultates the chest, and assembles the pertinent background information and the reports on diagnostic tests. In a coronary care unit the nurse may have a greatly expanded role, interpreting the data on an electrocardiographic tracing and adjusting medications.

■ OUTCOME CRITERIA: An accurate and complete assessment of cardiovascular function is an essential adjunct to a complete physical examination and is vital to the diagnosis and proper continuing care of a patient who has cardiovascular disease.

cardiovascular disease, any one of numerous abnormal conditions characterized by dysfunction of the heart and blood vessels. Some common kinds of cardiovascular disease are **atherosclerosis, cor pulmonale, rheumatic heart disease, syphilitic heart disease,** and **systemic hypertension.** In the United States cardiovascular disease is second to cancer as the leading cause of death, accounting for about 50 per cent of all deaths from disease annually. More than a quarter of a million persons under 65 years of age in the United States die each year from this disorder; about half of such deaths are attributed to atherosclerosis. The prevalent kinds of cardiovascular disease are the rheumatic, the syphilitic, and the traumatic varieties.

cardiovascular system, the network of structures, including the heart and the blood vessels, that pump and convey the blood throughout the body. The system includes thousands of miles of vessels, capillaries, and venules and is vital to maintaining homeostasis. Numerous control mechanisms of the system assure that the blood is delivered to the structures where it is most needed and at the proper rate. The system delivers nutrients and other essential materials to the fluids surrounding the cells and removes waste products which are conveyed to excretory organs, as the kidneys and the intestine. The cardiovascular system functions in close association with the respiratory system, transporting oxygen inhaled into the lungs and conveying carbon dioxide to the lungs for expiration. Sympathetic and parasympathetic impulses from the medulla and cardiac baroreceptors sensitive to changes in pressure control the function of the heart, which pumps the oxygenated blood carried by the arteries and receives deoxygenated blood from the veins. Cardiovascular diseases affect a large number of individuals throughout the world, and half a million Americans die each year from coronary diseases. A variety of factors, as diet, exercise, and stress, affect the cardiovascular system.

cardioversion, the restoration of the heart's sinus rhythm by delivery of a synchronized electrical shock through two metal paddles placed on the patient's chest. Cardioversion is used in the treatment of atrial fibrillation and in ventricular, nodal, and atrial arrhythmias.
■ METHOD: The synchronized electrical voltage is delivered by placing one of the insulated electrode paddles, covered with a thick layer of conductive paste, below the angle of the patient's left scapula; the other paddle is placed over the right parasternal area of the third intercostal space. The instrument is automatically preset to deliver an electrical discharge during the interval in which the normal cardiac impulse spreads through the bundle of His and its branches to initiate contraction (the QRS complex). The instrument is set initially to deliver five to ten watts per second, but if the normal rhythm does not resume, successive shocks of up to 400 watts per second are delivered. To prepare the patient for cardioversion, the physician's explanation of the procedure is reinforced, a signed informed consent is obtained, and diuretics and digitalis preparations are withheld for 24 to 72 hours as ordered. The patient's serum potassium level is checked for possible hypokalemia and a 12-lead electrocardiogram and rhythm strip are obtained. Nothing is given orally for six to eight hours before the procedure. Parenteral fluids are maintained and oxygen, delivered by mask or cannula, may be ordered. The patient voids and receives a sedative about an hour before cardioversion; dentures are removed. An emergency cart with cardiac drugs and airway equipment is placed at the bedside, and conductive gel, paste, or saline pads are applied to the electrode paddles. During and after cardioversion, observations are made of the patient's level of consciousness, pulse, respirations, and blood pressure; also noted are electrocardio-graphic changes, as return to sinus rhythm, atrial fibrillation, premature ventricular contractions, ventricular tachycardia, or cardiac standstill. Any signs of pulmonary embolus are noted. Following the procedure, the patient is maintained in a supine position in bed. The blood pressure, respirations, and apical pulse are checked every 15 minutes for an hour, then every four hours. Cardiac activity is monitored and oxygen is administered as ordered. The patient's skin areas exposed to the electrodes' gel or saline pads are washed with plain water, and a lanolin-based lotion is applied.
■ NURSING ORDERS: The nurse prepares the patient for cardioversion, assembles the necessary emergency equipment, and checks the vital signs during and after the procedure.
■ OUTCOME CRITERIA: Cardioversion is usually an effective method for restoring the heart's normal sinus rhythm.

carditis (kardai'tıs), an inflammatory condition of the muscles of the heart, usually resulting from infection. In most cases more than one layer of muscles is involved. Chest pain, cardiac arrhythmia, circulatory failure, and damage to the structures of the heart may occur. Kinds of carditis are **endocarditis, myocarditis, pericarditis.**

career ladder, (in nursing education) a pathway for upward mobility that begins with a course of study in practical nursing or a program that grants an associate degree in nursing. On completion of this basic level, the candidate may continue up the ladder, taking a baccalaureate program in nursing. After this, the person may continue on to a masters and a doctoral program.

care of the sick, (in public health nursing) the care of sick patients in their homes, as distinguished from health supervision. Public health nursing agencies are reimbursed for the nursing services rendered by the nurses according to the kind of service rendered, as a sick visit or a health supervision visit. Compare **health supervision.**

care plan. See **nursing care plan.**

caries (ker'iz), an abnormal condition of a tooth or a bone characterized by decay, disintegration, and destruction of the structure. Kinds of caries include **dental caries, radiation caries, spinal caries.**

carina, pl. **carinae.** any structure shaped like a ridge or keel, as the carina of the trachea, which projects from the lowest tracheal cartilage.

cariogenic, tending to produce caries.

carisoprodol, a skeletal muscle relaxant.
■ INDICATION: It is prescribed for the relief of muscle spasm.
■ CONTRAINDICATIONS: Porphyria or known hypersensitivity to this drug or to chemically similar drugs prohibits its use.
■ ADVERSE EFFECTS: Among the more serious adverse reactions are ataxia, drowsiness, pronounced weakness,

visual disturbances, mental confusion, and allergic reactions.

carminative (karmın′ətıv), **1.** of or pertaining to a substance that relieves flatulence and abdominal distention. **2.** a carminative agent that relieves gaseous distention and painful spasms, especially after meals. Volatile oils of anise, bitter almond, cinnamon, fennel, peppermint, spearmint, and wintergreen, which have a soothing effect passing through the stomach, were formerly used as carminatives, but they are rarely used in modern medicine except as flavoring agents.

carmine dye, a red coloring substance, produced by the addition of alum to an extract of cochineal, used for staining specimens in histology.

carmustine (karməs′tın), a lipid-soluble nitrosourea, used as a single agent or with other approved chemotherapeutic agents in the treatment of brain tumors, multiple myeloma, Hodgkin's disease, and non-Hodgkin's lymphomas. Also called **BCNU.**

carneous, having the quality of flesh.

carnivore, an animal belonging to the order *Carnivora,* classified as a flesheater, with appropriate teeth and a characteristically simple stomach and a short intestine for such a diet. – **carnivorous,** *adj.*

carotene, carotin, carrotene, carrotine (kær′ətin), a red or orange hydrocarbon found in carrots, sweet potatoes, milk fat, egg yolk, and leafy vegetables, as beet greens, spinach, and broccoli. Carotene is a provitamin and in the body is converted into vitamin A. An inability to utilize carotene results in vitamin A deficiency. See also **vitamin A.**

carotenemia (kær′ətıni′miə), the presence of carotene in the blood resulting in an abnormal yellow appearance of the plasma and skin. The conjunctivae are not discolored. Also called **pseudojaundice.** Compare **bilirubinemia.** See also **jaundice, icterus.**

carotenoid, carotinoid (kərot′ənoid), any of a group of red, yellow, or orange highly unsaturated pigments that are found in some animal tissue and in foods, as carrots, sweet potatoes, and leafy green vegetables. Many of these substances, as carotene, are necessary for the formation of vitamin A in the body, while others, including lycopene and xanthophyll, show no vitamin A activity.

carotenosis (kær′ətınou′sıs), See **carotenemia.**

carotid (kərot′ıd), of or pertaining to the carotid artery. See also **carotid body, carotid sinus.**

carotid body, a small structure containing neural tissue at the bifurcation of the carotid arteries. It monitors the oxygen content of the blood and assists in regulating respiration.

carotid body reflex, a normal chemical reflex initiated by a decrease in oxygen concentration in the blood and, to a lesser degree, by increased carbon dioxide and hydrogen ion concentrations that act on chemoreceptors at the bifurcation of the common carotid arteries and result in nerve impulses that cause the respiratory center in the medulla to increase respiratory activity. See also **aortic body reflex.**

carotid body tumor, a benign, round, firm growth that develops at the bifurcation of the common carotid artery. The tumor usually has no effect but it sometimes may cause dizziness, nausea, and vomiting, especially if it impedes the flow of blood as pressure is increased in the vascular system. It may be surgically excised in some cases.

carotid plexus, any one of three nerve plexuses associated with the carotid arteries. Compare **common carotid plexus, external carotid plexus, internal carotid plexus.**

carotid pulse, the pulse of the carotid artery, palpated by gently pressing a finger in the groove between the larynx and the sternocleidomastoid muscle in the neck.

carotid sinus, a dilatation of the arterial wall at the bifurcation of the common carotid artery. It contains sensory nerve endings from the vagus nerve that respond to changes in blood pressure.

carotid sinus reflex, the decrease in the heart rate as a reflex reaction from pressure on or within the carotid artery at the level of its bifurcation. This reflex starts in the sinus of the internal carotid artery. See also **carotid sinus syndrome.**

carotid sinus syndrome, a temporary loss of consciousness that sometimes accompanies convulsive seizures because of the intensity of the carotid sinus reflex when pressure builds in one or both carotid sinuses.

carotodynia (kərot′oudın′iə), a tenderness along the length of the common carotid artery.

-carp, a combining form meaning 'fruit': *archicarp, ascocarp, pericarp.*

carpal (kar′pəl), of or pertaining to the carpus, or wrist.

-carpal, a combining form referring to the wrist: *extracarpal, radiocarpal, trapeziometacarpal.*

carpal tunnel, a conduit for the median nerve and the flexor tendons, formed by the carpal bones and the flexor retinaculum.

carpal tunnel syndrome, a common painful disorder of the wrist and hand, induced by compression on the median nerve between the inelastic carpal ligament and other structures within the carpal tunnel. The syndrome is seen more often in women, especially in pregnant and in menopausal women. Symptoms may result from trauma, synovitis, or tumor, or may develop with rheumatoid arthritis, amyloidosis, agromegaly, or diabetes. The median nerve innervates the palm and the radial side of the hand; compression of the nerve causes weakness, pain with opposition of the thumb, and burning, tingling, or aching, sometimes radiating to the forearm and to the shoulder joint. Weakness and atrophy of muscles may increase from lack of use, impairing thumb and finger dexterity.

Pain may be intermittent or constant and is often most intense at night. Symptomatic treatment usually relieves mild symptoms of recent onset, but if the pain becomes disabling, the injection of corticosteroids often brings dramatic relief. Surgical division of the volar carpal ligament to relieve nerve pressure is usually curative. Nursing treatment includes emotional support, nocturnal splinting of the hand and forearm, elevation of the arm to relieve the swelling of soft tissue, and encouragement of mild wrist and finger movements to prevent atrophy of muscles.

carphenazine maleate, a phenothiazine anti-psychotic agent.
■ INDICATION: It is prescribed in the treatment of psychotic disorders.
■ CONTRAINDICATIONS: Parkinson's disease, concurrent administration of central nervous system depressants, liver or renal dysfunction, severe hypotension, or known hypersensitivity to this drug or to phenothiazine medication prohibits its use.
■ ADVERSE EFFECTS: Among the more serious adverse effects are hypotension, liver toxicity, a variety of extrapyramidal reactions, blood dyscrasias, and hypersensitivity reactions.

carpopedal spasm, a spasm of the hand, or thumbs, or foot, or toes that sometimes accompanies tetany.

carpus (kar′pəs), the wrist, made up of eight bones arranged in two rows. The proximal row consists of the scaphoid, lunate, triangular, and pisiform. The distal row consists of the trapezium, trapezoid, capitate, and hamate.

Carrel-Lindbergh pump (kərel′lınd′bərg). See **Lindbergh pump.**

carrier, 1. a person or animal who harbors and spreads an organism causing disease in others but who does not become ill. 2. one whose chromosomes carry a recessive gene.

Carrión's disease (kær′iounz′). See **bartonellosis.**

car sickness. See **motion sickness.**

cartilage, a nonvascular supporting connective tissue composed of various cells and fibers, found chiefly in the joints, the thorax, and various rigid tubes, as the larynx, trachea, nose, and ear. Temporary cartilage, as that comprising most of the fetal skeleton at an early stage, is later replaced by bone. Permanent cartilage remains unossified, except in certain diseases and, sometimes, in advanced age. Kinds of permanent cartilage are **hyaline cartilage, white fibrocartilage, yellow cartilage.** – **cartilaginous,** *adj.*

cartilage-hair hypoplasia, a genetic disorder, inherited as an autosomal recessive trait, characterized by dwarfism caused by hypoplasia of the cartilage, multiple skeletal abnormalities, and excessively sparse, short, fine, brittle hair that is usually light colored. The condition is found primarily among Amish people in the United States and Canada.

cartilaginous joint, a slightly movable joint in which

cartilage unites bony surfaces. Two types of articulation involving cartilaginous joints are synchondrosis and symphysis. Also called **amphiarthrosis, junctura cartilaginea.** Compare **fibrous joint, synovial joint.**

CARTOS, acronym for **computer-aided reconstruction by tracing of serial sections,** a technique in which serial, hand-drawn copies of electron micrographs are programmed on a computer for display on a television screen. The image can be manipulated for study of all dimensions of the structure.

caruncle (kar′əŋkəl), **caruncula** (kərəŋ′kyulə), a small, fleshy projection, as one of the lacrimal caruncles at the inner canthus of the eye or the hymenal caruncles that are the hymenal remnants.

carunculae hymenales, remnants of a ruptured hymen that appear as irregular projections of normal skin around the introitus to the vagina. Also called **hymeneal tags.**

caryo-, karyo-, a combining form meaning 'pertaining to a nucleus': *caryokinesis, caryophyllus.*

cascade, any process that develops in stages, with each stage dependent on the preceding one, often producing a cumulative effect.

cascara sagrada (kæskær′ə səgra′də), a stimulant cathartic prepared from the bark of the *Rhamnus purshiana* tree.
■ INDICATION: It is prescribed for constipation.
■ CONTRAINDICATIONS: Symptoms of appendicitis, intestinal obstruction or perforation, fecal impaction, or known hypersensitivity to this drug prohibits its use. It is not given to lactating mothers.
■ ADVERSE EFFECTS: Among the more serious adverse reactions are rectal bleeding, muscle cramps, dizziness, and laxative dependence.

caseation (kei′siei′shən), a form of tissue necrosis in which there is loss of cellular outline and the appearance is that of crumbly cheese. It is typical of tuberculosis. – **caseate,** *v.* **caseous,** *adj.*

caseation necrosis, necrosis that transforms tissue into a dry cheeselike mass.

case fatality rate, the number of deaths caused by any specific disease, expressed as a percentage of the total number of cases of the disease.

caseous (kei′siəs), cheeselike, describing the mixture of fat and protein that appear in some body tissues undergoing necrosis.

caseous fermentation, the coagulation of soluble casein through the action of rennin.

cast, 1. a stiff, solid dressing formed with plaster of Paris or other material around a limb or other body part to immobilize it during healing. 2. a mold of a part or all of a patient's teeth and internal jaw area for fitting prostheses or dentures. 3. a tiny structure formed by deposits of mineral or other substances on the walls of renal tubules, bronchioles, or other organs. Casts often appear in samples of urine or blood collected for laboratory examination. **4.** the deviation of an eye from the normal parallel lines of vision, as in strabismus.

Castellani's paint (kæs′tɪla′niz), a liquid applied topically to large areas of the skin, as a disinfectant for treatment of fungal infection. Castellani's paint consists of phenol, resorcinal, boric acid, acetone, and basic fuchsin. See also **paint.**

castor oil, an oil derived from *Ricinus communis,* used as a stimulant cathartic.
- INDICATIONS: It is prescribed for constipation and for a cleansing preparation of the bowel or colon prior to examination.
- CONTRAINDICATIONS: Symptoms of appendicitis, intestinal obstruction or perforation, and fecal impaction prohibit its use. It is not to be used during menstruation or pregnancy.
- ADVERSE EFFECTS: Among the most serious adverse reactions are rectal bleeding and laxative dependence. Nausea, abdominal cramps, and dizziness also may occur.

castration, the surgical excision of one or both testicles or ovaries, performed most frequently to reduce the production and secretion of certain hormones that may stimulate the proliferation of malignant cells in women with breast cancer and in men with cancer of the prostate. The patient must be informed that bilateral excision of the gonads causes sterility. See also **oophorectomy, orchiectomy.**

castration anxiety, **1.** the fantasized fear of injury or loss of the genital organs, often as the reaction to a repressed feeling of punishment for forbidden sexual desires. It may also be caused by some apparently threatening everyday occurrence, such as a humiliating experience, loss of a job, or loss of authority. **2.** a general threat to the masculinity or femininity of a person or an unrealistic fear of bodily injury or loss of power. Also called **anxiety complex.** See also **anxiety neurosis.**

castration complex. See **castration anxiety.**

casuistics, the recording and the study of the cases of any disease.

CAT (kæt), acronym for **computerized axial tomography.**

cata-, cat-, a combining form meaning 'down, under, against, with': *catabasis, catabolic, catacausis.*

catabasis (kətæb′əsɪs), *pl.* **catabases.** the phase in which a disease declines. — **catabatic,** *adj.*

catabiosis, the normal aging of cells. — **catabiotic,** *adj.*

catabolic activator protein. See **CAP.**

catabolism (kətæb′əlɪz′əm), a complex, metabolic process in which energy is liberated for use in work, energy storage, or heat production by the oxidation of carbohydrates, fats, and proteins. Carbon dioxide and water are produced as well as energy. Compare **anabolism.** — **catabolic,** *adj.*

catacrotism (kətæk′rətɪz′əm), an anomaly of the pulse,

characterized by a small additional wave in the descending limb of the pulse tracing. — **catacrotic,** *adj.*

catalepsy (kæt′əlep′si), an abnormal state characterized by a trancelike level of consciousness and postural rigidity. It occurs in hypnosis and in certain organic and psychological disorders, as schizophrenia, epilepsy, and hysteria.

catalysis (kətæl′əsɪs), an increase in the rate of any chemical reaction, caused by a chemical material that is neither part of the process itself nor consumed or affected by the reaction. Compare **negative catalysis.** See also **catalyst.** — **catalytic,** *adj.*

catalyst (kæt′əlɪst), a substance that influences the rate of a chemical reaction without being permanently altered by the process. Most catalysts, including enzymes in living organisms, accelerate chemical reactions; negative catalysts retard such reactions. See also **enzyme.**

-catalytic, a combining form meaning 'pertaining to a chemical reaction caused by an agent unchanged by the reaction': *allelocatalytic, autocatalytic, photocatalytic.* Also **-catalytical.**

catamnesis (kæt′æmni′sɪs), the medical history of a patient from the onset of an illness.

cataphylaxis (kæt′əfəlæk′sɪs), **1.** the migration of leukocytes and antibodies to the site of an infection. **2.** the deterioration of the natural defense system of the body. — **cataphylactic,** *adj.*

cataplexy (kæt′əplek′si), a condition characterized by sudden muscular weakness and hypotonia, caused by emotions, as anger, fear or surprise, often associated with narcolepsy. — **cataplectic,** *adj.*

Catapres, a trade name for an antihypertensive (clonidine hydrochloride).

cataract, an abnormal progressive condition of the lens of the eye, characterized by loss of transparency. A gray-white opacity can be seen within the lens, behind the pupil. Most cataracts are caused by degenerative changes, occurring most often after 50 years of age. The tendency to develop cataracts is inherited. Trauma, as a puncture wound, may result in cataract formation; less often, exposure to such poisons as dinitrophenol or naphthalene causes them. **Congenital cataracts** are usually hereditary but may be caused by viral infection during the first trimester of gestation. If cataracts are untreated, sight is eventually lost. At first vision is blurred; then, bright lights glare diffusely, and distortion and double vision may develop. Uncomplicated cataracts of old age (**senile cataracts**) are usually treated with excision of the lens and prescription of special contact lens or glasses. The soft cataracts of children and young adults may either be incised and drained or fragmented by ultrasound, followed by irrigation and aspiration of the fragments through a minute incision.

catarrh, *Obsolete.* inflammation of the mucous membranes with discharge, especially inflammation of the air passages of the nose and the trachea. — **catarrhal, catarrhous,** *adj.*

catarrhal dysentery. See **sprue.**

catastrophic care, a pattern of medical and nursing care that involves intensive, highly technical life-support care of an acutely ill or severely traumatized patient.

catastrophic health insurance, health insurance that awards benefits to pay for the cost of severe or lengthy disability or illness. Benefits on some policies are not paid until a specified minimum amount, paid by the insured, is exceeded. Most policies have a limit in total benefits paid, and payment for certain kinds of services may either be precluded or limited to a maximum idemnity.

catastrophic reaction, the uncoordinated response to a drastic shock or a sudden threatening condition, as often occurs in the victims of car crashes and disasters.

catatonia (kæt'ətou'niə), a state or condition characterized by conspicuous motor disturbance, manifested usually as immobility with extreme muscular rigidity or, less commonly, as excessive, impulsive activity. See also **catatonic schizophrenia.** — **catatonic,** *adj.*

catatonic schizophrenia, a form of schizophrenia characterized by alternating periods of extreme withdrawal and extreme excitement. During the withdrawal stage stupor, muscular rigidity, mutism, blocking, negativism, catalepsy, and cerea flexibilitas may be seen; during the period of excitement, purposeless and impulsive activity may range from mild agitation to violence. Either phase may last for a period of hours, days, or weeks, and the change to the alternate phase is usually abrupt and rapid. Treatment may include tranquilizers, an antidepressant or antianxiety drug, followed by long-term psychotherapy. See also **catatonia.**

cat-bite fever. See **cat-scratch fever.**

catchment area (kæch'mənt), the specific geographical area for which a particular institution, especially a mental health center, is responsible.

catch-up growth, an acceleration of the growth rate following a period of growth retardation owing to a secondary deficiency, as acute malnutrition or severe illness. The phenomenon, which is routinely seen in premature infants, involves rapid increase in weight, length, and head circumference and continues until the normal individual growth pattern is resumed. The severity, duration, and the developmental timing at which the deficiency occurs may result in some growth inadequacy or permanent deficit, especially in such tissue as the brain.

cat-cry syndrome, a rare, congenital disorder recognized at birth by a kittenlike cry which may prevail for weeks, then disappear. Other characteristics include low birth weight, microcephaly, "moon face," wide-set eyes, strabismus, and low-set misshaped ears. Infants are hypo-

tonic; heart defects and mental and physical retardation are common. Also called **cri du chat syndrome.**

catecholamine (kæt'əkəlæm'in), any one of a group of sympathomimetic compounds composed of a catechol molecule and the aliphatic portion of an amine. Some catecholamines are produced naturally by the body and function as key neurological chemicals. Catecholamines are also synthesized as drugs used in the treatment of various disorders, as anaphylaxis, asthma, cardiac failure, and hypertension. Some important endogenous catecholamines are dopamine, epinephrine and norepinephrine. Norepinephrine mediates a host of physiologic and metabolic responses that follow the stimulation of the sympathetic nerves. In response to stress, the adrenal medulla is stimulated, causing the elevation of epinephrine and norepinephrine concentrations in the circulation. Epinephrine dilates blood vessels to the skeletal muscles. Norepinephrine slightly constricts these blood vessels. Both compounds stimulate the myocardium. Dopamine is found primarily in the basal ganglia of the central nervous system (CNS), but dopaminergic nerve endings and specific receptors for this compound have been found in other CNS areas. The major functions of catecholamines and drugs that mimic their actions include the peripheral excitation of certain muscles, peripheral inhibition of certain muscles, cardiac excitation, metabolic actions, endocrine actions and CNS actions. Differences in the actions of the catecholamines depend on alpha and beta receptors in nerve terminals throughout the body. The brain contains separate neuronal systems that use dopamine, epinephrine, and norepinephrine. More than half of the catecholamine content of the CNS is dopamine, large quantities of which are found in the basal ganglia, the central nucleus of the amygdala, the median eminence, the olfactory tubercle and the restricted fields of the frontal cortex. The hypothalamus and certain zones of the limbic system contain relatively large amounts of norepinephrine, which is also found in lesser amounts in other brain areas. Neurons in the CNS that contain epinephrine are situated primarily in the medullary reticular formation. Catecholamines act directly on sympathetic effector cells by binding to receptors in cellular plasma membranes. Sympathomimetic drugs influence biochemical reactions and functional responses in all the tissues they effect.

cat-eye syndrome, a rare, congenital autosomal anomaly, marked by the presence of an extra, small chromosome 22 and pupils that resemble the vertical pupils of a cat. Anal atresia, heart abnormalities, and severe mental retardation are common.

categorical data, (in research) any data that are classified by name rather than by number, as race, religion, ethnicity, or marital status.

catgut, a nonabsorbable suture material, prepared from the intestines of sheep, used to close surgical wounds. Compare **chromic.**

catharsis (kəthar′sıs), **1.** a cleansing or purging. —**cathartic,** *n.* **2.** the therapeutic release of pent-up feelings and emotions by open discussion of ideas and thoughts. **3.** (in psychoanalysis) the process of bringing repressed ideas and feelings into the consciousness by the technique of free association, often in conjunction with hypnosis and the use of hypnotic drugs. Also called **psychocatharsis.** See also **abreaction.** —**cathartic,** *adj.*

cathartic (kəthar′tık), **1.** of or pertaining to a substance that causes evacuation of the bowel. **2.** a cathartic agent that promotes bowel evacuation by stimulating peristalsis, increasing the fluidity or bulk of intestinal contents, softening the feces, or lubricating the intestinal wall. The term *cathartic* implies a fluid evacuation; this is in contrast to *laxative,* which implies the elimination of a soft, formed stool. Cathartics that increase peristalsis, usually by irritating intestinal mucosa, include certain plant substances, as aloe, colocynth, croton oil, podophyllum senna, phenolphthalein, bisacodyl, and dehydrocholic acid. Saline cathartics, as sodium sulfate, magnesium sulfate, and magnesium hydroxide, dilute the intestinal contents by retaining water through osmotic forces. Suppositories containing sodium biphosphate, sodium acid pyrophosphate, and sodium bicarbonate induce defecation when the salts react to form carbon dioxide and the expanding gas stimulates peristalsis. Also called **coprogogue.** See also **laxative.** —**catharsis,** *n.*

-cathartic, a combining form meaning 'pertaining to cleaning': *cephalocathartic, emetocathartic, hematocathartic.*

catheter (kæth′ıtər), a hollow, flexible tube that can be inserted into a vessel or cavity of the body to withdraw or to instill fluids. Most catheters are made of soft plastic or rubber and may be used for treatment or diagnosis. Kinds of catheters include **acorn-tipped catheter, Foley's catheter, intrauterine catheter.**

Single-holed straight

Multiple-holed straight

Double-lumen cuffed (Foley)
CATHETERS

catheterization (kæth′ətərızei′shən), the introduction of a catheter into a body cavity or organ to inject or remove a fluid. The most common procedure is the insertion of a catheter into the bladder through the urethra for the relief of urinary retention and for emptying the bladder completely before surgery. It is also used when a urine specimen may otherwise be contaminated, as when a woman is menstruating. Self-catheterization is taught to those patients with neurogenic bladder. Sterile, aseptic techniques are necessary to prevent infection; trauma is also to be avoided, particularly to the male urethra and when the procedure is performed on children, who are frightened by the technique and cannot cooperate. For indwelling catheters, attention is given to maintaining continuous free drainage and to the increased possibility of infection. Frequent washing of the area surrounding the urinary meatus reduces the risk of infection and eliminates unpleasant odors and irritation. Kinds of catheterization are **cardiac catheterization, hepatic vein catheterization, laryngeal catheterization.** See also **Foley catheter.** —**catheterize,** *v.*

cathexis (kəthek′sıs), the conscious or unconscious attachment of emotional feeling and importance to a specific idea, person, or object. —**cathectic,** *adj.*

cathode ray, a stream of electrons emitted by the negative electrode of a gaseous discharge device when the cathode is bombarded by positive ions, as in a cathode ray tube, an oscilloscope, and a television picture tube. The ray itself is usually focused by a series of electromagnets that control its direction and position on a screen coated with a phosphor in order to create a visible pattern.

cathode ray oscilloscope, an instrument that produces a visual representation of electrical variations by means of the fluorescent screen of a cathode-ray tube. Oscilloscopes have many applications in medicine and in nursing, as the displaying of patients' brain waves and heart beats for monitoring and diagnostic purposes.

cation (kæt′aiən), a positively charged ion that in solution is attracted to the negative electrode.

cation exchange resin, any one of various insoluble organic polymers with high molecular weights that exchange their cations for other ions in solution. Cation exchange resins are used especially to restrict intestinal sodium absorption in patients with edema. Compare **anion exchange resin.**

catling, catlin, a long, sharp, double-edged knife used in amputation.

catoptric (kətop′trık), of or pertaining to a reflected image.

CAT scan. See **computerized axial tomography.**

cat-scratch fever, a disease that results from the scratch or bite of a healthy cat. Inflammation and pustules are found on the scratched skin and lymph nodes in the neck, head, groin, or axilla swell two weeks later. Although patients are rarely ill, fever and malaise may occur. No treatment is required. The cat-scratch skin test is available to help in the diagnosis. Also called **cat-scratch disease.**

cat's eye amaurosis, a monocular blindness, with a bright reflection from the pupil caused by a white mass in the vitreous humor resulting from inflammation or a malignant lesion.

caud-, a combining form meaning 'pertaining to a tail': *caudal, caudalward, caudocephalad.*

caudad (kɔ'dæd), toward the tail or end of the body, away from the head. Compare **cephalad.**

cauda equina, the lower end of the spinal cord at the first lumbar vertebrae and the bundle of lumbar, sacral, and coccygeal nerve roots that emerge from the spinal cord and descend through the spinal canal of the sacrum and coccyx before reaching the intervertebral foramina of their particular vertebrae. The cauda equina looks like a horse's tail.

caudal, signifying a position toward the distal end of the spine.

caudal anesthesia, the injection of a local anesthetic agent into the caudal portion of the spinal canal through the sacrum. It is performed in labor and delivery and in such procedures as culdoscopy and anorectal and genitourinary surgery. Caudal anesthesia has largely been replaced by epidural anesthesia because of the difficulty of controlling the level of anesthesia, the need for large volumes (10-15 ml) of anesthetic solution, a high, five to ten per cent rate of failure, frequent neurologic complications, arterial hypotension, and, in obstetrics, reduced force of labor. Other complications of caudal anesthesia include maternal infection and inadvertent injection into the fetus. See also **regional anesthesia.**

caudate, having a tail.

caudate process, a small elevation of tissue that extends obliquely from the lower extremity of the caudate lobe of the liver to the visceral surface of the right lobe. It separates the fossa for the gall bladder from the beginning of the fossa for the inferior vena cava.

caul, the intact amniotic sac surrounding the fetus at birth. The sac usually ruptures or is ruptured during the course of labor or delivery; when it remains intact it must be torn or cut to allow the baby to breathe. In the past, pieces of the caul were sold to sailors as a good luck token that would protect the bearer from death by drowning.

cauliflower ear, a thickened, deformed ear caused by repeated trauma, as suffered by boxers. Plastic surgery may be a means of restoring the normal appearance of the ear.

caumesthesia (kɔ'məsthi'źhə), an abnormal condition in which a patient has a low temperature but experiences a sense of intense heat. —**caumesthetic,** *adj.*

causalgia (kɔzæl'jə), a severe sensation of burning pain, often in an extremity, sometimes with local erythema of the skin. It is the result of injury to a peripheral sensory nerve.

causal hypothesis, (in research) a hypothesis that predicts a cause and effect relationship among the variables to be studied.

causal hypothesis testing study, (in nursing research) an experimental design used in testing a hypothesis that predicts a cause-and-effect relationship within the data to be studied.

causality (kɔzæl'ɪti), (in research) a relationship between one phenomenon or event (A) and another (B) in which A precedes and causes B and the direction of influence and the nature of the effect are predictable and reproducible and may be empirically observed. Causality is difficult to prove; some social scientists state that it is impossible to prove a causal relationship.

causal treatment. See **treatment.**

causation, (in law) the existence of a reasonable connection between the misfeasance, malfeasance, or nonfeasance of the defendant and the injury or damage suffered by the plaintiff. In a lawsuit in which negligence is alleged, the harm suffered by the plaintiff must be proven to result directly from the negligence of the defendant; causation must be demonstrated.

cause, any process, substance, or organism that produces an effect or condition.

CAUSN, abbreviation for **Canadian Association of University Schools of Nursing.**

CAUT, abbreviation for **Canadian Association of University Teachers.**

cautery (kɔ'təri), **1.** a device or agent that scars and burns the skin, as in the coagulation of tissue by heat or caustic substances. **2.** a destructive effect produced by a cauterizing agent.

cautery knife, a surgical knife that cuts tissue and cauterizes it to prevent bleeding. The knife is connected to an electrical source which generates the heat necessary for cauterization.

cav-, a combining form meaning 'hollow': *cavascope, cavernome, cavity.*

cavalry bone. See **rider's bone.**

Cavell (kəvel'), **Edith,** (1865-1915), an English nurse who trained at London Hospital. In 1907 she became the head of a nurses' training school in Brussels, with the task of raising nursing standards to match those of Britain. By 1912 the school offered a three-year intensive course and was associated with four hospitals in Brussels. After the Germans occupied Belgium in World War I, she nursed or sheltered more than 200 fleeing soldiers and helped them reach Holland; to her, this was an extension of her nursing: helping those in need. She was arrested by the Germans, tried, and shot on October 12, 1915. Her execution, which she met with courage and fortitude, brought her widespread fame and damaged Germany's reputation.

cavernoma (kæv'ərnou'mə), *pl.* **cavernomas, cavernomata.** See **cavernous hemangioma.**

cavernous, containing cavities or hollow spaces. See also **cavernous hemangioma.**

cavernous angioma. See **cavernous hemangioma.**

cavernous body of the clitoris. See **corpus cavernosum.**

cavernous body of the penis. See **corpus cavernosum.**

cavernous hemangioma, a benign, congenital tumor consisting of large, blood-filled, cystic spaces. The scalp, face, and neck are the most common sites, but these tumors have been found in the liver and other organs. Superficial cavernous hemangiomas are friable and easily infected if the skin is broken. Treatment includes observation, irradiation, sclerosing solutions, and surgery. Compare **capillary hemangioma, port-wine stain.**

cavernous lymphangioma. See **lymphangioma cavernosum.**

cavernous rale, an abnormal hollow, metallic sound heard during auscultation of the thorax. It is caused by contraction and expansion of a pulmonary cavity during respiration and indicates a pathological condition.

cavernous sinus, one of a pair of irregularly shaped, bilateral venous channels between the sphenoid bone of the skull and the dura mater. It is one of the five anterior inferior venous sinuses that drain the blood from the dura mater into the internal jugular vein. Like the other anterior inferior sinuses, the cavernous sinus has no valves. Coursing through the sinus are the oculomotor nerve, the trochlear nerve, the abducent nerve, the ophthalmic and the maxillary divisions of the trigeminal nerve, and the internal carotid artery. The cavernous sinus receives the superior and the inferior ophthalmic veins, some of the cerebral veins, and the sphenoparietal sinus, and joins the cavernous sinus from the opposite side through the intercavernous sinuses. The cavernous sinus drains into the inferior petrosal sinus, thence into the internal jugular vein.

cavernous sinus syndrome, an abnormal condition characterized by edema of the conjunctiva, the upper eyelid, and the root of the nose, and by paralysis of the third, the fourth, and the sixth nerves. It is caused by a thrombosis of the cavernous sinus.

cavernous sinus thrombosis, a syndrome, usually secondary to infections near the eye or nose, characterized by orbital edema, venous congestion of the eye, and palsy of the nerves supplying the extraocular muscles. The infection may spread to involve the cerebrospinal fluid and meninges. Treatment is with antibiotics and, sometimes, with anticoagulants. Prevention includes avoidance of squeezing pimples and other skin lesions in the area of the nose and central face.

cavitary, 1. denoting the presence of one or more cavities. 2. any entozoon having a body cavity or an alimentary canal.

cavitate, the act of rapidly forming and collapsing vapor pockets in a flowing fluid with low pressure areas, often causing damage to surrounding structures.

cavitation, 1. the formation of cavities within the body, as those formed in the lung by tuberculosis. 2. any cavity within the body, as the pleural cavities.

cavity, 1. a hollow space within a larger structure, as the peritoneal cavity or the oral cavity. 2. *Nontechnical.* a space in a tooth formed by dental caries.

cavogram (kæv'əgræm), an angiogram of the inferior or superior vena cava.

cavum (kei'vəm), *pl.* **cava** (kə'va). 1. any hollow or cavity. 2. the inferior or superior vena cava.

CBC, abbreviation for **complete blood count.**

CBF, abbreviation for *cerebral blood flow.*

CBS, abbreviation for **chronic brain syndrome.**

CCU, abbreviation for **coronary care unit.**

Cd, symbol for **cadmium.**

CDC, abbreviation for **Center for Disease Control.**

Ce, symbol for **cerium.**

CEA, abbreviation for **carcinoembryonic antigen.** *p172*

ceasmic (siæz'mɪk), pertaining to or characterized by a fissure or abnormal cleavage of parts.

ceasmic teratism, a congenital anomaly, caused by developmental arrest, in which parts of the body that should be fused remain in their fissured embryonic state, as in cleft palate.

cec-, a combining form meaning 'pertaining to a cecum': *cecitis, cecectomy, cecoplication.*

cecal, caecal (si'kəl), 1. of or pertaining to the cecum. 2. of or pertaining to the optic disc or the blind spot in the retina.

cecal appendix. See **vermiform appendix.**

Ceclor, a trade name for a cephalosporin antibiotic (cefaclor).

cecocolostomy, 1. a surgical operation that creates an anastomosis between the cecum and the colon. 2. the anastomosis produced by this operation.

cecofixation. See **cecopexy.**

cecoileostomy (si'koʊɪl'ios'təmi), a surgical operation that connects the ileum with the cecum. Also called **ileocecostomy.**

cecopexy, a surgical operation that fixes or suspends the cecum to correct its excessive mobility. Also called **cecofixation.**

cecostomy (sikos'təmi), the surgical construction of an opening into the cecum, performed as a temporary measure to relieve intestinal obstruction in a patient who cannot tolerate major surgery. Twenty-four hours before surgery, if time permits, a low residue diet is given with only clear liquids allowed. Cleansing enemas and antibiotics are prescribed to reduce the number of bacteria in the bowel. I.V. fluids and electrolytes are given, and a nasointestinal tube is inserted. With the patient under local anesthesia, a tube is inserted into the cecum to allow drainage of feces. The procedure may also be done to decompress the large bowel and prevent distention until peristalsis is restored after intestinal surgery. Postoperatively, the tube is connected to a drainage bottle. The nurse irrigates the cecostomy tube with saline solution as necessary, allowing the solution to flow in and out by gravity, if possible. Frequent changes of dressings are needed to keep the skin clean and dry. An ileostomy bag may be used. When edema and inflammation have subsided, the obstruction (usually cancer) is resected, the healthy sections of bowel reconnected, and the cecostomy closed. See also **abdominal surgery, intestinal obstruction.**

cecum (si'kəm), a cul-de-sac constituting the first part of the large intestine.

Cedilanid, a trade name for a cardiotonic (lanatoside C).

Cedilanid-D, a trade name for a cardiotonic (deslanoside).

CeeNU, a trade name for an antineoplastic (lomustine).

Ceepryn, a trade name for a topical anti-infective (cetylpyridinium chloride).

cefaclor, a cephalosporin antibiotic.

■ INDICATIONS: It is prescribed in the treatment of certain infections.

■ CONTRAINDICATIONS: Known hypersensitivity to cephalosporins prohibits its use. It is administered with caution to patients with a history of allergy to penicillins.

■ ADVERSE EFFECTS: Among the most serious adverse reactions are hypersensitivity reactions and severe diarrhea, nausea, and vomiting.

cefadroxil monohydrate, a cephalosporin antibiotic.

■ INDICATIONS: It is prescribed in the treatment of certain bacterial infections.

■ CONTRAINDICATIONS: Known hypersensitivity to cephalosporins prohibits its use. It is administered with caution to patients with a history of allergy to penicillins.

■ ADVERSE EFFECTS: Among the most serious adverse reactions are hypersensitivity reactions and severe diarrhea, nausea, and vomiting.

cefamandole nafate, a cephalosporin antibiotic.

■ INDICATIONS: It is prescribed in the treatment of certain bacterial infections.

■ CONTRAINDICATIONS: Known hypersensitivity to cephalosporins prohibits its use. It is administered with caution to patients with a history of allergy to penicillin.

■ ADVERSE EFFECTS: Among the most serious adverse reactions are various hypersensitivity reactions, phlebitis, suprainfection, and pain on intramuscular injection.

cefazolin sodium, a cephalosporin antibacterial.

■ INDICATIONS: It is prescribed in the treatment of a variety of infections.

■ CONTRAINDICATIONS: Known hypersensitivity to this

drug or to any cephalosporin medication prohibits its use. It is used with caution in patients who are allergic to penicillin.

■ ADVERSE EFFECTS: Among the more serious adverse reactions are pain at the site of injection and hypersensitivity reactions.

cefoxitin sodium, a cephalosporin antibiotic.

■ INDICATIONS: It is prescribed in the treatment of certain bacterial infections.

■ CONTRAINDICATIONS: Known hypersensitivity to cephalosporins prohibits its use. It is administered with caution to patients with a history of allergy to penicillins.

■ ADVERSE EFFECTS: Among the most serious adverse reactions are various hypersensitivity reactions, phlebitis, suprainfection, and pain on intramuscular injection.

cel-, coel-[1], a combining form meaning 'a cavity of the body': *celarium, celoschisis, celozoic.*

cel-, coel-[2], a combining form meaning 'a swelling or tumor, hernia': *celectome, celology, celosomia.*

-cele[1], a combining form meaning a 'tumor or swelling': *hematoscheocele, oodeocele, tracheocele.*

-cele[2], a combining form meaning a 'cavity': *paracele, orchidocele, syringocele.* Also **-coel, -coele.**

Celestone, a trade name for a glucocorticoid (betamethasone).

celiac artery, a thick visceral branch of the abdominal aorta, arising caudal to the diaphragm, usually dividing into the left gastric, the common hepatic, and the splenic arteries.

celiac disease, a chronic inability to tolerate foods containing gluten or wheat protein. The disease affects adults and young children, who suffer from abdominal distention, vomiting, diarrhea, muscle wasting, and extreme lethargy. A characteristic sign is a pale, foul-smelling stool that floats on water owing to its high fat content. There may be a secondary lactose intolerance, and it may become necessary to eliminate all milk products from the diet. Most patients respond well to a high-protein, high-calorie, gluten-free diet. Rice and corn are good substitutes for wheat, and any vitamin or mineral deficiencies can be corrected with oral preparations. Prognosis for full recovery is excellent. Failure to respond generally indicates misdiagnosis. Also called **celiac sprue, nontropical sprue.** Compare **malabsorption syndrome.**

celiac plexus. See **solar plexus.**

celiac rickets, arrested growth and osseous deformities resulting from malabsorption of fat and calcium. See **celiac disease, rickets.**

celio-, a combining form meaning 'pertaining to the abdomen': *celioma, celiopathy, celiorrhaphy.*

celiocolpotomy, an incision into the abdomen through the vagina.

celioma (si'liou'mə), *pl.* **celiomas, celiomata.** an abdomi-

Some major cell structures and their functions

Cell structures	Functions
Cytoplasmic membrane	Serves as the boundary of the cell, maintaining its integrity; protein molecules on outer surface of cytoplasmic membrane perform various functions, for example, they serve as markers that identify cells of each individual, receptor molecules for certain hormones and neurotransmitters provide means of communication between cells, receptor molecules for foreign proteins function to produce immunity
Endoplasmic reticulum (ER)	Serves as a cell's own circulatory system
Golgi apparatus	Synthesizes carbohydrate, combines it with protein, and packages the product as globules of glycoprotein
Mitochondria	Catabolism; ATP synthesis; a cell's "powerhouse"
Lysosomes	A cell's "digestive system"
Ribosomes	Synthesize proteins; a cell's "protein factory"
Nucleus	Dictates protein synthesis, thereby playing essential role in other cell activities, namely, active transport, metabolism, growth, and heredity
Nucleoli	Play essential role in the formation of ribosomes

nal neoplasm, especially a mesothelial tumor of the peritoneum.

celioscope. See **laparoscope.**

celiothelioma (si′lioʊθhi′lioʊ′mə), *pl.* **celiotheliomas, celiotheliomata.** a mesothelioma of the abdomen.

cell, the fundamental unit of all living tissue. Each cell consists of a nucleus, cytoplasm, and organelles surrounded by a cytoplasmic membrane. Within the nucleus are the nucleolus (containing RNA), and chromatin granules (containing protein and DNA) which develop into chromosomes, the determinants of hereditary characteristics. Organelles within the cytoplasm include the endoplasmic reticulum, ribosomes, the Golgi complex, mitochondria, lysosomes, and the centrosome. The specialized nature of body tissue reflects the specialized structure and function of its constituent cells.

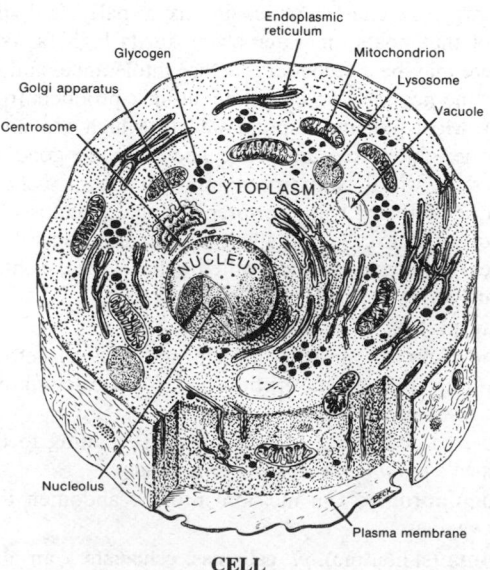

CELL

cella (sǝl′ǝ), *pl.* **cellae.** an enclosed space.

cell biology, the science that deals with the structures, living processes, and functions of cells, especially human cells.

cell body, the part of a cell that contains the nucleus and surrounding cytoplasm exclusive of any projections or processes, as the axon and dendrites of a neuron or the tail of a spermatozoon. This enlarged area is concerned more with the metabolism of the cell than with a specific function.

cell death, **1.** terminal failure of a cell to maintain the essential life functions. **2.** the point in the process of dying at which vital functions have ceased at the cellular level.

cell division, the continuous process by which a cell divides in four stages; prophase, metaphase, anaphase, and telophase. Preliminary to prophase the centrosome of the cell divides into two parts which become oriented at opposite poles of the nucleus. During the prophase, previously dispersed chromatin condenses into chromomeres strung along a threadlike chromonema composed of deoxyribonucleic acid. The chromonema then condenses into compact chromosomes. During metaphase, the chromosomes become oriented in the equatorial plate with a clear area directed toward the two centrosomes. Each chromosome meanwhile has doubled into chromatids attached to each other at the centromere. Each centromere divides during late metaphase and early anaphase. In telophase, the chromosomes form a compact mass, lose their individuality, and disperse into the chromatin of the intermitotic nucleus. Also called **mitosis.**

cell line, a colony of animal cells developed as a subculture from a primary culture.

cell-mediated immune response, a delayed type IV hypersensitivity reaction, mediated primarily by sensitized T cell lymphocytes as opposed to antibodies. Cell-mediated immune reactions are responsible for defense against certain bacterial, fungal, and viral pathogens, malignant cells, and other foreign protein or tissue.

cell-mediated immunity. See **cellular immunity.**

cell membrane, the outer covering of a cell, often having projecting microvilli and containing the cellular cytoplasm. The cell membrane is so thin and delicate it is barely visible with a light microscope and can be studied in detail only with an electron microscope. The membrane controls the exchange of materials between the cell and its environment by various processes, as osmosis, phagocytosis, pinocytosis, and secretion. Also called **plasma membrane.**

cell theory, the proposition that cells are the basic units of all living substance and that cellular function is the essential process of life.

cellular hypersensitivity reaction, type IV hypersensitivity. See **cell-mediated immune response.**

cellular immunity, the mechanism of acquired immunity characterized by the dominant role of small T cell lymphocytes. Cellular immunity is involved in resistance to infectious diseases caused by viruses and some bacteria, and in delayed hypersensitivity reactions, some aspects of resistance to cancer, certain autoimmune diseases, graft rejection, and certain allergies. Also called **cell-mediated immunity.** Compare **humoral immunity.**

cellular infiltration, the migration and grouping of cells within tissues throughout the body.

cellulitis, an infection of the skin characterized most commonly by local heat, redness, pain, and swelling, and occasionally by fever, malaise, chills, and headache. Abscess and tissue destruction usually follow if antibiotics are not taken. Damaged skin, poor circulation, and diabetes mellitus favor the development of cellulitis. Treatment in addition to appropriate antibiotics includes warm soaks and avoidance of pressure to the affected areas.

cellulose (sel′yulous), a colorless, insoluble, nondigestible, transparent solid carbohydrate that is the primary constituent of the skeletal substances of the cell walls of plants. In the diet it provides the bulk necessary for proper gastrointestinal functioning. Rich sources are fruits, as apples and bananas, legumes, bran, and green vegetables, especially celery. See also **dietary fiber.**

cell wall, the structure that covers and protects the cell membrane of some kinds of cells, as certain bacteria and all plant cells. The cell walls of plant cells are composed of cellulose.

celom. See **coelom.**

Celontin, a trade name for an anticonvulsant (methsuximide).

celosomia (si′losou′mia), a congenital malformation characterized by a fissure or the absence of the sternum and ribs and protrusion of the viscera.

celosomus (si′losou′mos), a fetus with celosomia.

celothelioma (si′louthi′liou′mə), *pl.* **celotheliomas, celotheliomata.** See **mesothelioma.**

Celsius (C) (sel′sias), denoting a temperature scale in which 0° is the freezing point of water and 100° is the boiling point of water at sea level. Also called **centigrade.** Compare **Fahrenheit.**

cement, 1. a sticky or mucilaginous substance that helps neighboring tissue cells stick together. 2. any of a variety of dental materials used to fill cavities or to hold bridgework or other dental prostheses in place. 3. a material used in the fixation of a prosthetic joint in adjacent bone, as methyl mathacrylate.

cementifying fibroma, a fibrous tumor containing masses of calcified tissue, occurring most frequently in the mandible of older people.

cementoblastoma (simen′toublæstou′mə), *pl.* **cementoblastomas, cementoblastomata.** an odontogenic fibrous tumor consisting of cells developing into cementoblasts but containing only a small amount of calcified tissue.

cementoma (si′mentou′mə), *pl.* **cementomas, cementomata.** an accumulation of cementum existing free at the apex of a tooth, probably caused by trauma rather than neoplastic growth.

cementum, the bonelike connective tissue that covers the roots of the teeth and helps to support them.

cen-, a combining form meaning 'common': *cenadelphus, cenesthesia, cenesthopathia.*

cenesthesia (si′nosfhi′žhə), **coenesthesia,** the general sense of existing, derived as the aggregate of all the various stimuli and reactions throughout the body at any specific moment to produce a feeling of health or of illness. Also called **cenesthesis, coenesthesis.**

cenesthesis, coenesthesis (sen′osfhi′sis). See **cenesthesia.**

ceno-, a combining form meaning 'new': *cenogenesis, cenophobia, cenopsychic.*

cenogenesis, coenogenesis, caenogenesis, kenogenesis, the development of structural characteristics that are absent in earlier forms of a species, as an adaptive response to environmental conditions. Compare **palingenesis.** – **cenogenetic, coenogenetic, caenogenetic,** *adj.*

cenophobia. See **kenophobia.**

censor, 1. a person who monitors or evaluates books, newspapers, plays, works of art, speech, or other means of expression in order to suppress certain kinds of information. 2. (in psychoanalysis) a psychic supression that allows unconscious thoughts to rise to consciousness only if they are heavily disguised.

cente-, a combining form meaning 'puncture': *centesis.*

center, centre, 1. the middle point of the body or geometric entity, equidistant from points on the periphery. 2. a group of neurons with a common function, as the accelerating center in the brain which controls the heartbeat.

Center for Disease Control (CDC), a federal agency of the United States government that provides facilities and services for the investigation, identification, prevention, and control of disease. It is concerned with all aspects of the epidemiology and the laboratory diagnosis of disease. Immunization programs, quarantine regulations and programs, laboratory standards, and community surveillance for disease are among the activities of the CDC, which is located in Atlanta, Georgia. Many state and local health workers and scientists receive training in specific techniques there. Formerly, the Communicable Disease Center, it was concerned only with communicable diseases; today its interests include environmental health, smoking, malnutrition, poisoning, and issues in occupational health.

centesis (senti′sis), a perforation or a puncture, as a paracentesis, abdominocentesis, or thoracocentesis.

centi-, a combining form meaning 'a hundred or a hundredth': *centibar, centiliter, centipoise.*

centigrade (C). See **Celsius.**

centimeter (cm) (sen′timi′tər), the metric unit of measurement equal to one hundredth of a meter, or .3937 inches.

centimeter-gram-second system (CGS, cgs), the internationally accepted scientific system of expressing length, mass, and time in basic units of centimeters, grams, and seconds. The CGS system is gradually being replaced by the Système Internationale d'Unites (SI) or the International System of Units based on the meter, kilogram, and second.

centipede bite, a wound produced by the poison claws and the first body segment of a centipede, an elongate arthropod with many pairs of legs. The bite of a few species, including *Scolopendra morsitans* in the southern United States, may cause painful local inflammation, fever, headache, vomiting, and dizziness.

central, of pertaining to, or situated at a center.

central amaurosis, blindness caused by a disease of the central nervous system.

central canal of spinal cord, the conduit that runs the entire length of the spinal cord and contains most of the 140 milliliters of cerebrospinal fluid in the body of the average individual. The central canal of the spinal cord lies in the center of the cord between the ventral and the dorsal gray commissures and extends cranialward into the medulla oblongata where it opens into the fourth ventricle of the brain. Caudalward, the canal runs into the filum terminale after forming a triangular, fusiform dilation about 10 mm long in the conus medullaris. Cerebrospinal fluid flows into the canal from the fourth ventricle of the brain, into the subarachnoid space around the spinal cord, and into the subarachnoid space around the brain. Subarachnoid hemorrhage may form blood clots that block drainage of the cerebrospinal fluid from the subarachnoid space. Lumbar puncture, often performed to obtain samples of cerebrospinal fluid for diagnostic purposes, draws fluid from the subarachnoid space around the spinal cord and not from the central canal. See also **lumbar puncture.**

central chondrosarcoma, a malignant cartilaginous tumor that forms inside a bone. Also called **enchondrosarcoma.**

central fissure. See **central sulcus.**

central implantation. See **superficial implantation.**

central lobe, one of the five lobes constituting each of the cerebral hemispheres, lying hidden in the depths of the lateral sulcus. The central lobe can be seen only if the lips of the sulcus are parted or cut away. The lips of the lateral sulcus are parts of the frontal, the parietal, and the temporal lobes and are separated by the rami of the lateral sulcus, thus constituting the frontal, the parietal, and the temporal opercula. With the opercula cut away, the insula appears as a triangular area with the limen insulae as the apex. Compare **frontal lobe, occipital lobe, parietal lobe, temporal lobe.**

central nervous system (CNS), one of the two main divisions of the nervous system of the body, consisting of the brain and the spinal cord. The central nervous system processes information to and from the peripheral nervous system and is the main network of coordination and control for the entire body. The brain controls many functions and sensations, as sleep, sexual activity, muscular movement, hunger, thirst, memory, and the emotions. The spinal cord extends various types of nerve fibers from the brain and acts as a switching and relay terminal for the peripheral nervous system. The 12 pairs of cranial nerves emerge directly from the brain. Sensory nerves and motor nerves of the peripheral system leave the spinal cord separately between the vertebrae but unite to form 31 pairs of spinal nerves containing sensory fibers and motor fibers. More than ten billion neurons constitute but one tenth of the brain cells, the other cells consisting of neuroglia. The neurons and the neuroglia form the soft, jellylike substance of the brain, which is supported and protected by the skull. Flowing through various cavities of the CNS, as the ventricles of the brain, the subarachnoid spaces of the brain and spinal cord, and the central canal of the spinal cord is the cerebrospinal fluid. This fluid helps to protect surrounding structures and affects the rate of respiration through changes in its content of carbon dioxide. The brain and the spinal cord are composed of gray matter and white matter. The gray matter contains primarily nerve cells and associated processes; the white matter consists of bundles of predominantly unmyelinated nerve fibers. The central nervous system develops from the embryonic neural tube, which first appears as the neural folds in the third week of pregnancy. The cavity of the neural tube is retained after birth in the ventricles of the brain and in the central canal of the spinal cord. Compare **peripheral nervous system**. See also **brain, spinal cord.**

central nervous system depressants, any drug that decreases the function of the central nervous system (CNS), as alcohol, barbiturates, and hypnotics. Such drugs can produce tolerance, physical dependence, and compulsive drug use. The compulsive use of barbiturates, benzodiazepines, and related drugs varies greatly and is believed to exceed that of the opiates. Depressants, especially the benzodiazepines, are the most widely prescribed drugs throughout the world. These substances depress excitable tissue throughout the CNS by stabilizing neuronal membranes, decreasing the amount of transmitter released by the nerve impulse, and generally depressing postsynaptic responsiveness and ion movement. The CNS is more affected by alcohol than any other body system, the effects generally proportional to the concentration of alcohol in the blood. Central nervous system depressants elevate the seizure threshold and can produce physical dependence in a relatively short period of time. All depressants are subject to abuse, and a recent marked increase in the use of illicitly procured depressants has been noted in some adolescent and preadolescent populations. The most abused depressants are the short-acting barbiturates, especially pentobarbital, secobarbital, glutethimide, methyprylon, and methaqualone. These substances have popular street names on the illicit market, as "reds" (secobarbital) and "yellows" (pentobarbital). Withdrawal of general CNS depressants that have been used in high doses for prolonged periods can be fatal to some individuals. Withdrawal treatment commonly involves the substitution of pentobarbital administered orally to produce a stabilization level followed by gradual reduction in dosage for a period of 10 days to 3 weeks.

central nervous system stimulant, a substance that quickens the activity of the central nervous system (CNS) by increasing the rate of neuronal discharge or by blocking an inhibitory neurotransmitter. Many natural and synthetic compounds stimulate the CNS but only a few are used therapeutically. Caffeine, a potent CNS stimulant, is used to help restore mental alertness and overcome respiratory depression, but it may cause nausea, nervousness, tinnitus, tremor, tachycardia, extra systoles, diuresis, and scintillating scotoma. Amphetamines, sympathomimetic amines with CNS-stimulating activity, are employed in treating narcolepsy and obesity, but these drugs have a high potential for abuse and may cause dizziness, restlessness, tachycardia, increased blood pressure, headache, mouth dryness, an unpleasant taste, gastrointestinal symptoms, and urticaria. Various amphetamines, especially methylphenidate, and deanol acetamidobenzoate, a precursor of acetylcholine, are prescribed for the hyperkinetic child syndrome. Doxapram, ethamivan, and nikethamide are used to stimulate the respiratory center and restore consciousness following anesthesia or in the treatment of acute sedative-hypnotic intoxication. Flurothyl is employed in convulsive therapy in psychiatry.

central nervous system syndrome (CNS syndrome), a constellation of neurologic and emotional signs and symptoms that results from a massive whole-body dosage of radiation. The syndrome includes hysteria and disorientation, increasing during the last 24 to 48 hours before death.

central nervous system tumor, a neoplasm of the brain or spinal cord that characteristically does not spread beyond the cerebrospinal axis, although it may be highly invasive locally and have widespread effects on body functions. Intracranial neoplasms are about four times more common than those arising in the spinal cord. From 20 to 40 per cent of brain tumors are metastatic lesions from primary cancer in the breast, lung, gastrointestinal tract, kidney, or a site of melanoma. See also **brain tumor, spinal cord tumor.**

central neuritis. See **parenchymatous neuritis.**

central placenta previa, placenta previa in which the placenta is implanted in the lower segment of the uterus and completely covers the internal os of the uterine cervix. In labor, as the cervix dilates, the placenta is gradually separated from the underlying blood vessels in the uterine lining, resulting in bleeding that usually begins slowly, is painless, and progresses to hemorrhage that is life-threatening to the mother and the baby. Caesarean section is usually performed to save the mother and the baby. The condition may be discovered before any bleeding occurs by ultrasound visualization or by digital palpation in the normal course of prenatal care.

central scotoma, an area of blindness or site of depressed vision involving the macula of the retina.

central stimulant. See **central nervous system stimulant.**

central sulcus, a cleft separating the frontal from the parietal lobes of brain. Also called **central fissure, fissure of Rolando.**

central venous pressure (CVP) monitor, a device for measuring and recording the venous blood pressure by means of an indwelling catheter and a pressure manometer. It is used to evaluate the right ventricular function, the right atrial filling pressure, and the capacity of the blood vessels.

central vision, vision that results from images falling on the macula of the retina.

centrencephalic (sen′trensɪfæl′ɪk), of, pertaining to, or involving the center of the encephalon.

centri-. See **centro-.**

centrifugal (sentrɪf′ugəl), **1.** denoting a force that is directed outward, away from a central point or axis, as the force that keeps the moon in its orbit around the earth. **2.** a direction away from the head.

centrifugal current, an electric current in the body with the positive pole near the nerve center and the negative pole at the periphery. Also called **descending current.**

centrifuge (sen'trɪfyuj'), a device for separating components of different densities contained in liquid by spinning them at high speeds. Centrifugal force causes the heavier components to move to one part of the container, leaving the lighter substances in another. — **centrifugal,** *adj.,* **centrifuge,** *v.*

centrilobular (sen'trəlob'yələr), of, pertaining to, or situated at the center of a lobule.

centriole (sen'trioul'), an intracellular organelle, usually as a component of the centrosome. Usually occurring in pairs, centrioles are associated with cell division and can be closely studied only with an electron microscope; under light microscope the centrioles appear as tiny dots. They are actually tiny cylinders positioned at right angles to each other, with walls consisting of nine bundles of fine tubules, three tubules to a bundle. The centriole measures approximately 150 millimicrons by 300 to 500 millimicrons. Numerous centrioles occur in some large cells, as the giant cells in bone marrow. The precise function of centrioles is still a mystery, but they appear to aid in the formation of the spindle that develops during mitosis.

centripetal (sentrɪp'ətəl), **1.** denoting an afferent direction, as that of a sensory nerve impulse traveling toward the brain. **2.** denoting the direction of a force pulling an object toward an axis of rotation or constraining an object to a specific curved path.

centripetal current, an electric current passing through the body from a peripheral positive electrode to a negative pole near the nerve center. Also called **ascending current.**

centro-, centri-, a combining form meaning 'center': *centrocecal, centrocinesia, centrosclerosis.*

centromere (sen'trəmir), the specialized, constricted region of the chromosome that joins the two chromatids to each other and attaches to the spindle fiber in mitosis and meiosis. During cell division the centromeres split longitudinally, half going to each of the new daughter chromosomes. The position of the centromere is constant for a specific chromosome and is identified accordingly as acrocentric, metacentric, subcentric, or telocentric. Also called **kinetochore, kinomere, primary constriction.** — **centromeric,** *adj.*

centrosome, a self-propagating cytoplasmic organelle present in animal cells and in those of some lower plants. The structure, which consists of the centrosphere and the centrioles, is located near the nucleus and functions as the dynamic center of the cell, especially during mitosis. Also called **cytocentrum, microcentrum, paranuclear body.**

centrosphere, the differentiated, condensed area of cytoplasm surrounding the centrioles in the centrosome of the cell.

centrum (sen'trəm), *pl.* **centra.** any kind of center, especially one related to a structure of the body, as the centrum semiovale of a cerebral hemisphere.

CEO, C.E.O., abbreviation for **Chief Executive Officer.**

cephal-. See **cephalo.**

cephalad (sef'əlæd), toward the head, away from the end, or tail. Compare **caudad.**

cephalalgia (sef'əlæl'jiə), headache, often combined with another word to indicate a specific type of headache, as histamine cephalalgia. See **histamine headache.**

cephalexin (sef'əlek'sɪn), a cephalosporin antibacterial.

■ INDICATIONS: It is prescribed orally in the treatment of certain infections.

■ CONTRAINDICATIONS: Known hypersensitivity to this drug or to any cephalosporin medication prohibits its use. It is used with caution in patients who are allergic to penicillin.

■ ADVERSE EFFECTS: Nausea, diarrhea, and hypersensitivity reactions may occur.

cephalhematoma (sef'əlhi'mətou'mə, sef'əlhem'ətou'mə), swelling owing to subcutaneous bleeding and accumulation of blood. It may begin to form in the scalp of a fetus during labor and enlarge slowly in the first few days after birth. It is usually a result of trauma, often from forceps. Large cephalhematomas may become infected, require surgical drainage, and take several months to resolve. Compare **caput succedaneum, molding.**

-cephalia, a combining form meaning '(condition of the) head': *hemicephalia, megacephalia, notancephalia.*

cephalic (sɪfæl'ɪk), of or pertaining to the head.

-cephalic, a combining form meaning 'relating to the head': *holocephalic, megalocephalic, postcephalic.*

cephalic presentation, a classification of fetal position in which the head of the fetus is at the uterine cervix. Cephalic presentation is usually further qualified by an indication of the part of the head presenting, as the occiput, bregma, or mentum.

cephalic vein, one of the four superficial veins of the upper limb. It begins in the dorsal venous network of the hand and winds upward to end in the axillary vein just caudal to the clavicle. It receives deoxygenated blood from the dorsal and the palmar surfaces of the forearm. Just distal to the antecubital fossa, it has a wide anastomosis with the median cubital vein. In the proximal third of the arm it passes between the pectoralis major and the deltoideus where it is accompanied by the thoracoacromial artery. Compare **basilic vein, dorsal digital vein, median antebrachial vein.**

cephalo-, cephal-, a combining form meaning 'pertaining to the head': *cephalocaudal, cephalocentesis, cephalogenesis.*

cephaloglycin (sef'əlouglai'sɪn), a cephalosporin antibiotic.

■ INDICATIONS: It is prescribed in the oral treatment of

certain infections. The use of this drug has been superseded by other cephalosporins.

■ CONTRAINDICATIONS: Known hypersensitivity to this drug or to cephalosporin medication prohibits its use. It is used with caution in patients who are allergic to penicillin.

■ ADVERSE EFFECTS: Diarrhea, gastrointestinal disturbances, and hypersensitivity reactions may occur.

cephalomelus (sef'əlom'ələs), a deformed individual with a structure resembling an arm or a leg protruding from the head.

cephalometry, scientific measurement of the head, as that performed in dentistry to determine appropriate orthodontic procedures for correcting malocclusions and other abnormal conditions. — **cephalometric,** *adj.*

cephalopagus (scf'əlop'əgəs), *pl.* **cephalopagi.** See **craniopagus.**

cephalopelvic disproportion (CPD), an obstetric condition in which a baby's head is too large or a mother's birth canal too small to permit normal labor or birth. In **relative CPD,** the size of the baby's head is within normal limits but larger than average or the size of the mother's birth canal is within normal limits but smaller than average, or both; relative CPD is often overcome by molding of the head, the forces of labor, or by the use of forceps to effect delivery. In **absolute CPD,** the baby's head is markedly or abnormally enlarged or the mother's birth canal is markedly or abnormally contracted, making vaginal delivery impossible.

cephaloridine, a cephalosporin antibiotic.

■ INDICATIONS: It is prescribed in the treatment of a variety of infections.

■ CONTRAINDICATIONS: Concurrent administration of medications causing nephrotoxicity or known hypersensitivity to this drug or to cephalosporin medication prohibits its use. It is used with caution in patients who are allergic to penicillin.

■ ADVERSE EFFECTS: Among the more serious adverse reactions are nephrotoxicity, pain at the site of injection, and hypersensitivity reactions.

cephalosporin (sef'əlouspor'ın), a semisynthetic derivative of an antibiotic originally derived from the microorganism *Cephalosporium acremonium.* Cephalosporins are similar in structure to penicillins except for a beta-lactam-dihydrothiazine ring in place of beta-lactam-thiazolidin in penicillin.

cephalothin sodium (sef'əlouθın), a cephalosporin antibacterial.

■ INDICATION: It is prescribed in the treatment of a variety of infections.

■ CONTRAINDICATIONS: Known hypersensitivity to this drug or to any cephalosporin medication prohibits its use. It is used with caution in patients who are allergic to penicillin.

■ ADVERSE EFFECTS: Among the more serious adverse reactions are pain at the site of injection and hypersensitivity reactions.

cephalothoracoiliopagus. See **synadelphus.**

cephalothoracopagus (sef'əlouθɔ'rəkop'əgəs), a conjoined twin fetal monster united at the head, neck, and thorax.

-cephaly, a combining form meaning a '(specified) condition of the head': *macrencephaly, platycephaly, trochocephaly.* Also **-cephalia.**

cephradine, a cephalosporin antibacterial.

■ INDICATIONS: It is prescribed in the treatment of certain bacterial infections.

■ CONTRAINDICATIONS: Known hypersensitivity to this drug or to any cephalosporin medication prohibits its use. It is used with caution in patients who are allergic to penicillin.

■ ADVERSE EFFECTS: Nausea, diarrhea, and hypersensitivity reactions may occur.

cer-, a combining form meaning 'wax': *ceraceous, cerate, cerumen.*

cerato-, a combining form meaning 'pertaining to the cornea or to horny tissue': *ceratocricoid, ceratohyal, ceratopharyngeus.* Also **kerato-.**

cercaria (sərker'iə), *pl.* **cercariae.** a minute, wormlike early developmental form of trematode. It develops in a freshwater snail, is released into the water, and swims toward the sun, rising to the surface of the water in the warmest part of the day. Cercariae enter the body of its next host by ingestion, by direct invasion through the skin, or through a cut or other break in the skin. Some cercariae of the genera *Schistosoma, Chlonorchis, Paragonimus, Fasciolopsis,* and *Fasciola* are known to infect man. They encyst and complete their development in various organs of the body. Each species tends to migrate to one organ, as *Fasciola hepatica,* which grows to become a liver fluke. See also **fluke, schistosomiasis.**

cerclage (sərklazh'), 1. an orthopedic procedure in which the ends of an oblique bone fracture or the chips of a broken patella are bound together with a wire loop or a metal band to hold the bone fragments in position until healed. 2. a procedure in which a taut silicone band is applied around the sclera to restore contact between the retina and the choroid when the retina is detached. 3. an obstetric procedure in which a nonabsorbable suture is used for holding the cervix closed to prevent spontaneous abortion in a woman who has an incompetent cervix. The band is usually released when the pregnancy is at full term to allow labor to begin. See also **incompetent cervix.**

cerea flexibilitas (sıri'ə flek'sıbıl'ıtæs'), a cataleptic state, frequently observed in catatonic schizophrenia, in which the limbs retain for an indefinite period of time the positions in which they are placed. Also called **flexibilitas cerea, waxy flexibility.** See also **catalepsy.**

cerebellar (ser′əbel′ər), of or pertaining to the cerebellum.

cerebellar angioblastoma, a tumor in the cerebellum composed of a mass of blood vessels. It may be cystic and is frequently associated with von Hippel-Lindau's disease.

cerebellar cortex, the superficial gray matter of the cerebellum covering the white substance in the medullary core and consisting of two layers, an external molecular layer and an internal granule cell layer. The layers are separated by an incomplete stratum of Purkinje cells. Also called **cortical substance of cerebellum.**

cerebellar cortical degeneration. See **alcoholic nutritional cerebellar degeneration.**

cerebellopontine (ser′əbel′oupon′tain), leading from the cerebellum to the pons varolii.

cerebellospinal (ser′əbel′ouspai′nəl), leading from the cerebellum to the spinal cord.

cerebellum (ser′əbel′əm), *pl.* **cerebellums, cerebella.** the part of the brain located in the posterior cranial fossa behind the brain stem. It consists of two lateral cerebellar hemispheres, or lobes, and a middle section called the vermis. Three pairs of peduncles link it with the brain stem. Its functions are concerned with coordinating voluntary muscular activity.

cerebr-, a combining form meaning 'pertaining to the cerebrum': *cerebralgia, cerebrocardiac, cerebropathy.*

cerebral, of or pertaining to the cerebrum.

-cerebral, a combining form referring to the brain: *craniocerebral, medicerebral, postcerebral.*

cerebral aneurysm, an abnormal localized dilatation of a cerebral artery, most commonly the result of congenital weakness of the media or muscle layer of the vessel wall. Cerebral aneurysms may also be caused by infection, as subacute bacterial endocarditis or syphilis, and by neoplasms, arteriosclerosis, and trauma. The most frequent sites are the middle cerebral, internal carotid, basilar, and anterior cerebral arteries, especially at bifurcations of vessels. Cerebral aneurysms may occur in infancy or old age and may be fusiform dilatations of the entire circumference of an artery or saccular outcroppings of the side of a vessel, which may be as small as a pinhead or as large as an orange but are usually the size of a pea.
■ OBSERVATIONS: Depending on its size and site, a cerebral aneurysm may cause headache, drowsiness, confusion, vertigo, facial weakness and pain, tinnitus, visual impairment, neck stiffness, and monoplegia or hemiplegia. Since about half the cases of cerebral aneurysm rupture, the patient is closely monitored for signs of subarachnoid hemorrhage and increased intracranial pressure. Few aneurysms rupture that are less than one cm in diameter.
■ INTERVENTION: The patient is placed in a bed, in which the head is raised at a 45° degree angle, and is maintained in a quiet, darkened environment. Antifibrinolytic, analgesic, anticonvulsant, antiemetic, or antihypertensive

medication, steroids, and parenteral fluids may be administered as ordered. The pulse, blood pressure, respiration, and neurologic status of the patient are checked frequently. Any sudden change in blood pressure or pupillary response is reported promptly. An icebag may be applied to relieve headache, and hypothermia or cooling measures may be indicated to reduce blood flow to the brain and decrease the risk of rupture of the aneurysm. The patient is turned gently every two to four hours and may need to be fed. Passive range of motion exercises to the extremities are performed to maintain function. A lumbar puncture, which can reveal rupture of the aneurysm if there is blood in the cerebrospinal fluid, and an angiogram, to show the site of the lesion, may be ordered; the contrast medium for angiography can be injected into the carotid artery but placement in a femoral artery is preferred because there is less risk of dislodging a carotid plaque. Surgery, if indicated, involves a craniotomy and the application of a silver clip to the neck of the aneurysm or the use of an electric current to produce thrombosis. If the base of the aneurysm is too large to be ligated, a coating containing methyl methacrylate may be applied to support the weakened artery. When craniotomy is contraindicated, the neurosurgeon may apply a special clamp to a common carotid artery to reduce blood flow to the site of the aneurysm if collateral vessels can supply enough blood to maintain vital brain functions.
■ NURSING CONSIDERATIONS: The patient with a cerebral aneurysm requires intensive care and as little stress as possible. The nurse limits the number of visitors and the length of visits but involves the family in the patient's care and instructions. The patient is almost certain to be anxious about the possibility of rupture of the aneurysm and resultant neurologic problems. This concern may be anticipated by the nurse in order to help the patient express the fear and adapt to the situation.

cerebral angiography, an x-ray procedure for visualizing the vascular system of the brain by injecting a radiopaque contrast material into a carotid, subclavian, brachial, or femoral artery and taking x rays at specific intervals in a series.

cerebral aqueduct, the narrow conduit, between the third and the fourth ventricles in the midbrain, which conveys the cerebrospinal fluid. Also called **aqueduct of Sylvius.**

cerebral cortex, a thin layer of gray matter on the surface of the cerebral hemisphere, folded into gyri with about two thirds of its area buried in fissures. It integrates higher mental functions, general movement, visceral functions, perception, and behavioral reactions. It has been classified many different ways, with reference according to supposed phylogenetic and ontogenetic differences, structure, cell, and fiber layers, and function areas. Research has described more than 200 areas on the basis of differences in myelinated fiber patterns and has defined 47 separate function areas with different cell designs. The precentral cortex or motor area has received special attention because its stimulation with electrodes causes voluntary muscle contractions. A motor speech area in the frontal operculum is better developed in the left hemisphere of right-handed persons, and its destruction causes motor aphasia or speech defects despite healthy, intact vocal organs. The surgical operation of lobotomy isolates the frontal area from the rest of the brain, especially the thalamus, and has been used in the treatment of severe psychoses. Stimulation of the frontal area affects circulation, respiration, pupillary reaction, and other visceral activity. Also called **pallium.**

cerebral dominance, the specialization of each of the two cerebral hemispheres in the integration and control of different functions. In 90 per cent of the population, the left cerebral hemisphere specializes in or dominates the ability to speak and write and the ability to understand spoken and written words. The areas that control these activities are situated in the frontal, parietal, and temporal lobes of the left hemisphere. In the other 10 per cent of the population, either the right hemisphere or both hemispheres dominate the speech and writing abilities. The right cerebral hemisphere dominates the integration of certain sounds other than those associated with speaking, as the sounds of coughing, laughter, crying, and melodies. The right cerebral hemisphere perceives tactual stimuli and visual spatial relationships better than the left cerebral hemisphere. See also **Brodmann's areas.**

cerebral embolism, a cerebrovascular accident caused by an embolus that blocks the flow of blood through the vessels of the cerebrum, resulting in tissue ischemia distal to the occlusion. See also **cerebrovascular accident.**

cerebral gigantism, an abnormal condition characterized by excessive weight and size at birth, accelerated growth during the first four or five years after birth without any increase in the level of growth hormone, and then reversion to normal growth. Some typical signs of this condition are prognathism, antimongoloid slant, dolichocephalic skull, moderate mental retardation, and impaired coordination.

cerebral hemisphere, one of the halves of the cerebrum. The two cerebral hemispheres are divided by a deep longitudinal fissure and are connected medially at the bottom of the fissure by the corpus callosum. Prominent grooves, subdividing each hemisphere into four lobes, are the central sulcus, the lateral fissure, and the parieto-occipital fissure. Each hemisphere also has a fifth lobe deep in the brian. The central fissure separates the frontal lobe from the parietal lobe. The lateral fissure separates the temporal lobe, which lies below the fissure, from the frontal and parietal lobes, which lie above it. The parieto-occipital fissure separates the occipital lobe from the two parietal lobes. The hemispheres consist of external gray substance internal white substance, and internal gray substance and are covered by cerebral cortexes at the surface. Recent research indicates that the right hemisphere functions in the perception of certain kinds of sound and may also function better than the left hemisphere at tactual perception and spatial relationships. The left hemisphere contains Broca's area which controls language functions in most individuals.

cerebral hemorrhage, a hemorrhage from a blood vessel in the brain. Three criteria are used to classify cerebral hemorrhages: location (subarachnoid, extradural, subdural), the kind of vessel involved (arterial, venous, capillary), and origin (traumatic, degenerative). Each kind of cerebral hemorrhage has its own clinical characteristics. Most cerebral hemorrhages occur in the region of the basal ganglia and are caused by the rupture of a sclerotic artery as a result of hypertension. Other causes of rupture include congenital aneurysm, cerebrovascular infarction, and head trauma.

■ OBSERVATIONS: Bleeding may lead to displacement or destruction of brain tissue and to medullary anemia. Extensive hemorrhage is usually fatal. Recovery from the condition, which occurs more often in men than in women, may be complete. Depending on the extent and the location of the damaged tissue, residual effects may include aphasia, diminished mental function, or disturbance of the function of a special sense.

■ INTERVENTION: Lumbar puncture may reveal blood in the spinal fluid. A CAT scan may be performed to locate the lesion and to differentiate the hemorrhage from an embolus or thrombus, or cerebral angiography may be utilized for these purposes. Surgery is often necessary to stop the bleeding in order to prevent death from medullary anemia or from greatly increased intracranial pressure. The person is kept immobile, with the body in a position that assures adequate blood flow to and from the head. Physical therapy and speech therapy may be necessary during convalescence.

■ NURSING CONSIDERATIONS: Initially, bedside care is directed towards the prevention of recurrence and of the sequelae of prolonged immobility. Special care is taken in the positioning of the head of the patient to avoid flexion of the head on the neck, which might impair circulation to the brain. Fastidious skin care to prevent decubiti and emotional support are required to keep the person comfortable and calm. During convalescence the nurse may be called on to assist the patient in developing self-help capabilities. See also **subarachnoid hemorrhage.**

cerebral localization, 1. the determination of various areas in the cerebral cortex associated with specific functions, as the 47 areas of Brodmann. 2. the diagnosis of a cerebral condition, as a brain lesion, by determining the area of the brain affected, a determination made by analysis of the signs manifested by the patient and of electroencephalograms.

cerebral nerve. See **cranial nerve.**

cerebral palsy, a motor function disorder caused by a permanent, nonprogressive brain defect or lesion present at birth or shortly thereafter. The neurologic deficit may result in spastic hemiplegia, monoplegia, diplegia, or quadriplegia, athetosis or ataxia, seizures, paresthesia, varying degrees of mental retardation, impaired speech, vision, and hearing. The disorder is usually associated with premature or abnormal birth and intrapartum asphyxia, causing damage to the nervous system. Abnormalities in breathing, sucking, swallowing, and responsiveness are usually apparent soon after birth, but the characteristic stiff, awkward movements of the infant's limbs may be overlooked for several months. Walking is usually delayed and, when attempted, the child manifests a typical scissors gait. The arms may be affected only slightly but the fingers are often spastic. Deep-tendon reflexes are exaggerated and there may be slurred speech, delay in acquiring sphincter control, and athetotic movements of the face and hands. Early identification of the disorder facilitates the handling of palsied infants and the initiation of an exercise and training program. Treatment is individualized and may include the use of braces, surgical correction of deformities, speech therapy, and various indicated drugs, as muscle relaxants and anticonvulsants. Also called **Little's disease.**

cerebral tabes. See **general paresis.**

cerebral thrombosis, a clotting of blood in any cerebral vessel, as the middle cerebral artery or the ascending parietal artery.

cerebriform carcinoma. See **medullary carcinoma.**

cerebritis (ser'əbrai'tıs), *Obsolete.* **1.** any inflammation of the cerebrum or brain. **2.** bacterial meningitis.

cerebrocerebellar atrophy, a deterioration of the cerebellum caused by certain abiotrophic diseases.

cerebroid (ser'əbroid), resembling the substance of the brain.

cerebroma (ser'əbrou'mə), *pl.* **cerebromas, cerebromata.** any unusual mass of brain tissue.

cerebromedullary tube. See **neural tube.**

cerebropathia psychia toxemia. See **Korsakoff's psychosis.**

cerebroretinal angiomatosis, a hereditary disease characterized by congenital, tumorlike vascular nodules in the retina and cerebellum. Similar spinal cord lesions, cysts of the pancreas, kidneys, and other viscera, seizures, and mental retardation may be present. Also called **Lindau-von Hippel disease, retinocerebral angiomatosis, von Hippel-Lindau disease.**

cerebrospinal (sıri'brouspai'nəl), of, pertaining to, or involving the brain and the spinal cord.

cerebrospinal fluid (CSF), the fluid that flows through and protects the four ventricles of the brain, the subarachnoid space, and the spinal canal. It is composed mainly of secretions of the choroid plexi in the lateral ventricles and in the third and the fourth ventricles of the brain. Openings in the roof of the fourth ventricle allow the fluid to flow into the subarachnoid spaces around the brain and the spinal cord. The flow of fluid is from the blood in the choroid plexi, through the ventricles, the central canal, the subarachnoid spaces, and back into the blood. The volume of cerebrospinal fluid in the adult is about 140 ml, including about 23 ml in the ventricles and 117 ml in the subarachnoid spaces of the brain and the spinal cord. Changes in the carbon dioxide content of CSF affect the respiratory center in the medulla, helping to control breathing. A brain tumor may press against the cerebral aqueduct and shut off the flow of the fluid from the third to the fourth ventricle, resulting in an accumulation of fluid in the lateral and the third ventricles, called internal hydrocephalus. Other blockages of the flow of cerebrospinal fluid, as those caused by blood clots, result in serious complications. Certain illnesses and various diagnoses may require microscopic examination and chemical analysis of CSF. Samples of the fluid may be removed by lumbar puncture between the third and the fourth lumbar vertebrae.

cerebrovascular (səri'brouvæs'kyulər), of or pertaining to the vascular system and blood supply of the brain.

cerebrovascular accident (CVA), an abnormal condition of the blood vessels of the brain characterized by occlusion by an embolus or cerebrovascular hemorrhage, resulting in ischemia of the brain tissues normally perfused by the damaged vessels. The sequelae of a cerebrovascular accident depend on the location and extent of ischemia. Paralysis, weakness, speech defect, aphasia, or death may occur. Symptoms remit somewhat after the first few days as brain swelling subsides. Physical therapy and speech therapy may restore much lost function.

cerebrum (ser'əbrəm, səri'brəm), *pl.* **cerebrums, cerebra.** the largest and uppermost section of the brain, divided by a central sulcus into the left and the right cerebral hemispheres. At the bottom of the groove the hemispheres are connected by the corpus callosum. The internal structures of the hemispheres merge with those of the diencephalon and further communicate with the brain stem through the cerebral peduncles. Each cerebral hemisphere is composed of the extensive outer cerebral cortex with its gray substance, the underlying semiovale with its white substance, the internal basal ganglia, and certain centrally and medially located structures comprising the rhinencephalon. The surface of the cerebrum is convoluted and lobed, each lobe bearing the name of the bone under which it lies. The cerebrum performs sensory functions, motor functions, and less easily defined integration functions associated with various mental activities. It generates a variety of electrical waves that may be recorded on an electroencephalogram to localize areas of brain dysfunction, to identify altered states of consciousness, or to establish brain death. Some of the other processes that are controlled or affected by the cerebrum are memory, speech, writing, and emotional response. See also **cerebral cortex.** – **cerebral,** *adj.*

cerium (Ce), a ductile, gray rare-earth element. Its atomic number is 58; its atomic weight is 140.13. A compound of cerium, cerium oxalate, is used as a sedative, an antiemetic, and an antitussive.

ceroid (sir′oid), a golden, waxy pigment appearing in the cirrhotic livers of some individuals, in the nervous system, and in the muscles. It is an insoluble, acid-fast, sudanophilic pigment.

ceroma (sirou′mə), *pl.* **ceromas, ceromata.** a neoplasm that has undergone waxy degeneration.

certificate-of-need or necessity, a statement or certificate issued by a governmental agency to the effect that a proposed construction or modification of a health facility will be needed at the time of its completion. The certificate is issued to the individual or group intending to build or modify the facility.

certification, 1. a process in which an individual, an institution, or an educational program is evaluated and recognized as meeting certain predetermined standards. Certification is usually made by a nongovernmental agency. The purpose of certification is to assure that the standards met are those necessary for safe and ethical practice of the profession or service. 2. (in nursing) a process in which the professional organization or association verifies the fact that a person who is licensed to practice has met the standards for specialty practice specified by the profession. The purpose of certification is to assure other professionals and the public that the person has mastered the skills necessary to practice a particular specialty and has acquired the standard body of knowledge common to that specialty.

certification for excellence, (in nursing) certification that recognizes professional achievement, advanced training, and superior performance in a special or subspecial field of practice.

certification in nursing, one of two processes in which a professional organization formally recognizes the right of a nurse to practice a subspecialty of nursing. One process, certification for excellence, bases recognition on professional achievement, advanced training, and superior performance. The second process, entry level certification, bases recognition on advanced training in a program approved by the certifying organization. Criteria vary according to the particular requirements of the professional organization but always require current licensure as a registered nurse and usually include an examination and certain educational or practice requirements. Submission

and evaluation of documented clinical practice and a statement of a philosophy of practice may also be required by some professional organizations.

certified milk, raw milk that is obtained, handled, and marketed in compliance with state health laws. The milk must be produced by disease-free cows, which are regularly inspected by a veterinarian and are milked by sterilized equipment in hygienic surroundings, contain less than a specified low bacterial count, and be not older than 36 hours when delivered.

Certified Nurse-Midwife (CNM), (according to the American College of Nurse-Midwives) "an individual educated in the two disciplines of nursing and midwifery, who possesses evidence of certification according to the requirements of the American College of Nurse-Midwives. Nurse-Midwifery practice is the independent management of care of essentially normal newborns and women, antepartally, intrapartally, postpartally, and/or gynecologically, occurring within a health care system which provides for medical consultation, collaborative management, or referral and is in accord with the Qualifications, Standards, and Functions for the Practice of Nurse-Midwifery as defined by the American College of Nurse-Midwives." See also **midwife.**

certified registered nurse anesthetist (CRNA). See **nurse anesthetist.**

certify, 1. to guarantee formally that certain requirements have been met based on expert knowledge of significant, pertinent facts. 2. to attest, by a legal process, that someone is insane. 3. to attest to the fact of someone's death in writing, usually on a form as required by local authority. 4. to declare that a person has satisfied certain requirements for membership or acceptance into a professional or other group. See also **board certification.** – **certification,** *n.,* **certifiable,** *adj.*

Cerubidine, a trade name for an antineoplastic (daunorubicin hydrochloride).

cerulean (siru′liən), sky-blue in color.

ceruloplasmin (siru′louplæz′min), a glycoprotein in plasma that transports 96 per cent of the plasma copper.

cerumen (siru′mən), earwax. Cerumen is a yellowish or brownish waxy secretion produced by vestigial apocrine sweat glands in the external ear canal. Excessive production or impaction of cerumen in the ear canal can cause discomfort, symptoms of hearing loss, and irritation leading to the development of infection. Removal of excess cerumen is accomplished by the local use of a wax softening agent followed by careful flushing with an ear syringe. A cerumen spoon is sometimes used to scoop out hard collections of old wax.

ceruminosis (siru′minou′sis), excessive buildup of cerumen or earwax in the external auditory canal.

ceruminous gland (siru′minəs), one of a number of tiny structures in the external ear canal, believed to be modified sweat glands. They secrete a waxy cerumen instead of watery sweat.

cervic-, a combining form meaning 'pertaining to the neck': *cervicectomy, cervicitis, cervicobrachial.*

cervical (sər'vɪkəl), **1.** of or pertaining to the neck or the region of the neck. **2.** of or pertaining to the constricted area of a necklike structure, as the neck of a tooth or the cervix of the uterus.

cervical abortion, spontaneous expulsion of a cervical pregnancy.

cervical adenitis, an abnormal condition characterized by enlarged, tender lymph nodes of the neck. It often occurs in association with acute infections of the throat.

cervical canal, the canal within the uterine cervix, which protrudes into the vagina. The uterine end of the canal is closed at the internal os and, in the nullipara, at the distal end by the external os. The canal is a passageway through which the menstrual flow escapes and, vastly dilated and effaced by labor, through which the infant must come to be delivered vaginally. Various diagnostic and therapeutic procedures require dilatation of the muscular cervix surrounding the canal, including endometrial biopsy, suction or surgical curettage, or radium implantation. Pelvic inflammatory disease is the result of the entry of pathogenic bacteria into the uterus through the cervical canal. Sperm must travel upward through the canal to reach the uterus and Fallopian tubes. The mucus that is secreted by endocervical glands changes in appearance and consistency through the menstrual cycle. For the first few days after menstruation little mucus is secreted. As ovulation approaches, increasing amounts of sticky, cloudy-white or yellowish secretions are seen. Around the time of ovulation, the volume of mucus increases and it becomes clear, slippery, and elastic, resembling the uncooked white of an egg. After ovulation the mucus becomes cloudy, thick, sticky, and progressively less profuse until menstruation supervenes to begin the cycle again.

cervical cancer, a neoplasm of the uterine cervix that can be detected in the early, curable stage by the Papanicolaou test. Factors associated with the development of cervical cancer are coitus at an early age, many sexual partners, genital herpesvirus infections, multiparity, and poor obstetric and gynecologic care. Early cervical neoplasia is usually asymptomatic, but there may be a watery vaginal discharge or occasional spotting of blood; advanced lesions may cause a dark, foul-smelling vaginal discharge, leakage from bladder or rectal fistulas, anorexia, weight loss, and back and leg pains. Pap smears of cervical cells are highly important in screening, but definitive diagnoses are based on colposcopic examination and cytologic study of specimens obtained by biopsy. Suitable sites for biopsy may be indicated by applying three per cent acetic acid to the cervix to accentuate characteristic changes in neoplastic epithelium or by using Schiller's test

in which an iodine solution stains normal cervical cells dark brown and does not stain the nongylcogen-producing cells of malignant epithelium. Cervical dysplasia may regress, persist, or progress to clinical disease, but carcinoma in situ is considered to be a precursor of invasive carcinoma. About 90 per cent of cervical tumors are squamous cell carcinomas, fewer than 10 per cent are adenocarcinomas, and others are mixtures of these kinds, or, in rare cases, sarcomas. Tumors on the surface of the cervix may be huge, polypoid masses while endophytic lesions tend to be small and hard; ulcerative lesions may cause extensive erosion. Cervical cancer invades the tissues of adjacent organs and may metastasize through lymphatic channels to distant sites, including the lungs, bone, liver, brain, and para-aortic nodes. Treatment depends on the kind and the extent of the malignancy, the age of the woman, and her general health. Also considered are her wishes in regard to maintaining her reproductive function. Carcinoma in situ may be treated by excisional conization or cryosurgery. Invasive tumors may be treated with radiotherapy or vaginal or abdominal hysterectomy.

cervical cap, a contraceptive device consisting of a small rubber cup fitted over the uterine cervix to prevent spermatozoa from entering the cervical canal. In some studies, its contraceptive effectiveness equals or exceeds that of the diaphragm. It may be more comfortable than the diaphragm and may be left safely on the cervix for days or weeks and remain effective. Accurate initial fitting by a trained person is necessary. Practice by the user may be required to manipulate the cap into proper position on the cervix. The cap has become a popular contraceptive in Great Britain and Europe among women who require nonsystemic, noninvasive means of preventing conception.

cervical carcinoma, a malignant neoplasm of the uterine cervix, one of the most common forms of cancer. Diagnosis is usually made with the Papanicolaou test of genital epithelial cells, direct examination of the cervix with a colposcope, or pathological microscopic examination of a specimen obtained by biopsy. Initial symptoms are a cervical discharge, bleeding, and, in some cases, pain. The tumor, a squamous cell lesion in about 95 per cent of the cases and an adenocarcinoma in approximately four per cent, may be exophytic, nodular, or ulcerating. Blood- or lymph-borne metastases may occur in any organ but are most frequent in the lungs, liver, and bones. Treatment of the primary tumor includes hysterectomy, removal of regional lymph nodes, and postoperative radiotherapy and chemotherapy when indicated. Genital herpes infection and coitus at an early age, especially with multiple partners, are associated with increased incidence of cervical carcinoma.

cervical disc syndrome, an abnormal condition characterized by compression or irritation of the cervical nerve roots in or near the intervertebral foramina before the roots divide into the anterior and the posterior rami. Cervical disc syndrome may be caused by ruptured intervertebral discs, degenerative cervical disc disease, or by cervical injuries. The form caused by ruptured cervical intervertebral discs or by degenerative disease may produce varying degrees of malalignment, causing nerve root compression. Most cervical disc syndromes owing to injuries involve hyperextension, which causes compression because of the anatomic structures involved. Flexion injuries in the cervical area do not result in nerve compression. Edema usually occurs in all cases of cervical disc syndrome. Pain, the most common symptom, usually emanates from the cervical area but may radiate down the arm to the fingers and increase with cervical motion. The pain may increase sharply with coughing, sneezing, or any radical movement. Other signs and symptoms associated with cervical disc syndrome may be paresthesia, headache, blurred vision, decreased skeletal function, and weakened hand grip. Physical examination may reveal varying degrees of muscular atrophy, sensory abnormalities, muscular weakness, and decreased reflexes. Radiographic examination may reveal a loss of normal lordosis associated with the cervical vertebrae and may also reveal some minor malalignment of the vertebrae. Nonsurgical intervention, which is usually a successful treatment, may include immobilization of the cervical vertebrae to decrease irritation and to provide rest for the traumatized area. Other treatment may include special exercises, heat therapy, and intermittent traction. Mild analgesics are usually successful in controlling the pain associated with cervical disc syndrome, especially when employed with immobilization. Surgery is usually recommended only when signs and symptoms persist despite nonsurgical treatment. The prognosis for this condition is usually good, but recurrence of symptoms is common. Also called **cervical root syndrome.** See also **ruptured intervertebral disc.**

cervical endometritis, an inflammation of the inner lining of the cervix uteri. See also **endometritis.**

cervical fistula, **1.** See **branchial fistula. 2.** an abnormal passage from the cervix to the vagina or bladder that may be caused by a malignant lesion, radiotherapy, surgical trauma, or injury during childbirth. A cervical fistula communicating with the bladder permits leakage of urine, causing irritation, odor, and embarrassment. When surgical repair is not possible, the patient is advised to take sitz baths, use a deodorizing douche or powder, as sodium borate, and to wear plastic pants or a protective apron.

cervical mucus method of family planning. See **ovulation method of family planning.**

cervical os. **1.** See **external cervical os. 2.** See **internal cervical os.**

cervical plexus, the network of nerves formed by the ventral primary divisions of the first four cervical nerves. Each nerve, except the first, divides into the superior branch and the inferior branch, and both branches unite to form three loops. The plexus is located opposite the cranial aspect of the first four cervical vertebrae, ventrolateral to the levator scapulae and the scalenus medius, and deep to the sternocleidomastoideus. It communicates with certain cranial nerves and numerous muscular and cutaneous branches.

cervical plexus anesthesia, nerve block at any point below the mastoid process from C_2 to the second cervical vertebra transverse process of the sixth cervical vertebra. This method is used for operations on the area between the jaw and clavicle. Complications may include Horner's syndrome, inadvertent stellate ganglion or brachial plexus block, vertebral artery bleeding, subarachnoid or peridural penetration, phrenic nerve block or palsy, or laryngeal nerve block, manifested by sudden hoarseness.

cervical polyp, an outgrowth of columnar epithelial tissue of the endocervical canal, usually attached to the wall of the canal by a slender pedicle. Often there are no symptoms, but multiple or abraded polyps may cause bleeding, especially with contact during coitus. Polyps are most common in women over 40 years of age. The etiology is not known. Treatment of a symptomatic polyp is removal by simple torsion, turning the polyp on its stalk while pulling gently until it tears off. Scant bleeding and prompt healing usually follow. The polyp is removed and sent to the laboratory for pathologic evaluation and histologic examination. Squamous metaplasia is a common finding; malignancy is rare. A Pap smear and endometrial biopsy may be performed at the same visit if other pathology is suspected.

cervical smear, a small amount of the secretions and superficial cells of the cervix, secured with a sterile applicator or special small wooden or plastic spatula from the external os of the uterine cervix. For a Pap smear, it is obtained from the squamo-columnar junction of the uterine cervix and from the vaginal vault and endocervical canal. The specimen is spread on a specially labeled glass slide and sent for cytologic examination by a special laboratory. For bacteriologic culture and identification, only the applicator is used; the specimen is spread on a glass slide and stained and examined under a microscope or placed in or on a culture medium and sent to a bacteriologic laboratory for culture and identification.

cervical tenaculum. See **tenaculum.**

cervical triangle, one of two triangular areas formed in the neck by the oblique course of the sternocleidomastoideus. The anterior triangle is bounded by the midline of the throat anteriorly, the sternocleidomastoideus laterally, and the body of the mandible superiorly. The posterior triangle is bounded by the clavicle inferiorly and by the borders of the sternocleidomastoideus and the trapezius superiorly.

cervical vertebra, one of the first seven segments of the vertebral column. They differ from the thoracic and the lumbar vertebrae by the presence of a foramen in each transverse process. The first, second, and seventh cervical vertebrae present exceptional features. The bodies of the four remaining cervical vertebrae are small, oval, and broader than the other three in transverse diameter and contain large, triangular foramens within their tranverse processes. Their spinous processes are short and bifid. The first cervical vertebra has no body, supports the head, and contains a smooth, oval facet for articulation with the dens of the second cervical vertebra. The dens extends from the cranial portion of the body of the second cervical vertebra which has a very large, strong spinous process with a bifid extremity. The seventh cervical vertebra has a very long, prominent spinous process that is nearly horizontal in direction and is often used as a palpable reference for locating the other cervical spines. Compare **coccygeal vertebra, lumbar vertebra, sacral vertebra, thoracic vertebra.** See also **vertebra.**

cervicitis (sər'vɪsaɪ'tɪs), acute or chronic inflammation of the uterine cervix. **Acute cervicitis** is the infection of the cervix marked by redness, edema, and bleeding on contact. Symptoms do not always occur but may include any or all of the following: copious, foul-smelling discharge from the vagina, pelvic pressure or pain, scant bleeding with intercourse, and itching or burning of the external genitalia. The principle causative organisms are: trichomonas, candida albicans, and hemophilus vaginalis. Diagnosis is by microscopic examination, confirmed, in some cases, by culture and Pap smear. Specific antimicrobial medication may be effective. Acute cervicitis tends to be a recurrent problem owing to re-exposure to the germ, undertreatment, or predisposing factors such as multiple sexual partners or poor nutritional status. **Chronic cervicitis** is a persistent inflammation of the cervix usually occurring among women in their reproductive years. Symptoms include a thick, irritating, malodorous discharge, that may, in severe cases, be accompanied by significant pelvic pain. The cervix looks congested and enlarged, nabothian cysts are often present, there are signs of eversion of the cervix and often old lacerations from childbirth. A Pap smear should be performed prior to treatment. Antibiotic treatment is seldom effective. The symptoms of mild chronic cervicitis may abate with topical treatment, but the underlying inflammatory condition will not change. The most effective treatments are hot or cold cautery. See also *Candida albicans,* **cautery, cervical cancer, cervical polyp, condylomatum accuminatum, nabothian cyst.**

cervico-, a combining form meaning 'neck': *cervicodynia, cervicolabial, cervicotomy.*

cervicodynia (sər'vɪkɔʊdɪn'iə), pain in the neck. Also called **trachelodynia.**

cervicofacial actinomycosis. See **actinomycosis.**

cervicolabial, of, pertaining to, or situated in the labial area of the neck of an incisor or a canine tooth.

cervicouterine (sər'vɪkɔʊyu'tərɪn), of, pertaining to, or situated at the cervix of the uterus.

cervicovesical, of or pertaining to the cervix of the uterus and the bladder.

cervix (sər'vɪks), the part of the uterus that protrudes into the cavity of the vagina. The cervix is divided into the supravaginal portion and the vaginal portion. The supravaginal portion is separated ventrally from the bladder by the parametrium, which attaches to the sides of the cervix and contains the uterine arteries. The vaginal portion of the cervix projects into the cavity of the vagina and contains the cervical canal and the internal and external os of the canal. The mucous membrane lining the endocervix is broken by numerous oblique ridges, deep glandular follicles, little cysts, and papillae.

ceryl alcohol, a fatty alcohol obtained from spermaceti, used as an emulsifying and stiffening agent.

cesium (Cs), an alkali metal element. Its atomic number is 55; its atomic weight is 132.9. Like other alkali metals cesium emits electrons when exposed to visible light and is used in photoelectric cells and in television cameras. The isotope cesium[137], which has a half-life of 33 years, has been used as a source of gamma rays in medical and industrial radiology.

cesspool fever, *Informal.* typhoid fever.

cestode (ses'toʊd). See **tapeworm.**

cestode infection. See **tapeworm infection.**

cestodiasis (ses'toʊdaɪ'əsɪs). See **tapeworm infection.**

cestoid (ses'tɔɪd), resembling a tapeworm.

Cetacaine, a trade name for a fixed-combination, anesthetic spray, containing several local anesthetics (benzocaine, butyl aminobenzoate, tetracaine), applied to mucous membranes.

cetyl alcohol, a fatty alcohol, derived from spermaceti, used as an emulsifier and stiffening agent. Also called **palmityl alcohol.**

cetylpyridinium chloride, an anti-infective used as a preservative in pharmaceutical preparations and as a topical cleanser.

■ INDICATION: It is prescribed prophylactically to prevent infection of the skin or mucous membranes.

■ CONTRAINDICATION: Known hypersensitivity to this drug is the only contraindication.

■ NOTE: It is inactivated by soap, serum, and tissue fluids; therefore, the surface of the skin must be clean and well rinsed.

C.E.U., abbreviation for **continuing education unit.**

Ce-Vi-Sol, a trade name for vitamin C (ascorbic acid).

cevitamic acid (si'væitæm'ık). See **ascorbic acid.**

Cf, symbol for **californium.**

C-F test, abbreviation for **complement-fixation test.**

CGS, cgs, abbreviation for **centimeter-gram-second (system).**

Ch[1], symbol for **Christchurch chromosome.**

Chaddock reflex, 1. an abnormal variation of the Babinski reflex, elicited by firmly stroking the side of the foot just distal to the lateral malleolus, characterized by extension of the great toe and fanning of the other toes. It is seen in pyramidal tract disease. 2. an abnormal reflex, induced by firmly stroking the ulnar surface of the forearm, characterized by flexion of the wrist and extension of the fingers in fanlike position. It is seen on the affected side in hemiplegia. Compare **Gordon reflex, Oppenheim reflex.** See also **Babinski's reflex.**

Chaddock's sign (chæd'əks), the extension of the big toe when the skin covering the malleolus is irritated, as in organic diseases affecting the corticospinal reflex paths. Also called **Chaddock's reflex.**

Chadwick's sign (chæd'wıks), the bluish coloration of the vulva and vagina that develops after the sixth week of pregnancy as a normal result of local venous congestion. It is an early sign of pregnancy.

chafe, an irritation of the skin by friction, as when rough material rubs against an unprotected area of the body.

chafing (chei'fıng), superficial irritation of the skin by friction.

Chagas-Cruz disease (chæg'əskruz'). See **Chagas' disease.**

Chagas' disease, a parasitic disease caused by *Trypanosoma cruzi* or by *Schizotrypanum cruzi,* transmitted to man by the bite of bloodsucking insects. It may occur in acute or chronic form. The acute form, which is common in children and rare in adults, is marked by a lesion at the site of the bite, by fever, weakness, enlarged spleen and lymph glands, edema of the face and legs, and tachycardia. This form resolves within four months unless complications, as encephalitis, develop. The chronic form may be manifested by cardiomyopathy, or by dilatation of the esophagus or colon. Often, infections are asymptomatic. Also called **American trypanosomiasis, Brazilian trypanosomiasis, Chagas-Cruz disease, Cruz trypanosomiasis, South American trypanosomiasis.** See also **trypanosomiasis.**

Chagres fever (chæg'rıs), an arbovirus infection transmitted to humans through the bite of a sandfly. The disease is rarely fatal and is characterized by fever, headache, and muscle pains of the chest or abdomen. There may be nausea and vomiting, giddiness, weakness, photophobia, and pain on moving the eyes. The infection subsides within a week. Supportive treatment includes analgesics, bed rest, and adequate fluid intake. The disease is most common in Central America.

chain, 1. a length of several units linked together in a linear pattern, as a polypeptide chain of amino acids or a chain of atoms forming a chemical molecule. 2. a group of individual bacteria linked together, as streptococci formed by a chain of cocci. 3. the serial relationship of certain structures essential to function, as the chain of ossicles in the middle ear. Each of the small bones moves successively in response to vibration of the tympanic membrane, thus transmitting the auditory stimulus to the oval window. See also **chain ligature.**

chain ligature, an interlocking ligature that ties off a pedicle at several places by passing a long thread through the pedicle at different points.

chain reaction, 1. (in chemistry) a reaction that produces a compound needed for the reaction to continue, as each product produced in the chain reactions of glycolysis which is essential for each succeeding reaction and the total catabolism of glucose. 2. (in physics) a reaction that perpetuates itself by the proliferating fission of nuclei and the release of atomic particles, which cause more nuclear fissions.

chain reflex, a series of reflexes, each stimulated by the preceding one.

chain stitch suture, a continuous surgical stitch in which each loop of the suture is secured by the next loop.

chalasia (kəlei'zhə), abnormal relaxation or incompetence of the cardiac sphincter of the stomach, resulting in reflux of the gastric contents into the esophagus with subsequent regurgitation. Conservative treatment in infancy includes feeding several small meals a day to avoid distention of the stomach and holding the baby upright while giving the feeding. The symptoms and treatment are similar to those of a hiatal hernia.

chalazion (kəlci'zion,) a small, localized swelling of the eyelid resulting from obstruction and retained secretions of the Meibomian glands. A nonmalignant condition, it often requires surgery for correction. Compare **hordeolum, sty.**

CHALAZION

chalice cell. See **goblet cell.**

chalkitis, an abnormal condition characterized by inflammation of the eyes, caused by rubbing the eyes with the hands after touching or handling brass. Also called **brassy eye.**

chalone (kei'loun), any one of numerous mitotic inhibitors that is elaborated by a tissue and functions within that tissue rather than affecting another tissue.

chamber, 1. a hollow but not necessarily an empty space or cavity in an organ, as in the anterior and posterior chambers of the eye or the atrial and ventricular chambers of the heart. 2. a room or closed space used for research or therapeutic purposes, as a decompression chamber or hyperbaric oxygen chamber.

Chamberlain's line, a line that extends from the posterior of the hard palate to the dorsum of the foramen magnum.

Chamberlen forceps, one of the earliest kinds of obstetric forceps.

chamaeprosopy (kæm'əpros'əpi), a facial appearance characterized by a low brow and a broad face with a facial index of 90 or less. —**chamaeprosopic,** adj.

CHAMPUS, abbreviation for **Civilian Health and Medical Programs for Uniformed Services.**

chancr-. See **cancr-.**

chancre (shæng'kər), 1. a skin lesion of primary syphilis that begins at the site of infection as a papule and develops into a red, bloodless, painless ulcer with a scooped-out appearance. It heals without treatment and leaves no scar. Two or more chancres may develop at the same time, occurring usually in the genital area but sometimes on the hands, face, or other body surface. The chancre teams with *Treponema pallidum* spirochetes and is highly contagious. 2. a papular lesion or ulcerated area of the skin that marks the point of infection of a nonsyphilitic disease, as tuberculosis. See also **chancroid, syphilis.**

chancroid (shæng'kroid), a highly contagious, local venereal ulcer caused by infection with a bacillus, *Haemophilus ducreyi.* It characteristically begins as a papule, usually on the skin of the external genitalia; it then grows and ulcerates, other papules form, and, if untreated, the bacillus spreads, causing buboes in the groin. An intradermal skin test is more reliable than smear and culture techniques in diagnosing this condition. Sulfa drugs are prescribed to treat chancroid. Because the lesion resembles syphilis and lymphogranuloma venereum, the diagnosis must be made before treatment in order to avoid obscuring simultaneous infections. Compare **chancre.**

change of life, *Informal.* the female climacteric; menopause.

channel, a passageway or groove that conveys fluid, as the central channels that connect the arterioles with the venules.

channel ulcer, a rare type of peptic ulcer found in the pyloric canal between the stomach and the duodenum. See also **peptic ulcer.**

chapped, pertaining to skin that is roughened, cracked, or reddened by exposure to cold or excessive surface evaporation. Stinging or burning sensations often accompany the disorder. Prevention is by protection against exposure to cold and wind. Treatment includes the avoidance of frequent washing, the replacement of soaps and detergents with super-fatted soaps, and the application of emollients. Compare **frostbite.** —**chap,** v.

character, the integrated composite of traits and behavioral tendencies that enable a person to react in a relatively consistent way to the customs and mores of society. Character, as contrasted with personality, implies volition and morality. Compare **personality.**

character analysis, a systematic investigation of the personality of an individual with special attention to psychological defenses and motivations, usually undertaken to improve behavior.

character disorder, a chronic, habitual, maladaptive, and socially unacceptable pattern of behavior and emotional response. The condition is usually accompanied by minimal feelings of anxiety. Also called **character neurosis.** See also **antisocial personality disorder.**

character neurosis. See **character disorder.**

charcoal. See **activated charcoal.**

Charcot-Bouchard aneurysm (sharkou'bushar'), a small, round aneurysm of a small artery of the cerebral cortex, which some authorities believe is the cause of massive cerebral hemorrhage. Charcot-Bouchard aneurysms often occur in individuals with very high blood pressure.

Charcot-Leyden crystal (sharkou'lei'dən), any one of the crystalline structures shaped like narrow, double pyramids found in the sputum of individuals suffering from bronchial asthma. The Charcot-Leyden crystals are protein compounds and occur in association with the fragmentation of eosinophils. Also called **asthma crystal, leukocytic crystal.**

Charcot-Marie-Tooth atrophy (sharkou'məri'tuth'), a progressive hereditary disorder characterized by degeneration of the peroneal muscles of the fibula, resulting in clubfoot, foot drop, and ataxia.

Charcot's fever (sharkouz'), a syndrome characterized by a recurrent fever, jaundice, and abdominal pain in the right upper quadrant occurring with inflammation of the bile ducts. It is caused by the intermittent impaction of a stone in the ducts.

Charcot's joint, See **neuropathic joint disease.**

charlatan, a totally unqualified individual posing as an expert, especially an individual pretending to be a physician. Also called **quack.** —**charlatanical,** adj.

Charles' law. See **Gay-Lussac's law.**

charley horse, a painful condition of the quadricep or hamstring muscles characterized by soreness and stiffness. It is the result of a strain, tear, or bruise of the muscle and is often associated with athletic activity. Compare **cramp.**

chart, 1. *Informal.* a patient record. 2. to note data in a patient record, usually at prescribed intervals.

charta (kar'tə), *pl.* **chartae.** a piece of paper, especially one treated with medicine, as for external application, or with a chemical for a special purpose, as litmus paper.

chauffeur's fracture, any fracture of the radial styloid, produced by a twisting or a snapping type injury.

Chaussier's areola (s̆housyeiz'), an areola of indurated tissue surrounding a malignant pustule.

CHC, abbreviation for *community health center.*

check ligament. See **alar ligament.**

check-up, a thorough study or examination of the health of an individual.

Chediak-Higashi syndrome (s̆hed'iækhɪga'shi), a congenital, autosomal disorder, characterized by partial albinism, photophobia, massive leukocytic inclusions, psychomotor abnormalities, recurrent infections, and early death. Antenatal diagnosis can be made by amniocentesis and tissue culture. Treatment includes antibiotics and transfusions.

cheek, a fleshy prominence, especially the fleshy protuberances on both sides of the face between the eye and the jaw and the ear and the nose and mouth. Also called **bucca.**

cheekbone. See **zygomatic bone.**

cheesewasher's lung, a lung disease caused by an allergic reaction to the mold of cheese. Avoidance of the causative agent assures prevention of the condition. No treatment is necessary.

cheil-. See **cheilo-.**

-cheilia, a combining form meaning '(condition of the) lips': *atelocheilia, dicheilia, xerocheilia.* Also **-chilia.**

cheilitis (kɑilai'tɪs), an abnormal condition of the lips characterized by inflammation and cracking of the skin. There are several forms including those caused by excessive exposure to sunlight, allergic sensitivity to cosmetics, and vitamin deficiency. Compare **cheilosis.**

cheilo-, cheil-, a combining form meaning 'pertaining to the lip': *cheiloangioscopy, cheilocarcinoma, cheiloplasty.*

cheilocarcinoma (kɑi'loukar'sɪnou'mə), *pl.* **cheilocarcinomas, cheilocarcinomata.** a malignant epithelial tumor of the lip.

cheiloplasty (kɑi'ləplæs'ti), surgical correction of a defect of the lip.

cheilorraphy (kɑilor'əfi), a surgical procedure that sutures the lip, as in the repair of a congenitally cleft lip or a lacerated lip.

cheilosis (kɑilou'sɪs), a disorder of the lips and mouth characterized by scales and fissures, resulting from a deficiency of riboflavin in the diet.

cheir-. See **cheiro-.**

cheiralgia (kɑiræl'jə), a pain in the hand, especially the pain associated with arthritis. **–cheiralgic,** *adj.*

-cheiria. See **-chiria.**

cheiro-, cheir-, a combining form meaning 'pertaining to the hand': *cheiragra, cheiromegaly, cheiroplasty.* Also **chir-, chiro-.**

cheiromegaly (kɑi'roumeg'əli), an abnormal condition characterized by excessively large hands. **–cheiromegalic,** *adj.*

cheiroplasty, an operation involving plastic surgery of the hand. **–cheiroplastic,** *adj.*

chelate (ki'leit), 1. (of a metal ion and two or more polar groups of a single molecule) to form a bond, thus creating a ringlike complex. 2. (in medicine) any compound composed of iron ions arranged in ring formations with polar groups of single molecules, used especially in chemotherapeutic treatments for metal poisoning. 3. of or pertaining to chelation.

chelating agent, a substance that promotes chelation. Chelating agents are used in the treatment of metal poisoning. See also **chelation.**

chelation (kilei'shən), a chemical reaction in which there is a combination with a metal to form a ring-shaped molecular complex in which the metal is firmly bound and sequestered. See also **chelating agent.**

cheloid (ki'loid). See **keloid.**

cheloidosis. See **keloidosis.**

chemical, 1. a substance composed of chemical elements or a substance produced by or used in chemical processes. 2. pertaining to chemistry.

chemical action, any process in which natural elements and compounds react with each other to produce a chemical change or a different compound, as hydrogen and oxygen, which combine to produce water.

chemical agent, any chemical power, active principle, or substance that can produce an effect in the body by interacting with various body substances, as aspirin, which produces an analgesic effect.

chemical antidote, any substance that reacts chemically with a poison to form a compound that is harmless. There are few true antidotes, and treatment of poisoning depends largely on eliminating the toxic agent before it can be absorbed by the body.

chemical burn, tissue damage caused by exposure to a strong acid or alkali, as phenol, creosol, mustard gas, or phosphorus. Emergency treatment includes washing the surface with copious amounts of water to remove the chemical and, if the damage is more than slight and superficial, immediate transport to a medical facility. See also **acid burn, acid poisoning, alkali burn, alkali poisoning.**

chemical cauterization, the corroding or burning of living tissue by a caustic chemical substance, as potassium hydroxide. Also called **chemocautery.**

chemical diabetes. See **latent diabetes.**

chemical equivalence, (of a drug or chemical) containing similar amounts of the same ingredients as another drug or chemical. See also **compendium.**

chemical gastritis, inflammation of the stomach caused by the ingestion of a chemical compound. Treatment is determined by the substance ingested. Gastric lavage is often advisable, but neither lavage nor emetics are administered in cases involving the most corrosive poisons. Compare **corrosive gastritis, erosive gastritis.**

chemical name, the exact designation of the chemical structure of a drug as determined by the rules of accepted systems of chemical nomenclature. For example, N,N-bis-(2-chloroethly)-N′-(3-hydroxypropyl) phosphordiamidic acid cyclic acid monohydrate is the chemical name of cyclophosphamide, a drug used in cancer chemotherapy.

chemical warfare, the waging of war with poisonous chemicals and gases.

cheminosis (kem′ənoʊ′sɪs), any disease caused by a chemical substance.

chemistry, the science dealing with the elements, their compounds, and the chemical structure and interactions of matter. Kinds of chemistry include **inorganic chemistry, organic chemistry.**

chemistry, normal values, the amounts of various substances in the normal human body, determined by testing a large sample of people presumed to be healthy. Normal values are expressed in ranges of numbers, and ranges vary from laboratory to laboratory. For example, a normal concentration of a substance in the blood might be expressed as 5 to 20 mg per 100 ml. Although variations from normal values may be highly significant tools in the diagnoses of certain diseases, in all cases an abnormal result must be cautiously interpreted. See also specific tests.

chemo-, a combining form meaning 'pertaining to a chemical or to chemistry': *chemo-antigen, chemobiotic, chemokinesis.*

chemocautery (ki′moʊkə′təri). See **chemical cauterization.**

chemodifferentiation, a stage in embryonic development that precedes and controls specialization and differentiation of the cells into rudimentary organs.

chemoreceptor (ki′moʊrɪsep′tər), a sensory nerve cell activated by chemical stimuli, as a chemoreceptor in the carotid that is sensitive to the P_{CO_2} in the blood, signaling the respiratory center in the brain to increase or decrease respiration.

chemoreflex (ki′moʊri′fleks), any reflex initiated by the stimulation of chemical receptors, as the carotid and aortic bodies, which respond to changes in carbon dioxide, hydrogen ion, and oxygen concentrations in the blood. See also **chemoreceptor.**

chemosis (kɪmoʊ′sɪs), an abnormal edematous swelling of the mucous membrane covering the eyeball and lining the eyelids that is usually the result of local trauma or infection. Chemosis may also occur in acute conjunctivitis. An obstruction of normal lymph flow, as might occur from growth of a tumor within the eye socket, may less commonly be found to be the cause of chemosis. Systemic disorders, as angioneurotic edema, anemia, and Bright's disease, may also cause the condition. Also called **conjunctival edema.**

chemostat (ki′məstæt′), a device which assures a steady rate of cell division in bacterial populations by maintaining a constant environment.

chemosurgery, the destruction of malignant, infected, or gangrenous tissue by the application of chemicals. The technique is used successfully to remove skin cancers.

chemotaxis (ki′moʊtæk′sɪs), a response involving movement that is positive (toward) or negative (away from) to a chemical stimulus.

chemotherapeutic index. See **therapeutic index.**

chemotherapy (unsealed radioactive), the oral or parenteral administration of a radioisotope, as iodine-131 (^{131}I) for the treatment of hyperthyroidism or thyroid cancer, phosphorus-32 (^{32}P) for leukemia or polycythemia vera, or gold-198 (^{198}Au) for lung cancer or peritoneal ascites resulting from widely disseminated carcinoma.

■ METHOD: Before unsealed radioactive chemotherapy is administered, the patient receives an explanation of the procedure and of the need for isolation during the half-life of the radioisotope (8.1 days for ^{131}I, 14 days for ^{32}P, and 2.7 days for ^{198}Au). The room in which the patient is isolated adjoins a private bathroom and is equipped with convenient furniture, a freshly made bed placed next to the building's outer wall, a functioning phone and television set, adequate lighting, reading and hobby materials, and containers for contaminated linen, dressings, and excreta. Radioactive tags are posted on the door. The patient's chart and individual radioactive badges, kept at the door, are worn by each staff member entering the room to record the amount of radiation exposure; pregnant staff members are not assigned to the patient's care. Disposable dishes, utensils, and trays are used for the patient's preferred diet, which is ordered before the isolation period. Prior to receiving the radioisotope, the patient bathes or showers and is assisted in notifying family and friends that visits are not allowed in the initial 24 hours of therapy and are thereafter limited to two hours if the person remains six feet or more from the patient. During isolation, the patient, if able, performs daily self-care measures and the staff member caring for the patient limits the time spent in the room by planning the observations and procedures to be accomplished beforehand. Urine excreted by a patient treated with ^{131}I is collected directly or via an indwelling catheter, in a lead-lined container, which is sent to the laboratory for assay of the radioisotope. Feces, sputum, and vomitus are placed in the toilet and decontaminated with a dropperful of a saturated solution of potassium iodide before the bowl is flushed. If excreta spill on the skin, the area is rinsed in running water for two minutes and washed in soap and water for an additional three minutes. If the bed or another surface in the room is contaminated with excreta, the radiation control officer is notified and the area is monitored before being cleaned. Dressings and bed linen are handled with rubber or plastic gloves; contaminated linens are placed in a hamper and trash in plastic bags, and they are not removed from the room until monitored with a Geiger-Müller counter. The staff member limits exposure by repositioning the debilitated patient with a turn sheet, by bathing only the soiled body areas, and by preparing and cutting food on the diet tray before entering the room. The patient treated with ^{131}I is observed for evidence of neck tenderness, changes in exophthalmia, a transient productive cough, hypoparathyroidism, hypothyroidism, and hyperthyroidism. Similar procedures of care are followed for the patient treated with ^{32}P, but since the beta rays emitted by this radionuclide are absorbed by the patient's body, there is no danger of external exposure. If ^{32}P is administered intravenously or injected into the body cavity, no special precautions are needed for disposal of excreta, but dressings and linen contaminated by seepage from wounds are placed in lead-lined containers, as is the vomitus of the patient who is given the radionuclide orally. Special precautions are required in caring for the patient treated with radioactive gold, which emits gamma and beta rays. After purple liquid ^{198}Au is injected into the body cavity, the patient is turned with a sheet every 15 minutes for two hours so that the radionuclide can spread. Dressings and cleansing tissues contaminated by the purple seepage from wounds are burned immediately; linen in contact with wounds is placed in special containers. The patient injected with ^{198}Au is usually terminally ill, and, if death occurs, a tag is placed on the body to alert the mortician to the presence of the radionuclide.

■ NURSING ORDERS: The nurse wears a radiation badge when entering the patient's room and limits exposure by performing planned procedures efficiently. Routine nursing functions are kept to a minimum, especially if the patient is ambulatory, but emotional support is provided in brief hourly visits at the door and via the intercommunication system. The nurse anticipates and fulfills the isolated patient's requests as promptly as possible, arranges diversional activities, and assures the patient that when a certain period of time has passed the patient will no longer be a source of radioactivity.

■ OUTCOME CRITERIA: Radioactive iodine usually counteracts hyperthyroidism and is frequently used in conjunction with surgery in the treatment of thyroid cancer. Radioactive phosphorus often controls polycythemia vera, but other agents are generally more effective in leukemia therapy. Radioactive gold is usually administered as a last resort in advanced lung cancer or peritoneal ascites resulting from malignant disease.

cherry angioma, a small, bright red, clearly circumscribed vascular tumor on the skin. It occurs most often on the trunk but may be found anywhere on the body. The lesion is very common; more than 85 per cent of people over the age of 45 have several cherry angiomas. Also called **capillary angioma, capillary hemangioma, De Morgan's spots, senile angioma.**

cherry red spot, an abnormal red circular area of the choroid, seen through the fovea centralis of the eye and surrounded by a contrasting white edema. It is associated with cases of infantile cerebral sphingolipidosis and sometimes appears in the late infantile form of amaurotic familial idiocy. Also called **Tay's spot.**

cherubism (ĉher'əbɪz'əm), an abnormal hereditary condition characterized by progressive bilateral swelling at the angle of the mandible, especially in children. In some cases of cherubism, the entire jaw swells and the eyes turn up, enhancing the cherubic facial appearance. The condition tends to regress during adult life.

chest. See thorax.

chest lead (lid), **1.** an electrocardiographic conductor in which the exploring electrode is placed on the chest or precordium. The indifferent electrode is placed on the patient's back for a CB (chest back) lead, on the front of the chest for a CF (chest front) lead, the left arm for a CL (chest left) lead, and on the right arm for a CR (chest right) lead. **2.** *Informal.* the tracing produced by such a lead on an electrocardiograph.

chest pain, a physical complaint that requires immediate diagnosis and evaluation. Chest pain may be symptomatic of cardiac disease, as angina pectoris, myocardial infarction, or pericarditis, or of disease of the lungs, as pleurisy, pneumonia, or pulmonary embolism or infarction. The source of chest pain may also be musculoskeletal, gastrointestinal, or psychogenic. Over 90 per cent of severe chest pain is caused by coronary disease, spinal root compression, or psychological disturbance. Because of its association with serious, life-threatening heart disease, chest pain causes extreme anxiety, which tends to mask other symptoms that would aid in diagnosis and treatment; reassuring the person being examined assists in proper diagnosis. Evaluation of chest pain requires determining the quality of the pain—dull, sharp, or crushing, locating the site of the pain—in the center or side of the chest, and determining how long the pain has persisted, how it has developed, and whether or not it has occurred in the past. The patient is asked to describe the spread of pain to other parts of the body and to identify factors, as exertion, emotional distress, movement, or deep breathing, that aggravate or relieve the pain. Specific cardiovascular conditions associated with chest pain are myocardial infarction, angina pectoris, pericarditis, and a dissecting aneurysm of the thoracic aorta. Musculoskeletal conditions include rib fractures, swelling of the rib cartilage, and muscle strain. Gastrointestinal conditions associated with chest pain include esophagitis, peptic ulcers, hernia of the diaphragm, and pancreatitis.

chest physiotherapy. See **chest wall percussion.**

chest tube, a catheter inserted through the thorax into the chest cavity for removing air or fluid. It is commonly used following chest surgery and lung collapse.

chest wall percussion. See **percussion.**

Cheyne-Stokes respiration (CSR) (chein′stouks′), an abnormal pattern of respiration, characterized by alternating periods of apnea and deep, rapid breathing. The respiratory cycle begins with slow, shallow breaths that gradually increase to abnormal depth and rapidity. Respiration gradually subsides as breathing slows and becomes shallower, climaxing in a 10- to 20-second period without respiration before the cycle is repeated. Each cyclical episode may last from 45 seconds to three minutes. The immediate cause of Cheyne-Stokes respiration is a complex alteration in the functioning of the respiratory center in the brain. Changes in blood gases, especially an increase in carbon dioxide, may be the proximal cause.

Alternatively, a direct reduction in the sensitivity of the respiratory center may occur in the presence of normal concentrations of blood gases, as seen in cerebral vascular disease, tumors of the brain stem, or as a result of severe head injury. The most common cause of an alteration in the blood chemistry that might induce CSR is congestive heart failure, especially in elderly patients with degenerative arterial disease. Bronchopneumonia or other respiratory diseases in elderly people may likewise induce Cheyne-Stokes breathing, and CSR may occur in an otherwise healthy person through hyperventilation or exposure to high altitudes. This pattern of breathing may also be induced by an overdose of a narcotic or hypnotic drug, and it occurs more frequently during sleep. Compare **Biot's respiration.**

-chezia, a combining form meaning '(condition of) defecation, especially involving the discharge of foreign substances': *dyschezia, hematochezia, pyochezia.* Also **-chesia.**

CHF, abbreviation for **congestive heart failure.**

Chiari-Frommel syndrome (kiær′ifrom′əl), a hormo-

Differential diagnosis of chest pain

Cause	Onset of pain	Characteristic of pain	Location of pain
Acute myocardial infarction	Sudden onset; lasts more than 30 minutes to 1 hour	Pressure, burning, aching, tightness, choking	Across chest; may radiate to jaws and neck and down arms and back
Angina	Sudden onset; lasts only a few minutes	Aches, squeezing, choking, heaviness, burning	Substernal: may radiate to jaws and neck and down arms and back
Dissecting aortic aneurysm	Sudden onset	Excruciating, tearing	Center of chest: radiates into back; may radiate to abdomen
Pericarditis	Sudden onset or may be variable	Sharp, knifelike	Restrosternal: may radiate up neck and down left arm
Pneumothorax	Sudden onset	Tearing, pleuritic	Lateral side of chest
Pulmonary embolus	Sudden onset	Crushing (but not always)	Lateral side of onset
Hiatus hernia	Sudden onset	Sharp, severe	Lower chest: upper abdomen
Gastrointestinal disturbance or cholecystitis	Sudden onset	Gripping, burning	Lower substernal and upper abdomen
Degenerative disc (cervical or thoracic spine) disease	Sudden onset	Sharp, severe	Substernal: may radiate to neck, jaw, arms, and shoulders
Degenerative or inflammatory lesions of shoulder, ribs, scalenus anterior	Sudden onset	Sharp, severe	Substernal: radiates to shoulder
Hyperventilation	Sudden onset	Vague	Vague

nal disorder that occurs after a pregnancy in which weaning does not spontaneously end lactation. The syndrome is usually the result of a decrease in pituitary gonadotropins and an excess of pituitary prolactin. Treatment includes observation, hormonal therapy, and investigation to confirm or rule out pituitary tumor.

Chiari's syndrome (kiar′iz).   See **Budd-Chiari syndrome.**

chiasm (kai′æzəm),   **1.** the crossing of two lines or tracts, as the crossing of the optic nerves at the optic chiasm. **2.** (in genetics) the crossing of two chromatids in the prophase of meiosis.   –**chiasmal, chiasmic,** *adj.*

chiasma (kaiæz′mə), *pl.* **chiasmata.**   (in genetics), the visible point of connection between homologous chromosomes during the first meiotic division in gametogenesis. The x-shaped configurations form during the late prophase stage and provide the means by which exchange of genetic material occurs. See also **crossing over.**   –**chiasmatic, chiasmic** *adj.*

chiasmatypy.   See **crossing over.**

chickenpox,   an acute, highly contagious viral disease

caused by a herpesvirus, varicella zoster virus (VZV). It occurs primarily in young children and is characterized by crops of pruritic vesicular eruptions on the skin. The disease is transmitted by direct contact with skin lesions or, more commonly, by droplets spread from the respiratory tract of infected persons, usually in the prodromal period or the early stages of the rash. The vesicular fluid and the scabs are infectious until entirely dry. Indirect transmission through uninfected persons or objects is rare. The diagnosis is usually made by physical examination and by the characteristic appearance of the disease. The virus may be identified by culture of the vesicle fluid. Also called **varicella.**

■ OBSERVATIONS: The incubation period averages two to three weeks, followed by slight fever, mild headache, malaise, and anorexia occurring about 24 to 36 hours before the rash begins. The prodromal period is usually mild in children but may be severe in adults. The rash, which is highly pruritic, begins as macules and progresses in a day or two to papules and, finally, to vesicles surrounding an

History	Pain worsened by	Pain relieved by	Other
40 to 70 years of age; may or may not have history of angina	Movement, anxiety	Nothing; no movement, stillness, position, or breath holding; only relieved by medication (morphine sulfate)	Shortness of breath, diaphoresis, weakness, anxiety
May have history of angina; circumstances precipitating; pain characteristic; response to nitroglycerin	Lying down, eating, effort, cold weather, smoking, stress, anger, worry, hunger	Rest, nitroglycerin	Unstable angina appears even at rest
Nothing specific except that pain is usually worse at onset			Blood pressure difference between right and left arms, murmur of aortic regurgitation
Short history of upper respiratory infection or fever	Deep breathing, trunk movement, maybe swallowing	Sitting up, leaning forward	Friction rub, paradoxical pulse over 10 mm Hg
None	Breathing		Dyspnea, increased pulse, decreased breath sounds, deviated trachea
Sometimes phlebitis	Breathing		Cyanosis, dyspnea, cough with hemoptysis
May have none	Heavy meal, bending, lying down	Bland diet, walking, antacids, semi-Fowler position	
May have none	Eating, lying down	Antacids	
May have none	Movement of neck or spine, lifting, straining	Rest, decreased movement	Pain usually on outer aspect of arm, thumb, or index finger
May have none	Movement of arm or shoulder	Elevation and arm support to shoulder, postural exercises	
Hyperventilation, anxiety, stress, emotional	Increased respiratory rate	Slowing of respiratory rate	Be *sure* hyperventilation is from nonmedical cause

erythematous base and containing clear fluid. Within 24 to 48 hours the vesicles turn cloudy and become umbilicated, are easily broken, and become encrusted. The lesions, which erupt in crops so that all three stages are present simultaneously, appear first on the back and chest and then spread to the face, neck, and limbs; they occur only rarely on the soles and palms. In severe cases, laryngeal or tracheal vesicles in the pharynx, larynx, and trachea may cause dyspnea and dysphagia. Prolonged fever, lymphadenopathy, and extreme irritability from pruritis are other symptoms. The symptoms last from a few days to two weeks.

■ INTERVENTION: Routine treatment consists of bed rest; antipyretics to reduce fever; applications of topical antipruritics, as wet compresses, calamine lotion, or a paste made from baking soda and water; or oral antihistamines, given for the relief of itching. Infected vesicles may be treated with neomycin-bacitracin, and systemic antibiotics may be given if the secondary bacterial infection is extensive. People who are susceptible and at risk for severe disease when exposed to the infection may be passively protected with zoster immune globulin (ZIG), immune serum globulin (ISG), or zoster immune plasma (ZIP). A preparation of the virus for active immunization is not yet available. Babies born to women who develop chicken pox within five days of delivery are especially likely to get a severe case of the disease. One attack of the disease confers permanent immunity, although recurring episodes of herpes zoster occur, especially in elderly or debilitated people, resulting from reactivation of the virus. Herpes zoster virus (HZV), like all herpesviruses, lies dormant in certain sensory nerve roots following primary infection.

■ NURSING CONSIDERATIONS: Chickenpox in childhood is usually benign. Few cases require hospitalization. It may be serious or fatal in immunocompromised people, as those receiving chemotherapy or radiotherapy for malignant disease, in those who have undergone organ transplantation, in those with congenital or acquired defects in cell-mediated immunity, or in those receiving high doses of steroids. Common complications are secondary bacterial infections, as abscesses, cellulitis, pneumonia, and sepsis, and hemorrhagic varicella (tiny hemorrhages which may occur in the vesicles or surrounding skin). Less common complications are encephalitis, Reye's syndrome, thrombocytopenia, and hepatitis.

chiclero's ulcer (chɪkler'ouz). See **American leishmaniasis.**

chief cell, **1.** Also called **zymogenic cell.** any one of the columnar epithelial cells or the cuboidal epithelial cells that line the gastric glands and secrete pepsin and the extrinsic factor, which is needed for the absorption of vitamin B_{12} and the normal development of red blood cells. Anemia is caused by the absence of intrinsic factor. **2.** any one of the epithelioid cells with pale-staining cyto-

plasm and a large nucleus containing a prominent nucleolus. Cords of such cells form the main substance of the pineal body. **3.** Also called **principal cell.** any one of the polyhedral epithelial cells, within the parathyroid glands, which contain pale, clear cytoplasm and a vesicular nucleus.

chief complaint, a subjective statement made by a patient describing the patient's most significant or serious symptoms or signs of illness or dysfunction.

Chief Executive Officer (CEO, C.E.O.), the most senior official of an organization or institution.

chief resident, a senior resident physician who acts temporarily as the clinical and administrative director of the house staff in a department of the hospital. The period of duty varies depending on the size of the department, the length of the residency, and the number of house staff.

chief surgeon, a surgeon appointed or elected head of the surgeons on the staff of a health-care facility.

chigger (chɪg'ər), the larva of a mite found in tall grass and weeds. It sticks to the skin and causes irritation and severe itching. Also called **harvest mite.**

chigoe (chɪg'ou), **1.** a flea found in tropical and subtropical America and Africa. The pregnant female flea burrows into the skin of the feet, causing an inflammatory condition that may lead to spontaneous amputation of a toe. Also called **burrowing flea, jigger, sand flea. 2.** See **chigger.**

chikungunya encephalitis (chɪk'əngən'yə), an arbovirus infection characterized by a high fever that begins abruptly, muscle aches, a rash, and pain in the joints. It is transmitted by the bite of a mosquito and occurs mainly in Africa, Asia, and on some of the Pacific islands, including Guam. The fever may last for a week then rise again after a remission of several days. Pain in the joints may continue after other symptoms have ceased. Supportive nursing care and symptomatic relief are the only treatments.

chilblain (chɪl'blein), redness and swelling of the skin owing to excessive exposure to cold. Burning, itching, blistering, and ulceration, similar to a thermal burn, may occur. Treatment includes protection against cold and injury, gentle warming, and avoidance of tobacco. Also called **pernio.** Compare **frostbite.**

child, *pl.* **children. 1.** a young person of either sex between the time of birth and adolescence; a boy or girl. **2.** an unborn or recently born human being; fetus, neonate, infant. **3.** an offspring or descendant; a son or daughter or a member of a particular tribe or clan. **4.** one who is like a child or immature. – **childish, childlike,** *adj.*

child abuse, the physical, sexual, or emotional maltreatment of a child. It may be overt or covert and often results in permanent physical or psychiatric injury, mental impairment, or, sometimes, death. Child abuse occurs predominantly with children less than three years of age and is the result of multiple and complex factors involving both the parents and the child, compounded by various stressful environmental circumstances, as poor socioeconomic conditions, inadequate physical and emotional support within the family, and any major life change or crisis, especially those crises arising from marital strife. Parents at high risk for abuse are characterized as having unsatisfied needs, difficulty in forming adequate interpersonal relationships, unrealistic expectations of the child, and a lack of nuturing experience, often involving neglect or abuse in their own childhoods. Predisposing factors among children include the temperament, personality, and activity level of the child, order of birth in the family, sensitivity to parental needs, and a need for special physical or emotional care resulting from illness, premature birth, or congenital or genetic abnormalities. Identification of abused children or potential child abusers is a major concern for all health care workers. Obvious physical marks on a child's body, as burns, welts, or bruises, and signs of emotional distress, including symptoms of failure to thrive, are common indications of some degree of neglect or abuse. Often, x rays to detect healed or new fractures of the extremities or diagnostic tests to identify sexual molestation are necessary. If abuse is suspected, the nurse is required to make the necessary report. Special counseling services or support groups, as Parents Anonymous, exist to help families in which a child is

---

Guidelines for identifying potential child abusers

One or both parents were often abused as children.
   Studies indicate over 90% of abusive parents were abused children.
Parents tend to be lonely adults, attracted to each other as they search for loving parent figures.
Extreme personal and social isolation. These parents lack group and community integration and most often lack family support.
Unstable marital relationship. Parents lack positive feedback and support.
Low self-esteem.
Parent-child role reversal. The parents want the infant to meet their unfulfilled needs for mothering.
Unrealistic expectations of infants. Parents expect children to act older.
Parents unable to reach out and ask for help.

Special traits that make a child vulnerable to abuse

Usually young child, under 3 years of age.
Something different about child (i.e., pregnancy or delivery uncomfortable, child unwanted, premature birth).
Child is extremely irritable or cries often.
Birth order. Most often the first or last child is abused.

---

abused. The nurse can play a significant role in preventing abuse by promoting a positive parent-child relationship, especially in the neonatal period, by teaching parents proper child care and disciplinary techniques, and by explaining normal child development and behavior so that parents can formulate realistic guidelines for discipline. Compare **child neglect.** See also **battered child syndrome.**

child-bearing period, the reproductive period in a woman's life, from puberty to menopause. It is the time during which she is physiologically able to conceive children.

childbed fever. See **puerperal fever.**

childbirth. See **birth.**

child development, the various stages of physical, social, and psychological growth that occur from birth through adulthood. See also **adolescence, development, growth, infant, neonatal period, psychosexual development, psychosocial development, toddler.**

childhood, 1. the period in human development that extends from birth until the onset of puberty. 2. the state or quality of being a child. See also **development, growth.**

childhood polycystic disease (CPD). See **polycystic kidney disease.**

childhood schizophrenia, a form of schizophrenia, occurring before the onset of puberty, resulting from organic brain damage or from environmental conditions. It is characterized by autistic withdrawal into fantasy, obsessional attachments, failure to communicate verbally, repetitive gestures, emotional unresponsiveness, and a severely impaired sense of identity. Two kinds of childhood schizophrenia are **early infantile autism** and **symbiotic infantile psychotic syndrome.**

child neglect, the failure by parents or guardians to provide the basic needs of a child by physical or emotional deprivation that interferes with normal growth and development or that places the child in jeopardy. Compare **child abuse.** See also **failure to thrive, maternal deprivation syndrome.**

child psychology, the study of the mental, emotional, and behavioral development of infants and children.

child welfare, any service sponsored by the community or special organizations that provide for the physical, social, or psychological care of children in need of it.

-chilia. See **-cheilia.**

chill, 1. the sensation of cold due to exposure to a cold environment. 2. an attack of shivering with pallor and a feeling of coldness, often occurring at the beginning of an infection and accompanied by a rapid rise in temperature.

Chilomastix (kaī'loumæs'tīks), a genus of flagellate protozoa, as *Chilomastix mesnili,* a nonpathogenic intestinal parasite of man.

chimera (kɪmir'ə, kaimir'ə), an organism carrying cell populations derived from different zygotes of the same or of different species. It may be a natural phenomenon, as in a bone marrow graft. Compare **mosaic.**

chimney-sweeps' cancer. See **scrotal cancer.**

Chinese restaurant syndrome, a syndrome consisting of tingling and burning sensations of the skin, facial pressure, headache, and chest pain that occurs immediately after eating food containing monosodium glutamate, frequently used in Chinese cooking.

chip, 1. a relatively small piece of a bone or tooth. 2. to break off or cut away a small piece.

chip fracture, any small fragmental fracture, usually one involving a bony process near a joint.

chir-. See **chiro-.**

chirality. See **handedness.**

-chiria, 1. a combining form meaning a '(specified) condition involving hands': *acephalochiria, atelochiria, dichiria.* 2. a combining form meaning a '(specified) condition involving stimulus and its perception': *allochiria, dyschiria, synchiria.* Also **-cheiria.**

chiro-, chir-. See **cheiro-.**

chiropodist (kɪrop'ədɪst, ʃhɪrop'ədɪst), a health professional trained to diagnose and treat diseases and other disorders of the feet. A chiropodist may be awarded a degree of D.S.C. (Doctor of Surgical Chiropody) or Pod.D. (Doctor of Podiatry) after completing at least two years of premedical studies and four years of study in an accredited college of podiatry. Internship is optional, but a graduate must pass an examination and receive a state license before being allowed to practice. After a refresher course, a D.S.C. or a Pod.D. may be granted the postgraduate degree D.P.M. (Doctor of Podiatric Medicine). Also called **podiatrist.**

chiropody (kɪrop'ədi, ʃhɪrop'ədi), the study of minor disorders of the feet and the practice of treating these disorders. Practitioners trained in chiropody are licensed to practice by the various states but do not hold a medical degree or license.

chiropractic (kaɪ'roupræk'tɪk), a system of therapy based on the theory that the state of a person's health is determined in general by the condition of his nervous system. In most cases treatment provided by chiropractors involves the mechanical manipulation of the spinal column. Some practitioners employ radiology for diagnosis and use physiotherapy and diet in addition to spinal manipulation. Chiropractic does not employ drugs or surgery, the primary basis of treatment used by medical physicians. A chiropractor is awarded the degree of Doctor of Chiropractic, or D.C., after completing at least two years of premedical studies followed by four years of training in an approved chiropractic school.

-chirurgia. See **-surgery.**

chisel fracture, any fracture in which there is an oblique detachment of a bone fragment from the head of the radius.

chi square (χ^2) (kaɪ'), (in statistics) a statistical test for an association between observed data and expected data represented by frequencies. The test yields a statement of the probability of the obtained distribution having occurred by chance alone.

Chlamydia (kləmɪd'iə), 1. a microorganism of the genus *Chlamydia.* 2. a genus of microorganisms that live as intracellular parasites, have a number of properties in common with gram-negative bacteria, and are currently classified as specialized bacteria. Two species of *Chlamydia* have been recognized; both are pathogenic to humans. *Chlamydia trachomatis,* an organism that lives in the conjunctiva of the eye and the epithelium of the urethra and cervix, is responsible for inclusion conjunctivitis, lymphogranuloma venereum, and trachoma. *Chlamydia psittaci* is an organism that infects birds and causes a type of pneumonia in humans. See also **psittacosis.** – **chlamydial,** *adj.*

Chlamydia psittaci. See *Chlamydia.*

Chlamydia trachomatis. See *Chlamydia.*

chloasma (klouæz'mə), tan or brown pigmentation, particularly of the forehead, cheeks, and nose, commonly associated with pregnancy or the use of oral contraceptives. The hyperpigmentation may be permanent or may disappear only to recur with subsequent pregnancies or use of oral contraceptives. Also called **mask of pregnancy, melasma.**

chlor-, a combining form meaning 'green': *chloremia, chlorephidrosis, chlorine.*

chloracne (klɔræk'ni), a skin condition characterized by small, black follicular plugs and papules on exposed surfaces, especially on the arms, face, and neck of workers in contact with chlorinated compounds, as cutting oils, paints, varnishes, and lacquers. Avoidance of contact with chlorinated compounds or the use of protective garments prevents the condition.

chloral camphor, a mixture of equal parts of camphor and chloral hydrate, used externally as a sedative.

chloral hydrate, a sedative and hypnotic.

■ INDICATIONS: It is prescribed for the relief of insomnia, anxiety, or tension.

■ CONTRAINDICATIONS: Liver or kidney dysfunction or known hypersensitivity to this drug prohibits its use.

■ ADVERSE EFFECTS: Among the more serious adverse reations are gastrointestinal disturbances, skin rash, paradoxical excitement, and hypotension.

chlorambucil, an alkylating agent.

■ INDICATIONS: It is prescribed in the treatment of a variety of malignant neoplastic diseases, including chronic lymphocytic leukemia and Hodgkin's disease.

■ CONTRAINDICATIONS: Bone marrow depression or known hypersensitivity to this drug prohibits its use. It is not given during the first trimester of pregnancy or within 28 days of chemotherapy or radiation therapy.

■ ADVERSE EFFECTS: Among the more serious adverse

reactions are bone marrow depression, gastrointestinal disturbance, skin rash, and hepatotoxicity.

chloramphenicol, an antibacterial and antirickettsial.

- INDICATIONS: It is prescribed in the treatment of a wide variety of serious infections.
- CONTRAINDICATIONS: Mild or unidentified infections, pregnancy, lactation, or known hypersensitivity to this drug prohibits its use.
- ADVERSE EFFECTS: Among the more serious adverse reactions are blood dyscrasias, bone marrow depression, and aplastic anemia.

chlorcyclizine hydrochloride (klɔrsai′klızin), an antihistamine that has been used for rhinitis, sinusitis, and hayfever. As a cream, it is also used for skin conditions.

chlordane poisoning. See **chlorinated organic insecticide poisoning.**

chlordantoin (klɔrdæn′touin), an antifungal.

- INDICATIONS: It is prescribed in the treatment of candidiasis of the vagina and the skin.
- CONTRAINDICATION: Known hypersensitivity to this drug prohibits its use.
- ADVERSE EFFECTS: Among the more serious adverse reactions are irritation and allergic reactions.

chlordiazepoxide (klɔr′daiei′zəpok′said), a minor tranquilizer.

- INDICATIONS: It is prescribed in the treatment of anxiety and nervous tension.
- CONTRAINDICATIONS: Psychosis, acute narrow angle glaucoma, or known hypersensitivity to this drug prohibits its use.
- ADVERSE EFFECTS: Among the more serious adverse reactions are withdrawal symptoms occurring on discontinuation of treatment. Drowsiness and fatigue commonly occur.

-chloric, a combining form meaning 'referring to or containing chlorine': *hydrochloric, hyperchloric, perchloric.*

chloride (klɔr′aid), a compound in which the negative element is chlorine. Chlorides are salts of hydrochloric acid, the most common being sodium chloride (table salt).

chlorinated organic insecticide poisoning, poisoning resulting from the inhalation, ingestion, or absorption of DDT and other insecticides containing chlorophenothane, as heptachlor, dieldrin, and chlordane. It is characterized by vomiting, weakness, malaise, convulsions, tremors, ventricular fibrillation, respiratory failure, and pulmonary edema. Treatment includes control of the neurological and neuromuscular symptoms with phenobarbitol and gastric lavage, instillation of a demulcent and absorbent like sodium sulfate or charcoal in the stomach, parenteral fluids, and supportive therapy as indicated by monitoring vital functions. Also called **DDT poisoning.**

chlorine (Cl), a yellowish-green, gaseous element of the halogen group. Its atomic number is 17; its atomic weight is 35.453. It has a strong, distinctive odor, is irritating to the respiratory tract, and is poisonous if ingested or inhaled. It occurs in nature chiefly as a component of sodium chloride in sea water and in salt deposits. It is used as a bleach and as a disinfectant to purify water for drinking or for use in swimming pools. Chlorine compounds in general use include many solvents, cleaning fluids, and chloroform. Most of the solvents and cleaning fluids containing chlorine are toxic when inhaled or ingested. Chloroform was formerly in general use as an anesthetic.

chlormezanone, an antianxiety agent.

- INDICATIONS: It is prescribed for mild anxiety and for nervous tension.
- CONTRAINDICATION: Known hypersensitivity to this drug prohibits its use.
- ADVERSE EFFECTS: Among the most serious adverse reactions are hypersensitivity and sedation. Dizziness, nausea, and rashes often occur.

chloroform (klɔr′əfɔrm), a nonflammable, volatile liquid that was the first inhalation anesthetic to be discovered. Because of ease of administration—often just a medicine dropper and a handkerchief face mask—it is still the principal general anesthetic in many underdeveloped countries, where anesthesia equipment for the newer agents is not available. Chloroform is a dangerous anesthetic drug: a difference of only 10 per cent in drug-plasma levels can result in hypotension, myocardial and respiratory depression, cardiogenic shock, ventricular fibrillation, coma, and death. Delayed poisoning, even weeks after apparently complete recovery, is not unusual, and serious ocular damage is frequently reported.

chloroformism, 1. the habit of inhaling chloroform for its narcotic effect. 2. the anesthetic effect of chloroform.

chloroguanide hydrochloride, an antimalarial.

- INDICATIONS: It is prescribed in the prophylaxis of malaria.
- CONTRAINDICATIONS: Hypersensitivity to the drug prohibits its use. It is prescribed with caution during pregnancy, especially in the first trimester.
- ADVERSE EFFECTS: Among the more serious adverse reactions are megaloblastic anemia, anorexia, and weight loss, usually occurring with prolonged prophylactic use.

chloroleukemia (klɔr′ouluki′miə), a kind of myelogenous leukemia in which specific tumor masses are not seen at autopsy but body fluids and organs are green. See also **myelogenous leukemia.**

chlorolymphosarcoma (klɔr′oulım′fousarkou′mə), *pl.* **chlorolymphosarcomas, chlorolymphosarcomata.** a greenish neoplasm of myeloid tissue occurring in patients with myelogenous, leukemia. The mononuclear cells in the peripheral blood are believed to be lymphocytes rather than myeloblasts, as found with chloroma.

chloroma (klɔrou′mə), *pl.* **chloromas, chloromata.** a malignant, greenish neoplasm of myeloid tissue occurring anywhere in the body in patients with myelogenous leukemia. The green pigment, primarily myeloperoxidase (verdoperoxidase), has no definite metabolic function. The tumor tissue fluoresces bright red under ultraviolet light. Also called **granulocytic sarcoma, green cancer.**

Chloromycetin, a trade name for an antibacterial and antirickettsial (chloramphenicol).

chloromyeloma (klɔr'oumaĭ'əlou'mə). See **chloroma.**

chlorophyll (klɔr'əfĭl), a plant pigment capable of absorbing light and converting it to energy for the oxidation and reduction involved in the photosynthesis of carbohydrates. Chlorophylls a and b are found in green plants; chlorophyll c occurs in brown algae, and chlorophyll d occurs in red algae. See also **photosynthesis.**

chlorophyll test. See **Boas' test.**

chloroprocaine (klɔr'ouprou'kein), a local anesthetic with a chemical structure similar to procaine.

chloroquine (klɔr'əkwain), an antimalarial.
- INDICATIONS: It is prescribed in the treatment of malaria, rheumatoid arthritis, some forms of lupus erythematosus, and photoallergic reactions.
- CONTRAINDICATIONS: Retinal or visual field changes, porphyria, or known hypersensitivity to this drug prohibits its use.
- ADVERSE EFFECTS: Among the more serious adverse reactions are gastrointestinal disturbances, headache, visual disturbances, and pruritus.

chlorosis (klɔrou'sĭs), *Archaic.* an iron deficiency anemia of young women characterized by hypochromic, microcytic erythrocytes and a small reduction in the total number of erythrocytes. See also **anemia.**

chlorothiazide, a diuretic and antihypertensive.
- INDICATIONS: It is prescribed in the treatment of hypertension and edema.
- CONTRAINDICATIONS: Anuria or known hypersensitivity to thiazide medication or to sulfonamide derivatives prohibits its use.
- ADVERSE EFFECTS: Among the more serious adverse reactions are hypokalemia, hyperglycemia, and hyperuricemia. Hypersensitivity reactions may occur.

chlorotrianisene, an estrogen.
- INDICATIONS: It is prescribed in the treatment of postpartum breast engorgement, menopausal symptoms, and prostatic cancer.
- CONTRAINDICATIONS: Liver dysfunction, thromboembolic disorders, unusual vaginal bleeding, known or suspected pregnancy, suspected estrogen dependent neoplastic disease, or known hypersensitivity to this drug prohibits its use.
- ADVERSE EFFECTS: Among the more serious adverse reactions are gastrointestinal distress, breakthrough bleeding, and, in men, gynecomastia, decreased libido, and impotence.

chlorpheniramine maleate, an antihistamine.

- INDICATIONS: It is prescribed in the treatment of a variety of hypersensitivity reactions, including rhinitis, skin rash, and pruritus.
- CONTRAINDICATIONS: Asthma or known hypersensitivity to this drug prohibits its use. It is not given to newborn infants or nursing mothers.
- ADVERSE EFFECT: Among the more serious adverse reactions are skin rash, hypersensitivity reactions, and tachycardia. Drowsiness and dry mouth commonly occur.

chlorpromazine (klɔrprou'məzin), a phenothiazine tranquilizer and antiemetic.
- INDICATIONS: It is prescribed in the treatment of psychotic disorders, severe nausea and vomiting, and intractable hiccups.
- CONTRAINDICATIONS: Parkinson's disease, concurrent administration of central nervous system depressants, liver or renal dysfunction, severe hypotension, or known hypersensitivity to this drug or to other phenothiazine medication prohibits its use.
- ADVERSE EFFECTS: Among the more serious adverse effects are hypotension, liver toxicity, a variety of extrapyramidal reactions, blood dyscrasias, and hypersensitivity reactions.

chlorpropamide, an oral antidiabetic.
- INDICATION: It is prescribed in the treatment of mild, stable adult onset diabetes mellitus.
- CONTRAINDICATIONS: Liver or kidney dysfunction or known hypersensitivity to this drug prohibits its use.
- ADVERSE EFFECTS: Among the most serious adverse reactions are hematologic derangements and jaundice. Gastrointestinal distress and rashes are common adverse effects.

chlorprothixene (klɔr'prouthĭk'sin), a thioxanthine antipsychotic agent.
- INDICATIONS: It is prescribed in the treatment of psychotic disorders.
- CONTRAINDICATIONS: Parkinson's disease, concurrent administration of central nervous system depressants, liver or renal dysfunction, severe hypotension, or known hypersensitivitity to this drug prohibits its use.
- ADVERSE EFFECTS: Among the more serious adverse effects are hypotension, liver toxicity, a variety of extra pyramidal reactions, blood dycrasias, and hypersensitivity reactions.

chlortetracycline hydrochloride, an antibiotic.
- INDICATIONS: It is prescribed in the treatment of a variety of infections.
- CONTRAINDICATIONS: Renal or liver dysfunction, pregnancy, early childhood, or known hypersensitivity to this drug or to other tetracycline medication prohibits its use.
- ADVERSE EFFECTS: Among the more serious adverse effects are gastrointestinal disturbances, phototoxicity, potentially serious suprainfections, and hypersensitivity re-

actions. Discoloration of teeth may occur in children exposed to this drug in utero or before eight years of age.

chlorthalidone, a diuretic.

- INDICATIONS: It is prescribed in the treatment of high blood pressure and edema.
- CONTRAINDICATIONS: Anuria or known hypersensitivity to this drug, to other thiazide medication, or to sulfonamide derivatives prohibits its use.
- ADVERSE EFFECTS: Among the more serious adverse reactions are hypokalemia, hyperglycemia, hyperuricemia, and hypersensitivity reactions.

Chlor-Trimeton, a trade name for an antihistamine (chlorpheniramine maleate).

chlorzoxazone (klɔrzok′səzoun), a skeletal muscle relaxant.

- INDICATION: It is prescribed for the relief of muscle spasm.
- CONTRAINDICATION: Known hypersensitivity to this drug is the only contraindication.
- ADVERSE EFFECTS: Among the more serious adverse reactions are jaundice and gastrointestinal bleeding.

choana (kou′ənə), pl. choanae. 1. a funnel-shaped channel. 2. See **posterior nares.**

choanal atresia (kou′ənəl), a congenital anomaly in which a bony or membranous occlusion blocks the passageway between the nose and pharynx. The condition, which is caused by the failure of the nasopharyngeal septum to rupture during embryonic development, can result in serious ventilation problems in the neonate, and providing an oral airway or endotracheal intubation may be necessary. The defect is usually repaired surgically shortly after birth.

choke, to interrupt respiration by compression or obstruction of larynx or trachea.

choke damp. See **damp.**

choked disc. *Informal.* papilledema.

chokes, a respiratory condition, occurring in decompression sickness, characterized by shortness of breath, substernal pain and a nonproductive cough caused by bubbles of gas in the blood vessels of the lungs.

choking, the condition in which a respiratory passage is blocked by constriction of the neck, an obstruction in the trachea, or swelling of the larynx. It is characterized by sudden coughing and a red face that rapidly becomes purple. The person cannot breathe and clutches his throat. Emergency treatment requires removal of the obstruction and resuscitation if necessary. See also **Heimlich maneuver.**

chol-. See **chole-.**

cholangeostomy (kɒulæn′jios′təmi), a surgical operation to form an opening in a bile duct.

cholangiogram (kɒulæn′jiəgræm′), an x-ray picture of the biliary duct system obtained after the injection of an appropriate radiopaque material. See also **cholangiography.**

cholangiography (kɒulæn′jiog′rəfi), a special roentgenographic test procedure for outlining the major bile ducts by the intravenous injection or the direct instillation of a radiopaque contrast material.

- METHOD: For intravenous cholangiography the contrast agent is given slowly by vein, and x rays are taken of the region of the gall bladder. If the gall bladder has not been removed, a fatty meal may then be given and further x rays taken to show contraction of the gall bladder. Operative and postoperative cholangiography employ the injection of contrast material into the common bile duct via a drainage T-tube inserted during surgery, the purpose being to discover any small, residual gallstones. In percutaneous transhepatic cholangiography the contrast material is injected through a long needle or needle-catheter, which is introduced directly through the skin into the substance of the liver. Endoscopic retrograde cholangiography is accomplished by cannulating the ampulla of Vater through a flexible fiberoptic duodenoscope and instilling radiopaque material directly into the common bile duct.
- NURSING ORDERS: Intravenous cholangiography cannot be used in the presence of severe liver disease or jaundice, because the dye will not be concentrated and excreted into the bile. The patient fasts, and fluids are restricted overnight. An early morning cleansing enema is given, usually followed by a sedative. The patient is warned about a brief period of a burning sensation that occurs as the dye is injected. For percutaneous transhepatic cholangiography, sedative premedication is often ordered and a local anesthetic injected at the site of needle puncture. Appropriate evaluation for bleeding tendencies must be carried out prior to percutaneous transhepatic cholangiography. Bile peritonitis is occasionally a complication of T-tube or percutaneous cholangiography, and close nursing observation is essential after the test is completed. For endoscopic retrograde cholangiography, nothing is given by mouth after midnight, an explanation is given to the patient, dentures are removed, and, to permit administration of medications, intravenous infusion is begun. The endoscope is passed with the patient in the left lateral position; then patient is turned to the prone position, the ampulla is cannulated, the dye is injected, and films are taken. Vital signs are observed and the patient is given a light meal in 2 to 4 hours following the procedure.
- OUTCOME CRITERIA: The resulting cholangiograms from any of these procedures are examined for unobstructed outlining of the biliary system. Calculi may be noted as shadows within the opaque medium. See also **cholecystography.**

cholangiohepatoma (kɒulæn′jiouhep′ətou′mə), pl. **cholangiohepatomas, cholangiohepatomata.** a neoplasm in which there is an abnormal mixture of liver cord cells and bile ducts.

cholangiolitis (kəlæn'jiəlai'tɪs), an abnormal condition characterized by inflammation of the fine tubules of the bile duct system, which may cause cholangiolitic cirrhosis. – **cholangiolitic,** *adj.*

cholangioma (koulæn'jiou'mə), *pl.* **cholangiomas, cholangiomata.** a neoplasm of the bile ducts.

cholangitis (kou'lænjai'tɪs), inflammation of the bile ducts, caused either by bacterial invasion or by obstruction of the ducts by calculi or a tumor. The condition is characterized by severe right upper quadrant pain, jaundice (if an obstruction is present), and intermittent fever. Blood tests reveal an elevated level of serum bilirubin. Diagnosis is made by oral cholecystogram or intravenous cholangiogram. Treatment is with antibiotics for infection and with surgery for acute obstruction. See also **biliary calculus.**

chole-, chol-, cholo-, a combining form meaning 'pertaining to the bile': *cholecystectomy, cholelithotomy, cholesterase.*

cholecalciferol (kou'lɪkælsɪf'ərɔl). See **vitamin D.**

cholecystectomy (kou'lɪsɪstek'təmi), the surgical removal of the gall bladder, performed to treat cholelithiasis and cholecystitis. Surgery may be delayed while the acute inflammation is treated. A cholecystogram is done to confirm the diagnosis, and an electrocardiogram and tests of hepatic function may be ordered. The prothrombin level is evaluated and, if it is low, vitamin K is given. Under general anesthesia, the gall bladder is excised and the cystic duct ligated; the common duct is searched and any stones found are removed. A T-tube is left in place to ensure adequate bile drainage; a Penrose drain may be left in a separate stab wound to prevent the formation of an abcess. The most common complication is a disruption of the hepatic or other ducts of the biliary system, requiring surgical correction. Wound infection, hemorrhage, bile leakage, and jaundice may also occur. A nasogastric tube is left in place postoperatively until bowel function has returned and food can be tolerated. See also **cholecystitis, cholelithiasis.**

cholecystitis (kou'lɪsɪstai'tɪs), acute or chronic inflammation of the gall bladder. **Acute cholecystitis** is usually caused by a gallstone that cannot pass through the cystic duct. Pain is felt in the right upper quadrant of the abdomen, accompanied by nausea, vomiting, eructation, and flatulence. Diagnosis is usually made with oral cholecystogram, useful in ruling out acute appendicitis, intestinal obstruction, peptic ulcer, and other upper abdominal disorders. Surgery is the preferred mode of treatment. **Chronic cholecystitis,** the more common type, has an insidious onset. Pain, often felt at night, may follow a fatty meal. Complications include biliary calculi, pancreatitis, and carcinoma of the gall bladder. Again, surgery is the

preferred treatment. See also **biliary calculus, cholecystectomy, cholelithiasis.**

cholecystogram (kou'lɪsɪs'təgræm), an x ray of the gall bladder, made after the ingestion or injection of a radiopaque substance, usually a contrast material containing iodine.

cholecystography (kou'lɪsɪstog'rəfi), an x-ray examination of the gall bladder. At least 12 hours prior to the study the patient has a fat-free meal and ingests a contrast material containing iodine, usually in the form of tablets; it may also be given intravenously. The iodine, which is opaque to x rays, is excreted by the liver into the bile in the gall bladder. Following the procedure, the patient consumes a fatty meal or cholecystokinin, which stimulates the gall bladder to contract, expelling bile and contrast material into the bile duct. Additional x rays are taken about an hour later. The test is useful in the diagnosis of cholecystitis, cholelithiasis, tumors, and the differential diagnosis of a mass in the upper right quadrant of the stomach.

cholecystokinin (kol'ɪsɪs'təkai'nɪn), a hormone, produced by the mucosa of the upper intestine, that stimulates contraction of the gall bladder and the secretion of pancreatic enzymes.

choledocholithiasis (kouled'oukou'lɪthai'əsɪs). See **biliary calculus.**

choledocholithotomy (kouled'oukou'lɪfhot'əmi), a surgical operation to make an incision in the common bile duct to remove a stone.

Choledyl, a trade name for a theophylline derivative (oxtriphylline), used as a bronchodilator.

cholelithiasis (kou'lɪlɪthai'əsɪs), the presence of gallstones in the gall bladder. The condition affects about 20 per cent of the population over age 40 and is more prevalent in women and in persons with cirrhosis of the liver. Many patients complain of unlocalized abdominal discomfort, eructation, and intolerance to certain foods. Other patients will have no symptoms at all. In patients with severe attacks of biliary pain associated with cholelithiasis, cholecystectomy is recommended to prevent such complications as cholecystitis, cholangitis, and pancreatitis. See also **biliary calculus, cholecystitis.**

cholelithic dyspepsia (kou'lɪlɪfh'ɪk), an abnormal condition characterized by sudden attacks of indigestion associated with the dysfunction of the gallbladder. See also **dyspepsia.**

cholelithotomy (kou'lɪlɪfhot'əmi), a surgical operation to remove gallstones through an incision in the gallbladder.

cholera (kol'ərə), an acute bacterial infection of the small intestine, characterized by severe diarrhea and vomiting, muscular cramps, dehydration, and depletion of electrolytes. The disease is spread by water and food that have been contaminated by feces of persons previously infected. The symptoms are caused by toxic substances produced by the infecting organism, *Vibrio cholerae*. The profuse, watery diarrhea, as much as a liter an hour, depletes the body of fluids and minerals. Complications include circulatory collapse, cyanosis, destruction of kidney tissue, and metabolic acidosis. Mortality is as high as 50 per cent if the infection remains untreated. Treatment includes the administration of antibiotics that destroy the infecting bacteria and the restoration of normal amounts of fluids and electrolytes with intravenous solutions. A cholera vaccine is available for people traveling to areas where the infection is endemic. Other preventive measures include drinking only boiled or bottled water and eating only cooked foods. See also *Vibrio cholerae, Vibrio gastroenteritis.*

choleragen (kol′ərəjɪn), an exotoxin, produced by the cholera vibrio, that stimulates the secretion of electrolyte and water into the small intestine in Asiatic cholera, draining the fluids of the body and weakening the patient.

cholera vaccine, an active immunizing agent.
■ INDICATION: It is prescribed as an immunization against cholera.
■ CONTRAINDICATIONS: Immunosuppression, acute infection, concomitant administration of corticosteroids, or known hypersensitivity to this drug prohibits its use.
■ ADVERSE EFFECTS: The most serious adverse reaction is anaphylaxis.

choleretic (kou′lɔret′ɪk), **1.** stimulating the production of bile either by cholepoiesis or by hydrocholeresis. **2.** a choleretic agent.

choleric (kol′ərɪk, kəler′ɪk), having a hot temper or an irascible nature.

cholestasis (kou′lɪstei′sɪs), interruption in the flow of bile through any part of the biliary system, from liver to duodenum. It is essential for the physician to discover whether the cause is within the liver (intrahepatic) or outside it (extrahepatic). Intrahepatic causes include hepatitis, drug and alcohol use, metastatic carcinoma, and pregnancy. Extrahepatic causes may be an obstructing calculus or tumor in the common bile duct or carcinoma of the pancreas. Symptoms of both types of cholestasis include jaundice, pale and fatty stools, dark urine, and intense itching over the skin. If liver disease is suspected, liver biopsy can confirm the suspicion, and attempts can be made to treat the underlying disorder. Extrahepatic cholestasis usually requires surgery. See also **cholestatic hepatitis.** — **cholestatic,** *adj.*

cholestatic hepatitis (kou′lɪstæt′ɪk), inflammation of the liver due to hepatitis infection that causes interruption of the flow of bile in the intrahepatic ducts. Signs are persistent jaundice, itching, and elevated alkaline phosphatase. These signs usually abate when the hepatitis remits. See also **cholestasis, hepatitis.**

cholesteatoma (koules′tiətou′mə), a cystic mass composed of epithelial cells and cholesterol that is found in the middle ear and occurs as a congenital defect or as a serious complication of chronic otitis media. The mass may occlude the middle ear, or enzymes produced by it may destroy the adjacent bones, including the ossicles. Surgery is required to remove a cholesteatoma. See also **otitis media.**

cholesteatoma tympani, a growth formed by shed squamous epithelial cells in the middle ear. It is associated with chronic infection.

cholesterase (kəles′təreis′), an enzyme in the blood and other tissues, that forms cholesterol and fatty acids by hydrolyzing cholesterol esters.

cholesteremia (koules′təri′miə). See **cholesterolemia.**

cholesterin (kəles′tərɪn). See **cholesterol.**

cholesterol (kəles′tərol), a fat-soluble crystalline steroid alcohol found in animal fats and oils, egg yolk, and widely distributed in the body, especially in the bile, blood, brain tissue, liver, kidneys, adrenal glands, and myelin sheaths of nerve fibers. It facilitates the absorption and transport of fatty acids and acts as the precursor for the synthesis of vitamin D at the surface of the skin. It also acts for the synthesis of the various steroid hormones, including cortisol, cortisone, and aldosterone in the adrenal glands and of the sex hormones progesterone, estrogen, and testosterone. It sometimes crystallizes in the gall bladder to form gallstones. Cholesterol is found almost exclusively in foods of animal origin and is continuously synthesized in the body, primarily in the liver and the adrenal cortex. Increased levels of serum cholesterol may be associated with the pathogenesis of atherosclerosis. Also called **cholesterin.** See also **high density lipoprotein, low density lipoprotein, vitamin D.**

cholesterolemia, **1.** the presence of excessive amounts of cholesterol in the blood. **2.** the abnormal condition of having excessive amounts of cholesterol in the blood. Also called **cholesteremia.**

cholesteroleresis (kəles′tərɔler′ɪsɪs), the increased elimination of cholesterol in the bile.

cholesterol metabolism, the sum of the anabolic and catabolic processes in the synthesis and degradation of cholesterol in the body. Ingested cholesterol is quickly absorbed. It is also synthesized in the liver and can be synthesized by most other tissues of the body. As more cholesterol is ingested, less is synthesized. Cholesterol is removed from the body by conversion in the liver and excretion in the bile.

cholesterolopoiesis (kəles′tərɔloupoii′sɪs), the elaboration of cholesterol by the liver.

cholesterolosis (kəles′tərɔlou′sɪs), an abnormal condition, found in about 5 percent of patients with chronic cholecystitis, in which there are deposits of cholesterol within large macrophages in the submucosa of the gall bladder. This produces a spotty appearance, sometimes referred to as a strawberry gall bladder. Cholesterolosis is often associated with gallstones and may be asymptomatic or accompanied by biliary colic. See also **cholecystitis.**

cholestyramine resin, an ion-exchange resin and antihyperlipoproteinemic agent.

■ INDICATIONS: It is prescribed for hyperlipoproteinemia and for pruritus resulting from partial biliary obstruction.

■ CONTRAINDICATIONS: Complete biliary obstruction or known hypersensitivity to this drug prohibits its use.

■ ADVERSE EFFECTS: Among the more serious adverse reactions are fecal impaction, gastrointestinal disturbances, and depletion of vitamins A, D, and K. Constipation is common.

-cholia, a combining form meaning '(condition of the) bile': *albuminocholia, syncholia, uricocholia.* Also **-choly.**

choline (kou′lin), one of the B complex vitamins, essential for the metabolism of fats in the body. It is a primary component of acetylcholine, the neurotransmitter, and functions with inositol as a basic constituent of lecithin. It prevents the deposition of fats in the liver and facilitates the movement of fats into the cells. The richest sources of choline are liver, kidneys, brains, wheat germ, brewer's yeast, and egg yolk. Deficiency leads to hepatic cirrhosis, resulting in bleeding stomach ulcers and impaired kidney function, hypertension, high blood levels of cholesterol, and atherosclerosis and arteriosclerosis. See also **inositol, lecithin.**

cholinergic, 1. of or pertaining to nerve fibers that elaborate acetylcholine at the myoneural junctions. 2. the tendency to transmit or to be stimulated or to stimulate by the elaboration of acetylcholine. Compare **adrenergic.**

cholinergic blocking agent, any agent that blocks the action of acetylcholine and substances similar to acetylcholine. Such agents, in effect, block the action of cholinergic nerves which transmit impulses by the release of acetylcholine at their synapses.

cholinergic crisis, a pronounced muscular weakness and respiratory paralysis caused by excessive acetylcholine, often apparent in patients suffering from myasthenia gravis as a result of overmedication with anticholinesterase drugs.

cholinergic nerve, a nerve that releases the neurotransmitter acetylcholine at its synapse. The cholinergic nerves include all the preganglionic sympathetic and the preganglionic parasympathetic nerves, the postganglionic parasympathetic nerves, the somatic motor nerves to skeletal muscles, and some nerves to sweat glands and to certain blood vessels.

cholinergic stimulant. See **cholinergic.**

cholinergic urticaria, an abnormal and usually transient vascular reaction of the skin, often associated with sweating in susceptible individuals subjected to stress, strong exertion, or hot weather. The condition is charac-

terized by small, pale, itchy papules surrounded by reddish areas; it is caused by the action of acetylcholine on mast cells.

cholinesterase (kou′lınes′təreis), an enzyme that acts as a catalyst in the hydrolysis of acetylcholine to choline and acetate.

cholo-. See **chole-.**

Cholografin, a trade name for a diagnostic dye (iodipamide), used in radiology.

-choly. See **-cholia.**

-chomic. See **-chrome**[1].

chondr-. See **chondro-.**

chondral (kon′drəl), of or pertaining to cartilage.

chondrectomy (kondrek′təmi), the surgical excision of a cartilage.

chondri-. See **chondro-.**

-chondria, 1. a combining form meaning a 'condition involving granules in cell composition': *lipochondria, mitochondria, plastochondria.* 2. a combining form meaning an 'abnormal preoccupation with worry about disease': *hypochondria.*

chondriocont (kon′driɔukont′), a threadlike or rod-shaped mitochondrion.

chondriome, chondrioma, the total mitochondria content of a cell, taken as a unit.

chondriomite, a single granular mitochondrion or a group of such organelles appearing in a chain formation.

chondriosome. See **mitochondrion.**

chondritis, any inflammatory condition affecting the joints.

chondro-, chondr-, chondri-, a combining form meaning 'pertaining to cartilage': *chondroblast, chondroclast, chondrocostal.*

chondroadenoma (kon′drouæd′ınou′mə), *pl.* **chondroadenomas, chondroadenomata.** See **adenochondroma.**

chondroangioma (kon′drouæn′jiou′mə), *pl.* **chondroangiomas, chondroangiomata.** a benign, mesenchymal tumor containing vascular and cartilaginous elements.

chondroblast (kon′droublæst), any one of the cells that develops from the mesenchyma and forms cartilage. Also called **chondroplast.**

chondroblastoma (kon′droublæstou′mə), *pl.* **chondroblastomas, chondroblastomata.** a benign tumor, derived from precursors of cartilage cells, that develops most frequently in epiphyses of the femur and humerus, especially in young men. The lesions may contain scattered areas of calcification and necrosis. Also called **Codman's tumor.**

chondrocalcinosis (kon′droukæl′sınou′sıs), an arthritic disease in which calcium deposits are found in the peripheral joints. Chondrocalcinosis, which resembles gout, is often found in patients over 50 who have osteoarthritis or diabetes mellitus. Aspiration of synovial fluid from the affected joints reveals crystals of calcium salts. Inflammation and pain may be relieved by intra-articular injections of hydrocortisone and by anti-inflammatory medications. Prognosis for recovery is excellent. Also called **pseudogout.** Compare **gout, gouty arthritis.**

chondrocarcinoma (kon'drɔukar'sɪnou'mə), *pl.* **chondrocarcinoma, chondrocarcinomata.** a malignant epithelial tumor in which there is cartilaginous metaplasia.

chondroclast, a giant multinucleated cell associated with the resorption of cartilage. —**chondroclastic,** *adj.*

chondrocostal (kon'drɔukos'təl), of or pertaining to the ribs and the costal cartilages.

chondrocyte (kon'drəsait), any one of the polymorphic cells that form the cartilage of the body. Each chondrocyte contains a nucleus, a relatively large amount of clear cytoplasm, and the common organelles, as mitochondria. —**chondrocytic,** *adj.*

chondrodystrophia calcificans congenita, an inherited defect characterized by many small opacities in the epiphyses of the long bones. This sign is present on x ray films of the newborn. Dwarfism, contractures, cataracts, mental retardation, and short stubby fingers develop as the infant grows into childhood. Also called **chondrodystrophia fetalis calcificans, Conradi's disease.**

chondrodystrophy (kon'drɔudɪs'trəfi), a group of disorders in which there is abnormal conversion of cartilage to bone, particularly in the epiphyses of the long bones. Patients are dwarfed, with normal trunks and shortened extremities. See also **achondroplasia.**

chondroendothelioma (kon'drɔuen'douthi'liou'mə), *pl.* **chondroendotheliomas, chondroendotheliomatas.** a benign mesenchymal tumor containing cartilaginous and endothelial components.

chondrofibroma (kon'drɔufaibrou'mə), *pl.* **chondrofibromas, chondrofibromata.** a fibrous tumor containing cartilaginous components.

chondrogenesis (kon'drɔujen'ɪsɪs), the development of cartilage. —**chondrogenetic,** *adj.*

chondroid (kon'drɔid), resembling cartilage.

chondrolipoma (kon'drɔulɪpou'mə), *pl.* **chondrolipomas, chondrolipomata.** a benign mesenchymal tumor containing fatty and cartilaginous components.

chondroma (kondrɔu'mə), *pl.* **chondromas, chondromata.** a benign, fairly common tumor of cartilage cells that grows slowly within cartilage (enchondroma) or on the surface (ecchondroma). Kinds of chondromas are **joint chondroma, synovial chondroma.** See also **ecchondroma, enchondroma.** —**chondromatous,** *adj.*

-chondroma, a combining form meaning a 'benign cartilaginous tumor': *hyaloenchondroma, osteochondroma, sarcoenchondroma.*

chondromalacia (kon'drɔuməlei'shiə), a softening of cartilage. **Chondromalacia fetalis** is a lethal congenital form of the condition in which the stillborn infant is born with soft and pliable limbs. **Chondromalacia patellae** occurs in young adults after knee injury and is characterized

by swelling and pain and by degenerative changes, which are revealed on examination by x ray.

chondromalacia fetalis. See **chondromalacia.**

chondromalacia patellae. See **chondromalacia.**

chondroma sarcomatosum. See **chondrosarcoma.**

chondromatosis (kon'drɔumətou'sɪs), a condition characterized by the presence of many cartilaginous tumors. A kind of chondromatosis is **synovial chondromatosis.**

chondromere, a cartilaginous, embryonic vertebra and its costal component.

chondromyoma (kon'drɔumaiou'mə), *pl.* **chondromyomas, chondromyomata.** a benign mesenchymal tumor containing myomatous and cartilaginous tissue.

chondromyxofibroma (kon'drɔumɪk'soufaibrou'mə), a benign tumor that develops from cartilage-forming connective tissue. The lesion, typically a firm, grayish-white, somewhat rubbery mass, tends to occur in the knee and small bones of the foot and may be confused with chondrosarcoma. Also called **chondromyxoid fibroma.**

chondromyxoid (kon'drɔumɪk'sɔid), composed of cartilaginous and myxoid elements.

chondromyxoid fibroma. See **chondromyxofibroma.**

chondrophyte (kon'drəfait'), an abnormal mass of cartilage that may develop at the articular surface of a bone. —**chondrophytic,** *adj.*

chondroplast (kon'drɔuplæst). See **chondroblast.**

chondroplasty (kon'drəplæs'ti), the surgical repair of cartilage.

chondrosarcoma (kon'drɔusarkɔu'mə), *pl.* **chondrosarcomas, chondrosarcomata.** a malignant neoplasm of cartilaginous cells or their precursors that occurs most frequently on long bones, the pelvic girdle, and the scapula. The characteristic tumor is a large, smooth, lobulated growth composed of nodules of hyaline cartilage that may show slight to marked calcification. Kinds of chondrosarcomas are **central chondrosarcoma, mesenchymal chondrosarcoma.** Also called **chondroma sarcomatosum.** —**chondrosarcomatous,** *adj.*

chondrosarcomatosis (kon'drɔusar'koumətou'sɪs), a condition characterized by multiple, malignant cartilaginous tumors.

chondrosis, 1. the development of the cartilage of the body. 2. a cartilaginous tumor.

chondrotomy (kondrot'əmi), a surgical procedure for dividing a cartilage.

chord-, a combining form meaning 'string, cord': *chordoblastoma, chordoma, chordotomy.*

chordal canal. See **notochordal canal.**

chorda spinalis. See **spinal cord.**

chorda umbicalis. See **umbilical cord.**

chordee (kɔr'di, kɔr'dei), a congenital defect of the genitourinary tract resulting in a ventral curvature of the penis, caused by a fibrous band of tissue instead of normal skin along the corpus spongiosum. The condition is often associated with hypospadias and is surgically corrected in early childhood. The goals of surgery are to improve the appearance of the genitalia cosmetically for psychological reasons, to construct an organ that allows the boy to void in a standing position, and to produce a sexually adequate organ.

chordencephalon (kord′ensef′əlon), the portion of the central nervous system that develops in the early weeks of pregnancy from the neural tube and includes the mesencephalon, the rhombencephalon, and the spinal cord. The chordencephalon is segmented and divided into the alar and the basal plates. The alar plate becomes the sensory portion of the gray substance of the spinal cord; the basal plate becomes the motor portion of the gray substance. – **chordencephalic,** *adj.*

chorditis (kordai′tis), **1.** inflammation of a spermatic cord. **2.** inflammation of the vocal cords or of the vocal folds.

chordoid (kor′doid), resembling the notocord or notochordal tissue.

chordoma (kordou′mə), *pl.* **chordomas, chordomata.** a rare, congenital tumor of the brain developing from the fetal notochord. It is usually located in the midline, behind the sella, and is slow growing but highly invasive. Surgical removal is rarely possible.

chordotomy (kordot′əmi), an operation in which the anterolateral tracts of the spinal cord are surgically divided to relieve pain.

chorea (kori′ə), a condition characterized by involuntary, purposeless, rapid motions, as flexing and extending the fingers, raising and lowering the shoulders, or grimacing. In some forms the person is also irritable, emotionally unstable, weak, restless, and fretful. See also **chorea gravidarum, Huntington's chorea, Sydenham's chorea.** – **choreic,** *adj.*

-chorea, a combining form meaning a '(specified) nervous disorder': *hemichorea, monochorea, orthochorea.*

chorea gravidarum, a form of chorea occurring during a first pregnancy subsequent to an episode of Sydenham's chorea in childhood. Similar symptoms may develop in a woman taking oral contraceptives.

chorea minor. See Sydenham's chorea.

choreiform (kəri′əform′), resembling the rapid jerky movements associated with chorea.

chorio-, a combining form meaning 'pertaining to the protective fetal membrane': *chorioblastosis, choriocele, chorioma.*

chorioadenoma (kor′iouæd′inou′mə), *pl.* **chorioadenomas, chorioadenomata.** an epithelial cell tumor of the outermost fetal membrane that is intermediate in the malignant development of a hydatid mole to invasive choriocarcinoma.

chorioadenoma destruens, an invasive hydatidiform mole in which the chorionic villi of the mole penetrate

into the myometrium and parametrium of the uterus and metastasize to distant parts of the body, most commonly to the lungs. Also called **invasive mole, malignant mole, metastasizing mole.**

chorioallantoic graft, the grafting of tissue onto the chorioallantoic membrane of the egg of a hen to improve the environment for embryonic growth.

chorioamnionic (kor′iouæm′niot′ik), of or pertaining to the chorion and the amnion.

chorioblastoma (kor′ioublæstou′mə). See **choriocarcinoma.**

choriocarcinoma (kor′ioukar′sinou′mə), *pl.* **choriocarcinomas, choriocarcinomata.** an epithelial malignancy of fetal origin that develops from the chorionic portion of the products of conception, usually from a hydatiform mole. Less frequently it develops following an abortion, during a normal or ectopic pregnancy, or from a genital or extragenital teratoma. The primary tumor usually appears in the uterus as a soft, dark red, crumbling mass. It may invade and destroy the uterine wall and metastasize through lymph or blood vessels, forming secondary hemorrhagic and necrotic tumors in the vaginal wall, vulva, lymph nodes, lungs, liver, and brain. The urine often contains much more chorionic gonadotropin than is expected in pregnancy. The hormone level returns to normal when the tumor is completely removed. This form of cancer, which is more common in older than in younger women, responds to chemotherapy with cytotoxic drugs, as methotrexate. Rarely, a choriocarcinoma may arise in a teratoma of the testis, mediastinum, or pineal gland, and chemotherapy is not usually effective in treating these tumors. Also called **chorioblastoma, chorioepithelioma, chorionic carcinoma, chorionic epithelioma.**

choriocele (kor′iəsil′), a hernia or protrusion of the tissue of the choroid layer of the eye.

chorioepithelioma (kor′iouep′ithi′liou′mə). See **choriocarcinoma.**

choriogenesis (kor′ioujen′əsis), the development of the chorion, which is first evident in the first month of pregnancy, after the trophoblast anchors to the uterine tissue and extends primary villi into the intervillous space. The chorion at first contains fluid and loose filaments of extraembryonic mesoderm. As pregnancy proceeds, the amnion grows into the chorionic space and obliterates it. The chorion continues to expand to accommodate the fetus and serves as the outer barrier between the fetus and the uterus. – **choriogenetic,** *adj.*

choriomeningitis (kor′ioumeninjai′tis). See **lymphocytic choriomeningitis.**

chorion (kor′ion), (in biology) the outermost extraembryonic membrane composed of trophoblast lined with mesoderm. It develops villi about two weeks after fertilization and is vascularized by allantoic vessels a week later. It gives rise to the placenta and persists until birth as the outer of the two layers of membrane containing the amniotic fluid and the fetus.

-chorion, a combining form meaning a 'membrane': *allantochorion, omphalochorion, prochorion.*

chorionic carcinoma. See **choriocarcinoma.**

chorionic epithelioma. See **choriocarcinoma.**

chorionic gonadotropin, a chemical component of the urine of pregnant women or pregnant mares. See **gonadotropin.**

chorionic plate, the part of the fetal placenta that gives rise to chorionic villi, attaching to the uterus during the early stage of formation of the placenta.

chorioretinitis (kɔr'iouret'ınai'tıs), an inflammatory condition of the choroid and retina of the eye, usually as a result of parasitic or bacterial infection. It is characterized by blurred vision, photophobia, and distorted images.

chorioretinopathy (kɔr'iouret'ənop'əłhi), a noninflammatory process caused by disease that involves the choroid and the retina.

choroid (kɔr'oid), a thin, highly vascular membrane covering the posterior five sixths of the eye between the retina and sclera.

choroidal malignant melanoma, a tumor of the choroid coat that grows into the vitreous humor, causing detachment and degeneration of the overlying retina. Typically mound-shaped or mushroom-shaped, the neoplasm may break through the sclera and present under the conjunctiva.

choroiditis (kɔr'oidai'tıs), an inflammatory condition of the choroid membrane of the eye. See also **chorioretinitis.**

choroidocyllitis (kɔroi'dousılai'tıs), an abnormal condition characterized by inflammation of the choroid and the ciliary processes.

choroid plexectomy (pleksek'təmi), a surgical procedure for the reduction of cerebrospinal fluid production in the ventricles of the brain in hydrocephalus, usually in the newborn. The procedure involves transcortical entry of the lateral ventricles to coagulate or to excise the choroid plexuses and seeks to correct a communicating type of hydrocephalus.

choroid plexus, any one of the tangled masses of tiny blood vessels contained within the third, the lateral, and the fourth ventricles of the brain. The choroid plexus of the third ventricle is part of the roof of the anterior commissure of the third ventricle, lying above the interventricular foramen. The choroid plexus of the lateral ventricle is continuous with the choroid plexus of the third ventricle, extending from the interventricular foramen, through the body of the ventricle, to the rostral end of the inferior horn. The choroid plexus of the fourth ventricle, on each side, is an elongated tuft of blood vessels extending through the roof of the ventricle.

Christmas factor. See **factor IX.**

Christchurch chromosome (Ch¹), an abnormally small acrocentric chromosome of the G group, involving any members of chromosome pairs 21 or 22, in which the short arms are missing or partially deleted. The aberration is associated with chronic lymphocytic leukemia but has also been found in patients with various other defects. See also **Philadelphia chromosome.**

Christmas disease. See **hemophilia.**

-chroia, a combining form meaning '(condition of) coloration': *cacochroia, cyanochroia, xanthochroia.*

chrom-. See **chromo-.**

chromaffin (krou'məfın), having an affinity for strong staining with chromium salts, especially strong staining of the cells of the adrenal, the coccygeal, and the carotid glands, certain cells of the adrenal medulla, and the cells of the paraganglions. Also called **chromaphil.**

chromaffin body. See **paraganglion.**

chromaffin cell, any one of the special cells comprising the paraganglia and connected to the ganglia of the celiac, the renal, the suprarenal, the aortic, and the hypogastric plexuses. Chromaffin cells are also sometimes found in association with other sympathetic plexuses. The chromaffin cells of the adrenal medulla secrete two catecholamines, epinephrine and norepinephrine, which affect smooth muscle, cardiac muscle, and glands in the same way as sympathetic stimulation, increasing and prolonging sympathetic effects. The chromaffin cells of the adrenal medulla are especially active in response to stress and the associated reception of nerve impulses from the hypothalamus. These impulses synapse with the chromaffin cells in the adrenal medulla and stimulate them to increase hormonal production, about 80 per cent of which is epinephrine, the rest, norepinephrine.

chromaffinoma (kroumæf'ınou'mə). See **pheochromocytoma.**

chromaphil. See **chromaffin.**

-chromasia, 1. a combining form meaning '(condition of) color (as cells, skin)': *allochromasia, hyperchromasia, oligochromasia.* 2. a combining form meaning '(condition of the) stainability of tissues': *amblychromasia, anisochromasia, anochromasia.*

chromatic, 1. of or pertaining to color. 2. stainable by a dye. 3. Also, **chromatinic.** of or pertaining to chromatin.

-chromatic, a combining form meaning the 'staining properties of tissues and microorganisms': *lithochromatic, orthochromatic, panchromatic.*

chromatic dispersion, the splitting of light into its various component wavelengths or frequencies, as with a prism, to separate and study the different colors.

chromatid (krou'mətıd), one of the two identical threadlike filaments of a chromosome. It results from the self-replication of the chromosome during interphase, is held together by a common centromere, and, during mitosis and meiosis, divides longitudinally to form daughter chromosomes.

chromatin (krou'mətɪn), the material within the cell nucleus from which the chromosomes are formed. It consists of fine, threadlike strands of deoxyribonucleic acid attached to a protein base, usually histone; it is readily stained with basic dyes; and it occurs in two different forms, euchromatin and heterochromatin, which are distinguishable during the phases of the cell cycle by variant degrees of staining depending on the amount of dispersion or coiling that occurs. During cell division, portions of the chromatin condense and coil to form the chromosomes. A kind of chromatin is **sex chromatin**. Also called **chromoplasm, karyotin.** See also **chromatid, euchromatin, heterochromatin.** – **chromatinic,** *adj.*

chromatin-negative, pertaining to or descriptive of the nuclei of cells that lack sex chromatin, specifically characteristic of the normal male.

chromatin nucleolus. See **karyosome.**

chromatin-positive, pertaining to or descriptive of the nuclei of cells that contain sex chromatin, specifically characteristic of the normal female.

chromatism (krou'mətɪz'əm), 1. an abnormal condition characterized by hallucinations in which the affected individual sees colored lights. 2. abnormal pigmentation.

chromato-, chromat-, 1. a combining form meaning 'pertaining to color': *chromatism, chromatogram, chromatopsia.* 2. See **chromo-.**

chromatogram (kroumæt'əgræm), 1. the record produced by the separation of gaseous substances or dissolved chemical substances moving through a column of absorbent material which filters out the various absorbates in different layers. 2. any graphic record produced by any chromatographic method.

chromatography (krou'mətog'rəfi), any one of several processes for separating and analyzing various gaseous or dissolved chemical materials according to differences in their absorbency with respect to a specific substance and according to their different pigments. Some kinds of chromatography are **column chromatography, displacement chromatography, gas chromatography, ion-exchange chromatography, paper chromatography.** – **chromatographic,** *adj.*

chromatopsia (krou'mətop'siə), 1. an abnormal condition characterized by a visual defect that makes colorless objects appear tinged with color. 2. Also called **color blindness.** an abnormal condition characterized by the imperfect perception of various colors. It may be caused by a deficiency in one or more of the retinal cones or from defective nerve circuits that convey color-associated impulses to the cerebral cortex. The most common defect in color sense is the inability to distinguish red from green, a defect evident in about 10 per cent of men and one per cent of women. Everyone is color-blind in very dim light because the color-discriminating cones of the retina are insufficiently stimulated to function. In very dim light only the retinal rods, which have the capacity to distinguish black from white, are sufficiently stimulated to function. Some color-blind persons may not be able to see red and green or blue and yellow; others cannot perceive any color, seeing everything as gray. Very few individuals are color-blind to blue. Compare **chromesthesia.**

-chrome[1], a combining form meaning a 'coloring substance within a cell or chemical compound': *cytochrome, hemochrome, serochrome.* Also **-chromatic, -chromic.**

-chrome[2], a combining form distinguishing 'chromium alloys': *hallachrome, nichrome, nicochrome.*

-chromemia, a combining form meaning '(condition of the) hemoglobin in the blood': *hyperchromemia, lipochromemia, polychromemia.*

chromesthesia (krou'mɪsθi'ʒə), 1. the color sense that depends on the mixture of wavelengths in the light that enters the eye and the response of the three different special types of retinal cones associated with color vision. One type of cone responds to green light, a second type to red light, a third to blue light. The human eye can distinguish hundreds of different colors which are combinations of the three basic light wavelengths for red, green, and blue. Some of the retinal cones can be stimulated by the whole visual spectrum, and variable stimulation of all the cones can produce all the color sensations known to humans. Changes in the pigments within the cones affect color vision, and defects in the cones cause various kinds of color blindness. 2. an abnormal condition characterized by the confusion of other senses, as taste and smell, with imagined sensations of color. Compare **chromatopsia.**

chromhidrosis (krou'mɪdrou'sɪs), a rare, functional disorder in which apocrine sweat glands secrete colored sweat. The sweat may be yellow, blue, green, or black and often also fluoresces. A known cause is occupational exposure to copper, catechols, or ferrous oxide. Industrial nurses should be aware of this benign condition.

-chromia, a combining form meaning a 'state or condition of pigmentation': *metachromia, normochromia, orthochromia.*

-chromic, 1. a combining form meaning the '(specified) number of colors seen by the eye': *bichromic, hexachromic, tetrachromic.* 2. a combining form meaning a '(specified) color of the blood indicating the hemoglobin content': *hypochromic, normochromic.* 3. a combining form meaning the 'staining ability of bacteria and tissues': *bathochromic, hemochromic, perchromic.* 4. a combining form meaning a '(specified) skin color as indicative of disease': *heterochromic, pleiochromic, xantochromic.* Also **-chromatic.**

chromic myopia (krou'mɪk), a kind of color blindness characterized by the ability to distinguish colors only of those objects that are close to the eye.

chromium (Cr), a hard, brittle, metallic element. Its atomic number is 24. Its atomic weight is 51.9; it does not occur naturally in pure form but exists in combination with iron and oxygen in chromite, a mineral found chiefly in Africa, Albania, Russia, and Turkey. Chromium strongly resists corrosion and is used extensively to plate other metals and harden steel, and, in combination with other elements, to form colored compounds. Stainless steels are more than 10 per cent chromium and strongly resist rusting. Traces of chromium occur in plants and animals, and there is evidence this element may be important in human nutrition, especially in carbohydrate metabolism. Some experts estimate that the safe and adequate daily intake of chromium ranges from 0.1 to 0.2 mg, depending on the age of the individual. Workers in chromite mines are susceptible to pneumoconiosis caused by the inhalation of chromite dust particles that lodge in the lung.

chromo-, chrom-, a combining form meaning 'pertaining to color': *chromocrinia, chromocyte, chromotrichia.* Also **chromato-.**

chromobacteriosis (krou'moubæktir'iou'sis), an extremely rare, usually fatal systemic infection caused by a gram-negative bacillus *Chromobacterium violaceum,* found in fresh water in tropical and subtropical regions, which enters the body through a break in the skin. The disease is characterized by sepsis, multiple liver abscesses, and severe prostration. Early diagnosis, surgical drainage of abscesses, and the administration of chloramphenicol markedly improve the chance of survival.

chromoblastomycosis (krou'moublæs'toumaikou'sis), an infectious skin disease caused by any of a variety of fungi and characterized by the appearance of pruritic, warty nodules that develop in a cut or other break in the skin. What may first appear as a small dull red lesion gradually develops into a large ulcerated growth. Over a period of weeks or months, additional warty growths may appear elsewhere on the skin along the path of lymphatic drainage. Treatment includes surgical excision and, in some cases, topical application of antibiotics. Also called **chromomycosis, verrucous dermatitis.** See also **mycosis,** specific fungal infections.

chromocenter (krou'mousen'tər). See **karyosome.**

chromolipid (krou'moulip'id), **chromolipoid** (krou'-moulip'oid). See **lipochrome.**

chromomere (krou'məmir), 1. any of the series of beadlike structures that lie along the chromonema of a chromosome during the early stages of cell division. The position of each chromomere is relatively constant for each chromosome and probably reflects the coiling pattern of the DNA molecule for the particular chromosome. Also called **idiomere.** 2. See **granulomere.**

chromomycosis. See **chromoblastomycosis.**

chromonema (krou'məni'mə), **chromoneme,** *pl.* **chromonemata.** the coiled filament along which the chromomeres lie that forms the central part of the chromatid of the chromosome during cell division. See also **chromosome.** – **chromonemal, chromonematic, chromonemic,** *adj.*

chromophilic (krou'məfil'ik), denoting a cell, tissue, or microorganism that is easily stained, particularly certain leukocytes. Compare **chromophobic.**

chromophobe adenoma (krou'məfoub), a tumor of the anterior pituitary, composed of cells that are chromophobic and do not stain with acidic or basic dyes. The lesion may be associated with hypopituitarism.

chromophobia (krou'məfou'biə), 1. the resistance of certain cells and tissues to stains. 2. a morbid aversion to colors. – **chromophobe,** *n.*

chromophobic (krou'məfou'bik), denoting a cell, tissue, or microorganism that is not easily stained, particularly certain cells of the anterior lobe of the pituitary gland. Compare **chromophilic.**

chromophobic adenoma (krou'məfou'bik), a tumor of the pituitary gland composed of cells that do not stain with acid or basic dyes. Diabetes insipidus and other conditions resulting from deficiency of one or more pituitary hormones are associated with this tumor.

chromoplasm (krou'məplæz'əm). See **chromatin.**

chromosomal aberration, any change in the structure or number of any of the chromosomes for a given species, which can result in anomalies of varying severity. In man, a number of physical disabilities and disorders are directly associated with chromosomal defects of both the autosomes and the sex chromosomes, including Down's syndrome, Turner's syndrome, and Kleinfelter's syndrome. The incidence for most of the chromosomal disorders is significantly higher than that for the single gene disorders. See also specific trisomy syndromes.

chromosomal nomenclature, a standard nomenclature that serves to identify the complement of chromosomes in an individual according to the number of chromosomes, sex, and the deletion or addition of a specific chromosome or part of a chromosome. Complement in a normal female is recorded as 46,XX and for a normal male, 46,XY. The addition or deletion of a chromosome is identified by number, if it can be identified, as 47,XY, 21 +. If the particular chromosome cannot be identified, the group is recorded, as 47,XY, G +. The short arm of a chromosome is designated "p," the long arm is "q," and a translocation "t".

chromosome (krou'məsoum), any one of the threadlike structures in the nucleus of a cell that function in the transmission of genetic information. Each consists of a double strand of the nucleoprotein deoxyribonucleic acid (DNA), which is coiled into a helix formation and attached to a protein base, usually a histone. The genes, which contain the genetic material that controls the inheritance of traits, are arranged in a linear pattern along the entire length of each DNA strand. Chromosomes are readily stainable with basic dyes and can be seen easily during cell division when they are compactly coiled and in their most condensed state. During interphase, the chromosomes disperse into chromatin and undergo self-replication, forming identical chromatids that separate during mitosis so that each new cell receives a full set of chromosomes. Each species has a characteristic number of chromosomes in the somatic cell, which in man is 46 and includes 22 homologous pairs of autosomes and one pair of sex chromosomes, with one member of each pair being derived from each parent. A standard nomenclature has been developed that identifies individual chromosomal complements according to the size of the chromosome and the position of the centromere as determined during mitotic metaphase. The morphologically paired auto-somes are separated into seven groups and numbered from 1 to 22, with 1 through 3 being designated group A; 4 and 5, group B; 6 through 12, group C; 13 through 15, group D; 16 through 18, group E; 19 and 20, group F; and 21 and 22, group G. The chromosomes are arranged according to decreasing length, followed by the sex chromosome complement, in the usual karyotype representation. Chromosomal aberrations are designated by indicating the total chromosomal number, sex complement, and the group or specific chromosome in which the addition or deletion occurs. For example, 47,XY,G+ indicates a male with an extra chromosome in the G group; 47,XX,21+ shows a female with an extra chromosome 21, or Down's syndrome. Kinds of chromosomes include **accessory chromosome, Christchurch chromosome, daughter chromosome, gametic chromosome, giant chromosome, homologous chromosomes, Philadelphia chromosome, sex chromosome, somatic chromosome, W chromosome, Z chromosome.** See also **centromere, chromatid, chromatin, Denver classification, gene, karyotype, mitosis.** — **chromosomal,** *adj.*

chromosome banding. See **banding.**

chromosome coil, the spiral formed by the coiling of two or more chromonemata of the chromatid within the chromosome.

chromosome complement, the normal number of chromosomes found in the somatic cell of any given species. In humans it is 46, consisting of 22 pairs of homologous autosomes and one pair of sex chromosomes.

chromosome mapping. See **mapping.**

chromosome puff, a band of accumulated chromatic material located at a specific site on a giant chromosome. It is indicative of gene activity, specifically DNA and

HUMAN CHROMOSOMAL PAIRS

Analysis of human chromosomes

Size	Position of centromere	Group	Autosomes	Sex chromosomes	Male	Female
Large	Metacentric or submetacentric	A	1, 2, 3		6	6
Large	Submetacentric	B	4, 5		4	4
Medium	Metacentric and submetacentric	C	6, 7, 8, 9, 10, 11, 12	X	15	16
Medium	Acrocentric (subterminal)	D	13, 14, 15		6	6
Small	Metacentric and submetacentric	E	16, 17, 18		6	6
Smallest	Metacentric	F	19, 20			
Small	Acrocentric (subterminal)	G	21, 22	Y	5	4
				TOTAL	46	46

The table also has a spanning header "Description of chromosomes" over Size and Position of centromere, and "Number of chromosomes in all body (somatic) cells" over Male and Female.

RNA synthesis, for the particular locus. Such bands appear at certain chromosomal locations within a given tissue at specific developmental stages in insects and are significant for studying the mode of genetic transmission.

chromosome walking, the process by which overlapping molecular clones that span large chromosomal intervals are isolated.

chromotrope (krou'mətroup), **1.** a component of tissue that stains metachromatically with metachromatic dyes. **2.** any one of several dyes differentiated by numerical suffixes. – **chromotropic,** *adj.*

chron-. See **chrono-.**

-chrone. See **-chronia.**

-chronia, 1. a combining form meaning '(condition of) processes with respect to time': *isochronia, heterochronia, synchronia.* **2.** a combining form meaning '(condition of) chronaxy between muscle and nerve': *isochronia.* **3.** a combining form meaning the 'time of formation of a part or tissue': *heterochronia, synchronia.* Also **-chrone.**

chronic (kron'ik), (of a disease or disorder) developing slowly and persisting for a long period of time, often for the remainder of the lifetime of the patient. Glaucoma is an example of a disease that may develop gradually and insidiously or that may occur as an acute disorder marked by sudden severe pain, requiring emergency treatment. Compare **acute.**

chronic alcoholic delirium. See **Korsakoff's psychosis.**

chronic alcoholism, a pathological condition resulting from the habitual use of alcohol in excessive amounts. The syndrome involves complex cultural, psychological, social, and physiological factors and usually impairs an individual's health and his ability to function normally in society. Symptoms of the disease include anorexia, diarrhea, weight loss, neurological and psychiatric disturbances (most notably depression), and fatty deterioration of the liver, sometimes leading to cirrhosis. Treatment depends on the severity of the disease and its resulting complications; hospitalization may be necessary. Nutritional therapy, use of tranquilizers in the detoxification process, use of disulfiram as an aid to continued abstinence, and psychotherapy are all methods of treatment. Alcoholism often goes unrecognized in patients admitted to the hospital for care following an accident, or for esophagitis, gastritis, peripheral neuropathy, anemia, or depression, all of which are secondary effects of their alcoholism. If alcoholism is not diagnosed and treated, the patient will not recover. The nurse usually spends more time with a patient than the doctor does and is in a better position to discover the condition and to observe signs of withdrawal; the nurse should inform the physician responsible in order that detoxification, sedation, and other treatment can be instituted. If the patient is to undergo an operation, it is imperative that the anesthesiologist be notified of the alcoholism. Alcoholism is a family disease, and the nurse can be instrumental in guiding the patient's family to seek treatment. Long-term support for the alcoholic and his family is offered by such organizations as Alcoholics Anonymous, Al-Anon, Alateen, and rehabilitation facilities for alcoholism. Compare **acute alcoholism.**

chronic appendicitis, 1. a type of appendicitis characterized by thickening or scarring of the vermiform appendix, caused by previous inflammation. **2.** an obsolete term formerly used to describe chronic pain in the appendiceal area without any evidence of inflammation.

chronic brain syndrome (CBS), an abnormal condition that is caused by impairment of the cerebral tissue function, characterized by loss of memory and disorientation. It may occur in dementia paralytica, cerebral arteriosclerosis, brain trauma, and Huntington's chorea.

chronic bronchitis, a very common debilitating respiratory disease, characterized by greatly increased production of mucus by the glands of the trachea and bronchi and resulting in a cough with expectoration for at least three months of the year for more than two consecutive years.

■ OBSERVATIONS: The condition has a strong association with smoking and occupational and environmental pollutants. Formerly seen almost exclusively in males, the disease is becoming more common in women who smoke. Productive cough, often with wheezing, is a universal feature, followed by progressive dyspnea on exertion, repeated purulent respiratory infections, airway narrowing and obstruction, and, often, respiratory failure. Cor pulmonale with right ventricular heart failure is a common result. Some patients develop secondary polycythemia due to chronic hypoxemia. Acute attacks of respiratory distress with rapid, labored respirations, prolonged expiratory phase, prominent cough, and cyanosis has led to these patients being called 'blue bloaters.' Common laboratory findings include elevated hematocrit, hypoxemia with or without respiratory acidosis, abnormal liver function tests due to right heart failure and hepatic congestion, pathogenic bacteria in the sputum, abnormal pulmonary function tests, and, often, chest x-ray signs of increased broncial markings and emphysema.

■ INTERVENTION: Broad-spectrum antibiotics, as ampicillin or erythromycin, are usually prescribed during acute exacerbations of symptoms. Bronchodilators, as theophylline or metaproterenol, as well as sympathomimetic drugs as terbutaline, are prescribed to prevent worsening of the condition. Heart failure is managed with sodium restriction, diuretics, and sometimes digitalis.

■ NURSING CONSIDERATIONS: A major effort should be made to have the patient discontinue smoking and avoid exposure to toxic inhalants as hair sprays, aerosol insecticides, and occupational irritants and poisons. Patients with chronic bronchitis should be immunized against influenza and pneumococcal infections. The use of low-flow oxygen in the home may require patient education and monitoring. Exercise, especially walking, chest physiotherapy, and postural drainage are often indicated, and nurses may give instruction to patients and their families in these therapeutic programs. See also **asthma, chroninc obstructive pulmonary disease, cor pulmonale, emphysema, respiratory failure.**

chronic care, a pattern of medical and nursing care that focuses on long-term care of people with chronic diseases or conditions, either at home or in a medical facility. It includes care specific to the problem, as well as other measures to encourage self-care, to promote health, and to prevent loss of function.

chronic carrier, an individual who acts as host to pathogenic organisms for an extended period of time without displaying any signs of disease.

chronic cervicitis. See **cervicitis.**

chronic cholecystitis. See **cholecystitis.**

chronic chorea. See **Huntington's chorea.**

chronic cystic mastitis. See **fibrocystic disease.**

chronic disease, a disease that persists over a long period of time as compared with the course of an acute disease. The symptoms of chronic disease are usually less severe than those of the acute phase of the same disease. Chronic disease may result in complete or partial disability.

chronic gastritis. See **gastritis.**

chronic glomerulonephritis, a noninfectious disease of the glomerulus of the kidney characterized by proteinuria, hematuria, edema, and decreased production of urine. Of unknown cause, it is asymptomatic for years: the symptoms develop slowly, but the disease progresses to kidney failure. Transplantation and dialysis are the only treatments available. See also **acute glomerulonephritis, subacute glomerulonephritis, uremia.**

chronic idiopathic thrombocytopenic purpura. See **idiopathic thrombocytopenic purpura.**

chronic interstitial nephritis. See **interstitial nephritis.**

chronic intestinal ischemia. See **intestinal angina.**

chronic lingual papillitis, an inflammatory disorder of the tongue, sometimes extending to the buccal mucosa and palate, characterized by irregularly scattered red patches, thinning of the lingual papillae, severe burning pain, and shedding of epidermal tissue. The disorder affects middle-aged individuals, especially women, and occurs in attacks alternating with remissions lasting weeks or months. Also called **Moeller's glossitis.**

chronic lymphocytic leukemia (CLL), a neoplasm of blood-forming tissues, characterized by a proliferation of small, long-lived lymphocytes, chiefly B-cells, in bone marrow, blood liver, and in lymphoid organs. CLL is rare under the age of 35, increases in frequency with age, and is more common in men than in women. The disease has

an insidious onset and progresses to cause malaise, easy fatigability, anorexia, weight loss, nocturnal sweating, lymphadenopathy, and hepatosplenomegaly. Most patients can continue normal activities for years; 25 per cent die of unrelated diseases. No treatment is curative, but remissions may be induced by chemotherapy with chlorambucil and glucocorticoids or by thymic, splenic, or total body irradiation.

chronic mastitis. See **mastitis.**

chronic mucocutaneous candidiasis, an abnormal condition and rare form of candidiasis, characterized by lesions of the skin, viral infections, and recurrent respiratory tract infections. This disease usually occurs during the first year of life but can develop as late as the 20s. It affects both men and women and is associated with an inherited defect of the cell-mediated immune system and apparently allows autoantibodies to develop against target organs. The humoral immune system functions normally in this disease. Chronic mucocutaneous candidiasis may affect the skin, the mucous membranes, the nails, and the vagina, usually causing large circular lesions. The onset of infections associated with the disease may precede endocrinopathy.

■ OBSERVATIONS: Chronic mucocutaneous candidiasis may affect the skin, the mucous membranes, the nails, and the vagina, usually causing large, circular lesions. Associated viral infections may lead to endocrinopathy and hepatitis. Infections of the mouth, nose, and palate may cause problems with speech and eating. Tetany and hypocalcemia are the most common symptoms associated with the endocrinopathy and are usually confined to the involved organ. Other complications associated with chronic mucocutaneous candidiasis may include diabetes, Addison's disease, hypothyroidism, and pernicious anemia. Some patients also develop psychiatric problems because of disfigurements and extensive endocrinal disorders. Diagnosis of this disease usually includes laboratory tests, which commonly show a normal T cell count and normal immunological responses to antigens other than *Candida albicans.* The endocrinopathy associated with this disease may include nonimmunologic aberrations, as hypocalcemia, abnormal hepatic function, hyperglycemia, iron deficiency, and abnormal vitamin B_{12} absorption. Other immunodeficiency diseases associated with chronic *Candida* infection must be excluded by diagnosis. Such immunodeficiency diseases as DiGeorge's syndrome, ataxiatelangiectasia, and severe combined immunodeficiency disease all cause serious immunologic defects. Required after diagnosis of chronic mucocutaneous candidiasis are evaluations of numerous functions of the patient, as adrenal, gonadal, pancreatic, parathyroid, pituitary, and thyroid functions. Chronic mucocutaneous candidiasis is progressive and usually leads to endocrinopathy.

■ INTERVENTION: Chronic mucocutaneous candidiasis resists treatment with topical antifungal agents, miconazole, and nystatin. Endocrinopathies associated with the disease must be treated individually by hormone replacement; some success in this regard has been reported with experimental injections of thymosin and levamisole. Most success in treating severe cases has been with transfer factor from a *Candida*-positive donor, with intravenous amphotericin B. Some success may also be possible against systemic infection with amphotericin B, but that agent is highly nephrotoxic. Some patients respond fairly well to fetal thymus transplants. Plastic surgery may also be part of the treatment to aid patients in coping with disfigurements caused by the disease. Treatment may also include iron replacement by oral or by intramuscular administration.

■ NURSING CONSIDERATIONS: Patients with chronic mucocutaneous candidiasis must be closely monitored for signs of other associated diseases, as Addison's disease, diabetes, hepatitis, and pernicious anemia. Patients suffering psychologically from disfigurements associated with the disease often respond positively to the counsel, encouragement, and kindness of the nursing staff. If amphotericin B is involved in the treatment, the patient must be carefully monitored for renal function, because amphotericin B is nephrotoxic. Patients benefit from calm explanations about the progressive manifestations of the disease and the importance of regular endocrinologic checkups.

chronic myelocytic leukemia (CML), a malignant neoplasm of blood-forming tissues, characterized by a proliferation of granular leukocytes and, often, of megakaryocytes. The disease occurs most frequently in older people and begins insidiously. Its progress is marked by malaise, fatigue, heat intolerance, bleeding gums, purpura, skin lesions, weight loss, hyperuricemia, abdominal discomfort, and massive splenomegaly. Differential blood count and bone marrow biopsies are performed to aid in the diagnosis. The alkaline phosphate activity of the leukocytes is low, and the Philadelphia chromosome is present in myeloblasts in most patients with CML. Therapy with an oral alkylating agent is usual, but advanced CML is refractory to chemotherapy. Also called **granulocytic leukemia, myelogenous leukemia, myeloid leukemia, splenomedullary leukemia, splenomyelogenous leukemia.**

chronic obstructive pulmonary disease, a progressive and irreversible condition characterized by diminished inspiratory and expiratory capacity of the lungs. The person complains of dyspnea with physical exertion, of difficulty in inhaling or exhaling deeply, and, sometimes, of a chronic cough. The condition may result from chronic bronchitis, pulmonary emphysema, asthma, or chronic bronchiolitis and is aggravated by cigarette smoking and air pollution.

chronic (open-angle) glaucoma. See **glaucoma.**

chronic pain, pain that continues or recurs over a prolonged period, caused by various diseases or abnormal conditions, as rheumatoid arthritis. Chronic pain is often less intense than the acute pain. The person with chronic pain does not display increased pulse and rapid respiration because these autonomic reactions to pain cannot be sustained for long periods. A characteristic of many persons with chronic pain is their impulse to control their surroundings. They cannot control their disease so they seek to control other people and their environment and are often labeled 'uncooperative' or 'manipulative.' Others with chronic pain may withdraw from their environment and concentrate solely on their affliction, totally ignoring their family, their friends, and external stimuli. Some of the factors that can complicate the treatment of persons with chronic pain are scarring, continuing psychologic stress, and medication. Compare **acute pain.** See also **pain intervention, pain mechanism.**

chronic pyelonephritis. See **pyelonephritis.**

chronic tuberculous mastitis, a rare infection of the breast resulting from extension of tuberculosis of underlying ribs. The condition is also characterized by multiple sinus tracts and the presence of tuberculosis elsewhere in the body.

chrono-, chron-, a combining form meaning 'pertaining to time': *chronognosis, chronophobia, chronotropism.*

chronograph, a device that records small intervals of time, as a stopwatch. — **chronographic,** *adj.*

chronologic, chronological, 1. arranged in time sequence. 2. of or pertaining to chronology.

chronological age, the age of an individual expressed as a period of time that has elapsed since birth, as the age of an infant, which is expressed in hours, days, or months, and the age of children and adults, which is expressed in years.

chrysiasis (krəsaī'əsis), an abnormal condition characterized by the deposition of gold in the tissues of the body. Also called **auriosis.**

chrysotherapy (kris'outher'əpi), the treatment of any disease with gold salts. — **chrysotherapeutic,** *adj.*

Churg-Strauss syndrome (cȟərg'straus'), an allergic disorder marked by granulomotosis, most often of the lungs.

Chvostek's sign, an abnormal spasm of the facial muscles elicited by light taps on the facial nerve in patients who are hypocalcemic. It is a sign of tetany.

Chvostek-Weiss sign (χvoš'tekvaīs'). See **Chvostek's sign.**

chyl-. See **chylo-.**

chyle (kaīl), the cloudy liquid products of digestion taken up by the small intestine. Consisting mainly of emulsified fats, chyle passes through fingerlike projections in the small intestine, called lacteals, and into the lymphatic system for transport to the venous circulation at the thoracic duct in the neck. Also called **chylus. chylous,** *adj.*

chyli-. See **chylo-.**

-chylia, a combining form meaning '(condition of the) digestive juices': *dyschylia, euchylia, polychylia.*

chyliform ascites. See **chylous ascites.**

chylo-, chyl-, chyli-, a combining form meaning 'pertaining to chyle': *chylocyst, chylophonic, chylosis.*

chyloid (kaī'loid), resembling the chyle that fills the lacteals of the small intestine during the digestion of fatty foods.

chylomicron (kaī'loumaī'kron), the largest of the lipoproteins. Chylomicrons primarily consist of triglycerides with small amounts of cholesterol, phospholipids, and protein. They are synthesized in the gastrointestinal tract and carry dietary glycerides from the intestinal mucosa via the thoracic duct into the plasma and, ultimately, to sites of utilization in the tissues. The remnant chylomicron particles are removed by the liver.

chylosus ascites. See **chylous ascites.**

chylothorax (kaī'louthor'æks), the effusion of chyle from the thoracic duct into the pleural space. The cause is usually a traumatic injury to the neck or a tumor which invades the thoracic duct. Treatment is directed at repairing damage to the duct.

chylous ascites, an abnormal condition characterized by an accumulation of chyle in the peritoneal cavity. Chylous ascites results from an obstruction of the thoracic duct that may be caused by a tumor or by a destructive lesion resulting in rupture of a lymph vessel. Also called **ascites adiposus, chylosus ascites, chyliform ascites, fatty ascites, milky ascites.** See also **ascites.**

chyluria (kaīlur'iə), a condition characterized by the milky appearance of the urine owing to the presence of chyle.

chylus (kaī'ləs). See **chyle.**

chyme (kaīm), the viscous, semifluid contents of the stomach present during digestion of a meal. Chyme then passes through the pylorus into the duodenum, where further digestion occurs.

-chymia, a combining form meaning '(condition of) partly digested food in the duodenum': *achymia, ischochymia, oligochymia.* Also **-chymy.**

chymosin (kaī'məsɪn). See **rennin.**

chymotrypsin (kaī'moutrɪp'sɪn), **1.** a proteolytic enzyme, produced by the pancreas, that catalyzes the hydrolysis of casein and gelatin. **2.** a yellow crystalline powder prepared from an extract of ox pancreas, used in treating digestive disorders in which the enzyme is present in less than normal amounts or is totally lacking.

chymotrypsinogen (kaī'moutrɪpsɪn'əjɪn), a substance, produced in the pancreas, that is the precursor to the enzyme chymotrypsin. It is converted to chymotrypsin by trypsin.

-chymy. See **-chymia.**

Ci, abbreviation for **curie.**

C.I., 1. abbreviation for **color index. 2.** abbreviation for *Colour Index.*

cibophobia (si'bəfou'biə), an abnormal aversion to food or to eating.

cicatricial ectropion (sɪk'ətrɪsh'əl), See **ectropion.** See also **cicatrix.**

cicatricial stenosis, the narrowing of a duct or tube owing to the formation of scar tissue.

cicatrix (sɪk'ətrɪks, sɪkeɪ'trɪks), *pl.* **cicatrices** (sɪk'ətraɪ'sɪz). scar tissue that is avascular, pale, contracted, and firm following the earlier phase of skin-healing characterized by redness and softness. **– cicatrize,** *v.*

cicutism (sɪk'yutɪz'əm), poisoning due to water hemlock, resulting in cyanosis, dilated pupils, convulsions, and coma.

CID, abbreviation for **cytomegalic inclusion disease.**

-cide, a combining element meaning 'killing': *amebicide, herbicide, protozoacide.* Also **-cid.**

cigarette drain, a surgical drain fashioned from a section of gauze or surgical sponge drawn into a tube of gutta-percha.

ciguatera poisoning (si'gwater'ə), a nonbacterial food poisoning that results from eating large fish contaminated with the ciguatera toxin. Any of over 300 varieties of fresh or frozen fish from the Caribbean or South Pacific have been implicated, but the sporadic nature of the outbreaks of poisoning is not understood. Characteristic of ciguaterra poisoning are vomiting, diarrhea, tingling or numbness of extremities and the skin around the mouth, itching, muscle weakness, and pain. Cold liquids feel hot to the surfaces of the mouth and throat. No specific treatment has been developed.

cili-, 1. a combining form meaning 'pertaining to an eyelid': *ciliectomy, cilioretinal, cilioscleral.* **2.** a combining form meaning 'pertaining to an eyelash': *ciliary, cilium.* **3.** a combining form meaning 'pertaining to a minute vibratile': *ciliated, ciliogenesis.*

cilia (sɪl'iə), *sing.* **cilium. 1.** the eyelids or eyelashes. **2.** small, hairlike processes on the outer surfaces of some cells, aiding metabolism by producing motion, eddies, or current in a fluid. **– ciliary,** *adj.*

ciliary body, the thickened part of the vascular tunic of the eye that joins the iris with the anterior portion of the choroid. It is composed of the ciliary crown, ciliary processes and folds, ciliary orbiculus, ciliary muscle, and a basal lamina.

ciliary canal, the spaces of the iridocorneal angle.

ciliary gland, one of the numerous tiny, modified sweat glands arranged in several rows near the free margins of the eyelids. The apertures of the glands lie near the attachments of the eyelashes. Acute localized bacterial infection of one or more of the ciliary glands causes external sties. Also called **gland of Zeiss.** Compare **tarsal gland.**

ciliary margin, the peripheral border of the iris, continuous with the ciliary body.

ciliary movement, the waving motion of the hairlike processes projecting from the epithelium of the respiratory tract and from certain microorganisms.

ciliary muscle, a semitransparent, circular band of smooth muscle fibers attached to the choroid of the eye, the chief agent in adjusting the eye to view near objects. It draws the ciliary process centripetally, relaxing the suspensory ligament of the crystalline lens and allowing the lens to become more convex. It consists of meridional fibers and circular fibers and is thickest anteriorly. The circular fibers close to the circumference of the iris are well developed in hypermetropic eyes but are rudimentary or absent in myopic eyes.

ciliary process, any one of about 80 tiny fleshy projections on the posterior surface of the iris, forming a frill around the margin of the crystalline lens of the eye. The larger ciliary processes are about 2.5 cm long and are more regularly arranged than the smaller ones. The processes comprise one of the two zones of the ciliary body of the eye and are formed by infolding of the various layers of the choroid. They are attached anteriorly to the orbicularis ciliaris and posteriorly to the suspensory ligament of the crystalline lens. See also **ciliary body.**

ciliary reflex. See **accommodation reflex.**

ciliary ring, a small grooved band of tissue, about 4 mm wide, that forms the posterior part of the ciliary body of the eye. It extends from the ora serrata of the retina to the ciliary processes and is thicker near the ciliary processes, owing to the thickness of the ciliary muscle.

ciliary zone, an outer circular area on the anterior surface of the iris, separated from the inner circular area by the angular line. The ciliary zone contains the stroma of the iris. Compare **zonula ciliaris.**

Ciliata (sıl′ia′tə), a class of protozoa of the subphylum Ciliophora, characterized by cilia throughout the life cycle. The class includes the subclasses Euciliata and Protociliata. The only significant ciliate in humans is the intestinal parasite *Balantidium coli.*

ciliate (sıl′ııt), of or having cilia, as certain epithelial cells of the body or protozoa of the class Ciliata.

ciliated epithelium, any epithelial tissue that projects cilia from its surface, as portions of the epithelium in the respiratory tract.

ciliospinal reflex (sıl′iouspaı′nəl), a normal brain-stem reflex initiated by scratching or pinching the skin of the back of the neck, resulting in dilatation of the pupil. Also called **pupillary-skin reflex.**

cimetidine, a histamine H_2-receptor antagonist.

■ INDICATIONS: It is prescribed to inhibit the production and secretion of acid in the stomach in the treatment of duodenal ulcer, pancreatitis, and hypersecretory conditions.

■ CONTRAINDICATION: Known hypersensitivity to this drug prohibits its use.

■ ADVERSE EFFECTS: Among the more serious adverse reactions are diarrhea, dizziness, rash, confusion (usually in elderly patients given large doses), and gynecomastia.

Cimex lectularius (lek′chuler′iəs). See **bedbug.**

Cinchocaine (sın′koukein), a trade name for a local anesthetic (dibucaine hydrochloride).

cinchona (sıngkou′nə,sınkou′nə, sınchou′nə), the dried bark of the stem or root of species of *Cinchona,* containing the alkaloids quinine and quinidine.

cinchonism, a condition resulting from excessive ingestion of cinchona bark or its alkaloid derivatives. Cinchonism is characterized by deafness, headache, ringing in the ears, and signs of cerebral congestion. See also **quinine.**

cine-, kine-, a combining form meaning 'pertaining to movement': *cineangiogram, cinefluorography, cineradiography.* Also **kinesio-.**

cineangiocardiogram (sın′iæn′jioukar′diəgræm′), a radiograph of the cardiovascular system obtained by special instruments that employ a combination of x-ray, fluoroscopic, and motion-picture techniques.

cineangiocardiography (sın′iæn′jioukar′diog′rəfi), the filming of fluorescent images of the cardiovascular system by using a combination of fluoroscopic, x-ray, and motion-picture techniques. See also **cineradiography.**

cineangiogram (sın′iæn′jiəgræm′), a movie film record of a blood vessel or of a portion of the cardiovascular system, obtained by injecting a patient with a nontoxic radiopaque medium and filming the action of the vessels through which it courses.

cineangiograph (sın′iæn′jiəgræf′), a special movie camera for recording fluorescent images of the cardiovascular system.

cinefluorography. See **cineradiography.**

cinematics. See **kinematics.**

cineradiography (sın′ırei′diog′rəfi), the filming with a movie camera of the images that appear on a fluorescent screen, especially those images of body structures that have been injected with a nontoxic, radiopaque medium for diagnostic purposes. Cineradiography incorporates the techniques of cinematography, fluoroscopy, and radiography and is an important diagnostic technique. Also called **cinefluorography, cineroentgenofluorography.** See also **cineangiocardiography.**

cineroentgenofluorography. See **cineradiography.**

-cinesis. See **-kinesis.** Also **-cinesia.**

cingulate (sıng′gyəlıt), **1.** having a zone or a girdle, usually with transverse markings. **2.** of or pertaining to a cingulum.

cingulate sulcus (sıŋ'gyulıt). See **callosomarginal fissure.**

cingulectomy (sıŋ'gyulek'təmi), the surgical excision of a portion of the cingulate gyrus in the frontal lobe of the brain, and the immediately surrounding tissue.

cingulotomy (sıŋ'gyulot'əmi), a procedure in brain surgery to alleviate intractable pain by producing lesions in the tissue of the cingulate gyrus of the frontal lobe. The operation interrupts the fibers of the white matter in the gyrus by the stereotactic application of heat or cold.

cinnamon, the aromatic inner bark of several species of *Cinnamomum,* a tree native to the East Indies and China. Saigon cinnamon is commonly used as a carminative, an aromatic stimulant, or as a spice. **– cinnamanic,** *adj.*

circadian rhythm (sər'kədi'ən, sərkæd'iən), a pattern based on a 24-hour cycle, especially the repetition of certain physiologic phenomena, as sleeping and eating.

circinate (sər'sıneit), having ring-shaped outline or formation; annular.

circle, (in anatomy) a circular or nearly circular structure of the body, as the circle of Willis and circle of Zinn. **– circular,** *adj.*

circle of Carus. See **curve of Carus.**

circle of Willis, a vascular network at the base of the brain, formed by the interconnection of the internal carotid, anterior cerebral, posterior cerebral, anterior communicating, and posterior communicating arteries.

CircOlectric (COL) bed, a trade name for an electronically controlled bed that can be vertically rotated 210° and permits vertical alteration of the position of the bed patient from prone to supine. This type of bed is used especially in orthopedics and in the treatment of patients with severe burns. The bed consists of a strong aluminum circular frame supporting an anterior and a posterior straight frame within the exterior aluminum circle. The patient is "sandwiched" and secured between the two straight frames during rotation, the anterior frame covering the patient's chest and abdomen, the posterior frame covering the patient's back. The COL bed is equipped with an electric motor operated by a toggle switch with "up" and "down" positions and by a lever button. Moving the switch to the "up" position and depressing the lever button rotates the circular bed frame clockwise, thus changing the vertical orientation of the patient. Moving the toggle switch to the "down" position and depressing the lever button rotates the the circular frame counterclockwise. Release of the lever button stops rotation. If electric power fails, the COL bed can be operated by a hand crank inserted into the control box. The anterior frame of the COL bed is secured to the posterior mattress by tightening the nut on the stud at each end of the frame. The stud at the head end is tightened first. The anterior frame footboard is adjusted gently against the patient's feet and the nut tightened on the foot end stud.

The forehead support is moved to just above brow level and the chin support is moved to just below the level of the upper lip. The distance between the frames is adjusted by pulling the adjusting knobs on the anterior support bar and lowering the anterior frame until it rests on the patient's chest. Many orthopedists caution about the use of the COL bed for patients with unstable spines and the dangers of vertical turning of the bed in the managment of such patients. Another disadvantage of the COL bed can be the development of "CircOlectric feet," when a patient without protective sensations may get decubiti from the pressure of the footboard against the feet and from the posterior mattress resting on the heels when the patient is prone. These pressure complications can be prevented if the attending staff takes proper precautions to eliminate the pressure on the dorsum of the feet by releasing the footplate after turning the patient prone and by repositioning the footplate before turning the patient supine. An additional hazard of the COL bed is the height of the frame and the absence of any high-low electrical adjustment mechanism. Patients that are elderly, postanesthesia, or heavily sedated may be injured by falling from the bed unless they are properly secured with safety belts. The COL bed has many safety features including caster locks to stabilize the mechanism when it is being operated and permanent stops to prevent the bed from rotating beyond 210°. The bed also has two stops that may be engaged by levers to prevent the bed from rotating past the sitting position and from rotating past the standing position. Some of the greatest advantages of the COL bed are its versatility in changing bed patient position, the accommodation for patient transfer to walkers, and the capability for gradually orienting the cardiovascular patient to a vertical position prior to walking. The COL bed also permits greater patient comfort during position changes essential to postoperative treatment for orthopedic surgery, controlled weight-bearing for patients after hip surgery, and easy mobilization of elderly pa-

CIRCOLECTRIC BED

tients who may be at lesser risk in a COL bed than they would be with 5 to 7 days bedrest in a regular hospital bed. Compare **Foster bed, hyperextension bed, Stryker wedge frame.**

circuit, a course or pathway, particularly one through which an electrical current passes. Current passes through a closed or continuous circuit and stops if the circuit is open, interrupted, or broken.

circular bandage, a bandage wrapped around an injured part, usually a limb.

circular fold, one of the numerous annular projections in the small intestine. They vary in size and frequency in the duodenum, the jejunum, and the ileum, and are formed by mucous and submucous tissue. Most of the folds make less than a full turn around the inside circumference of the intestine, but others spiral through the lumen, making as many as three turns. Also called **plica circularis, valve of Kerkring.**

circulation, movement of an object or substance through a circular course so it returns to its starting point, as in the circulation of blood through the circuitous network of arteries and veins.

circulation time, normal, the time required for blood to flow from one part of the body to another. Timing a particle of blood involves injecting a traceable dye or radioisotope into a vein and timing its reappearance in an artery at the point of injection. Alternatively, a tastable substance like saccharin can be injected, and the time it takes to travel to the tongue can be noted.

circulatory failure, failure of the cardiovascular system to supply the cells of the body with a volume of blood adequate to meet the metabolic demands of the cells. The condition results from abnormal function of the myocardium, as in myocardial infarction; from an inadequate circulatory volume of blood, as with hemorrhage; or from collapse of the peripheral vascular system, as in gram-negative septicemia. See also **shock.**

circulatory system, the network of channels through which the nutrient fluids of the body circulate.

circulus arteriosus minor, the small artery encircling the outer circumference of the iris.

circum-, a combining form meaning 'around': *circumanal, circumgemmal, circumvascular.*

circumanal (sər'kəmei'nəl), of or pertaining to the area surrounding the anus.

circumcision, a surgical procedure in which the prepuce of the penis, or, rarely, the prepuce of the clitoris is excised. Circumcision is widely performed on newborn boys despite the demonstrable lack of medical benefit and the small but significant risk of serious or lethal complications, as hemorrhage, urethral injury, or postoperative infection. These problems occur as often as the penile diseases of uncircumcised adults that circumcision is intended to prevent. The operation is performed on newborns without anesthesia, using one of several kinds of clamp. Circumcision is sometimes performed on adult males in the treatment of phymosis and balanitis. Ritual circumcision is required by the religions of approximately one sixth of the population of the world.

circumduction (sər'kəmdək'shən), **1.** the circular movement of a limb or of the eye. **2.** the motion of the head of a bone within an articulating cavity, as the hip joint. The bone circumscribes a conical space, the apex of which is in the cavity and the base of which is described by the distal end of the bone. Circumduction is one of the four basic kinds of motion allowed by various joints of the skeleton and is a combination of abduction, adduction, extension, and flexion. Compare **angular movement, gliding, rotation.** See also **joint.**

circumferential fibrocartilage, a structure made of fibrocartilage, in which fibrocartilaginous rims surround the margins of various articular cavities, as the glenoid labra of the hip and the shoulder. The rims deepen such cavities and protect their edges. Compare **connecting fibrocartilage, interarticular fibrocartilage, stratiform cartilage.**

circumferential implantation. See **superficial implantation.**

circumoral (sər'kəmor'əl), of or pertaining to the area of the face around the mouth.

circumscribed scleroderma. See **Addison's keloid.**

circumvallate papilla (sər'kəmvæl'ɪt). See under **papilla.**

circus movement, 1. an unusual and involuntary rolling or somersaulting, owing to injured neurological mechanisms that control body posture, as the cerebral peduncles or the vestibular apparatus. **2.** an unusual circular gait caused by injury to the brain or to basal nerve centers. **3.** a mechanism associated with the excitatory wave of the atrium of the heart and atrial flutter or fibrillation. The wave travels a circular path characterized by a gap between the refractory and the excitatory tissue, usually resulting in conduction of only a fraction of the impulses to the ventricle.

cirrhosis (sɪrou'sɪs), a chronic degenerative disease of the liver in which the lobes are covered with fibrous tissue, the parenchyma degenerates, and the lobules are infiltrated with fat. Gluconeogenesis, detoxification of drugs and alcohol, bilirubin metabolism, vitamin absorption, gastrointestinal function, hormonal metabolism, and other functions of the liver deteriorate. Blood flow through the liver is obstructed, causing back pressure and leading to portal hypertension and esophageal varices. Eventually, unless the cause of the disease is removed, hepatic coma, gastrointestinal hemorrhage, and kidney failure usually occur. Cirrhosis is most commonly the result of chronic alcohol abuse but can be the result of nutritional deprivation or hepatitis or other infection. The symptoms of cirrhosis are the same regardless of the cause: nausea, flatulence, anorexia, weight loss, ascites, light-colored stools, weakness, abdominal pain, varicosities and spider angiomas. Diagnosis is made definitively by biopsy, but x ray, physical examination, and several blood tests of liver function are serially performed to monitor the course of the disease. Treatment usually includes a balanced diet, as rich in protein as can be tolerated, vitamins (especially folic acid), rest, and total abstinence from alcohol. The liver has remarkable ability to regenerate, but recovery may be very slow. Kinds of cirrhosis are **biliary cirrhosis, fatty cirrhosis, posthepatic cirrhosis.** See also **hepatic coma.** – **cirrhotic,** *adj.*

cirsoid aneurysm (sər′soid). See **racemose aneurysm.**

cis configuration, cis arrangement, cis position (sis), (in genetics) **1.** the presence of the dominant alleles of two or more pairs of genes on one chromosome and the recessive alleles on the homologous chromosome. **2.** the presence of the mutant genes of a pair of pseudoalleles on one chromosome and the wild-type genes on the homologous chromosome. Compare **coupling** def. 2, **trans configuration.**

cisplatin, an antineoplastic.

■ INDICATIONS: It is prescribed in the treatment of metastatic testicular and ovarian tumors.

■ CONTRAINDICATIONS: Preexisting renal dysfunction, myelosuppression, hearing impairment, or known hypersensitivity to this drug or other drugs containing platinum prohibits its use.

■ ADVERSE EFFECTS: Among the most serious adverse reactions are nephrotoxicity, ototoxicity, myelosuppression, severe nausea, anorexia, vomiting, and allergic reactions.

cisterna (sistər′nə), *pl.* **cisternae.** a cavity that serves as a reservoir for lymph or other body fluids. Kinds of cisternae include **cisterna chyli, cisterna subarachnoidea.**

cisterna chyli, a dilatation at the beginning of the thoracic duct, situated ventral to the body of the second lumbar vertebra, on the right side of and dorsal to the aorta. It receives the two lumbar lymphatic trunks and the intestinal lymphatic trunk.

cisternal puncture, the insertion of a needle into the cerebellomedullary cistern to withdraw cerebrospinal fluid for examination. The puncture is made between the atlas and the occipital bone.

cisterna subarachnoidea, any one of many small subarachnoid spaces that serve as reservoirs for cerebrospinal fluid.

cistron (sis′tron), a fragment or portion of DNA that codes for a specific polypeptide. It is the smallest unit functioning as a transmitter of genetic information. Also called **gene.** – **cistronic,** *adj.*

cisvestitism (sisves′titiz′əm), the practice of wearing attire appropriate to the sex of the individual involved but not suitable to the age, occupation, or status of the wearer, as when a male bookkeeper impersonates a male police officer by wearing a police uniform.

Citanest Hydrochloride, a trade name for a local anesthetic (prilocaine hydrochloride).

citrate (sit′reit, sai′treit), **1.** any salt or ester of citric acid. **2.** the act of treating with a citrate or citric acid. – **citration,** *n.*

citric acid (sit′rik), a white, crystalline, organic acid soluble in water and alcohol. It is extracted from citrus fruits, especially lemons and limes, or obtained by fermentation of sugars and is used as a flavoring agent in foods, carbonated beverages, and certain pharmaceutical products, especially laxatives. It is also used as a preventive of scurvy. See also **ascorbic acid, scurvy.**

citrin (sit′rin), a crystalline flavonoid concentrate that is used as a source of bioflavonoid.

citrovorum factor (sitrov′ərəm). See **folinic acid.**

Civilian Health and Medical Programs for Uniformed Services (CHAMPUS), a health-care insurance system for military dependents and members of the military services when certain kinds of care are not available through the usual military medical service. CHAMPUS is the first, and one of the few, federal third-party reimbursement systems that will pay for care rendered by nurse-midwives and nurse practitioners.

CJPH, abbreviation for *Canadian Journal of Public Health.*

Cl, symbol for **chlorine.**

claims-made policy, a professional liability insurance policy that covers the holder for the period in which a claim of malpractice is made. The alleged act of malpractice may have occurred at some previous time, but the policy insures the holder when the claim is made. Compare **occurrence policy.**

clairsentience (klersen′shəns). See **clairvoyance.**

clairvoyance (klervoi′əns), **clairvoyancy** (klervoi′ənsi), the power or ability to perceive or to be aware of objects or events without the use of the physical senses. Also called **clairsentience.** See also **extrasensory perception, parapsychology, telepathy.**

clairvoyant (klervoi′ənt), **1.** of, pertaining to, or characterized by clairvoyance. **2.** one who possesses the powers of clairvoyance.

clamp, an instrument with serrated tips and locking handles, used for gripping, holding, joining, supporting, or compressing an organ or vessel. In surgery, clamps generally are used for hemostasis.

clamp forceps. See **pedicle clamp.**

clang association (klæŋ), **klang association,** the mental connection between dissociated ideas made because of similarity in the sounds of the words used to describe the ideas. The phenomenon occurs frequently in the manic phase of bipolar disorder.

clapping, (in massage) the procedure of making percussive movements on the body of a patient by lowering the cupped palms alternately in a series of rapid, stimulating blows. In this procedure the movement of the hands is from the wrist. Clapping stimulates the circulation and refreshes the skin and is often done to improve the comfort of bedridden patients, especially during the administration of a bed bath.

clarify, (in chemistry) to clear a turbid liquid by allowing any suspended matter to settle, by adding a substance that precipitates any suspended matter, or by heating. **– clarification,** n.

Clark's rule, a method of calculating the approximate pediatric dosage of a drug for a child using the formula: [weight (in pounds)/150] × adult dose. See **Cowling's rule.**

clas-, a combining form meaning 'a piece broken off': *clasmatocyte, clasmatodendrosis, clasmatosis.*

-clasia, a combining form meaning a '(specified) condition involving crushing or breaking up': *aortoclasia, collodoclasia, osteoclasia.*

clasmocytic lymphoma. See **histiocytic malignant lymphoma.**

clasp, 1. (in dentistry) a sleevelike fitting that is fastened over a tooth to hold a partial denture in place. 2. (in surgery) any device for holding tissues together, especially bones.

clasp-knife reflex, an abnormal sign in which a spastic limb resists passive motion and then suddenly gives way, similar to the blade of a jackknife. It is an indication of damage to the pyramidal tract.

classical Caesarean section, a method for surgically delivering a baby through a vertical midline incision of the upper segment of the uterus. For many practitioners this is the fastest method of Caesarean delivery, but it is attended with a weaker scar and, because the upper segment is thicker and more vascular, there is more bleeding during surgery than from the low cervical Caesarean section. Compare **extraperitoneal Caesarean section.** See also **Caesarean section.**

classical conditioning, a form of learning in which a previously neutral stimulus comes to elicit a given response through associative training. Also called **respondent conditioning.** See also **conditioned reflex.**

classic apraxia. See **ideomotor apraxia.**

classic typhus. See **epidemic typhus.**

classification, (in research) a process in data collection and analysis in which data are grouped according to previously determined characteristics. **– classify,** v.

-clast, a combining form meaning 'something that breaks': *angioclast, cranioclast, myeloclast.*

-clastic, a combining form meaning 'causing disintegration': *hemoclastic, histoclastic, lipoclastic.*

claudication, 1. a lameness or a limping. 2. an intermittent limp.

claustrophobia, a morbid fear of being in or becoming trapped in enclosed or narrow places. The phenomenon is observed more often in women than in men and generally can be traced to some traumatic situation involving enclosed spaces, usually occurring in childhood. Treatment consists of psychotherapy to uncover the cause of the phobic reaction, followed by behavior therapy, specifically systematic desensitization or flooding technique.

claustrum (klɔs'trəm), *pl.* **claustra.** 1. a barrier, as a membrane that partially closes an aperture. 2. Also called **claustrum of insula.** a thin sheet of gray matter, composed chiefly of spindle cells, situated lateral to the external capsule of the brain and separating the internal capsule from white matter of the insula.

clavicle (klæv'ıkəl), a long, curved, horizontal bone just above the first rib, forming the ventral portion of the shoulder girdle. It articulates medially with the sternum and laterally with the acromion of the scapula and accommodates the attachment of numerous muscles. It starts to ossify before any other bone in the body and does not totally unite with the sternum until about the twenty-fifth year. It is shorter, thinner, less curved, and smoother in the female than in the male and is thicker, more curved, and more prominently ridged for muscle attachment in persons performing consistent, strenuous manual labor.

clavicular notch (kləvık'yulər), one of a pair of oval depressions at the superior end of the sternum. Each clavicular notch is situated on one side of the sternum and articulates with the clavicle from the same side.

clavus (klei'vəs, kla'vəs). See **corn.**

clawfoot. See **pes cavus.**

clawhand, a hand fixed in a position of acute flexion. Also called **main en griffe.**

claw-type traction frame, an orthopedic apparatus that holds various pieces of traction equipment, as the pulleys, the ropes and the weights by which traction is applied to various parts of the body or by which various parts of the body are suspended. It consists of two metal uprights, one at the head of the bed and the other at the foot. Both the uprights are secured by claw-type attachments and support an overhead metal bar secured by metal clamps. Compare **I.V.-type traction frame, Balkan traction frame.**

clearance, the removal of a substance from the blood via the kidneys. Kidney function can be tested by measuring the amount of a specific substance excreted in the urine in a given length of time.

clear cell, 1. a type of cell found in the parathyroid gland that does not take on a color with the ordinary tissue stains used for microscopic examination. 2. the principal cell of most renal-cell carcinomas and, occasionally, of ovarian and parathyroid tumors. 3. a specific type of epidermal cell, probably of neural origin, that has a dark-staining nucleus but clear cytoplasm with hematoxylin and eosin stain.

clear cell carcinoma, **1.** a malignant tumor of the tubular epithelium of the kidney. Characteristically, the malignant cells contain abundant clear cytoplasm. See also **renal cell carcinoma.** **2.** an uncommon ovarian neoplasm characterized by cells with clear cytoplasm.

clear cell carcinoma of the kidney. See **renal cell carcinoma.**

clear liquid diet, a diet that supplies fluids and provides minimal residue. It consists primarily of dissolved sugar and flavored liquids, as ginger ale, sweetened tea or coffee, fat-free broth, plain gelatin desserts, and strained fruit juices. The diet is nutritionally inadequate and is usually prescribed for a limited amount of time, as one day, postoperatively.

cleavage, **1.** the series of repeated mitotic cell divisions occurring in the ovum immediately following fertilization to form a mass of cells that transforms the single-celled zygote into a multicellular embryo capable of growth and differentiation. At this initial stage, as the zygote remains uniform in size, the cleavage cells, or blastomeres, become smaller with each division. **2.** the act or process of cleaving or splitting, primarily the splitting of an complex molecule into two or more simpler molecules. Kinds of cleavage include **determinate cleavage, equal cleavage, indeterminate cleavage, partial cleavage, total cleavage, unequal cleavage.**

cleavage cavity. See **blastocoele.**

cleavage cell. See **blastomere.**

cleavage fracture, any fracture that splits cartilage with the avulsion of a small piece of bone from the distal portion of the lateral condyle of the humerus.

cleavage line, any one of a number of linear striations in the skin that delineate the general structural pattern and tension of the subcutaneous fibrous tissue. They correspond closely to the crease lines on the surface of the skin and are present in all areas of the body but are visible only in certain sites, as the palms of the hands and soles of the feet. The lines follow a characteristic pattern for each region of the body, although they vary with body configuration; they are consistent in persons of the same build regardless of age. In general, the lines run obliquely, lying in the direction in which the skin stretches the least, perpendicular to the direction of the greatest stretch. Incisions made parallel to these lines heal with much less scarring than those made perpendicular to them. To a certain degree, cleavage lines determine the direction and arrangement of lesions in skin diseases. Also called **Langer's line.**

cleavage nucleus. See **segmentation nucleus.**

cleavage plane, **1.** the area in a fertilized ovum where cleavage takes place; the axis along which any cell division occurs. **2.** any plane within the body where organs or structures can be separated with minimal damage to surrounding tissue.

cleft, **1.** divided. **2.** a fissure, especially one that originates in the embryo, as the branchial cleft or the facial cleft.

cleft foot, an abnormal condition in which the division between third and fourth toes extends into the metatarsum of the foot.

cleft lip. See **harelip.**

cleft lip repair, the surgical correction of a unilateral or bilateral congenital interruption of the upper lip, usually resulting from the embryologic failure of the median nasal and maxillary processes to unite.

■ METHOD: A cleft lip may sometimes be repaired during the infant's first 48 hours of life, but some surgeons follow a "rule of ten" and perform the operation when the child is ten weeks old, weighs ten or more pounds, and has a hemoglobin of at least ten gm per 100 ml. Preoperatively, elbow restraints, used to prevent the infant from touching the incision, are prepared in the proper size and are sent to the operating room with the patient. Postoperatively, the infant is maintained with ventilatory support as necessary until respirations are normal and is observed for respiratory stridor or obstruction, excessive bleeding, separation of the incision, and redness under the elbow restraints. The wire bow applied to the infant's upper lip and taped to the cheeks to prevent tension on the sutures is kept in place; if it becomes loose it is reapplied using tincture of benzoin. The infant is given clear liquids and juices through an Asepto syringe or special feeding unit; parenteral fluids are administered until the oral intake is adequate; milk products, solids, and a nipple or pacifier are not allowed. The diet and manner of feeding may vary, but the infant is fed while held with the head up or is placed in a cardiac chair and burped after the intake of each ounce of food. The intake and output of fluids are measured. The elbow restraints are worn at all times except when range of motion exercises are performed, one arm at a time, with skin care is administered to that limb. The saline dressing on the lip is kept moist and is changed at least every 12 hours.

■ NURSING ORDERS: The nurse administers preoperative and postoperative care and prepares for the infant's discharge by ensuring that the parents understand the proper diet and feeding schedule and technique, by emphasizing the importance of using elbow restraints, and by explaining the importance of maintaining motion and skin integrity of the arms, of avoiding injury to the surgical area, and of reporting symptoms of infection, including separation of the incision, excessive swelling, redness, bleeding, and drainage.

■ OUTCOME CRITERIA: Modern surgical techniques permit remarkable repair of cleft lips, but in some cases a second operation is required to eliminate the scar.

cleft palate, a congenital defect characterized by a fissure in the midline of the palate, resulting from the failure of the two sides to fuse during embryonic development. The fissure may be complete, extending through both the hard and soft palates into the nasal cavities, or it may show any degree of incomplete or partial cleft. The condition, which occurs approximately once in every 2,500 live births and affects females more than males, is often associated with a cleft in the upper lip. Together, these abnormalities are the most common of the craniofacial malformations, accounting for half of the total number of defects. Feeding is best accomplished with special feeding devices. Surgical repair of the defect is usually not begun until the first or second year of life and is usually performed in steps. Care of the child requires a team approach that includes a plastic surgeon, orthodontist, dentist, nurse, speech and hearing therapists, and social workers. Long-term, postoperative problems, including speech impairment and hearing loss, improper tooth development and alignment, chronic respiratory and ear infections, and varying levels of emotional and social maladjustment, may be largely avoided by modern techniques and reconstructive surgery. See also **harelip.**

cleft palate repair, the surgical correction of a congenital fissure in the midline of the partition separating the oral and nasal cavities. Palatine clefts range from a simple separation in the uvula to an extensive fissure involving the soft and hard palate and extending forward unilaterally or bilaterally through the alveolar ridge. A cleft lip often accompanies a cleft palate. Repair of a cleft palate is usually undertaken in the child's second year.
■ METHOD: Before surgery, properly sized elbow restraints to prevent the child from touching the mouth are prepared and sent to the operating room with the patient. Postoperatively, the youngster is kept in a moist oxygen-rich environment using a Croupette or other tent device until respirations are normal and is observed for signs of airway obstruction or excessive bleeding. Parenteral fluids are administered until the oral intake is adequate. Clear liquids and juices are given by cup only; straws, nipples, pacifiers, utensils, or toys may not be put in the mouth. Milk products and solids are contraindicated, but the kind of feeding ordered may vary. The child is fed in a high chair, when possible, and a bib is used to accommodate drooling. Only circumoral mouth care is administered; the teeth are not brushed. The intake and output of fluids are measured. The elbow restraints are worn continuously, except when daily range of motion exercises are performed and skin care is administered, to one arm at a time. With improvement, the child is permitted to walk as tolerated.
■ NURSING ORDERS: Prior to discharge the nurse ensures that the parents understand the required diet, the need to feed by cup only, to use elbow restraints, to maintain the motion and skin integrity of the arms, and to avoid injury to the mouth. The nurse reminds the parents to administer the required medication in the proper dosage and on schedule and to report symptoms of incision infection, as drainage, mouth odor, or bleeding.
■ OUTCOME CRITERIA: Depending on the extent and nature of a cleft palate, it may be repaired in one or in several operations. Some experts believe that early repair of a defect in the bony palate can lead to structural malrelations and advise delaying the operation until the child is between five and seven and has achieved more bone growth. Successful repair often greatly improves the child's oronasopharyngeal physiology, speech, and appearance.

cleft uvula, an abnormal congenital condition in which the uvula is split into two halves owing to the failure of the posterior palatine folds to unite.

cleido-, cleid-, a combining form meaning 'pertaining to the clavicle': *cleidocostal, cleidocranial, cleidomastoid.*

cleidocranial dysostosis, a rare, abnormal hereditary condition characterized by defective ossification of the cranial bones and by the complete or partial absence of the clavicles. It is transmitted as an autosomal dominant trait. The defective ossification of the cranial bones delays the closing of the cranial sutures and results in large fontanels. The complete or partial absence of the clavicles allows the shoulders to be brought together. This condition also involves dental and vertebral anomalies. Also called **cleidocranial dysplasia.** See also **dysostosis.**

cleidocranial dysplasia. See **cleidocranial dysostosis.**

cleidocranial dystrophia (klaɪ′doukreɪ′niəl). See **cleidocranial dysostosis.**

Cleocin, a trade name for an antibacterial (clindamycin).

cleptomania. See **kleptomania.**

click, (in cardiology) an extra heart sound that occurs during systole. See also **ejection click, systolic click.**

client, 1. a person who is recipient of a professional service. 2. a recipient of health care regardless of the state of health. 3. a recipient of health care who is not ill or hospitalized. 4. a patient.

client-centered therapy, a nondirective method of group or individual psychotherapy, originated by Carl Rogers, in which the role of the therapist is to listen to and then reflect or restate without judgment or interpretation the words of the client. The goal of the therapy is personal growth achieved by the client's increased awareness and understanding of his attitudes, feelings, and behavior.

client interview. See **patient interview.**

climacteric (klaɪmæk′tərɪk). See **menopause.**

climacteric melancholia. See **involutional melancholia.**

climate, a composite of the prevailing weather conditions that characterizes any particular geographical region. Various phenomena constitute climate, as air pressure, temperature, precipitation, sunshine, and humidity –all health factors considered in the diagnosis and treatment of certain illnesses, especially those affecting respiration. – **climatic,** *adj.*

clindamycin hydrochloride, an antibacterial.

■ INDICATIONS: It is prescribed in the treatment of certain serious infections.

■ CONTRAINDICATIONS: Hypersensitivity to this drug or to lincomycin prohibits its use.

■ ADVERSE EFFECTS: Among the more serious adverse reactions are colitis, severe gastrointestinal disturbances, and hypersensitivity reactions.

clinic, **1.** a department in a hospital where persons not requiring hospitalization may receive medical care. Formerly it was called a dispensary. **2.** a group practice of doctors, as the Mayo Clinic. **3.** a meeting place for doctors and medical students where instruction can be given at the bedside of a patient or in a similar setting. **4.** a seminar or other scientific medical meeting. **5.** a detailed published report of the diagnosis and treatment of a health care problem.

-clinic, a combining form meaning 'places set aside for medical treatment': *policlinic, polyclinic, psychoclinic.*

clinical, **1.** of or pertaining to a clinic. **2.** of or pertaining to direct, bedside medical care. **3.** of or pertaining to materials or equipment used in the care of a sick person.

clinical cytogenetics, the branch of genetics that studies the relationship between chromosomal abnormalities and pathological conditions.

clinical diagnosis, a diagnosis made on the basis of knowledge obtained by medical history and physical examination alone, without benefit of laboratory tests or x rays.

clinical genetics, a branch of genetics that studies inherited disorders and investigates the possible genetic factors that may influence the occurrence of any pathological condition. Also called **medical genetics.**

clinical laboratory, a laboratory in which tests directly related to the care of patients are performed. Such laboratories use material obtained from patients for testing, as compared with research laboratories where animal and other sources of test material are also used.

clinical nurse specialist (CNS), a registered nurse who holds a master of science degree in nursing (M.S.N.) and who has acquired advanced knowledge and clinical skills in a specific area of nursing and health care. The CNS, as a practitioner, assumes a leadership role in the distribution of clinical care to a specific patient population while interacting within the total health care delivery system. The unique functions of the CNS are based on clinical expertise and judgment and include caring for patients, delegating responsibility, teaching other staff members, and influencing and affecting change with re-

spect to the needs of the patient and family and the total health care delivery system.

clinical-pathological conference, a teaching conference in which a case is presented to a clinician who then demonstrates the process of reasoning that leads to his diagnosis. A pathologist then presents an anatomical diagnosis, based on the study of tissue removed at surgery or obtained in autopsy. Often the students will have been asked to suggest a diagnosis based on the same information presented to the clinician. A discussion usually follows that serves to demonstrate the origin of errors present in any of the diagnoses offered. The pathologist's diagnosis is usually the definitive one. The clinical-pathological conference is the model for the long series called 'case-reports' in the *New England Journal of Medicine* and is a part of the curricula of most medical schools.

clinical pathology, the laboratory study of disease by a pathologist using techniques appropriate to the specimen being studied. Among the many branches of clinical pathology are hematology, bacteriology, chemistry, and serology.

clinical pelvimetry, a process used to assess the size of the birth canal by means of the systematic vaginal palpation of specific bony landmarks in the pelvis and an estimation of the distances between them. Internal pelvic diameters are not accessible to direct measurement; they must be inferred. Clinical pelvimetry is usually performed by a midwife or an obstetrician during the first prenatal examination of a pregnant woman. Findings are commonly recorded in terms such as 'adequate,' 'borderline,' or 'inadequate,' rather than in centimeters or inches. Compare **x-ray pelvimetry.** See also **birth canal, cephalopelvic disproportion, contraction, dystocia.**

clinical psychology, the branch of psychology concerned with the diagnosis, treatment, and prevention of personality and behavioral disorders.

clinical research center, an organization, often associated with a medical school or a teaching hospital, that studies, analyzes, correlates, and describes medical cases. Such centers usually have extensive laboratory facilities and specialized staffs of physicians and medical technicians. Clinical research centers often offer free or very inexpensive diagnoses and treatment for patients participating in various research programs and often produce significant new medical information distributed through articles, journals, reports, seminars, and lectures. Funding for such facilities may come from minimal fees for various medical services and from grants.

clinical specialist, a doctor or nurse having advanced training in a particular field of practice, as a nurse-midwife, pediatrician, or radiologist.

Clinitest (klĭn′ĭtest′), a trademark for reagent tablets used to test for the presence of reducing sugars, as glucose, in the urine. The tablets contain copper sulfate, and the procedure is a modified version of Benedict's test.

clino-, a combining form meaning 'to bend or make lie down': *clinodactyl, clinostatic, clinostatism.*

clinocephaly (klai'nousef'əli), **clinocephalism,** a congenital anomaly of the head in which the upper surface of the skull is concave. — **clinocephalic, clinocephalous,** *adj.*

clinodactyly (klai'noudæk'təli), **clinodactylism,** a congenital anomaly characterized by abnormal lateral or medial bending of one or more fingers or toes. — **clinodactylic, clinodactylous,** *adj.*

Clinoril, a trade name for an anti-inflammatory (sulindac).

-clinous, a combining form meaning 'pertaining to ancestry': *matriclinous, matroclinous, patroclinous.*

clioquinol. See **iodochlorhydroxyquin.**

clip, a surgical device used for grasping the skin to align the edges of a wound and to stop bleeding, especially of the smaller blood vessels. It is also used in radiography for localization.

Clistin, a trade name for an antihistamine (carbinoxamine maleate).

clitoris (klɪt'əris), the vaginal erectile structure homologous to the corpora cavernosa of the penis. It consists of two corpora cavernosa within a dense layer of fibrous membrane, joined along their inner surfaces by an incomplete fibrous septum. It is situated beneath the anterior commissure, partially hidden between the anterior extremities of the labia minora.

CLL. See **chronic lymphocytic leukemia.**

cloaca (klouei'kə), *pl.* **cloacae. 1.** (in embryology) the end of the hindgut before the developmental division into the rectum, the bladder, and the primitive genital structures. **2.** (in pathology) an opening into the sheath of tissue around a necrotic bone.

cloacal membrane, a thin sheath that separates the internal and external portions of the cloaca in the developing embryo. It is formed from endoderm and ectoderm and closes the fetal anus during early prenatal development; it later ruptures and is absorbed so that the anal canal becomes continuous with the rectum. Also called **anal membrane.**

cloacal septum. See **urorectal septum.**

clocortolone pivalate, a topical corticosteroid.
■ INDICATION: It is used topically as an anti-inflammatory agent.
■ CONTRAINDICATIONS: Viral and fungal diseases of the skin or local impairment of circulation prohibits its use.
■ ADVERSE REACTIONS: Among the more serious adverse reactions are various systemic side effects that may occur from prolonged or excessive application. Local irritation of the skin may occur.

Cloderm, a trade name for a glucocorticoid (clocortolone pivalate).

clofibrate (klou'fəbreit), an antihyperlipoproteinemic.
■ INDICATIONS: It is prescribed in the treatment of high blood levels of cholesterol, triglycerides, or both.
■ CONTRAINDICATIONS: Liver or kidney dysfunction, pregnancy, lactation, biliary cirrhosis, or known hypersensitivity to this drug prohibits its use.
■ ADVERSE EFFECTS: Among the more serious adverse reactions are nausea, diarrhea, weight gain, and a syndrome resembling influenza. This drug interacts with many other drugs.

Clomid, a trade name for a nonsteroidal fertility drug (clomiphene citrate).

clomiphene citrate (klou'məfin), a nonsteroidal antiestrogen that acts to stimulate ovulation.
■ INDICATIONS: It is prescribed principally in the treatment of anovulation and oligo-ovulation in women.
■ CONTRAINDICATIONS: Abnormal vaginal bleeding, liver dysfunction, or known hypersensitivity to this drug prohibits its use.
■ ADVERSE EFFECTS: Among the more serious adverse reactions are enlargement of the ovaries, blurred vision, gastric upset, rashes, and abdominal pain.

clomiphene stimulation test (klou'mɪfin), a test used to evaluate gonadal function in males who show signs of abnormal pubertal development. Clomiphene, a nonsteroid analog of estrogen, stimulates the hypothalamic-pituitary system to raise FSH and LH levels of the blood. Failure to respond to clomiphene indicates hypothalamic-pituitary disease, possibly a pituitary tumor. In women, the drug clomiphene citrate stimulates ovulation and is used to treat anovulatory infertility. See also **gonadotropins.**

clonal selection theory, (in immunology) a theory of antibody formation proposed by Sir M. Burnet, stating that preprogrammed, or precommitted, clones of lymphoid cells that are produced in the fetus are capable of interacting with a limited number of antigenic determinants with which the host may come in contact. Any precommitted immunocompetent cells that encounter the specific antigen in utero are destroyed or suppressed so that entire clones are eliminated or inactivated. This, in effect, removes the cells programmed to become endogenous autoantigens and prevents the development of autoimmune diseases, leaving intact those cells capable of reacting with exogenous antigens.

clonazepam (klounæz'ɪpæm), an anticonvulsant.
■ INDICATIONS: It is prescribed in the prevention of seizures in petit mal epilepsy and other convulsive disorders.
■ CONTRAINDICATIONS: Liver disease, acute narrow-angle glaucoma, or known hypersensitivity to this drug or to other benzodiazepine drugs prohibits its use. It is not given during lactation.
■ ADVERSE EFFECTS: Among the more serious adverse

reactions are anemia, coma, palpitations, mental and respiratory depression, muscle weakness, and shortness of breath.

clone, a group of genetically identical cells or organisms derived from a single common cell or organism through mitosis.

-clonia, a combining form meaning '(condition involving) spasms': *logoclonia, myoclonia, polyclonia.*

clonidine hydrochloride (klou′nədin), an antihypertensive.

■ INDICATION: It is prescribed for the reduction of high blood pressure.

■ CONTRAINDICATIONS: Known hypersensitivity to this drug prohibits its use.

■ ADVERSE EFFECTS: Among the more serious adverse reactions are a withdrawal syndrome occurring on discontinuation of the medication, characterized by tachycardia, a rapid increase in blood pressure, and anxiety. Drowsiness and dry mouth commonly occur.

Clonopin, a trade name for an anticonvulsant (clonazepam).

Clonorchis sinensis (klounor′kıs sınen′sıs), the Chinese or Oriental liver fluke, a form of tapeworm that is acquired by humans who eat raw or imperfectly cooked fish that is the intermediate host of the parasite. The fluke exists in a dormant stage as a cercaria, encysted in the skin of a fish and unable to continue its life cycle until ingested by a warmblooded animal in which the larvae mature and produce eggs. The eggs are excreted in the feces of the host to enter water where the new generation evolves first in aquatic snails and then in fish. In human hosts, the liver fluke lives in the bile ducts and gall bladder, causing chronic liver disease with enlargement of the liver, diarrhea, edema, and, eventually, death. Also called *Opisthorchis sinensis.*

clonus (klou′nəs), an abnormal pattern of neuromuscular activity, characterized by rapidly alternating involuntary contraction and relaxation of skeletal muscle. Compare **tonus.** – **clonic,** *adj.*

C-loop, a surgically formed loop of bowel with a C-shape.

clorazepate dipotassium, a minor tranquilizer.

■ INDICATIONS: It is prescribed in the treatment of anxiety and nervous tension.

■ CONTRAINDICATIONS: Psychosis, acute narrow angle glaucoma, or known hypersensitivity to this drug prohibits its use.

■ ADVERSE EFFECTS: Among the more serious adverse reactions are withdrawal symptoms occurring on discontinuation of treatment. Drowsiness and fatigue commonly occur.

closed amputation, a kind of amputation in which one or two broad flaps of muscular and cutaneous tissue are retained to form a cover over the end of the bone. It is only performed when no infection is present. A rigid dressing may be applied and the patient fitted for a prosthesis immediately after surgery. Compare **open amputation.** See also **amputation.**

closed-chain, (in organic chemistry) of or pertaining to a compound in which the carbon atoms are bonded together to form a closed ring. Also called **carbocyclic.**

closed drainage. See **drainage.**

closed wound suction, any one of several techniques for draining potentially harmful fluids, as blood, pus, serosanguineous fluid, and tissue secretions from surgical wounds. Such fluids interfere with the healing of wounds and often promote infection. Postoperative drainage aids the healing process by removing dead spaces where extravascular fluids collect and helps draw healing tissues together. Many surgical authorities prefer closed wound suction to other wound drainage methods, as pressure bandages and wicks, because it minimizes danger of infection. Closed wound suction is often an important part of postoperative treatment and may be accomplished with a variety of reliable devices that create a gentle negative pressure to drain away undesirable exudates. The uses of closed wound suction are as varied as the different surgical procedures. The technique is used as an aid to many operations, as mastectomies, augmentations, plastic and reconstructive procedures, and urological and urogenital procedures. Closed wound suction devices usually consist of disposable transparent containers attached to suction tubes and portable suction pumps. After thoroughly irrigating the wound to remove blood clots and debris, the surgeon inserts the perforated wound tubing into the wound and brings it out through healthy tissue, approximately 5 cm from the incision line. When silicone tubing is used, the tube is passed through a stab wound made adjacent to the surgical wound. With the drainage tubing brought out away from the incision line, the closed wound suction system remains completely closed. Air cannot infiltrate the wound and cause contamination. When the suction tube has been inserted, the wound is closed and a light dressing is applied. Since the tubing drains most fluids, the dressing usually does not require frequent changing. Closed wound suction usually continues postoperatively for two or three days or until the wound stops exuding fluid. The surgeon then removes the suction tubing, and all drainage components of the suction device are discarded. The transparent tubing and reservoir are checked regularly while the suction is functioning as a precaution against clogging and to monitor the volume of exudate drawn from the wound. In some individuals closed wound suction systems can also accommodate antibiotic drips, which are connected to accessory tubing placed within the wound beside the suction tube. Closed wound suction also allows irrigation of the wound with special flow controls to permit a periodic change in the flow direction of solutions.

clostridial (klostrɪd′iəl),   of or pertaining to an anaerobic spore-forming bacteria of the genus *Clostridium.*

clostridial myonecrosis. See **myonecrosis.**

Clostridium,   a genus of spore-forming, anaerobic bacteria of the Bacillaceae family: *Clostridium bifermentans* causes gas gangrene and is found in feces and garbage; *C. botulinum* causes botulism; *C. perfringens* causes food poisoning, cellulitis, and wound infections; *C. tetani* is the cause of tetanus.

closure,   the surgical closing of a wound by suture. See also **flask closure, velopharyngeal closure.**

clot. See **blood clot.**

clotrimazole,   an antifungal.
■ INDICATIONS: It is prescribed in the treatment of a variety of superficial fungal infections and for candidal vulvovaginitis.
■ CONTRAINDICATION: Known hypersensitivity to this drug prohibits its use. It is not prescribed for ophthalmic use; contact with eyes is avoided.
■ ADVERSE EFFECTS: The most serious adverse reactions are severe hypersensitivity reactions of the skin.

clotting. See **blood clotting.**

clotting time,   the time required for blood to form a clot, tested by collecting 4 ml of blood in a glass tube and examining it for clot formation. The first appearance of a clot is noted and timed. This simple test has been used to diagnose hemophilias, but it will not detect mild coagulation disorders. Its chief application is in monitoring anticoagulant therapy. Also called **coagulation time.**

cloud baby,   a newborn who appears well and healthy but is a carrier of infectious bacterial or viral organisms. The infant may contaminate the surrounding environment with airborne droplets from the respiratory tract forming clouds of the organisms. A cloud baby may be the source of a nursery epidemic, especially one caused by a staphylococcal organism.

clove,   the dried flower bud of *Eugenia caryophyllata.* It contains the lactone caryophyllin and a volatile oil used as a dental analgesic, a germicide, and a salve. Clove is also used as a spice and a carminative against nausea, vomiting, and flatulence.

cloverleaf nail,   a surgical nail shaped in cross section like a cloverleaf, used especially in the repair of fractures of the femur.

cloverleaf skull deformity,   a congenital defect characterized by a trilobed skull resulting from the premature closure of multiple cranial sutures during embryonic development. The condition is associated with hydrocephalus, facial anomalies, and skeletal deformities. Also called **kleeblattschädel deformity syndrome.**

cloxacillin sodium,   an antibacterial.
■ INDICATIONS: It is prescribed in the treatment of certain serious infections, primarily those caused by penicillin resistant strains of staphylococci.
■ CONTRAINDICATIONS: Known hypersensitivity to this drug or to any penicillin prohibits its use.
■ ADVERSE EFFECTS: Among the more serious adverse reactions are gastrointestinal discomfort, rash, and hypersensitivity reactions.

clubbing,   an abnormal enlargement of the distal phalanges, usually associated with cyanotic heart disease or advanced chronic pulmonary disease but sometimes occurring with biliary cirrhosis, colitis, chronic dysentery, and thyrotoxicosis. The mechanism whereby diminished oxygen tension in the blood causes clubbing is not understood. Clubbing occurs in all the digits but is most easily seen in the fingers. Advanced clubbing is obvious but early clubbing is difficult to diagnose. Clubbing is present if the transverse diameter of the base of the fingernail is greater than the transverse diameter of the most distal joint of the digit. The affected phalange is full, fleshy and quite vascular; the skin may be excoriated.

clubfoot,   a congenital deformity of the foot, sometimes resulting from intrauterine constriction and characterized by unilateral or bilateral deviation of the metatarsal bones of the forefoot. Ninety-five per cent of clubfoot deformities are **equinovarus,** characterized by medial deviation and plantar flexion of the forefoot, but a few are **calcaneo valgus,** characterized by lateral deviation and dorsiflexion. Treatment depends on the extent and rigidity of the deformity. Splints and casts in infancy may produce complete correction; surgery in several steps may be necessary to achieve normal function. See also **Denis-Browne splint, talipes.**

cluster analysis,   (in statistics) a complex technique of data analysis of numerical scale scores that produces clusters of variables related to one another. The technique is performed using a computer.

cluster headache. See **histamine headache.**

cluttering,   a speech defect characterized by a rapid, confused, nervous delivery with uneven rhythmical patterns and the omission or transposition of various letters or syllables. The condition is commonly associated with other language disorders, as difficulty in learning to speak, read and spell, and with various personality and behavior problems.

Cm,   symbol for **curium.**

CMAJ,   abbreviation for *Canadian Medical Association Journal.*

CMHC,   abbreviation for **community mental health center.**

CML,   abbreviation for **chronic myelocytic leukemia.**

CMV,   abbreviation for **cytomegalovirus.**

CNA,   abbreviation for **Canadian Nurses' Association.**

CNATS,   abbreviation for **Canadian Nurses' Association Testing Service.**

-cnemia, a combining form meaning '(condition of the) leg below the knee': *bucnemia, cacocnemia, microcnemia.*

CNF, abbreviation for **Canadian Nurses' Foundation.**

CNM, abbreviation for **Certified Nurse-Midwife.**

CNP. See **community nurse practitioner.**

CNRS, abbreviation for **Canadian Nurses' Respiratory Society.**

CNS, 1. abbreviation for **central nervous system.** 2. abbreviation for **clinical nurse specialist.**

CNS syndrome. See **central nervous system syndrome.**

Co, symbol for **cobalt.**

co-, a combining form meaning 'together, with': *coadaptation, coagulate, coarctate.* Also **col-, com-, con-, cor-.**

CO₂, symbol for **carbon dioxide.**

coagulase (kɔuæg′yuleis), an enzyme produced by bacteria, particularly the *Staphylococcus aureus,* that promotes the formation of thrombi.

coagulation (kɔuæg′yulei′shən). See **blood clotting.**

coagulation factor, one of thirteen factors in the blood, the interactions of which are responsible for the process of blood clotting. The factors, using standardized numerical nomenclature, are factor I, fibrinogen; factor II, prothrombin; factor III, tissue thromboplastin; factor IV, calcium ions; factors V and VI, proaccelerin or labile factors; factor VII, proconvertin or stable factor; factor VIII, antihemophilic globulin; factor IX, plasma thromboplastin component (PTC); factor X, Stuart factor; factor XI, plasma thromboplastin antecedent (PTA); factor XII, Hageman factor or glass factor; factor XIII, fibrin stabilizing factor or Laki-Lorand factor. See also **blood clotting, coagulation, hemophilia.**

coagulation necrosis. See **necrosis.**

coagulation time. See **clotting time.**

coagulopathy (kɔuæg′yəlop′əthi), a pathological condition affecting the ability of the blood to coagulate.

coal tar, a topical antieczematic.

■ INDICATIONS: It is prescribed in the treatment of chronic skin diseases, as eczema and psoriasis.

■ CONTRAINDICATION: Known hypersensitivity to this drug prohibits its use.

■ ADVERSE EFFECTS: Among the most serious adverse effects are skin irritation and local hypersensitivity reactions.

Four stages of blood coagulation

Intrinsic thromboplastin system (thromboplastin derived from plasma)	Extrinsic thromboplastin system (thromboplastin derived from tissues)

Stage I: Formation of thromboplastin

Platelet factor (PF) released to react with AHF and PTC in presence of PTA, Hageman factor, factors V and X, and calcium ions

Duration: 3 to 5 minutes

Bypassed

AHF
PTC
PF
$X \xrightarrow[\text{Factor V}]{\text{Calcium}^{++}}$ Plasma thromboplastin
Hageman factor
PTA

Stage II: Conversion of inactive prothrombin

Reaction requiring thromboplastin, calcium ions, and accessory factors (factors V and X for both tissue and plasma thromboplastin, factor VII with tissue thromboplastin)

Note: Both thromboplastin systems must function for normal coagulation

Duration: 8 to 15 seconds

Prothrombin $\xrightarrow[\text{Calcium}^{++}, \text{V, X}]{\text{Plasma thromboplastin}}$ Thrombin   Prothrombin $\xrightarrow[\text{Calcium}^{++}, \text{V, VII, X}]{\text{Tissue thromboplastin}}$ Thrombin

Stage III: Conversion of fibrinogen to fibrin

As soon as any thrombin formed, soluble fibrinogen converted to insoluble fibrin

Duration: less than 1 second

Fibrinogen $\xrightarrow{\text{Thrombin}}$ Fibrin $\xrightarrow[\text{Calcium}^{++}]{\text{FSF}}$ Stabilized fibrin

Stage IV: Lysis of clot

Fibrinolysin (plasmin) acts on fibrin to dissolve it

Fibrin $\xrightarrow[\text{Fibrinolysin (plasmin)}]{}$ Lysis

coal worker's pneumoconiosis. See **anthracosis.**

coaptation splint (kou'æptei'ʃən), a small splint fitted to a fractured limb to prevent overriding of the fragments of bone. A longer splint usually covers the small one to provide for more support and fixation of the entire limb.

coarct (kouarkt'), the act of narrowing or constricting, especially the lumen of a blood vessel.

coarctation (kou'arktei'ʃən), a stricture or contraction of the walls of a vessel as the aorta.

coarctation of the aorta, a congenital cardiac anomaly characterized by a localized narrowing of the aorta, which results in increased pressure proximal to the defect and decreased pressure distal to it. Symptoms of the condition are directly related to the pressure changes created by the constriction. The most common site of coarctation is just beyond the origin of the left subclavian artery from the aorta, resulting in high blood pressure in the upper extremities and head and low blood pressure in the lower extremities. Clinical manifestations include dizziness, headaches, fainting, epistaxis, reduced or absent femoral pulses, and muscle cramps in the legs from tissue anoxia during increased exercise. Diagnosis is based on characteristic pressure changes in the upper and lower body and specific radiological findings, including notching of the lower ribs, left ventricular hypertrophy, and dilatation of the aorta proximal to the stricture. A murmur may or may not be present. Surgical repair is recommended for minor defects because of the high incidence of untreated complications, including aortic rupture, hypertension, infective endocarditis, subarachnoid hemorrhage, and congestive heart failure. See also **congenital cardiac anomaly.**

coarse, (in physiology) involving a wide range of movements, as those associated with tremors and other involuntary movements of the skeletal muscle.

coarse fremitus, a rough, loud, tremulous vibration of the chest wall noted on palpation of the chest during a physical examination as the person inhales and exhales. It is most common in pulmonary conditions characterized by consolidation.

coat, 1. a membrane that covers the outside of an organ or part. 2. one of the layers of a wall of an organ or part, especially a canal or a vessel.

cobalamin (koubɒl'əmɪn), a generic term for the vitamin B_{12} group. See also **cyanocobalamin.**

cobalt (Co), a metallic element that occurs in the minerals cobaltite, smaltite, and linnaeite. Its atomic number is 27; its atomic weight is 58.9. Extensive deposits of cobalt minerals are found in Ontario, Canada. Pure cobalt is obtained by reducing the oxide with alumium or with carbon. It is used in special alloys, as Alnico. Cobalt is a component of vitamin B_{12}, is found in most common foods, and is readily absorbed by the gastrointestinal tract. Research has established that this element is common in the human diet, but the precise daily intake requirement is not known, and cobalt deficiency in humans is not known. The administration of cobalt in the form of cobaltous chloride has been successful in some patients with certain types of anemia because of the capacity of cobalt to produce polycythemia. Accidental intoxication by cobaltous chloride, especially in children, may produce cyanosis, coma, and death. Certain amounts of cobalt stimulate the production of erythropoietin, but the exact mechanisms of this process are not completely understood. Large doses of cobalt depress erythrocyte production. It is believed that in stimulating the production of erythropoietin cobalt inhibits enzymes involved in oxidative metabolism and that erythropoietin increases as the result of tissue hypoxia. The only disease for which some experts still advocate the use of cobalt is normochromic, normocytic anemia associated with renal failure. The radioisotope Co^{60} emits gamma rays and is often used as an encapsulated radiation source in the treatment of cancer.

cobalt-60 (^{60}Co), (in radiotherapy) a radioactive isotope of the silver-white metallic element cobalt with a mass number of 60 and a half-life of 5.2 years. ^{60}Co emits high energy gamma rays and is the most frequently used radioisotope in radiotherapy. In ^{60}Co machines, the high-energy radioactive source is stored in a position well shielded by lead or uranium.

Cobefrin, a trade name for a vasoconstrictor (nordefrin), used as an adjunct to anesthesia.

coca, one of two South American shrubs, native to the Andes. The leaves are dried and then chewed for their stimulant effect by some of the people of the region. It is a natural source of cocaine.

cocaine hydrochloride, a white crystalline powder used as a local anesthetic. It was originally derived from coca leaves but is now prepared synthetically.

■ INDICATIONS: In solution the drug is an effective topical anesthetic commonly used in the examination and treatment of the eye, ear, nose, and throat. The vasoconstrictive action of the drug slows bleeding and limits absorption. Prolonged or frequent use may damage the mucous membranes.

■ CONTRAINDICATIONS: Cocaine is incompatible with all alkaloid precipitants, mercurials, and silver nitrate. Central nervous system overstimulation may result from use with monoamine oxidase inhibitors, amphetamines, or guanethidine. Combination with epinephrine or norepinephrine can lead to cardiac arrhythmias or ventricular fibrillation. Cocaine is not given to patients with severe cardiovascular disease, thyrotoxicosis, hypotension, or hypertension.

■ ADVERSE REACTIONS: Among the most serious adverse reactions are excitement, depression, euphoria, restlessness, tremors, vertigo, nausea, vomiting, hypotension, hypertension, abdominal cramps, exophthalmia, mydriasis, peripheral vascular collapse, tachypnea, tachycardia, chills, fever, coma or death from respiratory failure.

■ NOTE: Cocaine hydrochloride solution should be freshly made; it deteriorates rapidly on standing and cannot be heat sterilized. Cocaine is a Schedule II drug under the Controlled Substances Act.

cocci-, cocco-, a combining form meaning 'seed; pertaining to a sperical bacterial cell': *coccobacillus, coccogenous, coccoid.*

coccidioidomycosis (koksɪd'ɪɔɪ'dɔumaɪkou'sɪs), an infectious fungal disease caused by the inhalation of spores of the bacterium *Coccidioides immitis,* which is carried on windborne dust particles. The disease is endemic in hot, dry regions of the southwestern United States and Central and South America. Primary infection is characterized by symptoms resembling those of the common cold or influenza. Secondary infection, occurring after a period of remission and lasting from weeks to years, is marked by low-grade fever, anorexia and weight loss, cyanosis, dyspnea, hemoptysis, and arthritic pain in the bones and joints. The diagnosis is made by learning that the patient was living in or visiting an endemic area and by identifying *C. immitis* in sputum, exudate, or tissue. Treatment usually consists of bed rest and the administration of antibiotics. Also called **desert fever, desert rheumatism, San Joaquin fever, valley fever.**

coccidiosis, a parasitic disease of tropical and subtropical regions caused by the ingestion of oocysts of the protozoa *Isospora belli* or *I. hominis.* Symptoms include fever, malaise, abdominal discomfort, and watery diarrhea. The infection is usually self-limited, lasting one to two weeks, but occasionally it persists, resulting in malabsorption syndrome and, rarely, death. No specific therapy has been found. Compare **coccidioidomycosis.**

cocco-. See **cocci-.**

coccus (kok'əs), *pl.* **cocci.** a bacterium that is round, spherical, or oval in shape, as gonococcus, pneumococcus, staphylococcus, streptococcus. — **coccal,** *adj.*

-coccus, a combining form meaning a 'berry-shaped organism': *dermococcus, enterococcus, pneumonococcus.*

coccyg-, coccygo-, a combining form meaning 'coccyx': *coccygeal, coccygectomy, coccygodynia.*

coccygeal vertebra, one of the four segments of the vertebral column that fuse in the adult to form the coccyx. They are considered rudimentary vertebrae and have no pedicles, laminae, or spinous processes. Compare **cervical vertebra, lumbar vertebra, sacral vertebra, thoracic vertebra.** See also **coccyx, vertebra.**

coccygeus (koksɪj'iəs), one of two muscles in the pelvic diaphragm. Stretching across the pelvic cavity like a hammock, it is a triangular sheet of muscle and tendinous fibers, dorsal to the levator ani, arising from the spine of the ischium and from the sacrospinous ligament. It inserts into the coccyx and into the sacrum, is innervated by

branches of the pudendal plexus, which contain fibers from the fourth and the fifth sacral nerves, and it acts to draw the coccyx ventrally, helping to support the pelvic floor. Compare **levator ani.**

coccygodynia (kok'sɪgoudɪn'iə), a pain in the coccygeal area of the body.

coccyx (kok'sɪks), *pl.* **coccyges** (koksaɪ'jiz, kok'sɪjiz). the beaklike bone joined to the sacrum by a disc of fibrocartilage at the base of the vertebral column. It is formed by the union of three to five rudimentary vertebrae. The pieces of the coccyx fuse together in men at an earlier period in life than in women. In men and in women, the coccyx becomes fused with the sacrum by the sixth decade of life. The coccyx is freely movable on the sacrum during pregnancy. — **coccygeal** (koksɪj'iəl), *adj.*

cochineal (koch'ɪnil'), a red dye prepared from the dried female insects of the species *Coccus cacti* containing young larvae. During the preparation of the dye the larvae are extracted with an aqueous solution of alum, and the resulting dye is used in coloring medicines.

cochlea (kok'liə), a conical bony structure of the inner ear, perforated by numerous apertures for passage of the cochlear division of the acoustic nerve. Part of a complex tubular network called the osseous labyrinth, it is a spiral tunnel about 30 mm long with two full and three quarter turns, resembling a tiny snail shell. — **cochlear,** *adj.*

cochlear canal (kok'liər), a bony spiral tunnel within the cochlea of the internal ear. About 30 mm long, it narrows gradually in diameter as it rises to the apex of the cochlea. It contains one opening that communicates with the tympanic cavity, a second that connects with the vestibule, and a third that leads to a tiny canal opening on the inferior surface of the temporal bone.

cochlear duct. See **cochlear canal.**

cockscomb papilloma, a benign, small red lesion that may project from the uterine cervix during pregnancy; it regresses after delivery.

cocktail, *Informal.* an unofficial mixture of drugs, usually in solution, combined to achieve a specific purpose. See also **Brompton's cocktail.**

Coco-Diazine, a trade name for an antibacterial (sulfadiazine).

Coco-Quinine, a trade name for an antimalarial (quinine sulfate).

code, 1. (in law) a published body of statutes, as a civil code. 2. a collection of standards and rules of behavior, as a dress code. 3. a symbolic means of representing information for communication or transfer, as a genetic code. 4. a system of notation that allows information to be transmitted rapidly, as Morse code, or in secrecy, as a cryptographic code. 5. See also **no-code.** *Informal.* A discreet signal used to summon a special team to resuscitate a patient, as in "code zero, 3 west" announced over a public address system to bring the team to the west wing of the third floor without alarming patients or visitors.

codeine, a narcotic analgesic and antitussive.

- INDICATIONS: It is used to treat mild to moderate pain, to treat diarrhea, and as an antitussive.
- CONTRAINDICATION: Known hypersensitivity to this drug prohibits its use.
- ADVERSE EFFECTS: Among the most serious adverse reactions are constipation, nausea, drowsiness, and allergic reactions. High doses are associated with respiratory and circulatory depression. The drug is potentially addicting.

codeine phosphate, a narcotic analgesic and antitussive.

- INDICATIONS: It is prescribed to suppress cough and to relieve pain.
- CONTRAINDICATION: Known hypersensitivity to opiates is the only contraindication.
- ADVERSE EFFECTS: Among the more serious adverse reactions are depression of the central nervous system, paradoxical excitement, and drug dependence.

code team, a specially trained and equipped team of doctors, nurses, and technicians that is available to provide cardiopulmonary resuscitation when summoned by a code set by the institution. A code team usually includes a physician, registered nurse, respiratory therapist, and pharmacist. The members may work in any department or unit of the hospital. A schedule is made that ensures a full team on duty at all times.

cod liver oil, a pale-yellow, fatty oil extracted from the fresh livers of the codfish and other related species. It is a rich source of vitamins A and D, useful in the treatment of nutritional deficiency of those vitamins or of conditions owing to abnormal absorption of calcium and phosphorus. The oil must be stored in a cool, dark place or it becomes rancid. See also **osteomalacia, rickets, tetany.**

Codman's tumor. See **chondroblastoma.**

codominant, of or pertaining to the alleles or to the trait resulting from the full expression of both alleles of a pair in a heterozygote, as the AB or MN blood group antigens. — **codominance,** n.

codominant inheritance, the transmission of a trait or condition in which both alleles of a pair are given full expression in a heterozygote, as in the AB or MN blood group antigens and the leukocyte antigens.

codon (kou'don), a unit of three adjacent nucleotides along a DNA or messenger RNA molecule that designates a specific amino acid in the polypeptide chain during protein synthesis. Each codon consists of a specific section of the DNA molecule so that the order of the codons along the molecule determines the sequence of the amino acids in each protein. See also **genetic code.**

coefficient, a mathematical relationship between factors that can be used to measure or evaluate a characteristic under specified conditions. An example is the **oxygen util-**

ization **coefficient,** which measures the amount of oxygen in a patient's venous blood in terms of the proportion of oxygen in his arterial blood.

coel- 1. See **cel-.** 2. a combining form meaning 'pertaining to the colon': *colalgia, colauxe, colectasia.*

-coel. See **-cele**[2].

-coele. See **-cele**[2].

coelenteron, pl. **coelentera.** 1. See **archenteron.** 2. the digestive cavity of those animals having only two germ layers, as the hydra and jelly fish.

coelom, coeloma, coelome, celom, pl. **coeloms, coelomata.** the body cavity of the developing embryo. It is situated between the layers of mesoderm and in mammals gives rise to the pericardial, pleural, and peritoneal cavities. A kind of coelom is **extraembryonic coelom.** Also called **somatic cavity.** — **coelomic, celomic,** adj.

coelosomy, a congenital anomaly characterized by the protrusion of the viscera from the body cavity.

coenesthesia. See **cenesthesia.**

coenesthesis. See **cenesthesis.**

coenogenesis. See **cenogenesis.**

coenzyme (kouen'zaim), a nonprotein substance that combines with an apoenzyme to form a complete enzyme or holoenzyme. Coenzymes include some of the vitamins, as B_1 and B_2 and have smaller molecules than enzymes. Coenzymes are dialyzable and heat stable and usually dissociate easily from the protein portions of the enzymes with which they combine. See also **acetylcoenzyme-A.**

coffee, the dried and roasted ripe seeds of *Coffea arabica, C. liberica,* and *C. robusta* trees that may have originated in Africa but now grow in almost all tropical areas. Coffee contains the alkaloid caffeine and is the basis for a stimulating drink useful in treating the common headache, chronic asthma, and opium poisoning.

coffee-and . . . , (in psychiatric nursing) a method of treatment for chronically ill psychiatric outpatients. Patients meet on a regular schedule, with professional staff, in a quasi-social environment for mutual support and encouragement of the patients. Coffee and something to eat may be served.

coffee ground vomitus, dark brown vomitus the color and consistency of coffee grounds, composed of gastric juices and old blood and indicative of slow upper gastrointestinal bleeding. Compare **hematemesis.**

coffee worker's lung, a respiratory condition caused by an allergic reaction to the dust of the coffee bean. See also **organic dust.**

Cogentin, a trade name for an antiparkinsonian (benztropine mesylate).

cognition, the mental process characterized by knowing, thinking, learning, and judging. Compare **conation.** — **cognitive,** adj.

cognitive development, the developmental process by which an infant becomes an intelligent person, acquiring, with growth, knowledge and the ability to think, learn, reason, and abstract. Jean Piaget demonstrated the orderly sequence of this process from early infancy through childhood. See also **psychosexual development, psychosocial development.**

cognitive dissonance,   a state of tension resulting from a discrepancy in a person's emotional and intellectual frame of reference for interpreting and coping with his environment. It usually occurs when new information contradicts existing assumptions or knowledge.

cognitive function,   an intellectual process by which one becomes aware of, perceives, or comprehends ideas. It involves all aspects of perception, thinking, reasoning, and remembering. Compare **conation.**

cognitive learning,   learning that is concerned with acquisition of problem-solving abilities and with intelligence and conscious thought.

cognitive psychology,   the study of the development of thought, language, and intelligence in infants and children.

cognitive therapy,   any of the various methods of treating mental and emotional disorders that help a person change attitudes, perceptions, and patterns of thinking. Therapeutic approaches include behavior therapy, existential therapy, Gestalt therapy, and transactional analysis.

cogwheel rigidity,   an abnormal rigor in muscle tissue, characterized by jerky movements when the muscle is passively stretched. Some authorities believe cogwheel rigidity masks a muscular tremor that is not evident until the affected muscle is manipulated.

cohere,   to stick together, as similar molecules of a common substance. – **coherent,** *adj.*

coherence,   **1.** the property of sticking together, as the molecules within a common substance. **2.** (in psychology) the logical pattern of expression and thought evident in the speech of a normal, stable individual.

cohesive termini,   (in molecular genetics) the complementary single-stranded ends projecting from a double-stranded DNA segment that can be joined to introduced fragments. Also called **sticky ends.**

cohort,   (in statistics) a collection or sampling of individuals who share a common characteristic, as the same age or the same sex.

cohort study,   (in research) a study concerning a specific subpopulation, as the children born between December and May in 1975 and the children born in the same months in 1955. See also **prospective study.**

coil.   *Informal.* See **intrauterine device.**

coiled tubular gland,   one of the many multicellular glands that contain one coiled, tube-shaped secretory portion, as the sweat glands.

coil spring contraceptive diaphragm,   a kind of contraceptive diaphragm in which the flexible metal spring that forms the rim is a coiled, circular spring that is heavier than a flat spring but lighter than an arcing spring. The rubber dome of the diaphragm is approximately 1½ inches deep, and the diameter of the rubber covered rim is from 5½ to 10 cm. Ten sizes, in increments of 0.5 cm, allow the clinician to fit the diaphragm to the individual woman. The kind of spring and the size of the rim in millimeters is stamped on the rim, as, for example, 75 mm coil spring. This kind of diaphragm is prescribed for a woman whose vaginal musculature offers good support, whose uterus is not acutely retroflexed or anteflexed, and whose vagina, neither very long nor very short, has a deeper than usual arch behind the symphysis pubis. The coil spring diaphragm is lighter than an arcing spring and, if it is well fitted and conforms to the woman's vaginal contour, it is effective and comfortable to use. Compare **arcing spring contraceptive diaphragm, flat spring contraceptive diaphragm.** See also **contraceptive diaphragm fitting.**

coition (kouĭsh′ən).   See **coitus.**

coitus (kou′ĭtəs),   the sexual union of two people of opposite sex in which the penis is introduced into the vagina for copulation, typically resulting in mutual excitation, often orgasm. Also called **coition.** – **coital,** *adj.*

coitus interruptus.   See **withdrawal method.**

col-,   **1.** a combining form meaning 'pertaining to the colon': *colalgia, colauxe, colectasia.* **2.** See **co-.**

Colace,   a trade name for a stool softener (dioctyl sodium sulfosuccinate).

colation,   the act of filtering or straining, as urine is often strained for medical examination.

COL bed.   See **CircOlectric (COL) bed.**

ColBENEMID,   a trade name for a fixed-combination antigout drug containing a gout suppressant (colchicine) and a uricosuric (probenecid).

colchicine (kol′chəsin),   a gout suppressant.

■ INDICATIONS: It is prescribed in the treatment of acute gout and prophylaxis of recurrent gouty arthritis.

■ CONTRAINDICATIONS: Ulcer, ulcerative colitis, or known hypersensitivity to this drug prohibits its use. The drug is highly toxic and is not given to elderly, debilitated patients or to those people who have chronic renal, hepatic, cardiovascular, or gastrointestinal disease.

■ ADVERSE EFFECTS: Among the most serious adverse reactions are severe gastrointestinal distress including diarrhea with blood, bone marrow depression, peripheral neuritis, liver dysfunction, and alopecia.

cold,   **1.** the absence of heat. **2.** Also called **common cold.** a contagious viral infection of the upper respiratory tract, usually caused by a strain of rhinovirus. It is characterized by rhinitis, tearing, low-grade fever, and malaise and is treated symptomatically with rest, mild analgesia, decongestants, and an increased intake of fluids.

cold abscess, a site of infection that does not show common signs of heat, redness, and swelling.

cold agglutinin, a nonspecific antibody, found on the surface of red blood cells in certain diseases, that may cause clumping of the cells at temperatures below 4°C and may cause hemolysis. Mycoplasma pneumonia, infectious mononucleosis, and many lymphoproliferative disorders are associated with cold agglutinins.

cold bath, a bath in which the water temperature is approximately 10° to 18°C or 50° to 65°F, used primarily to reduce body temperature.

cold-blooded, unable to regulate body heat, as fishes, reptiles, and amphibians that have internal temperatures that are close to the temperatures of the environments in which they live. Also called **poikilothermic.** Compare **warm-blooded.**

cold cautery. See **cryocautery.**

cold hemoglobinuria. See **hemoglobinuria.**

cold injury, any of several abnormal and often serious physical conditions caused by exposure to cold temperatures. See also **chilblain, frostbite, hypothermia, immersion foot.**

cold pressor test, a test for the tendency to develop essential hypertension. One hand of the individual is immersed in ice-water for about 60 seconds. An excessive rise in the blood pressure or an unusual delay in the return of normal blood pressure when the hand is removed from the water is believed to indicate that the individual has a proclivity for hypertension.

cold-sensitive mutation, a genetic alteration resulting in a gene that functions at a high temperature and not at a low temperature.

cold sore. See **herpes simplex.**

colectomy (kəlek'təmi), surgical excision of part or all of the colon, performed to treat cancer of the colon or severe chronic ulcerative colitis. For several days before surgery, a low residue diet is prescribed. Antibiotics and cleansing enemas are given to reduce the number of bacteria in the bowel. Parenteral fluids and electrolytes are given, and a nasointestinal tube passed. Under general anesthesia the colon is removed. The nurse gives postoperative care as for any abdominal surgery. The nasointestinal tube is connected to suction and remains in place until bowel sounds are heard. See also **abdominal surgery.**

Colestid, a trade name for an antihyperlipoproteinemic (colestipol hydrochloride).

colestipol hydrochloride, an antihyperlipoproteinemic that acts by sequestering bile acids in the intestine, thus preventing the absorption of fats.

■ INDICATIONS: It is prescribed in the treatment of hypercholesterolemia and xanthoma.

■ CONTRAINDICATIONS: Biliary obstruction or known hypersensitivity to this drug prohibits its use.

■ ADVERSE EFFECTS: Among the more serious adverse reactions are skin rash, fecal impaction, and a deficiency of vitamins A, D, and K. Constipation may occur.

colic, 1. sharp visceral pain resulting from torsion, obstruction, or smooth-muscle spasm of a hollow or tubular organ, as a ureter or the intestines. Kinds of colic include **biliary colic, infantile colic, renal colic.** 2. of or pertaining to the colon. – **colicky,** *adj.*

colicinogen (kol'ısın'əjın), an episome in some strains of *Escherichia coli* that induces secretion of a colicin, a protein lethal to other strains of the bacterium. Specific colicins attach to specific receptors on the cell membrane and impair the synthesis of macromolecules or the production of energy. Also called **colicinogenic factor.**

coliform (kol'ıfɔrm), 1. of or pertaining to the colonaerogenes group, or the *Escherichia coli* species of microorganisms, constituting most of the intestinal flora in humans and other animals. 2. having the characteristic of a sieve or cribriform structure, as some of the porous bones of the skull.

colistimethate sodium, an antibacterial.

■ INDICATIONS: It is prescribed in the treatment of gastrointestinal infections caused by certain gram-negative microorganisms.

■ CONTRAINDICATIONS: Known hypersensitivity to this drug or to polymyxin B prohibits its use.

■ ADVERSE EFFECTS: Among the more serious adverse reactions are nephrotoxicity and neurotoxicity, including neuromuscular blockade.

colistin sulfate, an antibacterial.

■ INDICATIONS: It is prescribed topically in the treatment of infections of the outer ear, and systemically for serious gram negative infections.

■ CONTRAINDICATION: Known hypersensitivity to this drug prohibits its use.

■ ADVERSE EFFECTS: Among the more serious systemic reactions are respiratory arrest, renal toxicity, and neuromuscular blockade.

colitis, an inflammatory condition of the large intestine, either one of the episodic, functional, irritable bowel syndromes or one of the more serious chronic, progressive, inflammatory bowel diseases. Irritable bowel syndrome is characterized by bouts of colicky pain and diarrhea or constipation, often owing to emotional stress. Treatment includes stress reduction and adherence to a diet that may include bland foods and less roughage than in a usual diet. Because individuals with colitis may be irritated by different substances, the diet is individualized to avoid known irritants. Kinds of irritable bowel syndrome are **spastic colon, mucous colitis.** Inflammatory bowel disease is characterized by abcess formation, severe diarrhea, bleeding, and ulceration of the mucosa of the intestine. Weight loss and pain are significant. Steroids, fluids, electrolytes, antibiotics, and careful attention to diet are the usual modes of therapy. Most of the diseases of this group are of unknown etiology. Kinds of inflammatory bowel disease include **Crohn's disease, ulcerative colitis.** – **colitic,** *adj.*

collagen (kol′əjĭn), a substance consisting of bundles of tiny reticular fibrils, which combine to form the white glistening inelastic fibers of the tendons, the ligaments, and the fascia. – **collagenous,** *adj.*

collagen disease, any one of the various abnormal conditions characterized by extensive disruption of the connective tissue, as inflammation and fibrinoid degeneration. Some collagen diseases are polyarteritis nodosa, disseminated lupus erythematosus, rheumatic fever, rheumatoid coronary arteritis, and ankylosing spondylitis. Such disorders may also cause coronary problems which are often controlled with glucocorticoids.

collagenoblast (kəlæj′ənoublæst′), a cell that differentiates from a fibroblast and functions in the formation of collagen. It can also transform into cartilage and bone tissue by metaplasia.

collagenous fiber, any one of the tough, white fibers that constitute much of the intercellular substance and the connective tissue of the body. Collagenous fibers contain the protein collagen and are often arranged in bundles which strengthen the tissues in which they are imbedded.

collagen vascular disease, any of a group of acquired disorders which have in common diffuse immunologic and inflammatory changes in small blood vessels and connective tissue. The cause of most of these diseases is unknown. Hereditary factors and deficiencies, environmental antigens, infections, allergies, and antigen-antibody complexes in various combinations are probably involved. Common features of most of these entities include arthritis, skin lesions, iritis and episcleritis, pericarditis, pleuritis, subcutaneous nodules, myocarditis, vasculitis, and nephritis. Often associated also are Coombs test-positive hemolytic anemia, thrombocytopenia, leukopenia, B and T cell abnormalities, antinuclear antibodies, cryoglobulins, rheumatoid factors, false-positive serologic tests for syphilis, alterations in serum complement, and immunologic abnormalities. The diseases usually included in this category are mixed connective tissue disease, necrotizing vasculitis, polyarteritis nodosa, polymyositis, relapsing polychondritis, rheumatic fever, rheumatoid arthritis, scleroderma, Sjögren's syndrome, and systemic lupus erythematosus. Also called **connective tissue disease.**

collapse, 1. *Nontechnical.* a state of extreme depression or a condition of complete exhaustion owing to physical or to psychosomatic problems. 2. an abnormal condition characterized by shock. 3. the abnormal sagging of an organ or the obliteration of its cavity.

collar, any structure that encircles another, usually around its neck, as the periosteal bone collars that form around the diaphyses of young bones.

collarbone. See **clavicle.**

collateral, 1. secondary or accessory. 2. (in anatomy) a small branch, as any one of the arterioles or venules in the body.

collateral fissure, a fissure separating the subcalcarine and the subcollateral gyri of the cerebral hemisphere.

collecting tubule, any one of the many relatively large straight tubules of the kidney that funnel urine into the renal pelivis. The collecting tubules drain the urine from the distal convoluted tubules in the renal cortex and descend into the renal medulla before connecting with each other at various intervals along the path to the renal pelvis. The collecting tubules play an important role in maintaining the fluid balance of the body by allowing water to osmose through their membranes into the interstitial fluid in the renal medulla. Antidiuretic hormone in the blood makes the collecting tubules permeable to water. If no antidiuretic hormone is present in the blood, the membranes of the collecting tubules are practically impermeable to water. See also **Bowman's capsule, kidney.**

collective unconscious, (in analytic psychology) that portion of the unconscious common to all mankind. Also called **racial unconscious.** See also **analytic psychology.**

collector, (in medicine) a device with various modifications, used for collecting secretions from the bronchi and the esophagus for bacteriological and cytological examination.

college, 1. an organization of individuals with common professional training and interests, as the American College of Nurse-Midwives, the American College of Cardiology, or the American College of Surgeons. 2. an institution of higher learning.

Colles' fascia (kol′iz), the deep layer of the subcutaneous fascia of the perineum, constituting a distinctive structure in the urogenital region of the body. It is a strong, smooth sheet of tissue containing elastic fibers which give it a characteristic yellow tint. Ventrally, it is continuous with the deep layer of the subcutaneous abdominal fascia and fills a groove between the scrotum and the thigh or between the labium and the thigh; medially, it joins the superficial layer of the subcutaneous perineal fascia to form the dartos tunic of the scrotum or to form the thick fascial sheath of the labium; laterally, it firmly adheres to the ischiopubic ramus; and dorsally, it dips toward the ischiorectal fossa and attaches firmly to deep perineal fascia. In the anal region of the perineum Colles' fascia adheres to both the superficial layer and the deep layer of the subcutaneous fascia.

Colles' fracture (kol′iz), a fracture of the radius at the epiphysis within one inch of the joint of the wrist, easily recognized by the dorsal and lateral position of the hand that it causes.

colligative (kol′ɪgeɪ′tɪv), (in physical chemistry) of or pertaining to those properties of matter that depend on the number of particles, as molecules and ions, rather than the chemical properties of any substance. One such colligative property is the pressure of a specific volume of gas.

collimator, a device for limiting particles of radiation to parallel paths, used to restrict the beam of a radiotherapy machine to a specified area.

colliquation (kol′ɪkweɪ′zhən), the degeneration of a tissue of the body to a liquid state, usually associated with necrotic tissue.

colliquative (kol′ɪkweɪ′tɪv), characterized by the profuse discharge of fluid, as suppurating wounds and structures of the body that are infected.

collision tumor, a tumor formed as two separate growths, developing close to each other, join. See also **carcinoma.**

collodion (kəlou′diən), a clear or a slightly opaque, highly inflammable liquid composed of pyroxylin, ether, and alcohol. It dries to a strong, transparent film that is used as a surgical dressing.

collodion baby, an infant whose skin at birth is covered with a scaly, parchmentlike membrane. See also **harlequin fetus, lamellar exfoliation of the newborn.**

colloid (kol′oid), a state or division of matter in which large molecules or aggregates of molecules that do not precipitate and that measure between 1 and 100 nanometers are dispersed in another medium. In a suspension colloid the particles are insoluble and the medium may be solid, liquid, or gas. In an emulsion colloid, the particles are usually water and the medium is any of several complex hydrophilic, organic substances that become evenly dispersed among the particles of water. Compare **solution, suspension.**

colloid bath, a bath taken in water that contains such substances as bran, gelatin, and starch, used to relieve irritation and inflammation. See also **emollient bath.**

colloid carcinoma, a former term for mucinous carcinoma.

colloid chemistry, the science dealing with the composition and nature of chemical colloids.

colloid goiter, a greatly enlarged, soft thyroid gland in which the follicles are distended with colloid.

colo-, colon-, a combining form meaning 'pertaining to the colon': *colocolic, colodyspepsia, cololysis.*

coloboma (kol′əbou′mə), *pl.* **colobomas, colobomata.** a congenital or pathologic defect in the ocular tissue of the body, usually affecting the iris, ciliary body, or choroid by forming a cleft that extends inferiorly. Colobomas are usually the result of the failure of part of the fetal fissure to close. — **colobomatous,** *adj.*

-coloboma, a combining form meaning the 'absence or defect of an ocular tissue affecting function, especially of the iris': *blepharocoloboma, iridocoloboma, pseudocoloboma.*

colon, the portion of the large intestine extending from the cecum to the rectum. It has four segments: ascending colon, transverse colon, descending colon, and sigmoid colon. — **colonic,** *adj.*

colon-. See colo-.

-colon, a combining form meaning the 'part of the large intestine between the cecum and rectum': *cecocolon, megacolon, paracolon.*

-colonic, a combining form meaning 'relating to the colon': *pericolonic, rectocolonic, vesicocolonic.*

colonic fistula (kəlon′ɪk), an abnormal passage from the colon to the surface of the body or an internal organ or structure. In regional enteritis, chronic inflammation may lead to the formation of a fistula between two adjacent loops of bowel. An external opening from the colon to the surface of the abdomen may be created surgically following the removal of a malignant or severely ulcerated segment of the bowel.

colon stasis. See **atonia constipation.**

colony, **1.** (in bacteriology) a mass of microorganisms in a culture that originates from a single cell. Some kinds of colonies, according to different configurations, are smooth colonies, rough colonies, and dwarf colonies. **2.** (in cell biology) a mass of cells in a culture or in certain experimental tissues, as a spleen colony.

colony counter, a device used for counting colonies of bacteria growing in a culture and usually consisting of an illuminated, transparent plate that is divided into sections of known area. Petri dishes containing colonies of bacteria are placed over the plate and the colonies counted according to the number within the areas viewed.

-color, a combining form meaning 'hue or hues': *cuticolor, tricolor, versicolor.*

Colorado tick fever, a relatively mild, self-limited arbovirus infection transmitted to man by the bite of a tick. It is most prevalent in the spring and summer months throughout the Rocky Mountains, particularly in Colorado. Symptoms, occurring in two phases separated by a period of remission, include chills, fever, headache, pain in the eyes, legs, and back, and sensitivity to light. Treatment is supportive; analgesics can be given for headache and other pains. Also called **American mountain fever.** Compare **Rocky Mountain spotted fever.**

color blindness, an abnormal condition characterized by an inability to clearly distinguish colors of the spectrum. In most cases it is not a blindness but a weakness in perceiving them distinctly. There are two forms of color blindness. **Daltonism** is the most common form and is characterized by an inability to distinguish reds from greens. It is an inherited, sex-linked disorder. **Total color blindness,** or **achromatic vision,** is characterized by an inability to perceive any color at all. Only white, gray, and black are seen. It may be the result of a defect in or the absence of the cones in the retina.

color dysnomia (dısnou′miə), an inability to name colors despite an ability to match and distinguish them. It may be caused by expressive dysphasis.

colorectal cancer (kou′lərek′təl), a malignant neoplastic disease of the large intestine, characterized by melena, by a change in bowel habits, and by the passing of blood. Malignant tumors of the large bowel usually occur after the age of 50, are slightly more frequent in women than in men, and are almost as common as lung cancer in the United States. The high incidence of colorectal cancer in the western world, as contrasted with the low incidence in Japan and rural Africa, suggests that a diet high in refined carbohydrates and beef and low in roughage may be an etiologic factor. The risk of large bowel cancer is increased in chronic ulcerative colitis, diverticulosis, villous adenomas, and especially in familial polyposis of the colon. People who have inhaled asbestos fibers or who have been irradiated are more likely than others to develop colorectal cancer. In the vermiform appendix, carcinoid is the most common tumor. Most lesions of the large bowel are adenocarcinomas; one half arise in the rectum, one fifth in the sigmoid colon, approximately one sixth in the cecum and ascending colon, and the rest in other sites. Rectal tumors may cause pain, bleeding, and a feeling of incomplete evacuation; they may metastasize slowly through lymphatic channels and veins, and, occasionally, prolapse through the anus. Typical napkin ring tumors in the sigmoid and descending colon constrict the intestinal lumen, causing partial obstruction and the production of flat or pencil-shaped stools. Malignant lesions in the ascending colon are usually large growths that may be palpable on physical examination; they generally cause severe anemia, nausea, and alternating constipation and diarrhea. The diagnosis of colorectal cancer is based on digital rectal examination, testing for blood in the stool, proctosigmoidoscopic examination of the sigmoid, and x-ray studies of the gastrointestinal tract following a barium enema. Suspicious polyps may be removed for histologic study, often through a sigmoidoscope or colposcope or by a laparotomy. Surgical treatment of colorectal cancer may involve a wide resection of the lesion, the surrounding colon, and the attached tissues, with an end-to-end anastomosis of the remaining intestinal segments whenever possible. Tumors of the lower two thirds of the rectum usually require removal of the entire rectum by abdomino-perineal resection and the creation of a permanent colostomy. Transanal electric coagulation is currently being studied and tried in the treatment of certain rectal cancers. Irradiation may be administered preoperatively and postoperatively as palliative therapy for inoperable tumors or as the sole method of treating certain rectal cancers. Chemotherapy with 5-fluorouracil infused

intraluminally in the bowel at surgery and intravenously after surgery may be used as adjunctive treatment. Combinations of 5-fluorouracil, the nitrosourea CeeNU, and vincristine may offer palliation of the symptoms of the disease.

colorimetry (kəl′ərɪm′ɪtri), **1.** measurement of the intensity of color in a fluid or substance. See also **spectrophotometry. 2.** measurement of color in the blood by using of a colorimeter to determine hemoglobin concentration. The technique is useful only for gross screening purposes, as it is not exact and interpretation is subjective. **– colorimetric,** *adj.*

color index (C.I.), the ratio between the concentration of hemoglobin and the number of red blood cells in any given sample of blood. The color index is computed by dividing the concentration of hemoglobin, expressed as a percentage of normal concentration, by the approximate number of red blood cells, expressed as a percentage of a normal concentration of 5 million red cells per cubic millimeter. The average color index is about 0.85. Compare *Colour Index.*

color vision, a recognition of color as the result of changes in the pigments of the cones in the retina which react to varying intensities of red, green, and blue light. The exact mechanisms of color vision are not completely understood, but many experts believe they depend on three specialized types of cones, each type responding to red, green, or blue light. Some retinal cones respond to the entire visual spectrum.

colostomate (kəlos′təmeit), a person who has undergone a colostomy.

colostomy, surgical creation of an artificial anus on the abdominal wall by incising the colon and bringing it out to the surface, performed for cancer of the colon and benign obstructive tumors. A colostomy may be single-barreled, with one opening, or double-barreled, with distal and proximal loops open onto the abdomen. The latter is performed when the lower bowel is completely blocked or in paraplegia to simplify daily management. A temporary colostomy may be done to divert feces from an inflamed area; it is repaired when the inflammation subsides. Preoperative nursing care focuses on teaching the patient what to expect following surgery. A high-calorie, low-residue diet is given; an antibiotic, usually Neomycin, is prescribed to reduce the bacterial count in the bowel, and enemas are given until returns are clear. The surgery is done under general anesthesia. Immediate postoperative care is the same as for abdominal surgery. The color of the stoma is checked: a dark blue-black color (rather than bright red) indicates a circulation block, and the surgeon is notified. Saline irrigations are begun on the fourth or fifth day.

colostomy irrigation, a procedure used by colostomates to clear the bowel of fecal matter and to help establish an evacuation schedule.

■ METHOD: Daily irrigation may be ordered beginning seven to ten days following the operation, and the patient is involved in assisting in the procedure as soon as possible. In preparation for self-care, the technique is explained in a step-by-step manner and irrigation is carried out with the equipment the patient will use at home. In the hospital the procedure is performed as the patient sits in bed in a semi- or high-Fowler's position or on a commode, if ambulatory; at home the individual will probably find a toilet more convenient. A catheter, lubricated with petroleum jelly, is gently inserted in the stoma to a depth of about three inches; the catheter tip is advanced only as far as it will go easily and is never forced. If it is not accepted the stoma is usually dilated by gently inserting and rotating a gloved, lubricated finger approximating the size of the opening. An irrigating bag containing 500 to 1,000 ml of warm solution is held 12 to 18 inches above the stoma, and the fluid is allowed to flow slowly into the colon. If the patient complains of cramps, the catheter is clamped for a few minutes before the flow is resumed. The fluid is retained for several minutes and then drained through outlet tubing into a basin or commode. From 30 to 45 minutes is allowed for draining; if the return is slow the patient is asked to lean forward or move from side to side; the abdomen may be massaged. The character and amount of the return flow is noted. A dehydrated patient may retain some fluid.

■ NURSING ORDERS: The nurse performs and teaches colostomy irrigation, ensures that the patient knows how to carry out the procedure correctly and where to purchase the necessary equipment. The person is urged to report any symptoms of obstruction or prolapse of the stoma. A public health nurse is available in many areas for home visits if help is needed.

■ OUTCOME CRITERIA: Many colostomates establish a regular schedule of evacuation with irrigation, but the procedure may be unsatisfactory for patients with a liquid or semisoft fecal stream, for patients who, prior to the operation, had a tendency to develop diarrhea under stress, or for patients with irregular bowel habits.

colostrum (kəlos′trəm), the fluid secreted by the breast during pregnancy and the first days postpartum before lactation begins, consisting of immunologically active substances and white blood cells, water, protein, fat, and carbohydrate in a thin, yellow, serous fluid.

Colour Index (C.I.), a publication of dyers, colorists, and textile chemists that specifies all the standard industrial pigments and stains according to five-digit numbers associated with chemical coloring materials, as methylene blue is assigned number 52015. Compare **color index.**

colpo-, colp-, a combining form meaning 'pertaining to the vagina': *colpocele, colpocystitis, colpodynia.* Also **kolpo-, kysth, kystho-.**

colpohysterectomy, vaginal hysterectomy. See **hysterectomy.**

columbium, former name for **niobium.**

column chromatography, the process of separating and analyzing a group of substances according to the differences in their absorption affinities for a given absorbent as evidenced by pigments deposited during filtration through the same absorbent contained in a glass cylinder or tube. The substances are dissolved in a liquid which is passed through the absorbent. The absorbates move down the column at different rates and leave behind a band of pigments which is subsequently washed with a pure solvent to "develop" discrete pigmented bands that constitute a chromatograph. The cylinder of absorbent is then pushed from the tube, and the individual bands are either separated with a knife or further diluted with the pure solvent and collected in the bottom of the tube for analysis. Effective column chromatography depends on the selection of the appropriate absorbent and solvent and a flow rate that is slow enough to allow complete diffusion of the absorbates from the solvent to the absorbent and the retardation of the absorbates according to their different affinities for the absorbent. Compare **gas chromatography, ion-exchange chromatography.**

Coly-Mycin M, a trade name for an antibacterial (colistimethate sodium).

Coly-Mycin S, a trade name for an antibacterial (colistin sulfate).

com-. See **co-.**

coma, a state of profound unconsciousness, characterized by the absence of spontaneous eye movements, response to painful stimuli, and vocalization. The person cannot be aroused. Coma may be the result of trauma, space-occupying brain tumor, hematoma, toxic condition, acute infectious disease with encephalitis, vascular disease, poisoning, or intoxication.

-coma, 1. a combining form meaning '(condition of) profound unconsciousness': *narcoma, semicoma.* 2. a combining form meaning '(condition of) torpor': *agrypnocoma.*

combat fatigue, any of a variety of psychoneurotic mental disorders, usually temporary but sometimes leading to permanent neurosis, resulting from exhaustion, the stress of combat, or the cumulative emotions and psychological strain of warfare or similar situations. It is characterized by anxiety, depression, irritability, memory and sleep disorders, and various related symptoms. Also called **combat neurosis, war neurosis.** See also **post-traumatic stress disorder, shell shock.**

combat neurosis. See **combat fatigue.**

Combid, a trade name for a gastrointestinal fixed-combination drug containing an anticholinergic (isopropamide iodide) and a phenothiazine antipsychotic (prochlorper-azine).

combined anesthesia. See **balanced anesthesia.**

combined system disease, a disorder of the nervous system caused by a deficiency of vitamin B_{12} that results in pernicious anemia and degeneration of the spinal cord and peripheral nerves, marked by increased difficulty in walking, a feeling of vibration in the legs, and a loss of sense of position. Also known as **subacute combined degeneration of the spinal cord.** See also **pernicious anemia, vitamin B_{12}.**

combining form, a component of a word, usually derived from Latin or Greek, that is the base or main stem of the word. It is usually found in combination with a root, prefix, suffix, or all three, as in the words *arthralgia, encephalitis, hepatomegaly,* and *oliguria,* the combining forms are *arthr-, -algia, en-, -cephal-, -itis, hepato-, -megaly, olig-,* and *-uria.*

comedo (kom′ɪdou), *pl.* **comedones** (komɪdou′niz). blackhead, the basic lesion of acne vulgaris, caused by an accumulation of keratin and sebum within the opening of a hair follicle. It is dark owing to the effect of oxygen on sebum, not to the presence of dirt.

comedocarcinoma (kom′ɪdoukar′sɪnou′mə), *pl.* **comedo-carcinomas, comedocarcinomata.** a malignant intraductal neoplasm of the breast, in which the central cells degenerate and may be easily expressed from the cut surface of the tumor. As the growth is confined in the mammary ducts, the prognosis is better than in cases of invasive breast lesions.

comfort, alteration in: pain, a nursing diagnosis accepted by the Fourth National Conference on the Classification of Nursing Diagnoses. The etiology of the condition includes injury by biological, chemical, physical, or psychological agents. The defining characteristic is the verbal or nonverbal communication by the client of the presence of pain, including behavior that is self-protective; a narrowed focus that is indicated by an altered time perception, withdrawal from social contact, or impaired thought processes; distraction behavior, marked by moaning, crying, pacing, restlessness, or the seeking out of other people or activities; a facial mask of pain, recognized by eyes that appear dull and lusterless, a 'beaten' look, fixed or scattered facial movements, or grimace; alteration in muscle tone, ranging from listlessness to rigidity; and autonomic responses to increasing pain, including diaphoresis, changes in the blood pressure and pulse rate, pupillary dilatation, and an increased or decreased rate of respiration. See also **nursing diagnosis.**

comfort measure, any action taken to promote comfort of the patient, as a back rub, a change in position, or the prewarming of a stethoscope or a bedpan.

-comma, a combining form meaning a 'piece of a structure': *inocomma, myocomma, osteocomma.*

command automatism, a condition characterized by an abnormal responsiveness to commands, usually followed without critical judgment, as may be seen in hypnosis and various mental states. See also **automatism.**

commensal (kəmen′səl), (of two different organisms) living together in an arrangement that is not harmful to either and may be beneficial to both. Some bacteria in the digestive tract of humans aid in the processing of food and produce B vitamins needed for normal health while causing no harm. Compare **parasite, synergist.**

comminuted fracture, a fracture in which there are several breaks in the bone, creating two or more fragments.

commissurotomy (kom′ɪʃʊrot′əmi), the surgical division of a fibrous band or ring connecting corresponding parts of a body structure. A commissurotomy is commonly performed to separate the thickened, adherent leaves of a stenosed mitral valve.

commitment, 1. See also **institutionalize.** the placement or confinement of an individual in a specialized hospital or other institutional facility. 2. See also **certification.** the legal procedure of admitting a mentally ill person to an institution for psychiatric treatment. The process varies from state to state but usually involves judicial or court action based on medical evidence certifying that the person is mentally ill. 3. a pledge or contract to fulfill some obligation or agreement, used especially in some forms of psychotherapy or marriage counseling.

common bile duct, the duct formed by the juncture of the cystic duct and hepatic duct.

common carotid plexus, a network of nerves on the common carotid artery, supplying sympathetic fibers to the head and the neck, with branches that accompany the cranial blood vessels. The common carotid plexus is formed by the internal and external carotid plexuses and by the cervical ganglia of the sympathetic system. Compare **external carotid plexus, internal carotid plexus.**

common cold. See **cold.**

common hepatic artery, the visceral branch of the celiac trunk of the abdominal aorta, passing to the pyloris and dividing into five branches, the gastroduodenal, right gastric, right hepatic, left hepatic, and middle hepatic.

common iliac artery, a division of the abdominal aorta, starting to the left of the fourth lumbar vertebra, passing caudally about 5 cm, and dividing into external and internal iliac arteries. The right common iliac artery is somewhat longer than the left.

common iliac node, a node in one of the seven groups of parietal lymph nodes serving the abdomen and the pelvis. The nodes are arranged in clusters of about five nodes lying along the dorsal aspect of the common iliac artery. They drain the internal and the external iliac nodes and pass their efferents to the lateral aortic nodes. Compare **external iliac node, internal iliac node, iliac cir-**

cumflex node. See also **lymph, lymphatic system, lymph node.**

common iliac vein, one of the two veins that are the sources of the inferior vena cava, formed by the union of the internal and the external iliac veins, ventral to the sacroiliac articulation. The right common iliac vein runs almost vertically, ascends dorsal and lateral to its corresponding artery, and is shorter than the left common iliac vein. The left common iliac vein ascends more obliquely, at first to the medial side of the corresponding artery and then dorsal to the right common iliac vein. Each common iliac vein receives the iliolumbar and, in some individuals, the lateral sacral veins. The left common iliac vein also receives the middle sacral vein. Neither of the common iliacs contains valves. Compare **external iliac vein, internal iliac vein.**

communicable, contagious; transmissible by direct or indirect means, as a communicable disease.

communicable disease, any disease transmitted from one person or animal to another directly, by contact with excreta or other discharges from the body, or indirectly, via substances or inanimate objects, as contaminated drinking glasses, toys, or water, or via vectors, as flies, mosquitoes, ticks, or other insects. To control a communicable disease it is important to identify the organism, prevent its spread to the environment, protect others against contamination, and treat the infected person. Many communicable diseases, by law, must be reported to the health department. Kinds of communicable diseases include those caused by bacteria, chlamydia, fungi, parasites, rickettsiae, and viruses. Also called **contagious disease.** See also **infectious disease.**

Communicable Disease Center, former name of the Center for Disease Control.

communicating hydrocephalus. See **hydrocephalus.**

communication, any process in which a message containing information is transferred, especially from one person to another, via any of a number of media. Communication may be verbal or nonverbal; it may occur directly, as in a face-to-face conversation or with the observation of a gesture; or it may occur remotely, spanning space and time, as in writing and reading or in making or playing back a recording. Communication is basic to all nursing and contributes to the development of all therapeutic relationships.

communication channels, (in communication theory) any gesture, action, sound, written word, or visual image used in transmitting messages.

communication, impaired verbal, a nursing diagnosis accepted by the Fourth National Conference on the Classification of Nursing Diagnoses. The etiology of the condition includes decreased circulation to the brain; a physical barrier to speech, as a brain tumor, laryngectomy, tracheostomy, or intubation; an anatomical deficit, as a cleft palate; a psychological barrier, as a psychosis or lack of stimuli; a cultural difference; or a developmental or age-related factor. The defining characteristics of the condition include slurring, stuttering, difficulty in forming words or sentences, difficulty in expressing thoughts verbally, inappropriate verbalization, dyspnea, or disorientation. The critical defining characteristics, one of which must be present for the diagnosis to be made, are an inability to speak the dominant language of the culture, a difficulty in speaking or verbalizing, or the absence of speech. See also **nursing diagnosis.**

communication theory, a theory that describes a model of a system of communication consisting of a source of information (the sender), a transmitter, a communication channel, a source of noise (interference), a receiver, and a purpose for the message.

community health nursing, a field of nursing that is a blend of primary health care and nursing practice with public health nursing. The community health nurse conducts a continuing and comprehensive practice that is preventive, curative, and rehabilitative. The philosophy of care is based on the belief that care directed to the individual, the family, and the group contributes to the health care of the population as a whole. The community health nurse is not restricted to the care of a particular age or diagnostic group. Participation of all consumers of health care is encouraged in the development of community activities which contribute to the promotion, education, and maintenance of good health. These activities require comprehensive health programs that pay special attention to social and ecological influences and specific populations at risk.

community medicine, a branch of medicine that is concerned with the health of the members of a community, municipality, or region. The emphasis in community medicine is on the early diagnosis of disease, the recognition of environmental and occupational hazards to good health, and the prevention of disease in the community.

community mental health center (CMHC), a community-based center that provides comprehensive mental health services, including ambulatory and inpatient care. The specific services to be provided are specified in an act of Congress, the Community Mental Health Centers Act; these requirements have been updated periodically. The costs of consultation and educational services, instruction, development, and initial operation of the facility are provided by the federal government. The organization, management, and operation of CMHCs are specified by the Act. Consumer representation in each of these areas is required.

community nurse practitioner (CNP), a nurse who has completed a post-baccalaureate program in community nursing.

community psychiatry, the branch of psychiatry concerned with the development of an adequate and coordinated program of mental health care for residents of specified catchment areas. See also **community mental health center.**

companionship, (in psychiatric nursing) the assignment of a staff member or of another patient to stay with a disturbed patient to provide support and to protect the patient from self-harm or the harming of others. In constant companionship, the disturbed patient is accompanied in all activities until the companion is convinced the patient has regained control.

comparative anatomy, the study of the morphology and function of all living animals. A comparison of the forms indicates a progression on a scale from the simplest to the most highly specialized animals. The adult stage of animals that are lower in the scale resembles the immature stages of many animals that are higher in the scale. See also **applied anatomy, ontogeny, phylogeny.**

comparative embryology, the study of the similarities and differences among various organisms during the embryologic period of development.

comparative psychology, 1. the study of human behavior as it relates to or differs from animal behavior. 2. the study of the psychological and behavioral differences among various peoples.

compatibility, 1. the quality or state of existing together in harmony; congruity. 2. the orderly, efficient integration of the elements of one system with those of another. 3. the formation of a stable chemical or biochemical system, specifically in medication, so that two or more drugs can be administered at the same time without producing undesired side effects or without canceling or changing the therapeutic effects of the others. 4. (in immunology) the degree to which the body's defense system will tolerate the presence of foreign material, as transfused blood, grafted tissue, or transplanted organs, without an immune reaction; usually complete compatibility exists between identical twins. 5. (in blood grouping or crossmatching) the lack of reaction between blood groups so that there is no agglutination when the red blood cells of one sample are mixed with the serum of another sample; no reaction from transfused blood. — **compatible,** *adj.*

Compazine, a trade name for a phenothiazine (prochlorperazine), used as an antiemetic and antipsychotic.

compendium (kəmpen′diəm), *pl.* **compendia.** a collected body of information on the standards of strength, purity, and quality of drugs. The official compendia in the United States are the *United States Pharmacopoeia,* the *Homeopathic Pharmacopoeia of the United States,* the *National Formulary,* and their supplements. See also **formulary.**

compensated gluteal gait, one of the more common abnormal gaits associated with a weakness of the gluteus medius. It is a variation of the Trendelenburg gait and involves the dropping of the pelvis on the unaffected side of the body during the walking cycle between the moment of heelstrike on the affected side and the moment of heelstrike on the unaffected side. The compensated gluteal gait is also characterized by the dropping of the entire trunk downward and sideways over the affected hip and a short step on the unaffected side. In a compensated gait the trunk is forcibly thrown laterally during the weight-bearing or stance phase in the movement of the affected lower limb. This lateral movement is the result of an attempt to shift a significant portion of body weight above and outside the center of rotation of the affected hip. During this movement the erector spinae and the quadratus lumborum of the involved side function to lift the whole weight of the pelvis and the opposite lower extremity off the ground to allow the uninvolved leg to clear during its swing phase.

compensated heart failure, an abnormal cardiac condition in which heart failure is compensated for by normal compensatory mechanisms, as increased sympathetic adrenergic stimulation of the heart, fluid retention with increased venous return, increased end-diastolic ventricular volume and fiber length, and hypertrophy. Compensation may also occur through the administration of digitalis glycosides, with associated improved myocardial function, or by diuresis. However, diuretics may relieve only the symptoms of pulmonary and peripheral congestion and merely appear to compensate for the ventricular function, which remains severely abnormal.

compensating current, an electric current that neutralizes the intensity of a muscle current.

compensation, a complex defense mechanism that allows one to avoid the unpleasant or painful emotional stimuli that result from a feeling of inferiority or inadequacy. This is accomplished by any of several patterns of behavior, for example, one in which an extraordinary effort is spent in overcoming a handicap, one in which the quality lacking is scorned ("sour grapes"), one in which hard work and excellent performance in one field are substituted for a lack of ability in another, or one in which a fantasy of excellence, achievement, or perfection replaces awareness of a weakness or failure. See also **overcompensation.**

compensation neurosis, an unconscious process by which one prolongs the symptoms resulting from an injury or disease in order to receive secondary gains, especially money. Compare **malingering.**

competence, (in embryology) the total capacity of an embryonic cell to react to determinative stimuli in various ways of differentiation. A kind of competence is **embryonic competence.** See also **potency.**

competitive antagonist. See **antimetabolite.**

competitive identification, the unconscious modeling of one's personality on that of another as a means of outdoing or bettering the other person. See also **identification.**

complaint, 1. (in law) a pleading by a plaintiff made under oath to initiate a suit. It is a statement of the formal charge and the cause for action against the defendant. For a minor offense, the defendant is tried on the basis of the complaint. A more serious felony prosecution requires an indictment with evidence presented by a state's attorney. **2.** *Informal.* any ailment, problem, or symptom identified by the client, patient, member of the person's family, or other knowledgeable person. The chief complaint is often the reason that the person has sought health care.

complement, one of eleven complex, enzymatic, serum proteins. In an antigen-antibody reaction, complement causes lysis. Complement is also involved in other physiological reactions including anaphylaxis and phagocytosis. See also **antibody, antigen, antigen-antibody reaction, immune globulin.**

complement abnormality, an unusual condition characterized by deficiencies or by dysfunctions of any of the nine functional components of the enzymatic proteins of blood serum. The components are labeled C1 through C9. Intensive research currently seeks to determine the relationship between complement abnormalities or deficiencies and numerous disorders, and, theoretically, any of the nine complement components may be lacking. The most common abnormalities are C2 and C3 deficiencies and C5 familial dysfunction. Patients with complement deficiencies or with complement dysfunctions may be more susceptible to infections and to collagen vascular diseases. Some patients with lupus erythematosus or dermatomyositis have displayed complement abnormalities. Studies indicate that primary complement deficiencies may be inherited. Secondary complementary deficiencies may stem from immunologic reactions, as drug-induced serum disease, which depletes complement. Complement deficiencies may be associated with other illnesses, as acute streptococcal glomerulonephritis and acute systemic lupus erythematosus.

■ OBSERVATIONS: Increased susceptibility to systemic bacterial infection is associated with C2 and C3 deficiencies and with C5 familial dysfunction. Chronic renal failure and lupus erythematosus may also be associated with C2 deficiency. Signs of C5 dysfunction are malaise, diarrhea, and seborrheic dermatitis. It is difficult and often expensive to diagnose complement abnormalities, but some indications are EKG conduction abnormalities, detection of complement and immunoglobulin in the walls of blood vessels in glomerulonephritis, cerebrospinal fluid pleocytosis, increased erythrocyte sedimentation rate, and the presence in urine of RBCs, RBC casts, and protein.

■ INTERVENTION: Replacement of complement-fixing antibodies and the control of infection and associated illnesses are part of the standard treatment of complement abnormalities. The patient with complement deficiency or dysfunction commonly receives transfusions of fresh plasma to replace antibodies. Bone marrow transplants and injections of gamma globulin may also be employed, but bone marrow transplant carries the risk of a fatal graft-versus-host reaction. Complement abnormalities may usually be temporarily corrected by replacement therapy, but no permanent cure is yet available.

■ NURSING CONSIDERATIONS: Authorities recommend careful monitoring of patients with complement abnormalities, especially patients who receive gamma globulin injections. The gamma globulin is injected into a large muscle mass and massaged well after each injection. More than one site is usually selected if the dosage is more than 1.5 ml. If frequent doses are ordered, the injection sites are rotated. With plasma infusions, careful matching of leukocytes for HL-A cell types is important to prevent graft-versus-host reaction and other undesirable responses. Bone marrow transplants require close monitoring for transfusion reactions and are usually followed by instructions to the patient for scrupulous hygiene, prompt treatment of the smallest wound, and avoidance of crowds or persons with active infections. Renal infections require meticulous monitoring of intake and output, tests for serum electrolytes and acid-base balance, and observation for symptoms of renal failure. Neurologic damage resulting from infection is cause for special alertness to detect early signs of ataxia or slight changes in mental activity.

complemental inheritance, the acquisition or expression of a trait or condition from the presence of two independent pairs of nonallelic genes. Both of the genes must be present for the characteristic to appear in the phenotype.

complementary gene, either member of two or more nonallelic gene pairs that interact to produce an effect not expressed in the absence of any of the pairs. Also called **reciprocal gene.**

complement fixation, an immunologic reaction in which an antigen combines with an antibody and its complement, causing the complement factor to become inactive or "fixed." The complement fixation reaction can be tested in the laboratory by exposing the patient's serum to antigen, complement, and specially sensitized red blood cells. Complement fixation tests are widely used to detect antibodies for infectious diseases, especially syphilis and viral illnesses. See also **complement, immune system, immunity, Wassermann test.**

complement-fixation test (C-F test), any serological test in which complement-fixation is detected, indicating the presence of a particular antigen. Specific C-F tests are used to aid in the diagnosis of amebiasis, Rocky Mountain spotted fever, trypanosomiasis, and typhus. The Wasserman test is a C-F test for syphilis.

complete abortion, termination of pregnancy in which the conceptus is expelled or removed in its entirety. Because no products of conception remain in the uterus, surgical evacuation is not necessary. Compare **incomplete abortion.**

complete blood count (CBC), a determination of the number of red and white blood cells per cubic millimeter of blood. A complete blood count is one of the most routinely performed tests in a clinical laboratory and one of the most valuable screening and diagnostic techniques. The count can be performed manually by staining a smear of blood on a slide and counting the different types of cells under a microscope. Most laboratories use an electronic counter for reporting numbers of red and white blood cells. Platelets are more difficult to count automatically, and many laboratories continue to do this manually. Examining a stained slide of blood yields useful information about red cell morphology. Each type of white cell can be represented as a percentage of the total number of white cells observed. This is called a differential count. Many electronic blood counters also automatically determine hemoglobin or hematocrit and include this value in the complete blood count. Also see **differential white blood cell count, erythrocyte morphology, hematocrit, hemoglobin.**

complete breech, a fetal presentation in which the nates present with the legs folded on the thighs and the thighs on the abdomen. The position of the fetus is the same as in a normal vertex presentation, but upside down.

complete fistula, an abnormal passage from an internal organ or structure to the surface of the body or to another internal organ or structure.

complete fracture, a bone break that completely disrupts the continuity of osseous tissue across the entire width of the bone involved.

complete health history, a health history that includes a history of the present illness, a health history, social history, occupational history, sexual history, and a family health history. See also **health history.**

complete rachischisis, a rare congenital fissure of the entire vertebral column and spinal cord, resulting from the failure of the embryonic neural tube to close. The condition is characterized by flaccid paralysis and impaired sensations. It is often accompanied by other birth defects, as cleft palate, hare-lip, and hydrocephalus, and is frequently fatal. Also called **rachischisis totalis, holorachischisis.** See also **spina bifida.**

complex, 1. a group of items, as chemical molecules, that are related in structure or function, as the iron and protein portions of hemoglobin or the cobalt and protein portions of vitamin B_{12}. 2. a combination of signs and symptoms of disease that forms a syndrome. 3. (in psychology) a group of associated ideas with strong emotional overtones affecting a person's attitudes.

complex fracture, a closed fracture in which the soft tissue surrounding the bone is severely damaged.

complex protein, a protein that contains a simple protein and at least one molecule of another substance, as a glycoprotein, nucleoprotein, or hemoglobin.

compliance, fulfillment by the patient of the care-giver's prescribed course of treatment.

component, a significant part of a larger unit.

component drip set, a device used for delivering intravenous fluids, especially whole blood. It includes plastic tubing and a combination drip-chamber and filter. Compare **component syringe set, microaggregate recipient set, straight-line blood set, Y-set.**

component syringe set, a device used for delivering intravenous fluids. It includes plastic tubing, two slide clamps, a Y-connector and a syringe. The component syringe set may be used in various procedures, as in the transfusion of platelets and in the transfusion of cryoprecipitates. In such transfusions the component syringe set is used primarily to avoid clogging the intravenous line. Compare **component drip set, microaggregate recipient set, straight-line blood set, Y-set.**

component therapy, a kind of transfusion in which specific blood components are administered instead of whole blood. Packed red cells or platelet-rich plasma suspensions may be transfused in larger quantities than would be possible if whole blood were used. More sophisticated processing provides fibrinogen or antihemophilic globulin solutions for administration in therapeutic amounts in excess of what might be given with conventional blood transfusion therapy. Compare **plasmaphoresis.** See also **packed cells, pooled plasma.**

compound, 1. (in chemistry) a substance composed of two or more different elements, chemically combined in definite proportions, that cannot be separated by physical means. 2. any substance composed of two or more different ingredients. 3. To make a substance by combining ingredients, as a pharmaceutical. 4. denoting an injury characterized by multiple factors, as a compound fracture.

compound aneurysm, a localized dilatation of an arterial wall in which some of the layers are distended and others are ruptured or dissected. Also called **mixed aneurysm.**

compound fracture, a fracture in which the broken end or ends of the bone have torn through the skin. Also called **open fracture.**

compound melanocytoma. See **benign juvenile melanoma.**

compound monster, a fetus in which some of the parts or organs are duplicated but not fully developed.

compound tubuloalveolar gland, one of the many multicellular glands with more than one secretory duct that contains both tube-shaped and sac-shaped portions, as the salivary glands.

comprehensive care. See **holistic health care.**

compress, a soft pad, usually made of cloth, used to apply heat, cold, or medications to the surface of a body area. A compress also may be applied over a wound to help control bleeding. Compare **dressing.**

compression, the act of pressing, squeezing, or otherwise applying pressure to an organ, tissue, or body area. An intracranial tumor or hemorrhage may cause compression of brain tissue. Kinds of pathological compression include **compression fracture,** in which bone surfaces are forced against each other, causing a break, and **compression paralysis,** marked by paralysis of a body area due to pressure on a nerve.

compression fracture, a bone break, especially in a short bone, that disrupts osseous tissue and collapses the affected bone. The bodies of vertebrae are often sites of compression fractures.

compression neuropathy, any of several disorders involving damage to sensory nerve roots or peripheral nerves, caused by mechanical pressure or localized trauma and characterized by paresthesia, weakness, or paralysis. The carpal, peroneal, radial, and ulnar nerves are most commonly involved. Compare **neuritis.** See also **paresthesia, pressure palsy.**

compressor naris, the transverse part of the nasalis muscle that serves to depress the cartilage of the nose and to draw the ala toward the septum. Compare **dilatator naris.**

compromised host, a person who is less than normally able to resist infection, owing to immunosuppressive therapy, immunologic defect, severe anemia, or concurrent disease or condition, including metastatic malignancy, cachexia, or severe malnutrition.

compulsion, an irresistible, repetitive, irrational impulse to perform an act that is usually contrary to one's ordinary judgments or standards yet results in overt anxiety if it is not completed. The impulse is usually the result of an obsession. A kind of compulsion is **repetition compulsion.** See also **obsession.** – **compulsive,** *adj.*

compulsive idea, a recurring, irrational idea that persists in the mind, usually resulting in an irresistible urge to perform some inappropriate act. Also called **imperative idea.**

compulsive personality, a type of character structure in which there is a pattern of chronic and obsessive adherence to rigid standards of conduct. The person is usually excessively conscientious and inhibited, is extremely inflexible, has an extraordinary capacity for work, and lacks a normal ability to relax and to relate to other people. The compulsive person is likely to follow repetitive patterns of behavior, as snapping the fingers, crossing the legs, tapping the foot, or refusing to walk on cracks in the sidewalk and often leads an impoverished emotional life, being dominated by a need for order, cleanliness, punctuality, rules, and systems. See also **compulsive personality disorder, obsessive-compulsive neurosis.**

compulsive personality disorder, a condition in which an irrational preoccupation with order, rules, ritual, and detail interferes with everyday functioning and normal behavior. The disorder is characterized by an excessive devotion to work, a pathological adherence to a definite set of rules or system of behavior, and a persistent, compulsive following of specific rituals. The person cannot make decisions when faced with unexpected situations and cannot take pleasure in the normal activities of daily life. Psychotherapy is the usual treatment and may include behavior therapy with desensitization and flooding in order to reduce maladaptive anxiety. See also **compulsive personality, obsessive-compulsive neurosis.**

compulsive polydipsia, a neurotic, compelling urge to drink excessive amounts of liquid. The condition is psychogenic; it is not caused by any organic dysfunction or physical deprivation. Extreme cases can result in death from water intoxication and electrolyte imbalance. See also **polydipsia.**

compulsive ritual, a series of acts a person feels must be carried out even though he recognizes the behavior to be useless and inappropriate. Failure to complete the acts results in extreme tension or anxiety. See also **obsessive-compulsive neurosis.**

computerized axial tomography (CAT), (in radiology) a technique in which an EMI scanner, comprising an x-ray tube, two scintillation detectors, a line printer, teletyper, and a computer and magnetic disc unit, is used to attain a series of detailed visualizations of the tissues of brain at any depth desired. The procedure is painless, noninvasive, and requires no special preparation. The head is scanned in two planes simultaneously at various angles. The computer calculates tissue absorption, displays a printout of the numerical values and produces a visualization of the tissues that demonstrates the densities of the various intracranial structures. Tumor masses, infarctions, bone displacement, and accumulations of fluid may be detected. Also called **computerized transverse axial tomography.**

con-. See **co-.**

CONA, abbreviation for **Canadian Orthopedic Nurses' Association.**

conation (kounei'shən), the mental process characterized by desire, impulse, volition, and striving. Compare **cognition.** – **conative,** *adj.*

concentrate, 1. to decrease the bulk of a liquid and increase its strength per unit of volume by the removal of inactive ingredients through evaporation or other means.

2. a substance, particularly a liquid, that has been strengthened and reduced in volume through such means.

concentric, describing two or more circles that share a common center.

concentric fibroma, a fibrous tumor surrounding the uterine cavity.

concept, a construct or abstract idea or thought that originates and is held within the mind. – **conceptual,** *adj.*

conception, **1.** the beginning of pregnancy, usually taken to be the instant that a spermatozoon enters an ovum. **2.** the act or process of fertilization. **3.** the act or process of creating an idea or notion. **4.** the idea or notion created; a general impression resulting from the interpretation of a symbol or set of symbols.

conception control. See **contraception.**

conceptive, **1.** able to become pregnant. **2.** pertaining to or characteristic of the mental process of forming ideas or impressions.

conceptual framework, a group of concepts that are broadly defined and systematically organized to provide a focus, a rationale, and a tool for the integration and interpretation of information. Usually expressed abstractly using word models, a conceptual framework is the basis for many theories, as communication theory and general systems theory.

conceptus (kənsep′təs), the products of conception; the fertilized ovum and its enclosing membranes at all stages of intrauterine development, from the time of implantation to birth. See also **embryo, fetus.**

concordance, (in genetics) the expression of one or more specific traits in both members of a pair of twins. Compare **discordance.** – **concordant,** *adj.*

concrete thinking, a stage in the development of the cognitive thought processes in the child. During this phase thought becomes increasingly logical and coherent so that the child is able to classify, sort, order, and organize facts but is incapable of generalizing or dealing in abstractions. Problem solving is accomplished in a concrete, systematic fashion based on what is perceived, keeping to the literal meaning of words, as the word 'horse' applying to a particular animal and not to horses in general. In Piaget's classification, this stage occurs between 7 and 11 years of age, is preceded by syncretic thinking, and is followed by abstract thinking.

concurrent nursing audit. See **nursing audit.**

concurrent validity, validity of a test or a measurement tool that is established by concurrently applying a previously validated tool or test to the same phenomena, or data base, and comparing the results. Concurrent validity is achieved if the results are the same or similar at a statistically significant level. See also **validity.**

concussion, **1.** a violent jarring or shaking, as caused by a blow or an explosion. **2.** *Informal.* **brain concussion.**

condensed milk, a thick liquid prepared by the evaporation of half of the water content of cow's milk and the addition of sugar. The final product contains 40 to 50 per cent sugar and is used to prepare desserts and confectionery.

condition, **1.** a state of being, specifically in reference to physical and mental health or well-being. **2.** anything that is essential for or that restricts or modifies the appearance or occurrence of something else. **3.** to train the body or mind, usually through specific exercises and repeated exposure to a particular state or thing. **4.** (in psychology) to subject a person or animal to conditioning or associative learning so that a specific stimulus will always elicit a particular response. See also **classical conditioning.**

conditioned avoidance response, a learned reaction that is performed either consciously or unconsciously in order to avoid an unpleasant or painful stimulus or to prevent such stimuli from occurring.

conditioned escape response, a learned reaction that is performed either consciously or unconsciously in order to stop or to escape from an aversive stimulus.

conditioned reflex, a reflex developed gradually by training in association with a specific, repeated external stimulus. An example of a conditioned reflex is Pavlov's experiment in which a dog salivates at the ringing of a bell if over a period of time every feeding is preceded by the bell-ringing stimulus.

conditioned response, an automatic reaction to a stimulus that does not normally elicit such response but which has been learned through training. Such responses can be physical or psychological and are produced by repeated association of some physiological function or behavioral pattern with an unrelated stimulus or event. In Pavlov's classic experiments, dogs learned to associate the ringing of a bell with feeding time so that they would salivate at the sound of the bell regardless of whether or not food was given to them. Also called **acquired reflex, behavior reflex, conditioned reflex, trained reflex.** Compare **unconditioned response.** See also **classical conditioning.**

conditioning, a form of learning based on the development of a response or set of responses to a stimulus or series of stimuli. Kinds of conditioning are **classical conditioning, instrumental conditioning, operant conditioning.**

condom, a soft, flexible sheath that covers the penis and prevents semen from entering the vagina in sexual intercourse, used to avoid infection and as a contraceptive. Condoms are made of plastic, rubber, or skin. Also called **prophylactic,** *Informal.* **rubber.**

conduction (kəndək′shən), **1.** (in physics) **a.** a process in which heat is transferred from one substance to another owing to a difference in temperature **b.** a process in which energy is transmitted through a conductor. **2.** (in physiology) the process by which a nerve impulse is transmitted.

conduction anesthesia, a loss of sensation, especially pain, in a region of the body, produced by injecting a local anesthetic along the course of a nerve or nerves to inhibit the conduction of impulses to and from the area supplied by that nerve or nerves. Also called **block anesthesia, nerve block anesthesia.**

conduction aphasia, a dissociative speech phenomenon in which there is no difficulty in comprehending words seen or heard and in which there is no dysarthria, yet the patient has problems in self expression. The patient may substitute words similar in sound or meaning to the correct ones, but is unable to repeat from dictation, to spell, and to read aloud. The patient is alert and aware of the deficit. A common cause is an embolus in a branch of the middle cerebral artery. The nurse should try to reduce tension and frustration in the patient, encourage socialization, find the best means of communication for the patient, use simple language and direct questions requiring simple answers, and help the family to understand the problem and deal with it. See also **aphasia.**

conductive hearing loss, a form of hearing loss in which sound is inadequately conducted through the external or middle ear to the sensorineural apparatus of the inner ear. Sensitivity to sound is diminished, but clarity (interpretation of the sound) is not changed. If volume is increased to compensate for the loss, hearing is normal. Compare **sensorineural hearing loss.**

condylar fracture, any fracture of the round end of a hinge joint, usually occurring at the distal end of the humerus or at the distal end of the femur, frequently detaching a small bone fragment that includes the condyle.

condyle (kon′dāil), a rounded projection at the end of a bone that anchors muscle ligaments and articulates with adjacent bones.

-condyle, a combining form meaning a 'knucklelike projection on a bone': *entepicondyle, epicondyle, entocondyle.* Also **-condylus.**

condyloid joint, a synovial joint in which a condyle is received into an elliptical cavity, as the wrist joint. A condyloid joint permits no axial rotation but allows flexion, extension, adduction, abduction, and circumduction. Also called **articulatio ellipsoidea.** Compare **pivot joint.**

condyloma (kon′dīlou′mə), *pl.* **condylomata.** a wartlike growth on the anus, vulva, or glans penis.

condyloma latum, *pl.* **condylomata lata.** a flat, moist, papular growth that appears in secondary syphilis in the coronal sulcus of the perineum or on the glans penis.

condylomatum acuminatum, a soft, wartlike or papillomatous growth common on the warm and moist skin and mucous membrane of the genitalia. It is caused by a virus and is transmitted by sexual contact. Also called **acuminate wart, venereal wart.**

-condylus. See **-condyle.**

cone, 1. a photoreceptor cell in the retina of the eye that enables a person to visualize colors. There are three kinds of retinal cones, one for each of the colors, blue, green, and red; other colors are seen by stimulation of more than one type of cone. 2. **cone of light,** a triangular reflection observed during an ear examination when the light of an otoscope is focused on the image of the malleus. 3. a cone-shaped device attached to radiological equipment to focus x rays on a small target of tissue. See also **cone biopsy.** — **conic, conical,** *adj.*

cone biopsy, surgical removal of a cone-shaped segment of cervix, including both epithelial and endocervical tissue. General anesthesia is used. The cone of tissue is excised and examined microscopically to establish a precise diagnosis, usually to confirm or evaluate a positive Papanicolaou test. Postoperatively, hemorrhage sometimes occurs. If bleeding occurs 7 to 10 days later, suturing is required. See also **biopsy, cone.**

cone of light, 1. See **cone** def. 2. 2. the group of light rays entering the pupil of the eye and forming an image on the retina.

confabulation, the fabrication of experiences or situations, often recounted in a detailed and plausible way in order to fill in and cover up gaps in the memory. The phenomenon occurs principally as a defense mechanism and is most commonly seen in alcoholics, especially those who have Korsakoff's psychosis. Also called **fabrication.**

configurationism (konfig′yurei′Shəniz′əm). See **Gestalt psychology.**

confinement, 1. a state of being held or restrained within a specific place in order to hinder or minimize activity. 2. the final phase of pregnancy during which labor and childbirth occur; parturition. See also **puerperium.**

conflict, 1. a mental struggle, either conscious or unconscious, resulting from the simultaneous presence of opposing or incompatible thoughts, ideas, goals, or emotional forces, like impulses, desires, or drives. 2. a painful state of consciousness caused by the arousal of such opposing forces and the inability to resolve them; a kind of stress found to a certain degree in every person. 3. (in psychoanalysis) the unconscious emotional struggle between the demands of the id and those of the ego and superego or between the demands of the ego and the restrictions imposed by society. Kinds of conflict include **approach-approach conflict, approach-avoidance conflict, avoidance-avoidance conflict, extrapsychic conflict, intrapsychic conflict.**

confluence of the sinuses (kon′fluəns), the wide junction of the superior sagittal, the straight, and the occipital sinuses with the two large transverese sinuses of the dura mater. The right tranverse sinus ususlly receives most of the blood from the superior sagittal sinus, and the left transverse sinus receives the blood from the straight sinus. The confluence is one of six posterior superior sinuses of the dura matter, draining blood from the section and an inner bulging granular section.

confusion, a mental state characterized by disorientation regarding time, place, or person, causing bewilderment, perplexity, lack of orderly thought, and inability to choose or act decisively. It is usually symptomatic of an organic mental disorder, but it may accompany severe emotional stress and various psychological disorders. – **confusional,** *adj.*

confusional insanity. See **amentia.** See **Stearn's alcoholic amentia.**

congenital, present at birth, as a congenital anomaly or defect.

congenital absence of sacrum and lumbar vertebrae, an abnormal condition present at birth and characterized by varying degrees of deformity, ranging from the absence of the lower segment of the coccyx to the absence of the entire sacrum and all lumbar vertebrae. Congenital absence of the sacrum and the lumbar vertebrae is relatively rare. Lesser degrees of this anomaly may present so few signs that marked deformities are not present, and the condition may not be diagnosed unless accidentally found on radiographic examination. More severe forms display gross deformities and neurologic deficits. Signs and symptoms of the more severe kinds may include short stature, flattened buttocks, muscle paralysis to varying degrees, muscle atrophy in the lower extremities, foot deformities, contractures of the hips and the knees, and varying degrees of loss of sensation, especially sensation distal to the knees. The treatment varies greatly for the congenital absence of the sacrum and the lumbar vertebrae and depends on severity. Surgical intervention may be reconstructive or may involve disarticulation procedures at various spinal levels and subsequent fusion of the remaining vertebrae. Depending on the severity, many patients with this anomaly may be surgically provided with enough stability to sit and to walk with assistance. The most severe forms are usually fatal.

congenital adrenal hyperplasia. See **adrenogenital syndrome.**

congenital amputation, the absence of a fetal limb or part at birth, previously attributed to amputation by constricting bands in utero but now regarded as a developmental defect.

congenital anomaly, any abnormality present at birth, particularly a structural one, which may be inherited genetically, acquired during gestation, or inflicted during parturition. Also called **birth defect.**

congenital cardiac anomaly, any structural or functional abnormality or defect of the heart or great vessels existing from birth. Congenital heart disease is a major cause of neonatal distress and is the most common cause of death in the newborn other than problems related to prematurity. The incidence of congenital cardiovascular

anomalies is 8 to 10 per 1,000 live births, with the mortality rate greatest in the neonatal period. Approximately 90 per cent of all deaths from congenital heart disease occur during the first year of life. Congenital heart defects may result from genetic causes, primarily single gene mutations and chromosomal aberrations, or from environmental factors, as maternal infection or exposure to radiation or noxious substances during pregnancy. Most defects are probably owing to some interaction between genetic and environmental factors that results in arrested embryonic development. Congenital heart anomalies are classified broadly according to the resulting alteration in circulation as acyanotic, in which no unoxygenated blood mixes in the systemic system, or cyanotic, in which unoxygenated blood enters the systemic system. The general effects of cardiac malformations on cardiovascular functioning are increased cardiac workload, involving either systolic or diastolic overloading, increased pulmonary vascular resistance, inadequate systemic cardiac output, and decreased oxygen saturation from the shunting of unoxygenated blood directly into the systemic system. The general physical symptoms of these pathophysiological alterations are growth retardation, decreased exercise tolerance, recurrent respiratory infections, dyspnea, tachypnea, tachycardia, cyanosis, tissue hypoxia, and murmurs, all of which vary in severity depending on the type and degree of the defect. Kinds of congenital cardiac anomalies include **aortic stenosis, atrial septal defect, coarctation of the aorta, patent ductus arteriosus, pulmonic stenosis, tetralogy of Fallot, transposition of the great vessels, tricuspid atresia, truncus arteriosus, ventricular septal defect.**

(See next page for illustration)

congenital cloaca. See **persistent cloaca.**

congenital condition, a physical or mental defect existing in a person at birth owing to heredity, environmental influence during pregnancy, or an effect induced during labor. Kinds of congenital conditions include **Down's syndrome, hydrocephalus.** Compare **genetic.** See also **birth defect.**

congenital dermal sinus, a channel present at birth, extending from the surface of the body and passing between the bodies of two adjacent lumbar vertebrae to the spinal canal.

congenital dislocation of the hip, a congenital orthopedic defect in which the head of the femur does not articulate with the acetabulum, owing to an abnormal shallowness of the acetabulum. Treatment consists of maintaining continuous abduction of the thigh so that the head of the femur presses into the center of the shallow cavity causing it to deepen. Also called **congenital dysplasia of the hip, congenital subluxation of the hip.** See also **Frejka splint.**

congenital dysplasia of the hip. See **congenital dislocation of the hip.**

congenital glaucoma, a rare form of glaucoma affecting infants and young children, resulting from a congenital closure of the iridocorneal angle by a membrane that obstructs the flow of aqueous humor and increases the intraorbital pressure. The condition is progressive, usually bilateral, and may damage the optic nerve. It may be corrected surgically. Also called **buphthalmos, hydrophthalmos.**

congenital goiter, an enlargement of the thyroid gland at birth or caused by a congenital deficiency of enzymes required for the production of thyroxine.

congenital heart disease. See **congenital cardiac anomaly.**

congenital hypoplastic anemia. See **Diamond-Blackfan syndrome.**

congenital megacolon. See **Hirschsprung's disease.**

congenital nonspherocytic hemolytic anemia, a large group of blood disorders made up of a number of similar inherited diseases, each with a deficiency of one of the enzymes of red cell glycolysis. Most are associated with varying degrees of hemolysis but all are less severe and are to be differentiated from the more serious disorder associated with spherocytosis. Compare **spherocytic anemia.** See also **sickle cell anemia.**

congenital polycystic disease (CPD). See **polycystic kidney disease.**

congenital pulmonary arteriovenous fistula, a direct connection between the arterial and venous systems of the lung present at birth that results in a right-to-left shunt and permits unoxygenated blood to enter systemic circulation. The anomaly is probably caused by faulty development of the network of vessels covering the embryonic lungs and is often accompanied by hereditary hemorrhagic telangiectasis (Rendu-Osler-Weber disease). The fistula may be single or multiple and may occur in any

Normal

Coarctation of aorta
(aortic lumen is narrowed)

Patent ductus arteriosus
(blood tends to bypass lungs)

Atrial septal defect
(oxygenated and unoxygenated blood mix)

Ventral septal defect
(blood passes from left
to right ventricle)

Tetralogy of Fallot
(1) Narrowing of pulmonary artery
or valve, (2) ventricular septal
defect, (3) overriding aorta,
(4) hypertrophied right ventricle

COMMON CONGENITAL CARDIAC ANOMALIES

part of the lung; if it is in an accessible site, surgical correction is the only effective method of treatment.

congenital scoliosis, an abnormal condition present at birth, characterized by a lateral curvature of the spine, resulting from specific congenital rib and vertebral anomalies. The etiological and the pathological characteristics of congenital scoliosis are divided into six categories. Category I is associated with partial unilateral failure of the formation of a vertebra. Category II is associated with complete unilateral failure of the formation of a vertebra. Category III is associated with bilateral failure of segmentation with the absence of disc space. Category IV is associated with the unilateral failure of segmentation with the unsegmented bar. Category V is associated with the fusion of ribs. Category VI is associated with any condition not covered in the other categories. Category IV scoliosis seems to progress more rapidly and cause the greatest degree of deformity. The degree of obvious deformity caused by congenital scoliosis depends on the cause of the disease. The deformity increases with growth and age, usually progressing slowly during periods of slow growth of the trunk of the body. Diagnosis of the specific congenital anomaly may be confirmed by radiographic examination. The specific rate of progression of many congenital curvatures cannot be predicted. There may be little correlation between the rate of progression and the severity of the curvature at the time of diagnosis. Treatment of congenital scoliosis may be surgical or nonsurgical. Some kinds of nonsurgical treatment techniques are exercise programs and the use of orthotic devices, as scoliosis splints, a Milwaukee brace, a Risser localizer, or a turnbuckle cast. Surgical intervention in this disease may involve an anterior or a posterior spinal fusion. In a few individuals with this disease, additional surgical procedures, as spinal osteotomy or halo traction, may be required.

congenital short neck syndrome, a rare congenital malformation of the cervical spine in which the cervical vertebrae are fused, usually in pairs, into one mass of bone, resulting in decreased neck motion and decreased cervical length, sometimes with neurologic involvement. The posterior portion of the laminar arches in the cervical area is not fully developed, resulting in spina bifida in the cervical region, usually involving the lower cervical vertebrae and, in some cases, one or more of the upper thoracic vertebrae. Congenital short neck syndrome is often associated with a cervical rib or with hemivertebrae. Neurologic complications, as nerve root compression and peripheral nerve symptoms, are secondary to deformities of the vertebral bodies. The extreme shortness of the neck is the most common sign of this deformity, which allows only limited motion, lateral bending, and rotation. When the deformity involves nerve root compression, symptoms of peripheral nerve involvement, as pain or a burning

sensation, may be evident, accompanied by paralysis, hyperesthesia, or paresthesia. Involvement of the spinal cord may present signs of abnormalities of lower extremities with associated signs of an upper motor lesion. Congenital short neck syndrome may require no treatment. Mild associated symptoms may be alleviated with traction, cast application, or cervical collars. Surgery may be required to relieve neurologic manifestations. Also called **Klippel-Feil syndrome.**

congenital subluxation of the hip. See **congenital dislocation of the hip.**

congestion, abnormal accumulation of fluid in an organ or body area. The fluid is usually blood, but it may be bile or mucus.

congestive atelectasis, severe pulmonary congestion characterized by diffuse injury to alveolar-capillary membranes, resulting in hemorrhagic edema, stiffness of the lungs, difficult ventilation, and respiratory failure. Fulminating sepsis, especially when gram-negative organisms are involved, is the most common cause, but congestive atelectasis may occur following trauma, near drowning, aspiration of gastric acid, paraquat ingestion, inhalation of corrosive chemicals, as chlorine, ammonia, or phosgene, or the use of certain drugs, including barbiturates, chlordiazepoxide, heroin, methadone, propoxyphene, and salicylates. This serious pulmonary disorder may also be caused by diabetic ketoacidosis, fungal infections, high altitudes, pancreatitis, tuberculosis, and uremia. Management of congestive atelectasis consists of treatment of the underlying cause, frequent changes of the patient's position to promote drainage, careful dehydration, assistance with ventilation, and the use of bronchodilators and steroids. Also called **adult respiratory distress syndrome, hemorrhagic lung, pump lung, stiff lung, wet lung.**

congestive heart failure (CHF), an abnormal condition characterized by circulatory congestion caused by cardiac disorders, especially myocardial infarction of the ventricles. This condition usually develops chronically in association with the retention of sodium and water by the kidneys. Humoral agents which significantly affect such retention include renin, angiotensin, aldosterone, vasopressin, estrogen, and norepinephrine. Acute congestive heart failure may develop following myocardial infarction of the left ventricle and cause a significant shift of blood from the systemic to the pulmonary circulation before the typical retention of sodium and water occurs. Pulmonary congestion in this situation may be caused by mechanical obstruction at the left mitral valve or by ventricular failure, impairing the ventilatory function of the lungs. Ischemia also may affect the respiratory muscles, producing chest pains difficult to distinguish from the pains of myocardial infarction. Common symptoms of congestive heart failure include dyspnea, high venous pressure, prolonged circulation time, peripheral edema, and decreased vital capacity. Confirming diagnosis of congestive heart failure often depends on distinguishing this condition from the congested systemic state associated with rapid infusions, severe anemia, and chronic renal insufficiency. Such distinction is often made on the basis of cardiac catheterization, which, in the case of congestive heart failure, reveals an insufficient rise in cardiac output during exercise and a significant rise in cardiac output after the administration of digitalis. Treatment of this condition includes prolonged rest and the administration of oxygen, digitalis, and diuretics.

Congolian red fever. See **murine typhus.**

-conia, a combining form meaning 'small particles in the (specified) fluid or part of the body': *chondroconia, otoconia, statoconia.*

conical papilla. See **papilla.**

conjoined manipulation, the use of both hands in obstetric and gynecological procedures, with one positioned in the vagina, and the other on the abdomen.

conjoined tendon. See **inguinal falx.**

conjoined twins, two fetuses developed from the same ovum who are physically united at birth. The defect ranges from a superficial anatomical union of varying extent between equally or nearly equally formed fetuses to one in which only a part of the body is duplicated or in which a small, incompletely developed fetus, or parasite, is attached to a more fully formed one, the autosite. Conjoined twins result when separation of the blastomeres in early embryonic development does not occur until a late cleavage phase and is incomplete, causing the fused condition. Viability depends on the extent of the fusion and the degree of development of the fetuses. See also **Siamese twins.**

conjugated estrogen, a mixture of sodium salts of estrogen sulfates, chiefly those of estrone, equilin, and 17-alpha-dihydroequilin, blended to approximate the average composition of estrogenic substances in the urine of pregnant mares. Conjugated estrogens may be prescribed to relieve postmenopausal vasomotor symptoms, as hot flushes, for the treatment of atrophic vaginitis, female hypogonadism, and primary ovarian failure, and for palliation in advanced prostatic carcinoma and metastatic breast cancer in selected patients. The drug, in conjunction with other therapeutic measures, may also retard the progress of postmenopausal osteoporosis. Continued use of estrogens increases the risk of endometrial carcinoma, gall-bladder disease, and thromboembolic disorders; because of the danger of damage to the fetus, all female sex hormones are contraindicated during pregnancy. Among the adverse effects of conjugated estrogens are breakthrough bleeding, breast tenderness, nausea, headache, water retention, and acneiform skin eruptions.

conjugated protein, a compound that contains a protein molecule united to a nonprotein substance.

conjugation (kon'jʊgei'shən), (in genetics) a form of sexual reproduction in unicellular organisms in which the gametes temporarily fuse so that genetic material can transfer from the donor male to the recipient female, where it is incorporated, recombined, and then passed on to the progeny through replication.

conjugon (kon'jʊgon), an episome that induces bacterial conjugation.

conjunctiva (kon'jəngktai'və), the mucous membrane lining the inner surfaces of the eyelids and anterior part of the sclera. The **palpebral conjunctiva** lines the inner surface of the eyelids and is thick, opaque, and highly vascular. The **bulbar conjunctiva** is loosely connected, thin, and transparent, covering the sclera of the anterior third of the eye.

conjunctival edema. See **chemosis.**

conjunctival reflex, a protective mechanism for the eye in which the eyelids close whenever the conjunctiva is touched. Compare **corneal reflex.**

conjunctival test, a procedure used to identify offending allergens by instilling the eye with a dilute solution of the allergenic extract. A positive reaction in the allergic patient causes tearing and redness of the conjunctiva within 5 to 15 minutes. See also **allergy testing.**

conjunctivitis (kənjəngk'tɪvai'tɪs), inflammation of the conjunctiva, caused by bacterial or viral infection, allergy, or environmental factors. Red eyes, a thick discharge, sticky eyelids in the morning, and inflammation without pain are characteristic. The cause may be found by microscopic examination or bacteriologic culture of a specimen of the discharge. Choice of treatment depends on the causative agent and may include antibacterial agents, antibiotics, or corticosteroids. See also **choroiditis, uveitis.**

CONJUNCTIVITIS

connecting fibrocartilage, a disc of fibrocartilage found between many joints, especially those with limited mobility, as the spinal vertebrae. Each disc is composed of concentric rings of fibrous tissue separated by cartilaginous laminae. The disc swells outward if it is compressed by the vertebrae above or below. Compare **circumferential fibrocartilage, interarticular fibrocartilage, stratiform fibrocartilage.**

connective tissue, tissue that supports and binds other body tissue and parts. It derives from the mesoderm of the embryo and is dense, containing large numbers of cells and large amounts of intercellular material. The intercellular material is composed of fibers in a matrix or ground substance which may be liquid, gelatinous, or solid, as in bone and cartilage. Connective tissue fibers may be collagenous or elastic. The matrix or ground material surrounding fibers and cells is not composed of living material, as protoplasm, but is nonetheless a dynamic substance, varying with the general condition of the body, susceptible to its own special diseases, and transporting materials for metabolism, nutrition, and waste elimination. The most common cell in connective tissue is the histiocyte or microphage. Mast cells, plasma cells, and white blood cells are also found in connective tissue throughout different parts of the body. Red blood cells are not usually found in connective tissue unless blood vessels have been injured. Kinds of connective tissue are **bone, cartilage, fibrous connective tissue.**

connective tissue disease. See **collagen vascular disease.**

Conn's syndrome (konz), a disorder of the adrenal cortex, owing to an adenoma – often unilateral – or, rarely, to adrenal carcinoma or hyperplasia. The resultant hypersecretion of aldosterone may cause hypernatremia, hypervolemia, and hypokalemic alkalosis, with weakness, parathesias, tetany, and transient paralysis.

Conor's disease. See **Marseilles fever.**

Conradi's disease (konra′diz). See **chondrodystrophia calcificans congenita.**

conscience, 1. the moral, self-critical sense of what is right and wrong. 2. (in psychoanalysis) the superego.

conscious, 1. (in neurology) capable of responding to sensory stimuli; awake, alert; aware of one's external environment. 2. (in psychiatry) that part of the psyche or mental functioning in which thoughts, ideas, emotions, and other mental content are in complete awareness. Compare **preconscious, unconscious.**

conscious sedation. See **awake anesthesia.**

consecutive angiitis, an inflammatory condition of blood or lymph vessels resulting from a similar process in surrounding tissues.

consensual light reflex, a normally present crossed reflex in which light directed at one eye causes the opposite pupil to contract. See also **light reflex.**

consensual reaction to light, the constriction of the pupil of one eye when the other eye is illuminated. Stimulation of either optic nerve causes constriction of both pupils. In monocular blindness the pupil of the blind eye reacts consensually with stimulation of the seeing eye but does not cause constriction of the pupil of either eye. Compare **direct reaction to light.**

consensus sequence, (in molecular genetics) a sequence in a strand of RNA nucleotides that is used as a site for the insertion of a splice of an RNA sequence from another source into the segment.

conservation of energy, (in physics) a law stating that

in any closed system the total amount of energy is constant.

conservation of matter, (in physics) a law stating that matter can neither be created nor destroyed and that the amount of matter in the universe is finite. Also called **conservation of mass.** See also **conservation of energy.**

conservation principles of nursing, a conceptual framework for nursing that is directed toward maintaining the wholeness or integrity of the patient when the normal ability to cope is disturbed or exceeded by stress. Nursing intervention is determined by the patient's need to conserve energy and to maintain structural, personal, and social integrity. The patient is perceived as a person whose wholeness is threatened by stress. Subjective and objective indicators of stress are assessed by the nurse, the stimuli for the stress are identified, and the level of integrity in each area is evaluated. The nurse acts as a 'conservationist.'

conservative treatment. See **treatment.**

consolidation, 1. the combining of separate parts into a single whole. 2. a state of solidification. 3. (in medicine) the process of becoming solid, as when the lungs become firm and inelastic in pneumonia.

constipation, difficulty in passing stools or an incomplete or infrequent passage of hard stools. There are many causes, both organic and functional. Among the organic causes are intestinal obstruction, diverticulitis, and tumors. Functional impairment of the colon may occur in elderly or bedridden patients who fail to respond to the urge to defecate. For constipation that is not organically caused, the nurse can encourage a liberal diet of fruits, vegetables, and plenty of water. The patient should be encouraged to exercise moderately, if possible, and to develop regular, unhurried bowel habits. See also **atonia constipation.** – **constipated,** *adj.*

constitutional psychology, the study of the relationship of individual psychological makeup to body morphology and organic functioning.

constitutional symptom. See **symptom.**

constriction ring, a band of contracted uterine muscle that forms a stricture around part of the fetus during labor, usually following premature rupture of the membranes and sometimes impeding labor. The uterine wall is thickened in the zone of the ring and is not prone to rupture. Compare **pathologic retraction ring.**

constructional apraxia, a form of apraxia characterized by the inability to copy drawings or to manipulate objects to form patterns or designs.

constructive aggression, an act of self-assertiveness in response to a threatening action for purposes of self-protection and preservation. See also **aggression.**

construct validity, validity of a test or a measurement tool that is established by demonstrating its ability to identify the variables that it proposes to identify. See also **validity.**

consumption, *Obsolete.* tuberculosis.

contact, 1. the touching or bringing together of two surfaces, as those of upper and lower teeth; often used attributively, as in contact dermatitis and contact lens. **2.** the bringing together either directly or indirectly, as through the handling of food or clothing, of two individuals so as to allow the transmission of an infectious organism from one to the other. **3.** a person who has been exposed to an infectious disease.

contact dermatitis, skin rash resulting from exposure to a primary irritant or to a sensitizing antigen. In the first, or nonallergic, type, a primary irritant, as an alkaline detergent or an acid, causes a lesion similar to a thermal burn. Emergency treatment is to drench liberally and immediately with water. In the second, or allergic type, sensitizing antigens, on first exposure, result in an immunologic change in certain lymphocytes. Subsequent exposure to the antigen causes the lymphocytes to release irritating chemicals leading to inflammation, edema, and vesiculation. Poison ivy and nickel dermatitis are common examples of this delayed hypersensitivity reaction. The diagnosis can be aided by patch testing with suspected antigens. Treatment includes avoidance of the irritant or sensitizer, topical corticosteroid preparations, and soothing or drying lotions. In severe cases, systemic corticosteroids may be used. Also called **dermatitis venenata.** Compare **atopic dermatitis.** See also **delayed hypersensitivity.**

contact factor. See **factor XII.**

contact lens, a small, curved, glass or plastic lens shaped to fit the person's eye and to correct refraction. Contact lenses float on the precorneal tear film and must be inserted, removed, cleaned, and stored as directed to avoid damage or infection to the eyes.

contagious, communicable, as a disease that may be transmitted by direct or indirect contact. — **contagion,** *n.*

contagious disease. See **communicable disease.**

content validity, validity of a test or a measurement owing to the use of previously tested items or concepts within the tool. See also **validity.**

context, (in communications theory) the setting, meaning, and language of a message. If a message is interpreted (decoded) without strict regard for these limits, it will be taken out of context.

continent ileostomy, an ileostomy that drains into a surgically created pouch or reservoir in the abdomen. Involuntary discharge of intestinal contents is prevented by a nipple valve created from the ileum.

■ METHOD: After surgery, the pouch is kept relatively empty by means of a catheter placed in it at surgery. It is removed a week or two afterward, depending on the status of intestinal function and wound healing. Once the indwelling catheter is removed, the pouch is drained by periodically inserting a catheter through the stoma into the pouch through the valve. The length of time allowed to elapse between catheterizations is gradually lengthened as the capacity of the pouch increases to between 500 and 1000 ml. Six months after surgery, drainage may be necessary only three or four times a day. The patient learns to recognize a feeling of fullness that indicates the need for drainage. When the patient is seated on the toilet, the dressing over the stoma is removed, and the tip of a French size 28 to 32 catheter is lubricated and inserted into the stoma. The distal end of the catheter is in a receptacle or in the toilet, at least 30 cm below the stoma. The lubricated tip of the catheter is advanced carefully through the stoma. Resistance is usually felt at a depth of about 5 cm where the valve covers the opening to the pouch. Flow usually begins when the tip of the catheter has passed the valve, at a distance of approximately 7.5 cm from the stoma. Drainage may take up to 15 minutes to complete.

■ OUTCOME CRITERIA: The patient may expect to be able to care for the stoma and to manage the drainage of the pouch before discharge from the hospital. A continent ileostomy has several advantages, including the avoidance of unpleasant odors, and the convenience of not having to use a colostomy or ileostomy bag.

■ NURSING ORDERS: After surgery the patient is usually instructed to add foods one at a time. High-fiber foods and those that cause gas formation are particularily likely to be problematic. Thick secretions may be thinned by the injection of a little water into the pouch through the catheter. The stoma may be covered with a three-inch square cut from a disposable diaper. It is important to teach the patient to avoid irritation of the skin around the stoma. Nonallergenic tape may be used to hold the pad in place. After healing, if there is no danger of a blow to the abdomen, a pad is often not necessary. After surgery, activity is resumed as the patient is able. There is no reason for activity to be curtailed once healing is complete and the person feels well.

contingency contracting, a formal agreement between a psychotherapist and a patient undergoing behavior therapy regarding the consequences of certain actions by both parties.

contingency management, any of a group of techniques used in behavior therapy that attempts to modify a behavioral response by controlling the consequences of that response. Kinds of contingency management include **contingency contracting, shaping, token economy.**

continuing education, (in nursing) formal, organized, educational programs designed to promote the knowledge, skills, and professional attitudes of nurses. The programs are usually short-term and specific; a certificate may be offered for completion of a course and a number of continuing education units (C.E.U.s) may be conferred. Continuing education is required for relicensure in many states. It is not to be confused with academic, degree-granting programs, as advanced education or postgraduate education.

continuing education unit (C.E.U.), *U.S.* a point awarded to a professional person by a professional organization for having attended an educational program relevant to the goals of the organization. A value is established for the course, and that number of points is given. Many states require professionals in the various fields of medicine and nursing to obtain a specific number of C.E.U.'s annually for relicensure.

continuous anesthesia, a method for maintaining regional nerve block in anesthesia for surgical operations or labor in which an anesthetic solution drips either at intervals or at a low rate of flow. Barbiturates or other central nervous system depressant drugs are used. The procedure is named according to the area infiltrated: continuous spinal, caudal, epidural, peridural, or lumbar. Also called **fractional anesthesia.**

continuous bath, a bath of long duration, ranging from a few hours to several weeks or months, in tepid water. The procedure takes place in specially designed tubs that have flowing water and extensions to which a hammock can be attached. The patient has a waterproof pillow to support the head and a harness around the chest to maintain position and provide for safety.

continuous fever, a fever that persists steadily for a prolonged period of time. Compare **intermittent fever.**

continuous positive airway pressure (CPAP), (in respiratory therapy) ventilation assisted by a flow of air delivered at a constant pressure throughout the respiratory cycle. It is performed for patients who can initiate their own respirations but who are not able to maintain adequate arterial oxygen levels without assistance. CPAP may be given through a ventilator and endotracheal tube, through a nasal cannula, or into a hood over the patient's head. Respiratory distress syndrome in the newborn is often treated with CPAP. Also called **continuous positive pressure breathing.** Compare **positive end expiratory pressure.**

continuous positive pressure breathing (CPPB). See **continuous positive airway pressure.**

continuous tremor, fine, rhythmic, purposeless movements that persist during rest but sometimes disappear briefly during voluntary movements. The pill-rolling movements and trembling seen in Parkinson's disease are typical continuous tremors. Compare **intention tremor.** See also **tremor.**

continuous tub bath, a therapeutic bath, usually prescribed in the treatment of some dermatologic conditions, in which the patient lies supported in a medicated solution of tepid water.

■ METHOD: The bath is prepared as for a medicated tub bath. The patient is immersed in the water, and a towel saturated with the solution is placed over the torso. The patient may wear a loin cloth, and a harness is fitted comfortably around the chest and under the shoulders and head to hold the head safely out of the water as the patient sleeps or dozes. A pillow or folded towel is placed over the wide supporting straps under the head and neck to add to the patient's comfort. A board is placed on top of the tub from the patient's shoulders to the end of the tub, and a sheet is draped over it. A bell for calling for assistance, a container of drinking water with a flexible straw, and any other materials that may be needed are placed on the board.

■ NURSING CONSIDERATIONS: The method and the reason for the treatment is explained to the patient. Privacy is maintained; close supervision by a nurse is available throughout the treatment.

■ OUTCOME CRITERIA: The patient is observed for any febrile reaction, rapid or weak pulse, faintness, or increased severity of symptoms, as itching, burning, or pain. The solution is changed completely every four hours, the linen is changed twice a day, and the harness is changed once a day.

■ OUTCOME: The procedure is psychologically trying and may be physically unpleasant for the patient. Psychosocial support and attention to making the patient as comfortable as possible improves the patient's tolerance for the procedure.

continuum (kəntin′yuəm), *pl.* **continua. 1.** a continuous series or whole. **2.** (in mathematics) a system of real numbers.

contra-, a combining form meaning 'against': *contraception, contralateral, contraparetic.*

contraception (kon′trəsep′shən), a process or technique for the prevention of pregnancy by means of a medication, device, or method that blocks or alters one or more of the processes of reproduction in such a way that sexual union can occur without impregnation. Kinds of contraception are **cervical cap, condom, diaphragm, intrauterine contraceptive device, natural family planning, oral contraceptive, spermatocide, sterilization.** Also called **birth control, conception control, family planning, planned parenthood.**

contraceptive diaphragm, a contraceptive device consisting of a hemisphere of thin rubber bonded to a flexible ring, inserted in the vagina together with spermaticidal jelly or cream. Fitted between the pubic symphysis and the posterior fornix of the vagina, the diaphragm cups the cervix in a pool of spermaticide so that spermatozoa cannot enter the uterus, thus preventing conception. The rate of failure of the diaphragm method of contraception is approximately 5 to 10 unplanned pregnancies in one hundred women using the method properly for one year. The principal advantages of the diaphragm are that it has no systemic effects and that it needs to be used only during coitus. The most often reported disadvantages are that it is messy, that it is uncomfortable for some people, and that insertion may interfere with spontaneity or continuity in making love. Diaphragms are manufactured in seven standard sizes from 60 mm to 90 mm in diameter. Kinds of diaphragms are **arcing spring, coil spring, flat spring**. Also called **diaphragm**.

contraceptive diaphragm fitting, a procedure, performed in an office or clinic, in which a contraceptive diaphragm is selected according to the clinical assessment of certain anatomical factors specific to the woman being fitted, including the size of the vagina, the position of the uterus, the depth of the arch behind the symphysis pubis, and the degree of support afforded by the muscles surrounding the vagina. See also **arcing spring contraceptive diaphragm, coil spring contraceptive diaphragm, flat spring contraceptive diaphragm.**

■ METHOD: A vaginal and pelvic examination is performed to determine the appropriate kind of diaphragm and to estimate the size of the vagina. Fitting rings, which are available in various sizes and styles, or sets of actual diaphragms may be used for the fitting. With experience the clinician becomes able to choose a size with which to begin the fitting that is close to the best size for the woman being fitted. The ring or the rim of the diaphragm is lubricated, the rim is drawn together, and the diaphragm is inserted (domeside down) and directed upward toward the sacrum. As it enters the vagina, the posterior aspect of the rim is directed into the posterior fornix of the vagina, behind the cervix; the anterior rim is placed in the arch above and behind the symphysis. A digital examination is done to check that the cervix is covered; through the rubber dome it feels like a nose or a great toe with a dimple or depression in its center. When, by trial and error, the correct size has been determined, the woman is instructed in the technique of inserting it herself and checking its placement. A model may be used before she tries self-insertion. Squatting or standing with one foot on a low stool or chair, she is shown how to apply the correct amount of contraceptive cream or jelly in the dome and around the rim and how to place her hands on the diaphragm for easiest insertion. After she has inserted the diaphragm in her vagina, the clinician checks its placement. The woman may then remove and replace the diaphragm for practice.

■ OUTCOME CRITERIA: The diaphragm method of contraception is subject to great variation in effectiveness, largely owing to inconsistent or incorrect use of the device by the woman. After a woman has used it for several years, the pregnancy rate is as low as 2 to 3 pregnancies per 100 woman years. The pregnancy rate may be much greater, regardless of the perfect and consistent practice of the user, if the woman has a second or third degree uterine prolapse, a second or third degree cystocele, or an acute displacement of the uterus (severe anteversion, anteflexion, retroversion or retroflexion), or if the diaphragm is too small or the wrong kind, allowing spermatozoa to reach the cervix from around and under a loose fitting rim. Hypersensitivity to the spermicidal cream or jelly used in conjunction with the diaphragm sometimes occurs; another product containing different ingredients may not cause any allergic reaction. The method causes no other major adverse reactions.

■ NURSING CONSIDERATIONS: Careful and thorough instruction in the correct use of the contraceptive diaphragm is essential to its acceptance and use and, therefore, to its effectiveness in preventing pregnancy. Adequate time must be allowed for a diaphragm fitting. The woman is shown how to examine the dome for holes, tears, or weak spots and how to use the spermicidal cream or jelly. She is told to leave the diaphragm in place for at least 6 to 8 hours after coitus and never to have sexual intercourse without it, as pregnancy has been known to occur at all times during the menstrual cycle in women who have had coitus only once during the cycle. A new fitting is necessary if the woman gains or loses more than 20 pounds or if she has an abortion or a vaginal delivery. If the woman has not been sexually active prior to the fitting, the fit is re-evaluated after a month or two of sexual activity has passed. After use the diaphragm is washed and dried, powdered with a powder that doesn't contain perfume or talc, and stored in a dry container, preferably the plastic case in which it was dispensed. The diaphragm is checked for signs of weakness or for holes or tears within two years of the initial prescription. Often, the prescription is written with instructions to the pharmacist to give one refill of the prescription, in case of loss or destruction of the diaphragm.

contraceptive effectiveness, the effectiveness of a method of contraception in preventing pregnancy. For clinical purposes it combines the theoretical effectiveness of the device, medication, or method and the use effectiveness. It is sometimes represented as a percentage but more accurately as the number of pregnancies per 100 woman-years. The average pregnancy rate for a couple that is sexually active is 90 per 100 woman-years. A contraceptive method that results in a pregnancy rate of less than 10 pregnancies per 100 woman-years is considered highly effective. See also **pregnancy rate, woman-year.**

contraceptive method, any act, device, or medication for avoiding conception or a viable pregnancy. See also **cervical cap, condom, diaphragm, intrauterine device, natural family-planning method, oral contraceptive, spermatocide, sterilization.** *(See next page for table)*

contract, 1. an agreement or a promise that meets certain legal requirements, including competence of both or all parties to the contract, proper lawful subject matter, mutuality of agreement, mutuality of obligation, and consideration (the giving of something of value in payment

Summary of methods of conception control

Method	Action	Safety-effectiveness	Effects	Contraindications

Oral contraceptive ("The Pill")
Combination pill: each pill contains progestin and estrogen; schedule: one pill daily for 21 days, then discontinue for 7 days; placebo may be advised for last 7 days; pill cycle started and repeated on fifth day after onset of menstrual flow
	Inhibit ovulation by suppression of pituitary gonadotropin
	Produce cervical mucus that is hostile to sperm
	Modify tubal transport of ovum
	May have effect on endometrium to make implantation unlikely
		100% effective if taken accurately
		Failure results from failure to take pill regularly
		If woman forgets to take pill one day, she can "make up" by taking two pills next day
		Chances of pregnancy increased if pill is missed for even 1 day
		Highly acceptable to users; easy to take
		Linked with mortality caused by thromboembolus phenomena
		Does not alter fertility
			Useful
			Relief of dysmenorrhea in 60% to 90% of cases
			Relief of premenstrual tension
			Regulation of menstrual cycles
			Relief of acne in 80% to 90% of cases
			Improved feeling of well-being
			Minor (side effects usually decrease after third cycle)
			Weight gain
			Breast tenderness
			Headaches
			Corneal edema
			Nausea
			Breakthrough bleeding
			Hypertension
			Major side effects
			Thromboembolus disorders
			May also decrease lactation in breast-feeding women
				Undiagnosed vaginal bleeding
				Breast or pelvic cancer
				Liver disease
				Cardiovascular disease
				Renal disease
				Thyroid disease
				Diabetes
				Uterine fibroid tumors
				Use with caution if history of:
				    Epilepsy
				    Multiple sclerosis
				    Porphyria
				    Otosclerosis
				    Asthma

Intrauterine contraceptive device (IUD or IUCD) Small objects of various shapes made of plastic, nylon, or steel inserted into uterus; most have nylon string attached that protrudes from cervix into vagina; inserted using aseptic technique; follow-up visits in 1 month, then individualized EXAMPLES Lippes loop Saf-T-Coil Birnberg bow Margulies coil Hall-Stone ring Copper T Copper seven	Unknown Probably modifies endometrium or myometrium to prevent inflammation Probably hastens tubal transport of ovum	Easily inserted, highly effective: 97% to 99% Can be inserted any time during cycle; presence of menstrual flow rules out early pregnancy Can be inserted immediately postpartum, but expulsion rate is higher Can be left in place indefinitely Effectiveness highly dependent on knowing IUD remains in place; women need to be taught to feel for string after each period Spontaneous expulsion occurs most often during menstruation (expulsion rates: 10% to 20%) Failure rate (pregnancy) 1.5% to 3% during first year of use; rate declines thereafter Does not alter fertility	Uterine cramping Heavy menstrual flow Irregular menses NOTE: Usually disappear in 2 to 3 months Problems Infection: usually minor and occurs soon after insertion Perforation of uterus: varies with types of device; highest rates in first 6 weeks postpartum; usually occurs at time of insertion	Current infection of reproductive tract Uterine fibroids Undiagnosed vaginal bleeding

Summary of methods of conception control—cont'd

Method	Action	Safety-effectiveness	Effects	Contraindications
Diaphragm (with spermicidal foam, cream, jelly) Rubber dome attached to flexible metal ring; inserted into vagina to cover cervix; available in various sizes (require careful fitting); self-inserted by user; inner surface of diaphragm coated with spermicide before insertion; inserted at least 2 hours before intercourse and left in place at least 6 hours after intercourse	Provides mechanical barrier to sperm Spermicidal preparation destroys large number of sperm	97% to 98% effective if fitted properly and used correctly Requires sustained motivation for repeated insertion and removal Refitting necessary after childbirth, abortion, surgery of cervix and vagina, or weight change of 10 lb or more	None	Severe uterine prolapse
Condom ("rubber," "safes," "prophylactics") Thin, flexible plastic worn over penis; available without prescription; does not require medical supervision	Provides mechanical barrier to prevent sperm from entering vagina Prevents spread of venereal diseases	Effectiveness increased with use of diaphragm by woman Effectiveness decreased by tearing or slipping of condom during intercourse Failure rate 10% to 15%	None	None
Natural family planning (ovulation, symptothermal) Periodic abstinence from intercourse during fertile periods of menstrual cycle; days 12 to 16 before expected date of menstruation are possible ovulating days; because sperm can survive up to 48 hours, days 11, 17, and 18 added to fertile period	Sexual abstinence around time of ovulation	Safe 65% to 85% effective Fertile period varies; precise time of ovulation not known Effectiveness increased with calculation of fertile period, high motivation to prevent pregnancy, determination of basal body temperature	Frustration Lack of sexual gratification during period of abstinence	Irregular menstrual cycles Medical contraindications to pregnancy
Chemical contraceptive (jellies, creams, foams, suppositories) Applied inside vagina by means of plunger-type applicator or aerosol spray	Contains spermicidal ingredients Partial barrier to entrance of sperm into cervix	Effectiveness increased when used with diaphragm or condom Easily available without prescription Effectiveness depends on dispersion of substance within vagina	None	None

for the obligation undertaken). **2.** to make such an agreement or promise. **–contractual,** *adj.*

contractile ring dysphagia, an abnormal condition characterized by difficulty in swallowing, owing to an overreactive interior esophageal sphincteric mechanism that induces painful sticking sensations under the lower sternum. Compare **dysphagia lusoria, vallecular dysphagia.**

contraction, 1. (in labor) a rhythmic tightening of the musculature of the upper uterine segment that begins mildly and becomes very strong late in labor, occurring as frequently as every two minutes, and lasting over a minute. Contractions decrease the size of the uterus and squeeze the fetus through the birth canal. **2.** abnormal smallness of the birth canal or part of it, a cause of dystocia. **Inlet contraction** exists if the anteroposterior diameter is 10.0 cm or less, or if the transverse diameter is 11.5 cm or less. **Midpelvic contraction** exists if the sum of the measurements in centimeters of the interspinous diameter (normally 10.5 cm) and the posterior sagittal diameter (normally 5.0 cm) is 13.5 cm or less. **Outlet contraction** exists if the intertuberous diameter is 8.0 cm or less. See also **pelvimetry.**

contracture, an abnormal, usually permanent condition of a joint, characterized by flexion and fixation and caused by atrophy and shortening of muscle fibers or by loss of the normal elasticity of the skin, as from the formation of extensive scar tissue over a joint. See also **Volkmann's contracture.**

contraindication (kon'trɑin'dəkei'shən), a factor that prohibits the administration of a drug or the performance of a procedure in the care of a specific patient, as pregnancy is a contraindication for the prescription of tetracycline, immunosuppression is a contraindication for vaccination, and complete placenta previa is a contraindication for vaginal delivery.

contrast bath, a bath in which the patient alternately immerses a part of the body, usually the hands or feet, in hot and cold water for a specified period of time. The procedure is used to increase the blood flow to a particular area.

contrast enema. See **barium enema.**

contrast medium, a radiopaque substance injected into the body to facilitate roentgen imaging of internal structures that otherwise are difficult to visualize on x rays.

contribution, (in law) a right of a defendant who has been required to pay a judgment to demand that others who are equally liable for the plaintiff's injuries contribute a share of the payment.

control, to exercise restraint or maintain influence over a situation, as in self-control, the conscious limitation or suppression of impulses.

control group. See **group.**

controlled association, 1. a direct connection of relevant ideas as the result of a specific stimulus. 2. a process of bringing repressed ideas into the consciousness in response to words spoken by a psychoanalyst. Also called **word association.**

controlled hypotension. See **deliberate hypotension.**

controlled ventilation, the use of an intermittent positive pressure breathing unit or other respirator that has an automatic cycling device that replaces spontaneous respiration. Some units measure expired volume, nebulize medication or fluids in the air, exert negative pressure at the end of the expiration, or have a variety of alarms.

control of hemorrhage, the limitation of the flow of blood from a break in the wall of a blood vessel.
■ METHOD: Some of the methods for controlling hemorrhage are direct pressure, use of a tourniquet, or application of pressure on pressure points proximal to the wound. Direct pressure with a thick compress is applied in such a way that the edges of the wound are brought together. A tourniquet is applied proximal to the site of bleeding only in the most drastic emergency, for the limb may then have to be sacrificed owing to tissue anoxia caused by the use of the tourniquet. Pressure is applied to a pressure point by using firm manual pressure over the main artery supplying the wound. Points used to obtain the pulse may be used as pressure points to stop hemorrhage. See also **tourniquet.**
■ OUTCOME CRITERIA: Signs of continued bleeding, tachycardia, cold sweat, decreasing blood pressure, and anxiety on the part of the patient alert the nurse to the probability that bleeding has begun again or that replacement fluids administered after the hemorrhage are not adequate. The person is kept calm and quiet; if the fluid balance is promptly restored, recovery is usual. Excessive loss of blood leads to anoxia of all the tissues of the body, including the brain and vital organs, and causes death.
■ NURSING ORDERS: The flow of blood to an area is limited by restricting activity, elevating the part, and applying pressure. Specific treatment depends on the cause of the hemorrhage and the condition of the patient. In addition to intravenous infusion equipment and fluids, the nurse may anticipate the need for vasopressor drugs, ventilatory assistance, central venous pressure monitoring equipment, and materials for obtaining and recording the blood pressure and urinary output. If signs of shock are present the patient may be placed supine at a 45° angle to the pelvis, with the knees straight and the pelvis slightly higher than the chest. The head may be supported with a pillow. If the Trendelenburg's position is used, a pillow is placed under the left shoulder to maximize filling of the right atrium of the heart and to maintain an open airway. The person may be given oxygen, and the central venous pressure may be measured to determine the need for replacement of fluid volume. Sudden, severe hemorrhage with signs of shock usually is treated with intravenous infusion of fluids and a transfusion of blood. The application of additional warmth to the skin is not recommended, as heat increases the metabolism and the need for oxygen.

contusion, an injury that does not break the skin, caused by a blow to the body and characterized by swelling, discoloration, and pain. The immediate application of cold may limit the development of a contusion. Also called **bruise.**

convalescence, the period of recovery after an illness, injury, or surgery.

convalescent home. See **extended care facility.**

convection, (in physics) the transfer of heat through a gas or liquid by the circulation of heated particles.

convergent evolution, the development of similar structures or functions within widely differing phylogenetic species in response to similar environmental conditions.

convergent strabismus. See **esotropia.**

conversion, an unconscious defense mechanism by which emotional conflicts ordinarily resulting in anxiety are repressed and transformed into symbolic physical symptoms having no organic basis. Loss of sensation, paralysis, pain, or other dysfunction of the nervous system are the most common somatic expressions of conversion.

conversion disorder, a kind of hysterical neurosis in which emotional conflicts are repressed and converted into sensory, motor, or visceral symptoms having no underlying organic cause, as blindness, anesthesia, hypesthesia, hyperesthesia, parasthesia, involuntary muscular movements (as tics or tremors), paralysis, aphonia, mutism, hallucinations, catalepsy, choking sensations, and respiratory difficulties. The person who has conversion disorder is usually indifferent to the symptoms yet firmly believes the condition exists. Causal factors include a conscious or unconscious desire to escape from or avoid some unpleasant situation or responsibility or to obtain sympathy or some other secondary gain. Treatment usually consists of psychotherapy. Also called **conversion hysteria, conversion reaction.**

conversion hysteria. See **conversion disorder.**

conversion reaction. See **conversion disorder.**

convulsion, a sudden, violent involuntary contraction of a group of muscles that may be paroxysmal and episodic, as in a seizure disorder, or transient and acute, as following a head concussion. A convulsion may be clonic or tonic, focal, unilateral, or bilateral.

Cooley's anemia. See **thalassemia.**

cooling, reducing body temperature by the application of a hypothermia blanket, cold moist dressings, ice packs, or an alcohol bath. Subnormal body temperature may be induced to reduce metabolic function before some kinds of surgery. Very high fevers of any etiology may be treated in part by reduction of the fever with cooling techniques. See also **alcohol bath, hypothermia, hypothermia blanket.**

Coombs' test (kumz). See **antiglobulin test.**

cooperative play, any organized play among a group of children in which activities are planned for the purpose of achieving some goal. It usually occurs among older children. Compare **associative play, parallel play, solitary play.**

coordinated reflex, a sequence of muscular actions occurring in a purposeful, orderly progression, as the act of swallowing.

coping, a process by which a person deals with stress, solves problems, and makes decisions. The process has two components, cognitive and noncognitive. The cognitive component includes the thought and learning necessary to identify the source of the stress. The cognitive components are automatic and focus on relieving the discomfort. Many defense mechanisms fall into this category. While sometimes useful, noncognitive measures may fail to relieve the stress because the response may be inappropriate, may have the wrong effect, and, as it replaces cognitive coping measures, may prevent the person from learning more about the cause and a better solution for the problem.

coping ability, the degree to which an individual is able to adapt to any stress encountered in the activities of daily life, whether of a physical or psychological nature, through the use of both conscious and unconscious mechanisms. Abnormal behavior patterns result when such demands or problems cannot be adequately met.

coping, family: potential for growth, a nursing diagnosis accepted by the Fourth National Conference on the Classification of Nursing Diagnoses. The etiology of the problem is the need for self-actualization that occurs when a person's basic needs have been satisfied and the adaptive tasks required by the client's health problem have been mastered. The defining characteristics of the family's potential for growth in this area are the family's expressed wish to discuss the impact of the situation on the client's own life and values, interest in meeting with others in similar situations, and choice of healthful options available to the client. See also **nursing diagnosis.**

coping, ineffective family: compromised, a nursing diagnosis accepted by the Fourth National Conference on the Classification of Nursing Diagnoses. The diagnosis refers to a lack or absence of emotional and psychological support for the client that is usually available from a family member or other supportive person, a deficiency that causes further difficulty for the client in coping with the current health problem. The etiology of the situation may be inadequate or faulty understanding of the health problem by the supportive person, or it may result from temporary preoccupation with emotional conflicts on the part of the supportive person. Illness or health problems may cause changes in roles, resulting in temporary disorganization of the network of family and friends who may become exhausted by the demands of filling the needs of the client. Many situational crises may interrupt or prevent adequate expression of support for the client, and the client may be able to give little support in return. The defining characteristics of ineffective compromised family coping include expression by the client that support is lacking or expression by the supportive person that fear, anticipatory grief, anxiety, or other reaction is interfering with the ability to give support to the client. A frank statement of an inadequate understanding of the health problem from the client or supportive person may be made. Objectively, the nurse may observe that the support given is inadequate, that the communication between the parties is limited and unsatisfactory, or that the supportive person offers help that is disproportionate to the need. See also **nursing diagnosis.**

coping, ineffective family: disabling, a nursing diagnosis accepted by the Fourth National Conference on the Classification of Nursing Diagnoses. The diagnosis refers to the detrimental attitudes and behavior of a family, a family member, or other person who is important to the client. The etiology of the problem is often the disablement of the significant person by grief, anxiety, guilt, hostility, or despair. The defining characteristics of this kind of ineffective family coping include neglect in the care of the client, intolerance, rejection or abandonment, adoption of the symptoms of the client, disregard of the client's needs, and marked distortion of reality in regard to the client's health problem. See also **nursing diagnosis.**

coping, ineffective individual, a nursing diagnosis accepted by the Fourth National Conference on the Classification of Nursing Diagnoses. The etiology of the problem includes situational crises, maturational or developmental crises, or personal vulnerability. The defining characteristics include an inability to meet the expectations of a role, an inability to meet one's basic needs, or an alteration in ability to participate in society. The critical defining characteristics, one of which must be present for the diagnosis to be made, are an inability to ask for help, an inability to solve problems, and verbalization of the inability to cope. Other characteristics that may be present are destructive behavior, inappropriate or excessive use of defense mechanisms, a change in patterns of communication, verbal manipulation, and a greater than expected incidence of accidents and illness. See also **nursing diagnosis.**

copper (Cu), a malleable, reddish-brown, metallic element. Its atomic number is 29; its atomic weight is 63.54. Copper occurs in a pure state in nature and in many ores. It is a component of several important enzymes in the body and is essential to good health. Copper deficiency in the body is rare because only 2 to 5 mg daily, easily obtained from a variety of foods, is sufficient for a proper balance. Copper accumulates in individuals with Wilson's disease, primary biliary cirrhosis, and, occasionally, in chronic extrahepatic biliary tract obstruction. Copper is an excellent conductor of heat and electricity, a valuable component of numerous alloys, and it may be compounded with arsenic to form insecticides. Copper sulfate solution is commonly used to test for reducing agents, as glucose, in the urine. See also **ceruloplasmin, hepatolenticular degeneration.**

copperhead, a poisonous pit viper found in the southeastern United States. This reddish-brown, darkly banded snake is responsible for nearly 40 per cent of the snake bites in the United States, though few of its bites are fatal. Pain, swelling, fang marks, and a bruise are usually present. Immediate treatment includes placing a constricting band above the bite, tight enough to prevent lymphatic and superficial venous flow from the wound to the general circulation, but not tight enough to stop deep arterial and venous flow to the limb. The fang marks are incised, the venom is sucked out, and free bleeding is allowed. The victim should be taken to a medical facility and given antivenin if necessary. The medication is usually needed only for children and older people. See also **coral snake, cottonmouth.**

Copper Kettle, a trade name for a kind of vaporizer used in the circuits of an anesthesia machine to mix the carrier gas and the volatile anesthetic liquid to form an anesthetizing vapor.

copro-, copr-, a combining form meaning 'pertaining to feces': *coprodaeum, coprolalia, coprolith.* Also **kopr-, kopra-.**

coprogogue (kop'rəgog'). See **cathartic.**

coproporphyria (kop'roupourfir'iə), a rare, hereditary, metabolic disorder in which large quantities of nitrogenous substances, called porphyrins, are excreted in the urine. Attacks, with varying gastrointestinal and neurologic symptoms, may be precipitated by certain drugs, including barbiturates, sulfonamides, and steroids. Patients are often helped by a high carbohydrate diet. See also **coproporphyrin, porphyria.**

coproporphyrin (kop'roupour'firin), any of the nitrogenous organic substances normally excreted in the feces that are products of the breakdown of bilirubin from hemoglobin decomposition.

cor-. See **co-.**

coracoid process, the thick, curved extension of the superior border of the scapula, to which the pectoralis minor is attached. Compare **acromion.**

coral snake, a poisonous snake with transverse red, black, and yellow bands, native to the southern United States. Bites are rare; pain is not always present, but neuromuscular and respiratory effects may be severe. Coral snake antivenin and oxygen are the usual treatments.

Coramine, a trade name for a respiratory stimulant (nikethamide).

cord, any long, rounded, flexible structure. The body contains many different cords, as the spermatic, vocal, spinal, nerve, umbilical, and hepatic cords. Cords serve many different purposes, depending on location, kind of enclosed cells, and body parts or tissue involved. –**cordal,** *adj.*

corditis (kordai'tis), an abnormal inflammation of the spermatic cord, accompanied by pain in the testis, often caused by an infection originating in the urethra or by tumor, hydrocele, or varicocele. Injury to the groin often causes hematoma of the cord. Inflammatory conditions of the testis may lead to swelling and tenderness.

Cordran, a trade name for a glucocorticoid (flurandrenolide).

core-, coro-, a combining form meaning 'pertaining to the pupil of the eye': *coreclisis, corectasis, corectopia.*

core gender identity. See **gender identity.**

Corgard, a trade name for a beta-adrenergic blocking agent (nadolol).

-coria¹, a combining form meaning '(condition of the) sense of satiety': *acoria, hypercoria, saccharacoria.*

-coria², a combining form meaning '(condition of the) pupil': *anisocoria, diplocoria, platycoria.*

Cori's disease (kɔr'iz), a rare type of glycogen storage disease, in which a missing enzyme results in abnormally large deposits of glycogen in the liver, skeletal muscles, and heart. Signs are an enlarged liver, hypoglycemia, acidosis, and, occasionally, stunted growth. Symptoms can be controlled by giving the patient frequent, small meals rich in carbohydrate and protein. Also called **Forbes' disease, glycogenosis, glycogen storage disease, type III.** See also **glycogen storage disease.**

corium (kɔr'iəm), the layer of skin, just below the epidermis, consisting of papillary and reticular layers and containing blood and lymphatic vessels, nerves and nerve endings, glands, and hair follicles.

corkscrew esophagus, a neurogenic disorder in which normal peristaltic contractions of the esophagus are replaced by spastic movements occurring spontaneously or with swallowing or gastric acid reflux. Difficulty in swallowing, weight loss, severe pain over the upper chest, and a characteristic corkscrew image on x-ray pictures are the symptoms usually present. Management may include the use of antispasmodic drugs, avoidance of cold fluids, surgical dilatation, or myotomy. Compare **achalasia.**

cork worker's lung, a lung disease caused by an allergic reaction to cork dust. Also called **suberosis.** See also **organic dust.**

-cormia, a combining form meaning an 'abnormal development of the trunk of the body': *camptocormia, nanocormia, schistocormia.* Also **-cormy.**

corn, a horny mass of condensed epithelial cells overlying a bony prominence. Corns result from chronic friction and pressure. The conical shape of the corn compresses the underlying dermis, making it thin and tender. Corns can become soft and macerated by perspiration. Treatment includes relief of the mechanical pressure and surgical paring or chemical peeling of the excess keratin. Also called **clavus.** Compare **callus.**

cornea, the convex, transparent, anterior part of the eye, comprising one sixth of the outermost tunic of the eye bulb. It is a fibrous structure with five layers: the anterior corneal epithelium, continuous with that of the conjunctiva; the anterior limiting layer (Bowman's membrane); the substantia propria; the posterior limiting layer (Descemet's membrane); and the endothelium of the anterior chamber (keratoderma). It is dense, uniform in thickness, and nonvascular, and it projects like a dome beyond the sclera, which forms the other five sixths of the eye's outermost tunic. The degree of corneal curvature varies in different individuals and in the same person at different ages, the curvature being more pronounced in youth than in advanced age.

-cornea, a combining form meaning 'condition of the cornea': *entocornea, mesocornea, microcornea.*

corneal abrasion, the rubbing off of the outer layers of the cornea.

CORNEAL ABRASION

corneal grafting, transplantation of corneal tissue from one human eye to another, performed to improve vision in corneal scarring or distortion or to remove a perforating ulcer. Preoperative preparation includes constricting the pupil with a miotic drug, as pilocarpine. Under local anesthesia the affected area is excised; an identical section of clear cornea is cut from the donor eye and sutured in place, using an operating microscope. Cataract surgery may be performed at the same time. Postoperatively, the eye is covered with a protective metal shield, and the patient is cautioned to avoid coughing, sneezing, sudden movement, or lifting. The dressing is changed daily and antibiotics are instilled. A complication that may occur after several weeks is a clouding over of the graft, owing to the body's rejection of foreign tissue. Corticosteroid drugs administered immediately postoperatively may prevent the reaction. Healing is slow, and the sutures are usually left in place for one year. Also called **keratoplasty.**

corneal loupe, (in ophthalmology) a loupe designed especially for examining the cornea.

corneal reflex, a portective mechanism for the eye in which the eyelids close when the cornea is touched. This reflex is mediated by the ophthalmic division of the fifth cranial nerve and may be used as a test of integrity of that nerve branch. People who wear contact lenses may have a diminished or absent corneal reflex. Compare **conjunctival reflex.**

cornification (kɔr'nɪfɪkei'ʃən), thickening of the skin by a buildup of dead, keratinized epithelial cells.

corn pad, a device that helps relieve the pressure and the pain of a corn by transferring the pressure to surrounding, unaffected areas. Corn pads are constructed of pliable fabric and fashioned in various ways to accommodate different conditions. Some common kinds of corn pads are the foam toe cap, the foam toe sleeve, the soft corn shield, and the hard corn shield.

cornual pregnancy, an ectopic pregnancy that implants in the portion of the Fallopian tube that is within the horn of the uterus. Also called **interstitial pregnancy.** See also **ectopic pregnancy.**

coro-. See **core-.**

corona (kərou′nə), **1.** a crown. **2.** a crownlike projection or encircling structure, as a process extending from a bone. — **coronoid,** *adj.*

coronal plane (kərou′nəl). See **frontal plane.**

coronal suture, the serrated transverse suture between the frontal bone and the parietal bone on each side of the skull.

corona radiata, *pl.* **coronae radiatae. 1.** a network of fibers that weaves through the internal capsule of the cerebral cortex and intermingles with the fibers of the corpus callosum. **2.** an aggregate of cells that surrounds the zona pellucida of the ovum.

coronary, 1. (in anatomy) **a.** of or pertaining to encircling structures, as the coronary arteries. **b.** of or pertaining to the heart. **2.** *Nontechnical.* myocardial infarction or occlusion.

coronary arteriovenous fistula, an unusual congenital abnormality characterized by a direct communication between a coronary artery, usually the right, and the right atrium or ventricle, the coronary sinus, or the vena cava. There may be a left-to-right shunt of small magnitude causing no symptoms, but a large shunt may result in growth failure, limited exercise tolerance, dyspnea, and anginal pain. Possible complications with a large shunt are bacterial endocarditis, rupture of an aneurysmal fistula, thrombus formation causing occlusion or distal embolization, and, in rare cases, pulmonary hypertension and congestive heart failure. A loud continuous murmur heard at the lower or midsternal border of the heart suggests a coronary arteriovenous fistula; the diagnosis may be confirmed by coronary arteriography or aortography. Closure of the fistulous tract is a safe surgical procedure with excellent long-term results.

coronary artery, one of a pair of arteries that branch from the aorta, including the left and the right coronary arteries. As these vessels and their branches supply the heart, any dysfunction or disease that affects them can cause serious, sometimes fatal complications. Coronary arterial anastomoses occur throughout the heart and are especially numerous within the interventricular and interatrial septums, at the apex of the heart, at the crux, over the anterior surface of the right ventricle, and between the sinus node artery and the other atrial arteries. These anastomoses are more numerous and large in the epicardium than in the endocardium, and they provide important collateral circulation in the recovery of patients who suffer coronary occlusions. The branches of the coronary arteries are affected by many different disorders, as embolic, neoplastic, inflammatory, and noninflammatory diseases.

coronary artery disease, any one of the abnormal conditions which may affect the arteries of the heart and produce various pathological effects, especially the reduced flow of oxygen and nutrients to the myocardium. Any of the coronary artery diseases, as coronary atherosclerosis, coronary arteritis, or fibromuscular hyperplasia of the coronary arteries, may produce the common characteristic symptom of angina pectoris, which, however, may also be associated with cardiomyopathy in which the coronary arteries are normal. The most common kind of coronary artery disease is coronary atherosclerosis, which has increased dramatically in the last 50 years and is now the leading cause of death in the Western world. Epidemiological studies show marked regional differences in the incidence and prevalence of coronary atherosclerosis. The disease is not necessarily part of the aging process. It affects more men than women and occurs more often in Caucasians, the middle-aged, the elderly, and individuals from affluent countries. Coronary atherosclerosis affects more premenopausal women today than in the past, possibly because of the pathological effects of increased cigarette smoking by women, stressful sedentary jobs, and the use of oral contraceptives. Studies over the last 30 years confirm that coronary atherosclerosis occurs most frequently in populations with regular diets high in calories, total fat, saturated fat, cholesterol, and refined carbohydrates. The risk of developing coronary atherosclerosis and the risk of death from the disease is two to six times greater among cigarette smokers than nonsmokers and appears to be proportional to the number of cigarettes smoked per day. Significantly less risk is associated with pipe and cigar smoking. Hypertension is also a prime risk factor in atherosclerosis. Some studies show the combination of cigarette smoking and cholesterol level above 275 mg/100 ml increases the coronary risk fourteen to sixteen times. Research also has implicated other factors as possibly contributing to the risk of atherosclerosis. Some of these are coffee intake, alcohol intake, deficiencies of vitamins C and E, water hardness, hypoxia, carbon monoxide, social overcrowding, climate, and viruses. Atherosclerosis develops with the formation of fatty fibrous plaques that narrow the lumen of the coronary arteries and may lead to thrombosis and myocardial infarction. Although no single cause of atherosclerosis has been found, the development of the disease is closely associated with the plasma lipids and the lipoproteins that transport the plasma lipids from one tissue to another. The plasma lipids, composed chiefly of cholesterol, triglyceride, phospholipid, and free fatty acids are insoluble in water. The major classes of lipoproteins are chylomicra, very-low-density lipoproteins, low-density lipoproteins, high-density lipoproteins, and the free fatty acid-albumin complex.

■ OBSERVATIONS: Angina pectoris, the classic symptom of coronary artery disease, results from infarction and myocardial ischemia. Angina is usually described as a crushing substernal pain that radiates to the left arm, neck, jaw, and shoulder blade. In affected individuals, angina commonly follows physical exertion, emotional excitement, or exposure to cold. Angina may be stable, unstable, or decubitus. The frequency and the duration of stable angina are predictable, and this type of pain may be relieved with nitrates and rest. Unstable angina occurs more often and lasts longer than stable angina. Decubitis angina may recur even when the affected individual is resting. Prolonged, intense angina commonly indicates myocardial infarction with possible fatal mechanical failures and arrythmias. Diagnosis of coronary artery disease is usually based on patient history, especially a history with characteristic risk factors. Other diagnostic procedures are EKG during angina, treadmill or bicycle exercise tests, coronary angiography, and myocardial perfusion imaging.

■ INTERVENTION: Treatment of the patient with coronary artery disease concentrates on reducing myocardial oxygen demand or on increasing oxygen supply. Therapy commonly includes the administration of nitrates, as nitroglycerin, isosorbide dinitrate, or propranolol. Coronary artery bypass surgery may use vein grafts to obviate obstructive lesions. Angioplasty to relieve occlusion by compressing fatty deposits in coronary arteries with no calcification may also be performed. The prevalence of coronary artery disease highlights the importance of preventive measures, as the reduction of caloric intake for the obese patient; reduction of salt, fats, and cholesterol; regular exercise; abstention from smoking; and reduction of stress. Other preventive measures include the control of hypertension, reduction of elevated serum cholesterol and triglyceride levels, and reduction of dangers of blood clots and platelet aggregation. Hypertension may be controlled with sympathetic blocking agents, as propranolol. Serum cholesterol and triglyceride levels may be reduced with hypolipidemic drugs, as clofibrate. Clinical trials with various antithrombotic drugs seek to reduce the danger of blood clots from platelet aggregation. Further studies may determine the efficacy of aspirin in the prevention of platelet plugs as the predominant form of arterial thrombi. Aspirin inhibits the aggregation of platelets but may not retard their adherence to the walls of blood vessels.

■ NURSING CONSIDERATIONS: Nursing care of the patient with coronary artery disease involves monitoring of blood pressure and heart rate, taking of EKGs during anginal episodes, and administration of nitrates, as nitroglycerin. Meticulous maintenance of pulmonary artery catheters and of I.V.- and endotracheal tubes often associated with treatment is important. Nurses are especially alert to signs of ischemia and arrhythmias and, before the patient is discharged, stress the importance of following the prescribed regimens of diet, medication, and exercise.

coronary artery fistula, a congenital anomaly characterized by an abnormal communication between a coronary artery and the right side of the heart or the pulmonary artery.

coronary bypass, open-heart surgery in which a prosthesis or a section of a blood vessel is grafted onto one of the coronary arteries and connected to the ascending aorta, bypassing a narrowing or blockage in a coronary artery. The operation is performed in coronary artery disease to improve the blood supply to the heart muscle, to reduce the workload of the heart, and to relieve anginal pain. Coronary arteriography pinpoints the areas of obstruction preoperatively. Under general anesthesia, and utilizing a heart-lung machine, one end of a 15 to 20 cm prosthesis or segment of saphenous vein from the patient's leg is grafted to the ascending aorta, and the other end is sutured to the clogged coronary artery at a point distal to the stoppage. The internal mammary artery may also be used as graft tissue. Usually, double or triple grafts are done for multiple areas of blockage. Postoperatively, close observation in a coronary intensive care unit or surgical recovery unit is essential to ensure adequate ventilation and cardiac output. The systolic blood pressure is not allowed to drop more than 10 mm of Hg below the preoperative baseline, nor is it allowed to rise significantly, as hypertension can rupture a graft site. Arrhythmias occur frequently and are treated with lidocaine, procainamide, or digitalis, given intravenously, or by electrical cardioversion. The patient is usually discharged within 10 to 14 days. Nearly 20 per cent of cases are associated with thrombosis within the first year following surgery; 20 to 25 per cent are associated with closure of the graft within the first year, making the surgery controversial.

coronary care nursing, the nursing care provided in a hospital in a coronary care unit. Nursing in this setting requires technical knowledge, judgment, and skills as well as an ability to give emotional support to patients and their families during the acute stage of cardiac dysfunction.

coronary care unit (CCU), a specially equipped hospital area designed for the treatment of patients with sudden, life-threatening cardiac conditions, as acute coronary thrombosis. Such units contain resuscitation and monitoring equipment and are staffed by personnel especially trained and skilled in recognizing and immediately responding to cardiac emergencies with cardiopulmonary resuscitation techniques, the administration of antiarrhythmic drugs, and other appropriate therapeutic measures.

coronary occlusion, an obstruction of any one of the coronary arteries, usually caused by progressive atherosclerosis and sometimes complicated by thrombosis. Coronary occlusions are rarely caused by embolisms, arteritis, or by dissecting aneurysms. More often, an obstruction of a coronary artery develops gradually from the accumulation of fatty, fibrous plaques which narrow the arterial lumen, reduce the blood flow, and lead to myocardial infarction. In certain heart diseases arterial spasms may narrow the lumen of a coronary artery, blocking blood flow, and causing the characteristic signs of myocardial infarction, as crushing substernal pain that radiates to the arms, jaw, and neck. Atherosclerosis, which commonly develops in high-flow, high-pressure arteries is associated with numerous factors, including family history, hypertension, obesity, smoking, diabetes mellitus, stress, sedentary occupations, and high serum cholesterol and triglyceride levels. Occlusions that lead to myocardial infarction are common, and mortality is high when treatment is delayed. Almost half the sudden deaths caused by myocardial infarction occur before the affected individual is hospitalized, often within one hour of the onset of symptoms. If treatment begins immediately after the onset of symptoms, the prognosis significantly improves. Occlusion of the circumflex branch of the left coronary artery causes a lateral wall infarction. Occlusion of the anterior descending branch of the left coronary artery causes an infarction of the anterior heart wall. Occlusion of the right coronary artery or one of its branches causes a posterior wall infarction. Many patients who suffer coronary occlusions recover because of fast treatment and collateral circulation provided by extensive arterial anastomoses of the heart. The reasons why the arterial anastomoses function for collateral circulation in some patients with occlusions and not in others are apparently associated with individual differences in arterial pressure and configurations of the arterial anastomoses. In normal hearts, the coronary anastomoses are usually straight or gently curving; in hearts with coronary occlusion, the arterial anastomoses are twisted and tortuous. Occlusions of the sinus node artery and the main coronary artery proximal to the origin of the sinus node branch commonly cause infarctions of the atrium and the sinus node and lead to atrial arrhythmias. Coronary occlusions that produce posterior myocardial infarction cut off the blood supply to the atrioventricular node, resulting in characteristic signs, as fainting and syncope during angina. Treatment of coronary occlusion and associated myocardial infarction often includes the administration of lidocaine or other antiarrhythmic drugs, nitroglycerin to relieve pain, oxygen, bed rest, and the implanting of a temporary pacemaker.

coronary sinus, the wide venous channel, about 2.25 cm long, situated in the coronary sulcus and covered by muscular fibers from the left atrium. It drains five coronary veins through a single semilunar valve. They are the great cardiac vein, the small cardiac vein, the middle cardiac vein, the posterior vein of the left ventricle, and the oblique vein of the left atrium.

coronary thrombosis, a development of a thrombus which blocks a coronary artery, often causing myocardial infarction and death. Coronary thromboses commonly develop in segments of arteries with atherosclerotic lesions, thus supporting the opinion of many authorities that atherosclerosis favors the development of thrombi.

coronary vein, one of the veins of the heart that drain blood from the capillary beds of the myocardium through the coronary sinus into the right atrium. A few small coronary veins that collect blood from a small area in the right ventricle drain directly into the right atrium.

coronavirus (kor'ənəvaī'rəs), a member of a family of viruses that includes several types capable of causing acute respiratory illnesses.

coroner, a public official who investigates the causes and circumstances of a death occurring within a specific legal jurisdiction or territory, especially a death that may have resulted from unnatural causes. Also called **medical examiner.**

coronoid fossa, a small depression in the distal, dorsal surface of the humerus that receives the coronoid process of the ulna when the forearm is flexed.

coronoid process of mandible, a prominence on the anterior surface of the ramus of the mandible to which each temporal muscle attaches.

coronoid process of ulna, a wide, flaring projection of the proximal end of the ulna. The proximal surface of the process forms the lower part of the trochlear notch.

corpor-, a combining form meaning 'pertaining to the body': *corpora, corporeal, corporic.*

cor pulmonale (kor pul'mənæl'i), an abnormal cardiac condition characterized by hypertrophy of the right ventricle of the heart owing to hypertension of the pulmonary circulation. Pulmonary hypertension associated with this condition is caused by some disorder of the pulmonary parenchyma or of the pulmonary vascular system between the origin of the left pulmonary artery and the entry of the pulmonary veins into the left atrium. Chronic cor pulmonale commonly increases the size of the right ventricle of the heart, because the right ventricle cannot accommodate an increase in pressure as easily as the left ventricle. In some patients, however, the disease also increases the size of the left ventricle. Some of the diseases associated with cor pulmonale include cystic fibrosis, myasthenia gravis, myopathies, and pulmonary arteritis. Approximately 85 per cent of patients with cor pulmonale have chronic obstructive pulmonary disease; 25 per cent of patients with emphysema eventually develop cor pulmonale. Pulmonary capillary destruction and pulmonary vasoconstriction decrease the cross-sectional area of the pulmonary vascular bed, increasing pulmonary vascular resistance and causing pulmonary hypertension. The right ventricle dilates and hypertrophies to compensate for the extra work required in forcing blood through the lungs. To compensate for the low oxygen content associated with cor pulmonale, the bone marrow produces more red blood cells, causing erythrocytosis. Right ventricular failure results when blood viscosity increases and further aggravates pulmonary hypertension, increasing the hemodynamic load on the right ventricle. Cor pulmonale accounts for about 25 per cent of all types of heart failure and is most prevalent in populations where the incidence of cigarette smoking and chronic obstructive pulmonary disease is high. The disease affects middle-aged and elderly men more than women. Cor pulmonale in children may be a complication of cystic fibrosis, hemosiderosis, scleroderma, neurological diseases affecting respiratory muscles, or disorders of the respiratory control center.

■ OBSERVATIONS: Some of the early signs of cor pulmonale include chronic cough, exertional dyspnea, fatigue, wheezing, and weakness. As the disease progresses, dyspnea may become more severe and other signs, as tachypnea, orthopnea, and edema may emerge. Signs of this condition and right ventricular failure may include dependent edema, distended neck veins, hepatojugular reflux, and tachycardia. A weak pulse and hypotension may result from decreased cardiac output, and chest examination may reveal various signs, depending on the cause of the condition. In chronic obstructive pulmonary disease, auscultation may reveal rales, rhonchi, and diminished breath sounds. When cor pulmonale is secondary to obstruction of the upper airway or to damage of CNS respiratory centers, auscultation may reveal a right ventricular lift, a gallop rhythm, and a systolic pulmonic click. A pansystolic murmur, which intensifies on inspiration, may indicate tricuspid insufficiency. The patient with cor pulmonale may also experience fluctuating levels of drowsiness and consciousness. Diagnosis of the condition may be confirmed by measurements of pulmonary artery pressure by pulmonary artery catheterization. Systolic pressures of the right ventricle and the pulmonary arteries are usually more than 30 mm Hg in cor pulmonale, and the diastolic pressure of the pulmonary arteries is usually more than 15 mm Hg. Other diagnostic indicators commonly associated with this condition are an echocardiograph or an angiograph indicating right ventricular enlargement, a chest x ray showing large pulmonary arteries, and arterial oxygen pressure of less than 70 mm Hg and not more than 90 mm Hg. The EKG with cor pulmonale frequently shows arrhythmias, as ventricular and premature atrial contractions, and may also show right bundle branch block, right axis deviation, pronounced P waves and inverted T wave in the right precordial leads, and hypertrophy of the right ventricle. The hematocrit in cor pulmonale is often greater than 50 per cent.

■ INTERVENTION: The treatment of cor pulmonale seeks to reduce hypoxia, increase exercise tolerance, and correct the functional defect whenever possible. The prognosis is usually poor, because cor pulmonale commonly develops as the result of chronic obstructive pulmonary disease and other irreversible conditions. Treatment includes bed rest, the administration of digitalis glycoside, antibiotics to fight any respiratory infection, oxygen therapy, low-salt diet, restricted fluid intake, diuretics, and anticoagulants. Oxygen may be administered by mask or by cannula in concentrations from 24 to 40 per cent, depending on arterial oxygen pressure. A tracheotomy may be performed to open an obstructed upper airway, and mechanical ventilation may be used in acute cases. A phlebotomy may be performed to reduce red cell mass.

■ NURSING CONSIDERATIONS: Nursing care in the treatment of cor pulmonale commonly requires careful diet planning with frequent small meals, because the patient may tire easily during regular feedings. The nurse often helps to prevent edema by limiting the daily fluid intake of the patient to between 1,000 and 2,000 ml. It is important to monitor closely the serum potassium levels of the patient receiving diuretics, since low-serum potassium levels can increase the risk of arrthymias associated with digitalis. Digitalis toxicity is often a danger and may be indicated by anorexia, nausea, vomiting, and the observance by the patient of yellow halos surrounding visual images. Nurses commonly instruct the patient to check the radial pulse before ingesting any digitalis glycoside and to report any changes in pulse rate. The frequent repositioning of bed patients with cor pulmonale helps to prevent atelectasis. The nursing responsibility also usually includes respiratory care, including oxygen therapy, the periodic measuring of arterial blood gases, and monitoring for signs of respiratory failure, pulse rate changes, labored respirations, and exertional fatigue levels. Before the patient is discharged from the hospital, nurses instruct the patient on personal maintenance, especially the detection of pitting edema of the extremities. The cor pulmonale patient being discharged can also benefit from instructions about breathing exercises, the importance of reporting early signs of infection, the dangers of mingling with crowds, especially during the flu season, and the danger of using nonprescribed medications, especially sedatives which can depress the ventilatory drive.

corpus (kɔr′pəs), *pl.* **corpora.** See **body.**

corpuscle, corpuscule, (in anatomy) **1.** any cell of the body. **2.** a red or white blood cell. — **corpuscular,** *adj.*

corpus luteum, *pl.* **corpora lutea.** an anatomical structure on the surface of the ovary, consisting of a spheroid of yellowish tissue 1 to 2 cm in diameter that grows within the ruptured ovarian follicle following ovulation. The pleated wall of the collapsed follicle is made up of several layers of granulosa cells that grow toward the center of the cavity to form the structure. During the reproductive years of a woman's life, a corpus luteum forms after every ovulation. It acts as a short-lived endocrine organ that secretes progesterone which serves to maintain the decidual layer of the endometrium in the richly vascular state necessary for implantation and pregnancy. If conception occurs, the corpus luteum grows and secretes increasing amounts of progesterone. It reaches its maximum function and size (2 to 3 cm) at 10 to 12 weeks of gestation. It persists, slowly diminishing in size, and function until 6 months after the onset of gestation. During the two weeks prior to menstruation, the corpus luteum secretes progesterone in decreasing amounts, atrophies, undergoes fibrotic degeneration, and becomes a pale spot (corpus albicans) on the surface of the ovary.

corpus vitreum. See **vitreous humor.**

corrective exercise, a program of physical therapy to restore normal function to diseased, defective, or injured parts of the body. Also called **therapeutic exercise.** See also **exercise, osteopathy.**

correlation, (in statistics) a relationship between variables that may be negative (inverse), positive, or curvilinear. Correlation is measured and expressed using numerical scales.

correlative differentiation, (in embryology) specialization or diversification of cells or tissues caused by an inductor or other external factor. Also called **dependent differentiation.**

Corrigan's pulse, a bounding pulse in which a great surge is felt followed by a sudden and complete absence of force or fullness in the artery. This kind of pulse occurs in excited emotional states, in various abnormal cardiac conditions, including patent ductus arteriosus, and as a result of systemic arteriosclerosis.

corrosion of surgical instruments, the rusting of surgical instruments or the gradual wearing away of their polished surfaces owing to oxidation and the action of contaminants. Though minimized by the use of stainless steel alloys in the fabrication of the instruments, corrosion persists as a problem, even when cleaning procedures seem more than adequate. It usually occurs because of inadequate cleaning and drying of surgical instruments after use, the use of sterilizing solutions that eat into the surface, overexposure to such solutions, or a faulty autoclave. Cleanliness is the single most important factor in preventing corrosion. Any foreign material, either organic or inorganic, on the surface of stainless steel is likely to promote corrosion, and microscopic examinations often reveal foreign material and chlorides from cleaning solutions scattered over the surface of cleaned and sterilized instruments. A good soap and rubbing is required and a soft brush is often needed. Instruments must then be rinsed and dried. Instruments must be disassembled after use and thoroughly cleaned and dried before they are reassembled. Assembled instruments will corrode if they are stored with trapped moisture. An efficient method of removing corrosive products from inaccessible places on an instrument is to soak it in a mixture of equal parts of ethyl alcohol and aqueous ammonia. After soaking in this solution for about 12 hours, corrosive products may be rinsed or lightly brushed away. Polishing in the manufacturing process of surgical instruments is one of the steps that reduces corrosion. Box locks often corrode because they are more inaccessible than other parts of surgical instruments and their intersurfaces are not polished. Certain quaternary ammonium chlorides are effective cold sterilizing agents because they are both potent germicides and powerful detergents. The chloride ions in such compounds are corrosive. Corrosion during autoclaving will occur if the autoclave is not functioning properly, if corrosive materials are in contact with the instruments, or if tap water instead of distilled water is used to generate steam. Also, autoclaves in which a lot of corrosion occurs may have leaking valves. The bleaches and detergents remaining in laundered cloths and wrappings for autoclaving instruments may also cause corrosion, their chemical activity increased by high autoclave temperatures. The more chromium in the stainless steel alloys of which surgical instruments are made, the more resistant the instruments to corrosion. Carbon, which hardens such alloys, also reduces their resistance to corrosion. Most corrosion of surgical instruments is superficial and may be removed by soaking in a solution of ammonia and alcohol or by repolishing by the manufacturer.

corrosive, 1. eating away a substance or tissue, especially by chemical action. 2. an agent or substance that eats away a substance or tissue. —**corrode,** v., **corrosion,** n.

corrosive gastritis, an acute inflammatory condition of the stomach caused by the ingestion of an acid, alkali, or other corrosive chemical in which the lining of the stomach is eaten away by the corrosive substance. The amount of tissue destruction and recommended treatment depend on the nature of the corrosive agent and the extent of exposure. Compare **chemical gastritis, erosive gastritis.** See also **acid poisoning, alkali poisoning.**

corrugator (kor'yugei'tər). See **corrugator supercilii.**

corrugator supercilii, one of the three muscles of the eyelid. Arising from the medial end of the supercilliary arch and inserting into the skin above the orbital arch, it is innervated by temporal and zygomatic branches of the facial nerve and functions to draw the eyebrow downward and inward, as if to frown. Also called **corrugator.** Compare **levator palpebrae superioris, orbicularis oculi.**

Cortef, a trade name for a glucocorticoid (cortisol).

Cortef Acetate, a trade name for a glucocorticoid (cortisol acetate).

Cortef Fluid, a trade name for a glucocorticoid (cortisol cypionate).

cortex (kor'teks), *pl.* **cortices** (kor'tısiz). the outer layer of a body organ or other structure, as distinguished from the internal substance.

cortic-, a combining form meaning 'pertaining to the cortex or bark': *corticipetal, corticobulbar, corticothalamic.*

cortical apraxia. See **motor apraxia.**

cortical audiometry. See **audiometry.**

cortical blindness, blindness that results from a lesion in the visual center of the cerebral cortex of the brain.

cortical fracture, any fracture that involves the cortex of the bone.

cortical substance of cerebellum. See **cerebellar cortex.**

corticosteroid (kor'tıkoustir'oid), any one of the natural or the synthetic hormones associated with the adrenal cortex, which influences or controls key processes of the body, as carbohydrate and protein metabolism, electrolyte and water balance, and the functions of the cardiovascular system, the skeletal muscle, the kidneys, and other organs. The corticosteroids synthesized by the adrenal glands include the glucocorticoids and the mineralocorticoids. The principal glucocorticoids are cortisol and corticosterone. The only physiologically important mineralocorticoid in humans is aldosterone. The glucocorticoids tend to cause the cells of the body to shift from carbohydrate catabolism to fat catabolism, to accelerate the breakdown of proteins to amino acids, and to help maintain normal blood pressure. The secretion of these hormones increases during stress, especially that produced by anxiety and severe injury. Chronic overproduction of these substances is associated with various disorders, as Cushing's syndrome. A high blood-level of glucocorticoids markedly increases the number of eosinophils and decreases the size of lymphatic tissues, especially the thymus and the lymph nodes. The decrease in lymphocytes retards antibody formation and affects the immune system of the body. Aldosterone is the most powerful of the natural mineralocorticoids in the regulation of electrolyte balance, especially in the balance of sodium and potassium. Cortisol induces sodium retention and potassium excretion but not as effectively as aldosterone. The effects of the corticosteroids on the cardiovascular system, which are not precisely understood, are most evident in hypocorticism when the reduction in blood volume, accompanied by increased viscosity, may cause hypotension and cardiovascular collapse. The absence of corticosteroids increases capillary permeability, decreases the vasomotor response of the small vessels, and reduces cardiac size and output. The skeletal muscles require adequate amounts of the corticosteroids to function normally; excessive amounts cause them to function abnormally. Cortisol and its synthetic analogs can prevent or reduce inflammation by inhibiting edema, leukocytic migration, disposition of collagen, and other complications associated with inflammatory processes. The anti-inflammatory powers of synthetic hormones can be dangerous, however, because they mask the disease process and prevent accurate observation of its progress. Pharmacological doses of glucocorticosteroids retard bone growth of children and inhibit cell division in various developing structures, as the gastric mucosa, liver, lung, and brain. Glucocorticoids are absorbed from sites of local application, as synovial spaces, the conjunctival sac, and the skin. When large areas of the skin are involved or when the administration is prolonged, absorption may cause systemic effects, including adrenocortical suppression. Corticosteroids may be administered orally, parenterally, or topically. Toxic effects may result from the too rapid withdrawal of such drugs after prolonged therapy or from the continued use of large doses. Toxic effects associated with prolonged corticosteroid therapy include fluid and electrolyte imbalance, hyperglycemia and glycosuria, increased susceptibility to infections, myopathy, arrested growth, ecchymoses, Cushing's syndrome, acne, and behavioral disturbances. The increased susceptibility to infection associated with corticosteroids is not specific for any particular pathogen, and those patients who develop infections while undergoing corticosteroid therapy are usually treated concomitantly with appropriate antibacterial agents. Peptic ulceration occurs in some patients undergoing corticosteroid therapy, and some patients receiving large doses of these drugs develop myopathy, characterized by weakness of the proximal musculature of the arms and the legs and of associated shoulder and pelvic muscles. Corticosteroid therapy may also produce behavioral changes, as schizophrenia, suicidal tendencies, nervousness, and insomnia.

corticotropin (kor'tıkətrou'pin). See **adrenocorticotropic hormone.**

cortisol, a steroid hormone occurring naturally in the body and produced synthetically for pharmacologic use. Also called **hydrocortisone.**

■ INDICATION: It is prescribed as an anti-inflammatory agent.

■ CONTRAINDICATIONS: Fungal infections or known hypersensitivity to this drug prohibits its systemic use. Viral or fungal infections of the skin, impaired circulation, or known hypersensitivity to this drug prohibits its topical use.

■ ADVERSE EFFECTS: Among the more serious adverse reactions to the systemic administration of this drug are gastrointestinal, endocrine, neurologic, fluid, and electrolyte disturbances. A variety of hypersensitivity reactions may occur from topical administration of this drug.

cortisone, a glucocorticoid.

■ INDICATION: It is prescribed as an anti-inflammatory agent.

■ CONTRAINDICATIONS: Fungal infections or known hypersensitivity to this drug prohibits its systemic use. Viral or fungal infections of the skin, impaired circulation, or known hypersensitivity to this drug prohibits its topical use.

■ ADVERSE EFFECTS: Among the more serious adverse reactions to the systemic administration of the drug are gastrointestinal, endocrine, neurologic, fluid, and electrolyte disturbances. A variety of skin reactions may occur from topical administration of this drug.

Corti's organ (kɔr'tiz), a small, spiral structure within the cochlea of the internal ear, containing hair cells in contact with the acoustic nerve. Also called **spiral organ of Corti.**

Cortisporin, a trade name for a topical fixed-combination drug containing a glucocorticoid (hydrocortisone) and three antibacterials (neomycin sulfate, polymyxin B sulfate, and gramicidin).

Corynebacterium (kɔr'ınibæktir'iəm), a common genus of rod-shaped, curved bacilli having many species. The most common pathogenic species is *Corynebacterium diphtheriae,* the cause of diphtheria.

coryza (kərai'zə). See **rhinitis.**

coryza spasmodica. See **hay fever.**

Cosmegen, a trade name for an antineoplastic (dactinomycin).

cosmetic surgery, reconstruction of cutaneous or underlying tissues of the face and neck, performed to correct a structural defect, remove a scar, birthmark, or some normal evidence of aging. A local anesthetic is usually sufficient. Kinds of cosmetic surgery include **rhinoplasty, rhytidoplasty.** Compare **plastic surgery.**

cosmic radiation, high-energy particles with great penetrating power originating in outer space and reaching the earth as normal background radiation. The rays consist partly of high-energy atomic nuclei.

cost-. See **costi-.**

costal cartilage. See **cartilage.**

cost analysis, an analysis of the disbursements of a given activity, agency, department, or program.

cost-benefit ratio, a ratio that represents the relationship of the cost of an activity to the benefit of its outcome or product.

cost cap, *Informal.* a limit on the amount of money that an agency, department, or institution may spend.

cost center, a department, division, or other subunit of an institution established within its accounting system so that the income and expenses of the subunit can be separated from the income or expenses of other centers and monitored for cost and benefit.

cost control, the process of monitoring and regulating of the expenditure of funds by an agency or institution. Budgets, reports, and cost-accounting procedures are performed to achieve cost control.

cost effectiveness, the extent to which an activity is thought to be as valuable as it is expensive, as a public assistance program that gives vouchers for nutritious foods in pregnancy would be shown to be cost effective if it were to prevent the costly incidence of perinatal morbidity.

Costen's syndrome (kos'tənz). See **temporomandibular joint pain-dysfunction syndrome.**

costi-, cost-, costo-, a combining form meaning 'pertaining to a rib': *costicartillage, costicervical, costifluous.*

costochondral (kos'təkon'drəl), of or pertaining to a rib and its cartilage.

costotransverse articulation, any one of 20 gliding joints between the ribs and associated vertebrae, except for the eleventh and twelfth ribs. The five ligaments that associate with each costotransverse joint are the articular capsule, the superior costotransverse ligament, the posterior costotransverse ligament, the ligament of the neck of the rib, and the ligament of the tubercle of the rib.

costovertebral (kos'touvər'təbrəl), of or relating to a rib and the vertebral column.

costovertebral angle (CVA), one of two angles that outline a space over the kidneys. The angle is formed by the lateral and downward curve of the lowest rib and the vertical column of the spine itself. CVA tenderness to percussion is a common finding in pyelonephritis and other infections of the kidney and adjacent structures.

Cotazym, a trade name for an enzyme (pancrelipase).

cot death. See **sudden infant death syndrome.**

cotton-mill fever. See **byssinosis.**

cottonmouth, a poisonous pit viper commonly found near water and swamps of the southeastern part of the United States. The first symptoms of the bite of a cottonmouth are swelling, edema, and pain. Antivenin and oxygen are the usual treatments. Also called **water moccasin.**

Cotton's fracture, a trimalleolar fracture involving medial, lateral, and posterior malleoli.

cotyloid cavity. See **acetabulum.**

cough, a sudden, audible expulsion of air from the lungs. Coughing is preceded by inspiration, the glottis is partially closed, and the accessory muscles of expiration contract to expel the air forcibly from the respiratory passages. Coughing is an essential protective response that serves to clear the lungs, bronchi, or trachea of irritants and secretions or to prevent aspiration of foreign material into the lungs. It is a common symptom of diseases of the chest and larynx. Chronic coughing may be indicative of tuberculosis, lung cancer, bronchiectasis, or bronchitis. Otitis medea, subdiaphragmatic irritation, congestive heart failure, and mitral valve disease may be associated with episodes of severe chronic coughing. Coughing is a reflex action which may be induced voluntarily and, to some extent, voluntarily inhibited. The cough reflex center is located in the medulla of the brain.

It responds to stimulation transmitted by the glossopharyngeal or vagus nerve. The reflex is initiated by chemical or mechanical irritation of the pharynx, larynx or tracheobronchial tree. Since the function of coughing is to clear the respiratory tract of secretions, it is important that the cough bring out accumulated debris. Where it does not, because of weakness or inhibition of the force of the cough because of pain, instruction and assistance in effective coughing and deep-breathing exercises are required. Persons with chronic coughs may obtain symptomatic relief through environmental controls that reduce irritants in the air and provide humidification. Medication may be supplied to dilate the bronchi, liquefy secretions, and increase expectoration. Rest, increased fluid intake, and adequate nutrition are necessary. Antitussive medications are sometimes prescribed in the treatment of a cough in the absence of mucus or congestion.

cough fracture, any fracture of a rib, usually the fifth or the seventh rib, caused by violent coughing.

coulomb (ku'loum), the meter-per-kilogram-per-second unit of electricity equal to the quantity of charge transferred in one second across a conductor in which there is a constant current of one ampere.

Coulomb's law, (in physics) a law stating that the force of attraction or repulsion between two electrically charged bodies is directly proportional to the strength of the electrical charges and inversely proportional to the square of the distance between them.

Coulter counter (koul'tər), a trade name for an electrical device that rapidly identifies, sorts, and counts the various kinds of cells present in a small specimen of blood.

Coumadin, a trade name for an anticoagulant (warfarin sodium).

coumarin, an anticoagulant.
- INDICATIONS: It is prescribed for prophylaxis and treatment of thrombosis and embolism.
- CONTRAINDICATIONS: Known hypersensitivity to the drug prohibits its use. It is not used in situations where there is a risk of hemorrhage.
- ADVERSE EFFECTS: The most serious adverse reaction is hemorrhage. Many other drugs interact with this drug to increase or decrease its effect.

count, a computation of the number of objects or elements present per unit of measurement. Kinds of counts include **Addis count, bacteria count, blood count, platelet count.**

counterclaim, (in law) a claim made by a defendant establishing a cause for action in his favor against the plaintiff. The purpose of a counterclaim is to oppose or detract from the plaintiff's claim or complaint.

countertraction, a force that counteracts the pull of traction, especially in orthopedics, as the force of body weight owing to the pull of gravity. Orthopedic counter-traction may also be obtained by altering the angle of the body force in relation to the pull of traction, as by elevating the foot of the bed with shock blocks to attain the Trendelenburg's position. The magnitude of countertraction depends on the amount of force needed to counteract the pull of the traction and is usually developed gradually by methodically changing the position of a patient and by adding or by removing weights from weight hangers.

countertransference, the conscious or unconscious emotional response of a psychotherapist or psychoanalyst to a patient. See also **transference.**

coup (ku), any blow or stroke or the effects of such a blow to the body, usually used with a French word identifying a type of stroke: **1. coup de sabre,** a wound resembling a sword cut. **2. coup de soleil.** See **sunstroke. 3. coup sur coup,** administration of a drug in small amounts over a short period of time rather than in a single larger dose. **4. contre coup,** an injury most often associated with a blow to the skull in which the force of the impact is transmitted through the skull bones to the opposite side of the head where the bruise, fracture, or other sign of injury appears.

coupling, 1. the act of coming together, joining or pairing. 2. (in genetics) the situation in linked inheritance in which the nonalleles of two or more mutant genes are located on the same chromosome and are close enough so that they are likely to be inherited together. Compare **repulsion.** See also **cis configuration.**

Courvoisier's law (kurvwa'zieiz), a law stating that the gall bladder is smaller than usual if a gallstone blocks the common bile duct and that it is dilated if the common bile duct is blocked owing to a cause other than a gallstone, as cancer of the pancreas.

Couvelaire uterus (ku'vəleir), a hemorrhagic process in uterine musculature that may accompany severe abruptio placenta. Extravasated blood effuses between the muscle fibrils and under the uterine peritoneum. The uterus takes on a purplish color and does not contract well. Also called **uteroplacental apoplexy.** See also **abruptio placenta.**

Cowling's rule, a method of calculating the approximate pediatric dosage of a drug for a child using the formula: (age at next birthday/24) × adult dose. See **Clark's rule.**

Cowper's gland (kau'pərz), either of two round, pea-sized glands embedded in the urethral sphincter of the male. Normally yellow in color, they consist of several lobes with ducts that join and form a single excretory duct. Also called **bulbourethral gland.** Compare **Bartholin's gland.**

cowpox, a mild infectious disease characterized by a pustular rash, caused by the vaccinia virus transmitted to humans from infected cattle. Cowpox infection usually confers immunity to smallpox, owing to the similarity of the variola and vaccinia viruses. See also **smallpox, vaccinia, variola.**

coxa (kok′sə), *pl.* **coxae.** the head of the femur and the acetabulum of the innominate bone; the hip joint.

coxa adducta. See **coxa vara.**

coxa flexa. See **coxa vara.**

coxal articulation, the ball-and-socket joint of the hip, formed by the articulation of the head of the femur into the cup-shaped cavity of the acetabulum. It involves seven ligaments and permits very extensive movements, as flexion, extension, adduction, abduction, circumduction, and rotation. Also called **hip joint.** Compare **shoulder joint.**

coxa magna, an abnormal widening of the head and neck of the femur.

coxa plana. See **Perthes' disease.**

coxa valga, a hip deformity in which the angle formed by the axis of the head and neck of the femur and the axis of its shaft is significantly increased.

coxa vara, a hip deformity in which the angle formed by the axis of the head and neck of the femur and the axis of its shaft is decreased. Also called **coxa adducta, coxa flexa.**

coxa vara luxans, a fissure or crack in the neck of the femur with dislocation of the head, caused by coxa vara.

coxsackievirus (kuksa′ki), any of 30 serologically different enteroviruses associated with a variety of symptoms and primarily affecting children during warm weather. The coxsackieviruses resemble the virus responsible for poliomyelitis, particularly in size; both are picornaviruses. Among the diseases associated with coxsackievirus infections are herpangina, hand, foot, and mouth disease, epidemic pleurodynia, myocarditis, pericarditis, aseptic meninigitis, and several exanthems. There is no known preventive measure except isolation of infected persons, and the treatment is generally directed toward relief of symptoms. See also **viral infection.**

CPAP, abbreviation for **continuous positive airway pressure.**

CPD, 1. abbreviation for **cephalopelvic disproportion.** 2. abbreviation for **childhood polycystic disease.** See **polycystic kidney disease.** 3. abbreviation for **congenital polycystic disease.** See **polycystic kidney disease.**

CPHA, abbreviation for the **Canadian Public Health Association.**

CPK, abbreviation for *creatinine phosphokinase.* See **Duchenne's muscular dystrophy.**

CPPB, abbreviation for **continuous positive pressure breathing.**

CPPV, abbreviation for **continuous positive pressure ventilation.**

CPR, abbreviation for **cardiopulmonary resuscitation.**

CPRAM, abbreviation for *controlled partial rebreathing anesthesia method.*

CPT, abbreviation for **current procedural terminology.**

Cr, symbol for **chromium.**

CR, abbreviation for *controlled respiration.*

crab louse, a species of body louse, *Phthirus pubis,* that infests the hairs of the genital area and is often transmitted between persons by venereal contact. Also called *Pediculosis pubis, Informal.* **crab.** See also **pediculosis.**

cradle cap, a common seborrheic dermatitis of infants consisting of thick, yellow, greasy scales on the scalp. Treatment includes oil or ointment to soften the scales and frequent shampoos.

cramp, 1. a spasmodic and often painful contraction of one or more muscles. 2. a pain resembling a muscular cramp. Kinds of cramps include **cane-cutter's cramp, fireman's cramp, miner's cramp, stoker's cramp, writer's cramp.** See also **charley horse, dysmenorrhea, heat cramp, wryneck.**

-crania, a combining form meaning '(condition of the) skull or head': *diastematocrania, hemicrania, platycrania.*

cranial arachnoid. See **arachnoid membrane.**

cranial arteritis. See **temporal arteritis.**

cranial nerves, the twelve pairs of nerves emerging from the cranial cavity through various openings in the skull. Beginning with the most anterior they are designated by Roman numerals and named (I) olfactory, (II) optic, (III) oculomotor, (IV) trochlear, (V) trigeminal, (VI) abducens, (VII) facial, (VIII) acoustic, (IX) glossopharyngeal, (X) vagus, (XI) accessory, (XII) hypoglossal. The cranial nerves are attached to the base of the brain and carry impulses for such functions as smell, vision, ocular movement, pupil contraction, muscular sensibility, general sensibility, mastication, facial expression, glandular secretion, taste, cutaneous sensibility, hearing, equilibrium, swallowing, phonation, tongue movement, head movement, and shoulder movement. Certain cranial nerves, particularly V, VII, and VIII, contain two or more distinct functional components considered as independent nerves by some authorities. In this category the masticatory nerve would be separated from the trigeminal (V), the glossopalatine from the facial (VII), and the equilibratory from the acoustic (VIII), making 15 pairs in all. Some anatomists also classify the terminal nerve as the first cranial. A short couplet is a common aid for memorizing the names of the 12 cranial nerves in proper sequence, the first letter of each word in the couplet corresponding to the first letter of the appropriate nerve: On old Olympus' towering top/A Finn and German viewed a hop. Also called **cerebral nerves.** See also specific nerve.

cranio-, a combining form meaning 'pertaining to the skull or cranium': *craniobuccal, craniognomy, craniosacral.*

craniocele (krei′niousil′). See **encephalocele.**

craniodidymus, a two-headed fetal twin monster in which the bodies are fused.

craniofacial dysostosis, an abnormal hereditary condi-

Surface anatomy   Sensory nuclei   Motor nuclei

CRANIAL NERVES

see p 394 Taber's (Edition 15)

tion characterized by acrocephaly, exophthalmos, hypertelorism, strabismus, parrot-beaked nose, and hypoplastic maxilla with relative mandibular prognathism. This condition is transmitted as an autosomal dominant trait. See also **dysostosis.**

craniohypophyseal xanthoma (krei′niouhai′poufiz′iəl), a condition in which cholesterol deposits are formed around the hypophyses of the bones, as in Hand-Schüller-Christian disease.

craniopagus (krei′niop′əgəs), conjoined twins that are united at the heads. Fusion can occur at either the frontal, occipital, or parietal regions. Also called **cephalopagus.**

craniopharyngeal (krei′nioufərın′jiəl), of or pertaining to the cranium and the pharynx.

craniopharyngeal duct tumor. See **craniopharyngioma.**

craniopharyngioma (krei′nioufərın′jiou′mə), *pl.* **craniopharyngiomas, craniopharyngiomata.** a congenital pituitary tumor, appearing most often in children and adolescents, that arises in cells derived from Rathke's pouch or the hypophyseal stalk. The lesion, a solid or cystic body ranging in size from 1 to 8 cm, may expand into the third ventricle or the temporal lobe, frequently becoming calcified. The tumor may interfere with pituitary function, damage the optic chiasm, disrupt hypothalamic control of the autonomic nervous system, and result in hydrocephalus. Increased intracranial pressure, severe headaches,

vomiting, stunted growth, defective vision, irritability, somnolence, and infantile genitalia are often associated with the lesion in children. Development of the tumor after puberty usually results in amenorrhea in women and loss of libido and potency in men. Also called **ameloblastoma, craniopharyngeal duct tumor, pituitary adamantoma, Rathke's pouch tumor.**

craniostenosis (krei′nioustənou′sis), a congenital deformity of the skull resulting from premature closure of the sutures between the cranial bones. The severity of the malformation depends on which sutures close, at what point in the developmental process the closure occurred, and the success or failure of the other sutures to compensate by expansion. Impaired brain growth may or may not be involved. The most common form of the condition is permanent closure of the sagittal suture with anteroposterior elongation of the skull. Surgery is generally indicated when multiple sutures are fused in order to relieve cerebral pressure and may be performed for cosmetic reasons. See also **brachycephaly, oxycephaly, plagiocephaly, scaphocephaly.** – **craniostenotic,** *adj.*

craniostosis (krei′niostou′sis), premature ossification of the sutures of the skull, often associated with other skeletal defects. The sutures close before or soon after birth. If not surgically corrected, the growth of the skull is inhibited, the head is deformed, and the eyes and brain are often damaged. Also called **craniosynostosis.**

craniosynostosis (krei'niousai'nəstou'sis). See **craniostosis.**

craniotabes (krei'nioutei'biz), benign, congenital thinness of the top and back of the skull of a newborn, common because the rate of brain growth exceeds the rate of calcification of the skull during the last month of gestation. The bones feel brittle when pressed by an examiner's fingers. The condition disappears with normal nutrition and growth but may persist in infants who develop rickets.

craniotomy (krei'niot'əmi), any surgical opening into the skull, performed to relieve intracranial pressure, to control bleeding, or to remove a tumor. X rays of the skull are taken preoperatively and a CAT scan or an electroencephalogram is done to establish the diagnosis. The entire head is shaved and cleansed. Parenteral corticosteroids are given to reduce cerebral edema; mannitol and urea are administered to promote diuresis and decrease intercranial pressure. Narcotics are not given, as they depress cerebral function. Neuroleptic drugs that sedate but do not narcotize the patient may be combined with local anesthesia, or general anesthesia may be given. A semicircular skin incision is made just above the hairline, a series of burr holes are made and connected with a cut, and the flap of bone is removed. The meninges are incised, and the brain is exposed. The flap may be replaced after surgery or left off temporarily to prevent the build-up of pressure from the cerebral edema. Postoperatively, if the cerebral area is involved, the head of the patient's bed is elevated to 45° to reduce the risk of hemorrhage and edema; if the cerebellum or brain stem is affected the patient is kept flat. The dressing is checked frequently for yellowish drainage of cerebrospinal fluid. Any moist areas are reinforced with sterile materials to avoid infection. Frequent observation of neurologic signs, including the level of consciousness, speech, and strength, is essential.

cranium (krei'niəm), the bony skull that holds the brain. It is composed of eight bones: frontal, occipital, sphenoid, and ethmoid bones, and paired temporal and parietal bones. – **cranial,** *adj.*

-cranium, a combining form meaning 'referring to the skull': *chondrocranium, desmocranium, endocranium.*

crankcase spool catheter, a special, elastic catheter stored within a plastic spool to facilitate its insertion, especially for hyperalimentation. Most experts recommend the indirect method of venipuncture for insertion of this kind of catheter, usually into a peripheral vein that connects with the subclavian vein. When fully inserted, the crankcase spool catheter is usually lodged in the subclavian vein. The catheter is highly flexible and each revolution of the crankcase spool feeds about five inches of the catheter into the vein involved. When the crankcase spool catheter is fully inserted, an x-ray exposure is made of the insertion area to confirm its correct placement. The venipuncture site for insertion is prepared, dressed, and taped in the same manner as any other venipuncture site. The crankcase spool catheter is less irritating than a regular catheter, allows greater limb movement, and minimizes the risk of thrombosis. It may, however, cause complications, as occlusion, phlebitis, infection, and catheter sensitivity. Occlusion of the vein, a common risk, is usually countered by flushing the vein with dilute streptokinase. If the patient develops phlebitis and receives proper treatment, the catheter may be left in place. Infection, usually evidenced by purulent drainage at the insertion site, is accompanied by an elevated white blood cell count. In cases of such infection the attending physician may order an antibiotic or the removal of the catheter. Catheter sensitivity, evidenced by fever and phlebitis, may require removal of the catheter.

crash cart, a cart carrying emergency equipment, as analgesics, antiseptics, suction devices, sutures, scalpels, surgical needles, sponges, swabs, retractors, hemostats, forceps, trachea tubes, and often a defibrillator. Hospital emergency rooms and intensive care units usually have several crash carts equipped according to prescribed specifications. Efficient, effective emergency care often depends on the careful provisioning of crash carts and the precise knowledge of their layouts.

-crasia, 1. a combining form meaning '(condition of a) mixture, good or bad': *eucrasia, orthocrasia, spermacrasia.* 2. a combining form meaning a '(specified) condition involving loss of control': *copracrasia, uracrasia.*

-cratia, a combining form meaning '(condition of) incontinence': *scatacratia, scoracratia, uracratia.*

cravat bandage, a triangular bandage, folded lengthwise. It may be used as a circular, figure-of-eight, or spiral bandage to control bleeding or to tie splints in place.

crawling reflex. See **symmetric tonic neck reflex.**

C-reactive protein (CRP), a protein not normally detected in the serum but present in many acute inflammatory conditions and with necrosis. CRP appears in the serum before the erythrocyte sedimentation rate begins to rise, often within 24 to 48 hours of the onset of inflammation. After a myocardial infarction, it is present in 24 hours, begins to fall three days later, and is absent after two weeks. Acute rheumatic fever is monitored with serial estimations of CRP, as the serum level of the protein is the most sensitive indicator of rheumatic activity. Bacterial infections and widespread neoplastic disease are also associated with C-reactive protein in the serum. CRP disappears when an inflammatory process is suppressed by salicylates and steroids, or both. Also called **serum C-reactive protein.**

cream, 1. the portion of milk rich in butterfat. 2. any fluid mixture of thick consistency. Creams are often used as a method of applying medication to the surface of the body. Compare **ointment**.

crease, an indentation or margin formed by a doubling back of tissue, as the folds or creases on the palm of the hand and sole of the foot.

creat-, a combining form meaning 'pertaining to flesh': *creaton, creatorrhea, creatotoxism.*

creatine (kri'ətin, kri'ətin), an important nitrogenous compound produced by metabolic processes in the body. Combined with phosphorus it forms high-energy phosphate. In normal metabolic reactions the phosphorus is yielded to combine with a molecule of adenosine diphosphate to produce a molecule of the very high energy molecule adenosine triphosphate. See also **creatinine**.

creatine kinase, an enzyme in muscle, brain, and other tissues that catalyzes the transfer of a phosphate group from adenosine triphosphate to creatine, producing adenosine diphosphate and phosphocreatine.

creatinine (kriæt'min, kriæt'inin), a substance formed from the metabolism of creatine, commonly found in blood, urine, and muscle tissue. See also **creatine**.

creatinine phosphokinase (CPK). See **Duchenne's muscular dystrophy.**

creeping eruption, a skin lesion characterized by irregular, wandering red lines made by the burrowing larvae of hookworms and certain roundworms. The nurse instructs people not to walk barefoot where these parasites are known to be endemic. Antiparasitic treatment is specific to the organism. Also called **larva migrans.**

cremaster (krımæs'tər), a thin, muscular layer spreading out over the spermatic cord in a series of loops. It is a continuation of the obliquus internus. The muscle arises from the inguinal ligament and inserts into the crest of the pubis and into the sheath of the rectus abdominis. It is innervated by the genital branch of the genitofemoral nerve and functions to draw the testis up toward the superficial inguinal ring in response to cold or to stimulation of the nerve.

cremasteric reflex, a superficial neural reflex elicited by stroking the skin of the upper inner aspect of the thigh in a male. This normally results in a brisk retraction of the testis on the side of the stimulus. The reflex is lost in diseases of the pyramidal tract above the level of the first lumbar vertebra. See also **superficial reflex.**

crenation (krınei'shən), the formation of notches or leaflike, scalloped edges on an object. Red blood cells exposed to a hypertonic saline solution acquire a notched, shriveled surface because of the osmotic effect of the solution. They are then called crenated red blood cells. — **crenate, crenated,** *adj.*

creosote poisoning. See **phenol poisoning.**

crepitus (krep'itəs), **1.** flatulence or the noisy discharge of fetid gas from the intestine through the anus. **2.** a sound that resembles the crackling noise heard when rubbing hair between the fingers or throwing salt on an open fire. Crepitus is associated with gas gangrene, the rubbing of bone fragments, or the rales of a consolidated area of the lung in pneumonia. Also called **crepitation.**

cresc-, a combining form meaning 'to grow': *crescograph.*

CREST syndrome, acronym for **calcinosis, Raynaud's phenomenon, esophageal dysfunction, sclerodactyly,** and **telangiectasis,** which may occur for varying periods of time in patients with scleroderma.

cretin dwarf, a person in whom short stature is caused by infantile hypothyroidism and severe deficiency of thyroid hormone. Also called **hypothyroid dwarf.** See also **cretinism.**

cretinism (kri'təniz'əm), a condition characterized by severe congenital hypothyroidism and often associated with other endocrine abnormalities. Typical signs of cretinism include dwarfism, mental deficiency, puffy facial features, dry skin, a large tongue, umbilical hernia, and muscular incoordination. The disorder usually occurs in areas where the diet is deficient in iodine and where goiter is endemic. Early treatment with thyroid hormone generally promotes normal physical growth but may not prevent mental retardation. The use of iodized salt dramatically reduces the incidence of cretinism in a population. The condition is rare in the United States, but in some areas, including parts of Ecuador, the Himalayas, and Zaire, more than five per cent of the people are cretins. — **cretinoid, cretinous,** *adj.,* **cretin,** *n.*

Creutzfeldt-Jakob disease (kroits'feltya'kɔb), a rare, fatal encephalopathy caused by an as yet unidentified slow virus. The disease occurs in middle age, and symptoms are progressive dementia, dysarthria, muscle wasting, and various involuntary movements, as myoclonus and athetosis. Deterioration is obvious week to week. Death ensues, usually within a year. Transmission between humans is unusual but the disease has been observed years after exposure to needles, instruments, and electrodes previously used in the treatment of a patient with the disease. Isolation is not necessary. Special care in disposal or sterilization of potentially infective items is always necessary. Also called **Jakob-Creutzfeldt disease, spastic pseudoparalysis.**

crib death. See **sudden infant death syndrome.**

cribriform carcinoma. See **adenocystic carcinoma.**

crico-, a combining form meaning 'ring': *cricoderma, cricoid, cricoidectomy.*

cricoid (krai'koid), **1.** having a ring shape. **2.** a ring-shaped cartilage connected to the thyroid cartilage by the cricothyroid ligament at the level of the sixth cervical vertebra.

cricoid pressure, a technique to reduce the risk of the aspiration of stomach contents during induction of general anesthesia. The cricoid cartilage is pushed against the esophagus to prevent passive regurgitation. The technique cannot, however, stop vomiting that has begun. Cricoid pressure is applied prior to intubation, immediately after injection of the anesthetic drug or muscle relaxant.

cricopharyngeal (krai′koufərin′jiəl), of or pertaining to the cricoid cartilage and the pharynx.

cricopharyngeal incoordination, a defect in the normal swallowing reflex. The cricopharyngeus muscle ordinarily serves as a sphincter to keep the top of the esophagus closed except when the person is swallowing, vomiting, or belching. The trachea remains open for breathing, but air normally does not enter the esophagus during respiration. In swallowing, the reverse effect occurs and the larynx is closed while food slides past it into the esophagus, which is located immediately behind the larynx. When the somewhat complex series of neuromuscular actions is not properly coordinated as a result of disease or injury, the patient may choke, swallow air, regurgitate fluid into the nose, or experience discomfort in swallowing food. See also **dysphagia.**

cricothyrotomy (krai′koufhairot′əmi), an emergency incision into the larynx, performed to open the airway in a person who is choking. A small vertical midline cut is made just below the Adam's apple and above the cricoid cartilage. The incision is opened further with a transverse cut through the cricothyroid membrane, and the wound is spread open with a knife handle or other dilator. The new opening must be held open with a tube that is open at both ends to allow air to move in and out. The cartridge end of a ballpoint pen will suffice until a tracheostomy can be done. Compare **tracheostomy.**

cri du chat syndrome (kri du sha′). See **cat-cry syndrome.**

Crigler-Najjar syndrome (krig′lərnæj′ar), a congenital, familial, autosomal anomaly, in which glucuronide transferase, an enzyme, is deficient or absent. The condition is characterized by nonhemolytic jaundice, an accumulation of unconjugated bilirubin in the blood, and severe disorders of the central nervous system.

Crimean-Congo hemorrhagic fever (kraimi′ən korg′-gou), an arbovirus infection transmitted to humans through the bite of a tick, characterized by fever, dizziness, muscle ache, vomiting, headache, and other neurologic symptoms. After several days, in severe cases, bleeding from the skin and mucous membranes, particularly from the mouth and nose, bloody sputum or vomit, and blood-tinged feces may be seen. Transfusion may be necessary to replace lost blood; otherwise, treatment is symptomatic and supportive. There is no specific medication or therapy available for prevention or cure. It occurs mainly in the U.S.S.R., Asia, and Africa; agricultural workers are most often afflicted. See also **hemorrhagic fever.**

criminal abortion, the intentional termination of pregnancy under any condition prohibited by law. See also **induced abortion.**

criminal psychology, the study of the mental processes, motivational patterns, and behavior of criminals.

crin-, a combining form meaning 'to separate': *crinin*, *crinogenic*.

-crinia, a combining form meaning '(condition of) endocrine secretion': *hemocrinia, hypercrinia, neurocrinia*.

-crisia, 1. a combining form meaning a 'diagnosis': *acrisia, urocrisia*. 2. a combining form meaning a '(specified) condition of endocrine secretion': *hypercrisia, hyperendocrisia, hypocrisia*.

crisis, 1. a turning point for better or worse in the course of a disease, usually indicated by a marked change in the intensity of signs and symptoms. A crisis may be celiac, marked by an attack of watery diarrhea and vomiting leading, in turn, to dehydration; hepatic, characterized by intense pain in the region of the liver; or ocular, manifested by eye pain, a flow of tears, and sensitivity to light. 2. a turning point in events affecting the emotional state of a person, as death or divorce. See also **crisis intervention.**

crisis intervention, (in psychiatry) therapeutic intervention to help resolve a particular and immediate problem. No attempt is made at in-depth analysis. The goal is to restore in the person the level of functioning that existed before the current crisis.

crisis-intervention unit, a group trained in emergency medical treatment and in various methods for rendering psychiatric therapeutic assistance to a person or group of persons during a period of crisis, especially instances involving suicide attempts or drug abuse. Such networks are found within community hospitals, health care centers, or as specialized self-contained units, as suicide prevention centers, and operate 24 hours a day. The primary objective of such crisis assistance is to help the person cope with the immediate problem and to offer guidance and support for long-term therapy.

crisis theory, a conceptual framework for defining and explaining the phenomena that occur when a person faces a problem that appears to be insoluble. The theory is the basis of crisis therapy.

crisscross inheritance, the acquisition of genetic characteristics or conditions from the parent of the opposite sex.

crista supraventricularis (kris′tə su′prəven′trikyular′is), the muscular ridge on the interior dorsal wall of the right ventricle of the heart. It defines the limit of the arterial cone and extends toward the pulmonary trunk from the ventral cusp of the atrioventricular ring. Compare **moderator band.**

critical care. See **intensive care.**

critical organs, tissues that are the most sensitive to irradiation, as the gonads, lymphoid organs, and intestine. The skin, cornea, oral cavity, esophagus, vagina, cervix, and optic lens are the next most sensitive organs to irradiation.

CRNA. abbreviation for **certified registered nurse anesthetist.** See **nurse anesthetist.**

Crohn's disease (krōunz), a chronic inflammatory bowel disease of unknown etiology, usually affecting the terminal segment of the small intestine, the colon, or both structures. See also **colitis, ileitis.**

■ OBSERVATIONS: Crohn's disease is characterized by frequent attacks of diarrhea, severe abdominal pain, nausea, fever, chills, weakness, anorexia, and weight loss. Children with the disease often suffer retarded physical growth. The diagnosis of Crohn's disease is based upon clinical signs, x-ray studies using a contrast medium, and endoscopy. The disease is easily confused with ulcerative colitis, an inflammatory bowel disease affecting the colon and rectum.

■ INTERVENTION: Corticosteroids, antibiotics, and anti-inflammatory agents are used to control symptoms and to attempt to induce remission. In patients who are malnourished because of the disease, intravenous hyperalimentation is used to insure adequate intake of nutrients and to rest the bowel. Surgical removal of the diseased segment of the bowel provides some relief, but recurrence after surgery is likely.

■ NURSING CONSIDERATIONS: In many cases the inflammation extends to other areas of the bowel or to the stomach, duodenum, or mouth. Other complications are arthritis, ankylosing spondylitis, kidney and liver disease, and skin and eye disorders. The formation of fistulas from the diseased bowel to the anus, vagina, skin surface, or to other loops of bowel are common. Persons with Crohn's disease are hospitalized frequently and often become depressed owing to the relentless, painful character of the disease. Continued support and encouragement are essential in helping the patient maintain a hopeful outlook.

cromolyn sodium, an antiasthmatic that acts by decreasing allergic bronchospasm resulting from an inhaled allergen.

■ INDICATION: It is prophylactically prescribed in the treatment of bronchial asthma. The drug has no effect after an attack has begun.

■ CONTRAINDICATION: Known hypersensitivity to this drug prohibits its use.

■ ADVERSE EFFECTS: Bronchospasm, wheezing, nasal congestion, pharyngeal irritation, and other hypersensitivity reactions may occur.

Cronkhite-Canada syndrome, an abnormal familial condition characterized by gastrointestinal polyposis accompanied by ectodermal defects, as nail atrophy, alopecia, and excessive skin pigmentation. In some individuals it is also accompanied by protein-losing enteropathy, malabsorption, and deficiency of blood calcium, potassium, and magnesium.

cross, (in genetics) any method of crossbreeding or any individual, organism, or strain produced from crossbreeding. Kinds of crosses include **dihybrid cross, monohybrid cross, polyhybrid cross, trihybrid cross.**

crossbreeding, the production of offspring by the mating of individuals from different races or of plants and animals from different varieties, strains, or species; hybridization. See also **inbreeding.** –**crossbred,** adj.

crossed reflex, any neural reflex in which stimulation of one side of the body results in a response on the other side, as the consensual light reflex.

cross-eye. See **esophoria.**

cross fertilization, **1.** (in zoology), the union of gametes from different species or varieties in order to form hybrids. **2.** (in botany) the fertilization of the flower of one plant by the pollen from a different plant, as opposed to self-fertilization. Also called **allogamy.**

crossing over, the exchange of sections of chromatids between homologous pairs of chromosomes during the prophase stage of the first meiotic division. The process occurs through the formation of chiasmata and results in the recombination of genes. Also called **chiasmatypy.**

crossmatching of blood, a procedure used by blood banks to determine compatibility of a donor's blood with that of a recipient after the specimens have been matched for major blood type. Serum from the donor's blood is

Comparison of Crohn's disease and ulcerative colitis

	Crohn's disease	Ulcerative colitis
General appearance	Usually normal	May feel and look ill
Age	Bimodal: 20 to 30 years and 40 to 50 years	Mostly young adults
Area affected	Mainly the terminal ileum, cecum, and ascending colon (right side)	Colon only, primarily the descending colon (left side)
Extent of involvement	Segmental areas of involvement	Continuous, diffuse areas of involvement
Inflammation	Mostly submucosal	Mostly mucosal
Mucosal appearance	Cobblestone effect, granulomas	Ulcerations
Cancer potential	Normal incidence	Increased incidence
Character of stools	No blood; may have some fat; three to four semisoft per day	Blood present; no fat; frequent liquid stools
Reasons for surgery	Fistulas; intestinal obstruction	Poor response to medical therapy; hemorrhage, perforation
Complications	Fistulas; perianal disease; strictures, vitamin and iron deficiencies; perforation, fistulas to other organs	Pseudopolyps; hemorrhage; toxic megacolon; cachexia; perforation less often, causes peritonitis

mixed with red cells from the recipient's blood, and cells from the donor are mixed with serum from the recipient. If agglutination occurs, an antigenic substance is present, and the bloods are not compatible. If no agglutination occurs, the donor's blood may safely be transfused to the recipient. Compare **blood typing.** See also **ABO blood groups, Rh factor, transfusion, transfusion reaction.**

crossover, the result of the recombination of genes on homologous pairs of chromosomes during meiosis. See also **crossing over.**

cross-sectional anatomy, the study of the relationship of the structures of the body by the examination of cross sections of the tissue or organ. Compare **surface anatomy.**

crotamiton, a scabicide.

■ INDICATIONS: It is prescribed in treating scabies and other pruritic skin diseases.

■ CONTRAINDICATION: Known hypersensitivity to this drug prohibits its use. It is not applied near the eyes or on the mouth or raw skin.

■ ADVERSE EFFECTS: Among the most serious adverse reactions are irritation and allergic reactions of the skin.

croup (krup), an acute viral infection of the upper and lower respiratory tract that occurs primarily in infants and young children aged three months to three years following an upper respiratory tract infection. It is characterized by hoarseness, fever, a distinctive harsh, brassy cough, persistent stridor during inspiration, and varying degrees of respiratory distress resulting from obstruction of the larynx. The most common causative agents are the parainfluenza viruses, especially Type 1, followed by the respiratory syncytial viruses (RSV) and influenza A and B viruses. Also called **acute laryngotracheobronchitis, angina trachealis, exudative angina, laryngostasis.** Compare **acute epiglottitis.** – croupous, croupy, *adj.*

■ OBSERVATIONS: Transmission occurs by infection with airborne particles or by contact with infected secretions. Leukocytosis with an increased proportion of polymorphonuclear cells may be present at first, followed by leukopenia and lymphocytosis. A lateral neck x ray shows subepiglottic narrowing and a normal-sized epiglottis, which differentiate the condition from acute epiglottitis. Onset of the acute stage is rapid, usually occurs at night, and may be precipitated by exposure to cold air. The child becomes irritable, develops stridor, dyspnea, tachypnea, the characteristic barking cough, and, in severe cases, cyanosis or pallor. The child's condition often improves in the morning, but it may worsen at night.

■ INTERVENTION: Routine treatment consists of bed rest, adequate fluid intake, and the alleviation of airway obstruction to ensure adequate respiratory exchange. Children with mild infections are usually managed at home with supportive measures, as vaporizers, humidifiers, or steam from hot running water in an enclosed bathroom to reduce the spasm of the laryngeal muscles and to free

secretions. Hospitalization is indicated for children with high temperatures, progressive stridor and respiratory distress, and hypoxia, cyanosis, or pallor. Endotracheal intubation and tracheostomy may be necessary. Humidity and oxygen are usually prescribed. The vital signs are continuously monitored; a change in pulse and respiration may be early signs of hypoxia and impending airway obstruction. Arterial blood gas analysis is performed. Fluids are often given intravenously to reduce physical exertion and the possibility of vomiting, with its attendant increased risk of aspiration. Corticosteroids or other drugs, as expectorants, bronchodilators, and antihistamines, are rarely used, and sedatives are contraindicated, as they exert a depressant effect on the respiratory tract. Nebulized racemic epinephrine, administered diluted with water by a face mask aerosol, may provide temporary relief in the acute phase in some children.

■ NURSING CONSIDERATIONS: The primary focus of nursing care is to ease breathing by providing humidity and to maintain continuous monitoring and surveillance for signs of respiratory distress and impending airway obstruction, with intubation and tracheostomy equipment kept readily available. To conserve the child's energy and to reduce apprehension, the nurse encourages rest, disturbs the child as little as possible, remains in constant attendance, provides comfort with a familiar toy or other device, and encourages parental involvement whenever possible. Fever is usually reduced by the cool atmosphere of the mist tent; antipyretics are given as needed. To prevent chilling, frequent changes of clothing and bed linen are often necessary in the humid environment. The nurse also explains the condition to the parents and discusses appropriate care after discharge, including continued use of humidity and ensurance of adequate hydration and proper nutrition. In most children the condition is relatively mild and runs its course in three to seven days. The infection may spread to other areas of the respiratory tract and may cause complications, as bronchiolitis, pneumonia, and otitis media. The most serious complication is laryngeal obstruction, which may cause death. If a tracheostomy is required, as may happen with a small percentage of children, other complications, as infection, atelectasis, cannula occlusion, tracheal bleeding, granulation, stenosis, and delayed healing of the stoma, may develop.

Croupette (krupet'), a trade name for a device that provides cool humidification with the administration of oxygen or of compressed air, used especially in the treatment of pediatric patients. The Croupette consists of a nebulizer with attached tubing that connects with a canopy to enclose the patient and contain the humidifying mist. The environment of the patient may be cooled by adding ice to the ice compartment or by using a Croupette with its own refrigeration unit. This device is especially used with pediatric patients from 1 month to 10 years old to relieve hypoxia, liquefy secretions, and cool the environment of the patient. It is also often used in the treatment of the croup, bronchiolitis, cystic fibrosis, asthma, laryngitis, postoperative dehydration, and hyperpyrexia. The oxygen concentration obtainable is approximately 21 per cent to 60 per cent. Nursing care associated with this device usually involves assembling the unit, ensuring proper water level in the nebulizer, and adjusting the oxygen flow rate. The flow rate may be adjusted from 6 to 10 liters per minute or according to equipment specifications. Explaining the equipment and the humidifying treatment also helps to reassure the patient involved. Precautions in using the Croupette with a patient receiving periodic therapy involve ensuring that the flow of oxygen or compressed air is turned on when the canopy is placed over the patient and that the patient is carefully monitored throughout the therapy period. Some of the advantages of the Croupette are its capability for providing a cool, moist environment, its adaptability for the delivery of oxygen or the delivery of compressed air, and the ease of canopy installation. Croupette canopies are disposable. Some of the limitations associated with the device are that some Croupette units have awkward, bulky frames; nebulizer water reservoirs are usually small and require constant refilling; periodic refills of ice are required; and excess humidity may wet the bed linen and the patient.

crown, 1. the upper part of an organ or structure, as the upper portion of a tooth. 2. an artificial restoration that replaces the natural crown of a tooth.

CRP, abbreviation for **C-reactive protein.**

crucial bandage. See **T bandage.**

cruciate ligament of the atlas, a thin, bandlike ligament attaching the atlas to the base of the occipital bone above and the posterior surface of the body of the axis below.

crude birth rate, the number of births per 1,000 people in a population during one year. Compare **birth rate, refined birth rate, true birth rate.**

crur-, a combining form meaning 'pertaining to the leg': *crura, crural, crureus.*

crura anthelicis (krur'ə ænthel'ısıs), the two ridges on the external ear marking the superior termination of the anthelix and bounding the triangular fossa. Also called **crura of anthelix.**

crureus (kruri'əs). See **vastus intermedius.**

crus (krəs), *pl.* **crura** (krur'ə). 1. the leg, from knee to foot. 2. a structure resembling a leg, as crura anthelicis, crus cerebri.

crus cerebri, the ventral part of the cerebral peduncle, composed of the descending fiber tracts passing from the cerebral cortex to form the longitudinal fascicles of the pons. Also called **basis pedunculi cerebri.**

crush syndrome, 1. a severe, life-threatening condition caused by extensive crushing trauma, characterized by destruction of muscle and bone tissue, hemorrhage, and fluid loss resulting in hypovolemic shock, hematuria, renal failure, and coma. Massive supportive therapy, with fluids, electrolytes, antibiotics, analgesia, oxygen, and intensive care with close monitoring of all vital functions are usually necessary. 2. a severe complication of heroin-induced coma characterized by edema, vascular occlusion, and lymphatic obstruction.

crutch, a wooden or metal staff, the most common kind of which reaches from the ground almost to the axilla, to aid a person in walking. A padded, curved surface at the top fits under the arm; a grip in the form of a crossbar is held in the hand at the level of the palms to support the body. It is important that the person be taught how to use the crutches safely and how to achieve a stable and acceptable gait. Kinds of crutches include **axillary crutches, forearm crutches.**

Crutchfield tongs, an instrument inserted into the skull to hyperextend the head and neck of patients with fractured cervical vertebrae.

■ METHOD: The tongs are inserted into small bur holes drilled in each parietal region of the skull; the surrounding skin is sutured and covered with a collodion dressing. A weight of from 10 to 20 lbs. is suspended from a rope extending from the center of the tongs, over a pulley attached to head of the bed allowing the weights hang freely. The insertion sites of the tongs are inspected and cleaned every one to two hours; twice a day or as required, any formed crusts are removed with hydrogen peroxide. The patient is turned and assisted in deep breathing every other hour and is given scalp and skin care every two to four hours. The bed linen is kept dry and smooth, an air mattress or sheepskin is used, and back rubs are administered to prevent decubiti, especially of the scapulae, coccyx, and heels. Passive range-of-motion exercises of all extremities are performed. Sandbags may be used to prevent the patient from sliding to the head of the bed and the call bell is placed within easy reach. The immobilized patient receives food that is easy to swallow and is fed with care to prevent aspiration into the trachea; suction apparatus is kept at the bedside as an emergency measure.

■ NURSING ORDERS: The nurse maintains the patient's body alignment, checks the weight and traction apparatus, administers meticulous skin care, feeds the patient, and provides for other care as necessary.

■ OUTCOME CRITERIA: A patient may be immobilized by Crutchfield tongs for weeks before surgery is performed; during an operation on the cervical spine and cord, the tongs may be left in place to maintain the proper alignment.

crutch gait, a gait achieved by a person on crutches by alternately bearing weight on one or both legs and on the crutches. The gait selected and learned is determined by physical and functional abilities of the patient and on the diagnosis. In a three-point gait weight is borne on the noninvolved leg, then on both crutches, then on the good leg. Touchdown and progression to full-weight bearing on the involved leg are usual. Four-point gait gives stability but requires bearing weight on both legs. Each leg is used alternately with each crutch. Two-point gait characteristically uses each crutch with the opposing leg. The swing-to and swing-through gaits are often used by paraplegic patients with weight-supporting braces on the legs. Weight is borne on the supported legs; the crutches are placed one stride in front of the person who then swings to that point or through the crutches to a spot in front of them.

Cruz trypanosomiasis (kruz). See **Chagas' disease**.

cry, 1. a sudden, loud, voluntary or automatic vocalization in response to pain, fear, or a startle reflex. 2. weeping, because of pain or as an emotional response to depression or grief. 3. See **cri du chat syndrome**.

cry-. See **cryo-**.

crymo-. See **cryo-**.

cryo-, cry-, a combining form meaning 'pertaining to cold': *cryocautery, cryophilia, cryotolerant*. Also **crymo-**.

cryoanesthesia (kraɪ'ouæn'ɪsθhiʒhə), the freezing of a part to achieve adequate deadening of neural sensitivity to pain during brief minor surgical procedures.

cryocautery (kraɪ'ouko'təri), the application of any substance, as carbon dioxide, that destroys tissue by freezing. Also called **cold cautery**.

cryogen, a chemical that induces freezing, used to destroy diseased tissue without injury to adjacent structures. Cell death is caused by dehydration after cell membranes rupture. Kinds of cryogens include **carbon dioxide, freon, liquid nitrogen** and **nitrous oxide.** – **cryogenic,** *adj.*

cryoglobulin (kraɪ'ouglob'yulɪn), an abnormal plasma protein that precipitates and coalesces at low temperatures and dissolves and disperses at body temperature.

cryoglobulinemia (kraɪ'ouglob'yulɪni'miə), an abnormal condition in which cryoglobulins are present in the blood. Cryoglobulins may be found associated with multiple myeloma and angioneurotic edema.

cryonics, the techniques in which cold is applied for a variety of therapeutic goals, including brief local anesthesia, destruction of superficial skin lesions, and preservation of cells, tissue, organs or the entire body. – **cryonic,** *adj.*

cryoprecipitate. 1. any precipitate formed upon cooling a solution. 2. a preparation rich in factor VIII needed to restore normal coagulation in hemophilia. It is collected from fresh human plasma that has been frozen and thawed.

cryostat, a device used in surgical pathology that consists of a special microtome used for freezing and slicing sections of tissue for study by a surgical pathologist.

cryosurgery, use of subfreezing temperature to destroy tissue, as in the destruction of the ganglion of nerve cells in the thalmas in the treatment of Parkinson's disease, in the destruction of the pituitary gland to halt the progress of some kinds of metastic cancer, and in the treatment of various cancers and lesions of the skin. The process is also used in ophthalmology to cause the edges of a detached retina to heal and to remove cataracts. The coolant is circulated through a metal probe, chilling it to as low as −160°C, depending upon the chemical used. The moist tissues adhere to the cold metal of the probe and freeze. Cells are dehydrated as their membranes burst; they are eventually discarded or absorbed by the body. No specific postoperative nursing care is required.

cryotherapy (kraɪ'ouθer'əpi), a treatment using cold as a destructive medium. Cutaneous tags, warts, condylomata acuminatum, actinic keratosis, and dermatofibromas are some of the common skin disorders amenable to cryotherapy. Solid carbon dioxide or liquid nitrogen are applied briefly with a sterile cotton-tipped applicator. A blister forms, followed by necrosis. The procedure may be repeated.

crypt, a blind pit or tube on a free surface. Some kinds of crypts are **anal crypt, dental crypt, synovial crypt.**

crypt-. See **crypto-**.

cryptitis (kriptaɪ'tɪs), an inflammation of a crypt, usually a perianal crypt, often accompanied by pain, pruritus, and spasm of the sphincter. Treatment may include hot compresses, sitz-baths, antibiotics, or excision.

crypto-, crypt-, a combining form meaning 'hidden': *cryptocephalus, cryptocrystalline, cryptodidymus*. Also **krypto-**.

cryptocephalus, a malformed fetus that has a small, underdeveloped head. – **cryptocephalic, cryptocephalous,** *adj.,* **cryptocephaly,** *n.*

cryptococcosis (krip'toukokou'sɪs), an infectious disease caused by a fungus, *Cryptococcus neoformans,* which spreads through the lungs to the brain and central nervous system, skin, skeletal system, and urinary tract. The disease occurs in all parts of the world, but in North America it is most likely to afflict middle-aged men in the southeastern states. It is characterized by the development of nodules or tumors filled with a gelatinous material in visceral and subcutaneous tissues. Initial symptoms may include coughing or other respiratory effects because the lungs are a primary site of infection. After the fungus spreads to the meninges, neurologic symptoms may develop, including headache, blurred vision, and difficulty in speaking. The diagnosis is made by isolation and identification of the fungus in specimens of sputum, pus, or tissue biopsy. Amphotericin B and flucytosine may be administered in order to control the infection. Also called **Buschke's disease, European blastomycosis, torulosis.** See also *Cryptococcus,* specific fungal infections.

Cryptococcus (krɪp′toukok′əs), a genus of yeastlike fungi that reproduces by budding rather than by producing spores. Many nonpathogenic species of *Cryptococcus* are commonly found in the soil and on the skin and mucous membranes of people who are well. Certain pathogenic species exist; *C. neoformans* is the most important. See also **fungus, yeast.**

Cryptococcus neoformans, a species of yeastlike fungus that causes cryptococcosis, a potentially fatal infection which can affect the lungs, skin, and brain.

cryptodidymus (krɪp′toudɪd′əməs), conjoined twins in which one fetus is small, underdeveloped, and concealed within the body of the other, more fully formed autosite.

crypt of iris, any one of the small pits in the iris along its free margin encircled by the circulus arteriosus minor. Also called **crypt of Fuchs.**

cryptomenorrhea, an abnormal condition in which the products of menstruation are retained within the vagina owing to an imperforate hymen, or, less often, within the uterus owing to an occlusion of the cervical canal. Cryptomenorrhea is usually accompanied by subjective symptoms of menstruation with scant or absent flow and sometimes by severe pain. If the flow is completely obstructed, uterotubal reflux of menstrual flow into the pelvic cavity may cause peritonitis, pain, adhesions, and endometriosis. – **cryptomenorrheal,** *adj.*

cryptophthalmos (krɪp′təfthæl′məs), a developmental anomaly characterized by complete fusion of the eyelids, usually with defective formation or complete lack of the eyes.

cryptorchidism (krɪptor′kɪdɪz′əm), failure of one or both of the testicles to descend into the scrotum. If spontaneous descent does not occur by the age of one, hormonal injections may be given. If not successful, surgery, called orchipexy, will likely be performed before the boy is five. Also called **undescended testis.**

crystal, a solid inorganic substance, the atoms or molecules of which are arranged in a regular, repeating three-dimensional pattern. The shape of a crystal is determined by the nature and arrangement of the components. – **crystalline,** *adj.*

crystalline lens (krɪs′təlɪn, krɪs′təlaɪn), a transparent structure of the eye, enclosed in a capsule, situated between the iris and the vitreous humor, and slightly overlapped at its margin by the ciliary processes. The capsule of the lens is a transparent, elastic membrane that touches the free border of the iris anteriorly and is secured by the suspensory ligament of the lens. The circumference of the capsule recedes from the iris to form the posterior chamber of the eye. The lens is a transparent biconvex structure with the posterior surface more convex than the anterior. It is composed of a soft, cortical material, a firm nucleus, and concentric laminae and is covered anteriorly by transparent epithelium. In the fetus the lens is very

soft and has a slightly reddish tint; in the adult it is colorless and firm; in old age it becomes flattened, more dense, slightly opaque, and amber tinted. See also **eye.**

Crystodigin, a trade name for a cardiac glycoside (digitoxin).

Cs, symbol for **cesium.**

CSF, abbreviation for **cerebrospinal fluid.**

CSR, abbreviation for **Cheyne-Stokes respiration.**

CT, abbreviation for **computerized tomography.** See **computerized axial tomography.**

Cu, symbol for **copper.**

Cuban itch. See **alastrim.**

cuboid bone, the cuboidal tarsal bone on the lateral side of the foot, proximal to the fourth and fifth metatarsal bones. It articulates with the calcaneus, lateral cunciform, and fourth and fifth metatarsal bones, and, occasionally, with the navicular. Also called **os cuboideum.**

cuffed endotracheal tube, an endotracheal tube with a balloon at one end which may be inflated to tighten the fit of the tube in the lumen of the airway. The balloon forms a cuff that prevents gastric contents from passing along the sides of the tube into the lungs and gas from leaking back from the lungs. Hard or soft cuffs are in use. The pressure of a cuffed tube often causes sore throat after general anesthesia. In patients with tracheitis, arteriosclerosis, or general debility, overinflation of the cuff can cause contusion, hemorrhage, mucosal sloughing, or rupture.

cul-de-sac (kəl′dɔsæk), a blind pouch or cecum, as the conjunctival cul-de-sac and the dural cul-de-sac.

cul-de-sac of Douglas. See **rectouterine excavation.**

Cullen's sign, the appearance of faint, irregularly formed hemorrhagic patches on the skin around the umbilicus. The discolored skin is blue-black and becomes greenish-brown or yellow. Cullen's sign may appear one to two days after the onset of anorexia and the severe, poorly localized abdominal pains that are characteristic of acute pancreatitis. Cullen's sign is also present in massive upper gastrointestinal hemorrhage. Compare **Grey Turner's sign.** See also **pancreatitis.**

cult-, a combining form meaning 'to tend or cultivate': *cultivation, cultural, culture.*

culture medium. See **medium.**

culture procedure, (in bacteriology) any of several techniques for growing colonies of microorganisms in order to identify a pathogen and to determine which antibiotics are effective in combating the infection caused by the organism. Usually, a specimen is secured and a small amount is placed in or on one or more culture media, as different organisms are nourished by different nutrients and grow best at specific but different pH levels. The environment in which the media are held during observation is maintained at body temperature, and the ambient oxygen level is adjusted to achieve an aerobic or anaerobic state. All procedures are aseptic and all equipment is sterile to avoid accidental contamination of the media. As colonies appear in or on the media, small amounts of each (there are often several) are spread on other media to allow examination of a pure specimen of the microorganisms.

cumulative, increasing by incremental steps with an eventual total that may exceed the expected result.

cumulative action, 1. the increased activity of a therapeutic measure or agent when administered repeatedly, as the cumulative action of a regular exercise program. 2. the increased activity demonstrated by a drug when repeated doses accumulate in the body and exert a greater biological effect than the initial dose.

cumulative dose, the total dose that accumulates from repeated exposure to radiation or a radiopharmaceutical product.

cumulative gene. See **polygene.**

cune-, a combining form meaning 'pertaining to a wedge': *cuneate, cuneiform, cuneus.*

cuneate (kyu'nieit), (of tissue) wedge-shaped, used especially in describing cells of the nervous system.

cuneiform (kyuni'əform), (of bone and cartilage) wedge-shaped.

cuneiform bone. See **triangular bone.**

cup arthroplasty of the hip joint, the surgical replacement of the head of the femur by a metal or plastic mold to relieve pain and increase motion in arthritis or to correct a deformity. Under general anesthesia, the damaged or diseased bone is removed, and the acetabulum and the head of the femur are reshaped. A metal Vitallium cup is inserted between the two and becomes the articulating surface of the femur. Postoperatively, the patient's leg is suspended in traction to hold it in a position of abduction and internal rotation to keep the disc in place in the acetabulum. Continued abduction is necessary for six weeks. Possible complications include infection, thrombophlebitis, pulmonary embolism, and fat embolism. The patient receives extensive physical therapy; crutches are necessary to avoid bearing of full weight for six months, and an exercise program must be followed for several years. Compare **hip replacement.** See also **arthroplasty, knee replacement, osteoarthritis, plastic surgery.**

cupping and vibrating, the procedures to help remove mucus and fluid from the lungs by the use of the clinical nursing techniques of percussion and vibration to dislodge and mobilize the secretions.

■ METHOD: Cupping is performed by the rhythmic percussion of the affected segments of the lungs or bronchi by the cupped hands of the nurse. Cupping is begun gently and is increased in forcefulness as the patient tolerates increased percussion. Vibration is done by placing the nurse's hands over the affected area and shaking the arms from the shoulders, with the shaking sensation pro-

duced on the patient's chest comparable to the shaking that accompanies the chill of a fever. See also **postural drainage.**

■ OUTCOME CRITERIA: Thick, tenacious mucus is difficult to evacuate from the bronchi, the bronchioles, and the alveoli. As an adjunct to postural drainage, cupping and vibrating may greatly facilitate the clearing of the passages. The patient can breathe more deeply and with less effort, and the danger of pneumonia or atelectasis is reduced.

■ NURSING ORDERS: Cupping is never performed over breast tissue because it serves no purpose and causes discomfort. After head-down postural drainage with cupping and vibrating, the patient is helped to a position favorable for effective coughing and asked to breathe deeply at least three times and to cough at least twice.

cupric (kyu'prik), of or pertaining to copper in its divalent form, as cupric sulfate.

Cuprimine, a trade name for a chelating agent (penicillamine), used in treating poisoning by heavy metals.

cupulolithiasis (kyu'pyuloulɪthai'əsɪs), a severe, long-lasting vertigo brought on by movement of the head to certain positions. There are many possible causes, among them otitis media, ear surgery, or injury to the inner ear. In addition to extreme dizziness, signs are nausea, vomiting, and ataxia. There is no treatment except avoidance of the offending head positions. Also called **postural vertigo.**

curare (kyura'ri), a substance derived from tropical plants of the genus *Stryknos.* It is a potent muscle relaxant that acts by preventing transmission of neural impulses across the myoneural junctions. Large dosage can cause complete paralysis. Pharmacologic preparations of the substance are used as adjuncts to general anesthesia. The use of curare or other neuromuscular blocking agents requires respiratory and ventilatory assistance by a qualified anesthetist or anesthesiologist. See also **tubocurarine chloride.**

curariform (kyura'riform), (in pharmacology) 1. chemically similar to curare. 2. having the effect of curare.

Curarin (kyura'rɪn), a trade name for a nondepolarizing blocking agent (tubocurarine chloride), used as an adjunct to anesthesia.

curative treatment. See **treatment.**

cure, 1. restoration to health of a person afflicted with a disease or other disorder. 2. the favorable outcome of the treatment of a disease or other disorder. 3. a course of therapy, a medication, a therapeutic measure, or other remedy used in treatment of a medical problem, as faith healing, fasting, rest cure, work cure.

curet (kyuret'), 1. a surgical instrument shaped like a spoon or scoop for scraping and removing material or tissue from an organ, cavity, or surface. A curet may be blunt or sharp and is designed in a shape and size appropriate to its use. **2.** to remove tissue or debris with such a device. Kinds of curets include **Hartmann's curet.**

curettage (kyur′ətaźh′), scraping of material from the wall of a cavity or other surface, performed to remove tumors or other abnormal tissue or to obtain tissue for microscopic examination. Curettage also refers to clearing unwanted material from fistulas and areas of chronic infection. It may be performed with a blunt or a sharp curet or by suction.

curie (Ci, c) (kyur′i), a unit of radioactivity equal to 3.70×10^{10} disintegrations per second.

curium (Cm), a radioactive metallic element. Its atomic number is 96; its atomic weight is 247. Curium is an artificial element produced by bombarding plutonium with helium ions in a cyclotron. Numerous isotopes of curium are produced by bombarding lighter transuranium elements. Curium is so radioactive it glows in the dark.

Curling's ulcer, a duodenal ulcer that develops in people who have severe burns on the surface of the body. Also called **Curling's stress ulcer.** See also **milk therapy.**

current, 1. a flowing or streaming movement. **2.** a flow of electrons along a conductor in a closed circuit; an electric current. **3.** certain physiologic electrical activity and characteristics of blood circulation. Physiologic currents include abnerval current, action current, axial current, centrifugal current, centripetal current, compensating current, demarcation current, electrotonic current.

-current, a combining form meaning 'running, flowing, happening': *concurrent, excurrent, intercurrent.*

current of injury. See **demarcation current.**

Current Procedural Terminology (CPT), a system developed by the American Medical Association for standardizing the terminology and coding used to describe medical services and procedures.

Curschmann spiral (kurśh′man), one of the coiled fibrils of mucus occasionally found in the sputum of persons with bronchial asthma.

curvature myopia, a type of nearsightedness caused by refractive errors associated with an excessive curvature of the cornea.

curve, (in statistics) a straight or curved line used as a graphic method of demonstrating the distribution of data collected in a study or survey.

curve of Carus, the normal axis of the pelvic outlet. Also called **circle of Carus.**

curvilinear trend, (in statistics) a trend in which a graphic representation of the data yields a curved line. The value of the independent variable may be expressed as a polynomial coefficient, by a more complete mathematical expression, as a logistic curve, or by a smoothing process, as a moving average.

cushingoid (kuśh′ɪŋgoid), having the habitus and facies characteristic of Cushing's disease: fat pads on the upper

back and face, striae on the limbs and trunk, and excess hair on the face.

Cushing's disease (kuśh′ɪŋgz), a metabolic disorder characterized by the abnormally increased secretion of adrenocortical steroids caused by increased amounts of adrenocorticotropic hormone (ACTH) secreted by the pituitary, as by a pituitary adenoma. Excess adrenocortical hormones result in accumulations of fat on the chest, upper back, and face and in edema, hyperglycemia, increased gluconeogenesis, muscle weakness, purplish striae on the skin, decreased immunity to infection, osteoporosis with susceptibility to fracture of bones, acne, and facial hirsutism. Hyperglycemia resulting from Cushing's disease does not usually respond to treatment; diabetes mellitus may become a chronic condition. Therapy is aimed at removal or destruction of ACTH secreting tissue, most commonly by surgical or radiologic procedures. If this is not possible, the adrenal glands are totally or subtotally removed and pharmacologic preparations of adrenal steroids administered. Also called **hyperadrenalism.** Compare **Cushing's syndrome.**

Cushing's syndrome, a metabolic disorder resulting from the chronic and excessive production of cortisol by the adrenal cortex or by the administration of glucocorticoids in large doses for several weeks or longer. When occurring spontaneously, the syndrome represents a failure in the body's ability to regulate the secretion of cortisol or adrenocorticotropic hormone (ACTH). (Normally cortisol is produced only in response to ACTH, and ACTH is not secreted in the presence of high levels of cortisol.) The most common cause of the syndrome is a pituitary tumor that causes an increased secretion of ACTH. Also called **hyperadrenocorticism.** See also **Addison's disease, Cushing's disease, Nelson's syndrome.**

■ OBSERVATIONS: Characteristically, the patient with Cushing's syndrome has a decreased glucose tolerance, central obesity, round 'moon' face, supraclavicular fat pads, a pendulous, striae-covered pad of fat on the chest and abdomen, oligomenorrhea or decreased testosterone levels, muscular atrophy, edema, hypokalemia, and some degree of emotional change. The skin may be abnormally pigmented and fragile; minor infections may become systemic and long-lasting. Children with the disorder may stop growing. Occasionally, hypertension, kidney stones, and psychosis occur.

■ INTERVENTION: The objective of all treatment is reduction of the secretion of cortisol. The source of the excess ACTH is discovered by a series of tests that challenge the function of the adrenal and pituitary glands. Once known, the cause is treated. Most often, as the excess ACTH is the result of an adenoma of the anterior pituitary, x-ray irradiation or surgical excision of the tumor corrects the condition. If the condition is the result of medication, decreasing or changing the medication may alleviate the symptoms.

■ NURSING CONSIDERATIONS: In caring for children, the nurse normally observes height and weight, as rapidly developing obesity and failure to grow are suggestive of Cushing's syndrome. The patient with the syndrome may usually be reassured that treatment is largely successful and that the appearance may be expected to return to normal. Some of the medications used for some forms of the condition may cause nausea and anorexia, somnolence, and lethargy, and the patient is informed of this. Nursing care of the hospitalized patient with Cushing's syndrome is similar to that of Addison's disease and other endocrinologic disorders; weight and electrolyte and fluid balance are monitored, an adequate, balanced diet is urged, and emotional changes are observed with a goal of maintaining emotional equilibrium.

cusp, 1. a sharp projection or a rounded eminence that rises from the chewing surface of a tooth, as the two pyramidal cusps that arise from the premolars. 2. any one of the small flaps on the valves of the heart, as the ventral, dorsal, and medial cusps attached to the right atrioventricular valve.

cuspid valve (kəs′pɪd), either of two structures in the heart that control the flow of blood between the atria and the ventricles. The cuspid valves are the mitral, or bicuspid, valve with two flaps between the left atrium and the left ventricle, and the tricuspid valve with three main flaps between the right atrium and the right ventricle. Also called **atrioventricular valve.**

custodial care, services and care of a nonmedical nature provided on a long-term basis, usually for convalescent and chronically ill individuals. Kinds of custodial care include **board, room, personal assistance.**

cut, (in molecular genetics) a fissure or split in a double strand of DNA in contrast to a nick in a single strand. See also **nick.**

cut-, a combining form meaning 'pertaining to the skin': *cutaneous, cuticle, cuticularization.*

cutaneous (kyutei′niəs), of or pertaining to the skin.

cutaneous absorption, the taking up of substances through the skin.

cutaneous anaphylaxis, a localized, exaggerated reaction of hypersensitivity in the form of a wheal and flare caused by an antigen injected into the skin of a sensitized individual, generally used as a test of sensitivity to various allergens. Passive cutaneous anaphylaxis, the response to an intradermally injected antibody, is used in studies of antibodies that induce immediate reactions of hypersensitivity.

cutaneous horn, a hard, skin-colored projection of the epidermis, usually on the head or face. The lesion may be precancerous and is usually excised.

cutaneous larva migrans, a skin condition caused by a hookworm, *Ancylostoma braziliense,* a parasite of cats and dogs. Its ova are deposited in the ground with the feces of infected animals, develop into larvae, and invade the skin of people (particularly those who are barefoot). The larvae rarely develop into adult hookworms in the human body, but as the larvae migrate through the epidermis, a trail of inflammation follows the burrow causing severe pruritus. Secondary infections often occur if the skin has been broken by scratching. Topical application of a solution of thiabendazole usually eradicates the larvae. Also called **creeping eruption.**

cutaneous leishmaniasis. See **oriental sore.**

cutaneous lupus erythematosus. See **discoid lupus erythematosus.**

cutaneous membrane. See **skin.**

cutaneous papilloma, a small brown or flesh-colored outgrowth of skin, occurring most frequently on the neck of an older person. Also called **cutaneous tag, skin tag.**

cutaneous tag. See **cutaneous papilloma.**

cutdown, an incision into a vein with insertion of a polyethylene catheter for intravenous infusion. It is performed when an infusion cannot be started by venipuncture and in hyperalimentation therapy, when highly concentrated solutions are given via catheter into the superior vena cava. The skin is cleansed before the procedure; the incision is sutured, and a sterile dressing applied at its conclusion. See also **hyperalimentation, venipuncture.**

cuticle, 1. epidermis. 2. the sheath of a hair follicle. 3. the thin edge of cornified epithelium at the base of a nail.

cutis (kyu′tis). See **skin.**

cutis laxa, abnormally loose, relaxed skin owing to an absence of elastic fibers in the body, usually a hereditary condition.

cutis marmorata. See **livedo.**

CVA, 1. abbreviation for **cerebrovascular accident.** 2. abbreviation for **costovertebral angle.**

CVP monitor. See **central venous pressure monitor.**

cyan-. See **cyano-.**

cyanide poisoning, poisoning owing to the ingestion or inhalation of cyanide from such substances as bitter almond oil, wild cherry syrup, prussic acid, hydrocyanic acid, or potassium or sodium cyanide. Characterized by tachycardia, drowsiness, convulsion, and headache, cyanide poisoning may result in death within one to fifteen minutes. Treatment includes gastric lavage, amyl nitrite inhalation, oxygen, and sodium thiosulfate.

cyano-, cyan-, a combining form meaning 'blue': *cyanochroia, cyanocrystallin, cyanodermia.*

cyanocobalamin (saɪ′ənoukoubæl′əmɪn), a red, crystalline, water-soluble vitamin essential for the metabolism of protein, fats, and carbohydrates, normal blood formation, and neural function. It is the only vitamin that contains essential mineral elements and is the first substance containing cobalt that is found to be vital to life. It cannot be produced synthetically but can be obtained from cultures of *Streptomyces griseus*. Rich dietary sources are liver, kidney, meats, fish, and dairy products. Deficiency is usually owing to the absence of intrinsic factor, which is necessary for the absorption of cyanocobalamin from the gastrointestinal tract, and results in pernicious anemia and brain damage. Symptoms of deficiency include nervousness, neuritis, numbness and tingling in the hands and feet, poor muscular coordination, unpleasant body odor, and menstrual disturbances. Cyanocobalamin is used in the prophylaxis and treatment of pernicious anemia, tropical and nontropical sprue, and other macrocytic and megaloblastic anemias. It is nontoxic, even when administered in amounts greater than those recommended for therapeutic purposes. Also called **antipernicious anemia factor, extrinsic factor, LLD factor, vitamin B$_{12}$.** See also **intrinsic factor, pernicious anemia.**

cyanomethemoglobin (sai'ɔnoumethi'mɔglou'bɪn), a hemoglobin derivative formed during nitrite therapy for cyanide poisoning.

cyanosis (sai'ɔnou'sɪs), bluish discoloration of the skin and mucous membranes caused by an excess of deoxygenated hemoglobin in the blood or a structural defect in the hemoglobin molecule, as in methemoglobin. — **cyanotic,** *adj.*

Cyantin, a trade name for a urinary antibacterial (nitrofurantoin).

cycl-. See **cyclo-.**

cyclacillin, a penicillin antibiotic.
■ INDICATIONS: It is prescribed in the treatment of certain bacterial infections.
■ CONTRAINDICATIONS: Known hypersensitivity to penicillins prohibits its use.
■ ADVERSE EFFECTS: Among the most serious adverse reactions are hypersensitivity reactions and severe diarrhea and nausea. Skin rash also may occur.

Cyclaine, a trade name for a local anesthetic (hexylcaine hydrochloride).

cyclamate (sai'klɔmeit), an artificial, nonnutritive sweetener formerly used in the form of calcium or sodium salt. It was withdrawn from the market because it caused cancer in laboratory animals.

cyclandelate (saiklæn'dɔleit), a vasodilator.
■ INDICATIONS: It is prescribed in the treatment of peripheral vascular obstruction or spasm.
■ CONTRAINDICATIONS: Pregnancy or known hypersensitivity to this drug prohibits its use.
■ ADVERSE EFFECTS: Tachycardia, gastrointestinal distress, and flushing may occur.

Cyclapen, a trade name for a penicillin antibiotic (cyclacillin).

cycle. See **menstrual cycle.**

cyclencephaly (saik'lɔnsef'ɔli), a developmental anom-

aly characterized by the fusion of the two cerebral hemispheres. — **cyclencephalic, cyclencephalous,** *adj.,* **cyclencephalus,** *n.*

cyclic adenosine monophosphate, a cyclic nucleotide formed from adenosine triphosphate by the action of adenyl cyclase. This cyclic compound, known as the "second messenger," participates in the action of catecholomines, vasopressin, adrenocorticotropic hormone, and many other hormones. Also called **adenosine 3':5'-cyclic phosphate.**

cyclitis (sɪklai'tɪs), inflammation of the ciliary body causing redness of the sclera adjacent to the cornea of the eye.

cyclizine hydrochloride, an antihistamine.
■ INDICATION: It is prescribed in the treatment or prevention of motion sickness.
■ CONTRAINDICATIONS: Asthma or known hypersensitivity to this drug prohibits its use. It is not given to newborn infants or nursing mothers.
■ ADVERSE EFFECTS: Among the more serious adverse reactions are skin rash, hypersensitivity reactions, and tachycardia. Drowsiness and dry mouth commonly occur.

cyclo-, cycl-, a combining form meaning 'round, recurring'; often with reference to the eye: *cyclodialysis, cycloid, cyclops.*

cyclobenzaprine hydrochloride, a muscle relaxant.
■ INDICATION: It is prescribed in the treatment of muscle spasm.
■ CONTRAINDICATIONS: Hyperthyroidism, cardiac arrhythmia, cardiac failure, concomitant use of a monoamine oxidase inhibitor, or known hypersensitivity to this drug prohibits its use. It is used with caution in conditions in which anticholinergics are contraindicated.
■ ADVERSE EFFECTS: The most serious adverse effects are hypersensitivity reactions. Drowsiness, dry mouth, and dizziness commonly occur.

cyclocephaly. See **cyclopia.** — **cyclocephalic, cyclocephalous,** *adj.*

Cyclocort, a trade name for a glucocorticoid (amcinonide).

Cyclogyl, a trade name for an ophthalmic anticholinergic (cyclopentolate hydrochloride).

Cyclopar, a trade name for a broad spectrum antibiotic (tetracycline).

cyclopentolate hydrochloride, an ophthalmic anticholinergic.
■ INDICATION: It is prescribed to provide mydriasis and cycloplegia for diagnostic procedures in ophthalmology.
■ CONTRAINDICATIONS: Narrow-angle glaucoma or known hypersensitivity to this drug prohibits its use.
■ ADVERSE EFFECTS: Among the most serious adverse reactions are psychic disturbances and systemic anticholinergic effects, particularly in children. Local irritation and burning may also occur.

cyclophosphamide, an alkylating agent.
- INDICATIONS: It is prescribed in the treatment of a variety of neoplasms and as an immunosuppressant in organ transplants.
- CONTRAINDICATIONS: This drug is teratogenic in animals. It is not used during pregnancy; adequate methods of contraception should be considered for both males and females taking the drug. It is used with caution with impaired renal or hepatic function or with various blood disorders.
- ADVERSE EFFECTS: Among the more serious adverse reactions are anorexia, vomiting, alopecia, leukopenia, and potentially serious hemorrhagic cystitis.

cyclopia (saiklou′piə), a developmental anomaly characterized by fusion of the orbits into a single cavity containing one eye. The condition is usually combined with various other head and facial defects. Also called **cyclocephaly, synophthalmia.** — **cyclops,** n.

cycloplegia (sai′kləpli′jə), paralysis of the ciliary muscles, as induced by certain ophthalmic drugs to allow examination of the eye. — **cycloplegic,** adj., n.

cycloplegic (sai′kləpli′jik), **1.** of or pertaining to a drug or treatment that causes paralysis of the ciliary muscles of the eye. **2.** one of a group of anticholinergic drugs used to paralyze the ciliary muscles of the eye for ophthalmologic examination or surgery. Any of the cycloplegics may cause adverse effects in persons sensitive to anticholinergics.

cyclopropane (sai′klouprou′pein), a highly flammable and explosive potent anesthetic gas that gives good analgesia and skeletal muscle relaxation, with low toxicity, minimal adverse effects, and rapid induction and emergence. It has been largely replaced by the nonflammable halogenated hydrocarbons and is now used for anesthesia only when characteristics of other anesthetic agents contraindicate their use in a specific patient. Also called **trimethylene.**

cycloserine (sai′klouser′in), an antibiotic.
- INDICATIONS: It is prescribed in the treatment of active pulmonary and extrapulmonary tuberculosis.
- CONTRAINDICATIONS: Epilepsy, depression, severe anxiety, psychosis, severe renal insufficiency, excessive concurrent use of alcohol, or known hypersensitivity to this drug prohibits its use.
- ADVERSE EFFECTS: Among the most serious reactions are central nervous system toxicity, including tremor, drowsiness, convulsions, and psychotic changes.

Cyclospasmol, a trade name for a vasodilator (cyclandelate).

cyclothiazide, a diuretic and antihypertensive.
- INDICATIONS: It is prescribed in the treatment of hypertension and edema.
- CONTRAINDICATIONS: Anemia or known hypersensitivity to this drug, to other thiazide medication, or to sulfonamide derivatives prohibits its use.
- ADVERSE EFFECTS: Among the more serious adverse effects are hypokalemia, hyperglycemia, hyperuricemia, and hypersensitivity reactions.

cyclothymic disorder, a mild form of bipolar disorder.

cyclothymic personality, **1.** a personality characterized by extreme swings in mood from elation to depression. **2.** a person who has this disorder. Also called **bipolar disorder.**

cycrimine hydrochloride, an anticholinergic.
- INDICATION: It is prescribed in the treatment of Parkinson's disease.
- CONTRAINDICATIONS: Narrow angle glaucoma, asthma, obstruction of the genitourinary or gastrointestinal tract, severe ulcerative colitis, or known hypersensitivity to this drug prohibits its use.
- ADVERSE EFFECTS: Among the more serious adverse reactions are blurred vision, central nervous system effects, tachycardia, dry mouth, decreased sweating, and hypersensitivity reactions.

Cylert, a trade name for a central nervous system stimulant (pemoline).

cylindroma (sil′indrou′mə), pl. **cylindromas, cylindromata. 1.** Also called **adenocystic carcinoma.** a tumor characterized by cylinders of mucinous tissue in nests of epithelial cells. It may occur in the breast, salivary glands, or mucous glands of the respiratory tract. **2.** Also called **cylindromatous spiradenoma, trichobasalioma hyalinicum.** a benign neoplasm of the skin, usually of the scalp or face, developing from a hair follicle or sweat gland.

cylindromatous carcinoma. See **adenocystic carcinoma.**

cylindromatous spiradenoma. See **cylindroma,** def. 2.

cyno-, cyn-, a combining form meaning 'pertaining to dogs, doglike': cynobax, cynocephalic, cynophobia.

cyproheptadine hydrochloride, an antihistamine.
- INDICATIONS: It is prescribed in the treatment of a variety of hypersensitivity reactions, including rhinitis, skin rash, and pruritus.
- CONTRAINDICATIONS: Asthma or known hypersensitivity to this drug prohibits its use. It is not given to newborn infants or lactating mothers.
- ADVERSE EFFECTS: Among the more serious adverse reactions are skin rash, hypersensitivity reactions, and tachycardia. Drowsiness and dry mouth commonly occur.

Cyprus fever. See **brucellosis.**

cyst, a closed sac in or under the skin lined with epithelium and containing fluid or semisolid material, as a **sebaceous cyst.**

cyst-. See **cysto-.**

-cyst, a combining form meaning a 'pouch or bladder': enterocyst, microcyst, zoocyst. Also **-cystis.**

cystadenoma (sis′tædinou′mə), pl. **cystadenomas, cystadenomata. 1.** an adenoma associated with a cystoma.

2. an adenoma containing multiple cystic structures. The cysts may be serous, containing serum, or pseudomucinous, containing clear serous fluid or thick, viscid fluid.

cystectomy, a surgical procedure in which all or a part of the bladder is removed, as may be required in treating cancer of the bladder.

cysteine (sis'tin), an amino acid found in many proteins in the body, including keratin. It is a metabolic precursor of cystine.

cysti-. See **cysto-.**

cystic acne. See **acne conglobata.**

cystic carcinoma, a malignant neoplasm containing cysts or cystlike spaces. Tumors of this kind occur in the breast and ovary.

cystic duct, the duct through which bile from the gall bladder passes into the common bile duct.

cysticercosis (sis'tisərkou'sis), an infection and infestation by the larval stage of the pork tapeworm *Taenia solium.* The eggs are ingested and hatch in the intestine; the larvae invade the subcutaneous tissue, brain, eye, muscle, heart, liver, lung, and peritoneum. They attach themselves with two rows of hooklets, grow, mature, and become covered with a dense, fibrous capsule. The invasive, early phase of the infection is characterized by fever, malaise, muscle pain, and eosinophilia. Years later, epilepsy and personality change may appear if the brain is affected, and calcification and destruction of local structures are apparent in other infested areas of the body. Prophylaxis depends on avoiding ingestion of inadequately cooked, infected pork.

cystic fibroma, a fibrous tumor in which cystic degeneration has occurred.

cystic fibrosis, an inherited disorder of the exocrine glands, causing those glands to produce abnormally thick secretions of mucus. The glands most affected are those in the pancreas, the respiratory system, and the sweat glands. Cystic fibrosis is usually recognized in infancy or early childhood, occurring chiefly among Caucasians. When present in infancy, it may be preceded by meconium ileus, an obstruction of the small bowel by viscid stool. Other early signs are a chronic cough, frequent, foul-smelling stools, and persistent upper respiratory infections. The most reliable diagnostic tool is the sweat test, which shows elevations of both sodium and chloride. Since there is no known cure, treatment is directed at the prevention of respiratory infections, which are the most frequent cause of death. Mucolytic agents, bronchodilators, and mist tents are used to help liquefy the thick, tenacious mucus. Physical therapy measures, as postural drainage and breathing exercises, can also dislodge secretions. Broad spectrum antibiotics may be used prophylactically. The nurse's role is vital in instructing the family in health promotion and in all the aspects of care needed by the child. Life expectancy in cystic fibrosis

has improved markedly over the past several decades, and with early diagnosis and treatment, most patients can be expected to reach adulthood.

cystic goiter, an enlargement of the thyroid gland containing cysts resulting from mucoid or colloid degeneration.

cystic hygroma. See **cystic lymphangioma.**

cystic lymphangioma, a cystic growth formed by lymph vessels; usually congenital, it most frequently occurs in the neck, axilla, or groin of children. Also called **cystic hygroma, lymphangioma cysticum.**

cystic mole. See **hydatid mole.**

cystic myxoma, a tumor of the connective tissue that has undergone cystic degeneration.

cystic neuroma, a neoplasm of nerve tissue that has degenerated and become cystic. Also called **false neuroma.**

cystic tumor, a tumor with cavities or sacs containing a semisolid or a liquid material.

cystido-. See **cysto-.**

cystine, an amino acid found in many proteins in the body, including keratin and insulin. Cystine is a product of the metabolism of cysteine.

cystine storage disease. See **cystinosis.**

cystinosis (sis'tinou'sis), a congenital disease characterized by glucosuria, proteinuria, cystine deposits in the liver, spleen, bone marrow, and cornea, rickets, excessive amounts of phosphates in the urine, and retardation of growth. Also called **cystine storage disease, Fanconi's syndrome.** See also **cystine.**

cystinuria (sis'tinyur'iə), 1. abnormal presence in the urine of the amino acid cystine. 2. an inherited defect of the renal tubules, characterized by excessive urinary excretion of cystine and several other amino acids. The disorder is caused by an autosomal recessive trait which impairs cystine reabsorption by the kidney tubules. In high concentration cystine tends to precipitate in the urinary tract and form kidney or bladder stones. Treatment attempts to prevent the formation of stones or to dissolve them by increasing the volume of urine flow, decreasing the pH of the urine, and increasing the solubility of cystine. In addition to a large fluid intake, sodium bicarbonate, acetazolamide, and, in refractory cases, d-Penicillamine are sometimes prescribed.

-cystis, See **-cyst.**

cystitis (sistai'tis), an inflammatory condition of the urinary bladder and ureters, characterized by pain, urgency, and frequency of urination and by hematuria. It may be caused by a bacterial infection, calculus, or tumor. Depending upon the diagnosis, treatment may include antibiotics, increased fluid intake, bed rest, medications to control bladder wall spasms, and when necessary, surgery.

-cystitis, a combining form meaning an 'inflammation of the bladder or cyst': *epicystitis, gonecystitis, pericystitis.*

cysto-, cyst-, cysti-, a combining form meaning 'pertaining to the bladder, or to a cyst or sac': *cystocele, cystodynia, cystomyoma.* Also **cystido-.**

cystogram (sɪs'təgræm), a graphic record, usually a series of x-ray films, obtained as a part of any excretory urographic procedure, as in retrograde pyelography or retrograde cystoscopy.

cystoma (sɪstou'mə), *pl.* **cystomas, cystomata.** any tumor or growth containing cysts, especially one in or near the ovary.

-cystoma, a combining form meaning a 'cystic tumor': *enterocystoma, hydrocystoma, inocystoma.*

cystoscope, an instrument for examining and treating lesions of the urinary bladder, ureter, and kidney. It consists of an outer sheath with a lighting system, a viewing obturator, and a passage for catheters and operative devices. — **cystoscopic,** *adj.*

cystoscopic urography. See **retrograde cystoscopy.**

cystoscopy (saitos'kəpi), the direct visualization of the urinary tract by means of a cystoscope inserted in the urethra. For the examination the bladder is distended with air or water and the patient is in a fasting state, the procedure usually being performed under sedation or anesthesia with the patient in the lithotomy position. In addition to visualization, cystoscopy is used for obtaining biopsies of tumors or other growths and for the removal of polyps. After the examination the patient is observed for the common complications of trauma and signs of urinary infection. See also **cystoscope.** — **cystoscopic,** *adj.*

Cystospaz, a trade name for an anticholinergic (hyoscyamine).

cyt-, cyto-, a combining form meaning 'cell' or 'cytoplasm': *cytochrome, cytogenesis, cytosome.*

Cytadren, a trade name for an inhibitor of adrenocorticosteroid biosynthesis (aminoglutethimide).

cytarabine, an antineoplastic agent. Also called **arabinosylcitosine.**

■ INDICATIONS: It is prescribed in the treatment of acute and chronic myelocytic leukemia, acute lymphocytic leukemia, and erythroleukemia.

■ CONTRAINDICATIONS: Pre-existing bone marrow depression or known hypersensitivity to this drug prohibits its use.

■ ADVERSE EFFECTS: Among the most serious adverse reactions are bone marrow depression, stomatitis, phlebitis, liver toxicity, and fever. Gastrointestinal disturbances also may occur.

-cyte, a combining form meaning a 'cell' of a specified type: *gliacyte, hemacyte, plasmacyte.*

-cythemia, a combining form meaning a 'condition involving cells in the blood': *achroiocythemia, rhestocythemia, thrombocythemia.* Also **-cythaemia.**

cyto-. See **cyt-.**

cytoarchitectonic (sai'touar'kɪtekton'ɪk), pertaining to the cellular arrangement within a particular tissue or structure.

cytoarchitecture, the typical pattern of cellular arrangement within a particular tissue or organ, as in the cerebral cortex. — **cytoarchitectural,** *adj.*

cytobiotaxis (sai'toubai'outæk'sɪs). See **cytoclesis.** — **cytobiotactic,** *adj.*

cytoblast (sai'təblæst), *Obsolete.* the nucleus of a cell.

cytocentrum (sai'tousen'trəm). See **centrosome.**

cytocerastic (sai'tousəræs'tɪk). See **cytokerastic.**

cytochemism (sai'toukem'ɪzəm), the chemical activity within the living cell, specifically the various reactions to and affinity for chemical substances.

cytochemistry (sai'toukem'ɪstri), the study of the various chemicals within a living cell and their actions and functions.

cytocide, any substance that is destructive to cells. — **cytocidal,** *adj.*

cytoclesis (sai'toukli'sɪs), the influence exerted by one cell on the action of other cells; the vital principle of all living tissue. Also called **cytobiotaxis.** — **cytocletic,** *adj.*

cytoctony, the destruction of cells, specifically the killing of cells in culture by viruses.

cytode, the simplest type of cell, consisting of a protoplasmic mass without a nucleus, as a bacterium.

cytodieresis, (sai'toudaier'ɪsɪs) *pl.* **cytodiereses.** cell division, especially the phenomena involving the division of the cytoplasm. See also **meiosis, mitosis.** — **cytodieretic,** *adj.*

cytodifferentiation, (in embryology) **1.** a process by which embryonic cells acquire biochemical and morphological properties essential for specialization and diversification. **2.** the total and gradual transformation from an undifferentiated to a fully differentiated state.

cytogene (sai'təjin'), a particle within the cytoplasm of a cell that is self-replicating, derived from the genes in the nucleus, and capable of transmitting hereditary information. — **cytogenic,** *adj.*

cytogenesis (sai'toujen'ɪsɪs), the origin, development, and differentiation of cells. — **cytogenetic, cytogenic,** *adj.*

cytogeneticist (sai'toujinet'ɪsɪst), one who specializes in cytogenetics.

cytogenetics (sai'toujinet'ɪks), the branch of genetics that studies the cellular constituents concerned with heredity, primarily the structure, function, and origin of the chromosomes. One kind of cytogenetics is **clinical cytogenetics.** — **cytogenetic,** *adj.*

cytogenic gland, a glandular organ that secretes living cells, specifically the testes and ovary.

cytogenic reproduction, the formation of a new organism from a unicellular germ cell, either sexually through the fusion of gametes to form a zygote or asexually by means of spores.

cytogeny (saɪtoj′ɪni), **1.** cytogenetics. **2.** the origin and development of the cell. — **cytogenic, cytogenous,** *adj.*

cytogony (saɪtog′əni), cytogenic reproduction. — **cytogenic,** *adj.*

cytohistogenesis (saɪ′touhɪs′toujen′ɪsɪs), the structural development and formation of cells. — **cytohistogenetic,** *adj.*

cytohyaloplasm. See **hyaloplasm.**

cytoid, like or resembling a cell.

cytoid body, a small white spot on the retina of each eye that is seen by using an ophthalmoscope in examining the eyes of a patient affected with systemic lupus erythematosus.

cytokerastic (saɪ′toukəræs′tɪk), **cytocerastic,** pertaining to or characteristic of cellular development from a lower to a higher form or from a simple to more complex arrangement.

cytokinesis (saɪ′toukɪni′sɪs, saɪ′toukaɪni′sɪs), the division of the cytoplasm, exclusive of nuclear division, that occurs during the final stages of mitosis and meiosis to form daughter cells; the sum total of all the changes that occur in the cytoplasm during mitosis, meiosis, and fertilization. — **cytokinetic,** *adj.*

cytological map, the graphic representation of the location of genes on a chromosome, based on correlating genetic recombination testcrossing results with the structural analysis of chromosomes that have undergone such changes as deletions or translocations as detected by banding techniques.

cytologist (saɪtol′əjɪst), one who specializes in the study of cells, specifically one who uses cytological techniques in the differential diagnosis of neoplasms.

cytology, the study of cells, including their formation, origin, structure, function, biochemical activities, and pathology. Kinds of cytology are **aspiration biopsy cytology, exfoliative cytology.** — **cytologic, cytological,** *adj.*

cytolymph. See **hyaloplasm.**

cytolysin (saɪtol′ɪsɪn), an antibody that dissolves antigenic cells. Kinds of cytolysin are **bacteriolysin, hemolysin.**

cytolysis (saɪtol′ɪsɪs,) *pl.* **cytolyses.** the destruction or breakdown of the living cell, primarily by the disintegration of the outer membrane. A kind of cytolysis is **immune cytolysis.** — **cytolytic,** *adj.*

cytomegalic inclusion disease (CID) (saɪ′toumegæl′ɪk), an infection caused by the cytomegalovirus, one of the herpesviruses. It is primarily a congenitally acquired disease of newborn infants and is characterized by microcephaly, retarded growth, hepatosplenomegaly, hemolytic anemia, and pathological fracture of long bones. Also called **cytomegalovirus disease.** See also **TORCH syndrome.**

cytomegalovirus (CMV) (saɪ′toumeg′əlouvaɪ′rəs), a member of a group of species-specific herpesviruses with a wide variety of disease effects. It causes serious illness in newborns and in people being treated with immunosuppressive drugs and therapy, especially following an organ transplant. See also **cytomegalic inclusion disease, TORCH syndrome.**

cytomegalovirus (CMV) disease, **1.** See **cytomegalic inclusion disease.** **2.** a viral infection caused by the cytomegalovirus, characterized by malaise, fever, lymphadinopathy, pneumonia, hepatosplenomegaly, and superinfection with various bacteria and fungi as a result of the depression of immune response characteristic of herpesviruses.

Cytomel, a trade name for a thyroid hormone (liothyronine sodium).

cytometer (saɪtom′ɪtər), a device for counting and measuring the number of cells within a given amount of fluid, as blood, urine, or cerebrospinal fluid

cytometry (saɪtom′ɪtry), the counting and measuring of cells, specifically blood cells. — **cytometric,** *adj.*

cytomitome (saɪ′təmaɪ′toum), the fibrillary network within the cytoplasm of a cell, as contrasted with that in the nucleoplasm. See also **karyomitome.**

cytomorphology, the study of the various forms of cells and the structures contained within them. — **cytomorphologic, cytomorphological,** *adj.*, **cytomorphologist,** *n.*

cytomorphosis, *pl.* **cytomorphoses.** the various changes that occur within a cell during the course of its life cycle, from the earliest undifferentiated stage until destruction.

cyton, cytone (saɪ′tən, saɪ′toun), the cell body of a neuron or that portion containing the nucleus and its surrounding cytoplasm from which the axon and dendrites are formed.

cytophotometer (saɪ′toufətom′ɪtər), an instrument for measuring light density through stained portions of cytoplasm, used for locating and identifying chemical substances within cells.

cytophotometry (saɪ′toufətom′ɪtri), the identification of chemical substances within cells, using a cytophotometer. Also called **microfluorometry.** — **cytophotometric** (saɪ′toufou′təmet′rɪk), *adj.*

cytophysiology, the study of the biochemical processes involved in the functioning of an individual cell, as contrasted with the functioning of organs or tissues. — **cytophysiologic, cytophysiological,** *adj.*, **cytophysiologist,** *n.*

cytoplasm (saɪ′təplæz′əm), all of the substance of a cell other than the nucleus. See also **cell, nucleus.**

cytoplasmic inheritance, the acquisition of traits or conditions controlled by self-replicating substances within the cytoplasm, as mitochondria or chloroplasts, rather than by the genes on the chromosomes in the nucleus. The phenomenon occurs in plants and lower animals but has not yet been demonstrated in man.

Cytosar-U, a trade name for an antineoplastic (cytarabine).

cytotoxic anaphylaxis, an exaggerated reaction of hypersensitivity to an injection of antibodies specific for antigenic substances that occur normally on the surfaces of body cells.

cytotoxic drug, any pharmacological compound that inhibits the proliferation of cells within the body. Such compounds, as the alkylating agents and the antimetabolites, are designed to destroy abnormal cells selectively, while sparing as many normal cells as possible; they are commonly used in chemotherapy. Cytotoxic agents have a potential for producing teratogenesis, mutagenesis, and carcinogenesis.

cytotoxic hypersensitivity, an IgG or an IgM complement dependent, immediate-acting hypersensitive humoral response to foreign cells or to alterations of surface antigens on the cells. Direct and immediate destruction of cells occurs, as seen in hemolytic disease of the newborn and in severe transfusion reactions. Also called **type II hypersensitivity.** See also **immuneglobulin.**

cytotoxin, a substance that has a toxic effect on certain cells. — **cytotoxic,** *adj.*

cytotrophoblast (sāi'toutrof'əblæst), the inner layer of cells of the trophoblast of the early mammalian embryo that gives rise to the outer surface and villi of the chorion. Also called **Langhans' layer.** Compare **syncytiotrophoblast.** — **cytotrophoblastic,** *adj.*

Cytoxan, a trade name for an antineoplastic (cyclophosphamide).

D

D, 1. symbol for **diffusing capacity.** 2. symbol for **dead space gas.**

DA, abbreviation for **developmental age.**

D & C, abbreviation for **dilatation and curettage.**

dacarbazine, an alkylating agent used as an antineoplastic.
- INDICATION: It is prescribed primarily in the treatment of malignant melanoma.
- CONTRAINDICATION: Known hypersensitivity to this drug prohibits its use.
- ADVERSE EFFECTS: Among the more serious adverse reactions are bone marrow depression, gastrointestinal symptoms, alopecia, and fever.

Dacriose, a trade name for an isotonic ophthalmic irrigating solution containing boric acid, sodium carbonate, potassium chloride, benzalkonium chloride, and EDTA.

dacrocyst (dæk′rousɪst), a lacrimal sac at the medial angle of the eye, a normal anatomical feature.

dacry-. See **dacryo-.**

dacryo-, dacry-, a combining form meaning 'pertaining to tears'. *dacryocele, dacryolin, dacryorrhea.*

dacryocystectomy (dæk′rousɪstek′təmi), partial or total excision of the lacrimal sac.

dacryocystitis (dæk′rousɪstaɪ′tɪs), an infection of the lacrimal sac caused by obstruction of the nasolacrimal duct, characterized by tearing and discharge from the eye. In the acute phase, the sac becomes inflamed and painful. The disorder is nearly always unilateral and usually occurs in infants. Systemic administration of antibiotics is usual; local, topical treatment is seldom effective; and, rarely, a dacryocystorhinostomy may be required. Compare **dacryostenosis.**

DACRYOCYSTITIS

dacryocystorhinostomy (dæk′rousɪs′tourainos′təmi), a surgical procedure for restoring drainage into the nose from the lacrimal sac when the nasolacrimal duct is obstructed.

dacryostenosis (dæk′rioustɪnou′sɪs), an abnormal stricture of the nasolacrimal duct, occurring either as a congenital condition or as a result of infection or trauma. Dacryocystorhinostomy may be required to correct this condition. Compare **dacryocystitis.**

Dactil, a trade name for an anticholinergic (piperidolate hydrochloride).

dactinomycin, an antibiotic used as an antineoplastic agent.
- INDICATIONS: It is prescribed in the treatment of a variety of malignant neoplastic diseases, including Wilms' tumor and rhabdomyosarcoma in children.
- CONTRAINDICATIONS: Herpes zoster infection or known hypersensitivity to this drug prohibits its use.
- ADVERSE EFFECTS: Among the more serious adverse reactions are bone marrow depression, severe gastrointestinal disturbances, proctitis, alopecia, and ulcers of the mouth.

dactyl (dæk′tɪl), a digit (finger or toe). — **dactylic,** *adj.*

dactyl-, See **dactylo-.**

-dactyl, a combining form meaning 'digit (finger or toe)': *hermodactyl, pachydactyl, pentadactyl.*

-dactylia, a combining form meaning '(condition of the) fingers or toes': *ankylodactylia, heptadactylia, oligodactylia.* Also **-dactyly.**

dactylo-, dactyl-, a combining form meaning 'pertaining to a finger or toe': *dactylophasia, dactylospasm, dactylosymphysis.*

-dactyly. See **-dactylia.**

Dakin's solution, a formerly used antiseptic solution containing 0.4 to 0.5 per cent of sodium hypochlorite.

Dalmane, a trade name for a sedative-hypnotic (flurazepam hydrochloride).

daltonism (dɔl′tənɪz′əm), *Informal.* a form of color blindness characterized by an inability to distinguish the color red. It is genetically transmitted as a sex-linked autosomal recessive trait. Also called **protanopia.**

Dalton's law of partial pressures, (in physics) a law stating that the sum of the pressure exerted by a mixture of gases is equal to the total of the partial pressures that could be exerted by the gases if they were separated. See also **Avogadro's law, Boyle's law, Gay-Lussac's law.**

damages, (in law) a sum of money awarded to a plaintiff by a court as compensation for any loss, detriment, or injury to the plaintiff's person, property, or rights caused

301

by the malfeasance or negligence of the defendant. **Actual damages** are awarded to reimburse the plaintiff for the loss or injury sustained. **Nominal damages** are awarded to show that a legal wrong has been committed although no recoverable loss can be determined. **Punitive damages** exceed the actual cost of injury or damage and are awarded when the defendant has acted maliciously or in reckless disregard of the plaintiff's rights.

damp, a potentially lethal atmosphere in caves and mines. **Black damp** or **choke damp** is caused by absorption of the available oxygen by coal seams. **Fire damp** is composed of methane and other explosive hydrocarbon gases. **White damp,** is another name for carbon monoxide.

danazol, a synthetic androgen that acts to suppress the output of gonadotropins from the pituitary.

■ INDICATION: It is prescribed in the treatment of endometriosis.

■ CONTRAINDICATIONS: Genital bleeding, cardiac, liver, or kidney dysfunction, or known hypersensitivity to this drug prohibits its use. It is not used in pregnancy or during lactation.

■ ADVERSE EFFECTS: Among the most serious adverse reactions are weight gain, acne, edema, oily skin, and other androgenic effects.

dance reflex, a normal response in the neonate to simulate walking by a reciprocal flexion and extension of the legs when held in an erect position with the soles touching a hard surface. The reflex disappears by about three to four weeks of age and is replaced by controlled, deliberate movement. Also called **step reflex.**

dander, dry scales shed from the skin or hair of animals or feathers of birds that may cause allergy in some individuals.

dandruff, an excessive amount of scaly material composed of dead, keratinized epithelium shed from the scalp that may be a mild form of seborrheic dermatitis. Treatment with a keratolytic shampoo is usually recommended to soften and remove the scales.

dandy fever. See **dengue.**

Dandy-Walker cyst, a cystic malformation of the fourth ventricle of the brain, resulting from hydrocephalus. Diagnosis of the defect is made with CAT scan, with x rays and, less commonly, with a ventriculogram. See also **hydrocephalus, shunt.**

Danocrine, a trade name for an anterior pituitary suppressant (danazol).

Dantrium, a trade name for a skeletal muscle relaxant (dantrolene sodium), used as an adjunct to anesthesia.

dantrolene sodium, a skeletal muscle relaxant.

■ INDICATION: It is prescribed in the treatment of muscle spasticity resulting from injury to the spinal cord or cerebrum. It is not indicated in treatment of spasm from rheumatic disorders.

■ CONTRAINDICATIONS: Liver dysfunction or known hypersensitivity to this drug prohibits its use.

■ ADVERSE EFFECTS: The most serious adverse reaction is potentially fatal hepototoxicity. Common reactions include diarrhea, dizziness, fatigue, and muscular weakness.

dapsone, a bacteriostatic sulfone derivative.

■ INDICATIONS: It is prescribed in the treatment of leprosy and dermatitis herpetiformis.

■ CONTRAINDICATION: Known hypersensitivity to this drug prohibits its use.

■ ADVERSE EFFECTS: Among the more serious adverse reactions are hemolysis (particularly in people who have glucose-6-phosphate dehydrogenase deficiency, methemoglobinemia, nausea, anorexia, and skin rash).

Daraprim, a trade name for an antimalarial (pyrimethamine).

Darbid, a trade name for an anticholinergic (isopropamide iodide).

Darenthin, a trade name for bretylium tosylate.

Daricon, a trade name for an anticholinergic (oxyphencyclimine hydrochloride).

Darier's disease (der′ieiz). See **keratosis follicularis.**

dark-adapted eye, an eye in which the pupil has dilated, making it more sensitive to dim light.

darkfield illumination. See **darkfield microscopy.**

darkfield microscope, a microscope, with a special condenser and diaphragm, that scatters the light from the observed object, so that the object appears bright against a dark background and is more easily examined.

darkfield microscopy, examination with a darkfield microscope, in which the specimen is illuminated by a peripheral light source. Organisms in specimens that have been prepared for use with a darkfield microscope appear to glow against a dark background. The technique is used primarily to identify the syphilis spirochete. Also called **darkfield illumination, ultramicroscopy.**

Darvocet-N, a trade name for a fixed-combination drug containing an analgesic-antipyretic (acetaminophen) and an analgesic (propoxyphene napsylate).

Darvon, a trade name for an analgesic (propoxyphene hydrochloride).

Darvon Compound, a trade name for a fixed combination drug containing an analgesic (propoxyphene hydrochloride) and APC (aspirin, phenacetin, and caffeine).

Darvon-N, a trade name for an analgesic (propoxyphene napsylate).

Darwinian theory, the theory postulated by Charles Darwin that organic evolution results from the process of natural selection of those variants of plants and animals best suited to survive in their environmental surroundings. Also called **Darwinism.** Compare **Lamarckism.** –**Darwinian,** adj., n.

Darwinism. See **Darwinian theory.**

D.A.S.E., abbreviation for **Denver Articulation Screening Examination.**

DAT, abbreviation for *Dental Aptitude Test.* See **dentist.**

data, *sing.* **datum.** some pieces of information, especially those that are part of a collection of information to be used in an analysis of a problem, as the diagnosis of a health problem.

data analysis, (in research) the phase of a study that includes classifying, coding, and tabulating information needed to perform statistical or qualitative analyses according to the research design and appropriate to the data. Data analysis follows data collection and precedes interpretation or application of the data.

data base, a large store or bank of information, especially in a form that can be processed by computer.

data collection, (in research) the phase of a study that includes gathering of information and identification of sampling units as directed by the research design. Data collection precedes data analysis.

daughter chromosome, either of the paired chromatids that during the anaphase stage of mitosis separate and migrate to opposite ends of the cell prior to division. Each contains the complete genetic information of the original chromosome and was formed during interphase by the duplication of the DNA molecule.

daughter product. See **decay product.**

daunorubicin, an anthracycline antibiotic antineoplastic agent.
■ INDICATIONS: It is prescribed in the treatment of cancer, particularly leukemia and neuroblastoma.
■ CONTRAINDICATIONS: Pre-existing bone marrow depression or known hypersensitivity to this drug prohibits its use. It is not given to patients who have previously received a complete course of treatment with daunorubicin or duxorubicin.
■ ADVERSE EFFECTS: Among the most serious adverse reactions are bone marrow depression and cardiotoxicity. Gastrointestinal disturbances, stomatitis, and alopecia are common.

Davidson regimen (dei′vidsən), a method of treating chronic constipation in children, of developing regular bowel habits, and of identifying those with functional bowel disease or obstructive disorders. If necessary, the fecal impactions are removed by a series of hypertonic phosphate enemas. The child is then given in increasing doses mineral oil, until four or five loose bowel movements occur daily. The condition usually subsides within two to three weeks unless Hirschsprung's disease or other obstructive disorder is present. Some children, especially those under two years of age, require supplemental, fat-soluble vitamins to maintain proper nutrition. The regimen may be continued in children older than three years of age as a training procedure for developing regular bowel habits. The child is placed on a potty-chair at a specific time each day for 5 to 15 minutes and, as regular habits develop, the mineral oil is gradually withdrawn over a period of several weeks. See also **toilet training.**

day-care, a specialized program or facility that provides care for preschool children, usually within a group framework, either as a substitute for or extension of home care, particularly for single parents or for parents who are both employed outside the home. Day-care groups vary in size and function and range from casual neighborhood parent-supervised play groups to formal nursery schools or organized centers run by trained personnel. Most day-care programs incorporate a daily schedule of quiet play, outdoor activities, group games and projects, creative or educational play, and snack and rest periods. Group participation provides extensive opportunity for social, educational, and physical development, enables the child to learn how to cope with frustration, dissatisfaction, anger, and fear, especially fear of being separated from the parents, and may offer excellent preparation for entrance into elementary school.

db, abbreviation for **decibel.**

DBI, a trade name for an antidiabetic (phenformin hydrochloride).

DD, abbreviation for **developmental disability.**

DDAVP, a trade name for an antidiuretic (desmopressin acetate).

D.D.S., abbreviation for *Doctor of Dental Surgery.*

DDST, abbreviation for **Denver Developmental Screening Test.**

DDT (dichlorodiphenyltrichloroethane), a water-insoluble chlorinated hydrocarbon used worldwide as a major insecticide, especially in agriculture. In recent years knowledge of its adverse impact on the environment has led to restrictions in its use. In addition, because tolerance in formerly susceptible organisms develops rapidly, DDT has been largely replaced by organophosphate insecticides in the United States. It is still used as a pediculocide where large-scale delousing is justified, as in barracks and refugee camps. Its value as a scabicide is marginal, since scabies and crabs quickly become resistant to it. See also **scabicide.**

DDT poisoning. See **chlorinated organic insecticide poisoning.**

de-, a combining form meaning 'down or from': *deaquation, decartation, dedentition.*

D.E.A., 1. abbreviation for **Drug Enforcement Agency.** 2. abbreviation for *Drug Enforcement Administration.*

dead-end host, any animal from which a parasite cannot escape to continue its life cycle. Humans are dead-end hosts for trichinosis, because the larvae encyst in muscle and human flesh is unlikely to be a source of food for other animals susceptible to this parasite. Compare **definitive host, intermediate host, reservoir host.**

dead space, a cavity that remains after the incomplete closure of a surgical or traumatic wound, leaving an area in which blood can collect and delay healing. See also **anatomical dead space, physiological dead space.**

deaf, 1. unable to hear; hard of hearing. **2.** people who are unable to hear. — **deafness,** *n.*

deaf-and-dumb, the condition of being unable to hear or speak. See also **deaf-mute.**

deaf-mute, a person who is unable to hear or to speak because of disability of the brain or the organs of hearing and speech. Also called **deaf-and-dumb.**

deafness, a condition characterized by a partial or complete loss of hearing. In assessing deafness the patient's ears are examined for drainage, crusts, accumulation of cerumen, or structural abnormality. It is determined if the deafness is temporary or permanent and if the defect is congenital or a condition acquired in childhood, adolescence, or adulthood. The effect of aging, when applicable, is evaluated, and a psychosocial assessment is conducted to ascertain if the individual is well adjusted to deafness or reacts to the handicap with fear, anxiety, frustration, depression, anger, or hostility. In all cases the degree of loss and the kind of impairment causing the loss are determined. See also **conductive hearing loss, sensorineural hearing loss.**

■ OBSERVATIONS: Many conditions and diseases may result in deafness. More than six million people in the United States have some degree of bilateral hearing loss, and more than 50 per cent of those people are over 65 years old. The person with a slight hearing loss may be initially unaware of the problem and then, as the impairment increases, may tend to hide or deny it. Recognition, diagnosis, and early treatment may help to prevent further impairment and to avoid frustration, embarrassment, and danger for the person. An older person with hearing impairment usually has a sensorineural loss as well as a conductive hearing loss. High sounds are hard to hear and discernment of such letter sounds as 's' and 'f' becomes difficult. Speaking clearly and slowly, allowing the person to lip-read, is helpful, as are visual cues clear with enunciation; shouting is not. A severe or sudden hearing loss usually drives the person to seek help. If the loss is sudden, confusion, fear, and even panic are common. The person's speech becomes loud and slurred. There is new danger because the person can't hear horns, whistles, or sirens and has not developed any way to cope with the impairment safely. The congenitally deaf person needs special speech and language training before reaching school age. Most affected children also have a disturbance of visual perception and are more dependent and less mature emotionally and socially; also reading and writing are learned with more difficulty.

■ INTERVENTION: The treatment of deafness depends on the cause. Merely removing impacted cerumen from the external auditory canal may significantly improve hearing. Hearing aids, amplification of sound, or lip-reading may be useful. Speech therapy is useful in teaching a person to speak or helping a person to retain the ability to speak.

■ NURSING CONSIDERATIONS: Caring for a deaf person who is hospitalized for treatment of another problem requires certain adjustments in communication between nurse and patient. To communicate with the deaf patient who lip-reads, staff members speak slowly, enunciate distinctly, use simple phrases, and rephrase any statements that are not understood; the speaker avoids shouting, chewing gum or covering or obscuring the mouth in other ways while speaking. If the patient uses a hearing aid, its placement and operation are checked before the speaker begins to talk; the voice is modulated to a pitch that is comfortable for the patient, and the speaker stands or sits where the lips are visible to the deaf individual. If the patient uses sign language, an interpreter or another means of communication is sought; when a pad and pencil are used, a frequent practice with the newly deaf, the messages are written clearly in short, simple phrases, and adequate time is allowed for the patient to understand and answer. Because hospitalization increases the stress imposed by deafness and because persons with impaired hearing are acutely aware of movement and changes in light, the patient is maintained in a calm, nonstressful, and safe environment. The bed is located so that the patient can see the door. The call bell is placed within reach and is answered promptly and in person; if the patient's eyes are closed when approached, a gentle pat on the arm is used to arouse him without causing undue alarm. The patient is encouraged to express himself, to communicate with friends and relatives, and to participate in planning his own care. When possible, pictures are used to explain procedures or treatment. In addition to physical care, the nurse provides emotional support in frequent visits and communication with the deaf patient and suggests diversions, as working puzzles, playing cards, knitting, sewing, or various hobbies. In preparing the newly deaf patient for discharge, the nurse points out the availability of lip-reading or sign language classes, of organizations for the deaf, and of amplifiers and flashing lights for telephones and doorbells. The importance of a safe environment, of continuing the prescribed regimen of care of the ears, and of keeping outpatient appointments are stressed. If the patient is to wear a hearing aid, the nurse may assist in demonstrating its use and care.

dean, the chief executive and educational officer of a unit of a university, school, or college.

death, 1. apparent death, the cessation of life as indicated by the absence of heartbeat or respiration. **2. legal death,** the total absence of activity in the brain and central nervous system, the cardiovascular system, and the respiratory system as observed and declared by a physician. See also **cell death, crib death, fetal death, sudden infant death syndrome.**

death trance, a state in which a person appears to be dead.

debility (dɪbɪl′ɪti), feebleness, weakness, or loss of strength. See also **asthenia.**

debride (dɪbrid′), to remove dirt, foreign objects, damaged tissue, and cellular debris from a wound or a burn in order to prevent infection and to promote healing. In treating a wound, debridement is the first step in cleansing it; debridement also allows thorough examination of the extent of the injury. In treating a burn, debridement of the eschar may be performed in a hydrotherapy bath. —**debridement,** n.

Debrox, a trade name for a topical anti-infective (carbamide peroxide).

dec-, 1. a combining form meaning 'ten': *decagram, decaliter, decipara.* **2.** a combining form meaning 'tenth': *decigram, deciliter, decinormal.*

Decadron, a trade name for a glucocorticoid (dexamethasone).

Deca-Durabolin, a trade name for an androgen (nandrolone decanoate), used as an anabolic agent.

decalcification (dikæl′sɪfɪkei′ʃhən), loss of calcium salts from the teeth and bones caused by malnutrition, malabsorption, or other dietary or physiological factors. It may result, particularly in older people, from a diet that lacks adequate calcium. Malabsorption may be caused by a lack of vitamin D necessary for the absorption of calcium from the intestine, by an excess of dietary fats that can combine with calcium to form an indigestible soaplike compound, by the presence of oxalic acid that can combine with calcium to form a relatively insoluble calcium oxalate salt, or by a relative lack of acid in the digestive tract that can decrease the solubility of calcium. Other factors include the parathyroid hormone control of the calcium level in the bloodstream, the ratio of calcium to phosphorus in the blood, and the relative activity of osteoblast cells which form calcium deposits in the bones and teeth and osteoclast cells that absorb calcium from bones and teeth. Bone tissue tends to be maintained in quantities no greater than needed to meet current physical stress. Therefore, inactive and, particularly, bedridden people lose calcium from their bones; osteoclastic activity exceeds osteoblastic activity, and decalcification occurs. See also **calcium, mineral.**

decamethonium bromide (dek′əmɪthou′niəm), a skeletal muscle relaxant.

■ INDICATIONS: It is prescribed as an adjunct to anesthesia to induce skeletal muscle relaxation and to lessen skeletal muscle contractions in convulsions.

■ CONTRAINDICATIONS: Severe renal disease, myotonia, or known hypersensitivity to this drug or to other bromides prohibits its use.

■ ADVERSE EFFECTS: Among the more serious adverse reactions are ventricular arrhythmias, increased arterial pressure, and cardiac arrest.

decanoic acid (dek′ənou′ɪk). See **capric acid.**

Decapryn Succinate, a trade name for an antihistaminic (doxylamine succinate).

decay product, (in radiology) a stable or radioactive nuclide formed directly from the radioactive disintegration of a radionuclide or as a result of successive transformation in a radioactive series. Also called **daughter product.**

deceleration, a decrease in the speed or velocity of an object or reaction. Compare **acceleration.**

deceleration phase, (in obstetrics) the latter part of active labor characterized by a decreased rate of dilatation of the cervical os on a Friedman curve.

decerebrate rigidity (diser′əbreit). See **tonic labyrinthine reflex.**

decibel (db), a unit of measure of the intensity of sound. A decibel is one tenth of a bel; an increase of one bel is perceived as an approximate doubling of loudness.

decidua (dɪsɪj′uə), the epithelial tissue of the endometrium lining the uterus, especially that which envelops the conceptus during gestation and is shed in the puerperium, but also that which is shed during menstruation. Kinds of decidua are **decidua basalis, decidua capsularis, decidua vera.**

decidua basalis, the decidua of the endometrium in the uterus that lies beneath the implanted ovum. Also called **decidua serotina.**

decidua capsularis, the decidua of the endometrium of the uterus covering the implanted ovum. Also called **decidua reflexa.**

decidual endometritis, an inflammation or infection of any portion of the decidua during pregnancy. See also **endometritis.**

decidua menstrualis, the endometrium shed during menstruation.

decidua parietalis. See **decidua vera.**

decidua reflexa. See **decidua capsularis.**

decidua serotina. See **decidua basalis.**

decidua vera, the decidua of the endometrium lining the uterus except for those areas beneath and above the implanted and developing ovum called, respectively, the decidua basalis and the decidua capsularis.

deciduous dentition, the eruption of the first teeth, which are later replaced by the permanent teeth. The process usually begins between the sixth and eighth months of life with the appearance of the two lower incisors and is completed between two and three years of age with a total of 20 teeth. The deciduous teeth are shed in order of appearance and replaced by 32 permanent teeth. Also called **first dentition, primary dentition.** Compare

permanent dentition. See also **prediciduous dentition, teething.**

deciduous tooth, any one of the set of 20 teeth that appear during infancy, consisting of four incisors, two canines, and four molars in each jaw. Deciduous teeth start developing about the sixth week of fetal life as a thickening of the epithelium along the line of the future jaw. During the seventh week the epithelium splits longitudinally into the labial strand and the lingual strand. The labial strand forms the labiodental lamina. The lingual strand becomes the dental lamina which develops 10 enlargements in each jaw. The enlargements appear about the ninth week and correspond to the future deciduous teeth. In most individuals the first deciduous tooth erupts through the gum about six months after birth. Thereafter, one or more deciduous teeth erupt about every month until all 20 have appeared. The deciduous teeth are usually shed between the ages of 6 and 13, although the timing varies greatly from person to person. Also called **milk tooth.** Compare **permanent tooth.** See also **tooth.**

Declomycin, a trade name for an antibacterial (demeclocycline hydrochloride).

decoded message, (in communication theory) a message as translated by a receiver. If it is correctly interpreted within the context of the message as sent by the sender, the decoded message is the same as the encoded message; if it is not understood and interpreted as sent, it is not the same as the encoded message.

decoic acid (dɪkoʊ'ɪk). See **capric acid.**

decompression sickness, a painful, sometimes fatal syndrome caused by the formation of nitrogen bubbles in the tissues of divers, caisson workers, and aviators who move too rapidly from environments of higher pressure to those of lower pressure. Nitrogen breathed in air under pressure dissolves in tissue fluids. When ambient pressure is reduced too rapidly, nitrogen comes out of solution faster than it can be circulated to the lungs for expiration. Gaseous nitrogen then accumulates in the joint spaces and peripheral circulation, impairing tissue oxygenation. Disorientation, severe pain, and syncope follow. Treatment is by rapid return of the patient to an environment of higher pressure followed by gradual decompression. Death is more often caused by accident during syncope than by decompression sickness itself. Also called **the bends, caisson disease.** Compare **barotrauma.**

decongestant, 1. of or pertaining to a substance or procedure that eliminates or reduces congestion or swelling. 2. a decongestant drug. Antihistaminic agents, as chlorpheniramine maleate, and adrenergic drugs, as epinephrine, ephedrine, and phenylpropanolamine hydrochloride, that cause bronchodilation or vasoconstriction of nasal mucosa are used as decongestants. Respiratory tract congestion caused by bacterial infection is usually treated with an antibiotic, and nasal congestion produced by the common cold may be relieved by the inhalation of plain or mentholated steam.

decortication (dikɔr'tɪkei'šhən), (in medicine) the removal of the cortical tissue of an organ or structure, as the kidney, the brain, and the lung. —**decorticate,** v., adj.

decubitus (dɪkyu'bɪtəs), 1. a recumbent or horizontal position, as lateral decubitus which is lying on one side. 2. See also **decubitus care, a decubitus ulcer.**

decubitus care, the management and prevention of decubitus ulcers that occur most frequently on the sacrum, elbows, heels, outer ankles, inner knees, hips, shoulder blades, and ear rims of immobilized patients, especially those who are obese, elderly, or suffering from infections, injuries, or a poor nutritional state.

■ METHOD: Decubiti may be prevented by repositioning the immobile patient every two hours, by keeping the skin dry, and by inspecting pressure areas every four to six hours for signs of redness. Bed linen is kept dry and wrinkle-free; a sheet is used to lift the patient who is moved frequently from the bed but is not allowed to sit in one place for more than 30 minutes. A high-protein diet, vitamins, and iron may be ordered for vulnerable patients and a prophylactic measure is daily skin care, in which all areas are washed, rinsed, and dried thoroughly and lotion is gently rubbed on bony prominences. A thin layer of cornstarch or a noncaking powder is applied to areas showing excessive perspiration, and the perineal and perianal areas are washed with soap and water after each defecation and urination. Preventive devices include air mattresses, flotation mattresses, sheepskins, silicone pads, foam cushions for wheelchairs, and heel and elbow guards. Stage I decubiti, characterized by redness that is not relieved by circulatory stimulation or removal of pressure, and Stage II lesions, involving excoriation, vesiculation, or breaks in the skin, are treated similarly. The area is cleaned every eight hours as indicated with mild soap and water, dilute hydrogen peroxide, or normal saline solution and is blotted dry. To increase circulation the area is massaged gently and exposed every two to four hours for 15 minutes to air, sunlight, or a heat lamp. Magnesium aluminum hydroxide gel, karaya powder, tincture of benzoin, or povidone-iodine may be applied to the area, but if there is no improvement within 48 hours a different kind of dressing is tried. Pressure and irritation to excoriated areas are avoided at all times. Stage III decubiti, in which there is full-thickness skin loss, and Stage IV pressure ulcers that characteristically invade fascia, connective tissue, muscle, or bone, require more extensive treatment. The patient is turned every one to two hours and the lesion is irrigated with hydrogen peroxide and water every six to eight hours. The affected area is exposed to air for 15 to 30 minutes every two to four hours and to a heat lamp for 15 minutes every four to six hours. The ulcer may be incised, debrided, and covered with a nonadhering dressing secured by nonallergenic tape. Proteolytic enzyme preparations, antibiotics, magnesium aluminum hydroxide gel, or povidone-iodine may be applied to the wound, and granulated sugar dressings may be used after removal of necrotic tissue, though they are contraindicated in diabetic patients.

■ NURSING ORDERS: The nurse plays a major role in the prevention of decubiti and in their treatment if they occur, turning the patient at frequent intervals, applying the ordered medications and dressings to the lesions, and, in the administration of daily skin care, avoiding vigorous rubbing. The nurse conducts active or passive exercises with massage to the patient's extremities and, when indicated, prepares for incision and debridement of advanced ulcers.

■ OUTCOME CRITERIA: Decubiti are often resistant to treatment, and large areas of ulceration can be life-threatening, especially in a debilitated patient. Prompt and continued care of early lesions can prevent invasion of underlying tissue and promote healing.

decubitus ulcer, an inflammation, sore, or ulcer in the skin over a bony prominence. It results from ischemic hypoxia of the tissues owing to prolonged pressure on the part. Decubitus ulcers are most often seen in aged, debilitated, immobilized, or cachectic patients. The sores are graded by stages of severity: Stage I: The skin is red. With massage and relief of pressure, the color of the skin does not return to normal. Stage II: The skin is blistered, peeling, or cracked, though damage is still superficial. Stage III: The skin is broken; a full thickness of skin is lost, subcutaneous tissue may also be damaged, and a serous or bloody drainage may be seen. Stage IV: A deep, craterlike ulcer has formed. The full thickness of skin and the subcutaneous tissues are destroyed. Fascia, connective tissue, bone, or muscle underlying the ulcer are exposed and may be damaged. Prevention of decubitus ulcers is a cardinal aspect of nursing care; treatment is planned specific to the location and the extent of the condition.

■ OBSERVATIONS: Decubitus ulcers form most commonly on the skin over the shoulder blades, elbows, sacrum, hips, knees, ankles, and heels. The sores are likely to deepen and spread and become infected.

■ INTERVENTION: Nursing actions for the prevention of decubitus ulcers include keeping the skin dry, turning the patient at least every two hours, avoiding wrinkled or tight sheets, lifting instead of sliding the patient, massaging bony prominences with a lubricant at least once every four hours, and using pads, mattresses, flotation, and other devices designed to distribute the patient's weight over a larger body area. Exercise, movement, a high-protein diet, vitamins and minerals as needed, and scrupulous skin care all help to prevent the development of decubitus ulcers. Treatment of Stage I and Stage II lesions includes all of these preventive actions; in addition,

the ulcer is cleaned with soap and water, hydrogen peroxide and water, or normal saline solution three times a day. The sore should be dried by exposure to air and sunlight or by a heat lamp for fifteen minutes at least every four hours, with frequent checks to prevent burning. Sometimes oxygen is administered simultaneously to the sore. The patient is positioned so that no pressure is placed on the sore. A sterile dressing is applied over a preparation of magnesium aluminum hydroxide gel, karaya powder, A & D ointment, tincture of benzoin, or povidone-iodine. If the preparation is effective after 48 hours, its use is continued; if not, another is tried. Stage III and Stage IV decubitus ulcers require all of the care described for prevention and for the treatment of Stages I and II. Further treatment includes observation of the character and quantity of drainage and the irrigation of the ulcer with hydrogen peroxide and water at least every eight hours. Debridement and incision may be necessary. Dressings are changed at least every eight hours and may be placed over applications of granulated sugar, proteolytic enzymes, antibiotics, magnesium aluminum hydroxide gel, gold-leaf flakes, or povidone-iodine.

■ NURSING CONSIDERATIONS: Patients at risk for the development of decubitus ulcers receive preventive care. The nurse may elicit the cooperation and participation of the patient in a nursing-care plan that includes all preventive measures. The importance of frequent change of position, dryness, cleanliness, and good nutrition are emphasized.

decussate, to cross in the form of an 'X,' as certain nerve fibers from the retina cross at the optic chiasm. – decussation, n.

deep brachial artery, a branch of each of the brachial arteries, arising at the distal border of the teres major, passing deeply into the arm between the long and lateral heads of the triceps brachii, and supplying the humerus and the muscles of the upper arm. It has five branches: the ascending, radial collateral, middle collateral, muscular, and the nutrient. Also called **superior profunda artery.**

deep-breathing and coughing exercises, the exercises taught to a person to improve aeration or to maintain respiratory function, especially following prolonged inactivity or after general anesthesia. Incisional pain following surgery in the chest or abdomen inhibits normal respiratory excursion. See also **cupping and vibrating, postural drainage.**

■ METHOD: The person is assisted to a comfortable position, supine or sitting up. An analgesic is given prior to the exercises if pain is present. Inhalation through the nose and exhalation through the mouth are encouraged. Following a deep inhalation, with the incision supported, the patient is asked to cough. If pain prevents the person from producing a deep, effective cough, a series of short barklike coughs may be encouraged.

■ OUTCOME CRITERIA: When shallow breathing has replaced deep breathing, secretions tend to dry in the respiratory passages, causing damage to the mucous membranes lining the passages. Coughing and deep breathing serve to clear the dried or thick and viscid mucus, to allow moisturized air to enter the bronchi, bronchioles, and alveoli, and to expand the lungs and increase the exchange of gases, thereby improving ventilation.

■ NURSING ORDERS: The use of simple nursing techniques and patience and encouragement significantly improve the effectiveness of the exercises. Positioning increases comfort, allows the abdominal contents to fall away from the diaphragm, and encourages full expansion of the chest wall on inspiration. If an incision is present it may be supported with the hands or with a book or pillow held against the abdomen. The person is often reluctant to breathe deeply or to cough; adequate analgesia, encouragement, and a patient explanation to the person of the benefits may overcome that resistance. Various devices are available for use in respiratory exercises, as those used in atelactasis to strengthen the muscles used in expiration and to empty the air sacs of retained gas. Postural drainage is commonly performed concurrently with coughing and deep breathing exercises.

deep coma. See **coma.**

deep fascia, the most extensive of three kinds of fascia comprising an intricate series of connective sheets and bands that hold the muscles and other structures in place throughout the body, wrapping the muscles in gray, felt-like membranes. The deep fasciae comprise a continuous system, splitting and fusing in an elaborate network attached to the skeleton and divided into the outer investing layer, the internal investing layer, and the intermediate membranes. Compare **subcutaneous fascia, subserous fascia.**

deep palmar arch, the termination of the radial artery, joining the deep palmar branch of the ulnar artery in the palm of the hand.

deep sensation, the awareness or perception of pain, pressure, or tension in the deep layers of the skin, the muscles, tendons, or joints. Such sensations are conveyed to the brain via the spinal column. Compare **superficial sensation.**

deep temporal artery, one of the branches of the maxillary artery on each side of the head. It branches into the anterior portion and the posterior portion, both rising between the temporalis and the pericranium to supply the temporalis and to anastomose with the middle temporal artery. The anterior branch communicates with the lacrimal artery by small branches which pierce the zygomatic bone and the great wing of the sphenoid. Compare **middle temporal artery, superficial temporal artery.**

deep tendon reflex (DTR), a brisk contraction of a muscle in response to a sudden stretch induced by a sharp tap by a finger or rubber hammer on the tendon of

insertion of the muscle. Absence of the reflex may have been caused by damage to the muscle, the peripheral nerve, nerve roots, or the spinal cord at that level. A hyperactive reflex may indicate disease of the pyramidal tract above the level of the reflex arc being tested. Generalized hyperactivity of DTRs may be owing to hyperthyroidism. Kinds of DTRs include **ankle reflex, biceps reflex, brachioradialis reflex, patellar reflex, triceps reflex.** Also called **myotatic reflex, tendon reflex.** See also **hung-up reflex.**

deep vein, one of the many systemic veins that accompany the arteries, usually enclosed in a sheath that wraps both the vein and the associated artery. The larger arteries, as the axillary, the femoral, the popliteal, and the subclavian, are usually accompanied by only one deep vein. The deep veins accompanying the smaller arteries, as the brachial, the peroneal, and the radial, usually occur in pairs, one vein on each side of the artery. Various structures, as the skull, the vertebral column, and the liver, are served by less closely associated arteries and veins. Compare **superficial vein.**

deep x-ray therapy, the treatment of internal neoplasms, as Wilms' tumor of the kidney, Hodgkin's disease, and other cancers, with ionizing radiation from an external source. The dose delivered is determined according to the radiosensitivity, size, pathologic grade and differentiation of the tumor, the tolerance of normal surrounding tissue to irradiation, and the condition of the patient. Deep x-ray therapy frequently causes nausea, malaise, diarrhea, and skin reactions, as blanching, erythema, itching, burning, oozing, or desquamation, but with modern techniques the ray is beamed directly to the site, reducing side scatter, and the skin can be spared. Since tumor cells are hypoxic and are more effectively eradicated when they are well oxygenated, the patient may breathe hyperbaric oxygen or atmospheric oxygen with five per cent carbon dioxide during deep x-ray therapy.

deer-fly fever. See **tularemia.**

defamation, any communication, written or spoken, that is untrue and that injures the good name or reputation of another or that in any way brings that person into disrepute.

default judgment, (in law) a judgment rendered against a defendant because of the defendant's failure to appear in court or to answer the plaintiff's claim within the proper time.

defecation (def'ıkei'shən), the elimination of feces from the digestive tract through the rectum. See also **constipation, diarrhea, feces.** —**defecate,** v.

defecation reflex. See **rectal reflex.**

defendant, (in law) the party that is named in a plaintiff's complaint and against whom the plaintiff's allegations are made. The defendant must respond to the allegations.

defense mechanism, an unconscious, intrapsychic reaction that offers protection to the self from a stressful situation. Kinds of defense mechanisms include **compensation, conversion, dissociation, displacement, sublimation.** Also called **ego defense mechanism.**

deferent duct, the excretory duct of the testis. Also called **ductus deferens.**

defervescence (di'fərves'əns), the diminishing or disappearance of a fever. — **defervescent,** *adj.*

defibrillate (difai'brəleit, difib'rəleit), to stop fibrillation of the atria or the ventricles of the heart, usually by delivering an electric shock to the myocardium through the chest wall by the use of a defibrillator. — **defibrillation,** *n.*

defibrillation, the termination of atrial or ventricular fibrillation, usually accomplished by delivering a direct electrical countershock to the patient's precordium.

■ METHOD: Defibrillation by electrical countershock is a common emergency measure generally performed by a physician or specially trained nurse or paramedic. The electrode paddles of the defibrillator are covered with a conductive jelly or applied over wet saline sponges. One paddle is placed to the right of the upper sternum below the clavicle and the other is applied to the midaxillary line of the left lower rib cage. In another method, one paddle is placed over the precordium and the other is applied beneath the patient's chest. The defibrillator, usually a condenser discharge system, is set to deliver between 200 and 400 watts per second. Respiratory support is suspended during the shock but is promptly resumed. If one or two shocks fail to cause defibrillation, cardiopulmonary resuscitation (CPR) may be conducted until another shock is attempted. Before the procedure, the patient's level of consciousness, pulse, respirations, and electrocardiogram are observed. After defibrillation, the patient's level of consciousness, irritation or sloughing of the exposed skin of the chest, and electrocardiographic signs of the return of sinus rhythm, continued fibrillation, and the development of cardiac standstill are investigated. Blood pressure, apical pulse, and respirations are checked every five to ten minutes for four hours, and then every 30 to 60 minutes. CPR is initiated if no pulse is present. Cardiac activity is monitored; arterial blood gases may be determined, and oxygen with assisted ventilation may be ordered. Parenteral fluids are maintained and the patient's skin, which may be irritated by the shock, receives care by application of a lanolin-based lotion.

■ NURSING ORDERS: The nurse performs all the required procedures before and after defibrillation and makes certain that all equipment surrounding the patient is grounded.

■ OUTCOME CRITERIA: Successful defibrillation by electrical countershock can reverse life-threatening cardiac arrythmias, especially ventricular fibrillation.

defibrillator (difai'brilei'tər, difib'rilei'tər), a device that delivers an electrical shock at a preset voltage to the myocardium through the chest wall. It is used for restoring the normal cardiac rhythm and rate when the heart has stopped beating or is fibrillating.

deficiency disease, a condition resulting from the lack of one or more essential nutrients in the diet, from metabolic dysfunction, or from impaired digestion or absorption, excessive excretion, or increased biological requirements. Compare **malnutrition.** See also **avitaminosis.**

definitive, **1.** final; clearly established without doubt or question. **2.** (in embryology) fully formed in the final differentiation of a tissue, structure, or organ. Compare **primitive.** **3.** (in parasitology) of or pertaining to the host in which the parasite undergoes the sexual phase of its reproductive cycle.

definitive host, any animal in which the reproductive stages of a parasite develop. The female anopheles mosquito is the definitive host for malaria. Humans are definitive hosts for pinworms, schistosomes, and tapeworms. Also called **primary host.** Compare **dead-end host, intermediate host, reservoir host.** See also **host,** def. 1.

definitive treatment, any therapy generally accepted as a specific cure of a disease. Compare **expectant treatment, palliative treatment, supportive treatment.**

deformity, a condition of being distorted, disfigured, flawed, malformed, or misshapen, which may affect the body in general or any part of it and may be the result of disease, injury, or birth defect, as Arnold-Chiari deformity, in which a part of the brain protrudes through the base of the skull into the spinal canal, and seal-fin deformity, characterized by a deviation of the fingers as an effect of rheumatoid arthritis.

degenerative chorea. See **Huntington's chorea.**

degenerative disease, any disease in which there is deterioration of structure or function of tissue. Some kinds of degenerative disease are **arteriosclerosis, cancer, osteoarthritis.**

degenerative joint disease. See **osteoarthritis.**

deglutition (di'gluti∫'ən), swallowing.

deglutition apnea, the normal absence of respiration during swallowing.

dehydrate, **1.** to remove or lose water from a substance. **2.** to lose excessive water from the body. — **dehydration,** *n.*

dehydrated alcohol, a clear, colorless, highly hygroscopic liquid with a burning taste, containing at least 99.5 per cent ethyl alcohol by volume. Also called **absolute alcohol.**

dehydration, excessive loss of water from the body tissues. Dehydration is accompanied by a disturbance in the balance of essential electrolytes, particularly sodium, potassium, and chloride. Dehydration may follow prolonged fever, diarrhea, vomiting, acidosis, and any condition where there is rapid depletion of body fluids. It is of particular concern among infants and young children, since their electrolyte balance is normally precarious. Signs of dehydration include poor skin turgor, flushed dry skin, coated tongue, oliguria, irritability, and confusion. Normal fluid volume and balanced electrolyte values are the primary goals of therapy.

dehydration fever, a fever that frequently occurs in newborns, thought to be caused by dehydration. Also called **inanition fever.** Compare **inanition, starvation.**

déjà vu (*French* deiʐHAVY′), the sensation or illusion that one is encountering a set of circumstances or a place that was previously experienced. The phenomenon, which is normal in everyone but occurs more frequently or continuously in certain emotional and organic disorders, results from some unconscious emotional connection with the present experience. Compare **jamais vu, paramnesia.**

Dejerine-Sottas disease (deʐh′ərinsot′əz), a rare, congenital spinocerebellar disorder characterized by the development of palpable thickenings along peripheral nerves, degeneration of the peripheral nervous system, pain, paresthesia, ataxia, diminished sensation, and deep tendon reflexes. Diagnosis is made by a histological examination of a peripheral nerve. There is no specific treatment. Also called **interstitial hypertrophic neuropathy.**

Deladumone, a trade name for a fixed-combination drug containing an androgen (testosterone enanthate) and an estrogen (estradiol valerate).

Delalutin, a trade name for a progestin (hydroxyprogesterone caproate).

Delano, Jane A. (1862–1919), an American nurse who organized the American Red Cross Nursing Service, an organization formed to supply nurses to the military forces. In 1891 she became the director of the Nurses' Training School of the University of Pennsylvania and was later appointed the director of the Bellevue Hospital Training School for Nurses in New York, where she had been trained. On a trip to survey nursing conditions in Europe, she died following surgery for a mastoid infection at Base Hospital, Savenay, France, in March 1919.

Delatestryl, a trade name for an androgen (testosterone enanthate).

delayed dentition. See **retarded dentition.**

delayed echolalia, a phenomenon, commonly seen in schizophrenia, involving the meaningless, automatic repetition of overheard words and phrases. It occurs hours, days, or even weeks after the original stimulus.

delayed hypersensitivity reaction. See **cell-mediated immune response.**

delayed postpartum hemorrhage, hemorrhage occurring later than 24 hours after delivery. It is most often caused by retained fragments of the placenta, a laceration of the cervix or vagina that was not discovered or that was not completely sutured, or by subinvolution of the placental site within the uterus. Characteristics of delayed postpartum hemorrhage are heavy bleeding and signs of impending shock and anemia. The cause is diagnosed and treated. A laceration is closed with suture, retained fragments of placenta are removed, infection is treated with antibiotics, or the uterus is caused to contract by the administration of ergotrate or oxytocin. See also **postpartum hemorrhage.**

Delestrogen, a trade name for an estrogen (estradiol valerate).

deletion syndrome, any of a group of congenital autosomal anomalies that result from the loss of chromosomal genetic material, owing to breakage of a chromatid during cell division, as the cat-cry syndrome, which results from the absence of the short arms of chromosome 5.

Physical signs of dehydration

	Isotonic (loss of water and salt)	Hypotonic (loss of salt in excess of water)	Hypertonic (loss of water in excess of salt)
Skin			
Color	Gray	Gray	Gray
Temperature	Cold	Cold	Cold or hot
Turgor	Poor	Very poor	Fair
Feel	Dry	Clammy	Thickened
Mucous membranes	Dry	Slightly moist	Parched
Tearing and salivation	Absent	Absent	Absent
Eyeball	Sunken and soft	Sunken and soft	Sunken
Fontanel	Sunken	Sunken	Sunken
Body temperature	Subnormal or elevated	Subnormal	Subnormal or elevated
Pulse	Rapid	Very rapid	Moderately rapid
Respirations	Rapid	Rapid	Rapid
Behavior	Irritable to lethargic	Lethargic to comatose; convulsions	Marked lethargy with extreme hyper-irritability on stimulation

Delhi boil (del′i). See **oriental sore.**

deliberate hypotension, an anesthetic process in which a short-acting hypotensive agent like nitroprusside or trimethaphan is given to reduce blood pressure, thus bleeding, during surgery. The procedure facilitates surgery by making vessels and tissues more visible and reducing blood loss.

delinquency, 1. negligence or failure to fulfill a duty or obligation. 2. an offense, fault, misdemeanor, or misdeed; a tendency to commit such acts. See also **juvenile delinquency.**

delinquent, 1. characterized by neglect of duty or violation of law. 2. one whose behavior is characterized by persistent antisocial, illegal, violent, or criminal acts; a juvenile delinquent.

delirium (dilir′iəm), 1. a state of frenzied excitement or wild enthusiasm. 2. an acute organic mental disorder characterized by confusion, disorientation, restlessness, clouding of the consciousness, incoherence, fear, anxiety, excitement, and often illusions, hallucinations, usually of visual origin, and, at times, delusions. The condition is caused by disturbances in cerebral functions that may result from a wide range of metabolic disorders, including nutritional deficiencies and endocrine imbalances; postpartum or postoperative stress; the ingestion of several types of toxic substances, such as various gases, metals, or drugs, including alcohol; and any other causes of physical and mental shock or exhaustion. The symptoms are usually of short duration and reversible with treatment of the underlying cause, although in extreme cases, where the toxic condition is extremely severe or prolonged, permanent brain damage may occur. Bed rest in a quiet environment is essential. The delirious patient must be protected from accidents and self-injury. In prolonged cases, dehydration and vitamin deficiency may occur. Sedatives or tranquilizing drugs are often used to relieve excitability. Kinds of delirium include **acute delirium, delirium tremens, exhaustion delirium, senile delirium, traumatic delirium.** Compare **dementia.** – **delirious,** *adj.*

delirium tremens (DTs), an acute and sometimes fatal psychotic reaction caused by excessive intake of alcoholic beverages over a long period of time. The reaction may follow a prolonged alcoholic debauch without an adequate intake of food, occur during a period of abstinence, be precipitated by a head injury or infection, or result from the partial or total withdrawal of alcohol after prolonged drinking. Initial symptoms include loss of appetite, insomnia, and general restlessness, followed by agitation, excitement, disorientation, mental confusion, vivid and often frightening hallucinations, acute fear and anxiety, illusions and delusions, coarse tremors of the hands, feet, legs, and tongue, fever, increased heart rate, extreme perspiration, gastrointestinal distress, and precordial pain. The episode, which usually constituess a medical emergency, typically lasts from three to six days and is generally followed by a deep sleep. Treatment includes a quiet, nonstimulating environment in which the person is watched closely and protected from self-injury, not only during the period of delirium but, more importantly, during convalescence when depression and remorse often lead to attempted suicide. Extreme fatigue, pneumonia, respiratory infections, and heart failure are common complications, as are severe dehydration and nutritional deficiencies. Dietary supplements are often given; tube feeding and intravenous fluids may be needed. Sedatives and tranquilizing agents are useful for quieting the person. Compare **alcoholic hallucinosis, Stearns' alcoholic amentia.** See also **Korsakoff's psychosis.**

delivery, (in obstetrics) the birth of a child; parturition.

delta-1-testolactone. See **testolactone.**

Delta-Cortef, a trade name for a glucocorticoid (prednisolone).

delta rhythm. See **delta wave.**

delta wave, the slowest of the four types of brain waves, characterized by a frequency of 4 Hz and a relatively high voltage. Delta waves are "deep sleep waves" associated with a dreamless state from which an individual is not easily aroused. Also called **delta rhythm.** Compare **alpha wave, beta wave, theta wave.**

deltoid, 1. triangular. 2. of or pertaining to the deltoid muscle that covers the shoulder.

deltoideus (deltoi′diəs). See **deltoid muscle.**

deltoid muscle, a large, thick triangular muscle that covers the shoulder joint and abducts, flexes, extends, and rotates the arm. It arises from various surfaces on the clavicle, acromion, and scapula and inserts, with a thick tendon, into the humerus. Also called **deltoideus.**

delusion, a persistent, aberrant belief or perception held inviolable by a person even though it is illogical, unique, and probably wrong. Kinds of delusion include **delusion of being controlled, delusion of grandeur, delusion of persecution, nihilistic delusion, somatic delusion.** Compare **illusion.**

delusion of being controlled, the false belief that one's feelings, beliefs, thoughts, and acts are governed by some external force, as seen in various forms of schizophrenia. See also **delusion.**

delusion of grandeur, the gross exaggeration of one's importance, wealth, power, or talents, as seen in such disorders as megalomania, general paresis, and paranoid schizophrenia. See also **delusion.**

delusion of persecution, a morbid belief that one is being mistreated and harassed by unidentified enemies, as seen in paranoia and paranoid schizophrenia. See also **delusion.**

delusion of reference. See **idea of reference.**

delusion stupor, the state of lethargy and unresponsiveness observed in catatonic schizophrenia.

demarcation current, an electric current that flows from an uninjured to an injured end of a muscle. Also called **current of injury.**

Demazine, a trade name for a respiratory, fixed-combination drug containing an adrenergic (phenylephrine hydrochloride) and an antihistiminic (chlorpheniramine maleate).

deme (dim), a small, closely related interbreeding population of organisms or individuals, usually occupying a circumscribed area. Also called **genetic population.**

demecarium bromide, an ophthalmic anticholinesterase agent.
- INDICATION: It is prescribed in the treatment of open-angle glaucoma.
- CONTRAINDICATIONS: Active uveal inflammation, narrow-angle glaucoma, glaucoma associated with iridocyclitis, or known hypersensitivity to this drug prohibits its use.
- ADVERSE EFFECTS: Among the most serious adverse reactions are symptoms associated with systemic absorption of anticholinesterase agents, as bradycardia and diarrhea. Eye irritation, formation of cysts, and lens opacities also may occur.

demeclocycline hydrochloride, an antibiotic.
- INDICATIONS: It is prescribed in the treatment of a variety of infections.
- CONTRAINDICATIONS: Renal or liver dysfunction, pregnancy, early childhood, or known hypersensitivity to this drug or to other tetracycline medication prohibits its use.
- ADVERSE EFFECTS: Among the more serious adverse effects are gastrointestinal disturbances, phototoxicity, potentially serious suprainfections, and hypersensitivity reactions. Discoloration of teeth may occur in children exposed to the drug in utero or before eight years of age.

dementia (dimen'shə), a progressive, organic mental disorder characterized by chronic personality disintegration, confusion, disorientation, stupor, deterioration of intellectual capacity and function, and impairment of control of memory, judgment, and impulses. Dementia caused by drug intoxication, hyperthyroidism, pernicious anemia, paresis, subdural hematoma, benign brain tumor, hydrocephalus, insulin shock, and tumor of islet cells of the pancreas can be reversed by treating the condition; Alzheimer's disease, Pick's disease, Huntington's disease, and traumatic injuries to the brain are not amenable to treatment. Kinds of dementia include **Alzheimer's disease, dementia paralytica, dementia praecox, secondary dementia, senile dementia, toxic dementia.**

dementia paralytica. See **general paresis.**

dementia praecox (pri'koks), *Obsolete.* schizophrenia, especially developing in adolescence or early adulthood. See also **schizophrenia.**

Demerol, a trade name for a narcotic analgesic (meperidine).

Demerol Hydrochloride, a trade name for a narcotic analgesic (meperidine hydrochloride).

-demic, a combining form meaning 'relating to disease in a (specified) region': *interedemic, philodemic, prosodemic.*

demigauntlet bandage (dem'igont'lıt), a glovelike bandage covering only the hand and leaving the fingers free. See also **gauntlet bandage.**

demography (dəmog'rəfi), the study of human populations, particularly the size, distribution, and characteristics of members of population groups. Demography is applied in studies of health problems involving ethnic groups, populations of a specific geographic region, religious groups with special dietary restrictions, as Mormons or Seventh-Day Adventists, and members of population groups that may represent a typical cross-section of the entire nation, as in the continuing study of residents of Framingham, Massachusetts, by the National Institutes of Health. Compare **epidemiology.**

De Morgan's spots (dimor'gənz). See **cherry angioma.**

Demser, a trade name for an antihypertensive (metyrosine).

demulcent (diməl'sənt), **1.** any of several oily substances used for soothing and reducing irritation of surfaces that have been abraded or irritated. **2.** soothing, as a counter-irritant or balm.

Demulen, a trade name for an oral contraceptive containing an estrogen (ethinyl estradiol) and a progestin (ethynodiol diacetate).

demyelination (dimai'əlinei'shən), the process of destruction or removal of the myelin sheath from a nerve or a nerve fiber.

denatured alcohol, ethyl alcohol made unfit for ingestion by the addition of acetone or methanol, used as a solvent and in chemical processes.

dendr-, a combining form meaning 'pertaining to a tree or branches': *dendriceptor, dendroid, dendrophobia.*

-dendria, a combining form meaning the 'twiglike branching of nerve fibers': *oligodendria, telodendria, zoodendria.*

dendrite, a branching process that extends from the cell body of a neuron. Each neuron usually possesses several dendrites, which receive impulses that are conducted to the cell body. Compare **axon.**

dendritic (dendrit'ik), **1.** treelike, with branches that spread toward or into neighboring tissues, as dendritic keratitis. **2.** of or pertaining to a dendrite.

dendritic keratitis, a serious infection of the eye, characterized by an ulceration of the surface of the cornea resembling a tree with knobs at the ends of the branches. Photophobia, the sensation of a foreign body in the eye, pain, and conjunctivitis are usual. Treatment includes application of idoxuridine, chemical debridement with an iodine tincture, or surgical removal of the involved layer of corneal tissue cells. Untreated dendritic keratitis may result in permanent scarring of the cornea with impaired vision or blindness.

dendrodendritic synapse, a type of synapse in which a dendrite of one neuron comes in contact with a dendrite of another neuron.

-dendron, a combining form meaning a 'treelike formation': *neurodendron, telodendron, toxicodendron.*

dengue (den'gi, den'gei), **dengue fever,** an acute arbovirus infection transmitted to man by the Aëdes mosquito and occurring in tropical and subtropical regions. The disease usually produces a triad of symptoms: fever, rash, and severe head, back, and muscle pain. Manifestations of dengue usually occur in two phases, separated by a day of remission. In the first attack, the patient experiences fever, extreme weakness, headache, sore throat, muscle pains, and edema of the hands and feet. The second attack is marked by a return of fever and by a bright red scarlatinaform rash. Dengue is a self-limited illness, though it may take patients several weeks to recover. Treatment is symptomatic; analgesics may be given to relieve headache and other pains. Also called **Aden fever, bouquet fever, breakbone fever, dandy fever, solar fever.** See also *Aëdes,* **arbovirus.**

dengue hemorrhagic fever shock syndrome (DHFS), a grave form of dengue fever characterized by shock with collapse or prostration; cold, clammy extremities; a weak, thready pulse; respiratory distress; and all of the symptoms of dengue fever. Hemorrhage, bruises, small reddish spots indicating bleeding from skin capillaries, and bloody vomit, urine, and feces may occur and precede circulatory collapse. Treatment includes fluid and electrolyte replacement and fresh blood, plasma, or platelet transfusions as needed. Oxygen and sedatives may be administered. See also **breakbone fever, dandy fever, dengue.**

denial, 1. refusal or restriction of something requested, claimed, or needed, often resulting in physical or emotional deficiency. 2. an unconscious defense mechanism in which emotional conflict and anxiety are avoided by refusing to acknowledge those thoughts, feelings, desires, impulses, or external facts that are consciously intolerable.

Denis-Browne splint, a splint for the correction of talipes equinovarus (clubfoot) composed of a curved bar attached to the soles of a pair of high-top shoes. The splint is equipped with wing nuts, allowing abduction of each foot to be individualized. The splint is commonly applied nightly in late infancy after casting and manipulation have effectively reduced the deformity.

Denman's spontaneous evolution, a natural, unassisted turning of the fetus from the transverse presentation. The head rotates back and, as the breech descends, the shoulder ascends in the pelvis. The back of the fetus is generally posterior. Also called **Denman's method, Denman's spontaneous version.**

dens deciduus (denz). See **deciduous tooth.**

dense fibrous tissue, a fibrous connective tissue consisting of compact, strong, inelastic bundles of parallel collagenous fibers that have a glistening white color. Organized dense fibrous tissue comprises the tendons, the aponeuroses, and the ligaments; unorganized dense fibrous tissue comprises the fascial membranes, the dermis of the skin, the periosteum, and the capsules of organs. Compare **loose fibrous tissue.**

density, the amount of mass of a substance in a given volume. The greater the mass in a given volume, the greater the density. See also **mass, volume.**

density gradient, the variation of the concentration of a solute in a confined solution.

dens serotinus. See **wisdom tooth.**

dent-. See **dento-.**

denta-. See **dento-.**

dental, of or pertaining to a tooth or teeth.

dental alveolus, a tooth socket in the mandible or maxilla.

dental amalgam, an alloy of silver, tin, and mercury with small amounts of copper and sometimes zinc, used for filling teeth.

dental anesthesia, any of several anesthetic procedures used in dental surgery. The proliferation of injectable local anesthetics has largely replaced the use of inhalational general anesthesics, especially of nitrous oxide.

dental arch, the curving shape formed by the arrangement of a normal set of teeth.

dental assistant, a person who assists a dentist in the performance of generalized tasks, including chairside assistance, clerical work, reception, and some radiography and dental laboratory work.

dental canal. See **alveolar canal.**

dental caries, an abnormal destructive condition in a tooth, caused by the complex interaction of food, especially starches and sugars, with bacteria that form dental plaque. This material adheres to the surfaces of the teeth and provides the medium for the growth of bacteria and the production of organic acids that then cause breaks in the enamel sheath of the tooth. Enzymes produced by the bacteria then attack the protein component of the tooth. This process, if untreated, ultimately leads to the formation of deep cavities and the bacterial infection of the pulp chamber and nerves. Dental caries may be prevented by avoidance of sugar and carbohydrates in the diet, regular brushing and removal of food particles, from the surfaces and interstices of the teeth, fluoridation of drinking water, and the topical application of fluorides to the teeth. Removal of plaque by a dental hygienist is performed to eliminate the source of decay as well as to prevent infection and destruction of the peridontal tissues. Treatment of dental caries includes removal of the decayed material and the refilling of the cavity with an amalgam of silver or another restorative material. If the lesion has reached the nerve of the tooth, it may be necessary to remove the nerve tissue to alleviate pain, to prevent the spread of infection to the rest of the body, and to allow the continued use of the natural tooth. Alternatively, the entire tooth may be extracted. The development of dental caries in a debilitated patient is a concern because of the danger that infections of the teeth or gums might spread to the rest of the body. In addition, missing, decayed, or painful teeth inhibit mastication and lead to dietary changes which may in turn cause nutritional and digestive disorders. Kinds of dental caries include **active caries, arrested caries, primary caries, secondary caries.**

dental crypt, the space occupied by a developing tooth.

dental fistula, an abnormal passage from the apical periodontal area of a tooth to the surface of oral mucous membrane, permitting the discharge of inflammatory or suppurative material. Also called **alveolar fistula.**

dental floss, a waxed or unwaxed thread used to clean tooth surfaces and spaces between the teeth.

dental hygienist, a person with special training to provide dental services under the supervision of a dentist. Services supplied by a dental hygienist include dental prophylaxis, radiography, applying medications, and providing dental education at chairside and in the community.

dental papilla. See under **papilla.**

dental plaque. See **bacterial plaque.**

dental technician, a person who makes dental prostheses and orthodontic appliances as prescribed by a dentist. Kinds of dental prostheses made by dental technicians include full dentures, partial dentures, crowns, bridgework, and other dental restorations.

-dentate, a combining form meaning 'possessing teeth': *edentate, multidentate, tridentate.*

dentate fracture, any fracture that causes serrated bone ends that fit together like the teeth of gears.

denti-. See **dento-.**

dentia-. See **dento-.**

dentin, dentine, the chief material of teeth, surrounding the pulp and situated inside of the enamel and cementum. Harder and denser than bone, it consists of solid organic substratum infiltrated with lime salts.

dentin globule, a small spherical body in peripheral dentin, created by early calcification.

dentinoenamel (den'tınouınæm'əl), pertaining to both the dentin and the enamel of the teeth.

dentinogenesis (den'tınoujen'ısıs), the formation of the dentin of the teeth. —**dentinogenic,** *adj.*

dentinogenesis imperfecta, hereditary dysplasia of dentin of deciduous and permanent teeth in which brown, opalescent dentin overgrows and obliterates the pulp cavity and the teeth have short roots and wear rapidly. Early restorative dentistry is indicated. The condition is often associated with osteogenesis imperfecta and other congenital mesodermal dysplasias.

dentist, a person who is qualified by training and licensed by the state to practice dentistry. Training requires a minimum of two years, preferably four, in an undergraduate college and a satisfactory score on a Dental Aptitude Test (DAT), followed by three to four years at an approved dental college. After completing dental college, a dentist is awarded a degree of either Doctor of Dental Surgery (D.D.S.) or Doctor of Dental Medicine (D.M.D.), which are equivalent degrees. Dental internships and residencies are not required for general practice although written and practical examinations must be passed to obtain a state license. In various states, licensing requirements can be met by providing a certificate from the National Board of Dental Examiners in place of a written test and by taking the practical examination before a Regional Dental Examining Board rather than appearing before a state board. See also **dentistry.**

dentistry, the art of practicing the prevention and treatment of diseases and disorders of the teeth and surrounding structures of the oral cavity. Responsibilities include the repair and restoration of teeth and replacement of missing teeth, as well as the detection of signs of diseases, as tumors, that would require treatment by a physician. In addition to the general practice of dentistry, there are eight recognized specialties, each requiring additional training after graduation from a dental college: **endodontics, oral pathology, oral surgery, orthodontics, pedodontics, periodontics, prosthodontics,** and **public health dentistry.**

dentition, 1. See also **teething.** the development and eruption of the teeth. 2. the arrangement, number, and kind of teeth as they appear in the dental arch of the mouth. 3. the character of the teeth of an individual or species as determined by their form and arrangement. Kinds of dentition include **artificial dentition, deciduous dentition, mixed dentition, natural dentition, permanent dentition, precocious dentition, predeciduous dentition, retarded dentition.**

dento-, dent-, denta-, denti-, dentia-, a combining form meaning 'pertaining to a tooth or the teeth': *dentography, dentoidin, dentonomy.*

dentoalveolar abscess, the formation and accumulation of pus in a tooth socket or the jawbone around the base of a tooth. The pus results from a bacterial infection that is usually secondary to an infection or injury to the tooth or alveolar tissues. Also called **periapical abscess.**

denture (den'čhər), an artificial tooth or a set of artificial teeth not permanently fixed or implanted. Compare **fixed bridgework.**

denturist (den'čhərıst), a person who performs the same type of work as a dental technician but without a dentist's prescription, providing dental prostheses directly to clients. Denturists are more likely to be found in Canada than in the United States, where the practice is illegal in many states. See also **dental technician.**

Denver Articulation Screening Examination (D.A.S.E.), a test for evaluating the clarity of pronunciation in children between 2½ and 6 years of age. Each child's performance may be compared to a standardized norm for the age.

Denver classification, the system of identifying and classifying human chromosomes according to the criteria established at the Denver (1960), London (1963), and Chicago (1966) conferences of cytogeneticists. It is based on chromosome size and position of the centromere as determined during mitotic metaphase and is divided into seven major groups, designated A through G, which are arranged according to decreasing length. See also **karyotype.**

Denver Developmental Screening Test (DDST), a test for evaluating development in children from one month to six years of age. The developmental level of motor, social, and language skills may be discovered by comparing the child's performance to the average performance of other children. The score, or the developmental age, is expressed as a ratio in which the child's age is the denominator and the age at which the norm possesses skills equal to those of the child being tested is the numerator.

deodorant, 1. destroying or masking odors. 2. a substance that destroys or masks odors. Underarm deodorants are available as sprays, creams, solid gels, and liquids containing an antiperspirant, as aluminum chloride, aluminum hydroxyl, aluminum sulfate, or aluminum zirconyl hydroxychloride. These aluminum salts form an obstructive hydroxide gel in sweat ducts. Aluminum salts may produce an allergic reaction in some individuals and hydrolyzed aluminum chloride can cause local tissue necrosis. Some underarm deodorants contain antibacterial agents or fragrances. Vaginal deodorant sprays contain a fatty ester emollient, a masking fragrance, and an antimicrobial agent, as benzethonium chloride, chlorhexidine hydrochloride, or triacetin, and are often associated with allergic reactions. Room and breath deodorants contain masking agents, as various mints, pine, eucalyptus, lemon, lavender, rosemary, sassafras, or thyme. Ozone masks odors by decreasing olfactory sensitivity. Chlorophyll has a deodorizing action that is enhanced by croconic acid. Also called **antibromic.**

deodorized alcohol, a liquid, free of organic impurities, containing 92.5 per cent absolute alcohol.

deoxy-, desoxy-, a combining form meaning 'deoxidized or a reduction product of': *deoxygenation, desoxymorphine, desoxyribose.*

deoxyribonucleic acid, desoxyribonucleic acid (DNA) (diok'sīraī'bounuklī'ĭk), a large nucleic acid molecule, found principally in the chromosomes of the nucleus of a cell, that is the carrier of genetic information in living cells. The genetic information is coded in the sequence of the nitrogenous, molecular subunits that are constituents of the deoxyribonucleic acid molecule. See also **nucleic acid, ribonucleic acid.**

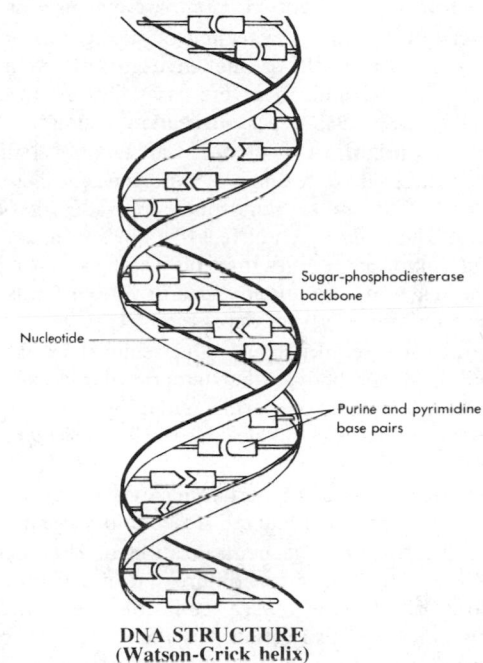

DNA STRUCTURE
(Watson-Crick helix)

Depakene, a trade name for an anticonvulsant (valproic acid).

dependence, the total psychophysical state of one addicted to drugs or alcohol who must receive an increasing amount of the substance in order to prevent the onset of abstinence symptoms.

dependency needs, the sum of the physical and emotional requirements of an infant for survival, including mothering, love, affection, shelter, protection, food, and warmth. Reliance on others to satisfy these needs decreases with age and maturity; continuance in later years, in overt or latent form, is indicative of a pathological emotional disorder. These needs may increase under stress, as during physical illness, in which case they do not reflect a psychopathological condition. Compare **emotional need.**

dependent, of or pertaining to a condition of being reliant upon someone or something else for help, support, favor, and other need, as a child is dependent on a parent, a narcotics addict is dependent upon a drug, or one variable is dependent on another variable. —**depend,** *v.,* **dependence,** *n.*

dependent differentiation. See **correlative differentiation.**

dependent variable, (in research) a factor that is measured to learn the effect of one or more independent variables, as in a study of the effect of preoperative nursing intervention on postoperative vomiting, vomiting is the dependent variable measured to determine the effect of the nursing intervention. Compare **independent variable.**

depersonalization, a feeling of strangeness or unreality concerning oneself or the environment, often resulting from anxiety and, in severe cases, leading to a neurotic reaction. See also **depersonalization disorder.**

depersonalization disorder, an emotional disturbance characterized by feelings of strangeness and unreality in which a dreamlike atmosphere pervades the consciousness. The body may not feel like one's own, and dramatic and important events may be watched with equanimity. The reaction is commonly seen in various forms of schizophrenia and in severe depression.

depilation (dep'ɪlei'Shən), the removal or extraction of hair from the body, either temporarily, by mechanical or chemical means or permanently, by electrolysis, which destroys the hair follicle. Also called **epilation.** — **depilate,** v.

depilatory, 1. of or pertaining to a substance or procedure that removes hair. 2. a depilatory agent.

depolarization, the neutralization of electrical polarity, as the reduction of ion differential of sodium and potassium across the nerve cells of the neuromuscular ionchons. See also **action potential.**

deposition, (in law) a sworn pretrial testimony given by a witness in response to oral or written questions and cross-examination. The deposition is transcribed and may be used for further pretrial investigation. It may also be presented at the trial if the witness cannot be present. Compare **discovery, interrogatories.**

depot, 1. any area of the body in which drugs or other substances are stored and from which they can be distributed. 2. (of a drug) injected or implanted to be slowly absorbed into the circulation.

depressant (dɪpres'ənt), 1. (of a drug) tending to decrease the function or activity of a system of the body. 2. such a drug, as a cardiac depressant or a respiratory depressant.

depressed fracture, any fracture of the skull in which fragments are depressed below the normal surface of the skull.

depression, 1. a depressed area, hollow, or fossa; downward or inward displacement. 2. a decrease of vital functional activity. 3. a mood disturbance characterized by feelings of sadness, despair, and discouragement resulting from and proportionate to some personal loss or tragedy. 4. an abnormal emotional state characterized by exaggerated feelings of sadness, melancholy, dejection, worthlessness, emptiness, and hopelessness that are inappropriate and out of proportion to reality. The overt manifestations, which are extremely variable, range from a slight lack of motivation and inability to concentrate to severe physiological alterations of body functions and may represent symptoms of a variety of mental and physical conditions, a syndrome of related symptoms associated with a particular disease, or a specific mental illness. The condition is neurotic when the precipitating cause is an intrapsychic conflict or a traumatic situation or event that is identifiable, even though the person is unable to explain the overreaction to it. The condition is psychotic when there is severe physical and mental functional impairment owing to some unidentifiable intrapsychic conflict; it is often accompanied by hallucinations, delusions, and confusion concerning time, place, and identity. Kinds of depression include **agitated depression, anaclitic depression, endogenous depression, involutional melancholia, reactive depression, retarded depression.** See also **bipolar disorder.** — **depressive,** adj.

depressor septi, one of the three muscles of the nose. Arising from the maxilla and inserting into the septum and the posterior aspect of the ala, it lies between the mucous membrane and the muscular structure of the lip and is a direct antagonist of the other muscles of the nose. It is innervated by buccal branches of the facial nerve and serves to draw the ala down, constricting the nostril. Compare **nasalis, procerus.**

depth electroencephalography. See **electroencephalography.**

depth perception, the ability to judge depth or the relative distance of objects in space and to orient one's position in relation to them. Binocular vision is essential to this ability.

depth psychology, any approach to psychology that emphasizes the study of personality and behavior in relation to unconscious motivation. See also **psychoanalysis.**

de Quervain's fracture (də kərveinz'), fracture of the navicular bone, with dislocation of the lunar bone.

de Quervain's thyroiditis, an inflammatory condition of the thyroid, characterized by swelling and tenderness of the gland, fever, dysphagia, fatigue, and severe pain in the neck, ears, and jaw. The disorder often occurs following a viral infection of the upper respiratory tract and tends to remit spontaneously and to recur several times. The diagnosis may be made by a radiologic scan showing depressed uptake of radioactive iodine in involved areas. Occasionally, a needle biopsy of the thyroid is performed. Treatment may include anti-inflammatory medication, as aspirin or thyroid hormone, if the condition continues for more than a few days. Corticosteroids are prescribed for prolonged or severe cases. Also called **giant cell thyroiditis, granulomatous thyroiditis, subacute thyroiditis.**

der-, a combining form meaning 'pertaining to the neck': *deradelphus, deradenitis, deranencephalia.*

derby hat fracture. See **dishpan fracture.**

derived protein, a metabolic product of protein hydrolysis, as proteose, peptone, or peptide.

-derm, a combining form meaning a 'skin': *angioderm, mucoderm, paraderm.*

-derma, **1.** a combining form meaning a '(specified) skin or covering': *chrysderma, micoderma, sarcoderma.* **2.** a combining form meaning a 'skin ailment or skin of a specified type': *rhinoderma, syphiloderma, vaselinoderma.*

derma-. See **dermato-.**

dermabrasion (dər'məbrei'zhən), a treatment for the removal of scars on the skin by the use of revolving wire brushes or sandpaper. An aerosol spray is used to freeze the skin for this procedure. Dermabrasion is used to reduce facial scars of severe acne and to remove pigment from undesired tattoos.

dermat-. See **dermato-.**

dermatitis (dər'mətai'tıs), an inflammatory condition of the skin, characterized by erythema and pain or pruritus. Various cutaneous eruptions occur and may be unique to a particular allergen, disease, or infection. The condition may be chronic or acute; treatment is specific to the cause. Some kinds of dermatitis are **actinic dermatitis, contact dermatitis, rhus dermatitis, seborrheic dermatitis.**

dermatitis exfoliativa neonatorum. See **Ritter's disease.**

dermatitis herpetiformis, a chronic, severely pruritic skin disease with symmetrically located groups of red, papulovesicular, vesicular, bullous, or urticarial lesions which leave hyperpigmented spots. It is occasionally associated with a malignancy of an internal organ or with celiac disease, patch, or IgA immunotherapy. Treatment may include a diet free of gluten and the administration of sulfone, dapsone, sulfapyridine, or antipruritic drugs.

dermatitis medicamentosa. See **drug eruption.**

dermatitis venenata. See **contact dermatitis.**

dermato-, derma-, dermat-, dermo-, a combining form meaning 'pertaining to the skin': *dermatobiasis, dermatocele, dermatocyst.*

dermatofibroma (dər'mətoufaibrou'mə), *pl.* **dermatofibromas, dermatofibromata.** a cutaneous nodule that is painless, round, firm, gray or red, and elevated. It is most commonly found on the extremities, requires no treatment, and is sometimes associated with systemic lupus erythematosus. Also called **fibrous histiocytoma.**

dermatographia (dər'mətougræf'iə), an abnormal skin condition characterized by wheals that develop from tracing on the skin with the fingernail or a blunted instrument. This condition makes the skin especially susceptible to irritation and may be associated with urticaria. Also called **autographism, dermatographism, Ebbecke's reaction.**

dermatologist, a physician specializing in disorders of the skin.

dermatology, the study of the skin, including the anatomy, physiology, and the pathology of the skin and the diagnosis and treatment of skin disorders.

dermatome, (in embryology) the part of the segmented mesodermal layer in the early developing embryo that originates from the somites and gives rise to the dermal layers of the skin. See also **somite.**

dermatomycosis (dər'mətoumaikou'sıs), a superficial, fungal infection of the skin, characteristically found on parts that are moist and protected by clothing, as the groin or feet. It is caused by a dermatophyte. See also **dermatophytosis.** — **dermatomycotic,** *adj.*

dermatomyositis (dər'mətoumaiousai'tıs), a disease of the connective tissues, characterized by pruritic or eczematous inflammation of the skin and tenderness and weakness of the muscles. Muscle tissue is destroyed and loss is often so severe that the person may become unable to walk or to perform simple tasks. Swelling of the eyelids and face and loss of weight are common manifestations. The cause is unknown, but in 15 per cent of cases the condition develops with an internal malignancy. Viral infection and antibacterial medication are also associated with an increased incidence of dermatomyositis.

Dermatophagoides farinae, a ubiquitous species of household dust mite responsible for allergic reactions in sensitive individuals. Protection against the microscopically small mite includes use of insecticides, vacuum cleaning, and control of the temperature and humidity. The mites thrive on skin scales, hair, pet foods, carpets, and bedding, in addition to ordinary house dust.

dermatophyte (dər'mətoufait', dərmæt'əfait'), any of several fungi that cause parasitic skin disease in humans. See also **dermatophytid,** specific fungal infections.

dermatophytid (dər'mətof'ıtıd, dər'mətoufai'tıd), an allergic skin reaction characterized by small vesicles and associated with dermatomycosis. The lesions result from sensitization to the infection elsewhere on the skin and do not contain fungi. See also **dermatomycosis, dermatophyte.**

dermatophytosis (dər'mətou'faitou'sıs), a superficial fungus infection of the skin, caused by *Microsporum, Epidermophyton,* or *Trichophyton* species of dermatophyte. On the trunk and upper extremities it is commonly called "ringworm" infection and is characterized by round or oval, scaly patches with slightly raised borders and clearing centers. On the feet small vesicles, cracking, itching, scaling, and often secondary bacterial infections occur and are commonly called "athlete's foot." Treatment includes topical antifungal agents, as tolnaftate, clotrimazole and undecylenic acid, and oral griseofulvin. Fingernails and toenails respond poorly to topical treatment. See also **tinea.**

dermatosis, any disorder of the skin, especially if not associated with inflammation. Compare **dermatitis.**

dermatosis papulosa nigra, a common abnormal skin condition in blacks consisting of multiple, tiny, benign, skin-colored or hyperpigmented papules on the cheeks. The lesions are permanent and increase in number with age.

-dermia, a combining form meaning a '(specified) skin condition': *allergodermia, carotenodermia, toxidermia.* Also **-derma.**

-dermic, 1. a combining form meaning 'related to the skin': *diadermic, epidermic, intradermic.* 2. a combining form meaning 'related to the variety of skin': *leptodermic, pachydermic, sarcodermic.* 3. a combining form meaning 'related to skin ailments': *leukodermic, toxicodermic, xerodermic.* 4. a combining form meaning 'related to a cell division process': *blastodermic, ectodermic, endodermic.*

dermis (dər'mıs). See **corium.**

-dermis, a combining form meaning 'tissue or skin': *hypodermis, endepidermis, osteodermis.*

dermo-. See **dermato-.**

dermographism (dərmog'rəfız'əm), an exaggerated response of the skin to stroking with a blunt instrument. Soon after such mild trauma a pale, raised wheal with a surrounding erythematous flare appears. Antihistamines may be prescribed to suppress this hypersensitivity.

dermoid (dər'mɔid), 1. of or pertaining to the skin. 2. *Informal.* a dermoid cyst.

dermoid cyst, a tumor, derived from embryonal tissues, that consists of a fibrous wall lined with epithelium and a cavity containing fatty material, and, frequently, hair, teeth, bits of bone, and cartilage. More than ten per cent of all ovarian tumors are dermoid cysts; usually benign, they may cause granulomatous peritonitis if they rupture. Kinds of dermoid cysts are **implantation dermoid cyst, inclusion dermoid cyst, thyroid dermoid cyst, tubal dermoid cyst.** Also called **organoid tumor, teratoid tumor.**

-dermoma, a combining form meaning a 'tumor of the skin layers': *epidermoma, monodermoma, tridermoma.*

DES, abbreviation for **diethylstilbestrol.**

descending aorta, the main portion of the aorta, consisting of the thoracic aorta and the abdominal aorta, that continues from the aortic arch into the trunk of the body and supplies many parts, as the esophagus, lymph glands, ribs, and stomach.

descending colon, the segment of the colon that extends from the end of the transverse colon at the splenic flexure on the left side of the abdomen down to the beginning of the sigmoid colon in the pelvis.

descending current. See **centrifugal current.**

descending oblique muscle. See **obliquus externus abdominis.**

descending urography. See **intravenous pyelography.**

descriptive anatomy, the study of the morphology and structure of the body by systems, as the vascular system and the nervous system. Each system is composed of similar tissues that are essential to a particular function.

descriptive embryology, the study of the changes that occur in cells, tissues, and organs during the progressive stages of prenatal development.

descriptive psychiatry, the study of external, readily observable behavior. Compare **dynamic psychiatry.**

Desenex, a trade name for a fixed-combination topical drug containing two antifungals (undecylenic acid and zinc undecylenate).

desensitization. See **systemic desensitization.**

desensitize, 1. (in immunology) to render an individual insensitive to any of the various antigens. 2. (in psychiatry) to relieve an emotionally disturbed person of the stress of phobias and neuroses by encouraging discussion of the anxieties and the stressful experiences that cause the emotional problems involved. 3. (in dentistry) to remove or reduce the painful response of vital, exposed dentin to irritating substances and temperature changes.

deserpidine (dısər'pədin), a rauwolfia alkaloid used as an antihypertensive.

■ INDICATIONS: It is prescribed for hypertension and for mild anxiety.

■ CONTRAINDICATIONS: Mental depression, peptic ulcer, ulcerative colitis, or known hypersensitivity to this drug prohibits its use.

■ ADVERSE EFFECTS: Among the more serious adverse reactions are orthostatic hypotension, potentially severe mental depression, and lethargy.

desert fever. See **coccidioidomycosis.**

desert rheumatism, a form of coccidioidomycosis characterized by pain in the bones and joints.

desipramine hydrochloride, a tricyclic antidepressant.

■ INDICATION: It is prescribed in the treatment of mental depression.

■ CONTRAINDICATIONS: Concomitant administration of monoamine oxidase inhibitors, recent myocardial infarction, or known hypersensitivity to this drug or to tricyclic medication prohibits its use. It is used with caution in patients who have seizure disorders or cardiovascular disease.

■ ADVERSE EFFECTS: Among the more serious adverse reactions are sedation, and gastrointestinal, cardiovascular, and neurologic reactions. This drug interacts with many other drugs.

deslanoside (dıslæn'əsaid), a cardiotonic.

■ INDICATIONS: It is prescribed for congestive heart failure and certain arrhythmias.

■ CONTRAINDICATIONS: Ventricular fibrillation, tachycardia, or known hypersensitivity to this drug prohibits its use.

■ ADVERSE EFFECTS: The most serious reactions are various cardiac arrhythmias.

-desma, a combining form meaning 'something bridging or connecting': *cytodesma, mesodesma, plasmodesma.*

desmo-, a combining form meaning 'pertaining to a ligament': *desmoma, desmorrhexis, desmotomy.*

desmocyte. See **fibroblast.** — **desmocytic,** *adj.*

desmoid tumor, a neoplasm in skeletal muscle and fascia that may occur in the head, neck, upper arm, abdomen, or lower extremities. The tumor is usually a firm, circumscribed, rubbery mass. Injury may be a factor in the development of this lesion, which is often regarded as overproliferation of scar tissue.

desmopressin acetate, an antidiuretic analog of vasopressin.

■ INDICATIONS: It is prescribed in the treatment of diabetes insipidus.

■ CONTRAINDICATION: Known hypersensitivity to this drug prohibits its use.

■ ADVERSE EFFECTS: Among the most serious adverse reactions are hyponatremia and water intoxication. Mild effects, as headache, cramps, and nasal congestion, also may occur.

desonide, a topical corticosteroid.

■ INDICATION: It is prescribed topically as an anti-inflammatory agent.

■ CONTRAINDICATIONS: Viral and fungal diseases of the skin, impaired circulation, or known hypersensitivity to this drug or to steroid medication prohibits its use.

■ ADVERSE EFFECTS: Among the more serious adverse reactions, usually occurring after prolonged or excessive application, are striae, hypopigmentation or local irritation of the skin, and various systemic effects.

desoximetasone, a topical corticosteroid.

■ INDICATION: It is prescribed topically as an anti-inflammatory agent.

■ CONTRAINDICATIONS: Viral and fungal diseases of the skin, impaired circulation, or known hypersensitivity to this drug or to other steroid medication prohibits its use.

■ ADVERSE EFFECTS: Among the more serious adverse reactions, usually occurring after prolonged or excessive application, are striae, hypopigmentation, or local irritation of the skin and various systemic effects.

desoxy-. See **deoxy-.**

desoxycorticosterone acetate (desok′sıkɔr′təkousti′-roun), a mineralocorticoid hormone.

■ INDICATIONS: It is prescribed in replacement therapy, in congenital adrenal hyperplasia, and in chronic primary adrenocortical insufficiency to prevent the excess loss of salt from the body.

■ CONTRAINDICATIONS: Hypertension, congestive heart failure, or known hypersensitivity to this drug prohibits its use.

■ ADVERSE EFFECTS: Among the more serious adverse reactions are excessive sodium and water retention and potassium loss, hypertension, edema, and heart failure.

Desoxyn, a trade name for a central nervous system stimulant (methamphetamine hydrochloride).

desoxyribonucleic acid (desok′sirai′bounukli′ık). See **deoxyribonucleic acid.**

desquamation (des′kwəmei′ʃhən), a normal process in which the cornified layer of the epidermis is sloughed in fine scales. Certain conditions, injuries, and medications accelerate desquamation and may cause peeling and the loss of deeper layers of the skin. Also called **exfoliation.** — **desquamate,** *v.,* **desquamative,** *adj.*

destructive aggression, an act of hostility unnecessary for self-protection or preservation, that is directed toward an external object or person. See also **aggression.**

detached retina. See **retinal detachment.**

detergent, 1. a cleansing agent. 2. cleansing. See also **surfactant.**

determinant evolution, the theory that evolution progresses according to a predetermined course. See also **orthogenesis.**

determinate cleavage, mitotic division of the fertilized ovum into blastomeres that are each destined to form a specific part of the embryo. If such cells are isolated, they are incapable of giving rise to an individual, complete embryo. Damage to or destruction of any of these cells results in a malformed organism. Also called **mosaic cleavage.** Compare **indeterminate cleavage.** See also **mosaic development.**

detrusor muscle (dıtru′zər, dıtru′sər), a complex of longitudinal fibers that form the external layer of the muscular coat of the bladder. These fibers arise from the posterior surface of the pubis, traverse the inferior surface of the bladder, descend along the fundus, and attach to the prostate in men and to the front of the vagina in women. Along the sides of the bladder the fibers pass obliquely and intersect. The detrusor muscle is supplied by branches from the internal iliac artery and innervated by medullated fibers from the third and fourth sacral nerves and by nonmedullated fibers from the hypogastric plexus.

deutero-, deuto-, a combining form meaning 'second': *deutero-albumose, deuteroconidium, deutero-elastose.*

deuteroplasm (du′tərouplæz′əm). See **deutoplasm.**

deuto-. See **deutero-.**

deutoplasm (du′təplæz′əm), **deuteroplasm,** the inactive elements of the protoplasm, primarily the stored nutritive material contained in the yolk.

DEV, abbreviation for **duck embryo vaccine.** See **rabies vaccine.**

development, 1. the gradual process of change and differentiation from a simple to a more advanced level of complexity. In man the physical, mental, and emotional capacities that allow complex adaptation to the environment and function within society are acquired through growth, maturation, and learning. Kinds of development include **arrested development, mosaic development, psychomotor development, psychosexual development, psychosocial development, regulative development. 2.** (in biology) the series of events that occur within an organism from the time of fertilization of the ovum to the adult stage. — **developmental,** *adj.*

developmental age (DA), an expression of a child's developmental progress stated in age and determined by standardized measurements, as of body size and dimensions, by social and psychological functioning, by observations of motor skills, and by the giving of mental and aptitude tests. Compare **achievement age, mental age.**

developmental agraphia, a deficiency in a child's ability to learn to form letters and to write. Other learning is normal, and the child usually has no musculoskeletal or neurologic problems.

developmental anatomy, the study of the differentiation and the growth of an organism from one cell to birth. Also called **embryology.**

developmental anomaly, any congenital defect that results from the interference with the normal growth and differentiation of the fetus. Such defects can arise at any stage of embryonic development, vary greatly in type and severity, and are caused by a wide variety of determining factors, including genetic mutations, chromosomal aberrations, teratogenic agents, and environmental factors. Developmental anomalies are classified either according to the organ system affected, as congenital heart defects, or according to the way in which the defect occurred, as developmental failure or arrest, failure to atrophy or subdivide, fusion, splitting, incorrect migration, and misplacement. Most developmental defects are apparent at birth, especially any structural malformation, but some, especially those involving the organ systems, do not become evident until days, weeks, or even years later.

developmental arrest. See **arrested development.**

developmental crisis, severe, usually transient, stress that occurs when a person is unable to complete the tasks of a psychosocial stage of development and is therefore unable to move on to the next stage. See also **psychosocial development.**

developmental disability (DD), a pathologic condition that starts developing before the age of 18. Most developmental disabilities persist throughout the life of the individual, although many can be effectively treated. See also **congenital condition.**

developmental horizon, any one of twenty-five stages in the development of the human embryo from the one-cell stage at conception to the morphologically and physiologically complex organism at the end of the seventh week of gestation.

developmental idiocy, *Obsolete.* Severe mental retardation resulting from arrest of brain development.

developmental model, **1.** a conceptual framework devised to be used as a guide in making a diagnosis, in understanding a developmental process, and in forming a prognosis for continued development. It has five components. The "identifiable state" describes the stage, level, phase, or period of the condition or process; the "shift in state" identifies qualities of change as progressive, sudden, abrupt, or recurrent; and the "form of progression" describes patterns of development as linear, spiral, or oscillating. The "force" that triggers the change or the step in development may be self-actualization or any form of stress. Development is ultimately constrained by the fifth component, "potentiality," the genetic and environmental potential for growth. **2.** (in nursing) a conceptual framework describing four stages, or processes, of development in the client during therapy. In the first stage, called orientation, the client begins a relationship with the nurse or other therapist and begins to clarify the problem with the help of the therapist. In the second stage, called identification, the client develops a sense of closeness and attachment to the therapist. During this period the client and the therapist work comfortably together. In the third stage, called exploitation, the client makes full use of the nursing services offered, begins to assume some control of the interactions, and becomes more independent. During the last stage, called resolution, the therapeutic relationship is terminated; the client is independent and no longer needs the nurse or therapist. With this model the nurse therapist may plan nursing interventions appropriate to the developmental level of the client. The developmental model is one of the earliest nursing models to be developed. It views the person as a psychobiological being whose needs are expressed in behavior and as one who is unique and capable of learning and changing. Health is viewed as a foward movement of personality development and other ongoing processes, reflected by the person's creative, constructive, and productive community living. Thus, the focus of nursing is to promote this foward movement by assisting the client in self-repair and self-renewal.

developmental quotient (DQ), the numerical expression of a child's developmental level as measured by dividing the developmental age by the chronological age and multiplying by 100. Compare **intelligence quotient.** See also **developmental age.**

developmental task, a physical or cognitive skill that a child must accomplish during a particular age period in order to continue developing, as walking, which precedes the development of a sense of autonomy in the toddler period.

deviate, (di'vīit), **1.** a person or an act that varies from that which is considered standard, as a social or sexual deviate, or that is within a statistical norm. **2.** (di'vīeit') to vary from that which is considered standard or within a statistical norm. — **deviant,** *adj.,* **deviation,** *n.*

deviated septum, a shifted medial partition of the nasal cavity, a condition affecting many adults. The nasal septum more commonly shifts to the left during normal growth but this deflection may be aggravated by a blow to the nose or by other trauma. A severe deflection of the septum may significantly obstruct the nasal passages and result in infection, sinusitis, shortness of breath, headache, or recurring nosebleeds. Severe septal deviation may be corrected by various surgical procedures, as rhinoplasty, or septoplasty. Postoperative care in such cases usually includes various measures, as the maintenance of nasal packing, the administration of sedatives, and the placement of ice packs around the affected area to reduce swelling.

deviation from normal, a quality, characteristic, symptom, or clinical finding that is different from what is commonly regarded as normal, as an elevated temperature, multiple gestation, or an extra digit.

device, an item other than a drug that has application in the healing arts. The term is generally used in reference to items used directly by, on, or in the patient rather than to items, as surgical instruments and other equipment used by health practitioners for diagnosis and treatment. Devices include orthopedic appliances, crutches, artificial heart valves, pacemakers, prostheses, wheel chairs, cervical collars, hearing aids, and eye glasses.

devil's grip. See **epidemic pleurodynia.**

dexamethasone, a glucocorticoid.
- INDICATIONS: It is prescribed in the treatment of a variety of inflammatory conditions.
- CONTRAINDICATIONS: Systemic fungal infections or known hypersensitivity to this drug prohibits its use.
- ADVERSE REACTIONS: Among the more serious adverse reactions are gastrointestinal, endocrine, neurologic, fluid, and electrolyte disturbances.

dexbrompheniramine maleate (deks′broum′fənɪr′əmin), an antihistamine.
- INDICATIONS: It is prescribed in the treatment of a variety of hypersensitivity reactions, including rhinitis, skin rash, and itching.
- CONTRAINDICATIONS: Asthma or known hypersensitivity to this drug prohibits its use. It is not prescribed for infants or lactating mothers.
- ADVERSE EFFECTS: Among the more serious adverse reactions are drowsiness, skin rashes, hypersensitivity reactions, tachycardia, and dry mouth.

dexchlorpheniramine maleate, an antihistamine.
- INDICATIONS: It is prescribed in the treatment of a variety of hypersensitivity reactions, including rhinitis, skin rash, and pruritus.
- CONTRAINDICATIONS: Asthma or known hypersensitivity to this drug prohibits its use. It is not given to newborn infants or lactating mothers.

- ADVERSE EFFECTS: Drowsiness, skin rash, hypersensitivity reactions, dry mouth, and tachycardia may occur.

Dexedrine, a trade name for a central nervous system stimulant (dextroamphetamine sulfate).

dextrality. See **right-handedness.**

dextran fermentation (dek′strən), the conversion of dextrose to dextran. Also called **LMD.**

dextran preparation, any of a group of solutions containing polysaccharides, water, and, in some preparations, electrolytes. These solutions are used as plasma-volume extenders in cases of hypovolemia from hemorrhage, dehydration, or other cause and are available for intravenous administration in several concentrations.

dextro-, a combining form meaning 'right': *dextrocardia, dextrocerebral, dextrogastria.*

dextroamphetamine sulfate, a central nervous system stimulant.
- INDICATIONS: It is prescribed in the treatment of narcolepsy and in the treatment of hyperkinetic disorders in children. It was formerly prescribed as an anorexiant in treating exogenous obesity.
- CONTRAINDICATIONS: Cardiovascular disease, glaucoma, hypertension, hyperthyroidism, agitation, history of drug abuse, concomitant administration of a monoamine oxidase inhibitor within 14 days, or known hypersensitivity to this drug prohibits its use.
- ADVERSE EFFECTS: Among the more serious adverse reactions are various manifestations of central nervous system excitation, increased blood pressure, arrhythmias and other cardiovascular effects, and nausea, anorexia, and drug dependence.

dextromethorphan hydrobromide, a nonnarcotic antitussive.
- INDICATION: It is prescribed for the suppression of nonproductive cough.
- CONTRAINDICATIONS: Use of a monomine oxidase inhibitor within the past 14 days or known hypersensitivity to this drug prohibits its use.
- ADVERSE EFFECT: The most serious adverse reaction is respiratory depression resulting from large doses.

dextrose and sodium chloride injection, a fluid, nutrient, and electrolyte replenisher. It is available for parenteral use in a variety of concentrations.

dextrose, a glucose available in various solutions for intravenous administration.
- INDICATIONS: It is prescribed to provide calories and fluid and to correct hypoglycemia.
- CONTRAINDICATIONS: Diabetic coma, intracranial or intraspinal hemorrhage, or delirium tremens prohibits its use.
- ADVERSE EFFECTS: Among the more serious adverse reactions are hyperglycemia, glycosuria, and phlebitis.

D.H.E.-45, a trade name for an alpha-adrenergic blocking agent (dihydroergotamine mesylate).

DHFS, abbreviation for **dengue hemorrhagic fever shock syndrome.**

dhobie itch (dou′bi), **1.** a fungal infection of the skin caused by *Tinea cruris* organisms, characterized by ringed lesions in the crural folds of the skin of the thighs, often followed by maceration and secondary infection. Warm, humid climate, tight clothing, and obesity aggravate the infection. Cold compresses may be applied to relieve symptoms, and griseofulvin is prescribed to eliminate the fungus. **2.** a form of contact dermatitis associated with the use of laundry marking fluids. Also called **eczema marginatum,** *Informal.* **jock itch, jockstrap itch.**

di-, **1.** a combining form meaning 'two, twice': *diacid, diamide, dimorphic.* **2.** Also **dia-.** a combining form meaning 'apart, through': *diuresis, diactinism.* **3.** a combining form meaning 'apart, away from': *diffraction, discission, divergent.*

dia-. See **di-.**

diabetes, **1.** a clinical condition characterized by the excessive excretion of urine. The excess may be caused by a deficiency of antidiuretic hormone (ADH), as in diabetes insipidus, or it may be the result of the hyperglycemia occurring in diabetes mellitus. **2.** diabetes mellitus. —**diabetic** *adj., n.*

diabetes insipidus (ɪnsɪp′ɪdəs), a metabolic disorder, characterized by extreme polyuria and polydipsia, owing to deficient production or secretion of the antidiuretic hormone (ADH) or an inability of the kidney tubules to respond to ADH. (Rarely, the symptoms are self-induced by an excessive water intake.) The condition may be acquired, familial, idiopathic, or nephrogenic.

■ OBSERVATIONS: The onset may be dramatic and sudden and urinary output may exceed 10 liters in 24 hours. The patient is usually well and comfortable except for the annoyance of frequent urination and a constant need to drink. A person with diabetes insipidus who is unconscious owing to trauma or surgery continues to produce massive quantities of urine. If fluids are not administered in adequate amounts the patient becomes severely dehydrated and hypernatremic.

■ INTERVENTION: In mild cases, no treatment is necessary. Vasopressin in an intramuscular injection or spray is effective. Oral hypoglycemic agents improve the response of the kidneys to the decreased amount of available ADH in some cases, and thiazide diuretics, by inducing a state of salt depletion, sometimes decrease the diuresis of water by as much as 50 per cent.

■ NURSING CONSIDERATIONS: Infants and small children are particularly vulnerable to serious circulatory disturbances when dehydrated; therefore, exceedingly careful monitoring is essential in cases where the condition is suspected, especially after head surgery or trauma.

diabetes mellitus (məlaɪ′təs) **(DM),** a complex disorder of carbohydrate, fat, and protein metabolism owing primarily to a relative or complete lack of insulin secretion by the beta cells of the pancreas. The disease is often familial but may be acquired, as in Cushing's syndrome, secondary to the administration of excessive glucocorticoid. See also **gestational diabetes, juvenile diabetes.**

■ OBSERVATIONS: The onset of diabetes mellitus is sudden in children and usually insidious in adults. Characteristically, the course is progressive and includes polyuria, polydipsia, weight loss, polyphagia, hyperglycemia, and glycosuria. The eyes, kidneys, nervous system, skin, and circulatory system may be affected, infections are common, and atherosclerosis often develops. In childhood and in the 'brittle,' advanced stage of the disease when no endogenous insulin is being secreted, ketoacidosis is a constant danger. The diagnosis is confirmed by glucose tolerance tests, history, and urinalysis.

■ INTERVENTION: The goal of treatment is to maintain insulin-glucose homeostasis. Mild, early, or late onset of the disease may be controlled by diet alone. In more severe diabetes, insulin is administered to keep blood glucose levels below the point where ketoacidosis is likely. Good control of diabetes may decrease the severity of the symptoms and the progression of the disease. The kind and amount of insulin given varies with the person's condition. Stress of any kind may require an adjustment in the dosage. See also **diabetic foot and leg care.**

■ NURSING CONSIDERATIONS: Diabetic patients need extensive teaching and emotional support. The nurse may help the person to accept the diagnosis, to understand the disease, and to learn self-administration of the medication. The person is also taught the need for continued medical supervision and dietary restriction, how to test the urine for sugar and interpret the results, recognize the signs of impending coma (restlessness, thirst, hot dry skin, rapid pulse, fruity odor to the breath, and nausea), and the signs of hypoglycemia and impending insulin shock (headache, nervousness, diaphoresis, thready pulse, and slurred speech). Certain safety precautions are emphasized; the patient should avoid infection, carry a supply of glucose at all times, wear a medical alert tag, and use sterile technique in giving self-medication.

(See next page for table)

diabetic, **1.** of or pertaining to diabetes. **2.** affected with diabetes. **3.** a patient with diabetes mellitus.

diabetic amaurosis, blindness associated with diabetes, caused by a proliferative, hemorrhagic form of retinopathy that is characterized by capillary microaneurysms and hard or waxy exudates. Cataracts also are common in adult onset diabetes, and, in juvenile onset diabetes, snowflake cataract may progress until the entire lens is milky white.

diabetic coma, a life-threatening condition occurring in diabetic patients, caused by inadequate treatment, failure to take prescribed insulin, or, most frequently, by infection, surgery, trauma, or other stress that increases the body's need for insulin. Without insulin to metabolize glucose, fats are burned for energy, resulting in ketosis and acidosis. The body's effort to counteract acidosis depletes the alkali reserve, causes a loss of sodium, chloride, potassium, and water, increases respirations (Kussmaul breathing) and urinary excretion, and leads to dehydration and generalized hypoxia. Warning signs of diabetic coma include a dull headache, fatigue, inordinate thirst, epigastric pain, nausea, vomiting, parched lips, a flushed face, and sunken eyes. The temperature usually rises and then falls; the systolic blood pressure drops and circulatory collapse may occur. Immediate treatment consists of administering insulin and replacing electrolytes and fluids to correct the acidosis and dehydration. Nonketotic coma may occur in patients with poorly controlled diabetes and high levels of blood glucose but no acetone in the urine. The plasma hyperosmolarity causes water to leave cells, and the dehydration of cerebral cells results in coma.

diabetic diet, a diet prescribed in the treatment of diabetes mellitus, usually containing limited amounts of sugar or readily available carbohydrates and increased amounts of proteins, complex carbohydrates, and unsaturated fats. Dietary regulation depends on the severity of the disease and on the type and extent of insulin therapy. The diet should be designed to prevent wide fluctuation in the amount of glucose in the blood in order to preserve pancreatic function and to prevent chronic diabetic complications. See also **diabetes mellitus, insulin.**

diabetic foot and leg care, the special attention given to prevent the circulatory disorders and infections that frequently occur in the lower extremities of diabetic patients.
■ METHOD: The patient's legs and feet are examined daily for signs of dry, scaly, red, itching, or cracked skin, blisters, corns, calluses, abrasions, infection, blueness and swelling around varicosities, and thickened, discolored nails. The feet are bathed daily in tepid water with mild or superfatted soap and are dried gently but thoroughly with a soft towel. A lanolin-based lotion is then applied, starting with the distal end of the toes; excess lotion is removed with a dry towel; vigorous rubbing and the use of alcohol preparations are avoided. The toenails are cut straight across above the level of soft tissue after the feet are soaked for three to five minutes in tepid water. The feet are also soaked in tepid water for several minutes before hardened areas are treated by applying soft soap and rubbing the area with a washcloth; calluses and corns are removed, and thickened, deformed nails are cut by a podiatrist. Prior to discharge, the patient is instructed to

Summary of differences between insulin reaction and diabetic ketoacidosis

Factors	Insulin reaction	Ketoacidosis
Onset	Rapid	Slow (days or weeks)
Precipitating factors		
Food	Insufficient	Excessive
Complications	None	Infection
Insulin	Excess	Too little
Exercise	Increased	Too little
Symptoms		
Thirst	Absent	Increased
Vomiting	Absent	Frequent
Hunger	Frequent	Absent
Abdominal pain	Absent	Frequent
Vision	Double	Dim
Signs		
Temperature	Normal or below	Elevated
Respirations	Normal	Hyperpnea (Kussmaul respiration), acetone odor to breath
Blood pressure	Normal or elevated	Lowered, may be in hypovolemic shock
Skin	Moist and pale	Hot, dry, and flushed
Dehydration	None	Loss of skin turgor, sunken eyeballs
Tremors	Frequent	Absent
Laboratory findings		
Urine		
Glycosuria	May be positive, but negative in second specimen	4+
Ketonuria	Negative	4+
Blood		
Sugar	Below normal	Elevated, usually above 200 mg/100 ml
Ketones	Normal	Elevated, usually 4+
Electrolytes	Normal	Decreased, except serum potassium

examine and bathe the feet daily according to the recommended method, to report abnormalities, to keep the feet dry at all times, to wear cotton socks or stockings with cotton feet, and to place clean lamb's wool or cotton between the toes if they perspire. The patient is cautioned to avoid foot and leg trauma, walking barefoot, scratching insect bites, using a hot-water bottle or heating pad on the lower extremities, getting sunburned, wearing constricting garments, remaining in the same position for long periods, sitting at more than a right-angle bend, and crossing the knees. The diabetic individual is advised to alternate the wearing of two pairs of rubber-soled, well-fitted shoes wide enough to prevent pressure and rubbing, to air each pair of shoes between use, and to break in new shoes gradually. The patient is urged to walk to tolerance daily, to plan exercise periods after meals, to bend and straighten the knees and rotate the ankles occasionally when sitting and, when standing, to shift weight from time to time and walk in place.

■ NURSING ORDERS: The nurse provides foot and leg care while the diabetic patient is hospitalized and gives instruction before the person is discharged.

■ OUTCOME CRITERIA: Meticulous care of the feet and legs can prevent serious complications to which diabetic patients are subject, including local infection, skin ulcers, cellulitis, and gangrene.

diabetic ketoacidosis, an acute, life-threatening complication of uncontrolled diabetes mellitus in which urinary loss of water, potassium, ammonium, and sodium results in hypovolemia, electrolyte imbalance, extremely high blood sugar levels, and the breakdown of free fatty acids causing acidosis, often with coma. Compare **insulin shock.**

■ OBSERVATIONS: The person appears flushed, has hot, dry skin, is restless, uncomfortable, agitated, diaphoretic, and has a fruity odor to the breath. Coma, confusion, and nausea are often noted. Juvenile diabetics and older diabetics who have no endogenous insulin are the most often affected. Untreated, the condition invariably proceeds to coma and death.

■ INTERVENTION: Intravenous insulin and hypotonic saline solution are administered immediately. Nasogastric intubation and bladder catheterization are usual. Blood glucose and ketone levels are determined hourly and electrolyte and acid-base balance are monitored frequently. Bicarbonate or potassium may be given in dosages dependent on the degree of acidosis. Plasma or a plasma expander may be necessary to prevent or correct shock owing to hypovolemia.

■ NURSING CONSIDERATIONS: The cause for the episode of ketoacidosis is sought. The most common precipitating factors are infection, gastrointestinal upset, alcohol consumption, and the patient's failure to take insulin. In childhood, diabetes characteristically begins suddenly and progresses rapidly; therefore, the diagnosis of juvenile di-

abetes is usually made when the child is brought to the hospital in diabetic ketoacidosis. The care of a patient in the hospital after an episode of ketoacidosis is the same as for diabetes mellitus.

diabetic retinopathy, a disorder of retinal blood vessels characterized by capillary microaneurysms, hemorrhage, exudates, and the formation of new vessels and connective tissue. The disorder occurs most frequently in patients with long-standing, poorly controlled diabetes. Repeated hemorrhage may result in permanent opacity of the vitreous humor, and blindness may eventually result. Photocoagulation of damaged retinal blood vessels by a laser beam may be performed to prevent hemorrhage from the vessels. Rarely, cloudy vitreus humor is surgically removed by vitrectomy.

diabetic treatment, therapy of diabetes mellitus by means of a low carbohydrate diet, insulin injections, or oral hypoglycemic agents, as chlorpropamide, acetohexamide, tolbutamide, and tolazamide.

diabetic xanthoma, an eruption of yellow papules or plaques on the skin in uncontrolled mellitus. The lesion disappears as the metabolic functions are stabilized and the disease is brought under control.

Diabinese, a trade name for an antidiabetic (chlorpropamide).

diacetic acid (daï'əsi'tık, daï'əset'ık). See **acetoacetic acid.**

diacondylar fracture (daï'əkon'dılər), any fracture that runs across the line of a condyle.

Diagnex blue test (daï'ægneks), a trade name for a test for the presence of hydrochloric acid in gastric secretions. Diagnex blue tablets, which contain the dye azuresin, are taken by mouth. If the urine appears blue it can be inferred that the stomach is secreting hydrochloric acid. See also **gastric analysis.**

diagnosis, *pl.* **diagnoses. 1.** identification of a disease or condition by a scientific evaluation of physical signs, symptoms, history, laboratory tests, and procedures. **2.** the name of a disease or condition. Kinds of diagnoses are **clinical diagnosis, differential diagnosis, laboratory diagnosis, nursing diagnosis, physical diagnosis.** —**diagnostic,** *adj.,* **diagnose,** *v.*

(See next page for table)

diagnostic, pertaining to a diagnosis.

Diagnostic and Statistical Manual of Mental Disorders **(DSM),** a manual, published by the American Psychiatric Association, listing the official diagnostic classifications of mental disorders. The *DSM* recommends the use of a multiaxial evaluation system as a holistic diagnostic approach consisting of five axes, each of which refers to a different class of information, including both mental and physical data. Axes I and II include all of the mental disorders, classified broadly as clinical syndromes and personality disorders; Axis III contains physical dis-

Diagnostic procedures

Test	Description	Purpose	Comments
Lumbar puncture (LP)	Long needle is inserted between L3 and L4 vertebrae into subarachnoid space; cerebrospinal fluid pressure is measured, and sample is collected for examination	Diagnostic—measures spinal fluid pressure, obtains cerebrospinal fluid for visualization and laboratory analysis Therapeutic—injection of medication, spinal anesthesia	Contraindicated for patients with increased intracranial pressure, infected skin over puncture site, when test does not contribute to diagnosis or treatment
Subdural tap	Needle is inserted into anterior fontanel or coronal suture	Helps rule out subdural effusions Relieves intracranial pressure	Requires shaving scalp Fluid removed is limited to no more than 15 ml from one side at each tap To and fro movement of needle is avoided to prevent laceration Pressure dressing applied after subdural tap Infant placed in semierect position after subdural tap to minimize leakage from site; avoid crying if possible
Ventricular puncture	Needle is inserted into lateral ventricle via anterior fontanel	Removes cerebrospinal fluid to relieve pressure	Used if lumbar puncture unsuccessful or contraindicated Should be performed by neurosurgeon Risk of intracerebral or ventricular hemorrhage
Electroencephalography	Records changes in electric potential of brain Electrodes are placed at various points on scalp and amplified Impulses are recorded by electromagnetic pen	Measures electric activity of cerebral cortex Detects electric abnormalities—diagnosis of seizures Used to determine brain death	Patient should rest quietly during procedure May require sedation Reduce external stimuli to a minimum during procedure
Computerized tomography	Pinpoint x-ray beam is directed on horizontal or vertical plane to provide series of "cuts" or "slices" that are fed into computer and assembled in image displayed on videoscreen and transferred to permanent record	Visualized horizontal and vertical cross section of brain at any axis Distinguishes density of various intracranial tissues and structures	Noninvasive procedure Requires sedation Can be done on outpatient basis
Brain scan	Intravenous injection of radioactive material that is counted and recorded after fixed time interval	Test material accumulates in areas where blood-brain barrier is defective Identifies focal brain lesions; for example, tumors, abscesses Positive uptake of material with encephalitis and subdural hematoma	Requires sedation in young or uncooperative children and intravenous infusion
Echoencephalography	Pulses of ultrasonic waves are beamed through head; echoes are recorded graphically	Identifies shifts in midline structures from their normal positions as a result of intracranial lesions	Simple, safe, rapid procedure
Pneumoencephalography	Introduction of oxygen or air into subarachnoid spaces via lumbar puncture	Visualizes entire ventricular system and subarachnoid spaces Identifies structural abnormalities Localizes intracranial lesions	Requires heavy sedation or anesthesia
Ventriculography	Air introduced into lateral ventricular system by direct ventricular tap in infants, burr hole in older children	Visualizes ventricular system Detects structural anomalies or localizes intracranial lesions Determines patency of ventricular system	May cause some trauma to brain
Cerebral angiography	Percutaneous injection of radiopaque substance into cerebral circulation via carotid system (or by reflux from cannulization of brachial or femoral arteries)	Outlines cerebral arteries and veins—determines size, location, and nature of cerebral vascular disorders and localizes tumors, abscesses, and other space-occupying lesions by detecting distortion of normal vascular patterns	Requires general anesthesia

continued.

Diagnostic procedures—cont'd

Test	Description	Purpose	Comments
Radiography	Skull films are taken from several projections—lateral, posterolateral, axial (submentoventrical), half-axial	Shows fractures, dislocations, spreading suture lines, and craniostenosis Shows degenerative changes, bone erosion, and calcifications	Simple, noninvasive procedure

orders and conditions; and Axes IV and V provide a coded outline of supplemental information on, for instance, psychosocial stressors and adaptive functioning, which may be useful for planning individual treatment and predicting its outcome. Each of the classifications of the mental disorders contains a code that provides a reference to the WHO *Classification of Diseases* and offers such useful diagnostic criteria as essential and associated features of the disorder, age at onset, course, impairment, complications, predisposing factors, prevalence, sex ratio, familial patterns, and differential diagnoses.

diagnostic anesthesia, a procedure in which analgesia is induced to depth adequate to comfortably permit performance of moderately painful diagnostic procedures of short duration. Awake anesthesia is often used for this purpose. See also **awake anesthesia.**

diagnostician, a person skilled and trained in making diagnoses.

diagnostic radiopharmaceutical, a radioactive drug administered to a patient as a diagnostic tracer to differentiate normal from abnormal anatomic structures or biochemical or physiological functions. Most diagnostic radioactive tracers indicate their position within the body by emitting gamma rays. By monitoring the emissions with a collimated external gamma-ray detector, the concentration of the tracer in different organs can be inferred and low-resolution images of the organs obtained. Tracers prepared with tritium, carbon-14, or phosphorus-32, which do not emit gamma rays, are used diagnostically by analyzing the concentration of the isotope in a metabolic end product in the patient's blood, urine, breath, or, in some cases, biopsy samples. When glucose containing ^{14}C is administered, the subsequent monitoring of $^{14}CO_2$ in the patient's breath can indicate the absorption of the compound, its metabolism, and elimination as a metabolic end product.

diagnostic related group (DRG), a designation in a system that classifies patients by age, diagnosis, and surgical procedure, producing 300 different categories used in predicting the use of hospital resources, including length of stay. The system is being tested for use in anticipating the cost of reimbursement to hospitals by studying the population served to improve the cash flow to the hospital. It is performed using grouped data about how much each particular DRG may be expected to cost in hospital services.

diakinesis (dai'əkını'sıs, dai'əkaini'sıs), the final stage in the first meiotic prophase in gametogenesis in which the chromosomes achieve maximum contraction and are ready to separate. The chiasmata and nucleolus disappear, the nuclear membrane degenerates, and the spindle fibers form in preparation for the formation of dyads. See also **diplotene, leptotene, pachytene, zygotene.**

Dialose, a trade name for a gastrointestinal, fixed-combination drug containing a stool softener (dioctyl sodium sulfosuccinate) and a laxative (sodium carboxymethylcellulose).

dialysate, a solution used in dialysis.

dialysis (daiæl'ısıs), 1. the process of separating colloids and crystalline substances in solution by the difference in their rate of diffusion through a semipermeable membrane. 2. a medical procedure for the removal of certain elements from the blood or lymph by virtue of the difference in their rates of diffusion through an external semipermeable membrane or, in the case of peritoneal dialysis, through the peritoneum. Dialysis may be used to remove poisons and excessive amounts of drugs, to correct serious electrolyte and acid-base imbalances, and to remove urea, uric acid, and creatinine in patients with chronic end-stage renal disease. Dialysis involves diffusion of particles from an area of high to lower concentration, osmosis of fluid across the membrane from an area of lesser to greater concentration of particles, and the ultrafiltration or movement of the fluid across the membrane as a result of an artifically created pressure differential. See also **hemodialysis, peritoneal dialysis.**

dialyzer (dai'əlai'zər), 1. a machine used in dialysis. 2. a semipermeable membrane or porous diaphragm in a dialysis machine. See also **hemodialysis, peritoneal dialysis.**

Diamond-Blackfan anemia. See **Blackfan-Diamond syndrome.**

Diamox, a trade name for a carbonic anhydrase inhibitor (acetazolamide), used as an adjunct in anticonvulsant therapy for certain seizure disorders and to reduce intraocular pressure in glaucoma.

Dianabol, a trade name for an androgen (methandrostenolone), used as an anabolic agent.

Dianeal, a trade name for a peritoneal dialysis solution containing dextrose and a number of electrolytes.

diapedesis (dai'əpıdi'sıs), the passage of blood corpuscles through the walls of the vessels that contain them.

diaper rash, a maculopapular and occasionally excoriated eruption in the diaper area of infants caused by irritation from feces, moisture, heat, or ammonia produced by the bacterial decomposition of urine. Secondary infection by monilia is common. Principles of treatment include frequent diaper changes, dryness, cleanliness, coolness, and ventilation of the affected area. Specific topical antimicrobial medication may be prescribed for secondary infection.

diaper restraint, a therapeutic device used especially in orthopedics for countertraction with lower extremity traction when other methods of countertraction are not effective. Diaper restraints are commonly used in treating children with orthopedic diseases and abnormalities and are designed to fit over the pelvic area like a diaper, with rings incorporated at each of four corners. A webbing strap is threaded through the rings and attached to the top side of the bedspring frame. Diaper restraints applied to incontinent patients are usually checked every half hour as a precaution against urinary tract infections that can develop from urinary wastes accumulating within such restraints. Diaper restraints are used with Russell traction and with split Russell traction if additional countertraction is required but are not usually used with other kinds of traction. Compare **jacket restraint, sling restraint.**

diaphanoscopy (daiæf′ənos′kəpi), examination of an internal structure with a diaphanoscope, an instrument that transilluminates body tissues.

diaphoresis (dai′əfəri′sis), the secretion of sweat, especially the profuse secretion associated with an elevated body temperature, physical exertion, exposure to heat, and mental or emotional stress. Sweating is centrally controlled by the sympathetic nervous system and is primarily a thermoregulatory mechanism, but the sweat glands on the palms and soles respond to emotional stimuli and do not participate in thermal sweating. The rate of sweating is generally not affected by water deficiency but it may be reduced by severe dehydration and diminishes when salt intake exceeds salt loss. Also called **sweating.** – **diaphoretic,** adj.

diaphoretic (dai′əfəret′ık). See **sudorific.**

diaphragm (dai′əfræm), **1.** (in anatomy) a domeshaped musculofibrous partition that separates the thoracic and the abdominal cavities. The convex cranial surface of the diaphragm forms the floor of the thoracic cavity and the concave surface forms the roof of the abdominal cavity. This partition is pierced by various openings through which pass different structures, as the aorta, esophagus, and vena cava. The diaphragm aids respiration by moving up and down. During inspiration it moves down and increases the volume of the thoracic cavity; during expiration it moves up, decreasing the volume. During deep inspiration and expiration the range of diaphragmatic movement in the adult is about 30 mm on the right side and about 28 mm on the left side. The height of this structure also varies with the degree of distension of the stomach and the intestines and with the size of the liver. It is innervated by the phrenic nerve from the cervical plexus. **2.** Informal. a contraceptive diaphragm. **3.** (in optics) an opening that controls the amount of light passing through an optical network. **4.** a thin, membranous partition, as that employed in dialysis. **5.** (in radiography) a metal plate with a small opening that limits the diameter of the radiographic beam.   – **diaphragmatic,** adj.

diaphragmatic hernia, the protrusion of part of the stomach through an opening in the diaphragm, most commonly an abnormally enlarged esophageal hiatus. The enlargement of the normal opening for the esophagus may be caused by trauma, congenital weakness, increased abdominal pressure, or relaxation of ligaments of skeletal muscles, and permits part of the stomach to slide into the thorax. A sliding hiatus hernia, one of the most common pathologic conditions of the upper gastrointestinal tract, may occur at any age but is most frequent in elderly and middle-aged people. Also called **hiatus hernia.**

■ OBSERVATIONS: Symptoms of diaphragmatic hernia vary but usually include heartburn after meals, when in a supine position, and on exertion, especially when bending forward. There may be regurgitation of food, dysphagia, abdominal distention after eating, belching, rumbling in the intestines, rapid breathing, and a dull epigastric pain radiating to the shoulder. The similarity of some of the symptoms to those of myocardial infarction may make the patient fearful and anxious. The continued reflux of gastric juice into the esophagus may lead to ulceration with bleeding and the formation of fibrous tissue. Gastric contents regurgitated during sleep may be aspirated into the lungs. Rarely, part of the cardiac portion of the stomach becomes incarcerated in the chest.

■ INTERVENTION: The patient is placed in bed in a semi-Fowler's position and raised to a high Fowler's position during and after small, frequent meals of a bland diet. The individual is encouraged to chew slowly and thoroughly, to drink one or two glasses of water with a meal (unless contraindicated), and to avoid smoking. The blood pressure, pulse, respirations, and temperature are monitored. Medication for pain, an antacid, as aluminum hydroxide gel, and diagnostic endoscopy and x rays may be ordered; to facilitate visualization of the hernia the patient may be placed in a Trendelenburg position during studies of barium swallowing. If symptoms are severe and persistent and if they are unrelieved by conservative measures, the hernia may be repaired surgically.

■ NURSING CONSIDERATIONS: Diaphragmatic hernias are very common, especially among older people in the hospital for other indications. The recurrence of the symptoms of diaphragmatic hernia may often be prevented by instructing the patient, before discharge, to have frequent, small bland meals, not to recline after eating, to lose weight (if indicated), not to smoke, and to avoid constipation. Serious complications and severe discomfort usually may be avoided by the patient if the instructions are observed.

diaphragmatic node, a node in one of three groups of thoracic parietal lymph nodes, situated on the thoracic side of the diaphragm and consisting of the anterior set, the middle set, and the posterior set of nodes. The anterior set includes about three nodes dorsal to the base of the xiphoid process and one or two nodes on either side near the junction of the seventh rib. The nodes dorsal to the xiphoid process receive afferent lymphatic vessels from the convex surface of the liver. The afferents of the nodes near the seventh rib drain the ventral side of the diaphragm. The efferents of the anterior set pass to the sternal nodes. The middle set of about three nodes on each side is close to the diaphragmatic entry of the phrenic nerves. Some of the nodes of the middle set on the right side lie within the pericardium. The afferents of the middle set drain parts of the diaphragm and the liver. The efferents of the middle set pass to the posterior mediastinal nodes. The posterior set of diaphragmatic nodes consists of a few nodes on the crura of the diaphragm, connecting with the lumbar nodes and the posterior mediastinal nodes. Compare **intercostal node, sternal node.** See also **lymphatic system, lymph node.**

diaphragm pessary. See **pessary.**

diaphragm stethoscope, an instrument for auscultation of bodily sounds. Originally designed by René Laënnec, it consists of a vibrating disc, or diaphragm, which transmits sound waves through tubing to two ear pieces. Also called **binaural stethoscope.** See also **stethoscope.**

diaphyseal aclasis (dai'əfɪz'iəl), a relatively rare abnormal condition that affects the skeletal system. Characterized by multiple exostoses or bony protrusions, it is hereditary, being transmitted as a dominant trait. Approximately half of the children of an individual with diaphyseal aclasis display varying degrees of its symptoms. The characteristic exostoses are radiographically and microscopically similar to osteochondromas. Evident involvement is diffuse, with the long bones usually affected more severely and more frequently than the short bones. Depending on the specific area involved, various angular or rotational deformities may result. Diaphyseal aclasis is usually bilateral and occurs more frequently in boys than in girls. Although this disease is hereditary, its signs and symptoms are not usually evident until the affected individual is two years of age or older. Children of a parent who has the disease are often routinely examined for symptoms. The major signs of the disease are the noticeable protrusions in the areas of the exostoses. Pain is not usually associated with the exostoses and, if present, is usually minimal. Deformities of the extremities may be evident, depending on the severity and the loca-

tion of the exostoses. Radiographic examination reveals a broadened metaphyseal area, and the specific lesion is exhibited by abnormal continuity and decreased density. Asymptomatic lesions characteristic of diaphyseal aclasis usually require little or no treatment other than continued observation. The lesions located near the joints that interfere with joint motion or impair neurovascular function may be surgically excised. Angular and rotational deformities caused by the lesions may require surgical correction to facilitate improved function. Inequalities in the length of lower extremities resulting from unilateral involvement may require epiphysiodesis. A relatively small number of these lesions may become malignant. Also called **hereditary deforming chondroplasia, multiple cartilaginous exostoses.**

diaphysis (daiæf'ɪsɪs), the shaft of a long bone, consisting of a tube of compact bone enclosing the medullary cavity.

Diapid, a trade name for a pituitary antidiuretic hormone (lypressin).

diarrhea, the frequent passage of loose, watery stools, generally the result of increased motility in the colon. The stool may also contain mucus, pus, blood, or excessive amounts of fat. Diarrhea is always a symptom of some underlying disorder. Conditions in which diarrhea is an important symptom are dysenteric diseases, malabsorption syndrome, lactose intolerance, irritable bowel syndrome, gastrointestinal tumors, and inflammatory bowel disease. In addition to stool frequency, patients may complain of abdominal cramps and generalized weakness. Untreated, diarrhea may lead to rapid dehydration and electrolyte imbalance and should be treated symptomatically until proper diagnosis can be made. Antidiarrheal preparations, as diphenoxylate (Lomotil) and paregoric, are helpful. If diarrhea is accompanied by vomiting, intravenous fluids may be necessary to prevent fluid depletion. See also **dehydration.** – **diarrheal, diarrheic,** *adj.*

diarthrosis (dai'arθrou'sɪs). See **synovial joint.**

Diasone Sodium Enterab, a trade name for a leprostatic antibacterial (sulfoxone sodium).

diastatic fermentation (dai'əstæt'ɪk), the conversion of starch to glucose by the enzyme ptyalin.

diasthesis (dai'asθi'sɪs), *pl.* **diastheses.** an inherited physical constitution predisposing to certain diseases or conditions, many of which are believed associated with the Y chromosome, because males appear to be more susceptible than females. A diasthesis may be bilious, indicating a familial tendency to develop gastrointestinal distress, or gouty, indicating a predisposition to the accumulation of urates in the tissues, particularly in mature males.

diastole (daiæs'təli), the period of time in the cardiac cycle between contractions of the ventricles during which blood enters the relaxed ventricular chambers from the atria. Diastole begins with the onset of the second heart sound and ends with the first heart sound. Compare **systole.** — **diastolic** (dai'əstol'ık), *adj.*

-diastole, a combining form referring to 'types and locations of the lower blood pressure measurement': *adiastole, hyperdiastole, prediastole.*

diastrophic dwarf, a person in whom short stature is caused by osteochondrodysplasia and is associated with various deformities of the bones and joints, including scoliosis, clubfoot, micromelia, hand defects, multiple joint contractures and subluxations, ear deformities, and cleft palate. The condition may be genetically related and transmitted as an autosomal recessive trait.

diathermy (dai'əthər'mi), a therapeutic procedure that employs high-frequency current, ultrasonic waves, or microwaves to raise slightly the temperature of deep tissues.

diazepam, a sedative and tranquilizer.
- INDICATIONS: It is prescribed in the treatment of anxiety, nervous tension, muscle spasm, and as an anticonvulsant.
- CONTRAINDICATIONS: Acute narrow angle glaucoma, psychosis, or known hypersensitivity to this drug or to any benzodiazepine medication prohibits its use.
- ADVERSE EFFECTS: Among the more serious adverse reactions are withdrawal symptoms resulting from discontinuation of treatment. Drowsiness and fatigue commonly occur.

diazoxide (dai'əzok'said), a vasodilator used as an antihypertensive.
- INDICATION: It is prescribed for the emergency reduction of blood pressure in malignant hypertension when drastic reduction of the diastolic blood pressure is required.
- CONTRAINDICATIONS: Compensatory hypertension or known hypersensitivity to this drug or other thiazides prohibits its use.
- ADVERSE EFFECTS: Among the more serious adverse reactions are sodium and water retention, hyperglycemia, and severe hypotension.
- NOTE: This drug is for intravenous use in hospitalized patients only. Severe hypotension may result.

Dibenzyline, a trade name for an alpha-adrenergic blocker (phenoxybenzamine hydrochloride).

dibromodulcitol. See **mitolactol.**

dibucaine, a topical anesthetic ointment.

DIC, abbreviation for **disseminated intravascular coagulation.**

dicalcium phosphate and calcium gluconate with vitamin D, a source of calcium and phosphorus.
- INDICATION: It is prescribed for hypocalcemia, especially in pregnancy and lactation.
- CONTRAINDICATIONS: Hypoparathyroidism or known hypersensitivity to any of the ingredients of this drug prohibits its use.

- ADVERSE EFFECTS: There are no known adverse reactions.

dicephaly, a developmental anomaly in which the fetus has two heads. — **dicephalous, dicephalic,** *adj.,* **dicephalus,** *n.*

dichlorodiphenyltrichloroethane. See **DDT.**

dichlorphenamide (dai'klorfen'əmaid), a carbonic anhydrase inhibitor.
- INDICATION: It is prescribed in the treatment of chronic glaucoma.
- CONTRAINDICATIONS: Liver and adrenocortical insufficiency, kidney failure, hyperchloremic acidosis, depressed sodium or potassium levels, pulmonary obstruction, Addison's disease, known or suspected pregnancy, or known hypersensitivity to this drug prohibits its use.
- ADVERSE EFFECTS: Among the more serious adverse reactions are anorexia, gastrointestinal disturbances, acidosis, ureteral calculus formation, and aplastic anemia.

dichorial twins (daikor'iəl), **dichorionic twins** (dai'korion'ık). See **dizygotic twins.**

dichotomy (daikot'əmi), a division or separation into two equal parts.

Dick test, a skin test for determining sensitivity to an erythrotoxin produced by the group A streptococci that cause scarlet fever. A skin test dose of the toxin is injected intradermally. An area of inflammation 1.0 cm in diameter indicates that the person is not immune, has no antitoxin, and therefore is susceptible to the toxin. Larger doses may then be given to induce immunity. Compare **Shultz-Carlton phenomenon.**

dicloxacillin sodium (dai'kloksəsıl'ın), an antibacterial.
- INDICATIONS: It is prescribed in the treatment of staphylococcal infections, especially those caused by penicillinase producing strains of staphylococci.
- CONTRAINDICATIONS: Known hypersensitivity to this drug or to any penicillin medication prohibits its use.
- ADVERSE EFFECTS: The most serious adverse effect is hypersensitivity reaction.

Dicodid, a trade name for an antitussive (hydrocodone bitartrate).

dicumarol, an anticoagulant.
- INDICATIONS: It is prescribed for the prophylaxis and treatment of thrombosis and embolism.
- CONTRAINDICATIONS: Risk of hemorrhage, peptic ulcer, ulcerative colitis, or known hypersensitivity to this drug prohibits its use.
- ADVERSE EFFECTS: Among the more serious adverse reactions are gastrointestinal disturbances, nausea, and diarrhea.

Dicurin Procaine, a trade name for a mercurial diuretic (merethoxylline procaine).

dicyclomine hydrochloride, an anticholinergic.
- INDICATION: It is prescribed as an adjunct to ulcer therapy.

■ CONTRAINDICATIONS: Narrow angle glaucoma, asthma, obstruction of the genitourinary or gastrointestinal tract, ulcerative colitis, or known hypersensitivity to this drug prohibits its use.

■ ADVERSE EFFECTS: Among the more serious adverse reactions are blurred vision, central nervous system effects, tachycardia, dry mouth, decreased sweating, and hypersensitivity reactions.

Didrex, a trade name for an anorexiant (benzphetamine hydrochloride).

Didronel, a trade name for a calcium regulator (etidronate disodium).

didym-, a combining form meaning 'pertaining to a testis': *didymalgia, didymitis, didymodynia.*

-didymus, 1. a combining form meaning a 'pair of twins joined at a (specified) part of the body': *gastrodidymus, thoracodidymus, vertebrodidymus.* 2. a combining form meaning a 'fetal monster with supernumerary organ(s)': *atlodidymus, opodidymus, pygodidymus.*

diecious, dioecious (daiˈshəs), an animal or plant that is sexually distinct, having either male or female reproductive organs.

diencephalon (daiˈensefˈəlon), the division of the brain between the telencephalon and the mesencephalon. It consists of the hypothalamus, thalamus, metathalamus, and the epithalamus and includes most of the third ventricle.

dienestrol (daiˈinesˈtrol), an estrogen.

■ INDICATIONS: It is prescribed in the treatment of atrophic vaginitis and kraurosis vulvae.

■ CONTRAINDICATIONS: Pregnancy, known or suspected cancer of the breast, thrombophlebitis, unusual vaginal bleeding, or known hypersensitivity to this drug prohibits its use.

■ ADVERSE EFFECTS: Among the more serious adverse reactions are increased risk of cancer, thrombophlebitis, hepatic adenoma, embolism, and gall bladder disease.

diet, 1. food and drink considered with regard to their nutritional qualities, composition, and effects on health. 2. nutrients prescribed, regulated, or restricted as to kind and amount for therapeutic or other purposes. 3. the customary allowance of food and drink regularly provided or consumed. Compare **nutrition.** See also specific diets. – **dietetic,** *adj.*

dietary allowances, the recommended allowances of essential nutrients formulated by the Food and Nutrition Board of the National Research Council to serve as a guide for planning the diet to maintain good nutrition in healthy individuals. In general the recommended allowances exceed average nutritional requirements and are lower than the amounts needed in disease or deficiency states.

dietary fiber, a generic term for the many nondigestible chemical substances found in plant cell walls and sur-

rounding cellular material, each with a different effect on the various gastrointestinal functions, as colon transit time, water absorption, and lipid metabolism. The main dietary fiber components are cellulose, lignin, hemicellulose, pectin, and gums. Foods high in dietary fiber are fruits, green leafy vegetables, as lettuce, spinach, celery, and cabbage, root vegetables, as carrots, turnips, and potatoes, and whole-grain cereals and breads. Also called **bulk, roughage.**

dietetic food, 1. a specially prepared low-calorie food, often containing artificial sweeteners. 2. a food prepared for any specific dietary need or restriction, as salt-free or vegetarian foods. See also **dietetics.**

dietetics (daiˈitetˈiks), the science of applying nutritional principles to the planning and preparation of foods and regulation of the diet in relation to both health and disease.

diethylcarbamazine citrate (daiethˈəlkarbæmˈəzin), an anthelmintic.

■ INDICATIONS: It is prescribed in the treatment of ascariasis, filariasis, onchocerciasis, loiasis, and tropical eosinophilia.

■ CONTRAINDICATION: Known hypersensitivity to this drug prohibits its use.

■ ADVERSE EFFECTS: Among the most serious adverse reactions are severe allergic reactions owing to the death of parasites.

diethyl ether. See **ether.**

diethylpropion hydrochloride, an appetite depressant.

■ INDICATION: It is prescribed in the treatment of exogenous obesity.

■ CONTRAINDICATIONS: Arteriosclerosis, hyperthyroidism, glaucoma, history of drug dependence, hypertension, concomitant administration of a monoamine oxidase inhibitor within 14 days, or known hypersensitivity to this drug prohibits its use.

■ ADVERSE EFFECTS: Among the more serious adverse reactions are restlessness and insomnia, increased blood pressure, arrhythmias, cardiovascular effects, nausea, dry mouth, and drug dependence.

diethylstilbestrol (DES), a synthetic hormone with estrogenic properties. Also called **stilbestrol.**

Dietl's crisis (diˈtəlz), a sudden, excruciating pain in the kidney, caused by distention of the renal pelvis, by the rapid ingestion of very large amounts of liquid, or by a kinking of a ureter that produces temporary occlusion of the flow of urine from the kidney. The pain may be accompanied by nausea, vomiting, hematuria, and general collapse. See also **hydronephrosis.**

differential diagnosis. See **diagnosis.**

differential growth, a comparison of the various increases in size or the different rates of growth of dissimilar organisms, tissues, or structures.

differential white blood cell count, an examination and enumeration of the distribution of leukocytes in a stained blood smear. The different kinds of white cells are counted and reported as a percentage of the total examined. Compare **complete blood count.** See also **erythrocyte morphology, hematocrit, hemoglobin, indices, red cell count, platelet count.**

differentiation, 1. (in embryology) a process in development in which unspecialized cells or tissues are systemically modified and altered to achieve specific and characteristic physical forms, physiologic functions, and chemical properties. Kinds of differentiation are **correlative differentiation, functional differentiation, invisible differentiation, self-differentiation.** 2. progressive diversification leading to complexity. 3. the acquisition of functions and forms different from those of the original. 4. the distinguishing of one thing or disease from another, as in differential diagnosis. – **differentiate,** v.

diffraction, the bending and scattering of wavelengths of radiation, as light, as the radiation passes around obstacles in its path. X-ray diffraction is utilized in the study of the internal structure of cells. The x rays are diffracted by cell parts into patterns which are indicative of chemical and physical structure. See also **refraction.**

diffuse fibrosing alveolitis. See **interstitial pneumonia.**

diffuse goiter, an enlargement of all parts of the thyroid gland.

diffuse hypersensitivity pneumonia, an immunologically mediated inflammatory reaction in the lungs induced by exposure to an allergen derived from a fungus, bird droppings, piscine, porcine, or bovine proteins, wood dust, or fur, or by an adverse reaction to a drug, as chlorpropamide, hydrochlorothiazide, mecamylamine, mephenesin, methotrexate, nitrofurantoin, para-aminosalicylic acid, or penicillin. The disorder is characterized by cough, fever, dyspnea, malaise, pulmonary edema, and infiltration of the alveoli with eosinophils and large mononuclear cells. Also called **allergic alveolitis, allergic interstitial pneumonitis, extrinsic allergic pneumonia, hypersensitivity pneumonitis, P.I.E. syndrome.**

diffuse lipoma. See **multiple lipomatosis.**

DIFFUSION

diffuse lipomatosis. See **multiple lipomatosis.**

diffusion, the process in which solid, particulate matter in a fluid moves from an area of higher concentration to an area of lower concentration, resulting in an even distribution of the particles in the fluid.

diffusion of gases, a natural process, essential in respiration, in which molecules of a gas pass from an area of high concentration to one of a lower concentration.

diflorasone diacetate, a topical corticosteroid.

■ INDICATION: It is prescribed topically as an anti-inflammatory agent.

■ CONTRAINDICATIONS: Viral and fungal diseases of the skin, impaired circulation, or known hypersensitivity to this drug or to other steroidal medication prohibits its use.

■ ADVERSE EFFECTS: Among the more serious adverse reactions, usually occurring after prolonged or excessive application, are striae, hypopigmentation, local irritation of the skin, and various systemic effects.

digastricus (daigæs′trɪkəs), one of four suprahyoid muscles having two parts, an anterior belly and a posterior belly. The anterior belly originates in the lower border of the mandible and inserts in the body and great cornu of the hyoid bone. It is innervated by fibers of the mandibular branch of the trigeminal nerve. It acts to open the jaw and to draw the hyoid bone forward. The posterior belly originates in the mastoid notch of the temporal bone and inserts in the body and great cornu of the hyoid bone. It is innervated by fibers of the mandibular branch of the facial nerve and acts to draw back and to raise the hyoid bone. Also called **digastric muscle.** Compare **geniohyoideus, mylohyoideus, stylohyoideus.**

DiGeorge syndrome (dɪjɔrj′), a congenital disorder characterized by severe immunodeficiency and structural abnormalities, including hypertelorism, notched, low-set ears, small mouth, downward slanting eyes, cardiovascular defects, and the absence of the thymus and parathyroid glands. Death, often from infection, usually occurs before age two. Rarely, transplantation of a human fetal thymus is performed. Also called **thymic parathyroid aplasia.**

digest, 1. to soften by heat and moisture. 2. to break into smaller parts and simpler compounds by mastication, hydrolysis, and the action of intestinal secretions and enzymes, especially in the way the body digests food for the absorption of nutrients required in metabolism. The small intestine digests food by enzymatic actions which produce absorbable amino acids, emulsified fat particles, and monosaccharides. 3. any material that results from digestion or hydrolysis.

digestion, the conversion of food into absorbable substances in the gastrointestinal tract. Digestion is accomplished through the mechanical and chemical breakdown of food into smaller and smaller molecules, with the help

Processes in the mechanics of digestion

Organ	Mechanical process	Nature of process
Mouth (teeth and tongue)	Mastication	Chewing movements—reduce size of food particles and mix them with saliva
	Deglutition	Swallowing—movement of food from mouth to stomach
Pharynx	Deglutition	
Esophagus	Deglutition	
	Peristalsis	Wormlike movements that squeeze food downward in tract; constricted ring forms first in one section, the next, etc., causing waves of contraction to spread along entire canal
Stomach	Churning	Forward and backward movement of gastric contents, mixing food with gastric juices to form chyme
	Peristalsis	Waves start in body of stomach about three times per minute and sweep toward closed pyloric sphincter; at intervals, strong peristaltic waves press chyme past sphincter into duodenum
Small intestine	Segmentation (mixing contractions)	Forward and backward (nonprogressive) movement within segment of intestine; purpose, to mix food and digestive juices thoroughly and to bring all digested food in contact with intestinal mucosa to facilitate absorption; purpose of peristalsis, on the other hand, to propel intestinal contents along digestive tract
	Peristalsis	
Large intestine		
Colon	Segmentation	Churning movements within haustral sacs
	Peristalsis	
Descending colon	Mass peristalsis	Entire contents moved into sigmoid colon and rectum; occurs three or four times a day, usually after a meal
Rectum	Defecation	Emptying of rectum, so-called bowel movement

of glands located both inside and outside the gut. — **digestive,** *adj.*

digestive fever, a slight rise in body temperature that normally accompanies the digestive process.

digestive gland, any one of the many structures that secretes reactive agents involved in the breaking down of food into the constituent absorbable substances needed for metabolism. Some kinds of digestive glands are the salivary glands, gastric glands, intestinal glands, liver, and pancreas. Some important secretions produced by different digestive glands are hydrochloric acid, bile, mucus, and various enzymes.

digestive system, the organs, structures, and accessory glands of the digestive tube of the body through which food passes from the mouth to the esophagus, stomach, and intestines. The accessory glands secrete the digestive enzymes, used by the digestive system to break down food substances in preparation for absorption into the blood stream before carrying the waste to the intestines for excretion.

digestive tube, a musculomembranous tube, about 9 meters long, extending from the mouth to the anus and lined with mucous membrane. Its various portions are the mouth, pharynx, esophagus, stomach, small intestine, and large intestine. The tube is part of the digestive system of the body which includes numerous accessory organs. Also called **alimentary canal.** See also **digestive system.**

digit-, a combining form meaning 'pertaining to a finger or toe': *digitate, digitigrade, digitoplantar.*

digital, 1. of or pertaining to a digit, that is, a finger or toe. 2. resembling a finger or toe. See also **digitate.**

digitalis, a cardiotonic.
■ INDICATIONS: It is prescribed in the treatment of congestive heart failure and certain cardiac arrhythmias.

■ CONTRAINDICATIONS: Ventricular fibrillation, ventricular tachycardia, or known hypersensitivity to this drug prohibits its use.

■ ADVERSE EFFECTS: The most serious reactions are various cardiac arrhythmias. *(See next page for table)*

digitalis glycoside. See **glycoside.**

digitalis therapy in children, the administration of a digitalis preparation to a child with a heart disorder in order to increase the force of myocardial contractions, produce a slower, more regular apical rate, and slow the transmission of impulses through the conduction system. Digitalis may be used in treating many cardiac disorders in children, including atrial fibrillation, atrial septal defect, coarctation of the aorta, congenital heart block, congestive heart failure, endocardial fibroelastosis, great vessel transposition, malformation of the tricuspid valve, myocarditis, paroxysmal atrial tachycardia, and patent ductus arteriosus.

■ METHOD: The completeness of the orders is ensured regarding the name of the digitalis preparation, the dosage in milligrams, the route and intervals of administration, and the pulse rate under which the drug is to be withheld. The dosage volume of the drug is carefully calculated by two people: two registered nurses, an RN and pharmacist, or an RN and physician. If the drug is to be given orally, the best method of ensuring that the child receives the full dose is determined, whether by spoon, nipple, or dropper. It is administered before feeding but is never mixed with the formula or food. Prior to each administration, the child's resting apical pulse is checked for rate and rhythm for a full minute; if the rate is slower than desired, if it is irregular or shows a rapid rise or fall,

Digitalis preparations

Generic name	Trade name	Digitalizing dose (time)	Maintenance dose	Route	Onset	Duration
Purple foxglove *(Digitalis purpurea)*						
Powdered digitalis	Digifortis Digiglusin	1 to 2 g (24 to 48 hr)	100 to 200 mg	Oral	Slow	Long
Digitoxin	Crystodigin Purodigin Digitaline Nati- velle Unidigin	1.5 mg (24 to 48 hr)	100 to 200 mg	Oral IV	Slow	Long
Gitalin	Gitaligin	4 to 6 mg (3 to 4 days)	0.5 mg	Oral	Fast	Moderate
White foxglove *(Digitalis lanata)*						
Digoxin	Lanoxin	1.5 mg 1.0 mg (12 to 24 hr)	0.125 to 0.5 mg	Oral IV IM	Fast	Moderate
Deslanoside	Cedilanid-D	1.6 mg (12 hr)	0.25 to 0.5 mg	IV IM	Fast	Short
Lanatoside C	Cedilanid	10 mg (4 days)	0.5 mg	Oral	Variable	Short
Acetyldigitoxin	Acylanid	1.6 to 2.2 mg (24 hr)	0.1 to 0.2 mg	Oral	Moderate	Short
Strophanthus gratus						
G-strophanthin	Ouabain	0.25 to 0.5 mg (12 to 24 hr)	—	IV	Fast	Short

if there are any signs of toxicity, as anorexia, nausea, vomiting, or if there are visual disturbances the drug is withheld and the problem is reported.

■ NURSING ORDERS: The nurse participates in calculating the dosage volume ordered, administers the drug, and observes for and reports any undesirable effects. Once the child's dosage is stabilized and before discharge, the nurse ensures that the parents understand the proper method, time, and purpose of administering the drug, as well as the need and the time to give the complete dose, when to withhold medication, and how to recognize and report signs of toxicity to the drug.

■ OUTCOME CRITERIA: In addition to promoting more forceful myocardial contractions and a slower, more regular apical beat, digitalis therapy can reduce venous pressure, improve pulmonary and systemic circulation, increase urinary output, reduce edema, and stop paroxysmal atrial tachycardia and atrial fibrillation.

digitate (dĭj′ĭteit), having fingers or fingerlike projections. See also **digital.**

digitate wart, a fingerlike, horny projection that arises from a pea-shaped base and occurs on the scalp or near the hairline. Like other kinds of warts, it is a benign viral infection of the skin and the adjacent mucous membrane. It may spontaneously disappear as the host individual develops an immune response, or it may require treatment, as by electrodesiccation and curettage.

digitoxin, a cardiac glycoside.

■ INDICATIONS: It is prescribed in the treatment of congestive heart failure and certain cardiac arrhythmias.

■ CONTRAINDICATIONS: Ventricular fibrillation, ventricular tachycardia, or known hypersensitivity to this drug prohibits its use.

■ ADVERSE EFFECTS: The most serious adverse reaction is cardiac arrhythmia.

digoxin (dĭjok′sĭn), a glycoside cardiotonic.

■ INDICATIONS: It is prescribed in the treatment of congestive heart failure and certain cardiac arrhythmias.

■ CONTRAINDICATIONS: Ventricular fibrillation, ventricular tachycardia, or known hypersensitivity to this drug prohibits its use.

■ ADVERSE EFFECTS: The most serious adverse reaction is cardiac arrhythmia.

diGuglielmo's disease (di′gulyel′mouz). See **erythroleukemia.**

diGuglielmo's syndrome. See **erythroleukemia.**

dihybrid (daï′haï′brid), (in genetics) pertaining to or describing a person, organism, or strain that is heterozygous for two specific traits, that is the offspring of parents differing in two specific gene pairs, or that is heterozygous for two particular traits or gene loci under consideration.

dihybrid cross, (in genetics) the mating of two individuals, organisms, or strains that have different gene pairs that determine two specific traits or in which two particular characteristics or gene loci are being followed.

dihydric alcohol, an alcohol containing two hydroxyl groups.

dihydroergotamine mesylate, an alpha-adrenergic blocking agent.

■ INDICATIONS: It is prescribed for migraine and for vascular headache.

■ CONTRAINDICATIONS: Cardiovascular disease, hypertension, liver or kidney dysfunction, sepsis, pregnancy, or known hypersensitivity to this drug prohibits its use.

■ ADVERSE EFFECTS: Among the more serious adverse reactions are gangrene and the toxicity of the ergot alkaloids.

dihydrotachysterol (daīhaī′droutəkıs′tərol), a rapid-acting form of vitamin D.

■ INDICATION: It is prescribed in the treatment of hypocalcemia resulting from hypoparathyroidism and pseudohypoparathyroidism.

■ CONTRAINDICATIONS: Hypercalcemia, hypocalcemia with kidney insufficiency, hyperphosphatemia, or known hypersensitivity to this drug or to vitamin D prohibits its use.

■ ADVERSE EFFECTS: The most serious adverse reaction is hypercalcemia. With overdosage, calcification of soft tissues, including those of the heart, or cardiovascular or kidney failure may occur.

diiodohydroxyquin (daīaī′ədouhaīdrok′səkwin), an amebicide.

■ INDICATION: It is prescribed in the treatment of intestinal amebiasis.

■ CONTRAINDICATIONS: Liver or thyroid disease or known hypersensitivity to this drug, hydroxyquinoline derivatives, or iodine prohibits its use.

■ ADVERSE EFFECTS: Among the most serious adverse reactions are myelo-optic neuropathy and thyroid enlargement. Occasionally, nausea, abdominal cramps, or pruritus ani occurs.

Dilantin, a trade name for an anticonvulsant (phenytoin).

dilatation (dıl′ətei′s̆hən), **1.** normal physiologic increase in the diameter of a body opening, blood vessel, or tube, as the widening of the pupil of the eye in response to decreased light or the widening of the opening of the uterine cervix during labor. **2.** artificial increase in the diameter of such an opening either by medication, as in the use of cycloplegic eye drops to open the pupil wide for examination of the retina, or by instrumentation as in the use of a dilator to open the uterine cervix to facilitate curettage. **3.** the diameter of the opening of the cervix in labor as measured on vaginal examination, expressed in centimeters or fingerbreadths, one fingerbreadth being ap-

proximately 2.0 cm. At full dilatation the diameter of the cervical opening is 10.0 cm. — **dilatate,** *v.*

Before labor   **Early effacement**

Complete effacement (100%)   **Complete dilatation (10 cm)**

CERVICAL EFFACEMENT AND DILATATION

dilatation and curettage (D & C), dilatation of the uterine cervix and scraping of the endometrium of the uterus, performed to diagnose disease of the uterus, to correct heavy or prolonged vaginal bleeding, or to empty uterine contents of the products of conception. It is also done to remove tumors, to rule out carcinoma of the uterus, to remove retained placental fragments postpartum or after an incomplete abortion, and to find the cause of infertility. Under a light, general anesthesia the cervix is dilated with a series of dilators of increasing size to allow the insertion of a curet into the uterus. Vaginal packing may sometimes be inserted to slow bleeding but is not usually recommended. It may be left in place for 24 hours. A sterile perineal pad is applied. Postoperative care requires emotional support appropriate to the clinical situation and close observation for hemorrhage, infection, or dysuria.

dilatator naris, the alar portion of the nasalis muscle that dilates the nostril. Compare **compressor naris.**

dilatator pupillae, a muscle that contracts the iris of the eye and dilates the pupil. It is comprised of radiating fibers that converge from the circumference of the iris toward the center and blend with fibers of the sphincter pupillae near the margin of the pupil. The dilatator pupillae is innervated by nerve fibers from the sympathetic system. Compare **sphincter pupillae.**

Dilaudid Hydrochloride, a trade name for a narcotic analgesic (hydromorphone hydrochloride).

Dilor, a trade name for a bronchodilator (dyphylline).

dimenhydrinate, an antihistamine.

■ INDICATIONS: It is prescribed in the treatment of nausea and motion sickness.

■ CONTRAINDICATIONS: Asthma or known hypersensitivity to this drug prohibits its use. It is not given to newborn infants or lactating mothers.

■ ADVERSE EFFECTS: Among the more serious adverse reactions are skin rash, hypersensitivity reactions, and tachycardia. Drowsiness and dry mouth are common.

dimer (dai′mər), a compound formed by the union of two radicals or two molecules of a simpler compound, as a polymer formed from two or more molecules of a monomer.

dimercaprol (dai′mərkæp′roul). See **British anti-lewisite.**

Dimetane, a trade name for an antihistamine (brompheniramine maleate).

Dimetapp, a trade name for a fixed-combination drug containing two decongestants (phenylephrine hydrochloride and phenylpropanolamine hydrochloride) and an antihistamine (brompheniramine maleate).

dimethindene maleate (daimeth′indin), an antihistamine.

■ INDICATIONS: It is prescribed in the treatment of a variety of hypersensitivity reactions, including rhinitis, skin reactions, and itching.

■ CONTRAINDICATIONS: The drug is not given to newborn infants or to lactating mothers. Asthma or known hypersensitivity to this drug prohibits its use.

■ ADVERSE EFFECTS: Drowsiness, skin rash, hypersensitivity reactions, dry mouth, and tachycardia commonly occur.

dimethoxymethylamphetamine (DOM), a psychedelic agent.

dimethyl carbinol (daimeth′il kar′binol). See **isopropyl alcohol.**

dimethyl sulfoxide (DMSO), an anti-inflammatory agent.

■ INDICATIONS: It is prescribed in the treatment of interstitial cystitis and is being investigated as a topical anti-inflammatory agent in orthopedic sports injuries.

■ CONTRAINDICATION: Known hypersensitivity to this drug prohibits its use.

■ ADVERSE EFFECTS: Among the most serious adverse reactions are gastrointestinal disturbances, photophobia, disturbance of color vision, and headache. A garlic-like body odor and taste in the mouth may occur. When applied to the skin it can cause local irritations.

dimethyl tubocurarine iodide. See **metocurine iodide.**

Dimitri disease (dimi′tri). See **encephalotrigeminal angiomatosis.**

dinoprost (dai′nəprost), a prostaglandin abortifacient.

■ INDICATION: It is prescribed to terminate a pregnancy during the second trimester.

■ CONTRAINDICATIONS: Acute pelvic inflammatory disease or known hypersensitivity to this drug prohibits its use.

■ ADVERSE EFFECTS: Among the more serious adverse reactions are cardiac arrhythmias, vomiting, and bronchospasm.

dinoprostone (dai′noupros′toun), a naturally occurring form of prostaglandin E_2 (PGE_2) administered in a vaginal suppository as an oxytocic agent.

■ INDICATIONS: It is prescribed to cause termination of pregnancy from 12 to 20 weeks of gestation, to evacuate the uterus following fetal death up to 28 weeks of gestation, in missed abortion, and in nonmetastatic gestational trophoblastic disease.

■ CONTRAINDICATIONS: Acute inflammatory disease, concurrent administration of oxytocin, or known hypersensitivity to this drug prohibits its use. It is used with caution in patients who have cardiac, pulmonary, hepatic, or renal disease, asthma, diabetes, or epilepsy or in patients who have had uterine surgery.

■ ADVERSE EFFECTS: Among the more serious reactions are wheezing, dyspnea, fever, vomiting, and diarrhea. Trauma to the cervix and to the lower uterine segment has occurred following administration of the drug owing to forceful expulsion of the uterine contents before full dilatation of the cervix.

dioctyl calcium sulfosuccinate. See **docusate.**

dioctyl sodium sulfosuccinate. See **docusate.**

dioecious. See **diecious.**

Diothane, a trade name for a local anesthetic (diperodon).

diovular (daiou′vyələr). See **binovular.**

diovulatory, routinely releasing two ova during each ovarian cycle. Compare **monovulatory.**

dioxybenzone, an ultraviolet screen.

■ INDICATION: It is prescribed to prevent burning from exposure to the sun.

■ CONTRAINDICATION: Known hypersensitivity to this drug prohibits its use. It should not come into contact with the eyes.

■ ADVERSE EFFECT: The only known adverse reaction is skin rash.

dioxyline phosphate, a synthetic antispasmodic and vasodilator.

■ INDICATIONS: It is prescribed for the relief of angina pectoris and for spasm of blood vessels in arms, legs, or lungs.

■ CONTRAINDICATION: Known hypersensitivity to this drug prohibits its use.

■ ADVERSE EFFECTS: Among the most serious adverse reactions are nauseau, dizziness, and flushing, which occur rarely.

Dipaxin, a trade name for an anticoagulant (diphenadione).

diphemanil methylsulfate (dɑ̄ifi′mənɪl), an anticholinergic.

■ INDICATION: It is prescribed as an adjunct to ulcer therapy.

■ CONTRAINDICATIONS: Narrow angle glaucoma, asthma, obstruction of the genitourinary or gastrointestinal tract, ulcerative colitis, or known hypersensitivity to this drug prohibits its use.

■ ADVERSE EFFECTS: Among the more serious adverse reactions are blurred vision, central nervous system effects, tachycardia, dry mouth, decreased sweating, and hypersensitivity reactions.

diphenadione (dɑ̄i′fənæd′ioun), an anticoagulant.

■ INDICATIONS: It is prescribed in the treatment of thrombosis and embolism.

■ CONTRAINDICATIONS: Hemorrhage or known hypersensitivity to this drug prohibits its use.

■ ADVERSE EFFECTS: The most serious adverse reaction is hemorrhage. This drug interacts with many other drugs.

diphenhydramine hydrochloride, an antihistamine.

■ INDICATIONS: It is prescribed in the treatment of a variety of hypersensitivity reactions, including rhinitis, skin rash, and pruritus, and in the treatment of motion sickness.

■ CONTRAINDICATIONS: Asthma or known hypersensitivity to this drug prohibits its use. It is not given to newborn infants or lactating mothers.

■ ADVERSE EFFECTS: Among the more serious adverse reactions are skin rash, hypersensitivity reactions and tachycardia. Drowsiness and dry mouth commonly occur.

diphenoxylate hydrochloride, an antidiarrheal.

■ INDICATIONS: It is prescribed in the treatment of diarrhea and intestinal cramping.

■ CONTRAINDICATIONS: Liver disease, antibiotic-associated diarrhea, or known hypersensitivity to this drug prohibits its use. It is not given to children under two years of age.

■ ADVERSE EFFECTS: Among the more serious adverse reactions are abdominal discomfort, intestinal obstruction, skin rash, and nausea.

diphenylhydantoin. See **phenytoin.**

diphenylpyraline hydrochloride (dɑ̄i′fenəlpɑ̄i′rəlin), an antihistamine.

■ INDICATIONS: It is prescribed in the treatment of a variety of hypersensitivity reactions, including rhinitis, skin rash, and pruritus.

■ CONTRAINDICATIONS: Asthma or known hypersensitivity to this drug prohibits its use. It is not given to newborn infants or lactating mothers.

■ ADVERSE EFFECTS: Among the more serious adverse reactions are skin rash, hypersensitivity reactions, and tachycardia. Drowsiness and dry mouth commonly occur.

diphtheria (dɪfthir′iə, dɪpfhir′iə), an acute, contagious disease caused by the bacterium *Corynebacterium diphtheriae,* characterized by the production of a systemic toxin and a false membrane lining of the mucous membrane of the throat. The toxin is particularly damaging to the tissues of the heart and central nervous system, and the dense pseudomembrane in the throat may interfere with eating, drinking, and breathing. The membrane may occur in other body tissues. Lymph glands in the neck swell and the neck becomes edematous. Untreated, the disease is often fatal, causing heart and kidney failure. Patients are usually hospitalized in isolation rooms. Treatment of the isolated patient may include administration of diphtheria antitoxin, antibiotics, bed rest, fluids, and an adequate diet. Tracheostomy is sometimes necessary. Recovery is slow, but it is usually complete. Immunization against diphtheria is available to all children in the United States and is usually given in conjunction with pertussis and tetanus immunization early in infancy. See also **Schick test.**

diphtheria and tetanus toxoids (DT), an active immunizing agent.

■ INDICATIONS: It is prescribed for immunization against diphtheria and tetanus.

■ CONTRAINDICATIONS: Immunosuppression, acute infection, or concomitant use of corticosteroids prohibits its use.

■ ADVERSE EFFECTS: The most serious adverse reaction is anaphylaxis.

diphtheria and tetanus toxoids and pertussis vaccine, an active immunizing agent.

■ INDICATIONS: It is prescribed for the routine immunization of children under six years of age against diphtheria, tetanus, and pertussis.

■ CONTRAINDICATIONS: Immunosuppressive therapy, active infection, or neurologic disorders prohibit its use.

■ ADVERSE EFFECT: The most serious adverse reaction is anaphylaxis.

diphtheria toxoid, an active immunizing agent.

■ INDICATION: It is prescribed for immunization against diphtheria.

■ CONTRAINDICATIONS: Immunosuppressive therapy, active infection, or neurologic disorders prohibit its use.

■ ADVERSE EFFECTS: The most serious adverse reaction is anaphylaxis.

diphtheroid (dɪf′thəroid′), 1. of or pertaining to diphtheria. 2. resembling the bacillus *Corynebacterium diphtheriae.*

Diphyllobothrium (dɑ̄ifɪl′oubofh′riəm), a genus of large, parasitic, intestinal flatworms having a scolex with two slitlike grooves. The species that most often infects humans is *Diphyllobothrium latum,* the fish tapeworm. See also **tapeworm infection.**

dipivefrin, an ophthalmic adrenergic.

■ INDICATIONS: It is prescribed in the treatment of open-angle glaucoma.

■ CONTRAINDICATIONS: Narrow-angle glaucoma or known hypersensitivity to this drug prohibits its use.

■ ADVERSE EFFECTS: Among the most serious adverse effects are reactive hyperemia, conjunctivitis, allergic reactions, and macular edema. Systemic reactions, as tachycardia, are possible.

diplegia (dɑipli'jə), bilateral paralysis of both sides of any part of the body or of like parts on the opposite sides of the body. A kind of diplegia is **facial diplegia**. Compare **hemiplegia.** – **diplegic,** *adj.*

diplo-, a combining form meaning 'double': *diplobacilli, diplococcus, diplokaryon.*

diplococcus (dɪp'loukok'əs), *pl.* **diplococci** (dɪp'loukok'sɑi). a coccus that occurs in pairs.

diploë (dɪp'loui), the loose bony tissue between the two tables of the cranial bones.

diploid (dɪp'loid), **1.** of or pertaining to an individual, organism, strain, or cell that has two complete sets of homologous chromosomes, as normally found in the somatic cells and the primordial germ cells before maturation. In humans the normal diploid number is 46. **2. diploidic (2n),** such an individual, organism, strain, or cell. Compare **haploid, tetraploid, triploid.**

diploidy (dɪp'loidi), the state or condition of having two complete sets of homologous chromosomes.

diplokaryon (dɪp'loukær'ion), a nucleus that contains twice the diploid number of chromosomes.

diploma program in nursing, an educational program that trains nurses in a hospital setting, usually in two or three years. The recipient of a diploma is eligible to take the national certifying examination to become a registered nurse. Diploma programs are being closed, as the professional nursing organizations have decided that today's professional nurse requires an academic background. In Canada, diploma programs are conducted in junior or community colleges, and hospital schools are being phased out, except in the Atlantic provinces.

diplomate (dɪp'ləmeit), an individual who has earned a diploma or certificate, especially a physician who has been certified by a specialty board. See also **board certified.**

diplonema (dɪp'ləni'mə), the looplike formation of the chromosomes in the diplotene stage of the first meiotic prophase of gametogenesis.

diplopagus (dɪplop'əgəs), conjoined twins that are more or less equally developed, although one or several internal organs may be shared.

diplopia (dɪplou'piə), double vision caused by defective function of the extraocular muscles or a disorder of the nerves that innervate the muscles. A transient episode of diplopia is usually of no clinical significance, indicating only a brief relaxation of the fusion mechanism of the central nervous system that maintains ocular straightness.

-diplopia, a combining form meaning '(condition of)

double vision': *amphodiplopia, amphoterodiplopia, monodiplopia.*

diplosomatia (dɪp'lousoumei'shə), **diplosomia,** a congenital anomaly in which fully formed twins are joined at one or more areas of their bodies.

diplotene (dɪp'lətin), the fourth stage in the first meiotic prophase in gametogenesis in which the tetrads exhibit chiasmata between the chromatids of the paired homologous chromosomes and genetic crossing over occurs. The chromosomes then begin to repel each other and separate longitudinally, forming loops. See also **diakinesis, leptotene, pachytene, zygotene.**

dipodia (dɑipou'diə), a developmental anomaly characterized by the duplication of one or both feet.

diprosopus (dɑipros'əpəs, dɑi'prəsou'pəs), a malformed fetus that has a double face showing varying degrees of development.

-dipsia, a combining form meaning '(condition of) thirst': *hydroadipsia, oligodipsia, polydipsia.* Also **-dipsy.**

dipsomania, an uncontrollable, often periodic craving for and indulgence in alcoholic beverages; alcoholism.

-dipsy. See **-dipsia.**

dipus (dɑi'pəs), conjoined twins that have only two feet.

dipygus (dɑipɑi'gəs, dɪp'əgəs), a malformed fetus that has a double pelvis, one of which is usually not fully developed.

dipyrone (dɑi'pɑiroun), an analgesic, antipyretic, and anti-inflammatory that was formerly used for pain and fever. Its use has been discontinued, except in rare cases of intractable fever, because the drug may cause fatal agranulocytosis.

direct calorimetry, the measurement of the amount of heat directly generated by any oxidation reaction, especially one involving a living organism. Compare **indirect calorimetry.**

direct contact, mutual touching of two individuals or organisms. Many communicable diseases may be spread by the direct contact between an infected individual and a healthy person. Some kinds of diseases that may be spread by direct contact are gonorrhea, impetigo, staphylococcal skin infections, and syphilis. Other infections are transmitted by insect or animal vectors, droplets, or contaminated food.

direct fracture, any fracture occurring at a specific point of injury that is a direct result of that injury.

direct generation. See **asexual generation.**

direct illumination. See **illumination.**

directive therapy, a psychotherapeutic approach in which the psychotherapist directs the course of therapy by intervening to ask questions and offer interpretations. Compare **nondirective therapy.** See also **psychoanalysis.**

direct lead, **1.** an electrocardiographic conductor in which the exploring electrode is placed directly on the surface of the exposed heart. **2.** *Informal.* a tracing produced by such a lead on an electrocardiograph.

direct patient care, (in nursing) care of a patient provided in person by a member of the staff. Direct patient care may involve any aspects of the health care of a patient, including treatments, counseling, self-care, patient education, and administration of medication.

direct percussion. See **percussion.**

direct reaction to light, the constriction of a pupil receiving increased illumination, as by a flashlight during an ophthalmologic examination. Compare **consensual reaction to light.**

direct relationship. See **positive relationship.**

dis-, **1.** a combining form meaning 'reversal or separation': *disacidify, dischronation, disinfect.* **2.** a combining form meaning 'duplication': *disdiaclast, dissogency, districhiasis.*

disadvantaged, **1.** any group of people who lack money, education, literacy, or another advantage. **2.** A euphemism for 'poor.'

disc, disk, **1.** a flat, circular platelike structure, as an articular disc or an optic disc. **2.** *Informal.* an intervertebral disc.

discharge, **1.** Also called **evacuate, excrete, secrete.** to release a substance or object. **2.** to release a patient from a hospital. **3.** to release an electric charge which may be manifested by a spark or surge of electricity from a storage battery, condenser, or other source. **4.** to release a burst of energy from or through a neuron. **5.** a release of emotions, often accompanied by a wide range of voluntary and involuntary reflexes, weeping, rage, or other emotional displays, called **affective discharge** in psychology. **6.** Also called **evacuate, excretion, secretion.** a substance or object discharged.

disciform keratitis, an inflammatory condition of the eye that often follows an attack of dendritic keratitis and is believed to be an immunologic response to an ocular herpes simplex infection. The condition is characterized by disclike opacities in the cornea, usually with inflammation of the iris. See also **herpesvirus.**

disco-, a combining form meaning 'pertaining to a disk, disk-shaped': *discophorous, discopathy, discoplacenta.*

discoblastula, a blastula formed from the partial cleavage that occurs in a fertilized ovum containing a large amount of yolk. It develops from the blastodisc and consists of a cellular cap, or blastoderm, separated from the uncleaved yolk mass by a small cavity, the blastocoele.

discocyte (dıs′kəsaıt), a mature, normal, erythrocyte, exhibiting one of its many steady-state configurations. It is a biconcave disc without a nucleus. Compare **echinocyte.**

discoid lupus erythematosus (DLE), a chronic, recurrent disease, primarily of the skin, characterized by red macules that are covered with scales and extend into follicles. The lesions are typically distributed in a butterfly

pattern covering the cheeks and bridge of the nose but may also occur on other parts of the body. On healing, the lesions atrophy and leave hyperpigmented or hypopigmented scars, and, if hairy areas are involved, alopecia may result. The cause of the disease is not established, but there is evidence that it may be an autoimmune disorder and some cases seem to be induced by certain drugs. It is at least five times more common in women than in men and occurs most frequently in the third and fourth decades of life. Treatment includes the use of a sunscreen lotion or ointment when exposure to sunlight cannot be avoided, the application of steroids to the lesions, and systemic antimalarial drugs, as hydroxychloroquinine; systemic corticosteroid agents may be used in severe cases. Also called **cutaneous lupus erythematosus.** See also **systemic lupus erythematosus.**

discoid meniscus, an abnormal condition characterized by a discoid rather than semilunar shape of the cartilaginous meniscus of the knee. The lateral meniscus is most often affected, although the medial meniscus may also become involved. The condition is a developmental anomaly, asymptomatic in the infant or in the young child, and occurs most frequently in children between the ages of six and eight. Common complaints are that a "clicking" occurs in the knee joint or that the knee joint gives way. These characteristics are often associated with an injury to the knee but also occur without any history of trauma. Examination demonstrates the "clicking," usually when the knee is moved from flexion to extension, during the last 15° to 20°. Surgical excision of the meniscus is seldom warranted in treating this benign condition.

discordance, (in genetics) the expression of one or more specific traits in only one member of a pair of twins. Compare **concordance.** – **discordant,** *adj.*

discovery, (in law) a pretrial procedure allowing one party to examine vital witnesses and documents held exclusively by the adverse party. Discovery is limited to materials, facts, and other resources that could not otherwise be reasonably expected to be discovered and that are necessary to the preparation of the case for trial. Also called **pretrial discovery.** Compare **deposition, interrogatories.**

discus (dıs′kəs). See **disc.**

discus interpubicus. See **interpubic disc.**

discus nervi optici. See **optic disc.**

disease, **1.** a condition of abnormal vital function involving any structure, part, or system of an organism. **2.** a specific illness or disorder characterized by a recognizable set of signs and symptoms, attributable to heredity, infection, diet, or environment. Compare **condition, diathesis.**

disengagement, an obstetrical manipulation in which the presenting part of the baby is dislodged from the maternal pelvis as part of an operative delivery. See also **Kielland rotation, version and extraction.**

dishpan fracture, a fracture that depresses the skull. Also called **derby hat fracture.**

disinfection, the process of killing pathogenic organisms or of rendering them inert.

disjunction, (in genetics) the separation of the paired homologous chromosomes during the anaphase stage of the first meiotic division or of the chromatids of a chromosome during anaphase of mitosis and the second meiotic division. Compare **nondisjunction.**

dislocation, the displacement of any part of the body from its normal position, particularly a bone from its normal articulation with a joint. See also **subluxation.** – **dislocate,** v.

dismiss, (in law) to discharge or dispose of an action, suit, or motion trial. – **dismissal,** n.

disodium edetate. See **edetate disodium.**

Disophrol, a trade name for a respiratory, fixed-combination drug containing an antihistamine (dexbrompheniramine maleate) and an adrenergic bronchodilator (pseudoephedrine sulfate).

disopyramide phosphate (dai′soupir′ɔmaid), a cardiac depressant.

■ INDICATIONS: It is prescribed in the treatment of premature ventricular contractions and ventricular tachycardia.

■ CONTRAINDICATIONS: Heart failure, pre-existing second- or third-degree heart block in the absence of a pacemaker, sick sinus syndrome, or known hypersensitivity to this drug prohibits its use.

■ ADVERSE EFFECTS: Among the more serious adverse reactions are severe hypotension, precipitation of heart failure, and aggravation of heart block. Dry mouth and constipation commonly occur.

disorganized schizophrenia, a form of schizophrenia characterized by an earlier age of onset, usually at puberty, and a more severe disintegration of the personality than occurs in other forms of the disease. Symptoms include inappropriate laughter and silliness; peculiar mannerisms, like facial grimaces; talking and gesturing to oneself; regressive, bizarre, and often obscene behavior; extreme social withdrawal; and fantastic and unsystematized hallucinations and delusions, which are usually of a sexual, religious, persecutory, or hypochondriacal nature. Also called **hebephrenia, hebephrenic schizophrenia.** See also **schizophrenia.**

disorient, to lose awareness or perception of space, time, or personal identity and relationships.

disorientation, a state of mental confusion characterized by inadequate or incorrect perceptions of place, time, or identity. Disorientation may occur in organic mental disorders, drug and alcohol intoxication, and, less commonly, following severe stress.

dispersing agent, a chemical additive used in pharmaceuticals to cause the even distribution of the ingredients throughout the product, as in dermatologic emulsions containing both oil and water. Dispersing agents commonly used in skin creams, lotions, and ointments include glyceryl monostearate, sodium lauryl sulfate, and polyethylene glycol derivatives, as polysorbate 80 and polyoxyl 40 stearate. Any of these agents may cause an allergic reaction or adverse effect.

dispersion medium. See **medium.**

displaced fracture, a traumatic bone break in which two ends of a fractured bone are separated from each other. The ends of broken bones in displaced fractures often pierce surrounding skin, as in an open fracture, or may be contained within the skin, as in a closed fracture.

displacement, 1. the state of being displaced or the act of displacing. 2. (in chemistry) a reaction in which an atom, molecule, or radical is removed from combination and replaced by another. 3. (in physics) the displacing in space of one mass by another, as the weight or volume of a fluid is displaced by a floating or submerged body. 4. (in psychiatry) an unconscious defense mechanism for avoiding emotional conflict and anxiety by transferring emotions, ideas, or wishes from one object to a substitute that is less anxiety-producing. Compare **sublimation.** See also **percolation.**

dissect, to cut apart tissues for visual or microscopic study using a scalpel, probe, or scissors. Compare **bisect.** – **dissection,** n.

dissecting aneurysm, a localized dilatation of an artery, most commonly the aorta, characterized by a longitudinal dissection between the outer and middle layers of the vascular wall. Aortic dissecting aneurysms occur most frequently in men between the ages of 40 and 60 and are, in more than 90 per cent of cases, preceded by hypertension. Blood entering a tear in the intimal lining of the vessel causes a separation of weakened elastic and fibromuscular elements in the medial layer and leads to the formation of cystic spaces filled with ground substance. Dissecting aneurysms in the thoracic aorta may extend into blood vessels of the neck. Rupture of a dissecting aneurysm may be fatal in less than an hour. Treatment consists of resection and replacement of the excised section of aorta with a synthetic prosthesis.

disseminated intravascular coagulation (DIC), a grave, coagulopathy resulting from the overstimulation of the body's clotting and anticlotting processes in response to disease or injury, as septicemia, acute hypotension, poisonous snake bites, neoplasms, obstetric emergencies, severe trauma, or extensive surgery and hemorrhage. The primary disorder initiates generalized intravascular clotting which, in turn, overstimulates fibrinolytic mechanisms, as a result the initial hypercoagulability is succeeded by a deficiency in clotting factors with hypocoagulability and hemorrhaging.

■ OBSERVATIONS: Widespread purpura on the chest and abdomen, reflecting fibrin deposits in capillaries, is a common first sign of DIC and is often followed by the appearance of hemorrhagic bullae, acral cyanosis, and focal gangrene in the skin and mucous membranes. There may be hemorrhages from incisions, catheter or injection sites, gastrointestinal bleeding, hematuria, pulmonary edema, pulmonary embolism, progressive hypotension, tachycardia, an absence of peripheral pulses, restlessness, convulsions, or coma. Laboratory studies generally show a marked deficiency of blood platelets, low levels of fibrinogen and other clotting factors, prolonged prothrombin and partial thromboplastin times, and abnormal erythrocyte morphology.

■ INTERVENTION: Treatment of the primary disorder is essential in the management of DIC. Heparin may be infused intravenously to prevent clot formation, but, since it may increase bleeding, it is not always used for surgical patients with DIC. Transfusions of whole blood, plasma, platelets, and other blood products are administered to replace depleted factors. Patients are maintained in a quiet, nonstressful environment and are protected from trauma and bleeding. The side rails of the bed are padded, foam or cotton swabs are used for mouth care, and, whenever possible, the use of tape or any invasive procedures that might cause bleeding is avoided.

■ NURSING CONSIDERATIONS: The care of a patient with life-threatening DIC is a challenge requiring monitoring of vital signs, observation for evidence of bleeding, extremely gentle handling, and the giving of considerable emotional support.

disseminated lupus erythematosus. See **systemic lupus erythematosus.**

disseminated multiple sclerosis. See **multiple sclerosis.**

dissent, (in law) a statement written by a judge who disagrees with the decision of the majority of the court. The dissent explicitly states the reasons for the dissenting judge's contrary opinion. – **dissenting,** *adj.*

dissimilar twins. See **dizygotic twins.**

dissociation, 1. the act of separating into parts or sections. 2. an unconscious defense mechanism by which an idea, thought, emotion, or other mental process is separated from the consciousness and thereby loses emotional significance. See also **dissociative disorder, dissociative reaction.** – **dissociative,** *adj.*

dissociative anesthesia, an anesthetic procedure characterized by analgesia and amnesia without loss of respiratory function or pharyngeal and laryngeal reflexes. This form of anesthesia may be used to provide analgesia during brief, superficial operative procedures or diagnostic processes. It is especially useful for people who are sensitive to general or local anesthetics or for those who, for

other reasons, may not be safely anesthetized with inhalant gases. Because the most commonly used drug is a hallucinogenic, ketamine hydrochloride, emergence may be accompanied by delirium, excitement, and confusion.

dissociative disorder, a type of hysterical neurosis in which emotional conflicts are so repressed that a separation or split in the personality occurs, resulting in an altered state of consciousness or a confusion in identity. Symptoms include amnesia, somnambulism, fugue, dream state, or multiple personality. The disorder is caused by an inability to cope with severe stress or conflict and usually occurs suddenly, following a situation catastrophic to the person. Treatment may include hypnosis, especially when amnesia is the primary symptom, psychotherapy, and antianxiety medication. Compare **conversion disorder.** See also **dissociation, dissociative reaction.**

dissociative reaction, a neurotic response to stress or emotional conflict characterized by some degree of personality disorganization with loss of affect and appropriate emotional response. In extreme cases it may lead to any of the dissociative disorders, as amnesia, fugue, or multiple personality. See also **dissociation, dissociative disorder.**

distal (dĭs′təl), 1. away from or being the farthest from a point of origin. 2. away from or being the farthest from the midline or a central point, as a distal phalanx, which is the bone at the end of a finger or toe. Compare **proximal.**

distal muscular dystrophy, a rare form of muscular dystrophy, usually affecting adults, characterized by moderate weakness and by wasting that begins in the arms and legs and then extends gradually to the proximal and facial muscles. Also called **Gowers' muscular dystrophy.**

distal phalanx, any one of the small distal bones in the third row of phalanges of the hand or the foot. Each one at the end of the fingers has a convex dorsal surface and a flat palmar surface, with a rough elevation at the end of the palmar surface that supports a fingernail and its sensitive pulp. Each distal phalanx of the toes is smaller and more flattened than that of a finger; it also has a rough elevation to support the toenail and its pulp. Also called **ungual phalanx.**

distal radioulnar articulation, the pivotlike articulation of the head of the ulna and the ulnar notch on the lower end of the radius, involving two ligaments. The joint allows rotation of the distal end of the radius around an axis which passes through the center of the head of the ulna. Also called **inferior radioulnar joint.** Compare **proximal radioulnar articulation.**

distal renal tubular acidosis (distal RTA), an abnormal condition characterized by excessive acid accumulation and bicarbonate excretion. It is caused by the inability of the distal tubules of the kidney to secrete hydrogen ions, thus decreasing the excretion of titratable acids and ammonium and increasing the urinary loss of potassium and bicarbonate. This condition may result in hypercalciuria and the formation of kidney stones. Treatment is as for renal tubular acidosis. **Primary distal RTA** occurs mostly in females, adolescents, older children, and young adults. It may occur sporadically or as the result of hereditary defects. **Secondary distal RTA** is associated with numerous disorders, as cirrhosis of the liver, malnutrition, starvation, and various genetic problems. Compare **proximal renal tubular acidosis.**

distress of the human spirit. See **spiritual distress.**

distributive analysis and synthesis, the system of psychotherapy used by the psychobiological school of psychiatry. It involves an extensive and systematic investigation and analysis of a person's total past experiences in order to discover the emotional factors underlying personality problems and how they can be synthesized into constructive behavioral patterns.

district, **1.** (in hospital nursing) a group of patients in an area of the unit for whom a head nurse or primary nurse is responsible, usually a subdivision of a ward unit. Patients are customarily assigned to a district on the basis of certain shared needs for nursing care. **2.** the area of a city or town assigned to a public health nurse.

district nurse. See **public health nurse.**

disulfiram, an alcohol deterrent.

■ INDICATIONS: It is prescribed as a deterrent to drinking alcohol in the treatment of chronic alcoholism. It causes severe intestinal cramping, diaphoresis, and nausea if alcohol is ingested.

■ CONTRAINDICATIONS: Alcoholic intoxication, recent or concomitant administration of metronidazole, paraldehyde, or alcohol, severe myocardial disease, coronary occlusion, psychosis, or known hypersensitivity to this drug prohibits its use.

■ ADVERSE EFFECTS: The most serious adverse reactions occur after alcohol is ingested, including optic neuritis, psychotic reaction, and polyneuritis. Drowsiness, headache, and skin rash may occur. This drug interacts with several other drugs.

disuse phenomena, the physical and the psychologic changes, usually degenerative, that result from the lack of use of a part of the body or a body system. Disuse phenomena are associated with confinement and immobility, especially in orthopedics. Individuals under treatment for fractures and other orthopedic disorders must often be confined to beds and immobilized in traction for long periods. Such patients are often deprived of interaction with the world around them and lose motivations, expectations, and even acquired abilities owing to lack of practice. Some studies have shown that young, healthy individuals confined to bed rest for even three hours experience disturbances of time sense and memory. Other individuals in similar circumstances have experienced tac-

tile, auditory, and visual hallucinations. Such disorientation is compounded by pain and therapeutic narcotic drugs commonly associated with the treatment of many illnesses and abnormal conditions. In hospital environments often requiring patients to drastically reduce physical and social movement during treatment and recuperation, many patients become egocentric, expecting other people to spend all their time and energy on them. Unable to interact with the normal world outside the hospital, many patients become less efficient in remembering, problem solving, and learning. The physical changes often induced by continued bed rest constitute problems affecting many key areas and systems of the body, as the skin, the musculoskeletal system, the gastrointestinal tract, the cardiovascular system, and the respiratory system. The skin of the patient on prolonged bed rest is commonly subjected to abnormal conditions, as pressure exerted by the bed, moisture, friction, and inadequate nutrition. Pressure exerted on the skin by the bed is slightly higher than capillary hydrostatic pressure, often causing problems in blood circulation and inadequate airing of the skin surface. Any pressure that causes collapse of the superficial capillaries will lead to ischemia and eventual tissue necrosis. Of particular interest to the orthopedic nurse is the phenomenon, accompanying disuse, that may prevent the neurologically impaired patient from feeling pain. This phenomenon may be the first sign of ischemia followed by a rapid breakdown of the skin. Some indications of skin ischemia are redness, pain, edema, and skin breakdown. Elderly patients are often more susceptible to skin breakdown because of possible poor nutrition, more restricted mobility, and generally poor skin condition. Younger patients may also develop ischemia if they are not sufficiently mobile. Tissue ischemia can occur in any individual in one or two hours. One of the biggest problems associated with extended bed rest or limited activity of a part of the body is disuse atrophy, which may affect the bones and muscles. The normal stress applied to these structures is important to their health and function. Unused muscles lose size and strength, often wasting away until they are unable to perform their vital functions of support and contraction. Another disuse phenomenon is contracture, which may result from constant flexion or extension of a body part by the patient on prolonged bed rest. Contractures are usually caused by flexion, because patients flex knees and hips whenever possible to relax muscles, especially when cold or in pain. The amputee often flexes the remaining portion of the affected limb for comfort or to reduce edema. Continued flexion in such circumstances may produce stiffness in the affected joint which, if not manipulated, may become permanently impaired. Prevention of contractures involves manipulation and various range-of-motion exercises, when possible. Constipation is a disuse phenomenon commonly developing from the weakening of abdominal muscles required for normal elimination of the bowel. This problem is often compounded by the horizontal position of the bed patient, dietary changes, and the administration of narcotics and anesthetic agents which slow peristalsis. The immobilized patient may experience bone demineralization owing to a restricted diet and decreased motility. Calcium and phosphorus are dependent on vitamin D for absorption from the gut and movement into the bones, and some nutritional experts describe calcium loss as a natural disuse phenomenon of bed rest. Muscle action is required to maintain the blood flow to the bones, and the immobilized patient may not be capable of sufficient muscular activity to assure such blood flow, with its attendant delivery of critical nutrients. The peak loss of calcium from the bones occurs in the fifth and the sixth weeks of bed rest. Disuse osteoporosis develops as the result of an imbalance between osteoblasts and osteoclasts; both types of cells proliferate during bed rest, but osteoclasts at a greater rate. Degeneration of bone matrix apparently occurs prior to osteoclastic resorption, causing the breakdown of the bony matrix and the resultant loss of minerals. The dangers of osteoporosis are pathologic fracture and softening of bones that can lead to deformity and pain in joints from calcium deposits. Calcium released from the bone enters the bloodstream and is deposited in the joints or carried to the kidneys for excretion in the urine. When the kidney cannot process the calcium fast enough, kidney stones develop which can block the ureters and cause kidney damage, glomerular degeneration, and acute pain. The pooling of respiratory secretions is another disuse phenomenon caused by the immotility and the horizontal position of the bed rest patient. When the individual lies down, secretions in the lungs tend to rest in the bronchioles unevenly, wetting the dependent side of the bronchioles and drying the other surfaces. The diameter of the bronchioles also decreases when the individual is supine, and a thicker coating of mucus develops, creating a riper medium for bacterial growth. Hypostatic pneumonia may result if the mucus is not removed. Prolonged bed rest also encourages certain cardiovascular problems, as venous stasis in the pelvis and the lower extremities, dehydration, and clot formation. Dehydration increases the risk of clot formation by increasing the viscosity of the blood. Some common therapeutic measures to deal with disuse phenomena are the improvement of diet and nutrition, proper positioning and regular movement of the bed rest patient, meticulous hygiene, scrupulous skin care, and positive social interaction with the patient.

Ditropan, a trade name for an antispasmodic (oxybutynin chloride).

Diucardin, a trade name for an antihypertensive and diuretic (hydroflumethiazide).

Diupres, a trade name for a fixed-combination drug containing a diuretic (chlorothiazide) and an antihypertensive (reserpine).

diuresis (dāi'yuri'sis), increased formation and secretion of urine. Diuresis is pronounced in conditions such as diabetes mellitus and diabetes insipidus. It is normal in the first 48 hours postpartum. Coffee, tea, certain foods, diuretic drugs, and some steroids cause diuresis.

diuretic, 1. (of a drug or other substance) tending to promote the formation and excretion of urine. **2.** a drug that promotes the formation and excretion of urine. The more than 50 diuretic drugs available for prescription in the United States and Canada are classified by chemical structure into several basic pharmacologic groups: anthralinics, ethacrynics, mercurials, steroids, sulfonamides, and thiazides. A diuretic medication may contain drugs from one or more of these groups. Diuretics are prescribed to reduce the volume of extracellular fluid in the treatment of many disorders, including hypertension, congestive heart failure, and edema. The particular drug to be prescribed is selected according to the action desired and the physical status of the patient. Hypersensitivity to sulfonamides prohibits use of this class of drug, and diabetes mellitus may be aggravated by thiazide medications; thus, the presence of a particular condition may prohibit the use of a particular agent. Several adverse reactions are common to all diuretics, including hypovolemia and electrolyte imbalance.
(See next page for table)

Diuril, a trade name for a diuretic (chlorothiazide).

divalent (dāiveil'ənt). See **bivalent.**

diversional activity, deficit, a nursing diagnosis accepted by the Fourth National Conference on the Classification of Nursing Diagnoses. The etiology of the situation includes a lack of diversion in the environment, long-term hospitalization, or frequent or prolonged treatment. The defining characteristics of the diagnosis include statements from the client that there is nothing to do or that everything is boring, but the usual diversions or hobbies pursued at home are not undertaken. See also **nursing diagnosis.**

diverticulitis (dāi'vərtık'yulāi'tıs), inflammation of one or more diverticula. The penetration of fecal matter through the thin-walled diverticula causes inflammation and abcess formation in the tissues surrounding the colon. With repeated inflammation, the lumen of the colon narrows and may become obstructed. During periods of inflammation, the patient will experience crampy pain, particularly over the sigmoid colon, fever, and leukocytosis. Barium enema and proctoscopy are performed to rule out carcinoma of the colon, which exhibits some of the same symptoms. Conservative treatment includes bed rest, intravenous fluids, antibiotics, and nothing by mouth. In acute cases, bowel resection of the affected part

Common diuretics and their effect on fluid and electrolyte balance

Generic name	Trade name	Method of administration	Peak effect	Probable effects on fluid and electrolyte balance
Thiazides				
Chlorothiazide	Diuril	Oral	4 hours	Hyponatremia Hypokalemia ↓ ECF volume Hyperglycemia Hyperuricemia
Hydrochlorothiazide	Esidrix HydroDIURIL	Oral	3 to 4 hours	Hypomagnesemia
Loop diuretics (act mainly on ascending loop of Henle)				
Furosemide	Lasix	IM or IV	½ hour	Hypokalemia Hyperuricemia
		Oral	2 to 4 hours	↓ ECF volume
Ethacrynic acid	Edecrin	Oral	2 to 4 hours	Hyponatremia
		IV	½ hour	
Aldosterone antagonist (opposes potassium-losing action of aldosterone)				
Spironolactone	Aldactone	Oral	72 hours	Hyperkalemia Hyponatremia
Potassium-conserving action				
Triamterene	Dyrenium	Oral	4 to 8 hours	Hyperkalemia
Osmotic agent				
Mannitol	Osmitrol	IV infused over 24-hour period	—	Hyponatremia Hypochloremia ↑ ECF volume

greatly reduces mortality and morbidity. Compare **diverticulosis.**

diverticulosis (dai'vərtɪk'yʊlou'sɪs), the presence of pouchlike herniations through the muscular layer of the colon, particularly the sigmoid colon. Diverticulosis affects increasing numbers of people over age 50 and may be the result of the modern, highly refined, low-residue diet. Most patients with this condition have few symptoms except for occasional bleeding from the rectum. The physician must exercise care in ruling out other reasons for bleeding, as carcinoma and inflammatory bowel disease. Barium enema and proctoscopic examination are used in establishing diagnosis. An increase in the dietary fiber can aid in propelling the feces through the colon. Hemorrhage from bleeding diverticula can become quite severe, and the patient may require surgery. Diverticulosis may lead to diverticulitis. See also **diverticulitis.**

diverticulum (dai'vərtɪk'yʊləm), pl. **diverticula.** a pouchlike herniation through the muscular wall of a tubular organ. A diverticulum may be present in the stomach, small intestine, or, most commonly, in the colon. See also **diverticulitis, diverticulosis, Meckel's diverticulum.** —**diverticular,** adj.

diving goiter, a large movable thyroid gland located at times above the sternal notch and at other times below the notch. Also called **plunging goiter, wandering goiter.**

division, 1. an administrative subunit in a hospital, as a division of medical nursing or a division of surgical nursing. 2. (in public health nursing) an area that encompasses several geographical districts.

Dix, Dorothea Lynde (1802–1887), an American humanitarian who achieved fame as a social reformer, primarily for her work in improving prison conditions and care of the mentally ill. During her lifetime, she helped to establish mental institutions in 30 states and in Canada. During the Civil War, she was appointed superintendent of army nurses for government hospitals.

dizygotic (dai'zaigot'ɪk), of or pertaining to twins from two fertilized ova. Compare **monozygotic.** See also **twinning.**

dizygotic twins (dai'zaigot'ɪk), two offspring born of the same pregnancy and developed from two ova that were released from the ovary simultaneously and fertilized at the same time. They may be of the same or opposite sex, differ both physically and in genetic constitution, and have two separate and distinct placentas and membranes, both amnion and chorion. The frequency of dizygotic twinning varies according to ethnic origin, the highest incidence being in the black race, the lowest in the Mongoloid, with the white races being intermediate; maternal age, the highest rate occurring when the mother is 35 to 39 years old; and heredity, showing an increase in the female genetic line rather than the male, although fathers may transmit the disposition toward double ovulation to their daughters. In general, the overall rate is two thirds dizygotic twinning to one third monozygotic. Also called **binovular twins, dissimilar twins, false twins, fraternal twins, heterologous twins.** Compare **monozygotic twins.**

dizziness, a sensation of faintness or an inability to maintain normal balance in a standing or seated position, sometimes associated with giddiness, mental confusion, nausea, and weakness. A patient who experiences dizziness should be carefully lowered to a safe position on a bed, chair, or floor because of the danger of injury from falling. Compare **syncope, vertigo.**

DLE, abbreviation for **discoid lupus erythematosus.**

DM, abbreviation for **diabetes mellitus.**

D.M.D., abbreviation for *Doctor of Dental Medicine.*

DMSO, abbreviation for **dimethyl sulfoxide.**

DNA, abbreviation for **deoxyribonucleic acid.**

DNA chimera, (in molecular genetics) a recombinant molecule of DNA composed of segments from more than one source.

DNA ligase, an enzyme that can repair breaks in a strand of DNA by synthesizing a bond between adjoining nucleotides. Under some circumstances the enzyme can join together loose ends of DNA strands, and, in some cases, it can repair breaks in RNA.

DNA nucleotidyltransferase. See **DNA polymerase.**

DNA polymerase, (in molecular genetics) an enzyme that catalyzes the assembly of deoxyribonucleoside triphosphates into DNA, with single-stranded DNA serving as the template. Also called **DNA nucleotidyltransferase.**

DNCB, abbreviation for *dinitrochlorobenzene.*

DNR, abbreviation for *do not resuscitate.* See **no-code.**

D.O., abbreviation for **Doctor of Osteopathy.**

Dobie's globule (dou′biz), a very small stainable body in the transparent disc of a muscle fiber.

dobutamine hydrochloride, a beta adrenergic stimulating agent.

■ INDICATIONS: It is prescribed to increase cardiac output in severe chronic congestive heart failure and as an adjunct in cardiac surgery.

■ CONTRAINDICATIONS: Idiopathic hypertrophic subaortic stenosis or known hypersensitivity to this drug prohibits its use. It is not recommended for use in pregnancy.

■ ADVERSE EFFECTS: Among the most serious adverse reactions are cardiovascular effects, including tachycardia, hypertension, arrythmias, and precipitation of angina. Nausea, vomiting, and headache also may occur.

Dobutrex, a trade name for a synthetic catecholamine (dobutamine hydrochloride), which stimulates beta-adrenergic receptors.

Dock, Lavinia Lloyd (1858–1956), an American public health nurse. Graduate of the Bellevue Hospital Training School for Nurses in New York, in 1886, she started a visiting nurse service in Norwalk, Connecticut, and then joined the New York City Mission before becoming an assistant to Isabel Hampton Robb at Johns Hopkins Hospital, in Baltimore. She returned to public health nursing when she joined the Henry Street Settlement in New York to work with Lillian Wald. She advocated an international public health movement and the improvement of education for nurses. With M. Adelaide Nutting, she wrote *History of Nursing,* a classic in nursing literature.

doctoral program in nursing, an educational program of study that offers preparation for a doctoral degree in the field of nursing designed to prepare nurses for advanced practice and research. Upon successful completion of the course of study the degree Ph.D. in nursing or D.S.N. (Doctor of Science in Nursing) is awarded. Higher standards of professional practice and the desire for scholarly achievement have caused nurses to work toward advanced educational degrees. Many nurses obtain a doctoral degree in fields ancillary to nursing, as the social or biological sciences, education, and the humanities. In Canada, there is no doctoral program in nursing.

Doctor of Medicine (M.D.). See **physician.**

Doctor of Osteopathy (D.O.). See **physician.**

docusate (dok′yuseit), a stool softener. Also called **dioctyl calcium sulfosuccinate, dioctyl sodium sulfosuccinate.**

■ INDICATION: It is prescribed in the treatment of constipation.

■ CONTRAINDICATIONS: Signs or symptoms of appendicitis; concomitant administration of mineral oil or known hypersensitivity to the drug prohibits its use.

■ ADVERSE EFFECTS: No serious adverse reactions are known.

Doehle bodies, inclusions in the cytoplasm of some leukocytes in May-Hegglin anomaly.

Döhle-Heller disease. See **syphilitic aortitis.**

Dolene, a trade name for an analgesic (propoxyphene hydrochloride).

dolicho-, a combining form meaning 'long': *dolichocephaly, dolichocolon, dolichomorphic.*

dolichocephaly (dol′əkousef′əli). See **scaphocephaly.**

doll's eye reflex, a normal response in newborns to keep the eyes stationary as the head is moved to the right or left. The reflex disappears as ocular fixation develops.

Dolophine Hydrochloride, a trade name for a narcotic analgesic (methadone hydrochloride).

DOM, abbreviation for **dimethoxymethylamphetamine.**

dome fracture, any fracture of the acetabulum, specifically involving a weight-bearing surface.

dominance, (in genetics) a basic principle stating that not all genes determining a given trait operate with equal vigor. If two genes at a given locus produce a different effect, as eye color, they compete for expression. The gene that is manifest is dominant; it masks the effect of the other gene, which is recessive. Compare **codominance.** See also **independent assortment.** —**dominant,** *adj.*

dominant gene, one that produces a phenotypic effect regardless of whether its allele is the same or different. Compare **recessive gene.**

Donath-Landsteiner syndrome, a rare blood disorder, marked by hemolysis minutes or hours after exposure to cold. Systemic symptoms include the passage of dark urine, severe pain in the back and legs, headache, vomiting, diarrhea, and moderate reticulocytosis. There may be temporary hepatosplenomegaly and mild hyperbilirubinemia following the onset of an attack. The condition may occur with congenital or acquired syphilis, in which case antisyphilitic treatment may be curative. Also called **paroxysmal cold hemoglobinuria.**

Don Juan, a seductive man who is sexually promiscuous.

Donnatal, a trade name for a gastrointestinal fixed-combination drug containing a sedative (phenobarbital) and three anticholinergics (hyoscyamine sulfate, atropine sulfate, and hyoscine hydrobromide), used to decrease the motility of the gastrointestinal tract.

donor, **1.** a human or other organism that gives living tissue to be used in another body, for example, blood for transfusion or a kidney for transplantation. **2.** a substance or compound that gives part of itself to another substance. Compare **acceptor.** See also **universal donor.**

Donovan bodies (don′əvən), encapsulated gram-negative rods of the species *Calymmato bacterium granulomatis,* present in the cytoplasm of mononuclear phagocytes obtained from the lesions of granuloma inguinale. They may be seen under the microscope in a Wright-stained smear of infected tissue. See also **granuloma inguinale.**

dopamine hydrochloride, a sympathomimetic catecholamine.

■ INDICATIONS: It is prescribed in the treatment of shock, hypotension, and low cardiac output.

■ CONTRAINDICATIONS: Pheochromocytoma, tachyarrhythmias, ventricular fibrillation, or known hypersensitivity to this drug prohibits its use.

■ ADVERSE EFFECTS: Among the more serious adverse reactions are arrhythmias, hypotension, hypertension, and tachycardia.

dopaminergic (dou′pəmɪnər′jɪk), having the effect of dopamine.

Dopar, a trade name for an antiparkinsonian (levodopa).

dope, *Slang.* morphine, heroin, or another narcotic, or marijuana or other substance illicitly bought, or sold, and often self-administered for sedative, hypnotic, euphoric, or other mood-altering purpose.

Doppler effect (dop′lər), the apparent change in frequency of sound or light waves emitted by a source as it moves away from or toward an observer. The frequency increases as the source moves toward the observer and decreases as it moves away, as the rising pitch of the whistle of an approaching train and the falling pitch of a departing train. The Doppler effect is also observed in electromagnetic radiations, as light and radio waves. See also **electromagnetic radiation, ultrasonography, wavelength.**

Dopram, a trade name for a respiratory stimulant (doxapram hydrochloride).

Dorantamin, a trade name for an antihistamine (pyrilamine maleate).

Dorbane, a trade name for a laxative (danthron).

Dorbantyl, a trade name for a fixed-combination drug containing a stool softener (dioctyl sodium sulfosuccinate) and a laxative (danthron).

Doriden, a trade name for a sedative (glutethimide).

Dornavac, a trade name for an enzyme (pancreatic dornase).

dorsal (dɔr′səl), pertaining to the back or posterior. Compare **ventral.** See also **dorsiflect.** — **dorsum,** *n.*

-dorsal, a combining form meaning 'the back of something' or 'the back': *predorsal, thoracodorsal, ventrodorsal.*

dorsal carpal ligament. See **retinaculum extensorum manus.**

dorsal digital vein, one of the communicating veins along the sides of the fingers. The veins from the adjacent sides of the fingers unite to form three dorsal metacarpal veins which end in a dorsal venous network on the back of the hand. Compare **basilic vein, cephalic vein, median antebrachial vein.**

dorsal interventricular artery, the arterial branch of the right coronary artery, branching to supply both ventricles. It runs down the dorsal sulcus two thirds of the way to the apex of the heart. Also called **right interventricular artery.**

dorsalis pedis artery, the continuation of the anterior tibial artery, starting at the ankle joint, dividing into five branches, and supplying various muscles of the foot and toes. Its branches are the lateral tarsal, medial tarsal, arcuate, first dorsal metatarsal, and deep plantar.

dorsalis pedis pulse, the pulse of the dorsalis pedis artery, palpable between the first and second metatarsal bones on the top of the foot. It can be felt in approximately 90 per cent of people.

dorsal lip, the marginal fold of the blastopore during gastrulation in the early stages of embryonic development of many animals. It marks the dorsal limit of the developing embryo, constitutes the primary organizer, gives rise to neural tissue, and corresponds to the primitive node in man and higher animals.

dorsal scapular nerve, one of a pair of supraclavicular branches from the roots of the brachial plexus. It arises from the fifth cervical nerve near the intervertebral foramen, pierces the scalenus medius, and runs dorsally and caudally to the vertebral border of the scapula. It supplies the rhomboideus major and the rhomboideus minor and sends a branch to the levator.

dorsi-. See **dorso-.**

dorsiflect (dɔr'sɪflekt), bending or flexing, as in the upward bending of the hand on the wrist or the foot on the ankle.

dorsiflexion (dɔr'sɪflek'shən), flexion toward the back, as accomplished by a muscle. See also **dorsiflexor.**

dorsiflexor (dɔr'sɪflek'sər), a muscle causing backward flexion of a part of the body, as the hand or foot.

dorsiflexor gait, an abnormal gait caused by the weakness of the dorsiflexors of the ankle. It is characterized by footdrop during the entire gait cycle and excessive knee and hip flexion to allow clearance of the involved extremity during the swing phase. The sole of the affected foot also slaps forcibly against the ground at the moment of heelstrike due to the inability of the dorsiflexor to decelerate the body weight as the heel strikes the ground. Compare **Trendelenburg gait.**

dorso-, dorsi-, a combining form meaning 'pertaining to a dorsum or to the back': *dorsocephalad, dorsomesial, dorsoscapular.*

dorsosacral position. See **lithotomy position.**

dosage, the regimen governing the size, frequency, and number of doses of a therapeutic agent to be administered to a patient.

dosage compensation, (in genetics) the mechanism that counterbalances the number of X-linked gene doses in the sex chromosomes so that they are equal in both the male, which has one X chromosome, and the female, which has two. In mammals this is accomplished by genetic activation of only one of the X chromosomes in the somatic cells of females. See also **Lyon hypothesis.**

dose, the amount of a drug or other substance to be administered at one time.

dose fractionation. See **fractionation,** def. 5.

dose rate, (in radiotherapy) the amount of delivered radiation absorbed per unit of time.

dose ratemeter, (in radiotherapy) an instrument for measuring the dose rate of radiation.

dose threshold, (in radiotherapy) the minimum amount of absorbed radiation that produces a detectable degree of a given effect.

dose to skin, (in radiotherapy) the amount of absorbed radiation at the center of the irradiation field on the skin. It is the sum of the dose in the air and the scatter from body parts.

dosimeter (dousɪm'ətər), an instrument to detect and measure accumulated radiation exposure. A pencil-sized ionization chamber with a self-reading electrometer is used to monitor exposure to personnel.

double-approach conflict. See **approach-approach conflict.**

double-avoidant conflict. See **avoidance-avoidance conflict.**

double-blind study, an experiment designed to test the effect of a treatment or substance using groups of experimental and control subjects in which neither the subjects nor the investigators know which treatment or substance is being administered to which group. In a double-blind test of a new drug, the substance may be identified to the investigators only by a code. The purpose of a double-blind study is to eliminate the risk of prejudgment by the participants, which could distort the results. A double-blind study may be augmented by a **cross-over experiment** in which experimental subjects unknowingly become control subjects, and vice versa, at some point in the study. See also **control, placebo.**

double blind technique, an experimental method of studying a drug or other medical treatment in which neither the investigators nor the subjects know which subjects are receiving the experimental drug or procedure and which are serving as controls. Typically, the control group receives a placebo which is indistinguishable from the substance or procedure being tested. The double blind technique is designed to eliminate bias in the interpretation of results.

double fracture, a fracture comprised of breaks or cracks in two places in a bone, resulting in more than two bone segments.

double gel diffusion. See **immunodiffusion.**

double innervation, innervation of effector organs by fibers of the sympathetic and parasympathetic divisions of the autonomic nervous system. The pelvic viscera, bronchioles, heart, eyes, and digestive system are all doubly innervated. The fibers of the two divisions operate at cross purposes to achieve a state of balance and to maintain the homeostatic condition of the body. The mode of action of each division varies: in some structures one division is stimulating and the other inhibiting; in others, separate fibers from each division act to stimulate and inhibit complementary function.

double monster, a fetus that has developed from a single ovum but has two heads, trunks, and multiple limbs. Also called **twin monster.**

double quartan fever, a form of malaria in which paroxysms of fever occur in a repeating pattern of two consecutive days followed by one day of remission. The pattern is usually the result of concurrent infections by two species of the genus *Plasmodium,* one causing paroxysms every 72 hours and the other every 48 hours. Compare **biduotertian fever.**

double setup, a nursing procedure in which an obstetric operating room is prepared for both vaginal delivery and Caesarean section. The circulating and scrub nurses lay out the equipment required for both procedures, possibly including a vacuum aspirator, forceps, and Caesarean section packs. The scrub nurse remains scrubbed until the infant is delivered but does not participate unless a Caesarean section is performed.

double vision. See **diplopia.**

douche (dū́sh), **1.** a procedure in which a liter or more of a solution of a medication or cleansing agent in warm water is introduced into the vagina under low pressure. The woman often performs the procedure herself. Semisitting in a bathtub she introduces the douche tip into the vagina and releases a clamp on the tubing connected to the douche bag, which is suspended two feet above the introitus. She allows the solution to flow in, while holding the lips of the vagina closed to retain the fluid. As the accumulation of fluid distends the vagina she clamps the tubing and, after a few minutes, allows the fluid to flow out. The process is repeated until the entire quantity of solution in the douche bag has been used. Douching may be recommended in the treatment of various pelvic and vaginal infections. **2.** to perform a douche.

doughnut pessary. See **pessary.**

Down's syndrome, a congenital condition characterized by varying degrees of mental retardation and multiple defects. It is the most common chromosomal abnormality of a generalized syndrome and is caused by the presence of an extra chromosome 21 in the G group, or in a small percentage of cases, by the translocation of chromosomes 14 or 15 in the D group and chromosomes 21 or 22. Also called **mongolism, mongoloid idiocy, trisomy G syndrome, trisomy 21.**

■ OBSERVATIONS: Down's syndrome occurs in approximately 1 in 600 to 650 live births and is associated with advanced maternal age, particularly over 35 years of age. The incidence is as high as 1 in 80 for offspring of women older than 40 years. In those cases caused by translocation, which is a genetic aberration that is hereditary rather than a chromosomal aberration caused by nondisjunction during cell division, the incidence is not associated with maternal age, and the risk is low, about 1 in 5 if the mother is the carrier and 1 in 20 if the father is the carrier. The condition, which can be diagnosed prenatally by amniocentesis, also occurs as a mosaic variant, in which there is a mixture of trisomy 21 and normal cells. Such patients have fewer physical defects and less severe retardation depending on the degree of mosaicism. Infants with the syndrome are small, hypotonic, with characteristic microcephaly, brachycephaly, a flattened occiput, and typical facies with a mongoloid slant to the eyes, depressed nasal bridge, low-set ears, and a large, protruding tongue that is furrowed and lacks the central fissure. The hands are short and broad with a transverse palmar or simian crease; the fingers are stubby and show clinodactyly, primarily of the fifth fingers; and the feet are broad and stubby with a wide space between the first and second toes and a prominent plantar crease. Other anom-

alies associated with the disorder are bowel defects, congenital heart disease, primarily septal defects, chronic respiratory infections, visual problems, abnormalities in tooth development, and susceptibility to acute leukemia. The most significant feature of the syndrome is mental retardation, which varies considerably, although the average IQ is in the range of 50 to 60 so that the child is generally trainable and in most instances can be reared at home. Those more severely affected are often institutionalized. The mortality rate is high within the first few years, especially in those children with cardiac anomalies. Those who survive tend to be shorter than average, stocky in build, show delayed or incomplete sexual development, and can live to middle or old age, although adults with Down's syndrome are prone to respiratory infections, pneumonia, and lung disease.

■ INTERVENTION: Care for the child with Down's syndrome involves several short- and long-term goals, depending on the severity of physical defects and the degree of mental impairment. Of immediate importance is the prevention of physical problems associated with the disorder, as respiratory infections, adequate nutrition and feeding difficulties because of the large protruding tongue, skin breakdown caused by the characteristic dry, cracked dermal condition, and positioning difficulties owing to the hypotonicity of muscles and hyperextensibility of the joints. Long-term intervention centers around carefully planned programs to promote optimal development, both in motor and mental skills. Since the developmental potential of a child with Down's syndrome is greatest during infancy, a stimulation program of exercise based on the child's ability and potential is mandatory for teaching gross motor skills.

■ NURSING CONSIDERATIONS: The primary role of the nurse is to offer support to the parents, to teach them how to provide adequate care, and to plan both short- and long-term programs that will realize the full physical and mental potential of the child. The nurse helps the parents to learn the child's limitations and to function within that range, periodically assesses the child's developmental progress, and advises parents on the various community programs and vocational classes that are available. Of utmost importance is that all family members understand that the child has the same basic needs as other children, as play, discipline, and social interaction. The nurse also functions in the genetic counseling of high-risk women and encourages those at risk to consider amniocentesis.

doxapram hydrochloride, a respiratory stimulant.

■ INDICATIONS: It is prescribed to improve respiratory function after anesthesia, in drug-induced central nervous system depression, and for chronic pulmonary disease associated with acute hypercapnia.

■ CONTRAINDICATIONS: Seizure disorder, pulmonary dis-

ease, coronary artery disease, hypertension, or known hypersensitivity to this drug prohibits its use.
■ ADVERSE EFFECTS: Among the more serious adverse reactions are convulsions, bronchospasm, and phlebitis.

doxepin hydrochloride (dok′səpın), a tricyclic antidepressant.
■ INDICATION: It is prescribed in the treatment of depression.
■ CONTRAINDICATIONS: Concomitant administration of monoamine oxidase inhibitors, recent myocardial infarction, seizure disorders, or known hypersensitivity to tricyclic medication prohibits its use.
■ ADVERSE EFFECTS: Among the more serious adverse reactions are gastrointestinal, cardiovascular, and neurologic disturbances. Sedation, dry mouth, and many drug interactions may occur.

doxorubicin hydrochloride, an anthracycline antibiotic.
■ INDICATIONS: It is prescribed in the treatment of a variety of malignant neoplastic diseases.
■ CONTRAINDICATIONS: Myelosuppression, heart disease, concurrent administration of daunorubicin, or known hypersensitivity to this drug prohibits its use.
■ ADVERSE EFFECTS: Among the more serious adverse reactions are myelosuppression and cardiomyopathy. Stomatitis, gastrointestinal disturbances, and alopecia commonly occur.

doxycycline, a tetracycline antibacterial.
■ INDICATIONS: It is prescribed in the treatment of a variety of infections.
■ CONTRAINDICATIONS: Renal or liver dysfunction or known hypersensitivity to this drug or to other tetracycline medication prohibits its use. It is not given during pregnancy or to children under eight years of age.
■ ADVERSE EFFECTS: Among the more serious adverse reactions are gastrointestinal disturbances, phototoxicity, potentially serious suprainfections, and hypersensitivity reactions. Discoloration of teeth may occur in children exposed to the drug in utero or under eight years of age.

doxylamine succinate (dok′sılæm′in), an antihistamine.
■ INDICATION: It is prescribed for the treatment of acute allergic symptoms produced by the release of histamine.
■ CONTRAINDICATIONS: Known hypersensitivity to this drug prohibits its use. It is not recommended for use during pregnancy or lactation and is not given to children under six years of age.
■ ADVERSE EFFECTS: Among the more serious reactions are sedation, ataxia, tachycardia, hemolytic anemia, and thrombocytopenia.

DPT vaccine, abbreviation for **diphtheria, tetanus toxoids and pertussis vaccine.**

DQ, abbreviation for **developmental quotient.**

dracontiasis (dræk′əntaı′əsıs). See **dracunculiasis.**

dracunculiasis (drækəŋ′kyulaı′əsıs), a parasitic infection caused by infestation by the nematode *Dracunculus mediniensis.* It is characterized by ulcerative skin lesions on the legs and feet that are produced by gravid female worms. People are infected by drinking contaminated water or eating contaminated shellfish. It is common in densely populated tropical and subtropical areas of the world. Also called **dracontiasis, guinea worm infection.**

Dracunculus medinensis (drəkəŋ′kyuləs mədi′nien′sıs), a parasitic nematode that causes dracunculiasis. Also called **fiery serpent.**

drainage, the removal of fluids from a body cavity, wound, or other source of discharge by one or more methods. **Closed drainage** is a system of tubing and other apparatus attached to the body to remove fluid in an airtight circuit that prevents environmental contaminants from entering the wound or cavity. **Open drainage** is drainage in which discharge is drained through an open-ended tube into a receptacle. **Postural drainage** is drainage in which gravity aids in the removal of fluid from the body by the positioning of the patient so discharge flows out, as through the trachea if the fluid source is in the lungs. **Suction drainage** is drainage in which a pump or other mechanical device is used to assist in extracting a fluid. **Tidal drainage** is drainage in which a body area is washed out by alternately flooding and then emptying it with the aid of gravity, a technique that may be used in treating a urinary bladder disorder.

drainage tube, a heavy-gauge catheter used for the evacuation of air or a fluid from a cavity or wound in the body. The tube may be attached to a suction device or simply allow flow by gravity into a receptacle.

dram (dræm), a unit of mass equivalent to an apothecaries' measure of 60 grains or $\frac{1}{8}$ ounce and to $\frac{1}{16}$ ounce or 27.34 grains avoirdupois.

Dramamine, a trade name for an antihistamine (dimenhydrinate), used as an antiemetic.

dramatic play, an imitative activity in which a child fantasizes and acts out various domestic and social roles and situations, as rocking a doll, pretending to be a doctor or nurse, or teaching school. It is the predominant form of play among preschool children.

drape, a sheet of fabric or paper, usually the size of a small bed sheet, for covering all or a part of a person's body during a physical examination or treatment. – **drape,** *v.*

drawing, *Informal.* a vague sensation of muscle tension.

dream, 1. a symbolically coherent sequence of ideas, thoughts, emotions, or images that pass through the mind during the rapid eye movement stage of sleep. 2. describing the sleeping state in which this process occurs. 3. a visionary creation of the imagination experienced during wakefulness. 4. (in psychoanalysis) the expression of thoughts, emotions, memories, or impulses repressed from the consciousness. **5.** (in analytic psychology) the wishes, emotions, and impulses that reflect the personal unconscious and the archetypes that originate in the collective unconscious. See also **dream analysis, dream state.**

dream analysis, a process of gaining access to the unconscious mind by means of examining the content of dreams, usually through the method of free association.

dream association, a relationship of thoughts or emotions discovered or experienced as a dream is remembered or analyzed. See also **dream analysis.**

dream state, a condition of altered consciousness in which a person does not recognize his environment and reacts in a manner opposed to his usual behavior, as by flight or an act of violence. The state is seen in epilepsy and certain neuroses. See also **automatism, fugue.**

drepanocytic anemia. See **sickle cell anemia.**

dress code, the standards set by an institution for the dress of the members of the institution.

dressing, a clean or sterile covering applied directly to wounded or diseased tissue for absorption of secretions, protection from trauma, administration of medications, or to stop bleeding. Kinds of dressings include **absorbent dressing, antiseptic dressing, occlusive dressing, pressure dressing, wet dressing.**

dressing forceps, a kind of forceps that has a narrow blade and blunt or notched teeth, designed for dressing wounds, removing drainage tubes, or extracting fragments of necrotic tissue.

Dressler's syndrome (dres'lərz), an autoimmune disorder that may occur several days after acute coronary infarction, characterized by fever, pericarditis, pleurisy, pleural effusions, and joint pain. It results from the body's immunologic response to a damaged myocardium and pericardium. Treatment usually includes intensive aspirin therapy and, in severe cases, corticosteroids. A similar syndrome may occur following cardiac surgery.

DRG, abbreviation for **diagnostic related group.**

drift, 1. antigenic drift, a change that occurs in a strain of virus so that variations appear periodically with alterations in antigenic qualities. **2. genetic drift,** random variations in gene frequency of a population from one generation to the next. **3.** (in dentistry) the movement of a tooth from one position in the jaw to another after the loss of a neighboring tooth.

Drinker respirator (drɪŋ'kər), an airtight respirator consisting of a metal tank that encloses the entire body, except for the head. Used for long-term therapy, it alternates positive and negative air pressure within the tank, providing artificial respiration by contracting and expanding the walls of the chest. Also called **artificial lung, iron lung.**

drip, 1. the process of a liquid or moisture forming and falling in drops. Kinds of drip are **nasal drip, postnasal drip. 2.** the slow but continuous infusion of a liquid into the body, as into the stomach or a vein. **3.** to infuse a liquid continuously into the body.

drip system, (in intravenous therapy) an apparatus for delivering specific volumes of intravenous solutions within predetermined periods of time and at a specific flow rate. See also **macrodrip, microdrip.**

Drisdol, a trade name for vitamin D_2 (ergocalciferol).

Drixoral, a trade name for a fixed-combination drug containing an antihistamine (dexbrompheniramine maleate) and a vasoconstrictor and bronchodilator (pseudoephedrine sulfate), used for the relief of congestion of the upper respiratory tract.

Drolban, a trade name for synthetic androgen (dromostanolone propionate), used in cancer therapy.

-drome, a combining form meaning 'that which runs' in a specified way: *dermadrome, heterodrome, syndrome.*

dromo-, a combining form meaning 'pertaining to running or conduction': *dromomania, dromophobic, dromotropic.*

dromostanolone propionate, an androgen.
- INDICATION: It is prescribed for female breast cancer.
- CONTRAINDICATIONS: It is not used for male breast cancer or in premenopausal women.
- ADVERSE EFFECTS: Among the more serious adverse reactions are masculinization, edema, and hypercalcemia.

droperidol (drəper'ədol), an antipsychotic, sedative drug of the butyrophenone group, used most commonly with a narcotic analgesic (fentanyl) in neuroleptanesthesia.

drop foot, a condition in which the foot is plantar flexed and cannot voluntarily be dorsiflexed. It is usually caused by damage to the peroneal nerve.

droplet infection, an infection acquired by the inhalation of pathogenic microorganisms suspended in particles of liquid exhaled, sneezed, or coughed by another infected person or animal. Some diseases spread by droplets are chickenpox, common cold, influenza, measles, and mumps.

dropped foot. See **footdrop.**

dropsy. *Obsolete.* See **hydrops.**

Drosophila (drousof'ilə), a genus of fly, including *Drosophila melanogaster,* the Mediterranean fruit fly, useful in genetics because of the large chromosomes found in its salivary glands and its sensitivity to environmental effects, as exposure to radiation.

drowning, asphyxiation owing to submersion in a liquid. See also **near-drowning.**

drug, 1. Also called **medicine.** Any substance taken by mouth, injected into a muscle, the skin, a blood vessel, or a cavity of the body, or applied topically to treat or prevent a disease or condition. **2.** *Informal.* a narcotic substance.

drug abuse, the use of a drug for a nontherapeutic effect, especially one for which it was not prescribed or intended. Some of the most commonly abused substances are alcohol, amphetamines, barbiturates, and methaqualone. Drug abuse may lead to organ damage, addiction, and disturbed patterns of behavior. Some illicit drugs, as lysergic acid diethylamide, and phencylidine hydrochloride, have no recognized therapeutic effect. Use of these drugs often incurs criminal penalty in addition to the potential for physical, social, and psychological harm. See also **drug addiction.**

drug action, the means by which a drug exerts a desired effect. Drugs are usually classified by their actions, as a vasodilator, prescribed to decrease the blood pressure, acts by dilating the blood vessels.

drug addiction, a condition characterized by an overwhelming desire to continue taking a drug to which one has become habituated through repeated consumption because it produces a particular effect, usually an alteration of mental activity, attitude, or outlook. Addiction is usually accompanied by a compulsion to obtain the drug, a tendency to increase the dose, a psychological or physical dependence, and detrimental consequences for the individual and society. Common addictive drugs are barbiturates, ethanol, and morphine and other narcotics, especially heroin, which has slightly greater euphorigenic properties than other opium derivatives. See also **alcoholism, drug abuse.**

drug allergy, hypersensitivity to a pharmacologic agent, manifested by reactions ranging from a mild rash to anaphylactic shock, depending on the individual, the allergen, and the dose. Allergic responses are frequently produced by contrast media containing iodine, aspirin, phenylbutazone, novobiocin, penicillin, and other antibiotics, but they may be caused by any drug.

drug dependence, a psychological craving for or a physiological reliance on a chemical agent, resulting from habituation, abuse, or addiction. See also **drug abuse, drug addiction.**

drug-drug interaction, a modification of the effect of a drug when administered with another drug. The effect may be an increase or a decrease in the action of either substance, or it may be an adverse effect that is not normally associated with either drug. The particular interaction may be the result of a chemical-physical incompatibility of the two drugs or a change in the rate of absorption or the quantity absorbed in the body, the binding ability of either drug, or an alteration in the ability of receptor sites and cell membranes to bind either drug.

Drug Enforcement Agency (D.E.A.), an agency of the Drug Enforcement Administration of the federal government, empowered to enforce regulations regarding the import or export of narcotic drugs and certain other substances or the traffic of these substances across state lines.

drug eruption, any skin lesion or rash caused by a drug taken internally. Also called **dermatitis medicamentosa.** See also **fixed drug eruption.**

drug fever, a fever caused by the pharmacologic action of a medication, its thermoregulatory action, a local complication of parenteral administration, or, most commonly, an immunologic reaction mediated by drug-induced antibodies. The onset of fever is usually between seven and ten days after the medication is begun; a return to normal is seen within two days of the discontinuance of the drug. The correct diagnosis of drug fever and the discontinuance of the medication are important to prevent further adverse reactions and to avoid possibly dangerous and expensive diagnostic and therapeutic interventions. See also **Jarisch-Herxheimer reaction.**

drug monograph, a statement that specifies the kinds and amounts of ingredients a drug or class of drugs may contain, the direction for the drug's use, the conditions in which it may be used, and contraindications.

dry catarrh, a dry cough, accompanied by almost no expectoration that occurs in severe coughing spells. It is associated with asthma and emphysema in older people.

dry dressing, a plain dressing containing no medication, applied directly to an incision or a wound to prevent contamination or trauma or to absorb secretions.

dry gangrene. See **gangrene.**

dry rale, an abnormal chest sound produced by air passing through a constricted bronchial tube. Compare **amphoric breath sound, atelectatic rale, bubbling rale.**

Drysdale's corpuscle (draiz′deilz), one of a number of transparent cells in the fluid of some ovarian cysts. Also called **Bennet's small corpuscle.**

dry skin, epidermis lacking moisture or sebum, often characterized by a pattern of fine lines, scaling, and itching. Causes include too frequent bathing, low humidity, decreased production of sebum in aging skin, and ichthyosis. Treatment includes decreased frequency of bathing, increased humidity, bath oils, emollients such as lanolin and glycerine, and hydrophilic ointments. Also called **xerosis.**

dry tooth socket, an inflamed condition of a tooth socket (alveolus) after extraction. Normally, a blood clot forms over the alveolar bone at the base of the tooth socket after an extraction. If the clot fails to form properly or becomes dislodged, the bone tissue is exposed to the environment and can become infected, a usually painful condition requiring analgesics and sedatives in addition to treatment to cure the infection. Also called **alveolitis.**

Dryvax, a trade name for an active immunizing agent (smallpox vaccine).

DSM, abbreviation for *Diagnostic and Statistical Manual of Mental Disorders.*

D.S.N., abbreviaition for *Doctor of Science in Nursing.*

DSR, abbreviation for **dynamic spatial reconstructor.**

DT. See **diphtheria and tetanus toxoids.**

dTc, abbreviation for *d-tubocurarine.*

DTIC-Dome, a trade name for an antineoplastic (dacarbazine).

DTR, abbreviation for **deep tendon reflex.**

DTs, abbreviation for **delirium tremens.**

DUB, **1.** See **dysfunctional uterine bleeding. 2.** a genetically determined human blood factor that is associated with immunity to certain diseases, as sickle cell anemia. The blood factors usually are numbered, as DUB-15 or DUB-40, depending upon their reactions with an antiserum. **3.** a strain of mice used in medical experiments.

Dubin-Johnson syndrome (du'bɪnjon'sən), a rare, chronic, hereditary hyperbilirubinemia, characterized by nonhemolytic jaundice, abnormal liver pigmentation, and abnormal function of the gall bladder. It is caused by an inability of the liver to excrete several organic anions.

Duchenne-Erb paralysis (dvshen'ərb'). See **Erb's palsy.**

Duchenne's disease (dushenz'), an eponym, after the French neurologist, for three different neurological conditions: **spinal muscular atrophy, bulbar paralysis,** and **tabes dorsalis.** The eponym is also strongly associated with the most common form of muscular dystrophy, **pseudohypertrophic (Duchenne's) muscular dystrophy.** See also **muscular dystrophy.**

Duchenne's muscular dystrophy, an abnormal congenital condition characterized by progressive symmetric wasting of the leg and pelvic muscles. This disease affects only males and accounts for 50 per cent of all muscular dystrophy diseases. It is an X-linked recessive disease that starts insidiously between the ages of 3 and 5 years and spreads from the leg and pelvic muscles to the involuntary muscles. Associated muscle weakness produces a waddling gait and pronounced lordosis. Muscles rapidly deteriorate and calf muscles become firm and enlarged. Affected children develop contractures, have difficulty climbing stairs, often stumble and fall, and display wing scapulae when they raise their arms. Such patients are usually confined to wheelchairs by the age of 12, and progressive weakening of cardiac muscle causes tachycardia and pulmonary problems. There is no correlation between the degree of muscular dystrophy and the severity of cardiac problems, but the electrocardiogram is abnormal in 40 to 90 per cent of the affected patients. The characteristic clinical finding is tachycardia persisting during sleep and often associated with arrhythmia and with cardiac enlargement. Certain distinctive electrocardiographic abnormalities, as tall R waves in the right precordial leads and deep Q waves in the limb leads may be present in affected family members and also in asymptomatic maternal carriers. The patients affected may also have cardiac murmurs, faint heart sounds, and chest pain, and suffer arrhythmias or infections that produce overt heart failure. Such complications, especially in the later stages of this disease, can cause sudden death.

Duchenne's muscular dystrophy usually results in death within 10 to 15 years of the onset of symptoms.

■ OBSERVATIONS: Abnormal cardiac signs may precede recognition of Duchenne's muscular dystrophy and may aid diagnosis based on other abnormalities of gait and voluntary movement. Typical medical and family history may also suggest the disease. Confirming diagnosis is usually aided by a muscle biopsy showing fat and connective tissue deposits. Electromyography is often used to help rule out neurogenic muscle atrophy by demonstrating viable muscle innervation. Laboratory results that indicate the disease include increased urinary creatinine excretion and increased serum levels of creatinine phosphokinase (CPK), lactic dehydrogenase (LDH), and transaminase. The CPK level often rises before muscular weakness becomes severe.

■ INTERVENTION: There is no successful treatment of the disease. Orthopedic appliances, exercise, physical therapy, and surgery to correct contractures can help preserve mobility. Involved doctors and nurses often caution family members who are carriers about the risk of transmitting this disease. No form of muscular dystrophy can be detected by amniocentesis, but this procedure can determine the sex of the fetus and is often recommended for carriers who are pregnant.

■ NURSING CONSIDERATIONS: Nursing care involves the psychologic support of the patient and the family and the encouragement of the patient to avoid long periods of bed rest and inactivity in order to to assure maximum physical activity. Splints, braces, grab bars, and overhead slings help the patient to exercise. A wheelchair helps to preserve mobility. Other devices that can increase comfort and help prevent footdrop include footboards, high-topped sneakers, and foot cradles. Nurses encourage the patient to maintain peer relationships and often encourage the parents to keep the child in school as long as possible. Nurses provide emotional support for the parents and the patient in coping with continuing changes in the patient's body and commonly refer parents to the Muscular Dystrophy Association for futher support and assistance.

duck embryo vaccine (DEV). See **rabies vaccine.**

duct, a narrow tubular structure, especially one through which material is secreted or excreted.

duct carcinoma, a neoplasm developed from the epithelium of ducts, especially in the breast or pancreas.

ductless gland, a gland lacking an excretory duct, as an endocrine gland, which secretes hormones into blood or lymph.

duct of Rivinus (rɪvi'nəs), one of the minor sublingual ducts. Compare **Bartholin's duct.**

duct of Wirsung (vir'suɳ). See **pancreatic duct.**

ductus (dək'təs), *pl.* **ductus.** a duct.

ductus arteriosus, a vascular channel in the fetus that joins the pulmonary artery directly to the descending aorta.

ductus deferens. See **deferent duct.**

ductus epididymidis, a tube into which the efferent ductules of the testes empty.

ductus venosus (venou′sıs), the vascular channel in the fetus passing through the liver and joining the umbilical vein with the inferior vena cava. Before birth, it carries highly oxygenated blood from the placenta to the fetal circulation. It closes shortly after birth as pulmonary circulation is established and as the vessels in the umbilical cord collapse and become occluded. See also **ductus arteriosus, foramen ovale.**

Duke diet. See **rice diet.**

Dulcolax, a trade name for a laxative (bisacodyl).

dumdum fever (dəm′dəm). See **kala-azar.**

dumping syndrome, the combination of profuse sweating, nausea, dizziness, and weakness experienced by patients who have had a subtotal gastrectomy. Symptoms are felt soon after eating, when the contents of the stomach empty too rapidly into the duodenum. A high-protein, high-calorie diet, with small meals taken frequently, should prevent discomfort and ensure adequate nutrition. See also **gastrectomy.**

Dunlop skeletal traction, an orthopedic mechanism that helps immobilize the upper limb in the treatment of the contracture or the supracondylar fracture of the elbow. The mechanism employs a system of traction weights, pulleys, and ropes. The system is attached to the bone involved with a pin or wire; it may be further secured by adhesive or nonadhesive skin traction components. Dunlop skeletal traction is usually applied unilaterally but may also be applied bilaterally. Compare **Dunlop skin traction.**

Dunlop skin traction, an orthopedic mechanism that helps immobilize the upper limb in the treatment of contracture and supracondylar fracture of the elbow. The mechanism employs a system of traction weights, pulleys, and ropes, usually applied unilaterally but sometimes bilaterally. Dunlop skin traction may be applied as adhesive skin traction or nonadhesive skin traction. Compare **Dunlop skeletal traction.**

duodenal (du′ədi′nəl), of or pertaining to the duodenum.

duodenal papilla. See under **papilla.**

duodenal ulcer, an ulcer in the duodenum, the most common type of peptic ulcer. See also **peptic ulcer.**

duodeno-, a combining form meaning 'pertaining to the duodenum': *duodenocolic, duodenohepatic, duodenostomy.*

duodenoscope (du′ədi′nəskoup), an endoscopic instrument, usually fiberoptic, for the visual examination of the duodenum.

duodenoscopy (du′ədənos′kəpi), the visual examination of the duodenum by means of an endoscope, usually a fiberoptic instrument.

duodenum (du′ədi′nəm, duod′ınəm), *pl.* **duodena, duodenums.** the shortest, widest, and most fixed portion of the small intestine, taking an almost circular course from the pyloric valve of the stomach so that its termination is close to its starting point. It is about 25 cm long and is divided into superior, descending, horizontal, and ascending portions. The superior portion is about 5 cm long and extends from the pylorus to the neck of the gall bladder. The descending portion is about 8 cm long and extends from the neck of the gall bladder at the level of the first lumbar vertebra to the cranial border of the fourth lumbar vertebra. The horizontal portion is about 6 cm long and passes from right to left, from the level of the fourth lumbar vertebra to the diaphragm. The ascending portion is about 3 cm long and rises on the left side of the aorta to the level of the second lumbar vertebra, turning ventrally to become the jejunum at the duodenojejunal flexure. Compare **jejunum, ileum.**

duplex inheritance. See **amphigonous inheritance.**

duplex transmission, the passage of a neural impulse in both directions along a nerve fiber.

Dupuytren's contracture (dʏpʏitRāz′), a progressive, painless thickening and tightening of subcutaneous tissue of the palm, causing the fourth and fifth fingers to bend into the palm and resist extension. Tendons and nerves are not involved. Although the condition begins in one hand, both will become symmetrically affected. Of unknown cause, it is most frequent in middle-aged males. Early surgical removal of the excess fibrous tissue will restore full use of the hand. Under general anesthesia, an incision is made into the palm, and the thickened tissue is excised carefully to avoid injury to adjacent ligaments.

Dupuytren's fracture. See **Galeazzi's fracture.**

Durabolin, a trade name for an anabolic steroid (nandrolone phenpropionate).

dura mater (dʊ′rə mei′tər, dyʊ′rə), the outermost and most fibrous of the three membranes surrounding the brain and spinal cord. The **dura mater encephali** covers the brain, and the **dura mater spinalis** covers the cord. See also **meninges.**

Duranest, a trade name for a local anesthetic (etidocaine hydrochloride).

duress, (in law) an action compelling another person to do what otherwise would not be done voluntarily. A consent form signed under duress is not valid.

dust, any fine, particulate, dry matter. Kinds of dust are **inorganic dust, organic dust.**

dust fever. See **brucellosis.**

Dutton's disease. See **Dutton's relapsing fever.**

Dutton's relapsing fever, an infection caused by a spirochete, *Borrelia duttoni,* which is transmitted by a soft tick, *Ornithodoros moubata,* found in human dwellings in tropical Africa. The spirochete enters the lesion through the tick bite, characteristically producing a high fever, chills, rapid heartbeat, headache, joint and muscle pain, vomiting, and neurological disorders. The symptoms recur in a pattern of remissions and peaks of fever and other effects. The infection is spread through the community as ticks bite infected people, thereby acquiring the spirochete for inoculation in others. Treatment with tetracycline is usually effective in curing the infection. Also called **Dutton's disease.** See also **relapsing fever.**

duty, (in law) an obligation owed by one party to another. Duty may be established by statute or other legal process, as by contract or oath supported by statute, or it may be voluntarily undertaken. Every person has a duty of care to all other people to avoid causing harm or injury by negligence.

Duverney's fracture (du'vərniz'), fracture of the ilium just below the anterior superior spine.

dwarf, **1.** an abnormally short, undersized person, especially one whose bodily parts are not proportional. **2.** Kinds of dwarfs include **achondroplastic dwarf, Amsterdam dwarf, asexual dwarf, ateliotic dwarf, bird-headed dwarf, Brissaud's dwarf, cretin dwarf, diastrophic dwarf, phocomelic dwarf, pituitary dwarf, primordial dwarf, rachitic dwarf, renal dwarf, Russell dwarf, sexual dwarf, Silver dwarf, thanatophoric dwarf.** Also called **nanus.** **2.** to prevent or retard normal growth.

dwarfism, the abnormal underdevelopment of the body, characterized predominantly by extreme shortness of stature, although the condition is associated with numerous other defects and may involve varying degrees of mental retardation. Dwarfism results from multiple causes, including genetic defects, endocrine dysfunction involving either the pituitary or thyroid glands, chronic diseases, as rickets, renal failure, and intestinal malabsorption defects, and psychosocial stress, as in the maternal deprivation syndrome. See also **dwarf.**

dwindles, *Informal.* a condition of physical deterioration involving several systems of the body, usually in an elderly person in multiple body systems.

Dwyer cable instrumentation, one of the two most common surgical methods for correcting the spinal curvature associated with scoliosis. The Dwyer cable method uses a mechanical device that assists in obtaining the curvature correction through an anterior approach and is used in association with spinal fusion. The device is inserted to assist in maintaining the corrected curvature while the fusion heals and is not usually removed unless there is postoperative indication of displacement or a pattern of associated symptoms. Dwyer cable instrumentation involves surgical intervention through the pulmonary cavity and the rib cage and involves a relatively greater surgical risk than a posterior approach. It is often inadequate to correct the spinal curvature involved and must

frequently be followed several weeks later by a posterior spinal fusion.

Dy, symbol for **dysprosium.**

dyad (dai'æd), (in genetics) one of the paired homologous chromosomes, which consist of two chromatids, that result from the division of a tetrad in the first meiotic division of gametogenesis. – **dyadic,** *adj.*

dyadic interpersonal communication, a process in which two people interact face-to-face as senders and receivers, as in a conversation.

Dyazide, a trade name for a fixed-combination drug containing two diuretic agents (triamterene and hydrochlorothiazide).

Dyclone, a trade name for a local anesthetic (dyclonine hydrochloride).

dydrogesterone (dai'drəjes'təroun), a progestin.

■ INDICATIONS: It may be prescribed in the treatment of abnormal uterine bleeding, menopausal vasomotor symptoms, Pickwickian syndrome, endometrial cancer, and contraception.

■ CONTRAINDICATIONS: Thrombophlebitis, breast cancer, missed abortion, known or suspected pregnancy, or known hypersensitivity to this drug prohibits its use.

■ ADVERSE EFFECTS: Among the more serious adverse reactions are thrombophlebitis, uterine fibroma, and embolism.

dye, **1.** to apply coloring matter to a substance. **2.** a chemical compound capable of imparting color to a substance to which it is applied. Various dyes are used in medicine as stains for tissues, test reagents, therapeutic agents, and to color pharmaceutical preparations.

Dymelor, a trade name for an antidiabetic (acetohexamide).

-dymia, a combining form meaning an 'abnormal condition of anomalous twins joined at part of their bodies': *cephalodymia, prosoposternodymia, sternodymia.*

-dynamia, a combining form meaning '(condition of) strength': *ataxiadynamia, hyperdynamia, plastodynamia.* Also **-dynamy.**

dynamic, tending to change or to encourage change, as a dynamic nurse-patient relationship. Compare **static.**

dynamic nurse patient relationship, a conceptual framework in which the interpersonal aspects of the nurse patient relationship are analyzed. The relationship is affected by many factors. Elements in the process include the behavior of the patient, the reaction of the nurse, and the actions of the nurse that are intended to aid the patient. Also examined are the means for validating nurses' perceptions and interpretations and for evaluating the effects of the nursing actions taken.

dynamic psychiatry, the study of motivational, emotional, and biological factors as determinants of human behavior.

dynamic spatial reconstructor (DSR), a kind of roentgenographic machine used in research permitting moving three-dimensional images of human organs to be examined visually and from any direction.

dynamo-, a combining form meaning 'pertaining to power or strength': *dynamogenesis, dynamometer, dynamophore.*

dynamometer (dæi'nəmom'ıtər), a device for measuring the amount of energy expended in the contraction of a muscle or a group of muscles, as a squeeze dynamometer which measures the force of the hand when squeezing the device.

-dynamy. See **-dynamia.**

Dynapen, a trade name for an antibacterial (dicloxacillin sodium).

dyphylline, a bronchodilator.

■ INDICATIONS: It is prescribed in the treatment of bronchospasm in acute bronchial asthma, bronchitis, and emphysema.

■ CONTRAINDICATIONS: It is used with caution in patients with peptic ulcer or cardiovascular disease. Known hypersensitivity to this or to other xanthines prohibits its use.

■ ADVERSE EFFECTS: Among the more serious adverse reactions are gastrointestinal distress, dizziness, tachycardia, headache, and palpitations.

Dyrenium, a trade name for a diuretic (triamterene).

dys-, a combining form meaning 'bad, painful, disordered': *dysadrenia, dysbolism, dysmnesia.*

dysadrenia, abnormal adrenal function characterized by decreased production of hormones, as in hypoadrenalism or hypoadrenocorticism, or by increased secretion of the products of the gland, as in hyperadrenalism or hyperadrenocorticism. Also called **dysadrenalism.**

dysarthria (dısar'thriə), difficult, poorly articulated speech, resulting from interference in the control over the muscles of speech, usually because of damage to a central or peripheral motor nerve.

dyschondroplasia (dıskon'droupleı'ʒə). See **enchondromatosis.**

dyscrasic fracture (dıskræz'ık), any fracture caused by the weakening of a specific bone owing to a debilitating disease.

dysentery (dıs'ınter'i), an inflammation of the intestine, especially of the colon, that may be caused by chemical irritants, bacteria, protozoa, or parasites. It is characterized by frequent and bloody stools, abdominal pain, and tenesmus. Dysentery is common in poverty-ridden areas of the world and in times of disaster and social disorganization when sanitary living conditions, clean food, and safe water are not available. See also **amebic dysentery, shigellosis.**

dysfunctional, (of a body organ or system) unable to function normally. — **dysfunction,** *n.*

dysfunctional uterine bleeding (DUB), uterine bleeding as a result of endocrine imbalance rather than a pathological condition.

dysgenesis (dısjen'ısıs), **dysgenesia** (dıs'jıni'ʒhə), **1.** defective or abnormal formation of an organ or part, primarily during embryonic development. **2.** impairment or loss of the ability to procreate. A kind of dysgenesis is **gonadal dysgenesis.** Compare **agenesis.** — **dysgenic,** *adj.*

dysgenics (dısjen'ıks), the study of those factors or situations that are genetically detrimental to the future of a race or species. Compare **eugenics.** — **dysgenic,** *adj.*

dysgenitalism (dısjen'ıtəlız'əm), any condition involving the abnormal development of the genital organs.

dysgraphia (dısgræf'iə), an impairment of the ability to write, owing to a pathological disorder. — **dysgraphic,** *adj.*

dyshidrosis (dıs'hıdrou'sıs, dıs'haidrou'sıs), a condition in which abnormal sweating occurs. Some kinds of dyshidrosis are **hyperhidrosis, miliaria, pompholyx.** Compare **anhidrosis.** — **dyshidrotic,** *adj.*

dyskeratosis (dıs'kerətou'sıs), an abnormal or premature keratinization of epithelial cells.

dyskinesia, an impairment of the ability to execute voluntary movements. — **dyskinetic,** *adj.*

dyslexia (dıslek'siə), an impairment of the ability to read, owing to a variety of pathological conditions, some of which are associated with the central nervous system. People with this condition often reverse letters and words, cannot adequately distinguish the letter sequences in written words, and have difficulty determining left from right. Some reading experts doubt that dyslexia is a pathological disorder and believe the condition represents a combination of reading problems, each of which should be isolated by specific tests. Some such problems cited by these authorities are poor vision, impaired hearing, emotional immaturity, lack of physical development, psychic stress, and inadequate reading instruction. — **dyslexic,** *adj.*

dysmaturity, **1.** the failure of an organism to develop, ripen, or otherwise achieve maturity in structure or function. **2.** the condition of a fetus or newborn being abnormally small or large for its age of gestation. Kinds of dysmaturity are **small-for-gestational age, large-for-gestational age.** Compare **postmature, premature.** — **dysmature,** *adj.*

dysmelia (dısmi'lyə), an abnormal congenital condition characterized by missing or shortened extremities of the body, associated with abnormalities of the spine in some individuals. It is caused by abnormal metabolism during the development of the embryonic limbs.

dysmenorrhea (dısmi'menəri'ə), pain associated with menstruation. Primary dysmenorrhea is menstrual pain that results from factors intrinsic to the uterus and the process of menstruation; it is extremely common, occurring at least occasionally in almost all women. If the painful episode is mild and brief, it is considered functional and normal and requires no treatment. In approximately 10 per cent of women, dysmenorrhea is sufficiently severe to cause episodes of partial or total disability. The etiology in most cases is poorly understood, various anatomic, neurohormonal, and psychosomatic abnormalities have been suggested. Pain occurs typically in the lower abdomen or back and is crampy, coming in successive waves —apparently in conjunction with intense uterine contractions and slight cervical dilatation. Pain usually begins just prior to, or at the onset of, menstrual flow and lasts a few hours to a day or more; but it may persist through the entire period in a few women. Pain is frequently associated with nausea, vomiting, and frequent bowel movements with intestinal cramping. Dizziness, fainting, pallor, and obvious distress may also be observed. Treatment with an antiprostaglandin provides relief for many women if begun 1 to 3 days premenstrually and continued through the first day of the menses. Oral contraceptive steroids are also effective for many women and are taken through the full monthly cycle. Potent analgesics or narcotics may be required by a few women. Secondary dysmenorrhea is menstrual pain that occurs secondary to specific pelvic abnormalities, as endometriosis, adenomyosis, chronic pelvic infection, chronic pelvic congestion, or degenerating fibroid tumors. Typically, the pain begins earlier in the cycle and lasts longer than the pain of primary dysmenorrhea. Painful bowel or bladder function may accompany the condition, depending on the location of the specific lesions. Diagnosis of the chief cause is made by pelvic examination, ultrasonography, laparoscopy, or laparotomy. Treatment, most often surgical, is directed at the specific organic disease involved.

dysmetria (dɪsmet'riə), an abnormal condition which prevents the affected individual from properly measuring distances associated with muscular acts and from controlling muscular action. See also **hypermetria, hypometria.**

dysostosis (dɪs'ostou'sɪs), an abnormal condition characterized by defective ossification, especially by defects in the normal ossification of fetal cartilages. Kinds of dysostoses include **cleidocranial dysostosis, craniofacial dysostosis, mandibulofacial dysostosis, metaphyseal dysostosis, Nager's acrofacial dysostosis.**

dyspareunia (dɪs'pəru'niə), an abnormal condition of women, in which sexual intercourse is accompanied by pain. The pain may result from abnormal conditions of the genitalia, dysfunctional psychophysiologic reaction to sexual union, forcible coition, or incomplete sexual arousal. See also **vaginismus.**

Dyspaz, a trade name for an anticholinergic (dicyclomine hydrochloride).

dyspepsia (dɪspep'siə), a vague feeling of gastric discomfort, felt after eating. There is an uncomfortable feeling of fullness, heartburn, bloating, and nausea. Dyspepsia is not a distinct condition, but it may be a sign of underlying intestinal disorder, as peptic ulcer, gall bladder disease, or chronic appendicitis. —**dyspeptic,** adj.

dysphagia, difficulty in swallowing, commonly associated with obstructive or motor disorders of the esophagus. Patients with obstructive disorders like esophageal tumor or lower esophageal ring are unable to swallow solids but can tolerate liquids. Persons with motor disorders, as achalasia, are unable to swallow solids or liquids. Diagnosis of the underlying condition is made through barium studies, the observed clinical signs, and evaluation of the patient's symptoms. See also **achalasia, corkscrew esophagus.**

dysphagia lusoria, an abnormal condition, characterized by difficulty in swallowing, caused by the compression of the esophagus from an anomalous right subclavian artery that arises from the descending aorta and courses behind the esophagus. Compare **contractile ring dysphagia, vallecular dysphagia.**

dysphasia (dɪsfei'jiə), an impairment of speech, not as severe as aphasia, usually the result of an injury to the speech area in the cerebral cortex of the brain. It may follow a stroke or brain tumor and may be accompanied by other language disorders, as dysgraphia. Compare **dysarthria.**

-dysplasia, a combining form meaning '(condition of) abnormal development': *chondrodysplasia, epidermodysplasia, osteomyelodysplasia.*

dyspnea (dɪspni'ə), a shortness of breath or a difficulty in breathing that may be caused by certain heart conditions, strenuous exercise, or anxiety. —**dyspneal, dyspneic,** adj.

dyspraxia (dɪspræk'siə), a partial loss of the ability to perform skilled, coordinated movements in the absence of any associated defect in motor or sensory functions. See also **apraxia.**

dysprosium (Dy), a rare-earth metallic element. Its atomic number is 66; its atomic weight is 162.50. Radioactive isotopes of dysprosium are used in radioisotope scanning, particularly in studies of the bones and joints.

dysraphia (dɪsrei'fiə), failure of a raphe to fuse completely, as in incomplete closure of the neural tube. Also called **status dysraphicus.**

dysreflexia (dɪs'rɪflek'siə), an abnormal neuromuscular condition characterized by abnormal motor response to stimuli that normally produce a specific response. —**dysreflexic,** adj.

dyssebacea (dɪsɪbei'shiə), a skin condition characterized by red, scaly, greasy patches on the nose, eyelids, scrotum, and labia. It results from a deficiency of vitamin B_2 and is most commonly associated with chronic alcoholism, liver disease, chronic diarrhea, and protein malnutrition. Also called *Informal.* **shark skin.**

dystocia (dɪstou'siə), abnormal labor, which occurs for one or more of the following reasons: the uterine expulsive powers are disordered, the birth passage is obstructed or contracted, or the size, shape, or position of the fetal passenger is abnormal. See also **contraction, presentation.**

dystonia musculorum deformans (dɪstou'niə məs'kyulɔr'əm dɪfɔr'mænz,) a rare abnormal condition characterized by intense, irregular torsion muscle spasms that contort the body. The muscles of the trunk, shoulder, and pelvis are commonly involved. This disease appears in several forms, generally classified as autosomal recessive or autosomal dominant. The cause of this disorder is not known; a biochemical dysfunction is suspected. The autosomal recessive form appears most often in Ashkenazic Jews and starts between the ages of 5 and 15, causing abnormalities of movement and speech. Muscle power and tone appear normal, but convulsive spasms make the involved muscles relatively useless. The autosomal recessive form of the disease commonly begins with intermittent spasmodic inversion of the foot, so that the affected individual has difficulty in placing the heel on the ground when walking and develops an odd, bowing gait. Lordosis and torsion of pelvis appear as the proximal muscles become more involved. Torticollis is often an early sign if the muscles of the neck and shoulder girdle are involved. The autosomal dominant form of the disease appears in early adult life, generally affects the axial musculature, and progresses more slowly than the autosomal recessive form. Some muscle-relaxing drugs, as the benzodiazepines, have been helpful in treating both forms of the condition. Mild cases have been successfully controlled for long periods with treatments that combine the use of muscle-relaxing drugs and psychotherapy. Some patients with this disease have also responded well for long periods to stereotactic thalamotomy, which, however, carries the risk of producing speech disorders.

dystrophy (dɪs'trəfi), any abnormal condition caused by defective nutrition. Also called **dystrophia.** — **dystrophic** (dɪstrof'ɪk), *adj.*

dysuria (dɪsyur'iə), painful urination, usually the result of a bacterial infection or obstructive condition in the urinary tract. The patient complains of a burning sensation when passing urine, and laboratory examination may reveal the presence of blood, bacteria, or white blood cells. Dysuria is a symptom of such conditions as cystitis, urethritis, prostatitis, urinary tract tumors, and some gynecological disorders. Compare **hematuria, pyuria.**

E

e-, a combining form meaning 'out from': *ebonation, egesta, emollient.*

E, symbol for **expired gas.**

E and GW, abbreviation for **Economic and General Welfare.**

ear, the organ of hearing, consisting of the internal, middle, and external ear.

earache, a pain in the ear, sensed as sharp, dull, burning, intermittent, or constant. The cause is not necessarily a disease of the ear since infections and other disorders of the nose, oral cavity, larynx, and temperomanidibular joint can produce referred pain in the ear. Also called **otalgia, otodynia.**

eardrop instillation, the instillation of a medicated solution into the external auditory canal of the ear. The patient is asked to turn the head to the side so that the ear being treated faces upward. The orifice is exposed, and the drops of medicine are directed toward the internal wall of the canal. The pinna is pulled up and back in a person over three years of age and down and back in a child younger than two or three years of age.

eardrops, a topical, liquid form of medication for the local treatment of various conditions of the ear, as inflammation or infection of the lining of the external auditory canal or impacted cerumen.

ear drum. See **tympanic membrane.**

Early and Periodic Screening Diagnosis and Treatment (EPSDT), a section of the Medicaid program that requires all states to maintain a program to determine the physical and mental defects of the children under 21 who are covered by the program and to provide short- and long-range treatment. See also **Medicaid.**

earth bath, the covering of a part of the body with warm sand or earth.

earwax. See **cerumen.**

East African Sleeping Sickness. See **Rhodesian trypanosomiasis.**

Eastern equine encephalitis (EEE). See **equine encephalitis.**

Eaton-agent pneumonia. See **mycoplasma pneumonia.**

Ebbecke's reaction (eb′eks). See **dermatographia.**

EBP, abbreviation for **epidural blood patch.**

EBV, abbreviation for **Epstein-Barr virus.**

ec-, a combining form meaning 'out of': *ecbolic, eccephalosis, ecchondroma.*

eccentric implantation, (in embryology) the embedding of the blastocyst within a fold or recess of the uterine wall, which then closes off from the main cavity.

ecchondroma (ek′əndrou′mə), a benign cartilaginous tumor that develops on the surface of a cartilage or under the periosteum of bone.

ecchondrosis (ek′əndrou′sıs). See **ecchondroma.**

ecchymosis (ek′ımou′sıs), *pl.* **ecchymoses.** discoloration of an area of the skin or mucous membrane owing to the extravasation of blood into the subcutaneous tissues as a result of trauma to the underlying blood vessels or to fragility of the vessel walls. Also called **bruise.** Compare **contusion, petechiae.**

eccrine (ek′rın), of or pertaining to a sweat gland that secretes outwardly through a duct to the surface of the skin. Compare **exocrine.**

eccrine gland (ek′rın), one of two kinds of sweat glands in the corium of the skin. Such glands are unbranched, coiled, and tubular, and they distributed throughout the dermal covering of the body. They promote cooling by evaporation of their secretion which is clear, has a faint odor, and contains water, sodium chloride, and traces of albumin, urea, and other compounds. Compare **apocrine gland.**

eccyesis (ek′saii′sıs). See **ectopic pregnancy.**

ECF, abbreviation for **extracellular fluid.**

ECG, **1.** abbreviation for **electrocardiogram. 2.** abbreviation for **electrocardiograph.**

-echia, a combining form meaning a 'condition of holding': *asynechia, blepharosynechia, synechia.*

echino-, a combining form meaning 'pertaining to spines, or spiny': *echinochroma, echinosis, echinostomiasis.*

echinococcosis (ekai′noukokou′sıs), a tissue infection, usually of the liver, caused by the larval stage of a tapeworm of the genus *Echinococcus.* Dogs are the principal hosts of the adult worm; sheep, cattle, rodents, and deer are the natural intermediate hosts for the larvae. Humans, especially children, can become infested with larvae by ingesting eggs shed in the stool of infected dogs. The disease is most common in countries where domestic animals are raised with the help of dogs. Clinical manifestations and prognosis vary, depending upon the tissue invaded and the extent of infestation. Diagnosis is made by skin tests for sensitivity, serologic tests, radiologic evidence of cyst formation, and identification of larval cysts in infected tissue. Surgical excision of the cysts is the only treatment available. The disease can be prevented by avoiding contact with infected dogs, deworming pet animals, and preventing dogs from eating carcasses of infected intermediate hosts. Also called **hydatid disease, hydatidosis.** See also **cysticerosis, tapeworm infection.**

Echinococcus (ĭkaī'noukok'əs), a genus of small tapeworms that infects primarily canines. Humans may become infected by handling pets that have eggs of the tapeworm on their hair. The eggs produce larvae which form hydatid cysts in the liver, lungs, abdominal cavity, or almost any other part of the human body. See also **hydatid cyst.**

echinocyte (ĭkaī'nəsaĭt). See **burr cell.**

echo, *Informal.* echoradiography.

echocardiography (ek'oukar'diog'rəfi), a diagnostic procedure for studying the structure and motion of the heart. Ultrasonic waves directed through the heart are reflected backward, or echoed, when they pass from one type of tissue to another, as from cardiac muscle to blood. The sound waves are transmitted from and received by a transducer and are recorded on a strip chart. Major diagnostic uses include the detection of atrial tumors and pericardial effusion, the measurement of the ventricular septa and the ventricular chambers, and the determination of mitral valve motion abnormalities and congenital lesions. Also called **ultrasonic cardiography.** See also **phonocardiograph, ultrasonography.**

echoencephalogram (ek'ouensef'ələgræm'), a recording produced by an echoencephalograph.

echoencephalography (ek'ouensef'əlog'rəfi), the use of ultrasound to study the intracranial structures of the brain. The technique is useful for showing ventricular dilatation and a major shift of midline structures as a result of an expanding lesion. See also **ultrasonography.** – **echoencephalographic,** *adj.*

echography (ekog'rəfi). See **ultrasonography.**

echolalia (ek'ouleĭ'liə, ek'ouleĭ'lyə), **1.** Also called **echophrasia.** (in psychiatry) the automatic and meaningless repetition of another's words or phrases, especially as seen in schizophrenia. A kind of echolalia is **delayed echolalia. 2.** (in pediatrics) a baby's imitation or repetition of sounds or words produced by others. It occurs normally in early childhood development. – **echolalic,** *adj.*

echophrasia (ek'oufreĭzhə). See **echolalia.**

echoradiography (ek'ourei'diog'rəfi), a diagnostic procedure using ultrasonography and various devices for the visualization of internal structures of the body.

echothiophate iodide, an anticholinesterase used for ophthalmic purposes.

■ INDICATIONS: It is prescribed for chronic open-angle glaucoma and accommodative esotropia.

■ CONTRAINDICATIONS: Uveal inflammation, most types of angle-closure glaucoma, or known hypersensitivity to this drug prohibits its use.

■ ADVERSE EFFECTS: Among the more serious adverse reactions are retinal detachment, nonreversible cataract, lens opacity, activation of iritis or uveitis, and iris cysts.

echovirus (ek'ouvaī'rəs), a picornavirus associated with many clinical syndromes but not identified as the causative organism of any specific disease. There are many echoviruses; most are harmless. Bacterial or viral disease may be complicated by echovirus infection, as seen in aseptic meningitis accompanying some severe bacterial and viral infections.

eclampsia (ĭklæmp'siə), the gravest form of toxemia of pregnancy, characterized by grand mal convulsion, coma, hypertension, proteinuria, and edema. The symptoms of impending convulsion often include anxiety, epigastric pain, headache, and blurred vision. The nurse is alert to persistently and extremely high blood pressure and to increasingly hyperactive deep-tendon reflexes, or clonus. Convulsions may be prevented by bed rest in a quiet, dimly lit room and parenteral administration of magnesium sulfate. The nurse attentively monitors the mother's general condition, blood pressure, and urine excretion, and the baby's heart rate. Treatment of a convulsion must include maintenance of the mother's airway, protection against self-injury, and administration of medication to check the convulsion and decrease the blood pressure. Once this is accomplished, delivery is indicated. Convulsions rarely occur in the puerperium. Complications of eclampsia include cerebral hemorrhage, pulmonary edema, renal failure, necrosis of the liver, abruptio placentae, hypofibrinogenemia, hemolysis, and retinal hemorrhages, sometimes with temporary blindness. Maternal mortality in eclampsia is 10 per cent; fetal mortality is 25 per cent. Eclampsia occurs in 0.2 per cent of pregnancies, and the cause is not known.

Eclipse, a trade name for a topical, fixed-combination drug containing an ultraviolet sun screen (padimate).

-ecoia, a combining form meaning '(condition of the) sense of hearing': *bradyecoia, dysecoia, oxyecoia.*

ecological chemistry, the study of chemical compounds synthesized by plants that influence ecology because of their toxic effects.

Econochlor, a trade name for an antibacterial and antirickettsial (chloramphenicol).

Economic and General Welfare (E and GW), a unit of the American Nurses' Association that works to upgrade the salaries, benefits, and working conditions of nurses.

Econopred, a trade name for a glucocorticoid (prednisolone acetate).

ecstasy, an emotional state characterized by exultation, rapturous delight, or frenzy. Compare **euphoria, mania.** – **ecstatic,** *adj.*

ECT, abbreviation for **electroconvulsive therapy.**

-ectasia, a combining form meaning '(condition of) dilation, extension, or distension of an organ': *esophagectasia, lymphectasia, pharyngectasia.* Also **-ectasis, -ectasy.**

-ectasis. See **-ectasia.**

-ectasy. See **-ectasia.**

ecthyma (ek'θɪmə), a deep, burrowing form of impetigo characterized by large pustules, crusts, and ulcerations surrounded by erythema. Staphylococci and streptococci are the offending bacteria, and the skin of the legs is most frequently affected. Treatment includes vigorous cleanliness, compresses of cool Burow's solution to soften and remove crusts, and penicillin or erythromycin given systemically. Compare **folliculitis, impetigo.**

ecto-, a combining form meaning 'outside': *ectoblast, ectocolon, ectodermal.*

ectoderm, the outermost of the three primary cell layers of an embryo. The ectoderm gives rise to the nervous system; the organs of special sense, as the eyes and ears; the epidermis; and epidermal tissue, as fingernails, hair, and skin glands; and the mucous membranes of the mouth and anus. See also **embryo, endoderm, mesoderm.** – **ectodermal, ectodermic,** *adj.*

ectodermal cloaca, a part of the cloaca in the developing embryo that lies external to the cloacal membrane and eventually gives rise to the anus and anal canal. Compare **endodermal cloaca.**

ectomorph (ek'təmɔrf'), a person whose physique is characterized by slenderness, fragility, and a predominance of structures derived from the ectoderm. Compare **endomorph, mesomorph.** See also **asthenic habitus.**

-ectomy, a combining form meaning the 'surgical removal' of something specified: *lobectomy, thrombectomy, thyroidectomy.*

ectoparasite (ek'toupær'əsait), (in medical parasitology) an organism that lives on the outside of the body of the host, as a louse.

-ectopia, a combining form meaning a 'condition in which a (specified) organ or part is out of its normal place': *corectopia, osteectopia, tarsectopia.*

ectopic (ektop'ɪk), **1.** (of an object or organ) situated in an unusual place, away from its normal location, as an ectopic pregnancy is a pregnancy that occurs outside the uterus. **2.** (of an event) occurring at the wrong time, as a premature heart beat or premature ventricular contraction.

ectopic myelopoiesis. See **extramedullary myelopoiesis.**

ectopic pregnancy, an abnormal pregnancy in which the conceptus implants outside the uterine cavity. Kinds of ectopic pregnancy are **abdominal pregnancy, interstitial pregnancy, ovarian pregnancy, tubal pregnancy.** Also called **eccyesis.**

ectopic teratism, a congenital anomaly in which one or more parts are misplaced, as dextrocardia, palatine teeth, and transposition of the great vessels.

ectotoxin. *Obsolete.* See **exotoxin.**

ectrodactyly, ectrodactylia, a congenital anomaly characterized by the absence of part or all of one or more of the fingers or toes. Also called **ectrodactylism.**

ectrogenic teratism, a congenital anomaly caused by developmental failure in which one or more parts or organs are missing.

ectrogeny (ektroj'əni), the congenital absence or defect of any organ or part of the body. – **ectrogenic,** *adj.*

ectromelia (ek'troumi'liə), the congenital absence or incomplete development of the long bones of one or more of the limbs. Kinds of ectromelia are **amelia, hemimelia, phocomelia.** – **ectromelic,** *adj.*, **ectromelus,** *n.*

ectropion (ektrou'piən), eversion, most commonly of the eyelid, exposing the conjunctival membrane lining the eyelid and part of the eyeball. The condition may involve only the lower eyelid or both eyelids. The cause may be paralysis of the facial nerve, or, in an older person, atrophy of the eyelid tissues. Compare **entropion.**

ECTROPION

ectrosyndactyly (ek'trousɪndæk'təli), **ectrosyndactylia,** a congenital anomaly characterized by the absence of some but not all of the digits, with those that are formed being webbed so as to appear fused.

eczema (ek'sɪmə), superficial dermatitis of unknown cause. In the early stage it may be pruritic, erythematous, papulovesicular, edematous, and weeping. Later it becomes crusted, scaly, thickened, and lichenified. Eczema is not a distinct disease entity. See also **atopic dermatitis, Kaposi's varicelliform eruption, nummular dermatitis.** – **eczematous,** *adj.*

eczema herpeticum, a generalized vesiculo-pustular skin disease caused by herpes simplex virus or vaccinia virus infection of a pre-existing rash like atopic dermatitis. Hospitalization is advisable because fatalities have occurred with this condition. Also called **Kaposi's varicelliform eruption.**

eczema marginatum. See **tinea cruris.**

eczematous conjunctivitis, conjunctival and corneal inflammation associated with multiple, tiny, ulcerated vesicles. The cause is believed to be a delayed hypersensitivity to bacterial protein. If untreated, the condition may lead to ingrowth of small blood vessels in the cornea, eventually obscuring vision. Treatment usually includes topical instillation of corticosteroids. Also called **phlyctenulosis.**

ED, abbreviation for **effective dose.**

ED50, symbol for **median effective dose.**

edaphon (ed'əfon), the composite of organisms that live in the soil. — **edaphic,** *adj.*

EDC, abbreviation for **expected date of confinement.**

Edecrin, a trade name for a diuretic (ethacrynic acid).

Edecrin Sodium, a trade name for a diuretic (ethacrynate sodium).

edema (ɪdi'mə), the abnormal accumulation of fluid in interstitial spaces of tissues, in the pericardial sac, intrapleural space, peritoneal cavity, or joint capsules. Edema may be caused by increased capillary fluid pressure, venous obstruction, as in varicosities, thrombophlebitis, or pressure from casts, tight bandages, or garters, congestive heart failure, overloading with parenteral fluids, renal failure, hepatic cirrhosis, hyperaldosteronism, as in Cushing's syndrome, corticosteroid therapy, and inflammatory reactions. Edema may also occur because of loss of serum protein in burns, draining wounds, fistulas, hemorrhage, nephrotic syndrome, or chronic diarrhea, in malnutrition, especially kwashiorkor, in allergic reactions, and in blockage of lymphatic vessels owing to malignant diseases, filariasis, or other disorders. Treatment of edema is directed to correction of the basic cause, but potassium-sparing diuretics may be administered to promote excretion of sodium and water and care is exercised in protecting edematous parts of the body from prolonged pressure, injury, and temperature extremes. When a limb is edematous because of venous stasis, elevating the extremity and applying an elastic stocking or sleeve facilitates venous return. See also **lymphedema.** — **edematous, edematose,** *adj.*

-edema, a combining form meaning 'swelling resulting from an excessive accumulation of serous fluid in the tissues of the body in (specified) locations': *cephaledema, dactyledema, papilledema.*

edetate (EDTA) (ed'əteit), one of several salts of edetic acid, including calcium disodium edetate and edetate disodium, used as a chelating agent in poisoning with heavy metals.

edetate disodium, a parenteral chelating agent.

■ INDICATIONS: It is prescribed for hypercalcemic crisis and for ventricular arrhythmia and heart block resulting from digitalis toxicity.

PITTING EDEMA

Causes of edema according to underlying physiological mechanism

Fluid pressure	Oncotic pressure
Increased capillary fluid pressure	*Decreased capillary oncotic pressure*
Increased venous pressure	Loss of serum protein
Vein obstruction	Burns, draining wounds, fistulas
Varicose veins	Hemorrhage
Thrombophlebitis	Nephrotic syndrome
Pressure on veins from casts, tight bandages, or garters	Chronic diarrhea
Increased total volume with decreased cardiac output	Decreased production of protein
Congestive heart failure	Malnutrition (kwashiorkor)
Fluid overloading	Cirrhosis of liver
Sodium and water retention: increased aldosterone caused by	
Decreased renal blood flow	*Increased interstitial oncotic pressure*
Congestive heart failure	Increased capillary permeability to protein
Renal failure	Burns
Increased production of aldosterone	Inflammatory reactions
Cushing's syndrome	Trauma
Aldosterone added to system	Infections
Corticosteroid therapy	Allergic reactions (hives)
Inability to destroy aldosterone	Blocked lymphatics: decreased removal of tissue fluid and protein
Cirrhosis of liver	Malignant diseases
	Surgical removal of lymph nodes
	Elephantiasis

■ CONTRAINDICATIONS: Hypocalcemia, kidney disease, or known hypersensitivity to this drug prohibits its use.

■ ADVERSE EFFECTS: Among the more serious adverse reactions are hypocalcemia, thrombophlebitis, kidney damage, and hemorrhage.

edetic acid (EDTA) (ɪdet'ɪk),   a chelating agent.

EDNA,   abbreviation for **Emergency Department Nurses' Association.**

edrophonium chloride,   a cholinesterase inhibitor that acts as an antidote to curare and is an aid in the diagnosis of myasthenia gravis.

■ INDICATIONS: It is prescribed in the treatment of curare toxicity, in the diagnosis of suspected myasthenia gravis, and to terminate paroxysmal supraventricular tachycardia.

■ CONTRAINDICATIONS: Obstruction of the gastrointestinal or urinary tract, hypotension, bradycardia, or known hypersensitivity to this drug prohibits its use.

■ ADVERSE EFFECTS: Among the most serious adverse reactions are respiratory paralysis, hypotension, bradycardia, and bronchospasm.

Edsall's disease,   a cramping condition that is the result of excessive exposure to heat. Also called **heat cramp.**

EDTA,   **1.** abbreviation for **edetate. 2.** abbreviation for **edetic acid.**

educational psychology,   the application of psychological principles, techniques, and tests to educational problems, as the determination of more effective instructional methods, the assessment of student advancement, and the selection of students for specialized programs.

Edward's syndrome,   a congenital autosomal disorder, occurring in about one in 3000 births and marked by small size and weight for gestational age, a long, narrow skull with a prominent occiput, flexion deformities of the fingers, cardiovascular abnormalities, and severe mental retardation. Infants with this condition seldom survive more than a few months. Also called **trisomy E syndrome.**

EEE,   abbreviation for **Eastern equine encephalitis.** See **equine encephalitis.**

EEG,   **1.** abbreviation for **electroencephalogram. 2.** abbreviation for **electroencephalography.**

EEOC,   abbreviation for **Equal Employment Opportunity Commission.**

E.E.S.,   abbreviation for an antibacterial (erythromycin ethylsuccinate).

ef-.   See **ex-.**

effacement,   the shortening of the vaginal portion of the cervix and thinning of its walls as it is stretched and dilated by the fetus during labor. When the cervix is fully effaced, the constrictive neck of the uterus is obliterated, the cervix being then continuous with the lower uterine segment. The extent of effacement, determined by vaginal examination, is expressed as a percentage of full effacement. See also **cervix, childbirth, dilatation, station.**

effective dose (ED),   the dosage of a drug that may be expected to cause a specific intensity of effect in the people to whom it is given.

effective half-life,   (in radiotherapy) the time required for a radioactive element in an animal body to be diminished 50 per cent as a result of the combined action of radioactive decay and biological elimination. The effective half-life (*ehl*) is equal to the product of the biological half-life (*bhl*) and the radioactive half-life (*rhl*) divided by the product of the biological half-life plus the radioactive half-life $ehl = (bhl \times rhl)/(bhl + rhl)$. See also **biological half-life.**

efferent (ef'ərənt),   directed away from a center, as certain arteries, veins, nerves, and lymphatics. Compare **afferent.**

efferent duct,   any duct through which a gland releases its secretions.

efficacy (ef'əkəsi),   (of a drug or treatment) the maximum ability of a drug or treatment to produce a result, regardless of dosage. Narcotics have a nearly identical efficacy but require various dosages to obtain the effect. Compare **potency.**

effleurage (ef'lərazh'),   a technique in massage in which long, light or firm strokes are used, usually over the spine and back. Fingertip effleurage is a light technique performed with the tips of the fingers in a circular pattern over one part of the body or in long strokes over the back or an extremity. Fingertip effleurage of the abdomen is a technique commonly used in the Lamaze method of natural childbirth. Compare **pétrissage, rolling effleurage.**

effort syndrome,   an abnormal condition characterized by chest pain, dizziness, fatigue, and palpitations. This condition is often associated with soldiers in combat but also occurs in other individuals. The symptoms of effort syndrome often mimic angina pectoris but are more closely connected to anxiety states. Some indications that pain and other symptoms are related to effort syndrome rather than angina pectoris include cold, moist hands, sighing respiration, and chest pain after, rather than during, exercise. In some patients effort syndrome may be directly and obviously related to psychological problems but angina may also be associated with anxiety, and positive diagnosis may require an exercise electrocardiograph. Other chest pains that mimic effort syndrome and angina may be caused by musculoskeletal problems, as inflammation of the costochondral junctions, fractured ribs, and cervical spondylosis. Also called **neurocirculatory asthenia.**

effraction (ɪfræk'shən),   a breaking open or weakening.

effusion (ɪfyu'zhən),   **1.** See also **edema, transudate.** the escape of fluid from blood vessels because of rupture or seepage, usually into a body cavity. The condition is usually associated with a circulatory or renal disorder and is often an early sign of congestive heart disease. The term may be associated with an affected body area, as pleural effusion. **2.** the outward spread of a bacterial growth.

EFM, abbreviation for **electronic fetal monitor.**

Efricel, a trade name for an adrenergic (phenylephrine hydrochloride).

Efudex, a trade name for an antineoplastic (fluorouracil).

egest (ijest′), to discharge or evacuate a substance from the body, especially the evacuation of unabsorbed residue of foods from the intestines. —**egesta,** *n. pl.,* **egestive,** *adj.*

ego (i′gou, eg′ou), **1.** the conscious sense of the self; those elements of a person, such as thinking, feeling, willing, and emotions, that distinguish the person as an individual. **2.** (in psychoanalysis) the part of the psyche that experiences and maintains conscious contact with reality and that tempers the primitive drives of the id and the demands of the superego with the social and physical needs of society. It represents the rational element of the personality, is the seat of such mental processes as perception and memory, and develops defense mechanisms against anxiety. See also **id, superego.**

ego-alien. See **ego-dystonic.**

ego analysis, (in psychoanalysis) the intensive study of the ego, especially the defense mechanisms.

ego boundary, (in psychiatry) a sense or awareness that there is a distinction between the self and others. In some psychoses the person does not have an ego boundary and cannot differentiate personal perceptions and feelings from other people's perceptions and feelings.

egocentric, **1.** regarding the self as the center, object, and norm of all experience and having little regard for the needs, interests, ideas, and attitudes of others. **2.** describing a person possessing these characteristics.

ego defense mechanism. See **defense mechanism.**

ego-dystonic (i′goudiston′ik, eg′oudiston′ik), describing those elements of a person's behavior, thoughts, impulses, drives, and attitudes at variance with the standards of the ego and inconsistent with the total personality. Also called **ego-alien, self-alien.** Compare **ego-syntonic.**

ego-dystonic homosexuality, a psychosexual disorder in which there is a persistent desire to change sexual orientation from homosexuality to heterosexuality. See also **homosexual.**

ego ideal, the image of the self to which a person aspires both consciously and unconsciously and against which he measures himself and his performance. It is usually based on a positive identification with the significant and influential figures of his early childhood years. See also **identification.**

egoism, **1.** Also called **egotism.** an overevaluation of the importance of the self expressed as a willingness to gain advantage at the expense of others. **2.** the belief that individual self interest is, or ought to be, the basic motive for all conscious behavior.

egoist, **1.** a person who seeks to satisfy his own interests at the expense of others. **2.** a person who believes in or follows the concept that all conscious action is justifiably motivated by self-interest. —**egoistic, egoistical,** *adj.*

ego libido, (in psychoanalysis) concentration of the libido on the self; self-love, narcissism.

egomania, a pathological preoccupation with the self and an exaggerated sense of one's own importance.

ego strength, (in psychotherapy) the ability to maintain the ego by a cluster of traits that together contribute to good mental health. The traits usually considered important include tolerance of the pain of loss, disappointment, shame, or guilt; forgiveness of those who have caused an injury, with feelings of compassion rather than anger and retaliation; acceptance of substitutes and the ability to defer gratification; persistence and perseverance in the pursuit of goals; openness, flexibility, and creativity in learning to adapt; and vitality and power in the activities of life. The psychiatric prognosis for a client correlates positively with his ego strength.

ego-syntonic (i′gousinton′ik, eg′ousinton′ik), those elements of a person's behavior, thoughts, impulses, drives, and attitudes that agree with the standards of the ego and are consistent with the total personality. Compare **ego-dystonic.**

egotism (i′gotiz′əm, eg′ətiz′əm), the overvaluation of the importance of the self and undervaluation or contempt of others. —**egotistic, egotistical,** *adj.*

egotist (i′gotist, eg′ətist), one who places too much importance on the self and is boastful, egocentric, and arrogant.

Egyptian ophthalmia. See **trachoma.**

EHD, abbreviation for **electrohemodynamics.**

Ehlers-Danlos syndrome (ei′lərzdæn′ləs), a hereditary disorder of connective tissue, marked by hyperplasticity of skin, tissue fragility, and hypermotility of joints. Minor trauma may cause a gaping wound with little bleeding. Sprains, joint dislocations, and synovial effusions are common; life expectancy is usually normal. Nursing management includes emotional support of the patient and the family, with emphasis on avoiding trauma in childhood.

eidetic (aidet′ik), **1.** pertaining to or characterized by the ability to visualize and reproduce accurately the image of objects or events previously seen or imagined. **2.** a person possessing such ability.

eidetic image, an unusually vivid, elaborate, and apparently exact mental image resulting from a visual experience and occurring as either a fantasy, dream, or memory. See also **image.**

eighth nerve. See **acoustic nerve.**

einsteinium (Es), a man-made transuranic metallic element. Its atomic number is 99; its atomic weight is 254. Einsteinium was first found in the debris from a hydrogen bomb explosion.

ejaculate (ɪjæk′yəlɪt), the semen discharged in a single emission. See also **ejaculation.** – **ejaculate,** (ɪjæk′yəleɪt) *v.*

ejaculation, the sudden emission of semen from the male urethra, usually occurring during copulation, masturbation, and nocturnal emission. It is a reflex action in two phases: first, sperm, seminal fluid, and prostatic and bulbourethral gland secretions are moved into the urethra; second, strong spasmodic peristaltic contractions force ejaculation. The sensation of ejaculation is called orgasm. The fluid volume of the ejaculate is usually between 2 and 5 ml; each ml usually contains 50,000,000 to 150,000,000 spermatozoa. – **ejaculatory,** *adj.*

ejaculatory duct, the passage through which semen enters the urethra.

ejection click, sharp clicking sounds from the heart, which may be caused by the sudden swelling of a pulmonary artery, the abrupt dilation of the aorta, or the forceful opening of the aortic cusps. Ejection clicks, often heard during examinations of individuals with septal defects and in cases of patent ductus arteriosis, are associated with high pulmonary resistance and hypertension, but are common and of no clinical significance in pregnant women and in many other healthy people.

ejection murmur. See **systolic murmur.**

Ekbom syndrome (ek′bom). See **restless legs syndrome.**

EKG, abbreviation for **electrocardiogram.**

elaborate, (in endocrinology) a process by which a gland synthesizes a complex substance from simpler substances and secretes it, usually under the stimulation of a tropic hormone from the pituitary gland. This process, regulated by a negative feedback system, serves to maintain homeostasis in body function. – **elaboration,** *n.*

Elase, a trade name for a topical, fixed-combination drug containing enzymes (fibrinolysin and desoxyribonuclease).

Elase with Chloromycetin, a trade name for a topical, fixed-combination drug containing Elase and an antibacterial (chloramphenicol).

elastance, **1.** the quality of recoiling or returning to an original form after the removal of pressure. **2.** the degree to which an air-filled or fluid-filled organ, as a lung, bladder, or blood vessel, can return to its original dimensions when a distending or compressing force is removed. **3.** the measurement of the unit volume of change in such an organ per unit of decreased pressure change. Compare **compliance.**

elastic bandage, a bandage of elasticized fabric that provides support and allows movement.

elastic band fixation, a method of treatment of fractures of the jaw using rubber bands to connect metal splints or wires which are attached to the maxilla and mandible. The rubber bands produce traction and bring the teeth into occlusion and proper alignment while the fracture is healing. Rubber bands are safer than rigid wires in the event of vomiting. See also **maxillomandibular fixation, nasomandibular fixation.**

elastic bougie, a flexible bougie that can be passed through angular or winding channels.

elastic cartilage. See **yellow cartilage.**

elasticity, the ability of tissue to regain its original shape and size after being stretched, squeezed, or otherwise deformed. Muscle tissue is generally regarded as elastic, because it is able to change size and shape and return to its original condition.

Elavil, a trade name for an antidepressant (amitriptyline hydrochloride).

elbow, the bend of the arm at the joint that connects the arm and forearm. Formed by the articulation of the ulna with the humerus, it is a common site of inflammation and disorders, as those incurred during participation in various sports.

elbow bone. See **ulna.**

elbow joint, the hinged articulation of the humerus, the ulna, and the radius. It is covered by a protective capsule associated with three ligaments and an extensive synovial membrane. The elbow joint allows flexion and extension of the forearm and accommodates the radioulnar articulation. Also called **articulatio cubiti.**

elbow reflex. See **triceps reflex.**

Eldopaque, a trade name for a dermatologic bleaching agent (hydroquinone).

elective, of or pertaining to a procedure that is performed by choice but that is not essential, as elective surgery.

elective abortion, induced termination of a pregnancy before the fetus has developed enough to live if born, deemed necessary by the woman carrying it and performed at her request. Commonly (but incorrectly) called **therapeutic abortion.** See also **induced abortion, therapeutic abortion.**

elective induction of labor. See **induction of labor.**

electrical burns, the tissue damage resulting from heat of up to 5000°C generated by an electrical current. The point of contact on the skin is burnt, and the muscle and subcutaneous tissues may be damaged. If the burn is severe, circulatory and respiratory failure may occur and are treated before the burn. Artificial ventilation and cardiac resuscitation are performed as the person is rapidly transported to a medical facility.

electrically stimulated osteogenesis, a bone regeneration process induced by surgically implanted electrodes conveying electrical current, especially at nonunion fracture sites. The process is effective due to the different electrical potentials within bone tissue. Viable nonstressed bone is electronegative in the metaphyseal regions and over a fracture callus and electropositive in the diaphyses and other less active regions. Electrical stimulation of fractures can accelerate osteogenesis, forming bone more quickly in the area of a surgically inserted negative electrode. The precise mechanisms by which electricity induces osteogenesis are not understood, but research shows that when cathodes are implanted at a fracture site and an electrical potential of less than one volt is applied, oxygen is consumed at the cathode and hydroxyl ions are produced, decreasing the oxygen tension of the local tissue and increasing the alkalinity. Low tissue oxygen tension encourages bone formation, which follows a predominantly anaerobic metabolic pathway. Studies of bone-forming junctions demonstrate that an alkaline pH exists in the zone of hypertrophic cells of the bone growth plate when calcification starts. Electrically stimulated osteogenesis can be achieved with a device that stimulates the fracture site electrically by means of several surgically implanted cathodes. Cathode pins are connected to an external power supply that delivers 20 microamperes to each pin. The cathodes are inserted and positioned in the fracture space with the aid of image intensification or other radiographic techniques. Other methods for applying electrical current to fractured bone involve open surgical procedures and the implantation of electrodes. The percutaneous technique involving the insertion of cathode pins is performed with a local anesthetic and usually involves less postoperative pain than open surgery methods. The number and the position of the cathodes in the percutaneous technique vary, depending on the bone involved. Generally two cathodes are used for nonunion fractures of small bones, as the medial malleolus or the carpal navicular. Three or more cathodes are used in the clavicle and the bones of the forearm. Four cathodes are used in the treatment of large bones, as the tibia, the femur, and the humerus. Cathodes are generally inserted from opposite directions into the nonunion site. If four cathodes are used, two are placed above and two below the fracture site, the exposed tips of the cathodes resting directly in the nonunion space. Patients who receive such treatment are routinely released from the hospital the day following the procedure, and the stimulation of their fractures continues during the healing period from a portable power supply strapped to the skin over the fracture site. The osteogenesis is radiographically monitored and, after about 12 weeks, the cathode pins are removed and the affected portion of the limb involved is placed in a weight-bearing cast. Use of the cathode-pin method of electrically stimulated osteogenesis is contraindicated in the treatment of pathological fractures owing to benign or to malignant tumors and in the treatment of congenital conditions, as congenital pseudarthrosis and osteogenesis imperfecta. The cathode-pin method is also contraindicated in the presence of active systemic infections, clinically active osteomyelitis, proven patient sensitivity to the nickel or chromium from which the pins are made, and synovial pseudarthrosis, unless the fluid-filled cavity at the nonunion site is excised before the cathode pins are inserted. The success rate of treatment with the percutaneous method of electrically stimulated osteogenesis is significantly reduced in nonunions in which the gap is wider than one-half the diameter of the bone involved.

electric blood warmer, an electrical device for heating blood before infusions, especially massive transfusions in which cold blood might put the patient into shock. The electric blood warmer includes a receptacle containing an electrical heater and space for the insertion of a disposable blood warming bag composed of parallel plastic tubes. The warmer is also equipped with a temperature indicator which shows when the heating bag reaches the proper temperature of 99°F (37.6°C). An intravenous Y-set is commonly employed in transfusions involving the electric blood warmer. The tubing of the warming bag is primed with normal saline solution. One lead of the warming bag is connected to the primed Y-set; the other lead is connected to the patient. Once the system is primed with normal saline solution, the line conveying the solution is clamped off, and blood is allowed to flow through the warming bag and into the vein of the patient. During transfusion, the electric blood warmer is attached to an I.V. pole or placed on a bedside table at mattress level. Authorities warn that the warming bag must be discarded after one use.

electric cautery. See **electrocautery.**

electric shock, a traumatic physical state caused by the passage of electric current through the body. It usually involves accidental contact with exposed parts of electrical circuits in home appliances and domestic power supplies but may also result from lightning or contact with high-voltage wires. About 1,000 persons in the United States die from electric shock each year. The damage electricity does in passing through the body depends on the intensity of the electrical current, the type of current, and the duration and the frequency of current flow. Alternating current (AC), direct current (DC), and mixed current cause different kinds and degrees of damage in passing through body tissues. High-frequency current produces more heat than low-frequency current and can cause burns, coagulation, and necrosis of affected body parts. Low-frequency current can burn tissues if the area of contact is small and concentrated. Severe electrical shock commonly causes unconsciousness, respiratory paralysis, muscle contractions, bone fractures, and cardiac disorders. Even small electrical currents passing through the heart can cause fibrillation. Treatment of this kind of electric shock commonly involves such measures as cardiopulmonary resuscitation, defibrillation, and the intravenous administration of electrolytes to help stabilize vital functions. See also **cardiogenic shock, hypovolemic shock.**

electric shock therapy (EST). See **electroconvulsive therapy.**

electro-, a combining form meaning 'pertaining to electricity': *electrobiology, electrocatalysis, electrolepsy.*

electroanalytical chemistry, the branch of chemistry concerned with the analysis of compounds using electric current to produce characteristic, observable change in the substance being studied. See also **chemistry.**

electrocardiogram (ECG, EKG), a graphic record produced by an electrocardiograph.

Correctly recorded ECG

Normal waveform

Suprasternal notch
Angle of Louis or sternal angle
Midclavicular line
Second rib
Second interspace
V_1
V_2
V_3
V_4
V_5
V_6

Landmarks for ECG 6 lead placement
ELECTROCARDIOGRAM (ECG)

electrocardiograph (ECG), a device used for recording the electrical activity of the myocardium to detect abnormal transmission of the cardiac impulse through the conductive tissues of the muscle. Electrocardiography allows diagnosis of specific cardiac abnormalities. Leads are affixed to certain anatomic points on the patient's chest, usually with an adhesive gel that promotes transmission of the electrical impulse to the recording device. The patient is positioned supine on an examining table and

asked to lie quietly during the test. — **electrocardiographic,** *adj.*

electrocardiographic-auscultatory syndrome. See **Barlow's syndrome.**

electrocardiograph lead, 1. an electrode placed on part of the body and connected to an electrocardiograph. **2.** a record, made by the electrocardiograph, that varies depending on the site of the electrode. Electrocardiography is generally performed using three peripheral leads and six leads placed on the precordium. The peripheral or extremity leads are designated I, II, and III, and the chest leads are designated V_1, V_2, V_3, V_4, V_5, and V_6 to indicate the points on the precordium on which the electrodes are placed.

electrocautery (ɪlek'trʊkɔ'tǝri), the application of a needle or snare heated by electrical current for the destruction of tissue, as for the removal of warts or polyps. Also called **electric cautery, galvanic cautery, galvanocautery.** See also **diathermy.**

electrocoagulation (ɪlek'trʊkʊæg'yʊleɪ'šhǝn), a therapeutic, destructive form of electrosurgery in which tissue is hardened by the passage of high-frequency current from an electric cautery. Also called **surgical diathermy.** Compare **electrodesiccation.**

electroconvulsive therapy (ECT), the induction of a brief convulsion by passing an electric current through the brain for the treatment of affective disorders, especially in patients resistant to psychoactive drug therapy. The patient is placed in a comfortable supine position with the limbs lightly restrained and with a padded tongue depressor between the back teeth, following premedication with succinylcholine to prevent fractures. Conductive paste is applied to the skin on both sides of the forehead where the electrodes are placed, and a 70 to 130 volt current is delivered for 0.1 to 0.5 of a second. The patient loses consciousness and undergoes tonic contractions for approximately ten seconds, followed by a somewhat longer period of clonic convulsions accompanied by apnea; on awakening the individual has no memory of the shock. ECT is usually administered three times a week for two months and is used primarily for the treatment of acute depression. Also called **electric shock therapy, electroshock therapy.**

electrocution, death caused by the passage of electric current through the body. See also **electric shock.**

electrodermal audiometry, a method of testing hearing in which a harmless electric shock is used to condition the subject to a pure tone; thereafter the tone, coupled with the anticipation of a shock, elicits a brief electrodermal response, which is recorded, and the lowest intensity of the sound producing the skin response is considered the subject's hearing threshold.

electrodesiccation (ɪlek'trʊdes'ɪkeɪ'šhǝn), a technique in electrosurgery in which tissue is destroyed by burning with an electric spark. It is used primarily for eliminating small superficial growths but may be used with curettage for eradicating abnormal tissue deeper in the skin in which case layers of skin may be burnt, then successively scraped away. The procedure is performed under local anesthesia.

electroencephalogram (EEG) (ɪlek'trouensef'ələgræm'), a graphic chart on which is traced the electrical potential produced by the brain cells, as detected by electrodes placed on the scalp. The resulting brain waves are called alpha, beta, delta, and theta rhythms, according to the frequencies they produce, which range from 2 to 12 cycles per second with an amplitude of up to 100 microvolts. Variations in brain-wave activity correlate with neurological conditions, psychological states, and level of consciousness. See also **encephalography.**

electroencephalograph (ɪlek'trouensef'ələgræf'), an instrument for receiving and recording the electrical potential produced by the brain cells. It consists of a vacuum tube amplifier that magnifies the electrical currents received through electrodes placed on the scalp and electromagnetically records the patterns on a graphic chart. See also **electroencephalography.**

electroencephalography (EEG) (ɪlek'trouensef'ələog'-rəfi), the process of recording brain-wave activity. Electrodes are attached to various areas of the patient's head with collodion. During the procedure the patient remains quiet, with eyes closed, and refrains from talking or moving, although, in certain cases, prescribed activities may be requested, especially hyperventilation. The test is used to diagnose seizure disorders, brain stem disorders, focal lesions, and impaired consciousness. During neurosurgery, the electrodes can be applied directly to the surface of the brain (intracranial electroencephalography) or placed within the brain tissue (depth electroencephalography) to detect lesions or tumors. See also **electroencephalogram.** – **electroencephalographic,** *adj.*

electrohemodynamics (EHD), a technique for noninvasively measuring the mechanical properties and hemodynamic characteristics of the vascular system, including arterial blood pressure, electrical impedance, blood flow, and resistance to blood flow.

electroimmunodiffusion. See **immunodiffusion.**

electrolysis, a process in which electrical energy causes a chemical change in a conducting medium, usually a solution or a molten substance. Electrodes, usually pieces of metal, induce the flow of electrical energy through the medium. Electrons enter the solution through the cathode and leave the solution through the anode. Negatively charged ions, or anions, are attracted to the anode; positively charged ions, or cations, are attracted to the cathode. Various conducting mediums are used, as solutions of copper, zinc, nickel, lead, and silver. Electrical energy passing through such solutions causes deposition of pure metal at the cathode. Passing electrical energy through solutions of alkali and alkaline-earth salts liberates hydrogen at the cathode. A metal anode causes metal ions to flow from the anode into the solution as the electrical current passes through the medium. An inert electrode, as one of platinum, may liberate an element, as oxygen, at the anode in an aqueous medium. A halogen salt solution liberates free bromine, chlorine, or iodine. Fluorine, which has a high oxidation potential, is not liberated by electrolysis. – **electrolytic,** *adj.*

Normal electrolyte content of body fluids*

Electrolytes (anions and cations)	Extracellular		Intracellular (mEq/liter)
	Intravascular (mEq/liter)	Interstitial (mEq/liter)	
Sodium (Na^+)	142	146	15
Potassium (K^+)	5	5	150
Calcium (Ca^{++})	5	3	2
Magnesium (Mg^{++})	2	1	27
Chloride (Cl^-)	102	114	1
Bicarbonate (HCO_3^-)	27	30	10
Protein ($Prot^-$)	16	1	63
Phosphate (HPO_4^-)	2	2	100
Sulfate (SO_4^-)	1	1	20
Organic acids	5	8	0

*The electrolyte level of the intravascular and interstitial fluids (extracellular) is approximately the same and sodium and chloride contents are markedly higher in these fluids, whereas potassium, phosphate, and protein contents are markedly higher in intracellular fluid.

electrolyte, an element or compound that, when melted or dissolved in water or other solvent, dissociates into ions and is able to conduct an electric current. Electrolytes differ in their concentrations in blood plasma, interstitial fluid, and cell fluid and affect the movement of substances between those compartments. Proper quantities of principal electrolytes and balance among them are critical to normal metabolism and function. For example, calcium (Ca^{++}) is necessary for the relaxation of skeletal muscle and contraction of cardiac muscle; potassium (K^+) is required for the contraction of skeletal muscle and relaxation of cardiac muscle. Sodium (Na^+) is essential in maintaining fluid balance. Certain diseases, conditions, and medications may lead to a deficiency of one or more electrolytes and to an imbalance among them, as certain diuretics and a low-sodium diet prescribed in hypertension may cause hypokalemic shock owing to a loss of potassium. Diarrhea may cause a loss of many electrolytes, leading to hypovolemia and shock, especially in infants. Careful and regular monitoring of electrolytes and intravenous replacement of fluid and electrolytes is part of the acute care in many illnesses. – **electrolytic,** *adj.*

electrolyte balance, the equilibrium between electrolytes in the body.

(See next page for table)

Fluid and electrolyte imbalances*

Imbalance	Clinical signs and symptoms	Therapy	Anticipate in
Dehydration	Thirst, anxiety, weight loss, poor skin turgor, slow vein filling, elevated temperature, tachycardia, dry mucous membranes, decreased level of consciousness, increased hematocrit, increased BUN, increased RBC concentration	Volume replacement	Any condition in which water output exceeds intake; vomiting, diarrhea
Edema	Weight gain exceeding 5%; rales; dyspnea; puffy eyelids, swollen ankles, bounding pulse	Salt-poor albumin, exchange resins, diuretics	Protein deficiency, venous obstruction, heart failure, obstructed lymphatics, toxin ingestion, liver disease, renal disease
Third space syndrome	Hypotension, tachycardia, peripheral vasoconstriction, oliguria, no weight loss, increased hematocrit with no evidence of fluid loss	Plasma, salts, water replacement, diuretics, paracentesis, thoracentesis	Ascites, cellulitis, crush injuries, vascular occlusion, intestinal obstructions
Hypokalemia	Weakness, flaccidity; diminished reflexes; weak pulse, hypotension; ECG changes—increased P wave amplitude, flat or inverted T waves, **ST** segment depression, prominent U wave, prolonged PR interval; dyspnea; nausea, vomiting; mental depression	Oral or IV potassium therapy	Long-term diuresis (i.e., thiazides), vomiting, diarrhea, draining fistulas, heat stroke, diabetic acidosis, alcoholism, malnutrition
Hyperkalemia	Muscle cramps; nausea, diarrhea, vomiting; weakness; hyperactivity; dizziness; paresthesias; ECG changes—early, high-peaked T waves, ST segment depressed, P wave disappears, later QRS widens, T waves taller, premature ectopic beat; escape beats, ventricular flutter, fibrillation, and standstill	$NaHCO_3$, mEq IV over 5 min; may repeat in 10 min NaCl: IV Calcium gluconate: 0.5 ml/kg of 10% solution over 2-4 min (do not give in central line) Infuse D/50 over 30-60 min with insulin Exchange resins: Kayexalate 20-50 gm in 100-200 ml of 20% sorbitol orally (repeat every 3-4 hr) or 50 mg with 50 gm sorbitol and 200 ml water as retention enema over 30-60 min Steroids Peritoneal dialysis or hemodialysis Glucose-insulin infusion: 2-4 gm glucose and 20-30 units insulin IV in 200-700 ml D/20/W over 30-60 min; or 1000 ml D/10/W with 90 mEq $NaHCO_3$ (infuse 300 ml over 30 min and remainder over 2-3 hr; give 25 units regular insulin SC at beginning of infusion)	Adrenal cortical insufficiency, acidosis, burns or other major tissue trauma, renal failure; overshooting IV or oral potassium
Hypocalcemia	Abdominal and muscle cramps, tetany, tingling of fingers and circumoral area, hyperactive reflexes, impaired mental functioning, laryngeal stridor, local or generalized seizures, ECG changes: prolonged QT interval caused by lengthened ST segment	IV calcium: 20-30 ml of 10% calcium gluconate IV over 10-15 min	Infections, burns, diarrhea, excessive use of citrated blood, pancreatitis, parathyroid malfunction
Hypomagnesemia	Positive Chvostek's sign, hyperactive reflexes, coarse tremors, seizures, disorientation, gait disturbances, choreiform or athetoid movements, stupor	Magnesium sulfate: 2 mEq/kg body weight IV over 4 hr at rate not exceeding 150 mg/min	Vomiting, diarrhea, enterostomal drainage, cirrhosis, diuretic therapy, delirium tremens
Hyponatremia	Heat cramps; general weakness and fatigue; decreased cardiac output; hypotension; fainting; lip and nailbed cyanosis; cool, clammy skin; scant urine output; elevated intracranial pressure with headache, confusion, agitation; seizures; coma	Hypertonic saline (do not give more than 300 ml in 4 hr; monitor plasma chloride and bicarbonate levels cautiously)	Salt deficit, cirrhosis, diabetic ketoacidosis, heart failure, hormonal disturbances, (e.g., ADH, ACTH), poorly managed diuretic therapy; diarrhea, perspiration

continued.

Fluid and electrolyte imbalances*—cont'd

Imbalance	Clinical signs and symptoms	Therapy	Anticipate in
Hypernatremia	Irritability, lethargy, coma, seizures, delirium, weakness, signs and symptoms of dehydration, high-pitched cry in infants	Balanced IV solution	Perspiration, fever, failure of thirst mechanism, inadequate water intake with high-protein feedings

*Unilateral contraction of facial muscle on facial nerve percussion (anterior to ear).

electrolyte solution, any solution containing electrolytes prepared for oral, parenteral, or rectal administration for the replacement or supplementation of ions necessary for homeostasis. The loss of potassium ion (K^+) by vomiting, diarrhea, or by the action of certain medications, including diuretics and corticosteroids, may be corrected by administering a solution high in potassium. Other electrolyte solutions containing combinations of calcium, sodium, phosphate, chloride, or magnesium may be given to treat acid-base disturbance, as seen in chronic renal dysfunction or diabetic ketoacidosis. The solutions are available in a wide range of balanced formulas for replacement or maintenance, and most include various trace minerals.

electromagnetic radiation, every kind of electrical and magnetic radiation, regarded as a continuous spectrum of energy that includes energy with the shortest wavelength (gamma rays, with a wavelength of 0.0011 angstrom) to that with the longest wavelength (long radio waves, with a wavelength of more than one million kilometers). The visible part of the electromagnetic spectrum is between 3,800 and 7,600 angstrom. Ultraviolet radiation occurs beyond the short-wave (violet) end of the visible spectrum, having a wavelength of less than 4,000 angstrom; x rays have a much shorter wavelength (from 0.05 to a few hundred angstrom). Infrared radiation occurs just beyond the longer-wave end of the visible spectrum, having a wavelength of 7,000 angstrom or more.

electromyogram (EMG) (ılek'troumaɪ'əgræm), a record of the intrinsic electrical activity in a skeletal muscle. Such data help in diagnosing neuromuscular problems and are obtained by applying surface electrodes or by inserting a needle electrode into the muscle and observing electrical activity with an oscilloscope and a loudspeaker. Some electromyograms show abnormalities, as spontaneous electrical potentials within the muscle under study, and help to pinpoint lesions of motor nerves. Electromyograms also measure electrical potentials induced by voluntary muscular contraction. See also **electroneuromyography.**

electron, 1. a negatively charged elementary particle that has a specific charge, mass, and spin. The number of electrons circling the nucleus of an atom is equal to the atomic number of the substance. Electrons may be shared or exchanged by two atoms; after the exchange the atom becomes an ion. 2. a negative beta particle emitted from a radioactive substance. See also **atom, element, ion, proton, neutron.**

electronarcosis (ılek'trounarkou'sıs), general anesthesia without the use of anesthetic gases or drugs. Narcosis is produced by passing an electric current through the brain, but adequate control and prevention of undesirable side effects, especially convulsions, remain a problem. The procedure is experimental.

electroneuromyography (ılek'trounʊr'oumaɪog'rəfi), a procedure for testing and recording neuromuscular activity by the electrical stimulation of nerves. The procedure involves the insertion of needle electrodes into any skeletal muscle being studied, applying electrical current to the electrodes, and observing and recording neuromuscular functions by means of instruments, as a cathode-ray oscilloscope and an appropriate recording device. The procedure helps in studying neuromuscular conduction, the extent of nerve lesions, and reflex responses. See also **electromyogram.**

electronic fetal monitor (EFM), a device that allows observation of the fetal heart rate and the maternal uterine contractions. It may be applied externally, in which case the fetal heart is detected by an ultrasound transducer on the abdomen and the uterine contractions by a pressure sensor applied to the abdomen. Internal monitoring of the fetal heart rate is accomplished via an electrode clipped to the fetal scalp; the amplitude, frequency, and duration of the uterine contractions are detected by the use of an intrauterine catheter.

electronic thermometer, a thermometer that registers temperature rapidly by electronic means.

electron microscope, an instrument, similar to an optical microscope, that scans cell surfaces with a beam of electrons, instead of visible light, creating an image that can be photographed or viewed on a fluorescent screen. Used to study very thin sections of tissue, the electron microscope has resolution and magnification 1,000 times greater than those of an optical microscope. Compare **scanning electron microscope.**

electron microscopy, a technique, using an electron miscroscope, in which a beam of electrons is focused by an electromagnetic lens and directed onto an extremely thin specimen. The electrons emerging are focused and directed by a second lens onto a fluorescent screen. The image produced is highly magnified and well resolved, but it is two-dimensional owing to the thinness of the specimen. Also called **transmission electron microscopy.** Compare **scanning electron microscopy, scanning transmission electron microscopy.**

electron scanning microscope. See **scanning electron microscope.**

electronystagmography (ɪlek′trouns′tægmog′rəfi), a method of assessing and recording eye movements by measuring the electrical activity of the extraocular muscles. See also **electroencephalogram, nystagmus.**

electrophoresis (ɪlek′troufəri′sɪs), the movement of charged suspended particles through a liquid medium in response to changes in an electric field. Charged particles of a given substance migrate in a predictable direction and at a characteristic speed. The pattern of migration can be recorded in bands on an electrophoretogram. The technique is widely used to separate and identify serum proteins and other biological substances. — **electrophoretic,** adj.

electrophoretogram (ɪlek′troufəret′ougræm). See **electrophoresis.**

electroshock therapy. See **electroconvulsive therapy.**

electrosleep therapy, a technique designed to induce sleep, especially in psychiatric patients, by administering a low amplitude pulsating current to the brain. The cathode is placed supraorbitally, and the anode is placed over the mastoid process; the current, which is discharged for 15 to 20 minutes, produces a tingling sensation, but not always sleep. The procedure, introduced by Soviet investigators, is repeated from five to 30 times. Electrosleep therapy is said to be beneficial for patients with anxiety, depression, gastric distress, insomnia, personality disorders, and schizophrenia, but double-blind studies have yielded contradictory results.

electrosurgery, surgery performed with various electrical instruments that operate on high-frequency electric current. Kinds of electrosurgery include **electrocoagulation, electrodesiccation, fulguration.**

electrotonic current, a current induced in a nerve sheath by an action potential within the nerve or an adjacent nerve.

element, one of more than 100 primary, simple substances that cannot be broken down by chemical means into any other substance. Each atom of any element contains a specific number of electrons orbiting the nucleus. The nucleus contains a variable number of neutrons. A **stable element** contains an equal number of neutrons and electrons and does not easily give up neutrons. A **radioactive element** does not contain a balanced number of electrons and neutrons, giving off neutrons readily. See also **atom, compound, molecule.**

element 104, a manmade, radioactive element, the twelfth transuranic element, as yet unnamed, and the first beyond the actinide series.

element 105, a manmade element, as yet unnamed; the thirteenth transuranic element.

eleo-, a combining form meaning 'pertaining to oil': *eleoma, eleomyenchysis, eleopten.* Also **oleo-.**

elephantiasis (el′əfəntai′əsɪs), the end-stage lesion of filariasis, characterized by tremendous swelling, usually of the external genitalia and the legs. The overlying skin becomes dark, thick, and coarse. Elephantiasis results from filiariasis that has lasted for many years. See also **filariasis.**

elephantoid fever. See **elephantiasis, filariasis.**

eleventh nerve. See **accessory nerve.**

elimination diet, a procedure for identifying a food or foods to which a person is allergic by successively omitting from the diet certain foods in order to detect those responsible for the symptoms.

elixir, a clear liquid containing water, alcohol, sweeteners, and flavors, used primarily as a vehicle for the oral administration of a drug.

Elixophyllin, a trade name for a smooth muscle relaxant (theophylline), used as a bronchodilator.

Elliot forceps. See **obstetric forceps.**

Elliot's position, a supine posture assumed by the patient on the operating table, with a support placed under the lower costal margin to elevate the chest. The position is used in gall bladder surgery.

elliptocytosis (ɪlɪp′tousaitou′sɪs), a mild abnormal condition of the blood that is characterized by increased numbers of elliptical or oval erythrocytes. Less than 15 per cent of the red cells appear in this form in normal blood; modest increases occur in a variety of anemias, including a rare congenital disorder, hereditary elliptocytosis, which may or may not be associated with a mild hemolytic anemia. Also called **ovalocytosis.** See also **acanthocytosis, congenital nonspherocytic hemolytic anemia, hereditary spherocytosis, sickle cell anemia.**

elope, *Informal.* to leave a locked psychiatric institution without notice or permission.

Elspar, a trade name for an antineoplastic (asparaginase).

em-, a combining form meaning 'in, on': *embolism, empasma, emphysis.* Also **en-.**

emaciation (ɪmei′shiei′shən), excessive leanness caused by disease or lack of nutrition.

Embden-Meyerhof pathway (emb′denmai′ərhof), a sequence of enzymatic reactions in the anaerobic conversion of glucose to lactic acid, producing energy in the form of adenosine triphosphate.

embolectomy, a surgical incision into an artery for the removal of an embolus or clot, performed as emergency treatment for arterial embolism. The operation is done within 4 to 6 hours of the onset of pain, if possible. Thrombi tend to lodge at the juncture of major arteries when the thrombi have broken away from a thrombophlebitis; more than half lodge in the aorta, in arteries of the lower extremities, in the common carotid arteries, or in the pulmonary arteries. Preoperatively, anticoagulants are administered, and an arteriogram is done to identify the affected artery. Under general anesthesia, a longitudinal incision is made in the artery, and the embolus is removed. Postoperatively, the blood pressure is maintained close to the level of the preoperative baseline, as a decrease might predispose to new clot formation. A frequent complication of the procedure is hemorrhage from small arteries that may have been clogged with the embolus but overlooked while tying larger bleeding vessels.

embolism, an abnormal circulatory condition in which an embolus travels through the bloodstream and becomes lodged in a blood vessel. The symptoms vary with the degree of occlusion that the embolism causes, the character of the embolus, and the size, nature, and location of the occluded vessel. Kinds of embolism include **air embolism, fat embolism.**

embolus, *pl.* **emboli.** a foreign object, a quantity of air or gas, a bit of tissue or tumor, or a piece of a thrombus that circulates in the bloodstream until it becomes lodged in a vessel. Kinds of emboli include **air embolus, fat embolus.** – **embolic, emboloid,** *adj.*

embryatrics (em'briæt'rɪks). See **fetology.**

embryectomy (em'briek'təmi), the surgical removal of an embryo, most commonly in an ectopic pregnancy.

embryo (em'briou), **1.** any organism in the earliest stages of development. **2.** in man, the stage of prenatal development between the time of implantation of the fertilized ovum about two weeks after conception until the end of the seventh or eighth week. The period is characterized by rapid growth, differentiation of the major organ systems, and development of the main external features. Compare **fetus, zygote.** – **embryonal, embryonoid, embryonic,** *adj.*

-embryo, a combining form meaning a 'fetus': *embryo, typembryo.*

embryoctony (em'briok'təni), the intentional destruction of the living embryo or fetus in utero. Also called **feticide.** See also **abortion.**

embryogenesis (em'brioujen'əsɪs), the process in sexual reproduction in which an embryo forms from the fertilization of an ovum. Also called **embryogeny.** See also **heterogenesis, homogenesis.** – **embryogenetic, embryogenic.** *adj.*

embryogeny (em'brioj'ini). See **embryogenesis.**

embryologic development, the various intrauterine stages and processes involved in the growth and differentiation of the conceptus from the time of fertilization of the ovum until the eighth week of gestation. The stages

are related to the biological status of the unborn child and are divided into two distinct periods. The first is embryogenesis, or the formation of the embryo, which occurs during the 10 days to two weeks following fertilization until implantation. The second period, organogenesis, involves the differentiation of the various cells, tissues, and organ systems and the development of the main external features of the embryo; it occurs from approximately the end of the second week through the eighth week of intrauterine life. The fetal stage follows these stages, beginning at about the ninth week of gestation. The entire process of the growth and development of the embryo and fetus is loosely called prenatal development. Embryogenesis is initiated shortly after fertilization by the formation of the zygote from the fusion of the pronuclei of the spermatozoon and the ovum. The zygote then divides by cleavage to form blastomeres, which eventually cluster into a solid mass of cells, called the morula, that are uniform in size, shape, and physiological capabilities. With continued division the cells become unequal in size and shape, and fluid accumulates between them to produce the blastocyst. This hollow ball of cells consists of an outer layer, the trophoblast, and a localized inner cluster, the inner cell mass, which protrudes into the cavity. The inner cell mass contains two formative layers that differentiate into the primary germ layers and develop into the embryo. The trophoblastic cells contain the enzymes and other substances necessary for the implantation of the blastocyst onto the uterine wall and the formation of the extraembryonic structures, as the chorion and the placenta. By the time of implantation and the beginning of organogenesis, the endoderm, ectoderm, and mesoderm germ layers have differentiated into the embryonic disc and have formed the amniotic cavity and yolk sac cavity. During this stage the embryo develops rapidly, changing from a flat, disclike shape into an elongated, cylindrical, curved mass that contains the primitive structures that will subsequently differentiate into all the organs and cavities of the body. By the fourth week of development the primitive body includes the neural tube, which will develop into the brain, spinal cord, and other neural tissue of the central nervous system; the notochord, which will be replaced by the vertebral column; the somites, which will segment into skeletal and muscle tissue; the nephrotomes, which will form the urogenital system; the gut, which will differentiate into the digestive and respiratory systems; the coelom, which will subdivide into separate cavities for the heart, lungs, and abdominal viscera; and the primitive heart and tiny spaces within the mesoderm that will become the vessels of the circulatory and lymphatic systems. At eight weeks of development, major differentiation of all the organs has occurred, and the main external features, as the eyes, ears, nose, mouth, and digits, are recognizable. The embryo is now remarkably humanlike in appearance and at this stage is called a fetus. For the remaining seven months of intrauterine life the primary changes in the fetus are growth, further tissue differentiation, elaboration of structural detail, and specialization of organs and systems. See also **prenatal development.**

embryologist, one who specializes in the study of embryology.

embryology (em'briol'əji), the study of the origin, growth, development, and function of an organism from fertilization to birth. Kinds of embryology include **comparative embryology, descriptive embryology, experimental embryology.** — **embryologic, embryological,** adj.

embryomorph (em'briəmorf'), any structure that resembles an embryo, especially a mass of tissue that may represent an aborted conceptus. — **embryomorphous,** adj.

embryonal adenomyosarcoma. See **Wilms' tumor.**

embryonal adenosarcoma. See **Wilms' tumor.** Also called **embryonal adenomyosarcoma.**

embryonal carcinoma, an extremely malignant neoplasm derived from germinal cells that usually develops in gonads, especially the testes. The tumor, a firm, nodular mass with many hemorrhagic areas, is characterized histologically by large, undifferentiated cells with indistinct borders, eosinophilic cytoplasm, and prominent nucleoli in pleomorphic nuclei. Bodies resembling a one- or two-week-old embryo are occasionally seen in these tumors. The neoplasm is relatively resistant to radiation therapy, and, early in its development, it metastasizes by way of lymph channels. Surgery and chemotherapy are usually included in the treatment. See also **choriocarcinoma.**

embryonal leukemia. See **stem cell leukemia.**

embryonate (em'briəneit'), **1.** impregnated; containing an embryo. **2.** of, pertaining to, or resembling an embryo.

embryonic abortion, 1. termination of pregnancy before the twentieth week of gestation. **2.** expelled products of conception before the twentieth week. Compare **fetal abortion.**

embryonic anideus. See **anideus.**

embryonic blastoderm, the area of the blastoderm that gives rise to the primitive streak from which the embryonic body develops. Compare **extraembryonic blastoderm.**

embryonic competence, the ability of an embryonic cell to react normally to the stimulation of an inductor allowing continued, normal growth or differentiation of the embryo.

embryonic disc, the thickened plate from which the embryo develops in the second week of pregnancy. Scattered cells from the border of the disc migrate to the space between the trophoblast and yolk sac and become the embryonic mesoderm. The disc develops from the ectoderm and endoderm. Also called **germ disc.**

embryonic layer, one of the three layers of cells in the embryo, the endoderm, the mesoderm, and the ectoderm.

From these layers of cells arise all of the structures and organs and parts of the body. The endoderm is the first to develop, followed by the ectoderm. During the third week of gestation the mesoderm arises between the ectoderm and the endoderm.

embryonic stage, (in embryology) the interval of time from the end of the germinal stage, at 10 days of gestation, to the end of the seventh week.

embryoniform (em'brion'ıform), resembling an embryo.

embryopathy (em'briop'əthi), any anomaly occurring in the embryo or fetus as a result of interference with normal intrauterine development. A kind of embryopathy is **rubella embryopathy.**

embryoplastic (em'briouplæs'tık), of or pertaining to the formation of an embryo, usually used with reference to cells.

embryotome (em'briətoum'), an instrument used in embryotomy.

embryotomy (em'briot'əmi), **1.** the dismemberment or mutilation of a fetus for removal from the uterus when normal delivery is not possible. **2.** the dissection of an embryo for examination and analysis.

embryotroph (em'briətrof), **embryotrophe** (em'-briətrouf), the liquefied uterine nutritive material, composed of glandular secretions and degenerative tissue, that nourishes the mammalian embryo until placental circulation is established. Also called **histotroph, histotrophic nutrition.** Compare **hemotroph.**

embryotrophy (em'briot'rəfi), the nourishment of the embryo. See also **embryotroph, hemotroph.** — **embryotrophic,** adj.

embryulcia (em'briəl'siə), the surgical removal of the embryo or fetus from the uterus.

emergence, a stage in the process of recovery from general anesthesia that includes spontaneous respiration, voluntary swallowing, and consciousness. See also **postoperative care.**

emergency, a serious situation that arises suddenly and threatens the life or welfare of a person or a group of people, as a natural disaster or a medical crisis.

emergency childbirth, a birth that occurs accidentally or precipitously in or out of the hospital, without standard obstetric preparations and procedures. Signs and symptoms of impending delivery include increased bloody show, frequent strong contractions, a desire on the part of the mother to bear down forcibly or her report that she feels like she is going to defecate, visible bulging of the bag of waters, or crowning of the baby's head at the vaginal introitus.

■ METHOD: If time permits, equipment is readied, but the delivery is not delayed for such preparations. Useful equipment includes sterile gloves, towels, bulb syringe, receiving blankets, scissors, two Kelly clamps, cord clamp or tie, and a basin for the placenta. The mother's vital signs are taken, and her baby's heart tones are listened to if time permits and if equipment is available. The mother is reassured that emergency deliveries are usually simple, and that all procedures and events will be explained. Despite her compelling urge to push and to deliver quickly, the mother is encouraged to ease the baby out slowly by not pushing and by blowing air forcibly out through pursed lips as she feels the strength of the urge building. As the head emerges it is supported but allowed to rotate naturally. A check is made immediately to determine whether or not the umbilical cord is wound around the neck. If it is, a gentle attempt is made to slip it over the baby's head; if it is too tight it is immediately clamped with two Kelly clamps placed two or three inches apart, cut between the clamps, and unwound from the neck. If the baby does not deliver immediately, mucus and fluid in the nose and the mouth are sucked out using a bulb syringe. The shoulders are delivered one at a time by guiding the head downward to deliver the anterior (upper) shoulder under the symphysis pubis, and then upward to deliver the posterior (lower) shoulder over the perineum. The rest of the baby is quickly born. If the membranes of the amniotic sac are intact, the sac is snipped or torn behind the baby's neck and peeled away from the face so the baby can breathe. If necessary, the nares, nasopharynx, and mouth may be suctioned with the bulb syringe, taking care not to slow the heart rate by stimulating the vagus nerve with the tip of the syringe on the back of the throat. The baby is kept warm and held with the head lower than the chest; it may be laid skin-to-skin on the mother's abdomen. The baby may thus be positioned, observed, and warmed in one place as the nurse or other helper covers mother and baby with a dry blanket or towel and continues to provide emergency care as necessary through the third stage of labor. There is no urgent need to cut the cord or to deliver the placenta. When desired, the cord may be cut by clamping it in two places several inches from the baby and cutting it between the clamps with sterile scissors. The cord clamp may be put on later. If possible, an Apgar score is assigned first at five minutes of age, then at ten. The placenta is ready to be delivered when the cord is seen to advance a few inches, the uterus becomes firmer and rises in the abdomen, and a small gush of bright red blood is seen coming from the vagina. The mother may help to expel it by bearing down. The placenta is lifted out of the vagina slowly, with care, so that all of the membranes are brought out with it. The placenta and membranes are kept for further evaluation. The uterus is massaged to ensure that it is well contracted, and the baby is put to breast if the mother wishes. The uterus is frequently palpated, and it is massaged when necessary. The baby is kept with the mother and observed for warmth, color, activity, and respiration. Following delivery of the placenta the perianal area is rinsed with warm sterile water and dried with a clean towel or cloth, and an ice pack and a sanitary pad or small towel are applied in such a way that the mother can hold them in place by bringing her legs together.

■ OUTCOME CRITERIA: Almost all births are normal and do not constitute true medical emergencies. If a mother is healthy and is not bleeding, if her vital signs are normal, and if the baby's heart tones are normal, there is no immediate cause for alarm, even if the birth is imminent. Emergency care is directed toward assuring that the baby breathes well and is kept warm, that the mother is protected from hemorrhage, and that her privacy is maintained. The nurse is likely to be the person who must initially evaluate the situation and decide whether to attempt to transfer or transport the mother or to prepare for emergency delivery. If a mother says the baby is coming, the attendant is advised to believe her and to act accordingly. Throughout the delivery and the third stage of labor, the nurse works to help the mother to feel calm, confident, and well cared for.

emergency department, (in a health care facility) a section of an institution that is staffed and equipped to provide rapid and varied emergency care, especially for those stricken with sudden and acute illness or those who are the victims of severe trauma.

Emergency Department Nurses' Association (EDNA), a national professional organization of emergency department nurses that defines and promotes emergency nursing practice. The Association, which was founded in 1970 and has more than 11,000 members, has written and implemented the Standards of Emergency Nursing Practice. The Association offers a certification examination and awards the designation Certified Emergency Nurse (CEN) to nurses who successfully complete it. EDNA publishes the *Journal of Emergency Nursing (JEN)* and *Continuing Education Core Curriculum of Emergency Nursing Practice.* The Association, which has its headquarters in Chicago, Illinois, works closely with its members and with related associations to define practice and to prepare professionals to practice in the area of emergency care.

emergency doctrine, (in law) a doctrine that assumes a person's consent to medical treatment when the person is in imminent danger and unable to give informed consent to treatment. Emergency doctrine assumes that the person would consent if able to do so.

Emergency Medical Service (EMS), a network of services coordinated to provide aid and medical assistance from primary response to definitive care, involving personnel trained in the rescue, stabilization, transportation, and advanced treatment of traumatic or medical emergencies. Linked by a communications system that operates on both a local and regional level, EMS is a tiered system of care which is usually initiated by citizen action in the form of a telephone call to an emergency number. Subsequent stages include the first medical responder, ambulance personnel, medium and heavy rescue equipment, and paramedic units, if necessary, continuing in the hospital with emergency room nurses, emergency room doctors, specialists, and critical care nurses and physicians. See also **emergency medical technician, emergency medical technician-advanced life support, emergency medical technician-intravenous, emergency medical technician-paramedic.**

Emergency Medical Technician-Advanced Life Support (EMT-ALS),   a third-level EMT. The EMT-ALS is certified in all the skills of the basic-level EMT and EMT-IV. Additionally, the EMT-ALS may administer certain medications following the orders of the hospital physician, with whom radio contact is maintained. An EMT-ALS is also trained in the use of advanced life support systems, including electrical defibrillation equipment. Compare **emergency medical technician, emergency medical technician-intravenous, emergency medical technician-paramedic.**

Emergency Medical Technician (EMT),   a person trained in and responsible for the administration of specialized emergency care and the transportation to a medical facility of victims of acute illness or injury. In addition to basic life support skills, the EMT is trained in extrication and disentanglement, operation of emergency vehicles, basic anatomy, basic assessment of injury or illness, triage, care for specific injuries and illnesses, environmental emergencies, childbirth, and transport of the patient. EMTs undergo ongoing training in new procedures and must qualify for recertification every two years. Kinds of EMTs are **emergency medical technician-advanced life support, emergency medical technician-intravenous, emergency medical technician-paramedic.** See also **emergency medical services.**

Emergency Medical Technician-Intravenous (EMT-I.V.),   a second-level emergency medical technician. The EMT-IV is trained and certified in intravenous therapy, endotracheal intubation, and the use of medical antishock trousers (MAST). Compare **emergency medical technician, emergency medical technician-advanced life support, emergency medical technician-paramedic.**

Emergency Medical Technician-Paramedic (EMT-P),   an advanced-level emergency medical technician. The EMT-P is certified in all the skills of EMTs of other levels, with additional training in pharmacology and the administration of emergency drugs. Compare **emergency medical technician, emergency medical technician-advanced life support, emergency medical technician-intravenous.**

emergency medicine,   a branch of medicine concerned with the diagnosis and treatment of conditions resulting from trauma or sudden illness. The patient's condition is stabilized, and care of the patient is transferred to the primary physician or to a specialist. Emergency medicine requires a broad interdisciplinary training in the physiology and pathology of all of the systems of the body.

emergency nursing,   nursing care provided to prevent imminent severe damage or death or to avert serious injury. Activities that exemplify emergency nursing are basic life support, cardiopulmonary resuscitation, and control of hemorrhage.

emergency room (E.R., ER),   a hospital area specially designed to receive and initially treat patients suffering from sudden trauma or medical problems, as accidental hemorrhage, poisoning, fracture, heart attack, and respiratory failure.

emergency theory,   (in physiology) a theory stating that when a person is faced with an emergency the adrenal medulla is stimulated by the sympathetic nervous system to release epinephrine which increases heart rate, raises blood pressure, reduces blood flow to viscera, and mobilizes blood glucose, preparing the body for flight from danger or for the fight to survive. See also **flight or fight reaction.**

emergent evolution,   the theory that evolution occurs in a series of major changes at certain critical stages and results from the total rearrangement of existing elements so that completely new and unpredictable characteristics appear within the species. See also **saltatory evolution.**

emesis (em′ɪsɪs).   See **vomit.**

Emete-con,   a trade name for an antiemetic (benzquinamide hydrochloride), used after anesthesia.

emetic (ɪmet′ɪk),   1. of or pertaining to a substance that causes vomiting. 2. an emetic agent. Apomorphine hydrochloride, acting through the central nervous system, induces vomiting 10 to 15 minutes after parenteral administration. Syrup of ipecac is used in the emergency treatment of drug overdosage and in certain cases of poisoning, but it can be cardiotoxic if it is absorbed and not vomited.

-emetic,   a combining form meaning 'pertaining to vomiting': *antiemetic, hematemetic, hyperemetic.* Also **-emetical.**

emetine hydrochloride,   a potent, parenteral antiamebic.

■ INDICATIONS: It is prescribed in the treatment of acute fulminating amebic dysentery, amebic abscesses, and amebic hepatitis.

■ CONTRAINDICATIONS: Previous emetine therapy within six to eight weeks, heart disease, polyneuropathy, kidney disease, or known hypersensitivity to this drug prohibits its use.

■ ADVERSE EFFECTS: Among the more serious adverse reactions are cardiovascular irregularities, hypotension, and neuromuscular effects.

Emetrol, a trade name for a fixed-combination drug containing fructose, glucose, and phosphoric acid, used to treat nausea and vomiting.

EMG, abbreviation for **electromyogram.**

EMG syndrome, a hereditary disorder transmitted as an autosomal recessive trait. Clinical manifestations include exophthalmos, macroglossia, and gigantism, often accompanied by visceromegaly, dysplasia of the renal medulla, and enlargement of the cells of the adrenal cortex. Also called **Beckwith-Wiedemann syndrome, exophthalmos-macroglossia-gigantism syndrome.**

EMI, abbreviation for *Electric and Musical Industries,* the British manufacturer of the first scanner produced for computerized axial tomography (CAT).

EMI scan. See **computerized axial tomography.**

-emia, -aemia, 1. a combining form meaning a '(specified) blood condition': *hypokinemia, panhyperemia, pyknemia.* **2.** a combining form meaning a 'blood condition involving a (specified) substance': *calcemia, iodemia, melitemia.* Also **-hemia, -haemia.**

emissary veins, the small vessels in the skull that connect the sinuses of the dura with the veins on the exterior of the skull through a series of anastomoses. The major emissary veins are the mastoid emissary vein, the parietal emissary vein, the internal carotid plexus, the rete canalis hypoglossi, the condyloid emissary vein, the rete foraminis ovalis, and the small veins passing through the foramen lacerum to connect the cavernous sinus with the pterygoid plexus. Also included in the emissary group is a vein passing through the foramen cecum, connecting the superior sagittal sinus with the veins of the nasal cavity.

Emivan, a trade name for an analeptic agent (ethamivan).

emmetropia, a state of normal vision characterized by the proper relationship between the refractive system of the eyeball and its axial length. This correlation assures that light rays entering the eye parallel to the optic axis are focused exactly on the retina. Compare **amblyopia, hypermetropia, myopia. – emmetropic,** *adj.*

emollient (ımol′yənt), a substance that softens tissue, particularly the skin and mucous membranes.

emollient bath, a bath taken in water containing an emollient, as bran, to relieve irritation and inflammation. See also **colloid bath.**

emotion, the affective aspect of consciousness as compared to volition and cognition. Physiologic alterations often occur with a marked change of emotion regardless of whether the feelings are conscious or unconscious, expressed or unexpressed. See also **emotional need, emotional response.**

emotional amalgam, an unconscious effort to deny or counteract anxiety.

emotional care of the dying patient, the compassionate, consistent support offered to help the terminally ill patient and the family cope with impending death. See also **stages of dying.**

■ METHOD: The professional person providing emotional support for the terminally ill encourages the expression of personal feelings, anxieties, and experiences regarding death, and empathizes with the patient and the family. The patient needs gentle, realistic care but all questions do not require answers, and the decision to tell the prognosis rests with the physician and family. To avoid conflicting statements, it is essential to know what the physician, other professionals, and family members tell the patient about the outcome. The terminally ill person may not express fear if it is sensed that others are unable to talk about dying. Effective support in terminal illness involves a nonjudgmental approach to the patient's relatives, an understanding of their problems, and efforts to assist them in the grieving process. The patient needs relief from pain, tender care, and continued attention through all the stages of dying: characteristically, a period of denial, followed by anger, bargaining, depression, and, finally, by acceptance. When the patient denies the prognosis and refuses to follow directions, the nursing staff does not interfere with or support the denial mechanism but spends time with the sick person and encourages self-care. During the stage of anger, often manifested by refusal of care and food and by abusive language and negative criticism of the staff, the patient is not allowed to indulge in physically harmful behavior but is encouraged to verbalize the anger. In the period in which the patient tries to make bargains, as "If I could live until . . . ," it is recognized that time is needed to accept death and that the person may appreciate discussing the importance of various events and people in earlier life. When depression, marked by apathy, insomnia, inability to concentrate, poor appetite, and weariness, sets in, efforts to cheer the patient or interrupt crying are inappropriate; the patient may want only the most beloved person to be present. In the final stage of acceptance, the patient usually experiences less pain and discomfort, seems peaceful and lacking in emotional affect, and appreciates care from people who are close and familiar.

■ NURSING ORDERS: The nurse has the major role in providing emotional care for the hospitalized, terminally ill patient and may help the family arrange for home care when it is possible and desirable for the person to die at home. The nurse may teach methods of care required at home, may assist the family in realizing the patient's need to live as normally and as long as possible, and may refer the family to the social service department and to community resources for assistance.

■ OUTCOME CRITERIA: Sensitive emotional support appropriate to the stage of dying may help the person to move more rapidly through the usual stages of acceptance of dying. The family usually goes through similar stages;

therefore, support and counseling by an experienced person may greatly enhance the quality of life of the patient and the patient's family.

emotional illness. See **mental disorder.**

emotional need, a psychological or mental requirement of intrapsychic origin, usually centering on such basic feelings as love, fear, anger, sorrow, anxiety, frustration, and depression and involving the understanding, empathy, and support of one person for another. Such needs normally occur in everyone but usually are increased during periods of excessive stress or physical and mental illness and during various stages of life, as infancy, early childhood, and old age. If these needs are not routinely met by appropriate, socially accepted means, they can precipitate psychopathological conditions. Appropriate measures common in nursing for anticipating and satisfying the emotional needs of patients in stress include physical closeness, especially remaining with the person during periods when the feeling is acute; empathic listening as the patient discusses the feeling; encouragement to talk; and planning activities that provide a constructive outlet for the feeling or the situation causing it. Compare **dependency needs.** See also **emotion.**

emotional response, a reaction to a particular intrapsychic feeling or feelings, accompanied by physiological changes that may or may not be outwardly manifest but that motivate or precipitate some action or behavioral response.

emotional support, the sensitive, understanding approach that helps patients accept and deal with their illnesses, communicate their anxieties and fears, derive comfort from a gentle, sympathetic, caring person, and increase their ability to care for themselves.

■ METHOD: Essential in providing emotional support is recognizing and respecting the individuality, personal preferences, and human needs of each patient. Understanding the sick role and appreciating the phsychological effects on the patient of the transition from health to illness are also important. The patient is encouraged to verbalize feelings and concerns and the attentive listener avoids interjecting clichés, as 'Don't worry,' 'Take it easy,' or 'Everything will be all right.' The nurse and other workers realize that the patient may express some fears but may act out others through anger, hostility, silence, or assumed joviality. Efforts to change the patient, negative criticism, a judgmental attitude, and facial expressions that may indicate rejection are carefully avoided. Opportunities to listen to the troubled patient and provide compassionate and realistic counseling and care are sought.

■ NURSING ORDERS: The nurse establishes means of communication, provides an atmosphere that invites the patient to discuss the worrisome feelings, and presents a caring attitude. This is especially important when the illness damages the person's body image or self-concept.

Care is administered by the nurse in a quiet, unhurried manner with the realization that a gentle touch is important and that the patient has a right to be informed of all procedures and their rationale.

■ OUTCOME CRITERIA: Emotional support often improves the patient's psychological—and physical—state, often enabling the patient to accept the illness and, adjust with less anxiety, to adjust and to cope with the changes required.

empathy (em'pəthi'), the ability to recognize and to some extent share the emotions and states of mind of another and to understand the meaning and significance of that person's behavior. It is an essential quality for effective psychotherapy. Compare **sympathy.** — **empathic,** *adj.,* **empathize,** *v.*

emphysema (em'fəsi'mə), an abnormal condition of the pulmonary system, characterized by overinflation and destructive changes of alveolar walls, resulting in a loss of lung elasticity and decreased gases. When emphysema occurs early in life, it is usually related to a rare genetic deficiency of serum alpha 1-antitrypsin, which inactivates the enzymes leukocyte collagenase and elastase. Acute emphysema may be caused by the rupture of alveoli by severe respiratory efforts, as in acute bronchopneumonia, suffocation, and whooping cough, and occasionally during labor. Chronic emphysema usually accompanies chronic bronchitis, a major cause of which is cigarette smoking. Emphysema is also seen following asthma or tuberculosis, conditions in which the lungs are overstretched until the elastic fibers of the alveolar walls are destroyed. In old age, the alveolar membranes atrophy and may collapse, resulting in large air-filled spaces with decreased total surface area of the pulmonary membranes.

■ OBSERVATIONS: The person may have shortness of breath, dyspnea, cough, cyanosis, orthopnea, unequal chest expansion, tachypnea, tachycardia, and an elevated temperature. Anxiety, carbon dioxide narcosis with a decreased pH, increased PCO_2 restlessness, confusion, weakness, anorexia, congestive heart failure, pulmonary edema, and respiratory failure are common in advanced cases.

■ INTERVENTION: The airway is kept open, and a low concentration of oxygen with humidification may be given for a prescribed number of minutes every hour. Bronchodilators, antibiotics, expectorants, and corticosteroids may be prescribed. Sedation is to be avoided, as most sedatives depress respiratory function. Postural drainage, cupping and vibration, and IPPB may improve pulmonary function.

■ NURSING CONSIDERATIONS: The patient is taught breathing exercises and encouraged to drink between 2,000 and 3,000 ml of fluids daily. Activity is encouraged to the limit of the patient's tolerance. Fatigue, constipation and upper respiratory tract infection and irritation are to be avoided. A respirator and oxygen equipment may be prescribed for the patient's use at home.

empiric, of or pertaining to a method of treating disease based on observations and experience without an understanding of the cause or mechanism of the disorder or the way the employed therapeutic agent or procedure effects improvement or cure. The empiric treatment of a new disease may be based on observations and experience gained in the management of analogous disorders. — **empirical,** *adj.*

empiricism, a form of therapy based on personal experience and the experience of other practitioners. — **empiric, empirical,** *adj.* — **empiricist,** *n.*

empiric treatment. See **treatment.**

Empirin, a trade name for a fixed-combination drug containing two analgesic-antipyretics (aspirin and phenacetin) and a central nervous system stimulant, (caffeine).

emprosthotonos (em'prosfhot'ənəs), a position of the body characterized by a forward, rigid flexure of the body at the waist. The position is the result of a prolonged, involuntary, muscle spasm that is most commonly associated with tetanus infection or strychnine poisoning.

empty-sella syndrome, an abnormal enlargement of the sella turcica in which no pituitary tumor is present; the gland may be smaller than normal, or it may be absent. Signs and symptoms of hormonal imbalance may be present, but some patients show no evidence of hypopituitarism or of any other endocrine abnormality. The condition is especially frequent in overweight, middle-aged, multiparous women. The diagnosis may be made by computerized axial tomography scan, skull x ray, or pneumoencephalography.

empyema (em'paii'mə, em'pii'mə), an accumulation of pus in a body cavity, especially the pleural space, as a result of bacterial infection, as pleurisy or tuberculosis. It is usually removed by surgical incision, aspiration, and drainage. Antibiotics are administered to correct the cause of the underlying infection.

-empyema, a combining form meaning an 'accumulation of pus, especially thoracic': *arthroempyema, pneumoempyema, typhloempyema.*

EMS, abbreviation for **Emergency Medical Service.**

EMT, abbreviation for **Emergency Medical Technician.**

EMT-ALS, abbreviation for **Emergency Medical Technician-Advanced Life Support.**

EMT-I.V., abbreviation for **Emergency Medical Technician-Intravenous.**

EMT-P, abbreviation for **Emergency Medical Technician-Paramedic.**

emulsify, to disperse a liquid into another liquid, making a colloidal suspension. Soaps and detergents emulsify by surrounding small globules of fat, preventing them from settling out. Bile acts as an emulsifying agent in the diges-

tive tract by dispersing ingested fats into small globules. — **emulsification,** *n.*

emulsion, 1. a system consisting of two immiscible liquids, one of which is dispersed in the other in the form of small droplets. 2. (in photography) a composition sensitive to actinic rays of light, consisting of one or more silver halides suspended in gelatin applied in a thin layer to film. — **emulsify,** *v.*

E-Mycin, a trade name for an antibacterial (erythromycin).

en-, a combining form meaning 'in, on': *enanthema, encelialgia, enostosis.* Also **em-.**

enamel, a hard white substance that covers the dentin of the crown of a tooth.

enamel hypocalcification, a hereditary dental defect in which the enamel of the teeth is soft and undercalcified in context yet normal in quantity, caused by defective maturation of the ameloblasts. The teeth are chalky in consistency, the surfaces wear down rapidly, and a yellow to brown stain appears as the underlying dentin is exposed. The condition affects both deciduous and permanent teeth. Compare **enamel hypoplasia.** See also **amelogenesis imperfecta.**

enamel hypoplasia, a developmental dental defect in which the enamel of the teeth is hard in context but thin and deficient in amount, caused by defective enamel matrix formation with a deficiency in the cementing substance. There is lack of contact between teeth, rapid breakdown of occlusive surfaces, and a yellowish brown stain that appears where the dentin is exposed. The condition, which affects both the deciduous and permanent teeth, is transmitted genetically or caused by environmental factors, as vitamin deficiency, fluorosis, exanthematous diseases, congenital syphilis, or injury or trauma to the mouth. Administration of tetracyclines during the second half of pregnancy or during tooth development in the child can also cause the condition. Compare **enamel hypocalcification.** See also **ameliogenesis imperfecta.**

enanthema (en'ænfhi'mə), an eruptive lesion from the surface of a mucous membrane. Also called **enanthem.**

Enarax, a trade name for a fixed-combination gastric antisecretory agent containing an anticholinergic (oxyphencyclimine hydrochloride) and a tranquilizer (hydroxyzine hydrochloride).

enarthrosis (en'arfhrou'sis). See **ball-and-socket joint.**

encapsulated, (of arteries, muscles, nerves, and other body parts) enclosed in fibrous or membranous sheaths. See also **capsule of Tenon, synovial sheath.** — **encapsulate,** *v.*

-encephalia, a combining form meaning '(condition of the) brain': *amyelencephalia, rhinencephalia, synencephalia.* Also **-encephaly.**

encephalitis (ensef'əlaı'tis), *pl.* **encephalitides.** an inflammatory condition of the brain. The cause is usually an arbovirus infection transmitted by the bite of an infected mosquito, but it may be the result of lead or other poisoning or of hemorrhage. **Post-infectious encephalitis** occurs as a complication of another infection, as chicken pox, influenza, or measles, or following smallpox vaccination. The condition is characterized by headache, neck pain, fever, nausea, and vomiting. Neurologic disturbances may occur, including seizures, personality change, irritability, lethargy, paralysis, weakness, and coma. The outcome depends on the cause, the age and condition of the person, and the extent of inflammation. Severe inflammation with destruction of nerve tissue may result in a seizure disorder, loss of a special sense or other permanent neurologic problem, or death. Usually, the inflammation involves the spinal cord and brain; hence, in most cases, a more accurate term is *encephalomyelitis*. See also **encephalomyelitis, equine encephalitis.**

encephalitis lethargica. See **epidemic encephalitis.**

encephalocele (ensef′əlasil′), protrusion of the brain through a congenital defect in the skull; hernia of the brain. See also **neural tube defect.**

encephalodysplasia, any congenital anomaly of the brain.

encephalogram, a radiograph of the brain made during encephalography.

encephalography (ensef′əlog′rəfi), radiographic delineation of the structures of the brain containing fluid after the cerebrospinal fluid is withdrawn and replaced by a gas, as air, helium, or oxygen. The procedure is used mainly for indicating the site of cerebrospinal fluid obstruction in hydrocephalus or the structural abnormalities of the posterior fossa. Because of the risks involved, it is used only when computerized tomography is not definitive. Kinds of encephalography are **pneumoencephalography, ventriculography.** Also called **air encephalography.** Compare **echoencephalography, electroencephalography.** — **encephalographic,** *adj.*

encephaloid carcinoma. See **medullary carcinoma.**

encephalomeningocele (ensef′əloumənɪŋ′gousil). See **meningoencephalocele.**

encephalomyelitis (ensef′əloumai′əlai′tɪs), an inflammatory condition of the brain and spinal cord characterized by fever, headache, stiff neck, back pain, and vomiting. Depending on the cause, the age and condition of the person, and the extent of the inflammation and irritation to the central nervous system, seizures, paralysis, personality changes, a decreased level of consciousness, coma, or death may occur. Sequelae, as seizure disorders or decreased mental ability may occur following severe inflammation that causes entensive damage to the cells and tissues of the nervous system. See also **equine encephalitis.**

encephalomyocarditis (ensef′əloumai′oukardai′tɪs), an infectious disease of the central nervous system caused by a group of small RNA picornaviruses. Rodents are a ma-

jor reservoir of the infection. Human illness ranges from asymptomatic infection to severe encephalomyelitis. Myocarditis is not a feature of infection in humans, and most victims recover promptly without sequelae. Treatment is supportive. See also **picornavirus.**

encephalopathy (ensef′əlop′əfhi), any abnormal condition of the structure or function of tissues of the brain, especially chronic, destructive, or degenerative conditions, as Wernicke's encephalopathy.

encephalotrigeminal angiomatosis, a congenital disorder characterized by a diffuse port wine stain of the face, angiomas of the leptomeninges and choroid, and late glaucoma, often associated with trigeminal nevi, calcified deposits in cerebral or meningeal tissue, mental retardation, epilepsy, and contralateral hemiplegia. Also called **Dimitri disease, Sturge-Weber syndrome.**

-encephaly. See **-encephalia.**

enchondroma (en′kəndrou′mə), *pl.* **enchondromas, enchondromata.** a benign, slowly growing tumor of cartilage cells that arises in the extremity of the shaft of tubular bones, usually in the hands or feet. The growth of the neoplasm, by cell proliferation and the accession of small satellite tumors, may distend the bone. Also called **enchondrosis, true chondroma.**

enchondromatosis (en′kəndrou′mətou′sis), a congenital disorder characterized by the proliferation of cartilage within the extremity of the shafts of several bones, causing thinning of the cortex and distortion in length. Also called **dyschondroplasia, multiple enchondromatosis, Ollier's disease, skeletal enchondromatosis.** See also **Maffucci's syndrome.**

enchondromatous myxoma, a tumor of the connective tissue, characterized by the presence of cartilage between the cells of connective tissue. See also **myxoma.**

enchondrosarcoma (enkon′drousarkou′mə). See **central chondrosarcoma.**

enchondrosis (en′kəndrou′sis). See **enchondroma.**

enchylema. See **hyaloplasm.**

-enchyma, a combining form meaning the 'liquid that nourishes tissue, or tissue itself': *karyenchyma, mesenchyma, sclerenchyma.*

encode, to translate a message, signal, or stimulus into a code.

encoded message, (in communication theory) a message as transmitted by a sender to a receiver.

encopresis (en′koupri′sis), fecal incontinence. — **encopretic,** *adj.*

encounter, (in psychotherapy) the interaction between a patient and a psychotherapist, as occurs in existential therapy, or among several members of a small group, as in encounter or sensitivity-training groups, in which emotional change and personal growth are brought about by the expression of strong feelings by the participants.

encounter group, (in psychology) a small group of people who meet to increase self-awareness, promote personal growth, and improve interpersonal communication. Members focus on becoming aware of their feelings and on developing the ability to express those feelings openly, honestly, and clearly. See also **group therapy, psychotherapy, sensitivity-training group.**

-ency, 1. a combining form meaning a 'quality or state': *deficiency, dependency.* **2.** a combining form meaning a 'person or thing in a state': *latency.* **3.** a combining form meaning an 'instance of a quality or state': *emergency.* Also **-ence, -ance, -ancy.**

encyst (ensɪst'), to form a cyst or capsule. See also **cyst.** – **encysted,** *adj.*

end-. See **endo-.**

endamebiasis, endamoebiasis (en'dəmibaiˈəsɪs). See **amebiasis.**

Endamoeba, Endameba (en'dəmiˈbə). See *Entamoeba.*

endarterectomy (en'dartərekˈtəmi), a surgical procedure which excises tunica intima of an artery which has become thickened by atherosclerosis.

endarteritis (en'dartəraiˈtɪs), an inflammatory disorder of the inner layer of one or more arteries, which may become partially or completely occluded.

endarteritis obliterans, an inflammatory condition of the lining of the arterial walls in which the intima proliferates, narrowing the lumen of the vessels and occluding the smaller vessels.

end bud, a mass of undifferentiated cells produced from the remnants of the primitive node and the primitive streak at the caudal end of the developing embryo after the formation of the somites is completed. In lower animals it gives rise to the tail or any other caudal appendage and part of the trunk; in man it forms the caudal portion of the trunk. Also called **tail bud.**

end bulb of Krause. See **Krause's corpuscle.**

Endecon, a trade name for a respiratory, fixed-combination drug containing an adrenergic (phenylpropanolamine hydrochloride) and an analgesic (acetaminophen).

endemic (endemˈɪk), (of a disease or microorganism) indigenous to a geographic area or population. See also **epidemic, pandemic.**

endemic goiter, an enlargement of the thyroid gland caused by the dietary intake of inadequate amounts of iodine. Iodine privation leads to diminished production and secretion of thyroid hormone by the gland. The pituitary gland, operating on a negative feedback system, senses the deficiency and secretes increased amounts of thyroid stimulating hormone, causing hyperplasia and hypertrophy of the thyroid gland. The goiter may grow during the winter months and shrink during the summer months when more iodine-bearing fresh vegetables are eaten. Initially, the goiter is diffuse; later, it becomes multinodular. Endemic goiter occurs occasionally in adolescents at puberty and widely in population groups in geographic areas in which limited amounts of iodine are present in the soil, water, and food. The use of iodized salt is the best prophylactic treatment. One injection of iodinated poppyseed oil provides a depot of potential iodide adequate for two to four years. Dessicated thyroid given orally may prevent further growth of adult goiters and may reduce the size of diffuse goiters. A large goiter may cause dysphagia, dyspnea, tracheal deviation, and cosmetic problems.

endemic typhus, a rickettsial infection transmitted by the bite of a rat flea infected with *Rickettsia typhi.* The disease, which is endemic to many areas of the world, is similar to epidemic typhus but less severe; the fever and rash last between 10 and 14 days. Permanent immunity follows infection. Treatment includes rest, an adequate intake of fluids, and tetracycline. A vaccine is available for people living in or intending to visit an area in which the disease is endemic. Also called **murine typhus.** Compare **Brill-Zinsser disease, epidemic typhus.**

endo-, end-, a combining form meaning 'inward, within': *endobiotic, endocranial, endognathion.* Also **ento-.**

endobronchial anesthesia, a procedure, rarely performed, in which anesthetic gas is administered into the bronchi.

endocardial cushion defect, any cardiac defect resulting from the failure of the endocardial cushions in the embryonic heart to fuse and form the atrial septum. See also **atrial septal defect, congenital cardiac anomaly.**

endocardial fibroelastosis (faiˈbrouiˈlæstouˈsɪs), an abnormal condition characterized by hypertrophy of the wall of the left ventricle and the development of a thick, fibroelastic endocardium. This condition often increases the ventricular capacity but sometimes decreases it. Some studies have incriminated the mumps virus in endocardial fibroelastosis, while other investigations refute such a connection.

endocarditis (en'doukardaiˈtɪs), an abnormal condition that affects the endocardium and the heart valves and is characterized by lesions caused by a variety of diseases. The kinds of endocarditis are bacterial endocarditis, nonbacterial endocarditis, and Libman-Sacks endocarditis. Untreated, all types of endocarditis are rapidly lethal, but they are often successfully treated by various antibacterial and surgical measures. With adequate treatment about 65 to 80 per cent of the patients with endocarditis survive.

endocardium (en'doukarˈdiəm), *pl.* **endocardia.** the interior lining of the heart, containing small blood vessels and a few bundles of smooth muscle. Compare **epicardium, myocardium.**

endocervicitis (en'dousər'vɪsaiˈtɪs), an abnormal condition characterized by inflammation of the epithelium and glands of the canal of the uterine cervix. See also **cervicitis.**

endocervix (en'dousər'vɪks), **1.** the membrane lining the canal of the uterine cervix. **2.** the opening of the cervix into the uterine cavity. —**endocervical,** *adj.*

endocrine fracture, any fracture that results from weakness of a specific bone due to an endocrine disorder, as hyperparathyroidism.

endocrine system, the network of ductless glands and other structures that elaborate and secrete hormones directly into the blood stream, affecting the function of specific target organs. Glands of the endocrine system include the thyroid and the parathyroid, the anterior pituitary, the posterior pituitary, the pancreas, the suprarenal glands, and the gonads. The pineal gland is also considered an endocrine gland because it is ductless, although its precise endocrine function is not established. The thymus gland, once considered an endocrine gland, is now classified in the lymphatic system. Various other organs have some endocrinologic function. Secretions from the endocrine glands affect various processes throughout the body, as metabolism, growth, and secretions from other organs. See also **exocrine.**

Names and locations of endocrine glands

Name	Location
Pituitary gland (hypophysis cerebri) and hypothalamus	Cranial cavity
Anterior lobe (adenohypophysis)	
Intermediate lobe (pars intermedia)	
Posterior lobe (neurohypophysis)	
Pineal gland (epiphysis)	Cranial cavity
Thyroid gland	Neck
Parathyroid glands	Neck
Thymus	Mediastinum
Adrenal glands	Abdominal cavity
Adrenal cortex	(retroperitoneal)
Adrenal medulla	
Islands of Langerhans	Abdominal cavity (pancreas)
Gastric and intestinal mucosa	Abdominal cavity
Ovaries	Pelvic cavity
Graafian follicle	
Corpus luteum	
Testes (interstitial cells)	Scrotum
Placenta	Pregnant uterus

endocrinologist (en'doukrɪnol'əjɪst), a physician who specializes in endocrinology.

endocrinology, the study of the anatomy, physiology, and pathology of the endocrine system and of the treatment of endocrine problems. —**endocrinologist,** *n.*

endoderm (end'ədərm), (in embryology) the innermost of the cell layers that develop from the embryonic disc of the inner cell mass of the blastocyst. From the endoderm

arises the epithelium of the trachea, bronchi, lungs, gastrointestinal tract, liver, pancreas, urinary bladder, urachus, pharynx, thyroid, tympanic cavity, tonsils, and parathyroid glands. The endoderm thus comprises the lining of the cavities and passages of the body and the covering for most of the internal organs. Compare **ectoderm, mesoderm.**

endodermal cloaca, a part of the cloaca in the developing embryo that lies internal to the cloacal membrane and gives rise to the bladder and urogenital ducts. Compare **ectodermal cloaca.** See also **urogenital sinus.**

endogenous depression, a major affective disorder characterized by a persistent dysphoric mood, anxiety, irritability, fear, brooding, appetite and sleep disturbances, weight loss, psychomotor agitation or retardation, decreased energy, feelings of worthlessness or guilt, difficulty in concentrating or thinking, occasional delusions and hallucinations, and thoughts of death or suicide. The disorder, which occurs in children, adolescents, and adults, may develop over a period of days, weeks, or months; episodes may occur in clusters or singly, separated by several years of normality. The causes of the disorder are multiple and complex and may involve biological, psychological, interpersonal, and sociocultural factors that lead to some unidentifiable intrapsychic conflict. Treatment includes the use of antidepressants and electroconvulsive therapy, followed by long-term psychotherapy. In severe cases, proper nursing care is needed for adequate nutrition, appropriate balance of fluid intake and output, good personal hygiene, and protection of the patient from self-injury. Also called **major depressive episode.** See also **bipolar disorder, depression.**

endogenous obesity, obesity resulting from dysfunction of the endocrine or metabolic systems. Compare **exogenous obesity.** See also **obesity.**

endolymph (en'dəlɪmf), the fluid in the membranous labyrinth of the internal ear. Compare **perilymph.**

endolymphatic duct, a passage joining an endolymphatic sac with a utricle and saccule.

endolymphatic hydrops. *Obsolete.* See **Ménière's disease.**

endometrial (en'doumi'triəl), **1.** of or pertaining to endometrium. **2.** of or pertaining to the uterine cavity.

endometrial cancer, a malignant neoplastic disease of the endometrium of the uterus most often occuring in the fifth or sixth decade of life. Some of the factors associated with an increased incidence of the disease are a medical history of infertility, anovulation, exogenous estrogen, uterine polyps, and a combination of diabetes, hypertension, and obesity. Abnormal vaginal bleeding, especially in a postmenopausal woman, is the cardinal symptom. There also may be lower abdominal and low back pain; a large, boggy uterus is often a sign of advanced disease. Less than half the patients with endometrial cancer have a positive Papanicolaou (Pap) test of the cervix and vagina, because the tumor cells rarely exfoliate in early stages of the lesion. A Pap test of cells removed from the endometrium obtained from jet washings of the uterine cavity provides more accurate data. Vacuum curettage is also used to extract endometrial cells for study, but the diagnostic technique most frequently recommended is a dilatation and curettage in which each section of the uterus is examined and curetted for biopsy specimens. Adenocarcinomas constitute roughly 90 per cent of all endometrial tumors; mixed carcinomas, sarcomas, and benign adenocanthomas comprise the rest. Endometrial lesions may spread to the cervix, but rarely invade the vagina. They metastasize to the broad ligaments, Fallopian tubes, and ovaries so frequently that bilateral salpingo-oophorectomy with abdominal hysterectomy is the usual treatment. Radiotherapy is usually administered preoperatively and postoperatively. High doses of a progestogen may be administered for palliation in advanced or inoperable cases.

endometrial hyperplasia, an abnormal condition characterized by overgrowth of the endometrium owing to sustained stimulation by estrogen (of endogenous or exogenous origin) that is not opposed by progesterone. Estrogens act as growth hormone for endometrium. Through a complex intercellular mechanism, endometrial cells bind estrogens preferentially and undergo changes characteristic of the proliferative phase of the menstrual cycle. If estrogen stimulation continues for three to six months without periodic cessation or counteractive progesterone stimulation, as occurs in anovulatory or perimenopausal women or in women receiving replacement estrogen without added progestogen, the endometrium becomes abnormally thickened and glandularized. Unremitting estrogen stimulation eventually causes cystic or adenomatous endometrial hyperplasia, the latter a premalignant lesion that undergoes malignant degeneration in approximately 25 per cent of women having it. The causative relationship between estrogen and endometrial hyperplasia is well established; there is implication but not proof that estrogen also provokes the change from hyperplasia to neoplasia and malignancy. Endometrial hyperplasia often results in abnormal uterine bleeding; such bleeding, particularly in older women, constitutes an indication for biopsy or curettage of the endometrium to establish histopathologic diagnosis and to rule out malignancy. A functioning estrogen-secreting tumor is suspected if the woman is not taking estrogen medication. Progestogen therapy is effective in reversing the abnormal histopathologic changes of endometrial hyperplasia; if hyperplasia is adenomatous, hysterectomy is commonly performed.

endometrial polyp, a pedunculated overgrowth of endometrium, usually benign. Polyps are a common cause of vaginal bleeding in perimenopausal women and are often associated with other uterine abnormalities, as endometrial hyperplasia or fibroids. They may occur singly or in clusters and are usually one cm or less in diameter, but they may become much larger and prolapse through the cervix. Treatment for the condition includes surgical dilatation and curettage.

endometriosis (en′dɔumi′triou′sɪs), an abnormal gynecologic condition characterized by ectopic growth and function of endometrial tissue. Precise incidence of the disease is unknown, but evidence of it is found in approximately 15 per cent of women who undergo pelvic laparotomy for other indications. Women of higher socioeconomic status and women who defer pregnancy are more likely to contract the disease. The average age of women found to have endometriosis is 37 years. The disease is uncommon among black women. Pregnancy has a definite but inconsistent influence in preventing or ameliorating the disease. The etiology of endometriosis is unknown; evidence suggests that the ectopic endometrium of endometriosis develops from vestigial tissue of the Wolfian or Müllerian ducts; other evidence strongly suggests that fragments of endometrium from the lining of the uterus are regurgitated during menstruation backward through the Fallopian tubes into the peritoneal cavity, where they attach, grow, and function. Fragments of this tissue, which is microscopically similar to or identical with endometrium having glands or glandlike structures, stroma, and areas of hemorrhage, may be found in the wall of the uterus or on its surface, in or on the tubes, ovaries, rectosigmoid, or pelvic peritoneum, or, occasionally, in remote, extrapelvic areas. Foci of endometriosis have been found in surgical scars, the umbilicus, the bowel, the lung, the eye, and the brain. When endometriosis occurs in a critical location, it may result in grave dysfunction of the organ involved or, rarely, in death; intestinal obstruction is a common complication. The lesions of pelvic endometriosis are typically small cystic structures a few millimeters in diameter that appear individually or in clusters as black nodules on the visceral and parietal peritoneum. Ovarian endometrial cysts, however, commonly grow to several centimeters in diameter. The endometrial tissue of endometriosis in both large and small lesions functions cyclically and undergoes periodic menstrual breakdown that results in bleeding within cysts, stretching of the cyst wall, and pain. Ovarian endometrial cysts containing menstruum that has become a thick, dark-brown liquid are called 'chocolate cysts.' The most characteristic symptom of endometriosis is pain, particularly dysmenorrhea and dyspareunia, but also dysuria, painful defecation, and suprapubic soreness. Pain is not always present, however, and its absence does not rule out the presence of the disease. Other common symptoms include premenstrual vaginal staining of blood, hypermenorrhea, and infertility. On pelvic examination, tender nodularity of the uterosacral ligaments is commonly found. Diagnosis is made by biopsy of tissue obtained from lesions found on culdoscopy, laparoscopy, or laparotomy. Some of the measures that have been recommended to prevent endometrial regurgitation include avoidance by examiners of forceful manipulation of the pelvic organs, particularly during a woman's menstruation, anteversion of retroverted uteri to provide better menstrual drainage, correction of cervical obstruction, and avoidance by women of prolonged deferral of pregnancy. Treatment of endometriosis in its milder forms may consist only of medication with analgesics and expectant follow-up, because many women will outgrow mild endometriosis or become pregnant. When the disease is more extensive, treatment is hormonal or surgical and is directed at reducing the size and number of lesions, relieving symptoms, and correcting infertility, if present. Prolonged suppression of ovulation may produce a hormonal milieu similar to pregnancy and result in partial or total regression of lesions; this condition of 'pseudopregnancy' may be brought about with Danazol, with estrogen and progestogen separately or in combination, or, less often, with androgen. Among women with endometriosis and infertility who undergo prolonged hormonal therapy, approximately 40 per cent become pregnant subsequent to treatment. Conservative surgery to preserve reproductive function entails excision or ablation of individual lesions, restoration of normal uterine and adnexal position, freeing of adhesions, and obliteration of the cul-de-sac, a most common site of endometrial implantation. Advanced endometriosis often requires surgery, including total abdominal hysterectomy and bilateral salpingo-oophorectomy to remove large lesions and to terminate cyclic ovarian stimulation on which endometrial growth depends so that retained lesions atrophy and heal.

endometritis (en'doumɪtrai'tɪs), an inflammatory condition of the endometrium, usually caused by bacterial infection, commonly gonococci or hemolytic streptococci. It is characterized by fever, abdominal pain, malodorous discharge, and enlargement of the uterus. It occurs most frequently following childbirth or abortion and in women fitted with an intrauterine contraceptive device. The diagnosis may be made by physical examination, history, laboratory analysis revealing an elevated white blood cell count, ultrasound, and bacteriologic identification of the pathogen. Treatment includes antibiotics, rest, analgesia, an adequate intake of fluids, and, if necessary, surgical drainage of a suppurating abscess, hysterectomy, or salpingo-oophorectomy. Endometritis may be mild and self-limited, chronic or acute, and unilateral or bilateral. It may result in sterility owing to scar formation occluding the passage of the Fallopian tubes. Septic abortion and puerperal fever are forms of endometritis that caused many deaths before antibiotics and asepsis became commonly available.

endometritis dessicans, *Obsolete.* endometritis characterized by ulceration and shedding of the endometrium of the uterus.

endometrium (en'doumi'triəm), the mucous membrane lining of the uterus, consisting of the stratum compactum, the stratum spongiosum, and the stratum basale. The endometrium changes in thickness and structure with the menstrual cycle. The stratum compactum and the stratum spongiosum comprise the pars funtionalis and are shed with each menstrual flow. The pars functionalis is known as the decidua during pregnancy, when it underlies the placenta. Compare **parametrium.**

endomorph, a person whose body build is characterized by a soft, round physique with a large trunk and thighs, tapering extremities, an accumulation of fat throughout the body, and a predominance of structures derived from the endoderm. Compare **ectomorph, mesomorph.** See also **pyknic.**

endoparasite (en'doupær'əsait'), (in medical parasitology) an organism that lives within the body of the host, as a tapeworm.

endophthalmitis (endolf'θælmai'tɪs), an inflammatory condition of the internal eye in which the eye becomes red, swollen, painful, and, sometimes, filled with pus. This condition may blur the vision and cause vomiting, fever, and headache. Endophthalmitis may result from bacterial or fungal infection, trauma, allergy, drug or chemical toxicity, or vascular disease. Depending on the cause, therapy requires surgical intervention or the administration of an antibiotic, atropine, or a corticosteroid. Also called **endophthalmia.**

endophthalmitis phacoanaphylactica (fæk'ouæn'-əfɪlæk'təkə), an abnormal condition characterized by an acute autoimmune reaction of the eye. It is caused by hypersensitivity of the eye to the protein of the crystalline lens and commonly occurs after trauma to the crystalline lens or after a cataract operation. Associated symptoms include swelling and inflammation of the eye, severe pain, and blurred vision. The substance of the lens is invaded by polymorphonuclear cells and mononuclear phagocytes. Sensitization of one eye often follows the extracapsular removal of the lens of the eye on the opposite side. Accurate diagnosis must differentiate between this condition and infectious endophthalmitis. Therapy is supportive and commonly includes the administration of corticosteroids and atropine. Refractory cases may require surgical removal of the lens. Compare **uveitis.**

endophytic (en'doufɪt'ɪk), of or pertaining to the tendency to grow inward, as an endophytic tumor that grows on the inside of an organ or structure.

endoplasmic reticulum, an extensive network of membrane-enclosed tubules in the cytoplasm of cells. The ultramicroscopic organelle, which can be seen only with an electron microscope, is classified as granular or rough-surfaced when ribosomes are attached to the surface of the membrane and agranular or smooth-surfaced when ribosomes are absent. The structure functions in the synthesis of proteins and lipids and in the transport of these metabolites within the cell.

endorphin (endôr'fĭn), any one of the neuropeptides composed of many amino acids, elaborated by the pituitary gland and acting on the central and the peripheral nervous systems to reduce pain. Endorphins isolated by researchers are alpha-endorphin, beta-endorphin, and gamma-endorphin, all chemicals producing pharmacological effects similar to morphine. Beta-endorphin has been isolated in the brain and in the gastrointestinal tract and seems to be the most potent of the endorphins. Beta-endorphin is composed of 31 amino acids which are identical to part of the sequence of 91 amino acids of the hormone beta-lipoprotein, also produced by the pituitary gland. Behavioral tests indicate that beta-endorphin is a powerful analgesic in humans and animals. Brain-stimulated analgesia in humans releases beta-endorphin into the cerebrospinal fluid. Compare **enkephalin.**

endorsement, a statement of recognition of the license of a health practitioner in one state by another state. An endorsement relieves the health practitioner of the necessity of going through the full licensing procedure of the state in which practice is to be undertaken.

endoscope, an illuminated optical instrument for the visualization of the interior of a body cavity or organ. Instruments are available in varying lengths, and the fiberoptic endoscope has great flexibility, reaching previously inaccessible areas. Although the endoscope is generally introduced through a natural opening in the body, it may also be inserted through an incision. Other instruments for viewing specific areas of the body include the bronchoscope, cystoscope, gastroscope, laparoscope, otoscope, and vaginoscope. See also **fiberoptics.** — **endoscopic,** adj.

endoscopic retrograde cholangiography, (in radiology) a diagnostic procedure for outlining the common bile duct. A flexible fiberoptic duodenoscope is placed in the common bile duct. A radio-opaque substance is instilled directly into the duct and serial x rays are taken. See also **cholangiography.**

endoscopy (endos'kəpi), the visualization of the interior of organs and cavities of the body with an endoscope. The procedure is indicated for the diagnosis of gastric ulcers with atypical radiologic features, to locate the source of upper gastrointestinal bleeding, to establish the presence and extent of varices in the lower esophagus and stomach in patients with liver disease, and to detect any abnormalities of the lower colon. For examination of the upper gastrointestinal tract, the stomach of the patient is lavaged with ice water through a large bore gastric tube, with the patient placed on the side to reduce the chance of aspiration. For examination of the lower colon, fecal material is removed by enema, laxative, or suppository. The patient is placed in the knee-chest position for the procedure and afterward is observed by the nurse for abdominal pain or rectal bleeding. Aseptic rather than sterile techniques are routinely followed. Endoscopy can also be used to obtain samples for cytological and histological examination and to follow the course of a disease, as the assessment of the healing of gastric and duodenal ulcers. See also **bronchoscopy, cystoscopy, gastroscopy, laparoscopy.** — **endoscopic,** adj.

endothelial myeloma, a malignant myeloma that develops in the bone marrow, occurring most frequently in the long bones. Pain, fever, and leukocytosis are characteristically present. Also called **Ewing's tumor.**

-endothelioma, a combining form meaning 'a tumor of endothelial tissue': hemendothelioma, lymphendothelioma.

endothelium (en'dŏuthil'iəm), the layer of squamous epithelial cells that lines the heart, the blood and the lymph vessels, and the serous cavities of the body. It is highly vascular, heals quickly, and is derived from the mesoderm.

endotoxin (en'dŏutok'sĭn), a toxin contained in the cell walls of some microorganisms, especially gram-negative bacteria, that is released when the bacterium dies and is broken down in the body. Fever, chills, shock, leukopenia, and a variety of other symptoms result, depending on the particular organism and the condition of the infected person.

endotracheal (en'dŏutrei'kiəl), within or through the trachea.

endotracheal anesthesia, inhalation anesthesia that is achieved by the passage of an anesthetic gas or mixture of gases through an endotracheal tube into the respiratory tract. General anesthesia is usually obtained by endotracheal anesthesia.

endotracheal intubation, the management of the patient with an airway catheter inserted through the mouth or nose into the trachea. An endotracheal tube may be used to maintain a patent airway, to prevent aspiration of material from the digestive tract in the unconscious or paralyzed patient, to permit suctioning of tracheobronchial secretions, or to administer positive pressure ventilation that cannot be given effectively by a mask. Endotracheal tubes may be made of rubber or plastic and usually have an inflatable cuff to maintain a closed system with the ventilator.

■ METHOD: The endotracheal tube is inserted via the mouth or nose through the larynx into the trachea; if the oral route is used, a bite block may be required to keep the patient from biting and obstructing the tube. Breath sounds are auscultated immediately after insertion and every hour or two hours thereafter to make certain the tube is properly positioned and is not obstructing one of the mainstem bronchi. Once the tube is correctly positioned, it is taped securely in place and checked for patency and slippage every 15 to 60 minutes. The trachea is suctioned every hour and irrigated with normal saline solution, if so ordered. The patient is usually on intermittent positive pressure breathing (IPPB) or a volume respirator with the cuff of the endotracheal tube inflated; if the patient can breathe independently, the trachea and mouth are suctioned, the cuff is deflated, and the respiratory rate and quality are checked hourly. The patient is turned every 1 to 2 hours, with the blood pressure and pulse checked every 2 to 4 hours. Parenteral fluids are administered as ordered; nothing is given orally; the intake and output of fluids are measured and recorded. The patient's level of consciousness is determined hourly and, if sufficiently conscious, a method of communication is established.

■ NURSING ORDERS: The nurse monitors the position and patency of the endotracheal tube, performs the necessary suctioning, inflates and deflates the cuff at appropriate times, and administers IPPB or support with the volume respirator. The nurse checks the vital signs at the ordered intervals and provides emotional support as well as physical care for the patient who is usually acutely ill, unable to communicate, and suffering from the discomfort of an endotracheal tube.

■ OUTCOME CRITERIA: Meticulous care of the patient with an endotracheal tube can result in the survival of a critically ill person.

endotracheal tube, a large-bore catheter inserted through the mouth or nose and into the trachea to a point above the bifurcation of the trachea proximal to the bronchi. It is used for delivering oxygen under pressure when ventilation must be totally controlled and in general anesthetic procedures. *(See next column for illustration)*

endoxin (endok′sin), an endogenous, recently discovered analog of digoxin, occurring naturally in man. It is a hormone that may regulate the excretion of salt.

Endrate, a trade name for a chelating agent (edetate disodium).

Enduron, a trade name for a diuretic and antihypertensive (methyclothiazide).

Enduronyl, a trade name for a cardiovascular, fixed-combination drug containing the diuretic (methyclothiazide) and an antihypertensive (deserpidine).

-ene, a combining form naming hydrocarbons: *ethidene, somnifene, xanthene.*

enema, a procedure in which a solution is introduced into the rectum for cleansing or therapeutic purposes. Enemas may be commercially packed disposable units or reusable equipment prepared just prior to use.

■ METHOD: The equipment is assembled; if reusable

Passage of endotracheal tube
via laryngoscope

Endotracheal tube in place

Nasotracheal intubation

ENDOTRACHEAL INTUBATION

equipment is to be used, an 18 to 20 French gauge catheter, a 2- to 3-foot length of tubing, an enema can, the solution, a clamp, and a thermometer are collected and brought to the bedside. If a disposable set is to be used, no other equipment is necessary. The patient is positioned in the left lateral knee-chest or dorsal position. After expelling air from the tubing, the tip of the catheter is lubricated. (Disposable units usually have prelubricated tips.) The patient is asked to bear down, as if to defecate, and the tip of the catheter is gently inserted 7.5 to 10 cm into the rectum, depending on the size of the patient and the purpose of the enema. The solution is allowed to flow from a height of 45 cm above the level of the hips, or, with some disposable enemas, the container is squeezed slowly to force the fluid into the rectum. The tip of the catheter or squeeze-bottle is withdrawn when all the solution has been administered, and light pressure is applied over the anus with a gauze pad. The fluid is held in by the patient for the prescribed length of time. It is then expelled as the patient sits on the toilet.

■ NURSING OBSERVATIONS: The reasons for performing the procedure and the steps to be taken are explained to the patient. The solution is warmed to 37.8° to 40.6°C in order to reduce the stimulation of intestinal peristalsis by a sudden change of temperature in the colon. The patient is warned that some discomfort may occur because the colon tends to contract when distended by the fluid. The enema is given slowly to avoid sudden distention that would cause peristalsis, or spasm, and increased discomfort. A call bell is kept within reach of the patient during expulsion of the enema because the discomfort of the procedure and the effort required to expel the enema may cause faintness. The color, consistency, and amount of material evacuated are evaluated. If reusable equipment is used, it is rinsed in cold water before being washed with warm soapy water and sterilized.

■ OUTCOME CRITERIA: Careful observation of the patient during the procedure, slow and gentle administration of the enema, evaluation of the results of the procedure, and a thorough explanation to the patient of all aspects of the procedure are important to achieve the desired effect of the enema.

energy, the capacity to do work or to perform vigorous activity. Compare **anergy.** – **energetic,** *adj.*

energy-protein malnutrition, a condition resulting from a diet deficient in both calories and proteins. Also called **protein-calorie malnutrition.** See also **marasmus, marasmic kwashiorkor.**

en face (ã fAs′), *French.* 'face-to-face.' a position in which the mother's face and the infant's face are approximately 8 inches apart, as when the mother holds the infant up in front of her face or when she nurses the child. Studies of maternal and infant bonding have shown that mothers seek eye-to-eye contact, and, if they are not stopped, they will instinctively move the baby to an en face position. In addition, infants have been shown to prefer a human face over other visual stimuli and to be best able to focus at a distance of 8 to 10 inches.

enflurane (en′flurein), a nonflammable anesthetic gas belonging to the ether family, used for induction and maintenance of general anesthesia in cases in which ethers are the drugs of choice. A halogenated volatile liquid, enflurane is administered through vaporizers specially calibrated for delivery via nitrous oxide or an oxygen-nitrous oxide mixture, permitting close control of dosage. Because excitement may occur on induction, a hypnotic dose of short-acting barbiturate is sometimes used for premedication. Adverse reactions may include seizure activity, muscle fasciculation, hypotension, cardiac arrhythmia, shivering, and elevated white blood count. Nausea and vomiting on emergence from anethesia sometimes occur.

engagement, (in obstetrics) **1.** fixation of the presenting part of the fetus in the maternal pelvis. The lowest part of the presenting part is at or below the level of the ischial spines. **2.** fixation of the fetal head in the maternal pelvis with the biparietal diameter of the head level with the ischial spines.

English position. See **lateral recumbent position.**

engrossment. See **bonding.**

Enisyl, a trade name for an amino acid (lysine hydrochloride).

enkephalin (enkef′əlin), one of two pentapeptides produced in the body that reduce pain. Researchers have isolated enkephalins in the pituitary gland, brain, and gastrointestinal tract. The enkephalins are methionine-enkephalin and isoleucine-enkephalin, each composed of five amino acids, four of which are identical in both compounds. It is believed that these two neuropeptides can depress neurons throughout the central nervous system. Axon terminals that release enkephalins are concentrated in the posterior horn of the gray matter of the spinal cord, in the central part of the thalamus, and in the amygdala of the limbic system of the cerebrum. Enkephalins inhibit neurotransmitters in the pathway for pain perception, thereby reducing the emotional as well as the physical impact of pain. Although it is not known exactly how these two neuropeptides function, many experts believe the enkephalins are not only natural pain killers but that they may be involved, with other neuropeptides, in the development of psychopathological behavior in some cases. Compare **endorphin.**

enomania (i′noumei′niə). See **oinomania.**

enophthalmos (en′əfthæl′məs), backward displacement of the eye in the bony socket, caused by traumatic injury or developmental defect. Ptosis may cause a false impression of enophthalmos. – **enophthalmic,** *adj.*

Enovid, a trade name for an oral contraceptive containing an estrogen (mestranol) and a progestin (norethyn-odrel).

ensiform process (en′sıfɔrm). See **xiphoid process.**

Ensure, a trade name for a lactose-free nutritional supplement containing protein, carbohydrate, and fat.

entamebiasis, entamoebiasis (en′təmibaı′əsıs). See **amebiasis.**

Entamoeba, Entameba (en′təmi′bə), a genus of intestinal parasite of which several species are pathogenic to humans. See also *Entamoeba histolytica.*

Entamoeba histolytica, a pathogenic species of ameba that causes amebic dysentery and hepatic amebiasis in man. See also **amebiasis, amebic dysentery, hepatic amebiasis.**

enter-. See **entero-.**

enteric fever. See **typhoid fever.**

enteric infection, a disease of the intestine owing to any infection. Symptoms similar to those caused by pathogens may be produced by chemical toxins in ingested foods and by allergic reactions to certain food substances. Among bacteria commonly involved in enteric infections are *Escherichia coli, Vibrio cholerae,* and several species of *Salmonella, Shigella,* and anaerobic streptococci. Enteric infections are characterized by diarrhea, abdominal discomfort, nausea and vomiting, and anorexia. There may be a significant loss of fluid and electrolytes as a result of severe vomiting and diarrhea. Nothing is offered by mouth until vomiting has ceased. At that time, a clear fluid diet may be given. In severe cases, an I.V. solution containing glucose, saline, and electrolytes may be administered. Medication for sedation and relief of abdominal cramps may be prescribed. Antibiotics may be recommended, depending upon the specific microorganism causing the infection.

entericoid fever, any febrile disease characterized by intestinal inflammation and dysfunction. See also **enteric infection, typhoid fever.**

enteritis (en′təraı′tıs), inflammation of the mucosal lining of the small intestine, resulting from a variety of causes—bacterial, viral, functional, and inflammatory. Involvement of small and large intestine is called **enterocolitis.** Compare **gastroenteritis.**

entero-, enter-, a combining form meaning 'pertaining to the intestines': *enteric, enterobiliary, enteroptosis.*

Enterobacter aerogenes (en′teroubæk′tər eroj′ıniz). See *Enterobacter cloacae.*

Enterobacter cloacae, a common species of bacterium found in human and animal feces, dairy products, sewage, soil, and water. It is rarely the cause of disease. Also called *Aerobacter aerogenes, Enterobacter aerogenes.*

enterobacterial (en′tıroubæktir′iəl), of or pertaining to a species of bacterium found in the digestive tract.

Enterobactericae (en′tıroubæktir′iei′sıı), a family of aerobic and anaerobic bacteria that includes both normal and pathogenic enteric microorganisms. Among the significant genera of the family are *Escherichia, Klebsiella, Proteus, Salmonella.*

enterobiasis (en′tıroubaı′əsıs), a parasitic infestation with *Enterobius vermicularis,* the common pinworm. The worms infect the large intestine, and the females deposit eggs in the perianal area, causing pruritis and insomnia. Reinfection commonly occurs by transfer of eggs to the mouth by contaminated fingers. Airborne transmission is possible, as eggs remain viable for two or three days in contaminated bedclothes. To make the diagnosis, the sticky side of an adhesive cellophane tape swab is pressed against the perianal skin and examined for eggs under a microscope. Therapy for the whole family may be necessary. Effective anthelmintics include piperazine, pyrantel pamoate, pyrvinium pamoate, and thiabendazole. Personal hygiene, including handwashing, is the best preventive measure. There appears to be little benefit from disinfection procedures for the home. Also called **oxyuriasis, pinworm.**

Enterobius vermicularis (en′tırou′biəs), a common parasitic nematode that resembles a white thread between one half and one centimeter long. Also called **pinworm, seatworm, threadworm.**

enterochromaffin cell (en′təroukroumæf′ın). See **argentaffin cell.**

enterokinase (en′tıroukaı′neis), an intestinal juice enzyme that activates the proteolytic enzyme in pancreatic juice by converting trypsinogen to trypsin.

enterolith (en′təroulıth), a stone or concretion found within the intestine. See also **calculus.**

enterolithiasis, the presence of enteroliths in the intestine.

enterostomy (en′təros′təmi), a surgical procedure that produces an artificial anus or fistula in the intestine by incision through the abdominal wall. Compare **colostomy.**

enterovirus (en′tərouvaı′rəs), a virus that multiplies primarily in the intestinal tract. Kinds of enteroviruses are **coxsackievirus, echovirus, poliovirus.** — **enteroviral,** *adj.*

ento-. See **endo-.**

entoderm. See **endoderm.**

Entozyme, a trade name for a gastrointestinal fixed-combination drug containing bile salts and the digestive enzymes (pancreatin and pepsin).

entrainment, a phenomenon observed in the microanalysis of sound films in which the speaker moves several parts of the body and the listener responds to the sounds by moving in ways that are coordinated with the rhythm of the sounds. Infants have been observed to move in time to the rhythms of adult speech but not to random noises or disconnected words or vowels. Entrainment is thought to be an essential factor in the process of maternal-infant bonding.

entropion (entrou′piən), turning inward or turning towards, usually a condition in which the eyelid turns inward toward the eye. **Cicatricial entropion** can occur in either the upper or lower eyelid as a result of scar tissue formation. **Spastic entropion** results from an inflammation or other factor that affects tissue tone. An inflammation of the eyelid may be the result of an infectious disease or irritation from an inverted eyelash. Compare **ectropion**. See also **blepharitis**.

ENTROPION

entropy (en′trəpi), the tendency of a system to go from a state of order to a state of disorder, expressed in physics as a measure of the part of the heat or energy in a thermodynamic system that is not available to perform work. Living organisms tend to go from a state of disorder to a state of order in their development and thus appear to reverse entropy. However, maintaining a living system requires the expenditure of energy leaving less energy available for work, with the result that the entropy of the universe is increasing.

enucleation (ınu′klieı′shən), **1.** removal of an organ or tumor in one piece. **2.** removal of the eyeball, performed in malignancy, severe infection, extensive trauma, or to control pain in glaucoma. Local or general anesthesia is used. The optic nerve and muscle attachments are cut; if possible, the surrounding layer of fascia is left with the muscles. A ball-shaped implant of silicone, plastic, or tantalum is inserted and the muscles are sutured around it, providing a permanent stump to give support and motion to an artificial eye. Postoperatively, pressure dressings are kept in place for one or two days to prevent hemorrhage. Other possible complications include thrombosis of nearby blood vessels, which may lead to infection, including meningitis.

Enuclene, a trade name for an ophthalmic, fixed-combination drug containing a detergent (tyloxapol) and a preservative (benzalkonium chloride).

enuresis (en′yuri′sıs), incontinence of urine, especially in bed at night.

environment, all of the many factors, as physical and psychological, that influence or affect the life and survival of a person. See also **biome, climate.** — **environmental,** *adj.*

environmental carcinogen, any one of many natural and synthetic substances which can cause cancer. Such agents, or oncogens, may be divided into chemical agents, physical agents, and certain hormones and viruses. Some environmental carcinogens are arsenic, asbestos, uranium, vinyl chloride, ionizing radiation, ultraviolet rays, x rays, and various coal tar derivatives. Carcinogenic effects of chemicals may be delayed as long as 30 years. Other carcinogens produce more immediate effects. Some studies indicate that the carcinogens in cigarette smoke are involved in 80 per cent of all lung cancers. Most carcinogens are unreactive or secondary carcinogens but are converted to primary carcinogens in the body. Research indicates that numerous factors, as heredity, affect the susceptibilities of different individuals to cancer-causing agents.

Enzactin, a trade name for a topical antifungal (triacetin).

enzygotic twins. See **monozygotic twins.**

enzyme, a protein produced by living cells that catalyzes chemical reactions in organic matter. Most enzymes are produced in minute quantities and catalyze reactions that take place within the cells. Digestive enzymes, however, are produced in relatively large quantities and act outside the cells in the lumen of the digestive tube.

eosin (i′əsın), a group of red, acidic xanthine dyes often used in combination with a blue-purple, basic dye, as hematoxylin, to stain tissue slides in the laboratory.

eosinophil (i′əsın′əfıl), a granulocytic, bi-lobed leukocyte somewhat larger than a neutrophil characterized by the large number of coarse, refractile, cytoplasmic granules that stain intensely with the acid dye, eosin. Eosinophils constitute 1 per cent to 3 per cent of the white blood cells of the body. They increase in number with allergy and some infections and decrease when steroid medications are being administered. See also **basophil, neutrophil.** – **eosinophilic,** *adj.*

eosinophilia (i′əsın′oufıl′iə), an increase in the number of eosinophils in the blood, accompanying many inflammatory conditions. Substantial increases are considered a reflection of an allergic response.

eosinophilic (i′əsın′əfıl′ık), **1.** the tendency of a cell, tissue, or organism to be readily stained by the dye eosin. **2.** of or pertaining to an eosinophilic leukocyte.

eosinophilic adenoma. See **acidophilic adenoma.**

eosinophilic enteropathy, a rare form of food allergy that is characterized by nausea, crampy abdominal pain, diarrhea, urticaria, an elevated eosinophil count in the blood, and eosinophilic infiltrates in the intestine. Diagnosis is made by an elimination diet; symptoms usually disappear when the offending food is removed from the diet.

eosinophilic granuloma, a growth characterized by numerous eosinophils and histiocytes, occurring as a single or multiple lesion in bone. Eosinophilic granulomas may also develop in the lung and occur most frequently in children and adolescents.

eosinophilic leukemia, a malignant neoplasm of leukocytes in which eosinophils are the predominant cells. It resembles chronic myelocytic leukemia but may have an acute course even though there are no blast forms in the peripheral blood.

eosinophilic pneumonia, inflammation of the lungs, characterized by infiltration of the alveoli with eosinophils and large mononuclear cells, pulmonary edema, fever, night sweats, cough, dyspnea, and weight loss. The disease may be caused by a hypersensitivity reaction to spores of fungi, plant fibers, wood dust, bird droppings, porcine, bovine, or piscine proteins, *Bacillus subtilus* enzyme in detergents, or certain drugs. Treatment consists of removal of the offending allergen and symptomatic and supportive therapy.

-eous, a combining form meaning 'like' something specified: *anedeous, cutaneous, osseous.*

ep-. See **epi-**.

ependymal glioma, a large, vascular, fairly solid glioma in the fourth ventricle.

ependymoblastoma (ıpen'dımoublæstou'mə), a malignant neoplasm composed of primitive cells of the ependyma. Also called **malignant ependymoma.**

ependymocytoma (ıpen'dımousaitou'mə). See **ependymoma.**

ependymoma (ıpen'dımou'mə), a neoplasm composed of differentiated cells of the ependyma. The tumor, which is usually a benign, pale, firm, encapsulated, somewhat nodular mass, commonly arises from the roof of the fourth ventricle and usually grows slowly. It may extend to the spinal cord. Primary lesions may also develop in the spinal cord. Also called **ependymocytoma.**

ephapse (cf'æps), a point of lateral contact between nerve fibers across which impulses are transmitted directly by electrical means through the membranes of the cells rather than across the synapse through the action of a neurotransmitter. Compare **synapse**. – **ephaptic,** *adj.*

ephaptic transmission (ıfæp'tık), the passage of a neural impulse from one nerve fiber to another through the nerve membrane by electrical means rather than across a synapse through the action of a neurotransmitter. The mechanism may be a factor in epileptic seizures because of the density of neurons in the brain. Compare **synaptic transmission.**

ephedrine, an adrenergic bronchodilator.

■ INDICATIONS: It is prescribed in the treatment of asthma and bronchitis and is used topically as a nasal decongestant.

■ CONTRAINDICATIONS: Concomitant administration of monoamine oxidase inhibitors, hypertension, cardiac artery disease, cardiac arrhythmia, or known hypersensitivity to this drug prohibits its use.

■ ADVERSE EFFECTS: Among the more serious adverse reactions are nervousness, insomnia, anorexia, and increased blood pressure.

ephemeral fever, any febrile condition lasting only 24 to 48 hours that is uncomplicated and of unknown etiology.

epi-, ep-, a combining form meaning 'on, upon': *epicanthus, epicostal, epidural.*

epiblast, 1. See **ectoderm**. 2. the primordial outer layer of the blastocyst or blastula, before differentiation of the germ layers, that gives rise to the ectoderm and contains cells capable of forming the endoderm and mesoderm. – **epiblastic,** *adj.*

epicanthus (ep'ıkæn'fhəs), a vertical fold of skin over the angle of the inner canthus of the eye. It may be slight or marked, covering the canthus and the caruncle. It is normal in oriental people and is of no clinical significance. Some infants with Down's syndrome have the folds. Also called **epicanthal fold, epicanthic fold.** – **epicanthal, epicanthic,** *adj.*

epicardium (ep'ıkar'dıəm), one of the three layers of tissue that form the wall of the heart. It is composed of a single sheet of squamous epithelial cells overlaying delicate connective tissue. The epicardium is the visceral portion of the serous pericardium and folds back upon itself to form the parietal portion of the serous pericardium. Compare **myocardium**. – **epicardial,** *adj.*

epicondylar fracture, any fracture that involves the medial or the lateral epicondyle of a specific bone, as the humerus.

epicondyle (ep'ıkon'daıl), a projection on the surface of a bone above its condyle. – **epicondylar,** *adj.*

epicondylitis (ep'ıkon'dılaı'tıs), a painful and sometimes disabling inflammation of the muscle and surrounding tissues of the elbow, owing to repeated strain on the forearm near the lateral epicondyle of the humerus, as from violent extension or supination of the wrist against a resisting force. The strain may result from activities, as tennis or golf, twisting a screwdriver, or carrying a heavy load with the arm extended. Treatment usually includes rest, injection of procaine with or without hydrocortisone, and, in some cases, surgery to release part of the muscle from the epicondyle. Also called **tennis elbow.**

epicranial aponeurosis, a fibrous membrane that covers the cranium between the occipital and frontal muscles of the scalp. Also called **galea aponeurotica.**

epicranium (ep'ıkreı'nıəm), the complete scalp, including the integument, the muscular sheets, and the aponeuroses. Compare **epicranius**. – **epicranial,** *adj.*

epicranius (ep'ıkreı'nıəs), the broad, muscular, and tendinous layer of tissue covering the top and the sides of the skull from the occipital bone to the eyebrows. It consists of broad, thin muscular bellies, connected by an extensive aponeurosis. Innervation of the epicranius by branches of the facial nerves can draw back the scalp, raise the eyebrows, and move the ears. Compare **epicranium.** See also **galea aponeurotica, occipitofrontalis, temperoparietalis.**

epidemic, **1.** affecting a significantly large number of people at the same time. **2.** a disease that spreads rapidly through a demographic segment of the human population, as everyone in a given geographic area, a military base, or similar population unit, or everyone of a certain age or sex, as the children or women of a region. **3.** a widespread disease that tends to occur periodically. Compare **endemic, epizootic, pandemic.**

epidemic encephalitis, any diffuse inflammation of the brain occurring in epidemic form. Some kinds of epidemic encephalitis are **influenzal encephalitis, Japanese B encephalitis, Russian spring-summer encephalitis, St. Louis encephalitis.** See also **encephalitis.**

epidemic hemoglobinuria. See **hemoglobinuria.**

epidemic hemorrhagic fever, a severe viral infection marked by fever and bleeding. The disorder develops rapidly, characterized initially by fever and muscle ache, possibly followed by hemorrhage, peripheral vascular collapse, hypovolemic shock, and acute kidney failure. The arbovirus or other pathogen is believed transmitted by mosquitoes, ticks, or mites. The pathophysiology of the hemorrhagic effect is uncertain, although it is assumed the disease organism causes the development of lesions in the lining of the capillaries. Among the various forms of epidemic hemorrhagic fevers are **Argentine hemorrhagic fever, Bolivian hemorrhagic fever, Dengue hemorrhagic fever, Lassa fever, yellow fever.** See also specific viral infections.

epidemic myalgia, a disease caused by coxsackie B virus, characterized by a sudden, acute chest or epigastric pain and fever lasting a few days, followed by complete, spontaneous recovery. Also called **Bornholm disease, devil's grip, epidemic myositis, epidemic pleurodynia.**

epidemic myositis. See **epidemic pleurodynia.**

epidemic parotitis. See **mumps.**

epidemic pleurodynia, an infection caused by a coxsackievirus, affecting mainly children. It is characterized by severe intermittent pain in the abdomen or lower chest, fever, headache, sore throat, malaise, and extreme myalgia. The symptoms may continue for weeks or subside after a few days and recur for a period of weeks. Treatment is symptomatic; complete recovery is usual. See also **Bornholm disease, coxsackievirus, viral disease.**

epidemic typhus, an acute, severe rickettsial infection characterized by prolonged high fever, headache, and a dark maculopapular rash that covers most of the body. The causative organism, *Rickettsia prowazekii,* is transmitted indirectly as a result of the bite of the human body louse; the pathogen is contained in feces of the louse and enters the body tissues as the bite is scratched. An intense headache and a fever reaching 40°C (104°F) begin after an incubation period of ten days to two weeks. The rash follows. Complications may include vascular collapse, renal failure, pneumonia, or gangrene. Mortality is high among older patients. Treatment may include chloramphenicol or tetracycline, aspirin, and supportive, symptomatic care. Also called **classic typhus, European typhus, jail fever, louse-borne typhus.** See also **rickettsia, typhus.**

epidemiology (ep′ɪdi′miol′əji), the study of the occurrence, distribution, and causes of health and disease in mankind. — **epidemiologic, epidemiological,** *adj.,* **epidemiologist,** *n.*

epiderm-, epidermo-, a combining form meaning 'of or pertaining to the epidermis': *epidermoid, epidermolysis, epidermolytic.*

epidermis (ep′ɪdər′mɪs), the superficial, avascular layers of the skin, made up of an outer, dead, cornified portion and a deeper, living, cellular portion. Epidermal cells gradually move outward to the skin surface, undergoing change as they migrate, until they are desquamated, as cornified flakes. Cells in various transitional stages make up the basal cell layer, the prickle cell layer, the granular layer, and the cornified layer. Altogether, these layers are between 0.5 mm and 1.1 mm in thickness. Also called **cuticle.** — **epidermal, epidermoid,** *adj.*

epidermoid carcinoma, a malignant neoplasm in which the tumor cells tend to differentiate in the manner of epidermal cells, then form horny cells called prickle cells.

epidermoid cyst, a common, benign, fluctuant, subcutaneous swelling lined by keratinizing epithelium and filled with a cheesy material composed of sebum and epithelial debris. The cyst is movable but attached to the skin by the remains of the duct of a sebaceous gland. Frequently, epidermoid cysts become infected. Treatment is surgical excision. Also called **sebaceous cyst, wen.** Compare **pilar cyst.**

epidermolysis bullosa, a group of rare, hereditary skin diseases in which vesicles and bullae develop, usually at sites of trauma. Severe forms may also involve mucous membranes and may leave scars and contractures on healing. Basal cell and squamous cell carcinomas sometimes develop in the scar tissue. Treatment is symptomatic.

epididymis (ep′ɪdɪd′ɪmɪs), one of a pair of long tightly coiled ducts that carry sperm by the millions from the seminiferous tubules of the testes to the vas deferens.

epididymitis (ep′ɪdɪd′ɪmaɪ′tɪs), acute or chronic inflammation of the epididymis. It may result from venereal disease, urinary tract infection, prostatitis, or prostatectomy. Symptoms include fever and chills, pain in the groin, and tender, swollen epididymis. Treatment includes bed rest, scrotal support, and antibiotics, as appropriate.

epididymo-orchitis (ep′ɪdɪd′ɪmoʊɔrkaɪ′tɪs), inflammation of the epididymis and of the testis. See also **epididymitis, orchitis.**

epidural (ep'ɪdur'əl),   outside the dura mater.

epidural anesthesia,   the process of achieving regional anesthesia of the pelvic, abdominal, genital or other area by the injection of a local anesthetic into the epidural space of the spinal column.

epidural blood patch,   a patch repairing a tear or a hole in the dura mater around the spinal cord. The tear is usually the result of needle puncture during spinal anesthesia or lumbar puncture. Spinal fluid leaks through the hole, resulting in a spinal headache. To form a seal, 10 to 15 ml of the patient's blood is injected into the epidural space. A clot forms, covering the hole and preventing further loss of fluid. The technique is used to treat persistent or severe spinal headache.

epidural space,   the space immediately surrounding the dura mater of the brain or spinal cord, beneath the periosteum of the cranium and the spinal column.

Epifrin,   a trade name for an adrenergic (epinephrine hydrochloride).

epigastric node (ep'ɪgæs'trɪk),   a node in one of the seven groups of parietal lymph nodes serving the abdomen and the pelvis, comprising about four nodes along the caudal portion of the inferior epigastric vessels. See also **lymph, lymphatic system, lymph node.**

epigenesis,   (in embryology) a theory of development in which the organism grows from a simple to more complex form through the progressive differentiation of an undifferentiated cellular unit. Compare **preformation.** – **epigenesist,** n. **epigenetic,** adj.

epiglottiditis (ep'ɪglot'ɪdaɪ'tɪs).   See **epiglottitis.**

epiglottis (ep'ɪglot'ɪs),   the cartilaginous structure that overhangs the larynx like a lid and prevents food from entering the larynx or the trachea while swallowing.

epiglottitis (ep'ɪglotaɪ'tɪs),   an inflammation of the epiglottis. Acute epiglottitis is a severe form of the condition, affecting primarily children. It is characterized by fever, sore throat, stridor, croupy cough, and an erythematous, swollen epiglottis. The child may become cyanotic and require an emergency tracheostomy to maintain respiration. The causative organism is usually *Haemophilus hemolyticus.* Antibiotics, rest, oxygen, and supportive care are usually included in treatment. Also called **epiglottiditis.**

epilating forceps (ep'ɪlei'tɪŋ),   a kind of small spring forceps, used for removing unwanted hair.

epilation (ep'ɪlei'ʃən).   See **depilation.**

epilepsy,   a group of neurological disorders characterized by recurrent episodes of convulsive seizures, sensory disturbances, abnormal behavior, loss of consciousness, or all of these. Common to all types of epilepsy is an uncontrolled electrical discharge from the nerve cells of the cerebral cortex. Although most epilepsy is of unknown cause, it may sometimes be associated with cerebral trauma, intracranial infection, brain tumor, vascular disturbances, intoxication, or chemical imbalance. Kinds of epilepsy include **grand mal epilepsy, Jacksonian epilepsy, petit mal epilepsy, psychomotor epilepsy.**

■ OBSERVATIONS: The frequency of attacks may range from several times a day to intervals of several years. In predisposed individuals, seizures may occur during sleep or after physical stimulation, as by a flickering light or sudden loud sound. Emotional disturbances also may be significant trigger factors. Some seizures are preceded by an aura, but others have no warning symptoms. Most epileptic attacks are brief. They may be localized or general, with or without clonic movements, and are often followed by drowsiness or confusion. Diagnosis is made by observation of the pattern of seizures and abnormalities on an electroencephalogram.

■ INTERVENTION: The kind of epilepsy determines the selection of preventive medication. Correctible lesions and metabolic causes are eliminated when possible. During an attack the patient should be protected from injury without being severely restrained.

■ NURSING CONSIDERATIONS: A nurse observing an epileptic attack, in addition to protecting the patient from injury, should carefully note and accurately describe the sequence of seizure activity. The patient and family must be fully informed and counseled about the disorder, the importance of regularly taking prescribed medication, never discontinuing treatment without professional advice, toxic effects of medication, wearing a medical identification tag, and continuing to live as normal a life as possible. Nurses also have a responsibility to help improve the public's attitude toward epilepsy and to correct misunderstanding which limits educational and occupational opportunities for patients with this diagnosis. See also **analeptic, anticonvulsant, aura, clonus, ictus, tonic.** – **epileptic,** adj., n.

epileptic mania,   *Obsolete.* a mood disorder characterized by attacks of violence that occur immediately preceding, following, or in place of an epileptic seizure. See also **epilepsy, mania.**

epileptic stupor,   the state of unawareness and unresponsiveness following an epileptic seizure.

epiloia (ep'ɪloi'ə).   See **tuberous sclerosis.**

epimysium (ep'ɪmɪz'iəm),   a fibrous sheath that enfolds a muscle and extends between the bundles of muscle fibers, as the perimysium. It is sturdy in some areas but more delicate in others, as those areas where the muscle moves freely under a strong sheet of fascia. The epimysium may also fuse with fascia that attaches a muscle to a bone.

Epinal,   a trade name for an adrenergic (epinephryl borate).

epinephrine (ep'ənef'rɪn),   an adrenergic vasoconstrictor.

■ INDICATIONS: It is prescribed in the treatment of anaphylaxis, acute bronchial spasm, and nasal congestion and to increase the effectiveness of a local anesthetic.

■ CONTRAINDICATION: Known hypersensitivity to this drug prohibits its use.

■ ADVERSE EFFECTS: Among the most serious adverse reactions are arrhythmias, increases in blood pressure, or rebound congestion (when used as a decongestant).

epinephryl borate, an adrenergic.

■ INDICATION: It is prescribed in the treatment of primary open-angle glaucoma.

■ CONTRAINDICATIONS: Narrow-angle glaucoma, aphakia, or known hypersensitivity to this drug prohibits its use. It is not given prior to peripheral iridectomy, and it is not administered to eyes that are capable of angle closure.

■ ADVERSE EFFECTS: Among the more serious adverse reactions are tachycardia, hypertension, headache, blurred vision, and allergic reaction.

epiphora (ɪpɪf′ərə). See **tearing.**

epiphyseal fracture, a fracture involving the epiphyseal growth plate of a long bone, resulting in separation or in fragmentation of the plate. Also called **Salter fracture.**

epiphysis (ɪpɪf′ɪsɪs), *pl.* **epiphyses.** the head of a long bone that is separated from the shaft of the bone by the epiphyseal plate until the bone stops growing, the plate is obliterated, and the shaft and the head become united. Compare **diaphysis.** – **epiphyseal,** *adj.*

epiphysis cerebri. See **pineal body.**

epiploic foramen, a passage between the peritoneal cavity and the omental bursa. It is lined with peritoneum and is approximately 3 cm in diameter.

epipygus (ep′əpaɪ′gəs). See **pygomelus.**

episcleritis (ep′ɪsklɛraɪ′tɪs), inflammation of the outermost layers of the sclera and of the tissues overlying the posterior portions of this tough, white outer coat of the eyeball.

episiotomy (ɪpi′zioɪt′əmi), a surgical procedure, usually required for forceps delivery, in which an incision is made in a woman's perineum to enlarge her vaginal opening for delivery, performed most often electively to prevent tearing of the perineum, to hasten or facilitate delivery of the baby, or to prevent stretching of perineal muscles and connective tissue thought to predispose to subsequent abnormalities of pelvic outlet relaxation, as cystocele, rectocele, and uterine prolapse; its prophylactic efficacy is debated. The incision into the vaginal and perineal tissue is closed with absorbable sutures that need not be removed. Deep incisions require closure in two or more layers. Immediate complications include hemorrhage and extension of the incision along the vaginal sulcus or into the anal sphincter or rectum. Delayed complications include hematoma and abscess. Application of cold packs to the perineum for several hours immediately postpartum minimizes swelling. Alternating applications later of heat and cold and warm sitz baths reduce discomfort, but sitz baths longer than ten minutes soften tissue and pro-

long healing. A mediolateral episiotomy is an episiotomy cut at an angle of approximately 45 degrees with the midline. Although it affords wide exposure for delivery, it is painful postpartum and is prone to hematoma and infection. A median or midline episiotomy is an incision in the perineum in the midline; although less painful postpartum, it affords less exposure for delivery and may extend into or through the anal sphincter and into the rectum.

episode, an incident or event that stands out from the continuity of everyday life, as an episode of illness or a traumatic episode in the course of a child's development. – **episodic,** *adj.*

episodic care, a pattern of medical and nursing care in which care is given to a person for a particular problem, without an ongoing relationship being established between the person and health care professionals. Emergency rooms provide episodic care.

episodic health history, an abbreviated form of the health history that is focused on the factors relevant to an illness or complaint that has been previously noted, as in a follow-up visit after a treatment or surgical procedure, or in the regular periodic visits for a chronic illness or condition. The current health status of the person is noted with an account of his health since the last visit as it pertains to the particular condition. An episodic health history is a partial history that serves to bring the data base up to date. In the patient's chart it may precede the progress notes made for the current visit.

episome (ep′ɪsoʊm), (in bacterial genetics) an extrachromosomal replicating unit that exists autonomously or functions with a chromosome. See also **colicinogen, conjugon, F factor, R factor.**

epispadias (ep′ɪspeɪ′diəs), a congenital defect in which the urethra opens on the dorsum of the penis at some point proximal to the glans. Treatment is directed at correcting or managing urinary incontinence, which occurs because the urinary sphincters are defective, and at permitting sexual function. The corresponding defect in women, fissure of the upper wall of the urethra, is quite rare. Compare **hypospadias.**

epistasis (ɪpɪs′təsɪs), (in genetics) a type of interaction between genes at different loci on a chromosome in which one is able to mask or suppress the expression of the other. The epistatic effect, which is nonallelic and therefore the opposite of the dominance relationship, may be caused by the presence of homozygous recessives at one gene pair, as occurs in the Bombay phenotype, or by the presence of a dominant allele that counteracts the expression of another dominant gene. Compare **dominance.** – **epistatic,** *adj.*

epistaxis (ep′ɪstæk′sɪs), bleeding from the nose caused by local irritation of mucous membranes, violent sneezing, fragility of the mucous membrane or of the arterial walls, chronic infection, trauma, hypertension, leukemia, vitamin K deficiency, or, most often, by picking of the nose. Also called **nosebleed.**

■ OBSERVATIONS: Epistaxis may result from rupture of tiny vessels in the anterior nasal septum; this occurs most frequently in early childhood and adolescence. In adults, it occurs more commonly in men than in women, may be severe in elderly persons, and may be accompanied by respiratory distress, apprehension, restlessness, vertigo, and nausea and may lead to syncope.

■ INTERVENTION: The patient suffering epistaxis is instructed to breathe through the mouth, to sit quietly with the head tilted slightly forward in order to prevent blood from entering the pharynx, and to avoid swallowing blood. The bleeding may be controlled by pinching the nose firmly with the fingers, by inserting a cotton ball soaked in a topical vasoconstrictor (as Neo-Synephrine) and applying pressure to the skin on both sides of the nose, occluding the blood supply to the nostrils, or by placing an ice compress over the nose. If bleeding continues, the clots may be removed by suction. The nasal mucosa may be anesthetized with topical lidocaine, cauterized with a silver nitrate stick or an electric cautery, and then sprayed with epinephrine. Severe bleeding, especially from the posterior nasal septum, may be treated by inserting packing, which generally is left in place for one to three days. During that period the patient is kept in a high Fowler's position, the placement of the packing is checked frequently, and a sedative, antibiotics, vitamins C and K, and a cool, nonirritating liquid diet may be ordered. Persistent or recurrent profuse epistaxis may be treated by ligating an artery supplying the nose, as the external carotid, ethmoid, or internal maxillary.

■ NURSING CONSIDERATIONS: The nurse administers first aid and ordered medication, assists in cauterization and nasal packing, checks the patient's blood pressure, pulse, and respiration every half hour until bleeding subsides, and then continues to check them every four hours. The nurse limits the patient's activity, avoids serving milk and hot liquids, encourages expectoration rather than swallowing of blood, and reports symptoms of respiratory distress, vertigo, and any bleeding. Before the patient is discharged, the nurse provides instruction on the prevention of epistaxis by using a vaporizer and applying petroleum jelly with a cotton swab gently to the mucous membrane lining the nostrils.

epistropheus (ep′ɪstrou′fiəs). See **axis.**

epithalamus (ep′ɪθæl′əməs), one of the five portions of the diencephalon. It includes the trigonum habenulae, the pineal body, and the posterior commissure. Compare **hypothalamus, metathalamus, subthalamus, thalamus.** – **epithalamic,** adj.

epithelioid leiomyoma, an uncommon neoplasm of smooth muscle in which the cells are polygonal in shape.

It usually develops in the stomach. Also called **bizarre leiomyoma, leiomyoblastoma.**

epithelioma (ep′ɪθhi′liou′mə), **1.** a neoplasm derived from the epithelium. **2.** Obsolete. any carcinoma.

-epithelioma, a combining form meaning a 'tumor of epithelial tissue': inoepithelioma, periepithelioma, trichoepithelioma.

epithelioma adamantinum. See **ameloblastoma.**

epithelioma adenoides cysticum. See **trichoepithelioma.**

epithelium (ep′ɪθhi′liəm), the covering of the internal and the external organs of the body, including the lining of vessels. It consists of cells bound together by connective material and varies in the number of layers and the kinds of cells. Epithelium in different parts of the body is made of simple squamous cells, simple cuboidal cells, and stratified columnar cells. The stratified squamous epithelium of the epidermis is comprised of five different cellular layers. – **epithelial,** adj.

epitope, an antigenic determinant that causes a specific reaction by an immunoglobulin. It consists of a group of amino acids on the surface of the antigen.

Epitrate, a trade name for an ophthalmic adrenergic (epinephrine bitartrate).

epitympanic recess, one of the two areas of the tympanic cavity, the other being the tympanic cavity proper. The recess is cranial to the tympanic membrane and contains the upper half of the malleus and greater part of the incus. Also called **the attic.**

epizootic, a disease or condition that occurs simultaneously in nearly all of the animals of a species in a geographical area.

Epontol, a trade name for a general anesthetic agent (propanidid).

epoophorectomy (ep′ouof′ərek′təmi), surgical removal of the epoophoron.

epoophoron (ep′ouof′əron), a structure that is situated in the mesosalpinx between the ovary and the uterine tube. It is composed of a few short tubules. The ends of the tubules converge in one direction toward the ovary and, in the opposite direction, open into a rudimentary duct. The epoophoron is a persistent portion of the embryonic mesonephric duct.

Eppy, a trade name for an adrenergic (epinephryl borate).

Eprolin, a trade name for vitamin E (alphatocopherol).

EPSDT, abbreviation for **Early and Periodic Screening Diagnosis and Treatment.**

Epsom salt. See **magnesium sulfate.**

Epstein-Barr virus (EBV) (ep′stainbar′), the herpesvirus that causes infectious mononucleosis.

Epstein's pearls, small, white, pearllike epithelial cysts that occur on both sides of the midline of the hard palate of the newborn baby. They are normal and usually disappear within a few weeks. Compare **Bednar's aphthae, thrush.**

epulis (ɪpyu′lɪs), any tumor or growth on the gingiva.

Equagesic, a trade name for a central nervous system fixed-combination drug containing analgesics (aspirin and ethoheptazine citrate) and a sedative (meprobamate).

equal cleavage, mitotic division of the fertilized ovum into blastomeres of identical size, as occurs in man and most mammals. Compare **unequal cleavage.**

Equal Employment Opportunity Commission (EEOC), a commission appointed by the President of the United States to administer the Civil Rights Act of 1964, particularly to investigate complaints of discrimination in employment in businesses engaged in interstate commerce. Discrimination based on race, color, creed, or national origin is forbidden, but certain kinds of employers and certain conditions of employment allow exceptions to the act. Women and men must both be considered for a position that both can perform, and men and women must be paid equal wages for equal work.

Equanil, a trade name for a sedative (meprobamate).

Equanitrate, a trade name for a cardiovascular, fixed-combination drug containing a vasodilator (pentaerythritol tetranitrate) and a sedative (meprobamate).

equatorial plate, the platelike configuration formed by the chromosomes at the center of the spindle during the metaphase stage of mitosis and meiosis.

equilibrium (i′kwɪlɪb′riəm), **1.** a state of balance or rest owing to the equal action of opposing forces, as calcium and phosphorus in the body. **2.** (in psychiatry) a state of mental or emotional balance.

equine encephalitis, an arbovirus infection, characterized by inflammation of the nerve tissues of the brain and spinal cord, with high fever, headache, nausea, vomiting, myalgia and neurologic symptoms, as visual disturbances, tremor, lethargy, and disorientation. The virus is transmitted by the bite of an infected mosquito. Horses are the primary host of the particular viruses that cause the infection; man is a secondary host. **Eastern equine encephalitis (EEE)** is a severe form of the infection. It occurs along the eastern seaboard of the United States and lasts longer and causes more deaths and residual morbidity than **Western equine encephalitis (WEE),** which occurs throughout the United States and results in a mild, brief illness, as does **Venezuelan equine encephalitis (VEE),** which is common in Central and South America, Florida, and Texas.

Er, symbol for **erbium.**

E.R., ER, abbreviation for **emergency room.**

erbium (Er), a rare-earth, metallic element. Its atomic number is 68; its atomic weight is 167.26.

Erb-Duchenne paralysis (erb′dyʃhen′). See **Erb's palsy.**

Erb's muscular dystrophy, a form of muscular dystro-

phy which first affects the shoulder girdle and, later, often involves the pelvic girdle. It is a progressively crippling disease with onset in childhood or adolescence and is usually inherited as an autosomal recessive trait. It affects both sexes. In males, differential diagnosis between Erb's muscular dystrophy and Duchenne's muscular dystrophy may be difficult.

Erb's palsy, a kind of paralysis caused by traumatic injury to the upper brachial plexus, occurring most commonly in childbirth from forcible traction during delivery. The signs of Erb's palsy include loss of sensation in the arm and paralysis and atrophy of the deltoid, the biceps, and the brachialis muscles. The arm on the affected side hangs loosely with the elbow extended and the forearm pronated. Treatment initially requires that the arm and shoulder be immobilized to allow the swelling and inflammation of the associated neuritis to resolve. Physical therapy and splinting may be necessary to improve function of the muscles and to prevent flexion contracture of the elbow. Also called **Erb-Duchenne paralysis.**

erectile (ɪrek′tɪl, ɪrek′tail), capable of being erected or raised to an erect position, usually applied in the description of spongy tissue of the penis or clitoris that becomes turgid and erectile when filled with blood. It also may be used when referring to the epidermal tissue involved in the appearance of "goose bumps" (horripilation) in response to fear, anger, cold, or other stimuli.

erectile myxoma, an angioma that contains areas of myxomatous tissue.

erectile tumor. See **cavernous hemangioma.**

erection, the condition of hardness, swelling, and elevation observed in the penis and to a lesser degree in the clitoris, usually due to sexual arousal but also occurring during sleep or as a result of physical stimulation. It occurs as additional blood enters the organ and blood pressure increases and is influenced by psychic and nerve stimulation. It is needed to enable the penis to enter the vagina and to emit semen. See also **ejaculation, nocturnal emission, priapism.**

erector spinae. See **sacrospinalis.**

erethistic idiocy (er′ɪθɪs′tɪk), *Obsolete.* severe mental retardation associated with continuous, purposeless activity and restlessness.

-ergasia, a combining form meaning 'interfunctioning of the mind and body': *cacergasia, dysgasia, orthergasia.*

ergastoplasm, a network of cytoplasmic structures that show basophilic-staining properties; granular endoplasmic reticulum. See **endoplasmic reticulum.**

-ergetic. See **-ergic.**

-ergic, a combining form meaning an 'effect of activity': *allergic, pathergic, telergic.* Also **-ergetic.**

ergo-, a combining form meaning 'pertaining to work': *ergodermatosis, ergomaniac, ergotropy.*

ergocalciferol (ər'goukælsɪf'ərɔl). See **calciferol**.

Ergomar, a trade name for an ergot alkaloid (ergotamine tartrate), used to treat migraine.

ergonomics, a scientific discipline devoted to the study and analysis of human work, especially as it is affected by individual anatomy, psychology, and other human factors. — **ergonomic,** *adj.*

ergonovine maleate (ər'gounou'vin, ər'gounou'vɪn), an oxytocic ergot alkaloid.

■ INDICATIONS: It is prescribed to contract the uterus in the treatment or prevention of postpartum or postabortion hemorrhage.

■ CONTRAINDICATIONS: Pregnancy, peripheral vascular disease, elevated blood pressure, or known hypersensitivity to this drug prohibits its use.

■ ADVERSE EFFECTS: Among the more serious adverse effects are hypertension, nausea, headache, blurred vision, and hypersensitivity reactions. Fetal death may occur if the drug is given in pregnancy.

ergosome. See **polysome**.

ergosterol (ərgos'tərəl), an unsaturated hydrocarbon of the vitamin D group isolated from yeast, mushrooms, ergot, and other fungi. When treated with ultraviolet irradiation it is converted into vitamin D_2. See also **calciferol, viosterol, vitamin D.**

ergot (ər'gət), (in pharmacology) the food storage body of a fungus, *Claviceps purpura*, which commonly infects rye and other cereal grasses. It contains ergotalkaloids.

ergot alkaloid, one of a large group of alkaloids derived from a common fungus that grows on rye and other grains throughout the temperate areas of the world. The alkaloids are divided into three groups; the amino acid alkaloids, typified by ergotamine; the dihydrogenated amino acid alkaloids, as dihydroergotamine; and the amine alkaloids, as ergonovine. Ergotamine and dihydroergotamine are not as effective oxytocics as ergonovine; therefore, ergonovine, given orally or intravenously is currently used in obstetrics to treat or prevent postpartum uterine atony and to complete an incomplete or missed, abortion. Ergotamine is prescribed to relieve migraine headache. It acts by reducing the amplitude of arterial pulsations in the external carotid branches of the cranial arteries. Dihydroergotamine was formerly used to improve cerebral blood flow in elderly patients in order to improve mental function but is no longer thought to be a useful or effective drug for that purpose. Contraindications to the use of any of the ergot alkaloids include peripheral vascular disease, coronary artery disease, hypertension, renal or hepatic dysfunction, and sepsis. Pregnancy prohibits use of the drugs because contractions of the uterus and decreased blood flow to the fetus may result, causing fetal death. Ergot poisoning may occur with prolonged or excessive use of the drug or by accidental ingestion of contaminated grain. Signs of toxicity are thirst, diarrhea, dizziness, chest pain, abnormal and variable rate of cardiac contraction, nausea and vomiting, digital paresthesia, severe cramping, and seizures. Tissue anoxia and gangrene of the extremities may occur, owing to prolonged vasoconstriction, if poisoning is severe.

ergotamine tartrate (ərgot'əmin), a vasoconstrictor and oxytocic.

■ INDICATIONS: It is prescribed in the treatment of migraine and postpartum uterine atony.

■ CONTRAINDICATIONS: Pregnancy, peripheral vascular disease, infectious disease, or known hypersensitivity to this drug prohibits its use.

■ ADVERSE EFFECTS: Among the more serious adverse reactions are vomiting, diarrhea, thirst, tingling of fingers and toes, and increased blood pressure. Fetal death may occur if the drug is administered to a woman during pregnancy.

ergotherapy, the use of physical activity and exercise in the treatment of disease. By extension, the therapy includes any procedure that increases the blood supply to a diseased or injured part, as massage or various types of hot baths. — **ergotherapeutic,** *adj.*

Ergotrate Maleate, a trade name for an ergot alkaloid (ergonovine maleate), used as an oxytocic.

-ergy, 1. a combining form meaning an 'action': *abioenergy, leukergy, synergy.* 2. a combining form meaning an 'effect or result': *allergy, anabolergy, pathergy.*

erosion, the wearing away or gradual destruction of a surface, as of a mucosal or epidermal surface as a result of inflammation, injury, or other effects, usually marked by the appearance of an ulcer. See also **necrosis**.

erosive gastritis, an inflammatory condition characterized by multiple erosions of the mucous membrane lining the stomach. Nausea, anorexia, pain, and gastric hemorrhage may occur. Treatment includes removal of the irritating substance, and supportive care includes intravenous fluids, electrolytes, and, if necessary, blood transfusion. See also **chemical gastritis, corrosive gastritis.**

erosive osteoarthritis. See **Kellgren's syndrome**.

-erotic, a combining form meaning 'pertaining to sexual love or desire': *anterotic, homoerotic, hysteroerotic.*

eroticism, erotism, 1. sexual impulse or desire. 2. the arousal or attempt to arouse the sexual instinct through suggestive or symbolic means. 3. the expression of sexual instinct or desire. 4. an abnormally persistent sexual drive. See also **anal eroticism, oral eroticism.**

eroto-, a combining form meaning 'pertaining to love or sexual desire': *erotogenic, erotopath, erotophobia.*

erotomania (irot'oumei'niə), *Obsolete.* a psychopathological state characterized by preoccupation with sexuality and sexual behavior.

erotomaniac (irot'oumei'niæk), *Obsolete.* a person displaying characteristics of erotomania.

error, (in research) a defect in the design of a study, in the development of measurements or instruments, or in the interpretation of the findings.

ERT, abbreviation for **external radiation therapy.**

eructation (i'rəktei'shən), the act of bringing up air from the stomach with a characteristic sound. Also called **belching.**

eruption, the rapid development of a skin lesion, especially of a viral exanthem or of the rash commonly accompanying a drug reaction.

eruptive fever, any disease characterized by fever and a rash.

eruptive xanthoma, a skin disorder associated with elevated triglyceride levels in the blood. Erythematous or pale raised papules suddenly appear in large numbers on the trunk, legs, arms, and buttocks.

ERV, abbreviation for **expiratory reserve volume.**

Erypar, a trade name for an antibacterial (erythromycin stearate).

erysipelas (er'ısıp'ələs), an infectious skin disease characterized by redness, swelling, vesicles, bullae, fever, pain, and lymphadenopathy. It is caused by a species of group A, beta-hemolytic streptococci. Treatment includes antibiotics, analgesics, and packs or dressings applied locally to the lesions.

erysipeloid (er'ısıp'əloid), an infection of the hands characterized by blue-red nodules or patches and, occasionally, by erythema. It is acquired by handling meat or fish infected with *Erysipelothrix rhusiopathiae.* The disease is self-limited, lasting about three weeks, but will respond to penicillin. Compare **erysipelas.**

erythema (er'ıthi'mə), redness or inflammation of the skin or mucous membranes that is the result of dilatation and congestion of superficial capillaries. Examples of erythema are nervous blushes and mild sunburn. See also **erythroderma, rubor.** – **erythematous,** *adj.*

erythema chronicum migrans, a skin lesion that begins as a small papule and spreads peripherally, extending by a raised, red margin and clearing in the center. It may be associated with **Lyme arthritis,** in which case it is caused by the bite of a small tick.

erythema infectiosum, an acute, benign infectious disease, mainly of children, characterized by fever and an erythematous rash beginning on the cheeks and appearing later on the arms, thighs, buttocks, and trunk. As the rash progresses, earlier lesions fade. Sunlight aggravates the eruption, which usually lasts about ten days. For a period of time the rash may reappear whenever the skin is irritated. Its cause is unknown, no treatment is necessary, and prognosis is excellent. The isolation of patients is not required. Also called **fifth disease.**

erythema marginatum, a variant of **erythema multiforme** seen in acute rheumatic fever, characterized by transient, disc-shaped, nonpruritic, reddened macules with raised margins.

erythema multiforme, a hypersensitivity syndrome characterized by polymorphous eruption of skin and mucous membranes. Macules, papules, nodules, vesicles, or bullae, and target, or bull's-eye-shaped lesions are seen. Erythema multiforme has been associated with many infections, collagen diseases, drug sensitivities, allergies, and pregnancy. Definitive and preventive treatment depends on finding the specific cause, but topical or systemic corticosteroids are helpful in most cases. A severe form of this condition is known as **Stevens-Johnson syndrome.**

erythema nodosum, a hypersensitivity vasculitis characterized by bilateral, reddened, tender, subcutaneous nodules on the shins and, occasionally, on other parts of the body. The nodules last for several days or weeks, never ulcerate, and are often associated with mild fever, malaise, and pains in muscles and joints. This condition may be seen with streptococcal infections, tuberculosis, sarcoid, leprosy, drug sensitivity, ulcerative colitis, and pregnancy. The prognosis is good, given appropriate treatment of the underlying disease. A course of corticosteroids is usually effective in diminishing the symptoms of this condition.

erythema perstans, a persistent local redness of the skin, often caused by a fixed drug eruption.

erythema toxicum neonatorum, a common skin condition of neonates characterized by a pink papular rash frequently superimposed with vesicles or pustules. The rash appears within 24 to 48 hours after birth, covers the thorax, abdomen, back, and diaper area, and disappears spontaneously after several days. A smear of the papules shows eosinophils rather than neutrophils to differentiate the condition from neonatal pustular melanosis. Also called **toxic erythema of the newborn,** *Informal.* **flea bites.**

erythrasma (er'ıthræz'mə), a bacterial skin infection of the axillary or inguinal regions, characterized by irregular, reddish-brown, raised patches. An asymptomatic disease, it is more common in diabetics and responds quickly to oral erythromycin. Compare **intertrigo, tinea cruris.**

erythrityl tetranitrate, a coronary vasodilator.

■ INDICATION: It is prescribed in the treatment of angina pectoris.

■ CONTRAINDICATION: It is used with caution when glaucoma is present. Known hypersensitivity to this drug prohibits its use.

■ ADVERSE EFFECTS: Among the most serious adverse reactions are hypotension, allergic reactions, headache, and flushing.

erythro-, a combining form meaning 'red': *erythroblast, erythroclast, erythrocyte.*

erythroblastosis fetalis, a type of hemolytic anemia that occurs in newborns as a result of maternal-fetal blood group incompatibility, specifically involving the Rh factor and the ABO blood groups. The condition is caused by an antigen-antibody reaction in the bloodstream of the infant resulting from the placental transmission of maternally formed antibodies against the incompatible antigens of the fetal blood. In Rh factor incompatibility, the hemolytic reaction occurs only when the mother is Rh negative and the infant is Rh positive. The isoimmunization process rarely occurs with the first pregnancy, but there is increased risk with each succeeding pregnancy. However, maternal sensitization to the Rh factor can be prevented by injection of a high-titer anti-Rh gamma globulin preparation following delivery or abortion of an Rh positive fetus. No sensitization may occur in situations in which a strong placental barrier prevents transfer of fetal blood into the maternal circulation. In about 10 to 15 per cent of sensitized mothers, there is no hemolytic reaction in the newborn. Clinical manifestations of the condition include severe anemia, jaundice, and enlargement of the liver and spleen, which, without intervention, can lead to hypoxia, cardiac failure, generalized edema, respiratory distress, and death. Prenatal diagnosis of the disease is confirmed through amniocentesis and analysis of bilirubin levels in amniotic fluid. Higher than normal levels result from the breakdown of hemoglobin from the lysed erythrocytes. Treatment consists of intrauterine transfusion when placental bilirubin levels progressively increase or immediate exchange transfusions following birth. Hemolytic reactions involving the ABO blood groups have similar manifestations but are generally less severe. See also **hydrops fetalis, hyperbilirubinemia of the newborn, rhesus factor.**

Erythrocin, a trade name for an antibacterial (erythromycin).

erythrocyte (erıth′rəsaıt′), a biconcave disc about 7 microns in diameter that contains hemoglobin confined within a lipoid membrane. The major cellular element of the circulating blood, its principal function is to transport oxygen. The number of cells per cu mm of blood is usually maintained between 4.5 and 5.0 million in men and between 4.0 and 4.5 million in women. It varies with age, activity, and environmental conditions. For example, an increase to a level of 8.0 million per cu mm can normally occur at over 10,000 feet above sea level. An erythrocyte normally lives for 110 to 120 days, at which time it is removed from the blood stream and broken down by the reticulo-endothelial system. New erythrocytes are produced at a rate of slightly more than one per cent a day; thus, a constant level is usually maintained. With acute blood loss, hemolytic anemia, or chronic oxygen deprivation, erythrocyte production may increase greatly. Erythrocytes originate in the marrow of the long bones. Maturation proceeds from a stem cell (promegaloblast) through the pronormoblast stage to the normoblast, the last stage before the mature adult cell develops. Kinds of erythro-

cyte include **discocyte, echinocyte, macrocyte, spherocyte.** Also called **red blood cell, red cell, red corpuscle.** Compare **normoblast, reticulocyte.** See also **erythropoiesis, hemoglobin.**

erythrocyte sedimentation rate (ESR), the rate at which red blood cells settle out in a tube of unclotted blood, expressed in millimeters per hour. Blood is collected in an anticoagulant and allowed to sediment in a calibrated glass column. At the end of one hour, the laboratory technician measures the distance the erythrocytes have fallen in the tube. Elevated sedimentation rates are not specific for any disorder but indicate the presence of inflammation. Inflammation causes an alteration of the blood proteins which makes the red blood cells aggregate, becoming heavier than normal. The speed with which they fall to the bottom of the tube corresponds to the degree of inflammation. Serial evaluations of erythrocyte sedimentation rate are useful in monitoring the course of inflammatory activity in rheumatic diseases and, when performed with a white blood cell count, can indicate infection. Certain noninflammatory conditions, as pregnancy, are also characterized by high sedimentation rates. Two methods are used. The Wintrobe ESR is performed in a 10 cm Wintrobe tube, and the Westergren ESR is performed in a 200 mm Westergren tube. Values are higher for women in both methods and vary according to the method used. Also called *Informal.* **sed rate.** See also **inflammation.**

erythrocytosis (erıth′rousaıtou′sıs), an abnormal increase in the number of circulating red cells. See also **polycythemia.**

erythroderma (erıth′rouder′mə), any dermatosis associated with abnormal redness of the skin. Compare **erythema, rubor.**

erythroleukemia (ırıth′roulukı′mıə), a malignant blood disorder characterized by a proliferation of erythropoietic elements in bone marrow, erythroblasts with bizarre, lobulated nuclei, and abnormal myeloblasts in peripheral blood. The disease may have an acute or chronic course. Also called **diGuglielmo's disease, diGuglielmo's syndrome, erythromyeloblastic leukemia.**

erythromelalgia (ırıth′roumılæl′jə), a rare disorder characterized by a paroxysmal dilation of the peripheral blood vessels. It occurs bilaterally, usually in the extremities, and is associated with burning, redness of the skin, and pain. — **erythromelalgic,** *adj.*

erythromycin, an antibacterial antibiotic.

■ INDICATIONS: It is prescribed in the treatment of many bacterial and mycoplasmic infections.

■ CONTRAINDICATIONS: Liver disease or known hypersensitivity to this drug prohibits its use.

■ ADVERSE EFFECTS: Among the more serious adverse effects are cholestatic hepatitis and hypersensitivity reactions.

erythromyeloblastic leukemia (ɪrɪth′roumæi′əloublæs′tɪk). See **erythroleukemia.**

erythrophobia (ɪrɪth′roufou′biə), **1.** an anxiety disorder characterized by an irrational fear of blushing or of displaying embarrassment. **2.** a neurotic symptom manifested by blushing at the slightest provocation. **3.** a morbid fear of or aversion to the color red. — **erythrophobic,** *adj.*

erythroplasia of Queyrat (ɪrɪth′rəplei′źhə), a premalignant lesion on the glans or corona of the penis. It is a well-circumscribed reddish patch on the skin. It is usually excised surgically.

erythropoiesis (ɪrɪth′roupoii′sɪs), the process of erythrocyte production involving the maturation of a nucleated precursor into a hemoglobin-filled, nucleus-free erythrocyte that is regulated by erythropoietin, a hormone produced by the kidney. See also **erythropoietin, hemoglobin, leukopoiesis.** — **erythropoietic,** *adj.*

erythropoietic porphyria (ɪrɪth′roupoiet′ɪk). See **porphyria.**

erythropoietin (ɪrɪth′roupoii′tɪn), a hormone synthesized in the liver and released into the bloodstream in response to anoxia. The hormone acts to stimulate and to regulate the production of erythrocytes and is thus able to increase the oxygen-carrying capacity of the blood.

Es, symbol for **einsteinium.**

escape beat, an automatic beat of the heart that occurs after an interval longer than the duration of the dominant heart beat cycle. Escape beats function as safety mechanisms, and anything that produces a pause in the prevailing heart cycle may allow an escape to occur. Some kinds of pauses in which escape beats occur are caused by sinoatrial (SA) block, atrioventricular (AV) block, extra systole, and the completion of a paroxysm of tachycardia. In the presence of atrial fibrillation, nodal escape beats present a unique diagnostic problem because fibrillation obviates any dominant heart beat cycle. In the electrocardiogram, the nodal escape beat commonly presents a QRS-T contour similar to that of the sinus beats but sometimes varies slightly from the dominant beats. Ventricular escape beats are associated with the late rather than the early occurrence of the usual ventricular beat patterns.

-escent, 1. a combining form meaning 'beginning to be': *alkalescent, convalescent, turgescent.* **2.** a combining form meaning 'emitting or reflecting light': *incandescent, iridescent, opalescent.*

eschar (es′kar), a scab or dry crust resulting from a thermal or chemical burn, infection, or excoriating skin disease. — **escharotic,** *adj.*

escharonodulaire (es′kærounod′yuler). See **Marseilles fever.**

Escherichia coli (eśhɪrai′kia kou′lai), a species of coliform bacteria of the family Enterobaccteriacae, normally present in the intestines and common in water, milk, and soil. *Escherichia coli* is the most frequent cause of urinary tract infection and is a serious pathogen in wounds. *E. coli* septicemia may rapidly result in shock and death owing to the action of an endotoxin released from the bacteria.

eserine (es′ərin, es′ərɪn). See **physostigmine.**

eserine sulfate. See **physostigmine.**

Esidrix, a trade name for a diuretic (hydrochlorothiazide).

-esis, a combining form meaning an 'action, process, or result of ': *enuresis, oxydesis, synthesis.*

Eskabarb, a trade name for an anticonvulsant and sedative-hypnotic (phenobarbital).

Eskalith, a trade name for an antidepressant (lithium carbonate).

Eskatrol, a trade name for a fixed-combination drug containing a central nervous system stimulant (dextroamphetamine sulfate) and a tranquilizer (prochlorperazine maleate), used as an appetite suppressant.

Esmarch's bandage (es′marks), an elastic bandage wrapped around an elevated limb to force blood out of the limb. It is used prior to certain surgical procedures to create a blood-free field.

eso-, a combining form meaning 'within': *esocataphoria, esogastritis, esotropia.*

esophageal cancer, a malignant neoplastic disease of the esophagus that occurs three times more frequently in men than in women and more often in Asia and Africa than in North America. Risk factors associated with the disease are heavy consumption of alcohol, smoking, betelnut chewing, Plummer-Vinson syndrome, hiatus hernia, or achalasia. Aflatoxin in moldy grain and peanuts or a dietary deficiency, especially of molybdenum, may be involved. Esophageal cancer does not often cause any symptoms in the early stages but in later stages causes painful dysphagia, anorexia, weight loss, regurgitation, cervical adenopathy, and, in some cases, a persistent cough. Left vocal cord paralysis and hemoptysis indicate an advanced state of the disease. The tumor may spread locally to invade the trachea, bronchi, pericardium, great blood vessels, and thoracic vertebrae or may metastasize to lymph nodes, the lungs, and the liver. Diagnostic measures include fluoroscopic observation of the esophagus as the patient swallows barium, fiberoptic esophagoscopy, and biopsy and cytologic examination of the primary lesion and regional nodes. Most esophageal tumors are poorly differentiated squamous cell carcinomas; adenocarcinomas occur less frequently and are usually found in the lower third of the esophagus as extensions of gastric cancer. Surgical treatment may require total or partial esophagectomy with the resected segment replaced by a Dacron graft or a section of the colon. If only the lower third of the esophagus is removed, the proximal end may be anastomosed to the stomach. A catheter inserted into the stomach through an incision or a nasogastric tube may be used to feed patients with inoperable esophageal cancer. Radiotherapy may eradicate early local tumors and may effectively palliate the symptoms of advanced lesion. Methotrexate given before irradiation may increase the chances of survival. See also **esophagectomy.**

esophageal lead, **1.** an electrocardiographic conductor in which the exploring electrode is placed within the lumen of the esophagus. It is used to detect sizable atrial deflections as an aid in identifying cardiac arrhythmias. **2.** *Informal.* a tracing produced by such a lead on an electrocardiograph.

esophageal varices, a complex of longitudinal, tortuous veins at the lower end of the esophagus, enlarged and swollen as the result of portal hypertension. These vessels are especially susceptible to ulceration and hemorrhage.

esophagectomy (ˌɪsof'əjek'təmi), a surgical procedure in which all or part of the esophagus is removed, as may be required to treat severe, recurrent, bleeding esophageal varices.

esophagitis (isof'əjai'tıs), inflammation of the mucosal lining of the esophagus, caused by infection, irritation from a naso-gastric tube, or, most commonly, backflow of gastric juice from the stomach. See also **gastroesophageal reflux.**

esophagus (ɪsof'əgəs), the muscular canal, about 24 cm long, extending from the pharynx to the stomach. It begins in the neck at the inferior border of the cricoid cartilage, opposite the sixth cervical vertebra, and descends to the cardiac sphincter of the stomach in a vertical path with two slight curves. It is the narrowest part of the digestive tube and is most constricted at its commencement and at the point where it passes through the diaphragm. The esophagus is composed of a fibrous coat, a muscular coat, and a submucous coat and is lined with mucous membrane. Also called **gullet.** — **esophageal,** *adj.*

esophoria (es'əfor'iə), deviation of the visual axis of one eye toward that of the other eye in the absence of visual stimuli for fusion. Also called **cross-eye.** Compare **esotropia.** — **esophoric,** *adj.*

esotropia (es'ətrou'piə), a kind of strabismus characterized by an inward deviation of one eye relative to the other eye. Also called **convergent strabismus, internal strabismus.** Compare **exotropia.** See also **strabismus.** — **esotropic,** *adj.*

ESP, abbreviation for **extrasensory perception.**

espundia (ɪspun'diə), a cutaneous form of American leishmaniasis most common in Brazil, caused by *Leishmania brasilensis.* See also **American leishmaniasis, leishmaniasis.**

ESR, abbreviation for **erythrocyte sedimentation rate.**

essential amino acid, an organic compound not synthesized in the body that is essential for nitrogen equilibrium in adults and optimal growth in infants and children. Adults require isoleucine, leucine, lysine, methionine, phenylalanine, threonine, tryptophan, and valine. Infants need these eight amino acids plus arginine and histidine. Cystine and tyrosine, limited substitutes respectively for methionine and phenylalanine, are considered quasi-essential. See also **amino acid.**

essential fatty acid, a polyunsaturated acid, linoleic, linolenic, and arachidonic, essential in the diet for the proper growth, maintenance, and functioning of the body. It is a precursor of the prostaglandins and has an important role in fat transport and metabolism and in maintaining the function and integrity of cellular membranes. It is also necessary for the normal functioning of the reproductive and endocrine systems and for the breaking up of cholesterol deposits on arterial walls. The best dietary sources are natural vegetable oils, as safflower, soy, and corn oils, margarines blended with vegetable oils, wheat germ, edible seeds, as pumpkin, sesame, and sunflower, poultry fat, and fish oils, especially cod-liver oil. Deficiency causes changes in cell structure and enzyme function resulting in decreased growth and other disorders. Symptoms include brittle and lusterless hair, nail problems, dandruff, allergic conditions, and dermatoses, especially eczema in infants. Excessive amounts may reduce the level of vitamin E in the tissues and cause other metabolic disturbances as well as abnormal weight gain.

essential fever, any fever of unknown etiology.

essential hypertension, an elevated systemic arterial pressure for which no cause can be found and which is often the only significant clinical finding. Elevated blood pressure is always considered a risk, and individuals with elevated pressures are at risk for cardiovascular disease. In examining patients with essential hypertension, clinicians consider the normal complex mechanisms that control pressure, as the arterial baroreflex, body fluid regulators, the renin-angiotensin system, and vascular autoregulation. These mechanisms are closely integrated, and it is not precisely clear how their impairment affects normotension and hypertension. Also called **benign hypertension.**

essential nutrient, the carbohydrates, proteins, fats, minerals, and vitamins necessary for growth, normal function, and body maintenance. These substances must be supplied by food, since most are not synthesized by the body in the quantities required for health.

essential thrombocythemia. See **thrombocytosis.**

essential tremor, an involuntary fine shaking of the hand, the head, and the face, especially during routine movements of the body. It is a familial disorder inherited as an autosomal dominant trait and appears during adolescence or in middle age, slowly progressing as a more pronounced disorder. The precise cause of this condition is not known, but it is believed to involve the central nervous system. Essential tremor is aggravated by activity and emotion and can be reduced in some patients by the administration of alcohol and mild sedatives, as propranolol and diazepam. Also called **familial tremor.** Compare **Parkinsonism.**

EST, abbreviation for **electric shock therapy.** See **electroconvulsive therapy.**

established name, the name assigned to a drug by the United States Adopted Names Council (USAN). The established name, generally shorter than the chemical name, is the name by which the drug is known to health practitioners. Also called **generic name.** See also **chemical name.**

Estar, a trade name for a coal tar preparation used to treat eczema.

ester (es'tər), a class of chemical compound formed by the bonding of an alcohol and one or more organic acids. Fats are esters, formed by the bonding of fatty acids with the alcohol glycerol.

ester-compound local anesthetic, any one of four potent local anesthetics slightly different in chemical structure from the amide group of local anesthetics. Tetracaine is the most commonly used. Kinds of ester-compound local anesthetics are **chloroprocaine, cocaine, procaine, tetracaine.**

esterified estrogen, an estrogen.
- INDICATIONS: It is prescribed in the treatment of menstrual irregularities, contraception, and menopausal symptoms.
- CONTRAINDICATIONS: Pregnancy, known or suspected breast cancer, thrombophlebitis, vaginal bleeding of unknown origin, or known hypersensitivity to this drug prohibit its use.
- ADVERSE EFFECTS: Among the more serious adverse reactions are gall bladder disease, thromboembolic disease, and a possible increase in risk of cancer.

esthesio-, a combining form meaning 'pertaining to feeling or to the perceptive faculties': *esthesiogenic, esthesioneure, esthesioscopy.*

-esthetic, a combining form meaning 'pertaining to a person's consciousness of something': *cenesthetic, photoesthetic, somatesthetic.* Also **-aesthetic, -esthetical, -aesthetical.**

Estinyl, a trade name for an estrogen (ethinyl estradiol).

Estrace, a trade name for an estrogen (estradiol).

estradiol (es'trədai'ɔl), the most potent naturally occurring human estrogen, also found in hog ovaries and in the urine of pregnant mares. Various esters of estradiol administered intramuscularly or orally are used as estrogens. See also **estrogen.**

Estradurin, a trade name for an antineoplastic estrogen (polyestradiol phosphate).

Estratab, a trade name for esterified estrogens.

Estratest, a trade name for a fixed-combination drug containing an androgen (methyltestosterone) and esterified estrogens.

Estraval, a trade name for an estrogen (estradiol valerate).

estriol (es'triɔl), a relatively weak, naturally occurring human estrogen found in high concentrations in urine. See also **estrogen.**

estrogen, one of a group of hormonal steroid compounds that promote the development of female secondary sex characteristics. Human estrogen is elaborated in the ovaries, adrenal cortices, testes, and fetoplacental unit. During the menstrual cycle estrogen renders the female genital tract suitable for fertilization, implantation, and nutrition of the early embryo. Pharmaceutical preparations of estrogen are used in oral contraceptives, to palliate postmenopausal breast cancer and prostatic cancer, to inhibit lactation, and to treat threatened abortion, osteoporosis, and ovarian disease. Estrogen is also prescribed to relieve discomforts of menopause, but its long-term, continued use increases the risk of endometrial carcinoma. Kinds of estrogen are **conjugated estrogens, equilin, esterified estrogens, estradiol, estriol, estrone.** – **estrogenic,** *adj.*

estrone (es'troun), an estrogen.
- INDICATIONS: It is prescribed in the treatment of menstrual cycle irregularities, prostatic cancer, menopausal vasomotor symptoms, and to prevent pregnancy.
- CONTRAINDICATIONS: Thrombophlebitis, abnormal genital bleeding, known or suspected pregnancy, or known hypersensitivity to this drug prohibits its use.
- ADVERSE EFFECTS: Among the more serious adverse reactions are thrombophlebitis, embolism, and hypercalcemia.

Estronol, a trade name for an estrogen (estrone).

ethacrynate sodium. See **ethacrynic acid.**

ethacrynic acid, a diuretic.
- INDICATION: It is prescribed to relieve the effects of edema.
- CONTRAINDICATIONS: Pregnancy, anuria, or known hypersensitivity to this drug prohibits its use. It is not given to infants.
- ADVERSE EFFECTS: Among the more serious adverse reactions are tetany, muscle weakness, cramps, and excessive diuresis. Hearing loss or deafness may occur.

ethambutol hydrochloride, a tuberculostatic antibiotic.
- INDICATION: It is prescribed in the treatment of pulmonary tuberculosis.
- CONTRAINDICATIONS: Optic neuritis or known hypersensitivity to this drug prohibits its use.
- ADVERSE EFFECTS: Among the most serious adverse reactions are diminished visual acuity and allergic reactions, as rashes.

Ethamide, a trade name for a carbonic anhydrase inhibitor (ethoxzolamide).

ethanoic acid (eth'ənou'ık). See **acetic acid.**

ethanol. See **alcohol.**

ethaverine hydrochloride, a smooth muscle relaxant.

■ INDICATIONS: It is prescribed to relieve spasm of the gastrointestinal or genitourinary tract, arterial vasospasm, and cerebral insufficiency.

■ CONTRAINDICATIONS: Liver disease, atrioventricular dissociation, or known hypersensitivity to this drug prohibits its use. It is used with caution in patients who have glaucoma.

■ ADVERSE EFFECTS: Among the more serious adverse reactions are hypotension, cardiac arrhythmia, and headache.

ethchlorvynol (eṭhklɔr'vɔnɔl), a sedative and hypnotic.

■ INDICATION: It is prescribed in the treatment of insomnia.

■ CONTRAINDICATIONS: Porphyria or known hypersensitivity to this drug prohibits its use.

■ ADVERSE EFFECTS: Among the most serious adverse reactions are allergic reactions, nausea, dizziness, aftertaste, and drug hangover.

ether, a nonhalogenated, volatile liquid used as a general anesthetic. Because ether is generally safe, and because it provides excellent analgesia and profound muscle relaxation, adjuncts to anesthesia, as narcotic analgesics and neuromuscular blocking agents, are often unnecessary. Ether has little depressant effect on the respiratory and cardiovascular systems but may cause hyperglycemia, decreased excretion of urine, decreased intestinal tone and motility, and transient abnormalities in the function of the liver. It has an irritating, pungent odor, is highly flammable and explosive, and frequently causes postoperative nausea and vomiting.

ethical drug, a drug available only by prescription and advertised only to physicians and other health professionals. Also called **prescription drug.**

ethinamate (ɪṭhɪn'ɔmeit), a sedative.

■ INDICATION: It is prescribed in the treatment of insomnia.

■ CONTRAINDICATIONS: Known hypersensitivity to this drug prohibits its use. It is not recommended for pregnant women or for people under 15 years of age.

■ ADVERSE EFFECTS: Among the more serious adverse reactions are thrombocytopenic purpura, physical and psychologic dependence, and skin rash.

ethinyl estradiol (eṭh'ɪnɪl), an estrogen.

■ INDICATIONS: It is prescribed in the treatment of menstrual cycle irregularities, prostatic cancer, for contraception, and to relieve menopausal vasomotor symptoms.

■ CONTRAINDICATIONS: Thrombophlebitis, abnormal genital bleeding, known or suspected pregnancy, or known hypersensitivity to this drug prohibits its use.

■ ADVERSE EFFECTS: Among the more serious adverse reactions are thrombophlebitis, embolism, and hypercalcemia.

ethionamide (eṭh'iɔnæm'æid), a tuberculostatic antibacterial.

■ INDICATION: It is prescribed for tuberculosis.

■ CONTRAINDICATIONS: Existing liver damage or known hypersensitivity to this drug prohibits its use.

■ ADVERSE EFFECTS: Among the more serious adverse reactions are skin rash, jaundice, and mental depression. Gastrointestinal side effects are common.

ethmoidal air cell (ɪṭhmɔi'dɔl), one of the numerous, small thin-walled cavities in the ethmoid bone of the skull, rimmed by the frontal maxilla, lacrimal, sphenoidal, and palatine bones. They are lined with mucous membrane continuous with that of the nasal cavity and lie between the upper part of the nasal cavities and the orbits. They are divided bilaterally into anterior, middle, and posterior cavities. The anterior and the middle cavities open into the middle meatus of the nose; the posterior cavities open into the superior meatus. The ethmoidal air cells start to develop at birth. Compare **frontal sinus, maxillary sinus, sphenoidal sinus.**

ethmoid bone, the very light and spongy bone at the base of the cranium, forming most of the walls of the superior part of the nasal cavity and consisting of four parts: a horizontal plate, a perpendicular plate, and two lateral labyrinths.

ethnocentrism, 1. a belief in the inherent superiority of the race or group to which one belongs. 2. a proclivity to consider other ethnic groups in terms of one's own racial origins.

Ethobral, a trade name for a sedative-hypnotic, fixed-combination drug containing three barbiturates, (phenobarbital, butabarbital sodium, and secobarbital sodium).

Ethocaine, a trade name for a local anesthetic (procaine hydrochloride).

ethoheptazine citrate, a non-narcotic analgesic.

■ INDICATION: It is prescribed to relieve mild to moderate pain.

■ CONTRAINDICATION: Known hypersensitivity to this drug prohibits its use.

■ ADVERSE EFFECTS: Among the most common adverse reactions are gastrointestinal distress and dizziness.

ethology, 1. (in zoology) the scientific study of the behavioral patterns of animals, specifically in their native habitat. 2. (in psychology) the empirical study of human behavior, primarily social customs, manners, and mores. — **ethologic, ethological,** adj., **ethologist,** n.

ethopropazine hydrochloride, a phenothiazine anticholinergic agent.

■ INDICATION: It is prescribed in the treatment of Parkinson's disease.

■ CONTRAINDICATIONS: Narrow angle glaucoma, asthma, obstruction of the genitourinary or gastrointestinal tract, severe ulcerative colitis, or known hypersensitivity to this drug or to phenothiazine medication prohibits its use.

■ ADVERSE EFFECTS: Among the more serious adverse effects are blurred vision, central nervous system effects, tachycardia, dry mouth, decreased sweating, and hypersensitivity reactions.

ethosuximide, an anticonvulsant.

■ INDICATION: It is prescribed in the treatment of petit mal epilepsy.

■ CONTRAINDICATIONS: Known hypersensitivity to this drug or to any succinimide medication prohibits its use.

■ ADVERSE EFFECTS: Among the more serious adverse reactions are blood dyscrasias, gastrointestinal disturbance, hemopoietic complications, and systemic lupus erythematosus.

ethotoin (ıfhoʊ′toʊɪn), an anticonvulsant.

■ INDICATIONS: It is prescribed in the treatment of grand mal and psychomotor seizures.

■ CONTRAINDICATIONS: Liver disease, hematologic disorders, or known hypersensitivity to this drug or to any hydantoin prohibits its use. It is not recommended for use during pregnancy or lactation.

■ ADVERSE EFFECTS: Among the more serious adverse reactions are nausea, fatigue, skin rash, and chest pain.

ethoxzolamide, a carbonic anhydrase inhibitor.

■ INDICATION: It is prescribed primarily in the treatment of certain types of glaucoma.

■ CONTRAINDICATIONS: Liver or kidney dysfunction, hyponatremia, hypokalemia, or known hypersensitivity to this drug prohibits its use.

■ ADVERSE EFFECTS: Among the most serious adverse reactions are bone marrow depression, kidney stones, and crystalluria. Fever and skin rash may also occur.

Ethrane, a trade name for an inhalational general anesthetic (enflurane).

Ethril, a trade name for an antibacterial (erythromycin stearate).

ethyl alcohol, See **alcohol.**

ethyl aminobenzoate. See **benzocaine.**

ethyl chloride, a topical anesthetic.

■ INDICATIONS: It is prescribed in the treatment of skin irritations and in minor skin surgery.

■ CONTRAINDICATIONS: Known hypersensitivity to this drug prohibits its use. It is not used on broken skin or on mucous membrane.

■ ADVERSE EFFECTS: Among the more serious adverse reactions are pain, muscle spasm, and, from excessive use, frostbite.

■ NOTE: It is highly flammable.

ethylestrenol, an anabolic steroid not currently available in the United States.

ethylnorepinephrine hydrochloride (efh′ɪlnɔrep′ɪnef′- rɪn), a bronchodilator.

■ INDICATION: It is prescribed in the treatment of bronchial asthma.

■ CONTRAINDICATIONS: Known hypersensitivity to this

drug or to other sympathomimetic medication prohibits its use.

■ ADVERSE EFFECTS: Among the more serious adverse reactions are increased or decreased blood pressure, palpitations, and an increase in heart rate.

ethyl oxide, a colorless highly volatile liquid solvent similar to diethyl ether. It is widely used in various pharmaceutical processes.

ethynodiol diacetate, a progestin that is used in combination with an estrogen as an oral contraceptive.

ethynodiol diacetate and ethinyl estradiol (efh′- ınoʊdaɪ′ɔl), an oral contraceptive.

■ INDICATION: It is prescribed for contraception.

■ CONTRAINDICATIONS: Thrombophlebitis, cardiovascular disease, breast or reproductive organ cancer, or known hypersensitivity to either ingredient prohibits its use.

■ ADVERSE EFFECTS: Among the more serious adverse reactions are thrombophlebitis, uterine fibroma, gall bladder disease, embolism, and hepatic lesions.

ethynodiol diacetate and mestranol, an oral contraceptive.

■ INDICATION: It is prescribed for contraception.

■ CONTRAINDICATIONS: Thrombophlebitis, cardiovascular disease, breast or reproductive organ cancer, or known hypersensitivity to either ingredient prohibits its use.

■ ADVERSE EFFECTS: Among the more serious adverse reactions are thrombophlebitis, uterine fibroma, gall bladder disease, embolism, and hepatic lesions.

-etic, a combining form used as the equivalent of *-ic* in forming adjectives: *enuretic, genetic, kinetic.*

etidronate disodium (ıtıd′rəneɪt), a regulator or calcium metabolism. Also called **sodium etidronate.**

■ INDICATIONS: It is prescribed in the treatment of Paget's disease, for heterotopic ossification caused by injury to the spinal cord, and after total hip replacement.

■ CONTRAINDICATIONS: There are no known contraindications.

■ ADVERSE EFFECTS: Among the more serious adverse reactions are bone pain at both Pagetic sites and previously asymptomatic sites, gastrointestinal disturbances, and elevated serum phosphate.

etiology (i′tiol′əji), 1. the study of all factors that may be involved in the development of a disease, including susceptibility of the patient, the nature of the disease agent, and the way in which the patient's body is invaded by the agent. 2. the cause of a disease. Compare **pathogenesis.**

etomidate (ıtom′ıdeɪt), a short-acting, investigational nonbarbiturate intravenous induction agent for general anesthesia. It is reported to have minimal adverse cardiovascular and respiratory effects, thus providing a greater margin of safety in patients at risk because of heart disease.

Etrafon, a trade name for a central nervous system fixed-combination drug containing a tranquilizer (perphenazine) and an antidepressant (amitriptyline hydrochloride).

eu-, a combining form meaning 'well, easily, good': *euangiotic, eucrasia, euthyroid.*

Eu, symbol for **europium.**

eucaryon. See **eukaryon.**

eucaryosis. See **eukaryosis.**

eucatropine hydrochloride (yukæt′rəpin), an ophthalmic anticholinergic.

■ INDICATION: It is prescribed for dilating the pupil in an ophthalmoscopic examination of the eye.

■ CONTRAINDICATIONS: Known hypersensitivity to this drug or to other anticholinergics prohibits its use.

■ ADVERSE EFFECTS: Among the most serious adverse reactions are tachycardia and severe constipation. Dry mouth, heat intolerance and other effects associated with systemic absorption of an anticholinergic agent may also occur.

euchromatin (yukroυ′mətɪn), that portion of chromosome material that is active in gene expression during cell division. It stains most deeply during mitosis when it is in a coiled, condensed state, and during each division of the cell it passes through a continuous cycle of condensation and dispersion. Compare **heterochromatin.** See also **chromatin** — **euchromatic,** *adj.*

euchromosome (yukroυ′mɔsoυm). See **autosome.**

eugamy (yu′gəmi), the union of those gametes that contain the same haploid number of chromosomes. — **eugamic,** *adj.*

eugenics (yujen′ɪks), the study of methods for controlling the characteristics of future human populations through selective breeding.

euglobulin, a "true" globulin (a protein insoluble in distilled water). This is only one of a number of different properties that have been used to classify proteins. Compare **albumin, cryoglobulin.** See also **plasma protein, electrophoresis.**

eukaryocyte, eucaryocyte (yukær′ioυsaɪt′), a cell with a true nucleus, found in all higher organisms and in some microorganisms, as amebae, plasmodia, and trypanosomes. Compare **prokaryocyte** — **eukaryotic,** *adj.*

eukaryon, eucaryon (yukær′ion), 1. a nucleus that is highly complex, organized, and surrounded by a nuclear membrane, usually characteristic of higher organisms. 2. an organism containing such a nucleus. Compare **prokaryon.**

eukaryosis, eucaryosis, the state of having a highly complex, organized nucleus surrounded by a nuclear membrane and containing organelles, as is characteristic of all organisms except bacteria, viruses, and blue-green algae. Compare **prokaryosis.**

eukaryote, eucaryote (yukær′iot), an organism having cells that contain a true nucleus. — **eukaryotic, eucaryotic,** *adj.*

eunuch (yu′nək), a male whose testicles have been removed. Symptoms such as a feminine voice and absence of facial hair can stem from the absence of male hormones prior to puberty. See also **secondary sex characteristics.**

eunuchoidism (yu′nəkoidɪz′əm), deficiency of the function of male hormone or of its formation by the testes. The deficiency leads to sterility and to abnormal tallness, small testes, deficient development of secondary sexual characteristics and of libido and potency.

euphoretic (yu′fəret′ɪk), 1. (of a substance or event) tending to produce a condition of euphoria. 2. a substance tending to produce euphoria, as LSD, mescaline, marijuana, and other hallucinogenic drugs.

euphoria (yufɔr′iə), 1. a feeling or state of well-being or elation. 2. an exaggerated or abnormal sense of physical and emotional well-being not based on reality or truth, disproportionate to its cause, and inappropriate to the situation, as commonly seen in the manic stage of bipolar disorder, in some forms of schizophrenia, in organic mental disorders, and in toxic and drug-induced states. Compare **ecstasy.**

euploid (yu′ploid), **euploidic,** 1. of or pertaining to an individual, organism, strain, or cell with a chromosome number that is an exact multiple of the normal, basic haploid number characteristic of the species, as diploid, triploid, tetraploid, or polyploid. Variation occurs through entire sets rather than individual chromosomes, so that there is a balanced number of chromosomes. 2. such an individual, organism, strain, or cell. Compare **aneuploid.**

euploidy (yu′ploidi), the state or condition of having a variation in chromosome number that is an exact multiple of the characteristic haploid number.

Eurax, a trade name for a scabicide (crotamiton).

European blastomycosis. See **cryptococcosis.**

European typhus. See **epidemic typhus.**

europium (Eu), a rare-earth, metallic element. Its atomic number is 63; its atomic weight is 151.96.

eury-, a combining form meaning 'wide, broad': *eurycephalic, eurygnathic, euryopia.*

eustachian tube (yustei′ʃən), a tube, lined with mucous membrane, that joins the nasopharynx and the tympanic cavity, allowing equalization of the air pressure in the inner ear with atmospheric pressure. Also called **auditory tube.**

euthanasia (yu′θənei′ʒə), deliberately bringing about the death of a person who is suffering from an incurable disease or condition, actively, by administering a lethal drug, or passively, by allowing the person to die by withholding treatment. Also called **mercy killing.**

Euthroid, a trade name for a thyroid hormone preparation (liotrix; a combination of T_4 and T_3).

Eutonyl, a trade name for an antihypertensive (pargyline hydrochloride).

Eutron, a trade name for a fixed-combination drug containing a diuretic (methyclothiazide) and the monoamine oxidase inhibitor (pargyline hydrochloride), used as an antihypertensive.

evacuate, 1. to discharge or to remove a substance from a cavity, space, organ, or tract of the body. 2. a substance discharged or removed from the body. —**evacuation,** n.

evaluating, (in five-step nursing process) a category of nursing behavior in which a determination is made and recorded regarding the extent to which the established goals of care have been met. To make this judgment the nurse estimates the degree of success in meeting the goals, evaluates the implementation of nursing measures, investigates the client's compliance with therapy, and records the client's response to therapy. The nurse evaluates effects of the measures used, the need for change in goals of care, the accuracy of the implementation of nursing measures, and the need for change in the client's environment or in the equipment or procedures used. The impact of the care or treatment on the client, the client's family, and the staff is evaluated, the accuracy of tests and measurements is checked, and the client's and the family's understanding of the information given them is evaluated. The client's expressed and observed response to care is recorded. Although evaluating is the final step of the five-step nursing process, following implementing, in practice, evaluating is integral to effective nursing practice at all steps of the process. See also **analyzing, assessing, planning.**

evaporated milk, homogenized whole milk from which 50 to 60 per cent of the water content has been evaporated. It is fortified with vitamin D, canned, and sterilized. When diluted with an equal amount of water, its nutritional value is comparable to that of fresh whole milk.

evaporation, the change of a substance from a solid or liquid state to a gaseous state. The process of evaporation is hastened by an increase in temperature and a decrease in atmospheric pressure. See also **boiling point.** —**evaporate,** v.

Evex, a trade name for esterified estrogens.

evocation, (in embryology) a specific morphogenetic change within a developing embryo that occurs as a result of the action of a single evocator. See also **induction.**

evocator, a specific chemical substance or hormone that is emitted from the organizer part of the embryonic tissue and acts as a morphogenetic stimulus in the developing embryo.

evoked potential, a tracing of a brain wave measured on the surface of the head at various places. The wave, unlike the waves seen on an electroencephalogram, is elic-ited by a specific stimulus. The stimulus may originate in the visual, auditory, or somatosensory areas normally evoked by the stimulus of the nervous system. The activity and function of the system may be monitored during surgery, while the patient is unconscious. The surgeon is thus able to avoid damage to the nerves during operative procedures. Evoked potentials are also used to diagnose multiple sclerosis and various disorders of hearing and of sight. Kinds of evoked potentials include **brain stem evoked auditory potential, somatosensory evoked potential, visual evoked potential.** See also **brain electrical activity mapping.**

evolution, 1. a gradual, orderly, and continuous process of change and development from one condition or state to another. It encompasses all aspects of life, including physical, psychological, sociological, cultural, and intellectual development, and involves a progressive advancement from a simple to a more complex form or state through the processes of modification, differentiation, and growth. 2. (in genetics) the theory of the origin and propagation of all plant and animal species, including man, and their development from lower to more complex forms through the natural selection of variants produced through genetic mutations, hybridization, and inbreeding. Kinds of evolution are **convergent evolution, determinant evolution, emergent evolution, organic evolution, orthogenic evolution, saltatory evolution.** —**evolutionist,** n.

Ewing's sarcoma (yu'ingz), a malignant tumor developing from bone marrow, usually in long bones or the pelvis. It occurs most frequently in adolescent boys and is characterized by pain, swelling, fever, and leukocytosis. The tumor, a soft, crumbly grayish mass that may invade surrounding soft tissues, is difficult to distinguish histologically from a neuroblastoma or a reticulum cell sarcoma. Radiotherapy often produces a dramatic initial response, but relapses are common. Surgical excision, often requiring amputation, may be recommended. Also called **Ewing's tumor.** See also **neuroblastoma, reticulum cell sarcoma.**

Ewing's tumor. See **endothelial myeloma.**

ex-, a combining form meaning 'away from, outside, without': *exacrinous, excoriation, exfoliato.*

exacerbation (igzæs′ərbei′shən), an increase in the seriousness of a disease or disorder as marked by greater intensity in the signs or symptoms of the patient being treated.

exanthem (igzæn′thəm), pl. **exanthemata.** a skin eruption, as the rash of any common infectious disease of childhood, as chickenpox, measles, roseola infantum, or rubella. Compare **enanthem.** —**exanthematous,** adj.

exanthem subitum. See **roseola infantum.**

exchange transfusion in the newborn, the introduction of whole blood in exchange for 75 to 85 per cent of an infant's circulating blood that is repeatedly withdrawn in small amounts and replaced with equal amounts of donor blood. The procedure is performed to improve the oxygen-carrying capacity of the blood in the treatment of erythroblastosis neonatorum by removing Rh and ABO antibodies, sensitized erythrocytes producing hemolysis, and accumulated bilirubin.

■ METHOD: A radiant heat warmer, pacifier, and cardiac and respiratory monitors are prepared, and resuscitative equipment and drugs, including oxygen, a mask, bag, suction apparatus, glucose, calcium, and sodium bicarbonate, are made readily available. The results of laboratory studies of the infant's bilirubin, hemoglobin, and calcium levels, hematocrit, blood culture, and random blood sugar test and the donor blood culture are checked. The donor blood is checked to make certain that it is not more than 48 hours old; if fresh whole blood is not used, stored blood is mixed in amounts as ordered with frozen plasma or plasmanate. Prior to exchange transfusion, nothing is administered by mouth for three to four hours, or the contents of the infant's stomach are aspirated. The baby's extremities are restrained; the blood is warmed as ordered and the physician is assisted with the insertion of an umbilical venous line, if one is not in place. The physician may administer albumin with the donor blood. The procedure may be carried out under phototherapy lights, and, unless contraindicated, the infant's parents may be in attendance. During the procedure the young patient is observed for bradycardia with less than 100 beats a minute, cyanosis, hypothermia, vomiting, aspiration, apnea, an air embolus, abdominal distention, or cardiac arrest. The respiratory and cardiac rates are checked every five minutes, the axillary temperature every 15 to 30 minutes. The integrity of all blood tubing connections is inspected periodically. The amount of blood withdrawn and infused is recorded and the physician is notified when each 100 ml of blood has been exchanged. A repetition of laboratory studies is requested as ordered for the last amount of blood removed from the infant. Following the procedure, the infant is observed for signs of tachycardia or bradycardia, tachypnea or bradypnea, hypothermia, lethargy, jitteriness, increasing jaundice, cyanosis, edema, dark urine, bleeding from the cord, convulsions, or complications as hemorrhage, hypocalcemia, heart failure, hypoglycemia, sepsis, acidosis, hyperkalemia, thrombus formation, or shock. The infant is maintained in a neutral thermal environment and is handled gently and minimally for the next two to four hours. The cardiac and respiratory rates are monitored every 15 minutes for four hours, then every 30 to 60 minutes for 24 to 48 hours or as ordered. The axillary temperature is checked every one to three hours for 48 hours and the cord is observed for bleeding every 5 to 15 minutes for one to two hours after the procedure. Feeding, by gavage or a bottle having a soft nipple with a large enough hole to ensure adequate

intake, is initiated four to six hours after the transfusion, as ordered; the infant is fed slowly and repositioned after each feeding. Intake and output of fluids are measured and ongoing care is provided as for all high-risk infants.

■ NURSING ORDERS: The nurse prepares the equipment and infant for the exchange transfusion, assists the physician in the insertion of the umbilical venous line, and monitors the baby during and after the procedure. The nurse offers the parents an explanation of the reason for the procedure and encourages them to participate in the infant's care as much as possible.

■ OUTCOME CRITERIA: An exchange transfusion is usually administered only to a high-risk infant, but the procedure often effectively counteracts the hemolytic anemia and hyperbilirubinemia associated with erythroblastosis neonatorum.

excise (iksaiz'), to remove completely, as in the surgical excision of the palatine tonsils. Compare **resect**. —**excision**, *n*.

excision, 1. the process of excising. 2. (in molecular genetics) the process by which a genetic element is removed from a strand of DNA.

exciting eye, (in sympathetic ophthalmia) the eye that is infected by the sympathizing eye, metastasis being by way of the blood stream or the lymphatics.

excoriation (ekskor'iei'shən), an injury to the surface of the skin or other part of the body caused by scratching or abrasion.

excrete, to evacuate a waste substance from the body, often via a normal secretion, as a drug may be excreted in breast milk. —**excretion**, *n*.

excretion, the process of eliminating, shedding, or getting rid of substances by body organs or tissues, as part of a natural metabolic activity. Excretion usually begins at the cellular level where water, carbon dioxide, and other waste products of cellular life are emptied into the capillaries. The epidermis excretes dead skin cells by shedding them daily. —**excrete**, *v*.

excretory, relating to the process of excretion, often used in combination with a term to identify an object or procedure associated with excretion, as in **excretory urography**.

excretory duct, a duct that is conductive but not secretory.

excretory urography. See **intravenous pyelography**.

executive physical, a physical examination including extensive laboratory, x-ray, and other tests that is provided periodically to management level personnel at company expense. Such examinations are often detailed, expensive, and overly complete.

exercise, 1. the performance of any physical activity for the purpose of conditioning the body, improving health, or maintaining fitness or as a means of therapy for correcting a deformity or restoring the organs and bodily functions to a state of health. **2.** any action, skill, or maneuver that exerts the muscles and is performed repeatedly in order to develop or strengthen the body or any of its parts. **3.** to use a muscle or part of the body in a repetitive way in order to maintain or develop its strength. The nurse constantly assesses the patient's needs and provides the proper type and amount of exercise, taking into account the patient's physical or mental limitations. Exercise has a beneficial effect on each of the body systems, although in excess it can lead to the breakdown of tissue and cause injury. Kinds of exercise are **active exercise, active assisted exercise, active resistive exercise, aerobic exercise, anaerobic exercise, corrective exercise, isometric exercise, isotonic exercise, muscle-setting exercise, passive exercise, progressive resistance exercise, range of motion exercise, underwater exercise.**

exercise electrocardiogram, (exercise ECG), a stress test that is important in the diagnosis of coronary artery disease. An exercise electrocardiogram is recorded as a person walks on a treadmill or pedals a stationary bicycle for a given length of time at a specific rate of speed. Abnormal changes in cardiac function may occur with exercise that were absent during rest.

exfoliation, peeling and sloughing off of dead skin layers. This is a normal process which may be exaggerated in certain skin diseases or after a severe sunburn. See also **desquamation, exfoliative dermatitis.** – exfoliative, *adj.*

exfoliative cytology, the microscopic examination of desquamated cells for diagnostic purposes. The cells are obtained from lesions, sputum, secretions, urine, and other material by aspiration, scraping, a smear, or washings of the tissue. Compare **aspiration cytology.**

exfoliative dermatitis, any inflammatory skin disorder in which there is excessive peeling or shedding of skin. The cause is unknown in about half of the cases. Known causes include drug reactions, scarlet fever, leukemia, lymphoma, and generalized dermatitis. Treatment is individualized, but care is essential to prevent secondary infection, to avoid further irritation, and to maintain fluid balance.

exhalation. See **expiration.**

exhale, to breathe out or to let out with the breath. – exhalation, *n.*

exhaustion delirium, a delirium that may result from prolonged physical or emotional stress, fatigue, or shock associated with severe metabolic or nutritional problems. See also **delirium.**

exhibitionism, **1.** the flaunting of oneself or one's abilities in order to attract attention. **2.** (in psychiatry) a psychosexual disorder occurring in men in which the repetitive act of exposing the genitals to unsuspecting women or girls in socially unacceptable situations is the preferred means of achieving sexual excitement and gratification. See also **paraphilia, scopophilia.** – exhibitionist, *n.*

existential-humanistic psychotherapy. See **humanistic-existential therapy.**

existential psychiatry, a school of psychiatry based on the philosophy of existentialism that emphasizes an analytical, holistic approach in which mental disorders are viewed as deviations within the total structure of an individual's existence rather than as caused by any biologically or culturally related factors.

existential therapy, a kind of psychotherapy that emphasizes the development of a sense of self-direction through choice, awareness, and acceptance of individual responsibility.

exit dose, (in radiotherapy) the amount of radiation at the surface of the body opposite the surface to which the beam is directed.

Exna, a trade name for a diuretic and antihypertensive (benzthiazide).

exo-, a combining form meaning 'outside, outward': *exocataphoria, exohysteropexy, exotoxin.*

exocoelom. See **extraembryonic coelom.**

exocrine (ek'səkrın), of or pertaining to the process of secreting outwardly through a duct to the surface of an organ or tissue or into a vessel, as a gland that secretes through a duct. Compare **endocrine.** See also **eccrine.**

exocrine gland, any one of the two kinds of multicellular glands that open on the surface of the skin through ducts in the epithelium, as the sweat glands and the sebaceous glands. Exocrine glands comprise simple glands having only one duct and compound glands having more than one duct.

exogenous depression. See **reactive depression.**

exogenous hyperlipemia. See **Type I hyperlipidemia.**

exogenous obesity, obesity owing to a caloric intake greater than needed to meet the metabolic needs of the body. Compare **endogenous obesity.** See also **obesity.**

exon (ek'son), (in molecular genetics) the part of a DNA molecule that produces the code for the final messenger RNA.

exonuclease (ek'sounu'klieis), (in molecular genetics) a nuclease that digests DNA from the ends of the strands.

exophoria (ek'səfɔr'iə), deviation of the visual axis of one eye away from that of the other eye, occurring in the absence of visual stimuli for fusion. Compare **exotropia.** – exophoric, *adj.*

exophthalmia (ek'softhæl'miə), an abnormal condition characterized by marked protrusion of the eyeballs, usually resulting from the increased volume of the orbital contents caused by a tumor, swelling associated with cerebral, intraocular, or intraorbital edema or hemorrhage, paralysis of or trauma to the extraocular muscles, or cavernous sinus thrombosis. It may also be caused by endocrine disorders, as hyperthyroidism and Graves' disease, by varicose veins within the orbit, or by injury to orbital bones. Visual acuity may be impaired in exophthalmia; keratitis, ulceration, infection, and blindness may also occur. Treatment depends on the underlying cause. The outcome depends on the cause and the stage at which the condition is detected and treatment is begun. Acute advanced exophthalmia is often irreversible. Also called **proptosis, protrusio bulbi.** — **exophthalmic,** *adj.*

exophthalmic goiter, exophthalmos occurring in association with goiter, as in Graves' disease.

exophthalmometer (ek'səfthælmom'ətər), an instrument used for measuring the degree of forward displacement of the eye in exophthalmos. The device allows measurement of the distance from the center of the cornea to the lateral orbital rim. This distance is rarely more than 18 mm.

exophthalmos, exophthalmus (ek'softhæl'məs), abnormal protrusion of one or both eyeballs caused by trauma, intracranial lesions, intraorbital disorders, or systemic disease, most commonly hyperthyroidism. Exophthalmos may occur in acromegaly, Cushing's disease, systemic amyloides, Wegener's granulomatosis, or as a result of leukemic infiltration into retrobulbar spaces, nasopharyngeal infection or tumor, or intraorbital inflammatory disease, tumor, or vascular anomaly, as ophthalmic artery aneurysm, arteriovenous malformation, hemangioma, or varices. Dark glasses or shields may be required to protect the cornea from abrasion. Long-standing exophthalmos may lead to drying, infection, or ulceration of the cornea. Treatment may include control of hyperthyroidism, the administration of prednisone, or, as a last resort, decompression of the orbit by lateral orbitotomy, transantral decompression, or transfrontal craniotomy. — **exophthalmic,** *adj.*

EXOPHTHALMOS

exophthalmos-macroglossia-gigantism syndrome. See **EMG syndrome.**

exophytic (ek'səfit'ik), of or pertaining to the tendency to grow outward, as an exophytic tumor that grows on the surface or exterior portion of an organ or structure.

exophytic carcinoma, a malignant, epithelial neoplasm that resembles a papilloma or wart.

exostosis (ek'səstou'sis), an abnormal, benign growth on the surface of a bone. — **exostosed, exostotic,** *adj.*

exotoxin (ek'sətok'sin), a toxin that is secreted or excreted by a living microorganism. Compare **endotoxin.**

exotropia (ek'sətrou'piə), strabismus characterized by the outward deviation of one eye relative to the other. Compare **esotropia.** See also **strabismus.** — **exotropic,** *adj.*

expectant treatment, applying therapeutic measures to relieve symptoms as they arise in the course of a disease rather than treating the cause of the illness itself. Some kinds of expectant treatment are amputations for gangrene in a patient with diabetes, coronary bypass procedures in a patient with generalized atherosclerosis, transplantation of tendons in a patient with severe rheumatoid arthritis. Compare **definitive treatment, palliative treatment, supportive treatment.**

expectation, (in nursing) **1.** anticipation by the staff of a client's behavior based on a knowledge and understanding of the client's abilities and problems. **2.** anticipation of the performance of the nursing staff, as role expectation.

expectation of life, the probable number of years a person will live after a given age, as determined by the mortality rate in a specific geographic area. It may be individually qualified by the person's condition or race, sex, age, or other demographic factor. Also called **life expectancy.**

expected date of confinement (EDC), the predicted date of a pregnant woman's delivery. Pregnancy lasts approximately 266 days or 38 weeks from the day of fertilization but is considered clinically to last 280 days, or 40 weeks, or 10 lunar months, or 9 $\frac{1}{3}$ calendar months from the first day of the last menstrual period (LMP). The EDC is usually calculated on the basis of 9 $\frac{1}{3}$ calendar months, but if a woman is certain that coitus occurred only once during the month and if she knows the date on which it occurred, the EDC may be calculated as 38 weeks from that date. In the absence of a special calendar or device for calculating the EDC, it is arrived at by counting back three months from the first day of the LMP and then adding seven days and one year; thus, if the first day of a woman's LMP is July 18, 1984, one counts back three months to April 18, 1984, then adds seven days and one year to arrive at an EDC of April 25, 1985. Because calendar months differ in length, this calculation may give a date that is a few days more or less than 280 days from the first day of the LMP, but it provides a very close approximation, and a trivial error will not be of clinical significance because of the variability of the actual durations of normal pregnancies. The expectant mother is advised that the EDC is only an estimate and that the chances are that she will give birth within two weeks before or, more commonly, after the calculated date.

expectorant, **1.** of or pertaining to a substance that promotes the ejection of mucus or other exudates from the lung, bronchi, and trachea. **2.** an agent that promotes expectoration by reducing the viscosity of pulmonary secretions or by decreasing the force with which exudates adhere to the lower respiratory tract. Expectorant drugs include acetycysteine, guaifenesin, terpin hydrate, and tyloxapol. – **expectorate,** *v.*

expectoration, the ejection of mucus, sputum, or fluids from the trachea and lungs by coughing or spitting.

experience rating, 1. a rating system used by an insurance company to set the premium to be paid by the insured, based on the risk to the insurance company of providing the insurance. Experience rating has led to very high malpractice premiums in some specialties and areas, for the insurance company calculates the premium on the basis of settlements made in all malpractice claims during a specified period. Experience rating is also used to set annual membership health maintenance fees in organizations in which the cost of providing the services in a previous accounting period is used to determine the premiums for the next fiscal year. 2. the rating that is used to calculate an insurance premium.

experimental design, (in research) a study design used to test cause-and-effect relationships between variables. The classic experimental design specifies an experimental group and a control group. The independent variable is administered to the experimental group and not to the control group, and both groups are measured on the same dependent variable. Subsequent experimental designs have used more groups and more measurements over longer periods of time.

experimental embryology, the study and analysis through experimental techniques of the factors, mechanisms, and relationships that determine and influence prenatal development.

experimental group. See **group.**

experimental medicine, a branch of the practice of medicine in which new drugs or treatments are evaluated for safety and efficacy in a clinical laboratory setting by using animals or, in certain cases, human subjects.

experimental physiology, a branch of the study of physiology in which the functions of various body systems are evaluated in a clinical laboratory setting by using animals or, in some cases, human subjects.

experimental psychology, the study of mental processes and phenomena by observation in a controlled environment using various tests, manipulations, and experiments.

experimental variable. See **independent variable.**

expert witness, a person who has special knowledge of a subject about which a court requests testimony. Special knowledge may be acquired by experience, education, observation, or study but is not possessed by the average person. An expert witness gives expert testimony or expert evidence. This evidence often serves to educate the court and the jury in the subject under consideration.

expiration, breathing out, normally a passive process, depending on the elastic qualities of lung tissue and the

thorax. Also called **exhalation.** Compare **inspiration.** – **expire,** *v.*

expiratory reserve volume (ERV), the maximum volume of gas that can be expired from the resting expiratory level. See also **vital capacity.**

expired gas (E), any gas exhaled from the lungs.

expression, 1. the indication of a physical or emotional state through facial appearance or vocal intonation. 2. the act of pressing or squeezing in order to expel something, as milk from the breast following pregnancy or the fetus from the uterus by exerting pressure on the abdominal wall. 3. (in genetics) the detectable effect or appearance in the phenotype of a particular trait or condition. See also **expressivity.** – **express,** *v.*

expressive aphasia. See **motor aphasia.**

expressivity, (in genetics) the variability with which basic patterns of inheritance are modified, both in degree and in variety, by the effect of a given gene in people of the same genotype. Polydactyly may be expressed as extra toes in one generation and extra fingers in another.

expulsive stage of labor, the second stage of labor, during which the mother's uterine contractions are accompanied by a bearing-down reflex. It begins after full dilatation of the cervix and continues to the complete delivery of the infant.

extended care facility, an institution devoted to providing medical, nursing, or custodial care for an individual over a prolonged period of time, as during the course of a chronic disease or during the rehabilitation phase after an acute illness. Kinds of extended care facilities are **intermediate care facility, skilled nursing facility.** Also called **convalescent home, nursing home.**

extended family, a family group consisting of the biological parents, their children, the parents' parents, and other family members. The extended family is the basic family group in many societies. Among its characteristics are increased exchange of information from experienced older members to less experienced younger ones, care of the older family members in the home by the younger ones, and care by the older people for the children of the younger members. Compare **nuclear family.**

extended insulin zinc suspension, a long-acting ultralente insulin that is slowly absorbed and slow to act.

Extendryl, a trade name for a fixed-combination nasal decongestant drug containing an adrenergic (phenylephrine hydrochloride), an antihistaminic (chlorpheniramine maleate), and an anticholinergic (methscopolamine nitrate).

extension, a movement allowed by certain joints of the skeleton that increases the angle between two adjoining bones, as extending the leg, which increases the angle between the femur and the tibia. Compare **flexion.**

extensor carpi radialis brevis (ɪksten'sər), one of the seven superficial muscles of the posterior forearm. Lying beneath the extensor carpi radialis longus, it arises from the lateral epicondyle of the humerus, from the radial collateral ligament of the elbow joint, and from various intermuscular septa. It inserts into the dorsal surface of the third metacarpal bone. The muscle is innervated by a branch of the radial nerve that contains fibers from the sixth and the seventh cervical nerves, and it functions to extend the hand. Compare **extensor carpi radialis longus, extensor carpi ulnaris, extensor digiti minimi.**

extensor carpi radialis longus, one of the seven superficial muscles of the posterior forearm. Arising from the lateral supracondylar ridge of the humerus,forearm. It arises from the lateral epicondyle of the humerus and inserts by a tendon into the ulnar side of the fifth metacarpal bone. It is innervated by a branch of the deep radial nerve, containing fibers from the sixth, seventh, and eighth cervical nerves, and functions to extend and adduct the hand. Compare **extensor carpi radialis brevis, extensor carpi radialis longus, extensor digiti minimi.**

extensor digiti minimi, one of the seven superficial muscles of the posterior forearm. Located on the medial side of the extensor digitorum, it is a slender muscle that arises from the common extensor tendon and joins the expansion of the extensor digitorum tendon on the back of the first phalanx of the little finger. It is innervated by a branch of the deep radial nerve that contains fibers from the sixth, seventh, and eighth cervical nerves, and it functions to extend the little finger. Compare **extensor carpi radialis brevis, extensor carpi radialis longus, extensor digitorum.**

extensor digitorum, one of the seven superficial muscles of the posterior forearm. Arising from the lateral epicondyle of the humerus, the intermuscular septa between it and adjacent muscles, and the antebrachial fascia, it divides distally into four tendons which pass through the extensor retinaculum and diverge on the back of the hand, inserting into the second and the third phalanges of the fingers. The muscle is innervated by a branch of the deep radial nerve that contains fibers from the sixth, seventh, and eighth cervical nerves, and it functions to extend the phalanges and, by continued action, the wrist. Also called **extensor digitorum communis.** Compare **extensor carpi radialis brevis, extensor carpi radialis longus, extensor digiti minimi.**

extensor digitorum communis. See **extensor digitorum.**

extensor digitorum longus, a penniform muscle located at the lateral part of the anterior leg. It is one of three anterior crural muscles and arises from the lateral condyle of the tibia, the anterior surface of the fibula, the deep surface of the fascia, and from intermuscular septa. Its distal tendon passes under the extensor retinacula and divides into four slips that insert into the second and third phalanges of the four lesser toes. The muscle is innervated by branches of the deep peroneal nerve containing fibers from the fourth and the fifth lumbar and first sacral nerves. It extends the proximal phalanges of the four small toes and dorsally flexes and pronates the foot. Compare **tibialis anterior.**

extensor retinaculum of the hand. See **retinaculum extensorum manus.**

external, 1. being on the outside or exterior of the body or an organ. 2. acting from the outside, as an external influence, or exogenous factor. 3. pertaining to the outward or visible appearance. Compare **internal.**

external absorption, the taking up of poisons, food, or other substances through the mucous membranes or the skin.

external acoustic meatus, the s-shaped canal of the external ear, comprised of bone and cartilage, extending from the auricle to the tympanic membrane. Also called **external auditory canal.**

external aperture of aqueduct of vestibule, an external opening for the small canal extending from the vestibule of the inner ear, located on the internal surface of the petrous part of the temporal bone lateral to the opening for the internal acoustic passage.

external aperture of canaliculus of cochlea, an external opening of the cochlear channel on the margin of the jugular opening in the temporal bone.

external aperture of tympanic canaliculus, the lower opening of the tympanic channel on the inferior surface of the petrous part of the temporal bone.

external auditory canal. See **external acoustic meatus.**

external carotid artery, one of a pair of arteries with eight major temporal or maxillary branches, rising from the common carotid arteries and supplying various parts and tissues of the head and neck.

external carotid plexus, a network of nerves around the external carotid artery, formed by the external carotid nerves from the superior cervical ganglion and supplying sympathetic fibers associated with branches of the external carotid artery. Compare **common carotid plexus, internal carotid plexus.**

external cervical os, an external opening of the uterus that leads into the cavity of the cervix. This opening, bounded by the ventral lip and the dorsal lip, is in the center of the rounded extremity of the cervix that projects into the cavity of the vagina. Compare **internal cervical os.**

external conjugate, the distance measured with obstetric calipers from the depression below the lowest lumbar vertebra posteriorly to the upper border of the symphysis anteriorly (usually about 21 cm). The external conjugate is roughly 8.5 cm greater than the obstetric conjugate, but the correlation is not consistent and the measurement is seldom used in modern obstetrics. Also called **Baudeloc que's diameter.**

external cuneiform bone. See **lateral cuneiform bone.**

external ear, the outer structure of the ear, consisting of the auricle and the external acoustic meatus. Sound waves are funneled through the external ear to the middle ear. Compare **internal ear, middle ear.**

external fertilization, the union of male and female gametes outside of the bodies from which they originated, as occurs in most fish.

external fistula, an abnormal passage between an internal organ or structure and the cutaneous surface of the body.

external iliac artery, a division of the common iliac artery descending into the thigh and becoming the femoral artery. The external iliac supplies the lower limb and is larger than the internal iliac, except in the fetus, where it is smaller. Compare **internal iliac artery.**

external iliac node, a node in one of the seven groups of parietal nodes serving the lymphatic system in the abdomen and the pelvis. About ten external iliac nodes, arranged in three groups, lie along the external iliac vessels. Their afferents drain lymph from numerous abdominal and pelvic structures, as the deep abdominal wall, the adductor region of the thigh, the prostate, and the vagina. Compare **common iliac node, iliac circumflex node, internal iliac node.** See also **lymph, lymphatic system, lymph node.**

external iliac vein, one of a pair of veins in the lower body that join the internal iliac vein to form the two common iliac veins. Each external iliac vein begins under the inguinal ligament, ascends along the brim of the lesser pelvis, and ends opposite the sacroiliac articulation by joining the internal iliac vein. In many individuals it contains at least one valve, and sometimes two. It receives the inferior epigastric vein, the deep iliac circumflex vein, and the pubic veins. Compare **internal iliac vein.**

external jugular vein, one of a pair of large vessels in the neck that receive most of the blood from the exterior of the cranium and the deep tissues of the face. Each external jugular vein is formed by the junction of the retromandibular vein with the posterior auricular vein and arises in the parotid gland on a level with the angle of the mandible. It runs perpendicularly down the neck and joins the subclavian vein lateral or ventral to the scalenus anterior. It contains two pairs of valves, the inferior pair at the junction with the subclavian vein and the superior pair, usually about four cm above the clavicle. A sinus lies between the two sets of valves. Compare **internal jugular vein.**

external oblique muscle. See **obliquus externus abdominis.**

external perimysium. See **epimysium.**

external pin fixation, a method of holding together the fragments of a fractured bone by employing transfixing metal pins through the fragments and a compression device attached to the pins outside the skin surface. Nursing care includes regular cleansing of the skin around the pins and, often, the application of antibiotic solutions or ointments. The pins are removed at a later procedure when the fracture is healed. Compare **internal fixation.**

external pterygoid muscle. See **pterygoideus lateralis.**

external radiation therapy (ERT), the therapeutic application of ionizing radiation from an external beam from a kilovoltage x-ray machine, a megavoltage cobalt-60 machine, or a supervoltage linear accelerator, cyclotron, or betatron. ERT is used most frequently in the treatment of cancer but may also be applied in the therapy of keloids and some dermatological conditions and in counteracting the body's physiological rejection of transplanted organs.

external shunt, a device for the passage of a body fluid from one compartment of the body to another, consisting of a tube or catheter or a series of such containers that passes over the surface of the body from one compartment or cavity to another. See also **hemodialysis, hydrocephalus.**

exteroceptive, pertaining to stimuli that originate from outside of the body or to the sensory receptors that they activate. Compare **interoceptive, proprioception.**

exteroceptor, any sensory nerve ending, as those located in the skin, mucous membranes, or sense organs, that responds to stimuli originating from outside of the body, as touch, pressure, or sound. Compare **interoceptor, proprioceptor.** See also **chemoreceptor, exteroceptive nervous system, receptor.**

extra-, a combining form meaning 'outside of, beyond, in addition to': *extrabronchial, extradural, extramarginal.*

extrabuccal feeding, the administration of nutrients by means other than the mouth. Also called **extraoral feeding.** See also **gavage, intravenous feeding.**

extracapsular fracture, any fracture that occurs near a joint but does not directly involve the joint capsule. This type of fracture is extremely common in the hip.

extracellular, occurring outside a cell or cell tissue, or in cavities or spaces between cell layers or groups of cells. About 40 per cent of the water in a human body is contained in extracellular fluids. See also **cell, edema, interstitial.**

extracellular fluid (ECF), the portion of the body fluid comprising the interstitial fluid and blood plasma. The adult body contains about 11.2 liters of interstitial fluid, constituting about 16 per cent of body weight, and about 2.8 liters of plasma, constituting about 4 per cent of body weight. Plasma and interstitial fluid are very similar chemically and, in conjunction with intracellular fluid, help control the movement of water and electrolytes throughout the body. Some of the important ionized components of extracellular fluid are protein, magnesium, potassium, chlorine, calcium, and certain sulfates.

extradural (ek'strədur'əl),   outside the dura mater.

extradural anesthesia,   anesthetic nerve block achieved by the injection of a local anesthetic solution into the space in the spinal canal outside the dura mater of the spinal cord, as in epidural, caudal, or paravertebral anesthesia.

extradural hemorrhage,   a hemorrhage of an area surrounding but outside of the dura of the brain or spinal cord.

extraembryonic blastoderm,   the area of the blastoderm that gives rise to the membranes that surround the embryo during gestation. Compare **embryonic blastoderm.** See also **allantois, amnion, chorion, yolk sac.**

extraembryonic coelom,   a cavity external to the developing embryo that forms between the mesoderm of the chorion and that covering the amniotic cavity and yolk sac. During early prenatal development, there is direct contact with the embryonic coelom at the umbilicus, but this junction is obliterated by the growth of the amnion and the closing of the body wall. Also called **exocoelom.**

extramedullary myeloma,   a plasma cell tumor that occurs outside of the bone marrow, usually affecting the visceral organs or the nasopharyngeal and oral mucosa. Also called **extramedullary plasmacytoma, peripheral plasma cell myeloma, plasma cell tumor.**

extramedullary myelopoiesis,   the formation and development of myeloid tissue outside of the bone marrow. Also called **ectopic myelopoiesis.**

extraocular (ek'straok'yulər),   outside the eye.

extraocular muscle palsy,   an abnormal condition characterized by paralysis of the extrinsic muscles of the eye, as the superior, inferior, medsial, and lateral rectus muscles, and the superior and the inferior oblique muscles.

extraoral feeding.   See **extrabuccal feeding.**

extraperitoneal Caesarean section,   a method for surgically delivering a baby through an incision in the lower uterine segment without entering the peritoneal cavity. The uterus is approached through the paravesicle space. This procedure is performed most often to avoid spread of infection from the uterus into the peritoneal cavity. It is somewhat slower to perform than the low cervical or classical Caesarean operations. See also **Caesarean section.**

extrapsychic conflict,   an emotional conflict usually occurring when one's inner needs and desires do not coincide with the restrictions of the environment or society. Compare **intrapsychic conflict.** See also **conflict.**

extrapyramidal (ek'strəpɪræm'ədəl),   **1.** of or pertaining to the tissues and structures of the brain that are associated with movement of the body, excluding motor neurons, the motor cortex, and the corticospinal and corticobulbar tracts. **2.** of or pertaining to the function of these tissues and structures.

extrapyramidal disease,   any of a large group of conditions characterized by involuntary movement, changes in muscle tone, and abnormal posture, as in tardive dyskinesia, chorea, athetosis, and Parkinson's disease.

extrapyramidal reaction,   a response to a treatment or a drug characterized by the signs of extrapyramidal disease. The reaction may persist or regress after discontinuation of the treatment or drug.

extrapyramidal system,   the part of the nervous system that includes the basal ganglia, substantia nigra, subthalamic nucleus, part of the midbrain, and the motor neurons of the spine. The extrapyramidal system controls and coordinates the motor activities required for locomotion and for stasis, body support, and posture. Also called **extrapyramidal tracts.**

extrapyramidal tracts,   the tracts of motor nerves from the brain to the anterior horns of the spinal cord, except for the fibers of the pyramidal tracts. Within the brain, extrapyramidal tracts comprise various relays of motoneurons between motor areas of the cerebral cortex, the basal ganglia, the thalamus, the cerebellum, and the brain stem. Research into the precise functions of these networks continues, and it is not yet known how some of them work. The extrapyramidal tracts are functional rather than anatomical units, comprising the nuclei and the fibers and excluding the pyramidal tracts. They especially control and coordinate the postural, static, supporting, and locomotor mechanisms and cause contractions of muscle groups in sequence or simultaneously. The extrapyramidal tracts include the corpus striatum, the subthalamic nucleus, the substantia nigra, and the red nucleus, together with their interconnections with the reticular formation, the cerebellum, and the cerebrum. Compare **pyramidal tract.**

extrasensory perception (ESP),   awareness or knowledge acquired without using the physical senses. See also **clairvoyance, parapsychology, telepathy.**

extrasystole (ek'trəsɪs'təli),   a premature atrial, ventricular, or cardiac contraction that does not change the fundamental rhythm of the heart.

extravasation (ɪkstræv'ɪzei'shən),   a passage or escape into the tissues, usually of blood, serum, or lymph. Compare **bleeding.** See also **exudate, transudate.**   — **extravasate,** v.

extraventricular hydrocephalus.   See **hydrocephalus.**

extraversion.   See **extroversion.**

extrinsic allergic alveolitis,   an inflammatory form of interstitial pneumonia that results from an immunological reaction in a hypersensitive person. The reaction may be provoked by a variety of inhaled organic dusts, often those containing fungal spores. The disease can be prevented by avoiding contact with the causative agents. Extrinsic allergic alveolitis is a disease in which classification is based solely on the character of the immune response rather than on its clinical manifestations. A wide variety of symptoms may occur, including asthma, fever, chills, malaise, and muscle aches, which usually develop four to six hours after exposure. On laboratory examination of the blood, leukocytosis is commonly found. Recovery is usually spontaneous. In an acute attack, corticosteroids may be given to diminish the inflammatory response. Kinds of extrinsic allergic alveolitis include **bagassosis, farmer's lung, humidifier or air conditioner lung, mushroom worker's lung, suberosis.** Also called **hypersensitivity pneumonitis.** See also **Arthus reaction.**

extrinsic allergic pneumonia. See **diffuse hypersensitivity pneumonia.**

extrinsic asthma, a form of asthma in which attacks are precipitated primarily by allergens to which the patient is sensitized. The initial onset usually occurs prior to the age of 30 years. Also called **allergic asthma, atopic asthma.** See also **asthma in children.**

extrinsic factor. See **cyanocobalamin.**

extroversion, extraversion, 1. the tendency to direct one's interests and energies toward external values or things outside the self. 2. the state of being totally or primarily concerned with what is outside the self. Compare **introversion.**

extrovert, extravert, 1. a person whose interests are directed away from the self and concerned primarily with external reality and the physical environment rather than with inner feelings and thoughts. This person is usually highly sociable, outgoing, impulsive, and emotionally expressive. 2. a person characterized by extroversion. 3. to direct one's interests to external values and those things outside the self. Compare **introvert.** – **extroversion,** n.

extrusion reflex, a normal response in infants to force the tongue outward when touched or depressed. The reflex begins to disappear by about three or four months of age. Before it fades, food must be placed well back in the mouth to be retained and swallowed. Constant protrusion of a large tongue may be a sign of Down's syndrome.

extubation, the process of withdrawing a tube from an orifice or cavity of the body. – **extubate,** v.

exuberant callus. See **heterotopic ossification.**

exudate (eks′yʊdeɪt), fluid, cells, or other substances that have been slowly exuded, or discharged, from cells or blood vessels through small pores or breaks in cell membranes. Perspiration is sometimes identified as an exudate.

exudative (ɪgzu′dətɪv), relating to the exudation or oozing of fluid and other materials from cells and tissues, usually as a result of inflammation or injury, used in the identification of a disease or disorder marked by signs of exudation, as exudative enteropathy.

exudative angina. See **croup.**

exudative enteropathy, diarrhea seen in diseases characterized by inflammation or destruction of intestinal mucosa. Crohn's disease, ulcerative colitis, tuberculosis, and some lymphomas cause an increase of plasma, blood, mucus, and protein to accumulate in the intestine, adding to fecal bulk and frequency. See also **diarrhea.**

eye, one of a pair of organs of sight, contained in a bony orbit at the front of the skull, embedded in orbital fat, and innervated by one of a pair of optic nerves from the forebrain. Associated with the eye are certain accessory structures, as the muscles, the fasciae, the eyebrow, the eyelids, the conjunctiva, and the lacrimal gland. The bulb of the eye is composed of segments of two spheres with nearly parallel axes that constitute the outside tunic and one of three fibrous layers enclosing two internal cavities separated by the crystalline lens. The smaller cavity anterior to the lens is divided by the iris into two chambers, both filled with aqueous humor. The posterior chamber is larger than the anterior chamber and contains the jellylike vitreous body which is divided by the hyaloid canal. The outside tunic of the bulb consists of the transparent cornea anteriorly, constituting one fifth of the tunic, and the opaque sclera posteriorly, constituting five sixths of the tunic. The intermediate vascular, pigmented tunic consists of the choroid, the ciliary body, and the iris. The internal tunic of nervous tissue is the retina. Light waves passing through the lens strike a layer of rods and cones in the retina creating impulses that are transmitted by the optic nerve to the brain. The transverse and the anteroposterior diameters of the eye bulb are slightly greater than the vertical diameter; the bulb in women is usually smaller than the bulb in men. Also called **bulbus oculi, eyeball.**

eyebrow, 1. the supraorbital arch of the frontal bone that separates the orbit of the eye from the forehead. 2. the arch of hairs growing along the ridge formed by the supraorbital arch of the frontal bone.

Eye-Cort, a trade name for a glucocorticoid (hydrocortisone acetate).

eyeground, the fundus of the eye. See also **funduscopy.**

eyelash, one of many cilia growing in double or triple rows along the border of the eyelids in front of a row of ciliary glands that are in front of a row of Meibomian glands.

eyelid, a movable fold of thin skin over the eye, with eyelashes and ciliary and Meibomian glands along its margin. It consists of loose connective tissue containing a thin plate of fibrous tissue lined with mucous membrane. The orbicularis oculi muscle and the oculomotor nerve control the opening and closing of the eyelid. The upper and lower eyelids are separated by the palpebral fissure. Also called **palpebra.**

eye memory. See **visual memory.**

F

f, 1. symbol for *breaths per unit time*. 2. symbol for *respiratory frequency*.

F, 1. symbol for **fluorine**. 2. abbreviation for **farad**.

F_1, (in genetics) the symbol for the first filial generation; the heterozygous offspring produced by the mating of two unrelated individuals or by the crossing of a homozygous dominant strain with a homozygous recessive.

F_2, (in genetics) the symbol for the second filial generation; the offspring produced by mating two members of the F_1 generation or, broadly, by crossing any two heterozygous strains.

FAAN, abbreviation for **Fellow of the American Academy of Nursing.**

fabrication. See **confabulation.**

Fabry's disease (fa'briz). See **angiokeratoma corporis diffusum.**

Fabry's syndrome. See **angiokeratoma corporis diffusum.**

F.A.C.C.P., abbreviation for **Fellow of the American College of Chest Physicians.**

face, 1. the front of the head from the chin to the brow, including the skin, muscles and structures of the forehead, eyes, nose, mouth, cheeks, and jaw. 2. the visage. 3. to direct the face toward something. See also **en face** —**facial,** *adj.*

face validity, the apparent validity of a test or measurement device as it is to be used in a particular study. See also **validity.**

facial artery, one of a pair of tortuous arteries that arise from the external carotid arteries, divide into four cervical and five facial branches, and supply various organs and tissues in the head. The cervical branches of the facial artery are the ascending palatine, tonsillar, glandular, and the submental. The facial branches are the inferior labial, superior labial, lateral nasal, and the angular.

facial diplegia, a rare neuromuscular condition characterized by bilateral paralysis of various muscles of the face.

facial muscle, one of numerous muscles of the face, seldom remaining distinct over its entire length because of a tendency to merge with a neighboring muscle at its termination or its attachment. The five groups of facial muscles include the muscles of the scalp, the extrinsic muscles of the ear, the muscles of the nose, and the muscles of the mouth. The platysma is one of the facial group but is described with the muscles of the neck. Also called **muscle of expression.**

facial nerve, either of a pair of mixed sensory and motor cranial nerves that arises from the brain stem at the base of the pons and divides just in front of the ear into its six branches, innervating the scalp, forehead, eyelids, muscles of facial expression, cheeks, and jaw. Also called **seventh nerve.**

facial paralysis, an abnormal condition characterized by the partial or the total loss of the functions of the facial muscles or the loss of sensation in the face. It may be caused by disease or by trauma. The degree of paralysis depends on the nerves affected. Brain injury above the facial nucleus usually does not block the innervation of the brow and the forehead muscles. Injury to the nucleus of the facial nerve or injury to its peripheral neurons paralyzes all the ipsilateral facial muscles. See also **Bell's palsy.**

facial perception, the ability to judge the distance and direction of objects through the sensation felt in the skin of the face. The phenomenon is commonly experienced by those who are blind and is rarely experienced in the dark by those with sight. Also called **facial vision.**

facial vein, one of a pair of superficial veins that drain deoxygenated blood from the superficial structures of the face. Each facial vein starts as the angular vein at the union of the frontal and the supraorbital veins and accompanies the facial artery, passing deep to the zygomaticus major and the zygomaticus minor, following the border of the masseter, curving around the mandible into the neck, and communicating with the anterior jugular vein and the external jugular vein to empty into the internal jugular vein. The facial vein anastomoses with the cavernous sinus through various veins, as the angular, the supraorbital, and the superior ophthalmic. As the vein has no valves that prevent the backflow of blood, infections of the skin near the nose and mouth may cause meningitis, because blood-borne organisms can reach the cavernous sinus through the anastomoses.

facial vision. See **facial perception.**

facilitation, 1. Compare **inhibition.** See also **summation.** the enhancement or reinforcement of any action or function so that it is carried out with increased ease. 2. (in neurology) the phenomenon whereby two or more afferent impulses that individually are not strong enough to elicit a response in a neuron can collectively produce a reflex discharge greater than the sum of the separate responses. **3.** (in neurology) the process of lowering the threshold action potential of a neuron by the repeated passage of an impulse along the same pathway. Also called **law of facilitation.**

facio-, a combining form meaning 'pertaining to the face': *faciocervical, faciolingual, facioplegia.*

F.A.C.O.G., abbreviation for *Fellow of the American College of Obstetricians and Gynecologists.* See **board certification.**

F.A.C.S. abbreviation for **Fellow of the American College of Surgeons.**

-faction, a combining form meaning a 'process of making': *bilifaction, chylifaction, liquefaction.*

factitial (fæktɪˈshəl), artificial or self-induced, as a factitial dermatitis.

factitial dermatitis, a skin rash caused by the patient, usually for secondary gain or as a manifestation of psychiatric illness.

-factive, a combining form meaning 'making': *liquefactive, stupefactive, vasofactive.* Also **-fying.**

factor I. See **fibrinogen.**

factor II. See **prothrombin.**

factor III. See **thromboplastin.**

factor IV, a designation for calcium as an element in the process of the coagulation of blood.

factor V, an unstable procoagulant that occurs in normal plasma but is deficient in the blood of parahemophiliacs. It is needed to rapidly convert prothrombin to thrombin. Some research indicates that during coagulation, factor V changes from an inactive agent to an active prothrombin accelerator. Also called **proaccelerin.**

factor VI, a hypothetical chemical agent which some suggest is derived from proaccelerin, or factor V, in the process of blood coagulation.

factor VII, a blood procoagulant present in the blood plasma synthesized in the liver by the action of vitamin K. Also called **proconvertin.**

factor VIII, a coagulation factor present in normal plasma but deficient in the blood of persons with hemophilia A.

factor IX, a coagulation factor present in normal plasma but deficient in the blood of persons with hemophilia B. Also called **Christmas factor.**

factor IX complex, a hemostatic containing factors II, VII, IX, and X.
■ INDICATIONS: It is prescribed in the treatment of hemophilia B and Christmas Disease.
■ CONTRAINDICATION: Liver disease with intravascular coagulation and fibrinolysis is the only contraindication.
■ ADVERSE EFFECTS: Among the more serious adverse

reactions are hepatitis, intravascular coagulation, circulatory collapse, and hypersensitivity reaction.

factor X, a coagulation factor which occurs in normal plasma but is deficient in some inherited defects in coagulation. Factor X and prothrombin are closely related; both are synthesized in the liver by the action of vitamin K. Also called **Stuart-Power factor.**

factor XI, a coagulation factor present in normal plasma. Deficiency results in prolonged coagulation time.

factor XII, a coagulation factor present in normal plasma. It triggers the formation of bradykinin and associated enzymatic reactions. It is required for rapid coagulation in vitro but is apparently not needed for hemostasis in vivo. It can be activated in the laboratory by contact with negatively charged surfaces, which can develop on glass and kaolin or on biological material, as collagen. Also called **activation factor, contact factor, glass factor, Hageman factor.**

factor XIII, a coagulation factor present in normal plasma that acts with calcium to produce an insoluble fibrin clot. Also called **fibrinase, fibrin stabilizing factor.**

Factorate, a trade name for human antihemophilic factor VIII.

factor searching study, (in nursing research) a study design that produces a qualitative, narrative description including categories or classifications of phenomena. It may be used to describe various aspects of nursing practice, characteristics of a population, or both. Factor searching is often a preliminary step in a study at a higher level of inquiry.

facultative (fækˈəlteɪˈtɪv), not obligatory; having the ability to adapt to more than one condition, as a facultative anaerobe.

facultative aerobe, an organism able to grow under anaerobic conditions that develops most rapidly in an aerobic environment. Compare **obligate aerobe.** See also **aerobe.**

facultative anaerobe, an organism able to grow under aerobic conditions that develops most rapidly in an anaerobic environment. Compare **obligate anaerobe.** See also **anaerobe, anaerobic infection.**

facultative parasite. See **parasite.**

faculty, 1. an ability to do something specific, as learn languages or remember names. **2.** any mental ability or power, as memory or thought. **3.** a department in an institution of learning or the people who teach in a department of such an institution.

faculty practice plan, a system in a medical school by which faculty members are able to increase the income to their department or themselves by practicing their specialty of medicine in a departmental practice in a school-controlled organization. Nursing school faculties are beginning to use the same device for retrieval of incomes from service.

Faget's sign (fæˈʒheiz'), a falling pulse rate associated with a constant temperature, or a constant pulse associated with a rising temperature. It is an unusual sign found in yellow fever. Also called **Faget's law.**

fagicladosporic acid (fæj'iklædˈousporˈik), a toxin produced by *Cladosporum epiphyllum,* a member of a genus of fungi that cause 'black spot' in stored meat, tinea negra, and black degeneration of the brain.

Fahrenheit, a scale for the measurement of temperature in which the boiling point of water is 212° and the freezing point of water is 32° at sea level. Compare **Celsius.**

failed forceps, an attempted mid-forceps operation that is abandoned because there is a greater degree of resistance to rotation or traction than anticipated, owing to cephalopelvic disproportion. Caesarean section is performed to deliver the infant. Compare **trial forceps** See also **cephalopelvic disproportion.**

failure to thrive, the abnormal retardation of the growth and development of an infant resulting from conditions that interfere with normal metabolism, appetite, and activity. Causative factors include chromosomal abnormalities, as in Turner's syndrome and the various trisomies; major organ system defects that lead to deficiency or malfunction; systemic disease or acute illness; physical deprivation, primarily malnutrition; and various psychosocial factors, as seen in severe cases of maternal deprivation syndrome. Metabolic disturbances of short duration, as occur during acute illness, usually have no long-term effects on development and are usually followed by a period of rapid growth. Prolonged nutritional deficiency may cause permanent and irreversible retardation of physical, mental, or social development.

faint, *Nontechnical.* **1.** to lose consciousness, as in a syncopal attack. **2.** a syncopal attack. See also **syncope.**

falciform body (fælˈsəform). See **sporozoite.**

falciparum malaria (fælsipˈərəm), the most severe form of malaria, caused by the protozoan *Plasmodium falciparum,* characterized by extremely grave systemic symptoms, mental confusion, enlarged spleen, edema, gastrointestinal symptoms, and anemia. Falciparum malaria does not last as long as other forms of malaria; if treatment is begun promptly, the disease may be mild and the recovery uneventful. Relapses are uncommon, but death may result from dehydration and anemia. The usual treatment is chloroquine, but patients known to have contracted malaria in an area that harbors drug-resistant *P. falciparum* are often treated with a combination of quinine, pyremethamine, and one of the sulfones or sulfanamides. Compare **quartan malaria, tertian malaria.** See also **algid malaria, blackwater fever, malaria.**

Fallopian tube (fəlouˈpiən), one of a pair of ducts opening at one end into the uterus and at the other end into the peritoneal cavity, over the ovary. Each tube serves as the passage through which an ovum is carried to the uterus and through which spermatozoa move out toward the ovary. The tube lies in the upper border of the broad ligament (the mesosalpinx). Each tube has four parts: the fimbriae, the infundibulum, the ampulla, and the isthmus. The fimbriae drape in fingerlike projections from the infundibulum over the ovary. Just proximal to the infundibulum is the ampulla, the widest portion of the tube. The ampulla is connected to the fundus of the uterus by the isthmus. Also called **oviduct, uterine tube.**

Fallot's syndrome (fælouz'). See **tetralogy of Fallot.** Also called **Fallot's tetralogy.**

fallout, the deposition of radioactive debris after a nuclear explosion. The debris from an atmospheric explosion of an atomic bomb may travel thousands of miles and be deposited over a large geographical area.

false anorexia. See **pseudoanorexia.**

false imprisonment, (in law) the intentional, unjustified, nonconsensual detention or confinement of a person for any length of time.

false labor. See **Braxton-Hicks contractions.**

false negative, an incorrect result of a diagnostic test or procedure that falsely indicates the absence of a finding, condition, or disease. The rate of occurrence of false negative results varies with the diagnostic accuracy and the specificity of the test or procedure. As the accuracy and specificity of a test increase, the rate of false negatives decreases. Certain tests are known to yield false negative results at a certain rate; in all tests, a small number will occur by chance alone. False negative results are more common than false positive results, because the person conducting the test is more likely to fail to observe a finding than to imagine seeing something that does not exist. Compare **false positive.**

false neuroma, 1. a neoplasm that does not contain nerve elements. **2.** a cystic neuroma.

false nucleolus. See **karyosome.**

false positive, a test result that wrongly indicates the presence of a disease or other condition the test is designed to reveal.

false rib. See **rib.**

false suture, an immovable fibrous joint in which rough articulating surfaces form the connection between certain bones of the skull. Two kinds of false sutures are **sutura plana, sutura squamosa.** Compare **true suture.**

false twins. See **dizygotic twins.**

false vocal cord, either of two thick folds of mucous membrane in the larynx separating the ventricle from the vestibule. Each fold encloses a narrow band of fibrous tissue (the ventricular ligament). Compare **vocal cord.**

falx (fælks, folks), *pl.* **falces** (fælˈsiz, folˈsiz). **1.** a sickle-shaped structure. **2.** sickle-shaped.

falx cerebelli, a small sickle-shaped process of the dura mater attached to the occipital bone above and projecting into the posterior cerebellar notch between the two cerebellar hemispheres.

falx cerebri, a tough membrane extending into and following along the longitudinal fissure of the two hemispheres of the cerebrum.

falx inguinalis, transverse and internal oblique muscles.

falx ligamentosa, the broad ligament of the liver.

familial, pertaining to a characteristic, condition, or disease that is present in some families and not others or that occurs in more family members than would be expected by chance. It is usually but not always hereditary. Compare **acquired, congenital, hereditary.**

familial cretinism, a rare genetic disorder characterized by hypothyroidism caused by an inborn error of metabolism resulting from a deficiency of the enzyme iodotrysine deiodinase, which interferes with thyroid hormone biosynthesis. Clinical manifestations include lethargy, stunted growth, and mental retardation. The condition, which is transmitted as an autosomal recessive trait, is treated by early administration of thyroid hormone.

familial hypercholesterolemia, an inherited disorder transmitted as a dominant trait and characterized by a high level of serum cholesterol, tendinous xanthomas, and early evidence of atherosclerosis, especially of the coronary arteries. Affected individuals at the age of 50 have three to ten times greater risk of ischemic heart disease than the general population. Cholesterol levels are elevated at birth, increase with age, and average 250 to 500 mg/100 ml in heterozygous adults and 500 to 1,000 mg/100 ml in adults who are homozygous for the gene. Xanthomas begin to appear at the age of 20 and occur most frequently on the Achilles tendon, extensor tendons of the hands, elbows, and tibial tuberosities. In Type IIa familial hypercholesterolemia, only low-density lipoprotein (LDL) is elevated, while in Type IIb, LDL and very low-density lipoprotein (VLDL) are increased. The disorder occurs in whites, blacks, and Orientals, and the prevalence of the gene in the United States is 1:1000. Treatment consists of a low-cholesterol and low-saturated-fat diet. Cholestyramine may be given to patients with Type IIa familial hypercholesterolemia but not to those with Type IIb. Also called **hypercholesterolemic xanthomatosis, type II hyperlipoproteinemia.**

familial iminoglycinuria. See **iminoglycinuria.**

familial juvenile nephronophthisis. See **medullary cystic disease.**

familial lipoprotein lipase deficiency. See **hyperchylomicronemia.**

familial osteochondrodystrophy. See **Morquio's disease.**

familial spinal muscular atrophy. See **Werdnig-Hoffmann disease.**

familial tremor. See **essential tremor.**

family, 1. a group of people related by heredity, as parents, children, and siblings. The term sometimes is broadened to include persons living in the same household or those related by marriage. 2. a group of persons having a common surname, as the Anderson family. 3. a category of animals or plants situated on a taxonomic scale between order and genus. Humans are members of the genus *Homo sapiens,* which is a part of the hominid family which, in turn, is a division of the primate order of mammals. See also **genetics, heredity.** – **familial,** *adj.*

family-centered care, primary health care that includes an assessment of the health of an entire family, identification of actual or potential factors that might influence the health of its members, and implementation of actions needed to maintain or improve the health of the unit and its members.

family-centered nursing care, nursing care directed toward improving the potential health of a family or any of its members by assessing individual and family health needs and strengths, by identifying problems influencing the health care of the family as a whole as well as those influencing the individual members, by utilizing family resources, by teaching and counseling, and by evaluating progress toward stated goals. See also **family nursing, generalized nursing.**

family ganging, an unethical medical practice in which the patient is encouraged or required to involve the entire family in a program of health care even if the other family members do not require such care. The practice enables the health care facility to obtain third-party compensation for all family members. Family ganging is often practiced in so-called Medicaid mills. See also **Medicaid.**

family health, (in a health history) an account of the health of the members of the immediate family. Hereditary and familial diseases are especially noted. The age and health of each person, the ages at death, and the causes of death are charted. The family health history is obtained from the patient or family in the initial interview and becomes a part of the permanent record.

family history, an essential portion of a patient's medical history in which the patient is asked about the health of the other members of the family in a series of specific questions, as "Has anyone in your family had tuberculosis? diabetes mellitus? breast cancer?," to discover any diseases to which the patient may be particularly vulnerable. Other questions, as those concerning the age, sex, relationships of others in the household, and the marital history of the patient may also be asked if the information has not been secured as part of the social history.

family medicine, the branch of medicine that is concerned with the diagnosis and treatment of health problems in people of either sex and any age. Practitioners of family medicine are often called family practice physicians, family physicians, or, formerly, general practitioners. They often act as the primary health-care providers, referring complicated problems to a specialist.

family nurse practitioner (FNP), a nurse practitioner possessing skills necessary for the detection and management of acute self-limiting conditions and management of chronic stable conditions. An FNP provides primary, ambulatory care for families in collaboration with primary care physicians. The FNP meets the needs of health and specified illness care by providing direct care and by guiding or counseling the family as required. Consultation, copractice, and referral to associated physicians occur in the course of the FNP's practice.

family physician, 1. a medical practitioner of the specialty of family medicine. 2. a general practitioner. 3. a family practice physician. See also **family medicine.**

family planning. See **contraception.**

family practice physician, a practitioner of family medicine, usually one who has completed a residency program in the specialty. See also **family medicine.**

family therapy, (in psychiatry) a therapeutic approach to the care of any one of the members of a family. The entire immediate family may meet together, usually with a male and a female therapist, in order to discover the dynamics of the situation, especially as it affects the disturbed, symptomatic family member.

famine fever. See **relapsing fever.**

FANCAP, *U.S.* a mnemonic device, for helping student nurses learn to assess, provide, and evaluate direct patient care. It stands for fluids, aeration, nutrition, communication, activity, and pain. Occasionally a variant, FANCAS, is substituted for FANCAP in which case the 'S' stands for stimulation.

Fanconi's syndrome (fænkou′niz), a rare, usually congenital disorder, characterized by aplastic anemia, bone abnormalities, olive-brown skin pigmentation, microcephaly, hypogenitalism, cystinosis, and abnormalities of renal tubular function, including glycosuria, phosphaturia, and bicarbonate wasting. A form of the syndrome acquired in adulthood is the result of heavy metal poisoning by cadmium, copper, lead, mercury, or uranium, by the ingestion of outdated tetracycline, or by other damage to the renal tubules. The condition may occur with Wilson's disease or follow transplantation of a kidney.

fantasy, 1. the unrestrained free play of the imagination; fancy. 2. a mental image, usually distorted or grotesque in nature, often the result of the action of drugs or a disease of the central nervous system. 3. the mental process of transforming undesirable experiences into imagined events or into a sequence of ideas in order to fulfill an unconscious wish, need, or desire or to give expression to unconscious conflicts, as a daydream.

farad (F) (fær′əd), a unit of capacitance that increases the potential difference between the plates of a capacitor by one volt with a charge of one coulomb.

Farber test, a microscopic examination of newborn meconium for lanugo and squamous cells. The fetus normally swallows amniotic fluid containing these large proteins which then pass through the digestive system to be excreted, usually after birth, in the first stools. The absence of hair or skin cells is suggestive of intestinal obstruction or atresia and requires further evaluation.

Far Eastern hemorrhagic fever, a form of epidemic hemorrhagic fever, indigenous to Asia, that is transmitted by a virus carried by an Asian rodent. The infection is characterized by chills, fever, headache, abdominal pain, nausea, vomiting, anorexia, and extreme thirst. Hypotensive shock may occur as the fever subsides. Thirst continues into the second week, oliguria develops, and the blood pressure returns to normal. Blood urea nitrogen levels increase hyperphosphatemia and hypercalcemia, and other complications occur. Diuresis follows the oliguric phase, resulting in an output of as much as eight liters a day of urine and in electrolyte imbalance. Mortality may be as high as 33 per cent. There is no specific treatment.

farmer's lung, a respiratory disorder caused by the inhalation of actinomycetes or other organic dusts from moldy hay. It is a form of hypersensitivity pneumonitis, affecting individuals who have developed antibodies to the mold spores. It is characterized by coughing, dyspnea, cyanosis, tachycardia, nausea, chills, and fever. Treatment may include cromolyn sodium and a corticosteroid.

far-sightedness. See **hyperopia.**

fasci-, a combining form meaning 'pertaining to a band or bundle of fibrous tissue': *fasciagram, fascicular, fasciitis.*

fascia (fæsh′iə), *pl.* **fasciae.** the fibrous connective tissue of the body that may be separated from other specifically organized structures, as the tendons, the aponeuroses, and the ligaments. It varies in thickness and density and in the amounts of fat, collagenous fiber, elastic fiber, and tissue fluid it contains. Kinds of fasciae are **deep fascia, subcutaneous fascia, subserous fascia.** — **fascial,** *adj.*

fascia bulbi, a thin membranous socket that envelops the eyeball from the optic nerve to the ciliary region and allows the eyeball to move freely. The fascia bulbi has a smooth inner surface, pierced by vessels and nerves, and fuses with the sheath of the optic nerve and with the sclera. The lower part of the membrane thickens into the suspensory ligament, which attaches to the zygomatic arch and the lacrimal bones. Also called **Tenon's capsule.**

fascial cleft, a place of cleavage between two contiguous fascial surfaces, as the deep fasciae and the subcutaneous fasciae. A fascial cleft is rich in fluid but poor in traversing fibers; thus, two fascial surfaces may move or be separated from each other easily. Compare **fascial compartment, fascial membrane lamination.**

fascial compartment, a part of the body that is walled off by fascial membranes, usually containing a muscle or group of muscles or an organ, as the heart is contained by the mediastinum. Compare **fascial cleft, fascial membrane lamination.**

fascial membrane lamination, a pad of connective tissue that contains fat and an occasional blood vessel or a lymph node. It is found where a fascial membrane splits into two sheets, as at the division of the outer cervical fascia above the sternum. Compare **fascial cleft, fascial compartment.**

fascia thoracolumbalis, the extensive subdivision of the vertebral fascia that sheaths the sacrospinalis muscle. It spreads caudally to become the glistening, white lumbar aponeurosis and the origin of the latissimus dorsi. Medially it attaches to the sacrum, laterally to the ribs and the intercostal fascia, and cranially to the ligamentum nuchae. Also called **lumbodorsal fascia.**

fascicle, a general term for a small bundle of nerve, muscle, or tendon fibers. Also called **fasciculus.**

fascicular neuroma, a neoplasm composed of myelinated nerve fibers. Also called **medullated neuroma.**

fasciculation (fæsik′yulei′shən), a localized, uncoordinated, uncontrollable twitching of a single muscle group innervated by a single motor nerve fiber or filament that may be palpated and seen under the skin. It results from a variety of drugs as a side effect with normal dosage or from an overdose, or it may be symptomatic of a number of disorders, including dietary deficiency, cerebral palsy, fever, neuralgia, polio, rheumatic heart disease, sodium deficiency, tic, or uremia. Fasciculation of the heart muscle is known as fibrillation. —**fascicular,** *adj.,* **fasciculate,** *v.*

fasciculus (fəsik′yələs), *pl.* **fasciculi.** a small bundle of muscle, tendon, or nerve fibers. The arrangement of fasciculi in a muscle is correlated with the power of the muscle and its range of motion. The patterns of muscular fasciculi are penniform, bipenniform, multipenniform, and radiated. —**fascicular,** *adj.*

fascioliasis (fæs′iɔulai′əsis), infection with the liver fluke *Fasciola hepatica,* characterized by epigastric pain, fever, jaundice, eosinophilia, urticaria, and diarrhea, with fibrosis of the liver a consequence of prolonged infection. It is acquired by ingestion of encysted forms of the fluke found on aquatic plants, as watercress. The disease is prevalent in many parts of the world, including southern and western United States. Bithionol, given orally, is the usual treatment.

fasciolopsiasis (fæs′iɔulopsai′əsis), an intestinal infection, prevalent in the Far East, characterized by abdominal pain, diarrhea, constipation, eosinophilia, ascites, and, sometimes, edema and caused by the fluke *Fasciolopsis buski.* The disease is usually acquired by eating contaminated water plants, as water chestnuts. It is easily treated with anthelmintics, as piperazine.

fascioscapulohumeral dystrophy (fæs′iɔuskæp′yu-louhyu′mərəl), an abnormal congenital condition and one of the main types of muscular dystrophy. It is characterized by progressive symmetric wasting of the skeletal muscles, especially the muscles of the face, the shoulders, and the upper arms, without any associated neural or sensory disorders. This disease is not usually fatal but spreads to all the voluntary muscles and commonly produces a pendulous lower lip and the absence of the nasolabial fold. It is an autosomal dominant disease that may be transmitted to males and females. Compare **Duchenne's muscular dystrophy.**

■ OBSERVATIONS: Fascioscapulohumeral dystrophy usually occurs before age 10 but may also develop during adolescence. Early symptoms include the inability to pucker the lips, abnormal facial movements when laughing or crying, facial flattening, winging of the scapulae, inability to raise the arms over the head, and, in infants, the inability to suckle. Diagnosis of this disease is based on the typical family and medical history and associated characteristic signs of abnormality. Confirming diagnosis is based on muscle biopsy showing abnormal deposits of fat and connective tissue. Electromyography may show attenuated electrical activity, an inconclusive sign when considered alone but helpful in ruling out neurogenic muscle atrophy.

■ INTERVENTION: No treatment can halt the progression of this disease and associated muscle impairment. Some measures that may help preserve mobility are physical therapy, surgery, and the use of orthopedic appliances.

■ NURSING CONSIDERATIONS: Nurses usually help preserve the mobility of the patient by assisting with therapeutic exercises. Encouragement and instruction can help the patient and the family deal with long-term care and adjustment. The individual with a dystrophy disorder often becomes constipated because activity is increasingly limited. High-protein, high-fiber diets and the use of stool softeners can help avoid constipation. Nurses often counsel family members who are carriers of the disease about the dangers of transmitting the disorder and refer patients who must learn new job skills to the appropriate agencies. Information about social services and financial assistance for patients and families is available from the Muscular Dystrophy Association, Inc.

fast, 1. resistant to change, especially to the action of a specific drug or chemical, as a staining agent. 2. to abstain from all or certain foods. See also **fasting.**

fast-acting insulin, one of a group of insulin preparations in which the onset of action is rapid, approximately one hour, and the duration of the action is relatively brief, approximately 6 to 14 hours. Kinds of fast-acting insulins include **insulin injection, prompt insulin zinc suspension.**

fastigium (fæstɪj′iəm), 1. the highest point in the course of a fever, or the most symptomatic point in the course of an illness. **2.** the angle at the top of the roof of the fourth ventricle in the brain.

Fastin, a trade name for an anorexiant (phentermine hydrochloride).

fasting, the act of abstaining from food for a specific period of time, usually for therapeutic or religious purposes.

fat, **1.** a substance composed of lipids or fatty acids and occurring in various forms or consistencies ranging from oil to tallow. **2.** a type of body tissue composed of cells containing stored fat (depot fat). Stored fat is usually identified as white fat, which is found in large cellular vesicles, or brown fat, which consists of lipid droplets. Stored fat contains more than twice as many calories per gram as sugars and serves as a source of quickly mobilized body energy. In addition, stored fat helps cushion and insulate vital organs. See also **adipose, obesity.**

fat cell lipoma. See **hibernoma.**

fat embolism, a serious circulatory condition characterized by the blocking of an artery by an embolus of fat that entered the circulatory system following the fracture of a long bone, or less commonly, after traumatic injury to adipose tissue or to a fatty liver. A systemic condition may occur following extensive trauma, because lipid metabolism is altered by the injury and causes release of free fatty acids resulting in vasculitis with obstruction of many small pulmonary and cerebral arteries. Fat embolism usually occurs suddenly 12 to 36 hours after the injury and is characterized by severe chest pain, pallor, dyspnea, tachycardia, delirium, prostration, and, in some cases, coma. Anemia and thrombocytopenia are common. Classic signs of systemic fat embolism are petechial hemorrhages on the neck, shoulders, axillae, and conjunctivae, appearing two or three days after the injury. There is no specific therapy for systemic fat embolism; the patient is placed in a high Fowler's position and given oxygen, digitalis, corticosteroids, blood transfusion, respiratory assistance, and other supportive care.

FA test. See **fluorescent antibody test.**

father complex, *Nontechnical.* a repressed desire for an incestuous relationship with one's father. See also **Oedipus complex.**

father fixation, an arrest in psychosexual development characterized by an abnormally persistent, close, and often paralyzing emotional attachment to one's father. Compare **mother fixation.** See also **Freudian fixation.**

fatigue, **1.** a state of exhaustion or a loss of strength or endurance, as may follow strenuous physical activity. **2.** loss of ability of tissues to respond to stimuli that normally evoke muscular contraction or other activity. Muscle cells generally require a refractory or recovery period after activity, during which time cells restore their energy supplies and excrete metabolic waste products. **3.** a sense of weariness or tiredness. **4.** an emotional state associated with extreme or extended exposure to psychic pressure, as in battle or combat fatigue. See also **lactic acid.**

fatigue fever, a benign episode of fever and muscle pain following overexertion. The symptoms are caused by an accumulation of the metabolic waste products of muscle contractions and may persist for several days.

fatigue fracture, any fracture that results from excessive physical activity and not from any specific injury, as commomly occurs in the metatarsal bones of runners.

fat metabolism, the biochemical process by which fats are broken down and elaborated by the cells of the body. Fats provide more food energy than carbohydrates; the catabolism of one gram of fat provides nine kilocalories of heat as compared with 4.1 kilocalories yielded in the catabolism of one gram of carbohydrate. Fat catabolism involves a series of chemical reactions, the last stages of which are similar to the final reactions of carbohydrate catabolism. Before the final reactions in fat catabolism can occur, fats must be hydrolyzed into fatty acids and glycerol. Conversion of glycerol provides a compound that can enter the citric acid cycle. Catabolism of fatty acids continues by beta-oxidation to produce acetyl-CoA, which also enters the citric acid cycle. The body synthesizes fats from fatty acids and glycerol or from compounds derived from excess glucose or from amino acids. Fat anabolism also includes the synthesis of complex compounds, as phospholipid, an important component of cell membranes. The body can synthesize only saturated fatty acids. Essential unsaturated fatty acids can be supplied only by the diet. Certain hormones, as insulin, growth hormone, adrenocorticotropic horomone, and the glucocorticoids control fat metabolism. Fat catabolism is inversely related to the rate of carbohydrate catabolism and in some conditions, as diabetes mellitus, the secretion of these hormones increases to counter a decrease in carbohydrate catabolism.

fatty acid, any of several organic acids produced by the hydrolysis of neutral fats. In a living cell a fatty acid occurs in combination with another molecule rather than in a free state. Essential fatty acids are unsaturated molecules that cannot be produced by the body and must therefore be included in the diet. Kinds of essential fatty acids are **arachidonic, linoleic, linolenic.** See also **saturated fatty acid, unsaturated fatty acid.**

fatty alcohol, a hydroxide of a hydrocarbon from the paraffin series.

fatty ascites. See **chylous ascites.**

fatty cirrhosis. See **cirrhosis.**

fatty liver, an accumulation of triglycerides in the liver. The causes include alcoholic cirrhosis, I.V. administration of drugs such as tetracycline and corticosteroids, and exposure to toxic substances, as carbon tetrachloride and yellow phosphorus. Fatty liver is also seen in kwashiorkor and is a rare complication of unknown etiology in late pregnancy. The symptoms are anorexia, hepatomegaly, and abdominal discomfort; fat cells can be seen under the microscope after liver biopsy. The condition is usually reversible after the underlying condition is corrected or the offending drug is withdrawn. See also **cirrhosis.**

fauces (fɔ'siz), the opening of the mouth into the pharynx. The anterior pillars of the fauces form the glossopalatine arch, and the posterior pillars form the pharyngopalatine arch.

favism (fa'vizəm), an acute hemolytic anemia caused by ingestion of the beans or inhalation of the pollen from the *Vicia faba (fava)* plant. Sensitive individuals show a deficiency of glucose-6-phosphate dehydrogenase, usually the result of a hereditary biochemical abnormality of the erythrocytes. Symptoms include dizziness, headache, vomiting, fever, jaundice, eosinophilia, and often diarrhea. The condition is found primarily in persons of southern Italian extraction and is treated by blood transfusion and avoidance of fava beans and pollen. See also **glucose-6-phosphate dehydrogenase deficiency.**

favus (fei'vəs), a fungal infection of the scalp, more common in children than adults. It is characterized by thick, yellow crusts with suppuration, a distinct, "mousy" odor, permanent scars, and alopecia. Rarely seen in the United States, it is common in the Middle East and Africa.

F.C.A.P., abbreviation for **Fellow of the College of American Pathologists.**

F.D.A., abbreviation for **Food and Drug Administration.**

Fe, symbol for **iron.**

fear, (in nursing) a nursing diagnosis accepted by the Fourth National Conference on the Classification of Nursing Diagnoses. The etiology of the problem is to be developed at a later conference. As a symptom, fear is analogous to anxiety about or to dread of a specific or real occurrence. The client is able to identify the object of the fear, which may itself range from mild apprehension to panic. See also **nursing diagnosis.**

fear-tension-pain syndrome, a concept formulated by Grantly Dick-Read, M.D., to explain the pain commonly expected and reported in childbirth. The concept proposes that mistaken cultural attitudes induce anxiety before labor and cause fear in labor. This fear causes muscular and psychological tension that interferes with the natural processes of dilatation and delivery, resulting in pain. He advocated education, exercise, and warm emotional and physical support in labor to counteract the syndrome, coining the term "natural childbirth" for a labor or delivery in which the well-trained woman joyfully, comfortably, and with a calm, cooperative attitude, participates in the natural experience. Elements of his method of psychophysical preparation for childbirth are incorporated into most other methods of natural childbirth. See also **Bradley method, Lamaze method.**

febri-, a combining form meaning 'pertaining to a fever': *febricant, febrifugal, febriphobia.*

febrifuge (feb'rifyuj). See **antipyretic.**

febrile (fi'bril, feb'ril), pertaining to or characterized by an elevated body temperature, as a febrile reaction to an infectious agent. — **febrility,** *n.*

-febrile, a combining form meaning 'pertaining to fever': *afebrile, nonfebrile, subfebrile.*

fecal fistula, an abnormal passage from the colon to the external surface of the body, discharging feces. Fistulas of this kind are usually created surgically in operations involving the removal of malignant or severely ulcerated bowel segments.

fecal impaction, an accumulation of hardened or inspissated feces in the rectum or sigmoid colon which the individual is unable to move. Diarrhea may be a sign of fecal impaction since only liquid material is able to pass the obstruction. Occasionally, fecal impaction may cause urinary incontinence due to pressure on the bladder. Treatment includes oil and cleansing enemas and manual breaking up and removal of the stool by a gloved finger. Persons who are dehydrated, nutritionally depleted, on long periods of bedrest, receiving constipating medications such as iron or opiates, or undergoing barium x rays are at risk of developing fecal impaction. Prevention includes adequate bulk food, fluids, exercise, regular bowel habits, privacy for defecation, and occasional stool softeners or laxatives. See also **constipation, obstipation.**

fecalith (fi'kəlith), a hard, impacted mass of feces in the colon. To allow evacuation, an oil retention enema is usually administered; if ineffective, manual removal can be performed. See also **atonia constipation, constipation.**

fecal softener, a drug that lowers the surface tension of the fecal mass, allowing the intestinal fluids to penetrate and soften the stool. Also called **stool softener.**

feces (fi'siz), waste or excrement from the digestive tract that is formed in the intestine and expelled through the rectum. Feces consist of water, food residue, bacteria, and secretions of the intestines and liver. Gross examination of feces for color, odor, quantity, and consistency and microscopic examination for the presence of blood, fat, mucus, or parasites are common diagnostic procedures. Also called **stool.** See also **defecation.** — **fecal,** *adj.*

fecundation (fi'kəndei'shən, fek'əndei'shən), impregnation or fertilization; the act of fertilizing. See also **artificial insemination.** — **fecundate,** *v.*

fecundity (fikən'diti), the ability to produce offspring, especially in large numbers and rapidly; fertility. — **fecund,** *adj.*

Federal Tort Claims Act, a statute passed in 1946 that allows the federal government to be sued for the wrongful action or negligence of its employees. The Act, for most purposes, eliminates the doctrine of governmental immunity, which formerly prohibited the bringing of a suit against the federal government.

Federal Trade Commission (FTC), an agency in the executive branch of the federal government created to promote trade and to prevent practices that restrain free enterprise and competition. In the area of health care, the Commission recently won a suit against the American Medical Association that prevented a continuation of the Association's ban on advertising. The FTC held that competition among physicians and the free choice of the consumer were impaired by the anti-advertising policy.

Federation Licensing Examination (FLEX), the standardized licensing examination for state licensure of physicians. Developed by the Federation of State Medical Boards of the United States, the examination is based on National Board of Medical Examiners test materials.

feeblemindedness. See **mental retardation.**

feedback, (in communication theory) information produced by a receiver and perceived by a sender that informs the sender about the receiver's reaction to the message. Feedback is a cyclic part of the process of communication that regulates and modifies the content of messages.

feeding, the act or process of taking or giving food or nourishment. Kinds of feeding include **artificial feeding, breastfeeding, extrabuccal feeding, forced feeding, sham feeding.**

fee-for-service, **1.** a charge made for a professional activity, as for a physical examination, the fitting of a contraceptive diaphragm, or the monitoring of a person's blood pressure. **2.** a system for the payment of professional services in which the practitioner is paid for the particular service rendered, rather than receiving a salary for providing professional services as needed during scheduled hours of work or time on call.

feel life, *Nontechnical.* to experience quickening.

Fehling's solution (fei′lingz), a solution containing cupric sulfate with sodium hydroxide and potassium sodium tartrate, used for testing for the presence of glucose and other reducing substances in the urine. Also called **Fehling's reagent.**

Fellow of the American Academy of Nursing (FAAN), a member of the American Academy of Nursing.

Fellow of the American College of Chest Physicians (F.A.C.C.P.), a physician who is a board-certified member of the **American College of Chest Physicians.**

Fellow of the American College of Surgeons (F.A.C.S.), a member of the American College of Surgeons, recognized by that professional organization as being qualified by education, training, and experience to practice surgery.

Fellow of the College of American Pathologists

(F.C.A.P.), a physician who is a member of the **College of American Pathologists.**

fellowship, a grant given to a person for study or training or to allow payment for work on a special project, but not for study toward a degree. It provides a salary and, in some cases, the miscellaneous expenses involved in the study, training, or project.

felon, a suppurative abscess on the distal phalanx of a finger.

felonious assault. **1.** See **felony.** **2.** See **assault.**

felony, (in criminal law) a crime declared by statute to be more serious than a misdemeanor and deserving of a more severe penalty. Conviction usually requires imprisonment in a penitentiary for longer than one year. Charges of murder, rape, burglary, and arson are tried as felonies in most cases. Compare **misdemeanor.**

Felty's syndrome (fel′tiz), hypersplenism occurring with adult rheumatoid arthritis, characterized by splenomegaly, leukopenia, and frequent infections. The etiology of the syndrome is unknown. Surgical resection of the spleen offers temporary improvement in about one half of the cases. See **hypersplenism.**

female, **1. a.** of or pertaining to the sex that becomes pregnant and bears children. **b.** feminine. **2.** a female person.

female catheterization, a procedure for removing urine by means of a urinary catheter introduced through the urinary meatus and urethra into the bladder. The procedure is performed to relieve distention if voluntary micturition is not possible (as after trauma or surgery), as a preparation for and during anesthesia, if a specimen of urine from the bladder is required, or if medication is to be instilled into the bladder. A straight catheter or a retention catheter with a ballon may be used. A French size 12 to 16 is usually selected for straight drainage.

■ METHOD: The necessary sterile equipment is obtained, including cotton swabs, a bowl for collecting the urine, a disposable catheter, a sponge stick for holding the swabs, a disinfectant for washing the urinary meatus and the perineal area adjacent to it, gloves, a lubricant for the catheter tip, and a drape. Often, a preassembled kit of disposable sterile equipment is available, leaving only the separately packaged catheter to be selected. The patient is positioned on her back, with the knees flexed and the legs abducted, and is then draped. A bright light is directed at the perineum. The nurse then scrubs her hands, dries them well, and opens the catheterization kit or tray carefully, not touching the inside of the wrapper or the contents. Sterile gloves are put on, and the tray is lifted and placed between the patient's legs. The small sterile drape in the kit is placed over the patient so that the window in it allows access to the urinary meatus. With the thumb and the forefinger, the labia are separated and the tissues are retracted, exposing the meatus. The area is cleansed from the front to the back using one pledget or swab for each stroke. Each pledget is discarded before beginning another stroke; three or more strokes are used, and the location of the meatus is verified while the area is cleaned. The labia is separated, the catheter is picked up approximately 4 cm from its tip, the tip is lubricated, and the end is placed in the basin. While the patient's attention is diverted, the catheter is inserted approximately 7.5 cm until the urine begins to flow. When the urine stops flowing, the bladder is gently massaged to empty it completely and the catheter is slowly withdrawn. A sterile sponge is gently pressed to the meatus to remove any lubricant and to dry the area. The urine is measured, and the odor, color, and any abnormal precipitate are noted. A specimen for bacteriologic culture and antibiotic sensitivity is often secured, labeled, and sent to the laboratory.

■ OUTCOME CRITERIA: Catheterization predisposes the urinary tract to infection, and traumatic catheterization further increases the risk. Care, gentleness, and asepsis are essential. If the bladder is distended with urine the first 1,000 cc may be withdrawn, the catheter clamped, and the physician consulted, as withdrawing more than that amount at once may cause damage to the bladder, chills, and shock. Certain conditions, including radical vulvectomy, postoperative swelling, or structural anomalies may obscure the urinary meatus. The indication for catheterization, the age of the patient, and the condition and size of the urethra affect the choice of catheter style and size.

■ NURSING ORDERS: Catheterization is usually ordered by a physician for an individual patient, or the conditions under which a catheterization is to be performed are stated in written standing orders. Catheterization is needlessly dreaded by many patients; careful explanation may allay the fears. Having the woman take a deep breath may cause the meatus to open slightly, revealing its presence, and asking her to bear down slightly may minimize the momentary discomfort that commonly accompanies the insertion of the catheter into the bladder. Voluntary micturition is almost always preferable, and the nurse encourages the woman to try to void spontaneously. Signs of infection are carefully observed. If a woman is to be catheterized more than twice, an indwelling catheter is usually preferred to a third catheterization.

female dietary allowance. See **dietary allowances.**

female reproductive system assessment, an evaluation of a patient's genital tract and breasts and an investigation of past and present disorders that may be factors in the individual's current gynecologic condition. See also **pelvic examination.**

■ METHOD: The patient is interviewed to determine if she has lower abdominal pain, cramps, vaginal bleeding, itching, swelling, redness, or a discharge that is mucoid, watery, frothy, or thick in consistency, and white, yellow, greenish, bloody, or brown in color. She is asked if she experiences pain on intercourse and pain or burning on urination. Observations are recorded of her general appearance, vital signs, weight, breast symmetry, texture, and lumps or bumps, nipple color, and the presence of a serous, bloody, or purulent nipple discharge. The abdomen is examined for contour, symmetry, stretch marks, scars, lesions, visible pulsations and peristaltic waves, and is auscultated for bowel sounds in each quadrant. Carefully noted are edema or redness of the external genitalia, cervix, and perineum, lumps or lesions on the labia majora, the size of the urethral orifice, the presence or absence of the hymenal ring, hymenal tags, perineal scars or excoriation, and a bloody, purulent, or odoriferous discharge. The normal mucoid secretion is distinguished from the thick, white, cheesy discharge typical of moniliasis, the frothy, yellow-green, watery liquid characteristic of trichomoniasis, and the thick, yellow-green or brown, and bloody drainage typical of upper genital tract infection. The patient's age at onset of menses, the duration, spacing, and regularity of cycles, the amount and character of the flow, the date of the last menstrual period, and associated symptoms, as pain and menorrhagia, are investigated. The complications and outcome of each of the patient's pregnancies, the kind of delivery, the incidence and outcome of any abortion, and the date of menopause and associated symptoms, as hot flashes and dry vaginal mucosa, are explored. It is determined if the patient suffers from a venereal disease, constipation, hemorrhoids, hypothyroidism or hyperthyroidism, Stein-Leventhal syndrome, hypertension, or blood dyscrasias or has a history of gynecologic or other major abdominal surgery or a serious illness, especially one related to the endocrine system. The patient's smoking habits, sexual activity, use of oral contraceptives or an intrauterine device, her experience with estrogen therapy, and family history of gynecologic diseases and deaths are reported in the assessment. Diagnostic procedures indicated by the history may include a manual examination, Pap test, a basal body temperature determination, culture of vaginal discharge, punch biopsy, endometrial biopsy, dilatation and curettage, cold-knife conization, laparoscopy, ultrasound study, and tubal insufflation. Laboratory studies that may be performed include determinations of levels of human chorionic gonadotropin, serum luteinizing and follicle-stimulating hormones, 17-ketosteroids, and corticosteroids, tests for venereal diseases, and thyroid function tests, as the basal metabolic rate and protein-bound iodine level.

■ NURSING ORDERS: The nurse conducts the interview, records observations of the patient, and collects the pertinent background information and the results of the diagnostic procedures and laboratory studies.

■ OUTCOME CRITERIA: A careful assessment of the patient's reproductive system is essential in establishing the diagnosis.

feminization, 1. the normal development or induction of female sex characteristics. 2. the induction of female sex characteristics in a genotypic male. Testicular feminization may be caused by the inability of target tissues to respond to endogenous or administered androgen; some cases seem related to an absent or inadequate conversion of testosterone to dihydrotestosterone, which presumably is the active form of the androgen. Feminization may also be caused by adrenocortical estrogen-secreting tumor, by failure of the liver to inactivate endogenous estrogens, as in advanced alcoholism, or by the administration of estrogen therapy for androgen-dependent neoplasms. Pseudohermaphroditism in males with an X and Y chromosome and a female phenotype may be caused by fetal hypogonadism and is often familial. Individuals with this defect usually have undescended or labial testes, a short, blind vaginal pouch, no uterus, well developed breasts, sparse or absent axillary and pubic hair, normal plasma levels of testosterone and follicle stimulating hormone, and increased concentrations of estradiol and luteinizing hormone. Treatment consists of orchiectomy because of the risk of cancer in gonads of these patients. Some testicular tumors may produce feminizing symptoms, and gynecomastia may be caused by Klinefelter's syndrome and by certain drugs, as reserpine, digitalis, meprobamate, and cimetidine. Compare **virilization.**

feminizing adrenal tumor, a rare neoplasm of the adrenal cortex, characterized in males by gynecomastia, hypertension, diffuse pigmentation, a high level of estrogen in urine, and loss of potency. Testicular atrophy frequently occurs, but the prostate and penis are usually normal in size. The tumor may be large enough to palpate or to be diagnosed by intravenous urography or arteriography. In most cases it is a carcinoma. Treatment includes surgical resection and chemotherapy with mitotane. In women, these tumors, which are extremely rare, are associated with precocious puberty.

Feminone, a trade name for an estrogen (ethinyl estradiol).

Femogen, a trade name for esterified estrogens.

femoral (fem′ərəl), of or pertaining to the femur or the thigh.

femoral artery, an extension of the external iliac artery into the lower limb, starting just distal to the inguinal ligament and ending at the junction of the middle and lower third of the thigh. It divides into seven branches and supplies various parts of the lower limb and trunk, as the groin and its organs. Its branches are the superficial epigastric, superficial iliac circumflex, superficial external pudendal, deep external pudendal, muscular, profundis femoris, and descending genicular.

femoral hernia, a hernia in which a loop of intestine descends through the femoral canal into the groin. Surgical repair, herniorrhaphy, is the usual treatment. See also **hernia.**

femoral nerve, the largest of the seven branches from the lumbar plexus and the main nerve of the anterior part of the thigh. It arises from the dorsal parts of the ventral primary divisions of the second, third, and fourth lumbar nerves, passes through the lateral, distal fibers of the psoas major, and descends between the psoas major and the iliacus under the cover of the transversalis fascia. Lateral to the femoral artery, it passes under the inguinal ligament, enters the thigh, and breaks into the muscular branches, the anterior cutaneous branches, the intermediate cutaneous nerve, the medial cutaneous nerve, the nerve to the pectineus, the nerve to the sartorious, the saphenous nerve, the branches to the quadriceps femoris, the articular branch to the hip joint, and the articular branches to the knee joint. Also called **anterior crural nerve.**

femoral pulse, the pulse of the femoral artery, palpated in the groin.

femoral torsion, an extreme lateral or a medial twisting rotation of the femur on its longitudinal axis, as may occur owing to the action of the gluteal muscles. Compare **tibial torsion.**

femoral vein, a large vein in the thigh originating in the popliteal vein and accompanying the femoral artery in the proximal two thirds of the thigh. Its distal portion lies lateral to the artery; its proximal portion deeper to the artery. About four cm below the inguinal ligament, it is joined by the deep femoral vein. Near its termination, it is joined by the great saphenous vein. It receives tributaries from the branches of the deep femoral artery and receives the medial and the lateral femoral circumflex veins. At the inguinal ligament it becomes the external iliac vein. The formal vein has four valves.

femur (fi′mər), the thigh bone, which extends from the pelvis to the knee. It is largely cylindrical and is the longest and strongest bone in the body. It has a large, round head that fits the acetabulum of the hip, and it displays a large neck and several prominences and ridges for muscle attachments. In an erect posture it inclines medially, bringing the knee joint near the line of gravity of the body. The degree of this inclination is usually greater in a woman than in a man. Also called **thigh bone.**

fenestra (fines′tra), *pl.* **fenestrae.** an aperture, especially in a bandage or cast, that is often cut out to relieve pressure or to administer regular skin care.

fenestration (fen′istrei′shən), 1. a surgical procedure in which an opening is created in order to gain access to the cavity within an organ or a bone. 2. an opening created surgically in a bone or organ of the body. Also called **window.** —**fenestrate,** *v.*

fenfluramine hydrochloride (fenflur′əmin), an anorectic agent.

■ INDICATION: It is prescribed to decrease the appetite in exogenous obesity.

■ CONTRAINDICATIONS: Glaucoma, alcoholism, severe hypertension, use of a monoamine oxidase inhibitor within 14 days, or known hypersensitivity to this drug or to other sympathomimetic medication prohibits its use.

■ ADVERSE EFFECTS: Among the more serious adverse reactions are drug dependence, diarrhea, mental confusion, and depression.

fenoprofen calcium, a nonsteroidal anti-inflammatory agent and analgesic.

■ INDICATIONS: It is prescribed in the treatment of arthritis and other painful inflammatory conditions.

■ CONTRAINDICATIONS: Renal dysfunction, upper gastrointestinal disease, or known hypersensitivity to this drug, to aspirin, or to nonsteroidal anti-inflammatory medication prohibits its use.

■ ADVERSE EFFECTS: Among the more serious adverse reactions are gastrointestinal disturbances, gastric or duodenal ulceration, dizziness, skin rash, and tinnitus. The drug interacts with many other drugs.

fentanyl, a potent, narcotic analgesic, used most commonly with the sedative and antipsychotic drug droperidol as an adjunct in anesthesia.

fentanyl citrate, a narcotic analgesic.

■ INDICATIONS: It is prescribed as an adjunct to general anesthesia, as a preoperative and postoperative analgesic, and as a component in neurolept anesthesia and analgesia.

■ CONTRAINDICATIONS: Myasthenia gravis, use of a monoamine oxidase inhibitor within 14 days, or known hypersensitivity to this drug prohibits its use.

■ ADVERSE EFFECTS: Among the more serious adverse reactions are drug dependence, hypotension, pruritus, respiratory depression, and laryngospasm.

fentanyl citrate and droperidol (fen′tənıl), a parenteral anesthetic.

■ INDICATIONS: It is given to induce neurolept anesthesia for various brief surgical or diagnostic procedures.

■ CONTRAINDICATIONS: Use of MAO inhibitors within 14 days or known hypersensitivity to either ingredient prohibits its use. It is used with caution in elderly and poor-risk patients, in patients with head injury or brain tumor, and in children younger than two years of age.

■ ADVERSE EFFECTS: Among the more serious adverse reactions are hypotension, respiratory depression, laryngospasm, and drug dependence.

Feosol, a trade name for a hematinic (ferrous sulfate).

-fer, a combining form meaning 'something that carries something': *parasitifer, sonifer, vaccinifer.*

Fergon, a trade name for a hematinic (ferrous gluconate).

fermentation (fər′mentei′šhən), a chemical change that is brought about in a substance by the action of an enzyme or microorganism, especially the anaerobic conversion of food stuffs to certain products. Kinds of fermentation are **acetic fermentation, alcoholic fermentation, ammoniacal fermentation, amylic fermentation, butyric fermentation, caseous fermentation, dextran fermentation, diastatic fermentation, lactic acid fermentation, propionic fermentation, storing fermentation, viscous fermentation.**

fermentative dyspepsia (fərmen′tətıv), an abnormal condition characterized by impaired digestion associated with the fermentation of digested food. See also **dyspepsia.**

fermium (Fm), a man-made transuranic metallic element. Its atomic number is 100; its atomic weight is 253. Fermium was first detected in the debris from a hydrogen bomb explosion.

-ferous, a combining form meaning 'producing or carrying' something specified: *lactiferous, sebiferous, tubiferous.*

ferr-. See **ferro-.**

ferri-. See **ferro-.**

ferritin (fer′ıtın), an iron compound found in the intestinal mucosa, the spleen, and the liver. It contains over 20 per cent iron and is essential for hematopoiesis.

ferro-, ferr-, ferri-, a combining form meaning 'pertaining to iron': *ferrocyanide, ferropectic, ferrosilicon.*

fertile, 1. capable of reproducing or bearing offspring. 2. of a gamete, capable of inducing fertilization or being fertilized. 3. prolific; fruitful; not sterile. —**fertility,** *n.,* **fertilize,** *v.*

fertile eunuch syndrome, a hypogonadotropic hormonal disorder occurring only in males in which the quantity of testosterone and follicle-stimulating hormone is inadequate for the inducement of spermatogenesis and the development of secondary sexual characteristics. If supplemental hormones are not prescribed, the affected person acquires the appearance of a eunuch.

fertile period, the time in the menstrual cycle during which fertilization may occur. Spermatozoa can survive for 48 to 72 hours; the ovum lives for 24 hours. Thus, the fertile period begins 2 to 3 days before ovulation and lasts for 2 to 3 days afterward. To increase the contraceptive effectiveness of natural family-planning methods, some allowance is made for the possibility of longer survival of the spermatozoa and the ovum, extending the length of the fertile period to 7 or 8 days. The fertile period may be identified by observation of the changes in the quantity and character of cervical mucus or of changes in the basal body temperature, or it may be deduced from a calendar record of six or more menstrual cycles, applying the fact that ovulation usually occurs fourteen days prior to menstruation.

fertility factor. See **F factor.**

fertilization, the union of male and female gametes to form a zygote from which the embryo develops. The process takes place in the Fallopian tube of the female when a spermatozoon, carried in the seminal fluid discharged during coitus, comes in contact with and penetrates the ovum. Rapid chemical changes in the membrane of the ovum prevent the entrance of additional spermatozoa. Penetration by the spermatozoon stimulates the completion of the second meiotic division and formation of the pronucleus in the ovum. Fusion and synapsis of the male and female pronuclei restore the diploid number of chromosomes to the germ cell, resulting in the determination of the sex of the zygote and of the characteristics inherited from each parent, and stimulate the initiation of development through cleavage. Kinds of fertilization include **cross fertilization, external fertilization, internal fertilization, self-fertilization.** See also **oogenesis, spermatogenesis.**

fertilization age. See **fetal age.**

fertilization membrane, a viscous membrane surrounding the fertilized ovum that prevents the penetration of additional spermatozoa. It is formed by granules from the cytoplasm of the fertilized ovum adhering to the vitelline membrane.

fertilizin (fərtil'ızın), a glycoprotein found on the plasma membrane of the ovum in various species. It was once thought that the specific agglutinizing receptor groups of the substance were complementary to antifertilizin, a substance extracted from the sperm, and were responsible for binding the spermatozoon to the ovum during the early stage of fertilization, but the theory has since been discarded. See also **acrosomal reaction.**

Festal, a trade name for a gastrointestinal fixed-combination drug containing a group of digestive enzymes and bile constituents.

fetal abortion, termination of pregnancy after the twentieth week of gestation but before the fetus has developed enough to live outside of the uterus. Compare **embryonic abortion.**

fetal age, the age of the conceptus computed from the time elapsed since fertilization. Also called **fertilization age.** Compare **gestational age.**

fetal attitude, the relationship of the fetal parts to each other, as in the "military" attitude, in which the fetal head is not flexed and the chin on chest is as usual but is held straight up. Compare **fetal position, fetal presentation.**

fetal circulation, the pathway of blood circulation in the fetus. Oxygenated blood from the placenta travels through the umbilical vein to the liver and the ductus venosus, which carries it to the inferior vena cava and right atrium. The blood enters the right atrium at a pressure sufficient to direct the flow across the atrium and through the foramen ovale into the left atrium; thus, oxy-genated blood is available for circulation through the left ventricle to the head and upper extremities. The blood returning from the head and arms enters the right atrium via the superior vena cava. It flows through the atrium at a relatively low pressure; passing the tricuspid valve the blood falls into the right ventricle, from which it is pumped through the pulmonary artery and the ductus arteriosus into the descending aorta for circulation to the lower parts of the body. A small amount of blood in the pulmonary artery is not shunted through the ductus and is carried to the lungs. The blood is returned to the placenta through the umbilical arteries.

Ductus arteriosus
Pulmonary artery
Foramen ovale
Ductus venosus
Umbilical vein
Intestine
Umbilicus
Umbilical arteries
Urachus

FETAL CIRCULATION

fetal distress, a compromised condition of the fetus, usually discovered during labor, characterized by a markedly abnormal rate or rhythm of myocardial contraction. Some patterns, as late decelerations of the fetal heart rate seen on records of electronic fetal monitoring, are indicative of fetal distress. If possible the cause of the situation is identified and corrected and the acid-base balance of the fetal blood is tested. Labor is allowed to continue if the pH is within normal range and if the abnormal pattern does not recur or persist. Caesarean section may be necessary if the fetus is markedly alkalotic or acidotic or if the cause of the problem cannot be corrected. If possible, the baby is stabilized before being delivered by giving the mother oxygen, increased fluids, or a narcotic antagonist, a vasopressor, or an agent to relax the uterus. A pediatrician is required to attend the birth of a distressed baby to manage resuscitation and care immediately after delivery.

fetal heart rate (FHR), the number of heartbeats in the fetus occurring in a given unit of time. The FHR varies in cycles of fetal rest and activity and is affected by many factors, including maternal fever, uterine contractions, maternal-fetal hypotension, and many drugs. The normal FHR is more than 100 beats per minute and less than 160 beats per minute. In labor the FHR is monitored with a fetoscope or an electronic fetal monitor to detect abnormal alterations in the rate, especially recurrent decelerations that continue past the end of uterine contractions.

fetal heart tones (fht), the pulsations of the fetal heart heard through the maternal abdomen in pregnancy. The rate, usually between 120 and 160 beats per minute, tends to increase briefly with or just following fetal movement.

fetal hydantoin syndrome (FHS), a complex of birth defects associated with prenatal maternal ingestion of hydantoin derivatives. Symptoms of FHS include microcephaly, hypoplasia or absence of nails on the fingers or toes, abnormal facies, mental and physical retardation, and cardiac defects. The syndrome occurs to some degree in 10 to 40 per cent of infants born of mothers for whom this anticonvulsant has been prescribed. Hydantoin sometimes appears to be associated with hemorrhage and, more rarely, with neural crest tumors in the newborn.

fetal hydrops, massive edema of the fetus or newborn, as in severe hemolytic disease of the newborn and in other rare hematologic and circulatory disorders of the fetus or newborn. Also called **hydrops fetalis.**

fetal lie. See **presentation.**

(See next column for illustration)

fetal lipoma. See **hibernoma.**

fetal monitor. See **electronic fetal monitor.**

Longitudinal   Oblique   Transverse

FETAL LIE PRESENTATION

fetal position, the relationship of the part of the fetus that presents in the pelvis to four quadrants of the maternal pelvis identified by initial L (left), R (right), A (anterior), and P (posterior). The presenting part is also identified by initial O (occiput), M (mentum), S (sacrum). If a fetus presents with the occiput directed to the posterior aspect of the mother's right side, the fetal position is right occiput posterior (ROP). Compare **fetal attitude, fetal presentation.**

fetal presentation, the part of the fetus that presents in the pelvis. Cephalic presentations include vertex, brow, and chin; breech presentations include frank breech, complete breech, and single or double footling breech. Shoulder presentations are rare and require Caesarean section or turning before vaginal delivery. Compound presentation involves the entry of more than one part in the true pelvis; most commonly a hand next to the head. See also **fetal attitude, fetal position.**

fetal stage, (in embryology) the interval of time from the end of the embryonic stage, at the end of the seventh week of gestation, to birth, 38 to 42 weeks after the first day of the last menstrual period.

Locking device
Drive tube
Electrode wires
Guide tube
Fetal scalp electrode
Reference electrode
Electrode

Locking device
Drive tube grip
Vaginal insertion

FETAL MONITORING

feti-, feto-, foeti-, foeto-, a combining form meaning 'fetus or fetal': *feticide, fetochorionic, fetoscope.*

feticide (fi′tɪsaid). See **embryoctony.**

fetish (fet′ɪsh), **1.** any object or idea given unreasonable or excessive attention or reverence. **2.** (in psychology), any inanimate object or any part of the body not of a sexual nature that arouses erotic feelings or fixation. The erotic symbology is unique to the fetishist and results from unconscious associations. — **fetishism,** *n.*

fetishist (fet′ɪshɪst), a person who believes in or receives erotic gratification from fetishes.

feto-. See **feti-.**

fetochorionic (fi′toukɔr′ion′ɪk), of or pertaining to the fetus and the chorion.

fetography (fitog′rəfi), roentgenography of the fetus in utero. See also **fetometry.**

fetology (fitol′əji), the branch of medicine that is concerned with the fetus in utero, including the diagnosis of abnormalities, congenital anomalies, the prevention of teratogenic influences, and the treatment of certain disorders. Also called **embryatrics.**

fetometry (fitom′ɪtri), the measurement of the size of the fetus, especially the diameter of the head and circumference of the trunk. A kind of fetometry is **roentgen fetometry.**

fetoplacental (fi′toupləsen′təl), of or pertaining to the fetus and the placenta.

fetoprotein (fi′touprou′tin), an antigen that occurs naturally in fetuses and occasionally in adults as the result of certain diseases. Leukemia, hepatoma, sarcoma, and other neoplasms are associated with **beta fetoprotein** in the blood of adults. An increased amount of **alpha fetoprotein** in the fetus is diagnostic for neural tube defects.

fetoscope (fi′təskoup), a stethoscope for auscultating the fetal heartbeat through the mother's abdomen.

fetoscopy, a procedure in which a fetus may be directly observed in utero, using a fetoscope introduced through a small incision in the abdomen under local anesthesia. Photographs of the fetus may be taken and amniotic fluid, fetal cells, or blood may be sampled for study for prenatal diagnosis of many congenital anomalies or genetic defects.

fetus, foetus, the unborn offspring of a viviparous animal after it has attained the particular form of the species, more specifically, the human child in utero following the embryonic period and the beginning of the development of the major structural features, usually from the eighth week after fertilization until birth. Kinds of fetuses include **fetus acardiacus, fetus anideus, calcified fetus, mummified fetus, parasitic fetus, sireniform fetus.** Compare **embryo.** See also **prenatal development.** — **fetal, foetal,** *adj.*

fetus acardiacus, fetus acardius. See **acardius.**

fetus amorphus, a shapeless conceptus in which there are no formed or recognizable parts.

fetus anideus. See **anideus.**

fetus in fetu, a fetal anomaly in which a small, imperfectly formed twin, incapable of independent existence, is contained within the body of the normal twin, the autosite.

fetus papyraceus, a twin fetus that has died in utero early in development and has been pressed flat against the uterine wall by the living fetus. Also called **paper-doll fetus, papyraceous fetus.**

fetus sanguinolentis (sæng′gwɪnəlen′tɪs), a fetus that has died in utero and is darkly colored and partly macerated.

FEV, abbreviation for **forced expiratory volume.**

fever, an abnormal elevation of the temperature of the body above 37°C (98.6°F) owing to disease. Fever results from an imbalance between the elimination and the production of heat. Exercise, anxiety, and dehydration may increase the temperature of healthy people. Infection, neurologic disease, malignancy, pernicious anemia, thromboembolic disease, paroxysmal tachycardia, congestive heart failure, crushing injury, severe trauma, and many drugs may cause the development of fever. No single therapy explains the mechanism whereby the temperature is increased. Fever has no recognized function in conditions other than infection. It increases metabolic activity by seven per cent per degree C, requiring a greater intake of food. Convulsions may occur in children whose fevers tend to rise abruptly, and delirium is seen with high fevers in adults and in children. Very high temperatures, as in heat stroke, may be fatal. The course of a fever varies with the cause and the condition of the patient and with the treatment given. The onset may be abrupt or gradual, and the period of maximum elevation, called the stadium or fastigium, may last for a few days or up to three weeks. The fever may resolve suddenly, by crisis, or gradually, by lysis. Certain diseases and conditions are associated with fevers that begin, rise, and fall in such characteristic curves that diagnosis may be made by studying a graphic record of the course of the fever. Also called **hyperpyrexia.** Kinds of fever include **constant fever, habitual fever, intermittent fever, relapsing fever.**

fever blister, a cold sore caused by herpesvirus I or II. Also called **herpes simplex.**

fever therapy. See **artificial fever.**

F factor, (in bacterial genetics) an episome present in conjugating male bacteria but absent in females. Also called **F element, fertility factor, sex factor.**

FHR, abbreviation for **fetal heart rate.**

FHS, abbreviation for **fetal hydantoin syndrome.**

fht, abbreviation for **fetal heart tones.**

fiberoptic bronchoscopy, the visual examination of the tracheobronchial tree through a fiberoptic bronchoscope.

Also called **bronchofibroscopy.** See also **bronchoscopy, fiberoptics.**

fiberoptic duodenoscope, an instrument for visualizing the interior of the duodenum, consisting of an eyepiece, a flexible tube incorporating bundles of coated glass or plastic fibers with special optical properties, and a terminal light. When the duodenoscope is introduced into the patient's mouth and threaded through the upper digestive tract to the duodenum, the light illuminates the internal structures and any lesions present, and the fiberoptic bundles transmit the image to the observer's eyepiece.

fiberoptics (fai′bərop′tiks), the technical process by which an internal organ or cavity can be viewed, using glass or plastic fibers to transmit light through a specially designed tube and reflect a magnified image. — **fiberoptic,** *adj.*

fiberscope, a flexible fiberoptic instrument having an inner shaft coated with light-conveying glass or plastic fibers for visualization of internal structures. Fiberscopes are specially designed for the examination of particular organs and cavities of the body and are used in bronchoscopy, endoscopy, and gastroscopy.

fibrillation, involuntary recurrent contraction of a single muscle fiber or of an isolated bundle of nerve fibers. Fibrillation of a chamber of the heart results in inefficient random contraction of that chamber and disruption of the normal sinus rhythm of the heart. Fibrillation is usually described by the part that is contracting abnormally, as atrial fibrillation or ventricular fibrillation.

fibrin (fai′brin), a stringy, insoluble protein, responsible for the semisolid character of a blood clot, that is a product of the action of thrombin on fibrinogen in the clotting process. Compare **fibrinogen.** See also **blood clotting, coagulation, fibrinolysis, thrombin.**

fibrinase (fai′brineis′). See **factor XIII.**

Fibrindex, a trade name for a local hemostatic (thrombin).

fibrinogen (faibrin′əjin), a plasma protein essential to the blood clotting process that is converted into fibrin by thrombin in the presence of calcium ions. Compare **fibrin.** See also **afibrinogenemia, blood clotting, fibrinolysis, thrombin.**

fibrinokinase (fai′brinoukai′neis), a nonwater-soluble enzyme in animal tissue that activates plasminogen. Also called **tissue activator, tissue kinase.**

fibrinolysin (fai′brinol′isin), a proteolytic enzyme that dissolves fibrin. It is formed from plasminogen in the blood plasma. Also called **plasmin.** See also **fibrinolysis.**

fibrinolysis (fai′brinol′isis), the continual process of fibrin decomposition by fibrinolysin that is the normal mechanism for the removal of small fibrin clots. It is stimulated by anoxia, inflammatory reactions, and other kinds of stress. — **fibrinolytic,** *adj.*

fibrinopeptide (fai′brinoupep′taid), a product of the ac-

tion of thrombin on fibrinogen. The enzymatic cleavage responsible for the release of this protein fragment produces fibrin as well as the fibrinopeptides A and B. The latter consist of short peptides derived from the N-terminal ends of the alpha and beta chains of the fibrinogen molecule. See also **fibrinogen, thrombin.**

fibrin stabilizing factor. See **factor XIII.**

fibro-, a combining form meaning 'pertaining to fiber': *fibroadipose, fibroblast, fibrolastosis.*

fibroadenoma (fai′brouæd′inou′mə), *pl.* **fibroadenomas, fibroadenomata.** a benign tumor of the breast composed of epithelial and fibroblastic tissue. It is nontender, encapsulated, round, movable, and firm. It occurs most frequently in women under 25 years of age and is caused by greater than usual amounts of estrogen. Surgical excision under local anesthesia and cytologic examination of the mass are usually performed to be sure it is not cancerous.

fibroangioma (fai′brouæn′jiou′mə), *pl.* **fibroangiomas, fibroangiomata.** a tumor composed of a mass of blood vessels and fibrous tissue.

fibroareolar tissue. See **areolar tissue.**

fibroblast, a flat, elongated undifferentiated cell in the connective tissue that gives rise to various precursor cells, as the chondroblast, collagenoblast, and osteoblast, that form the fibrous, binding, and supporting tissue of the body. Also called **desmocyte, fibrocyte.** — **fibroblastic,** *adj.*

fibroblastoma (fai′broublæstou′mə), *pl.* **fibroblastomas, fibroblastomata.** a tumor derived from a fibroblast, now differentiated as a fibroma or a fibrosarcoma.

fibrocarcinoma (fai′broukar′sinou′mə). See **scirrhous carcinoma.**

fibrocartilage (fai′broukar′təlij), cartilage that consists of a dense matrix of collagenous fibers. Of the three kinds of cartilage in the body, fibrocartilage has the greatest tensile strength. Fibrocartilaginous discs between the vertebrae help to cushion the jolts to which the vertebral column is continually subjected. See also **elastic cartilage, hyaline cartilage.** — **fibrocartilaginous,** *adj.*

fibrocartilaginous joint. See **symphysis.**

fibrocystic disease, 1. (of the breast) the presence of single or multiple cysts in the breasts. The cysts are benign and fairly common, yet must be considered potentially malignant and observed carefully for growth or change. Women with fibrocystic disease of the breast are at greater than usual risk of developing breast cancer later in life. The cysts can be aspirated and a biopsy performed. In most cases no treatment is required. The nurse must vigorously counsel women who have fibrocystic disease to examine their own breasts frequently. A woman is shown any cysts present, palpation is taught, and the importance of any change is emphasized. Reassurance should also be given that the condition is very common and usually not associated with cancer. Also called **chronic cystic mastitis. 2.** (of the pancreas) See **cystic fibrosis.**

fibrocyte (fai'brəsait). See **fibroblast.** − **fibrocytic,** *adj.*

fibroelastic tissue. See **fibrous tissue.**

fibroepithelial papilloma, a benign epithelial tumor containing extensive fibrous tissue. Also called **fibropapilloma.**

fibroepithelioma (fai'brouep'ıthi'liou'mə), *pl.* **fibroepitheliomas, fibroepitheliomata.** a neoplasm consisting of fibrous and epithelial components. A kind of fibroepithelioma is **premalignant fibroepithelioma.**

fibroid (fai'broid), **1.** having fibers. **2.** *Informal.* a fibroma or myoma, particularly of the uterus.

fibroid tumor. See **fibroma.**

fibroma *pl.* **fibromas, fibromata.** a benign neoplasm consisting largely of fibrous or fully developed connective tissue. See also specific fibroma.

-fibroma, a combining form meaning a 'benign tumor made up of fibrous tissue': *eulofibroma, hemangiofibroma, lymphangiofibroma.*

fibroma cavernosum, a tumor containing large vascular spaces and an excessive amount of fibrous tissue.

fibroma cutis, a fibrous tumor of the skin.

fibroma durum. See **hard fibroma.**

fibroma molle. See **soft fibroma.**

fibroma mucinosum, a fibrous tumor in which there is mucoid degeneration.

fibroma myxomatodes. See **myxofibroma.**

fibroma pendulum, a pendulous fibrous tumor of the skin.

fibroma sarcomatosum. See **fibrosarcoma.**

fibroma thecocellulare xanthomatodes. See **theca cell tumor.**

fibromyoma uteri. See **leiomyoma uteri.**

fibromyositis (fai'broumai'əsai'tıs), any one of a large number of disorders in which the common element is stiffness and joint or muscle pain, accompanied by localized inflammation of the muscle tissues and of the fibrous connective tissues. The condition may develop after climatic change, infection, or physical or emotional trauma. Fibromyositis may recur and become chronic. Treatment includes rest, heat, massage, salicylates, and, in severe cases, intra-articular injections of a corticosteroid and procaine. Kinds of fibromyositis include **lumbago, pleurodynia, torticollis.** See also **rheumatism.**

fibropapilloma. See **fibroepithelial papilloma.**

fibrosarcoma (fai'brousarkou'mə), *pl.* **fibrosarcomas, fibrosarcomata.** a sarcoma that contains connective tissue. It develops suddenly from small nodules on the skin; metastases often occur before the nodules begin to change.

fibrosing alveolitis (fai'brousıŋ), a severe form of alveolitis characterized by dyspnea and hypoxia, occurring in advanced rheumatoid arthritis and other autoim-

mune diseases. X-ray films show thickening of the alveolar septa and diffuse pulmonary infiltrates. See also **alveolitis.**

fibrosis (faibrou'sıs), **1.** a proliferation of fibrous connective tissue. The process occurs normally in the formation of scar tissue to replace normal tissue lost through injury or infection. **2.** an abnormal condition in which fibrous connective tissue spreads over or replaces normal smooth muscle or other normal organ tissue. Fibrosis is most common in the heart, lung, peritoneum, and kidney. See also **cystic fibrosis, fibrositis.**

fibrositis (fai'brəsai'tıs), an inflammation of fibrous connective tissue, usually characterized by a poorly defined set of symptoms, including pain and stiffness of the neck, shoulder, and trunk. Fibrositis usually develops in middle age. There are no objectively measurable signs on radiologic examination. The person is often tense and the etiology of the condition may be psychogenic. Salicylates, sedatives, tranquilizers, muscle relaxants, and intrarticular injection of a local anesthetic may be prescribed in treatment. Compare **fibromyositis.**

fibrous, consisting mainly of fibers or fiber-containing materials, as fibrous connective tissue. See also **fibrosis.**

-fibrous, a combining form meaning 'composed of fibrous tissue': *cellulofibrous, fibrofibrous, interfibrous.*

fibrous capsule, 1. the external layer of an articular capsule. It surrounds the articulation of two adjoining bones. **2.** the external, tough membranous envelope surrounding some visceral organs, as the liver. Compare **synovial membrane.**

fibrous dysplasia, an abnormal condition characterized by the fibrous displacement of the osseous tissue within the bones affected. The specific cause of fibrous dysplasia is unknown, but indications are that the disease is of developmental or congenital origin. The distinct kinds of fibrous dysplasia are monostotic fibrous dysplasia, polyostotic fibrous dysplasia, and polyostotic fibrous dysplasia with associated endocrine disorders. Any bone may be affected with monostotic fibrous dysplasia. The polyostotic type usually displays a segmental distribution of the involved bones, all of which show varying degrees of the characteristic fibrous replacement of the osseous tissue. The onset of fibrous dysplasia is usually during childhood, progressing beyond puberty and through adulthood. The onset of symptoms is usually during childhood although diagnosis may be delayed until adolescence or even early adulthood if symptoms are minimal. The initial signs may be a limp, a pain, or a fracture on the affected side. Girls affected may have an early onset of menses and breast development and early epiphyseal closure. Albright's syndrome is usually diagnosed on the basis of a triad of symptoms, including the polyostotic type of fibrous dysplasia, café-au-lait patches on the skin, and precocious puberty. Pathologic fractures are frequently associated with this process and angulation deformities may follow. The involved extremity may be shortened, and the classic 'shepherd's crook' deformity is common. Radiographic examination usually reveals a well-circumscribed lesion occupying all or a portion of the shaft of the long bone involved. Pathological fractures in patients with fibrous dysplasia usually heal with conservative treatment, but residual deformities often remain. When symptoms are mild and limited, this disease usually progresses slowly. Radiation therapy is not employed because it may provoke malignant degeneration. Biopsies are commonly performed if pain increases or if alterations are seen on radiographic examination.

fibrous goiter, an enlargement of the thyroid gland, characterized by hyperplasia of the capsule and connective tissue.

fibrous histiocytoma. See **dermatofibroma.**

fibrous joint, any one of many immovable joints, as those of the skull, in which a fibrous tissue or a hyaline cartilage connects the bones. The three kinds of articulation associated with fibrous joints are syndesmosis, satura, and gomphosis. Also called **junctura fibrosa, synarthrosis.** Compare **cartilaginous joint, synovial joint.**

fibrous thyroiditis, a disorder characterized by slowly progressive fibrosis of an enlarged thyroid with replacement of normal thyroid tissue by dense fibrous tissue. The gland eventually becomes fixed to the adjacent muscles, nerves, blood vessels, and trachea by means of this fibrous tissue. The disease occurs more frequently in women than in men and usually arises after the age of 40. Symptoms include a choking sensation, dyspnea, dysphagia, and hypothyroidism, but in some patients the gland functions normally. Treatment includes surgical excision and thyroid hormone administered postoperatively, as required. Also called **ligneous thyroiditis, Riedel's struma, Riedel's thyroiditis.**

fibrous tissue, the fibrous connective tissue of the body, consisting of closely woven elastic fibers and fluid-filled areolae. Also called **fibroelastic tissue.** Compare **areolar tissue.**

fibula (fib'yulə), the bone of the leg, lateral to and smaller than the tibia. In proportion to its length, it is the most slender of the long bones and presents three borders and three surfaces, attaching to various muscles, including the peronei longus and brevis and the soleus longus. Also called **calf bone.**

Fick principle (fik), a method for making indirect measurements, based on the law of conservation of mass. It is used specifically to determine cardiac output, in which the amount of oxygen uptake of each unit of blood as it passes through the lungs is equal to the oxygen concentration difference between arterial and mixed venous blood. Cardiac output is calculated by measuring the uptake of oxygen for a given period of time, noted as

ml per min, then dividing that ratio by the difference in oxygen saturation of arterial and mixed venous blood samples in ml per 100 ml of blood, and multiplying the total by 100.

Fick's Law, 1. (in chemistry and physics) an observed law stating that the rate at which one substance diffuses through another is directly proportional to the concentration gradient of the diffusing substance. **2.** (in medicine) an observed law stating that the rate of diffusion across a membrane is directly proportional to the concentration gradient of the substance on the two sides of the membrane and inversely related to the thickness of the membrane.

field fever, a form of leptospirosis caused by *Leptospira grippotypgosa,* affecting primarily agricultural workers. It is characterized by fever, abdominal pain, diarrhea, vomiting, stupor, and conjunctivitis. Also called **canefield fever, harvest fever.** See also **leptospirosis.**

fiery serpent, *Informal. Dracunculus medinesis.* See also **dracunculiasis.**

fifth disease. See **erythema infectiosum.**

fifth nerve. See **trigeminal nerve.**

FIGLU, abbreviation for **formiminoglutamic acid.**

figure-of-eight bandage, a bandage with successive laps crossing over and around each other like the figure eight. See also **bandage.**

fila-, a combining form meaning 'pertaining to a thread, or threadlike': *filacious, filamentous, filaria.*

filariasis (fil'ərai'əsis), a disease caused by the presence of filariae or microfilariae in the tissues of the body. Filarial worms are round, long, and threadlike and are common in most tropical and subtropical regions of the world. They tend to infest the lymph glands and channels after entering the body as microscopic larvae through the bite of a mosquito or other insect. The infection is characterized by occlusion of the lymphatic vessels, with swelling and pain of the limb distal to the blockage. After many years, the limb may become greatly swollen and the skin coarse and tough. Treatment is largely ineffective. The most effective means of combating infestation is mosquito control. See also **elephantiasis.**

filial generation, the offspring produced from a given mating or cross in a genetic sequence. See also F_1, F_2.

filiform bougie (fil'əfɔrm), an extremely thin bougie for passage through a narrow stricture, as a sinus tract.

filiform catheter, a catheter with a slender, threadlike tip that allows the wider portion of the instrument to be passed through canals that are constricted or irregular because of an obstruction or an angulation in the canal. It may bypass obstructions or dilate strictures.

filiform papilla. See under **papilla.**

film badge, a photographic film packet, sensitive to ionizing radiation, used for estimating the exposure of personnel working with x rays and other radioactive sources.

fimbrial tubal pregnancy, a kind of tubal pregnancy in which implantation occurs in the fimbriated distal end of one of the Fallopian tubes. See also **tubal pregnancy.**

finger, any of the digits of the hand. The fingers of the hand are composed of a metacarpal bone and three bony phalanges. Some anatomists regard the thumb as a finger, since its metacarpal bone ossifies in the same way as a phalange. Other anatomists regard the thumb as being composed of a metacarpal bone and two phalanges. The digits of the hand are anatomically numbered 1 to 5, starting with the thumb.

finger percussion. See **percussion.**

Finnish bath. See **Russian bath.**

Fiorinal, a trade name for a fixed-combination drug containing a sedative-hypnotic (butalbital), an analgesic, antipyretic, and anti-inflammatory (aspirin), an analgesic (phenacetin), and a central nervous system stimulant (caffeine).

fire damp. See **damp.**

fireman's cramp. See **heat cramp.**

first aid, the immediate care that is given to an injured or ill person prior to treatment by medically trained personnel. Attention is directed first to the most critical problems: evaluation of the patency of the airway, the presence of bleeding, and the adequacy of cardiac function. The patient is kept warm and as comfortable as possible. The conscious patient is reassured and is queried for significant details of his medical history, as diabetes, a known heart condition, or allergic reactions to drugs; if the patient is unconscious, a medical identification card, bracelet, or necklace is sought. The patient is moved as little as possible, particularly if there is a possibility of fracture. If there is vomiting, the patient's head is moved to a position for the vomitus to exit easily to avoid aspiration. See also **cardiopulmonary resuscitation, control of hemorrhage, emergency medicine, emergency nursing.**

first cuneiform. See **medial cuneiform bone.**

first dentition. See **deciduous dentition.**

first filial generation. See F$_1$.

first intention, See **intention.**

first metacarpal bone, the metacarpal bone of the thumb.

first nerve. See **olfactory nerve.**

fish tapeworm infection, an infection caused by the tapeworm *Diphyllobothrium latum* that is transmitted to humans when they eat contaminated raw or undercooked freshwater fish. Fish tapeworm infection is common in temperate zones throughout the world and is found in the Great Lakes region of the United States. See also **diphyllobothrium, tapeworm infection.**

fiss-, a combining form meaning 'pertaining to a split or cleft': *fissile, fissiparous, fissula.*

fission, **1.** the act or process of splitting or breaking up into parts. **2.** a type of asexual reproduction common in bacteria, protozoa, and other lower forms of life in which the cell divides into two or more equal components, each of which eventually develops into a complete organism. Kinds of fission are **binary fission, multiple fission.** **3.** Also called **nuclear fission.** (in physics) the splitting of the nucleus of an atom and subsequent release of energy.

fissiparous (fɪsɪp'ərəs), reproduced by fission.

fissural angioma, a tumor composed of a cluster of dilated blood vessels found in an embryonal fissure, especially on a lip, the face, or the neck.

fissure (fɪsh'ər), **1.** a cleft or a groove on the surface of an organ, often marking division of the organ into parts, as the lobes of the lung. **2.** a cracklike lesion of the skin, as an anal fissure. **3.** a lineal fault on a bony surface occurring during the development of a part, as a fissure in the enamel of a tooth. A fissure is usually deeper than a sulcus but, in the terminology of anatomy, *fissure* and *sulcus* are often used interchangeably. Also called **fissura.** Compare **sulcus.** —**fissured,** *adj.*

fissure fracture, any fracture in which a crack extends into the cortex of the bone but not through the entire bone.

fissure of Bichat (biSha'). See **transverse fissure.**

fissure of Rolando. See **central sulcus.**

fissure of Sylvius (sɪl'viəs). See **lateral cerebral sulcus.**

fistula (fɪs'chulə, fɪs'chyələ), *pl.* **fistulas, fistulae.** an abnormal passage from an internal organ to the body surface or between two internal organs, as a hepatopleural or pulmonoperitoneal fistula, caused by a congenital defect, injury, infection, the spreading of a malignant lesion, radiotherapy of a cancerous growth, or trauma during childbirth. Fistulas may occur in many sites from the gingiva to the anus and may be created for therapeutic purposes or to obtain body secretions for physiologic studies. An arteriovenous fistula is commonly created to gain access to the patient's bloodstream for the administration of hemodialysis. Anal fistulas resulting from rupture or drainage of abscesses may be treated by fistulectomy or fistulotomy and fistulas between the vagina and bladder, urethra, ureter, or rectum may be repaired surgically, but the results are not always successful. —**fistulous, fistular, fistulate,** *adj.*

FISTULA

fistula in ano. See **anal fistula.**

fit, **1.** *Nontechnical.* a paroxysm or seizure. **2.** the sudden onset of an episode of symptoms, as a fit of coughing. **3.** the manner in which one surface is aligned to another, as the fit of a denture to the gingiva and jaw.

Fitzgerald treatment. See **zone therapy.**

five-day fever, *Informal.* trench fever.

five-step nursing process, a nursing process comprising five broad categories of nursing behaviors: assessing, analyzing, planning, implementing, and evaluating. The nurse gathers information about the client, identifies the specific needs of the client, develops a plan of care with the client to answer these needs, implements the plan of care, and evaluates the effects of the implementation. The nurse involves the client, the client's family, and significant others in each step of the process to the greatest extent possible and compensates for and acknowledges the factors that might influence the provision of care by the nurse and staff. Implicit in the nursing process is a therapeutic and personal relationship between the nurse, the client, the client's family, and significant others.

fixating eye, (in strabismus) the normal eye that can be focused. Compare **squinting eye.**

fixation, (in psychoanalysis) an arrest at a particular stage of psychosexual development, as anal fixation. —**fixate,** *v.,* **fixated,** *adj.*

fixation muscle, a muscle that acts to hold a part of the body in appropriate position. Compare **antagonist, prime mover, synergist.**

fixative, **1.** any substance used to bind, glue, or stabilize. **2.** any substance used to preserve gross or histologic specimens of tissue for later examination.

fixed bridgework, a dental device incorporating artificial teeth permanently attached in the upper or the lower jaw.

fixed-combination drug, any of a group of multiple-ingredient preparations that provides concomitant administration of specific amounts of two or more drugs.

fixed coupling, an abnormality of the pulse in which a premature beat follows a normal heart beat in a recurrent, regularly irregular pattern.

fixed dressing, a dressing usually made of gauze impregnated with a hardening agent, as plaster of Paris, sodium silicate, starch, or dextrin, applied to support or immobilize a part of the body. The dressing is soaked in water, applied to the part to be immobilized, and allowed to harden. See also **cast.**

fixed drug eruption, a circumscribed skin lesion either persisting or recurring in the same location, caused by continuing or repeated exposure to a sensitizing drug.

fixed idea, **1.** a persistent, obsessional thought or notion. **2.** in certain mental disorders, especially obsessive-compulsive neurosis, a delusional idea that dominates mental activity and persists despite contrary evidence or rational refutation. Also called *idée fixe.*

fixed phagocyte. See **phagocyte.**

flaccid (flæk′sɪd), weak, soft, and flabby; lacking normal muscle tone, as flaccid muscles. —**flaccidity, flaccidness,** *n.*

flaccid bladder, a form of neurogenic bladder caused by interruption of the reflex arc associated with the voiding reflex in the spinal cord. It is marked by continual filling and occasional overfilling of the bladder, absence of bladder sensation, and inability to urinate voluntarily. It is most often produced by trauma. The bladder can be emptied by pressure to the area. Also called **atonic bladder, autonomous bladder, nonreflex bladder.** Compare **spastic bladder.**

flaccid paralysis, an abnormal condition characterized by the weakening or the loss of muscle tone. It may be caused by disease or by trauma affecting the nerves associated with the involved muscles. Compare **spastic paralysis.**

flagell-, a combining form meaning 'pertaining to a whiplike process, tapping': *flagellation, flagelliform, flagellospore.*

flagellant, a person who receives sexual gratification from the practice of flagellation.

flagellate (flæj′ɪlɪt, flæj′ɪleit′), a microorganism that propels itself by waving whiplike filaments or cilia behind its body, as *Trypanosoma, Leishmania, Trichomonas,* and *Giardia.* See also **protozoa.**

flagellation, **1.** the act of whipping, beating, or flogging. **2.** a type of massage administered by tapping the body with the fingers. See also **massage.** **3.** a type of sexual deviation in which a person is erotically gratified by being whipped or by whipping another. See also **masochism, sadism.** **4.** the arrangement of flagella on an organism; exflagellation.

Flagyl, a trade name for an antiprotozoal (metronidazole).

flail chest, a thorax in which multiple rib fractures cause instability in part of the chest wall and paradoxical breathing, with the lung underlying the injured area contracting on inspiration and bulging on expiration. The condition, if uncorrected, leads to hypoxia.

■ OBSERVATIONS: Flail chest is characterized by sharp pain, uneven chest expansion, shallow, rapid respirations, and decreased breath sounds. Tachycardia and cyanosis may be present and potential complications are atelectasis, pneumothorax, hemothorax, cardiac tamponade, shock, and respiratory arrest.

■ INTERVENTION: The treatment of choice is internal stabilization of the chest wall through the use of a volume-controlled ventilator with a cuffed tracheostomy tube or endotracheal tube. If the patient breathes against the automatic ventilator, a sedative and muscle relaxant may be ordered to achieve ventilatory control. Chest tubes may be required to remove air or fluid preventing expansion of the affected lung, and a nasogastric tube may be ordered to provide food and fluids. The patient's blood pressure, pulse, respirations, and breath sounds are checked every one to two hours, the rectal temperature every two to four hours, and arterial blood gases are determined as ordered. Traction is less frequently used in treating flail chest but may be applied by attaching a steel wire to the ribs or sternum under local anesthesia and connecting the wire to a rope, pulley, and weight.

■ NURSING CONSIDERATIONS: The patient with flail chest usually requires a long period of care involving frequent repositioning, scrupulous attention to the patency and cleanliness of the tracheostomy or endotracheal tube, skin care, oral hygiene, and emotional support. The nurse performs passive range-of-motion exercises to the extremities, explains the various procedures, and provides a pad and pencil or a magic slate so that the patient is able to communicate.

flame photometry, measurement of the wavelength of light rays emitted by excited metallic electrons exposed to the heat energy of a flame, used to identify characteristics in clinical specimens of body fluids. The intensity of the emitted light is proportional to the concentration of atoms in the fluid, and a quantitative analysis can be made on that basis. In the clinical laboratory, flame photometry is used to measure sodium, potassium, and lithium levels.

flapping tremor. See **asterixis.**

flare, 1. a red blush on the skin at the periphery of an urticarial lesion seen in immediate hypersensitivity reactions. 2. an expanding skin flush, spreading from an infective lesion or extending from the principal site of a reaction to an irritant. 3. the sudden intensification of a disease.

flask closure, (in dentistry) the joining of two halves of a flask that encloses and forms a denture base. Compare **closure, velopharyngeal closure.**

flat electroencephalogram, a graphic chart on which no tracings were recorded during electroencephalography, indicating a lack of brain-wave activity. Flat readings are indicative of death except in cases of profound hypothermia and central nervous system depression. Also called **isoelectric electroencephalogram.**

flatfoot, an abnormal but relatively common condition characterized by the flattening out of the arch of the foot. Also called **pes planus.**

flat spring contraceptive diaphragm, a kind of contraceptive diaphragm in which the flexible metal spring that forms the rim is a thin, light, flat band made of stainless steel. The rubber dome is approximately 1½ inches deep, and the diameter of the rubber-covered rim is between 5.5 and 10 cm. Ten sizes, in increments of 0.5 cm, allow the clinician to fit the diaphragm to each individual woman. The kind of spring and the size of the rim in millimeters is stamped on the rim, as, for example, 75 mm flat spring. This kind of diaphragm is prescribed for a woman whose vaginal musculature provides good support, whose uterus is in the normal position and not acutely retroflexed or anteflexed, and whose vagina, neither very long nor very short, has a shallow arch behind the symphysis pubis. The flat spring diaphragm offers protection equal to the other kinds of diaphragm if it is appropriate for the woman and is correctly fitted. It is preferred by many women because it is very light and comfortable to use. Compare **arcing spring contraceptive diaphragm, coil spring contraceptive diaphragm.** See also **contraceptive diaphragm fitting.**

flatus (flei′təs), air or gas in the intestine that is passed through the rectum. See also **aerophagia.**

flat wart. See **verruca plana.**

flav-, a combining form meaning 'yellow': *flavescens, flavin, flavism.*

flavone (flei′voun), a colorless, crystalline, flavonoid derivative and component of bioflavonoid that increases capillary resistance.

flavoxate hydrochloride, a smooth muscle relaxant.

■ INDICATION: It is prescribed for spastic conditions of the urinary tract.

■ CONTRAINDICATIONS: Gastrointestinal hemorrhage or obstruction, urinary tract obstruction, or known hypersensitivity to this drug prohibits its use.

■ ADVERSE EFFECTS: Among the more serious adverse reactions are nervousness, nausea, abdominal pain, fever, and tachycardia.

Flaxedil, a trade name for a neuromuscular blocking agent (gallamine triethiodide), used as an adjunct to general anesthesia.

flea, a wingless, bloodsucking insect of the order Siphonaptera, some species of which transmit arboviruses to humans by acting as host or vector to the organism.

COSMOPOLITAN RAT FLEA

flea bite, a small puncture wound produced by a bloodsucking flea. Certain species of fleas transmit plague, murine typhus, and probably tularemia.

flea-borne typhus. See **endemic typhus.**

-flect, a combining form meaning 'to bend': *anteflect, circumflect.*

Fleet Theophylline a trade name for a smooth muscle relaxant (theophylline ethanolamine), administered rectally as a bronchodilator.

FLEX, abbreviation for **Federation Licensing Examination.**

Flexeril, a trade name for a muscle relaxant (cyclobenzaprine hydrochloride).

flexibilitas cerea (flek'sɪbɪl'ɪtæs' sɪri'ə). See **cerea flexibilitas.**

Flexical, a trade name for a nutritional supplement containing protein, carbohydrate, and fat.

flexion (flek'shən), a movement allowed by certain joints of the skeleton that decreases the angle between two adjoining bones, as bending the elbow, which decreases the angle between the humerus and the ulna. Compare **extension.**

flexor carpi radialis, a slender, superficial muscle of the forearm that lies on the ulnar side of the pronator teres. It arises from the medial epicondyle, the fascia of the forearm, and from several intermuscular septa, and inserts by a long tendon into the base of the second metacarpal bone. Fibers of the muscle extend to the base of the third metacarpal bone. The flexor carpi radialis is innervated by a branch of the median nerve that contains fibers from the sixth and the seventh cervical nerves, and it functions to flex and to help abduct the hand. Compare **flexor carpi ulnaris, palmaris longus.**

flexor carpi ulnaris, a superficial muscle lying along the ulnar side of the forearm, that arises in a humeral and an ulnar head and inserts in a long tendon into the pisiform bone, extending by ligaments to the hamate and the fifth metacarpal bones. It is innervated by a branch of the ulnar nerve, which contains fibers from the eighth cervical and the first thoracic nerves. The flexor carpi ulnaris functions to flex and adduct the hand. Compare **flexor carpi radialis, palmaris longus.**

flexor digitorum sublimis. See **flexor digitorum superficialis.**

flexor digitorum superficialis, the largest superficial muscle of the forearm, lying on the ulnar side under the palmaris longus, arising by a humeral, an ulnar, and a radial head. The humeral head originates in the medial epicondyle of the humerus, the ulnar collateral ligament of the elbow joint, and in various intermuscular septa; the ulnar head originates in the medial side of the coronoid process; the radial head originates in the oblique line of the radius. The muscle separates into a superficial layer and a deep layer and inserts by four tendons into the second phalanx of the fingers. The flexor digitorum superficialis is innervated by branches of the median nerve that contains fibers from the seventh and the eighth

cervical and the first thoracic nerves. The muscle flexes the second phalanx of each finger and, by continued action, the hand. Also called **flexor digitorum sublimis.** Compare **flexor carpi radialis, flexor carpi ulnaris, palmaris longus, pronator teres.**

flexor retinaculum of the hand. See **retinaculum flexorum manus.**

flextime, flexitime, a system of staffing that allows the individualization of work schedules. A person working days might choose to work from 7 to 3, 10 to 5, or other hours. Full staffing must be maintained, but within the group flextime can be arranged. Use of the system tends to improve morale and decrease turnover.

flight into health, an abnormal but common reaction to an unpleasant physical sensation or symptom in which the person denies the reality of the feeling or observation, insisting that there is nothing wrong. See also **illness experience.**

flight or fight reaction, **1.** (in physiology) the reaction of the body to stress, in which the sympathetic nervous system and the adrenal medulla act to increase the cardiac output, dilate the pupils of the eyes, increase the rate of the heartbeat, constrict the blood vessels of the skin, increase the glucose and fatty acids in the circulation, and induce an alert, aroused mental state. **2.** (in psychiatry) a person's reaction to stress by either fleeing from a situation or remaining and attempting to deal with it.

floater, one or more spots that appear to drift in front of the eye, caused by a shadow cast on the retina by vitreous debris. Most floaters are benign and represent remnants of a network of blood vessels that existed prenatally in the vitreous cavity. The sudden onset of several floaters may indicate serious disease. Hemorrhage into the vitreous humor may cause a large number of big and little shadows and a red discoloration of vision. The cause is often traumatic injury, but spontaneous intraocular hemorrhage is seen in severe diabetes mellitus, hypertension, or increased intracranial pressure. Cancer, detachment of the retina, occlusion of a retinal vein, and other purely ocular diseases may also cause hemorrhage into the vitreous cavity. Inflammation of the retina resulting from chorioretinitis may cause entry of inflammatory cells into the vitreous humor. Inflammatory debris may adhere to the vitreous framework in netlike masses that are very disruptive of normal vision. Retinal detachment also causes a sudden appearance of lightninglike floaters and a diminished field of vision as a shower of red cells and pigment is released into the vitreous humor. Careful ophthalmologic examination through a well-dilated pupil is recommended for all people who experience a sudden occurrence of floaters, as each of the pathologic causes can be treated in the early stages and loss of vision can usually be avoided. *Technical name:* **muscae volitantes.**

floating head, unengaged fetal head. See also **ballottement, engagement.**

floating kidney, a kidney that is not securely fixed in the usual anatomic location, owing to congenital malplacement or traumatic injury. Compare **ptotic kidney.**

floating rib. See **rib.**

flocculant (flok′yulənt), an agent or substance that causes flocculation.

flocculation test (flok′yulei′shən), a serologic test in which a positive result depends on the degree of flocculent precipitation produced in the material being tested. Many tests for syphilis, including the VDRL slide test, are flocculation tests.

flocculent (flok′yulənt), clumped or tufted, as a cloud, or covered with a woolly, fuzzy surface. — **flocculate,** v., **flocculation, floccule,** n.

flood fever. See **typhus.**

flooding, a technique used in behavior therapy for the reduction of anxiety associated with various phobias. Exposure to a stimulus that usually provokes anxiety desensitizes a person to that stimulus, thereby reducing fear and anxiety. Also called **implosive therapy.** Compare **systemic desensitization.**

floppy infant syndrome, a general term for juvenile spinal muscular atrophies, including Werdnig-Hoffmann disease and Wohlfart-Kugelberg-Welander disease.

Floraquin, a trade name for an antiamebic (iodoquinol).

Florinef Acetate, a trade name for an adrenocortical steroid (fludrocortisone acetate).

Florone, a trade name for an anti-inflammatory agent (diflorasone diacetate).

Floropryl, a trade name for an inhibitor of cholinesterase (isoflurophate), used ophthalmically.

Flo-Trol clamp, a trade name of a triggerlike off-on control for intravenous and other infusion lines.

flowmeter. See **rotameter.**

flow sheet, (in a patient record) a graphic summary of several changing factors, especially the patient's vital signs or weight and the treatments and medications given. In labor, the flow sheet displays the progress of labor, including the centimeters of cervical dilatation, cervical effacement, position of the baby's head, the baby's heart rate, the frequency of contractions, the mother's temperature and blood pressure, and any medications given or procedures performed.

floxuridine (floksyur′ədin), an antineoplastic.

■ INDICATION: It is prescribed in the treatment of malignant neoplastic disease.

■ CONTRAINDICATIONS: Bone marrow depression, infection, poor nutritional state, or known hypersensitivity to this drug prohibits its use.

■ ADVERSE EFFECTS: Among the more serious adverse reactions are severe depression of the bone marrow and acute gastrointestinal disturbances, including nausea,

vomiting, diarrhea, and stomatitis. Alopecia and dermatitis commonly occur.

flu, *Informal.* **1.** influenza. **2.** any viral infection, especially of the respiratory or intestinal system.

Fluax, a trade name for an active immunizing agent (influenza virus vaccine).

flucytosine (flusai′təsin), an antifungal.

■ INDICATIONS: It is prescribed in the treatment of certain serious fungal infections.

■ CONTRAINDICATIONS: Known hypersensitivity to this drug prohibits its use. Close monitoring is required when administering this drug to patients with renal disorders or bone marrow depression.

■ ADVERSE EFFECTS: Among the more serious adverse reactions are gastrointestinal disturbances, including enterocolitis, abnormal liver function, hepatomegaly, and bone marrow depression.

fludrocortisone acetate (flu′droukor′təsoun), a mineralocorticosteroid.

■ INDICATIONS: It is prescribed in the treatment of Addison's disease and in salt-losing adrenogenital syndrome. It is not used as a glucocorticoid.

■ CONTRAINDICATIONS: Systemic fungal infections or known hypersensitivity to this drug prohibits its use.

■ ADVERSE EFFECTS: Among the more serious adverse reactions are salt and water retention. This drug has the potential for the adverse effects of glucocorticoids, including peptic ulcer, hyperglycemia, mental disturbances, and adrenal failure.

-fluent, a combining form meaning 'flowing': *diffluent, ossifluent.*

fluid, **1.** a substance, as a liquid or gas that is able to flow and to adjust its shape to that of a container because it is composed of molecules that are able to change positions with respect to each other without separating from the total mass. **2.** a body fluid, either intracellular or extracellular, that is involved in the transport of electrolytes and other vital chemicals to, through, and from tissue cells. See also **blood, lymph, cerebrospinal fluid.**

fluid dram. See **dram,** def. 2.

fluid ounce, a measure of liquid volume in the apothecaries' system, equal to 8 fluidrams or 29.57 ml. See also **apothecaries' measure, metric system.**

fluid volume deficit, actual, **1.** a nursing diagnosis accepted by the Fourth National Conference on the Classification of Nursing Diagnoses. The etiology of the condition is a failure of the body's homeostatic mechanisms that regulate the retention and excretion of body fluids. The defining characteristics of the problem are dilute urine, increased output of urine, and a sudden loss of body weight. Several other characteristics may be observed, including hypotension, increased pulse rate, decreased turgor, increased body temperature, hemoconcentration, weakness, and thirst. **2.** a nursing diagnosis accepted by the Fourth National Conference on the Classification of Nursing Diagnoses. The etiology of the condition is the active loss of excessive amounts of body fluid. The defining characteristics of the condition are decreased output of urine, high specific gravity of the urine, and output of urine that is greater than the intake of fluid into the body, a sudden loss of weight, hemoconcentration, and increased serum levels of sodium. Other characteristics that may be observed are increased thirst, alteration in the mental state, dryness of skin and mucous membranes, elevated temperature, and an increased pulse rate. See also **nursing diagnosis.**

fluke, a parasitic flatworm of the class Trematoda, including the genus *Schistosoma.* See also **schistosomiasis.**

flumethasone pivalate, a topical glucocorticoid.

■ INDICATION: It is prescribed as a topical anti-inflammatory agent.

■ CONTRAINDICATIONS: Viral and fungal diseases of the skin, impaired circulation, or known hypersensitivity to this drug or to steroid medication prohibits its use.

■ ADVERSE EFFECTS: Among the more serious adverse reactions, usually occurring after prolonged and excessive application, are striae, hypopigmentation, local irritation of the skin, and various systemic effects.

fluocinolone acetonide, a topical glucocorticoid.

■ INDICATION: It is prescribed as an anti-inflammatory agent.

■ CONTRAINDICATIONS: Impaired circulation, viral and fungal diseases of the skin, or known hypersensitivity to this drug or to other steroid medication prohibits its use.

■ ADVERSE EFFECTS: Among the more serious adverse reactions are systemic side effects resulting from prolonged use or excessive application. Various hypersensitivity reactions may occur.

fluocinonide (flu'ousın'ənaıd), a synthetic corticosteroid.

■ INDICATION: It is prescribed to reduce inflammation.

■ CONTRAINDICATIONS: Viral and fungal diseases of the skin, tuberculosis of the skin, or known hypersensitivity to this drug prohibits its use.

■ ADVERSE EFFECTS: Among the more serious adverse reactions are secondary infections, striae, miliaria, and contact dermatitis.

Fluonid, a trade name for a glucocorticoid (fluocinolone acetonide).

fluorescence (flures'əns), the emission of light of one wavelength (usually ultraviolet) when exposed to light of a different, usually shorter, wavelength, a property possessed by certain substances. Fluorescent substances that simultaneously absorb and emit light appear luminous. –**fluoresce,** *v.,* **fluorescent,** *adj.*

fluorescent antibody test (FA test), a test in which a fluorescent dye is used to stain an antibody for identification of clinical specimens. Fluorescent dyes conjugate with immunoglobulins without altering the antibody-antigen reaction, making the dyed organisms glow visibly when examined under a fluorescent microscope. The fluorescent antibody technique can be used to identify *Mycobacterium tuberculosis* and is used in the most common serologic screening test for syphilis. Kinds of fluorescent antibody tests include the **FTA-ABS test.** Also called **immunofluorescence test.**

fluorescent microscopy, examination with a fluorescent microscope equipped with a source of ultraviolet light rays, used to study specimens, as tissues or microorganisms, that have been stained with fluorescent dye. Also called **ultraviolet microscopy.** See also **fluorescent antibody test.**

Fluorescent Treponemal Antibody Absorption Test (FTA-ABS test), a serologic test for syphilis. See also **fluorescent antibody test.**

fluoridation (flɔ'ıdei'ʃən), the process of adding fluoride, especially to a public water supply, to reduce tooth decay. See also **fluoride.**

fluoride, a salt of hydrofluoric acid introduced into drinking water and applied directly to the teeth to prevent tooth decay.

Fluori-Methane, a trade name for a local anesthetic (fluoromethane vapocoolant spray).

fluorine (F) (flu'ərin), an element of the halogen family and the most reactive of the nonmetals. Its atomic number is 9; its atomic weight is 19. It occurs in nature only as a component of substances as fluorspar, cryolite, and phosphate rocks. It can be prepared by the electrolytic decomposition of hydrogen fluoride and in its pure form is a pale-yellow, flammable, toxic gas 1.6 times heavier than air. It is also a component of very stable fluorocarbons used in the manufacture of resins and plastics. As a component of fluorides it is widely distributed throughout the soils of the earth, enters plants, is ingested by humans, and absorbed from the gastrointestinal tract. Fluorides in the atmosphere and industrial dust are absorbed by the lungs and the skin. Relatively soluble compounds, as sodium fluoride, are almost completely absorbed by humans. The relatively insoluble compounds, as cryolite, are poorly absorbed. Small amounts of sodium fluoride are added to the water supply of many communities to harden the tooth enamel and decrease dental caries. Excessive amounts of fluoride can mottle enamel and cause osteosclerosis. Acute fluoride poisoning and death can result from the accidental ingestion of insecticides and rodenticides containing fluoride salts.

fluoroacetic acid (flur'ouəsi'tık, flur'ouəset'ık), a colorless, water-soluble, highly toxic compound that blocks the Krebs' citric acid cycle, causing convulsions and ventricular fibrillation. It is derived from a South African tree.

fluorometholone, a topical glucocorticoid.

■ INDICATION: It is prescribed as an anti-inflammatory agent.

■ CONTRAINDICATIONS: Impaired circulation, viral and fungal diseases of the skin, or known hypersensitivity to this drug or to steroid medication prohibits its use.

■ ADVERSE EFFECTS: Among the more serious adverse reactions are systemic side effects resulting from prolonged use or excessive application. Various hypersensitivity reactions may occur.

fluorometry (flᴜrom'ɪtri), measurement of fluorescence emitted by compounds when exposed to ultraviolet or other intense radiant energy. The atoms of certain substances produce fluorescence of a characteristic color and wavelength, enabling identification and quantification of several clinically significant compounds in biological specimens. Fluorometry is used to measure urinary estrogens, triglycerides, catecholamines, and other substances. While it is a highly sensitive method of analysis, test interference by other compounds, especially drugs, may limit its usefulness in some situations. — **fluorometric**, *adj.*

Fluoroplex, a trade name for a topical preparation of antineoplastic (fluorouracil).

fluoroscope (flᴜr'əskoup), a device used for the immediate projection of an x-ray image on a fluorescent screen for visual examination. — **fluoroscopic**, *adj.*

fluoroscopy (flᴜros'kəpi), a technique in radiology for visually examining a part of the body or the function of an organ using a fluoroscope. The technique offers immediate, serial images that are invaluable in many clinical situations, as in intrauterine fetal transfusion and cardiac catheterization.

fluorosis (flᴜrou'sɪs), the condition that results from excessive, prolonged ingestion of fluorine. Unusually high concentration of fluorine in the drinking water typically causes mottled discoloration and pitting of the enamel of the permanent and deciduous teeth in children whose teeth developed while maternal intake of fluorinated water was high. Severe chronic fluorine poisoning will lead to osteosclerosis and other pathological bone and joint changes in adults. See also **fluoridation, fluoride.**

fluorouracil (flu'ərouyur'əsɪl), an antineoplastic.

■ INDICATION: It is prescribed in the treatment of malignant neoplastic disease.

■ CONTRAINDICATIONS: Bone marrow depression, infection, poor nutritional status, or known hypersensitivity to this drug prohibits its use.

■ ADVERSE EFFECTS: Among the more serious adverse reactions are severe depression of the bone marrow and acute gastrointestinal disturbances, including nausea, vomiting, diarrhea, and stomatitis. Alopecia and dermatitis commonly occur.

Fluothane, a trade name for an inhalational general anesthetic (halothane).

fluoxymesterone (fluok'simes'təroun), an androgen.

■ INDICATIONS: It is prescribed in the treatment of testos-

terone deficiency, breast cancer in females, and delayed puberty in males.

■ CONTRAINDICATIONS: Male breast or prostate cancer, liver disease, known or suspected pregnancy, or known hypersensitivity to this drug prohibits its use.

■ ADVERSE EFFECTS: Among the more serious adverse reactions are anaphylaxis, hypercalcemia, and jaundice.

fluphenazine hydrochloride, a phenothiazine tranquilizer.

■ INDICATIONS: It is prescribed in the treatment of psychotic disorders.

■ CONTRAINDICATIONS: Parkinson's disease, concurrent administration of central nervous system depressants, liver or renal dysfunction, severe hypotension, or known hypersensitivity to this drug or to other phenothiazine medication prohibits its use.

■ ADVERSE EFFECTS: Among the more serious adverse effects are hypotension, liver toxicity, a variety of extrapyramidal reactions, blood dyscrasias, and hypersensitivity reactions.

fluprednisolone (flu'prednɪs'əloun), a glucocorticoid.

■ INDICATIONS: It is prescribed in the treatment of inflammatory and hypersensitivity reactions.

■ CONTRAINDICATIONS: Systemic fungal infections or known hypersensitivity to this drug prohibits its use.

■ ADVERSE EFFECTS: Among the more serious adverse reactions are gastrointestinal, endocrine, neurologic, and fluid and electrolyte disturbances.

flurandrenolide, a topical glucocorticoid.

■ INDICATION: It is prescribed as an anti-inflammatory agent.

■ CONTRAINDICATIONS: Impaired circulation, viral and fungal diseases of the skin, or known hypersensitivity to this drug or to steroid medication prohibits its use.

■ ADVERSE EFFECTS: Among the more serious adverse reactions are systemic side effects resulting from prolonged use or excessive application. Various hypersensitivity reactions may occur.

flurandrenolone. See **flurandrenolide.**

flurazepam hydrochloride (flᴜræz'əpæm), a benzodiazepine minor tranquilizer.

■ INDICATION: It is prescribed in the treatment of insomnia.

■ CONTRAINDICATION: Known hypersensitivity to this drug prohibits its use.

■ ADVERSE EFFECTS: Among the most serious adverse reactions are possibile physical and psychological dependence. Dizziness and drug hangover also may occur.

Fluress, a trade name for a topical ophthalmic fixed-combination drug containing the dye (fluorescein sodium) and the topical anesthetic (benoxinate hydrochloride).

Flurobate, a trade name for a glucocorticoid (betamethasone benzoate).

flush, 1. a blush or sudden reddening of the face and

neck. **2.** a sudden, subjective feeling of heat. **3.** a prolonged reddening of the face such as may be seen with fever, certain drugs, or hyperthyroidism. **4.** a sudden, rapid flow of water or other liquid.

flush device, a device for the accurate transmission of a pressure wave from a catheter to a transducer in an I.V. line.

fly, a two-winged insect of the order Diptera, some species of which transmit arboviruses to humans.

Fm, symbol for **fermium.**

FMET, abbreviation for **formylmethionine.**

FMG, abbreviation for **foreign medical graduate.**

FML, a trade name for a glucocorticoid (fluorometholone).

FNP, abbreviation for **family nurse practitioner.**

foam bath, a bath taken in water containing a saporin substance that covers the surface of the liquid and through which air or oxygen is blown to form the foam.

focal illumination. See **illumination.**

focal motor seizure. See **motor seizure.**

focal seizure, a transitory disturbance in motor, sensory, or autonomic function resulting from abnormal neuronal discharges in a localized part of the brain, most frequently motor or sensory areas adjacent to the fissure of Rolando. Focal motor seizures commonly begin as spasmodic movements in the hand, face, or foot and may spread progressively to other muscles to end in a generalized convulsion. Abnormal neuronal discharges arising in the motor area controlling mastication and salivation may be manifested by chewing, lip-smacking, swallowing movements, and by profuse salivation. Seizures originating in the eye-turning area of the brain may begin with a forced turning of the head and eyes away from the side of the focus or lesion. Abnormal electrical activity in the sensory strip of the cortex may be evident initially as a numb, prickling, tingling, or crawling feeling, and the neuronal discharge may spread to motor areas. Focal seizures may be caused by localized anoxia or a small lesion in the brain.

foeti-, foeto-. See **feti-.**

foetus. See **fetus.**

folacin (fol'əsɪn). See **folic acid.**

folate (fou'leit), **1.** a salt of folic acid. **2.** any of a group of substances found in some foods and in mammalian cells that act as coenzymes and promote the chemical transfer of single carbon units from one molecule to another.

Foley catheter (fou'li), a rubber catheter with a balloon tip to be filled with air or a sterile liquid after it has been placed in the bladder. This kind of catheter is used when continuous drainage of the bladder is desired, as in surgery, or when repeated urinary catheterization would be necessary if an indwelling catheter were not used. Sterile technique is used in placing the catheter. See also **catheterization.**

folic acid (fou'lɪk, fol'ɪk), a yellow, crystalline, water-soluble vitamin of the B complex group essential for cell growth and reproduction. It functions as a coenzyme with vitamins B_{12} and C in the breakdown and utilization of proteins and in the formation of nucleic acids and heme in hemoglobin. It also increases the appetite and stimulates the production of hydrochloric acid in the digestive tract. The vitamin is stored in the liver and may by synthesized by the bacterial flora of the gastrointestinal tract. Deficiency of the vitamin results in poor growth, graying hair, glossitis, stomatitis, gastrointestinal lesions, and diarrhea, and it may lead to megaloblastic anemia. Deficiency is caused by inadequate dietary intake of the vitamin, malabsorption, or metabolic abnormalities. Need for folic acid is increased as in pregnancy, infancy, and stress. Rich dietary sources include spinach and other green leafy vegetables, liver, kidney, asparagus, lima beans, nuts, and whole-grain cereals. It is both heat and light labile, and considerable loss of the vitamin occurs when it has been stored for a long period. The vitamin, which is nontoxic, is effective in treating the specific deficiency states and may be beneficial in alleviating menstrual problems and leg ulcers. Also called **folacin, pteroylglutamic acid.**

folie (fouli'), a mental disorder; any of a variety of psychopathological reactions. Kinds of folie include **folie à deux, folie circulaire, folie du doute, folie du pourquoi, folie gemellaire, folie musculaire, folie raisonnante.**

folie à deux (*French* Adœ'). See **shared paranoid disorder.**

folie circulaire (*French* sikkyleʀ'). See **bipolar disorder.**

folie du doute (*French* dʏdut'), an extreme obsessive-compulsive reaction characterized by persistent doubting, vacillation, repetition of a particular act or behavior, and pathological indecisiveness to the point of being unable to make even the most trifling decision.

folie du pourquoi (*French* dʏpuʀkwa'), a psychopathological condition characterized by the persistent tendency to ask questions, usually concerning unrelated topics.

folie gemellaire (*French* źhemeleʀ'), a psychotic condition occurring simultaneously in twins, sometimes in those not living together or closely associated at the time.

folie musculaire (*French* mʏskyleʀ'), severe chorea.

folie raisonnante (*French* ʀeizɔnant'), a delusional form of any psychosis.

folinic acid (foulɪn'ɪk), an active form of folic acid. Folinic acid is used in the treatment of megaloblastic anemias not caused by vitamin B_{12} deficiency and to counteract the toxic effects of antineoplastic folic acid antagonists, as methotrexate. Also called **citrovorum factor, leucovorin.**

Follestrol, a trade name for an estrogen (estrone).

follicle, a pouchlike depression, as the dental follicles that enclose the teeth before eruption or the hair follicles within the epidermis. — **follicular,** *adj.*

follicle stimulating hormone (FSH), a gonadotropin, secreted by the anterior pituitary gland, that stimulates the growth and maturation of Graafian follicles in the ovary and promotes spermatogenesis in the male. FSH releasing factor produced in the median eminence of the hypothalamus controls the release of FSH by the pituitary. Increasing amounts of FSH are secreted in the postmenstrual or resting phase of the menstrual cycle, causing a primordial follicle to develop into a mature Graafian follicle containing a mature ovum. The Graafian follicle produces estrogen which reaches a high level prior to ovulation and suppresses release of FSH. In males, FSH maintains the integrity of the seminiferous tubules and influences all the stages of spermatogenesis. FSH may be given in treating some conditions; it is derived from the urine of postmenopausal women and is called menotropins.

follicular adenocarcinoma, a neoplasm characterized by a follicular arrangement of cells that are usually derived from the thyroid gland. It is not especially malignant, but it has a greater tendency to metastasize distantly to the lungs and bones than the more common papillary adenocarcinoma of the thyroid. Surgery is the preferred treatment; if complete excision of the primary tumor is not feasible, radioiodine therapy is indicated. See also **medullary carcinoma, papillary adenocarcinoma.**

follicular goiter, an enlargement of the thyroid gland characterized by proliferation of the follicles and epithelial tissue.

folliculitis (foulɪk'yulaɪ'tɪs), inflammation of hair follicles, as in sycosis barbae.

folliculoma (foulɪk'yulou'mə). See **granulosa cell tumor.**

Follutein, a trade name for a placental hormone (chorionic gonadotropin).

fomentation (fou'mentei'shən), **1.** a topical treatment with a warm, moist application. **2.** a substance or poultice that is used as a warm, moist application.

fontanel, fontanelle (fon'tənel'), a space covered by tough membranes between the bones of an infant's cranium. The anterior fontanel, roughly diamond-shaped, remains palpable until about two years of age. The posterior fontanel, triangular in shape, closes about two months after birth. Increased intracranial pressure may cause a fontanel to become tense or bulge. A fontanel may be soft and depressed in the presence of dehydration.

food, 1. any substance, usually of plant or animal origin, consisting of carbohydrates, proteins, fats, and such supplementary elements as minerals and vitamins, that is ingested or otherwise taken into the body and assimilated to provide energy and to promote the growth, repair, and maintenance essential for sustaining life. **2.** nourishment in solid form as contrasted with liquid form. **3.** a particular kind of solid nourishment, such as breakfast food or snack food.

food allergy, a hypersensitive state resulting from the ingestion of a specific food antigen. Symptoms of sensitivity to specific foods include allergic rhinitis, bronchial asthma, urticaria, angioneurotic edema, dermatitis, pruritus, headache, labyrinthitis and conjunctivitis, nausea, vomiting, diarrhea, pylorospasm, colic, spastic constipation, mucous colitis, and perianal eczema. Food allergens are predominantly protein in nature. The most common foods causing allergic reactions are wheat, milk, eggs, fish and other sea foods, chocolate, corn, nuts, strawberries, chicken, pork, legumes, tomatoes, cucumbers, garlic, and citrus fruits. Foods that are rarely allergenic are rice, lamb, gelatin, peaches, pears, carrots, lettuce, artichokes, sesame oil, and apples. Diagnosis of a specific food allergy is obtained by a detailed food history, food diary, elimination diet, or cutaneous tests.

Food and Drug Administration (F.D.A.), a federal agency responsible for the enforcement of federal regulations regarding the manufacture and distribution of food, drugs, and cosmetics as protection against the sale of impure or dangerous substances.

food exchange list, a grouping of foods in which the carbohydrate, fat, and protein values are equal for the items listed. The list is used for meal planning in various diseases and deficiency states and was compiled by a joint committee of The American Dietetic Association, The American Diabetes Association, and the National Institutes of Health. The six groups of foods included on the list are milk, vegetables, fruits, bread, meat, and fats. Starchy vegetables are listed as bread exchanges; fish and cheese are meat exchanges.

food poisoning, any of a large group of toxic processes resulting from the ingestion of a food contaminated by toxic substances or by bacteria containing toxins. Kinds of food poisoning include **bacterial food poisoning, ciguatera poisoning, Minamato disease, mushroom poisoning, shellfish poisoning.** See also **botulism, ergot alkaloid, phalloidine poisoning, toadstool poisoning.**

foot, the distal extremity of the leg, consisting of the tarsus, the metatarsus, and the phalanges.

foot-and-mouth disease, a common epidemic picornavirus disease of farm animals in Europe, Asia, and Africa, which occasionally affects humans exposed to infected stock, hides, meat, or dairy products. Symptoms and signs in humans include headache, fever, malaise, and vesicles on tongue, oral mucous membranes, hands, and feet. Generalized pruritus and painful ulcerations may occur; however, the temperature soon falls, the lesions subside in about a week, and total healing without scars is complete by two or three weeks. Treatment is symptomatic. See also **picornavirus.**

footdrop, an abnormal neuromuscular condition of the lower leg and foot, characterized by an inability to dorsiflect, or invert, the foot owing to damage to the peroneal nerve.

-footed, a combining form meaning 'having feet' of a specified sort: *clubfooted, flatfooted, splayfooted.*

footling breech (fut'lɪŋ), an intrauterine position of the fetus in which one or both feet are folded under the buttocks at the inlet of the maternal pelvis, one foot presenting in a single footling breech, both feet in a double footling breech. Compare **frank breech.**

foot-pound, a unit for the measurement of work or energy. One foot-pound is the amount of work required to move one pound a distance of one foot in the same direction as that of the applied force.

for-, a combining form meaning 'pertaining to an opening': *foramen, foramina, foration.*

foramen (fɔrei'mɪn), *pl.* **foramina.** an opening or aperture in a membranous structure or bone, as the apical dental foramen and the carotid foramen.

foramen magnum, a passage in the occipital bone through which the spinal cord enters the spinal column.

foramen of Monro (monrou'), a passage between the lateral and third ventricles of the brain.

foramen ovale, an opening in the septum between the right and the left atria in the fetal heart. This opening provides a bypass for blood that would otherwise flow to the fetal lungs. Most of the blood from the inferior vena cava in the fetus flows through the foramen ovale into the left atrium. After birth, the foramen ovale functionally closes when the newborn takes the first breath and full circulation through the lungs begins. Complete closure of this opening takes about nine months, and the foramen ovale eventually becomes the fossa ovale in the wall of the right atrial septum. See also **ductus arteriosus.**

Forane, a trade name for a general anesthetic (isoflurane).

Forbes-Albright syndrome, an endocrine disease characterized by amenorrhea, prolactinemia, and galactorrhea, caused by an adenoma of the anterior pituitary. Diagnosis is made by x ray of the anterior pituitary and a blood test for prolactin. Surgical resection of the adenoma is usually indicated. See also **galactorrhea, pituitary gland.**

Forbes' disease. See **Cori's disease, glycogen storage disease.**

forbidden clone theory, a theory, associated with autoimmunity, based on the clonal evolution theory that at birth all the cells of the body that might react against the body have been eliminated, leaving only the cells that will react against foreign substances. The forbidden clone theory postulates that certain clone cells that can react against the body persist after birth and can be activated by a viral infection or by some metabolic change, especially if the viral organism is structurally similar to a body cell. The theory holds that the regular cells of the immune system attack only the virus, but the clone cells attack the tissues of the body. Compare **sequestered antigens theory.**

force, energy applied in such a way that it initiates motion, changes the speed or direction of motion, or alters the size or shape of an object.

forced expiratory volume (FEV), the volume of air that can be forcibly expelled in one second following full inspiration. See also **expiratory reserve volume.**

forced feeding, the administration of food by force, as nasal feeding, to persons who cannot or will not eat.

forceps, a pair of any of a large variety and number of surgical instruments, all of which have two handles or sides, each attached to a blade. The handles may be joined at one end, as a pair of tweezers, or the two sides may be separate to be conjoined in use, as obstetric forceps. Forceps are used to grasp, handle, compress, pull, or join tissue, equipment, or supplies. See specific forceps.

forceps delivery, an obstetric operation in which instruments are used to deliver a baby. It is performed to overcome dystocia, to quickly deliver a baby experiencing fetal distress or, most often, to shorten normal labor. Local or regional anesthesia is usual, as is episiotomy. Prerequisites to forceps delivery include full dilatation of the cervix, engagement of the fetal head, and certain knowledge of the position of the head. The blades of the forceps are introduced into the vagina one at a time and applied symmetrically to opposite sides of the baby's head; the handles of the forceps are brought together so that the head is held firmly between the blades; the head is rotated, if necessary, to the occiput anterior or occiput posterior position; and traction is applied so as to draw the head from the birth passage. When the head has been delivered the forceps are removed and the delivery completed manually. Forceps produce marks on a baby's head and face; unless application has been imperfect the marks are usually superficial and disappear in few days. Because Caesarean section is performed more often now than formerly, traumatic forceps deliveries are uncommon. Kinds of forceps delivery are **high forceps, low forceps, mid forceps.** Compare **failed forceps, forceps rotation, trial forceps.** See also **obstetric forceps.**

forceps rotation, an obstetric operation in which forceps are used to turn a baby's head that is arrested in transverse or posterior position in the birth canal. It may be performed to facilitate spontaneous birth or as the first step in a forceps delivery. Kinds of forceps rotation are **Kielland rotation, Scanzoni rotation.** Compare **forceps delivery, manual rotation.** See also **obstetric forceps.**

forceps tenaculum. See **tenaculum.**

fore-, a combining form meaning 'front or before': *forearm, foregut, forewaters.*

forebrain (fɔr'brein). See **prosencephalon.**

foregut, the cephalic portion of the embryonic alimentary canal. It consists of endodermal tissue and gives rise to the pharynx, esophagus, stomach, liver, pancreas, most of the small intestine, and the respiratory ducts. Compare **hindgut, midgut.**

foreign body, any object or substance found in the body in an organ or tissue in which it does not belong under normal circumstances, as a bolus of food in the trachea or a particle of dust in the eye.

foreign body obstruction, a disturbance in normal function or a pathologic condition caused by an object lodged in a body orifice, passage, or organ. Most cases occur in children who suddenly inhale or swallow a foreign object or insert it in a body opening. In adults, large boluses of hastily eaten food frequently lodge in the esophagus, causing coughing, choking, and, if the airway is obstructed, asphyxia. Forceful blows to the victim's back between the shoulder blades or the Heimlich maneuver may dislodge the bolus. Esophageal foreign bodies usually produce an immediate reaction, but occasionally children have a long asymptomatic period before signs of obstruction or infection are evident. Laryngeal foreign bodies usually cause hoarseness, wheezing, a palpatory thud, and dyspnea; a sharp object, as a chicken bone, may perforate the larynx and produce swelling and infection. Objects may be removed from the larynx, using a grasping forceps through a direct laryngoscope, with the patient under local or general anesthesia in the Trendelenburg position. A foreign body in the trachea may cause wheezing, an audible slap, coughing, and dyspnea; a small object may become lodged in a bronchus, producing coughing, which is often followed by an asymptomatic period before signs of obstruction and inflammation appear; vegetable foreign bodies produce earlier, more severe inflammatory symptoms than other objects. A bronchoscope with suitable forceps and general anesthesia are usually employed in removing bronchial foreign bodies, but thoracotomy may be required if the object is in the periphery of a lung. Objects that children sometimes insert in their nostrils may cause local obstruction, mild discomfort, or infection and may be removed by forceps or nasal suction. Needles and hairpins ingested by children often pass through the esophagus and stomach without incident but may become lodged at the turn of the duodenum and require removal by a magnetized nasogastric tube or by laporotomy; laxatives are contraindicated and, if tenderness, rigidity, pain, nausea, or vomiting ensues, immediate surgery is necessary. Coins, marbles, and closed safety pins usually pass through the digestive tract without creating problems; but bezoars of hair, vegetable fibers, or shellac concretions, sometimes found in the stomach of emotionally disturbed or retarded patients, may cause anorexia, nausea, and vomiting. These hairballs may be fragmented, using an endoscope, and removed by lavage; surgery may be required. Urethral inflammation and hematuria, sometimes caused by the introduction of a foreign body into the urethra during self-exploration, may be treated symptomatically.

foreign medical graduate (FMG), a physician trained in and graduated from a medical school outside the United States and Canada. United States citizens graduated from medical schools outside the United States and Canada are also classified as FMGs.

forensic medicine, a branch of medicine that deals with the legal aspects of health care.

forensic psychiatry, the branch of psychiatry that deals with legal issues and problems relating to mental disorders, especially the determination of insanity for legal purposes.

foreskin, a loose fold of skin that covers the end of the penis or clitoris. Its removal constitutes circumcision. The nurse observes for any interference with urination in infants. Also called **prepuce.**

forest yaws, a cutaneous form of American leishmaniasis, common in South and Central America, caused by *Leishmania guyanensis.* See also **American leishmaniasis, leishmaniasis.**

Forhistal Maleate, a trade name for an antihistaminic (dimethindene maleate).

-form, a combining form meaning 'having a (specified) shape or form': *linguiform, toruliform.* Also **-forme.**

formaldehyde (fərmæl'dəhaid), a toxic, colorless, foul-smelling gas that is soluble in water and used in that form as a disinfectant, fixative, or preservative.

formalin (fɔr'məlin), a clear solution of formaldehyde in water. A 37 per cent solution is used for fixing and preserving biological specimens for pathologic and histologic examination.

Formatrix, a trade name for a hormonal fixed-combination drug containing conjugated estrogens, an androgen (methyltestosterone), and a vitamin (ascorbic acid).

formic acid (fɔr'mik), a colorless, pungent liquid found in nature in nettles, in ants, and in other insects. It is prepared commercially from oxalic acid and glycerin and from the oxidation of formaldehyde. Formerly used as a vesicant, it no longer has any therapeutic applications.

formiminoglutamic acid (FIGLU) (fɔrmim'ınouglutæm'ık), a compound formed in the metabolism of histidine, occurring in urine in elevated levels in folic acid deficiency. Increased excretion of FIGLU may indicate folic acid deficiency.

formol (fɔr'mol). See **formaldehyde.**

formula, a simplified statement, generally using numerals and other symbols, expressing the constituents of a chemical compound, a method for preparing a substance, or a procedure for achieving a desired value or result. — **formulaic,** *adj.*

formulary, a listing of drugs intended to include a large enough range of drugs and sufficient information about them to enable health practitioners to prescribe treatment that is medically appropriate. Hospitals maintain formularies which list all drugs commonly stocked in the hospital pharmacy. Third-party organizations, as insurance companies, usually maintain formularies listing drugs for which the company will pay in settlement of claims. See also **compendium,** *United States Pharmacopeia.*

formulation, 1. a pharmacologic substance prepared according to a formula. 2. a systematic and precise statement of a problem, a theory, or a method of analysis in research.

formylmethionine (FMET) (fôr′mĭlməthī′ənin), (in molecular genetics) the first amino acid in a protein sequence.

fornication, (in law) sexual intercourse between two people who are not married to each other. The specific legal definition varies from jurisdiction to jurisdiction. In some, both persons are unmarried; in some, one is unmarried; in some, the charge is adultery rather than fornication if the woman is married, regardless of the man's marital status.

fornix (fôr′nĭks), *pl.* **fornices** (fôr′nĭsiz). an archlike structure or space, as the fornix cerebri, the superior or inferior conjunctival fornices, or the vaginal fornices.

Fort Bragg fever. See **pretibial fever.**

fortified milk, pasturized milk enriched with one or more nutrients, usually vitamin D, which has been standardized at 400 International Units per quart. Also called **fortified vitamin D milk.**

fossa (fos′ə), *pl.* **fossae.** a hollow or depression, especially on the surface of the end of a bone, as the olecranon fossa or the coronoid fossa.

Foster bed, a special bed used in the care and treatment of severely injured patients, especially those with spinal injuries. It consists of two Bradford frames mounted on a castered base and secured with locking bars to the head and foot assemblies. The assembly at each end is attached to a rotary bearing mechanism, permitting horizontal turning of the patient without moving the spine. The patient can be rotated to supine and prone positions while maintaining proper immobilization and alignment of injured body structures. The Foster bed is a horizontal turning frame that permits hyperextension and traction at each end of the frame and either end of the bed can be elevated to provide countertraction. It is used in postraumatic management of patients with spinal instability, with or without cord damage, and in the management of the postoperative patient with multilevel spinal fusion when weight-bearing or ambulation is contraindicated. The Foster bed is also used in many scoliosis centers for halo-femoral traction, preparatory to spinal procedures with Harrington roads and Dwyer instrumentation. This preoperative technique permits stretching of the paravertebral soft tissues on the concavity of the spinal curve prior to operative correction and fusion. The bed also allows techniques for maintaining continuous cervical traction in flexion for selected patients with unstable cervical neck problems. An outrigger attachment for the bed maintains a constant angle with the patient in the supine or prone position. The bed, which allows clockwise and counterclockwise rotation around its long axis is equipped with a convenient storage rack at the base of the bed and is available in three sizes. The weight of each frame is approximately 20 pounds and the bed can be turned by one person, although hospital and nursing officials recommend that two trained hospital staff members perform each turning to ensure the safety of the patient and the welfare of the nursing staff. Also, two safety straps are required to guard against slippage and to decrease the margin of human error. A pillow is placed over the patient's lower legs to prevent slippage in turning. The length of the canvas on the Foster bed must be adjusted to correspond with the size of the patient, so that correct ankle posture can be maintained when the patient is prone. The relative position of the patient on the posterior frame must correspond so that when the bedpan section is released, the buttocks of the patient will not sag and compromise the alignment of the lumbosacral spine. The anatomic landmark in this adjustment is the level of the trochanters, which should be even with the bottom edge of the torso canvas to prevent hyperextension of the lumbosacral spine. The turn sheet is placed under the patient's torso to adjust movement up and down the frame, without endangering proper alignment. Other safety precautions in caring for a patient confined to a Foster bed include the placement of I.V. and catheter tubing at the head and the foot of the frame before rotating the patient. A Foster bed patient with thoracotomy tubing must be rotated toward the chest tube side. A Foster bed patient recovering from anesthesia or heavy sedation is usually secured with a safety strap at thigh level to help prevent turning or falling. The prone position with the use of a reading board permits self-feeding by the patient and the participation in personal hygiene. Massage of the patient's forehead and chin areas toughens the skin and increases the patient's tolerance of the prone position. Foster bed patients sometimes display claustrophobia on being "sandwiched" between Foster frames, and skillful techniques to minimize the "sandwiching" time are needed to assure the greatest possible tranquility of the patient. Frequent sensory stimulation with patient-staff interaction, discussions, and games, and prism glasses that allow the patient to read and watch TV increase the person's comfort and tolerance of prolonged immobility. Compare **hyperextension bed, Stryker wedge frame.**

foulage (fulaźh′).   See **pétrissage**.

foundation,   a charitable organization usually established to allocate private funds to worthy projects or to provide other services.

four-forty (4-40),   a work schedule in which a person works four ten-hour days each week rather than five eight-hour days.

four-tailed bandage,   a narrow piece of cloth with two ties on each end for wrapping a joint, as an elbow or knee, or a prominence, as the nose or chin.

fourth nerve.   See **trochlear nerve**.

Fowler's position,   the posture assumed by the patient when the head of the bed is raised 18 or 20 inches and the individual's knees are elevated.

Fr,   symbol for **francium**.

fract-,   a combining form meaning 'pertaining to a breaking': *fractional, fractography, fracture*.

fractional anesthesia.   See **continuous anesthesia**.

fractional dilatation and curettage,   a diagnostic technique in which each section of the uterus is examined and curetted to obtain specimens of the endometrium from all parts of the uterus. It is often performed under regional anesthesia in the diagnosis of endometrial cancer.

fractionation,   **1.** (in neurology) a mechanism within the neural arch of the vertebrae whereby only a portion of the efferent nerves innervating a muscle reacts to a stimulus, even when the reflex requirement is maximal, so that there is a reserve of neurons to respond to additional stimuli. Through this phenomenon muscle tension is maintained. **2.** (in chemistry) the separation of a substance into its basic constituents, by using such procedures as fractional distillation or crystallization. **3.** (in bacteriology) the process of isolating a pure culture by successive culturing of a small portion of a colony of bacteria. **4.** (in histology) the process of isolating the different components of living cells by centrifugation. **5.** (in radiology) the process of administering a dose of radiation in smaller units over a period of time rather than in a single large dose in order to minimize tissue damage. Also called **dose fractionation, fractionation radiation**.

fractionation radiation.   See **fractionation**, def. 5.

fracture,   a traumatic injury to a bone in which the continuity of the tissue of the bone is broken. A fracture is classified by the bone involved, the part of that bone, and the nature of the break, as a comminuted fracture of the head of the tibia. Kinds of fracture include **butterfly fracture, comminuted fracture, complete fracture, compression fracture, displaced fracture, impacted fracture, incomplete fracture, segmental fracture, spiral fracture, undisplaced fracture**.
(See next page for illustration)

fracture-dislocation,   a fracture involving the bony structures of any joint, with associated dislocation of the same joint.

fractured rib,   a break in a bone of the thoracic skeleton caused by a blow or crushing injury or by violent coughing or sneezing. The ribs most commonly broken are the fourth to eighth, and, if the bone is splintered or the fracture is displaced, sharp fragments may pierce the lung, causing hemothorax or pneumothorax.
■ OBSERVATIONS: The patient with a fractured rib suffers pain, especially on inspiration, and usually breathes rapidly and shallowly. The site of the break is generally very tender to the touch, and the crackling of bone fragments rubbing together may be heard on auscultation. Breath sounds may be absent, decreased, or accompanied by rales and rhonchi. The location and nature of the fracture are determined by chest x rays and the patient is observed for signs of hemoptysis, hemothorax, flail chest, atelectasis, pneumothorax, and pneumonia.
■ INTERVENTION: Fractured ribs may be splinted with an elastic belt, an Ace bandage, or adhesive strapping; to prevent irritation the area may be shaved and painted with tincture of benzoin before the adhesive tape is applied. If hospitalization is required, the patient is placed in a semi-Fowler's position and the blood pressure, pulse, temperature, respirations, and breath sounds are checked every two to four hours. An analgesic may be ordered, but morphine sulfate is avoided. The patient is assisted in turning and is instructed in how to deep breathe, to cough, and to perform range-of-motion exercises of extremities. If strapping and analgesic medication fail to relieve pain, the physician may perform a regional nerve block by infiltrating the intercostal spaces above and below the fracture site with one per cent procaine.
■ NURSING CONSIDERATIONS: The nurse assists in splinting the chest, administers the ordered medication, and helps the patient to turn.

fragilitas ossium (frəjıl′ıtæs os′iəm).   See **osteogenesis imperfecta**.

fragmented fracture,   a fracture that results in multiple bone fragments.

frambesia (fræmbi′źhə).   See **yaws**.

Franceschetti's syndrome (fran′ćhəsket′iz),   a complete form of mandibulofacial dysostosis. See also **Treacher Collins' syndrome**.

francium (Fr),   a metallic element of the alkali metal group. Its atomic number is 87; its atomic weight is 223. Formed from the decay of actinium, all of its isotopes are radioactive and short-lived.

frank,   obvious or clinically evident, as the unequivocal presence of a condition or a disease.

frank breech,   an intrauterine position of the fetus in which the buttocks present at the maternal pelvic inlet, the legs are straight up in front of the body, and the feet are at the shoulders. Babies born in this position tend to hold their feet near their heads for some days after birth. Compare **complete breech, footling breech**.

FRACTURES

Frank-Starling relationship, an index for determing cardiac output, based on the length of the myocardial fibers at the onset of contraction. The force exerted per beat of the heart is directly proportional to the length of or degree of stretch of the myocardial fiber so that improved performance is the result of a longer initial fiber length or a larger diastolic ventricular volume. Since there are no adequate in vivo methods of measuring fiber length or diastolic volume, end-diastolic pressure is used as an index of volume or stretch. The cardiac output is plotted on a graph against atrial pressure. In congestive heart failure there is a shift in the curve to the right and downward. Also called **Frank-Starling mechanism.**

fraternal twins. See **dizygotic twins.**

fraud, (in law) the act of intentionally misleading or deceiving another person by any means so as to cause him legal injury, usually the loss of something valuable or the surrender of a legal right.

FRC, abbreviation for **functional residual capacity.**

FreAmine II, a trade name for a nutritional supplement containing protein, amino acids, and electrolytes.

freckle, a brown or tan macule on the skin usually resulting from exposure to sunlight. There is an inherited tendency to freckling, most frequently seen in persons with red hair. Freckles are harmless in themselves, but people who freckle easily should avoid excessive sun exposure or use protective sunscreen lotions because such individuals have a tendency to develop more serious actinic skin changes. Compare **lentigo.**

free association, 1. the spontaneous, consciously unrestricted association of ideas, feelings, or mental images. 2. spontaneous verbalization of thoughts and emotions entering the consciousness during psychoanalysis.

free clinic, a clinic or health program, usually located in a neighborhood setting, that provides health care for ambulatory patients at nominal or no cost.

free-floating anxiety, a generalized, persistent, pervasive fear that is not attributable to any specific object, event, or source. See also **anxiety, anxiety neurosis.**

free phagocyte. See **phagocyte.**

free thyroxine, the amount of the unbound, active thyroid hormone, thyroxine (T_4), circulating in the blood, measured by special laboratory procedures. See also **free thyroxine index.**

free thyroxine index, the amount of unbound, physiologically active thyroxine (T_4) in serum, determined by direct assay or, more frequently, calculated on the basis of an in vitro uptake test. In this test the uptake (by resin or charcoal) of labeled triiodothyronine (T_3) is measured; since T_3 is less strongly bound by serum, it is used rather than T_4. The free T_4 index is then obtained by multiplying the T_3 uptake by the total concentration of T_4 in serum.

Freiberg's infarction, an abnormal orthopedic condition characterized by the aseptic necrosis of bone tissue, most commonly affecting the head of the second metatarsal.

Frei test (fraī), a test performed to confirm a diagnosis of lymphogranuloma venereum. Killed antigen, originally derived from infected patients, is injected intradermally in one forearm, and a control material is injected into the other arm. If a red, thickened papule develops at the site of injection of antigen, the test is positive. See also *Chlamydia.*

Frejka splint, (freī'kə), a corrective device consisting of a pillow that is belted between the legs of a baby born with dislocated hips to maintain abduction and articulation of the head of the femur with the acetabulum. See also **congenital dysplasia of the hips.**

fremitus (frem'ītəs), a tremulous vibration of the chest wall that can be auscultated or palpated during physical examination. Kinds of fremitus include **bronchial fremitus, coarse fremitus, tactile fremitus, vocal fremitus.**

frenulum linguae. See **lingual frenum.**

frenum (frī'nəm), *pl.* **frenums, frena.** a restraining portion or structure. Also called **frenulum.**

frequency, 1. the number of repetitions of any phenomenon within a fixed period of time, as the number of heart beats per minute. 2. (in biometry) the proportion of the number of persons having a discrete characteristic to the total number of persons being studied. 3. (in electronics) the number of cycles of a periodic quantity, as alternating current, that occur in a period of one second. Electronic frequencies, formerly expressed in cycles per second, are now expressed in hertz for which the symbol is Hz.

Freudian, 1. of or pertaining to Sigmund Freud, his theories and doctrines, which stress the formative years of childhood as the basis for later psychoneurotic disorders, primarily through the unconscious repression of instinctual drives and sexual desires, and his system of psychoanalysis for treating such disturbances. 2. anything that is easily interpreted according to the theories of Freud or in psychoanalytic terms. 3. of or pertaining to the school of psychiatry based on Freud's teachings. 4. one who adheres to Freud's school of psychiatry. See also **psychoanalysis.**

Freudian fixation, an arrest in psychosexual development characterized by a firm emotional attachment to another person or object. Some kinds of Freudian fixation are **father fixation, mother fixation.**

Freudianism, Freudism, the school of psychiatry based on the psychoanalytic theories and psychotherapeutic methods of treating psychoneurotic disorders developed by Sigmund Freud and his followers. See also **psychoanalysis.**

friction, 1. See also **attrition.** the act of rubbing one object against another. 2. See also **massage.** a type of massage in which deeper tissues are stroked or rubbed, usually through strong circular movements of the hand.

friction burn, tissue injury caused by abrasion of the skin. See also **abrasion.**

friction rub, a dry, grating sound heard with a stethoscope during auscultation. It is a normal finding when heard over the liver and splenic areas. A pericardial friction rub auscultated over the pericardial area is suggestive of pericarditis; a pleural friction rub over the lungs may be present in heart or lung disease.

Friedländer's bacillus (frid'lendərz), a bacterium of the species *Klebsiella pneumonia,* associated with infection of the respiratory tract, especially lobar pneumonia.

Friedman curve (frid'mən), a graph depicting the progress of labor, prepared by labor attendants to facilitate detection of dysfunctional labor. Observations of cervical dilatation and fetal descent are plotted on the vertical axis against time on the horizontal axis. The labor curve is divided into latent and active phases, with the latter subdivided into latent, acceleration, maximum slope, and deceleration phases.

Friedreich's ataxia (frid'Raīχs), an abnormal condition characterized by muscular weakness, loss of muscular control, weakness of the lower extremities, and an abnormal gait. Friedreich's ataxia, which may be hereditary, exhibits both dominant and recessive inheritance patterns. The primary pathologic feature of the disease is pronounced sclerosis of the posterior columns of the spinal cord with possible involvement of the spinocerebellar tracts and the corticospinal tracts. Friedreich's ataxia usually affects individuals between the ages of 5 and 20. The highest incidence of onset is at puberty. The characteristically ataxic gait may progress to severe disability. Over a period of years a child affected by Friedrich's ataxia may also develop ataxia of the upper extremities and have difficulty performing simple maneuvers, as writing or handling silverware while eating. The characteristic gait of this disease is caused by a cavus deformity, or clawfoot.

The gait and the stance of the affected individual are unsteady. A positive Romberg's sign may be evident and Babinski's sign is present with absent or decreased deep reflexes. The condition may also cause slurred speech, head tremors, tachycardia, and cardiac failure. Thoracic scoliosis is present in approximately 80 to 90 per cent of the patients afflicted. All the signs and symptoms are progressive. There is no curative treatment for Friedreich's ataxia. Orthoses may be useful to varying degrees in the prevention of associated deformities and the maintenance of an ambulatory status. Correction of the foot deformity allows the patient to remain ambulatory as long as possible and is preferred when the lack of progression of the disease process is demonstrated, thereby reducing the potential for recurrence. Spinal fusion may correct the associated scoliosis. Death in the progression of this disease is usually owing to myocardial failure.

frigid, 1. lacking warmth of feeling; unemotional; unimaginative; without passion or ardor and stiff or formal in manner. 2. **Compare impotence.** See also **orgasm.** a woman who is unresponsive to sexual advances or stimuli, abnormally indifferent or averse to sexual intercourse, or unable to have an orgasm during sexual intercourse. – **frigidity,** n.

Fröhlich's syndrome (frou'lĭks). See **adiposogenital dystrophy.**

frôlement (frŏlmañ'), 1. the rustling type of sound often heard on auscultating the chest in diseases of the pericardium. 2. See also **massage.** a kind of massage that uses a light brushing stroke with the hand.

front-, a combining form meaning 'pertaining to the forehead, or front': *frontad, frontalis, frontonasal.*

frontal lobe, the largest of five lobes constituting each of the two cerebral hemispheres. It lies beneath the frontal bone, occupies part of the lateral, the medial, and the inferior surfaces of each hemisphere, and extends posteriorly to the central sulcus and inferiorly to the lateral fissure. The frontal lobe significantly influences personality and is associated with the higher mental activities, as planning, judgment, and conceptualizing. Research indicates that the right frontal and the right temporal lobes are associated with the nonverbal, specialized activities of the right cerebral hemisphere and that the left frontal and the left temporal lobes are associated with the verbal activities of the left cerebral hemisphere. The lateral surface of each frontal lobe contains the precentral, the superior, and the inferior sulci, which divide the lobe into the precentral, the superior, the middle, and the inferior frontal gyri. The left inferior frontal gyrus constitutes Broca's speech area and, in most individuals, is more convoluted than the right inferior frontal gyrus. An H-shaped orbital sulcus on the inferior surface of the frontal lobe divides its inferior surface into the medial, the anterior, the lateral, and the posterior orbital gyri. The olfactory sulcus on the inferior surface contains the olfactory tract and separates the gyrus rectus from the medial orbital gyrus. The medial surface of the frontal lobe is limited posteriorly by an imaginary line that extends downward and anteriorly to the corpus callosum from the intersection of the central sulcus with the superior margin of the lobe. The medial surface of the frontal lobe includes the superior frontal gyrus and part of the cingulate gyrus. The superior frontal gyrus extends posteriorly as the paracentral lobule into the parietal lobe of the hemisphere. Compare **central lobe, occipital lobe, parietal lobe, temporal lobe.**

frontal lobe syndrome, behavioral and personality changes observed following a neoplastic or traumatic frontal lobe lesion. The patient may become sociopathic, boastful, hypomanic, uninhibited, exhibitionistic, and subject to outbursts of irritability or violence; but in other cases the person may become depressed, apathetic, lacking in initiative, negligent about his personal appearance, and inclined to perseverate. Partial frontal lobectomy or leukotomy was formerly performed by some psychosurgeons to reduce drive in extremely disturbed psychotic patients, but the results were highly questionable.

frontal plane, any one of the vertical planes passing through the body from the head to the feet, perpendicular to the sagittal planes, dividing the body into front and back portions. Also called **coronal plane.** Compare **median plane, transverse plane.**

frontal sinus, one of a pair of small cavities in the frontal bone of the skull that communicates with the nasal cavity. The frontal sinuses, which are rarely symmetrical, are situated behind the superciliary arches. Each sinus measures approximately 3 cm in height, 2.5 cm in width, and 2.5 cm in depth and is lined with a mucous membrane that is continuous with that of the nasal cavity. A large frontal sinus may project over most of the orbit. Each sinus opens into the anterior part of the middle meatus through the frontonasal duct. The frontal sinuses are absent at birth, well developed between the seventh and eighth years, and reach their full size after puberty. Compare **ethmoidal air cell, maxillary sinus, sphenoidal sinus.**

frontal vein, one of a pair of superficial veins of the face, arising in the plexus of the forehead. Each frontal vein communicates with the frontal tributaries of the superficial temporal vein and lies near the vein of the opposite side as it courses toward the root of the nose. The two frontal veins communicate by a transverse vessel before joining the supraorbital veins. Compare **angular vein, facial vein.**

frontocortical aphasia (frən'toukɔr'tıkəl). See **motor aphasia.**

frostbite, traumatic effect of extreme cold on skin and subcutaneous tissues that is first recognized by distinct pallor of exposed skin surfaces, particularly the nose, ears, fingers, and toes. Vasoconstriction and damage to blood vessels impair local circulation and result in anoxia, edema, vesiculation, and necrosis. Gentle warming is appropriate first aid treatment; rubbing of the affected part is avoided. Later, therapy is similar to treatment of thermal burns. Iatrogenic frostbite is the result of excessive use of ethyl chloride sprays for local anesthesia for the relief of muscle and tendon strains. Compare **chilblain, immersion foot.**

frottage (frɔtaźh′), **1.** See **effleurage. 2.** sexual gratification obtained by rubbing against the clothing of another person, as can occur in a crowd.

frotteur (frɔtœr′), a person who obtains sexual gratification by the practice of frottage.

frozen section method, (in surgical pathology) a method used in preparing a selected portion of tissue for pathologic examination. The tissue is moistened and, fixed or unfixed, is rapidly frozen and cut by a microtome in a cryostat. This method is very rapid, allowing the pathologist to examine the specimen during a surgical procedure.

fructokinase (frək′toukai′neis), an enzyme that catalyzes the transfer of a phosphate group from adenosine triphosphate to D-fructose.

fructose (frək′tous, fruk′tous), a yellowish-to-white, crystalline, water soluble levorotatory ketose monosaccharide that is sweeter than sucrose and found in honey, several fruits, and combined in many disaccharides and polysaccharides. It is used as a preservative and in solution as an intravenous nutrient. In the absence of insulin it is metabolized or converted in the body to glycogen. Also called **fruit sugar, levulose.**

fructosuria (fruk′tousur′iə), presence of the sugar, fructose, in the urine. This harmless and asymptomatic condition is caused by the hereditary absence of the enzyme fructokinase, which normally helps metabolize fructose. Also called **levulosuria.**

fruit sugar. See **fructose.**

FSH, abbreviation for **follicle stimulating hormone.**

FTA-ABS test. See **Fluorescent Treponemal Antibody Absorption Test.**

FTC, abbreviation for **Federal Trade Commission.**

Fuadin, a trade name for an antischistosomal (stibophen).

fuchsin bodies. See **Russell's bodies.**

FUDR, a trade name for an antiviral and antineoplastic (floxuridine).

fugue (fyug), a state of dissociative reaction characterized by amnesia and physical flight from an intolerable situation. During the episode, the person appears normal and acts as though consciously aware of what may be very complex activities and behavior, but after the episode, the person has no recollection of the actions or behavior. The condition may last for only a few days or weeks, or it may continue for several years, during which the person wanders away from the customary environment, enters a new occupation, and undertakes an entirely different way of life. The syndrome appears to be caused by an inability to cope with a severe conflict or with a chronically stressful life situation. A form of fugue also occurs briefly following an epileptic seizure. See also **ambulatory automatism, automatism.**

fulcrum (ful′krəm, fəl′krəm), the stable point or the position on which a lever, as the ulna and the femur, turns in moving an object. Numerous common movements of the body, as raising the arm and walking, are combinations of lever actions involving fulcrums. The muscles of the body provide the forces that move the numerous bones acting as levers.

fulguration (fəl′gyurei′śhən). See **electrodesiccation.**

full bath, a bath in which the patient's body is immersed in water up to the neck.

full diet. See **regular diet.**

full liquid diet, a diet consisting only of liquids and foods that liquefy at body temperature. It includes milk, milk drinks, carbonated beverages, coffee, tea, strained fruit juices, broth, strained cream soup, raw eggs, cream, melted butter or margarine, strained precooked infant cereals in milk, thin custards, gelatin desserts, ice cream, sherbet, strained vegetables in soup, honey, syrups, sugar, and dry skim milk dissolved in liquids. The diet is prescribed following surgery, in some acute infections of short duration, in the treatment of acute gastrointestinal disorders, and for patients too ill to chew. See also **liquid diet.**

fulminating (fəl′minei′tıng), (of a disease or condition) rapid, sudden, severe, as an infection, fever, or hemorrhage. — **fulminant,** adj. **fulminate,** v.

Fulvicin, a trade name for an antifungal (griseofulvin).

fumagillin (fyu′məjıl′ın). See **helvolic acid.**

fumigacin (fyu′mıgei′sın). See **helvolic acid.**

function, **1.** an act, process, or series of processes that serve a purpose. **2.** to perform an activity or to work properly and normally.

functional contracture. See **hypertonic contracture.**

functional differentiation, (in embryology) the specialization or diversification as a result of the particular function of a cell or tissue.

functional disease, **1.** a disease that affects function or performance. **2.** a condition marked by signs or symptoms of an organic disease or disorder although careful examination fails to reveal any evidence of structural or physiological abnormalities. The symptoms of a functional disorder are as real as those of an organic disease. Headache, impotence, certain heart murmurs, and constipation may be symptoms of organic disease or of functional disease.

functional dyspepsia, an abnormal condition characterized by impaired digestion due to an atonic or to a neurologic problem. See also **dyspepsia.**

functional imaging, (in nuclear medicine) a diagnostic procedure in which a sequence of radiographic or scintillation camera images of the distribution of an administered radioactive tracer delineates one or more physiologic processes in the body.

functional impotence. See **impotence.**

functional residual capacity, (in anesthesiology) the volume of gas in the lungs at the end of a normal expiration.

fundal height, the height of the fundus, measured in centimeters from the top of the symphysis pubis to the highest point in the midline at the top of the uterus. Fundal height is measured at each prenatal visit with large, blunt calipers or with a tape measure. From the 20th to the 32nd weeks of pregnancy, the height in centimeters is equal to the gestation in weeks. Two measurements two weeks apart showing a deviation of more than 2 cm may indicate that the fetus is large or small for dates, that the estimated gestation is in error, or that the woman is carrying a multiple pregnancy.

fundamental needs of man, (in nursing education) the fourteen basic needs of man, as described in a curriculum for basic nursing. The needs are: respiration; nutrition; elimination; mobility, including posture and locomotion; sleep and rest; clothing; maintenance of normal body temperature; cleanliness; safety; communication; worship, according to the person's faith; work that is satisfying to the person; recreation and learning and discovery. Recognition and identification of a need precede and serve as the basis for a nurse's plan for care, taking into consideration that the need and the ability to cope with the need vary according to age, temperament, social and cultural status, and physical and intellectual ability.

fundamentals of nursing, the basic principles and practices of nursing as taught in educational programs for nurses. In a course called "the fundamentals of nursing," traditionally required in the first semester of the program, the student attends classes and gives care to selected patients. The emphasis of this phase of training is the acquisition by the student of the basic skills of nursing. Currently, nursing educators emphasize the importance of knowledge and understanding of the fundamental needs of man as well as competence in the basic skills as prerequisites to providing comprehensive nursing care.

fundus (fən′dəs), *pl.* **fundi** (fən′dɑi). the base or the deepest part of an organ; the portion farthest from the mouth of an organ, as the fundus of the uterus or the fundus of an eye.

funduscope (fən′dəskoup). See **ophthalmoscope.**

funduscopy (fəndəs′kəpi), the examination and study of the fundus of the eye by means of an ophthalmoscope. —**fundoscopic, funduscopic,** *adj.*

fundus microscopy, examination of the base of the interior of the eye using an instrument that combines an ophthalmoscope and a lens with high magnifying power for observing minute structures in the cornea and iris.

fundus reflex. See **light reflex.**

fungal infection, any inflammatory condition caused by a fungus. Most fungal infections are superficial and mild, though persistent and difficult to eradicate. Some, particularly in older, debilitated, or immunosuppressed people, may become systemic and life-threatening. Some kinds of fungal infections are **aspergillosis, blastomycosis, candidiasis, coccidioidomycosis, histoplasmosis.**

fungemia (fənji′miə), the presence of fungi in the blood. Compare **bacteremia, parasitemia, viremia.**

fungicide (fən′jisɑid), a drug that kills fungi. See also **antifungal,** def. 2. —**fungicidal,** *adj.*

fungiform papilla. See under **papilla.**

Fungizone, a trade name for an antifungal (amphotericin B).

fungus (fəŋ′gəs), *pl.* **fungi** (fən′jɑi). a simple parasitic plant that, lacking chlorophyll, is unable to make its own food and is dependent on other life forms. A simple fungus reproduces by budding; multicellular fungi reproduce by spore formation. Of the 100,000 identified species of fungi, 100 are common in man and 10 are pathogenic. See also **fungal infection.** —**fungal, fungous,** *adj.*

funiculitis (fənik′yulɑi′tis), any abnormal inflammatory condition of a cordlike structure of the body, as the spinal cord or spermatic cord.

funiculus umbilicalis. See **umbilical cord.**

funnel feeding, a technique in which liquids may be given orally to a patient who cannot move the lips or masticate, as may occur following surgery to the mouth or lips. A rubber tube attached to a funnel is placed in the mouth, usually at one corner, and a liquid is poured slowly through the funnel and tube into the mouth near the back of the tongue. The patient quickly learns to control the flow with sucking action and the position of the tongue. If the method is used for a weak or young infant, a rubber bulb or a large syringe may be used instead of a funnel. The bulb or syringe is compressed gently, slowly, and continuously to control the rate of flow and prevent choking.

Furacin, a trade name for a topical anti-infective (nitrofurazone).

Furadantin, a trade name for an antibacterial (nitrofurantoin).

furazolidone, an anti-infective and antiprotozoal.

■ INDICATIONS: It is prescribed for certain bacterial or protozoal infections of the gastrointestinal tract.

■ CONTRAINDICATIONS: Known hypersensitivity to this

drug prohibits its use. It is not given to children under one month of age and it is not used with drugs that are contraindicated with monoamine oxidase inhibitors.
- ADVERSE EFFECTS: Among the more serious adverse reactions are hemolytic anemia and fever; skin rash and abdominal pain sometimes occur.

furosemide (fyərou′səmɪd), a diuretic.
- INDICATIONS: It is prescribed in the treatment of hypertension and edema.
- CONTRAINDICATIONS: Anuria, pregnancy, lactation, electrolyte depletion, or known hypersensitivity to this drug prohibits its use.
- ADVERSE EFFECTS: Among the more serious adverse reactions are fluid and electrolyte imbalance.

Furoxone, a trade name for an anti-infective antiprotozoal (furazolidone).

furuncle (fyur′əŋkəl), a localized, suppurative staphylococcal skin infection originating in a gland or hair follicle, characterized by pain, redness, and swelling. Necrosis deep in the center of the inflamed area forms a core of dead tissue that will be spontaneously extruded, eventually resorbed, or surgically removed. To prevent spread of infection it is important to avoid irritating or squeezing the lesion. Treatment may include antibiotics, local moist heat, and, when there is definite fluctuation and the hard white core is evident, incision and drainage. Also called **boil.** – **furunculous,** *adj.*

furunculosis (fyurəŋ′kyulou′sɪs), an acute skin disease characterized by boils or successive crops of boils that are caused by staphylococci or streptococci.

-fuse, a combining form meaning 'to pour or flow': *diffuse, effuse, perfuse.*

fusimotor (fyu′zɪmou′tər), pertaining to the motor nerve fibers, or gamma efferent fibers, that innervate the intrafusal fibers of the muscle spindle.

fusion, 1. bringing together into a single entity, as in optical fusion. 2. the act of uniting two or more bones of a joint. 3. the surgical joining together of two or more spinal vertebrae, performed to stabilize a segment of the spinal column following severe trauma, a herniated disc, or degenerative disease. Under general anesthesia, the cartilage pads are removed from between the posterior portions of the involved vertebrae. Bone chips are cut from one of the patient's iliac crests and inserted in place of the cartilage, fusing the articulating surfaces into one segment of bone. Postoperative nursing care focuses on strict limitations of motion for the graft site until bony healing occurs. The patient's bed is completely flat; a Stryker frame may be used. In a standard bed, the patient is log-rolled from side to side to avoid twisting the trunk. The nurse observes the dressing for any drainage of spinal fluid. Ambulation takes place before sitting.

fusospirochetal disease, (fyu′zouspai′rouki′təl), any infection characterized by ulcerative lesions in which both a fusiform bacillus and a spirochete are found, as trench mouth or Vincent's angina.

-fy, a combining form meaning 'to make into' something specified: *acidify, decalcify, salify.*

-fying. See **-factive.**

G

Ga, symbol for **gallium.**

GA, abbreviation for **general anesthesia.**

GABA, abbreviation for **gamma-aminobutyric acid.**

gadolinium (Gd), a rare-earth metallic element. Its atomic number is 64; its atomic weight is 157.25.

gag reflex, a normal neural reflex elicited by touching the soft palate or posterior pharynx, the response being elevation of the palate, retraction of the tongue, and contraction of the pharyngeal muscles. The reflex is used as a test of the integrity of the vagus and glossopharyngeal nerves. Also called **pharyngeal reflex.**

gait, the manner or style of walking, including rhythm, cadence, and speed.

gait determinant, one of a number of the kinetic anatomic factors that govern the locomotion of an individual in the process of walking. Some authorities have defined pelvic rotation, pelvic tilt, knee and hip flexion, knee and ankle interaction, and lateral pelvic displacement as the main determinants of gait. Such descriptions are often important in analyzing and correcting pathological gaits of individuals afflicted by orthopedic diseases, deformities, or abnormal bone conditions.

galact-. See **galacto-.**

galacta-. See **galacto-.**

-galactia, a combining form meaning a 'condition involving secretion of milk': *cacogalactia, dysgalactia, oligogalactia.*

galacto-, galact-, galacta-, a combining form meaning 'pertaining to milk': *galactochloral, galactogen, galactorrhea.*

galactokinase (gəlæk′toʊkaɪ′neɪs), an enzyme that functions in the metabolism of glycogen. Galactokinase catalyzes a metabolic step involving the transfer of a high-energy phosphate group from a donor molecule to a molecule of galactose producing a molecule of D-galactose-1-phosphate.

galactokinase deficiency, an inherited disorder of carbohydrate metabolism in which galactokinase (an enzyme) is deficient or absent. As a result, dietary galactose is not metabolized, galactose accumulates in the blood, and cataracts usually develop rapidly. Food containing galactose, as milk and milk products, must be eliminated from the diet. Compare **lactase deficiency.**

galactophorous duct, a passage for milk in the lobes of the breast.

galactorrhea (gælæk′təri′ə), lactation not associated with childbirth or nursing. The condition is sometimes a symptom of a pituitary gland tumor. See also **Forbes-Albright syndrome.**

galactose (gəlæk′toʊs), a simple sugar found in the dextrorotatory form in lactose (milk sugar), nerve cell membranes, sugar beets, gums, and seaweed and, in the levorotatory form, in flaxseed mucilage. Prepared galactose, a white crystalline substance, is less sweet and less soluble in water than glucose but is similar in other properties.

galactosemia (gəlæk′toʊsi′miə), an inherited, autosomal recessive disorder of galactose metabolism, characterized by a deficiency of the enzyme galactose-1-phosphate uridyl transferase. Shortly after birth, an intolerance to milk is evident. Hepatosplenomegaly, cataracts, and mental retardation develop. Greater than normal amounts of galactose are present in the blood, the galactose tolerance test is abnormal, and the red cells show deficient galactose-1-phosphate uridyl transferase activity. Because the elimination of galactose from the diet results in the rapid amelioration of all symptoms except mental retardation, early diagnosis and prompt therapy are essential. Compare **diabetes mellitus, glycogen storage disease.** See also **galactose, inborn error of metabolism.**

galactosyl ceramide lipidosis, a rare, fatal, inherited disorder of lipid metabolism, present at birth. Infants become paralyzed, blind, deaf, and increasingly retarded, and eventually die of bulbar paralysis. There is no known treatment for the disorder, but it can be detected in pregnancy by amniocentesis. Also called **globoid leukodystrophy, Krabbe's disease.** Compare **Tay-Sachs disease.**

Galant reflex (gəlænt′), a normal response in the neonate to move the hips toward the stimulated side when the back is stroked along the spinal cord. The reflex disappears by about four weeks of age. Absence of the reflex may indicate spinal cord lesion. Also called **trunk incurvation reflex.**

galea aponeurotica. See **epicranial aponeurosis.**

Galeazzi's fracture (gæl′iæt′siz), a fracture of the distal radius accompanied by dislocation of the distal ulnar. Also called **Dupuytren's fracture.**

Galen's bandage (geɪ′lɪnz), a bandage for the head, consisting of a strip of cloth with each end divided into three pieces. The center of the cloth is placed on top of the head; the two strips in front are joined at the back of the neck; the two strips at the back are pulled up and fastened on the forehead; the remaining middle strips are fastened under the chin.

gall. See **bile.**

gallamine triethiodide, a neuromuscular blocking agent.

■ INDICATIONS: It is prescribed as a muscle relaxant as an adjunct to anesthesia.

■ CONTRAINDICATIONS: Myasthenia gravis, impaired kidney function, in patients where increased heart rate may be hazardous, or known hypersensitivity to this drug or to iodine prohibits its use.

■ ADVERSE EFFECTS: Among the most serious adverse reactions are risks associated with skeletal muscle relaxation, as respiratory depression and apnea, and tachycardia. Allergic reactions also may occur.

gall bladder, a pear-shaped excretory sac lodged in a fossa on the visceral surface of the right lobe of the liver. It serves as a reservoir for bile. About 8 cm long and 2.5 cm wide at its thickest part, it holds about 32 cu cm of bile. During digestion of fats, the gall bladder contracts, ejecting bile through the common bile duct into the duodenum. The gall bladder is divided into a fundus, body, and neck and is covered by the peritoneum. Obstruction of the biliary system by gallstones may lead to jaundice and pain. It is a common condition in overweight, middle-aged women and may require surgical excision.

gall bladder cancer, a malignant neoplasm of the bile reservoir, characterized by anorexia, nausea, vomiting, weight loss, progressively severe right upper quadrant pain, and, eventually, jaundice. Tumors of the gall bladder are predominantly adenocarcinomas; often associated with biliary calculi, they are three to four times more common in women than in men and rarely occur before the age of 40. Physical examination reveals an enlarged gall bladder in about half the cases. X rays may aid in making a diagnosis, but obstruction of the biliary duct by the cancer or the inability of the gall bladder to concentrate the radiopaque dye often prevents visualization of the lesion, and the diagnosis is usually made during a laporotomy. Complete removal of the gall bladder may be curative, but partial hepatectomy may be required because the liver is often a site of early metastases. Surgery is contraindicated if there are distant metastases, as frequently occur in the lungs, bone, and adrenal glands. Radiotherapy may be palliative; chemotherapy is usually ineffective.

gallium, a metallic element. Its atomic number is 31; its atomic weight is 69.72. The melting point of gallium is 29.8°C (88.6° F); it will melt if held in the hand. Because of its high boiling point (1983°C; 3602°F), it is used in high-temperature thermometers. Radioisotopes of gallium are used in total body scanning procedures. Many of its compounds are poisonous.

gallop, (in cardiology) a cardiac arrhythmia characterized by a low-pitched extra sound heard in diastole on auscultation of the heart during a physical assessment. The rhythm resembles the pattern produced as a horse's hooves strike the ground at a gallop. If the sound is heard early in diastole in a child or a young adult, it is a physiologic third heart sound and is of no clinical significance; in an older person with heart disease it is a ventricular gallop, a pathologic sound. An extra sound late in diastole is an atrial gallop. It indicates increased resistance to ventricular filling.

gallstone. See **biliary calculus.**

galvanic cautery. See **electrocautery.**

galvanocautery (gæl′vənɔukɔ′təri). See **electrocautery.**

gam-. See **gamo-.**

Gambian trypanosomiasis, a usually chronic form of African trypanosomiasis, caused by the parasite *Trypanosoma brucei gambiense.* An infected individual may have relatively mild symptoms for months or years before developing the neurologic symptoms of the terminal stage. Also called **West African sleeping sickness.** Compare **Rhodesian trypanosomiasis.** See also **African trypanosomiasis.**

Gamene, a trade name for a pediculicide and scabicide (gamma-benzene hexachloride).

gamet-. See **gameto-.**

gamete (gæm′it), **1.** a mature male or female germ cell that is capable of functioning in fertilization or conjugation and that contains the haploid number of chromosomes of the somatic cell. **2.** the ovum or spermatozoon. See also **meiosis.** — **gametic,** *adj.*

gametic chromosome, any of the chromosomes contained in the haploid cell, specifically the spermatozoon or ovum, as contrasted to those in the diploid, or somatic cell.

gameto-, gamet-, a combining form meaning 'reproductive cell': **gametocyte, gametophore, gamogenesis.**

gametocide (gəmi′tousæid), any agent that is destructive to gametes or gametocytes, specifically to the malarial gametocytes. — **gametocidal,** *adj.*

gametocyte (gəmi′təsait), (in genetics) any cell capable of dividing into or in the process of developing into a gamete, specifically an oocyte or spermatocyte.

gametogenesis (gæm′ɪtoujen′ɪsɪs), the maturation of gametes, which occurs through the process of meiosis. See also **oogenesis, spermatogenesis.** — **gametogenic, gametogenous,** *adj.*

gamma-aminobutyric acid (GABA) (gæm′əæmi′noubyutɪr′ɪk), an amino acid found in the brain and in bacteria, yeast, and green plants.

gamma-benzene hexachloride. See **lindane.**

Gammacorten, a trade name for a glucocorticoid (dexamethasone).

gamma efferent fiber, any of the motor nerve fibers that transmit impulses from the central nervous system to the intrafusal fibers of the muscle spindle. The gamma efferent fibers are responsible for deep tendon reflexes, spasticity, and rigidity but not for the degree of contractile response. They function in regulating the sensitivity of the spindle and the total tension of the muscle. See also **primary afferent fiber.**

Gammagee, a trade name for a passive immunizing agent (immune globulin).

gamma globulin. See **immune gamma globulin.**

gamma radiation, a very high frequency electromagnetic emission of photons from certain radioactive elements in the course of nuclear transition or from nuclear reactions. Gamma rays are more penetrating than alpha radiation and beta radiation but have less ionizing power and are not deflected in electric and magnetic fields. The wavelengths of gamma rays emitted by radioactive substances are characteristic of the radioisotopes involved and range from about 4×10^{-10} to 5×10^{-13} meters. High-voltage generators can produce x rays of a wavelength much shorter than that of most gamma rays. The depth to which gamma rays penetrate depends on their wavelengths and energy. Gamma radiation and other forms of radiation can injure, distort, or destroy body cells and tissue, especially cell nuclei, but controlled radiation is used in the diagnosis and treatment of various diseases. Gamma radiation can penetrate thousands of meters of air and several inches of soft tissue and bone. Sixty per cent of a dose of gamma radiation that enters the body tissue normally exits the same tissue. Radiation is an important form of therapy in the treatment of skin cancer and malignancies deep within the body. The ionizing effect of radiation affects all the cells of the body, but young, growing, and dividing cells are most susceptible. Radiation therapy seeks to destroy the nuclei of rapidly dividing cancer cells by bombarding the nuclei with selective doses of radiation that spare normal tissue. Any cell is vulnerable to injury if radiated while dividing, and the injury to the cells and tissue from radiation is basically the same, regardless of the type of radiant energy. There is no practical application of radiation in routine sterilization, but both heat and gamma radiation are employed to sterilize spacecraft. Body cells especially sensitive to radiation include lymphoid cells, bone marrow cells, cells that line the alimentary tract, and cells of the testes and the ovaries. Exposure of the entire body to sizable doses of radiation can cause acute radiation sickness. See also **ultraviolet radiation.**

gamma ray, an electromagnetic radiation of short wavelength emitted by the nucleus of an atom during a nuclear reaction. Composed of high-energy photons, gamma rays lack mass and an electric charge and travel at the speed of light. They are usually associated with beta rays (electrons ejected at high velocities from radioactive substances).

gammopathy (gæmop'əthi), an abnormal condition characterized by the presence of markedly increased levels of gamma globulin in the blood. Two different types of hypergammaglobulinemia can be distinguished. **Monoclonal gammopathy** is commonly associated with an electrophoretic pattern showing one sharp, homogenous electrophoretic band in the gamma globulin region. This reflects the presence of excessive amounts of one type of immunoglobulin secreted by a single clone of B cells. **Polyclonal gammopathy** reflects the presence of a diffuse hypergammaglobulinemia in which all immunoglobulin classes are proportionally increased. See also **Bence Jones protein, multiple myeloma.**

gamo-, gam-, a combining form meaning 'pertaining to marriage or sexual union': *gamobium, gamont, gamophagia.*

gamogenesis (gæm'oujen'ɪsɪs), sexual reproduction through the fusion of gametes. —**gamogenetic,** *adj.*

gamone (gæm'oun), a chemical substance secreted by the ova and spermatozoa that supposedly attracts the gametes of the opposite sex in order to facilitate union. Kinds of gamones are **androgamone, gynogamone.**

gampsodactyly (gæmp'soudæk'tɪli). See **clawfoot.**

Gamulin Rh, a trade name for a passive immunizing agent (immune human globulin).

-gamy, 1. a combining form meaning a '(specified) type of marriage': *endogamy, monogamy, pedogamy.* **2.** a combining form meaning 'possession of organs for reproduction': *cleistogamy, dichogamy, homogamy.* **3.** a combining form meaning a 'union for propagation': *hologamy, macrogamy, syngamy.*

gangli-. See **ganglio-.**

ganglia (gæŋ'gliə). See **ganglion.**

ganglio-, gangli-, a combining form meaning 'pertaining to a ganglion': *gangliocytoma, ganglioneuroma, ganglioplexus.*

ganglion (gæŋ'gliən), *pl.* **ganglia. 1.** a knot, or knotlike mass. **2.** one of the nerve cells, chiefly collected in groups outside the central nervous system. Individual cells and very small groups abound in association with alimentary organs. The two types of ganglia in the body are the sensory ganglia on the dorsal roots of spinal nerves and on the sensory roots of the trigeminal, facial, glossopharyngeal, and vagus nerves and the autonomic ganglia of the sympathetic and parasympathetic systems.

ganglionar neuroma, a tumor composed of nerve cells. Also called **ganglionated neuroma, ganglionic neuroma.**

ganglionic blocking agent, any one of a group of drugs prescribed to produce controlled hypotension, as required in certain surgical procedures or in emergency management of hypertensive crisis. The drugs act by occupying receptor sites on sympathetic and parasympathetic nerve endings of autonomic ganglia, preventing response of these nerves to the action of acetylcholine liberated by the presynaptic nerve endings. Trimethaphan and mecamylamine are the most commonly prescribed ganglionic blocking agents. They are used with great caution in treating patients who are affected with coronary, cerebrovascular, or renal insufficiency or who have a history of severe allergy. Adverse reactions to the drugs include sudden marked hypotension, paralytic ileus, urinary retention, constipation, visual disturbances, heartburn, and nausea.

ganglionic crest.   See **neural crest.**

ganglionic glioma,   a tumor composed of glial cells and ganglion cells that are nearly mature. See also **neuroblastoma.**

ganglionic neuroma.   See **ganglionar neuroma.**

ganglionic ridge.   See **neural crest.**

gangliosidosis type I.   See **Tay-Sachs disease.**

gangliosidosis type II.   See **Sandhoff's disease.**

gangrene,   necrosis or death of tissue, usually the result of ischemia (loss of blood supply), bacterial invasion, and subsequent putrefaction. The extremities are most often affected, but it can occur in the intestines and gall bladder. Internally, gangrene may be a complication of strangulated hernia, appendicitis, cholecystitis, or thrombosis of the mesenteric arteries to the gut. **Dry gangrene** is a late complication of diabetes mellitus that is already complicated by arteriosclerosis in which the affected extremity becomes cold, dry, and shriveled and eventually turns black. **Moist gangrene** may follow a crushing injury or an obstruction of blood flow by an embolism, tight bandages, or tourniquet. This form of gangrene has an offensive odor, spreads rapidly, and may result in death in a few days. **Gas gangrene,** caused by anaerobic bacteria of the genus *Clostridium,* is rapidly fatal if antibiotics are not prescribed early in the disease. In all types of gangrene, surgical debridement is necessary to remove the necrotic tissue before healing can progress. Cleanliness and the maintenance of good circulation are nursing considerations essential in preventing this condition. —**gangrenous,** *adj.*

gangrenous necrosis.   See **necrosis.**

gangrenous stomatitis.   See **noma.**

ganja (gan'ja).   *Slang.* See **cannabis.**

Gantanol,   a trade name for an antibacterial (sulfamethoxazole).

Gantrisin,   a trade name for an antibacterial (sulfisoxazole).

gap,   (in molecular genetics) a short, missing segment in one strand of double-stranded DNA.

Garamycin,   a trade name for an antibacterial (gentamicin sulfate).

Gardener's syndrome,   familial polyposis of the large bowel, with fibrous dysplasia of the skull, extra teeth, osteomas, fibromas, and epidermal cysts. The condition is inherited as a dominant trait, and malignancies occur more often than usual in families having this syndrome.

Gardner, Mary Sewell (1871–1961),   an American public health nurse who wrote the classic *Public Health Nurse.* She directed the Providence, Rhode Island, District Nursing Association and was instrumental in the development of the National Organization for Public Health Nursing and of public health nursing in the American Red Cross.

Gardner-Diamond syndrome,   a condition resulting from autoerythrocyte sensitization, marked by large, painful, transient ecchymoses that appear without apparent cause but often accompany emotional upsets, various collagen disorders, and abnormalities of protein metabolism. Treatment includes topical and systemic corticosteriods. Also called **autoerythrocite sensitization syndrome.**

gargle,   **1.** to hold and agitate a liquid at the back of the throat by tilting the head backward and forcing air through the solution. The procedure is used for cleansing or medicating the mouth and oropharynx. **2.** a solution used to rinse the mouth and oropharynx.

gargoylism (gar'goilız'əm).   See **Hurler's syndrome.**

Gartner's duct (gart'nərz),   one of two vestigial, closed ducts, each one parallel to a uterine tube.

gas,   an aeriform fluid possessing complete molecular mobility and the property of indefinite expansion. A gas has no definite shape and its volume is determined by temperature and pressure. Compare **liquid, solid.**

gas chromatography,   the separation and analysis of different substances according to their different affinities for a standard absorbent. In the process a gaseous mixture of the substances is passed through a glass cylinder containing the absorbent, which may be dampened with a nonvolatile liquid solvent for one or more of the gaseous components. As the mixture passes through the absorbent, each substance is absorbed to a different extent and leaves a characteristic pigment. The bands of different colors left when all the gaseous mixture has moved through the absorbent constitute a chromatograph for analysis. Compare **column chromatography, ion-exchange chromatography.**

gas embolism,   an occlusion of one or more small blood vessels, especially in the muscles, tendons, and joints, caused by expanding bubbles of gases. Gas emboli can rupture tissue and blood vessels, causing decompression sickness and death. This phenomenon commonly affects deep-sea divers who rise too quickly to the surface without adequate decompression. Gas emboli are most dangerous in the central nervous system because of associated neurologic changes, as syncope, paralysis, and aphasia. Such embolisms are extremely painful. The prevention and treatment of gas embolisms involve gradual decompression of atmospheric gases, especially nitrogen, that are dissolved in the blood.

gas exchange, impaired, a nursing diagnosis accepted by the Fourth National Conference on the Classification of Nursing Diagnoses. The etiology of the condition is an imbalance in ventilatory perfusion. The defining characteristics are confusion, restlessness, irritability, somnolence, hypercapnea, and hypoxia. See also **nursing diagnosis.**

gas gangrene, necrosis accompanied by gas bubbles in soft tissue following surgery or trauma. It is caused by anaerobic organisms, as various species of *Clostridia,* particularly, *C. perfringens.* Symptoms include pain, swelling, and tenderness of the wound area, moderate fever, tachycardia, and hypotension. The skin around the wound becomes necrotic and ruptures, revealing necrotic muscle. A characteristic finding is toxic delirium. If untreated, gas gangrene is rapidly fatal. Prompt treatment, including excision of gangrenous tissue and administration of penicillin G intravenously, saves 80 per cent of patients. The disease is prevented by proper wound care. Also called **anaerobic myositis.**

gasoline poisoning. See **petroleum distillate poisoning.**

gas scavenging system, the equipment and procedures used to eliminate anesthetic gases that escape into the atmosphere of the operating room. See also **trace gas.**

gaster-. See **gastro-.**

gastr-. See **gastro-.**

gastrectomy, surgical excision of all or, more commonly, part of the stomach, performed to remove a chronic peptic ulcer, to stop hemorrhage in the perforating ulcer, or to remove a malignancy. Preoperatively, a GI series is done and a nasogastric tube is introduced. Under general anesthesia, one half to two thirds of the stomach is removed, including the ulcer and a large area of acid-secreting mucosa. A gastroenterostomy is then done, joining the remainder of the stomach to the jejunum or duodenum. If a malignant tumor is found, the chest cavity is opened and the entire stomach is removed, along with the omentum and, usually, the spleen; the jejunum is anastomosed to the esophagus. Postoperatively, the nurse observes the drainage from the nasogastric suction tube for bright red blood, indicative of hemorrhage. The nurse encourages the person to breathe deeply and to cough. With the return of peristalsis, water is given orally, and, if tolerated without pain or nausea, the tube is removed. A temperature elevation or dyspnea may indicate a leakage of the oral liquids from the incision into the abdomen. Complications of gastrectomy include fullness and discomfort following meals, a marginal ulcer formed when gastric acids come into contact with the mucous membrane of the anastomosis of the jejunum, and painful contractions and vomiting of bile from a blockage of pancreatic juices and bile in the distal end of the duodenum. The diet gradually progresses to six small, bland meals a day, with 120 ml of fluid hourly between meals.

See also **dumping syndrome, gastroenterostomy, G.I. series, nasogastric tube, peptic ulcer.**

-gastria, a combining form meaning '(condition of) possessing a stomach or stomachs': *atretogastria, macrogastria, megalogastria.*

gastric, of or pertaining to the stomach.

-gastric, a combining form meaning a 'type of stomach or number of stomachs': *endogastric, paragastric, trigastric.*

gastric analysis, examination of the contents of the stomach, primarily to determine the quantity of acid present and incidentally to ascertain the presence of blood, bile, bacteria, and abnormal cells. A sample of gastric secretion is obtained via a nasogastric tube. The technique used varies according to the information desired. The total absence of hydrochloric acid is diagnostic of pernicious anemia. Patients with gastric ulcer and gastric cancer may secrete less acid than normal, while patients with duodenal ulcers secrete more. The composition and volume of the secretions may also provide diagnostic information. See also **Diagnex Blue test.**

gastric antacid. See **antacid.**

gastric atrophy. See **atrophic gastritis.**

gastric cancer, a malignancy of the stomach that is declining in incidence in the United States and western Europe. Dietary factors, as nitrates, smoked and salted fish and meats, and moldy foods containing aflatoxin, are thought to cause gastric cancer, but the etiology remains unknown. The incidence is higher in men than in women and peaks in the 50- to 59-year-old age group. The risk is increased in workers exposed to asbestos and in patients with pernicious anemia. Gastric ulcers may become malignant and those that do may have originated as ulcerating cancerous lesions. Symptoms of gastric cancer are vague epigastric discomfort, anorexia, weight loss, and unexplained iron-deficiency anemia; but many cases are asymptomatic in the early stages and metastatic enlargement of the left supraclavicular lymph node may be the first manifestation of a stomach lesion. Diagnostic measures include a test for occult blood in the stool, gastric analysis, x rays of the upper gastrointestinal tract following barium ingestion, examination of gastric mucosa with a flexible endoscope, biopsy, and cytologic studies of exfoliated tumor cells. Approximately 97 per cent of stomach tumors are adenocarcinomas that may be ulcerating, polypoid, diffuse and fibrous, or superficial spreading lesions; lymphomas and leiomyosarcomas account for less than 3 per cent. Radical subtotal gastrectomy with excision of contiguous involved tissues and reconstruction by anastomosing the remainder of the stomach to the duodenum or jejunum is usually recommended. Total gastrectomy is associated with high morbidity and mortality, and it usually leads to pernicious anemia. Radiotherapy and chemotherapy are usually not effective, but postoperative irradiation is recommended to control microscopic residual tumor; combinations of antineoplastic antimetabolites are used in treating advanced, metastatic gastric cancer.

gastric dyspepsia, an abnormal condition characterized by impaired digestion associated with a problem that originates in the stomach. See also **dyspepsia.**

gastric fistula, an abnormal passage into the stomach, communicating most frequently with an opening on the external surface of the abdomen. A gastric fistula may be created surgically to provide tube feeding for patients with severe esophageal disorders.

gastric intubation, a procedure in which a Levin tube or other small-caliber catheter is passed through the nose into the esophagus and stomach for the introduction into the stomach of liquid formulas to provide nutrition for unconscious patients or for premature or sick newborn infants. Medication or a contrast medium may be instilled for treatment or for radiologic examination. Gastric intubation is most often performed to remove the contents of the stomach in order to prevent post-surgical gastric distention, to prevent aspiration of gastric contents during general anesthesia, or to remove a poisonous substance and wash the stomach. See also **gastric lavage, Levin tube.**

gastric juice, digestive secretions of the gastric glands in the stomach, consisting chiefly of pepsin, hydrochloric acid, rennin, lipase, and mucin. The pH is strongly acid (0.9 to 1.5). Achlorhydria (a deficiency of hydrochloric acid in gastric juice) is present in pernicious anemia and stomach cancer. Excessive secretion of gastric juice may lead to mucosal irritation and to peptic ulcer. See also **achlorhydria, gastric analysis, gastric ulcer.**

gastric lavage, the washing out of the stomach with sterile water or a saline solution. The procedure is performed before and after surgery to remove irritants or toxic substances and prior to such examinations as endoscopy or gastroscopy. See also **irrigation.**

gastric motility, the spontaneous peristaltic movements of the stomach which aid in digestion, moving food through the stomach and out through the pyloric sphincter into the duodenum. Excess gastric motility causes pain that is usually treated with antispasmodic medication. Less than normal motility is common in labor, after general anesthesia, and as a side effect of some sedative hypnotics.

gastric node, a node in one of three groups of lymph glands associated with the abdominal and pelvic viscera supplied by branches of the celiac artery. The gastric nodes accompany the left gasric artery and are divided into the superior and inferior gastric nodes. Compare **hepatic node, pancreaticolienal node.**

gastric ulcer, a circumscribed erosion of the mucosal layer of the stomach that may penetrate the muscle layer and perforate the stomach wall. It tends to recur with stress and is characterized by episodes of burning epigastric pain, belching, and nausea, especially when the stomach is empty or after eating certain foods. Characteristically, antacid medication or milk quickly relieves the pain. Treatment includes medication to decrease the acidity and motility of the stomach and to relieve symptomatic stress. If perforation and hemorrhage occur, surgical resection of part of the stomach may be necessary. Also called **peptic ulcer.**

gastrin (gæs'trɪn), a polypeptide hormone, secreted by the pylorus, that stimulates the flow of gastric juice and contributes to the stimulus causing bile and pancreatic enzymes secretion.

gastritis (gæstraɪ'tɪs), an inflammation of the lining of the stomach which occurs in two forms. **Acute gastritis** may be caused by the ingestion of alcohol, aspirin, or other medications or by the presence of viral, bacterial, or chemical toxins. The symptoms—anorexia, nausea, vomiting, and discomfort after eating—usually abate after the causative agent has been removed. **Chronic gastritis** is usually a sign of underlying disease, as peptic ulcer, stomach cancer, Zollinger-Ellison syndrome, or pernicious anemia. Differential diagnosis is by endoscopy with biopsy. Kinds of gastritis include **antral gastritis, atrophic gastritis, hemorrhagic gastritis, hypertrophic gastritis.** Compare **peptic ulcer.**

Gastrix, a trade name for an anticholinergic (oxyphencyclimine hydrochloride).

gastro-, gaster-, gastr-, a combining form meaning 'pertaining to the stomach or abdomen': *gastroadynamia, gastrocolitis, gastrophrenic.*

gastrocnemius (gæs'trokni'miəs), the most superficial muscle in the posterior part of the leg. It arises by a lateral head and a medial head and forms the greater part of the calf. The lateral head arises from the lateral condyle of the femur and the capsule of the knee. The medial head arises from the medial condyle of the femur and from the capsule of the knee. The fibers of both heads insert into a broad aponeurosis which narrows distally to join the tendon of the soleus as part of the tendo calcaneus. Compare **soleus, plantaris.**

gastrocnemius gait, an abnormal gait associated with a weakness of the gastrocnemius. It is characterized by the dropping of the pelvis on the affected side at the last moment of the stance phase in the walking cycle, accompanied by the lagging or the slowness of forward pelvic movement.

gastrocoele (gæs'trousil). See **archenteron.**

gastrocolic omentum (gæs'troukol'ɪk). See **greater omentum.**

gastrocolic reflex, a mass peristaltic movement of the colon that often occurs when food enters the stomach. When an infant is fed, this reflex may result in a bowel movement.

gastrodidymus, conjoined, equally developed twins united at the abdominal region. Also called **omphalodidymus.**

gastrodisc. See **embryonic disc.**

gastroenteritis (gæs′trouen′tərai′tis), inflammation of the stomach and intestines accompanying numerous gastrointestinal disorders. Symptoms are anorexia, nausea, vomiting, abdominal discomfort, and diarrhea. The condition may be attributed to bacterial enterotoxins, bacterial or viral invasion, chemical toxins, or to miscellaneous conditions, as lactose intolerance. The onset may be slow, but more often it is abrupt and violent, with rapid loss of fluids and electrolytes from persistent vomiting and diarrhea. Hypokalemia and hyponatremia, acidosis, or alkalosis may develop. Treatment is supportive, employing bed rest, sedation, intravenous replacement of electrolytes, and antispasmodic medication to control vomiting and diarrhea. With a precise diagnosis, medication and treatment can be specific and curative, as an antitoxin that might be prescribed for gastroenteritis resulting from a bacterial endotoxin. After the acute phase, water may be given by mouth. If it produces no vomiting or diarrhea, clear fluids may be added, followed, if tolerated, by a bland diet.

gastroenterologist (gæs′trouen′tərol′əjist), a physician who specializes in gastroenterology.

gastroenterology (gæs′trouen′tərol′əji), the study of diseases affecting the gastrointestinal tract, including the stomach, intestines, gall bladder, and bile duct.

gastroenterostomy, surgical formation of an artificial opening between the stomach and the small intestine, usually at the jejunum. The operation is performed with a gastrectomy, to route food from the remainder of the stomach into the small intestine, or by itself, for perforating ulcer of the duodenum. A GI series is done preoperatively, and a nasogastric tube is inserted. Under general anesthesia, the jejunum is pulled up and anastomosed with the stomach. A new opening is then made for food to pass from the stomach directly into the jejunum. Pancreatic juices and bile are still secreted into the duodenum and pass through its distal end to the jejunum. Postoperatively, drainage from the nasogastric suction tube is observed for bright-red bleeding, indicative of hemorrhage. Deep breathing and coughing are encouraged. The nasogastric tube is removed when peristalsis returns and when water given orally does not cause pain or nausea. Temperature elevation or dyspnea may indicate a leakage of the fluids from the incision around the anastomosis. The diet is gradually increased to six small, bland meals a day, with 120 ml of fluids hourly between meals. Compare **gastrectomy.**

gastroesophageal (gæs′trouisof′əji′əl), of or pertaining to the stomach and the esophagus.

gastroesophageal hemorrhage. See **Mallory-Weiss syndrome.**

gastroesophageal reflux, a backflow of contents of the stomach into the esophagus that is often the result of incompetence of the lower esophageal sphincter. Gastric juices are acid and therefore produce burning pain in the esophagus. Repeated episodes of reflux may cause esophagitis, peptic esophageal stricture, or esophageal ulcer. In uncomplicated cases, treatment consists of elevation of the head of the bed, avoidance of acid-stimulating foods, and regular administration of antacids. In complicated cases, surgical repair may provide relief. See also **esophagitis, heartburn, hiatus hernia.**

gastrogavage (gæs′trougəvaźh′). See **gastrostomy feeding.**

gastrohepatic omentum. See **lesser omentum.**

gastrointestinal (gæs′trouintes′tinəl), of or pertaining to the organs of the gastrointestinal tract, from mouth to anus.

gastrointestinal allergy, an immediate reaction of hypersensitivity following the ingestion of certain foods or drugs. Gastrointestinal allergy differs from food allergy, which can affect organ systems other than the digestive system. Characteristic symptoms include itching and swelling of the mouth and oral passages, nausea, vomiting, diarrhea (sometimes containing blood), severe abdominal pain, and, if severe, anaphylactic shock. Treatment includes identification and removal of the allergen. In an acute attack epinephrine may be administered as a stimulant, and muscle relaxants may be given to reduce intestinal spasms causing abdominal pain. In childhood, gastrointestinal allergy is most often caused by hypersensitivity to cow's milk and is characterized by diarrhea and colicky pain, sometimes with vomiting, eczema, respiratory distress, and thrombocytopenia. See also **lactose intolerance.**

gastrointestinal bleeding, any bleeding from the gastrointestinal tract. The most common underlying conditions are peptic ulcer, esophageal varices, diverticulitis, ulcerative colitis, and carcinoma of the stomach and colon. Vomiting of bright red blood or the passage of coffee ground vomitus indicates upper gastrointestinal bleeding, usually from the esophagus, stomach, or upper duodenum. Aspiration of the gastric contents, lavage, and endoscopy are performed to determine the site and rate of bleeding. Tarry, black stools indicate a bleeding source in the upper gastrointestinal tract; bright red blood from the rectum usually indicates bleeding in the distal colon. Gastrointestinal bleeding is treated as a potential emergency. Patients may require transfusions or fluid replacement and are watched carefully for signs of shock and hypovolemia. In all patients, blood loss is evaluated and ability to coagulate is tested. See also **coffee ground vomitus, hematochezia, melena.**

gastrointestinal obstruction, any obstruction of the passage of intestinal contents, caused by mechanical blockage or failure of motility. Mechanical blockage may be caused by adhesions resulting from surgery or inflammatory bowel disease, an incarcerated hernia, fecal impaction, tumor, intussusception, or volvulus. Failure of motility may follow anesthesia, abdominal surgery, or occlusion of any of the mesenteric arteries to the gut. Symptoms vary with the cause of obstruction but generally include vomiting, abdominal pain, and increasing abdominal distention. Dehydration and prostration may follow. Characteristically, borborygmus is diminished or absent and abdominal guarding is prominent. A barium enema may be performed, but barium is never given by mouth in such cases because it would increase the volume of the obstruction. The objective of therapy is to remove the obstruction as quickly and safely as possible. A tube is inserted into the stomach or small intestine to aspirate contents and relieve distention. During these procedures, the person is monitored for proper fluid and electrolyte balance. Surgical intervention may be necessary. The nurse helps the person to understand that medication for pain can aggravate the condition by further decreasing motility of the gastrointestinal tract and that it may not be prescribed in the acute period, before the location and extent of the obstruction is discovered.

gastrointestinal system assessment, an evaluation of the patient's digestive system and symptoms.

■ METHOD: Discussion of symptoms is encouraged, and the patcint is asked if there is or has been pain or tenderness in the oral cavity, gums, tongue, lips, or abdomen, if there have been instances of dysphagia, belching, heartburn, anorexia, nausea, vomiting, constipation, diarrhea, or painful defecation. Information is elicited concerning any changes in eating, bowel habits, the color, character, frequency of stools and urine, the use of laxatives or enemas, the occurrence of fatigue, hemorrhoids, and edema of the extremities. The patient's general appearance, weight, and temperature are noted; the blood pressure, pulse and respirations are checked in the supine, sitting, and standing positions, and the urinary output and color are determined. The presence of allergies, stomatitis, halitosis, and the condition of the tongue, gums, oral mucosa, and teeth are recorded. The abdomen is examined for distention, rigidity, ascites, symmetry, hepatomegaly, keloid tissue, visible peristalsis, bowel sounds, masses, and the presence of an ostomy. The perianal area is inspected for its general condition, color, odor, hemorrhoids, the sclera for signs of jaundice, and the skin for pruritis, spider angioma, purpura, palmar erythema, peripheral edema, jaundice, and distended, tortuous blood vessels. Relevant to the assessment are the patient's concurrent endocrine, cardiovascular, and neurologic disorders, severe burns, psychologic problems, carci-

noma, alcohol or drug abuse, and previous gastrointestinal surgery and illnesses, as hepatitis, liver cirrhosis, or pancreatitis. The patient's personality type, attitude toward work, use of tobacco, antacids, laxatives, anticholinergics, steroids, antidiarrheals, antiemetics, sedatives, tranquilizers, barbiturates, antihypertensives, antibiotics, and aspirin are investigated. The family history, especially of gastrointestinal disease, carcinoma, and diabetes, is an important aspect of the evaluation. Diagnostic aids include a complete blood count, stool examination, prothrombin time, and determinations of levels of alkaline phosphatase, serum and urine bilirubin, serum glutamic oxaloacetic transaminase (SGOT), serum glutamic pyruvic transaminase (SGPT), lactic acid dehydrogenase (LDH), blood urea nitrogen, and serum lipase, cholinesterase, calcium, albumin, and glucose. Additional laboratory studies for the evaluation are the total protein level, a serum electrolyte profile, serum carotene, delta-xylose tolerance, galactose tolerance, hippuric acid, and bromosulphalein tests, the albumin-globulin ratio, serum flocculation and thymol turbidity tests, urobilinogen level, the polyvinylpyrrolidone (PVP) test for protein loss, Sulkowitch's test for calcium in urine, and Schilling's test for gastrointestinal absorption of vitamin B_{12}. Procedures that may be required for the diagnosis include upper GI, small bowel and gallbladder series, esophageal and gastric endoscopy and biopsy, scans of the liver and pancreas, biopsies of the liver, colon, or rectum, gastric analysis, sigmoidoscopy, abdominal x rays, fluoroscopy, percutaneous transhepatic cholangiography, splenoportography, and digital rectal examinations.

■ NURSING ORDERS: The nurse conducts the interview, records observations of the patient, and assembles the results of the diagnostic laboratory studies and procedures.

■ OUTCOME CRITERIA: A well-conducted assessment of the patient's gastrointestinal system is a valuable contribution to the diagnosis and plan of treatment.

gastropore. See **blastopore.**

gastroschisis (gæstros′kəsis), a congenital defect characterized by incomplete closure of the abdominal wall with protrusion of the viscera.

gastroscope, a fiberoptic instrument for examining the interior of the stomach. See also **fiberoptics.** —**gastroscopy,** *n.,* **gastroscopic,** *adj.*

gastroscopy (gæstros′kəpi), the visual inspection of the interior of the stomach by means of a gastroscope inserted through the esophagus. The flexible fiberoptic gastroscope has increased the visualization of the prepyloric antrum, but the fundus is still not visible. See also **endoscopy, fiberoptics.** —**gastroscopic,** *adj.*

gastrostomy, surgical creation of an artificial opening into the stomach through the abdominal wall, performed to feed a patient with cancer of the esophagus or one who is expected to be unconscious for a prolonged period. Under local anesthesia, the anterior wall of the stomach is drawn forward and sutured to the abdominal wall. A Foley catheter or other tube or a special prosthesis is then inserted into an incision in the stomach, and the opening is tightly sutured to prevent leakage of the contents of the stomach. The device is clamped, and opened when food is instilled. Postoperatively, glucose in water may be given; then a warm, blended formula is given every four hours. The skin is kept clean and dry around the site. Skin irritation indicates a leakage of gastric secretions and digestive enzymes. After two weeks the tube is withdrawn after feeding and reinserted before the next meal.

gastrostomy feeding, the introduction of a nutrient solution through a tube that has been surgically inserted into the stomach through the abdominal wall. Also called **gastrogavage.**

gastrothoracopagus (gæs′trouˈthɔr′əkop′əgəs), conjoined twins that are united at the thorax and abdomen.

gastrula (gæs′trulə), the early embryonic stage formed by the invagination of the blastula. The cup-shaped gastrula consists of an outer layer of ectoderm and an inner layer of mesentoderm which subsequently differentiates into the mesoderm and endoderm. See also **blastula, embryonic layer.**

-gastrula, a combining form meaning an 'embryonic stage following the blastula': *amphigastrula, discogastrula, paragastrula.*

gastrulation, the development of the gastrula in lower animals and the formation of the three germ layers in the embryo of man and higher animals. It is characterized by an extensive series of coordinated morphogenetic movements within the blastula or blastocyst by which the primitive body plan of the organism is established and by which the areas that later differentiate into various structures and organs are in their proper position for development.

gatch bed, a bed that has an adjustable joint, allowing the knees to be flexed and the legs supported.

Gaucher's disease (gouˈsheiz′), a rare, familial disorder of fat metabolism, owing to an enzyme deficiency, characterized by widespread reticulum cell hyperplasia in the liver, spleen, lymph nodes, and bone marrow. Beginning in infancy or early childhood, splenomegaly, hepatomegaly, and abnormal bone growth develop. Diagnosis is made through biopsy of the liver, spleen, or bone marrow. Mortality is high, but children who survive adolescence may live for many years. Also called **glucosyl cerebroside lipidosis.**

gauntlet bandage (gɔnt′lɪt), a glovelike bandage covering the hand and the fingers. See also **demigauntlet bandage.**

gauze, a transparent fabric of open weave and differing degrees of fineness, most often cotton muslin, used in surgical procedures and for bandages and dressings. It may be sterilized and permeated by an antiseptic or lotion. Kinds of gauze include **absorbable gauze, absorbent gauze, petrolatum gauze.** See also **bandage.**

gavage (gavaźh′), the process of feeding a patient through a nasogastric tube.

gavage feeding of the newborn, a procedure in which a tube passed through the nose or mouth into the stomach is used to feed a newborn infant with weak sucking, uncoordinated sucking and swallowing, respiratory distress, tachypnea, or repeated apneic spells.

■ METHOD: After the gastric tube is inserted, its placement is checked by instilling air and auscultating the stomach for air sounds or by immersing the proximal end of the tube in water (which bubbles if the distal end is misplaced in the infant's respiratory tract). During feeding, the infant is held in a low Fowler's position, preferably by the mother, and is restrained only if necessary. The feeding syringe is held six to eight inches above the infant's head and the flow is initiated by pressure on the plunger. As the formula is slowly instilled, the baby is stroked and is offered a pacifier to promote gravity flow, exert a calming effect, and reinforce the relationship between sucking and feeding. If the infant gags, spits, chokes, regurgitates, vomits, or becomes cyanotic, the rate of flow of formula is reduced and the feeding may be stopped. To prevent air from entering the stomach when the feeding is completed, the tube is pinched closed as it is withdrawn. The infant is burped gently by patting or rubbing the back and then positioned on the right side in the crib; postural drainage and percussion are avoided for at least an hour after feeding. The time, amount, and kind of feeding and the size of tube used are entered in the nursing care plan; if the amount of residual formula left in the infant's stomach at the time of the next feeding exceeds the quantity specified, the next feeding may be delayed or omitted.

■ NURSING ORDERS: The nurse administers intermittent gavage feeding to the infant, offers an explanation to the parents of the need for the procedure, and points out that nipple feedings may be instituted when the infant sucks on the gavage tube or pacifier, roots actively, shows good suck and swallow coordination, gains weight, and has a respiratory rate of less than 60 breaths per minute.

■ OUTCOME CRITERIA: Intermittent gavage feedings can enable the high-risk infant to survive.

gay, *Slang.* **1.** any person who is homosexual. **2.** of or pertaining to homosexuality.

Gay-Lussac's law (geiˈləsæks′), (in physics) a law stating that the volume of a specific mass of a gas will increase as the temperature is increased at a constant rate, determined by the volume of the gas at $0°C$ if the pressure remains constant. Also called **Charles' law.**

Gay Nurses' Alliance (GNA), a national organization of homosexual nurses.

gaze palsy, a partial or complete inability to move the eyes to all directions of gaze. A gaze palsy is often named for the absent direction of gaze, as a right lateral gaze palsy.

GBIA. See **Guthrie test.**

g.c., *Informal.* abbreviation for **gonococcus,** the causative organism of gonorrhea.

Gd, symbol for **gadolinium.**

Ge, symbol for **germanium.**

Geiger counter. See **Geiger-Müller counter.**

Geiger-Müller counter (gaɪ'gərmyl'ər), an electronic device that indicates the level of radioactivity of any substance by counting the number of subatomic particles, as electrons, emitted by a substance. The counter detects ionizing particles with a Geiger-Müller tube. As ionizing particles cross the tube they ionize the gas within the tube and cause an electrical discharge. Also called **Geiger counter.**

gel, a colloid that is firm even though it contains a large amount of liquid, used in many medicines as a demulcent, a vehicle for other drugs, an antacid, or an astringent, depending on the drug from which it is derived.

gelat-, a combining form meaning 'to freeze, congeal': *gelatigenous, gelatinoid, gelatum.*

gelatin film, absorbable, a hemostatic.
- INDICATIONS: It is used to attain hemostasis during surgery, particularly neurologic, thoracic, and ophthalmic procedures.
- CONTRAINDICATIONS: Infection or gross contamination of the surgical wound prohibits its use.
- ADVERSE EFFECTS: There are no known adverse reactions.

gelatiniform carcinoma. See **mucinous carcinoma.**

gelatinous carcinoma, a former term for **mucinous carcinoma.**

gelatin sponge, an absorbable local hemostatic.
- INDICATIONS: It is prescribed to control bleeding in various surgical procedures and in the treatment of decubitus ulcers to promote healing and hemostasis.
- CONTRAINDICATIONS: Frank infection, extensive and abnormal bleeding, postpartum bleeding, or menorrhagia prohibits its use.
- ADVERSE EFFECTS: There are no known adverse reactions.

gel diffusion. See **immunodiffusion.**

Gelfilm, a trade name for an absorbable, hemostatic gelatin film.

Gelfoam, a trade name for an absorbable hemostatic gelatin sponge.

Gelhorn pessary (gel'hɔrn). See **pessary.**

Gelusil, a trade name for a gastrointestinal, fixed-combi-

nation drug containing an antiflatulent (simethicone) and antacids (aluminum and magnesium hydroxide).

gemellary (jem'əler'i), of or pertaining to twins.

gemellipara (jem'əlɪp'ərə), a woman who has given birth to twins.

gemellology (jem'əlol'əji), the study of twins and the phenomenon of twinning.

gemin-, a combining form meaning 'pertaining to a twin, or double': *geminate, gemini, geminous.*

gemma (jem'ə), *pl.* **gemmae.** **1.** a budlike projection produced by lower forms of life during the budding process of asexual reproduction. **2.** any budlike or bulblike structure, as a taste bud or end bulb. —**gemmaceous,** *adj.*

gemmate (jem'eit), **1.** having buds or gemmae. **2.** to reproduce by budding.

gemmation (jemei'shən), the process of cell reproduction by budding. Also called **gemmulation.**

gemmiferous (jemif'ərəs), having buds or gemmae; gemmiparous.

gemmiform (jem'ɪfɔrm), resembling a bud or gemma.

gemmipara (jemɪp'ərə), an animal that produces gemmae or reproduces by budding, such as the hydra. —**gemmiparous,** *adj.*

gemmulation (jem'yʊlei'shən). See **gemmation.**

gemmule (jem'yʊl), (in genetics) **1.** the small, asexual reproductive structure produced by the parent during budding that eventually develops into an independent organism. **2.** (according to the early theory of pangenesis) any of the submicroscopic particles containing hereditary elements that are produced by each somatic cell of the parent, transmitted through the bloodstream to the gametes, and, after fertilization, give rise to cells and tissues that have the exact characteristics as those from which they originated. Compare **biophore.**

Gemonil, a trade name for an anticonvulsant (metharbital).

gen-, a combining form meaning 'to become or produce': *generic, genesiology, genus.*

-gen, **1.** a combining form meaning 'that which generates': *aerogen, proteinogen, venogen.* **2.** a combining form meaning 'that which is generated': *immunogen, ionogen, nitrogen.* Also **-gene.**

Genapax Tampon, a trade name for an anti-infective tampon (gentian violet).

gender, **1.** the classification of the sex of a person into male, female, or intersexual. **2.** the particular sex of a person. See also **sex.**

gender identity, the sense or awareness of knowing to which sex one belongs. The process begins in infancy, continues throughout childhood, and is reinforced during adolescence. Also called **core gender identity.**

gender identity disorder, a condition characterized by a persistent feeling of discomfort or inappropriateness concerning one's anatomical sex. The disorder typically begins in childhood with gender identity problems and is manifested in adolescence or adulthood as asexuality, homosexuality, transvestism, or transsexualism.

gender role, the expression of a person's gender identity; the image that a person presents to both himself and others demonstrating his maleness or femaleness.

gene, the biological unit of genetic material and inheritance. Since the concept of the gene was introduced with Mendelian genetics, it has undergone considerable modification and change and is still evolving as techniques for studying the molecular components of the cell are refined. The gene is now considered to be a particular nucleic acid sequence within a DNA molecule that occupies a precise locus on a chromosome and is capable of self-replication by coding for a specific polypeptide chain. In diploid organisms, which include man and other mammals, genes occur as paired alleles and function in numerous capacities, primarily as structural and regulative components in controlling the differentiation of the cells and tissues of the body. Kinds of genes include **complementary genes, dominant gene, lethal gene, mutant gene, operator gene, pleiotropic gene, recessive gene, regulator gene, structural gene, sublethal gene, supplementary genes, wild-type gene.** See also **chromosome, cistron, DNA, operon.**

-gene. See **-gen.**

gene library, (in molecular genetics) a collection of all of the genetic information of a specific species, obtained from cloned fragments.

general adaptation syndrome, the defense response of the body or the psyche to injury or prolonged stress, as described by Hans Selye. It consists of an initial stage of shock or alarm reaction, followed by a phase of increasing resistance or adaptation, utilizing the various defense mechanisms of the body or mind, and culminating in either a state of adjustment and healing or of exhaustion and disintegration. Also called **adaptation syndrome.** See also **post-traumatic stress disorder, stress.**

general anesthesia, the absence of sensation and consciousness as induced by various anesthetic agents, given primarily by inhalation or intravenous injection. Four kinds of nerve blocks attained by general anesthesia are sensory, voluntary motor, reflex motor, and mental. There are several levels of mental block: calmness, sedation, hypnosis, narcosis, and complete, potentially lethal depression of all vital regulatory functions of the medulla in the brain. The kind of anesthesia selected and the dose and route by which it is given depend on the indication for anesthesia. The depth of anesthesia is planned to allow the surgical procedure to be performed without the patient's experiencing pain or having any recall of the procedure. Endotracheal intubation and respiratory support are often necessary. General anesthesia may be administered only by a physician or a Certified Registered Nurse Anesthetist. See also **stages of anesthesia.**

generalized anaphylaxis, a severe reagin-mediated reaction to an allergen characterized by itching, edema, wheezing respirations, apprehension, cyanosis, dyspnea, pupillary dilation, a rapid, weak pulse, and falling blood pressure, that may rapidly result in shock and death. Systemic anaphylaxis, the most extreme form of hypersensitivity, may be caused by insect stings, proteins in animal sera, food, or certain drugs; parenterally administered penicillin and contrast media containing iodide are frequent causes of anaphylactic shock, especially in individuals with a history of allergies. An anaphylactic reaction is mediated by reaginic antibodies (IgE) that form in response to an initial sensitizing dose of an allergen and render the individual hypersensitive to the allergen by binding it to mast cells and basophils. A subsequent challenging dose of the allergen, causing the cells to degranulate and release histamine, bradykinin, and other vasoactive amines, produces anaphylaxis; the severity of the reaction depends on several factors, including the amount and route of entrance of the sensitizing and challenging

The three stages of the general adaptation syndrome

Alarm	Resistance stage	Exhaustion stage
Increased secretion of glucocorticoids and resultant changes	Glucocorticoid secretion returns to normal	Increased glucocorticoid secretion sometimes to higher levels than during alarm reaction
Increased activity of sympathetic nervous system	Sympathetic activity returns to normal	
Increased norepinephrine secretion by adrenal medulla	Norepinephrine secretion returns to normal	
"Fight or flight" syndrome of changes	"Fight or flight" syndrome disappears	
Low resistance to stressors	High resistance (adaptation) to stressor	Loss of resistance to stressor; may lead to death
Stress triad (hypertrophied adrenals, atrophied thymus and lymph nodes, bleeding ulcers in stomach and duodenum)		

doses of the allergen. Treatment of generalized anaphylaxis consists of an immediate subcutaneous or intramuscular injection of 1:1000 epinephrine hydrochloride, the administration of an antihistamine, as tripelennamine or diphenhydramine, and isoproterenol or aminophylline to relieve bronchial spasm. A vasopressor may be given to increase blood pressure and a corticosteroid to suppress the immune response. The patient's legs are elevated to counteract shock; oxygen may be administered by a positive pressure mask, and, if tracheal edema is present an endotracheal tube, may be inserted or a tracheostomy performed. See also **reagin-mediated disorder.**

generally recognized as effective (GRAE), one of the statutory criteria that must be met by a drug before it can be approved as a 'new drug.' Meeting these criteria relieves the manufacturer of the necessity of obtaining premarket approval as required by the Federal Food, Drug, and Cosmetic Act. To be recognized as effective, the drug must be, according to the Act, considered safe and effective by "experts qualified by scientific training and experience." See also **generally recognized as safe.**

general paralysis of the insane (GPI). *Obsolete.* See **general paresis.**

general paresis, an organic mental disorder resulting from chronic syphilitic infection, characterized by degeneration of the cortical neurons; progressive dementia, tremor, and speech disturbances; muscular weakness; and, ultimately, generalized paralysis. It is often accompanied by periods of exultation and delusions of grandeur. Treatment usually consists of large doses of penicillin without which the outcome is almost invariably progressive deterioration and death. Also called **cerebral tabes, dementia paralytica, general paralysis of the insane, paretic dementia, syphilitic meningoencephalitis.**

general practitioner (GP), a family practice physician. See also **family medicine.**

generation, 1. the act or process of reproduction; procreation. 2. a group of contemporary individuals, animals, or plants that are the same number of life cycles from a common ancestor. 3. the period of time between the birth of one individual or organism and the birth of its offspring. Kinds of generation include **alternate generation, asexual generation, filial generation, parental generation, sexual generation, spontaneous generation.**

generic, 1. of or pertaining to a genus. 2. of or pertaining to a substance, product, or drug that is not protected by trademark. 3. of or pertaining to the name of a kind of drug that is also the description of the drug, as penicillin or tetracycline.

generic equivalent, a drug product sold under its generic name, identical in chemical composition to one or more others sold under a trade name but not, necessarily, equivalent in therapeutic effect.

generic name, the official, established nonproprietary name assigned to a drug. A given drug is licensed under its generic name, and all manufacturers of the drug list it by its generic name. However, a drug is usually marketed under a trade name chosen by the manufacturer. See also **chemical name, established name.**

generic nursing program, a program to prepare people with no previous professional nursing experience for entry into the field of nursing, now usually used to distinguish baccalaureate programs from master's programs or practitioner programs.

-genesia, 1. a combining form meaning a '(specified) condition concerning information': *agenesia, morphogenesia, paragenesia.* 2. a combining form meaning 'the production or procreation of something (specified)': *algogenesia, palingenesia, syngenesia.* Also **-genesis.**

genesis, 1. the origin, generation, or developmental evolution of anything. 2. the act of producing or procreating. **– genetic,** *adj.*

-genesis. See **-genesia.**

gene splicing, (in molecular genetics) the process by which a segment of DNA is attached to or inserted in a strand of DNA from another source. In recombinant DNA technology genetic material from man and other mammals is spliced into bacterial plasmids.

genetic, 1. pertaining to reproduction, birth, or origin. 2. pertaining to genetics or heredity. 3. pertaining to or produced by a gene; inherited.

-genetic, 1. a combining form meaning 'pertaining to generation by (specified) agents': *gamogenetic, mitogenetic, spermatogenetic.* 2. a combining form meaning 'generating': *glycogenetic, ovigenetic, ureagenetic.* 3. a combining form meaning 'pertaining to something generated by a (specified) agent': *biogenetic, ideogenetic, phylogenetic.* Also **-genic, -genous, -geneous.**

genetic affinity, relationship by direct descent.

genetic code, the information carried by the DNA molecules that determines the specific amino acids and their arrangement in the polypeptide chain of each protein synthesized by the cell. The code represents the sequence of nucleotides along the DNA molecule of each chromosome, and, during transcription, this arrangement is synthesized in messenger RNA and carried from the nucleus to the cytoplasm of the cell where it is translated into protein at the site of the ribosomes. A unit of three consecutive nucleotides, or a codon, codes for each amino acid of the protein molecule. Any change in the code results in the incorrect arrangement of the amino acids in the protein, causing a mutation. See also **transcription, translation.**

genetic colonization, the process by which a parasite introduces into its host genetic information that induces the host to synthesize products solely for the use of the parasite.

genetic counseling, the process of determining the occurrence or risk of occurrence of a genetic disorder within a family and of providing appropriate information and advice about the courses of action that are available, whether care of a child already affected, prenatal diagnosis, termination of a pregnancy, sterilization, or artificial insemination is involved. Effective genetic counseling requires an accurate diagnosis of the condition, sometimes necessitating special biochemical or cytogenetic tests, because many of the some 2,000 known inherited disorders have similar clinical manifestations but totally different modes of inheritance; a careful, detailed family history, recorded in the form of a pedigree chart; and an understanding of genetic principles, especially a knowledge of the risks related to multifactorial inheritance. The most efficient counseling services consist of a group of specialists, including physicians, geneticists, psychologists, biochemists, cytologists, nurses, and social workers. It is especially important that nurses be alert to those situations in which persons may need genetic counseling, become familiar with facilities in the area that provide genetic counseling services, and help couples arrive at tentative decisions regarding future family planning or the care of a child with a genetic disorder. See also **genetic screening, prenatal diagnosis.**

genetic death, 1. the failure of an organism to survive as a result of its genetic makeup. 2. the removal of a gene or genotype from the gene pool of a population or a given familial descent because of sterility, failure of the individual or organism to reproduce, or death before sexual maturity.

genetic disorder. See **inherited disorder.**

genetic drift, the chance fluctuations in gene frequencies within a population. The smaller the population, the greater the tendency for variation within each generation, so that eventually small, isolated inbreeding groups become genetically quite different from the ancestors from which they derived. Also called **drift, random genetic drift.**

genetic engineering, the process of producing recombinant DNA so that the genotype and phenotype of organisms can be altered and controlled. Enzymes are used to break the DNA molecule into fragments so that genes from another organism can be inserted and the nucleotides rearranged in any desired sequence. Through genetic engineering such human proteins as the growth hormone, insulin, and interferon have been produced in bacteria by using the recombinant DNA technique. At present, genetic engineering represents a powerful tool for medical research and is possible only in microorganisms; but in the future, the technique may be applicable to higher organisms, with the possibility of controlling and eliminating genetic disorders and malformations in man.

genetic equilibrium, the state within a population at which the frequency of genes and genotypes does not change from generation to generation. The condition routinely occurs in a large interbreeding population in which mating is random and there are no or relatively few mutations. See also **Hardy-Weinberg equilibrium principle.**

genetic homeostasis, the maintenance of genetic variability within a population through adaptation to varied or changing environments and conditions of life as a result of shifts or resistance to shifts in gene frequencies.

genetic immunity. See **natural immunity.**

genetic isolate, a group of plants, animals, or individuals that are genetically separated by geographical, racial, social, cultural, or any other barriers that prevent them from interbreeding with those outside of the group. Depending on the size of the group and the amount of inbreeding that occurs, genetic isolates generally show an increased incidence of otherwise rare, inherited defects. See also **deme.**

geneticist, one who specializes in the study or application of genetics.

genetic load, the average number of accumulated detrimental genes per individual within a population, including those caused by mutation and selection within a recent generation and those inherited from ancestors. Genetic load is measured according to lethal equivalents.

genetic map, the graphic representation of the linear arrangement of genes on a chromosome and the relative distance between them, as expressed in map or morgan units. Also called **linkage map.**

genetic marker, any specific gene that produces a readily recognizable genetic trait that can be used in family and population studies or in linkage analysis. Also called **gene marker, marker gene.**

genetic polymorphism, the recurrence within a population of two or more discontinuous genetic variants of a specific trait in such proportions that they cannot be maintained simply by mutation, as the sickle cell trait, the Rh factor, and the blood groups. Compare **balanced polymorphism.**

genetic population. See **deme.**

genetics, 1. the science that studies the principles and mechanics of heredity, specifically the means by which traits are passed from parents to offspring and the causes of the similarities and differences between related organisms. 2. the total genetic makeup of a particular individual, family, group, or condition. Kinds of genetics are **clinical genetics, molecular genetics, population genetics.** See also **cytogenetics, Mendel's laws.**

genetic screening, the process of investigating a specific population of persons for the purpose of detecting the presence of disease, either incipient or overt, as the generalized screening of all newborn infants for phenylketonuria, of identifying those who possess defective genes, of gaining information concerning the incidence of a disorder in the population, and of providing reproductive information, specifically to those at risk, as the close relatives of persons affected with inborn errors of metabolism or those in certain ethnic groups who have a high incidence of a particular disease, specifically sickle cell anemia in blacks and Tay-Sachs disease in Ashkenazic Jews. When accompanied by education and counseling, mass screening programs can be effective in the management of genetic disorders. See also **genetic counseling.**

Genga's bandage (jeng'gəz). See **Theden's bandage.**

-genia, a combining form meaning '(condition or development of the) jaw': *microgenia, opisthogenia, progenia.*

-genic, 1. a combining form meaning 'causing, forming, producing': *collagenic, hemorrhagenic, phosphagenic.* 2. a combining form meaning 'produced by or formed from': *bacillogenic, coccigenic, pituitarigenic.* 3. a combining form meaning 'related to a gene': *intragenic, polygenic, trigenic.*

geniculate neuralgia, a severe, debilitating, inflammatory condition of the geniculate ganglion of the facial nerve, characterized by pain, loss of the sense of taste, facial paralysis, and a decrease in salivation and lacrimation. It sometimes follows herpes zoster infection. See also **Ramsay Hunt's syndrome.**

geniculate zoster. See **herpes zoster.**

geniohyoideus (ji'niouhaioi'diəs), one of the four suprahyoid muscles, arising from the symphysis menti of the lower jaw and inserting into the body of the hyoid bone. A narrow muscle, it is innervated by a branch of the first cervical nerve, and it acts to draw the hyoid bone and the tongue forward. Also called **geniohyoid muscle.** Compare **digastricus, mylohyoideus, stylohyoideus.**

genital herpes. 1. See **herpes genitalis.** 2. See **herpes simplex.**

genital reflex. See **sexual reflex.**

genitals, genitalia, the reproductive organs. — **genital,** *adj.*

genital stage, (in psychoanalysis) the final period in psychosexual development, beginning with adolescence and continuing through the adult years when the genitals are the predominant source of pleasurable stimulation. The most significant feature of this stage is direction of sexual interest not just toward self-satisfaction but toward the establishment of a stable and meaningful heterosexual relationship. See also **psychosexual development.**

genitourinary (GU), referring to the genital and urinary systems of the body, either the organ structures or functions or both. Also called **urogenital.**

genitourinary system. See **urogenital system.**

genome (ji'noum), the complete set of genes in the chromosomes of each cell of a particular organism.

genotype (ji'noutaip'), 1. the complete genetic constitution of an organism or group, as determined by the particular combination and location of the genes on the chromosomes. 2. the alleles situated at one or more sites on homologous chromosomes. The genetic information carried by a pair of alleles determines a specific characteristic or trait, usually designated by a letter or symbol, as AA when the alleles are identical and Aa when they are different. 3. a group or class of organisms having the same genetic makeup; the type species of a genus. Compare **phenotype.** — **genotypic,** *adj.*

-genous, a combining form meaning 'producing or produced by': *tetanigenous, thyroigenous, tuberculigenous.*

Gensoul's disease (zhansulz'). See **Ludwig's angina.**

gentamicin sulfate (jen'təmai'sın), an aminoglycoside antibiotic.

■ INDICATIONS: It is prescribed to relieve the effects of of severe infections caused by organisms sensitive to gentamicin.

■ CONTRAINDICATIONS: Concomitant administration of other potentially ototoxic drugs or known hypersensitivity to this drug or to other aminoglycoside medication prohibits its use. It is used with caution in patients having impaired renal function.

■ ADVERSE EFFECTS: Among the more serious adverse reactions are nephrotoxicity, auditory or vestibular ototoxicity, impairment of neuromuscular transmission, and hypersensitivity reactions.

gentian violet (jen'shon), an antibacterial anti-infective, antifungal, and anthelmintic.

■ INDICATIONS: It is prescribed in the treatment of pinworms, superficial infections of the skin, and vaginal infections.

■ CONTRAINDICATIONS: Known hypersensitivity to this drug prohibits its use. It is not applied to ulcerative lesions of the face.

■ ADVERSE EFFECTS: Among the most serious adverse reactions are permanent discoloration of the skin following topical exposure to the drug. Gastrointestinal distress and purple vomitus may occur following oral administration.

gentiotannic acid (jen'shiotæn'ık), a form of tannic acid once used as an astringent and in the treatment of burns but no longer recommended because the compound is hepatotoxic.

Gentran 40, a trade name for a plasma volume extender (dextran 40).

Gentran 75, a trade name for a plasma volume extender (dextran 75).

genuine issue, (in law) an issue that is upheld by substantial evidence. It is a real issue, not a false one or one that is subject to interpretation.

genupectoral position, knee-chest position. To assume the genupectoral position, the person kneels so that the weight of his body is supported by the knees and chest, with the abdomen raised. The head is turned to one side and the arms are flexed so that the upper part of the body can be supported in part by the elbows.

genus (ji'nəs), *pl.* **genera** (jen'ərə). a subdivision of a family of animals or plants. A genus usually is composed of several closely related species, but the genus *Homo sapiens* has only one species, humans. See also **family.**

genu valgum (ji'nu), a deformity in which the legs are curved inward so that the knees are close together, knocking as the person walks, with the ankles widely separated. Also called **knock-knee.**

genu varum, a deformity in which one or both legs are bent outward at the knee. Also called **bowleg.** Compare **genu valgum.**

-geny, a combining form meaning 'production, generation, origin': *homogeny, hylogeny, morphogeny.*

geo-, a combining form meaning 'pertaining to the earth, or soil': *geobiology, geophagia, geotropism.*

Geocillin, a trade name for an antibacterial (carbenicillin indanyl sodium).

geographic tongue, a disorder in which small white or yellowish plaques develop on the tongue, gradually enlarge, and desquamate in the center, leaving denuded red patches surrounded by thickened white borders that converge, forming figures with scalloped outlines. The disorder, which may persist for months or years, causes a burning or itching sensation, is aggravated by food, and is often associated with digestive problems, especially in children.

geometric mean. See **mean,** def. 3.

Geopen, a trade name for an antibacterial (carbenicillin disodium).

geotrichosis (ji'outrıkou'sıs), an abnormal condition associated with the fungus *Geotrichum candidum,* which may cause oral, bronchial, pharyngeal, and intestinal disorders. *Geotrichum candidum,* normally found in healthy individuals, the soil, and in dairy products, is not necessarily pathogenic. Geotrichosis most commonly occurs in immunosuppressed individuals and in diabetics. Bronchopulmonary complications associated with this disorder may produce a cough with thick, bloody sputum. Geotrichosis has produced allergic asthmatic reactions similar to allergic aspergillosis and a type of intestinal disorder characterized by abdominal pain, diarrhea, and rectal bleeding. Oral lesions that may develop from this disorder are commonly treated with a solution of gentian violet; associated abdominal lesions are treated with the oral administration of gentian violet capsules; associated pulmonary lesions are treated with the oral administration of potassium iodide.

geriatrician (jer'iətrıʃh'ən), a medical specialist in the field of geriatrics.

geriatrics (jer'iæt'rıks), the branch of medicine dealing with the physiology of aging and the diagnosis and treatment of diseases affecting the aged.

germ, 1. any microorganism, especially one that is pathogenic. 2. a unit of living matter able to develop into a self-sufficient organism, as a seed, spore, or egg. 3. (in embryology) the first stage in development, as a spermatozoon or other germ cell.

germanium (Ge), a metallic element with some nonmetallic properties. Its atomic number is 32; its atomic weight is 72.59.

German measles. See **rubella.**

germ cell, 1. a sexual reproductive cell in any stage of development, from the primordial embryonic form to the mature gamete. 2. an ovum or spermatozoon or any of their preceding forms. 3. any cell undergoing gametogenesis. Also called **gonoblast, gonocyte.** Compare **somatic cell.**

germ disc. See **embryonic disc.**

germicide, a drug that kills pathogenic microorganisms. See also **antibacterial,** def. 2, **antifungal,** def. 2, **antiviral,** def. 2. – **germicidal,** *adj.*

germinal (jər'mınəl), pertaining to or characteristic of a germ cell or to the early stages of development.

germinal disc. See **embryonic disc.**

germinal epithelium, 1. the epithelial layer covering the genital ridge from which the gonads are derived in early embryonic development. 2. the epithelial covering of the ovary, formerly thought to be the site of the formation of the oogonia. See also **oogenesis.**

germinal membrane. See **blastoderm.**

germinal nucleus. See **pronucleus.**

germinal pole. See **animal pole.**

germinal spot, the nucleolus of a mature oocyte, prior to fertilization. See also **oogenesis, ovum.**

germinal stage, (in embryology) the interval of time from fertilization to implantation during which the ovum undergoes cell division several times, travels to the uterus, and, in the form of a blastocyst, begins to implant itself in the endometrium. The germinal stage is over at about 10 days of gestation.

germinal vesicle, the nucleus of a mature oocyte prior to fertilization. Much larger than the nucleus of other cells, it initiates the completion of meiotic division after fertilization. See also **oogenesis, ovum.**

germination, 1. the initial growth and development of an organism from the time of fertilization to the formation of the embryo. 2. the sprouting of a spore or the seed of a plant. – **germinate,** *v.*

germ layer, one of the three primordial cell layers formed during gastrulation in the early stages of embryonic development from which the entire range of body tissue is derived. Each layer has the potentiality for forming different cellular types that differentiate into the various structures and organs of the body. See also **ectoderm, endoderm, mesoderm.**

germ nucleus. See **pronucleus.**

germ plasm, 1. the protoplasm of the germ cells containing the basic reproductive and hereditary material;

the sum total of the DNA in a particular cell or organism. The substance was first named by August Weismann to indicate the material that originates in the germ cell, produces new organisms, transmits hereditary characteristics, and passes in direct continuity to germ cells of succeeding generations. **2.** (in nontechnical use) germ cells in any stage of development together with the tissues from which they originated. Compare **somatoplasm.** See also **Weismannism.**

germ plasm theory. See **Weismannism.**

gero-, geronto-, a combining form meaning 'pertaining to old age or the aged': *gerocomia, gerodontology, geromarasmus.*

-gerontic, a combining form meaning 'pertaining to old age': *paragerontic, phylogerontic, ungerontic.* Also **-gerontal.**

geronto-. See **gero-.**

gerontology, the study of the aging process.

-gerous, a combining form meaning 'bearing or characterized by' something specified: *calcigerous, ovigerous, setigerous.*

gestalt (gəshtalt′), *pl.* **gestalts, gestalten** (gəshtalt′ən). a single physical, psychological, or symbolic configuration, pattern, or experience consisting of a number of elements, that has an effect as a whole different from that of the sum of its parts.

Gestaltism (gəshtalt′ızəm). See **Gestalt psychology.**

Gestalt psychology, a school of psychology, originating in Germany, that maintains that a psychological phenomenon is perceived as a total configuration or pattern, rising from the relationships among its constituent elements, rather than as discrete elements possessing attributes of their own, and that the pattern, or gestalt, cannot be derived from the summation of its constituents. Thus, learning is regarded as resulting from insight, defined as a process or reorganization, rather than from association or trial and error, and behavior is seen as an integrated response to a unitary situation rather than as a series of reflexes and sensations. Also called **configurationism, Gestaltism.** See also **gestalt.**

Gestalt therapy, a form of psychotherapy that stresses the unity of self-awareness, behavior, and experience. It incorporates elements of psychoanalytic, behavioristic, and humanistic-existential therapy. See **Gestalt psychology.**

gestate, 1. to carry a developing fetus in the womb. **2.** to grow and develop slowly toward maturity, as a fetus in the womb.

gestation, the length of pregnancy in viviparous animals; the period of time from the fertilization of the ovum until birth. Gestation varies with the species; in man the average duration is 266 days or approximately 280 days from the onset of the last menstrual period. See also **pregnancy.**

gestational age, the age of a fetus or a newborn, usually expressed in weeks dating from the first day of the mother's last menstrual period.

gestational diabetes, a disorder characterized by an impaired ability to metabolize carbohydrate, usually caused by a deficiency of insulin, occurring in pregnancy and disappearing after delivery but, in some cases, returning years later. There is evidence that placental lactogen and considerable destruction of insulin by the placenta play a role in precipitating gestational diabetes. Treatment consists of insulin injections, a high protein diet, and an adequate intake of calcium and iron, but no attempt is made to keep the patient's urine free of sugar. See also **diabetes mellitus.**

-geusia, a combining form meaning, '(condition of the) sense of taste': *glycogeusia, hemiageusia, parageusia.* Also **-geustia.**

-geustia. See **-geusia.**

GH, abbreviation for **growth hormone.**

GHRF, abbreviation for **growth hormone releasing factor.**

giant cell arteritis. See **temporal arteritis.**

giant cell carcinoma, a malignant epithelial neoplasm characteristically containing numerous very large anaplastic cells. A small percentage of adenocarcinomas of the lung and some liver tumors also contain such cells. Also called **carcinoma gigantocellulare.**

giant cell interstitial pneumonia. See **interstitial pneumonia.**

giant cell myeloma, a bone tumor of multinucleated giant cells that resembles osteoclasts scattered in a matrix of spindle cells. Myelomas of this kind may be benign or malignant and may cause pain, functional disability, and, in some cases, pathologic fractures. Also called **giant cell tumor of bone.**

giant cell thyroiditis. See **de Quervain's thyroiditis.**

giant cell tumor of bone. See **giant cell myeloma.**

giant chromosome, any of the excessively large chromosomes found in insects and the lower animals, specifically the lampbrush chromosome and polytene chromosome.

giant follicular lymphadenopathy (lımfæd′ınop′əthi). See **giant follicular lymphoma.**

giant follicular lymphoma, a nodular, well-differentiated, lymphocytic, malignant lymphoma in which many nodules distort the normal structure of a lymph node. Also called **Brill-Symmer's disease, giant follicular lymphadenopathy, Symmer's disease.**

giant hypertrophic gastritis, a rare disease characterized by large folds of nodular gastric rugae that may cover the wall of the stomach, causing anorexia, nausea, vomiting, and abdominal distress. X-ray or endoscopic examination or surgery may be necessary for diagnosis. The nurse usually recommends periodic re-examination because the disease is associated with an incidence of stomach cancer that is greater than normal.

Giardia (jiar'diə), a common genus of the flagellate protozoans. Many species of *Giardia* normally inhabit the digestive tract causing inflammation in association with other factors that produce rapid proliferation of the organism. See also **giardiasis**.

giardiasis (ji'ardai'əsis), an inflammatory, intestinal condition caused by overgrowth of the protozoan *Giardia lamblia*. The source of infection is usually untreated water contaminated with *G. lamblia* cysts. Also called **traveler's diarrhea**.

gibbus (gib'əs, jib'əs), **1.** a hump, swelling, or enlargement on a body surface, usually confined to one side. **2.** a convex spinal curvature that may occur after the collapse of a vertebral body as may result from a fracture or tuberculosis of the spine.

Gibraltar fever. See **brucellosis**.

Gibson walking splint (gib'sən), a kind of Thomas splint that allows a patient to be ambulatory.

Giemsa's stain (giem'zəz), an azure dye used as a stain in the microscopic examination of the blood for certain protozoan parasites, viral inclusion bodies, rickettsia, and, more routinely, in the preparation of a smear for a differential white cell count.

gigantic acid, an antibiotic substance derived from *Aspergillus giganteus,* a species of mold.

gigantism (jigæn'tizəm), an abnormal condition characterized by excessive size and stature, caused most frequently by hypersecretion of growth hormone (GH) and occurring to a lesser degree in hypogonadism and in certain genetic disorders. Gigantism with normal body proportions and normal sexual development usually results from hypersecretion of GH in early childhood. Hypogonadism, by delaying puberty and closure of the epiphyses, may lead to gigantism. Excessive linear growth often occurs in males with more than one Y chromosome, and it may accompany Klinefelter's syndrome, Marfan's syndrome, and some cases of generalized lipodystrophy. Children with cerebral gigantism are mentally retarded and have a large head and extremities and a clumsy gait. They grow rapidly during their first few years and then at a normal rate. Appropriate gonadal hormones may be administered to control abnormal growth of children with hypogonadism. The treatment of acromegalic gigantism is usually irradiation, but hypophysectomy may be indicated. See also **acromegaly, eunuchoidism**.

giganto-, a combining form meaning 'huge': *gigantoblast, gigantochromoblast, gigantocyte*.

Gilbert's syndrome, a benign, hereditary condition characterized by hyperbilirubinemia and jaundice. No treatment is required.

Gilchrist's disease (gil'krists). See **blastomycosis**.

Gilles de la Tourette syndrome (ẑhil'dələturet'), an

abnormal condition characterized by facial grimaces, tics, and involuntary arm and shoulder movements. In adolescence, the condition worsens; the child may grunt, snort, and shout involuntarily. Coprolalia often develops, to the consternation of the person and the people around the person afflicted. In adulthood the condition usually does not worsen; it comes and goes. Recently, treatment with dopamine antagonists has been found to be very effective, demonstrating an organic cause for this syndrome.

gingiva (jinjai'və), *pl.* **gingivae.** the gum of the mouth, a mucous membrane with supporting fibrous tissue that overlies the crowns of unerupted teeth and encircles the necks of those that have erupted. – **gingival,** *adj.*

gingival hyperplasia, overgrowth of the soft tissue of the gums, often seen in patients treated with phenytoin for epileptic seizures.

gingival papilla. See under **papilla**.

gingivectomy, surgical removal of infected and diseased gingival tissue, performed to arrest the development of pyorrhea. Under general anesthesia, all pockets around the teeth are scraped and hypertrophied tissue is removed. The exposed surface of the gum is covered with packing to prevent trauma while eating and to allow new epithelial tissue to cover and fill in the areas. Considerable bleeding and pain are associated with the procedure. Postoperatively, the patient is closely observed for signs that may indicate hemorrhage, as excess bleeding, frequent swallowing, or a rise in pulse rate. The packing is removed one week later.

gingivitis (jin'jivai'tis), a condition in which the gums are red, swollen, and bleeding. Most gingivitis is the result of poor oral hygiene and of the accumulation of bacterial plaque on the teeth, but it may be a sign of another condition, as diabetes mellitus, leukemia, or vitamin deficiency. It is common in pregnancy, usually painless, and may be acute or chronic. Frequent removal of plaque and regular visits to the dentist may be preventive. Compare **Vincent's infection**. See also **hypertrophic gingivitis**.

gingivo-, a combining form meaning 'pertaining to the gingiva': *gingivoglossitis, gingivolabial, gingivosis*.

gingivostomatitis (jin'jivoustou'mətai'tis), multiple, painful ulcers on the gums and mucous membranes of the mouth, the result of a herpesvirus infection. Seen most frequently in infants and young children, the condition usually subsides after a week, but, in rare cases, it may progress to a systemic viral infection. See also **herpes simplex**.

ginglymus joint (jin'gliməs). See **hinge joint**.

Giordano-Giovannetti diet (jorda'nou jou'vənet'i,) a low-protein, low-fat, high-carbohydrate diet with controlled potassium and sodium intake, used in chronic renal insufficiency and liver failure. Protein is given only in the form of essential amino acids so that the body will use excess blood urea nitrogen to synthesize the nonessential amino acids for the production of tissue protein. The foods included are eggs, small amounts of milk, low-protein bread, some fruits and vegetables low in potassium, as green beans, summer squash, cabbage, pears, grapefruit, and fresh or frozen blackberries, blueberries, and boysenberries. There are many modified forms of this diet depending on patient requirements and tolerance, usually varying in the amount and origin of the protein. Also called **Giovannetti diet.** See also **renal diet.**

Giovannetti diet. See **Giordano-Giovannetti diet.**

Gitaligin, a trade name for a cardiotonic (gitalin).

gitalin (jɪt′əlɪn), a combination of digitalis glycosides.

■ INDICATIONS: It is prescribed as a cardiotonic in the treatment of congestive heart failure, atrial fibrillation, and atrial tachycardia.

■ CONTRAINDICATIONS: Ventricular fibrillation, ventricular tachycardia, concomitant administration of calcium salts, or known hypersensitivity to this drug prohibits its use.

■ ADVERSE EFFECTS: The most serious adverse reactions are various cardiac arrhythmias.

glabrous skin, smooth, hairless skin.

gland, any one of many organs in the body, comprising specialized cells that secrete or excrete materials not related to their ordinary metabolism. Some glands lubricate; others, like the pituitary gland, produce hormones; hematopoietic glands, like the spleen, thyroid, and certain lymph nodes, take part in the production of blood.

Goblet cells (dark)

Simple tubular

Branched tubular

Compound
tubuloalveolar

Coiled tubular
GLAND TYPES

glanders (glæn′dərz), an infection caused by the bacillus *Pseudomonas mallei,* transmitted to humans from horses and other domestic animals. It is characterized by purulent inflammation of the mucous membranes and the development of skin nodules that ulcerate. If untreated with antibiotics, the infection may spread to the bones, liver, central nervous system, and other tissues and cause death. It is endemic in Africa, Asia, and South America but has been eradicated in Europe and North America.

gland of Montgomery. See **areolar gland.**

glands of Zeiss. See **ciliary gland.**

glandular carcinoma. See **adenocarcinoma.**

glandular fever. See **infectious mononucleosis.**

glandula vestibularis major. See **Bartholin's gland.**

glans, *pl.* **glandes. 1.** a general term for a small, rounded mass, or glandlike body. **2.** erectile tissue, as on the ends of the clitoris and the penis.

glans clitoridis. See **glans of clitoris.**

glans of clitoris, the erectile tissue at the end of the clitoris, continuous with the intermediate part of the vaginal vestibular bulbs. It comprises two corpora cavernosa enclosed in a dense, fibrous membrane and connected to the pubis and ischium. Also called **glans clitoridis.**

glans penis, the conical tip of the penis that covers the end of the corpora vavemosa penis and the corpus spongiosom like a cap. The urethral orifice is normally located at the center of the distal tip of the glans penis; the corona glandis, the widest part of the glans penis, is around the base of the proximal portion. A fold of dark, thin, hairless skin forms the foreskin covering the glans penis.

Glanzmann's disease (glants′manz). See **thrombasthenia.**

Glasgow Coma Scale (glæs′gou), a quick, practical, and standardized system for assessing the degree of conscious impairment in the critically ill and for predicting the duration and ultimate outcome of coma, primarily in patients with head injuries. The system involves three determinants: eye opening, verbal response, and motor response, all of which are evaluated independently according to a rank order that indicates the level of consciousness and degree of dysfunction. There are four grades of eye opening: spontaneous, which indicates that the arousal mechanisms in the brain stem are unimpaired, receives the highest score; opening in response to a verbal statement; opening in response to pain, which should be tested on the limbs, since facial pressure may cause eye closure; and no response. Verbal response has five grades: orientation is indicated by the patient's awareness of who he or she is, where he or she is, and why he or she is there, as well as the month and year; confused conversation is identified by the patient's verbal responses to questions accompanied by varying degrees of confusion and disorientation; inappropriate speech is indicated by the inability to sustain conversation, the shouting of intelligible words, and swearing; incomprehensible speech is identified by verbalization using unrecognizable 'words' and by speechlessness. Motor responses also have five grades of dysfunction: the patient obeys commands, with care being taken not to confuse the grasp reflex or postural adjustment for a response; a localizing response is the result of a painful stimulus to more than one site causing a limb to move; flexor responses may be slow or rapid; extension responses are usually associated with adduction, internal rotation of the shoulder, and pronation of the forearm; no response indicates hypotonia, and spinal transection must be ruled out. The degree of consciousness may vary from determinant to determinant and is assessed numerically by the best response. The results are plotted on a graph to provide a visual representation of the improvement, stability, or deterioration of a patient's level of consciousness, which is crucial to predicting the eventual outcome of coma. The sum of the numerical values for each parameter can also be used as an overall objective measurement, with 14 being indicative of no impairment, 3 being compatible with brain death, with 7 usually accepted as a state of coma. The test score can also function as an indicator for certain diagnostic tests or treatments, as the need for a CAT scan, intracranial pressure monitoring, and intubation. The scale has a high degree of consistency even when used by staff of varied experience.

glass factor. See **factor XII.**

glaucoma (glɔkou′mə, glaukou′mə), an abnormal condition of elevated pressure within an eye owing to obstruction of the outflow of aqueous humor. **Acute (angle-closure) glaucoma** occurs if the pupil in an eye with a narrow angle between iris and cornea dilates markedly, causing the folded iris to block the exit of aqueous humor from the anterior chamber. **Chronic (open-angle) glaucoma** is much more common, often bilateral; it develops slowly

---

Glasgow coma scale*

The Glasgow coma scale has been designed to quantitatively relate consciousness to motor responses, verbal responses, and eye opening. Coma is defined as no response and no eye opening. Scores of 7 or less on the Glasgow scale qualify as ''coma''; all scores of 9 or more do not qualify as ''coma.'' The examiner determines the *best* response the patient can make to a set of standardized stimuli. Higher points are assigned to responses that indicate increasing degrees of arousal.

  1. Best motor response. (Examiner determines the *best* response with *either* arm.)
    a. *6 points.* Obeys simple commands. Raises arm on request or holds up specified number of fingers. Releasing a grip (not grasping, which can be reflexive) is also an appropriate test.
    b. *5 points.* Localizes noxious stimuli. Fails to obey commands but can move either arm toward a noxious cutaneous stimulus and eventually contacts it with the hand. The stimulus should be maximal and applied in various locations, i.e., sternum pressure, or trapezius pinch.
    c. *4 points.* Flexion withdrawal. Responds to noxious stimulus with arm flexion but does not localize it with the hand.
    d. *3 points.* Abnormal flexion. Adducts shoulder, flexes and pronates arm, flexes wrist, and makes a fist in response to a noxious stimulus (decorticate rigidity).
    e. *2 points.* Abnormal extension. Adducts and internally rotates shoulder, extends forearm, flexes wrist, and makes a fist in response to a noxious stimulus (decerebrate rigidity).
    f. *1 point.* No motor response. Exclude reasons for no response; for example, insufficient stimulus or spinal cord injury.

  2. Best verbal response. (Examiner determines the *best* response after arousal. Noxious stimuli are employed if necessary.) Omit this test if the patient is dysphasic, has oral injuries, or is intubated. Place a check mark after other two test category scores after totaling to indicate omission of the verbal response section.
    a. *5 points.* Oriented patient. Can converse and relate who he is, where he is, and the year and month.
    b. *4 points.* Confused patient. Is not fully oriented or demonstrates confusion.
    c. *3 points.* Verbalizes. Does not engage in sustained conversation, but uses intelligible words in an exclamation (curse) or in a disorganized manner which is nonsensical.
    d. *2 points.* Vocalizes. Makes moaning or groaning sounds that are not recognizable words.
    e. *1 point.* No vocalization. Does not make any sound even in response to noxious stimulus.

  3. Eye opening. (Examiner determines the minimum stimulus that evokes opening of one or both eyes.) If the patient cannot realistically open the eyes because of bandages or lid edema, write ''E'' after the total test score to indicate omission of this component.
    a. *4 points.* Eyes open spontaneously.
    b. *3 points.* Eyes open to speech. Patient opens eyes in response to command or on being called by name.
    c. *2 points.* Eyes open to noxious stimuli.
    d. *1 point.* No eye opening in response to noxious stimuli.

*From Teasdale, G., and Jennett, B.: Assessment of coma and impaired consciousness: a practical scale, Lancet **2:**81-84, 1974.

and is genetically determined. The obstruction is believed to be within the canal of Schlemm. —**glaucomatous,** *adj.*

■ OBSERVATIONS: Acute glaucoma is accompanied by extreme ocular pain, blurred vision, a red eye, and a dilated pupil. Nausea and vomiting may occur. If untreated, acute glaucoma results in complete and permanent blindness within two to five days. Chronic glaucoma may produce no symptoms except for gradual loss of peripheral vision over a period of years. Sometimes headaches, blurred vision, and dull pain in the eye are present. Cupping of the optic discs may be noted on ophthalmoscopic examination. Halos around lights and central blindness are late manifestations. Both types have elevated intraocular pressure by tonometry.

■ INTERVENTION: Acute glaucoma is treated with eye drops to constrict the pupil and draw the iris away from the cornea, osmotic agents such as urea, mannitol, or glycerol given systemically to lower intraocular pressure, acetazolamide to reduce fluid formation, and surgical iridectomy to produce a filtration pathway for aqueous humor. Chronic glaucoma can usually be controlled with miotic eye drops such as pilocarpine. Other treatment includes carbonic anhydrase inhibitors, epinephrine eye drops, and timolol, a beta-adrenergic blocking agent.

■ NURSING CONSIDERATIONS: Persons who complain of tunnel vision or who bump into objects frequently should be referred for evaluation. Routine tonometry and ophthalmoscopic examinations are advised for all adults every three to five years. Nurses should remember that the use of mydriatic and cycloplegic eye drops, atropinelike drugs, and epinephrine in a person with a narrow anterior chamber angle is dangerous. Patients who have glaucoma are cautioned to avoid straining at defecation, to reduce excessive emotional and exertional stress, and to wear a medical identification tag. The nurse stresses the importance of regular eye examinations and the continuous use of medications prescribed for glaucoma.

Glaucon, a trade name for an adrenergic (epinephrine hydrochloride).

-glea, a combining form meaning a 'binding gelatinous medium': *ooglea, mesoglea, zooglea.* Also **-gloea.**

glia (gli′ə). See **neuroglia.**

gliadin (glaiʹədɪn), a protein substance, soluble in diluted alcohol, that is obtained from wheat and rye.

gliding, 1. a smooth, continuous movement. 2. the simplest of the four basic movements allowed by various joints of the skeleton. It is common to all movable joints and allows one surface to move smoothly over an adjacent surface, regardless of shape. Gliding is the only motion allowed by most of the wrist and the ankle joints. Compare **angular movement, circumduction, rotation.**

gliding joint, a synovial joint in which articulation of contiguous bones allows only gliding movements, as in the wrist and the ankle. The ligaments or the osseous processes around each gliding joint limit movements of

apposed plane surfaces or concavo-convex articulations. Also called **arthrodia, articulatio plana.**

glio-, a combining form meaning 'pertaining to the neuroglia, or a gluey substance': *gliococcus, gliosarcoma, gliosome.*

glioblastoma (glaiʹoublæstouʹmə). See **spongioblastoma.**

glioblastoma multiforme, a malignant, rapidly growing, pulpy or cystic tumor of the cerebrum or, occasionally, of the spinal cord. The lesion spreads with pseudopodlike projections. It is composed of a mixture of monocytes, pyriform cells, immature and mature astrocytes, and neural ectodermal cells with fibrous or protoplasmic processes. Also called **anaplastic astrocytoma, glioma multiforme.**

glioma (glaiouʹmə), *pl.* **gliomas, gliomata.** any of the largest group of primary tumors of the brain, composed of malignant glial cells. Kinds of gliomas are **astrocytoma, ependymoma, glioblastoma multiforme, medulloblastoma, oligodendroglioma.**

-glioma, a combining form meaning a 'tumor arising from the neuroglia': *angioglioma, fibroglioma, ganglioma.*

glioma multiforme. See **gliobastoma multiforme.**

glioma retinae. See **retinoblastoma.**

glioma sarcomatosum. See **gliosarcoma.**

glioneuroma (glaiʹounurouʹmə), *pl.* **glioneuromas, glioneuromata.** a neoplasm composed of nerve cells and elements of their supporting connective tissue.

gliosarcoma (glaiʹousarkouʹmə), *pl* **gliosarcomas, gliosarcomata.** a tumor composed of spindle-shaped cells in the delicate supporting connective tissue of nerve cells. Also called **glioma, glioblastoma, spongioblastoma, spongiocytoma.**

gliosarcoma retinae. See **retinoblastoma.**

Glisson's sling (glɪsʹənz), *Obsolete.* an apparatus with a collar for the neck and chin, which is attached to weights and a pulley and used for traction of the cervical spine.

-globinuria, a combining form meaning '(condition involving) the presence of complex proteins in the urine': *hemoglobinuria, methemoglobinuria, myoglobinuria.*

globin zinc insulin injection, a form of intermediate-acting lente insulin in a mixture with zinc chloride and a protein, globin, from beef hemoglobin. It is seldom used in current diabetic treatment regimens.

globoid leukodystrophy. See **galactosyl ceramide lipidosis.**

globule (globʹyul), a small spherical mass. Kinds of globules are **dentin globule, Dobie's globule, Marchi's globule, Margagni's globule, milk globule, myelin globule.**

globulin (globʹyulɪn), one of a broad category of simple proteins classified by solubility, electrophoretic mobility, and size. Compare **albumin.** See also **euglobulin, plasma protein, protein electrophoresis.**

globus hystericus, a transitory sensation of a lump in the throat that cannot be swallowed or coughed up, often accompanying emotional conflict or acute anxiety. The condition is thought to be due to a functional disturbance of the 9th cranial nerve and spasm of the inferior constrictor muscle that encircles the lower part of the throat. The physical exam tends to be normal, as does the barium esophagram.

globus pallidus, the smaller and more medial part of the lentiform nucleus of the brain, separated from the putamen by the lateral medullary lamina and divided into external and internal portions closely connected to the stratium, thalamus, and mesencephalon.

-gloea. See **-glea.**

glomangioma (gloʊmæn'jioʊ'mə), pl. **glomangiomas, glomangiomatas.** a benign tumor that develops from a cluster of blood cells in the skin. Also called **angiomyoneuroma, angioneuroma.**

glomerular (gloʊmer'yʊlər), of or pertaining to a glomerulus, especially a renal glomerulus.

glomerular capsule. See **Bowman's capsule.**

glomerular disease, any of a group of diseases in which the glomerulus of the kidney is affected. Depending on the particular disease, there may be hyperplasia, atrophy, necrosis, scarring, or deposits in the glomeruli. The symptoms may be abrupt in onset or slowly progressive. See also **glomerulonephritis.**

glomerulonephritis (gloʊmer'yʊloʊnɪfraɪ'tɪs), a noninfectious disease of the glomerulus of the kidney, characterized by proteinuria, hematuria, decreased urine production, and edema. Kinds of glomerulonephritis are **acute glomerulonephritis, chronic glomerulonephritis, subacute glomerulonephritis.**

glomerulus (gloʊmer'yʊləs), pl. **glomeruli. 1.** a tuft or cluster. **2.** a structure composed of blood vessels or nerve fibers, as a renal glomerulus.

glomus (gloʊ'məs), pl. **glomera** (glom'ərə). a small group of arterioles connecting directly to veins and having a rich nerve supply.

gloss-. See **glosso-.**

-glossia, 1. a combining form meaning the 'possession of a specified type or condition of tongue': *cacoglossia, megaloglossia, schistoglossia.* **2.** a combining form meaning the 'possession of a specified number of tongues': *aglossia, diglossia.*

glossitis (glosaɪ'tɪs), inflammation of the tongue. Acute glossitis, characterized by swelling, intense pain that may be referred to the ears, salivation, fever, and enlarged regional lymph nodes, may develop during an infectious disease or following a burn, bite, or other injury. Glossitis in which there is smooth atrophy of the surface and edges of the tongue is seen in pernicious anemia. Chronic superficial glossitis (Moeller's glossitis), in which irregular, bright red patches appear on the tip or sides of the tongue, occurs in middle-aged people, chiefly women. The condition causes pain or a burning sensation and sensitiv-

ity to hot or spicy foods; it often resists treatment. In congenital glossitis, there is a flat or slightly elevated patch or plaque anterior to the circumvallate papillae in the midline of the dorsal surface of the tongue.

glossitis parasitica. See **parasitic glossitis.**

glossitis rhomboidea mediana. See **median rhomboid glossitis.**

glosso-, gloss-, a combining form meaning 'pertaining to the tongue': *glossocele, glossodynia, glossoplegia.*

glossodynia (glos'oʊdɪn'iə), pain in the tongue, caused by acute or chronic inflammation, an abscess, or an ulcer.

glossodynia exfoliativa, a form of chronic glossitis, characterized by pain and sensitivity to spicy foods without any evidence of pathology. It occurs primarily in middle-aged women. Also called **Moeller's glossitis.**

glossohyal (glos'oʊhaɪ'əl), of or pertaining to the tongue and the horseshoe-shaped hyoid bone at the base of the tongue immediately above the thyroid cartilage. Also called **hyoglossal.**

glossolalia (glos'oʊleɪl'yə), speech in an unknown language, as "speaking in tongues" during a state of religious ecstasy when the message being transmitted through the speaker is believed to be a message from a celestial spirit or from God.

glossoncus (glosoŋ'kəs), a local swelling or general enlargement of the tongue.

glossopathy (glosop'əθi), a pathologic condition of the tongue, as acute inflammation caused by a burn, bite, injury, or infectious disease, enlargement resulting from congenital lymphangioma, or a disorder produced by mycotic infection, a malignant lesion, or a congenital anomaly.

glossopexy (glos'əpek'si), an adhesion of the tongue to the lip.

glossopharyngeal (glos'oʊfərɪn'jiəl), of or pertaining to the tongue and pharynx. See also **glossopharyngeal nerve.**

glossopharyngeal nerve, either of a pair of cranial nerves essential to the sense of taste, for sensation in some viscera, and for secretion from certain glands. The nerve has both sensory and motor fibers that pass from the tongue, parotid gland, and pharynx, communicate with the vagus nerve, and connect with two areas in the brain. Also called **nervus glossopharyngeus, ninth nerve.**

glossophytia (glos'əfɪt'iə), a condition of the tongue characterized by a blackish patch on the dorsum on which filiform papillae are greatly elongated and thickened like bristly hairs. The usually painless condition may be caused by heavy smoking, the extensive use of broad-spectrum antibiotics, or a mycosis in which *Cryptococcus* grows in symbiosis with *Nocardia.*

glossoplasty (glos'oʊplæs'ti), a surgical procedure or plastic operation on the tongue performed to correct a congenital anomaly, repair an injury, or restore a measure of function following excision of a malignant lesion.

glossoptosis (glos'optou'sıs), the retraction or downward displacement of the tongue.

glossopyrosis (glos'oupairou'sıs), a burning sensation in the tongue caused by chronic inflammation, by exposure to extremely hot or spicy food, or by psychogenic glossitis.

glossorrhaphy (glosor'əfi), the surgical suturing of a wound in the tongue.

glossotrichia (glos'ətrık'iə), a condition of the tongue characterized by a hairlike appearance of the papillae. Also called **hairy tongue.**

glott-, a combining form meaning 'pertaining to the glottis': *glottic, glottidas, glottis.*

glottis (glot'ıs), *pl.* **glottises, glottides. 1.** Also called **true glottis, rima glottidis.** a slitlike opening between the true vocal cords (plica vocalis). **2.** the phonation apparatus of the larynx, composed of the true vocal cords and the opening between them (rima glottidis). —**glottal, glottic,** *adj.*

glucagon (glu'kəgon), a hormone, produced by alpha cells in the islands of Langerhans, that stimulates the conversion of glycogen to glucose in the liver. Secretion of glucagon is stimulated by hypoglycemia and by the growth hormone of the anterior pituitary. A preparation of purified, crystallized glucagon is used in the treatment of certain hypoglycemic states. Also called **hyperglycemic-glycogenolytic factor.**

glucagonoma syndrome (glu'kəgonou'mə), a disease associated with a glucagon-secreting tumor of the islet cells of the pancreas, characterized by hyperglycemia, stomatitis, anemia, weight loss, and a characteristic rash.

gluco-, glyco-, a combining form meaning 'pertaining to sweetness or to glucose': *glucofuranose, glucokinetic, glucosuria.*

glucocorticoid (glu'koukor'təkoid), an adrenocortical steroid hormone that increases glyconeogenesis, exerts an anti-inflammatory effect, and influences many body functions. The most important of the three glucocorticoids is cortisol (hydrocortisone); corticosterone is less active, and cortisone is inactive until converted to cortisol. Glucocorticoids promote the release of amino acids from muscle, mobilize fatty acids from fat stores, and increase the ability of skeletal muscles to maintain contractions and avoid fatigue. In vitro, these hormones are known to stabilize mitochondrial and lysosomal membranes, increase the production of adenosine triphosphate, promote the formation of certain key enzymes in the liver, and decrease antibody production and the number of circulating eosinophils. A deficiency of glucocorticoids is characterized by hyperpigmentation of the skin, fasting hypoglycemia, weight loss, and apathy. An excess is associated with impaired glucose tolerance, thinning of the skin, ecchymosis, osteoporosis, poor wound healing, increased sus-ceptibility to infection, and obesity. Glucocorticoid secretion is stimulated by the adrenocorticotropic hormone of the anterior pituitary, which in turn is regulated by the corticotropin-releasing factor of the hypothalamus. Synthetic or semisynthetic glucocorticoids, derived chiefly from cortisol, include prednisone, prednisolone, dexamethasone, methylprednisolone, triamcinolone, and betamethasone. Compare **mineralocorticoid.**

glucose (glu'kous), a simple sugar found in certain foods, especially fruits, and a major source of energy occurring in human and animal body fluids. Glucose, when ingested or produced by the digestive hydrolysis of double sugars and starches, is absorbed into the blood from the intestines. Excess glucose in circulation is normally polymerized and stored in the liver and muscles as glycogen, which is depolymerized to glucose and liberated as needed. The determination of blood glucose levels is an important diagnostic test in diabetes and other disorders. Prepared glucose is a syrupy sweetening agent. Pharmaceutical preparations of glucose are widely used in the treatment of many disorders. See also **dextrose, glycogen.**

glucose 1-phosphate, an intermediate compound in carbohydrate metabolism.

glucose 6-phosphate, an intermediate compound in carbohydrate metabolism.

glucose-6-phosphate dehydrogenase (G-6-PD) deficiency, an inherited disorder characterized by red cells partially or completely deficient in glucose-6-phosphate dehydrogenase, a critical enzyme in aerobic glycolysis. The gene for this enzyme is sex-linked, and the defect is fully expressed in affected males despite a heterozygous pattern of inheritance. The disorder is associated with episodes of acute hemolysis under conditions of stress or in response to certain chemicals or drugs. The anemia that results is a kind of nonspherocytic hemolytic anemia. See also **congenital nonspherocytic hemolytic anemia.**

glucose tolerance test, a test of the body's ability to metabolize carbohydrates by administering a standard dose of glucose and measuring the blood and urine for glucose at regular intervals thereafter. The patient usually eats a high carbohydrate diet for the three days preceding the test and fasts the night before. A fasting blood glucose is obtained the next morning and then the patient drinks a 100-gram dose of glucose. Blood and urine are collected periodically for up to six hours. The glucose tolerance test is most often used to assist in the diagnosis of diabetes or other disorders that affect carbohydrate metabolism.

glucosuria (glu'kousur'iə), abnormal presence of glucose in the urine resulting from the ingestion of large amounts of carbohydrate or from a kidney disease, as nephrosis, or a metabolic disease, as diabetes mellitus. See also **glycosuria.** —**glucosuric,** *adj.*

glucosyl cerebroside lipidosis. See **Gaucher's disease.**

glue sniffing, the practice of inhaling the vapors of toluene, a volatile organic compound used as a solvent in certain glues. The glue is squeezed into a plastic bag, which is then placed over the nose and mouth. Intoxication and dizziness result. Prolonged accidental or occupational exposure or repeated recreational use may damage a variety of organ systems. Death has been reported from asphyxiation by the plastic bag.

glutamate, a salt of glutamic acid.

glutamic acid (glutæm′ık), a nonessential amino acid occurring widely in a number of proteins. Preparations of glutamic acid are used as aids for digestion.

glutamic acid hydrochloride, a gastric acidifier.

■ INDICATION: It is prescribed for hypoacidity.

■ CONTRAINDICATIONS: Hyperacidity, peptic ulcer, or known hypersensitivity to this drug prohibits its use.

■ ADVERSE EFFECT: The most serious adverse reaction is systemic acidosis resulting from overdose.

glutamic-oxaloacetic transaminase (GOT), an enzyme normally present in body serum and in certain body tissues, especially those of the heart and liver. This enzyme affects the intermolecular transfer of amino groups within the myocardium and may increase as the result of myocardial infarction and liver damage. Also called **serum glutamic-oxaloacetic transaminase.** Compare **glutamic-pyruvic transaminase.**

glutamic-pyruvic transaminase (GPT), an enzyme normally present in the serum and tissues of the body, especially the tissues of the liver. This enzyme may increase in persons with acute liver damage. Also called **serum glutamic-pyruvic transaminase.** Compare **glutamic-oxaloacetic transaminase.**

gluteal gait. See **Trendelenburg gait.**

gluteal tuberosity, a ridge on the lateral posterior surface of the thigh bone to which is attached the gluteus maximus.

gluten, the insoluble protein constituent of wheat and other grains. It is obtained from flour by washing out the starch and is used as an adhesive agent, giving to dough its tough, elastic character.

gluten enteropathy. See **celiac disease.**

glutethimide (gluteth′əmaɪd), a sedative.

■ INDICATIONS: It is prescribed in the treatment of anxiety and insomnia.

■ CONTRAINDICATION: Known hypersensitivity to this drug prohibits its use.

■ ADVERSE EFFECTS: Among the most serious adverse reactions are physical and psychological dependence. Rashes also may occur.

-glycemia, a combining form meaning a 'condition of sugar in the blood': *dysglycemia, hepatoglycemia, hyperglycemia.* Also **-glycaemia.**

glycerin, gylcerine, a sweet, colorless, oily fluid that is a pharmaceutical preparation of glycerol. Glycerin is used as a moistening agent for chapped skin, as an ingredient of suppositories for constipation, and as a sweetening agent and vehicle for drug preparations.

glycerol (glɪs′ərɔl), an alcohol that is a component of fats. Glycerol is soluble in ethyl alcohol and water. See also **glycerin.**

glycerol kinase, an enzyme in the liver and kidneys that catalyzes the transfer of a phosphate group from adenosin triphosphate to form adenosine diphosphate and L-glycerol-3-phosphate.

glyceryl alcohol. See **glycerin.**

glyceryl guaiacolate. See **guaifenesin.**

glyceryl triacetate. See **triacetin.**

glycine (glaɪ′sin), a nonessential amino acid occurring widely as a component of animal and plant proteins. Synthetically produced glycine is used in solutions for irrigation, in the treatment of various muscle diseases, and as an antacid and dietary supplement. See also **amino acid, protein.**

glyco-. See **gluco-.**

glycobiarsol, an antiamebic containing arsenic, formerly used to treat intestinal amebiasis.

glycocoll (glaɪ′kəkol). See **aminoacetic acid.**

glycogen (glaɪ′kəjɪn), a polysaccharide that is the major carbohydrate stored in animal cells. It is formed from glucose and stored chiefly in the liver and, to a lesser extent, in muscle cells. Glycogen is depolymerized to glucose and released into circulation as needed by the body. Also called **animal starch, hepatin, tissue dextrin.** See also **glucose.**

glycogenesis, the synthesis of glycogen from glucose.

glycogenosis (glaɪ′koʊjɪnoʊ′sɪs). See **glycogen storage disease.**

glycogen storage disease, any of a group of inherited disorders of glycogen metabolism. An enzyme deficiency causes glycogen to accumulate in abnormally large amounts in various parts of the body. Biopsy and chemical analysis reveal the missing enzyme. Also called **glyogenosis.**

glycogen storage disease, type I. See **von Gierke's disease.**

glycogen storage disease, type II. See **Pompe's disease.**

glycogen storage disease, type III. See **Cori's disease.**

glycogen storage disease, type IV. See **Andersen's disease.**

glycogen storage disease, type V. See **McArdle's disease.**

glycogen storage disease, type VI. See **Hers' disease.**

glycolic acid, a substance in bile, formed by glycine and cholic acid, that aids in digestion and absorption of fats. Glycolic acid is used as a food additive and a emulsifying agent.

glycolysis (glaikol′ɪsɪs), a series of enzymatically catalyzed reactions, occurring within cells, by which glucose and other sugars are broken down to yield lactic acid or pyruvic acid, releasing energy in the form of adenosine triphosphate. **Aerobic glycolysis** yields pyruvic acid in the presence of adequate oxygen. **Anaerobic glycolysis** yields lactic acid and does not require oxygen. See also **Krebs' citric acid cycle.**

glycopyrrolate (glaɪ′koupɪr′əleit), an anticholinergic.

■ INDICATION: It is prescribed as an adjunct to ulcer therapy.

■ CONTRAINDICATIONS: Narrow angle glaucoma, asthma, obstruction of the genitourinary or gastrointestinal tract, ulcerative colitis, or known hypersensitivity to this drug prohibits its use.

■ ADVERSE EFFECTS: Among the more serious adverse reactions are blurred vision, central nervous system effects, tachycardia, dry mouth, decreased sweating, and hypersensitivity reactions.

glycoside (glaɪ′kəsaid), any of several carbohydrates that yield a sugar and a nonsugar on hydrolysis. The plant *Digitalis purpurea* contains a glycoside used in the treatment of heart disease.

glycosuria (glaɪ′kousur′iə), abnormal presence of a sugar, especially glucose, in the urine. Glycosuria can result from the ingestion of large amounts of carbohydrate, or it may be the result of endocrine or renal disorders. It is a finding most routinely associated with diabetes mellitus. — **glycosuric,** *adj.*

glycosuric acid, a compound that is an intermediate product of the metabolism of tyrosine. It forms a melaninlike staining substance in the urine of people who have alkaptonuria.

glycyl alcohol. See **glycerin.**

Glyestrin, a trade name for esterified estrogens.

Glynazan, a trade name for a smooth muscle relaxant (theophylline sodium glycinate) used as a bronchodilator.

Glysennid, a trade name for a stimulant laxative (sennosides A and B).

gm, abbreviation for **gram.**

GMENAC, abbreviation for **Graduate Medical Education National Advisory Committee.**

GNA, abbreviation for **Gay Nurses' Alliance.**

gnath-. See **gnatho-.**

-gnathia, a combining form meaning a 'condition of the jaw': *brachygnathia, campylognathia, retrognathia.*

gnathic (næth′ɪk), of or pertaining to the jaw or cheek.

gnatho-, gnath-, a combining form meaning 'pertaining to the jaw': *gnathocephalus, gnathodynia, gnathoplasty.*

gno-, a combining form meaning 'to know or discern': *gnosia, gnosis.*

-gnomonic, a combining form meaning 'signs or experience in knowing or judging (a condition)': *pathognomonic, physiognomonic, thanatognomonic.* Also **-gnomonical.**

-gnomy, a combining form meaning the 'science or means of judging' something specified: *craniognomy, pathognomy, physiognomy.*

-gnosia, a combining form meaning a '(condition of) perceiving or recognizing': *acognosia, hypergnosia, topognosia.*

-gnosis, a combining form meaning 'knowledge': *acrognosis, diagnosis, topognosis.*

goblet cell, one of the many specialized cells that secrete mucus and form glands of the epithelium of the stomach, the intestine, and parts of the respiratory tract. Also called **beaker cell, chalice cell.** See also **gland.**

goiter, a hypertrophic thyroid gland, usually evident as a pronounced swelling in the neck. The enlargement may be associated with hyperthyroidism, hypothyroidism, or normal levels of thyroid function. The goiter may be cystic or fibrous, containing nodules or an increased number of follicles; it may surround a large blood vessel, or a part of the enlarged gland may be situated beneath the sternum or in the thoracic cavity. Treatment may include total or subtotal surgical removal, the administration of antithyroid drugs or radioiodine, or the use of thyroid hormone to block the hypothalamic-hypophyseal mechanism that releases thyroid-stimulating hormone. Following thyroidectomy, maintenance therapy with thyroid hormone may be required. See specific goiter. — **goitrous,** *adj.*

gold (Au), a yellowish, soft metallic element that occurs naturally as a free metal and as the telluride $AuAgTe_4$. Its atomic number is 79; its atomic weight is 197. Gold has been highly valued since antiquity and has been and is used for currency and ornamentation. It is usually hardened by alloying it with small amounts of nickel or copper. Gold is highly resistive to oxidation but can be dissolved in aqua regia and aqueous potassium cyanide. Gold salts, in which gold is attached to sulfur, are often used in the treatment, or chrysotherapy, of patients with rheumatoid arthritis but cause serious toxicity in about 10 per cent of patients and some toxicity in 25 to 50 per cent. See also **chrysotherapy.**

gold 198, a radioactive gold antineoplastic.

■ INDICATIONS: It is prescribed for cancer of the prostate, cervix, and bladder and for the reduction of fluid accumulation secondary to a cancer.

■ CONTRAINDICATIONS: Ulcerative tumors, pregnancy, lactation, or unhealed surgical wounds prohibit its use. It is not prescribed for patients under 18 years of age.

■ ADVERSE EFFECT: The most serious adverse reaction is radiation sickness.

gold compound, a drug containing gold salts, usually administered with other drugs in the treatment of rheumatoid arthritis. Gold is potentially toxic and is administered only under the supervision of a specialist in chrysotherapy. Toxic reactions range from mild dermatoses to lethal poisoning. Various radioisotopes of gold have been used in diagnostic radiology and in the radiologic treatment of certain malignant neoplastic diseases.

gold sodium thiomalate, an antirheumatic.

- INDICATION: It is prescribed for rheumatoid arthritis.

- CONTRAINDICATIONS: Severe debilitation, systemic lupus erythematosus, renal or liver disease, blood dyscrasias, Sjögren's syndrome (in rheumatoid arthritis), or known hypersensitivity to this drug or to other gold or heavy metal salts prohibits its use.

- ADVERSE EFFECTS: Among the most serious adverse reactions are various blood dyscrasias, renal damage, and allergic reactions. Dermatitis, stomatitis, and lesions of the mucous membranes also may occur.

gold therapy. See **chrysotherapy.**

Golgi apparatus, (gɔl'ji), one of many small membranous structures found in most cells, composed of various elements associated with the formation of carbohydrate side chains of glycoproteins, mucopolysaccharides, and other substances. Saccules within each structure migrate through the cell membrane and release substances associated with external and internal secretion. Also called **Golgi body, Golgi complex.**

Golgi body. See **Golgi apparatus.**

Golgi complex. See **Golgi apparatus.**

Golgi-Mazzoni corpuscles (goul'jimætzou'ni), a number of thin capsules enveloping terminal nerve fibrils in the subcutaneous tissue of the fingers. They have thicker cores than Pacini's corpuscles but are similar special sensory end organs. Compare **Pacini's corpuscles, Ruffini's corpuscles.**

gomphosis (gomfou'sis), *pl.* **gomphoses.** an articulation by the insertion of a conical process into a socket, as the insertion of a root of a tooth into an alveolus of the mandible or the maxilla. Gomphosis is not a connection between true bones but is considered a type of fibrous joint. Compare **sutura, syndesmosis.**

gon-. 1. See **gono-.** 2. See **gony-.**

gonad (gou'næd), a gamete-producing gland, as an ovary or a testis. – **gonadal,** *adj.*

gonadal dysgenesis, a general designation for a variety of conditions involving anomalies in the development of the gonads, as Turner's syndrome, hermaphroditism, and gonadal aplasia.

gonadotropin, gonadotrophin, a hormonal substance that stimulates the function of the testes and the ovaries. The gonadotropins follicle stimulating hormone and luteinizing hormone are produced and secreted by the anterior pituitary gland. In early pregnancy, chorionic gonadotropin is produced by the placenta. It acts to sustain the function of the corpus luteum of the ovary, forestalling menstruation and thus maintaining pregnancy. Gonadotropins are prescribed to induce ovulation in infertility that is caused by inadequate stimulation of the ovary by endogenous gonadotropic hormones. Excessive

stimulation of the ovary may result in vast enlargement of the gland, maturation of many follicles, multiple pregnancy, bleeding into the abdomen, and pain. – **gonadotropic, gonadotrophic,** *adj.*

-gonic, a combining form meaning 'agents, processes, or results of generation, reproduction, including the sexual': *dysgonic, endergonic, exergonic.*

gonio-, a combining form meaning 'pertaining to an angle': *goniocraniometry, goniometer, gonion.*

goniometry (gou'niom'ətri), a system of testing for various labyrinthine diseases which affect the sense of balance. One test uses a plank, one end of which may be raised to any desired height. The patient stands on the plank as one end is gradually raised, and the point where the patient can no longer maintain balance is noted. – **goniometric,** *adj.*

gono-, gon-, a combining form meaning 'pertaining to semen or seed': *gonococcin, gonophore, gonotome.*

gonoblast (gon'əblæst). See **germ cell.**

gonococcal pyomyositis, an acute inflammatory condition of a muscle caused by infection with a *Neisseria gonorrhoeae,* characterized by abscess formation and pain. It is an unusual form of gonorrhea and must be differentiated from sarcoma. The diagnosis is made by the discovery of the gonococcal diplococci within the abscess when a bacterial culture of a specimen is prepared following exploratory surgery. The person is then usually found to be asymptomatically infected in the urogenital organs. Antibiotic treatment, most often with ampicillin, is rapidly effective in curing the infection.

gonococcus (gon'əkok'əs), *pl.* **gonococci** (gon'əkok'sai). a gram-negative, intracellular diplococcus of the species *Neisseria gonorrhoeae,* the cause of gonorrhea.

gonocyte (gon'əsait). See **germ cell.**

gonorrhea, a common venereal disease most often affecting the genitourinary tract and, occasionally, the pharynx, conjunctiva, or rectum. Infection results from contact with an infected person or by contact with secretions containing the causitive organism *Neisseria gonorrhoeae.* – **gonorrheal, gonorrheic,** *adj.*

- OBSERVATIONS: Urethritis, dysuria, purulent, greenish-yellow urethral or vaginal discharge, red or edematous urethral meatus, and itching, burning, or pain around the vaginal or urethral orifice are characteristic. The vagina may be massively swollen and red and the lower abdomen may be tense and very tender. As the infection spreads, which is more common in women than in men, nausea, vomiting, fever, and tachycardia may occur as salpingitis, oophoritis, or peritonitis develops. Inflammation of the tissues surrounding the liver may also occur, causing pain in the upper right quadrant of the abdomen. Severe disseminated infection is also more common in women than in men and is characterized by signs of septicemia with polyarthritis, tender papillary lesions on the skin of the hands and feet, and inflammation of the tendons of the wrists, knees, and ankles. Gonoccocal ophthalmia involves infection of the conjunctiva and may lead to scarring and blindness. Gonorrhea is diagnosed by bacteriologic culture of the organism from a smear obtained from a specimen of exudate. In men a microscopic study of a gram-stained specimen of exudate that reveals gram-negative intracellular diplococci is diagnostic of gonorrheal infection, but this finding is not diagnostic in women.

■ INTERVENTION: Penicillin is used to treat uncomplicated gonorrhea. It is given, usually by intramuscular injection, one half hour after an oral dose of probenecid that acts to slow the excretion of the penicillin from the body. Oral treatment with a large, one-time dose of ampicillin is also held to be effective, and erythromycin or tetracycline is sometimes used to treat the infection, most commonly in people who are sensitive to penicillin and penicillinlike drugs. The client is tested one or two weeks after treatment to confirm eradication of the organism. The routine instillation of 1 per cent silver nitrate in the eyes of the newborn provides effective prophylaxis against infection in the newborn period that might otherwise result from contact with the infected secretions of an asymptomatic infected mother during vaginal delivery.

■ NURSING CONSIDERATIONS: It is important that the client's sexual contacts be treated. Before giving any antibiotic it is ascertained that the client does not have any known sensitivity to the drug being given and that equipment and drugs are available to treat any hypersensitivity reaction that may occur. The person is alerted to the fact that until it is proven that the microorganism has been eradicated, transmission of the infection is possible and therefore precautions against spread are recommended. It may also be appropriate to inform the client that use of condoms during coitus affords excellent protection against venereal infection.

gonorrheal conjunctivitis, a severe, destructive form of purulent conjunctivitis caused by the gonococcus *Neisseria gonorrhoeae*. Prompt treatment by the intravenous administration of antibiotics is required to prevent scarring of the cornea and blindness. Also called **ophthalmia neonatorum.**

gonorrheal salpingitis, 1. See **pelvic inflammatory disease.** 2. See **gonorrhea.**

gony-, gon-, a combining form meaning 'pertaining to a knee': *gonycampsis, gonyectyposis, gonyoncus.*

-gony, a combining form meaning 'birth or origin': *amphigony, merogony, zoogony.*

Goodell's sign (gudelz′), softening of the uterine cervix, a probable sign of pregnancy.

Goodpasture's syndrome, a chronic, relapsing pulmonary hemosiderosis, usually associated with glomerulonephritis and characterized by a cough with hemoptysis, dyspnea, anemia, and progressive renal failure. Mild forms of the syndrome may respond to corticosteroids or immunosuppressive drugs. Severe recurrent cases have a poor prognosis; hemodialysis and kidney transplantation are the only treatments.

Goodrich, Annie Warburton (1866–1954), an American nursing educator, instrumental in bringing nursing from an apprenticeship to a profession. She was superintendent of nurses at several New York hospitals before going to Teachers College, Columbia University, in 1914. In addition to teaching, she was associated with the Henry Street Settlement and the Nursing Department of the United States Army. In 1923 she became dean of the newly formed Yale School of Nursing at Yale University, bringing to nursing the same university rank as other professions.

gooseflesh. See **pilomotor reflex.**

Gordon reflex, 1. an abnormal variation of the Babinski reflex, elicited by compressing the calf muscles, characterized by extension of the great toe and fanning of the other toes. It is evidence of disease of the pyramidal tract. 2. an abnormal reflex, elicited by compressing the forearm muscles, characterized by flexion of the fingers or of the thumb and index finger. It is seen in diseases of the pyramidal tract. Compare **Chaddock reflex, Oppenheim reflex.** See also **Babinski's reflex.**

Gordon's elementary body, a particle found in tissues containing eosinophils once thought to be the viral cause of Hodgkin's disease. Also called **Gordon's encephalopathic agent.**

Gordon's encephalopathic agent. See **Gordon's elementary body.**

Gosselin's fracture (goslænz′), a V-shaped fracture of the distal tibia, extending to the ankle.

GOT, abbreviation for **glutamic-oxaloacetic transaminase.**

goundou (gun′du), a condition characterized by bony exostoses of the nasal and maxillary bones, usually occurring as a late sequela of yaws in people of Central and South America.

gout, a disease associated with an inborn error of uric acid metabolism that increases production or interferes with excretion of uric acid. Excess uric acid is converted to sodium urate crystals that precipitate from the blood and become deposited in joints and other tissues. Men are more often affected than women. The great toe is a common site for the accumulation of urate crystals. The condition can result in exceedingly painful swelling of a joint, accompanied by chills and fever. The symptoms are recurrent; episodes become longer each year. The disorder is disabling and, if untreated, can progress to the development of tophi and destructive joint changes. Treatment usually includes administration of colchicine, phenylbutazone, indomethacin or glucocorticoid drugs, a diet that excludes purine-rich foods, as organ meats, and may include surgical removal of tophi. Acquired gout is a condition having the signs and symptoms of gout but occurring as a result of another disorder or treatment for a different condition. Diuretic drugs can alter the concentration of uric acid so that uric acid salts precipitate from the blood and are carried to the joints. See also **Lesch-Nyhan syndrome, tophus.**

gouty arthritis. See **gout.**

Gowers' muscular dystrophy (gau'ərz). See **distal muscular dystrophy.**

GP, abbreviation for **general practitioner.**

G-6-PD deficiency, abbreviation for **glucose-6-phosphate dehydrogenase deficiency.**

GPI, *Obsolete.* abbreviation for **general paralysis of the insane.** See **general paresis.**

GPT, abbreviation for **glutamic-pyruvic transaminase.**

gr, abbreviation for **grain.**

Graafian follicle (græf'iən), a mature ovarian vesicle, measuring about 10 to 12 mm in diameter, that ruptures during ovulation to release the ovum. Many primary ovarian follicles, each containing an immature ovum about 35 μ in diameter, are imbedded near the surface of the ovary, just below the tunica albuginea. Under the influence of the follicle stimulating hormone from the adenohypophysis, one ovarian follicle ripens into a Graafian follicle during the proliferative phase of each menstrual cycle. The cells that form the Graafian follicle are arranged in a layer 3 to 4 cells thick around a relatively large volume of follicular fluid. Within the follicle the ovum grows to about 100 μ in diameter and, when the follicle ruptures, is swept into the fimbriated opening of the uterine tube. The cavity of the follicle collapses when the ovum is released, and the remaining follicular cells greatly enlarge to become the corpus luteum. If the ovum is fertilized, the corpus luteum grows and becomes the corpus luteum of pregnancy which, at the end of nine months, has a diameter of about 30 mm. As the ovarian follicle ripens into the Graafian follicle, it produces estrogen, which stimulates the proliferation of the endometrium and the enlargement of the uterine glands. The growing corpus luteum produces progesterone, which triggers endometrial gland secretion and prepares the uterus to receive the fertilized ovum. If the ovum is not fertilized, the Graafian follicle forms the corpus luteum of menstruation, which degenerates, leaving the small scarred corpus albicans.

gracile (græs'ıl), long, slender, and graceful.

gracilis (græs'ılıs), the most superficial of the five medial femoral muscles. A thin, flattened muscle that is broad proximally and narrow distally, it originates in a thin aponeurosis secured on the inferior aspect of the symphysis pubis and the superior half of the pubic arch. The muscle curves around the medial condyle of the tibia and inserts into the body of the tibia, distal to the condyle. It is innervated by a branch of the obturator nerve, which contains fibers from the third and fourth lumbar nerves, and it functions to adduct the thigh and flex the leg and to assist in the medial rotation of the leg after it is flexed. Compare **adductor brevis, adductor longus, adductor magnus, pectineus.**

gradient, 1. the rate of increase or decrease of measurable phenomenon, as temperature or pressure. 2. a visual representation of the rate of change of a measurable phenomenon; a curve.

gradient of approach, the inverse relationship between the distance from a positive stimulus and the tendency to approach it.

gradient of avoidance, the inverse relationship between the distance from a negative stimulus and the tendency to avoid it.

graduated bath, a bath in which the temperature of the water is slowly reduced.

graduated resistance exercise. See **progressive resistance exercise.**

graduate medical education, formal medical education pursued after receipt of M.D. or other professional degree in the medical sciences. Graduate medical education is usually obtained as an intern, resident, or fellow, or in continuing medical education programs.

Graduate Medical Education National Advisory Committee (GMENAC), a committee established by order of the Secretary of the Department of Health, Education and Welfare (now the Department of Health and Human Services) to study the manpower issues in medicine. The Committee issued its final report in September 1980. Among its conclusions were some regarding the supply of nurses in expanded roles, including nurse practitioners and nurse midwives.

Graduate Record Examination (GRE), an examination administered to graduates of institutions of higher learning. The scores are used as criteria for admission to masters and doctoral programs in many institutions and areas of specialization, including nursing. The examination tests verbal and mathematical aptitudes and abilities.

GRAE, abbreviation for **generally recognized as effective.**

graft, a tissue or an organ taken from a site or a person and inserted into a new site or person, performed to repair a defect in structure. The graft may be temporary, as an emergency skin transplant for extensive burns, or permanent, as the grafted tissue growing to become a part of the body. Skin, bone, cartilage, blood vessel, nerve, muscle, cornea, and whole organs, as the kidney or the heart, may be grafted. Preoperative care focuses on a high protein diet and vitamins to ensure optimum physical condition and on freedom from infection. Under general or local anesthesia the tissue is transferred and sutured into place. Rejection is the major complication: fever, pain in the graft area, and evidence of loss of function four to fifteen days after the procedure are indicative of rejection. Immunosuppressive drugs are given in large doses to suppress antibody production and rejection. Even if an early reaction is blocked, late rejection may occur a year or more after the graft is done. Also called **transplant.**

graft-versus-host reaction, a rejection response of certain grafts, especially bone marrow. It involves an incompatibility resulting from a deficiency in the immune response of some patients and is commonly associated with inadequate immunosuppressive therapy. Characteristic signs may include skin lesions with edema, erythema, ulceration, scaling, and loss of hair. Such reactions may also cause lesions of the joints and the heart and hemolytic anemia with a positive Coombs' reaction. The graft-versus-host reaction is similar to the Type IV reaction in hypersensitive individuals who receive tuberculin injections. Some experts believe that it involves certain immunologically active cells which originate as the result of defective tolerance mechanisms or as the result of somatic mutation of certain host cells. Also called **homologous disease.**

grain (gr), the smallest unit of mass in avoirdupois, troy, and apothecaries' weights, being the same in all and equal to 0.06479891 gram. The troy and apothecaries' ounces contain 480 grains; the avoirdupois ounce contains 437.5 grains.

grain itch, a skin condition caused by a mite that lives in grain or straw. The lesion consists of an intensely itchy, urticarial papule surmounted by a tiny vesicle.

gram (gm), a unit of mass in the metric system equal to 1/1000 of a kilogram, 15.432 grains, and 0.03 ounce avoirdupois.

-gram, 1. a combining form meaning a 'drawing': *cephalogram, mammogram, splenogram.* 2. a combining form meaning '1/1000 kilogram': *centigram, decagram, microgram.* Also **-gramme.**

gram calorie. See **calorie.**

gram-molecular weight, the molecular weight of a substance expressed in grams. See also **mole, molecular weight.**

gram-negative, having the pink color of the counterstain used in Gram's method of staining microorganisms. This property is a primary method of characterizing organisms in microbiology. Some of the most common gram-negative pathogenic bacteria are *Bacteroides fragilis, Brucella abortus, Escherichia coli, Haemophilus influenzae, Klebsiella pneumoniae, Neisseria gonorrhoeae, Proteus vulgaris, Pseudomonas aeroginosa, Salmonella typhi, Shigella dysenteriae, Yersinia pestis.*

gram-positive, retaining the violet color of the stain used in Gram's method of staining microorganisms. This property is a primary method of characterizing organisms in microbiology. Some of the most common kinds of gram-positive pathogenic bacteria are *Bacillus anthracis, Clostridium, Mycobacterium leprae, Mycobacterium tuberculosis, Staphylococcus aureus, Streptococcus pneumoniae, Streptococcus pyogenes.*

Gram's stain, the method of staining microorganisms using a violet stain, followed by an iodine solution, decolorizing with an alcohol or acetone solution, and counterstaining with safranin. The retention of either the violet color of the stain or the pink color of the counterstain serves as a primary means of identifying and classifying bacteria. Gram-positive organisms appear violet or blue; gram-negative organisms appear rose pink. Also called **Gram's method.**

grand rounds, a formal conference in which one usually expert person presents a lecture concerning a clinical issue intended to be educational for the listeners. Charts, tables, films, slides, tapes, and demonstrations are often used in presentation at grand rounds. Historically the patient was present. In some settings grand rounds may be formal teaching rounds conducted by an expert at the bedsides of selected patients.

grant, an award given to an institution, a project, or an individual usually consisting of a sum of money. A grant is given by a granting agency, the federal government, a foundation, private enterprise, or institution to provide financial support for research, service, or training. The applicant usually writes a formal application (proposal) for the grant, which is reviewed by the granting agency and compared to other proposals. The selected grantee is usually required to sign a contract with the agency, specifying the terms of the grant and the responsibilities of the grantee.

granul-, a combining form meaning 'pertaining to grains or granules': *granulase, granulocorpuscle, granulocytemia.*

granular, 1. macroscopically looking or feeling like sand. 2. microscopically appearing to have a few or many particles within or on its surface, as a stained granular leucocyte. — **granularity,** *n.*

granular conjunctivitis. See **trachoma.**

granular endoplasmic reticulum. See **endoplasmic reticulum.**

granulation tissue, any soft, pink, fleshy projections that form during the healing process in a wound not healing by first intention, consisting of many capillaries surrounded by fibrous collagen. Overgrowth of granulation tissue results in proud flesh growing to protrude above the skin. See also **pyogenic granuloma.**

granulocyte (græn′yuləsait′), one of a group of leukocytes characterized by the presence of cytoplasmic granules. Kinds of granulocytes are **basophil, eosinophil, neutrophil.** Compare **agranulocyte.**

granulocyte transfusion, the use of specially prepared leukocytes for the treatment of severe granulocytopenia and prophylactically for the prevention of serious infection in leukemic patients or those receiving cancer chemotherapy. The procedure has the same risks as a blood transfusion. Also called **buffy coat transfusion.**

granulocytic leukemia. See **acute myelocytic leukemia, chronic myelocytic leukemia.**

granulocytic sarcoma. See **chloroma.**

granulocytopenia (græn'yulousai'toupi'niə), an abnormal condition of the blood, characterized by a decrease in the total number of granulocytes. Also called **neutropenia.** Compare **granulocytosis.** See also **leukopenia.** – **granulocytopenic,** *adj.*

granuloma (græn'yulou'mə), *pl.* **granulomas, granulomata.** a mass of nodular granulation tissue resulting from inflammation, injury, or infection. It is composed of capillary buds and growing fibroblasts. Granulomas may resolve spontaneously, become gangrenous, spread, or remain as a focus of infection. Treatment depends on the cause and probable course of the particular granuloma.

-granuloma, a combining form meaning a 'tumor-like mass or nodule of granulation tissue': *paragranuloma, ulcerogranuloma, xanthogranuloma.*

granuloma annulare, a self-limited, chronic skin disease of unknown cause, consisting of reddish papules and nodules arranged in a ring and most commonly seen on the distal portions of the extremities in children. No treatment is necessary.

granuloma gluteale infantum, a skin condition of the neonate characterized by large, elevated bluish or brownish-red nodules on the buttocks, often occurring as a secondary reaction to the application of strong steroid salves over a period of time. The lesions routinely disappear within a couple of months after the use of the preparations is discontinued.

granuloma inguinale, a venereal disease characterized by ulcers of the skin and subcutaneous tissues of the groin and genitalia. It is caused by infection with *Calymmatobacterium granulomatis,* a small gram-negative rod-shaped bacillus, transmitted by sexual contact. The diagnosis is made by the microscopic examination and identification of characteristic 'safety-pin'-shaped bodies in the cytoplasm of phagocytes taken from a lesion and dyed with Wright's stain. Untreated, the lesions spread, deepen, multiply, and become secondarily infected. Streptomycin is usually effective in treatment of the infection. All persons that have or are suspected of having granuloma inguinale are also tested for syphilis, as concurrent infection is common.

granulomatosis (græn'yuloumətou'sis), a condition or disease characterized by the development of granulomas, as **berylliosis, pulmonary granulomatosis, Wegener's granulomatosis.**

granulomatous colitis. See **Crohn's disease.**

granulomatous ileitis. See **Crohn's disease.**

granulomatous lymphoma. See **Hodgkin's disease.**

granulomatous thyroiditis. See **de Quervain's thyroiditis.**

granulosa cell carcinoma. See **granulosa cell tumor.**

granulosa cell tumor, a fleshy ovarian tumor with yellow streaks that originates in cells of the primordial membrana granulosa and that may grow to an extremely large size. It may be associated with the excessive production of estrogen, resulting in endometrial hyperplagia and menorrhagia.

-graph, 1. a combining form meaning the 'product of drawing or writing': *hemophotograph, micrograph, retinograph.* 2. a combining form meaning a 'machine for making something drawn': *clonograph, pneumograph, scopograph.*

-grapher, a combining form meaning 'one who writes about' something specified: *nosographer, syphilographer.*

-graphia, a combining form meaning a 'psychological abnormality revealed through handwriting': *dysantigraphia, echographia, palingraphia.*

grapho-, a combining form meaning 'pertaining to writing': *graphocatharsis, graphomania, graphophobia.*

graphospasm, muscle cramping and pain in the hand and forearm resulting from prolonged writing. Also called **writer's cramp.**

-graphy, a combining form meaning a 'kind of printing': *arteriography, cardiography, dermagraphy.*

GRAS, abbreviation for *generally recognized as safe.*

grasp reflex, a pathological reflex induced by stroking the palm or sole with the result that the fingers or toes flex in a grasping motion. The reflex occurs in diseases of the premotor cortex. In young infants the tonic grasp reflex is normal: when an examiner strokes the infant's palms, the examiner's fingers are grasped so firmly that the child can be lifted into the air.

grass. *Slang.* See **cannabis.**

Graves' disease, a disorder characterized by pronounced hyperthyroidism usually associated with an enlarged thyroid gland and exophthalmos. The etiology is unknown but the disease is familial and may be autoimmune; antibodies to thyroglobulin or to thyroid microsomes are found in more than 60 per cent of patients with the disorder. Graves' disease, which is five times more common in women than in men, occurs most frequently between the ages of 20 and 40 and often arises following an infection or physical or emotional stress. Typical signs are nervousness, a fine tremor of the hands, weight loss, fatigue, breathlessness, palpitations, heat intolerance, increased metabolic rate and gastrointestinal motility. There may be an enlarged thymus, generalized hyperplasia of the lymph nodes, blurred or double vision, localized edema, atrial arrhythmias, and osteoporosis. The diagnosis may be established by tests that measure thyroxine and triiodothyronine levels in serum. If necessary, radioactive iodine uptake in the gland may be tested. Treatment may include prescription of antithyroid drugs, as methimazole, propylthiouracil, and iodine preparations, or subtotal thyroidectomy. Radioactive iodine may be administered, but hospitalization for a few days is recommended for patients treated with a large dose. In patients with inadequately controlled Graves' disease, infection or stress may precipitate a life-threatening thyroid storm. Also called **exophthalmic goiter, thyrotoxicosis, toxic goiter.**

gravid (græv′ɪd), pregnant; carrying fertilized eggs or a fetus. – **gravidity, gravidness,** *n.*

gravid-, a combining form meaning 'pertaining to pregnancy, or pregnant': *gravida, graviditas, gravidocardiac.*

gravida 1. See **primigravida.**

gravida 2. See **secundigravida.**

-gravida, a combining form meaning 'pregnant woman with (specified) quantity of pregnancies': *nonigravida, plurigravida, unigravida.*

gravity, the heaviness or weight of an object resulting from the universal effect of the attraction between any body of matter and any planetary body. The force of the attraction depends on the relative masses of the bodies and on the distance between them.

gray baby syndrome, a toxic condition in neonates, especially premature infants, caused by a reaction to chloramphenicol. Because the body's mechanisms for detoxification and excretion of drugs are immature, the infant has limited ability to conjugate and thus eliminate the chloramphenicol. The name of the condition comes from a characteristic ashen-gray cyanosis, which is accompanied by abdominal distention, hypothermia, vomiting, respiratory distress, and vascular collapse. The condition, which is fatal if the drug is continued, can be prevented by conservative dosages of the drug and by restricting its use in women during late pregnancy or labor (since chloramphenicol readily crosses the placental barrier) and in lactating mothers.

gray hepatization. See **hepatization.**

gray matter. See **gray substance.**

gray substance, the gray tissue that makes up the inner core of the spinal column, arranged in two large lateral masses connected across the midline by a narrow commissure. Each lateral portion of the gray substance splays outward, forming the posterior and anterior horns of the spinal cord. The horns consist primarily of cell bodies of interneurons and cell bodies of motoneurons. The quantity of gray substance varies greatly at different levels of the cord, and its shape is characteristic at each level. In the thoracic region, the gray substance is small in comparison with surrounding white substance; in the cervical and the lumbar regions it is larger; and in the conus medullaris its proportion to the white substance is the greatest. Nuclei in the gray matter of the spinal cord

function as centers for all spinal reflexes. Also called **gray matter.** Compare **white substance.** See also **spinal cord, spinal nerves.**

GRE, abbreviation for **Graduate Record Examination.**

great auricular nerve, one of a pair of cutaneous branches of the cervical plexus, arising from the second and the third cranial nerves. It winds around the border of the sternocleidomastoideus, perforates the deep fascia, and ascends on the surface of the muscle before dividing into the anterior branch and the posterior branch. The anterior branch is distributed to the skin of the face over the parotid gland, communicating within the gland with the facial nerve. The posterior branch supplies the skin of the mastoid process and the back of the auricula. It also communicates with the smaller occipital nerve, the auricular branch of the vagus nerve, and the posterior auricular branch of the facial nerve.

great calorie. See **calorie.**

great cardiac vein, one of the five tributaries of the coronary sinus, beginning at the apex of the heart and ascending along the anterior interventricular sulcus to the base of the ventricles. It then curves left in the coronary sulcus, reaches the back of the heart, and opens into the left part of the coronary sinus. It receives various tributaries from the left atrium, as the large left marginal vein, which ascends along the left margin of the heart. The great cardiac vein drains the blood through its tributaries from the capillaries of the myocardium. Compare **middle cardiac vein, oblique vein of the left atrium, posterior vein of the left ventricle, small cardiac vein.**

greater multangular. See **trapezium.**

greater omentum, a filmy, transparent extension of the peritoneum, draping the transverse colon and coils of the small intestine. It is attached along the greater curvature of the stomach and the first part of the duodenum, and between its two layers contains blood vessels and fat pads. Between the stomach and the colon the greater omentum forms the gastrocolic ligament, which contains the right and the left gastroepiploic blood vessels near the greater curvature of the stomach. The greater omentum is a very movable structure that spreads easily into areas of trauma, often sealing hernias and walling off infections that would otherwise cause general peritonitis, as can occur from a ruptured vermiform appendix. Also called **gastrocolic omentum.** Compare **lesser omentum.**

greater trochanter, a large projection of the thigh bone to which are attached various muscles, including the gluteus medius, gluteus maximus, and obturator internus. The greater trochanter projects from the angle formed by the neck and the body of the thigh bone.

greater vestibular gland. See **Bartholin's gland.**

great saphenous vein, one of a pair of the longest veins in the body, containing 10 to 20 valves along its course through the leg and the thigh before ending in the femoral vein. It begins in the medial marginal vein of the dorsum of the foot, ascends anterior to the tibial malleolus and up the medial side of the leg in relation to the saphenous nerve. It runs posterior to the medial condyles of the tibia and the femur and passes through the hiatus saphenus just before joining the femoral vein. It contains more valves in the leg than in the thigh and receives many cutaneous veins and numerous tributaries, as those from the sole of the foot. Near the saphenous hiatus it is joined by the superficial epigastric vein, the superficial epigastric circumflex, and the superficial external pudendal veins. Compare **common iliac vein, femoral vein.**

green cancer. See **chloroma.**

green journal, *Informal.* **1.** *American Journal of Medicine.* **2.** *American Journal of Psychiatry.* **3.** *Obstetrics and Gynecology.* Each is so named for the color of its cover. Compare **grey journal, yellow journal.**

Greenough microscope. See **stereoscopic microscope.**

greenstick fracture, an incomplete fracture in which the bone is bent but fractured only on the outer arc of the bend. Children are particularly likely to have greenstick fractures. Immobilization is usually effective, and healing is rapid. See also **fracture.**

grenade-thrower's fracture, a fracture of the humerus caused by violent muscular contraction.

grey journal, *Informal. The American Journal of Obstetrics and Gynecology;* so named for the color of its cover. Compare **green journal, yellow journal.**

Grey Turner's sign, bruising of the skin of the loin in acute hemorrhagic pancreatitis. Also called **Turner's sign.**

grief, a nearly universal pattern of physical and emotional responses to bereavement, separation, or loss. The physical components are similar to those of fear, hunger, rage, and pain. Stimulation of the sympathetic portion of the autonomic nervous system causes increased heart and respiratory rates, dilatation of the pupils, sweating, bristling of the hair, increased flow of blood to the muscles, and increased reserves of energy. Digestion is slowed. The emotional components proceed in stages from alarm to disbelief and denial, to anger and guilt, to finding a source of comfort, and, finally, to adjustment to the loss. The way in which a grieving person behaves is greatly affected by the culture in which the person has been raised.

grief process. See **grief reaction.**

grief reaction, a complex of somatic and psychological symptoms associated with some extreme sorrow or loss, specifically the death of a loved one. Somatic symptoms include feelings of tightness in the throat and chest with choking and shortness of breath, abdominal distress, lack of muscular power, and extreme tiredness and lethargy. Psychological reactions involve a generalized awareness of mental anguish and discomfort accompanied by feelings of guilt, anger, hostility, extreme restlessness, inability to

concentrate, and the lack of capacity to initiate and maintain organized patterns of activities. Such symptoms may appear immediately following a crisis or they may be delayed, exaggerated, or apparently absent, depending on the degree of involvement of the relationship and the physical and mental status of the person. Although both the somatic and psychological reactions have the potential for developing into pathological conditions, appropriate adaptive behavior and normal responses, as sobbing or talking about the dead person or tragedy, are methods of working through the acute grief and lead to successful resolution of the crisis. Most acute grief reactions are resolved within four to six weeks, although the period varies and may be much longer, especially in cases of unexpected and sudden death. Intervention by health-care professionals, especially nurses, is necessary when individuals exhibit maladaptive behavioral patterns that avoid the resolution of grief and can lead to morbid reactions, including such accepted psychosomatic illnesses as asthma and ulcers. Also called **grief process.** See also **death, parental grief.**

grieving, anticipatory, a nursing diagnosis accepted by the Fourth National Conference on the Classification of Nursing Diagnoses. The etiology of the condition is to be developed at a later conference. The defining characteristics of the problem include the potential loss of something or someone important, expressions of distress, denial of potential loss, anger, guilt or sorrow, and changes in eating habits, sleep patterns, activity level, libido, and patterns of communication. See also **nursing diagnosis.**

grieving, dysfunctional, a nursing diagnosis accepted by the Fourth National Conference on the Classification of Nursing Diagnoses. The etiology of the problem is an actual or perceived loss of someone or something of great importance to the client. The defining characteristics of the problem include expressions of distress or a denial of the loss; grief, anger, sadness, and weeping; changes in patterns and habits of sleeping, eating, and dreaming; and alterations in libido and activity levels. The lost person or object is idealized, past experience is relived, and concentration and purposeful work are diminished. The client has a labile affect and seems to regress developmentally.

griffe des orteils (grif′deizɔrtei′). See **pes cavus.**

Grifulvin, a trade name for an antifungal (griseofulvin).

grinder's asthma, a condition characterized by asthmatic symptoms caused by inhalation of fine particles produced by industrial grinding processes. Also called **grinder's disease.** See also **pneumoconiosis.**

grinder's disease. See **grinder's asthma.**

grippe (grɪp). See **influenza.**

Grisactin, a trade name for an antifungal (griseofulvin).

griseofulvin (grɪs′ioufəl′vɪn), an antifungal.

■ INDICATIONS: It is prescribed in the treatment of certain infections of the skin, hair, and nails.

■ CONTRAINDICATIONS: Liver dysfunction, porphyria, or known hypersensitivity to this drug prohibits its use.

■ ADVERSE EFFECTS: The most serious adverse reactions are blood dyscrasias. Headache, gastrointestinal symptoms, and rashes also may occur.

groin, each of two areas where the abdomen joins the thighs.

Grönblad-Strandberg syndrome (groun′blædstrænd′bərg), an autosomal recessive disorder of connective tissue characterized by premature aging and breakdown of the skin, gray or brown streaks on the retina, and hemorrhagic arterial degeneration, including retinal bleeding that causes loss of vision. Angina pectoris and hypertension are common; weak pulse, episodic claudication, and fatigue with exertion may affect the extremities. The prognosis depends upon vessel involvement, but life expectancy is shortened by the condition. Treatment is symptomatic. Also called **pseudoxanthoma elasticum.**

groove, a shallow, linear depression in various structures throughout the body, as those that form channels for nerves along the bones, those in bones for the insertion of muscles, and those between certain areas of the brain.

gross, 1. macroscopic, as *gross anatomy,* from the study of organs or parts of the body large enough to be seen with the naked eye, or *gross pathology,* from the study of tissue changes without magnification by a microscope. 2. large or obese. Compare **microscopic.**

ground itch, pruritic macules, papules, and vesicles secondary to penetration of the skin by hookworm larvae, prevalent in tropical and subtropical climates. It may be prevented by wearing shoes and by establishing sanitary disposal of feces. See also **hookworm.**

ground substance. See **matrix.**

group, (in research) any set of items or groups of people under study. An **experimental group** is studied to determine the effect of an event, a substance, or a technique. A **control group** serves as a standard or reference for comparison with an experimental group. A control group is similar to the experimental group in number and is identical in specified characteristics, as sex, age, annual income, parity, or other factors. Subjects meeting the study criteria are selected from a larger group at random or by a protocol that ensures nonbiased selection.

group therapy, the application of psychotherapeutic techniques within a small group of emotionally disturbed persons who, usually under the leadership of a psychotherapist, discuss their problems in an attempt to promote individual psychological growth and favorable personality change. The procedure provides opportunities for treating a greater number of people in a shorter period of time than would be possible with individual therapy, and it is used in clinics, in institutions, and in private practice.

Group therapy has been found to be particularly effective in the treatment of various addictions. A kind of group therapy is **psychodrama.** See also **Gestalt therapy, psychotherapy, self-help group, transactional analysis.**

growing pains, 1. rheumaticlike pains that occur in the muscles and joints of children or adolescents as a result of fatigue, emotional problems, postural defects, and other causes that are not related to growth and that may be symptoms of various disorders. 2. emotional and psychological problems experienced during adolescence.

growth, 1. an increase in the size of an organism or any of its parts, as measured in increments of weight, volume, or linear dimensions, that occurs as a result of hyperplasia or hypertrophy. 2. the normal progressive anatomical, physiological, psychological, intellectual, social, and cultural development from infancy to adulthood as a result of the gradual and normal processes of accretion and assimilation. The total of the numerous changes that occur during the lifetime of an individual constitute a dynamic and complex process that involves many interrelated components, notably heredity, environment, nutrition, hygiene, and disease, all of which are subject to a variety of influences. In childhood, growth is categorized according to approximate age at which distinctive physical changes usually appear and at which specific developmental tasks are achieved. Such stages include the prenatal period, infancy, early childhood, including the toddler and the preschool child, middle childhood, and adolescence. There are two periods of accelerated growth: the first twelve months, in which the infant triples in weight, grows approximately 50 per cent of the height at birth, and undergoes rapid motor, cognitive, and social development; the second, in the months around puberty, when the child approaches adult height and secondary sexual characteristics emerge. Physical growth may be abnormally accelerated or slowed by a defect in the hypophyseal or pituitary gland. 3. any abnormal localized increase of the size or number of cells, as in a tumor or neoplasm. 4. a proliferation of cells, specifically a bacterial culture or mold. Compare **development, differentiation, maturation.**

growth failure, a lack of normal physical and psychological development as a result of genetic, nutritional, pathological, or psychosocial factors. See also **failure to thrive, maternal deprivation syndrome.**

growth hormone (GH), a single-chain peptide secreted by the anterior pituitary gland in response to growth hormone releasing factor (GHRF) from the hypothalamus. GH promotes protein synthesis in all cells, increases fat mobilization and use of fatty acids for energy, and decreases utilization of carbohydrate. Growth effects depend on the presence of thyroid hormone, insulin, and carbohydrate. Somatomedins, proteins produced chiefly in the liver, play a vital role in GH-induced skeletal growth, but the hormone cannot cause elongation of long bones after the epiphyses close, so that stature does not increase after puberty. GH accelerates the transport of specific amino acids into cells, stimulates the synthesis of messenger RNA and ribosomal RNA, influences the activity of several enzymes, increases the storage of phosphorus and potassium, and promotes a moderate retention of sodium. The secretion of GH, controlled almost exclusively by the central nervous system, occurs in bursts with more than half the total daily amount released during early sleep. Somatostatin, an anterior pituitary regulating hormone produced in the hypothalamus, inhibits GH secretion. A deficiency of GH causes dwarfism; an excess results in gigantism or acromegaly. Also called **somatotropic hormone, somatotropin.** See also **acromegaly, dwarfism, gigantism, somatostatin.**

growth hormone-release-inhibiting hormone. See **somatostatin.**

growth hormone releasing factor (GHRF), somatotropin-releasing factor released by the hypothalamus. Also called **somatoliberin.**

Grünfelder's reflex (grɪn'feldərz), an involuntary dorsal flexion of the great toe with a fanlike spreading of the other toes, caused by continued pressure on the posterior lateral fontanel. The reflex occurs in children who have middle-ear disease.

grunting, abnormal, short audible gruntlike breaks in exhalation that often accompany severe chest pain. The grunt occurs as the glottis briefly stops the flow of air, halting the movement of the lungs and their surrounding or supporting structures. Grunting is most often heard in a person who has pneumonia, pulmonary edema, or fractured or bruised ribs. Atelectasis in the newborn also causes grunting owing to the effort required for the baby to fill the lungs.

GU, abbreviation for **genitourinary.**

guaiacol poisoning. See **phenol poisoning.**

guaifenesin, glyceryl guaiacolate, a white to slightly gray powder with a bitter taste and faint odor, widely used as an expectorant. Guaifenesin increases the flow of fluid in the respiratory tract, reducing the viscosity of bronchial and tracheal secretions and facilitating their removal by the cough reflex and ciliary action.

guanethidine sulfate, an antihypertensive.

■ INDICATION: It is prescribed in the treatment of moderate and severe hypertension.

■ CONTRAINDICATIONS: Heart failure, concomitant administration of monoamine oxidase inhibitors, pheochromocytoma, or known hypersensitivity to this drug prohibits its use.

■ ADVERSE EFFECTS: Among the more serious adverse reactions are orthostatic hypotension, salt and water retention, bradycardia, diarrhea, and an inability to ejaculate.

guaranine (gwərə'nın). See **caffeine.**

guardian ad litem (æd' lai'təm), (in law) a person who is appointed by a court to prosecute or defend a suit for an infant or an incapacited person. A guardian ad litem is sometimes appointed when a person's life is in imminent danger and that person refuses treatment.

Guedel's signs, a system for describing the stages and planes of anesthesia during an operative procedure.

■ STAGE I (amnesia and analgesia) begins with the administration of anesthesia and continues to the loss of consciousness. Respiration is quiet, though sometimes irregular, and reflexes are still present.

■ STAGE II (delirium or excitement) begins with the loss of consciousness and includes the onset of total anesthesia. During this stage the patient may move his limbs, chatter incoherently, hold his breath, or become violent. Vomiting, with the attendant danger of aspiration, may occur. No avoidable stimulation is allowed at this stage; the patient is brought to Stage III as quickly and smoothly as possible.

■ STAGE III (surgical anesthesia) begins with establishment of a regular pattern of breathing and total loss of consciousness and includes the period during which signs of respiratory or cardiovascular failure first appear. This stage is divided into four planes: At *plane 1* all movements cease and respiration is regular and "automatic." Eyelid reflexes are lost, but eyeball movements are marked. Pharyngeal reflexes disappear, but laryngeal and peritoneal reflexes are still present. Tonicity of the abdominal muscles can be judged by the tonicity of the extraocular muscles. At *plane 2* the eyeballs become fixed centrally, conjunctivae lose their luster, and intercostal muscle activity diminishes. Respiration remains regular, with reduced tidal volume, and does not change in quality or rate in response to incision. Intubation no longer causes laryngospasm. At *plane 3* intercostal paralysis occurs, and respiration becomes solely diaphragmatic. The pupils no longer react to light, and total muscle relaxation is achieved. At *plane 4* deep anesthesia is achieved, with the cessation of spontaneous respiration and the absence of sensation.

■ STAGE IV (premortem) signals danger. This stage is characterized by pupils that are maximally dilated and skin that is cold and ashen. Blood pressure is extremely low, often unmeasurable, and the brachial pulse is feeble or entirely absent. Cardiac arrest is imminent. Anesthesia is reduced, the lungs are manually ventilated with 100 per cent oxygen, and the reservoir bag is continually emptied.

Guérin's fracture (geiræz'), a fracture of the maxilla. Also called **LeFort I fracture.**

Guillain-Barré syndrome (giyæ'bærei'), an idiopathic, peripheral polyneuritis occurring between 1 and 3 weeks after a mild episode of fever associated with a viral infection or with immunization. Symmetrical pain and weakness affect the extremities, and paralysis may develop. The neuritis may spread, ascending to the trunk and involving the face, arms, and thoracic muscles. The course of the disease is variable; some people may have minimal symptoms while others may have symptoms severe enough to require critical nursing care, including respiratory assistance and a circ-o-lectric bed. The disease resolves itself completely in a few weeks or a few months. There is no treatment other than supportive care. Also called **acute febrile polyneuritis, acute idiopathic polyneuritis, infectious polyneuritis.**

guilty, (in criminal law) a verdict by the court, finding that to a moral certainty it is beyond reasonable doubt that the defendant committed the crime and is responsible for the offense as charged.

Guinea worm infection. See **dracunculiasis.**

gullet. See **esophagus.**

gum, 1. a sticky excretion from certain plants. 2. See **gingiva.**

gumboil, an abscess of the gingiva and periosteum resulting from injury, infection, or dental decay. The gum is characteristically red, swollen, and tender. The abscess may rupture spontaneously, or it may require incision. Treatment may include antibiotics and hot mouthwashes. Also called **parulis.**

gum camphor. See **camphor.**

gumma (gəm′ə), *pl.* **gummas, gummata.** 1. a granuloma, characteristic of tertiary syphilis, varying from one millimeter to one centimeter in diameter. It is usually encapsulated and contains a central necrotic mass surrounded by inflammatory and fibrotic zones of tissue. Infectious organisms of the genus *Treponema* may be found in a gumma. The lesion may be localized or diffuse, occurring on the trunk, legs, and face and on various internal organs, especially the liver. A ruptured gumma results in a shallow ulcer that heals slowly. 2. a soft granulomatous lesion sometimes occurring with tuberculosis.

gunshot fracture, a fracture caused by a bullet or similar missile.

Gunther's disease (gən′thərz), a rare congenital disorder of porphyrin metabolism that is associated with sunlight-induced skin lesions. See also **porphyria.**

gurgling rale, an abnormal coarse sound heard during auscultation, especially over large cavities or over a trachea nearly filled with secretions.

gurry (gər′i), *Slang.* the detritus incident to physical trauma or surgery, including body fluids, secretions, and tissue.

Gurvich radiation. See **mitogenetic radiation.**

gustatory organ (gəs′tətor′i). See **taste bud.**

gut, 1. intestine. 2. *Informal.* digestive tract. 3. suture material manufactured from the intestines of sheep.

Guthrie test (gəth′ri), a screening for phenylketonuria used to detect the abnormal presence of phenylalanine

metabolites in the blood. A small amount of blood is obtained and placed in a medium with a strain of *Bacillus subtilis,* a bacterium that cannot grow without phenylalanine. If phenylalanine metabolites are present the bacteria reproduce and the test is positive, indicating that the subject has phenylketonuria. In most states, this test is done twice on all infants, once before discharge from the hospital and again at two weeks of age. See also **phenylketonuria.**

guttate psoriasis, an acute form of psoriasis consisting of teardrop-shaped, red, scaly patches measuring 3 to 10 mm all over the body. A beta-hemolytic streptococcal pharyngitis or other upper respiratory infection may precipitate this reaction in susceptible individuals. Adequate treatment is essential to prevent a more severe form of psoriasis. Compare **pustular psoriasis.** See also **psoriasis.**

GVS, a trade name for a topical anti-infective (gentian violet).

gymno-, a combining form meaning 'pertaining to nakedness': *gymnocarpus, gymnocyte, gymnospore.*

gyn, 1. *Informal.* abbreviation for **gynecology.** 2. abbreviation for **gynecologist.**

gyn-. See **gyneco-.**

gynandrous (gainæn′drəs, jinæn′drəs), describing a man or a woman who has some of the physical characteristics usually attributed to the other sex, as a female pseudohermaphrodite. —**gynandry,** *n.*

gyne-. See **gyneco-.**

-gyne, a combining form meaning '(specified) female characteristics': *androgyne, epigyne, trichogyne.* Also **-gyn.**

gyneco-, gyn-, gyne-, gyno-, a combining form meaning 'pertaining to a woman or the female sex': *gynecoid, gynecomasia, gynotermon.*

gynecoid pelvis, a type of pelvis characteristic of the normal female and associated with the smallest incidence of fetopelvic disproportion. The inlet is nearly round, the sacrum is parallel to the posterior aspect of the symphysis pubis, the sidewalls are straight and the ischial spines are blunt and do not encroach on the space in the true pelvis. It is the ideal pelvic type for childbirth.

gynecologic examination. See **pelvic examination.**

gynecologist (gai′nəkol′əjist, jin′ekol′əjist), a physician who specializes in gynecology.

gynecology (gai′nəkol′əji, jin′əkol′əji), a branch of medicine concerned with the health care of women, including their sexual and reproductive function and the diseases of their reproductive organs, except diseases of the breast that require surgery. Unlike most specialities in medicine, gynecology encompasses surgical and nonsurgical expertise. It is almost always studied and practiced in conjunction with obstetrics. —**gynecologic, gynecological,** *adj.*

gynecomastia (gai′nəkoumæs′tia, jin′ikoumæs′tiə), **gynecomasty,** an abnormal enlargement of one or both breasts in men. The condition is usually temporary and benign. It may be caused by hormonal imbalance, tumor of the testis or pituitary, medication with estrogens or steroidal compounds, or failure of the liver to inactivate circulating estrogen, as in alcoholic cirrhosis. Less commonly, the gynecomastia may be caused by a hormone-secreting tumor of the breast, lung, or other organ. It tends to remit spontaneously, but, if marked, may be corrected surgically for cosmetic or psychologic reasons. Biopsy may be performed to rule out the presence of cancer. Malignant neoplastic gynecomastia is usually inoperable and only briefly responsive to chemotherapy.

Gyne-Lotrimin, a trade name for an antifungal (clotrimazole).

gynephobia (gai'nəfoʊ'biə, jɪn'əfoʊ'biə), an anxiety disorder characterized by a morbid fear of women or by a morbid aversion to the society of women. It is an obsessive, phobic phenomenon occurring almost entirely in men and may usually be traced to some frightening experience involving women that occurred in childhood. Treatment consists of psychotherapy to uncover the causative emotional conflict, followed by behavior therapy, specifically systemic desensitization and flooding to reduce anxiety.

Gynergen, a trade name for an ergot alkaloid (ergotamine tartrate), used to treat migraine.

Gynetone, a trade name for a hormonal fixed-combination drug containing an estrogen (ethinyl estradiol) and an androgen (methyltestosterone).

-gynic, a combining form meaning 'relating to the human female': *hologynic, monogynic, polygonic.*

gyno-. See **gyneco-.**

gynogamone (gai'noʊgæm'oʊn), a gamone secreted by the female gamete.

Gynorest, a trade name for a progestin (dydrogesterone).

-gynous, a combining form meaning 'pertaining to female characteristics': *androgynous.* Also **-gynic.**

-gyria, a combining form meaning '(condition of the) development of the convolutions of the cerebral cortex': *oculogyria, polymicrogyria, ulegyria.*

gyri cerebri, the convolutions of the outer surface of the cerebral hemisphere, separated from each other by sulci, most of which appear during the sixth or seventh months of fetal life.

gyrus (jai'rəs), *pl.* **gyri.** one of the tortuous convolutions of the surface of the brain caused by infolding of the cortex. See also **gyri cerebri.**

H

H, chemical symbol for **hydrogen.**

habit, **1.** a customary or particular practice, manner, or mode of behavior. **2.** an involuntary pattern of behavior or thought. **3.** *Archaic.* appearance or physique. Also called **habitus. 4.** the habitual use of drugs or narcotics. See also **habit spasm, habit training.**

habit spasm, an involuntary twitching or tic usually involving a small muscle group of the face, neck, or shoulders and resulting in movements like spasmodic blinking or rapid jerking of the head to the side. The movements are often generated by emotional conflicts rather than being caused by any organic disorder. They may serve as a release for tension or anxiety.

habit training, the process of teaching a child how to adjust to the demands of the external world by forming certain habits, primarily those related to eating, sleeping, elimination, and dress.

habitual abortion, spontaneous termination of three successive pregnancies before the twentieth week of gestation. Habitual abortion can result from chronic infection, abnormalities of the conceptus, maternal hormonal dysfunction, or uterine abnormalities as cervical incompetence. See also **cerclage, incompetent cervix.**

habitual fever. See **habitual hyperthermia.**

habitual hyperthermia, a condition of unknown cause occurring in young females, characterized by body temperatures of 99.0° to 100.5°F regularly or intermittently for years, associated with fatigue, malaise, vague aches and pains, insomnia, bowel disturbances, and headaches. No organic cause can be found; the diagnosis is usually made only after a prolonged period of study and observation. No specific treatment is recommended. Reassurance and psychotherapy offer the best relief. Also called **habitual fever.**

habituation, **1.** an acquired tolerance from repeated exposure to a particular stimulus. **2.** Also called **negative adaptation.** a decline and eventual elimination of a conditioned response by repetition of the conditioned stimulus. **3.** Compare **addiction.** psychological and emotional dependence on a drug, tobacco, or alcohol resulting from the repeated use of the substance but without the addictive, physiological need to increase dosage.

habitus (hæb′ɪtəs), describing a person's appearance or physique, as an athletic habitus.

Haeckel's law (hek′əlz). See **recapitulation theory.**

-haemia. See **-emia.**

Haemophilus (himof′ɪləs), a genus of gram-negative pathogenic bacteria, frequently found in the respiratory tract of man and other animals, as *Haemophilus influenzae,* which causes influenza and one form of meningitis, *H. haemolyticus,* a hemolytic species pathogenic in the upper respiratory tract of man, and *H. ducreyi,* which causes chancroid. *Haemophilus* species are generally sensitive to tetracyclines and sulfonamides.

Haemophilus influenzae, a small, gram-negative, nonmotile, parasitic bacterium that occurs in two forms, encapsulated and nonencapsulated, and in six types, a, b, c, d, e, and f. Almost all infections are caused by encapsulated type b organisms. *Haemophilus influenzae* is found in the throats of 30 per cent of healthy, normal people. In children and in debilitated older people severe destructive inflammation of the larynx, trachea, and bronchi may result from infection. Subacute bacterial endocarditis and purulent meningitis may also be caused by it. Secondary infection by *H. influenzae* occurs in influenza and in many other respiratory diseases. Immunization is available by inoculation with anti-Haemophilus influenzae serum.

hafnium (Hf), a hard, brittle, silver-gray metallic element of the first transition group. Its atomic number is 72; its atomic weight is 178.49 Elements in this group show some nonmetallic chemical characteristics.

Hagedorn's needle (ha′gədɔrnz), a flat surgical needle with a cutting edge near its point and a very large eye at the other end.

Hageman factor (HF) (hægəmən). See **factor XII.**

hair, a filament of keratin consisting of a root and a shaft formed in a specialized follicle in the epidermis. There are two stages of hair development: **anagen,** the active growing stage, and **telogen,** the resting, or club, stage. Scalp hair grows at an average rate of one mm every three days, body and eyebrow hair at a much slower rate. Hair plucking does not stop hair growth. See also **hirsutism, lanugo.**

hair matrix carcinoma. See **basal cell carcinoma.**

hair pulling. See **trichotillomania.**

hairy-cell leukemia, an uncommon neoplasm of blood-forming tissues, characterized by pancytopenia, a massively enlarged spleen, and the presence in blood and bone marrow of reticulum cells with many fine projections on their surface. The disease occurs six times more frequently in men than in women, usually appears in the fifth decade with an insidious onset and a variable course marked by anemia, thrombocytopenia, and spontaneous bruising. A tartrate-resistant acid phosphate isoenzyme found in hairy cells may aid in the diagnosis. Splenectomy may control the cytopenia and some cases may improve with chemotherapy using vincristine and prednisone. Also called **leukemic reticuloendotheliosis.**

hairy tongue, a dark, pigmented overgrowth of the filiform papillae of the tongue that is a benign and frequent side effect of some antibiotics. The condition gradually subsides, and no treatment is indicated.

halcinonide, a topical glucocorticoid.

■ INDICATION: It is prescribed topically as an anti-inflammatory agent.

■ CONTRAINDICATIONS: Viral and fungal diseases of the skin, impaired circulation, or known hypersensitivity to this drug or to steroid medication prohibits its use.

■ ADVERSE EFFECTS: Among the more serious adverse effects are skin reactions and systemic side effects occurring from prolonged or excessive application.

Haldol, a trade name for a tranquilizer (haloperidol).

Haldrone, a trade name for a glucocorticoid (paramethasone acetate).

half-life, radioactive half-life, the time required for a radioactive substance to lose 50 per cent of its activity through decay. Each radionuclide has a unique half-life. See also **biological half-life, effective half-life.**

half-sibling, one of two or more children who have at least one parent in common; a half brother or half sister. Also called **half-sib.**

halfway house, a specialized treatment facility, usually for psychiatric patients who no longer require complete hospitalization but who need some care and time to adjust to living independently.

halitosis (hæl'ıtou'sıs), offensive breath resulting from poor oral hygiene, dental or oral infections, the ingestion of certain foods, as garlic or alcohol, use of tobacco, or some systemic diseases, as the odor of acetone in diabetes and ammonia in liver disease.

Hallpike caloric test, a method for evaluating the function of the vestibule of the ear in people with vertigo or hearing loss. Irrigation of the ears with cool and warm water or air mimics the stimulus of turning in the vestibular apparatus, causing nystagmus. Nystagmus can then be evaluated, and specific disorders of the vestibule may be diagnosed. See also **nystagmus.**

hallucination, a sensory perception that does not result from an external stimulus. It can occur in any of the senses and is classified accordingly as auditory, gustatory, olfactory, tactile, or visual. Kinds of hallucinations are **hypnagogic hallucination, lilliputian hallucination, stump hallucination.** – **hallucinate,** v.

hallucinogen (həlu'sənəjen', hæl'əsın'əjın, hæl'yəsın'əjın), a substance that causes excitation of the central nervous system, characterized by hallucination, mood change, anxiety, sensory distortion, delusion, depersonalization, increased pulse, temperature, and blood pressure, and dilation of the pupils. Psychic dependence may occur, and depressive or suicidal psychotic states may result from the ingestion of hallucinogenic substances. Some kinds of hallucinogens are **lysergic acid diethylamide (LSD), mescaline, peyote, phencyclidine, psilocybin.**

hallucinosis (hælu'sınou'sıs), a pathological mental state in which awareness consists primarily or exclusively of hallucinations. A kind of hallucinosis is **alcoholic hallucinosis.**

hallux (hæl'əks), pl. **halluces** (hæl'yusiz). the great toe.

hallux rigidus, a painful deformity of the great toe, limiting motion at the metatarsophalangeal joint.

hallux valgus, a deformity in which the great toe is angulated away from the midline of the body toward the other toes; in some cases the great toe rides over or under the other toes.

halo cast, an orthopedic device used to help immobilize the neck and head. It incorporates the trunk, usually with shoulder straps, and an apparatus by means of an outrigger within the cast to secure pins to a band around the skull. The halo cast is used to help the healing of cervical injuries, cervical dislocations, and for postoperative positioning and immobilization following cervical surgery.

halo effect, the beneficial effect of an interview or other encounter, as may occur in the course of a research project or a health-care visit. The halo effect cannot be attributed to the content of the interview or to any specific act or treatment; it is the result of indefinable interpersonal factors present in the interaction.

halofenate (hæl'oufi'neit), an antihyperlipoproteinemic and uricosuric, not currently on the market in the U.S.

Halog, a trade name for a topical glucocorticoid (halcinonide).

halogenated hydrocarbon, a volatile liquid used for general anesthesia, administered in combination with nitrous oxide or oxygen, or both. Nausea, vomiting, laryngospasm, and pharyngeal irritation are less severe and frequent when this anesthesia is used. Because the secretion of mucus is reduced, premedication with atropine and scopolamine may be reduced. Kinds of halogenated hydrocarbons are **enflurane, halothane, isoflurane, methoxyflurane, trichoroethylene.**

haloperidol (hæl'ouper'ədɔl), a butyrophenone tranquilizer.

■ INDICATIONS: It is prescribed in the treatment of psychotic disorders and in the control of Tourette's syndrome.

■ CONTRAINDICATIONS: Parkinson's disease, concurrent administration of central nervous system depressants, liver or renal dysfunction, severe hypotension, or known hypersensitivity to this drug prohibits its use.

■ ADVERSE EFFECTS: Among the more serious adverse effects are hypotension and a variety of extrapyramidal and hypersensitivity reactions.

haloprogin (hei′louprou′jın), an antibacterial and antifungal.

■ INDICATIONS: It is prescribed in the treatment of susceptible fungal infections, including athlete's foot.

■ CONTRAINDICATION: Known hypersensitivity to this drug prohibits its use.

■ ADVERSE EFFECTS: Among the most serious adverse reactions are exacerbation of existing lesions, formation of vesicles, and pruritus.

Halotestin, a trade name for an androgen (fluoxymesterone).

Halotex, a trade name for an antibacterial (haloprogin).

halothane (hæl′əθein), an inhalation anesthetic.

■ INDICATIONS: It is prescribed for induction and maintenance of general anesthesia.

■ CONTRAINDICATION: It is not recommended for obstetrical anesthesia unless uterine relaxation is required.

■ ADVERSE EFFECTS: Among the more serious adverse reactions are hepatic necrosis, cardiac arrest or arrhythmia, hypotension, nausea, and emesis.

Halsted's forceps (hæl′stedz), **1.** Also called **mosquito forceps.** a small, pointed hemostatic forceps. **2.** a forceps with slender jaws for grasping arteries and other blood vessels.

hamamelis water (hæm′əmi′lıs). See **witch hazel,** def 2.

hamate bone (hæm′eit), a carpal bone that rests on the fourth and fifth metacarpal bones and projects a hooklike process, the hamulus, from its palmar surface. Its dorsal surface is rough for ligamentous attachment. The hamate bone articulates with the lunate proximally, the fourth and fifth metacarpal distally, the triangular medially, and the capitate laterally. Also called **os hamatum, unciform bone.**

Hamman-Rich syndrome (hæm′ənrich), progressive interstitial pulmonary fibrosis of unknown origin, accompanied by right-sided heart disease and cor pulmonale. Anorexia, fatigue, weight loss, and vague chest pains are common symptoms. The syndrome may be acute and rapidly progressive or chronic and slowly developing. Treatment includes use of corticosteroids, control of infections, and relief of specific symptoms.

hammertoe, a foot digit permanently flexed at the midphalangeal joint, resulting in a clawlike appearance. The anomaly may be present in more than one digit but is most common in the second toe.

hamstring muscle, any one of three muscles at the back of the thigh; medially, the semimembranosus and the semitendinosus and laterally, the biceps femoris.

hamstring reflex, a normal deep tendon reflex elicited by tapping one of the hamstring tendons behind the knee, resulting in contraction of the tendon and flexion of the

knee. The patient should be lying in the supine position with the knee and hip partially flexed and the leg supported by the examiner's hand. An accentuated hamstring reflex may result from a lesion of the pyramidal system above the level of the fourth lumbar nerve root. See also **deep tendon reflex.**

hamstring tendon, one of the three tendons from the three hamstring muscles in the back of the thigh. The one lateral and the two medial hamstring tendons connect the hamstring muscles to the knee.

hand, the part of the upper limb distal to the forearm. It is the most flexible part of the skeleton and has a total of 27 bones, eight forming the carpus, five forming the metacarpus, and 14 comprising the phalangeal section. Also called **manus.**

handedness, voluntary or involuntary preference for use of either the left or right hand. The preference is related to cerebral dominance, with left-handedness corresponding to dominance of the right side of the brain and vice versa. Also called **chirality, laterality.**

hand-foot syndrome. See **sickle cell crisis.**

handicapped, referring to a person who has a congenital or acquired mental or physical defect that interferes with normal functioning of the body system or the ability to be self-sufficient in modern society.

Hand-Schüller-Christian syndrome (hænd′shu′lərkrıs′-chən), *Obsolete.* a triad of symptoms, exopthalmos, diabetes insipidus, and bone destruction, which may occur in any of several disorders. See also **eosinophilic granuloma, Letterer-Siwe syndrome.**

hanging drop preparation, a technique used for the examination and identification of certain microorganisms, as spirochetes or trichomonads. The technique requires a cover slip, a microscope, and a special slide that has a central concavity. A specimen suspected of containing the microorganism is diluted with a sterile isotonic solution. A drop of this fluid mixture is placed on a glass cover slip, which is then inverted carefully and placed over the slide so that the drop is hanging from the slip into the concavity in the slide. The delicate structures and the method of movement characteristic of the species may then be viewed through the microscope. An ordinary glass slide can be prepared for hanging drop examination by making a ring of petroleum jelly on the slide and inverting a cover slip bearing the drop of solution over the ring.

hangman's fracture, a fracture of the posterior elements of the cervical vertebrae with dislocation of C2 or C3.

hangnail, a piece of partially disconnected epidermis of the cuticle or nail fold. Tearing the skin fragment causes a red, painful, easily infected sore. Early treatment is to trim the hangnail close with nail clippers. For inflamed situations an antibiotic ointment and protective bandage are used.

Hankow fever (hæŋ′kau). See **schistosomiasis.**

Hanot's disease (hænouz′), primary biliary cirrhosis. See **biliary cirrhosis.**

Hansen's disease. See **leprosy.**

-haphia. See **-aphia.**

haploidy (hæp′lɔidi), the state or condition of having only one complete set of nonhomologous chromosomes. – **haploid,** *adj.*

hapten (hæp′ten), **haptene** (hæp′tin), a nonproteinaceous substance that acts as an antigen by combining with particular bonding sites on an antibody. Unlike a true antigen, it does not induce the formation of antibodies. A hapten bonded to a carrier protein may induce an immune response.

haptoglobin (hæp′touglou′bın), a plasma protein whose only known function is to bind free hemoglobin. The quantity of haptoglobin is increased in certain chronic diseases and inflammatory disorders and is decreased or absent in hemolytic anemia. Compare **transferrin.** See also **hemoglobinemia, hemoglobinuria.**

hardening of the arteries. See **arteriosclerosis.**

hard fibroma, a neoplasm composed of fibrous tissue in which there are few cells. Also called **fibroma durum.**

hard money, *Informal.* (in a university, school, or agency) income from stable sources as an endowment, tuition, or fees.

hardness of x rays, the relative penetrating power of x rays. In general, the shorter the wavelength, the harder the radiation.

hard palate, the bony portion of the roof of the mouth, continuous posteriorly with the soft palate and bounded anteriorly and laterally by the alveolar arches and the gums. The palatine process of the maxilla and the horizontal portion of the palatine bone form the bony support for the hard palate which is covered by periosteum and by the mucous membrane of the mouth. A linear raphe along its middle line ends anteriorly in a small papilla, which corresponds with the incisive canal. On each side and anterior to the raphe, the mucous membrane is thick, pale in color, and corrugated. Posteriorly the mucous membrane is thin, smooth, and of a deeper color. The hard palate is covered with squamous epithelium and furnished with numerous palatal glands lying between the mucous membrane and the surface of the bone. Compare **soft palate.**

Hardy-Weinberg equilibrium principle, the mathematical relationship between the frequency of genes and the resulting genotypes in populations. In a large interbreeding population characterized by random mating, Mendelian inheritance, and the absence of migration, mutation, and selection, the ratio of individuals homozygous for a dominant gene to those heterozygous to those ho-

mozygous for a recessive gene is 1:2:1, at which point equilibrium is established; and the frequency of genes and genotypes remains relatively unchanged from generation to generation. See also **genetic equilibrium.**

harelip, a congenital anomaly consisting of one or more clefts in the upper lip resulting from the failure in the embryo of the maxillary and median nasal processes to close. Treatment is surgical repair in infancy. See also **cleft palate.**

hare's eye. See **lagophthalmos.**

harlequin color, a transient flushing of the skin on the dependent side with pallor of the upward side. Commonly seen in normal young infants, it disappears as the child matures.

harlequin fetus, an infant whose skin at birth is completely covered with thick, horny scales that resemble armor and are divided by deep red fissures. The condition is the most severe form of lamellar exfoliation of the newborn, and the infant is stillborn or dies within a few days of birth. Also called **ichthyosis fetus.**

Harmonyl, a trade name for an antihypertensive (deserpidine).

Harris tube, a tube used for gastric and intestinal decompression. It is a mercury weighted, single lumen tube that is passed through the nose and carried through the alimentary tract by gravity. The amount of mercury in the soft bag surrounding the tube varies from 2 to 5 ml according to the age, size, and condition of the patient. The location of the tube is followed by fluoroscopy, and its final placement is also checked. The tube is lubricated before the procedure is begun, and the patient is positioned in such a way that gravity can aid advancement of the tube through the alimentary tract.

Hartmann's curet (hart′manz), a curet used for the removal of adenoids. See also **curet.**

Hartnup disease (hart′nəp), a recessive genetic metabolic disorder characterized by pellagralike skin lesions, transient cerebellar ataxia, and hyperaminoaciduria, caused by defects in intestinal absorption and renal reabsorption of neutral amino acids. Bacterial degradation of unabsorbed amino acids in the gut leads to the absorption of breakdown products and their appearance in urine; the unavailability of tryptophan leads to a deficiency of niacin, the antipellagra vitamin. Common symptoms of the disease are dry, scaly, well-circumscribed skin lesions, glossitis, stomatitis, diarrhea, psychiatric problems, and pronounced photosensitivity; brief exposure to the sun may cause erythema, edema, and vesiculation. Treatment consists of oral nicotinamide and a diet containing proteins composed of more easily absorbed small peptides.

Harvard pump, a small pump that can be adjusted to deliver small amounts of medication in solution through an intravenous infusion set. It is commonly used to administer oxytocin in the induction or augmentation of labor. Compare **Abbot pump.**

harvest fever. See **leptospirosis.**

harvest mite. See **chigger.**

Hashimoto's disease (ha'shimou'touz), an autoimmune thyroid disorder, characterized by the production of antibodies in response to thyroid antigens and the replacement of normal thyroid structures with lymphocytes and lymphoid germinal centers. The disease shows a marked hereditary pattern, but it is 20 times more common in women than in men. It occurs most frequently between the ages of 30 and 50 but may arise in young children. The thyroid, typically enlarged, pale yellow, and lumpy on the surface, shows dense lymphocytic infiltration, and the remaining thyroid tissue frequently contains small empty follicles. The goiter is usually asymptomatic, but occasionally patients complain of dysphagia and a feeling of local pressure. The thymus is usually enlarged, and regional lymph nodes often show hyperplasia. A definitive diagnosis can be made if a fluorescent scan shows a decrease or absence of thyroid-stable iodine and if a hemagglutination test for thyroid antigens is positive. Replacement therapy with thyroid hormone is indicated for patients with thyroid deficiency and can prevent further enlargement of the goiter. Also called **Hashimoto's struma, Hashimoto's thyroiditis, lymphadenoid goiter, lymphocytic thyroiditis, struma lymphomatosa.**

hashish (hashish', hæshish'). See **cannabis.**

Haverhill fever (hei'vərıl), a febrile disease, caused by infection with *Streptobacillus moniliformis,* transmitted by the bite of a rat. The spirochetelike bacterium is normally present in rat saliva. Characteristically the wound from the bite heals, but within 10 days fever, chills, vomiting, headache, muscle and joint pain, and a rash appear. Treatment with antibiotics is effective. *S. moniliformis* is identified by laboratory analysis using fluorescent antibody screening. Also called **streptobacillary ratbite fever.**

Haversian canal (hævər'shən), one of the many tiny longitudinal canals in bone tissue, averaging about 0.05 mm in diameter. Each contains blood vessels, connective tissue, nerve filaments, and, occasionally, lymphatic vessels. The canals are interconnected and part of an intricate network. See also **Haversian canaliculus, Haversian system, Volkmann's canal.**

Haversian canaliculus, any one of the many tiny passages radiating from the lacunae of bone tissue to larger Haversian canals. See also **Haversian system.**

Haversian system, a circular district of bone tissue, consisting of lamellae in the bone around a central canal. See also **Haversian canal, Haversian canaliculus, Volkmann's canal.**

Hawthorne effect, a general, unintentional, but usually beneficial effect on a person, a group of people, or the function of the system being studied. The Hawthorne ef-

fect is the effect of an encounter, as with an investigator or health-care provider, or of a change in a program or facility, as by painting an office or changing the lighting system. The Hawthorne effect is likely to confound the results of a study or investigation, as it is usually present and difficult to identify. It was named for a study in industrial management at the Hawthorne facility of the Western Electric Company.

hay fever, *Informal.* an acute seasonal allergic rhinitis stimulated by tree, grass, or weed pollens. See **allergic rhinitis.**

hazard, a condition or phenomenon that increases the probability of a loss arising from some danger that may result in injury or illness. —**hazardous,** *adj.*

Hb A, abbreviation for **hemoglobin A.**

Hb C, abbreviation for **hemoglobin B.**

Hb F, abbreviation for **hemoglobin F.**

HBIG, abbreviation for **hepatitis B immune globulin.**

Hb S, abbreviation for **hemoglobin S.**

HBsAG, abbreviation for **hepatitis B surface antigen.** See **Australia antigen.**

Hb S-C, abbreviation for **hemoglobin S-C.**

HCG, abbreviation for *human chorionic gonadotropin.* See **chorionic gonadotropin.**

He, symbol for **helium.**

headache, a pain in the head from any cause. Also called **cephalalgia.** Kinds of headaches include **functional headache, migraine headache, organic headache, sinus headache, tension headache.**

head and neck cancer, any malignant neoplasms of the upper aerodigestive tract, facial features, and structures in the neck, presenting as masses, ulcerations, or flat lesions that usually produce early symptoms. Tumors of the oral cavity, lips, and tongue characteristically begin as a swelling or nonhealing ulcer and are most commonly epidermoid carcinomas that occur in men over 60; predisposing factors are chronic alcoholism, heavy use of tobacco, poor oral hygiene, syphilis, and Plummer-Vinson syndrome. Nasal and paranasal sinus malignancies, most often epidermoid cancers, cause a bloody discharge, obstruction in breathing, and facial and dental pain. Nasopharyngeal tumors, predominantly squamous cell and undifferentiated carcinomas occurring most frequently in Orientals, are associated with nasal obstruction, serous otitis media, hearing loss, lymphadenopathy, and cranial nerve involvement. Oropharyngeal and tonsillar neoplasms, usually squamous cell carcinomas and less frequently lymphomas, produce dysphagia, pain, dyspnea, and trismus. Most hypopharyngeal and laryngeal tumors are carcinomas that cause hoarseness, dysphagia, dyspnea, cough, and cervical adenopathy. Salivary gland carcinomas occur most frequently in the parotid gland and may cause facial palsy. Cancer of the mandible, including extremely painful osteosarcoma and, often, painless giant cell tumor, Ewing's sarcoma, and ameloblastoma, may erode through the gingiva, producing an intraoral ulcer, and may cause pathologic fractures. Ear neoplasms involve the auricle in most cases, usually occur in persons over 50, and are most commonly squamous cell carcinomas that cause pain, deafness, and facial nerve paralysis. Cancers of the lacrimal glands, lacrimal sacs, and parathyroid glands are rare, but hypercalcemia, hypercalcinuria, kidney stones, and renal and bone diseases are associated with parathyroid carcinoma. Tumors of the eye, as malignant melanoma in patients over 50 and retinoblastoma in children, are also rare. Head and neck tumors are diagnosed by clinical examination, x rays, tomograms, biopsies, arteriograms, supravital staining of lesions, and cytologic studies. Surgery and radiotherapy are the primary treatment modalities, but their use may cause problems with swallowing and speaking; the effectiveness of chemotherapy is limited by the poor nutritional status of many patients with head or neck lesions. Plastic surgery and various prostheses are often essential in correcting deformities and restoring functions in patients who have undergone the excision or radiotherapy of a head or neck tumor. See also specific cancer.

head, eye, ear, nose and throat (HEENT), a specialty in medicine concerned with the anatomy, physiology, and pathology of the head, the eyes, ears, nose, and throat and with the diagnosis and treatment of disorders of those structures.

head injury, any traumatic damage to the head resulting from penetration of the skull or from too rapid inertial acceleration or deceleration of the brain within the skull. Blood vessels, nerves, and meninges are torn; bleeding, edema and ischemia may result. Meningeal infection is a grave and frequent complication of fracture of the bones of the paranasal sinuses. See also **concussion.**

head kidney. See **pronephros.**

head nurse, the clinical and administrative leader of the nurses working in a given geographical division of an institution, usually a floor, ward, or unit. The responsibilities of a head nurse may include directing nursing care activities, scheduling of staff, evaluation of nursing personnel, and hiring, firing, or promoting staff nurses. The head nurse may also be responsible for budget preparation and general clinical leadership. The head nurse acts as liaison in the communication between the nursing staff and others, including physicians, institutional personnel, and nursing educators.

head process, a strand of cells that extends forward from the primitive node in the early stages of embryonic development in vertebrates. It is the precursor of the notochord and forms the primitive axis around which the embryo develops. Also called **notochordal plate.**

Heaf test (hif), a tuberculin skin test using a multiple puncture technique. See also **tuberculin test.**

healing, the act or process in which the normal structural and functional characteristics of health are restored to diseased, dysfunctional, or damaged tissues, organs, or systems of the body.

health, a condition of physical, mental, and social well-being and the absence of disease or other abnormal condition. It is not a static condition; constant change and adaptation to stress result in homeostasis. René Dubos, often quoted in nursing education, says, "The states of health or disease are the expressions of the success or failure experienced by the organism in its efforts to respond adaptively to environmental challenges." See also **high-level wellness, homeostasis.**

health assessment, an evaluation of the health status of an individual by performing a physical examination after obtaining a health history. Various laboratory tests may also be ordered to confirm a clinical impression or to screen for dysfunction. The depth of investigation and the frequency of the assessment varies with the condition and age of the client and the facility in which the assessment is performed. A significant part of the health assessment is counseling and education that may explain aspects of anatomy, physiology, and pathophysiology and that introduces or affirms the general tenets of a healthful way of life. The person's response to any dysfunction present is observed and noted. The techniques of the health assessment include: palpation, percussion, auscultation, and inspection, including sight, sound, and smell.

health behavior, an action taken by a person to maintain, attain, or regain good health and to prevent illness. Health behavior reflects a person's health beliefs. Some common health behaviors are exercising regularly, eating a balanced diet, and obtaining necessary inoculations.

health belief model, a conceptual framework that describes a person's health behavior as an expression of his health beliefs. The model was designed to predict a person's health behavior, including the use of health services, and to justify intervention to alter maladaptive health behavior. Components of the model include the person's own perception of susceptibility to a disease or condition, the likelihood of contracting that disease or condition, the person's perception of the severity of the consequences of contracting the condition or the disease, the perceived benefits of care and barriers to preventive behavior, and the internal or external stimuli that result in appropriate health behavior by the person.

health care consumer, any actual or potential recipient of health care, as a patient in a hospital, a client in a community mental health center, or a member of a prepaid health maintenance organization.

health care delivery system, the complete network of agencies, facilities, and all providers of health care in a specified geographical area. Nursing services are integral to all levels and patterns of care, and nurses form the largest number of providers in a health care system.

health-care industry, the complex of preventive, remedial, and therapeutic services provided by hospitals and other institutions, nurses, doctors, dentists, government agencies, voluntary agencies, noninstitutional care facilities, pharmaceutical and medical equipment manufacturers, and health insurance companies.

health certificate, a statement signed by a health care provider that attests to the state of health of a person.

health consumer. See **health care consumer.**

health culture, a system that attempts to explain and treat sickness and to maintain health. Health cultures are part of the larger culture or tradition of a people. It may be a popular or folk system, or it may be a technical or scientific one.

health education, an educational program directed to the general public that attempts to improve, maintain, and safeguard the health of the community.

health history, (in nursing and medicine) a collection of information obtained from the client and from other sources concerning the person's physical status and psychological, social, and sexual functions. The history provides a data base upon which a plan for management of the diagnosis, treatment, care, and follow-up of the person may be made. The first part of the history describes the present illness (PI), including its signs and symptoms, onset and character, and any factors or behaviors that aggravate or ameliorate the symptoms. The patient's own words often serve as the best description and may be quoted. The second part of the history comprises an account of previous illnesses, conditions, allergies, transfusions, immunizations, screening tests, and hospitalizations. An occupational history, describing the person's work and exposure to stress, toxins, radiation, or other occupational hazards, may be included. The effect of the current illness on the person's work is also noted. A social history is taken in which the person's social, cultural, and familial milieux are outlined, focusing on aspects that might have an effect on the current illness. In some instances a sexual history may be relevant. A review of systems may follow or be incorporated into the health history. Kinds of history include **complete health history, episodic health history, interval health history.** Also called **medical history.** See also **occupational history, review of systems, sexual history, social history.**

health maintenance, a program or procedure planned to prevent illness, to maintain maximal function, and to promote health. It is central to health care, especially to nursing care at all levels (primary, secondary, and tertiary) and in all patterns (preventive, episodic, acute, chronic, and catastrophic).

Health Maintenance Organization (HMO), a type of group health care practice that provides basic and supplemental health maintenance and treatment services to voluntary enrollees who prepay a fixed periodic fee that is set without regard to the amount or kind of services received. Some of the first HMOs, Kaiser-Permanente among them, have demonstrated that high quality medical care can often be provided at less expense by such a system than by other health care systems. In addition to diagnostic and treatment services, including hospitalization and surgery, an HMO often offers supplemental services, as dental, mental, and eye care and prescription drugs. Federal financial support for the establishment of HMOs was provided under Title XIII of the 1973 U.S. Public Health Service Act.

health physics, the study of the effects of ionizing radiation on the body and the methods for protecting people from the undesirable effects of the radiation. Health physics is concerned with the development and evaluation of methods, techniques, materials, and procedures to be used to protect people from these untoward effects.

health policy, 1. a statement of a decision regarding a goal in health care and a plan for achieving that goal, as, in order to prevent an epidemic, a program for innoculating a population is developed and implemented. 2. a field of study and practice in which the priorities and values underlying health resource allocation are determined.

health professional, any person who has completed a course of study in a field of health, as a registered nurse, physical therapist, or physician. The person is usually licensed by a governmental agency or certified by a professional organization.

health provider, any individual who provides health services to health care consumers.

health resources, all materials, personnel, facilities, funds, and anything else that can be utilized for providing health care and services.

health screening, a program designed to evaluate the health status and potential of an individual person. In the process it may be found that a person has a particular disease or condition or is at greater than normal risk of developing it. Health screening may include taking a personal and family health history and performing a physical examination or tests, laboratory tests, or radiologic examination and may be followed by counseling, education, referral, or further testing.

health supervision, (in public health nursing) a visit made to a patient in his home for the purpose of health teaching, counseling, or monitoring the status of the patient's health rather than for physical care. Compare **care-of-the-sick.**

health systems agency (HSA), an agency established under the terms of the National Health Planning and Resources Development Act of 1974. Health planning agencies are intended to provide networks of health planning and resource development services in each of several health service areas established by the Act. Health systems agencies are nonprofit and include private organizations, public regional planning bodies, or local governmental agencies and consumers. See also **health systems plan.**

health systems plan, a plan in which the long-range health goals of a health services area are specified. Health systems plans are prepared by health systems agencies. See also **health policy.**

hearing aid, a device used to increase the intensity of sound.

heart, the muscular, cone-shaped organ, about the size of a clenched fist, that pumps blood throughout the body and beats normally about 70 times per minute by coordinated nerve impulses and muscular contractions. Enclosed in pericardium, the heart rests on the diaphragm between the lower borders of the lungs, occupying the middle of the mediastinum. It is covered ventrally by the sternum and the adjoining parts of the third to the sixth costal cartilages. The organ is about 12 cm long, 8 cm wide at its broadest part, and 6 cm thick. The weight of the heart in men averages between 280 and 340 gm and in women, between 230 and 280 gm. The layers of the heart, starting from the outside, are the epicardium, the myocardium, and the endocardium. The epicardium includes the visceral pericardium and a layer of fibroelastic connective tissue interspersed with fat. The myocardium is composed of layers and bundles of cardiac muscle laced by blood vessels. The endocardium is continuous with the endothelial lining of the blood vessels and is composed of squamous endothelium. The chambers of the heart include two ventricles with thick muscular walls, making up the bulk of the organ, and two atria with thin muscular walls. A septum separates the ventricles and extends between the atria, dividing the heart into the right and the left sides. The left side of the heart pumps oxygenated blood from the pulmonary veins into the aorta and on to all parts of the body. The right side of the heart pumps deoxygenated blood, received through the venae cavae, into the pulmonary arteries. The sinoatrial node in the right atrium of the heart initiates the cardiac impulse, causing the atria to contract. The atrioventricular node in the septal wall of the right atrium spreads the impulse over the bundle of His, causing the ventricles to contract. Both atria contract almost simultaneously, followed quickly by the nearly simultaneous contraction of the ventricles. The valves of the heart include the tricuspid valve between the right atrium and the right ventricle, the mitral valve between the left atrium and the left ventricle, the aortic valve at the exit of the left ventricle, and the pulmonary valve at the exit of the right ventricle. The sinoatrial node of the pulse sets the rate. Other factors affecting the pulse are emotion, exercise, hormones, temperature, pain, and stress.

heartburn, a painful burning sensation in the esophagus just below the sternum. Heartburn is usually caused by

HUMAN HEART
(cross-section)

the reflux of gastric contents into the esophagus but may be caused by gastric hyperacidity or peptic ulcer. Antacids relieve the symptoms but do not cure the heartburn. Also called **pyrosis.** See also **hiatus hernia, reflux esophagitis.**

heart failure, a condition in which the heart cannot pump enough blood in relation to the venous return and the metabolic requirements of body tissues. Extreme exertion may cause heart failure in individuals with normal hearts if there is a discrepancy between the needs of the body and the volume of blood pumped by the heart. Heart failure may be generally classified as cardiac mechanical failure, myocardial failure, and arrhythmic failure. Most forms of heart failure are caused by atrial failure or by ventricular failure, and many patients develop heart failure from more than one cause. Many of the symptoms associated with heart failure are caused by the dysfunction of organs other than the heart, especially the lungs, kidneys, and liver. Ventricular dysfunction is usually the basic disorder in congestive heart failure and often triggers compensatory mechanisms that preserve cardiac output but produce symptoms and signs, as dyspnea, orthopnea, rales, and edema. Heart failure is closely associated with many forms of heart disease and is commonly diagnosed only after the diagnosis of heart disease. Most kinds of heart disease initially affect the left side of the heart, and clinicians commonly divide associated heart failure into left-heart failure and right-heart failure.

Peripheral edema occurs in connection with right-heart failure and dyspnea in connection with left-heart failure. The adjustments of the body to heart failure are divided into the acute adjustments, the subacute adjustments, and the chronic adjustments, depending on how long the adjustment takes. The acute adjustments involve numerous complex mechanisms, the most important of which increase autonomic sympathetic excitation to the heart and most of the arteries and veins. The stimulation of the peripheral arteries helps to maintain arterial pressure. The stimulation of the veins helps to increase venous tone and venous pressure. The increased venous pressure aids venous return, ventricular filling, and the diastolic stretching of the ventricular fibers. The subacute adjustments of the body to heart failure mainly involve those mechanisms which cause the kidneys to retain salt and water, resulting in increased blood volume. The localization of edema produced by the excess fluid and salt depends on various hydrostatic factors, as the position of the patient. The main chronic adjustment of the body to heart failure is hypertrophy of the ventricular myocardium, apparently owing to a chronic increase in the tension of the myocardial fibers. Current studies indicate that heart failure in infants and children is usually owing to congenital heart disease, but it may also be caused by myocarditis and ectopic tachycardia. The most frequent cause of congestive heart failure between birth and one week of age is aortic atresia. Between the ages of one week and one month, the most common causes are coarctation of the aorta and transposition of the great vessels, followed in order of causative frequency by endomyocardial disease, ventricular septal defect, and patent ductus arteriosis. Between the ages of three and six months, endomyocardial disease is the most common cause of cardiac failure, followed in frequency by ventricular septal defect, patent ductus arteriosus, total anomalous pulmonary venous return, coarctation of the aorta and transposition of the great vessels. From birth to six months of age, paroxysmal atrial tachycardia may cause acute catastrophic heart failure without other evidence of heart disease. The most common causes of heart failure between the ages of five and fifteen are acute rheumatic myocarditis, acute glomerulonephritis, and congenital heart disease, especially ventricular septal defect, atrial septal defect, and patent ductus arteriosus. Heart failure during early life is rarely caused by secundum-type atrial septal defect, congenital valve disease, or acquired valve disease. Rheumatic mitral disease and aortic valve disease frequently cause congestive heart failure in young adults. Mitral valve disease, especially mitral stenosis, is the most common cause of heart failure and affects more young women than men. Other heart diseases that may affect young adults are nonrheumatic myocardial disease and congenital heart disease. The common causes of heart failure after age 40

are coronary atherosclerosis with myocardial infarction, diastolic hypertension in which the pressure is usually above 110 mm Hg, valvular heart disease, pulmonary disease, and diffuse myocardial disease. Some individuals may suffer heart failure caused by a combination of congenital heart disease and acquired disease. After age 50, a common cause of heart failure, especially in men, is calcific aortic stenosis. Some of the behavioral and environmental factors that may cause heart failure in asymptomatic patients with heart disease are sudden extraordinary effort, increased work load, excessive dietary intake of sodium, sudden emotional upset, and the administration of excessive volumes of intravenous fluids. Some signs of heart failure based on physical examination may be divided into those signs caused by the effects of cardiac failure on other organs and those signs of cardiac failure that are associated with the heart, the arteries, and the veins. Some of the extracardiac signs are ascites, bronchial wheezing, hydrothorax, edema, enlargement of the liver, moist rales, and splenomegaly. Some of the cardiac signs associated with heart failure are abnormalities in the jugular venous pulsation and the carotid pulse, and abnormal cardiographic tracings of the apex wave. The treatment for heart failure commonly involves the reduction of the workload of the heart, the administration of certain drugs, as digitalis, to increase myocardial contractility and cardiac output, salt-free diets, diuretics, and surgical intervention. Many patients with heart failure, especially elderly patients, become constipated and require laxatives, as mineral oil, milk of magnesia, and cascara sagrada. In acute heart failure, a complex autonomic response and local regulatory mechanisms redistribute the available blood flow, and body tissues receiving less blood than required may use anaerobic metabolism or withdraw more oxygen from each unit of available blood. The sudden onset of acute pulmonary edema associated with some cases of heart failure is a life-threatening condition requiring immediate treatment. Acute pulmonary edema may develop in patients with chronic heart failure owing to atherosclerosis and old infarcts or in patients with normal hearts who develop ectopic tachycardia or pulmonary embolism. Acute pulmonary edema may sometimes be confused with bronchial asthma, and caution is required in the administration of appropriate drugs. Aminophylline and oxygen are used in therapy for both pulmonary edema and acute asthma.

heart-lung machine, an apparatus consisting of a pump and an oxygenator that takes over the functions of the heart and lungs, especially during cardiac surgery. The blood is shunted from the venous system through an oxygenator and returned to the arterial circulation.

heart massage. See **cardiac massage.**

heart murmur, an abnormal sound heard during auscultory examination of the heart, caused by the flow of

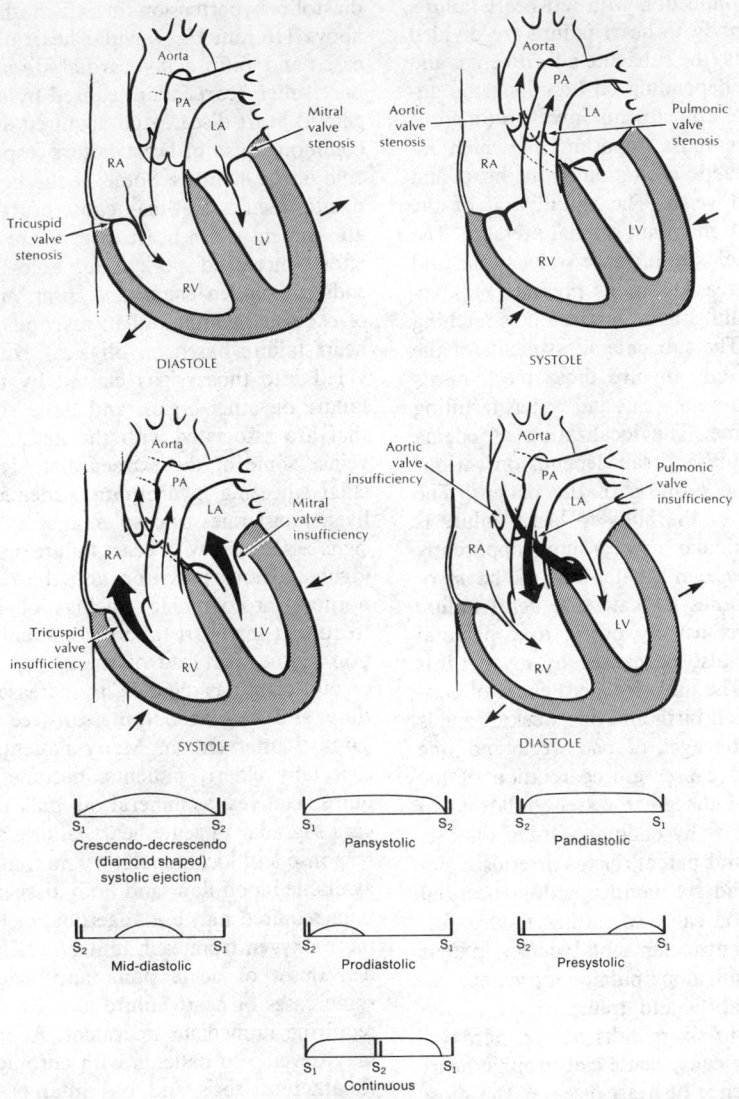

HEART MURMURS

blood into a chamber or through a valve or by a valve opening or closing. A murmur is classified by the time of its occurrence during the cardiac cycle, the duration, and the intensity of the sound on a scale of I to V. For example, a moderately loud murmur that begins at the beginning of systole and ends just as systole ends might be described as a grade III/V pansystolic murmur. Also noted is the part of the heart over which the murmur is heard and any parts to which it radiates. In general, many systolic murmurs are benign and of no significance, but some signal cardiac pathophysiology. Most diastolic murmurs are pathologic.

heart rate, the pulse, calculated by counting the number of contractions of the cardiac ventricles per unit of time. Tachycardia is a heart rate of more than 100 beats per minute; bradycardia is a heart rate of fewer than 60 beats per minute. See also **pulse.**

heart sound, a noise produced within the heart during the cardiac cycle that can be heard over the precordium and may reveal abnormalities in cardiac structure or function. Cardiac auscultation is performed systematically from apex to base of the heart or from base to apex, using a stethoscope to listen initially with the diaphragm and then with the bell of the instrument. The first heart sound

(S_1), a dull, prolonged 'lub,' occurs with the closure of the mitral and tricuspid valves and marks the onset of ventricular systole; the mitral valve sound is loudest at the apex of the heart and that of the tricuspid valve at the left fourth intercostal space. The second heart sound (S_2), a short, sharp 'dup,' occurs with the closing of the aortic and pulmonic valves at the beginning of ventricular diastole; the aortic valve closure is heard loudest on the right side and that of the pulmonic valve is most distinct on the left side over the second intercostal space. A weak, low-pitched, dull third heart sound (S_3) is sometimes heard and is thought to be caused by vibrations of the walls of the ventricles when they are suddenly distended by blood from the atria. S_3, which is heard most clearly at the apex of the heart with the bell of a stethoscope, is called a ventricular or diastolic gallop; it may be normal in children, adolescents, or very thin adults, or it may be a sign of congestive heart failure or hypertension causing left ventricular failure. A fourth heart sound (S_4), which may be heard with the stethoscope's bell at the apex of the heart during expiration, is caused by vibrations of the atria following contraction. Called an atrial or presystolic gallop, S_4 is usually a sign of pathology, as myocardial infarction or impending heart failure from another cause. Asynchronous closure of cardiac valves may result in split heart sounds. An S_1 split occurs in right bundle branch block, mitral stenosis, and tricuspid valve dysfunction associated with pulmonary hypertension. S_2 splits may occur in normal inspiration but may also indicate septal defects, pulmonic stenosis, or other mechanical problems. Brief, periodic endocardial murmurs may indicate various disorders. A murmur characteristic of incompetency of the mitral orifice is loudest at the cardiac apex, a murmur characteristic of tricuspid incompetency is loudest at the ensiform cartilage, and a murmur typical of obstruction of the pulmonic orifice is loudest at the left second intercostal space near the sternum. Systolic and diastolic murmurs that are loudest at the junction of the right second costal cartilage and sternum indicate problems in the aortic orifice, and a presystolic murmur over the body of the heart may be the result of mitral orifice obstruction. A phonocardiogram recorded simultaneously with the electrocardiogram shows the relationships between heart sounds and electrical events. S_1 begins midway in the QRS complex; during this interval the mitral and tricuspid valves close, the pulmonic and aortic valves open, and ejection of blood from the right ventricle begins. Left ventricular ejection occurs between S_1 and S_2, which begins immediately after the T wave and is signaled by closure of the aortic valve, followed by closure of the pulmonic valve and opening of the tricuspid and mitral valves. S_3 occurs between the T and P wave on the EKG at the end of the rapid-filling phase of the ventri-

cles, and S_4 begins at the peak of the P wave during vibrations of the atria.

heart surgery, any surgical procedure involving the heart, performed to correct acquired or congenital defects, to replace diseased valves, to open or bypass blocked vessels, or to graft a prosthesis or a transplant in place. Two major types of heart surgery are performed, closed and open. The closed technique is done through a small incision, without using the heart-lung machine. In the open technique the heart chambers are open and fully visible, and blood is detoured around the surgical field by the heart-lung machine. Preoperative care focuses on the correction of metabolic imbalances and cardiac and pulmonary ailments and on diagnostic and laboratory tests. General anesthesia is used, the chest cavity is opened, and the heart-lung machine is connected. Hypothermia may also be used to reduce the metabolic rate and the need of the tissues for oxygen. The heart is opened and the defect is corrected. Postoperatively, constant observation is required in an intensive care unit for signs of hemorrhage, shock, fibrillation, arrhythmia, sudden chest pain, and pulmonary edema. The blood pressure, all pulses, respirations, and venous and pulmonary artery pressures are monitored. If the blood pressure is high enough to assure cerebral profusion, the head of the patient's bed is lifted to a semi-Fowler's position to encourage chest drainage and lung expansion. Oxygen is given via the endotracheal tube for 18 to 24 hours. The chest tube is cleared hourly to dislodge clots; urinary output and temperature are noted hourly; and intravenous infusions and blood transfusions are often given. Small doses of a narcotic will help to control pain and allow coughing and deep breathing. Antibiotics are given to prevent infection. The mortality rate is highest during the first 48 hours following surgery. Kinds of heart surgery include **Blalock-Taussig procedure, coronary bybass, endarterectomy, mitral commissurotomy.** See also **arrhythmia, fibrillation, heart-lung machine, hypothermia, pulmonary edema.**

heart valve, one of the four structures within the heart that control the flow of blood by opening and closing with each heartbeat. The valves include two semilunar valves, the mitral valve, and the tricuspid valve. The valves permit the flow of blood in only one direction, and any one of the valves may become defective permitting the backflow associated with heart murmurs. Also called **cardiac valve.** See also **heart.**

heat cramp, any cramp in the arm, leg, or abdomen caused by depletion in the body of both water and salt owing to heat exhaustion. It usually occurs after vigorous physical exertion in an extremely hot environment or under other conditions that cause profuse sweating and depletion of body fluids and electrolytes. Also called **cane-cutter's cramp, fireman's cramp, miner's cramp, stoker's cramp.** See also **heat exhaustion.**

heated nebulization, a method of inhalation therapy using a heating device with a nebulizer that produces a spray with a higher water content than that of a cold atomizer. The mist may be administered through a mask or in a tent. Croup in infancy is often treated with a heated nebulizer.

heat exhaustion, an abnormal condition characterized by weakness, vertigo, nausea, muscle cramps, and loss of consciousness, caused by depletion of body fluid and electrolytes resulting from exposure to intense heat or the inability to acclimatize to heat. Body temperature is near normal; blood pressure may drop but usually returns to normal as the person is placed in a recumbent position; the skin is cool, damp, and pale. The person usually recovers with rest and replacement of water and electrolytes. Compare **heat hyperpyrexia.** See also **heat cramp.**

heat hyperpyrexia, a severe and sometimes fatal condition resulting from the failure of the temperature-regulating capacity of the body, caused by prolonged exposure to the sun or to high temperatures. Reduction or cessation of sweating is an early symptom. Body temperature of 105°F or higher, tachycardia, hot and dry skin, headache, confusion, unconsciousness, and convulsions may occur. Treatment includes cooling, sedation, and fluid replacement. Also called **heatstroke, siriasis, sunstroke.** See also **hyperpyrexia.** Compare **heat exhaustion.**

heat labile. See **thermolabile.**

heat rash, a finely papular or vesicular inflammation of the skin resulting from prolonged exposure to heat and high humidity. Tingling and prickling sensations are common. Prevention and treatment include cool, dry temperatures, ventilation, and absorbent powders. See also **miliaria, prickly heat.**

heatstroke. See **heat hyperpyrexia.**

heaves, **1.** a chronic respiratory disease of horses, similar to human pulmonary emphysema, characterized by wheezing, coughing, and dyspnea on exertion. The causes of the condition are unknown. **2.** *Informal.* vomiting and retching.

heavy metal, a metallic element with a specific gravity five or more times that of water. The heavy metals are cadmium, cerium, chromium, cobalt, copper, gallium, gold, iron, lead, manganese, mercury, nickel, platinum, silver, tellurium, thallium, tin, uranium, vanadium, and zinc. Small amounts of many of these elements are common and necessary in the diet. Large amounts of any of them may cause poisoning.

heavy metal poisoning, poisoning caused by the ingestion, inhalation, or absorption of various toxic heavy metals. Kinds of heavy metal poisoning include **antimony poisoning, arsenic poisoning, cadmium poisoning, lead poisoning, mercury poisoning.**

heavy vaginal bleeding. See **vaginal bleeding.**

Heb-Cort, a trade name for a glucocorticoid (cortisol).

hebephrenia (hi′bəfri′niə). See **disorganized schizophrenia.**

hebephrenic schizophrenia. See **disorganized schizophrenia.**

Heberden node (hi′bərdən), an abnormal cartilaginous or bony enlargement of a distal interphalangeal joint of a finger, usually occurring in degenerative diseases of the joints. Compare **Bouchard's node.**

hebetude (heb′ıtud′), a state of dullness or lethargy, characteristic of some forms of schizophrenia.

heboid paranoia (heb′oid). See **paranoid schizophrenia.**

-hedonia, a combining form meaning '(condition of) pleasure, cheerfulness': *anhedonia, hyphedonia, parhedonia.*

-hedron, a combining form meaning a 'geometrical figure with (specified) sides': *decahedron, octahedron, polyhedron.*

Hedulin, a trade name for an anticoagulant (phenindione).

heel, the posterior part of the foot, formed by the largest tarsal bone, the calcaneus.

heel-knee test, a method of assessing coordination of movements of the extremities. In the test the patient, lying prone, is asked to touch the knee of one leg with the heel of the other.

heel-shin test, a method of assessing coordination of movements of the extremities. In the test the patient, lying prone, is asked to pass the heel of one leg slowly down the shin of the other leg from the knee to the ankle.

HEENT, abbreviation for **head, eyes, ears, nose** and **throat.**

Hegar's sign (hei′garz), a softening of the isthmus of the uterine cervix early in gestation. It is a probable sign of pregnancy.

height, the vertical measurement of a structure, organ, or other object from bottom to top, when it is placed or projected in an upright position.

Heimlich maneuver (haim′lık), an emergency procedure for dislodging a bolus of food or other obstruction from the trachea to prevent asphyxiation. The choking person is grasped from behind by the rescuer whose fist, thumb side in, is placed just below the victim's sternum with the other hand placed firmly over the fist. The rescuer then pulls his fist firmly and abruptly into the epigastrium forcing the obstruction up the trachea. If repeated attempts do not free the airway, an emergency tracheotomy may be necessary.

(See next page for illustration)

Helen, Sister (Helen Bowden), a nurse who received her education in England and became the first director of the newly formed Bellevue Hospital Training School for Nurses in New York, in 1873. Although she had not trained under Florence Nightingale, she set up the Bellevue school along Nightingale's principles. She was a member of the All Saints Sisterhood. After several years

HEIMLICH MANEUVER

at Bellevue, having established one of the leading nursing schools in the United States, she went to South Africa.

Heliodorus' bandage (hi′liədor′əs). See **T bandage.**

helium (He), a colorless, odorless, gaseous element; the second lightest element after hydrogen. Its atomic number is 2; its atomic weight is 4. Helium is one of the rare or inert gases and does not usually combine with other elements. Most of the commercial helium in the world comes from natural gas reservoirs in Texas and Louisiana where it is recovered after natural gas has been liquefied. It is produced in nature by the decay of radioactive elements and is produced in the sun from hydrogen. It occurs in the atmosphere in the ratio of 5 parts per million. Helium is used industrially in arc-welding, refining, and other processes. Because of its lightness and lack of flammability it is also used to lift airships and balloons. The main physiological and medical uses of helium are in respiratory therapy and testing and the prevention of nitrogen narcosis and decompression sickness in hyperbaric environments. A mixture of 80 per cent helium and 20 per cent oxygen is commonly breathed by deep-sea divers to prevent gas embolisms and by patients undergoing treatment to clear obstructed respiratory tracts. Problems associated with such uses involve the high velocity of acoustic transmission in helium and the high thermal conductivity of the gas. These characteristics produce voice distortions and hypothermia in persons who inhale it.

Helium is one third as soluble in lipids as nitrogen, which accounts for its preferred use in hyperbaric atmospheres, as those associated with deep-sea diving. The low density of helium reduces the effort of breathing any gas mixture of which it is a component. Helium is used in pulmonary-function testing to calculate the diffusing and residual capacities of the lungs.

helix, a coiled, spirallike formation characteristic of many organic molecules, as deoxyribonucleic acid (DNA).

Hellin's law, Hellin-Zeleny law, a generalized formula for calculating the ratio of multiple births in any population, stating that if twin births occur at the rate of $1:N$, then the rate of triplet births is approximately $1:N^2$, quadruplets $1:N^3$, quintuplets $1:N^4$, and so on, with the exponent of N being once less than the number in the multiple set. The constant N varies greatly with population, although it was originally set at 89 when the law was formulated. In general, twin births occur approximately once in every 80 pregnancies.

helminth (hel′mınth), a worm, especially one of the pathogenic parasites of the division Metazoa fluke, including flukes, tapeworms, and roundworms.

-helminth, a combining form meaning 'worm': *nemathelminth, platyhelminth.*

helminthiasis (hel′mınthai′əsıs), a parasitic infestation of the body by helminths that may be cutaneous, visceral, or intestinal. Ascariasis, bilharziasis, filariasis, hookworm, and trichinosis are common forms of the disease.

helper T cell. See **T cell.**

Helsinki accords, a declaration signed by the representatives of thirty-five member nations of the Conference on Security and Cooperation in Europe in Helsinki, Finland, on August 1, 1975. The declared goals of the nonbinding document comprised four principal aspects of European security: economic cooperation, humanitarian issues, contact between the East and West and provision for a later follow-up conference (held in Belgrade in 1978). Follow-up conferences were planned in part to allow the member nations to monitor each other's performance on humanitarian issues, as the right to self-determination of all people and respect for the fundamental freedoms, including thought, conscience, and religion or belief, without regard to race, language, sex, or religion. The Helsinki accords grew from the precedent set by the judgments at the trials of the Nuremberg tribunals—that crimes against humanity are offenses subject to criminal prosecution. The principal and the practice of informed consent in health care grew from this precedent. Also called **Helsinki Declaration.** See also **Nuremberg tribunals.**

helvolic acid (helvol′ık), an antibiotic, derived from the mold *Aspergillus fumigatus,* formerly used as an amebicide. Also called **fumagillin, fumigacin.**

hemadsorption (hi′mædsorp′shən, hem′adsorp′shən), a process in which a substance or an agent, as certain viruses and bacilli, adheres to the surface of an erythrocyte. The process occurs naturally or it may be induced for laboratory identification of bacteriologic specimens.

hemagglutination (hi'məglu'tɪneı'ŝhən, hem'əglu'tɪneı'ŝhən), an antigen-antibody reaction resulting in the agglutination of red cells. See **ABO blood groups.**

hemangioblastoma (hımæn'jiɔublæstou'mə), *pl.* **hemangioblastomas, hemangioblastomata.** a brain tumor composed of a proliferation of capillaries and of disorganized clusters of capillary cells or angioblasts.

hemangioendothelioma (hımæn'jiɔuen'douthi'liou'mə), *pl.* **hemangioendotheliomas, hemangioendotheliomata.** a tumor, consisting of endothelial cells, that grows around an artery or a vein. It may become malignant. Also called **angioendothelioma.**

hemangioma (hımæn'jiou'mə), *pl.* **hemangiomas, hemangiomata.** a benign tumor consisting of a mass of blood vessels. Kinds of hemangiomas include **capillary hemangioma, cavernous hemangioma, nevus flammeus.**

hemangioma simplex. See **strawberry hemangioma.**

hemangiosarcoma (hımæn'jiousarkou'mə), *pl.* **hemangiosarcomas, hemangiosarcomata.** a malignant neoplasm composed of endothelial and fibroblastic tissues that proliferate and eventually surround vascular channels. Also called **malignant hemangioendothelioma.**

hematemesis (hi'mətem'əsıs, hem'ətem'əsıs), vomiting of bright, red blood, indicating rapid upper gastrointestinal bleeding, commonly associated with esophageal varices or peptic ulcer. The rate and the source of bleeding are determined by endoscopic examination. Any blood found in the stomach is removed by nasogastric suction. Treatment requires replacement of blood by transfusion and administration of intravenous fluids for maintenance of fluid and electrolyte balance. Vasoconstrictors may sometimes be infused at the site of bleeding. Surgery may be necessary. The patient is usually very anxious and needs quiet, warmth, and reassurance. See also **gastrointestinal bleeding.**

hematocrit (hımæt'ʃoukrɪt), a measure of the packed cell volume of red cells, expressed as a percentage of the total blood volume. The normal range is between 43 per cent and 49 per cent in men, and between 37 per cent and 43 per cent in women. See also **complete blood count.**

hematolmyelia, the appearance of frank blood in the fluid of the spinal cord.

hematologist (hi'mətol'əjıst, hem'ətol'əjıst), a medical specialist in the field of hematology.

hematology (hi'mətol'əji, hem'ətol'əji), scientific medical study of blood and blood-forming tissues. — **hematologic, hematological,** *adj.*

hematoma (hi'mətou'mə, hem'ətou'mə), *pl.* **hematomas, hematomata.** a collection of extravasated blood trapped in the tissues of the skin or in an organ, resulting from trauma or incomplete hemostasis after surgery. Initially,

there is frank bleeding into the space; if the space is limited, pressure slows and eventually stops the flow of blood. The blood clots, serum collects, the clot hardens, the mass becomes palpable to the examiner and is often painful to the patient. A hematoma may be drained early in the process and bleeding arrested with pressure or, if necessary, with surgical ligation of the bleeding vessel. Considerable blood may be lost, and infection is a serious complication.

-hematoma, a combining form meaning a 'swelling containing blood': *cephalhematoma, episiohematoma, othematoma.*

hematopoiesis (hi'mətoupoii'sıs, hem'ətoupoii'sıs), the normal formation and development of blood cells in the bone marrow. In severe anemia and other hematologic disorders, cells may be produced in organs outside the marrow (extramedullary hematopoiesis). See also **erythropoiesis.** — **hematopoietic,** *adj.*

hematuria (hi'mətyur'iə, hem'ətem'əsıs), abnormal presence of blood in the urine. Hematuria is symptomatic of many renal diseases and disorders of the genitourinary system. Microscopic examination of the urine, culture and sensitivity of the urine and physical examination of the person are usually performed. — **hematuric,** *adj.*

heme (him), the pigmented, iron-containing, non-protein portion of the hemoglobin molecule. There are four heme groups in a hemoglobin molecule, each consisting of a cyclic structure of four pyrrole residues, called protoporphyrin, and an atom of iron in the center. Heme binds and carries oxygen in the red blood cells, releasing it to tissues that give off excess amounts of CO_2. Compare **porphobilinogen.** See also **hemoglobin, protoporphyrin.**

hemeralopia (hem'ərəlou'piə), an abnormal visual condition in which bright light causes blurring of vision. Hemeralopia is an unpleasant side effect of certain anticonvulsant medications, including trimethadione, prescribed in treating children affected with petit mal epilepsy. — **hemeralopic,** *adj.*

-hemia. See **-emia.**

hemiacephalus, a fetal monster in which the brain and most of the cranium are lacking. See also **anencephaly.**

hemiazygous vein (hem'iəzæi'gəs), one of the tributaries of the azygous vein of the thorax. It starts in the left ascending lumbar vein, enters the thorax through the left crus of the diaphragm, ascends on the left side of the vertebral column as high as the ninth thoracic vertebra, and passes dorsal to the aorta to enter the azygous. The hemiazygous vein receives about four of the caudal intercostal veins, the left subcostal vein, and some of the esophageal and the mediastinal veins.

hemicellulose (hem'isel'yulous), any of a group of polysaccharides that constitute the chief part of the skeletal substances of the cell walls of plants and resemble cellulose but are more soluble and more easily extracted and decomposed. See also **dietary fiber.**

hemicephalia, a congenital anomaly characterized by the absence of the cerebrum, caused by severe arrest of brain development in the fetus. The cerebellum and basal ganglia are usually present, at least in rudimentary form.

hemicephalus, a fetal monster with congenital absence of the cerebrum.

hemicrania, **1.** a headache, usually migraine, that affects only one side of the head. **2.** a congenital anomaly characterized by the absence of half of the skull in the fetus; incomplete anencephaly.

hemiectromelia, a congenital anomaly characterized by the incomplete development of the limbs on one side of the body. — **hemiectromelus,** *n.*

hemignathia, a congenital anomaly characterized by incomplete development of the lower jaw on one side of the face. — **hemignathus,** *n.*

hemihyperplasia, overdevelopment or excessive growth of one half of a specific organ or part or of all the organs and parts on one side of the body.

hemihypoplasia, partial or incomplete development of one half of a specific organ or part or of all the organs and parts on one side of the body.

hemikaryon (hem′ikær′ion), a cell nucleus that contains the haploid number of chromosomes, as that of the gametes. Compare **amphikaryon.** — **hemikaryotic,** *adj.*

hemimelia, a developmental anomaly characterized by the absence or gross shortening of the lower portion of one or more of the limbs. The condition may involve either or both of the bones of the distal arm or leg and is designated according to whichever is absent or defective, as fibular, radial, tibial, or ulnar hemimelia. See also ectromelia, phocomelia.

hemipagus (hemip′əgəs), conjoined symmetrical twins who are united at the thorax.

hemiplegia (hem′ipli′jə), paralysis of one side of the body. Kinds of hemiplegia are **cerebral hemiplegia, facial hemiplegia, infantile hemiplegia, spastic hemiplegia.** Also called **unilateral paralysis.** Compare **diplegia.** — **hemiplegic,** *adj.*

hemisomus (hem′isou′məs), a fetus or individual in which one side of the body is malformed or defective.

hemisphere, **1.** half of a sphere or globe. **2.** the lateral half of the cerebrum or of the cerebellum. — **hemispherical,** *adj.*

hemiteras (hem′iter′əs), *pl.* **hemiterata.** any individual with a congenital malformation that is not so severe or disabling as to be classified as a monstrous or teratic condition. — **hemiteratic,** *adj.*

hemivertebra, an abnormal condition characterized by the congenital failure of a vertebra to develop completely, possibly caused by the complete failure of the growth center of one vertebral body. Usually half of the vertebra

involved is completely or partially developed and the other half is absent. One or more vertebrae may be involved, the different conditions producing varying degrees of balanced or unbalanced scoliosis. As a result of the developmental abnormality of the spine a wedge-shaped vertebra develops, and adjacent vertebral bodies expand to fit the deformity or tilt to accommodate wedge-shaped articulation. Hemivertebra may be classified according to the degree of developmental failure of involved vertebral growth centers. There may be involvement of two vertebral bodies in which growth centers on the same side fail to develop, resulting in moderate to severe unbalanced congenital scoliosis, or there may be involvement of two vertebral bodies in which growth centers fail to develop on opposite sides, creating balanced congenital scoliosis. Singular hemivertebra may pose few if any signs and symptoms. Depending on the degree of congenital scoliosis involved, any associated deformity may become more apparent with growth. Other types of hemivertebra, especially those involving unbalanced congenital scoliosis, usually progress markedly with growth and have a relatively poor prognosis unless early spinal fusion prevents further spinal curvature. No treatment may be required for the form of the condition associated with balanced congenital scoliosis.

hemizygote, an individual, organism, or cell that has only one of a pair of genes for a specific characteristic. Such traits are expressed regardless of whether the genes transmitting them are dominant or recessive, as with the X-linked genes on the single X chromosome in males, which have no alleles on the Y chromosome. — **hemizygosity,** *n.,* **hemizygous, hemizygotic,** *adj.*

hemoblastic leukemia. See **stem cell leukemia.**

hemochromatosis (hi′moukrou′mətou′sis, hem′oukrou′-mətou′sis), a rare disease of iron storage, characterized pathologically by excess iron deposits throughout the body. Hepatomegaly, skin pigmentation, diabetes mellitus, and cardiac failure may occur. The disease most often develops in men over forty years old and as a complication of some hemolytic anemias requiring multiple blood transfusions. Compare **hemosiderosis.** See also **iron metabolism.**

hemocytoblastic leukemia. See **stem cell leukemia.**

hemodialysis (hi′moudaiæl′əsis, hem′oudaiæl′əsis), a procedure in which impurities or wastes are removed from the blood, used in treating renal insufficiency and various toxic conditions. The patient's blood is shunted from the body through a machine for diffusion and ultrafiltration and then returned to the patient's circulation. Hemodialysis requires access to the patient's blood stream, a mechanism for the transport of the blood to and from the dialyzer, and a dialyzer. See also **arteriovenous fistula, external shunt.** *(See next page for illustration)*

■ METHOD: Access may be achieved by an external shunt

or an arteriovenous fistula. The external shunt is constructed by inserting two cannulas through the skin into a large vein and a large artery. When dialysis is not being performed the cannulas are joined, allowing the blood to flow from artery to vein. When dialysis is being performed the cannulas are separated, allowing the arterial blood to flow to the dialyzer and the dialyzed blood to return from the dialyzer to the circulation through the cannula in the vein. An arteriovenous fistula is created by the anastomosis of a large vein to an artery. Large-bore needles are threaded into superficial vessels enlarged by the increased flow caused by the fistula. Various dialyzers may be used. The procedure takes from 3 to 7 or 8 hours and may be necessary daily in acute situations or 2 or 3 times a week in chronic renal failure.

■ NURSING OBSERVATIONS: A decrease in the flow of blood through the shunt may result in clotting; therefore, any factor that may result in a slowing of the flow is to be avoided. Some of these factors are systemic hypotension, infection of the shunt or fistula, compression of the shunt or fistula, thrombophlebitis, and prolonged inflation of a blood pressure cuff. Infection is avoided in the area around an external shunt by placing a sterile dressing over the shunt and changing the dressing daily. Before the procedure is begun the patient is told how long the procedure will take, what pain or discomfort may be expected, what will be felt afterward, what food or activity will be allowed during the procedure, and whether or not family or friends may be present during treatment. Headache and nausea are common, especially during the procedure and for a few hours afterward. The patient usually feels the best on the day following hemodialysis. Rest, an antiemetic, and a mild analgesic may make the procedure more comfortable. Most patients need emotional support and some physical assistance during hemodialysis. The physical status of the patient is monitored frequently throughout; blood pressure, pulse, and blood tests for electrolyte and acid-base balance are performed. Normal saline may be administered to counteract hypotension that occurs as a result of a rapid removal of fluid from the intravascular compartment. The patient is weighed before and after the treatment to determine the amount of fluid lost during the procedure. An anticoagulant is usually given to prevent coagulation of the blood in the dialyzer, cannulas, or catheters; to prevent hemorrhage, protamine sulfate may be given after the procedure to reverse the effect of the anticoagulant. Any treatment that causes tissue trauma, as dental extraction, venipuncture, or intramuscular injection, is not recommended during or immediately following dialysis.

■ OUTCOME CRITERIA: Infection and clotting of the shunt or erosion of the skin around the shunt are frequent complications of the external shunt; therefore, the method utilizing an arteriovenous fistula is more common. The

discomfort before, during, and just after dialysis, the prolonged time of relative immobility during the procedure, and the dietary restrictions necessary in renal insufficiency all place considerable stress on the patient. Adjustments in the patterns of daily life are necessary and require the assistance of professionals with experience and training in the field.

External shunt

Arteriovenous fistula

HEMODIALYSIS

hemodialyzer (hi′moudai′ələi′zər, hem′ɔudai′ələi′zər). See **dialyzer.**

Hemofil, a trade name for human antihemophilic factor.

hemoglobin, a complex protein-iron compound in the blood that carries oxygen to the cells from the lungs and carbon dioxide away from the cells to the lungs. Each erythrocyte contains between 200 and 300 molecules of hemoglobin, each molecule of hemoglobin contains several molecules of heme, and each molecule of heme can carry one molecule of oxygen. Hemoglobin is normally present in the blood at a concentration within a range of 12 to 16 gm/dl in women and 13.5 to 18 gm/dl in men. In an atmosphere of high concentrations of oxygen, as in the lungs, hemglobin binds with oxygen to form oxyhemoglobin. In an atmosphere of low concentrations of oxygen, as in the peripheral tissues of the body, oxygen is replaced by carbon dioxide to form carboxyhemoglobin. Hemoglobin then releases the carboxyhemoglobin in the lungs for excretion and more oxygen is picked up for transport to the cells. Hemoglobin has a precise structure consisting of two different chains made of 141 and 146 amino acids. The absence, replacement, or addition of only one amino acid modifies the properties of the hemoglobin. Such alterations are genetically mediated and may be associated with severe pathology, as in sickle cell disease. See also **carboxyhemoglobin, heme, oxyhemoglobin.**

hemoglobin A (Hb A), a normal hemoglobin. Also called **adult hemoglobin.** Compare **hemoglobin F.** See also **hemoglobin variant, hemoglobinopathy.**

hemoglobin C (Hb C) disease, a genetic blood disorder characterized by a moderate, chronic hemolytic anemia and associated with the presence of hemoglobin C, an abnormal form of the red cell pigment. Hemoglobin C is inherited as an autosomal codominant gene and, in the homozygous form, is the only kind of hemoglobin found in the blood. In the heterozygous form, hemoglobin C trait, there is no anemia or increased blood hemolysis. Target cells may be seen in microscopic examination of a blood smear. Abnormal hemoglobin C is accompanied by an approximately equal amount of its normal counterpart, hemoglobin A. See also **hemoglobinopathy, hemoglobin variant.**

hemoglobinemia (hi′mouglou′bini′mia, hem′ɔglou′bini′-mia), presence of free hemoglobin in the blood plasma.

hemoglobin F (Hb F), the normal hemoglobin of the fetus, most of which is broken down in the first days after birth and replaced by hemoglobin A. Small amounts are produced throughout life.

hemoglobinopathy (hi′mouglou′binɒp′ɒfhi, hem′ouglou′-binɒp′ɒfhi), any of a group of inherited disorders characterized by variation of the structure of the hemoglobin molecule. The alteration appears as the substitution of one or more amino acids in the globin portion of the molecule at selected positions in the two alpha or two beta polypeptide chains. More than 100 variants have been described and identified. Only hemoglobins S, C, and D are seen regularly. The abnormality may occur in the heterozygous or the homozygous form. In the heterozygous form, the normal adult pigment, hemoglobin A, and its variant both appear in the red cell; there may be little or no clinical manifestation of disease. In the homozygous form, only the variant hemoglobin is present, and the characteristic symptoms of that hemoglobinopathy appear. Mixed heterozygous forms are also known to occur. These are characterized by the absence of the normal hemoglobin A and the presence of two or three hemoglobin variants. Kinds of hemoglobinopathies include **hemoglobin C disease, hemoglobin D disease, hemoglobin S/C disease, sickle cell anemia, thalassemia.** Compare **thalassemia.** See also **fetal hemoglobin, hemoglobin, sickle cell thalassemia, sickle cell trait.**

hemoglobin S (Hb S), an abnormal type of hemoglobin, characterized by the substitution of the amino acid valine for glutamic acid in the B chain of the hemoglobin molecule. It moves more slowly and is much less soluble than hemoglobin A. As the abnormal molecules become deoxygenated, owing to decreased oxygen tension in the peripheral circulation, they tend to become sickle-shaped, to move slowly, to clump together, and to hemolyze. If the proportion of Hb S to Hb A is large, as in sickle cell disease, anemia, local thrombosis, and infarction may occur. See also **sickle cell anemia, sickle cell crisis.**

hemoglobin S-C (Hb S-C) disease, a genetic blood disorder in which two different abnormal alleles, one for hemoglobin S and one for hemoglobin C, are inherited. The disorder is characterized by a clinical course considerably less severe than sickle cell anemia despite the absence of normal hemoglobin. See also **hemoglobin C disease, hemoglobinopathy, sickle cell thalassemia.**

hemoglobinuria (hi′mouglou′binyur′ia, hem′ouglou′-binyur′ia), an abnormal presence in the urine of hemoglobin that is unattached to red blood cells. Hemoglobinuria can result from various autoimmune diseases or episodic hemolytic disorders. It can be diagnosed using a dipstick reagent that is sensitive to free hemoglobin. Kinds of hemoglobinuria include **cold hemoglobinuria, march hemoglobinuria, paroxymal hemoglobinuria.**

hemoglobin variant, any type of hemoglobin other than hemoglobin A. All variants are characterized by an alteration in the sequence of amino acids in the polypeptide chains of globin contained in the hemoglobin molecule. These variations are genetically determined and, depending on the kind and extent of change, result in altered physical and chemical function of the red blood cells. See also **hemoglobin C, hemoglobinopathy, hemoglobin S.**

hemolysin (himol′əsin), any one of the numerous substances which lyse or dissolve red blood cells. Hemolysins are produced by strains of many kinds of bacteria, including some of the staphlococci and streptococci. They are also contained in venoms and in certain vegetables. Bacterial hemolysins are divided into those that are filterable and those that cluster around the bacterial colony on a culture medium containing red blood cells. Hemolysins appear to aid the invasive power of bacteria. See also **hemoglobin, hemolysis.**

hemolysis (himol′isis), the breakdown of red blood cells and the release of hemoglobin. It occurs normally at the end of the life span of a red cell, but it may occur under a variety of other circumstances, including certain antigen-antibody reactions, metabolic abnormalities of the red cell that significantly shorten its life span, and mechanical trauma, as in hemodialysis, cardiac prosthesis, or exposure to snake venoms. Dilution of the blood by intravenous administration of excessive amounts of hypotonic solutions, which cause progressive swelling and eventual rupture of the erythrocyte, also results in hemolysis. See also **hemolytic anemia, transfusion reaction.** — **hemolytic,** *adj.*

hemolytic anemia, a disorder characterized by the premature destruction of red blood cells. Anemia may be minimal or absent, reflecting the ability of the bone marrow to increase production of red blood cells. The condition may occur in association with some infectious diseases, with certain inherited red cell disorders, or as a response to drugs or other toxic agents. Compare **aplastic anemia, congenital nonspherocytic hemolytic anemia, myelophthisic anemia.** See also **anemia, hemolysis, spherocytosis.**

hemolytic uremia syndrome, a rare kidney disorder marked by renal failure, microangiopathic hemolytic anemia, and platelet deficiency. The syndrome, the etiology of which is unknown, usually occurs in infancy.

hemophilia (hi'moufi'lia, hem'afi'lia), an inherited disorder characterized by excessive bleeding. It exists as two distinct, but clinically indistinguishable entities, hemophilia A and hemophilia B. Hemophilia A, the classic form, is the result of a deficiency or absence of antihemophilic factor VIII, a trace protein that acts to accelerate the conversion of prothrombin to thrombin through the formation of thromboplastin. Hemophilia B (Christmas disease) represents a deficiency of plasma thromboplastin component, another plasma protein active in the formation of thromboplastin. The clinical severity of the disorder varies markedly with the extent of the deficiency. Greater than usual loss of blood during dental procedures, epistaxis, hematoma, and hemarthrosis are common problems in hemophilia. Severe internal hemorrhage and hematuria are less common. See also **specific factors.** —**hemophiliac,** *n.,* **hemophilic,** *adj.*

Defective gene is found on X chromosome.
When faulty X chromosome is present in a male,
the male will be a hemophiliac.

Ⓧ Y

When faulty X chromosome is present in a female,
she will be a carrier of hemophilia.

Ⓧ X

In conception between a normal male and a carrier
female, four possibilities arise:

Ⓧ X ——————— X Y

| Ⓧ Y | X Y | Ⓧ X | X X |

Hemophiliac son (mother's carrier X) / Normal son (mother's good X chromosome) / Carrier daughter (mother's carrier X and father's X) / Normal daughter (mother's good X and father's X)

X X ——— Ⓧ Y

X Y ——— Ⓧ X

In conception between a hemophiliac male and a normal female,
son will be normal but daughter will be carrier.

HEMOPHILIA INHERITANCE PATTERN

hemophilia A, a hereditary blood disorder, transmitted as an X-linked recessive trait, caused by a deficiency of coagulation factor VIII. Hemophilia A is considered the classical type of hemophilia in contrast to hemophilia B and hemophilia C, which may be less severe. See also **coagulation factor, hemophilia.**

hemophilia B, a hereditary blood disorder, transmitted as an X-linked recessive trait, caused by a deficiency of factor IX, the plasma thromboplastin component. The condition is clinically similar to but less severe than hemophilia A. Also called **Christmas disease.** See **coagulation factor, hemophilia.**

hemophilia C, a hereditary blood disorder, transmitted as an X-linked recessive trait, caused by a deficiency of factor XI, the plasma thromboplastin antecedent. The condition is clinically similar to but may be less severe than hemophilia A. Also called **Rosenthal's syndrome.** See also **coagulation factor, hemophilia.**

hemoptysis (hɪmop'tɪsɪs), coughing up of blood from the respiratory tract. Blood-streaked sputum often occurs in minor upper respiratory infections or in bronchitis. More profuse bleeding may indicate *Aspergillus* infection, lung abcess, tuberculosis, or bronchogenic carcinoma. X-ray examination, endoscopy, and bronchoscopy are often used to diagnose hemoptysis. Treatment of significant hemoptysis includes monitoring the patient for signs of shock, preventing asphyxiation, and localizing and stopping the bleeding. Antibiotics and antitussives may be given. The frightened patient may be calmed by quiet and warmth; sedatives and tranquilizers are not given because of their tendency to depress respiration. Compare **hematemesis.**

hemorrhage, a loss of a large amount of blood in a short period of time, either externally or internally. Hemorrhage may be arterial, venous, or capillary.

■ OBSERVATIONS: Symptoms of massive hemorrhage are related to hypovolemic shock: rapid, thready pulse; thirst; cold, clammy skin; sighing respirations; dizziness; syncope; pallor; apprehension; restlessness; and hypotension. If bleeding is contained within a cavity or joint, pain will develop as the capsule or cavity is stretched by the rapidly expanding volume of blood.

■ INTERVENTION: All effort is directed toward stopping the hemorrhage. If hemorrhage is external, pressure is applied directly to the wound or to the appropriate pressure points. The part of the body that is wounded may be elevated. Ice, applied directly to the wound, may slow bleeding by causing vasoconstriction. Body temperature may be maintained by keeping the person covered and flat. If an extremity is wounded, and if the bleeding is severe, a tourniquet may be applied proximal to the wound.

■ NURSING CONSIDERATIONS: A tourniquet is not applied if there is any other way to stanch the flow, because the risk is great that the limb will not survive the hypoxia induced by obstruction of the supply of blood. The tourniquet is not removed until surgical repair of the wound is possible.

Internal bleeding requires prompt medical intervention. The patient is kept warm and quiet. –**hemorrhagic,** *adj.*

hemorrhagic diathesis, an inherited predisposition to any one of a number of abnormalities characterized by excessive bleeding. See also **Fanconi's syndrome, hemophilia, von Willebrand's disease.**

hemorrhagic familial angiomatosis. See **hereditary hemorrhagic telangiectasia.**

hemorrhagic fever, an arbovirus infection, characterized by fever, chills, headache, malaise, and respiratory or gastrointestinal symptoms, followed by capillary hemorrhages, and, in severe infection, oliguria, kidney failure, hypotension, and, possibly, death. Many forms of the disease occur in specific geographical areas. Some kinds of hemorrhagic fever are **Argentinian hemorrhagic fever, dengue fever, Far Eastern hemorrhagic fever.**

hemorrhagic gastritis, a form of acute gastritis usually caused by a toxic agent, as alcohol, aspirin or other drugs, or bacterial toxins that irritate the lining of the stomach. If bleeding is significant, vasoconstrictors and ice water lavage of the stomach may be necessary. Nausea, vomiting, and epigastric distress may persist after the irritant is removed. Treatment is symptomatic; the nurse usually includes identification of the irritant and dietary counseling for a patient with hemorrhagic gastritis.

hemorrhagic lung. See **congestive atelectasis.**

hemorrhagic scurvy. See **infantile scurvy.**

hemorrhagic shock, a state of physical collapse and prostration associated with the sudden and rapid loss of significant amounts of blood. Severe traumatic injuries often cause such blood losses, which, in turn, produce low blood pressure in affected individuals. Death occurs within a relatively short time unless transfusion quickly restores normal blood volume. Hemorrhagic shock often accompanies secondary shock. Compare **primary shock.**

hemorrhoid, a varicosity in the lower rectum or anus owing to congestion in the veins of the hemorrhoidal plexus.

■ OBSERVATION: Internal hemorrhoids originate above the internal sphincter of the anus. If they become large enough to protude from the anus, they become constricted and painful. Small internal hemorrhoids may bleed with defecation. External hemorrhoids appear outside the anal sphincter. They are usually not painful and bleeding does not occur unless a hemorrhoidal vein ruptures or thromboses.

■ INTERVENTION: Treatment includes local application of a topical medication to lubricate, anesthetize, and shrink the hemorrhoid; sitz baths and cold or hot compresses are also soothing. The hemorrhoids may require sclerosing by injection, or ligation, or excision by a surgical procedure. Ligation is increasingly the preferred treatment: it is sim-

ple, effective, and does not require anesthesia. The hemorrhoid is grasped with a forceps and a rubber band is slipped over the varicosity, causing tissue necrosis and sloughing of the hemorrhoid, usually within one week.

■ NURSING CONSIDERATIONS: Straining to defecate, constipation, and prolonged sitting contribute to the development of hemorrhoids. The client is counseled in ways to avoid these predisposing factors. As pregnancy is associated with an increased incidence of hemorrhoids, the pregnant woman, in particular, is advised to avoid constipation.

hemosiderin (hi'mousɪd'ərɪn, hem'ousɪd'ərɪn), an iron-rich pigment that is a product of red-cell hemolysis. Iron is often stored in this form.

hemosiderosis (hi'mousɪd'ərou'sɪs, hem'ousɪd'ərou'sɪs), an abnormal deposition of iron in a variety of tissues, usually in the form of hemosiderin. It is often associated with diseases involving chronic, extensive destruction of red blood cells, as thalassemia major. Compare **hemochromatosis, sideroblastic anemia.** See also **ferritin, iron transport, transferrin.**

hemostasis (himos'təsɪs, hi'məsteɪ'sɪs), the termination of bleeding by mechanical or chemical means or by the complex coagulation process of the body, consisting of vasoconstriction, platelet aggregation, and thrombin and fibrin synthesis. See also **platelet, thrombus, vasoconstriction.**

hemostat (hi'məstæt, hem'əstæt). See **Halsted's forceps.**

hemostatic, of or pertaining to a procedure, device, or substance that arrests the flow of blood. Direct pressure, tourniquets, and surgical clamps are mechanical hemostatic measures. Cold applications are hemostatic and include the use of an ice bag on the abdomen to halt uterine bleeding and irrigation of the stomach with an iced solution to check gastric bleeding. Gelatin sponges, solutions of thrombin, and microfibrillar collagen, which causes the aggregation of platelets and the formation of clots, are used to arrest bleeding in surgical procedures. Aminocaproic acid is administered orally or intravenously in the treatment of excessive bleeding caused by systemic hyperfibrinolysis. Phytonadione is used for the prevention and treatment of hemorrhagic disease in newborn infants and for the treatment of prothrombin deficiency induced by anticoagulants or other drugs.

hemostatic forceps (hi'məstæt'ɪk, hem'əstæt'ɪk). See **artery forceps.**

hemothorax (hi'mouθɔr'æks, hem'ouθɔr'æks), an accumulation of blood and fluid in the pleural cavity, between the parietal and visceral pleura, usually the result of trauma. Hemothorax may also be caused by the rupture of small blood vessels owing to inflammation from pneumonia, tuberculosis, or tumors. Shock from hemorrhage, pain, and respiratory failure follows if emergency care is not available. *(See next page for illustration)*

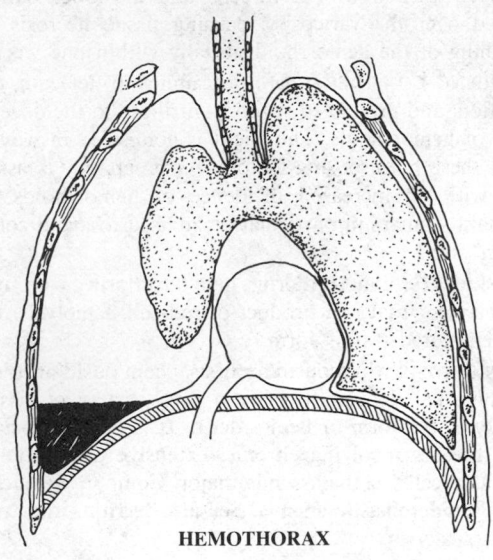

HEMOTHORAX

hemotroph (hi′mətrof), **hemotrophe** (hi′mətrouf), the total nutritive substances supplied to the embryo from the maternal circulation following the development of the placenta. Also called **hemotrophic nutrition.** Compare **embryotroph.** – **hemotrophic,** *adj.*

hemotrophic nutrition. See **hemotroph.**

Henle's fissure (hen′liz), one of many patches of connective tissue between the muscle fibers of the heart.

Henoch-Schönlein purpura (hei′nɔχʃhœn′laɨn), a self-limited hypersensitivity vasculitis, chiefly of children, characterized by purpuric skin lesions that appear predominantly on the lower abdomen, buttocks, and legs, and usually associated with pain in the knees and ankles. Other joint involvement, gastrointestinal bleeding, and hematuria are also common findings. The disease lasts up to six weeks and has no sequelae if renal involvement is not severe. Immunosuppressive drugs, as corticosteroids, may help the nephropathy. Also called **anaphylactoid purpura, Schönleinhenoch purpura.**

Henry's law, (in physics) a law stating that the solubility of a gas in a liquid is proportional to the pressure of the gas if the temperature is constant and if the gas does not chemically react with the liquid.

Hensen's knot, Hensen's node. See **primitive node.**

Hensen's node. See **primitive node.**

hen worker's lung. See **pigeon breeder's lung.**

heparin (hep′ərɪn), a naturally occurring mucopolysaccharide that acts in the body as an antithrombin factor to prevent intravascular clotting. It is produced by basophils and mast cells, which are found in large numbers in the connective tissue surrounding capillaries, particularly in the lungs and liver. In the form of its sodium salt, heparin is used therapeutically as an anticoagulant. See also **heparin sodium.**

heparin sodium, an anticoagulant.

■ INDICATIONS: It is prescribed in the treatment and prophylaxis of a variety of thromboembolic disorders.

■ CONTRAINDICATIONS: Known hypersensitivity to this drug prohibits its ues. It is not given in situations in which frequent monitoring of the coagulation status of the patient's blood is not possible.

■ ADVERSE EFFECTS: The most serious adverse reaction is hemorrhage. Vasospastic disorders may occur.

hepat-. See **hepato-.**

-hepatia, a combining form meaning '(condition of the) liver or its functioning': *anhepatia, dyshepatia, hypohepatia.*

hepatic (hɪpæt′ɪk), of or pertaining to the liver.

hepatic adenoma, a rapidly growing liver tumor that may become very large and may rupture, causing a lethal internal hemorrhage. It is sometimes called a 'pill tumor' because of its frequent association with the use of oral contraceptives.

hepatic amebiasis, enlargement and tenderness of the liver that often occurs in association with amebic dysentery, owing to inflammation resulting from infection with *Entamoeba histolytica.* See also **amebiasis,** *Entamoeba histolytica.*

hepatic coma, a neuropsychiatric manifestation of extensive liver damage owing to chronic or acute liver disease. Either endogenous or exogenous waste toxic to the brain is not neutralized in the liver before being shunted back into the peripheral circulation of the blood, or substances required for cerebral function are not synthesized in the liver and, therefore, are not available to the brain. The condition is characterized by variable consciousness, lethargy, stupor, and coma; a tremor of the hands, personality change, memory loss, hyperreflexia, and hyperventilation. Respiratory alkalosis, mania convulsions, and death may occur. The outcome varies according to the pathogenesis of the condition and the treatment. Treatment in most cases includes cleansing enemas, low-protein diet, parenteral hydration with a balanced electrolyte solution, and specific treatment for the underlying cause. Also called **portal-systemic encephalopathy.** See also **cirrhosis, hepatitis.**

hepatic cord, a mass of cells, arranged in irregular radiating columns and plates, spreading outward from the central vein of the hepatic lobule. The cells are many-sided and contain one or, sometimes, two distinct nuclei. Many such cords join to form the parenchyma of the lobule. Each cell usually contains granules, some of which are protoplasmic while others consist of glycogen, fat, or an iron compound. Also called **hepatic cells.**

hepatic fistula, an abnormal passage from the liver to another organ or body structure.

hepatic node, a node in one of three groups of lymph glands associated with the abdominal and the pelvic viscera supplied by branches of the celiac artery. The hepatic nodes are divided into the hepatic and subpyloric groups. The hepatic group, on the stem of the hepatic artery, extends along the common bile duct, between the two layers of the lesser omentum, as far as the porta hepatis. The subpyloric group comprises about five nodes closely relating to the division of the gastroduodenal artery. Both groups receive afferents from the stomach, the duodenum, the liver, the gall bladder, and the pancreas. Their efferents join the celiac set of preaortic nodes. Compare **gastric node, pancreaticolienal node.**

hepatico-. See **hepato-.**

hepatic porphyria. See **porphyria.**

hepatic vein catheterization, the introduction of a long, fine catheter into a hepatic venule for the purpose of recording intrahepatic venous pressure. The catheter is inserted through a vein in the arm and is passed through the right atrium, the inferior vena cava, and hepatic vein into the small hepatic vessel.

hepatin (hep′ətin). See **glycogen.**

hepatitis (hep′ətai′tis), an inflammatory condition of the liver, characterized by jaundice, hepatomegaly, anorexia, abdominal and gastric discomfort, abnormal liver function, clay-colored stools, and dark urine. The condition may be caused by bacterial or viral infection, parasitic infestation, alcohol, drugs, toxins, or transfusion of incompatible blood. It may be mild and brief or severe, fulminant, and life-threatening. The liver usually is able to regenerate its tissue, but severe hepatitis may lead to cirrhosis and chronic liver dysfunction. See also **viral hepatitis.**

hepatitis A, a form of infectious viral hepatitis caused by the hepatitis A virus, characterized by slow onset of signs and symptoms. The virus may be spread by direct contact or through contaminated food or water. The infection most often occurs in young adults and is usually followed by complete recovery. See **viral hepatitis.**

hepatitis B, a form of viral hepatitis caused by the hepatitis B virus, characterized by rapid onset of acute symptoms and signs. The virus is transmitted in contaminated serum in blood transfusion or by the use of contaminated needles and instruments. The infection may be severe and result in prolonged illness, destruction of liver cells, cirrhosis, B or death. Also called **serum hepatitis.** See **viral hepatitis.**

hepatitis B immune globulin (HBIG), a passive immunizing agent.

■ INDICATION: It is prescribed for post-exposure prophylaxis against infection by the hepatitis B virus.

■ CONTRAINDICATIONS: Known hypersensitivity to the drug or to gamma globulin prohibits its use.

■ ADVERSE EFFECTS: Among the most serious adverse reactions are severe hypersensitivity reactions. Pain and inflammation at the site of injection also may occur.

hepatitis B surface antigen (HBsAG). 1. See **Australia antigen.**

hepatization (hep′ətizei′s̆hən), transformation of lung tissue into a solid mass resembling the liver, as in early pneumococcal pneumonia in which consolidation and effusion of red blood cells in the alveoli produce **red hepatization.** In later stages of pneumococcal pneumonia, when white blood cells fill the alveoli, the consolidation becomes **gray hepatization.**

hepato-, hepat-, a combining form meaning 'pertaining to the liver': *hepatobiliary, hepatocarcinogenic, hepatocellular.* Also **hepatico.**

hepatocarcinoma (hep′ətoukar′simou′mə). See **malignant hepatoma.**

hepatocellular carcinoma. See **malignant hepatoma.**

hepatoduodenal ligament (hep′ətoudu′ədi′nəl, hep′ətouduod′inəl), the portion of the lesser omentum between the liver and the duodenum, containing the hepatic artery, the common bile duct, the portal vein, lymphatics, and the hepatic plexus of nerves. These structures are enclosed within a fibrous capsule between the two layers of the ligament. Compare **hepatogastric ligament.**

hepatogastric ligament (hep′ətougæs′trik), the portion of the lesser omentum between the liver and the stomach. Compare **hepatoduodenal ligament.**

hepatojugular reflux (hep′ətoujəg′yulər), an increase in jugular venous pressure when pressure is applied for 30 to 60 seconds over the abdomen, suggestive of right-sided heart failure.

hepatolenticular degeneration (hipæt′oulentik′yulər), an abnormal condition associated with defective copper metabolism in the body, characterized by decreased serum ceruloplasmin and copper levels and increased secretion of urinary copper. Individuals with this condition develop tissue deposits of copper associated with hepatic cirrhosis, deep marginal pigmentation of the cornea, and extensive degeneration of the central nervous system, especially the basal ganglions. Also called **Wilson's disease.**

hepatoma (hep′ətou′mə), *pl.* **hepatomas, hepatomata.** a primary malignant tumor of the liver characterized by hepatomegaly, pain, hypoglycemia, weight loss, anorexia, ascites, and the presence of alphafetoprotein in the plasma. It occurs most frequently in association with hepatitis or cirrhosis of the liver and, geographically, in those parts of the world where the microtoxin, aflatoxin, is commonly found.

hepatomegaly (hep′ətoumeg′əli), abnormal enlargement of the liver that is usually a sign of liver disease. It is often discovered by percussion and palpation as part of a physical examination: the liver is easily palpable below the ribs and is tender to the touch. Hepatomegaly may be caused by hepatitis or other infection, fatty infiltration, as in alcoholism, biliary obstruction, or malignancy.

hepatotoxic, potentially destructive of liver cells. — **hepatotoxicity,** *n.*

hepatotoxicity (hep'ətoutoksıs'ıti), the tendency of an agent, usually a drug or alcohol, to have a destructive effect on the liver. — **hepatotoxic,** *adj.*

hept-. See **hepta-.**

hepta-, hept-, a combining form meaning 'seven': *heptachromic, heptadactylia, heptavalent.*

heptachlor poisoning (hep'təklɔr'). See **chlorinated organic insecticide poisoning.**

heptaploid (hep'təplɔid), **heptaploidic.** See **polyploid.**

herald patch. See **pityriasis rosea.**

herb bath, a medicinal bath taken in water containing a decoction of aromatic herbs.

herbicide poisoning, a poisoning caused by the ingestion, inhalation, or absorption of a substance intended for use as a weed killer or defoliant. Most of the commonly used agricultural herbicides, as alachlor, isopropylamine salt of glyphosate, and trifluralin, are only mildly toxic. If ingested, an emetic or gastric lavage is administered. Some herbicides contain extremely toxic substances; poisoning is characterized by dysphagia, burning stomach pain, throat constriction, diarrhea, or other severe symptoms. The substance is identified, the victim is rapidly taken to a medical facility, and therapy specific to the poison is promptly instituted.

hereditability, the degree to which a given trait is controlled by inheritance.

hereditary, pertaining to a characteristic, condition, or disease transmitted from parent to offspring; inborn; inherited. Compare **acquired, congenital, familial.**

hereditary ataxia, one of a group of inherited degenerative diseases of the spinal cord, cerebellum, and, often, other parts of the nervous system, characterized by tremor, spasm, wasting of muscle, skeletal change, and sensory disturbances resulting in impaired motor activity. Kinds of hereditary ataxia include **ataxia telangiectasia, Friedreich's ataxia.**

hereditary brown enamel. See **amelogenesis imperfecta.**

hereditary deforming chondroplasia. See **diaphyseal aclasis.**

hereditary disorder. See **inherited disorder.**

hereditary disorder, heritable disorder. See **inherited disorder.**

hereditary elliptocytosis. See **elliptocytosis.**

hereditary enamel hypoplasia. See **amelogenesis imperfecta.**

hereditary essential tremor. See **essential tremor.**

hereditary hemorrhagic telangiectasia. See **Osler-Weber-Rendu syndrome.**

hereditary hyperuricemia. See **Lesch-Nyhan syndrome.**

hereditary multiple exostoses, a rare, familial, dyschondroplastic disease in which bony protruberances form on the shafts of the long bones and eventually develop into caps of cartilage covering the ends of the bones. The affected joints lose their mobility and the bones stop growing. The disease begins in childhood and has no cure. Very rarely, a chondrosarcoma may develop from the cap of an exostosis. See also **Ollier's dyschondroplasia.**

hereditary opalescent dentin. See **dentinogenesis imperfecta.**

hereditary protoporphyria. See **porphyria.**

hereditary spherocytosis. See **spherocytic anemia.**

hereditary tyrosinemia. See **tyrosinemia.**

heredity, 1. the process by which particular traits or conditions are genetically transmitted from parents to offspring, resulting in resemblance of individuals related by descent. It involves the separation and recombination of genes during meiosis and fertilization and the further interaction of developmental influences and genetic material during embryogenesis. 2. the total genetic constitution of an individual; the sum of the qualities inherited from ancestors and the potentialities of transmitting these qualities to offspring.

heredo-, a combining form meaning 'hereditary': *heredobiologic, heredosyphilitic, heredotrophedema.*

heredofamilial tremor (her'ıdoufəmıl'yəl). See **essential tremor.**

Hering-Breuer reflexes, inhibitory and excitatory impulses that maintain the rhythm of respiration and prevent the overdistension of alveoli. The impulses originate in stretch receptors of the bronchi and bronchioles, travel via afferent fibers of the vagus nerves to the medullary respiratory centers, and back by motor neurons to the respiratory muscles of the chest. Hering-Breuer reflexes are well developed at birth. They are stimulated by distension of the airway, increased intratracheal pressures, or pulmonary inflation. The inflation reflex stops inspiration and stimulates expiration; the deflation reflex inhibits expiration and brings on inspiration. These reflexes are hyperactive in conditions of restrictive ventilatory insufficiency.

hermaphrodism (hərmæf'rədız'əm). See **hermaphroditism.**

hermaphroditism (hərmæf'rədaitız'əm), rare condition in which both testicular and ovarian tissue exist in the same person, the testicular tissue containing semeniferous tubules or spermatozoa and the ovarian tissue containing follicles or corpora albicantia. The condition results from a chromosomal abnormality. Also called **hermaphrodism.** Compare **pseudohermaphroditism.**

hernia, protrusion of an organ through an abnormal opening in the muscle wall of the cavity that surrounds it. A hernia may be congenital, may result from the failure of certain structures to close after birth, or may be acquired later in life owing to obesity, muscular weakness, surgery, or illness. Kinds of hernia include **abdominal hernia, femoral hernia, hiatus hernia, inguinal hernia, umbilical hernia.** See also **herniorrhaphy.**

herniated disc, a rupture of the fibrocartilage surrounding an intervertebral disc, releasing the nucleus pulposus that cushions the vertebrae above and below. The resultant pressure on spinal nerve roots may cause considerable pain and damage the nerves. The condition most frequently occurs in the lumbar region. Also called **herniated nucleus pulposus, ruptured intervertebral disc, slipped disc.**

herniated intervertebral disc. See **herniated disc.**

herniated nucleus pulposus. See **herniated disc.**

herniation, a protrusion of a body organ or portion of an organ through an abnormal opening in a membrane, muscle, or other tissue. See also **hernia, hiatus.**

herniorraphy, the surgical repair of a hernia.

heroin, a morphinelike drug with no currently acceptable medical use in the United States. Heroin is included in Schedule I of the Comprehensive Drug Abuse Prevention and Control Act of 1970. As covered in this legislation, it may not be obtained by prescription but only for research and instructional use or for chemical analysis by application to the Drug Enforcement Administration of the Department of Justice. Heroin, like other opium alkaloids, can produce analgesia, respiratory depression, gastrointestinal spasm, and physical dependence. It produces its major effects on the central nervous system (CNS) and the bowel and alters the endocrine and the autonomic nervous systems. The binding sites for heroin are widely distributed in the CNS, especially throughout the limbic system, thalamus, striatum, hypothalamus, midbrain, and spinal cord. Illicitly obtained heroin is commonly used by individuals who become addicted and have a higher death rate than nonaddicts of similar age. Some studies conducted in the United States and England have shown that the majority of heroin users are relatively young people who have been introduced to the drug by friends and first start using heroin out of curiosity but continue because of its euphoric effects. Such individuals commonly show similar patterns of behavior, social adjustment, and health impairment. Heroin use in the United States reached epidemic proportions during the 1960s and, in 1971, became a major cause of death in New York City among males between the ages of 15 and 35. The problem abated somewhat during the 1970s but has apparently increased and spread from the larger cities to the smaller communities across the country. Initial street use of the drug commonly involves sniffing powdered heroin, which is absorbed through the mucous membranes of the nasopharynx and the respiratory tract. Other methods of self-administration include subcutaneous injection and intravenous injection. Heroin, which loses much of its analgesic power when taken orally, is more powerful than morphine and acts more rapidly. It is hydrolyzed to morphine by the body and becomes concentrated in the parenchymatous tissues, skeletal muscle, and brain. Heroin administered intravenously is almost immediately effective and produces reactions that last from 3 to 6 hours. Many users liken the initial sensation to a sexual orgasm. Heroin addicts may spend as much as $300 daily for the drug and inject themselves every 3 to 6 hours. Repeated use of this drug produces tolerance to most of the acute narcotic effects; physical dependence develops concurrently with tolerance. Withdrawal from heroin after relatively few exposures commonly produces acute abstinence syndrome. Withdrawal signs are usually observed shortly before the next planned dose and commonly include anxiety, restlessness, irritability, and craving for another dose. Other withdrawal signs that may appear 8 to 15 hours after the last dose include lacrimation, perspiration, yawning, and restless sleep. On awakening from such sleep the severely addicted heroin user may experience withdrawal signs, as vomiting, pain in the bones, diarrhea, convulsions, and cardiovascular collapse. Withdrawal signs usually peak at between 36 and 48 hours and gradually subside during the following 10 days. Associated anxiety and depression may persist for months in many heroin addicts under treatment. Most authorities consider such addiction a complex disease caused by heroin-induced neurochemical disturbances in combination with deep psychological and social factors. A variety of diluents, as quinine, are used to dissolve street heroin for subcutaneous and intravenous injection. Toxic diluents in combination with unhygienic administration and other unhealthy factors are responsible for more than half the fatalities associated with the illegal use of opiates. The most frequent disorders associated with injections of adulterated heroin are tetanus, skin abscesses, cellulitis, and thrombophlebitis. Heroin-connected pulmonary complications may include pneumonia, infarction, and tuberculosis. Neurologic disorders stemming from the use of street heroin may include transverse myelitis, peripheral nerve lesions, and fibrosing chronic myopathy. Women heroin addicts who become pregnant often give birth to premature babies who are highly susceptible to toxemia. Relapses of heroin addicts during withdrawal treatment are common and protracted abstinence signs, as altered blood pressure and pulse rate, anxiety, and depression, may persist for months. Methadone is commonly used as a substitute drug in the treatment of heroin addiction. Also being studied is the effectiveness of the synthetic methadone congener, alpha acetyl methadol which can prolong opiate effects for 72 hours. Numerous outpatient programs staffed by former opiate users seek to provide psychological and therapeutic support for addicts trying to break their drug habits. Some of these programs are Synanon, Daytop Village, and Phoenix House. Research and community-supported psychotherapy projects continue to seek more effective treatment methods for addicts, many of whom are successfully rehabilitated. Enforced abstinence from heroin and other opiates in penal institutions has been much less effective in rehabilitating addicts, and most authorities propose a combination of medically prescribed withdrawal psychotherapeutic procedures and rehabilitative programs as the most promising approach.

herpangina (hər′pænjai′nə), a viral infection, usually of young children, characterized by sore throat, headache, anorexia, and pain in the abdomen, neck, and extremities. Febrile convulsions and vomiting may occur in infants. Papules or vesicles may form in the pharynx and on the tongue, the palate, or the tonsils. The lesions evolve into shallow ulcers which heal spontaneously. The disease usually runs its course in less than a week. Treatment is symptomatic. The cause is often infection by a strain of coxsackievirus.

herpes genitalis, an infection caused by Type 2 herpes simplex virus (HSV2), usually transmitted by sexual contact, that causes painful vesicular eruptions on the skin and mucous membranes of the genitalia of males and females. When acquired during pregnancy, HSV2 may be transmitted through the placenta to the fetus and to the newborn by direct contact with infected tissue during birth.

■ OBSERVATIONS: In the male, herpes genitalis infections may resemble penile ulcers. A small group of vesicular lesions surrounded by erythematous tissue may occur on the glans or prepuce. The lesions erupt into superficial ulcers that often heal in five to seven days, although they also may become the sites of secondary infections. The lesions are painful and are often associated with a burning sensation, urinary dysfunction, fever, malaise, and swelling of the lymph glands in the inguinal area. The female patient may exhibit the same or similar systemic effects, and members of both sexes may complain of painful sexual intercourse. In the female, herpes genitalis lesions are likely to appear as multiple superficial eruptions on the surfaces of the cervix, vagina, or perineum. There may be a discharge from the cervix. Vaginal lesions may appear as mucous patches with grayish ulcerations. Laboratory tests from smears of fluid taken from the base of lesions show a positive Tzanck reaction with multiple nucleated giant cells which distinguishes HSV2 infections from other venereal diseases. HSV2 tends to recur.

■ INTERVENTION: Treatment of uncomplicated herpes genitalis is mainly symptomatic. An attack of the disease is generally self-limiting. Lesions may be cleansed with soap and water, where feasible, to limit the risk of secondary infections, and drying medications may be applied to lesions that rupture or ooze. Secondary infections are treated with appropriate antibiotics. Except for experi-

mental antiviral drugs, there are no specific cures or vaccines for the control of HSV2 infections.

■ NURSING CONSIDERATIONS: The nurse exercises extreme caution in contacts with infected patients. Smears for laboratory analysis are obtained by cleansing fresh vesicles with alcohol and removing fluid from the base of lesions with a cotton swab or wooden applicator. Rubber gloves are worn and the hands washed after contact to prevent transfer of virus particles from vesicles to other skin or mucous membranes of the patient or other individuals. Transfer of the virus to the cornea or conjunctiva results in herpetic keratitis. Primary infections that develop in pregnant women may progress to viremia and a marked incidence of mortality and morbidity in the fetus. Active HSV2 lesions within three weeks of delivery usually require that the infant be delivered by Caesarean section to avoid dangerous neonatal herpesvirus infection.

herpes gestationis, a generalized, pruritic, vesicular or bullous rash appearing in the second or third trimester of pregnancy and disappearing several weeks postpartum. The lesions often recur with succeeding pregnancies and are associated with premature birth and increased fetal mortality. The disease closely resembles erythema multiforme.

herpes labialis. See **herpes simplex.**

herpes simplex, an infection caused by a herpes simplex virus (HSV), which has an affinity for the skin and nervous system and usually produces small, transient, irritating, and sometimes painful fluid-filled blisters on the skin and mucous membranes. HSV 1 (oral herpes, herpes labialis) infections tend to occur in the facial area, particularly around the mouth and nose; HSV 2 (herpes genitalis) infections are usually limited to the genital region.

■ OBSERVATIONS: The initial symptoms of a herpes simplex infection usually include burning, tingling, or itching sensations about the edges of the lips or nose within a week or two after contact with an infected person. Several hours later, small red papules develop in the irritated area, followed by the eruption of small vesicles, or fever blisters, filled with fluid. Several small vesicles may merge to form a larger blister. The vesicles generally are associated with itching, pain, or similar discomfort. Other effects often include a mild fever and enlargement of the lymph nodes in the neck. Laboratory analysis of the vesicular fluid usually shows the presence of herpesvirus particles and the absence of pyogenic bacteria. Within a week after the onset of symptoms, thin yellow crusts form on the vesicles as healing begins. In skin areas that are moist or protected or in severe cases, healing may be delayed. HSV 2 infections in adolescence are associated with an increased incidence of cervical cancer in adulthood.

■ INTERVENTION: Treatment of herpes simplex is symptomatic. The lesions may be washed gently with soap and water to reduce the risk of secondary infection. Otherwise, topical applications of drying medications, as camphor or alcohol solutions, may speed healing, but they are very painful. Where secondary infections have begun, appropriate antibiotics are prescribed.

■ NURSING CONSIDERATIONS: Because herpesviruses are extremely contagious, the nurse follows all appropriate procedures in contacts with patients to avoid acquiring the infection and carrying it to other persons. Washing the hands and wearing rubber gloves while working about the mouth of a patient help prevent transmission of the virus. Once acquired, the virus tends to remain latent in the skin or tissues of the nervous system and may be reactivated by a variety of stimuli, including a febrile illness, physical or emotional stress, exposure to sunlight, or ingestion of certain foods or drugs. Topical sunscreen preparations offer some protection against exposure to the sun, and patients are advised to avoid repeated exposure to stimuli to which they have a known sensitivity. The complications of herpetic infections may include encephalitis, herpes simplex keratitis, and gingivostomatitis. In cases involving system complications, antibiotics, blood transfusions, I.V. solutions, and other therapeutic measures may be required. In uncomplicated cases, the herpes attack is usually self-limiting and runs its course in three weeks or less.

herpesvirus hominis (hər'pizvaï'rəs). See **herpes simplex.**

herpes zoster, an acute infection caused by the varicellazoster virus (VZV), affecting mainly adults and characterized by the development of painful vesicular skin eruptions that follow the underlying route of cranial or spinal nerves inflamed by the virus.

■ OBSERVATIONS: Distribution of the pain and vesicular eruptions is usually unilateral, although both sides of the body may be involved. Any sensory nerve may be affected, but the virus in most cases tends to invade the posterior root ganglia associated with thoracic and trigeminal nerves. The pain, which may be constant or intermittent, superficial or deep, usually precedes other effects and may mimic other disorders, as appendicitis or pleurisy. Early symptoms may include gastrointestinal disturbances, malaise, fever, and headache. The vesicles usually evolve from small red macules along the path of a nerve, and the skin of the area is hypersensitive. All of the lesions may appear within a period of hours, but they most often develop gradually over a period of several days. The macules vesiculate and, after about three days, become turbid with cellular debris. Usually, at the end of the first week, the vesicules develop crusts. The symptoms may persist for three to five weeks, but in most cases they diminish after two weeks.

■ INTERVENTION: Treatment is primarily symptomatic

and includes application of calamine lotion or similar medications to relieve itching and administration of analgesics for pain symptoms. Cool compresses may be applied to the affected skin areas. Topical corticosteroids may be prescribed for severe cases and for elderly patients who are potential candidates for a common sequela of postherpetic neuralgia. Surgical intervention to excise an affected nerve may be advised in cases of severe pain that fail to respond to more conservative treatment.

■ NURSING CONSIDERATIONS: The nurse encourages bed rest during the early stages of zoster infection, when fever and other systemic effects occur. Irritation of the vesicles may be exacerbated by contact with clothing or bed linen. The use of nonadherent dressings and of cradles to prevent direct contact of affected skin areas with irritating fabrics relieves discomfort. Older patients are most susceptible to complications, as exhaustion and postherpetic neuralgia, which may persist for several months after the skin lesions have cleared. Other complications are geniculate zoster, with involvement of the ear, face, and soft palate, and ophthalmic herpes zoster, which can result in corneal damage. An attack of herpes zoster does not confer immunity, but most patients recover without permanent effects except for occasional scarring at sites of severe vesicular lesions. Evidence indicates VZV remains latent in the body of a person once infected, and a person lacking varicella immunity can acquire chickenpox from a herpes zoster patient. Also called **shingles.** See also **herpesvirus, hominis, varicellazoster virus.**

herpes zoster oticus, an infection caused by a herpesvirus that involves the eighth nerve ganglia and geniculate ganglion, causing severe pain in the external ear structures and pain or paralysis along the facial nerve. The disease also may result in hearing loss and vertigo. The vertigo is usually transient but the hearing loss and facial paralysis may be permanent. There may be vesicular eruptions along the external ear canal and ear pinna. Treatment is generally symptomatic, with diazepam administered for vertigo, analgesics for pain, and corticosteroids for other symptoms.

herpes zoster virus (HZV). See **chickenpox.**

herpetiform (hərpet'ıform), having clusters of vesicles; resembling the skin lesions of some herpesvirus infections. See also **herpes simplex, herpes zoster.**

Herplex, a trade name for an antiviral (idoxuridine).

Hers' disease, an uncommon metabolic disorder of glycogen storage, characterized by hepatomegaly and an accumulation of abnormally large amounts of glycogen in the liver owing to its inability to break down glycogen. The condition is inherited as an autosomal, recessive trait. There is no known treatment. Also called **glycogen storage disease, type VI.** See also **glycogen storage disease.**

hertz (Hz), a unit of measurement of wave frequency equal to one cycle per second (cps).

hesperidin (hesper'ɪdɪn), a crystalline flavone glycoside found in bioflavonoid and occurring in most citrus fruits, especially in the spongy casing of oranges and lemons.

hetacillin, a penicillinase sensitive penicillin antibiotic that has no antibacterial activity until it is converted into ampicillin in the body.

■ INDICATIONS: It is prescribed in the treatment of certain infections.

■ CONTRAINDICATIONS: Known hypersensitivity to this drug or to any penicillin medication prohibits its use. Severe impairment of kidney function or a history of hypersensitivity reactions, as eczema, asthma, or hives, require that the drug be administered with caution.

■ ADVERSE EFFECTS: Among the more serious adverse reactions are diarrhea, gastrointestinal distress, skin rash, and hypersensitivity reactions.

hetastarch, a plasma-volume extender.

■ INDICATIONS: It is prescribed as an adjunct in shock and leukophoresis.

■ CONTRAINDICATIONS: Severe bleeding, severe heart or kidney dysfunction with oliguria or anuria, or known hypersensitivity to this drug prohibits its use.

■ ADVERSE EFFECTS: Among the more serious adverse reactions are influenzalike symptoms, muscle pain, edema, and anaphylaxis.

heter-. See **hetero-.**

heterauxesis (het'ərɔksi'sɪs). See **allometric growth.**

hetero-, heter-, a combining form meaning 'pertaining to another': *heteroalbumose, heterochronia, heterogamy.*

heteroallele (het'ərouəlil'), one of a set of genes located at a specific locus on homologous chromosomes that differs from the other of the pair, resulting in a mutation. – **heteroallelic,** *adj.*

heteroblastic, developing from different germ layers or kinds of tissue rather than from a single type. Compare **homoblastic.**

heterocephalus, a malformed fetus that has two heads of unequal size. – **heterocephalous, heterocephalic,** *adj.*

heterochromatin (het'əroukrou'mətɪn), that portion of chromosome material that is inactive in gene expression but may function in controlling metabolic activities, transcription, and cell division. It stains most intensely during the interphase stage and usually remains in a condensed state throughout the cell cycle. It consists of two types, constitutive heterochromatin, which occurs in the centromeric region of the chromosome and is characteristic of the Y chromosome, and facultative heterochromatin, which is present in the inactivated X chromosome of the mammalian female. Compare **euchromatin.** See also **chromatin** – **heterchromatic,** *adj.*

heterochromatinization, the transformation of genetically active euchromatin into genetically inactive heterochromatin; the inactivation of one of the X chromosomes in the mammalian female during the early stages of embryogenesis. See also **Lyon hypothesis.**

heterochromosome (het'əroukrou'məsoum), a sex chromosome. See also **heterotypical chromosomes.** – **heterochromosomal,** *adj.*

heterodidymus. See **heterodymus.**

heteroduplex (het'əroudu'pleks), (in molecular genetics) a DNA molecule in which the two strands are derived from different individuals, with the result that some pairs or blocks of base pairs may not match.

heterodymus, heterodidymus, a conjoined twin fetus in which the parasitic element consist of a head, neck, and thorax attached to the thoracic wall of the autosite.

heteroeroticism (het'ɪrouɪrot'ɪsɪz'əm), sexual feeling or activity directed toward another individual. Also called **alloeroticism, heteroerotism.** Compare **autoeroticism.**

heteroerotism (het'ɪrouer'ətɪz'əm). See **heteroeroticism.**

heterogamete, a gamete that differs considerably in size and structure from the one with which it unites, specifically denoting those of higher organisms as opposed to those of lower plants and animals. Compare **anisogamete, isogamete.**

heterogamy, 1. sexual reproduction in which there is fusion of dissimilar gametes, usually differing in size and structure. The word is used primarily to denote the reproductive processes of higher organisms as opposed to certain lower plants and animals. Compare **anisogamy, isogamy.** 2. reproduction by the alternation of sexual and asexual generations; heterogenesis. – **heterogamous,** *adj.*

heterogeneous, 1. consisting of dissimilar elements or parts; unlike; incongruous. 2. not having a uniform quality throughout. Compare **homogeneous.** – **heterogeneity,** *adj.*

heterogenesis (het'əroujen'əsis), 1. Also called **heterogeny, heterogony.** reproduction that differs in successive generations, as the alternation of sexual with asexual reproduction, so that offspring have characteristics different from those of the parents. In the asexual stage, it often involves one or more parthenogenic or hermaphroditic generations, often with various hosts, as in the case of many trematode parasites. 2. asexual generation. 3. abiogenesis. Compare **autogenesis, homogenesis.** See also **metagenesis.** – **heterogenetic, heterogenic,** *adj.*

heterogenous, derived or developed from another source or from two different sources.

heterogeny (het'əroj'əni). See **heterogenesis.**

heterograft (het'ərougræft'), tissue from another species used as a temporary graft in certain cases, as in treating a severely burned patient when sufficient tissue from the patient or from a tissue bank is not available. It is quickly rejected but provides a cover for the burn for the first few days, reducing the amount of fluid loss from the open wound. Also called **zenograft.** Compare **homograft.**

heterologous insemination. See **artificial insemination donor.**

heterologous tumor, a neoplasm consisting of tissue different from that of its site.

heterologous twins. See **dizygotic twins.**

heterophil test, a test for the presence of heterophil antibodies in the serum of patients suspected of having infectious mononucleosis, based on an agglutination reaction between heterophil antibodies in a person's serum and heterophil antigen, a normal component of sheep erythrocytes. This antibody eventually appears in the serum of more than 80 per cent of the patients with mononucleosis, hence is highly diagnostic of the disease. See also **Epstein-Barr virus.**

heteroploid (het'ərəploid), **heteroploidic,** 1. of or pertaining to an individual, organism, strain, or cell that has a variation in the number of whole chromosomes characteristic for the somatic cell of the species. The change may involve entire sets of chromosomes or the addition or loss of single whole chromosomes. 2. such an individual, organism, strain, or cell. See also **aneuploid, euploid.**

heteroploidy (het'ərəploi'di), the state or condition of having an abnormal number of chromosomes, either more or less than that characteristic of the somatic cell of the species.

heterosexual, 1. a person whose sexual desire or preference is for people of the opposite sex. 2. of or pertaining to sexual desire or preference for people of the opposite sex. — **heterosexuality,** n.

heterosexual panic, an acute attack of anxiety resulting in the frantic pursuit of heterosexual activity in response to unconscious or latent homosexual impulses. Compare **homosexual panic.**

heterosis (het'ərou'sis), the superiority of first-generation hybrid plants and animals in respect to one or more traits when compared to either of the parent strains or to corresponding inbred strains. Also called **hybrid vigor.**

heterotopic ossification, a nonmalignant overgrowth of bone, frequently occurring after a fracture, that is sometimes confused with certain bone tumors when visualized on x-ray film. Also called **exuberant callus, myositis ossificans.**

heterotypic (het'əroutip'ik), **heterotypical,** pertaining to or characteristic of a type differing from the usual or the normal, specifically applied to the first meiotic division of germ cells in gametogenesis as distinguished from the second or mitotic division. Compare **homeotypic.**

heterotypical chromosomes, any unmatched pair of chromosomes, specifically the sex chromosomes.

heterotypic mitosis, the division of bivalent chromosomes, as occurs in the first meiotic division of germ cells in gametogenesis; a reduction division. Compare **homeotypic mitosis.**

heterozygosis (het'ərouzaigou'sis), 1. the formation of a zygote by the union of two gametes that have dissimilar pairs of genes. 2. the production of hybrids through crossbreeding. — **heterozygotic,** adj.

heterozygous (het'ərəzai'gəs), having two different genes at corresponding loci on homologous chromosomes. An individual who is heterozygous for a particular characteristic has inherited a gene for that characteristic from one parent and the alternative gene from the other parent. A person heterozygous for a genetic disease caused by a dominant gene, as Huntington's chorea, manifests the disorder. An individual heterozygous for a hereditary disorder produced by a recessive gene, as sickle cell anemia, is asymptomatic or exhibits reduced symptoms of the disease. The offspring of a heterozygous carrier of a genetic disorder have a 50 per cent chance of inheriting the gene associated with the trait. Compare **homozygous.**

Hetrazan, a trade name for an anthelmintic (diethylcarbamazine citrate).

heuristic (hyuris'tik), 1. serving to stimulate interest for further investigation. 2. a teaching method in which the student is encouraged to learn through independent research and investigation. 3. a method of argument that postulates what is to be proved.

hex-, hexa-, a combining form meaning 'six': *hexabasic, hexavaccine, hexhydric.*

hexa-. See **hex-.**

Hexa-Betalin, a trade name for vitamin B_6 (pyridoxine hydrochloride).

hexachlorophene, a topical anti-infective and detergent.
- INDICATIONS: It is used as an antiseptic scrub and as a disinfectant for inanimate objects.
- CONTRAINDICATION: Known hypersensitivity to this drug is the only contraindication.
- ADVERSE EFFECTS: Among the more serious adverse reactions are skin rash and neurologic abnormalities.
- NOTE: The skin should be rinsed thoroughly to prevent systemic absorption.

Hexadrol, a trade name for a glucocorticoid (dexamethasone).

hexafluorenium bromide, an inhibitor of plasma choline terase.
- INDICATIONS: It is used an adjunct to anesthesia to prolong the skeletal muscle relaxation caused by succinylcholine.
- CONTRAINDICATIONS: Known hypersensitivity to this drug or to bromides prohibits its use.
- ADVERSE EFFECTS: Among the more serious adverse reactions are excessive prolongation of muscle relaxation and resultant apnea, allergic reactions, and hypotension.

Hexalet, a trade name for a urinary antibacterial (methenamine sulfosalicylate).

hexamethylenamine. See **methenamine.**

hexamethylmelamine, an experimental antineoplastic

which has been used to treat bronchogenic, cervical, and ovarian carcinomas.

hexaploid (hek′səploid), **hexaploidic.** See **polyploid.**

hexenmilch (hek′sənmɪlχ). See **witch's milk.**

hexestrol (hekses′trol), an estrogen.

■ INDICATIONS: It is prescribed in the treatment of menstrual cycle irregularities, menopausal symptoms, and to prevent pregnancy.

■ CONTRAINDICATIONS: Thrombophlebitis, abnormal genital bleeding, known or suspected pregnancy, or known hypersensitivity to this drug prohibits its use.

■ ADVERSE EFFECTS: Among the more serious adverse reactions are thrombophlebitis, malignant neoplasms, embolisms, and hypercalcemia.

hexobarbital, a short-acting barbiturate.

■ INDICATIONS: It is prescribed as an hypnotic and as a short-acting sedative.

■ CONTRAINDICATIONS: Porphyria, liver dysfunction, or known hypersensitivity to this drug prohibits its use.

■ ADVERSE EFFECTS: Among the most serious adverse reactions are respiratory depression, paradoxical excitement, porphyria, allergic reactions, and drug dependence.

hexocyclium methylsulfate, an anticholinergic.

■ INDICATION: It is prescribed as an adjunct to ulcer therapy.

■ CONTRAINDICATIONS: Narrow angle glaucoma, asthma, obstruction of the genitourinary or gastrointestinal tract, ulcerative colitis, or known hypersensitivity to this drug prohibits its use.

■ ADVERSE EFFECTS: Among the more serious adverse reactions are blurred vision, central nervous system effects, tachycardia, dry mouth, decreased sweating, and hypersensitivity reactions.

hexokinase (hek′səkai′neis), an enzyme that catalyzes the transfer of a phosphate group from adenosine triphosphate to D-glucose.

Hf, symbol for **hafnium.**

HFPPV, abbreviation for *high-frequency positive-pressure ventilation.*

Hg, symbol for **mercury.**

hiatus (haiei′təs), a usually normal opening in a membrane or other body tissue. — **hiatal,** *adj.*

hiatus hernia, protrusion of a portion of the stomach upward through the diaphragm. The condition occurs in about 40 per cent of the population, and most people display few, if any, symptoms. The major difficulty in symptomatic patients is gastroesophageal reflux, the backflow of the acid contents of the stomach into the esophagus. Diagnosis is made easily on x ray. Surgical treatment is usually unnecessary, and efforts should be directed toward alleviating the discomfort associated with reflux. See also **gastroesophageal reflux, heartburn.**

hibernoma (hai′bərnou′mə), *pl.* **hibernomas, hibernomata.** a benign tumor, usually on the hips or the back, composed of fat cells that are partly or entirely of fetal origin. Also called **fat cell lipoma, fetal lipoma.**

hiccup, hiccough, a characteristic sound that is produced by the involuntary contraction of the diaphragm, followed by rapid closure of the glottis. Hiccups have a variety of causes, including indigestion, rapid eating, certain types of surgery, and epidemic encephalitis. Most episodes of hiccups do not persist longer than a few minutes, but recurrent and prolonged attacks sometimes occur. The condition is most often seen in men. Sedatives are used in extreme cases. Also called **singultus.**

hickory stick fracture. See **greenstick fracture.**

hidradenitis (hai′drædənai′tis). See **hydradenitis.**

hidro-, a combining form meaning 'pertaining to sweat or a sweat gland': *hidrocystoma, hidrosadenitis, hidroschesis.*

hidrosis (hɪdrou′sɪs, haidrou′sɪs), sweat production and secretion. Compare **anhidrosis, dyshidrosis, hyperhidrosis.** — **hidrotic,** *adj.*

hier-. See **hiero-.**

hiero-, hier-, a combining form meaning 'pertaining to the sacrum, or to religion': *hierolisthesis, hieromania, hierotherapy.*

high blood pressure. See **hypertension.**

Detection and confirmation

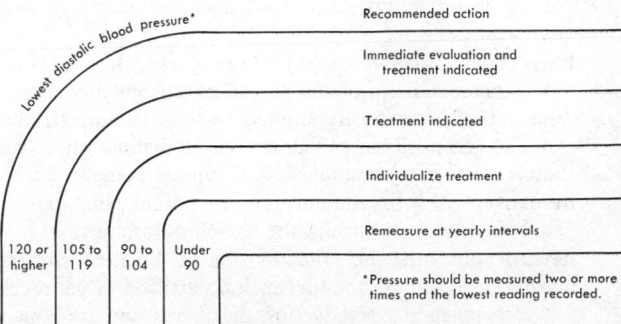

Follow-up recommendations
HIGH BLOOD PRESSURE

high-density lipoprotein, a plasma protein containing relatively more protein and less cholesterol and triglycerides. It may serve to stabilize very low-density lipoprotein and is involved in transporting cholesterol and other lipids from the plasma to the tissues.

high energy phosphate compound, a chemical compound containing a high-energy bond between phosphoric acid residues and certain organic substances. When the bond is hydrolyzed, a large amount of energy is released. Adenosine triphosphate is the most powerful and ubiquitous of the high energy phosphate compounds found in the body. All of these compounds liberate energy to fuel muscle contraction, active transport across cell membranes, and the synthesis of many substances in the body.

highest intercostal vein, one of a pair of veins that drain the blood from the upper two or three intercostal spaces. The right vein descends and opens into the azygous vein. The left vein crosses the arch of the aorta and opens into the left brachiocephalic vein, usually receiving the left bronchial vein.

high forceps, an obstetric operation in which forceps are used to deliver a baby whose head is not engaged in the birth canal. The procedure is considered hazardous and is generally condemned. Compare **low forceps, mid forceps.** See also **forceps delivery, obstetric forceps.**

high-Fowler's position, placement of the patient in a semi-sitting position by raising the head of the bed more than twenty inches.

high-level wellness, a concept of optimal health that emphasizes the integration of body, mind, and environment to maximize the function of an individual.

high-potassium diet, a diet that contains foods rich in potassium, including all leafy green vegetables, brussels sprouts, citrus fruits, bananas, dates, raisins, legumes, meats, and whole grains. It is indicated for any condition resulting in the loss of extracellular fluid, as acute diarrhea, congenital renal alkalosis, aldosteronism, hypokalemia, hypertension, and diabetic coma. It is also indicated for patients receiving thiazide or corticosteroid therapy.

high-protein diet, a diet that contains large amounts of protein, consisting largely of meats, fish, milk, legumes, and nuts. It may be indicated in protein depletion from any cause, as a preoperative preparation, in nephrotic syndromes, or in hepatic disorders. It may be contraindicated in liver failure or when function of the kidneys is so impaired that added protein could result in azotemia and acidosis.

high-risk infant, any neonate, regardless of birth weight, size, or gestational age, who, because of preconceptual, prenatal, natal, or postnatal conditions or circumstances that interfere with the normal birth process or impede adjustment to extrauterine growth and develop-ment, has a greater than average chance of morbidity or mortality, especially within the first 28 days of life. See also **neonatal period, premature infant.**

high-vitamin diet, a dietary regimen that includes a variety of foods that contain therapeutic amounts of all of the vitamins necessary for the metabolic processes of the body. It is often ordered in combination with other therapeutic diets containing larger than usual amounts of protein or calories, especially when treating severe or chronic infection, malnutrition, or vitamin deficiency.

Hill-Burton Act, a 1946 amendment to the U.S. Public Health Service Act authorizing grants to states for surveying their hospital and public health center needs and for the planning and construction of additional facilities. Subsequent amendments authorized federal funding for as much as two thirds of the cost of construction projects and broadened the scope of the legislation to include diagnostic and treatment centers, long-term treatment centers, and nursing homes and to aid in modernization of existing hospitals. Also called **Hospital Survey and Construction Act.**

Hill-Burton programs, a cluster of programs created by legislation included in the National Health Planning and Resources Development Act of 1974. The programs allow federal monetary assistance for modernization of health facilities, construction of outpatient health centers, construction of inpatient facilities in underserved areas, and the conversion of existing health care facilities for the provision of new health services.

hilus (hai'ləs), *pl.* **hili.** a depression or pit at that part of an organ where vessels and nerves enter.

hindgut, the caudal portion of the embryonic alimentary canal. Consisting of endodermal tissue, it is formed by the development of the tail fold and eventually gives rise to part of the small and large intestines, rectum, bladder, and urogenital ducts. Compare **foregut, midgut.** See also **cloaca.**

hind kidney. See **metanephros.**

hinge joint, a synovial joint providing a connection in which articular surfaces are closely molded together in a manner that permits extensive motion in one plane. The distal bone of a hinge joint seldom moves in the same plane as that of the axis of the proximal bone. The interphalangeal joints are hinge joints. Also called **ginglymus joint.** Compare **gliding joint, pivot joint.**

hip. See **coxa.**

hip bath. See **sitz bath.**

hip joint. See **coxal articulation.**

hippocampal fissure, a fissure reaching from the posterior aspect of the corpus callosum to the tip of the temporal lobe.

Hippocrates (hɪpok'rətiz), a Greek physician born about 460 B.C. on the island of Cos, a center for the worship of Æsculapius. Called the "Father of Medicine," Hippocrates introduced a scientific approach to healing by seeking physical causes for disease rather than magic or mythical relationships employed by members of the Æsculapian cults of the time. He also compiled case records of illnesses, including results of treatments administered, and developed the art of ethical bedside care. See also **Æsculapius, Hippocratic Oath.**

Hippocrates' bandage. See **capeline bandage.**

Hippocratic Oath (hɪp′əkræt′ɪk), an oath, attributed to Hippocrates, that serves as an ethical guide for the medical profession. It is traditionally incorporated into the graduation ceremonies of medical colleges and reads as follows:

I swear by Apollo the physician, by Æsculapius, Hygeia and Panacea, and I take to witness all the gods, and all the goddesses, to keep according to my ability and my judgment the following Oath:

To consider dear to me as my parents him who taught me this art; to live in common with him and if necessary to share my goods with him; to look upon his children as my own brothers, to teach them this art if they so desire without fee or written promise; to impart to my sons and the sons of the master who taught me and the disciples who have enrolled themselves and have agreed to the rules of the profession, but to these alone, the precepts and the instruction. I will prescribe regimen for the good of my patients according to my ability and my judgment and never do harm to anyone. To please no one will I prescribe a deadly drug, nor give advice which may cause his death. Nor will I give a woman a pessary to procure abortion. But I will preserve the purity of my life and my art. I will not cut for stone, even for patients in whom the disease is manifest; I will leave this operation to be performed by practitioners (specialists in this art). In every house where I come I will enter only for the good of my patients, keeping myself far from all intentional ill-doing and all seduction, and especially from the pleasures of love with women or with men, be they free or slaves. All that may come to my knowledge in the exercise of my profession or outside of my profession or in daily commerce with men, which ought not to be spread abroad, I will keep secret and will never reveal. If I keep this oath faithfully, may I enjoy my life and practice my art, respected by all men and in all times; but if I swerve from it or violate it, may the reverse be my lot. See also **Æsculapius, Hippocrates.**

hip replacement, replacement of the hip joint with an artificial ball and socket joint, performed to relieve a chronically painful and stiff hip in advanced osteoarthritis, an improperly healed fracture, or degeneration of the joint. Antibiotic therapy is begun preoperatively, and the patient is taught to walk with crutches. General anesthesia is used, the femoral head, neck, and part of the shaft are removed, and the contours of the socket are smoothed. A prosthesis of a durable, hard metal alloy or stainless steel is shaped to resemble a femur and head of a femur and is attached to the femur with screws or an acrylic cement; a metal or a plastic acetablum is implanted. Postoperatively, the patient is placed in traction. The affected leg is kept abducted and in straight alignment with pillows; external rotation of the leg must be prevented. The nurse observes nerve function and circulation in the leg frequently during the first postoperative day. Support hose may be ordered and anticoagulant therapy begun. The most frequent complications are infection requiring removal of the new joint, or its dislocation. Ambulation begins gradually, with frequent short walks. Sitting for more than an hour is to be avoided, and hip flexion beyond 90° may cause dislocation of the prosthesis. The patient continues an exercise program after discharge to maintain functional motion of the hip joint and to strengthen the abductor muscles.

Hiprex, a trade name for a urinary antibacterial (methenamine hippurate).

Hirschsprung's disease (hɪrsh′sprʊɳgz), the congenital absence of autonomic ganglia in the smooth-muscle wall of the colon, resulting in poor or absent peristalsis in the involved segment of colon, accumulation of feces, and dilation of the bowel (megacolon). Symptoms include intermittent vomiting, diarrhea, and constipation. The abdomen may become distended to several times its normal size. The condition is usually diagnosed in infancy, but it may not be recognized until much later in childhood, when there is anorexia, lack of urge to defecate, distention of the abdomen, and poor health. Diagnosis is confirmed by barium enema; biopsy of the affected tissue shows the absence of ganglia. Surgical repair in early childhood is usually successful. A temporary colostomy is performed and the aganglionic portion of the bowel is resected. The colostomy is almost always reversed a few months later. Also called **congenital megacolon.**

Distended
sigmoid colon

Aganglionic portion

Rectum

HIRSCHSPRUNG'S DISEASE

hirsutism (hər'sutɪz'əm), excessive body hair in a masculine distribution owing to heredity, hormonal dysfunction, porphyria, or medication. Treatment of the specific cause will usually stop growth of more hair. Excess hair may be removed by dermabrasion, electrolysis, chemical depilation, shaving, plucking, or rubbing with pumice. Fine facial hair may be most effectively minimized by bleaching. Also called **hypertrichosis.** – **hirsute,** *adj.,* **hirsuteness,** *n.*

hirsutoid papilloma of the penis (hər'sutoid), a condition characterized by clusters of small, white papules on the coronal edge of the glans penis. Also called **papillomatosis coronal penis, pearly penile papules.**

His bundle (hɪs). See **bundle of His.**

Hispril, a trade name for an antihistaminic (diphenylpyraline hydrochloride).

hist-. See **histo-.**

histamine (hɪs'təmin, lɪs'təmin), a compound, found in all cells, produced by the breakdown of histidine. It is released in allergic, inflammatory reactions and causes dilation of capillaries, decreased blood pressure, increased secretion of gastric juice, and constriction of smooth muscles of the bronchi and uterus.

histamine headache, a headache associated with the release of histamine from the body tissues and marked by symptoms of dilated carotid arteries, fluid accumulation under the eyes, tearing or lacrimation, and rhinorrhea (runny nose). Symptoms include sudden sharp pain on one side of the head, involving the facial area from the neck to the temple. Treatment includes the use of preparations of antihistamines and ergot that help constrict the arteries. Also called **cluster headache, Horton's histamine cephalalgia.** See also **cephalalgia.**

-histechia, a combining form meaning a 'tissue retaining a (specified) substance': *cholesterohistechia, glycohistechia, uratohistechia.*

histiocyte. See **macrophage.**

histiocytic leukemia (hɪs'tiəsɪt'ɪk). See **monocytic leukemia.**

histiocytic malignant lymphoma, a lymphoid neoplasm containing undifferentiated primitive cells or differentiated reticulum cells. Also called **clasmocytic lymphoma, reticulum cell sarcoma.**

histiocytosis X (hɪs'tiousaitou'sɪs eks'), *Obsolete.* a cluster of conditions encompassing benign eosinophilic granuloma and several malignant lymphomatous diseases.

histiotypic growth (hɪs'tioutɪp'ɪk), the uncontrolled proliferation of cells, as occurs in bacterial cultures and molds. Compare **organotypic growth.**

histo-, hist-, a combining form meaning 'pertaining to tissue': *histoclastic, histohematin, histonectomy.*

histocompatibility antigens, a group of genetically determined antigens on the surface of many cells. Histocompatibility antigens are the cause of most graft rejections that occur in organ transplantation. See also **isoantigen, histocompatibility locus.**

histocompatibility locus, a set of positions on a chromosome that are occupied by a complex of genes that govern several tissue antigens. Together, the loci and the genes comprise the human leukocyte antigen complex.

histogram (hɪs'təgræm), (in research) a graph showing the values of one or more variables plotted against time or against frequency of occurrence. A graph of a patient's temperature, pulse, and respiration is an example of a histogram.

histography (hɪstog'rəfi), the process of describing or creating visualizations of tissues and cells. – **histographer,** *n.,* **histographic,** *adj.,* **histographically,** *adv.*

histoid neoplasm, a growth that resembles the tissues in which it originates. Compare **organoid neoplasm.**

histologist (hɪstol'əjɪst), a medical scientist who specializes in the study of histology. See also **histology.**

histology (hɪstol'əji), **1.** the science dealing with the microscopic identification of cells and tissue. **2.** the structure of organ tissues, including the composition of cells and their organization into various body tissues. – **histologic, histological,** *adj.,* **histologically,** *adv.*

histone (hɪs'toun), any of a group of strongly basic, low molecular weight proteins that are soluble in water, insoluble in dilute ammonia, and combine with nucleic acid to form nucleoproteins. They are found in the cell nucleus, especially of glandular tissue, where they form a complex with deoxyribonucleic acid in the chromatin and function in regulating gene activity. Histones also interfere with coagulation of the blood and have been isolated from the urine of patients with leukemia and febrile conditions.

Histoplasma capsulatum (hɪs'touplæz'mə), a dimorphic fungal organism that is a single budding yeast at body temperature and a mold at room temperature. The causative organism in histoplasmosis, it is common in the Mississippi River Valley. The fungus, spread by airborne spores from soil contaminated with excreta from infected birds, acts as a parasite on the cells of the reticuloendothelial system.

histoplasmosis (hɪs'touplæzmou'sɪs), an infection caused by inhalation of spores of the fungus *Histoplasma capsulatum.* **Primary histoplasmosis** is characterized by fever, malaise, cough, and lymphadenopathy. Spontaneous recovery is usual; small calcifications remain in the lungs and affected lymph glands. **Progressive histoplasmosis,** the sometimes fatal, disseminated form of the infection, is characterized by ulcerating sores in the mouth and nose, enlargement of the spleen, liver, and lymph nodes, and severe and extensive infiltration of the lungs. Infection confers immunity; a histoplasmin skin test may be performed to identify people who may safely work with contaminated soil. The disease is most common in the Mississippi and Ohio Valleys.

history, 1. a record of past events. 2. a systematic account of the medical and psychosocial occurrences in a patient's life and of factors in family, ancestors, and environment that may have a bearing on the patient's present condition.

history of present illness, an account obtained during the interview with the patient of the onset, duration, and character of the present illness as well as of any acts or factors that aggravate or ameliorate the symptoms. The patient is asked what is believed to be the cause of the symptoms and whether or not a similar condition has occurred in the past.

histotroph (hɪs′tətrof), histotrophe (hɪs′tətrouf). See **embryotroph.**

histotrophic nutrition. See **embryotroph.**

histrionic personality, a personality characterized by behavioral patterns and attitudes that are overreactive, emotionally unstable, overly dramatic, and self-centered, exhibited as a means of attracting attention, consciously or unconsciously. Also called **hysterical personality.** See also **histrionic personality disorder.**

histrionic personality disorder, a disorder characterized by dramatic, reactive, and intensely exaggerated behavior, which is typically self-centered and results in severe disturbance in interpersonal relationships that can lead to psychosomatic disorders, depression, alcoholism, and drug dependency. Symptoms include emotional excitability, such as irrational angry outbursts or tantrums; abnormal craving for activity and excitement; overreaction to minor events; manipulative threats and gestures; egocentricity; inconsiderateness; inconsistency; and continuous demand for reassurance because of feelings of helplessness and dependency. A person having this disorder is perceived by others as vain, demanding, superficial, self-centered, and self-indulgent. The disorder is more prevalent in women than in men and is treated by various psychotherapies, depending on the individual and the severity of the condition.

hives, *Nontechnical.* pruritic eruption of the skin, typically consisting of small elevated wheals with a blanched center and surrounding redness. The individual lesions often fade within hours but may recur, as in chronic urticaria. Many cases of hives are precipitated immunologically by certain foods or drugs. Acute hives are characterized by capillary dilation in the dermis, leading to a loss of fluid into the tissues. Capillary dilation is caused by the release of vasoactive mediators, including histamine, kinin, and the slow, reactive substance of anaphylaxis, as a result of the antigen-antibody reaction. Treatment includes antihistamines and removal of the stimulus or allergen, if possible. Cholinergic urticaria is a kind of hives that appears as small wheals surrounded by a large axon flare. It may be caused by emotional stress, exposure to heat, or exercise. Also called **urticaria.** Compare **angioedema.**

m₂O. See **water.**

HLA. See **human leukocyte antigen.**

HLA-A, abbreviation for *human leukocyte antigen A.* See **human leukocyte antigen.**

HLA-B, abbreviation for *human leukocyte antigen B.* See **human leukocyte antigen.**

HLA-D, abbreviation for *human leukocyte antigen D.* See **human leukocyte antigen.**

HLA-L, abbreviation for *human leukocyte antigen L.* See **human leukocyte antigen.**

HMO. See **Health Maintenance Organization.**

HMS Liquifilm, a trade name for an ophthalmic preparation containing a glucocorticoid (medrysone).

Ho, symbol for **holmium.**

Hô, symbol for **null hypothesis.**

hod-, a combining form meaning 'pertaining to pathways': *hodology, hodoneuromare.*

Hodgkin's disease (hoj′kɪnz), a malignant disorder characterized by painless, progressive enlargement of lymphoid tissue, usually first evident in cervical lymph nodes; splenomegaly; and the presence of Reed-Sternberg cells, large, atypical histiocytes with multiple or hyperlobulated nuclei and prominent nucleoli. Symptoms include anorexia, weight loss, generalized pruritus, low-grade fever, night sweats, anemia, and leukocytosis. The disease is diagnosed in about 7,100 Americans annually, causes approximately 1,700 deaths a year, affects twice as many males as females, and usually develops between the ages of 15 and 35. The diagnosis is established by blood studies, x rays, lymphangiograms, lymph node biopsies, and ultrasonic and computerized tomographic scans. Total lymphoid radiotherapy, using a covering mantle to protect other organs, is the treatment of choice for early stages of the disease; combination chemotherapy is the treatment for advanced disease. Long-term remissions are achieved in more than half the patients treated, and 60 to 90 per cent of those with localized disease may be cured. It is widely held that Hodgkin's disease may start as an inflammatory or infectious process and then become a neoplasm; according to another theory it may be an immune disorder. Clusters of cases have been reported but there is no conclusive evidence of a causative infectious agent, and the etiology of the disease remains an enigma.

Hoffmann's atrophy (hɔf′manz). See **Werdnig-Hoffmann disease.**

Hoffmann's reflex, an abnormal reflex elicited by sudden, forceful flicking of the nail of the index, middle, or ring finger, resulting in flexion of the thumb and of the middle and distal phalanges of one of the other fingers. It is not a very reliable sign of pyramidal tract disease above the level of the seventh or eighth cervical and first thoracic vertebra. Also called **Hoffmann's sign.**

hol-. See **holo-.**

holandric (holæn′drɪk), **1.** designating genes located on the nonhomologous portion of the Y chromosome. **2.** of or pertaining to traits or conditions transmitted only through the paternal line. Compare **hologynic.**

holandric inheritance, the acquisition or expression of traits or conditions only through the paternal line, transmitted by genes carried on the nonhomologous portion of the Y chromosome. Compare **hologynic inheritance.**

holism, wholism (hou′lɪzəm), a philosophical concept in which an entity is seen as more than the sum of its parts. Holism is prominent in current approaches to psychology, biology, nursing, medicine, and other scientific, sociologic, and educational fields of study and practice.

holistic, wholistic (houlɪs′tɪk), of or pertaining to the whole; considering all factors, as holistic medicine.

holistic health care, a system of comprehensive or total patient care that considers the physical, emotional, social, economic, and spiritual needs of the person, the response to the illness, and the impact of the illness on the person's ability to meet self-care needs. Holistic nursing is the modern nursing practice that expresses this philosophy of care. Also called **comprehensive care.**

holmium (Ho), a rare-earth metallic element. Its atomic number is 67; its atomic weight is 164.93.

holo-, hol-, a combining form meaning 'entire, or pertaining to the whole': *holodiastolic, holomastigote, holotonia.*

holoacardius (hou′louəkar′diəs), a separate, grossly defective monozygotic twin fetus, usually represented by a shapeless, nonformed mass, in which the heart is absent and the circulation in utero is accomplished totally by the heart of the viable twin through a vascular shunt.

holoacardius acephalus, a grossly defective separate twin fetus that lacks a heart, a head, and most of the upper portion of the body.

holoacardius acormus, a grossly defective, separate twin fetus in which the trunk is malformed and little more than the head is recognizable.

holoacardius amorphus, a malformed separate twin fetus in which there are no recognizable or formed parts.

holoblastic (hol′əblæs′tɪk), of or pertaining to an ovum that contains little or no yolk and undergoes total cleavage. Compare **meroblastic.**

Holocaine Hydrochloride, a trade name for a local anesthetic agent (phenacaine hydrochloride).

holocephalic (hou′lousɪfæl′ɪk), a malformed fetus in which several parts are deficient although the head is complete.

holodiastolic (hol′oudai′astol′ɪk). See **pandiastolic.**

hologynic (hol′oujɪn′ɪk), **1.** designating genes located on attached X chromosomes. **2.** of or pertaining to traits or conditions transmitted only through the maternal line. Compare **holandric.**

hologynic inheritance, the acquisition or expression of traits or conditions only through the maternal line, transmitted by genes located on attached X chromosomes. The phenomenon is not known to occur in man. Compare **holandric inheritance.**

holoprosencephaly (hol′oupros′ensef′əli), a congenital defect caused by the failure of the prosencephalon to divide into hemispheres during embryonic development. It is characterized by multiple midline facial defects, including cyclopia in severe cases. It can also be caused by an extra chromosome in the 13-15 or D group, manifesting as one of many developmental defects. See also **trisomy 13.** – **holoprosencephalic, holoprosencephalous,** *adj.*

holorachischisis (hol′ourəkis′kisis). See **complete rachischisis.**

holosystolic (hol′ousɪstol′ɪk). See **pansystolic.**

Holtzman inkblot technique (hoults′mən), a modification of the Rorschach test in which many more pictures of inkblots are used, the subject is permitted only one response to each design, and the scoring is predominantly objective rather than subjective.

Homan's sign (hou′mənz), pain in the calf with dorsiflexion of the foot, indicating thrombophlebitis or thrombosis.

homatropine methylbromide, an anticholinergic.

■ INDICATIONS: It is prescribed as an antispasmodic and as a cycloplegic and mydriatic medication in ophthalmic procedures.

■ CONTRAINDICATIONS: Narrow angle glaucoma, asthma, obstruction of the genitourinary or gastrointestinal tract, ulcerative colitis, or known hypersensitivity to this drug prohibits its use.

■ ADVERSE EFFECTS: Among the more serious adverse reactions are blurred vision, central nervous system effects, tachycardia, dry mouth, decreased sweating, and hypersensitivity reactions.

home care, a health service provided in the client's place of residence for the purpose of promoting, maintaining, or restoring health or minimizing the effects of illness and disability. Service may include such elements as medical, dental, and nursing care, speech and physical therapy, the homemaking services of a home health aide, or the provision of transportation. The level of care needed is determined by an assessment of the nature and extent of care needed and by the ability of the patient's family and friends to assume responsibility for the care needed. Nursing may be provided by a registered nurse, licensed practical nurse, or a home health aide. Some hospitals have home care services that include regular visits by a nurse and a physician to patients in their homes.

home health agency, an organization that provides health care in the home. Medicare certification for a home health agency is dependent on the providing of skilled nursing services and of at least one additional therapeutic service.

home maintenance management: impaired, a nursing diagnosis accepted by the Fourth National Conference on the Classification of Nursing Diagnoses. This diagnosis describes the situation in which a client is unable to maintain a safe, healthy home environment without help. The etiology may include any of the following: disease or injury of a member of the family or household, disorganization of the family, inadequate finances, lack of knowledge of community or neighborhood resources, impaired or disordered emotional or cognitive function, inadequate support from others, lack of knowledge, or lack of role models competent in home maintenance. Among the defining characteristics reported by the client and other members of the household are difficulty in maintaining the home in a comfortable condition, a need for help from the outside in maintaining the home, and the existence of debt or a financial crisis. Among the defining characteristics that may be observed in the home are disorder, an offensive odor, an inappropriate temperature, lack of necessary equipment or supplies, and the presence of rodents or vermin. The critical defining characteristics, at least one of which must be present for the diagnosis to be made, are unwashed or unavailable cooking utensils, clothes, or linens; the presence of accumulations of dirt, food, waste, and refuse; exhausted or distressed family or household members; and repeated infections and infestations owing to lack of hygiene. See also **nursing diagnosis.**

homeo-, homoeo-, homoio-, a combining form meaning 'sameness, similarity': *homeochrome, homeomorphus, homeothermal.*

Homeopathic Pharmacopoeia of the United States, one of the three official drug compendia specified in the Federal Food, Drug, and Cosmetic Act. See also **compendium, National Formulary, United States Pharmacopoeia.**

homeopathist (hou'miop'əθist), a physician who practices homeopathy.

homeopathy (hou'miop'əθi), a system of therapeutics based on the theory that "like cures like." The theory was advanced in the late 18th century by Dr. Samuel Hahnemann, who believed that a large amount of a particular drug may cause symptoms of a disease and moderate dosage may reduce those symptoms; thus, some disease symptoms could be treated by very small doses of medicine. In practice, homeopathists dilute drugs with milk sugar in ratios of 1 to 10 to achieve the smallest dose of a drug that seems necessary to control the symptoms in a patient and prescribe only one medication at a time. Compare **allopathy.** – **homeopathic,** *adj.*

homeostasis (hou'miəstei'sis), a relative constancy in the internal environment of the body, naturally maintained by adaptive responses that promote healthy survival. Various sensing, feedback, and control mechanisms function to effect this steady state which depends, in a sense, on every part of the body always knowing what all the other parts are doing. Some of the key control mechanisms are the reticular formation in the brain stem and the endocrine glands. Some of the functions controlled by homeostatic mechanisms are the heartbeat, hematopoiesis, blood pressure, body temperature, electrolytic balance, respiration, and glandular secretion. – **homeostatic,** *adj.*

homeotypic (hou'mioutip'ik), **homeotypical,** pertaining to or characteristic of the regular or usual type, specifically applied to the second meiotic division of germ cells in gametogenesis as distinguished from the first meiotic division. Compare **heterotypic.**

homeotypic mitosis, the equational division of chromosomes, as occurs in the second meiotic division of germ cells in gametogenesis. Compare **heterotypic mitosis.**

homiothermal. See **warmblooded.**

homo-, 1. a combining form meaning 'the same' *homocentric, homodont, homolysis.* 2. a combining form meaning 'the addition of one CH_2 group to the main compound': *homocheldonine, homocystine, homoquinine.*

homoblastic, developing from the same germ layer or a single type of tissue. Compare **heteroblastic.**

homochronous inheritance, the appearance of traits or conditions in the offspring at the same age as they appeared in the parents.

homocystinuria (hou'mousis'tinyur'iə), a rare biochemical abnormality characterized by the abnormal presence of homocystine, an amino acid, in the blood and urine, caused by any of several enzyme deficiencies in the metabolic pathway of methionine to cystine. Inherited as an autosomal recessive trait, the clinical signs of the disease are similar to Marfan's syndrome, including mental retardation, osteoporosis leading to skeletal abnormalities, dislocated lenses, and thromboembolism. Treatment may include a diet low in methionine and supplementation with large doses of vitamin B_6. Long term results of treatment are not available. – **homocystinuric,** *adj.*

homoeo-. See **homeo-.**

homogeneous, 1. consisting of similar elements or parts. 2. having a uniform quality throughout. Compare **heterogeneous.** – **homogeneity,** *adj.*

homogenesis, reproduction by the same process in succeeding generations so that offspring are similar to the parents. Compare **heterogenesis.**

homogenetic, 1. of or pertaining to homogenesis. 2. homogenous, def. 2.

homogenized milk, pasteurized milk that has been mechanically treated to reduce and emulsify the fat globules so that the cream cannot separate and the protein is more digestible.

homogenous, 1. homogeneous. 2. having a likeness in form or structure because of a common ancestral origin. Compare **heterogenous.** 3. homoplasy.

homogentisic acid (hou′moujentɪs′ɪk). See **glycosuric acid.**

homogeny, 1. homogenesis. 2. a likeness in structure or form owing to a common ancestral origin. Compare **homoplasy.**

homoio-. See **homeo-.**

homolog (hom′əlog), **homologue** (həmol′əgəs), 1. any organ corresponding in function, origin, and structure to another organ, as the flippers of a seal which correspond to human hands. 2. (in chemistry) one of a series of compounds, each formed by an added common element, as CO, carbon monoxide, is followed by CO_2, carbon dioxide, with the addition of an oxygen atom. — **homologous,** adj.

homologous chromosomes, any two chromosomes in the diploid complement of the somatic cell that are identical in size, shape, and gene loci. In man there are 22 pairs of homologous chromosomes and one pair of sex chromosomes, with one member of each pair being derived from the mother and the other from the father. Any deviation in the size, number, or genetic makeup of the chromosomes results in defects or disorders of varying severity in the affected individual.

homologous disease. See **graft-versus-host reaction.**

homologous insemination. See **artificial insemination husband.**

homologous tumor, a neoplasm made up of cells resembling those of the tissue in which it is growing.

homonymous hemianopia (həmon′ɪməs hem′iənou′piə), blindness or defective vision in the right or left halves of the visual fields of both eyes.

homoplasy, having a likeness in form or structure acquired through similar environmental conditions or parallel evolution rather than because of common ancestral origin. Compare **homogeny.** — **homoplastic,** adj.

homosexual, 1. of, pertaining to, or denoting the same sex. 2. a person who is sexually attracted to members of the same sex. Compare **heterosexual.** See also **lesbian.**

homosexual panic, an acute attack of anxiety based on unconscious conflicts concerning gender identity and a fear of being homosexual. Compare **heterosexual panic.**

homothermal (hou′məfhər′məl). See **warm-blooded.**

homovanillic acid (hou′mouvənɪl′ɪk), a terminal metabolite of dopamine, norepinephrine, and serotonin that occurs in normal urine as a phenolic compound. A high level of homovanillic acid, representing an increased breakdown of its precursors, is found in the cerebrospinal fluid of patients in hepatic coma.

homozygosis (hou′mouzaɪgou′sɪs), 1. the formation of a zygote by the union of two gametes that have one or more pairs of identical genes. 2. the production of purebred organisms or strains through the process of inbreeding.

homozygous (hou′məzaɪ′gəs), having two identical genes at corresponding loci on homologous chromosomes. An individual who is homozygous for a particular characteristic has inherited from each parent one of two identical genes for that characteristic. A person homozygous for a genetic disease caused by a pair of recessive genes, as sickle cell anemia manifests the disorder, and his or her offspring have a 100 per cent chance of inheriting the gene for the disease. Compare **heterozygous.**

homunculus (houmənɜ′kyales), pl. **homunculi.** 1. a dwarf in which all the body parts are proportionally developed and in which there is no deformity or abnormality. 2. (in early embryological theories of development, primarily preformation) a minute and complete human being contained in each of the germ cells which after fertilization grows from the microscopic to normal size; by extension, the human fetus. 3. a small anatomical model of the human form; a manikin, specifically, one believed to have been produced by an alchemist and placed in a flask. 4. (in psychiatry) a little man created by the imagination who possesses magical powers.

hookworm, Nontechnical. a nematode of the genera Ancylostoma, Necator, or Urcinaria. Most hookworm infections in the Western Hemisphere are caused by the species Necator Americanus.

hordeolum (hordi′ɔləm), a furuncle of the margin of the eyelid originating in the sebaceous gland of an eyelash. Treatment includes hot compresses and antibiotic ophthalmic preparations; it occasionally requires incision and drainage. Also called **sty.** Compare **chalazion.**

HORDEOLUM

horizon, a specific stage of human embryonic development based on the appearance and ultimate formation of certain anatomical characteristics. The classification comprises 23 stages, each lasting two to three days, beginning with the fertilization of the ovum and ending seven to nine weeks later with the initiation of the fetal period of intrauterine life.

horizontal fissure of the right lung, a cleft that marks the separation of the upper and middle lobes of the right lung.

horizontal transmission, the spread of an infectious agent from one person or group to another, usually through contact with contaminated material, such as sputum or feces.

horm-, a combining form meaning 'to urge or stimulate': hormesis, hormonal, hormothyrin.

hormic psychology, (in psychology) the school that

stresses the purposive, goal-oriented nature of human behavior. Also called **hormism.**

hormism. See **hormic psychology.**

hormone, a complex chemical substance produced in one part or organ of the body that initiates or regulates the activity of an organ or a group of cells in another part of the body. Hormones secreted by the endocrine glands are carried through the blood stream to the target organ. Secretion of these hormones is regulated by other hormones, by neurotransmitters, and by a negative feedback system in which an excess of target organ activity signals a decreased need for the stimulating hormone. This principal is integral to oral contraceptive pills. A steady supply of estrogen and progesterone in the medication causes a reduction in the secretion of the pituitary hormones that ordinarily stimulate the ovary to develop the follicle, release the egg, and secrete the estrogen and progesterone. Other hormones are released by organs for local effect, most commonly in the digestive tract.

-hormone, 1. a combining form meaning a 'chemical substance possessing a regulatory effect' classified by source: *necrohormone, phytohormone, zoohormone.* 2. a combining form meaning a 'chemical substance possessing a regulatory effect' classified by activity affected: *cytohormone, neurohormone, parathormone.*

Hormonin, a trade name for a hormonal, fixed-combination drug containing estrogens (estriol, estrone, and estradiol).

Horner's syndrome, a neurologic condition characterized by miotic pupils, ptosis, and facial anhidrosis, resulting from a lesion in the spinal cord, with damage to a cervical nerve. In the case of traumatic injury, the person is carried prone or supine with as little movement as possible.

horny layer. See **stratum corneum.**

horripilation. See **pilomotor reflex.**

horse serum, immune serum prepared from the blood of a horse, especially tetanus antitoxin. As many people are sensitive to horse serum, a skin test for sensitivity is usually performed prior to immunization. Tetanus immune globulin prepared from human immune serum is preferred.

horseshoe fistula, an abnormal, semicircular passage in the perianal area with both openings on the surface of the skin.

Hortega cells (ortei′gə). See **microglia.**

Horton's arteritis (hor′tənz). See **temporal arteritis.**

Horton's headache. See **migrainous cranial neuralgia.**

Horton's histamine cephalalgia. See **histamine headache.**

hospice (hos′pis), a system of family-centered care designed to assist the chronically ill person to be comfortable and to maintain a satisfactory life style through the terminal phases of dying. Hospice care is multidiscipli-

nary and includes home visits, professional medical help available on call, teaching and emotional support of the family, and physical care of the client. Some Hospice programs provide care in a center as well as in the home.

hospital-acquired infection. See **nosocomial infection.**

hospitalism, the physical or mental effects of hospitalization or institutionalization on patients, especially infants and children in whom the condition is characterized by social regression, personality disorders, and stunted growth. See also **anaclitic depression.**

Hospital Survey and Construction Act. See **Hill-Burton Act.**

host, 1. an organism in which another, usually parasitic organism is nourished and harbored. A **primary,** or **definitive host** is one in which the adult parasite lives and reproduces. A **secondary,** or **intermediate host** is one in which the parasite exists in its nonsexual, larval stage. A **reservoir host** is a primary animal host for organisms that are sometimes parasitic in man and from which humans may become infected. 2. the recipient of a transplanted organ or tissue. Compare **donor.**

hot bath, a bath in which the temperature of the water is gradually raised to about 106°F.

hot flash, a transient sensation of warmth experienced by some women during or after menopause. Hot flashes result from autonomic vasomotor disturbances that accompany changes in the neurohormonal activity of the ovaries, hypothalamus, and pituitary. The exact etiologic mechanism is not known. Most menopausal women do not experience hot flashes; among those who do, the frequency, duration, and intensity of flashes vary widely. Though physically harmless, the symptom may be extremely disturbing or, rarely, disabling. Hot flashes may be alleviated by cyclic administration of exogenous estrogen.

hot-line, a means of contacting a trained counselor or specific agency for help with a particular problem, as a rape hot-line or a battered-child hot-line. The person needing help calls a telephone number and speaks to a counselor who remains anonymous and who offers emotional support, specific recommendations for action, and referral to other medical, social, or community services. Such services are usually maintained by volunteers who answer phones 24 hours a day, seven days a week.

hot spot, (in molecular genetics) a site in a gene sequence at which mutations occur with an unusually high frequency.

housemaid's knee, a chronic inflammation of the bursa in front of the kneecap, characterized by redness and swelling. It is caused by prolonged and repetitive pressure of the knee on a hard surface.

house organ, a publication designed for distribution to the employees or members of an institution or business. A house organ may be prepared by a staff within the institution or business, or it may be prepared by an outside agency for the institution or business.

house physician, a physician on call and immediately available in a hospital or other health care facility.

house surgeon, a surgeon on call and immediately available on the premises of a hospital.

housewives eczema, *Nontechnical.* contact dermatitis of the hands caused and exacerbated by their frequent immersion in water and by the use of soaps and detergents.

Houston's valves (hyus'tənz). See **plicae transversales recti.**

Howell-Jolly bodies, spherical and granular inclusions in the erythrocytes observed on microscopic examination of stained blood smears. They are most commonly seen in people who have hemolytic or pernicious anemia, leukemia, thalassemia, or congenital absence of the spleen and in those who have had a splenectomy.

HPL, abbreviation for **human placental lactogen.**

h.s., (in prescriptions) abbreviation for *hora somni,* a Latin phrase meaning 'bedtime.'

HSA, abbreviation for **health systems agency.**

HSV, abbreviation for *herpes simplex virus.* See **herpes genitalis, herpes simplex.**

Hubbard tank, a large tank in which a patient may be immersed in order to perform underwater exercise. The mechanism provides superficial heat and is generally used for exercising the trunk and lower limbs. See also **whirlpool bath.**

Hüerthle cell adenoma, a benign tumor of the thyroid gland composed of large cells with granular eosinophilic cytoplasm (Hüerthle cells). Compare **Hüerthle cell carcinoma.**

Hüerthle cell carcinoma, a malignant neoplasm of the thyroid gland composed of Hüerthle cells. Tumors of this kind, which occur more often in women than in men, are encapsulated and resemble adenomas, but they are locally invasive. See also **Hüerthle cell adenoma.**

Hüerthle cell tumor, a neoplasm of the thyroid gland composed of large cells with granular eosinophilic cytoplasm (Hüerthle cells); it may be benign (Hüerthle cell adenoma) or malignant (Hüerthle cell carcinoma).

Humafac, a trade name for human antihemophilic factor.

human bite, a wound caused by the piercing of skin by human teeth. Bacteria are usually present, and serious infection often follows. The area is thoroughly washed, using an antiseptic, and rinsed well. The wound is examined frequently and appropriate antibiotic therapy instituted, if necessary.

human chorionic gonadotropin (HCG). See **chorionic gonadotropin.**

human investigations committee, a committee established in a hospital, school, or university to review appli-

cations for research involving human subjects to protect the rights of the people to be studied. Also called **human subjects review committee.**

humanistic-existential therapy, a kind of psychotherapy that promotes self-awareness and personal growth by stressing current reality and by analyzing and altering specific patterns of response to help realize the potential of a person. This process may be facilitated in a group setting, where additional aspects of problems are revealed through interaction with others. Kinds of humanistic-existential psychotherapy are **client-oriented therapy, existential therapy, Gestalt therapy.** Also called **existential-humanistic psychotherapy.**

humanistic nursing model, a conceptual framework in which the nurse-patient relationship is analyzed as a human-to-human event rather than a nurse-to-client interaction. The nurse makes therapeutic use of herself, understanding the effects of nursing actions. Four phases are recognized in the development of the therapeutic relationship. The encounter phase is followed by the phase in which the identities of the nurse and patient emerge. The nurse empathizes and then sympathizes with the patient. The meaning of the patient's experience is important; hope and suffering are seen as central to that experience. Self-knowledge and self-awareness on the part of the nurse are essential. Nursing intervention proceeds in five steps: observation of the need for intervention; validation of this observation; determination of the ability of the nurse to meet the necessity for referral; formulation of a plan for meeting the need; and evaluation of the degree to which the need was met.

humanistic psychology, a branch of psychology that emphasizes a person's struggle to develop and maintain an integrated, harmonious personality as the primary motivational force in human behavior. See also **self-actualization.**

human leukocyte antigen (HLA), any one of four significant genetic markers identified as specific loci on chromosome 6. They are HLA-A, HLA-B, HLA-L, and HLA-D. Each locus has several genetically determined alleles; each of these is associated with certain diseases or conditions, as HLA-B27 is usually present in people who have ankylosing spondylitis. The HLA system is used to assess tissue compatibility. White blood cells are used for testing. Perfect tissue compatibility exists only between identical twins.

human placental lactogen (HPL), a protein hormone secreted by the placenta that helps to promote growth.

human subjects investigation committee. See **human investigation committee.**

Humatin, a trade name for an antiamebic (paromomycin sulfate).

humeral (hyu'mərəl). See **humerus.**

humeral articulation. See **shoulder joint.**

humerus (hyu′mərəs), *pl.* **humeri.** the largest bone of the upper arm, comprising a body, a head, and a condyle. The body is almost cylindrical proximally, prismatic and flattened distally, and has two borders and three surfaces. The nearly hemispherical head articulates with the glenoid cavity of the scapula and has a constriction called the surgical neck, frequently the seat of a fracture. The condyle at the distal end has several depressions into which articulate the radius and ulna. Also called **arm bone.** – **humeral,** *adj.*

humidifier lung, a type of hypersensitivity pneumonitis common among workers involved with refrigeration and air-conditioning equipment. The antigens to which the hypersensitive reaction occurs are genera of the fungi *Micropolyspora* and *Thermoactinomyces.* Symptoms of the acute form of the disease include chills, cough, fever, dyspnea, anorexia, nausea, and vomiting. The chronic form of the disease is characterized by fatigue, chronic cough, weight loss, and dyspnea on exercise. Also called **air conditioner lung.** See also **pneumonitis.**

humoral immunity (hyu′mərəl), one of the two forms of immunity that respond to antigens like bacteria and foreign tissue. Humoral immunity is the result of the development and the continuing presence of circulating antibodies carried in the immunoglobulins IgA, IgB, and IgM. Circulating antibodies are produced by the plasma cells of the reticuloendothelial system. Compare **cellular immunity.**

humoral response, one of a broad category of hypersensitivity reactions. Humoral responses are mediated by B cell lymphocytes and occur in type I, type II, and type III hypersensitivity reactions. Compare **cell-mediated immunity.**

Humorsol, a trade name for an ophthalmic anticholinesterase agent (demecarium bromide).

hung-up reflex, a deep tendon reflex in which, after a stimulus is given and the reflex action takes place, there is a slow return of the limb to its neutral position. This prolonged relaxation phase is characteristic of the reflexes in patients with hypothyroidism. See also **deep tendon reflex.**

Hunner's ulcer (hən′ərz). See **interstitial cystitis.**

Hunter's canal. See **adductor canal.**

Hunter's syndrome (hən′tərz), a hereditary defect in mucopolysaccharide metabolism affecting only males, characterized by dwarfism, kyphosis, gargoylism, and mental retardation. It is transmitted as an X-linked recessive trait. Females who carry the gene can be identified by biochemical tests, and known carriers may choose to abort if amniocentesis reveals a male fetus, as males born of women who carry the trait have a 50 per cent chance of having the syndrome. Also called **MPS II.** See also **mucopoly-saccharidosis.**

Huntington's chorea, a rare, abnormal hereditary condition characterized by chronic, progressive chorea and mental deterioration that terminates in dementia. An individual afflicted with the condition usually shows the first signs in the fourth decade of life and dies about 15 years later. The condition is transmitted as an autosomal trait. Also called **chronic chorea, degenerative chorea.**

Hurler's syndrome (hər′lərz), a type of mucopolysaccharidosis, transmitted as an autosomal-recessive trait, that results in severe mental retardation. The onset of the symptoms of Hurler's syndrome occurs within the first few months of life. Characteristic signs of the disease are enlargement of the liver and the spleen, often with cardiovascular involvement. Facial characteristics of individuals affected by Hurler's syndrome include a low forehead and enlargement of the head, sometimes resulting from hydrocephalus. Corneal clouding is common and the neck is short. Marked kyphosis is apparent at the dorsolumbar level, and the hands and the fingers are short and broad. Flexion contractures are common with this disease. Hurler's syndrome usually results in death during childhood from cardiac complications or pulmonary disorders. Also called **MPSI.** See also **mucopolysaccharidosis.**

husband-coached childbirth. See **Bradley method.**

Hutchinson's disease (həch′ɪnsənz). See **angioma serpiginosum.**

Hutchinson's freckle (həch′ɪnsənz), a tan patch on the skin that grows slowly, becoming mottled, dark, thick, and nodular. The lesion is usually seen on one side of the face of an elderly person. Local excision is recommended as it often becomes malignant. Also called **lentigo maligna.**

Hutchinson's teeth, a characteristic of congenital syphilis in which the permanent incisor teeth are peg-shaped, widely spaced, and notched at the end with a centrally placed crescent-shaped deformity.

Hutchinson's triad, the intersterstitial keratitis, notched teeth, and deafness characteristic of congenital syphilis.

Hutchison type neuroblastoma, a neuroblastoma that has metastasized to the cranium.

hyal-. See **hyalo-.**

hyaline cartilage, the gristly, elastic connective tissue comprised of specialized cells in a translucent, pearly-blue matrix. Hyaline cartilage thinly covers the articulating ends of bones, connects the ribs to the sternum, and supports the nose, trachea, and part of the larynx. It is covered by a membranous perichondrium, except where it coats the ends of bones, and tends to calcify in advanced age. Compare **yellow cartilage, white fibrocartilage.**

hyaline membrane disease. See **acute respiratory distress syndrome of the newborn.**

hyaline thrombus, a translucent, colorless mass consisting of hemolyzed erythrocytes.

hyalo-, hyal-, a combining form meaning 'resembling glass': *hyaloenchondroma, hyaloplasm, hyaloid.*

hyaloid artery (haɪ'ɔlɔid), an embryonic blood vessel that branches to supply the vitreous body of the eye and develops part of the blood supply to the capsula vasculosa lentis. The hyaloid artery disappears from the fetus in the ninth month of pregnancy, leaving a vestigial remnant which persists in the adult as a narrow passage through the vitreous body from the optic disc to the posterior surface of the crystalline lens.

hyaloplasm (haɪ'ɔlouplæz'əm), the portion of the cytoplasm that is clear and more fluid, as opposed to the granular and reticular part. Also called **cytohyaloplasm, cytolymph, enchylema, hyalotome, interfilar ma..s, interfibrillar mass of Flemming, paramitome, paraplasm.**

hyalotome. See **hyaloplasm.**

hyaluronic acid (haɪ'əluron'ɪk), a mucopolysaccharide formed by the polymerization of acetylglucosamine and glucuronic acid, occurring in vitreous humor, synovial fluids, and various tissues. Known as the cement substance of tissues, it forms a gel in intercellular spaces.

hyaluronidase (haɪ'əlyuron'ədeis), an enzyme that hydrolyzes hyaluronic acid.

- INDICATIONS: It is prescribed to increase the absorption and dispersion of other parenteral drugs, for hypodermoclysis, and for improving resorption of radiopaque agents.
- CONTRAINDICATIONS: Acute inflammation or infection or known hypersensitivity to this drug prohibits its use.
- ADVERSE EFFECT: The most serious adverse reaction is hypersensitivity.

Hyazyme, a trade name for an enzyme (hyaluronidase).

Hybephen, a trade name for a gastrointestinal, fixed-combination drug containing anticholinergics (atropine sulfate, methscopolamine hydrobromide, and hyoscyamine hydrobromide) and a sedative-hypnotic (phenobarbital).

hybrid, 1. an offspring produced from mating plants or animals from different species, varieties, or genotypes. 2. of or pertaining to such a plant or animal.

hybridization, 1. the process of producing hybrids by crossbreeding. 2. (in molecular genetics) the process of combining single-stranded nucleic acids whose base composition is identical but whose base sequence is different to form stable double-stranded duplex molecules. The technique involves the fragmentation and separation of the double-stranded molecules by heating, then recombination through cooling. The resulting hybrids can be of a DNA-DNA, DNA-RNA, or RNA-RNA nature.

hybrid vigor. See **heterosis.**

Hycodan, a trade name for a fixed-combination drug containing an anticholinergic (homatropine methylbromide) and an antitussive (hydrocodone bitartrate), used for cough relief.

Hycomine, a trade name for a fixed-combination drug containing an adrenergic (phenylpropanolamine hydrochloride) and an antitussive (hydrocodone bitartrate), used to treat coughs.

hydantoin (haɪdæn'touɪn), any one of a group of anticonvulsant medications, chemically and pharmacologically similar to the barbiturates, that act to limit seizure activity and reduce the spread of the abnormal electrical excitation from the focus of the seizure. A primary drug in the management of almost all forms of epilepsy, the most common hydantoin in current use is phenytoin, formerly known as diphenylhydantoin. Toxic effects of the drug include cardiovascular collapse and central nervous system depression when it is given in excessive dosage intravenously, as may occur in the emergency treatment of status epilepticus. Chronic toxicity, which is related to the dosage and the route of administration, may result in behavioral change, gastrointestinal disturbance, osteomalacia, gingival hyperplasia, or megaloblastic anemia. Hypersensitivity reactions are rare but serious. Frequent observation for the blood concentrations of hydantoin are necessary. Seizures are usually controlled at a level of 10 µg/ml; higher levels of concentration are associated with toxic effects. Phenytoin interacts with many drugs, including chloramphemicol, dicumarol, disulfiram, isoniazid, salicylates, phenylbutazone, and some sulfonamides. The interaction usually has the adverse effect of increasing the concentration of phenytoin in the blood, resulting in toxicity. Phenytoin is sometimes also prescribed in the treatment of trigeminal neuralgia and cardiac arrhythmias.

hydatid (haɪ'dətɪd), a cyst or cystlike structure that usually is filled with fluid, especially the cyst formed around the developing scolex of the dog tapeworm *Echinococcus granulosus.* Humans and sheep can become hosts to the larval stage by ingesting the eggs. Hydatid cysts may be identified by palpation; they occur most commonly in the liver. An acute anaphylactoid allergic reaction may occur if the cyst ruptures. See also **hydatidiform mole, hydatidosis.** – **hydatidiform,** *adj.*

hydatid cyst, a cyst in the liver that contains larvae of the tapeworm *Echinococcus granulosus,* whose eggs are carried from the intestinal tract to the liver via the portal circulation. Patients are generally asymptomatic, except for hepatomegaly and a dull ache over the right upper quadrant of the adbomen. Radiologic tests are employed in diagnosis, and since no medical treatment is available, surgical removal of the cyst is indicated. Compare **hydatidiform mole.**

hydatid disease. See **echinococcosis.**

hydatidiform mole (haɪ'dətɪd'ɪfɔrm). See **hydatid mole.**

hydatid mole, an intrauterine neoplastic mass of grapelike enlarged chorionic villi occurring in approximately one in 1,500 pregnancies in the United States and eight times more frequently in some oriental countries. Molar pregnancies are more common in older and younger women than in those between the ages of 20 and 40. The cause of the degenerative disorder is not known; it may be the result of a primary ovular defect, an intrauterine abnormality, or nutritional deficiency. Characteristic signs of the condition are extreme nausea, uterine bleeding, anemia, hyperthyroidism, an unusually large uterus for the length of pregnancy, absence of fetal heart sounds, and edema and high blood pressure. Diagnostic measures include ultrasonography, amniography, and serial bioassay of chorionic gonadotropin in the blood. In most cases the mole is discovered when abortion is threatened or in progress. Oxytocin may be used to stimulate the evacuation of a mole that is not spontaneously aborted, and curettage is usually performed several days later to be certain that no molar tissue remains in the uterus. It is important that pregnancy be avoided for at least one year and that assays for chorionic gonadotropin be performed to minimize the risk of developing trophoblastic choriocarcinoma. Also called **hydatidiform mole.** See also **trophoblastic disease.**

hydatidosis (hai'dətɪdou'sɪs),   infestation with the tapeworm *Echinococcus granulosus.* See also **hydatid cyst.**

Hydeltrasol,   a trade name for a glucocorticoid (prednisolone sodium phosphate).

Hydeltra T.B.A.,   a trade name for a glucocorticoid (prednisolone tebutate).

Hydergine,   a trade name for a fixed-combination drug containing various ergot alkaloids.

hydr-. See **hydro-.**

hydradenitis, hidradenitis (hai'drædənai'tɪs),   an infection or inflammation of the sweat glands.

hydralazine hydrochloride (haidræl'əzin),   a vasodilator.

■ INDICATION: It is prescribed in the treatment of high blood pressure.

■ CONTRAINDICATIONS: Coronary artery disease, mitral valvular rheumatic heart disease, or known hypersensitivity to this drug prohibits its use.

■ ADVERSE EFFECTS: Among the more serious adverse reactions are headache, anorexia, tachycardia, gastrointestinal disturbances, and a syndrome resembling lupus erythematosus.

hydramnios (haidræm'niəs),   an abnormal condition of pregnancy characterized by an excess of amniotic fluid. It occurs in less than one per cent of pregnancies and is diagnosed by palpation, ultrasound, or x-ray examination. It is associated with maternal disorders, including toxemia of pregnancy and diabetes mellitus. Some fetal disorders, including anomalies of the gastrointestinal tract, respiratory tract, and cardiovascular system may interfere with normal exchange of amniotic fluid, resulting in hydramnios. Fetal hydrops and multiple gestation are also associated with the condition. The incidence of pre-

mature rupture of the membranes, premature labor, and perinatal mortality are increased. Periodic amniocentesis may be necessary. Also called **hydramnion, polyhydramnios.** Compare **acute hydramnios, oligohydramnios.**

hydrargyrism (haidrar'jɪrɪz'əm).   See **mercury poisoning.**

Hydrazol,   a trade name for a carbonic anhydrase inhibitor (acetazolamide).

Hydrea,   a trade name for an antimetabolite (hydroxyurea).

hydremic ascites,   an abnormal accumulation of fluid within the peritoneal cavity accompanied by hemodilution, as in protein-calorie malnutrition. See also **ascites.**

-hydria,   a combining form meaning 'level of fluid in the body': *histohydria, isohydria, oligohydria.*

hydro-, hydr-,   a combining form meaning 'pertaining to water or hydrogen': *hydroadipsia, hydrocele, hydropexis.*

hydroa (haidrou'ə),   an unusual vesicular and bullous skin condition of childhood that recurs each summer following exposure to sunlight, sometimes accompanied by itching and lichenification. Hydroa usually disappears soon after puberty. Treatment includes use of sunscreen preparations and the avoidance of exposure to sunlight.

hydrocarbon,   any one of a large group of organic compounds, the molecules of which are composed of hydrogen and carbon, most of which are derived from petroleum.

hydrocephalus, hydrocephaly,   a pathological condition characterized by an abnormal accumulation of cerebrospinal fluid, usually under increased pressure, within the cranial vault and subsequent dilatation of the ventricles. Interference with the normal flow of cerebrospinal fluid may be caused by increased secretion of the fluid, obstruction within the ventricular system (noncommunicating or intraventricular hydrocephalus), or defective reabsorption from the cerebral subarachnoid space (communicating or extraventricular hydrocephalus), resulting from developmental anomalies, infection, trauma, or brain tumors.   **—hydrocephalic,** *adj., n.*

■ OBSERVATIONS: The condition may be congenital with rapid onset of symptoms or it may progress slowly so that neurological manifestations do not appear until early to late childhood or even until early adulthood. In infants, the head grows at an abnormal rate with separation of the sutures, bulging fontanelles, and dilated scalp veins, the face becomes disproportionately small, and the eyes appear depressed within the sockets. Typical behavior includes irritability with lethargy and vomiting, opisthotonos, lower-extremity spasticity, and failure to perform normal reflex actions. If the condition progresses, lower brain stem function is disrupted, the skull becomes enormous, the cortex is destroyed, and the infant displays somnolence, seizures, and cardiopulmonary obstruction, usually not surviving the neonatal period. At later onset, after the cranial sutures have fused and the skull has formed, symptoms are primarily neurological and include headache, edema of the optic disc, strabismus, and loss of muscular coordination. Hydrocephalus in infants is suspected when head growth is observed to be in excess of the normal rate. In all age groups diagnosis is confirmed by such procedures as cerebrospinal fluid examination, computerized axial tomography, air encephalography, arteriography, and echoencephalography.

■ INTERVENTION: Treatment consists almost exclusively of surgical intervention to correct the ventricular obstruction, reduce the production of cerebrospinal fluid, or shunt the excess fluid by ventricular bypass to the right atrium of the heart or to the peritoneal cavity. Surgically treated hydrocephalus with continued neurosurgical and medical management has a survival rate of approximately 80 per cent, although prognosis depends largely on the cause of the condition. Hydrocephalus is frequently associated with myelomeningocele, in which case there is a less favorable prognosis.

■ NURSING CONSIDERATIONS: Primary care of the child with hydrocephalus consists of maintaining adequate nutrition, proper positioning and support to prevent extra strain on the neck, and assistance with diagnostic evaluation and procedures. Postoperatively, in addition to routine care and observation to prevent complications, especially infection, the nurse gives support to the parents and teaches them how to care for a child with a functioning shunt, specifically how to recognize signs that indicate shunt malfunction or infection and how to pump the shunt.

hydrochloric acid, a compound consisting of hydrogen and chlorine. Hydrochloric acid is secreted in the stomach and is a major component of gastric juice.

hydrochlorothiazide, a diuretic and antihypertensive.

■ INDICATIONS: It is prescribed in the treatment of hypertension and edema.

■ CONTRAINDICATIONS: Anuria or known hypersensitivity to this drug, to other thiazide medication, or to sulfonamide derivatives prohibits its use.

■ ADVERSE EFFECTS: Among the more serious adverse effects are hypoglycemia, hyperglycemia, hyperuricemia, and hypersensitivity reactions.

Hydrocil, a trade name for a laxative (psyllium hydrophilic muciloid).

hydrocodone bitartrate, a narcotic antitussive.

■ INDICATION: It is prescribed in the treatment of cough.

■ CONTRAINDICATIONS: Drug dependence or known hypersensitivity to this drug prohibits its use.

■ ADVERSE EFFECTS: Among the more serious adverse reactions are drug dependence and respiratory and circulatory depression.

hydrocortisone. See **cortisol.**

hydrocortisone acetate. See **cortisol.**

hydrocortisone cyclopentylpropionate. See **cortisol.**

hydrocortisone sodium succinate. See **cortisol.**

hydrocortisone valerate, a topical corticosteroid.

■ INDICATION: It is used topically as an anti-inflammatory agent.

■ CONTRAINDICATIONS: Viral and fungal diseases of the skin that occur where circulation is impaired or known hypersensitivity to steroids prohibits its use.

■ ADVERSE REACTIONS: Among the more serious adverse reactions are various systemic side effects that may occur from prolonged or excessive use. Local irritation of the skin may occur.

Hydrocortone, a trade name for a glucocorticoid (cortisol).

HydroDiuril, a trade name for a diuretic (hydrochlorothiazide).

hydroflumethiazide, a diuretic and antihypertensive.

■ INDICATIONS: It is prescribed in the treatment of hypertension and edema.

■ CONTRAINDICATIONS: Anuria or known hypersensitivity to this drug, to other thiazide medication, or to sulfonamide derivatives prohibits its use.

■ ADVERSE EFFECTS: Among the more serious adverse effects are hypokalemia, hyperglycemia, hyperuricemia, and hypersensitivity reactions.

hydrogen (H), a gaseous, univalent element. Its atomic number is 1; its atomic weight is 1.008. It is the simplest and the lightest of the elements and is normally a colorless, odorless, highly inflammable diatomic gas. It occurs in pure form only sparsely in the earth and the atmosphere but is plentiful in the sun and in many stars and nebulae. Hydrogen is a component of numerous compounds, many of them produced by the body. As a component of water, hydrogen is crucial in the metabolic interaction of acids, bases, and salts within the body and in the fluid balance necessary for the body to survive. Hydrogen makes it possible for water, which serves as a host to many body functions, to dissolve the many different substances on which the body depends, as oxygen and food substances. Hydrogen makes possible the process of hydrolysis by which compounds unite with water and split into simpler compounds.

hydrogenation (hai′drəjɪnei′shən, haidroj′ɪnei′shən). See **reduction.**

hydrogen peroxide, a topical anti-infective.

■ INDICATIONS: It is prescribed to cleanse open wounds, as a mouthwash, and to aid in the removal of cerumen in the external ear.

■ CONTRAINDICATIONS: Irritations to skin or mucous membranes or known hypersensitivity to this agent prohibits its use.

■ ADVERSE EFFECTS: There are no known adverse effects.

Hydrolose, a trade name for a laxative (methylcellulose).

hydrolysis (haidrol′ısıs), the chemical alteration or decomposition of a compound with water.

hydrometer (haidrom′ıtər), a device which determines the specific gravity or density of a liquid by a comparison of its weight with that of an equal volume of water. A calibrated, hollow glass device is placed in the liquid being examined, and the depth to which the device settles in the liquid is noted.

hydromorphone hydrochloride, a narcotic analgesic.
- INDICATION: It is used to treat moderate to severe pain.
- CONTRAINDICATIONS: It is used with caution in many conditions, including head injuries, asthma, impaired renal or hepatic function, or unstable cardiovascular status. Known hypersensitivity to this drug prohibits its use.
- ADVERSE EFFECTS: Among the most serious adverse reactions are drowsiness, dizziness, nausea, constipation, respiratory and circulatory depression, and drug addiction.

hydronephrosis (hai′drounefrou′sıs), distention of the pelvis and calyces of the kidney by urine that cannot flow past an obstruction in a ureter. Ureteral obstruction may be caused by a tumor, a calculus lodged in the ureter, inflammation of the prostate gland, or edema owing to a urinary tract infection. The person may experience pain in the flank, and, in some cases, hematuria, pyuria, and hyperpyrexia. Intravenous pyelography, cytoscopy, or retrograde pyelography may be used in diagnosis. Surgical repair or removal of the obstruction may be necessary. Prolonged hydronephrosis will result in atrophy and eventual loss of kidney function. See also **urinary calculi.** – **hydronephrotic,** *adj.*

hydrophobia (hai′droufou′biə), 1. *Nontechnical.* rabies. 2. a morbid, extreme fear of water.

hydrophthalmos (hai′drɔfthæl′məs). See **congenital glaucoma.**

Hydropres, a trade name for a fixed-combination drug containing a diuretic (hydrochlorothiazide) and an antihypertensive (reserpine).

hydrops (hai′drops), an abnormal accumulation of clear, watery fluid in a body tissue or cavity, as a joint, Graafian follicle, Fallopian tube, the abdomen, middle ear, or gall bladder. Hydrops in the entire body may occur in infants born with thalassemia or severe Rh sensitization. Formerly called **dropsy.**

hydrops fetalis, massive edema in the fetus or newborn, usually in association with severe erythroblastosis fetalis. Severe anemia and effusions of the pericardial, pleural, and peritoneal spaces also occur. The condition usually leads to death, even with immediate exchange transfusions following delivery.

hydroquinone (hai′droukwın′oun), a dermatologic bleaching agent.
- INDICATION: It is prescribed to reduce pigmentation of the skin in certain skin conditions in which an excess of melanin causes hyperpigmentation.
- CONTRAINDICATION: Sunburn, prickly heat, other irritation of the skin, or known hypersensitivity to this drug prohibits its use.
- ADVERSE EFFECTS: Among the more serious adverse reactions are tingling, erythema, burning, and severe inflammation of the skin.

hydrosalpinx (hai′drousæl′pıŋks), an abnormal condition of the Fallopian tube in which the tube is cystically enlarged and filled with clear fluid, the end result of an infection that has previously occluded the tube at both ends. The purulent material produced by the infection undergoes liquefaction during resolution of the acute phase of the inflammatory process.

hydrostatic pressure, the pressure exerted by a liquid.

hydrous wool fat. See **lanolin.**

hydroxyamphetamine hydrobromide, an adrenergic and mydriatic.
- INDICATIONS: It is prescribed for dilatation of the pupil for ophthalmoscopy and as a diagnostic aid in Horner's syndrome.
- CONTRAINDICATIONS: Narrow-angle glaucoma or known hypersensitivity to this drug prohibits its use.
- ADVERSE EFFECTS: Among the more serious adverse reactions are increased intraocular pressure and photophobia.

hydroxybenzene (haidrok′sıben′zin). See **carbolic acid.**

hydroxychloroquine sulfate, an antiprotozoal, antirheumatic drug that is also a suppressant of lupus erythematosus and of polymorphous light eruption.
- INDICATIONS: It is prescribed in the treatment of malaria and for the suppression of acute paroxysmal attacks of the disease, in the treatment of extra-intestinal, usually hepatic, amebiasis, and in the reduction of symptoms of lupus erythematosus and rheumatoid arthritis.
- CONTRAINDICATIONS: Concurrent use of other 4-aminoquinolones or of gold salts or a known hypersensitivity to this drug or to other 4-aminoquinolones prohibits its use. It is used with caution in people affected with alcoholism, blood dyscrasia, severe neurologic disorder, retinal or visual field damage, psoriasis, or porphyria. The drug is not usually recommended in pregnancy as it has been associated with damage to the central nervous system of the fetus.
- ADVERSE EFFECTS: Among the many severe adverse reactions are retinopathy, corneal opacity, polyneuritis, seizure, agranulocytasis, and hepatitis. The incidence and severity of these and many other adverse effects increase with the dosage and prolonged duration of treatment.

hydroxyl (OH) (haidrok′sıl), a radical compound containing an oxygen atom and a hydrogen atom.

hydroxyurea (haidrok′sıyuri′ə), an antineoplastic.

■ INDICATIONS: It is prescribed in the treatment of a variety of neoplasms.

■ CONTRAINDICATIONS: Bone marrow depression or known hypersensitivity to this drug prohibits its use. It is not be given to women who are or might become pregnant.

■ ADVERSE EFFECTS: The most serious adverse reaction is bone marrow depression. Gastrointestinal disturbances and dermatitis also may occur.

hydroxyzine hydrochloride (hǎidrok′səzin), a minor tranquilizer.

■ INDICATIONS: It is prescribed to relieve anxiety, nervous tension, and motion sickness.

■ CONTRAINDICATION: Known hypersensitivity to this drug is the only contraindication.

■ ADVERSE EFFECTS: No serious adverse reactions have been observed. Decreased mental alertness is sometimes seen.

hygroscopic humidifier, a humidifying device attached to the tubing circuit of a mechanical ventilator or anesthesia gas machine to maintain a constant rate of humidity in the patient's trachea.

Hygroton, a trade name for a diuretic (chlorthalidone).

hymen, a fold of mucous membrane, skin, and fibrous tissue at the introitus of the vagina. It may be absent, small, thin and pliant, or, rarely, tough and dense, completely occluding the introitus. When the hymen is ruptured, small rounded elevations remain. See also **canunculae hymenales.**

Hymenolepis (hǎi′mɪnol′ɪpɪs), a genus of intestinal tapeworms infesting man, as *Hymenolepis nana,* the dwarf tapeworm, and *H. diminuta.* Heavy infestation by *H. nana* may cause abdominal pain, bloody stools, and disorders of the nervous system, especially in children. Contaminated food spreads the disease, which is endemic in the United States. Quinacrine hydrochloride or hexylresorcinol is used to treat the infestation.

hyoglossal (hǎi′ouglos′əl). See **glossohyal.**

hyoid bone, a single bone suspended from the styloid processes of the temporal bones. The body of the hyoid is square and flat, its ventral surface convex and angled cranially. Two greater wings of the bone attach to the lateral thyroid ligaments, and the body of the bone attaches to various muscles, as the hypoglossus and the sternohyoideus. The hyoid is palpable in the neck. Also called **lingual bone, os hyoideum.**

hyoscine (hǎi′əsin), scopolamine.

hyoscine hydrobromide. See **scopolamine hydrobromide.**

hyoscyamine (hǎi′əsai′əmin), an anticholinergic.

■ INDICATIONS: It is prescribed in the treatment of hypermotility of the gastrointestinal and the lower urinary tracts.

■ CONTRAINDICATIONS: Narrow angle glaucoma, asthma, obstruction of the genitourinary or gastrointestinal tracts, severe ulcerative colitis, or known hypersensitivity to this drug prohibits its use.

■ ADVERSE EFFECTS: Among the more serious adverse reactions are blurred vision, central nervous system effects, tachycardia, dry mouth, decreased sweating, and hypersensitivity reactions.

hyp-. See **hypo-.**

hyper-, a combining form meaning 'excessive, above, or beyond': *hyperacidaminuria, hyperalkalinity, hyperechema.*

Hyperab, a trade name for a passive immunizing agent (rabies immune globulin).

hyperactivity. See **attention deficit disorder.**

hyperadrenalism. See **Cushing's disease.**

hyperadrenocorticism (hǎi′pərədri′noukər′tɪsɪz′əm). See **Cushing's syndrome.**

hyperaldosteronism (hǎi′pəræl′doustɪrou′nɪzəm, hǎi′pərældos′tɪrəniz′əm). See **aldosteronism.**

hyperalimentation (hǎi′pəræl′ɪmentei′shən), **1.** overfeeding or the ingestion or administration of a greater than optimal amount of nutrients in excess of the demands of the appetite. **2.** See **total parenteral nutrition.**

hyperammonemia (hǎi′pəræm′ouni′miə), abnormally high levels of ammonia in the blood. Ammonia is produced in the intestine, absorbed into the blood, and detoxified in the liver. If there is an increased production of ammonia or a decreased ability to detoxify it, levels of ammonia in the blood may increase. Untreated, the condition leads to asterixis, vomiting, lethargy, coma, and death.

hyperbetalipoproteinemia (hǎi′pərbei′təlɪp′ouprou′tini′miə), type II hyperlipoproteinemia, a genetic disorder of lipid metabolism, in which there are abnormally high levels of serum cholesterol, and xanthomas appear on the tendons of the heels, knees, and fingers. There is a marked tendency to develop atherosclerosis and early myocardial infarction, especially among males. Treatment attempts to reduce blood cholesterol levels in the hope of lowering the risk of early death from heart disease. The person is usually counseled to avoid most meats, eggs, milk products, and all saturated fats and is encouraged to eat fish, grains, fruits, vegetables, poultry, and unsaturated fats. Exercise may be recommended, and drugs may be prescribed in some cases. See also **cholesterolemia.**

hyperbilirubinemia (hǎi′pərbɪl′ɪru′bɪni′miə), greater than normal amounts of the bile pigment bilirubin in the blood, often characterized by jaundice, anorexia, and malaise. Hyperbilirubinemia is most often associated with liver disease or biliary obstruction, but it also occurs when there is excessive destruction of red blood cells, as in hemolytic anemia. Treatment is specific to the underlying condition. About half of all newborn infants develop physiologic jaundice owing to the normal hemolysis of fetal erythrocytes. Most infants require no treatment.

When bilirubin levels are high, treatment includes phototherapy and hydration. See also **jaundice.**

hyperbilirubinemia of the newborn (hai′pərbil′iru′bini′-miə), an excess of bilirubin in the blood of the neonate, resulting from hepatic dysfunction. It is usually caused by a deficiency of an enzyme, owing to physiologic immaturity, or by increased hemolysis, especially from blood group incompatibility, which, in severe cases, can lead to kernicterus. Also called **neonatal hyperbilirubinemia.** See also **breast milk jaundice, cholestasis, Crigler-Najjar syndrome, Dubin-Johnson syndrome, erythroblastosis fetalis, Gilbert's disease, kernicterus, Rotor syndrome.**

■ OBSERVATIONS: Serum bilirubin levels are elevated in the normal newborn because the concentration of circulating erythrocytes is greater and because infants have a decreased ability to conjugate and excrete bilirubin owing to a lack of the enzyme glucuronyl transferase, to reduced albumin concentration, and to a lack of intestinal bacteria. Jaundice appears when blood levels of bilirubin exceed 5 mg/100 ml, usually not before 24 hours in full-term neonates. Clinically observable jaundice or serum bilirubin levels exceeding 5 mg/100 ml within the first 24 hours of life are abnormal and indicate a pathologic cause of hyperbilirubinemia. In erythroblastosis fetalis, jaundice is evident shortly after birth and bilirubin levels rise rapidly. Severely affected infants also show hepatosplenomegaly and signs of anemia, which quickly worsen, causing decreased oxygen-carrying capacity that may lead to cardiac failure and shock. Early symptoms of kernicterus are lethargy, poor feeding, and vomiting, followed by severe neurologic excitation or depression, including tremors, twitching, convulsion, opisthotonos, a high-pitched cry, hypotonia, diminished deep-tendon reflexes, and the absence of Moro and sucking reflexes. Brain damage generally does not occur at serum bilirubin levels below 20 mg/100 ml. Factors like metabolic acidosis, lowered albumin levels, hypoxia, hypothermia, free fatty acids, and certain drugs, especially salicylates and sulfonamides, increase the risk at much lower levels. The mortality may reach 50 per cent. Sequelae of kernicterus include mental retardation, minimal brain dysfunction, cerebral palsy, delayed or abnormal motor development, hearing loss, ataxia, athetosis, perceptual problems, and behavioral disorders.

■ INTERVENTION: Such preventive measures as frequent feedings during the first 6 to 12 hours of life to increase gastrointestinal motility have little justification. Infants with mild jaundice require no treatment, only observation. Phototherapy is the usual treatment for severe or increasing hyperbilirubinemia. If hyperbilirubinemia is caused by increased hemolysis owing to blood group incompatibility, exchange transfusion is the standard procedure. It is usually indicated if laboratory analysis reveals a positive Coombs' test, a hemoglobin concentration of

the cord blood below 12 g/100 ml, or a bilirubin level of 20 mg/100 ml or more in a full-term infant or 15 mg/100 ml or more in a premature infant. Phototherapy may be used in conjunction with exchange transfusion, except in Rh incompatiblity. If used immediately after the initial exchange transfusion, phototherapy may remove enough bilirubin from the tissues to make subsequent transfusions unnecessary. Pharmacologic management, as the use of barbiturates to stimulate protein synthesis which, in turn, increases albumin for conjugating bilirubin and promotes hepatic glucuronyl transferase synthesis, is indicated in some instances, although this form of therapy is controversial because of the known side effects of the drugs.

■ NURSING CONSIDERATIONS: An initial concern is to identify high-risk infants who may develop hyperbilirubinemia and kernicterus. The nurse may monitor the serum bilirubin levels and observe for evidence of jaundice, anemia, central nervous system irritability, and such conditions as acidosis, hypoxia, and hypothermia. In erythroblastosis fetalis, exchange transfusion may be necessary. The amounts of blood infused and withdrawn, the vital signs, and any signs of exchange reactions are noted. Resuscitative equipment is kept available. Optimal body temperature is maintained: hypothermia increases oxygen and glucose consumption, causing metabolic acidosis, and hyperthermia damages the donor's erythrocytes, causing an elevation in the amount of free potassium that may lead to infant cardiac arrest. After the procedure, a sterile dressing is applied to the catheter site. See also **phototherapy in the newborn.**

hypercalcemia (hai′pərkælsi′miə), greater than normal amounts of calcium in the blood, most often resulting from excessive bone resorption and release of calcium, as occurs in hyperparathyroidism, metastatic tumors of bone, Paget's disease, and osteoporosis. Clinically, people with hypercalcemia are confused and have anorexia, abdominal pain, and muscle pain and weakness. Extremely high levels of blood calcium may result in shock, kidney failure, and death. Hypercalciuria is also found in most patients with elevated blood calcium. Prednisone, diuretics, isotonic saline, and other drugs may be used in treatment. – **hypercalcemic,** *adj.*

hypercalcinuria. See **hypercalciuria.**

hypercalciuria (hai′pərkæl′siyur′iə), the presence of abnormally great amounts of calcium in the urine, resulting from conditions such as sarcoid, hyperparathyroidism, or certain types of arthritis, characterized by augmented bone resorption. Immobilized patients are often hypercalciuric. Some people absorb more calcium than is normal and therefore excrete greater than normal amounts into their urine. Concentrated amounts of calcium in the urinary tract may form kidney stones. Treatment is directed toward correcting any underlying disease condition and limiting dietary intake of calcium. Also called **hypercalcinuria.** Compare **hypercalcemia.** — **hypercalciuric,** *adj.*

hypercapnia (haī'pərkæp'niə), greater than normal amounts of carbon dioxide in the blood. Also called **hypercarbia.**

hypercarbia. See **hypercapnia.**

hypercholesterolemia (haī'pərkəles'tərouli'miə), a condition in which greater-than-normal amounts of cholesterol are present in the blood. High levels of cholesterol and other lipids may lead to the development of atherosclerosis. Hypercholesterolemia may be reduced or prevented by avoiding saturated fats, which are found in red meats, eggs, and dairy products.

hypercholesterolemic xanthomatosis (haī'pərkəles'tıroli'mık). See **familial hypercholesterolemia.**

hyperchromic, having a greater density of color or pigment.

hyperchylomicronemia (haī'pərkai'loumaī'krouni'miə), type I hyperlipoproteinemia, a rare congenital deficiency of an enzyme essential to fat metabolism. Fat accumulates in the blood as chylomicrons. The condition affects children and young adults, who develop xanthomas (fatty deposits) in the skin, hepatomegaly, and abdominal pain. Pancreatitis is the most significant complication. Strict limitation of dietary fat may allow the person to avoid discomfort and complications. Also called **familial lipoprotein lipase deficiency.**

hypercoagulability, a tendency of the blood to coagulate more rapidly than is normal.

hyperdactyly (haī'pərdæk'tıli), **hyperdactylia, hyperdactylism.** See **polydactyly.**

hyperdiploid (haī'pərdıp'loid), **hyperdiploidic.** See **hyperploid.**

hyperdynamic syndrome, a cluster of symptoms that signal the onset of septic shock, often including a shaking chill, rapid rise in temperature, flushing of the skin, galloping pulse, and alternating rise and fall of the blood pressure. This is a medical emergency that requires expert medical support in a hospital. Emergency measures include keeping the patient warm and elevating the feet to assist venous return. Usually, it is ordered that nothing be given by mouth and that the patient's head be turned to avoid aspiration if there is vomiting. See **septic shock.**

hyperemesis gravidarum (haī'pərem'ısıs), an abnormal condition of pregnancy characterized by protracted vomiting, weight loss, and fluid and electrolyte imbalance. If severe and intractable, brain damage, liver and kidney failure, and death may result. The cause of the condition is not known; an increase in chorionic gonadotropins or other hormones, an immunologic sensitivity to products of conception, or aggravation of preexisting emotional conflicts has been suggested, but a causal relationship has not been proven. It occurs in approximately three of every thousand pregnancies, its incidence having diminshed in recent years.

■ OBSERVATIONS: Women are frightened of and uncomfortable and embarrassed about their illness. Dehydration results in dry mucous membranes, decreased skin elasticity, a rapid pulse, and falling blood pressure. The specific gravity of the urine rises and the volume of urine excreted falls. The hematocrit is elevated because of hemoconcentration. Loss of electrolytes in vomitus leads to metabolic acidosis with hypokalemia, hypochloremia, and hyponatremia. Severe potassium deficit alters myocardial function; the electrocardiogram may show prolonged P-R and Q-T intervals and inverted T waves. In addition to weight loss, undernourishment causes fever, ketosis, and acetonuria. Severe vitamin B deficiency may result in encephalopathy manifested by confusion and, eventually, coma. Laboratory analyses of blood indicate increased concentrations of metabolic products normally cleared from the blood by the liver and kidneys. Forceful vomiting may cause retinal hemorrhages that impair vision and gastroesophageal tears that bleed and result in hematemesis or melena.

■ INTERVENTION: Effective therapy arrests vomiting and achieves rehydration, adequate nutrition, and emotional stabilization. Women are placed at bed rest. Antiemetics safe for the fetus are administered. Fluids, electrolytes, nutrients, and vitamins are given parenterally if the woman is unable to retain fluids by mouth. The fetal heart rate is measured frequently. Psychiatric consultation and therapy are sometimes beneficial. Termination of pregnancy is curative but almost never required.

■ NURSING CONSIDERATIONS: Visitors are encouraged; formerly recommended isolation is not desirable. Sympathetic listening and supportive, nonjudgmental care are provided. The woman and her family are told often that the prognosis is excellent for both mother and baby. She is weighed regularly and her weight is accurately recorded, for the best evidence of recovery is steady weight gain.

hyperemia (haī'pəri'miə), increased blood in part of the body, caused by increased blood flow, as in the inflammatory response, local relaxation of arterioles, or obstruction of the outflow of blood from an area. Skin overlying a hyperemic area usually becomes reddened and warm. — **hyperemic,** *adj.*

hyperextension, (of a joint) a position of maximum extension.

hyperextension bed, a bed used in pediatric orthopedics to maintain any correction achieved by suspension of a body part and to increase the range of motion of the hips following an operative muscle release procedure. The hyperextension bed may be purchased or it may be converted from a regular hospital bed. Removal of the mattress from a regular hospital bed and the addition of three half mattresses allows sufficient height to permit alternating prone and supine positions and the concomitant alternating flexion and extension of the hips. The bilateral extremities of the patient, in casts, are suspended over the lower half of the bed with rings and traction apparatus. The position of the patient's hips is alternated at two-hour intervals; abduction and adduction can be controlled by the position of the pulleys. Restraints are required to maintain the child in position so that the horizontal, gluteal folds are even with the bottom edge of the stacked mattresses. Also called **Schwartz bed.** Compare **Foster bed, Stryker wedge frame.**

hyperextension suspension, an orthopedic procedure used in the postoperative positioning of hip muscles. The procedure uses traction equipment, including metal frames, ropes, and pulleys to relieve the weight of the lower limbs and to position properly the muscles of the hip, without applying traction to the lower limbs involved. The ropes used to suspend the lower limbs in this procedure are attached by rings to long leg casts encasing the lower limbs of the patient. Compare **balanced suspension, lower extremity suspension, upper extremity suspension.**

hypergenesis, excessive growth or overdevelopment. The condition may involve the entire body, as in gigantism, or any particular part or it may result in the formation of extra parts, as the development of additional fingers or toes. — **hypergenetic,** *adj.*

hypergenetic teratism, a congenital anomaly in which there is excessive growth of a part or organ or the entire body, as in gigantism.

hyperglycemia (hai′pərglaisi′miə), a greater than normal amount of glucose in the blood. Most frequently associated with diabetes mellitus, the condition may occur in newborns, after the administration of glucocorticoid hormones, and with an excess infusion of intravenous solutions containing glucose, especially in poorly monitored, long-term hyperalimentation. Compare **hypoglycemia.**

hyperglycemic-glycogenolytic factor (hai′pərglaisi′-mıkglai′koujen′əlıt′ık). See **glucagon.**

hyperhidrosis (hai′pərhıdrou′sıs, hai′pərhaidrou′sıs), excessive perspiration, often caused by heat, hyperthyroidism, strong emotion, menopause, or infection. Symptomatic therapy usually includes topical antiperspirants and may involve surgery to remove axillary sweat glands.

hyperkalemia (hai′pərkəli′miə), greater than normal amounts of potassium in the blood. This condition is seen frequently in acute renal failure. Early signs are nausea, diarrhea, muscle weakness. As potassium levels increase, marked cardiac changes are observed in the ECG. Treatment of severe hyperkalemia includes the intravenous administration of sodium bicarbonate, calcium salts, and dextrose. Hemodialysis is used if these measures fail.

hyperkalemic periodic paralysis. See **adynamia episodica hereditaria.**

hyperkeratosis (hai′pərker′ətou′sıs), **1.** overgrowth and thickening of the cornea. **2.** overgrowth of the cornified epithelial layer of the skin. See also **callus, corn.**

hyperkinesis (hai′pərkıni′sıs). See **attention deficit disorder.**

hyperkinetic (hai′pərkınet′ık), hyperactive. See **hyperactivity.**

hyperlipoproteinemia (hai′pərlıp′ouprou′tini′miə), any of a large group of inherited and acquired disorders of lipoprotein metabolism characterized by greater than normal amounts of certain lipoproteins and cholesterol in the blood. The treatment includes diet to control obesity; diet may reduce lipoprotein levels in the blood. Medication and other treatment vary according to the specific metabolic defect, its cause, and its prognosis.

hypermagnesemia (hai′pərmæg′nısi′miə), a greater than normal amount of magnesium in the plasma, found in people with kidney failure and in those who use a large quantity of drugs containing magnesium, as antacids. Toxic levels of magnesium cause cardiac arrhythmias and depression of deep tendon reflexes and respiration. Treatment often includes intravenous fluids, a diuretic, and hemodialysis.

hypermenorrhea. See **menorrhagia.**

hypermetria (hai′pərmi′triə), an abnormal condition, a form of dysmetria, characterized by a dysfunction of the power to control the range of muscular action, resulting in movements which overreach the intended goal of the affected individual. Compare **hypometria.**

hypermetropia, hypermetropy, See **hyperopia.**

hypermorph (hai′pərmɔrf′), (in genetics) a mutant gene that shows an increased activity in the expression of a trait. Compare **amorph, antimorph, hypomorph.**

hypernatremia (hai′pərnætri′miə), greater than normal concentration of sodium in the blood, caused by excessive loss of water and electrolytes owing to polyuria, diarrhea, excessive sweating, or inadequate water intake. When water loss is caused by kidney dysfunction, urine is profuse and dilute. If water loss is not through the kidneys, as in diarrhea and excessive sweating, the urine is scanty and highly concentrated. People with hypernatremia may become mentally confused, have seizures, and lapse into coma. The treatment is restoration of fluid and electrolyte balance by mouth or by I.V. infusion. Care must be taken to restore water balance slowly, since further electrolyte imbalances may occur. In diabetes insipidus, the pituitary hormone vasopressin (ADH) will control excessive water loss through the kidneys. See also **diabetes insipidus.**

hyperopia (hai′pərou′piə), farsightedness, a condition resulting from an error of refraction in which rays of light entering the eye are brought into focus behind the retina. Also called **hypermetropia, hypermmetropy.**

(See next page for illustration)

Shortened
eyeball
Normal
eyeball

FARSIGHTED EYE
(HYPEROPIA)

BICONVEX LENS

HYPEROPIA

hyperparathyroidism (hai'pərpær'əthai'roidız'əm), an abnormal endocrine condition characterized by hyperactivity of any of the four parathyroid glands with excessive secretion of parathyroid hormone (PTH) that results in increased resorption of calcium from the skeletal system and increased absorption of calcium by the kidneys and gastrointestinal system. The condition may be primary, originating in one or more of the parathyroid glands, or secondary, resulting from an abnormal hypocalcemia-producing condition in another part or system of the body causing a compensatory hyperactivity of the parathyroid glands.

■ OBSERVATIONS: Hypercalcemia in primary hyperparathyroidism results in dysfunction of most of the systems of the body. In the kidneys, tissue calcifies, calculi form, and renal failure may ensue. In the bones and joints, osteoporosis develops, causing pain and fragility; fractures, synovitis and pseudogout often occur. In the gastrointestinal tract chronic, piercing epigastric pain may develop owing to pancreatitis. Hematemesis, anorexia, and nausea may be seen if peptic ulceration occurs. In the neuromuscular system generalized weakness and atrophy develop if the condition is not corrected, and changes in the central nervous system result in alteration of consciousness, coma, psychosis, abnormal behavior, and disturbances of personality. Secondary hyperparathyroidism may result in many of these signs of calcium imbalance and in various abnormalities of the long bones, as in rickets. The diagnosis of primary hyperparathyroidism is made by laboratory findings of increased levels of PTH and calcium in the blood and by the characteristic appearance of the bones on x-ray films. Calcium in the blood and urine and chloride and alkaline phosphotase in the blood are present in excessive amounts; phosphorus is present in the serum in less than normal amounts.

■ INTERVENTION: Primary parathyroidism that is the result of an adenoma of one of the glands is treated by excision of the tumor; other causes of primary disease might require excision of up to one half of the glandular tissue. Dietary intake of calcium may be limited, and diuretics that promote urinary excretion of calcium and sodium may be administered. Postoperatively, calcium levels in the blood may drop rapidly to dangerously low levels if frequent laboratory evaluations are not made and supplemental calcium is not given as required. Secondary hyperparathyroidism is treated by treating the underlying cause of hypertrophy of the gland. Vitamin D is frequently given, and peritoneal dialysis may be necessary to remove excess calcium from the circulation.

■ NURSING CONSIDERATIONS: Frequent laboratory evaluations of blood levels of calcium, phosphorus, potassium, and magnesium are necessary throughout the course of treatment. Because fractures occur easily and are common, great care is taken to avoid trauma for the patient. Intravenous hydration is usually performed to dilute the concentration of calcium, and the lungs are auscultated and percussed regularly to detect pulmonary edema in its earliest stages. Tetany is a warning sign of severe hypoglycemia; calcium gluconate is kept available for immediate use postoperatively. Walking and moving about cause pain to the patient but accelerate healing of the affected bones and are therefore encouraged.

hyperparathyroidism, an abnormal endocrine condition in which an excess of parathyroid hormone (PTH) is secreted by the parathyroid gland. Excessive amounts of circulating PTH result in hypercalcemia, owing to increased resorption of calcium and phosphate from the bones, increased resorption of calcium, and loss of phosphates via the kidneys, and increased resorption of both elements from the gastrointestinal tract.

hyperphenylalaninemia (hai'pərfen'ılæl'ənıni'miə), an abnormally high concentration of phenylalanine in the blood. This symptom may be the result of one of several defects in the metabolic process of breaking down phenylalanine. See also **phenylketonuria.**

hyperphoria (hai'pərfor'iə), the tendency of an eye to deviate upward.

hyperpigmentation (hai'pərpıg'məntei'shən), unusual darkening of the skin. Causes include heredity, drugs, exposure to the sun, and adrenal insufficiency. Compare **hypopigmentation.** See also **chloasma, melanocyte-stimulating hormone.**

hyperplasia (hai'pərplei'zhə), an increase in the number of cells. Compare **hypertrophy, hypoplasia.**

hyperplastic endometritis, *Obsolete.* endometritis with endometrial hyperplasia.

hyperploid (hai'pərploid), **hyperploidic,** 1. of or pertaining to an individual, organism, strain, or cell that has one or more chromosomes in excess of the basic haploid number or of an exact multiple of the haploid number characteristic of the species. The result is unbalanced sets of chromosomes, which are referred to as hyperdiploid, hypertriploid, hypertetraploid, and so on, depending on the number of multiples of the haploid chromosomes they contain. **2.** such an individual, organism, strain, or cell. Compare **hypoploid.** See also **trisomy.**

hyperploidy (hai'pərploi'di), any increase in chromosome number that involves individual chromosomes rather than entire sets, resulting in more than the normal haploid number characteristic of the species, as in Down's syndrome. Compare **hypoploidy.**

hyperpnea, hyperpnoea (hai'pərpni'ə), a deep, rapid, or labored respiration. It occurs normally with exercise, and abnormally with pain, fever, hysteria, or any condition in which the supply of oxygen is inadequate, as cardiac disease and respiratory disease. Compare **dyspnea, hypopnea, orthopnea.** – **hyperpneic, hyperpnoic,** adj.

hyperptyalism (hai'pərtai'əliz'əm). See **ptyalism.**

hyperpyrexia (hai'pərpairek'siə), an extremely elevated temperature sometimes occurring in acute infectious diseases, especially in young children. Malignant hyperpyrexia, characterized by a rapid rise in temperature, tachycardia, tachypnea, sweating, rigidity, and blotchy cyanosis, occasionally occurs in patients undergoing general anesthesia. A high temperature may be reduced by sponging the body with tepid water and alcohol, by giving a tepid tub bath, hypothermia treatment, or by administering antipyretic medication, as aspirin or acetaminophen. – **hyperpyretic,** adj.

hypersensitivity, an abnormal condition characterized by an excessive reaction to a particular stimulus. See also **allergy.** – **hypersensitive,** adj.

hypersensitivity pneumonitis. See **extrinsic allergic alveolitis.**

hypersensitivity reaction, an inappropriate and excessive response of the immune system to a sensitizing antigen. The antigenic stimulant is an allergen. There are several factors that determine the degree of an allergic response: the responsiveness of the host to the allergen, the amount of allergen, the kind of allergen, its route of entrance into the body, the timing of the exposures, and the site of the allergen-immune mediator reaction. Hypersensitivity reactions are classified by the components of the immune system involved in their mediation. Humoral reactions, mediated by the circulating B lymphocytes, are immediate and include three types: anaphylactic hypersensitivity, cytotoxic hypersensitivity, and immune system hypersensitivity. Cellular reactions, mediated by the T lymphocytes, are delayed, cell-mediated hypersensitivity reactions.

hypersomnia (hai'pərsom'niə), **1.** sleep of excessive depth or abnormal duration, usually caused by psychological rather than physical factors and characterized by a state of confusion upon awakening. **2.** extreme drowsiness, often associated with lethargy. **3.** a condition characterized by periods of deep, long sleep. Compare **narcolepsy.**

hypersplenism (hai'pərsplen'izəm), a syndrome consisting of splenomegaly and a deficiency of one or more types of blood cells. The numerous causes of this syndrome include the lymphomas, the hemolytic anemias, malaria, tuberculosis, and various connective tissue and inflammatory diseases. People complain of abdominal pain on the left side and often experience fullness after eating very little, because the greatly enlarged spleen is pressing against the stomach. On physical examination the enlarged spleen is felt and abnormal bruits (vascular sounds) are heard with a stethoscope over the epigastric area. Treatment of the underlying disorder may cure the syndrome. Splenectomy is usually performed only in treating the hemolytic anemias or when splenic enlargement is severe and the danger of vascular accident is significant. See also **splenectomy.**

Hyperstat, a trade name for a vasodilator (diazoxide).

hypertelorism (hai'pərtel'əriz'əm), a developmental defect characterized by an abnormally wide space between two organs or parts. A kind of hypertelorism is **ocular hypertelorism.** Compare **hypotelorism.**

Hypertensin, a trade name for a vasoconstrictor (angiotensin amide).

hypertension, a common, often asymptomatic disorder characterized by elevated blood pressure persistently exceeding 140/90 Hg. Essential hypertension, the most frequent kind, has no single identifiable cause, but the risk of the disorder is increased by obesity, a high sodium level in serum, hypercholesterolemia, and a family history of high blood pressure. Known causes of hypertension include adrenal disorders, as aldosteronism, Cushing's syndrome, and pheochromocytoma, thyrotoxicosis, toxemia of pregnancy, and chronic glomerulonephritis. The incidence of hypertension is higher in men than in women and is twice as great in blacks as in whites. Persons with mild or moderate hypertension may be asymptomatic or may experience suboccipital headaches, especially on rising, tinnitus, lightheadedness, easy fatigability, and palpitations. With sustained hypertension arterial walls become thickened, inelastic, and resistant to blood flow and, as a result, the left ventricle becomes distended and hypertrophied in its efforts to maintain normal circulation. Inadequate blood supply to the coronary arteries may cause angina or myocardial infarction. Left ventricular hypertrophy may lead to congestive heart failure. High blood pressure associated with hypersecretion of catecholamines in pheochromocytoma is often accompanied by anxiety attacks, palpitation, profuse sweating, pallor, nausea, and, in some cases, pulmonary edema. Malignant hypertension, characterized by a diastolic pressure higher than 120 mm Hg, severe headaches, blurred vision, and confusion, may result in fatal uremia, myocardial infarction, congestive heart failure, or a cerebral vascular accident. Drugs used to treat hypertension include diuretics, as furosemide and thiazide derivatives; vasodilators, as hydralazine and praxosin; sympathetic nervous system (SNS) depressants, as rauwolfia alkaloids; SNS inhibitors, as guanethidine and methyldopa; and ganglionic blocking agents, as clonidine and propranolol. Patients with high blood pressure are advised to follow a low-sodium, low-saturated fat diet, to reduce calories to control obesity, to exercise, avoid stress, and take adequate rest. See also **blood pressure.**

hypertensive crisis, a sudden severe increase in blood pressure to a level exceeding 200/120 mm Hg, occurring most frequently in untreated hypertension and in patients who have stopped taking prescribed antihypertensive medication.

■ OBSERVATIONS: Characteristic signs include severe headache, vertigo, diplopia, tinnitus, nosebleed, twitching muscles, tachycardia or other cardiac arrhythmia, distended neck veins, narrowed pulse pressure, nausea, and vomiting. The patient may be confused, irritable, or stuporous and the condition may lead to convulsions, coma, myocardial infarction, renal failure, cardiac arrest, or stroke.

■ INTERVENTION: Treatment consists of antihypertensive drugs, administered intravenously or intramuscularly, and diuretics and may include the use of anticonvulsants, sedatives, and antiemetics, if indicated. The patient is usually placed on a cardiac monitor in a bed with the head elevated and is maintained in a quiet environment. The diet is low in calories, and sodium and fluids may be restricted. As the condition improves the patient is permitted progressive ambulation but is carefully observed for symptoms of orthostatic hypotension, as pallor, diaphoresis, or faintness.

■ NURSING CONSIDERATIONS: A major concern in caring for patients who have suffered a hypertensive crisis is observing and reporting any sign of hypotension. In preparation for discharge the nurse advises the patient to recognize symptoms of any dramatic increase or decrease in blood pressure, to adhere to the prescribed diet and medication, and to avoid fatigue, heavy lifting, smoking, and stressful situations.

hypertetraploid (hai'pərtet'rəploid), **hypertetraploidic.** See **hyperploid.**

hyperthermia, 1. a higher-than-normal body temperature induced therapeutically or iatrogenically. 2. *Nontechnical.* malignant hyperthermia.

hypertonic (hai'pərton'ik), (of a solution) having a greater concentration of solute than another solution, hence exerting more osmotic pressure than that solution, as a hypertonic saline solution that contains more salt

than is found in intra- and extracellular fluid. Cells shrink in a hypertonic solution.

hypertonic contracture, prolonged muscle contraction owing to continuous nerve stimulation in spastic paralysis. Anesthesia or sleep eliminates this condition. Also called **functional contracture.**

hypertrichosis (hai'pərtrikou'sis). See **hirsutism.**

hypertriglyceridemia (hai'pərtraiglis'əridi'miə). See **hyperchylomicronemia.**

hypertriploid (hai'pərtriploid), **hypertriploidic.** See **hyperploid.**

hypertrophic angioma. See **hemangioendothelioma.**

hypertrophic catarrh, a chronic condition characterized by inflammation and discharge from a mucous membrane, accompanied by the thickening of the mucosal and submucosal tissue. Compare **atrophic catarrh.** See also **catarrh.**

hypertrophic endometritis, *Obsolete.* endometritis with endometrial hyperplasia.

hypertrophic gastritis, an inflammatory condition of the stomach characterized by epigastric pain, nausea, vomiting, and distention. It is differentiated from other forms of gastritis by the presence of prominent rugae (folds), enlarged glands, and nodules on the wall of the stomach. This condition often occurs with peptic ulcer, Zollinger-Ellison syndrome, or gastric hypersecretion. See also **gastritis.**

hypertrophic gingivitis. See **gingivitis.**

hypertrophy (haipər'trəfi), an increase in the size of a cell or a group of cells and thus, an increase in the size of an organ. Compare **atrophy, hyperplasia.** — **hypertrophic,** *adj.*

Hypertussis, a trade name for a passive immunizing agent (pertussis immune globulin).

hyperuricemia (hai'pəryur'isi'miə). See **gout.**

hyperventilation, a pulmonary ventilation rate that is greater than that metabolically necessary for the exchange of respiratory gases. It is the result of an increased frequency of breathing, an increased tidal volume, or a combination of both, and causes excessive intake of oxygen and the blowing off of carbon dioxide. Hypocapnia and respiratory alkalosis then occur, leading to chest pain, dizziness, faintness, numbness of the fingers and toes, and psychomotor impairment. Causes of hyperventilation include asthma or early emphysema; increased metabolism owing to exercise, fever, hyperthyroidism, or infections; lesions of the central nervous system, as in cerebral thrombosis, encephalitis, head injuries, or meningitis; hyposia or metabolic acidosis; hormones and drugs, as epinephrine, progesterone, salicylates; difficulties with mechanical respirators; and psychogenic factors, as acute anxiety or pain. Compare **hypoventilation.**

hypervitaminosis (hai'pərvai'təminou'sis), an abnormal condition resulting from excessive intake of toxic amounts of one or more vitamins, especially over a long period of time. Serious effects may result from overdosage of vitamins A, D, E, or K, but rarely with the water-soluble vitamins. Compare **avitaminosis**. See also specific vitamins.

hypesthesia (hɪp'ɪsθhi'ʒhə), an abnormal weakness of sensation in response to stimulation of the sensory nerves. Touch, pain, heat, and cold are poorly perceived. Also called **hypoesthesia**. – **hypesthetic**, *adj.*

hypha (hai'fə), *pl.* **hyphae**. the threadlike structure of the mycelium in a fungus.

hyphema (haifi'mə), **hyphemia** (haifi'miə), a hemorrhage into the anterior chamber of the eye, usually caused by a blunt or percussive injury. Bedrest and a sedative are indicated. The patient is treated by an ophthalmologist who evaluates the need for evacuation of the blood, the use of mydriatic or miotic medications or a carbonic anhydrase inhibitor. Glaucoma may result from recurrent bleeding.

hypnagogic hallucination, one that occurs in the period between wakefulness and sleep. See also **hallucination**.

hypnagogue (hɪp'nəgog), an agent or substance that tends to induce sleep or the feeling of dreamy sleepiness, as occurs prior to falling asleep. See also **hypnotic**. – **hypnagogic**, *adj.*

hypo-, hyp-, a combining form meaning 'under, beneath, or deficient': *hypocalcia, hypomastia, hyposynergia.*

hypnoanalysis, the use of hypnosis as an adjunct to other techniques in psychoanalysis.

hypnosis, a passive, trancelike state that resembles normal sleep during which perception and memory are altered, resulting in increased responsiveness to suggestion. The condition is usually induced by the monotonous repetition of words and gestures while the subject is completely relaxed. Susceptibility to hypnosis varies from person to person. Hypnosis is used in some forms of psychotherapy and psychoanalysis to gain access to the subconscious, in behavior modification programs to help a person stop overeating or smoking or to end other unwanted behavior, or in medicine to reduce pain and promote relaxation.

hypnotherapy, the use of hypnosis as an adjunct to other techniques in psychotherapy.

-hypnotic, a combining form meaning 'pertaining to hypnosis': *anhypnotic, autohypnotic, posthypnotic.*

hypnotic trance, an artificially induced sleeplike state, as in hypnosis.

hypnotism, the study or practice of inducing hypnosis.

hypnotist, one who practices hypnotism.

hypnotize, 1. to put into a state of hypnosis. 2. to fascinate, entrance, or control through personal charm.

hypo-, a combining form meaning 'beneath, deficient', or, in chemistry, 'lacking oxygen': *hypochlorite, hypodermic, hypodontia.*

hypoacidity (hai'pouəsɪd'ɪti), an abnormal condition characterized by a decreased secretion of hydrochloric acid. It is usually secondary to another condition, as pernicious anemia or carcinoma of the stomach.

hypoadrenalism. See **Addison's disease**.

hypoalimentation (hai'pouæl'ɪmentei'ʃhən), a condition of insufficient or inadequate nourishment.

hypobetalipoproteinemia (hai'poubei'təlɪp'ouprou'-tini'miə), an inherited disorder in which there are less than normal amounts of beta-lipoprotein in the serum. Blood lipids and cholesterol are present at less than the expected levels regardless of dietary intake of fats. There are no clinical signs, and treatment is unnecessary. Compare **hyperbetalipoproteinemia**.

hypocalcemia (hai'poukælsi'miə), a deficiency of calcium in the serum that may be caused by hypoparathyroidism, vitamin D deficiency, kidney failure, acute pancreatitis, or inadequate plasma magnesium and protein. Mild hypocalcemia is asymptomatic. Severe hypocalcemia is characterized by cardiac arrhythmias and tetany with hyperparesthesia of the hands, feet, lips, and tongue. The underlying disorder is diagnosed and treated and calcium is given by mouth or by intravenous infusion. Hypocalcemia is also seen in dysmature newborns, in infants born of diabetic mothers, or in normal babies delivered by normal mothers after a long or stressful labor and delivery. It is recognized by vomiting, twitching of extremities, poor muscle tone, high-pitched crying, and difficulty in breathing. See also **tetany**. – **hypocalcemic**, *adj.*

hypochlorous acid (hai'pouklor'əs), a greenish-yellow liquid derived from an aqueous solution of lime. An unstable compound that decomposes to hydrochloric acid and water, hypochlorous acid is used as a bleaching agent and disinfectant.

hypochondria (hai'pəkon'driə). See **hypochondriasis**.

hypochondriacal neurosis. See **hypochondriasis**.

hypochondriasis (hai'poukəndrai'əsɪs), **hypochondria**, 1. a chronic, abnormal concern about the health of the body. 2. Also called **hypochondriacal neurosis**. A disorder characterized by extreme anxiety, depression and an unrealistic interpretation of real or imagined physical symptoms as indications of a serious illness or disease despite rational medical evidence that no disorder is present. The condition is caused by some unresolved intrapsychic conflict and may involve a specific organ, as the heart, lungs, or eyes, or several body systems at various times or simultaneously. In severe cases, the distorted body-mind relationship is so strong that actual symptoms and disease may develop. Treatment usually consists of psychotherapy to uncover the underlying emotional conflict. – **hypochondriac**, *adj., n.,* **hypochondriacal**, *adj.*

hypochromic (hai'pəkrou'mɪk), having less than normal

color, usually describing a red blood cell and characterizing anemias associated with decreased synthesis of hemoglobin. Compare **normochromic**. See also **hypochromic anemia, red cell indices.**

hypochromic anemia, any of a large group of anemias characterized by a decreased concentration of hemoglobin in the red blood cells. See also **anemia, red cell indices.**

hypocytic leukemia (hai'pəsɪt'ɪk). See **subleukemic leukemia.**

hypodermatoclysis (hai'poudər'mətok'ləsɪs). See **hypodermoclysis.**

hypodermic, of or pertaining to the area below the skin, as a hypodermic injection.

hypodermic needle, a short, thin, hollow needle that attaches to a syringe for injecting a drug or medication under the skin or into vessels and for withdrawing a fluid, as blood, for examination.

hypodermoclysis (haipoudərmok'lɪsɪs), **hypodermatoclysis** (hai'poudərmətok'lɪsɪs), the injection of an isotonic or hypotonic solution into subcutaneous tissue to supply the patient with a continuous and large amount of fluid, electrolytes, and nutrients. The procedure is used to replace the loss of or inadequate intake of water and salt during illness or surgery or following shock or hemorrhage and is performed only when the patient is unable to take fluids intravenously, orally, or rectally. The rate of absorption into the circulatory system is increased with the addition to the solution of the enzyme hyaluronidase. The most common sites of administration are the anterior thighs, the abdominal wall along the crest of the ilium, below the breasts in women, and directly over the scapula in children; sites should be changed when multiple infusions are given. The patient is placed in a comfortable position, since the procedure takes a long time. The nurse observes for signs of circulatory collapse, respiratory difficulty, and edema at the site of injection. Also called **interstitial infusion, subcutaneous infusion.**

hypodiploid (hai'poudɪp'lɔid), **hypodiploidic.** See **hypoploid.**

hypoesthesia (hai'pouɪsθhi'ʒhə). See **hypesthesia.** —**hypoesthetic,** *adj.*

hypogammaglobulinemia (hai'pougæm'əglob'yulmi'miə), a less-than-normal concentration of gamma globulin in the blood, usually the result of increased protein catabolism or the loss of protein in the urine, as in nephrosis. The condition is associated with a decreased resistance to infection. Compare **agammaglobulinemia.**

hypogastric artery. See **internal iliac artery.**

hypoglossal nerve, either of a pair of cranial nerves essential for swallowing and for moving the tongue. Each nerve has four major branches, communicates with the vagus nerve, and connects to nucleus XII in the brain. Also called **nervus hypoglossus, twelfth nerve.**

hypoglycemia (hai'pouglaisi'miə), a less-than-normal amount of glucose in the blood, usually caused by administration of too much insulin, excessive secretion of insulin by the islet cells of the pancreas, or by dietary deficiency. The condition may result in weakness, headache, hunger, visual disturbances, ataxia, anxiety, personality changes, and if untreated, delirium, coma, and death. The treatment is the administration of glucose in orange juice by mouth if the person is conscious or in an intravenous glucose solution if the person is unconscious. Compare **diabetic coma.**

hypoglycemic agent, any of a large heterogeneous group of drugs prescribed to decrease the amount of glucose circulating in the blood. Hypoglycemic agents include insulin, the sulfonylureas, and the biguanides. Insulin in its various forms is given parenterally and acts by increasing the utilization of carbohydrates and the metabolism of fats and protein. The sulfonylureas, including tolbutamide, tolinamide, chlorpropamide, and acetohexamide, act by stimulating the release of endogenous insulin from the pancreas. The biguanides, of which only phenformin has been recently prescribed, act by potentiating the action of endogenous insulin, augmenting the utilization of glucose by the peripheral cells of the body. Phenformin has been recently removed from the market in the United States, primarily because of its tendency to cause lactic acidosis. The adverse reactions of any hypoglycemic agent and contraindications for its prescription depend on the class of drug and the condition of the patient.

hypoglycemic shock treatment. See **insulin-shock treatment.**

hypokalemia (hai'poukəli'miə), a condition in which an inadequate amount of potassium, the major intracellular cation, is found in the circulating blood stream. Hypokalemia is characterized by abnormal EKG, weakness, and flaccid paralysis and may be caused by starvation, treatment of diabetic acidosis, adrenal tumor, or diuretic therapy. Mild hypokalemia may resolve itself when the underlying disorder is corrected. Severe hypokalemia may be treated by the administration of potassium chloride, orally or parenterally, and by a diet high in potassium. Compare **hyperkalemia.** See also **electrolyte balance.**

hypokalemic alkalosis, a pathologic condition resulting from the accumulation of base or the loss of acid from the body associated with a low level of serum potassium. The retention of alkali or the loss of acid occurs primarily in extracellular fluid, but the pH of intracellular fluid may also be subnormal. See also **hypokalemia.**

hypolipemia (hai'poulɪpi'miə). See **hypolipoproteinemia.**

hypolipoproteinemia (hai'poulɪp'ouprou'tini'miə), a group of rare, hereditary defects of lipid metabolism that result in varying complexes of signs. These include abnormal transport of triglycerides in the blood, low levels of high-density lipoproteins, high levels of low-density lipoproteins, and abnormal deposition of lipids in the body, especially in the kidneys and the liver. In some of the syndromes ocular, intestinal, and neurologic effects are also present. Kinds of hypolipoproteinemias are **abetalipoproteinemia (Bassen-Kornzweig syndrome), hypobetalipoproteinemia, lecithin-cholesterol acyltransferase deficiency, Tangier disease.**

hypomagnesemia (hai'poumæg'nɪsi'miə), an abnormally low concentration of magnesium in the blood plasma, resulting in nausea, vomiting, muscle weakness, tremors, tetany, and lethargy. Mild hypomagnesemia is usually the result of inadequate absorption of magnesium in the kidney or intestine, although it is also seen after prolonged parenteral feeding and during lactation. A more severe form is associated with malabsorption syndrome, protein malnutrition, and parathyroid disease. Magnesium salts to correct the deficiency may be given orally or by I.V. infusion.

hypomania (hai'pəmei'niə), a psychopathological state characterized by optimism, excitability, a marked hyperactivity and talkativeness, heightened sexual interest, quick anger and irritability, and a decreased need for sleep. — **hypomaniac,** *n.,* **hypomanic,** *adj.*

hypometria (hai'pəmi'triə), an abnormal condition, a form of dysmetria, characterized by a dysfunction of the power to control the range of muscular action, resulting in movements which fall short of the intended goals of the affected individual. Compare **hypermetria.**

hypomorph, (in genetics) a mutant allele that has a reduced effect on the expression of a trait but at a level too low to result in abnormal development. Also called **leaky gene.** Compare **amorph, antimorph, hypermorph.**

hyponatremia (hai'pounætri'miə), a less than normal concentration of sodium in the blood, caused by inadequate excretion of water or by excessive water in the circulating blood stream. In a severe case, the person may develop water intoxication, with confusion and lethargy, leading to muscle excitability, convulsions, and coma. Restoration of fluid and electrolyte balance may be accomplished by intravenous infusion of a balanced solution.

hypopharyngeal (hai'poufərɪn'jiəl), 1. of, pertaining to, or involving the hypopharynx. 2. situated below the pharynx.

hypophosphatasia (hai'poufos'fətei'ʒhə), congenital absence of alkaline phosphatase, an enzyme essential to the calcification of bone tissue. Affected newborns vomit, grow slowly, and often die in infancy. Children who survive have numerous skeletal abnormalities and are dwarfs. There is no known treatment.

hypophosphatemic rickets (hai'poufos'fəti'mɪk), a rare familial disorder in which there is impaired resorption of phosphate in the kidneys and poor absorption of calcium in the small intestine, resulting in osteomalacia, retarded growth, skeletal deformities, and pain. Treatment includes the prescription of phosphate and vitamin D, to be taken by mouth.

hypophyseal cachexia (hai'pəfɪz'iəl). See **panhypopituitarism.**

hypophyseal dwarf. See **pituitary dwarf.**

hypophysectomy (haipof'əsek'təmi), surgical removal of the pituitary gland. It may be performed to slow the growth and spread of endocrine-dependent malignant tumors of the breast, ovary, or prostate gland, to halt deterioration of the retina in diabetes, or to excise a pituitary tumor. The gland is removed only if other treatment, as x-ray therapy, radioactive implants, or cryosurgery, fails to destroy all pituitary tissue. General anesthesia is given, a craniotomy is performed, and the gland is completely removed. Postoperative nursing care is as for a craniotomy. Hormone levels, including thyroid stimulating hormone, adrenocorticotropic hormone, and antidiuretic hormone, are monitored and replacement therapy is begun as needed. Urinary output is measured every two hours for several days, and an amount in excess of 300 ml in any two-hour period is reported. The patient is closely monitored for early signs of thyroid crisis, Addisonian crisis, electrolyte imbalance, hemorrhage, and meningitis. — **hypophysectomize,** *v.*

hypophysis cerebri. See **pituitary gland.**

hypopigmentation (hai'poupɪg'məntei'ʃhən), unusual lack of skin color, seen in albinism or vitiligo. Compare **hyperpigmentation.**

hypoplasia (hai'pəpleiʒhə), **hypoplasty** (hai'pouplæs'ti), incomplete or underdevelopment of an organ or tissue, usually owing to a decrease in the number of cells. Kinds of hypoplasia are **cartilage-hair hypoplasia, enamel hypoplasia.** Compare **aplasia, hyperplasia.** See also **oligomeganephronia, osteogenesis imperfecta.** — **hypoplastic,** *adj.*

hypoplasia of the mesenchyme. See **osteogenesis imperfecta.**

hypoplastic anemia, a broad category of anemias characterized by decreased production of red blood cells. Compare **aplastic anemia, polycythemia.** See also **anemia.**

hypoplastic dwarf. See **primordial dwarf.**

hypoploid (hai'pəploid), 1. Also called **hypoploidic.** of or pertaining to an individual, organism, strain, or cell that has fewer than the normal haploid number or an exact multiple of the haploid number of chromosomes characteristic of the species. The result is unbalanced sets of chromosomes, which are referred to as hypodiploid, hypotriploid, hypotetraploid, and so on, depending on the number of multiples of the haploid chromosomes they contain. 2. such an individual, organism, strain, or cell. Compare **hyperploid.** See also **monosomy.**

hypoploidy (hai'pəploi'di), any decrease in chromosome number that involves individual chromosomes rather than entire sets, resulting in fewer than the normal haploid number characteristic of the species, as in Turner's syndrome. Compare **hyperploidy.**

hypopnea (hai̇pop′niə), shallow or slow respiration. In well-conditioned athletes it is normal and is accompanied by a slow pulse; otherwise, it is characteristic of damage to the brain stem, in which case it is accompanied by a rapid, weak pulse and is a grave sign.

hypoproteinemia (hai̇′pouprou′tini′miə), a disorder characterized by a decrease in the amount of protein in the blood to an abnormally low level, accompanied by edema, nausea, vomiting, diarrhea and abdominal pain. It may be caused by an inadequate dietary supply of protein, by intestinal lymphangiectasia, or by renal failure. See also **intestinal lymphangiectasia.**

hypoprothrombinemia (hai̇′pouprouthrom′bini′miə), an abnormal reduction in the amount of prothrombin (factor II) in the circulating blood, characterized by poor clot formation, longer bleeding time, and possible hemorrhage. The condition is usually the result of inadequate synthesis of prothrombin in the liver, most often the result of a deficiency of vitamin K owing to severe liver disease or to anticoagulant therapy with the drug dicoumarol. See also **blood clotting.**

hypoptyalism (hai̇′poutai̇′əliz′əm), a condition in which there is a decrease in the amount of saliva secreted by the salivary glands. Compare **hyperptyalism.**

hypopyon, an accumulation of pus in the anterior chamber of an eye, appearing as a gray fluid between the cornea and the iris. It may occur as a complication of conjuctivitis, herpetic keratitis, or corneal ulcer.

hyposensitization. See **immunotherapy.**

hypospadias (hai̇′pəspei̇′diəs), a congenital defect in which the urinary meatus is on the underside of the penis. Incontinence does not occur because the sphincters are not defective. The opening may be off center or anywhere along the underside of the penis or on the perineum. Surgical correction is performed as necessary for cosmetic, urologic, or reproductive indications. A corresponding defect in women is rare but recognized by the location of the urinary meatus in the vagina. Compare **epispadias.**

hypotelorism (hai̇′poutel′əriz′əm), a developmental defect characterized by an abnormally decreased distance between two organs or parts. A kind of hypotelorism is **ocular hypotelorism.** Compare **hypertelorism.**

hypotension (hai̇′pouten′ʃhən), an abnormal condition in which the blood pressure is not adequate for normal perfusion and oxygenation of the tissues. An expanded intravascular space, a decreased intravascular volume, or a diminished cardiac thrust may be the cause.

hypotensive anesthesia. See **deliberate hypotension.**

hypotetraploid (hai̇′poutet′rəploid), **hypotetraploidic.** See **hypoploid.**

hypothalamic amenorrhea, cessation of menses caused by disorders that inhibit the hypothalamus from initiating the cycle of neurohormonal interactions of the brain, pituitary, and ovary necessary for ovulation and subsequent menstruation. Examples of causes are stress, anxiety, and acute weight loss. See **amenorrhea.**

hypothalamus (hai̇′pəthæl′əməs), a portion of the diencephalon of the brain, forming the floor and part of the lateral wall of the third ventricle. It activates, controls, and integrates the peripheral autonomic nervous system, endocrine processes, and many somatic functions, as body temperature, sleep, and appetite. – **hypothalamic,** *adj.*

hypothermia (hai̇′pouthər′miə), **1.** an abnormal and dangerous condition in which the temperature of the body is below 35°C, usually owing to prolonged exposure to cold. Respiration is shallow and slow, and the heart rate is faint and slow. The person is very pale and may appear to be dead. People who are very old or very young, people who have cardiovascular problems, and people who are hungry, tired, or under the influence of alcohol are most susceptible to hypothermia. Treatment includes slowly warming the person. Hospitalization is necessary for evaluating and treating any metabolic abnormalities that may result from hypothermia. **2.** the deliberate and controlled reduction of body temperature with cooling mattresses or ice as preparation for some surgical procedures.

hypothermia blanket, a covering used to conserve heat in the body of a patient suffering from hypothermia.

hypothermia therapy, the reduction of a patient's body temperature to counteract high prolonged fever caused by an infectious or neurologic disease, or, less frequently, as an adjunct to anesthesia in heart or brain surgery.

■ METHOD: Hypothermia may be produced by placing crushed ice around the patient, by immersing the body in ice water, by autotransfusing blood after it is circulated through coils submerged in a refrigerant, or, most commonly, by applying cooling blankets or vinyl pads containing coils through which cold water and alcohol are circulated by a pump. The cooling unit is placed in an open area; any kinks or twists in the tubing are removed and the blanket is checked for leaks. The patient is wrapped in bath blankets and then covered with the cooling blanket; the patient's temperature, registered by means of a probe inserted in the rectum, is read and recorded before hypothermia is initiated, every five minutes until the desired reduction is achieved, and then every 15 minutes. The blood pressure, pulse, respirations, and neurologic status are checked every five to ten minutes until the temperature is stabilized, then every 30 minutes for two hours, every four hours in the next 24 hours, and subsequently as required. Every one to two hours the patient is assisted in turning, coughing, and deep breathing. At similar intervals the chest is auscultated for breath sounds, and oral, nose, and skin care are administered; the skin is lubricated with oil or lotion before and during the procedure. An indwelling catheter is connected to a closed gravity drainage system, as ordered, and fluid intake and output are measured; if less than 30 ml of urine per hour is excreted the physician is notified. If the patient's temperature is less than 90°F (32.2°C), his gag reflex is tested before any oral fluids or foods are administered. Naso-oral suction is performed as indicated; body alignment is maintained, and a passive or active range of motion exercises is performed every four hours. Since shivering increases body heat, medication for its prevention, as chlorpromazine hydrochloride, may be ordered. The patient is observed for medication reactions, decreased blood pressure, bradycardia, arrhythmias, bradypnea, respiratory failure, unequal pupils, increased intracranial pressure, changes in consciousness, intestinal ileus, and frostbite. Any changes in skin color or signs of edema and induration are reported to the physician immediately. At the termination of hypothermia, the cooling blanket is replaced by regular blankets and the patient usually warms at his own rate. As the patient's temperature approaches normal, the warming blankets are removed, but the temperature probe remains in place until the body temperature is stable.

■ NURSING ORDERS: The nurse administers hypothermia, carefully monitoring the patient's vital signs and any evidence of complications.

■ OUTCOME CRITERIA: Hypothermia used in the treatment of high fever associated with generalized severe infections reduces body heat by decreasing metabolism and also inhibits the multiplication of the etiologic pathogenic organisms. Patients with a high temperature caused by a neurologic disease may be maintained in a state of mild hypothermia (87° to 95°F or 30.6° to 35°C) for as long as five days. The procedure is successful if the fever is broken and complications do not occur.

hypothesis (haipoth′isis), (in research) a statement derived from a theory that predicts the relationship among variables representing concepts, constructs, or events. Kinds of hypotheses include **causal hypothesis, null hypothesis, predictive hypothesis.**

hypothyroid dwarf. See **cretin dwarf.**

hypotonic (haĭ′pəton′ĭk), (of a solution) having a smaller concentration of solute than another solution, hence exerting less osmotic pressure than that solution, as a hypotonic saline solution that contains less salt than is found in intra- or extracellular fluid. Cells expand in a hypotonic solution.

hypotriploid (haĭ′poutrĭp′loid), **hypotriploidic.** See **hypoploid.**

hypoventilation, an abnormal condition of the respiratory system, characterized by cyanosis, clubbing of the fingers, polycythemia, increased carbon dioxide arterial tension, Cheyne-Stokes breathing, and generalized decreased respiratory function. It occurs when the volume of air which enters the alveoli and takes part in gas exchanges is not adequate for the metabolic needs of the body. Hypoventilation may be caused by uneven distribution of inspired air, as in bronchitis, obesity, neuromuscular or skeletal disease affecting the thorax, decreased response of the respiratory center to carbon dioxide, and by reduced functional lung tissue, as in atelectasis, emphysema, and pleural effusion. The result of hypoventilation is hypoxia, hypercapnia, pulmonary hypertension with cor pulmonale, and respiratory acidosis. Treatment includes weight reduction in cases of obesity, artificial respiration, and tracheostomy.

hypovitaminosis (haĭ′pouvaĭ′təmĭnou′sĭs). See **avitaminosis.**

hypovolemic shock, a state of physical collapse and prostration caused by massive blood loss, circulatory dysfunction, and inadequate tissue perfusion. The loss of about one fifth of total blood volume in the affected individual can produce this condition. The common signs include low blood pressure, feeble pulse, clammy skin, tachycardia, rapid breathing, and reduced urinary output. The associated blood losses may stem from gastrointestinal bleeding, internal hemorrhage, external hemorrhage, or excessive reduction of intravascular plasma volume and body fluids. Disorders that may cause hypovolemic shock are dehydration from excessive perspiration, severe diarrhea, or protracted vomiting, intestinal obstruction, peritonitis, acute pancreatitis, and severe burns, which deplete body fluids. Associated effects may include metabolic acidosis with the accumulation of lactic acid, irreversible cerebral and renal damage, and disseminated intravascular coagulation. Treatment of hypovolemic shock focuses on prompt replacement of blood and fluid volumes, identification of bleeding sites, and the control of bleeding. Without fast aggressive treatment there is further collapse that can cause death. Compare **cardiogenic shock.**

hypoxemia (haĭ′poksĭ′mĭə), an abnormal deficiency of oxygen in the arterial blood. Symptoms of acute hypoxemia are cyanosis, restlessness, stupor, coma, Cheyne-Stokes breathing, or apnea, increased blood pressure, tachycardia, and an initial increase in cardiac output which later falls, resulting in hypotension and ventricular fibrillation or asystole. Chronic hypoxemia stimulates red cell production by the bone marrow, leading to secondary polycythemia. Hypoxemia caused by decreased alveolar oxygen tension or underventilation improves with oxygen therapy. Hypoxemia resulting from shunting of blood from the right side of the heart to the left side of the heart without exchange of gases in the lungs is treated with bronchial hygiene and positive and expiratory pressure therapy. Compare **hypoxia.** See also **anoxia, asphyxia.**

hypoxia, an inadequate, reduced tension of arterial oxygen, characterized by cyanosis, tachycardia, hypertension, peripheral vasoconstriction, dizziness, and mental confusion. Mild hypoxia stimulates the peripheral chemoreceptors to increase heart and respiratory rates. However, the central mechanisms that regulate breathing fail in severe hypoxia, leading to irregular respiration, Cheyne-Stokes breathing, apnea, and respiratory and cardiac failure. Increased sensitivity to the depressant effect on the respiratory system by certain drugs is common in chronic hypoxia, resulting in severe depression or apnea from relatively small doses of opiates. If the amounts of oxygen are not adequate for aerobic cellular metabolism, energy is provided by anaerobic pathways that are less efficient and that produce metabolites other than carbon dioxide. The tissues most sensitive to hypoxia are the brain, heart, pulmonary vessels, and liver. Treatment may include cardiotonic and respiratory stimulant drugs, oxygen therapy, mechanical ventilation, and frequent analysis of blood gases. Compare **hypoxemia.** See also **anoxia, chemoreceptor, hyperventilation, respiratory center.**

hypsi-, a combining form meaning 'high': *hypsicephalia, hypsiconchous, hypsistaphylie.*

hypso-, a combining form meaning 'pertaining to height': *hypsonosus, hypsophobia, hypsotherapy.*

hyssibrachycephaly (hɪs'ɪbræk'ɪsef'əli), the condition of having a skull that is high with a broad forehead. See also **brachycephaly, oxycephaly.** —**hyssibrachycephalic,** *adj., n.*

hyssicephaly (hɪs'ɪsef'əli). See **oxycephaly.**

hyster-. See **hystero-.**

hysterectomy, surgical removal of the uterus, performed to remove fibroid tumors of the uterus, to treat chronic pelvic inflammatory disease, severe recurrent endometrial hyperplasia, uterine hemorrhage, and precancerous and cancerous conditions of the uterus. Types of hysterectomy include total hysterectomy, in which the uterus and cervix are removed and radical hysterectomy, in which ovaries, oviducts, lymph nodes and lymph channels are removed with the uterus and cervix. Menstruation ceases after either type is performed. A vaginal douche may be given preoperatively. Under general or spinal anesthesia the uterus is excised and removed, either through the abdominal wall or, if plastic repair of vaginal structures is needed, through the vagina. One or both ovaries and oviducts may be removed at the same time. Postoperatively, the nurse will frequently observe the abdominal dressing, if present, for bleeding. Food and oral fluids are restricted to prevent abdominal distention. Toe to knee elastic stockings or bandages are reapplied twice a day to give snug, even support and to prevent circulatory stasis. The lower half of the bed is kept flat and the patient is

instructed to avoid sharply flexing the thighs or knees, since thrombophlebitis of the blood vessels of the pelvis and upper thigh is a frequent complication. Low back pain or scanty urine may indicate a ligated ureter. Compare **hysterosalpingo-oophorectomy.** —**hysterectomize,** *v.*

hysteria, 1. a general state of tension or excitement in a person or a group, characterized by unmanageable fear and temporary loss of control over the emotions. 2. *Obsolete.* a psychoneurosis, now commonly called **hysterical neurosis.**

hysterical fever, an abnormal rise in body temperature without general symptoms, often seen in hysterical neurosis.

hysterical mania, a mood disorder characterized by symptoms of hysteria and mania.

hysterical neurosis, a form of psychoneurosis in which extreme excitability and anxiety resulting from an underlying emotional conflict are converted either into physical symptoms having no organic basis or into states of altered consciousness or identity. Kinds of hysterical neurosis are **conversion disorder, dissociative disorder.**

hysterical personality. See **histrionic personality.**

hysterical trance, a somnambulistic state occurring as a symptom of hysterical neurosis.

hysteric amaurosis, monocular or, more rarely, binocular blindness occurring following an emotional shock and lasting for hours, days, or months.

hysteric apepsia. See **anorexia nervosa.**

hysteric lethargy, a sleep induced by hypnosis. See also **hypnosis, lethargy.**

hystero-, hyster-, a combining form meaning 'pertaining to the uterus': *hysterocarcinoma, hysterocleisis, hysterolith.*

hysterolaparotomy (hɪs'təroulæp'ərot'əmi), abdominal hysterectomy or hysterotomy.

hysterosalpingogram (hɪs'tərousælpɪŋ'gougræm), an x-ray film of the uterus and the Fallopian tubes using gas or a radiopaque substance introduced through the cervix to allow visualization of the cavity of the uterus and the passageway of the tubes. A blockage of a structure is demonstrated on the film as the radiopaque substance cannot pass to the more distal structures and escape from the ends of the tubes into the peritoneal cavity. Serial hysterosalpingograms are useful in the diagnosis of the cause of infertility.

hysterosalpingo-oophorectomy, surgical removal of one or both ovaries and oviducts along with the uterus, performed most commonly to treat malignant neoplastic disease of the reproductive tract and chronic endometriosis. To avoid the severe symptoms of sudden menopause, a portion of one ovary is left, unless a malignancy is present. Under general anesthesia the uterus, one or both oviducts, and one or both ovaries are removed. If both ovaries are removed and no malignancy is present, estrogen-replacement therapy is often begun immediately. Elastic stockings or bandages are applied to the legs twice a day to prevent circulatory stasis because thrombophlebitis of the blood vessels of the pelvis or thigh is a frequent complication. The lower half of the bed is kept flat, and the patient instructed to avoid sharply flexing the thighs or knees. Low back pain or scanty urine may indicate a ligated ureter. Compare **hysterectomy**.

hysteroscopy, direct visual inspection of the cervical canal and uterine cavity through a systeroscope, performed to examine the endometrium, to secure a specimen for biopsy, to remove an intrauterine device, or to excise cervical polyps. Under spinal anesthesia the endoscope is passed through the vagina and into the uterus, and the surrounding tissues are examined. The nurse keeps the patient flat in bed for the next eight hours. The procedure is contraindicated in pregnancy, acute pelvic inflammatory disease, chronic upper genital tract infection, recent uterine perforation, and known or suspected cervical malignancy. — **hysteroscope,** *n.,* **hysteroscopic,** *adj.*

hysterotomy, surgical incision of the uterus, performed as a method of abortion in a pregnancy beyond the first trimester of gestation in which a saline-injection abortion was incomplete, or in which a tubal sterilization is to be done with the abortion. Under general or spinal anesthesia the lower segment of the uterus is incised, and the products of conception are withdrawn. Postoperative care includes close observation for excessive vaginal bleeding.

Hytakerol, a trade name for a calcium regulator (dihydrotachysterol).

Hytone, a trade name for a glucocorticoid (hydrocortisone), used in a topical ointment for the relief of dermatitis.

Hz, abbreviation for **hertz.**

HZV, abbreviation for *herpes zoster virus.* See **chicken pox.**

I

-i, a plural-forming element used in native and later scientific Latin words: *bacilli, bronchi, plumbi* and in scientific terms derived through Latin from Greek: *encephali, pylori, tympani.*

I, 1. symbol for **inspired gas.** 2. symbol for **iodine.**

-ia, a combining form meaning a 'specified condition (disease)': *athrombia, phrenoblabia, pontobulbia.*

I.A.D.R., abbreviation for **International Association for Dental Research.**

-iasis, 1. a combining form meaning a 'disease produced' by something specified: *cestodiasis, dicroeliasis, myiasis.* 2. a combining form meaning a 'disease producing (specified) characteristics': *elephantiasis, leontiasis, lithiasis.*

-iatria. See **-iatry.**

-iatric, a combining form meaning 'relating to medical treatment': *neuropsychiatric, orthopsychiatric, pithiatric.* Also **-iatrical.**

-iatrician. See **-iatrist.**

-iatrist, a combining form meaning a 'physician': *hydriatrist, pediatrist, podiatrist.* Also **-iatrician.**

iatro-, a combining form meaning 'pertaining to a physician or to treatment': *iatrogenic, iatrophysics, iatrotechnics.*

iatrogenic (yæt'roʊgen'ɪk), caused by treatment or diagnostic procedures. An iatrogenic disorder is a condition caused by medical personnel or procedures or through exposure to the environment of a health care facility. —**iatrogenesis,** *n.*

-iatry, a combining form meaning a '(specified) type of medical treatment': *andriatry, pediatry, pithiatry.* Also **-iatria.**

ibuprofen (aɪbyu'prəfɪn), a nonsteroidal anti-inflammatory agent.

■ INDICATIONS: It is prescribed in the treatment of rheumatoid and osteo-arthritis conditions.

■ CONTRAINDICATIONS: Renal dysfunction, disorders of the gastrointestinal tract, or known hypersensitivity to this drug, to other nonsteroidal anti-inflammatory drugs, or to aspirin prohibits its use.

■ ADVERSE EFFECTS: Among the more serious adverse reactions are gastrointestinal disturbances, gastric or duodenal ulceration, dizziness, skin rash, and tinnitus. The drug interacts with many other drugs.

-ic, -ac, a combining form meaning 'pertaining to, similar to': *allelic, cadaveric, hypochondriac.*

IC, abbreviation for **inspiratory capacity.**

ICD, abbreviation for **International Classification of Diseases.**

ICDA, abbreviation for **International Classification of Disease,** adapted for use in the United States.

ichthammol (ɪk'θəmɔl), a topical anti-infective used for treating certain skin diseases.

ichthyo-, a combining form meaning 'pertaining to fish': *ichthyocolla, ichthyophagy, ichthyotoxic.*

Ichthyol, a trade name for a topical anti-infective (ichthammol).

ichthyosis (ɪk'θioʊ'sɪs), any of several inherited dermatologic conditions in which the skin is dry, hyperkeratotic, and fissured, resembling fish scales. It usually appears at or shortly after birth and may be part of one of several rare syndromes. Some types respond temporarily to bath oils, topical retinoic acid, or propylene glycol. A rare, acquired variety occurs in adult life accompanying a lymphoma or multiple myeloma. —**ichthyotic,** *adj.*

ichthyosis congenita. See **lamellar exfoliation of the newborn.**

ichthyosis fetalis. See **lamellar exfoliation of the newborn.**

ichthyosis fetus. See **harlequin fetus.**

ichthyosis simplex. See **ichthyosis vulgaris.**

ichthyosis vulgaris (ɪk'θioʊ'sɪs), a hereditary skin disorder characterized by large, dry, dark scales that cover the face, neck, scalp, ears, back, and extensor surfaces but not the flexor surfaces of the body. The condition is transmitted as an autosomal dominant trait; not present at birth, it appears several months to one year afterward. Management consists of topical application of emollients and the use of keratolytic agents to facilitate removal of the scales. Also called **ichthyosis simplex.** See also **sex-linked ichthyosis.**

-ician, a combining form meaning a 'specialist in a field': *clinician, pediatrician, technician.*

ICN, abbreviation for **International Council of Nurses.**

ICP, abbreviation for **intracranial pressure.**

-ics, a combining form meaning the 'systematic formulation of a body of knowledge': *bionomics, osmics, psychics.*

I.C.S., abbreviation for **International Congress of Surgeons.**

ICSH, abbreviation for **interstitial-cell-stimulating hormone.** See **luteinizing hormone.**

icterus (ık′tərəs),   jaundice. See also **hyperbilirubinemia.** — **icteric,** *adj.*

ictus (ık′təs), *pl.* **ictuses, ictus. 1.** a seizure. **2.** a cerebrovascular accident. — **ictal, ictic,** *adj.*

ICU,   abbreviation for **intensive care unit.**

id, 1. (in psychoanalysis) the part of the psyche, functioning in the unconscious, that is the source of instinctive energy, impulses, and drives. It is based on the pleasure principle and has strong tendencies toward self-preservation. Compare **ego, superego. 2.** the true unconscious.

-id, 1. a combining form meaning a 'structural element of teeth': *protoconid, talonid, trigonid.* **2.** a combining form meaning a '(specified) body or particle': *cuspid, rhabdoid, sporid.*

-ide,   a combining form naming binary compounds composed of a metallic and a nonmetallic element: *chloride, monoxide, sulfide.*

idea,   any thought, concept, intention, or impression that exists in the mind as a result of awareness, understanding, or other mental activity. Kinds of ideas include **autochthonous idea, compulsive idea, dominant idea, fixed idea, idea of influence, idea of persecution, idea of reference.**

idea of influence,   an obsessive delusion, often seen in paranoid disorders, that external forces or persons are controlling one's thoughts, actions, and feelings.

idea of persecution,   an obsessive delusion, often seen in paranoid disorders, that one is being threatened, discriminated against, or mistreated by other persons or by external forces.

idea of reference,   an obsessive delusion that the statements or actions of others refer to oneself, usually taken to be depreciatory, often seen in paranoid disorders. Also called **delusion of reference, referential idea.**

ideational apraxia,   a condition in which the conceptual process is lost, often owing to a lesion in the submarginal gyrus of the parietal lobe. The individual is unable to formulate a plan of movement and does not know the proper use of an object owing to a lack of perception of its purpose. There is no loss of motor movement, but the reason for the movement is confused. Also called **sensory apraxia.** See also **apraxia.**

idée fixe (French ideifiks′).   See **fixed idea.**

identical twins.   See **monozygotic twins.**

identification,   an unconscious defense mechanism by which a person patterns his personality on that of another person, assuming the person's qualities, characteristics, and actions. The process is a normal function of personality development and learning, and it contributes to the acquisition of interests and ideals. Kinds of identification are **competitive identification, positive identification.**

identity crisis,   a period of disorientation concerning an individual's sense of self and role in society, occurring most frequently in the transition from one stage of life to the next. Identity crises are most common during adolescence, when a sudden increase in the strength of internal drives combined with greater peer pressure and parents' or society's expectations of more mature behavior often results in conflicts. The youngster may become confused about personal worth, abilities, values, goals, choice of vocation, and place in the world. The erosion of family life, social fluidity, mobility of the population, and changes in the relationships between the sexes all contribute to an increased incidence of identity crises. Although confusion regarding one's identity is usually considered an adolescent problem, it also is widespread among elderly people who lose their status in the community and their position as head of a family.

ideokinetic apraxia.   See **ideomotor apraxia.**

ideomotor apraxia,   the inability to translate an idea into motion, resulting from some interference with the transmission of the appropriate impulses from the brain to the motor centers. There is no loss of the ability to perform an action automatically, as tying the shoelaces, but the action cannot be performed on request. The condition is often owing to diffuse cortical disease. Also called **classic apraxia, ideokinetic apraxia, limb-kinetic apraxia, transcortical apraxia.** See also **apraxia.**

ideophobia (ai′diəfou′biə),   an anxiety disorder characterized by the irrational fear or distrust of ideas or reason. See also **phobia.**

idio-,   a combining form meaning 'pertaining to self or to something separate': *idiocratic, idioneurosis, idioventricular.*

idiomere.   See **chromomere.**

idiopathic (ıd′ioupæfh′ık),   without a known cause. An **idiopathic disease** may have a recognizable pattern of signs and symptoms; it may be curable, but its cause is not known.

idiopathic disease,   a disease that arises without an apparent or known cause.

idiopathic multiple pigmented hemorrhagic sarcoma. See **Kaposi's sarcoma.**

idiopathic scoliosis,   an abnormal condition characterized by a lateral curvature of the spine. It is the most common type of scoliosis, evident in 70 per cent of all patients with scoliosis and up to 80 per cent of those with structural scoliosis. It may occur at any age, but three types are commonly associated with certain age groups. The infantile type affects one- to three-year-olds. The juvenile type affects three- to ten-year-olds. The adolescent type affects preadolescents and adolescents. The main factors in diagnosing idiopathic scoliosis are the degree, balance, and rotational component of the curvature. The rotational component may contribute to rib cage deformities and impingement on the pulmonary and the cardiac systems. The most common type is the adolescent type. Early diagnosis is difficult because the associated curvature is often hidden by clothing, and many states have started scoliosis screening programs for the early detection of this condition. The signs commonly associated with scoliosis include unlevel shoulders, a prominent scapula, a prominent breast, a prominent flank area, an unlevel or a prominent hip, poor posture, and an obvious curvature. During diagnosis it is necessary to view the patient from the front, from the back, and while the patient is bending. Other signs that may be associated with idiopathic scoliosis are occasional transient pain and fatigue and decreased pulmonary function. Radiographic films of the spine in the bending position are important in ascertaining the flexibility of the curvature and the potential of spontaneous correction. Neurologic deficits are commonly associated with severe curvature and vary according to the extent to which the curvature has impinged on the spinal cord. Some signs of such impingement are reflex, sensation, and motor alterations of the lower extremities. Nonsurgical intervention commonly employs observation, an exercise program, and a Milwaukee brace. Observation and an exercise program often suffice, the observation implemented by frequent physical examinations and radiographic monitoring of the progress of the curvature. Exercise programs are designed to promote the maximum correction possible, as indicated by the degree of flexibility shown in the initial x-ray examination. Observation and the exercise program are employed with patients who have a curvature under 15° to 20°. Greater degrees of curvature usually require the use of a Milwaukee brace in addition to observation and an exercise program. The Milwaukee brace, which is usually worn 23 hours a day, is used to control the progress of the curvature. The exercise program is implemented when the adolescent is out of the brace, and additional exercises are performed while in the brace. Surgical intervention may be required if the curvature has progressed to 40° or more at the time of diagnosis or if a slightly lesser degree of curvature exists with a high degree of rotational component or imbalance. Approximately 5 to 10 per cent of patients with idiopathic scoliosis require surgical intervention, which involves fusing of the involved vertebrae to prevent progress of the deformity. Preoperative traction, as Cotrel traction and halo-femoral traction, may also be used to encourage gradual tissue alterations and to decrease postoperative complications. The patient involved may be placed in Cotrel traction for a period of 5 to 10 days preoperatively. If halo-femoral traction is used, the patient may be placed in traction 1 to 3 weeks preoperatively. Some physicians apply a preoperative cast to their patients with idiopathic scoliosis to achieve immobilization and adjustment, especially if surgery must be postponed for a considerable period following diagnosis. Common surgical intervention techniques for this condition are Harrington rod instrumentation technique and Dwyer cable instrumentation technique, the former being more common. Initial postoperative immobilization is achieved with a posterior plaster shell, a Milwaukee brace, or a windowed cast. A Stryker frame, Foster frame, or CircOlectric bed may also be utilized. Blood replacement may be required postoperatively, and appropriate intravenous therapy is usually employed for several days. Additional postoperative immobilization by means of cast therapy is often required for 8 to 12 months or until the bony union of the fused area is absolutely assured. The usual type of cast in this application is a Risser localizer cast, applied with a degree of traction. The Risser turnbuckle cast may also be used when instrumentation has not been employed. A Milwaukee brace or a plastic body jacket may be used when less immobilization is desired.

idiopathic thrombocytopenic purpura (ITP), bleeding into the skin and other organs owing to a deficiency of platelets. **Acute ITP,** a disease of children, may follow a viral infection, lasts a few weeks to a few months, and usually has no residua. **Chronic ITP,** more common in adolescents and adults, begins more insidiously and lasts longer. Antibodies to platelets have been in patients with ITP; the condition may be transmitted to the fetus if a pregnant woman develops it. Treatment includes corticosteroids and splenectomy. See also **thrombocytopenia, thrombocytopenic purpura.**

idiopathy, any primary disease that arises without an apparent cause. —**idiopathic,** *adj.*

idiosyncrasy (ɪd′iousɪn′krəsi), **idiocrasy** (ɪd′iok′rəsi), **1.** a physical or behavioral characteristic or manner that is unique to an individual or to a group. **2.** an individual's unique hypersensitivity to a particular drug, food, or other substance. See also **allergy.** —**idiosyncratic,** *adj.*

idiot, *Obsolete.* a severely retarded person having an intelligence quotient of less than 20, incapable of developing beyond the mental age of three or four years. Compare **imbecile, moron.** See also **mental retardation.** —**idiocy,** *n.,* **idiotic,** *adj.*

idiot savant (sævant′), *pl.* **idiot savants** (*French.* **idiots savants).** an individual with severe mental retardation who is nonetheless capable of performing certain unusual mental feats, primarily those involving music, puzzle-solving, or the manipulation of numbers.

-idium, a noun-forming combining form: *coracidium, parorchidium, thrombidium.*

idoxuridine (ɪdoksyur′ədin), an ophthalmic antiviral.

■ INDICATION: It is prescribed for herpes simplex keratitis.

■ CONTRAINDICATIONS: Deep ulceration of the cornea or known hypersensitivity to this drug prohibits its use.

■ ADVERSE EFFECTS: Among the more serious adverse reactions are visual disturbances.

-iform, a combining form meaning 'in the form of': *amebiform, bulbiform, nucleiform.*

Ig, abbreviation for **immunoglobulin.**

IgA, abbreviation for **immunoglobulin A.**

IgA deficiency, a selective lack of immunoglobulin A, the most common type of immunoglobulin deficiency, appearing in about 1 in 400 individuals. Immunoglobulin A is a major protein antibody in the saliva and the mucous membranes of the intestines and the bronchi. It protects against bacterial and viral infections. A deficiency of immunoglobulin A is associated with autosomal dominant or with autosomal recessive inheritance, and with autoimmune abnormalities. The IgA deficiency is common in patients with rheumatoid arthritis and in patients with systemic lupus erythematosus. Many individuals with this deficiency have normal numbers of peripheral blood lymphocytes with IgA receptors and normal amounts of other immunoglobulins. Normality accompanied by IgA deficiency suggests that the B-lymphocytes of the involved patient may not secrete IgA. In some patients with this deficiency, T cells seem to depress the synthesis of IgA. ■ OBSERVATIONS: Symptoms of IgA deficiency are often lacking in patients whose humoral immune systems may be compensating for low IgA with extra amounts of IgM to assure adequate defenses. Common symptoms are respiratory allergies associated with chronic sinopulmonary infection, gastrointestinal diseases, as celiac disease and regional enteritis, autoimmune diseases, as rheumatoid arthritis, systemic lupus erythematosus, and chronic hepatitis, malignant tumors, as squamous cell carcinoma of the lungs, recticulum cell sarcoma, and thymona. The age of onset varies. Some children with IgA deficiency may begin to synthesize the immunoglobulin spontaneously when their recurrent infections wane and their conditions improve. Diagnoses of IgA-deficient patients depend on the results of tests which commonly show normal IgE and IgM levels while IgA levels are below 5 mg/dl in serum. Cell-mediated reponse and circulating B cells commonly appear normal, although tests may indicate autoantibodies and antibodies against IgG, IgM, and cow's milk. T cell interferon production may be decreased in some patients with IgA deficiency, increasing the chances of infection. ■ INTERVENTION: There is no known cure for selective IgA deficiency; treatment usually involves the effort to control associated diseases, as respiratory and gastrointestinal infections. ■ NURSING CONSIDERATIONS:The patient with IgA deficiency should not receive gamma globulin because associated sensitization may cause anaphylaxis during administration of blood products. When the IgA deficient patient requires a blood transfusion, the risk of any harmful reaction can be reduced by using washed red blood cells. Using the cross-matched blood of an IgA deficient donor in such a transfusion is considered a safer method and completely avoids the risk of an adverse reaction. The

IgA deficiency is a lifelong condition and patients with this disorder are commonly instructed to identify its symptoms and to seek treatment promptly.

IgD, abbreviation for **immunoglobulin D.**

IgE, abbreviation for **immunoglobulin E.**

IgG, abbreviation for **immunoglobulin G.**

IgM, abbreviation for **immunoglobulin M.**

Ikwa fever. See **trench fever.**

-il, a combining form meaning a 'substance related to another': *benzil, uracil, uramil.* Also **-ile.**

10-ile. See **-il.**

ileitis (ıl′iaı′tıs). See **Crohn's disease.**

ileo-, a combining form meaning 'pertaining to the ileum': *ileocecum, ileorectostomy, ileotomy.*

ileocecal valve, the valve between the ileum of the small intestine and the cecum of the large intestine. The valve consists of two flaps which project into the lumen of the large intestine, just above the vermiform appendix, allowing the contents of the intestine to pass only in a forward direction.

ileocecostomy (ıl′iɔusikos′təmi). See **cecolieostomy.**

ileocolic node (ıl′iɔukol′ık), a node in one of three groups of superior mesenteric lymph glands, forming a chain of approximately 15 nodes around the ileocolic artery. They tend to form in two main groups, one near the duodenum, the other on the lower part of the ileocolic artery. The chain breaks into several groups where the artery divides into its terminal branches. The ileocolic nodes receive afferents from the jejunum, ilieum, cecum, vermiform appendix, ascending colon, and transverse colon. Their efferents pass to the preaortic nodes. Compare **mesenteric node, mesocolic node.**

ileostomate (ıl′ios′təmeit), a person who has undergone an ileostomy.

ileostomy (ıl′ios′təmi), surgical formation of an opening of the ileum onto the surface of the abdomen, through which fecal matter is emptied. The operation is performed in advanced or recurrent ulcerative colitis, Crohn's disease, or cancer of the large bowel. A low-residue diet is given preoperatively and is reduced to fluids 24 hours before surgery to decrease intestinal residue. Intestinal antibiotics are given to decrease the bacterial count. A nasogastric or intestinal tube is passed. The diseased portion of the large bowel is removed in a permanent ileostomy; occasionally, the distal and proximal segments of bowel may be reconnected after ulcerated areas have healed. A loop of the proximal ileum is then brought out onto the abdomen and sutured in place, and a stoma is formed. A pouch may be made with part of the terminal ileum, in which the open end is woven through the rectus muscles to form a valve and then opens onto the abdomen. Postoperatively, the patient wears a temporary disposable bag to collect the semiliquid fecal matter, which begins to drain once peristalsis is restored and the tube is removed. Since the secretions contain digestive enzymes which can ulcerate the skin around the stoma, the nurse ensures that nothing leaks from the bag. The nurse instructs the patient how to apply and care for the stoma and the colostomy bag. If a pouch is present, it is irrigated or drained three or four times a day through a small irrigating catheter through the valve. Compare **colostomy**. See also **enterostomy, ostomy irrigation, stoma.**

ileum (il′iəm), the distal portion of the small intestine, extending from the jejunum to the cecum. It has a few small circular folds and numerous clusters of lymph nodes. It ends in the right iliac fossa, opening into the medial side of the large intestine. —**ileac, ileal,** *adj.*

ileus (il′iəs), an obstruction of the intestines, as an adynamic ileus caused by immobility of the bowel, or a mechanical ileus in which the intestine is blocked by mechanical means.

-iliac, a combining form meaning 'the ilium': *occipitoiliac, subiliac, vertebroiliac.*

iliac circumflex node (il′iæk), a node in one of the seven clusters of parietal lymph nodes of the abdomen. This node is one of a group found along the course of the deep iliac circumflex vessels. Compare **common iliac node, external iliac node, internal iliac node.** See also **lymph, lymphatic system, lymph node.**

iliac fascia, the portion of the endoabdominal fascia that is attached with the iliacus to the crest of the ilium and passes under the inguinal ligament into the thigh.

iliacus (ilai′əkəs), a flat, triangular muscle that covers the inner curved surface of the iliac fossa. It arises from the inner aspect of the superior iliac crest, from the anterior and the iliolumbar ligaments, and from the sacrum. It joins the psoas major to form the iliopsoas at the inguinal ligament. The iliacus is innervated by branches of the femoral nerve that contain fibers from the second and the third lumbar nerves. It acts to flex and laterally rotate the thigh. Compare **psoas major, psoas minor.**

ilio-, a combining form meaning 'of or pertaining to the ilium or flank': *iliocostal, iliolumbar, iliometer.*

iliofemoral (il′ioufem′ərəl), of or pertaining to the ilium and femur.

ilioinguinal (il′iouiŋg′gwinəl), of or pertaining to the hip and inguinal regions.

iliolumbar ligament, one of a pair of ligaments forming part of the connection between the vertebral column and the pelvis. Each iliolumbar ligament attaches to a transverse process of the fifth lumbar vertebra and passes to the base of the sacrum.

iliopsoas (il′iousou′əs), one of the pair of muscle complexes that flexes the thigh and the lumbar vertebral column. Each complex is comprised of the psoas major, the psoas minor, and the iliacus, although the psoas minor is often absent. The psoas major is a long fusiform muscle, arising from certain lumbar vertebrae and inserting into

the femur. The iliacus is a flat, triangular muscle arising from the iliac fossa and inserting into the femur and the tendon of the psoas major. The psoas minor is a long slender muscle ventral to the psoas major.

ilium (il′iəm), *pl.* **ilia,** one of the three bones that make up the innominate bone. The ilium forms part of the acetabulum and provides attachment for several muscles, including the obturator internus, the gluteals, the iliacus, and the sartorius. The ilium is divided into the body, which forms less than two fifths of the acetabulum, and the ala, which is the large, winglike portion of the greater pelvis. The ala contains the iliac fossa and the greater sciatic notch and presents various prominences for muscle attachment, as the iliac crest, the anterior superior and the posterior superior iliac spines, and the anterior inferior and the posterior inferior iliac spines. Compare **ischium, pubis.** —**iliac,** *adj.*

illness, an abnormal process in which aspects of the social, physical, emotional, or intellectual condition and function of a person are diminished or impaired, compared to that person's previous condition.

illness experience, the process of being ill, comprised of five stages: phase I, experiencing a symptom; phase II, assuming a sick role; phase III, making contact for health care; phase IV, being dependent (a patient); and phase V, recovering or being rehabilitated. Each stage is characterized by certain decisions, behaviors, and end points. During phase I, in which a symptom is experienced, the person decides that something is wrong and tries to remedy the situation. Phase I ends with the person accepting the reality of the symptom, no longer delaying any action toward help or denying the symptom (flight into health). During phase II the person decides that the illness is real and that care is necessary. Advice, guidance, and validation are sought. This gives the person permission to act sick and to be excused temporarily from usual obligations. The outcome of this phase is acceptance of the role —or denial of its necessity. In phase III professional advice is sought; authoritative declarations identify and validate the illness and legitimize the sick role. The person usually asks for help and negotiates for treatment. Denial may still occur and the patient may 'shop' further for medical care or may accept the illness, the medical authority, and the plan for treatment. In phase IV professional treatment is performed and accepted by the person, who is now perceived as a patient. At any time during this phase the dependent patient may develop ambivalent feelings and may decide to reject the treatment, the care giver, and the illness. More often, care is accepted with ambivalence. The patient has a particular need to be informed and to be given emotional support during this phase. During phase V, the last stage of the illness experience, the patient relinquishes the sick role. The usual tasks and roles are resumed to the greatest degree possible. Some people do not willingly give up the sick role, becoming, in their own eyes, chronically ill or, for secondary gain, they malinger, acting sick. Most people accept the recovery and work toward rehabilitation.

illumination, the lighting up of a part of the body or of an object under a microscope for the purpose of examination. **— illuminate,** *v.*

illusion, a false interpretation of an external sensory stimulus, usually visual or auditory, as a mirage in the desert or voices on the wind. Compare **delusion, hallucination.**

Ilopan, a trade name for a precursor of coenzyme A (dexpanthenol).

Ilosone, a trade name for an antibacterial (erythromycin estolate).

im-, **1.** a combining form in chemistry indicating the bivalent group > NH: *imadyl, imide, imperialine.*

I.M.A., abbreviation for **Industrial Medical Association.**

image, **1.** a representation or visual reproduction of the likeness of someone or something, as a painting, photograph, or sculpture. **2.** an optical representation of an object, as that produced by refraction or reflection. **3.** a person or thing that closely resembles another; semblance. **4.** a mental picture, representation, idea, or concept of an objective reality. **5.** (in psychology) a mental representation of something previously perceived and subsequently modified by other experiences resulting from intrapsychic or extrapsychic stimuli, or both. Kinds of images include **body image, eidetic image, memory image, mental image, motor image, tactile image.**

imagery, (in psychiatry) the formation of mental concepts, figures, ideas; any product of the imagination. In mentally disturbed persons these images are often bizarre and delusional.

imagination, **1.** the ability to form, or the act or process of forming mental images or conscious concepts of things that are not immediately available to the senses. **2.** (in psychology) the ability to reproduce images or ideas stored in the memory by the stimulation or suggestion of associated ideas or to regroup former ideas and concepts to form new images and ideas concerned with a particular goal or problem. See also **fantasy.**

imaging, the formation of a mental picture or representation of someone or something using the imagination. See also **fantasy.**

imago (ɪmeɪ′gou), (in analytic psychology) an unconscious, usually idealized mental image of a significant individual in a person's early, formative years. See also **identification.**

Imavate, a trade name for an antidepressant (imipramine hydrochloride).

imbalance, **1.** lack of balance between opposing muscle groups, as in the imbalance of extraocular muscles, leading to strabismus. **2.** an abnormal balance of fluid and electrolytes in the body tissues. **3.** an unequal distribution of subjects in a population group, as an only girl in a large family of boys. **4.** a person with mental abilities that are remarkable in one area but deficient in others, as an idiot savant.

imbecile, *Obsolete.* a moderately retarded person having an intelligence quotient of 20 to 49, incapable of developing beyond a mental age of seven or eight years. Compare **idiot, moron.** See also **mental retardation.** **— imbecile, imbecilic,** *adj.,* **imbecility,** *n.*

imbricate (ɪm′brɪkeɪt), to build a surface with overlapping layers of material. Surgeons may imbricate with layers of tissue when closing a wound or other opening in a body part. **— imbrication,** *n.*

Imferon, a trade name for an injectable hematinic (iron dextran).

imido-, a combining form indicating the presence in a chemical compound of the bivalent group > NH: *imidogen.*

imino-, a combining form indicating the presence of the bivalent group > NH attached to a nonacid radical: *imino-urea.*

iminoglycinuria, a benign familial condition characterized by the abnormal urinary excretion of the amino acids glycine, proline, and hydroxyproline.

imipramine hydrochloride, a tricyclic antidepressant.
- INDICATION: It is prescribed in the treatment of mental depression.
- CONTRAINDICATIONS: Concomitant administration of monoamine oxidase inhibitors, recent myocardial infarction, cardiovascular disease or seizure disorder, or known hypersensitivity to this drug or to other tricyclic medication prohibits its use.
- ADVERSE EFFECTS: Among the more serious adverse reactions are sedation, gastrointestinal disturbances, and cardiovascular and neurologic reactions. This drug interacts with many other drugs.

immediate auscultation, a method of examining a patient by placing an ear or stethoscope on the skin directly over the body part being studied.

immediate hypersensitivity, an allergic reaction that occurs within minutes after exposure to an allergen.

immediate hypersensitivity reaction. See **hypersensitivity reaction.**

immediate percussion. See **percussion.**

immediate post-traumatic automatism, a post-traumatic state in which a person acts spontaneously and automatically without having any recollection of the behavior.

immersion, the placing of a body or an object into water or other liquid so that it is completely covered by the liquid. **— immerse,** *v.*

immersion foot, an abnormal condition of the feet characterized by damage to the muscles, nerves, skin and blood vessels, caused by prolonged exposure to dampness or by prolonged immersion in cold water. See also **frostbite.**

imminent abortion. See **inevitable abortion.**

immiscible (ımıs′əbəl), not capable of being mixed, as oil and water. Compare **miscible.**

immune complex hypersensitivity, an IgG or IgM complement dependent, immediate acting humoral hypersensitivity to certain soluble antigens. An intradermal skin test results in erythema and edema within three to eight hours and an acute inflammatory reaction with an increase in polymorphonuclear leukocytes. It is seen in serum sickness, Arthus reaction, and glomerulonephritis. Also called **type III hypersensitivity.** Compare **anaphylactic hypersensitivity, cell-mediated hypersensitivity, cytotoxic hypersensitivity.**

immune cytolysis, cell destruction mediated by a particular antibody in conjunction with complement.

immune gamma globulin, passive immunizing agents obtained from pooled human plasma. Also called **immune globulin.** See also **immunoglobulin G.**

■ INDICATIONS: It is prescribed for immunization against measles, poliomyelitis, chickenpox, serum hepatitis following transfusion, hepatitis A, agammaglobulinemia, and hypogammaglobulinemia.

■ CONTRAINDICATION: Known hypersensitivity to gamma globulins prohibit its use.

■ ADVERSE EFFECTS: Among the more serious adverse reactions are pain and inflammation at the site of injection and allergic reactions.

immune globulin. See **immune gamma globulin.**

immune human globulin, a sterile solution of globulins, used as a passive immunizing agent, derived from adult human blood.

immune serum. See **antiserum.**

immune serum globulin, (ISG). **1.** See **chickenpox.** **2.** See **immune human globulin.** **3.** See **immunoglobulin antibody.**

immune response, a defense function of the body that produces antibodies to destroy invading antigens and malignancies. Important components of the immune system and response are immunoglobulins, lymphocytes, phagocytes, complement, properdin, the migratory inhibitory factor, and interferon. Antigens, which are largely foreign protein macromolecules, trigger the immune response during interaction with countless cells of the reticuloendothelial system of the body. The kinds of immune response are humoral immune response, involving B-lymphocytes or B cells, and cell-mediated immune response, involving T-lymphocytes or T cells. The B cells and the T cells derive from the hemopoietic stem cells, which originate in the embryonic yolk sac. Every normal baby is born with many different clones of B cells in the bone marrow, the lymph nodes, and the spleen. All the cells of each clone synthesize a specific antibody with a different sequence of amino acids from that of any of the other numerous clones of B cells. The receptor sites on the surface membranes of the B cells are the combining sites of immunoglobulin molecules. The classes of immunoglobulins, identified by letter names, are M, G, A, E, and D. Immunoglobulin M, the antibody that immature B cells synthesize and incorporate in their cytoplasmic membranes, is the predominant antibody produced after initial contact with an antigen. The T cells develop in the thymus gland and proliferate with antigen receptors on their surface membranes. The T cells assist in the antigen-antibody reaction of the B cells and control the cell-mediated response associated with the reduction of tissue inflammation. The cell-mediated response is also effective against fungi, viruses, and tumors and is the major reaction in the rejection of organ transplants. In transplant surgery, certain methods, as the administration of appropriate drugs and radiation, suppress transplant rejection. The T cells have little or no immunoglobulin on their surfaces and always maintain their leukocyte structure. They are divided into circulating T cells, noncirculating T cells, and memory T cells. Circulating T cells function within circulating fluids; noncirculating T cells include those that produce lymphokines and selectively migrate to inflamed tissue sites. Memory T cells recognize antigens as foreign and mobilize tissue macrophages in the presence of the migratory inhibitory factor. Humoral immune response protects the body against bacterial and viral infections through the stimulation of antibodies associated with the B cells. Plasma cells, which derive from B cells through the stimulation of antigens, secrete trillions of antibody molecules that aid the humoral immune response. Such molecules recognize microinvaders of the body as "foreigners" when the antigens bind to them. The antigen-antibody reaction may transform the toxic antigen into a harmless substance, or it may agglutinate antigens, allowing macrophages and other phagocytes to digest large numbers of antigens at one time. The antigen-antibody reactions of the humoral immune response also activate the complement in the blood serum, which triggers a nonspecific series of chemical reactions to amplify the humoral immune response. Activated discrete plasma proteins C_1 to C_3 in the complement system cause lysis of the antigenic cell and opsonize the antigen for phagocytosis. Humoral immune response may begin immediately with antigen contact or may be delayed for as long as 48 hours. The speed of humoral response is demonstrated in anaphylaxis. Other proteins associated with the immune response are properdin and interferon. Properdin provides an alternate process for activating complement. Interferon is synthesized by body cells after viral invasion acts to combat viruses and may retard the growth of cancer cells. Humoral immune response and cell-mediated immune response immunity are interdependent. The former can influence the function of T cells and the latter the function of B cells. Humoral and cell-mediated immunity can be natural or acquired. Natural immunity, or genetically inherited resistance to specific infectious organisms, can be affected by diet, mental health, environment, metabolism, and the virulence of invading pathogens.

immune system, a biochemical complex which protects the body against pathogenic organisms and other foreign bodies. The system incorporates the humoral immune response, which produces antibodies to react with specific antigens, and the cell-mediated response, which uses T-cells to mobilize tissue macrophages in the presence of a foreign body. The immune system also protects the body from invasion by creating local barriers and inflammation. The local barriers provide chemical and mechanical defenses through the skin, the mucous membranes, and the conjunctiva. Inflammation draws polymorphonuclear leukocytes and neutrophils to the site of injury where these phagocytes engulf the invading organism. The humoral response and the cell-mediated response develop if these first-line defenses fail or are inadequate to protect the body. The humoral immune response is especially effective against bacterial and viral invasions and employs B-cells that produce appropriate antibodies. The principal organs of the immune response system include the bone marrow, the thymus, and the lymphoid tissues. The system also employs peripheral organs, as the lymph nodes, the spleen, and the lymphatic vessels. The antigen-antibody reactions of the immune system activate the complement system, which removes antigens from the body. The complement system contains several discrete proteins which function to produce lysis of the antigenic cells. The humoral response may begin immediately on invasion by the antigen or may start as long as 48 hours later.

immunity, 1. (in civil law) exemption from a duty or an obligation generally required by law, as an exemption from taxation, exemption from penalty for wrongdoing, or protection against liability. 2. the quality of being insusceptible to or unaffected by a particular disease or condition. —**immune,** *adj.*

immunization, a process by which resistance to an infectious disease is induced or augmented.

immunodeficient (ɪmyu'noudɪfɪsh'ənt), an abnormal condition of the immune system in which cellular or humoral immunity is inadequate and resistance to infection is decreased. Kinds of immunodeficient conditions are **hypogammaglobulinemia, lymphoid aplasia.**

immunodiagnosis. See **serological diagnosis.**

immunodiagnostic (ɪmyu'noudai'əgnos'tɪk), pertaining to or characterizing a diagnosis based on an antigen-antibody reaction. In many cases, a tumor releases a discrete antigenic substance into the blood; detection of a particular antigen can provide an immunodiagnostic sign of the presence of the tumor associated with that antigen.

immunodiffusion (ɪmyu'noudɪfyu'zhən), a technique for the identification and quantification of any of the immunoglobulins. It is based on the presence of a visible precipitate that results from an antigen-antibody combination under certain circumstances. **Gel diffusion** is a technique that involves evaluation of the precipitin reaction in a clear gel, seen when an antigen placed in a hole in the agarose diffuses evenly into the medium. An obvious ring forms where the antigen meets the antibody. **Electroimmunodiffusion** is a gel diffusion to which an electric field is applied, accelerating the reaction. **Double gel diffusion** is a technique that permits identification of antibodies in mixed specimens. In an agar plate, antigen is placed in one well, antibody in another. Antigen and antibody diffuse out of their wells. In mixed antigen specimens, each antigen-antibody combination forms a separate line; observation of the location, shape, and thickness of a line permits identification and quantification of the antibody.

immunoelectrodiffusion (ɪmyu'noʊɪlek'troʊdɪfyu'zhən). See **immunodiffusion.**

immunoelectrophoresis (ɪmyu'noʊɪlek'troʊfəri'sɪs), a technique that combines electrophoresis and immunodiffusion to separate and allow identification of complex proteins. The proteins in the test serum are spread out in agar and separated by electrophoresis. Wells or troughs are then cut into the agar, and aliquots of antibody are placed in the troughs and allowed to diffuse toward the separated proteins. A visible precipitin will form in a series of arcs in the agar when an antigen-antibody reaction occurs. The shape and location of each arc are specific for known proteins. Unusual arcs are representative of abnormal or unknown protein. Although the density of the precipitation corresponds to the concentration of protein in each electrophoretic band, immunoelectrophoresis does not accurately quantify the amount of protein in the test serum. — **immunoelectrophoretic,** *adj.*

immunofluorescence (ɪmyu'noʊflʊres'əns), a technique used for the rapid identification of an antigen by exposing it to known antibodies tagged with the fluorescent dye fluorescein and observing the characteristic antigen-antibody reaction of precipitation. As the fluorescent antibody reacts with its specific antigen, the precipitate appears luminous in the ultraviolet light projected by a fluorescent microscope. Many of the most common infectious organisms can be identified using this technique. Among them are *Candida albicans, Haemophilus influenzae, Neisseria gonorrhae, Shigella, Staphylococcus aureus,* and several viruses, including rabies virus and many enteroviruses. See also **fluorescent microscopy.** — **immunofluorescent,** *adj.*

immunofluorescence test. See **fluorescent antibody test.**

immunofluorescent microscopy. See **fluorescent microscopy, immunofluorescence.**

immunogen (ɪmyu'nəjɪn), any agent or substance capable of provoking an immune response or producing immunity. —**immunogenic,** *adj.*

immunoglobulin A (IgA), one of the five classes of humoral antibodies produced by the body and one of the most prevalent. It is found in all secretions of the body and is the major antibody in the mucous membrane lining the intestines and in the bronchi, saliva, and tears. IgA combines with a protein in the muscosa and defends body surfaces against invading microorganisms. Research indicates that it protects body tissues by seeking out foreign microorganisms and triggering an antigen-antibody reaction. Compare **immunoglobulin D, immunoglobulin E, immunoglobulin G, immunoglobulin M.**

immunoglobulin antibody, any of five structurally and antigenically distinct antibodies present in the serum and external secretions of the body. In response to specific antigens, immunoglobulins are formed in the bone marrow, spleen, and all lymphoid tissue of the body except the thymus. Kinds of immunoglobulins are **IgA, IgE, IgG, IgM, IgP.** Also called **immune serum globulin.** See also **antibody, antigen, immunity.**

immunoglobulin D (IgD), one of the five classes of humoral antibodies produced by the body. It is a specialized protein found in small amounts in serum tissue. The precise function of IgD is not known, but it increases in quantity during allergic reactions to milk, insulin, penicillin, and various toxins. Compare **immunoglobulin A, immunoglobulin E, immunoglobulin G, immunoglobulin M.**

immunoglobulin E (IgE), one of the five classes of humoral antibodies produced by the body. It is concentrated in the lung, the skin, and the cells of mucous membranes. It provides the primary defense against environmental antigens and is believed to be responsive to immunoglobulin A. IgE reacts with certain antigens to release certain chemical mediators which cause Type I hypersensitivity reactions characterized by wheal and flare. Compare **immunoglobulin A, immunoglobulin D, immunoglobulin G, immunoglobulin M.**

immunoglobulin G (IgG), one of the five classes of humoral antibodies produced by the body. It is a specialized protein synthesized by the body in response to invasions by bacteria, fungi, and viruses. IgG crosses the placenta and protects against red cell antigens and white cell antigens. Compare **immunoglobulin A, immunoglobulin D, immunoglobulin E, immunoglobulin M.**

immunoglobulin M (IgM), one of the five classes of humoral antibodies produced by the body and the largest in molecular structure. It is the first immunoglobulin the body produces when challenged by antigens and is found in circulating fluids. IgM triggers the increased production of immunoglobulin G and the complement fixation required for effective antibody response. It is the dominant antibody in ABO incompatibilities. Compare **immunoglobulin A, immunoglobulin D, immunoglobulin E, immunoglobulin G.**

immunologist, a specialist in immunology.

immunology, the study of the reaction of tissues of the immune system of the body to antigenic stimulation.

immunomodulator, a substance that acts to alter the immune response by augmenting or reducing the ability of the immune system to produce specifically modified serum antibodies or sensitized cells that recognize and react with the antigen that initiated their production. Corticosteroids, cytotoxic agents, thymosin, and the immunoglobulins are among the immunomodulating substances. Some immunomodulating substances are naturally present in the body; some of these are available in various pharmacologic preparations. —**immunomodulation,** *n.*

immunosuppression (ɪmyu'nousəpreSH'ən), **1.** the administration of agents that significantly interfere with the ability of the immune system to respond to antigenic stimulation by inhibiting cellular and humoral immunity. Corticosteroid hormones given in large amounts, cytotoxic drugs, including antimetabolites and alkylating agents, antilymphocytic serum (ALS), and irradiation may result in immunosupression. Immunosuppression may be deliberate, as in preparation for bone marrow or other transplantation to prevent rejection by the host of the donor tissue, or incidental, as often results from chemotherapy for the treatment of cancer. **2.** an abnormal condition of the immune system characterized by markedly inhibited ability to respond to antigenic stimuli. —**immunosuppressed,** *adj.*

immunosuppressive (ɪmyu'nousəpres'ɪv), **1.** of or pertaining to a substance or procedure that lessens or prevents an immune response. **2.** an immunosuppresive agent. The immunosuppressive drugs used most frequently to prevent homograft rejection are the cytotoxic purine antimetabolite azathioprine, the alkylating agent cyclophosphamide, and the adrenocoricosteroid prednisone. Methotrexate, cytarbine, dactinomycin, thioguanine, and antilymphocyte globulin are also potent immunosuppressives. The use of some of these agents is being explored for the treatment of autoimmune diseases, as systemic lupus erythematosus, and for many other disorders.

immunotherapy, a special treatment of allergic responses which administers increasingly large doses of the offending allergens to gradually develop immunity. Immunotherapy is based on the premise that low doses of the offending allergen will bind with IgG to prevent an allergic reaction by damping the action of IgE by fostering the synthesis of the blocking IgG antibody. The individual who is exposed to the offending allergen develops an amount of blocking antibody in proportion to the extent of the exposure. The blocking antibody binds to the circulating antigen and seems to decrease the allergic response, or it eliminates the allergic response by producing an immunologic tolerance toward the antigen. In immunotherapy low doses of the offending allergen are gradually increased throughout the year or during a 3- to 6-month period before the allergy season starts; it usually continues until the patient shows no significant allergic response for 2 to 5 years. Also called **hyposensitization.** — **immunotherapeutic,** *adj.*

Imodium, a trade name for an intestinal antiperistaltic (loperamide hydrochloride), used as an antidiarrheal agent.

impacted, tightly or firmly wedged in a limited amount of space. — **impact,** *v.,* **impaction,** *adj.*

impacted fracture, a bone break in which the adjacent fragmented ends of the fractured bone are mashed together.

impedance audiometry. See **audiometry.**

impedance plethysmography, a technique for detecting blood vessel occlusion that determines volumetric changes in the limb by measuring changes in its girth as indicated by changes in the electrical impedance of mercury-containing silastic tubes in a pressure cuff. The method is based on the principle that any circumferential rate of change in a limb segment is directly proportional to the volumetric rate of change, which in turn reflects occlusion of venous and arterial blood flow. However, the technique does not accurately indicate the presence or absence of partially obstructing thrombi in major vessels.

imperative conception, a thought or impression that appears spontaneously in the mind and cannot be eliminated, as an obsession.

imperative idea. See **compulsive idea.**

imperforate (ımpər′fərıt), lacking a normal opening in a body organ or passageway. An infant may be born with an imperforate anus. Compare **perforate.**

imperforate anus, any of several congenital, developmental malformations of the anorectal portion of the gastrointestinal tract.

■ OBSERVATION: The most common form is anal agenesis, in which the rectal pouch ends blindly above the surface of the perineum. An anal fistula is present in 80 to 90 per cent of cases. Other forms include anal stenosis, in which the anal aperture is small, and anal membrane atresia, in which the anal membrane covers the aperture creating an obstruction.

■ INTERVENTION: The defect is usually discovered at birth; inspection reveals an absence of the anus or the presence of a thin translucent membrane covering it. Digital and endoscopic examination allows identification of the anatomic character of the malformation. X-ray examination is performed to outline the rectal pouch. A radiopaque marker is placed at the usual site of the anus, and the infant is held upside down. Air moving through the intestines into the distal portion of the bowel or the rectum is visible on the x-ray film. Anal stenosis is treated with daily digital dilatation begun in the hospital and continued at home by the parents. An imperforate anal membrane is excised, and digital dilatation is performed daily as the skin heals. Surgical reconstruction is performed to treat anal agenesis in infants in whom the pouch is below the puborectalis of the levator ani; an anus is created surgically by an anoplasty. Anal atresia in which the pouch at the end of the bowel is high above the perineum may require a colostomy.

■ NURSING CONSIDERATIONS: Often it is the nurse who identifies the anal malformation, as the thermometer cannot be inserted during the routine newborn assessment. A newborn who does not pass any stool in the first 24 hours requires further evaluation for the possibility of the defect. The passage of meconium from the vagina or urinary meatus clearly indicates the presence of anal fistula and usually occurs in association with an imperforate anus. Postoperative care in the newborn treated surgically for any of these conditions requires scrupulous perineal care.

impermeable, (of a tissue, membrane, or film) preventing the passage of a substance through it.

impetigo (ım′pətaı′goʊ), a streptococcal, a staphylococcal, or a combined infection of the skin beginning as focal erythema and progressing to pruritic vesicles, erosions, and honey-colored crusts. Lesions usually form on the face and spread locally. The disorder is highly contagious by contact with the discharge from the lesions. Acute glomerulonephritis is an occasional complication. Treatment includes thorough cleansing with antibacterial soap and water, compresses of Burow's solution, removal of crusts, and topical or oral antibiotics. Essential to prevent spread of infection are treatment of the sores, use of individual wash cloths and linens, and the need for scrupulous hand washing. — **impetiginous,** *adj.*

implant, 1. (in radiotherapy) an encapsulated radioactive substance embedded in tissue for therapy. Seeds containing iodine-125 may be implanted permanently in prostate and chest tumors and seeds of iridium-192 in ribbons or wire may be embedded temporarily in head and neck cancers. Sealed sources of cesium-137 or radium-226 may be implanted in the body cavity temporarily in the treatment of gynecological malignancies; strontium-90 in sealed sources may be embedded for a brief period (usually less than two minutes) in the treatment of eye tumors; needles containing radium-226 may be used as temporary interstitial implants. Patients with radioactive implants are isolated from other patients whenever possible. 2. (in surgery) material inserted or grafted into an organ or structure of the body. The implant may be of tissue, as in a blood vessel graft, or of an artificial substance, as in a hip prosthesis, a cardiac pacemaker, or a container of radioactive material.

implantation, (in embryology) the process involving the attachment, penetration, and embedding of the blastocyst in the lining of the uterine wall during the early stages of prenatal development. The degree of invasiveness required for an adequate maternal-fetal exchange varies greatly among species. In man, the process occurs over a period of a few days, beginning about the seventh or eighth day following fertilization, and consists of the complete embedding of the conceptus within the uterine endometrium. Kinds of implantation include **eccentric implantation, interstitial implantation, superficial implantation.** Also called **nidation.**

implantation dermoid cyst, a tumor derived from embryonal tissues, caused by an injury that forces part of the ectoderm into the body.

implementation, a deliberate action performed to achieve a goal, as carrying out a plan in caring for a patient. — **implement,** *v.*

implementing, (in five-step nursing process) a category of nursing behavior in which the actions necessary for accomplishing the health care plan are initiated and completed. Implementing includes the performance or assisting in the performance of the client's activities of daily living; counseling and teaching the client or the client's family; giving care to achieve therapeutic goals and to optimize the achievement of health goals by the client; supervising and evaluating the work of staff members; and recording and exchanging information relevant to the client's continued health care. The client may require assistance in performing certain activities of daily living. The nurse helps the client to maintain optimal function, while instituting measures for the client's comfort as necessary. The nurse helps the client and the client's family to recognize and manage the emotional and psychological stress attendant on the client's condition and facilitates the relationships of the client, client's family, staff, and other significant people. Correct principles, procedures, and techniques of health care are taught, and the client is informed about the current status of health. If necessary, the client or the client's family is referred to a health or social resource in the community. Care is given to achieve therapeutic goals, including acting to compensate for adverse reactions; using preventive and precautionary measures and correct technique in administering care; preparing the client for surgery, delivery, or other procedure; or initiating life-saving measures for emergency situations. Care is given to the client in a manner and to a degree that best promotes attainment of the goals by the client by providing an environment that is conducive to attaining the goals; by adjusting the care given according to the

client's needs; by stimulating and motivating the client to achieve independence; by encouraging the client to comply with and accept the regimen of care; and by compensating for the staff reactions to factors that influence the relationship with the client and the therapy planned. Implementing follows planning and precedes evaluating in the five-step nursing process. See also **analyzing, assessing.**

implosion, 1. a bursting inward. 2. Also called **flooding.** a psychiatric treatment for people disabled by phobias and anxiety in which the person is desensitized to anxiety-producing stimuli by repeated intense exposure in imagination or reality, until the stimuli are no longer stressful. — **implode,** *v.*

implosive therapy. See **flooding.**

impotence, 1. weakness. 2. inability of the adult male to achieve penile erection or, less commonly, to ejaculate having achieved an erection. Several forms are recognized. **Functional impotence** has a psychologic basis. **Anatomic impotence** results from physically defective genitalia. **Atonic impotence** involves disturbed neuromuscular function. Poor health, age, drugs, and fatigue can inhibit normal sexual function. Also called **impotency.** Compare **infertility.** — **impotent,** *adj.*

impotency. See **impotence.**

impregnate, 1. to inseminate and make pregnant; to fertilize. 2. to saturate or mix with another substance. — **impregnable,** *adj.,* **impregnation,** *n.*

impression, 1. (in dentistry and prosthetic medicine) a mold of a part of the mouth or other part of the body from which a replacement or prosthesis may be formed. 2. (in the medical record) the examiner's diagnosis or assessment of a problem, disease, or condition. 3. a strong sensation or effect on the mind, intellect, or feelings.

imprinting, (in ethology) a special type of learning that occurs at critical points during the early stages of development in animals. It involves behavioral patterning and social attachment, is characterized by rapid acquisition and irreversibility, and is usually species-specific, although animals exposed to members of a different species during this short period may become attached to and identify with that particular species instead of their own. The degree to which imprinting occurs in human development has not been determined. See also **bonding.**

imprisonment, (in law) the act of confining, detaining, or arresting a person or in any way restraining personal liberty and preventing free exercise of movement. Imprisonment may be in a prison or other special facility, but every confinement is an imprisonment.

impulse, 1. (in psychology) a sudden, irresistible, often irrational inclination, urge, desire, or action resulting from a particular feeling or mental state. 2. (in physiology) the electrochemical process involved in neural transmission. Also called **nerve impulse, neural impulse.** —**impulsive,** *adj.*

impulsion, an abnormal, irrational urge to commit an unlawful or socially unacceptable act.

Imuran, a trade name for an immunosuppressive (azathioprine).

IMV, abbreviation for **intermittent mandatory ventilation.**

In, symbol for **indium.**

in-, **1.** a combining form meaning 'of or pertaining to fibers': *inaxon, inemia, initis.* **2.** a combining form meaning 'in, on': *incineration, indigitation, induced.* **3.** a combining form meaning 'not': *inaction, inassimilable, incompetence.*

-in, **1.** a combining form meaning an 'antibiotic': *bacitracin, penicillin, streptomycin.* **2.** a combining form meaning a 'pharmaceutical product': *aspirin, Empirin, niacin.* **3.** a combining form meaning a 'chemical compound': *albumin, gelatin, palmitin.* **4.** a combining form meaning an 'enzyme': *emulsin, pepsin, myrosin.* Also **-ine.**

inactive colon, hypotonicity of the bowel resulting in decreased contractions and propulsive movements and a delay in the normal 12-hour transit time of luminal contents from cecum to anus. Colonic inactivity may be caused by acquired or congenital megacolon, aging, anticholinergic drugs, depression, faulty habits of elimination, inadequate fluid intake, lack of exercise, a low-residue or starvation diet, neuroendocrine response to surgical stress, prolonged bed rest, or a neurologic disease, as diabetic visceral neuropathy, multiple sclerosis, parkinsonism, and spinal cord lesions. Normal motility of the colon is frequently compromised by the continued use of laxatives. Acquired megacolon, characterized by an abnormally large, inactive bowel and chronic constipation, is common in retarded children and adults with chronic mental illness. In congenital megacolon (Hirschsprung's disease) congenital absence of myenteric innervation in a distal segment of the colon results in loss of motility and causes massive dilatation of the proximal segment of the large bowel and extreme constipation. The disorder is more common in males than females and in severe cases retards growth. Treatment of colonic inactivity includes a stimulus-response training program to establish regular bowel habits, the use of stool softeners and hydrophilic colloids to increase fecal bulk, and a diet containing adequate roughage.

inadequate personality, a personality characterized by a lack of physical stamina, emotional immaturity, social instability, poor judgment, reduced motivation, ineptness —especially in interpersonal relationships—and an inability to adapt or react effectively to new or stressful situations.

inanimate, not alive; lacking signs of life.

inanition (ɪn'ənɪ́sh'ən), **1.** an exhausted condition resulting from lack of food and water or a defect in assimila-

tion; starvation. **2.** a state of lethargy characterized by a loss of vitality or vigor in all aspects of social, moral, and intellectual life.

inanition fever, a temporary, mild, febrile condition of the newborn in the first few days after birth, usually caused by dehydration.

inborn, innate; acquired or occurring during intrauterine life, with reference to both normally inherited traits and developmental or genetically transmitted anomalies. See also **congenital, hereditary, inborn error of metabolism.**

inborn error of metabolism, one of many abnormal metabolic conditions caused by an inherited defect of a single enzyme or other protein. Though people with such diseases are each defective in only protein, they generally display a large number of physical signs that are characteristic of the genetic trait. The diseases are rare. Kinds of inborn errors of metabolism include **phenylketonuria (PKU), Tay-Sachs disease, Lesch-Nyan syndrome, galactosemia,** and **glucose-6-phosphate dehydrogenase deficiency.**

■ OBSERVATIONS: Inborn errors of metabolism may be detected in the fetus in utero by the examination of squamous and blood cells obtained by amniocentesis and fetoscopy. Laboratory tests after birth often show higher than normal levels of particular metabolites in the blood and urine, as phenylpyruvic acid and phenylalanine in PKU and galactose in galactosemia. The values are higher in homozygous than in heterozygous carriers. Physical stigmata of the various defects are usually seen only in homozygous carriers.

■ INTERVENTION: Treatment for some pathological inborn errors may be initiated by removing dietary precursors of the nondegradable metabolite in order to prevent its accumulation, as removal of dietary phenylalanine in PKU and galactose in galactosemia are effective in preventing the development of symptoms if treatment is begun early. In those cases of inborn errors of metabolism in which the nondegradable metabolite is endogenous, as in the mucopolysaccharidoses, there is no treatment available.

inborn reflex. See **unconditioned response.**

inbreeding, the production of offspring by the mating of closely related individuals, organisms, or plants; self-fertilization is the most extreme form, which normally occurs in certain plants and lower animals. The practice provides a greater chance for recessive genes for both desirable and undesirable traits to become homozygous and to be expressed phenotypically. In man, the amount of inbreeding in a specific population is largely controlled by tradition and cultural practices. In plants and animals, inbreeding is a standard method for developing desirable genotypes and pure lines. Compare **outbreeding.**

incarcerate, to trap, imprison, or confine, as a loop of intestine in an inguinal hernia. See also **hernia.**

incest, sexual intercourse between members of the same family who are so closely related as to be legally prohibited from marrying one another by reason of their consanguinity. – **incestuous,** *adj.*

incidence, 1. the number of times an event occurs. 2. (in epidemiology) the number of new cases in a particular period of time. Incidence is often expressed as a ratio, in which the number of cases is the numerator and the population at risk is the denominator. See also **rate.**

incipient, coming into existence; an initial stage; beginning to appear or to become apparent, as a symptom or disease.

incisor, one of the eight front teeth, four in each dental arch, that first appear as milk teeth during infancy, are replaced by permanent incisors during childhood, and last until old age. The crown of the incisor is chisel-shaped and has a sharp cutting edge. Its labial surface is convex, smooth, and highly polished, its lingual surface is concave and, in many individuals, is marked by an inverted V-shaped basal ridge near the gum of the upper arch. The neck of the incisor is constricted. The root is single, long, and conical. The upper incisors are larger and stronger than the lower incisors and are directed obliquely downward and forward. Compare **canine tooth, molar, premolar.**

inclusion, 1. the act of enclosing or the condition of being enclosed. 2. a structure within another, as inclusions in the cytoplasm of the cells.

inclusion conjunctivitis, an acute, purulent, conjunctival infection caused by *Chlamydia* organisms. It occurs in two forms: bilateral chemosis, redness, and purulent discharge characterize the infection in infants; the adult variety is unilateral, less severe, less purulent, and associated with preauricular lymphadenopathy. Local instillation of antibiotics is effective treatment. Also called **swimming pool conjunctivitis.**

inclusion dermoid cyst, a tumor derived from embryonal tissues, caused by the inclusion of a foreign tissue when a developmental cleft closes.

incoherent, 1. disordered; without logical connection; disjointed; lacking orderly continuity or relevance; inharmonious. 2. unable to express one's thoughts or ideas in an orderly, intelligible manner, usually as a result of emotional stress.

incompatible, unable to coexist. A tissue transplant may be rejected because recipient and donor antibody factors are incompatible.

incompetence, lack of ability. Body organs that do not function adequately may be described as incompetent. Kinds of incompetence include **aortic incompetence, ileocecal incompetence, valvular incompetence.** – **incompetent,** *adj.*

incompetent cervix, (in obstetrics) a condition characterized by dilatation of the cervical os of the uterus before term without labor or contractions of the uterus. Miscarriage or premature delivery may result. Incompetent cervix is treated prophylactically by a Shirodkar or other procedure in which the cervix is held closed by a surgically implanted suture.

incomplete abortion, termination of pregnancy in which the products of conception are not entirely expelled or removed, often causing hemorrhage that may require surgical evacuation by curettage, oxytocics, and blood replacement. Infection is also a frequent complication of incomplete abortion. Compare **complete abortion.**

incomplete fistula. See **blind fistula.**

incomplete fracture, a bone break in which the crack in the osseous tissue does not completely traverse the width of the affected bone but may angle off in one or more directions.

incontinence (inkon'tinəns), the inability to control urination or defecation. Urinary incontinence may be caused by cerebral clouding in the aged, infection, lesions in the brain or spinal cord, damage to peripheral nerves of the bladder, or injury to the sphincter or perineal structures, sometimes occurring in childbirth. Treatment includes bladder retraining, the implantation of an artificial sphincter, and the use of internal or external drainage devices. Stress incontinence precipitated by coughing, straining, or heavy lifting occurs more often in women than in men and may be treated by exercises involving tightening and relaxing perineal and gluteal muscles. Fecal incontinence may result from relaxation of the anal sphincter or by central nervous system or spinal cord disorders and may be treated by a program of bowel training. A Bradford frame with an opening for a bedpan or urinal may be used for bedridden incontinent patients. See also **bowel training.** – **incontinent,** *adj.*

increment, 1. an increase or gain. 2. the act of growing or increasing. 3. the amount of an increase or gain. – **incremental,** *adj.*

increto-, a combining form meaning 'of or pertaining to internal secretions': *incretodiagnosis, incretogenous, incretology.*

incrustation, hardened exudate, scale, or scab.

incubation period, 1. the time between exposure to a pathogenic organism and the onset of symptoms of a disease. 2. the time required to induce the development of an embryo in an egg or to induce the development and replication of tissue cells or microorganisms being grown in culture media or other special laboratory environment.

incubator, an apparatus used to provide a controlled environment, especially a particular temperature. Other environmental components, as darkness, light, oxygen, moisture, or dryness may also be provided, as in an incubator for the cultivation of eggs or microorganisms in a laboratory or an incubator for premature infants.

incud-, a combining form meaning 'of or pertaining to an anvil (the incus)': *incudectomy, incudiform, incudomalleal.*

incudectomy (ɪn'kyudek'təmi), surgical removal of the incus, performed to treat conductive deafness owing to necrosis of the tip of the incus. Local or general anesthesia is used. The defective incus is excised and replaced with a bone chip graft so that sound vibrations are again transmitted. Postoperatively, the nurse instructs the patient to change position slowly to avoid dizziness, to avoid blowing the nose and sneezing, and to report any fever, headache, dizziness or pain in the ear.

incus (ɪŋ'kəs), one of the three ossicles in the middle ear, resembling an anvil. It communicates sound vibrations from the malleus to the stapes. Compare **malleus, stapes.** See also **middle ear.**

IND, abbreviation for **investigational new drug.**

indandione derivative, one of a small group of oral anticoagulants designed for long-term therapeutic use in patients who cannot tolerate other oral anticoagulants. The indandiones are difficult to control and may cause grave adverse effects, including severe renal and hepatic toxicity, agranulocytosis, and leukopenia. For this reason coumarin derivatives are preferred. Regular evaluations of prothrombin are necessary. Extreme fatigue, sore throat, chills, and fever are signs of impending toxicity and require discontinuation of the drug.

indentation, a notch, pit, or depression in the surface of an object, as toothmarks on the tongue or skin. — **indent,** *v.*

independence, **1.** Also called **independency.** the state or quality of being independent; autonomy; free from the influence, guidance, or control of a person or a group. **2.** a lack of requirement or reliance on another for physical existence or emotional needs. — **independent,** *adj.*

independent assortment, (in genetics) a basic principle stating that the members of a pair of genes are randomly distributed in the gametes, independent of the distribution of other pairs of genes. See also **dominance, segregation.**

independent practice, (in nursing) the practice of certain aspects of professional nursing which are encompassed by applicable licensure and law and require no supervision or direction from others. Nurses in independent practice may have an office in which they see patients and charge fees for service. In all nursing settings, state practice acts define certain aspects of nursing practice which are independent and may define those which must be done only under supervision or direction of another individual, usually a physician.

independent variable, (in research) a variable that is controlled by the researcher and evaluated by its measurable effect on the dependent variable or variables, as in a study of the effect of nursing intervention on postopera-tive vomiting, nursing intervention is the independent variable evaluated by its effect on the incidence of postoperative vomiting. Also called **experimental variable, predictor variable.** Compare **dependent variable.**

Inderal, a trade name for a beta-adrenergic blocking agent (propranolol).

indeterminate cleavage, mitotic division of the fertilized ovum into blastomeres that have similar developmental potential and, if isolated, can give rise to a complete individual embryo. Also called **regulative cleavage.** Compare **determinate cleavage.** See also **regulative development.**

index case, **1.** See **propositus.** **2.** (in epidemiology) the first case of a disease as contrasted with the appearance of subsequent cases.

Index Medicus, an index published monthly by the National Library of Medicine, which lists articles from the medical literature from throughout the world by subject and by author. An annual edition, the *Cumulative Index Medicus,* is published yearly; it contains all 12 issues of the *Index Medicus.*

index myopia, a kind of nearsightedness owing to a variation in the index of refraction of the media of the eye.

Indian Health Service, a bureau within the Department of Health and Human Services for providing public health and medical services to native Americans in the United States.

Indian tick fever. See **Marseilles fever.**

indication, a reason to prescribe a medication or perform a treatment, as a bacterial infection may be an indication for the prescription of a specific antibiotic or as appendicitis is an indication for appendectomy. — **indicate,** *v.*

indicator, a tape, paper, tablet, or any other substance that is used to test for a particular reaction because it changes in a predictable visible way. Also called **reagent.** Some kinds of indicators are **autoclave indicator, dipsticks, litmus paper.**

indigenous (ɪndɪj'ənəs), native to or occurring naturally in a specified area or environment, as certain species of bacteria in the human digestive tract.

indigestion. See **dyspepsia.**

indirect anaphylaxis, an exaggerated reaction of hypersensitivity to a person's own antigen that occurs because the antigen has been altered in some way.

indirect calorimetry, the measurement of the amount of heat generated in an oxidation reaction by determining the intake or consumption of oxygen or by measuring the amount of carbon dioxide or the amount of nitrogen released and translating these quantities into a heat equivalent. Compare **direct calorimetry.**

indirect division. See **mitosis.**

indirect ophthalmoscope, an ophthalmoscope with a biconvex lens that produces a reversed direct image.

indirect percussion. See **percussion.**

indium (In), a silvery metallic element with some non-metallic chemical properties. Its atomic number is 49; its atomic weight is 114.82. It is used in electronic semiconductors.

individual immunity, a form of natural immunity not shared by most other members of the race and species. It is rare and probably occurs as the result of the person having had an infection that went unrecognized. Compare **racial immunity, species immunity.**

individual psychology, a modified system of psychoanalysis, developed by Alfred Adler, that views maladaptive behavior and personality disorders as resulting from a conflict between the desire to dominate and feelings of inferiority. See also **inferiority complex.**

Indocin, a trade name for an anti-inflammatory agent (indomethacin).

Indoklon, a trade name for an inhalation anesthetic agent (flurothyl).

indoleacetic acid (ɪn′dɒuləsi′tɪk, ɪn′dɒuləset′ɪk), a major terminal metabolite of tryptophan, present in very small amounts in normal urine and excreted in elevated quantities by patients with carcinoid tumors.

indomethacin, a nonsteroidal anti-inflammatory agent.
- INDICATIONS: It is prescribed in the treatment of arthritis and certain other inflammatory conditions.
- CONTRAINDICATIONS: Upper gastrointestinal disease or known hypersensitivity to this drug or to aspirin prohibits its use. It is not given to children under 15 years of age or to pregnant or lactating women.
- ADVERSE EFFECTS: The most serious adverse reaction is peptic ulcers. Gastrointestinal upset, dizziness, tinnitus, and rashes also may occur.

induce, to cause or stimulate the start of an activity, as an enzyme induces a metabolic activity. See also **induced fever.** – **inducer, induction,** *n.*

induced abortion, an intentional termination of pregnancy before the fetus has developed enough to live if born. Twenty to fifty per cent of pregnancies are terminated deliberately, at the request of the mother or for medical indications—during the first trimester by curettage, or during the second trimester by induction of labor or hysterotomy. Termination of pregnancy by a trained person under proper conditions is safe. Unskilled abortions can be extremely hazardous because of the susceptibility of the uterus to infection and laceration. Puerperal sepsis and hemorrhage after criminal abortion have been leading causes of maternal death.

induced fever, a deliberate elevation of body temperature by application of heat or by inoculation with a fever-producing organism in order to kill heat-sensitive pathogens.

induced hypotension. See **deliberate hypotension.**

induced lethargy, a trancelike state produced during hypnosis. See also **hypnosis, lethargy.**

induced trance, a somnambulistic state resulting from a hysterical neurosis or hypnotism.

induction, (in embryology) the process of stimulating and determining morphogenetic differentiation in a developing embryo through the action of chemical substances transmitted from one to another of the embryonic parts. See also **evocation.**

induction of anesthesia, all portions of the anesthetic process that occur prior to attaining the desired level of anesthesia, including premedication with a sedative, hypnotic, tranquilizer, or curariform adjunct to anesthesia, intubation, administration of oxygen, and administration of the anesthetic.

induction of labor, an obstetric procedure in which labor is initiated artificially by means of amniotomy or the administration of oxytocics. It is performed electively or for fetal or maternal indications. Elective induction is carried out for the convenience of the mother or the obstetrician, often to avert the possibility of delivery outside of the hospital when labor is judged to be imminent and the mother is expected to have an unusually rapid birth. Elective inductions are performed less often now than in the past. Prerequisites for elective induction are a term gestation, a fetal weight of at least 2,500 gm, a cervix judged ready to dilate, a vertex presentation, and engagement of the presenting part of the fetus in the pelvis. Errors in the estimation of gestational age and fetal weight may result in the delivery of an unexpectedly immature or low-birthweight infant. Indicated induction is performed when the risk of induction is judged to be less than that of continuing the pregnancy in such conditions as premature rupture of the membranes, severe maternal diabetes, and intractable pre-eclampsia. Surgical induction is effected by amniotomy, often with stripping of the membranes and digital stretching of the cervix; it is very often carried out in conjunction with medical induction. Medical induction is achieved through the administration of pitocin, almost always by intravenous infusion, in a carefully controlled manner using microdrip equipment or an infusion pump. Beginning with very small amounts of pitocin in an intravenous solution, the dosage is increased by gradual increments of the rate or concentration of infusion until effective labor is established. Pitocin can be administered by buccal lozenge or by subcutaneous or intramuscular injection, but these methods are less controllable and are considered less safe than the intravenous method. Prostaglandins are now used to induce labor more often than formerly, particularly for therapeutic abortions in the second trimester. With intravenous pitocin inductions, a secondary, piggyback infusion without medication is usually attached to the tubing so that an unmedicated infusion can be maintained if pitocin is stopped. Electronic fetal and uterine monitoring is usually instituted during induction of labor to avoid hyperstimulation of the uterus and fetal distress. Ideally, induced labor mimics natural labor, but in practice this is not usually achieved. Longer and harder contractions commonly occur. In addition to unexpected fetal immaturity, complications of induction of labor include umbilical cord prolapse following amniotomy, tumultuous labor, tetanic uterine contractions, rupture of the uterus, placental abruption, fetal maternal hypotension, water intoxication, postpartum uterine atony and hemorrhage, and fetal asphyxia, hypoxia, or death. If the induction fails to produce effective labor, Caesarean section is often required to prevent the adverse sequelae of the procedures used in the induction. For this reason, it is usually recommended that induction of labor not be attempted unless delivery must be accomplished to avoid severe fetal or maternal morbidity.

inductor (ɪndək′tər),   (in embryology) a tissue or cell that emits a chemical substance that stimulates some morphogenetic effect in the developing embryo. See also **evocator, organizer.**

induration,   hardening of a tissue, particularly the skin, owing to edema, inflammation, or infiltration by a neoplasm.   – **indurated,** *adj.*

Industrial Medical Association (I.M.A.),   a professional organization whose members are concerned with the identification, prevention, diagnosis, and treatment of disorders associated with technology and industry.

industrial psychology,   the application of psychological principles and techniques to the problems of business and industry, including the selection of personnel, the motivation of workers, and the development of training programs.

indwelling catheter,   any catheter designed to be left in place for a prolonged period. See also **self-retaining catheter.**

-ine,   a combining form meaning a 'chemical substance': *chlorine, pyrroline, strychnine.*

inert,   **1.** not moving or acting, as inert matter. **2.** (of a chemical substance) not taking part in a chemical reaction or acting as a catalyst, as neon or an inert gas. **3.** (of a medical ingredient) not active pharmacologically; serving only as a bulking, binding, or sweetening agent or other excipient in a medication.

inert gas,   a chemically inactive gaseous element. The inert gases are argon, helium, krypton, neon, radon, and xenon. Also called **noble gas.**

inertia,   **1.** the tendency of a body at rest to remain at rest unless acted upon by an outside force, and the tendency of a body in motion to remain at motion in the direction in which it is moving unless acted upon by an outside force. **2.** an abnormal condition characterized by a general inactivity or sluggishness, as colonic inertia or uterine inertia.

inevitable abortion,   a condition of pregnancy in which spontaneous termination is imminent and cannot be prevented. It is characterized by bleeding, uterine cramping, dilatation of the cervix, and presentation of the conceptus in the cervical os. If heavy bleeding supervenes, immediate evacuation of the uterus may be required. The point at which an inevitable abortion becomes an incomplete abortion is of medicolegal interest because of the statutory difference between spontaneous and induced abortion. In clinical practice precise differentiation is seldom practicable. Compare **incomplete abortion, imminent abortion, threatened abortion.**

infant,   **1.** a child who is in the earliest stage of extrauterine life, a time extending from birth to approximately 12 months of age, when the baby is able to assume an erect posture; some extend the period to 24 months of age. **2.** (in law) a person not of full legal age; a minor. **3.** of or pertaining to infancy; in an early stage of development.   – **infantile,** *adj.*

infant death,   the death of a live-born infant before one year of age.

infant botulism,   an intoxication from neurotoxins produced by *Clostridium botulinum* that occurs in children less than six months of age. The condition is characterized by severe hypotonicity of all muscles, constipation, lethargy, and feeding difficulties, and it may lead to respiratory insufficiency. The botulism neurotoxin is usually found in the gastrointestinal tract rather than in the blood, indicating that it is probably produced in the gut rather than ingested, although the epidemiology and pathophysiology of the syndrome are not clearly understood. Treatment is supportive, including optimal management of fluids, electrolytes, and nutrition. Ventilatory support may also be necessary. There is no evidence that antitoxin therapy is helpful and it is usually not recommended.

infant death,   the death of a live-born infant before one year of age.

infant feeder,   a device for feeding small or weak infants who cannot suck hard enough to nurse from the breast or to get milk from a bottle. The feeder resembles a bulb syringe with a long soft nipple on the end. The bulb is squeezed slowly and gently, permitting the baby to suck and swallow without great effort and preventing the escape of fluid into the infant's trachea, where it might cause asphyxiation or aspiration pneumonia.

infant feeding.   See **bottle feeding, breast feeding.**

infanticide (ɪnfæn′tɪsaɪd),   **1.** the killing of an infant or young child. The act is usually a psychotic reaction often associated with severe depression, as occurs in bipolar disorder and, occasionally, in extreme postpartum disturbances. Infanticide may become a neurotic obsession among mothers who do not want the baby or who do not feel physically, mentally, or emotionally capable of caring for or coping with the infant. **2.** one who takes the life of an infant or young child. — **infanticidal,** *adj.*

infantile, **1.** of, relating to, or characteristic of infants or infancy. **2.** lacking maturity, sophistication, or reasonableness. **3.** affected with infantilism. **4.** being in a very early stage of development.

infantile arteritis, a disorder in infants and young children characterized by inflammation of many arteries in which atherosclerotic lesions are rarely present.

infantile autism, a disability characterized by abnormal emotional, social, and linguistic development in a child. It may result from organic brain dysfunction, in which case it occurs before the age of three years, or it may be associated with childhood schizophrenia, in which case the autism occurs later, but before the onset of adolescence. The autistic child remains fixed at one of the consecutive stages through which a normal infant passes as it develops. If the condition is the result of organic brain disease, the child appears to be unable to proceed beyond the current stage of development, though there is no regression to an earlier stage. If the condition accompanies schizophrenia in later childhood, regression occurs. Treatment includes psychotherapy, often accompanied by play therapy.

infantile celiac disease. See **celiac disease.**

infantile cerebral sphingolipidosis. See **Tay-Sachs disease.**

infantile dwarf, a person whose mental and physical development is greatly retarded as a result of various causes, as genetic or developmental defects.

infantile eczema. See **atopic dermatitis.**

infantile paralysis. See **poliomyelitis.**

infantile pellagra. See **kwashiorkor.**

infantile scurvy, a nutritional disease caused by an inadequate dietary supply of vitamin C, most commonly occurring because cow's milk, unfortified with vitamin C, is the principal food in an infant's diet. Families are counseled to feed their children foods rich in vitamin C or to use a formula supplemented with this vitamin. Also called **Barlow's disease, hemorrhagic scurvy.** See also **ascorbic acid, citric acid, scurvy.**

infantile spinal muscular atrophy. See **Werdnig-Hoffmann disease.**

infantilism (ɪn'fəntəlɪz'əm), **1.** Compare **progeria.** a condition in which various anatomical, physiological, and psychological characteristics of childhood persist in the adult. It is characterized by mental retardation, underdeveloped sexual organs, and, usually small stature. **2.** a condition, usually of psychological rather than organic origin, characterized by speech and voice patterns in an older child or adult that are typical of very young children.

infant mortality, the statistical rate of infant death during the first year after live birth, expressed as the number of such births per 1000 live births in a specific geographical area or institution in a given period of time. Neonatal mortality accounts for 70 per cent of infant mortality.

infant of addicted mother, a newborn infant showing withdrawal symptoms, usually within the first 24 hours of life, most commonly caused by maternal antepartum dependence on heroin, methadone, diazepam, phenobarbital, and alcohol.

■ OBSERVATIONS: Characteristic symptoms include tremors, irritability, hyperactive reflexes, increased muscle tone, twitching, increased mucus production, nasal congestion, respiratory distress, excessive sweating, elevated temperature, vomiting, diarrhea, and dehydration. The infants cry shrilly, often sneeze, frantically suck their fists but feed poorly, and frequently yawn but have difficulty falling asleep. They are usually pale, are often born with nose and knee abrasions, and are subject to convulsions.

■ INTERVENTION: The infant is kept warm, snugly swaddled in a padded crib, and is exposed to minimal visual, auditory, and tactile stimulation. The baby is handled only when necessary and is then held firmly, close to the body. Parenteral fluid therapy and drugs, as paregoric, phenobarbital, chlorpromazine, or diazepam, may be administered. Small, frequent feedings of concentrated formula are usually ordered, and before each feeding the infant's nasopharynx is suctioned. If the buttocks become excoriated because of diarrhea, a paste of zinc oxide and karaya powder is applied and if the infant's flailing about is likely to cause abrasions, bony prominences of the body may be protected with light padding and the hands with the mitts of the infant shirt.

■ NURSING CONSIDERATIONS: These high-risk infants require special attention, and it is important for the mother to be encouraged to participate in her baby's care as soon as possible. The nurse may help to promote parent-child bonding.

infant psychiatry, the branch of psychiatry that specializes in the diagnosis, etiology, and treatment of the psychopathological syndromes and symptoms of infants. Such conditons are associated with early pathology, tactile hypersensitivity, and homeostatic disorders and include poor infant-parent attachment, infantile autism, anaclitic depression, avoidance reaction, persistent stranger and separation anxiety, early signs of aggression, hyperactivity, cyclic vomiting, and disturbances in sleeping, eating, and elimination.

infarct (ɪnfarkt'), a localized area of necrosis in a tissue, vessel, organ, or part resulting from tissue anoxia caused by an interruption in the blood supply to the area, or, less frequently, by circulatory stasis produced by the occlusion of a vein that ordinarily carries blood away from the area. An infarct may resemble a red swollen bruise, owing to hemorrhage and an accumulation of blood in the area. Some infarcts are pale and white, owing to a lack of circulation to the area. Kinds of infarct include **anemic infarct, calcareous infarct, cicatrized infarct, hemorrhagic infarct, uric acid infarct.** — **infarcted,** *adj.*

infarction (ınfark′shən), **1.** the development and formation of an infarct. **2.** an infarct. Kinds of infarction include **myocardial infarction, pulmonary infarction.**

infect, to transmit a pathogen that may induce development of an infectious disease in another person.

infected abortion, a spontaneous or induced termination of an immature pregnancy in which the products of conception have become infected, causing fever, and requiring antibiotic therapy and evacuation of the uterus. Compare **septic abortion.**

infection, **1.** the invasion of the body by pathogenic microorganisms which reproduce and multiply, causing disease by local cellular injury, secretion of a toxin, or antigen-antibody reaction in the host. **2.** a disease caused by the invasion of the body by pathogenic microorganisms. Compare **infestation.** — **infectious,** *adj.*

infectious, **1.** capable of causing an infection. **2.** caused by an infection.

infectious hepatitis. See **hepatitis A.**

infectious mononucleosis, an acute herpesvirus infection caused by the Epstein-Barré virus (EBV). It is characterized by fever, sore throat, swollen lymph glands, atypical lymphocytes, splenomegaly, hepatomegaly, abnormal liver function, and bruising. The disease is usually transmitted by droplet infection but is not highly or predictably contagious. Young people are most often affected. In childhood, the disease is mild and usually unnoticed; the older the person, the more severe the symptoms are likely to be. Infection confers permanent immunity. Treatment is primarily symptomatic, with enforced bed rest to prevent serious complications of the liver or spleen, analgesics to control pain, and saline gargles for throat discomfort. Rupture of the spleen may occur, requiring immediate surgery and blood transfusion. See also **Epstein-Barr virus, viral infection.**

infectious myringitis, an inflammatory, contagious condition of the ear drum owing to viral or bacterial infection, characterized by the development of painful vesicles on the drum. Also called **bullous myringitis.**

infectious nucleic acid, DNA or, more commonly, viral RNA that is able to infect the nucleic acid of a cell and to induce the host to produce viruses.

infectious parotitis. See **mumps.**

infectious polyneuritis. See **Guillain-Barré syndrome.**

inferomedial, located below and toward the center.

infective tubulointerstitial nephritis, an acute inflammation of the kidneys caused by an infection by *Escherichia coli* or other pyogenic pathogen. The condition is characterized by chills, fever, nausea and vomiting, flank pain, dysuria, proteinuria, and hematuria. The kidney may become enlarged and portions of the renal cortex may be destroyed. Infection is usually the result of bacterial contamination of a urinary catheter, but it may occur in any condition characterized by urinary stasis.

inferior, **1.** situated below or lower than a given point of reference, as the feet are inferior to the legs. **2.** of poorer quality or value. Compare **superior.**

inferior alveolar artery, an artery that descends with the inferior alveolar nerve from the first or mandibular portion of the maxillary artery to the mandibular foramen on the medial surface of the ramus of the mandible. It enters the mandibular canal and runs through to the first premolar tooth where it divides into the mental and incisor branches. Also called **arteria alveolaris inferior.**

inferior aperture of minor pelvis, an irregular aperture bounded by the coccyx, the sacrotuberous ligaments, part of the ischium, the sides of the pubic arch, and the pubic symphysis.

inferior aperture of thorax, an irregular opening bounded by the twelfth thoracic vertebra, the twelfth ribs, and the edge of the costal cartilages as they meet the sternum.

inferior conjunctival fornix, the space in the fold of conjunctiva created by the reflection of the conjunctiva covering the eyeball and the lining of the lower eyelid.

inferior gastric node, a node in one of two groups of gastric lymph glands, lying between the two layers of the lesser omentum along the pyloric half of the greater curvature of the stomach. Compare **hepatic node, superior gastric node.**

inferiority complex, **1.** a feeling of fear and resentment resulting from a sense of being physically inadequate, characterized by a variety of abnormal behaviors. **2.** (in psychoanalysis) a complex characterized by striving for unrealistic goals owing to an unresolved Oedipus complex. **3.** *Informal.* a feeling of being inferior.

inferior maxillary bone. See **mandible.**

inferior mesenteric node, a node in one of the three groups of visceral lymph glands serving the viscera of the abdomen and the pelvis. The inferior mesenteric nodes are associated with the branches of the inferior mesenteric artery and are divided into a group of small nodes along the branches of the left colic and sigmoid arteries, another group in the sigmoid mesocolon, and a pararectal group touching the muscular coat of the rectum. The inferior mesenteric nodes drain the descending colon, the iliac and sigmoid parts of the colon, and the upper part of the rectum. Their efferents pass to the preaortic nodes. Compare **gastric node, superior mesenteric node.**

inferior mesenteric vein, the vein in the lower body that returns the blood from the rectum, the sigmoid colon, and the descending colon. It begins in the rectum as the superior rectal vein, ascends through the lesser pelvis, and continues upward as the inferior mesenteric vein. It passes dorsal to the pancreas and opens into the lienal vein. It receives the sigmoid veins from the sigmoid colon and the iliac colon and the left colic vein from the descending colon and the left colic flexure. Compare **superior mesenteric vein.**

inferior orbital fissure, a groove in the inferolateral wall of the orbit that contains the infraorbital and zygomatic nerves and the infraorbital vessels.

inferior phrenic artery, a small, visceral branch of the abdominal aorta, arising from the aorta itself, the renal artery, or the celiac artery. It divides into the medial and lateral branches and supplies the diaphragm. A few vessels of the inferior vena cava stem from the lateral branch of the right phrenic artery. Some branches of the left phrenic artery supply the esophagus.

inferior radioulnar joint. See **distal radioulnar articulation.**

inferior sagittal sinus, one of the six venous channels of the posterior dura mater, draining blood from the brain into the internal jugular vein. It is a cylindrical sinus contained in the posterior portion of the free margin of the falx cerebri, increases in size as it courses posteriorly, and ends in the straight sinus. It receives deoxygenated blood from several veins from the falx cerebri and, in some individuals, a few veins from the cerebral hemispheres. Compare **straight sinus, superior sagittal sinus, transverse sinus.**

inferior subscapular nerve (səbskæp′yulər), one of two small nerves on opposite sides of the back that arise from the posterior cord of the brachial plexus. It supplies the distal part of the subscapularis and ends in the teres major. Compare **superior subscapular nerve.**

inferior thyroid vein, one of the few veins that arise in the venous plexus on the thyroid gland and form a plexus ventral to the trachea, under the sternothyroidei. A left vein descends from this plexus to join the left brachiocephalic trunk; a right vein descends obliquely to open into the right brachiocephalic vein at its junction with the superior vena cava. The inferior thyroid veins contain valves at their terminations and receive the esophageal, the tracheal, and the inferior laryngeal veins.

inferior ulnar collateral artery, one of a pair of branches of the deep brachial arteries, arising about 5 cm from the elbow, passing inward to form an arch with the deep brachial artery, and carrying blood to the muscles of the forearm. Compare **superior ulnar collateral artery.**

inferior vena cava, the large vein that returns deoxygenated blood to the heart from parts of the body below the diaphragm. It is formed by the junction of the two common iliac veins at the right of the fifth lumbar vertebra and ascends along the vertebral column, pierces the diaphragm and opens into the right atrium of the heart. As it passes through the diaphragm it receives a covering of serous pericardium. The inferior vena cava contains a semilunar valve that is rudimentary in the adult but very large and important in the fetus. The vessel receives blood from the two common iliacs, the lumbar veins, and the testicular veins. Compare **superior vena cava.**

infero-, a combining form meaning 'low': *inferolateral, inferomedian, inferoposterior.*

inferolateral (ɪn′fəroulæt′ərəl), located below and to the side. Compare **inferomedial.**

infest, to attack, invade, and subsist on the skin or in the internal organs of a host. Compare **infect.**

infestation, the presence of animal parasites in the environment or on the skin or in the hair of a host.

inflammation, the protective response of the tissues of the body to irritation or injury. Inflammation may be acute or chronic; its cardinal signs are redness (rubor), heat (calor), swelling (tumor), and pain (dolor), accompanied by loss of function. The process begins with a brief increase in vascular permeability. The second stage is prolonged and consists of sustained increase in vascular permeability, exudation of fluids from the vessels, clustering of leukocytes along the vessel walls, phagocytosis of microorganisms, deposition of fibrin in the vessel, disposal of the accumulated debris by macrophages, and, finally, the migration of fibroblasts to the area and the development of new, normal cells. The severity, timing, and local character of any particular inflammatory response depend on the cause, the area affected, and the condition of the host. Histimine, kinins, and various other substances mediate the inflammatory process.

inflammatory bowel disease. See **ulcerative colitis.**

inflammatory fracture, a fracture of bone tissue weakened by inflammation.

inflatable pessary. See **pessary.**

influenza, a highly contagious infection of the respiratory tract caused by a myxovirus and transmitted by airborne droplet infection. It occurs in isolated cases, epidemics, and pandemics. Symptoms include sore throat, cough, fever, muscular pains, and weakness. The incubation period is brief (from one to three days), and the onset is usually sudden, with chills, fever, and general malaise. Treatment is symptomatic and usually involves bed rest, aspirin, and drinking of fluids. Fever and constitutional symptoms distinguish influenza from the common cold. Complete recovery in from three to ten days is the rule, but bacterial pneumonia may occur among high-risk patients, as the elderly, the very young, and people who have chronic pulmonary disease. Three main strains of influenza virus have been recognized: type A, type B, and type C. New strains of the virus emerge at regular intervals and are named according to their geographic origin. **Asian flu** is a type A influenza. Yearly vaccination with the currently prevalent strain of influenza virus is recommended for elderly or debilitated persons. Also called **grippe, la grippe,** *Informal.* **flu.**

influenza virus vaccine, an active immunizing agent.

■ INDICATION: It is prescribed for immunization against influenza.

■ CONTRAINDICATIONS: Acute infection or allergy to eggs prohibits its use.

■ ADVERSE EFFECTS: Among the more serious adverse reactions are anaphylaxis and Guillain-Barré syndrome.

informed consent, permission obtained from a patient to perform a specific test or procedure. Informed consent is required prior to performing most invasive procedures and prior to admitting a patient to a research study. The document used must be written in a language understood by the patient and be dated and signed by the patient and at least one witness. Included in the document are clear, rational statements that describe the procedure or test, the risk to the patient, the expected benefits to the patient, the natural anticipated consequences of not allowing the test or procedure, and the alternative procedures or diagnostic aids that are available. Also required is a statement that care will not be withheld if the patient does not consent; informed consent is voluntary. By law, informed consent must be obtained more than a given number of days or hours prior to certain procedures, including therapeutic abortion and sterilization, and must always be obtained when the patient is fully competent.

infra-, a combining form meaning 'situated, formed, or occurring beneath': *infraclavicular, infracortical, infratemporal.*

infraction fracture, a pathologic fracture characterized by a small radiolucent line and most commonly associated with a disorder of metabolism.

infranodal block (ɪn'frənoʊ'dəl), a type of arterioventricular (A-V) block in which an impairment of the stimulatory mechanism of the heart causes blockage of the impulse in the bundle if His or in both bundle branches after leaving the A-V node. The condition is often the result of arteriosclerosis, degenerative diseases, a defect in the conduction system, or tumor; it is most often seen in older patients. Symptoms include frequent episodes of fainting and a pulse rate of between 20 and 50 beats per minute. Diagnosis is made by an electrocardiogram, which shows intraventricular conduction disturbances during sinus rhythm and distinguishes nodal from infranodal block. The usual therapy is the implantation of a pacemaker of the demand type. See also **atrioventricular block, cardiac conduction defect, Adams-Stokes syndrome.**

infrared radiation, electromagnetic radiation in which the wavelengths are longer than those of visible light waves and shorter than those of radio waves. Infrared radiation striking the body surface is perceived as heat.

infrared therapy, treatment by exposure to various wavelengths of infrared radiation. Hot water bottles and heating pads of all kinds emit long-wave infrared radiation; incandescent lights emit short-wave infrared radiation. Infrared treatment is performed to relieve pain and to stimulate circulation of blood.

infusion, 1. Compare **injection, instillation, insufflation. a.** the introduction of a substance, as a fluid, electrolyte, nutrient, or drug, directly into a vein or interstitially by means of gravity flow. Sterile techniques are maintained, the equipment is periodically checked for mechanical difficulties, and the patient is observed for swelling at the site of injection and for cardiac or respiratory difficulties. **b.** the substance introduced into the body by infusion. **2.** the steeping of a substance, as an herb, in order to extract its medicinal properties. **3.** the extract obtained by the steeping process. — **infuse,** *v.*

infusion pump, an apparatus designed to deliver measured amounts of a drug through injection over a period of time. Some kinds of infusion pumps can be implanted surgically.

ingrown hair, a hair that fails to follow the normal follicle channel to the surface, with the free end becoming embedded in the skin. The hair then acts like a foreign body, and inflammation and suppuration follow.

ingrown toenail, a toenail whose free distal margin grows or is pressed into the skin of the toe, causing an inflammatory reaction. Granulation tissue may develop and secondary infection is common. Treatment includes wider shoes, proper trimming of the nail, and various surgical procedures to narrow the nail or to reduce the size of the lateral nail fold.

inguinal (ɪŋ'gwɪnəl), of or pertaining to the groin.

inguinal falx, the inferior terminal portion of the common aponeurosis of the obliquus internus abdominis and the transverse abdominis. It is inserted into the crest of the pubis, just under the superficial inguinal ring, and strengthens that part of the anterior abdominal wall. The width and the strength of the inguinal falx vary. Also called **conjoined tendon.**

inguinal hernia, a hernia in which a loop of intestine enters the inguinal canal, sometimes filling, in a male, the entire scrotal sac. An inguinal hernia is usually repaired surgically to prevent the herniated segment from becoming strangulated, gangrenous, or obstructive, thereby blocking passage of waste through the bowel. Seventy-five to eighty per cent of all hernias are inguinal hernias. See also **hernia.**

inguinal node, one of approximately 18 nodes in the group of lymph glands in the upper femoral triangle of the thigh. These nodes are divided into the superficial inguinal nodes and the subinguinal nodes. Compare **anterior tibial node, popliteal node.**

inguino-, a combining form meaning 'of or pertaining to the groin': *inguinocrural, inguinodynia, inguinoscrotal.*

INH. Abbreviation for **isoniazid.**

inhalation administration of medication, the administration of a drug by inhalation of the vapor released from a fragile ampoule packed in a fine mesh that is crushed for immediate administration. Amyl nitrate and ammonia act quickly and are often used in this way. The medication is absorbed into the circulation through the mucous membrane of the nasal passages. Vaporized medication is also given by inhalation. See also **inhalation therapy.**

inhalation analgesia, the occasional administration of anesthetic gas during the second stage of labor to reduce pain. Consciousness is retained to allow the woman to follow instructions and to avoid the adverse effects of general anesthesia.

inhalation anesthesia, surgical narcosis achieved by the administration of an anesthetic gas or a volatile anesthetic liquid via a carrier gas. Although general anesthesia by gas inhalation has been used to permit surgical operations for over a century, the mechanism by which these anesthetics obtund the pain centers of the brain is not yet understood. Administration of an inhalation anesthetic is usually preceded by intravenous or intramuscular administration of a short-acting sedative or hypnotic drug, often a barbiturate. The procedure almost always requires endotracheal intubation. Among the principal inhalation anesthetics are nitrous oxide, cyclopropane, ethylene, halothane, enflurane, fluroxene, methoxyflurane, trichloroethylene, and isoflurane. Some other inhalation anesthetics, including chloroform, ether, and ethyl chloride, are rarely used in the United States because of adverse effects, potential toxicity, or the possibility of explosion.

inhalation therapy, a treatment in which a substance is introduced into the respiratory tract with inspired air. Oxygen, water, and various drugs may be administered using techniques of inhalation therapy. The goals of treatment are varied, as improved strength of respiratory function in a bedridden patient, bronchodilatation in an asthmatic, or liquefaction of mucus in a person with chronic obstructive lung disease.

inhale, to breathe in or to draw in with the breath. — **inhalation,** n.

inherent, inborn, innate; natural to an environment. Compare **indigenous.**

inheritance, (in genetics) **1.** the acquisition or expression of traits or conditions by transmission of genetic material from parents to offspring. **2.** the sum total of the genetic qualities or traits transmitted from parents to offspring; the total genetic makeup of the fertilized ovum. Kinds of inheritance include **alternative inheritance, amphigonous inheritance, blending inheritance, codominant inheritance, complemental inheritance, crisscross inheritance, cytoplasmic inheritance, holandric inheritance, hologynic inheritance, homochronous inheritance, maternal inheritance, Mendelism, monofactorial inheritance,** **multifactorial inheritance, supplemental inheritance.** — **inherited,** adj. **inherit,** v.

inherited disorder, any disease or condition that is genetically determined and involves either a single gene mutation, multifactorial inheritance, or a chromosomal aberration. Also called **genetic disorder, hereditary disorder.**

inhibiting hormone. See **hormone.**

inhibition, **1.** the act or state of inhibiting or of being inhibited; restrained; prevented; held back. **2.** (in psychology) the unconscious restraint of a behavioral process, usually resulting from the social or cultural forces of the environment; the condition inducing such restraint. **3.** (in psychoanalysis) the process in which the superego prevents the conscious expression of an unconscious instinctual drive, thought, or urge. **4.** (in physiology) restraining, checking, or arresting the action of an organ or cell or the reducing of a physiological activity by an antagonistic stimulation. **5.** (in chemistry) the stopping or slowing down of the rate of a chemical reaction.

inhibitory, tending to stop or slow a process, as a neuron that suppresses the intensity of a nerve impulse. Compare **induce.**

Inhiston, a trade name for an antihistamine (pheniramine maleate).

inio-, a combining form meaning 'of or pertaining to the occiput': iniodymus, iniopagus, iniops.

inion (ĭn'ĭən), the most prominent point of the back of the head, where the occipital bone protrudes the farthest.

initial contact stance stage, one of the five stages in the stance phase of walking or gait, specifically associated with the moment when the foot touches the ground or floor, and the leg prepares to accept the weight of the body. The initial contact stance stage figures in the diagnoses of many abnormal orthopedic conditions and is often correlated with electromyographic studies of the muscles used in walking, as the pretibial muscle and the gluteus maximus. Compare **loading response stance stage, midstance, preswing stance stage, terminal stance.** See also **swing phase of gait.**

initiation codon (kou'don), (in molecular genetics) the triplet of nucleotides, usually adenine-uracil-guanine (AUG) or, in some cases, guanine-uracil-guanine (GUG), that code for formylmethionine, the first amino acid in protein sequences. Also called **start codon.**

injection, **1.** Compare **infusion, instillation, insufflate.** **a.** the act of forcing a liquid into the body by means of a syringe. Injections are designated according to the anatomical site involved; the most common are intra-arterial, intradermal, intramuscular, intravenous, and subcutaneous. Parenteral injections are usually given for therapeutic reasons, although they may be used diagnostically. Sterile technique is maintained. **b.** the substance injected. **2.** redness and swelling observed in the physical examination of a part of the body, caused by dilation of the blood vessels

Ventrogluteal area (intramuscular)

Glutens medius area

Deltoid muscle area

Vastus lateralis area
(lateral view of right thigh)

Anterolateral muscle area

Mid-anterior thigh area

INJECTION SITES

secondary to an inflammatory or infectious process. – **inject**, *v.*

injection technique. See specific injection technique.

injury: potential for, a nursing diagnosis accepted by the Fourth National Conference on the Classification of Nursing Diagnoses. The etiology of the condition may be somatic (internal) or environmental (external). The somatic factors may be biological, chemical, physiological, psychological, or developmental; the environmental factors may be biological, chemical, physiological, psychological, or interpersonal. The defining characteristics of a somatic potential for injury include abnormal sensory function, autoimmune condition, malnutrition, hemoglobinopathy or other abnormal hematologic condition, broken skin, developmental abnormality, or psychological dysfunction. The defining characteristics of an environmental potential for injury include lack of immunization; presence of pathogenic microorganisms, chemical pollutants, poisons, alcohol, nicotine, or food additives; modes of transportation; physical aspects of the community, buildings, equipment, or facilities; nosocomial agents; nonavailability of assistance; and various psychological factors. Three subcomponents of this diagnosis have been developed: poisoning, potential for; suffocation, potential for; and trauma, potential for. See also **nursing diagnosis.**

inlet contraction. See **contraction.**

in loco parentis (ɪn lou'kou pəren'tɪs), *Latin.* 'in the place of the parent.' The assumption by a person or institution of the parental obligations of caring for a child without adoption.

innate, 1. existing in or belonging to a person from birth; inborn; hereditary; congenital. 2. a natural and essential characteristic of something or someone; inherent. 3. originating in or produced by the intellect or the mind.

innate immunity. See **natural immunity.**

inner cell mass, a cluster of cells localized around the animal pole of the blastocyst of placental mammals from which the embryo develops. See also **trophoblast.**

inner ear. See **internal ear.**

innervation apraxia. See **motor apraxia.**

innidation (in'aidei'shən). See **nidation.** — **innidate,** *v.*

innocent, benign, innocuous, or functional; not malignant, as an innocent heart murmur.

inoculate, to introduce a substance (inoculum) into the body to produce or to increase immunity to the disease or condition associated with the substance. It is introduced by making multiple scratches in the skin after placing a drop of the substance on the skin, by puncture of the skin with an implement bearing multiple short tines, or by intradermal, subcutaneous, or intramuscular injection.

inoculum (inok'yuləm), *pl.* **inocula.** a substance introduced into the body to cause or to increase immunity to a specific disease or condition. It may be a toxin, a live, attenuated, or killed virus or bacterium, or an immune serum. Also called **inoculant.** See also **immune system.**

inorganic, (in chemistry) any chemical compound that does not contain carbon.

inorganic acid, a compound containing no carbon that is made up of hydrogen and an electronegative element. Some organic acids, as carbonic acid, contain carbon dioxide.

inorganic chemistry, the study of the properties and reactions of all chemical elements and compounds other than hydrocarbons.

inorganic dust, dry, finely powdered particles of an inorganic substance, especially dust, which, when inhaled, can cause abnormal conditions of the lungs. See also **anthracosis, asbestosis, berylliosis, pneumoconiosis, silicosis.**

inosine (in'əsin, in'əsain', in'əsin), a nucleoside, derived from animal tissue, especially intestines, originally used in food processing and flavoring and now under investigation in studies of cancer and virology chemotherapy. See also **inosiplex.**

inosiplex, a form of inosine that acts as a stimulator of the immune system. It is currently under investigation for use in cancer therapy and in the treatment of herpesvirus and rhinovirus infections.

inositol (inou'sətoul, inos'ətoul, inou'sətol), an isomer of glucose which occurs widely in plant and animal cells. Although inositol has no current therapeutic use, it may be an essential cell constituent.

inpatient, 1. a patient who has been admitted to a hospital or other health-care facility for at least an overnight stay. 2. of or pertaining to the treatment or care of such a patient or to a health-care facility to which a patient may be admitted for twenty-four hour care. Compare **outpatient.**

insect bite, the bite of any parasitic or venomous arthropod as a louse, flea, mite, tick, or arachnid. Many arthropods inject venom that produces poisoning or severe local reaction, saliva that may contain viruses, or substances that produce mild irritation. The degree of irritation of an insect's bite is affected by the design and shape of its mouthparts: a horsefly, for example, makes a short lateral and coarse wound, while a tick takes hold with its backward curved teeth, making its removal difficult. Spiders inflict a sharp pinprick bite that may remain unnoticed until the injected venom has begun to produce a painful reaction. Treatment of a bite depends on the species of insect, the reaction to the bite, and the risk of sequelae from it. First-aid treatment is generally symptomatic and includes ice or cold packs, careful cleaning of the wound and antihistamines or specific antivenin as necessary.

insecticide, a chemical agent that kills insects.

insecticide poisoning. See **chlorinated organic insecticide poisoning.**

insensible perspiration, the loss of fluid from the body by evaporation, as normally occurs during respiration. A small amount of perspiration is continually excreted by the sweat glands in the skin; the portion that evaporates before it may be observed also contributes to insensible perspiration. Also called **insensible water loss.**

insensible water loss. See **insensible perspiration.**

insertion, (in anatomy) the place of attachment, as of a muscle to the bone it moves.

in-service education, a program of instruction or training that is provided by an agency or institution for its employees. The program is held in the institution or at the agency and is intended to increase the skills and competence of the employees in a specific area. In-service education may be a part of any program of staff development.

insidious (ɪnsɪd′iəs), of, pertaining to, or describing a development that is gradual, subtle, or imperceptible. Certain chronic diseases, as glaucoma, can develop insidiously with symptoms that are not detected by the patient until the disorder is established. Compare **acute.**

insight, 1. the capacity of comprehending the true nature of a situation or of penetrating an underlying truth. 2. an instance of penetrating or comprehending an underlying truth, primarily through intuitive understanding. 3. (in psychology) a type of self-understanding encompassing both an intellectual and emotional awareness of the unconscious nature, origin, and mechanisms of one's attitudes, feelings, and behavior. It is one of the most important goals of psychotherapy and, with integration, leads to modification of maladaptive behavioral patterns. See also **integration.**

in situ (ɪn saɪ′tu, sɪt′u), 1. in the natural or usual place. 2. describing a cancer that has not metastasized or invaded neighboring tissues, as carcinoma in situ.

insoluble, unable to be dissolved, usually in a specific solvent, as a substance that is insoluble in water.

insomnia, chronic inability to sleep or to remain asleep throughout the night; wakefulness; sleeplessness. The condition is caused by a variety of physical and psychological factors, including emotional stress, physical pain and discomfort, disturbances in cerebral function, like toxic delirium and senile dementia, drug abuse and drug dependence, psychosomatic disorders, neuroses, psychoses, and psychological problems that produce anxiety, irrational fears, and tensions. Treatment may include medication with sedatives, tranquilizers, or hypnotics, psychotherapy, and exercise.

insomniac, 1. a person with insomnia. 2. pertaining to, causing, or associated with insomnia. 3. characteristic of or occurring during a period of sleeplessness.

inspiration, the act of drawing air into the lungs in order to exchange oxygen for carbon dioxide, the end product of tissue metabolism. The major muscle of inspiration is the diaphragm, the contraction of which creates a negative pressure in the chest, causing the lungs to expand and air to flow inward. Additional muscles aiding inspiratory efforts are the external intercostals, scaleni, scapular elevators, and sternocleidomastoids. Since expiration is usually a passive process, these muscles of inspiration alone perform normal respiration. Lungs at maximal inspiration have an average total capacity of 5500 to 6000 ml of air. See also **inspiratory reserve volume.**

inspiratory, of or pertaining to inspiration.

inspiratory capacitis, the total volume of air that can be inhaled. It is the sum of the inspiratory reserve and tidal volumes and is measured by means of a spirometer.

inspiratory capacity, the maximum volume of gas that can be expired from the resting expiratory level; the tidal volume and the inspiratory reserve volume.

inspiratory reserve volume, the maximum volume of gas that can be inspired from the end-tidal inspiratory level.

inspissate (ɪnspɪs′eɪt), (of a fluid) to thicken or harden through the absorption or evaporation of the liquid portion, as milk in an inspissated milk duct.

instillation, 1. a procedure in which a fluid is slowly introduced into a cavity or passage of the body and allowed to remain for a specific length of time before being drained or withdrawn. It is performed to expose the tissues of the area to the solution, to warmth or cold, or to a drug or substance in the solution. 2. a solution so introduced. Compare **infusion, injection, insufflate.** – **instill,** v.

instinctive reflex. See **unconditioned response.**

institutionalize, to place a person in an institution for psychological or physical treatment or for the protection of the person or society. – **institutionalization,** n., **institutionalized,** adj.

institutional licensure, a proposed procedure in which licensure for almost all health professions would be abandoned and the responsibility for assessing professional competence would fall to the health care facility where the health professional is employed. Proponents of the procedure maintain that health needs would be better and more flexibly served. Opponents maintain that knowledge, judgment, and competency are the products of a good basic education in the profession and that educators cannot teach the profession without a set of standardized expectations, as are now provided by government-controlled licensing procedures and certifying examinations. In addition, health care facilities may not have the expertise or resources necessary to evaluate the various kinds of health care providers.

institutional review board (IRB), a federally approved committee that reviews all research proposals prior to submission of requests for funding to federal government granting agencies.

instrument, a surgical tool or device designed to perform a specific function, as cutting, dissecting, grasping, holding, retracting, or suturing. Surgical instruments are usually made of steel and are specially treated to be durable, heat-resistant, rust-resistant, and stain-proof. Proper care of surgical instruments is essential and includes correct use, careful handling, inspection for defects, adequate and appropriate sterilization, and proper labeling, dating, and storage. Some kinds of instruments are **clamp, needle holder, retractor, speculum.**

instrumental conditioning. See **operant conditioning.**

instrumentation, the use of instruments for treatment and diagnosis.

insufficiency, inability to perform a necessary function adequately. Some kinds of insufficiency are **adrenal insufficiency, aortic insufficiency, ileocecal insufficiency, pulmonary insufficiency, valvular insufficiency.**

insufflate (ɪnsəf′leɪt), to blow a gas or powder into a tube, cavity, or organ to allow visual examination, to remove an obstruction, or to apply medication. See also **Rubin's test**.

insul-, a combining form meaning 'of or pertaining to an island, or island-shaped': *insula, insulin, insuloma*.

insulin, **1.** a naturally occurring hormone secreted by the beta cells of the islands of Langerhans in the pancreas in response to increased levels of glucose in the blood. The hormone acts to regulate the metabolism of glucose and the processes necessary for the intermediary metabolism of fats, carbohydrates, and proteins. Insulin lowers blood glucose levels and promotes transport and entry of glucose into the muscle cells and other tissues. Inadequate secretion of insulin results in hyperglycemia, hyperlipemia, ketonemia, and azoturia and in the characteristic signs of diabetes mellitus, including polyphagia, polydipsia, and polyuria, and, eventually, lethargy and weight loss. Uncorrected severe deficiency of insulin is incompatible with life. **2.** a pharmacologic preparation of the hormone administered in treating diabetes mellitus. The various preparations of insulin available for prescription vary in promptness, intensity, and duration of action. They are termed rapid-acting, intermediate-acting and long-acting. Most forms of insulin drugs are given by subcutaneous injection in individualized dosage schedules. Adverse reactions include hypoglycemia and insulin shock from excess dosage and hyperglycemia and diabetic ketoacidosis from inadequate dosage. Many drugs interact with insulin, among them the monoamine oxidase inhibitors, corticosteroids, salicylates, thiazide diuretics, and phenytoin. Fever, stress, infection, pregnancy, surgery, and hyperthyroidism may significantly increase insulin requirements; liver disease, hypothyroidism, vomiting, and renal disease may decrease the need for insulin. Urine or blood tests for glucose and ketones are performed to determine the need for adjustment of the dosage or of the schedule of administration.

insulin injection, a fast-acting, regular insulin, prescribed in the treatment of diabetes mellitus when the

INSULIN INJECTION SITES

desired action is prompt, intense, and short-acting. Insulin injection prepared from zinc insulin crystals is slightly longer-acting than the amorphous noncrystalline form of this type of insulin preparation. Insulin injection is the only form of insulin suitable for intramuscular administration. Also called **regular insulin.**

insulin kinase, an enzyme, assumed to be present in the liver, that activates insulin.

insulinogenic, promoting the production and release of insulin by the islands of Langerhans in the pancreas.

insulinoma (ɪn′sulɪnou′mə), *pl.* **insulinomas, insulinomata.** a benign tumor of the insulin-secreting cells of the islands of Langerhans. Surgical resection of the tumor may be possible, thus limiting the development of hypoglycemia. Also called **insuloma, islet cell adenoma.** Compare **islet cell tumor.**

Action of insulin preparations

Type of insulin	Time of onset	Peak of action	Duration of action
Rapid acting			
Crystalline zinc	Within 1 hour	2 to 4 hours	5 to 8 hours
Regular	Within 1 hour	2 to 4 hours	4 to 6 hours
Semilente	Within 1 hour	6 to 10 hours	12 to 16 hours
Intermediate acting			
Globin zinc	2 to 4 hours	6 to 10 hours	18 to 24 hours
NPH	2 to 4 hours	8 to 12 hours	28 to 32 hours
Lente	2 to 4 hours	8 to 12 hours	28 to 30 hours
Slow acting			
Ultralente	Within 8 hours	16 to 24 hours	36+ hours

insulin shock, hypoglycemic shock caused by an overdose of insulin, a decreased intake of food, or excessive exercise. It is characterized by sweating, trembling, chilliness, nervousness, irritability, hunger, hallucination, numbness, and pallor. Uncorrected, it will progress to convulsions, coma, and death. Treatment requires an immediate dose of glucose. Compare **ketoacidosis.**

insulin-shock treatment, the injection of large, convulsion-producing doses of insulin, administered as a therapeutic measure in psychoses, especially schizophrenia. Electroconvulsive therapy is currently administered more commonly than insulin-shock and is used chiefly for manic-depressive psychosis. Also called **hypoglycemic shock treatment.**

insulin tolerance test, a test of the body's ability to utilize insulin, in which insulin is given and blood glucose is measured at regular intervals. Thirty minutes after the insulin is given, blood glucose is usually lower but not less than half of the fasting glucose level. Glucose levels usually return to normal after about 90 minutes. In people with hypoglycemia, the glucose levels may drop lower and be slower to return to normal.

insuloma (ɪn'syəlou'mə), pl. **insulomas, insulomata.** See **insulinoma.**

intake, Informal. **1.** the process in which a person is admitted to a clinic or hospital or is signed in for an office visit. The reason for the visit and various identifying data about the patient are noted. Certain preliminary, routine procedures may be performed, as obtaining a blood pressure reading or a urine specimen. In some clinical settings, the intake may also include obtaining such additional information as the patient's basic health history and previous source of care. **2.** (in nursing) the amount of food or fluids ingested in a given period of time, measured and noted as ccs or gms per shift or in 8 or 24 hours.

Intal, a trade name for an antiasthmatic (cromolyn sodium).

integral dose, (in radiotherapy) the total amount of energy absorbed by a patient or object during exposure to radiation. Also called **volume dose.**

integrating dose meter, (in radiotherapy) an ionization chamber, usually designed to be placed on the patient's skin, with a measuring system for determining the total radiation administered during an exposure. A device may be included to terminate the exposure when the desired value is reached.

integration, **1.** the act or process of unifying or bringing together. **2.** (in psychology) the organization of all elements of the personality into a coordinated, functional whole that is in harmony with the environment, one of the primary goals in psychotherapy. It involves the assimilation of insight and the coordination of new and old data, experiences, and emotional reactions so that an ef-

fective change can occur in behavior, thinking, or feeling. See also **insight.** – **integrate,** v.

integration of self, one of the components of high-level wellness. It is a prerequisite for the achievement of maturity and is characterized by the integration of mind, body, and spirit into one harmoniously functioning unit.

integument (ɪnteg'yumənt), a covering or skin. – **integumentary,** adj.

integumentary system, the skin and its appendages, hair, nails, and sweat and sebaceous glands. See also **integument.**

integumentary system assessment, an evaluation of the general condition and any abnormalities of a patient's integument and of factors that may contribute to the presence of a dermatologic disorder.

■ METHOD: The nurse askes if the patient suffers from itching, pain, rashes, blisters, or boils, if the skin usually is dry, oily, thin, rough, bumpy, or puffy, if it feels hot or cold, if it peels, changes in color, or if it is marked with dark liver (aging) spots. Observations are made of the intactness, turgor, elasticity, temperature, cleanliness, odor, wetness or dryness, and color of the skin. Cyanosis of the lips, circumoral area, mucous membranes, earlobes, or nailbeds, jaundice of the sclera, pale conjunctivae, the distribution of pigment, and evidence of plethora are noted. Indications of rashes, edema, needle marks, insect bites, scabies, acne, sclerema, decubiti, uremic frost on the beard or eyebrows, or pressure areas over bony prominences, are recorded. The nails are examined for brittleness, lines, a convex ram's horn or concave spoon shape, and the condition of surrounding tissue, including clubbing of the fingers and toes. The existence and characteristics of maculae, papules, vesicles, pustules, bullae, hives, warts, moles, ulcers, scars, keloids, petechiae, lipomas, crusts of dried exudate, flakes of dead epidermis, excoriations, blackheads, or a chancre are noted. The patient's exposure to parasites, to internal allergens in food and drugs, and to external allergens in cosmetics, soaps, topical medication, and plants, as well as a family history of allergies is investigated. The patient's currently used medication, creams, lotions, ointments, hygienic measures, and sexual practices are ascertained. Diagnostic aids contributing to the evaluation are skin and lesion cultures, punch biopsies, skin tests for allergies, a lupus erythematosus preparation, and a blood culture.

■ NURSING ORDERS: the nurse conducts the interview to obtain subjective data on the patient's condition, makes the necessary observations, and assembles the background information and the results of the diagnostic tests.

■ OUTCOME CRITERIA: A well-conducted assessment of the patient's integument is a valuable aid in diagnosing a dermatologic disorder.

intellect, **1.** the power and ability of the mind for knowing and understanding, as contrasted with feeling or with willing. **2.** a person possessing a great capacity for thought and knowledge.   **—intellectual,** *adj., n.*

intellectualization, (in psychiatry) a defense mechanism in which reasoning is used as a means of blocking a confrontation with an unconscious conflict and the emotional stress associated with it.

intelligence, **1.** the potential ability and capacity to acquire, retain, and apply experience, understanding, knowledge, reasoning, and judgment in coping with new experiences and in solving problems. **2.** the manifestation of such ability. See also **intelligence quotient.** **—intelligent,** *adj.*

intelligence quotient, (IQ), a numerical expression of a person's intellectual level as measured against the statistical average of his age group. It is determined by dividing the mental age, derived through psychological testing, by the chronological age and multiplying the result by 100. Average IQ is considered to be 100. See also **mental retardation.**

intelligence test, any of a variety of standarized tests designed to determine the mental age of an individual by measuring the relative capacity to absorb information and to solve problems. These tests are routinely used by the medical profession to diagnose and determine degrees of mental retardation and to aid in the planning of therapeutic programs for such persons. Two kinds of intelligence tests are **Stanford-Binet, Wechsler-Bellevue scale.** Compare **achievement test, aptitude test, personality test, psychological test.**

intensive care, constant, complex, detailed health care as provided in various acute life-threatening conditions, as multiple trauma, severe burns, myocardial infarction, or following certain kinds of surgery. Special training is often necessary to provide intensive care. Care is most frequently given in an intensive care unit equipped with various advanced machines and devices for treating and monitoring the patient. Also called **critical care.**

intensive care unit (ICU), a hospital unit in which patients requiring close monitoring and intensive care are housed for as long as needed. An ICU contains highly technical and sophisticated monitoring devices and equipment, and the staff in the unit is educated to give critical care as needed by the patients. A large tertiary care facility usually has separate units specifically designed for the intensive care of adults, infants, children or newborns or for other groups of patients requiring a certain kind of treatment.

intention, a kind of healing process: healing by **first intention** is the primary union of the edges of a wound, progressing to complete scar formation without granulation; healing by **second intention** is wound closure in which the edges are separated, granulation tissue develops to fill the gap, and, finally, epithelium grows in over the granulations, producing a larger scar than results from healing by first intention.

intention tremor, fine, rhythmic, purposeless movements that tend to increase during voluntary movements. Compare **continuous tremor.** See also **tremor.**

inter-, a combining form meaning 'situated, formed, or occurring between': *interacinar, intercalary, intercartilaginous.*

interaction processes, a component of the theory of effective practice. The processes consist of a series of interactions between a nurse and a client. The series occurs in a sequence of actions and reactions until the client and the nurse both understand what is wanted and the desired behavior or act is achieved. The processes are not used in Canada.

interarticular fibrocartilage, one of four kinds of fibrocartilage, consisting of flattened fibrocartilaginous plates between the articular cartilage of the most active joints, as the sternoclavicular, wrist, and knee joints. The synovial surfaces extend over the fibrocartilaginous plates and attach to surrounding ligaments. The fibrocartilaginous plates absorb shocks and increase mobility. Compare **circumferential fibrocartilage, connecting fibrocartilage, stratiform fibrocartilage.**

intercalary (intər'kələr'i, in'tərkæl'əri), occurring between two others, as the absence of the middle part of a bone with the proximal and the distal parts present.

intercalate (intər'kəleit), to insert between adjacent surfaces or structures. **—intercalation,** *n.*

intercapillary glomerulosclerosis, an abnormal condition characterized by degeneration of the renal glomeruli. It is associated with diabetes and often produces albuminuria, nephrotic edema, hypertension, and renal insufficiency. Also called **Kimmelstiel-Wilson's disease.**

interchange. See **reciprocal translocation.**

interconceptional gynecological care, health care of a woman during her reproductive years, between pregnancies, and after six weeks following delivery. Papanicolaou testing for cervical cancer, breast and pelvic examinations, evaluation of general health, and laboratory determination of glucosuria and proteinuria and of the hematocrit or hemoglobin are common and routine aspects of interconceptional care. Testing and treatment for pelvic, vaginal, or genital infections may be required. A contraceptive method may also be discussed, taught, prescribed, or provided. Ordinarily, the basic examination is performed annually. The method of contraception may be adjusted or changed at interim visits; infections or other complaints are investigated, diagnosed, and treated as symptoms appear. Interconceptional care is increasingly given by nurse practitioners or nurse midwives who follow protocols for treatment and referral formulated in consultation with a supervising gynecologist.

intercondylar fracture (ın'tərkon'dılər), a fracture of the tissue between condyles.

intercostal, of or pertaining to the space between two ribs.

intercostal bulging, the visible bulging of the soft tissues of the intercostal spaces that occurs when increased expiratory effort is needed to exhale, as in asthma, cystic fibrosis, or obstruction of a respiratory passage by a foreign body. Compare **retraction of the chest.**

intercostal node, a node in one of three groups of thoracic parietal lymph nodes situated near the dorsal parts of the intercostal spaces and associated with lymphatic vessels that drain the posterolateral area of the chest. The efferent vessels from the nodes in the caudal four or five spaces form a descending trunk which opens into the dilated origin of the thoracic duct. The efferents from the nodes in the upper intercostal spaces on the left side connect with the thoracic duct; those on the right side end in the right lymphatic duct. Compare **diaphragmatic node, sternal node.** See also **lymphatic system, lymph node.**

intercourse, *Informal.* sexual intercourse. See **coitus.**

intercristal, of or pertaining to the space between two crests.

intercurrent disease, a disease that develops in the course of another disease.

interfibrillar mass of Flemming. See **hyaloplasm.**

interfilar mass. See **hyaloplasm.**

interior mesenteric artery, a visceral branch of the abdominal aorta, arising just above the division into the common iliacs and supplying the left half of the transverse colon, all of the descending and iliac colons, and most of the rectum. It has left colic, sigmoid, and superior rectal branches.

interkinesis (ın'tərkını'sıs, ın'tərkaini'sıs), the interval between the first and second nuclear divisions in meiosis. See also **interphase.**

interlobular duct, any duct connecting or draining the lobules of a gland.

interlocked twins, interlocking twins, monozygotic twins so positioned in the uterus that the neck of one becomes entwined with that of the other during presentation so that vaginal delivery is not possible. Such interlocking occurs when one fetus is a breech presentation and the other a vertex presentation.

intermediate-acting insulin, a preparation of the antidiabetic principle of beef pancreas or pork pancreas modified by interaction with zinc under specific chemical conditions and having an intermediate range of action. The action of semilente insulin begins within an hour of injection, reaches a peak in six to ten hours, and lasts for 12 to 16 hours. Three other intermediate-acting preparations begin to act two to four hours after injection; globin zinc insulin reaches a peak in six to ten hours and lasts

for 18 to 24 hours; neutral protamine Hagedorn insulin (NPH) has a peak action in eight to 12 hours and a duration of action of 28 to 32 hours, while lente insulin has a similar peak interval and a slightly shorter duration of action. See also **insulin.** Compare **long-acting insulin, short-acting insulin.**

intermediate care, a level of medical care for certain chronically ill or disabled individuals in which room and board are provided but skilled nursing care is not. Title XI of U.S. Medicaid legislation mandates standards and federal subsidies for intermediate care of the recipients of public assistance.

intermediate cell mass. See **nephrotome.**

intermediate cuneiform bone, the smallest of the three cuneiform bones of the foot, located between the medial and the lateral cuneiform bones. It has six surfaces, is attached to various ligaments, and articulates with the navicular, medial, and lateral cuneiform bones and with the second metatarsal. Also called **middle cuneiform bone, second cuneiform bone.**

intermediate host, any animal in which the larval or intermediate stages of a parasite develop. Certain snails are intermediate hosts for liver flukes and schistosomes. Humans are intermediate hosts for malaria parasites. Also called **secondary host.** Compare **dead-end host, definitive host, reservoir host.** See also **host,** def. 1.

intermediate mesoderm. See **nephrotome.**

intermenstrual, of or pertaining to the time between menstrual periods.

intermenstrual fever, the normal, slight elevation of temperature that marks ovulation, usually occurring about 14 days before the onset of menses.

intermittent, occurring at intervals; alternating between periods of activity and inactivity, as rheumatoid arthritis, which is marked by periods of signs and symptoms followed by periods of remission.

intermittent fever, a fever that recurs in cycles of paroxysms and remissions, as in malaria. Kinds of intermittent fever include **bidoutertian fever, double quartan fever, quartan fever.**

intermittent mandatory ventilation (IMV), a method of respiratory therapy in which the patient is allowed to breathe independently and then at certain prescribed intervals a ventilation machine forces him to take a breath either under positive pressure or in a measured volume. Compare **continuous positive pressure breathing, intermittent positive pressure breathing.** See also **respiratory therapy.**

intermittent positive pressure breathing. See **IPPB.**

intermittent positive pressure breathing unit. See **IPPB unit.**

intermittent positive pressure ventilation. See **IPPB.**

intern, interne, 1. a physician in the first postgraduate year, learning medical practice under supervision before beginning a residency program. **2.** any immediate post-graduate trainee in a clinical program. **3.** to work as an intern.

internal, within or inside. — **internally,** *adv.*

internal aperture of tympanic canaliculus, the upper opening of the tympanic channel in the temporal bone, leading to the tympanum.

internal carotid artery, each of two arteries starting at the bifurcation of the common carotid arteries, opposite the cranial border of the thyroid cartilage, through which blood circulates to many structures and organs in the head. Each artery includes cervical, petrous, cavernous, and cerebral portions and divides into 11 branches. There are no branches from the cervical portion. The four branches from the petrous portion are the caroticotympanic, the artery of the pterygoid canal, the cavernous, and the hypophyseal. The five branches from the cavernous portion are the ganglionic, anterior meningeal, ophthalmic, anterior cerebral, and the middle cerebral. The two branches from the cerebral portion are the posterior communicating and the anterior choroidal.

internal carotid plexus, a network of nerves on the internal carotid artery, formed by the internal carotid nerve. The internal carotid plexus supplies sympathetic fibers to the branches of the internal carotid artery, the tympanic plexus, the nerves of the cavernous sinus, and the cranial parasympathetic ganglia through which the fibers pass. Compare **common carotid plexus, external carotid plexus.**

internal cervical os, an internal opening of the uterus that corresponds to the slight constriction or isthmus of that organ about midway in its length. The internal cervical os separates the body of the uterus from the cervix. Compare **external cervical os.**

internal cuneiform bone. See **medial cuneiform bone.**

internal ear, the complex inner structure of the ear, communicating directly with the acoustic nerve, transmitting sound vibrations from the middle ear through the fluid-filled network of three semicircular canals joining at a vestibule connected to the cochlea. It has two parts: the osseous labyrinth and the membranous labyrinth. Also called **inner ear, labyrinth.**

internal fertilization, the union of gametes within the body of the female after insemination. See also **artificial insemination.**

internal fistula, an abnormal passage between two internal organs or structures.

internal fixation, any method of holding together the fragments of a fractured bone without the use of appliances external to the skin. After open reduction of the fracture, smooth or threaded pins, Kirschner wires, screws, plates attached by screws, or medullary nails may be used to stabilize the fragments. In some instances the device is removed at a later operation, but sometimes it may remain in the body permanently. Compare **external pin fixation.**

internal iliac artery, a division of the common iliac artery, supplying the walls of the pelvis, the pelvic viscera, the genital organs, and part of the medial thigh. The pattern of its branches is the most variable of any artery in the body. Its ten most common branches are umbilical, inferior vesical, middle rectal, uterine, obturator, internal pudendal, iliolumbar, lateral sacral, superior gluteal, and inferior gluteal. In the fetus, the internal iliac artery is twice as large as the external iliac and is the direct continuation of the common iliac artery. After birth, the internal iliac becomes smaller than the external iliac. Also called **hypogastric artery.** Compare **external iliac artery.**

internal iliac node, a node in one of seven groups of parietal lymph nodes serving the abdomen and the pelvis. The internal iliac nodes surround the internal iliac vessels and receive lymphatic vessels corresponding to the branches of the internal iliac artery. Their afferent vessels drain lymph from the pelvic viscera, the buttocks, and dorsal portions of the thighs. Their efferents end in the common iliac nodes. Compare **external iliac node, iliac circumflex node.** See also **lymph, lymphatic system, lymph node.**

internal iliac vein, one of the pair of veins in the lower body that join the external iliac vein to form the two common iliac veins. Each internal iliac vein begins at the greater sciatic foramen, ascends dorsal to its corresponding artery, and, at the pelvic brim joins the external iliac vein. It receives various tributaries, as the superior gluteal, the inferior gluteal, the internal pudendal, the obturator, the lateral sacral, the middle rectal, the dorsal veins of the penis, the vesical, the uterine, and the vaginal. Compare **external iliac vein.**

internalization, the process of adopting within the self, either unconsciously or consciously through learning and socialization, the attitudes, beliefs, values, and standards of another person or, more generally, of the society or group to which one belongs. See also **socialization.**

internal jugular vein, one of a pair of veins in the neck. Each vein collects blood from one side of the brain, the face, and the neck, and both unite with the subclavian vein to form the brachiocephalic vein. The left internal jugular vein is usually smaller than the right, and each vein contains a pair of valves located about 2.5 cm above its termination. The thoracic duct on the left side and the right lymphatic duct on the right side drain into the junction of the internal jugular and the subclavian veins. Each internal jugular vein is continuous with the transverse sinus in the posterior part of the jugular foramen at the base of the skull where, in some people, the vein forms a jugular bulb. Just above the termination is the inferior bulb. Compare **external jugular vein.**

internal medicine, the branch of medicine concerned with the study of the physiology and pathology of the internal organs and with the medical diagnosis and treatment of disorders of these organs.

internal oblique muscle. See **obliquus internus abdominis.**

internal podalic version and total breech extraction. See **version and extraction.**

internal pterygoid muscle. See **pterygoideus medialis.**

internal respiratory nerve of Bell. See **phrenic nerve.**

internal strabismus. See **esotropia.**

internal thoracic artery, one of a pair of arteries that arise from the first portions of the subclavian arteries, descend to the margin of the sternum, and divide into the musculophrenic and superior gastric arteries at the level of the sixth intercostal space, supplying the pectoral muscles, the breasts, the pericardium, and the abdominal muscles. Each artery has eight branches: pericardiophrenic, mediastinal, thymic, sternal, anterior intercostal, perforating, musculophrenic, and superior epigastric.

internal thoracic vein, one of a pair of veins that accompanies the internal thoracic artery, receiving tributaries that correspond to those of the artery. It forms a single trunk which runs up on the medial side of the artery and ends in the corresponding brachiocephalic vein. The superior phrenic vein usually opens into the internal thoracic vein.

International Association for Dental Research (I.A.D.R.), an international organization concerned with research in dentistry and the exchange of information regarding such research.

International Classification of Diseases (ICD), an official list of categories of diseases, physical and mental, issued by the World Health Organization (WHO). It is used primarily for statistical purposes in the classification of morbidity and mortality data. Any nation belonging to WHO may adjust the classification to meet specific needs, as in the United States, the *ICD-9-CM,* a clinical modification of the 1975 revision, *ICD-9,* was adopted in order to provide additional data required by clinicians, research workers, epidemiologists, medical record librarians, and administrators of inpatient, outpatient, and community programs. See also *Diagnostic and Statistical Manual of Mental Disorders.*

International Classification of Disease (ICDA), a classification system adapted for use in the United States by the United States Public Health Service from the parent system developed by the World Health Organization. The system is used in categorizing and indexing hospital records. Each disease is listed as belonging to a major section, as infectious disease or neoplastic disease, and then further coded into major disease categories and subdivisions. The system is updated every ten years.

International Congress of Surgeons (I.C.S.), an international professional organization of surgeons.

International Council of Nurses (ICN), the oldest international health organization. It is a federation of nurses' associations from 93 nations and was one of the first health organizations to develop strict policies of nondiscrimination based on nationality, race, creed, color, politics, sex, or social status. The objectives of the ICN include promotion of national associations of nurses; improvement of standards of nursing and competence of nurses; improvement of the status of nurses within their countries; and provision of an authoritative international voice for nurses. The following ICN definition of the nurse is accepted internationally and serves as a pattern in developing nursing practice and nursing education throughout the world: "A nurse is a person who has completed a program of basic education and is qualified and authorized in her/his country to practice nursing. Basic nursing education is a formally recognized program of study which provides a broad and sound foundation for the practice of nursing and for post-basic education which develops specific competency. At the first level, the educational program prepares the nurse, through study of behavior, life and nursing sciences and clinical experience, for effective practice and direction of nursing care, and for the leadership role. The first level nurse is responsible for planning, providing and evaluating nursing care in all settings for the promotion of health, prevention of illness, care of the sick and rehabilitation; and functions as a member of the health team. In countries with more than one level of nursing personnel, the second level program prepares the nurse, through study of nursing theory and clinical practice, to give nursing care in co-operation with and under the supervision of a first level nurse." The ICN is active in the World Health Organization (WHO), the United Nations Educational, Scientific, and Cultural Organization (UNESCO), and other international organizations.

International Red Cross Society, an international philanthropic organization, based in Geneva, Switzerland, concerned primarily with the humane treatment and welfare of the victims of war and calamity and with the neutrality of hospitals and medical personnel in times of war. See also **American Red Cross.**

International System of Units, a system for the standardization of the measurement of certain substances, including some antibiotics, vitamins, enzymes, and hormones. An International Unit (I.U.) of substance is the amount that produces a specific biological result. Each I.U. of a substance has the same potency and action as another unit of the same substance.

International Unit (I.U., IU), a unit of measure in the International System of Units.

internist, a physician who specializes in internal medicine.

interoceptive (ɪn'tərousep'tɪv), pertaining to stimuli originating from within the body regarding the functioning of the internal organs or to the receptors they activate. Compare **exteroceptive, proprioception.**

interoceptor, any sensory nerve ending located in cells in the viscera that responds to stimuli originating from within the body regarding the function of the internal organs, as digestion, excretion, and blood pressure. Compare **exteroceptor, proprioceptor.** See also **interoceptive nervous system, receptor.**

interparietal fissure. See **intraparietal sulcus.**

interperiosteal fracture (ɪn'tərper'ios'tiəl), an incomplete fracture in which the periosteum is not disrupted.

interpersonal therapy, a kind of psychotherapy that views faulty communications, interactions, and interrelationships as basic factors in maladaptive behavior. A kind of interpersonal therapy is **transactional analysis.**

interphase, the metabolic stage in the cell cycle during which the cell is not dividing, the chromosomes are not individually distinguishable, and such biochemical and physiological activities as DNA synthesis occur. The stage follows telophase of one division and extends to the beginning of prophase of the next division. See also **interkinesis.**

interpubic disc, the fibrocartilaginous plate connecting the opposed surfaces of the pubic bones at the pubic symphysis. Varying in thickness, it is strengthened by interlacing fibers and often contains a cavity that usually appears after the tenth year of life. Also called **discus interpubicus.**

interrogatories, (in law) a series of written questions submitted to a witness or other person having information of interest to the court. The answers are transcribed and are sworn to under oath. Interrogatories are used during pretrial preparation as a means of discovery. They differ from depositions in that there is no opportunity for cross-examination. Compare **discovery, deposition.**

intersex, 1. any individual who has anatomical characteristics of both sexes or whose external genitalia are ambiguous or inappropriate for either the normal male or female. 2. See **intersexuality.** See also **hermaphrodite, pseudohermaphrodite.**

intersexuality, the condition in which an individual has both male and female anatomical characteristics to varying degrees or in which the appearance of the external genitalia is ambiguous or differs from the gonadal or genetic sex. See also **hermaphroditism, pseudohermaphroditism.** – **intersexual,** *adj.*
■ OBSERVATIONS: Any disturbance in the normal sequence of sex determination during embryonic development, including sex chromosome aberrations, abnormal differentiation of the gonads or ductal systems, or hormonal imbalance, which may result in situations in which the phenotypic sex differs from the genotypic sex. Those conditions characterized by ambiguous or inappropriate genitalia are apparent at birth, but others, as Turner's syndrome or Kleinfelter's syndrome, may not be diagnosed until later as a result of delayed development or infertility. There are conditions producing ambiguous genitalia in the newborn that require prompt evaluation and attention: the masculinized female, or female pseudohermaphrodite, of which the most common type is congenital adrenal hyperplasia, caused by an inherited deficiency in the enzymes of adrenal corticoid synthesis; the incompletely masculinized male, or male pseudohermaphrodite, produced as an inherited X-linked recessive or autosomal dominant trait and caused by a deficiency in any of the enzymes needed for testosterone biosynthesis or the unresponsiveness of genital structures to testosterone; the true hermaphrodite, which is rare; and mixed gonadal dysgenesis, in which affected infants are sex chromosomal mosaics. In cases of sexual ambiguity at birth, several diagnostic tests are performed to determine gender assignment. These include a buccal smear to determine the presence or absence of sex chromatin, which is found only in the female; gonadal biopsy; chromosomal analysis, to detect chromosomal abnormalities and the precise genetic sex; endoscopic and x-ray contrast studies to show the presence, absence, or nature of internal genital structures; and biochemical tests to measure adrenocortical function.
■ INTERVENTION: Sex determination should be made as soon as possible after birth to minimize medical, social, and psychological problems. The primary criterion for the choice of gender is the infant's anatomy rather than genetic sex, although diagnostic tests are performed to assist in gender selection. Usually, female pseudohermaphrodites are reared as females with early genital reconstruction and corticosteroid treatment throughout life. Male intersex conditions caused by developmental abnormalities are usually treated surgically to establish male genital appearance and function. In instances of ambiguous genitalia, it is most often recommended that the infant be reared as a female because the outcome of surgical and medical treatment is likely to be better.
■ NURSING CONSIDERATIONS: Gender determination of an infant whose sex is doubtful constitutes more of a psychological and social problem rather than a medical emergency. Such situations are always highly emotional for the parents, who are often overwhelmed by feelings of guilt and shame, and a great deal of support and encouragement are needed. Of special importance is the education of the family about the abnormality, primarily what measures can be undertaken immediately and what will be involved in the long-term management of the condition. The nurse also helps the parents to set realistic goals

for the child, depending on the severity of the condition and the degree of medical and surgical treatment possible.

interspinal ligament, one of many thin, narrow membranous ligaments that connect adjoining spinous processes and extend from the root of each process to the apex. The interspinal ligaments meet the ligamenta flava ventrally and the supraspinal ligament dorsally and are only slightly developed in the neck.

interspinous, of or pertaining to the space between any spinous processes.

interstitial (ɪnˈtərstɪsh′əl), of or pertaining to the space between tissues, as interstitial fluid.

interstitial cystitis, an inflammation of the bladder, believed to be associated with an autoimmune or allergic response. The bladder wall becomes inflamed, ulcerated, and scarred, causing frequent, painful urination. Hematuria often occurs. Treatment may include distention of the bladder and cauterization of the ulcers or weekly lavage of the bladder until the inflammation clears. Both procedures are performed under anesthesia. Corticosteroids are often prescribed to control inflammation. Ulceration is rarely severe enough to require cystectomy with urinary diversion. The condition occurs most often in women of middle age and may resemble the early stages of cancer of the bladder. Cystoscopy and biopsy are required for a diagnosis. Also called **Hunner's ulcer.**

interstitial emphysema, a form of emphysema in which air or gas escapes into the interstitial tissues of the lung following a penetrating injury or as the result of a rupture in an alveolar wall. As the alveoli must be decompressed, there is danger that the pleura will be torn, resulting in a pneumothorax. The condition is diagnosed by chest x ray. See also **emphysema, pneumothorax.**

interstitial fluid, an extracellular fluid that fills the spaces between most of the cells of the body and provides a substantial portion of the liquid environment of the body. Formed by filtration through the blood capillaries, it is drained away as lymph. It closely resembles blood plasma in composition but contains less protein. Compare **intracellular fluid, lymph, plasma.**

interstitial growth, an increase in size by hyperplasia or hypertrophy within the interior of a part or structure that is already formed. Compare **appositional growth.**

interstitial hypertrophic neuropathy. See **Dejerine-Sottas disease.**

interstitial implantation (ɪnˈtərstɪsh′əl), (in embryology) the complete embedding of the blastocyst within the endometrium of the uterine wall.

interstitial infusion. See **hypodermoclysis.**

interstitial keratitis, an uncommon inflammation within the layers of the cornea, the first symptom of which is a diffuse haziness. Blood vessels may grow into the area and cause permanent opacities. Its causes are syphilis, tuberculosis, leprosy, and vascular hypersensitivity. Treatment is specific to the infection or condition.

interstitial myositis. See **myositis.**

interstitial nephritis, inflammation of the interstitial tissue of the kidney, including the tubules. The condition may be acute or chronic. **Acute interstitial nephritis** is an immunologic, adverse reaction to certain drugs, often sulfonamide or methicillin. Acute renal failure, fever, rash, and proteinuria are characteristic of this condition. Most people regain normal function of the kidneys when the offending drug is removed. **Chronic interstitial nephritis** is a syndrome of interstitial inflammation and structural changes, sometimes associated with such conditions as ureteral obstruction, pyelonephritis, exposure of the kidney to a toxin, rejection of a transplant, and certain systemic diseases. Gradually, renal failure, nausea, vomiting, weight loss, fatigue, and anemia develop. Acidosis and hyperkalemia may follow. The nurse watches carefully for signs of electrolyte imbalance, dehydration, and hypovolemia, especially if there is frequent vomiting. Fluids and electrolytes may be replaced intravenously. Treatment includes correction of the underlying cause. If the cause is an obstruction of the urinary tract, rapid recovery may follow removal of the obstruction; in other cases hemodialysis and kidney transplantation may be necessary.

interstitial plasma cell pneumonia. See **pneumocystosis.**

interstitial pneumonia, a diffuse, chronic inflammation of the lungs beyond the terminal bronchioles, characterized by fibrosis and collagen formation in the alveolar walls and by the presence of large mononuclear cells in the alveolar spaces. The symptoms of this condition are progressive dyspnea, clubbing of the fingers, cyanosis, and fever. The disease may result from a hypersensitive reaction to busulphan, chlorambucil, hexamethonium, or methotrexate. Interstitial pneumonia may also be an autoimmune reaction, since it often accompanies celiac disease, rheumatoid arthritis, Sjögren's syndrome, and systemic sclerosis. X rays of the lungs show patchy shadows and mottling, as in bronchopneumonia. Later stages of the disease reveal bronchiectasis, dilatation of the bronchi, and shrinkage of the lungs. Treatment includes bed rest, oxygen therapy, and corticosteroids. Most patients die within six months to a few years, usually from cardiac or respiratory failure. Also called **diffuse fibrosing alveolitis, giant cell interstitial pneumonia, Hamman-Rich syndrome, interstitial.** Compare **bronchopneumonia.**

interstitial pregnancy. See **ectopic pregnancy.**

interstitial tubal pregnancy, a kind of tubal pregnancy in which implantation occurs in the proximal, interstitial portion of one of the Fallopian tubes. See also **tubal pregnancy.**

intertransverse ligament, one of many fibrous bands connecting the transverse processes of vertebrae. In the cervical region, intertransverse ligaments consist of a few scattered fibers; in the thoracic region, they are rounded cords intimately connected with the deep muscles of the back; in the lumbar region, they are thin and membranous.

intertrigo (ın'tərtraɪ'gou), an erythematous irritation of opposing skin surfaces due to friction. Common sites are the axillae, the folds beneath large or pendulous breasts, and the inner aspects of the thighs. Maceration and monilial infection may complicate the picture if the area is also warm and moist. Prevention is by weight reduction, powdering, cleansing, and antifungal topical medication when necessary. – **intertriginous,** *adj.*

intertrochanteric crest (ın'tərtrou'kænter'ık), one of a pair of ridges along the thigh bones, curving obliquely from the greater to the lesser trochanter. Immediately distal to the crest a slight ridge, the linea quadrata, receives the insertion of the quadratus femoris and a few fibers of the adductor magnus.

intertrochanteric fracture, a fracture characterized by a crack in the tissue of the proximal femur between the greater and the lesser trochanters.

intertrochanteric line, a line that runs across the anterior surface of the thigh bone from the greater to the lesser trochanter, winding around the medial surface, and ending in the linea aspera. The proximal half of the intertrochanteric line is the attachment for the iliofemoral ligament; the distal half holds the vastus medialis muscle.

interval health history, a kind of health history that notes the general condition of a client during the period between visits and is not limited to facts relevant to a particular condition. The interval health history provides an ongoing account of a person's health, serving to bring the data base up to date.

intervention, any act performed to prevent harm from occurring to a client or to improve the mental, emotional, or physical function of a client. A physiologic process may be monitored or enhanced, or a pathologic process may be arrested or controlled. See also **nursing intervention.**

intervertebral (ın'tərvər'təbrəl), of or pertaining to the space between any two vertebrae, as the fibrocartilaginous discs.

intervertebral disc, one of the fibrous discs found between each of the spinal vertebrae, except the axis and the atlas. The discs vary in size, shape, thickness, and number depending on the location in the back and on the particular vertebrae they separate.

intervertebral fibrocartilage. See **intervertebral disc.**

intervertebral foramen, any of the passages between adjacent vertebrae through which the spinal nerves and vessels pass.

intervillous space (ın'tərvıl'əs), one of many spaces between the chorionic villi of the endometrium of the gravid uterus, beneath the placenta. The intervillous spaces act as small resevoirs for oxygenated maternal blood from which the fetal circulation may take up the nutrients and gases by osmosis, hydrostatic pressure, and diffusion. The spaces form early in gestation, when the trophoblastic layer of the embryo embeds itself in the wall of the uterus.

intestinal absorption, the passage of the products of digestion from the lumen of the small intestine into the blood and lymphatic vessels in the wall of the gut. The surface area of the intestine is greatly increased by the presence of fingerlike projections, called villi, each of which contains capillaries and a lymphatic vessel, or lacteal. Most dissolved nutrients pass quickly into the capillary bed for transport through the portal circulation to the liver. Lipids enter the lymphatic channels, which eventually rejoin the venous circulation at the thoracic duct in the neck.

intestinal amebiasis. See **amebic dysentery.**

intestinal angina, chronic vascular insufficiency of the mesentery caused by atherosclerosis and resulting ischemia of the smooth muscle of the small bowel. Abdominal pain or cramping after eating, constipation, melena, malabsorption, and weight loss are characteristic of the condition. Also called **chronic intestinal ischemia.**

intestinal apoplexy, the sudden occlusion of one of the three principal arteries to the intestine by an embolism or a thrombus. This condition leads rapidly to necrosis of intestinal tissue and is often fatal. Treatment is usually surgical: the occlusion is removed, and, often, the affected portion of the bowel is resected. See also **atherosclerosis.**

intestinal dyspepsia, an abnormal condition characterized by impaired digestion associated with a problem that originates in the intestines. See also **dyspepsia.**

intestinal fistula, an abnormal passage from the intestine to an external abdominal opening or stoma, usually created surgically for the exit of feces following removal of a malignant or severely ulcerated segment of the bowel. See also **colostomy.**

intestinal infarction. See **intestinal strangulation.**

intestinal flu, a viral gastroenteritis, usually caused by infection by an enterovirus. It is characterized by abdominal cramps, diarrhea, nausea, and vomiting. Outbreaks may be sporadic or epidemic, and the disease usually is mild and self-limited. Treatment is symptomatic. Control of diarrhea may be achieved with antidiarrheal medication and a diet limited to clear fluids. See also **enteric infection, gastroenteritis.**

intestinal juices, the secretions of glands lining the intestine.

intestinal lymphangiectasia. See **hypoproteinemia.**

intestinal obstruction, any obstruction that results in failure of the contents of the intestine to pass through the lumen of the bowel. The most common cause is a mechanical blockage resulting from adhesions, impacted feces, tumor of the bowel, hernia, intussusception, volvulus, or the strictures of inflammatory bowel disease. Obstruction may also be the result of paralytic ileus. Obstruction of the small bowel may cause severe pain, vomiting of fecal matter, dehydration, and eventually, a drop in blood pressure. Obstruction of the colon causes less severe pain, marked abdominal distention, and constipation. X-ray examination reveals the level of obstruction and its cause. Treatment includes the evacuation of intestinal contents by means of an intestinal tube. Surgical repair is sometimes necessary. Fluid balance and electrolyte balance are restored by carefully monitored intravenous infusion. Non-narcotic analgesics are usually prescribed in order to avoid the decrease in intestinal motility that often accompanies the administration of narcotic analgesics. Also called *Informal.* **ileus.** See also **hernia, intussusception, volvulus.**

intestinal strangulation, the arrest of blood flow to the bowel, resulting in edema, cyanosis, and gangrene of the affected loop of bowel. This condition is usually caused by a hernia, intussusception, or volvulus. Early signs of intestinal strangulation resemble those of intestinal obstruction, but peritonitis, shock, and the presence of a tender mass in the abdomen are important in making a differential diagnosis. In addition to surgery, treatment includes the immediate correction of fluid and electrolyte imbalance. Also called **intestinal infarction.**

intestinal tonsil, one of a group of lymphatic nodules forming a single layer in the mucous membrane of the ileum opposite the mesenteric attachment. They are oval patches about one cm wide and extend for about four cm along the intestine. In most individuals they appear in the distal ileum but also appear in the jejunum of a few individuals Also called **Peyer's patches.** Compare **lingual tonsil, palatine tonsil, pharyngeal tonsil.**

intestine, the portion of the alimentary canal extending from the pyloric opening of the stomach to the anus. It includes the small and large intestines.   —**intestinal,** *adj.*

intima (ɪn'tɪmə), *pl.* **intimae.** the innermost layer of a structure, as the lining membrane of an artery, vein, lymphatic, or organ.   —**intimal,** *adj.*

intolerance, a condition characterized by an inability to absorb or metabolize a nutrient or medication. Exposure to the substance may cause an adverse reaction, as in lactose intolerance. Compare **allergy, atopic.**

intoxication, **1.** the state of being poisoned by a drug or other toxic substance. **2.** the state of being inebriated owing to an excessive consumption of alcohol. **3.** a state of mental or emotional hyperexcitability, usually euphoric.

intoxication amaurosis, loss of vision occurring without an apparent ophthalmic lesion, caused by a systemic poison, as alcohol or tobacco.

intra-, a combining form meaning 'situated, formed, or occurring within': *intrabronchial, intracutaneous, intramatrical.*

intra-aortic balloon pump, a counterpulsation device that provides temporary cardiac assist in the management of refractory left ventricular failure, as may follow myocardial infarction or occur in preinfarction angina. The balloon is attached to a catheter inserted in the aorta and is automatically inflated during diastole and deflated during systole.

intra-articular (ɪn'trəartɪk'yulər),   within a joint.

intra-articular fracture, a fracture involving the articular surfaces of a joint.

intra-articular injection, the injection of a medication into a joint space, usually to reduce inflammation, as in bursitis or fibromyostis. Using the same technique, fluid may be withdrawn from the joint space in abnormal, excessive accumulations of fluid in a joint, secondary to trauma or inflammation.

intra-articular ligament, a ligament that forms part of the joints between 16 of the 24 ribs, dividing the joints into two cavities, each containing a synovial membrane. Each intra-articular ligament consists of a short, flattened band of fibers inside the joint, attached by one extremity to the rib and by the other to the intervertebral disc. Intra-articular ligaments are not present in the joints of the first, tenth, eleventh, and twelfth ribs, each of which has only one synovial cavity. Compare **radiate ligament.**

intra-atrial (ɪn'trəei'triəl),   within an atrium in the heart.

intra-atrial block (ɪn'trəei'triəl),   delayed or abnormal conduction within the atria, identified on an electrocardiogram by a prolonged and often notched P wave.

intracanalicular fibroma (ɪn'trəkæn'əlɪk'yulər),   a tumor containing glandular epithelium and fibrous tissue, occurring in the breast.

intracanicular papilloma (ɪn'trəkənɪk'yulər),   a benign warty growth in certain glands, especially the breast.

intracapsular fracture (ɪn'trəkæp'sulər),   a fracture within the capsule of a joint.

intracardiac catheter (ɪn'trəkar'diæk).   See **cardiac catheter.**

intracardiac lead, **1.** an electrocardiographic conductor in which the exploring electrode is placed within one of the cardiac chambers, usually by means of cardiac catheterization. **2.** *Informal.* a tracing produced by such a lead on an electrocardiograph.

intracartilaginous ossification (ɪn'trəkar'təlæj'ɪnəs). See **ossification.**

intracatheter, a thin, flexible plastic catheter introduced and threaded into a blood vessel to infuse blood, fluid, or medication. Also called *Informal.* **intracath.**

intracavitary therapy, a kind of radiotherapy in which one or more radioactive sources are placed, usually with the help of an applicator or holding device, within a body cavity in order to irradiate the walls of the cavity or adjacent tissues.

intracellular fluid (in'trəsel'yulər), a fluid within cell membranes throughout most of the body, containing dissolved solutes which are essential to electrolytic balance and to healthy metabolism. Compare **interstitial fluid, lymph, plasma.**

intracerebral (in'trəsiri'brəl), within the tissue of the brain, inside the bony skull.

intracistronic (in'trəsistron'ik), within a cistron.

intracranial (in'trəkrei'niəl), within the cranium.

intracranial aneurysm, any aneurysm of any of the cerebral arteries. Rupture of an intracranial aneurysm results in mortality approaching 50 per cent, and there is a high risk of recurrence in survivors of a rupture. Characteristics of the condition include sudden severe headache, stiff neck, nausea, vomiting, and, sometimes, loss of consciousness. Some forms of intracranial aneurysm may be treated surgically. Kinds of intracranial aneurysms include **berry aneurysm, fusiform aneurysm, mycotic aneurysm.**

intracranial electroencephalography. See **electroencephalography.**

intractable, having no relief, as a symptom or a disease that remains unrelieved by the therapeutic measures employed.

intracutaneous (in'trəkyutei'niəs), within the layers of the skin.

intracystic papilloma (in'trəsis'tik), a benign epithelial tumor formed with a cystic adenoma.

intradermal test, a procedure used to identify suspected allergens by subcutaneously injecting the patient with small amounts of extracts of the suspected allergens. The injections are made at spaced intervals, usually in the forearm or in the scapular region. The patient is concurrently injected with the diluent alone as a control procedure. The test is positive if, within 15 to 30 minutes, the injection of extract produces a wheal surrounded by erythema and the control injection produces no symptoms. The intradermal test is started with highly diluted solutions, and, if the initial test is negative, the procedure is repeated with stronger solutions. This gradual method is used to prevent a systemic reaction, which is more of a risk with intradermal testing than with other kinds of allergy testing, as the scratch test. Intradermal testing tends to be more accurate than the scratch test and is often performed if scratch test results are negative or unclear. Intradermal testing also limits to between 20 and 30 the number of suspected allergens that can be examined simultaneously in the skin of one patient. Also called

subcutaneous test. Compare **patch test, scratch test.** See also **conjunctival test, use test.**

intraductal carcinoma, a frequently large neoplasm occuring most often in the breast. The lesion on cross section usually shows well differentiated tumor cells in calcified and dilated ducts of the breast.

intradural lipoma, a fatty tumor in or beneath the dura mater of the spine or sacrum that tends to infiltrate the dorsal column and roots of spinal nerves, causing pain and dysfunction.

intraepidermal carcinoma, a neoplasm of squamous epidermal cells that does not proliferate into the basal area and often occurs at many sites simultaneously. The lesions, which enlarge slowly without healing at the center, are resistant to chemotherapy and to radiation. Also called **Bowen's disease, Bowen's precancerous dermatosis, precancerous dermatitis.**

intracpithelial carcinoma. See **carcinoma in situ.**

intramembranous ossification. See **ossification.**

intramuscular injection, the introduction of a hypodermic needle into a muscle to administer a medication.

■ METHOD: The equipment is selected and the medication drawn up into the syringe. The site that has been selected is prepared by cleansing with alcohol or acetone. The sites most commonly used are the upper, outer quadrant of the gluteal area, the ventrogluteal area, the vastus lateralis of the thigh, or the deltoid muscle. The skin is stretched between the thumb and forefinger. The needle is introduced at a 90-degree angle with a quick thrust and advanced as necessary—not as far as the hub of the needle, but deep into the muscle. The plunger is withdrawn slightly to be sure that the needle has not been placed in a blood vessel. The solution is injected slowly, the needle is withdrawn, and the injection site is massaged.

■ NURSING ORDERS: If the gluteal area is chosen, the patient is asked to lie prone with ankles bent and feet curved in so that the toes of each foot are directed toward the opposite foot to relax the gluteal muscles, thus making the injection less painful. Injection in deltoid muscles is more painful than in other sites and is avoided if possible. The ventral gluteal area and the vastus lateralis are the preferred injection sites in infants. Care is taken not to hit the femur with the tip of the needle when injecting into the vastus lateralis. Needles and syringes are always disposed of in a safe way; they are usually destroyed.

■ OUTCOME CRITERIA: Infection may result from nonaseptic technique; care is taken not to contaminate the needle before injection. Certain medications can cause tissue necrosis if injected into the subcutaneous tissues. Many medications may be given intravenously or intramuscularly, but the intravenous dose may be much smaller; inadvertent injection into a blood vessel could result in severe systemic reactions of an overdose. Not uncommonly, biologicals may leave a knot in the muscle that is not painful and that subsides slowly over several weeks or months, though it may cause concern in the patient or the young patients' parents. The lump should not grow larger or become more painful—if it does, it may be assumed that an abcess has formed.

90°

INTRAMUSCULAR INJECTION

intraocular pressure, the internal pressure of the eye, regulated by resistance to the flow of aqueous humor through the fine sieve of the trabecular meshwork. Contraction or relaxation of the longitudinal muscles of the ciliary body affects the size of the apertures in the meshwork. In older persons, the trabecular meshwork may become sclerotic and obstructed, preventing the normal flow of aqueous humor from passing out at the proper rate and causing an increase in the intraocular pressure. See also **glaucoma.**

intraparietal sulcus, an irregular groove on the convex surface of the parietal lobe that marks the division of the inferior and superior parietal lobules. Also called **interparietal fissure.**

intrapartal care, care of a pregnant woman from the onset of labor to the completion of the third stage of labor with the expulsion of the placenta. See also **antepartal care, newborn intrapartal care, postpartal care.**
■ METHOD: The signs and symptoms of true labor are observed. Uterine contractions increase in frequency, duration, and strength. Pressure of the presenting part of the fetus causes dilatation and effacement of the cervix, producing a bloody discharge called 'bloody show.' A physical examination of the mother is performed, urine is measured regularly through labor and tested for ketones, protein, glucose, and specific gravity and a microhematocrit is often done. The position, attitude, and presentation of the fetus is ascertained by abdominal palpation. The cervical effacement and dilatation and the station of the presenting part of the fetus are determined periodically by vaginal examination, using careful aseptic technique. If the amniotic sac has broken, the color, character, and quantity of the amniotic fluid is noted. The fetal heart rate is counted, and variations are noted in relation to the timing and intensity of contractions. See also **emergency childbirth.**
■ NURSING CONSIDERATIONS: Emotional support and

measures to increase physical comfort are provided by the nurse throughout labor and delivery. Asepsis is maintained, the progress of labor is monitored, and the well-being of the fetus and the mother are continually observed. Following delivery of the infant the mother is observed for hemorrhage; the uterine fundus may need to be massaged to cause it to contract. The placenta is weighed and examined for completeness. The episiotomy, if performed, or any laceration that occurred is usually repaired after delivery of the placenta. Depending on the mother's preference and condition and the policy of the maternity service, the infant may be placed in a warmer or on the mother's abdomen. The mother and infant are observed for a brief period in the delivery area before being transferred to the postpartum unit.
■ OUTCOME CRITERIA: During labor and delivery several danger signs alert the observer to problems. These danger signs include strong, continuous uterine contractions, marked variation of the fetal heart rate, sudden, excessive fetal movement, continuous abdominal pain with increased fundal height, vaginal bleeding, protrusion of the umbilical cord, a large amount of amniotic fluid, meconium-stained amniotic fluid, or an elevation or drop in the mother's temperature, pulse, or blood pressure. Observation for these danger signs is important in providing intrapartal care, but normal spontaneous vaginal delivery of a healthy baby from a healthy mother is the usual outcome of this period.

intrapartal period, the period spanning labor and birth.

intraperiosteal fracture (in'traper'ios'tiəl), a fracture that does not rupture the periosteum.

intrapsychic conflict, an emotional conflict within oneself. See also **conflict.**

intrasocial idiocy, *Obsolete.* a state of mental retardation in which the person is capable of undertaking some form of regular occupation.

intrathecal (in'trəthi'kəl), of or pertaining to a structure, process, or substance within a sheath, as the cerebrospinal fluid within the theca of the spinal canal.

intrathoracic goiter, an enlargement of the thyroid gland that protrudes into the thoracic cavity.

intrauterine contraceptive device (IUCD). See **intrauterine device.**

intrauterine device (IUD) (in'trəyu'tərin), a contraceptive device consisting of a bent strip of radiopaque plastic with a fine monofilament tail that is inserted and left in the uterine cavity for the purpose of altering the physiology of the uterus and Fallopian tubes in order to prevent pregnancy. The mechanism of action is not known. Insertion is performed during or just after menstruation when the cervix is slightly open and menstruation assures that a pregnancy does not exist. The tail string of the IUD is left projecting a few centimeters from the cervix. By feeling the string with her finger from time to time the wearer can be sure the device is in place. The string also provides a hold for removing the IUD. The rate of failure for the IUD method of contraception is approximately 2 to 4 unplanned pregnancies in 100 women using the device for one year. IUDs develop complications, the most serious being infection. Such infections occurring in pregnancy may be overwhelming and lethal; therefore, the IUD is removed if pregnancy is suspected. Some other complications are cervicitis, perforation of the uterus, salpingitis causing sterility, ectopic pregnancy, abortion, embedding of the device in the wall of the uterus, endometritis, bleeding, pain, cramping, undetected expulsion, and irritation of the penis. Women who do not have complications using an IUD are commonly able to retain the device safely for several years, or indefinitely. Also called **intrauterine contraceptive device,** *Informal.* **coil, loop.**

intrauterine fracture, a fracture that occurs during fetal life.

intrauterine growth curve, a line on a standardized graph representing the mean weight for gestational age through pregnancy to term. It provides a method for classifying infants according to their state of maturity and fetal development.

intrauterine growth retardation, an abnormal process in which the development and maturation of the fetus is impeded or delayed by genetic factors, maternal disease, or fetal malnutrition caused by placental insufficiency. See also **small-for-gestational-age infant.**

intravenous, of or pertaining to the inside of a vein, as of a thrombus or an injection, infusion, or catheter.

intravenous bolus, a relatively large dose of medication administered intravenously in a short period of time, usually within 1 to 30 minutes. The intravenous bolus is commonly used when administration of a medication is needed quickly, as in an emergency, when administering drugs that cannot be diluted, as many cancer chemotherapeutic drugs, and when the therapeutic purpose is to achieve a peak drug level in the bloodstream of the patient. The intravenous bolus is not used when the medication involved must be diluted in a large-volume parenteral before entering the bloodstream or when the rapid administration of a medication, as potassium chloride, could be life-threatening. The intravenous bolus is normally not used for patients with decreased cardiac outputs, decreased urinary outputs, pulmonary congestion, or systemic edema. Such patients have decreased tolerances to medications, which therefore must be diluted more than usual and administered at slower rates. A wristwatch with a second hand is recommended for the timing of all intravenous bolus injections. The amount of medication to be delivered per minute is determined by dividing the total amount of medication to be injected by the prescribed time for delivery. The intravenous bolus site is prepared

with an appropriate antiseptic and the site entered with a venipuncture needle. A winged-tip needle is used for administering an intravenous bolus because it is small enough to lessen the risk of collapsing the vein and causing trauma and is more stable than a syringe needle. If a primary intravenous line is already established, the intravenous bolus is administered by mixing the prescribed drug with the appropriate amount of diluent, after first determining whether the drug is compatible with the primary I.V. solution. Also called **intravenous push.**

intravenous cholangiography, (in diagnostic radiology) a procedure for outlining the major bile ducts. A radio-opaque contrast material is injected intravenously and serial x rays are taken. See also **cholangiography.**

intravenous controller, any one of several devices that automatically deliver intravenous fluid at selectable flow rates, usually between 1 and 69 drops per minute. The controller is commonly equipped with a rate selector, drop sensor, drop indicator, and a drop alarm. When the infusion does not flow at the prescribed rate, the drop alarm emits a visual and an audible signal. The intravenous controller works by gravity so that the I.V. container must be placed at least 30 inches above the venipuncture site. The controller cannot exert the positive pressure of a true pump and is not recommended for the delivery of highly viscous fluid or for keeping an arterial line open. Compare **intravenous peristaltic pump, intravenous piston pump, intravenous syringe pump.**

intravenous fat emulsion, a preparation of 10 per cent fat administered intravenously to help maintain the weight of an adult patient or the weight and growth of a younger patient. Such fat emulsions are prepared from refined soy-bean oil and egg-yolk phospholipids and may contain such major fatty acids as linoleic, oleic, palmitic, and linolenic acids. The intravenous fat emulsion is isotonic and may be administered into a peripheral vein but is not mixed with other solutions employed in parenteral alimentation. Intravenous fat emulsions are often administered when hyperalimentation is not sufficient to maintain adequate treatment of a patient or when the patient needs calories but cannot tolerate the high percentage of dextrose contained in hyperalimentation solutions. Such emulsions may also be administered to patients who need more essential fatty acids than are contained in hyperalimentation solutions or to patients who need general nutritional improvement, especially postoperative patients. Intravenous fat emulsions are not administered to patients suffering from disturbances of normal fat metabolism, as hyperlipemia, from severe hepatic diseases, blood coagulation defects caused by decreased blood-platelet counts, pulmonary diseases, lipoid nephrosis, hepatocellular damage, bone marrow dyscrasia, or to patients being treated with anabolic inhibitory drugs. If possible, the intravenous fat emulsion is usually administered during the daytime hours so that the patient may follow a normal eating pattern with rest during the night and a lower nocturnal urinary flow. Once the primary intravenous line has been established, intravenous fat emulsions are usually administered with the aid of an electronic control device to maintain an even flow rate and avoid any fatty-acid overload. The patient's fluid intake and output are regularly measured during the delivery of such an emulsion, and daily blood studies are conducted to determine the level of free-floating triglycerides. Hepatic function tests are performed if the patient receives consecutive intravenous fat emulsion infusions over a long period of time. Immediate adverse reactions or those that may occur up to 2 ½ hours after the onset of the infusion may include temperature rise, flushing, sweating, pressure sensations over the eyes, nausea, vomiting, headache, chest and back pains, dyspnea, and cyanosis. Delayed adverse reactions or those that may occur within 10 days of the onset of such infusions may include hepatomegaly, splenomegaly, thrombocytopenia, focal seizures, hyperlipemia, hepatic damage, jaundice, hemorrhagic diathesis, and gastroduodenal ulcer.

intravenous feeding, the administration of nutrients through a vein or veins.

intravenous infusion, **1.** a solution administered intravenously through an infusion set that includes a plastic or glass vacuum bottle or bag containing the solution and tubing connecting the bottle to a catheter or a needle in the patient's vein. **2.** the process of administering a solution intravenously. Swelling of the limb around and distal to the site of injection may indicate that the tip of the catheter or needle is in the subcutaneous tissue, and not in the vein. The fluid may be infiltrating the tissue spaces. It is withdrawn and the limb is elevated. Redness, swelling, heat, and pain around the vein at the site of injection or proximal to it may indicate thrombophlebitis. The infusion is discontinued and the inflammatory condition is treated. The infusion is usually begun again at another site. See also **venipuncture.**

intravenous infusion filter, any one of the numerous devices used in helping to ensure the purity of an intravenous solution. Intravenous filters strain the intravenous solution to remove such contaminants as dissolved impurities (detergents, proteins, and polysaccharides), extraneous salts, microorganisms, particles, precipitates, and undissolved drug powders. Any such contaminants may complicate the intravenous therapy and the recovery of the patient involved. Some filters are built into the primary intravenous tubing; others must be attached. Manufacturers' instructions come with most filters to assure proper use. One of the main criteria for selecting a filter is the assurance that the filter is not too fine for the intravenous solution to be strained. Filters that are too fine will clog. The size of filter membranes vary from 5 microns to 0.22 microns. Filters of 1 to 5 microns will remove most particulate debris but not most fungi or bacteria. Filters that are 0.45 microns or less will remove fungi and most bacteria; filters that are 0.22 microns will remove all fungi and bacteria but will also reduce the flow rate of the intravenous solution, which is crucial when rapid delivery is required. Aseptic techniques are essential in attaching all filters to the intravenous delivery system. Once attached, filters must be primed according to manufacturers' instructions. Most filters should be upright to function properly, but some filters must be inverted. See also **needle filter.**

intravenous infusion technique, the calculations for determining the delivery rate of intravenous (I.V.) fluid for the individual patient and the necessary spiking of the container and priming of the tubing prior to venipuncture and administration of the fluid.

■ METHOD: The rate at which solution is to be adminis-

Solutions for intravenous use

Type of solution	Contents of solutions								
	Cations (mEq/liter)					Anions (mEq/liter)			Glucose (g/liter)
	Na^+	K^+	Ca^{++}	Mg^{++}	NH_4^+	Cl^-	HCO_3^- lactate	PO_4^-	
5% dextrose in water									50
10% dextrose in water									100
Normal saline (0.9%)	154					154			
3% saline	513					513			
Ringer's solution	147	4	4			155			
5% dextrose in Ringer's lactate	130	4	3			109	28		50
Ringer's lactate	130	4	3			109	28		
Ammonium chloride (0.9%)					170	170			
Sodium lactate 1/6 molar	167						167		
5% dextrose in 0.2% saline	34					34			50

tered by intravenous infusion can be determined from this formula:

$$\frac{\text{Total amount of solution (in ml)}}{\text{Period over which delivered (in hrs)}} = \text{rate (in ml) per hr.}$$

Thus, if 1,000 ml are to be delivered in 8 hrs:

$$\frac{1000}{8} = 125 \text{ ml per hr}$$

To determine which drip system to use, the following formula is useful:

$$\frac{\text{drops per ml x amount of solution (in ml) per hr}}{60 \text{ min}} = \text{drops per min.}$$

Thus, if a macrodrip system of 15 drops per one ml is

$$\frac{15}{60} \times 125 = 31 \text{ drops per min.}$$

used, following the preceding example:
Or, if a microdrip system (60 drops per ml) is used:

$$\frac{60}{60} \times 125 = 125 \text{ drops per min.}$$

The hands are washed thoroughly before assembling the container of I.V. solution, the I.V. pole, and proper tubing with the flow clamp placed in a position directly beneath the drip chamber and clamped. If a bottle with a rubber stopper is used the protective metal cap is removed, and, with the bottle held securely on a stable surface, the spike of the tubing is pushed firmly into the stopper. To spike an I.V. bottle with an indwelling vent and latex diaphragm, the metal cap and diaphragm are removed and the spike is inserted into the nonvented hole; if a hiss, indicating a vacuum, is not heard the bottle is contaminated and is discarded. Nonvented tubing is used with this kind of bottle. A plastic bag of I.V. fluid is hung on a hook for spiking; the cap is removed by pulling it smoothly to the right, and a nonvented spike is inserted into the port using one quick, even motion to prevent the escape of fluid. An I.V. bag with a firm, easily grasped port with a lip to prevent touch contamination may be spiked before hanging by grasping the port firmly; squeezing the bag may expel air and is carefully avoided. After the hanging bag or bottle is spiked, the drip chamber is gently squeezed until it is half full before the tubing is primed. The end of the tubing is held over a sink or wastebasket as the protective cap is removed, and the cap is kept uncontaminated for reuse. The flow clamp is released, and the tubing is allowed to fill with fluid until all air bubbles are expelled; if a backcheck valve is on the tubing, the valve is inverted during priming. The flow clamp is then closed, the protective cap is replaced, and the tubing is looped over the I.V. pole so that it is out of the way during venipuncture. Once the needle or intracatheter is inserted and connected to the tubing, the fluid container is hung securely from the I.V. pole or a hook at a height three feet above the insertion site. The flow clamp is opened and adjusted to deliver the proper rate of delivery of fluid by counting the number of drops entering the drip chamber in a minute. Throughout the administration of I.V. fluid the rate of flow is checked periodically and any necessary readjustments of the clamp are made.

■ NURSING ORDERS: The nurse assembles the apparatus for the I.V. infusion, spikes the fluid container, primes the tubing, calculates the proper rate for the patient, and ensures that the rate of delivery and asepsis are maintained. The nurse carefully observes the patient for signs of circulatory overload, as a bounding pulse, engorged peripheral veins, dyspnea, cough, and pulmonary edema, indicating that the infusion rate is too rapid and requires adjustment.

■ OUTCOME CRITERIA: I.V. solutions administered to maintain normal body fluid levels and the electrolyte balance do not overload the circulation when delivered at the flow rate required by the individual patient.

intravenous injection, a hypodermic injection into a vein for the purpose of instilling a single dose of medication, withdrawing blood, or beginning an intravenous infusion of blood, medication, or a fluid solution, as saline or dextrose in water. See also **venipuncture.**

INTRAVENOUS INJECTION

intravenous peristaltic pump, any one of several devices for administering intravenous fluids by exerting pressure on the I.V. tubing rather than on the fluid itself. Most peristaltic pumps operate with normal I.V. tubing and deliver fluid at a selectable drop-per-minute rate. This device typically can infuse between 1 and 99 drops of intravenous fluid per minute and is equipped with a drop sensor, rate selector, power switch indicator lamp, and drop indicator and alarm. The drop indicator flashes whenever a drop of intravenous fluid passes the drop sensor. The drop alarm beeps when the infusion does not flow at the prescribed rate. Compare **intravenous controller, intravenous piston pump, intravenous syringe pump.**

intravenous piston pump, any one of several devices that accurately control the infusion of intravenous fluids by piston action. Most intravenous piston pumps can be operated by battery as well as by electric current and require special tubing. Some models are portable. Intravenous piston pumps are commonly equipped with controls that allow selectable flow rates and indicators that display flow rates, dose limits, and cumulative fluid volumes. Such pumps commonly monitor the patient's skin for infiltration by intravenous fluid and are equipped with infiltration and flow alarms. The intravenous piston pump monitors the actual volume of intravenous fluid administered instead of counting drops of fluid. Hence, its accuracy is not affected by drop size, temperature, or fluid viscosity. The pump is designed to reduce the delivery rate to a keep-vein-open rate if the proper flow rate or the dose limit is exceeded. The pump also stops delivery of the intravenous fluid if the I.V. line is clogged or if infiltration is detected. Compare **intravenous controller, intravenous peristaltic pump, intravenous syringe pump.** See also **infiltration detector.**

intravenous pump, a pump designed to regulate the rate of flow of a fluid given intravenously through an intracatheter or a scalp vein needle. See also **Abbot pump, Harvard pump.**

intravenous push. See **intravenous bolus.**

intravenous pyelography (IVP), a technique in radiology for examining the structures and evaluating the function of the urinary system. A contrast medium is injected intravenously, and serial x rays are taken as the medium is cleared from the blood by glomerular filtration. The renal calyces, renal pelvis, ureters, and urinary bladder are all visible on the x-ray films. Tumors, cysts, stones, and many structural and functional abnormalities may be diagnosed using this technique. A cathartic or an enema is usually given the day before the procedure, since the kidneys lie retroperitoneally and gas or fecal material in the bowel may prevent visualization of the urinary tract. The person is given nothing by mouth from midnight preceding the test in order to induce a moderate state of dehydration, thereby allowing concentration of the contrast medium in the collecting structures. The client may also be asked to void immediately prior to injection of the dye in order to avoid dilution of the medium in the bladder. Also called **descending urography, excretory urography.**

intravenous syringe pump, any one of several devices which automatically compress a syringe plunger at a controlled rate. Such devices are used with disposable syringes that can deliver blood, medications, or nutrients by intravenous, arterial, or subcutaneous routes. Intravenous syringe pumps can deliver small volumes of fluid at rates as low as 0.01 ml/hr and are often used in the treatment of infants. They are ideal for keeping arterial lines open and are usually battery-operated and portable. They are especially useful in treating ambulatory patients. Compare **intravenous controller, intravenous peristaltic pump, intravenous piston pump.**

intravenous urography. See **intravenous pyelography (IVP).**

intraventricular (ɪn'trəventrɪk'yulər), of or pertaining to the space within a ventricle.

intraventricular heart block, an interruption of the cardiac stimulus as it passes over the ventricles, seen as a prolonged QRS complex on an electrocardiogram. It is usually caused by decreased conduction in the branches of the bundle of His.

intraventricular hydrocephalus. See **hydrocephalus.**

intrinsic, a natural or inherent part or quality.

intrinsic asthma, a nonseasonal, nonallergic form of asthma, usually first occurring later in life than allergic asthma, that tends to be chronic and persistent rather than episodic. The precipitating factors include inhalation of irritating pollutants in the atmosphere, as dust particles, smoke, aerosols, strong cooking odors, paint fumes, and other volatile substances. Bronchospasm may also occur in cold, damp weather, after the sudden inhalation of cold, dry air, and after physical exercise or violent coughing or laughing. Respiratory infections, as the common cold, and psychological factors, as anxiety, may also induce an attack. Compare **allergic asthma.** See also **asthma in children.**

intrinsic factor, a substance secreted by the gastric mucosa that is essential for the intestinal absorption of vitamin B_{12}. Intrinsic factor forms a bond with molecules of vitamin B_{12} (cobalamin) and transports them across the membranes of the ileum. A deficiency of intrinsic factor, owing to gastrectomy, myxedema, or atrophy of the gastric mucosa, results in pernicious anemia. See also **pernicious anemia.**

intro-, a combining form meaning 'into or within': *introgastric, introjection, introsusception.*

introitus (ɪntrou'ɪtəs), an entrance or orifice to a cavity or a hollow tubular structure of the body, as the vaginal introitus.

intron (ɪn'tron), (in molecular genetics) a sequence of base pairs in DNA that interrupts the continuity of genetic information. Some genes contain a number of long intervening sequences.

Intropin, a trade name for an adrenergic (dopamine hydrochloride).

introspection, 1. the act of examining one's own thoughts and emotions by concentrating on the inner self. 2. a tendency to look inward and view the inner self. —**introspective,** *adj.*

introversion, intraversion, 1. the tendency to direct one's interests, thoughts, and energies inward or toward things concerned only with the self. 2. the state of being totally or primarily concerned with one's own intrapsychic experience. Compare **extroversion.**

introvert, 1. a person whose interests are directed inward and who is shy, withdrawn, emotionally reserved, and self-absorbed. 2. to turn inward or to direct one's interests and thoughts toward oneself. Compare **extrovert.** See also **egocentric.** —**introversion,** *n.*

intubation, passage of a tube into a body aperture, specifically, the insertion of a breathing tube through the mouth or nose or into the trachea to ensure a patent airway for the delivery of an anesthetic gas or oxygen. **Blind intubation** is the insertion of a breathing tube without the use of a laryngoscope. Kinds of intubation are **endotracheal intubation, nasogastric intubation.**

intussusception (ɪn′təsəsep′shən), prolapse of one segment of bowel into the lumen of another segment. This kind of intestinal obstruction may involve segments of the small intestine, the colon, or the terminal ileum and cecum. Intussusception occurs most often in infants and small children and is characterized by abdominal pain, vomiting, and bloody mucus in the stool. Barium enema is used to confirm the diagnosis, and surgery is usually necessary to correct the obstruction. See also **intestinal obstruction.**

inulin (ɪn′yulɪn), a diagnostic aid used in tests of kidney function, specifically glomerular filtration.

inulin clearance, a test of the rate of filtration of a starch, inulin, in the glomerulus of the kidney. Inulin is given by mouth, and the glomerular filtration rate can be estimated from the length of time needed for the inulin to appear in the urine.

inundation fever. See **scrub typhus.**

invagination, 1. a condition in which one part of a structure telescopes into another part, as the intestine during peristalsis. If the invagination is extensive or involves a tumor or polyps, it may cause an intestinal obstruction, and surgery is indicated. 2. surgery for repair of a hernia by replacing the contents of the hernial sac in the abdominal cavity. General or spinal anesthesia may be used. No upper respiratory infection, chronic cough, or allergy with sneezing can be present, for it will weaken the repair. Postoperatively, the nurse checks for retention of urine. See also **hernia, intestinal obstruction, peristalsis.** – **invaginate,** v.

invariable behavior, behavior that results from physiologic response to a stimulus and is not modified by individual experience, as a reflex. Compare **variable behavior.**

invasion of privacy, (in law) the violation of another person's right to be left alone and free from unwarranted publicity and intrusion.

invasive, characterized by a tendency to spread, infiltrate, and intrude.

invasive carcinoma, a malignant neoplasm composed of epithelial cells that infiltrate and destroy surrounding tissues.

invasive mole. See **chorioadenoma destruens.**

inverse anaphylaxis, an exaggerated reaction of hypersensitivity induced by an antibody rather than by an antigen. Also called **reverse anaphylaxis.**

inverse relationship. See **negative relationship.**

inverse square law, a law stating that the amount of radiation emitted is inversely proportional to the square of the distance between the source and the irradiated surface, as a person two feet from a patient being treated with radium is exposed to four times more radiation than he would be exposed to at four feet.

Inversine, a trade name for a ganglionic blocking agent (mecamylamine hydrochloride).

inversion, 1. an abnormal condition in which an organ is turned inside out, as a uterine inversion. 2. a chromosomal defect in which two or more segments of a chromosome break off and become separated. They rejoin the chromosome in the wrong order, causing the genes carried on one arm of the chromosome to be in a position and sequence different from those on the other arm.

invert, a homosexual.

investigational new drug (IND), a drug not yet approved for marketing by the Food and Drug Administration and available only for use in experiments to determine its safety and effectiveness. The use of an investigational new drug in human subjects requires approval by the Food and Drug Administration of an application that includes reports of animal toxicity tests, descriptions of proposed clinical trials, and a list of the investigators and their qualifications.

invisible differentiation, (in embryology) a fixed determination for specialization and diversification that exists in embryonic cells but is not yet visibly apparent. See also **chemodifferentiation.**

in vitro (ɪn vi′trou), (of a biological reaction) occurring in laboratory apparatus. Compare **in vivo.**

in vivo (ɪn vi′vou), (of a biological reaction) occurring in a living organism. Compare **in vitro.**

in vivo tracer study, (in nuclear medicine) a diagnostic procedure in which a series of radiograms of an administered radioactive tracer as it passes through a compartment in the patient's body demonstrates normal or abnormal structures or processes. A strip chart recording of an in vivo tracer study, as a radionuclide angiocardiogram, shows the passage of the tracer through the central circulation.

involucrum (ɪn′vəlu′krəm), pl. **involucra.** a sheath or coating, as that encasing a sequestrum of necrotic bone.

involuntary, occurring without conscious control or direction. See also **autonomy.**

involuntary muscle. See **smooth muscle.**

involuntary nervous system. See **visceral nervous system.**

involution, 1. a normal process characterized by a decrease in the size of an organ owing to a decrease in the size of its cells, as postpartum involution of the uterus. 2. (in embryology) a developmental process in which a group of cells grows over the rim at the border of the organ or part and, rolling inward, rejoins the organ or part to form a tube, as in the heart or bladder.

involutional depression. See **involutional melancholia.**

involutional melancholia, a state of depression occurring during the climacteric. The disorder begins gradually and is characterized by pessimism, irritability, insomnia, loss of appetite, feelings of anxiety, and an increase in motor activity, ranging from mere restlessness to extreme agitation. In the rare instances where treatment is necessary, antidepressant drugs, electroconvulsive treatment, and various forms of psychotherapy may be used. Also called **climacteric melancholia, involutional depression, involutional psychosis.** See also **depression.**

involutional psychosis. See **involutional melancholia.**

inward aggression, destructive behavior that is directed against oneself. See also **masochism.**

-io, a noun-forming combining form: *abrasio, evulsio, injectio.*

ioderma (ai′oudər′mə), **iododerma** (aiou′doudər′mə), a skin rash caused by a hypersensitivity to ingested iodides. The lesions may be acneiform, bullous, or fungating. Treatment requires removal of iodides from the diet.

iodinated ^{125}**I serum albumin** (ai′ədɪnei′ted), a sterile, buffered isotonic solution containing radioiodinated normal human serum adjusted to provide not more than one millicurie of radioactivity per milliliter in diagnostic tests of blood volume and cardiac output.

iodine (I), a nonmetallic element of the halogen group. Its atomic number is 53; its atomic weight is 128.90. Iodine is a bluish-black solid that becomes a violet vapor upon heating without going through a liquid phase. An essential micronutrient or trace element, almost 80 per cent of the iodine present in the body is in the thyroid gland, mostly in the form of thyroglobulin. Iodine deficiency can result in goiter or cretinism. Iodine is found in seafoods, iodized salt, and some dairy products. Radioisotopes of iodine are used in radioisotope scanning procedures and in palliative treatment of cancer of the thyroid.

iodize, to treat or impregnate with iodine or an iodide. Table salt is iodized to prevent the occurrence of goiter in areas with insufficient iodine in the drinking water. Iodized oil, a viscous liquid with the odor of garlic, has been used as a contrast medium in roentgenology.

iodo-, a combining form meaning 'of or pertaining to iodine': *iododerma, iodogenic, iodolography.*

iodochlorhydroxyquin (aiou′dəklərhaidrok′səkwɪn), an antiamebic and topical anti-infective.

■ INDICATIONS: It is prescribed in the treatment of eczema, athlete's foot, and other fungal infections.

■ CONTRAINDICATIONS: The presence of tuberculosis or viral skin conditions or known hypersensitivity to this drug or to iodine prohibits its use.

■ ADVERSE EFFECTS: The most serious adverse reaction is irritation to sensitive skin.

iodoform, a topical anti-infective used as an antiseptic.

iodopsin (ai′oudop′sɪn), a photosensitive chemical in the cones of the retina, which reacts in association with other chemicals and plays a part in color vision. Iodopsin is more stable when exposed to bright light than rhodopsin, which is found in the rods of the retina. Color vision, a synthesis of red, green, and blue light, is induced by changes within the pigments of different types of cones during a photochemical process in which coded nerve impulses are sent to the brain. Research continues into color vision, and the exact role of iodopsin is still unknown.

ion (ai′ən, ai′on), an atom or group of atoms that has acquired an electric charge through the gain or loss of an electron or electrons.

-ion[1], a combining form meaning an 'electrically charged particle': *anion, cation, ion.*

-ion[2], a noun-forming combining form: *endognation, osteopedion, parhelion.*

Ionamin, a trade name for an anoretic (phentermine).

ion-exchange chromatography, the process of separating and analyzing different substances according to their affinities for chemically stable but very reactive synthetic exchangers, which are composed largely of polystyrene and cellulose. The process uses an absorbent containing ionizing groups and accommodates the exchange of ions between a solution of substances to be analyzed and the absorbent. Ion-exchange chromatography is often used to separate components of nucleic acids and proteins elaborated by various structures throughout the body. Different ions deposited in the absorbent during the exchange produce bands of different colors, which constitute a chromatograph. Compare **column chromatography, gas chromatography.**

ionization, the process in which a neutral atom or molecule gains or loses electrons and thus acquires a negative or positive electric charge. Ionization occurs when atoms or molecules dissociate in solution or when those of gases dissociate in an electric field. Ionizing radiation produces ionization in its passage through matter.

ionize (ai′ənaiz), to separate or change into ions. See also **ion.** – **ionization,** *n.*

ionizing energy, the average energy lost by ionizing radiation in producing an ion pair in a gas. In air, the value is approximately 33.73 electron-volts (eV).

ionizing radiation, high-energy electromagnetic waves (as x rays and gamma rays,) and particulate rays, (as alpha particles, beta rays, electrons, neutrons, positrons, protons, and heavy nuclei), that dissociate substances in their paths into ions. The spatial distribution of the ionization depends on the kind of radiation, its penetrating power, the location of the source, and the nature of the irradiated material. High energy x rays penetrate deeply, most beta particles penetrate only a few millimeters, and alpha particles penetrate only a fraction of a millimeter, but they all produce intense ionization along their tracks. Ionizing radiation directly affects living organisms by killing cells or retarding their development; its indirect effects include the production of gene mutations and chromosome breaks. Animal tissues containing elements with relatively high atomic weights, as calcium in bones and teeth, absorb much higher doses from a given radiation than are absorbed by soft tissue.

Iowa trumpet, a kind of needle guide used in performing a pudendal block. It consists of a long thin cylinder through which a needle may be passed. A ring is attached to the proximal end of the guide, allowing the operator to hold it securely.

ipecac, an emetic.
- INDICATIONS: It is prescribed to cause emesis in certain types of poisoning and drug overdose.
- CONTRAINDICATIONS: Known hypersensitivity to this drug prohibits use. It is not used in unconscious patients or for poisoning by petroleum distillates, strong alkalis, acids, or strychnine.
- ADVERSE EFFECT: The most serious adverse reaction is cardiotoxicity if vomiting does not occur and the substance is retained.
- NOTE: If vomiting does not occur, the ipecac is recovered by gastric lavage.

ipomea (ɪpəmiʹə), a resin prepared from the dried root of *Ipomoea orizabensis,* formerly used as a cathartic.

IPPB, abbreviation for **intermittent positive pressure breathing.** a form of assisted or controlled respiration produced by a ventilatory apparatus in which compressed gas is delivered under positive pressure into the person's airways until a preset pressure is reached. Passive exhalation is allowed through a valve and the cycle begins again as the flow of gas is triggered by inhalation.
- METHOD: The use of the IPPB unit involves the combined efforts of the physician, inhalation therapist or technician, and the nurse. Orders for the specific pressure and volume and the use of nebulizing or other attachments are ordered individually. The equipment is tested and is introduced to the patient by the inhalation therapist. The nurse observes that the patient closes the lips around the mouthpiece and does not allow air to escape from the nose or mouth during inspiration and that the therapy is effective. Also called **intermittent positive pressure ventilation.**
- OUTCOME CRITERIA: Ventilation may be greatly improved by the use of the IPPB unit. Secretions may be thinned and cleared and the passages may be humidified, allowing greater comfort and a better exchange of gases.
- NURSING ORDERS: The patient may require reassurance that the machine will automatically shut off the flow of air at the end of inspiration and encouragement to relax and allow the lungs to be completely filled by the machine. The patient is cautioned not to manipulate any of the controls.

IPPB (intermittent positive pressure breathing) unit,
a pressure-cycled ventilator for providing a flow of air into the lungs at a predetermined pressure. As the pressure is attained, the flow is stopped, pressure is released, and the patient exhales. The device is used to prevent postoperative atelectasis, to promote full expansion of the lungs, to improve oxygenation, and to administer nebulized medications into the respiratory passages.

IPPV, abbreviation for *intermittent positive pressure ventilation.* See **IPPB.**

IQ, abbreviation for **intelligence quotient.**

Ir, symbol for **iridium.**

iralgia (ɪrælʹjə), **iridalgia** (ɪrɪdælʹjə), *Obsolete.* any pain or inflammation in the iris. **iralgic, iridalgic,** *adj.*

IRB, abbreviation for **institutional review board.**

iridectomy, surgical removal of part of the iris of the eye, performed most often to restore drainage of the aqueous humor in glaucoma or to remove a foreign body or a malignant tumor. General anesthesia is used. An incision is made through the cornea, and the iris is grasped with forceps or a hook and drawn out through the incision. The area involved is cut away and the elastic iris is allowed to slip back into place. Atropine and an antibiotic are instilled, and a dressing and a shield are applied. Postoperatively, the patient is observed for signs of local hemorrhage or excessive pain.

iridium (Ir), a silvery-bluish metallic element. Its atomic number is 77; its atomic weight is 192.2.

irido-, a combining form meaning 'of or pertaining to the iris, or to a colored circle': *iridocele, iridokeratitis, iridoplegia.*

iridotomy, a surgical incision into the iris of the eye, performed to relieve occlusion of the pupil, to enlarge the pupil in cataract extraction, or to treat postoperative glaucoma. Local or general anesthesia is used. An incision is made through the cornea, and a cut is made transversely across the sphincter fibers of the iris. Atropine and an antibiotic are instilled, and a dressing and shield are applied. Postoperatively, the dressing is observed for signs of drainage. Excessive pain is abnormal. See also **iridectomy, iris.**

iris, a circular, contractile disc suspended in aqueous humor between the cornea and the crystalline lens of the eye and perforated by a circular pupil. The periphery of the iris is continuous with the ciliary body and is connected to the cornea by the pectinate ligament. The iris divides the space between the lens and the cornea into an anterior and a posterior chamber. In the adult, the two chambers communicate through the pupil but are separated in the fetus, up to the seventh month, by the membrana pupillaris. The involuntary muscle of the iris is composed of circular fibers and radiating fibers. Dark pigment cells under the translucent tissue of the iris are variously arranged in different people to produce different colored irises. The pigment is absent in albinos. In blue eyes the pigment cells are confined to the posterior surface of the iris but in gray eyes, brown eyes, and black eyes the pigment cells appear in the anterior layer of epithelium and in the stroma. See also **dilatator pupillae, sphincter pupillae.** —**iridic,** *adj.*

iritis, an inflammatory condition of the iris of the eye characterized by pain, lacrimation, photophobia, and, if severe, diminished visual acuity. On ophthalmic examination the eye looks cloudy, the iris bulges, and the pupil is contracted. The underlying cause is treated if known, but the condition is most often idiopathic. The pupil is dilated, usually with atropine, and a corticosteroid may be prescribed to reduce inflammation. If the inflammation is allowed to continue and the pupil left constricted, permanent scarring may occur, causing an opacity over the lens and diminished vision.

IRITIS

iron (Fe), a common metallic element essential for the synthesis of hemoglobin. It is used as a hematinic in the form of its salts and complexes, as ferrocholinate, ferrous fumarate, gluconate, sulfate, and iron-dextran.

iron-deficiency anemia, a microcytic, hypochronic anemia caused by inadequate supplies of iron needed to synthesize hemoglobin, characterized by pallor, fatigue, and weakness. Laboratory diagnosis includes hemoglobin, hematocrit, transferrin, and serum iron evaluation. Iron deficiency may be the result of an inadequate dietary supply of iron, of poor absorption of iron in the digestive system, or of chronic bleeding. Compare **hemolytic anemia, hypoplastic anemia.** See also **anemia, iron metabolism, red cell indices.**

iron dextran, a hematinic.

■ INDICATIONS: It is prescribed in the treatment of iron-deficiency anemia not responsive to oral iron therapy.

■ CONTRAINDICATIONS: Early pregnancy, anemias other than iron-deficiency anemia, or known hypersensitivity to this drug prohibits its use.

■ ADVERSE EFFECTS: Among the more serious adverse effects are severe hypersensitivity reactions, including fatal anaphylaxis. Inflammation or phlebitis at the site of injection, arthralgia, headache, gastrointestinal distress, fever, and lesser hypersensitivity reactions may occur.

iron lung. See **Drinker respirator.**

iron metabolism, a series of processes involved in the entry of iron into the body through its absorption, its transport and storage throughout the body, its utilization for the formation of hemoglobin and other iron compounds, and its eventual excretion. Iron normally enters the body through the epithelium of the intestinal mucosa, being oxidized from ferrous to ferric iron in the process. The rate at which iron enters is modulated by this absorption mechanism. When iron stores are high, iron no longer passes through, but, instead, is trapped by the mucosal cells of the intestine to be eliminated upon their death. Once iron enters the blood, it is in a closed system in which, attached to transferrin, it cycles between the plasma and the reticuloendothelial or erythropoietic system. Plasma iron is delivered to the normoblast for hemoglobin synthesis where it remains up to four months, trapped in the hemoglobin molecules of a mature red cell. Senescent red cells then deteriorate and break down. The iron is released from the hemoglobin by the reticuloendothelial system to reenter the transport pool for recycling. The normal iron distribution in a 70 kg adult (male) totals approximately 3.7 gm with more than 65 per cent of this in circulating hemoglobin. Another 27 per cent is found in the storage pool as hemosiderin or ferritin. The body normally conserves iron so well that loss, usually only through the feces, is normally limited to about 1 mg/day. This amount is easily provided by a dietary intake of only 10 mg/day. Iron deficiency may follow extended intervals of inadequate iron intake (especially in women) or after excessive blood loss. Iron overload sometimes occurs in disorders in which normal regulation of absorption of iron is impaired. It is most commonly produced iatrogenically through the parenteral administration of large amounts of iron or blood for therapeutic purposes. See also **anemia.**

iron-rich food, a nutrient containing a relatively large amount of iron. The best source of dietary iron is liver, with oysters, clams, heart, kidney, lean meat, and tongue as second choices. Leafy green vegetables are the best plant sources. See also **iron, iron-deficiency anemia.**

iron salts poisoning, poisoning caused by overdosage of ferric or ferrous salts, characterized by vomiting, bloody diarrhea, cyanosis, and gastric and intestinal pain. Therapy includes gastric lavage, administration of an emetic, deferoxamine, and supportive therapy as indicated by the severity of the symptoms.

iron transport, the process whereby iron is carried from its entry point into the body, the intestinal mucosa, to the various sites of utilization and storage. Transferrin binds with free iron and shuttles it to storage and utilization sites. Transferrin becomes attached to exogenous iron entering through the intestinal villi or to iron reentering the plasma from the sinusoids of the spleen. The iron is then released to the normoblasts and the transferrin is freed for additional transport functions that may, to a small extent, involve iron stored as ferritin or hemosiderin. Compare **transferrin.** See also **hemosiderosis, iron metabolism.**

irradiation, exposure to any form of radiant energy like heat, light, or x-ray. Radioactive sources of radiant energy, such as x-rays or isotopes of iodine or cobalt, are used diagnostically to examine internal body structures, utilizing knowledge of the ways in which various tissues absorb or reflect radioactive emissions. The same or similar sources of radioactivity in larger amounts are used to destroy microorganisms or tissue cells that have become cancerous. Infrared or ultraviolet light may be used to produce heat in body tissues to relieve pain and soreness or to treat acne, psoriasis, or other skin ailments. Ultraviolet light is also used to identify certain bacteria and toxic molds. See also **radiation sickness, radioactivity, ultraviolet.** – **irradiate,** v.

irreducible, unable to be returned to the normal position or condition, as an irreducible hernia. See also **incarcerate.**

irreversible coma. See **brain death.**

irrigation, the process of washing out a body cavity or wounded area with a stream of water or other fluid. It is also used to cleanse a tube or drain inserted into the body, as an in-dwelling catheter. The procedure is most commonly performed with water, saline, aminoacetic acid, or antiseptic solutions on the eye, ear, throat, vagina, and urinary tract. Gentle pressure is applied in the introduction of the fluid, except in the debridement of wounds, and the solution is removed from internal cavities through suction or by drainage. See also **lavage.** – **irrigate,** v.

irrigator, an apparatus with a flexible tube for flushing or washing out a body cavity.

irritable bowel syndrome, abnormally increased motility of the small and large intestines, generally associated with emotional stress. Most of those affected are young adults, who complain of diarrhea and, occasionally, pain in the lower abdomen. The pain is usually relieved by moving the bowels. In diagnosing irritable bowel syndrome, other more serious conditions, as dysentery, lactose intolerance, and the inflammatory bowel diseases must be ruled out. Because there is no organic disease present in irritable bowel syndrome, no specific treatment is necessary. Many persons benefit from the use of bulk-producing agents in the diet, because bulk tends to stabilize the water content of the stool. Antidiarrheal drugs are helpful in decreasing the frequency of stool. Although this is a functional disorder, patients experience pain and discomfort and need emotional support. Mild tranquilizers or antidepressants are sometimes given to relieve anxiety or depression. Also called **mucous colitis, spastic colon.**

IRV, abbreviation for *inspiratory reserve volume.* See **pulmonary function test.**

ischemia (iski'miǝ), decreased blood supply to a body organ or part. Some causes of ischemia are arterial embolism, atherosclerosis, thrombosis, vasoconstriction. Compare **infarction.** – **ischemic,** adj.

ischemic contracture. See **Volkmann's contracture.**

ischemic lumbago, a pain in the lower back and buttocks caused by vascular insufficiency, as in occlusion of the abdominal aorta.

ischemic pain, the unpleasant, often excruciating sensation associated with ischemia, resulting from peripheral vascular disease, from decreased blood flow owing to constricting orthopedic casts, or from insufficient blood flow owing to surgical trauma or accidental injury. Ischemic pain caused by occlusive arterial disease is often severe and may not be relieved, even with narcotics. The individual with peripheral vascular disease may experience ischemic pain only while exercising because the metabolic demands for oxygen cannot be met by the occluded flow of blood. The ischemic pain of partial arterial occlusion is not as severe as the abrupt, excruciating pain associated with a complete blocking of the artery, as by an embolism. The ischemic pain caused by the pressure of an orthopedic cast is difficult to differentiate from the acute pain caused by surgical intervention, because both types of pain may be localized rather than diffused, as is the pain caused by trauma. Compare **incisional pain.** See also **pain intervention, pain mechanism.**

ischio-, a combining form meaning 'of or pertaining to the ischium, or to the hip': *ischioanal, ischiodidymus, ischiopagus.*

ischium (is'kiǝm), pl. **ischia.** one of the three parts of the hip bone, joining the ilium and the pubis to form the acetabulum. The ischium comprises the dorsal part of the hip bone and is divided into the body of the ischium, which forms two fifths of the acetabulum, and the ramus, which joins the inferior ramus of the pubis. The spine of the ischium provides attachment for various muscles, as the gemellus superior, the coccygeus, and the levator ani. The greater sciatic notch above the spine transmits the superior and the inferior gluteal vessels and various nerves, as gluteal nerves, the sciatic nerve, and the nerves to the obturator internus and the quadratus femoris. A notch below the spine of the ischium transmits various ligaments, vessels, and nerves for other parts. The large dorsal tuberosity of the ischium provides attachment for various muscles, as the adductor longus, the semimembranosus, the biceps femoris, and the semitendinosus. Compare **ilium, pubis.**

ISG, abbreviation for **immune serum globulin.**

Ishihara color test (ish'iha'rǝ), a test of color vision using a series of plates on which are printed round dots in a variety of colors and patterns. People with normal color vision are able to discern specific numbers or patterns on the plates; the inability to pick out a given number or shape is symptomatic of a specific deficiency in color perception.

island fever. See **scrub typhus.**

islands of Langerhans (lɑrŋ'gərhænz), clusters of cells within the pancreas that produce insulin, glucagon, and pancreatic polypeptide. They form the endocrine portion of the gland and their hormonal secretions released into the blood stream are balanced, important regulators of sugar metabolism. The islands of Langerhans are scattered throughout the pancreas; the beta cells, which secrete insulin, usually appear in the center of each of the lobules. Alpha cells secrete glucagon, and pancreatic- peptide cells secrete pancreatic peptide. The cells comprising the islands are arranged in plates interspersed by capillaries. Also called **islets of Langerhans.**

islet adenoma. See **insulinoma.**

islet cell adenoma. See **insulinoma.**

islet cell tumor, any tumor of the islands of Langerhans.

islets of Langerhans. See **islands of Langerhans.**

-ism, -ismus, a combining form meaning 'condition of, practice of, theory of': *hyperthyroidism, hypopituitarism, strabismus.*

Ismelin, a trade name for an antihypertensive (guanethidine sulfate).

iso-, a combining form meaning 'equal': *isobar, isochromatic, isohydria.*

isoagglutinin (ai'souəglu'tɪnɪn), an antibody that causes agglutination of erythrocytes in other members of the same species that carry an isoagglutinogen on their erythrocytes. Also called **isohemagglutinin.** Compare **isoagglutinogen.** See also **ABO bloodgroups, antibody.**

isoagglutinogen (ai'souəglutɪn'əjɪn), an antigen that causes the agglutination of erythrocytes in others of the same species that carry a corresponding isoagglutinin in their serum. Also called **isohemagglutinin.** Compare **agglutinin.** See also **ABO blood groups.**

isoamyl alcohol (ai'souæm'ɪl). See **amyl alcohol.**

isoantibody, an antibody to isoantigens found in other members of the same species. See also **autoimmune disease, tissue typing.**

isoantigen (ai'souæn'tɪjɪn), a substance that interacts with isoantibodies in other members of the same species. Compare **autoantigen, autoimmune disease.** See also **antigen, isoagglutinogen.**

isobar (ai'səbar), (in nuclear medicine) one of a group of nuclides having the same total number of neutrons and protons in the nucleus but so proportioned as to result in different values of the atomic number.

isobutyl alcohol (ai'soubyu'tɪl), a clear, colorless liquid that is miscible with ethyl alcohol or ether.

isocarboxazid, a monoamine oxidase inhibitor.

■ INDICATION: It is prescribed in the treatment of mental depression.

■ CONTRAINDICATIONS: Liver or kidney dysfunction, congestive heart failure, pheochromocytoma, concomitant use of a sympathomimetic drug or foods high in tryptophan or tyramine, or known hypersensitivity to this drug prohibits its use.

■ ADVERSE EFFECTS: Among the more serious adverse reactions are hyperactivity, cardiac arrhythmia, hypotension, vertigo, dryness of mouth, constipation, and blurred vision. Monoamine oxidase inhibitors produce many adverse drug interactions.

isodose chart, (in radiotherapy) a graphic representation of the distribution of radiation in a medium; lines are drawn through points receiving equal doses. Isodose charts are determined for x rays traversing the body, for radium applicators used in intracavitary or interstitial treatment, and for working areas where x rays or radionuclides are employed.

isoelectric electroencephalogram. See **flat electroencephalogram.**

isoetharine, a bronchodilator. See **isoetharine mesylate.**

isoetharine hydrochloride, a bronchodilator. See **isoetharine mesylate.**

isoetharine mesylate, a beta-adrenergic bronchodilator.

■ INDICATIONS: It is prescribed in the treatment of bronchial asthma, bronchitis, and emphysema.

■ CONTRAINDICATIONS: A history of cardiac arrhythmias or known hypersensitivity to this drug or to sympathomimetic medications prohibits its use.

■ ADVERSE EFFECTS: Among the more serious adverse reactions are palpitations, tachycardia, arrhythmias, vertigo, nervousness, and headache.

isoflurophate, a cholinesterase inhibitor.

■ INDICATIONS: It is prescribed in the treatment of open-angle glaucoma and esotropia.

■ CONTRAINDICATIONS: Uveal inflammation or known hypersensitivity to this drug or to other organophosphates prohibits its use.

■ ADVERSE EFFECTS: Among the more serious adverse reactions are systemic cholinergic effects, visual disturbances, a paradoxical increase in intraocular pressure, and, with long-term administration, the development of cataracts.

isogamete (ai'sougæm'it), a reproductive cell of the same size and structure as the one with which it unites. Compare **anisogamete.** – **isogametic,** *adj.*

isogamy (aisog'əmi), sexual reproduction in which there is fusion of gametes of the same size and structure, as in certain algae, fungi, and protozoa. Compare **anisogamy, heterogamy.** – **isogamous,** *adj.*

isogenesis, isogeny, development from a common origin and according to similar processes. – **isogenetic, isogenic,** *adj.*

isohemagglutinin (ai'souhi'məglu'tının, ai'souhem'əglu'- tının). See **isoagglutinin**.

Isolette, a trade name for a self-contained incubator unit that provides a controlled heat, humidity, and oxygen microenvironment for the isolation and care of premature and low birth-weight neonates. The apparatus is made of a clear plastic material and has a large door and portholes for easy access to the infant with a minimum of heat and oxygen loss. A servocontrol mechanism constantly monitors the infant's temperature and controls the heat within the unit.

isoleucine (ai'soulu'sin), an amino acid, occurring in most dietary proteins, that is essential for proper growth in infants and for nitrogen balance in adults. See also **amino acid, protein.**

isomethcptene hydrochloride, an antispasmodic and vasoconstrictor drug that is a component in some fixed-combination drugs used to treat migraine.

isometric (ai'səmet'rık), maintaining the same length or dimension.

isometric exercise, a form of active exercise that increases muscle tension by applying pressure against stable resistance. This may be accomplished by opposing different muscles in the same individual, as by pressing the hands together or by making a limb push or pull against an immovable object. There is no joint movement and the length of the muscle remains unchanged, but muscle strength and tone are maintained or improved. Compare **isotonic exercise.** See also **exercise.**

isometric growth, an increase in size of different organs or parts of an organism at the same rate. Compare **allometric growth.**

isoniazid (INH) (ai'sənai'əzıd), a tuberculostatic antibacterial.
- INDICATION: It is prescribed in the treatment of tuberculosis caused by mycobacteria sensitive to the drug.
- CONTRAINDICATIONS: Liver disease, a previous history of a hepatotoxic reaction to isoniazid, or known hypersensitivity to this drug prohibits its use.
- ADVERSE EFFECTS: Among the more serious adverse reactions in long-term treatment are hepatoxicity and peripheral neuropathy. Rashes, fever, and central nervous system effects commonly occur.

isopentoic acid (ai'soupentou'ık). See **isovaleric acid.**

isophane insulin suspension, a modified form of protamine zinc insulin suspension. It is an intermediate-acting insulin that is a stable, commonly prescribed preparation. Also called **NPH insulin.**

isophosphamide, an antineoplastic, currently under investigation, that is a derivative of cyclophosphamide. See also **cyclophosphamide.**

isopropamide iodide, an anticholinergic.
- INDICATION: It is prescribed as an adjunct to ulcer therapy.

- CONTRAINDICATIONS: Narrow angle glaucoma, asthma, obstruction of the genitourinary or gastrointestinal tract, ulcerative colitis, or known hypersensitivity to this drug prohibits its use.
- ADVERSE EFFECTS: Among the more serious adverse reactions are blurred vision, central nervous system effects, tachycardia, dry mouth, decreased sweating, and hypersensitivity reactions.

isopropanol (ai'souprou'pənol). See **isopropyl alcohol.**

isopropylacetic acid (ai'souprou'pıləsi'tık, ai'souprou'- pıləset'ık). See **isovaleric acid.**

isopropyl alcohol (ai'souprou'pıl), a clear, colorless, bitter aromatic liquid that is miscible with water, ether, chloroform, and ethyl alcohol. A solution of approximately 70 per cent isopropyl alcohol in water is used as a rubbing compound. Also called **avantin, dimethyl carbinol, isopropanol.** See also **alcohol, ethyl alcohol.**

isopropylaminoacetic acid. See **valine.**

isoproterenol hydrochloride (ai'souprəter'ənol), a beta-adrenergic stimulant.
- INDICATIONS: It is used as a bronchodilator and as a cardiac stimulant.
- CONTRAINDICATIONS: Cardiac arrhythmia or known hypersensitivity to this drug prohibits its use.
- ADVERSE EFFECTS: Among the more serious adverse reactions are arrhythmias, tachycardia, hypotension, and intensification of angina.

Isopto Atropine, a trade name for an anticholinergic (atropine sulfate).

Isopto Carbachol, a trade name for a cholinergic (carbachol).

Isopto Carpine, a trade name for a cholinergic (pilocarpine hydrochloride).

Isopto Cetamide, a trade name for an antibacterial (sulfacetamide sodium).

Isopto Eserine, a trade name for a cholinergic (physostigmine salicylate).

Isopto Frin, a trade name for an adrenergic (phenylephrine hydrochloride).

Isopto Homatropine, a trade name for an anticholinergic (homatropine hydrobromide).

Isopto Hyoscine, a trade name for an anticholinergic (scopolamine hydrobromide).

Isordil, a trade name for an antianginal agent (isosorbide dinitrate).

Isordil with Phenobarbital, a trade name for a cardiovascular fixed-combination drug containing an antianginal agent (isosorbide dinitrate) and a sedative-hypnotic (phenobarbital).

isosmotic (ai'sozmot'ık). See **isotonic.**

isosorbride dinitrate, an antianginal agent.
- INDICATIONS: It is prescribed as a coronary vasodilator in the treatment of angina pectoris and congestive heart failure.

■ CONTRAINDICATION: Known hypersensitivity to this drug prohibits its use.

■ ADVERSE EFFECTS: The most serious reaction is occasional marked hypotension. Flushing, headache, and dizziness also may occur.

isotonic (ai'səton'ık), (of a solution) having the same concentration of solute as another solution, hence exerting the same amount of osmotic pressure as that solution, as an isotonic saline solution that contains an amount of salt equal to that found in the intra- and extracellular fluid. Also called **isosmotic.**

isotonic exercise, a form of active exercise in which the muscle contracts and causes movement. Throughout the procedure there is no significant change in the resistance so that the force of the contraction remains constant. Such exercise greatly improves joint mobility and helps to improve muscle strength and tonality. Compare **isometric exercise.** See also **exercise.**

isotope (ai'sətoup), one of two or more forms of a chemical element having almost identical properties: they have the same number of protons in the atomic nucleus and the same atomic number, but they differ in the number of their nuclear neutrons and atomic weights. Carbon (C^{12}) has six nuclear neutrons, while its isotope C^{14} has eight. Many hundreds of radioactive isotopes are used in diagnostic and therapeutic procedures.

isotopic tracer (ai'sətop'ık), an isotope or artificial mixture of isotopes of an element incorporated into a sample to permit observation of the course of the element, alone or in combination, through a chemical, physical, or biological process. The observations may be made by measuring the radioactivity or the abundance of the isotope.

isovaleric acid (ai'souvələr'ık), a combustible, toxic compound with a disagreeable taste and odor, found in tobacco, valerian, oil of hops, and cheese, in sweat of the feet, and in urine in smallpox, typhus, and hepatitis. Commercially produced isovaleric acid is used in perfumes, flavors, and certain drugs. Also called **isopentoic acid, isopropylacetic acid.**

isoxsuprine hydrochloride, a peripheral vasodilator.

■ INDICATIONS: It is prescribed for the symptomatic relief of cerebrovascular insufficiency and to improve the circulation in arteriosclerosis, Raynaud's disease, and Buerger's disease.

■ CONTRAINDICATION: Known hypersensitivity to this drug is the only contraindication.

■ ADVERSE EFFECTS: Among the more serious adverse reactions are tachycardia, hypotension, and dermatitis.

-ist, a combining form meaning a 'practitioner of a science': *audiologist, pharmacist, psychosomaticist.*

isthmus (ıs'məs), *pl.* **isthmuses, isthmi.** a narrow connection between two larger bodies or parts, as the isth-mus of the auditory tube in the ear, which connects the bony and the cartilaginous parts of the tube.

Isuprel, a trade name for a beta-adrenergic stimulant (isoproterenol).

itch, 1. to feel a sensation, usually on the skin, that makes one want to scratch. 2. a tingling, annoying sensation on an area of the skin that makes one want to scratch it, as may be caused in some people by rhus dermatitis, a mosquito bite, or an allergic reaction. 3. the pruritic condition of the skin caused by infestation with the parasitic mite *Sarcoptes scabiei.* —**itchy,** *adj.*

-ite, 1. a combining form meaning 'compounds': *nitrite, phosphite, sulfite.* 2. a combining form meaning a 'body part': *chondriomite, osteite, zygoite.*

ithy-, a combining form meaning 'straight': *ithylordosis, ithyokyphosis.*

-itic, a combining form meaning 'of or related to something specified': *encephalitic, nephritic, syphilitic.*

-itis, a combining form meaning an 'inflammation of a (specified) organ': *carditis, cecitis, sarcitis.*

ITP, abbreviation for **idiopathic thrombocytopenic purpura.** *Rx splenectomy*

I.U., IU, abbreviation for **International Unit.**

IUCD, abbreviation for **intrauterine contraceptive device.** See **intrauterine device.**

IUD, abbreviation for **intrauterine device.**

-ium, a combining form used to name metallic elements: *aluminum, radium, sodium.*

I.V., 1. abbreviation for **intravenous. 2.** *Informal.* equipment consisting of a bottle of fluid, infusion set with tubing, and an intracatheter, used in intravenous therapy. 3. intravenous administration of fluids or medication by injection into a vein.

IVAC pump, a trade name for a portable intravenous pump that electronically regulates and monitors the flow of fluid. It is usually attached to the I.V. stand. See also **intravenous pump.**

ivory bones. See **osteopetrosis.**

IVP, abbreviation for **intravenous pyelography.**

I.V. push, a technique in which a bolus of medication or a large volume of intravenous fluid is given rapidly via intravenous injection or infusion. Methergine may be given in this way to cause immediate contraction of the uterus in postpartum hemorrhage. See also **intravenous injection.**

I.V.-type traction frame, a metal support that holds traction equipment consisting of two metal uprights, one at each end of the bed, which support an overhead metal bar. Each upright is clamped to a horizontal bar that fits into holders inserting at the corners of the bed. Compare **claw-type traction frame.** See also **traction frame.**

Ixodes (ıksou′diz), a genus of parasitic hard-shelled ticks associated with the transmission of a variety of arbovirus infections, as Rocky Mountain spotted fever.

ixodi-, a combining form meaning 'of or pertaining to ticks': *ixodiasis, ixodism.*

ixodid (ıksod′ıd, ıksou′dıd), of or pertaining to hard ticks of the family Ixodidae.

-ize, a combining form meaning 'do, treat, cause': *anesthetize, canalize, fertilize.*

J

jacket, a supportive or confining therapeutic casing or garment for the torso. Some kinds of jackets are **Minerva jacket, plaster-of-Paris jacket, Sayre's jacket.**

jacket restraint, an orthopedic device used to help immobilize the trunk of a patient in traction and to discourage the patient from sitting up in bed. The jacket restraint is attached to both sides of the bedspring frame by means of buckled webbing straps that are sewn into the side seams of the restraint. The jacket restraint may be used with most kinds of traction but is not usually used with Dunlop skin traction or Dunlop skeletal traction, Bryant traction, halo-femoral traction, or halo-pelvic traction. Compare **diaper restraint, sling restraint.**

jackknife position, an anatomic position in which the patient is placed on the back in a semi-sitting position, with the thighs flexed on the abdomen. Examination and instrumentation of the male urethra is facilitated by this position.

Jacob's membrane (jei'kəbz), the outermost of the nine layers of the retina, composed of rods and cones interacting directly with the optic nerve.

Jacquemier's sign (źhakmyeiz'), a deepening of the color of the vaginal mucosa just below the urethral orifice. It may sometimes be noted after the fourth week of pregnancy, but it is not a reliable sign of pregnancy.

jact-, a combining form meaning 'to throw': *jactatio, jactation, jactitation.*

jail fever. See **epidemic typhus.**

Jakob-Creutzfeldt disease (ya'kəbkrɔits'felt). See **Creutzfeldt-Jakob disease.**

JAMA, abbreviation for *Journal of the American Medical Association.*

jamais vu (źhʌmei vʏ'), *French.* the sensation of being a stranger when with a person one knows or when in a familiar place. The phenomenon occurs occasionally in normal people but more frequently in people who have temporal lobe epilepsy. Compare **déjà vu.**

Janeway lesion, a small erythematous or hemorrhagic macule occurring on the palms or soles, sometimes diagnostic of subacute bacterial endocarditis.

janiceps (jæn'əseps), a conjoined, twin fetal monster in which the heads are fused, with the faces looking in opposite directions. The faces and bodies of both twins may be fully formed or one member may be only partially formed and act as a parasite on the more fully developed fetus.

Jansen's disease. See **metaphyseal dysostosis.**

Japanese B encephalitis. See **Japanese encephalitis.**

Japanese encephalitis, a severe epidemic infection of brain tissue seen in East Asia and Japan, characterized by shaking chills, paralysis, and weight loss, and caused by a group of B arboviruses transmitted by mosquitoes. Mortality may be as high as 33 per cent. Various neurologic and psychiatric sequelae are common. There is no specific treatment. Also called **Japanese B encephalitis.**

Japanese flood fever. See **scrub typhus.**

Japanese river fever. See **scrub typhus.**

JAPHA, abbreviation for *Journal of the American Public Health Association.*

Jarisch-Herxheimer reaction (ja'rɪśhhərks'haimər), a sudden transient fever and exacerbation of skin lesions observed several hours after administration of penicillin or other antibiotics in the treatment of syphilis, leptospirosis, or relapsing fever. The effect lasts less than 24 hours and requires no treatment.

Jarotzky's treatment (jərot'skiz), therapy of gastric ulcer using a bland diet consisting of egg whites, fresh butter, bread, milk, and noodles.

jaundice, a yellow discoloration of the skin, mucous membranes, and sclerae of the eyes, caused by greater-than-normal amounts of bilirubin in the blood. Persons with jaundice may also experience nausea, vomiting, and abdominal pain and may pass dark urine. Jaundice is a symptom of many disorders, including liver disease, biliary obstruction, and the hemolytic anemias. Newborns commonly develop physiological jaundice, which disappears after a few days. Rarer disorders causing jaundice are Crigler-Najjar syndrome and Gilbert's syndrome. Useful diagnostic procedures include a clinical evaluation of the signs and symptoms, tests of liver function, techniques for direct or indirect visualization as x ray, CAT scan, ultrasound, endoscopy or exploratory surgery, and biopsy. Also called **icterus.** See also **hyperbilirubinemia.** −**jaundiced,** *adj.*

jaw jerk. See **jaw reflex.**

jaw reflex, an abnormal reflex elicited by tapping the chin with a rubber hammer while the mouth is half open and the jaw muscles are relaxed. A quick snapping shut of the jaw implies damage to the area of cerebral cortex governing motor activity of the fifth cranial nerve. Also called **jaw jerk.**

JCAH, abbreviation for **Joint Commission on Accreditation of Hospitals.**

jeco-, a combining form meaning 'of or pertaining to the liver': *jecolein, jecoral, jecorin.*

Jefferson fracture, a fracture characterized by bursting of the ring of the atlas.

jejuno-, a combining form meaning 'of or pertaining to the jejunum': *jejunocecostomy, jejunocolostomy, jejunotomy.*

jejunoileitis (jɪju'nɔʊɪl'iaɪ'tɪs). See **Crohn's disease.**

jejunum (jɪju'nəm), *pl.* **jejuna.** one of the three portions of the small intestine, connecting proximally with the duodenum and distally with the ileum. The jejunum has a slightly larger diameter, a deeper color, and a thicker wall than the ileum, and contains heavy, circular folds that are absent in the lower part of the ileum. The jejunum also has larger villi than the ileum. Compare **ileum.** — **jejunal,** *adj.*

jellyfish sting, a wound caused by skin contact with a jellyfish, a sea animal with a bell-shaped gelatinous body and suspended numerous long tentacles containing stinging structures. In most cases a tender, red welt develops on the affected skin. In some cases, depending on the sensitivity of the person and the particular species of jellyfish, severe localized pain and nausea, weakness, excessive lacrimation, nasal discharge, muscle spasm, perspiration, and dyspnea may occur. Treatment includes carefully removing any tentacles and applying a compress of alcohol, aromatic spirits of ammonia, or Dakin's solution. Calcium gluconate may be administered to control muscle spasms.

Jendrassik's maneuver (yendra'shɪks), (in neurology) a diagnostic procedure in which the patient hooks the flexed fingers of the two hands together and forcibly tries to pull them apart. While this tension is being exerted, the lower extremity reflexes are tested, particularly the patellar reflex.

jet lag, a condition characterized by fatigue, insomnia, and sluggish body functions caused by disruption of the normal circadian rhythm resulting from air travel across several time zones.

jigger. See **chigoe.**

Job-Basedow phenomenon, thyrotoxicosis occurring when dietary iodine is given to a patient with endemic goiter in an area of environmental iodine deficiency. It is presumed that iodine deficiency protects some patients with endemic goiter from developing thyrotoxicosis. The phenomenon may also occur when large doses of iodine are given to patients with nontoxic multinodular goiter in areas with sufficient environmental iodine. There is a danger of inducing the phenomenon if iodine containing drugs, as x-ray contrast media, are administered to elderly patients with nontoxic multinodular goiter.

jock itch. See **tinea cruris.**

jogger's heel, a painful condition, common among joggers and distance runners. It is characterized by bruising, bursitis, fasciitis, or calcaneal spurs, caused by repetitive and forceful strikes of the heel on the ground. Judicious selection of well-fitting running shoes and avoidance of running on hard surfaces are recommended to avoid occurrence or recurrence of the condition. Rest, heat, or corticosteroid medication or aspirin may be recommended.

joint, any one of the connections between bones. Each is classified according to structure and movability as fibrous, cartilaginous, or synovial. Fibrous joints are immovable, cartilaginous joints slightly movable, and synovial joints freely movable. Typical immovable joints are those connecting most of the bones of the skull with a sutural ligament. Typical slightly movable joints are those connecting the vertebrae and the pubic bones. Most of the joints in the body are freely movable and allow gliding, circumduction, rotation, and angular movement. Also called **articulation.** See also **cartilaginous joint, fibrous joint, synovial joint.**

(See next page for illustration)

joint and several liability, (in law) a condition in which several persons share the liability for a plaintiff's injury and may be found liable individually or as a group.

joint appointment, **1.** a faculty appointment to two institutions within a university or system, as to the schools of nursing and medicine of the same university. **2.** (in academic nursing) the appointment of a member of the faculty of a university to a clinical service of an associated service institution. A psychiatric nurse might hold appointment in a university as an assistant professor and might also be a clinical nurse specialist in a service institution. The practice of joint appointments is said to have begun at Case-Western Reserve University, University Hospital. See also **unification model.**

joint audit. See **nursing audit.**

joint chondroma, a cartilaginous mass that develops in the synovial membrane of a joint.

Joint Commission on Accreditation of Hospitals (JCAH), a private, nongovernmental agency that establishes guidelines for the operation of hospitals and other health-care facilities, conducts accreditation programs and surveys, and encourages the attainment of high standards of institutional medical care. Members of the JCAH include representatives from the American Medical Association, American College of Physicians, and American College of Surgeons.

joint fracture, a fracture of the articular surfaces of the bony structures of a joint.

jointly exhaustive categories, categories on a research instrument that are sufficiently complete to allow every possible subject, factor, or variable to be classified and assigned to a category.

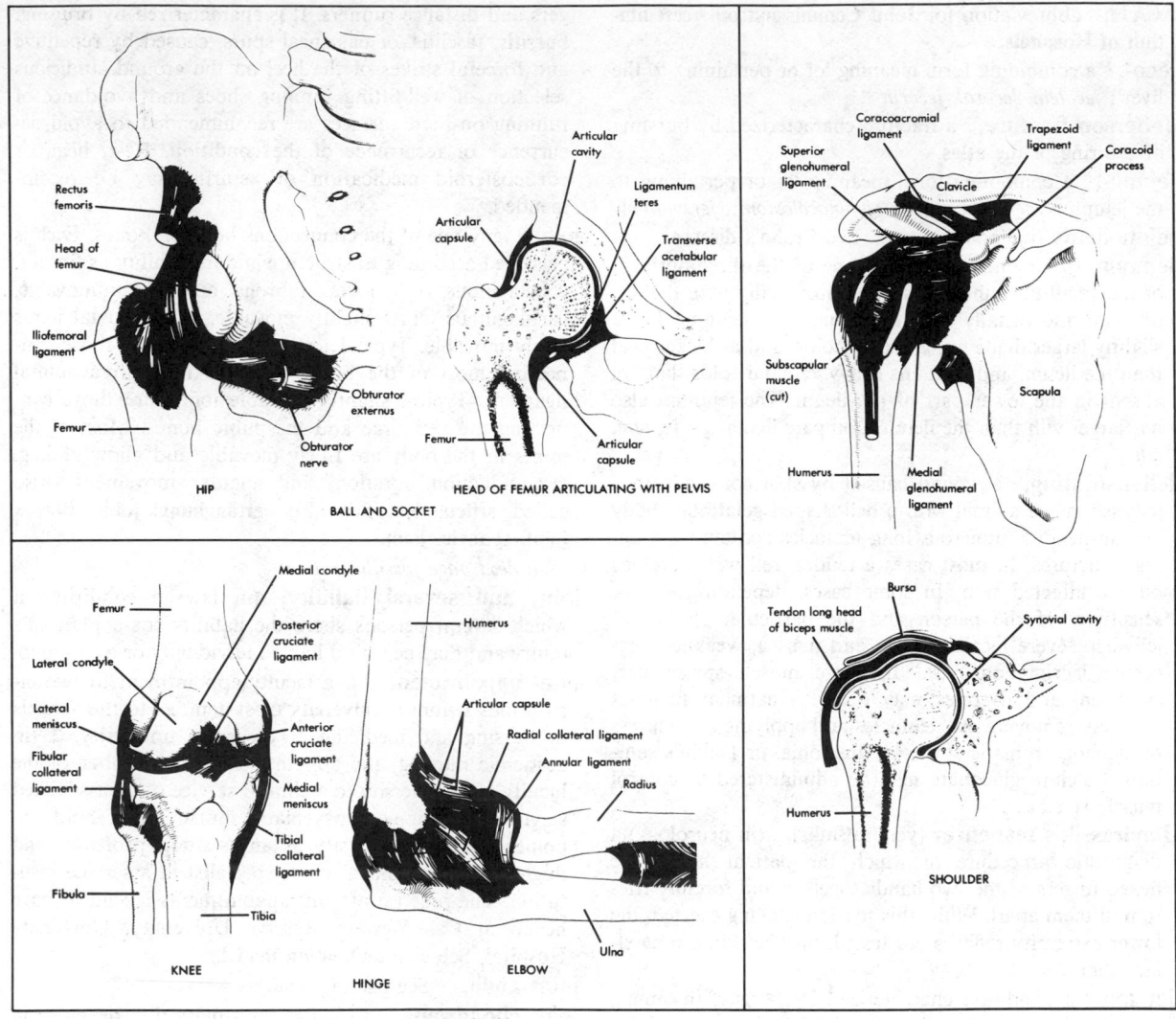

JOINTS

joint practice, **1.** the practice of a physician and a nurse practitioner, usually private, who work as a team, sharing responsibility for a group of patients. **2.** (in inpatient nursing) the practice of making joint decisions about patient care by committees of the physicians and nurses working on a division.

Jones criteria, a standardized set of guidelines for the diagnosis of rheumatic fever, as recommended by the American Heart Association. See also **rheumatic fever.**

judgment, (in law) **1.** the final decision of the court regarding the case before it. **2.** the reason given by the court for its decision; an opinion. **3.** an award, penalty, or other sentence of law given by the court.

judgment call, *Slang.* a decision based on experience,

especially a judgment that resolves a serious problem in which the data are inconclusive or equivocal.

jug-, a combining form meaning 'yoke': *jugal, jugum.*

jugu-, a combining form meaning 'throat or neck': *jugular, jugulation.*

jugular foramen, one of a pair of openings between the lateral part of the occipital bone and the petrous part of the temporal bones in the skull. The foramen transmits the inferior petrosal sinus, the transverse sinus, some meningeal branches of the occipital and ascending pharyngeal arteries and the glossopharyngeal, vagus, and accessory nerves.

juice, any fluid secreted by the tissues of animals or plants. In humans, it usually refers to the secretions of the digestive glands. Kinds of juices include **gastric juice, intestinal juice, pancreatic juice.**

jumping gene, (in molecular genetics) a unit of genetic information associated with a segment of DNA that can move from one position in the genome to another.

junction nevus, a hairless, flat or slightly raised, brown skin blemish arising from pigment cells at the epidermal-dermal junction. A junction nevus may be found anywhere on the surface of body. All nevi of the palms and soles and all pigmented nevi in early childhood are of this type. Malignant change may be signaled by increase in size, hardness or darkening, bleeding, or the appearance of satellite discoloration around the nevus. Junction nevi undergoing these changes and lesions found in areas subject to trauma should be removed.

junctura cartilaginea (kar'tɪləjɪn'ɪə). See **cartilaginous joint.**

junctura fibrosa. See **fibrous joint.**

junctura synovialis. See **synovial joint.**

Jungian psychology (yuŋ'ɪən). See **analytic psychology.**

Junin fever. See **Argentinian hemorrhagic fever.**

junk, *Slang.* heroin.

justo major, *Archaic.* atypically large, as a woman's bony pelvis.

juvenile, 1. a young person; youth; child; youngster. **2.** of, pertaining to, characteristic of, or suitable for a young person; youthful. **3.** physiologically underdeveloped or immature. **4.** denoting psychological or intellectual immaturity; childish.

juvenile alveolar rhabdomyosarcoma, a rapidly growing tumor of striated muscle with a grave prognosis, occurring in children and adolescents, chiefly in the extremities.

juvenile angiofibroma. See **nasopharyngeal angiofibroma.**

juvenile delinquency, persistent antisocial, illegal, or criminal behavior by children or adolescents to the degree that it cannot be controlled or corrected by the parents, it endangers others in the community, and it becomes the concern of a law enforcement agency. Such behavioral patterns are characterized by aggressiveness, destructiveness, hostility, and cruelty and occur more frequently in boys than in girls. Causative factors typically involve poor parent-child relationships, especially parental rejection, indifference, and apathy, and unstable family environments where disciplinary methods are lax, erratic, overly strict, or involve harsh physical punishment. Traditional punitive treatments, primarily correctional institutions and reform schools, usually aggravate rather than remedy the situation. More progressive approaches, such as foster-home placement, work and recreational programs, and various community and family counseling services, have been more successful. Behavior therapy and other forms of psychotherapy, often involving the parents as well as the child, are also used as modes of treatment and prevention. See also **antisocial personality disorder, behavior disorder.**

juvenile delinquent, a person who performs illegal acts and who has not reached an age at which treatment as an adult can be accorded under the laws of the community having jurisdiction.

juvenile diabetes, an inability to metabolize carbohydrate caused by an overt insulin deficiency, occurring in children and characterized by polydipsia, polyuria, polyphagia, loss of weight, diminished strength, and marked irritability. The onset is usually rapid, but approximately one third of the patients have a remission within three months; this stage may continue for days or years, but diabetes then progresses quickly to a state of total dependence on insulin. Occasionally, the disease is asymptomatic and is discovered only by postprandial hyperglycemia or glucose tolerance tests. Juvenile diabetes tends to be unstable and brittle, with the patients quite sensitive to insulin and physical activity and liable to develop ketoacidosis. Recent evidence suggests that juvenile onset diabetes may be caused by environmental factors, as a virus. See also **diabetes mellitus.**

juvenile kyphosis. See **Scheuermann's disease.**

juvenile lentigo. See **lentigo.**

juvenile-onset diabetes. See **juvenile diabetes.**

juvenile rheumatoid arthritis. See **Still's disease.**

juvenile xanthogranuloma, a skin disorder characterized by groups of yellow, red, or brown papules or nodules on the extensor surfaces of the arms and legs, and in some cases on the eyeball, meninges, and testes. The lesions typically appear in infancy or early childhood and usually disappear in a few years.

juxta-, a combining form meaning 'near': *juxtaglomerular, juxtangina, juxtaposition.*

K

K, symbol for **potassium.**

Kafocin, a trade name for an antibacterial (cephaloglycin).

kak-, a combining form meaning 'bad': *kakidrosis, kakosmia.*

Kakke disease (kak′kei). See **beriberi.**

kala-azar (ka′ləəzar′), a disease caused by the protozoan, *Leishmania donovani,* transmitted to humans, particularly to children, by the bite of the sand fly. Kala-azar occurs primarily in Asia, parts of Africa, several South and Central American countries, and in the Mediterranean region. The liver and spleen are the main sites of infection; signs and symptoms include anemia, hepatomegaly, splenomegaly, irregular fever, and emaciation. Patients with kala-azar are also susceptible to secondary bacterial infections. Untreated, the disease has an extremely high mortality rate. Treatment includes sodium antimony gluconate, blood transfusions (for anemia), bed rest, and adequate nutrition. Also called **Assam fever, black fever, dumdum fever, ponos, visceral leishmaniasis.** See also **leishmaniasis.**

Kalavert, a trade name for a nutritional supplement containing potassium chloride, sodium chloride, dextrose, and fructose.

kali-, a combining form meaning 'of or pertaining to potassium': *kaliemia, kaligenous, kalium.*

kanamycin (kæn′əmaɪ′sɪn), an antibacterial substance derived from *Streptomyces kanamyceticus.*

kanamycin sulfate, an aminoglycoside antibiotic.

■ INDICATIONS: It is prescribed in the treatment of certain severe infections.

■ CONTRAINDICATIONS: Concomitant administration of ototoxic drugs or known hypersensitivity to this drug or to other aminoglycoside antibiotics prohibits its use. It is used with caution in patients having impaired renal function.

■ ADVERSE EFFECTS: Among the more serious adverse reactions are nephrotoxicity, vestibular and auditory ototoxicity, neuromuscular blockade, and hypersensitivity reactions.

Kantrex, a trade name for an antibacterial (kanamycin sulfate).

Kanulase, a trade name for a gastrointestinal, fixed-combination drug containing various antiflatulent ingredients.

Kaochlor, a trade name for an electrolyte-replacement solution (potassium chloride).

kaodzera (ka′odzi′rə). See **Rhodesian trypanosomiasis.**

kaolin (kei′əlɪn), an adsorbent used internally to treat diarrhea, often in combination with pectin. Kaolin in an ointment base is also used topically as an absorbent and a protective emollient.

Kaon, a trade name for the electrolyte-replacement solution (potassium gluconate).

Kaopectate, a trade name for an antidiarrheal fixed-combination drug containing an adsorbent (kaolin) and an emollient (pectin).

Kaposi's sarcoma (kæp′əsiz), a malignant, multifocal neoplasm of reticuloendothelial cells that begins as soft, brownish or purple papules on the feet and slowly spreads in the skin, metastasizing to the lymph nodes and viscera. It occurs most often in Jewish, Italian, and Negro men and is occasionally associated with diabetes or malignant lymphoma. Radiotherapy and chemotherapy are usually recommended. Also called **idiopathic multiple pigmented hemorrhagic sarcoma, multiple idiopathic hemorrhagic sarcoma.**

Kaposi's varicelliform eruption. See **eczema herpeticum.**

kaps-. See **caps-.**

karaya powder, a dried form of *Sterculia urens* or other species of *Sterculia,* used as a bulk cathartic. Like other bulk-forming agents, karaya powder reduces the intraluminal rectosigmoid pressure and helps relieve symptoms in patients with irritable bowel disease and diverticular disease of the colon. Relief of pain and other symptoms may occur progressively over several months. Because of its ability to absorb water and form an emollient intestinal mass, karaya powder also may be useful in relieving the symptoms of acute diarrhea and in modifying the effluent in the patient with an ileostomy or a colostomy. The use of such a bulk-forming cathartic may also increase the loss of sodium, potassium, and water in such patients. With some individuals the use of karaya powder may cause allergic reactions, as urticaria, rhinitis, dermatitis, and asthma. Methylcellulose has largely replaced this drug in modern use.

Kardex (kar′deks), a trade name for a card-filing system that allows quick reference to the particular needs of each patient for certain aspects of nursing care. Included on the card may be a schedule of medications, level of activity allowed, ability to perform basic self-care, diet, any special problems, a schedule of treatments and procedures, and a care plan. The Kardex is updated as necessary and is usually kept at the nurses' station.

karyenchyma (kær′ieng′kimə). See **karyolymph.**

karyo-, a combining form meaning 'of or pertaining to a nucleus': *karyochrome, karyokinesis, karyolymph.*

karyogamy (kær′iog′əmi), the fusion of cell nuclei, as in conjugation and zygosis. – **karyogamic,** *adj.*

karyogenesis (kær′ioujen′isis), the formation and development of the nucleus of a cell. – **karyogenetic,** *adj.*

karyokinesis (kær′ioukini′sis, kær′ioukaini′sis), the division of the nucleus and equal distribution of nuclear material during mitosis and meiosis. The process involves the four stages of prophase, metaphase, anaphase, and telophase, and it precedes the division of the cytoplasm. Also called **karyomitosis.** See also **cytokinesis.** – **karyokinetic,** *adj.*

karyoklasis, karyoclasis (kær′iok′ləsis), **1.** the disintegration of the cell nucleus or nuclear membrane. **2.** the interruption of mitosis. – **karyoklastic, karyoclastic,** *adj.*

karyology (kær′iol′əji), the branch of cytology that concentrates on the study of the cell nucleus, especially the structure and function of the chromosomes. – **karyologic, karyological,** *adj., ***karyologist,** *n.*

karyolymph (kær′iəlimf′), the clear, usually nonstaining, fluid substance of the nucleus. It consists primarily of proteinaceous, colloidal material in which the nucleolus, chromatin, linin, and various submicroscopic particles are dispersed. Also called **karyenchyma, nuclear hyaloplasm, nuclear sap, nucleochyme.** – **karyolymphatic,** *adj.*

karyolysis (kær′iol′isis), the dissolution of the cell nucleus. It occurs normally, both as a form of necrobiosis and during the generation of new cells through mitosis and meiosis.

karyolytic (kær′iəlit′ik), **1.** of or pertaining to karyolysis. **2.** that which causes the destruction of the cell nucleus.

karyomere (kær′iəmir′), **1.** a saclike structure containing an unequal portion of the nuclear material following atypical mitosis. **2.** a segment of the chromosome. See also **chromomere.**

karyometry, the measurement of the nucleus of a cell. – **karyometric,** *adj.*

karyomit (kær′iəmit′), a single chromatin fibril of the network within the nucleus of a cell.

karyomitome (kær′iom′itoum), the fibrillar chromatin network within the nucleus of a cell. Also called **karyoreticulum.**

karyomitosis (kær′ioumaitou′sis, kær′ioumitou′sis). See **karyokinesis.**

karyomorphism, the shape or form of a cell nucleus, especially that of the leukocyte. – **karyomorphic,** *adj.*

karyon, the nucleus of a cell. – **karyontic,** *adj.*

karyophage, an intracellular protozoan parasite that destroys the nucleus of the cell it infects. – **karyophagic, karyophagous,** *adj.*

karyoplasm (kær′iouplæz′əm). See **nucleoplasm.** – **karyoplasmic,** *adj.*

karyoplasmic ratio. See **nucleocytoplasmic ratio.**

karyopyknosis (kær′ioupiknou′sis), the state of a cell in which the nucleus has shrunk and the chromatin has condensed into solid masses, as in cornified cells of stratified squamous epithelium. – **karyopyknotic,** *adj.*

karyoreticulum (kær′iouritik′yuləm). See **karyomitome.**

karyorrhexis (kær′iərek′sis), the fragmentation of chromatin and distribution of it throughout the cytoplasm as a result of nuclear disintegration. – **karyorrhectic,** *adj.*

karyosome (kær′iəsoum′), a dense irregular mass of chromatin filaments in the cell nucleus. It is often seen during interphase and may be confused with the nucleolus because of similar staining properties. Also called **chromocenter, chromatin nucleolus, false nucleolus, prochromosome.**

karyospherical (kær′iousfer′ikəl), **1.** of or pertaining to a nucleus that is spherical in shape. **2.** such a nucleus.

karyostasis (kær′ios′təsis), the resting stage of the nucleus between cell division. See also **interphase.** – **karyostatic,** *adj.*

karyotheca (kær′iəthi′kə), the membrane that encloses a cell nucleus. – **karyothecal,** *adj.*

karyotin (kær′iou′tin). See **chromatin.**

karyotype (kær′iətaip′), **1.** the total morphological characteristics of the somatic chromosome complement of an individual or species, described in terms of number, form, size, and arrangement within the nucleus, as determined by a microphotograph taken during the metaphase stage of mitosis. **2.** a diagrammatic representation of the chromosome complement of an individual or species, arranged in pairs in descending order of size and according to the position of the centromere. See also **Denver classification.** – **karyotypic,** *adj.*

kat-, a combining form meaning 'down, against': *katadidymus, katakinetomeric, katolysis.* Also **kata-, cat-, cata-.**

katadidymus, conjoined twins that are united in the lower portion of the body and separated at the top.

Kavrin, a trade name for a smooth-muscle relaxant (papaverine hydrochloride).

Kawasaki disease (ka′wasa′ki). See **mucocutaneous lymph node syndrome.**

Kay Ciel, a trade name for an electrolyte-replacement solution (potassium chloride).

Kayser-Fleischer ring (kai′zərflai′shər), a gray-green to red-gold pigmented ring at the outer margin of the cornea, pathognomonic of hepatolenticular degeneration, a rare progressive disease caused by a defect in copper metabolism and transmitted as an autosomal recessive trait. The disease is characterized by cerebral degenerative changes, liver cirrhosis, splenomegaly, involuntary movements, muscle rigidity, psychic disturbances, and dysphagia.

K cell. See **null cell.**

Kedani fever. See **scrub typhus.**

kefir, kephir (kef′ər), a slightly effervescent, acidulous beverage prepared from the milk of cows, sheep, or goats through fermentation by kefir grains, which contain yeasts and lactobacilli. It is an important source of the bacteria necessary in the gastrointestinal tract to synthesize vitamin K.

Keflex, a trade name for an antibacterial (cephalexin).

Keflin, a trade name for an antibiotic (cephalothin).

Kefzol, a trade name for an antibacterial (cefazolin sodium).

Kegel exercises (keg′əl). See **pubococcygeus exercises.**

Keith-Flack node (kith′flæk′). See **sinoatrial node.**

kel-, a combining form meaning 'of or pertaining to a tumor': *kelectome, keloid, keloplasty.*

Kellgren's syndrome (kel′grinz), a form of osteoarthritis affecting the proximal and distal interphalangeal joints, the first metatarsophalangeal and carpometacarpal joints, the knees, and the spine. The absence of rheumatoid factor and rheumatoid nodules and the lack of systemic involvement differentiate this syndrome from rheumatoid arthritis. Also called **erosive osteoarthritis.**

Kelly's pad, a horseshoe-shaped, inflatable rubber drainage pad used in a bed or on the operating table.

keloid, cheloid (ki′loid), overgrowth of collagenous scar tissue at the site of a wound of the skin. The new tissue is elevated, rounded, and firm, with irregular, clawlike margins. Young women and blacks are particularly susceptible to keloid formation. Most keloids flatten and become less noticeable over a period of years. Types of therapy include solid carbon dioxide, liquid nitrogen, intralesional corticosteroid injections, radiation, and surgery. Treatment may worsen the condition and should be performed only by skilled professionals. — **cheloidal, keloidal,** *adj.*

keloidosis (ki′loidou′sis), **cheloidosis,** habitual or multiple formation of keloids.

Kemadrin, a trade name for an antiparkinsonian skeletal-muscle relaxant (procyclidine hydrochloride).

Kempner rice-fruit diet (kemp′nər). See **rice diet.**

Kenacort Diacetate, a trade name for a glucocorticoid (triamcinolone diacetate).

Kenalog, a trade name for a glucocorticoid (triamcinolone acetonide).

Kenny treatment. See **Sister Kenny's treatment.**

keno-, a combining form meaning 'empty': *kenophobia, kenotoxin, kenotron.*

kenogenesis. See **cenogenesis.**

kenophobia, cenophobia, the morbid fear of large and open spaces; agoraphobia.

Kenya fever. See **Marseilles fever.**

kephal-. See **cephal-.**

kephir. See **kefir.**

kera-, a combining form meaning 'horn': *keracele, keraphyllocele.*

kerat-, kerato-, **1.** a combining form meaning 'horny, cornified': *keratolysis, keratoma, keratonosis.* **2.** a combining form meaning 'cornea, corneal': *keratoiritis, keratoleukoma, keratome.*

keratectomy, surgical removal of a portion of the cornea, performed to excise a small, superficial lesion that does not warrant a corneal graft. Local anesthesia is used. The scar is excised, and an antibiotic is injected under the conjunctiva. A topical steroid is given, and a light pressure dressing is applied. Postoperatively, the dressings are changed daily. Corneal epithelium grows rapidly, filling a small surgical area in about 60 hours.

keratic (kəræt′ik), **1.** of or pertaining to keratin. **2.** of or pertaining to the cornea.

keratic precipitate, a group of inflammatory cells deposited on the endothelial surface of the cornea after trauma or inflammation, sometimes obscuring vision.

keratitis (ker′ətai′tis), any inflammation of the cornea. Kinds of keratitis include **dendritic keratitis, interstitial keratitis, keratoconjunctivitis sicca,** and **trachoma.** Compare **keratopathy.** — **keratic,** *adj.*

kerato-, a combining form meaning 'of or pertaining to the cornea, or to horny tissue': *keratocele, keratocentesis, keratoderma.* Also **cerato-.**

keratoacanthoma (kər′ətouæk′ænθou′mə), *pl.* **keratoacanthomas, keratoacanthomata.** a benign, rapidly growing, flesh-colored papule of the skin with a central plug of keratin. The lesion is most common on the face or the back of the hands and arms. It disappears spontaneously in four to six months, leaving a slightly depressed scar. Biopsy is often necessary to differentiate it from a squamous carcinoma.

keratoconjunctivitis (ker′ətoukənjəngk′tivai′tis), inflammation of the cornea and the conjunctiva. Kinds of keratoconjunctivitis include **eczematous conjunctivitis, epidemic keratoconjunctivitis,** and **keratoconjunctivitis sicca.**

keratoconjunctivitis sicca, dryness of the cornea owing to a deficiency of tear secretion in which the corneal surface appears dull and rough, and the eye feels gritty and irritated. The condition may be associated with erythema multiforme, Sjögren's syndrome, trachoma, and vitamin A deficiency. Methylcellulose artificial tears may give some relief.

keratoconus (ker′ətoukou′nəs), a noninflammatory protrusion of the central part of the cornea. More common in females, it may cause marked astigmatism; contact lenses usually restore visual acuity. The cause of the condition is unknown.

keratomalacia (ker'ətoumələi'shə), a condition, characterized by xerosis and ulceration of the cornea, resulting from severe vitamin A deficiency. It commonly occurs as a secondary result of diseases that affect vitamin A absorption or storage, as ulcerative colitis, celiac syndrome, cystic fibrosis, or sprue. Also at risk are infants and children who are given dilute formula, who are malnourished, or who are allergic to whole milk and are fed skimmed milk, which is a poor source of vitamin A. Early symptoms include night blindness, photophobia, swelling and redness of the eyelids, and drying, roughness, pain, and wrinkling of the conjunctiva. In advanced deficiency, Bitôt's spots appear, the cornea becomes dull, lusterless, and hazy and, without adequate therapy, it eventually softens and perforates, resulting in blindness. Treatment consists of vitamin A supplements determined by the severity of the condition, although prolonged daily administration of large doses, especially to infants, may result in hypervitaminosis. An adequate diet containing whole milk and foods high in vitamin A or carotenes prevents the condition. See also **vitamin A.**

keratomycosis linguae (ker'ətoumaikou'sɪs). See **parasitic glossitis.**

keratopathy (ker'ətop'əthɪ), any noninflammatory disease of the cornea. Compare **keratitis.**

keratoplasty, a procedure in ophthalmologic surgery in which an opaque portion of the cornea is excised.

keratosis (ker'ətou'sɪs), any skin condition in which there is overgrowth and thickening of the cornified epithelium. Kinds of keratosis are **actinic keratosis** and **seborrheic keratosis.** —**keratotic,** *adj.*

keratosis follicularis, an uncommon, hereditary skin disorder characterized by keratotic papules that coalesce to form brown or black, crusted, wartlike patches. These vegetations may spread widely, ulcerate, and become covered with a purulent exudate. Treatment includes large doses of vitamin A orally, topical vitamin A acid cream, and oral or topical corticosteroids. Also called **Darier's disease.**

keratosis seborrheica. See **seborrheic keratosis.**

kerauno-, a combining form meaning 'of or pertaining to lightning': *keraunoneurosis, keraunophobia.*

kerion (ki'rion), an inflamed, boggy granuloma that develops as an immune reaction to a superficial fungus infection in association with *Tinea capitas* of the scalp. The lesion heals within a short time without treatment.

kernicterus, an abnormal toxic accumulation of bilirubin in the brain tissues owing to hyperbilirubinemia. See also **hyperbilirubinemia of the newborn.**

kerosene poisoning, a toxic condition caused by the ingestion of kerosene or the inhalation of its fumes. Symptoms following ingestion include drowsiness, fever, a rapid heartbeat, tremors, and severe pneumonitis if the fluid is aspirated. Vomiting is not induced. Treatment for ingestion usually includes one or two oz. of vegetable oil to prevent absorption of the kerosene in the stomach and gastric lavage with copious amounts of water, a three per cent sodium bicarbonate solution or normal saline. Treatment for poisoning by inhalation includes fresh air, oxygen, and respiratory assistance if necessary. See also **petroleum distillate poisoning.**

Ketaject, a trade name for a general anesthetic (ketamine hydrochloride).

Ketalar, a trade name for a general anesthetic (ketamine hydrochloride).

ketamine hydrochloride (ki'təmin), a nonbarbiturate general anesthetic administered parenterally to achieve dissociative anesthesia. Because ketamine hydrochloride does not cause muscle relaxation, intubation is usually not required. Ketamine hydrochloride is particularly useful for brief, minor surgical procedures and for the induction of inhalation anesthesia in pediatric, geriatric, and disturbed patients. Hallucinations, confusion, and disorientation may occur on emergence from anesthesia. Other potential disadvantages attending use of this drug include increased blood pressure, increased cerebrospinal fluid pressure, increased intracranial pressure, and a tendency toward potentiation of the effects of alcohol, barbiturates, and narcotics. See also **dissociative anesthesia.**

Ketanest, a trade name for a general anesthetic agent (methoxyflurane).

keto-, a combining form indicating possession of the carbonyl group :C:O: *ketoheptose, ketolysis, ketonuria.*

ketoacidosis (ki'touæs'ɪdou'sɪs), acidosis accompanied by an accumulation of ketones in the body, resulting from faulty carbohydrate metabolism. It occurs primarily as a complication of diabetes mellitus and is characterized by a fruity odor of acetone on the breath, mental confusion, dyspnea, nausea, vomiting, dehydration, weight loss, and, if untreated, coma. Emergency treatment includes the administration of insulin and I.V. fluids and the evaluation and correction of electrolyte imbalance. Nasogastric intubation and bladder catheterization may be required if the patient is comatose. Before discharge of the patient from the hospital, the nurse carefully reviews the diet, activity, urine testing, and insulin schedule prescribed, emphasizing to the patient that ketoacidosis may be life threatening and is largely avoidable by strict adherence to the patient's prescribed diabetic regimen. Compare **insulin shock.** See also **diabetes mellitus, ketosis.** —**ketoacidotic,** *adj.*

ketoaciduria (ki'touæs'ɪdyur'iə), presence in the urine of excessive amounts of ketone bodies, occurring as a result of uncontrolled diabetes mellitus, starvation, or any other metabolic condition in which fats are rapidly catabolized. The condition can be diagnosed with a dipstick reagent or acetone test tablet. Also called **ketonuria.** See also **Acetest, ketosis.** — **ketoaciduric,** *adj.*

ketone alcohol, an alcohol containing the ketone group.

ketone bodies, normal metabolic products, B-hydroxylbutyric acid and aminoacetic acid, from which acetone may arise spontaneously. The two acids are products of lipid pyruvate metabolism, via acetyl CoA in the liver, and are oxidized by the muscles. Excessive production of these bodies leads to their excretion in urine, as in diabetes mellitus. Also called **acetone bodies.**

ketonuria (ki′toʊnyʊr′iə). See **ketoaciduria.**

ketosis (kɪtoʊ′sɪs), the abnormal accumulation of ketones in the body as a result of a deficiency or inadequate utilization of carbohydrates. Fatty acids are metabolized instead, and the end products, ketones, begin to accumulate. This condition is seen in starvation, occasionally in pregnancy, if the intake of protein and carbohydrates is inadequate, and, most frequently, in diabetes mellitus. It is characterized by ketonuria, loss of potassium in the urine, and a fruity odor of acetone on the breath. Untreated, ketosis may progress to ketoacidosis, coma, and death. See also **diabetes mellitus, ketoacidosis, starvation.** — **ketotic,** *adj.*

Kew Gardens spotted fever. See **rickettsialpox.**

kg, abbreviation for **kilogram.**

kidney, one of a pair of bean-shaped urinary organs in the dorsal part of the abdomen, one on each side of the vertebral column. The cranial extremities of the kidneys are on a level with the cranial border of the twelfth thoracic vertebra, the caudal extremities on a level with the third lumbar vertebra. In most individuals, the right kidney is more caudal than the left. Each kidney is about 11 cm long, 6 cm wide, and 2.5 cm thick. In men, each kidney weighs from 125 to 170 gm; in women, each kidney weighs from 115 to 155 gm. In the newborn, the kidneys are about three times as large in proportion to the body weight as in the adult. The kidneys produce and eliminate urine through a complex filtration network and reabsorption system comprising more than two million nephrons. The nephrons are composed of glomeruli and renal tubules that filter blood under high pressure, removing urea, salts, and other soluble wastes from blood plasma and returning the purified filtrate to the blood. More than 2,500 pints of blood pass through the kidneys every day, entering the kidneys through the renal arteries and leaving through the renal veins. All the blood in the body passes through the kidneys about 20 times every hour but only about one fifth of the plasma is filtered by the nephrons during that period. The kidneys remove water as urine and return water that has been filtered to the blood plasma, thus helping to maintain the water balance of the body. Hormones, especially the antidiuretic hormone (ADH), produced by the pituitary gland, control the function of the kidneys in regulating the water content of the body. ADH reaches the renal tubules in the blood and stimulates the reabsorption of water from the filtrate into the blood. If water intake is inadequate to compensate for the water lost in perspiration and in respiration, the change in concentration in the blood is detected by the brain and the pituitary gland releases more ADH, thus reducing the loss of water in urine. If the blood is too dilute, the pituitary gland reduces the secretion of ADH, producing a large flow of dilute urine to restore the water balance.

kidney cancer, a malignant neoplasm of the renal parenchyma or renal pelvis. Factors associated with an increased incidence of disease are exposure to aromatic hydrocarbons or tobacco smoke and the use of drugs containing phenacetin. A long asymptomatic period may precede the onset of the characteristic symptoms, which include hematuria, flank pain, fever, and the detection of a palpable mass. Diagnostic measures include urinalysis, excretory urography, nephrotomography, ultrasonography, renal arteriography, and microscopic and cytologic studies of cells from the renal pelvis. Adenocarcinoma of the renal parenchyma accounts for 80 per cent of kidney tumors, occurring twice as frequently in men as in women; transitional cell or squamous cell carcinomas in the renal pelvis account for approximately 15 per cent and are equally frequent in men and women. Radical nephrectomy with lymph node dissection is usually recommended for tumors of the parenchyma; nephroureterectomy is usually recommended for operable tumors of the renal pelvis. Radiotherapy may be used preoperatively or postoperatively and as palliation for inoperable tumors. Chemotherapeutic agents that may induce temporary remission are cyclophosphamide, bleomycin, hydroxyurea, and vinblastine. See also **Wilms' tumor.**

kidney disease, any one of a large group of conditions including infectious, inflammatory, obstructive, vascular, and neoplastic disorders of the kidney. Characteristics of kidney disease are hematuria, persistent proteinuria, pyuria, edema, dysuria, and pain in the flank. Specific symptoms vary with the type of disorder, for example: hematuria with severe, colicky pain suggests obstruction by a kidney stone; hematuria without pain may indicate renal carcinoma; proteinuria is generally a sign of disease in the glomerulus, or filtration unit of the kidney; pyuria indicates infectious disease; and edema is characteristic of the nephrotic syndrome. Diagnosis of kidney disease is made after laboratory tests and other procedures have been performed. Among the special tests for kidney disorders are excretory urography, intravenous pyelography, tests of the glomerular filtration rate, biopsy, and ultrasound examination. Treatment depends upon the type of kidney disease diagnosed. Some forms of advanced kidney disease may lead to renal failure, coma, and death unless hemodialysis is started. See also **glomerulonephritis, nephrotic syndrome, renal calculus, renal failure.**

kidney failure, *Informal.* renal failure.

kidney machine. 1. See **artificial kidney. 2.** See **hemodialyzer.**

kidney stone. See **urinary calculus.**

Kielland forceps (kilʹənd). See **obstetric forceps.**

Kielland rotation, an obstetric operation in which Kielland's forceps are used in turning the head of the fetus from an occiput posterior or occiput transverse position to an occiput anterior position. It is performed most commonly to correct an arrest in the active stage of labor. The rotation is done at the midplane of the pelvis. As it is associated with increased harm to the mother and to the baby, Caesarean section is often preferred. See also **forceps delivery, obstetric forceps.**

killer cell. See **null cell.**

kilo-, a combining form meaning 'one thousand': *kilocalorie, kilogram, kilometer.*

kilogram (kg) (kilʹəgræm), a unit for the measurement of mass in the metric system. One kilogram is equal to 1,000 grams or to 2.2046 pounds avoirdupois.

kilogram calorie. See **calorie.**

Kimmelstiel-Wilson's disease. See **intercapillary glomerulosclerosis.**

KI-N, a trade name for an expectorant and an iodine supplement (potassium iodide).

kinase (kaiʹneis), **1.** an enzyme that catalyzes the transfer of a phosphate group or another high-energy molecular group to an acceptor molecule. Each of these kinases is named for its receptor, as acetate kinase, fructokinase, hexokinase. **2.** an enzyme that activates a pre-enzyme (zymogen). Each of these kinases is named for its source, as bacterial kinase, enterokinase, fibrinokinase, insulin kinase, staphylokinase, streptokinase, streptokinase-streptodornase, urokinase.

kine-. See **kinesio-.**

kinematics (kɪnʹəmætʹɪks, kaiʹnəmætʹɪks), (in physiology) the geometry of the motion of the body without regard to the forces acting to produce the motion. Kinematics deals with the description and the measurement of body motion and the means of recording it. Recordings of body motions are defined in one-plane relationships, although natural motions of the body often occur in more than one plane. Kinematics considers the motions of all body parts relative to the segments of the part involved in the motion and not necessarily in relation to the standard anatomical position, as the movements of the fingers are considered in relation to the midline of the hand, not the midline of the body. The most common types of motions studied in kinematics are flexion, extension, adduction, abduction, internal rotation, and external rotation. Kinematics is especially important in orthopedics and rehabilitation medicine. Also called **cinematics.** Compare **kinetics.**

kinesio-, a combining form meaning 'of or pertaining to movement': *kinesiology, kinesioneurosis, kinesiotherapy.* Also **kine-.**

kinesiology (kɪniʹsiolʹəji, kaɪniʹsiolʹəji, kɪniʹziolʹəji, kaɪniʹziolʹeji), the scientific study of muscular activity and of the anatomy, physiology, and mechanics of the movement of body parts.

-kinesis, 1. a combining form meaning an 'activation': *angiokinesis, lymphokinesis, thrombokinesis.* **2.** a combining form meaning a 'division (of cells)': *catakinesis, diakinesis, heterokinesis.* Also **-cinesia, -cinesis, -kinesia.**

kinesthetic memory, the recollection of movement, weight, resistance, and position of the body or parts of the body.

-kinetic, 1. a combining form meaning 'pertaining to motion': *akinetic, parakinetic, synkinetic.* **2.** a combining form meaning 'pertaining to a (specified) agent causing motion': *chemokinetic, ideokinetic, photokinetic.* **3.** a combining form meaning 'referring to kinesis': *astrokinetic, biokinetic, catakinetic.* **4.** a combining form meaning 'referring to activation of a body part by a (specified) agent': *angiokinetic, gametokinetic, gonadokinetic.* Also **-cinetic, -cinetical, -kinetical.**

kinetics (kɪnetʹɪks, kaɪnetʹɪks), (in physiology) the study of the forces that produce, arrest, or modify the motions of the body. Newton's first and third laws of inertia are especially applicable to kinetics. Newton's first law states that bodies at rest tend to stay at rest and bodies in motion tend to keep moving. Newton's third law states that action and reaction are equal in magnitude but opposite in direction. These two laws are applicable to the forces produced by muscles of the body which act on joints. The reaction forces of the muscles contribute to the equilibrium and the motion of the body. Compare **kinematics.**

kineto-, a combining form meaning 'movable': *kinetochore, kinetogenic, kinetoplasm.*

kinetochore (kɪnetʹəkɔr). See **centromere.**

kinetotherapeutic bath (kɪnetʹoᴜferʹəpyuʹtɪk), a bath in which underwater exercises are performed in order to strengthen weak or partially paralyzed muscles.

kino-, a combining form meaning 'of or pertaining to movement': *kinoplasm, kinosphere, kinotoxin.*

kinomere (kɪnʹəmir). See **centromere.**

kinship model family group, a family unit comprised of the biological parents and their offspring. It is like a nuclear family but is more closely tied to an extended family. Characteristics of this family group include dominance by the maternal grandmother, who raises the children and makes most of the decisions, clearly delineated sex roles, and resistance to change.

kiono-. See **ciono-.**

Kirschner's wire (kərsh'nərz), a threaded or smooth metallic wire available in three diameters and 22.86 cm long. The wire is used in internal fixation of fractures or for skeletal traction.

kiting, *Informal.* the improper and illegal practice of altering a drug prescription to indicate that more of a drug was prescribed than was actually ordered by the physician. Kiting may be done by a patient seeking greater quantities of drugs, especially narcotics, than the physician prescribed, or may be done by the pharmacist to increase reimbursement from a third party, as the involved insurance company.

klang association. See **clang association.**

Klebsiella (kleb'ziel'ə, kleb'siel'ə), a genus of diplococcal bacteria that appear as small, plump rods with rounded ends. Several respiratory diseases, including bronchitis, sinusitis, and some forms of pneumonia, are caused by infection by species of *Klebsiella.*

Klebs-Loeffler bacillus (klebz'lef'lər). See *Corynebacterium diphtheriae.*

kleeblattschädel deformity syndrome. See **cloverleaf skull deformity.**

Kleine-Levine syndrome (klain'ləvin'), a disorder of unknown etiology often associated with psychotic conditions, characterized by episodic somnolence, abnormal hunger, and hyperactivity. The episodes of sleep may last for several hours or days and are followed by confusion on awakening. There is no specific treatment. Compare **narcolepsy.**

klepto-, a combining form meaning 'of or pertaining to theft or stealing': *kleptohemodeipnonism, kleptolagnia, kleptomania.*

kleptolagnia (klep'toulæg'niə), sexual excitement or gratification produced by stealing.

kleptomania, cleptomania, a neurosis characterized by an abnormal, uncontrollable, and recurrent urge to steal. The objects, taken not for their monetary value, immediate need, or utility but because of a symbolic meaning usually associated with some unconscious emotional conflict, are usually given away, returned surreptitiously, or kept and hidden. People who have the condition experience an increased sense of tension before committing the theft and intense gratification during the act. Afterward, they display signs of depression, guilt, and anxiety over the possibility of being apprehended and losing status in society. In less severe cases, the impulse is expressed by the continuous borrowing of objects and not returning them. Treatment usually consists of psychotherapy to uncover the underlying emotional problems. **—kleptomaniac,** *n.*

Klinefelter's syndrome (klain'feltərz), a syndrome of gonadal defects, appearing in males, with an extra X chromosome in at least one cell line. Characteristics are small, firm testes, long legs, gynecomastia, poor social adaptation, subnormal intelligence, chronic pulmonary disease, and varicose veins. The severity of the abnormalities increases with greater numbers of X chromosomes. The most common abnormality is a 47 XXY karyotype. Men with the karyotype XXXXY have marked congenital malformations and mental retardation.

Klippel-Feil syndrome (klip'əlfail'). See **congenital short neck syndrome.**

K-Lor, a trade name for an electrolyte replacement solution (potassium chloride).

Klorvess, a trade name for an electrolyte replenisher (potassium chloride).

K-Lyte/Cl, a trade name for an electrolyte replacement solution (potassium chloride).

kneading, a grasping, rolling, and pressing movement, as is used in massaging the muscles. See also **massage.**

knee, a joint complex that connects the thigh with the lower leg. It consists of three condyloid joints, 12 ligaments, 13 bursae, and the patella. Two of the condyloid joints comprising the knee are between the condyles of the femur and the corresponding menisci and condyles of the tibia. The third condyloid joint within the knee is a partially arthrodial joint between the patella and the femur. The motion of this joint is not a simple gliding motion, because the articular surfaces of the bones involved are not mutually adapted to each other. The ligaments of the knee include the articular capsule, the patellar, the oblique popliteal, the arcuate popliteal, the tibial collateral, the fibular collateral, the anterior cruciate, the posterior cruciate, the medial and the lateral menisci, the transverse ligament, and the coronary ligament. Four of the bursae of the knee are located in front, four laterally, and five medially. The largest bursa is the prepatellar bursa between the patellar ligament and the skin. The painful condition 'housemaid's knee' is caused by inflammation of the prepatellar bursa. The knee is relatively unprotected by surrounding muscles and is often injured by blows, sudden stops, and turns, especially those associated with sports. Ligamental tears of the knee joint are extremely common in athletes and produce a variety of signs and symptoms, as effusion surrounding the knee joint, varying degrees of edema, differences in the shape of the knee joint, tenderness on palpation, crepitation, instability of the knee joint, and possible ecchymosis. Radiographic examination may reveal varying degrees of displacement from ligamental tears, but the primary ligamentous injuries are not visible on x-ray films. Ligamental tears are a form of sprain and are treated according to the degree of trauma. Mild tears involving only a few fibers usually do not require any treatment and heal with time. Moderate ligamental tears require protective treatment, with rest essential to healing. Aspiration of excessive joint fluid and compression of the joint may be performed to control swelling. Sports injuries of this kind are commonly taped in a special way or treated with splints. Surgical intervention is often necessary to repair severe ligamentous tears, and postoperative exercises are prescribed to strengthen knee structures. Torn menisci are very common sports injuries and can cause severe pain, limping, edema, and greatly reduced motion. Surgical intervention, as a meniscectomy, may be required. Various orthopedic conditions, as arthritis, commonly affect the knee, especially in elderly individuals, and require continuing treatment and special maintenance.

knee-ankle interaction, one of the five major kinetic determinants of gait that helps to minimize the displacement of the center of gravity of the body during the walking cycle. The knee and the foot work simultaneously to lower the center of gravity of the body. When the heel of the foot is in contact with the ground, the foot is dorsiflexed and the knee is fully extended so that the associated limb is at its maximum length with the center of gravity at its lower point. Plantar flexion of the foot with the initiation of knee flexion maintains the center of gravity in its forward progression at about the same level, also helping to minimize the vertical displacement of the center of gravity. Knee-ankle interaction is often a factor in the diagnosis and treatment of various orthopedic diseases, deformities, and abnormal conditions, and in the analysis and the correction of pathological gaits. Compare **knee-hip flexion, lateral pelvic displacement, pelvic rotation, pelvic tilt.**

knee cap. See **patella.**

knee chest position. See **genupectoral position.**

knee-hip flexion, one of the five major kinematic determinants of gait, which allows the passage of body weight over the supporting extremity during the walking cycle. Knee-hip flexion occurs during the stance and the swing phases of the cycle. The knee first locks into extension as the heel of the weight-bearing limb strikes the ground, and is unlocked by final flexion and initiation of the swing phase in the walking cycle. Hip flexion is synchronized with these movements which help to minimize the vertical displacement of the center of gravity of the body in the act of walking. Knee-hip flexion is often a factor in the diagnosis and treatment of various orthopedic diseases, deformities, and abnormal conditions and in the analysis and correction of pathological gaits. Compare **knee-ankle interaction, lateral pelvic displacement, pelvic rotation, pelvic tilt.**

knee-jerk reflex. See **patellar reflex.**

knee joint, the complex, hinged joint at the knee, regarded as three articulations in one, comprising condyloid joints connecting the femur and the tibia and a partly arthrodial joint connecting the patella and the femur. The knee joint and its ligaments permit flexion, extension, and, in certain positions, medial and lateral rotation. It is a common site for sprain and dislocation. Also called **articulatio genus.**

knee replacement, the surgical insertion of a hinged prosthesis, performed to relieve pain and restore motion to a knee severely affected by osteoarthritis, rheumatoid arthritis, or trauma. Under inhalation anesthesia, the diseased surfaces are removed and a two-piece metallic hinge is cemented into the medullary cavities of the femur and tibia. Postoperatively, the knee is held in a position of maximum extension, usually with a plaster cast. Progressive exercise and whirlpool baths are prescribed through physical therapy. Possible complications include infection, fat embolism, peroneal nerve palsy, loosening of the prosthesis, and flexion contractures. To prevent contractures, the nurse cautions the patient to keep the leg extended in bed; a blanket roll along the femur prevents external rotation. The mobility and range of motion of the joint increase slowly. See also **arthroplasty, hip replacement, osteoarthritis, plastic surgery.**

knife needle, a slender surgical knife with a needle point, used in the discission of a cataract and in other ophthalmic procedures, as goniotomy and goniopuncture.

knock-knee. See **genu valgum.**

knot, (in surgery) the interlacing of the ends of a ligature or suture so that they remain in place without slipping or becoming detached. The ends of the suture are passed twice around each other before being pulled taut to make a simple surgeon's knot. For additional stability, the ends may be recrossed and a second simple knot made over the first. There are many kinds of knots, some of which are interlocking.

knowledge deficit, a nursing diagnosis accepted by the Fourth National Conference on the Classification of Nursing Diagnoses. The etiology of the condition may be a lack of exposure to information, a lack of ability to recall the information, a misinterpretation of the information, a cognitive or perceptual limitation in the ability to learn or to understand the information, a lack of interest in acquiring the information, or an unfamiliarity with the resources necessary to gain the information. The defining characteristics of the knowledge deficit include a statement by the person that the deficit exists, an observed failure on the part of the client to follow through on instructions, the observation of an inadequate performance by the client on a test, or the observation of inappropriate or exaggerated behavior on the part of the client. See also **nursing diagnosis.**

Kocher's forceps (kou'kərz), a kind of surgical forceps that has notched jaws, interlocking teeth, and thick, curved or straight, powerful handles.

Koch's postulates (kouks), the prerequisites for establishing that a specific microorganism causes a particular disease. The conditions are: (1) the microorganism must be observed in all cases of the disease; (2) the microorganism must be isolated and grown in pure culture; (3) microorganisms from the pure culture, when inoculated into a susceptible animal, must reproduce the disease; (4) the microorganism must be observed in and recovered from the experimentally diseased animal.

Koebner phenomenon (koub′nər), the development of isomorphic lesions at the site of an injury occurring in psoriasis, lichen nitidus, lichen planus, and verruca plana.

koilo-, a combining form meaning 'hollow or concave': *koilonychia, koilorrhachic, koilosternia.*

koilonychia (koi′lounɪk′iə), spoon nails; a condition in which nails are thin and concave from side to side. It is usually familial but may occur with iron-deficiency anemia and Raynaud's phenomenon.

koinoni-, a combining form meaning 'of or pertaining to a community': *koinonia, koinoniphobia.*

kolpo-. See **colpo-.**

koly-, a combining form meaning 'to hinder': *kolypeptic, kolyphrenia, kolyseptic.*

kon-, a combining form meaning 'of or pertaining to dust': *konometer, koniocortex.*

Konakion, a trade name for a vitamin (phytonadione).

Konyne, a trade name for a hemostatic (factor IX complex).

Koplik's spots (kop′lıks), small red spots with bluish-white centers on the lingual and buccal mucosa, characteristic of measles. The rash of measles usually erupts a day or two after the appearance of Koplik's spots.

kopr-. See **copro-.**

kopra-. See **copro-.**

Korotkoff sounds (korot′kof), sounds heard during the taking of blood pressure using a sphygmomanometer and stethoscope. As air is released from the cuff, pressure on the brachial artery is reduced, and the blood is heard pulsing through the vessel. See also **blood pressure, diastole, sphygmomanometer, systole.**

Korsakoff's psychosis (kor′səkofs), a form of amnesia often seen in chronic alcoholics, characterized by a loss of short-term memory and an inability to learn new skills. The person is usually disoriented and confabulates to conceal the condition. The cause of the condition can often be traced to degenerative changes in the thalamus owing to a deficiency of B complex vitamins, especially thiamine and B_{12}. Compare **Wernicke's encephalopathy.**

kosher (kou′shər), conforming to or prepared in accordance with the dietary or ceremonial laws of Judaism.

Krabbe's disease (kræb′iz). See **galactosyl ceramide lipidosis.**

Kraske position (kras′ke), an anatomical position in which the patient is prone, with hips flexed and elevated, head and feet down. The position is used for renal surgery, as it enlarges the costovertebral angle, allowing the surgeon to have optimal access to the kidneys.

kraurosis (krorou′sis), a thickening and shriveling of the skin. See also **kraurosis vulvae.**

kraurosis vulvae, a skin disease of aged women characterized by dryness, itching, and atrophy of the external genitalia. It is a condition that exhibits a predisposition to leukoplakia and carcinoma of the vulva. See also **lichen sclerosis et atrophicus.**

Krause's corpuscles, a number of sensory end organs in the conjunctiva of the eye, mucous membranes of the lips and tongue, epineurium of nerve trunks, the penis and the clitoris, and the synovial membranes of certain joints. Krause's corpuscles are tiny cylindrical oval bodies with a capsule formed by the expansion of the connective tissue sheath of a medullated fiber. They contain a soft, semifluid core in which the axon terminates either in a bulbous extremity or in a coiled mass. Also called **end bulbs of Krause.** Compare **Golgi-Mazzoni corpuscles, Pacini's corpuscles.**

Krebs' citric acid cycle (krebz), a sequence of enzymatic reactions involving the metabolism of carbon chains of sugars, fatty acids, and amino acids to yield carbon dioxide, water, and high-energy phosphate bonds. The cycle is initiated when pyruvate combines with coenzyme A (CoA) to form a two-carbon unit, acetyl CoA, which enters the cycle by combining with four-carbon oxaloacetic acid to form six-carbon citric acid. In subsequent steps isocitric acid, produced from citric acid, is oxidized to oxalsuccinic acid, which loses carbon dioxide to form alpha-ketoglutaric acid. Succinic acid, resulting from the oxidative decarboxylation of alpha-ketoglutraic acid, is oxidized to fumaric acid, and its oxidation regenerates oxalacetic acid which condenses with acetyl CoA, closing the cycle. The Krebs' cycle provides a major source of adenosine triphosphate energy and also produces intermediate molecules that are starting points for a number of vital metabolic pathways. Also called **tricarboxylic acid cycle.** See also **acetylcoenzyme A.**

Krukenberg's tumor (kru′kənbərgz), a neoplasm of the ovary that is a metastasis of a gastrointestinal malignancy, usually stomach cancer. Cytologic examination reveals mucoid degeneration and many large cells shaped like signet rings. Also called **carcinoma mucocellulare.**

krypto-. See **crypto-.**

Kulchitsky-cell carcinoma (kulčhit′skisel′). See **carcinoid.**

Kulchitsky's cell (kəlčhıt′skiz). See **argentaffin cell.**

Küntscher nail (kunt′shər), a stainless steel nail used in orthopedic surgery for the fixation of fractures of the long bones, especially the femur. Also called **Küntscher intramedullary nail.**

Kupffer's cells (kup′fərz), specialized cells of the reticuloendothelial system lining the sinusoids of the liver. The function of Kupffer's cells is to filter bacteria and other small, foreign proteins out of the blood.

kuru (ku′ru), a slow, progressive, fatal viral infection of the central nervous system seen only in natives of the New Guinea Highlands. The incubation period may be 30 or more years, but death usually occurs within months of the onset of symptoms. Characteristic of kuru are ataxia and decreased coordination progressing to paralysis, dementia, slurring of speech, and visual disturbances. Transmission of the disease is probably the result of cannibalism, as brain tissue from infected people produces the disease when inoculated in primates in the laboratory and incidence of the disease has declined with the decline of cannibalism.

Kussmaul breathing (kus′maul), abnormally deep, very rapid sighing respirations characteristic of diabetic acidosis.

Kveim reaction, a reaction used in a diagnostic test for sarcoidosis, based on an intradermal injection of antigen derived from a lymph node known to be sarcoid. If a noncaseating granuloma appears on the skin at the test site in four to eight weeks, the reaction is said to be positive, evidence that the patient has sarcoidosis.

kwashiorkor (kwash′ior′kor), a malnutrition disease, primarily of children, caused by severe protein deficiency, usually occurring when the child is weaned from the breast. Because calorie rich starches like breadfruit are available, the child does not lose weight as dramatically and does not look as sick as a marasmic child, who lacks protein and calories. Eventually the following symptoms occur: retarded growth, changes in skin and hair pigmentation, diarrhea, loss of appetite, nervous irritability, edema, anemia, fatty degeneration of the liver, necrosis, dermatoses, and fibrosis, often accompanied by infection and multivitamin deficiencies. Because dietary fats are poorly tolerated in kwashiorkor, a skimmed milk formula is used in initial feedings, followed by additional foods until a full, well-balanced diet is achieved. Also called **infantile pellagra, malignant malnutrition.** See also **marasmic kwashiorkor, marasmus.**

Kwell, a trade name for a pediculicide and scabicide (gamma benzene hexachloride).

Kyasanur forest disease, an arbovirus infection transmitted by the bite of a tick that is harbored by shrews and other forest animals in western tropical India. Characteristics of the infection include fever, headache, muscle ache, cough, abdominal and eye pain, and photophobia. Treatment is symptomatic.

kymo-, a combining form meaning 'of or pertaining to waves': *kymograph, kymoscope, kymotrichous.*

kyno- a combining form meaning 'of or pertaining to dogs': *kynocephalus, kynophobia.*

kypho-, a combining form meaning 'of or pertaining to a hump': *kyphoscoliosis, kyphosis, kyphotone.*

kyphoscoliosis (kai′fouskou′liou′sis), an abnormal condition characterized by an anteroposterior curvature and a lateral curvature of the spine. It occurs in children and adults, often associated with cor pulmonale. Compare **kyphosis, scoliosis.** —**kyphoscoliotic,** *adj.*

kyphosis (kaifou′sis), an abnormal condition of the vertebral column, characterized by increased convexity in the curvature of the thoracic spine as viewed from the side. Kyphosis may be caused by rickets or tuberculosis of the spine. Adolescent kyphosis is usually self-limiting and often undiagnosed, but if the curvature progresses there may be moderate back pain. Conservative treatment consists of spine-stretching exercises and sleeping without a pillow, with a board under the mattress. A modified Milwaukee brace may be used for severe kyphosis, and, rarely, spinal fusion may be required. —**kyphotic,** *adj.*

KYPHOSIS

kysth-. See **colpo-.**
kystho-. See **colpo-.**
kyto-. See **cyto-.**

L

L, symbol for **lung.**

La, symbol for **lanthanum.**

label, (in radiology and immunology) **1.** a substance with a special affinity for an organ, tissue, cell, or microorganism in which it may become deposited and fixed. **2.** the process of depositing and fixing a substance in an organ, tissue, cell, or microorganism.

labeled compound, a chemical substance in which part of the molecules are labeled with a radionuclide so that observations of the radioactivity or isotopic composition make it possible to follow the compound or its fragments through physical, chemical, or biological processes.

labeling, the providing of information on a drug, food, device, or cosmetic to the purchaser or user. The information may be in any one of various forms, including printing on a carton, stick-on label, package insert, and monograph. Regulations for labeling are provided by the Food and Drug Administration. The label must contain directions for use, unless such directions are exempted by regulation, as well as warnings or contraindications. It may not contain false or misleading information.

labia, *sing.* **labium. 1.** the fleshy, liplike edges of an organ or tissue. **2.** the folds of skin at the opening of the vagina.

-labial, a combining form meaning 'of or pertaining to lips': *alveolabial, glossolabial, maxillolabial.*

labia majora (major'ə), *sing.* **labium majus** (mei'jəs). two long lips of skin one on each side of the vaginal orifice outside the labia minora. They extend from the anterior labial commissure to the posterior labial commissure and form the lateral boundaries of the pudendal cleft. Each labium contains areolar tissue, fat, and a thin layer of nonstriated muscle. In some women the outer surface of each lip may be covered with coarse pubic hair. The embryologic derivation of the labia majora and the scrotum are homologous.

labia minora (minor'ə), *sing.* **labium minus** (mi'nəs). two folds of skin between the labia majora, extending from the clitoris backward on both sides of the vaginal orifice, ending between it and the labia majora. Anteriorly, each labium divides into an upper and a lower division. The upper divisions pass above the clitoris and meet to form the preputium clitoridis; the lower divisions pass beneath the clitoris and unite to form the frenulum of the

clitoris. Opposed surfaces of the labia minora contain sebaceous follicles.

labile (lei'bil), **1.** unstable; characterized by a tendency to change or to be altered or modified. **2.** (in psychiatry) describing a personality characterized by rapidly shifting or changing emotions, as in bipolar disorder and certain types of schizophrenia; emotionally unstable. —**lability,** *n.*

-labile, a combining form meaning 'unstable, subject to change': *frigolabile, siccolabile, thixolabile.*

labio-, a combining form meaning 'of or pertaining to the lips, particularly the lips of the mouth': *labiocervical, labiodental, labiomental.*

labioglossolaryngeal paralysis. See **bulbar palsy.**

labor, the time and the processes that occur during parturition from the beginning of cervical dilatation to the delivery of the placenta. See also **childbirth.**

(See next page for illustration)

labor, abnormal. See **dystocia.**

laboratory, 1. a facility, room, building, or part of a building in which scientific research, experimentation, testing, or other investigative activities are carried out. **2.** of or pertaining to a laboratory.

laboratory diagnosis. See **diagnosis.**

laboratory error, any error made by the personnel in a clinical laboratory in the performance of a test, the interpretation of the data, or in reporting or recording the results. Laboratory error must always be considered a possible explanation for findings that are at variance with the composite clinical condition of the patient or that are widely divergent from previous laboratory tests.

laboratory medicine, the branch of medicine in which specimens of tissue, fluid, or other body substance is examined outside of the person, usually in the laboratory. Some fields of laboratory medicine are **chemistry, eytology, hematology, histology,** and **pathology.**

laboratory test, a procedure, usually conducted in a laboratory, that is intended to detect, identify, or quantify one or more significant substances, evaluate organ functions, or establish the nature of a condition or disease. Laboratory tests range from quite simple to extremely sophisticated. In modern medical practice, they are commonly used to help establish or confirm a diagnosis and often aid in the management of disease.

labor coach, a person who assists a woman in labor and delivery by closely attending to her emotional needs and by encouraging her to use properly the breathing patterns, concentration techniques, body positions, and massage techniques that were taught in a program of psychophysical preparation for childbirth. The goal of a labor coach is to minimize the need for pharmacologic pain relief used to decrease or eliminate the use of analgesia or anesthesia. Usually, the coach is the father of the baby or a close friend of the mother, but a professional labor coach, often a registered nurse specially trained in a method, may fill the role. See also **monitrice.**

labored breathing, abnormal respiration characterized by evidence of increased effort, including use of the accessory muscles of respiration of the chest wall, stridor, grunting, or nasal flaring.

labyrinth. See **internal ear.**

labyrinthitis, inflammation of the labyrinthine canals of the inner ear, resulting in vertigo.

labyrinthus osseus. See **osseus labyrinth.**

laceration, 1. the act of tearing or lacerating. 2. a torn, jagged wound. —**lacerate,** *v.,* **lacerated,** *adj.*

lacri-, lachry-, a combining form meaning 'of or pertaining to tears': *lacrimalin, lacrimator, lacrimotomy.*

Engagement

Descent with flexion

Internal rotation

Extension

External rotation

LABOR MECHANISMS

lacrimal, lachrymal (læk′rɪməl), of or pertaining to tears.

lacrimal apparatus, a network of structures of the eye that secrete tears and drain them from the surface of the eyeball. These parts include the lacrimal glands, the lacrimal ducts, the lacrimal sacs, and the nasolacrimal ducts.

lacrimal bone, one of the smallest and most fragile bones of the face, located at the anterior part of the medial wall of the orbit. It unites with the maxilla to form the lacrimal fossa, which lodges the lacrimal duct.

lacrimal caruncle, the small, reddish, fleshy protuberance that fills the triangular space between the medial margins of the upper and the lower eyelids. It contains sebaceous and sudoriferous glands and secretes a whitish substance that collects in the corner of the eye.

lacrimal duct, one of two channels through which tears pass from the lacrimal lake to the lacrimal sac of each eye.

lacrimal fistula, an abnormal communication from a tear duct or sac to the surface of the eye or eyelid.

lacrimal gland, one of a pair of glands situated superior and lateral to the eye bulb in the lacrimal fossa. It is an oval structure about the size of an almond and is divided into an orbital part and a palpebral part. The orbital part is connected to the periosteum of the orbit by a few fibrous bands and rests on the tendons of the recti superioris and the recti lateralis, which separate the gland from the eye bulb. The palpebral part is separated from the orbital part by a fibrous septum and projects into the back portion of the upper eyelid. The gland has about 10 ducts which run obliquely beneath the conjunctiva and open along the upper and lateral half of the superior conjunctival fornix. The watery secretion from the gland consists of the tears, slightly alkaline and saline, that moisten the conjunctiva.

lacrimal papilla, the small conical elevation on the medial margin of each eyelid, supporting an apex pierced by the punctum lacrimale through which tears emerge to moisten the conjunctiva.

lacrimal sac, the dilated end of each of the two nasolacrimal ducts. Each sac is lodged in a deep groove formed by the lacrimal bone and the frontal process of the maxilla. The sac is oval and about 13 mm long. Its upper end is closed and rounded, its lower end continuous with the nasolacrimal duct. The lacrimal sacs fill with tears secreted by the lacrimal glands and conveyed through the lacrimal ducts.

lacrimation, lachrymation (læk′rɪmei′šhən). **1.** the normal continuous secretion of tears by the lacrimal glands. **2.** an excessive amount of tear production, as in crying or weeping.

lact-. See **lacto-.**

lactalbumin (læk′təlbyu′mɪn), a simple, highly nutritious protein found in milk. It is similar to serum albumin. See also **albumin, serum albumin.**

lactase, an enzyme that catalyzes the hydrolysis of alpha-D-galactoside to D-galactose. Lactase is concentrated in the kidney, liver, and intestinal mucosa. Also called beta-galactosidase.

lactase deficiency, a congenital abnormality in which the amount of the enzyme lactase is deficient, resulting in the inability to digest lactose. The deficiency occurs in infancy in severe form and persists throughout life. In adults, a relative deficiency may appear as a natural process of aging; it occurs more frequently in persons of Asiatic and African heritage. Lactase deficiency may result from subtotal gastrectomy, any disease of the small intestine in which structural changes occur, as tropical sprue, ulcerative colitis, infectious hepatitis, and kwashiorkor, or from malnutrition. See also **lactose intolerance.**

lactation, the process of the synthesis and secretion of milk from the breasts in the nourishment of an infant or child. See also **breast milk.**

lacteal (læk′tiəl), of or pertaining to milk.

lacteal fistula, an abnormal passage opening into a lacteal duct.

lacteal gland, one of the many central lymphatic capillaries in the villi of the small intestine. It opens into the lymphatic vessels in the submucosa. The capillary is filled with chyle that turns milky white during the absorption of fat.

lactic, referring to milk and milk products. See also **lactic acid, lactose.**

lactic acid, a three-carbon organic acid produced by anaerobic respiration. There are three forms: L-lactic acid in muscle and blood is a product of glucose and glycogen metabolism; D-lactic acid is produced by the fermentation of dextrose by a species of micrococcus; DL-lactic acid is a racemic mixture found in the stomach, in sour milk, and in certain other foods, as sauerkraut, prepared by bacterial fermentation. Also called **alpha-hydroxypropionic acid.** See also **glycolysis.**

lactic acid fermentation, 1. the production of lactic acid from sugars by various bacteria. **2.** the souring of milk.

lactic dehydrogenase (LDH). See **Duchenne's muscular dystrophy.**

lactiferous (læktɪf′ərəs), of or pertaining to a structure that produces or conveys milk, as the tubules of the breasts.

lactiferous duct, one of many channels carrying milk from the lobes of each breast to the nipple.

lactin. See **lactose.**

Lactinex, a trade name for a gastrointestinal, fixed-combination drug containing antidiarrheals (*Lactobacillus acidophilus* and *Lactobacillus bulgaricus*).

lacto-, lact-, a combining form meaning 'of or pertaining to milk': *lactobacillus, lactopeptin, lactotoxin.*

Lactobacillus (læk'toubəsɪl'əs), any one of a group of nonpathogenic, gram-positive, rod-shaped bacteria that produce lactic acid from carbohydrates. Many species are normally found in the human intestinal tract and vagina.

lactogen (læk'təjɪn), a drug or other substance that enhances the production and secretion of milk. —**lactogenic,** *adj.*

lactogenic hormone. See **prolactin.**

lacto-ovo-vegetarian (læk'touou'vouvej'əteir'iən), one whose diet consists primarily of foods of vegetable origin and also includes some animal products, as eggs, milk, and cheese but no meat, fish, or poultry. Also called **ovo-lacto-vegetarian.**

lactose, a disaccharide found in milk. On hydrolysis lactose yields the monosaccharides glucose and galactose. Lactose is used as a laxative, as a diuretic, and as a component of formulas for infants. Also called **lactin, milk sugar.** See also **sugar.**

lactose intolerance, a sensitivity disorder resulting in the inability to digest lactose owing to a deficiency of or defect in the enzyme lactase. Symptoms of the disorder are bloating, flatus, nausea, diarrhea, and abdominal cramps. The diet is adjusted according to the tolerance level, restricting such foods as milk, cheese, butter, margarine, and any products containing milk, as cakes, ice cream, cream soups, and sauces. See **lactase deficiency.**

lacto-vegetarian (læk'touvej'əteir'iən), one whose diet consists of milk and milk products in addition to foods of vegetable origin but does not include eggs, meat, fish, or poultry.

lacuna (ləkyu'nə), *pl.* **lacunae. 1.** a small cavity within a structure, especially bony tissue. **2.** a gap, as in the field of vision.

lacus lacrimalis (lei'kəs), a triangular space separating the medial ends of the upper and the lower eyelids. It is an extension of the medial canthus and contains the lacrimal caruncle.

lae-. See **le-.**

Laënnec's catarrh (lei'əneks'), a form of bronchial asthma characterized by the discharge of small, round, viscous, beadlike bodies of sputum. These bodies, **Laënnec's pearls,** are formed in the bronchioles and appear in the asthmatic's expectorated bronchial secretions.

Laënnec's cirrhosis, See **cirrhosis.**

Laënnec's pearls. See **Laënnec's catarrh.**

laevo-. See **levo-.**

lagen-, a combining form meaning 'flasklike': *lagena, lageniform.*

-lagnia, a combining form meaning a 'sexual predilection': *osmolagnia, pyrolagnia, scoptolagnia.* Also **-lagny.**

lagophthalmos (læg'əfthæl'məs), an abnormal condition in which an eye may not be fully closed owing to a neurologic or muscular disorder. Also called **hare's eye.**

la grippe (lə grɪp). See **influenza.**

laked blood (leikt), blood that is clear, red, and homogenous owing to hemolysis of the red blood cells, as may occur in poisoning and severe, extensive burns.

lal-, lalio-, lalo-, a combining form meaning 'talk, babble': *laliatry, lalognosis, lalopathology.*

-lalia, a combining form meaning a 'disorder of speech': *agitolalia, eschrolalia, oxylalia.*

laliophobia (lei'lioufou'biə), a morbid dread of talking caused by fear and anxiety that one will stammer or stutter. **laliophobic,** *adj.*

lallation (lælei'shən), **1.** babbling, repetitive, unintelligible utterances, like the babbling of an infant, and the mumbled speech of schizophrenics, alcoholics, and the severely mentally retarded. **2.** a speech disorder characterized by a defective pronunciation of words containing the sound "l" or by the use of the sound "l" in place of the sound "r." Compare **lambdacism, rhotacism.**

lalo-. See **lal-.**

Lamarckism (ləmar'kızəm), the theory postulated by French naturalist Jean Baptiste de Lamarck that organic evolution results from structural changes in plants and animals that are caused by adaptation to environmental conditions, and that these acquired characteristics are transmitted to offspring. Also called **Lamarckianism, Lamarck's theory.** Compare **Darwinism.** —**Lamarckian,** *adj., n.*

Lamaze method (ləmaz'), a method of psychophysical preparation for childbirth developed in the 1950's by a French obstetrician, Fernand Lamaze. It is based on the work of Pavlov and Nicolaïev with hypnosis and stimulus-response conditioning in Russia before 1950. The method was popularized in the United States by Marjorie Karmel who wrote the book, *Thank you, Dr. Lamaze,* based on her experience delivering a child in Paris under the care of Dr. Lamaze. The first program was established at Mt. Sinai Hospital in New York City under the direction of Marjorie Karmel, Elizabeth Bing, a British physical therapist, and Dr. Alan Guttmacher. In 1960, the American Society for Psychoprophylaxis in Obstetrics was founded. The Lamaze method soon became the most often used method of natural childbirth. It requires classes, practice at home, and coaching during labor and delivery, often by a trained coach called a 'monitrice.' The classes, given during pregnancy, teach the physiology of pregnancy and childbirth, exercises to develop strength in the abdominal muscles and control of isolated muscles of the vagina and perineum, and techniques of breathing and relaxation to promote control and relaxation during labor. The woman is conditioned by repetition and practice to dissociate herself from the source of a stimulus by concentration on a focal point, by consciously relaxing all muscles, and by breathing in a special way at a particular rate—thereby training herself not to pay attention to the stimuli associated with labor. The kind and rate of breathing changes with the advancing stages of labor. During the early part of the first stage of labor, when the uterine cervix is dilated less than 5 cm and the contractions occur every 2 to 4 minutes, last 40 to 60 seconds, and are of mild to moderate strength, the mother does slow chest breathing during contractions. Her fingers may rest lightly on her lower ribs to feel them rise and fall. The abdominal wall does not move with respiration. She may perform an effleurage, or rhythmic fingertip massage, of her lower abdomen during the contractions. The rate of respiration is 10 or fewer breaths a minute, increasing to 12 per minute as labor intensifies. A deep "cleansing breath" is taken before and after each contraction. During the active part of the first stage of labor up to the transition to the second stage, the cervix is from 5 cm to nearly fully dilated, the interval between contractions is from 1½ to 4 minutes, and the duration of contractions is from 45 to 90 seconds. (The interval decreases and the intensity and duration increase as labor progresses.) During contractions, the mother breathes quietly and shallowly in her chest. The rate of her breathing varies with the strength of the contractions, increasing during a contraction to as fast as once a second at the peak and slowing to every 6 seconds as the uterus relaxes. She is coached to concentrate on the focal point she has selected, to perform the effleurage of her abdomen, to relax her perineal and vaginal muscles, and to take a cleansing breath at the beginning and end of each contraction. At the end of the first stage of labor, when the cervix is almost completely dilated and the contractions are strong, occurring every 1½ to 2 minutes and lasting 60 to 90 seconds, the mother begins to feel the urge to bear down and push during contractions. She avoids pushing before full dilatation by combining several light, shallow breaths in the chest with short puffing exhalations as the urge increases during the contractions. During the second stage of labor, the cervix is fully dilated and contractions are strong, frequent, and expulsive. The mother's head and shoulders are supported on pillows. During contractions, she is helped to draw her legs back, flexing the thighs against the abdomen, holding them behind the lower thigh with her hands. Her chin is tucked on her chest, the air is blocked from escaping from her lungs, her perineum is relaxed, and she bears down forcibly. Depending on the length of the contraction, several pushes of 10 to 15 or more seconds may be possible during the contraction. As the baby's head crowns, she is asked to pant lightly so that the head may be born slowly. The advantages of the method include the need for little or no analgesia for relief of pain and participation in the labor by the mother, giving her a great sense of self-satisfaction at delivery. Compare **Bradley method, Read method.**

lambdacism (læm′dəsɪz′əm), a speech disorder characterized by a defective pronunciation of words containing the sound "l," or by the excessive use of the sound, or by the substitution of the sound "r" for "l." Compare **lallation, rhotacism.**

lambdoidal suture (læmdɔɪ′dəl), the serrated connection between the occipital bone and the parietal bones of the skull. It is continuous with the occipitomastoid suture between the occipital and the mastoid portions of the temporal bones.

lamella (ləmɛl′ə), pl. **lamellae. 1.** a thin leaf or plate, as of bone. **2.** a medicated disc, prepared from glycerin and an alkaloid, for insertion under the eyelid.

lamellar exfoliation of the newborn, a congenital skin disorder transmitted as an autosomal recessive trait in which a parchmentlike, scaly membrane that covers the infant peels off within 24 hours of birth. Complete healing or a progressively less severe process of reforming and shedding of the scales then occurs. Also called **ichthyosis congenita, ichthyosis fetalis, lamellar desquamation of the newborn, lamellar ichthyosis of the newborn.** See also **collodion baby, lamellar ichthyosis.**

lamin-, a combining form meaning 'layer': *laminagram, laminated, laminotomy.*

lamina (læm′ɪnə), pl. **laminae.** a thin flat plate, as the lamina of the thyroid cartilage that overlays the structure on each side.

laminated thrombus, a thrombus comprised of an aggregation of blood platelets, fibrin, clotting factors, and cellular elements, arranged in layers apparently formed at different times.

laminectomy, surgical chipping away of the bony arches of one or more vertebrae, performed to relieve compression of the spinal cord, as caused by a bone displaced in an injury or as the result of degeneration of a disc, or to reach and remove a displaced intervertebral disc. With the patient prone and under general anesthesia, the laminae are removed and the underlying problem corrected. Spinal fusion may be necessary for stability of the spine if several laminae are removed. After surgery, the bed is kept flat to hold the patient's spine in correct alignment. If the procedure was a cervical laminectomy the patient is observed for signs of respiratory distress owing to cord edema. Motor function and sensation in the extremities are evaluated every two to four hours for 48 hours. The dressing is examined frequently for hemorrhage or leakage of cerebrospinal fluid. A sheet is used to logroll the patient without twisting the spine or hips. Ambulation often begins three to five days after surgery. **—laminectomize,** v.

lampbrush chromosome, an excessively large type of chromosome found in the oocytes of many lower animals.

It has long, threadlike projecting loops, giving it a hairy, brushlike appearance. See also **giant chromosome.**

lampro-, a combining form meaning 'clear': *lamprophonia, lamprophonic.*

lanatoside C (lænæt′əsaid), a cardiotonic.

■ INDICATIONS: It is prescribed where digitalis action is required, as for congestive heart failure and cardiac arrhythmias.

■ CONTRAINDICATIONS: Ventricular tachycardia or known hypersensitivity to this drug prohibits its use.

■ ADVERSE EFFECTS: Among the more serious adverse reactions are irregular or slow pulse, nausea, tiredness, and loss of appetite.

lance, to incise a furuncle or an abscess to release accumulated pus. A topical anesthetic is applied, the lesion is incised, and the pus is drained. A drain is inserted if the infection is deep. The bacteria involved are most often staphylococci. The nurse uses aseptic technique; soiled dressings are wrapped in paper to be burned. An antibiotic is given systemically if the boil is facial to prevent infection from spreading into the cranial sinuses. Infected drainage is kept off surrounding skin to prevent a recurrence. The nurse teaches the patient and family stringent handwashing techniques.

Lancefield's classification, a serologic classification of streptococci based on their antigenic characteristics. The bacteria are divided into 13 groups by the identification of their pathologic action. Group A contains most of the streptococci that cause infection in humans. Groups B to T are less pathogenic and are often present without causing disease. Most are hemolytic; of those, the beta subgroup is the most likely to be the cause of infection.

Lancereaux's diabetes (læn′sərouz), a chronic disease of carbohydrate metabolism characterized by marked emaciation. See also **diabetes mellitus.**

lancet, **1.** *Obsolete.* a very small, pointed, surgical knife, sharp on both sides. **2.** a short pointed blade used to obtain a drop of blood for a capillary sample. It has a guard above the blade that prevents deep incision, and it is usually disposable.

lancinating (læn′sinei′tıŋ), sharply cutting or tearing, as lancinating pain.

Landau reflex (læn′dau), a normal response of infants when held in a horizontal prone position to maintain a convex arc with the head raised and the legs slightly flexed. The reflex is poor in those with floppy-infant syndrome and exaggerated in hypertonic and opisthotonic infants.

landmark position, the correct placement of the hands on the chest in cardiopulmonary resuscitation. See also **cardiopulmonary resuscitation.**

Landsteiner's classification (lænd′stai′nərz), the classification of blood groups A, B, AB, and O on the basis of the presence or absence of the two agglutinogens A and B on the erythrocytes in human blood.

Langer's line (læŋ′ərz). See **cleavage line.**

Langhans' layer (laŋ′hans). See **cytotrophoblast.**

lano-, a combining form meaning 'of or pertaining to wool': *lanolin, lanonol, lanosterol.*

lanolin, a fatlike substance from the wool of sheep. It contains about 25 per cent water as a water-in-oil emulsion and is used as an ointment base and an emollient for the skin. Also called **hydrous wool fat.**

Lanoxin, a trade name for a cardiotonic (digoxin).

lanthanum (La), a rare-earth metallic element. Its atomic number is 57; its atomic weight is 138.91.

lanugo (lænyu′gou), **1.** the soft, downy hair covering a normal fetus, beginning with the fifth month of life and almost entirely shed by the ninth month. **2.** the fine, soft hair covering all parts of the body except palms, soles, and areas where other types of hair are normally found. Also called **vellus hair.**

lanulous (læn′yuləs), downy or covered with short, fine wooly hair, as the skin of a fetus. Also called **lanugo.**

laparo-, a combining form meaning 'of or pertaining to the loin or flank': *laparocele, laparocolectomy, laparorrhaphy.*

laparoscope (læp′ərəskoup′), a type of endoscope, consisting of an illuminated tube with an optical system, that is inserted through the abdominal wall for examining the peritoneal cavity. Also called **celioscope, peritoneoscope.** – **laparoscopic,** *adj.,* **laparascopy,** *v.*

laparoscopy (læp′əros′kəpi), the examination of the abdominal cavity with a laparoscope through a small incision in the abdominal wall. The procedure is also used for examining the ovaries and Fallopian tubes and as a gynecologic sterilization technique for fulgurating the oviducts. Also called **abdominoscopy.** See also **endoscopy, laparoscope.**

laparotomy, any surgical incision into the peritoneal cavity, usually performed under general or regional anesthesia, often on an exploratory basis. Before surgery, a complete blood count, a type and cross-match of blood, and a urinalysis are done; the skin is shaved and cleansed from the nipple line to the pubis. A barbiturate may be given at bedtime. Food and fluids by mouth are not given after midnight. Shortly before surgery, a barbiturate or tranquilizer and a narcotic are usually given, with an anticholinergic agent such as atropine. If the intestine is to be opened, a nasogastric tube is passed. Frequent observation of vital signs and drainage systems is essential. Intake and output of fluids are recorded. The patient is turned and helped to cough and breathe deeply every hour; medication is given as needed for relief of pain. Some kinds of laparotomy are **appendectomy, cholecystectomy, colostomy.** – **laparotomize,** *v.*

-lapse, a combining form meaning 'a slip': *collapse, prolapse, relapse.*

large calorie. See **calorie.**

large-for-gestational-age (LGA) infant, an infant whose fetal growth was accelerated and whose size and weight at birth fall above the ninetieth percentile of appropriate-for-gestational-age infants, whether delivered prematurely, at term, or later than term. Factors other than genetic influences that cause accelerated intrauterine growth include maternal diabetes mellitus and Beckwith's syndrome. LGA infants born of diabetic mothers are generally obese and plethoric, with very pink skin and red, shiny cheeks. They are often listless and limp, feed poorly, and become hypoglycemic within the first few hours. A major problem is that preterm LGA infants, because of their size, are not recognized as high-risk neonates with immature organ system development. Often these infants develop respiratory distress syndrome because pulmonary maturation occurs later in gestation. In cases of Beckwith's syndrome, the infant is characterized by gigantism, macroglossia, omphalocele or umbilical hernia, and visceromegaly. Compare **small-for-gestational-age infant.**

large intestine, the portion of the digestive tract comprising the cecum, appendix, the ascending, transverse, and descending colons, and the rectum. The ileocecal valve separates the ceccum from the ileum.

Largon, a trade name for a sedative (propiomazine hydrochloride).

Larodopa, a trade name for an antiparkinsonian (levodopa).

Larotid, a trade name for an antibacterial (amoxicillin hydrochloride).

larva migrans (mai'grænz). See **cutaneous larva migrans, visceral larva migrans.**

laryng-. See **laryngo-.**

laryngeal cancer, a malignant neoplastic disease characterized by a tumor arising from the epithelium of the structures of the larynx. Laryngeal tumors are almost 20 times more common in men than in women and occur most frequently between the ages of 50 and 70. Chronic alcoholism and heavy use of tobacco increase the risk of developing the cancer. Persistent hoarseness is usually the first sign; advanced lesions may cause a sore throat, dyspnea, dysphagia, and unilateral cervical adenopathy. Diagnostic measures include direct laryngoscopy, biopsy, and radiologic examination, including tomographic studies and chest films. Malignant tumors of the larynx are epidermoid carcinomas. Radiation is generally recommended for small lesions; total laryngectomy, often combined with radiotherapy, is indicated for extensive lesions. Following the operation, many persons with laryngectomies learn esophageal speech; some use an electric larynx, and

a few undergo surgical reconstruction. See also **laryngectomy.**

laryngeal catheterization, the insertion of a catheter into the larynx for the purpose of removing secretions or introducing gases.

laryngeal prominence. See **Adam's apple.**

laryngectomy, surgical removal of the larynx, performed to treat cancer of the larynx. Before surgery, the patient is referred to a speech pathologist to discuss esophageal speech and prostheses. Antibiotics are usually administered to reduce the risk of infection. Under regional or general anesthesia, the trachea is sutured to the skin, as in a tracheostomy, to ensure an adequate airway. In a partial laryngectomy only the vocal cords are removed, and the tracheostomy is closed within several days. If the malignancy is extensive the entire larynx is removed, along with the thyroid cartilage and epiglottis; the tracheostomy is permanent, and a laryngectomy tube left in place. After surgery the patient is observed for excessive coughing or any vomiting of blood, and the laryngectomy tube is kept free of mucus. A humidifier or vaporizer is useful to decrease coughing and the production of mucus. I.V. fluids are given, and liquid feedings may be given via nasogastric tube; oral fluids begin after one week. A magic slate is useful for communication between patient, staff, and family. The laryngectomy tube is removed three to six weeks after surgery. Compare **neck dissection, radical neck dissection.** —**laryngectomize,** *v.*

laryngismus (lær'ɪnjɪz'məs), spasm of the larynx. Laryngismus stridulus, a condition characterized by sudden laryngeal spasm with a crowing sound on inspiration and the development of cyanosis, occurs in inflammation of the larynx, in connection with rickets, and as an independent disease. The relatively small larynx of the infant and young child is susceptible to spasm when infected or irritated and readily becomes partially or totally obstructed.

laryngitis, inflammation of the mucous membrane lining the larynx, accompanied by edema of the vocal cords with hoarseness or loss of voice, occurring as an acute disorder caused by a cold, by irritating fumes, by sudden temperature changes or as a chronic condition resulting from excessive use of the voice, heavy smoking, or exposure to irritating fumes. In acute laryngitis, there may be a cough, and the throat usually feels scratchy and painful. The patient is advised to remain in an environment with an even temperature, to avoid talking and exposure to tobacco smoke, and to inhale steam containing aromatic vapors, as tincture of benzoin, oil of pine, or menthol. Acute laryngitis may cause severe respiratory distress in children under the age of five because the relatively small larynx of the young child is subject to spasm when irritated or infected and readily becomes partially or totally obstructed. The youngster may develop a hoarse, barking cough and an inspiratory stridor and may become restless, gasping for air. Treatment consists of the administration of copious amounts of vaporized cool mist. Chronic laryngitis may be treated by removal of irritants, avoidance of smoking, voice rest, correction of faulty voice habits, cough medication, steam inhalations, and spraying the throat with an astringent antiseptic, as hexylresorcinol.

laryngo-, laryng-, a combining form meaning 'of or pertaining to the larynx': *laryngocentesis, laryngograph, laryngometry.*

laryngopharyngitis (ləriŋˈgoʊfærˈɪnjaiˈtɪs), inflammation of the larynx and pharynx. See also **laryngitis, pharyngitis.**

laryngopharynx (ləriŋˈgoʊfærˈɪŋks), one of the three regions of the throat, extending from the hyoid bone to its termination in the esophagus. Compare **nasopharynx, oropharynx.** —**laryngopharyngeal,** (ləriŋˈgoʊfərɪnˈjiəl) *adj.*

laryngostasis (ləriŋˈgoʊsteiˈsɪs). See **croup.**

laryngotracheobronchitis (LTB), (ləriŋˈgoʊtreiˈkioʊbroŋkaiˈtɪs), an inflammation of the major respiratory passages, usually causing hoarseness, nonproductive cough, and dyspnea. Among the causes are infection by coxsackieviruses, echoviruses, *Haemophilus influenzae,* and *Corynebacterium diphtheriae.* Treatment includes steam inhalations, cough suppressants, and, for bacterial infections, appropriate antibiotics. See also **croup.**

larynx (lærˈɪŋks), the organ of voice that is part of the air passage connecting the pharynx with the trachea. It produces a large bump in the neck called the Adam's apple and is larger in men than in women although remaining the same size in men and women until puberty. The larynx forms the caudal portion of the anterior wall of the pharynx and is lined with mucous membrane that is continuous with that of the pharynx and the trachea. The larynx extends vertically to the fourth, fifth, and sixth cervical vertebrae and is somewhat higher in the female and during childhood. It is composed of three single cartilages and three paired cartilages, all connected together by ligaments and moved by various muscles. The single cartilages are the thyroid, cricoid, and epiglottis. The three paired cartilages are the arytenoid, corniculate, and cuneiform. The larynx is broad above and narrow and cylindrical at its caudal extremity. —**laryngeal,** *adj.*

Lasan, a trade name for an antipsoriatic (anthralin).

laser, acronym for *light amplification by stimulated emission of radiation,* a source of intense radiation of the visible, ultraviolet, or infrared portions of the spectrum. It is produced by exposing a large number of electrons to a high energy level in a gaseous, solid, or liquid medium. The electrons emit very narrow beams of light, all of one wavelength and parallel to each other. Lasers are used in

surgery to divide or to cause adhesions or to destroy or to fix tissue in place. Also called **optical maser.**

Laserdil, a trade name for a coronary vasodilator (isosorbide dinitrate).

Lasix, a trade name for a diuretic (furosemide).

Lassa fever (laˈsə), a highly contagious disease caused by a virulent arenavirus. It is characterized by fever, pharyngitis, dysphagia, and ecchymoses. Pleural effusion, edema and renal involvement, mental disorientation, confusion, and death from cardiac failure often ensue. Stringent precautions are taken against the spread of infection. Supportive, symptomatic care is the only treatment available.

late dyspituitary eunuchism. See **acromegalic eunuchoidism.**

latency stage, (in psychoanalysis) a period in psychosexual development occurring between early childhood and puberty when sexual motivation and expression are repressed or transferred, through sublimation, to the feelings and behavioral patterns expected as typical of the age. The manifestations of this stage are culturally influenced and vary greatly. See also **psychosexual development.**

latent, dormant; existing as a potential, as tuberculosis may be latent for extended periods of time and become active under certain conditions.

latent carcinoma. See **occult carcinoma.**

latent diabetes, a mild disorder of carbohydrate metabolism characterized by hyperglycemia or hyperinsulinemia only when stress loads of glucose are administered. Also called **chemical diabetes.** See also **diabetes mellitus.**

latent heart failure, an abnormal condition characterized by inadequacy that is not apparent during rest but becomes evident under conditions of increased stress, as that produced by exercise, fever, and emotional excitement. During stress situations the heart affected by latent failure is unable to pump an adequate supply of blood in relation to venous return and the metabolic needs of body tissues and structures.

latent period, (in radiology) an interval of seeming inactivity between the time of exposure to an injurious dose of radiation and the response.

latent phase, the early stage of labor that is characterized by irregular, infrequent, and mild contractions and little or no dilatation of the cervix or descent of the fetus. Also called **prodromal labor.** See also **Friedman curve.**

latent schizophrenia, a form of schizophrenia characterized by the presence of mild symptoms of the disease. Latent schizophrenics have no previous history of psychotic schizophrenic episodes but do have a preexisting susceptibility to the disease in its overt form. Also called **borderline schizophrenia, pseudoneurotic schizophrenia, pseudopsychopathic schizophrenia.** See also **schizophrenia, schizotypal personality disorder.**

lateral aortic node, a lumbar lymph node in any of three clusters of nodes serving the pelvis and abdomen. The right lateral aortic nodes are situated partly ventral to the inferior vena cava, near the termination of the renal vein, and partly dorsal to the inferior vena cava on the right crus of the diaphragm. The left lateral aortic nodes form a chain on the left side of the abdominal aorta, ventral to the origin of the psoas major and ventral to the right crus of the diaphragm. The afferents from both sides drain various structures, as the testes, ovaries, kidneys, and lateral abdominal muscles. Most of the efferents from the lateral aortic nodes converge to form the right and the left lumbar trunks, which join the cisterna chyli. Compare **preaortic node, retroaortic node.**

lateral aperture of the fourth ventricle, an opening between the end of each lateral recess of the fourth ventricle and the subarachnoid space.

lateral cerebral sulcus, a deep cleft marking the division of the temporal, frontal, and parietal lobes of brain. Also called **fissure of Sylvius.**

lateral cuneiform bone, one of the three cuneiform bones of the foot, located in the center of the front row of tarsal bones between the intermediate cuneiform bone medially, the cuboid bone laterally, the scaphoid bone posteriorly, and the third metatarsal anteriorly. It also articulates with the second and fourth metatarsals. Also called **external cuneiform bone, third cuneiform bone.**

lateral geniculate body, one of two elevations of the lateral posterior thalamus receiving visual impulses from the retina via the optic nerves and tracts and relaying the impulses to the calcarine cortex.

lateral humeral epicondylitis, inflammation of the tissue at the lower end of the humerus at the elbow joint, caused by the repetitive flexing of the wrist against resistance. It may result from athletic activity or manual manipulation of tools or other equipment. Pain radiates from the elbow joint. Treatment includes rest, correction of body mechanics, infiltration of a long-acting anesthetic, or serial injections of hydrocortisone, depending on the severity of the condition. Surgery is rarely indicated. Also called **tennis elbow.**

laterality. See **handedness.**

lateral pectoral nerve, one of a pair of branches from the brachial plexus that, with the medial pectoral nerve, supplies the pectoral muscles. It lies lateral to the axillary artery and arises from the lateral cord of the plexus or from the anterior divisions of the superior and the middle trunks just before they unite into the cord. It passes above to the first part of the axillary artery and the axillary vein, gives a filament to the inferior pectoral branch, pierces the clavipectoral fascia, and ends on the deep surface of the clavicular and the cranial sternocostal parts of the pectoralis major. Compare **medial pectoral nerve.**

lateral pelvic displacement, one of the five major ki-

netic determinants of gait that helps to synchronize the rhythmic movements of walking. It is produced by the horizontal shift of the pelvis or by relative hip abduction. It is often a factor in the diagnosis and treatment of various orthopedic diseases, deformities, and abnormal conditions, and in the analysis and the correction of dysfunctional gaits. Compare **knee-ankle interaction, knee-hip flexion, pelvic rotation, pelvic tilt.**

lateral recumbent position, the posture assumed by the patient lying on the left side with the right thigh and knee drawn up. Also called **English position, obstetrical position.**

lateral rotation, a turning away from the midline of the body. Compare **medial rotation.** See also **rotation.**

lateral umbilical fold, a fold in the peritoneum produced by a slight protrusion of the inferior epigastric artery and the interfoveolar ligament. The lateral umbilical fold is about 3 cm lateral to the middle umbilical fold. Also called **plica umbilicalis lateralis.**

latero-, a combining form meaning 'of or pertaining to the side': *laterodeviation, lateroduction, laterotorsion.*

late systolic murmur. See **systolic murmur.**

latex fixation test, a serologic test used in the diagnosis of rheumatoid arthritis in which antigen-coated latex particles agglutinate with rheumatoid factors in a slide specimen of serum or synovial fluid. If positive, the screening slide test is followed by titration. Also called **RA latex test, RF test.** See also **rheumatoid factor.**

Lathrop, Rose Hawthorne (1851–1926), an American nurse, who was a daughter of Nathaniel Hawthorne. She established a home in New York for incurable cancer patients, mostly those who were poor and who were not accepted in hospitals because of the nature of their disease. Later, she became a member of the Third Order of St. Dominic and founded the order of sisters called Servants of Relief for Incurable Cancer. The order founded hospitals wherever there was sufficient need and offered quality care to their patients.

latissimus dorsi, one of a pair of large triangular muscles on the thoracic and lumbar areas of the back. The base of the triangle inserts through lumbar aponeuroses to the spines of lumbar and sacral vertebrae and in the supraspinous ligaments, posterior iliac crest, and the lower four ribs. The fibers of the muscle twist as they pass the scapula and converge at the base of the intertubercular groove of the humerus. The latissimus dorsi extends, adducts, and rotates the arm medially, draws the shoulder back and down, and, with the pectoralis major, draws the body up when climbing. It is innervated by the thoracodorsal nerve. Compare **levator scapulae, rhomboideus major, rhomboideus minor, trapezius.**

LATS, abbreviation for **long-acting thyroid stimulator.**

LATS-P, abbreviation for **long-acting thyroid stimulator protector.**

laughing gas, *Informal.* nitrous oxide, a side effect of which is laughter or giggling when administered in less than anesthetizing amounts.

lavage (ləvaźh′), **1.** the process of washing out an organ, usually the bladder, bowel, paranasal sinuses, or stomach for therapeutic purposes. **2.** to perform a lavage. Kinds of lavage are **blood lavage, gastric lavage, peritoneal dialysis.** See also **irrigation.**

law, 1. (in a field of study) a rule, standard, or principle that states a fact or a relationship between factors, as Dalton's law regarding partial pressures of gas or Koch's law regarding the specificity of a pathogen. **2. a.** a rule, principle, or regulation established and promulgated by a government to protect or to restrict the people affected. **b.** the field of study concerned with such laws. **c.** the collected body of the laws of a people, derived from custom and from legislation.

law of definite composition, (in chemistry) a law stating that a given compound is always made of the same elements present in the same proportion.

law of facilitation. See **facilitation.**

law of independent assortment. See **Mendel's laws.**

law of segregation. See **Mendel's laws.**

law of universal gravitation, (in physics) a law stating that the force with which bodies are attracted to each other is directly proportional to the masses of the objects and inversely proportional to the square of the distance by which they are separated. See also **gravity, mass.**

lawrencium (Lw), a man-made transuranic metallic element. Its atomic number is 103; its atomic weight is 257.

laxative, 1. of or pertaining to a substance that causes evacuation of the bowel by a mild action. **2.** a laxative agent that promotes bowel evacuation by increasing the bulk of the feces, by softening the stool, or by lubricating the intestinal wall. Compare **cathartic.**

lay referral system, an illness referral system through which a person passes from the first recognition of an abnormality to an announcement to the family, to members of the community, then to traditional or culturally recognized healers, and then to the regular medical system that includes nurses and physicians. Depending on the culture and the medical care available, some steps may be omitted.

lazy colon. See **atonia constipation.**

LBW, abbreviation for **low birth weight.**

LD, abbreviation for *lethal dose.*

LD50, (in toxicology) the amount of a substance sufficient to kill one half of the population of test subjects.

LDH, abbreviation for *lactic dehydrogenase.* See **Duchenne's muscular dystrophy.**

L-dopa (el′dou′pə). See **levodopa.**

L.E., abbreviation for *lupus erythematosus.* See **systemic lupus erythematosus.**

lead (Pb) (led), a common soft, blue-gray, metallic element. Its atomic number is 82; its atomic weight is 207.19. In its metallic form, lead is used as a protective shielding against x rays. Lead is poisonous, a characteristic that has led to a reduction in the use of lead compounds as pigments for paints and inks.

lead (lid), an electrical connection attached to the body to record electrical activity, especially of the heart or brain. See also **electrocardiograph, electroencephalograph.**

lead equivalent (led), (in radiology) the thickness of lead required to achieve the same shielding effect against radiation, under specified conditions, as that provided by a given material.

lead pipe fracture (led), a fracture that compresses the bony tissue at the point of impact and creates a linear fracture on the opposite side of the bone involved.

lead poisoning (led), a toxic condition caused by the ingestion or inhalation of lead or lead compounds. Many children have developed the condition as a result of eating flaked lead paint. Poisoning also occurs from the ingestion of water from lead pipes, lead salts in certain foods and wines, the use of pewter or earthenware glazed with a lead glaze, and the use of leaded gasoline for cleaning. Inhalation of lead fumes is common in industry. The acute form of intoxication is characterized by a burning sensation in the mouth and esophagus, colic, constipation, or diarrhea, mental disturbances, and paralysis of the extremities, followed in severe cases by convulsions and muscular collapse. Chronic lead poisoning, which is characterized by extreme irritability, anorexia, and anemia, may progress to the acute form. If ingested, treatment commences with gastric lavage with magnesium or sodium sulfate. All cases call for fluid therapy followed by chelation with intramuscular injection of calcium disodium edetate, or for severe cases, British anti-lewisite. Encephalopathy must be anticipated in children with lead poisoning.

leakage radiation, radiation, exclusive of the primary beam, that is emitted through the housing of equipment used in radiation therapy.

leaky gene. See **hypomorph.**

learning, 1. the act or process of acquiring knowledge or some skill by means of study, practice, or experience. **2.** knowledge, wisdom, or a skill acquired through systematic study or instruction. **3.** (in psychology) the modification of behavior through practice, experience, or training. See also **conditioning.**

learning disability, an abnormal condition often affecting children of normal or above-average intelligence, characterized by difficulty in learning such fundamental procedures as reading, writing, and numerical calculation. The condition may result from psychological or organic causes and is usually related to slow development of perceptual motor skills. See also **attention deficit disorder, dysgraphia, dyslexia.**

leather-bottle stomach. See **linitis plastica.**

Leber's congenital amaurosis (lei′bərz), a rare kind of blindness or severely impaired vision caused by a defect transmitted as an autosomal recessive trait and occurring at birth or shortly thereafter. The eyes appear normal externally, but pupillary constriction to light is sluggish or absent and retinal pigment is degenerated. Pendular nystagmus, photophobia, cataract, and keratoconus may be present and the ophthalmic disorder may be associated with mental retardation and epilepsy. One kind of Leber's amaurosis results in complete blindness, but with a second kind the pathology does not progress and the patient has very slight vision. Also called **amaurosis congenita of Leber.**

Leboyer method of delivery (ləbɔiyei′), an approach to the delivery of an infant formulated by the French obstetrician, Charles Leboyer. It has four aspects: a gentle, controlled delivery in a quiet, dimly lit room, avoidance of pulling on the head, avoidance of overstimulation of the infant's sensorium, and encouragement of maternal-infant bonding. The goal of the method is to minimize the trauma of birth by gently and pleasantly introducing the newborn to life outside the womb. Unnecessary intervention in the process of birth is eschewed. Following delivery, the baby is gently laid on the mother's abdomen, the back is massaged as the cord stops pulsating, and, when regular spontaneous respirations are established the baby is gently supported in a warm tub of water by the father. Many birth centers and obstetric services in the United States have found that no adverse effects result from this method. Some studies in France have suggested superior psychological, social, and intellectual development in young children delivered by this method. Compare **Bradley method, Lamaze method, Read method.**

lecithin (les′ıthın), any of a group of phospholipids common in plants and animals. Lecithins are found in the liver, nerve tissue, semen, and in smaller amounts in bile and blood. They are essential for the metabolism of fats and are used in the processing of foods, pharmaceutical products, cosmetics, and inks. Rich dietary sources are soybeans, egg yolk, and corn. Deficiency leads to hepatic and renal disorders, high serum cholesterol levels, atherosclerosis, and arteriosclerosis. See also **choline, inositol.**

lecitho-, a combining form meaning 'of or pertaining to the yolk of an egg, or to the ovum': *lecithoblast, lecithoprotein, lecithovitellin.*

Ledercillin VK, a trade name for an antibacterial (penicillin V potassium).

Lee-White, a method of determining the length of time required for a clot to form in a test tube of venous blood. It is not specific for any coagulation disorder but is often used to monitor coagulation during heparin therapy. Because normal values and precise methodology vary, instructions are provided by most laboratories. See also **clotting time.**

LeFort I fracture (ləfɔrt′). See **Guérin's fracture.**

left atrioventricular valve. See **mitral valve.**

left brachiocephalic vein, a vessel, about 6 cm long, that starts in the root of the neck at the junction of the internal jugular and the subclavian veins on the left side and runs obliquely across the thorax to join the right brachiocephalic vein and form the superior vena cava. The left brachiocephalic vein, which is longer than the right, receives various tributaries, as the vertebral vein, the internal thoracic vein, and the inferior thyroid vein. Also called **left innominate vein.** Compare **right brachiocephalic vein.**

left common carotid artery, the longer of the two common carotid arteries, springing from aortic arch and having cervical and thoracic portions. The cervical portion passes obliquely from the level of the sternoclavicular articulation to the cranial border of the thyroid cartilage, dividing into the left internal and the left external carotid arteries. Compare **right common carotid artery.**

left coronary artery, one of a pair of branches from the ascending aorta, arising in the left posterior aortic sinus, dividing into the left interventricular artery and the circumflex branch, supplying both ventricles and the left atrium. Compare **right coronary artery.**

left-handedness, a natural tendency to favor the use of the left hand in performing tasks. Also called **sinistrality.** See also **cerebral dominance, handedness.**

left-heart failure, an abnormal cardiac condition characterized by the impairment of the left side of the heart and by elevated pressure and congestion in the pulmonary veins and capillaries. Left-heart failure is usually related to right-heart failure, because both sides of the heart are part of a circuit and the impairment of one side will eventually affect the other. However, research indicates that experimentally produced pure failure of one ventricle may produce significant hemodynamic and biochemical abnormalities of the opposite ventricle, even without the usual signs of failure. In "pure" left-heart failure, the body retains significant amounts of sodium and water and consequently develops peripheral edema without clinical evidence of right-heart failure. Also called **left-sided failure.** Compare **right-heart failure.**

left hepatic duct, the duct that drains the bile from the left lobe of the liver into the common bile duct.

left innominate vein. See **left brachiocephalic vein.**

left lymphatic duct. See **thoracic duct.**

left pulmonary artery, the shorter and smaller of two arteries conveying venous blood from the heart to the lungs, rising from the pulmonary trunk, connecting to the left lung, and tending to have more separate branches than the right pulmonary artery. In the fetus it is larger and more important than the right pulmonary artery because it provides the ductus arteriosus. Compare **right pulmonary artery.**

left subclavian artery, an artery, divided into three parts, that arises from the aortic arch dorsal to the left common carotid at the level of the fourth thoracic vertebra, ascends to the root of the neck, arching laterally to the scalenus anterior, and forms six main branches to supply the vertebral column, spinal cord, ear, and brain. The short second portion lies dorsal to the scalenus anterior and forms the arch described by the vessel. The third portion runs from the scalenus anterior to the first rib where it becomes the axillary artery. Also see **subclavian artery.** Compare **right subclavian artery.**

left ventricle, the thick-walled chamber of the heart that pumps blood through the aorta and the systemic arteries, the capillaries, and back through the veins to the right atrium. It has walls about three times thicker than those of the right ventricle and contains a mitral valve with two flaps that controls the flow of blood from the right atrium. The left ventricle occupies about half the diaphragmatic surface of the heart and is longer and more conical than the right ventricle, narrowing caudally to form the apex. The chordae tendinae of the left ventricle are thicker, stronger, and less numerous than those in the right ventricle. See also **heart.**

left ventricular failure, heart failure in which the left ventricle fails to contract forcefully enough to maintain a normal cardiac output and peripheral perfusion. Pulmonary congestion and edema develop from back pressure of accumulated blood in the left ventricle. Signs include breathlessness, pallor, sweating, and peripheral vasoconstriction. The heart is usually enlarged. A prominent third heart sound (gallop), normal in children and young adults, is a sign of left ventricular failure in older adults with heart disease. Hypertension is common and may be a causative factor or a result of pulmonary edema. Treatment includes meperidine or morphine for sedation, diuretics, digitalis, and rest.

legal death. See **death.**

leg cylinder cast, an orthopedic device of plaster of Paris or fiberglass to immobilize the leg in treating fractures in the legs from the ankle to the upper thigh. It is especially used for fractures and dislocations of the knee, for the soft tissue trauma round the knee, for postoperative positioning and immobilization of the knee, and for correction or maintenance of correction of deformities of the knee. The long leg cast may be used for these same conditions rather than the leg cylinder cast because it encases the foot and assures greater immobilization.

Legg-Calvé-Perthès' disease (leg′kælvei′pərtes′). See **Perthès' disease.**

Legionella pneumophilia (li′jǝnel′ǝ nu′moufil′iǝ, nu′-moufi′lyǝ), a small, fastidious, gram-negative, rod-shaped bacterium that is the causative agent in **Legionnaire's disease.**

legionellosis (li′jǝnɪlou′sɪs). See **Legionnaire's disease.**

Legionnaire's disease, an acute bacterial pneumonia caused by infection with *Legionella pneumophilia* and characterized by an influenzalike illness followed within a week by high fever, chills, muscle aches, and headache. The symptoms may progress to dry cough, pleurisy, and sometimes diarrhea. Usually the disease is self-limited, but mortality has been 15 to 20 per cent in a few localized epidemics. Contaminated air-conditioning cooling towers and moist soil may be a source of organisms. Person-to-person contagion has not occurred. Treatment includes supportive care and erythromycin. Also called **legionellosis.**

leio-, lio-, a combining form meaning 'smooth': *leiodermia, leiodystonia, leiomyofibroma.*

leiomyoblastoma (lai′oumai′oublæstou′mǝ). See **epithelioid leiomyoma.**

leiomyofibroma (lai′oumai′oufaibrou′mǝ), *pl.* **leiomyofibromas, leiomyofibromata.** a tumor consisting of smooth-muscle cells and fibrous connective tissue, commonly occurring in the uterus in middle-aged women. See also **fibroid.**

leiomyoma (lai′oumaiou′mǝ), *pl.* **leiomyomas, leiomyomata.** a benign tumor most commonly occurring in the stomach, esophagus, or small intestine. Surgical resection is necessary only in the rare case in which the tumor undergoes central necrosis, causing sudden and possibly severe hemorrhage.

leiomyoma cutis, a neoplasm of the smooth muscles that raise the hair. The lesion is characterized by many small, tender, red nodules.

leiomyoma uteri, a benign neoplasm of the smooth muscle of the uterus that is characteristically firm, well-circumscribed, round, and gray-white, and, under the microscope, shows a pattern of whorls. Multiple tumors of this kind develop most often in the myometrium and occur most frequently in women between the ages of 30 and 50 years. Also called **fibromyoma uteri, myoma previum,** *Informal.* **fibroids.**

leipo-. See **lipo-.**

Leishman-Donovan body (lish′mǝndon′ǝvɪn), an intracellular, nonflagellated protozoan parasite that causes visceral and cutaneous leishmaniasis.

Leishmania (lishmei′niǝ), a genus of protozoan parasites. These organisms are transmitted to man by any of several species of sand flies.

leishmaniasis (lish′mǝnai′ǝsɪs, laish′mǝnai′ǝsɪs), infection with any species of protozoan of the genus *Leishmania.* The diseases caused by these organisms may be cutaneous or visceral. Diagnosis is made by microscopic identification of the intracellular, nonflagellated protozoan on a Giemsa-stained smear taken from a cutaneous lesion or visceral biopsy. Kinds of leishmaniasis are **American leishmaniasis. kala-azar, oriental sore.** See also **leishmania.** — **leishmanial,** *adj.*

Lemiserp, a trade name for an antihypertensive (reserpine).

-lemma, a combining form meaning a 'confining membrane': *axiolemma, epilemma, neurolemma.*

lemo-, **1.** a combining form meaning 'of or pertaining to plague': *lemography, lemology.* **2.** a combining form meaning 'of or pertaining to the gullet': *lemoparalysis, lemostenosis.*

length of stay (LOS), the period of time a patient remains in a hospital or other health-care facility as an inpatient.

lens, **1.** a curved transparent piece of plastic or glass that is shaped, molded, or ground to refract light in a specific way, as in eyeglasses, microscopes, or cameras. **2.** *Informal.* the crystalline lens of the eye. — **lenticular,** *adj.*

lens capsule, the clear thin elastic capsule that surrounds the lens of the eye. Also called **capsule of the lens.**

lens implant, an artifical lens of clear polymethylmethacrylate that is usually implanted at the time of cataract extraction but may also be used for patients with extreme myopia, diplopia, ocular albinism, and certain other abnormalities. The operation may be performed with a local anesthetic, as lidocaine, but general anesthesia is often preferred, especially for patients with vitreous humor in the anterior chamber. Eyedrops containing an antibiotic, as neomycin, are applied preoperatively to prevent infection, and several times a day for a number of weeks postoperatively. Following extraction of the cataract, the lens is inserted through a corneal incision; it may be held in place in the anterior chamber by extremely fine sutures to the iris or, if the lens is implanted into the capsular sac, a miotic agent, as pilocarpine, is used to prevent the iris from dilating too widely, which would allow the implant to slip. The implanted lens does not cause the problems with abnormal peripheral vision associated with cataract spectacles, and it produces only 2 per cent larger images on the retina than the normal lens, compared with a 24 per cent enlargement produced by cataract spectacles and an 8 per cent enlargement produced by contact lenses. A high rate of complications is reported in implant surgery, and the procedure is contraindicated for patients with diabetes mellitus or uveitis.

Lente Iletin, a trade name for an antidiabetic (insulin zinc suspension).

Lente Insulin, a trade name for an antidiabetic (insulin zinc suspension).

lentigo (lentai′gou), *pl.* **lentigenes** (lentɪj′əniz). a tan or brown macule on the skin brought on by sun exposure, usually in a middle-aged or older person. Another variety, called **juvenile lentigo,** is unrelated to sunlight and appears in children two to five years of age, before the onset of freckles. The melanin pigment in a lentigo is at a deeper level of the epidermis than in a freckle. Both types are benign and no treatment is necessary. Compare **freckle.**

lentigo maligna. See **Hutchinson's freckle.**

leontiasis ossea (li′ontai′əsis os′iə). See **megalocephaly.**

lepido-, a combining form meaning 'of or pertaining to a flake or scale': *lepidoma, lepidosis.*

LE prep, abbreviation for **lupus erythematosus preparation.**

lepro-, a combining form meaning 'of or pertaining to leprosy': *leprologist, lepromatous, leprosarium.*

lepromatous leprosy. See **leprosy.**

lepromin test (leprou′mɪn), a skin sensitivity test used to distinguish between the lepromatous and tuberculoid forms of leprosy. The test consists of intradermal injection of lepromin, which is prepared from heat-sterilized Mycobacterium leprae. The appearance of a palpable nodule in eight to ten days is indicative of the tuberculoid form of leprosy. As no nodule appears in the lepromatous form, the test is not diagnostic of leprosy. The test is used only to follow the course of the disease. See also **leprosy.**

leprosy, a chronic, communicable disease, caused by *Mycobacterium leprae,* that may take either of two forms, depending on the degree of immunity of the host. **Tuberculoid leprosy,** seen in those with high resistance, presents as thickening of cutaneous nerves and anesthetic, saucershaped skin lesions. **Lepromatous leprosy,** seen in those with little resistance, involves many systems of the body, with widespread plaques and nodules in the skin, iritis, keratitis, destruction of nasal cartilage and bone, testicular atrophy, peripheral edema, and involvement of the reticuloendothelial system. Blindness may result. Death is rare unless amyloidos or tuberculosis occur concurrently. Contrary to traditional belief, leprosy is not very contagious, and prolonged, intimate contact is required for it to be spread between individuals. Children are more susceptible than adults. Plastic surgery, physical therapy, and psychotherapy are often necessary. Treatment with sulfones, as dapsone, continued for several years usually results in improvement of skin lesions, but recovery from nerve impairment is limited. The disease is found mostly in underdeveloped tropical and subtropical countries. In the United States, patients may be referred to the U.S. Public Health Service leprosarium in Carville, Louisiana. BCG vaccine may protect against leprosy. Also called **Hansen's disease.** See also *Mycobacterium.* — **lepromatous, leprotic, leprous,** *adj.*

-lepsia. See **-lepsy.**

-lepsis. See **-lepsy.**

-lepsy, a combining form meaning a 'seizure': *deolepsy, electrolepsy, pyknolepsy.* Also **-lepsia, -lepsis.**

-leptic, a combining form meaning 'pertaining to a (specified) type of seizure': *cataleptic, epileptic, hypnoleptic.*

lepto-, a combining form meaning 'thin, or delicate': *leptocephalia, leptocyte, leptosome.*

leptocyte (lep'təsaɪt). See **target cell.**

leptocytosis (lep'tousaɪtou'sɪs). See **thalassemia.**

leptomeninges (lep'toumɪnɪn'jiz), the arachnoid membrane and the pia mater, two of the three layers covering the spinal cord. Compare **meninges.**

leptonema (lep'təni'mə), the threadlike chromosome formation in the leptotene stage in the first meiotic prophase of gametogenesis before the beginning of synapsis.

leptospirosis (lep'touspairou'sɪs), an acute infectious disease caused by several serotypes of the spirochete *Leptospira interrogans,* transmitted in the urine of wild or domestic animals, especially rats and dogs. Human infections arise directly from contact with an infected animal's urine or tissues or indirectly from contact with contaminated water or soil. Clinical symptoms may include jaundice, hemorrhage into the skin, fever, chills, and muscular pain. The spirochete can be isolated from the urine or blood during the acute stage of the disease, and antibodies can be found in the patient's blood during convalescence. Treatment with antibiotics, usually penicillin or tetracycline, may be effective if they are administered during the first few days of the disease. Fluid and electrolyte replacement is essential if jaundice or other signs of severe illness are present. The disease is usually short-lived and mild, but severe infections can damage the kidneys and the liver. Blood pressure and vital signs should be monitored, and the patient's urine should be disposed of carefully to prevent spread of the organism. The most serious form of the disease is called **Weil's disease.** Also called **autumn fever.** See also **nanukayami.**

leptotene (lep'tətin), the initial stage in the first meiotic prophase in gametogenesis in which the chromosomes become visible as single thin filaments. See also **diakinesis, diplotene, pachytene, zygotene.**

Leriche syndrome (lərish'), a vascular disorder marked by gradual occlusion of the terminal aorta, intermittent claudication in the buttocks, thighs, or calves, absence of pulsation in femoral arteries, pallor and coldness of the legs, gangrene of the toes, and, in men, impotence. Symptoms are the result of chronic tissue hypoxia owing to inadequate arterial perfusion of the affected areas. Treatment may include endarterectomy, embolectomy, or synthetic bypass graft at the bifurcation of the aorta.

lesbian, 1. a female homosexual. 2. of or pertaining to the sexual preference or desire of one woman for another. —**lesbianism,** *n.*

Lesch-Nyhan syndrome (leʃ'naɪ'hæn), a hereditary disorder of purine metabolism, characterized by mental retardation, self-mutilation of the fingers and lips by biting, impaired renal function, and abnormal physical development. It is transmitted as a recessive, sex-linked trait.

lesion, any visible, local abnormality of the tissues of the body, as a wound, sore, rash, or boil. A lesion may be described as benign, cancerous, gross, occult, or primary. *(See next page for table)*

lesser multangular bone. See **trapezoid bone.**

lesser occipital nerve, one of a pair of cutaneous branches of the cervical plexus, arising from the second cervical nerve, curving around the sternocleidomastoideus, and ascending along the side of the head behind the ear to supply the skin. It communicates with the greater occipital and the great auricular nerves and with the posterior auricular branch of the facial nerve.

lesser omentum, a membranous extension of the peritoneum from the peritoneal layers covering the ventral and the dorsal surfaces of the stomach and the first part of the duodenum. The lesser omentum extends from the porta of the liver to the diaphragm where the layers separate to enclose the end of the esophagus. It also forms two ligaments, one associated with the liver, the other with the duodenum. Also called **gastrohepatic omentum, small omentum.**

lesser trochanter, one of a pair of conical projections at the base of the neck of the femur, providing insertion of the tendon of psoas major. Compare **greater trochanter.**

let-down, a sensation in the breasts of lactating women that often occurs as the milk flows into the ducts, as when the infant begins to suck or when the mother hears the baby cry or even thinks of nursing the child.

let-down reflex. See **milk-ejection reflex.**

leth-, a combining form meaning 'of or pertaining to forgetfulness': *letheomania, letheral, lethologica.*

lethal, capable of causing death.

lethal equivalent, any recessive gene carried in the heterozygous state that, if homozygous, would be lethal and result in the death of the individual or organism before being transmitted. It is estimated that man carries from three to eight lethal equivalents or any combination of many genes, each with slightly deleterious effects, that are equivalent to three to eight recessive genes.

lethal gene, any gene that produces a phenotypic effect that causes the death of the organism at some stage of development from fertilization of the egg to advanced age. The gene may be dominant, incompletely dominant, or recessive. In humans, examples of diseases caused by lethal genes are Huntington's chorea, which is transmitted as an autosomal dominant, and sickle cell anemia, which shows recessive lethality. Compare **sublethal gene.** See also **lethal equivalent.**

lethargic encephalitis. See **epidemic encephalitis.**

lethargy, 1. the state or quality of being indifferent, apathetic, or sluggish. 2. stupor or coma resulting from disease or hypnosis. Kinds of lethargy include **hysteric lethargy, induced lethargy, lucid lethargy.** —**lethargic,** *adj.*

Types of skin lesions

Observed skin changes	Differentiation	Term	Example
Change in color or texture			
Spot	Circumscribed, flat, color change	Macule	Freckle
Discoloration, (reddish-purple)	Bleeding beneath the surface, injury to tissue	Contusion	Bruise
Soft whitening	Caused by repeated wetting of skin	Maceration	Between toes after soaking
Flake	Dry cells of surface	Scale	Dandruff, psoriasis
Roughness from dried fluid	Dry exudate over lesions	Crust	Eczema, impetigo
Roughness from cells	Leathery thickening of outer skin layer	Lichenification	Callus on foot
Change in shape			
Fluid-filled lesions	Less than 1 cm, clear fluid	Vesicle	Blister, chickenpox
	Greater than 1 cm, clear fluid	Bulla	Large blister, pemphigus
	Small, thick yellowish fluid (pus)	Pustule	Acne
	Semisolid	Cyst	Sebaceous cyst
Solid mass, *cellular* growth	Less than 5 mm	Papule	Small mole, raised rash
	5 mm to 2 cm	Nodule	Enlarged lymph node
	Greater than 2 cm	Tumor	Benign or malignant tumor
	Excess connective tissue over scar	Keloid	Overgrown scar
Swelling of tissue	Generalized swelling; fluid between cells	Edema	Inflammation, swelling of feet
	Circumscribed surface edema, transient, some itching	Wheal	Allergic reaction
Breaks in skin surfaces			
Oozing, scraped surface	Loss of superficial surface of skin	Abrasion	"Floor burn," scrape
Scooped-out depression	Loss of deeper layers of skin	Ulcer	Decubitus, stasis ulcer
Superficial linear skin breaks	Scratch marks, frequently by fingernails	Excoriations	Scratching
Linear crack or cleft	Slit or splitting of skin layers	Fissure	Athlete's foot
Jagged cut	Tearing of skin surface	Laceration	Accidental cut by blunt object
Linear cut, edges approximated	Cutting by sharp instrument	Incision	Knife cut
Vascular lesions			
Small, flat, round, purplish-red spot	Intradermal or submucous hemorrhage	Petechia	Bleeding tendency, vitamin C deficiency
Spiderlike, red, small	Dilatation of capillaries, arterioles, or venules	Telangiectasis	Liver disease, vitamin B deficiency
Discoloration, reddish-purple	Escape of blood into tissue	Ecchymosis	Trauma to blood vessels

Letterer-Siwe syndrome (let′ərərzi′və), any of a poorly classified group of malignant neoplastic diseases of unknown etiology, characterized by histiocytic elements. The syndrome, which is fatal, occurs in infancy and is not familial. Anemia, hemorrhage, splenomegaly, lymphadenopathy, and localized tumefactions over bones are usually present.

leucine (lu′sin), a white, crystalline amino acid essential for optimal growth in infants and nitrogen equilibrium in adults. It cannot be synthesized by the body and is obtained by the hydrolysis of protein during pancreatic digestion. An inherited defect in one of the enzymes involved in the process results in a rare disorder called maple syrup urine disease. See also **leucinosis, maple syrup urine disease.**

leucinosis (lu′sınou′sıs). See **maple syrup urine disease.**

leuco-. See **leuko-.**

leucovorin (lukov′ərın). See **folinic acid.**

leucovorin calcium, an antianemic.

■ INDICATIONS: It is prescribed in the treatment of an overdose of a folic acid antagonist and certain cases of megaloblastic anemia.

■ CONTRAINDICATIONS: Anemia owing to vitamin B_{12} deficiency or known hypersensitivity to this drug prohibits its use.

■ ADVERSE EFFECTS: Hypersensitivity reactions may occur.

leukemia, a malignant neoplasm of blood-forming organs characterized by diffuse replacement of bone marrow with proliferating leukocyte precursors, abnormal numbers and forms of immature white cells in circulation, and infiltration of lymph nodes, the spleen, liver, and other sites. Aproximateley 20,500 new cases in adults and 2,500 in children are diagnosed annually in the United States, and the disease causes about 15,900 deaths a year. Males are affected twice as frequently as females. The etiology of leukemia is not clear, but it may result from exposure to ionizing radiation, benzene, or other chemicals that are toxic to bone marrow. The risk of the disease is increased in individuals with Down's syndrome, Fanconi's anemia, ataxia-telangiectasia, Bloom's syndrome, or some other forms of congenital aneuploidy, and in an identical twin of a leukemia patient. Leukemia is classified according to the predominant proliferating cells, the clinical course, and the duration of the disease. Acute leukemia usually has a sudden onset and rapidly progressess from early signs, as fatigue, pallor, weight loss, and easy bruising, to fever, hemorrhages, extreme weakness, bone or joint pain, and repeated infections. Chronic leukemia develops slowly, and signs similar to those of the acute forms of the disease may not appear for years. Diagnoses of acute and chronic forms are made by blood tests and bone-marrow biopsies. Involved marrow may range in color from muddy red-brown to pale gray, and changes are usually first evident in the vertebrae, ribs, sternum, and pelvis. The most effective treatment includes intensive combination chemotheraphy, the use of antibiotics to prevent infections, and blood transfusions to replace red cells and platelets. The overall five-year survival rate is 14 per cent. Also called **leukocythemia.** See also **acute childhood leukemia.** – **leukemic, leukemoid,** *adj.*

-leukemia, a combining form meaning an 'increased number of leukocytes in the tissues and/or in the blood': *chloroleukemia, erythroleukemia, hypoleukemia.*

leukemia cutis, a condition in which yellow-brown, red, or purple nodular lesions and diffuse infiltrations or large accumulations of leukemic cells develop in the skin. It may be general or localized, usually in the skin of the face. Also called **lymphoderma perniciosa.**

leukemic reticuloendotheliosis. See **hairy-cell leukemia.**

leukemoid (luki'moid), resembling leukemia.

leukemoid reaction, a clinical syndrome resembling leukemia in which the white blood cell count is elevated in response to an allergy, inflammatory disease, infection, poison, hemorrhage, burn, or other causes of severe physical stress. Compare **leukemia.**

Leukeran, a trade name for an antineoplastic (chlorambucil).

leuko-, a combining form meaning 'of or pertaining to a white corpuscle, or white': *leukoblast, leukomaine, leukoplakia.* Also **leuco-.**

leukocyte (lu'kəsait'), a white blood cell, one of the formed elements of the circulating blood system. There are five types of leukocytes, classified by the presence or absence of granules in the cytoplasm of the cell. The agranulocytes are lymphocytes and monocytes. The granulocytes are neutrophils, basophils, and eosinophils. White cells are able to squeeze through intracellular spaces by diapedesis and migrate by ameboid movements. Leukocytes are larger than erythrocytes, measuring 8μ to 20μ in diameter. A cubic millimeter of normal blood usually contains 5,000 to 12,000 leukocytes. Among the most important functions of the leukocytes are phagocytosis of bacteria, fungi, and viruses, detoxification of toxic proteins that may result from allergic reactions and cellular injury, and the development of immunities. Also called **white blood cell, white corpuscle.** Compare **erythrocyte, platelet.** See also **leukocytopenia. leukocytosis.** – **leukocytic,** *adj.*

leukocythemia (lu'kousaithi'miə). See **leukemia.**

leukocytic crystal. See **Charcot-Leyden crystal.**

leukocytosis (lu'kousaitou'sis), an abnormal increase in the number of circulating white blood cells. An increase often accompanies bacterial, but not usually viral infections. The normal range is 5,000 to 10,000 white cells per cu mm of blood. Leukemia may be associated with a white blood cell count as high as 500,000 to 1 million per cu mm of blood, the increase being either equally or disproportionately distributed among all types. Kinds of leukocytosis include **basophilia, eosinophilia, neutrophilia.** Compare **leukemia, leukemoid reaction, leukopenia.** See also **leukocyte.**

leukoderma (lu'koudər'miə), localized loss of skin pigment owing to any of a number of specific causes. Compare **vitiligo.**

leukoerythroblastic anemia (lu'kouerith'roublæs'tik), an abnormal condition in which there are large numbers of immature white and red blood cells. It is characteristic of some anemias that occur as a result of the replacement of normal bone marrow with malignant tumor. See also **myelofibrosis, myeloid metaplasia, myelophthisic anemia.**

leukonychia (lu'kounik'iə), a benign, congenital condition in which the nails are pure white. Trauma, infection, and many systemic disorders can cause white spots or streaks on nails.

leukopenia (lu'kəpi'niə), an abnormal decrease in the number of white blood cells to fewer than 5,000 cells per cu mm. It may be caused by an adverse drug reaction, radiation poisoning, or other pathological conditions and may affect one or all kinds of white blood cells. The two most common forms of leukopenia are neutrophilic leukopenia and lymphocytic leukopenia. Compare **leukocytosis.** See also **aplastic anemia, leukocyte.** – **leukopenic,** *adj.*

leukopenic leukemia. See **subleukemic leukemia.**

leukophlegmasia (lu'kɒuflegmei'ziə). See **phlegmasia alba dolens.**

leukophoresis (lu'kɒufəri'sıs), a laboratory procedure in which white blood cells are separated by electrophoresis for identification and an evaluation of the types of cells and their proportions.

leukoplakia (lu'kɒuplei'kiə), a precancerous, slowly developing change in a mucous membrane characterized by thickened, white, firmly attached patches that are slightly raised and sharply circumscribed. They may occur on the penis or vulva; those appearing on the lips and buccal mucosa are associated with pipe smoking. Malignant potential is evaluated by microscopic study of biopsied tissue. Compare **lichen planus.** See also **lichen sclerosis et atrophicus.**

leukopoiesis (lu'kɒupɒii'sıs), the process by which white blood cells form and develop. Neutrophils, basophils, and eosinophils are produced in myeloid tissue in the bone marrow. Lymphocytes and monocytes are almost all normally derived from hemocytoblasts in lymphoid tissue, but a few develop in the marrow. —**leukopoietic,** *adj.*

leukorrhea (lu'kəri'ə), a white discharge from the vagina. Normally, vaginal discharge occurs in regular variations of amount and consistency during the course of the menstrual cycle. A greater than usual amount is normal in pregnancy and a decrease is to be expected after delivery, during lactation, and after menopause. An irritating, pruritic, copious, foul-smelling, green or yellow discharge may indicate vaginal or uterine infection or other pathology of gynecologic origin. Leukorrhea is the most common reason for women to seek gynecologic care. See also **vaginal discharge.**

leukotomy. See **lobotomy.**

leukotoxin (lu'kətok'sın), a substance that can inactivate or destroy leukocytes. —**leukotoxic,** *adj.*

levallorphan tartrate, a narcotic antagonist.
■ INDICATION: It is prescribed in the treatment of severe narcotic-induced respiratory depression.
■ CONTRAINDICATIONS: Mild respiratory depression, narcotic addiction, or known hypersensitivity to this drug prohibits its use.
■ ADVERSE EFFECTS: Among the more serious adverse reactions are myosis, dysphoria, dizziness, respiratory depression, and, in high dosage, hallucinations and disorientation.

levamisole, a new drug used as an anthelmintic agent against a wide variety of nematodes. It is also under investigation as a stimulant of the immune system that may be effective in the prophylaxis and treatment of bacterial and viral infections.

levamphetamine, levamfetamine, an isomer of amphetamine, formerly used as an anorexiant.

levarterenol bitartrate. See **norepinephrine bitartrate.**

levator (lɪvei'tər), *pl.* **levators** (lev'ətɔr'iz). **1.** a muscle that raises a structure of the body, as the levator ani raises parts of the pelvic diaphragm. **2.** a surgical instrument used to lift depressed bony fragments in fractures of the skull and other bones.

levator ani, one of a pair of muscles of the pelvic diaphragm that stretches across the bottom of the pelvic cavity like a hammock, supporting the pelvic organs. It is a broad, thin muscle that separates into the pubococcygeus and the iliococcygeus. It originates from the ramus of the pubic bone, the spine of the ischium, and a band of fascia between the pubis and the ischium; it inserts into the last two segments of the coccyx, the anococcygeal raphe, the sphincter ani externus, and the central tendinous point of the perineum. The left and right levator ani muscles are divided ventrally but converge as a single sheet across the midline dorsally, forming most of the pelvic diaphragm. The levator ani is innervated by branches of the pudendal plexus, which contains fibers from the fourth sacral nerve, and it functions to support and slightly raise the pelvic floor. The pubococcygeus draws the anus toward the pubis and constricts it. Compare **coccygeus.**

levator palpebrae superioris, one of the three muscles of the eyelid, also considered a muscle of the eye. It is thin and flat and rises from the small wing of the sphenoid. It splits into three lamellae: the superficial lamella extends to the upper eyelid; the middle lamella inserts into the superior tarsus; and the deep lamella is attached to the conjunctiva. It is innervated by the oculomotor nerve, raises the upper eyelid, and is the antagonist of the orbicularis oculi. Compare **corrugator supercilii, orbicularis oculi.**

levator scapulae, a muscle of the dorsal and lateral aspects of the neck. It arises from the axis and the atlas, and it inserts in the third and fourth cervical vertebrae. It is innervated by the third and fourth cervical nerves and acts to raise the scapula and pull it toward the midline.

LeVeen shunt, a tube that is surgically implanted to connect the peritoneal cavity and the superior vena cava to drain an accumulation of fluid in the peritoneal cavity in cirrhosis of the liver, right-sided heart failure, or cancer of the abdomen. Before surgery, a sodium-restricted diet and diuretics are given to decrease sodium and water retention. Under general anesthesia, a silicone-rubber tube is inserted under the subcutaneous tissue from the peritoneum to the superior vena cava. As the patient inhales, the fluid pressure in the peritoneal cavity rises and that in the blood vessel falls, allowing peritoneal fluid to enter the shunt valve. After surgery the patient is closely observed for signs of occlusion of the shunt, gastrointestinal bleeding, or leakage of peritoneal fluid from the incision. Excessive dilution of the blood may lead to abnormalities of coagulation.

level of inquiry, (in nursing research) one of the levels in a rank-ordered system of classification and organization of the questions to be answered in a research study. The level of inquiry is determined by an analysis of the theory to be developed or tested and the kinds of data to be collected. Studies that describe comprise the first level while those that explain comprise the second level. Those that prescribe or predict are the most difficult to answer or to support.

levels of care, a classification of health care service levels by the kind of care given, the number of people served, and the people providing the care. Kinds of health care service levels are **primary health care, secondary health care, tertiary health care.**

lever, (in physiology) any one of the numerous bones and associated joints of the body that act together as a lever so that force applied to one end of the bone to lift a weight at another point tends to rotate the bone in the direction opposite from that of the applied force. The basic components of a lever are the fulcrum, the force arm, the weight arm, and the force moment. A first-class lever, as the hip, has a fulcrum between the weight and the applied force. A third-class lever, as that situated at all the joints of the upper and the lower extremities of the body, accommodates forces between the fulcrum and the weight. The body contains few second-class levers in which the force arm is longer than the weight arm. The muscles of the body produce the forces that move the levers. The body uses its third-class levers for speed and first-class levers to gain either force or speed, depending on the force applied to the weight arm. The moment of force produced by the weight of any body part involved in a lever action can be determined if the center of gravity of the part is known. Charts are available that list the center of gravity of various body parts.

Lévi-Lorain dwarf (lei′vilɔRæ′). See **pituitary dwarf.**

Levin tube (lev′ɪn), a #16 French, plastic catheter, used in gastric intubation, that has a closed, weighted tip and an opening on the side. Compare **Miller-Abbott tube.** See also **gastric intubation.**
(See next column for illustration)

levitation, (in psychiatry) a hallucinatory sensation of floating or rising in the air. —**levitate,** *v.*

levo-, a combining form meaning 'left': *levocardia, levoclination, levotorsion.*

levodopa (li′vɔudou′pə), an antiparkinsonian.
■ INDICATIONS: It is prescribed in the treatment of Parkinson's disease, juvenile forms of Huntington's disease, and chronic manganese poisoning.
■ CONTRAINDICATIONS: Narrow-angle glaucoma, concomitant use of a monoamine oxidase inhibitor, suspected melanoma, or known hypersensitivity to this drug prohibits its use.
■ ADVERSE EFFECTS: Among the more serious adverse reactions are severe gastrointestinal disturbances, hypo-

LEVIN TUBE

tension, various movement disorders, emotional changes, cardiac arrhythmia, and anorexia.

levodopa and carbidopa, an antiparkinsonian.
■ INDICATION: It is prescribed in the treatment of Parkinson's disease.
■ CONTRAINDICATIONS: Narrow angle glaucoma, concomitant administration of a monoamine oxidase inhibitor, suspected melanoma, or known hypersensitivity to this drug prohibits its use.
■ ADVERSE EFFECTS: Among the more serious adverse reactions are gastrointestinal disturbances, hypotension, various dystonic symptoms, emotional changes, and arrhythmias.

Levo-Dromoran, a trade name for a narcotic analgesic (levorphanol tartrate).

Levophed Bitartrate, a trade name for an adrenergic (levarterenol bitartrate).

Levoprome, a trade name for an analgesic (methotrimeprazine).

levopropoxyphene napsylate, an antitussive.
■ INDICATION: It is prescribed for cough.
■ CONTRAINDICATIONS: Its use is prohibited during the first trimester of pregnancy, following surgery, or in cases of known hypersensitivity to this drug.
■ ADVERSE EFFECTS: Among the more serious adverse reactions are skin rash, muscle tremor, and vomiting.

levorphanol tartrate, a narcotic analgesic.
■ INDICATIONS: It is prescribed for pain and preoperative analgesia.
■ CONTRAINDICATIONS: Alcoholism, asthma, increased

intracranial pressure, respiratory depression, anoxia, or known hypersensitivity to this drug prohibits its use.

■ ADVERSE EFFECTS: Among the more serious adverse reactions are drug dependence, orthostatic hypotension, cardiac arrhythmia, and retention of urine.

levothyroxine sodium, a thyroid hormone.

■ INDICATION: It is prescribed in the treatment of hypothyroidism.

■ CONTRAINDICATIONS: Recent myocardial infarction, normal thyroid function, or known hypersensitivity to this drug prohibits its use.

■ ADVERSE EFFECT: The most serious adverse reaction is angina.

Levsin, a trade name for an anticholinergic (hyoscyamine sulfate).

Levsinex, a trade name for an anticholinergic (hyoscyamine sulfate).

levulose (lev′yəlous). See **fructose.**

levulosuria (lev′yulousur′iə). See **fructosuria.**

lewisite (lu′ısait), 2-chlorovinyl arsine; a poisonous gas, used in World War I, that causes irritation of the lungs, dyspnea, damage to the tissues of the respiratory tract, tears, and pain.

-lexia, a combining form meaning 'reading': *alexia, bradylexia, dyslexia.*

Leyden-Moebius muscular dystrophy (lai′dənmœ′bius). See **pelvifemoral muscular dystrophy.**

Leydig cell tumor (lai′dıg), a generally benign neoplasm of interstitial cells of a testis that may cause gynecomastia in adults and precocious sexual development if the lesion occurs before puberty. The tumor is usually a circumscribed, lobulated, palpable mass.

Leydig's cells (lai′dıgz), cells of the interstitial tissue of the testes that secrete testosterone.

LFT, abbreviation for **liver function test.**

LGA, abbreviation for **large-for-gestational-age.**

LGV. See **lymphogranuloma venereum.**

LH, abbreviation for **luteinizing hormone.**

Lhermitte's sign (leir′mıts), sudden, transient, electriclike shocks spreading down the body when the head is flexed forward, occurring chiefly in multiple sclerosis but also in compression disorders of the cervical spinal cord.

Li, symbol for **lithium.**

liability, 1. something one is obligated to do or an obligation required to be fulfilled by law, usually financial in nature. 2. the amount of money required to fulfill a financial obligation.

libel, a false accusation written, printed, or typewritten, or presented in a picture or a sign that is made with malicious intent to defame the reputation of a person who is living or the memory of a person who is dead, resulting in public embarrassment, contempt, ridicule, or hatred.

libidinal development. See **psychosexual development.**

libidinous, libidinal, 1. pertaining to or belonging to the libido. 2. having or characterized by sexual desire. − **libidinize,** *v.*

libido (libi′dou, libai′dou), 1. the psychic energy or instinctual drive associated with sexual desire, pleasure, or creativity. 2. (in psychoanalysis) the instinctual drives of the id. 3. lustful desire or striving. Kinds of libido are **bisexual libido, ego libido.**

Libman-Sacks endocarditis (lib′mənsæks′), an abnormal condition and the most common manifestation of lupus erythematosus, characterized by verrucous lesions which develop near the heart valves but rarely affect valvular action. The lesions usually are dry and granular, with a pink or tawny color, contain basophilic cellular debris, and develop in the angle of the atriventricular valves and at the base of the mitral valve.

Libman-Sacks syndrome (lib′mənsæks′), a typical verrucous endocarditis occurring with systemic lupus erythematosus. Also called **Libman-Sacks disease.**

Librax, a trade name for a gastrointestinal, fixed-combination drug containing an anticholinergic (clidinium bromide) and a sedative (chlordiazepoxide hydrochloride).

Libritabs, a trade name for an antianxiety agent (chlordiazepoxide).

Librium, a trade name for an antianxiety agent (chlordiazepoxide).

licensed practical nurse (LPN), *U.S.* a person trained in basic nursing techniques and direct patient care who practices under the supervision of a registered nurse. The course of training usually lasts one year. In Canada an LPN is called a nursing assistant. Also called *U.S.* **licensed vocational nurse.**

licensed psychologist, a person who has earned a Ph.D. in psychology from an accredited graduate school and has completed two to three years of postgraduate training with special emphasis on the diagnosis and treatment of psychological disorders. Also called **clinical psychologist.** See also **psychotherapist.**

licensed vocational nurse (LVN). See **licensed practical nurse.**

licensure, the granting of permission by a competent authority (usually a governmental agency) to an organization or individual to engage in a practice or activity that would otherwise be illegal. Kinds of licensure include the issuing of licenses for general hospitals or nursing homes, for health professionals, as physicians, and for the production or distribution of biological products. Licensure is usually granted on the basis of education and examination rather than performance. It is usually permanent, but a periodic fee, demonstration of competence, or continuing education may be required. Licensure may be revoked by the granting agency for incompetence, criminal acts, or other reasons stipulated in the rules governing the specific area of licensure.

lichenification (laiken'ıfıkei'shən), thickening and hardening of the skin, often resulting from the irritation caused by repeated scratching of a pruritic lesion. –**lichenified**, *adj.*

lichen nitidus, a rare skin disorder characterized by numerous flat, glistening, pale, discrete papules measuring two to three mm in diameter. Also called **Pinkus' disease.**

lichen planus, a nonmalignant, chronic, pruritic skin disease of unknown cause, characterized by small, flat, purplish papules or plaques having fine, gray lines on the surface. Common sites are flexor surfaces of wrists, forearms, ankles, abdomen, and sacrum. On mucous membranes the lesions appear gray and lacy. Nails may have longitudinal ridges. Episodes of disease activity, of which there are numerous variations, may last for months and may recur. Compare **leukoplakia.**

lichen sclerosis et atrophicus, a chronic skin disease characterized by white, flat papules with an erythematous halo and black, hard follicular plugs. In advanced cases, the papules tend to coalesce into large, white patches of thin, pruritic skin. Lesions often occur on the torso and, almost inevitably, in the anogenital regions, in which case the disease is called kraurosis vulvae. Corticosteroids are applied topically to reduce itching.

lichen simplex chronicus, a form of neurodermatitis characterized by a patch of pruritic, confluent papules. Psychogenic factors and mechanical trauma, as scratching, contribute to its chronicity. Treatment may include topical or intralesional application of corticosteroids to relieve the pruritis.

lid. See **eyelid.**

Lidaform-HC, a trade name for a topical, fixed-combination drug containing a glucocorticoid (hydrocortisone acetate), a topical anti-infective (iodochlorhydroxyquin), and a local anesthetic (lidocaine)

Lida-Mantle-HC, a trade name for a topical, fixed-combination drug containing a glucocorticoid (hydrocortisone acetate) and a local anesthetic (lidocaine).

Lidex, a trade name for a glucocorticoid (fluocinonide).

lidocaine hydrochloride (lai'dəkein), a local anesthetic agent.

■ INDICATIONS: It is prescribed as a local anesthetic for topical administration to skin or to mucous membranes. It is used parenterally as an antiarrhythmic agent.

■ CONTRAINDICATIONS: Known hypersensitivity to this drug prohibits its topical use. Heart block or known hypersensitivity to this drug prohibits its systemic use.

■ ADVERSE EFFECTS: Among the more serious adverse reactions to the systemic administration of the drug are central nervous system disturbances, hypotension, bradycardia, and cardiac arrest. A variety of hypersensitivity reactions may occur from topical administration of this drug. Eating and drinking is avoided for one hour after topical application of this drug to the pharynx or the esophagus.

Lidosporin, a trade name for an otic, fixed-combination drug containing an antibacterial (polymyxin B sulfate) and a local anesthetic (lidocaine hydrochloride).

lie detector, an electronic device or instrument used to detect lying or anxiety in regard to specific questions. A commonly used lie detector is the polygraph recorder which senses and records pulse, respiratory rate, blood pressure, and perspiration. Some experts hold that certain patterns indicate the presence of anxiety, guilt, or fear, emotions that are likely to occur when the subject is lying.

lien. See **spleen.** –**lienal,** *adj.*

lienal vein, a large vein of the lower body that unites with the superior mesenteric vein to form the portal vein. It returns blood from the spleen and arises from about six large tributaries which unite to form the single vessel passing from left to right across the superior, dorsal part of the pancreas. It receives the short gastric veins, the left gastroepiploic vein, the pancreatic veins, and the inferior mesenteric veins. Also called **splenic vein.**

lieno-, a combining form meaning 'of or pertaining to the spleen': *lienomalacia, lienomedullary, lienopathy.*

life costs, the mortality, morbidity, and suffering associated with a given disease or medical procedure.

life expectancy. See **expectation of life.**

life science, the study of the laws and properties of living matter. Some kinds of life science are **anatomy, bacteriology, biology.** Compare **physical science.**

ligament, 1. Compare **tendon.** one of many predominantly white, shiny, flexible bands of fibrous tissue binding joints together and connecting various bones and cartilages. Such ligaments are slightly elastic and composed of parallel collagenous bundles. When part of the synovial membrane of a joint, they are covered with fibroelastic tissue which blends with surrounding connective tissue. Yellow elastic ligaments, as the ligamenta flava, connect certain parts of adjoining vertebrae. 2. See also **broad ligament.** A layer of serous membrane with little or no tensile strength, extending from one visceral organ to another, as the ligaments of the peritoneum. Also called **ligamentum.** –**ligamentous,** *adj.*

ligamenta flava, the bands of yellow elastic tissue connecting the laminae of adjacent vertebrae from the axis to the first segment of the sacrum. They are thin, broad, and long in the cervical region, thicker in the thoracic region, and thickest in the lumbar region. They help to hold the body erect.

ligamental tear, a complete or a partial tear of a ligamentous structure connecting and surrounding the bones of a joint, caused by an injury to the joint, as by a sudden twisting motion or by a forceful blow.

■ OBSERVATIONS: Ligamental tears may occur at any joint

but are most common in the knees. The pathologic features of ligamental tears of the knee are dependent on the location and severity of the injury. The most common ligaments involved in knee injuries are the medial, lateral, and posterior ligaments and the anterior and posterior cruciate ligaments. Usually, the injury involves more than one structure because of the way in which the structures connect with and support each other.

■ INTERVENTION: Treatment depends on the severity of the injury. A mild injury may cause little damage with tenderness, swelling, and pain with stress. Rest, compression, applications of heat and cold, elevation, and early use, are usually recommended. Injection of an anti-inflammatory agent may be desirable. Treatment for a moderate injury in which few fibers have been completely torn is protective. In addition to the above measures, the joint is aspirated and supported. Treatment for a severe, complete tear is restorative. This may be by immobilization followed by physical therapy, or if necessary, by surgical repair.

■ NURSING CONSIDERATIONS: Ligamental tears of the knee joint are extremely common in young adults and are associated with sports injuries. Good physical condition may help prevent many injuries, and proper care during healing is necessary to prevent permanent disability, which is often accompanied by instability, stiffness, or pain in the joint.

ligament of the neck of the rib, one of five ligaments of each costotransverse joint, consisting of short, strong fibers passing from the neck of the rib to the transverse process of the adjacent vertebra. Also called **middle costotransverse ligament.**

ligament of the tubercle of the rib, one of the five ligaments of each costotransverse joint, comprised of a short, thick fasciculus passing obliquely from the transverse process of a vertebra to the tubercle of the associated rib. Compare **ligament of the neck of the rib.**

ligamentum (lɪg′əmen′təm), *pl.* **ligamenta.** See **ligament.**

ligamentum latum uteri. See **broad ligament.**

ligamentum nuchae, the fibrous membrane that reaches from the external occipital protuberance and median nuchal line to the spinous process of the seventh vertebra. A fibrous lamina from the ligament attaches to the posterior tubercle of the atlas and to the spinous processes of the cervical vertebrae, forming a septum between muscles on either side of the neck.

ligation (laɪgeɪ′shən), tying off of a blood vessel or duct with a suture or wire ligature performed to stop or prevent bleeding during surgery, to stop spontaneous or traumatic hemorrhage, or to prevent passage of material through a duct, as in tubal ligation or to treat varicosities. In venous ligation, the saphenous vein is tied above the varicosed portion, and the distal portions are removed. General anesthesia is used. After surgery, the nurse ob-

serves the patient's feet and legs for circulatory impairment; the foot of the bed is raised to encourage venous return. Ambulation is begun the day of surgery, with elastic bandages for firm support. Analgesics are given as necessary for pain and discomfort. See also **ligature, saphenous vein, tubal ligation, varicose veins.** —**ligate,** *v.*

ligature, 1. a suture. 2. a wire, as used in orthodontia.

ligature needle, a long, thin, curved needle used for passing a suture underneath an artery for ligation of the vessel.

light, 1. electromagnetic radiation of the wavelength and frequency that stimulate visual receptor cells in the retina to produce nerve impulses that are perceived as vision. 2. electromagnetic radiation with wavelengths shorter than ultraviolet light and longer than infrared light, the range of visible light.

light bath, the exposure of the patient's uncovered skin to the sun or to actinic light rays from an artificial source for therapeutic purposes.

light diet, a diet suitable for convalescent or bed-ridden patients taking little or no exercise. It consists of simple, moderate quantities of soft-cooked and easily digested foods, including meats, potatoes, rice, eggs, pasta, some fruits, refined cereals, and breads. It avoids all highly seasoned and fried foods.

lightening, a subjective sensation reported by many women late in pregnancy as the fetus settles lower in the pelvis, leaving more space in the upper abdomen. The diaphragm, no longer restricted by the fundus of the uterus beneath it, can move down more fully during inspiration, allowing deeper breaths to be taken. The stomach, too, is less compressed so the woman can comfortably eat more food at a sitting. The profile of the abdomen changes with lightening, as the round, full uterus is visibly lower. The baby is then said to have 'dropped.'

light reflex, the mechanism by which the pupil of the eye becomes more or less open in response to direct or consensual pupillary stimulation. Also called **pupillary reflex.** Compare **consensual light reflex.** See also **consensual reaction to light.**

light vaginal bleeding. See **vaginal bleeding.**

ligneous (lɪg′niəs), woody or resembling wood in texture or other characteristics.

ligneous thyroiditis. See **fibrous thyroiditis.**

lignin (lɪg′nɪn), a polysaccharide that with cellulose and hemicellulose forms the chief part of the skeletal substances of the cell walls of plants. It provides bulk in the diet necessary for the proper gastrointestinal functioning. See also **dietary fiber.**

lilliputian hallucination (lɪl′ɪpyu′shən), one in which things seem smaller than they actually are. See also **hallucination.**

limb, 1. an appendage or extremity of the body, as an

arm or leg. **2.** a branch of an internal organ, as a loop of a nephron.

limb-girdle muscular dystrophy, a form of muscular dystrophy transmitted as an autosomal recessive trait. The characteristic weakness and degeneration of the muscles begins in the shoulder girdle or in the pelvic girdle. The condition is progressive, regardless of the area in which it is first manifest. Kinds of limb-girdle muscular dystrophy are **pelvifemoral muscular dystrophy, scapulohumeral muscular dystrophy.**

limbic system, a group of structures within the rhinencephalon of the brain that are associated with various emotions and feelings, as anger, fear, sexual arousal, pleasure, and sadness. The structures of the limbic system are the cigulate gyrus, the isthmus, the hippocampal gyrus, the uncas, and the hippocampus. The structures connect with various other parts of the brain, as the septum and the hypothalamus. Unless the limbic system is modulated by other cortical areas, periodic attacks of uncontrollable rage may occur in some individuals. The function of the system is poorly understood.

limb-kinetic apraxia. See **ideomotor apraxia.**

lime, 1. any of several oxides and hydroxides of calcium. The various kinds of lime have many uses, including the treatment of sewage, purification of water and refining of sugar, and the manufacture of materials like plaster and fertilizers. **2.** a citrus fruit yielding a juice with a high ascorbic acid content. Lime juice was one of the first effective agents to be used in the treatment of scurvy. See also **ascorbic acid, scurvy.**

limo , a combining form meaning 'of or pertaining to hunger': *limophthisis, limosis, limotherapy.*

limp, an abnormal pattern of ambulation in which the two phases of gait are markedly asymmetric. See also **stance phase of gait, swing phase of gait.**

LINAC, abbreviation for **linear accelerator.**

Lincocin, a trade name for an antibacterial (lincomycin).

Lincocin Hydrochloride, a trade name for an antibacterial (lincomycin hydrochloride).

lincomycin hydrochloride, an antibiotic.
■ INDICATIONS: It is prescribed in the treatment of certain infections.
■ CONTRAINDICATIONS: Known hypersensitivity to this drug or to clindamycin prohibits its use.
■ ADVERSE EFFECTS: Among the more serious adverse reactions are diarrhea and the development of life-threatening pseudomembranous colitis owing to suprainfection.

lincomycin hydrochloride monohydrate. See **lincomycin hydrochloride.**

lincomycin monohydrate. See **lincomycin hydrochloride.**

lindane (lĭn′dein), gamma benzene hexachloride.
■ INDICATIONS: It is prescribed in the treatment of pediculosis and scabies.

■ CONTRAINDICATIONS: It is not usually given to infants or pregnant women and is not applied to the face. Known hypersensitivity to this drug prohibits its use.
■ ADVERSE EFFECTS: Among the most serious adverse reactions are neurological damage and aplastic anemia. Given topically, irritation of eyes, skin, and mucosa may occur.

Lindau-von Hippel disease (lĭn′dau von hĭp′əl). See **cerebroretinal angiomatosis.**

Lindbergh pump, a pump used to preserve an organ of the body by perfusing its tissues with oxygen and other essential nutrients, usually during the transport of an organ from a donor to a recipient. Also called **Carrel-Lindbergh pump.**

line, a stripe, streak, or narrow ridge, often imaginary, that serves to connect anatomical reference points or to separate various parts of the body, as the hair line or nipple line. Also called **linea.**

linea (lĭn′iə). See **line.**

linea alba, the portion of the anterior abdominal aponeurosis in the middle line of the abdomen, representing the fusion of three aponeuroses into a single tendinous band extending from the xiphoid process to the symphysis pubis. It contains the umbilicus. Compare **linea semilunaris.**

linea arcuata, the curved tendinous band in the sheath of the rectus abdominis below the umbilicus. It is usually derived from the aponeurosis of the transversus abdominis or the obliquus internus, sometimes from both those muscles. It inserts into the linea alba. Compare **linea semilunaris.**

linea aspera, the posterior crest of the thigh bone, extending proximally into three ridges to which are attached various muscles, including the glutcus maximus, pectineus, and iliacus.

linear accelerator (LINAC), an apparatus for accelerating charged subatomic particles used in radiotherapy, physics research, and in the production of radionuclides. In a linear accelerator a pulsed electron beam generated by an electron gun passes through a straight long vacuum tube containing alternating hollow electrodes. The electrodes are so arranged that when their high-frequency potentials are properly varied, the particles passing through the vacuum-tube waveguide receive successive increments of energy. The electrons are stopped abruptly by a heavy metal target at the end of the waveguide and are directed by a collimator to deliver supervoltage x rays to the patient receiving radiotherapy.

linear fracture, a fracture that extends parallel to the long axis of a bone but does not displace the bone tissue.

linea semilunaris, the slightly curved line on the ventral abdominal wall, approximately parallel to the median line and lying about halfway between the median line and the side of the body. It marks the lateral border of the rectus abdominis and can be seen as a shallow groove when that muscle is tensed. Compare **linea alba.**

lingu-, a combining form meaning 'of or pertaining to the tongue': *linguiform, lingulectomy, linguodental.*

lingua (lɪng'gwə). See **tongue.**

lingual artery, one of a pair of arteries that arises from the external carotid arteries, divides into four branches, and supplies the tongue and surrounding muscles. The branches of the lingual artery are the suprahyoid, dorsal lingual, sublingual, and the deep lingual.

lingual bone. See **hyoid bone.**

lingual frenum, a band of tissue that extends from the floor of the mouth to the inferior surface of the tongue. Also called **frenulum linguae.**

lingual goiter, a tumor at the back of the tongue formed by an enlargement of the primordial thyrolingual duct.

lingual papilla. See **papilla.**

lingual tonsil, a mass of lymphoid follicles near the root of the tongue. Each follicle forms a rounded eminence containing a small opening leading into a funnel-shaped cavity surrounded by lymphoid tissue.

lingua villosa nigra. See **parasitic glossitis.**

liniment, a preparation, usually containing an alcoholic, oily, or soapy vehicle, that is rubbed on the skin as a counterirritant.

linitis (lɪnai'tɪs), inflammation of cellular tissue of the stomach as in linitis plastica, seen frequently in adenocarcinoma of the stomach. The layer of connective tissue of the stomach becomes fibrotic and thick, and the stomach wall becomes shrunken and rigid.

linitis plastica, a diffuse fibrosis and thickening of the wall of the stomach, resulting in a rigid, inelastic organ. Causes of this condition include infiltrating undifferentiated carcinoma, syphilis, and Crohn's disease involving the stomach. Also called **leather-bottle stomach.**

linkage, 1. See also **synteny.** (in genetics) the location of two or more genes on the same chromosome so that they do not segregate independently during meiosis but tend to be transmitted together as a unit. The closer the loci of the genes, the more likely they are to be inherited as a group and associated with a specific trait, while the farther apart they are, the greater the chance that they will be separated by crossing over and carried on homologous chromosomes. The concept of linkage, which opposes the independent assortment theory of Mendelian genetics, led to the foundation of the modern chromosome theory of genetics. 2. (in psychology) the association between a stimulus and the response it elicits. 3. (in chemistry) the bond between two atoms or radicals in a chemical compound or the lines used to designate valency connections between the atoms in structural formulas.

linkage group, (in genetics) a group of genes located on the same chromosome that tends to be inherited as a unit.

Theoretically, without crossing over, all of the genes on a given chromosome constitute a linkage group and are equal to the number of autosomes in the haploid cell.

linkage map. See **genetic map.**

linked genes, genes that are located on the same chromosome and whose position is close enough so that they tend to be transmitted as a linkage group.

linker, (in molecular genetics) a small segment of synthetic DNA having a place on its surface that can be ligated to DNA fragments in cloning. Some linkers are commercially available.

linoleic acid (lɪn'əli'ɪk), a colorless to straw-colored essential fatty acid with two unsaturated bonds, occurring in linseed and safflower oils. Commercially produced linoleic acid is used in margarine, animal feeds, emulsifying agents, soaps, and drugs.

lio-. See **leio-.**

liothyronine sodium (lai'outhai'rənin), a synthetic thyroid hormone.

■ INDICATIONS: It is prescribed in the treatment of primary hypothyroidism, simple goiter, and secondary hypothyroidism.

■ CONTRAINDICATIONS: Hyperthyroidism, thyrotoxicosis, acute myocardial infarction, or known hypersensitivity to this drug prohibits its use. It is used with caution in patients with diabetes mellitus or cardiovascular disease.

■ ADVERSE EFFECTS: Among the serious adverse reactions, usually owing to overdosage, are thyrotoxicosis, nausea, vomiting, hypertension, nervousness, and loss of weight.

liotrix (lai'ətrɪks), a uniform mixture of the thyroid hormones T_3 and T_4.

■ INDICATIONS: It is prescribed in the treatment of hypothyroid conditions.

■ CONTRAINDICATIONS: Most diseases and abnormal conditions of the myocardium or known hypersensitivity to this drug prohibits its use.

■ ADVERSE EFFECTS: Among the more serious adverse reactions are symptoms of thyrotoxicosis, including tachycardia, nervousness, insomnia, and fever.

lip-, lipo-, combining form meaning 'fat': *lipase, lipodystrophy, lipoma.*

lipase (lai'peis, lɪp'eis), any of several enzymes, produced by the organs of the digestive system, that catalyze the breakdown of lipids through the hydrolysis of the linkages between fatty acids and glycerol in triglycerides and phospholipids. See also **fat, fatty acid, glycerol, phospholipid, triglyceride.**

lipectomy (lɪpek'təmi), an excision of subcutaneous fat, as from the abdominal wall. Also called **adipectomy.**

lipemia (lɪpi'miə), a condition in which increased amounts of lipids are present in the blood, a normal occurance after eating.

lipid, any of a class of greasy organic substances insoluble in water but soluble in alcohol, chloroform, ether, and other solvents. Lipids are stored in the body and serve as an energy reserve. Kinds of lipids are **fatty acid, phospholipid, steroid, wax.**

lipidosis (lɪp'ɪdou'sɪs), a general term including several rare familial disorders of fat metabolism. The chief characteristic of these disorders is the accumulation of abnormal levels of certain lipids in the body. Kinds of lipidoses are **Gaucher's disease, Krabbe's disease, Niemann-Pick disease, Tay-Sachs disease.**

Lipivas, a trade name for an antihyperlipoproteinemic (halofenate).

lipo-. See **lip-.**

lipocele (lɪp'əsil). See **adipocele.**

lipochondrodystrophy. See **Hurler's syndrome.**

lipochrome (lɪp'əkroum), any of the naturally occurring pigments that contain a lipid, as carotene.

lipodystrophia progressiva, an abnormal accumulation of fat around the buttocks and thighs and a progressive, symmetrical disappearance of subcutaneous fat from areas above the pelvis and on the face. Also called **lipomatosis atrophicans.**

lipodystrophy (lɪp'oudɪs'trəfi), any abnormality in the metabolism or deposition of fats. Kinds of lipodystrophy are **bitrochanteric lipodystrophy, insulin lipodystrophy, intestinal lipodystrophy.**

lip of hip fracture, a fracture of the posterior lip of the acetabulum, often associated with displacement of the hip.

lipogranuloma (lɪp'ougræn'yulou'mə), pl. **lipogranulomas, lipogranulomata.** a nodule of necrotic, fatty tissue associated with granulomatous inflammation or with a foreign-body reaction around a deposit of injected material containing an oily substance.

Lipo-Hepin, a trade name for an anticoagulant (heparin sodium).

lipoic acid (lɪpou'ɪk), a bacterial growth factor found in liver and yeast.

lipoid (lɪp'oid), any substance that resembles a lipid.

Lipo-Lutin, a trade name for a progestin (progesterone).

lipoma (lɪpou'mə), pl. **lipomas, lipomata.** a benign tumor consisting of mature fat cells. Also called **adipose tumor.** See also **multiple lipomatosis.** — **lipomatous,** adj.

-lipoma, a combining form meaning a 'tumor made up of fatty tissue': angiolipoma, fibrolipoma, osteolipoma.

lipoma annulare colli, a diffuse, symmetrical accumulation of fat around the neck, not a true lipoma. Also called **Madelung's neck.**

lipoma arborescens, a fatty tumor of a joint, characterized by a treelike distribution of fat cells.

lipoma capsulare, a benign neoplasm characterized by the abnormal presence of fat cells in the capsule of an organ.

lipoma cavernosum. See **angiolipoma.**

lipoma diffusum renis. See **lipomatous nephritis.**

lipoma dolorosa. See **lipomatosis dolorosa.**

lipoma fibrosum, a fatty tumor containing masses of fibrous tissue.

lipoma myxomatodes. See **lipomyxoma.**

lipoma sarcomatode. See **liposarcoma.**

lipomatosis (lɪp'oumətou'sɪs), a disorder characterized by abnormal tumorlike accumulations of fat in body tissues.

lipomatosis atrophicans. See **lipodystrophia progressiva, lipomatosis.**

lipomatosis dolorosa, a disorder characterized by the abnormal accumulation of painful or tender fat deposits. Also called **lipoma dolorosa.**

lipomatosis gigantea, a condition characterized by massive deposits of fat.

lipomatosis renis. See **lipomatous nephritis.**

lipomatous myxoma, a tumor containing fatty tissue that arises in connective tissue.

lipomatous nephritis, a rare condition in which the renal nephrons are replaced by fatty tissue. Kidney failure may result. Also called **lipoma diffusum renis, lipomatosis renis.**

lipomyxoma (lɪp'oumɪksou'mə), pl. **lipomyxomas, lipomyxomata.** a myxoma that contains fat cells. Also called **lipoma myxomatodes.**

lipoprotein (lɪp'ouprou'tin), a conjugated protein in which lipids form an integral part of the molecule. They are synthesized primarily in the liver, contain varying amounts of triglycerides, cholesterol, phospholipids, and protein, and are classified according to their composition and density. Practically all of the plasma lipids are present as lipoprotein complexes. Kinds of lipoproteins are **chylomicrons, high-density lipoproteins, low-density lipoproteins, very low-density lipoproteins.** See also **proteolipid.**

liposarcoma (lɪp'ousarkou'mə), pl. **liposarcomas, liposarcomata.** a malignant growth of primitive fat cells. Also called **lipoma sarcomatode.**

liposis (lɪpou'sɪs). See **lipomatosis.**

-lipsis, a combining form meaning 'to leave, fail, omit': eclipsis, ellipsis, menolipsis. Also **-lipse.**

Liquaemin Sodium, a trade name for an anticoagulant (heparin sodium).

Liquamar, a trade name for an anticoagulant (phenprocoumon).

liquefaction, the process in which a solid or a gas is made liquid.

liquid, a state of matter, intermediate between solid and gas, in which the substance flows freely with little application of force and assumes the shape of the vessel in which it is contained. Compare **fluid.** See also **gas, solid.**

liquid diet, a diet consisting of foods that can be served in liquid or strained form plus custard, ice cream, pudding, tapioca, and soft-cooked eggs. It is prescribed in acute infections, in acute inflammatory conditions of the gastrointestinal tract, and for patients unable to consume soft or semifluid foods, usually following surgery. See also **full liquid diet.**

liquid glucose, a thick, syrupy, odorless, colorless or yellowish liquid obtained by the incomplete hydrolysis of starch primarily consisting of dextrose with dextrins, maltose, and water. It is used as a flavoring agent and may be used as a food, chiefly in treating dehydration.

liquor amnii. See **amniotic fluid.**

liquorice, licorice, a dried root of gummy texture from the leguminous plant *Glycyrrhiza glabra*. It has a sweet, astringent taste and is used as a flavoring agent in medicines, especially in cough syrups and laxatives, confectionery, and tobacco.

Lisfranc's fracture (lɪsfraŋks′), a fracture-dislocation of the foot in which one or all of the proximal metatarsals are displaced.

Listeria monocytogenes (monˈousaitojˈmiz), a common species of gram-positive, motile bacillus that causes listeriosis.

listeriosis (lɪstirˈiouˈsɪs), **listerosis** (lɪsˈtərouˈsɪs), an infectious disease caused by a genus of gram-positive motile bacteria that are nonsporulating. *Listeria monocytogenes* infects shellfish, birds, spiders, and mammals in all areas of the world, but infection in man is uncommon. Transmitted by direct contact from infected animals to man, by inhalation of dust, or by contact with mud, sewage, or soil contaminated with the organism, it is characterized by circulatory collapse, shock, endocarditis, hepatosplenomegaly, and a dark red rash over the trunk and the legs. Fever, bacteremia, malaise, and lethargy are commonly seen. Newborns and immunosuppressed, debilitated older patients are more vulnerable to infection than are immunocompetent children and young or middle-aged adults. The signs of infection and the severity of the disease vary according to the site of infection and the age and condition of the patient. Pregnant women characteristically experience a mild, brief episode of illness but fetal infection acquired through the placental circulation in utero is usually fatal. Infection in the newborn apparently results from exposure to the organism in the birth canal of an infected mother. Meningitis and encephalitis occur in 75 per cent of cases. Treatment may include ampicillin, penicillin, tetracycline, or erythromycin, given intramuscularly or intravenously. If infection is suspected in a pregnant woman, treatment is begun immediately, even before bacteriologic culture of the blood, spinal fluid, or vaginal secretions can confirm the diagnosis. All secretions from the patient may contain the organism.

Liston's forceps (lɪs′tənz), a kind of bone-cutting forceps.

lith. See **litho-.**

-lith, a combining form meaning 'a calculus': *pneumolith, ptyalith, tonsillolith.*

Lithane, a trade name for an antidepressant (lithium carbonate).

lithiasis (lɪfhaiˈəsɪs), the formation of calculi in the hollow organs or ducts of the body. Calculi are formed of mineral salts and may irritate, inflame, or obstruct the organ in which they form or lodge. Lithiasis occurs most commonly in the gall bladder, kidney, and lower urinary tract. Lithiasis may be asymptomatic, but more often the condition is extremely painful. Surgery may be necessary if the stones cannot be excreted spontaneously. Lower urinary tract calculi often can be dissolved. See also **biliary calculus, cholelithiasis, renal calculus, urinary calculus.**

lithium (Li), a silvery-white alkali metal occurring in various compounds, as petalite and spodumene. Its atomic number is 3; its atomic weight is 6.940. Lithium is the lightest known metal and one of the most reactive elements. Traces of lithium ion occur in animal tissue, and it abounds in many alkaline mineral-spring waters. Its salts are used in the treatment of manias, but the mechanisms by which these compounds help to stabilize psychological moods are not understood. Lithium carbonate is the salt approved for psychiatric use in the United States; it has been effective in the prevention of recurrent attacks of manic-depressive illnesses. It has helped to correct sleep disorders in manic patients, apparently by suppressing the rapid eye movement phases of sleep. Therapeutic concentrations of lithium have no observable psychotropic effects on normal individuals. In manic patients, lithium salts also produce high-voltage slow waves in the electroencephalograph, often with superimposed beta waves. An important feature of the lithium ion is its relatively small gradient of distribution across biological membranes. Although it can replace sodium in supporting a nerve cell action potential, it cannot adequately prime the sodium pump and maintain membrane potentials. Lithium ions are quickly and almost completely absorbed from the gastrointestinal tract, producing peak concentrations in plasma within 2 to 4 hours. The ion first spreads through the extracellular fluid and then gradually disperses in varying concentrations through different tissues. The ion passes slowly through the blood-brain barrier and, when a steady state is achieved, the concentration of lithium in the cerebrospinal fluid is about 40 per cent of the lithium concentration in the plasma. About 95 per cent of a single dose of lithium salts is eliminated in the urine. The lithium ion has such a low therapeutic index that safe treatment requires daily determination of plasma concentrations. Intoxication may result if levels rise beyond peak concentrations, which can be two to three times higher than steady-state concentrations. Acute intoxication by lithium may cause seizure and death. Side effects may include polyuria, polydipsia, and benign enlargement of the thyroid. Mixed and inconclusive results have followed lithium treatment of disorders other than manias, as premenstrual tension, alcoholism, episodic anger, and anorexia nervosa. Patients suffering severe manic attacks are hospitalized so that they can receive proper medical maintenance; treatments start with large doses of antipsychotic drugs, which are followed by the gradual and safe introduction of lithium therapy. Ideally, lithium treatment is prescribed only for patients with normal sodium intake and normal heart and kidney function.

lithium carbonate, an antimanic agent.
- INDICATION: It is prescribed in the treatment of manic episodes of manic-depressive disorder.
- CONTRAINDICATIONS: It is used with caution in the presence of renal or cardiovascular disease and is not recommended for children under twelve years of age. Known hypersensitivity to this drug prohibits its use.
- ADVERSE EFFECTS: Among the most serious adverse reactions are renal damage, polydipsia and polyuria, and impairment of mental and physical abilities. Retention of sodium and fluid may occur.

litho-, lith-, a combining form meaning 'of or pertaining to a stone, or to a calculus': *litholysis, lithomyl, lithophone.*

Lithonate, a trade name for an antidepressant (lithium carbonate).

Lithonate S, a trade name for an antimanic (lithium citrate).

lithopedion (lɪth'əpi'diən), **lithopedium** (lɪth'əpi'diəm), a fetus that has died in utero and has become calcified or ossified. Also called **calcified fetus, ostembryon, osteopedion.**

lithotomy (lɪfhot'əmi), the surgical excision of a calculus, especially one from the urinary tract.

lithotomy forceps, a forceps for the extraction of a calculus, usually from the urinary tract.

lithotomy position, the posture assumed by the patient lying supine with the hips and the knees flexed and the thighs abducted and rotated externally. Also called **dorsosacral position.**

lithotriptor (lɪfh'ətrɪp'tər). See **lithotrite.**

lithotrite (lɪfh'ətrait'), an instrument for crushing a stone in the urinary bladder. Also called **lithotriptor.** —**lithotrity,** *n.*

litigant (lɪt'əgənt), (in law) a party to a lawsuit. See also **defendant, plaintiff.**

litigate, (in law) to carry on a suit or to contest.

litigious paranoia, a form of paranoia in which the person seeks legal proof or justification for his systematized delusions.

litmus paper, absorbent paper coated with litmus, a blue dye, that is used to determine pH. Acid substances or solutions turn litmus from blue to red. Alkaline substances or solutions do not cause a change in color.

litter, a stretcher.

Little's disease. See **cerebral palsy.**

Litzmann's obliquity (lɪts'manz). See **asynclitism.**

live birth, the birth of an infant, irrespective of the duration of gestation, that exhibits any sign of life, as respiration, heartbeat, umbilical pulsation, or movement of voluntary muscles. A live birth is not always a viable birth.

livedo (lɪvi'dou), a blue or reddish mottling of the skin, worse in cold weather and probably owing to arteriolar spasm. One form, **livedo reticularis,** is characterized by a reddish-blue, netlike discoloration and may be associated with lupus erythematosus, dermatomyositis, rheumatoid arthritis, or various types of arteritis. **Cutis marmorata** is a transient form of livedo.

livedo reticularis. See **livedo.**

livedo vasculitis. See **segmented hyalinizing vasculitis.**

liver, the largest gland of the body and one of its most complex organs: more than 500 of its functions have been identified. It is divided into four lobes, contains as many as 100,000 lobules, and is served by two distinct blood supplies. The hepatic artery conveys oxygenated blood to the liver, and the hepatic portal vein conveys nutrient-filled blood from the stomach and the intestines. At any given moment the liver holds about one pint of blood or approximately 13 per cent of the total blood supply of the body. Some of the major functions performed by the liver are the production of bile by hepatic cells, the secretion of glucose, proteins, vitamins, fats, and most of the other compounds used by the body, the processing of hemoglobin for vital use of its iron content, and the conversion of poisonous ammonia to urea. Bile from the liver is stored in the gall bladder, which is connected to the liver by connective tissue, in the hepatic duct, and in numerous blood vessels. The liver is located in the cranial, right portion of the abdominal cavity, occupying almost the entire right hypochondrium, the greater part of the epigastrium, and, in many individuals, extends into the left hypochondrium as far as the mammary line. The liver develops in the embryo as a hollow projection from the ventral surface of the primitive gut, which eventually becomes the descending portion of the duodenum. The adult liver in men weighs about 1.5 kg; in women, about 1.3 kg. It has a soft, solid consistency, is shaped like an irregular hemisphere, and is dark reddish-brown in color. The right lobe of the liver is much larger than the left lobe or the caudate and the quadrate lobes. The ventral portion of the liver is separated by the diaphragm from the sixth to the tenth ribs on the right side and from the seventh and the eighth costal cartilages on the left side. It is completely covered by peritoneum except along the line of attachment of the falciform ligament. The dorsal part of the organ is wide and rounded on the right but narrow on the left, and the central section has a deep concavity which fits the vertebral column and the crura of the diaphragm. The liver attaches to the diaphragm by the coronary and the triangular ligaments. During the descent of the diaphragm in deep breathing, the liver rolls forward, shifting the inferior border downward where it can be felt through the abdominal wall. The tiny lobules of the organ are composed of polyhedral hepatic cells. These communicate with small ducts that connect with larger ducts to form the left and the right hepatic ducts which emerge on the caudal surface of the liver. The left and the right hepatic ducts converge to form the single hepatic duct, which conveys the bile to the duodenum and to the gall bladder for storage. The liver cells produce about one pint of bile daily. They also detoxify numerous ingested substances, as alcohol, nicotine, and other poisons, as well as various toxic substances produced by the intestine. See also **gall bladder.**

liver biopsy, a diagnostic procedure in which a special needle is introduced into the liver under local anesthesia to obtain a specimen for pathologic examination.

■ METHOD: Before a liver biopsy is performed by the physician, the procedure is explained to the patient, whose baseline vital signs are recorded and who is taught how to inhale and hold the breath during insertion of the needle. After the patient's possible allergy to the local anesthetic is checked and results of bleeding, clotting, and prothrombin tests are obtained, an analgesic or sedative is administered as ordered. On completion of the biopsy, pressure is applied to the site for 15 minutes; the patient is positioned on the right side for the first two hours and remains in a supine position in bed for the next 22 hours. The blood pressure, pulse, and respirations are checked every 15 minutes for the first hour, then every 30 minutes for the next two hours, and subsequently every four hours or as ordered. The biopsy site is observed every 30 minutes for bleeding, swelling, or increased pain; epigastric or referred shoulder pain may occur. Analgesia and Vitamin K may be given as ordered and the recumbent patient is assisted with eating and other activities as needed.

■ NURSING ORDERS: The nurse reinforces explanations of the biopsy and its purpose, provides care before and after the procedure, and closely observes the patient for postbiopsy complications, as intraperitoneal hemorrhage, shock, and pneumothorax.

■ OUTCOME CRITERIA: An uneventful liver biopsy is a valuable aid in establishing a diagnosis of hepatic disease, including primary and metastatic malignant neoplastic disease.

liver breath. See **fetor hepaticus.**

liver cancer, a malignant neoplastic disease of the liver, occurring most frequently as a metastasis from another malignancy. Primary liver cancer is common in Africa and Southeast Asia but relatively uncommon in the United States. Primary tumors are six to ten times more prevalent in men than in women, develop most often in the sixth decade of life, and are associated with cirrhosis of the liver in 70 per cent of the cases. Other risk factors include hemochromatosis, schistosomiasis, exposure to vinyl chloride or arsenic, and possibly nutritional deficiencies. Alcoholism may be a predisposing factor, but nonalcoholic cirrhosis is a greater risk than alcoholic cirrhosis. Aflatoxins in moldy grain and peanuts appear to be linked to high rates of hepatocellular carcinoma in parts of Africa. Characteristics of liver cancer are abdominal bloating, anorexia, weakness, dull upper abdominal pain, ascites, mild jaundice, and a tender enlarged liver; in some cases tumor nodules are palpable on the liver surface. Diagnostic procedures include radioisotope scan, needle biopsy, and various laboratory studies of liver function. An elevated level of alkaline phosphatase, increased retention of sulfobromophthalein, and the presence of alpha-fetoprotein in the blood suggest liver cancer. All primary liver tumors are adenocarcinomas, classified as hepatomas when derived from hepatic cells and cholangiomas if they originate in cells of the bile duct. They form large single nodules or satellite nodules surrounding a central lesion and are found more often in the right lobe than in the left. Primary lesions spread centrifugally in the liver, invade the portal vein and lymphatic vessels, and metastasize to lymph nodes, the lungs, brain, and other sites. Total hepatic lobectomy is the treatment of choice for primary tumors; because the liver is able to regenerate, 80 per cent of it may be resected. Systemic chemotherapy or methotrexate and 5-fluorouracil infused through a catheter in the hepatic artery may result in temporary tumor regression. Irradiation is very destructive to liver cells and not very toxic to tumor cells in the liver.

liver cell carcinoma. See **malignant hepatoma.**

liver disease, any one of a group of disorders of the liver. The most important diseases in this group are cirrhosis, cholestasis, and viral and toxic hepatitis. Characteristics of liver disease are jaundice, anorexia, hepatomegaly, ascites, and impaired consciousness. The exact diagnosis of liver disease is made through a combination of laboratory tests and clinical findings. See also **cholestasis, cirrhosis, hepatitis.**

liver flap. See **asterixis.**

liver function test, a test used to evaluate various functions of the liver—for example, metabolism, storage, filtration, and excretion. Kinds of liver function tests include **alkaline phospatase, bromsulfalein test, prothrombin time, serum bilirubin, serum glutamic pyruvic transaminase.**

liver scan, a noninvasive technique of visualizing the size, shape, and consistency of the liver by the intravenous injection of a radioactively labeled compound that is readily taken up and trapped in the Kupffer cells of the liver. The radiation emitted by the compound is recorded by a radiation detector and can be photographed with a scintillation camera or filmed with x ray. Liver scans are most useful for diagnosing three-dimensional lesions as abscesses or tumors.

liver spot, *Nontechnical.* a senile lentigo or actinic keratosis.

lizard, a scaly-skinned reptile with a long body and tail and two pairs of legs. The large Gila monster of Arizona, New Mexico, and Utah, and the beaded lizard of Mexico are the only lizards known to be venomous. The symptoms of their bites and the recommended treatment are similar to those of the bites from moderately poisonous snakes.

LLD factor. See **cyanocobalamin.**

LMD. See **dextran preparation.**

L.M.D., abbreviation for **local medical doctor,** used by house staff or others to distinguish a patient's primary physician from university faculty, attending specialist, physicians, or house staff. Also called **P.M.D.**

LMP, abbreviation for *last menstrual period.*

loading response stance stage, one of the five stages of the stance phase of walking or gait, specifically associated with the moment when the leg reacts to and accepts the weight of the body. The loading response stance stage is one of the factors in the diagnoses of many abnormal orthopedic conditions and is often studied in conjunction with analyses of the electromyographic activity of the muscles used in walking. Compare **initial contact stance stage, midstance, preswing stance stage, terminal stance.**

loads, *Slang.* a fixed combination of a sedative hypnotic, glutethimide, and a major narcotic analgesic, codeine. The medications are taken orally by drug abusers for a euphoric effect reported to be similar to that produced by heroin, but longer lasting. Addiction is increasingly common. Toxicity may develop, characterized by nystagmus, slurred speech, seizures, coma, pulmonary edema, or sudden apnea and death. Detoxification of an addicted person is managed under close medical supervision with methadone and phenobarbital, as sudden withdrawal can cause death.

Loa loa, a parasitic worm of Western and Central Africa that causes loiasis.

lobar bronchus, a bronchus extending from a primary bronchus to a segmental bronchus into one of the lobes of the right or left lung.

lobar pneumonia, a severe infection of one or more of the five major lobes of the lungs which, if untreated, eventually results in consolidation of lung tissue. The disease is characterized by fever, chills, cough, rusty sputum, rapid shallow breathing, cyanosis, nausea, vomiting, and pleurisy. *Streptococcus pneumoniae* is the usual cause but *Klebsiella pneumoniae, Haemophilus influenzae,* and other streptococci can produce the disease. If the diagnosis is made early, appropriate antibiotic therapy is highly successful. Complications include lung abscess, atelectasis, empyema, pericarditis, and pleural effusion. Precautions against spread of the contagious disease are important. Because the fatality rate in the elderly and those with underlying systemic illness is high, prophylactic polyvalent pneumococcal vaccine is recommended for them. Compare **bronchopneumonia.**

lobe, 1. a roundish projection of any structure. 2. a portion of any organ, demarcated by sulci, fissures, or connective tissue, as the lobes of the brain, liver and lungs. −**lobar, lobular,** *adj.*

-lobe, a combining form meaning a 'rounded prominence': *gonilobe, multilobe, sublobe.*

lobectomy, a type of chest surgery in which a lobe of a lung is excised, performed to remove a malignant tumor and to treat uncontrolled bronchiectasis, trauma with hemorrhage, or intractable tuberculosis. Any respiratory infection is cleared before surgery; smoking is forbidden; administration of antibiotics is begun. General anesthesia is administered via an endotracheal tube. The chest cavity is entered through a long back-to-front incision, and the diseased lobe is removed. A large caliber tube remains in the wound and is connected to a water-sealed drainage system. Oxygen is given during the first 24 hours after surgery. The vital signs are closely monitored, coughing and deep breathing are encouraged hourly, blood transfusion may be given, and I.V. fluids are continued. Care is taken that the chest tube remain open and that the drainage system be sealed and functional. The chest tube is removed two to three days after surgery. Some compensatory emphysema is expected as the remaining lung tissue overexpands to fill the new space. −**lobectomize,** *v.*

lobotomy, a neurosurgical procedure in which the nerve fibers in the bundle of white matter in the frontal lobe of the brain are severed to interrupt the transmission of various affective responses. Severe intractable depression and pain are among the indications for the operation. It is rarely performed because it has many unpredictable and undesirable effects, including personality change, aggression, socially unacceptable behavior, incontinence, apathy, and lack of consideration for others. As lobotomy is simple to perform it was overused in the treatment of mental patients in the past. A cannula is passed through the bony orbit of the eye and a wire loop is inserted through the cannula to the cingulum. The nerve fibers are severed with the wire loop. Also called **leukotomy.**

lobster-claw deformity. See **bidactyly.**

lobular carcinoma, a neoplasm that often forms a diffuse mass and accounts for a small percentage of breast tumors.

lobule (lob'yul), a small lobe, as the soft, lower, pendulous part of the external ear. −**lobular,** *adj.*

loc-, a combining form meaning 'place': *locomotor, locum, locus.*

local, 1. of or pertaining to a small circumscribed area of the body. 2. of or pertaining to a treatment or drug applied locally. 3. *Informal.* a local anesthetic.

local anesthesia, the direct administration of a local anesthetic agent to tissues to induce the absence of sensation in a small area of the body. Brief surgical or dental procedures are the most common indications for local anesthesia. The anesthetic may be applied topically to the surface of the skin or membrane or injected subcutaneously through an intradermal weal. The principal drawbacks to the use of local anesthesia are the incidence of allergic reactions to certain agents, especially the "-caine" drugs, and the occasional difficulty encountered in achieving adequate anesthesia. The advantages include low cost, ease of administration, low toxicity, and safety—a conscious patient can cooperate and does not require respiratory support or intubation. To avoid general anesthesia, major surgical procedures are occasionally performed under local anesthesia. The tissues are anesthetized layer by layer, as the surgeon approaches the deeper structures of the body. Regional anesthesia has largely replaced this procedure. In all cases, the recommended dosage of any agent is the smallest possible to achieve the desired effect, as toxicity is directly related to the total amount of drug given rather than to the initial amount or the concentration of the agent used. Each anesthetic agent also carries a recommended maximum allowable dose that is not safely exceeded. Compare **general anesthesia, regional anesthesia, topical anesthesia.**

local anesthetic, a substance used to reduce or eliminate neural sensation, specifically pain, in a limited area of the body. Local anesthetics act by blocking transmission of nerve impulses. More than one hundred drugs are available for local anesthesia; they are classified as members of the alcohol-ester or the amineamide family. Differences among various trade products often may be no more than a slight chemical variation, but even these variations may cause a difference of action and effect. Principal representatives of the alcohol-ester group are phenols and benzyl, ethyl, and salicylic alcohol; these have generally been replaced by the less toxic esters (chloroprocaine, cocaine, procaine, tetracaine) and the amides (dibucaine, bupivacaine, lidocaine, mepivacaine, prilocaine, etidocaine). Specific preparations are available for use for topical administration, for infiltration, and for various kinds of regional administration, including field block, regional nerve block, epidural nerve block, and spinal nerve block. Any substance sufficiently potent to induce local anesthesia has potential for causing adverse side effects, ranging from easily reversible dermatitis to lethal anaphylaxis or simultaneous respiratory and cardiac arrest. Among the factors that are involved in an adverse reaction to a local anesthetic are hypersensitivity to the drug, the vascularity of the injection site, the speed with which the drug is given, the rapidity of action of the drug, and the presence of epinephrine in the solution. Serious adverse results have occurred when the operator has failed to notice that the local anesthetic contains epinephrine in solution. A person might be able to tolerate the local agent without adverse reaction but might be dangerously hypersensitive to the epinephrine. Some people who are sensitive to local anesthetics of the amide group, which are broken down in the liver, can tolerate local anesthetics of the ester group, which are broken down in the plasma. Vasopressors should also be at hand in case of hypotension or other forms of circulatory depression. A patient who has a severe adverse reaction to a particular local anesthetic is advised to avoid this class of drug in the future.

localization audiometry. See **audiometry.**

localization film, (in radiotherapy) a diagnostic film taken to confirm a treatment portal or to view the position of an intracavitary or interstitial implant, especially for the purpose of computing the dose delivered.

localized scleroderma. See **Addison's keloid.**

localizing symptom. See **symptom.**

local symptom. See **symptom.**

lochia (lou′kiə), the discharge that flows from the vagina following childbirth. During the first three or four days postpartum, the lochia is red (**lochia rubra**) and is made up of blood, endometrial decidua, and fetal lanugo, vernix, and sometimes meconium, small shreds of placental tissue and membranes. After the third day the amount of blood diminishes, the placental site exudes serous material and lymph, and the lochia becomes darker and thinner (**lochia fusca**), and then serous (**lochia serosa**) as evacuation of particulate material is completed. During the second week white blood cells and bacteria appear in large numbers along with fatty, mucinous decidual material, causing the lochia to appear yellow (**lochia flava** or **purulenta**). During the third week and thereafter, as endometrial epithelialization progresses, the amount of lochia decreases markedly and takes on a seromucinous consistency and a gray-white color (**lochia alba**). Cessation of the flow of lochia at about six weeks is usual. —**lochial,** *adj.*

locked twins. See **interlocked twins.**

lockjaw, *Informal.* tetanus.

locomotor ataxia. See **tabes dorsalis.**

Locorten, a trade name for a glucocorticoid (flumethasone pivalate).

loculate (lok′yuleit), divided into small spaces or cavities.

loculus (lok′yuləs), a small chamber, pocket, or cavity, as the interior of a polyp.

locum tenens (lou′kəm ten′inz), a temporary substitute for a physician who is away from his practice.

locus, a specific place or position, as the locus of a particular gene on a chromosome.

locus of infection, a site in the body where an infection originates.

Löffler's syndrome (lef'lərz), a benign, idiopathic disorder marked by episodes of pulmonary eosinophilia, transient opacities in the lungs, anorexia, breathlessness, fever, and weight loss. Recovery is spontaneous and prompt.

Loestrin, a trade name for an oral contraceptive containing an estrogen (ethinyl estradiol) and a progestin (norethindrone acetate).

Lofenalac, a trade name for a commercial milk-substitute formula that is low in phenylalamine and used for infants with phenylketonuria. It is made from hydrolyzed casein, and is supplemented with tyrosine and fortified with added fat, carbohydrate, minerals, and vitamins to balance the formula. A common problem with the formula is diarrhea, which may appear after the first few feedings but generally disappears in a few days.

log-, logo-, a combining form meaning 'word, speech, thought': *logagnosia, logopathy, logorrhea.*

loga-, a combining form meaning 'of or pertaining to the whites of the eyes': *logadectomy, logaditis, logadoblennorrhea.*

-logia. See **-logy.**

logo-, a combining form meaning 'of or pertaining to words or speech': *logomania, logoneurosis, logopathy.*

log-roll, a maneuver used to turn a reclining patient from one side to the other or completely over without flexing the spinal column. The arms of the patient are folded across the chest and the legs extended. A draw sheet under the patient is manipulated by attending nursing personnel to facilitate the procedure.

-logy, a combining form meaning 'a science': *mammalogy, metabology, nealogy.* Also **-logia.**

loiasis (louæi'əsɪs), a form of filariasis caused by the worm *Loa loa,* which may migrate for 10 to 15 years in subcutaneous tissue, producing localized inflammation known as Calabar swellings. Occasionally, the migrating worms may be visible beneath the conjunctiva. The disease is acquired through the bite of an infected African deer fly. Treatment with diethylcarbamazine usually results in cure and may also be successful as prophylaxis. See also **filariasis, onchocerciasis.**

loin, a part of the body on each side of the spinal column between the false ribs and the hip bones.

Lomotil, a trade name for an antidiarrheal fixed-combination drug containing an antiperistaltic (diphenoxylate hydrochloride) and an anticholinergic (atropine sulfate).

lomustine, an antineoplastic alkylating agent.

■ INDICATION: It is prescribed in the treatment of a variety of malignant neoplastic diseases.

■ CONTRAINDICATIONS: Known hypersensitivity to this drug prohibits its use.

■ ADVERSE EFFECTS: Among the more serious adverse reactions are bone marrow depression, nausea, and vomiting.

Lonalac, a trade name for a low-sodium, nutritional supplement.

long-acting drug, a pharmacologic agent with a prolonged effect owing to a formulation resulting in the slow release of the active principle or the continued absorption of small amounts of the dosage of the drug over an extended period.

long-acting insulin, a preparation of the antidiabetic principle of beef pancreas or pork pancreas modified by an interaction with zinc under specific chemical conditions and supplied as a suspension with a prolonged action. An injection of the preparation takes effect within eight hours, reaches a peak of action in 16 to 24 hours, and has a duration of action of more than 36 hours. Also called **slow-acting insulin, ultralente insulin.** See also **insulin.** Compare **intermediate-acting insulin, short-acting insulin.**

long-acting thyroid stimulator (LATS), an immunoglobulin, probably an autoantibody, that exerts a prolonged stimulatory effect on the thyroid gland, causing rapid growth of the gland and excess activity of thyroid function resulting in hyperthyroidism. It is found circulating in the blood of 50 per cent of people affected with Graves' disease.

long arm cast, an orthopedic cast applied to immobilize upper extremities from the hand to the upper arm. It is used in the treatment of fractures of the forearm and the elbow, fractures of the humerus, for postoperative positioning of the distal arm, the elbow, or the upper arm, and for correction or for maintenance of correction of deformities of the distal arm, the wrist, or the elbow. Compare **short arm cast.**

long leg cast, an orthopedic cast applied to immobilize the leg from the toes to the upper thigh. It is used in treating fractures and dislocations of the knee, for postoperative positioning and immobilization of the knee, distal leg, and ankle, and for correction or for maintenance of correction of the foot, distal leg, and knee. Compare **short leg cast.**

long leg cast with walker, an orthopedic cast applied to immobilize the lower extremities from the toes to the upper thigh in treating certain fractures of the leg. This type of cast is the same as the long leg cast but incorporates a rubber walker, allowing the patient to walk while the leg is encased in the cast and when weight-bearing ambulation is allowed.

long-term memory, the ability to recall sensations, events, ideas, and other information for long periods of time without apparent effort.

long thoracic nerve, one of a pair of supraclavicular branches from the roots of the brachial plexus. It arises by three roots, from the fifth, the sixth, and the seventh cervical nerves. Its fibers from the fifth and the sixth cervical nerves join just after they pierce the scalenus medius and are united with its fibers from the seventh cervical nerve at the level of the first rib. Compare **phrenic nerve.**

Loniten, a trade name for an antihypertensive (minoxidil).

loop. Informal. See **intrauterine device.**

loop diuretic. See **diuretic.**

loop of Henle (hen′li), the U-shaped portion of a renal tubule, consisting of a thin descending limb and a thick ascending limb.

loose fibrous tissue, a constrictive, pliable fibrous connective tissue consisting of interwoven elastic and collagenous fibers, interspersed with fluid-filled areolae. It is found in adipose tissue, areolar tissue, reticular tissue, and fibroelastic tissue. Compare **dense fibrous tissue.**

Lo/Ovral, a trade name for an oral contraceptive containing an estrogen (ethinyl estradiol) and a progestin (norgestrel).

loperamide hydrochloride, an antiperistaltic.
■ INDICATION: It is prescribed in the treatment of diarrhea.
■ CONTRAINDICATIONS: Known hypersensitivity to this drug prohibits its use. It is not given to patients in whom constipation must be avoided.
■ ADVERSE EFFECTS: Among the most serious reactions are abdominal pain, constipation, nausea, and vomiting.

loph-, a combining form meaning 'of or pertaining to a ridge': *lophius, lophodont, lophotrichous.*

Lopressor, a trade name for a beta-adrenergic receptor blocking agent (metoprolol tartrate).

lorazepam (lɔreɪ′zəpæm), a benzodiazepine tranquilizer.
■ INDICATIONS: It is prescribed as a minor tranquilizer in the treatment of anxiety, nervous tension, and insomnia.
■ CONTRAINDICATIONS: Acute glaucoma, psychosis, or known hypersensitivity to this drug or to any benzodiazepine prohibits its use.
■ ADVERSE EFFECTS: Among the more serious adverse reactions are drowsiness and fatigue. Withdrawal symptoms may occur on discontinuation of the drug, especially following prolonged use or high dosage.

lordosis (lɔrdoʊ′sɪs), **1.** the normal curvature of the lumbar and cervical spine, seen as an anterior concavity if the person is observed from the side. **2.** an abnormal, increased degree of curvature of any part of the back.

(See next column for illustration)

Lorfan, a trade name for a narcotic antagonist (levallorphan tartrate).

LORDOSIS

Loridine, a trade name for an antibacterial (cephaloridine).

LOS, abbreviation for **length of stay.**

loss of consortium, (in law) a claim for damages sought in recompense for the loss of conjugal relations, including society, affection, and assistance, and impairment or loss of sexual relations. Loss of consortium may be charged against a person whose negligence or malfeasance caused injury to the spouse or against a person who caused a marriage to break up.

lotion, a liquid preparation applied externally to protect the skin or to treat a dermatologic disorder.

Lotrimin, a trade name for an antifungal (clotrimazole).

Lotusate, a trade name for a barbiturate (talbutal).

Lou Gehrig's disease. See **amyotrophic lateral sclerosis.**

loupe (lup), a magnifying lens mounted in a frame worn on the head, as used to examine the eyes.

louse, *pl.* **lice.** a small, wingless, parasitic insect that is the carrier of such diseases as relapsing fever and typhus. Lice are common parasites on the skin and may cause intense pruritus. See also **pediculosis.**

HUMAN BODY LOUSE

louse bite, a minute puncture wound produced by a louse, that may transmit typhus, trench fever, and relapsing fever. Secondary infection may result from scratching the affected area. Head and body lice are the most common and are frequently found among school children. Washing and bathing, application of an approved insecticide, and the washing or cleaning of clothes and bed linens are recommended procedures for treatment and prophylaxis against spread of the infestation. See also **pediculosis.**

louse-borne typhus. See **epidemic typhus.**

low back pain, local, or referred pain at the base of the spine caused by a sprain, strain, osteoarthritis, ankylosing spondylitis, a neoplasm, or a prolapsed intervertebral disc. Low back pain is a common complaint and is often associated with poor posture, obesity, sagging abdominal muscles, or sitting for prolonged periods of time.

■ OBSERVATIONS: Pain may be localized and static; it may be accompanied by muscle weakness or spasms; or it may radiate down the back of one or both legs, as in sciatica. It may be initiated or increased by coughing, sneezing, rising from a seated position, lifting, stretching, bending, or turning. To guard against the pain, the person may decrease the range of motion of the spine. If an intervertebral disc is prolapsed, deep pressure over the interspace generally causes pain, and flexion of the hip elicits sciatic pain when the knee is extended but not when the knee is flexed (Lasègue's sign).

■ INTERVENTION: The patient is placed in a semi-Fowler's position on a firm mattress with the knees flexed and supported. Analgesics, muscle relaxants, and tranquilizers may be administered, and dry or moist heat is applied. Diagnostic x rays; pelvic traction; and physiotherapy, consisting of hydrotherapy, diathermy, or the application of hot paraffin; and a myelogram may be performed if a herniated disc is suspected. When the acute pain subsides, the patient may increase activity as tolerated, fatigue is avoided, and a corset or back brace may be ordered. The patient is instructed to use a straight-backed chair, not to sit with legs crossed or extended on a footstool, and to sleep on the side or back with knees flexed and a small pillow under the head. Before discharge the patient is advised to maintain a normal weight, to follow the ordered exercise program, to wear flat-heeled shoes, and to avoid constipation by using natural laxatives, if required.

■ NURSING CONSIDERATIONS: The nurse encourages the person to follow the recommended regimen. Correct body mechanics, adequate and appropriate exercise, and the elimination of excess weight are emphasized.

low-birth-weight (LBW) infant, an infant whose weight at birth is less than 2,500 gm, regardless of gestational age. These babies are at risk for the development of hypoxia during labor, hypoglycemia after birth, and growth retardation in childhood, especially if the condition is the result of prolonged placental insufficiency, maternal malnutrition, or drug addiction. Many low-birth-weight infants have no problems and develop normally,

their smallness being genetic or idiopathic or the problem that caused their slowed growth being mild or brief.

low blood, *Informal.* anemia.

low-calcium diet, a diet that restricts the use of calcium and that eliminates most of the dairy foods, all breads made with milk or dry skimmed milk, and deep-green leafy vegetables. It is prescribed for people who form renal calculi. Meats, including beef, lamb, pork, veal, and poultry, fish, vegetables, legumes, and fruits are recommended.

low-caloric diet, a diet that is prescribed to limit the intake of calories, usually to cause a reduction in body weight. Such diets may be designated as 800 calorie, 1,000 calorie, or other specific numbers of calories. Exchange lists may be used to allow the patient to select preferred foods from groups of foods categorized as carbohydrate, protein, and fat.

low cervical Caesarean section, a method for surgically delivering a baby through a transverse incision in the thin supracervical portion of the lower uterine segment, behind the bladder and the bladder flap. This incision bleeds less during surgery and heals with a stronger scar than the higher vertical scar of the classical Caesarean section. Compare **extraperitoneal Caesarean section.** See also **Caesarean section.**

low-cholesterol diet, a diet that restricts foods containing animal fats and saturated fatty acids, as egg yolk, cream, butter, milk, muscle and organ meats, and shellfish and concentrates on poultry, fish, vegetables, fruits, cottage cheese, and polyunsaturated fats. The diet is indicated for persons with high serum cholesterol levels, cardiovascular disorders, obesity, hyperlipidemia, hypercholesterolemia, or hyperlipoproteinemia. Also called **low-saturated-fat diet.**

low-density lipoprotein, a plasma protein containing relatively more cholesterol and triglycerides than protein. It is derived in part, if not completely, from the intravascular breakdown of the very low-density lipoproteins. The high cholesterol content may account for its greater atherogenic potential as compared to the very low-density lipoproteins and chylomicrons.

lower extremity suspension, an orthopedic procedure used in the treatment of bone fractures and in the correction of orthopedic abnormalities of the lower limbs. The procedure uses traction equipment, including metal frames, ropes, and pulleys, to relieve the weight of the lower limb involved rather than to exert traction pull. Lower extremity suspension may be either unilateral or bilateral and is used in the postoperative, posttraumatic, or postreduction control of edema. Compare **balanced suspension, hyperextension suspension, upper extremity suspension.**

lower motor neuron paralysis, an injury to or lesion in the spinal cord that damages the cell bodies or axons, or both, of the lower motor neurons, which are located in the anterior horn cells and the spinal and peripheral nerves. If complete transection of the spinal cord occurs, voluntary muscle control is totally lost. In partial transection, function is altered in varying degrees, depending on the areas innervated by the nerves involved. In lower motor neuron paralysis the reflex arcs are permanently damaged, causing decreased muscle tone and flaccidity, diminished or absent reflexes, absence of pathological reflexes, local twitching of muscle groups, and progressive atrophy of the atonic muscles. Compare **upper motor neuron paralysis.**

lower respiratory infection.   See **respiratory tract infection.**

lower respiratory tract,   one of the two divisions of the respiratory system. The lower respiratory tract includes the left and the right bronchi and the lungs where the exchange of oxygen and carbon dioxide occurs during the respiratory cycle. The bronchi divide into smaller bronchioles in the lungs, the bronchioles divide into alveolar ducts, the ducts into alveolar sacs, and the sacs into alveoli. The alveolar sacs and the alveoli present a total lung surface of about 850 square feet for the exchange of oxygen and carbon dioxide, which occurs between the most internal alveolar surface and the tiny capillaries surrounding the external alveolar wall. The lower respiratory tract is a continuation of the upper respiratory tract and is a common site of infections, obstructive conditions, and neoplastic disease. Compare **upper respiratory tract.** See also **lung.**

low-fat diet,   a diet containing limited amounts of fat and consisting chiefly of easily digestible foods of high carbohydrate content. It includes all vegetables, lean meats, fish, fowl, pasta, cereals, whole wheat or enriched bread. Egg yolk and fatty meats are restricted. Cream, fried foods, foods prepared in oil, gravy, cheese, peanut butter, and olives are among the foods omitted. The diet may be indicated in gall bladder disease and malabsorption syndromes.

low fat milk,   milk containing one to two per cent fat, making it an intermediate in fat content between whole and skimmed milk.

low forceps,   an obstetric operation in which forceps are used to deliver a baby whose head is on the pelvic floor. The procedure is performed most often as an elective procedure to shorten normal labor and to control delivery, usually in conjunction with anesthesia and episiotomy. It is commonly required for the delivery of mothers whose expulsive powers have been weakened by analgesia, anesthesia, or fatigue. Also called **outlet forceps, prophylactic forceps.** Compare **high forceps, mid forceps, natural childbirth, spontaneous delivery.** See also **forceps delivery, obstetric forceps.**

low-grade fever,   a temperature that is above 98.6°F but lower than 100.4°F for 24 hours.

Lown-Ganong-Levine syndrome (loun'gənoŋ'ləvin'), a disorder of the atrioventricular (AV) conduction system, marked by ventricular pre-excitation. Part or all of the AV nodal connection is bypassed by an abnormal AV connection from the atrial muscle to the bundle of His. The condition may be discovered by routine ECG or may be seen in association with paroxysmal atrial arrhythmias, supraventricular tachycardia, atrial flutter, and fibrillation. Treatments include the use of antiarrhythmic drugs, as quinidine sulfate, procainamide, and propranolol, surgical interruption of the abnormal AV pathway, and implantation of a pacemaker. Compare **Wolff-Parkinson-White syndrome.**

low-residue diet,   a diet that will leave a minimal residue in the lower intestinal tract after digestion and absorption. It consists of tender meats, poultry, fish, eggs, white bread, pasta, simple desserts, clear soups, tea, and coffee. Omitted are highly seasoned or fried foods, all fruits and fruit juices, raw vegetables, whole grain cereals and bread, nuts, jams, and, usually, milk. The diet is prescribed in cases of diverticulosis and diverticulitis, gastrointestinal irritability or inflammation, and before and after gastrointestinal surgery. Since it is lacking in calcium, iron, and vitamins, it should be used only for a limited period of time.

low-salt diet.   See **low-sodium diet.**

low-saturated-fat diet.   See **low-cholesterol diet.**

low-sodium diet,   a diet that restricts the use of sodium chloride plus other compounds containing sodium, as baking powder or soda, monosodium glutamate, sodium citrate, sodium propionate, and sodium sulfate. It is indicated in hypertension, edematous states (especially when associated with cardiovascular disease), renal or liver disease, and therapy with corticosteroids. The degree of sodium restriction depends on the severity of the condition. Foods included in the diet are eggs, skimmed milk, beef, poultry, lamb, pork, veal, fish, potatoes, green beans, broccoli, asparagus, peas, salad ingredients, and fresh fruits. Many flavoring extracts, spices, and herbs can be used to add taste to the diet. Foods to be avoided include fresh or canned shellfish, ham, bacon, frankfurters, luncheon meats, sausage, cheese, salted butter or margarine, any breads or cereals made with salt, beets, carrots, celery, sauerkraut, spinach, and most canned or frozen foods —unless prepared without sodium. Also to be avoided are many drugs, as laxatives, sedatives, and alkalizers, which contain sodium, and drinking water from a source using a water softener, since this appliance adds sodium to the water. Also called **low-salt diet, salt-free diet, sodium-restricted diet.**

loxapine,   a tranquilizer.

■ INDICATION: It is prescribed in the treatment of schizophrenia.

■ CONTRAINDICATIONS: Parkinson's disease, concurrent administration of central nervous system depressants, liver or kidney dysfunction, severe hypotension, or known hypersensitivity to this drug prohibits its use.

■ ADVERSE EFFECTS: Among the more serious adverse effects are hypotension, liver toxicity, a variety of extrapyramidal reactions, and hypersensitivity reactions.

Loxitane, a trade name for a tranquilizer (loxapine hydrochloride).

loxo-, a combining form meaning 'oblique': *loxophthalmus, loxotic, loxotomy.*

lozenge. See **troche.**

LP, abbreviation for **lumbar puncture.**

LPN, abbreviation for **licensed practical nurse.**

LSD, abbreviation for **lysergic acid diethylamide.** See **lysergide.**

LTB, abbreviation for **laryngotracheobronchitis.** See **croup.**

Lu, symbol for **lutetium.**

luc-, a combining form meaning 'of or pertaining to light': *lucifugal, lucipetal, lucotherapy.*

-lucent, a combining form meaning 'light-admitting': *radiolucent, roentgenolucent, translucent.*

lucid (lu′sɪd), clear, rational, and able to be understood. See also **lucid interval.**

lucid interval, a period of relative mental clarity between periods of irrationality, especially in organic mental disorders, as delirium and dementia.

lucid lethargy, a mental state characterized by a loss of will; hence, an inability to act, even though the person is conscious and intellectual function is normal. See also **lethargy.**

Ludiomil, a trade name for an antidepressant (maprotiline hydrochloride).

Ludwig's angina (lud′vɪgz), acute streptococcal cellulitis of the floor of the mouth. It is treated with penicillin.

lue-, a combining form meaning 'of or pertaining to syphilis': *luetic, luetin, luetism.*

Luer's Lok syringe (lu′ərz), a glass syringe for injection having a simple metal lock mechanism that securely holds the needle in place. Also called **Luer's syringe.**

lues (lu′iz). See **syphilis.**

-luetic, a combining form meaning 'pertaining to syphilis': *antiluetic, heredoluetic, paraluetic.* Also **-luic.**

luetic aortitis (luet′ɪk). See **syphilitic aortitis.**

Lufyllin, a trade name for a smooth-muscle relaxant (dyphylline).

Lugol's solution, an aqueous solution of iodine (5%) and potassium iodide (10%).

-luic. See **-luetic.**

lukewarm bath, a bath in which the temperature of the water is between 90° and 96°F.

lumbago (lembei′gou), pain in the lumbar region caused by a muscle strain, rheumatoid arthritis, osteoarthritis, or a herniated intravertebral disc. Ischemic lumbago, characterized by pain in the lower back and buttocks, is caused by vascular insufficiency, as in terminal aortic occlusion. See also **low back pain.**

lumbar (ləm′bər, ləm′bar), of or pertaining to the part of the body between the thorax and the pelvis.

lumbar nerves, the five pairs of spinal nerves rising in the lumbar region. They become increasingly large the more caudal their location and pass laterally and downward under the cover of the psoas major or between its fasciculi. The first three lumbar nerves and the larger part of the fourth are connected by communicating loops and, in many individuals, communicate with the twelfth thoracic nerve, forming the lumbar plexus. The ventral primary divisions of the lumbar nerves give rise to muscular branches which supply the psoas major and the quadratus lumborum before the nerves enter the lumbar plexus. The smaller section of the fourth lumbar nerve joins the fifth lumbar nerve to form the lumbosacral trunk which comprises part of the sacral plexus. Only the first two lumbar nerves extend white rami to the sympathetic trunk. All lumbar nerves receive gray rami. The lumbar ganglia follow no fixed pattern and massive fusions of ganglia are common. When occurring independently, the lumbar ganglia lie on the bodies corresponding vertebrae or intervertebral discs caudally. The ganglion on the second lumbar vertebra is the largest, the most constant, and the most easily palpated.

lumbar node, a node in one of the seven groups of parietal lymph nodes serving the abdomen and the pelvis. The lumbar nodes are very numerous and are divided into the lateral aortic nodes, the preaortic nodes, and the retroaortic nodes. They receive the afferents from many different structures, as the kidneys, the internal reproductive organs, the lateral abdominal muscles, and certain vertebrae, and pass efferents that form lymphatic trunks. Compare **sacral node.** See also **lymph, lymphatic system, lymph node.**

lumbar plexus, a network of nerves formed by the ventral primary divisions of the first three and the greater part of the fourth lumbar nerves. It is located on the inside of the posterior abdominal wall, either dorsal to the psoas major or among its fibers and ventral to the transverse processes of the lumbar vertebrae. The plexus develops from the splitting of various lumbar nerves. The first lumbar nerve splits into the cranial and the caudal branches. The cranial branch forms the iliohypogastric and the ilioinguinal nerves. The caudal branch unites with a branch from the second lumbar nerve to form the genitofemoral nerve. The rest of the second nerve and the third and the fourth nerves each split into a small ventral and a large dorsal section. The ventral portions unite to form the obturator nerve. The dorsal portions of the second and the third nerves each divide into two smaller branches to form the lateral femoral cutaneous nerve and two larger branches which join the dorsal portion of the fourth lumbar nerve to form the femoral nerve. Part of the fourth lumbar nerve joins the fifth lumbar nerve in the lumbosacral trunk. The branches of the lumbar plexus are the iliohypogastric nerve, the ilioinguinal nerve, the genitofemoral nerve, the lateral femoral cutaneous nerve, the obturator nerve, the accessory obturator nerve, and the femoral nerve. The iliohypogastric, the ilioninguinal, and the genitofemoral nerves supply the caudal part of the abdominal wall. The lateral femoral cutaneous, the obturator, the accessory obturator, and the femoral nerves supply the anterior thigh and the middle of the leg. The accessory obturator nerve is present in only 20 per cent of individuals and comes from the third and the fourth lumbar nerves. Compare **sacral plexus.**

lumbar puncture (LP), the introduction of a hollow needle and stylet into the subarachnoid space of the lumbar portion of the spinal canal. Using strict aseptic technique, it is performed in various therapeutic and diagnostic procedures. Diagnostic indications include measuring of cerebrospinal fluid (CSF) pressure, obtaining CSF for laboratory analysis, evaluating the canal for the pressure of a tumor, and injecting air, oxygen, or a radiopaque substance for radiographic visualization of the structures of the nervous system of spinal canal and meninges and brain. Therapeutic indications for lumbar puncture include removing blood or pus from the subarachnoid space, injecting sera or drugs, withdrawing CSF to reduce intracranial pressure, introducing a local anesthetic to induce spinal anesthesia, and placing a small amount of the patient's blood in the subarachnoid space to form a clot to patch a rent or hole in the dura in order to prevent leak of CSF into the epidural space. ■ METHOD: The skin over the interspace of the third and fourth lumbar vertebrae is cleansed. A fenestrated sterile drape is placed over the back, the window over the puncture site. The needle is inserted through the interspace to the subarachnoid space and the stylet is withdrawn. If the needle is in the proper place, clear, strawcolored CSF will begin to drip out through the needle. Depending on the indication for the procedure, various techniques follow. The pressure of the CSF may be measured using a manometer attached to a catheter and stopcock or fluid may be withdrawn, visually examined, and sent to the laboratory for chemical or bacteriologic analysis. ■ OUTCOME CRITERIA: Lumbar puncture is contraindicated if the procedure will not contribute to the diagnosis or treatment of the illness, if intracranial tumor is suspected and there is evidence of greatly increased intracranial pressure, if there are signs of infection at the site of puncture, or, in order to avoid a second puncture, if encephalography or myelography is planned in the near future. Infection, leakage of CSF, headache, nausea, vomiting, dysuria, or signs of meningeal irritation occur in approximately 25 per cent of patients. ■ NURSING ORDERS: The nurse is often responsible for obtaining the patient's written permission for the physician to perform a lumbar puncture. The patient, if apprehensive, is given a sedative one half hour before the procedure. The techniques to be used and the treatments to be given or the information to be obtained are explained. The person is placed in a lateral recumbent position, the back as near the edge of the bed as possible. The legs are flexed on the thighs, the thighs are flexed on the abdomen, and the head and shoulders are bent down, curving the spine convexly to afford the greatest space between the vertebrae. If the person is hirsute, a dry shave of the lumbar area is performed prior to draping the area. Following the procedure, significant signs to be observed by the nurse include pain, change in mentation or alertness, leakage of CSF from the puncture site, fever, and urinary retention. The patient is usually kept flat in bed, often in a prone position, for 4 to 6 hours after the procedure.

lumbar subarachnoid peritoneostomy, a surgical procedure for draining cerebrospinal fluid in hydrocephalus, usually in the newborn. It spares the kidney but is a somewhat less effective method than a lumbar subarachnoid ureterostomy. The procedure may be used when a temporary shunt is needed. First a lumbar laminectomy is performed, then a polyethylene tube is passed from the subarachnoid space around the flank and into the peritoneum. This procedure is performed to correct a communicating type of hydrocephalus.

lumbar subarachnoid ureterostomy, a surgical procedure for draining excess cerebrospinal fluid though the ureter to the bladder in hydrocephalus, usually in the newborn. The procedure first completes a lumbar laminectomy and a left nephrectomy, after which a polyethylene tube is passed from the lumbar subarachnoid space through the paraspinal muscles and into the free ureter. The procedure is performed to correct a communicating type of hydrocephalus.

lumbar veins, four pairs of veins that collect blood by dorsal tributaries from the loins and by abdominal tributaries from the walls of the abdomen. They receive veins from the vertebral plexus, pass ventrally around the vertebrae, dorsal to the psoas major, and end in the inferior vena cava. The left lumbar veins are longer than the right and pass dorsal to the aorta. The lumbar veins are connected by the ascending lumbar vein which runs ventral to the transverse processes of the lumbar vertebrae.

lumbar vertebra, one of the five largest segments of the movable part of the vertebral column, distinguished by the absence of a foramen in the transverse process and by vertebral bodies without facets. The body of each lumbar vertebra is flattened or slightly concave superiorly and inferiorly and is deeply constricted ventrally at the sides. The spinous process of each is thick, broad, and somewhat quadrilateral. The body of the fifth lumbar vertebra is much deeper ventrally then dorsally, and in some individuals, is defective, tending to weaken the spinal column. Compare **cervical vertebra, coccygeal vertebra, sacral vertebra, thoracic vertebra.**

lumbo-, a combining form meaning 'of or pertaining to the loins': *lumbocolostomy, lumbocostal, lumbosacral.*

lumbodorsal fascia. See **fascia thoracolumbalis.**

lumbosacral plexus (ləm'bousei'krəl), the combination of all the ventral primary divisions of the lumbar, the sacral, and the coccygeal nerves. The lumbar and the sacral plexuses supply the lower limb. The sacral nerves also supply the perineum through the pudendal plexus and the coccygeal area through the coccygeal plexus. See also **lumbar plexus, sacral plexus.**

lumen (lu'min), *pl.* **lumina, lumens.** 1. a cavity or the channel within any organ or structure of the body. 2. a unit of luminous flux that equals the flux emitted in a unit solid angle by a point source of one candle intensity. —**lumenal, luminal,** *adj.*

lumin-, a combining form meaning 'of or pertaining to light': *luminescence, luminiferous, luminophore.*

Luminal, a trade name for an anticonvulsant and sedative-hypnotic (phenobarbital).

Luminal Sodium, a trade name for an anticonvulsant and sedative-hypnotic (phenobarbital sodium).

lumpectomy (ləmpek'təmi), surgical excision of a tumor without removal of large amounts of surrounding tissue or adjacent lymph nodes.

lumpy jaw, *Nontechnical.* actinomycosis of cows, caused by infection with *Actinomyces bovis* and not communicable to man.

lun-, a combining form meaning 'of or pertaining to the moon': *lunacy, lunate, lunatism.*

lunate bone, the carpal bone in the center of the proximal row of carpal bones between the scaphoid and triangular bones. It articulates with five bones, the radius proximally, the capitate and the hamate distally, the scaphoid laterally, and the triangular medially. Also called **os lunatum, semilunar bone.**

lung, one of a pair of light, spongy organs in the thorax, constituting the main component of the respiratory system. The two highly elastic lungs are the main mechanisms in the body for inspiring air from which oxygen is extracted for the arterial blood system and for exhaling carbon dioxide dispersed from the venous system. The lungs are composed of lobes that are smooth and shiny on their surface. The right lung contains three lobes; the left lung two lobes. Each lung is composed of an external serous coat, a subserous layer of areolar tissue, and the parenchyma. The serous coat comprises the thin, visceral pleura. The subserous areolar tissue contains many elastic fibers and invests the entire surface of the organ. The parenchyma is composed of secondary lobules divided into primary lobules, each of which consists of blood vessels, lymphatics, nerves, and an aveolar duct connecting with air spaces. The color of the lungs at birth is pinkish-white, and darkens in later life. The coloring is from carbon granules deposited in the areolar tissue near the surface of the lung. The carbon deposits increase with age and are more abundant in men than women. The lungs of men are usually heavier than the lungs of women and usually have a greater capacity. The quantity of air that can be exhaled from the lungs after the deepest inspiration averages 3,700 cc. Each lung is conical and has an epex, a base, three borders, and two surfaces. The apex is rounded and extends into the root of the neck about 4 cm above the first rib. The base of the lung is broad and concave, rests upon the convex surface of the diaphragm, and with the diaphragm, moves up during expiration and down during inspiration. The surfaces of the lungs are partially concave, with a cardiac impression that cradles the heart. The bronchial arteries supply blood to nourish the lungs and are derived from the ventral side of the thoracic aorta or from the aortic intercostal arteries. The bronchial vein is formed at the root of the lung. Most of the blood supplied by the bronchial arteries is returned by the pulmonary veins.

lung cancer, a pulmonary malignancy attributable to cigarette smoking in 75 per cent of cases. Other predisposing factors are exposure to asbestos, acronitrile, arsenic, beryllium, chromium, chloromethyl ether, coal products, ionizing radiation, iron oxide, mustard gas, nickel, petroleum, uranium, and vinyl chloride. Lung cancer develops most often in scarred or chronically diseased lungs, and is usually far advanced when detected, as brain metastases may precede the detection of the primary lesion in the lung. Symptoms of lung cancer include persistent cough, dyspnea, purulent or blood-streaked sputum, chest pain, and repeated attacks of bronchitis or pneumonia. Diagnostic measures include x rays, fluoroscopy, tomography, bronchography, angiography, cytologic studies of sputum, bronchial washings or brushings, and needle biopsy. Epidermoid cancers and adenocarcinomas each account for approximately 30 per cent of lung tumors, about 25 per cent are small or oat-cell carcinomas, and 15 per cent are large-cell anaplastic cancers. Epidermoid tumors tend to remain in the thorax, but other lung lesions metastasize widely; oat-cell carcinomas usually invade bone marrow, and large-cell cancers frequently metastasize to mediastinal nodes and gastrointestinal mucosa. Surgery is the most effective treatment, but only half the cases are operable at the time of diagnosis and of these 50 per cent are not resectable. Thoracotomy is contraindicated if metastases are found in contralateral or scalene lymph nodes. Irradiation is used to treat localized lesions and unresectable intrathoracic tumors and as palliative therapy for metastatic lesions. Radiotherapy may also be administered postoperatively to destroy remaining tumor cells and may be combined with chemotherapy. Cures and remissions are obtained in some cases treated with chemotherapeutic agents, as cyclophosphamide, procarbazine, methotrexate, adriamycin, and bleomycin. Chemotherapy is especially indicated for oat-cell carcinoma. Postoperatively, bacillus Calmette-Guérin vaccine is administered to some patients with early stage lung cancer.

lung compliance, a measure of the ease of expansion by the lungs and thorax during respiratory movements. It is determined by pulmonary volume and elasticity, a high degree of compliance indicating a loss of elastic recoil of the lungs, as in old age or emphysema. Decreased compliance of the lungs occurs in conditions when greater pressure is needed for changes of volume, as in atelectasis, edema, fibrosis, pneumonia, or absence of surfactant. Dyspnea on exertion is the main symptom of diminished lung compliance. See also **breathing, expiratory reserve volume, residual volume, vital capacity.**

lupoid hepatitis (lu′poid). *Obsolete.* See **hepatitis.**

lupus, 1. *Nontechnical.* lupus erythematosus. 2. *Obsolete.* any chronic skin condition in which ulcerative lesions spread over the body over a long period of time. —**lupoid,** *adj.*

lupus erythematosus (LE), See **systemic lupus erythematosus.**

lupus erythematosus preparation (LE prep), a laboratory test for lupus erythematosus in which normal neutrophils are incubated with a specimen of the patient's serum resulting in the appearance of large, spherical, phagocytized inclusions within the neutrophils if the patient has lupus erythematosus.

lupus vulgaris, a rare cutaneous form of tuberculosis in which areas of the skin become ulcerated and heal slowly, leaving deeply scarred tissue. The disease is not related to lupus erythematosus.

Luride, a trade name for a chemical prophylactic (sodium fluoride) which reduces dental caries.

lusus naturae (lu′səs nətur′i), a congenital anomaly; teratism.

luteal (lu′tiəl), of or pertaining to the corpus luteum or its functions or effects.

luteal phase, (of the menstrual cycle) the second half of the cycle during which the corpus luteum is stimulated by luteinizing hormone to produce progesterone. This hormone causes the endometrium to develop from the proliferative to the secretory state, becoming a rich, dense wall suitable for nidation by a fertilized ovum. If fertilization does not occur, progesterone secretion slowly diminishes, until approximately 14 days after ovulation the

amount has decreased to a level that is not adequate for maintenance of the endometrium, and menstruation occurs.

lutein (lu′tiin), a yellow-red, crystalline, carotenoid pigment found in plants with carotenes and chlorophylls and also in animal fats, egg yolk, the corpus luteum, or any lipochrome.

luteinizing hormone (LH), a glycoprotein hormone, produced by the anterior pituitary, that stimulates the secretion of sex hormones by the ovary and the testes and is involved in the maturation of spermatozoa and ova. In men, it induces the secretion of testosterone by the interstitial cells of the testes. Testosterone, together with follicle stimulating hormone (FSH), induces the maturation of seminiferous tubules and stimulates them to produce sperm. In females, LH, working together with FSH, stimulates the growing follicle in the ovary to secrete estrogen. High concentrations of estrogen stimulate the release of a surge of LH, which stimulates ovulation. LH then induces the development of the ruptured follicle into the corpus luteum, which continues to secrete estrogen and progesterone. See also **menstrual cycle.**

luteoma (lu′tiou′mə), *pl.* **luteomas, luteomata. 1.** a granulosa-theca-cell tumor whose cells resemble those of the corpus luteum. **2.** Also called **pregnancy luteoma.** a unilateral or bilateral nodular hyperplasia of ovarian lutein cells, occasionally developing during the last trimester of pregnancy.

luteotropin. See **prolactin.**

lutetium (Lu), a rare-earth metallic element. Its atomic number is 71; and its atomic weight is 174.97.

LVN, abbreviation for **licensed vocational nurse.** See **licensed practical nurse.**

Lw, symbol for **lawrencium.**

lyco-, a combining form meaning 'of or pertaining to a wolf': *lycomania, lycorexia.*

lycopene (lai′kəpin), a red, crystalline, unsaturated hydrocarbon that is the carotenoid pigment in tomatoes and various berries and fruits. It is considered the primary substance from which all natural carotenoid pigments are derived.

lying-in, 1. designating the time before, during, and after childbirth. 2. designating a hospital that provides care for women in childbirth and the puerperium. 3. the condition of being in confinement, or childbed.

Lyme arthritis, an acute, recurrent inflammatory disease, involving one or a few joints, believed to be transmitted by an unidentified tickborne virus. The condition was originally described in the community of Lyme, Connecticut, but has also been reported in other parts of the northeastern United States and, sporadically, in other countries. Knees, other large joints, and temperomandibular joints are most commonly involved, with local heat and swelling. Chills, fever, headache, malaise, and erythema chronicum migrans, an expanding annular, erythematous skin eruption, often precede the joint manifestations. Occasionally cardiac conduction abnormalities, aseptic meningitis, or Bell's palsy are associated conditions. Symptoms appear in recurrent episodes, lasting usually about a week, at intervals of from one to several weeks, declining in severity over a two- or three-year period. There is no significant permanent joint damage. Treatment includes salicylates for joint symptoms and corticosteroids to reduce cardiac and neurological manifestations.

lymph, a thin opalescent fluid originating in many organs and tissues of the body that is circulated through the lymphatic vessels and filtered by the lymph nodes. Lymph enters the blood stream at the junction of the internal jugular and subclavian veins. It contains chyle, a few erythrocytes, and variable numbers of leukocytes, most of which are lymphocytes. It is otherwise similar to plasma. See also **chyle.**

lymph-. See **lympho-.**

-lymph, a combining form meaning a 'clear body fluid': *hemolymph, neurolymph, perilymph.*

lymphadenitis (lımfæd'ınai'tıs, lım'fədınai'tıs), an inflammatory condition of the lymph nodes, usually the result of systemic neoplastic disease or bacterial infection or other inflammatory condition. The nodes may be enlarged, hard, smooth or irregular, red, and may feel hot. The location of the affected node is indicative of the site or origin of disease.

lymphangiectasia (lımfæn'jiektei'źhə), dilatation of lymphatic vessels, characterized by diarrhea, steatorrhea, and protein malabsorption. It usually results from obstruction, as in pelvic tuberculosis, mesenteric node metastases, and certain protozoan diseases.

lymphangioma (lımfæn'jiou'mə), *pl.* **lymphangiomas, lymphangiomata.** a benign, yellowish-tan tumor on the skin, composed of a mass of dilated lymph vessels. It is often removed by excision or electrocoagulation for cosmetic reasons. Also called **angioma lymphaticum.** See also **angioma.**

lymphangioma cavernosum, a tumor formed by dilated lymphatic vessels and filled with lymph that is often mixed with coagulated blood. The lesion, which is often congenital, may cause extensive enlargement of the affected tissue, especially of the tongue and lips. Also called **cavernous lymphangioma.**

lymphangioma circumscriptum, a benign skin lesion that develops from superficial hypertrophic lymph vessels. Most commonly seen in young children, it is characteristically pigmented and may grow to several centimeters in diameter.

lymphangioma cysticum. See **cystic lymphangioma.**

lymphangioma simplex, a growth formed by moderately dilated lymph vessels in a circumscribed area, chiefly on the skin.

lymphangitis (lım'fænjai'tıs), an inflammation of one or more lymphatic vessels, usually resulting from an acute streptococcal infection of one of the extremities. It is characterized by fine red streaks extending from the infected area to the axilla or groin, and by fever, chills, headache, and myalgia. The infection may spread to the bloodstream. Penicillin and hot soaks are usually prescribed; aseptic technique is important to avoid contagion.

lymphatic, 1. of or pertaining to the lymphatic system of the body, consisting of a vast network of tubes transporting lymph. 2. any one of the vessels associated with the lymphatic network.

lymphatic capillary plexus, one of the numerous networks of lymphatic capillaries that collect lymph from the intercellular fluid and constitute the beginning of the lymphatic system. The lymphatic vessels arise from the capillary plexuses, which vary in size and number in different regions and organs of the body. The capillary networks do not contain lymphatic valves as do the vessels. The plexuses are especially abundant in the dermis of the skin but also lace many other areas as the mucous membranes of the repiratory and digestive systems, testes, ovaries, liver, kidneys and heart. See also **lymphatic system.**

lymphatic leukemia. See **acute lymphocytic leukemia, chronic lymphocytic leukemia.**

lymphatic nodule. See **Malpighian body.**

lymphatic system, a vast, complex network of capillaries, thin vessels, valves, ducts, nodes, and organs that helps to protect and maintain the internal fluid environment of the entire body by producing, filtering, and conveying lymph and by producing various blood cells. The lymphatic network also transports fats, proteins, and other substances to the blood system and restores 60 per cent of the fluid that filters out of the blood capillaries into interstitial spaces during normal metabolism. The peripheral parts of the lymphatic complex do not directly communicate with the venous system into which the lymph flows, but the endothelium of the veins at the junction of the blood and the lymphatic networks is continuous with the endothelium of the lymphatic vessels. Small semilunar valves throughout the lymphatic network help to control the flow of lymph and, at the junction with the venous system, prevent venous blood from flowing into the lymphatic vessels. The lymph collected from throughout the body drains into the blood through two ducts situated in the neck. Various body dynamics, as respiratory pressure changes, muscular contractions, and movements of organs surrounding lymphatic vessels combine to pump the lymph through the lymphatic system. The thoracic duct that rises into the left side of the neck is the major vessel of the lymphatic system and conveys lymph from the whole body, except for the right quadrant, which is served by the right lymphatic duct. Lymphatics have a beaded appearance because of sinuses associated with the many valves in the vessels. They resemble veins but have more valves, thinner walls, and contain lymph nodes. The lymphatics are so thin and transparent that the lymph they contain can be seen moving through these delicate tubules in a living body. Special techniques are required, however, to examine the lymphatic system closely. The lymphatic capillaries, which are the beginning of the system, abound in the dermis of the skin, forming a continuous network over the entire body, except for the cornea. The system also includes specialized lymphatic organs, as the tonsils, the thymus, and the spleen. The lymphatics of the intestine contain a special substance, especially during the digestion of fatty foods. Lymph flows into the general cirulation through the thoracic duct at a rate of about 125 ml per hour during routine exertion. The rate may jump to as high as 1,800 ml per hour during vigorous exercise. See also **lymph, lymph node, spleen, thymus.**

lymphedema (lim'fidi'mə), a primary or secondary disorder characterized by the accumulation of lymph in soft tissue and swelling, caused by inflammation, obstruction, or removal of lymph channels. Congenital lymphedema (Milroy's disease) is a hereditary disorder characterized by chronic lymphatic obstruction. Lymphedema praecox occurs in adolescence, chiefly in females, and causes puffiness and swelling of the lower limbs, apparently because of hyperplastic development of lymph vessels. Secondary lymphedema may follow surgical removal of lymph channels in mastectomy, obstruction of lymph drainage caused by malignant tumors, or the infestation of lymph vessels with adult filarial parasites. Lymphedema of the lower extremities begins with mild swelling of the foot, gradually extends to the entire limb, and is aggravated by prolonged standing, pregnancy, obesity, warm weather, and the menstrual period. There is no cure for the disorder, but lymph drainage from the extremity can be improved if the patient sleeps with the foot of the bed elevated four to eight inches, wears an elastic stocking, and takes moderate exercise regularly. Light massage in the direction of the lymph flow and thiazide diuretics may be prescribed; constricting clothing and salty or spicy foods that increase thirst are contraindicated. Surgery may be performed to remove hypertrophied lymph channels and disfiguring tissue. — **lymphedematous, lymphedematose,** *adj.*

lymph node, one of the many, small oval structures that filter the lymph, fight infection, and in which there are formed lymphocytes, monocytes, and plasma cells. The lymph nodes are of different sizes, some as small as pinheads, others as large as lima beans. Each node is enclosed in a capsule, is composed of a lighter colored cortical portion and a darker medullary portion, and consists of closely packed lymphocytes, reticular connective tissue laced by trabeculae, and three kinds of sinuses, subcapsular, cortical, and medullary. Lymph flows into the node through afferent lymphatic vessels that open into the subcapsular sinuses. Efferent lymphatic vessels arise from the medullary sinuses of the node and emerge through a small peripheral hilum that also receives blood vessels. The sinuses and meshes of reticular fibers retard the flow of lymph to which lymphocytes are added from germinal centers within the node that multiply those cells by mitosis. Most lymph nodes are clustered in areas, as the mouth, the neck, the lower arm, the axilla, and the groin. The lymphatic network and nodes of the breast are especially crucial in the diagnosis and treatment of breast cancer in women. Cancer cells from a "primary" breast tumor often spread through the lymphatic system to other parts of the body. Also called **lymph gland.**

lympho-, lymph-, a combining form meaning 'of or pertaining to the lymph': *lymphoduct, lymphography, lymphomatous.*

lymphoblastic lymphoma. See **poorly differentiated lymphocytic malignant lymphoma.**

lymphoblastic lymphosarcoma. See **poorly differentiated lymphocytic malignant lymphoma.**

lymphoblastoma (lim'foublæstou'mə). See **poorly differentiated lymphocytic malignant lymphoma.**

lymphocyte (lim'fəsait), one of two kinds of small, agranulocytic leukocytes, originating from fetal stem cells and developing in the bone marrow. Lymphocytes normally comprise 25 per cent of the total white blood cell count but increase in number in response to infection. They occur in two forms: **B cells** and **T cells.** Each develops uniquely, and each has its own function. B cells circulate in an immature form and synthesize antibodies for insertion into their own cytoplasmic membranes. They reproduce mitotically, each of the clones displaying identical antibodies on their surface membranes. When an immature B cell is exposed to a specific antigen the cell is activated, traveling to the spleen or to the lymph nodes, differentiating, and rapidly producing **plasma cells** and **memory cells.** Plasma cells synthesize and secrete copious amounts of antibody. Memory cells do not secrete antibody, but if re-exposure to the specific antigen occurs, they develop into antibody-secreting plasma cells. The function of the B cell is to search out, identify, and bind with specific antigens. T cells are lymphocytes that have circulated through the thymus gland and have differentiated to become thymocytes. When exposed to an antigen, they divide rapidly and produce large numbers of new T cells sensitized to that antigen. T cells are often called 'killer cells' because they secrete immunologically essential chemical compounds and assist B cells in destroying foreign protein. T cells also appear to play a significant role in the body's resistance to the proliferation of cancer cells. See also **lymphokine.**

lymphocytic choriomeningitis, an arenavirus infection of the meninges and the cerebrospinal fluid, caused by the lymphocytic choriomeningitis virus and characterized by fever, headache, and stiff neck. The infection occurs primarily in young adults, most often in the fall and winter months. Recovery usually takes place within two weeks.

lymphocytic leukemia. See **acute lymphocytic leukemia, chronic lymphocytic leukemia.**

lymphocytic lymphoma. See **well-differentiated lymphocytic malignant lymphoma.**

lymphocytic lymphosarcoma. See **well-differentiated lymphocytic malignant lymphoma.**

lymphocytic thyroiditis. See **Hashimoto's disease.**

lymphocytoma (lɪm'foʊsaɪtoʊ'mə). See **well-differentiated lymphocytic malignant lymphoma.**

lymphocytopenia (lɪm'foʊsaɪ'təpi'niə), a smaller than normal number of lymphocytes in the peripheral circulation, occurring as a primary hematologic disorder or in association with nutritional deficiency, malignancy, or infectious mononucleosis. See also **agranulocyte.**

lymphoderma perniciosa. See **leukemia cutis.**

lymphoepithelial carcinoma. See **lymphoepithelioma.**

lymphoepithelioma (lɪm'foʊep'ɪthi'liou'mə), a poorly differentiated neoplasm developing from the epithelium overlying lymphoid tissue in the nasopharynx. It occurs most frequently in young Oriental people. Also called **lymphoepithelial carcinoma.**

lymphogenous leukemia (lɪmfoj'ɪnəs). See **acute lymphocytic leukemia, chronic lymphocytic leukemia.**

lymphogranuloma venerum (LGV), an infection caused by a strain of the bacterium *Chlamydia trachomatis.* It is characterized by ulcerative genital lesions, marked swelling of the lymph nodes in the groin, headache, fever, and malaise. Ulcerations of the rectal wall occur less commonly. The disease is transmitted by coitus and is diagnosed by isolating the organism from an infected node, demonstrating LGV antibodies by serologic blood test or by a Frei intradermal test. Tetracycline is usually prescribed for the patient and for any person with whom there has been sexual contact. When changing dressings aseptic technique is used. Also called **lymphopathia venerum.** See also *Chlamydia.*

lymphoid leukemia (lɪm'foɪd). See **acute lymphocytic leukemia, chronic lymphocytic leukemia.**

lymphoidocytic leukemia (lɪmfoɪ'dəsɪt'ɪk). See **stem cell leukemia.**

lymphokine (lɪm'foʊkaɪn), one of the chemical factors produced and released by T-lymphocytes that attract macrophages to the site of infection or inflammation and prepare them for attack. Kinds of lymphokines include **chemotactic factor, lymphotoxin, migration-inhibitory factor, mitogenic factor.**

lympholysis (lɪmfol'əsɪs), cellular destruction of lymphocytes, especially of certain lymphocytes in the process of an immune response. —**lympholytic,** *adj.*

lymphoma (lɪmfoʊ'mə), *pl.* **lymphomas, lymphomata.** a neoplasm of lymphoid tissue that is usually malignant but, in rare cases, may be benign. The various lymphomas differ in degree of cellular differentiation and content, but the manifestations are similar in all types. Characteristically, the appearance of a painless, enlarged lymph node or nodes in the neck is followed by weakness, fever, weight loss, and anemia. With widespread involvement of lymphoid tissue, the spleen and liver usually enlarge, and gastrointestinal disturbances, malabsorption, and bone lesions frequently develop. Men are more likely than women to develop lymphoid tumors. Treatment for lymphoma includes intensive radiotherapy and chemotherapy. Kinds of lymphoma include **Burkitt's lymphoma, giant follicular lymphoma, histiocytic malignant lymphoma, Hodgkin's disease, mixed cell malignant lymphoma.** —**lymphomatoid,** *adj.*

-lymphoma, a combining form meaning a 'tumor or neoplastic disorder of lymphoid tissue': *adenolymphoma, angiolymphoma, cystadenolymphoma.*

lymphoma staging, a system for classifying lymphomas according to the stage of the disease for the purpose of appropriate treatment. Stage I is characterized by the involvement of a single lymph node region or one extralymphatic organ or site and Stage II by the involvement of two or more lymph node regions on the same side of the diaphragm or a localized involvement of an extralymphatic organ or site plus one or more node regions on the same side of the diaphragm. In Stage III lymph nodes on both sides of the diaphragm are affected, and there may be involvement of the spleen or localized involvement of an extralymphatic organ or site. Stage IV is typified by diffuse or disseminated involvement of one or more extralymphatic organs or sites with or without associated lymph node involvement.

lymphopathia venerum (lɪm'foʊpæth'iə). See **lymphogranuloma venerum.**

lymphopenia (lɪm'foʊpi'niə). See **lymphocytopenia.**

lymphoreticulosis, subacute granulomatous inflammation of lymphoid tissue with proliferation of reticuloendothelial cells, occurring most commonly as the result of a cat scratch. No causative agent is known. The disorder is characterized by the formation of an ulcerated papule at the site of the scratch, and by fever and tender lymphadenopathy, sometimes progressing to suppuration. Also called **cat-scratch fever.**

lymphosarcoma (lɪm'foʊsarkoʊ'mə). *pl.* **lymphosarcomas, lymphosarcomata.** See **non-Hodgkin's lymphoma.**

lymphosarcoma cell leukemia, a malignancy of blood-forming tissues characterized by many lymphosarcoma cells in the peripheral circulation that tend to infiltrate surrounding tissues. These cells are extremely immature and larger and more reticulated than lymphocytes. The disease may accompany lymphoma or exist as a separate entity with more bone marrow involvement than is found in lymphoma.

lyo-, a combining form meaning 'dissolved': *lyogel, lyophobe, lyotropic.*

Lyon hypothesis, (in genetics) a hypothesis stating that only one of the two X chromosomes in a female is functional, the other having become inactive early in development. A female is mosaic in regard to X chromosomes; some are from her father, some from her mother. Sex-linked genes may therefore appear on some of her cells and not on others.

lypressin (laɪpres'ɪn), an antidiuretic and vasoconstrictor.

■ INDICATION: It is prescribed in diabetes insipidus to decrease urinary water loss.

■ CONTRAINDICATION: Vascular disease or known hypersensitivity to this drug prohibits its use.

■ ADVERSE EFFECTS: Among the most serious adverse reactions are angina (in people with vascular disease), nausea, cramping, and marked facial pallor.

lysergide (laɪsər'jaɪd), a psychotomimetic, semisynthetic derivate of ergot that acts at multiple sites in the central nervous system from the cortex to the spinal cord. In susceptible individuals, as little as 20 to 25 μg of the potent drug may cause pupillary dilation, increased blood pressure, hyperreflexia, tremor, muscle weakness, piloerection, and increased body temperature. Larger doses also produce dizziness, drowsiness, paresthesia, euphoria or dysphoria, and synesthesias; colors may be heard, sounds visualized, and time is felt to pass slowly. Psychological dependence may develop and use of lysergide is associated with significant hazards, as panic, serious depression, paranoid behavior, and prolonged psychotic episodes. Treatment of lysergide intoxication involves 'talking down' the patient and administering antianxiety agents or barbiturates. It has been proposed but not approved for use as an adjunct to psychotherapy, in the treatment of alcoholism, and to relieve pain in terminal cancer patients. See also **hallucinogen.** Also called **LSD, lysergic acid diethylamide,** *Slang.* **acid.**

-lysin, a combining form meaning a 'cell-dissolving antibody': *antilysin, betalysin, paralysin.*

lysine (laɪ'sin, laɪ'sɪn), an essential amino acid needed for proper growth in infants and for maintenance of nitrogen balance in adults. See also **amino acid, protein.**

lysine intolerance, a congenital disorder resulting in the inability to utilize the essential amino acid lysine owing to an enzyme deficiency or defect. The disorder is characterized by weakness, vomiting, and coma and is treated by adjusting the protein content of the diet, restricting those foods especially high in lysine. See also **lysinemia.**

lysinemia (laɪ'sɪni'miə), a condition caused by an inborn error of metabolism and resulting in the inability to utilize the essential amino acid lysine owing to an enzyme defect or deficiency. It is characterized by muscle weakness and mental retardation. Treatment consists of a diet that controls the intake of lysine by reducing proteins and including such foods as fruits, vegetables, and rice.

lysine monohydrochloride, a salt of the amino acid lysine, used as a dietary supplement to increase the utilization of vegetable proteins, as corn, rice, and wheat.

lysis (laɪ'sɪs), **1.** destruction or dissolution of a cell or molecule through the action of a specific agent. Cell lysis is frequently caused by a lysin. **2.** gradual diminution in the symptoms of a disease. Compare **crisis.**

-lysis, a combining form meaning a 'breaking down or detachment': *cytolysis, dialysis, osteolysis.*

lyso-, a combining form meaning 'of or pertaining to dissolution': *lysocephalin, lysotype, lysozyme.*

Lysodren, a trade name for an antineoplastic (mitotane).

lysosome (laɪ'səsoum), a cytoplasmic, membrane-bound particle that contains hydrolytic enzymes that function in intracellular digestive processes. The organelles are found in most cells but are particularly prominent in leukocytes and in the cells of the liver and kidney. If the hydrolytic enzymes are released into the cytoplasm, they cause self-digestion of the cell so that lysosomes may play an important role in certain self-destructive diseases characterized by the wasting of tissue, as muscular dystrophy.

lysso-, a combining form meaning 'of or pertaining to rabies, or hydrophobia': *lyssodexis, lyssoid, lyssophobia.*

Lysthenon (lɪs'θənon), a trade name for a depolarizing blocking agent (succinylcholine chloride), used as an adjunct to general anesthesia.

-lyte, a combining form meaning a 'substance capable of or resulting from decomposition': *ampholyte, cytolyte, sarcolyte.*

lytes (laɪts), *Informal.* electrolytes, especially the levels of potassium, sodium, phosphorus, magnesium, and calcium in the blood, as determined by laboratory testing.

-lytic, a combining form meaning 'pertaining to or effecting decomposition': *fibrillolytic, leukolytic, myelolytic.*

lytic cocktail, an informal name for an anesthetic compound of chlorpromazine, meperidine, and promethazine that blocks the autonomic nervous system, depresses the circulatory system, and induces neuroplegia.

Lytren, a trade name for a nutritional supplement containing various electrolytes.

-lyze, a combining form meaning 'to produce decomposition': *bacteriolyze, hemolyze, paralyze.* Also **-lyse.**

M

m, abbreviation for **meter.**

M, abbreviation for **metastasis** in the TNM system for staging malignant neoplastic disease. See also **cancer staging.**

ma, abbreviation for **milliampere.**

MA, abbreviation for **mental age.**

Maass, Clara (1876–1901), an American nurse. After training and working at the Newark German Hospital, which has since been renamed for her, she volunteered for military service at the outbreak of the Spanish-American War. After working at Army camps where soldiers were dying of yellow fever, she volunteered to go to Havana to participate in the experiments being done to determine the cause of that disease. She was bitten by a mosquito and ten days later died of yellow fever. She was one of the first nurses to be inducted into the Hall of Fame of the American Nurses' Association.

MAC, abbreviation for **minimum alveolar concentration.**

MAC AWAKE, the time at which a patient recovering from general anesthesia is able to respond rationally to questions and verbal instructions.

macerate (mæs′ıreit), to soften something solid by soaking. —**maceration,** *n.*

machupo. See **Bolivian hemorrhagic fever.**

macrencephaly, macroencephaly (mæk′rənsef′əli), a congenital anomaly characterized by abnormal largeness of the brain. See also **macrocephaly.** —**macrencephalic, macroencephalic,** *adj., n.*

macro-, a combining form meaning 'large, or abnormal size': *macrobiosis, macrocardius, macrophage.* Also **makro-.**

macroblepharia (mæk′roublıfer′iə), the condition of having abnormally large eyelids.

macrocephaly (mæk′rousef′əli), **macrocephalia,** a congenital anomaly characterized by abnormal largeness of the head and brain in relation to the rest of the body, resulting in some degree of mental and growth retardation. The head is more than two standard deviations above the average circumference size for age, sex, race, and period of gestation, with excessively wide fontanelles; the facial features are usually normal. The condition may be caused by some defect in formation during embryonic development, or it may be the result of progressive degeneration processes, as Schilder's disease, Greenfield's disease, or congenital lipoidosis. In macrocephaly there is symmetrical overgrowth at the head without increased intracranial pressure, as differentiated from hydrocephalus in which the lateral, asymmetrical growth of the head is caused by excessive accumulation of cerebrospinal fluid, usually under increased pressure. Specific diagnostic tests may be necessary to differentiate the two conditions. Treatment is primarily symptomatic, with nursing care concentrated specifically on helping parents learn to care for a brain-damaged child. Also called **megalocephaly.** Compare **microcephaly.** See also **hydrocephalus.** —**macrocephalic, macrocephalous,** *adj.,* **macrocephalus,** *n.*

macrocyte (mæk′rəsait), an abnormally large, mature erythrocyte usually exceeding 9 μ in diameter. It is most commonly seen in megaloblastic anemia. Compare **microcyte.** See also **macrocytic anemia.** —**macrocytic,** *adj.*

macrocytic, (of a cell) larger than normal, as the erythrocytes in macrocytic anemia.

macrocytic anemia (mæk′rousıt′ık), a disorder of the blood characterized by impaired erythropoiesis and the abnormal presence of large, fragile, red blood cells in the circulation. Macrocytic anemia is most often the result of a deficiency of folic acid and vitamin B_{12}.

macrocytosis (mæk′rousaitou′sıs), an abnormal proliferation of macrocytes in the peripheral blood.

Macrodantin, a trade name for a urinary antibacterial (nitrofurantoin).

Macrodex, a trade name for a plasma expander (dextran 70).

macrodrip, (in intravenous therapy) an apparatus that is used to deliver measured amounts of intravenous solutions at specific flow rates based on the size of drops of the solution. The size of the drops is controlled by the fixed diameter of a plastic delivery tube. The drops delivered by a macrodrip are larger than those delivered by a microdrip. Different macrodrips deliver 10, 15, or 20 drops per milliliter of solution. Macrodrips are not usually used to deliver a small amount of intravenous solution or to keep a vein open, because the time between drips is so long that a clot may form at the tip of the intravenous catheter. Compare **microdrip.**

macroelement. See **macronutrient.**

macroencephaly (mæk′rouensef′əli). See **macrencephaly.**

macrogamete, a large, nonmotile female gamete of certain thallophytes and sporozoa, specifically the malarial parasite *Plasmodium.* It corresponds to the ovum of the higher animals and is fertilized by the smaller, motile male gamete. See also **microgamete.**

macrogametocyte, an enlarged merozoite that undergoes meiosis to form the mature female gamete during the sexual phase of the life cycle of certain thallophytes and sporozoa, specifically the malarial parasite *Plasmodium*. Macrogametocytes are found in the red blood cells of a person infected with the malarial parasite, but they must be ingested by a female *Anopheles* mosquito to complete the maturation process and develop into a macrogamete.

macrogenitosomia (mæk'roujen'ɪtousou'miə), a congenital condition in which the genitalia are abnormal owing to an excess of androgen during fetal development. It is characterized in boys by enlarged external genitalia and in girls by pseudohermaphroditism.

macroglobulinemia (mæk'rouglob'yulɪni'miə), a form of monoclonal gammopathy in which a large immunoglobulin (IgM) is vastly overproduced by the clones of a plasma B cell in response to an antigenic signal. Increased viscosity of the blood may result in circulatory impairment, weakness, neurologic disorders, and fatigue. Normal immunoglobulin synthesis is decreased and the person is susceptible to infection, particularly bacterial pneumonia and septicemia. Also called **Waldenström's macroglobulinemia.** See also **multiple myeloma.**

macroglossia (mæk'rouglos'iə), a congenital anomaly characterized by excessive size of the tongue, as seen in certain syndromes of congenital defects, including Down's syndrome.

macrognathia (mæk'rounei'fhiə), an abnormally large growth of the jaw. Compare **micrognathia.** —**macrognathic,** *adj.*

macronucleus (mæk'rounu'kliəs), 1. a large nucleus. 2. (in protozoa) the larger of two nuclei in each cell; it governs cell metabolism and growth as opposed to the micronucleus, which functions in sexual reproduction.

macronutrient (mæk'rounu'triənt), a chemical element required in relatively large quantities for the normal physiological processes of the body. Macronutrients include carbon, hydrogen, oxygen, nitrogen, potassium, sodium, calcium, chloride, magnesium, phosphorus, and sulfur. Also called **macroelement, major element.** Compare **micronutrient.**

macrophage (mæk'rəfeij), any phagocytic cell of the reticuloendothelial system including Kupffer cell in the liver, splenocyte in the spleen, and histocyte in the loose connective tissue. See also phagocyte, reticuloendothelial system.

macrosomia. See **gigantism.**

macula (mæk'yulə), *pl.* **maculae.** a small pigmented area or a spot that appears separate or different from the surrounding tissue.

macula cerulea, *pl.* **maculae cerulea.** See **blue spot,** def. 1.

macula lutea, an oval yellow spot at the center of the retina 2 mm from the optic nerve. It contains a pit, no blood vessels, and the fovea centralis. Central vision occurs when an image is focused directly on the fovea centralis of the macula lutea. Also called *Informal.* **macula.**

macule (mæk'yul), 1. Compare **papule.** a small, flat blemish or discoloration that is flush with the skin surface. Examples are the rashes of measles and roseola. 2. a gray scar on the cornea that is visible without magnification. —**macular,** *adj.*

Madelung's neck (mæd'ələŋz). See **lipoma annulare colli.**

mad hatter's disease. See **mercurialism.**

Madura foot (mæj'urə), a progressive, destructive, tropical fungal infection of the foot. Also called **maduromycosis.**

maduromycosis (mæj'uroumaikou'sis). See **Madura foot.**

mafenide acetate, a topical anti-infective.

■ INDICATION: It is prescribed in the treatment of burns.

■ CONTRAINDICATIONS: Known hypersensitivity to this drug or to sulfonamide prohibits its use.

■ ADVERSE EFFECTS: Among the more serious adverse effects are hypersensitivity reactions and suprainfections particularly by *Candida albicans*.

Maffucci's syndrome (mæfu'ʧhiz), a condition characterized by enchondromatosis and multiple cutaneous or visceral hemangiomas.

Magendie's law. See **Bell's law.**

magic bullet approach, 1. a therapeutic or diagnostic method that makes use of a specific mechanistic connection between a drug and a disease or organ. 2. (in clinical medicine) the administration of a specific drug to cure or ameliorate a given disease or condition. 3. (in traditional diagnostic radiology) the administration of a specific dye to facilitate the visualization by x ray of a given organ, as the intravenous injection of a specific dye for renal studies. 4. (in nuclear medicine) the administration of a specific radionuclide tagged to an appropriate carrier to provide a scintillation camera image of a given organ or structure, as the use of a substance containing phosphate and technetium for bone scanning.

magnesia magma. See **milk of magnesia.**

magnesium (Mg), a silver-white mineral element. Its atomic number is 12; its atomic weight is 24.32. Magnesium occurs abundantly in nature, always in combination with other elements, in sea water, bones, seeds, in the chlorophyll in the green parts of plants, and in minerals, as magnesite, dolomite, and carnalite. It is obtained chiefly by the electrolysis of fused salts containing magnesium chloride or by the thermal reduction of magnesia and is used in photography, metallurgy, and in various medicines, as magnesium sulfate. Magnesium is the second most abundant cation of the intracellular fluids in the body and is essential for many enzyme activities. It also is important to neurochemical transmissions and muscular excitability. The body of the average 145-pound adult contains about 2,000 mEq of magnesium, about 50 per cent of which is in the bones, 45 per cent existing as intracellular cations, and about 5 per cent in the extracellular fluid. Intracellular concentrations of magnesium range from 5 to 30 mEq per kilogram, depending on the type of tissue. The concentration of magnesium in plasma is 1.5 to 2.2 mEq per liter, with about two thirds as free cation and one third bound to plasma proteins. Very little is known about the exchange of magnesium between the plasma, the intracellular capsule, and the bone. About 30 per cent of the magnesium in the skeleton represents an exchangeable pool. The average adult in the United States ingests between 20 and 40 mEq of magnesium daily, and about one third of the quantity ingested is absorbed from the gastrointestinal tract. Absorption occurs in the upper small bowel by means of an active process closely related to the transport system for calcium. Magnesium is excreted mainly by the kidney and 3 to 5 per cent of the magnesium is excreted in the urine. Most of the reabsorption of magnesium takes place in the proximal tubules of the kidney. Renal excretion of magnesium increases during diuresis induced by ammonium chloride, glucose, and organic mercurials. Diuretic therapy can cause hypomagnesemia. Small amounts of magnesium are excreted in milk and in the saliva. The element influences many enzymes in the body and is a cofactor of all enzymes participating in phosphate transfer reactions involving adenosine triphosphate and other nucleotide triphosphates as substrates. It is also essential to the interaction of intracellular particles and the binding of macromolecules to subcellular organelles, as the binding of messenger RNA to ribosomes. Magnesium affects the central nervous, neuromuscular and cardiovascular systems. Hypomagnesemia increases central nervous system irritability and may cause disorientation, convulsions, and psychosis. Some researchers report abnormally high concentrations of magnesium in the plasma of manic-depressive and schizophrenic individuals and abnormally low magnesium concentrations in the plasma of patients with endogenous and neurotic depressions. Magnesium tends to depress the action of skeletal muscle, and excessive magnesium inhibits the release of acetylcholine by motor-nerve impulses. Insufficient magnesium in extracellular fluid increases the release of acetylcholine, increases muscular excitability, and can cause tetany. Excess magnesium in the body can slow the heartbeat, and concentrations of magnesium greater than 15 mEq per liter can produce cardiac arrest in diastole. Excess magnesium also causes vasodilation by directly affecting the blood vessels and by ganglionic blockade. Hypomagnesemia can cause changes in cardiac muscles and skeletal muscle and can cause nephrocalcin-

osis. Some of the abnormal conditions that can produce hypomagnesemia are diarrhea, steatorrhea, chronic alcoholism, and diabetes mellitus. Hypomagnesemia may also be associated with newborns and infants who are fed cow's milk or artificial formulas, apparently because of the high phosphate-magnesium ratio in such diets. Hypomagnesemia is often treated with parenteral fluids containing magnesium sulfate or magnesium chloride. Hypermagnesemia is usually due to renal insufficiency and is manifested by hypotension, electrocardiogram changes, muscle weakness, sedation, and a confused mental state.

magnesium sulfate, a salt of magnesium.

■ INDICATIONS: It is prescribed parenterally to prevent seizures, especially in pre-eclampsia, and orally to treat constipation and heartburn and to correct deficiency of magnesium in the body.

■ CONTRAINDICATIONS: It is used with caution with renal impairment or hypersensitivity to the drug. Respiratory depression, severe cardiac myopathy, heart block, or symptoms of appendicitis or fecal impaction prohibits its use.

■ ADVERSE EFFECTS: The most serious adverse reaction is circulatory collapse from excessive serum concentrations of magnesium. Respiratory depression, confusion, and muscle weakness also may occur.

magnet reflex, a pathologic reflex seen in an animal that has had its cerebellum removed. If the animal is placed on its back and its head is strongly flexed, all four limbs will flex. Then light pressure by a finger on a toepad causes contraction of limb extensor muscles so that if the finger is slowly removed the limb appears to follow the finger.

Mahoney, Mary Eliza (1845-1926), the first American black nurse. She did private nursing in the Boston area and was active in furthering intergroup relationships and in improving the role of the black nurse in the community. A medal in her name, established after her death, was first presented in 1936; it is given to a black nurse in recognition of an outstanding contribution to the profession.

main en griffe (mänägrif′). See **clawhand.**

Majocchi's granuloma, a rare type of tinea corporis, mainly affecting the lower legs. It is caused by the fungus *Trichophyton,* which infects the hairs of the affected site and raises spongy granulomas. The lesions persist for three to four months and are gradually absorbed, or they necrose, often leaving deep scars. Also called **trichophytic granuloma.**

major affective disorder, any of a group of psychotic disorders characterized by severe and inappropriate emotional responses, by prolonged and persistent disturbances of mood and related thought distortions, and by other symptoms associated with either depressed or manic states, as occurs in bipolar disorder, depression, and involutional melancholia. The disorder is usually episodic but may be chronic or cyclical, as in the case of bipolar disorder; it is not caused by any organic dysfunction of the brain.

major depressive episode. See **endogenous depression.**

major element. See **macronutrient.**

major medical insurance, insurance coverage designed to offset the costs of prolonged or catastrophic illness and injury. Most major medical insurance policies are written to pay a certain percentage of costs up to predetermined figure, beyond which payment is in full up to a maximum amount, at which payment ceases. Many require the insured to pay in full a specified initial, or deductible amount.

major renal calyx. See **renal calyx.**

major surgery, any surgical procedure that requires general anesthesia or respiratory assistance. Compare **minor surgery.**

makro-. See **macro-.**

mal (mæl), *French.* an illness or disease, as grand mal or petit mal.

mal-, a combining form meaning 'abnormal': *maladjustment, malalignment, malignant.*

malabsorption (mæl′æbsɔrp′s̆hən, mæl′æbzɔrp′s̆hən), impaired absorption of nutrients from the gastrointestinal tract. It occurs in celiac disease, sprue, dysentery, diarrhea, and other disorders and may result from an inborn error of metabolism, malnutrition, or any chemical or anatomic condition of the digestive system that prevents normal absorption. See **inborn error of metabolism, malnutrition.**

malabsorption syndrome, a complex of symptoms resulting from disorders in the intestinal absorption of nutrients, characterized by anorexia, weight loss, bloating of the abdomen, muscle cramps, bone pain, and steatorrhea. Anemia, weakness, and fatigue occur because iron, folic acid, and vitamin B_{12} are not absorbed in sufficient amounts. Among the many conditions causing this syndrome are gastric or small-bowel resection, celiac disease, tropical sprue, Whipple's disease, intestinal lymphangiectasia, and cystic fibrosis. Treatment and prognosis are determined by the underlying condition. See also **celiac disease, cystic fibrosis, intestinal lymphangiectasia, tropical sprue.**

malacia (məlei′s̆hə), **1.** a morbid softening or a sponginess in any part or any tissue of the body. **2.** a craving for spicy foods, as mustard, hot peppers, or pickles. — **malacic,** *adj.*

-malacia, a combining form meaning the 'softening of tissue': *cardiomalacia, esophagomalacia, tracheomalacia.*

malaco-, a combining form meaning 'a condition of abnormal softness': *malacoplakia, malacosarcosis, malacosteon.*

maladaptation, faulty intrapersonal adaptation to stress or change. It may involve a failure to make necessary changes in the desires, values, needs, and attitudes or an inability to make necessary adjustments in the external world. Illness often provokes maladaptive behavior that increases the problems accompanying the illness.

malaise, a vague feeling of bodily weakness or discomfort, often marking the onset of disease.

malar (mei′lər), of or pertaining to the cheek or the cheek bone.

malaria (məler′iə), a serious infectious illness caused by four species of the protozoan genus *Plasmodium,* characterized by chills, fever, anemia, an enlarged spleen, and a tendency to recur. The disease is transmitted from human to human by a bite from an infected *Anopheles* mosquito. Malarial infection can also be spread by blood transfusion from an infected patient or by the use of an infected hypodermic needle. Although the endemic disease is limited largely to tropical areas of South and Central America, Africa, and Asia, a number of new cases have been brought to the U.S. in recent years by refugees, military personnel returning from Southeast Asia, and travelers to malarial areas. *Plasmodium* parasites penetrate the erythrocytes of the human host, where they mature, reproduce, and burst out periodically. Malarial paroxysms occur at regular intervals, coinciding with the development of a new generation of parasites in the body. Because the life cycle of the infecting parasite varies according to species, the clinical patterns of chills and fever differ as do the course and severity of the disease. Bouts of malaria usually last from one to four weeks, with attacks occurring less frequently as the disease progresses. Relapse is common, and the disease can persist for years. Diagnosis is made by demonstrating the *Plasmodium* parasite in a blood smear. The organism is most likely to be seen in the blood during an acute attack. The exact species of *Plasmodium* must be identified, as the treatment and prognosis will vary according to the strain found. Chloroquine, given orally or intramuscularly, is the drug of choice for all but those strains of *Plasmodium* resistant to chloroquine, which are treated with a combination of quinine, pyrimethamine, and one of the sulfonamides or sulfones. Modern antimalarial drugs can suppress symptoms or cure malaria completely. Symptoms of headache, nausea, muscle ache, and high fever can be relieved with cold compresses and aspirin and fluids. Through the use of insecticides and by destroying the swampy habitat of *Anopheles,* the disease has been eliminated from most parts of the world where it has been endemic. Worldwide eradication of the disease has not been possible, however, and insecticide-resistant mosquitoes and drug-resistant protozoa have arisen. Prophylaxis with antimalarial drugs is still important for those visiting endemic areas. The use of netting and mosquito repellent is also encouraged. See also **blackwater fever, falciparum malaria, quartan malaria, tertian malaria.** — **malarial,** *adj.*

malarial hemoglobinuria. See **blackwater fever.**

malathion poisoning, a toxic condition caused by the ingestion or absorption through the skin of malathion, an organophosphorus insecticide. Symptoms include vomiting, nausea, abdominal cramps, headache, dizziness, weakness, confusion, convulsions, and respiratory difficulties. Treatment includes immediate intravenous administration of atropine, followed by pralidoxime chloride, gastric lavage, a saline cathartic, respiratory assistance, and oxygen. Malathion is much less toxic than parathion and is the only organophosphorus insecticide approved for household use.

malaxation. See **petrissage.**

Malayan pit viper venom. See **ancrod.**

mal del pinto (mæl'delpɪn'tou). See **pinta.**

male, **1. a.** of or pertaining to the sex that fertilizes the female to beget children. **b.** masculine. **2.** a male person.

male dietary allowance. See **dietary allowances, table of recommended daily dietary allowances.**

male reproductive system assessment, an evaluation of the condition of the patient's genitalia, reproductive history, and past and present genitourinary infections and disorders.

■ METHOD: In a relaxed, professional interview the procedures to be conducted are explained and the patient is reassured that his privacy will be scrupulously maintained. He is questioned about his offspring, sexual activity, the existence of nocturia, urgency, frequency, dysuria, urethral discharge, hernia, genital sores, discomfort or pain in the groin, lower back, or legs, and past treatment for epididymitis, gonorrhea, herpes genitalis, hydrocele, nonspecific urethritis, orchitis, prostatitis, syphilis, and varicocele. The examiner, while inspecting the genitalia, wears rubber gloves to prevent infection. The penis is examined for swelling, inflammation, and lesions, as herpes vesicles or a syphilitic sore, chancre, or scar. Anomalies that may be noted include hypospadias or epispadias, resulting from failed closure of the urethra, elongation of the foreskin constricting the urinary meatus, or swelling of the glans caused by a retracted, tight foreskin. The urethral orifice is inspected for a purulent or bloody discharge, and the scrotum is observed for symmetry and shape; in elderly or debilitated men the scrotum may be elongated and flat. The normally smooth testes, epididymes and spermatic cords are palpated for the presence of beading, varicosities, and the size, location, and consistency of any scrotal mass; fluid felt around the testes may be seen by darkening the room and illuminating the scrotum with a flashlight. The patient is asked to cough or bear down to reveal a hernia, and the abdomen is palpated above the symphysis pubis to determine if the bladder is distended. The inguinal lymph nodes are palpated, and the amount and distribution of pubic hair is observed. The prostate may be examined with the patient in the Sims' knee-chest position or lithotomy position, but, when possible, it is preferable for the patient to stand bent at a right angle over a table as the examiner's well-lubricated gloved forefinger sweeps the rectal circumference and palpates the lobes and medial sulcus of the gland. The size, consistency, and any localized nodule suggesting a neoplasm of the normally smooth, firm prostate are carefully noted, and the findings are recorded as on a clock dial with the symphysis pubis representing 12 o'clock. When additional studies are indicated, a smear is prepared from the first urine voided following massage of the prostate. Enzyme tests showing elevated phosphatase levels in serum suggest prostate cancer, but a diagnosis is usually established by a biopsy. Tissue may be obtained by a perineal, transurethal, or transrectal needle biopsy, but the most accurate method is an open perineal biopsy, which permits identification of the suspect lesion and the removal of multiple specimens. The assessment includes laboratory studies of discharge from the penis. A gram-stained smear usually confirms or rules out a diagnosis of gonorrhea, and a fluorescent-tagged antibody method may be required if the result is equivocal. Cultures may be needed to determine whether nonspecific urethritis is caused by *Escherichia coli, Pseudomonas, Staphylococcus, Streptococcus,* or organisms of other pathogenic genera. Syphilis may be diagnosed by the Veneral Disease Research Laboratory serologic test, but the Fluorescent Treponemal Antibody-Absorption test is the most sensitive and specific diagnostic measure. If infertility is a problem, examinations of multiple semen samples are conducted; each specimen collected after three days of abstinence is inspected in the laboratory to determine if the volume of the ejaculate approximates the normal 3.5 ml average and if the semen has a pH of 7.7 and a sperm count of 60 to 150 million per ml.

■ NURSING ORDERS: The nurse conducts the interview and examination, assembles the results of laboratory studies, and urges the patient to inform his sex partner, or partners, if an infectious disease is diagnosed. Throughout the assessment the nurse recognizes that the patient may be reluctant to discuss his symptoms and activities and be sensitive about the necessary procedures.

■ OUTCOME CRITERIA: A careful, understanding evaluation of the male patient's reproductive system helps to establish the diagnosis and plan the treatment and aids in allaying the patient's anxiety. The assessment also serves as a public health measure by encouraging the reporting of a sexually transmitted disease to the patient's contacts and proper authorities.

male sexual dysfunction, impaired or inadequate ability of a man to carry on his sex life to his own satisfaction. Symptoms, often psychologic in origin, include difficulties in starting and maintaining an erection, premature ejaculation, inability to ejaculate, and even loss of desire. Men are often so ashamed of the problem that they ask the physician to treat a "prostate problem," hoping that the covert message becomes clear. Compare **female sexual dysfunction.** See also **sexuality.**

malfeasance (mælfi'zəns), performance of an unlawful, wrongful act. Compare **misfeasance, nonfeasance.**

malformation, an anomalous structure in the body. See also **birth defect, congenital anomaly.**

malgaigne of pelvis (mælgei'nyə), trauma involving multiple pelvic fractures, including fracture of the wing of the ilium or sacrum and fracture of the ipsilateral pubic rami, with associated upper displacement of the hemipelvis.

malicious prosecution, (in law) a suit begun in malice and pursued without sufficient cause. It is usually an action for damages. Malicious prosecution is a wrongful civil proceeding, and a person who takes an active part in initiating or continuing it is subject to liability.

malignant (məlɪg'nənt), **1.** Also called **virulent.** tending to become worse and cause death. **2.** describing a cancer that is anaplastic, invasive, and metastatic. —**malignancy,** *n.*

malignant ependymoma. See **ependymoblastoma.**

malignant hemangioendothelioma. See **hemangiosarcoma.**

malignant hepatoma, a malignant tumor of the liver. Primary liver cancer is relatively rare in the United States, occurring one sixth to one fifth as often as in Africa and the Far East. The only effective treatment is surgical excision of the tumor. This is often not feasible, as the tumors grow rapidly and spread through both lobes of the liver. The prognosis is poor. Also called **hepatocarcinoma, hepatocellular carcinoma, liver cell carcinoma.**

malignant hypertension, an abnormal condition and the most lethal form of both essential hypertension and secondary hypertension. It is a fulminating condition, characterized by severely elevated blood pressure, that commonly damages the intima of small vessels, the brain, retina, heart, and kidneys. It affects more blacks than whites and may be caused by a variety of factors, as stress, genetic predisposition, obesity, the use of tobacco, the use of oral contraceptives, high intake of sodium chloride, a sedentary life-style, and aging. Many patients with this condition exhibit signs of hypokalemia, alkalosis, and aldosterone secretion rates even higher than those associated with primary aldosteronism.

malignant hyperthermia (MH), an autosomal dominant trait characterized by often fatal hyperthermia with rigidity of the muscles occurring in affected people exposed to certain anesthetic agents, particularly halothane, succinylcholine, and methoxyflurane. Treatment includes the administration of Dantrolene or 100 per cent oxygen,

cooling procedures, and the correction of acidosis and hyperkalemia. People who have malignant hyperthermia are informed of their condition and advised that one half of their first-degree relatives are likely to have the trait.

malignant malnutrition. See **kwashiorkor.**

malignant mesenchymoma, a sarcoma that contains two or more cellular elements, not including fibrous elements; a mixed cell sarcoma.

malignant mole. See **malignant melanoma.**

malignant neoplasm, a tumor that tends to grow, invade, and metastasize. It usually has an irregular shape and is composed of poorly differentiated cells. If untreated it may be expected to result in the death of the organism. The degree to which a neoplasm is malignant varies with the kind of tumor and the condition of the patient.

malignant neuroma. See **neurosarcoma.**

malignant pustule. See **anthrax.**

malignant tumor, a neoplasm that characteristically invades surrounding tissue, metastasizes to distant sites, and contains anaplastic cells. A malignant tumor may be expected to result in the death of the host if remission or treatment do not intervene.

malingering, a willful and deliberate feigning of the symptoms of a disease or injury to gain some consciously desired end. Compare **compensation neurosis.** —**malinger,** *v.,* **malingerer,** *n.*

malleolus (məli'ələs), *pl.* **malleoli.** a rounded bony process, as the protuberance on each side of the ankle.

mallet fracture, avulsion fracture of the dorsal base of a distal phalanx of the hand or foot, involving the associated extensor apparatus and causing dropped flexion of the distal segment.

malleus (mæl'iəs), one of the three ossicles in the middle ear, resembling a hammer with a head, neck, and three processes. It is connected to the tympanic membrane and transmits sound vibrations to the incus, which communicates with the stapes. Compare **incus, stapes.** See also **middle ear.**

Mallory-Weiss syndrome, a condition characterized by massive bleeding following a tear in the mucous membrane at the junction of the esophagus and the stomach. The laceration is usually caused by protracted vomiting, most commonly in alcoholics or in persons whose pylorus is obstructed. The esophageal tear is located by esophagoscopy or arteriography. Surgery is usually necessary to stop the bleeding. After repair, the prognosis is excellent.

malnutrition, any disorder concerning nutrition. It may result from an unbalanced, insufficient, or excessive diet or to the impaired absorption, assimilation, or utilization of foods. Compare **deficiency disease.**

malocclusion (mæl'əklu'ʐhən), abnormal contact of the

teeth of the upper jaw with the teeth of the lower jaw. See also **occlusion.**

malonic acid (məlou′nık), a white, crystalline, highly toxic substance used as an intermediate compound in the production of barbiturates.

Malpighian body (mælpıg′iən), **1.** the renal corpuscle, which includes a glomerulus with Bowman's capsule. **2.** lymphoid tissue surrounding the arteries of the spleen. Also called **lymphatic nodule.**

Malpighian corpuscle, one of a number of small, round, deep-red bodies in the cortex of the kidney, each communicating with a renal tubule. Malphigian corpuscles average about 0.2 mm in diameter, each capsule composed of two parts: a central glomerulus and a glomerular capsule. The corpuscles are thought to be part of a filter system through which nonprotein components of blood plasma enter the tubules for urinary excretion. Also called **Malpighian body, renal corpuscle.**

malpractice, (in law) professional negligence that is the proximate cause of injury or harm to a patient, resulting from a lack of professional knowledge, experience, or skill that can be expected in others in the profession or from a failure to exercise reasonable care or judgment in the application of professional knowledge, experience, or skill.

Malta fever. See **brucellosis.**

malt worker's lung, a respiratory disorder acquired by occupational exposure to fungi-laden particles of moldy barley grain or malt. See also **organic dust.**

malunion (mælyu′nyən), an imperfect union of previously fragmented bone or other tissue.

mamm-, a combining form meaning 'of or pertaining to the breast': *mammectomy, mammogram, mammotropic.*

mammary duct. See **lactiferous duct.**

mammary gland, one of two discoid, hemispherical glands on the chest of mature females, present in rudimentary form in children and in males. Glandular tissue forms a radius of lobes containing alveoli, each lobe having a system of ducts for the passage of milk from the alveoli to the nipple. The central portion of the breast is filled with glandular tissue; the periphery is made up mostly of adipose tissue. The left breast is usually larger than the right. Also called **breast, mamma.** See also **lactation.**

mammary papilla. See **nipple.**

mammillary body, either of the two small round masses of gray matter in the hypothalamus located close to one another in the interpeduncular space.

mammogram, an x-ray film of the soft tissues of the breast.

mammography, radiography of the soft tissues of the breast to allow identification of various benign and malignant neoplastic processes.

mammoplasty, plastic reshaping of the breasts, performed to reduce or lift enlarged or sagging breasts, to enlarge small breasts, or to reconstruct a breast after removal of a tumor. Antibiotic therapy is started before surgery. General anesthesia is used for all types of mammoplasty. To reduce the size of the breasts and raise them, excess tissue is removed from the underside of the breasts; the breast is then lifted and the nipple brought through an opening in an overhanging skin flap. To enlarge a breast, a thin plastic sac of silicone fluid is inserted in a pouch formed beneath the breast on the chest wall. The complications after surgery are infection and, with the use of implants, rejection reaction of tissues to the foreign body. The nurse observes the nipples for signs of vascular insufficiency or congestion, applies a firm supporting breast binder, and instructs the patient not to use her arms to lift herself. The patient stays prone in semi-Fowler's position, with elbows at her sides. Pain may be severe in the first days after surgery.

mammothermography, a diagnostic procedure in which thermography is used for examining the breast to detect abnormal growths. Compare **mammography.** See also **thermography.**

man-, a combining form meaning 'of or referring to the hand': *manoptoscope, manual, manudynamometer.*

-mancy, a combining form meaning 'divination in, through, or by': *hidromancy, labiomancy, uromancy.* Also **-mantia.**

Mandelamine, a trade name for an antibacterial (methenamine mandelate).

mandible (mæn′dıbəl), a large bone constituting the lower jaw. It contains the lower teeth and consists of a horizontal portion, a body, and two perpendicular rami that join the body at almost right angles. The body of the mandible is curved, somewhat resembling a horseshoe, and has two surfaces and two borders. The external surface is marked by the symphysis menti, indicating the junction of the two halves of the mandible in the fetus. Each ramus is topped by the anterior coronoid process and the posterior condyle, prominences separated by the mandibular notch. The superior border of the mandible contains sockets for the 16 lower teeth. The inferior border provides a groove for the facial artery. The mandible and its rami provide attachment for various muscles, as the masseter, temporalis, pterygoideus lateralis, digastricus, mentalis, genioglossi, geniohyoidei, and mylohyoideus. Also called **inferior maxillary bone.** Compare **maxilla.** — **mandibular,** *adj.*

mandibular sling, the connection between the mandible and the maxilla, formed by the masseter and the pterygoideus at the angle of the mandible. When the mouth is opened and closed the mandible moves around a center of rotation formed by the mandibular sling and the sphenomandibular ligament.

mandibulofacial dysostosis, an abnormal hereditary condition characterized by antimongoloid slant of the palpebral fissures, colomboma of the lower lid, micrognathia and hypoplasia of the zygomatic arches, and microtia. Evidence indicates that this disorder is transmitted as an autosomal dominant trait. The condition occurs in the complete form as Franceschetti's syndrome and in the incomplete form as Treacher Collins syndrome. See also **dysostosis.**

Mandol, a trade name for a cephalosporin antibiotic (cefamandole nafate).

maneuver, 1. an adroit or skillful manipulation or procedure. **2.** (in obstetrics) a manipulation of the fetus performed to aid in delivery.

manganese (Mn), a common metallic element found in trace amounts in tissues of the body. Its atomic number is 25; its atomic weight is 54.938.

mani-, a combining form meaning 'mental aberration': *mania, maniaphobia, manigraphy.*

mania, a mood disorder characterized by an expansive emotional state, extreme excitement, excessive elation, hyperactivity, agitation, overtalkativeness, flight of ideas, increased psychomotor activity, fleeting attention, and sometimes violent, destructive, or self-destructive behavior. It is manifested in the major affective disorders, specifically as the manic phase of bipolar disorder, and in certain organic mental disorders, as delirium and dementia. Kinds of mania include **Bell's mania, dancing mania, epileptic mania, hysterical mania, periodical mania, puerperal mania, transitory mania.** — maniac, *n., adj.,* maniacal, *adj.*

-mania, a combining form meaning a '(specified) state of mental disorder': *desanimania, enosimania, tristimania.*

-maniac, 1. a combining form meaning a 'person exhibiting a type of psychosis': *kleptomaniac, narcomaniac, toxicomaniac.* **2.** a combining form meaning a 'person revealing an inordinate interest in something': *ergomaniac, nymphomaniac, opiomaniac.*

-manic, 1. a combining form meaning a '(specified) psychosis': *choromanic, melomanic, poriomanic.* **2.** a combining form meaning a 'mental state like mania': *hyomanic, melomanic, submanic.*

manic depressive, a person with or exhibiting the symptoms of bipolar disorder.

manic-depressive psychosis. See **bipolar disorder.**

manipulation, the skillful use of the hands in therapeutic or diagnostic procedures, as palpation, reducing a dislocation, turning the position of the fetus, or various treatments in physical therapy and osteopathy. A kind of manipulation is **conjoined manipulation.** See also **massage.**

mannitol, an osmotic diuretic.

■ INDICATIONS: It is prescribed to promote diuresis, to decrease intraocular and intracranial pressure, to promote the excretion of poisons and other toxic wastes, and to evaluate renal function.

■ CONTRAINDICATIONS: Pulmonary edema, dehydration, or known hypersensitivity to this drug prohibits its use.

■ ADVERSE EFFECTS: Among the more serious adverse reactions are pulmonary edema, heart failure, hyponatremia, headache, vomiting, and confusion.

manometer (mənom'ıtər), a device for measuring the pressure of a fluid, consisting of a tube that is marked with a scale and contains a relatively incompressible fluid. The level of the fluid in the tube varies with the pressure of the fluid being measured. Kinds of manometer are **aneroid manometer, sphygmomanometer.**

Mansil, a trade name for a schistosicide (oxamniquine).

Mantadil, a trade name for a topical, fixed-combination drug containing a glucocorticoid (hydrocortisone acetate) and an antihistaminic (chlorcyclizine hydrochloride).

-mantia. See **-mancy.**

Mantoux test (mæntu'), a tuberculin skin test that consists of intradermal injection of a purified protein derivative of the tubercle bacillus. A hardened, raised red area of 8 to 10 mm, appearing 24 to 72 hours after injection, is a positive reaction. This method is the most reliable means of testing tuberculin sensitivity. See also **tuberculin test.**

manual rotation, an obstetric maneuver in which a baby's head is turned by hand from a transverse to an antero-posterior position in the birth canal to facilitate delivery. Compare **forceps rotation.**

manubriosternal articulation (mənu'brıoustər'nəl), the fibrocartilaginous connection between manubrium and the body of the sternum. This joint usually closes by the age of 25 years. Compare **xiphisternal articulation.**

manubrium (mənu'briəm), one of the three bones of the sternum, presenting a broad quadrangular shape which narrows caudally at its articulation with the superior end of the body of the sternum. The pectoralis major and the sternocleidomastoideus are attached to the manubrium. Compare **xiphoid process.** — manubrial, *adj.*

manus (mei'nəs), *pl.* manus. See **hand.**

many-tailed bandage, 1. a broad, evenly shaped bandage with both ends split into strips of equal size and number. As the bandage is placed on the abdomen, chest, or limb, the ends may be overlapped. **2.** an irregularly shaped bandage with torn or cut ends which are tied together. See also **scultetus bandage.**

MAO, abbreviation for **monoamine oxidase.**

MAO inhibitor. See **monoamine oxidase inhibitor.**

Maolate, a trade name for a skeletal-muscle relaxant (chlorphenesin carbamate).

MAP, abbreviation for **mean arterial pressure.**

map distance. See **map unit.**

maple bark disease, a hypersensitivity pneumonitis caused by exposure to the mold *Cryptostroma corticale,* found in the bark of maple trees. In the susceptible person, the condition may be acute, accompanied by fever, cough, dyspnea, and vomiting, or it may be chronic, characterized by fatigue, weight loss, dyspnea on exertion, and a productive cough. Although differential diagnosis may be difficult, a good occupational history may reveal the cause and the source of exposure. In an acute or severe case, a short course of prednisone may be used to control the symptoms; avoiding exposure to the bark prevents further reaction.

maple syrup urine disease,   an inherited metabolic disorder in which an enzyme necessary for the breakdown of the amino acids lysine, leucine, and isoleucine is lacking. The disease is usually diagnosed in infancy, being recognized by the characteristic maple-syrup odor of the urine and by hyperreflexia. Stress, fever, infection, and the ingestion of lysine, leucine, or isoleucine aggravate the condition. Treatment includes a diet avoiding these amino acids and, rarely, dialysis or transfusion.

mapping,   (in genetics) the process of locating the relative position of genes on a chromosome through the analysis of genetic recombination. Distances between genes in a linkage group are expressed in map or morgan units. Also called **chromosome mapping.**

maprotiline hydrochloride,   an antidepressant similar to the tricyclics.

■ INDICATION: It is prescribed for the treatment of mental depression.

■ CONTRAINDICATIONS: It is used with caution in conditions where anticholinergics are contraindicated, in seizure disorders, and in patients with cardiovascular disorders. Concomitant administration of monoamine oxidase inhibitors, recent myocardial infarction, or known hypersensitivity to this drug prohibits its use.

■ ADVERSE EFFECTS: Among the more serious adverse reactions are sedation and anticholinergic side effects. A variety of gastrointestinal, cardiovascular, and neurological (including convulsions) reactions may occur. The drug, like the tricyclics, is involved in many potential drug interactions.

map unit,   (in genetics) an arbitrary unit of measure used to designate the distance between genes on a chromosome. It is calculated from the percentage of recombination that occurs between specific genes so that one per cent of crossing over represents one unit on a genetic map or approximately the number of new combinations that can be detected. The measurement is accurate only for small distances, since double crossovers do not appear as new recombinations. Also called **map distance.** See also **morgan.**

marasmic kwashiorkor,   a malnutrition disease, primarily of children, resulting from the deficiency of both calories and protein. The condition is characterized by severe tissue wasting, dehydration, loss of subcutaneous fat, lethargy, and growth retardation.

marasmic thrombus,   an aggregation of blood platelets, fibrin, clotting factors, and cellular elements formed in infants with marasmus. Marasmic thrombus is often a terminal event in cachexia.

marasmus (məræz′məs),   a condition of extreme malnutrition and emaciation, occurring chiefly in young children, that is characterized by progressive wasting of subcutaneous tissue and muscle. It results from a lack of adequate calories and proteins and is seen in failure-to-thrive children and in starvation. Less commonly, marasmus occurs as a result of an inability to assimilate or utilize protein owing to a defect in metabolism. Care of the marasmic child involves the reestablishment of fluid and electrolyte balance, followed by the slow and gradual addition of foods as they are tolerated. Stimulation appropriate to the developmental age should be provided. As much of the care of the child as possible should be given consistently by one person, as it must be assumed that the physically starved child has also been emotionally deprived. See also **failure to thrive, kwashiorkor.**

marathon encounter group,   an intensive group experience that accelerates self-awareness and promotes personal growth and behavioral change through the continuous interaction of group members for a period ranging from 16 to more than 40 hours. See also **encounter group.**

Marax,   a trade name for a respiratory, fixed-combination drug containing a smooth-muscle relaxant (theophylline), an adrenergic (ephedrine sulfate), and a tranquilizer (hydroxyzine hydrochloride).

marble bones.   See **osteopetrosis.**

Marburg-Ebola virus disease (mar′bɔrgeb′ələ),   a serious febrile disease characterized by rash and severe gastrointestinal hemorrhages. An epidemic in Marburg, Germany, in 1967, was apparently contracted from imported monkeys. In 1976, in the Ebola River District of Zaire and Sudan, an explosive epidemic occurred with a mortality of 85 per cent. This disease may be transmitted to hospital personnel by improper handling of contaminated needles or from hemorrhagic lesions of patients. The diagnosis is made by serologic abnormalities. There is no effective treatment.

Marcaine Hydrochloride,   a trade name for a local anesthetic (bupivacaine hydrochloride).

march foot,   an abnormal condition of the foot owing to excessive use, as in a long march. The forefoot is swollen and painful, and one or more of the metatarsal bones may be broken. See also **stress fracture.**

march fracture.   See **metatarsal stress fracture.**

march hemoglobinuria,   a rare, abnormal condition, characterized by the presence of hemoglobin in the urine, that occurs following strenuous physical exertion or prolonged exercise, as marching or distance running. See also **hemolysis.**

Marchiafava-Micheli disease (mar′kyəfa′vəmɪkei′li), a rare disorder of unknown etiology characterized by episodic hemoglobinuria, occurring usually, but not always, at night.

Marchi's method (mar′kiz), a laboratory staining procedure for demonstrating degenerated nerve fibers. The tissue specimen is first fixed in a solution of potassium bichromate, which prevents normal nerve fibers from being stained with osmic acid; osmic acid is then applied as a definitive stain for abnormal nerve fibers.

Marcus Gunn pupil sign, paradoxical dilation of the pupils in an ophthalmologic examination in response to afferent visual stimuli. In a dark room a beam of light is moved from one eye to the other. Normal meiosis is caused by the consensual pupil reaction when the normal eye is illuminated; but as the light is moved to the opposite, abnormal eye, the direct reaction to light is weaker than the consensual reaction; hence both pupils dilate.

Marezine Hydrochloride, a trade name for an antiemetic (cyclizine hydrochloride).

Marfan's syndrome (marfanz′), an abnormal condition characterized by elongation of the bones, often with associated abnormalities of the eyes and the cardiovascular system. Marfan's syndrome is inherited as an autosomal-dominant trait. The disease causes major pathologic musculoskeletal disturbances, as muscular underdevelopment, ligamentous laxity, joint hypermobility, and bone elongation. With Marfan's syndrome pathologic alterations of the cardiovascular system appear to produce fragmentation of the elastic fibers in the media of the aorta, which may lead to aneurysm. Ocular changes associated with the disease include a variety of disorders, including dislocation of the lens. Cardiac and ocular involvement occurs in approximately half of the patients affected. The disease affects men and women equally, elongating the limbs so that most adult patients with the disease are over six feet tall. The extremities of individuals with Marfan's syndrome are very long and spiderlike, with greatly extended metacarpals, metatarsals, and phalanges. The skulls of such patients are usually asymmetric. Pectus excavatum is common and a lateral curvature of the spine may develop and increase during years of rapid vertebral growth with kyphoscoliosis developing to varying degrees. The severe ligamental laxity and the joint hypermobility associated with Marfan's syndrome may be seen by radiographic examination and often results in pes valgus and genu recurvatum. No specific treatment is advocated for Marfan's syndrome and symptomatic management of the associated problems is the usual alternative. Resulting deformities, as kyphoscoliosis, may be treated with orthoses or other surgical procedures, as indicated. Also called **arachnodactyly.**

marginal peptic ulcer, an ulcer that develops postoperatively at the surgical anastomosis of the stomach and jejunum. See also **peptic ulcer.**

marginal placenta previa, placenta previa in which the placenta is implanted in the lower uterine segment, with its margin touching or spreading to some degree over the internal os of the uterine cervix. During labor, as the cervix dilates, bleeding may occur from the separation of the edge of the placenta from the uterus beneath it. Bleeding may be so scant as to pose no clinical problem. In some cases frank severe hemorrhage may occur, but the pressure of the presenting part of the baby is often sufficient to act as a tamponade, arresting the hemorrhage. Diagnosis of marginal placenta previa may be suggested by the apparent location of the placenta on ultrasonic visualization. Caesarean section is not usually necessary. See also **placenta previa.**

marginal rale. See **atelectatic rale.**

Marie-Strumpell disease (məri′strəm′pəl). See **ankylosing spondylitis.**

marijuana. See **cannabis.**

mark, any nevus or birthmark.

marker gene. See **genetic marker.**

Marplan, a trade name for an antidepressant (isocarboxazid).

marrow. See bone **marrow.**

Marseilles fever, a disease endemic around the Mediterranean, in Africa, the Crimea, and India, caused by *Rickettsia conorii* transmitted by the brown dog tick (*Rhipicephalus sanguineus*). Characteristic symptoms are chills, fever, an ulcer covered with a black crust at the site of the tick bite, and a rash appearing on the second to fourth day. Also called **boutonneuse fever, Bruch's disease, Conor's disease, escharonodulaire, Indian tick fever, Kenya fever.**

marsupialize, to form a pouch surgically in order to treat a cyst when simple removal would not be effective, as in a pancreatic or a pilonidal cyst. Under general or local anesthesia, the cyst sac is opened and emptied. Its edges are sutured to adjacent tissues, and a drain is left in place. Secretions decrease over a period of several months and may eventually cease.

Martorell's disease (martərelz′). See **aortic arch syndrome.**

Martorell's syndrome. See **Takayasu's arteritis.**

masculine, having the characteristics of a male. —**masculinization,** n., **masculinize,** v.

masculinization. See **adrenal virilism, virilization.**

mask, 1. to obscure, as symptomatic treatment that may mask the development of a disease. 2. to cover, as a skin-toned cosmetic that may mask a pigmented nevus. 3. a cover worn over the nose and mouth to prevent inhalation of toxic or irritating materials, to control delivery of oxygen or anesthetic gas, or (by medical personnel) to shield a patient during aseptic procedures from pathogenic organisms normally exhaled from the respiratory tract.

masking, 1. the covering or concealing of a disorder by a second condition, as when a person begins a weight-loss diet while an undiagnosed wasting disease such as cancer has developed. The loss of body weight is attributed to the diet, masking the disease and delaying diagnosis and treatment. **2.** the unconscious display of a personality trait that conceals a behavioral aberration.

masking agent, a cosmetic preparation for covering nevi, surgical scars, and other blemishes. Masking agents are generally composed of a flesh-colored pigment in a lotion or cream base.

mask of pregnancy. See **chloasma.**

Maslow's hierarchy of need, (in sociology) a hierarchical categorization of the basic needs of man. The most basic needs on the scale are the physiologic or biologic, as the need for air, food, or water. Of second priority are the safety needs, including protection and freedom from fear and anxiety. The subsequent order of needs in the hierarchical progression are the need to belong, to love, and to be loved; the need for self-esteem; and ultimately, the need for self-actualization. To progress from one need to another the more basic need must first be satisfied.

masochism, pleasure or gratification derived from receiving physical, mental, or emotional abuse. The maltreatment may be inflicted by another person or by oneself. Compare **sadism.** – **masochist,** *n.,* **masochistic,** *adj.*

masochist, a person deriving pleasure or gratification from masochistic acts or abuse. See also **masochism.**

mass, 1. the physical property of matter that gives it weight and inertia. **2.** (in pharmacology) a mixture from which pills are formed. **3.** an aggregate of cells clumped together as a tumor. Compare **weight.** See also **inertia.**

massage, the manipulation of the soft tissue of the body through stroking, rubbing, kneading, or tapping, to increase circulation, to improve muscle tone, and to relax the patient. The procedure is performed either with the bare hands or through some mechanical means, as a vibrator. The most common sites for massage are the back, knees, elbows, and heels. Care is taken not to massage inflamed areas, particularly of the extremities, because of the danger of loosening blood clots; open wounds and areas of rash, tumor, or excessive sensitivity are avoided. The procedure is performed with the patient prone or on the side, comfortably positioned, with an emollient lotion or cream applied to the area to be massaged. The nurse's hands are warm, and excessive pressure is avoided so as not to cause pain or injury. Kinds of massage are **cardiac massage, effleurage, flagellation, friction, fréolement, petrissage, tapotement, vibration.**

-massage, a combining form meaning a 'therapeutic kneading of the body': *electromassage, hydromassage, phonomassage.*

masseter (mæsi'tər), the thick, rectangular muscle in the cheek that functions to close the jaw. It is one of the four muscles of mastication and consists of a superficial portion and a deep portion, each arising from the zygomatic arch and inserting into the mandible. The deep portion is the smaller and more muscular of the two parts. The masseter is innervated by the masseteric nerve from the mandibular division of the trigeminal nerve.

mass reflex, an abnormal condition, seen in patients with transection of the spinal cord, characterized by a widespread nerve discharge, resulting in flexor muscle spasms, incontinence of urine and feces, priapism, hypertension, and profuse sweating.

■ OBSERVATIONS: A mass reflex may be triggered by scratching or other painful stimulus to the skin, overdistention of the bladder or intestines, cold weather, prolonged sitting, or emotional stress. Muscle spasms may be so violent as to throw the patient off a bed or stretcher.

■ INTERVENTION: Medications to reduce mass reflexes include diazepam, dantraline, chlordiazepoxide, and meprobamate. Hubbard baths and exercises in warm water also help. Occasionally chordotomy, rhizotomy, peripheral nerve transaction, or tenotomy may be necessary.

■ NURSING CONSIDERATIONS: Nurses should avoid stimulating areas that trigger mass reflexes and should be prepared to accept them when they occur and to explain the cause to the patient. It is important to prevent decubitus ulcers and bladder infections in paraplegic and quadriplegic patients as they may also serve as triggers to initiate mass reflexes. Siderails should be kept up on the bed and restraining straps secured to transportation stretchers and Stryker frames. Psychotherapeutic counseling may also help reduce stress and the frequency of mass reflexes.

mass spectrometer, an analytic instrument for identifying a substance by sorting a stream of charged particles (ions) according to their mass. The sorting is usually accomplished by deflecting a stream of charged particles into a semicircular path as it enters a magnetic field and ultimately strikes a photographic plate or a photomultiplier tube sensor.

mass spectrometry, (in chemistry) a technique for the analysis of a substance in which the constituents are identified and quantified using a mass spectrometer. See also **spectrometry, spectrophotometry.**

mast-. See **masto.**

mastalgia (mæstæl'jə), pain in the breast caused by congestion or 'caking' during lactation, an infection, fibrocystic disease, especially during or prior to menstruation, or advanced cancer. The early stages of breast cancer are rarely accompanied by pain. – **mastalgic,** *adj.*

mast cell, a constituent of connective tissue containing large basophilic granules that bear heparin, serotonin, bradykinin, and histamine. These substances are freed from the mast cell in response to injury and infection.

mast cell leukemia, a malignant neoplasm of leukocytes characterized by many connective tissue mast cells in circulating blood.

mastectomy, the surgical removal of one or both breasts, performed to remove a malignant tumor. In a simple mastectomy, only breast tissue is removed. In a radical mastectomy, some of the muscles of the chest are removed with the breast and with all lymph nodes in the axilla. In a modified radical mastectomy, the large muscles of the chest which move the arm are preserved. Under general anesthesia, a biopsy of tissue taken from the tumor is performed if this was not previously done. If the specimen shows a malignancy, the tumor and adjacent tissues are removed in one piece. After surgery, a drainage catheter is placed in the wound. The nurse inspects the wound for swelling or excessive bleeding and encourages the patient to take deep breaths and to cough at frequent intervals. The affected arm is positioned with the hand pointed upwards or on pillows so that the hand is higher than the lower arm, with the lower arm above heart level. Hand and wrist movements and flexion and extension of the elbow are begun within 24 hours and performed regularly. No abduction or external rotation of the upper arm is permitted before the tenth day. An elastic bandage and, later, a pressure gradient elastic sleeve are used to reduce edema of the arm. The patient is fitted with a prosthesis when the wound is completely healed. Emotional support and counseling are essential. See also **modified radical mastectomy, radical mastectomy, simple mastectomy.** – **mastectomize,** *v.*

master problem list, (in a problem-oriented medical record) a list of a client's problems that serves as an index to the client's record. Each problem, the date the problem was first noted, the treatment, and the outcome are added to the master problem list as each becomes known. Thus, the master problem list provides an on-going guide for reviewing the health status of the client and for planning care for the client.

master's degree program in nursing, a postgraduate program in a school of nursing, based in a university setting, that grants the degree Master of Science in Nursing (M.S.N.) to successful candidates. Most programs include theory of nursing and techniques in nursing research as integral parts of the curriculum. The degree may be awarded for work in maternal-newborn nursing, medical-surgical nursing, pediatric nursing, psychiatric nursing or in other fields of nursing. Nurses with this degree often work in leadership roles in clinical nursing, as consultants in various settings, in faculty positions in schools of nursing, and as nurse practitioners in the various specialties.

-mastia. See **-mazia.**

mastication (mæs′tɪkeɪ′ʃən), chewing, tearing, or grinding food with the teeth while it becomes mixed with saliva. See also **bolus, digestion, ptyalin.**

mastitis (mæstaɪ′tɪs), an inflammatory condition of the breast, usually caused by streptococcal or staphylococcal infection. **Acute mastitis,** most common in the first two months of lactation, is characterized by pain, swelling, redness, axillary lymphadenopathy, fever, and malaise. If untreated or inadequately treated, abscesses may form. Antibiotics, rest, analgesia, and warm soaks are usually prescribed. Usually, breast feeding may continue. **Chronic tuberculous mastitis** is rare; when it occurs it represents

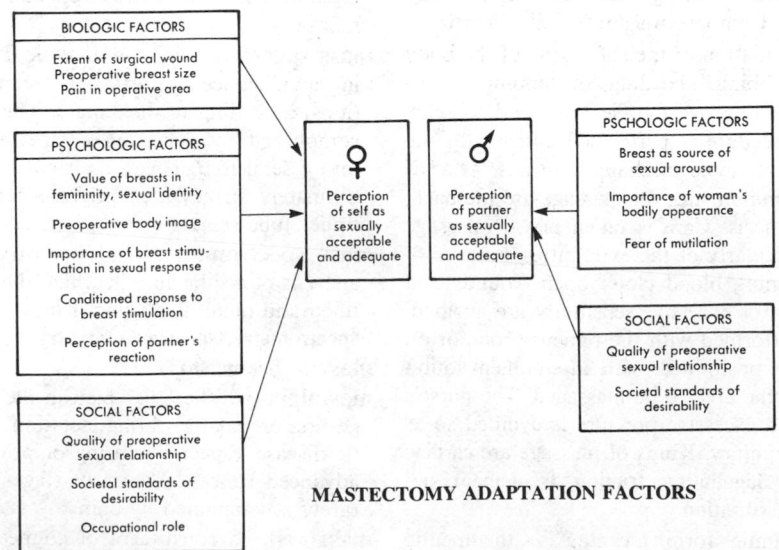

MASTECTOMY ADAPTATION FACTORS

extension of tuberculosis from the lungs and ribs beneath the breast.

masto-, mast-, a combining form meaning 'of or pertaining to the breast': *mastochondroma, mastologist, mastoplasia.*

mastocytosis, local or systemic overproduction of mast cells, which, in rare instances, may infiltrate liver, spleen, bones, the gastrointestinal system, and skin. Systemic mastocytosis may precede mast cell leukemia.

mastoid (mæs'toid), **1.** of or pertaining to the mastoid process of the temporal bone. **2.** breast-shaped.

mastoidectomy, surgical excision of a portion of the mastoid part of the temporal bone, performed to treat chronic suppurative otitis media or mastoiditis when systemic antibiotics are ineffective. Entry is made through the ear canal or from behind the ear. In a simple mastoidectomy, under general anesthesia, infected bone cells are removed and the eardrum is incised to drain the middle ear. Topical antibiotics are then instilled in the ear. In a radical procedure, the eardrum and most middle ear structures are removed; the stapes is left intact so a hearing aid may be used. The opening to the eustachian tube is plugged. In a modified radical procedure, the eardrum and the middle ear structures are saved, and the patient will hear better than after a radical mastoidectomy. After surgery any bright red blood on the dressing may indicate hemorrhage. A stiff neck or disorientation may signal the onset of meningitis. Dizziness is usual and may be expected to last for several days.

mastoiditis (mæs'toidai'tis), an infection of one of the mastoid bones, usually an extension of a middle ear infection, characterized by earache, fever, headache, and malaise. The infection is difficult to treat, often requiring antibiotics administered intravenously for several days. Children are most often affected. Residual hearing loss may follow the infection.

mastoid process, the conical projection of the caudal, posterior portion of the temporal bone, serving as the attachment for various muscles, including the sternocleidomastoideus, splenius capitis, and longissimus capitis. A hollow section of the process contains air cells which are distinguished from a large, irregular tympanic antrum in the superior anterior portion of the process. See also **temporal bone.**

masturbation, sexual activity in which the penis or clitoris is stimulated, usually to orgasm, by means other than coitus. It is performed, at least occasionally, by most people and is considered to be normal and harmless. Also called, in men, **onanism.** — **masturbate,** *v,* **masturbatic, masturbatory,** *adj.*

-masty. See **-mazia.**

matched group. See **group.**

materia (mətir'iə), matter or material, as materia medica.

material fact, (in law) a fact that establishes or refutes an element essential to the complaint, or charge, or to the defense. The presence of a material fact in a case being tried precludes granting of a summary judgment.

materia medica, **1.** the study of drugs and other substances used in medicine, their origins, preparation, uses, and effects. **2.** a substance or a drug used in medical treatment.

Materna 1.60, a trade name for an antenatal multivitamin supplement with calcium and iron.

maternal and child health (MCH) services, various facilities and programs organized for the purpose of providing medical and social services for mothers and children. Medical services include prenatal, postnatal, family planning care, and pediatric care in infancy.

maternal-child attachment. See **maternal-infant bonding.**

maternal-child separation syndrome. See **separation anxiety.**

maternal deprivation syndrome, a condition characterized by developmental retardation that occurs as a result of physical or emotional deprivation. It is seen primarily in infants. Typical symptoms include lack of physical growth, with weight below the third percentile for age and size, malnutrition, pronounced withdrawal, silence, apathy, and irritability, and a characteristic posture and body language, featuring unnatural stiffness and rigidity with a slow response reaction to others. Causes of the syndrome are usually multiple and complex, involving such factors as parental indifference, emotional instability or insecurity of the mother, lack of or delayed development of the mother-child attachment process, unrealistic expectations or disappointment concerning the sex, appearance, or adaptability of the child, or unfavorable socioeconomic conditions within the family. Treatment often requires hospitalization, especially in cases of severe malnutrition. Care includes assessment of the family situation, and treatment often involves psychotherapy, counseling, or special nursing instruction to help the parents learn to deal with and provide for the child. The nature and extent of the effects of the condition on later physical, emotional, intellecutal, and social development vary considerably and depend on the age at which deprivation occurs, the degree and duration of the situation, the constitutional makeup of the child, and the substituted care that is provided. Emotionally deprived children often remain below normal in intellecutal development, fail to learn acceptable social behavior, and are unable to form trusting, meaningful relationships with others. In severe cases of early and prolonged deprivation, the damage to an infant may be irreversible. See also **failure to thrive.**

maternal effect. See **maternal inheritance.**

maternal-infant bonding, the complex process of attachment of a mother to her newborn baby. Disastrous effects of the disruption or absence of this attachment have long been known. The specific steps in its development and the factors that disturb or encourage it have been identified and described by anthropologists, pediatricians, nurses, midwives, and sociologists. Two principal investigators are Marshal Klaus, M.D. and John Kennel, M.D. In their book, *Parental-Infant Bonding,* they state: "This original mother-infant bond is the wellspring for all the infant's subsequent attachments and is the formative relationship in the course of which the child develops a sense of himself. Throughout his lifetime, the strength and character of this attachment will influence the quality of all future bonds to other individuals." The process begins before birth as the parents plan for the pregnancy and then discover that the mother is pregnant. The mother feels fetal movement, begins to accept the fetus as an individual, and makes plans for the baby after birth. In the first minutes and hours after birth, a sensitive period occurs during which the baby and the mother become intimately involved with each other via behaviors and stimuli that are complementary and that provoke further interactions. The mother touches the baby and holds it en face to achieve eye-to-eye contact. The infant looks back eye to eye. The mother speaks in a quiet, high-pitched voice. The mother and the baby move in turn to the voice and sounds of the other, a process known as entrainment; it can be likened to a dance. The infant's movements constitute a response to the mother's voice, and she is encouraged to continue the process. The secretion of oxytocin and prolactin by the maternal pituitary gland is stimulated by the baby's sucking or licking of the mother's breasts; T and B lymphocytes and macrophages are given to the baby in the mother's milk, promoting resistance to infection. The child is also colonized by the normal flora of the mother's skin and nasal passages, improving the baby's ability to fend off infection. Physically, the mother provides her body heat for the baby's warmth and comfort. Thus, the extended contact in the newborn period satisfies physical as well as emotional needs of the mother and baby. Kennel and Klaus make the following recommendations to enhance the development of maternal-infant bonding: the special needs of the mother are assessed before delivery, the parents are given classes to prepare them for labor, delivery, and the puerperium, and discussions are held regarding the stresses of pregnancy and the postpartum period. In labor and delivery, a companion is encouraged to stay with the mother. After the baby is born, silver nitrate drops are not placed in the baby's eyes until the mother and the baby have had time to be together en face, with eye contact for an extended period of time, as the drops cause a film to form over the eyes, dimming vision. During the first hour after birth the parents and the infant are not separated and are given as much privacy as possible. Skin-to-skin contact is

encouraged; various methods may be used to maintain an ambient temperature adequate to maintain the baby's temperature. On the postpartum unit the mother and the baby are kept together for at least five hours a day, but optimally for 24 hours a day in a 24-hour rooming-in unit. The entire family is allowed to visit. The mother has responsibility for the care of her baby, with consultation available from a midwife or a nurse. The staff does not criticize the mother's performance, as it is to the baby's inestimable benefit that the mother believes her baby is the best, most beautiful, perfect baby in the world and that she feels able to care for her baby. Many changes in facilities, in staff training, and in hospital policy are needed to give every mother and infant the chance to bond fully in the early days of their life together.

maternal inheritance, the transmission of traits or conditions controlled by cytoplasmic factors within the ovum that are not self-replicating and are determined by genes within the nucleus. An example of such a characteristic is the direction of coiling in the shells of snails. Also called **maternal effect.**

maternity cycle, the antepartal, intrapartal, and postpartal periods of pregnancy and the puerperium, from conception to six weeks after birth.

maternity nursing, nursing care of women and their families during pregnancy, parturition, and through the first days of the puerperium. Increasingly, postpartum maternity nursing includes the supervision of the mothers' care of their newborns in rooming-in units and may include care of normal newborns in the nursery when they are not with their mothers. Maternity nursing requires extensive instruction of the mothers in the usual behavior and needs of a newborn, expected patterns of growth and development of the infant during the first week, and in details of care needed by the mother during the first weeks after birth. Breastfeeding, bottlefeeding, baby baths, perineal care, nutrition, and danger signs of the puerperium are usually taught by the maternity nurse. Observation for abnormal conditions, as thrombophlebitis, mastitis and other infections, and pre-eclampsia are daily on-going concerns of the maternity nurse on the postpartum unit. Intrapartum maternity nursing involves the care of mothers in labor and delivery, as well as high risk technical nursing, emotional support in labor and delivery, and the customary on-going observation for abnormal signs or symptoms. Often, pregnant women with medical problems associated with pregnancy are cared for on a special high-risk antepartum unit by specially trained maternity nurses.

matrifocal family (mæt′rɪfoʊ′kəl), a family unit comprised of a mother and her children. Biologic fathers have a temporary place in the family during the first years of the children's lives, but they maintain a more permanent position in their own original families. Common characteristics of this kind of family include living at a subsistence level, owing to irregular employment of the fathers and unreliable economic support from them, and child care by older female relatives so that the mother of the children is free to work.

matrix, 1. an intercellular substance, 2. Also called **ground substance.** a basic substance from which a specific organ or kind of tissue develops. 3. a form used in shaping a tooth surface in dental procedures.

Matropinal, a trade name for a gastrointestinal, fixed-combination drug containing an anticholinergic (homatropine methylbromide) and a sedative-hypnotic (phenobarbital).

matter, 1. anything that has mass and occupies space. 2. any substance not otherwise identified as to its constituents, as gray matter, pus, or serum exuding from a wound.

Matulane, a trade name for an antineoplastic (procarbazine hydrochloride).

maturation, 1. the process or condition of attaining complete development. In man, the unfolding of full physical, emotional, and intellectual capacities that enable a person to function at a higher level of competency and adaptability within the environment. 2. See also **meiosis, oogenesis, spermatogenesis.** the final stages in the meiotic formation of germ cells in which the number of chromosomes in each cell is reduced to the haploid number characteristic of the species. 3. suppuration. —**maturate,** v.

mature, 1. to become fully developed, to ripen. 2. fully developed or ripened.

mature cell leukemia. See **polymorphocytic leukemia.**

maturity, 1. a state of complete growth or development, usually designated as the period of life between adolescence and old age. 2. the stage at which an organism is capable of reproduction.

maturity-onset diabetes, diabetes mellitus arising in adults, usually after the age of fifty. See also **diabetes mellitus.**

Maxibolin, a trade name for an anabolic (ethylestrenol).

Maxidex, a trade name for a glucocorticoid (dexamethasone).

maxilla (mæksɪl′ə), pl. **maxillae.** one of a pair of large bones that form the upper jaw, consisting of a pyramidal body and four processes: the zygomatic, frontal, alveolar, and palatine.

-maxilla, a combining form meaning the 'upper jaw or the bones composing it': *intermaxilla, submaxilla, supermaxilla.*

maxillary artery, either of two larger terminal branches of the external carotid arteries that rise from the neck of the mandible near the parotid gland and divide into three branches, supplying the deep structures of the face.

maxillary sinus, one of the pair of large air cells forming a pyramidal cavity in the body of the maxilla. The apex of each sinus extends into the zygomatic arch, and its floor, formed by the aveolar process, is usually 1 to 10 ml below the floor of the nose. In the adult the volume of the sinus averages 14.75 cu cm. The mucous membrane of the sinus is continuous with that of the nasal cavity; an opening in the medial wall of the sinus communicates with the middle meatus. In the fourth month of gestation the embryonic sinus appears as a shallow groove on the medial surface of the bone but does not reach full size until after the second teething. Compare **ethmoidal air cell, frontal sinus, sphenoidal sinus.**

maxillary vein, one of a pair of deep veins of the face, accompanying the maxillary artery and passing between the condyle of the mandible and the sphenomandibular ligament. Each maxillary vein is formed by the confluence of veins in the pterygoid plexus and joins the superficial temporal vein to form the retromandibular vein. Each maxillary vein is a tributary of the internal jugular and the external jugular veins.

maxillofacial prosthesis, a prosthetic replacement for part, or all, of the upper jaw, nose, or cheek. It is applied when surgical repair alone is inadequate.

maxillomandibular fixation (mæksɪl′oumændɪb′yulər), stabilization of fractures of the face or jaw by temporarily connecting the maxilla and mandible by wires, elastic bands, or metal splints. See also **elastic band fixation, nasomandibular fixation.**

maximal breathing capacity, the amount of gas exchanged per minute with maximal rate and depth of respiration.

maximal expiratory flow rate (MEFR), the rate of the most rapid flow of gas from the lungs during the expiratory phase of respiration.

maximum inspiratory pressure (MIP), the maximum pressure within the alveoli of the lungs that occurs during the inspiratory phase of respiration.

maximum permissible dose equivalent, (in radiotherapy) the greatest amount of radiation that a person or a specific body part is allowed to receive in a given period of time.

Maxitrol, a trade name for an ophthalmic, fixed-combination drug containing a glucocorticoid (dexamethasone) and antibacterials (neomycin sulfate and polymyxin B sulfate).

Mayer's reflex (mei′ərz), a normal reflex elicited by grasping the ring finger and flexing it at the metacarpalphalangeal joint of a subject whose hand is relaxed with thumb abducted. The normal response is adduction and apposition of the thumb. The reflex is absent in disease of the pyramidal system.

May-Hegglin anomaly, an inherited hematologic condition characterized by leukopenia, giant platelets, and Doehle bodies. The condition is usually benign but may be associated with a decreased ability of the blood to coagulate. Compare **Pelger-Huet anomaly.**

Mayo scissors (mei′ou). See **scissors.**

-mazia, a combining form meaning '(condition of the) breasts': *macromazia, pleomazia, polymazia.* Also **-mastia, -masty.**

mazindol (mei′zındoul), an anorectic.

■ INDICATION: It is prescribed to decrease the appetite in the treatment of exogenous obesity.

■ CONTRAINDICATIONS: Glaucoma, history of drug abuse, concomitant use of a monoamine oxidase inhibitor, or known hypersensitivity to this drug prohibits its use.

■ ADVERSE EFFECTS: Among the more serious adverse reactions are insomnia, palpitation, dizziness, dry mouth, tachycardia, and hypersensitivity reactions.

mazo-, a combining form meaning 'of or pertaining to the breast': *mazodynia, mazology, mazopexy.*

MBC, abbreviation for **maximal breathing capacity.**

MBD, abbreviation for **minimal brain dysfunction.** See also **attention deficit disorder.**

mc, abbreviation for **millicurie.**

mC, abbreviation for **millicoulomb.**

McArdle's disease (mıkar′dəlz), an inherited metabolic disease in which abnormally large amounts of glycogen accumulate in skeletal muscle. It is milder than other glycogen storage diseases, characterized only by muscle weakness and cramping after exercise. There is no known treatment. Also called **glycogen storage disease, type V.** See also **glycogen storage disease.**

MCAT, abbreviation for **Medical College Aptitude Test.**

McBurney's point, a site of extreme sensitivity in acute appendicitis, situated in the normal area of the appendix about two inches below the right anterior superior spine of the ilium, on a line between that spine and the umbilicus.

McBurney's sign, a reaction of the patient indicating severe pain and extreme tenderness when McBurney's point is palpated. Such a reaction indicates appendicitis.

mcg, abbreviation for **microgram.**

MCH, 1. abbreviation for **mean corpuscular hemoglobin.** 2. abbreviation for **maternal and child health.**

MCHC, abbreviation for **mean corpuscular hemoglobin concentration.**

mCi, mc, abbreviation for **millicurie.**

McManus, R. Louise (1885–), an American nurse and writer who established the first national testing service for the nursing profession, currently the second largest educational testing program in the nation. She was also instrumental in developing a means of evaluating the nursing programs of community and junior colleges, and she established a center for training in research in nursing at Teachers College, Columbia University.

McMurray's sign, an audible click heard when rotat-

ing the tibia on the femur, indicating injury to meniscal structures.

MCTD, abbreviation for **mixed connective tissue disease.**

MCV, abbreviation for **mean corpuscular volume.**

M.D., abbreviation for *Doctor of Medicine.* See **physician.**

mean, 1. occupying a position midway between two extremes of a set of values or data. 2. **arithmetic mean,** a value that is derived by dividing the total of a set of values by the number of items in the set. 3. **geometric mean,** a value that is between the first and last of a set of values organized in a geometric progression.

mean arterial pressure (MAP), the arithmetic mean of the blood pressure in the arterial portion of the circulation.

mean corpuscular hemoglobin (MCH), an estimate of the amount of hemoglobin in an average erythrocyte, derived from the ratio between the amount of hemoglobin and the number of erythrocytes present in a specimen. The normal MCH is between 28 and 32 picograms of hemoglobin per red blood cell. See also **hypochromic anemia, iron-deficiency anemia.**

mean corpuscular hemoglobin concentration (MCHC), an estimation of the concentration of hemoglobin in grams per 100 ml of packed red blood cells, derived from the ratio of the hemoglobin to the hematocrit. The normal MCHC is between 32 per cent and 36 per cent.

mean corpuscular volume (MCV), an evaluation of the average volume of each red cell, derived from the ratio of the volume of packed red cells (the hematocrit) to the total number of red blood cells. The normal MCV is between 82 and 92 cu microns.

measles, an acute, highly contagious, viral disease involving the respiratory tract and characterized by a spreading maculopapular cutaneous rash that occurs primarily in young children who have not been immunized. Measles is caused by a paramyxovirus and is transmitted by direct contact with droplets spread from the nose, throat, and mouth of infected persons, usually in the prodromal stage of the disease. Indirect transmission by uninfected persons or by contaminated articles is unusual. Diagnosis is confirmed by the identification of Koplik spots on the buccal mucosa and by bacteriologic culture or serologic examination. Also called **morbilli, rubeola.** See also **roseola infantum, rubella.**

■ OBSERVATIONS: An incubation period of 7 to 14 days is followed by the prodromal stage, characterized by fever, malaise, coryza, cough, conjunctivitis, photophobia, anorexia, and the pathognomonic Koplik's spots, which appear one to two days before onset of the rash. Pharyngitis and inflammation of the laryngeal and tracheobronchial mucosa develop, the temperature may rise to 103 or 104 degrees, and there is marked granulocytic leukopenia. The papules of the rash first appear as irregular brownish-pink spots around the hairline, the ears, and the neck, then spread rapidly, within 24 to 48 hours, to the trunk and extremities, becoming red, maculopapular, and dense, giving a blotchy appearance. Within three to five days, the fever subsides, and the lesions flatten, turn a brownish color, and begin to fade, causing a fine desquamation, especially over heavily affected areas.

■ INTERVENTION: Routine treatment consists of bed rest, antipyretics, antibiotics to control secondary bacterial infection, and, when necessary, application of calamine lotion, corn starch solution, or cool water to relieve itching. Preventive measures include active immunization with measles virus vaccine after the infant is one year old. Passive immunization with immune serum globulin is recommended for unvaccinated individuals exposed to the disease. One attack of the disease confers lifelong immunity.

■ NURSING CONSIDERATIONS: Bed rest, isolation, and quiet activity are recommended as long as fever and rash persist. Aspirin, fluids, cool sponge baths, nose drops, and cough medication may be necessary to counteract fever and respiratory symptoms. Bright sunlight may be irritating to the eyes. Special attention is given to the care and cleansing of the eyes and skin, especially in cases of severe papular eruption. An important nursing function is instruction of the parents in the proper home care of the child, as most cases are not serious enough to require hospitalization. The disease is usually benign, and mortality is rare. Complications sometimes occur, the most common of which are otitis media, pneumonia, bronchiolitis, obstructive laryngitis, laryngotracheitis, and, occasionally, encephalitis and appendicitis. Rarely, but most gravely, the virus causes subacute sclerosing panencephalitis several years after the acute attack of measles has occurred.

measles and rubella virus vaccine live, an active immunizing agent.

■ INDICATIONS: It is prescribed for immunization against measles and rubella.

■ CONTRAINDICATIONS: Immunosuppression, concomitant administration of corticosteroids, tuberculosis, known or suspected pregnancy, hypersensitivity to neomycin, neoplasms of the lymphatic system or bone marrow, or active infection prohibits its use. It should not to be given for three months following the use of whole blood, plasma, or immune serum globulin, or for one month before of after immunization with other live virus vaccines, except mumps vaccine.

■ ADVERSE EFFECT: The most serious adverse reaction is anaphylaxis.

measles immune globulin. See **immune globulin.**

measles, mumps, and rubella virus vaccine live, an active immunizing agent.

■ INDICATION: It is prescribed for simultaneous immunization against measles, mumps, and rubella.

■ CONTRAINDICATIONS: Immunosuppression, concomitant administration of corticosteroids, tuberculosis, hypersensitivity to neomycin, neoplasms of the lymphatic system or bone marrow, known or suspected pregnancy, or acute infection prohibits its use. It is not given for three months following the use of whole blood, plasma, or immune serum globulin, and it is not given for one month before or after immunization with other live virus vaccines.

■ ADVERSE EFFECT: The most serious adverse reaction is anaphylaxis.

measurement, the determination, expressed numerically, of the extent or quantity of a substance, energy, or time. See also **international unit, metric system.**

meatorrhaphy (mi'ətor'əfi), the suturing of the cut end of the urethra to the glans penis after surgery to enlarge the urethral meatus.

meatoscopy (mi'ətos'kəpi), the visual examination of any meatus, especially the urethra, usually performed with the aid of a speculum.

meatus (miei'təs), pl. **meatuses, meatus.** an opening or tunnel through any part of the body, as the external acoustic meatus that leads from the external ear to the tympanic membrane.

Mebaral, a trade name for an anticonvulsant and sedative (mephobarbital).

mebendazole, an anthelmintic.

■ INDICATIONS: It is prescribed in the treatment of pinworm, whipworm, roundworm, and hookworm infestations.

■ CONTRAINDICATIONS: Pregnancy or known hypersensitivity to this drug prohibits its use.

■ ADVERSE EFFECTS: Among the most serious adverse reactions are abdominal pain and diarrhea.

mecamylamine hydrochloride, a ganglionic blocking agent.

■ INDICATION: It is prescribed in the management of hypertensive cardiac disease.

■ CONTRAINDICATIONS: Coronary or cerebrovascular insufficiency, recent myocardial infarction, uremia, pyelonephritis, glaucoma, or known hypersensitivity to this drug prohibits its use.

■ ADVERSE EFFECTS: Among the most serious adverse reactions are orthostatic hypotension, paralytic ileus, urinary retention, and cycloplegia. The incidence of side effects is very high because the drug reduces all autonomic activity.

mechanical advantage, (in physiology) the ratio of the output force developed by the muscles to the input force applied to the body structures that the muscles move, especially the ratio of these forces associated with the body structures that act as levers. Variations in the sizes of muscles and the lengths of bones in different individuals partially account for the different mechanical advantages from one body type to another and their different physical capabilities, as speed and strength.

mechanical vector. See **vector.**

mechanism of labor. See **cardinal movements of labor.**

mechano-, a combining form meaning 'mechanical': *mechanocyte, mechanotherapy, mechanothermy.*

mechanoreceptor (mek'ənoʊrɪsep'tər), any sensory nerve ending that responds to mechanical stimuli, as touch, pressure, sound, and muscular contractions. See also **proprioceptor.**

mechlorethamine hydrochloride, an antineoplastic alkylating agent.

■ INDICATIONS: It is prescribed in the treatment of a variety of neoplasms.

■ CONTRAINDICATIONS: Bone marrow depression, pregnancy, infection, or known hypersensitivity to this drug prohibits its use.

■ ADVERSE EFFECTS: Among the most serious adverse reactions are bone marrow depression and inflammation owing to extravasation at the site of injection. Nausea, vomiting, and alopecia also may occur.

Meckel's diverticulum (mek'əlz), an anomalous sac protruding from the wall of the ileum between 30 and 90 cm from the ileocecal sphincter. It is congenital, resulting from the incomplete closure of the yolk stalk, and occurs in 1 to 2 per cent of the population. The diverticulum is usually asymptomatic, but the condition is suggested by signs of appendicitis in infancy, by sudden and painless bleeding, usually in childhood, or by symptoms of intestinal obstruction. Symptomatic diverticula are most commonly resected. Surgical resection of asymptomatic diverticula is also recommended to avoid diverticulitis, obstruction, and blood loss, which may occur. Many Meckel's diverticula are discovered incidentally during surgery for other causes and on post mortem examination.

Meclan, a trade name for an antibacterial (meclocycline sulfosalicylate).

meclizine hydrochloride, an antihistamine.

■ INDICATIONS: It is prescribed in the prevention and treatment of motion sickness.

■ CONTRAINDICATIONS: Newborn infants and lactating mothers are not given this drug. Asthma or known hypersensitivity to this drug prohibits its use.

■ ADVERSE EFFECTS: Among the more serious adverse effects are drowsiness, skin rash, hypersensitivity reactions, dry mouth, tachycardia, and nervousness.

meclofenamate sodium, an anti-inflammatory agent.

■ INDICATIONS: It is prescribed in the treatment of rheumatoid arthritis and osteoarthritis.

■ CONTRAINDICATIONS: Known hypersensitivity to aspirin or to nonsteroidal anti-inflammatory drugs prohibits

its use. It is used with caution in patients having upper gastrointestinal disease or impaired renal function.

■ ADVERSE EFFECTS: Among the more serious adverse reactions are gastrointestinal distress, peptic ulcers, dizziness, rashes, and tinnitus. This drug interacts with many other drugs.

Meclomen, a trade name for an anti-inflammatory agent (meclofenamate sodium).

mecocephaly (mek'oʊsef'əli). See **scaphocephaly.**

meconium (mɪkoʊ'niəm), a material that collects in the intestines of a fetus and forms the first stools of a newborn. It is thick and sticky in consistency, usually greenish to black in color, and composed of secretions of the intestinal glands, some amniotic fluid, and intrauterine debris, as bile pigments, fatty acids, epithelial cells, mucus, lanugo, and blood. With ingestion of breast milk or formula and the proper functioning of the gastrointestinal tract, the color, consistency, and frequency of the stools change by the third or fourth day after the initiation of feedings. The presence of meconium in the amniotic fluid during labor may indicate fetal distress.

meconium ileus, obstruction of the small intestine in the newborn caused by impaction of thick, dry, tenacious meconium, usually at or near the ileocecal valve. Symptoms include abdominal distention, vomiting, failure to pass meconium within the first 24 to 48 hours after birth, and rapid dehydration with associated electrolyte imbalance. The condition results from a deficiency in pancreatic enzymes and is the earliest manifestation of cystic fibrosis. In uncomplicated cases in which perforation, volvulus, or atresia does not occur, the obstruction may be relieved by giving enemas with a contrast medium, as a hypertonic solution of meglumine diatrizoate and sodium diatrizoate, under fluoroscopy. Fluid loss is replaced intravenously to prevent dehydration. If two to three enemas do not dislodge the obstruction, surgery is necessary. See also **meconium plug syndrome.**

meconium plug syndrome, obstruction of the large intestine in the newborn caused by thick, rubbery meconium that may fill the entire colon and part of the terminal ileum. Symptoms include failure to pass meconium within the first 24 to 48 hours following birth, abdominal distention, and vomiting if complete intestinal blockage occurs. A barium enema will indicate the plug and in most cases will dislodge it from the bowel wall. Subsequent gentle saline enemas may be needed to expel the plug. The condition may be an indication of Hirschsprung's disease or cystic fibrosis. See also **meconium ileus.**

M.E.D., abbreviation for *minimal effective dose* or *minimal erythema dose.*

medcard, (in nursing) a small card listing the name, dose, and schedule of administration of each patient's medications, used in dispensing medication to each patient.

MEDEX, 1. an educational program accredited by the A.M.A. for training military personnel with medical experience to become physician's assistants. 2. a physician's assistant who have gained medical experience during military service and further training in a physician's assistant program.

medi-, a combining form meaning 'middle': *medialecithal, medicinerea, mediotarsal.*

medial, 1. situated or oriented toward the midline of the body. 2. pertaining to the media, the middle layer of a blood vessel wall. Also called **mesial.**

medial antebrachial cutaneous nerve, a nerve of the arm that arises from the medial cord of the brachial plexus, medial to the axillary artery. Near the axilla it passes a filament to supply the skin over the biceps almost as far as the elbow. It descends on the ulnar side of the arm medial to the brachial artery, pierces the deep fascia with the basilic vein about the middle of the arm, and divides into the anterior branch and the ulnar branch. The anterior branch is the larger of the two branches and continues on the anterior part of the ulnar side of the arm, distributes filaments to the skin as far as the wrist, and communicates with the palmar cutaneous branch of the ulnar nerve. The ulnar branch descends on the medial side of the basilic nerve as far as the wrist, innervates the skin, and communicates with branches of the ulnar nerve. Compare **medial brachial cutaneous nerve.**

medial arteriosclerosis. See Monckeberg's atherosclerosis.

medial brachial cutaneous nerve, a nerve of the arm arising from the medial cord of the brachial plexus and distributed to the medial side of the arm. It passes through the axilla, pierces the deep fascia in the middle of the arm, and supplies the skin of the arm as far as the olecranon. Compare **medial antebrachial cutaneous nerve.**

medial cuneiform bone, the largest of three cuneiform bones of the foot, situated on the medial side of the tarsus, between the scaphoid bone and the first metatarsal. It serves as the attachment for various ligaments, the tendons of the tibialis anterior, and the peroneus longus. It articulates with the scaphoid, the intermediate cuneiform, and the first and second metatarsals. Also called **internal cuneiform bone.**

medial geniculate body, either of the two areas on the posterior dorsal thalamus, relaying auditory impulses from the lateral lemniscus to the auditory cortex.

medial pectoral nerve, a branch of the brachial plexus, that, with the lateral pectoral nerve, supplies the pectoral muscles. It arises from the medial cord of the plexus, medial to the axillary artery, passes between the axillary artery and the axillary vein, and joins the lateral pectoral nerve to form a loop around the artery before ending deep in the pectoralis minor. The loop branches to supply the pectoralis minor and the pectoralis major. Compare **lateral pectoral nerve.**

medial rotation, a turning toward the midline of the body. Compare **lateral rotation.** See also **rotation.**

median, (in statistics) the number representing the middle value of the scores in a sample. In an odd number of scores arrayed in ascending order, it is the middle score; in an even number of scores so arrayed, it is the average between the two central scores.

median antebrachial vein (æn'tibrei'kiəl), one of the superficial veins of the upper limb that drains the venous plexus on the palmar surface of the hand. It ascends on the ulnar side of the anterior forearm and, at its terminus, joins the median cubital vein. In many individuals it divides into two vessels, one joining the basilic vein, the other joining the cephalic vein distal to the elbow. One of the veins of the median cubital complex commonly anastomoses with the deep veins of the forearm. The anastomosis holds the superficial vein in place and makes it a practical choice for venipuncture. Compare **basilic vein, cephalic vein, dorsal digital vein.**

median aperture of fourth ventricle, an opening between the lower part of the roof of the fourth ventricle and the subarachnoid space.

median atlantoaxial joint, one of three points of articulation of the atlas and the axis. The median atlantoaxial joint is a pivot articulation between the dens and ring of the atlas and involves five ligaments. It allows rotation of the axis and the skull, the extent of rotation limited by the alar ligaments.

median basilic vein, one of the superficial veins of the upper limb, often formed as one of two branches from the median cubital vein. The median basilic vein courses across the palmar surface of the forearm near the elbow and is commonly used for venipuncture, phlebotomy, or intravenous infusion. Compare **basilic vein.**

median effective dose (ED50), the dosage of a drug that may be expected to cause a specific intensity of effect in one half of the subjects to whom it is given.

median glossitis. See median rhomboid glossitis.

median lethal dose (MLD), (in radiotherapy) the amount of radiation that kills 50 per cent of the individuals in a large group of animals or organisms within a specified period of time. Also called **LD50.**

median nerve, one of the terminal branches of the brachial plexus that extends along the radial portions of the forearm and the hand and supplies various muscles and the skin of these parts. It arises from the brachial plexus by two large roots, one from the lateral and one from the medial cord. The roots unite to form the trunk of the nerve which courses down the arm with the brachial artery. In the forearm it passes between the two heads of the pronator teres and passes through the flexor retinaculum into the palm of the hand, where it is covered only by the skin and the palmar aponeurosis. Emerging from the retinaculum it is enlarged and flattened and splits into digital and muscular branches. The median nerve usually has no branches above the elbow, but in some individuals the nerve to the pronator teres arises there. The median nerve gives off a few articular branches to the elbow joint and muscular branches to the forearm, the anterior interosseous nerve, the palmar branch, the muscular branch in the hand, the first, second, and third palmar digital nerves, and the proper digital nerves. Compare **musculocutaneous nerve, radial nerve, ulnar nerve.**

median palatine suture, the line of junction between the horizontal portions of the palatine bones that extends from both sides of the skull to form the posterior part of the hard palate.

median plane, a vertical plane that divides the body into right and left halves and passes approximately through the sagittal suture of the skull. Compare **frontal plane, sagittal plane, transverse plane.**

median rhomboid glossitis, a red, depressed, diamond-shaped area on the dorsum of the tongue, frequently irritated by alcohol, hot drinks, or spicy foods. The condition is most often seen in adult males and may be caused by candidiasis.

median toxic dose (TD50) the dosage that may be expected to cause a toxic effect in one half of the subjects to whom it is given.

mediastinum (mi'diəstai'nəm), *pl.* **mediastina.** a portion of the thoracic cavity in the middle of the thorax, between the pleural sacs containing the two lungs. It extends from the sternum to the vertebral column and contains all the thoracic viscera, except the lungs. It is enclosed in a thick extension of the thoracic subserous fascia and is divided into the cranial portion and the caudal portion by a plane extending from the sternal angle to the caudal border of the fourth thoracic vertebra. The caudal portion is divided into the anterior mediastinum, ventral to the pericardium, the middle mediastinum, containing the pericardium, and the posterior mediastinum, dorsal to the pericardium. —**mediastinal,** *adj.*

mediate, 1. to cause a change to occur, as in stimulation by a hormone. 2. to settle a dispute, as in collective bargaining. 3. situated between two places, things, parts, or terms. 4. (in psychology) an event that follows upon one process or event and precedes another, as, in the process of cognition, perception follows stimulation and precedes thinking. —**mediating,** *adj.,* **mediator,** *n.*

Mediatric, a trade name for a nutritional supplement containing multivitamins, minerals, hormones, and a central-nervous-system stimulant (methamphetamine hydrochloride).

Medicaid, a federally funded, state-operated program of medical assistance to people with low incomes, authorized by Title XIX of the Social Security Act. Under broad federal guidelines, the individual states determine benefits, eligibility, rates of payment, and methods of administration.

Medicaid mill, *Informal.* a health program or facility that solely or primarily serves persons eligible for Medicaid. Such facilities are found mainly in depressed areas where there are few other health services.

medical center, 1. a health care facility. 2. a hospital, especially one staffed and equipped to care for many patients and for a large number of kinds of diseases and dysfunction using sophisticated technology.

Medical College Aptitude Test (MCAT), an examination taken by persons applying to medical school, the score on this examination being an important criteria for acceptance. Basic science, intellectual ability, and mathematical and verbal aptitude and knowledge are tested.

medical examiner. See **coroner.**

medical genetics. See **clinical genetics.**

medical history. See **health history.**

medical indigency, the lack of financial reserves adequate to pay for medical care, especially in a person or family able to manage other expenses.

medical induction of labor. See **induction of labor.**

medical model, the traditional approach to the diagnosis and treatment of illness as practiced by physicians in the western world since the time of Koch and Pasteur. The physician focuses on the defect, or dysfunction, within the person, using a problem-solving approach. The medical history and the physical examination and diagnostic tests provide the basis for the identification and treatment of a specific illness. The medical model is thus focused on the physical and biological aspects of specific diseases and conditions. Nursing differs from the medical model in that the patient is perceived primarily as a social person relating to his environment; nursing care is formulated on the basis of a nursing assessment that assumes multiple causes for the problems experienced by the person.

medical staff, all physicians, dentists, and health professionals responsible for providing health care in a hospital or other health-care facility. Medical staff personnel may be full-time or part-time, employed by the facility, or simply affiliated, that is, not employees.

medical-surgical nursing, the nursing care of people whose conditions or disorders are treated pharmacologically or surgically.

Medical Women's International Association (M.W.I.A.), an international professional organization of women physicians.

Medicare, federally funded national health insurance for certain persons over the age of 65. The program is administered in two parts. Part A provides basic protection against costs of medical, surgical, and psychiatric hospital care. Part B is a voluntary medical insurance program financed in part from federal funds and in part from premiums contributed by persons enrolled in the program. Medicare enrollment is offered to persons aged 65 or older who are entitled to receive Social Security or railroad retirement benefits. Other persons over 65, as federal employees and aliens, may not be eligible. Medicare was authorized by Title XVIII of the Social Security Act of 1965.

medicated bougie, 1. a bougie containing a medicated agent. 2. *Obsolete.* a suppository.

medicated tub bath, a therapeutic bath in which medication is dispersed in water, usually in the treatment of dermatologic disorders.

■ METHOD: The amount of medication and the amount and temperature of the water are specified in the order for the bath. The water is run, the medication is added, and the solution is stirred with a bath thermometer to disperse the medication in the water while testing the temperature. The temperature is usually between 35.6°C and 37.8°C but may be as high as 39.4°C, as in the treatment of psoriasis vulgaris. Most medicated baths are prescribed as half-hour treatments. A folded towel or waterproof pillow is placed behind the head, and a towel is draped over the shoulders to add to the patient's comfort. In certain conditions, the patient may be asked to scrub affected areas with a brush and washcloth; in others, the patient is instructed not to scrub at all. After the bath the skin is patted dry and any ointment, cream, or other topical prescription is applied.

■ NURSING ORDERS: The reason for the treatment is explained to the patient, and instructions are given not to get out of the tub without assistance and not to add water without calling the nurse. If the patient is to scrub the affected areas, the necessary equipment is brought to the bath. The tub is thoroughly scrubbed and rinsed before and after the treatment.

■ OUTCOME: The medicated bath is usually soothing, relaxing, and comforting for the patient. Close attention to fully instructing the patient and to assuring comfort during the procedure improves the patient's compliance with the treatment.

medication, 1. a drug or other substance that is used as a medicine. 2. the administration of a medicine.

medicinal treatment, therapy of disorders based chiefly on the use of appropriate pharmacologic agents.

medicine, 1. a drug or a remedy for illness. 2. the art and science of the diagnosis, treatment, and prevention of disease and the maintenance of good health. 3. the art or technique of treating disease without surgery. Two major divisions of medicine are academic medicine and clinical medicine. Some of the many branches of medicine include **environmental medicine, family medicine, forensic medicine, internal medicine, physical medicine.** — **medical,** *adj.*

medicolegal, of or pertaining to both medicine and law. Medicolegal considerations are a significant part of the process of making many patient care decisions and in determining definitions and policies regarding the treatment of mentally incompetent people and minors, the performance of sterilization or therapeutic abortion, and the care of terminally ill patients. Medicolegal considerations, decisions, definitions, and policies provide the framework for informed consent, professional liability, and many other aspects of current practice in the health care field.

Medihaler-Epi, a trade name for an adrenergic (epinephrine bitartrate).

Medihaler-Ergotamine, a trade name for an analgesic (ergotamine tartrate).

Mediterranean anemia. See **thalassemia.**

Mediterranean fever. See **brucellosis.**

medium, *pl.* **media.** a substance through which something moves or through which it acts. A **contrast medium** is a substance that has a density different from that of body tissues, permitting visual comparison of structures when used with imaging techniques such as x ray. A **culture medium** is a substance that provides a nutritional environment for the growth of microorganisms or cells. A **dispersion medium** is the substance in which a colloid is dispersed. A **refractory medium** is the transparent tissues and fluid of the eye that refract light.

MEDLARS, a computerized literature retrieval service of the National Library of Medicine in Bethesda, Maryland. MEDLARS contains more than 4,500,000 references to medical articles found in professional journals and books published since 1966. The references are made available on request to more than 1,000 hospitals, universities, and government agencies throughout the world by means of a network of computer terminals. The references are filed in 15 data bases, including MEDLINE, TOXLINE, CHEMLINE, RTECS, CANCERLIT, and EPILEPSYLINE. See also **MEDLINE.**

MEDLINE, a National Library of Medicine computer data base that covers approximately 600,000 references to biomedical journal articles published in the current and two preceding years. The files duplicate the contents of the monthly and annual volumes of the *Unabridged Index Medicus,* also published by the National Library of Medicine, which indexes medical reports from 3,000 professional journals in more than 70 countries. See also **MEDLARS.**

Medrol, a trade name for a glucocorticoid (methylprednisolone).

Medrol Acetate, a trade name for a glucocorticoid (methylprednisolone acetate).

Medrol Enpak, a trade name for a glucocorticoid (methylprednisolone acetate).

medroxyprogesterone acetate,   a progestin.

■ INDICATION: It is prescribed in the treatment of menstrual disorders due to hormone imbalance.

■ CONTRAINDICATIONS: Known or suspected pregnancy, thrombophlebitis, embolism, stroke, liver dysfunction, cancer of the breast or genitals, abnormal vaginal bleeding, missed abortion, or known hypersensitivity to this drug prohibits its use.

■ ADVERSE EFFECTS: Among the more serious adverse reactions are thrombophlebitis, pulmonary embolism, stroke, hepatitis, and cerbral thrombosis.

medrysone,   an ophthalmic glucocorticoid.

■ INDICATIONS: It is prescribed for various inflammatory conditions of the eye.

■ CONTRAINDICATIONS: Concurrent viral, fungal, or tubercular infections of the eye or known hypersensitivity to this drug prohibits its use.

■ ADVERSE EFFECTS: Among the more serious adverse reactions are aggravation of glaucoma, damage to the optic nerve, and exacerbation of viral or fungal infections of the eye.

medulla (mɪdəl′ə), *pl.* **medullas, medullae. 1.** the most internal part of a structure or organ, as the spinal medulla. See also **marrow. 2.** *Informal.* medulla oblongata.

medulla oblongata,   the most vital part of the entire brain, continuing as the bulbous portion of the spinal cord just above the foramen magnum and separated from the pons by a horizontal groove. It is one of three parts of the brain stem and contains mostly white substance with some mixture of gray substance. The medulla contains the cardiac, the vasomotor, and the respiratory centers of the brain, and medullary injury or disease often proves fatal. Compare **mesencephalon, pons.**

medullary (med′əler′i, mɪdəl′əri, med′yəler′i), **1.** of or pertaining to the medulla of the brain. **2.** of or pertaining to the bone marrow. **3.** of or pertaining to the spinal cord and central nervous system. Also called **medullar.**

medullary carcinoma,   a soft, malignant neoplasm of the epithelium containing little or no fibrous tissue. A small percentage of breast and thyroid tumors are medullary carcinomas. Also called **carcinoma medullare, carcinoma molle, encephaloid carcinoma.**

medullary cystic disease,   a chronic familial disease of the kidney, characterized by the slow onset of uremia. The disease appears in young children or adolescents, who pass large volumes of dilute urine with greater than normal amounts of sodium. Hemodialysis is the usual treatment for the disease as the uremia progresses and becomes severe. See also **uremia.**

medullary fold.   See **neural fold.**

medullary groove.   See **neural groove.**

medullary plate.   See **neural plate.**

medullary sponge kidney,   a congenital defect of the kidney, leading to cystic dilation of the collecting tubules.

Persons with this defect often develop a kidney stone or an infection of the kidney owing to urinary stasis. The condition is diagnosed using urographic techniques. Treatment includes drugs to acidify the urine and a diet low in calcium and high in fluids to discourage formation of stones.

medullary tube.   See **neural tube.**

medulla spinalis.   See **spinal cord.**

medullated neuroma.   See **fascicular neuroma.**

medulloblastoma (mɪdəl′oublæstou′mə),   a poorly differentiated malignant neoplasm composed of tightly packed cells of spongioblastic and neuroblastic lineage. The tumor usually arises in the cerebellum, occurs most frequently between the ages of five and nine years, and affects more boys than girls. Although medulloblastomas are extremely radiosensitive, they grow rapidly, and radiotherapy usually prolongs life for only one or two years.

medulloepithelioma (mədəl′ouep′ɪthi′liou′mə).   See **neurocytoma.**

mefenamic acid (mef′ənæm′ɪk),   a nonsteroidal anti-inflammatory agent and analgesic.

■ INDICATION: It is prescribed in the treatment of mild to moderate pain.

■ CONTRAINDICATIONS: Gastrointestinal ulceration or inflammation, impaired renal function, or known hypersensitivity to this drug prohibits its use. It is used with caution in asthmatics.

■ ADVERSE EFFECTS: Dyspepsia and diarrhea are the most common adverse effects. Other gastrointestinal symptoms, dizziness, drowsiness, or skin rash occasionally occur. Rarely, serious blood dyscrasias occur.

mefloquine (mef′ləkin),   an antimalarial, not currently available in the United States, that has been shown to be effective in the prophylaxis and treatment of chloroquine-resistant falciparum and vivax malaria.

Mefoxin,   a trade name for a cephalosporin antibiotic (cefoxitin sodium).

MEFR,   abbreviation for **maximal expiratory flow rate.**

mega-, megalo-, mego-,   a combining form meaning 'great or huge': *megacardia, megacoccus, megadyne.*

megabladder (meg′əblæd′ər).   See **megalocystis.**

megacaryocyte (meg′əkær′iəsaits′),   an extremely large bone marrow cell measuring between 35 and 160 cu μ in diameter and having a nucleus with many lobes. Megacaryocytes are essential for the production and proliferation of platelets in the marrow and are normally not present in the circulation blood. See also **platelet.** — **megacaryocytic,** *adj.*

Megace,   a trade name for an antineoplastic (megestrol acetate).

megacolon (meg′əkou′lən),   massive, abnormal dilation of the colon that may be congenital, toxic, or acquired. **Congenital megacolon** (Hirschsprung's disease) is caused by the absence of autonomic ganglia in the smooth-muscle wall of the colon. **Toxic megacolon** is a grave complication of ulcerative colitis and may result in perforation of the colon, septicemia, and death. Surgery is the usual treatment for toxic and congenital megacolon. **Acquired megacolon** is the result of a chronic refusal to defecate, usually occurring in children who are psychotic or mentally retarded. The colon becomes dilated by an accumulation of impacted feces. Laxatives, enemas, and psychiatric treatment are often necessary. See also **Hirschsprung's disease.**

megaesophagus (meg'əɪsof'əgəs), abnormal dilation of the lower segments of the esophagus owing to distention resulting from the failure of the cardiac sphincter to relax and allow the passage of food into the stomach. See also **achalasia.**

megakaryocytic leukemia (meg'əkær'ɪousɪt'ɪk), a rare malignancy of blood-forming tissue in which megakaryocytes proliferate abnormally in the bone marrow and circulate in the blood in relatively large numbers.

megalencephaly (meg'əlɪnsef'əli), a condition characterized by pathologic overgrowth of the brain. In some cases generalized cerebral hyperplasia is associated with mental retardation or a brain disorder, as epilepsy. Also called **macrencephaly, macroencephaly.** — **megalencephalic, megalencephalous,** *adj.*

-megalia. See **-megaly.**

megalo-. See **mega-.**

megaloblast (meg'əloublæst'), an abnormally large nucleated immature erythrocyte that develops in large numbers in the bone marrow and is plentiful in the circulation in many anemias owing to deficiency of vitamin B_{12}, folic acid, or intrinsic factor. Effective treatment is the intramuscular injection of vitamin B_{12}. — **megaloblastic,** *adj.*

megaloblastic anemia, a hematologic disorder characterized by the production and peripheral proliferation of immature, large, and dysfunctional erythrocytes. Megaloblasts are usually associated with severe pernicious anemia or folic acid deficiency anemia.

megalocephaly (meg'əlousef'əli). See **macrocephaly.**

megalocystis (meg'əlousɪs'tɪs), an abnormal condition occurring primarily in female children, characterized by an enlarged and thin-walled bladder. Reduction of the size of the bladder or diversion of the flow of urine through the ileum may be surgically performed to correct this condition. Also called **megabladder.**

megalomania (meg'əloumei'niə), an abnormal mental state characterized by delusions of grandeur in which one believes himself to be a person of great importance, power, fame, or wealth. See also **mania.**

megaloureter (meg'əlouyuri'tər), an abnormal condition characterized by marked dilation of one or both ureters, resulting from dysfunctional peristaltic action of the smooth muscle in the ureters. Treatment may include surgical resection.

-megaly, a combining form meaning an 'enlargement of a (specified) body part': *cardiomegaly, dactylomegaly, gastromegaly.* Also **-megalia.**

megestrol acetate (məjes'troul), an antineoplastic progestational agent.

■ INDICATIONS: It is prescribed to treat endometrial cancer and, more commonly, to palliate advanced endometrial and breast cancer.

■ CONTRAINDICATION: Hypersensitivity to the drug is the only contraindication.

■ ADVERSE EFFECTS: There are no known serious adverse reactions.

mego-. See **mega.**

megrim (mi'grɪm). See **migraine.**

Meibomian cyst (maibou'miən). See **chalazion.**

Meibomian gland, one of several sebaceous glands that secrete sebum from their ducts on the posterior margin of each eyelid. The glands are embedded in the tarsal plate of each eyelid. Also called **tarsal gland, palpebral gland.**

Meigs' syndrome (megz), ascites and hydrothorax associated with a fibroma of the ovaries or other pelvic tumor.

meio-. See **mio-.**

meiocyte (mai'əsait), any cell undergoing meiosis.

meiogenic (mai'əjen'ɪk), producing or causing meiosis.

meiosis (maiou'sɪs), constriction of the pupil of the eye, resulting from contraction of the ciliary muscle. — **meiotic** (maiot'ɪk), *adj.*

(See next page for illustration)

meiotic division. See **meiosis.**

Meissner's corpuscle (mais'nər). See **tactile corpuscle.**

mel-, a combining form meaning 'limb, member': *melalgia, melomelus, melosalgia.*

melancholia (mel'æŋkou'liə), 1. extreme sadness; melancholy. 2. *Obsolete.* the major affective depressive disorder. See also **bipolar disorder, depression.**

melancholia agitata, *Obsolete.* a state of depression in which psychomotor excitement is a prominent symptom. See also **agitated depression, bipolar disorder.**

melancholia simplex, *Obsolete.* a mild state of depression. See also **bipolar disorder.**

melancholia stuporosa, *Obsolete.* a state of depression in which stupor in varying degrees is often accompanied by hallucinations. See also **bipolar disorder, stupor.**

melanin (mel'ənɪn), a black or dark brown pigment which occurs naturally in the hair, skin, and in the iris and choroid of the eye. See also **melanocyte.**

melano-, a combining form meaning 'black': *melanoderm, melanoleukoderma, melanophore.*

melanocyte (mel'ənousait, məlæn'ousait), a body cell capable of producing melanin. Such cells are distributed throughout the basal cell layer of the epidermis and form melanin pigment from tyrosine, an amino acid. Melanin granules are then transferred to adjacent basal cells and to hair. Melanocyte-stimulating hormone from the pituitary controls the amount of melanin produced.

melanocyte-stimulating hormone (MSH), a polypeptide hormone, secreted by the anterior pituitary gland, that controls the intensity of pigmentation in pigmented cells. It is synthesized on the same large precursor polypeptide as adrenocorticotrophic hormone and the enkephalins.

melanoderma (mel'ənoudər'mə), any abnormal darkening of the skin caused by increased deposits of melanin or by the salts of iron or silver.

melanoma (mel'ənou'mə), any of a group of malignant neoplasms, primarily of the skin, that are composed of melanocytes. Most melanomas develop from a pigmented nevus over a period of several months or years and occur most commonly in fair-skinned people having light-colored eyes. Any black or brown spot having an irregular border, pigment appearing to radiate beyond that border, a red, black, and blue coloration observable upon close examination, or a nodular surface is suggestible of mela-

noma and is usually excised for biopsy. Prognosis depends on the kind of melanoma, its size and depth, its location, and the age and condition of the patient. Kinds of melanoma are **amelanotic melanoma, benign juvenile melanoma, lentigo-maligna melanoma, nodular melanoma, primary cutaneous melanoma, superficial spreading melanoma, unpigmented melanoma.**

melanotrichia linguae. See **parasitic glossitis.**

melasma (melæz'mə). See **chloasma.**

melatonin (mel'ətou'nɪn), the only hormone secreted into the blood stream by the pineal gland. It has marked diurnal rhythm; blood levels are up to ten times greater at night than during the day. The hormone appears to inhibit numerous endocrine functions, including the gonadotropic hormones, and to decrease the pigmentation of the skin. When injected, exogenous melatonin causes drowsiness. Decreased secretion of melatonin occurs when calcification or tumor formation destroys or damages the pineal gland. A marked decrease results in precocious puberty, especially in boys, and in diabetes insipidus, hypogonadism, and optic atrophy.

MEIOSIS

melena (məli′nə), abnormal, black, tarry stool containing digested blood. It usually results from bleeding in the upper gastrointestinal tract and is often a sign of peptic ulcer or small bowel disease. See also **gastrointestinal bleeding.**

meli-, a combining form meaning 'sweet, or related to honey': *melicera, melitagra, melitoptyalism.*

-melia, a combining form meaning '(condition of the) limbs': *acromelia, dolichomelia, phocomelia.*

melioidosis (mel′iɔidou′sɪs), an uncommon infection of man caused by the gram-negative bacillus, *Malleomyces pseudomallei.* Acute **melioidasis** is fulminant and usually characterized by pneumonia, empyema, lung abscess, septicemia, and liver or spleen involvement. Chronic **melioidosis** is associated with osteomyelitis, multiple abscesses of the internal organs, and the development of fistulas from the abscesses. The disease, most commonly seen in China and Southeast Asia, is acquired by direct contact with infected animals. Human-to-human transmisson is unlikely. Treatment using chloramphenicol, sulfonamides, or tetracycline for several months is usually successful.

Mellaril, a trade name for a tranquilizer (thioridazine).

melphalan (mel′fəlæn), an antineoplastic alkylating agent.

■ INDICATIONS: It is prescribed in the treatment of malignant neoplastic diseases, including multiple myeloma.

■ CONTRAINDICATIONS: Pregnancy, recent exposure to antineoplastic medication or to radiation, or known hypersensitivity to this drug prohibits its use.

■ ADVERSE EFFECTS: Among the more serious adverse reactions are bone marrow depression, nausea, and vomiting.

membrana tectoria, the broad, strong ligament covering the dens and helping to connect the axis to the occipital bone of the skull. Also called **occipitoaxial ligament.** Compare **alar ligament, apical dental ligament.**

membrana tympani. See **tympanic membrane.**

membrane, a thin layer of tissue that covers a surface, lines a cavity, or divides a space, as the abdominal membrane that lines the abdominal wall and Descemet's membrane between the substantia propria and the endothelium of the cornea. The principal kinds of membranes are **mucous membrane, serous membrane, synovial membrane, cutaneous membrane.**

membranous labyrinth, a network of three fluid-filled, membranous, semicircular ducts suspended within the bony semicircular canals of the inner ear, associated with the sense of balance. The ducts, which contain endolymph, follow the contours of the bony canals and are about one fourth the diameter of the canals.

membranous stomatitis. See **pseudomembranous stomatitis.**

memory, 1. the mental faculty or power that enables one to retain and to recall, through unconscious associative processes, previously experienced sensations, impressions, ideas, concepts, and all information that has been consciously learned. 2. the reservoir of all past experiences and knowledge that may be recollected or recalled at will. 3. the recollection of a past event, ideas, sensations, or previously learned knowledge. Kinds of memory include **affect memory, anterograde memory, kinesthetic memory, long-term memory, screen memory, short-term memory, visual memory.** See also **amnesia, déjà vu.**

memory cell. See under **lymphocyte.**

memory image, a sensation, impression, or sense perception as it is recalled in the memory.

-men, a combining form meaning a 'condition or result of a (specified) action': *flumen, lumen, semen.*

menadiol sodium diphosphate, a water-soluble analog of vitamin K. See **menadione.**

menadione (men′ədɑi′oun), an analog of vitamin K.

■ INDICATIONS: It is prescribed in the treatment of vitamin K deficiency and hypoprothrombinemia (other than the hereditary type).

■ CONTRAINDICATIONS: It is not indicated in pregnancy, for anticoagulant overdose, or to counteract heparin. Known hypersensitivity to this drug prohibits its use.

■ ADVERSE EFFECTS: Among the most serious adverse reactions are kernicterus in the newborn and hemolytic anemia in glucose-6-phosphate dehydrogenase deficient individuals. Gastrointestinal upset, rashes, and headaches also may occur.

menadione sodium bisulfite, a water-soluble analog of vitamin K. See **menadione.**

menaphthone (mənæf′thoun). See **menadione.**

menarche (menar′ki), the first menstruation and the commencement of cyclic menstrual function. It usually occurs between the ages of 9 and 17. See also **pubarche.**

mendelevium (Mv), a manmade element in the actinide group. Its atomic number is 101. The atomic weight of its most stable isotope is 256. It is the ninth transuranic element.

Mendelian genetics (mendi′liən). See **Mendel's laws.**

Mendelism (men′dəlɪz′əm), **Mendelianism** (mendi′-liənɪz′əm), the concept of inheritance derived from the application of Mendel's laws. —**Mendelian,** *adj.*

Mendel's laws, Mendelian laws, the basic principles of inheritance based on the breeding experiments of garden peas by the 19th-century Austrian monk Gregor Mendel. These are usually stated as two laws, commonly called the law of segregation and the law of independent assortment. According to the first, each characteristic of a species is represented in the somatic cells by a pair of units, now known as genes, which separate during meiosis so that each gamete receives only one gene for each trait. In any monohybrid crossing, the possible ratio for the phenotypic expression of a particular dominant characteris 3:1, while the ratio of pure dominants to dominant hybrids to pure recessives is 1:2:1. According to the second law, the members of a gene pair on different chromosomes segregate independently from other pairs during meiosis, so that the gametes show all possible combinations of factors. Genes on the same chromosome are affected by linkage and segregate in blocks according to the amount of crossing over that occurs, a discovery made after Mendel. Also called **Mendelian genetics.** See also **chromosome, crossing over, dominant, gene, linkage, meiosis, recessive gene.**

Mendelson's syndrome (men′dəlsənz), a respiratory condition caused by the chemical pneumonia resulting from the aspiration of acid gastric contents into the lungs. It usually occurs when a person vomits when inebriated, when stuporous from anesthesia, or when unconscious, as during a seizure.

Menest, a trade name for esterified estrogens.

Ménétrier's disease (mei′neitrieirz′). See **giant hypertrophic gastritis.**

-menia, a combining form meaning '(condition of) menstrual activity': *catamenia, ischomenia, pausimenia.*

Ménière's disease (meinyeirz′), a chronic disease of the inner ear characterized by recurrent episodes of vertigo, progressive unilateral nerve deafness, and tinnitus. Also called **Ménière's syndrome, paroxysmal labyrinthine vertigo.**
■ OBSERVATIONS: The cause is unknown although occasionally the condition follows middle ear infection or trauma to the head. There also may be associated nausea, vomiting, and profuse sweating. Attacks last from a few minutes to several hours.
■ INTERVENTION: Treatment includes a low-salt diet and the administration of dimenhydrinate, diphenhydramine, or atropine sulfate. In severe cases, surgery on the labyrinth or vestibular nerve or ultrasonic labyrinthectomy may be necessary.
■ NURSING CONSIDERATIONS: Since sudden movements often aggravate the vertigo, the patient will usually prefer to move at a self-determined rate, although walking without assistance should not be undertaken. Siderails should be in place on the bed at all times.

meningeal hydrops (mɪnɪn′jiəl). See **pseudotumor cerebri.**

meninges (mɪnɪn′jiz), *sing.* **meninx** (mi′ɪŋks, men′ɪŋks), any one of the three membranes that enclose the brain and the spinal cord, comprising the dura mater, the pia mater, and the arachnoid. The pia mater and the arachnoid can become inflamed by bacterial meningitis, causing serious complications which may be life threatening. —**meningeal,** *adj.*

meningioma (mɪnɪn′jiou′mə), *pl.* **meningiomas, meningiomata.** a mesenchymal fibroblastic tumor of the membranes enveloping the brain and spinal cord. Meningio-

mas often grow slowly, are usually vascular, and occur most commonly near the superior longitudinal transverse and cavernous sinuses of the dura mater of the brain. The tumors may be nodular, plaquelike, or diffuse lesions that invade the skull, causing bone erosion and compression of brain tissue. Meningiomas usually occur in adults, in some cases following a head injury.

meningism (mɪnɪn′jɪzəm), an abnormal condition characterized by irritation of the brain and the spinal cord and by symptoms that mimic those of meningitis. In meningism, however, there is no actual inflammation of the meninges.

meningitis, any infection or inflammation of the membranes covering the brain and spinal cord. It is usually purulent and involves the fluid in the subarachnoid space. Compare **encephalitis.**
■ OBSERVATIONS: It is characterized by severe headache, vomiting, and pain and stiffness in the neck. The most common causes are bacterial infection with *Streptococcus pneumoniae, Neisseria meningitides,* or *Haemophilus influenzae.* Aseptic meningitis may be caused by other kinds of bacteria, by chemical irritation, neoplasm, or by viruses. Many of these diseases are benign and self-limited, as meningitis caused by strains of coxsackievirus or echovirus. Others are more severe, as those involving arboviruses, herpesviruses, or poliomyelitis viruses. Yeasts such as *Candida* and fungi such as *Cryptococcus* may cause a severe, often fatal, meningitis. Tuberculous meningitis, invariably fatal if untreated, may result in a variety of neurological abnormalities even with the best treatment available.
■ INTERVENTION: Bacterial meningitis is treated promptly with antibiotics specific for the causative organism; they are administered intravenously or intrathecally. Except for adenine arabinoside, recommended for herpes simplex meningitis, there is no specific therapy available for viral infections of the meninges. Antifungal medications, like amphotericin B, given intravenously or intrathecally for several weeks may prevent death from fungal meningitis, but serious neurological sequelae may occur.
■ NURSING CONSIDERATIONS: Constant skilled nursing attention is necessary to ensure early recognition of rising intracranial pressure, to prevent aspiration in the event of convulsive seizures, and to avoid airway obstruction. Except for the first day or two of meningococcal disease, strict isolation procedures are unnecessary. Intravenous fluids and nasogastric tube feeding may be necessary for a prolonged period. Sedatives and narcotic analgesics may obscure important neurological signs in addition to depressing vital functions.

meningo-, a combining form meaning 'pertaining to membranes covering the brain or spinal cord or to other membranes': *meningocele, meningococcus, meningopathy.*

meningocele (mĭnĭng′gousil′), a saclike protrusion of either the cerebral or spinal meninges through a congenital defect in the skull or the vertebral column. It forms a hernial cyst that is filled with cerebrospinal fluid but does not contain neural tissue. The anomaly is designated a cranial meningocele or spinal meningocele, depending on the site of the defect; it can be easily repaired by surgery. See also **myelomeningocele, neural tube defect.**

meningococcal polysaccharide vaccine, either of two active immunizing agents against group A and group C meningococcal organisms.

■ INDICATION: It is prescribed for immunization against meningococcal meningitis.

■ CONTRAINDICATIONS: Immunosuppression or acute infection prohibits its use.

■ ADVERSE EFFECT: The most serious adverse reaction is anaphylaxis.

meningococcemia (mĭnĭng′goukoksi′miə). See **Rocky Mountain spotted fever.**

meningococcus (mĭnĭng′goukok′əs), pl. **meningococci** (mĭnĭng′goukok′sai). a bacterium of the genus *Neisseria meningitidis,* a nonmotile, gram-negative diplococcus, frequently found in the nasopharynx of asymptomatic carriers, that may cause septicemia or epidemic cerebrospinal meningitis. Meningococcal infections are not highly communicable; however, crowded conditions, as may be found in army camps, concentrate the number of carriers and reduce individual resistance to the organism. Hemorrhagic skin lesions are significant clues to the diagnosis. Stained smears of these lesions or of cerebrospinal fluid must be examined quickly as meningococci are fragile and lyse easily. Early treatment with appropriate antibiotics, as penicillin G, is essential for cure. Several meningococcal vaccines are available. See also **meningitis.** — **meningococcal,** *adj.*

meningoencephalocele (mĭnĭng′gouensef′əlousil′), a saclike cyst containing brain tissue, cerebrospinal fluid, and meninges that protrudes through a congenital defect in the skull. The anomaly may or may not contain portions of the ventricular system and is commonly associated with defects in the brain. Also called **encephalomeningocele.** See also **neural tube defect.**

meningomyelocele (mĭnĭng′goumai′əlousil′). See **myelomeningocele.**

meniscectomy (men′isek′təmi), surgical excision of one of the crescent-shaped cartilages of the knee joint, performed when a torn cartilage results in chronic pain and in instability or locking of the joint. Under low spinal or general anesthesia, the torn cartilage is freed and removed, and an elastic compression bandage is applied. After surgery, the leg is kept elevated to reduce swelling and exercises are performed to maintain muscle strength. Crutch walking usually begins about the fourth day and full ambulation about the 12th day.

meniscocystosis (mĭnĭs′kousaitou′sis). See **sickle cell anemia.**

meniscus (mĭnĭs′kəs), 1. the interface between a liquid and air. 2. a lens with both convex and concave aspects. 3. a curved, fibrous cartilage in the knees and other joints.

Menke's kinky hair syndrome (men′kiz), a familial disorder affecting the normal absorption of copper from the intestine, characterized by the growth of sparse, kinky hair. Infants with the syndrome suffer cerebral degeneration, retarded growth, and early death. Early diagnosis and intravenous administration of copper may prevent irreversible damage.

meno-, a combining form meaning 'of or related to the menses': *menolipsis, menopause, menorrhea.*

menometrorrhagia (men′oumet′rourci′jiə), excessive menstrual and uterine bleeding other than that caused by menstruation. It is a combination of metrorrhagia and menorrhagia and may be a sign of a urogenital malignancy, especially cancer of the cervix.

menopause (men′əpoz), strictly, the cessation of menses, but commonly used to refer to the period of the female climacteric. Menses stop naturally with the decline of cyclic hormonal production and function between the ages of 45 and 60, but may stop earlier in life as a result of illness or the surgical removal of the uterus or both ovaries. As the production of ovarian estrogen and pituitary gonadotropins decreases, ovulation and menstruation become less frequent and eventually stop. Fluctuations in the circulating levels of these hormones occur as the levels decline. Hot flashes are the only nearly universal symptom of the menopause. They can often be controlled with estrogen but are seldom so severe as to require therapy and will cease in time without hormonal treatment. Occasionally, heavy irregular bleeding occurs at this time, usually associated with myomata (fibroids) or other uterine pathology. Estrogens given in large parenteral doses may be effective, but hysterectomy is sometimes required for control of the bleeding. Formerly—and incorrectly—emotional and psychological turmoil was expected with the menopause and attributed to it. Symptoms of this sort that are coincidental with the cessation of the menses are unusual and are not attributable to it. The nurse can be of help to her patients, menopausal or not, by encouraging them to identify properly the source of their discomfort, by counseling, and by referral to an appropriate specialist.

menorrhagia (men′ərei′jiə), abnormally heavy or long menstrual periods. Menorrhagia occurs occasionally during the reproductive years of most women's lives. If the condition becomes chronic, anemia from recurrent excessive blood loss may result. Abnormal bleeding following menopause always warrants investigation to rule out malignancy. Menorrhagia is a relatively common complication of benign uterine fibromyomata; it may be so severe, or intractable, as to require hysterectomy. Also called **hypermenorrhea.** Compare **oligomenorrhea, metrorrhagia.** — **menorrhagic,** *adj.*

menostasis (mɪnos′təsɪs), an abnormal condition in which the products of menstruation cannot escape the uterus or vagina owing to stenosis, an occlusion of the cervix, or the introitus of the vagina. An imperforate hymen is a rare cause of menostasis. — **menostatic,** *adj.*

Menotabs, a trade name for conjugated estrogens.

menotropins, a preparation of gonadotropic hormones from the urine of postmenopausal women.

■ INDICATION: It is prescribed with chorionic gonadotropin to induce ovulation.

■ CONTRAINDICATIONS: Elevated gonadotropin levels in the urine, thyroid or adrenal dysfunction, pituitary tumor, abnormal bleeding, ovarian cysts, pregnancy, or known hypersensitivity to this drug prohibits its use.

■ ADVERSE EFFECTS: Among the more serious adverse reactions are ovarian hyperstimulation syndrome, hemoperitoneum, arterial thromboembolism, multiple gestation, and possible birth defects.

Menrium, a trade name for a fixed-combination drug for menopausal symptoms, containing esterified estrogens and a sedative (chlordiazepoxide).

menses (men′siz), the normal flow of blood and decidua that occurs during menstruation. The first day of the flow of the menses is the first day of the menstrual cycle.

menstrual cycle, the recurring cycle of change in the endometrium during which the decidual layer of the endometrium is shed, then regrows, proliferates, is maintained for several days, and sheds again at menstruation. The average duration of menstruation is 5 days; the average length of the cycle, from the first day of bleeding of one cycle to the first of another, is 28 days. The length, duration, and character vary greatly among women. Menstrual cycles begin at menarche and end with menopause.

menstrual phase, the final of the four phases of the menstrual cycle, the one in which menstruation occurs. The necrotic mucosa of the endometrium is shed, leaving the stratum basale; bleeding, primarily from the spiral arteries, occurs. The average blood loss is 30 ml. For convenience, the days of the menstrual cycle are counted from the first day of the menstrual phase. Compare **luteal phase, secretory phase.**

menstrual sponge, a small natural sponge or a piece of a sponge of synthetic material to which a loop of string is attached. It is inserted in the vagina to absorb the menstrual flow and is removed by pulling the string. It may be washed, squeezed dry, and reused as necessary through menstruation. Menstrual sponges are not commonly used and are not easily available.

ment-, a combining form meaning 'mind': *mental, menticide, mentimeter.*

mental[1], **1.** of, relating to, or characteristic of the mind or psyche. **2.** existing in the mind; performed or accomplished by the mind. **3.** of, relating to, or characterized by a disorder of the mind.

mental[2], of or pertaining to the chin.

mental age (MA), the age level at which one functions intellectually, as determined by standardized psychological and intelligence tests and expressed as the age at which that level is average. Compare **achievement age.** See also **developmental age.**

mental deficiency. See **mental retardation.**

mental disorder, any disturbance of emotional equilibrium, as manifested in maladaptive behavior and impaired functioning, caused by genetic, physical, chemical, biological, psychological, or social and cultural factors. Also called **emotional illness, mental illness, psychiatric disorder.**

mental handicap, any mental defect or characteristic resulting from a congenital abnormality, traumatic injury, or disease that impairs normal intellectual functioning and prevents a person from participating normally in activities appropriate for his particular age group. See also **mental retardation.**

mental health, a relative state of mind in which a person who is healthy is able to cope with and adjust to the recurrent stresses of everyday living in an acceptable way.

Mental Health Association (MHA), a voluntary, nonprofessional agency dedicated to the improvement of mental health facilities and services in community clinics and hospitals, the recruitment and training of volunteers, and the promotion of mental health legislation. Formerly called the **National Association for Mental Health.**

mental health nursing. See **psychiatric nursing.**

mental health service, any one of a group of government, professional, or lay organizations operating at a community, state, national, or international level to aid in the prevention and treatment of mental disorders. See also **community mental health center.**

mental hygiene, the study concerned with the development of healthy mental and emotional habits, attitudes, and behavior and with the prevention of mental illness. Also called **psychophylaxis.**

mental illness. See **mental disorder.**

mental image, any concept or sensation produced in the mind through memory or imagination.

mentality, **1.** the functional power and the capacity of the mind. **2.** intellectual character.

mental retardation, a disorder characterized by subaverage general intellectual function with deficits or impairments in the ability to learn and to adapt socially. The cause may be genetic, biological, psychosocial, or sociocultural. The disorder, which is twice as prevalent among men as among women, is classified according to the intelligence quotient as: borderline, IQ 71 to 84; mild, IQ 50 to 70; moderate, IQ 35 to 49; severe, IQ 20 to 34; and profound, IQ below 20. Treatment consists of educational programs and training specific to the level of retardation. Emphasis is placed on preventive measures, such as genetic counseling, amniocentesis, and general health care for pregnant women and for the baby following delivery, especially for the socially disadvantaged and other high-risk groups. Also called *Obsolete.* **feeblemindedness, mental deficiency.** See also **Down's syndrome, Hurler's syndrome, phenylketonuria, Tay-Sachs disease.**

mental status, the degree of competence shown by a person in intellectual, emotional, psychological, and personality functioning as measured by psychological testing with reference to a statistical norm. See also **mental status examination.**

mental status examination, a diagnostic procedure for determining the mental status of a person. The trained interviewer poses certain questions in a carefully standardized manner and evaluates the verbal responses and behavioral reactions.

mentation (mentei'shən), any mental activity, including conscious and unconscious processes.

menthol, a topical antipruritic with a cooling effect that relieves itching. It is an ingredient in many topical creams and ointments.

mentholated camphor, a mixture of equal parts of camphor and menthol, used as a local counterirritant.

-mentia, a combining form meaning '(condition of the) mind': *dementia, moramentia, pseudodementia.*

mentum (men'təm), the chin, especially of the fetus.

mepenzolate bromide, an anticholinergic agent.
- INDICATIONS: It is prescribed in the treatment of gastrointestinal hypermotility and as an adjunct in treating peptic ulcer.
- CONTRAINDICATIONS: Narrow angle glaucoma, asthma, obstruction of the genitourinary or gastrointestinal tract, severe ulcerative colitis, or known hypersensitivity to this drug prohibits its use.
- ADVERSE EFFECTS: Blurred vision, central nervous system effects, tachycardia, dry mouth, decreased sweating, or hypersensitivity reactions may occur.

Mepergan, a trade name for a central-nervous-system fixed-combination drug containing a narcotic analgesic (meperidine hydrochloride) and an antihistaminic (promethazine hydrochloride).

Mepergan Fortis, a trade name for a central-nervous-system, fixed-combination drug containing a narcotic analgesic (meperidine hydrochloride) and an antihistaminic (promethazine hydrochloride).

meperidine hydrochloride, a narcotic analgesic.
- INDICATIONS: It is used to treat moderate to severe pain and as preoperative medication to relieve pain and allay anxiety.
- CONTRAINDICATIONS: It is used with caution in many

conditions, including head injuries, asthma, impaired renal or hepatic function, or unstable cardiovascular status. Concomitant use of a monoamine oxidase inhibitor or known hypersensitivity to this drug prohibits its use.
- ADVERSE EFFECTS: Among the most serious adverse reactions are drowsiness, dizziness, nausea, constipation, sweating, respiratory and circulatory depression, and drug addiction.

mephenesin (mɪfen'ɪsɪn), a skeletal muscle relaxant.
- INDICATIONS: It is prescribed in the relief of muscle spasm.
- CONTRAINDICATIONS: There are no known contraindications.
- ADVERSE EFFECTS: Among the untoward adverse reactions are vertical nystagmus, diplopia, lassitude, and asthenia. Administering the drug after meals or with milk or fruit juice may avoid gastrointestinal problems, as nausea and vomiting.

mephenytoin (mɪfen'ətou'ɪn), an anticonvulsant.
- INDICATIONS: It is prescribed for the control of seizures in epilepsy when less toxic medications have not been effective.
- CONTRAINDICATIONS: It is not usually recommended in pregnancy. Known hypersensitivity to this drug or to any hydantoin prohibits its use.
- ADVERSE EFFECTS: Among the most serious adverse reactions are morbilliform rash, fever, hepatotoxicity, and various blood dyscrasias. The frequent occurrence of adverse reactions limits the use of this drug.

mephobarbital (mef'oubar'bɪtæl), an anticonvulsant and sedative.
- INDICATIONS: It is prescribed in the treatment of anxiety, nervous tension, insomnia, and epilepsy.
- CONTRAINDICATIONS: Porphyria or known hypersensitivity to this drug or to barbiturates prohibits its use.
- ADVERSE EFFECTS: Among the more serious adverse reactions are drug dependence, deficiency in Vitamin D, paradoxical excitement, skin rash, and gastrointestinal disturbance.

Mephyton, a trade name for a vitamin (phytonadione).

meprednisone, a glucocorticoid.
- INDICATIONS: Glucocorticoids are prescribed in the treatment of a large number of inflammatory conditions.
- CONTRAINDICATIONS: Systemic fungal infections or known hypersensitivity to this drug prohibits its use. It is used with caution in many conditions.
- ADVERSE EFFECTS: Among the more serious adverse reactions are a large number of gastrointestinal, endocrine, neurologic, fluid and electrolyte disturbances.

meprobamate (mɪprou'bəmeit), a sedative.
- INDICATIONS: It is prescribed in the treatment of anxiety and tension and as a muscle relaxant.
- CONTRAINDICATIONS: Intermittent porphyria or known hypersensitivity to this drug or to the chemically related

drugs tybamate, mebutamate, and carisoprodol prohibits its use.

■ ADVERSE EFFECTS: Among the most serious adverse reactions are exacerbation of intermittent porphyria, augmentation of effects of other central nervous system depressants, and various allergic reactions. Drowsiness and ataxia commonly occur.

mEq, abbreviation for **milliequivalent.**

-mer, a combining form meaning 'part, portion': *isomer, monomer.* Also **-mere.**

meralgia (mɪræl'jə), the presence of pain in the thigh.

meralgia paresthetica (pær'esθhet'ɪkə), a condition characterized by pain, paresthesia, and numbness on the lateral surface of the thigh in the region supplied by the lateral femoral cutaneous nerve. The cause of the condition is ischemia of the nerve owing to its entrapped position in the inguinal ligament.

mercaptomerin sodium (mər'kæptom'ərɪn), a diuretic rarely used because other diuretics with fewer adverse effects are available.

mercaptopurine, an antineoplastic and immunosuppressive.

■ INDICATIONS: It is prescribed in the treatment of a variety of malignant neoplastic diseases, including acute lymphocytic leukemia.

■ CONTRAINDICATIONS: Known hypersensitivity to this drug prohibits its use.

■ ADVERSE EFFECTS: Among the more severe adverse reactions are bone marrow depression and acute gastrointestinal disturbances, including nausea, vomiting, diarrhea, and stomatitis.

Mercodol W/Decapryn, a trade name for an antitussive, fixed-combination drug containing adrenergics (phenylephrine hydrochloride and etafedrine hydrochloride), an antihistaminic (doxylamine succinate), and an antitussive (codeine phosphate).

mercurial (mərkyur'iəl), **1.** of or pertaining to mercury, particularly a medicine containing the element mercury. **2.** an adverse effect associated with the administration of a mercurial medication, as a mercurial tremor owing to mercury poisoning.

mercurial diuretic, any one of several diuretic agents that contain mercury in an organic chemical form. Only two are recognized for use, mercaptomerin and mercaluride. Mercurial diuretics inhibit tubular reabsorption of sodium and chloride and the excretion of potassium but do not produce diuresis in patients who are in metabolic alkalosis. The principal use for the drugs is in treating edema of cardiac origin, ascites associated with cirrhosis, or oliguria in the nephrotic stage of glomerulonephritis. Response usually begins within one to two hours and lasts for 12 hours. Immediate fatal reactions have occurred, usually owing to ventricular failure following intravascular injection and transient high concentration of

mercury in the blood. Flushing, urticaria, fever, and nausea and vomiting are common side effects. Thrombocytopenia, neutropenia, agranulocytosis, systemic mercury poisoning, and severe hypersensitivity reactions are among the more serious adverse effects of the mercurial diuretics: the drugs are contraindicated for use in the presence of renal insufficiency or acute nephritis. Because of the toxicity of these drugs, current practice usually recommends their replacement with more convenient and less toxic diuretics, as furosemide or ethacrynic acid.

mercurialism (mərkyur'iəlɪz'əm). See **mercury poisoning.**

-mercuric, a combining form meaning 'molecules of bivalent mercury or its compounds': *phenylmercuric, potassiomercuric, trimercuric.*

mercury (Hg), a metallic element. Its atomic number is 80; its atomic weight is 200.6. It is the only common metal that is liquid at room-temperature, and it occurs in nature almost entirely in the form of its sulfide, cinnabar. Mercury is produced commercially and is used in thermometers, barometers, and other measuring instruments. It forms many poisonous compounds. The air, soil, and water in many areas of the world have become contaminated by mercury because of the burning of fossil fuels that contain the element and because of the greater use of mercury in industry and agriculture. The major toxic forms of this metal are mercury vapor, mercuric salts, and organic mercurials. Elemental mercury is only mildly toxic when ingested, because it is poorly absorbed. The vapor of elemental mercury, however, is readily absorbed through the lungs and enters the brain before it is oxidized. The kidneys retain mercury longer than any of the other body tissues.

mercury poisoning, a toxic condition caused by the ingestion or inhalation of mercury or a mercury compound. The chronic form, resulting from inhalation of the vapors or dust of mercurial compounds or from repeated ingestion of very small amounts, is characterized by irritability, excessive saliva, loosened teeth, gum disorders, slurred speech, tremors, and staggering. Symptoms of acute mercury poisoning appear in a few to 30 minutes and include a metallic taste in the mouth, thirst, nausea, vomiting, severe abdominal pain, bloody diarrhea, and renal failure which may result in death. The presence of mercury in the body is determined by a urine test. Treatment may include gastric lavage with milk and egg white or sodium bicarbonate, chelation with British anti-lewisite (BAL), and fluid therapy. Free mercury as in thermometers, is not absorbed in the gastrointestinal tract, but as it is very volatile, hazardous vapors may penetrate ordinary toxic dust respirators, causing poisoning by inhalation. Mercury compounds are found in agricultural fungicides and in certain antiseptics and pigments; they are used extensively in industry. Industrial wastes containing mercury have been identified in some areas, and seafood from contaminated waters have caused serious public health problems. Also called **hydrargyrism, mercurialism.** See also **Minamata disease.**

mercy killing. See **euthanasia.**

merergasia (mer'ərgei'źhə), a mild mental incapacity characterized by some emotional instability and some anxiety. — **merergastic,** adj.

merethoxylline procaine, a diuretic.

■ INDICATION: It is prescribed in the treatment of edema.

■ CONTRAINDICATIONS: Nephritis, ulcerative colitis, dehydration, or known hypersensitivity to mercury, procaine, or theophylline prohibits its use.

■ ADVERSE EFFECTS: Among the most serious adverse reactions are renal failure and hemorrhagic colitis following prolonged use and ventricular fibrillation after I.V. administration. Gastrointestinal symptoms, rashes, other allergic symptoms, and electrolyte disturbances also may occur.

-meria, a combining form meaning '(condition of) parts': *platymeria, polymeria.*

merisis (mer'ɪsɪs), an increase in size as a result of cell division and the addition of new material rather than of cell expansion. Also called **multiplicative growth.** Compare **auxesis.** See also **hyperplasia.**

mero-, a combining form meaning 'part': *meroacrania, merocyte, meropia.*

meroblastic (mer'əblæs'tɪk), pertaining to or characterizing an ovum that contains a large amount of yolk and in which cleavage is restricted to a part of the cytoplasm. Compare **holoblastic.**

meromelia (mer'əmil'yə), a general designation for the congenital absence of any part of a limb. It is used in reference to such conditions as adactyly, hemimelia, or phocomelia. Compare **amelia.**

merozoite (mer'əzou'ɑit), an organism produced from segmentation of a schizont during the asexual reproductive phase of the life cycle of a sporozoan, specifically the malarial parasite *Plasmodium.* Merozoites can either continue the asexual phase of the life cycle by developing into trophozoites and repeating the process of schizogony, or they can differentiate into male and female gametes and enter the sexual stage. See also *Plasmodium.*

mersalyl and theophylline, a diuretic.

■ INDICATION: It is prescribed in the treatment of edema.

■ CONTRAINDICATIONS: Nephritis, ulcerative colitis, dehydration, severe liver disease, or known hypersensitivitiy to mercury or theophylline prohibits its use.

■ ADVERSE EFFECTS: Among the most serious adverse reactions are renal failure and hemorrhagic colitis after prolonged use. Gastrointestinal symptoms, rashes and other allergic reactions, and electrolyte disturbances also may occur.

■ NOTE: It is not to be given subcutaneously.

Merthiolate, a trade name for a topical anti-infective (thimerosal).

Meruvax, a trade name for an active immunizing agent (live rubella virus vaccine).

Mesantoin, a trade name for an anticonvulsant (mephenytoin).

mescaline (mes'kəlin, mes'kəlin), a psychoactive, poisonous alkaloid derived from a colorless alkaline oil in the flowering heads of the cactus *Lophophora williamsii.* Closely related chemically to epinephrine, mescaline causes heart palpitations, diaphoresis, pupillary dilation, and anxiety. The drug, taken in capsules or dissolved in a drink, produces visual hallucinations, as color patterns and spatial distortions, but it does not ordinarily induce disorientation. North American Indians used mescaline in ceremonial feasts to produce euphoria and a feeling of ecstasy. Also called **peyote.**

mesencephalon (mes'ensef'əlon), one of the three parts of the brain stem, lying just below the cerebrum and just above the pons. It consists primarily of white substance with some gray substance around the cerebral aqueduct. A red nucleus lies within the reticular formation of the mesencephalon and contains the terminations of fibers from the cerebellum and the frontal lobe of the cerebral cortex. The ventral part of the mesencephalon is formed by the cerebral peduncles; the dorsal part is formed by the corpora quadrigemina. The cerebral peduncles are two twisted masses of white substance that extend from the pons to the undersurface of the cerebral hemispheres. Deep within the mesencephalon are nuclei of the third and the fourth cranial nerves and the anterior part of the fifth cranial nerve. The mesencephalon also contains nuclei for certain auditory and certain visual reflexes. Also called **midbrain.** — **mesencephalic** (mes'ensɪfæl'ɪk), adj.

mesenchymal chondrosarcoma (meserg'kəməl), a malignant cartilaginous tumor that develops in many sites.

mesenchymoma (mez'ənkɪmou'mə), a mixed mesenchymal neoplasm composed of two or more cellular elements, not usually associated and fibrous tissue. See also **benign mesenchymoma, malignant mesenchymoma.**

mesenteric adenitis. See **adenitis.**

mesenteric node, a node in one of three groups of superior mesenteric lymph glands serving parts of the intestine. An average of 125 mesenteric nodes in three different groups lie between the layers of the mesentery. The first group lies close to the wall of the small intestine, among the terminal twigs of the superior mesenteric artery. The second group is located in relation to the loops and primary branches of the artery. The third group lies along the trunk of the artery. The mesenteric nodes receive afferents from the jejunum, ileum, cecum, vermiform appendix, ascending colon, and transverse colon. Their efferents pass to the preaortic nodes. Compare **ileocolic node, mesocolic node.**

mesentery proper, a broad, fan-shaped fold of peritoneum connecting the jejunum and the ileum with the dorsal wall of the abdomen. The root of the mesentery proper is about 15 cm long and is connected to certain structures ventral to the vertebral column. The intestinal border of the mesentery proper is about 6 m long and separates to enclose the intestine. The cranial part of the mesentery is narrow but widens to about 20 cm and suspends the small intestine and various nerves and arteries. Compare **sigmoid mesocolon, transverse mesocolon.**

mesial (mi′ziəl). See **medial.**

meso-, 1. a combining form meaning 'middle': *mesocardium, mesocecum, mesoderm.* 2. a combining form meaning 'inactive or without effect on polarized light': *mesomerism, meson, mesoporphyrin.*

mesocolic node (mez′oukol′ık), a node in one of three groups of superior mesenteric lymph glands, proliferating between the layers of the transverse mesocolon, close to the transverse colon. They are best developed near the right and the left colic flexures and receive afferents from the jejunum, ileum, cecum, vermiform appendix, ascending colon, and transverse colon. Their efferents pass to the preaortic nodes. Compare **mesenteric node.**

mesocolopexy (mes′oukou′ləpek′si), suspension or fixation of the mesocolon.

mesoderm, (in embryology) the middle of the three cell layers of the developing embryo. It lies between the ectoderm and the endoderm. Bone, connective tissue, muscle, blood, vascular and lymphatic tissue, and the pleurae of the pericardium and peritoneum are all derived from the mesoderm.

mesoglia (mesog′liə). See **microglia.**

mesometritis (mes′oumıtrai′tıs). See **myometritis.**

mesomorph (mez′əmorf), a person whose physique is characterized by a predominance of muscle, bone, and connective tissue, structures which develop from the mesodermal layer of the embryo. Compare **ectomorph, endomorph.**

mesonephric duct, (in embryology) a duct that, in the male, gives rise to the ducts of the reproductive system (ductus epididymidis, ductus deferens, seminal vesicle, ejaculatory duct). In the female, it persists vestigially as **Gartner's duct.** Also called **Wolffian duct.**

mesonephric tubule, any of the embryonic renal tubules comprising the mesonephros. They function as excretory structures during the early embryonic development of man and other mammals but are later incorporated into the reproductive system. In males the tubules give rise to the efferent and aberrant ductules of the testes, the appendix epididymis, and paradidymis, and in females to the epoophoron, paroophoron, and vesicular appendices. All of the structures are vestigial except the efferent ductules of the testes.

mesonephron, *pl.* **mesonephra.** See **mesonephros.**

mesonephros, mesonephron, *pl.* **mesonephroi, mesonephra.** the second type of excretory organ to develop in the vertebrate embryo. It consists of a series of twisting tubules that arise from the nephrogenic cord caudal to the pronephros and that at one end form the glomerulus and at the other connect with the excretory mesonephric duct. The organ is the permanent kidney in lower animals, but in man and various other mammals it is functional only during early embryonic development and is later replaced by the metanephros, although the duct system is retained and incorporated into the male reproductive system. Also called **middle kidney, Wolffian body.** See also **metanephros, pronephros.** − **mesonephric, mesonephroid,** *adj.*

Mesopin, a trade name for an anticholinergic (homatropine methylbromide).

mesoridazine besylate, a phenothiazine tranquilizer.

■ INDICATIONS: It is prescribed in the treatment of psychotic disorders, behavioral problems in mental deficiency, and alcoholism.

■ CONTRAINDICATIONS: Parkinson's disease, concurrent administration of central nervous system depressants, liver or renal dysfunction, severe hypotension, or known hypersensitivity to this drug or to other phenothiazine medications prohibits its use.

■ ADVERSE EFFECTS: Among the more serious adverse effects are hypotension, liver toxicity, a variety of extrapyramidal reactions, persistent tardive dyskinesia, blood dyscrasias, and hypersensitivity reactions.

mesosalpinx (mez′ousæl′pıŋks), the cephalic, free border of the broad ligament in which the uterine tubes lie.

mesothelioma (mez′ouθhi′liou′mə), *pl.* **mesotheliomas, mesotheliomata.** a rare, malignant tumor of the mesothelium of the pleura or peritoneum, associated with earlier exposure to asbestos. The lesion, composed of spindle cells or fibrous tissue, may form thick sheets covering the viscera. The prognosis is poor. Also called **celothelioma.**

messenger RNA (mRNA), (in molecular genetics) an RNA fraction which transmits information from DNA to the protein-synthesizing ribosomes of cells.

Mestinon, a trade name for a neuromuscular blocking agent (pyridostigmine), used as an adjunct to anesthesia and in the treatment of myasthenia gravis.

mestranol (mes′trənoul), an estrogen prescribed in fixed-combination drugs with a progestin as an oral contraceptive. It is not marketed alone.

MET, abbreviation for **metabolic equivalent.**

meta-, 1. a combining form meaning 'change or exchange': *metabasis, metallaxis, metamorphosis.* 2. a combining form meaning 'after or next': *metachemical, metapneumonic, metapsychics.* 3. a combining form meaning 'the 1, 3 position in derivative of benzine': *metacetone, metachloridine, metacresol.*

metabolic (met′əbol′ık), of or pertaining to **metabolism.**

metabolic acidosis, acidosis in which excess acid is added to the body fluids or bicarbonate is lost from them. In starvation and in uncontrolled diabetes mellitus, glucose is not present or is not available for oxidation for cellular nutrition. The plasma bicarbonate of the body is used up in neutralizing the ketones that result from the breakdown of body fat for energy that occurs in compensation for the lack of glucose. Metabolic acidosis also occurs when oxidation takes place without adequate oxygen, as in heart failure or shock. Severe diarrhea, renal failure, and lactic acidosis also may result in metabolic acidosis. Hyperkalemia often accompanies the condition.

metabolic alkalosis, an abnormal condition characterized by the significant loss of acid in the body or by increased levels of base bicarbonate. The reduction of acid may be caused by excessive vomiting, insufficient replacement of electrolytes, hyperadrenocorticism, and Cushing's disease. A decrease in base bicarbonate may be caused by various problems, as the ingestion of excessive bicarbonate of soda and other antacids during the treatment of peptic ulcers, and by the administration of excessive intravenous fluids containing high concentrations of bicarbonate. Severe, untreated metabolic alkalosis can lead to coma and death. Compare **respiratory alkalosis.** See also **metabolic acidosis, respiratory acidosis.**

■ OBSERVATIONS: Signs and symptoms of metabolic alkalosis may include apnea, headache, lethargy, irritability, nausea, vomiting, and atrial tachycardia. Confirmation of the diagnosis is commonly based on laboratory findings that show a blood pH level greater than 7.45, a carbonic acid concentration greater than 29 mEq/l, and alkaline urine. The electrocardiogram of a patient with this condition may show atrial tachycardia with a low T wave merging with a P wave.

■ INTERVENTION: Treatment seeks to eliminate the underlying cause of alkalosis and may include the intravenous administration of ammonium chloride to release hydrogen chloride and restore chloride levels. Potassium chloride and normal saline solutions usually replace fluid losses from gastric drainage but are contraindicated in patients with associated congestive heart failure.

■ NURSING CONSIDERATIONS: Nurses closely monitor the status of the patient and cautiously administer any prescribed intravenous solutions. The intravenous administration of ammonium chloride is usually contraindicated in patients with liver or kidney disease. Too rapid infusion of ammonium chloride may hemolyze the red blood cells, and excessive dosage may overcorrect alkalosis and cause acidosis. The fluid intake and output of the patient are carefully noted, and the respiration rate is regularly checked. Decreased respiratory rate indicates an effort to compensate for alkalosis.

metabolic disorder, any pathophysiologic dysfunction that results in a loss of metabolic control of homeostasis in the body.

metabolic equivalent (MET), the amount of oxygen consumed per kilogram of body weight per minute when at rest.

metabolic rate, the amount of energy liberated or expended in a given unit of time. Energy is stored in the body in energy-rich phosphate compounds (adenosine triphosphate, adenosine monophosphate, and adenosine diphosphate) and in proteins, fats, and complex carbohydrates. See also **basal metabolic rate.**

metabolic respiratory quotient (R), the ratio of production of CO_2 to the corresponding consumption of O_2. The values of R change according to the fuel being burned; thus, as fat contains relatively little O_2 compared to glucose, the R of fat is lower than that of glucose, while the R of protein is between that of glucose and fat.

metabolism, the aggregate of all chemical processes that take place in living organisms, resulting in growth, generation of energy, elimination of wastes, and other bodily functions as they relate to the distribution of nutrients in the blood after digestion. Metabolism takes place in two steps: anabolism, the constructive phase, in which smaller molecules (as amino acids) are converted to larger molecules (as proteins); and catabolism, the destructive phase, in which larger molecules (as glycogen) are converted to smaller molecules (as pyruvic acid). Exercise, elevated body temperature, hormonal activity, and digestion can increase the metabolic rate, which is the rate determined when a person is at complete rest, physically and mentally. The metabolic rate is customarily expressed (in Calories) as the heat liberated in the course of metabolism. See also **acid-base metabolism, anabolism, basal metabolism, catabolism.** —**metabolic,** adj.
(See next page for table)

metabolite (mɪtæb'əlait), a substance produced by metabolic action or necessary for a metabolic process. An essential metabolite is one required for a vital metabolic process.

metacarpus (met'əkar'pəs), the middle portion of the hand, consisting of five slender bones numbered from the thumb side, metacarpals I through V. Each metacarpal consists of a body and two extremities. —**metacarpal,** adj., n.

metacentric (met'əsen'trɪk), pertaining to a chromosome in which the centromere is located near the center so that the arms of the chromatids are of approximately equal length. Compare **acrocentric, submetacentric, telocentric.**

metagenesis (met'əjen'ɪsɪs), the regular alternation of sexual with asexual methods of reproduction within the same species. —**metagenetic, metagenic,** adj.

Metahydrin, a trade name for a diuretic and antihypertensive (trichlormethiazide).

metal, any element that conducts heat and electricity, is

Metabolism

Food	Anabolism	Catabolism
Carbohydrates	Temporary excess changed into glycogen by liver cells in presence of insulin; stored in liver and skeletal muscles until needed and then changed back to glucose True excess beyond body's energy requirements converted into adipose tissue; stored in various fat depots of body	Oxidized, in presence of insulin, to yield energy (4.1 kcal per gram) and wastes (carbon dioxide and water) $C_6H_{12}O_6 + 6\ O_2 \rightarrow$ Energy $+ 6\ CO_2 + 6\ H_2O$
Fats	Built into adipose tissue; stored in fat depots of body	Fatty acids $\qquad\qquad$ Glycerol $\quad\downarrow$ (beta-oxidation) $\qquad\quad\downarrow$ (glycolysis) Acetyl-CoA $\leftrightarrows$ Ketones $\quad\downarrow$ (tissues; citric acid cycle) $\qquad$ Acetyl-CoA Energy (9.3 kcal per gram) $+ CO_2 + H_2O$
Proteins	Temporary excess stored in liver and skeletal muscles Synthesized into tissue proteins, blood proteins, enzymes, hormones	Deaminated by liver forming ammonia (which is converted to urea) and keto acids (which are either oxidized or changed to glucose or fat)

malleable and ductile, and forms positively charged ions (cations) in solution.

metal fume fever, an occupational disorder caused by the inhalation of fumes of metallic oxides and characterized by symptoms similar to those of influenza. The condition occurs among workers engaged in welding, metal fabrication, casting, and other occupations dealing with the manipulation of metals. Access to fresh air and treatment of the symptoms usually alleviate the condition. Also called **brassfounder's ague, zinc chill.** Compare **siderosis.**

metamorphopsia (met'əmɔrfop'siə), a defect in vision in which objects are seen as distorted in shape, resulting from disease of the retina or imperfection of the media.

metamorphosis, a change in shape or structure, especially a change from one stage of development to another, as the transition from the larval to the adult stage.

metamyelocyte (met'əmai'əlousait), a stage in the development of the granulocyte series of leukocytes. It is intermediate between the myelocyte stage and the mature granulocyte. See also **leukocyte, myeloblast, myelocyte.**

Metandren, a trade name for an androgen (methyltestosterone).

metanephrine (met'ənef'rɪn), one of the two principal urinary metabolites of epinephrine and norepinephrine in the urine, the other being vanillylmandelic acid. The 24-hour normal value for total metanephrine is < 1.3 mg. Normally, less than 1.3 mg of metanephrine is excreted in 24 hours.

metanephrogenic (met'ənef'rəjen'ɪk), capable of forming the metanephros, or fetal kidney.

metanephron, *pl.* **metanephra.** See **metanephros.**

metanephros, metanephron, *pl.* **metanephroi, metanephra.** the third, and permanent, excretory organ to develop in the vertebrate embryo. It consists of a complex structure of secretory and collecting tubules that develop into the kidney and are formed later than the mesonephros from the caudal end of the nephrogenic cord and the mesonephric duct. In most mammals there is limited functional use of the metanephric kidney during fetal life, since waste materials are transferred across the placenta to the mother for elimination. Also called **hind kidney.** See also **kidney, mesonephros, pronephros.**

metaphase (met'əfeiz), the second of the four stages of nuclear division in mitosis and in each of the two divisions of meiosis, during which the chromosomes become arranged in the equatorial plane of the spindle to form the equatorial plate, with the centromeres attached to the spindle fibers in preparation for separation. See also **anaphase, interphase, meiosis, mitosis, prophase, telophase.**

metaphyseal dysostosis (mɪtæf'ɪzi'əl, met'əfɪz'iəl), an abnormal condition that affects the skeletal system and is characterized by a disturbance of the mineralization of the metaphyseal area of the bones, resulting in dwarfism. Metaphyseal dysostosis is classified as the Gansen type, Schmidt type, Spahar-Hartmann type, or cartilage-hair hypoplasia. The Gansen type is characterized by metaphyseal alterations similar to those of achondroplasia but not involving the skull or the epiphyses of the long bones. The Schmidt type of metaphyseal dysostosis is characterized by developmental changes from the weight-bearing age to approximately five years. The metaphyseal alterations associated with the Schmidt type are similar to those of achondroplasia, resulting in moderate dwarfism. The Spahar-Hartmann type is characterized by skeletal changes and severe genu varum. Cartilage-hair hypoplasia is characterized by severe dwarfism and hair that is sparse, short, and brittle. Mental retardation is not usually associated with metaphyseal dysostosis. Radiographic examination of all types of the disease reveals characteristic widening of the metaphyses of the tubular bones, with normal diaphyseal and epiphyseal ossification centers. Treatment is supportive and symptomatic with no specific modality.

metaphyseal dysplasia, an abnormal condition characterized by disordered modeling of the cylindrical bones. The involvement of this disease is limited to the long bones and displays a characteristic radiographic image of the 'Erlenmeyer flask' deformity in which the metaphyseal circumference is enlarged and the medullary area of the affected bone is reduced. Metaphyseal dysplasia most often affects the distal femur or the proximal tibia.

Metaprel, a trade name for a bronchodilator (metaproterenol sulfate).

metaproterenol sulfate (met′əprouter′ınɔl), a bronchodilator.
- INDICATIONS: It is prescribed in the treatment of bronchial asthma.
- CONTRAINDICATIONS: Arrhythmias associated with tachycardia or known hypersensitivity to this drug prohibits its use.
- ADVERSE EFFECTS: Among the more serious adverse reactions are tachycardia, hypertension, and cardiac arrest.

metaraminol bitartrate, an adrenergic vasopressor.
- INDICATIONS: It is prescribed in the treatment of hypotension and shock.
- CONTRAINDICATIONS: Known hypersensitivity to this drug prohibits its use. It is not used with cyclopropane or halothane anesthesia or as the sole drug for hypovolemic hypotension.
- ADVERSE EFFECTS: Among the more serious adverse reactions are cardiac arrythmia, tissue necrosis at the site of injection, hypertension, tremors, and nausea.

metastasis (mətæs′təsıs), pl. **metastases** (mətæs′təsis). 1. the process by which tumor cells are spread to distant parts of the body. Because malignant tumors have no enclosing capsule, cells may escape, become emboli, and be transported by the lymphatic circulation or the blood stream to implant on lymph nodes and other organs far from the primary tumor. 2. a tumor that develops in this way. —**metastatic,** adj., **metastasize,** v.

metastasizing mole. See **chorioadenoma destruens.**

metastatic ophthalmia. See **sympathetic ophthalmia.**

metastic ophthalmia. See **sympathetic ophthalmia.**

metatarsal (met′ətar′səl), 1. of or pertaining to the metatarsus of the foot. 2. any one of the five bones comprising the metatarsus.

metatarsalgia (met′ətarsæl′jə), a painful condition around the metatarsal bones caused by an abnormality of the foot or recalcification of degenerated heads of metatarsal bones. Also called **Morton's foot, Morton's neuroma, Morton's toe.**

metatarsal stress fracture, a break or rupture of a metatarsal bone, resulting from prolonged running or walking. The condition is often difficult to diagnose with x-ray films. Also called **fatigue fracture, march fracture.**

metatarsus, a part of the foot, consisting of five bones numbered I to V, from the medial side. Each bone has a long, slender body, a wedge-shaped proximal end, a convex distal end, and flattened, grooved sides for the attachment of ligaments. The metatarsal bones articulate with the tarsus proximally and the first row of phalanges distally. —**metatarsal,** adj.

Metatensin, a trade name for a cardiovascular, fixed-combination drug containing a diuretic (trichlormethiazide) and an antihypertensive (reserpine).

metathalamus (met′əθæl′əməs), one of five parts of the diencephalon. It is composed of a medial geniculate body and a lateral geniculate body on each side. The medial geniculate body acts as a relay station for nerve impulses between the inferior brachium and the auditory cortex. The lateral geniculate body is an oval bulge at the posterior end of the thalamus, which accommodates the terminal ends of the fibers of the optic tract. Compare **epithalamus, hypothalamus, metathalamus, subthalamus.** —**metathalamic,** adj.

metaxalone, a skeletal muscle relaxant.
- INDICATION: It is prescribed as an adjunct in the treatment of acute skeletal muscle spasm.
- CONTRAINDICATIONS: Significantly impaired renal or hepatic function, susceptibility to drug-induced hemolytic anemia, or known hypersensitivity to this drug prohibits its use.
- ADVERSE EFFECTS: Among the more serious adverse reactions are hemolytic anemia, leukopenia, and liver dysfunction. Gastrointestinal disturbances, dizziness, and nervousness may occur.

Metchnikoff theory, a theory that living cells ingest microorganisms. The theory proved correct, as seen in the process of phagocytosis and the ingestion of injurious microbes by leukocytes.

meteorism, accumulation of gas in the abdomen or the intestine.

meteorotropism (mi′tiərətrou′pizəm), a reaction to meteorological influences shown by various biological occurrences, as sudden death, attacks of arthritis, and angina. —**meteorotropic,** adj.

-meter, a combining form meaning a 'measuring instrument': anesthesimeter, ionometer, scopometer. Also **-metre.**

meter (m), a metric unit of length equal to 39.37 inches.

methacycline hydrochloride, a tetracycline antibiotic.
- INDICATIONS: It is prescribed in the treatment of a variety of infections.
- CONTRAINDICATIONS: Renal or liver dysfunction, preg-

nancy, early childhood, or known hypersensitivity to this drug or to other tetracycline medications prohibits its use.
■ ADVERSE EFFECTS: Among the more serious adverse reactions are gastrointestinal disturbances, phototoxicity, potentially serious suprainfections, and hypersensitivity reactions. Discoloration of teeth may occur in children exposed to the drug in utero or before eight years of age.

methadone, a synthetic narcotic analgesic.
■ INDICATIONS: It is prescribed for relief of severe pain, for treatment in detoxification, and in treatment programs for opiate-addicted patients.
■ CONTRAINDICATIONS: It is used with caution in many conditions, including head injuries, asthma, impaired renal or hepatic function, or unstable cardiovascular status. Known hypersensitivity to the drug prohibits its use.
■ ADVERSE EFFECTS: Among the more serious adverse reactions are drowsiness, dizziness, nausea, constipation, respiratory and circulatory depression, and drug addiction.

methadone hydrochloride, a narcotic analgesic used for anesthesia or as a substitute for heroin, permitting withdrawal without development of acute abstinence syndrome. Methadone does not produce marked euphoria, sedation, or narcosis. It is not given to pregnant women or to people with liver disease.

methallenestril, an estrogen.
■ INDICATIONS: It is prescribed in the treatment of menstrual cycle irregularities, menopausal symptoms, and to prevent pregnancy.
■ CONTRAINDICATIONS: Thrombophlebitis, liver dysfunction, unusual vaginal bleeding, or known hypersensitivity to this drug prohibits its use.
■ ADVERSE EFFECTS: Among the more serious adverse reactions are thrombophlebitis, porphyria, embolisms, and jaundice.

methamphetamine hydrochloride, a central stimulant.
■ INDICATIONS: It is prescribed in the treatment of narcolepsy and hyperkinesis and to reduce the appetite in exogenous obesity.
■ CONTRAINDICATIONS: Glaucoma, arteriosclerosis, cardiovascular disease, hypertension, hyperthyroidism, history of drug abuse, concomitant use of monoamine oxidase inhibitor, or known hypersensitivity to this drug or to other sympathomimetic drugs prohibits its use.
■ ADVERSE EFFECTS: Among the more serious adverse reactions are various manifestations of central nervous system excitation, increase in blood pressure, arrythmia and other cardiovascular effects, nausea, and drug dependence.

methampyrone. See **dipyrone.**

methandrostenolone (meθhæn′drousten′əloun), an androgen.
■ INDICATION: It is prescribed primarily in the treatment of osteoporosis.

■ CONTRAINDICATIONS: Cancer of the male breast or prostate, cardiac, renal, or hepatic disease, nephrosis, pregnancy, or known hypersensitivity to this drug prohibits its use.
■ ADVERSE EFFECTS: Among the more serious adverse reactions are various endocrine effects, depending on age of the patient. Hirsutism and masculinization is seen in women, and nausea and jaundice are not uncommon.

methanol, a clear, colorless, toxic, liquid distillate of wood miscible with water, alcohol, and ether. It is widely used as a solvent and in the production of formaldehyde. Ingestion of methanol paralyzes the optic nerve and may cause death. Also called **wood alcohol.**

methanol-extractable residue, an immunotherapeutic substance, prepared from a methanol-extracted fraction of the bacillus Calmette-Guérin (BCG). It is given to prevent or delay recurrences of Stage II malignant melanoma after surgery and to prolong drug-induced remissions in acute myelocytic leukemia.

methantheline bromide, an anticholinergic.
■ INDICATIONS: It is prescribed in the treatment of peptic ulcer and a wide variety of other gastrointestinal disorders.
■ CONTRAINDICATIONS: Narrow angle glaucoma, asthma, obstruction of the genitourinary or the gastrointestinal tract, severe ulcerative colitis, or known hypersensitivity to this drug prohibits its use.
■ ADVERSE EFFECTS: Among the more serious adverse effects are blurred vision, central nervous system disturbances, tachycardia, dry mouth, decreased sweating, and hypersensitivity reactions.

methapyrilene hydrochloride, an antihistamine.
■ INDICATIONS: It is prescribed in the treatment of a variety of hypersensitivity reactions, including rhinitis, dermatitis and pruritus.
■ CONTRAINDICATIONS: Asthma or known hypersensitivity to this drug prohibits its use. It is not given to newborn infants or lactating mothers.
■ ADVERSE EFFECTS: Among the more serious adverse reactions are skin rash, hypersensitivity reactions, and tachycardia. Drowsiness and dry mouth commonly occur.

methaqualone (meθhæk′wəloun), a sedative-hypnotic.
■ INDICATIONS: It is prescribed in the treatment of anxiety and insomnia.
■ CONTRAINDICATIONS: It is not given to children or to pregnant women. Known hypersensitivity to this drug prohibits its use.
■ ADVERSE EFFECTS: Among the more serious adverse reactions are gastrointestinal distress, drug hangover, peripheral neuropathy, loss of inhibition, and drug dependence.

metharbital, an anticonvulsant.
■ INDICATION: It is prescribed in the treatment of epilepsy.

■ CONTRAINDICATIONS: Porphyria or known hypersensitivity to barbiturates prohibits its use. It is prescribed with caution in pregnancy or hepatic impairment.

■ ADVERSE EFFECTS: Among the more serious adverse reactions are ataxia, irritability in children, and confusion in elderly patients. Rashes and other allergic reactions also may occur.

methazolamide, a carbonic anhydrase inhibitor.

■ INDICATION: It is prescribed in the treatment for glaucoma.

■ CONTRAINDICATIONS: Hyponatremia, hypokalemia, Addison's disease, severe pulmonary obstruction, adrenocortical insufficiency, or known hypersensitivity to this drug prohibits its use.

■ ADVERSE EFFECTS: Among the more serious adverse effects are drowsiness, paresthesia, hypersensitivity reactions, and acidosis.

methdilazine (methdil'azin), a phenothiazine antihistamine.

■ INDICATION: It is prescribed to relieve itching.

■ CONTRAINDICATIONS: Asthma, glaucoma, or known hypersensitivity to this drug or to phenothiazine medication prohibits its use. It is not given to newborn infants or lactating mothers.

■ ADVERSE EFFECTS: Among the more serious adverse reactions are bone marrow depression and extrapyramidal reactions. Dry mouth and sedation commonly occur.

methemoglobin (methi'məglou'bın, methem'əglou'bın), a form of hemoglobin in which the iron component has been oxidized from the ferrous to the ferric state. Methemoglobin cannot carry oxygen and so contributes nothing to the oxygen-transporting capacity of the blood. Methemoglobin is a product of the various oxidative reactions that constitute normal metabolic activity. Normally present in only trace amounts (about one per cent) in the blood, it is maintained at this level by an active enzymatic-reducing capability, the NADH-methemoglobin reductase system present in all normal red cells. See also **hemoglobin.**

methenamine, a urinary antibacterial.

■ INDICATION: It is prescribed in the treatment of urinary tract infections.

■ CONTRAINDICATIONS: Liver or kidney dysfunction or known hypersensitivity to this drug or to mandelic acid prohibits its use.

■ ADVERSE EFFECTS: Among the most serious adverse reactions are severe gastrointestinal disturbances and rashes.

Methergine, a trade name for an oxytocic (methylergonovine maleate).

methicillin sodium, a penicillinase-resistant penicillin antibiotic.

■ INDICATION: It is prescribed primarily in the treatment of severe penicillinase-producing staphylococcal infection.

■ CONTRAINDICATIONS: Known hypersensitivity to this drug or to any penicillin prohibits its use.

■ ADVERSE EFFECTS: Among the more serious adverse reactions are phlebitis at the site of injection, nephritis, and allergic reactions.

methimazole, an inhibitor of thyroid hormone synthesis.

■ INDICATIONS: It is prescribed in the treatment of hyperthyroidism, in preparation for subtotal thyroidectomy, or for radioactive iodine therapy.

■ CONTRAINDICATION: Known hypersensitivity to this drug prohibits its use.

■ ADVERSE EFFECTS: Among the more serious adverse reactions are blood dyscrasias (particularly granulocytopenia) and hypersensitivity reactions resembling lupus erythematosus. Skin rash, pruritus, and gastrointestinal distress commonly occur.

methixene hydrochloride, an anticholinergic agent.

■ INDICATIONS: It is prescribed in the treatment of hypermotility or spasms of the gastrointestinal tract.

■ CONTRAINDICATIONS: Narrow angle glaucoma, asthma, obstruction of the genitourinary or gastrointestinal tract, severe ulcerative colitis, or known hypersensitivity to this drug prohibits its use.

■ ADVERSE EFFECTS: Among the more serious adverse reactions are blurred vision, central nervous system effects, tachycardia, dry mouth, decreased sweating, and hypersensitivity reactions.

methocarbamol, a skeletal muscle relaxant.

■ INDICATION: It is prescribed in the treatment of skeletal muscle spasm.

■ CONTRAINDICATIONS: Renal dysfunction, central nervous system depression, or known hypersensitivity to this drug prohibits its use.

■ ADVERSE EFFECTS: Among the more serious adverse reactions are hypotension and tachycardia. Drowsiness, dizziness, vertigo, and nausea may occur.

method, a technique or procedure for producing a desired effect, as a surgical procedure, a laboratory test, or a diagnostic technique.

methodology, 1. a system of principles or methods of procedure in any discipline, as education, research, diagnosis, or treatment. —**methodological,** *adj.* 2. the section of a research proposal in which the methods to be used are described. The research design, the population to be studied, and the research instruments, or tools, to be used are discussed in the methodology.

methohexital sodium (Brevital sodium) (meth'ouhek'-sıtɔl), an intravenous barbiturate.

■ INDICATION: It is prescribed for the induction of anesthesia in short surgical procedures as a supplement to other anesthetics.

■ CONTRAINDICATIONS: Porphyria, status asthmaticus, or known hypersensitivity to this drug or to any barbiturate prohibits its use.

■ ADVERSE EFFECTS: Among the more serious adverse reactions are respiratory depression, skin rash, and cardiovascular dysfunction.

methotrexate, an antineoplastic antimetabolite.

■ INDICATIONS: It is prescribed in the treatment of severe psoriasis and a variety of malignant neoplastic diseases.

■ CONTRAINDICATIONS: Blood dyscrasias, severe renal or hepatic impairment, or known hypersensitivity to this drug prohibits its use.

■ ADVERSE EFFECTS: Among the more serious adverse reactions are diarrhea, ulcerative stomatis, bone marrow depression, hepatotoxicity, and skin rash.

methotrimeprazine (meth′outræimep′rəzin), a phenothiazine analgesic.

■ INDICATION: It is prescribed for the relief of moderate to severe pain in bedridden patients.

■ CONTRAINDICATIONS: Concurrent administration of antihypertensives, hypotension, renal or hepatic disease, or known hypersensitivity to this drug or to phenothiazine medication prohibits its use.

■ ADVERSE EFFECTS: Among the more serious adverse reactions are orthostatic hypotension, dizziness, dry mouth, and mental confusion.

methoxamine hydrochloride, an adrenergic that acts as a vasoconstrictor.

■ INDICATION: It is prescribed for use during anesthesia to maintain blood pressure and in the treatment of paroxysmal supraventricular tachycardia.

■ CONTRAINDICATIONS: It is not recommended for use as a vasoconstrictor with local anesthetics. Known hypersensitivity to this drug prohibits its use.

■ ADVERSE EFFECTS: Among the most serious adverse reactions are hypertension, severe headache, and vomiting.

methoxsalen, a pigmentation agent.

■ INDICATIONS: It is used topically to enhance pigmentation or for repigmentation in vitiligo.

■ CONTRAINDICATIONS: Liver impairment, concomitant use of a drug that may cause photosensitization, or known hypersensitivity to this drug prohibits its use.

■ ADVERSE EFFECTS: Among the most serious adverse reactions are central nervous system effects and burns. Gastrointestinal discomfort and allergic reactions also may occur.

methoxyphenamine hydrochloride, a beta-adrenergic agent.

■ INDICATIONS: It is prescribed in the treatment of bronchial asthma and hypersensitivity reactions.

■ CONTRAINDICATIONS: Cardiac arrythmias, concomitant administration of monoamine oxidase inhibitors, coronary artery disease, or known hypersensitivity to this drug prohibits its use.

■ ADVERSE EFFECTS: Among the more serious adverse reactions are tachycardia and cardiac arrythmias.

methscopolamine bromide, an anticholinergic.

■ INDICATIONS: It is prescribed in the treatment of hypermotility of the gastrointestinal tract and as an adjunct in treating peptic ulcer.

■ CONTRAINDICATIONS: Narrow angle glaucoma, asthma, obstruction of the genitourinary or gastrointestinal tract, severe ulcerative colitis, or known hypersensitivity to the drug prohibits its use.

■ ADVERSE EFFECTS: Blurred vision, central nervous system effects, tachycardia, dry mouth, decreased sweating, or hypersensitivity reactions may occur.

methsuximide (methsək′sımæid), an anticonvulsant.

■ INDICATION: It is prescribed in the treatment of refractory petit mal epilepsy.

■ CONTRAINDICATIONS: Known hypersensitivity to this drug or to any succinimide prohibits its use.

■ ADVERSE EFFECTS: Among the more serious adverse reactions are blood dyscrasias, liver and kidney damage, and systemic lupus erythematosus.

methyclothiazide (meth′əklouthæi′əzaid), a diuretic and antihypertensive.

■ INDICATIONS: It is prescribed in the treatment of hypertension and edema.

■ CONTRAINDICATIONS: Anemia or known hypersensitivity to this drug, to other thiazide medications, or to sulfonamide derivatives prohibits its use.

■ ADVERSE EFFECTS: Among the more serious adverse reactions are hypokalemia, hyperglycemia, hyperuricemia, and hypersensitivity reactions.

methyl alcohol. See **methanol.**

methylbenzethonium chloride, a topical anti-infective.

■ INDICATIONS: It is prescribed for the prevention and treatment of diaper rash and other dermatoses.

■ CONTRAINDICATION: Known hypersensitivity to this drug is the only contraindication.

■ ADVERSE EFFECTS: There are no known adverse reactions. Local skin irritation may occur.

methylcellulose, a bulk-forming laxative.

■ INDICATION: It is prescribed in the treatment of constipation.

■ CONTRAINDICATIONS: Appendicitis, acute surgical abdomen, intestinal adhesions, obstruction or ulceration, or known hypersensitivity to this drug prohibits its use.

■ ADVERSE EFFECTS: The most serious adverse reactions are intestinal obstruction and fecal impaction if insufficient fluids are ingested.

methyldopa, an antihypertensive.

■ INDICATION: It is prescribed for the reduction of high blood pressure.

■ CONTRAINDICATION: Liver dysfunction or known hypersensitivity to this drug prohibits its use.

■ ADVERSE EFFECTS: Among the more serious adverse reactions are liver toxicity and blood dyscrasias. Sedation, dry mouth, nasal stuffiness, and postural hypotension may occur.

methylene blue, a bluish-green crystalline substance used as a histological stain and as a laboratory indicator. It is also used in the treatment of cyanide poisoning and methemoglobinemia.

methylergonovine maleate, a synthetic ergot alkaloid.
- INDICATIONS: It is prescribed as an oxytocic to prevent or to treat postpartum uterine atony, hemorrhage, or subinvolution.
- CONTRAINDICATIONS: It is not prescribed during pregnancy or given intravenously, except in life-threatening situations. Hypertension, toxemia, or known hypersensitivity to ergot alkaloids prohibits its use.
- ADVERSE EFFECTS: Among the most serious adverse reactions are convulsions and death. Hypertension, nausea, blurred vision, and headaches also may occur. Adverse effects are more common after I.V. administration.

methylphenidate hydrochloride, a central nervous system stimulant.
- INDICATIONS: It is prescribed in the treatment of hyperkinesis in children and in the treatment of narcolepsy in adults.
- CONTRAINDICATIONS: Glaucoma, severe anxiety, tension, mental depression, or known hypersensitivity to this drug prohibits its use. It is not given to children under six years of age.
- ADVERSE EFFECTS: Among the more serious adverse reactions are nervousness, insomnia, and anorexia. Hypersensitivity reactions and tachycardia may occur.

methylprednisolone, a glucocorticoid.
- INDICATIONS: It is prescribed in the treatment of inflammatory conditions, including rheumatic fever and rheumatoid arthritis.
- CONTRAINDICATIONS: Fungal infections or known hypersensitivity to this drug prohibits its systemic use. Viral or fungal infections of the skin, impaired circulation, or known hypersensitivity to this drug prohibits its topical use.
- ADVERSE EFFECTS: Among the more serious adverse reactions to the systemic administration of the drug are gastrointestinal, endocrine, neurologic, fluid, and electrolyte disturbances. A variety of skin reactions may occur from topical administration of this drug.

methylrosaniline chloride. See **gentian violet.**

methyl salicylate, a counterirritant and analgesic balm.
- INDICATIONS: It is prescribed externally for minor pain of muscles and joints.
- CONTRAINDICATIONS: It is not recommended for children. Known hypersensitivity to salicylates prohibits its use.
- ADVERSE EFFECTS: Among the more serious adverse reactions are minor skin reaction and possible systemic salicylate poisoning from absorption of the drug when applied externally.

methyltestosterone (mefh′ɪltestos′təroun), an androgen.

- INDICATIONS: It is prescribed in the treatment of testosterone deficiency, osteoporosis, and female breast cancer and to stimulate growth, weight gain, and red blood cell production.
- CONTRAINDICATIONS: Cancer of the male breast or prostate, cardiac, renal, or hepatic disease, hypercalcemia, known or suspected pregnancy, lactation, or known hypersensitivity to this drug prohibits its use.
- ADVERSE EFFECTS: Among the more serious adverse reactions are hypercalcemia, edema, irreversible masculinization of female patients, and jaundice.

methyprylon (mefh′əprai′lon), a sedative and hypnotic.
- INDICATION: It is prescribed in the treatment of insomnia.
- CONTRAINDICATIONS: It is not given to children under three months of age. Known hypersensitivity to this drug prohibits its use.
- ADVERSE EFFECTS: Among the most serious adverse reactions are physical dependence and paradoxical excitement. Dizziness, headache, rash, and gastrointestinal upset also may occur.

methysergide maleate (mefh′ɪsər′jaid), a vasoconstrictor.
- INDICATION: It is prescribed for relief of migraine headache.
- CONTRAINDICATIONS: Pregnancy, severe infection, liver or kidney dysfunction, cardiovascular or lung disease, or known hypersensitivity to this drug prohibits its use. It is not recommended for use in children.
- ADVERSE EFFECTS: Among the more serious adverse reactions are retroperitoneal fibrosis, hallucinations, abnormally low white cell count, pulmonary and cardiac complications, hemolytic anemia, leg cramps, and pain in the chest, abdomen, back, hands, or feet.

Meticortelone Acetate, a trade name for a glucocorticoid (prednisolone acetate).

Meticorten, a trade name for a glucocorticoid (prednisone).

metoclopramide hydrochloride (met′əklou′prəmaid), a gastrointestinal stimulant.
- INDICATIONS: It is prescribed to stimulate motility and to increase the tone of gastric contractions of the upper gastrointestinal tract.
- CONTRAINDICATIONS: Epilepsy, concomitant use of drugs that cause extrapyramidal reactions, pheochromocytoma, gastrointestinal hemorrhage, obstruction, or perforation, or known hypersensitivity to this drug prohibits its use.
- ADVERSE EFFECTS: Among the more serious adverse reactions are extrapyramidal reactions, usually in children, and gastrointestinal disturbances. Drowsiness and allergic reactions with a rash also may occur.

metocurine iodide, a potent neuromuscular blocking agent. Also called **dimethyl tubocurarine iodide.**

■ INDICATIONS: It is given to produce flaccid paralysis as an adjunct to anesthesia, to reduce muscle spasm in tetanus, and to assist controlled ventilation.

■ CONTRAINDICATIONS: Asthma or known hypersensitivity to this drug or to iodides prohibits its use. It is given only by medical personnel trained and equipped to maintain assisted mechanical ventilation.

■ ADVERSE EFFECTS: Among the more serious adverse reactions are hypotension, respiratory or circulatory depression, and bronchospasm.

metolazone (mətou'ləzoun), a diuretic and antihypertensive.

■ INDICATIONS: It is prescribed for the treatment of edema and high blood pressure.

■ CONTRAINDICATIONS: Anuria or known hypersensitivity to this drug, to thiazides, or to sulfonamide drugs prohibits its use.

■ ADVERSE EFFECTS: Among the more serious adverse reactions are hypokalemia, hyperglycemia, hyperuricemia, and various allergic reactions.

'me-too' drug, *Informal.* a drug product that is similar, identical, or closely related to a drug for which a manufacturer has obtained a new drug application. The drug is placed on the market by a company or companies other than the holder of the new drug application. On the assumption that the new drug has been recognized as safe and effective, clinical trials required of the original manufacturer are not required of the new supplier, but information regarding the manufacture, bioavailability, and labeling of the product is required to complete the abbreviated procedure for approval by the Food and Drug Administration.

metopic (mətou'pɪk), of or pertaining to the forehead.

metopo-, a combining form meaning 'of or related to the forehead': *metopodynia, metopopagus, metopoplasty.*

metoprolol tartrate, an antiadrenergic (beta-receptor).

■ INDICATION: It is prescribed in the treatment of hypertension.

■ CONTRAINDICATIONS: Bradycardia, cardiogenic shock, overt cardiac failure, bronchospastic disease, or known hypersensitivity to this drug prohibits its use.

■ ADVERSE EFFECTS: Among the more serious adverse reactions are fatigue, bradycardia, bronchospasms, and gastrointestinal upset.

metr-, a combining form meaning 'measure': *metrechoscopy, metric, metrology.*

metra-. See **metro-.**

metralgia (mɪtræl'jiə), tenderness or pain in the uterus. Also called **metrodynia.**

Metrazol, a trade name for a central nervous system stimulant (pentylenetetrazol).

Metreton, a trade name for a glucocorticoid (prednisolone sodium phosphate).

-metria[1], a combining form meaning '(condition of the) ability to measure muscular acts': *dysmetria, hypermetria, hypometria.*

-metria[2], a combining form meaning '(condition of the) uterus': *ametria, atretometria, dimetria.*

metric, of or pertaining to a system of measurement that uses the meter as a basis. See also **metric system.**

metric equivalent, any value in metric units of measurement that equals the same value in English units, as 2.54 centimeters equal 1 inch or 1 liter equals 1.0567 quarts.

metric system, a decimal system of measurement based on the meter (39.37 inches) as the unit of length, on the gram (15.432 grams) as the unit of weight or mass, and, as a derived unit, on the liter (0.908 U.S. dry quart or 1.0567 U.S. liquid quart) as the unit of volume.

METRIC SYSTEM PREFIXES, MULTIPLES, SUBMULTIPLES

Prefix	Symbol	Power	Multiple, Submultiple
tera	T	10^{12}	1,000,000,000,000
giga	G	10^9	1,000,000,000
mega	M	10^6	1,000,000
kilo	k	10^3	1,000
hecto	h	10^2	100
deca	da	10^1	10
(single unit)			1
deci	d	10^{-1}	0.1
centi	c	10^{-2}	0.01
milli	m	10^{-3}	0.001
micro	μ	10^{-6}	0.000001
nano	n	10^{-9}	0.000000001
pico	p	10^{-12}	0.00000000001
femto	f	10^{-15}	0.000000000000001
atto	a	10^{-18}	0.000000000000000001

metritis (mɪtrai'tɪs), inflammation of the walls of the uterus. Also called **uteritis.** Kinds of metritis are **endometritis, parametritis.** See also **puerperal metritis.**

metro-, metra-, a combining form meaning 'of or related to the uterus': *metrocele, metrofibroma, metromalacoma.*

metrodynia (mi'troudin'iə), tenderness or pain in the uterus. Also called **metralgia.**

metronidazole, an antimicrobial.

■ INDICATIONS: It is prescribed in the treatment of amebiasis, trichomonas, and certain bacterial infections.

■ CONTRAINDICATIONS: First trimester of pregnancy, blood dyscrasias, organic disease, central nervous system disorders, or known hypersensitivity to this drug prohibits its use.

■ ADVERSE EFFECTS: Among the more serious adverse reactions are severe gastrointestinal distress, dizziness, neutropenia, and neurologic disturbances. A metallic taste in the mouth is commonly noted.

-metropia, a combining form meaning '(condition of the) refraction of the eye': *allometropia, antimetropia, isometropia.* Also **-metropy.**

metrorrhagia (met′rourei′jiə), uterine bleeding other than that caused by menstruation. It may be caused by uterine lesions and may be a sign of a urogenital malignancy, especially cervical cancer.

-metry, a combining form meaning the 'process of measuring something' specified: *oncometry, pelvimetry, symmetry.* Also **-metria.**

Metubine, a trade name for a neuromuscular blocking agent (metocurine iodide), used as an adjunct to anesthesia.

Metubine Iodide, a trade name for a skeletal muscle relaxant (metocurine iodide), used as an adjunct to anesthesia.

Metycaine Hydrochloride, a trade name for a local anesthetic (piperocaine hydrochloride).

metyrosine (mɔtir′əsin), an antihypertensive.
■ INDICATION: It is prescribed in the treatment of pheochromocytoma.
■ CONTRAINDICATION: Known hypersensitivity to this drug prohibits its use.
■ ADVERSE EFFECTS: Among the more serious adverse reactions are extrapyramidal reactions, including tremor, drooling, and crystalluria. Sedation is common and diarrhea and anxiety may occur.

Metzenbaum scissors (mets′ɔnbɑum). See **scissors.**

Meuse fever (myuz). See **trench fever.**

MeV, mev, abbreviation for *million electron volts,* the equivalent of 3.82×10^{-14} small calories, or 1.6×10^{-6} ergs.

mevalonate kinase, an enzyme in the liver and in yeast that catalyzes the transfer of a phosphate group from adenosine triphosphate to produce adenosine diphosphate and 5-phosphomevalonate.

Meynet's node (meineiz′), any one of the numerous nodules that may develop within the capsules surrounding joints and in tendons affected by rheumatic diseases, especially in children.

mfd, abbreviation for one **microfarad.**

M.F.D., abbreviation for *minimal fatal dose.*

mg, abbreviation for **milligram.**

Mg, symbol for **magnesium.**

MH, abbreviation for **malignant hyperthermia.**

MHA, abbreviation for **Mental Health Association.**

MI, abbreviation for **myocardial infarction.**

MicaTin, a trade name for an antifungal (miconazole nitrate).

miconazole nitrate (maikon′əzoul), an antifungal.
■ INDICATIONS: It is used topically in the treatment of certain fungal infections of the skin and vagina and parenterally to treat systemic fungal infections.

■ CONTRAINDICATION: Known hypersensitivity to this drug prohibits its use.
■ ADVERSE EFFECTS: Among the more serious adverse reactions to topical or vaginal application are irritation, burning, and maceration of the skin. When used systemically, nausea, pruritus, phlebitis, and anemia may occur.

micr-. See **micro-.**

micrencephalon (mai′krənsef′əlon), **1.** See also **microcephaly.** an abnormally small brain. **2.** *Obsolete.* the cerebellum. – **micrencephalic,** *adj., n.*

micrencephaly, micrencephalia. See **microcephaly.**

micro-, micr-, a combining form meaning 'small': *microadenopathy, microanalysis, microglossia.* Also **mikro.**

microaerotonometer, an instrument for measuring the volume of gases in the blood.

microaggregate recipient set, a device composed of plastic components for the intravenous delivery of large volumes of stored whole blood or of packed blood cells. The components of the set include the plastic tubing, the roller clamp, and the special filter that prevents the microaggregates or deteriorated red blood cells of stored whole blood from entering and clogging the circulatory system of the patient. The plastic tubing of this device has a larger lumen than the tubing of most other intravenous sets, hence allows the blood to be delivered more rapidly. Compare **component drip set, component syringe set, straight-line blood set, Y-set.**

microaneurysm, a microscopic aneurysm characteristic of thrombotic purpura.

microangiopathy, a disease of the small blood vessels, as diabetic microangiopathy, in which the basement membrane of capillaries thickens and thrombotic microangiopathy, in which thrombi form in the arterioles and the capillaries.

microbe, a pathogenic microorganism. – **microbial,** *adj.*

-microbe, a combining form meaning a 'small living organism': *aeromicrobe, inframicrobe, ultramicrobe.*

-microbic, a combining form meaning 'referring to or consisting of microbes': *amicrobic, monomicrobic, polymicrobic.*

microbiology, the branch of biology concerned with the study of microorganisms, including algae, bacteria, viruses, protozoa, fungi, and rickettsiae.

microbrachia (mai′kroubrei′kiə), a developmental defect characterized by abnormal smallness of the arms. – **microbrachius,** *n.*

microcentrum (mai′krousen′trəm). See **centrosome.**

microcephaly (mai′krousef′əli), **microcephalia, microcephalism,** a congenital anomaly characterized by abnormal smallness of the head in relation to the rest of the body and by underdevelopment of the brain, resulting in some degree of mental retardation. The head is more than two standard deviations below the average circumference size for age, sex, race, and period of gestation, and it has a narrow, receding forehead, a flattened occiput, and a pointed vertex. The facial features are generally normal. The condition may be caused by an autosomal recessive disorder, a chromosomal abnormality, a toxic stimulus, as irradiation, chemical agents, or maternal infection during prenatal development, or any trauma, especially during the third trimester of pregnancy or early infancy. There is no treatment, and nursing care is primarily supportive and educational, helping parents learn to care for a brain-damaged child. Compare **macrocephaly**. — **microcephalic, microcephalous**, *adj.*, **microcephalic, microcephalus**, *n.*

microcheiria, microchiria (maĭ′kroukaĭ′riə), a developmental defect characterized by abnormal smallness of the hands. The condition is usually associated with other congenital malformations or with bone and muscle disorders.

microcirculation, the flow of blood throughout the system of smaller vessels of the body, those with a diameter of 100 microns or less.

microcurie (μCi, μc), a unit of radiation equal to one-millionth (10^{-6}) of a curie.

microcyte (maĭ′krəsaĭt), an abnormally small erythrocyte with a mean corpuscular volume less than 80 μ, often occurring in iron-deficiency and other anemias.

microcytic, (of a cell) smaller than normal, as the erythrocytes in microcytic anemia.

microcytic anemia, a hematologic disorder characterized by abnormally small erythrocytes, usually associated with chronic blood loss or a nutritional anemia, as iron deficiency anemia. Compare **macrocytic anemia**.

microcytosis (maĭ′krousaĭtou′sıs), a hematologic condition characterized by erythrocytes that are smaller than normal. Microcytosis and hypochromatosis are usual in iron-deficiency anemia. — **microcytic**, *adj.*

microdactyly (maĭ′kroudæk′təli), a developmental defect characterized by abnormal smallness of the fingers and toes. The condition is usually associated with bone and muscle disorders, as progressive myositis ossificans.

microdrip (maĭ′kroudrıp′), (in intravenous therapy) an apparatus for delivering relatively small, measured amounts of intravenous solutions at specific flow rates. The microdrip device usually consists of plastic tubing designed to allow small drops of solution to pass into the primary intravenous tubing through a clear plastic housing. A microdrip is usually used to deliver small volumes of solution over a long time. With a microdrip 60 drops deliver 1 ml of solution. Compare **macrodrip**.

microelement. See **micronutrient**.

microencapsulation, a laboratory technique used in the bioassay of hormones in which certain antibodies are encapsulated with a perforated membrane, resembling a whiffle ball. The antibodies cannot escape, but hormones that bind with the antibodies may enter the structure to bind with them. Technicians then can measure the amount of hormone present in the specimen. The technique is used for encapsulating unstable enzymes and in the preparation of some drugs in slow- or timed-release forms.

microfarad (mfd), a unit of capacitance that equals one millionth of a farad.

microfilaria (maĭ′kroufıler′iə), *pl.* **microfilariae**. the prelarval form of any filarial worm. Certain blood-sucking insects ingest these forms from an infected host, and the microfilariae then develop in the body of the insect and become infective larvae. See also **dracontiasis, filariasis, loiasis, onchocerciasis**, *Wuchereria*.

microfluorometry (maĭ′krouflurom′ıtri, maĭ′krouflɔrom′-ıtri). See **cytophotometry**. — **microfluorometric**, *adj.*

microgamete, the small, motile male gamete of certain thallophytes and sporozoa, specifically the malarial parasite *Plasmodium*. It corresponds to the sperm of the higher animals and unites in conjugation with the larger, nonmotile female gamete. See also **macrogamete**.

microgametocyte, an enlarged merozoite that undergoes meiosis to form the mature male gamete during the sexual phase of the life cycle of certain thallophytes and sporozoa, specifically the malarial parasite *Plasmodium*. Microgametocytes are found in the red blood cells of a person infected with the malarial parasite, but they must be ingested by a female *Anopheles* mosquito to complete the maturation process and develop into a microgamete.

microgenitalia, a condition characterized by abnormally small external genitalia.

microglia (maĭkrog′liə), small migratory interstitial cells that form part of the central nervous system. They have various forms and slender, branched processes. Microglia serve as phagocytes which collect waste products of the nerve tissue of the body. Also called **Hortega cells, mesoglia**.

micrognathia (maĭ′krounei′ɾhiə), underdevelopment of the jaw, especially the mandible. Compare **macrognathia**. — **micrognathic**, *adj.*

microgram (mgm, μgm), a unit of measurement of mass equal to one millionth (10^{-6}) of a gram. See also **gram**.

microgyria (maĭ′kroujaĭ′riə), a developmental defect of the brain in which the convolutions are abnormally small, resulting in structural malformation of the cortex. The condition is usually associated with mental retardation and physical defects. Also called **polymicrogyria**.

microgyrus (maĭ′kroujaĭ′rəs), *pl.* **microgyri**. an underdeveloped, malformed convolution of the brain.

microhm, a unit of electrical resistance equal to one millionth of an ohm.

microinvasive carcinoma, a squamous epithelial neoplasm that has penetrated the basement membrane, the first stage in invasive cancer. It is most frequently diagnosed in the uterine cervix, but the lesion is difficult to demonstrate. Some oncologists often prefer to designate the lesion as either invasive or in situ. See also **carcinoma in situ.**

microliter (μl), a unit of liquid volume equal to one millionth of a liter.

microlith, a small rounded mass of mineral matter or calcified stone.

micromelic dwarf, a dwarf whose limbs are abnormally short.

micrometer (maikrom′itər), 1. an instrument used for measuring small angles or distances on objects being observed through a microscope or telescope. 2. a unit of measurement, commonly referred to as a *micron,* that is one thousandth (10^{-3}) of a millimeter.

micromicro- ($\mu\mu$), a combining form meaning '10^{-12}': *micromicron.*

micromyeloblastic leukemia (mai′kroumai′əloublæs′tik), a malignant neoplasm of blood-forming tissues, characterized by the proliferation of small myeloblasts distinguishable from lymphocytes only by special staining techniques and microscopic examination.

micron (μ, **mu**) (mai′kron), 1. a metric unit of length equal to one millionth of a meter. 2. (in physical chemistry), a colloidal particle with a diameter of between 0.2 and 10 microns.

Micronor, a trade name for an oral contraceptive containing a progestin (norethindrone).

micronucleus, 1. a small or minute nucleus. 2. (in protozoa) the smaller of two nuclei in each cell; it functions in sexual reproduction as opposed to the macronucleus, which governs cell metabolism and growth. 3. See **nucleolus.**

micronutrient (mai′krounu′triənt), an organic compound, as a vitamin, or a chemical element, as zinc or iodine, essential only in minute amounts for the normal physiological processes of the body. Also called **microelement, minor element, trace element.**

microorganism, any tiny, usually microscopic entity capable of carrying on living processes. It may be pathogenic. Kinds of microorganisms include **bacteria, fungi, protozoa, viruses.**

micropenis (mai′krəpi′nis). See **microphallus.**

microphage (mai′krəfeij), a neutrophil capable of ingesting small things, as bacteria. Compare **macrophage.** —**microphagic,** *adj.*

microphallus (mai′krəfæl′əs), an abnormally small penis. When observed in the newborn the nurse examines the child for other signs of ambiguous genitalia. Also called **micropenis.** See also **ambiguous genitalia.**

microphthalmos (mai′krəfthæl′məs), **microphthalmia,** a developmental anomaly characterized by abnormal smallness of one or both eyes. When the condition occurs in the absence of other ocular defects, it is called pure microphthalmos or nanophthalmos. —**microphthalmic,** *adj.,* **microphthalmus,** *n.*

microplasia. See **dwarfism.**

micropodia, a developmental anomaly characterized by abnormal smallness of the feet. The condition is often associated with other congenital malformations or with bone and skeletal disorders.

microprosopus (mai′krouprou′səpəs, mai′krouprəsou′-pəs), a fetus in which the face is abnormally small or underdeveloped.

micropsia (maikrop′siə), a condition of vision by which a person perceives objects smaller than they really are. —**microptic,** *adj.*

microscopic, 1. of or pertaining to a microscope. 2. very small; visible only when magnified and illuminated by a microscope.

microscopic anatomy, the study of the microscopic structure of the tissues and cells. Kinds of microscopic anatomy are **cytology, histology.**

microscopy (maikros′kəpi), a technique for observing minute materials using a microscope. Kinds of microscopy include **darkfield microscopy, electron microscopy, immunofluorescent microscopy.**

microsomia, the condition of having an abnormally small and underdeveloped yet otherwise perfectly formed body with normal proportionate relationships of the various parts. See also **primordial dwarf.**

microtome (mai′krətoum), a device that cuts specimens of tissue prepared in paraffin blocks into extremely thin slices for microscopic study by a surgical pathologist.

micturate (mik′ĉhureit). See **urination.**

micturition (mik′ĉhuri′ŝhən). See **urination.**

micturition reflex, a normal reaction to a rise in pressure within the bladder, resulting in contraction of the bladder wall and relaxation of the urethral sphincter. Voluntary inhibition normally prevents incontinence, with urination occurring on withdrawal of this inhibition.

midbrain. See **mesencephalon.**

midclavicular line (mid′kləvik′yulər), (in anatomy) an imaginary line that extends downward over the trunk from the midpoint of the clavicle, dividing each side of the anterior chest into two parts. The left midclavicular line is an important marker in describing the location of various cardiac phenomena, including the point of maximum impulse.

middle cardiac vein, one of the five tributaries of the coronary sinus that drains blood from the capillary bed of the myocardium. It starts at the apex of the heart, rises in the posterior interventricular sulcus, receives tributaries from both ventricles, and ends in the right extremity of the coronary sinus. Compare **great cardiac vein, small cardiac vein.**

middle costotransverse ligament. See **ligament of the neck of the rib.**

middle cuneiform bone. See **intermediate cuneiform bone.**

middle ear, the tympanic cavity and the auditory ossicles contained in an irregular space in the temporal bone. It is separated from the external ear by the tympanic membrane. The auditory tube carries air from the posterior pharynx into the middle ear.

middle kidney. See **mesonephros.**

middle lobe syndrome, localized atelectasis of the middle lobe of the right lung, characterized by chronic infection, cough, dyspnea, wheezing, and obstructive pneumonitis. Asymptomatic obstruction of the bronchus may occur. The condition is caused by enlargement of the surrounding cuff of lymphatic glands, owing to nonspecific or tuberculous inflammation during childhood. The middle lobe bronchus is thus compressed, with bronchiectasis developing in the obstructed part of the lung. Treatment includes antituberculosis chemotherapy, corticosteroids, or surgical excision. See also **atelectasis.**

middle mediastinum, the widest part of the mediastinum containing the heart, ascending aorta, lower half of the superior vena cava, pulmonary trunk, and phrenic nerves. It is one of three caudal portions of the mediastinum. Compare **anterior mediastinum, posterior mediastinum, superior mediastinum.**

middle plate. See **nephrotome.**

middle sacral artery, a small, visceral branch of the abdominal aorta, descending to the fourth and fifth lumbar vertebrae, the sacrum, and the coccyx. Minute branches are said to supply the posterior surface of the rectum.

middle suprarenal artery, one of a pair of small, visceral branches of the abdominal aorta, arising opposite the superior mesenteric artery, and supplying the suprarenal gland.

middle temporal artery, one of the branches of the superficial temporal artery on each side of the head. It arises just above the zygomatic arch, pierces the temporal fascia, branches to the temporalis, and anastomoses with the deep temporal branches of the maxillary artery. Compare **deep temporal artery, superficial temporal artery.**

middle umbilical fold, the fold of peritoneum over the urachal remnant within the abdomen. Approximately 3 cm lateral to the middle umbilical fold is the lateral umbilical fold. Between the lateral and the middle folds is the medial umbilical fold. Also called **plica umbilicalis mediana.**

mid forceps, an obstetric operation in which forceps are applied to the head of the baby when the head has reached the midplane of the mother's pelvis. An episiotomy is usually performed, and local, regional, or inhalation anesthesia is provided. In some cases, as severe fetal distress, mid forceps may be the most rapid and the safest means of delivery, but astute selection of cases, skill, and experience are essential. Difficult mid forceps delivery is likely to more traumatic to the baby and the mother than

Caesarean section. Compare **high forceps, low forceps.** See also **failed forceps, forceps delivery, obstetric forceps, trial forceps.**

midgut, the middle portion of the embryonic alimentary canal. It consists of endodermal tissue, is connected to the yolk sac during early prenatal development, and eventually gives rise to some of the small intestine and part of the large intestine. Compare **foregut, hindgut.**

midline episiotomy. See **episiotomy.**

midpelvic contraction. See **contraction.**

Midrin, a trade name for a central-nervous-system, fixed-combination drug containing an adrenergic (isometheptene mucate), an hypnotic (dichloralphenazone), and an analgesic (acetaminophen), used in the treatment of migraine headaches.

midsagittal plane. See **cardinal sagittal plane.**

midstance, one of the five stages in the stance phase of walking, or gait, directly associated with the period of single-leg support of body weight or the period during which the body advances over the stationary foot. During midstance the tibialis posterior and the flexor hallucis longus display their greatest activity. The midstance phase is considered in the diagnosis of many abnormal orthopedic conditions and in the analysis of the associated weaknesses of certain muscles and muscle groups. Compare **initial contact stance stage, loading response stance stage, preswing stance stage, terminal stance.** See also **swing phase of gait.**

midwife, 1. (in traditional use) a person who assists women in childbirth. 2. (according to the International Confederation of Midwives, World Health Organization, and Federation of International Gynecologists and Obstetricians) "a person who, having been regularly admitted to a midwifery educational program fully recognized in the country in which it is located, has successfully completed the prescribed course of studies in midwifery and has acquired the requisite qualifications to be registered and/or legally licensed to practice midwifery." Among the responsibilities of the midwife are supervision of the woman's pregnancy, labor, delivery, and puerperium. The midwife conducts the delivery independently, cares for the newborn, procures medical assistance when necessary, executes emergency measures as required, and may practice in a hospital, clinic, maternity home, or in a woman's home. The midwife, whose practice may include wellchild care, family planning, and some aspects of gynecology, is often an important source of health counseling in the community. 3. a lay-midwife. 4. a nurse-midwife or Certified Nurse Midwife.

migraine, recurring vascular headache characterized by a prodromal aura, unilateral onset, and severe pain, photophobia, and autonomic disturbances during the acute phase, which may last for hours or days. The disorder occurs more frequently in women than in men and a predisposition to migraine may be inherited. The exact mechanism responsible for the disorder is not known but the head pain is related to dilation of extracranial blood vessels, which may be the result of chemical changes that cause spasms of intracranial vessels. A greatly increased amount of a vasodilating polypeptide related to bradykinin is found in tissue fluid of patients during migraine attacks. Allergic reactions, excess carbohydrates, iodine-rich foods, alcohol, bright lights, or loud noises may trigger attacks, which often occur during a period of relaxation following physical or psychic stress. An impending attack may be heralded by visual disturbances, as flashing lights or wavy lines, by a strange taste or odor, numbness, tingling, vertigo, tinnitus, or a feeling that part of the body is distorted in size or shape. The acute phase may be accompanied by nausea, vomiting, chills, polyuria, sweating, facial edema, irritability, and extreme fatigue. After an attack the individual often has dull head and neck pains and a great need for sleep. Aspirin seldom provides relief during an attack, but ergotamine tartrate preparations that constrict cranial arteries can usually prevent the headache from developing if administered early in the onset as an injection, suppository, or tablet. Ergotamine tartrate is also available combined with other drugs, as caffeine, phenobarbital, and belladonna; migrane patients unable to tolerate ergot preparations may use other analgesics, including acetaminophen, phenacetin, and propoxyphene. Also called **hemicrania, megrim.**

migrainous cranial neuralgia (mæigreiˈnəs), a variant of migraine, characterized by closely spaced episodes of excruciating, throbbing, unilateral headaches often accompanied by dilation of temporal blood vessels, flushing, sweating, lacrimation, nasal congestion or rhinorrhea, ptosis, and facial edema. Repeated episodes usually occur in clusters within a few days or weeks and may be followed by a relatively long remission period. A typical attack begins abruptly without prodromal signs, as a burning sensation in an orbit or temple, and the resulting radiating intense pain may last an hour or two. Histamine diphosphate injected subcutaneously in persons subject to these headaches produces symptoms identical to those occurring in a spontaneous attack. The pain may be relieved by antihistamines, and ergotamine tartrate preparations may be helpful if administered at the onset of an attack. Also called **cluster headache, histamine headache, Horton's headache.** See also **migraine.**

migratory gonorrheal polyarthritis. See **migratory polyarthritis.**

migratory ophthalmia. See **sympathetic ophthalmia.**

migratory polyarthritis, arthritis progressively affecting a number of joints and finally settling in one or more, occurring in patients with gonorrhea and developing a few days to a few weeks following the onset of gonorrheal urethritis. The patient usually has a moderate fever and

one to five days of migratory polyarthralgia with variable signs of inflammation. In more prolonged episodes, initially arthritic sites may clear as new areas are affected, but persistently involved joints are usually severely inflamed and swollen. Large joints are most affected; after the swelling subsides the overlying skin may peel. Treatment with penicillin or tetracycline generally produces some response in 24 to 72 hours. Also called **migratory gonorrheal polyarthritis.**

migratory thrombophlebitis, an abnormal condition in which multiple thromboses appear here and there in both superficial and deep veins. It may be associated with malignancy, especially carcinoma of the pancreas, often preceding other evidence of cancer by several months. Pulmonary embolism is uncommon with this condition. Also called **thrombophlebitis migrans.** See also **thrombophlebitis.**

mikro-. See **micro-.**

Mikulicz's syndrome (mɪkˈyuliĉˈɪz), an abnormal bilateral enlargement of the salivary and lacrimal glands, found in a variety of diseases, including leukemia, tuberculosis, and sarcoidosis. Also called **Mikulicz's disease.**

mild, a quality of gentleness, subtlety, or low intensity, as a mild infection.

milia (milˈiə), minute, white cysts of the epidermis caused by obstruction of hair follicles and eccrine sweat glands. One variety is seen in newborn infants and disappears within a few weeks. Another type is found primarily on the faces of middle-aged women. Milia may be treated with an abrasive cleanser or by incision and drainage. Compare **miliaria.**

milia neonatorum, a normal dermatologic condition characterized by minute epidermal cysts consisting of keratinous debris that occur on the face and, occasionally, the trunk of the newborn. They are eliminated by normal desquamation of the skin within a few weeks following birth and leave no scars.

miliaria (milˈierˈiə), minute vesicles and papules, often with surrounding erythema, caused by occlusion of sweat ducts during times of exposure to heat and high humidity. Back-up pressure may cause sweat to escape into adjacent tissue producing itching and prickling. Prevention and treatment include cool environment, ventilation, colloidal baths, and dusting powders. Also called **prickly heat.** Compare **milia.**

miliary (milˈierˈi), describing a condition marked by the appearance of very small lesions the size of millet seeds, as miliary tuberculosis, which is characterized by tiny tubercules throughout the body.

miliary carcinosis, a condition characterized by the presence of numerous cancerous nodules resembling miliary tubercles.

miliary tuberculosis, extensive dissemination by the bloodstream of tubercle bacilli. In children it is associated with high fever, night sweats, and, often, meningitis, pleural effusions, or peritonitis. A similar illness may occur in adults but with a less abrupt onset and, occasionally, with weeks or months of nonspecific symptoms, as weight loss, weakness, and low-grade fever. Multiple small opacities resembling millet seeds may be evident on chest x ray. The liver, spleen, bone marrow, and meninges are often affected. The tuberculin test may be negative, and diagnosis is made by biopsy of the infected tissue or organ. Combined drug therapy with isoniazid and rifampin or with isoniazid and streptomycin is usually successful if the diagnosis is not delayed. Concurrent tuberculous meningitis makes the prognosis less favorable. See also *Mycobacterium,* **tuberculosis.**

milieu (milyœ′), *pl.* **milieus, milieux.** *French.* the environment, surroundings, or setting. Kinds of milieus are **milieu extérieur, milieu intérieur.**

milieu extérieur (eksteiryœʀ′), *French.* the external or physical surroundings of an organism, including the social environment, especially the home, school, and recreational facilities, that plays a dominant role in personality development.

milieu intérieur (ãteiryœʀ′), *French.* the basic concept in physiology, originated by Claude Bernard, that multicellular organisms exist in an aqueous internal environment composed of the blood, lymph, and interstitial fluid that bathes all cells and provides a medium for the elementary exchange of nutrients and waste material. All fundamental processes necessary for the maintenance and life of the tissue elements are dependent on the stability and balance of this environment.

milieu therapy, a type of psychotherapy in which the total environment is utilized in treating mental and behavioral disorders. It is primarily conducted in a hospital or other institutional setting where the entire facility acts as a therapeutic community. The emphasis is on providing pleasant physical surroundings, structured activities, and a stable social environment where behavioral modification and personal growth are promoted through patient-group interaction, staff support and understanding, and a total, humanistic approach. Individual daily routines and treatment modalities, such as drug therapy, occupational therapy, and sensitivity training, are determined by the patient's emotional and interpersonal needs. Also called **situation therapy.**

milk, a liquid secreted by the mammary glands or udders of animals that suckle their young. After breast feeding, people consume the milk of the cow as well as that of many other animals, including the goat, camel, mare, reindeer, llama, and yak. Milk is a basic food containing carbohydrate (in the form of lactose), protein (mainly casein, with small amounts of lactalbumin, and lactoglobulin), suspended fat, the minerals calcium and phosphorous, the vitamins riboflavin, niacin, thiamine, A, and,

when the milk is fortified, vitamin D. It is a valuable nutrient for adults and nearly a complete food for infants, especially breast milk. Milk does not contain a significant amount of iron; its ascorbic acid content depends on the amount ingested by the mother or by the animal producing the milk. Some individuals show a sensitivity reaction to milk owing to a deficiency of the enzyme lactase. See also **breast milk.**

milk baby, an infant with iron-deficiency anemia caused by ingestion of excessive amounts of milk and the delayed or inadequate addition of iron-rich foods to the diet. Milk babies are overweight, have pale skin and poor muscle development, and are highly susceptible to infection. See also **anemia.**

milk bath, a bath taken in milk for cosmetic or emollient reasons.

milk-ejection reflex, a normal reflex in a lactating woman elicited by tactile stimulation of the nipple, resulting in release of milk from the glands of the breast. This reflex requires intact nerve connections from nipple to hypothalamus and the release of the hormone, oxytocin, from the posterior pituitary into the bloodstream. Also called **let-down reflex.** See also **oxytocin.**

milker's nodule, a smooth, brownish-red papilloma of the fingers or palm that begins as a macule and progresses through a vesicular stage to become a nodule. The disease is acquired from pustular lesions on the udder of a cow infected with poxvirus. No treatment is necessary because immunity is produced after primary infection.

milk fever, *Nontechnical.* postpartum fever that begins with the onset of lactation. It was formerly considered a normal reaction to lactation. Maternal temperature during the puerperium does not normally exceed 99°F; higher elevations usually indicate infection.

milk globule, a spherical droplet of fat in milk that tends to separate out as cream.

milking, a procedure used to express the contents of a duct or tube, to test for tenderness, or to obtain a specimen for study. The examiner compresses the structure with a finger and moves the finger firmly along the duct or tube to its opening. Also called **stripping.**

milk leg. See **phlegmasia alba dolens.**

milk of magnesia, a laxative and antacid containing magnesium hydroxide.

■ INDICATIONS: It is prescribed to relieve constipation and acid indigestion.

■ CONTRAINDICATIONS: Renal impairment, symptoms of appendicitis, or known hypersensitivity to the drug prohibits its use.

■ ADVERSE EFFECTS: Among the most serious adverse reactions are diarrhea and hypermagnesemia, usually occurring in patients who have impaired renal function.

milkpox. See **alastrim.**

milk sugar. See **lactose.**

milk therapy, a nutritional treatment used in the therapy of Curling's ulcer in patients who have been severely burned. Cool, homogenized milk is administered in doses of one to two ounces every hour through a nasogastric tube. After instillation the tube is clamped for five minutes and then unclamped. Milk remaining in the stomach is allowed to flow into a basin. As the milk is better absorbed and tolerated feedings are increased to 150 ml of milk/kg of body weight daily. The interval between feedings is gradually lengthened to four hours. As the condition improves, the nasogastric tube is withdrawn, and milk may be continued by mouth.

milk tooth. See **deciduous tooth.**

milky ascites. See **chylous ascites.**

Miller-Abbott tube, a long, small-caliber, double-lumen catheter, used in intestinal intubation for decompression. It has several openings on the side of its tip and a balloon above the tip. Compare **Harris tube.** See also **gastric intubation.**

milli-, a combining form meaning '1/1000th part': *milliampere, millibar, milliliter.*

milliampere (ma), a unit of electrical current that is one thousandth of an ampere.

millicoulomb (mC), a unit of electrical charge that is one thousandth of a coulomb.

millicurie (mCi, mc), a unit of radioactivity that is equal to one thousandth of a curie, or 3.70×10^7 disintegrations per second.

milliequivalent (mEq), the number of grams of solute dissolved in one milliliter of a normal solution.

milligram (mg), a metric unit of weight equal to one thousandth (10^{-3}) of a gram.

milliliter (ml), a metric unit of volume that is one thousandth (10^{-3}) of a liter.

millimeter (mm), a metric unit of length equal to one thousandth (10^{-3}) of a meter.

millimicrogram (mμgm), one thousandth (10^{-3}) of a microgram, or one billionth (10^{-9}) of a gram. Also called **nanogram.**

millimole (mmol), a unit of metric measurement of mass that is equal to one thousandth (10^{-3}) of a mole.

milliosmol (mɪl'ioz'moul), a unit of measure representing the concentration of an ion in a solution, expressed in milligrams per liter divided by atomic weight. See also **osmol, osmolality, osmolarity.** — **milliosmolar,** *adj.*

millipede (mɪl'ɪpid'), a many-legged, wormlike arthropod. Certain species squirt irritating fluids that may cause dermatitis.

millirad, one thousandth (10^{-3}) of a rad, a unit of measurement of absorbed dose of ionizing radiation.

milliroentgen (mR, mr) (mɪl'rent'gən, mɪl'rent'jən), a unit of radiation that is equal to one thousandth (10^{-3}) of a roentgen.

millivolt (mV, mv), a unit of electromotive force equal to one thousandth of a volt.

Milontin, a trade name for an anticonvulsant (phensuximide).

Milpath, a trade name for a gastrointestinal, fixed-combination drug containing an anticholinergic (tridihexethyl chloride) and a sedative (meprobamate).

Milprem, a trade name for a hormonal, fixed-combination drug containing conjugated estrogens and a sedative (meprobamate).

Miltown, a trade name for a sedative (meprobamate).

Miltrate, a trade name for a cardiovascular, fixed-combination drug containing a vasodilator (pentaerythritol tetranitrate) and a sedative (meprobamate).

Milwaukee brace, an orthotic device that helps to immobilize the torso and the neck of a patient in the treatment or correction of spinal scoliosis, lordosis, or kyphosis. It is usually constructed of strong but light metal and fiberglass supports lined with rubber to protect against abrasion. Milwaukee braces, which may be employed in the treatment of orthopedic bed patients or ambulatory patients, commonly connect cervical supports, rib supports, and hip supports with rigid bars of metal that hold the trunk and the neck erect while controlling cervical flexion and hip movements.

-mimesis, a combining form meaning 'simulation, imitation': *necromimesis, neuromimesis, pathomimesis.*

-mimetic, a combining form meaning 'pertaining to simulation of (specified) effects': *andromimetic, neuromimetic, vagomimetic.*

-mimia, a combining form meaning '(condition of) ability to express thought through gestures': *macromimia, paramimia, pathomimia.*

mimic spasm, involuntary, stereotyped movements of a small group of muscles, as of the face. The spasm is usually psychogenic and may be aggravated by stress or anxiety but is generally controllable momentarily. Multiple grimacing and blinking mimic spasms occur in Gilles de la Tourette's syndrome. Also called **tic.**

min, abbreviation for **minim.**

Minamata disease (mɪn'əma'tə), a severe, degenerative, neurologic disorder caused by the ingestion of seed grain heated with alkyl compounds of mercury or of seafood taken from waters polluted with industrial wastes contaminated by soluble mercuric salts. It is most often seen in those Japanese who eat seafood from Minamata Bay. Mercury passes the placental barrier, causing the congenital form of the disease. Symptoms may not appear for several weeks or months; they include paresthesia of the mouth and extremities, tunnel vision, difficulties with speech, hearing, muscular coordination, and concentration, weakness, emotional instability, and stupor. Continued ingestion causes serious damage to the renal tubules and corrosion of the gastrointestinal tract. Acute cases may result in coma and death. See also **mercury poisoning.**

mind, 1. the part of the brain that is the seat of mental activity and that enables one to know, reason, understand, remember, think, feel, and to react and adapt to surroundings and all external and internal stimuli. 2. the totality of all conscious and unconscious processes of the individual that influence and direct mental and physical behavior. 3. the faculty of the intellect or understanding in contrast to emotion and will. See also **brain, intellect, psyche.**

mine damp. See **damp.**

mineral, 1. an inorganic substance occurring naturally in the earth's crust, having a characteristic chemical composition and (usually) crystalline structure. 2. (in nutrition) a mineral is usually referred to by the name of a metal, nonmetal, radical, or phosphate rather than by the name of the compound of which it is a part, and it is ingested as a compound, like sodium chloride (table salt), rather than as a free element. Minerals play a vital role in regulating many bodily functions.

mineral deficiency, the inability to utilize one or more of the mineral elements essential in human nutrition because of a genetic defect, malabsorption dysfunction, or the lack of that mineral in the diet. The symptoms and manifestations vary, depending on the specific function or functions of the element in promoting growth and maintaining body health. Minerals are constituents of all the body tissues and fluids, and they are important factors in maintaining physiological processes. They act as catalysts in nerve response, muscle contraction, and the metabolism of nutrients in foods, they regulate electrolyte balance and hormonal production, and they strengthen skeletal structures. All mineral deficiencies are treated by adding the specific element to the diet, either in supplementary form or in the appropriate foods. See also specific minerals.

mineralization, the addition of any mineral to the body.

mineralocorticoid, a hormone, secreted by the adrenal cortex, that maintains normal blood volume, promotes sodium and water retention, and increases urinary excretion of potassium and hydrogen ions. Aldosterone, the most potent mineralocorticoid in regard to electrolyte balance, and corticosterone, a glucocorticoid as well as mineralocorticoid, act on the distal tubules of the kidneys to enhance the reabsorption of sodium into the plasma. Aldosterone secretion is stimulated by angiotensin, the polypeptide formed by the action of renin, which is released by juxtaglomerular cells of the kidneys when serum sodium levels fall. Hypersecretion of aldosterone causes expansion of extracellular fluid, hypertension, hypokalemia, alkalosis, and a slight increase in plasma sodium. Hyposecretion of the hormone results in hypotension, circulatory collapse, hyperkalemia, and severe

sodium loss; without aldosterone an adult may secrete as much as 25 gm of sodium a day. Trauma and stress increase mineralocorticoid secretion. The synthetic mineralocorticoids desoxycorticosterone, which does not influence carbohydrate metabolism, and fluorocortisone, which also has glucocorticoid activity, are used in treating the salt-losing, adrenogenital syndrome and the severe corticoid deficiency characteristic of Addison's disease. See also **glucocorticoid.**

mineral oil, a laxative, stool softener, emollient, and pharmaceutic aid used as a solvent.

■ INDICATIONS: It is prescribed to prevent constipation, to treat mild constipation, to prepare the bowel for surgery or examination, and as a solvent for various preparations.

■ CONTRAINDICATIONS: Symptoms of appendicitis, fecal impaction, obstruction or perforation of the intestinal tract, pregnancy, or known hypersensitivity to this drug prohibits its use.

■ ADVERSE EFFECTS: Among the more serious adverse reactions are laxative dependence, lipid pneumonitis, fat-soluble vitamin deficiency, and abdominal cramps.

miner's cramp. See **heat cramp.**

miner's elbow, an inflammation of the olecranon bursa, caused by resting the weight of the body on the elbow, as in hewing for coal. The condition is sometimes seen in school children who lean on their elbows. Compare **lateral humeral epicondylitis.** See also **bursitis.**

miner's pneumoconiosis. See **anthracosis.**

Minerva cast (mĭnər'və), an orthopedic cast applied to the trunk and the head, with spaces cut out for the face area and the ears. The section encasing the trunk extends to the sternum and the distal rib border anteriorly and across the distal rib border posteriorly. The cast is used for immobilizing the head and part of the trunk in the treatment of torticollis, cervical injuries, and cervical spinal infections. It is not used as frequently as it once was because of advancement in the field of orthotics.

Minerva jacket, a cast extending from the chin to the hips, applied for support and immobilization of the cervical and thoracic spine, especially after a fracture.

minim, (min), a measurement of volume in the apothecaries' system, originally one drop (of water). Sixty minims equal one fluid dram. One minim equals 0.06 milliliters.

minimal brain dysfunction (MBD). See **attention deficit disorder.**

minimum alveolar concentration (MAC), the smallest amount of a gas detected and measured in the alveoli of the lungs.

Minipress, a trade name for an antihypertensive (prazosin hydrochloride).

Minocin, a trade name for an antibacterial (minocycline hydrochloride).

minocycline hydrochloride (min'əsaı'klin), a tetracycline antibiotic active against bacteria, rickettsia, and other organisms.

■ INDICATIONS: It is prescribed in the treatment of a variety of infections.

■ CONTRAINDICATIONS: Its use must be used with caution with renal or hepatic dysfunction. Known hypersensitivity to this or other tetracyclines prohibits its use.

■ ADVERSE EFFECTS: Among the more serious adverse reactions are gastrointestinal disturbances, phototoxicity, vestibular toxicity, potentially serious suprainfections, and various allergic reactions. Use during pregnancy or in children under 8 years of age may result in discoloration of teeth.

minor, (in law) a person not of legal age; beneath the age of majority. Minors usually cannot consent to their own medical treatment unless they are substantially independent from their parents, are married, support themselves, or satisfy other requirements as provided by statute.

minor element. See **micronutrient.**

minor renal calyx. See **renal calyx.**

minor surgery, any surgical procedure that does not require general anesthesia or respiratory assistance.

minoxidil, a vasodilator.

■ INDICATION: It is prescribed in the treatment of severe refractory hypertension.

■ CONTRAINDICATIONS: Pheochromocytoma or known hypersensitivity to this drug prohibits its use.

■ ADVERSE EFFECTS: Among the most serious adverse reactions are tachycardia, pericardial effusion, cardiac tamponade, salt and water retention, and excessive hair growth. Gastrointestinal disturbances also may occur.

Mintezol, a trade name for an anthelmintic (thiabendazole).

mio-, a combining form meaning 'less': *miolecithal, mioplasmia, miosphygmia.* Also **meio-.**

Miocel, a trade name for an ophthalmic, fixed-combination drug containing cholinergics (pilocarpine hydrochloride and physostigmine salicylate).

Miochol, a trade name for a parasympathetic blocking agent (acetylcholine chloride).

miosis (maıoʊ'sıs), **1.** contraction of the sphincter muscle of the iris, causing the pupil to become smaller. Certain drugs and stimulation of the pupillary light reflex by an increase in light result in miosis. **2.** an abnormal condition characterized by excessive constriction of the sphincter muscle of the iris, resulting in very small, pin point pupils. Compare **mydriasis.** — **miotic,** *adj.*

Miostat, a trade name for a cholinergic (carbachol).

miotic, **1.** of or pertaining to miosis. **2.** causing constriction of the pupil of the eye. **3.** any substance or pharmaceutical, as pilocarpine, that causes constriction of the

pupil of the eye. Such agents are used in the treatment of glaucoma. — **miosis,** *n.*

MIP, abbreviation for **maximum inspiratory pressure.**

miracidium (mır'əsıd'iəm), *pl.* **miracidia.** the ciliated larva of a parasitic trematode that hatches from an egg and can survive only by penetrating and further developing within a host snail, whereupon the larva further develops into a maternal sporocyte that produces more larvae.

Miradon, a trade name for an anticoagulant (anisindione).

mirage, an optical illusion caused by the refraction of light through air layers of different temperatures, as the illusionary sheets of water that seem to shimmer over hot stretches of hot sand and pavement. This phenomenon is caused by horizontal light waves being bent upwards from the layer of heated air directly over the hot surface. Wind rippling the air layers may produce surprising changes in the shapes and sizes of such mirages. Individuals under severe stress are especially susceptible to interpreting these optical phenomena in bizarre, unrealistic ways.

miscarriage. See **spontaneous abortion.**

miscible, able to be mixed or mingled with another substance. Compare **immiscible.**

misdemeanor, (in criminal law) an offense that is considered less serious than a felony and carries with it a lesser penalty, usually a fine or imprisonment for less than one year. Conviction for a misdemeanor does not prohibit the person from holding public office or from practicing a licensed occupation.

misfeasance (mısfi'zəns), an improper performance of a lawful act, especially in a way that might cause damage or injury. Compare **malfeasance, nonfeasance.**

miso-, a combining form meaning 'hatred of': *misocainia, misogyn, misopedia.*

misogamy (mısog'əmi), an aversion to marriage. — **misogamic, misogamous,** *adj.,* **misogamist,** *n.*

misogyny (mısoj'ıni), an aversion to women. — **misogynist,** *n.,* **misogamic,** *adj.*

misopedia (mısoʊpi'diə), an aversion to children. — **misopedic,** *adj.,* **misopedist,** *n.*

missed abortion, a condition in which a dead, immature embryo or fetus is not expelled from the uterus for two or more months. The uterus diminishes in size and symptoms of pregnancy abate; infection and disorders of the clotting of the mother's blood may follow. The fetus and placenta may become necrotic or, less commonly, the fetus becomes calcified and the rest of the products of conception are resorbed.

missile fracture, a penetration fracture caused by a projectile, as a bullet or a piece of shrapnel.

Mistura C, a trade name for a cholinergic (carbachol).

Mistura D, a trade name for an adrenergic (phenylephrine hydrochloride).

Mistura E, a trade name for an adrenergic (epinephrine hydrochloride).

Mistura P, a trade name for a cholinergic (pilocarpine hydrochloride).

mite, a minute arachnid with a flat, almost transparent body and four pairs of legs. Many species of these relatives of ticks and spiders are parasitic, including the chigger and *Sarcoptes scabei,* which cause localized pruritus and inflammation. Some female mites burrow into the skin and lay eggs which hatch into larvae; the movements of the larvae cause intense itching. See also **scabies.**

mite typhus. See **scrub typhus.**

Mithracin, a trade name for an antineoplastic (mithramycin).

mithramycin, an antineoplastic.

■ INDICATIONS: It is prescribed primarily in the treatment of malignant tumors of the testis. It is also prescribed in the treatment of hypercalcemia.

■ CONTRAINDICATIONS: Clotting disorders, thrombocytopenia, kidney or liver dysfunction, bone marrow depression, or known hypersensitivity to this drug prohibits its use.

■ ADVERSE EFFECTS: Among the more serious adverse reactions are thrombocytopenia and clotting defects. Nausea and stomatitis commonly occur.

mithridatism (mĭth′rədei′tĭzəm). See **tachyphylaxis.**

mito-, a combining form meaning 'threadlike': *mitochondria, mitokinetic, mitoplasm.*

mitochondrion (mäi′toukon′drion), *pl.* **mitochondria.** a small rodlike, threadlike, or granular organelle, within the cytoplasm, that functions in cellular metabolism and respiration and occurs in varying numbers in all living cells except bacteria, viruses, blue-green algae, and mature erythrocytes. It consists of two sets of membranes, a smooth outer one and a convoluted inner one, arranged in folds to form projections, or cristae, that extend into the matrix. Mitochondria provide the principal source of cellular energy through oxidative phosphorylation and adenosine triphosphate synthesis. They also contain the enzymes involved with electron transport and the citric and fatty acid cycles. Mitochondria are self-replicating and contain an extranuclear source of DNA, RNA polymerase, transfer RNA, and ribosomes. Also called **chondriosome.** – **mitochondrial,** *adj.*

mitogen (mäi′təjĭn, mĭt′əjĭn), an agent that triggers mitosis. – **mitogenic,** *adj.*

mitogenesia (mäi′toujĭni′žə), the production by or formation resulting from mitosis.

mitogenesis (mäi′toujen′ĭsĭs), the induction of mitosis in a cell. – **mitogenetic,** *adj.*

mitogenetic radiation, mitogenic radiation, the force or specific energy that is supposedly given off by cells undergoing division. It may, in turn, stimulate the process of mitosis in other cells. Also called **Gurvich radiation.**

mitogenic factor, a kind of lymphokine that is released from activated T lymphocytes and stimulates the production of normal unsensitized lymphocytes.

mitolactol (mäi′tələk′tol), an antineoplastic currently used investigationally for a variety of neoplasms, including Hodgkin's disease. It may be used in combination with doxorubicin. Also called **dibromodulcitol.**

mitome (mäi′toum), the reticular network found within the cytoplasm and nucleoplasm of the cell. See also **cytomitome, karyomitome.**

mitomycin, an antineoplastic antibiotic.

■ INDICATIONS: It is prescribed in the treatment of a variety of malignant neoplastic diseases.

■ CONTRAINDICATIONS: Clotting deficiency, thrombocytopenia or known hypersensitivity to this drug prohibits its use.

■ ADVERSE EFFECTS: The most serious adverse reaction is bone marrow depression. Gastrointestinal disturbances, alopecia, and skin reactions commonly occur.

mitosis (mæitou′sĭs, mĭtou′sĭs), a type of cell division that occurs in somatic cells and results in the formation of two genetically identical daughter cells containing the diploid number of chromosomes characteristic of the species. It consists of the division of the nucleus through the four stages of prophase, metaphase, anaphase, and telophase, during which the two chromatids of the chromo-

MITOSIS

somes separate and migrate to opposite ends of the cell, followed by the division of the cytoplasm. Mitosis is the process by which the body produces new cells for both growth and repair of injured tissue. Kinds of mitosis are **heterotypic mitosis, homeotypic mitosis, multipolar mitosis,** pathologic mitosis. Also called **indirect division.** Compare **meiosis.** See also **interphase.** — **mitotic** (maitot′ik, mitot′-ik), *adj.*

mitotane (mai′tətein), an antineoplastic which destroys normal and neoplastic adrenal cortical cells.

■ INDICATION: It is prescribed in the treatment of carcinoma of the adrenal cortex.

■ CONTRAINDICATION: Known hypersensitivity to this drug is the only contraindication.

■ ADVERSE EFFECTS: Among the more serious adverse reactions are gastrointestinal symptoms, lethargy, and adrenal insufficiency.

mitotic figure, any chromosome or chromosome aggregation during any of the stages of mitosis.

mitotic index, the number of cells per unit (usually one thousand) undergoing mitosis during a given time. The ratio is used primarily as an estimation of the rate of tissue growth.

mitral (mai′trəl), 1. of or pertaining to the mitral valve of the heart. 2. shaped like a miter.

mitral gradient, the difference in pressure in the left atrium and left ventricle during diastole.

mitral stenosis. See **mitral valve stenosis, valvular heart disease.**

mitral valve, one of the four valves of the heart, situated between the left atrium and the left ventricle; the only valve with two, rather than three flaps. The mitral valve allows blood to flow from the left atrium into the left ventricle but prevents blood from flowing back into the atrium. Ventricular contraction in systole forces the blood against the valve, closing the two flaps and assuring the flow of blood from the ventricle into the pulmonary artery and the aorta. The ventral flap of the mitral valve is longer than the dorsal flap. Also called **bicuspid valve, left atrioventricular valve.** Compare **semilunar valve, tricuspid valve.**

mitral valve stenosis, an obstructive lesion in the mitral valve of the heart caused by adhesions on the leaflets of the valve, usually the result of recurrent episodes of rheumatic endocarditis. Hypertrophy of the left atrium develops and may be followed by right-sided heart failure and pulmonary edema (cor pulmonale). Reduced cardiac output characteristically produces fatigue, dyspnea, orthopnea, and cyanosis. Surgical correction of the defective valve may be necessary. The valve may be freed of the adhesions in a comminsurotomy, or it may be replaced by a prosthetic valve.

mittelschmerz (mit′əlshmerts), abdominal pain in the region of an ovary during ovulation, which usually occurs midway through the menstrual cycle. Present in many women, mittelschmerz is useful for identifying ovulation, thus pinpointing the fertile period of the cycle.

mixed anesthesia. See **balanced anesthesia.**

mixed aneurysm. See **compound aneurysm.**

mixed cell malignant lymphoma, a lymphoid neoplasm containing lymphocytes and histiocytes (macrophages).

mixed-cell sarcoma, a tumor consisting of two or more cellular elements, excluding fibrous tissue. Also called **malignant mesenchymoma.**

mixed connective tissue disease (MCTD), a systemic disease characterized by the combined symptoms of various collagen diseases, as synovitis, polymyositis, scleroderma, and systemic lupus erythematosus. This condition involves a high concentration of antibodies of ribonucleoprotein and may produce arthralgia, inflammation of the muscles, nondeforming arthritis, swollen hands, esophageal hypomotility, and reduced diffusing capacity of the lungs. Treatment often includes the administration of corticosteroids. Recurrence is common when the steroid medication is discontinued.

mixed dentition, a phase of dentition during which some of the teeth are permanent and some are deciduous.

mixed glioma, a tumor, composed of glial cells, that contains more than one kind of cell, the most common being nonneural cells of ectodermal origin.

mixed leukemia, a malignancy of blood-forming tissues characterized by the proliferation of eosinophilic, neutrophilic, and basophilic granulocytes, in contrast to one predominant cell line, as in lymphocytic or monocytic leukemia.

mixed lymphocyte culture (MLC) reaction, an assay of the function of the T cell lymphocytes, primarily used for histocompatibility testing prior to grafting.

mixed porphyria. See **variegate porphyria.**

mixed tumor, a growth composed of more than one kind of neoplastic tissue, especially a complex embryonal tumor of local origin.

-mixia. See **-mixis.**

-mixis, a combining form meaning a '(specified) means of conjugation': *amphimixis, automixis, endomixis.* Also **-mixia, -mixie, -mixy.**

mixture, 1. a substance composed of ingredients that are not chemically combined and do not necessarily occur in a fixed proportion. 2. (in pharmacology) a liquid containing one or more medications in suspension. The proportions of the ingredients are specific to each mixture. Compare **compound, solution.**

-mixy. See **-mixis.**

ml, abbreviation for **milliliter.**

MLC, abbreviation for *mixed lymphocyte culture.* See **mixed lymphocyte culture reaction.**

MLD, abbreviation for **median lethal dose.**

mm, abbreviation for **millimeter.**

MMEF, abbreviation for **maximal midexpiratory flow.**

mmol, abbreviation for **millimole.**

Mn, symbol for **manganese.**

mne-, a combining form meaning 'of or pertaining to memory': *mnemic, mnemism, mnemonic.*

-mnesia, a combining form meaning '(condition or type of) memory': *acousmatamnesia, ecmnesia, logamnesia.*

-mnestic, a combining form meaning 'pertaining to memory': *amnestic, anamnestic, catamnestic.* Also **-mnesic.**

Mo, symbol for **molybdenum.**

Moban, a trade name for an antipsychotic agent (molindone).

Mobidin, a trade name for an analgesic (magnesium salicylate).

mobility, impaired physical, a nursing diagnosis accepted by the Fourth National Conference on the Classification of Nursing Diagnoses. The etiology of the condition may be a decrease in the person's strength or endurance, the presence of pain or discomfort, impaired cognition or perception, depression or severe anxiety, or impaired neuromuscular or musculoskeletal function. The defining characteristics of the condition include an inability to achieve a functional level of mobility in the environment, a reluctance to move, a limited range of motion of the limbs or extremities, a decrease in the strength or control of the musculoskeletal system, abnormal or impaired ability to coordinate movements, or any of a large number of imposed restrictions on movement, as medically required bedrest or traction. It is suggested that the limitation of injury be ranked from "0" – completely independent, to "4" – dependent, does not participate in any activity. See also **nursing diagnosis.**

-mobility. See **-motility.**

Mobitz I heart block, second degree or partial atrioventricular (AV) block in which the PR interval increases progressively until the propagation of an atrial impulse does not occur and the corresponding ventricular beat drops out. After the pause the PR interval shortens to within the normal range. Symptoms include fatigue, dizziness, and, in some cases, syncope. Mobitz I block is often caused by abnormal conduction of the cardiac impulse at the AV junction proximal to the bundle of His and may be precipitated by increased vagal tone, occurring spontaneously, after carotid sinus pressure, or following digitalis therapy. It may be a complication of inferior myocardial infarction but is usually a transitory condition requiring no treatment. Also called **Wenchebach heart block.**

Mobitz II heart block, second degree or partial atrioventricular block, characterized by the sudden nonconduction of an atrial impulse and a periodic dropped beat without prior lengthening of the P-R interval. This kind of block usually results from impaired conduction in the bundle of His and may be caused by anterior myocardial infarction, myocarditis, drug toxicity, electrolyte disturbances, rheumatoid nodules, and various degenerative diseases. Syncopal attacks, occurring without warning when the patient is upright or recumbent, are common in Mobitz II block, which may be transient or suddenly progress to complete block. Long-term therapy requires the implantation of a pacemaker.

mode, a value or term in a set of data that occurs more frequently than other values or terms.

model, (in nursing research) a symbolic representation of the interrelations exhibited by the phenomena within a system or a process. The model is presented as a conceptual framework or a theory that explains the phenomena and allows predictions to be made about a patient or a process. An equation is analagous to a model in mathematics. Nursing models usually describe person, environment, health, and nursing.

modeling, a technique used in behavior therapy in which a person learns a desired response by observing it performed.

moderator band, a thick bundle of muscle in the central part of the right ventricle of the heart. Missing in some individuals and varying in size in different persons, it usually contains part of the atrioventricular conduction bundle. Also called **trabecula septomarginalis.**

Moderil, a trade name for an antihypertensive (rescinnamine).

Modicon, a trade name for an oral contraceptive containing an estrogen (ethinyl estradiol) and a progestin (norethindrone).

modified milk, cow's milk in which the protein content has been reduced and the fat content increased to correspond to the composition of breast milk. See also **formula, infant.**

modified radical mastectomy, a surgical procedure in which a breast is completely removed with the underlying pectoralis minor and some of the adjacent lymph nodes. The pectoralis major is not excised. The operation is performed in treating early and well-localized malignant neoplasms of the breast. It appears to be as curative as the more extensive radical mastectomy when the tumor meets these criteria. Care of the woman before and after a modified radical mastectomy is similar to that for a radical mastectomy. Compare **radical mastectomy, simple mastectomy.**

Moeller's glossitis (mœ'lərz), a form of chronic glossitis, characterized by burning or pain in the tongue and an increased sensitivity to hot or spicy foods. Also called **glossodynia exfoliativa.** See also **glossitis.**

mogi-, a combining form meaning 'difficult, or with difficulty': *mogiarthria, mogigraphia, mogilalia.*

moiety (mɔi'ɪti), a part of a molecule that exhibits a particular set of chemical and pharmacological characteristics.

moist gangrene. See **gangrene.**

mol. See **mole².**

molar, 1. any one of the 12 molar teeth, six in each dental arch, three located posterior to the premolar teeth.

The crown of each molar is nearly cubical, convex on its buccal surface and its lingual surface and flattened on its surfaces of contact. It is surmounted by four or five cusps separated by cruciate depressions and has a large rounded neck. Each of the upper molars has three roots, two of which are buccal, the other being lingual. The roots of the third upper molar are more or less fused. The lower molars are larger than the upper and each has two roots, an anterior, almost vertical root, and a posterior root directed almost obliquely backward. The roots of the third lower molar tend to fuse. **2.** See also **mole.** of or pertaining to the gram molecular weight of a substance.

molar pregnancy, pregnancy in which a hydatid mole develops from the trophoblastic tissue of the early embryonic stage of development. The signs of pregnancy are all exaggerated: the uterus grows more rapidly than is normal, morning sickness is often severe and constant, blood pressure is likely to be elevated, and blood levels of chorionic gonadotropins are extremely high. The uterus must be evacuated, as the mole may develop into a malignant trophoblastic disease, choriocarcinoma. See also **hydatid mole.**

molar solution, a solution that contains one mole of solute per liter of solution.

mold¹, **1.** a fungus. **2.** a growth of fungi.

mold², a hollow form for casting or shaping an object, as a prosthesis.

molding, the natural process by which a baby's head is shaped during labor as it is squeezed into and through the birth passage by the forces of labor. The head often becomes quite elongated, and the bones of the skull may be caused to overlap slightly at the suture lines. The biparietal diameter of the head may be compressed as much as 0.5 cm without intracranial damage. Most of the changes caused by molding resolve themselves during the first few days of life. Compare **caput succedaneum.** See also **cephalhematoma.**

mole¹, **1.** *Informal.* a pigmented nevus. **2.** *Informal.* (in obstetrics) a hydatidiform mole.

mole², **mol,** the standard unit used to measure the amount of a substance. A mole of a substance is the amount containing the same number of elementary particles (atoms, electrons, ions, molecules, or other particles) as there are atoms in 0.012 kg of carbon 12. — **molar,** *adj.*

molecular genetics, the branch of genetics that focuses on the chemical structure and the functions, replication, and mutations of the molecules involved in the transmission of genetic information, as DNA and RNA. Molecular genetics is concerned with the arrangement of genes on DNA, the double helix molecule's replication and transcription into RNA, and the way RNA directs the formation of proteins. See also **recombinant DNA.**

molecular weight, the total of the atomic weights of the atoms in a molecule. See also **atom, atomic weight, molecule.**

molecule, the smallest unit that exhibits the properties of an element or compound. A molecule is composed of two or more atoms that are chemically combined. See also **atom, compound.**

molindone hydrochloride, an antipsychotic agent.

■ INDICATION: It is prescribed in the treatment of schizophrenia.

■ CONTRAINDICATIONS: Severe central nervous system depression or known hypersensitivity to this drug prohibits its use.

■ ADVERSE EFFECTS: Among the most serious adverse reactions are extrapyramidal reactions, hypotension, sedation, and other reactions characteristic of the phenothiazine antipsychotics.

molluscum (mələs′kəm), any skin disease having soft, rounded masses or nodules. See also **molluscum contagiosum.**

molluscum contagiosum (kəntei′jiou′səm), a disease of the skin and mucous membranes, caused by a poxvirus and found all over the world. It is characterized by scattered white papules. Palms of the hands and soles of the feet are not affected. The disease most frequently occurs in children and in adults with an impaired immune response. It is transmitted from person to person by direct or indirect contact and lasts up to three years, although individual lesions persist for only six to eight weeks. Diagnosis is easily made by electron microscopy. Curettage or electrical or chemical dessication helps to clear the lesions, but untreated lesions eventually resolve spontaneously without scarring.

molybdenum (Mo), a grayish metallic element. Its atomic number is 42; its atomic weight is 95.94. Molybdenum is poisonous if ingested in large quantities.

Mönckeberg's arteriosclerosis, a form of arteriosclerosis in which extensive calcium deposits are found in the media of the artery with little obstruction of the lumen. Also called **medial arteriosclerosis.**

Monday morning fever. See **byssinosis.**

Mongolian spot, a benign, bluish-black macule, between two and eight cm, occurring over the sacrum and on the buttocks of some newborns. It is especially common in blacks, American Indians, Southern Europeans, and Orientals and usually disappears during early childhood.

mongolism. See **Down's syndrome.**

mongoloid idiocy. See **Down's syndrome.**

Monilia (mənil′iə). See *Candida albicans.* — **monilial,** *adj.*

monilial vulvovaginitis. See **candidiasis.**

moniliasis (mon′ilai′əsis). See **candidiasis.**

Monistat, a trade name for an antifungal (miconazole nitrate).

monitor, 1. to observe and evaluate a function of the body closely and constantly. 2. a mechanical device that provides a visual or audible signal or a graphic record of a particular function, as a cardiac monitor or a fetal monitor.

monitrice, a labor coach, usually a registered nurse, who is specially trained in the Lamaze method of childbirth. The coach provides emotional support and leads the mother through labor and delivery, using the specific techniques for breathing, concentration, and massage taught by the Lamaze method in classes for the psychophysical preparation for childbirth.

mono-, a combining form meaning 'one': *monobacillary, monodal, mononeuritis.*

monoamine, an amine containing one amine group.

monoamine oxidase (MAO), an enzyme that catalyzes the oxidation of amines. Also called **amino oxidase.** See also **monoamine oxidase inhibitor.**

monoamine oxidase (MAO) inhibitor, any of a chemically heterogeneous group of drugs used primarily in the treatment of depression. These drugs also exert an anti-anxiety effect, especially anxiety associated with phobia. The effects of the drugs vary greatly from patient to patient, and their specific actions leading to clinical benefits are poorly understood. Among the most common adverse effects are drowsiness, dry mouth, orthostatic hypotension, and constipation. Overdosage may cause tremor, euphoria, or manic behavior. MAO inhibitors interact with many drugs and with foods containing large amounts of the amino acid tyromine. Ingestion of these foods by a person taking a MAO inhibitor is likely to cause a severe hypertensive episode associated with headache, palpitations, and nausea. Among these foods are cheeses, red wine, smoked or pickled herring, beer, and yogurt. Patients taking MAO inhibitors are given a list of foods to avoid. Among the drugs that interact with MAO inhibitors are dopamine, meperidine, and the indirect acting sympathemimetics, one of which, ephedrine, is an ingredient in many common cold remedies. MAO inhibitors are also sometimes used in the treatment of migraine headache and hypertension.

monobasic acid (mon′oubei′sik), an acid with only one replaceable hydrogen atom, as hydrochloric acid (HCl).

monobenzone, a depigmenting agent.
■ INDICATIONS: It is prescribed in the treatment of abnormal skin pigmentation, as in disseminated vitiligo. It is not to be used for more trivial conditions, as freckles.
■ CONTRAINDICATION: Known hypersensitivity to this drug prohibits its use.
■ ADVERSE EFFECTS: The most serious adverse reaction is excessive and irreversible hypopigmentation. Common reactions are irritation and allergic reactions of the skin.

monoblast (mon′oblæst), a large, immature monocyte. Certain of the leukemias are characterized by greatly in-

creased production of monoblasts in the marrow and by the abnormal presence of these forms in the peripheral circulation. Compare **megaloblast, myeloblast.** See also **bone marrow, leukocyte.** – **monoblastic,** *adj.*

monoblastic leukemia, a progressive malignancy of blood-forming organs, characterized by the proliferation of monoblasts and monocytes. The disease occurs in children and adults and develops late in the course of a small but significant number of cases of plasma cell myeloma. Also called **monocytic leukemia, Schilling's leukemia.**

monocephalus. See **syncephalus.**

monochorial twins (mon′oukɔr′iəl), **monochorionic twins.** See **monozygotic twins.**

monoclonal (mon′əklou′nəl), of, pertaining to, or designating a group of identical cells or organisms derived from a single cell.

monoclonal gammopathy. See **gammopathy.**

monocyte (mon′əsait), a large mononuclear leukocyte, 13 μ to 25 μ in diameter with an ovoid or kidney-shaped nucleus, containing lacy, linear chromatin material and abundant gray-blue cytoplasm filled with fine, reddish and azurophilic granules. See also **monocytosis.**

monocytic leukemia (mon′əsit′ik), a malignancy of blood-forming tissues in which the predominant cells are monocytes. The disease has an erratic course characterized by malaise, fatigue, fever, anorexia, weight loss, splenomegaly, bleeding gums, dermal petechiae, anemia, and unresponsiveness to therapy. There are two forms: **Schilling's leukemia,** in which most of the cells are monocytes that probably arise from the reticuloendothelial system, and the more common **Naegeli's leukemia,** in which a large number of the cells resemble myeloblasts. Also called **histiocytic leukemia.**

monocytosis (mon′ousaitou′sis), an increased proportion of monocytic white blood cells in the circulation.

monofactorial inheritance (mon′oufæktor′iəl), the acquisition or expression of a trait or condition that is dependent on the transmission of a single specific gene. Compare **multifactorial inheritance.**

monohybrid, pertaining to or describing an individual, organism, or strain that is heterozygous for the only one specific trait or that is heterozygous for the single trait or gene locus under consideration.

monohybrid cross, the mating of two individuals, organisms, or strains that have different gene pairs for only one specific trait or in which only one particular characteristic or gene locus is being followed.

monohydric alcohol, an alcohol containing one hydroxyl group.

monomer (mon′əmər), a molecule that repeats itself to form a polymer, as the molecules of fibrin monomer which polymerize to form fibrin in the blood-clotting process. – **monomeric,** *adj.*

monomphalus (mənom'fələs), conjoined twins that are united at the umbilicus. Also called **omphalopagus.**

mononeuritis multiplex (mon'ounurai'tis). *Obsolete.* See **multiple mononeuropathy.**

mononeuropathy (mon'ounurop'əfhi), any disease or disorder that affects a single nerve trunk. Some common causes of disorders involving single nerve trunks are electrical shock, radiation, and fractured bones that may compress or lacerate nerve fibers. Casts and tourniquets that are too tight may also damage a nerve by compression or by ischemia. Accidental injection of penicillin and other medications into the sciatic nerve can seriously injure the nerve, especially if the injected medication is an oil-based drug. The peripheral nerve trunks are especially vulnerable to compression and entrapment.

mononucleosis (mon'ounu'kliou'sis), 1. an abnormal increase in the number of mononuclear leukocytes in the blood. 2. See **infectious mononucleosis.**

monophasic, having one phase, part, aspect, or stage.

monoploid, monoploidic (mon'əploid). See **haploid.**

monopodial symmelia. See **sympus monopus.**

monopus (mon'əpəs), a fetus or individual with the congenital absence of a foot or leg.

monorchid (monor'kid), a man who has monorchism.

monorchidism (monor'kidiz'əm). See **monorchism.**

monorchism (mon'orkiz'əm), a condition in which only one testicle has descended into the scrotum. Also called **monorchidism.** See also **cryptorchidism. — monorchidic,** *adj.*

monosome (mon'əsoum), 1. the unpaired sex chromosome. 2. the single, unpaired chromosome in monosomy.

monosomy (mon'əsou'mi), a chromosomal aberration characterized by the absence of one chromosome from the normal diploid complement; in humans, the momosomic cell contains 45 chromosomes and is designated $2n - 1$, as occurs in the XO condition in Turner's syndrome. Compare **trisomy. — monosomic,** *adj.*

monosomy X. See **Turner's syndrome.**

monotropy (mənot'rəpi), a concept named by J. Bowlby, describing the phenomenon in which a mother appears to be able to bond with only one infant at a time. The concept is used by Marshall Klaus and John Kennell in their studies of maternal-infant bonding in mothers of twins. When one twin is taken home from the hospital earlier than the other, the mother often reports that she does not feel that the baby discharged later is hers. The second baby to reach the home is much more likely to fail to thrive or to be neglected or abused. Nurses working in intensive care nurseries and adoption homes are also known to become attached to only one child at a time. Monotropy may also explain a mother's common tendency to dress twins alike, in effect making them one. **— monotropic,** *adj.*

monounsaturated fatty acid (mon'ouənsæʧ'urei'tid). See **unsaturated fatty acid.**

monovular, (monou'vyələr), **mono-ovular,** See **uniovular.**

monovulatory (mənou'vyələtor'i), routinely releasing one ovum during each ovarian cycle. Compare **diovulatory.**

monozygotic (MZ), pertaining to or developed from a single fertilized ovum, or zygote, as occurs in identical twins. Compare **dizygotic. — monozygosity,** *n.,* **monozygous,** *adj.*

monozygotic twins, two offspring born of the same pregnancy and developed from a single fertilized ovum that splits into equal halves during an early cleavage phase in embryonic development, giving rise to separate fetuses. Such twins are always of the same sex, have the same genetic constitution, possess identical blood groups, and closely resemble each other in physical, psychological, and mental characteristics. Monozygotic twins may have single or separate placentas and membranes, depending on the time during development when division occurred. Monozygotic twinning occurs with relatively uniform frequency in all races, is unaffected by heredity, and represents approximately one third of all twin births. Also called **enzygotic twins, identical twins, true twins, uniovular twins.** Compare **dizygotic twins.** See also **Siamese twins.**

monster, a fetus that is grossly malformed and usually nonviable. Kinds of monsters include **compound monster, double monster, single monster.**

monstrosity, 1. the state or condition of having severe congenital defects. 2. anything that deviates greatly from the normal; a monster or teras.

Monteggia's fracture (montej'əz), fracture of the proximal third of the proximal half of the ulna, associated with radial dislocation or rupture of the annular ligament and resulting in the angulation or overriding of ulnar fragments.

Montercaux fracture (mon'tərkou'), a fracture of the neck of the fibula associated with the diastasis of ankle mortise.

Montgomery's gland (montgum'əriz). See **areolar gland.**

Montgomery's tubercle, one of several sebaceous glands on the areolae of the breasts. The tubercles normally enlarge during pregnancy. The sebaceous material that is secreted from the ducts of the glands to the skin of each areola serves to lubricate and protect the breast from infection and trauma during breast feeding.

moon face, a condition characterized by a rounded, puffy face, occurring in people treated with large doses of corticosteroids, as those with rheumatoid arthritis or acute childhood leukemia. The features return to normal when the medication is stopped.

moor bath, a bath taken in water containing earth from a swamp.

Moore's fracture, a fracture of the distal radius with associated dislocation of the ulnar head, resulting in the securement of the styloid process under the annular ligaments of the wrist.

MOPP, an acronym for a combination drug regimen used in the treatment of cancer, containing three antineoplastics, Mustargen (mechlorethamine), Oncovin (vincristine sulfate), procarbazine hydrochloride (Matulane), and prednisone (a glucocorticoid). MOPP is prescribed in the treatment of Hodgkin's disease.

morbid anatomy. See **pathological anatomy.**

morbidity 1. an illness or an abnormal condition of quality. 2. (in statistics) a. the rate at which an illness or abnormality occurs, calculated by dividing the entire number of people in a group by the number in that group who are affected with the illness or abnormality. b. the rate at which an illness occurs in a particular area or population.

morbilli (mɔrbɪl'ai). See **measles.**

morbilliform (mɔrbɪl'ɪfɔrm), describing a skin condition that resembles the erythematous, maculopapular rash of measles.

Morgagni's globule (mɔrgan'yiz), a minute opaque sphere that may form between the eye lens and its capsule, especially in cataract.

Morgagni's tubercle, one of several small, soft nodules on the surface of each of the areola in women. The tubercles are produced by large sebaceous glands just under the surface of the areolae. They secrete a bacteriostatic, lubricating substance during pregnancy and lactation.

morgan, (in genetics) a unit of measure used in mapping the relative distances between genes on a chromosome. The measurement, named after the biologist Thomas Hunt Morgan, uses the total crossover value as the basic unit so that one morgan equals 100 per cent crossing over or one centimorgan equals one per cent recombination. One centimorgan is also equal to one map unit.

-moria, a combining form meaning '(condition of) dementia': *monomoria, phantasmatomoria.*

morning-after pill, *Informal.* A large dose of an estrogen given orally, over a short period of time, to a woman within 24-72 hours after sexual intercourse to prevent conception, most commonly in an emergency situation such as rape or incest. The woman is warned that the medication may cause the formation of clots, severe nausea and vomiting, and teratogenic and carcinogenic effects on the fetus if pregnancy already exists or if contraception fails. See also **diethystilbestrol.**

morning sickness. *Nontechnical.* See **nausea and vomiting of pregnancy.**

moron, *Obsolete.* a retarded person having an IQ between 50 and 70 and incapable of developing beyond the mental age of 12 years. Compare **idiot, imbecile.** See also **mental retardation.**

moronism, moronity, *Obsolete.* the condition of being a moron.

Moro reflex (mɔr'ou), a normal mass reflex in a young infant elicited by a sudden loud noise or by striking the table next to the child, resulting in flexion of the legs, an embracing posture of the arms, and usually a brief cry. Also called **startle reflex.**

morph-, a combining form meaning 'form or shape': *morphallaxis, morphea, morphogenesis.*

-morph, a combining form meaning 'something possessing a (specified) form': *endomorph, hypomorph, neomorph.*

morphea (mɔr'fiə), localized scleroderma consisting of patches of yellowish or ivory-colored, rigid, dry, smooth skin. It is more common in females and rarely progresses to a generalized or systemic form of sclerosis.

-morphia, a combining form meaning a 'condition of form': *pantamorphia, prosopodysmorphia, theromorphia.* Also **-morphy.**

morphine sulfate, a narcotic analgesic.

■ INDICATION: It is prescribed to reduce pain.

■ CONTRAINDICATIONS: Drug dependence or known hypersensitivity to this drug prohibits its use.

■ ADVERSE EFFECTS: Among the more serious adverse reactions are increased intracranial pressure, cardiovascular disturbances, respiratory depression, and drug dependence.

-morphism, a combining form meaning the 'condition of having a (specified) shape': *amorphism, isomorphism, pedomorphism.*

morphogenesis (mɔr'fəjen'ɪsɪs), **morphogeny** (mɔrfoj'ɪni), the development and differentiation of the structures and the form of an organism, specifically the changes that occur in the cells and tissue during embryonic development.

morphogenetic (mɔr'foujɪnet'ɪk), **morphogenic** (mɔr'fəjen'ɪk), (in embryology) of or pertaining to a substance or hormone that acts as an evocator in differentiation.

morphogeny, See **morphogenesis.**

morphology, the study of the physical shape and size of a specimen, plant, or animal. — **morphologic,** *adj.*

-morphosis, a combining form meaning a 'development or change': *chemomorphosis, epimorphosis, heteromorphosis.*

Morquio's disease (mɔrki'ouz), a familial form of mucopolysaccharidosis that results in abnormal musculoskeletal development in childhood. Dwarfism, hunchback, enlarged sternum, and knock-knees may occur. The disease may first be evident as the child, learning to walk, displays an abnormal, waddling gait.

morrhuate sodium injection (mɔr'ueit), a sclerosing agent.

■ INDICATION: It is prescribed for varicose veins.

■ CONTRAINDICATIONS: It is not used if deep veins are occluded, inflamed, or infected. Known hypersensitivity to this drug prohibits its use.

■ ADVERSE EFFECTS: Among the more serious adverse effects are allergic reactions, including anaphylaxis.

mortality, 1. the condition of being subject to death. 2. the death rate, which reflects the number of deaths per unit of population in any specific region, age group, disease, or other classification, usually expressed as deaths per 1,000, 10,000, or 100,000.

mortar, a cup-shaped vessel in which materials are ground or crushed by a pestle in the preparation of drugs.

Morton's foot (mɔr'tənz). See **metatarsalgia.**

Morton's neuroma. See **metatarsalgia.**

Morton's plantar neuralgia, a severe throbbing pain that affects the anastomotic nerve branch between the medial and the lateral plantar nerves. Also called *Obsolete.* **Morton's plantar neuroma.**

Morton's plantar neuroma, *Obsolete.* See **Morton's plantar neuralgia.**

Morton's toe. See **metatarsalgia.**

morula (mɔr'ələ), *pl.* **morulas, morulae,** a solid, spherical mass of cells resulting from the cleavage of the fertilized ovum in the early stages of embryonic development. It represents an intermediate stage between the zygote and the blastocyst and consists of blastomeres that are uniform in size, shape, and physiological capabilities. – **morular,** *adj.*

-morula, a combining form meaning a 'clump of blastomeres formed by cleavage of a fertilized ovum': *amphimorula, archimorula, pseudomorula.*

mosaic, 1. (in genetics) an individual or organism that developed from a single zygote but that has two or more kinds of cell populations in regard to genetic constitution. Such a condition results from a mutation, crossing-over, or, more commonly in humans, nondisjunction of the chromosomes during early embryogenesis, which causes a variation in the number of chromosomes in the cells. The type of chromosomal aberration and its ratio depend on whether nondisjunction occurred in the first or later mitotic divisions of the zygote. Since monosomic cells are nonviable, except in X monosomic conditions, most mosaic conditions in humans represent a mixture of normal and trisomic cells, regardless of whether an autosome or the sex chromosomes are involved. The degree of clinical involvement depends on the type of tissue containing the abnormality and may vary from near normal to full manifestation of a syndrome, as Down's syndrome or Turner's syndrome. Compare **chimera.** See also **monosomy, sex chromosome mosaic, trisomy.** 2. (in embryology) a fertilized ovum that undergoes determinate cleavage. See also **mosaic development.**

mosaic bone, bone tissue appearing to be made up of many tiny pieces cemented together, as seen upon microscopic examination of an x-ray film of the affected bone. It is characteristic of Paget's disease of the bone.

mosaic cleavage. See **determinate cleavage.**

mosaic development, a kind of embryonic development occurring in the blastocyst. The fertilized ovum undergoes determinate cleavage, developing according to a precise, unalterable plan in which each blastomere has a characteristic position, limited developmental potency, and is a precursor of a definite part of the embryo. Damage to or destruction of these cells results in a defective organism. Compare **regulative development.**

mosaicism (mouzei'ɪsɪz'əm), (in genetics) a condition in which an individual or an organism that develops from a single zygote has two or more cell populations that differ in genetic constitution. Most commonly seen in man is a variation in the number of chromosomes in the cells, which may involve either a particular autosome, as in Down's syndrome, or the sex chromosomes, as in Turner's syndrome and Kleinfelter's syndrome. See also **mosaic, sex chromosome mosaic.**

mosaic wart, a group of contiguous plantar warts.

mosquito bite, a bite of a bloodsucking arthropod of the subfamily Culicidae that may result in a systemic allergic reaction in a hypersensitive person, an infection, or, most often, a pruritic wheal. Mosquitoes, which are attracted to hosts by moisture, carbon dioxide, estrogens, sweat, or warmth, are vectors of many infectious diseases.

mosquito forceps. See **Halsted's forceps,** def. 1.

Mössbauer spectrometer (məs'bauər, mœs'bauər), an instrument that can detect small changes between an atomic nucleus and its environment, as caused by changes in temperature, pressure, or chemical state. The device is used in chemical and physical research with applications in medicine.

mot-, a combining form meaning 'of or related to movement': *motoneuron, motorgraphic, motoricity.*

mother fixation, an arrest in psychosexual development characterized by an abnormally persistent, close, and often paralyzing emotional attachment to one's mother. Compare **father fixation.** See also **Freudian fixation.**

motile (mou'tɪl), capable of spontaneous but unconscious or involuntary movement. – **motility,** *n.*

-motility, a combining form meaning the 'condition of being capable of movement': *cardiomotility, hypermotility, supermotility.* Also **-mobility.**

motion sickness, a condition caused by erratic or rhythmic motions in any combination of directions, as in a boat or a car. Severe cases are characterized by nausea, vomiting, vertigo, and headache, mild cases by headache and general discomfort. Various antihistamines are used prophylactically. Kinds of motion sickness are **air sickness, car sickness, seasickness** (*mal de mer*).

motivational conflict, a conflict resulting from the arousal of two or more motives that direct behavior toward incompatible goals. Kinds of motivational conflict include **approach-approach conflict, approach-avoidance conflict, avoidance-avoidance conflict.** See also **motivation.**

motor, 1. of or pertaining to motion, the body apparatus involved in movement, or the brain functions that direct purposeful activities. 2. of or pertaining to a muscle, nerve, or brain center that produces or subserves motion.

-motor, a combining form meaning 'pertaining to the effects of activity in a body part': *nervimotor, psychomotor, viscerimotor.*

motor aphasia, the inability to utter remembered words, owing to a cerebral lesion in the inferior frontal gyrus (Broca's motor speech area) of the left hemisphere in right-handed individuals. The condition most commonly is the result of a stroke. The patient knows what to say but cannot articulate the words. Patients with motor aphasia sometimes use expletives, suggesting that emotionally charged expressions may be controlled by the right hemisphere. Also called **ataxic aphasia, expressive aphasia, frontocortical aphasia, verbal aphasia.**

motor apraxia, the inability to carry out planned movements or to handle small objects, although the proper use of the object is recognized. The condition results from a lesion in the premotor frontal cortex on the opposite side of the affected limb. Also called **cortical apraxia, innervation apraxia.** See also **apraxia.**

motor area, a portion of the cerebral cortex that includes the precentral gyrus and the posterior part of the frontal gyri and that causes the contraction of the voluntary muscles upon stimulation with electrodes. It corresponds to Brodmann's areas IV and VI and is characterized histologically by the absence of the granular layer in the cortex. It contains the giant pyramidal cells of Betz in layer V. Normal voluntary activity requires associations between the motor area and other parts of the cortex; removal of the motor area from one cerebral hemisphere causes paralysis of voluntary muscles, especially of the opposite side of the body. Various parts of the motor area are associated with different body structures, as the lower limb, the face, the mouth, and the hand. The parts associated with more delicate, complicated movements, as those of the hand, are larger than those associated with more general movements.

motor end plate, a broad band of terminal fibers of the motor nerves of the voluntary muscles. Motor nerves derived from the cranial and spinal nerves enter the sheaths of striated muscle fibers, lose their myelin sheaths, and ramify like the roots of a tree. In forming the motor end plate, the neurilemma of the nerve fiber merges with the sarcolemma of the muscle, and the axon synapses with the muscle fibers.

motor fiber, one of the fibers in the spinal nerves that transmit impulses to muscle fibers.

motor image, a visual concept of one's bodily movements, real or imagined.

motor nerve, a nerve consisting of efferent fibers that conduct impulses away from the brain or the spinal cord to one of the muscles or one of the organs. Compare **sensory nerve.** See also **nervous system.**

motor neuron, motoneuron (mou′tounur′on), one of various kinds of nerve cells that transmit nerve impulses from the brain or from the spinal cord to muscular or glandular tissue. According to location, some kinds of motor neurons are the peripheral motor neurons and the upper motor neurons.

motor neuron paralysis, an injury to the spinal cord that causes damage to the motor neurons and results in various degrees of functional impairment depending on the site of the lesion. See **lower motor neuron paralysis, upper motor neuron paralysis.**

motor point, 1. a point at which a motor nerve enters the muscle it innervates. 2. a point at which electrical stimulation will cause contraction of a muscle. Compare **motor end plate.** See also **motor nerve, nervous system.**

motor seizure, a transitory disturbance in brain function caused by abnormal neuronal discharges that arise initially in a localized motor area of the cerebral cortex. The manifestations depend on the site of the abnormal electrical activity, as tonic contractures of the thumb, caused by excessive discharges in the motor area of the cortex controlling the first digit, or chewing movements resulting from discharges in the lower part of the motor strip controlling mastication. The disturbance may spread, or it may end in a shower of clonic movements or a generalized convulsion. Also called **focal motor seizure.**

motor sense, the feeling or perception enabling a person to accomplish a purposeful movement, presumably achieved by evoking a sensory engram or memory of the pattern for that specific movement. Proprioceptive signals transmitted by feedback pathways through the cerebellum and sensory areas of the motor cortex are compared with the engram and modify the movement. Experiments with animals show that a movement cannot be performed if the corresponding sensory area of the brain is removed; if the motor area is removed the movement is accomplished by using a different group of muscles.

motor unit, a functional structure consisting of a motor neuron and the muscle fibers it innervates.

Motrin, a trade name for an anti-inflammatory (ibuprofen).

mountain fever. 1. See **brucellosis.** 2. See **Colorado tick fever.** 3. See **Rocky Mountain spotted fever.**

mountain tick fever. 1. See **Rocky Mountain spotted fever.** 2. See **Colorado tick fever.**

mouse-tooth forceps, a kind of dressing forceps that

has one or more fine sharp points on the tip of each blade. The tips turn in, and the delicate teeth interlock.

mouth,   **1.** the nearly oval oral cavity at the anterior end of the digestive tube, bounded anteriorly by the lips and containing the tongue and the teeth. It consists of the vestibule and the mouth cavity proper. The vestibule, situated in front of the teeth, is bounded externally by the lips and the cheeks, internally by the gums and the teeth. The vestibule receives the secretion from the parotid salivary glands and communicates, when the jaws are closed, with the mouth cavity proper by an aperture on each side behind the molar teeth and by narrow clefts between opposing teeth. The mouth cavity proper is bounded ventrally and laterally by the alveolar arches and the teeth, communicates dorsally with the pharynx by the ischmium faucium, and is roofed by the hard and the soft palates.

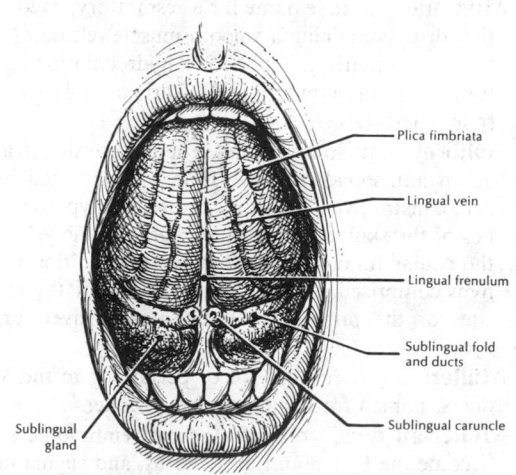

MOUTH STRUCTURES

The tongue forms the greater part of the floor of the cavity. The rest of the floor is formed by the reflection of the mucous membrane from the sides and the bottom of the tongue to the gum lining the inner part of the mandible. The mouth cavity proper receives the secretion from the submandibular and the sublingual salivary glands. **2.** an orifice.

mouth-to-mouth resuscitation, a procedure in artificial resuscitation, performed most often with cardiac massage. The victim's nose is sealed by pinching the nostrils closed, the head is extended, and air is breathed by the rescuer through the mouth into the lungs. See also **cardiopulmonary resuscitation.**

mouth-to-nose resuscitation, a procedure in artificial resuscitation in which the mouth of the victim is covered and held closed and air is breathed through the victim's nose. See also **mouth-to-mouth resuscitation.**

moxibustion (mok′səbəs′chən), a method of producing analgesia or altering the function of a system of the body achieved by igniting moxa, wormwood, or other combustible, slow-burning substance and holding it as near the point on the skin as possible without causing pain or burning. It is also sometimes used in conjunction with acupuncture.

M.P.D., abbreviation for **maximum permissible dose.**

M.P.H., abbreviation for *Master of Public Health.*

MPS, abbreviation for **mucopolysaccharidosis.**

MPS I, abbreviation for *mucopolysaccharidosis I.* See **Hurler's syndrome.**

MPS II, abbreviation for *mucopoly saccharidosis II.* See **Hunter's syndrome.**

mR, mr, abbreviation for **milliroentgen.**

MS, abbreviation for **multiple sclerosis.**

M.S.,   **1.** abbreviation for *Master of Science.* **2.** abbreviation for *Master of Surgery.*

MSH, abbreviation for *melanocyte-stimulating hormone.*

M.S.N., abbreviation for *Master of Science in Nursing.* See *master's degree program in nursing.*

M.T., abbreviation for **Medical Technologist.**

mu, μ, symbol for **micron.**

Much's granules (muχs), granules and rods, found in tuberculosis sputum, that stain with gram stain but not by the usual methods for acid-fast bacilli.

mucin (myu′sɪn), a mucopolysaccharide, the chief ingredient in mucus. Mucin is present in most glands that secrete mucus and is the lubricant protecting body surfaces from friction or erosion.

mucinous adenocarcinoma. See **mucinous carcinoma.**

mucinous carcinoma, an epithelial neoplasm with a sticky gelatinous consistency owing to the copious mucin secreted by its cells. Also called **colloid carcinoma, gelatiniform carcinoma, gelatinous carcinoma.**

mucocutaneous (myu′koukyutei′niəs), of or pertaining to the mucous membrane and the skin.

mucocutaneous leishmaniasis. See **American leishmaniasis.**

mucocutaneous lymph node syndrome, an acute, febrile illness, primarily of young children, characterized by inflamed mucous membranes of the mouth, "strawberry tongue," cervical lymphadenopathy, polymorphous rash on the trunk, and edema, erythema, and desquamation of the skin on the extremities. Other commonly associated findings include arthralgia, diarrhea, otitis, pneumonia, photophobia, meningitis, and electrocardiographic changes. The cause is unknown, no environmental or geographic factors have been discovered, and person-to-person transmission is unproven. Treatment includes aspirin in large doses, which may be prescribed over a long period of time, and supportive care. Also called **Kawasaki disease.**

mucoepidermoid carcinoma, a malignant neoplasm of glandular tissues, especially the ducts of the salivary glands. The tumor contains mucinous and epidermoid squamous cells.

mucoid (myu′koid), 1. Also called **myxoid.** resembling mucus. 2. any one of a group of mucuslike proteins derived from an animal source. The mucoids differ from the mucins in solubility; they are precipitated by acetic acid. Kinds of mucoids are **colloids, ovomucoid.**

mucolytic (myu′kəlıt′ık), capable of dissolving mucus.

mucomembranous (myu′koumem′brənəs), of or pertaining to a mucous membrane, as that of the small intestine or the bladder.

Mucomyst, a trade name for a mucolytic (acetylcysteine), used as an adjunct to anesthesia and as adjuvant therapy for patients with abnormal, viscid or inspissated mucous secretions.

mucopolysaccharidosis (MPS) (myu′koupol′isæk′əridou′sis), pl. **mucopolysaccharidoses.** one of a group of genetic disorders characterized by greater than normal accumulations of mucopolysaccharides in the tissues, with other symptoms specific to each type. The disorders are numbered MPS I through MPS VII, and each type has a specific eponym. In all types, there is pronounced skeletal deformity (especially of the face), mental and physical retardation, and decreased life expectancy. The disorders may be detected before birth by testing fetal cells present in amniotic fluid. After birth, diagnosis is established through urine testing, skeletal changes observed on x ray, and family history. There is no successful treatment. Kinds of mucopolysaccharidosis include **Hunter's syndrome (MPS II), Hurler's syndrome (MPS I).**

mucoprotein (myu′kouprou′tin, myu′kouprou′tiin), a compound, present in all connective and supporting tissue, that contains mucopolysaccharides as prosthetic groups and is relatively resistant to denaturation.

mucopurulent (myu′koupyur′yələnt), characteristic of a combination of mucus and pus.

mucormycosis. See **zygomycosis.**

mucosa (myukou′sə), pl. **mucosae.** mucous membrane. —**mucosal,** adj.

mucous (myu′kəs), of or pertaining to mucus or the secretion of mucus.

-mucous, a combining form meaning 'containing or composed of mucous': *fibromucous, puromucous, seromucous.*

mucous colitis. See **irritable bowel syndrome.**

mucous membrane, any one of four major kinds of thin sheets of tissue that cover or line various parts of the body. Mucous membranes line cavities or canals of the body that open to the outside, as the linings of the mouth, the digestive tube, the respiratory passages, and the genitourinary tract. It consists of a surface layer of epithelial tissue covering a deeper layer of connective tissue and protects the underlying structure, secretes mucus, and absorbs water, salts, and other solutes. Compare **serous membrane, skin, synovial membrane.**

mucous plug, (in obstetrics) a collection of thick mucus in the uterine cervix that is often expelled at the onset of dilatation of the cervix, just before labor begins or in its early hours. The plug may be dry and firm, following the shape of the endocervical canal, but, more often, it is semifluid and mucoid, streaked with blood.

mucous shreds. See **shreds.**

mucous tumor. See **myxoma.**

mucoviscidosis (myu′kouvis′idou′sis). See **cystic fibrosis.**

mucus, the viscous, slippery secretions of mucous membranes and glands, containing mucin, white blood cells, water, inorganic salts, and exfoliated cells. —**mucoid,** *adj.,* **mucous,** *adj.*

mud bath, the application of warm mud to the body for therapeutic purposes.

Mudrane, a trade name for a respiratory, fixed-combination drug containing a smooth-muscle relaxant (theophylline), an adrenergic (ephedrine hydrochloride), an expectorant (potassium iodide), and a sedative-hypnotic (phenobarbital).

mulibrey nanism, a rare genetic disorder, transmitted as an autosomal recessive trait, characterized by dwarfism, constrictive pericarditis, muscular hypotonia, anomalies of the skull and face, and characteristic yellow dots in the ocular fundus. The name of the condition is an acronym comprised of the first two letters of the anatomical sites of the principal defects: muscle, liver, brain, and eyes.

Müllerian (myler′iən), of or pertaining to the Müllerian ducts, named for Johannes Peter Müller.

Müllerian duct, one of a pair of embryonic ducts that become the Fallopian tubes, uterus, and vagina in females and that atrophy in males.

Mull-Soy. See **Neo-Mull-Soy.**

multi-, a combining form meaning 'many': *multicapsular, multifamilial, multipara.*

multicentric mitosis. See **multipolar mitosis.**

multifactorial, of, pertaining to, or characteristic of any condition or disease resulting from the interaction of many factors, specifically the interaction of several genes, usually polygenes, with or without the involvement of environmental factors. Many disorders, as spina bifida, neural tube defects, and Hirschsprung's disease, are considered to be multifactorial.

multifactorial inheritance, the tendency to develop a characteristic, disease, or condition that is genetic and environmental, as stature, blood pressure, or neural tube defect.

multi-infarct dementia (məl'tiin'farkt), a form of organic brain disease characterized by the rapid deterioration of intellectual functioning, caused by vascular disease. Symptoms include emotional lability, disturbances in memory, abstract thinking, judgment, and impulse control, and focal neurological impairment, such as gait abnormalities, pseudobulbar palsy, and paresthesia. The condition is more prevalent in men than in women and may be caused by a cerebrovascular accident with cerebrovascular insufficiency or by intracerebral hemorrhage. See also **dementia, senile psychosis.**

multipenniform (məl'tipen'ıfɔrm), (of a bodily structure) having a shape resembling a pattern of many feathers, especially the pattern formed by the muscular fasciculi that converge to several tendons. Compare **bipenniform, penniform.**

multiphasic screening, a technique of screening populations for diseases in which there is combined use of a battery of screening tests. The technique serves to identify any of several diseases being screened for in a population that is apparently healthy.

multiple benign cystic epithelioma. See **trichoepithelioma.**

multiple cartilaginous exostoses. See **diaphyseal aclasis.**

multiple enchondromatosis. See **enchondromatosis.**

multiple endocrine adenomatosis. See **adenomatosis.**

multiple factor. See **polygene.**

multiple fission, cell division in which the nucleus first divides into several equal parts followed by the division of the cytoplasm into as many cells as there are nuclei. It is the common form of asexual reproduction in certain unicellular organisms, as a sporozoan. Compare **binary fission.**

multiple fracture, 1. a fracture extending several fracture lines in one bone. 2. the fracture of several bones at one time or from the same injury.

multiple gene. See **polygene.**

multiple idiopathic hemorrhagic sarcoma. See **Kaposi's sarcoma.**

multiple lipomatosis, a rare, inherited disorder characterized by discrete, localized, subcutaneous deposits of fat in the tissues of the body. This fat is not available for metabolic use, even in starvation.

multiple mononeuropathy, an abnormal condition characterized by dysfunction of several individual nerve trunks. It may be caused by various diseases, as necrotizing angiopathy, uremia, diabetes mellitus, and some inflammatory immunologic disorders. Also called *Obsolete.* **mononeuritis multiplex.**

multiple myeloma, a malignant neoplasm of the bone marrow. The tumor, composed of plasma cells, destroys osseous tissue, especially in flat bones, causing pain, fractures, and skeletal deformities, including spinal curvature. Characteristically, there are abnormal proteins in the plasma and urine, anemia, weight loss, pulmonary complications secondary to rib fractures, and kidney failure. Also called **multiple plasmacytoma of bone, myelomatosis, plasma cell myeloma.**

multiple myositis. See **polymyositis.**

multiple neuroma. See **neuromatosis.**

multiple peripheral neuritis, acute or subacute disseminated inflammation or degeneration of symmetrically distributed peripheral nerves, characterized initially by numbness, tingling in the extremities, hot and cold sensations, and slight fever, progressing to pain, weakness, diminished reflexes, and in some cases flaccid paralysis. The disorder may be caused by toxic substances, as antimony, arsenic, carbon monoxide, copper, lead, mercury, nitrobenzol, organophosphates, and thallium, or various drugs, including diphenylhydantoin, isoniazid, nitrofurantoin, thalidomide, and vincristine. Multiple peripheral neuritis may occur in alcoholism, arteriosclerosis, beriberi, chronic gastrointestinal disease, diabetes, leprosy, pellagra, porphyria, rheumatoid arthritis, systemic lupus erythematosus, and many infectious diseases. Therapy consists of removal of the toxic agent or treatment of the causative disease, rest, and medication for pain. Guillain-Barré syndrome sometimes occurs following an influenza vaccination. Also called **peripheral polyneuritis.** See also **Guillain-Barré syndrome.**

multiple personality, an abnormal condition in which the organization of the personality is fragmented. It is characterized by the presence of two or more distinct subpersonalities. Also called **split personality.**

multiple personality disorder, a dissociative disorder characterized by the existence of two or more distinct, clearly differentiated personality structures within the same individual, any of which may dominate at a particular time. Each personality is a complex unit with separate, well-developed emotional and thought processes, behavior patterns, and social relationships. The various subpersonalities are usually dramatically different from one another and may or may not be aware of the existence of the others. Often, complex interrelationships exist between the personalities, with one functioning on a conscious level and the other or others on a subconscious level. Transition from one subpersonality to another is usually sudden and associated with psychosocial stress. The dominance of a particular subpersonality may last from a few minutes to several years. The condition, most often diagnosed in female adolescents or young adults, primarily results from intrapsychic conflicts that are so deep-seated that the only solution is to separate the conflicting parts of the psyche into separate autonomous personality systems. Classic examples of the disorder are extremely rare; various symptoms, but not the complete entity, are apparent in some schizophrenic patients. Treatment may include hypnosis or psychotropic medication and long-term psychotherapy aimed at uncovering the emotional conflicts that precipitated the development and maintenance of the various subpersonalities. See also **dissociative disorder, hysterical neurosis.**

multiple plasmacytoma of bone. See **multiple myeloma.**

multiple sclerosis (MS), a progressive disease characterized by disseminated demyelination of nerve fibers of the brain and spinal cord. It begins slowly, usually in young adulthood, and continues throughout life with periods of exacerbation and remission. The first signs are paresthesias, or abnormal sensations in the extremities or on one side of the face. Other early signs are muscle weakness, vertigo, and visual disturbances, as nystagmus, diplopia (double vision), and partial blindness. Later in the course of disease, there may be extreme emotional lability, ataxia, abnormal reflexes, and difficulty in urinating. Because many other conditons affect the nervous system and produce similar symptoms, the diagnosis of MS is difficult to make. A history of exacerbation and remission of symptoms and the presence of greater than normal amounts of protein in cerebrospinal fluid are characteristic. As the disease progresses, the intervals between exacerbations grow shorter, and disability becomes greater. There is no specific treatment for the disease; corticosteroids and other drugs are used to treat the symptoms accompanying acute episodes. Physical therapy may help to postpone or prevent specific disabilities. The patient is encouraged to live as normal and active a life as possible. Also called **disseminated multiple sclerosis.**

multiple self-healing squamous epithelioma. See **keratoacanthoma.**

multiplicative growth. See **merisis.**

multipolar mitosis, cell division in which the spindle has three or more poles and results in the formation of a corresponding number of daughter cells. Also called **multicentric mitosis, pluripolar mitosis.** See also **trisomy.**

multisource drug, a drug that can be purchased under any of several trade names from different manufacturers or distributors. See also **generic equivalent, generic name.**

multivalent (məl'tɪveɪ'lənt), **1.** (in chemistry) the capacity of an element to combine with three or more univalent atoms. **2.** (in immunology) able to act against more than one strain of organism. Compare **valence.**

mummified fetus, a fetus that has died in utero and has shriveled and dried up.

mumps, an acute viral disease, characterized by a swelling of the parotid glands, caused by a paramyxovirus. It is most likely to affect children between 5 and 15 years of age, but it may occur at any age. In adulthood the infection may be severe. Passive immunity from maternal antibodies usually prevents this disease in children under one year of age. The incidence of mumps is highest during the late winter and early spring. The mumps paramyxovirus lives in the saliva of the affected individual and is transmitted in droplets or by direct contact. The virus is present in the saliva from six days before to nine days after the onset of the swelling of the parotid gland. The time of maximum communicability is believed to be the 48-hour period immediately preceding the start of parotid swelling. The prognosis in mumps is good, but the disease sometimes involves complications, as arthritis, pancreatitis, myocarditis, oophoritis, and nephritis. About half of the men with mumps-induced orchitis suffer some atrophy of the testicles, as the condition is usually unilateral, but sterility rarely results. Also called **epidemic parotitis, infectious parotitis.**

■ OBSERVATIONS: The common symptoms of mumps usually last for about 24 hours and include anorexia, headache, malaise, and low-grade fever. These signs are commonly followed by earache, parotid gland swelling and a temperature of 101° to 104°F (38.3° to 40°C). The patient also experiences pain when drinking acidic liquids or when chewing. The salivary glands may also become swollen. Complications, as epididymo-orchitis and mumps meningitis, may develop. About 25 per cent of the postpubertal males who contract mumps develop epididymo-orchitis with associated testicular swelling and tenderness that may persist for several weeks. Mumps meningitis develops in 10 per cent of the patients with mumps and occurs in three to five times as many males as females. Diagnosis of mumps is usually based on typical symptoms, especially parotid gland swelling. If the parotid gland is not swollen, confirming diagnosis may be based on serologic antibody tests.

■ INTERVENTION: The treatment of mumps commonly includes the respiratory isolation of the patient and the administration of analgesics, antipyretics, and a fluid intake adequate to prevent dehydration associated with fever and anorexia. Intravenous fluids may be administered to the patient who can't swallow as the result of severe parotitis.

■ NURSING CONSIDERATIONS: The patient is confined to bed and may be given antipyretics and tepid sponge baths to reduce fever. Patients with mumps are also encouraged to drink fluids and to avoid spicy foods and those that require considerable chewing. During the acute phase of the disease, the nurse is especially alert to any signs of central nervous system involvement, as nuchal rigidity and altered consciousness. All cases of mumps are routinely reported to local health authorities. Nurses aid public health education by stressing the importance of immunization with live attenuated mumps virus for individuals the at age of 15 months and for susceptible persons, especially males who are approaching puberty or who are past puberty. Immunization within 24 hours of exposure may prevent the disease or may minimize its effects.

Mumpsvax, a trade name for an active immunizing agent (live mumps virus vaccine).

mumps virus vaccine live, an active immunizing agent.

■ INDICATION: It is prescribed for immunization against mumps.

■ CONTRAINDICATIONS: Immunosuppression, concomitant use of corticosteroids, acute infection, pregnancy, Known hypersensitivity to chicken proteins, neomycin, or to this drug prohibits its use.

■ ADVERSE EFFECTS: Among the most serious adverse effects are fevers, parotitis, and allergic reactions.

Munchausen's syndrome (mən'chauzınz), an unusual condition characterized by habitual pleas for treatment and hospitalization for a symptomatic but imaginary acute illness. The affected person may logically and convincingly present the symptoms and history of a real disease. Symptoms resolve with treatment, but the person may seek further treatment for another imaginary disease. Also called **pathomimicry.**

Murchison fever. See **Pel-Ebstein fever.**

murine typhus, an acute arbovirus infection caused by *Rickettsia typhi* and transmitted by the bite of an infected flea. It is characterized by headache, chills, fever, myalgia, and rash. After an 8- to 16-day incubation period, fever develops and lasts about twelve days. A dull-red, maculopapular rash, mainly on the trunk, appears about the fifth day and lasts for four to eight days. Recovery is usually rapid and complete, but death has occurred in elderly or debilitated people. Weil-Felix and complement fixation tests aid in the diagnosis. Chloramphenicol or tetracycline is usually prescribed in treatment. Prevention involves the elimination of the rodents that are the natural host of the organism and the use of appropriate insecticides to control fleas. Also called **endemic typhus, fleaborne typhus, new world typhus, rat typhus, urban typhus.** Compare **epidemic typhus, Rocky Mountain spotted fever.**

murmur, a low pitched fluttering or humming sound, as a heart murmur.

Murocoll, a trade name for an ophthalmic, fixed-combination drug containing an adrenergic (epinephrine bitartrate) and an astringent (zinc sulfate).

Murray Valley encephalitis, an acute inflammatory disease of the brain, once epidemic in Australia's Murray Valley, characterized by convulsions, muscle rigidity, high fever, mental confusion, and coma. It is considered identical to Australian X disease, which is caused by a neurotropic herpeslike virus.

muscae volitantes (məs'i vol'ıtæn'tiz). See **floater.**

muscarinic (məs'kərın'ık), stimulating the postganglionic parasympathetic receptor.

muscle, a kind of tissue comprised of fibers that are able to contract, causing and allowing movement of the parts and organs of the body. Muscle fibers are richly vascular, irritable, conductive, and elastic. There are two basic kinds, striated muscle and smooth muscle. Striated muscle, which comprises all skeletal muscles except for the myocardium, is long and voluntary; it responds very quickly to stimulation and is paralyzed by interruption of its innervation. Smooth muscle, which comprises all visceral muscles, is short and involuntary; it reacts slowly to all stimuli and does not entirely lose its tone if innervation is interrupted. The myocardium is sometimes classified as a third (cardiac) kind of muscle, but it is basically a striated muscle that does not contract as quickly as the striated muscle of the rest of the body, and it is not completely paralyzed if it loses its neural stimuli. See also **cardiac muscle, smooth muscle, striated muscle.**

muscle albumin, albumin present in muscle.

muscle of expression. See **facial muscle.**

muscle relaxant, a chemotherapeutic agent that reduces the contractility of muscle fibers. Curare derivatives and succinylcholine compete with acetylcholine and block neural transmission at the myoneural junction. These drugs are used during anesthesia, in the management of patients undergoing mechanical ventilation, and in shock therapy, to reduce muscle contractions in pharmacologically or electrically induced seizures. Quinine sulfate, prescribed for the prevention and treatment of nocturnal leg cramps, reduces muscle tension by increasing the refractory period of muscle fibers and by decreasing the excitability of the motor end plate. Several drugs that relieve muscle spasms act at various levels in the central nervous system: baclofan inhibits monosynaptic and polysynaptic reflexes at the spinal level; cyclobenzaprine acts primarily in the brain stem; chlorzoxazone inhibits multisynaptic arcs in the spinal cord and subcortical areas of the brain; and the benzodiazepines reduce muscle tension, chiefly by acting on reticular neuronal mechanisms that control muscle tone. Dantrolene acts directly on muscles in reducing contraction and apparently achieves its effect by interfering with the release of calcium from the sarcoplasmic reticulum.

muscle-setting exercise, a method of maintaining muscle strength and tonality by alternately contracting and relaxing a skeletal muscle or any group of muscles without moving the associated part of the body. Such activity is useful in preventing atrophy of the muscles, especially in patients with conditions involving the joints.

muscular, 1. of or pertaining to a muscle. 2. characteristic of well-developed musculature.

muscular branch of the deep brachial artery, one of several similar branches of the deep brachial artery, supplying certain arm muscles, as the coracobrachialis, biceps brachii, and brachialis.

muscular dystrophy, a group of genetically transmitted diseases characterized by progressive atrophy of symmetrical groups of skeletal muscles without evidence of involvement or degeneration of neural tissue. In all forms of muscular dystrophy there is an insidious loss of strength with increasing disability and deformity, although each type differs in the groups of muscles affected, the age of onset, the rate of progression, and the mode of genetic inheritance. The basic etiology is unknown but appears to be an inborn error of metabolism. Serum creatine phosphokinase is increased in affected individuals and acts as a diagnostic aid, especially in asymptomatic children in families at risk. Diagnostic confirmation is made by muscle biopsy, electromyography, and genetic pedigree. Treatment of the muscular dystrophies consists primarily of supportive measures, as physical therapy and orthopedic procedures to minimize deformity. The main types of the disease are pseudohypertrophic (Duchenne) muscular dystrophy, limb-girdle muscular dystrophy, and facioscapulohumeral (Landouzy-Dejerine) muscular dystrophy. Rarer forms include Becker's muscular dystrophy, distal muscular dystrophy, ocular myopathy, and myotonic muscular dystrophy. See also **myotonic myopathy.**

muscular sarcoidosis, sarcoidosis of the skeletal muscles in which there is interstitial inflammation, fibrosis, atrophy, and damage of the muscle fibers, as sarcoid tubercles form within and replace normal muscle cells. See also **sarcoidosis.**

muscular tumor. See myoma.

musculocutaneous nerve (məs′kyuloukyutei′niəs), one of the terminal branches of the brachial plexus. It is formed on each side by division of the lateral cord of the plexus into two branches. It pierces the coracobrachialis and crosses to the lateral side of the arm, where it pierces the deep fascia just above the elbow and continues into the forearm as the lateral antebrachial cutaneous nerve. Various branches and filaments supply different structures, as the biceps, the brachialis, the humerus, and the skin of the forearm. The branches of the musculocutaneous nerve are the coracobrachialis branch, the muscular branches, an articular filament to the elbow joint, a filament to the humerus, the lateral antebrachial cutaneous

nerve, the anterior branch, and the dorsal branch. Compare **median nerve, radial nerve, ulnar nerve.**

musculoskeletal (məs′kyulouskel′itəl), of or pertaining to the muscles and the skeleton.

musculoskeletal system assessment, an evaluation of the condition and functioning of the patient's muscles, joints, and bones and of factors which may contribute to abnormalities in these body structures.

■ METHOD: The patient is questioned about any pain and edema in muscles, joints, and bones, weakness in extremities, limitations in movements and activities, unsteadiness on the feet, fatigability, insomnia, anorexia, weight loss, and feelings of frustration. The individual's general appearance, age, blood pressure, pulse, respirations, body alignment, ability or inability to move in bed, gait, need for assistance in walking, handgrip, range of motion, and internal and external rotation of extremities are observed. The presence of contractures, deformities, paralysis, contusions, lacerations, wounds, footdrop, wristdrop, paralysis, crutches, brace, cast, prosthesis, cane, walker, decubiti, allergies, skin rash, or tenseness is noted. It is ascertained whether the patient can perform activities of daily living, is able to sit up, turn, and use the trapeze in bed, if constipation is a complaint, and if the individual is independent or dependent. Concurrent diseases or conditions investigated include injury to the spinal cord, nerve impairment, cerebrovascular accident, rheumatoid arthritis, osteoarthritis, bursitis, polyneuritis, multiple sclerosis, muscular dystrophy, myasthenia gravis, fracture, ruptured disc, Ménière's disease, and labyrinthitis. It is determined if the patient previously had orthopedic or spinal surgery, poliomyelitis, hemiplegia, cerebral palsy, parkinsonism, a cerebrovascular accident, ataxia, syphilis, hyperparathyroidism, osteoporosis, rickets, osteomalacia, tuberculosis, alcoholism, and impaired vision or hearing. A family history of carcinoma, diabetes, or tuberculosis, the patient's involvement in a hazardous job or recreation, history of previous accidents, and the use of tobacco or medications, as steroids, sedatives, tranquilizers, analgesics, antimalarials, acetylsalicylic acid, or indomethacin, are determined. Laboratory studies important for the assessment are assays of serum and urine calcium and phosphorus and of alkaline phosphatase serum level. Diagnostic procedures that may be required include x rays of bones, arthrograms, myelograms, arteriograms, arthroscopy, biopsies of bone or muscle, incision and drainage of joints, and electromyograms of muscles.

■ NURSING ORDERS: The nurse conducts the interview to obtain subjective data, makes the necessary observations of the patient, and assembles the information on concurrent and previous disorders, the family history, the patient's social and medication background, and the results of laboratory studies and diagnostic procedures.

■ OUTCOME CRITERIA: A meticulous assessment of the

patient's musculoskeletal system is a valuable aid in diagnosis, in planning the course of therapy, and in predicting the prognosis.

musculospiral nerve (məs'kyʊlospai'rəl). See **radial nerve.**

mushroom, the fruiting body of the fungus of the class Basidomycetes, especially those of the edible order Agaricales, commonly known as the field mushrooms or meadow mushrooms. Although mushrooms contain some protein and minerals, they are composed largely of water and are of limited nutritional value. Fungal poisoning is caused by ingestion of mushrooms of the genus *Amanita,* in particular *A. muscaria* and *A. phalloides.* Symptoms, caused by toxic peptides, may appear within a few minutes of ingestion and consist of severe abdominal pain, vomiting, extreme nausea, salivation, sweating, diarrhea, excessive thirst, coma, and, occasionally, convulsion. Extensive damage to the liver, kidneys, and central nervous system may occur. Some mushrooms, especially *Psilocybe mexicana,* contain substances that produce hallucinatory states.

mushroom poisoning, a toxic condition caused by the ingestion of certain mushrooms, particularly two species of the genus *Amanita.* Muscarine in *Amanita muscaria* produces intoxication in from a few to 120 minutes. Symptoms include lacrimation, salivation, sweating, vomiting, labored breathing, abdominal cramps, diarrhea, and, in severe cases, convulsions, coma, and circulatory failure. Atropine is usually administered in treatment. More deadly but slower acting phalloidine in *A. phalloides* and *A. verna* causes similar symptoms as well as liver damage, renal failure, and death in 30 to 50 per cent of the cases. Treatment includes emptying the stomach by gastric lavage with a weak solution of tannic acid or of potassium permanganate, followed by a saline purgative. Intensive care, as for kidney or liver failure, and hemodialysis may reduce mortality. In some people, the consumption of alcohol complicates mushroom poisoning and the combination has the effect of disulfiram.

mushroom worker's lung, a type of hypersensitivity pneumonitis common among workers in the mushroom-growing industry. The antigens to which the hypersensitive reactions occur are genera of the fungi *Micropolyspora* and *Thermoactinomyces.* Spores of these fungi are found in the postspawning compost used to grow mushrooms. Symptoms of the acute form of the disease include chills, cough, fever, dyspnea, anorexia, nausea, and vomiting. The chronic form of the disease is characterized by fatigue, chronic cough, weight loss, and dyspnea on exercise.

music therapy, a form of adjunctive psychotherapy in which music is used as a means of recreation and communication, especially with autistic children, and as a means to elevate the mood of depressed and psychotic patients.

mustard gas, a poisonous gas used in chemical warfare during World War I. It causes corrosive destruction of the skin and mucous membranes, often resulting in permanent respiratory damage and death.

Mustargen Hydrochloride, a trade name for an antineoplastic (mechlorethamine hydrochloride).

mutagen (myu'təjın), any chemical or physical environmental agent that induces a genetic mutation or increases the mutation rate. —**mutagenic,** *adj.,* **mutagenicity,** *n.*

mutagenesis (myu'təjen'əsıs), the induction or occurrence of a genetic mutation. See also **teratogenesis.**

Mutamycin, a trade name for an antineoplastic (mitomycin).

mutant gene, any gene that has undergone a change, as the loss, gain, or exchange of genetic material, which affects the normal transmission and expression of a trait. Such genes can become inactive or show reduced, increased, or antagonistic activity. See also **amorph, antimorph, hypermorph, hypomorph.**

mutation, an unusual change in genetic material occurring spontaneously or by induction. The alteration changes the original expression of the gene. Genes are stable units, but when a mutation occurs it is transmitted to future generations. —**mutate,** *v.,* **mutational,** *adj.*

mutism (myu'tızəm), the inability or refusal to speak. The condition may result from an unconscious response to emotional conflict and confusion and is most commonly observed in patients who are catatonic, stuporous, hysterical, or depressed. A kind of mutism is **akinetic mutism.**

muton (myu'ton), (in molecular genetics), the smallest DNA segment whose alteration can result in a mutation.

mutually exclusive categories, categories on a research instrument that are sufficiently precise to allow each subject, factor, or variable to be classified in only one category.

mV, mv, abbreviation for **millivolt.**

Mv, symbol for **mendelevium.**

mV̇O₂, symbol for **myocardial oxygen consumption.**

MVV, abbreviation for *maximal voluntary ventilation.* See **maximal breathing capacity.**

M.W.I.A., abbreviation for **Medical Women's International Association.**

my-. See **myo-.**

myalgia (maiæl'jə), diffuse muscle pain, usually accompanied by malaise, occurring in many infectious diseases, as brucellosis, dengue, influenza, leptospirosis, measles, malaria, relapsing fever, rheumatic fever, salmonellosis, tick-borne hemorrhagic fevers, toxoplasmosis, trichinosis, tularemia, and poliomyelitis. Myalgia occurs in arteriosclerosis obliterans, fibrositis, fibromyositis, Guillain-Barré syndrome, hyperparathyroidism, hypoglycemia, hypothyroidism, muscle tumor, myoglobinuria, myositis, and renal tubular acidosis. Various drugs that may cause myalgia include amphotericin B, carbenoxolone, chloroquinine, clofibrate, and corticosteroids. See also **epidemic myalgia.** — **myalgic,** *adj.*

myalgic asthenia, a condition characterized by a general feeling of fatigue and muscular pain, often resulting from or associated with psychological stress.

Myambutol, a trade name for an antibacterial (ethambutol hydrochloride).

myasthenia gravis, an abnormal condition characterized by the chronic fatigability and weakness of muscles, especially in the face and throat, as a result of a defect in the conduction of nerve impulses at the myoneural junction.

■ OBSERVATIONS: Muscular fatigability in myasthenia gravis is caused by the inability of receptors at the myoneural junction to depolarize because of a deficiency of acetylcholine; hence, the diagnosis may be made by administering an anticholinesterase drug and observing improved muscle strength and stamina. The onset of symptoms is usually gradual, with ptosis of the upper eyelids, diplopia, and weakness of the facial muscles. The weakness may then extend to other muscles innervated by the cranial nerves, particularly the respiratory muscles. Muscular exertion aggravates the symptoms, which typically vary over the course of the day. The disease occurs in younger women more often than in older women and in men over 60 years of age more often than in younger men.

■ INTERVENTION: Anticholinesterase drugs are given. The Tensilon test is used to determine the optimal maintenance dose. Neostigmine or pyridostigmine is the drug most often used.

■ NURSING CONSIDERATIONS: Physical activity is restricted and bed rest encouraged. Anticholinesterase drugs are usually administered before meals, and the patient is monitored for toxic side effects. Myasthenic crisis may require emergency respiratory assistance. The patient's diet may have to be adjusted if the ability to chew and swallow is affected.

myasthenia (maiˈəsfhiˈniə), a condition characterized by an abnormal weakness of a muscle or a group of muscles that may be the result of a systemic myoneural disturbance, as in myasthenia gravis, or of a local circulatory inadequacy, as in intermittent claudication. — **myasthenic,** *adj.*

myasthenia gravis crisis, acute exacerbation of the muscular weakness characterizing the disease, triggered by infection, surgery, emotional stress, or an overdose or insufficiency of anticholinesterase medication.

■ OBSERVATIONS: Typical signs and symptoms include respiratory distress progressing to periods of apnea, extreme fatigue, increased muscular weakness, dysphagia, dysarthria, and fever. The patient may be anxious, restless, irritable, unable to move the jaws or to raise one or

both eyelids. If the condition is caused by anticholinesterase toxicity, there may be anorexia, nausea, vomiting, abdominal cramps, diarrhea, excessive salivation, sweating, lacrimation, blurred vision, vertigo, and muscle cramps and spasms, as well as general weakness, dysarthria, and respiratory distress.

■ INTERVENTION: Initial treatment is directed to maintaining patency of the airway. Oxygen with assisted or controlled ventilation is administered, as a tracheostomy may be performed and bronchoscopy may be indicated. The patient is placed in a bed in which the head is elevated 30 degrees. The withdrawal or reduction of anticholinergic drugs may be ordered, or they may be given to differentiate the kind of crisis. Respiratory secretions and saliva are suctioned and blood pressure, pulse, and respiration are carefully observed. The chest is auscultated and the rectal temperature is taken every two to four hours; cooling measures may be necessary. Parenteral fluids, antibiotics, nasogastric feeding, and the insertion of an indwelling catheter with closed gravity drainage may be ordered. The patient is turned every two hours and given mouth and skin care every two to four hours; the lips are kept well lubricated and decubiti are avoided by using an air mattress or sheepskin and by keeping the skin dry at all times. If an eyelid is affected, the eye may be covered with a patch; crusts are removed whenever required, and soothing eyedrops may be administered. To enable the patient to communicate, the call bell and a pad and pencil or magic slate are placed within reach. When the acute crisis subsides, the patient may progress from clear liquids to a soft diet but may require help in eating. Nourishment is offered between meals and a daily intake of up to 2,000 ml of fluids is encouraged. Walking as tolerated and other activities are planned at the time of the maximum effect of medication. Active or passive range-of-motion exercises of all extremities are performed several times a day, but rest periods are maintained to avoid fatigue and relapse.

■ NURSING CONSIDERATIONS: Before discharge the patient is instructed on the importance of taking the prescribed medication with milk, crackers, or bread at the scheduled time and of reporting toxic side effects and symptoms of recurrent or progressive disease. The nurse points out the need to maintain a regular diet, to exercise to tolerance, to rest, and to avoid infections and exposure to hot or cold weather as well as the use of alcohol and tobacco. The nurse's help in planning a schedule that conserves energy for essential activities can enable the patient to be relatively independent and self-sufficient.

myc-. See **myco-.**

mycelium (maiˈsiˈliəm), *pl.* **mycelia.** a mass of interwoven, branched, threadlike filaments which make up most fungi. Also called **hypha.**

mycetismus (mai'sıtız'məs),　mushroom poisoning.

myceto-.　See **myco-.**

mycetoma (mai'sətou'mə),　a serious fungal infection involving skin, subcutaneous tissue, fascia, and bone. One kind of mycetoma is **Madura foot.**

Mychel,　a trade name for an antibacterial and antirickettsial (chloramphenicol).

Mycifradin Sulfate,　a trade name for an antibacterial (neomycin sulfate).

Mycitracin,　a trade name for a topical, fixed-combination drug containing antibacterials (polymyxin B sulfate and neomycin sulfate).

myco-, myc,　a combining form meaning 'related to fungus': *mycobacteriosis, mycohemia, mycophage.* Also **myceto-, myko.**

mycobacteria (mai'koubæktir'iə),　acid-fast microorganisms belonging to the genus *Mycobacterium.* — **mycobacterial,** *adj.*

mycobacteriosis (mai'koubæk'tiriou'sıs),　a tuberculosislike disease caused by mycobacteria other than *Mycobacterium tuberculosis.*

Mycobacterium (mai'koubæktir'iəm),　a genus of rod-shaped, acid-fast bacteria having two significant pathogenic species: *Mycobacterium leprae* causes leprosy; *M. tuberculosis* causes tuberculosis.

Mycolog,　a trade name for a topical fixed-combination drug containing a glucocorticoid (triamcinolone acetonide), two antibacterials (neomycin sulfate and gramicidin), and an antifungal (nystatin).

mycology (maikol'əji),　the study of fungi and fungoid diseases. — **mycologic, mycological,** *adj.,* **mycologist,** *n.*

mycomyringitis.　See **myringomycosis.**

mycophenolic acid (mai'koufınou'lık),　a bacteriostatic and fungistatic crystalline antibiotic obtained from *Pencillium brevi compactum* and related species.

Mycoplasma (mai'kouplæz'mə),　a genus of ultramicroscopic organisms lacking rigid cell walls and considered to be the smallest free-living organisms. Some are saprophytes, some are parasites, and many are pathogens. One species is a cause of mycoplasma pneumonia, tracheobronchitis, pharyngitis, and bullous myringitis. Also called **pleuropneumonialike organism.**

mycoplasma pneumonia,　a contagious disease of children and young adults caused by *Mycoplasma pneumoniae,* characterized by a 9- to 12-day incubation period and followed by symptoms of an upper respiratory infection, dry cough, and fever. Also called **Eaton-agent pneumonia, primary atypical pneumonia, viral pneumonia, walking pneumonia.** See also **cold agglutinin.**

■ OBSERVATIONS: Harsh or diminished breath sounds and fine inspiratory rales are frequently heard. Pulmonary infiltrates visible on chest x ray may resemble bacterial or viral pneumonia and may persist for three weeks in untreated cases. Rarely, complications, as sinusitis, pleurisy, polyneuritis, myocarditis, or Stevens-Johnson syndrome, may follow the pneumonia. In untreated adults prolonged cough, weakness, and malaise are common. Diagnosis is suggested by physical examination and by observation of the clinical course and elevated cold agglutinins and is confirmed by a complement fixation test. Prognosis is favorable.

■ INTERVENTION: Erythromycin or tetracycline, bedrest, a high-protein diet, and an adequate intake of fluids are recommended. It is important that infants and people for whom a respiratory illness would be a particular hazard avoid or be protected from contact with patients having mycoplasma pneumonia.

mycosis (maikou'sıs),　any disease caused by a fungus. Some kinds of mycoses are **athlete's foot, candidiasis, coccidioidomycosis.** — **mycotic,** *adj.*

mycosis fungoides (fəŋgoi'diz),　a rare, chronic, lymphomatous skin malignancy resembling eczema or a cutaneous tumor that is followed by microabscesses in the epidermis and lesions simulating those of Hodgkin's disease in lymph nodes and viscera. The condition is considered a distinctive entity by some specialists and a cutaneous manifestation of a malignant lymphoma by others.

Mycostatin,　a trade name for an antifungal (nystatin).

mycotic aneurysm,　a localized dilatation in the wall of a blood vessel caused by the growth of a fungus, usually occurring as a complication of bacterial endocarditis. Also called **bacterial aneurysm.**

Mydriacyl,　a trade name for a cycloplegic mydriatic (tropicamide).

mydriasis (mıdrai'əsıs),　**1.** dilation of the pupil of the eye caused by contraction of the dilator muscle of the iris, a muscular sheath that radiates outward like the spokes of a wheel from the center of the iris around the pupil. With a decrease in light or the pharmacologic action of certain drugs the dilator acts to pull the iris outward, enlarging the pupil. **2.** an abnormal condition characterized by contraction of the dilator muscle, resulting in widely dilated pupils. Compare **miosis.** — **mydriatic** (mıd'riæt'ık), *adj.*

mydriatic cycloplegic agent,　any one of several ophthalmic pharmaceutical preparations that dilate the pupil and paralyze the ocular muscles of accommodation. These drugs are used in diagnostic ophthalmoscopic and refractive examination of the eye, before and after various procedures in eye surgery, in some tests for glaucoma, in the treatment of anterior uveitis, and in treating certain kinds of glaucoma. Blurred vision, thirst, flushing, fever, and rash may occur. In children and elderly people, ataxia, somnolence, delirium, and hallucination may occur but are rare. Among these drugs are atropine, cyclopentolate, homatropine, scopolamine and tropicamide; they are prepared in solution for topical ophthalmic application.

Mydriatic and cycloplegic drugs

Drug	Form and concentration	Duration of effect
Mydriatics		
Phenylephrine (Neo-Synephrine)	Eyedrops, 1% to 10%	12 hours
Epinephrine (Epitrate)	Eyedrops, 1% to 2%	12 hours
Cycloplegics		
Atropine sulfate	Eyedrops, 1% to 3%	2 to 4 weeks
	Ointment, 1%	
Scopolamine (hyoscine)	Eyedrops, 0.25% to 0.5%	1 to 3 weeks
Homatropine hydrobromide	Eyedrops, 0.5% to 3%	1 to 2 days
	Ointment, 1% to 3%	
Cyclopentolate hydrochloride (Cyclogyl)	Eyedrops, 0.5% to 1%	4 to 12 hours
Tropicamide (Mydriacyl)	Eyedrops, 0.5% to 1%	2 to 8 hours

myel-.   See myelo-.

myelacephalus, a fetal monster, usually a separate monozygotic twin, whose form and parts are barely recognizable; a slightly differentiated amorphous mass.   — **myelacephalous,** *adj.*

myelatelia (mai'ələti'liə), any developmental defect involving the spinal cord.

myelauxe (mai'ɔlɔk'si), a developmental anomaly characterized by hypertrophy of the spinal cord.

-myelia, a combining form meaning '(condition of the) spinal cord': *atelomyelia, hydromyelia, syringomyelia.*

myelin (mai'əlın), a substance constituting the sheaths of various nerve fibers throughout the body. It is largely composed of fat, which gives the fibers a white, creamy color.   — **myelinic,** *adj.*

myelinated (mai'əlınei'tıd), (of a nerve) having a myelin sheath.

myelination (mai'əlınei'šhən), the process of furnishing or taking on myelin.

myelin globule, a fatlike droplet found in some sputum.

myelinic, of or pertaining to myelin.

myelinic neuroma, a neuroma neoplasm composed of myelinated nerve fibers.

myelinization (mai'əlın'ızei'šhən), development of the myelin sheath around a nerve fiber.

myelinogenesis (mai'əlın'oujen'ısıs). See myelinization.   — **myelinogenetic,** *adj.*

myelinolysis (mai'əlınol'ısıs), a pathological process that dissolves the myelin sheaths around certain nerve fibers, as those of the pons in alcoholic and undernourished people who are afflicted with central pontine myelinolysis.

myelin sheath, a segmented, fatty lamination composed of myelin that wraps the axons of many nerves in the body. In myelinated peripheral nerves, the sheaths are composed of Schwann cells. The myelin sheaths around the central nerve fibers are composed of oligodendroglia. Their lipoid content gives these coverings a whitish appearance. In the peripheral nerves the sheaths are interrupted every 1 to 2 cm by the nodes of Ranvier, which occur only rarely in the fibers of the central nervous system. The usual thickness of the myelin sheath is between 2 and 10 microns. Various diseases, as multiple sclerosis, can destroy these myelin wrappings.

myelitis (mai'əlai'tıs), an abnormal condition characterized by inflammation of the spinal cord with associated motor or sensory dysfunction. Some kinds of myelitis are **acute transverse myelitis,** **leukomyelitis, poliomyelitis.**   — **myelitic,** *adj.*

myelo-, myel-, a combining form meaning 'related to marrow': *myeloblast, myelocyte, myelomenia.*

myeloblast, one of the earliest precursors of the granulocytic leukocytes. The cytoplasm appears light blue, scanty, and nongranular when seen in a stained blood smear through a microscope. The nucleus contains distinct chromatin material in strands, together with several nucleoli. In certain leukemias, a marked increase in myeloblasts is observed in the marrow and in the peripheral blood. Compare **megaloblast, myelocyte, normoblast.** See also **myelocytic leukemia.** — **myeloblastic,** *adj.*

myeloblastemia (mai'əloublæsti'miə). See **myeloblastosis.**

myeloblastic leukemia, a malignant neoplasm of blood-forming tissues, characterized by many myeloblasts in the circulating blood and tissues. The disease may be a terminal event in the course of chronic granulocytic leukemia.

myeloblastomatosis (mai'əloublæs'toumətou'sıs), abnormal, localized clusters of myeloblasts in the peripheral circulation.

myeloblastosis (mai'əloublæstou'sıs), the abnormal presence of myeloblasts in the circulation.

myelocele (mai'əlousıl'), a saclike protrusion of the spinal cord through a congenital defect in the vertebral column. See also **myelomeningocele, neural tube defect.**

myeloclast (mai'əlouklæst'), a cell that breaks down the myelin sheaths of nerves of the central nervous system.

myelocyst (mai'əlousıst'), any benign cyst that is formed from the rudimentary medullary canals that give rise to the vertebral canal during embryonic development.

myelocystocele (mai'əlousıs'təsil'), a protrusion of a cystic tumor containing spinal cord substance through a defect in the vertebral column. See also **myelomeningocele, neural tube defect, spina bifida.**

myelocystomeningocele (mai'əlousɪs'toumənɪŋ'gousil'), a protrusion of a cystic tumor containing both spinal cord substance and meninges through a defect in the vertebral column. See also **myelomeningocele, neural tube defect, spina bifida.**

myelocyte (mai'elousait'), an immature white blood cell normally found in the bone marrow, being the first of the maturation stages of the granulocytic leukocytes. When stained and microscopically examined, granules typical of the granulocytic series are seen in the cytoplasm. The nuclear material of the myelocyte is denser than that of the myeloblast, but it lacks a definable membrane. The cell is flat and contains increasing numbers of granules as the maturation process progresses. These cells appear in the circulating blood only in certain forms of leukemia. Compare **myeloblast.** See also **myelocytic leukemia.** — **myelocytic,** adj.

myelocythemia (mai'əlousaɪθi'miə), an abnormal presence of myelocytes in the circulating blood, as in myelocytic leukemia.

myelocytic leukemia, a disorder characterized by the unregulated and excessive production of myelocytes of the granulocytic series. As many as several hundred thousand per cu mm may be seen. Also called **granulocytic leukemia, myelogenous leukemia.** Compare **leukemoid reaction, lymphatic leukemia.** See also **leukocytosis.**

myelocytoma (mai'əlousaɪtou'mə), a localized cluster of myelocytes in the peripheral vasculature that may occur in myelocytic leukemia.

myelocytosis (mai'əlousaɪtou'sɪs). See **myelocythemia.**

myelodiastasis (mai'əloudaiæs'təsɪs), disintegration and necrosis of the spinal cord.

myclodysplasia, a general designation for the defective development of any part of the spinal cord. The term is used primarily to describe abnormalities without gross superficial defects, especially of the lower segment, specifically spina bifida occulta.

myelofibrosis (mai'əloufaɪbrou'sɪs). See **myeloid metaplasia.**

myelogenesis, 1. See also **neural tube formation.** the formation and differentiation of the nervous system during prenatal development, in particular the brain and spinal cord. 2. See also **myelinization.** the development of the myelin sheath around the nerve fiber.

myelogenous (mai'əloj'ənəs), pertaining to the cells produced in bone marrow or to the tissue from which such cells originate. — **myelogenetic, myelogenic,** adj.

myelogenous leukemia. See **acute myelocytic leukemia, chronic myelocytic leukemia.**

myelogeny, the formation and differentiation of the myelin sheaths of nerve fibers during the prenatal development of the central nervous system.

myelogram (mai'əlougræm'), 1. an x ray taken following the injection of a radiopaque medium into the subarachnoid space to demonstrate any distortions of the spinal cord, spinal nerve roots, and the subarachnoid space. 2. a graphic representation of a count of the different kinds of cells in a stained preparation of bone marrow.

myelography (mai'əlog'rəfi), a radiographic process by which the spinal cord and the spinal subarachnoid space are viewed and photographed after the introduction of a contrast medium, as air or an absorbable contrast substance. It is used to identify and study spinal lesions caused by trauma or disease. — **myelographic,** adj.

myeloid (mai'əloid), 1. of or pertaining to the bone marrow. 2. of or pertaining to the spinal cord. 3. of or pertaining to myelocytic forms that do not necessarily originate in the bone marrow.

myeloid leukemia. See **acute myelocytic leukemia, chronic myelocytic leukemia.**

myeloid metaplasia, a disorder in which bone marrow tissue develops in abnormal sites. Characteristics of the condition are anemia, splenomegaly, immature blood cells in the circulation and hematopoesis occurring in the liver and spleen. Myeloid metaplasia may be secondary to carcinoma, leukemia, polycythemia vera, or tuberculosis. The primary form is also called **agnogenic myeloid metaplasia, myelofibrosis.**

myeloidosis (mai'əloidou'sɪs), an abnormal condition characterized by general hyperplasia of the myeloid tissue. See also **Hodgkin's disease, multiple myeloma.**

myeloma (mai'əlou'mə), an osteolytic neoplasm consisting of a profusion of cells typical of the bone marrow. It may develop simultaneously in many sites, causing extensive areas of patchy destruction of the bone. The tumor, which is usually grayish-red, occurs most frequently in the ribs, vertebrae, pelvic bones, and flat bones of the skull. Intense pain and spontaneous fractures are common. The tumor is radiosensitive and local lesions are curable. Kinds of myeloma are **endothelial myeloma, extramedullary myeloma, giant cell myeloma, multiple myeloma, osteogenic myeloma.**

-myeloma, a combining form meaning a 'tumor composed of cells normally found in bone marrow': *globomyeloma, lymphomyeloma, orchiomyeloma.*

myelomalacia (mai'əloumɘlei'ſhiə), abnormal softening of the spinal cord, caused primarily by inadequate blood supply.

myelomatosis (mai'əloumɘtou'sɪs). See **multiple myeloma.**

myelomeningocele (mai'əloumənɪŋ'gousil'), a developmental defect of the central nervous system in which a hernial sac containing a portion of the spinal cord, its meninges, and cerebrospinal fluid protrudes through a congenital cleft in the vertebral column. The condition is caused primarily by the failure of the neural tube to close during embryonic development, although in some instances it may result from the reopening of the tube from an abnormal increase in cerebrospinal fluid pressure. Also called **meningomyelocele. See also neural tube defect, spinal bifida.**

■ OBSERVATIONS: The defect, which occurs in approximately two in every 1,000 live births, is readily apparent and easily diagnosed at birth. Although the opening may be located at any point along the spinal column, the anomaly characteristically occurs in the lumbar, low thoracic, or sacral region and extends for three to six vertebral segments. The saclike structure may be covered with a thin layer of skin or with a fine membrane that can be easily ruptured, increasing the risk of meningeal infection. The severity of neurological dysfunction is directly related to the amount of neural tissue involved, which can be roughly estimated by the degree of the transillumination of the mass. Usually the condition is accompanied by varying degrees of paralysis of the lower extremities, by musculoskeletal defects, as clubfoot, flexion and joint deformities, or hip dysplasia, and by anal and bladder sphincter dysfunction, which can lead to serious genitourinary disorders. Hydrocephalus, frequently related to the Arnold-Chiari malformation, is the most common anomaly associated with myelomeningocele and occurs in approximately 90 per cent of the cases in which the spinal lesion is located in the lumbosacral region. In most cases, hydrocephalus is apparent at birth, although it may appear shortly afterward. Supplementary diagnostic procedures include x rays of the spine, skull, and chest to determine the extent of the vertebral defect and the presence of other malformations in other organ systems, a computerized axial tomographic scan of the brain to establish the ventricular size and the presence of any structural congenital anomalies, and laboratory examinations, especially urine analysis, culture, blood urea nitrogen evaluation, and creatinine clearance determination.

■ INTERVENTION: Supportive care and surgery are the only treatments for myelomeningocele and they require a multidisciplinary approach involving specialists from neurology, neurosurgery, urology, pediatrics, orthopedics, rehabilitation, and physical therapy, as well as intensive nursing care. Initial treatment involves prevention of infection and assessment of neurological involvement. Immediate surgical repair is essential if the defect is leaking cerebrospinal fluid. However, surgical intervention may not be appropriate if neurologic involvement is extreme, if the lesion is infected, or if associated problems, as hydrocephalus, are severe. When surgical repair of the spinal defect is recommended, associated problems are managed by appropriate measures, including shunt procedures for correction of hydrocephalus; antibiotic therapy to reduce the incidence of meningitis, urinary tract infec-

tions, and pneumonia; casting, bracing, traction, and surgical techniques for correction of hip, knee, and foot deformities; and prevention and treatment of renal complications. Although improved surgical techniques and other treatment modalities have significantly increased the survival rate, these procedures cannot alter the major physical disability and deformity, mental retardation, and chronic urinary tract and pulmonary infections that afflict these children for life, nor can they alter the financial and emotional burden on and within the family. Prognosis is determined by the severity of neurologic involvement and the number of associated anomalies. With proper care and long-term maintenance, most children can survive and do well. Early death is usually caused by central nervous system infection or by hydrocephalus, while mortality in later childhood is caused by urinary tract infection, renal failure, complications from shunt therapy, or pulmonary disease.

■ NURSING CONSIDERATIONS: Care of the child with a spinal defect entails both immediate and long-term nursing goals. Immediate care centers on the prevention of local infection and trauma by careful handling and positioning of the infant, applying sterile moist dressings to the membranous sac, avoiding fecal contamination and breakdown of sensitive skin areas, and maintaining warmth, proper nutrition, and adequate hydration and electrolyte balance. Gentle range of motion exercises are carried out to prevent or minimize hip and lower extremity deformity. An important function of the nurse is to involve the parents in the care of the infant as soon as possible and to teach them the essential procedures for adequate home care, including how to observe for signs of complications. The nurse also helps the parents in long-term management by planning activities appropriate to the developmental age and physical limitations of the child, by providing information for teaching all family members about the condition, and, if appropriate, by assisting with placement in schools that can accommodate the special needs of handicapped children.

myelomere (mī′əloumir′), any of the embryonic segments of the brain or spinal cord during prenatal development.

myelomonocytic leukemia (mī′əloumon′əsit′ik). See **monocytic leukemia.**

myelopathic anemia. See **myelophthisic anemia.**

myelopathy (mī′əlop′əthi), 1. any disease of the spinal cord. 2. any disease of the myelopoietic tissues.

myelophthisic anemia (mī′əloutiz′ik), a disorder attributed to several pathological processes that displace the hemopoietic tissues of the bone marrow. It is characterized by anemia and the appearance of immature granulocytes and nucleated erythroid elements in the peripheral blood. Also called **myelopathic anemia.** Compare **leukoerythroblastic anemia.**

myelopoiesis (mai'əloupoii'sıs), the formation and development of the bone marrow or the cells that originate from it. A kind of myelopoiesis is **extramedullary myelopoiesis.** – **myelopoietic,** *adj.*

myeloradiculodysplasia (mai'əlourədık'yəloudısplei'Źhə), any developmental abnormality of the spinal cord and spinal nerve roots. See also **myelomeningocele, neural tube defect.**

myeloschisis (mai'əlos'kəsıs), a developmental defect characterized by a cleft spinal cord that results from the failure of the neural plate to fuse and form a complete neural tube. See also **neural tube defect, neural tube formation, myelomeningocele, rachischisis, spina bifida.**

myesthesia (mai'esthi'Źhə), perception of any sensation in a muscle, as touch, direction, proprioception, contraction, relaxation, or extension.

myiasis (mai'əsıs), infection or infestation of the body by the larvae of flies, usually through a wound or an ulcer, but, rarely, through the intact skin.

myitis (maiai'tıs). See **myositis.**

myko-. See **myco-.**

Mylaxen, a trade name for a cholinesterase inhibitor (hexafluorenium bromide), used as an adjunct to anesthesia.

Myleran, a trade name for an antineoplastic (busulfan).

Mylicon, a trade name for an antiflatulent (simethicone).

mylohyoideus (mai'louhaioi'diəs), one of a pair of flat triangular muscles that form the floor of the cavity of the mouth. One of the four suprahyoid muscles, immediately superior to the digastricus, it arises from the whole length of the mylohyoid line of the mandible and inserts into the hyoid bone. It is innervated by the mylohyoid nerve and acts to raise the hyoid bone and the tongue. Also called **mylohyoid muscle.** Compare **digastricus, geniohyoideus, stylohyoideus.**

myo-, my-, a combining form meaning 'relating to muscle': *myocardia, myocele, myolipoma.*

myocardial infarction (MI), an occlusion of a coronary artery, caused by atherosclerosis or an embolus that results in a necrotic area in the vasculature myocardium.

■ OBSERVATIONS: The onset of MI is characterized by a crushing, viselike chest pain that may radiate to the left arm, neck, or epigastrium and sometimes simulates the sensation of acute indigestion or a gall bladder attack. The patient usually becomes ashen, clammy, short of breath, faint, and anxious and often feels that death is imminent. Typical signs are tachycardia, a barely perceptible pulse, low blood pressure, an elevated temperature, cardiac arrhythmia, and electrocardiographic evidence of elevation of the ST segment and Q wave. Laboratory studies usually show an increased sedimentation rate, leukocytosis, and elevated serum levels of creatine phosphokinase, lactic dehydrogenase, and glutamic-oxaloacetic transaminase. Potential complications in MI are pulmo-

nary or systemic embolism, pulmonary edema, shock, and cardiac arrest.

■ INTERVENTION: Emergency treatment of MI may require cardiopulmonary resuscitation before the patient is admitted to an intensive cardiac care unit and placed on a cardiac monitor. In the acute phase oxygen, cardiotonic drugs, antiarrhythmic agents, and anticoagulants are usually administered and sedatives and analgesics may be indicated. Blood pressure, temperature, respiration, and apical pulse are checked frequently. Parenteral fluids may be administered; iced drinks and cold foods are avoided and the patient is usually served a low-sodium, low cholesterol diet. Stool softeners and laxatives may be indicated to prevent straining.

■ NURSING CONSIDERATIONS: The nurse's role in helping the patient and family understand the nature and treatment of the disease is extremely important. Prior to discharge, discussions regarding the need to adhere to the prescribed diet and medication, to limit activities, to rest at regular periods, and to avoid caffeine, nicotine, large meals, and emotional stress can facilitate the patient's convalescence.

myocardiopathy (mai'oukar'diop'əthi), any disease of the myocardium. Also called **cardiomyopathy.**

myocarditis (mai'oukardai'tıs), an inflammatory condition of the myocardium caused by viral, bacterial, or fungal infection, serum sickness, rheumatic fever, chemical agent, or as a complication of a collagen disease. Myocarditis most frequently occurs in an acute viral form and is self-limited, but it may lead to acute heart failure. Management includes treatment of the cause, analgesia, oxygen, anti-inflammatory agents, constant monitoring, and rest to prevent shock or heart failure.

myocardium (mai'oukar'diəm), a thick, contractile, middle layer of uniquely constructed and arranged muscle cells that forms the bulk of the heart wall. The myocardium contains a minimum of other tissue, except for the blood vessels, and is covered interiorly by the endocardium. The contractile tissue of the myocardium is composed of fibers with the characteristic cross striations of muscular tissue. The fibers, which are about one third as large in diameter as those of skeletal muscle and which contain more sarcoplasm, branch frequently and are interconnected to form a network that is continuous except where the bundles and the laminae are attached at their origins and insertions into the fibrous trigone of the heart. The bundles of myocardial fibers are spiral-shaped; the individual muscle fibers contain fibrillae which are more concentrated at the periphery of each fiber. The central cores of the fibers contain the nuclei and may also contain concentrated sarcoplasm rich in sarcosomes. Myocardial muscle fibers also contain characteristic intercalated discs. Electron microscope studies reveal that these discs represent cell boundries and may cross an entire fiber in a straight line or may be arranged in a steplike configuration. Myocardial muscle contains less connective tissue than skeletal muscle. The fibers of the connective tissue are covered by a delicate fibrillar net with few elastic fibers. Collagenous fibers run between the muscular bundles and the associated blood vessels. Specially modified fibers of myocardial muscle constitute the conduction system of the heart, including the sinoatrial node, the atrioventricular node, the atrioventricular bundle, and the Purkinje fibers. Most of the myocardial fibers function to contract the heart. Contraction involves the action of calcium ions and sodium ions and a complex electrochemical process still not precisely understood. Defects in the kinetics of intracellular calcium may cause myocardial dysfunctions in patients with heart failure. The metabolic processes of the myocardium are almost exclusively aerobic and constantly supply the heart muscle with high-energy phosphate bonds for mechanical and chemical functions. The heart uses free fatty acids as its predominant fuel as well as important quantities of glucose, lactate, pyruvate, and ketone bodies and a very small amount of amino acids. Many key enzymatic reactions of the heart, as the citric acid cycle and oxidative phosphorylation, take place in the highly concentrated myocardial sarcosomes. The major anaerobic processes of glycolysis occur in the sarcoplasm. The process of oxidative phosphorylation produces adenosine triphosphate, the immediate energy source for myocardial contraction. Oxygen, which significantly affects contractibility, is the most important metabolic nutrient for the myocardium, which consumes from 6.5 to 10.0 ml/100 gm of tissue per minute. Without this oxygen supply, myocardial contractions decrease in a few minutes. Ventricular pressure and heart rate together determine myocardial oxygen consumption. The heart normally extracts about 70 per cent of the oxygen reaching it by the coronary arteries. This leaves only about 30 per cent in coronary sinus blood and limits the amount of additional oxygen the heart can extract from its blood supply. In heart failure owing to hypertension, valvular heart disease, or coronary atherosclerosis, the myocardial oxygen consumption per gram of tissue is usually normal, but the total oxygen consumption per minute often increases significantly because the weight of the heart often increases with such diseases. Myocardial oxygen consumption increases in hyperthyroidism and decreases in hypothyroidism. The myocardium maintains a relatively constant level of glycogen in the form of sarcoplasmic granules. Hypoxia rapidly depletes this supply and produces lactate and hexosemonophosphate. In anemia, the total consumption of myocardial oxygen may significantly increase because of increased hemodynamic demands resulting from the disorder. Myocardial hypertrophy may develop if the anemia is chronic. — **myocardial,** *adj.*

Myochrysine, a trade name for an antirheumatic (gold sodium thiomalate).

myoclonus (mīok′lənəs), a spasm of a muscle or a group of muscles. — **myoclonic,** *adj.*

myodiastasis (mī′oudaiæs′təsis), an abnormal condition in which there is separation muscle bundles.

myoedema (mī′oʊidi′mə), *pl.* **myoedemas, myoedemata.** muscle edema. Compare **myxedema.**

myofacial pain-dysfunction syndrome. See **temporomandibular pain-dysfunction syndrome.**

myogelosis (mī′oʊjɪloʊ′sɪs), a condition in which there are hardened areas or nodules within muscles, especially the gluteal muscles. There are no serious consequences of this condition and no treatment is necessary.

myoglobin (mī′əgloʊ′bɪn), a ferrous globin complex consisting of one heme molecule containing one iron molecule attached to a single globin chain. Myoglobin is found in muscle and is responsible for the red color of that tissue and for its ability to store oxygen.

myokinase (mī′oʊkaɪ′neis). See **adenylate kinase.**

myoma, *pl.* **myomas, myomata.** a common, benign fibroid tumor on the uterine muscle. It develops most frequently after the age of 30 in women, especially black women, who have never been pregnant. Menorrhagia, backache, constipation, dysmenorrhea, dyspareunia, and other symptoms develop proportionate to the size, location, and rate of growth of the tumor. Obstruction of a ureter may result if a large myoma compresses it. A myoma may be associated with sterility if it blocks the Fallopian tube, with abortion if it interferes with fetal growth, or with difficult childbirth and hemorrhage if it is in or near the cervix. Also called *Informal.* **fibroid.**

myoma previum. See **leiomyoma uteri.**

myoma striocellulare. See **rhabdomyoma.**

myomeningocele (mī′oʊmɪnɪŋ′goʊsil), an abnormal saclike protrusion from the spine of a segment of the meninges and the spinal cord. It is caused by the defective closure of the neural tube during the first trimester of pregnancy. The sac associated with this abnormality commonly protrudes from the lumbosacral, area and, less frequently, from the sacral area, the thoracic area, or the cervical area. Depending on the level of protrusion, the myomeningocele may cause permanent neurological defects, including paralysis and incontinence. Associated problems may include cyanosis, ulceration, clubfoot, and knee contractions. About 90 per cent of the affected patients develop hydrocephalus. Others may develop Arnold-Chiari syndrome, spinal curvature, and mental retardation. Compare **meningocele, spina bifida.**

■ OBSERVATIONS: Myomeningocele is usually obvious on examination and is easily distinguished from meningocele. The sac of myomeningocele does not transilluminate; the sac of meningocele does. Sensory and motor function can usually be determined by neurologic examination. Prenatal amniocentesis can detect myomeningocele, and it is recommended for all pregnant women who have delivered a child with a neural tube defect.

■ INTERVENTION: Surgical closure of the myomeningocele sac is the common treatment and is supported by appropriate measures to develop the independence of the patient and to prevent further problems. A shunt is often required to relieve associated hydrocephalus. Surgery can place the myomeningocele tissues back inside the spinal column but usually cannot repair neurological damage already sustained. Urinary and fecal incontinence are common.

■ NURSING CONSIDERATIONS: The treatment and care requires the cooperation of nurses, neurosurgeons, orthopedists, urologists, social workers, and the parents of the patient. Emotional support and counseling are necessary in helping the parents accept and adjust to the associated diagnoses and preoperative and postoperative procedures. The patient is handled carefully to avoid exerting pressure on the myomeningocele sac and is placed in the prone position. The head circumference is measured daily and meticulous skin care to the lesion, the buttocks, and the genitalia is performed to prevent infection. The bladder is emptied at regular intervals. Glycerin suppositories and manual pressure on the abdomen are common aids to prevent bowel obstruction. For more information about spinal disorders the patients may be referred to the Spina Bifida Association of America.

myomere (mai'oumir). See **myotome**. —**myomeric,** *adj.*

myometritis (mai'oumɪtrai'tɪs), an inflammation or infection of the myometrium of the uterus.

myometrium (mai'oumi'triəm), *pl.* **myometria.** the muscular layer of the wall of the uterus. The fibers of the myometrium course around the uterus horizontally, vertically, and diagonally.

myonecrosis (mai'ounekrou'sɪs), the death of muscle fibers. **Progressive,** or **clostridial myonecrosis** is caused by the anaerobic bacteria of the genus *Clostridium.* Seen in deep wound infections, progressive myonecrosis is accompanied by pain, tenderness, a brown serous exudate, and a rapid accumulation of gas within the tissue of the muscle. The affected muscle turns a blackish-green color. Treatment includes thorough wound debridement, I.V. administration of penicillin, and the use of hyperbaric oxygen therapy to destroy the anaerobe and to promote healing.

myoneural (mai'ounur'əl), of or pertaining to a muscle and its associated nerve, especially to nerve endings in muscles.

myoneural junction. See **neuromuscular junction.**

myopathy (maiop'əthi), an abnormal condition of skeletal muscle characterized by muscle weakness, wasting, and histological changes within muscle tissue, as seen in any of the muscular dystrophies. A myopathy is distinct from a muscle disorder caused by nerve dysfunction. The specific diagnosis of any myopathy is made using tests of serum enzymes, electromyography, and muscle biopsy. See also **muscular dystrophy.** —**myopathic,** *adj.*

myope (mai'oup), an individual who is nearsighted or afflicted with myopia.

myophosphorylase deficiency glycogenosis. See **McArdle's disease.**

myopia (maiou'piə), a condition of nearsightedness caused by the elongation of the eyeball or by an error in refraction so that parallel rays are focused in front of the retina. Some kinds of myopia are **chronic myopia, curvature myopia, index myopia, pathologic myopia.** Also called **short sight.** See also **second sight.** —**myopic,** *adj.*

MYOPIA

myorrhaphy, suturing of a wound in a muscle.

myorrhexis (mai'ərek'sɪs), a tearing in any muscle. —**myorrhectic,** *adj.*

myosarcoma (mai'ousarkou'mə), a malignant tumor of muscular tissue.

myosin (mai'əsɪn), a protein that makes up close to half of the proteins that occur in muscle tissue. The interaction of myosin and actin is essential for muscle contraction.

myositis (mai'əsai'tɪs), inflammation of muscle tissue, usually of the voluntary muscles. Causes of myositis include infection, trauma, and infestation by parasites. Kinds of myositis include **epidemic myositis, interstitial myositis, parenchymatous myositis, polymyositis, traumatic myositis.** Also called **myitis.** Compare **fibrositis.**

myositis fibrosa (faibrou'sə), an uncommon inflammation of the muscles, characterized by abnormal formation of connective tissue. Also called **interstitial myositis.** See also **myositis.**

myositis ossificans (əsɪf'əkænz), a rare, inherited disease in which muscle tissue is replaced by bone. It begins in childhood, with stiffness in the neck and back and progresses to rigidity of the spine, trunk, and limbs. The administration of diphosphonates may prevent the abnormal deposition of bone, but there is no cure once it has occurred. Metabolism of calcium and phosphate remains normal throughout the course of the disease. Compare **myositis.**

myositis purulenta (pyur'ələn'tə), any bacterial infection of muscle tissue. This condition may result in the formation of an abscess or multiple abscesses.

myositis trichinosa (trɪk'ənou'sə), inflammation of the muscles resulting from infection by the parasite *Trichinella spiralis.* See also **trichinosis.**

myostasis (mai'oustei'sɪs), an abnormal condition of weakened muscle in which there is a relatively fixed length of muscle fibers in the relaxed state. In normal muscle the force of contraction is greatest at the resting length of the muscle; in myostasis the resting length is shorter than normal, and there is a shorter acting length in which the contractile force can work. — **myostatic,** *adj.*

myostroma (mai'əstrou'mə), the framework of muscle tissue.

myotatic reflex (mai'outæt'ɪk). See **deep tendon reflex.**

myotenotomy, division of the whole or part of a muscle by cutting through its main tendon.

myotome (mai'ətoum), **1.** Also called **myomere.** The muscle plate of an embryonic somite that develops into a voluntary muscle. **2.** a group of muscles innervated by a single spinal segment. **3.** an instrument for cutting or dissecting a muscle.

myotomic muscle, any of the numerous muscles of the trunk of the body, derived from the myotomes and divided into the deep muscles of the back and the thoracoabdominal muscles.

myotomy (maiot'əmi), the cutting of a muscle, performed to gain access to underlying tissues or to relieve constriction in a sphincter, as in severe esophagitis or pyloric stenosis. Under general anesthesia, a longitudinal cut is made through the sphincter muscle but not through the mucosa lining the stomach. See also **abdominal surgery.**

Myotonachol, a trade name for a cholinergic (bethanechol chloride).

myotonia (mai'ətou'niə), any condition in which a muscle or a group of muscles do not readily relax after contracting. — **myotonic** *adj.*

myotonia atrophica (eitrof'ɪkə). See **myotonic muscular dystrophy.**

myotonia congenita (konjen'ɪtə), a rare, mild, and nonprogressive form of myotonic myopathy evident early in life. The only effects of the disorder are hypertrophy and stiffness of the muscles. Also called **Thomsen's disease.**

myotonic muscular dystrophy, a severe form of muscular dystrophy marked by ptosis, facial weakness, and dysarthria. Weakness of the hands and feet precedes that in the shoulders and hips. Myotonia of the hands is usually present. Electromyography is helpful in establishing the diagnosis. Although there is no specific treatment, active and passive exercises are used to alleviate symptoms. Also called **myotonia atrophica, Steinert's disease.**

myotonic myopathy, any of a group of disorders characterized by increased skeletal muscle tone and decreased relaxation of muscle after contraction. Kinds of myotonic myopathy include **myotonia congenita, myotonic muscular dystrophy.**

Myprozine, a trade name for an antifungal agent (natamycin), used topically in the treatment of corneal infections.

myria-, a combining form meaning 'a great number': *myriapod.*

myringa (mɪrɪŋ'gə). See **tympanic membrane.**

myringectomy (mɪr'ɪnjek'təmi), excision of the tympanic membrane.

myringitis (mɪr'ɪnjai'tɪs), inflammation or infection of the tympanic membrane.

myringo-, a combining form meaning 'related to the tympanic membrane': *myringodectomy, myringoplasty, myringoscope.*

myringomycosis (mɪrɪŋ'goumaikou'sɪs), a fungal infection of the tympanic membrane. Also called **mycomyringitis.**

myringoplasty (mərɪŋ'gouplæs'ti), surgical repair of perforations of the eardrum with a tissue graft, performed to correct hearing loss. Under local or general anesthesia, the openings in the eardrum are enlarged, and the grafting material is sutured over them. Topical antibiotics are applied and then a packing of absorbable gelatin sponge is applied to hold the graft in position. After surgery, an antihistamine with an ephedrine derivitive is given. The nurse keeps the outer ear clean and dry. Debris is removed by gentle suctioning about 12 days after surgery. See also **myringotomy.**

myringotomy (mɪr'ɪŋgot'əmi), surgical incision of the eardrum, performed to relieve pressure and release pus from the middle ear. Antibiotics are given before surgery and continued afterwards. The drum is incised and cultures are taken; fluid is gently suctioned from the middle ear. Ear drops may be instilled to improve drainage. The nurse cautions against putting cotton in the canal, since the ear must drain freely. The outer ear is kept clean and dry; careful handwashing is essential to prevent infection. If pain increases, the procedure may have to be repeated. Severe headache or disorientation must be reported. See also **myringoplasty.**

Mysoline, a trade name for an anticonvulsant (primidone).

mysophobia, misophobia (mi′səfou′biə), an anxiety disorder characterized by an overreaction to the slightest uncleanliness, or an irrational fear of dirt, contamination, or defilement. — **mysophobic, misophobic,** *adj.*

Mytelase Chloride, a trade name for a cholinergic (ambenonium chloride).

Mytrate, a trade name for an adrenergic (epinephrine bitartrate).

myxo-, a combining form meaning 'relating to mucus': *myxoblastoma, myxocyte, myxoma.*

myxofibroma (mɪk′soufaibrou′mə), a fibrous tumor that contains myxomatous tissue.

myxoma (mɪksou′mə), a neoplasm of the connective tissue, characteristically composed of stellate cells in a loose mucoid matrix crossed by delicate reticulum fibers. These tumors may grow to enormous size and are usually pale gray, soft, and jellylike; they may occur under the skin but are also found in bones, the genitourinary tract, and the retroperitoneal area. Some have exceeded 30 cm in diameter. — **myxomatous,** *adj.*

-myxoma, a combining form meaning a 'soft tumor made up of primitive connective tissues': *adenomyxoma, gliomyxoma, lipomyxoma.*

myxoma fibrosum. Also called **myxofibroma.**

myxoma sarcomatosum. See **myxosarcoma.**

myxopoiesis (mɪk′soupoii′sɪs), the production of mucus.

myxosarcoma (mɪk′sousarkou′mə), a sarcoma that contains some myxomatous tissue. Also called **myxoma sarcomatosum.**

myxovirus (mɪk′souvai′rəs), any of a group of medium-sized RNA viruses which are further divided into ortho-myxoviruses and paramyxoviruses. Infection with these viruses is usually transmitted by the respiratory secretions of an infected host. Some kinds of myxoviruses are the viruses that cause influenza, mumps, and parainfluenza.

MZ, abbreviation for **monozygotic.**

N

n, 2n, 3n, 4n, symbols for the haploid, diploid, triploid, and tetraploid number of chromosomes in a cell, organism, strain, or individual.

N, 1. abbreviation for **normal.** 2. See also **cancer staging.** abbreviation for **node** in the TNM system for staging malignant neoplastic disease. 3. symbol for **nitrogen.**

N, abbreviation for **node** in TNM system for staging malignant neoplastic disease. See also **cancer staging.**

Na, chemical symbol for **sodium.**

N₂O, symbol for **nitrous oxide.**

NAACOG, abbreviation for **Nurses Association of the American College of Obstetrics and Gynecology.**

Nabothian cyst (nabou'tiən), a cyst formed in a Nabothian gland of the uterine cervix. It is a common finding on routine pelvic examination of women of reproductive age, especially in women who have borne children. The cyst, which is pearly white and firm, seldom results in adverse or pathologic effects.

Nabothian gland, one of many small, mucus-secreting glands of the uterine cervix.

Nactisol, a trade name for a fixed-combination drug containing an anticholinergic antispasmodic (poldine methylsulfate) and a barbiturate (butabarbital), used in the treatment of peptic ulcer.

nadolol, a beta-adrenergic blocking agent.

■ INDICATIONS: It is prescribed for long-term management of angina pectoris and for hypertension.

■ CONTRAINDICATIONS: Bronchial asthma, sinus bradycardia, and greater than first-degree conduction block, cardiogenic shock, overt cardiac failure, or known hypersensitivity to this drug prohibits its use.

■ ADVERSE EFFECTS: Among the more serious adverse reactions are bronchospasm, bradycardia, precipitation of heart failure, cardiac arrythmia, masking of signs of hypoglycemia in diabetics, fatigue, and lethargy. Gastrointestinal disturbances, rashes and other allergic reactions also may occur.

Naegeli's leukemia (nei'gəliz). See **monocytic leukemia.**

nafcillin sodium, an antibacterial.

■ INDICATIONS: It is prescribed in the treatment of infections caused by penicillinase-producing staphylococci.

■ CONTRAINDICATIONS: Known hypersensitivity to this drug or to other penicillins prohibits its use.

■ ADVERSE EFFECTS: Among the more serious adverse

reactions are hypersensitivity reactions, nausea, and vomiting.

Nägele's obliquity. See **asynclitism.**

Nägele's rule (nei'gələz), a method for calculating the estimated date of delivery based on a mean length of gestation. Three months are subtracted from the first day of the last normal menstrual period, and seven days are added to that date. See also **estimated day of confinement.**

Nager's acrofacial dysostosis (nei'gərz), an abnormal cogenital condition characterized by limb deformities, as radioulnar synostosis, hypoplasia, and the absence of the radius or of the thumbs. Compare **cleidocranial dysostosis, craniofacial dysostosis, mandihbulofacial dysostosis.**

Nahrungs Einheit Milch (nem) (na'rungz ain'haitmilχ), a nutritional unit in Pirquet's system of feeding that is equivalent to one gram of breast milk.

nail, a flattened, elastic structure with a horny texture at the end of a finger or a toe. Each nail is comprised of a root, body, and free edge at the distal extremity. The root fastens the nail to the finger or the toe by fitting into a groove in the skin and is closely molded to the surface of the corium. The nail matrix beneath the body and the root projects longitudinal vascular ridges, which are easily visible through the translucent tissue of the body. The matrix firmly attaches the body of the nail to the underlying connective tissue. The whitish lunula near the root contain irregularly arranged papillae which are less firmly attached to the connective tissue than the rest of the matrix. The cuticle is attached to the surface of the nail just ahead of the root. The superficial horny part of the nail consists of the thick stratum lucidum, the thin stratum corneum, which forms the eponychium overlapping the lunula, and the stratum mucosum. The nails grow longer by proliferation of the cells in the stratum germinativum at the root. They grow thicker from proliferation of that part of the stratum germinativum underlying the lunula. Also called **unguis.**

Naldecon, a trade name for a fixed-combination drug containing two adrenergics (phenylpropanolamine hydrochloride and phenylephrine hydrochloride) and two antihistamines (chlorpheniramine maleate and phenyltoloxamine citrate).

Nalfon, a trade name for an anti-inflammatory agent (fenoprofen calcium).

nalidixic acid, an antibacterial.

■ INDICATIONS: It is prescribed in the treatment of certain urinary tract infections.

■ CONTRAINDICATIONS: Renal or hepatic insufficiency, a history of convulsive disorders, or known hypersensitivity to this drug prohibits its use.

■ ADVERSE EFFECTS: Among the more serious adverse reactions are mild neurological disturbances, gastrointestinal disturbances, and hemolytic anemia in glucose-6-phosphate dehydrogenase deficiency. Convulsions and increased cranial pressure may occur. Among the more serious reactions are increased intracranial pressure, seizures, hemolytic anemia in people affected with glucose-6-phosphate dehydrogenase deficiency, and gastrointestinal and neurological disturbances.

Nalline Hydrochloride, a trade name for a narcotic antagonist (nalorphine hydrochloride).

naloxone hydrochloride, a narcotic antagonist.

■ INDICATIONS: It is prescribed for complete or partial reversal of narcotic depression or for acute narcotic intoxication.

■ CONTRAINDICATION: Known hypersensitivity to this drug prohibits its use.

■ ADVERSE EFFECTS: Among the most serious adverse reactions when given to narcotic dependent patients are side effects associated with narcotic withdrawal.

NANB, abbreviation for **non-A, non-B, hepatitis.**

nandrolone decanoate (næn′drəloun), an androgen.

■ INDICATIONS: It is prescribed in the treatment of testosterone deficiency, osteoporosis, and female breast cancer and to stimulate growth, weight gain, and the production of red cells.

■ CONTRAINDICATIONS: Cancer of the male breast or prostate, liver disease, pregnancy or suspected pregnancy, or known hypersensitivity to this drug prohibits its use.

■ ADVERSE EFFECTS: Among the most serious adverse effects are various endocrine disturbances, depending on the age of the patient. Hirsutism, acne, liver toxicity, and electrolyte imbalances also occur.

nandrolone phenpropionate, an anabolic steroid with androgenic properties.

■ INDICATIONS: It is prescribed in the treatment of osteoporosis, in certain anemias, in metastatic breast cancers of women, and for protein-sparing effects in many situations.

■ CONTRAINDICATIONS: Carcinoma of the breast in males and some females, pregnancy, nephrosis, or known hypersensitivity to this drug prohibits its use.

■ ADVERSE EFFECTS: Among the more serious adverse reactions are hirsutism, acne, various endocrine effects depending on the age and sex of the patient, masculinization, liver dysfunction, hypercalcemia in women taking the drug for breast cancer, and fluid and salt retention.

nanism (nei′nɪzəm, næn′ɪzəm), an abnormal smallness or underdevelopment of the body; dwarfism. Kinds of na-

nism are **mulibrey nanism, Paltauf's nanism, pituitary nanism, renal nanism, senile nanism, symptomatic nanism.** Also called **nanosomia.** — **nanus,** *n.*

nano-, a combining form meaning 'small, or related to smallness or dwarfism': *nanocephalia, nanocormia, nanomelia.*

nanocephalic dwarf. See **bird-headed dwarf.**

nanocephaly (nei′nousef′əli, næn′ousef′əli), **nanocephalia, nanocephalism,** a developmental defect characterized by abnormal smallness of the head. — **nanocephalous,** *adj.,* **nanocephalus,** *n.*

nanocormia (nei′noukɔr′miə, næn′oukɔr′miə), a developmental defect characterized by abnormal and disproportionate smallness of the trunk of the body in comparison to the head and limbs. — **nanocormus,** *n.*

nanocurie (nC, nc) (nei′noukyuri, næn′oukyur′i), a unit of radiation equal to one billionth of a curie.

nanogram See **millimicrogram.**

nanomelia (nei′noumi′liə, næn′oumi′liə), a developmental defect characterized by abnormally small limbs in comparison to the size of the head and trunk. — **nanomelous,** *adj.,* **nanomelus,** *n.*

nanophthalmos (nei′nofthæl′məs, næn′ofthæl′məs), **nanophthalmia,** the condition in which one or both eyes are abnormally small, although other ocular defects are not present. See also **microphthalmos.**

nanosomia, nanosoma. See **nanism.**

nanosomus, a person of extremely short stature; a dwarf.

nanukayami (na′nukaya′mi), an acute, infectious disease caused by one of the serotypes of the spirochete *Leptospira* that is indigenous to Japan. See also **leptospirosis.**

nanus, 1. a dwarf. 2. a pygmy. — **nanoid,** *adj.*

nape, the back of the neck.

naphazoline hydrochloride (nəfæz′əlin), an adrenergic vasoconstrictor.

■ INDICATIONS: It is prescribed in the treatment of nasal congestion and as an ophthalmic vasoconstrictor.

■ CONTRAINDICATIONS: Glaucoma or known hypersensitivity to this drug or abnormal sensitivity to sympathomimetic drugs prohibits its use.

■ ADVERSE EFFECTS: Among the most serious adverse reactions are those associated with systemic absorption, including sedation and cardiovascular effects. Irritation to mucosa and rebound congestion also may occur.

naphthalene poisoning, a toxic condition, caused by the ingestion of naphthalene or paradichlorobenzene, that may cause nausea, vomiting, headache, abdominal pain, spasm, and convulsions. Treatment may include induced emesis, lavage, a saline cathartic, and sodium bicarbonate. Blood transfusion and fluid replacement may be necessary. Diazepam is indicated for the control of involuntary muscular contractions. Naphthalene and paradichlorobenzene are common ingredients in mothballs and moth crystals; paradichlorobenzene is also used as an insecticide in agriculture.

naphthol camphor, a syrupy mixture of two parts of camphor and one part betanaphthol, used externally as an antiseptic.

naphthol poisoning. See **phenol poisoning.**

napkin-ring tumor, a tumor that encircles a tubular structure of the body, usually impairing its function and constricting its lumen to some degree. These tumors are typical of colorectal cancer of the sigmoid colon.

NAP-NAP, abbreviation for **National Association of Pediatric Nurse Associates/Practitioners.**

N.A.P.N.E.S., abbreviation for **National Association for Practical Nurse Education and Services.**

Naprosyn, a trade name for a nonsteroidal anti-inflammatory, antipyretic, and analgesic (naproxen).

naproxen, a nonsteroidal anti-inflammatory agent.
- INDICATION: It is prescribed for the relief of inflammatory symptoms of arthritis.
- CONTRAINDICATIONS: Impaired renal function, gastrointestinal disease, or known hypersensitivity to this drug, to aspirin, or to nonsteroidal anti-inflammatory drugs prohibits its use.
- ADVERSE EFFECTS: Among the more serious adverse reactions are gastrointestinal disorders and peptic ulcers. Dizziness, rashes, and tinnitus commonly occur. This drug interacts with many other drugs.

Naqua, a trade name for a diuretic and antihypertensive (trichlormethiazide).

Naquival, a trade name for an antihypertensive, fixed-combination drug containing a diuretic (trichlormethiazide) and an antihypertensive (reserpine).

Narcan, a trade name for a narcotic antagonist (naloxone hydrochloride).

narcissism (nar′sɪsɪz′əm), **1.** an abnormal interest in oneself, especially in one's own body and sexual characteristics; self-love. **2.** (in psychoanalysis) sexual self-interest that is a normal characteristic of the phallic stage of psychosexual development, occurring as the infantile ego acquires a libido. Narcissism in the adult is abnormal, representing fixation at this stage of development or regression to it. Compare **egotism.** See also **narcissistic personality, narcissistic personality disorder.**

narcissistic personality, a personality characterized by behavior and attitudes that indicate an abnormal love of the self. Such a person is self-centered and self-absorbed, is extremely unrealistic concerning his attributes and goals, vacillates between overidealizing and devaluing others, and, in general, assumes that he is entitled to more than is reasonable in his relationships with others. Compare **narcissism.**

narcissistic personality disorder, a condition characterized by an exaggerated sense of self-importance and uniqueness, an abnormal need for attention and admiration, preoccupation with grandiose fantasies concerning the self, and disturbances in interpersonal relationships, usually involving the exploitation of others and a lack of empathy for them. Symptoms include depression, egocentricity, self-consciousness, inconsiderateness, inconsistency, preoccupation with grooming and remaining youthful, and intense concern with psychosomatic pains and illnesses. Treatment consists of various psychotherapeutic procedures, depending on the individual and the severity of the condition. See also **histrionic personality disorder.**

narco-, a combining form meaning 'related to stupor or a stuporous state': *narcolepsy, narcomania, narcotic.*

narcoanesthesia (nar′kouæn′ɪsthi′žə). See **basal anesthesia.**

narcolepsy (nar′kəlep′si), a syndrome characterized by sudden sleep attacks, cataplexy, sleep paralysis, and visual or auditory hallucinations at the onset of sleep. The syndrome begins in adolescence or young adulthood and persists throughout life. Its cause is unknown, and no pathological lesions are found in the brain. Persons with narcolepsy experience an uncontrollable desire to sleep, sometimes many times in one day. Episodes may last from a few minutes to several hours. Momentary loss of muscle tone occurs during waking hours (cataplexy), or while the person is asleep. Narcolepsy may be difficult to diagnose because all persons with the disorder do not experience all four symptoms. EEG or other brain studies may be used to distinguish narcolepsy from an intracranial mass or encephalitis. Amphetamines and other stimulant drugs are prescribed effectively to prevent the attacks. – **narcoleptic,** *adj.*

narcoleptic (nar′kəlep′tɪk), **1.** of or pertaining to a condition or substance that causes an uncontrollable desire for sleep. **2.** a narcoleptic drug. **3.** a person suffering from narcolepsy.

narcosis (narkou′sɪs), a state of insensibility or stupor caused by narcotic drugs. See also **narcotic.**

narcotic, (in pharmacology) **1.** of or pertaining to a substance that produces insensibility or stupor. **2.** a narcotic drug. Narcotic analgesics, derived from opium or produced synthetically, alter perception of pain; induce euphoria, mood changes, mental clouding, and deep sleep; depress respiration and the cough reflex; constrict the pupils; and cause smooth muscle spasm, decreased peristalsis, emesis, and nausea. Repeated use of narcotics may result in physical and psychological dependence. Among the narcotic drugs administered clinically for relief of pain are butorphanol tartrate, hydromorphone hydrochloride, morphine sulfate, pentazocine lactate, and meperidine hydrochloride. These drugs act by binding to opiate receptors in the central nervous system; narcotic antagonists, as naloxone hydrochloride, which is used in treating narcotic overdosage, apparently displace opiates from receptor sites.

-narcotic, a combining form meaning 'pertaining to analgesic or soporific drugs': *antinarcotic, prenarcotic, pseudonarcotic.* Also **-narcotical.**

narcotic analgesic. See **analgesic.**

narcotic antagonist, a drug that is used primarily in the treatment of narcotic-induced respiratory depression. The narcotic antagonists nalorphine, levallorphan, and naloxone are usually administered parenterally. See also **antagonist drug.**

narcotic antitussive. See **antitussive.**

Nardil, a trade name for an antidepressant (phenelzine sulfate).

nares (neir'iz), *sing.* **naris.** the pairs of anterior openings and posterior openings in the nose that allow the passage of air from the nose to the pharynx and the lungs during respiration. See also **anterior nares, posterior nares.**

nas-. See **naso-.**

nasal, of or pertaining to the nose and the nasal cavity. — **nasally,** *adv.*

nasal cavity, one of a pair of cavities that open on the face through the pear-shaped anterior nasal aperture and communicate with the pharynx. Each cavity is narrower at the top than at the bottom.

nasal decongestant, a drug that provides temporary relief of nasal symptoms in acute and chronic rhinitis and sinusitis. Most are over-the-counter products compounded with a small amount of vasoconstrictor, as ephedrine or phenylephrine. An antihistamine may enhance the value of a nasal decongestant in allergic rhinitis, and a corticosteroid may reduce inflammation. Prolonged use or dosage greater than recommended on the package label may cause rebound vasodilation and severe congestion.

nasal drip, a method of slowly infusing liquid into a dehydrated infant by means of a catheter inserted through the nose down the esophagus.

nasal fossa, one of the pair of approximately equal chambers of the nasal cavity, that are separated by the nasal septum, open externally through the nostrils, and internally into the nasopharynx through the choanae. Each fossa is divided into an olfactory region, consisting of the superior nasal concha and part of the septum, and a respiratory region, constituting the rest of the chamber. Overhanging the three meatuses of each fossa on the lateral wall are the corresponding superior, middle, and inferior nasal conchae. The superior meatus extends obliquely about half way along the superior border of the middle concha. The middle meatus continues into the atrium and bulges on the lateral wall at the bulla ethmoidalis. The inferior meatus courses below and lateral to the inferior nasal concha and contains the opening of the nasolacrimal duct. The olfactory region is located in the most superior part of the fossa and contains olfactory cells, olfactory nerves, and olfactory hairs. The respiratory region is lined with mucous membrane, numerous glands, nerves, a plexus of dilated veins, and blood spaces. The plexus is easily irritated, causing the membrane to swell, blocking the meatuses and the openings of sinuses.

nasal glioma, a neoplasm characterized by the ectopic growth of neural tissue in the nasal cavity.

nasal instillation of medication, the instillation of a medicated solution into the nostrils by drops from a dropper or by an atomized spray from a squeeze bottle. Drops are instilled in each nostril as the patient's neck is hyperextended and the head tilted back over the edge of the bed. The patient's mouth should remain open during the procedure, and the head should stay in the tilted back position for several minutes to allow spread of the medication through the nasal passages. Nasal spray is administered to the patient in a sitting position. The patient is asked to expectorate any solution that runs down the posterior nares into the throat.

nasalis (neizæl'is), one of the three muscles of the nose, divided into a transverse part and an alar part. The transverse part arises from the maxilla and covers the bridge of the nose; the alar part attaches at one end to the greater alar cartilage and at the other end to the skin at the end of the nose. The transverse part serves to depress the cartilaginous portion of the nose and to draw the alar toward the septum. The alar part serves to dilate the nostril. The nasalis is innervated by buccal branches of the facial nerve. Compare **depressor septi, procerus.**

nasal septum, the partition dividing the nostrils. It is composed of bone and cartilage covered by mucous membrane.

nasal sinus, any one of the numerous cavities in various bones of the skull, lined with ciliated mucous membrane continuous with that of the nasal cavity. The membrane is very sensitive; easily irritated, it may cause swelling that blocks the sinuses. The nasal sinuses are divided into frontal sinuses, ethmoidal air cells, sphenoidal sinuses, and maxillary sinus. Also called **air cells of the nose.**

nascent, **1.** just born; beginning to exist; incipient. **2.** (in chemistry) pertaining to any substance liberated during a chemical reaction, which, because of its uncombined state, is more reactive.

nasion (nei'zion), **1.** the anthropometric reference point at the front of the skull where the midsagittal plane intersects a horizontal line tangential to the highest points in the superior palpebral sulci. **2.** the depression at the root of the nose that indicates the frontonasal suture.

naso-, nas-, a combining form meaning 'of or pertaining to the nose': *nasociliary, nasolabial, nasonnement.*

nasogastric feeding (nei'zougæs'trik), the process of introducing nutrients in a liquid form directly into the stomach via a nasogastric tube. Also called **gavage feeding**. See also **nasogastric intubation**.

nasogastric intubation, the placement of a nasogastric tube through the nose into the stomach in order to relieve gastric distention by removing gas, gastric secretions, or food; to instil medication, food, or fluids; or to obtain a specimen for laboratory analysis. After surgery and in any condition in which the person is able to digest food but not eat it, the tube may be introduced and left in place for tube feeding until the ability to eat normally is restored.

■ METHOD: A French size 12 to 18 plastic or rubber catheter is selected. The procedure is explained to the patient. If the catheter is rubber it is soaked in ice water to stiffen and lubricate it. The patient is placed in an upright sitting position, and a towel or bib is placed over the chest. The necessary length of tube is marked off; it is the same as the distance from the tip of the nose to the xiphoid process. The tip of the tube may be lubricated with a water-soluble lubricating jelly, but, if a specimen is to be obtained for cytologic study, water or saline solution is preferred. The tube is grasped and held 7.5 cm from the tip and is placed in the nostril, where it is advanced forward and downward. When it has been passed 7.5 cm it is in the pharynx. The patient is then asked to bend the neck forward, to take shallow, rapid breaths, and to help advance the tube by swallowing. The placement of the tube is checked after it has been inserted the predetermined distance to be sure that the tube is in the stomach and not in the lungs. This may be done in several ways: fluoroscopy allows visualization of the placement; gastric contents may be aspirated; or air may be injected with a syringe through the tube and heard through a stethescope as the air enters the stomach. Another simple technique is to place the end of the tube in water; if air bubbles are seen rhythmically flowing from the tube, it is probably in the trachea and not in the stomach.

■ OUTCOME CRITERIA: For the patient's comfort, the tube is selected to fit well and to be suitable for the purpose of the procedure: a tight fit is irritating to the tissues, and a small tube might not allow the prescribed formula to pass through. The tube is accepted most easily with the full cooperation of the patient. Resistance, gagging, and wincing may be minimized by explaining the procedure, by a slow steady progress, and by proper lubrication of the tube and positioning of the patient.

■ NURSING ORDERS: In many hospitals a physician inserts the tube the first time; in most hospitals, the nurse inserts it thereafter. Oral hygiene is performed regularly and the tube, if left in place, is carefully secured with adhesive tape to the nose and to the cheek or jaw. Orders for tube feeding usually include the amount and timing of feeding as well as the concentration and, sometimes, the ingredients of the formula. The formula is refrigerated

and then warmed in bowl of warm water. If the person is unconscious or unresponsive, suction equipment is kept at hand. An exact record of the feedings is kept.

NASOGASTRIC INTUBATION

nasogastric tube, any tube passed into the stomach through the nose. See **nasogastric intubation**.

nasolabial reflex (nei′zoulei′biəl), a sudden backward movement of the head, arching of the back, and extension and stretching of the limbs that occurs in infants in response to a light touch to the tip of the nose with an upward sweeping motion. The reflex disappears by about five months of age.

nasolacrimal (nei′zoulæk′rıməl), of or pertaining to the nasal cavity and associated lacrimal ducts.

nasolacrimal duct, a channel that carries tears from the lacrimal sac to the nasal cavity.

nasomandibular fixation (nei′zoumændıb′yulər), a type of maxillomandibular fixation to stabilize fractures of the jaw by using maxillomandibular splints connected to a wire through a hole drilled in the anterior nasal spine of the maxillary bone. It has been used particularly in edentulous patients. See also **maxillomandibular fixation**.

nasopharyngeal angiofibroma (nei′zoufərın′jiəl), a benign tumor of the nasopharynx, consisting of fibrous connective tissue with many vascular spaces. The tumor usually arises in puberty and is more common in boys than in girls. Typical signs are nasal and eustachian tube obstruction, adenoidal speech, and dysphagia. Also called **juvenile angiofibroma, nasopharyngeal fibroangioma**.

nasopharyngeal cancer, a malignant neoplastic disease of the nasopharynx. Depending on the site of a nasopharyngeal tumor, there may be nasal obstruction, otitis media, hearing loss, sensory or motor nerve damage, bony destruction of the skull, or deep cervical lymphadenopathy. Diagnostic measures include nasopharyngoscopy, biopsy, and radiologic examination of the skull with tomographic studies. Squamous cell and undifferentiated carcinomas are the most common lesions. Nasopharyngeal cancer occurs rarely in the United States and very frequently in southern China. Exposure to dusts of nickel, chromium, wood, and leather and to isopropyl oil increases the risk of developing nasopharyngeal cancer. High titers of antibodies to the Epstein-Barr virus are found in Chinese patients with the cancer, and there is evidence of genetic susceptibility, as a certain histocompatibility antigen is associated with the disease and multiple cases occur in some families. Radiation is the most effective therapy and 5-fluorouracil and adriamycin are also used.

nasopharyngeal fibroangioma. See **nasopharyngeal angiofibroma.**

nasopharyngoscopy (nei′zoufær′ɪŋgos′kəpi), a technique in physical examination in which the nose and throat are visually examined using a laryngoscope, a fiberoptic device, a flashlight, and a dilator for the nares. – **nasopharyngoscopic,** *adj.*

nasopharynx (nei′zoufær′ɪŋks), one of the three regions of the throat, situated behind the nose and extending from the posterior nares to the level of the soft palate. On the posterior wall of the nasopharynx, opposite the posterior nares, are the pharyngeal tonsils. Swollen or enlarged pharyngeal tonsils can fill the space behind the posterior nares and may completely block the passage of air from the nose into the throat. Compare **laryngopharynx, oropharynx.** See also **tonsil.** – **nasopharyngeal,** (nei′-zoufərɪn′jiəl) *adj.*

nasotracheal tube, a catheter inserted into the trachea through the nasal cavity and the pharynx. It is commonly used to administer oxygen and in other respiratory therapy.

NASOTRACHEAL TUBE

natal, 1. of or pertaining to birth. 2. of or pertaining to the nates, or buttocks.

natamycin, an ophthalmic antifungal. Also called **pimaricin.**
■ INDICATIONS: It is prescribed in the treatment of fungal keratitis, blepharitis, and conjunctivitis.
■ CONTRAINDICATION: Known hypersensitivity to this drug prohibits its use.
■ ADVERSE EFFECTS: No adverse effects have been reported other than a rare case of conjunctival chemosis and hyperemia.

nates (nei′tiz), *sing.* **natis,** the large fleshy protuberances at the lower posterior portion of the torso comprising fat and the gluteal muscles. Also called **buttocks.**

National Association for Mental Health. See **Mental Health Association.**

National Association for Practical Nurse Education and Services (N.A.P.N.E.S.), a national professional organization concerned with the education of practical nurses and with the services provided by licensed practical nurses.

National Association of Pediatric Nurse Associates/ Practitioners (NAP-NAP), a national organization of nurses who are prepared by training or experience to give primary care to pediatric patients. NAP-NAP works in conjunction with the American Academy of Pediatrics.

National Bureau of Standards (NBS), a federal agency in the Department of Commerce that sets accurate measurement standards for commerce, industry, and science in the United States. The NBS compares and coordinates its standards with those of other countries and provides research and technical service to improve computer science, materials technology, building construction, and consumer product safety. The Bureau also provides measurement services and standards for other federal agencies and for state and local governments.

National Eye Institute (NEI), a division of the National Institutes of Health. NEI was established in 1968 to support research in the normal functioning of the human eye and visual system, the pathology of visual disorders, and the rehabilitation of the visually handicapped. See also **eye, vision.**

National Formulary (***N.F.***), a publication containing the official standards for the preparation of various pharmaceuticals not listed in the *United States Pharmacopoeia.* It is revised every five years.

National Health Service Corps (NHSC), a program of the United States Public Health Service (USPHS) in which health care personnel are placed in areas that are underserved. The Corps was established by the Emergency Health Personnel Act of 1970. The provisions of Act are updated as needed. Nurses, physicians, and dentists serve in rural and urban areas, usually as employees of local health care agencies. The USPHS pays most of the salary of each corps member.

National Institute of Child Health and Human Development (N.I.C.H.H.D.), the Institute in the National Institutes of Health that is concerned with all aspects of the growth, development, and health of the children of the United States.

National Institutes of Health (N.I.H.), an agency within the United States Public Health Service made up of several institutions and constituent divisions, including the Bureau of Health Manpower Education, the National Library of Medicine, the National Cancer Institute, and several research institutes and divisions.

National League for Nursing (NLN), an organization concerned with the improvement of nursing education, nursing service, and the delivery of health care in the United States. Among its many activities are accreditation of nursing programs at all levels, preadmission and achievement tests for nursing students, and compilation of statistical data on nursing manpower and on trends in health-care delivery. It acts as the testing service for the State Board Test Pool Examinations for registered and practical nurse licensure. The Research Division and the Public Affairs Office are among the other sections of NLN. A monthly refereed journal, *Nursing and Health Care,* is the official publication of the organization.

National Male Nurses' Association (NMNA), a national organization that promotes the interests and practice of male nurses.

National Student Nurses' Association (NSNA), a national organization of students in the field of nursing. Among its purposes are the improvement of nursing education to improve health care, to aid in the development of the student nurse, and to encourage optimal achievement in the professional role of the nurse and the health care of people. It publishes a journal, *Imprint,* five times a year, participates in legislative activities at all levels, and gives scholarships, awards, and career workshops.

natriuresis (nei'triuri'sis), the excretion of greater-than-normal amounts of sodium in the urine, as from the administration of natriuretic diuretic drugs or from various metabolic or endocrine disorders. – **natriuretic,** *adj.*

natriuretic (nei'trıyuret'ık), **1.** of or pertaining to the process of natriuresis. **2.** a substance that inhibits the resorption of sodium ions from the glomerular filtrate in the kidneys, thus allowing more sodium to be excreted with the urine.

natural childbirth, labor and parturition accomplished by a mother with little or no medical intervention. It is generally considered the optimal way of giving birth and being born, safest for the baby and most satisfying for the mother. Prerequisites include normal gestation, an adequate birth canal, strong maternal motivation, physical and emotional preparation, and constant and intensive support of the mother during labor and birth. See also **Lamaze method, prepared childbirth.**

natural dentition, the entire array of natural teeth in the dental arch at any given time, consisting of deciduous or permanent teeth or a mixture of the two. See also **tooth.**

natural family-planning method, any one of several methods of family planning that does not rely on a medication or a device for effectiveness in avoiding pregnancy. Some of the methods are also used to pinpoint the time of ovulation in order to increase the chance of fertilization when artificial insemination or extraction of an oocyte for in vitro fertilization is to be performed. Natural family-planning methods require thorough instruction, the cooperation and self-motivation of the couple, and the diligent, accurate observation and recording of the data relevant to the method. Kinds of natural family-planning include **basal body temperature method of family planning, calendar method of family planning, ovulation method of family planning, symptothermal method of family planning.**

natural immunity, a usually innate and permanent form of immuntiy to a specific disease. Kinds of natural immunity include **individual immunity, racial immunity, species immunity.** Also called **genetic immunity, innate immunity.**

naturally acquired immunity. See **acquired immunity.**

natural network, (in psychiatric nursing) a patient's natural contacts in the community, including church and social groups, friends, family, and occupation that support the person's function outside the hospital environment.

natural selection, the natural evolutionary processes by which those organisms best suited for adaptation to the environment tend to survive and propagate the species while those unfit are eliminated. Compare **artificial selection.**

Naturetin, a trade name for a diuretic and antihypertensive (bendroflumethiazide).

naturopath (nei'churəpæth, næch'urəpæth'), a person who practices naturopathy.

naturopathy (nei'churop'əthi, næch'urop'əthi), a system of therapeutics based on natural foods, regular exercise, and the avoidance of medications. Advocates believe that illness can be healed by the natural processes of the body.

Nauheim bath (nau'haim), a bath taken in water through which carbon dioxide is bubbled, followed by systematic exercises, used in the treatment of cardiac conditions. The procedure is named after the natural waters of Bad-Nauheim, Germany.

nausea (nɔ'ziə, nɔ'zhə), a sensation often leading to the urge to vomit. Common causes are sea and other motion sicknesses, early pregnancy, intense pain, emotional stress, gall bladder disease, food poisoning, and various enteroviruses. – **nauseate,** *v.,* **nauseous,** *adj.*

nausea and vomiting of pregnancy, a common condition of early pregnancy, characterized by recurrent or persistent nausea, often in the morning, that may result in vomiting, weight loss, anorexia, general weakness, and malaise. The etiology of the condition is poorly understood. It usually does not begin before the sixth week after the last menstrual period and ends by the twelfth to the fourteenth week of pregnancy. Symptomatic relief is often obtained by eating small, easily digested meals frequently and by not allowing the stomach to be empty. In the past, antiemetic drugs were routinely prescribed for this complaint, but this practice is currently reserved for severe cases. Nausea and vomiting after the sixteenth week is an unusual complication of pregnancy, called persistent nausea and vomiting of pregnancy. If severe and intractable, hyperemesis gravidarum may ensue. Also called *Nontechnical.* **morning sickness.**

Navane, a trade name for a tranquilizer (thiothixene).

navel, the depression in the abdomen at the point of insertion of the umbilical cord in the fetus. It interrupts the linea alba about halfway between the infrasternal notch and the pubic symphysis. It is located at the level of the interspace of the third and the fourth lumbar vertebrae.

navicular (nəvɪk'yulər), having the shape of a boat, as the navicular bone in the wrist.

navicular bone. See **scaphoid bone.**

Nb, symbol for **niobium.**

NBS standard, (in nuclear medicine) a radioactive source standardized, or certified, or both, by the National Bureau of Standards.

nC, nc, abbreviation for **nanocurie.**

N-CAP, abbreviation for **Nurses Coalition for Action in Politics.**

NCI, abbreviation for the *National Cancer Institute.* See **National Institutes of Health**

Nd, abbreviation for **neodymium.**

ne-, See **neo-.**

Ne, symbol for **neon.**

near-drowning, a pathological state in which the victim has survived exposure to circumstances that usually cause drowning. Cardiopulmonary resuscitation is performed immediately; hospitalization is always indicated. The return of consciousness does not necessarily assure recovery. Intensive supportive therapy may be required for up to several days. Compare **drowning.** See also **hypothermia.**

nearest neighbor analysis, (in molecular genetics) a biochemical method used to estimate the frequency with which pairs of bases are located next to one another.

near-sightedness. See **myopia.**

Nebcin, a trade name for an antibacterial (tobramycin sulfate).

nebula, *pl.* **nebulae. 1.** a slight corneal opacity or scar that seldom obstructs vision and that can be seen only by oblique illumination. **2.** a murkiness in the urine. **3.** an oily concoction that is applied with an atomizer.

nebulize (neb'yulaɪz'), to vaporize or disperse a liquid in a fine spray.

nebulizer, a device for producing a fine spray. Intranasal medications are often administered by a nebulizer. Also called **atomizer.**

NEC, abbreviation for **necrotizing enterocolitis.**

neck, a constricted section, as the part of the body that connects the head with the trunk. Other such constrictions are the neck of the humerus and the neck of the femur.

neck dissection, surgical removal of the cervical lymph nodes, performed to prevent the spread of malignant tumors of the head and neck. Under general anesthesia, the cervical chain of lymph nodes with their lymphatic channels is removed in one mass to prevent the spread of cancer cells. After surgery, the patient is observed closely for signs of hemorrhage and difficulty in breathing. Compare **radical neck dissection.**

neck-righting reflex, 1. an involuntary response in newborns in which turning the head to one side while the infant is supine causes rotation of the shoulders and trunk in the same direction. The reflex enables the child to roll over from the supine to prone position. Absence of the reflex or persistence beyond about 10 months of age may indicate central nervous system damage. **2.** any tonic reflex associated with the neck that maintains body orientation in relation to the head.

necro-, a combining form meaning 'of or pertaining to death or a corpse': *necrobiosis, necronectomy, necrophilia.*

necrobiosis lipoidica, a skin disease characterized by thin, shiny, yellow to red plaques on the shins or forearms. Telangiectases, crusting, and ulceration of these plaques may occur. Necrobiosis lipoidica is usually associated with diabetes mellitus and occurs most often in women. Treatment includes precise control of the diabetes and, possibly, intralesional application of corticosteroids.

necrolysis (nekrol'ɪsɪs), disintegration or exfoliation of dead tissue. Compare **necrosis.** – **necrolytic,** *adj.*

necrophilia, 1. a morbid liking for being with dead bodies. **2.** a morbid desire to have sexual contact with a dead body, usually of men to perform a sexual act with a dead woman. – **necrophile, necrophiliac,** *n.*

necropsy (nek'ropsi). See **autopsy.**

necroscopy (nɪkros'kəpi). See **autopsy.**

necrosis (nɪkrou'sɪs), localized tissue death that occurs in groups of cells in response to disease or injury. In **coagulation necrosis,** blood clots block the flow of blood, causing tissue ischemia distal to the clot; in **gangrenous necrosis,** ischemia combined with bacterial action causes putrefaction to set in. See also **gangrene.**

necrotizing angiitis (æn'jiaɪ'tɪs). See **periarteritis nodosa.**

necrotizing enteritis, acute inflammation of the small and the large intestine by the bacterium *Clostridium perfringens,* characterized by severe abdominal pain, bloody diarrhea, and vomiting. Some people recover completely, some survive with chronic bowel obstruction, and some die of perforation of the intestine, dehydration, peritonitis, or septicemia.

necrotizing enterocolitis (NEC), an acute inflammatory bowel disorder that occurs primarily in preterm or low-birth-weight neonates. It is characterized by ischemic necrosis of the gastrointestinal mucosa that may lead to perforation and peritonitis. The cause of the disorder is unknown, although it appears to be a defect in host defenses with infection resulting from normal gastrointestinal flora rather than from invading organisms. See also **enteritis.**

■ OBSERVATIONS: Significant predisposing factors of the condition include prematurity, hypovolemia, respiratory distress syndrome, sepsis, an indwelling umbilical catheter, exchange transfusion, and feeding with hyperosmolar or high-caloric formulas. The condition results from a reflex shunting of blood away from the gastrointestinal tract, which leads to convulsive vasoconstriction of the mesenteric vessels supplying the intestines. The diminished blood supply interferes with the normal production of mucus and with other bowel functions and results in severe necrosis with bacterial invasion of the bowel wall. Bottle-fed infants are more susceptible to the disorder, possibly because formula lacks the immunoglobulin A antibodies and macrophages, found in breast milk, that may protect the gastrointestinal mucosa from damage and bacterial invasion. Initial symptoms, which usually develop after several days of life, include temperature instability (usually hypothermia), lethargy, poor feeding, vomiting of bile, abdominal distention, blood in the stools, and decreased or absent bowel sounds. Signs of deterioration are apnea, pallor, hyperbilirubinemia, oliguria, abdominal tenderness, erythema and edema of the anterior abdominal wall or palpable masses, with eventual respiratory failure leading to death. Diagnosis is confirmed by x-ray visualization of the intestine or by the presence of increased peritoneal fluid or pneumoperitoneum.

■ INTERVENTION: Treatment includes discontinuing oral feeding, beginning intravenous infusion, abdominal decompression by nasogastric suction, hydration, plasma or whole blood transfusion, and administration of broad-spectrum antibiotics (usually ampicillin, gentamicin, or kanamycin). With routine supportive management, improvement usually occurs within 48 to 72 hours. Oral feedings usually are not resumed for 10 days to two weeks. Total parenteral nutrition is necessary during that period. Surgical resection of the affected bowel segment may be necessary, especially if signs of intestinal perforation or peritonitis develop. If a large portion of bowel is affected, an ileostomy or colostomy may be necessary. Stenosis of the involved bowel segment may present later complications.

■ NURSING CONSIDERATIONS: The primary concern of the nurse is to observe high-risk, formula-fed infants for early symptoms of necrotizing enterocolitis, especially for difficulty in feeding, bile-stained regurgitation, bloody stools, temperature variations, or a distended, shiny abdomen. Once the diagnosis is confirmed, the nurse initiates nasogastric intubation for abdominal decompression and continues to monitor the baby constantly for dehydration and electrolyte balance. In addition to the ordered laboratory tests, daily weight is taken. Infants who are unable to take fluids by mouth require special oral care. Glycerin and lemon swabs reduce dryness, and a pacifier or a nipple stuffed with gauze helps to meet the infant's need to suck. Parents are encouraged to visit and are helped to meet the emotional needs of the infant and to provide tactile, auditory, and visual stimulation. The nurse explains the usual course of the disease, the medical and nursing procedures, and keeps the parents informed of the infant's progress. Frequent visits to the care unit facilitate family-infant relationships, and provide the nurse with an opportunity to teach proper care techniques prior to discharge. Also called **pseudomembranous enterocolitis.**

necrotizing vasculitis, an inflammatory condition of blood vessels, characterized by necrosis, fibrosis, and proliferation of the inner layer of the vascular wall, in some cases resulting in occlusion and infarction. Necrotizing vasculitis may occur in rheumatoid arthritis and is common in systemic lupus erythematosus, periarteritis nodosa, and progressive systemic sclerosis. The condition is usually treated with corticosteroids.

needle bath, a shower in which fine jets of water are sprayed over the body.

needle biopsy, the removal of a segment of living tissue for microscopic examination by inserting a hollow needle through the skin or the external surface of an organ or tumor and rotating it within the underlying cellular layers. See also **aspiration biopsy.**

needle filter, a device, usually made of plastic, used for filtering medications that are drawn into a syringe before administration. Some syringe needles are equipped with built-in filters; other filters are separate units that are attached to the needle before use. Manufacturers' instructions are usually supplied with such devices. Needle filters are commonly disposable items designed for one-time applications.

negative, 1. (of a laboratory test) indicating that a substance or a reaction is not present. 2. (of a sign) indicating on physical examination that a finding is not present, often meaning that there is no pathologic change. 3. (of a substance) tending to carry or carrying a negative chemical charge.

negative adaptation. See **habituation.**

negative anxiety, (in psychology) an emotional and psychological condition in which anxiety prevents a person's normal functioning and interrupts the person's ability to perform the usual activities of daily living.

negative catalysis, a decrease in the rate of any chemical reaction caused by a substance that is neither part of the process itself nor consumed nor affected by the reaction. Compare **catalysis.** See also **catalyst.**

negative feedback, 1. (in physiology) a decrease in function in response to a stimulus, as the secretion of follicle-stimulating hormone decreases even as the amount of circulating estrogen increases. 2. *Informal.* a critical, derogatory, or otherwise negative response from one person to what another person has communicated.

negative pi meson (pion), a form of electromagnetic radiation emitted from a proton linear accelerator. In the treatment of certain tumors, negative pi meson particles are beamed at the tumor; the atomic nuclei of malignant cells take in the radioactive particles and explode, scattering intensely radioactive subatomic particles through the adjacent malignant tissue.

negative pi meson (pion) radiotherapy, a form of radiotherapy using a negative pi meson (pion) beam emitted by a proton linear accelerator. Pion radiotherapy requires fewer rad and has a 60 per cent greater biologic effect than conventional, x-radiation techniques. It may also have less effect on normal tissue near the tumor. Some locally advanced neoplasms, especially those of the prostate, are destroyed. Gliomas and advanced cancers of the head and neck may also be well controlled with pion radiotherapy. Moderately acute toxicity occurs with treatment; chronic toxicity is minimal.

negative pressure, less-than-ambient atmospheric pressure, as in a vacuum, at an altitude above sea level, or in a hypobaric chamber. Some ventilators have a negative cycle that may help stimulate or cycle exhalation in controlled ventilation in IPPB therapy.

negative relationship, (in research) an inverse relationship between two variables; as one variable increases the other decreases. Also called **inverse relationship.** Compare **positive relationship.**

negativism, a behavioral attitude characterized by opposition, resistance, the refusal to cooperate with even the most reasonable request, and the tendency to act in a contrary manner. The resulting response may be passive, as the immobile, rigid postures observed in catatonic schizophrenia, or active, as in a belligerent, impulsive, or capricious act, like lowering the arms when asked to raise them or sitting down when asked to stand.

NegGram, a trade name for an antibacterial (nalidixic acid).

negligence, (in law) the commission of an act that a prudent person would not have done or the omission of a duty that a prudent person would have fulfilled, resulting in injury or harm to another person. In particular, in a malpractice suit, a professional person is negligent if harm to a client results from such an act or such failure to act, but it must be proved that other prudent persons of the same profession would ordinarily have acted differently under the same circumstances. Thus, negligence may be misfeasance, malfeasance, or nonfeasance.

negligence per se, (in law) a finding of negligence rendered in judgment of a professional action or inaction in violation of a statute or so at odds with common sense that beyond any doubt no prudent person would have been guilty of it.

NEI, abbreviation for **National Eye Institute.**

Neisseria gonorrhoeae, a gram-negative, nonmotile, diplococcal bacterium usually seen microscopically as flattened pairs within the cytoplasm of neutrophils. It is the causative organism of gonorrhea. Also called **gonococcus.**

Neisseria meningitidis. See **meningococcus.**

NEJM, abbreviation for *New England Journal of Medicine.*

Nelson's syndrome, an endocrine disorder that may follow adrenalectomy for Cushing's disease. It is characterized by a marked increase in the secretion of ACTH and MSH by the pituitary gland. Treatment includes irradiation to decrease pituitary function and, in some cases, hypophysectomy. See also **Cushing's disease.**

nem, abbreviation for **Nahrungs Einheit Milch** (German for "nutritional unit milk").

-nema, a combining form meaning a 'threadlike stage in the development of chromosomes': *chromonema, plasmonema, uronema.*

nemato-, a combining form meaning 'pertaining to a nematode, or to a threadlike structure': *nematoblast, nematocide, nematodiasis.*

nematode (nem′ətoud), a multicellular, parasitic animal of the phylum Nematoda. All roundworms belong to the phylum, including *Ancylostoma duodenale, Ascaris lumbricoides, Enterobius vermicularis, Necator americanus, Strongyloides stercoralis,* and several other species.

Nembutal, a trade name for a barbiturate (pentobarbital), used as an adjunct to anesthesia.

-nemia. See **-anemia.**

neo-, ne-, a combining form meaning 'new': *neobiogenesis, neocyte, neonatal.*

neoantigen, a new specific antigen that develops in a cell infected by oncogenic virus; which it appears following infection by SV40.

neobehaviorism, a school of psychology based on the general principles of behaviorism but broader and more flexible in concept. It stresses experimental research and laboratory analyses in the study of overt behavior and in various subjective phenomena that cannot be directly observed and measured, as fantasies, love, stress, empathy, trust, and personality. See also **behaviorism.**

neobehaviorist, a disciple of the school of neobehaviorism.

Neobiotic, a trade name for an antibacterial (neomycin sulfate).

neoblastic, of or pertaining to a new tissue or development within a new tissue.

Neo-Cort-Dome, a trade name for a topical, fixed-combination drug containing a glucocorticoid (hydrocortisone) and an antibacterial (neomycin sulfate).

Neo-Cortef, a trade name for a topical, fixed-combination drug containing a glucocorticoid (hydrocortisone acetate) and an antibacterial (neomycin sulfate).

NeoDecadron, a trade name for a topical, fixed-combination drug containing a glucocorticoid (dexamethasone phosphate) and an antibacterial (neomycin sulfate).

Neo-Delta-Cortef, a trade name for a topical, fixed-combination drug containing a glucocorticoid (prednisolone acetate) and an antibacterial (neomycin sulfate).

neodymium (Nd), a rare earth element. Its atomic number is 60; its atomic weight is 144.27.

Neo-Hydeltrasol, a trade name for a topical, fixed-combination drug containing a glucocorticoid (prednisolone sodium phosphate) and an antibacterial (neomycin sulfate).

neologism (niol′əjız′əm), **1.** a newly coined word or term. **2.** (in psychiatry) a word coined by a psychotic or a delirious patient that is meaningful only to the patient.

Neo-Medrol, a trade name for a topical, fixed-combination drug containing a glucocorticoid (methylprednisolone) and an antibacterial (neomycin sulfate).

Neo-Mull-Soy, a trade name for a commercial milk-substitute formula that is lactose free, used for infants with galactosemia and persons with lactose intolerance. It is made from a soy isolate base and supplemented with added nutrients, especially vitamins and minerals. See also **Nutramigen, Pro Sobee, Soyalac.**

neomycin sulfate, an aminoglycoside antibiotic.
■ INDICATIONS: It is prescribed in the treatment of infections of the intestine, in hepatic coma, and, topically, in the treatment of skin infections.
■ CONTRAINDICATIONS: Renal dysfunction, intestinal obstruction, or known hypersensitivity to this drug or to any aminoglycoside medication prohibits its use.
■ ADVERSE EFFECTS: Among the more serious adverse reactions are nausea, vomiting, diarrhea, malabsorption, or suprainfection. Prolonged treatment in patients with impaired renal function may result in the toxicities of systemic aminoglycosides. Hypersensitivity reactions may occur with topical administration of this drug.

neon (Ne), a colorless, odorless gaseous element and one of the inert gases. Its atomic number is 10; its atomic weight is 20.2. Neon has no compounds and occurs in the atmosphere in the ratio of about 18 parts per million. Some minerals and meteorites contain traces of this element. It is prepared commercially by the fractional distillation of liquefied air and is one of the first components to boil off. Neon is an excellent conductor of electricity which ionizes the gas and causes it to emit a reddish-orange glow; this characteristic makes neon useful in devices to warn against electric current overload.

Neonatal Behavior Assessment Scale, a scale for evaluating and assessing an infant's alertness, motor maturity, irritability, consolability, and interaction with people. It is used as a tool for the evaluation of the neurologic condition as well as the behavior of a newborn infant. Using the scale, the individuality of an infant may be demonstrated for parents, and some researchers theorize that the quality of the parent-child relationship may be predicted.

neonatal breathing, respiration in newborn infants which begins when pulmonary fluid in the lungs is expelled by mechanical compression of the thorax during delivery and by resorption from the alveoli into the bloodstream and lymphatics. As air enters the lungs, the chest and lungs recoil to a resting position, but forceful inspirations are necessary to keep the lungs inflated. These forces come from changes in blood gas tension, strong Hering-Breuer reflexes, temperature, and tactile stimuli. Irregular fetal breathing movements, which occur during rapid-eye-movement sleep, may be observed as early as 13 weeks of gestation. At birth, the peripheral and central chemoreceptors are very active, and newborns are highly sensitive to carbon dioxide during the first weeks. However, control of rhythm is not fully developed at birth.

neonatal death, the death of a live-born infant during the first 28 days after birth. Early neonatal death is usually considered to be one that occurs during the first 7 days. Compare **infant death, perinatal death.**

neonatal developmental profile, an evaluation of the developmental status of a newborn infant based on three examinations, a gestational age inventory, a neurologic examination, and a Neonatal Behavior Assessment score.

neonatal hyperbilirubinemia. See **hyperbilirubinemia of the newborn.**

neonatal intensive care unit (NICU), a hospital unit containing a variety of sophisticated mechanical devices and special equipment for the management and care of premature and seriously ill newborn infants. The unit is staffed by a team of nurses and neonatologists who are highly trained in the pathophysiology of the newborn.

neonatal mortality, the statistical rate of infant death during the first 28 days after live birth, expressed as the number of such deaths per 1,000 live births in a specific geographic area or institution in a given period of time.

neonatal period, the interval from birth to 28 days of age. It represents the time of the greatest risk to the infant; approximately 65 per cent of all deaths that occur in the first year of life happen during this four-week period.

neonatal pustular melanosis, a transient skin condition of the neonate characterized by vesicles present at birth that become pustular. The lesions contain neutrophils rather than eosinophils as seen in erythema toxicum neonatorum, and they disappear within 72 hours, leaving dark spots that gradually fade by about three months of age.

neonatal thermoregulation, the regulation of the body temperature of a newborn infant, which may be affected by evaporation, conduction, radiation, and convection.

■ METHOD: To prevent the loss of body heat through evaporation, the infant is patted dry with a warm towel immediately after birth. Loss of heat by conduction is prevented by wrapping the baby in a warm blanket or wrapping a warm blanket over him as he lies on his mother's skin and by warming all equipment that is to be used to touch, cover, or examine the infant. Loss of heat by radiation can be minimized by placing the baby under a radiant heater, on a warmed, padded surface, skin-to-skin with the mother. Loss of body heat by convection is prevented by avoiding drafts, air-conditioning vents, and low ambient temperatures. Infant bassinettes have high sides to prevent cross drafts.

■ OUTCOME CRITERIA: The axillary temperature is normally between 36.5° and 37°C, and the rectal temperature is normally one degree higher than the axillary temperature.

■ NURSING ORDERS: The infant is kept covered and protected from any means of heat loss. As the surface area of the head of a newborn is proportionally large when compared to the body, heat loss from the head may be great; therefore, a cap or fold of blanket is placed around the head. Progressive family centered maternity services, in which the practice after delivery is to place the infant skin-to-skin with the mother, often provide caps made of stockinet. An over-head radiant heater is rolled to the delivery bed to maintain a warm ambient temperature for the infant.

neonatal tyrosinemia. See **tyrosinemia.**

neonate (ni′əneit), an infant from birth to four weeks of age. —**neonatal,** adj.

neonatology (ni′ounətol′əji), the branch of medicine that concentrates on the care of the neonate and specializes in the diagnosis and treatment of the disorders of the newborn infant. —**neonatologic, neonatological** adj., **neonatologist** n.

neoplasia (ni′ouplei′ʒhə), the new and abnormal development of cells which may be benign or malignant. —**neoplastic,** adj.

neoplasm (ni′ouplæz′əm), any abnormal growth of new tissue, benign or malignant. See also **benign, malignant.** —**neoplastic,** adj.
(See next page for table)

neoplastic fracture, a fracture resulting from weakened bone tissue caused by neoplasm or by a malignant growth. Also called **pathologic fracture.**

Neosporin, a trade name for a topical, fixed-combination drug containing antibacterials (polymyxin B sulfate, neomycin sulfate, and bacitracin zinc).

neostigmine bromide (ni′oustıg′min), a cholinergic.

■ INDICATION: It is prescribed in the treatment of myasthenia gravis.

■ CONTRAINDICATIONS: Bowel obstruction, urinary tract infection, or known hypersensitivity to this drug or to other bromides prohibits its use.

■ ADVERSE EFFECTS: Among the more serious adverse reactions are severe respiratory depression, hyperptyalism, and intestinal cramps.

Neo-Synephrine Hydrochloride, a trade name for a vasoconstrictor (phenylephrine hydrochloride).

neoteny (niot′əni), the attainment of sexual maturity during the larval stage of development, as in certain amphibians, especially salamanders.

Neothylline, a trade name for a smooth-muscle relaxant (dyphylline).

Neotrizine, a trade name for an antibacterial (trisulfapyrimidine).

nephelometer (nef′əlom′ıtər), an apparatus used to determine the concentration of solids suspended in a liquid or a gas, as may be used to determine the number of bacteria in a specimen. See also **nephelometry.**

nephelometry (nef′əlom′ıtri), a technique of determining the concentration of solids suspended in a liquid or a gas by use of a nephelometer. —**nephelometric, nephelometrical,** adj.

nephr-. See **nephro-.**

nephrectomy, the surgical removal of a kidney, performed to remove a tumor, drain an abcess, or treat hydronephrosis. Before surgery, the fluid intake is increased to improve the excretion of waste products. The blood is typed and cross-matched for transfusion. Under general anesthesia, the kidney is approached through either a flank or a thoraco-abdominal incision and is removed. If the thoracic cavity is opened, a chest tube is inserted and connected to water-seal drainage. Hemostats may be left in place with handles extending out through the incision, preventing the patient from lying on the affected side. The nurse observes carefully for rapid pulse, restlessness, sweating, and a drop in blood pressure. The urinary output is measured hourly, and fluid intake and body weight are closely monitored. Deep breathing is difficult because the incision is close to the diaphragm; intermittent positive pressure breathing apparatus is used

Classification of neoplasms

Parent tissue	Benign tumor	Malignant tumor
Epithelium		
Skin and mucous membrane	Papilloma	Squamous cell carcinoma
	Polyp	Basal cell carcinoma
		Transitional cell carcinoma
Glands	Adenoma	Adenocarcinoma
	Cystadenoma	
Endothelium		Endothelioma
Blood vessels	Hemangioma	Hemangioendothelioma
		Angiosarcoma
Lymph vessels	Lymphangioma	Lymphangiosarcoma
		Lymphangioendothelioma
Bone marrow		Multiple myeloma
		Ewing's sarcoma
		Leukemia
		Lymphosarcoma
Lymphoid tissue		Reticulum cell sarcoma (difficult to classify because of cell embryology)
		Lymphatic leukemia
Connective tissues		
Embryonic fibrous tissue	Myxoma	Myxosarcoma
Fibrous tissue	Fibroma	Fibrosarcoma
Adipose tissue	Lipoma	Liposarcoma
Cartilage	Chondroma	Chondrosarcoma
Bone	Osteoma	Osteogenic sarcoma
Synovial membrane	Synovioma	Synovial sarcoma
Muscle tissue		
Smooth muscle	Leiomyoma	Leiomyosarcoma
Striated muscle	Rhabdomyoma	Rhabdomyosarcoma
Nerve tissue		
Nerve fibers and sheaths	Neuroma	Neurogenic sarcoma
	Neurinoma (neurilemoma)	
	Neurofibroma	Neurofibrosarcoma
Ganglion cells	Ganglioneuroma	Neuroblastoma
Glia cells	Glioma	Glioblastoma
		Spongioblastoma
Meninges	Meningioma	
Pigmented neoplasms		
Melanoblasts	Pigmented nevus	Malignant melanoma
		Melanocarcinoma
Miscellaneous		
Placenta	Hydatidiform mole	Chorionepithelioma (choriocarcinoma)
	Dermoid cyst	Embryonal carcinoma
		Embryonal sarcoma
		Teratocarcinoma

to drain secretions. The nurse reports at once any sudden shortness of breath, a sign of spontaneous pneumothorax that may occur if the pleura was accidentally nicked during surgery.

-nephric, a combining form meaning 'of or referring to the kidneys': *archinephric, cardionephric, splenonephric.*

nephritis (nefrai′tis), any one of a large group of diseases of the kidney characterized by inflammation and abnormal function. Kinds of nephritis include **acute nephritis, glomerulonephritis, hereditary nephritis, interstitial nephritis, parenchymatous nephritis, suppurative nephritis.**

nephro-, nephr-, a combining form meaning 'of or related to the kidneys': *nephroblastoma, nephrogram, nephrorrhagia.*

nephroangiosclerosis (nef′rouæn′jiousklərou′sis), necrosis of the renal arterioles, associated with hypertension. This condition is present in a small number of hypertensive individuals between the ages of 30 and 50. Early signs of the condition are headaches, blurring of vision, and a diastolic blood pressure greater than 120 mm Hg. Examination of the retina reveals hemorrhages, vascular exudates, and papilledema. The heart is usually enlarged, especially the left ventricle. Proteins and red blood cells are found in the urine. Heart failure and kidney failure may occur if the disease remains untreated. Treatment includes measures to lower blood pressure using diet and antihypertensive medications. Hemodialysis is used when preventive measures have failed. Also called **malignant hypertension.** See also **hypertension, renal failure.**

nephroblastoma (nef′roublæstou′mə). See **Wilms' tumor.**

nephrocalcinosis (nef′roukæl′sınou′sıs), an abnormal condition of the kidneys in which deposits of calcium form in the parenchyma at the site of previous inflammation or degenerative change. Infection, hematuria, anal colic, and decreased function of the kidney may occur.

nephrogenic (nef′roujen′ık), 1. generating kidney tissue. 2. originating in the kidney.

nephrogenic ascites, the abnormal presence of fluid in the peritoneal cavity of persons undergoing hemodialysis for renal failure. The cause of this type of ascites is unknown. See also **ascites.**

nephrogenic cord, either of the paired longitudinal ridges of tissue that lie along the dorsal surface of the coelom in the early developing vertebrate embryo. It is formed from the fusion of the nephrotome tissue and gives rise to the structures comprising the embryonic urogenital system. See also **mesonephros, metanephros, pronephros.**

nephrogenic diabetes insipidus, an abnormal condition in which the kidneys do not concentrate the urine, resulting in polyuria, polydipsia, and very dilute urine. The secretion of antidiuretic hormone (ADH) by the pituitary is normal, and all kidney function is normal except that there is no response to ADH. See also **diabetes insipidus.**

nephrogenous (nəfroj′ənəs), of or pertaining to the formation and development of the kidneys.

nephrolith, a calculus formed in a kidney. —**nephrolithic,** adj.

nephrolithiasis (nef′roulıfhai′əsıs), a disorder characterized by the presence of calculi in the kidney. See also **urinary calculus.**

nephrology, the study of the anatomy, physiology, and pathology of the kidney. —**nephrologic, nephrological,** adj.

nephrolytic, of or pertaining to the destruction of the structure and function of a kidney.

-nephroma, a combining form meaning a 'tumor of the kidney or area of the kidney': epinephroma, paranephroma.

nephromere. See **nephrotome.**

nephron (nef′ron), **nephrone** (nef′roun), a structural and functional unit of the kidney, resembling a microscopic funnel with a long stem and two convoluted sections. Each kidney contains about 1.25 million nephrons, each consisting of the renal corpuscle, the loop of Henle, and the renal tubules. Each renal corpuscle consists of the glomerulus of renal capillaries enclosed within the Bowman's capsule. The renal corpuscles and the convoluted portions of the renal tubules are located in the cortex of the kidney. The renal medulla contains the loops of Henle and the collecting tubules. Urine is formed in the renal corpuscles and in the renal tubules by filtration, reabsorption, and secretion. See also **kidney, renal corpuscle.**

nephronophthisis (nef′rounof′fhısıs). See **medullary cystic disease.**

nephropathy (nefrop′əfhi), any disorder of the kidney, including inflammatory, degenerative, and sclerotic conditions. See also **kidney disease.**

nephropexy (nef′rəpek′si), a surgical operation to fixate a floating or ptotic kidney.

nephroptosis (nef′roptou′sıs), a downward displacement or dropping of a kidney.

nephrorrhaphy (nefror′əfi), an operation that sutures a floating kidney in place.

nephrosclerosis (nef′rouskları′sıs). See **nephroangiosclerosis.**

nephrosis (nefrou′sıs). See **nephrotic syndrome.**

nephrostoma, nephrostome, pl. **nephrostomata, nephrostomes.** the funnel-shaped ciliated opening of the excretory tubules into the coelom of the early developing vertebrate embryo. —**nephrostomic,** adj.

nephrotic syndrome, an abnormal condition of the kidney characterized by marked proteinuria, hypoalbuminemia, and edema. It occurs in glomerular disease, thrombosis of a renal vein, and as a complication of many systemic diseases, diabetes mellitus, amyloidosis, systemic lupus erythematosus, and multiple myeloma. The nephrotic syndrome occurs in a severe, primary form characterized by anorexia, weakness, proteinuria, hypoalbuminuria, and edema. Treatment and prognosis depend on the underlying cause of disease. Patients with primary nephrotic syndrome usually respond favorably to corticosteroids. Diuretics are used to control edema, and dialysis may be necessary. Also called **nephrosis.**

nephrotome, a zone of segmented mesodermal tissue in the developing vertebrate embryo lying along each side of the body dorsal to the abdominal cavity between the somite-forming dorsal mesoderm and the unsegmented lateral-plate mesoderm. It is the primordial tissue for the urogenital system and gives rise to the nephrogenic cord. Also called **intermediate cell mass, intermediate mesoderm, middle plate, nephromere.** See also **mesonephros, metanephros, pronephros.**

nephrotomy, a surgical procedure in which an incision is made in the kidney.

nephrotoxic, toxic or destructive to a kidney.

nephrotoxin, a toxin with specific destructive properties for the kidneys.

Neptazane, a trade name for a carbonic anhydrase inhibitor (methazolamide).

neptunium (Np), a transuranic, metallic element. Its atomic number is 93; its atomic weight is 237. Although neptunium is considered a man-made element, traces of natural neptunium have been found in uranium ores.

nerve, one or more bundles of fibers outside the central nervous system that connect the brain and the spinal cord with other parts of the body. Nerves transmit afferent impulses from receptor organs toward the brain and the spinal cord and efferent impulses peripherally to the effector organs. Each nerve consists of an epineurium enclosing fasciculi of nerve fibers, each fasciculus surrounded by its own sheath of connective tissue. Individual nerve fibers, which are microscopic, consist of formed elements within a matrix of protoplasm and are wrapped in a neurilemmal sheath. Inside the neurilemma are nerve fibers, also enclosed in a myelin sheath, derived from the neurilemmal cells. See also **axon, dendrite, neuroglia, neuron.**

nerve accommodation, the ability of nerve tissue to adjust to a constant source and intensity of stimulation so that some change in either intensity or duration of the stimulus is necessary in order to elicit a response beyond the initial reaction. Accommodation is probably owing to reduced sodium ion permeability, which causes an increased threshold intensity and subsequent stabilization of the resting membrane potential.

nerve block anesthesia. See **conduction anesthesia.**

nerve compression, a pathological event that causes harmful pressure on one or more nerve trunks, resulting in nerve damage and muscle weakness or atrophy. Any nerve that passes over a rigid prominence is vulnerable, and the degree of damage depends on the magnitude and the duration of the compressive force. Various factors may contribute to susceptibility, as inherited predisposition, malnutrition, trauma, and disease. Various activities associated with routine occupations may unduly compress especially vulnerable nerves as the median nerve, the radial nerve, the femoral nerve, and the plantar nerves. Rest and the cessation or modification of causative activities often heal nerve damage owing to compression. Surgery may be required to correct more severe cases. Compare **nerve entrapment.**

nerve entrapment, an abnormal condition and type of mononeuropathy, characterized by nerve damage and muscle weakness or atrophy. The peripheral nerve trunks of the body are especially vulnerable to entrapment in which repeated compression results in significant impairment. Nerves that pass over rigid prominences or through narrow bony and fascial canals are particularly prone to entrapment. The common signs of this disorder are pain and muscular weakness. Nerve damage by entrapment occurs more often when adjacent joints are affected by swelling and inflammation, as in rheumatoid arthritis, pregnancy, and acromegaly. Signs of nerve entrapment may also develop after repeated bruising of certain nerves by various activities involving repeated motions, as those associated with knitting and prolonged walking. One of the most common types of entrapment is **carpal tunnel syndrome.** Compare **nerve compression.**

nerve growth factor (NGF), a protein resembling insulin whose hormonelike action affects differentiation, growth, and maintenance of neurons.

nerve impulse. See **impulse.**

nervous breakdown, *Informal.* any mental condition that markedly interferes with and disrupts normal functioning.

nervous system, the extensive, intricate network of structures that activates, coordinates, and controls all the functions of the body. It is divided into the central nervous system, composed of the brain and the spinal cord, and the peripheral nervous system, which includes the cranial nerves and the spinal nerves. These morphological subdivisions combine and communicate to innervate the somatic and the visceral parts of the body with the afferent and the efferent nerve fibers. Afferent fibers carry sensory impulses to the central nervous system; efferent fibers carry motor impulses from the central nervous system to the muscles and other organs. The somatic fibers are associated with the bones, the muscles, and the skin. The visceral fibers are associated with the internal organs, the blood vessels, and the mucous membranes. Various functions throughout the nervous system are coordinated through a vast complex of tiny structures, as neurons, axons, dendrites, and ganglia. Compare **parasympathetic nervous system, sympathetic nervous system, visceral nervous system.**

nervus abducens. See **abducent nerve.**

nervus accessorius. See **accessory nerve.**

nervus facialis. See **facial nerve.**

nervus glossopharyngeus. See **glossopharyngeal nerve.**

nervus hypoglossus. See **hypoglossal nerve.**

nervus oculomotorius. See **oculomotor nerve.**

nervus olfactorius. See **olfactory nerve.**

nervus opticus. See **optic nerve.**

nervus terminalis. See **terminal nerve.**

nervus trigeminus. See **trigeminal nerve.**

nervus trochlearis. See **trochlear nerve.**

nervus vagus. See **vagus nerve.**

Nesacaine, a trade name for a long-acting local anesthetic (chloroprocaine), used in regional anesthetic block.

nettle rash, a fine, urticarial eruption resulting from skin contact with nettle, a common weed. It is characterized by stinging and itching that lasts from a few minutes to several hours.

networking, 1. (in psychiatric nursing) the process of developing a set of agencies and professional personnel that are able to create a system of communication and support for psychiatric patients, usually those newly discharged from inpatient psychiatric facilities. Kinds of networks include **natural network, professional network. 2.** a network of supportive contacts or services, as the Women's Health Network.

Neufeld nail (noi'felt), an orthopedic nail with a v-shaped tip and shank used for fixating an intertrochanteric fracture. The nail is driven into the neck of the femur until it reaches a round metal plate screwed onto the side of the femur. The nail is secured to a receptacle on the plate. Also called **Neufeld angled nail.**

neur-. See **neuro-.**

neural (nur'əl), of or pertaining to nerve cells and their processes.

-neural, a combining form meaning 'of or relating to a nerve or nerves': *epineural, epithelioneural, myoneural.* Also **-neuric.**

neural canal. See **neurocoele.**

neural crest, the band of ectodermally derived cells that lies along the outer surface of each side of the neural tube in the early stages of embryonic development. The cells migrate laterally throughout the embryo and give rise to certain spinal, cranial, and sympathetic ganglia. Also called **ganglionic crest, ganglionic ridge.** See also **neural tube formation.**

neural ectoderm, the part of the embryonic ectoderm that develops into the neural tube. Also called **neuroderm.** See also **neural tube formation.**

neural fold, either of the paired longitudinal elevations resulting from the invagination of the neural plate in the early developing embryo. The folds unite to enclose the neural groove and form the neural tube. Also called **medullary fold.** See also **neural tube formation.**

neuralgia (nuræl'jə), an abnormal condition characterized by severe stabbing pain, caused by a variety of disorders affecting the nervous system. — **neuralgic,** *adj.*

neural groove, the longitudinal depression that occurs between the neural folds during the invagination of the neural plate to form the neural tube in the early stages of embryonic development. Also called **medullary groove.** See also **neural tube formation.**

neural impulse. See **impulse.**

neural plate, a thick layer of ectodermal tissue that lies along the central longitudinal axis of the early developing embryo and gives rise to the neural tube and subsequently to the brain, spinal cord, and other tissues of the central nervous system. Also called **medullary plate.** See also **neural tube formation.**

neural tube, the longitudinal tube, lying along the central axis of the early developing embryo, that gives rise to the brain, spinal cord, and other neural tissue of the central nervous system. It consists of thick ectodermal tissue and is formed by the fusion of the neural folds, resulting from the invagination of the neural plate. Failure of the tube to close results in a number of congenital defects. Also called **cerebromedullary tube, medullary tube,** See also **neural tube defect, neural tube formation.**

neural tube defect, any of a group of congenital malformations involving defects in the skull and spinal column that are caused primarily by the failure of the neural tube to close during embryonic development. In some instances, the cleft results from an abnormal increase in cerebrospinal fluid pressure on the closed neural tube during the first trimester of development. The defect may occur at any point along the neural axis or extend the entire length of the spinal column, as in holorachischisis. The amount of deformity and disability depends on the degree of neural involvement, the most severe defect being complete cranioschisis, or the total absence of the skull and defective brain development. Other cerebral dysplasias resulting from the failure of the cranial end of the neural tube to fuse are meningoencephalocele and cranial meningocele. These defects, usually accompanied by severe mental and physical disorders, occur most often in the occipital region of the skull but may also occur in the frontal or basal regions. Most neural tube malformations are caused by incomplete fusion of one or more laminae of the vertebral column, with varying degrees of tissue protrusion and neural involvement. Such anomalies include rachischisis, spinal bifida, myelocele, myelomeningocele, and meningocele. In all of these conditions there is constant risk of rupture of the saclike protrusion and danger of meningeal infection. Often, immediate surgical repair is necessary. Many of the major neural tube defects can be determined prenatally by ultrasonic scanning of the uterus and by the presence of elevated concentrations of alpha-fetoprotein levels in the amniotic fluid. Such diagnostic tests are performed during the 14th to 16th week of gestation so that termination of the pregnancy is possible.

neural tube formation, the various processes and stages involved in the embryonic development of the neural tube, which subsequently differentiates into the brain, the spinal cord, and other neural tissue of the central nervous system. The primitive tube originates from a flat, single layer of ectodermal tissue that extends longitudinally along the middorsal line of the embryonic disc from the area of the primitive streak forward to the cephalic extremity. This tissue, called the neural plate, grows rapidly and becomes striated and thickened. The rate of growth is greater along the midplane than at the margin, resulting in the invagination of the cells and formation of a hollow groove, the neural groove, bounded on either side by the elevated neural folds. With continued cell division the groove becomes deeper and the folds thicken so that they eventually meet and fuse, converting the neural groove into the neural tube. The closing of the neural tube occurs first at the midpoint and progresses both toward the caudal and the cephalic regions. At the cephalic end the tube expands into a large vesicle with three subdivisions that differentiate into the forebrain (prosencephalon), the midbrain (mesencephalon), and the hindbrain (rhombencephalon). The epithelium of the wall of the tube develops into the various tissues of the nervous system. The caudal portion of the tube subsequently forms the spinal cord. Along the outer surface of the neural tube is a thin layer of ectodermal cells that extend the entire length of the structure. These primordial cells migrate to other parts of the developing embryo and give rise to cranial and spinal ganglia and to certain cells of the autonomic nervous system. Failure of any part of the neural tube to close during early embryonic development results in a number of congenital defect. See also **neural tube defect.**

neurasthenia (nur′əsˈthi′niə), **1.** an abnormal condition characterized by nervous exhaustion and a vague functional fatigue that often follows depression. **2.** (in psychiatry) a stage in the recovery from a schizophrenic experience, during which the patient is listless and apparently unable to cope with routine activities and relationships. –**neurasthenic,** *adj.*

-neure, a combining form meaning a 'nerve cell': *ganglioneure, myoneure, sporadoneure.* Also **-neuron.**

neurenteric canal (nur′ənterˈik), a tubular passage between the posterior part of the neural tube and the archenteron in the early embryonic development of lower animals. It corresponds to the notochordal canal of man and the higher animals. Also called **archenteric canal, blastoporic canal, Braun's canal.**

-neuria, a combining form meaning a '(specified) condition involving nerves': *acystineuria, ovariodysneuria.*

neurilemma, neurolemma (nur′əlemˈə), a layer of cells composed of one or more Schwann cells that encloses the segmented myelin sheaths of peripheral nerve fibers. Each myelinated nerve fiber has a neurilemma cell for each internodal segment between the nodes of Ranvier. The cell nucleus is a flattened oval that lies in a small depression in the myelin. The nerve fibers of the brain and the spinal cord are not enclosed by neurilemma. Also called **Schwann's sheath.** –**neurilemmal, neurilemmatic, neurilemmatous,** *adj.*

neurilemoma (nur′ɪlɪmouˈmə). See **schwannoma.**

neurinoma (nur′ɪnouˈmə), *pl.* **neurinomas, neurinomata. 1.** a tumor of the nerve sheath. It is usually benign but may undergo malignant change. A kind of neurinoma is **acoustic neurinoma.** See also **schwannoma. 2.** a neuroma.

neuritis (nurai′tɪs), *pl.* **neuritides.** an abnormal condition characterized by inflammation of a nerve. Some of the signs of this condition are neuralgia, hyperthesia, anesthesia, paralysis, muscular atrophy, and defective reflexes.

neuro-, neur-, a combining form meaning 'of or pertaining to nerves': *neuroclonic, neurohormone, neuromast.*

neuroblast, any embryonic cell that develops into a functional neuron; an immature nerve cell. –**neuroblastic,** *adj.*

neuroblastoma (nur′oublæstouˈmə), *pl.* **neuroblastomas, neuroblastomata.** a highly malignant tumor composed of primitive ectodermal cells derived from the neural plate during embryonic life. The tumor may originate in any part of the sympathetic nervous system, but it is most common in the adrenal medulla of young children. Neuroblastomas metastasize early and widely to lymph nodes, liver, lung, and bone. Symptoms may include an abdominal mass, respiratory distress, and anemia, depending on the site of the primary tumor and metastases, and hormonally active adrenal lesions may cause irritability, flushing, sweating, hypertension, and tachycardia. Prior to metastasis, treatment with radical surgery, deep irradiation, and chemotherapy are often successful. Spontaneous remissions may occur with the tumor undergoing maturation and forming a benign ganglioneuroma. A kind of neuroblastoma is **Pepper syndrome.**

neurocele. See **neurocoele.**

neurocentral, pertaining to the centrum and the developing vertebrae in the early stages of embryology.

neurocentrum, the embryonic mesodermal tissue that subsequently gives rise to the vertebrae. See also **sclerotome.**

neuro check, *Nontechnical.* a brief neurologic assessment, usually performed in the triage of patients in an emergency situation or on admission to an emergency service. The level of consciousness is evaluated as alert and oriented, lethargic, stuporous, or comatose. The movements of the extremities are determined to be voluntary or involuntary. The color, temperature, and turgor of the skin are noted. The pupils of the eyes are observed for equality of dilation, reactivity to light, and ability to accommodate. See also **neurologic assessment.**

neurocirculatory asthenia, a psychosomatic disorder characterized by nervous and circulatory irregularities, including dyspnea, palpitation, giddiness, vertigo, tremor, precordial pain, and increased susceptibility to fatigue. The symptoms often result from or are associated with psychological stress.

neurocoele, neurocele, neurocoel (nur′əsil), a system of cavities in the central nervous system of man and other vertebrate animals. It consists of the ventricles of the brain and the central canal of the spinal cord, which originate from the neural tube during early embryonic development. Also called **neural canal.**

neurocytoma (nu′rousaitouˈmə), a tumor composed of undifferentiated nerve cells that are usually ganglionic. Also called **neuroma.**

neuroderm. See **neuroectoderm.** –**neurodermal,** *adj.*

neurodermatitis (nur′oudər′mətai′tis), a nonspecific, pruritic skin disorder seen in anxious, nervous individuals. Excoriations and lichenification are found on easily accessible, exposed areas of the body such as the forearms and forehead. Sometimes loosely (and incorrectly) applied to **atopic dermatitis**.

neuroectoderm, the part of the embryonic ectoderm that gives rise to the central and peripheral nervous systems, including some glial cells. — **neuroectodermal,** *adj.*

neuroepithelial tumor (nur′ouep′ıfhi′liəl). See **neuroepithelioma**.

neuroepithelioma (nu′rouep′ıfhi′liou′mə). An uncommon neoplasm of neuroepithelium in a sensory nerve. Also called **neuroepithelial tumor**.

neurofibroma (nur′oufæıbrou′mə), *pl.* **neurofibromas, neurofibromata.** a fibrous tumor of nerve tissue resulting from the abnormal proliferation of Schwann cells. Multiple growths of this type in the peripheral nervous system are often associated with extensive abnormalities in other tissues. See also **neurofibromatosis**.

neurofibromatosis (nur′oufaı′broumətou′sis), a congenital condition transmitted as an autosomal dominant trait, characterized by numerous neurofibromas of the nerves and skin, by café-au-lait spots on the skin, and, in some cases, by developmental anomalies of the muscles, bones, and viscera. Many large, pedunculated soft-tissue tumors may develop, as exemplified by the "Elephant Man." Bone changes may result in skeletal deformities, especially curvature of the spine. Neurofibromas may develop in the alimentary tract, bladder, endocrine glands, and cranial nerves. The disorder occurs in one of 2,500 to 3,000 live births; sometimes it is associated with meningocele, spina bifida, or epilepsy. Also called **multiple neuroma, neuromatosis, von Recklinghausen's disease.**

neurogen (nur′ojen), **1.** See **neurotransmitter. 2.** a substance within the early developing embryo that stimulates the primary organizer to initiate the formation of the neural plate, which gives rise to the primary axis of the body.

neurogenesis, the development of the tissue of the nervous system. — **neurogenetic,** *adj.*

neurogenic arthropathy, an abnormal condition associated with neural damage, characterized by the gradual and usually painless degeneration of a joint. One of the major causes of this condition is believed to be a minor injury which is disregarded by the affected individual because of a lack of sensation in the injured tissue. Inadequate rest and care aggravate such injuries and prevent proper healing. See also **Charcot's joint.**

neurogenic bladder, dysfunctional urinary bladder caused by lesion of the nervous system. Treatment is aimed at enabling the bladder to empty completely and regularly, preventing infection, controlling incontinence, and preserving kidney function. Kinds of neurogenic bladder are **spastic bladder, reflex bladder, flaccid bladder.** Also called **neuropathic bladder.**

neurogenic fracture, a fracture resulting from the destruction of the nerve supply to a specific bone.

neuroglia (nurog′liə), one of the two main kinds of cells comprising the nervous system. It performs the less specialized functions of the nerve network. Kinds of neuroglia include **astrocytes, oligodendroglia, microglia.** Compare **neuron.** — **neuroglial,** *adj.*

neurohormonal regulation, regulation of the function of an organ or a gland by the combined effect of neurologic and hormonal activity.

neurohumor (nur′ouhyu′mər), one of the chemical substances, formed and transmitted by a neuron, that is essential for the activity of adjacent neurons or nearby organs or muscles. Kinds of neurohumoral substances are **acetylcholine, dopamine, epinephrine, norepinephrine, serotonin.** — **neurohumoral,** *adj.*

neurohypophyseal hormone, a hormone secreted by the posterior pituitary gland. Kinds of neurohypophyseal hormones are **oxytocin, vasopressin.** See also **pituitary gland.**

neurohypophysis (nur′ouhaıpof′ısis), the posterior lobe of the pituitary gland that is the source of antidiuretic hormore (ADH) and oxytocin. Nervous stimulation controls the release of both substances into the blood. The neurohypophysis releases ADH when stimulated by the hypothalamus by an increase in the osmotic pressure of extracellular fluid in the body. The hormone acts on the cells in the distal and the collecting tubules of the kidneys, making them more permeable to water and reducing the volume of urine. The neurohypophysis releases oxytocin under appropriate stimulation from the hypothalamus. Oxytocin produces powerful contractions of the pregnant uterus and causes milk to flow from lactating breasts. Stimulation of the nipples of the breast by a nursing infant triggers the release of this hormone. Also called **posterior pituitary gland.** Compare **adenohypophysis.**

neurolemma. See **neurilemma.**

neurolepsis, an altered state of consciousness, as induced by a neuroleptic agent, characterized by quiescence, reduced motor activity and anxiety and by indifference to the surroundings. Sleep may occur, but usually the person can be roused and can respond to commands. Drugs that produce neurolepsis may be administered with a narcotic analgesic to produce neurolept analgesia, or with an anesthetic to produce neurolept anesthesia.

neurolept. See **neuroleptic.**

neurolept analgesia, a form of analgesia achieved by the concurrent administration of a neuroleptic and an analgesic. Anxiety, motor activity, and sensitivity to painful stimuli are reduced; the person is quiet and indifferent to the environment and surroundings. Sleep may or may not occur, but the patient is not unconscious and is able to respond to commands. If nitrous oxide in oxygen is also administered, neurolept analgesia can be converted to neurolept anesthesia. Droperidol and fentynal are often administered together to achieve neurolept anesthesia.

neurolept anesthesia, a form of anesthesia achieved by the administration of a neuroleptic agent, a narcotic analgesic, and nitrous oxide in oxygen. Induction of anesthesia is slow, but consciousness returns quickly after the inhalation of nitrous oxide is stopped.

neuroleptic, neurolept, 1. of or pertaining to neurolepsis. 2. a drug that causes neurolepsis, as the butyrophenone derivative, droperidol.

neurologic assessment, an evaluation of the patient's neurologic status and symptoms.

■ METHOD: If alert and orientated, the patient is asked about instances of weakness, numbness, headaches, pain, tremors, nervousness, irritability, or drowsiness. Information is elicited regarding loss of memory, periods of confusion, hallucinations, and episodes of loss of consciousness. The patient's general appearance, facial expression, attention span, responses to verbal and painful stimuli, emotional status, coordination, balance, cognition, and ability to follow commands are noted. If the patient is disoriented, stuporous, or comatose, demonstrated signs of these states are recorded. Observations are made of the skin color and temperature, pupillary size, equality, dilation, and reactions to light, the respiratory rate, rhythm, and quality, as well as of chest movements and breath sounds. The pulse is checked; the ears and nose are examined for possible drainage; the strength of the handgrip is tested; and the extremities' sensations, voluntary and involuntary motions are assessed. The urinary output is determined for evidence of polyuria and the patient's speech is evaluated for signs of slurring and aphasia. Included in the record are concurrent diseases, as hypertension, cancer, and coarctation of the aorta, past illnesses associated with head trauma, seizures, motor, sensory, or emotional disturbances, loss of consciousness, and neurologic, medical or surgical procedures. Pertinent to the assessment are the patient's sleep pattern, medication, personality changes, relationships with family and friends, and a family history of seizures, stroke, mental illness, tumors, or sudden death. Diagnostic aids that may be required for a complete evaluation are a lumbar puncture, complete blood count, myelogram, echoencephalogram, brain scan, computerized tomogram and determinations of glucose, fluid, and electrolyte levels.

■ NURSING ORDERS: The nurse may conduct the interview to obtain subjective data, examines the patient, and assembles the pertinent background information and the results of the diagnostic tests.

■ OUTCOME CRITERIA: A careful neurologic assessment is an important aid to the neurologist in establishing a diagnosis and the course of treatment.

neurologic examination, a systematic examination of the nervous system, inducing an assessment of mental status, of the function of each of the cranial nerves, of sensory and neuromuscular function, of the reflexes, and of proprioception and other cerebellar functions.

neurologist, a physician who specializes in neurology.

neurology (nurol'əji), the field of medicine that deals with the nervous system and its disorders. — **neurologic, neurological,** *adj.* **neurologist,** *n.*

neuroma (nurou'mə), *pl.* **neuromas, neuromata.** a benign neoplasm composed chiefly of neurons and nerve fibers, usually arising from a nerve tissue. It may be relatively soft or extremely hard and vary in size from 1 to 15 or more centimeters. Pain radiating from the lesion to the periphery of the affected nerve is usually intermittent but may become continuous and severe. Kinds of neuromas include **acoustic neuroma, cystic neuroma, false neuroma, multiple neuroma, myelinic neuroma, neuroma cutis, nevoid neuroma, traumatic neuroma.**

-neuroma, a combining form meaning a 'tumor made up of nerve cells and fibers': *angiomyoneuroma, inoneuroma, myoneuroma.*

neuroma cutis, a neoplasm in the skin that contains nerve tissue and that may be extremely sensitive to painful stimuli.

neuroma telangiectodes. See **nevoid neuroma.**

neuromatosis (nur'oumətou'sis), a neoplastic disease characterized by numerous neuromas. Also called **multiple neuroma.** See also **neurofibromatosis.**

neuromuscular (nur'oumən'kyulər), of or pertaining to the nerves and the muscles.

neuromuscular blocking agent, a chemical substance that interferes locally with the transmission or reception of impulses from motor nerves to skeletal muscles. Nondepolarizing agents, as metocurine, pancuronium, and tubocurarine, competitively block the transmitter action of acetylcholine at the postjunctional membrane. Depolarizing blocking agents, as succinylcholine chloride, compete with acetylcholine for cholinergic receptors of the motor end plate. Neuromuscular blocking agents are used to induce muscle relaxation in anesthesia, endotracheal intubation, and electroshock therapy and as adjuncts in the treatment of tetanus, encephalitis, and poliomyelitis. Neuromuscular blocking drugs can cause bronchospasm, hyperthermia, hypotension, or respiratory paralysis and are used with caution, especially in patients with myasthenia gravis, renal, hepatic, or pulmonary impairment, and in elderly and debilitated individuals. See also **muscle relaxant.**

neuromuscular junction, the area of contact between the ends of a large myelinated nerve fiber and a fiber of skeletal muscle. Also called **myoneural junction.** See also **motor end plate, myelin, nerve.**

neuromuscular spindle, any one of a number of small bundles of delicate muscular fibers, enclosed by a capsule, in which sensory nerve fibers terminate. The spindles vary in length from 0.8 to 5 mm, accommodating as many as four large myelinated nerve fibers which pierce the capsule and lose their myelin sheaths. The nerve fibers end as naked axons encircling the intrafusal fibers with flattened expansions or ovoid disks.

neuromyal transmission, the passage of excitation from a motor neuron to a muscle fiber at the myoneural junction.

neuromyelitis (nʊr'oʊmaɪ'əlaɪ'tɪs), an abnormal condition characterized by inflammation of the spinal cord and peripheral nerves.

neuron, neurone (nʊr'on), the basic nerve cell of the nervous system, containing a nucleus within a cell body and extending one or more processes. Neurons are classified according to the direction in which they conduct impulses and according to the number of processes they extend. Sensory neurons transmit nerve impulses to the spinal cord and the brain. Motor neurons transmit nerve impulses from the brain and the spinal cord to the muscles and the glandular tissue. Multipolar neurons, the bipolar neurons, and the unipolar neurons are classified according to the number of processes they extend to the different kinds of neurons. Multipolar neurons have one axon and several dendrites, as do most of the neurons in the brain and the spinal cord. Bipolar neurons, which are less numerous than the other types, have only one axon and one dendrite. Unipolar neurons are embryonic structures which originate as bipolar bodies but fuse dendrites and axons into a single fiber that stretches for a short distance from the cell body before separating again into the two processes. All neurons have at least one axon and one or more dendrites and have a slightly gray color when clustered, as in the brain and the spinal cord. As the carriers of nerve impulses, neurons function according to electrochemical processes involving positively charged sodium and potassium ions and the changing electrical potential of the extracellular and the intracellular fluid of the neuron.

-neuron. See **-neure.**

neuronitis (nʊr'ənaɪ'tɪs), an abnormal condition characterized by inflammation of a nerve or a nerve cell, especially the cells and the roots of the spinal nerves.

neuropathic bladder. See **neurogenic bladder.**

neuropathic joint disease, a chronic, progressive, degenerative disease of one or more joints, characterized by swelling, instability of the joint, hemorrhage, heat, and atrophic and hypertrophic changes in the bone. Pain is usually less severe than would be expected by the appearance of the joint on an x-ray film. The disease is the result of an underlying neurologic disorder, as tabes dorsalis from syphilis, diabetic neuropathy, leprosy, or congenital absence or depression of pain sensation. Early recognition of the disease and prophylactic protection of the joint may prevent further damage in some cases. Surgical reconstruction is not usually effective because healing is slow. Amputation may be necessary. Also called **Charcot's joint.**

neuropathy (nʊrop'əfhi), any abnormal condition characterized by inflammation and degeneration of the peripheral nerves, as that associated with lead poisoning. —**neuropathic,** *adj.*

neuroplegia (nʊr'oʊpli'jiə), nerve paralysis owing to disease, injury, or the effect of neuroleptic drugs, administered to achieve **neurolept analgesia** or **neurolept anesthesia.** See also **lytic cocktail.**

neuropore, the opening at each end of the neural tube during early embryonic development. The closure of these apertures as the tube grows and differentiates occurs with such precision that they are used to indicate horizons XI and XII in the systematic anatomical charting of human embryonic development. Kinds of neuropores are **anterior neuropore, posterior neuropore.** See also **horizon, neural tube formation.**

neurosarcoma (nʊr'oʊsarkoʊ'mə), a malignant neoplasm composed of nerve tissue, connective tissue, and vascular tissue. Also called **malignant neuroma.**

neurosis, **1.** any faulty or inefficient way of coping with anxiety or inner conflict, usually involving the use of an unconscious defense mechanism, that may ultimately lead to a neurotic disorder. **2.** *Informal.* an emotional disturbance other than psychosis. See also **neurotic disorder, neurotic process.**

-neurosis, a combining form meaning a 'disease of the nerves' or a 'mental disorder': *angioneurosis, psychoneurosis, synneurosis.*

neurosurgery, any surgery involving the brain, spinal cord, or peripheral nerves. Brain surgery is performed to treat a wound, remove a tumor or foreign body, relieve pressure in intracranial hemorrhage, excise an abcess, treat Parkinsonism, or relieve pain. Before surgery skull x rays and a ventriculogram or an arteriogram may be taken; a diagnostic electroencephalogram, lumbar tap, or brain scan may be necessary. A blood type and crossmatch is done. Parenteral corticosteroids are given if cerebral edema is present, and urea may be given to reduce intracranial pressure. Narcotics and hypnotics are avoided, and the nurse must confirm any that are ordered. No enemas are given. Light general or local anesthesia is used, occasionally with hypothermia. After surgery, the nurse observes carefully both vital signs and changes in the level of consciousness, speech, and strength. Any yellowish drainage from the wound may be cerebrospinal fluid and is reported immediately. Sterile dressing technique is essential. Kinds of brain surgery include craniotomy, lobotomy, hypophysectomy. Surgery of the spine is performed to correct a defect, remove a tumor, repair a ruptured intervertebral disc, or relieve pain. Before surgery x rays are taken and a blood type and cross-match is done. General anesthesia or a spinal block is used. After surgery, the nurse keeps the bed flat and the patient's spine in good alignment. Return of sensation and motor function are monitored carefully. Kinds of spinal surgery include fusion, laminectomy. Surgery on the peripheral nerves is performed to remove a tumor, relieve pain, or reconnect a severed nerve. Local anesthesia is used. After surgery, the nurse observes closely the return of sensation to the area. One kind of nerve surgery is **sympathectomy**.

neurosyphilis (nur'ousıf'əlıs), infection of the central nervous system by syphilis organisms, which may invade the meninges and cerebrovascular system. If the brain tissue is affected, general paresis may result; if the spinal cord is infected, tabes dorsalis may result. See also **syphilis,** *Treponema pallidum.* – **neurosyphiltic,** *adj.*

neurotendinous spindle, a capsule containing enlarged tendon fibers, found chiefly near the junctions of tendons and muscles. One or more nerve fibers pierce the side of the capsule and lose their medullary sheaths; the axons subdivide and terminate between the tendon fibers in irregular discs or varicosities. Also called **organ of Golgi.**

neurotic, 1. of or pertaining to neurosis or to a neurotic disorder. 2. pertaining to the nerves. 3. one who is afflicted with a neurosis. 4. *Informal.* an emotionally unstable person.

-neurotic, 1. a combining form meaning 'pertaining to a (specified) abnormal condition of the nerves': *angioneurotic, aponeurotic, vasoneurotic.* 2. a combining form meaning 'pertaining to (psycho)neurosis': *hyperneurotic, psychoneurotic, unneurotic.*

neurotic disorder, any mental disorder characterized by a symptom or group of symptoms that a person finds distressing, unacceptable, and alien to his personality, as severe anxiety, obsessional thoughts, and compulsive acts, and that produces psychological pain or discomfort disproportionate to the reality of the situation. Although the person's ability to function may be markedly impaired, his behavior generally remains within acceptable social norms and his perception of reality is unaffected. There is no proof of organic cause. The disturbance is relatively long-lasting, cannot be considered simply a reaction to stress, and may recur if untreated. Kinds of neurotic disorders include **anxiety neurosis, compulsive-obsessive neurosis, psychosexual disorder, somatoform disorder.** See also **neurosis, neurotic process.**

neurotic illness. See **neurotic disorder.**

neurotic process, (in psychology) a process in which unconscious conflicts lead to feelings of anxiety. Defense mechanisms are employed to avoid these uncomfortable feelings, and personality disturbance and the symptoms of neurosis ensue.

neurotoxic (nur'outok'sık), having a poisonous effect on nerves and nerve cells, as when ingested lead degenerates peripheral nerves.

neurotoxin (nur'outok'sın), a toxin that acts directly on the tissues of the central nervous system, traveling along the axis cylinders of the motor nerves to the brain. The toxin may be secreted in the venom of certain snakes, or it may be present on the spines of a shell or in the flesh of fish or shellfish; it may be produced by certain bacteria or by the cellular disintegration of certain bacteria.

neurotransmitter (nur'outrænz'mıtər), any one of numerous chemicals that modify or result in the transmission of nerve impulses between synapses. Neurotransmitters are released from synaptic knobs into synaptic clefts and bridge the gap between presynaptic and postsynaptic neurons. Each vesicle within a synaptic knob stores as many as 10,000 neurotransmitter molecules. When a nerve impulse reaches a synaptic knob, thousands of neurotransmitter molecules squirt into the synaptic cleft and bind to specific receptors. This flow allows an associated diffusion of potassium and sodium ions which causes an action potential. Excitatory neurotransmitters decrease the negativity of postsynaptic membrane potentials; inhibitory neurotransmitters increase such potentials. Kinds of neurotransmitters include **acetylcholine, gamma-aminobutyric acid, norepinephrine.**

neurula (nur'ələ), *pl.* **neurulas, neurulae.** an early embryo during the period of neurulation when the nervous system tissue begins to differentiate. The embryo at this level of growth represents a third stage in embryonic development, following the morula and blastocyst stages in man and the higher animals and the blastula and gastrula stages in lower animals. In man, the neurula stage occurs from about 19 to 26 days after fertilization.

neurulation, the development of the neural plate and the processes involved with its subsequent closure to form the neural tube during the early stages of embryonic development. See also **neural tube formation.**

neutral, the state exactly between two opposing values, qualities, or properties, as, in electricity, a neutral state is one in which there is neither a positive nor a negative charge or, in chemistry, a neutral state is one in which a substance is neither acid nor alkaline. See also **acid, base, pH.**

neutralization, the interaction between an acid and a base that produces a solution that is neither acidic nor basic. The usual products of neutralization are a salt and water.

neutral thermal environment, an environment created by any method or apparatus to maintain the normal body temperature in order to minimize oxygen consumption and caloric expenditure, as in an incubator or Isolette for a premature, sick, or low-birth-weight infant. See also **incubator, Isolette.**

neutron, (in physics) an elementary particle that is a constituent of the nuclei of all elements except hydrogen. It has no electrical charge and is approximately the same size as a proton.

neutron activation analysis, the analysis of elements in a specimen, performed by exposing it to neutron irradiation to convert many elements to a radioactive form in which they can be identified by measuring their emissions of radiation. The method is applicable, to a limited extent, to human and animal studies.

neutropenia (nu'trɔupi'niə), an abnormal decrease in the number of neutrophils in the blood. The decrease may be relative or absolute. Neutropenia is associated with acute leukemia, infection, rheumatoid arthritis, vitamin B_{12} deficiency, and chronic splenomegaly. Compare **leukopenia.** See also **neutrophil.**

neutrophil (nu'trəfil), a polymorphonuclear granular leukocyte that stains easily with neutral dyes. Its nucleus, which stains dark blue, contains three to five lobes connected by slender threads of chromatin; its cytoplasm contains fine, inconspicuous granules. Neutrophils are the circulating white blood cells essential for phagocytosis and proteolysis in which bacteria, cellular debris, and solid particles are removed and destroyed. An increase in neutrophils is the most common form of leukocytosis and may result from many causes, including acute infection, intoxication, hemorrhage, and malignant neoplastic disease. See also **granulocyte, neutrophilic leukocyte, polymorphonuclear leukocyte.**

neutrophilic leukemia. See **polymorphocytic leukemia.**

nevoid amentia (ni'void). See **Sturge-Weber syndrome.**

nevoid neuroma, a tumor of nerve tissue that contains numerous small blood vessels. Also called **neuroma telangiectodes.**

nevus (ni'vəs), a pigmented, congenital skin blemish that is usually benign but, rarely, may become cancerous. Any change in color, size, or texture, or any bleeding or itching of a nevus deserves investigation. Also called **birthmark, mole.** See also **blue nevus, junction nevus, nevus flammeus.**

nevus flammeus (nev'əs flæm'iəs), a flat, capillary hemangioma that is present at birth and that varies in color from pale red to deep reddish purple. It is most commonly seen on the occiput and rarely causes any problems. If the lesion is on any other part of the body, it tends to be darker colored and, unlike the scalp lesions, does not regress spontaneously. These lesions are most often seen on the face. The depth of the color depends on whether the superficial, middle, or deep dermal vessels are involved. On the face, the lesion persists and develops a thick verrucous nodular surface. Nevus flammeus is usually unilateral, following the distribution of a cutaneous nerve. If the lesion is on the middle of the face, Sturge-Weber disease is suspected. Treatment is not often satisfactory. Cosmetic creams are used to cover the lesion and electrodessication or cryotherapy is sometimes performed, especially to improve the verrucous surface appearance. Laser therapy may eventually offer the best results, but, to date, it is an experimental treatment. Also called **port-wine stain.**

newborn, 1. recently born. 2. a recently born infant; neonate.

newborn intrapartal care, care of the newborn in the delivery area during the time after birth before the mother and infant are transferred to the postpartum unit.

■ METHOD: The nasopharynx and mouth may be suctioned to remove excess mucus as the head is born. Depending on the preference and the condition of the mother and the policies of the maternity service, the baby may then be placed on the mother's abdomen and covered with a warm, dry blanket or taken by the nurse to an infant warmer. Apgar scores are assigned at one minute of age and at five minutes of age; less commonly, another is assigned at 10 minutes of age. The baby is handled gently and quietly; bright lights are often avoided, and maternal contact is encouraged.

■ NURSING CONSIDERATIONS: The nurse is usually the first person to observe and examine the baby. Most newborns are healthy and normal; if abnormal function is observed expert assistance may be summoned as emergency measures, including tracheal suction with a deLee mucous trap and administration of oxygen by ventilator or mask, are initiated. If there are no problems the nurse may instill silver nitrate drops in the conjunctival sacs of the eyes, trim and clamp the umbilical cord, administer an injection of vitamin K, obtain footprints for identification, and diaper and wrap the baby. If the baby needs to be transferred to a nursery or special care facility, the nurse accompanies the infant and acts as the initial liaison for the mother with the nursery.

■ OUTCOME: Most infants born at term are healthy and do not need any medical intervention. Hemorrhage from the umbilical cord, difficult respiration, imperforate anus, endocrine dysfunction, and various other abnormal conditions may occur, but if a baby has good color, is alert, can cry and suck, urinate, defecate, and respond to sound and light, the nurse may reassure the mother that the baby is almost invariably healthy and normal. The individuality of each infant is remarkable and may be pointed out to the mother.

new drug, a drug for which the Food and Drug Administration requires premarketing approval. A new drug is generally regarded as one for which safety and effectiveness has not yet been demonstrated for its prescribed use.

New England Journal of Medicine (*NEJM*), a professional medical journal that publishes findings of medical research and articles about controversial political and ethical issues in the practice of medicine.

new growth, a neoplasm or tumor.

New World leishmaniasis. See **American leishmaniasis.**

new world typhus. See **typhus.**

Nezelof's syndrome (nez'əlofs), an abnormal condition characterized by absent T-cell function, deficient B-cell function, fairly normal immunoglobulin levels, and little or no specific antibody production. The cause of Nezelof's syndrome is unknown. It affects both male and female siblings, indicating the possibility of a genetic disorder transmitted as an autosomal recessive trait, but not all individuals with this disease have a positive family history. The disease may be caused by a cytogenic dysfunction of the stem cells, resulting in deficiencies of T-cells and B-cells. Another theory is that the disorder is caused by underdevelopment of the thymus gland and the consequent inhibition of T-cell development. Still another holds that the disease results from the failure to produce or to secrete thymic humoral factors, especially thymosin.

■ OBSERVATIONS: Nezelof's syndrome causes progressively severe, recurrent, and eventually fatal infections. Signs that often appear in infants or in children up to four years of age include recurrent pneumonia, otitis media, chronic fungal infections, upper respiratory tract infections, diarrhea, and hepatosplenomegaly. The disease may also enlarge the lymph nodes and the tonsils. These structures may also be totally absent in infants with the disease. Involved patients may also develop a tendency toward malignancy. Infection may cause sepsis, which is the usual cause of death. Symptoms that often suggest Nezelof's syndrome also include weight loss and poor eating habits. Definite diagnostic evidence of the disease includes defective B-cell and T-cell immunity despite a normal number of circulating B cells, a moderate to high rise in the number of T cells, a deficiency or an increase in one or more immunoglobulins, a nonreactive Schick test after DPT immunization, a reduced or an absent antibody reaction after specific antigen immunization, no thymus shadow on a chest x ray, thymus-dependent regions with abnormal lymphoid structure, and a decrease in the number of lymphocytes in the blood.

■ INTERVENTION: Initial supportive treatment of Nezelof's syndrome may include monthly injections of gamma globulin or monthly infusions of fresh frozen plasma and the heavy use of antibiotics to fight infection. The plasma infusions are especially beneficial if the patient cannot produce specific immunoglobulins. Cell-mediated immune function associated with T cells can usually be temporarily restored within weeks by a fetal thymus transplant. Repeated transplants are required to maintain the immunity. Cell-mediated immunity can be only partially restored with either transfer factor therapy or repeated injection of thymosin. Histocompatible bone marrow transplants have been used in treating this disease, but effective evaluation of this treatment method is incomplete.

■ NURSING CONSIDERATIONS: The nursing role in treating this disease is essentially supportive. The injection site for gamma globulin in a large muscle mass is massaged after the injection, and injection sites are rotated and recorded to prevent tissue damage. Gamma globulin doses greater than 1.5 ml are divided and injected into more than one site. The nursing role is also one of instruction and support for the parents of children affected by Nezelof's syndrome. Nurses commonly instruct parents on how to recognize the signs of infection and explain the dangers of allowing the affected child to become exposed to infection.

N.F., abbreviation for *National Formulary.*

NGF, abbreviation for **nerve growth factor.**

NGU, abbreviation for **nongonococcal urethritis.**

NHSC, abbreviation for **National Health Service Corps.**

Ni, symbol for **nickel.**

niacin (naï'əsin), a white, crystalline, water-soluble vitamin of the B complex group usually occurring in various plant and animal tissues as nicotinamide. It functions as a coenzyme necessary for the breakdown and utilization of all major nutrients and is essential for a healthy skin, normal functioning of the gastrointestinal tract, maintenance of the nervous system, and synthesis of the sex hormones. It may also be effective in improving circulation and reducing high blood cholesterol levels. Rich dietary sources of both niacin and its precursor tryptophan are meats, poultry, fish, liver, kidney, eggs, nuts, peanut butter, brewer's yeast, and wheat germ. Symptoms of deficiency include muscular weakness, general fatigue, loss of appetite, various skin eruptions, halitosis, stomatitis, insomnia, irritability, nausea, vomiting, recurring headaches, tender gums, tension, and depression. Severe deficiency results in pellagra. The vitamin is not stored in the body and any excess in the diet is excreted. Also called **nicotinic acid.** See also **pellagra.**

N.I.C.H.H.D., abbreviation for **National Institute of Child Health and Human Development.**

nick, (in molecular genetics) a fissure or split in a single strand of DNA that can be made with the enzyme deoxyribonuclease or with ethidium bromide.

nickel (Ni), a silvery-white metallic element. Its atomic number is 28; its atomic weight is 58.71. Large numbers of people are allergic to nickel. Nickel causes more cases of allergic contact dermatitis than all other metals combined. Many cases occur from exposure to jewelry, coins, buckles, and snaps and to continued use of "carbonless" business forms. Nickel carbonyl, a volatile liquid, may produce serious lung damage if inhaled. See also **contact dermatitis.**

nickel dermatitis, an allergic contact dermatitis owing to the metal, nickel. Exposure comes usually from jewelry, wristwatches, metal clasps, and coins. Sweating increases the degree of rash. Treatment includes avoidance of exposure to nickel and reduction of perspiration. See also **contact dermatitis.**

nick translation, a method of labeling DNA in the laboratory by using the enzyme DNA polymerase.

niclosamide (nɪklou′səmaɪd), an anthelmintic prescribed in the treatment of tapeworm infestations. It is currently classified as an investigational drug and is available from the Center for Disease Control. Also called **Yomesan.**

Nicobid, a trade name for two coenzymes (niacin and niacinamide), used as a vitamin supplement.

Niconyl, a trade name for an antibacterial (isoniazid).

nicotinamide. See **niacinamide.**

nicotine, a colorless, rapidly acting toxic substance in tobacco that is one of the major contributors to the ill effects of smoking. It is used as an insecticide in agriculture and as a parasiticide in veterinary medicine. Ingestion of large amounts causes salivation, nausea, vomiting, diarrhea, headache, vertigo, slowing of the heartbeat and, in acute cases, paralysis of respiratory muscles. Treatment includes gastric lavage with a weak solution of potassium permanganate, followed by activated charcoal, and the administration of artificial respiration and oxygen, as needed. Pentobarbitol is used to control convulsions, ephedrine for hypotension, and autonomic blocking agents to control visceral symptoms.

nicotine poisoning, poisoning from intake of nicotine. Nicotine poisoning is characterized by stimulation of the central and autonomic nervous systems followed by depression of these systems. In fatal cases, death occurs from respiratory failure.

nicotinic acid. See **niacin.**

nicotinyl alcohol (nɪk′ɔti′nəl), an alcohol used as a vasodilator, in the form of its tartrate salt, in the treatment of peripheral vascular disease, vascular spasm, varicose ulcers, decubital ulcers, chilblains, Ménière's syndrome, and vertigo.

NICU, abbreviation for **neonatal intensive care unit.**

nidation (naɪdei′ʃən), the process by which an embryo burrows into the endometrium of the uterus. Also called **implantation.** See also **placenta, uterus.**

Niemann-Pick disease (ni′manpɪk′), an inherited disorder of lipid metabolism in which there are accumulations of sphingomyelin in the bone marrow, spleen, and lymph nodes. The disease, which in the United States and Canada is most common among Jewish people, begins in infancy or childhood and is characterized by enlargement of liver and spleen, anemia, lymphadenopathy, and progressive mental and physical deterioration. There is no effective treatment, and children with the disease usually die within a few years of the onset of symptons.

night blindness, an abnormal reduction in vision in darkness, resulting from a decreased synthesis of rhodopsin, vitamin A deficiency, retinal degeneration, or a congenital defect. Also called **nyctalopia.**

Nightingale, Florence (1820–1910), the founder of modern nursing. After limited formal training in nursing in Germany and Paris, she became superintendent in 1853 of a small hospital in London. Her outstanding success in reorganizing the hospital led to a request by the British government to head a mission to the Crimea, where Britain was fighting a war with Russia. She arrived in November, 1854, with 38 nurses to find 5000 men crowded into dilapidated buildings, filthy, mostly without beds, lacking adequate food and medical supplies. Through superhuman efforts, often working 20 hours on the wards and then sending off a stream of letters to England to obtain money and supplies and to mobilize the government to act, she brought order out of chaos. After her return to England, in 1856, she wrote *Notes on Hospitals* and *Notes on Nursing* and founded a training school for nurses at St. Thomas' Hospital, where she attracted well-educated, dedicated women. The graduates became matrons of the most important hospitals in Great Britain, thus raising the standards of nursing across the nation and eventually around the world. Although she was, by now, bedridden much of the time, she carried on her work on the sanitary reform of India, conducted a study of midwifery, helped to establish visiting nurse service, and worked for the reform of the poor laws in which she proposed separate institutions for the sick, the insane, the incurable, and children. After Longfellow wrote *Santa Filomena,* she became known as "The Lady with The Lamp," and the Nightingale Pledge, named after her, embodies her ideals and has inspired thousands of young graduating nurses.

Nightingale ward, a kind of hospital ward designed by Florence Nightingale, that revolutionized hospital design. The number of beds allowed in a ward of given size was limited to permit the circulation of air and for general cleanliness and the comfort of patients. Three sides of the ward were windowed to admit light and fresh air. Although multiple-bed wards are now obsolete in hospital design, the concerns and the benefits that impelled Miss Nightingale to create them remain central to hospital planning.

nightmare, a dream occurring during rapid eye movement sleep that arouses feelings of intense, inescapable fear, terror, distress, or extreme anxiety and that usually awakens the sleeper. Compare **pavor nocturnus, sleep terror disorder.**

night vision, a capacity to see dimly lit objects. It stems from a chemophysical phenomenon associated with the retinal rods. The rods contain the highly light-sensitive chemical rhodopsin, or visual purple, which is essential for the conduction of optic impulses in subdued light.

Night vision is sharpest at the periphery of the retina because of the concentration of rods. Night vision may be diminished by a deficiency of vitamin A, an important component of rhodopsin.

nigrites linguae. See **parasitic glossitis.**

N.I.H., abbreviation for **National Institutes of Health.**

nihilistic delusion, a persistent denial of the existence of particular things or of everything, including oneself, as seen in various forms of schizophrenia. A person who has such a delusion may believe that he lives in a shadow or limbo world or that he died several years ago and that only his spirit, in a vaporous form, really exists. See also **delusion.**

nikethamide (naiketh'əmaid), a central nervous system stimulant.

■ INDICATIONS: It is prescribed as an analeptic in the treatment of depression of the central nervous and respiratory systems.

■ CONTRAINDICATION: Known hypersensitivity to this drug prohibits its use.

■ ADVERSE EFFECTS: Among the most serious adverse reactions at high doses are tachycardia, hypertension, muscle spasm, and convulsions. Burning and itching are common.

Nikolsky's sign (nɪkol'skiz), easy separation of the epidermis from the basal cell layer by rubbing apparently normal skin areas; found in phemphigus and a few other bullous diseases.

Nilstat, a trade name for an antifungal (nystatin).

90-90 traction. See **traction, 90-90.**

ninth nerve. See **glossopharyngeal nerve.**

niobium (Nb), a silver-gray metallic element. Its atomic number is 41; its atomic weight is 92.906. Formerly called **columbium.**

nipple, a small cylindrical, pigmented structure that projects just below the center of each breast. The tip of the nipple has about 20 tiny openings to the lactiferous ducts. The skin of the nipple is surrounded by the lighter pigmented skin of the areola. The depth of pigmentation of the nipple and areola in nulliparas varies from rosy pink to brown, depending on the complexion of the individual. In pregnancy, the skin of the nipple darkens but loses some of its pigmentation when lactation is completed. Stimulation of the nipple in men and women causes the structure to become erect through the contraction of radiating smooth muscle bundles in the surrounding areola. In women the nipple enlarges somewhat and becomes more sensitive after puberty.

nipple cancer, an inflammatory malignant neoplasm of the nipple and areola that is usually associated with carcinoma in deeper breast structures. It represents only a small percentage of breast cancers and usually begins in the nipple and spreads to the areola. Also called **Paget's disease of the nipple.**

nipple discharge, spontaneous exudation of material from the nipple that may be normal, as colostrum in pregnancy, or that may be a sign of endocrinologic, neoplastic, or infectious disease.

nipple protector. See **nipple shield.**

nipple shield, a device to protect the nipples of a lactating woman. The shield is usually made of soft latex, is 4 or 5 cm wide, and has a tab on one side with which the mother may hold it. The baby nurses from a nipple at the center of the shield. It is most often used to allow sore or cracked nipples to heal while maintaining lactation. Also called **nipple protector.**

Nipride, a trade name for a direct-acting vasodilator (sodium nitroprusside), used as an adjunct to anesthesia.

niridazole (nɪrɪd'əzoul), an antischistosomal available only from the Center for Disease Control.

Nissl body (nɪs'əl), any one of the large granular structures in the cytoplasm of nerve cells that stains with basic dyes and contains ribonucleoprotein.

nit, the egg of a parasitic insect, particularly a louse. It may be found attached to human or animal hair or to clothing fiber. See also **pediculosis.**

Nitoman, a trade name for a serotonin antagonist (tetrabenazine methanesulfonate), used in the treatment of Huntington's chorea and other hyperkinetic movement disorders. It is not approved for use or available in the United States.

nitric acid (nai'trɪk), a colorless, highly corrosive liquid that may give off suffocating brown fumes of nitrogen dioxide on exposure to air. Traces of nitric acid are found in rain water during a thunderstorm. Commercially prepared nitric acid is a powerful oxidizing agent used in photoengraving and metallurgy, in the manufacture of explosives, fertilizers, dyes, and drugs, and, occasionally, as a cauterizing agent for the removal of warts.

nitrite, an ester or salt of nitrous acid, used as a vasodilator and antispasmodic. Among the most widely used nitrites in medicine are amyl, ethyl, potassium, and sodium nitrite.

nitro-, a combining form indicating presence of the group -NO_2: *nitrobenzol, nitrofuran, nitromethane.*

nitrobenzene poisoning, a toxic condition caused by the absorption into the body of nitrobenzene, a pale yellow, oily liquid used in the manufacture of aniline, shoe dyes, soap, perfume, and artificial flavors. Nitrobenzene, especially its vapors, is extremely toxic. Exposure in industry is usually by inhalation of the fumes or by absorption through the skin. Symptoms of acute poisoning include headache, drowsiness, nausea, ataxia, cyanosis, and in extreme cases respiratory failure. Contaminated clothing is removed and the skin is washed with vinegar, followed by soap and water. Oxygen, blood transfusion, and, in severe cases, hemodialysis may be required. Ingestion is treated with gastric lavage with weak acetic acid, followed by the administration of liquid petrolatum, a saline cathartic, and oxygen and blood transfusion if indicated. Chronic exposure to nitrobenzene may cause headache, fatigue, loss of appetite, and anemia.

Nitro-Bid, a trade name for a coronary vasodilator (nitroglycerin), used as an antianginal agent.

nitrofuran, one of a group of synthetic antimicrobials used to treat infections caused by protozoa or by certain gram-positive or gram-negative bacteria. The precise mechanism by which nitrofurans exert their antimicrobial effects is not known. Three of these agents are commonly prescribed. Nitrofurazone is used topically to treat superficial wounds and infections, particularly burns. Systemic toxicity is not seen when the drug is used in this way, although allergic skin reactions may occur. Furazolidone is used to treat bacterial and protozoal diarrhea and enteritis. Nitrofurantoin is used to treat urinary tract infections caused by *Escherichia coli* and other enteric pathogens of the urinary tract. Systemic administration of nitrofurans is associated with many side effects, the most common being nausea and diarrhea. Serious side effects include polyneuropathies and several hypersensitivity reactions, including pneumonitis and blood dyscrasias. Nitrofurans can cause hemolytic anemia in glucose-6-phosphate dehydrogenase deficient people.

nitrofurantoin (naɪ′troʊfyʊræn′toʊɪn), a urinary antibacterial.
■ INDICATIONS: It is prescribed in the treatment of certain urinary tract infections.
■ CONTRAINDICATIONS: Kidney dysfunction or known hypersensitivity to this drug prohibits its use. It is not given to children under one month of age or to pregnant or lactating women.
■ ADVERSE EFFECTS: Among the most serious adverse reactions is hypersensitivity pneumonitis, which can lead to fibrosis, neurotoxicity, and hemolytic anemia in glucose-6-phosphate dehydrogenase deficient individuals. Gastrointestinal disturbances and fever are common.

nitrofurazone, a topical antibacterial.
■ INDICATIONS: It is prescribed in the prophylaxis and treatment of infection in second- and third-degree burns and in the treatment of infections of the skin and mucous membranes.
■ CONTRAINDICATION: Known hypersensitivity to this drug prohibits its use.
■ ADVERSE EFFECTS: Among the most serious adverse reactions are severe allergic reactions and suprainfections.

nitrogen (N), a gaseous nonmetallic element. Its atomic number is 7; its atomic weight is 14.008. Nitrogen constitutes approximately 78 per cent of the atmosphere and is a component of all proteins and a major component of most organic substances. Nitrogen is found in mineral compounds, as saltpeter, and is the seventeenth most abundant element in the earth's crust. Compounds of nitrogen are essential constituents of all living organisms, the proteins and the nucleic acids being especially basic to all life forms. Nitrogen forms a series of oxides and oxyacids, the most important of which is nitric acid. It also unites with hydrogen to form ammonia and with many metallic elements to form nitrides. Nitrogen is essential to the synthesis of proteins that the body must have, particularly nitrogen-containing compounds or amino acids derived directly or indirectly from plant food. Nitrogen follows a cycle from atmospheric gas into nitrogen-fixing bacteria, into green vascular plants, into humans and animals, and, by decay or in excreted nitrogenous wastes, as urea, back into the soil. Denitrifying bacteria in the soil break down nitrogenous compounds and release gaseous nitrogen. During a 24-hour period in a healthy individual the nitrogen excreted in the urine, feces, and perspiration, together with the nitrogen retained in dermal structures, as the skin and hair, equals the nitrogen consumed in food and drink. The process of protein metabolism accounts for this nitrogen balance. When protein catabolism exceeds protein anabolism, the amount of nitrogen in the urine exceeds the amount of nitrogen consumed in foods, producing a negative nitrogen balance or a state of tissue wasting. A positive nitrogen balance exists in the body when the nitrogen intake in foods is greater than that excreted in urine. Conditions usually associated with positive nitrogen balance are those in which protein anabolism is proceeding faster than protein catabolism, as in conditions associated with growth, pregnancy, and convalescence from a tissue-wasting illness. Nitrogen is a component of nitrous oxide or laughing gas, which is sometimes used as an anesthetic. Nitrous oxide is a colorless, nonflammable, sweet-tasting gas. Three liters of nitrogen may be eliminated from the lungs and tissues in the first hour of anesthesia if a nitrous oxide/oxygen mixture is inspired. Precautions are taken to exhaust this nitrogen from the breathing circuit if high concentrations of both oxygen and nitrous oxide are desired. Nitrous oxide takes effect quickly and allows a fast recovery from anesthesia but is not considered suitable for prolonged surgery or for surgery requiring deep muscle relaxation. It must be administered with oxygen or air to prevent anoxia. Nitrogen is a component of nitrogen dioxide, which is irritating to the lungs and can cause pulmonary edema. Nitrogen dioxide can be released from silage and may produce symptoms of pulmonary damage in workers who perform ensilage tasks. Some studies indicate that measurable changes in pulmonary function occur when healthy individuals are exposed to nitrous oxide concentrations of 2 to 3 parts per million. Nitrogen is also a component of nitric and nitrous acids. Organic nitrates or polyol esters of nitric acid, as nitroglycerin, and organic nitrites or esters of nitric acid, as amyl nitrite, are effective vasodilators often used in relieving angina, but exactly how they function in dilating arterial and venous smooth muscle is not yet understood.

nitrogen balance, the relationship between the nitrogen taken into the body, usually as food, and the nitrogen excreted from the body in urine and feces. Most of the body's nitrogen is incorporated into protein. Positive nitrogen balance, which occurs when the intake of nitrogen is greater than its excretion, implies tissue formation. Negative nitrogen balance, which occurs when more nitrogen is excreted than is taken in, indicates wasting or destruction of tissue.

nitrogen fixation, the process by which free nitrogen in the atmosphere is converted by biological or chemical means to ammonia and to other forms usable by plants and animals. Biological nitrogen fixation is the more important process and is accomplished by microorganisms in the soil, either free-living or in close association with root nodules of certain plants. In contrast, chemical nitrogen fixation, as used in industry, requires extremely high temperatures and pressures.

nitrogen mustard. See **mechlorethamine hydrochloride.**

nitroglycerin, a coronary vasodilator.

■ INDICATION: It is prescribed for the prevention or relief of angina pectoris.

■ CONTRAINDICATION: Known hypersensitivity to this drug prohibits its use.

■ ADVERSE EFFECTS: Among the most serious adverse reactions are hypotension, flushing, headache, and syncope.

nitromersal, an organic mercurial antiseptic that is not a highly effective germicide, sometimes used for the disinfecting of surgical instruments and as an antiseptic on the skin and mucous membranes.

nitroprusside sodium (nai'troupros'aid). See **sodium nitroprusside.**

nitroso-, a combining form indicating presence of the group -N:O: *nitrosobacteria, nitrososubstitution.*

nitrosourea (naitrou'souyuri'ə), one of a group of alkylating drugs used as an antineoplastic drug in the chemotherapy of brain tumors, multiple myeloma, Hodgkin's disease, chronic leukemias, lymphomas, myelomas, and cancers of the breast and ovaries. They have been less successful in therapy for cancers of the lungs, head, neck, and gastrointestinal tract. Like other alkylating agents, they have severe toxic effects, including bone marrow depression. Nausea and vomiting are almost always present. Safe use during pregnancy has not been established, and animal studies have generally shown teratogenicity and embryotoxicity. Carmustine and lomustine are typical examples of this group. See also **alkylating agent.**

Nitrospan, a trade name for a coronary vasodilator (nitroglycerin).

Nitrostat, a trade name for a coronary vasodilator (nitroglycerin).

nitrous oxide (N_2O), a gas used as an anesthetic in dentistry, surgery, and childbirth. It provides light anesthesia and is delivered in various concentrations with oxygen. Nitrous oxide alone does not provide deep enough anesthesia for major surgery, for which it is supplemented with other anesthetic agents. It is often given for induction of anesthesia, preceded by the administration of a barbiturate or an analgesic narcotic. Nitrous oxide is neither explosive nor flammable, and recovery is rapid. It is not administered to patients with hypoxemia, respiratory disease, or intestinal occlusion.

NLN, abbreviation for **National League for Nursing.**

NMNA, abbreviation for **National Male Nurses' Association.**

NMR, abbreviation for **nuclear magnetic resonance.**

No, symbol for **nobelium.**

nobelium (No), a man-made, transuranic metallic element. Its atomic number is 102; its atomic weight is 254.

noble gas. See **inert gas.**

Nocardia (noukar'diə), a genus of gram-positive aerobic bacteria, some species of which are pathogenic, as *Nocardia asteroides* which causes maduromycosis. See also **nocardiosis.**

nocardiosis (noukar'diou'sis), infection with *Nocardia asteroides,* an aerobic gram species of actinomycetes, characterized by pneumonia, often with cavitation, and by chronic abcesses in the brain and subcutaneous tissues. The organism enters via the respiratory tract and spreads by the bloodstream, especially in Cushing's syndrome. Surgical drainage of abscesses and sulfonamide therapy for 12 to 18 months cures between 50 and 60 per cent of the cases treated.

no-code, a note written in the patient record and signed by a qualified, usually senior or attending physician, instructing the staff of the institution not to attempt to resuscitate a particular patient in the event of cardiac or respiratory failure. This instruction is usually given only when a person is so gravely ill that death is imminent and inevitable. Also called **DNR.** See also **code,** def. 5.

noctambulation. See **somnambulism.**

Noctec, a trade name for a sedative-hypnotic (chloral hydrate).

nocturia (noktur'iə), urination, particularly excessive urination at night. While it may be a symptom of renal disease, it may occur in the absence of disease in persons who drink excessive amounts of fluids, particularly alcohol or coffee, before bedtime or in those with prostatic disease. It may occur in older patients, who may have excess fluids that are mobilized by lying down at night. Also called **nycturia.** Compare **enuresis.**

nocturnal, 1. pertaining to or occurring during the night. 2. describing an individual or animal that is active at night and sleeps during the day.

nocturnal emission, involuntary emission of semen

during sleep, usually in association with an erotic dream. Also called **wet dream.**

nocturnal paroxysmal dyspnea, an abnormal condition of the respiratory system, characterized by sudden attacks of shortness of breath, profuse sweating, tachycardia, and wheezing that waken the person from sleep. The paroxysms may be induced by nightmares, noises, or coughing. The condition is usually associated with heart failure or pulmonary edema. Characteristically, the attack is relieved by getting up and opening a window. See also **dyspnea.**

nod-, a combining form meaning 'knot': *nodal, nodose, nodulus.*

nodal bradycardia. See **bradycardia.**

node, **1.** a small rounded mass. **2.** a lymph node.

nodular, (of a structure or mass) small, firm, and knotty. See also **node, nodule.**

nodular circumscribed lipomatosis, a condition in which many circumscribed, encapsulated lipomas are distributed around the neck symmetrically, randomly, or like a collar. The adipose deposits may be painful and tender.

nodular cutaneous angiitis, an inflammatory condition of small arteries accompanied by lesions of the skin.

nodular melanoma, a melanoma that is uniformly pigmented, usually bluish-black and nodular and sometimes surrounded by an irregular halo of pale, unpigmented skin. The lesion is always raised and may be dome-shaped or polypoid. It is most often found in adults in middle age.

nodule, **1.** a small node. **2.** a small nodelike structure.

-noia, a combining form meaning '(condition of the) mind or will': *aponoia, hypernoia, hyponoia.*

Noludar, a trade name for a sedative (methyprylon).

Nolvadex, a trade name for a nonsteroidal antiestrogen (tamoxifen).

noma (nou′mə), an acute, necrotizing ulcerative process involving mucous membranes of mouth or genitalia. The condition is most commonly seen in children with poor nutrition and hygiene. There is rapid-spreading and painless destruction of bone and soft tissue accompanied by a putrid odor. Fusospirochetal organisms have been implicated. Healing eventually occurs but often with disfiguring defects. Also called **acute necrotizing ulcerative mucositis, gangrenous stomatitis.**

-noma, a combining form meaning a 'spreading, invasive gangrene': *müllerianoma, pelidnoma.*

nomenclature (nou′mɪnkleɪ′ćhər, noumen′kləćhər), a consistent, systematic method of naming used in a scientific discipline to denote classifications and to avoid ambiguities in names, as binomial nomenclature in biology and chemical nomenclature in chemistry.

-nomia, a combining form meaning 'aphasia involving names or naming ability': *anomia, paranomia, dysnomia.*

Nomina Anatomica, the book of official international nomenclature for anatomy as designated by the International Congress of Anatomists.

nominal damages. See **damages.**

nomo-, a combining form meaning 'of or relating to usage or law': *nomogenesis, nomogram, nomotopic.*

nomogram (nom′əgræm, nou′məgræm), **1.** a graphic representation, by any of various systems, of a numerical relationship. **2.** a graph on which a number of variables is plotted so that the value of a dependent variable can be read on the appropriate line when the values of the other variables are given.

WEST NOMOGRAM

-nomy, a combining form meaning 'received knowledge in a field': *pathonomy, physionomy, psychonomy.*

non-, a combining form meaning 'nine': *nonan, nonigravida, nonipara.*

non-A, non-B, (NANB) hepatitis, viral hepatitis that is caused by a virus antigenically separate from the serologic strains that cause hepatitis A or hepatitis B. It accounts for more than 90 per cent of the cases of post-transfusion hepatitis in the United States, occurring primarily in people receiving multiple transfusions. NANB hepatitis is usually milder than types A or B but is otherwise clinically indistinguishable from them. The treatment is the same as for other forms of viral hepatitis.

nonadhesive skin traction, one of two kinds of skin traction in which the therapeutic pull of traction weights is applied with foam-backed traction straps that do not stick to the skin over the body structure involved. Nonadhesive skin traction straps may be easily removed to facilitate skin care and are usually used when continuous traction is not required. The straps spread the traction pull over a wide area of skin surface, thus decreasing the vulnerability of the patient to skin breakdown. Compare **adhesive skin traction.**

nonbacterial thrombic endocarditis, one of the three main types of endocarditis, characterized by various kinds of lesions that affect the heart valves. Some studies indicate that this disease may be the first step in the development of bacterial endocarditis and that the lesions involved cause peripheral arterial embolisms resulting in death. This disease equally affects men and women between ages of 18 and 90, causes heart murmurs in about 30 per cent of the cases, and most often affects the valves on the left side of the heart. There is no successful treatment of nonbacterial thrombic endocarditis, but anticoagulation therapy may be employed to reduce the incidence of peripheral arterial embolism. See also **Libman-Sacks endocarditis.**

noncommunicating hydrocephalus. See **hydrocephalus.**

noncompliance, a nursing diagnosis accepted by the Fourth National Conference on the Classification of Nursing Diagnoses. The specific nature of the noncompliance is to be specified, as noncompliance: medications. The etiology of noncompliance is an informed decision on the part of the client not to adhere to a therapeutic suggestion owing to a health belief, a cultural or spiritual value, or a problem in the relationship between the provider of the recommendation and the client. The defining characteristics of noncompliance include objective tests that show noncompliance, observation of physical or psychological signs that demonstrate lack of compliance, or a failure to keep appointments. The critical defining characteristic, which must be present for the diagnosis to be made, is an observation of the client's failure to adhere to a recommendation or a statement by the client or knowledgeable other person that the recommendations are not being followed. See also **nursing diagnosis.**

nondirective therapy, a psychotherapeutic approach in which the psychotherapist refrains from giving advice or interpretation as the client is helped to identify conflicts and to clarify and understand his feelings and values. Compare **directive therapy.** See also **client-centered therapy.**

nondisjunction, failure of homologous pairs of chromosomes to separate during the first meiotic division or of the two chromatids of a chromosome to split during anaphase of mitosis or the second meiotic division. The result is an abnormal number of chromosomes in the daughter cells. Compare **disjunction.** See also **monosomy, trisomy.**

nonfat milk. See **skimmed milk.**

nonfeasance (nonfi′zəns), a failure to perform a task, duty, or undertaking that one has agreed to perform or that one had a legal duty to perform. Compare **malfeasance, misfeasance.** See also **negligence.**

nongonococcal urethritis (NGU), an infectious condition of the urethra in males that is characterized by mild dysuria and a scanty to moderate amount of penile discharge. The discharge may be white or clear, thin or mucoid, or, less often, purulent. The infection is often caused by the obligate intracellular parasite *Chlamydia trachomatis.* The diagnosis of NGU is made by excluding a diagnosis of gonococcal urethritis by microscopic examination and bacteriologic culture of the exudate. Untreated NGU may result in urethral stricture, epididymitis, proctitis, and chronic inflammation of the urethra. Women exposed to the exudate during coitus may develop a hyperthropic erosion of the cervix and purulent cervical mucus. An infant in passing through the cervix and vagina of a mother infected with *C. trachomatis* may develop conjunctivitis and nasopharyngeal infection in the first few days after birth and pneumonia at three to four months. Most cases of NGU are successfully treated with tetracycline or erythromycin. Sexual contacts are treated whether or not they are symptomatic. Nearly fifty per cent of all cases of urethritis are nongonococcal.

non-Hodgkin's lymphoma, any kind of malignant lymphoma except Hodgkin's disease. Also called **lymphosarcoma.**

noninvasive, (in health care) of or pertaining to a diagnostic or therapeutic technique that does not require the skin to be broken or a cavity or organ of the body to be entered, as obtaining a blood pressure reading by auscultation with a stethoscope and sphygmomanometer.

nonosteogenic fibroma (non′ostiəjen′ık), a common bone lesion in which there is degeneration and proliferation of the medullary and cortical tissue, usually near the ends of the diaphyses of the large long bones, especially those of the lower extremities. Frequently it does not cause any symptoms and is only discovered during x rays of the skeleton for other reasons.

nonparametric test of significance, (in statistics) one of several tests that use a qualitative approach to analyze rank order data and incidence data that cannot be assumed to have a normal distribution. Kinds of nonparametric tests of significance include **chi-square test, Mann-Whitney U test, Spearman rank order correlation test.**

nonproductive cough, a sudden, noisy expulsion of air from the lungs that may be caused by irritation or inflammation and does not remove sputum from the respiratory tract. Expectorants, as ammonium chloride, ammonium carbonate, sodium iodide, potassium iodide, ipecac, and terpin hydrate increase respiratory tract secretions and may result in productive coughing when administered to patients with respiratory infections. If suppression of coughing is required, antitussives that depress the cough reflex may be prescribed, including codeine or dextromethorphan. Intratracheal suctioning may be necessary when secretions cause severe respiratory difficulty and coughing is unproductive. Compare **productive cough.**

nonrapid eye movement (NREM). See **sleep.**

nonreflex bladder. See **flaccid bladder.**

nonsense mutation. See **amber mutation.**

nonsexual generation. See **asexual generation.**

nonspecific urethritis (NSU), inflammation of the urethra not known to be caused by a specific organism. Onset of symptoms is often related to sexual intercourse. Its acute phase is seldom seen in women, but its chronic phase is a common urologic difficulty among them. The condition is noted by urethral discharge in men and by reddening of the urethral mucosa in women. Treatment with antibiotics is not often successful. See also **nongonoccal urethritis.**

nontoxic, not poisonous. Also called **atoxic.**

nontropical sprue, a malabsorption syndrome resulting from an inborn inability to digest foods that contain gluten. See also **celiac disease.**

nonulcerative blepharitis, a form of blepharitis characterized by greasy scales on the margins of the eyelids around the lashes and hyperemia and thickening of the skin. Nonulcerative blepharitis is often associated with seborrhea of the scalp, eyebrows, and the skin behind the ears.

Noonan's syndrome, a hypergonadotropic disorder, occurring only in males, characterized by short stature, low-set ears, webbing of the neck, and cubitus valgus. Testicular function may be normal, but fertility is often decreased. The number and morphology of the chromosomes are normal. The cause is unknown. See also **Turner's syndrome.**

norepinephrine (nor'epɪnef'rɪn), an adrenergic hormone that acts to increase blood pressure by vasoconstriction but does not affect cardiac output. It is synthesized naturally by the adrenal medulla and is available also as a drug, levarterenol, given to maintain the blood pressure in acute hypotension secondary to trauma, heart disease, or vascular collapse.

norepinephrine bitartrate (nor'epənef'rɪn), an adrenergic vasoconstrictor.
■ INDICATIONS: It is prescribed in the treatment of cardiac arrest and in certain acute hypotensive states.
■ CONTRAINDICATIONS: Hypovolemia, vascular thrombosis, or known hypersensitivity to this drug prohibits its use. It is not used in conjunction with cyclopropane or halothane anesthesia.

■ ADVERSE EFFECTS: Among the more serious adverse reactions are local tissue necrosis at the site of injection, bradycardia, headache, and hypertension.

norethindrone (nɔreth'ɪndroun), a progestin.
■ INDICATIONS: It is prescribed in the treatment of abnormal uterine bleeding and endometriosis and is a component in oral contraceptive medications.
■ CONTRAINDICATIONS: Thrombophlebitis, liver dysfunction, unusual vaginal bleeding, breast cancer, missed abortion, or known hypersensitivity to this drug prohibits its use. It is not recommended for use during pregnancy.
■ ADVERSE EFFECTS: Among the more serious adverse reactions are breakthrough bleeding, amenorrhea, gastrointestinal disturbances, breast changes, and masculinization of the female fetus.

norethindrone acetate and ethinylestradiol (nɔreth'ɪndroun), an oral contraceptive.
■ INDICATIONS: It is prescribed for contraception, endometriosis, and hypermenorrhea.
■ CONTRAINDICATIONS: Thrombophlebitis, cardiovascular disease, breast or reproductive organ cancer, unusual vaginal bleeding, gall bladder disease, liver tumor, or known hypersensitivity to this drug prohibits its use. It is not given to women over 40 years of age or during lactation, pregnancy, or suspected pregnancy. It is given with caution to women who smoke.
■ ADVERSE EFFECTS: Among the more serious adverse reactions are thrombophlebitis, uterine fibroma, porphyria, embolism, jaundice, and cerebrovascular accident.

Norflex, a trade name for a skeletal muscle relaxant and antihistamine (orphenadrine citrate).

Norgesic Forte (nɔrji'zɪk fɔrt'), a trade name for a fixed-combination drug containing a muscle relaxant with anti-cholinergic activity (orphenadrine citrate) and APC (aspirin, phenacetin, and caffeine), used for the relief of mild to moderate pain of acute musculoskeletal disorders.

norgestrel (nɔrjes'trəl), a progestin.
■ INDICATIONS: It is prescribed alone or in combination with estrogen as a contraceptive.
■ CONTRAINDICATIONS: Thrombophlebitis, liver dysfunction, unusual vaginal bleeding, breast cancer, missed abortion, or known hypersensitivity to this drug prohibits its use.
■ ADVERSE EFFECTS: Among the more serious adverse reactions are amenorrhea, dysfunctional uterine bleeding, breast changes, and masculinization of a female fetus.

Norinyl, a trade name for an oral contraceptive containing a progestin (norethindrone) and an estrogen (mestranol).

Norisodrine Hydrochloride, a trade name for an adrenergic (isoproterenol hydrochloride).

Norlac, a trade name for a nutritional supplement containing multivitamins, calcium, and iron.

Norlestrin, a trade name for an oral contraceptive containing an estrogen (ethinyl estradiol) and a progestin (norethindrone acetate).

Norlutin, a trade name for a progestin (norethindrone).

norm, a measure of a phenomenon generally accepted as the ideal standard performance against which other measures of the phenomenon may be measured.

norma basalis, the inferior surface of the base of the skull with the mandible removed, formed by the palatine bones, the vomer, the pterygoid processes, and parts of the sphenoid and temporal bones.

normal, 1. describing a standard, average, or typical example of a set of objects or values. 2. describing a chemical solution in which one liter contains one gram of a substance or the equivalent in replaceable hydrogen ions.

-normal, a combining form meaning 'relating to a norm': *centinormal, decanormal, prenormal.*

normal diet. See **regular diet.**

normal dwarf. See **primordial dwarf.**

normal human serum albumin, an isotonic preparation of pooled human serum albumin for treating hypoproteinemia, hypovolemia, and threatened or existing shock.

normoblast (nor′məblæst), a nucleated cell that is the normal precursor of the adult circulating erythrocyte. The developmental stages include the pronormoblast, the basophilic normoblast, the polychromatic normoblast, and the orthochromatic normoblast. After the extrusion of the nucleus of the normoblast, the young erythrocyte becomes known as a reticulocyte. See also **reticulocyte.** – **normoblastic,** *adj.*

normochromic (nor′məkrou′mɪk), (of a blood cell) having normal color, usually because it contains an adequate amount of hemoglobin. Compare **hypochromic.** See also **red cell indices.**

normocyte (nor′məsait), an ordinary, normal, adult red blood cell of average size having a diameter of 7 μ. Compare **macrocyte, microcyte.** – **normocytic,** *adj.*

Normosol = M in D5W, a trade name for a balanced solution of 5 per cent dextrose in water with electrolytes.

normotensive, of or pertaining to the condition of having normal blood pressure. – **normotension,** *n.*

Norpace, a trade name for an antiarrhythmic cardiac depressant (disopyramide phosphate).

Norpramin, a trade name for an antidepressant (desipramine hydrochloride).

Nor-Q-D, a trade name for an oral contraceptive containing a progestin (norethindrone), but no estrogen.

North American blastomycosis, an infection caused by inhaling the fungus *Blastomyces dermatitidis.* It may resemble bacterial pneumonia, and x-ray films of the chest may show cavities. Painless, well-demarcated, verrucous or ulcerated skin lesions occur on the face and hands. Occasionally, lesions of the oral mucous membrane may be mistaken for squamous-cell carcinoma. The disease may progress to involve bones and the brain; many viscera are infected in fatal cases. Diagnosis is made by microscopic examination of body secretions. Treatment is amphotericin B, given intravenously, or, in severe cases, a combination of amphotericin B and sulfonamides. The disease has been reported in Africa as well as North America and occurs more frequently in males. Compare **paracoccidioidomycosis.**

North Asian tick-borne rickettsiosis, an infection, acquired in the Eastern Hemisphere, caused by *Rickettsia siberica,* transmitted by ticks, and resembling Rocky Mountain spotted fever. Usual findings include a generalized maculopapular rash involving palms and soles, fever, and lymph node enlargement. It is rarely fatal and responds quickly to treatment with chloramphenicol. No vaccine is available; prevention depends on avoidance of tick bites.

North Asian tick typhus. See **Siberian tick typhus.**

nortriptyline hydrochloride, a tricyclic antidepressant.
■ INDICATION: It is prescribed in the treatment of mental depression.
■ CONTRAINDICATIONS: Concomitant administration of monoamine oxidase inhibitors, recent myocardial infarction, or known hypersensitivity to this drug or to other tricyclic medications prohibits its use. It is used with caution in patients having a seizure disorder or a cardiovascular disease.
■ ADVERSE EFFECTS: Among the more serious adverse effects are sedation and gastrointestinal, cardiovascular, and neurologic reactions. This drug interacts with many other drugs.

nose, the structure that protrudes from the anterior portion of the skull and serves as a passageway for air to and from the lungs. The nose filters the air, warming, moistening, and chemically examining it for impurities that might irritate the mucous lining of the respiratory tract. The nose also serves as the organ of smell, and it aids the faculty of speech. It consists of an internal portion and an external portion. The external portion, which protrudes from the face, is considerably smaller than the internal portion, which lies over the roof of the mouth. The hollow interior portion is separated into a right cavity and a left cavity by a septum. Each cavity is divided into the superior, middle, and inferior meati by the projection of nasal conchae. The external portion of the nose is perforated by two nostrils and the internal portion by two posterior nares. The pairs of sinuses that drain into the nose are the frontal, maxillary, ethmoidal, and sphenoidal sinuses. Ciliated mucous membrane lines the nose, closely adhering to the periosteum. The mucous membrane is continuous with the skin through the nares and with the mucous membrane of the nasal part of the pharynx through the choanae. The mucous membrane contains the olfactory cells which connect with the olfactory nerves.

nosebleed, abnormal hemorrhage from the nose. Emergency responses to nosebleed include seating the patient upright with the head thrust forward to prevent swallowing of blood. Pressure with both thumbs directly under the nostril and above the lips may block the main artery supplying blood to the nose. Alternatively, pressure with both forefingers on each side of the nostril often slows bleeding by blocking the main arteries as well as their branches. Continued bleeding may require the insertion of cotton or other absorbent material within the nostril and reapplication of pressure. Cold compresses on the nose, lips, and the back of the head may help control hemorrhage. Continued bleeding may require cautery. Also called **epistaxis.**

noso-, a combining form meaning 'of or relating to disease': *nosochthonography, nosogeny, nosophobe.*

nosocomial (nos'əkou'miəl), of or pertaining to a hospital.

nosocomial infection, an infection acquired during hospitalization, often caused by *Candida albicans, Escherichia coli,* hepatitis viruses, herpes zoster virus, *Pseudomonas,* or *Staphylococcus.* Also called **hospital-acquired infection.**

nosology (nousol'əji), the science of classifying diseases. See also **nomenclature.**

nostrils. See **anterior nares.**

notch, an indentation or a depression in a bone or other organ, as the auricular notch or the cardiac notch.

notifiable, pertaining to certain conditions, diseases, and events that must, by law, be reported to a governmental agency, as birth, death, smallpox, and certain other communicable diseases and to certain violations of public health regulations.

noto-, a combining form meaning 'of or related to the back': *notochord, notogenesis, notomyelitis.*

notochord, an elongated strip of mesodermal tissue that originates from the primitive node and extends along the dorsal surface of the developing embryo beneath the neural tube, forming the primary longitudinal skeletal axis of the body of all chordates. In man and other vertebrate animals, the structure is replaced by vertebrae, although a remnant of it remains as part of the nucleus pulposus of the intervertebral discs. See also **neural tube.** — **notochordal,** *adj.*

notochordal canal, a tubular passage that extends from the primitive pit into the head process during the early stages of embryonic development in mammals. It perforates the splanchnopleure layer so that there is a temporary connection between the yolk sac and the amnion. Also called **chordal canal.**

notochordal plate. See **head process.**

notogenesis, the formation of the notochord. — **notogenetic,** *adj.*

notomelus (nətom'ələs), a congenital malformation in which one or more accessory limbs are attached to the back.

nourish, to furnish or supply the essential foods or nutrients for maintaining life.

nourishment, 1. the act or process of nourishing or being nourished. 2. any substance that nourishes and supports the life and growth of living organisms.

Novacain, a trade name for a local anesthetic (procaine hydrochloride).

Novahistine, a trade name for a fixed-combination drug containing an antihistamine (chlorpheniramine maleate) and an adrenergic decongestant (propanolamine).

novobiocin, an antibiotic produced by the growth of *Streptomyces niveus* and other species formerly used in the treatment of infections caused by certain cocci and other gram-positive organs. Because of the toxicity of the drug there are no current valid indications for its therapeutic use.

Novrad, a trade name for an antitussive (levopropoxyphene napsylate).

noxious (nok'šhəs), harmful, injurious, or detrimental to health.

Np, symbol for **neptunium.**

NPH Iletin, a trade name for an insulin suspension (isophane).

NPH Insulin, a trade name for an insulin suspension (isophane).

n-propyl alcohol (en'prou'pıl), a clear, colorless liquid used as a solvent for resins.

NREM, abbreviation for **nonrapid eye movement.** See **sleep.**

NSNA, abbreviation for **National Student Nurses' Association.**

NSU. abbreviation for **nonspecific urethritis.**

Nubain, a trade name for a synthetic analgesic (nalbuphine hydrochloride), used as an adjunct to anesthesia.

nucha (nu'kə), *pl.* **nuchae.** the nape, or back of the neck. — **nuchal,** *adj.*

nuchal cord, an abnormal but common condition in which the umbilical cord is wrapped around the neck of the fetus in utero or of the baby as it is being born. It is usually possible to slip the loop or loops of cord gently over the child's head. Sometimes it is a single loose loop, and the shoulders may deliver through it. If it is tight, it may be clamped in two places and cut with sterile, blunt tipped scissors. The condition occurs in more than 25 per cent of deliveries, more often with long cords than with short ones.

nucle-. See **nucleo-.**

-nuclear, a combining form meaning 'of or referring to the nucleus': *circumnuclear, endonuclear, multinuclear.*

nuclear family, a family unit consisting of the biologic parents and their offspring. The nuclear family is a relatively recent product of western society. Dissolution of a marriage results in dissolution of the nuclear family. The nuclear family unit is less efficient than an extended family unit in providing information and vital services to family members, as in child rearing, child care, and care of older family members. As is most often the kind of family from which doctors, nurses, social workers, teachers, and other professional people come, it is not surprising that the nuclear family is often regarded as the norm for family style. Allowances must be made for bias in a professional's attitude toward other kinds of family units that may answer the needs and expectations of other groups of people. Compare **extended family, matrifocal family.**

nuclear fission. See **fission.**

nuclear hyaloplasm. See **karyolymph.**

nuclear isomer, one of two or more nuclides with the same number of neutrons and protons in the nucleus (the same atomic number, or Z, and the same atomic mass, or A) but existing in different energy states.

nuclear magnetic resonance, spectra emited by phosphorus in body tissues as measured and imaged on phosphorus nuclear magnetic resonance instruments.

nuclear sap. See **karyolymph.**

nucleic acid (nukli′ık), a polymeric compound of high molecular weight composed of nucleotides, each consisting of a purine or pyrimidine base, a ribose or deoxyribose sugar, and a phosphate group. Nucleic acids are involved in energy storage and release and in the determination and transmission of genetic characteristics. Kinds of nucleic acid are **deoxyribonucleic acid, ribonucleic acid.** See also **nucleotide.**

nucleo-, nucle-, a combining form meaning 'of or related to a nucleus': *nucleochylema, nucleokeratin, nucleolus.*

nucleocapsid (nu′klioukæp′sıd), a viral enclosure consisting of a capsid or protein coat that encloses nucleic acid. Some viruses consist solely of bare nucleocapsids; others have more complex enclosures.

nucleochylema (nu′klioukaili′mə), the ground substance of the nucleus, as distinguished from that of the cytoplasm.

nucleochyme (nu′kliəkaim′). See **karyolymph.**

nucleocytoplasmic (nu′kliousai′touplæz′mık), of or relating to the nucleus and cytoplasm of a cell.

nucleocytoplasmic ratio, the ratio of the volume of a nucleus of a cell to the volume of the cytoplasm. The proportion is usually constant for a specific cell type and an increase is indicative of malignant neoplasms. Also called **karyoplasmic ratio, nucleoplasmic ratio.**

nucleohistone (nu′kliouhıs′toun), a complex nucleoprotein that consists of deoxyribonucleic acid and a histone. It is the basic constituent of the chromatin in the cell nucleus.

nucleolar organizer, a part of the nucleus of the cell, thought to consist of heterochromatin, that is responsible for the formation of the nucleolus. Also called **nucleolar zone, nucleolus organizer.**

nucleolar zone. See **nucleolar organizer.**

nucleolus (nukli′ələs), *pl.* **nucleoli** (nukli′əlai). any one of the small, dense structures composed largely of ribonucleic acid and situated within the cytoplasm of cells. Nucleoli are essential in the formation of ribosomes which synthesize cell proteins.

nucleoplasm (nu′kliəplæz′əm), the protoplasm of the nucleus as contrasted with that of the cell. Also called **karyoplasm.** Compare **cytoplasm.** – **nucleoplasmic,** *adj.*

nucleoplasmic ratio. See **nucleocytoplasmic ratio.**

nucleoside monophosphate kinase, a liver enzyme that catalyzes the transfer of a phosphate group from adenosine triphosphate, producing adenosine diphosphate and a nucleoside diphosphate.

nucleosome (nu′kliəsoum′), any one of the repeating nucleoprotein units consisting of histones forming a complex with deoxyribonucleic acid that appear as the beadlike structures at distinct intervals along the chromosome.

nucleotide (nu′kliətaid), any one of the compounds into which nucleic acid is split by the action of nuclease. A nucleotide consists of a phosphate group, a pentose sugar, and a nitrogenous base. Chains of such structures form deoxyribonucleic acid molecules essential for life.

nucleus (nu′kliəs, nyu′kliəs), 1. the central controlling body within a living cell, usually a spherical unit enclosed in a membrane and containing genetic codes for maintaining life systems of the organism and for issuing commands for growth and reproduction. 2. a group of nerve cells of the central nervous system having a common function, as supporting the sense of hearing or smell. 3. the center of an atom about which electrons rotate. 4. the central element in an organic chemical compound or class of compounds. – **nuclear,** *adj.*

nucleus pulposus, the central portion of each intervertebral disc, consisting of a pulpy elastic substance that loses some of its resiliency with age. In elderly persons, the nucleus pulposus may be suddenly compressed by unusual exertion or by trauma and squeeze out through the annular fibrocartilage, causing a herniated disc and extreme pain.

nuclide (nu′klaid), a species of atom characterized by the number of protons and neutrons, energy content, and mass of its nucleus, capable of existing for a measurable time, generally greater than 10^{10} seconds. A kind of nuclide is a **radionuclide.**

null cell, a lymphocyte that develops in the bone marrow, and lacks the characteristic surface markers of the B and T lymphocytes. It represents a small proportion of the lymphocyte population. Stimulated by the presence of antibody, cells of this kind can apparently attack certain cellular targets directly and are known as 'killer,' or K cells. Compare **B cell, T cell.** See also **cytotoxin, immune globulin.**

null hypothesis (N_0), (in research) a hypothesis that predicts that no difference or relationship exists among the variables studied that could not have occurred by chance alone.

nullipara (nəlɪp'ərə), *pl.* **nulliparae.** a woman who has not delivered a viable infant. In the chart the designation 'para O' indicates nulliparity. —**nulliparity,** *n.,* **nulliparous,** *adj.*

numbness, a partial or total lack of sensation in a part of the body, resulting from any factor that interrupts the transmission of impulses from the sensory nerve fibers. Numbness is often accompanied by tingling.

nummular dermatitis (nəm'yələr), a skin disease characterized by coin-shaped, vesicular, or scaling eczemalike lesions on the forearms and the front of the calves. The cause is unknown.

Numorphan Hydrochloride, a trade name for a narcotic analgesic (oxymorphone hydrochloride).

Nupercainal, a trade name for a local anesthetic (dibucaine hydrochloride).

Nuremberg tribunal, an international tribunal planned and implemented by the United Nations War Crimes Commission to detect, apprehend, try, and punish persons accused of war crimes. In preparation for the prosecution of the war criminals, the War Department of the United States caused Andrew Ivy, M.D., to devise a set of principles to govern the participation of human beings in medical research. The principle and practice of informed consent was reinforced by the precedent set in the trials in which Nazi physicians were declared guilty of crimes against humanity in performing experiments on human beings who were not volunteers and did not consent. See also **Helsinki accords.**

nurse, 1. a person educated and licensed in the practice of nursing; one who is concerned with "the diagnosis and treatment of human responses to actual or potential health problems" (American Nurses' Association). The practice of the nurse includes data collection, diagnosis, planning, treatment, and evaluation within the framework of the nurse's singular concern with the person's response to the problem, rather than to the problem itself. The concerns of the nurse are thus broader and less discreet and circumscribed than the traditional concerns of medicine. In a cooperative participatory relationship with the client or patient, the nurse acts to promote, maintain, or restore the health of the person; wellness is the goal. A collegial collaborative relationship with other health professionals who share a mission and a common database furthers the practice of nursing. Guided by humanitarian,

ethical principles, the nurse practices in a personal, nurturing, and protective manner that promotes health in all ways. The nurse may be a generalist or a specialist and, as a professional, is ethically and legally accountable for the nursing activites performed and for the actions of others to whom the nurse has delegated responsibility. **2.** to provide nursing care. See also **five-step nursing process, nursing, registered nurse.**

nurse anesthetist, a registered nurse qualified by advanced training in an accredited program in the speciality of nurse anesthesia to manage the anesthetic care of the patient in certain surgical situations.

nurse-client interaction, any process in which a nurse and a client exchange or share information, verbally or nonverbally. It is fundamental to communication and is an essential component of the nursing assessment.

nurse-client relationship, a therapeutic relationship between a nurse and a client built on a series of interactions and developing over time. All interactions do not develop into relationships but may nonetheless be therapeutic. The relationship differs from a social relationship in that it is designed to meet the needs only of the patient. Its structure varies with the context, the client's needs, and the goals of the nurse and the client. Its nature varies with the context, including the setting, the kind of nursing, and the needs of the patient. The relationship is dynamic and uses cognitive and affective levels of interaction. It is time-limited and goal-oriented and has three phases. During the first phase, the phase of establishment, the nurse establishes the structure, purpose, timing, and context of the relationship and expresses an interest in discussing this initial structure with the client. Data collection for the nursing care plan continues and basic goals for the relationship are stated. During the middle, developmental phase of the relationship, the nurse and the client get to know each other better and test the structure of the relationship in order to be able to trust one another. The nurse is careful to assess correctly the degree of dependency that is necessary for the particular patient. Plans may be devised for improved ways of coping with problems and achieving goals. The nurse is alert to the danger of losing objectivity during this phase. The last phase, termination, ideally occurs when the goals of the relationship have been accomplished, when both the client and the nurse feel a sense of resolution and satisfaction. Often this is not possible because the nurse is transferred or the patient discharged; in either case both may be left with a feeling of frustration.

nurse clinician, a nurse who is prepared to identify and diagnose problems of clients by using the expanded knowledge and skills gained by advanced study in a specific area of nursing practice. The specialist may function independently within standing orders or protocols and collaborates with associates to implement a plan of care that is focused on the client.

Nurse Corps, the branch within each of the armed services comprised of the nurses within that service, as the Army Nurse Corps. In each of the armed services, the members of the Nurse Corps have the rank, title, responsibilities, and status of officer.

nurse educator, a registered nurse whose primary area of interest, competence, and professional practice is the education of nurses.

nurse practice act, a statute enacted by the legislature of any of the states or by the appropriate officers of the districts or possessions. The act delineates the legal scope of the practice of nursing within the geographical boundaries of the jurisdiction.

nurse practitioner, a nurse who by advanced training and clinical experience in a branch of nursing, as in a master's degree program in nursing, has acquired expert knowledge in the special branch of practice. See specific kinds of nurse practitioner.

nursery diarrhea, diarrhea of the newborn. In nurseries, outbreaks of diarrhea caused by *Escherichia coli, Salmonella,* echoviruses, or adenoviruses are potentially life-threatening to the infant. The neonate may be infected at the time of birth by organisms from the mother's stool or infected later by organisms spread by the hands of hospital personnel. Fluid loss is the most serious aspect of the disease, leading to dehydration and electrolyte imbalance. Care includes maintaining fluid and electrolyte balance and administration of antibiotics, if appropriate. Good hand-washing technique, use of disposable nursing bottles and nipples, and early isolation of infected infants reduce the possibility of such outbreaks.

nurse's aide, a person who is employed to carry out basic nonspecialized tasks in the care of a patient, as bathing and feeding, making beds, and transporting patients. Many hospitals offer extensive training and orientation programs for newly hired nurse's aides and in-service education for continued training.

Nurses' Association of the American College of Obstetrics and Gynecology (NAACOG), a national organization of nurses who work in obstetrics and gynecology. It functions in close association with the American College of Obstetrics and Gynecology.

Nurses' Coalition for Action in Politics (N-CAP), an organization that works in association with the American Nurses' Association. It raises funds for political contributions to candidates for public office at the state and national levels.

nurse's registry, an employment agency or listing service for nurses who wish to work in a specific area of nursing, usually for a short period of time or on a per diem basis.

nurses' station, an area in a clinic, unit, or ward in a health-care facility that serves as the administrative center for nursing care for a particular group of patients. It is usually centrally located and may be staffed by a ward secretary or clerk who assists with paper work and telephone and other communication. Before going on duty nurses usually meet there to receive daily assignments, to review the patients' charts, and to update the Kardex. In a critical care unit of a large teaching hospital, the nurses' station may also contain panels of visual display terminals that allow centralized monitoring of many patients and may also have computer terminals that allow access to information in the patients' records or to a data bank of clinical information. In other parts of a hospital, the nurses' station is equipped in any of various ways appropriate to the care of the patients in that area or unit.

nurse therapist model, (in psychiatric nursing research) a theoretical framework to clarify the role of the mental health nurse. Techniques from traditional and contemporary modes of treatment, including transactional analysis and crisis intervention, may be used singly or in various combinations. The nurse therapist chooses the technique or techniques after using the model to examine the nurse-client interaction, the feedback, and the goal of the interaction.

nursing, 1. the practice in which a nurse assists "the individual, sick or well, in the performance of those activities contributing to health or its recovery (or to a peaceful death) that he would perform unaided if he had the necessary strength, will or knowledge. And to do this in such a way as to help him gain independence as rapidly as possible." (Virginia Henderson) 2. "the diagnosis and treatment of human responses to actual or potential health problems," American Nurses' Association. There are four principal characteristics that further define nursing care. The phenomena that concern nurses; the use of theories to observe the need for nursing intervention and to plan nursing action; the nursing action taken; and an evaluation of the effects of the actions relative to the phenomena. This definition of nursing provides a framework for the nursing process including data collection, diagnosis, planning, treatment, and evaluation. The nursing process is supported by standards of nursing practice that are congruent with the definition and that provide more specific guidelines for practice. These standards include systematic, continuous collection of data concerning the health status of the client in recorded form that is accessible and that may be communicated. A nursing diagnosis is derived from the data collected. A plan for nursing care incorporates goals derived from the nursing diagnosis and the priorities and approaches to achieve the goals as indicated by the nursing diagnosis. Nursing actions, which are selected and performed with the client's participation, provide for the promotion, maintenance, or restoration of the health of the client and serve to maximize the health care abilities of the client. The progress or lack of progress toward the goal is mutually determined by the client and the nurse, resulting in reassessment, reordering of priorities, establishment of new goals, and revision of the plan for nursing care. Nursing touches on, intersects with, and complements other professional roles in health care, addressing itself to a wide range of health-related responses in people who are well and in those who are not. Nursing seeks to diagnose and treat the response to the problem; thus the concerns of nursing are less circumscribed and discrete than those of other health-related professions. These concerns include: limitations of the client's self-care ability; impaired ability to function in any fundamental area, as sleeping, breathing, eating, maintaining circulation, pain; anxiety, fear, loneliness, grief, or other physical or emotional problems related to health, illness, or treatment; impaired social or intellectual processes; impaired ability to make decisions and choices; alteration of self-image as required by the change in health; dysfunctional perception of health or health-care activities; extra demands posed by such normal life processes as birth, growth, or death; and difficulty in affiliative relationships. Various concepts, principles, processes, and actions, developed and examined in nursing research, guide the steps in the nursing process, from initial observation and diagnosis through evaluation based on intrapersona, interpersonal, and systems theories. The boundary for nursing practice is not static: it tends to move outward as the needs and capacities of society change. Collegial, collaborative practice with other health-care professions further softens the boundaries of nursing practice. All health-care professionals share a mission and a scientific data base, and to some degree their practices overlap. At its core, nursing is nurturative, generative, and protective; preventive care is a part of every nurse's practice. Nurses value independence and self-respect; they are guided by an ethical and humanitarian philosophy in which every human being deserves respect regardless of racial, social, cultural, sexual, economic, religious or other factors. The nurse practices in the context of a relationship with the client, family, or group that is professional and yet close, in an interpersonal sense. The function of a nurse involves the physical intimacy of laying-on of hands; compassion and constant recognition of the person's dignity are essential. Nursing is practiced by specialists and by generalists; generalists provide most nursing care; specialists, having added to their knowledge of an organized and systematized body of knowledge and competencies, practice in specialized areas of nursing. Nursing care is given to people at all stages of life, in the home, hospital, place of employment, school, or other environment where nursing care is needed. Nurses are ethically and legally accountable for their practice and for the actions of others to whom they have delegated responsibility. **3.** the professional practice of a nurse. **4.** the process of acting as a nurse, of providing care that encourages and promotes the health of the person being served.

nursing assessment, an identification by a nurse of the needs, preferences, and abilities of a patient. Assessment follows an interview with and observation of a patient by the nurse and considers the symptoms and signs of the condition, the patient's verbal and nonverbal communication, medical and social history, and any other information available. Among the physical aspects assessed are vital signs, skin color and condition, motor and sensory nerve function, nutrition, rest, sleep, activity, elimination, and conciousness. Among the social and emotional factors assessed are religion, occupation, attitude toward hospital and health care, mood, emotional tone, and family ties and responsibilities. Assessment is extremely important as it provides the scientific basis for a complete nursing care plan.

nursing assistant, *Canada.* a person trained in basic nursing techniques and direct patient care who practices under the supervision of a registered nurse.

nursing audit, a thorough investigation designed to identify, examine, or verify the performance of certain specified aspects of nursing care using established criteria. A **concurrent nursing audit** is performed during ongoing nursing care. A **retrospective nursing audit** is performed after discharge from the care facility, using the patient's record. Often, a nursing audit and a medical audit are performed collaboratively, resulting in a **joint audit.**

nursing-bottle caries, a dental condition that occurs in children between the ages of 18 months and 3 years as a result of being given giving a bottle at bedtime, resulting in prolonged exposure of the teeth to milk or juice. Caries are formed because pools of milk or juice in the mouth break down to lactic acid and other decay-causing substances. Preventive measures include elimination of the bedtime feeding or substitution of water for milk or juice in the nighttime bottle. Also called **bottle-mouth syndrome.**

nursing care of the patient with fever, the observation and treatment of a person with an elevated temperature.

■ METHOD: The patient is observed for symptoms of fever, as tachycardia; a full, bounding pulse or a weak, thready pulse; rapid breathing; hot, dry, hyperemic skin; chills; headache; diaphoresis; restlessness; delirium; dehydration; tremors; convulsions; and coma. Treatment may include the administration of antibiotic, antipyretic and sedative drugs. If the temperature is extremely high, an alcohol sponge bath, cooling tub bath, a cold wet sheet, ice packs, or hypothermia may be ordered. The patient's temperature is checked every two to four hours. Antipyretic and sedative therapy is continued as ordered and, if necessary, cooling measures are reinstituted; the room temperature is reduced, and air currents are increased by a fan. Increased amounts of fluids are given orally or parenterally, physical activity is reduced, and the skin is exposed to air.

■ NURSING ORDERS: The nurse observes and records the symptoms accompanying fever, administers the ordered medication and cooling measures, reassures the patient, and explains the importance of therapy and of drinking adequate fluids.

■ OUTCOME CRITERIA: Antipyretic drugs and cooling measures usually reduce the temperature, but the patient usually requires additional fluids and treatment for the underlying cause of the fever.

nursing care plan, a plan that is based on a nursing assessment and a nursing diagnosis, devised by a nurse. It has four essential components: identification of the nursing care problems and a statement of the nursing approach to solve those problems; the statement of the expected benefit to the patient; the statement of the specific actions by the nurse that reflect the nursing approach and achieve the goals specified; the evaluation of the patient's response to nursing care, and the readjustment of that care as required. The nursing care plan is begun when the patient is admitted to the health service, and, following the initial nursing assessment, a diagnosis is formulated and nursing orders are developed. The goal of the process is to ensure that nursing care is consistent with the patient's needs and progress toward self-care. A written nursing care plan should be a part of every patient's chart; an abbreviated form should be available for quick reference, as in a Rand or Kardex file. See also **diagnosis, nursing assessment, nursing orders.**

nursing diagnosis, a statement of a health problem or of a potential problem in the client's health status that a nurse is licensed and competent to treat. Four steps are required in the formulation of a nursing diagnosis. A database is established by collecting information from all available sources, including interviews with the client and the client's family, a review of any existing records of the client's health, observation of the response of the client to any alterations in health status, a physical assessment, and a conference or consultation with others concerned in the care of the client. The database is continually updated. The second step includes an analysis of the client's responses to the problems, healthy or unhealthy, and a classification of those responses as psychological, physiological, spiritual, or sociological. The third step is the organization of the data so that a tentative diagnostic statement can be made that summarizes the pattern of problems discovered. The last step is the confirmation of the sufficiency and accuracy of the database by evaluation of the appropriateness of the diagnosis to nursing intervention and by the assurance that, given the same information, most other qualified practitioners would arrive at the same nursing diagnosis. In use, each diagnostic category has three parts: the term that concisely describes the problem, the probable etiology of the problem, and the defining characteristics of the problem. A number of nursing diagnoses have been identified and are listed as accepted by the National Group on Classification of Nursing Diagnoses, updated and refined at periodic meetings of the group. The nursing diagnoses accepted at the Fourth National Conference are:

airway clearance, ineffective

bowel elimination, alteration in: constipation

bowel elimination, alteration in: diarrhea

bowel elimination, alteration in: incontinence

breathing pattern, ineffective

cardiac output, alteration in: decreased

comfort, alteration in: pain

communication, impaired verbal

coping, ineffective individual

coping, ineffective family: compromised

coping, ineffective family: disabling

coping, family: potential for growth

diversional activity, deficit

fear

fluid volume deficit, actual

fluid volume deficit, potential

gas exchange, impaired

grieving, anticipatory

grieving, dysfunctional

home maintenance management: impaired

injury: potential for

knowledge deficit

mobility, impaired physical

noncompliance

nutrition, alteration in: less than body requirements

nutrition, alteration in: more than body requirements

nutrition, alteration in: potential for more than body requirements

parenting, alteration in: actual or potential

rape-trauma syndrome

self-care deficit: feeding, bathing/hygiene, dressing/grooming, toileting

self-concept, disturbance in: body image, self-esteem, role performance, personal identity

sensory perceptual alteration: visual, auditory, kinesthetic, gustatory, tactile, olfactory

sexual dysfunction

skin integrity, impairment of: actual

skin integrity, impairment of: potential

sleep pattern disturbance

spiritual distress (distress of the human spirit)

thought processes, alteration in

tissue perfusion, alteration in: cerebral, cardiopulmonary, renal, gastrointestinal, peripheral

urinary elimination, alteration in patterns

violence, potential for: self-directed or directed at others

In addition to the accepted diagnoses listed above, eight others were developed and approved by the Fifth National Conference:

activity intolerance

anxiety

family processes, alterations in

fluid volume, alteration in: excess

health maintenance, alteration in

oral mucous membrane, alterations in

powerlessness

social isolation

nursing goal, a general goal of nursing involving activities that are desirable but difficult to measure, as self-care, good nutrition, and relaxation. Compare **nursing objective.**

nursing home. See **extended care facility.**

nursing intervention, any act by a nurse that implements the nursing care plan or any specific objective of that plan, as turning a comatose patient to avoid the development of decubitus ulcers or teaching injection technique to a person with diabetes before discharge from the hospital. The patient may require intervention in the form of support, limitation, medication, or treatment for the current condition or to prevent the development of further stress. As stress increases, the need to adapt and the need for nursing intervention increase. See also **adaptation, stress.**

nursing intervention model, (in nursing research) a conceptual framework used to determine appropriate nursing interventions. The model is a holistic representation of the client and the health care system. The client's physiological, psychological, sociocultural, and developmental status, the client's stressors and ability to react to them, and the levels and patterns of available health care are observed. The goal is to learn what nursing interventions would be most effective for the particular problem within the particular health care system.

nursing objective, a specific aim planned by a nurse to decrease a person's stress, or improve the ability to adapt, or both. A nursing objective may be physical, emotional, social, or cultural and may involve the person's family and friends and other patients. It is the purpose of any specific nursing order or nursing intervention. Some common nursing objectives are adequate understanding by the patient of certain details of the condition, adequate and comfortable daily elimination, a certain amount of rest, a balanced diet, and participation in specific items of self-care. Nursing objectives, contrasted with nursing goals, can be measured. Compare **nursing goal.**

nursing observation, an objective, holistic evaluation made by a nurse of the various aspects of a client's condition. It includes the person's general appearance, emotional affect, and nutritional status, habits, and preferences, as well as body temperature, skin condition, and any obvious abnormal processes, including those complained of by the client. The client's religious preference, ethnic background, and familial relationships are also noted. Compare **nursing assessment, nursing intervention.**

nursing orders, specific instructions for implementing the nursing care plan, including the patient's preferences, timing of activities, details of health education necessary for the particular patient, role of the family, and plans for care after discharge. Nursing orders must be signed by the professional nurse who writes them. They should not duplicate the orders of the medical staff or of other members of the health team.

nursing process, the process that serves as an organizational framework for the practice of nursing. It encompasses all of the steps taken by the nurse in caring for a patient: data collection, diagnosis, planning, treatment, and evaluation. The rationale for each step is founded in nursing theory. The process requires a systematic approach to a nursing assessment of the person's situation, including an evaluation and reconciliation of the perceptions by the person, the person's family, and the nurse. A plan for the nursing actions to be taken may then be made and, with the participation of the person and the person's family, the plan may be set. The plan developed with the person and the person's family is then implemented. Evaluation of the outcome is performed with the person and the person's family. The steps follow each other at the start of the process but may need to be taken concurrently in some situations. The process does not reach completion with evaluation; the steps are begun again, allowing recurrent evaluation of the assessment, plan, goals, and actions. See also **five-step nursing process, nursing.**

nursing process model, a conceptual framework in which the nurse-patient relationship is the basis of the nursing process. The nursing process is represented as dynamic and interpersonal, the nurse and the patient being affected by each other's behavior and by the environment around them. Each successful two-way communication is termed a 'transaction' and can be analyzed to discover the factors that promote transactions. The constraints that the various systems in the environment (personal, interpersonal, and social) place on the development of the relationship are also examined. The nurse views the patient as a person with whom to communicate in order to have transactions that achieve defined adaptive objectives toward the goal of health.

nursing research, a detailed process in which a systematic study of a problem in the field of nursing is performed. One basic approach requires the following steps: formulation of the problem; review of the literature; development of a theory; formation of a hypothesis or hypotheses; definition of variables; determination of a method for weighting and counting variables; selection of a research design; choice of a population; plan for the analysis of the data; determination of interpretation; and plan for promulgation of the results. Nursing research is practice- or discipline-oriented and is essential for the continued development of the scientific aspects of professional nursing.

Nursing Research, a bimonthly refereed journal containing papers and other materials concerning nursing research. The goal of the journal is to stimulate research in nursing.

nursing rounds, chart rounds, walking rounds, teaching rounds, or grand rounds that are held specifically for nurses and that focus on nursing care problems. See also **rounds.**

nursing specialty, a nurse's particular professional field of practice, as surgical, pediatric, obstetric, or psychiatric nursing. Compare **subspecialty.**

nursing supervisor, a nurse whose function is the administrative and clinical leadership of the nursing service of a division of a health care facility, as a nursing supervisor of maternal and infant care nurses.

nursology (nərsol′əji), a conceptual framework for the study and practice of nursing. It requires the nurse to interact with the patient in an 'authentic' way, without aloofness and the distance of professionalism; the nurse must take the risk of caring. The patient as a person is perceived as a 'subject' rather than an 'object'; the relationship is described as 'intersubjective,' and the parties to the relationship as 'nurse-nursed.' As a method, nursology requires that the nurse cut through the defenses and fears that prevent self-knowledge. The nurse tries to know the patient on an intuitive, subjective level and then, using reflection, on an objective, scientific level. The nurse recognizes that each person has an 'angular view' of the whole truth; comparison of the views of others is necessary for a perspective that allows a synthesis, often paradoxical but closer to the truth than any one person's angular view. The nurse must then struggle with the multiple views to arrive at a final synthesis. This process is called a progression from "we to paradoxical one." Nursology is intended to provide a model for nursing methods and for research. The nurse and the patient have the opportunity to grow, while the science of nursing may emerge from the 'angular' investigations and syntheses.

Nursoy, a trade name for a hypoallergenic nutritional supplement for infants.

nutation, the act of nodding, especially involuntary nodding as occurs in some neurologic disorders.

Nutramigen, a trade name for a milk-substitute formula that is prepared from a soy isolate base and is lactose free, prescribed for infants with galactosemia and as a protein supplement for people with lactose intolerance. See also **Neo-Mull-Soy, Pro Sobee, Soyalac.**

nutri-, a combining form meaning 'of or related to nourishment': *nutriceptor, nutrient, nutritorium.*

nutrient, a substance that provides nourishment and affects the nutritive and metabolic processes of the body.

nutrient artery of the humerus, one of a pair of branches of the deep brachial arteries, arising near the middle of the arm and entering the nutrient canal of the humerus.

nutriment, any substance that nourishes and aids the growth and the development of the body. See also **food.**

nutrition, 1. nourishment. 2. the sum of the processes involved in the taking in of nutrients and in their assimilation and utilization for proper body functioning and maintenance of health. The successive stages include ingestion, digestion, absorption, assimilation, and excretion. 3. the study of food and drink as related to the growth and maintenance of living organisms.

nutritional-alcoholic cerebellar degeneration. See **alcoholic-nutritional cerebellar degeneration.**

nutritional anemia, a disorder characterized by the inadequate production of hemoglobin or erythrocytes owing to nutritional deficiency of iron, folic acid, or vitamin B_{12}, or other nutritional disorders. See also **iron deficiency anemia, megaloblastic anemia, pernicious anemia.**

nutritional care, the substances, procedures, and setting involved in assuring the proper intake and assimilation of nutriments, especially for the hospitalized patient.

■ METHOD: Depending on the patient's condition, nutritional requirements may be provided by regular meals with menus selected from the ordered diet, by tube feeding, or by parenteral hyperalimentation. Meals are served on attractive trays in an environment conducive to eating; distasteful procedures are avoided before and after mealtime. Patients who are unable to feed themselves are assisted, and abnormal intake of food is recorded and reported. Supplemental nourishment when indicated and fluids are offered between meals. The nutritional assessment includes observations of the patient's appetite, food preferences, height, weight, measurements of the head, arms, abdomen, and skinfold thickness, the skin color and turgor, and the condition of the mouth, eyes, and hair. Any cutaneous lesions, thyroid enlargement, dental caries, loose teeth, ill-fitting dentures, gum problems, nausea, vomiting, dehydration, diarrhea, or constipation are noted.

■ NURSING ORDERS: The nurse sees that food is presented attractively, offers a wash cloth and mouthwash before and after meals, and, when necessary, feeds the patient to maintain an adequate intake. If indicated, as in obese patients or those with disorders requiring a highly restricted diet, the nurse restricts the intake of food as ordered. Tube feedings are administered as ordered.

■ OUTCOME CRITERIA: Obvious good health, a normal weight, and the absence of gastrointestinal symptoms usually indicate that the individual's nutritional requirements are being fulfilled.

nutrition, alteration in: less than body requirements, a nursing diagnosis accepted by the Fourth National Conference on Nursing Diagnoses. The etiology of the condition is an inability, based on psychological, biological, or economic factors, to ingest or to digest food or to absorb nutrients in sufficient quantity for the maintenance of normal health. The defining characteristics of the condition may include loss of weight, reported intake of less food than is recommended, evidence or report of a lack of food, lack of interest in food, aversion to eating, alteration in the taste of food, feelings of fullness immediately after eating small quantities, abdominal pain with no other explanation, sores in the mouth, diarrhea or steatorrhea, pallor, weakness, and loss of hair. See also **nursing diagnosis.**

nutrition, alteration in: more than body requirements, a nursing diagnosis accepted by the Fourth National Conference on the Classification of Nursing Diagnoses. The etiology of the condition is an excessive intake of food in relation to the metabolic needs of the body. The defining characteristics of the condition include overweight, sedentary activity level, and dysfunctional eating habits, including eating in response to internal cues other than hunger. See also **nursing diagnosis.**

nutrition alteration in: potential for more than body requirements, a nursing diagnosis accepted by the Fourth National Conference on the Classification of Nursing Diagnoses. The etiology of the condition may be an inherited or familial predisposition to overweight, an excessive intake of calories during adolescence and other periods of rapid growth, frequent, closely spaced pregnancies, dysfunctional psychological conditioning in regard to food, or membership in a lower socioeconomic group. The defining characteristics of the problem may include the use of solid foods as a significant part of the diet before the age of five months, the use of food as a reward, an observed increase in the baseline weight at the onset of each pregnancy, or dysfunctional eating patterns, as eating in response to external cues such as social situations or the time of day. The critical defining characteristics which must be present for the diagnosis to be made include reported or observed obesity in one or both parents and rapidly increasing percentiles in measurement of the infant's or child's weight as compared to others of the same age. See also **nursing diagnosis.**

nutritionist, one who studies and applies the principles and science of nutrition.

Nutting, Mary Adelaide (1858–1947), a Canadian-born American nursing educator and reformer. As head of Johns Hopkins School of Nursing in Baltimore, beginning in 1894, she improved course content, and teaching facilities, instituted the six-months preparatory course, reduced the 12-hour day to eight hours, and abolished the monthly payment system to students. At Teachers College, Columbia University, she created and developed the Department of Nursing and Health and became the first professor of nursing in the world. With Lavinia Dock, she wrote *History of Nursing,* a classic in nursing literature.

nyctalopia (nĭk′tə-lou′pĭə), poor vision at night or in dim light, associated with vitamin A deficiency and pigmentary degeneration of the retina. Also called **night blindness.** — **nyctalopic,** *adj.*

nycto-, a combining form meaning 'pertaining to night or darkness': *nyctohemeral, nyctophilia, nyctophobia.*

nyctophobia (nĭk′toufou′bĭə), an anxiety reaction characterized by an obsessive, irrational fear of darkness.

nycturia (nĭktur′ĭə). See **nocturia.**

Nydrazid, a trade name for an antibacterial (isoniazid).

nylidrin hydrochloride (nĭl′ĭdrĭn), a peripheral vasodilator.

■ INDICATIONS: It is prescribed in the treatment of peripheral vascular disease and circulatory disturbances of the inner ear.

■ CONTRAINDICATIONS: Acute cardiac disease, paroxysmal tachycardia, thyrotoxicosis, progressive angina pectoris, or known hypersensitivity to this drug prohibits its use.

■ ADVERSE EFFECTS: The most serious adverse reaction is hypotention with dizziness, tachycardia, nausea, and weakness.

Nylmerate, a trade name for an antimicrobial (phenylmercuric nitrate).

nympho-, a combining form meaning 'of or pertaining to the labia minora': *nymphocaruncular, nymphohymeneal, nymphoncus.*

nymphomania, a psychosexual disorder of women characterized by an insatiable desire for sexual satisfaction, often resulting from an unconscious conflict concerning personal adequacy. Compare **satyriasis.** See also **psychosexual disorder.**

nymphomaniac, 1. a person with or displaying characteristics of nymphomania. 2. of, pertaining to, or exhibiting nymphomania. — **nymphomaniacal,** *adj.*

Nystaform, a trade name for a topical, fixed-combination drug containing an antifungal (nystatin) and a topical anti-infective (iodochlorhydroxyquin).

nystagmus (nĭstæg′məs), involuntary, rhythmic movements of the eyes; the oscillations may be horizontal, vertical, rotary, or mixed. Jerking nystagmus, characterized by faster movements in one direction than in the opposite direction, is more common than pendular nystagmus, in which the oscillations are approximately equal in rate in both directions. Jerking nystagmus occurs normally when an individual watches a moving object, but, on other occasions, it may be a sign of barbiturate intoxication or of labyrinthine-vestibular, vascular, or neurologic disease. Labyrinthine-vestibular nystagmus, most frequently rotary, is usually accompanied by vertigo and nausea. Vertical nystagmus is considered pathognomonic of disease of the brainstem's tegmentum, and nystagmus occurring only in the abducting eye is said to be a sign of multiple sclerosis. Seesaw nystagmus, in which one eye moves up and other down, may be seen in bilateral hemianopia. Pendular nystagmus occurs in albinism, various diseases of the retina and refractive media, and in miners, following many years of working in darkness; in miners, the eye movements are very rapid, increase on upward gaze, and are often associated with vertigo, head tremor, and photophobia. Electronystagmography, used in testing for vestibular disease and in evaluating patients with vertigo, hearing loss, or tinnitus, records changes in the electrical field around the eyes when nystagmus is induced by douching cold or warm water into the external auditory canal; this test causes nystagmus in normal individuals and a diminished or absent reaction in patients with labyrinth disorder. Also called **nystaxis.** — **nystagmic,** *adj.*

nystatin (nis′tətin), an antifungal antibiotic.

■ INDICATION: It is prescribed in the treatment of fungal infections of the gastrointestinal tract, vagina, and skin.

■ CONTRAINDICATION: Known hypersensitivity to this drug is the only contraindication.

■ ADVERSE EFFECTS: There are no known serious adverse reactions. Mild gastrointestinal distress and mild skin reactions may occur.

nystaxis (nistæk′sis). See **nystagmus.**

O

O, symbol for **oxygen.**

O₂, symbol for **oxygen.**

oario-. See **ovario-.**

OASHDI, abbreviation for **Old Age, Survivors, Disability and Health Insurance Program,** as provided by the Social Security Act.

oat cell carcinoma, a malignant, usually bronchogenic epithelial neoplasm consisting of small, tightly packed, round, oval, or spindle-shaped epithelial cells that stain darkly and contain neurosecretory granules and little or no cytoplasm. Tumors produced by these cells do not form bulky masses but usually spread along submucosal lymphatics. One third of all malignant tumors of the lung are of this type. Usually surgical resection is not possible, and chemotherapy and radiation therapy are not effective in treatment; thus, the prognosis is poor. Also called **small cell carcinoma.**

OB, **1.** *Informal.* abbreviation for **obstetrics.** **2.** *Informal.* abbreviation for **obstetrician.**

ob-, a combining form meaning 'against, in front of': *obdormition, obduction, obtuse.* Also **oc-.**

Obedrin-LA, a trade name for a sustained-release central nervous system stimulant (methamphetamine hydrochloride)

Obegyn, a trade name for a hematinic, fixed-combination drug containing iron and vitamins.

obesity, an abnormal increase in the proportion of fat cells in the subcutaneous tissues of the body. Obesity may be exogenous or endogenous.

Obetrol, a trade name for a fixed-combination drug containing central-nervous-system stimulants (dextroamphetamine and amphetamine).

objective, **1.** a goal. **2.** of or pertaining to a phenomenon or clinical finding that is observed; not subjective. An objective finding is often described in health care as a sign, as compared to a symptom, which is a subjective funding.

objective data collection, the process in which data relating to the client's problem are obtained by an observer through direct physical examination, including observation, palpation, and auscultation, and by laboratory analyses and radiologic and other studies. Compare **subjective data collection.**

obligate (ob′lıgıt, ob′lıgeıt), characterized by the ability to survive only in a particular set of environmental conditions, as an obligate parasite, which can survive only within the host organism. Compare **facultative.**

obligate aerobe, an organism that cannot grow in the absence of oxygen. Compare **facultative aerobe.** See also **aerobe.**

obligate anaerobe, an organism that cannot grow in the presence of oxygen, as *Clostridium tetani, C. botulinum,* and *C. perfringens.* Compare **facultative anaerobe.** See also **anaerobe, anaerobic infection.**

obligate parasite. See **parasite.**

oblique, a slanting direction or any variation from the perpendicular or the horizontal.

oblique bandage, a circular bandage applied spirally in slanting turns, usually to a limb.

oblique fissure of the lung, **1.** the groove marking the division of the lower and the middle lobes in the right lung. **2.** the groove marking the division of the upper and the lower lobes in the left lung.

oblique fracture, a fracture that cracks a bone at an oblique angle.

oblique illumination. See **illumination.**

obliquus externus abdominis, one of a pair of muscles that are the largest and the most superficial of the five anterolateral muscles of the abdomen. A broad, thin, four-sided muscle that arises by eight fleshy digitations from the lower eight ribs and by the broad abdominal aponeurosis, it inserts in the iliac crest and the linea alba. It is innervated by branches of the eighth through the twelfth intercostal nerves and by the iliohypogastric and ilioinguinal nerves. It acts to compress the contents of the abdomen and assists in micturition, defecation, emesis, parturition, and forced expiration. Both sides acting together serve to flex the vertebral column, drawing the pubis toward the xiphoid process. One side alone functions to bend the vertebral column laterally and to rotate it, drawing the shoulder of the same side forward. Also called **descending oblique muscle, external oblique muscle.** Compare **obliquus internus abdominis, pyramidalis, rectus abdominis, transversus abdominis.**

obliquus internus abdominis, one of a pair of anterolateral muscles of the abdomen, lying under the obliquus externus abdominis in the lateral and ventral part of the abdominal wall. Smaller and thinner than the obliquus externus abdominis, it arises from the inguinal ligament, the iliac crest, and the lower portion of the lumbar apo-

759

neurosis. It inserts into the last three or four ribs and into the linea alba. The obliquus internus abdominis functions to compress the abdominal contents and assists in micturition, defecation, emesis, parturition, and forced expiration. Both sides acting together serve to flex the vertebral column, drawing the costal cartilages toward the pubis. One side acting alone acts to bend the vertebral column laterally and rotate it, drawing the shoulder of the opposite side downward. Also called **ascending oblique muscle, internal oblique muscle.** Compare **obliquus externus abdominis, pyramidalis, rectus abdominis, transversus abdominis.**

Obotan, a trade name for a central-nervous-system stimulant (dextroamphetamine tannate).

Obron-6, a trade name for a nutritional supplement containing multivitamins, calcium, and iron.

observation, 1. the act of watching carefully and attentively. 2. a report of what is seen or noticed, as a **nursing observation.**

obsession, a persistent thought or idea with which the mind is continually and involuntarily preoccupied and which suggests an irrational act. The thought cannot be eliminated by logic or reason and usually gives rise to a compulsion. See also **compulsion, obsessive-compulsive reaction.** —**obsessive,** *adj.*

obsessional personality, a type of personality in which persistent, intrusive, irrational, uncontrollable, and unwanted thoughts lead to compulsive actions. The thoughts may consist of single words, simple ideas or desires, images, ruminations, or, more commonly, a complex train of ideas referring to past events and completed actions or to anticipated events and future actions. A person with an obsessional personality is punctual, orderly, meticulous, and dependable, is dominated by feelings of inadequacy, insecurity, and guilt, and is highly vulnerable to threat, worry, indecision, overscrupulousness, and excessive anxiety.

obsessive-compulsive, 1. characterized by or relating to the tendency to perform repetitive acts or rituals, usually as a means of releasing tension or relieving anxiety. 2. describing a person who has an obsessive-compulsive neurosis.

obsessive-compulsive neurosis, a neurotic condition characterized by the inability to resist or stop the intrusion of persistent, irrational, and uncontrollable urges, ideas, thoughts, or fears contrary to the person's standards or judgments. The disorder usually appears after adolescence, resulting from fear, feelings of guilt, and anticipation of punishment. Treatment may consist of psychotherapy to uncover the basic fears and to help the person distinguish objective dangers from imagined dangers. Also called **obsessive-compulsive reaction, psychasthenia.**

obsessive-compulsive personality, a type of personality in which there is an uncontrollable need to perform certain acts or rituals. This behavior is manifested in many forms and may range from mildly stylized personal habits, as repeating certain words or phrases before undertaking a particular act or ritually counting and touching, to more serious compulsive acts, as the continous washing of hands or changing of clothes. A person with this kind of personality is usually orderly, meticulous, punctual, dependable, and scrupulous, though with a tendency to be rigid, stubborn, and pedantic. When the acts or rituals become irrational and exaggerated, they reduce the flexibility of behavior and interfere with everyday functioning in society, becoming neurotic reactions.

obsessive-compulsive reaction. See **obsessive-compulsive neurosis.**

obstetrical position. See **lateral recumbent position.**

obstetric anesthesia, any of various procedures used to provide anesthesia for childbirth. It includes local anesthesia for episiotomy or episiotomy repair, regional anesthesia for labor or delivery, as by paracervical block or pudendal block, or, for a wider block—epidural, caudal, or saddle block. Anesthesia for Caesarean section may be achieved with an epidural block or by general anesthesia. Light inhalation anesthesia with a mixture of nitrous oxide and oxygen is commonly given when forceps are required or when a difficult vaginal delivery is expected.

obstetrician, a physician who specializes in obstetrics.

obstetric forceps, forceps used to assist delivery of the fetal head. They vary in weight, length, shape, and mechanism of action, but all consist of a pair of instruments comprising a handle, a shank, and a blade. The blade is curved and, sometimes, fenestrated. The shank is long enough to allow the blade to reach the fetal head. The several styles of forceps are designed to assist in various clinical situations. The station of the fetus in the pelvis, the position of the head in relation to the pelvis, the size of the fetus, and the preference of the operator all affect the choice of forceps. Kinds of obstetrical forceps include **Barton forceps, Elliot forceps, Kielland forceps, Simpson forceps.** See also **forceps delivery.**

obstetrics, the branch of medicine concerned with pregnancy and childbirth, including the study of the physiologic and pathologic function of the female reproductive tract and the care of the mother and fetus throughout pregnancy, childbirth, and the immediate postpartum period. —**obstetric, obstetrical,** *adj.*

obstipation (ob'stɪpei'shən), 1. a condition of extreme and persistent constipation caused by obstruction in the intestinal or eliminatory system. See also **constipation.** 2. a process of blocking. —**obstipant,** *n.,* **obstipate,** *v.*

obstruction, 1. something that blocks or clogs. 2. the act of blocking or preventing passage. 3. the condition of being obstructed or clogged. —**obstruct,** *v.,* **obstructive,** *adj.*

obstructive anuria, an abnormal urologic condition characterized by an almost complete absence of urination and caused by an obstruction of the urinary tract. See also **anuria.**

obstructive jaundice. See **cholestasis.**

obtund (obtənd′), **1.** to deaden pain. **2.** to render insensitive to unpleasant or painful stimuli by reducing the level of consciousness, as by anesthesia or a strong narcotic analgesic. — **obtundation, obtundity,** *n.,* **obtunded, obtundent,** *adj.*

obtundation, the use of an agent that soothes and reduces irritation or pain by blocking sensibility at some level of the central nervous system, as in the preoperative use of anesthesia, the use of narcotics to control pain, and the giving of a tranquilizer as a calming agent.

obturator (ob′tərei′tər, ob′tyərei′tər), **1.** a device used to block a passage or a canal or to fill in a space, as a prosthesis implanted to bridge the gap in the roof of the mouth in a cleft palate. **2.** *Nontechnical.* an obturator muscle or membrane.

obturator externus, the flat, triangular muscle covering the outer surface of the anterior wall of the pelvis. It arises in several pelvic structures, including the rami of the pubis and the ramus of each ischium, and inserts into the trochanteric fossa of the femur. The obturator externus is innervated by a branch of the obturator nerve, which contains fibers of the third and the fourth lumbar nerves, and it functions to rotate the thigh laterally. Compare **obturator internus.**

obturator foramen, a large opening on each side of the lower portion of the innominate bone, formed posteriorly by the ischium, superiorly by the illium, and anteriorly by the pubis.

obturator internus, a muscle that covers a large area of the inferior aspect of the lesser pelvis, where it surrounds the obturator foramen. It arises from the superior and the inferior rami of the pubis, the ischium, and the obturator membrane and inserts into the greater trochanter of the femur. It is innervated by a special nerve from the sacral plexus, which contains fibers from the lumbosacral trunk and the first and the second sacral nerves, and it functions to rotate the thigh laterally and to extend and abduct the thigh when it is flexed. Compare **obturator externus, piriformis.**

obturator membrane, a tough fibrous membrane that covers the obturator foramen of each side of the pelvis.

obturator muscle, a muscle of the pelvis and upper leg that acts to rotate the leg laterally.

oc-. See **ob-.**

occipital (oksɪp′ɪtəl), **1.** of or pertaining to the occiput. **2.** situated near the occipital bone, as the occipital lobe of the brain.

occipital artery, one of a pair of tortuous branches from the external carotid arteries that divides into six branches and supplies parts of the head and scalp. Each terminal portion at the vertex of the skull is accompanied by the greater occipital nerve.

occipital bone, the cuplike bone at the back of the skull, pierced by a large opening called the foramen magnum that communicates with the vertebral canal. Its inner surface is divided into four fossae. The occipital bone articulates with the two parietal bones, the two temporal bones, the sphenoid, and the atlas.

occipital lobe, one of the five lobes of each cerebral hemisphere, occupying a relatively small pyramidal portion of the occipital pole. The occipital lobe lies beneath the occipital bone and presents medial, lateral, and inferior surfaces. The medial surface is bounded anteriorly by the pareitooccipital sulcus and the preoccipital notch and is divided by the posterior calcarine sulcus into the wedge-shaped cuneus and the lingual gyrus. The lateral surface of the lobe is divided by the lateral sulcus into the superior and the inferior occipital gyri. An imaginary transverse line across the preoccipital notch limits the inferior surface. Compare **central lobe, frontal lobe, parietal lobe, temporal lobe.**

occipital sinus, the smallest of the cranial sinuses and one of six posterior superior venous channels associated with the dura mater. It is located in the attached margin of the falx cerebelli, courses around the foramen magnum by several small channels, communicates with the posterior internal vertebral venous plexuses, and ends in the confluence of the sinuses. Compare **inferior sagittal sinus, occipital sinus, straight sinus, superior sagittal sinus.**

occipitoaxial ligament (oksɪp′ɪtouæk′siəl). See **membrana tectoria.**

occipitobregmatic (oksɪp′ɪtoubregmæt′ɪk), of or pertaining to the occiput and the bregma.

occipitofrontal (oksɪp′ɪtoufrən′təl), of or pertaining to the occiput and the frontal bone of the skull.

occipitofrontalis (oksɪp′ɪtoufrəntæl′ɪs), one of a pair of thin, broad muscles covering the top of the skull, consisting of an occipital belly and a frontal belly connected by an extensive aponeurosis. The frontal belly originates at the galea aponeurotica and inserts in the skin of the eyebrows and the nose. The occipital belly originates in the superior nuchal line of the occipital bone and inserts at the galea aponeurotica. The occipitofrontalis is innervated by the facial nerve. It is the muscle that draws the scalp and raises the eyebrows. Compare **temporoparietalis.**

occipitoparietal fissure. See **parieto-occipital sulcus.**

occiput (ok′sɪpət), *pl.* **occiputs, occipita** (oksɪp′ɪtə). the back part of the head. Also called **occiput cranii.**

occiput cranii. See **occiput.**

occlusal trauma (əklu′səl), injury to a tooth and surrounding structures caused by malocclusive stresses.

occlusion, a blockage in a canal, vessel, or passage of the body. — **occlude,** *v.,* **occlusive,** *adj.*

occlusion rim, an artificial dental structure with occluding surfaces attached to temporary or permanent denture bases, used for recording the relation of the maxilla to the mandible and for positioning the teeth. Also called **bite block.**

occlusive dressing (əklu'sɪv), a dressing that prevents air from reaching a wound or lesion and that retains moisture, heat, body fluids, and medication. It may consist of a sheet of thin plastic affixed with transparent tape. See also **dressing.**

occult, hidden or difficult to observe directly, as occult prolapse of the umbilical cord or occult blood.

occult blood, a minute or hidden quantity of blood that can be detected only by means of a chemical test or by microscopic or spectroscopic examination. Occult blood is often present in the stools of patients with gastrointestinal lesions.

occult carcinoma, a small carcinoma that does not cause overt symptoms. It may remain localized and be discovered only incidentally at autopsy following upon death owing to another cause, or it may metastasize and be discovered in the diagnostic study of the resulting metastatic disease. Also called **latent carcinoma.**

occult fracture, a fracture that cannot be initially detected by radiographic examination but may be evident radiographically weeks later. It is accompanied by the usual signs of pain and trauma and may produce soft tissue edema.

occupational accident, an accidental injury to an employee that occurs in the workplace. Occupational accidents account for over 95 per cent of occupational disabilities. In most cases the injured worker is eligible for compensation.

occupational asthma, an abnormal condition of the respiratory system resulting from exposure in the workplace to allergenic or other irritating substances. The condition is most common among persons working with detergents, Western red cedar, cotton, flax, hemp, grain, flour and stone. See also **asthma, byssinosis, occupational lung disease.**

occupational disability, a condition in which a worker is unable to perform the functions required to complete a job satisfactorily, owing to an occupational disease or an occupational accident.

occupational disease, a disease that results from a particular employment, usually from the effects of long-term exposure to specific substances or of continuous or repetitive physical acts.

occupational history, a portion of the health history in which questions are asked about the person's occupation, source of income, effects of the work on worker's health or the worker's health on the job, the duration of the job, and to what degree the occupation satisfies the person. Any adverse effects known to be associated with the work or the place of work are investigated by further questions by the interviewer, as a tennis player might be asked about musculoskeletal problems or a taxi driver about function of the urinary tract.

occupational lung disease, any one of a group of abnormal conditions of the lungs caused by the inhalation of dusts, fumes, gases, or vapors in an environment where a person works. See also **chronic obstructive pulmonary disease, metal fume fever, occupational asthma, silo fillers' disease.**

occupational neurosis, a neurotic disorder in which various symptoms occur that prevent the activities required by the occupation, as in writer's cramp. The symptoms are not caused by the occupation; rather, they serve as an expression of a neurotic conflict.

occupational therapist, a person who practices occupational therapy and who may be licensed, registered, certified, or otherwise regulated by law.

occupational therapy, a subdivision of physical medicine in which handicapped or convalescing patients are trained in vocational skills and activities of daily life through a program designed to satisfy the specific needs of the patient while providing diversion and exercise.

occurrence policy, a professional liability insurance policy that covers the holder during the period an alleged act of malpractice occurred. Occurrence policies are said to have a 'long tail,' because the statute of limitations on malpractice allegations is unlimited. Thus, an individual could be sued years after an event had taken place. If the individual held an occurrence type of malpractice policy, there would be protection under that policy; under a claims-made policy there would not be protection unless the policy were current.

ochre mutation. See **amber mutation.**

ochronosis (ou'krənou'sɪs), a condition characterized by the deposition of brown-black pigment in connective tissue and cartilage, often caused by alkaptonuria or poisoning with phenol. Bluish macules may be noted on the sclera, fingers, ears, nose, genitalia, buccal mucosa, and axillae. The urine may be dark-colored. See also **alkaptonuria.**

octaploid, octaploidic (ok'təploid). See **polyploid.**

Octin, a trade name for an alpha adrenergic-agent (isometheptene) which has been used to treat migraine.

ocular (ok'yulər), **1.** of or pertaining to the eye. **2.** an eyepiece of an optical instrument.

ocular hypertelorism, a developmental defect involving the frontal region of the cranium, characterized by an abnormally widened bridge of the nose and increased distance between the eyes. The condition is often associated with other cranial and facial deformities and some degree of mental retardation. Also called **orbital hypertelorism.**

ocular hypotelorism, a developmental defect involving the frontal region of the cranium, characterized by a narrowing of the bridge of the nose and an abnormal decrease in the distance between the eyes, with resulting convergent strabismus. The condition is often associated with other cranial and facial deformities, primarily microcephaly and trigonocephaly, and some degree of mental retardation. Also called **orbital hypotelorism.**

ocular myopathy, slowly progressive weakness of ocular muscles, characterized by decreased mobility of the eye and drooping of the upper lid. The disorder may be unilateral or bilateral and may be caused by damage to the oculomotor nerve, an intracranial tumor, or a neuromuscular disease.

ocular spot, an abnormal opacity in the eye. A shower of red and black dots may be seen in the eye following hemorrhage of a retinal vessel; opacities in the crystalline lens are characteristic in cataracts. In asteroid hyalitis, often associated with diabetes, small white spherical and stellate opacities are found in the vitreous humor; these bodies consist of calcium soaps and sparkle when examined with a light.

oculo-, a combining form meaning 'of or pertaining to the eye': *oculofacial, oculomycosis, oculopathy.*

oculogyric crisis (ok'yuloujai'rɪk), a paroxysm in which the eyes are held in a fixed position, usually up and sideways, for minutes or several hours, often occurring in postencephalitic patients with signs of parkinsonism. In some cases the eyes are held down or sideways and there may be spasm or closing of the lids. Oculogyric crises may be precipitated by emotional stress, and patients with the disorder frequently show psychiatric symptoms.

oculomotor nerve, either of a pair of cranial nerves essential for eye movements, supplying certain extrinsic and intrinsic eye muscles. They pass through the superior orbital fissure, connecting to the brain in nucleus III. Also called **nervus oculomotorius, third nerve.**

Ocusert Pilo, a trade name for a cholinergic (pilocarpine).

O.D., abbreviation for *oculus dexter,* a Latin phrase meaning 'right eye.'

-ode[1], a combining form meaning a 'type of (specified) electrical conductor': *anode, cathode, electrode.*

-ode[2], a combining form meaning 'like in form' of something specified: *cytode, icterode, sarcode.*

odont-. See **odonto-.**

-odontia, a combining form meaning a 'form, condition, or mode of treatment of the teeth': *periodontia, prosthodontia, radiodontia.*

odontiasis (ou'dontai'əsɪs), the process of cutting teeth; teething.

-odontic, 1. a combining form meaning 'pertaining to the size of teeth': *isodontic, macrodontic, mesodontic.* 2. a combining form meaning 'pertaining to type of dental treatment': *gerodontic, orthodontic, pedodontic.*

odontitis (ou'dontai'tɪs), abnormal enlargement of a tooth, usually resulting from an inflammation of the odontoblasts (cells responsible for dentine formation) rather than of the mature, or erupted tooth. It may be caused by infection, tumor, or trauma.

odonto-, odont-, a combining form meaning 'of or pertaining to the teeth': *odontoblast, odontopathy, odontotechny.*

odontogenesis imperfecta. See **dentinogenesis imperfecta.**

odontogenic (oudon'toujen'ɪk), 1. generating teeth. 2. developing in tissues which produce teeth.

odontogenic fibroma, a benign neoplasm of the jaw derived from the embryonic part of the tooth germ, dental follicle, or dental papilla or developing later from the periodontal membrane.

odontogenic fibrosarcoma, a malignant neoplasm of the jaw that develops in a mesenchymal component of a tooth or tooth germ.

odontogenic myxoma, a rare tumor of the jaw, that apparently develops from the mesenchyme of the tooth germ.

odontoid ligament. See **alar ligament.**

odontoid vertebra. See **axis.**

odontology (ou'dontol'əji), the scientific study of the anatomy and physiology of the teeth and of the surrounding structures of the oral cavity.

odor, a scent or smell. The sense of smell is activated when airborne molecules stimulate the first cranial nerve.

-odyne, a combining form meaning 'referring to, treating pain': *acesodyne, anodyne, biodyne.*

-odynia, a combining form meaning a 'state of pain in a (specified) location': *coccyodynia, odontodynia, uterodynia.*

odyno-, a combining form meaning 'pain': *odynolysis, odynophagia, odynopoeia.*

odynophagia (od'ɪnoufei'jə), a severe sensation of burning, squeezing pain while swallowing, caused by irritation of the mucosa or a muscular disorder of the esophagus, as gastroesophageal reflux, bacterial or fungal infection, tumor, achalasia, or chemical irritation.

oenomania. See **oinomania.**

Ogen, a trade name for an estrogen (piperazine estrone sulfate).

OH, symbol for **hydroxyl.**

OHF, abbreviation for **Omsk hemorrhagic fever.**

ohm, a unit of measurement of electrical resistance. One ohm is the resistance of a conductor in which an electrical potential of one volt produces a current of one ampere.

-oi, a plural-forming element in borrowings from Greek: *auloi, catanephroi, mesonephroi.* Also **-i.**

-oid[1], a combining form meaning 'resembling' something specified: *alkaloid, spheroid, trochoid.*

-oid², a combining form meaning 'having the form or appearance of': *cuboid, lambdoid, ovoid.*

oiko-, a combining form meaning 'house': *oikofugic, oikology, oikophobia.*

oil, any of a large number of greasy liquid substances not miscible in water. Oil may be fixed or volatile and is derived from animal, vegetable, or mineral matter.

oinomania (oi'noumei'niə), **enomania, oenomania** (i'noumei'niə), **1.** *Archaic.* a periodic, irresistible craving for alcohol, especially wine. **2.** delirium tremens.

ointment, a semisolid, externally applied preparation, usually containing a drug. Various ointments are used as local analgesic, anesthetic, anti-infective, astringent, depigmenting, irritant, and keratolytic agents. Also called **salve, unction, unguent.**

-ol¹, a combining form designating a member of the alcohol group: *ethanol, methanol, naphthol.*

-ol², a combining form meaning an 'oil': *benzol, furol, petrol.* Also **-ole.**

-ola, a combining form meaning, a 'singular diminutive of the noun named': *arteriola, neurovariola, taeniola.*

Old Age, Survivors, Disability and Health Insurance Program, a benefit program, administered by the Social Security Administration, that provides cash benefits to workers who are retired or disabled, their dependents, and survivors. This part of the program is commonly referred to as Social Security. The program also provides health insurance benefits for people over 65 and for disabled people under 65. This part of the program is commonly referred to as Medicare. See also **Medicare.**

Old World leishmaniasis. See **oriental sore.**

oleandomycin (ou'liæn'doumai'sın). See **troleandomycin.**

olecranon (oulek'rənon), a proximal projection of the ulna that forms the point of the elbow and fits into the olecranon fossa of the humerus when the forearm is extended. The anterior surface of the olecranon forms part of the trochlear notch that articulates with the humerus. Also called **olecranon process.**

olecranon bursa, the bursa of the elbow.

olecranon fossa, the depression in the posterior surface of the humerus that receives the olecranon of the ulna when the forearm is extended. Compare **coronoid fossa.**

olecranon process. See **olecranon.**

oleic acid (ouli'ık), a colorless, liquid, monounsaturated fatty acid occurring in almost all natural fats. Commercial oleic acid is used in soaps, cosmetics, ointments, lubricants, and food additives.

oleo-, a combining form meaning 'of or pertaining to oil': *oleocreosote, oleodistearin, oleoresin.* Also **eleo-.**

oleometer (ou'liom'ıtər), a device for measuring the purity of oils.

oleovitamin (ou'liouvai'təmın), a preparation of fish-liver oil or edible vegetable oil that contains one or more of the fat-soluble vitamins or their derivatives.

oleovitamin A, an oily preparation, usually fish-liver oil or fish-liver oil diluted with an edible vegetable oil, containing the natural or synthetic form of vitamin A. See also **vitamin A.**

oleovitamin D₂. See **calciferol.**

olfactory (olfæk'təri), of or pertaining to the sense of smell. – **olfaction,** *n.*

olfactory anesthesia. See **anosmia.**

olfactory center, the part of the brain responsible for the subjective appreciation of odors, a complex group of neurons located near the junction of the temporal and parietal lobes.

olfactory foramen, one of several openings in the cribiform plate of the ethmoid bone.

olfactory nerve, one of a pair of nerves associated with the sense of smell. The olfactory nerve is cranial nerve I and is composed of numerous fine filaments that ramify in the mucous membrane of the olfactory area. The fibers of the olfactory nerve are nonmedullated and unite into fasciculi which form a plexus under the mucous membrane and rise in grooves or canals in the ethmoid bone. The fibers pass into the skull and form synapses with the dendrites of the mitral cells. The area in which the olfactory nerves arise is situated in the most superior portion of the mucous membrane that covers the superior nasal concha. The olfactory sensory endings are modified epithelial cells and the least specialized of the special senses. The olfactory nerves connect with the olfactory bulb and the olfactory tract, which are components of the portion of the brain associated with the sense of smell.

olig-. See **oligo-.**

oligo-, olig-, a combining form meaning 'few, little': *oligocholia, oligodontia, oligosialia.*

oligodactyly (ol'ıgoudæk'tıli), **oligodactylism, oligodactylia,** a congenital anomaly characterized by the absence of one or more of the fingers or toes. – **oligodactylic,** *adj.*

oligodendroblastoma (ol'ıgouden'droublæstou'mə). See **oligodendroglioma.**

oligodendroglioma (ol'ıgouden'drougliaiou'mə), *pl.* **oligodendrogliomas, oligodendrogliomata.** an uncommon brain tumor composed of nonneural ectodermal cells that usually form part of the supporting connective tissue around nerve cells. The lesion, a firm, reddish-gray mass with calcified spots and a distinct margin, may grow to a large size. It develops most often in frontal, parietal, and paraventricular sites but may also occur in the cerebellum. Also called **oligodendroblastoma.**

oligodontia (ol'ıgoudon'Sha), a genetically determined dental defect characterized by the development of fewer than the normal number of teeth.

oligogenic (ol'ıgoujen'ık), of or pertaining to hereditary characteristics produced by one or only a few genes.

oligomeganephronia (ol'ɪgoumeg'ənefrou'niə), a type of congenital renal hypoplasia associated with chronic renal failure in children. The condition is characterized by a decreased number of functioning nephrons and hypertrophy of other renal elements without the presence of aberrant tissue. Also called **oligomeganephronic renal hypoplasia**. — **oligomeganephronic**, *adj.*

oligomeganephronic renal hypoplasia. See **oligomeganephronia**.

oligomenorrhea, abnormally light or infrequent menstruation. — **oligomenorrheic**, *adj.*

oligopnea, oligopnoea (ol'ɪgopni'ə). See **hypopnea**. — **oligopneic, oligopnoic**, *adj.*

oligospermia (ol'ɪgouspər'miə), insufficient spermatozoa in the semen. Compare **azoospermia**.

oliguresis (ol'ɪgyuri'sɪs). See **oliguria**.

oliguria (ol'ɪgyur'iə), a diminished capacity to form and pass urine so that the end products of metabolism cannot be excreted efficiently. It is usually caused by imbalances in bodily fluids and electrolytes, by renal lesions, or by urinary tract obstruction. Also called **oliguresis**. Compare **anuria**. — **oliguric**, *adj.*

olivopontocerebellar (ol'ɪvoupon'touser'ɪbel'ər), of or pertaining to the olivae, the middle peduncles, and the cerebellum.

Ollier's disease (ol'ieiz'). See **enchondromatosis**.

Ollier's dyschondroplasia, a rare disorder of bone development in which the epiphyseal tissue responsible for growth spreads through the bones, causing abnormal irregular growth and, eventually, deformity. The long bones and the ilia are most often affected. Orthopedic procedures to correct deformities may be necessary and helpful, but invalidism is the usual prognosis. A kind of dyschondroplasia is **hereditary multiple exostoses**. Also called **multiple enchondromatosis**.

oma-. See **omo-**.

-oma, a combining form meaning a 'tumor': *capsuloma, lymphadenoma, neurinoma*.

omental bursa, a cavity in the peritoneum behind the stomach, the lesser omentum, and the lower border of the liver and in front of the pancreas and duodenum.

omentum, *pl.* **omenta, omentums**. an extension of the peritoneum that enfolds one or more adjacent organs in the stomach. See also **greater omentum, lesser omentum**. — **omental**, *adj.*

omission, (in law) intentional or unintentional neglect to fullfull a duty required by law.

Omnipen, a trade name for an antibacterial (ampicillin).

omo-, oma-, a combining form meaning 'of or pertaining to the shoulder': *omoclavicular, omodynia, omohyoid*.

omphal-. See **omphalo-**.

omphalo-, omphal-, a combining form meaning 'of or related to the navel': *omphalocele, omphaloma, omphalosite*.

omphaloangiopagus (om'fəlouæn'jiop'əgəs). See **allantoidoangiopagus**.

omphalocele (om'fəlousil'), congenital herniation of intra-abdominal viscera through a defect in the abdominal wall around the umbilicus. The defect is usually closed surgically soon after birth.

omphalodidymus. See **gastrodidymus**.

omphalogenesis, the formation of the umbilicus or yolk sac during embryonic development. — **omphalogenetic**, *adj.*

omphalomesenteric artery. See **vitelline artery**.

omphalomesenteric circulation. See **vitelline circulation**.

omphalomesenteric duct. See **yolk stalk**.

omphalomesenteric vein. See **vitelline vein**.

omphalopagus (om'fəlop'əgəs). See **monomphalus**.

omphalosite, the underdeveloped parasitic member of unequal conjoined twins united by the vessels of the umbilical cord. The omphalosite has no heart, derives its blood supply from the placenta of the autosite, and is incapable of independent existence after birth.

OMS, abbreviation for **Organisation Mondiale de la Santé**. See **World Health Organization**.

Omsk hemorrhagic fever (OHF) (ɔmsk), an acute infection, seen in regions of the U.S.S.R., caused by an arbovirus transmitted by the bite of an infected tick or by handling infected muskrats. The disease is characterized by fever, headache, epistaxis, gastrointestinal and uterine bleeding, and other hemorrhagic manifestations. Treatment is supportive; recovery usually occurs.

-on, 1. a combining form meaning an 'elementary atomic particle': *electron, nucleon, proton*. 2. a combining form meaning a 'unit': *magneton, photon*. 3. a combining form meaning a '(nonmetallic) chemical element': *carbon, krypton, silicon*.

onanism. See **masturbation**.

onchocerciasis (on'kousərkaɪ'əsɪs), a form of filariasis common in Central and South America and in Africa, characterized by subcutaneous nodules, pruritic rash, and eye lesions. It is transmitted by the bites of black flies that deposit microfilariae under the skin. The microfilariae migrate to the subcutaneous tissue and eyes, and fibrous nodules develop around the developing adult worms. Hypersensitive reactions to the dying microfilariae include extreme pruritus, a cellulitislike rash, lichenification, depigmentation, and rarely, elephantiasis. Involvement of the eye may include keratitis, iridocyclitis, and, rarely, blindness from choroidoretinitis. Diagnosis is made by demonstrating microfilariae by skin biopsy or in the eye by slit lamp. Treatment is diethylcarbamazine for the microfilariae and surgical excision of nodules to remove adult worms. Protective clothing and control of black flies with DDT are the best preventives. Also called **river blindness**.

onco-, a combining form meaning 'of or pertaining to a swelling, tumor, or mass': *oncogenesis, oncograph, oncotomy.*

oncogenesis (on'koujen'ısıs), the process initiating and promoting the development of a neoplasm. Compare **carcinogenesis, sarcomagenesis, tumorigenesis.** — **oncogenic,** *adj.*

oncogenic virus (ong'kəjen'ık), a virus that is able to cause the development of a malignant neoplastic disease. Over one hundred oncogenic viruses have been identified. In the laboratory, oncogenic viruses have been inoculated and grown in all major groups of animals, including primates. Many, especially the 'slow viruses' (as the one that causes kuru), are thought to cause cancer in humans, but this is not yet proven.

oncologist (ongkol'əjıst), a physician who specializes in the study and treatment of neoplastic diseases, particularly cancer.

oncology (ongkol'əji), the branch of medicine concerned with the study of tumors.

Oncology Nursing Society (ONS), an organization of nurses interested or specialized in nursing of the patient with cancer. The national publication of the ONS is *Oncology Nursing Forum.*

Oncovin, a trade name for an antineoplastic (vincristine sulfate).

oncovirus (ong'kouvai'rəs), a member of a family of viruses associated with leukemia and sarcoma in animals and, possibly, in humans.

Ondine's curse (ondinz'), an eponym for apnea owing to loss of automatic control of respiration. The term refers to a syndrome in patients with marked sensitivity to retained carbon dioxide. A defect in the central chemoreceptor responsiveness to carbon dioxide leaves the patient with hypercapnia and hypoxemia, although fully able to breathe voluntarily. This condition may result in the Pickwickian syndrome or the sleep-apnea syndrome, and it may be one cause of sudden infant death syndrome. Ondine's curse may occur as a result of drug overdose, as with opioids; following bulbar poliomyelitis or encephalitis; or after surgery involving the brain stem or the higher segments of cervical cord, as in cervical cordotomy for intractable pain.

-one, a combining form designating organic compounds: *acetone, ketone, quinone.*

one-and-a-half spica cast, an orthopedic cast used for immobilizing the trunk of the body cranially to the nipple line, one leg caudally as far as the toes, and the other leg caudally as far as the knee. For stability, a diagonal crossbar connects the parts of the cast encasing the legs. This type of cast is used for immobilization during convalescence after healing of surgical hip repair or a fractured femur and for the correction and the maintenance of correction of a hip deformity. Compare **bilateral long leg spica cast, unilateral long leg spica cast.**

oneiro-, a combining form meaning 'of or related to a dream': *oneirodynia, oneirology, oneiroscopy.*

ONS, abbreviation for **Oncology Nursing Society.**

ontogenesis (on'toujen'ısıs). See **ontogeny.** — **ontogenetic,** *adj.*

ontogenetic, ontogenic, 1. of, relating to, or acquired during ontogeny. 2. an association based on visible morphological characteristics and not necessarily indicative of a natural evolutionary relationship.

ontogeny (ontoj'ıni), the life history of one organism from a single-celled ovum to the time of birth, including all phases of differentiation and growth. Compare **phylogeny.**

onych-. See **onycho-.**

onychia (ounık'iə), inflammation of the nail bed. Compare **paronychia.**

-onychia, a combining form meaning a 'condition of the finger- or toenails': *celonychia, melanonychia, pachyonychia.*

onycho-, onych-, a combining form meaning 'of or related to the nails': *onychogenic, onychohelcosis, onychopathology.*

onychogryphosis (on'ıkougrıfou'sıs), thickened, curved, clawlike overgrowth of fingernails or toenails.

onycholysis (on'ıkol'ısıs), separation of a nail from its bed, beginning at the free margin, associated with psoriasis, dermatitis of the hand, fungal infection, *Pseudomonas* infection, and many other conditions.

onychomycosis (on'ıkoumaikou'sıs), any fungus infection of the nails.

oo-, a combining form meaning 'of or pertaining to an egg or ovum': *ooblast, oocytase, ootid.*

ooblast (ou'əblæst), the primodial germ cell from which the mature ovum is developed.

oocenter (ou'əsen'tər). See **ovocenter.**

oocyst (ou'əsıst), a stage in the development of any sporozoan in which after fertilization a zygote is produced that develops about itself an enclosing cyst wall. Oocysts of malarial parasites are found in the stomachs of infected mosquitoes. Oocysts of toxoplasma organisms are excreted in the feces of infected cats. Compare **oocyte.**

oocyte (ou'əsait'), a primordial or incompletely developed ovum.

oocytin (ou'əsai'tın), the substance in a spermatozoon that stimulates the formation of the fertilization membrane after penetration of an ovum.

oogamy (ouog'əmi), 1. sexual reproduction by the fertilization of a large, nonmotile female gamete by a smaller, actively motile male gamete, as occurs in certain algae and the malarial parasite *Plasmodium.* 2. heterogamy. Compare **isogamy.** — **oogamous,** *adj.*

oogenesis (ou'əjen'ısıs), the process of the growth and

maturation of the female gametes, or ova. Development begins during intrauterine life when the primordial germ cells within the epithelium of the fetal ovarian cortex give rise to precursor oogonia. By the time of birth, the oogonia have multiplied and developed into primary oocytes, each surrounded by a layer of epithelial cells that together form the primordial follicle. These have entered the prophase stage of the first meiotic division and remain suspended in this state until sexual maturity is reached. Then at monthly intervals one or sometimes two of the primary oocytes are stimulated simultaneously by the anterior pituitary hormones and the maturation of the follicle to continue meiotic division, forming a large secondary oocyte and a much smaller nonfunctional first polar body. The second meiotic division begins at about the time of ovulation and remains suspended in the prophase stage until fertilization stimulates the completion of the process, resulting in one large mature ovum, or ootid, and either one or three smaller secondary polar bodies that soon disintegrate. The ootid contains a pronucleus with the haploid number of maternal chromosomes that will fuse with the pronucleus of the spermatozoon to form the zygote. If fertilization does not occur, the ovum disintegrates and is discharged with the menses. The female infant is born with the entire number of primary oocytes that will function throughout reproductive life. Only a fraction of these survive until puberty and only a small percentage will be ovulated. Follicles containing the primary oocytes are found in varying stages of development in the ovary of the sexually mature woman. Egg and sperm formation differ considerably in the number and size of gametes resulting from gametogenesis, the total number of gametes produced in a lifetime, and the time sequence for the initiation of the meiotic divisions and the completion of the cycle. Also called **ovogenesis.** Compare **spermatogenesis.** See also **meiosis, menstrual cycle, ovulation.** — **oogenetic,** *adj.*

oogonium (ou′əgou′niəm), *pl.* **oogonia.** the precursor cell from which an oocyte develops in the fetus during intrauterine life. It is derived from primordial germ cells, multiplies rapidly during gestation, and near the time of birth enters the prophase stage of the first meiotic division to form the primary oocyte. Also called **ovogonium.** See also **oogenesis.**

ookinesis (ou′əkini′sis, ou′əkaini′sis), **ookinesia** (ou′əkini′źhə, ou′əkaini′źhə), the mitotic phenomena occurring in the nucleus of the egg cell during maturation and fertilization. See also **oogenesis.** — **ookinetic,** *adj.*

ookinete, the motile elongated zygote that is formed by the fertilization of the macrogamete during the sexual reproductive phase of the life cycle of a sporozoan, specifically the malarial parasite *Plasmodium.* It penetrates the lining of the stomach of the female *Anopheles* mosquito

and attaches to the outer wall, where it forms an oocyst and gives rise to sporozoites.

oolemma (ou′əlem′ə). See **zona pellucida.**

oophor-. See **oophoro-.**

oophorectomy (ou′əfərek′təmi), the surgical removal of one or both ovaries, performed to remove a cyst or tumor, excise an abcess, treat endometriosis, or, in breast cancer, to remove the source of estrogen, which stimulates some kinds of cancer. If both ovaries are removed, sterility results and menopause is abruptly induced; in premenopausal women one ovary or a portion of one ovary may be left intact unless a malignancy is present. The operation often accompanies a hysterectomy. Regional or general anesthesia is used. Unless a malignancy is present, estrogen may be given to treat the unpleasant side effects of the abrupt onset of menopause. Also called **ovariectomy.**

oophoritis (ou′əfərai′tis), an inflammatory condition of one or both ovaries, usually occurring with salpingitis.

oophoro-, oophor-, a combining form meaning 'of or pertaining to the ovary': *oophorocytosis, oophorogenous, oophoroma.* Also **ootheco-.**

oophorosalpingectomy (ou′əfor′əsæl′pinjek′təmi), the surgical removal of one or both ovaries and the corresponding oviducts, performed to remove a cyst or tumor, excise an abcess, or treat the condition of endometriosis. In a bilateral procedure the patient becomes sterile and menopause is induced. General anesthesia is used. Estrogen therapy may be started after bilateral surgery unless a malignancy is present to relieve the unpleasant side effects of the abrupt onset of menopause.

ooplasm (ou′əplæz′əm), the cytoplasm of the egg, or ovum, including the yolk in lower animals. Also called **ovoplasm.**

oosperm (ou′əsperm), a fertilized egg; the cell resulting from the union of the pronuclei of the spermatozoon and the ovum following fertilization; a zygote.

ootheco-. See **oophoro-.**

ootid (ou′ətid), the mature ovum after penetration by the spermatozoon and completion of the second meiotic division but prior to the fusion of the pronuclei to form the zygote. It is one of the four cells resulting from oogenesis, the other three being nonfunctional secondary polar bodies, and corresponds to the four spermatid cells derived from spermatogenesis. See also **meiosis, oogenesis.**

opaque, 1. of or pertaining to a substance or surface that neither transmits nor allows the passage of light. 2. neither transparent nor translucent.

-ope, a combining form meaning a 'person having an eye defect': *asthenope, hyperope, protanope.*

open amputation, a kind of amputation in which a straight, guillotine cut is made without skin flaps. Open amputation is performed if an infection is probable or developing or has been recurrent. The cross section is left open for drainage, and skin traction is applied to prevent retraction. Antibiotic therapy is begun, and surgical closure is completed when the infection clears. Compare **closed amputation.** See also **amputation, gangrene.**

open drainage. See **drainage.**

open-drop anesthesia, the oldest and simplest anesthetic technique. A volatile liquid anesthetic agent is dripped, one drop at a time, onto a porous cloth or mask held over the patient's face. Chloroform and ether are the major general anesthetics adaptable to open-drop administration. Some psychologists believe that open-drop anesthesia can be a traumatic experience to a child and, therefore, consider this form of anesthesia ill-advised in pediatric use. It is not currently used in developed countries.

open fracture. See **compound fracture.**

operant, any act or response occurring without an identifiable stimulus. The result of the act or response determines whether or not it is repeated.

operant conditioning, a form of learning used in behavior therapy in which the person undergoing therapy is rewarded for the correct response and punished for the incorrect response. Also called **instrumental conditioning.**

operating microscope, a binocular microscope used in delicate surgery, especially surgery of the eye or ear. The standing type of operating microscope has a motorized zoom system operated by a foot pedal that quickly changes the magnification. The operating microscope that attaches to a surgeon's head has interchangeable oculars for different magnifications. Also called **surgical microscope.**

operating room (O.R.), 1. a room in a health care facility in which surgical procedures requiring anesthesia are performed. 2. *Informal.* a suite of rooms or an area in a health care facility in which patients are prepared for surgery, undergo surgical procedures, and recover from the anesthetic procedures required for the surgery.

operation, any surgical procedure, as an appendectomy or a hysterectomy.

operative cholangiography, (in diagnostic radiology) a procedure for outlining the major bile ducts. It is performed during surgery by injecting a radio-opaque contrast material directly into these ducts. It is usually performed to detect residual calculi in the biliary tract. See also **cholangiography.**

operator gene, (in molecular genetics) a genetic unit that regulates the transcription of structural genes in its operon. The operator gene serves as the starting point in the coding sequence and interacts with a repressor protein in controlling the activity of structural genes.

operculum (ɔupər'kyuləm), *pl.* **opercula, operculums.** a lid or covering, as the mucous plug that blocks the cervix of the gravid uterus or the temporal operculum of the cerebral temporal hemisphere that overlaps the insula as

an extension of the superior surface of the temporal lobe. — **opercular,** *adj.*

operon (op'əron), (in molecular biology) a segment of DNA consisting of an operator gene and one or more structural genes with related functions controlled by the operator gene in conjunction with a regulatory gene. See also **operator gene, regulatory gene.**

-ophidia, a combining form meaning 'venomous snakes': *thanatophidia, toxicophidia.*

Ophthaine, a trade name for a local anesthetic (proparacaine hydrochloride 0.5%) solution, used in ophthalmic procedures.

ophthalm-. See **ophthalmo-.**

ophthalmia (ofħæl'miə), severe inflammation of the conjunctiva or of the deeper parts of the eye. Some kinds of ophthalmia are **ophthalmia neonatorum, sympathetic ophthalmia, trachoma.**

-ophthalmia, a combining form meaning a 'pathological or anatomical condition of the eye': *allophthalmia, echinophthalmia, polemophthalmia.*

ophthalmia neonatorum (ni'ounɔtɔr'əm), a purulent gonococcal conjunctivitis and keratitis of the newborn resulting from exposure of the eyes to infected maternal secretions as the baby passes through the vagina at birth. Routine prophylaxis by the topical instillation of a 1 per cent solution of silver nitrate or an antibiotic ointment in the conjuntival sac of every newborn has largely eradicated the infection. When necessary, intravenous antibiotic therapy given in the hospital for several days is effective, and recovery is usually complete.

ophthalmic (ofħæl'mɪk), of or pertaining to the eye.

-ophthalmic, a combining form meaning 'referring to, near, or for the eye': *exophthalmic, periophthalmic, podophthalmic.*

ophthalmic administration of medication, the administration of a drug by instillation of a cream or ointment or by drops of a liquid preparation in the conjunctival sac. The correct strength and amount of the drug are selected, and the medication is instilled in the eye or eyes as directed. The order usually specifies O.D. for right eye, O.S. for left eye, or O.U. for each eye. Ophthalmic preparations are often refrigerated for storage but are given at room temperature. Cloudiness or sedimentation in a liquid may indicate deterioration of the drug. For administration, the patient is positioned comfortably, lying back on a bed or examining table or sitting up with the neck hyperextended. The cul-de-sac of the conjunctival sac is exposed by gentle traction on the tissue just below the lower eyelid. The medication is placed in the sac as the patient is instructed to look away from the point of instillation. The dispenser is not allowed to touch the eye, and the medication is not placed directly on the cornea. The eyelid is slowly released, and the patient is asked to roll the eye around a few times to spread the medication over the entire surface of the eye.

ophthalmic herpes zoster. See **herpes zoster.**

ophthalmo-, ophthalm-, a combining form meaning 'of or pertaining to the eye': *ophthalmodynia, ophthalmolith, ophthalmostat.*

ophthalmologist (of'thælmol'əjist), a physician who specializes in ophthalmology.

ophthalmology (of'thælmol'əji), the branch of medicine concerned with the study of the physiology, anatomy, and pathology of the eye and the diagnosis and treatment of disorders of the eye. — **ophthalmologic, ophthalmological,** *adj.*

ophthalmoplegia (ofthæl'məpli'jə), an abnormal condition characterized by paralysis of the motor nerves of the eye. Bilateral lateral ophthalmoplegia of rapid onset is associated with acute myasthenia gravis, acute thiamin deficiency, botulism, and acute inflammatory cranial polyneuropathy. These diseases are potentially very destructive and require prompt attention. In some patients with myopathic ophthalmoplegia structural abnormalities and biochemical disorders may be evident in limb muscles. Ophthalmoplegia is also associated with ocular dystrophy.

ophthalmoscope, a device for examining the interior of the eye. It includes a light, a mirror with a single hole through which the examiner may look, and a dial holding several lenses of varying strengths. The lenses are selected to allow clear visualization of the structures of the eye at any depth. If the patient or the examiner ordinarily requires extensive correction of a refractive error, the examination may require that the corrective lenses normally worn be worn for the examination.

ophthalmoscopy (of'thælmos'kəpi), the technique of using an ophthalmoscope to examine the eye.

Ophthochlor, a trade name for an ophthalmic preparation of the antibacterial and antirickettsial (chloramphenicol).

Ophthocort, a trade name for an ophthalmic, fixed-combination drug containing a glucocorticoid (hydrocortisone acetate) and antibacterials (chloramphenicol and polymyxin B sulfate).

-opia, a combining form meaning a '(specified) visual condition': *boopia, nonopia, senopia.* Also **-opy, -opsia, -opsy.**

opiate, 1. a narcotic drug that contains opium, derivatives of opium, or any of several semi-synthetic or synthetic drugs with opium-like activity. 2. *Informal.* any soporific or narcotic drug. 3. of or pertaining to a substance that causes sleep or relief of pain. Also called **opioid.**

-opic, a combining form meaning 'kind of vision or visual defect': *cyclopic, hemeralopic, nyctalopic.* Also **-opical.**

opinion, (in law) 1. a statement by the court, usually in writing, of the reasoning behind its decision or judgment in a particular case. 2. a statement prepared for a client by an attorney that represents the attorney's understanding of the law as it pertains to a legal question posed by the client.

opistho-, a combining form meaning 'backward or relating to the back': *opisthognathism, opisthoporeia, opisthotonos.*

opisthorchiasis (ou'pisthorkai'əsis), infection with one of two species of liver flukes commonly found in the Philippines, India, Thailand, and Laos. Symptoms and signs are similar to those caused by *Clonorchis sinensis.* Carcinoma of the intrahepatic bile ducts may be a late complication. Treatment is unsatisfactory. The disease is prevented by avoiding eating raw or inadequately cooked freshwater fish.

Opisthorchis sinensis (ou'pisthor'kis sinen'sis). See *Clonorchis sinensis.*

opisthotonos, a prolonged severe spasm of the muscles causing the back to arch acutely, the head to bend back on the neck, the heels to bend back on the legs, and the arms and hands to flex rigidly at the joints.

opium, a milky exudate from the unripe capsules of *Papaver somniferum* and *Papaver album* yielding 9.5 per cent or more of anhydrous morphine. It is a narcotic analgesic, a hypnotic, and an astringent. Opium contains several alkaloids, including codeine, morphine, and papaverine. See also **codeine, morphine sulfate, papaverine hydrochloride, opium tincture, paregoric.**

opium alkaloid, one of several alkaloids isolated from the milky exudate of the unripe seed pods of *Papaver somniferum,* a species of poppy indigenous to the Near East. Three of the alkaloids, codeine, papaverine, and morphine, are used clinically for the relief of pain, but their use entails the risk of physical or psychological dependence. Morphine is the standard against which the analgesic effect of newer drugs for relief of pain are measured. The opium alkaloids and their semisynthetic derivatives, including heroin, act on the central nervous system, producing analgesia, change in mood, drowsiness, and mental slowness. The effects in a person who has pain are usually pleasant; euphoria and pain-free sleep are not uncommon, but nausea and vomiting sometimes occur. In usual doses, the analgesic effects are achieved without loss of consciousness. Morphine and its surrogates appear to relieve the discomfort of the original sensation and the person's reaction to the sensation; thus the actual pain diminishes, and what remains of it is less distressing to the patient. The opium alkaloids have several other effects on the various systems of the body: coughing is suppressed; the electrical activity pattern of the brain resembles that of sleep; the pupils constrict; respiration is depressed in rate, minute volume, and tidal exchange; the secretory activity and motility of the gastrointestinal tract are diminished; and biliary and pancreatic secretions are reduced. The use of morphine as an antidiarrheal preceded its use as an analgesic by hundreds of years. Prepared in a tincture, it remains the most effective constipating agent available.

opium tincture, an analgesic and antidiarrheal.

■ INDICATIONS: It is prescribed in the treatment of intestinal hyperactivity, cramping, and diarrhea.

■ CONTRAINDICATIONS: Drug dependence, the presence of toxic matter in the bowel, or known hypersensitivity to this drug prohibits its use.

■ ADVERSE EFFECTS: Among the more serious adverse reactions are drug dependence, toxic megacolon, and central nervous system depression.

Oppenheim reflex, a variation of the Babinski reflex, elicited by firmly stroking downward on the anterior and medial surfaces of the tibia, characterized by extension of the great toe and fanning of other toes. It is a sign of pyramidal tract disease. Compare **Chaddock reflex, Gordon reflex.** See also **Babinski' reflex.**

Oppenheim's disease (op'ənhaimz), a rare congenital disease of infants, characterized by flabby, atonic muscles, especially in the legs, and absent or extremely sluggish deep reflexes. The infant seems paralyzed during its first few months of life and almost a third of the patients do not survive for a year. Also called **amyotonia congenita, myotonia congenita.**

opportunistic infection, 1. an infection caused by normally nonpathogenic organisms in a host whose resistance has been decreased by such disorders as diabetes mellitus or cancer or by a surgical procedure, as a cerebrospinal fluid shunt or a cardiac or urinary tract catheterization. 2. an unusual infection with a common pathogen, as cellulitis, meningitis, otitis media.

-opsia. See **-opia.**

opsonin (op'sənɪn), an antibody or complement split product which, on attaching to foreign material, microorganism, or other antigen, enhances phagocytosis of that substance by leukocytes and other macrophages. **– opsonize,** v.

opsonization (op'sənɪzei'shən), the process by which opsonins render bacteria more susceptible to phagocytosis by leukocytes.

Optef, a trade name for an ophthalmic preparation containing a glucocorticoid (hydrocortisone).

-opter, a combining form referring to 'measurement of vision': *myodiopter, oxyopter, phoropter.*

opti-. See **opto-.**

optic, of or pertaining to the eyes or to sight. **– optical,** *adj.*

-optic, a combining form meaning 'pertaining to vision': *bioptic, panoptic, preoptic.*

optical maser. See **laser.**

optic atrophy, wasting of the optic disc resulting from degeneration of fibers of the optic nerve and optic tract.

In primary optic atrophy the disc is white and sharply margined, the central depression (physiologic cup) is enlarged, and the optic foramen of the sclera is clearly seen. In secondary atrophy the disk is gray, its margins are blurred, the depression is filled in, and the foramen is difficult to detect. Optic atrophy may be caused by a congenital defect, inflammation, occlusion of the central retinal artery or internal carotid artery, by alcohol, arsenic, lead, tobacco, or other toxic substances. Degeneration of the disc may accompany arteriosclerosis, diabetes, glaucoma, hydrocephalus, pernicious anemia, and various neurologic disorders.

optic cup, a two-layered embryonic cavity that develops in early pregnancy. The optic cup is completed by the seventh week with the closing of the choroidal fissure. The cup initially develops from the infolding of the optic vesicle after the vesicle separates from the embryonic ectoderm. The cells of the optic cup differentiate to form the retina that first develops its layers of rods and cones in the central portion of the cup, growing as the layer gradually spreads toward the cup margin. The outer layer of the cup persists as the pigmented layer of the retina; the inner layer develops the nervous elements and the supporting fibers of the retina. Compare **optic stalk.**

optic disc, the small blind spot on the surface of the retina, located about 3 mm to the nasal side of the macula. It is the only part of the retina which is insensitive to light. At its center the porus opticus marks the point of entrance of the central artery of the retina. Also called *Informal.* **blind spot, discus nervi optici.**

optic glioma, a tumor composed of glial cells. It develops slowly on the optic nerve or in the optic chiasm, causing loss of vision, and is often accompanied by secondary strabismus, exophthalmos, and ocular paralysis.

optician, a person who grinds and fits eyeglass and contact lenses by prescription. To become an optician, a person must graduate from high school and complete a four- or five-year apprenticeship. In some states licensure is required.

optic nerve, either of a pair of cranial nerves consisting mainly of coarse, myelinated fibers that arise in the retinal ganglionic layer, traverse the thalamus, and connect with the visual cortex. At the optic chiasm the fibers from the inner or nasal half of the retina cross to the optic tract of the opposite side. The remaining fibers from the temporal or outer half of each retina are uncrossed and pass to the visual cortex on the same side. The visual cortex functions in the perception of light and shade and in the perception of objects. Optic radiations conduct impulses from the geniculate bodies in the cerebral hemispheres to the visual cortices. The optic nerve is divided into portions within the bulb, orbit, optic canal, and cranial cavity. The intraocular portion of the nerve is about 1 mm long and contains unmyelinated fibers which become myelinated after passing through the lamina cribosa. The orbital portion of the nerve, about 3.5 mm in diameter and about 25 mm long, is invested by sheaths derived from the dura, the arachnoid, and the pia mater. The portion of the nerve within the optic canal lies superior to the ophthalmic artery, and the three sheaths are fused to each other, to the nerve, and to the periosteum of the bone, securing the nerve and preventing it from being forced back and forth in the foramen. The intracranial portion of the nerve rests on the anterior portion of the cranial sinus in close proximity to the internal carotid artery. The optic nerve is cranial nerve II and develops from a diverticulum of the laterial portion of the forebrain. The optic nerve fibers therefore correspond to a tract of fibers within the brain rather than to the other cranial nerves.

optico-. See **opto-.**

optic papilla. See **papilla.**

optics, **1.** (in physics) a field of study that deals with the electromagnetic radiation of wavelengths shorter than radio waves but longer than x rays. **2.** (in physiology) a field of study that deals with vision and the process by which the functions of the eye and the brain are integrated in the perception of shapes, patterns, movements, spatial relationships, and color. — **optic, optical,** *adj.*

optic stalk, one of a pair of slender embryonic structures that become the optic nerve. In the embryo the optic stalk develops during the second week and attaches the optic vesicle to the wall of the brain. The stalk becomes complete during the seventh week of pregnancy when the choroidal fissure closes and is later converted into the optic nerve when nerve fibers fill the cavity of the stalk. Most of the fibers are centripetal and grow backward into the stalk from the nerve cells of the retina. A few fibers grow into the stalk from the brain. About the tenth week after birth the fibers of the optic nerve receive their myelin sheaths. Compare **optic cup.**

optic system assessment, an evaluation of the patient's eyes, vision, and current and past disorders or injuries that may be responsible for abnormalities in the individual's optic system.

■ METHOD: The patient is interviewed to determine if vision is blurred, double, decreased, or absent in one or both eyes, or diminished peripherally at night or in bright light. The interviewer asks if halos or lights are seen and if the patient collides with unfamiliar objects, is unable to distinguish objects held too close or too far, if the eyes water, itch, feel tender, painful, or fatigued, and if an injury to the eye, face, or head has occurred. Observations are made of the patient's general appearance, vital signs, kind of eyeglasses or contact lenses worn, the amount of tearing, ability to blink, tendency to rub the eyes, and visual acuity. Evidence is recorded of conjunctivitis, drainage, optic hemorrhage, edema or ptosis of the eyelids, exophthalmos, strabismus, nystagmus, scleral edema, chalazion, lacerations, contusions, or a foreign body in the eye. Carefully noted are signs of aging, glaucoma, cataract, retinal detachment, and the presence of multiple sclerosis, diabetes mellitus, myasthenia gravis, gonorrhea, thyroid dysfunction, sinus problems, or cerebral trauma or tumors. The patient's report of previous eye operations or treatments, head or face trauma, arteriosclerosis, glomerulonephritis, retinal degeneration, episodes of coma, therapy with oxygen, and drug misuse are investigated, as well as a family history of glaucoma or diabetes. Also explored are the possibility that the patient has a hazardous job or recreation and note is made of any safety precautions taken, the individual's misuse of alcohol, and use of medication. especially antibiotics, antiemetics, miotics, mydriatics, and acetazolamide. Diagnostic aids for the evaluation include a test of visual fields, x rays of the orbit and skull, an ophthalmoscopic examination, tonometry, brain scan, and microscopic studies of conjunctival scrapings.

■ NURSING ORDERS: The nurse conducts the interview, makes the observations of the patient, and assembles the pertinent background data and the results of the diagnostic procedures.

■ OUTCOME CRITERIA: A careful assessment of the patient's eyes, vision, and of certain aspects of the medical, family, and social history is a significant aid in establishing the diagnosis of an optic system disorder.

Optimyd, a trade name for an ophthalmic, fixed-combination drug containing a glucocorticoid (prednisolone sodium phosphate) and an antibacterial (sulfacetamide sodium).

opto-, a combining form meaning 'visible, or pertaining to vision or sight': *optoblast, optometer, optostriate.* Also **opti-, optico-.**

optometrist, a person who practices optometry. An optometrist is awarded the degree of Doctor of Optometry (O.D.) after completion of at least two years of college, followed by four years in an approved college of optometry. A state examination and license are also required. See also **optician, optometry.**

optometry, the practice of testing the eyes for visual acuity, prescribing corrective lenses, and recommending eye exercises. See also **optician.**

OPV, abbreviation for **oral poliovirus vaccine.**

O.R., OR, abbreviation for **operating room.**

oral, of or pertaining to the mouth. Compare **buccal, parenteral.**

oral administration of medication, the administration of a tablet, a capsule, an elixir, or a solution or other liquid form of medication by mouth. Adequate water to lubricate the solid forms or to dilute the liquid forms is given for swallowing with the medication. Preparations with a disagreeable taste may be given with something of sufficient flavor to disguise the bad taste. Substances that are harmful to the teeth are given through a straw. People who have difficulty swallowing pills or capsules may find if easier to swallow the medication if they look up as they swallow. Kinds of oral administration of medication are **buccal administration of medication, sublingual administration of medication.**

oral airway, a curved tubular device of rubber, plastic, or metal placed in the oropharynx during general anesthesia to maintain free passage of air and keep the tongue from falling back and obstructing the trachea. The artificial airway is not removed until the patient begins to awaken and regains pharyngeal, cough, and swallowing reflexes.

oral cancer, a malignant neoplasm on the lip or in the mouth, occurring at an average age of 60 with a frequency eight times higher in men than in women. Predisposing factors in the etiology of the disease are alcoholism, heavy use of tobacco, poor oral hygiene, ill-fitting dentures, syphilis, Plummer-Vinson syndrome, betel nut chewing, and, in lip cancer, overexposure to sun and wind and the smoking of pipes. Premalignant leukoplakia or erythroplasia or a painless nonhealing ulcer may be the first sign of oral cancer; localized pain usually appears later, but lymph nodes may be involved early in the course. Diagnostic measures include digital examination, biopsy, exfoliative cytology, x rays of the mandible, and chest films to detect metastatic lung lesions. Almost all oral tumors are epidermoid carcinomas; adenocarcinomas occur occasionally, sarcomas and metastatic lesions from other sites are rare. Small primary lesions may be treated by excision or irradiation and more extensive oral tumors by surgery, with removal of involved lymph nodes and preoperative or postoperative radiotherapy. Among chemotherapeutic agents administered palliatively for inoperable or recurrent lesions are methotrexate, 5-fluorouracil, bleomycin, and adriamycin.

oral character, (in psychoanalysis) a kind of personality exhibiting patterns of behavior originating in the oral phase of infancy, characterized by optimism, self-confidence, and carefree generosity reflecting the pleasurable aspects of the stage or pessimism, futility, anxiety, and sadism as manifestations of frustrations or conflicts occurring during the period. See also **oral stage, psychosexual development.**

oral contraceptive. See **contraception.**

oral eroticism, oral erotism, (in psychoanalysis) libidinal fixation at or regression to the oral stage of psychosexual development, often reflected in such personality traits as passivity, insecurity, and oversensitivity. Compare **anal eroticism.** See also **oral character.**

oral herpes. See **herpes simplex.**

oral hygiene, the condition or practice of maintaining

the tissues and structures of the mouth. Oral hygiene includes brushing the teeth to remove food particles, bacteria, and plaque; massaging the gums with a tooth brush, dental floss, or water irrigator to stimulate circulation and remove foreign matter; and cleansing of dentures and ensuring their proper fit to prevent irritation. Dependent or unconcious patients are assisted in maintaining a healthy oral condition. Such care includes lubricating the lips and cleaning the inside of the cheeks, the roof of the mouth, and the tongue. In addition, the nurse checks for loose teeth that might be swallowed or aspirated.

oral poliovirus vaccine (OPV), an attenuated preparation of live poliovirus that confers immunity to poliomyelitis. Also called **Sabin vaccine.**

■ INDICATION: It is routinely prescribed for immunization against poliomyelitis.

■ CONTRAINDICATIONS: Immunosuppression, concomitant use of corticosteroids, cancer, immunoglobulin abnormalities, or acute infection prohibits its use.

■ ADVERSE EFFECTS: Adverse effects are uncommon. Cases of vaccine-induced paralytic disease have occurred but are very rare.

oral sadism, (in psychoanalysis) a sadistic form of oral eroticism, manifested by such behavior as biting, chewing, and other aggressive impulses associated with eating habits. Compare **anal sadism.**

oral stage, (in psychoanalysis) the initial stage of psychosexual development, occurring in the first 12 to 18 months of life when the feeding experience and other oral activities are the predominant source of pleasurable stimulation. Experiences encountered during this stage determine to a great extent later attitudes concerning food, love, acceptance and rejection, and many other aspects of interpersonal relationships and behavioral patterns. Pleasurable experiences associated with suckling may lead to oral eroticism in adulthood, unpleasant experiences may lead to extreme aggression and such patterns as smoking, overeating, excessive talking, or sarcasm and may be a pervasive influence or underlying determinant in addictive disorders. See also **oral character, psychosexual development.**

Orap, a trade name for an investigational antipsychotic (pimozide).

Orasone, a trade name for a glucorticoid (prednisone).

Ora-Testryl, a trade name for an androgen (fluoxymesterone).

Oratrol, a trade name for a carbonic anhydrase inhibitor (dichlorphenamide).

orbicularis ciliaris (ɔrbık′yʊlarʹıs), one of the two zones of the ciliary body of the eye, extending from the ora serrata of the retina to the ciliary processes at the margin of the iris. The orbicularis ciliaris is about 4 millimeters wide and increases in thickness as it approaches the ciliary processes.

orbicularis oculi, the muscular body of the eyelid comprising the palpebral, orbital, and lacrimal muscles. It arises from the nasal part of the frontal bone, from the frontal process of the maxilla in front of the lacrimal groove, and from the anterior surface of the medial palpebral ligament. The palpebral muscle functions to close the eyelid gently; the orbital muscle functions to close it more energetically, as in winking. Also called **obicularis palpebrarum.** Compare **corrugator, levator palpebrae superioris.**

orbicularis oris, the muscle surrounding the mouth, consisting partly of fibers derived from other facial muscles, as the buccinator, that are inserted into the lips, and partly of fibers proper to the lips. It is innervated by buccal branches of the facial nerve and serves to close and purse the lips.

orbicularis palpebrarum. See **orbicularis oculi.**

orbicularis pupillary reflex, a normal phenomenon elicited by forceful closure of the eyelids or attempting to close them while they are held apart, resulting first in constriction and then dilatation of the pupil.

orbit, one of a pair of bony, conical cavities in the skull that accommodate the eyeballs and associated structures, as the eye muscles, the nerves, and the blood vessels. The medial walls of the orbits are approximately parallel with each other and with the middle line, but the lateral walls diverge widely. The roof of each orbit is formed by the orbital plate of the frontal bone and the small wing of the sphenoid bones. The trochlear fovea of the orbital roof accommodates the cartilaginous pulley of the obliquus superior oculi, and the lacrimal fossa in the roof cradles the lacrimal gland. The superior orbital fissure between the roof and the lateral wall of the orbit admits various nerves, as the oculomotor, trochlear, and ophthalmic division of the trigeminal and the abducent nerves. The openings that communicate with each orbit are the optic foramen, the superior and the inferior orbital fissures, the supraorbital foramen, the infraorbital canal, the anterior and the posterior ethmoidal foramina, the zygomatic foramen, and the canal for the nasolacrimal duct. — **orbital,** *adj.*

orbital aperture, an opening in the cranium to the orbit of the eye.

orbital fat, a semifluid cushion of fat that lines the bony orbit supporting the eye. Traumatic loss of the fat causes a sunken appearance of the eye. Replacement of the fat by tumor or abnormal tissue may be discovered on ophthalmologic examination. The examiner gently presses on the front of the eyes through the eyelids. Normally each eye may be displaced .5 cm into the socket.

orbital hypertelorism. See **ocular hypertelorism.**

orbital hypotelorism. See **ocular hypotelorism.**

orbital pseudotumor, a specific inflammatory reaction of the orbital tissues of the eye, characterized by exoph-

thalmos and edematous congestion of the eyelids. The etiology is unknown.

orchi-. See **orchio-.**

orchidectomy (ɔr'kɪdek'təmi), a surgical procedure to remove one or both testes. It may be indicated for serious disease or injury to the testis or to control cancer of the prostate by removing a source of androgenic hormones. Also called **orchiectomy.**

orchido-. See **orchio-.**

orchiectomy. See **orchidectomy.**

orchio-, orchi-, a combining form meaning 'of or pertaining to the testes': *orchiocatabasis, orchiopathy, orchioscirrhus.* Also **orchido-.**

orchiopexy (ɔr'kiɔupek'si), an operation to mobilize an undescended testis, bring it into the scrotum, and attach it so that it will not retract. Sometimes a suture is attached to the lower scrotum and taped to the inner thigh. The nurse must be careful not to disturb this tension attachment.

orchis (ɔr'kɪs). See **testis.**

orchitis (ɔrkaɪ'tɪs), inflammation of one or both of the testes, characterized by swelling and pain, often caused by mumps, syphilis, or tuberculosis. Symptomatic treatment includes support and elevation of the scrotum, cold packs, and analgesics. — **orchitic,** *adj.*

orciprenaline sulfate. See **metaproterenol sulfate.**

Oretic, a trade name for a diuretic (hydrochlorothiazide).

Oreticyl, a trade name for an antihypertensive, fixed-combination drug containing a diuretic (hydrochlorothiazide) and an antihypertensive (deserpidine).

Oreton, a trade name for an androgen (testosterone).

Oreton Methyl, a trade name for an androgen (methyltestosterone).

Oreton Propionate, a trade name for an androgen (testosterone propionate).

-orexia, a combining form meaning '(condition of the) appetite': *cynorexia, dysorexia, hyperorexia.*

orexigenic (ɔrek'sɪjen'ɪk), a substance that increases or stimulates the appetite.

oreximania (ɔrek'sɪmei'niə), a condition characterized by a greatly increased appetite and excessive eating resulting from an unrealistic or exaggerated fear of becoming thin. Compare **anorexia nervosa.**

orexis (ɔrek'sɪs), 1. desire, appetite, 2. the aspect of the mind involving feeling and striving as contrasted with the intellectual aspect.

orf, a viral skin disease acquired from sheep, characterized by painless vesicles which may progress to red, weeping nodules, and, finally, to crusting and healing. Treatment is not necessary because the condition is self-limited, and active infection results in immunity.

organ, a structural part of a system of the body that is comprised of tissues and cells that enable it to perform a particular function, as the liver, spleen, the digestive organs, reproductive organs, or organs of special sense. Each one of the paired organs can function independently of the other. The liver, pancreas, spleen, and brain may maintain normal or near normal function with over 30 per cent of the organ damaged, destroyed, or excised. Also called **organon, organum.** – **organic,** *adj.*

organ albumin, albumin characteristic of a particular organ.

organelle (ɔr′gənel′, ɔr′gənel), **organella** (ɔr′gənel′ə), 1. any one of various particles of living substance bound within most cells, as the mitochondria, the Golgi complex, the endoplastic reticulum, the lysosomes, and the centrioles. 2. any one of the tiny organs of protozoa associated with locomotion, metabolism, and other processes.

organic, 1. Compare **inorganic.** any chemical compound containing carbon. 2. of or pertaining to an organ.

-organic, a combining form meaning 'related to the internal organs of the body': *enorganic, homorganic, psychorganic.*

organic brain syndrome. See **organic mental disorder.**

organic chemistry, the branch of chemistry concerned with the composition, properties, and reactions of chemical compounds containing carbon.

organic dust, dried particles of plants, animals, fungi or bacteria that are fine enough to be windborne. Many kinds of organic dust cause various respiratory disorders if inhaled. See also **asthma, bagassosis, byssinosis, hay fever, rose fever.**

organic evolution, the theory that all existing forms of animal and plant life have descended with modification from previous, simpler forms or from a single cell; the origin and perpetuation of species.

organic mental disorder, any psychological or behavioral abnormality associated with transient or permanent brain dysfunction caused by a disturbance of the physiological functioning of brain tissue, as may occur with cerebral arteriosclerosis, lead poisoning, or many other pathologic conditions. Also called **organic brain syndrome.**

organic motivation. See **physiological motivation.**

Organisation Mondiale de la Santé (OMS) (ɔrgʌnizasyɔ̃′ mɔ̃dyal′ də lʌ sãtei′). See **World Health Organization.**

organism, an individual living animal or plant able to carry on life functions through mutually dependent organs or organelles.

organization center, a focal point within the developing embryo from which the organism grows and differentiates. In vertebrates this point is the chordamesoderm of the dorsal lip of the blastopore.

organizer, (in embryology) any part of the embryo that induces morphologic differentiation in some other part. Those parts that are formed and in turn give rise to other parts are classified as organizers of the second degree,

third degree, and so on as the embryo develops in complexity. Kinds of organizers include **nucleolar organizer, primary organizer.**

organo-, a combining form meaning 'of or pertaining to an organ or organs': *organofaction, organogenesis, organoleptic.*

organ of Giraldes. See **paradidymis.**

organ of Golgi. See **neurotendinous spindle.**

organogenesis, (in embryology) the formation and differentiation of organs and organ systems during embryonic development. In man the period extends from approximately the end of the second week through the eighth week of gestation. During this time the embryo undergoes rapid growth and differentiation and is extremely vulnerable to environmental hazards and toxic substances. Any interference with the sequential processes involved with organogenesis causes an arrest in development and results in one or more congenital anomalies. Also called **organogeny.** See also **embryological development, prenatal development.** – **organogenetic,** *adj.*

organogeny. See **organogenesis.**

organoid, 1. resembling an organ. 2. any structure that resembles an organ in appearance or function, specifically an abnormal tumor mass. 3. See **organelle.**

organoid neoplasm, a growth that resembles a body organ. Compare **histoid neoplasm.**

organoid tumor. See **teratoma.**

organotherapy (ɔrgæn′oʊθer′əpi), the treatment of disease by administering animal endocrine glands or their extracts. Whole glands are no longer implanted, but substances derived from animal organs are widely used. Also called **Brown-Séquard's treatment.** – **organotherapeutic,** *adj.*

organotypic growth (ɔr′gænoʊtɪp′ɪk), the controlled reproduction of cells, as occurs in the normal growth of tissues and organs. Compare **histiotypic growth.**

orgasm, the sexual climax, a series of strong, involuntary contractions of the muscles of the genitalia experienced as exceedingly pleasurable, set off by sexual excitation of critical intensity. – **orgasmic,** *adj.*

orient, 1. to make someone aware of new surroundings, including people and their roles, the layout of a facility, and its routines, rules, and services. New patients oriented to a hospital as are new staff to a hospital unit. 2. to help a person become aware of a situation or simply of reality, as when a patient recovers from anesthesia. – **orientation,** *n.,* **oriented,** *adj.*

oriental sore, a dermatologic disease caused by the parasite *Leishmania tropica,* transmitted to man by the bite of the sand fly. This form of leishmaniasis, characterized by ulcerative lesions, occurs primarily in Africa, Asia, and some Mediterranean countries. Oriental sore causes no systemic symptoms, but the sores are susceptible to secondary infections. Treatment options include infrared therapy and injection of ulcers with sodium antimony gluconate. Also called **Aleppo boil, cutaneous leishmaniasis, Delhi boil, Old World leishmaniasis, tropical sore.** See also **leishmaniasis.**

orientation, (in molecular genetics) the insertion of a fragment of genetic material into a vector so that the placement of the fragment is in the same direction as the genetic map of the vector (the n orientation) or in the opposite direction (the u orientation).

orifice (ɔr'ɪfɪs), the entrance or the outlet of any cavity in the body. Also called **ostium.** – **orificial,** *adj.*

ori gene (ɔr'i), (in molecular genetics) the site or region in which DNA replication starts.

origin, the more fixed end of a muscle attachment. Compare **insertion.**

Orimune, a trade name for an active immunizing agent (live oral poliovirus vaccine).

Orinase, a trade name for an oral sulfanylurea antidiabetic (tolbutamide).

Ornade, a trade name for a fixed-combination drug containing an adrenergic decongestant (phenylpropanolamine hydrochloride), an antihistamine (chlorpheniramine maleate), and an anticholinergic (isopropamide iodide), used for the relief of symptoms of upper respiratory tract congestion.

Ornithodoros (ɔr'nɪθod'ərəs), a genus of ticks, some species of which are vectors for the spirochetes of relapsing fevers.

ornithosis (ɔr'nɪθou'sɪs). See **psittacosis.**

oro-, 1. a combining form meaning 'of or pertaining to the mouth': *orolingual, oromaxillary, oropharynx.* 2. Also **orrho.** a combining form meaning 'the watery part of the blood or serum': *orodiagnosis, orosin, orotherapy.*

oropharynx (ɔr'oufær'ɪŋks), one of the three anatomical divisions of the pharynx. It extends behind the mouth from the soft palate above to the level of the hyoid bone below and contains the palatine tonsils and the lingual tonsils. Compare **laryngopharynx, nasopharynx.** – **oropharyngeal,** *adj.*

Oroya fever. See **bartonellosis.**

orphenadrine citrate, a skeletal muscle relaxant with anticholinergic and antihistaminic activity.

■ INDICATION: It is prescribed in the treatment of severe muscle strain.

■ CONTRAINDICATIONS: Myasthenia gravis, contraindications of anti-cholinergic agents, or known hypersensitivity to this drug prohibits its use.

■ ADVERSE EFFECTS: Among the most serious adverse reactions are those associated with anticholinergic activity, as dry mouth and tachycardia, and allergic reactions.

orphenadrine hydrochloride, an anticholinergic and antihistaminic agent.

■ INDICATION: It is prescribed in the treatment of parkinsonism.

■ CONTRAINDICATIONS: Myasthenia gravis or other condition that contraindicates the use of anticholinergic agents or a known sensitivity to this drug prohibits its use.

■ ADVERSE EFFECTS: Among the most serious adverse reactions are anti-cholinergic side effects and allergic reactions.

orrho-, a combining form meaning 'of or pertaining to serum': *orrhomeningitis, orrhoreaction, orrhorrhea.* Also **oro-.**

ortho-, a combining form meaning 'straight, normal, correct': *orthobiosis, orthodontist, orthotopic.*

orthoboric acid (ɔr'θoubɔr'ɪk). See **boric acid.**

orthodontia. See **orthodontics.**

orthodontics (ɔr'θədon'tɪks), the specialty of dentistry concerned with the diagnosis and treatment of malocclusion and irregularities of the teeth.

orthodromic conduction (ɔr'θədrom'ɪk), the conduction of a neural impulse in the normal direction, from a synaptic junction or a receptor forward along an axon to its termination with depolarization.

orthogenesis, the theory that evolution is controlled by intrinsic factors within the organism and progresses according to a predetermined course rather than in several directions as a result of natural selection and other environmental factors. – **orthogenetic,** *adj.*

orthogenic, 1. of or pertaining to orthogenesis; orthogenetic. 2. of or pertaining to the treatment and rehabilitation of children who are mentally or emotionally disturbed. See also **orthopsychiatry.**

orthogenic evolution, change within an animal or plant induced solely by an intrinsic factor, independent of any environmental elements. Also called **bathmic evolution.**

orthomyxovirus (ɔr'θoumɪk'souvai'rəs), a member of a family of viruses that includes several organisms responsible for human influenza infection.

Ortho-Novum, a trade name for an oral contraceptive containing an estrogen (mestranol) and a progestin (norethindrone).

orthopantogram (ɔr'θoupæn'təgræm), an x ray showing a panoramic view of the entire dentition, alveolar bone, and other contiguous structures on a single film, taken extraorally.

orthopedic nurse, a nurse whose primary area of interest, competence, and professional practice is in orthopedic nursing.

orthopedics, the branch of medicine devoted to the study and treatment of the skeletal system, its joints, muscles, and associated structures.

orthopedic traction, a procedure in which a patient is maintained in a device attached by ropes and pulleys to weights that exert a pulling force on an extremity or body part while countertraction is maintained. Traction is applied most often to reduce and immobilize fractures but it also is used to overcome muscle spasm, to stretch adhesions, to correct certain deformities, and to help release arthritic contractures. Traction may be applied directly to the skin by attaching the rope-pulley-weight system to bands of adhesive, moleskin, or foam rubber or to a splint affixed to the affected limb; side arm traction is a kind of skin traction used to align a fractured humerus following open reduction. Skeletal traction is exerted directly on a bone in which a wire or pin is inserted under anesthesia in the open reduction of a fracture; the ends of the pin protruding through the skin on both sides of the bone are covered with corks and attached to a metal U-shaped spreader or bow, which in turn is attached to the traction rope. Skin or skeletal traction applied to a lower extremity by a balanced suspension apparatus, as the Thomas splint and Pearson's attachment, permits the patient to move more freely in bed since the leg is balanced with countertraction and any slack in traction caused by the patient's movements is taken up by the suspension apparatus. Bryant's traction for treating fractures of the femur shaft in young children uses a suspension apparatus to hold the youngster's legs at right angles to the body. A girdle that fits over the iliac crests and pelvis is used in the application of traction to relieve low back pain and a cervical halter is employed in applying traction to reduce neck pain; cervical traction may also be used when a fracture of the cervical spine is suspected. See specific devices and specific kinds of traction.

■ METHOD: To maintain the required constant pull, the traction ropes are kept taut, free to ride over the pulleys, and securely tied to the weights that hang free — away from the bed and off the floor. Countertraction is maintained by elevating the patient's bed under the body part to which traction is applied and a pull exerted in the opposite direction; a chest restraint sheet may be applied to the patient in side arm traction for countertraction if necessary. During the initial stages of traction, the involved extremity is checked every two hours for quality of the distal pulse, color, warmth, motion, sensation, and swelling. Blood pressure, temperature, pulse, and respirations are recorded every four hours until stable. Pain is controlled and the patient is positioned as ordered. If the patient is in balanced suspension, abduction of the leg and a 20° angle between the thigh and bed are maintained; the heel is kept free of the sling under the calf. A harness restraint is used to prevent a child in Bryant's traction from turning over, and the youngster's buttocks are raised slightly from the mattress. Bed linen is changed only as necessary and an air mattress is used when required. Every two hours the patient is helped to cough and deep-breathe; bony prominences are massaged, but vigorous rubbing is avoided. Lotion is applied to the skin, which is periodically inspected for signs of redness, abra-

sions, blisters, dryness, itching, excoriation, and pressure areas; special attention is given to the pin insertion sites of the patient in skeletal traction. The patient is observed every four hours for neurologic signs, as tingling, numbness, loss of sensation or motion, for thrombophlebitis in the involved extremity, and for evidence of a pulmonary blood clot or fat embolus, as indicated by decreased breath sounds, fever, tachypnea, diaphoresis, pallor, bloody or purulent sputum, and tachycardia. Oral hygiene is administered every four hours and, unless contraindicated, a daily intake of 2,500 to 3,000 ml of fluids is encouraged. As the patient's condition improves, the position is changed every four hours; if the kind of traction permits and if the upper extremities are not involved, a trapeze is added to the bed. The patient is taught to perform range of motion exercises with the uninvolved extremities, dorsiflexion and plantar flexion of the ankles, and isometric exercises, as gluteal and abdominal contraction. A high-protein, low-carbohydrate diet is served, and vitamin and iron therapy may be ordered. The immobilized patient uses a flat, fracture bedpan and usually requires stool softeners or a mild laxative.

■ NURSING ORDERS: The patient in traction often needs extensive physical care and emotional support. The person is encouraged to verbalize feelings and concerns about prolonged hospitalization and absence from work or school. To the greatest degree possible, the nurse encourages the patient to participate in self-care and to engage in diversions, as handicrafts, reading, watching television, and listening to the radio.

■ OUTCOME CRITERIA: The healthy young adult or adolescent in traction for the treatment of a fracture usually has an uneventful recovery, but diligent attention and nursing care are necessary to avoid the formation of decubitus ulcers, infection, constipation, and other sequelae of immobility.

orthopedist, a specialist in orthopedics. Also called *Informal.* **orthopod.**

orthopnea (ɔrʃhop'niə), an abnormal condition in which a person must sit or stand in order to breathe deeply or comfortably. It occurs in many disorders of the cardiac and respiratory systems, as asthma, pulmonary edema, emphysema, pneumonia, and angina pectoris. See also **dyspnea.** —**orthopneic,** *adj.*

orthopod, *Informal.* an orthopedist.

orthopsychiatry, the branch of psychiatry that specializes in correcting incipient and borderline mental and behavioral disorders, especially in children, and in developing preventive techniques to promote mental health and emotional growth and development. See also **mental hygiene.**

orthoptic (ɔrʃhop'tɪk), **1.** of or pertaining to normal binocular vision. **2.** of or pertaining to a procedure or technique for correcting the visual axes of eyes improperly coordinated for binocular vision.

orthoptic examination, an ophthalmoscopic examination of the binocular function of the eyes. A stereoscopic instrument presents a slightly different picture to each eye. The examiner notes the degree to which the pictures are combined by the normal process of fusion. If the person has diplopia separate pictures are seen. If the person has suppression amblyopia only one picture is seen. Stereoscopic training may improve binocular vision in some conditions.

orthosis (orthou'sis), a force system designed to control, correct, or compensate for a bone deformity, deforming forces, or forces absent from the body. Orthosis often involves the use of special braces. **orthotic,** (orthot'ik) *adj., n.*

orthostatic albuminuria. See **orthostatic proteinuria.**

orthostatic hypotension, abnormally low blood pressure occurring when an individual assumes the standing posture. Also called **postural hypotension.**

orthostatic proteinuria, presence of protein in the urine of some people, especially teenagers, who have been standing. It disappears when they recline and is of no pathologic significance. Also called **orthostatic albuminuria, postural albuminuria, postural proteinuria.**

orthotonos (orthot'onos), a straight, rigid posture of the body caused by a tetanic spasm, usually owing to strychnine poisoning or tetanus infection. The neck and all other parts of the body are in a position of extension but not as severely as in opisthotonos. Compare **emprosthotonos.**

Orthoxine Hydrochloride, a trade name for an adrenergic bronchodilator (methoxyphenamine hydrochloride).

Ortolani's test (or'tola'niz), a procedure used to evaluate the stability of the hip joints in newborns and infants. The baby is placed on his back, the hips and knees are flexed at right angles and abducted until the lateral aspects of the knees are touching the table. The examiner's fingers are extended along the outside of the thighs, with the thumbs grasping the insides of the knees. Internal and external rotation are attempted, and symmetry of mobility is evaluated. A click or a popping sensation (Ortolani's sign) may be felt if the joint is unstable, because the head of the femur moves out of the acetabulum under pressure from the examiner's hands during rotation and abduction. See also **congenital dislocation of the hip.**

os (os). See **bone.**

-os, a combining form signaling singular nouns: *biologos, hepatomphalos, megophthalmos.*

Os, symbol for **osmium.**

O.S., abbreviation for *oculus sinister,* a Latin phrase meaning 'left eye.'

os calcis (kæl'sis). See **calcaneus.**

os capitatum. See **capitate bone.**

oscheo-, a combining form meaning 'of or pertaining to the scrotum': *oscheocele, oscheolith, oscheoma.*

os cuboideum. See **cuboid bone.**

-ose, **1.** a combining form meaning a 'carbohydrate': *cellulose, lactose, sucrose.* **2.** a combining form meaning a 'primary product of hydrolysis': *albumose, nucleose, myoproteose.*

Osgood-Schlatter disease (oz'gudshlæt'ər), inflammation or partial separation of the tibial tubercle caused by chronic irritation, usually secondary to overuse of the quadriceps muscle. The condition is seen primarily in muscular, athletic adolescent boys and is characterized by swelling and tenderness over the tibial tubercle that increase with exercise or any activity that extends the leg. Treatment consists primarily of preventing further irritation during the healing process and may necessitate complete immobilization of the knee in a cast. Any residual nonunion of a proximal fragment after healing may require surgical excision. Also called **Osgood's disease, Schlatter's disease, Schlatter-Osgood disease.**

os hamatum. See **hamate bone.**

os hyoideum. See **hyoid bone.**

-osis, **1.** a combining form meaning a '(specified) action, process, or result': *homeosis, narcosis, zygosis.* **2.** a combining form meaning a 'pathological condition': *calcicosis, psittacosis, varicosis.*

Osler's disease (ous'lərz). See **Osler-Weber-Rendu disease.**

Osler's nodes (ous'lərz), tender, reddish or purplish subcutaneous nodules of the soft tissue on the ends of fingers or toes, seen in subacute bacterial endocarditis and usually lasting only one or two days.

Osler-Weber-Rendu syndrome (ous'lərweb'ərrandu'), a vascular anomaly, inherited as an autosomal dominant trait, characterized by hemorrhagic telangiectasia of skin and mucosa. Small red-to-violet lesions are found on the lips, the oral and nasal mucosa, the tongue, and the tips of fingers and toes. The thin, dilated vessels may bleed spontaneously or as a result of only minor trauma, and this condition becomes progressively more severe. Bleeding from superficial lesions is often profuse and may result in severe anemia. No specific treatment is known, but accessible, bleeding lesions may be treated with pressure, styptics, and topical hemostatics. Transfusions may be indicated for acute hemorrhage, and iron deficiency anemia may require continuous treatment. Also called **hereditary hemorrhagic telangiectasia, Rendu-Osler-Weber syndrome.**

os lunatum. See **lunate bone.**

os magnum. See **capitate bone.**

-osmia, a combining form meaning '(condition of the) sense of smell': *dysosmia, hemianosmia, merosmia.*

Osmitrol, a trade name for a diagnostic aid and osmotic diuretic (mannitol).

osmium (Os), a hard, grayish, pungent-smelling metallic element. Its atomic number is 76; its atomic weight is 190.2. Used to produce alloys of extreme hardness, it is highly toxic.

osmo-, **1.** a combining form meaning 'of or pertaining to odors': *osmoceptor, osmodysphoria, osmonosology.* **2.** a combining form meaning 'pertaining to an impulse, or to osmosis': *osmophilic, osmosology, osmotaxis.*

osmolality (oz′moulæl′ɪti), the osmotic pressure of a solution expressed in osmols or milliosmols per kilogram of water. Compare **osmolarity.**

osmolar (osmou′lər), of or pertaining to the osmotic characteristics of a solution of one or more molecular substances, ionic substances, or both, expressed in osmols or milliosmols.

osmolarity (os′moulær′ɪti), the osmotic pressure of a solution expressed in osmols or milliosmols per kilogram of the solution. Compare **osmolality.**

osmole (os′moul), the quantity of a substance in solution in the form of molecules, ions, or both (usually expressed in grams) that has the same osmotic pressure as one mole of an ideal nonelectrolyte. **– osmolal,** *adj.*

osmometry, a field of study that deals with the phenomenon of osmosis and the measurement of osmotic forces. **– osmometric,** *adj.*

osmosis (ozmou′sɪs, osmou′sɪs), the movement of a pure solvent, as water, through a semipermeable membrane from a solution that has a lower solute concentration to one that has a higher solute concentration. The membrane is impermeable to the solute but is permeable to the solvent. The rate of osmosis depends on the concentration of solute, the temperature of the solution, the electrical charge of the solute, and the difference between the osmotic pressures exerted by the solutions. Movement across the membrane continues until the concentrations of the solutions equalize.

OSMOSIS

osmotic diuresis, diuresis owing to the presence of certain nonabsorbable substances in tubules of the kidney, as mannitol, urea, or glucose.

osmotic fragility, a sensitivity to change in osmotic pressure characteristic of red blood cells. Exposed to a hypotonic concentration of sodium in a solution, red cells take in increasing quantities of water, swell until the capacity of the cell membrane is exceeded, and burst. Exposed to a hypertonic concentration of sodium in a solution, red cells give up intracellular fluid, shrink, and break up. Laboratory findings of exceptional fragility or resistance may be diagnostic of certain conditions.

osmotic pressure, **1.** the pressure exerted on a semipermeable membrane separating a solution from a solvent, the membrane being impermeable to the solutes in the solution and permeable only to the solvent. **2.** the pressure exerted on a semipermeable membrane by a solution containing one or more solutes that cannot penetrate the membrane, which is permeable only by the solvent surrounding it. See also **osmosis.**

os naviculares pedis. See **scaphoid bone.**

-osphresia, a combining form meaning a 'condition of the sense of smell': *anosphresia, hyperosphresia, oxyosphresia.* Also **-osphrasia.**

osphresio-, a combining form meaning 'of or pertaining to odors': *osphresiolagnia, osphresiology, osphresiophilia.*

oss-, a combining form meaning 'of or pertaining to bone': *osseocartilaginous, ossicle, ossific.*

osseous labyrinth, the bony portion of the internal ear, composed of three cavities: the vestibule, the semicircular canals, and the cochlea, transmitting sound vibrations from the middle ear to the acoustic nerve. All three cavities contain perilymph, in which a membranous labyrinth is suspended. Also called **labyrinthus osseus.** Compare **membranous labyrinth.**

ossicle (os′ɪkəl), a small bone, as the malleus, the incus, or the stapes, ossicles of the inner ear. **– ossicular,** *adj.*

ossification (os′ɪfɪkei′šhən), the development of bone. **Intramembranous ossification** is that preceded by membrane, as in the process initially forming the roof and the sides of the skull. **Intracartilaginous ossification** is that preceded by rods of cartilage, as that forming the bones of the limbs.

ossifying fibroma, a slow-growing, benign neoplasm of bone, occurring most often in the jaws, especially the mandible. The tumor is composed of bone that develops within fibrous connective tissue.

ostealgia, any pain that is associated with an abnormal condition within a bone, as osteomyelitis. **– ostealgic,** *adj.*

osteanagenesis. See **osteoanagenesis.**

osteitis (os′tiai′tɪs), an inflammation of bone, caused by infection, degeneration, or trauma. Swelling, tenderness, dull aching pain, and redness in the skin over the affected bone are characteristic of the condition. Some kinds of osteitis are **osteitis deformans, osteitis fibrosa cystica.** See also **osteomyelitis, Paget's disease.**

osteitis deformans. See **Paget's disease.**

osteitis fibrosa cystica, an inflammatory degenerative condition in which normal bone is replaced by cysts and fibrous tissue. It is usually associated with hyperparathyroidism.

osteitis fibrosa disseminata. See **Albright's syndrome.**

ostembryon (ostem′brion). See **lithopedion.**

osteo-, a combining form meaning 'of or pertaining to bone': osteoanesthesia, osteocele, osteopathy.

osteoanagenesis, osteanagenesis (os′tiɔuæn′ɔjen′ɔsɪs), the regeneration or formation of bone tissue.

osteoarthritis (os′tiɔuɑrθrɑi′tɪs), a form of arthritis in which one or many joints undergo degenerative changes, including subchondral bony sclerosis, loss of articular cartilage, and proliferation of bone and cartilage in the joint, forming osteophytes. Inflammation of the synovial membrane of the joint is common late in the disease. The most common form of arthritis, its cause is unknown but may include chemical, mechanical, genetic, metabolic, and endocrine factors. Emotional stress often aggravates the condition. Usually, it begins with pain after exercise or use of the joint. Stiffness, tenderness to the touch, crepitus, and enlargement develop and deformity, subluxation, and synovial effusion may eventually occur. Involvement of the hip, knee, or the spine causes more disability than osteoarthritis of other areas. Treatment includes rest of the involved joints, heat, and anti-inflammatory drugs. Systemic corticosteroids are contraindicated, but intra-articular injections of corticosteroids may give relief. Surgical treatment is sometimes necessary and may reduce pain and greatly improve the function of a joint. Hip replacement, joint debridement, fusion, and decompression laminectomy are some of the surgical procedures used in treating advanced osteoarthritis. Compare **rheumatoid arthritis.**

osteoblast, a cell that originates in the embryonic mesenchyme and, during the early development of the skeleton, differentiates from a fibroblast to function in the formation of bone tissue. Osteoblasts synthesize the collagen and glycoproteins to form the matrix and, with growth, develop into osteocytes. Also called **osteoplast.** See also **ossification.** — **osteoblastic,** *adj.*

osteoblastoma (os′tiɔublæstou′mɔ), *pl.* **osteoblastomas, osteoblastomata.** a small, benign, fairly vascular tumor of poorly formed bone and fibrous tissue, occurring most frequently in the vertebrae, femur, tibia, or bones of the upper extremities in children and young adults. The lesion causes pain, erosion, and resorption of native bone. When feasible, excision is the preferred treatment. Also called **osteoid osteoma.**

osteochondrodystrophy (os′tiɔukon′droudɪs′trɔfi). See **Morquio's disease.**

osteochondroma (os′tiɔukondrou′mɔ), a benign tumor made of bone and cartilage.

osteochondrosis (os′tiɔukondrou′sɪs), a disease affecting the ossification centers of bone in children, initially characterized by degeneration and necrosis, followed by regeneration and recalcification. Kinds of osteochondrosis include **Legg-Calvé-Perthe's disease, Osgood-Schlatter's disease, Scheuermann's disease.**

osteoclasia (os′tiɔuklei′ziɔ), **1.** the destruction and absorption of bony tissue by osteoclasts, as during growth or the healing of fractures. **2.** the degeneration of bone through disease. See also **osteolysis.**

osteoclasis, the intentional surgical fracture of a bone to correct a deformity. Also called **osteoclasty.** — **osteoclastic,** *adj.*

osteoclast, 1. Also called **osteophage.** See also **ossification.** a large type of multinucleated bone cell that functions in the development and periods of growth or repair, as the breakdown and resorption of osseous tissue. During bone healing of fractures, or during certain disease processes, osteoclasts excavate passages through the surrounding tissue by enzymatic action. Osteoclasts become activated in the presence of parathyroid hormone and also in a lymphokine substance produced by lymphocytes in such diseases as multiple myeloma and malignant lymphomas. **2.** a surgical instrument used in the fracturing or refracturing of bones for therapeutic purposes, as correction of a deformity.

osteoclastic, 1. pertaining to or of the nature of osteoclasts. **2.** destructive to bone.

osteoclastoma (os′tiɔuklæstou′mɔ), *pl.* **osteoclastomas, osteoclastomata.** a giant cell tumor of the bone, occurring most frequently at the end of a long bone and appearing as a mass surrounded by a thin shell of new, periosteal bone. The lesion may be benign but is more often malignant. It causes local pain, loss of function, and, in some cases, weakness followed by pathologic fracture. Also called **giant cell myeloma, giant cell tumor of bone.**

osteoclasty. See **osteoclasis.**

osteocyte, a bone cell; a mature osteoblast that has become embedded in the bone matrix. It occupies a small cavity and sends out protoplasmic projections that anastomose with those of other osteoblasts to form a system of minute canals within the bone matrix. — **osteocytic,** *adj.*

osteodystrophy, any generalized defect in bone development, usually associated with disturbances in calcium and phosphorus metabolism and renal insufficiency, as in renal osteodystrophy. Also called **osteodystrophia.**

osteogenesis, osteogeny, the origin and development of bone tissue. See also **ossification.** — **osteogenetic, osteogenic,** *adj.*

osteogenesis imperfecta, a genetic disorder involving defective development of the connective tissue. It is inherited as an autosomal dominant trait and is characterized by abnormally brittle and fragile bones that are easily fractured by the slightest trauma. Also called **brittle bones, fragilitas ossium, hypoplasia of the mesenchyme, osteopsathyrosis.**

■ OBSERVATIONS: In its most severe form, the disease may be apparent at birth, when it is known as osteogenesis imperfecta congenita. The newborn has multiple fractures that have occurred in utero and is usually severely deformed, owing to imperfect formation and mineralization of bone. Most infants die shortly after birth, although a few survive as deformed dwarfs with normal mental development if no head trauma has occurred. If the disease has a later onset, it is called osteogenesis imperfecta tarda and usually runs a milder course. Symptoms generally appear when the child begins to walk, but they become less severe with age and the tendency to fracture decreases and often disappears after puberty. Other manifestations of the condition include blue sclerae, translucent skin, hyperextensibility of ligaments, hypoplasia of the teeth, recurrent epistaxis, excess diaphoresis, mild hyperpyrexia, and a tendency to bruise easily and to develop otosclerosis with hearing loss. There is a broad expressivity of the disease so that the number and extent of pathological features may range from minimal to severe involvement.

■ INTERVENTION: There is no known cure for the disease. Treatment is predominantly supportive; extreme care must be taken in handling patients, especially infants who are severely affected, to prevent fractures. In many children oral administration of magnesium oxide may decrease the fracture rate as well as the diaphoresis, hyperpyrexia, and constipation associated with the condition.

■ NURSING CONSIDERATIONS: The primary function of the nurse is to educate the parents about the disease, especially the extent of the child's limitations, and to help them plan suitable activities that will promote optimum growth and development and, at the same time, protect the child from harm. Genetic counseling is also part of the goals of long-term care.

osteogenic, osteogenous, composed of or originating from any tissue involved in the development, growth, or repair of bone.

osteogenic sarcoma. See **osteosarcoma.**

osteogeny. See **osteogenesis.**

osteoid (os'tioid), of, pertaining to, or resembling bone.

osteoid osteoma. See **osteoblastoma.**

osteolysis (os'tiol'əsis), the degeneration and dissolution of bone, caused by disease, infection, or ischemia. The condition commonly affects the terminal bones of the hands and feet, as in acro-osteolysis, and is seen in disorders involving blood vessels, as in Raynaud's disease, scleroderma, and systemic lupus erythematosus. — **osteolytic,** adj.

osteoma (os'tiou'mə), pl. **osteomas, osteomata.** a tumor of bone tissue.

-osteoma, a combining form meaning a 'tumor composed of bone tissue, usually benign': endosteoma, myosteoma, periosteoma.

osteomalacia (os'tiouməlei'shə), an abnormal condition of the lamellar bone, characterized by a loss of calcification of the matrix resulting in softening of the bone, accompanied by weakness, fracture, pain, anorexia, and weight loss. The condition is the result of an inadequate amount of phosphorus and calcium available in the blood for mineralization of the bones. This deficiency may be caused by a diet lacking these minerals or vitamin D, or by a lack of exposure to sunlight, hence an inability to synthesize vitamin D, or by a metabolic disorder causing malabsorption. Osteomalacia results from and also complicates many diseases and conditions. Treatment usually includes the administration of the necessary vitamins and minerals and therapy appropriate for the underlying disorder. See also **hyperparathyroidism, Paget's disease, rickets.**

osteomyelitis (os'tioumai'əlai'tis), local or generalized infection of bone and bone marrow, usually caused by bacteria introduced by trauma or surgery, by direct extension from a nearby infection, or via the bloodstream. Staphylococci are the most common causative agents.

■ OBSERVATIONS: The long bones in children and the vertebrae in adults are the commonest sites of infection as a result of hematogenous spread. Persistent, severe, and increasing bone pain, tenderness, guarding on movement, regional muscle spasm and fever suggest this diagnosis. Draining sinus tracts may accompany post-traumatic osteomyelitis or osteomyelitis from a contiguous infection. Specific diagnosis and selection of therapy depend on bacterial examination of bone, tissue, or pus.

■ INTERVENTION: Treatment includes bed rest and parenteral antibiotics for several weeks. Surgery may be necessary to remove necrotic bone and tissue, to obliterate cavities, to remove infected prosthetic appliances, and to apply prostheses to stabilize affected parts. Chronic osteomyelitis may persist for years with exacerbations and remissions despite treatment.

■ NURSING CONSIDERATIONS: Any drainage is disposed of with the usual precautions against contamination. Absolute rest of the affected part may be necessary, with a careful positioning using pillows and sandbags for good alignment. During the early phase of infection, pain is extremely severe and extraordinary gentleness in moving and manipulating the infected part is essential. — **osteomyelitic,** adj.

osteon (os'tion), the basic structural unit of compact bone, consisting of the haversian canal and its concentric rings of 4 to 20 lamellae. Most of the units run with the long axis of the bone.

-osteon, a combining form meaning 'bone': melacosteon, otosteon, pleurosteon. Also **-osteum.**

osteonecrosis (os'tiounəkrou'sɪs), the destruction and death of bone tissue, as from ischemia, infection, malignant neoplastic disease, or trauma. — **osteonecrotic,** *adj.*

osteopath, osteopathist, a physician specialized in osteopathy.

osteopathy (os'tiop'əthi), a therapeutic approach to the practice of medicine that utilizes all the usual forms of medical therapy and diagnosis, including drugs, surgery, and radiation, but that places greater emphasis on the role of the relationship of the organs and the musculoskeletal system than is done in medicine. Osteopathic physicians recognize and correct structural problems using manipulation. The process is important in both the diagnosis and the treatment of health problems. See also **Doctor of Osteopathy.** — **osteopathic,** *adj.*

osteopedion (os'tioupi'dion). See **lithopedion.**

osteopetrosis, an inherited disorder characterized by a generalized increase in bone density, probably caused by faulty bone resorption resulting from a deficiency of osteoclasts. In its most severe form, transmitted as an autosomal recessive condition, there is obliteration of the bone marrow cavity, causing severe anemia, marked deformities of the skull, and compression of the cranial nerves, which may result in deafness and blindness and lead to an early death. A milder, benign form, transmitted as an autosomal dominant trait, is characterized by short stature, fragile bones that fracture easily, and a proneness to develop osteomyelitis. Also called **Albers-Schönberg disease, ivory bones, marble bones, osteosclerosis fragilis.** — **osteopetrotic,** *adj.*

osteophage. See **osteoclast.**

osteoplast. See **osteoblast.**

osteopoikilosis, an inherited condition of the bones, transmitted as an autosomal dominant trait, characterized by multiple areas of dense calcification throughout the osseous tissue, producing a mottled appearance on x-ray examination. It is a benign condition, usually without symptoms, and of unknown cause. Also called **osteosclerosis fragilis congenita.** — **osteopoikilotic,** *adj.*

osteoporosis, a disorder characterized by abnormal rarefaction of bone, occurring most frequently in postmenopausal women, in sedentary or immobilized individuals, and in patients on long-term steroid therapy. The disorder may cause pain, especially in the lower back, pathologic fractures, loss of stature, and various deformities. Osteoporosis may be idiopathic or secondary to other disorders, as thyrotoxicosis or the bone demineralization caused by hyperparathyroidism. Estrogen therapy is often used for the prevention and management of postmenopausal osteoporosis, but use of the hormone carries the risk of endometrial cancer.

osteopsathyrosis (os'tiopsæth'ərou'sɪs). See **osteogenesis imperfecta.**

osteosarcoma (os'tiousarkou'mə), a malignant bone tumor composed of anaplastic cells derived from mesenchyme. Also called **osteogenic sarcoma.**

osteosclerosis, an abnormal increase in the density of bone tissue. The condition occurs in a variety of disease states, is commonly associated with ischemia, chronic infection, and tumor formation, and may be caused by faulty bone resorption as a result of some abnormality involving the osteoclasts. See also **achondroplasia, osteopetrosis, osteopoikilosis.** — **osteosclerotic,** *adj.*

osteosclerosis fragilis. See **osteopetrosis.**

osteosclerosis fragilis congenita. See **osteopoikilosis.**

-osteum. See **-osteon.**

ostium (os'tiəm), *pl.* **ostia.** See **orifice.** — **ostial,** *adj.*

ostium primum defect. See **atrial septal defect.**

ostium secundum defect. See **atrial septal defect.**

ostomate (os'təmeit), a person who has undergone an ostomy.

ostomy (os'təmi), *Informal.* a surgical procedure in which an opening is made to allow the passage of urine from the bladder or of intestinal contents from the bowel *(See next page for table)*

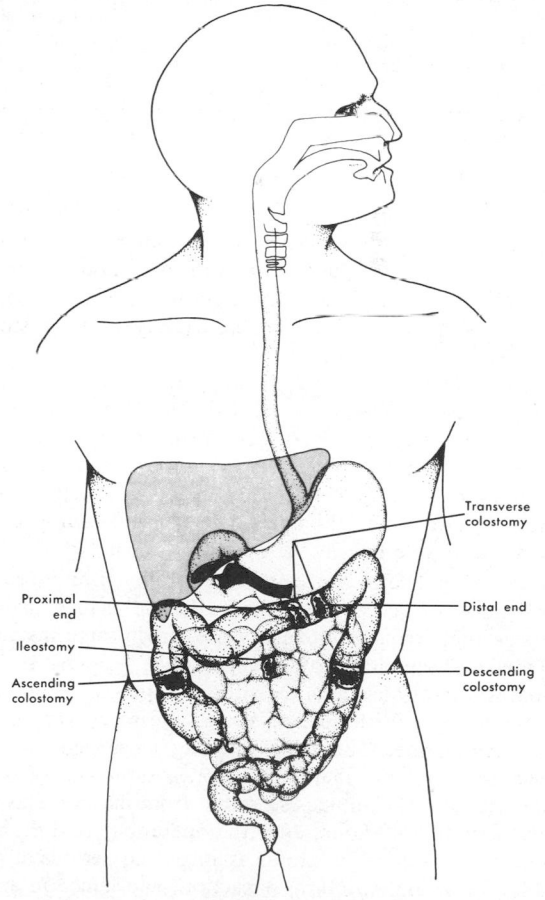

OSTOMY SITES

Comparative aspects of ileostomy and colostomy in preparation for teaching

Skin care	Stoma functioning	Usual drainage	Appliance	Control	Complications
Ileostomy Immediate protection of surrounding skin to prevent autodigestion (appliance to fit within 3 mm [⅛ inch] of stoma) Skin care to include: Wash and dry area well Use "barrier" between appliance and skin	Within 48 hours mucus produced Within 3 weeks stoma size shrinks to allow for fit of permanent appliance	Continuous liquid fecal stream	Will require a permanent set	Essentially none Control may *not* be achieved with irrigations	Excessive loss of water and electrolytes Stricture or inversion of stoma Skin excoriation and autodigestion Bleeding from decrease of vitamin K Undernutrition
Permanent colostomy Immediate protection of surrounding skin to prevent excoriation (appliance to fit within 6 mm [¼ inch] of stoma) Skin care to include: Wash and dry area well Use "barrier" between appliance and skin	Same as ileostomy	Sigmoid colostomy: formed stool Transverse colostomy: semiliquid to semiformed stool Ascending (right colon) colostomy: liquid fecal stream	Temporary set until control is achieved Use of a permanent set will depend on stool formation Permanent set is generally necessary	Irrigations and modifications in diet Modifications in diet (irrigations may assist in control) Same as ileostomy	Stricture or inversion of stoma Skin excoriation *(Candida)* Dehydration if water loss excessive

to an incision or stoma surgically created in the wall of the abdomen. An ostomy procedure may be performed to correct an anatomic defect or to relieve an obstruction in the urinary or intestinal tract. Each procedure is named for the anatomic location of the ostomy, as a colostomy, ceceostomy, or cystostomy.

ostomy care, the management and support of a patient with a surgical opening created in the bladder, ileum, or colon for the temporary or permanent passage of urine or feces, necessitated by carcinoma, intestinal obstruction, trauma, or severe ulceration distal to the site of the incision. In most cases the opening is covered with a temporary disposable bag in the operating room.

■ METHOD: The patient with a colostomy or an ileostomy is helped to accept the stoma and the change in body image that frequently causes grief, or, in some instances, denial. Discussions of the person's feelings are encouraged and questions regarding the procedure and possible changes in the person's life style are answered in a positive manner. The disposable bag is changed whenever necessary and the character, color, and amount of drainage are observed; mucus secretion from the stoma usually begins within 48 hours after the operation, fecal drainage within 72 hours. The stoma is inspected periodically for color, bleeding, stricture, retraction, and infection and is measured every other day to determine the size of the

permanent appliance that is to be used as soon as the condition of the opening permits. Each time the temporary or permanent appliance is changed, the skin around the stoma is washed with soap and water, rinsed thoroughly, and patted dry with a clean towel. If the skin is irritated or excoriated, karaya powder, alone or mixed with an ointment, is spread over the area before the appliance is reinstalled. An adhesive substance may be used to maintain a tight seal with the appliance, and deodorant drops, aspirin, or various bismuth or chlorophyll preparations are added to the ostomy bag to control odor. The diet is planned according to the kind of ostomy; ileostomates require food high in sodium and potassium, as bananas, citrus juices, molasses, and cola, and are advised to avoid fried, highly seasoned, and rich foods, nuts, raisins, raw fruits other than bananas, and anything that produces gas or causes diarrhea. Gas-producing foods, as cabbage, beans, broccoli, cauliflower, and corn, foods causing disturbing odors, as onions, eggs, and fish, and sharp condiments are contraindicated; a low-residue diet is ordered for most ostomates. The fluid intake is carefully maintained.

■ NURSING ORDERS: Prior to discharge, each step in the care of the stoma and surrounding skin is rehearsed with the patient, using the equipment that will be available at home. Appropriate diet instruction is provided, emphasizing the need to eat adequate meals regularly, to chew slowly, and to avoid extremely hot and very cold food. The patient is urged to establish a regular pattern of evacuation, and to report any signs of wound infection or obstruction, as nausea, vomiting, decreased drainage from the stoma, abdominal distention, and cramps. Normal daily activity is encouraged.

■ OUTCOME CRITERIA: The ability of the patient to adjust to the ostomy procedures and equipment is greatly affected by the nursing care received in the days following surgery. A positive, patient, and matter-of-fact approach, sensitive emotional support, and thorough teaching of self-care measures are essential aspects of ostomy nursing care.

ostomy irrigation, a procedure for cleansing, stimulating, and regulating evacuation of an artificially created orifice. Fluids used in irrigation include tap water and saline or medicated solutions. Necessary equipment includes properly sized irrigator tips, catheters, drainage bags that allow for insertion of the catheter, an irrigation container, and shields to prevent leakage. Loop and double-barrel colostomies require a sequential irrigation of the proximal loop, distal loop, and rectum in order to prevent the accumulation of discharge.

os trapezium. See **trapezium.**

os trapezoideum. See **trapezoid bone.**

os triquetrum. See **triangular bone.**

ot-. See **oto-.**

otalgia (ōutæl′jiə), pain in the ear. Also called **otodynia, otoneuralgia.**

OTC, abbreviation for *over-the-counter,* describing a drug available without a prescription from a physician.

Othello syndrome, a psychopathological condition, characterized by suspicion of a spouse's infidelity and by morbid jealousy. This condition may be accompanied by rage and violence and is frequently associated with paranoia.

-otia, a combining form meaning '(condition of the) ear': *melotia, microtia, synotia.*

otic, of or pertaining to the ear. Also called **auricular.**

-otic[1], **1.** a combining form meaning 'pertaining to part of the ear': *entotic, epitotic, prootic.* **2.** a combining form meaning 'pertaining to an area spatially related to the ear': *opisthotic, parotic, periotic.* **3.** a combining form meaning 'pertaining to a bone spatially related to the ear': *basiotic, prootic, sphenotic.*

-otic[2], **1.** a combining form meaning 'pertaining to a (specified) action or condition': *antidotic, biotic, osmotic.* **2.** a combining form meaning pertaining to a disease condition': *anthracotic, mycotic, neurotic.* **3.** a combining form meaning 'pertaining to an increase (of something specified)': *hematotic, morphotic, zymotic.*

otics (ōu′tĭks, ŏt′ĭks), a group of drugs used locally to treat inflammation of the external ear canal or to remove excess cerumen.

otitic barotrauma (ōutĭt′ĭk). See **barotrauma.**

otitis (ōutaī′tĭs), inflammation or infection of the ear. Kinds of otitis are **otitis externa, otitis interna, otitis media.**

otitis externa, inflammation or infection of the external canal or the auricle of the external ear. Major causes are allergy, bacteria, fungi, viruses, and trauma. Allergy to nickel or chromium in earrings, to chemicals in hair sprays, cosmetics, hearing-aids, and medications, particularly sulfonamides and neomycin, is common. *Staphylococcus aureus, Pseudomonas aeruginosa,* and *Streptococcus pyogenes* are common bacterial causes. Herpes simplex and herpes zoster viruses are frequently implicated. Eczema, psoriasis, and seborrheic dermatitis also may affect the external ear. Abrasions of the ear canal may become infected, and excessive swimming may wash out protective cerumen, remove skin lipids, and lead to secondary infection. Otitis externa is more prevalent during hot, humid weather. Folliculitis is particularly painful in the external auditory meatus and is a common occupational hazard in nurses, owing to irritation by the earpieces of stethoscopes. Treatment includes oral analgesics, thorough local cleansing, topical antimicrobials to treat infection, or topical corticosteroids to reduce inflammation. Prevention includes measures to reduce maceration of the skin and to avoid trauma.

otitis interna. See **labyrinthitis.**

otitis media, inflammation or infection of the middle ear, a common affliction of childhood. Acute otitis media is most often caused by *Hemophilus influenzae* or *Streptococcus pneumoniae.* Chronic otitis media is usually caused by gram-negative bacteria, as *Proteus, Klebsiella,* and *Pseudomonas.* Allergy, *Mycoplasma,* and several viruses also may be etiologic factors. Otitis media is often preceded by an upper respiratory infection.

■ OBSERVATIONS: Organisms gain entry to the middle ear through the eustachian tube. The small diameter and horizontal orientation of the tube in infants predisposes them to infection. Obstruction of the eustachian tube and accumulation of exudate may increase pressure within the middle ear, forcing infection into the mastoid bone or rupturing the tympanic membrane. Symptoms of acute otitis media include a sense of fullness in the ear, diminished hearing, pain, and fever. Usually, only one ear is affected. Squamous epithelium may grow in the middle ear through a rupture in the tympanic membrane, and development of a cholesteatoma and deafness may occur if repeated infections cause an opening to persist. Pneumoccoccal otitis media may spread to the meninges.

■ INTERVENTION: Accurate diagnosis of the causative microorganism is important for selection of effective antimicrobial therapy. Treatment also includes analgesics, local heat, nasal decongestants, needle aspiration of secretions collected behind the membrane, and myringotomy.

■ NURSING OBSERVATIONS: Parents are taught to recognize and watch for early warning signs of otitis media. The use of vaporizers and decongestants is often recommended during an upper respiratory tract infection as prophylaxis against otitis media.

oto-, ot-, a combining form meaning 'of or pertaining to the ear': *otoantritis, otoblennorrhea, otocyst.*

Otobione, a trade name for an otic, fixed-combination drug containing a glucocorticoid (hydrocortisone) and antibacterials (neomycin sulfate and polymyxin B sulfate).

otocephalus (ou'tousef'ələs), a fetus with otocephaly.

otocephaly (ou'tousef'əli), a congenital malformation characterized by the absence of the lower jaw, defective formation of the mouth, and union or close approximation of the ears on the front of the neck. See also **agnathocephaly.** – **otocephalic, otocephalous,** *adj.*

Otocort, a trade name for an otic, fixed-combination drug containing a glucocorticoid (hydrocortisone), the antibacterials (neomycin sulfate and polymyxin B sulfate), the analgesic (antipyrine), and the local anesthetic (dibucaine).

otodynia (ou'toudın'iə). See **otalgia.**

otolith-righting reflex (ou'təlıthrai'tıng), an involuntary response in newborns in which tilting of the body when the infant is in an erect position causes the head to return to the upright position. The reflex enables the infant to raise the head and is important for development of later gross motor skills. Absence of the reflex may indicate central nervous system damage.

otoneuralgia (ou'tounuræl'jə). See **otalgia.**

otoplasty (ou'təplæs'ti), a common procedure in reconstructive plastic surgery in which, for cosmetic reasons, some of the cartilage in the ears is removed to bring the auricle and pinna closer to the head.

Otoreid-HC, a trade name for an otic, fixed-combination drug containing a glucocorticoid (hydrocortisone) and antibacterials (neomycin sulfate and polymyxin B sulfate).

otorrhea, any discharge from the external ear. Otorrhea may be serous, sanguinous, purulent, or contain cerebrospinal fluid. – **otorrheal, otorrheic, otorrhetic,** *adj.*

otosclerosis (ou'tousklərou'sıs), a hereditary condition of unknown cause in which irregular ossification in the bony labyrinth of the inner ear, especially of the stapes, occurs, causing tinnitus, then deafness. The deafness is usually first noticed between the ages of 11 and 30. Women are affected twice as often as men. The condition may worsen in pregnancy. Stapedectomy is usually successful in permanently restoring hearing. Also called **otospongiosis.**

otoscope (ou'təskoup'), an instrument used to examine the external ear, the eardrum, and, through the eardrum,

the ossicles of the middle ear. It consists of a light, a magnifying lens, and a device for insufflation.

ototoxic (ou'toutok'sık), (of a substance) having a harmful effect on the eighth cranial nerve or the organs of hearing and balance. Common ototoxic drugs include the aminoglycoside antibiotics, aspirin, furosemide, and quinine.

Otrivin, a trade name for an adrenergic vasoconstrictor (xylometazoline hydrochloride), used as a nasal decongestant.

O.U., abbreviation for *oculus uterque,* a Latin phrase meaning 'each eye.'

ouabain (wəbai'ən), a cardiotonic.

■ INDICATIONS: It is prescribed in the treatment of congestive heart failure and certain atrial arrhythmias.

■ CONTRAINDICATIONS: Arrhythmias or known hypersensitivity to this drug prohibits its use.

■ ADVERSE EFFECTS: Among the more serious adverse reactions are nausea, vomiting, visual disturbances, and arrhythmias.

ounce (oz.), a unit of weight equal to $\frac{1}{16}$ of a pound avoirdupois.

-ous, a combining form meaning an 'element or compound with a valence lower than the corresponding one ending in *-ic*': *cuprous, ferrous, hypochlorous.* Also **-eous.**

outbreeding, the production of offspring by the mating of unrelated individuals, organisms, or plants, which can lead to superior hybrid traits or strains. Compare **inbreeding.** See also **heterosis.**

outcome, the condition of a client at the end of therapy or of a disease process, including the degree of wellness and the need for continuing care, medication, support, counseling, or education.

outcome data, data collected to evaluate the capacity of a client to function at a level described in the outcome statement of a nursing care plan or in standards for client care.

outcome measure, a measure of the quality of medical care, the standard on which is made the assessment of the expected end result of the intervention employed.

outlet contraction. See **contraction.**

outlet contracture, an abnormally small pelvic outlet. It may be anteroposterior or transverse and is of significance in childbirth as it may impede or prevent the passage of a baby through the birth canal. Anteroposterior contracture owing to fixation of the coccyx may sometimes be overcome by the force of labor, freeing the bones and allowing them to move back. Significant narrowing of the space between the ischial tuberosities is unlikely to be overcome and is most commonly associated with a heavy, android type of pelvis.

outlet forceps. See **low forceps.**

outpatient, 1. a patient, not hospitalized, who is being treated in an office, clinic, or other ambulatory care facility. **2.** of or pertaining to a health-care facility for patients who are not hospitalized or to the treatment or care of such a patient. Compare **inpatient.**

ovale malaria. See **tertian malaria.**

ovalocytosis (ouvei′lousaitou′sis). See **elliptocytosis.**

ovari-. See **ovario-.**

-ovaria, a combining form meaning '(condition of the) ovary or ovarial activity': *anovaria, hyperovaria, hyperovaria.*

ovarian, of or pertaining to the ovary.

ovarian artery, a slender branch of the abdominal aorta, arising caudal to the renal arteries, and supplying an ovary. Compare **testicular artery.**

ovarian cancer, a malignant neoplastic disease of the ovary, occurring most frequently in women between the ages of 40 and 60 and occasionally in young adolescents. Risk factors in adults are a history of infertility, nulliparity or low parity, repeated spontaneous abortion, delayed childbearing, a family history of ovarian cancer, and Peutz-Jeghers syndrome. Ovarian tumors are usually advanced before any symptoms appear. Regular yearly pelvic examinations after the age of 40 contribute significantly to early diagnosis and the possibility of curative treatment. Characteristic of the disease as it advances are abdominal swelling and discomfort, abnormal vaginal bleeding, weight loss, dysuria or abnormal frequency of urination, constipation, and a palpable ovarian mass, especially in postmenopausal women. Ultrasonography and computerized axial tomography are useful in the diagnosis, but laparotomy and surgical exploration are required to determine the extent and character of the tumor. In many cases the cancer spreads over the surface of the peritoneum, and, early in the course of the lesion, tumor cells invade the lymphatic vessels under the diaphragm and the para-aortic nodes. Many kinds of tumors may arise in the ovary. About 85 per cent are epithelial in origin, with papillary serous tumors the most common, followed by mucinous, endometroid, and undifferentiated solid cancers. The surgery recommended for ovarian cancer is total abdominal hysterectomy and bilateral salpingo-oophorectomy with omentectomy. Postoperative radiotherapy is used to control residual tumor, and antineoplastic agents are used to treat metastatic lesions. Among the effective chemotherapeutic drugs are chlorambucil, cyclophosphamide, fluorouracil, hexamethylmelamine, melphalen, and thiotepa.

ovarian carcinoma, a malignant neoplasm of the ovaries rarely detected in the early stage and usually far advanced when diagnosed. It occurs frequently in the fifth decade of life. The most fatal, common gynecologic tumor, ovarian cancer appears to be increasing in the United States. Risk factors of the disease are infertility, nulliparity, endometriosis, Group A blood type, previous irradiation of pelvic organs, and exposure to chemical carcinogens, as asbestos and talc. After an insidious onset and asymptomatic period, the tumor may become evident as a palpable abdominal or pelvic mass accompanied by irregular or excessive menses or postmenopausal bleeding. In advanced cases the patient may have ascites, edema of the legs, and pain in the abdomen and the backs of the legs. A pap smear may show malignant cells if the tumor is advanced; an ultrasonic examination can demonstrate an ovarian mass but does not distinguish between a benign and malignant lesion. A CAT scan may be useful in detecting ovarian cancer, but a definitive diagnosis requires surgical exploration. Most ovarian carcinomas are papillary or serous, followed in frequency by mucinous, endometroid, and undifferentiated cancers. Approximately half the tumors diagnosed are inoperable. Treatment of resectable lesions consists of total abdominal hysterectomy, removal of both ovaries and tubes, omentectomy, and biopsies of any suspicious sites, especially in the liver and diaphragm. Postoperative supervoltage irradiation of the pelvis and para-aortic lymph nodes is recommended; the instillation of radioisotopes is used in some cases. Chemotherapeutic agents that may be administered postoperatively include chlorambucil, cyclophosphamide, melphalen, and thiotepa.

ovarian cyst, a globular sac filled with fluid or semisolid material that develops in or on the ovary. It may be transient and physiologic or pathologic. Kinds of ovarian cysts include **chocolate cyst, corpus luteum cyst, dermoid cyst.**

ovarian varicocele, a varicose swelling of the veins of the uterine broad ligament. Also called **pelvic varicocele.**

ovarian vein, one of a pair of veins that emerge from convoluted plexuses in the broad ligament near the ovaries and the uterine tubes. The veins from each plexus ascend and unite to form single veins. The right ovarian vein opens into the inferior vena cava, the left ovarian vein into the renal vein. In some individuals the ovarian veins contain valves and greatly enlarge during pregnancy. Compare **testicular vein.**

ovariectomy (ouver′iek′təmi). See **oophorectomy.**

ovario-, ovari-, a combining form meaning 'of or pertaining to the ovary': *ovariocentesis, ovariosteresis, ovariotubal.* Also **oario-, ootheco-.**

ovary, one of the pair of female gonads found on each side of the lower abdomen, beside the uterus, in a fold of the broad ligament. At ovulation, an egg is extruded from a follicle on the surface of the ovary under the stimulation of the gonadotrophic hormones, follicle stimulating hormone (FSH), and luteinizing hormone (LH). The mature ovarian follicle secretes the hormones estrogen and progesterone that regulate the menstrual cycle by a negative feedback system in which an increase in estrogen decreases the secretion of FSH by the pituitary gland and an increase in progesterone decreases the secretion of LH.

Each ovary is normally firm and smooth and resembles an almond in size and shape. The ovaries are homologous to the testes.

Ovcon, a trade name for an oral contraceptive containing an estrogen (ethinyl estradiol) and a progestin (norethindrone acetate).

overcompensation, an exaggerated attempt to overcome a real or imagined physical or psychological deficit. The attempt may be conscious or unconscious. See also **compensation.**

overload, 1. a burden greater than the capacity of the system designed to move or process it. 2. (in physiology) any factor or influence that stresses the body beyond its natural limits and impairs its health.

overoxygenation, an abnormal condition in which the oxygen concentration in the blood and other tissues of the body is greater than normal, and the carbon dioxide concentration is less than normal. The condition is characterized by a fall in blood pressure, decreased vital capacity, fatigue, errors in judgment, paresthesia of the hands and feet, anorexia, nausea and vomiting, and hyperemia.

over the counter, (of a drug) available to the consumer without a prescription.

overweight, more than normal in body weight after adjustment for height, body build, and age.

ovi-. See ovo-.

oviduct (ou'vɪdəkt'). See **Fallopian tube.**

oviferous (ouvif'ərəs), bearing or capable of producing ova (egg cells).

oviparous (ouvip'ərəs), giving birth to young by laying eggs. Compare **ovoviviparous, viviparous.**

oviposition (ou'vɪpəziŝh'ən), the act of laying or depositing eggs by the female member of oviparous animals.

ovipositor (ou'vɪpos'ɪtər), a specialized organ, found primarily in insects, for depositing eggs on plants or in the soil.

ovo-, ovi-, a combining form meaning 'of or pertaining to an egg, or to ova': ovoglobulin, ovoplasm, ovotestis.

ovocenter (ou'vəsen'tər), the centrosome of a fertilized ovum. Also called **oocenter.**

ovoflavin (ou'vəflei'vɪn), a riboflavin derived from the yolk of eggs.

ovogenesis (ou'vəjen'ɪsɪs). See **oogenesis.** – **ovogenetic, ovogenic,** adj.

ovoglobulin (ou'vəglob'yulɪn), a globulin derived from the white of eggs.

ovogonium (ou'vəgou'niəm). See **oogonium.**

ovo-lacto-vegetarian (ou'voulæk'touvej'ɪter'iən). See **lacto-ovo-vegetarian.**

ovomucin (ou'vəmyu'sɪn), a glycoprotein derived from the white of eggs.

ovomucoid (ou'vəmyu'koid), of or pertaining to a glycoprotein, similar to mucin, derived from the white of eggs.

ovoplasm (ou'vəplæz'əm). See **ooplasm.**

ovotestis (ou'vətes'tɪs), a gonad that contains both ovarian and testicular tissue; a hermaphroditic gonad. – **ovotesticular,** adj.

ovovitellin (ou'vouvitel'ɪn). See **vitellin.**

ovoviviparous (ou'vouvaivɪp'ərəs), bearing young in eggs that are hatched within the body, as some reptiles and fishes. Compare **oviparous, viviparous.**

Ovral, a trade name for an oral contraceptive containing a progestin (norgestrel) and an estrogen (ethinyl estradiol).

Ovrette, a trade name for an oral contraceptive containing a progestin (norgestrel).

ovulation, expulsion of an ovum from the ovary upon spontaneous rupture of a mature follicle as a result of cyclic ovarian and pituitary endocrine function. It usually occurs on the fourteenth day following the first day of the last menstrual period and often causes brief, sharp lower abdominal pain on the side of the ovulating ovary. – **ovulate,** v.

ovulation method of family planning, a natural method of family planning that uses observation of changes in the character and quantity of cervical mucus as a means of determining the time of ovulation during the menstrual cycle. As pregnancy occurs with fertilization of an ovum extruded from the ovary at ovulation, the method is used to increase or decrease the woman's chance of becoming pregnant by causing or avoiding insemination by spontaneous or artificial means during the fertile period associated with ovulation. The cyclic changes in gonadotropic hormones, especially estrogen, cause changes in the quantity and character of cervical mucus. In the first days after menstruation, scant thick mucus is secreted by the cervix. These "dry days" are "safe days," with ovulation several days away. The quantity of mucus then increases; it is pearly-white and sticky, becoming clearer and less sticky as ovulation approaches; these "wet days" are "unsafe days." During and just after ovulation the mucus is clear, slippery, and elastic; it resembles the uncooked white of an egg. The day on which this sign is most apparent is the "peak day," probably the day preceding ovulation. The four days following the "peak day" are "unsafe": fertilization might occur. By the end of the four days, the mucus becomes pearly-white and sticky again and progressively decreases in quantity until menstruation supervenes to begin a new cycle. Essential to the effectiveness of this method are thorough instruction by a family planning counselor, and strong self-motivation in the couple. During the first cycle, abstinence may be necessary to allow observation of the mucus without the confusing addition of semen or contraceptive foam, cream, or jelly, if being used. Daily close monitoring of the mucus is necessary even after several cycles because the length of the "safe" and "unsafe" periods and the time of ovulation vary from cycle to cycle, as they do from woman to woman. Postpartally, and during lactation, the method is not effective until the menses have become regular. Effectiveness of the method in identifying the most fertile days of the cycle is augmented by using the basal body temperature method. This combined method is called the symptothermal method of planning. Proponents of the ovulation method claim the benefits of low cost, naturalness, and effectiveness. Detractors emphasize a limited public health application of the method, stating that it requires extensive teaching and self-motivation and that its effectiveness is limited by the ability of the user to observe correctly and diligently the changes in the cervical mucus. Abstinence may be necessary for up to ten days by a woman whose menstrual cycles are long or are of irregular length. Also called **cervical mucus method of family planning.**

Ovulen, a trade name for an oral contraceptive containing an estrogen (mestranol) and a progestin (ethynodiol diacetate).

ovum, *pl.* **ova. 1.** an egg. **2.** a female germ cell extruded from the ovary at ovulation.

oxacillin sodium, a penicillinase resistant penicillin antibiotic.

■ INDICATIONS: It is prescribed in the treatment of severe infections caused by penicillinase-producing staphylococci.

■ CONTRAINDICATIONS: Known hypersensitivity to this drug or to any other penicillin prohibits its use.

■ ADVERSE EFFECTS: Among the most serious effects are anaphylaxis and other less severe allergic reactions, gastrointestinal disturbances, and pruritus ani and vulvae.

Oxaine, a trade name for a topical anesthetic (oxethazaine).

Oxalid, a trade name for an anti-inflammatory and antirheumatic (oxyphenbutazone).

oxaluric acid (ok′səlur′ik), a compound derived from uric acid or from parabonic acid, which occurs in normal urine.

oxamniquine (oksæm′nəkwin), an antischistosomal.

■ INDICATION: It is prescribed in the treatment of infection caused by *Schistosoma mansoni.*

■ CONTRAINDICATIONS: Renal failure, congestive heart failure, or known hypersensitivity to this drug prohibits its use.

■ ADVERSE EFFECTS: Among the more serious adverse reactions are dizziness, drowsiness, and convulsions, particularly in patients with a history of epilepsy.

oxandrolone, an androgen.

■ INDICATIONS: It is prescribed in the treatment of testosterone deficiency, osteoporosis, female breast cancer, and for the stimulation of growth, weight gain, and red blood cell production.

■ CONTRAINDICATIONS: Cancer of the male breast or prostate, liver disease, pregnancy or suspected pregnancy, or known hypersensitivity to this drug prohibits its use.

■ ADVERSE EFFECTS: Among the more serious adverse reactions are hirsutism, acne, liver toxicity, electrolyte imbalances, and various endocrine effects in some patients.

oxazepam (oksei′zəpæm), a minor tranquilizer.

■ INDICATIONS: It is prescribed to relieve anxiety and nervous tension.

■ CONTRAINDICATIONS: Acute narrow angle glaucoma, psychotic disorders, or known hypersensitivity to this drug prohibits its use.

■ ADVERSE EFFECTS: Among the more serious adverse reactions are withdrawal symptoms resulting from discontinuation of treatment. Dizziness and fatigue commonly occur.

-oxemia, a combining form meaning a '(specified) state of oxygen in the blood': *anoxemia, hyperoxemia, hypoxemia.*

-oxia, a combining form meaning '(condition of) oxygenation': *anoxia, asthenoxia, hypoxia.*

oxidation, (in chemistry) **1.** any process in which the oxygen content of a compound is increased. **2.** any reaction in which the positive valence of a compound or a radical is increased owing to a loss of electrons. **– oxidize,** *v.*

oxidize, (of an element or compound) to combine or cause to combine with oxygen, to remove hydrogen, or to increase the valence of an element through the loss of electrons. **– oxidation,** *n.,* **oxidizing,** *adj.*

oxidizing agent, a compound that readily gives up oxygen and attracts hydrogen from another compound. In chemical reactions an oxidizing agent acts as an acceptor of electrons, thereby increasing the valence of an element.

oxolinic acid, an antibacterial.

■ INDICATIONS: It is prescribed in the treatment of urinary tract infections caused by gram-negative pathogens.

■ CONTRAINDICATIONS: A history of convulsive disorders or known hypersensitivity to this drug prohibits its use. It is not given to infants or to women during pregnancy or lactation.

■ ADVERSE EFFECTS: Among the more serious adverse reactions are central nervous system stimulation, insomnia, and gastrointestinal distress.

Oxsoralen, a trade name for a pigmentation agent (methoxsalen).

oxtriphylline (oks′trəfil′in), a bronchodilator.

■ INDICATIONS: It is prescribed in the treatment of bronchial asthma, bronchitis, and emphysema.

■ CONTRAINDICATIONS: Known hypersensitivity to this drug or other xanthine derivatives prohibits its use. It is used with caution in patients with ulcer or with coronary disease for whom cardiac stimulation might be harmful.

■ ADVERSE EFFECTS: Among the more common adverse

reactions are gastrointestinal distress, palpitations, nervousness, and insomnia.

oxy-, **1.** a combining form meaning 'sharp, quick, or sour': *oxyblepsia, oxycephalia, oxyecoia.* **2.** a combining form indicating the presence of oxygen in a compound: *oxyacanthine, oxycamphor, oxyquinoline.*

Oxy-5, a trade name for a keratolytic (benzoyl peroxide).

oxybenzene (ok'siben'zin). See **carbolic acid.**

oxybutynin chloride, an anticholinergic.

■ INDICATION: It is prescribed in the treatment of neurogenic bladder.

■ CONTRAINDICATIONS: Glaucoma, obstruction of the gastrointestinal or urinary tract, ulcerative colitis, paralytic ileus, toxic megacolon, or known hypersensitivity to this drug or to other anticholinergics prohibits its use.

■ ADVERSE EFFECTS: Among the more serious adverse effects are decreased sweating, urinary retention, blurred vision, tachycardia, and severe allergic reactions.

Oxycel, a trade name for a local hemostatic (oxidized cellulose).

oxycephaly (ok'sisef'əli), **oxycephalia,** a congenital malformation of the skull in which premature closure of the coronal and sagittal sutures results in accelerated upward growth of the head, giving it a long, narrow appearance with the top pointed or conical in shape. The cephalic index is over 75. Also called **acrocephaly, hyssicephaly, steeple head, steeple skull, tower head, tower skull, turricephaly.** See also **craniostenosis.** — **oxycephalus,** *n.,* **oxycephalous,** *adj.*

oxycodone hydrochloride, a narcotic analgesic.

■ INDICATION: It is used to treat moderate to severe pain.

■ CONTRAINDICATIONS: It is used with caution in many conditions, including head injuries, asthma, impaired renal or hepatic function, or unstable cardiovascular status. Known hypersensitivity to this drug prohibits its use.

■ ADVERSE EFFECTS: Among the most serious adverse reactions are drowsiness, dizziness, nausea, constipation, respiratory and circulatory depression, and drug addiction.

oxygen (O), a tasteless, odorless, colorless gas essential for human respiration. In anesthesia, oxygen functions as a carrier gas for the delivery of anesthetic agents to the tissues of the body. It is given by mask at a rate of flow and concentration appropriate to the physical status of the patient, the surgical procedure, and the anesthetic agent being administered. In respiratory therapy, oxygen is administered to increase the amount of oxygen and thus to decrease the amount of other gases circulating in the blood.

■ CONSIDERATIONS: Overdose of oxygen can cause irreversible toxicity in people with pulmonary abnormalities, especially when complicated by chronic carbon dioxide retention. Prolonged administration of high concentrations of oxygen may cause irreversible damage to infants' eyes. Oxygen itself is not flammable or explosive, but because an oxygen-rich environment is favorable to fire and explosion, flame or electric spark must be avoided when oxygen is being administered.

oxygenation, the process of combining or treating with oxygen. — **oxygenate,** *v.*

oxygen mask, a device used to administer oxygen. It is shaped to fit snugly over the mouth and nose and may be secured in place with a strap or held with the hand. The mask has inspiratory and expiratory valves allowing oxygen to be inhaled or pumped into the respiratory tract and carbon dioxide to be exhaled into the environment. Oxygen flows at a prescribed rate through a catheter to the mask, often through a soft rubber bag that can be pumped by hand.

oxygen tension, the force with which oxygen molecules that are physically dissolved in blood are constantly trying to escape, expressed as partial pressure (PO_2). The tension at any instant is related to the amount of oxygen physically dissolved in plasma; the larger amount carried in chemical combination with hemoglobin serves as a reservoir that releases oxygen molecules to physical solution when the tension decreases and that stores additional molecules of the gas when the tension increases.

oxygen therapy, any procedure in which oxygen is administered to a person in order to relieve hypoxia.

■ METHOD: Of the many methods for providing oxygen therapy, the one selected depends upon the condition of the patient and the cause of hypoxia. Low or moderate amounts of oxygen may be supplied to postoperative patients by a nasal catheter or cannula. Low concentrations, precisely measured, may be delivered to patients with chronic obstructive lung disease by a Venturi mask. If hypoxia is the result of impaired cardiac function, a high concentration of oxygen may be delivered by a nonrebreathing or partial rebreathing mask. Humidity and drugs in aerosol form may be given with oxygen using a variety of devices, as a Croupette, aerosol face mask, or T-piece.

■ RATIONALE: Oxygen therapy may be used in the treatment of any condition that results in hypoxia. Although there are several kinds of hypoxia, all result in hypoxemia. The administration of oxygen may relieve hypotension, cardiac arrythmias, tachypnea, headache, disorientation, nausea, and agitation characteristic of hypoxia, as well as restore the ability of the cells of the body to carry on normal metabolic function.

■ NURSING CONSIDERATIONS: Thorough and careful observation of the patient's need for oxygen and his response to therapy are important. The concentration of oxygen received by the patient must not be assumed by the rate and concentration at which it is delivered: a person whose respirations are rapid and shallow receives more oxygen than does a person breathing deeply and slowly. Many clinical situations require frequent laboratory evaluations of the levels of arterial blood gases. The adverse effects of oxygen therapy include respiratory depression, absorption atelectasis, alveolar collapse, alveolar edema, pulmonary congestion, intra-alveolar hemorrhage, hyaline membrane formation, pain, retrolental fibroplasia, and disturbance of the central nervous system with seizures and, possibly, death. Thorough knowledge of the equipment used and of the condition being treated enables the nurse to care safely and effectively for the patient who requires oxygen.

oxygen transport, the process by which oxygen is absorbed in the lungs by the hemoglobin in circulating deoxygenated red cells and carried to the peripheral tissues. This process is made possible by a special characteristic of hemoglobin, i.e., the ability to combine with large quantities of oxygen present at a high concentration, as in the lungs, and to release this oxygen when the concentration is low, as in the peripheral tissues. See also **hemoglobin.**

oxyhemoglobin (ok′sihi′məglou′bɪn, ok′sihem′əglou′bɪn), the product of the combining of hemoglobin with oxygen. It is a loosely bound complex that dissociates easily when there is a low concentration of oxygen.

Oxylone, a trade name for a glucocorticoid (fluorometholone).

oxymetazoline hydrochloride (ok′simətæz′əlin), a decongestant.

■ INDICATION: It is prescribed in the treatment of nasal congestion.

■ CONTRAINDICATIONS: Hyperthyroidism, diabetes, use of a monoamine oxidase inhibitor within 14 days, or known hypersensitivity to this drug prohibits its use.

■ ADVERSE EFFECTS: Among the more serious adverse reactions are rebound congestion, central nervous system stimulation, and, in children, a severe shocklike syndrome with coma, hypotension, and bradycardia.

oxymetholone, an androgen.

■ INDICATIONS: It is prescribed in the treatment of testosterone deficiency, osteoporosis, and female breast cancer and for the stimulation of growth, weight gain, and red blood cell production.

■ CONTRAINDICATIONS: Cancer of the male breast or prostate, liver disease, pregnancy or suspected pregnancy, or known hypersensitivity to this drug prohibits its use.

■ ADVERSE EFFECTS: Among the more serious adverse reactions are hirsutism, acne, liver toxicity, electrolyte imbalances, and, depending on the age of the patient, various endocrine effects.

oxymorphone hydrochloride, a narcotic analgesic.

■ INDICATIONS: It is prescribed to reduce moderate to severe pain, as a preoperative medication, and to support anesthesia.

■ CONTRAINDICATION: Drug dependence or known hypersensitivity to this drug prohibits its use.

■ ADVERSE EFFECTS: Among the more serious adverse reactions are drug dependence and respiratory or circulatory depression.

oxyopia (ok′siou′piə), **oxyopy** (ok′siou′pi), unusual acuteness of vision. A person with normal (20/20) vision when standing 20 feet from the standard Snellen eye chart can read the seventh line of letters, each of which is an eighth of an inch high, while an individual with oxyopia can read smaller letters at that distance.

oxyphenbutazone, a nonsteroidal anti-inflammatory agent and antirheumatic.

■ INDICATIONS: It is prescribed in the treatment of arthritis, bursitis, and other inflammatory conditions.

■ CONTRAINDICATIONS: Impaired hepatic or renal function, a history of gastric ulcer, blood dyscrasias, stomatitis, hypertension and edema, or known hypersensitivity to this drug or to other phenylbutazone medication prohibits its use.

■ ADVERSE EFFECTS: Among the more serious adverse reactions are fluid retention and blood dyscrasias. Gastrointestinal irritation and nausea commonly occur. This drug interacts with many other drugs.

oxyphencyclimine hydrochloride, an anticholinergic.

■ INDICATION: It is prescribed in the treatment of peptic ulcer.

■ CONTRAINDICATIONS: Glaucoma, obstruction of the gastrointestinal or urinary tract, ulcerative colitis, paralytic ileus, toxic megacolon, or known hypersensitivity to this drug or to other anticholinergics prohibits its use.

■ ADVERSE EFFECTS: Among the more serious adverse effects are decreased sweating, urinary retention, circulatory or respiratory depression, and severe hypersensitivity reactions.

oxyphenonium bromide, an anticholinergic.

■ INDICATION: It is prescribed in the treatment of peptic ulcer.

■ CONTRAINDICATIONS: Glaucoma, obstruction of the gastrointestinal or urinary tract, ulcerative colitis, paralytic ileus, toxic megacolon, or known hypersensitivity to this drug or to other anticholinergics prohibits its use.

■ ADVERSE EFFECTS: Among the more serious adverse effects are decreased sweating, urinary retention, tachycardia, blurred vision, and severe hypersensitivity reactions.

oxytetracycline, a tetracycline antibiotic.

■ INDICATIONS: It is prescribed in the treatment of bacterial and rickettsial infections.

■ CONTRAINDICATIONS: Pregnancy, early childhood, or known hypersensitivity to this or to other tetracyclines prohibits its use. The drug is used with caution in patients who have renal or liver dysfunction.

■ ADVERSE EFFECTS: Among the more serious adverse

reactions are gastrointestinal disturbances, phototoxicity, potentially serious suprainfections, and various hypersensitivity reactions. Discoloration of teeth may occur in children exposed to the drug in utero or before eight years of age.

oxytetracycline calcium, a tetracycline antibiotic.

oxytocic (ok'sɪtou'sɪk), **1.** of or pertaining to a substance that is similar to the hormone oxytocin. **2.** any one of numerous drugs that stimulate the smooth muscle of the uterus to contract. The administration of an oxytocic can initiate and enhance rhythmic uterine contraction at any time, but relatively high doses are required for such responses in early pregnancy. These drugs are often used to initiate labor at term. Oxytocic agents commonly used include oxytocin, certain prostaglandins, and the ergot alkaloids. These drugs are used to induce or augment labor, control postpartum hemorrhage, correct postpartum uterine atony, produce uterine contractions after Caesarean section or other uterine surgery, and induce therapeutic abortion. Considerable controversy surrounds the use of oxytocics to induce labor. The United States Food and Drug Administration has ruled that oxytocin is not indicated for elective termination of pregnancy and should be used only in cases where continued pregnancy is seen as a greater risk to the mother or to the fetus than the risk of drug-induced labor. These drugs are used with extreme caution in parturients with severe hypotension and hypertension, partial placenta previa, cephalopelvic disproportion, or grand multiparity. The risk of using these agents is much higher in mothers who have undergone recent uterine surgery or who have suffered recent sepsis or trauma. The most serious adverse reaction is sustained tetanic contraction of the uterus resulting in fetal hypoxia or in rupture of the uterus.

oxytocin (ok'sɪtou'sɪn), an oxytocic.

■ INDICATIONS: It is prescribed to stimulate contractions in inducing or augmenting labor, and to contract the uterus to control postpartum bleeding.

■ CONTRAINDICATIONS: Cephalopelvic disproportion, unfavorable fetal position, or known hypersensitivity to this drug prohibits its use.

■ ADVERSE EFFECTS: Among the more serious adverse reactions are tetanic contraction, jaundice, uterine rupture, and fetal anoxia.

oxytocin challenge test, a stress test for the assessment of intrauterine function of the fetus and the placenta. It is performed to evaluate the ability of the fetus to tolerate continuation of pregnancy or the anticipated stress of labor and delivery. A dilute intravenous infusion of oxytocin is begun, monitored by a meter or regulated by an infusion pump. The uterine activity is monitored with a tocodynamometer, and the fetal heart rate is moni-

tored with an ultrasonic sensor as the uterus is stimulated to contract by the oxytocin. The amount of solution infused is increased as necessary to cause the uterus to contract for 30 to 40 seconds three times every ten minutes. The fetal heart rate is observed for variability and for the timing of any marked variation from the normal in relation to uterine contractions. Decelerations of the fetal heart rate in certain repeating patterns may indicate fetal distress. One quarter of the infants diagnosed by this method as being in distress are normal; therefore, other tests of fetal well-being are recommended before performing an emergency Caesarean section or induction of labor.

oxyuriasis (ok'siyuraɪ'əsɪs). See **enterobiasis.**

Oxyuris vermicularis. See *Enterobius vermicularis.*

ozena (ouzi'nə), a condition of the nose characterized by atrophy of the nasal chonchae and mucous membranes. Symptoms include crusting of nasal secretions, discharge, and, especially, a very offensive odor. Ozena may follow chronic inflammation of the nasal mucosa.

ozone, a form of oxygen characterized by molecules having three atoms. Ozone is formed when oxygen is electrically charged, as might occur in a lightning storm. Ozone is used as a bleaching, cleaning, and oxidizing agent and has a faint, chlorinelike odor.

ozone shield, the layer of ozone that hangs in the atmosphere from 20 to 40 miles above the surface of the earth and protects the earth from excessive ultraviolet radiation. Some experts warn that the manufacture of various chemicals, as chlorofluorocarbons used as propellants in aerosol sprays and the effects of high-flying jet aircraft are destroying this protective layer and allowing excessive amounts of ultraviolet radiation to penetrate the earth's atmosphere, thus subjecting humans to increased dangers of skin cancer and other health problems. Some chemistry experts and federal health officials warn that an additional threat comes from nitrous oxide in nitrogenous fertilizers rising into the atmosphere and reacting unfavorably with the ozone shield. Other experts say the depletion of the ozone layer by chlorofluorocarbons may be offset by the release of carbon dioxide into the atmosphere from the combustion of fuels. One study indicates that ozone concentration has actually increased 6 per cent since monitoring was begun more than 50 years ago. The ozone shield is implicated in certain health problems that affect some air travelers. See also **ozone sickness.**

ozone sickness, an abnormal condition caused by the inhalation of ozone that may seep into jet aircraft at altitudes over 40,000 feet. It is characterized by headaches, chest pains, itchy eyes, and sleepiness. Exactly why and how ozone causes this condition is not known. It is more prevalent early in the year and occurs more often over the Pacific Ocean.

P

P, 1. symbol for **gas partial pressure**. See **partial pressure**.
2. symbol for **phosphorus**.

P₁, (in genetics) symbol for **parental generation**.

pa, abbreviation for **physician's assistant**.

PABA, abbreviation for **para-aminobenzoic acid**.

Pabalate-SF, a trade name for a central nervous system fixed-combination drug containing analgesics (potassium salicylate and potassium aminobenzoate), used to alleviate the pain of arthritis in people who require low-sodium regimens.

Pabanol, a trade name for an ultraviolet screen (para-aminobenzoic acid).

pabulum (pæb'yələm), any substance that is food or nutrient.

pacemaker, an electrical apparatus used for maintaining a normal sinus rhythm of myocardial contraction by electrically stimulating the heart muscle. A pacemaker may be permanent, emitting the stimulus at a constant and fixed rate, or it may fire only on demand, when the heart does not spontaneously contract at a minimum rate. Also called **cardiac pacemaker**.

pachometer (pækom'ətər). See **pachymeter**.

pachy-, a combining form meaning 'thick': *pachyaria, pachycephaly, pachymucosa*.

pachycephaly (pæk'isef'əli), an abnormal thickness of the skull, as in acromegaly. Also called **pachycephalia**. —**pachycephalic, pachycephalous,** *adj.*

pachydactyly (pæk'idæk'təli), an abnormal thickening of the fingers or the toes. —**pachydactylic, pachydactylous,** *adj.*

pachymeter (pækim'ətər), an instrument used to measure thickness, especially of thin structures, as a membrane or a tissue. Also called **pachometer**.

pachynema (pæk'mi'mə), the postsynaptic tetradic chromosome formation that occurs in the pachytene stage of the first meiotic prophase of gametogenesis.

pachyonychia congenita (pæk'iounik'iə), a congenital deformity characterized by abnormal thickening and raising of the nails on the fingers and the toes, and hyperkeratosis of the palms of the hands and the soles of the feet. The papillae of the tongue also atrophy, causing a whitish coating over the lingual surface.

pachytene (pæk'itin), the third stage in the first meiotic prophase of gametogenesis in which the paired homologous chromosomes form tetrads. The bivalent pairs become short and thick and intertwine so that four chromatids are visible. See also **diakinesis, diplotene, leptotene, zygotene**.

pacifier, 1. an agent that soothes or comforts. 2. a nipple-shaped object used by infants and children for sucking. Such devices can be dangerous if they are too small or poorly constructed, as the entire object or part of it can be aspirated or lodged in the pharynx or trachea and obstruct the passage of air. The safest pacifiers are constructed in one piece, are large enough so that only the nipple fits into the mouth, and have a handle that can be easily grasped.

Pacinian corpuscle (pəsin'iən). See **Pacini's corpuscles**.

Pacini's corpuscles, a number of special sensory end organs resembling tiny white bulbs, each attached to the end of a single nerve fiber in the subcutaneous, submucous, and subserous connective tissue of many parts of the body, especially the palm of the hand, sole of the foot, genital organs, joints, and in the pancreas. They average about 3 mm in diameter, contain numerous concentric layers around a central core, and in cross section resemble an onion. Also called **Pacinian corpuscles**. Compare **Golgi-Mazzoni corpuscles, Krause's corpuscles**.

pack, 1. a treatment in which the entire body or a portion of it is wrapped in wet or dry towels or in ice for various therapeutic purposes, as with cold packs for the reduction of high temperatures and swellings or for inducing hypothermia during certain surgical procedures, especially heart surgery and organ transplants. 2. a tampon. 3. (in dentistry) the act of applying a dressing or cement to a surgical wound. 4. (in dentistry) a surgical dressing to cover a wound or to fill the cavity left from a tooth extraction, especially an extraction of a wisdom tooth.

package insert, a leaflet that, by order of the FDA, must be placed inside the package of every prescription drug. In it, the manufacturer is required to describe the drug, to state its generic name, and to give the applicable indications, contraindications, warnings, precautions, adverse effects, form, dosage, and administration.

packed cells, a preparation of blood cells separated from liquid plasma, often administered in severe anemia to restore adequate levels of hemoglobin and red cells without overloading the vascular system with excess fluids. See also **bank blood, pooled plasma**.

pad, **1.** a mass of soft material used to cushion shock, prevent wear, or absorb moisture, as the abdominal pads used to absorb discharges from abdominal wounds or to separate viscera and improve accessibility during abdominal surgery. **2.** (in anatomy) a mass of fat that cushions various structures, as the infrapatellar pad lying below the patella between the patellar ligamant, the head of the tibia, and the femoral condyles.

paedogenesis. See **pedogenesis.**

Paget's disease (pæj'ıts), a common, nonmetabolic disease of bone of unknown cause, usually affecting middle-aged and elderly people, characterized by excessive bone destruction and unorganized bone repair.

■ OBSERVATIONS: Most cases are asymptomatic or mild; however, bone pain may be the first symptom. Bowed tibias (saber shins), kyphosis, and frequent fractures are owing to the soft, abnormal bone in this condition. Enlargement of the head, headaches, and warmth over involved areas owing to increased vascularity are additional features. The serum alkaline phosphatase is often markedly elevated and there is increased urinary calcium and hydroxyproline. The x-ray picture of areas of decreased bone density adjacent to sites of increased density is characteristic. Radioactive bone scans help locate regions of active disease. Complications include fractures, kidney stones if the patient is immobilized, heart failure, deafness or blindness owing to pressure from bony overgrowth, and osteosarcoma.

■ INTERVENTION: No treatment is necessary for mild cases. A high-protein, high-calcium diet, unless the patient is immobilized, is recommended. Parenteral synthetic salmon calcitonin may help the patient temporarily. Diphosphonates and mithramycin are also effective but require close monitoring for side effects.

■ NURSING CONSIDERATIONS: Immobilization of the patient is avoided, if possible, to prevent hypercalcemia and kidney stones. Observation for neurological signs and symptoms and prompt reporting of changes may help to avert irreversible nerve damage. Also called **osteitis deformans.**

Paget's disease of the nipple. See **nipple cancer.**

Pagitane Hydrochloride, a trade name for an anticholinergic (cycrimine hydrochloride).

pagophagia (pei'goufei'jiə), an abnormal condition characterized by a craving to eat enormous quantities of ice. It is associated with a lack of nutrient iron. — **pagophagic, pagophagous,** *adj.*

-pagus, a combining form meaning 'conjoined twins': *craniopagus, pyropagus, thoracopagus.*

pain, **1.** an unpleasant sensation caused by noxious stimulation of the sensory nerve endings. It is a cardinal symptom of inflammation and is valuable in the diagnosis of many disorders and conditions. Pain may be mild or severe, chronic, acute, lancinating, burning, dull, or sharp,

precisely or poorly localized, or referred. See also **referred pain.**

pain and suffering, (in law) an element in a claim for damages that allows recovery for the mental and physical pain, suffering, distress, and trauma that an individual has endured as a result of injury.

pain assessment, an evaluation of the factors that alleviate or exacerbate a patient's pain.

■ METHOD: The patient is asked to describe the cause of the pain, if known, its intensity, location, and duration, the events preceding it, and the pattern usually followed for handling pain. Severe pain causes pallor, cold perspiration, piloerection, dilated pupils, and increases in the pulse, respiratory rate, blood pressure, and muscle tension. When brief, intense pain subsides, the pulse may be slower and the blood pressure lower than before the pain began. If pain occurs frequently or is prolonged, the pulse rate and blood pressure may not increase markedly, and, if pain persists for many days, there may be an increased production of eosinophils and 17-ketosteroids and greater susceptibility to infections. The patient's statements regarding pain, the tone of voice, speed of speech, cries, groans, or other vocalizations, facial expressions, body movements, or tendency to withdraw are all noted. Pertinent background information in the assessment includes a record of the patient's chronic conditions, previous surgery, and any illnesses that caused pain, the patient's experiences with relatives and friends in pain, the role or position of the patient in the family structure, and the patient's use of alcohol and medications.

■ NURSING ORDERS: The nurse establishes a relationship with the patient and uses individual counseling or group situations to teach the person about pain and how to modify the anxiety associated with it. Analgesics ordered for the patient are administered by the nurse before the pain becomes intense, for this increases their effectiveness. In addition to helping promote rest and relaxation, the nurse decreases noxious stimuli, provides other pleasant sensory input, and helps to distract the patient by using guided imagery, walking, watching television, or reading. If the patient believes that certain acceptable measures alleviate pain, the nurse uses them.

■ OUTCOME CRITERIA: Dramatic relief of intense or chronic pain is often difficult to accomplish, but the patient can be helped to learn to handle pain effectively and to function fairly normally.

pain evaluation, the clinical assessment of the pain experienced by an individual, used as an aid in the diagnosis and the treatment of disease and trauma. Responses to pain vary widely among individuals and depend on many different physical and psychological factors, as specific diseases and injuries and the health, pain threshold, fear and anxiety, and the cultural background of the individual involved, as well as the way different individuals express their pain experiences. Some important factors in pain evaluation are nonverbal expressions of pain, as moaning and groaning, the clenching of fists, and the rubbing of painful areas. Other evaluation factors are the intensity, the location, the duration, and the pattern of pain. Key aspects in evaluating pain intensity are the size of the pain area, the tenderness within the pain area, and the effects of movement and pressure on the pain. Duration of pain is considered in terms of hours, days, weeks, months, or years. Pain patterns are associated with various sensations as burning, pricking, aching, rhythmic throbbing, and the effects on the sympathetic and the parasympathetic nervous systems. Also considered in pain evaluation are the past experiences of the individual experiencing the pain, especially any distinction between sudden, new pain and chronic pain. Evaluation includes the meanings the individual may attach to pain, as a test of character, a penance, or as a sign of worsening illness. Such interpretations may affect the intensity of pain and mask its significance. Also called **pain assessment.** See also **pain intervention, pain mechanism.**

pain intervention, the relief of the painful sensations experienced in suffering the physiologic and the psychologic effects of disease and trauma. Effective pain intervention depends on proper evaluation of the type of pain the patient is experiencing, the physical and the psychological origins of the pain, and the behavioral patterns commonly associated with different kinds of pain. The most common method of pain intervention is the administration of narcotics, as morphine, but many authorities believe that the exclusive use of pain-killing drugs without consideration and implementation of psychological aids is too narrow an approach. There are few patients without a psychogenic overlay on the physical experience of pain, and comprehensive pain intervention employs methods and procedures that incorporate both psychological and physical measures. Methods of pain intervention for acute pain are different from those for chronic pain. Acute pain, occurring in the first 24 to 48 hours after surgery, is often difficult to relieve, and narcotics seldom relieve all such pain. Some authorities believe that the individual who has undergone repeated surgical operations has a decreased tolerance for pain. The type of pain intervention usually depends on the description of the pain by the individual experiencing it. Mild pain may best be relieved by comfort measures and the distraction afforded by television, visitors, reading, and other passive activities. Moderate pain may best be relieved by a combination of comfort measures and drugs. Cognitive dissonance, often employed to dampen moderate pain, encourages the patient to reflect on pleasant experiences and describe them to health-care personnel. Intervention to relieve severe pain often includes the administration of narcotics, purposeful interaction between the patient and attending hospital personnel, reduction of environmental stimuli, increased comfort measures, and "waking imagined analgesia," in which the patient is encouraged to concentrate on and become distracted by former pleasant experiences, as relaxing on a beach surrounded by cool ocean water. In the alleviation of all types of pain, dampening or decreasing stimuli that create pain is the chief goal. Pain often increases in a cold room because the muscles of the patient tend to contract; but the local application of cold, as with an ice pack, often alleviates pain by reducing swelling. Pain intervention seeks to reduce the effects of other factors that compound pain, as fatigue and anxiety. Coping with pain becomes increasingly difficult as the patient becomes more tired. Sensory restriction may increase pain, because it blocks otherwise effective distraction; overstimulation may cause fatigue and anxiety, thus increasing pain. Religious beliefs may be effective in helping the patient to decrease pain or increase tolerance if the pain is viewed by the patient as requiring self-discipline or as a catharsis for past transgressions. Religious beliefs, however, may increase pain if the patient interprets the pain as punishment and relates the severity of the pain with the gravity of transgressions or faults. Pain intervention by the use of drugs includes the administration of mild nonnarcotic analgesics and of much more potent and potentially addictive opioids, as morphine. Opioid analgesics administered for the relief of pain, cough, or diarrhea provide only symptomatic treatment and are used cautiously in the care of patients with acute or chronic diseases. Opioids may obscure the symptoms or the progress of the disease, and repeated daily administration of any opioid will eventually produce some tolerance to the therapeutic effects of the drug as well as some physical dependence on the dosage. The risk of developing psychological and physical dependency on any drug is always present, especially with opioids. In usual doses, opioids relieve suffering by altering the emotional component of the painful experience as well as by effecting analgesia. Some care givers are so concerned about the addictive dangers of opioids that they tend to prescribe initial doses that are too low or too infrequent to alleviate pain. A typical dose of 10 mg of morphine relieves postoperative pain in only two thirds of patients. Some patients may require considerably more than the average dose of an opioid to experience adequate pain relief. Some other patients with more rapid metabolisms may require such drugs at shorter intervals. Many drugs are appropriate substitutes for the potent opioids morphine and codeine. Some of the effective semisynthetic substitutes are hydrocodone, dihydrocodeine, and meperidine. Morphine and related opioids may produce unwanted side effects, as nausea, vomiting, dizziness, and constipation. Rarely, a patient treated with an opioid may become delirious. Some patients may also develop increased sensitivity to pain after the opioid has worn off. Allergic reactions to opioids, as urticaria and other skin rashes, rarely occur, although contact dermatitis in nurses and pharmaceutical workers has been reported. Patients with reduced blood volume are more susceptible to the hypotensive effect of morphine and related drugs. Opioids are used with extreme caution in obese patients and in those with head injuries, emphysema, or other problems associated with decreased respiratory function. In patients with prostatic hypertrophy, morphine may cause acute urinary retention, requiring repeated catheterization. Pain intervention in the treatment of terminal illnesses employs numerous drugs that relieve pain and produce euphoria and tranquility in patients who would otherwise suffer greatly. Analgesic mixtures of opioids and alcoholic solutions may be prescribed. Nerve block by the injection of alcohol, chordotomy, and other neurosurgical interventions may sometimes be employed. See also **pain evaluation.**

pain mechanism,   the psychosomatic network that communicates unpleasant sensations and the perceptions of noxious stimuli throughout the body, most commonly in association with physical disease and trauma involving tissue damage. Many studies of the pain mechanism have resulted in numerous theories as to how it functions, and such research continues; but variations in pain are so numerous and individual responses so diverse that a precise understanding of the subject still eludes health professionals. Some theories about the pain mechanism that have evolved are the gate control theories and the pattern theories. One of the biggest problems in pain research is that the actual cause of pain originating at the peripheral level is poorly understood. Some authorities believe that bradykinin and histamine, two chemical substances elaborated by the body, cause pain. Recently discovered painkillers produced naturally by the body are the enkephalins and the endorphins. Some studies indicate that the enkephalins are ten times as potent as morphine in reducing pain. It is known that once histamine and some other naturally occurring chemical substances are released in the body, pain sensations travel along fast-conducting nerve fibers and slow-conducting nerve fibers. These pain-transmitting neuropathways communicate the pain sensation to the dorsal root ganglia of the spinal cord and synapse with certain neurons in the posterior horns of the gray matter. The pain sensation is then transmitted to the reticular formation and the thalamus by neurons that form the anterolateral spinothalamic tract and is then conveyed to various areas of the brain, as the cortex and the hypothalamus, by synapses at the thalamus. The immediate reaction to pain is transmitted over the reflex arc by sensory fibers in the dorsal horn of the spinal cord and by synapsing motor neurons in the anterior horn. This anatomic pattern of sensory and motor neurons allows the individual to move quickly at the touch of some harmful stimulus, as extreme heat or cold. Nerve impulses alerting the individual to move away from such stimuli are simultaneously sent along efferent nerve fibers from the brain. The most recent pain theories incorporate the emotional component as an important factor in the pain mechanism. Past experiences, anxiety, and motivations greatly affect the pain sensations of everyone, and the fear of pain is second only to the fear of death for most people. It is known that fear and anxiety often intensify pain.

pain receptor,   any one of the many free nerve endings throughout the body that warn of potentially harmful changes in the environment, as excessive pressure or temperature. The free nerve endings constituting most of the pain receptors occur chiefly in the epidermis and in the epithelial covering of certain mucous membranes. They also appear in the stratified squamous epithelium of the cornea, in the root sheaths and in the papillae of the hairs, and around the bodies of sudoriferous glands. The terminal ends of pain receptors consist of unmyelinated nerve fibers which often anastomose into small knobs between the epithelial cells. Any kind of stimulus, if it is intense enough, can stimulate the pain receptors in the skin and the mucosa, but only radical changes in pressure and certain chemicals can stimulate the pain receptors in the viscera. Referred pain results only from stimulation of pain receptors located in deep structures, as the viscera, the joints, and the skeletal muscles but never from pain receptors in the skin.

pain spot,   any spot on the skin where a stimulus can produce pain.

paint,   **1.** to apply a medicated solution to the skin, usually over a wide area. **2.** a medicated solution that is applied in this way. Kinds of paint include **antiseptics, germicides, sporicides.** See also **Castellani's paint.**

pain threshold,   the point at which a stimulus, usually one associated with pressure or temperature, activates pain receptors and produces a sensation of pain. Individuals with low pain thresholds experience pain much sooner and faster than individuals with higher pain thresholds; the reaction to stimulation of pain receptors varies with individuals.

palatal,   **1.** of or pertaining to the palate. **2.** of or pertaining to the lingual surface of a maxillary tooth.

palate,   a structure that forms the roof of the mouth. It is divided into the hard palate and the soft palate.   —**palatal, palatine,** *adj.*

palatine,   of or pertaining to the palate.

palatine arch,   the vault-shaped muscular structure forming the soft palate between the mouth and the nasopharynx. An opening in the arch connects the mouth with the oropharynx; the uvula is suspended from the middle of the posterior border of the arch.

palatine bone, one of a pair of bones of the skull, forming the posterior part of the hard palate, part of the nasal cavity, and the floor of the orbit of the eye. It resembles a letter "L" and consists of horizontal and vertical parts and three processes.

palatine ridge, any one of the four to six transverse ridges on the anterior surface of the hard palate.

palatine suture, one of a number of thin wavy lines marking the joining of the palatine processes that form the hard palate. See also **median palatine suture, transverse palatine suture.**

palatine tonsil, one of a pair of almond-shaped masses of lymphoid tissue between the palatoglossal and the palatopharyngeal arches on each side of the fauces. They are covered with mucous membrane and contain numerous lymph follicles and various crypts.

palatitis, an inflammation of the hard palate.

palato-, a combining form meaning 'of or pertaining to the palate': *palatoglossal, palatography, palatomaxillary.*

palato-, a combining form meaning 'of the palate': *palatoproximal, palatoschisis, palatouvularis.*

palatomaxillary, of or pertaining to the palate and the maxilla.

palatonasal, of or pertaining to the palate and the nose.

paleo-, a combining form meaning 'old': *paleocerebellar, paleogenesis, paleostriatum.*

paleogenesis. See **palingenesis.**

paleogenetic, 1. a trait or structure of an organism or species that originated in a previous generation. 2. relating to the development of such a trait or structure.

pali-. See **palin-.**

palilalia, an abnormal condition characterized by the increasingly rapid repetition of the same word or phrase.

palin-, pali-, a combining form meaning 'again': *palindromia, palinesthesia, palingenesis.*

palindrome (pæl′ɪndrōm′), (in molecular genetics) a segment of DNA in which identical, or almost identical, sequences of bases run in opposite directions.

palingenesis, 1. the regeneration of a lost part. 2. the hereditary transmission of ancestral structural characteristics, especially abnormalities, in successive generations. Also called **paleogenesis.** Compare **cenogenesis.** — **palingenetic, palingenic,** *adj.*

palladium (Pd), a hard, silvery metallic element. Its atomic number is 46; and its atomic weight is 106.4. Highly resistant to tarnish and corrosion, palladium is used in high-grade surgical instruments and in dental inlays, bridgework, and orthodontic appliances.

palliate (pæl′ieit), to soothe or relieve. — **palliation,** *n.,* **palliative,** *adj.*

palliative treatment, therapy designed to relieve or reduce intensity of uncomfortable symptoms but not to produce a cure. Some kinds of palliative treatment are the use of narcotics to relieve pain in a patient with advanced cancer, the creation of a colostomy to bypass an inoperable obstructing lesion of the bowel, and the debridement of necrotic tissue in a patient with metastatic malignancy. Compare **definitive treatment, expectant treatment, supportive treatment.**

pallidum (pæl′ɪdəm). See **globus pallidus.**

pallium (pæl′iəm). See **cerebral cortex.**

pallor, an unnatural paleness or absence of color in the skin.

palm, the lower side of the hand, between the wrist and the bases of the fingers, when the hand is held horizontal with the thumb in medial position. — **palmar,** *adj.*

palmar aponeurosis, fascia surrounding the muscles of the palm. Also called **palmar fascia.**

palmar crease, a normal groove across the palm of the hand.

palmar fascia. See **palmar aponeurosis.**

palmaris longus, a long, slender, superficial, fusiform muscle of the forearm, lying on the medial side of the flexor carpi radialis. It arises from the medial epicondyle of the humerus by a tendon from the intermuscular septa between it and the adjacent muscles and from the antebrachial fascia. It inserts by a long, thin tendon into the flexor retinaculum and into the palmar aponeurosis. A tendinous slip of the muscle is often found extending to the thumb. The palmaris longus is innervated by a branch of the median nerve, which contains fibers from the sixth and the seventh cervical nerves, and it functions to flex the hand. Compare **flexor carpi radialis, flexor carpi ulnaris.**

palmar metacarpal artery, one of several arteries arising from the deep palmar arch, supplying the fingers.

palmar reflex, a reflex that curls the fingers when the palm of the hand is tickled.

palmature, an abnormal condition in which the fingers are webbed.

palm-chin reflex. See **palmomental reflex.**

palmityl alcohol. See **cetyl alcohol.**

palmomental reflex, an abnormal neurological sign, elicited by scratching the palm of the hand at the base of the thumb, characterized by contraction of the muscles of the chin and corner of the mouth on the same side of the body as the stimulus. It is occasionally seen in normal individuals but an exaggerated reflex may be seen in pyramidal tract disease, latent tetany, increased intracranial pressure, and central facial paresis. Also called **palm-chin reflex.**

palpable, perceivable by touch.

palpation, a technique used in physical examination in which the examiner feels the texture, size, consistency, and location of certain parts of the body with the hands. — **palpable,** *adj.,* **palpate,** *v.*

palpatory percussion, a technique in physical examination in which the vibrations produced by percussion are evaluated by using light pressure of the flat of the examiner's hand.

palpebra (pæl'pəbrə), *pl.* **palpebrae.** See **eyelid.**

palpebral commissure. See **canthus.**

palpebral fissure, the opening between the margins of the upper and lower lids.

palpebral gland (pæl'pəbrəl, pælpi'brəl, pælpeb'rəl). See **Meibomian gland.**

palpebra superior, *pl.* **palpebrae superiores.** the upper eyelid, larger and more movable than the lower eyelid and furnished with an elevator muscle.

palpebrate, 1. to wink or blink. 2. having eyelids.

palpeleral conjunctiva. See **conjunctiva.**

palpitate, to pulsate rapidly, as in the unusually fast beating of the heart under various conditions of stress and in patients with certain heart problems.

palpitation, a pounding or racing of the heart, associated with normal emotional responses or with certain heart disorders. Some people may complain of pounding hearts and display no evidence of heart disease, while others, with serious heart disorders, may not detect associated abnormal palpitations. Some patients complain of palpitations after receiving digitalis medication, because it increases the force of heart contractions. Many healthy individuals become concerned and describe as palpitations the normal sounds of their hearts against their pillows when they lie down to sleep.

palsy (pol'zi), an abnormal condition characterized by paralysis. Some kinds of palsy are **Bell's palsy, cerebral palsy.**

Paltauf's dwarf (pal'taufs). See **pituitary dwarf.**

Paltauf's nanism, dwarfism associated with excessive production or growth of lymphoid tissue.

Paludrine Hydrochloride, a trade name for an antimalarial (chloroguanide hydrochloride), used in the prophylaxis of malaria.

Pamine, a trade name for an anticholinergic (methscopolamine bromide).

PAMP, abbreviation for *pulmonary arterial mean pressure.*

pampiniform, having the shape of a tendril.

pampinform body. See **epoophoron.**

pan-, a combining form meaning 'all': *panacea, pancarditis, pandemic.*

panacea (pæn'əsi'ə), 1. a universal remedy. 2. an ancient name for a herb or a liquid potion with healing properties.

panacinar emphysema (pænæs'ənər), a form of emphysema that affects all lung areas by causing dilation and atrophy of the alveoli and by destroying the vascular bed of the lung. Also called **panlobular emphysema.**

Panafil, a trade name for a topical, fixed-combination drug containing an enzyme (papain).

panarthritis, an abnormal condition characterized by the inflammation of many joints of the body. — **panarthritic,** *adj.*

pancake kidney, a congenital anomaly in which the left and right kidneys are fused into a single mass in the pelvis. The fused kidney has two collecting systems and two ureters and frequently becomes obstructed because of its abnormal position.

pancarditis, an abnormal condition characterized by inflammation of the entire heart, including the endocardium, myocardium, and pericardium.

Pancoast's syndrome, 1. a combination of various signs associated with a tumor in the apex of the lung. The signs include neuritic pain in the arm, an x-ray shadow at the apex of the lung, atrophy of the muscles of the arm and the hand, and Horner's syndrome. The signs are caused by the damaging effects of the tumor on the brachial plexus. 2. an abnormal condition caused by osteolysis in the posterior part of one or more ribs, sometimes involving associated vertebrae.

Pancoast's tumor (pæn'kousts). See **pulmonary sulcus tumor.**

pancolectomy, the excision of the entire colon, requiring also an ileostomy.

pancreas, a fish-shaped, greyish-pink gland that stretches transversely across the posterior abdominal wall in the epigastric and hypochondriac regions of the body and secretes various substances, as digestive enzymes, insulin, and glucagon. It is divided into a head, a body, and a tail. The head of the gland, divided from the body by a small constriction, is tucked into the curve of the duodenum. The tapered left extremity of the organ forms the tail. In adults, the pancreas is about 13 cm long and weighs more in a man than it does in a woman. A compound racemose gland composed of exocrine and endocrine tissue, it contains a main duct that runs the length of the organ, draining smaller ducts and emptying into the duodenum at the major duodenal papilla, the same site that accommodates the exit of the common bile duct. About a million cellular islets or islands of Langerhans are embedded between the exocrine units of the pancreas. Beta cells of the islands secrete insulin, which helps control carbohydrate metabolism. Alpha cells of the islets secrete glucagon which counters the action of insulin. The acinar units of the pancreas secrete digestive enzymes.

pancreatectomy (pæŋ'kriətek'təmi), the surgical removal of all or part of the pancreas, performed to remove a cyst or tumor, treat pancreatitis, or repair trauma. The resection is done under general anesthesia; the gastrointestinal tract is reconstructed, usually with an anastomosis between the common bile duct and the upper jejunum. Drains are left in the wound. After surgery the patient is given a low-sugar, low-fat diet. If the entire pancreas is removed, a brittle type of diabetes develops, requiring precise management of both diet and insulin dosage. A frequent complication is the formation of a fistula in the pancreatic bile duct, allowing digestive enzymes to contact adjacent tissues.

-pancreatic, a combining form meaning the 'pancreas or a condition of the pancreas or adjacent organs': *hepaticopancreatic, lienopancreatic, splenopancreatic.*

pancreatic cancer, a malignant neoplastic disease of the pancreas, characterized by anorexia, flatulence, weakness, dramatic weight loss, epigastric or back pain, jaundice, pruritus, a palpable abdominal mass, the recent onset of diabetes, and clay-colored stools if the pancreatic ducts are obstructed. Insulin-secreting tumors of islet cells cause hypoglycemia, especially in the morning. Nonfunctioning islet cell lesions produce gastrin, causing symptoms of peptic ulcer, or, in some cases, acute diarrhea and hypokalemia, and achlorhydria, the result of the lesion's elaboration of secretin. Diagnostic measures include barium x-ray studies of the stomach and duodenum, transhepatic cholangiography, laboratory evaluation of liver function, coeliac arteriography, and computerized axial tomography. Exploratory laparotomy is often required for a definitive diagnosis. About 90 per cent of pancreatic tumors are adenocarcinomas; two thirds are in the head of the pancreas. Most tumors are not resectable at the time of diagnosis, but localized cancers in the pancreas may be treated by partial pancreatectomy with excision of the common bile duct, duodenum, and distal part of the stomach. Functioning islet cell lesions may be excised or treated with streptozotocin, an antibiotic toxic to beta cells of the pancreas. Total gastrectomy is recommended for nonfunctioning islet-cell tumors that are accompanied by peptic ulcer disease. Radiotherapy or chemotherapy with 5-fluorouracil or mitomycin-C may offer temporary palliation, but cancer of the pancreas has a poor prognosis: few people live for more than a year following diagnosis. Pancreatic cancer occurs three to four times more often in men than in women. Though uncommon, it is increasing in incidence in the industrialized areas of the world. People who smoke more than 10 to 20 cigarettes a day, who have diabetes mellitus, or who have been exposed to polychlorinated biphenyl compounds are at increased risk of developing pancreatic cancer.

pancreatic diverticulum, one of a pair of membranous pouches arising from the embryonic duodenum. These two diverticula later form the pancreas and its ducts.

pancreatic dornase, an enzyme from beef pancreas that has been used as a mucolytic for upper respiratory infections and cystic fibrosis.

pancreatic duct, the primary secretory channel of the pancreas. Also called **duct of Wirsung.**

pancreatic enzyme, any one of the enzymes secreted by the pancreas in the process of digestion. The most important are trypsin, chymotrypsin, steapsin, and amylopsin. See also **pancreatic juice.**

pancreatic hormone, any one of several chemical compounds secreted by the pancreas, associated with the regulation of cellular metabolism. Major hormones secreted by the pancreas are insulin, glucagon, and pancreatic polypeptide. Insulin and glucagon are secreted by different types of cells within the alpha and beta cells of the islands of Langerhans; pancreatic polypeptide is secreted by a group of glandular cells arranged in a halo around each island of Langerhans.

pancreatic insufficiency, a condition characterized by inadequate production and secretion of pancreatic hormones or enzymes, usually occurring secondary to a disease process destructive of pancreatic tissue. Nutritional malabsorption, anorexia, poorly localized upper abdominal or epigastric pain, malaise, and severe weight loss often occur. Alcohol-induced pancreatitis is the most common form of the condition. Supportive care, specific treatment of the cause of the condition, and replacement or augmentation of the absent or lacking substances are usually recommended as therapy for pancreatic insufficiency.

pancreatic juice, the fluid secretion of the pancreas, produced by the stimulation of food in the duodenum. Pancreatic juice contains water, protein, inorganic salts, and enzymes. The juice is essential in breaking down proteins into their amino acid components, in reducing dietary fats to glycerol and fatty acids, and in converting starch to simple sugars.

pancreaticolienal node (pæn'kriæt'ɪkoulāii'nəl), a node in one of three groups of lymph glands associated with branches of the abdominal and the pelvic viscera that are supplied by branches of the celiac artery. The pancreaticolienal nodes accompany the splenic artery along the posterior surface and the upper border of the pancreas. Their afferents, which originate from the stomach, the spleen, and the pancreas, join the celiac group of preaortic nodes. Also called **splenic gland.** Compare **gastric node, hepatic node.**

pancreatin (pæŋ'kriətin'), a concentrate of pancreatic enzymes from swine or beef cattle.

■ INDICATIONS: It is prescribed as an aid to digestion to replace endogenous pancreatic enzymes in cystic fibrosis and following pancreatectomy.

■ CONTRAINDICATIONS: Known hypersensitivity to this drug or to pork or beef protein prohibits its use.

■ ADVERSE EFFECTS: There are no known serious adverse reactions. High doses may cause nausea or diarrhea.

pancreatitis (pæn'kriətai'tis), an inflammatory condition of the pancreas that may be acute or chronic. **Acute pancreatitis** is generally the result of damage to the biliary tract, as by alcohol, trauma, infectious disease, or certain drugs. It is characterized by severe abdominal pain radiating to the back, fever, anorexia, nausea, and vomiting. There may be jaundice if the common bile duct is obstructed. The development of pseudocysts or abscesses in pancreatic tissue is a serious complication. Treatment includes nasogastric suction to remove gastric secretions. To prevent any stimulation of the pancreas, nothing is given by mouth. Intravenous fluids and electrolytes are administered, and nonmorphine derivatives are given to relieve pain. Acute pancreatitis is associated with a mortality of 50 per cent. The causes of **chronic pancreatitis** are similar to those of the acute form. When the cause is alcohol abuse, there may be calcification and scarring of the smaller pancreatic ducts. There is abdominal pain, nausea, and vomiting, as well as steatorrhea and creatorrhea, owing to the diminished output of pancreatic enzymes. Pancreatic insulin production may be diminished, and some patients develop diabetes mellitus. Treatment includes analgesics for pain and subtotal pancreatectomy when pain is intractable. A pancreatic extract is given orally to replace the missing enzymes; vitamin supplements are essential. Both forms of pancreatitis are diagnosed by history, physical examination, radiologic studies, endoscopy, and laboratory analysis of the amount of pancreatic enzymes in the blood.

pancreatoduodenectomy (pæn'kriæ'toudu'oudənek'-təmi), a surgical procedure in which the head of the pancreas and the loop of duodenum that surrounds it are excised. The operation is performed to remove the periampullary masses occurring in certain forms of biliary tract cancer.

pancreatography (pæŋ'kriətog'rəfi), visualization of the pancreas or its ducts by means of x rays and contrast media injected into the ducts at surgery or via an endoscope or by means of ultrasonography, computerized tomography, or radionuclide imaging.

pancreatolith, a stone or calculus in the pancreas.

pancrelipase (pæŋ'krəlip'eis), an enzyme concentrate derived from hogs.

■ INDICATIONS: It is prescribed as an aid to digestion to replace endogenous pancreatic enzymes in cystic fibrosis and chronic pancreatitis and following pancreatectomy.

■ CONTRAINDICATIONS: Known hypersensitivity to this drug or to pork protein prohibits its use.

■ ADVERSE EFFECTS: There are no known serious adverse reactions. High doses may cause nausea or diarrhea.

pancuronium bromide, a skeletal muscle relaxant.

■ INDICATIONS: It is prescribed as an adjunct to anesthesia and mechanical ventilation.

■ CONTRAINDICATIONS: It is used with caution in patients with myasthenia gravis, renal and hepatic disease, and in pregnancy. Known hypersensitivity to this drug or to other bromides prohibits its use.

■ ADVERSE EFFECTS: The most serious adverse reaction is prolonged muscle relaxation and respiratory depression.

pancytopenia, (pæn'saitəpi'niə), an abnormal condition characterized by a marked reduction in the number of all of the cellular elements of the blood, the red blood cells, white blood cells, and platelets. See also **anemia, aplasia.** – **pancytopenic,** adj.

p and a, abbreviation for percussion and auscultation, as noted in the patient's chart following physical examination of the chest. See **auscultation, percussion.**

pandemic, (of a disease) occurring throughout the population of a country, a people, or the world.

pandiastolic, of or pertaining to the complete diastole. Also called **holodiastolic.**

panencephalitis (pæn'ensef'əlai'tis), inflammation of the entire brain characterized by an insidious onset, a progressive course with deterioration of motor and mental functions, and evidence of a viral etiology. Subacute sclerosing panencephalitis is an uncommon childhood disease thought to be caused by a 'slow' latent measles virus following recovery from a previous infection. Most of the patients are younger than 11 and many more boys than girls are affected. The disease results in ataxia, myoclonus, atrophy, cortical blindness, and mental deterioration. Antiviral drugs, immunosuppressants, and interferon inducers are sometimes administered, but the disease is usually fatal. Microscopic studies of postmortem brain tissue often reveal intracellular inclusion bodies resembling the nucleocapsids of paramyxoviruses. Rubella panencephalitis, a rare disease of adolescents, follows a chronic progressive course marked by motor and mental deterioration and sometimes resembles juvenile paresis. Inclusion bodies are not found in brain cells, but the pathology is similar to the mineralization found in infantile congenital rubella and antibodies to the virus are present.

panendoscope, a cystoscope that allows a wide view of the interior of the bladder.

panesthesia, the total of all sensations experienced by an individual at one time. Compare **cenesthesia.**

pangenesis, a Darwinian theory that every cell and particle of a parent reproduces itself in progeny.

Panheprin, a trade name for an anticoagulant (heparin sodium).

panhypopituitarism (pænhai'poupitu'itəriz'əm), generalized insufficiency of pituitary hormones, resulting from damage to or deficiency of the gland. **Prepubertal panhypopituitarism,** a rare disorder usually associated with a suprasellar cyst or craniopharyngioma, is characterized by dwarfism with normal body proportions, subnormal sexual development, and insufficient thyroid and adrenal function. Diabetes insipidus is frequently present; there may be bitemporal hemianopia or complete blindness; skin is often yellow and wrinkled, but mentality is usually unimpaired. X rays show delayed fusion of the epiphyses, suprasellar calcification, and, frequently, destruction of the sella turcica. The condition is treated with cortisone, thyroid and sex hormones, and, if available, human growth hormone. Postpubertal panhypopituitarism may be caused by postpartum pituitary necrosis, resulting from thrombosis of pituitary circulation during or after delivery. Characteristic signs of the disorder are failure to lactate, amenorrhea, weakness, cold intolerance, lethargy, loss of libido and of axillary and pubic hair. There may be bradycardia or hypotension, and progression of the disorder leads to premature wrinkling of the skin and atrophy of the thyroid and adrenal glands. Treatment consists of the administration of ACTH, thyroid stimulating hormone, and hormones of the target organs. Also called **hypophyseal cachexia, pituitary cachexia, Simmonds' disease.**

panhysterectomy (pæn′hɪstərek′təmi), complete surgical removal of the uterus, cervix, Fallopian tubes, and ovaries. Compare **subtotal hysterectomy, total hysterectomy.** See also **hysterectomy.**

panic, an intense, sudden, and overwhelming fear or feeling of anxiety that produces terror and immediate physiological changes that result in paralyzed immobility or senseless, hysterical behavior.

panic disorder. See **anxiety neurosis.**

panivorous (pənɪv′ərəs), of or pertaining to the practice of subsisting exclusively on bread. —**panivore,** n.

panlobular emphysema. See **panacinar emphysema.**

Panmycin Hydrochloride, a trade name for an antibacterial and antiprotozoal (tetracycline hydrochloride).

panniculus, pl. **panniculi.** a membranous layer, the many sheets of fascia covering various structures in the body.

pannus (pæn′əs), an inflamed lymphatic gland that is not suppurating.

panophthalmitis (pæn′ofthəlmɑi′tɪs), an inflammation of the entire eye, usually caused by virulent pyogenic organisms, as strains of meningococci, pneumococci, streptococci, anthrax bacilli, and clostradia. Initial symptoms are pain, fever, headache, drowsiness, edema, and swelling. As the infection progresses, the iris appears muddy and gray, the aqueous humor becomes turbid, and precipitates form on the posterior surface of the cornea. Treatment consists of intensive systemic and local antibiotic therapy; evisceration of the globe or excision of the eye may be required, but excision is contraindicated if surrounding tissues are infected.

Panoxyl, a trade name for a keratolytic (benzoyl peroxide).

panphobia, panophobia, pantophobia, an anxiety disorder characterized by an irrational, vague fear or apprehension of some pervading or unknown evil; a generalized fear. —**panophobic,** adj.

panphobic melancholia, Obsolete. a state of depression characterized by an irrational dread or pervading fear of everything. See also **bipolar disorder, phobia.**

Panrexin-M, a trade name for an anorexic (phendimetrazine tartrate).

pansystolic, of or pertaining to the entire systole. Also called **holosystolic.**

pansystolic murmur. See **systolic murmur.**

pant-. See **panto-.**

Panteric, a trade name for an enzyme (pancreatin).

panthenol (pæn′thənol), an alcohol converted in the body to pantothenic acid, a vitamin in the B complex.

panto-, pant-, a combining form meaning 'all, the whole': *pantophobia, pantoscopic, pantosomatous.*

Pantocaine, a trade name for a local anesthetic (tetracaine hydrochloride).

pantograph, a jointed device for copying a plane figure to any desired scale.

Pantolax (pæn′təlæks′), a trade name for a depolarizing blocking agent (succinylcholine chloride), used as an adjunct to general anesthesia.

Pantopon, a trade name for a narcotic analgesic, fixed-combination drug containing hydrochlorides of opium alkaloids.

pantothenic acid (pæn′təfhen′ɪk), a member of the vitamin B complex. It is widely distributed in plant and animal tissues and may be an important element in human nutrition.

pantothenyl alcohol. See **panthenol.**

Panwarfin, a trade name for an anticoagulant (warfarin sodium).

PaO₂, symbol for **arterial partial pressure of oxygen.**

papain (pəpei′in), an enzyme from the fruit of *Carica papaya,* the tropical melon tree. It has been prescribed for enzymatic debridement of wounds and promotion of healing.

Papanicolaou test, a simple smear method of examining stained exfoliative cells. It is used most commonly to detect cancers of the cervix, but it may be used for tissue specimens from any organ. A smear is usually obtained during a routine pelvic examination. The technique permits early diagnosis of cancer and has contributed to a lower death rate from cervical cancer. The findings are usually reported descriptively and grouped into the following classes: Class I, only normal cells seen; Class II, atypical cells consistent with inflammation; Class III, mild dysplasia; Class IV, severe dysplasia, suspicious cells; Class V, carcinoma cells seen. Also called *Informal.* **Pap test.**

papaverine hydrochloride, a smooth muscle relaxant.
■ INDICATIONS: It is prescribed in the treatment of cardiovascular or visceral spasms.
■ CONTRAINDICATIONS: Complete atrioventricular heart block or known hypersensitivity to this drug prohibits its use.
■ ADVERSE EFFECTS: The most serious adverse reaction is jaundice.

paper chromatography, the separation of a mixture into its components by filtering it through a strip of special paper.

paper-doll fetus. See **fetus papyraceus.**

papilla (pəpɪl′ə), *pl.* **papillae.** a small nipple-shaped projection, as the conoid papillae of the tongue and the papillae of the corium which extend from collagen fibers, the capillary blood vessels, and sometimes the nerves of the dermis. —**papillary,** *adj.*

papilla of Vater. See under **papilla.**

papillary, of or pertaining to a papilla.

papillary adenocarcinoma, a malignant neoplasm characterized by small papillae of vascular connective tissue covered by neoplastic epithelium that project into follicles, glands, or cysts. The tumor is most common in the ovaries and thyroid gland. Also called **polypoid adenocarcinoma.**

papillary adenocystoma lymphomatosum, an unusual tumor, consisting of epithelial and lymphoid tissues, that develops in the area of the parotid and submaxillary glands. Also called **adenolymphoma, Warthin's tumor.**

papillary adenoma, a benign epithelial tumor in which the membrane lining the glandular tissue forms papillary processes that project into the alveoli or grow out of the surface of a cavity.

papillary carcinoma, a malignant neoplasm characterized by many fingerlike projections. It is the most common type of thyroid tumor.

papillary duct, any one of the thousands of straight collecting renal tubules that descend through the medulla of the kidney and join with others to form the common ducts opening into the renal papillae. Compare **Henle's loop.** See also **kidney.**

papillary muscle, any one of the rounded or conical muscular projections attached to the chordae tendineae in the ventricles of the heart. The papillary muscles vary in number but the two main ones are the anterior papillary muscle and the posterior papillary muscle. The papillary muscles are associated with the atrioventricular valves which they help to open and close. Compare **chorda tendinea, trabecula carnea.**

papillary tumor. See **papilloma.**

papillate, marked by papillae or nipplelike prominences.

papilledema, *pl.* **papilledemas, papilledemata.** swelling of the optic disc, visible on ophthalmoscopic examination of the fundus of the eye, caused by increased intracranial pressure. The meningeal sheaths that surround the optic nerves from the optic disc are continuous with the meninges of the brain; therefore, increased intracranial pressure is transmitted forward from the brain to the optic disc in the eye to cause the swelling.

papilliform, shaped like a papilla.

papillitis (pæp′ɪlai′tɪs), **1.** an abnormal condition characterized by the inflammation of a papilla, as the lacrimal papilla. **2.** an abnormal condition characterized by the inflammation of a renal papilla.

papilloma (pæp′ɪlou′mə), a benign epithelial neoplasm characterized by a branching or lobular tumor. Kinds of papilloma are **basal cell papilloma, cockscomb papilloma, cutaneous papilloma, fibroepithelial papilloma, hirsutoid papilloma of the penis, intracanalicular papilloma, intracystic papilloma, villous papilloma.** Also called **papillary tumor.**

-papilloma, a combining form meaning an 'epithelial tumor': *fibropapilloma, myxopapilloma, polypapilloma.*

papillomatosis (pæp′ɪloumətou′sɪs), an abnormal condition in which there is widespread development of nipplelike growths.

papillomatosis coronal penis. See **hirsutoid papilloma of the penis.**

papillomavirus (pæp′ɪlou′məvai′rəs), the virus that causes warts in humans.

papillophlebitis (pæp′ɪloufləbai′tɪs), See **retinal-vein occlusion.**

papovavirus (pæp′əvəvai′rəs), one of a group of small DNA viruses, some of which may be potentially cancer-producing. The human wart is caused by a kind of papovavirus, but it very rarely undergoes malignant transformation. Kinds of papovaviruses are **papilloma papovavirus, polyoma papovavirus, SV-40 papovavirus.**

pappataci (pap′ata′chi). See **phlebotomus fever.**

pappus, the first growth of beard, characterized by downy hairs.

Pap smear, *Informal.* a specimen of exfoliated, epithelial cells and cervical mucus collected during a pelvic exam for cytologic evaluation according to the Papanicolaou cytologic classification.

Pap test, *Informal.* Papanicolaou test.

papular scaling disease, any of a group of skin disorders in which there are discrete, raised, dry, scaling lesions. Also called **papulosquamous disease.** Some kinds of papular scaling diseases are **lichen planus, pityriasis rosea, psoriasis.**

papulation, the development of papules.

papule (pæp′yul), a small, solid, raised skin lesion less than one cm in diameter, as the lesions of lichen planus and nonpustular acne. Compare **macule.** —**papular,** *adj.*

papulosquamous disease. See **papular scaling disease.**

papyraceous, having a paperlike quality.

papyraceous fetus. See **fetus papyraceus.**

Paquelin's cautery (pæk′əlɪnz), a cauterizing device consisting of a platinum loop through which a heated hydrocarbon is passed.

par, a pair, specifically a pair of cranial nerves, as the par nonum or the ninth pair.

PAR, abbreviation for **pulmonary arteriolar resistance.**

par-, a combining form meaning 'aside, beyond, apart from, against': *parabacteria, parotid, parumbilical.*

para-, par-, a combining form meaning 'similar, beside': *paronchia, parotid, parasympathetic.*

-para, 1. a combining form meaning a 'woman who has given birth to children in a number of pregnancies': *bipara, nonipara, unipara.* 2. a combining form meaning a 'female of any species producing a number or type of egg or offspring': *nymphipara, ovovipara, pipipara.*

para-aminobenzoic acid (PABA) (pær′əæmi′noubenzou′ık), a substance often occurring in association with the vitamin B complex, found in cereals, eggs, milk, and meat and present in detectable amounts in blood, urine, spinal fluid, and sweat. It is widely used as a sunscreen that forms a partial chemical conjugation with constituents of the horny layer and that resists removal by water and sweat. PABA is a sulfonamide antagonist and may be an effective agent for the treatment of scleroderma, dermatomyositis, and pemphigus.

para-aminosalicylic acid (PAS, PASA), a bacteriostatic agent.

■ INDICATIONS: It is prescribed for the treatment of pulmonary and extrapulmonary tuberculosis.

■ CONTRAINDICATION: Known hypersensitivity to the drug prohibits its use.

■ ADVERSE EFFECTS: Among the most serious reactions are nausea, vomiting, diarrhea, and abdominal pain. Fever, skin eruptions, and other kinds of hypersensitivity reactions, goiter, hypokalemia, and acidosis may occur.

paracentesis (pær′əsenti′sıs), a procedure in which fluid is withdrawn from a cavity of the body. An incision is made in the skin and a hollow trocar, cannula, or catheter is passed through the incision into the cavity to allow outflow of fluid into a collecting device. Paracentesis is most commonly performed to remove excessive accumulations of ascitic fluid from the abdomen.

paracervical block, a form of regional anesthesia in which a local anesthetic is injected into the area on each side of the uterine cervix that contains the plexus of nerves innervating the uterine cervix. Effective anesthesia for active labor is often achieved. The duration of the anesthetic effect depends on the agent used. Transient maternal hypotension sometimes occurs following paracervical block, usually owing to inadvertent intravascular injection of the anesthetic.

paracoccidiodal granuloma (pær′əkoksıd′ioi′dəl). See **paracoccidioidomycosis.**

paracoccidioidomycosis (pær′əkoksıd′ioi′doumaikou′sıs), a chronic, occasionally fatal, fungous infection caused by *Paracoccidioides brasiliensis,* characterized by ulcers of the oral cavity, larynx, and nose; large, draining lymph nodes; cough; dyspnea; weight loss; and skin, genital, and intestinal lesions. The disease occurs only in Mexico and Central and South America and is acquired by inhalation of spores of the fungus. The diagnosis is made by microscopic examination of a smear prepared from a lesion. Treatment requires several years of sulfonamides or, in severe cases, intravenous amphotericin B followed by oral sulfonamides. Also called **paracoccidioidal granuloma, South American blastomycosis.** Compare **North American blastomycosis.**

paradichlorobenzene poisoning (pær′ədaiklɔr′əben′zin). See **naphthalene poisoning.**

paradidymal, 1. pertaining to the paradidymis. 2. beside the testis.

paradidymis, *pl.* **paradidymides.** a rudimentary structure in the male, situated on the spermatic cord of the epididymis, that consists of vestigial remains of the caudal part of the embryonic mesonephric tubules. A similar vestigial structure, the paroophoron is found in the female. Also called **organ of Giraldes, parepididymis.** See also **aberrant ductule, appendix epididymis.**

Paradione, a trade name for an anticonvulsant (paramethadione).

paraffin bath, the application of heat to a specific area of the body through the use of paraffin. The part is quickly immersed in heated liquid wax and then withdrawn so that the wax solidifies to form an insulating layer. The procedure is repeated until the layer is 5 to 10 mm thick, and then the entire area is wrapped in an insulating fabric, as a loose-fitting plastic bag or paper towels. The technique is effective for heating traumatized or inflamed areas, especially the hands, feet, and wrists, and is used primarily for patients with arthritis and rheumatism or any joint condition. Also called **wax bath.**

Paraflex, a trade name for a skeletal-muscle relaxant (chlorzoxazone).

Parafon Forte, a trade name for a fixed-combination drug containing an analgesic-antipyretic (acetaminophen) and a skeletal muscle relaxant (chlorzoxazone), used for the relief of painful musculoskeletal conditions.

paraganglion, *pl.* **paraganglia.** any one of the small groups of chromaffin cells associated with the ganglia of the sympathetic nerve trunk and situated outside the adrenal medulla, most often near the sympathetic ganglia along the aorta and its branches. The paraganglia are also connected with the ganglia of the celiac, renal, suprarenal, aortic, and hypogastric plexuses. The paraganglia secrete the hormones epinephrine and norepinephrine. Also called **chromaffin body.** See also **chromaffin cell.**

paragonimiasis (pær′əgon′ımai′əsıs), chronic infection with the lung fluke *Paragonimus westermani,* occurring most commonly in Asia. It is characterized by hemoptysis, bronchitis, and, occasionally, abdominal masses, pain and diarrhea, or cerebral involvement with paralysis, ocular pathology, or seizures. The disease is acquired by ingesting cysts in infected freshwater crabs or crayfish, the intermediate hosts. Adequate cooking of shellfish prevents the disease. Bithionol, given orally is the usual treatment.

parainfluenza virus, a myxovirus with four serotypes, causing respiratory infections in infants and young children, and, less commonly, in adults. Types 1 and 2 parainfluenza viruses may cause laryngotracheobronchitis or croup; type 3 is a cause of croup, tracheobronchitis, bronchiolitis, and bronchopneumonia in children; types 1, 3, and 4 are associated with pharyngitis and the common cold. Compare **influenza.**

Paral, a trade name for a sedative-hypnotic (paraldehyde).

paraldehyde (pəræl'dəhaid), a clear, colorless, strong-smelling liquid obtained by the polymerization of acetaldehyde with a small amount of sulfuric acid. Paraldehyde is used as a solvent and may be administered orally, intravenously, intramuscularly, or rectally to induce hypnotic states or sedation.

parallel play, a form of play among a group of children, primarily toddlers, in which each one engages in an independent activity that is similar to but not influenced by or shared with the others. Compare **cooperative play.** See also **associative play, solitary play.**

paralysis, *pl.* **paralyses.** an abnormal condition characterized by the loss of muscle function or the loss of sensation. It may be caused by a variety of problems, as trauma, disease, and poisoning. Paralyses may be classified according to etiology, muscle tone, distribution, or the part of the body affected. See also **flaccid paralysis, spastic paralysis.** – **paralytic,** *adj.*

paralysis agitans. See **Parkinson's disease.**

-paralytic, a combining form meaning 'pertaining to paralysis': *antiparalytic, aparalytic, subparalytic.*

paralytic dementia. See **paresis,** def. 2.

paralytic ileus, a decrease in or absence of intestinal peristalsis that may occur following abdominal surgery or peritoneal injury or in connection with severe pyelonephritis, ureteral stone, fractured ribs, myocardial infarction, extensive intestinal ulceration, heavy-metal poisoning, porphyria, retroperitoneal hematomas, especially those associated with fractured vertebrae, or any severe metabolic disease. The most common overall cause of intestinal obstruction, paralytic ileus is mediated by a hormonal component of the sympathoadrenal system.

■ OBSERVATIONS: Paralytic ileus is characterized by abdominal tenderness and distention, absence of bowel sounds, lack of flatus, and by nausea and vomiting. There may be fever, decreased urinary output, electrolyte imbalance, dehydration, and respiratory distress. The loss of fluids and electrolytes may be extreme, and, unless they are replaced, the condition may lead to hemoconcentration, hypovolemia, renal insufficiency, shock, and death.

■ INTERVENTION: The patient is kept in bed in a low Fowler's position and nothing is given by mouth. An intestinal tube is inserted as a nasogastric tube into the duodenum and connected to intermittent suction; it is not taped to the nose and the patient is positioned to facilitate the advancement of the tube, which is checked every 30 to 60 minutes. The character of gastrointestinal drainage is monitored every two to four hours, and any increase or decrease in the amount or changes in the color or consistency is reported. Bowel sounds, blood pressure, pulse, and respirations are checked every two to four hours and rectal temperature every four hours. Abdominal girth is measured every two hours and report is made of any increase. Parenteral fluids with electrolytes and medication to promote peristalsis are administered as ordered; intake and output are measured and, if less than 30 ml of urine is excreted per hour, the physician is informed. The patient is helped to turn and deep-breathe every two to four hours and is given oral hygiene every one to two hours. Active or passive range of motion exercises are performed every four hours. When intestinal output increases and bowel sounds return, the intestinal tube may be clamped and small amounts of warm tea or a carbonated beverage may be given. If pain, distention, or cramps do not recur the intestinal tube may be removed but a rectal tube, or an enema may be ordered to relieve distention.

■ NURSING CONSIDERATIONS: The concerns of the nurse include monitoring and reporting the signs of paralytic ileus and its potential complications, ensuring that the patient is as comfortable as possible, and explaining to the patient the purpose of the intestinal tube. The nurse instructs the patient to avoid mouth breathing, because swallowed air can increase distention.

paralytic shellfish poisoning. See **shellfish poisoning.**

paramedic, a person who acts as an assistant to a physician or in place of a physician, especially a person in the military, trained in emergency medical procedures. – **paramedical,** *adj.*

paramedical personnel, health-care workers other than physicians, dentists, podiatrists, and nurses who have special training in the performance of supportive health care tasks. Kinds of paramedical personnel are **ambulance attendants, audiologists, x-ray technologists.**

paramesonephric duct (pær'əmez'ounef'rık), one of a pair of embryonic ducts that develops into the uterus and the uterine tubes. Also called **Müllerian duct.**

parameter (pəræm'ıtər), **1.** a value or constant used to describe or measure a set of data representing a physiological function or system, as in the use of acid-base relationships of the blood as parameters for evaluating the function of a patient's respiratory system. **2.** a statistical value of a population group. **3.** *Informal, not in technical use.* **a.** any standard against which something is measured. **b.** limits or boundary.

paramethadione (pær'əmeθ'ədai'oun), an anticonvulsant.

■ INDICATION: It is prescribed for the prevention of seizures in petit mal epilepsy.

■ CONTRAINDICATIONS: Blood dyscrasias, severe renal or hepatic impairment, or known hypersensitivity to this drug prohibits its use.

■ ADVERSE EFFECTS: Among the more serious adverse reactions are exfoliative dermatitis, blood dyscrasias, and hepatitis. Sedation, hemerolopia, and moderate neutropenia may occur.

paramethasone acetate, a glucocorticoid.

■ INDICATIONS: It is prescribed in the treatment of inflammatory and allergic conditions.

■ CONTRAINDICATIONS: Systemic fungal infections or known hypersensitivity to this drug prohibits its use.

■ ADVERSE EFFECTS: Among the more serious adverse reactions are gastrointestinal, endocrine, and neurologic disturbances and fluid and electrolyte imbalance.

parametric imaging, (in nuclear medicine) a diagnostic procedure in which an image of an administered radioactive tracer is derived according to a mathematical rule, as by the division of one image by another.

parametritis (pær'əmətraɪ'tɪs), an inflammatory condition of the tissue of the structures around the uterus. See also **pelvic inflammatory disease.**

parametrium (pær'əmi'triəm), *pl.* **parametria.** the lateral extension of the uterine subserous connective tissue into the broad ligament. Compare **endometrium, myometrium.**

paramitome (pær'əmaɪ'toum). See **hyaloplasm.**

paramnesia (pær'æmni'ʒə), **1.** a perversion of memory in which one believes he remembers events and circumstances that never actually occurred. **2.** a condition in which words are remembered and used without the comprehension of their meaning. Compare **déjà vu.**

paramyxovirus (pær'əmɪk'souvaɪ'rəs), a member of a family of viruses that includes the organisms that cause parainfluenza, measles, mumps, and some respiratory infections.

paranasal (pær'ənei'zəl), situated near or alongside the nose, as the paranasal sinuses.

paranasal sinus, one of the air cavities in various bones around the nose, as the frontal sinus in the frontal bone lying deep to the medial part of the superciliary ridge and the maxillary sinus within the maxilla between the orbit, the nasal cavity, and the upper teeth. Compare **confluence of the sinuses, occipital sinus.**

parangi (pəræn'ji). See **yaws.**

paranoia (pær'ənoi'ə), **paranoea** (pær'əni'ə), (in psychiatry) a disorder characterized by an elaborate system of thinking with delusions of persecution and grandeur usually centered on one major theme, as a financial matter, a job situation, an unfaithful spouse, or other problem. The delusional system typically develops slowly and progressively over a period of months or years, becoming intricate, logical, and highly organized, with the result that it

can be most convincing. The person appears perfectly normal in his conduct, conversation, thinking patterns, and emotional responses aside from the delusions. Associated symptoms include suspiciousness, seclusion, stubbornness, resentfulness, aloofness, hostility, aggressiveness, dominating or grandiose attitudes, and unrealistic expectations. Causal factors are predominantly psychosocial in nature, as inadequate socialization during childhood, poor development of interpersonal relationships, and sexual maladjustment, and do not involve genetic or biochemical alterations. Persons with the disorder are highly resistant to available methods of treatment, although individual or group psychotherapy and behavior therapy may be effective in the early stages. Kinds of paranoia include **acute hallucinatory paranoia, alcoholic paranoia, litigious paranoia, querulous paranoia.** Compare **paranoid schizophrenia.**

paranoiac (pær'ənoi'æk), **paranoeac, 1.** a person afflicted with or exhibiting characteristics of paranoia. **2.** of or pertaining to paranoia.

paranoia hallucinatoria (hælu'sɪnətɔr'iə). See **acute hallucinatory paranoia.**

paranoia quaerula (kwer'yulə). See **querulous paranoia.**

paranoid (pær'ənoid), **1.** pertaining to or resembling paranoia. **2.** a person afflicted with a paranoid disorder. **3.** *Informal.* a person who is overly suspicious or exhibits persecutory trends or attitudes.

paranoid disorder, any of a large group of mental disorders characterized by an impaired sense of reality and persistent delusions. Kinds of paranoid disorders include **acute paranoid disorder, paranoia, shared paranoid disorder.**

paranoid ideation, an exaggerated belief or suspicion, usually not of a delusional nature, that one is being harassed, persecuted, or treated unfairly.

paranoid personality, a personality characterized by paranoia.

paranoid personality disorder, a disorder characterized by extreme suspiciousness and distrust of others to the degree that one blames them for one's mistakes and failures and goes to abnormal lengths to validate prejudices, attitudes, or biases. Symptoms include hypersensitivity, rigidity, hostility, stubbornness, envy, exaggerated self-importance, extreme argumentativeness, tenseness, and lack of passive, sentimental, or tender feelings. The condition is more commonly diagnosed in men than in women. The disorganization of the personality in this condition is less severe than in paranoid schizophrenia.

paranoid reaction, a psychopathological condition of the aged, characterized by the gradual formation of delusions, usually of a persecutory nature and often accompanied by related hallucinations. Other manifestations of senile degeneration, as memory loss and confusion, do not usually accompany the reaction and the individual maintains orientation for time, place, and person.

paranoid schizophrenia, a form of schizophrenia characterized by persistent preoccupation with illogical, absurd, and changeable delusions, usually of a persecutory, grandiose, or jealous nature, accompanied by related hallucinations. The symptoms include extreme anxiety, exaggerated suspiciousness, aggressiveness, anger, argumentativeness, hostility, and violence. The condition occurs most frequently during middle age. Current therapy is not usually effective. Also called **heboid paranoia.** Compare **paranoia.** See also **schizophrenia.**

paranoid state, a transitory abnormal mental condition characterized by illogical thought processes and generalized suspicion and distrust, with a tendency toward persecutory ideas or delusions.

paranuclear body. See **centrosome.**

parapertussis (pær'əpərtəs'ıs), an acute bacterial respiratory infection caused by *Bordetella parapertussis,* having symptoms closely resembling those of pertussis. It is usually milder than pertussis, although it can be fatal. It is possible to be infected with both *B. parapertussis* and *B. pertussis* at the same time. A parapertussis vaccine is available and may be given in combination with pertussis vaccine.

parapharyngeal abscess (pær'əfərın'jiəl), a suppurative infection of tissues adjacent to the pharynx, usually a complication of acute pharyngitis or tonsillitis. Infection may spread to the jugular vein where it may cause thrombophlebitis and septic emboli. Systemic antibiotics and surgical drainage may be required. Also called **parapharyngeal space abscess.** Compare **peritonsillar abscess, retropharyngeal abscess.** See also **tonsillitis.**

paraphilia (pær'əfıl'iə, pær'əfil'yə), sexual perversion or deviation; a condition in which the sexual instinct is expressed in ways that are socially prohibited or unacceptable or are biologically undesirable, as the use of an inanimate object for sexual arousal, sexual activity with another person that involves real or simulated suffering or humiliation, or sexual relations with a nonconsenting partner. Kinds of paraphilia include **exhibitionism, fetishism, pedophilia, transvestism, voyeurism, zoophilia.** – **paraphiliac,** *adj., n.*

paraphimosis (pær'əfæimou'sıs), a condition characterized by an inability to replace the foreskin in its normal position after it has been retracted behind the glans penis. Caused by a narrow or inflamed foreskin, the condition may lead to gangrene. Circumcision may be required. Compare **phimosis.**

paraplasm, 1. See **hyaloplasm. 2.** any abnormal growth or malformation. – **paraplasmic,** *adj.*

paraplastic, 1. misshapen or malformed. **2.** showing abnormal formative power; of the nature of a paraplasm.

paraplegia (pær'əpli'jə), an abnormal condition charac-

terized by motor or sensory loss in the lower limbs. This condition may or may not involve the back and abdominal muscles and may cause either complete or incomplete paralysis. The incidence of this disorder in men is double that in women and is highest between the ages of 16 and 35. About 50 per cent of approximately 11,000 spinal cord injuries reported each year in the United States involve paraplegia. Such injuries commonly occur as the result of automobile and motorcycle accidents, sporting accidents, falls, and gunshot wounds. Paraplegia less commonly results from nontraumatic lesions, as scoliosis and spina bifida. – **paraplegic,** *adj., n.*

■ OBSERVATIONS: The signs and symptoms of paraplegia may develop immediately from trauma and include the loss of sensation, motion, and reflexes below the level of the lesion. Depending on the level of the lesion and whether damage to the spinal cord is complete or incomplete, the patient may lose bladder and bowel control and develop sexual dysfunctions. An incomplete spinal cord injury does not usually inhibit circumanal sensation, voluntary toe flexion, or sphincter control. A complete spinal cord injury destroys sensation and voluntary muscle control and usually causes the permanent loss of muscle function distal to the injury. Diagnosis is based on clinical history, neurologic examination, and x rays. Various laboratory tests are performed, as a complete blood count, prothrombin time, electrolyte, evaluation, and urinalysis.

■ INTERVENTION: The treatment of paraplegia seeks to restore proper spine alignment, stabilize the injured spinal area, decompress any involved neurological structures, and rehabilitate the patient as quickly as possible. At the accident scene, when spinal cord injury is suspected, the patient must not be moved until strapped and stabilized on a board. Such stabilization helps to prevent permanent damage to any injured spinal structures. A Foley catheter is commonly inserted to assure uninterrupted urine drainage. Treatment may also include the administration of drugs, as nitrofurantoin to prevent bladder infection and vitamin C to minimize infection by acidifying the urine. A laminectomy may be performed if bone fragments are pressing on the spinal cord. Drugs, as baclofen, may be administered to relieve any muscle spasms associated with dysfunction of the upper motor neurons.

■ NURSING CONSIDERATIONS: Nursing care in paraplegic cases commonly includes the proper positioning and maintenance of the patient on a Stryker frame or a Circ-Olectric bed, proper wound care following a laminectomy, catheter and skin care, and meticulous monitoring of intake and output. When the paraplegic patient progresses from bed rest to a wheelchair, the nurse is alert to any signs of orthostatic hypotension. Special binders and antiembolism hose are used to help the patient adjust to the transition from bed to wheelchair. Other treatment may include the administration of a high-bulk diet and suppositories to prevent constipation. The patient and family benefit from counseling and encouragement during the rehabilitation period, especially if the patient develops psychologic problems associated with the difficult adjustment to paraplegia. Accurate assessment of paralysis is often not possible until a year after the injury.

parapsoriasis (pær'əsərai'əsis), a group of chronic skin diseases resembling psoriasis, characterized by maculopapular, erythematous, scaly eruptions without systemic symptoms. Parapsoriasis is resistant to all treatment.

parapsychology, a branch of psychology concerned with the study of psychic phenomena, like clairvoyance, extrasensory perception, and telepathy.

paraquat poisoning (pær'əkwot'), a toxic condition caused by the ingestion of paraquat dichloride, a highly poisonous pesticide. Characteristically, progressive pulmonary fibrosis and damage to the esophagus, kidneys, and liver develop several days following ingestion. Once fibrosis begins, death is inevitable, usually within three weeks. The mechanism of action of the poison is unknown. Most often, poisoning results from accidental occupational exposure. There is considerable concern that the inhalation of the smoke of marijuana treated with the herbicide may cause intoxication, but no clinical syndrome resulting from such exposure has been documented.

parasite, 1. an organism living in or on and obtaining nourishment from another organism. A **facultative parasite** may live on a host but is capable of living independently. An **obligate parasite** is one that depends entirely on its host for survival. 2. in conjoined twins, the less complete twin who derives support from the more complete twin. — **parasitic,** *adj.*

parasitemia (pær'əsaiti'miə), the presence of parasites in the blood. Compare **bacteremia, fungemia, viremia.**

parasitic fetus, the smaller, usually malformed member of conjoined, unequal, or asymmetrical twins that is attached to and dependent upon the more normal fetus for growth and development. Compare **autosite.**

parasitic fibroma, a pedunculated uterine fibroid deriving part of its blood supply from the omentum.

parasitic glossitis, a mycosis of the tongue, characterized by a black or brown furry patch on the posterior dorsal surface composed of hypertrophied filiform papillae that measure about 1.0 cm in length and are easily broken. The condition, caused by *Cryptococcus linguae-pilosasae* in symbiosis with *Nocardia lingualis,* produces no discomfort and may be treated with a simple mouthwash. The patch may disappear spontaneously and later reappear. Also called **anthracosis linguae, black hairy tongue, black tongue, glossitis parasitica, glossophytia, keratomycosis linguae, lingua villosa nigra, melanotrichia linguae, nigrites linguae.**

parasitic thrombus, an aggregation of bodies and spores of malarial parasites formed in the vessels of the brain in cerebral malaria.

parasympathetic, of or pertaining to the craniosacral division of the autonomic nervous system, consisting of the oculomotor, facial, glossopharyngeal, vagus, and pelvic nerves. The actions of the parasympathetic division are mediated by the release of acetylcholine and primarily involve the protection, conservation, and restoration of body resources. Preganglionic parasympathetic fibers, which emerge from the hypothalamus, other brain areas, and sacral segments of the spinal cord, form synapses in ganglia located near or in the walls of the organs to be innervated. Reactions to parasympathetic stimulation are highly localized and tend to counteract the adrenergic effects of sympathetic nerves. Parasympathetic fibers slow the heart, stimulate peristalsis, promote the secretion of lacrimal, salivary, and digestive glands, induce bile and insulin release, dilate peripheral and visceral blood vessels, constrict the pupils, esophagus, and bronchioles, and relax sphincters during micturition and defecation. Postganglionic parasympathetic fibers extend to the uterus, vagina, oviducts, and ovaries in females, and to the prostate, seminal vesicles, and external genitalia in males, innervating blood vessels of pelvic organs in both sexes; stimulation of these nerves causes vasodilation in the clitoris and labia minora and erection of the penis.

parasympathetic nervous system. See **autonomic nervous system.**

parasympatholytic (pær'əsim'pæfhəlit'ik). See **anticholinergic.**

parasympatholytic drug. See **anticholinergic.**

parasympathomimetic (pær'əsim'pəfhoumimet'ik), 1. of, or pertaining to a substance producing effects similar to those caused by stimulation of a parasympathetic nerve. 2. an agent whose effects mimic those resulting from stimulation of parasympathetic nerves, especially the effects produced by acetylcholine. The parasympathomimetic drugs include bethanecol chloride, neostigmine bromide, neostigmine methylsulfate, and pyridostigmine bromide, variously used to treat myasthenia gravis, acute postoperative and postpartum nonobstructional urinary retention, and to reverse or antagonize the action of nondepolarizing muscle relaxants. Also called **cholinergic.**

parasympathomimetic drug. See **cholinergic.**

parataxic distortion (pær'ətæk'sik), a defense mechanism in which current interpersonal relationships are perceived and judged according to a mode of reference established by an earlier experience. See also **transference.**

parathion poisoning (pær'əthai'on), a toxic condition caused by the ingestion, inhalation, or absorption through the skin of the highly toxic organophosphorus insecticide parathion. Symptoms include nausea, vomiting, abdominal cramps, confusion, headache, lack of muscular control, convulsions, and dyspnea. Treatment calls for close observation and for immediate intravenous administration of atropine, followed by pralidoxime chloride and oxygen.

parathyroid gland, one of several small structures, usually four in number, attached to the dorsal surfaces of the lateral lobes of the thyroid gland. The parathyroid glands secrete parathyroid hormone, which helps to maintain the level of blood calcium concentration and assures normal neuromuscular irritability, blood clotting, and cell membrane permeability. Each parathyroid gland has the appearance of an oval, brownish-red disc and measures about 6 mm by 4 mm. The parathyroids are divided, according to their location, into the superior parathyroids and the inferior parathyroids. The superior parathyroids, usually two in number, are commonly situated, one on each side, on the caudal border of the cricoid cartilage beside the junction of the pharynx and the esophagus. The inferior parathyroids, also usually two in number, may be situated on the caudal edge of the lateral lobes of the thyroid gland, just caudal to the gland, or adjacent to one of the inferior thyroid veins. These glands are composed of intercommunicating columns of cells bound by connective tissue with a rich supply of capillaries. Parathyroid hypofunction usually causes tetany, which can be treated by the administration of calcium salts or parathyroid extracts.

parathyroid hormone (PH), a hormone secreted by the parathyroid glands that acts to maintain a constant concentration of calcium in the extracellular fluid. The hormone regulates absorption of calcium from the gastrointestinal tract, mobilization of calcium from the bones, deposition of calcium in the bones, and excretion of calcium in the breast milk, feces, sweat, and urine. Surgical removal of the parathyroid glands, as may inadvertently occur in thyroidectomy, results in hypocalcemia, leading to anorexia, tetany, seizures, and death if not corrected. See also **hypoparathyroidism.**

parathyroid injection, bovine parathyroid hormone.

■ INDICATION: It is prescribed to regulate blood levels of calcium, especially in the treatment of hypoparathyroidism with tetany.

■ CONTRAINDICATIONS: Hypercalcemia, tetany not caused by hypoparathyroidism, hypercalciuria, or known hypersensitivity to this drug prohibits its use.

■ ADVERSE EFFECTS: Among the most serious adverse reactions are hypercalcemia and allergic reactions.

paratrooper fracture, a fracture of the distal tibia and its malleolus, commonly occurring when an individual jumps from an elevated platform, as the back of a truck, or parachutes from an airplane and lands feet first on the ground, subjecting the ankles to extreme force.

paratyphoid fever, a bacterial infection, caused by any

Salmonella species other than *S. typhi,* characterized by symptoms resembling typhoid fever, although somewhat milder. See also **rose spots,** *Salmonella,* **salmonellosis, typhoid fever.**

paraurethral duct, one of two ducts that drain the bulbourethral glands into the vestibule of the vagina. Also called **Skene's duct.**

paravaccinia (pær'əvæksın'iə). See milker's nodule.

Paredrine, a trade name for an adrenergic (hydroxyamphetamine hydrobromide).

paregoric, a camphorated tincture of opium.

■ INDICATIONS: It is prescribed in the treatment of diarrhea and as an analgesic.

■ CONTRAINDICATIONS: Known hypersensitivity to this drug or to any opium derivative prohibits its use.

■ ADVERSE EFFECTS: There are usually no adverse reactions. Occasionally, gastrointestinal disturbances, including constipation, occur.

parenchyma (pəreng'kımə), the tissue of an organ as distinguished from supporting or connective tissue.

parenchymatous neuritis (pær'ıngkım'ətəs), any inflammation affecting the substance, axons, or myelin of the nerve. Also called **axial neuritis, central neuritis.** See also **neuritis.**

parent, a mother or father; one who bears offspring. —**parental,** *adj.*

parental generation (P₁), the initial cross between two varieties in a genetic sequence; the parents of any individual, organism, or plant belonging to an F₁ generation.

parental grief, the behavioral reactions that characterize the grieving process and result in the resolution of the loss of a child from expected or unexpected death. All persons who survive the loss of a loved one normally experience symptoms of both somatic and psychological distress, as feelings of guilt and hostility accompanied by changes in usual patterns of conduct, depending on the individual's response to the awareness of the loss. When the death of a child is expected from terminal illness, there is time for anticipatory grieving, so that parents can evaluate their relationship with the child, set priorities for the duration of time involved, and prepare for the actual death of the child. In such cases, parental grieving begins with the discovery of the diagnosis of a life-threatening condition. Parents' adjustment to the diagnosis involves a complete cycle of reactions that extends over an indefinite period of time, depending on the severity and nature of the disease. The immediate reaction is shock and disbelief, followed by acute grief at the anticipation of losing the child. Periods of depression, anger, hope, fear, and anxiety alternate during induction therapy, remission, and maintenance of the disease as parents learn to accept and cope with the situation. Heightened anticipatory grieving recurs during episodes of relapse and the parents experience increased fear, depression, and the final acceptance of death during the terminal stages of the illness. Although families can prepare themselves for the expected loss, at the time of death there is a period of acute grief, during which parents need to express their deep sorrow and anger. An extended phase of mourning follows, with the eventual resolution of grief and integration into society. In sudden, unexpected death, parents are denied the advantages of anticipatory grief and, because of the lack of time to prepare, usually have extreme feelings of guilt and remorse. The nurse can especially help such parents to assess their feelings so that they can work through them and progress through the resolution of grief and the mourning process, which in unexpected death takes a much longer period of time. The function of the nurse during all phases of parental grief is primarily supportive, and the degree of intervention depends on the family's strengths and weaknesses in coping with the crisis. Nurses can act directly, or they can help to find other potential sources of support for the parents, as extended family members, other parents who have lost children, or specific community services or agencies. A large part of the nursing support involves helping families explore new ways of coping, not only to meet the present crisis but to grow and change. Always an important nursing consideration is the education of the parents about all aspects of the child's illness, especially in terminal conditions. See also **death, grief reaction.**

parent-child relationship. See **maternal-infant bonding**

parenteral (pəren'tərəl), not in or through the digestive system. —**parenterally,** *adv.*

parenteral absorption, the taking up of substances within the body by structures other than the digestive tract.

parenteral nutrition, the administration of nutrients by a route other than through the alimentary canal, as subcutaneously, intravenously, intramuscularly, intradermally. The parenteral fluids usually consist of physiological saline with glucose, amino acids, electrolytes, vitamins, and medications. They are not nutritionally complete but maintain fluid and electrolyte balance during the immediate postoperative period and in other conditions, as shock, coma, malnutrition, and chronic renal and hepatic failures. See also **total parenteral nutrition.**

parent figure, 1. a parent or a substitute parent or guardian who cares for a child, providing the physical, social, and emotional requirements necessary for normal growth and development. 2. a person who symbolically represents an ideal parent, having those attributes that one conceptualizes as necessary for forming the perfect parent-child relationship.

parent image, a conscious and unconscious concept that a child forms concerning the roles and characteristics of the personality of the mother and father. See also **imago, primordial image.**

parenting, alteration in: actual or potential, a nursing diagnosis accepted by the Fourth National Conference on the Classification of Nursing Diagnoses. This diagnosis includes any maladjustment or marked potential for maladjustment of a mother or father to the role of parent. The etiology of the problem may be complex and may involve several factors, as lack of an available role model, lack of support, interruption of the process of bonding in the newborn period, unrealistic expectations for the self, the infant, or the partner, mental or physical illness, the presence of financial, legal, or cultural stressors, a lack of knowledge, limited cognitive ability, multiple pregnancies, or a death in the family concurrent with the birth or early infancy of the new baby. The defining characteristics of the condition are also multiple and may include constant complaints about the sex or the appearance of the new child; verbal self-assessment of inadequacy in the parental role; expressed disgust about the bodily functions of the child; failure to keep health care appointments for the child; inconsistent disciplinary practices; slow growth and development in the child; and an observed need on the part of the parent to receive approval from others. The critical defining characteristics, at least one of which must be present to make the diagnosis, include an observed lack of actions that demonstrate attachment to the child, inattentiveness to the needs of the child, inappropriate caretaking behavior, especially in toilet training and in sleep and feeding patterns, and a history of abuse or abandonment of the child. See also **nursing diagnosis.**

Parents Anonymous, a self-help group for parents who have abused their children or who feel that they are prone to maltreat them. The organization offers support and guidance, provides a forum for discussing mutual problems, and furnishes distressed parents with a positive mechanism for coping with anger by talking to another member rather than by releasing their emotions on the child. See also **child abuse.**

parepididymis, *pl.* **parepididymides.** See **paradidymis.**

paresis (pəri'sis, pær'isis), 1. slight or partial paralysis related in some cases to local neuritis. 2. a late manifestation of neurosyphilis, characterized by generalized paralysis, tremulous incoordination, transient seizures, Argyll Robertson pupils, and progressive dementia caused by degeneration of cortical neurons. Paresis resulting from untreated syphilis usually develops in the third to fifth decades but may occur at an early age in patients with congenital syphilis. Also called **dementia paralytica, general paresis, paralytic dementia.** —**paretic,** *adj.*

Parest, a trade name for a sedative-hypnotic (methaqualone hydrochloride).

paretic dementia (pəret'ik). See **general paresis.**

pareunia (pəru'niə). See **coitus.**

Pargel, a trade name for a gastrointestinal fixed-combination drug containing an adsorbant (kaolin) and a protectant (pectin).

pargyline hydrochloride (par′jəlin), a monoamine oxidase (MAO) inhibitor used as an antihypertensive.

■ INDICATION: It is prescribed in the treatment of moderate to severe hypertension.

■ CONTRAINDICATIONS: As with all MAO inhibitors contraindications include pheochromocytoma, malignant hypertension, hyperthyroidism, renal failure, concomitant use of sympathomimetic drugs, foods high in tyramine, alcoholic beverages, or hypersensitivity to this drug prohibits its use. It is not given to children under 12 years of age.

■ ADVERSE EFFECTS: Among the most serious adverse reactions are hepatotoxicity, orthostatic hypotension, hyperexcitability, constipation, and dry mouth. MAO inhibitors produce many adverse drug interactions.

paries (peir′iiz), *pl.* **parietes** (pərai′itiz). the wall of an organ or cavity in the body. —**parietal,** *adj.*

parietal (pərai′itəl), **1.** of or pertaining to the outer wall of a cavity. **2.** of or pertaining to the parietal bone of the skull, as the parietal lobe of the brain.

parietal bone, one of a pair of bones that form the sides of the cranium. Each parietal bone has two surfaces, four borders, and four angles and articulates with five bones: the opposite parietal, occipital, frontal, temporal, and sphenoid.

parietal lobe, a portion of each cerebral hemisphere that occupies the parts of the lateral and the medial surfaces that are covered by the parietal bone. On the lateral surface of the hemisphere the parietal lobe is separated from the frontal lobe by the central sulcus and from the temporal lobe by an imaginary line that extends from the posterior ramus of the lateral sulcus toward the occipital pole. On the parietal lobe the postcentral sulcus runs parallel with the central sulcus, so that the postcentral gyrus lies between them. The intraparietal sulcus extends posteriorly from the middle of the postcentral sulcus toward the occipital pole and joins the transverse occipital sulcus near the occipital pole. The part of the parietal lobe posterior to the postcentral sulcus is divided by the horizontal intraparietal sulcus into the superior and the inferior parietal lobules. On the medial surface of the hemisphere the parietooccipital sulcus separates the parietal and the occipital lobes. Compare **central lobe, frontal lobe, occipital lobe, temporal lobe.**

parietal lymph node, one of the small oval glands that filter the lymph coursing through the lymphatic vessels in the walls of the thorax or through the lymphatic vessels associated with the larger blood vessels of the abdomen and the pelvis. The parietal lymph nodes of the thorax include the sternal nodes, intercostal nodes, and diaphragmatic nodes. The parietal lymph nodes of the abdomen and pelvis include the common iliac nodes, epigastric nodes, external iliac nodes, iliac circumflex nodes, internal iliac nodes, lumbar nodes, and sacral nodes. See also **lymph, lymphatic system, lymph node.**

parietal pain, a sharp sensation of distress in the parietal pleura, aggravated by respiration and thoracic movements and caused by pneumonia, empyema, pneumothorax, asbestosis, tuberculosis, neoplasm, or the accumulation of fluid resulting from heart, liver, or kidney disease. Noxious stimuli do not cause pain in the visceral pleura. Pain arising from the parietal pleura lining the chest wall is perceived over the involved area, but that arising from the central part of the diaphragm is referred to the posterior shoulder area; pain from the costal portions of the diaphragm is referred to the adjacent thoracic wall.

parietal peritoneum, the portion of the largest serous membrane in the body that lines the abdominal wall. Compare **visceral peritoneum.** See also **peritoneal cavity.**

parieto-occipital, of or pertaining to the parietal and the occipital bones or lobes.

parieto-occipital sulcus, a groove on each cerebral hemisphere marking the division of the parietal and occipital lobes of the brain. Also called **occipitoparietal fissure.**

Parinaud's syndrome (pær′ənouz), a term often used to refer to conjunctivitis that is usually unilateral, follicular, and followed by enlargement of the preauricular lymph nodes and tenderness. The syndrome is frequently caused by infection with a species of the microorganism *Leptothrix.* It may also be associated with other infections, as tularemia, cat-scratch fever, and lymphogranuloma venereum. Also called **ophthalmoplegia, Parinaud's oculoglandular syndrome.**

parity, **1.** (in obstetrics) the classification of a woman by the number of live-born children and still-births she has delivered at more than 28 weeks of gestation. Commonly, parity is noted with the total number of pregnancies and represented by the letter "P" or the word "para." A para 4 (P4) gravida 5 (G5) has had four deliveries after 28 weeks and one abortion or miscarriage before 28 weeks. Currently, a more complete system is in use in which the total number of pregnancies is followed by the number of deliveries at term, the number of premature infants, the number of abortions or miscarriages before 28 weeks gestation, and the number of children living at present. This system may be written as TPAL. **2.** (in epidemiology) the classification of a woman by the number of live-born children she has delivered.

parkinsonism, a neurologic disorder characterized by tremor, muscle rigidity, hypokinesia, a slow shuffling gait, difficulty in chewing, swallowing, and speaking, caused by various lesions in the extrapyramidal motor system. Signs and symptoms of parkinsonism resemble those of idiopathic Parkinson's disease and may develop during or following acute encephalitis and in syphilis, malaria, and poliomyelitis. Parkinsonism frequently occurs in patients treated with antipsychotic drugs, as amitriptyline, chlorpromazine, fluphenazine, loxapine, thioridazine, and other phenothiazine derivatives. See also **Parkinson's disease.**

Parkinson's disease, a slowly progressive, degenerative, neurologic disorder characterized by resting tremor, pill rolling of the fingers, a masklike facies, shuffling gait, forward flexion of the trunk, and muscle rigidity and weakness. It is usually an idiopathic disease of persons over the age of 60, though it may occur in younger persons, especially following acute encephalitis or carbon dioxide, metallic, or other poisoning. Typical pathologic changes are destruction of neurons in basal ganglia, loss of pigmented cells in the substantia nigra, and depletion of dopamine in the caudate nucleus, putamen, and pallidum, structures in the neostriatum which normally contain high levels of the neurotransmitter dopamine. Signs and symptoms of Parkinson's disease, which include drooling, increased appetite, intolerance to heat, oily skin, emotional instability, and defective judgment, are increased by fatigue, excitement, and frustration. Intelligence is rarely impaired. Palliative and symptomatic treatment of the disease focuses on correcting the imbalance between depleted dopamine and abundant acetylcholine in the striatum, since dopamine normally appears to inhibit excitatory cholinergic activity in this brain area. Levodopa, a dopamine precursor which crosses the blood-brain barrier, may be used, but many patients experience side effects, as nausea, vomiting, insomnia, orthostatic hypotension, and mental confusion. Carbidopa-levodopa, which contains an inhibitor of the enzyme dopa decarboxylase, limits peripheral metabolism of levodopa and thus causes fewer side effects. Anticholinergic drugs, as benztropine mesylate, biperiden, procyclidine, and trihexyphenidyl, may be used as therapeutic agents but often cause ataxia, blurred vision, constipation, dryness of the mouth, mental disturbances, slurred speech, and urinary urgency or retention. Amantadine hydrochloride, an antiviral drug with antiparkinsonian activity, promotes the accumulation of dopamine in extracellular or synaptic sites, but the therapeutic effectiveness may not last more than three months in some patients; side effects, as mental confusion, visual disturbances, and seizures, occur infrequently. Patients with the disease are encouraged to continue to work and remain active as long as possible and to prevent the spine from bending forward by lying prone on a firm mattress and by walking with the hands folded behind the back. Hand tremor is less apparent if the patient grasps the arms of the chair when seated. Some patients may be treated by surgical procedures in which cautery, excision, or the injection of alcohol or liquid nitrogen is used to destroy portions of the globus

pallidus to relieve rigidity or of the thalamus to alleviate tremor. Also called **paralysis agitans.**

Parlodel, a trade name for a dopamine receptor against bromocriptine mesylate.

Parnate, a trade name for an antidepressant (tranylcypromine sulfate).

paromomycin sulfate (pær'əmoumai'sɪn), an oral antiamebic aminoglycoside antibiotic.

■ INDICATION: It is prescribed in the treatment of intestinal amebiasis.

■ CONTRAINDICATIONS: Intestinal inflammation, intestinal obstruction, or known hypersensitivity to this drug prohibits its use.

■ ADVERSE EFFECTS: Among the most serious reactions are gastrointestinal distress and diarrhea.

paronychia (pær'ɔnɪk'iə), an infection of the fold of skin at the margin of a nail. Treatment includes hot compresses or soaks, antibiotics, and, possibly, surgical incision and drainage. Compare **onychia.**

paroophoritis (pær'ouof'ərai'tɪs), 1. inflammation of the paroophoron. 2. inflammation of the tissues surrounding the ovary.

paroophoron (pær'ouof'ɔron), a small vestigial remnant of the mesonephros, consisting of a few rudimentary tubules lying in the broad ligament between the epoophoron and the uterus. It is most evident in very young girls. Compare **epoophoron.**

parotid duct (pɔrot'ɪd), a tubular canal, about 7 cm long, that extends from the anterior part of the parotid gland to the mouth. It crosses the masseter after leaving the parotid gland, pierces the buccinator, runs for a short distance obliquely forward between the buccinator and the mucous membrane of the mouth, and opens on the oral surface of the cheek through a small opening opposite the second upper molar tooth. As the parotid duct crosses the masseter, it receives the duct from the accessory portion of the parotid gland. The duct, which has a thick wall, is about four millimeters in diameter over most of its length but narrows considerably at the opening into the mouth. Also called **Stensen's duct.** See also **parotid gland.**

parotid gland, one of the largest pair of salivary glands that lie at the side of the face just below and in front of the external ear. The main part of the gland is superficial, somewhat flattened and quadrilateral, and lies between the ramus of the mandible, the mastoid process, and the sternocleidomastoideus. It is wide superiorly and reaches nearly to the zygomatic arch, inferiorly tapering near the angle of the mandible. The rest of the gland is wedge-shaped and extends deeply toward the pharyngeal wall. It is enclosed in a capsule continuous with the deep cervical fascia. The parotid duct starts at the anterior part of the gland and opens on the inside of the cheek opposite the second upper molar. Compare **sublingual gland, submandibular gland.** See also **salivary gland.**

parotitis (pær'ətai'tıs), inflammation or infection of one or both parotid salivary glands. See also **mumps.**

-parous, a combining form meaning 'pertaining to the quantity of offspring produced simultaneously or to the method of gestation': *quadriparous, uniparous, viviparous.*

parovarium. See **epoöphoron.**

paroxysm (pær'əksız'əm), **1.** a marked, usually episodic increase in symptoms. **2.** a convulsion, fit, seizure, or spasm. — **paroxysmal,** *adj.*

paroxysmal cold hemoglobinuria (PCH), a rare autoimmune disorder characterized by hemolysis and hematuria, associated with exposure to cold.

paroxysmal hemoglobinuria, the sudden passage of hemoglobin in urine, occurring following local or general exposure to low temperatures, as in paroxysmal cold hemoglobinuria. See also **Marchiafava-Micheli disease.**

paroxysmal labyrinthine vertigo. See **Menière's disease.**

paroxysmal nocturnal dyspnea (P.N.D.), a disorder characterized by sudden attacks of respiratory distress, usually occurring after several hours of sleep in a reclining position, most commonly caused by pulmonary edema resulting from congestive heart failure. The attacks are often accompanied by coughing, a feeling of suffocation, cold sweat, and tachycardia with a gallop rhythm. Sleeping with the head propped up on pillows may prevent dyspneic paroxysms at night, but treatment of the underlying cause is required to prevent fluid from accumulating in the lungs.

paroxysmal nocturnal hemoglobinuria (PNH), a disorder characterized by intravascular hemolysis and hemoglobinuria. It occurs in irregular episodes of several days duration, especially at night. The basic defect in the red blood cell is an unusual sensitivity to lysis by complement or a deficiency or absence of acetylcholinesterase. The etiology of the condition is unknown, but it is seen in association with abnormalities of the function of the bone marrow. Occurring predominantly in adults between 25 and 45 years of age, it is characterized by abdominal pain, back pain, and headache. Its course may be complicated by thrombotic episodes and by iron deficiency, owing to excessive loss of hemoglobin. Therapy includes blood transfusion and the oral or parenteral administration of iron. Corticosteroids are sometimes employed and found useful; treatment of thromboses may require anticoagulant therapy.

parrot fever. See **psittacosis.**

parry fracture (pær'i). See **Monteggia's fracture.**

pars (parz), a part, as the pars abdominalis esophagi. Also called **part.**

Parsidol, a trade name for an antiparkinsonian (ethopropazine hydrochloride).

part, a portion of a larger area, as the condylar part of the occipital bone. Also called **pars.**

part-, a combining form meaning 'of or related to childbirth': *parturient, parturifacient, parturiometer.*

parthenogenesis (par'thənoujen'əsıs), a type of nonsexual reproduction in which an organism develops from an unfertilized ovum, as in many lower animals. Initiation of the development of the unfertilized ovum may be artificially induced through mechanical or chemical stimulation. — **parthenogenetic, parthenogenic,** *adj.*

partial breech extraction. See **assisted breech.**

partial cleavage, mitotic division of only part of a fertilized ovum into blastomeres, usually the activated cytoplasmic portion surrounding the nucleus; restricted division. Compare **total cleavage.** See also **meroblastic.**

partial placenta previa, placenta previa in which the placenta is implanted in the lower uterine segment and partially covers the internal os of the uterine cervix. As the cervix dilates in labor, the portion of the placenta that lies over the cervix is separated, causing bleeding from the villous spaces of the uterine wall. Depending on the degree of separation, the bleeding may be scant or severe, resulting in hemorrhage that is life-threatening to the mother and the baby. Treatment may require Caesarean section if the pressure of the presenting part of the baby is not sufficient to tamponade the bleeding site, stopping the hemorrhage. Diagnosis of partial placenta previa may be made before bleeding occurs by ultrasonic visualization or digital palpation in the course of prenatal examination. See also **placenta previa.**

partial pressure, the pressure exerted by any single gas in a mixture of gases.

partial thromboplastin time (PTT), a test for detecting coagulation defects of the intrinsic system by adding activated partial thromboplastin to a sample of test plasma and to a control sample of normal plasma. The time required for the formation of a clot in test plasma is compared with that in the normal plasma. A delayed clotting time suggests an abnormality in one or more factors of the intrinsic system. If indicated, specific factor abnormalities can be identified by exposing the test plasma to a series of plasma samples with known factor deficiencies and observing for coagulation, which occurs only if the test plasma provides the missing clotting factors. Partial thromboplastin time is one of the basic tests used to measure specific factor activity and to detect hemophilias. It can also be used to monitor the activity of the anticoagulant, heparin. Also called **PTT.** Compare **prothrombin time.** See also **hemostasis.**

-partite, a combining form meaning 'having the (specified) number of parts': *bipartite, tripartite, quadripartite.*

parturition (par'tyuısh'ən), the process of giving birth.

parulis (pəru'lıs). See **gumboil.**

PAS, PASA, abbreviation for **para-aminosalicylic acid.**

Pascal's principle, (in physics) a law stating that a confined liquid transmits pressure applied to it from an external source equally in all directions. Pascal's principle provides the basis for all hydraulic devices.

passive-aggressive personality, a personality characterized by passivity and aggression in which forceful actions or attitudes are expressed in an indirect, nonviolent manner, such as pouting, obstructionism, procrastination, inefficiency, stubbornness, and forgetfulness. Compare **aggressive personality, passive-dependent personality.** See also **passive-aggressive personality disorder.**

passive-aggressive personality disorder, a disorder characterized by the indirect expression of resistance to occupational or social demands, resulting in persistent, pervasive ineffectiveness, lack of self-confidence, poor interpersonal relationships, and pessimism that can lead, in severe cases, to major depression, alcoholism, or drug dependence. The behavior often reflects an unexpressed hostility or resentment stemming from a frustrating interpersonal or institutional relationship on which an individual is overdependent. Treatment may consist of behavior therapy or any of the various psychotherapeutic procedures, depending on the individual and the severity of the condition.

passive algolagnia. See **masochism.**

passive anaphylaxis. See **antiserum anaphylaxis.**

passive-dependent personality, a personality characterized by helplessness, indecisiveness, and a tendency to cling to and seek support from others. Compare **aggressive personality, passive-aggressive personality.**

passive euthanasia, the practice of allowing terminally ill and mortally injured individuals to die without taking exceptional or heroic measures to prolong their lives, as connecting their organic systems to artificial devices, which may sustain heart beats and brain waves but offer no hope for natural survival. Legal authorities, church leaders, philosophers, and commentators on ethics and morality usually treat passive euthanasia differently from active euthanasia.

passive exercise, repetitive movement of a part of the body as a result of an externally applied force or the voluntary effort of the muscles controlling another part of the body. Compare **active exercise.** See also **aerobic exercise, anaerobic exercise.**

passive immunity, a form of acquired immunity resulting from antibodies that are transmitted naturally through the placenta to a fetus or through the colostrum to an infant or artificially by injection of antiserum for treatment or prophylaxis. Passive immunity is not permanent and does not last as long as active immunity.

passive movement, the moving of parts of the body by an outside force without voluntary action or resistance by the individual. Compare **active movement.**

passive play, play in which a person does not participate actively. For younger children such activity may include watching and listening to others, observing other children or animals, listening to stories, or looking at pictures. Older children are passively entertained by games and toys that require concentration and intellectual skill, as chess, reading, listening to music, or watching television. Compare **active play.**

passive smoking, the inhalation by nonsmokers of the smoke from other people's cigarettes, pipes, and cigars. The amount of such ambient smoke inhaled by a nonsmoker is small compared to that inhaled by tobacco users, but research provides increasing evidence that passive smoking can aggravate respiratory illnesses and contribute to more serious illnesses, as cancer, and can injure the health of nonsmoking spouses and of infants and unborn babies. Studies also show that individuals with chronic heart and lung diseases and allergies to tobacco can be adversely affected by passive smoking.

passive transfer test. See **Prausnitz-Küstner test.**

passive transport, the movement of small molecules across the membrane of a cell by diffusion. Passive transport occurs when the chemicals outside a cell become concentrated and start moving into the cell, changing the intracellular equilibrium. Passive transport is essential to various processes of metabolism, as the intake of digestive products by the cells lining the intestines. Compare **active transport, osmosis.**

passive tremor, an involuntary trembling occurring when the person is at rest, one of the signs of Parkinson's disease. Also called **resting tremor.**

Pasteurella (pæs'tərel'ə), a genus of gram-negative bacilli or coccobacilli, including species pathogenic to man and domestic animals. The plague bacillus, *Pasteurella pestis,* is now called *Yersinia pestis. P. tularensis,* which causes tularemia, is now called *Francisella tularensis.* Pasteurella infections may be transmitted to man by animal bites.

pasteurization, the process of applying heat, usually to milk or cheese, for a specified period of time for the purpose of killing or retarding the development of pathogenic bacteria. **—pasteurize,** *v.*

pasteurized milk, milk that has been treated by heat to destroy pathogenic bacteria. By law, pasteurization requires a temperature of 145°F to 150°F for not less than 30 minutes, followed by a temperature of 161°F for 15 seconds, followed by immediate cooling.

past health, (in a health history) an overall summary of the person's general health to date, including past injuries, allergies, surgical procedures, immunizations, hospitalizations, and obstetric and psychiatric history. The past health history is obtained from the person or the person's family at the initial interview and becomes part of the permanent record.

Patau's syndrome, a complex of birth defects owing to trisomy of chromosome 13 and occurring in approximately one in five thousand births. Affected newborns are tiny, prone to apneic spells, severely mentally retarded, and have a variety of physical abnormalities, as cleft lip, cleft palate, deafness, and cardiovascular and brain anomalies. Approximately 70 per cent die before reaching the age of six months, and fewer than 20 per cent survive beyond the first year. Also called **trisomy D syndrome.**

patch test, a skin test for identifying allergens, especially those causing contact dermatitis. The suspected substance (food, pollen, animal fur, etc.), is applied to an adhesive patch that is placed on the patient's skin. Another patch, with nothing on it, serves as a control. After a certain period of time (usually 24 to 48 hours), both patches are removed. If the skin under the suspect patch is red and swollen and the control area is not, the test is said to be positive, and the subject is probably allergic to that substance. Compare **Prausnitz-Küstner test, radio-alergosorbent test.**

patek. See **yaws.**

patella (pətel′ə), a flat, triangular bone at the front of the knee joint, having a pointed apex that attaches to the ligamentum patellae. The convex, anterior surface of the bone is perforated for the passage of nutrient vessels and covered by an expansion from the tendon of the quadriceps femoris. Also called **knee cap.**

patellar ligament, the central portion of the common tendon of the quadriceps femoris. The ligament is a strong, flat, ligamentous band, about 8 cm long, attached proximally to the apex and the adjoining margins of the patella and distally to the tuberosity of the tibia. Its superficial fibers are continuous over the front of the patella with those of the tendon of the quadriceps femoris.

patellar reflex, a deep tendon reflex, elicited by a sharp tap on the tendon just distal to the patella, normally characterized by contraction of the quadriceps muscle and extension of the leg at the knee. The reflex is hyperactive in disease of the pyramidal tract above the level of the second lumbar vertebra. Also called **knee-jerk reflex, quadriceps reflex.** See also **deep tendon reflex.**

patent, the condition of being open and unblocked, as a patent airway or a patent anus.

patent ductus arteriosus (PDA), an abnormal opening between the pulmonary artery and the aorta caused by failure of the fetal ductus arteriosus to close after birth. The defect, which is seen primarily in premature infants, allows blood from the aorta to flow into the pulmonary artery and to recirculate through the lungs where it is reoxygenated and returned to the left atrium and left ventricle, causing an increased workload on the left side of the heart and increased pulmonary vascular congestion and resistance. Clinical manifestations include cardiomegaly, especially of the left atrium and left ventricle, dilated

ascending aorta, bounding pulses from increased systolic pressure, tachycardia, and a typical machinery-like murmur that is heard during all of systole and most of diastole. Characteristic auscultatory and radiological findings are sufficient to confirm diagnosis so that cardiac catheterization is not necessary. Correction is delayed until the child is old enough to tolerate surgery and to allow time for spontaneous closure. Untreated complications include congestive heart failure, pulmonary vascular disease, calcification of the ductal site, and infective endocarditis. See also **congenital cardiac anomaly.**

paternal engrossment. See **bonding.**

Paterson-Kelly syndrome, a condition of the digestive system associated with iron deficiency anemia, characterized by the development of esophageal webs in the upper esophagus, making swallowing of solids difficult. The webs are easily ruptured during esophagoscopy and tube feeding and can produce hemorrhage. When the hemoglobin count is improved, the webs disappear. Also called **Plummer-Vinson syndrome.**

path-. See **patho-.**

-path, 1. a combining form meaning 'one suffering from a (specified) illness': *cardiopath, endocrinopath, neuropath.* 2. a combining form meaning 'one who treats illness by a (specified) system': *dermopath, naprapath, naturopath.*

-pathetic, a combining form meaning 'pertaining to emotions': *antipathetic, apopathetic, sympathetic.* Also **-pathetical.**

Pathibamate, a trade name for a gastrointestinal, fixed-combination drug containing an anticholinergic (tridihexethyl chloride) and a sedative (meprobamate).

-pathic, 1. a combining form meaning 'referring to an illness or affected part of the body': *angiopathic, encephalopathic, hemopathic.* 2. a combining form meaning 'referring to a form or system of treatment': *homeopathic, naturopathic, physiopathic.*

Pathilon, a trade name for an anticholinergic (tridihexethyl chloride).

Pathilon with Phenobarbital, a trade name for a gastrointestinal, fixed-combination drug containing Pathilon and a sedative-hypnotic (phenobarbital).

patho-, path-, a combining form meaning 'of or related to disease': *pathocrinia, pathoformic, pathography.*

pathogen (pæth′əjən), any microorganism capable of producing disease. — **pathogenic,** *adj.*

pathogenesis, the source or cause of an illness or abnormal condition.

pathognomonic (pəthog′nəmon′ik), (of a sign or symptom) specific to a disease or condition, as Koplik's spots on the buccal and lingual musosa, which are indicative of measles.

pathognomonic symptom. See **symptom.**

pathologic absorption, the taking up by the blood of an excretory or morbid substance.

pathological anatomy, (in applied anatomy) the study of the structure and morphology of the tissues and cells of the body as related to disease.

pathological diagnosis, a diagnosis arrived at by an examination of the substance and function of the tissues of the body, especially of the abnormal developmental changes in the tissues by histologic techniques of tissue examination.

pathologic fracture. See **neoplastic fracture.**

pathologic mitosis, any cell division that is atypical, asymmetrical, or multipolar and results in the unequal number of chromosomes in the nuclei of the daughter cells. It is indicative of malignancy, as occurs in cancer and the genetic anomalies.

pathologic myopia, a type of progressive nearsightedness characterized by changes in the fundus of the eye, posterior staphyloma, and deficient corrected acuity.

pathologic retraction ring, a ridge that may form around the uterus at the junction of the upper and lower uterine segments during the prolonged second stage of an obstructed labor. The lower segment is abnormally distended and thin, while the upper segment is abnormally thick. The ring which may be seen and felt abdominally, is a warning of impending uterine rupture. Also called **Bandl's ring.** Compare **physiologic retraction ring, constriction ring.**

pathologist, a physician who specializes in the study of disease, usually in a hospital, school of medicine, or research institute or laboratory. A pathologist usually specializes in autopsy, clinical, or surgical pathology.

pathology, 1. the study of the characteristics, causes, and effects of disease, as observed in the structure and function of the body. 2. **cellular pathology,** the study of cellular changes in disease. 3. **clinical pathology,** the study of disease by the use of laboratory tests and methods. – **pathologic,** *adj.*

pathomimicry. See **Munchausen's syndrome.**

pathophysiology, the study of the biological and physical manifestations of disease as they correlate with the underlying abnormalities and physiologic disturbances. Pathophysiology does not deal directly with the treatment of disease; rather, it explains the processes within the body that result in the signs and symptoms of a disease. – **pathophysiologic,** *adj.*

pathway, 1. a network of neurons that provides a transmission route for nerve impulses from any part of the body to the spinal cord and the cerebral cortex or from the central nervous system to the muscles and organs. Neural pathways in the body are the somatic sensory pathways and the somatic motor pathways. 2. a chain of chemical reactions that produces various compounds in critical sequence, as the Embden-Meyerhof pathway.

-pathy, 1. a combining form meaning a 'suffering or illness' of a specified sort: *gynecopathy, nephropathy, psy-*chopathy. 2. a combining form meaning a 'therapy for suffering': *homeopathy, osteopathy.*

patient, 1. a recipient of a health-care service. 2. a health-care recipient who is ill or hospitalized. 3. a client in a health-care service.

patient day (P.D.), a unit in a system of accounting used by health care facilities and health care planners. Each day represents a unit of time during which the services of the institution or facility were used by a patient, thus fifty patients in a hospital for one day would represent fifty patient days.

patient interview, a systematic interview of a patient, the purpose of which is to obtain information that can be used to develop an individualized plan for care. Also called **client interview.**

patient mix, 1. the distribution of demographic variables in a patient population, often represented by the percentage of a given race, age, sex, or ethnic derivation. 2. the distribution of indications for admission in a patient population, as surgical, maternity, or trauma.

patient record, a collection of documents that provides a record of each episode in which a person visited or sought treatment and received care or a referral for care from a health care facility. The record is confidential and is usually held by the facility, and the information in it is released only to the person, or with the person's written permission. It contains the initial assessment of the person's health status, the health history, laboratory reports of tests performed, notes by nurses and physicians regarding the daily condition of the person, and notes by consultants, as well as order sheets, medication sheets, admission records, discharge summaries, and other pertinent data. A problem-oriented medical record also contains a master problem list. The patient record is often a collection of papers held in a folder, but, increasingly, hospitals are computerizing the records after every discharge, making the past record available on visual display terminals. Also called *Informal.* **chart.**

Patient's Bill of Rights, a list of patient's rights promulgated by the American Hospital Association. It offers some guidance and protection to patients by stating the responsibilities that a hospital and its staff have toward patients and their families during hospitalization, but it is not a legally binding document.
(See next page for table)

Paul's tube, a large-bore glass drainage tube with a projecting rim, used in performing an enterostomy. Also called **Paul-Mixter tube.**

Pautrier microabscess (pɔ'triei), an accumulation of intensely staining mononuclear cells in the epidermis, characterizing malignant lymphoma of the skin, especially mycosis fungoides. See also **mycosis fungoides.**

Pauwel's fracture (pɑu'əlz), a fracture of the proximal femoral neck with varying degrees of angulation.

Pavabid, a trade name for a smooth-muscle relaxant (papaverine hydrochloride).

Pavacap, a trade name for a smooth-muscle relaxant (papaverine hydrochloride).

paraffin method, (in surgical pathology) a method used in preparing a selected portion of tissue for pathologic examination. The tissue is fixed, dehydrated, and infiltrated and embedded in paraffin, forming a block that is cut with a microtome into slices 8 μm thick. This method, which is more commonly used than the frozen-section method, is slower and therefore not used during surgery.

Paveril Phosphate, a trade name for a vasodilator (dioxyline phosphate).

Paverine, a trade name for a smooth muscle relaxant (papaverine hydrochloride).

pavor (pei'vor), a reaction to a frightening stimulus characterized by excessive terror. Kinds of pavor are **pavor diurnus, pavor nocturnus.**

pavor diurnus (daiər'nəs), a sleep disorder occurring in children during daytime sleep in which they cry out in alarm and awaken in fear and panic. See also **sleep terror disorder.**

pavor nocturnus (noktər'nəs), a sleep disorder occurring in children during nighttime sleep that causes them to cry out in alarm and awaken in fear and panic. See also **nightmare, sleep terror disorder.**

Pavulon, a trade name for a neuromuscular blocking agent (pancuronium bromide), used as an adjunct to anesthesia.

Payr's clamp (pai'ərz), a clamp used in gastrointestinal surgery.

Pb, symbol for **lead.**

PBI, abbreviation for **protein-bound iodine.**

PC, abbreviation for **professional corporation.**

PCH, abbreviation for **paroxysmal cold hemoglobinuria.**

Pco_2, symbol for **partial pressure of carbon dioxide.** See **partial pressure.**

PCP, abbreviation for **phencyclidine hydrochloride.**

Pd, symbol for **palladium.**

P.D., abbreviation for **patient day.**

PDA, abbreviation for **patent ductus arteriosus.**

PDR, abbreviation for *Physician's Desk Reference.*

PE, abbreviation for **pulmonary embolism.**

P1E1, P2E1, P3E1, P4E1, P6E1, trade names for ophthalmic fixed-combination drugs containing a cholinergic (pilocarpine hydrochloride) and an adrenergic (epinephrine bitartrate). The numbers indicate the per cent of each ingredient in the solution; for example, P2E1 contains 2 per cent pilocarpine HCl and 1 per cent epinephrine bitartrate.

Péan's forceps (peianz'), *Obsolete* a basic hemostatic clamp.

pearly penile papules. See **hirsutoid papilloma of the penis.**

pearly tumor. See **cholesteatoma.**

Pearson's product movement correlation, (in statistics) a statistical test of the relationship between two variables measured in interval or ratio scales. Correlations computed fall between $+1.00$ and -1.00.

pecilo-. See **poikilo-.**

pectin, a gelatinous substance found in fruits and succulent vegetables that is used as the setting agent for jams and jellies and as an emulsifier and stabilizer in many foods. It also adds to the diet bulk necessary for proper gastrointestinal functioning. See also **dietary fiber.**

pectineus (pektin'iəs), the most anterior of the five medial femoral muscles. It arises from the pectineal line and inserts in a rough line on the femur extending distally and caudally from the lesser trochanter to the linea aspera. The muscle is innervated by a branch of the femoral nerve containing fibers from the second, the third, and the fourth lumbar nerves, and it functions to flex and adduct the thigh and to rotate it medially. Compare **adductor brevis, adductor longus, adductor magnus, gracilis.**

pector-, a combining form meaning 'of or pertaining to the breast': *pectoralgia, pectoriloquy, pectorophony.*

pectoralis major, a large muscle of the upper chest wall that acts on the joint of the shoulder. Thick and fan-shaped, it arises from the clavicle, the sternum, the cartilages of the second to the sixth ribs, and the aponeurosis of the obliquus externus abdominis. It inserts by a flat wide tendon into the crest of the greater tubercle of the humerus. The pectoralis major is innervated by the medial and lateral pectoral nerves from the brachial plexus, which contain fibers from the fifth, sixth, seventh, and eighth cervical nerves and by fibers from the first thoracic nerve. The pectoralis major serves to flex, adduct, and medially rotate the arm in the shoulder joint.

pectoralis minor, a thin, triangular muscle of the upper chest wall beneath the pectoralis major. The base arises from the third, fourth, and fifth ribs on their upper, outer surfaces. It inserts as a flat tendon into the corocoid process of the scapula. The pectoralis minor is innervated by the medial pectoral nerve from the brachial plexus, which contains fibers from the eighth cervical and the first tho-

racic nerves, and it functions to rotate the scapula, to draw it down and forward, and to raise the third, the fourth, and the fifth ribs in forced inspiration. Compare **pectoralis major, subclavius.**

ped-. See **pedo-.**

-ped, **1.** a combining form meaning a 'creature possessing feet of a (specified) sort or quantity': *biped, quadruped.* **2.** a combining form meaning 'possessing feet of a (specified) sort or quantity': *taliped.* Also **-pede.**

-pedal. See **-pedic**[1].

pederosis, paederosis (ped'ərou'sis). See **pedophilia.**

pedia-, ped-, pedo-, a combining form meaning 'of or pertaining to a child': *pediatric, pediatrician, pediatrics.*

-pedia, a combining form meaning 'compendium of knowledge': *orthopedia, pharmacopedia, logopedia.* Also **-paedia.**

Pediaflor, a trade name for a dental preparation (sodium fluoride), used as prophylaxis against dental caries in children.

Pedialyte, a trade name for a nutritional supplement containing various electrolytes.

Pediamycin, a trade name for an antibacterial (erythromycin ethylsuccinate).

pediatric anesthesia, a subspecialty of anesthesiology dealing with the anesthesia of neonates, infants, and children up to the age of 12.

pediatric dosage, the determination of the correct amount, frequency, and total number of doses of a medication to be administered to a child or infant. Such variables as the age, weight, body surface area, and the ability of the child to absorb, metabolize, and excrete the medication must be considered as well as the expected action of the drug, possible side effects, and potential toxicity. Various formulas have been devised to calculate pediatric dosage from a standard adult dose, although the most reliable method is to use the proportional amount of body surface area to body weight, based on one of the formulas. See also **Clark's rule, Cowling's rule, Young's rule.**

pediatric hospitalization, the confinement of a child or infant in a hospital for diagnostic testing or therapeutic treatment. Regardless of age or the degree of illness or injury, hospitalization constitutes a major crisis in the life of a child, and the emotional trauma elicits various behavioral reactions that the nurse must recognize and be prepared to cope with in order to facilitate recovery. The dominant factors influencing stress, which vary according to the child's developmental age, previous experience with illness, and the seriousness of the condition, include separation from the parents and familiar environment, disruption of routine patterns of daily life, loss of independence, and worry about bodily injury or painful experiences. The nurse can minimize stress by preparing the child and family through prehospital counseling; by encouraging active parental participation in the care of the child through rooming-in facilities or frequent visits; by maintaining as normal a daily routine as possible, especially with eating, sleeping, hygiene, and play activities; by explaining all hospital procedures and the immediate and long-term prognosis in terms that the child can easily understand; and by providing support and guidance for parents and siblings. The nurse may also use the hospital experience to foster an improved parent-child relationship and to teach other members of the family about proper health care. Emergency admission greatly increases the emotional trauma of hospitalization, making the role of the nurse in counteracting negative reactions even more significant.

pediatrician (pi'diətrɪʃ'ən), **pediatrist** (pi'diæt'rɪst), a physician who specializes in pediatrics.

pediatric nurse practitioner (PNP), a nurse practitioner who, by advanced study and clinical practice, as in a master's degree program in pediatric nursing, has gained expert knowledge in the nursing care of infants and children. See also **pediatric nursing.**

pediatric nursing, the branch of nursing concerned with the care of infants and children. Pediatric nursing requires knowledge of normal psychomotor, psychosocial, and cognitive growth and development as well as of the health problems and needs of people in this age group. Preventive care and anticipatory guidance are integral to the practice of pediatric nursing. See also **pediatric nurse practitioner.**

pediatric nutrition, the maintenance of a proper, well-balanced diet, consisting of the essential nutrients and the adequate caloric intake necessary to promote growth and sustain the physiological requirements at the various stages of development. Nutritional needs vary considerably with age, level of activity, and environmental conditions, and they are directly related to the rate of growth. In the prenatal period, growth is totally dependent on adequate maternal nutrition. During infancy the need for calories, especially in the form of protein, is greater than at any postnatal period because of the rapid increase in both height and weight. From the toddler through the preschool and middle childhood years, growth is uneven and occurs in spurts, with a subsequent fluctuation in appetite and calorie consumption. In general, the average child expends 55 per cent of energy on metabolic maintenance, 25 per cent on activities, 12 per cent on growth, and 8 per cent on excretion. The accelerated growth phase during adolescence demands greater nutritional requirements, although food habits are often influenced by emotional factors, peer pressure, and fad diets. Inadequate nutrition, especially during critical periods of growth, results in retarded development or illness, as anemia from deficiency of iron or scurvy from deficiency of vitamin C. An important function of the nurse is to give nutritional guidance and teach good eating habits. A special problem is overfeeding in the early childhood years, which may lead to obesity or hypervitaminosis. See also **dietary allowances,** specific vitamins.

pediatrics, a branch of medicine concerned with the development and care of children. Its specialties are the particular diseases of children and their treatment and prevention. — **pediatric,** *adj.*

pediatric surgery, the special preparation and care of the child undergoing surgical procedures for injuries, deformities, or disease. In addition to the usual fears and emotional trauma of illness and hospitalization, the child is especially concerned about being anesthetized. Younger children worry more about what will happen to them and how they will feel after awakening from anesthesia, whereas the older child fears the operation itself and possible death, the loss of control while under anesthesia, and any change in body image or mutilation of parts. The role of the nurse is to prepare the child psychologically and physically for the particular surgical procedure and any postoperative reactions, to offer support to the parents and involve them as much as possible in the care, both before and after surgery, and to explain immediate and long-term prognoses. See also **pediatric hospitalization.**

-pedic[1], a combining form meaning 'of or pertaining to children or their treatment': *gymnopedic, orthopedic.* Also **-paedic.**

-pedic[2], a combining form meaning 'referring or pertaining to the feet': *arthrosteopedic, talipedic, velocepedic.* Also **-pedal.**

pedicle clamp (ped'ɪkəl), a locking surgical forceps used for compressing blood vessels or pedicles of tumors during surgery. Also called **clamp forceps.**

pediculicide (pɪdɪk'yulɪsaɪd'), any of a group of drugs that kill lice.

pediculosis (pədɪk'yulou'sɪs), infestation with blood-sucking lice. **Pediculosis capitis** is infestation of the scalp with lice. **Pediculosis corporis** is infestation of the skin of the body with the lice. **Pediculosis palpebrae** is infestation of the eyelids and eyelashes with lice. **Pediculosis pubis** is infestation of the pubic hair region with lice. See also **crab louse, louse.**

■ OBSERVATIONS: Infestation with lice causes intense itching, often resulting in excoriation of the skin and secondary bacterial infection. Frequently, only the eggs of the lice may be seen. Body lice lay eggs in the seams of clothing; crab and head lice attach their eggs to hairs. Lice are spread by direct contact with infested clothing, people, or toilet seats. Body lice may transmit certain diseases, among them relapsing fever, typhus, and trench fever.

■ INTERVENTION: Treatment includes the topical use of 1 per cent lindane as shampoo, lotion, or cream, or of malathion 0.5 per cent lotion. After applying the pediculocide, the eggs are combed out of the hair with a fine-toothed comb. Lice and eggs on the eyelashes require topical treatment with an ophthalmic ointment containing 0.25 per cent physostigmine. Infestation sometimes may be prevented by avoiding contact with the organism and by washing and ironing any clothing or bedding that may be infested.

Pediculosis pubis. See **crab louse.**

pedigree, 1. line of descent; lineage; ancestry. 2. (in genetics) a chart that shows the genetic makeup of a person's ancestors, used in the Mendelian analysis of an inherited characteristic or disease in a particular family. Specific stylized symbols, usually plain and shaded or partially shaded squares and circles, are used, respectively, to designate normal males and females, those affected by the disease or trait, and those who are heterozygote carriers. The generations are numbered with Roman numerals at the left with the most recent at the bottom, and members within each generation are designated by Arabic numerals from left to right according to age, the oldest at the left. The inquiry begins with the siblings of the affected person and proceeds to the parents and grandparents and any of their immediate relatives. See also **Punnett square.**

pedo-[1], a combining form meaning 'of or related to a child': *pedodontics, pedogenesis, pedophilia.*

pedo-[2], **ped-, pedia-,** a combining form meaning 'of or pertaining to the foot': *pedodynamometer, pedograph, pedopathy.*

pedodontics (ped'ədon'tıks), a field of dentistry devoted to the diagnosis and the treatment of dental problems affecting children.

pedogenesis, paedogenesis (pı'doujen'əsıs), the production of offspring by young or larval forms of animals, often by parthenogenesis, as in certain amphibians. — **pedogenetic,** *adj.*

pedophilia, paedophilia (ped'əfıl'ıə, ped'əfıl'yə), 1. an abnormal interest in children. 2. (in psychiatry) a psychosexual disorder in which the fantasy or act of engaging in sexual activity with prepubertal children is the preferred or exclusive means of achieving sexual excitement and gratification. It may be heterosexual or homosexual. Also called **pederosis.** See also **paraphilia.** — **paedophilic, pedophilic,** *adj.*

peds, *Informal.* pediatrics.

peduncle (pıdəŋ'kəl), a stemlike connecting part, as the pineal peduncle or a peduncle graft. — **peduncular, pedunculate,** *adj.*

PEEP, abbreviation for **positive end expiratory pressure.**

Peeping Tom. See **voyeur.**

peer review, (in nursing) an appraisal by professional coworkers of equal status of the way an individual nurse conducts practice, education, or research. The appraisal uses accepted standards as measures against which performance is weighed. See also **Professional Standards Review Organization.**

Peganone, a trade name for an anticonvulsant (ethotoin).

Pel-Ebstein fever (pel'eb'stin), a recurrent fever, occurring in cycles of several days or weeks, characteristic of Hodgkin's disease or malignant lymphoma. Also called **Murchison fever.**

Pelger-Huët anomaly (pel'gərhyu'ət), an inherited disorder characterized by granulocytes with unusually coarse nuclear material and a dumbbell-shaped or peanut-shaped nuclei. Normal nuclear segmentation does not seem to occur, but there are no associated findings. See also **band.**

pell-, a combining form meaning 'of or pertaining to the skin': *pellagra, pellicle, pellicular.*

pellagra (pəlei'grə, pəlæg'rə), a disease resulting from a deficiency of niacin or tryptophan or a metabolic defect that interferes with the conversion of the precursor tryptophan to niacin. It is frequently seen in individuals whose diet consists primarily of maize, which is deficient in tryptophan. It is characterized by scaly dermatitis, especially of the skin exposed to the sun, glossitis, inflammation of the mucous membranes, diarrhea, and mental disturbances, including depression, confusion, disorientation, hallucination, and delirium. Treatment and prophylaxis consist of administration of niacin and tryptophan, usually in conjunction with other vitamins, particularly thiamine and riboflavin, and a well-balanced diet containing foods rich in these nutrients, as liver, eggs, milk, and meat. Kinds of pellagra are **pellagra sine pellagra, typhoid pellagra.** Compare **kwashiorkor.** — **pellagrous,** *adj.*

pellagra sine pellagra, a form of pellagra in which the characteristic dermatitis is not present. See **pellagra.**

pelo-, a combining form meaning 'of or pertaining to mud': *pelohemia, pelology, pelotherapy.*

pelvic, of or pertaining to the pelvis.

pelvic brim, the curved top of the bones of the hip extending from the anterior superior iliac crest in front on one side around and past the sacrum to the crest on the other side. Below the brim is the pelvis.

pelvic cellulitis, bacterial infection of the parametrium, occurring after childbirth or spontaneous therapeutic abortion. It represents an extension of infection via the blood vessels and lymphatics from a primary wound infection in the external genitalia, perineum, vagina, cervix, or uterus. It is characterized by fever, uterine subinvolution, chills and sweats, abdominal pain that spreads laterally, and, if untreated, by the formation of a large abscess and by signs of peritonitis. It is seen most commonly between the third and the ninth days after delivery or abortion. Treatment includes an antibiotic, bed rest, intravenous fluids, and drainage of any abscess that forms. Oxytocics may be given to augment involution.

pelvic classification, 1. a process in which the anatomic and spatial relationships of the bones of the pelvis are evaluated, usually to assess the adequacy of the pelvic structures for vaginal delivery. Caldwell-Moloy's system of classification is the one most commonly used. **2.** one of the types in a classification system of the pelvis.

pelvic congestion syndrome, an abnormal gynecologic condition characterized by chronic low back pain, dysuria, dysmenorrhea, vague lower abdominal pain, vaginal discharge, and dyspareunia. The cause of the symptoms is not understood; formerly it was thought that the vascular bed of the area was distended with blood, but this has not been demonstrated. Women between 25 and 45 years of age are most often affected.

pelvic diaphragm, the caudal aspect of the body wall, stretched like a hammock across the pelvic cavity and comprised of the levator ani and the coccygeus muscles. It holds the abdominal contents, supports the pelvic viscera, and is pierced by the anal canal, the urethra, and the vagina. It is reinforced by fasciae and muscles associated with these structures and with the perineum.

pelvic examination, a diagnostic procedure in which the external and internal genitalia are physically examined using inspection, palpation, percussion, and auscultation. It is performed regularly throughout a woman's life, usually every one to three years.

■ METHOD: The woman empties her bladder, disrobes, and puts on an examining gown. She is made as comfortable as possible in the dorsal lithotomy position, her feet in stirrups and her buttocks at the very edge of the foot of the examining table, and is then draped. Breast examination is often carried out at this point, prior to the pelvic examination, and the lower abdomen is palpated. Particular attention is paid to the suprapubic area to detect any masses extending from the pelvis above the symphysis and to the groin to detect inguinal lymphadenopathy or hernia. If a mass is felt, percussion may be performed to delineate it. If pregnancy is suspected, palpation and percussion of the uterus and auscultation of fetal heart tones are attempted. The examiner then moves to the stool at the foot of the table between the patient's legs. The labia majora are spread apart to permit inspection of the clitoris, the urethral meatus, the labia minora, and the vaginal vestibule. Any swelling, discoloration, lesion, scar, cyst, discharge, or bleeding is noted. Skene's and Bartholin's glands and ducts are palpated and milked, and any secretions expressed are evaluated and a specimen is spread on culture media. The tone of the perineal and paravaginal musculature is assessed. Cystocele, rectocele, or varying degrees of uterine descensus may be observed as the woman is asked to bear down. Because lubricating jelly interferes with cytologic and bacteriologic studies, the speculum examination is usually performed without using the jelly. The speculum is warmed, lubricated with warm water, and introduced gradually. The examiner is careful to direct the speculum along the axis of the vagina, which is at an angle of approximately forty-five degrees to the axis of the table if the woman is lying flat. The speculum may need to be moved lightly from side to side in order to slip it over the vaginal rugae. The woman is advised that she may feel a stretching sensation; the speculum is gently opened and its position is adjusted to hold the vaginal folds out of the way to reveal the cervix. The color and condition of the vaginal epithelium are observed and the position, size, and quality of the superficial epithelium are evaluated. Specimens for bacteriologic study are obtained before the Pap test. For the Pap test, scrapings of the endocervix and the cervix and a sample of the vaginal secretions are secured on a Pap stick and an applicator and lightly spread on labeled glass slides. The slides are immediately sprayed with a fixative or dipped in it. The speculum is then closed, rotated slightly, removed from the vagina and rinsed or placed directly in a germicidal solution. In the bimanual part of the examination, two gloved fingers are well lubricated and inserted slowly and gently into the vagina. The examiner uses the opposite hand to apply pressure to the lower abdomen in several positions and directions to bring the uterus, tubes, and ovaries into positions in which they may be felt. The size, shape, position, mobility, and consistency of the organs and tissues are evaluated, and any tenderness or discomfort is noted. Rectal or rectovaginal examination is then performed. Prior to the insertion of a finger in the anus, lateral pressure is applied to the sphincter and the woman is urged to bear down lightly to relax the muscle and minimize discomfort.

■ OUTCOME CRITERIA: Pelvic examination may demonstrate many pelvic abnormalities and diseases. Cytologic and bacteriologic specimens are conveniently obtained. A pelvic examination cannot be satisfactorily performed without the cooperation of the woman being examined; inadequate relaxation, obesity, extensive scarring, pelvic tenderness, and heavy vaginal discharge may also preclude an adequate examination.

■ NURSING ORDERS: Minor unthoughtfulness or inadvertent movement may cause tension and make the examination more difficult for the woman and for the examiner. Instruments, culture materials, a light, drapes, and a gown are all made ready beforehand. The table, instruments, and drapes are clean and warm. Materials from previous examinations are not in evidence. The woman is forewarned of what to expect at each step of the examination. Gentleness and quietness are exercised at all times. Upon completion of the examination the woman is helped to slide well back on the table before sitting up. Syncope following pelvic examination is uncommon but not rare; there is risk of injury should the patient faint and fall from the examining table. The woman is observed briefly after sitting up before being left alone. She is then given tissues, a sanitary napkin or tampon, and a private area in which to dress.

pelvic inferior aperture.   See **pelvic outlet.**

pelvic inflammatory disease (PID),   any inflammatory condition of the female pelvic organs, especially one caused by bacterial infection.

■ OBSERVATIONS: Characteristics of the condition include fever, foul-smelling vaginal discharge, pain in the lower abdomen, abnormal uterine bleeding, pain with coitus, and tenderness or pain in the uterus, affected ovary, or Fallopian tube on bimanual pelvic examination. If an abscess has already developed, a soft, tender, fluid-filled mass may be palpated.

■ INTERVENTION: The cause of the inflammatory process is determined and treated. A specimen of cervical mucus is obtained for bacteriologic identification and antibiotic sensitivity. A sonogram may be useful in visualizing an abscess or fluid-filled Fallopian tube. Bed rest and antibiotics are usually prescribed, but surgical drainage of an abscess may be required. Severe, fulminating PID may necessitate hysterectomy to avoid fatal septicemia. If the cause is infection by gonococci or chlamydiae, the woman's sexual partners are also treated with antibiotics.

■ NURSING CONSIDERATIONS: The full course of prescribed antibiotics is taken. Inadequate therapy may result in chronic PID or in the formation of an abscess. If an abscess has already developed, PID may become chronic and recurrent. Severe PID is usually very painful: the woman may be prostrate and require narcotic analgesia. Recurrent or severe PID often results in scarring of the Fallopian tubes, obstruction, and infertility.

pelvic inlet,   (in obstetrics) the inlet to the true pelvis, bounded by the sacral promontory, the horizontal rami of the pubic bones, and the top of the symphysis pubis. As the infant must pass through the inlet to enter the true pelvis and to be born vaginally, the anteroposterior, transverse, and oblique dimensions of the inlet are important measurements to be made in assessing the pelvis in pregnancy. There are three anteroposterior diameters: the true conjugate, the obstetric conjugate, and the diagonal conjugate. The true conjugate can be measured only on x ray, as it extends from the sacral promontory to the top of the symphysis pubis. Its normal measurement is 11 or more cm. The obstetric conjugate is the shortest of the three, as it extends from the sacral promontory to the thickest part of the pubic bone. It measures 10 or more cm. The diagonal conjugate is the most easily and commonly assessed, as it extends from the lower border of the symphysis pubis to the sacral promontory. It normally measures 11.5 or more cm. The inlet is said to be contracted when any of these diameters is smaller than normal. The anteroposterior diameters are shorter than normal in the small gynecoid and platypellard pelvis. The transverse diameter of the inlet is bounded by the inferior border of the walls of the iliac bones and is measured at the widest point. It is normally close to 13.5 cm but may

be less in the small gynecoid pelvis and anthropoid pelvis. The oblique diameters of the pelvis extend from the juncture of the sacrum and ilium to the emminence on the ilium on the opposite side of the pelvis. Each oblique diameter measures nearly 13 cm. This dimension is smaller than normal in the small gynecoid and platypelloid pelves. See also **android pelvis, anthropoid pelvis, gynecoid pelvis, platypelloid pelvis.**

pelvic kidney.   See **ptotic kidney.**

pelvic minilaparotomy (mĭn′ĭlăp′ərot′əmi),   a surgical operation in which the lower abdomen is entered through a small, suprapubic incision, performed most often for tubal sterilization but also for diagnosis and treatment of eccyesis, ovarian cyst, endometriosis, and infertility. It may be performed as an alternative to laparoscopy, often on an outpatient basis. Compare **laparoscopy.** See also **bilateral tubal ligation, sterilization.**

■ METHOD: General, regional, or local anesthesia is administered. The patient is placed in the supine position and the abdomen is prepared with antiseptic solution and draped with sterile drapes. Often, pelvic examination is performed, and a device with a long handle is inserted into the uterus or attached to the cervix; the handle extends from the vagina and provides a means of manipulating the uterus during surgery. An incision a few centimeters long is made, usually transversely, in the suprapubic fold of skin in the midline, and is then carried down through the fat and fascia, between the rectus abdominis muscles, and into the peritoneal cavity. Bleeders are ligated, and a small self-retaining retractor is placed in the incision. The smallness of the incision permits intraperitoneal palpation with one or, at most, two fingers. With the placement of small packs to exclude the bowel from the operative field, the various pelvic structures can usually be exposed, inspected, and palpated. A laparoscope may be used for visualization. Each uterine tube is brought up into the incision and the sterilization or other procedure is performed. After hemostasis is assured each tube is replaced in its anatomic position and the incision is closed in layers. A small, sterile dressing is applied, and the vaginal instruments are removed.

■ OUTCOME CRITERIA: Because the abdomen is entered under direct vision in minilaparotomy, the risk of injury by the trocar, inherent in laparoscopy, is reduced. Minilaparotomy can be performed in the presence of pelvic adhesions or other abnormalities that may preclude laparoscopy. Minilaparotomy affords direct rather than telescopic observation of the pelvic viscera, so there are likely to be fewer blind spots. Tissues are directly palpated and surgery is performed in hand. The abdominal cavity need not be distended with gas, and the risks of limitation of diaphragmatic excursion and vagotonia from peritoneal distention are avoided. Often, minilaparotomy may be performed faster and less expensively than laparoscopy. Though small, the minilaparotomy incision is considerably larger than is the usual laparoscopy incision. It is, therefore, less pleasing cosmetically, as well as more painful in the postoperative period. Minilaparotomy is often performed on an outpatient basis, although some women require brief postoperative hospitalization.

■ NURSING ORDERS: The prospect of sterilization and its effects may add to the anxiety of undergoing surgery; therefore, preoperatively and postoperatively the woman may require emotional support and information in answer to her questions. As incisional pain in the postoperative period may mask the pain of intraperitoneal bleeding, vital signs are monitored frequently. Tachycardia, and hypotension that are not alleviated by analgesia may be signs of hemorrhage or injury to the bowel. Prior to discharge, outpatients are carefully instructed in the postoperative danger signs and in the proper care of the incision at home. Arrangements are made for follow-up examination.

pelvic outlet, the space surrounded by the bones of the lower portion of the true pelvis. In men, the shape of the pelvic outlet is narrower than in women, but this is of no clinical significance. In women, the shape and size of the pelvis varies and is of importance in childbirth. The shapes are classified by the length of the diameters as compared to each other and by the thickness of the bones. The diameters of the outlet are the anteroposterior, from the symphysis pubis to the coccyx, and the intertuberous, laterally from one to the other ischial tuberosity. See also **pelvic classification.**

pelvic pain, pain in the pelvis, as occurs in appendicitis, oophoritis, and endometritis. The character and onset of pelvic pain and any factors that alleviate or aggravate it are significant in making a diagnosis.

pelvic pole, the end of the axis at which the breech of the fetus is located.

pelvic rotation, one of the five major kinematic determinants of gait, involving the alternate rotation of the pelvis to the right and the left of the central axis of the body. The usual pelvic rotation occurring at each hip joint in most healthy individuals is approximately 4° to each side of the central axis. Pelvic rotation occurs during the stance phase of gait and involves a medial to lateral circular motion. With normal locomotion or walking considered a progressive sinusoidal movement, pelvic rotation serves to minimize the vertical displacement of the center of gravity of the body during the act of walking. Analysis of pelvic rotation is often a factor in diagnosing various orthopedic diseases, deformities, and abnormal bone conditions and in the correction of pathological gaits. Compare **knee-ankle interaction, knee-hip flexion, lateral pelvic displacement, pelvic tilt.**

pelvic tilt, one of the five major kinematic determinants of gait that lowers the pelvis on the side of the swinging

lower limb during the walking cycle. Through the action of the hip joint the pelvis tilts laterally downward, adducting the lower limb in the stance phase of gait and abducting the opposite extremity in the swing phase of gait. The knee joint of the non-weight-bearing limb flexes during its swing phase to allow the pelvic tilt, which helps minimize the vertical displacement of the center of gravity of the body, thus conserving energy during walking. Pelvic tilt is often a factor in the diagnosis and treatment of various orthopedic diseases, deformities, and abnormal conditions and in the analysis and the correction of pathological gaits. Compare **knee-ankle interaction, knee-hip flexion, lateral pelvic displacement, pelvic rotation.**

pelvic varicocele. See **ovarian varicocele.**

pelvifemoral, of or pertaining to the structures of the hip joint, especially the muscles and the area around the bony pelvis and the head of the femur that make up the pelvic girdle.

pelvifemoral muscular dystrophy, a form of limb-girdle muscular dystrophy that begins in the pelvic girdle. Also called **Leyden-Moebius muscular dystrophy.**

pelvimetry (pelvim′itri), the act or process of determining the dimensions of the bony birth canal. Kinds of pelvimetry are **clinical pelvimetry, x-ray pelvimetry.**

pelvis (pel′viz), *pl.* **pelves.** the lower portion of the trunk of the body, composed of four bones, the two innominate bones laterally and ventrally and the sacrum and coccyx posteriorly. It is divided into the greater or false pelvis and the lesser or true pelvis by an oblique plane passing through the sacrum and the pubic symphysis. The greater pelvis is the expanded portion of the cavity situated cranially and ventral to the pelvic brim. The lesser pelvis is situated distal to the pelvic brim, and its bony walls are more complete than those of the greater pelvis. The inlet and outlet of the pelvis have three important diameters, anteroposterior, oblique, and transverse. The pelvis of a woman is usually less massive but wider and more circular than that of a man. – **pelvic,** *adj.*

pemoline (pem′əlin), a central nervous system stimulant.

■ INDICATION: It is prescribed in the treatment of attention-deficit disorder in children.

■ CONTRAINDICATION: Known hypersensitivity to this drug prohibits its use.

■ ADVERSE EFFECTS: Some of the more serious adverse reactions are insomnia, gastrointestinal disturbances, rash, convulsions, and hallucinations.

pemphigoid (pem′figoid), a bullous disease resembling pemphigus, distinguished by thicker-walled bullae arising from erythematous macules or urticarial bases. Oral lesions are uncommon. It may rarely be associated with an internal malignancy. Spontaneous remission occasionally occurs after several years. Treatment is usually with oral corticosteroids. Compare **pemphigus.**

pemphigus (pem′fɪgəs, pemfai′gəs), an uncommon, serious disease of the skin and mucous membranes, characterized by thin-walled bullae arising from apparently normal skin or mucous membrane. The bullae rupture easily, leaving raw patches. The person loses weight, becomes weak, and is subject to major infections. Treatment with corticosteroids and other immunosuppressive medications has changed the prognosis of this disease from an almost universally fatal one to a controllable problem compatible with a nearly normal life. The cause is unknown. Compare **pemphigoid.**

Pen A, a trade name for an antibacterial (ampicillin).

Penapar VK, a trade name for an antibacterial (penicillin V potassium).

Penbritin, a trade name for an antibacterial (ampicillin).

Penbritin-S, a trade name for an antibacterial (ampicillin sodium).

pendular nystagmus, an undulating involuntary movement of the eyeball.

penetrance, (in genetics) a variable factor that modifies basic patterns of inheritance. It is the regularity with which an inherited trait is manifest in the person who carries the gene. If a gene always produces its effect on the phenotype, it is fully and completely penetrant. Achondroplasia is caused by a fully penetrant gene; if the gene is present achondroplasia results. If a gene produces its effect less frequently than 100 per cent of the time it is not fully penetrant. Retinoblastoma develops in 90 per cent of the children carrying the gene; in 10 per cent of children, the gene is nonpenetrant. – **penetrant,** *adj.*

penfluridol, an investigational antipsychotic drug, chemically similar to pimozide.

-penia, a combining form meaning a '(specified) deficiency': *glycopenia, lipopenia, thyropenia.*

penicillamine (D-penicillamine), a chelating agent.

■ INDICATIONS: It is prescribed to bind with and remove metals from the blood in the treatment of heavy metal (especially lead) poisoning, in cystinuria, and in Wilson's disease. It is also prescribed as a palliative in the treatment of sclerosis and rheumatoid arthritis when other medications have failed.

■ CONTRAINDICATIONS: Known hypersensitivity to this drug or penicillamine-related aplastic anemia prohibits its use. It is not given during pregnancy or to patients who have kidney dysfunction.

■ ADVERSE EFFECTS: Among the more serious adverse reactions are fever, rashes, and blood dyscrasias. Severe bone marrow depression and immune disorders have been associated with long term use of this drug. D-penicillamine is less toxic than the L-form and much of the reported toxicity is due to the use of the L or DL forms.

penicillic acid (pen′ɪsɪl′ɪk), an antibiotic compound isolated from various species of the fungus *Penicillium.*

penicillin, any one of a group of antibiotics derived from cultures of species of the fungus *Penicillium* or produced semisynthetically. Various penicillins administered orally or parenterally for the treatment of bacterial infections exert their antimicrobial action by inhibiting the biosynthesis of cell wall mucopeptides during active multiplication of the organisms. Penicillin G (benzylpenicillin), a widely used therapeutic agent for meningococcal, pneumococcal, and streptococcal infections, syphilis, and a number of other diseases, is rapidly absorbed when injected intramuscularly or subcutaneously, but it is inactivated by gastric acid and hydrolyzed by penicillinase produced by most strains of *Staphylococcus aureus.* Penicillin V (phenethicillin) is also active against gram-positive cocci, with the exception of penicillinase-producing staphylococci, and, since it is resistant to gastric acid, it is effective when administered orally. Penicillins resistant to the action of the enzyme penicillinase (beta-lactamase) are cloxacillin, dicloxacillin, methicillin, nafcillin, and oxacillin. Ampicillin, carbenicillin, and hetacillin are broad-spectrum penicillins that are active against gram-negative organisms, including *Escherichia coli, Hemophilus influenzae, Neisseria gonorrhoeae, Proteus mirabilis,* and species of *Pseudomonas.* Hypersensitivity reactions are common in patients receiving penicillin and may appear in the absence of prior exposure to the drug, presumably because of unrecognized exposure to a food or other substance containing traces of the antibiotic. The most common hypersensitivity reactions are rash, fever, and bronchospasm, followed in frequency by vasculitis, serum sickness, and exfoliative dermatitis. Some patients develop severe erythema multiforme accompanied by headache, fever, arthralgia, and conjunctivitis (Stevens-Johnson syndrome); the most frequent cause of anaphylactic shock is an injection of penicillin.

penicillinase (pen′əsɪl′əneis), an enzyme elaborated by certain bacteria, including many strains of staphylococci, which inactivates penicillin and thereby promotes resistance to the antibiotic. A purified preparation of penicillinase, derived from cultures of saprophytic, spore-forming *Bacillus cereus,* is used in the treatment of adverse reactions to penicillin. Also called **beta-lactamase.**

penicillinase-producing staphylococci, strains of staphylococcal organisms that elaborate the penicillin inactivating enzyme penicillinase (beta-lactamase) and thereby resist the bacteriocidal action of the antibiotic.

penicillinase-resistant antibiotic, an antimicrobial agent that is not rendered inactive by penicillinase, an enzyme produced by certain bacteria, especially by strains of staphylococci. The semisynthetic penicillins, cloxacillin sodium, dicloxacillin sodium, methicillin sodium, nafcillin sodium, and oxacillin sodium, resist the action of penicillinase and are used in treating infections caused by staphylococci that elaborate the enzyme.

penicillinase-resistant penicillin, one of the semisynthetic penicillins derived from *Penicillium,* a genus of mold. Among these drugs are cloxacillin sodium, dicloxacillin sodium, methicillin sodium, nafcillin sodium, and oxacillin sodium. They are not inactivated by the enzyme penicillinase (beta-lactamase), which is produced by certain strains of staphylococci. These resistant antibiotics are used in treating infections caused by organisms that elaborate the enzyme.

penicillin G, an antibacterial.
■ INDICATIONS: It is prescribed in the treatment of many infections.
■ CONTRAINDICATIONS: Known hypersensitivity to this drug or to any penicillin prohibits its use.
■ ADVERSE EFFECTS: Among the more serious adverse effects are allergic reactions that vary from minor skin rashes to anaphylaxis. Nausea and diarrhea occur frequently.

penicillin G benzathine, a long-acting, depot form of penicillin.
■ INDICATIONS: It is used in the treatment of group A beta-hemolytic streptococcal pharyngitis, group A beta-hemolytic streptococcal pyoderma, and syphilitic infection occurring outside the central nervous system. It is given by deep intramuscular injection to achieve steady concentrations in the plasma and to slow systemic absorption from the repository in the muscle over a period of 12 hours to several days.
■ CONTRAINDICATION: Hypersensitivity to this drug or to other penicillins prohibits its use.
■ ADVERSE EFFECTS: The most serious adverse reaction is anaphylaxis. The most common side effects are maculopapular rash, urticarial rash, fever, bronchospasm, vasculitis, serum sickness, and exfoliative dermatitis.

penicillin phenoxymethyl. See **penicillin V.**

penicillin V, an antibacterial.
■ INDICATIONS: It is prescribed in the treatment of susceptible infections.
■ CONTRAINDICATION: Known hypersensitivity to this drug or to any penicillin prohibits its use.
■ ADVERSE EFFECTS: Among the more serious adverse reactions are anaphylaxis and urticaria.

penicilliosis (pen'ısıl'iou'sis), pulmonary infection caused by fungi of the genus *Penicillium.*

Penicillium (pen'ısıl'iəm), a genus of fungi, some species of which have been tentatively linked to disease in man. Penicillin G is obtained from *Penicillium chrysogenum* and *P. notatum.*

penile cancer, a rare malignancy of the penis occurring in uncircumcised men and associated with genital herpesvirus infection and poor personal hygiene. Smegma may be a causative factor, but the specific substance and mechanism are unknown. Leukoplakia or the flat-topped papules of balanitis xerotica obliterans may be pre-malignant lesions, and the velvety, red, painful papules of Queyrat's erythroplasia are penile squamous cell carcinoma in situ. Cancer of the penis usually presents as a local mass or a bleeding ulcer and metastasizes early in its course. Surgical treatment involves partial or total amputation of the penis and excision of inguinal nodes and adjacent tissue when necessary. Radiotherapy is often used preoperatively and postoperatively. Methotrexate or bleomycin may also be administered, especially in metastatic disease.

penis, the external reproductive organ of a man, homologous with the clitoris of a woman. It is attached with ligaments to the front and sides of the pubic arch and is composed of three cylindrical masses of cavernous tissue covered with skin. The corpora cavernosa penis surround a median mass called the corpus spongiosum penis, which contains the greater part of the urethra. The subcutaneous fascia of the penis is directly continuous with that of the scrotum, which contains the testes.

-pennate, a combining form meaning 'having feathers': *bipennate, pennate, unipennate.*

penniform (pen'ıfɔrm), of or pertaining to the shape of a feather, especially the patterns of muscular fasciculi that correlate with the range of motion and the power of muscles. Penniform fasciculi converge on one side of certain tendons. Muscles with more fasciculi have greater power but less range of motion than muscles with fewer fasciculi. Compare **bipenniform, multipenniform.**

Pensyn, a trade name for an antibacterial (ampicillin).

pent-, penta, a combining form meaning 'five': *pentaploid, pentose, pentoside.*

pentaerythritol tetranitrate (pen'tɔerıfh'rɔtol), a coronary vasodilator.
■ INDICATION: It is prescribed for the relief of angina pectoris.
■ CONTRAINDICATION: Known hypersensitivity to this drug prohibits its use.
■ ADVERSE EFFECTS: Among the most serious reactions are hypotension and allergic reactions. Headaches and flushing also may occur.

pentamidine, an antiprotozoal that is available only from the Center for Disease Control. It is sometimes prescribed in the treatment of trypanosomiasis and leishmaniasis, but, owing to its extreme toxicity, other agents are usually prescribed.

pentaploid, (pen'tɔploid). **pentaploidic.** See **polyploid.**

pentazocine hydrochloride (pentei'zɔsin), an analgesic.
■ INDICATION: It is prescribed for the relief of moderate to severe pain.
■ CONTRAINDICATION: Known hypersensitivity to this drug prohibits its use. It is administered with caution to patients with head injury or those with a history of drug abuse and dependency.
■ ADVERSE EFFECTS: Nausea and dizziness commonly oc-

cur. Other minor problems include constipation, euphoria, and drowsiness. High dosage may cause respiratory and circulatory depression. This drug can precipitate acute withdrawal symptoms in narcotic-dependent individuals.

pentazocine lactate. See **pentazocine hydrochloride.**

Penthrane, a trade name for a general anesthetic (methoxyflurane).

Pentids, a trade name for an antibacterial (penicillin G potassium).

pentobarbital, a sedative and hypnotic.
- INDICATIONS: It is prescribed as a preoperative sedative, in the treatment of insomnia, and in the control of acute convulsive disorders.
- CONTRAINDICATIONS: Porphyria or known hypersensitivity to this drug or to other barbiturates prohibits its use. It is used with caution in patients having impaired liver function or a history of dependence on sedative or hypnotic drugs.
- ADVERSE EFFECTS: Among the more serious adverse reactions are respiratory or circulatory depression, paradoxical excitement, jaundice, or various hypersensitivity reactions. Nausea and hangover-like symptoms may be seen.

pentobarbital sodium, a sedative-hypnotic.
- INDICATION: It is prescribed in the treatment of insomnia.
- CONTRAINDICATIONS: Known hypersensitivity to barbiturates or previous addiction to sedative hypnotic drugs prohibits its use.
- ADVERSE EFFECTS: Among the most serious adverse reactions are effects attributable to depression of various systems of the body and physical dependence resulting in withdrawal symptoms on discontinuance.

pentosuria (pen'tǝsur'iǝ), a rare condition, in which pentose is found in the urine, caused by a genetically transmitted error of metabolism.

Pentothal Sodium, a trade name for a barbiturate drug (thiopental sodium), used as a general anesthetic and as an anesthetic adjuvant.

pentylenetetrazol, a central nervous system stimulant.
- INDICATIONS: It is prescribed as an analeptic to stimulate the respiratory, vagal, and vasomotor centers of the brain and to increase cerebral blood flow, especially in geriatric patients.
- CONTRAINDICATIONS: Epilepsy and low convulsive threshold prohibit its use.
- ADVERSE EFFECTS: Among the more serious adverse reactions are convulsion, confusion, and anorexia.

Pen-Vee, a trade name for an antibacterial (penicillin V).

Pen-Vee K, a trade name for an antibacterial (penicillin V potassium).

Pepper syndrome, a neuroblastoma of the right adrenal gland that usually metastasizes to the liver.

peps-, a combining form meaning 'of or pertaining to digestion': *pepsin, pepsiniferous, pepsitensin.* Also **pept-.**

-pepsia, a combining form meaning a 'state of the digestion': *anapepsia, colodyspepsia, oligopepsia.* Also **-pepsy.**

pepsin (pep'sin), an enzyme secreted in the stomach that catalyzes the hydrolysis of protein. Preparations of pepsin obtained from pork and beef stomachs are sometimes used as digestive aids. See also **enzyme, hydrolysis.**

pept-. See **peps-.**

peptic, of or pertaining to digestion or to the enzymes and secretions essential to digestion.

-peptic, 1. a combining form meaning 'pertaining to digestion': *apeptic, kolypeptic, proteopeptic.* 2. a combining form meaning 'pertaining to a (specified) condition of digestion': *dyspeptic, eupeptic, hyperpeptic.*

peptic ulcer, a sharply circumscribed loss of the mucous membrane of the stomach or duodenum or of any other part of the gastrointestinal system exposed to gastric juices containing acid and pepsin.
- OBSERVATION: Peptic ulcers may be acute or chronic. Acute lesions are almost always multiple and superficial. They may be totally asymptomatic and usually heal without scarring or other sequelae. Chronic ulcers are true ulcers: they are deep, single, persistent, and symptomatic; the muscular coat of the wall of the organ does not regenerate; a scar forms, marking the site, and the mucosa may heal completely. Peptic ulcers are caused by a combination of poorly understood factors, including an excessive secretion of gastric acid, inadequate protection of the mucous membrane, stress, heredity, and the taking of certain drugs, including the corticosteroids, certain antihypertensives, and anti-inflammatory medications. Characteristically, ulcers cause a gnawing pain in the epigastrium that does not radiate to the back, is not aggravated by a change in position, and has a temporal pattern that mimics the diurnal rhythm of gastric acidity.
- INTERVENTION: Symptomatic relief is provided with antacids and frequent, small, bland meals. The underlying cause is treated if known. Cimetidine is a new and effective drug that blocks the formation of gastric acid, but it is associated with serious adverse effects. Anticholinergic medications may slow gastric motility and diminish pain in some patients. Hemorrhage owing to perforation of the muscle and blood vessels may require surgical resection of the damaged area. The diagnosis and evaluation of peptic ulcer involves serial x-ray studies using a contrast medium, endoscopy, and analysis of the contents of the stomach and duodenum. A definitive diagnosis is important because the early signs of cancer of the stomach and duodenum are like those of peptic ulcer.
- NURSING CONSIDERATIONS: The patient is reassured that in most cases the ulcers heal completely and that the

pain may be controlled with simple measures. The nurse emphasizes the correct use of antacids and the other medications that have been prescribed. It is usually recommended that the patient eat frequent small meals consisting of foods known to be nonirritating. For many, but not all patients, fatty, highly spiced, heavy, or fibrous foods are likely to provoke pain. The use of tobacco and alcohol is discouraged.

peptide (pep'tæid), a compound composed of two or more amino acids joined by peptide bonds. See also **amino acid, polypeptide, protein.**

per-, **1.** a combining form meaning 'throughout, or completely': *peracephalus, perfuse, permeable.* **2.** a combining form meaning 'a large amount (in chemical terms)' or to designate a combination of an element in its highest valence: *peracetate, peracid, perhydride.*

Percaine, a trade name for a local anesthetic (dibucaine hydrochloride).

perceived severity, (in health belief model) a person's perception of the seriousness of the consequences of contracting a disease. Compare **perceived susceptibility.**

perceived susceptibility, (in health belief model) a person's perception of the likelihood of contracting a disease. Compare **perceived severity.**

percentage depth dose, (in radiotherapy) the amount of radiation delivered at a specified dose, expressed as a percentage of the skin dose.

percephalus, *pl.* **percephali.** a fetus or individual with a malformed head.

percept (pər'sept), the mental impression of an object that is perceived through the use of the senses.

perception, **1.** the conscious recognition and interpretation of sensory stimuli through unconscious associations, especially memory, that serve as a basis for understanding, learning, and knowing or for the motivation of a particular action or reaction. **2.** the end result or product of the act of perceiving. Kinds of perception include **depth perception, extrasensory perception, facial perception, stereognostic perception.** – **perceptive, perceptual,** *adj.*

perceptivity, the ability to receive sense impressions; perceptiveness.

perceptual defect, any of a broad group of disorders or dysfunctions of the central nervous system that interfere with the conscious mental recognition of sensory stimuli. Such conditions are caused by lesions at specific sites in the cerebral cortex that may result from any illness or trauma affecting the brain at any age or stage of development. Impairment of mental activity, cognitive processes, and emotional responses may be diffuse, as occurs in organic mental disorders, as the psychoses, delirium, and dementia and in attention deficit disorder, or they may be manifested focally, as in aphasia, apraxia, epilepsy, disor-

ders of memory, cerebrovascular disorders, and various intercranial neoplasms.

perchloromethane (pərklour'oumeth'ein). See **carbon tetrachloride.**

Percodan, a trade name for a central-nervous-system, fixed-combination drug containing narcotic analgesics (oxycodone hydrochloride and oxycodone terephthalate).

Percogesic, a trade name for a respiratory, fixed-combination drug containing an antihistaminic (phenyltoloxamine citrate) and an analgesic (acetaminophen).

percolation, **1.** the act of filtering any liquid through a porous medium. **2.** (in pharmacology) the removal of the soluble parts of a crude drug by passing a liquid solvent through it.

Percorten Acetate, a trade name for an adrenocortical steroid (desoxycorticosterone acetate).

percussion, a technique in physical examination used to evaluate the size, borders, and consistency of some of the internal organs and to discover the presence and evaluate the amount of fluid in a cavity of the body. **Immediate,** or **direct percussion** refers to percussion performed by striking the fingers directly on the body surface; **indirect, mediate,** or **finger percussion** involves striking a finger of one hand on a finger of the other hand as it is placed over the organ. See also **pleximeter, plexor.** – **percuss,** *v.,* **percussable,** *adj.*

Correct hand placement   Correct technique

PERCUSSION

percussor, a small, hammerlike diagnostic tool having a rubber head that is used to tap the body lightly in percussion. Also called **plexor.** See also **percussion.**

percutaneous (pər'kyutei'niəs), (of a procedure) performed through the skin, like the aspiration of fluid from a space below the skin using a needle, catheter, and syringe or the instillation of a fluid in a cavity or space by similar means.

percutaneous catheter placement, (in arteriography) the technique in which an intracatheter is introduced through the skin into an artery and placed at the place or structure to be studied. The puncture site is infiltrated with a local anesthetic. A special needle is inserted into the artery, and a long, flexible spring guide is passed through the needle for approximately 15 cm. The needle is then removed, the catheter is advanced to the desired position, and the guide is withdrawn. Selective angiography and other diagnostic procedures are performed using this technique. The catheter is withdrawn at the end of the procedure.

percutaneous transhepatic cholangiography, (in diagnostic radiology) a procedure for outlining the major bile ducts. A radiopaque contrast material is injected via a needle or a catheter introduced through the skin into the liver.

percutaneous transluminal coronary angioplasty (PTCA), a technique in the treatment of atherosclerotic coronary heart disease and angina pectoris in which one or more plaques in the arteries of the heart are flattened against the arterial walls, resulting in improved circulation. The procedure involves threading a catheter through the vessel to the atherosclerotic plaque and inflating and deflating a small balloon at the tip of the catheter several times, then removing the catheter. The procedure is performed under x-ray or ultrasonic visualization. When it is successful, the plaques remain compressed and the symptoms of heart disease, including the pain of angina, are decreased. The alternative to this treatment is coronary by-pass surgery, which is more expensive and dangerous and requires longer hospitalization.

Perez reflex (pɪrez'), the normal response of an infant to cry, flex the limbs, and elevate the head and pelvis when supported in a prone position with a finger pressed along the spine from the sacrum to the neck. Persistence of the reflex beyond the age of six months may indicate brain damage.

perforate, 1. to pierce, punch, puncture, or otherwise make a hole. 2. riddled with small holes. 3. (of the anus) having a normal opening; not imperforate. —**perforation,** n.

perforating fracture, an open fracture caused by a projectile, making a small surface wound.

Pergonal, a trade name for human menopausal gonadotropin.

peri-, a combining form meaning 'around': *periaxial, pericardial, pericolitis.*

Periactin Hydrochloride, a trade name for an antihistaminic and antipruritic (cyproheptadine hydrochloride).

perianal abscess, a focal, purulent, subcutaneous infection in the region of the anus. Treatment includes hot soaks, antibiotics, and, possibly, incision and drainage. If a rectal fistula or sinus track is found to be the cause of recurrent perianal abscesses, surgical excision is usually performed.

periapical (per'iæp'ɪkəl, per'iei'pɪkəl), of or pertaining to the tissues around the apex of a tooth, including the periodontal membrane and the alveolar bone.

periapical abscess, an infection around the root of a

tooth, usually a result of spread from dental caries. The abscess may extend into nearby bone, causing osteomyelitis, or, more often, it may spread to soft tissues causing cellulitis and a swollen face, or it may perforate into the oral cavity or maxillary sinus. There may be associated fever, malaise, and nausea. Treatment includes drilling into the pulp of the tooth to establish drainage and relieve pain, followed by antibiotics and later root canal therapy or tooth extraction.

periapical infection, infection surrounding the root of a tooth, often accompanied by toothache.

periarteritis (per'iar'tərai'tɪs), an inflammatory condition of the outer coat of one or more arteries and the tissue surrounding the vessel. Kinds of periarteritis are **periarteritis nodosa, syphilitic periarteritis.**

periarteritis gummosa. See **syphilitic periarteritis.**

periarteritis nodosa, a progressive, polymorphic disease of the connective tissue that is characterized by numerous large and palpable or visible nodules in clusters along segments of middle-sized arteries, particularly near points of bifurcation. This process causes occlusion of the vessel, resulting in regional ischemia, hemorrhage, necrosis, and pain. The early signs of the disease include tachycardia, fever, weight loss, and pain in the viscera. Kidney, lung, and intestinal involvement are common. Other systems and organs of the body may also be affected. Periarteritis nodosa is treated with corticosteroid medication and sometimes with cytotoxic drugs. The rate of survival four years after diagnosis is approximately fifty per cent.

pericardial artery, one of several small vessels branching from the thoracic aorta, supplying the dorsal surface of the pericardium.

pericardial tamponade. See **cardiac tamponade.**

pericardiocentesis (per'ɪkar'diousɪntɪ'sɪs), **pericardicentesis,** a procedure for drawing fluid in the pericardial space between the serous membranes by surgical puncture and aspiration of the pericardial sac.

pericarditis (per'ɪkardai'tɪs), an inflammation of the pericardium owing to trauma, malignant neoplastic disease, infection, uremia, myocardial infarction, collagen disease, or idiopathic causes.

■ OBSERVATIONS: Two stages are observed if treatment in the first stage does not halt progress of the condition to the extremely grave second stage. The first stage is characterized by fever, substernal chest pain that radiates to the shoulder or neck, dyspnea and a dry, nonproductive cough. On examination a rapid and forcible pulse, a pericardial friction rub, and a muffled heart beat over the apex are noted. The patient becomes increasingly anxious, tired, and orthopneic. During the second stage, a serofibrinous effusion develops within the pericardium, restricting cardiac activity; the heart sounds become muffled, weak, and distant on auscultation. A bulge is visible on the chest over the precordial area. If the effusion is purulent, owing to bacterial infection, a high fever, sweats, chills, and prostration also occur.

■ INTERVENTION: The person is kept in bed, and the head of the bed is elevated 45 degrees to decrease dyspnea. Hypothermia treatment may be necessary to reduce the temperature. An antibiotic or antifungal and analgesic may be ordered. Oxygen and parenteral fluids are usually given, vital signs are evaluated, and the chest is auscultated frequently. Pericardiocentesis or percardiotomy may be performed to remove accumulated fluid or to make a diagnosis.

■ NURSING CONSIDERATIONS: Emotional support of a patient being treated for pericarditis requires remaining with the person if anxiety is present and explaining all procedures thoroughly. During recovery, rest periods are planned and the person is urged to avoid fatigue and exposure to upper respiratory infections. The patient is told that symptoms of recurrence, including a fever, chest pain, and dyspnea, are to be reported.

pericardium (per′ıkar′diəm), *pl.* **pericardia.** a fibroserous sac that surrounds the heart and the roots of the great vessels. It consists of the serous pericardium and the fibrous pericardium. The serous pericardium consists of the parietal layer, which lines the inside of the fibrous pericardium, and the visceral layer, which adheres to the surface of the heart. Between the two layers is the pericardial space containing a few drops of pericardial fluid, which lubricates opposing surfaces of the space and allows the heart to move easily during contraction. Injury or disease may cause fluid to exude into the space, causing a wide separation between the heart and the outer pericardium. The fibrous pericardium, which constitutes the outermost sac and is composed of tough, white fibrous tissue lined by the parietal layer of the serous pericardium, fits loosely around the heart and attaches to large blood vessels emerging from the top of the heart but not to the heart itself. It is relatively inelastic and protects the heart and the serous membranes. If pericardial fluid or pus accumulates in the pericardial space, the fibrous pericardium cannot stretch, causing a rapid increase of pressure around the heart. – **pericardial,** *adj.*

pericholangitis (per′əkoʊlænjaɪ′tɪs), an inflammatory condition of the tissues surrounding the bile ducts in the liver. Pericholangitis is a complication of ulcerative colitis and is characterized by a recurrent fever, chills, jaundice, and, possibly, portal hypertension. Treatment of the ul-

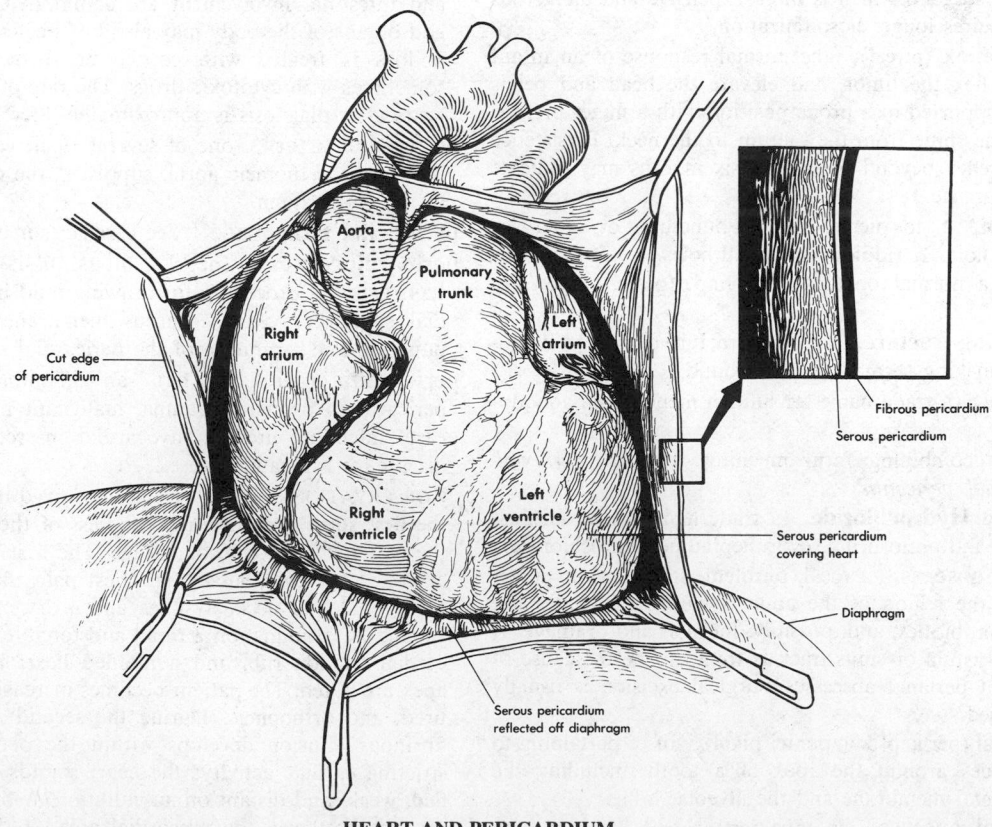

HEART AND PERICARDIUM

cerative colitis has little effect on the liver disease. See also **ulcerative colitis.**

Peridial, a trade name for a peritoneal dialysis solution containing various electrolytes and dextrose in varying concentrations.

peridural anesthesia (per'ıdur'əl). See **epidural anesthesia.**

perifolliculitis (per'ifolık'yulai'tıs), inflammation of the tissue surrounding a hair follicle. Compare **folliculitis.**

perikaryon (per'ıkær'ıon), the cytoplasm of a cell body exclusive of the nucleus and any processes, specifically the cell body of a neuron. —**perikaryontic,** adj.

perilymph (per'ılımf), the clear fluid separating the osseous labyrinth from the membranous labyrinth in the internal ear. Compare **endolymph.**

perinatal (per'ınei'təl), of or pertaining to the time and process of giving birth or being born.

perinatal death, 1. the death of a fetus weighing more than 1,000 gm at 28 or more weeks of gestation. 2. the death of an infant between birth and the end of the neonatal period.

perinatal mortality, the statistical rate of fetal and infant death, including stillbirths, from 28 weeks of gestation to the end of the neonatal period of 4 weeks after birth. Perinatal mortality is usually expressed as the number of deaths per 1,000 live births in a specific geographical area or program, in a given period of time.

perinatal physiology, the physiology of the process of giving birth or being born.

perinatologist, a physician who specializes in the practice of perinatology.

perinatology, a branch of medicine concerned with the study of the anatomy and physiology of the mother and her unborn and newborn infant and with the diagnosis and treatment of disorders occurring in them during pregnancy, childbirth, and the puerperium. —**perinatologic, perinatological,** adj.

perineal care, a cleansing procedure prescribed for cleansing the perineum after various obstetric and gynecologic procedures. Sterile or clean perineal care may be prescribed. See also **postpartum perineal care.**
■ METHOD: In the sterile procedure, the cleansing strokes always move from the vulva toward the anus and from the midline out. After each stroke, the disposable washcloth or pledget is discarded, and a new one is used for the next stroke. In sterile perineal care, a sterile basin, gloves, forceps, pledgets, and pitcher or measure containing solution are used. The draped patient is assisted into position on her back with a bedpan or on a disposable pad beneath her buttocks, and 200 to 300 ml of solution are poured over the vulva. Then pledgets moistened with the solution are used to cleanse the area more thoroughly. The pledgets are held with sterile forceps or a sterile gloved hand. The area is dried using sterile pledgets and

the bedpan is removed. The patient then changes position and lies on her side for cleansing and drying of the posterior area, always using strokes moving away from the perineal area. In providing clean perineal care, disposable washcloths, soap, and a basin or a squeeze-bottle of warm water are used. A fresh, disposable washcloth is used for each stroke. The strokes are always from anterior to posterior. Soap may be used. A fresh pad or cloth is used to remove the soap and for each drying stroke. The patient then rolls to one side and the posterior area is cleansed and dried in the same way.
■ OUTCOME CRITERIA: Sterile and clean perineal care are practiced to remove secretions or dried blood from a wound and to avoid contaminating the urethral and vaginal areas or perineal wounds with fecal matter or urine.
■ NURSING ORDERS: Perineal care is given at prescribed intervals and after urination and defecation.

perincorrhaphy (per'əniɔr'əfi), a surgical procedure in which an incision, tear, or defect in the perineum is repaired by suturing.

perineotomy (per'əniot'əmi), a surgical incision into the perineum. See also **episiotomy.**

perineum (per'ıni'əm), the part of the body situated dorsal to the pubic arch and the arcuate ligaments, ventral to the tip of the coccyx, and lateral to the inferior rami of the pubis and the ischium and the sacrotuberus ligaments. The perineum supports and surrounds the distal portions of the urogenital and gastrointestinal tracts of the body. In the female, the central fibrous perineal body between the vagina and the anus is larger than in the male, and the bulbospongiosus, which is a sphincter around the orifice of the vagina and a cover over the clitoris, does not exist in the male perineum. In men and women, the muscles are innervated by the perineal branch of the pudendal nerve. —**perineal,** adj.

period, Nontechnical. menses.

periodic, (of an event or phenomenon) recurring at regular or irregular intervals. —**peridocity,** n.

periodical mania, Obsolete. a mood disorder in which successive attacks of mania of various duration occur at regular intervals. See also **mania.**

periodic apnea of the newborn, a normal condition in the full-term newborn infant characterized by an irregular pattern of rapid breathing followed by a brief period of apnea, usually associated with rapid eye movement (REM) sleep. Apnea in the newborn not associated with REM sleep or with periodic breathing is ominous because it is symptomatic of intracranial bleeding, seizure activity, infection, pneumonia, hypoglycemia, drug depression, or various cardiac defects. See also **sudden infant death syndrome.**

periodic breathing. See **Cheyne-Stokes respiration.**

periodic deep inspiration, (in respiratory therapy) periodic deep forced inspiration of compressed gas or air in controlled ventilation. Many ventilators can be set to provide a selected number of deep respirations each hour. The process helps to prevent atelectasis. Also called **sigh.**

periodontal (per′ioudon′təl), of or pertaining to the area around a tooth, as the peridontium.

periodontal disease, disease of the tissues around a tooth, as an inflammation of the periodontal membrane or periodontal ligament.

periodontics, periodontia, a branch of dentistry concerned with the diagnosis, treatment, and prevention of diseases of the periodontium. —**periodontic, periodontal,** *adj.*

periodontist, a dentist who specializes in periodontics.

periodontitis (per′ioudontai′tis), inflammation of the periodontium, which includes the periodontal ligament, the gingiva, and the alveolar bone. See also **periodontal, periodontal disease, periodontics.**

periorbita (per′ior′bitə), the periostium of the orbit of the eye. It is continuous with the dura mater and the sheath of the optic nerve and extends a process at the margin of the orbit to form the orbital septum. The periorbita is loosely connected to the bones of the orbit, from which it can be easily detached.

periosteum (per′ios′tiəm), a fibrous vascular membrane covering the bones, except at their extremities. It consists of an outer layer of collagenous tissue containing a few fat cells and an inner layer of fine elastic fibers. Periosteum is permeated with the nerves and blood vessels that innervate and nourish underlying bone. The membrane is thick and markedly vascular over young bones but thinner and less vascular in later life. Bones that lose periosteum through injury or disease usually scale or die.

peripheral, of or pertaining to the outside, surface, or surrounding area of an organ or other structure.

peripheral acrocyanosis of the newborn, a normal, transient condition of the newborn, characterized by pale cyanotic discoloration of the hands and feet, especially the fingers and toes. The blueness fades as the baby begins to breathe easily but returns if the baby is allowed to get chilled.

peripheral glioma. See **schwannoma.**

peripheral nervous system, the motor and sensory nerves and ganglia outside the brain and spinal cord. The system consists of 12 pairs of cranial nerves, 31 pairs of spinal nerves, and the various branches of the 43 pairs in body organs. Sensory, or afferent peripheral nerves transmitting information to the central nervous system and motor, or efferent peripheral nerves carrying impulses from the brain usually travel together but separate at the cord level into a posterior sensory root and an anterior motor root. Fibers innervating the body wall are designated somatic and those supplying internal organs are termed visceral. The autonomic system includes the peripheral nerves involved in regulating cardiovascular, respiratory, endocrine, and other automatic body functions. Nerves in the sympathetic or thoracolumbar division of the autonomic system secrete norepinephrine and cause peripheral vasoconstriction, cardiac acceleration, coronary artery dilation, bronchodilation, and inhibition of peristalsis. Parasympathetic nerves constitute the craniosacral division of the autonomic system, secrete acetylcholine, and cause peripheral vasodilation, cardiac inhibition, bronchoconstriction, and stimulate peristalsis. Injury to a peripheral nerve results in loss of movement and sensation in the area innervated distal to the lesion.

peripheral plasma cell myeloma. See **plasmacytoma.**

peripheral polyneuritis. See **multiple peripheral neuritis.**

peripheral vascular disease, any abnormal condition which affects the blood vessels outside the heart and the lymphatic vessels. Different kinds and degrees of peripheral vascular disease are characterized by a variety of signs and symptoms, as numbness, pain, pallor, elevated blood pressure, and impaired arterial pulsations. Various causative factors include obesity, cigarette smoking, stress, sedentary occupations, and numerous metabolic disorders. Peripheral vascular disease in association with bacterial endocarditis may involve emboli in terminal arterioles and produce gangrenous infarctions of various distal parts of the body, as the tip of the nose, the pinna of the ear, the fingers, and the toes. Large emboli may occlude peripheral vessels and cause atherosclerotic occlusive disease. Treatment of severe cases may require amputation of gangrenous body parts. Less severe peripheral vascular problems may be treated by eliminating causative factors, especially cigarette smoking, and by the administration of various drugs, as salicylates and anticoagulants. Some kinds of peripheral vascular disease are **arteriosclerosis, atherosclerosis.**

peripheral vision, a capacity to see objects that reflect light waves falling on areas of the retina distant from the macula.

peristalsis (per′istol′sis, per′istal′sis), the coordinated, rhythmic, serial contraction of smooth muscle that forces food through the digestive tract, bile through the bile duct, and urine through the ureters.

peritoneal cavity, the potential space between the parietal and the visceral layers of the peritoneum. Normally, the two layers are in contact. The peritoneal cavity is divided by a narrow constriction into a greater sac and a lesser sac. The greater sac is the peritoneal cavity and the lesser sac is the omental bursa. The omental bursa is associated with the dorsal surface of the stomach and the surrounding structures. See also **epiploic foramen.**

peritoneal dialysis, a dialysis procedure performed to correct an imbalance of fluid or of electrolytes in the blood or to remove toxins, drugs, or other wastes normally excreted by the kidney. The peritoneum is used as a diffusible membrane. Peritoneal dialysis may be performed nightly for chronically ill children while they sleep and may also be carried out regularly at home. It is contraindicated in patients with extensive intra-abdominal adhesions, localized peritoneal infection, and gangrenous or perforated bowels, although peritonitis may itself sometimes be treated by peritoneal lavage and antibiotics, using peritoneal dialysis.

■ METHOD: Under local anesthesia, a many-eyed catheter is sutured in place and a sterile dressing is applied. The catheter is connected to the inflow and outflow tubing with a "Y" connector and the air in the tubing is displaced by the dialysate to avoid introducing air into the peritoneal cavity. The amount and the kind of dialysate and the length of time for each exchange cycle vary with the age, size, and condition of the patient. There are three phases in each cycle. During inflow, the dialysate is introduced into the peritoneal cavity. During equilibration, the dialysate remains in the peritoneal cavity; by means of osmosis, diffusion, and filtration, the needed electrolytes pass to the blood stream via the vascular peritoneum to the blood vessels of the abdominal cavity, and the waste products pass from the blood vessels through the vascular peritoneum into the dialysate. During the third phase, called outflow, the dialysate is allowed to drain from the peritoneal cavity by gravity.

■ NURSING ORDERS: The fluid is warmed to body temperature before instillation, and heparin antibiotics or other additives may be added to the dialysate. The patient's fluid balance, respirations, pulse, blood pressure, temperature, aAnd mental state are frequently evaluated, and blood glucose and electrolytes are tested regularly. The amount of fluid instilled and the amount and character of the fluid drained are noted. Bacteriologic cultures of the drainage are performed regularly, and a low-sodium, high-carbohydrate, high-fat, 20- to 40-gm protein diet is usually given. Medication for pain may be necessary. The need for dialysis and the techniques, dangers, and advantages of peritoneal dialysis are explained to the patient and the patient's family.

■ OUTCOME CRITERIA: Peritoneal dialysis may result in several complications, including perforation of the bowel, peritonitis, atelectasis, pneumonia, pulmonary edema, hyperglycemia, hypovolemia, hypervolemia, and adhesions. Peritonitis, the most common problem, is usually caused by failure to use aseptic technique and is characterized by fever, cloudy dialysate, leukocytosis, and abdominal discomfort. Dialysis may usually be continued while the infection is treated with antibiotics which are given systemically or intraperitoneally. Atelectasis and pneumonia may result from compression of the thoracic cavity, with decreased respiratory excursion and blood flow to the bases of the lungs caused by an excessive volume of dialysate in the peritoneal cavity. Dyspnea, tachypnea, rales, and

tachycardia require reevaluation of the amount of dialysate, the raising of the head of the bed, and respiratory therapy to prevent atelectasis and pneumonia. As diabetics are at risk of developing hyperglycemia, serum and urine glucose levels are monitored, and, if necessary, sorbitol may be substituted for glucose in the dialsyate. If dialysate fluid is retained in the peritoneal cavity, hypervolemia may occur, predisposing the patient to pulmonary edema and congestive failure. If the dialysate is removed too rapidly or if the dialysate used is a hypotonic glucose solution, hypovolemia may result. Adhesions often develop because of local irritation to the surrounding tissues caused by the intraperitoneal catheter.

peritoneal dialysis solution, a solution of electrolytes and other substances that is introduced into the peritoneum to remove toxic substances from the body.

peritoneoscope (per'ɪtənɪ'əskoup'). See **laparoscope.**

peritoneum (per'ɪtənɪ'əm), an extensive serous membrane that covers the entire abdominal wall of the body and is reflected over the contained viscera. It is divided into the parietal peritoneum and the visceral peritoneum. In men, the peritoneum is a closed membranous sac. In women, it is perforated by the free ends of the uterine tubes. The free surface of the peritoneum is smooth mesothelium lubricated by serous fluid which permits the viscera to glide easily against the abdominal wall and against one another. The mesentery of the peritoneum fans out from the main membrane to suspend the small intestine. Other parts of the peritoneum are the transverse mesocolon, the greater omentum, and the lesser omentum. —**peritoneal,** adj.

peritonitis (per'ɪtənaī'tɪs), an inflammation of the peritoneum produced by bacteria or irritating substances introduced into the abdominal cavity by a penetrating wound or perforation of an organ in the gastrointestinal tract or the reproductive tract. Peritonitis is caused most commonly by rupture of the vermiform appendix but also occurs following perforations of intestinal diverticuli, peptic ulcers, gangrenous gall bladders, gangrenous obstructions of the small bowel, or incarcerated hernias, as well as ruptures of the spleen, liver, ovarian cyst, or Fallopian tube, especially in ectopic pregnancy. In some cases peritonitis is secondary to the release of pancreatic enzyme, bile, or digestive juices of the upper gastrointestinal tract, and there are reports of postoperative peritonitis caused by cornstarch used to powder surgical gloves. The genera most frequently identified as causative agents in peritonitis are *Escherichia coli, Bacteroides, Fusobacterium,* anaerobic and aerobic streptococci; *Klebsiella* and *Proteus* are uncommon and *Clostridium, Staphylococcus aureus,* and gonococci are rare. Pneumococci occasionally found in peritonitis in girls are thought to enter the abdominal cavity via the vagina and Fallopian tubes.

■ OBSERVATIONS: Characteristic signs and symptoms of

peritonitis include abdominal distention, rigidity and pain, rebound tenderness, decreased or absent bowel sounds, nausea, vomiting, and tachycardia. The patient has chills and fever, breathes rapidly and shallowly, is anxious, dehydrated, unable to defecate, and may vomit fecal material. Leukocytosis, an electrolyte imbalance, and hypovolemia are usually present, and shock and heart failure may ensue.

■ INTERVENTION: The patient is placed in bed in a semi-Fowler's position with the knees flexed to facilitate breathing and localize pus in the lower abdomen. Oxygen, parenteral fluids with electrolytes, large doses of antibiotics, and emetics are administered as ordered. A nasogastric or nasointestinal tube is passed for intermittent suctioning; an indwelling catheter is inserted and a rectal tube may be used. Measurements are made of the intake and output of fluids, and the character, color, odor, and amount of drainage are noted. Blood pressure, apical pulse, and respiration are checked every one to two hours; at similar intervals the patient is turned and instructed in coughing and deep breathing. Rectal temperature, bowel sounds, and abdominal distention are checked every two to four hours. Pain is controlled with analgesia, and the dehydrated patient, whose lips tend to be dry and cracked, receives frequent mouth care. Paracentesis may be performed to withdraw ascitic fluid that is turbid or purulent in pyogenic peritonitis. Repair of the perforation or rupture responsible for the infection may be indicated, but surgery is usually delayed until the patient is stabilized. Patients who respond to antibiotic therapy receive a liquid diet when the nasogastric tube is removed and bowel sounds return and gradually progress to a diet appropriate for the disorder that caused the peritonitis.

■ NURSING CONSIDERATIONS: The patient acutely ill with peritonitis is usually very apprehensive and needs constant care.

peritonsillar abscess, an infection of tissue between the tonsil and pharynx, usually following acute follicular tonsillitis. The symptoms include dysphagia, pain radiating to the ear, and fever. Redness and swelling of the tonsil and adjacent soft palate are present. Treatment includes penicillin, warm saline irrigation, incision and drainage with suction if there is no spontaneous rupture of the abscess, and, sometimes, tonsillectomy. Also called **quinsy.** Compare **parapharyngeal abscess, retropharyngeal abscess.** See also **tonsillitis.**

Peritrate, a trade name for a vasodilator (pentaerythritol tetranitrate).

periungual (per'iərɳ'gwəl), of or pertaining to the area around the fingernails or the toenails.

perivascular goiter (per'ɪvæs'kyulər), an enlargement of the thyroid gland surrounding a large blood vessel.

perivitelline (per'ɪvɪtel'ɑin), surrounding the vitellus or yolk mass.

perivitelline space, the space between the ovum and the zona pellucida of mammals into which the polar bodies are released at the time of maturation. In some animals it is a fluid-filled space that separates the fertilization membrane from the vitelline membrane surrounding the ovum after the penetration of the spermatozoon.

perlèche (pərlesh'). See cheilosis.

permanent dentition, the eruption of the 32 permanent teeth, beginning with the appearance of the first permanent molars at about six years of age. The process is completed by age 12 or 13 except for the four wisdom teeth, which do not erupt until 18 to 25 years of age, or later. Also called **secondary dentition.** Compare **deciduous dentition.** See also **tooth.**

permanent tooth, one of the set of 32 teeth that appear during and after childhood and last until old age. In each jaw they include four incisors, two canines, four premolars, and six molars. They are divided into the permanent teeth, which replace the 20 deciduous teeth of infancy, and the superadded teeth, which include 12 molars, three on each side of the upper and lower jaws. The permanent teeth start to develop in the ninth week of fetal life with the thickening of the epithelium along the line of the future jaw. They develop from the embryonic dental lamina and dental germ tissue. As the ten permanent teeth develop in the fetus they recede into the substance of the gum behind the deciduous teeth. The permanent teeth start to calcify soon after birth; the teeth in the lower jaw proceeding somewhat faster than those in the upper jaw. The permanent first molar in the lower jaw calcifies just after birth; the permanent incisors and the canines, approximately six months later; the premolars during the second year; the second molar, at about the end of the second year, and the third molar, at about the twelfth year. The permanent teeth erupt first in the lower jaw; the first molars in about the sixth year; the two central incisors, about the seventh year; the two lateral incisors, about the eighth year; the first premolars, about the ninth year; the second premolars, about the tenth year; the canines, between the eleventh and the twelfth years; the second molars, between the twelfth and the thirteenth years; the third molars, between the seventeenth and the twenty-fifth years. The eruption of each corresponding permanent tooth in the upper jaw lags only slightly behind that of the corresponding permanent tooth in the lower jaw. The third molars in many people are badly oriented or so deeply buried in bone that they must be surgically removed. In some individuals, one or all four of the third molars may not develop completely. Compare **deciduous tooth.** See also **tooth.**

Permapen, a trade name for an antibacterial (penicillin G benzathine).

permissible dose, (in radiotherapy) the amount of radiation that may be received by an individual in a specified period of time with the expectation of no significantly harmful results.

Permitil, a trade name for a tranquilizer (fluphenazine hydrochloride).

pernicious anemia (pərnɪʃ'əs), a progressive, megaloblastic, macrocytic anemia, affecting mainly older people, that results from a lack of intrinsic factor essential for the absorption of vitamin B_{12}. The maturation of red blood cells in bone marrow becomes disordered, the posterior and lateral columns of the spinal cord deteriorate, the white blood cell count is reduced, and the polymorphonuclear leukocytes become multilobed. Extreme weakness, numbness and tingling in the extremities, fever, pallor, anorexia, and loss of weight may occur. The condition is usually treated with vitamin B_{12} injection and with folic acid and iron therapy.

pernio (pər'niou). See **chilblain.**

pero-, a combining form meaning 'maimed or deformed': *perobrachius, perodactylus, peromelus.*

perobrachius (pi'roubrei'kiəs), a fetus or individual with deformed arms.

perochirus (pi'roukai'rəs), a fetus or individual with malformed hands.

perocormus (pi'roukor'məs). See **perosomus.**

perodactylus (pi'roudæk'tələs), a fetus or an individual with a deformity of the fingers or the toes, especially the absence of one or more digits.

perodactyly, perodactylia, a congenital anomaly characterized by a deformity of the digits, primarily the complete or partial absence of one or more of the fingers or toes.

peromelia (pər'əmi'liə), **peromely** (pərom'əli), a congenital anomaly characterized by the malformation of one or more of the limbs. — **peromelus,** *n.*

peroneal, of or pertaining to the outer part of the leg, over the fibula and the peroneal nerve.

peroneal muscular atrophy, an abnormal condition characterized by the symmetrical weakening or atrophy of the foot and the ankle muscles and by hammertoes. This disease is a dominantly inherited condition and occurs in a hypertrophic neuropathy form or in a neuronal form. The hypertrophic neuropathy form results in demyelination of nerve fibers and characteristic onion-bulb formations. Affected individuals usually have high plantar arches and an awkward gait, caused by weak ankle muscles. In the neuronal form, this condition usually starts in the second decade of life and causes muscle weaknesses similar to those associated with the hypertrophic neuronal form. Both forms of the disease may also involve mild sensory loss in the lower limbs. Affected individuals may be helped by corrective surgery and leg braces that stabilize weak ankle joints.

peroneus brevis (per'əni'əs), the smaller of the two lateral muscles of the leg, lying under the peroneus longus. The peroneus brevis arises from the fibula and inserts into the fifth metatarsal bone. Innervated by a branch of the superficial peroneal nerve, it contains fibers from the fourth and the fifth lumbar and the first sacral nerves. It pronates and plantar flexes the foot. Compare **peroneus longus.**

peroneus longus, the more superficial of the two lateral muscles of the leg. It arises from the head and the body of the fibula, converges to a long tendon that crosses the sole of the foot, and inserts into the first metatarsal bone and the medial cuneiform bone. The peroneus longus is innervated by a branch of the peroneal nerve, containing fibers from the fourth and the fifth lumbar and the first sacral nerves. The muscle pronates and plantar flexes the foot. Compare **peroneus brevis.**

peronia (pɪrou'niə), a congenital malformation or developmental anomaly.

peropus (pɪrou'pəs), a fetus or individual with malformed feet, often in association with some defect of the legs.

perosomus (pi'rousou'məs), a fetus or individual whose body, especially the trunk, is severely malformed. Also called **perocormus.**

perosplanchia (pi'rousplæŋk'iə), a congenital anomaly characterized by the malformation of the viscera.

peroxide (pərok'said). See **hydrogen peroxide.**

perphenazine, an antipsychotic.

■ INDICATIONS: It is prescribed in the treatment of psychotic disorders and in the control of severe nausea and vomiting in adults.

■ CONTRAINDICATIONS: Parkinson's disease, the concurrent administration of central nervous system depressants, liver or renal dysfunction, severe hypotension, or known hypersensitivity to any phenothiazine prohibits its use.

■ ADVERSE EFFECTS: Among the more serious adverse reactions are hypotension, liver toxicity, a variety of extrapyramidal reactions, blood dyscrasias, and various hypersensitivity reactions.

PERRLA, acronym for *pupils equal, round, react to light, accommodation.* In the process of performing an assessment of the eyes, the size and shape of the pupils, their reaction to light, and their ability to accommodate are evaluated. If all findings are normal, the acronym is noted in the account of the physicial examination.

Persadox, a trade name for a keratolytic (benzoyl peroxide).

Persadox HP, Persadox with twice the amount of benzoyl peroxide.

Persa-Gel, a trade name for a keratolytic (benzoyl peroxide).

Persantine, a trade name for a coronary vasodilator (dipyridamole).

persistent cloaca, a congenital anomaly in which the intestinal, urinary, and reproductive ducts open into a common cavity resulting from the failure of the urorectal septum to form during prenatal development. Also called **congenital cloaca.**

Persistin, a trade name for a central-nervous-system, fixed-combination drug containing analgesics (aspirin and salicylsalicylic acid).

persona (pərsou′nə), *pl.* **personae** (pərsou′ni). (in analytic psychology) the personality façade or role that a person assumes and presents to the outer world in order to satisfy the demands of the environment or society or as an expression of some intrapsychic conflict. The persona masks the person's inner being or unconscious self. Compare **anima.** See also **archetype.**

personal and social history, (in a health history) an account of the personal and social details of a person's life that serve to identify the person. Place of birth, religion, race, marital status, number of children, military status, occupational history, and place of residence are the usual components of this part of the history, but it may often include other information, as education, current living situation, and smoking, alcohol, and drug habits. The personal and social history is obtained at the initial interview and becomes a part of the permanent record.

personality, **1.** the composite of the behavioral traits and attitudinal characteristics by which one is recognized as an individual. **2.** the pattern of behavior each person evolves, both consciously and unconsciously, as a means of adapting to a particular environment and its cultural, ethnic, national, and provincial standards.

personality disorder, any of a large group of mental disorders characterized by rigid, inflexible, and maladaptive behavior patterns that impair a person's ability to function in society by severely limiting his adaptive potential. Such a disorder, which is generally recognized during childhood or adolescence, tends to continue through adulthood. Some kinds of personality disorders are **antisocial personality disorder, histrionic personality disorder, paranoid personality disorder, passive-aggressive personality disorder, schizoid personality disorder.** Also called **character disorder.**

personality test, any of a variety of standardized tests used in the evaluation or assessment of various facets of personality structure, emotional status, and behavioral traits. Compare **achievement test, aptitude test, intelligence test, psychological test.**

personal orientation, **1.** a continually evolving process in which a person determines and evaluates the relationships that appear to exist between the person and other people. **2.** the assessment derived by a person regarding those relationships.

personal unconscious, (in analytic psychology) the thoughts, ideas, emotions, and other mental phenomena acquired and repressed during one's lifetime. Compare **collective unconscious.**

perspiration, **1.** the act or process of perspiring; the excretion of fluid by the sweat glands through pores in the skin. **2.** the fluid excreted by the sweat glands. It consists of water containing sodium chloride, phosphate, urea, ammonia, and other waste products. Perspiration serves as a mechanism for excretion and for regulating body temperature. Abnormal amounts of perspiration usually result from organic causes but may also be precipitated by severe emotional stress. Kinds of perspiration are **insensible perspiration, sensible perspiration.** See also **diaphoresis, sweat.**

Perthes' disease (peʀtes′), osteochondrosis of the head of the femur in children, characterized initially by epiphyseal necrosis or degeneration followed by regeneration or recalcification. Also called **coxa plana, Legg-Calvé-Perthes' disease, pseudocoxalgia, Waldenström's disease.**

Pertofrane, a trade name for an antidepressant (desipramine hydrochloride).

pertussis (pərtəs′ɪs), an acute, highly contagious respiratory disease characterized by paroxysmal coughing that ends in a loud whooping inspiration. It occurs primarily in infants and in children less than four years of age who have not been immunized. The causative organism, *Bordetella pertussis,* is a small, nonmotile, gram-negative coccobacillus. A similar organism, *B. parapertussis,* causes a less severe form of the disease called parapertussis. Also called **whooping cough.**

■ OBSERVATIONS: Transmission occurs directly by contact or by inhalation of infectious particles, usually spread by coughing and sneezing, and indirectly through freshly contaminated articles. Diagnosis consists of positive identification of the organism in nasopharyngeal secretions. The initial stages of the disease are difficult to distinguish from bronchitis or influenza. A fluorescent antibody staining technique specific for the *B. pertussis* is an accurate means of early diagnosis. The incubation period averages 7 to 14 days, followed by 6 to 8 weeks of illness divided into three distinct stages: catarrhal, paroxysmal, and convalescent. Onset of the catarrhal stage is gradual, usually beginning with coryza, sneezing, a dry cough, a slight fever, listlessness, irritability, and anorexia. The cough becomes paroxysmal after 10 to 14 days and occurs as a series of short rapid bursts during expiration followed by the characteristic whoop, a hurried, deep inhalation that has a high-pitched crowing sound. There is usually no fever, and the respiratory rate between paroxysms is normal. During the paroxysm there is marked facial redness or cyanosis and vein distention, the eyes may bulge, the tongue may protrude, and the facial expression usually indicates severe anxiety and distress. Large amounts of a viscid mucus may be expelled during or following paroxysms, which occur from four to five times a day in mild cases to as many as 40 to 50 times a day in severe cases. Vomiting frequently occurs after the paroxysms because of gagging or choking on the mucus. In infants, choking may be more common than the characteristic whoop. This stage lasts from four to six weeks, with the attacks being most frequent and severe during the first one to two weeks, then gradually declining and disappearing. During the convalescent stage, a simple persistent cough is usual. For a period of up to two years following the initial attack, paroxysmal coughing may accompany respiratory infections.

■ INTERVENTION: Routine treatment consists of bed rest, a good diet, and adequate amounts of fluid. Erythromycin or another antibacterial may be prescribed to reduce contagiousness or to control secondary infection. Hospitalization may be necessary for infants and children with severe or prolonged paroxysms and for those with dehydration or other complications. Oxygen may be needed to relieve dyspnea and cyanosis; intravenous therapy may be necessary when prolonged vomiting interferes with adequate nutrition. Intubation is rarely necessary but may be lifesaving in infants if the thick mucus cannot be easily suctioned from the air passages. Pertussis immune globulin is available, but its efficacy has not been established and its use is not recommended. Active immunization is recommended with pertussis vaccine, usually in combination with diphtheria and tetanus toxoids in a series of three injections. One attack of the disease usually confers immunity, although some second, usually mild episodes have occurred.

■ NURSING CONSIDERATIONS: Severe paroxysms in an infant may require oxygen, suction, and intubation. The child needs to be kept calm and protected from respiratory irritants like dirt, smoke, or dust. Overstimulation, noise, or excitement may precipitate paroxysms. A good diet and adequate fluids are encouraged through frequent, small feedings. Common complications of the disease include bronchopneumonia; atelectasis; bronchiectasis; emphysema; otitis media; convulsions; hemorrhage, including subarachnoid, subconjunctival, and epistaxis; weight loss; dehydration; hernia; prolapsed rectum; and asphyxia, especially in infants.

pertussis immune globulin, a passive immunizing agent against whooping cough.

■ INDICATION: It is prescribed for immunization against whooping cough.

■ CONTRAINDICATION: Known hypersensitivity to this drug prohibits its use.

■ ADVERSE EFFECTS: Among the more serious adverse reactions is anaphylaxis.

pertussis vaccine, an active immunizing agent.

■ INDICATION: It is prescribed for immunization against pertussis when the administration of diphtheria, pertussis, tetanus vaccine is contraindicated.

■ CONTRAINDICATIONS: Thrombocytopenia or known hypersensitivity to the vaccine prohibits its use.

■ ADVERSE EFFECTS: Among the most serious adverse reactions are severe allergic reactions, pain and induration at the site of injection, and fever.

perversion, 1. any deviation from what is considered normal or natural. 2. the act of causing a change from what is normal or natural. 3. *Informal.* (in psychiatry) any of a number of sexual practices that deviate from what is considered normal adult behavior. See also **paraphilia.**

pervert, 1. *Informal.* a person whose sexual pleasure is derived from stimuli almost universally regarded as unnatural, as a fetishist or sadomasochist; a paraphiliac. 2. one whose sexual behavior deviates from a social or statistical norm but is not necessarily pathological.

pes cavus, a deformity of the foot characterized by an excessively high arch with hyperextension of the toes at the metatarsophalangeal joints, flexion at the interphalangeal joints, and shortening of the Achilles tendon. The condition may be present at birth or appear later owing to contractures or an imbalance of the muscles of the foot, as in neuromuscular diseases such as Friedreich's ataxia or peroneal muscular atrophy. Surgical treatment is indicated in severe cases, especially in childhood, although in milder forms the pain from the excessive pressure under the metatarsal heads can be relieved by sponge rubber or leather insoles fitted into the shoes. Also called **clawfoot, gampsodactyly, griffe des orteils, talipes cavus.**

pes planus. See **flatfoot.**

pessary (pes′əri), a device inserted in the vagina to treat uterine prolapse, uterine retroversion, or cervical incompetence. It is employed in the treatment of women whose advanced age or poor general condition precludes procedures required for surgical repair. A vaginal cream containing estrogen is usually prescribed to cause the vaginal epithelium to thicken and become more resistant to irritation from the pessary. Pessaries are also used in younger women in evaluating symptomatic uterine retroversion: if pelvic pain is relieved by anteversion of the uterus with the pessary in place and returns when retroversion recurs after the pessary is removed, retroversion is demonstrated to be the cause of pain, and surgical uterine suspension can be expected to provide long-term relief. The pessary is also used in the management of cervical incompetence in pregnancy. It holds the uterus in a forward position in which intra-abdominal and intrauterine pressure cause less stress on the neck of the womb. A pessary must be removed, usually daily, for cleaning. The woman may do this herself, or it may be done by someone else if she is disabled. Left in place, the pessary is likely to cause severe irritation, leading to vaginal infection. A **Smith-Hodge pessary** is a rubber or vinyl covered wire rectangle that fits between the pubic bone and the posterior vaginal fornix, supporting the uterus and holding the cervix in a posterior position. A **Gelhorn pessary** is an inflexible device made of lucite in the form of a large collar button. It has a canal through the stem that allows drainage of vaginal secretions. The large end of the pessary is placed deep in the vagina, the small end of the stem protruding at the introitus. A **doughnut pessary** is a permanently inflated flexible rubber doughnut that is inserted to support the uterus by blocking the canal of the vagina. An **inflatable pessary** is a collapsible rubber doughnut to which is attached a flexible stem containing a rubber valve. The pessary is inserted collapsed, inflated with a bulb similar to that of a sphygmomanometer, and deflated for removal. A **Bee-cell pessary** is a soft rubber cube: in each face of the cube is a conical depression that acts as a suction cup when the pessary is in the vagina. A **diaphragm pessary** is a contraceptive diaphragm used for uterovaginal support. A similar device of somewhat heavier construction is sometimes used. A **stem pessary** is a slim curved rod that is fitted into the cervical canal for uterine positioning. It is rarely used today.

pessimism, the inclination to anticipate the worst possible results from any action or situation or to emphasize unfavorable conditions, even when progress or gain might reasonably be expected. – **pessimist,** *n.*

pesticide poisoning, a toxic condition caused by the ingestion or inhalation of a substance used for the eradication of pests. Kinds of pesticide poisoning include **malathion poisoning, parathion poisoning.** See also **herbicide poisoning, insecticide poisoning, rodenticide poisoning.**

pestis (pes'tis). See **bubonic plague.**

PET, abbreviation for **positron emission tomography.**

petalo-, a combining form meaning 'of or related to a leaf': *petalobacteria, petalococcus.*

petechiae (piti'kii), *sing.* **petechia.** tiny purple or red spots that appear on the skin as a result of minute hemorrhages within the dermal or submucosal layers. Petechiae range from pinpoint to pinhead size and are flush with the surface. Compare **ecchymosis.** – **petechial,** *adj.*

petechial fever (pɪti'kiəl), any febrile illness accompanied by small petechiae on the skin, as seen in the late stage of typhoid fever.

petit mal (pət'i mæl'), an epileptic seizure characterized by a sudden, momentary loss of consciousness occasionally accompanied by minor myoclonus of the neck or upper extremities, slight symmetrical twitching of the face, or a loss of muscle tone. The seizures usually occur many times a day without a warning aura and are most frequent in children and adolescents, especially at the time of puberty. The patient experiencing a typical seizure has a vacant facial expression and ceases all voluntary motor activity; with the rapid return of consciousness, the patient may resume conversation at the point of interruption without realizing what occurred. During and between seizures, the patient's electroencephalogram shows three cycle-per-second spike and wave discharges. Anticonvulsant drugs used to prevent petit mal attacks include clonazepam, ethosuximide, methsuximide, paramethadione, phensuximide, trimethadione, and valproic acid. See also **epilepsy.**

P.E.T.N., a trade name for a vasodilator (pentaerythritol tetranitrate).

petr-, a combining form meaning 'of or pertaining to stone': *petrifaction, petroleum, petrous.*

pétrissage (pei'trısaźh'), a technique in massage in which the skin is gently lifted and squeezed. Pétrissage promotes circulation and relaxes the muscles. Compare **effleurage, rolling effleurage.**

Petrogalar, a trade name for a cathartic (mineral oil).

petrolatum gauze (pet'rəlei'təm), absorbent gauze permeated with white petrolatum.

petroleum distillate poisoning, a toxic condition caused by the ingestion or inhalation of a petroleum distillate, as fuel oil, lubricating oil, glue used in making model airplanes or the like, and various solvents. Nausea, vomiting, chest pain, dizziness, and severe depression of the central nervous system characterize the condition. Severe or fatal pneumonitis may occur if the substance is aspirated, therefore induced emesis is contraindicated. Gastric lavage with water, a saline cathartic, and oxygen, if required, are recommended. See also **gasoline poisoning, kerosene poisoning.**

petrosphenoidal fissure (pe'trousfinoi'dəl), a fissure on the floor of the cranial fossa between the posterior edge of the great wing of the sphenoid bone and the petrous part of the temporal bone.

Peutz-Jeghers syndrome, an inherited disorder, transmitted as an autosomal dominant trait, characterized by multiple intestinal polyps, and abnormal mucocutaneous pigmentation, usually over the lips and buccal mucosa. If obstruction or bleeding occurs, surgical removal of the polyps may be indicated.

-pexia. See **-pexis.**

-pexis, a combining form meaning 'a fixation of' something specified: *glycopexis, hemopexis, splenopexis.* Also **-pexia, -pexy.**

-pexy. See **-pexis.**

Peyer's patches (pai'ərz), groups of lymph nodes in the terminal ileum near its junction with the colon opposite to the juncture of the mesentery. In certain infectious diseases, as typhoid fever, they become ulcerated and enlarged.

peyote (peiou'ti), 1. a cactus from which a hallucinogenic drug, mescaline, is derived. 2. mescaline.

Peyronie's disease (peirouniz'), a disease of unknown cause resulting in fibrous induration of the corpora cavernosa of the penis. An association with Dupuytren's contracture of the palm has been recognized. The chief symptom of Peyronie's disease is painful erection. Palliative treatment includes radiation therapy and intralesional corticosteroid injections. There is no known cure.

PfiKlor, a trade name for an electrolyte replacement solution (potassium chloride).

Pfizer-E, a trade name for an antibacterial (erythromycin stearate).

Pfizerpen-AS, a trade name for an antibacterial (penicillin G procaine).

Pfizerpen G, a trade name for an antibacterial (penicillin G potassium).

Pfizerpen VK, a trade name for an antibacterial (penicillin V potassium).

PFT, abbreviation for **pulmonary function test.**

PG, abbreviation for **prostaglandin.**

PGY, abbreviation for *postgraduate year,* describing medical school graduates during their postgraduate training as interns (PGY-1, first year), residents (PGY-2, 3, 4), or fellows (PGY-4, 5).

pH, a scale representing the relative acidity (or alkalinity) of a solution, in which a value 7.0 is neutral, below 7.0 is acid, and above 7.0 is alkaline. The numerical pH value indicates the relative concentration of hydrogen atoms in the solution compared to that of a standard solution; it is equal to the negative log of the hydrogen ion concentration expressed in moles per liter. See also **acid, acid-base balance.**

PH, abbreviation for **parathyroid hormone.**

phaco-, a combining form meaning 'of or related to a lens': *phacocele, phacocyst, phacoglaucoma.* Also **phako-.**

phacomalacia (fæk'oumalei'ʃha), an abnormal condition of the eye in which the lens of the eye becomes soft, owing to the presence of a soft cataract.

phacomatosis (fæk'oumatou'sis). See **phakomatosis.**

phage (feij). See **bacteriophage.**

-phage, a combining form meaning 'something that eats' the matter specified: *hemophage, mycophage, osteophage.* Also **-phag.**

-phagia, 1. a combining form meaning an 'eating of a substance': *autophagia, chthonophagia, creophagia.* 2. a combining form meaning 'desire for food': *amylophagia, monophagia, osteophagia.*

phago-, a combining form meaning 'of or pertaining to eating or ingestion': *phagocyte, phagokaryosis, phagology.*

phagocyte (fæg'əsait), a cell that is able to surround, engulf, and digest microorganisms and cellular debris. **Fixed phagocytes,** which do not circulate, include the fixed macrophages and the cells of the reticuloendothelial system. **Free phagocytes,** which circulate in the blood stream, include the leukocytes and the free macrophages. —**phagocytic,** *adj.*

phagocytosis (fæg'əsaitou'sis), the process by which certain cells engulf and dispose of microorganisms and cell debris.

-phagy, a combining form meaning the 'practice of eating' something specified: *bacteriophagy, biophagy, coprophagy.* Also **-phagia.**

-phakia, a combining form meaning a 'lens': *aphakia, microphakia, pseudophakia.*

phako-. See **phaco-.**

phakomatosis (fæk'oumatou'sis), **phacomatosis,** *pl.* **phakomatoses.** (in opthalmology) a hereditary syndrome characterized by benign tumorlike nodules of the eye, skin, and brain. The four disorders designated phakomatoses are neurofibromatosis (Recklinghausen's disease), tuberous sclerosis (Bourneville's disease), encephalotrigeminal angiomatosis (Sturge-Weber syndrome), and cerebroretinal angiomatosis (von Hippel-Lindau disease).

-phalangia, a combining form meaning a 'condition of the bones of the fingers or toes': *bradyphalangia, symphalangia, triphalangia.*

phalanx (fei'læŋks), *pl.* **phalanges** (fəlæn'jiz). any one of the 14 tapering bones comprising the fingers of each hand and the toes of each foot. They are arranged in three rows at the distal end of the metacarpus and the metatarsus. The fingers each have three phalanges; the thumb has two. The toes each have three phalanges; the great toe has two. The phalanges of the foot are smaller and less flexible than those of the hand.

phall-. See **phallo-.**

phallic stage, (in psychoanalysis) the period in psychosexual development occurring between the ages of three and six years when emerging awareness and self-manipulation of the genitals are the predominant source of pleasurable experience. Fixation at this stage may lead to extreme aggressiveness in adulthood, or it may be a precipitating factor in the development of psychosexual disorders. See also **psychosexual development.**

phallo-, phall-, a combining form meaning 'of or related to the penis': *phallocampsis, phallodynia, phalloplasty.*

phalloidine, phalloidin (fæloi'din), a poison present in the mushroom *Amanita phalloides.* Ingestion of phalloidine results in bloody diarrhea, vomiting, severe abdominal pain, kidney failure, and liver damage. Approximately fifty per cent of phalloidine poisonings are fatal.

phallus. See **penis.**

-phane, a combining form meaning a 'thing with a (specified) appearance': *diaphane, rhodophane, xanthophane.* Also **-phan.**

phanero-, a combining form meaning 'visible or apparent': *phanerogenetic, phaneromania, phaneroplasm.*

phantom limb syndrome, a phenomenon common after amputation of a limb in which sensation or discomfort is experienced in the missing limb. In some people severe pain persists. See also **pseudesthesia.**

phantom tumor, a swelling resembling a tumor, usually caused by muscle contraction or gaseous distention of the intestines.

phao-. See **pheo-.**

pharmaceutical, 1. of or pertaining to pharmacy or drugs. 2. a drug.

pharmaceutical chemistry, the science dealing with the composition and preparation of chemical compounds used in medical diagnoses and therapies.

pharmacist, a specialist in formulating and dispensing medications. Pharmacists are licensed by the various states to practice pharmacy.

pharmaco-, a combining form meaning 'of or related to drugs or medicine': *pharmacochemistry, pharmacomania, pharmacopsychosis.*

pharmacogenetics (far′məkoujɪnet′ɪks), the study of the effect that the genetic factors belonging to a group or to an individual have on the response of the group or the individual to certain drugs.

pharmacokinetics, (in pharmacology) the study of the action of drugs within the body, including the routes and mechanisms of absorption and excretion, the rate at which a drug's action begins and the duration of the effect, the biotransformation of the substance in the body, and the effects and routes of excretion of the metabolites of the drug.

pharmacological treatment. See **treatment.**

pharmacologist, a specialist in pharmacology.

pharmacology, the study of the preparation, properties, uses, and actions of drugs.

pharmacopoeia, pharmacopeia (far′məkəpi′ə), 1. a compendium containing descriptions, recipes, strengths, standards of purity, and dosage forms for selected drugs. 2. the available stock of drugs in a pharmacy. 3. the total of all authorized drugs available within the jurisdiction of a given geographical or political area.

pharmacy, 1. the study of preparing and dispensing drugs. 2. a place for preparing and dispensing drugs.

-pharmic, a combining form meaning 'related to drugs and medicinal remedies': *alexipharmic, antipharmic, polypharmic.*

pharyng-. See **pharyngo-.**

pharyngeal aponeurosis, a sheet of connective tissue just beneath the mucosa of the pharynx.

pharyngeal bursa, a blind sac at the base of the pharyngeal tonsil.

pharyngeal reflex. See **gag reflex.**

pharyngeal tonsil, one of two masses of lymphatic tissue situated on the posterior wall of the nasopharynx behind the posterior nares. During childhood these masses often swell and block the passage of air from the nasal cavity into the pharynx, preventing the child from breathing through the nose.

pharyngitis (fær′ɪnjai′tɪs), inflammation or infection of the pharynx, usually causing symptoms of a sore throat. Some causes of pharyngitis are diphtheria, herpes simplex virus, infectious mononucleosis, and streptococcal infection. Specific treatment depends upon the cause. Symptoms may be relieved by analgesic medication, drinking warm or cold liquids, or saline irrigation of the throat. See also **strep throat.**

pharyngo-, pharyng-, a combining form meaning 'of or related to the pharynx': *pharyngocele, pharyngoglossus, pharyngorrhagia.*

pharyngoconjunctival fever (fərɪŋ′goukon′jəŋktai′vəl), an adenovirus infection characterized by fever, sore throat, and conjunctivitis. An epidemic illness, particularly prevalent in summer, that is spread by droplet infection and direct contact. Contaminated water in lakes and swimming pools is a common source of infection. Also called **swimming pool conjunctivitis.** See also **adenovirus.**

pharynx, the throat, a tubular structure about 13 cm long that extends from the base of the skull to the esophagus and is situated just in front of the cervical vertebrae. The pharynx serves as a passageway for the respiratory and digestive tracts and changes shape to allow the formation of various vowel sounds. The pharynx is composed of muscle, is lined with mucous membrane, and is divided into the nasopharynx, the oropharynx, and the laryngopharynx. It contains the openings of the right and the left auditory tubes, the openings of the two posterior nares, the fauces, the opening into the larynx, and the opening into the esophagus. It also contains the pharyngeal tonsils, the palatine tonsils, and the lingual tonsils. Also called **throat.** See also **larynx.**

phase microscope, a microscope with a special condenser and objective containing a phase-shifting ring which allows the viewer to see small differences in refraction indexes as differences in image intensity or contrast. The phase microscope is used especially for examining transparent specimens, as living or unstained cells and tissues.

phase of maximum slope, the time of rapid cervical dilatation and rapid fetal descent in the active phase of labor. See **Friedman curve.**

-phasia, a combining form meaning a 'speech disorder': *acataphasia, agitophasia, logaphasia.*

phasic (fei′zık), referring to a process proceeding in stages or phases.

-phasic, a combining form meaning 'relating to a speech disorder': *aphasic, endophasic, paraphasic.*

-phasis, a combining form meaning 'speech, utterance': *allophasis, heterophasis, paraphasis.* Also **-phasia, -phasy.**

-phasy. See **-phasis.**

Phelantin, a trade name for a central-nervous-system, fixed-combination drug containing an anticonvulsant (phenytoin), a stimulant (methamphetamine hydrochloride), and a sedative-hypnotic (phenobarbital).

Phe-Mer-Nite, a trade name for an antimicrobial (phenylmercuric nitrate).

Phemerol Chloride, a trade name for a topical anti-infective (benzethonium chloride.)

-phemia, a combining form meaning a '(specified) disorder of speech': *dysphemia, paraphemia, spasmophemia.*

phen-, a combining form indicating derivation from benzene: *phenacitin, phenicate, phenobarbitone.*

phenacemide (fɪnæs′əmaɪd), an anticonvulsant.
- INDICATION: It is prescribed in the treatment of severe epilepsy, particularly mixed forms of psychomotor seizures refractory to other drugs.
- CONTRAINDICATIONS: Pregnancy, previous personality disturbances, or known hypersensitivity to this drug prohibits its use.
- ADVERSE EFFECTS: Among the more serious adverse reactions are aplastic anemia, acute psychosis, paranoid and depressive reactions, nephritis, and hepatitis.

phenacetin (fɪnæs′ɪtɪn), an analgesic.
- INDICATIONS: It is prescribed to relieve pain and to reduce fever.
- CONTRAINDICATION: Known hypersensitivity to this drug prohibits its use.
- ADVERSE EFFECTS: Among the more serious adverse reactions are hepatic necrosis, fever, and skin rash.

Phenaphen, a trade name for an analgesic-antipyretic (acetaminophen).

phenazopyridine hydrochloride, a urinary tract analgesic.
- INDICATION: It is prescribed to reduce the pain of cystitis.
- CONTRAINDICATIONS: Renal insufficiency or known hypersensitivity to this drug prohibits its use.
- ADVERSE EFFECTS: Among the more serious adverse reactions are gastrointestinal disturbances.

phencyclidine hydrochloride (PCP) (fensaɪ′klɪdin), a piperidine derivative administered parenterally to achieve neurolept anesthesia. Because of its marked hallucinogenic properties, it is now rarely used in the United States.

phendimetrazine tartrate (fen′daɪmet′rəzin), a sympathomimetic amine used as an anorectic agent.
- INDICATION: It is prescribed to decrease the appetite in the treatment of exogenous obesity.
- CONTRAINDICATIONS: Cardiovascular disease, hypertension, hyperthyroidism, glaucoma, nervousness, a history of drug abuse, concomitant administration of central nervous system stimulants or monoamine oxidase inhibitors, or known hypersensitivity to this drug prohibits its use.
- ADVERSE EFFECTS: Among the more serious adverse reactions are central nervous system stimulation, elevated blood pressure, insomnia, and dry mouth.

-phene, a combining form denoting members of the phenol group: *camphene, phlobaphene, phosphene.* Also **-phen.**

phenelzine sulfate, a monoamine oxidase (MAO) inhibitor.
- INDICATION: It is prescribed in the treatment of mental depression.
- CONTRAINDICATIONS: Liver dysfunction, congestive heart failure, pheochromocytoma, concomitant use of sympathomimetic drugs or foods high in tryptophan or tyramine, or known hypersensitivity to this drug prohibits its use.
- ADVERSE EFFECTS: Among the most serious adverse reactions are orthostatic hypotension, vertigo, constipation, blurred vision, headache, overactivity, and dryness of mouth. MAO inhibitors produce many adverse drug interactions.

Phenergan, a trade name for a phenothiazine derivative (promethazine), used as an adjunct to anesthesia.

Phenergan Compound, a trade name for a respiratory, fixed-combination drug containing an adrenergic (pseudoephedrine hydrochloride), an antihistaminic (promethazine hydrochloride), and an analgesic (aspirin).

phenic acid (fi′nɪk). See **carbolic acid.**

phenindione (fənɪn′dioun), an anticoagulant.
- INDICATIONS: It is prescribed for prophylaxis and treatment of thrombosis and embolism in a variety of situations.
- CONTRAINDICATIONS: Known hypersensitivity to this drug prohibits its use. It is not used in situations where there is a risk of hemorrhage.
- ADVERSE EFFECTS: The most serious adverse reaction is hemorrhage. Many other drugs interact with this drug to increase or decrease its effect.

pheniramine maleate (fənir′əmin, fənir′əmɪn), an antihistamine.
- INDICATIONS: It is prescribed in the treatment of a variety of hypersensitivity reactions, including rhinitis, skin rash, and pruritus.
- CONTRAINDICATIONS: Asthma or known hypersensitivity to this drug prohibits its use. It is not given to newborn infants or lactating mothers.
- ADVERSE EFFECTS: Among the more serious adverse reactions are drowsiness, skin rash, and hypersensitivity reactions. Dry mouth and tachycardia commonly occur.

phenmetrazine hydrochloride, a sympathomimetic amine used as an anorectic agent.
- INDICATION: It is prescribed to reduce the appetite in treating exogenous obesity.
- CONTRAINDICATIONS: Cardiovascular disease, hypertension, hyperthyroidism, glaucoma, history of drug abuse, concomitant use of a central-nervous-system stimulant, or a monoamine oxidase (MAO) inhibitor, or known hypersensitivity to this drug or other sympathomimetic drugs prohibits its use. It is not recommended for children under 12 years of age.
- ADVERSE EFFECTS: Among the most serious adverse re-

actions are central nervous system stimulation, elevated blood pressure, insomnia, dry mouth, and others common to this class of drug.

phenobarbital, a barbiturate anticonvulsant and sedative-hypnotic.

■ INDICATIONS: It is prescribed in the treatment of a variety of seizure disorders and as a long-acting sedative.

■ CONTRAINDICATIONS: Porphyria or known hypersensitivity to this drug or other barbiturates prohibits its use.

■ ADVERSE EFFECTS: Among the most serious adverse reactions are ataxia, porphyria, paradoxical excitement, drowsiness, occasional rashes, and, rarely, blood dyscrasias. It is involved in many drug interactions.

phenocopy (fi′noʊkop′i), a phenotypic trait or condition that is induced by nongenetic factors but closely resembles a phenotype usually produced by a specific genotype. The trait is neither inherited nor transmitted to offspring. Such conditions as deafness, cretinism, mental retardation, and congenital cataracts are caused by mutant genes but can also result from a number of different agents, as the rubella virus in the case of congenital cataracts. Phenocopies may present problems in genetic screening and genetic counseling so that all exogenous factors must be ruled out before any congenital trait or defect is labeled hereditary.

phenol (fi′nol), 1. a highly poisonous, caustic, crystalline chemical derived from coal tar or plant tar or manufactured synthetically. It has a distinctive, pungent odor and, in solution, is a powerful disinfectant, commonly called carbolic acid. 2. Any of a large number and variety of chemical products closely related in structure to the alcohols and containing a hydroxyl group attached to a benzene ring. The phenols are components in dyes, plastics, disinfectants, and in antimicrobials and other drugs, including salicylic acid.

Phenolax, a trade name for a laxative (phenolphthalein).

phenol camphor, an oily mixture of camphor and phenol, used as an antiseptic and toothache remedy.

phenolphthalein (fi′noʊlthæl′in, fi′noʊlthei′lin), a laxative.

■ INDICATION: It is prescribed in the treatment of constipation.

■ CONTRAINDICATIONS: Symptoms of appendicitis, acute surgical abdomen, fecal impaction, intestinal obstruction or perforation, or known hypersensitivity to this drug prohibits its use.

■ ADVERSE EFFECTS: Among the most serious adverse reactions are abdominal cramping and pain, allergic reaction (particularly of the skin), dehydration, and laxative dependence.

phenol poisoning, corrosive poisoning owing to the ingestion of compounds containing phenol, as carbolic acid, creosote, creosol, guaiacol, and naphthol. Characteristic of phenol poisoning are burns of the mucous membranes,

weakness, pallor, pulmonary edema, convulsion, and respiratory, circulatory, cardiac, and renal failure. In treatment, the skin around the mouth and nose are washed, as are any external burns; the mouth, throat, esophagus, and stomach are lavaged with water and charcoal. Oxygen, intravenous fluids, electrolytes, and pain medication may be necessary. Rarely, esophageal stricture may develop as a complication of extensive tissue damage.

phenomenon, a sign that is often associated with a specific illness or condition and is, therefore, diagnostically important.

phenothiazine, any of a group of drugs which have a three ring structure in which two benzene rings are linked by a nitrogen and a sulfur. They represent the largest group of antipsychotic compounds in clinical medicine. Of the many phenothiazines and their congeners that are used as adjuncts to general anesthesia, antiemetics, major tranquilizers (antipsychotic agents), and antihistamines the most widely used are the two prototypes, chlorpromazine and prochlorperazine; closely related are trimeprazine and triflupromazine. This group of drugs has largely revolutionized the practice of psychiatric medicine. Unlike the barbiturates, which act exclusively on the central nervous system (CNS), the phenothiazines exert significant influence on many organ systems of the body at once; for example, they exert antiadrenergic, anticholinergic, and antihistaminic activity. The effects on the CNS differ according to individual drug and patient status. All phenothiazines are withheld from patients with severe CNS depression or epilepsy and are given with caution to those with liver disease. These drugs are not recommended for use in pregnancy. See also specific drugs.

phenotype, 1. the complete observable characteristics of an organism or group, including anatomical, physiological, biochemical, and behavioral traits, as determined by the interaction of both genetic makeup and environmental factors. 2. a group of organisms that resemble each other in appearance. Compare **genotype.** −**phenotypic,** *adj.*

Phenoxene, a trade name for an anticholinergic and antiparkinsonian (chlorphenoxamine hydrochloride).

phenoxy-, a combining form indicating the presence of a chemical group composed of phenyl and an atom of oxygen: *phenoxycaffeine.*

phenoxybenzamine hydrochloride, an antihypertensive.

■ INDICATIONS: It is prescribed in the control of hypertension and sweating in pheochromocytoma. If tachycardia is excessive, concomitant administration of propranolol may be necessary.

■ CONTRAINDICATIONS: Hypotension or known hypersensitivity to this drug prohibits its use.

■ ADVERSE EFFECTS: Among the more serious adverse

reactions are severe hypotension, tachycardia, and gastrointestinal irritation.

phenoxymethyl penicillin. See **penicillin V.**

phenprocoumon (fen'prouku'mən), an anticoagulant.

■ INDICATIONS: It is prescribed in the treatment and prophylaxis of thrombosis and embolism in a variety of clinical situations.

■ CONTRAINDICATIONS: Known hypersensitivity to this drug prohibits its use. It is not used in clinical situations in which there is a risk of hemorrhage.

■ ADVERSE EFFECTS: The most serious adverse reaction is hemorrhage. Many other drugs interact with this drug to either increase or decrease its effect.

phensuximide, an anticonvulsant.

■ INDICATION: It is prescribed to prevent seizures in petit mal epilepsy.

■ CONTRAINDICATIONS: Known hypersensitivity to this drug or to any succinimide prohibits its use.

■ ADVERSE EFFECTS: Among the most serious adverse reactions are blood dyscrasias and a systemic lupus-like syndrome. Common reactions are gastrointestinal disturbances and central nervous system depression with drowsiness or dizziness.

phentermine hydrochloride (fen'tərmin), a sympathomimetic amine used as an anorexic agent.

■ INDICATION: It is prescribed to decrease the appetite in the treatment of obesity.

■ CONTRAINDICATIONS: Arteriosclerosis, cardiovascular disease, hypertension, glaucoma, hyperthyroidism, or known hypersensitivity to this drug or to other sympathomimetic drugs prohibits its use.

■ ADVERSE EFFECTS: Among the more serious adverse reactions are restlessness, insomnia, tachycardia, increased blood pressure, and dry mouth.

phentolamine hydrochloride, an antiadrenergic.

■ INDICATIONS: It is prescribed in the control of symptoms of pheochromocytoma prior to and during surgery and for dermal necrosis and sloughing following extravasation of parenteral norepinephrine.

■ CONTRAINDICATIONS: History of myocardial infarction, angina, coronary artery disease, or known hypersensitivity to this drug prohibits its use.

■ ADVERSE EFFECTS: Among the more serious adverse reactions are severe hypotension, tachycardia, cardiac arrhythmias, anginal pain, and hypotension.

Phenurone, a trade name for an anticonvulsant (phenacemide).

phenylacetic acid (fen'ıləsi'tık), a metabolite of phenylalanine excreted in urine in conjugation with glutamine.

phenylalanine (fen'ılæl'ənin), an essential amino acid necessary for the normal growth and development of infants and children and for normal protein metabolism throughout life. It is abundant in milk, eggs, and other common foods. See also **phenylketonuria.**

phenylalaninemia (fen'ılælənıni'miə), the presence of phenylalanine in the blood. See also **hyperphenylalaninemia.**

phenylbutazone, a nonsteroidal anti-inflammatory agent.

■ INDICATIONS: It is prescribed in the treatment of severe symptoms of arthritis, bursitis, and other inflammatory conditions.

■ CONTRAINDICATIONS: Impaired renal or hepatic function, a history of upper gastrointestinal problems, blood dyscrasia, stomatitis owing to other drugs, hypertension, edema, or known hypersensitivity to this drug or to oxyphenbutazone prohibits its use.

■ ADVERSE EFFECTS: Among the more serious adverse reactions are fluid retention and potentially serious blood dyscrasias. Gastrointestinal irritation and nausea commonly occur. This drug interacts with many other drugs.

phenyl carbinol. See **benzyl alcohol.**

phenylephrine hydrochloride, an alpha-adrenergic agent.

■ INDICATIONS: It is prescribed to maintain blood pressure and is used locally as a nasal or ophthalmic vasoconstrictor.

■ CONTRAINDICATIONS: Narrow angle glaucoma, concomitant administration of monoamine oxidase inhibitors, or known hypersensitivity to this drug prohibits its use.

■ ADVERSE EFFECTS: Among the more serious adverse reactions to the systemic administration of this drug are arrhythmias and an excessive rise in blood pressure. Anxiety, congestion, and hypersensitivity reactions may occur from local administration of this drug.

phenylethyl alcohol, a colorless, fragrant liquid with a burning taste, used as a bacteriostatic agent and preservative in medicinal solutions. Also called **benzyl carbonol.**

phenylic acid (fənıl'ık). See **carbolic acid.**

phenylic alcohol. See **carbolic acid.**

phenylketonuria (PKU) (fen'əlki'tounyur'iə, fi'nəlki'-tounyur'iə), abnormal presence of phenylketone and other metabolites of phenylalanine in the urine, characteristic of an inborn metabolic disorder caused by the absence or a deficiency of phenylalanine hydroxylase, the enzyme responsible for the conversion of the amino acid phenylalanine into tyrosine. Accumulation of phenylalanine is toxic to brain tissue. Untreated individuals have very fair hair, eczema, a mousy odor of the urine and skin, and progressive mental retardation. Treatment consists of a diet free of phenylalanine. Phenylketonuria occurs approximately once in 16,000 births in the United States. Most states require a screening test for all newborns. See also **Guthrie test.** —**phenylketonuric,** adj.

phenylmercuric nitrate, a topical antiseptic.

■ INDICATIONS: It is prescribed as an antiseptic in skin diseases and for preoperative disinfection.

■ CONTRAINDICATIONS: Known hypersensitivity to this drug or to other compounds containing mercury prohibits its use.

■ ADVERSE EFFECTS: Among the more serious adverse reactions are local hypersensitivity with rash and irritation. Systemic mercury intoxication may occur with frequent and widespread use.

phenyl methanol. See **benzyl alcohol.**

phenylpropanolamine hydrochloride (fen'əlprou'pə-nol'əmin), a sympathomimetic amine.

■ INDICATION: It is prescribed to relieve nasal congestion.

■ CONTRAINDICATIONS: Hypertension, coronary artery disease, concomitant administration of monoamine oxidase inhibitors, or known hypersensitivity to this drug prohibits its use.

■ ADVERSE EFFECTS: Among the more serious adverse reactions are nervousness, insomnia, anorexia, and increased blood pressure.

phenylpyruvic acid (fen'ɪlpæiru'vɪk), a product of the metabolism of phenylalanine. The presence of phenylpyruvic acid in the urine is indicative of phenylketonuria.

phenylpyruvic amentia. See **phenylketonuria.**

phenyltoloxamine citrate (fen'ɪltəlok'səmin, fi'nɪltəlok'-səmin), an antihistamine usually used in a fixed-combination drug with an analgesic.

Phenylzin, a trade name for an ophthalmic, fixed-combination drug containing an adrenergic (phenylephrine hydrochloride) and an astringent (zinc sulfate).

phenytoin (fen'ətou'ɪn, fen'ətou'ɪn), an anticonvulsant.

■ INDICATIONS: It is prescribed as an anticonvulsant in grand mal and psychomotor seizure disorders and as an antiarrhythmic agent, particularly in digitalis-induced arrhythmias.

■ CONTRAINDICATIONS: Known hypersensitivity to this drug or to other hydantoins prohibits its use. It is used with caution in patients with a history of hepatic or hematologic abnormalities and in the presence of certain arrhythmias.

■ ADVERSE EFFECTS: Among the more serious adverse reactions are ataxia, nystagmus, hypersensitivity reactions, and gingival hyperplasia. Rarely, a variety of severe reactions occur. This drug interacts with many other drugs.

pheo-, a combining form meaning 'dusky': *pheochrome, pheochromoblast, pheophytin.* Also **phao-.**

pheochromocytoma (fi'oukrou'mousæitou'mə), pl. **pheochromocytomas, pheochromocytomata.** a vascular tumor of chromaffin tissue of the adrenal medulla or sympathetic paraganglia, characterized by hypersecretion of epinephrine and norepinephrine, causing persistent or intermittent hypertension. Typical signs include headache, palpitation, sweating, nervousness, hyperglycemia, nausea, vomiting, and syncope. There may be weight loss,

myocarditis, cardiac arrhythmia, and heart failure. The tumor occurs most frequently in young people, and only a small percentage of the lesions are malignant. The diagnosis may be established by laboratory assays showing increased catecholamines and their metabolites in urine and by pressor tests; intravenously injected histamine causes a sharp increase in blood pressure of patients with pheochromocytoma and the administration of phentolamine produces a marked decrease. Surgical excision is the usual treatment; patients with nonresectable tumors may be treated with adrenergic blocking agents or with methyl tyrsine, an experimental drug that reduces norepinephrine production.

pheromone (fer'əmoun'), a hormonal substance secreted by an individual that elicits a particular response from another individual of the same species.

phil-, a combining form meaning 'having an affinity for': *philanthropist, philocatalase, philoneism.*

-phil, a combining form meaning 'of that which combines with or is stained by': *chromaphil, hydrophil, lipophil.* Also **-philic, -philous.**

Philadelphia chromosome, a translocation of the long arm of chromosome 22, often seen in the abnormal myeloblasts, erythroblasts, and megakaryoblasts of patients who have chronic myelocytic leukemia.

-philia, 1. a combining form meaning a 'tendency towards an action': *calciphelia, cryophilia, spasmophilia.* 2. a combining form meaning 'abnormal appetite for a thing': *carcinophilia, lygophilia, necrophilia.* Also **-phily.**

-philous, a combining form meaning 'having an affinity for': *calciphilous, chromophilous, cyanophilous.*

-phily, 1. a combining form meaning a 'fondness for something': *necrophily.* 2. a combining form meaning an 'affinity for something': *hydrophily, photophily, xerophily.*

phimosis (faɪmou'sɪs), tightness of the prepuce of the penis that prevents the retraction of the foreskin over the glans. The condition is usually congenital but may be the result of infection. Circumcision is the usual treatment. An analogous condition of the clitoris occurs rarely. Compare **paraphimosis.** See also **phimosis vaginalis.**

phimosis vaginals (væj'ɪnei'lɪs), congenital narrowness or closure of the vaginal opening.

pHisoHex, a trade name for a detergent containing a topical anti-infective (hexachlorophene).

phleb-. See **phlebo-.**

phlebitis. See **thrombophlebitis.**

phlebo-, phleb-, a combining form meaning 'of or related to a vein or veins': *phlebocarcinoma, phlebograph, phlebostenosis.*

phlebogram (fleb'əgræm), 1. an x-ray film obtained by phlebography. 2. a graphic representation of the venous pulse, obtained by phlebograph. Also called **venogram.**

phlebograph (fleb'əgræf), a device for producing a graphic record of the venous pulse.

phlebography (fləbog′rəfi), **1.** the technique of preparing an x-ray image of veins injected with a radiopaque contrast medium. **2.** the technique of preparing a graphic record of the venous pulse by means of a phlebograph. Also called **venography.**

phlebothrombosis (fleb′ouθrombou′sɪs), an abnormal venous condition in which a clot forms within a vein, usually owing to hemostasis, hypercoagulability, or occlusion. In contrast to thrombophlebitis, the wall of the vein is not inflamed.

phlebotomus fever, an acute, mild infection, caused by one of five distinct arboviruses transmitted to man by the bite of an infected sandfly, characterized by rapidly developing fever, headache, eye pain, conjunctivitis, myalgia, and, occasionally, a macular or urticarial rash. Aseptic meningitis may also occur. The disease is widespread in hot, dry areas where sandflies abound, and it has been seen in Panama and Brazil. Phlebotomus fever is self-limited, no fatalities have been recorded, and no specific therapy is available. Bed rest, fluids, and aspirin are recommended. A second attack may occur a few weeks after the first. Also called **pappataci, sandfly fever, three day fever.**

phlebotomy (fləbot′əmi), the incision of a vein for the letting of blood, as in collecting blood from a donor. Phlebotomy is the chief treatment for polycythemia vera and may be performed every six months, or more frequently if required. The procedure is sometimes used to decrease the amount of circulating blood and pulmonary engorgement in acute pulmonary edema. At one time phlebotomy was practiced for almost every disorder. Also called **venesection.**

phleg-. See **phlogo-.**

phlegm (flem), thick mucus secreted by the tissues lining the respiratory passages.

phlegmasia (flegmei′zhə), *Obsolete.* an inflammation.

phlegmasia alba dolens, thrombophlebitis of the femoral vein, resulting in edema of the leg and pain. It may occur after childbirth or after a severe febrile illness.

phlegmasia cerulea dolens, a severe form of thrombosis of a deep vein, usually the femoral vein. The condition is acute and fulminating and is usually accompanied by vast edema and cyanosis of the limb distal to the occluding thrombosis.

phlegmonous gastritis, a rare but severe form of gastritis, involving the connective tissue layer of the stomach wall. It occurs as a complication of systemic infection, peptic ulcer, cancer, surgery, or other severe stress and represents an acute abdominal emergency. Treatment includes surgery, antibiotics, and analgesics.

phlogo-, phleg-, a combining form meaning 'of or related to inflammation': *phlogocyte, phlogogen, phlogoxelotism.*

phlyctenular keratoconjunctivitis, an inflammatory condition of the cornea, characterized by tiny, ulcerating nodules, seen most often in children as a response to allergens found in tuberculin, gonococci, monilia, or various parasites. Vitamin deficiency may be a factor. The condition responds to topical corticosteroids, but corneal scars may remain. Also called **phlyctenulosis, scrofulous keratitis.** See also **eczematous conjunctivitis.**

phlyctenulosis (flɪk′tenyʊlou′sɪs). See **phyctenular keratoconjunctivitis.**

phob-, a combining form meaning 'of or pertaining to fear or morbid dread': *phobia, phobic, phobophobia.*

-phobe, a combining form meaning 'one who fears' something specified: *dermatophobe, heliophobe, nosophobe.* Also **-phobiac, -phobist.**

phobia, an anxiety disorder characterized by an obsessive, irrational, and intense fear of a specific object, as an animal or dirt, of an activity, as meeting strangers or leaving the familiar setting of the home, or of a physical situation, as heights and open or closed spaces. Typical manifestations of phobia include faintness, fatigue, palpitations, perspiration, nausea, tremor, and panic. The fear, which is out of proportion to reality, usually results from some early painful or unpleasant experience involving the particular object or situation, or it may arise from displacing an unconscious conflict to an external object or situation to which it is symbolically related. The irrational, compelling need to avoid the feared object or situation can interfere with customary daily activities, often resulting in complex alterations in life patterns and interpersonal relationships. Although the individual usually recognizes the inappropriateness of the reaction, he is powerless to overcome the fear until the repressed conflict is recognized, usually through extensive psychotherapy. Treatment also consists of behavior therapy to reduce the maladaptive anxiety resulting from the fear by altering the behavioral response. Some kinds of phobias are **agoraphobia, claustrophobia, gynephobia, laliophobia, photophobia, simple phobia, social phobia, zoophobia.** Also called **phobic disorder, phobic neurosis, phobic reaction.** Compare **compulsion.** – **phobiac,** *n.,* **phobic,** *adj.*

-phobia, a combining form meaning 'abnormal fear' of the object, experience, or place specified: *agoraphobia, claustrophobia, nyctophobia.*

phobiac (fou′biæk′), a person who exhibits or is afflicted with a phobia.

-phobiac. See **-phobe.**

-phobic, 1. a combining form meaning 'exhibiting or possessing an aversion for or fear of (something)': *Anglophobic, necrophobic, zoophobic.* **2.** a combining form meaning the 'absence of a strong affinity': *chromophobic, gentianophobic, osmiophobic.* Also **-phobous.**

phobic disorder. See **phobia.**

phobic neurosis. See **phobia.**

phobic reaction. See **phobia.**

phobic state, a condition characterized by extreme anxiety resulting from the excessive, irrational fear of a particular object, situation, or activity. See also **phobia.**

-phobist. See **-phobe.**

-phobous. See **-phobic.**

phocomelia (fou'koumi'liə), a developmental anomaly characterized by the absence of the upper portion of one or more of the limbs so that the feet or hands or both are attached to the trunk of the body by short, irregularly shaped stumps, resembling the fins of a seal. The condition, caused by interference with the embryonic development of the long bones, is rare and is seen primarily as a side effect of the drug thalidomide taken during early pregnancy. Also called **seal limbs.** Compare **amelia.** — **phocomelic,** adj.

phocomelic dwarf, a dwarf in whom the long bones of any or all of the extremities are abnormally short.

phocomelus (foukom'ələs), an individual who has phochomelia.

phon-. See **phono-.**

-phone, 1. a combining form meaning a 'device for transmitting sound': *auriphone, ossiphone, osteophone.* 2. a combining form meaning a 'device for monitoring body sounds': *miophone, sphygmophone, stethophone.*

phonic, of or pertaining to voice, sounds, or speech.

-phonic, a combining form meaning 'sounds made in a (specified) part of the body': *bronchiophonic, leptophonic, organophonic.*

phono-, phon-, a combining form meaning 'of or related to sound, often specifically the sound of the voice': *phonocardiograph, phonopathy, phonopsia.*

phonocardiogram, a graphic recording obtained from a phonocardiograph.

phonocardiograph (fou'noukar'diəgræf), an electroacoustical device that produces graphic heart sound recordings, used in the diagnosis and monitoring of heart disorders. This instrument produces phonocardiograms by using a system of microphones and associated recording equipment. One microphone is usually placed on the chest near the base of the heart; another is positioned on the chest over the apex of the heart. The microphone placed over the base of the heart records the timing of the aortic and the pulmonary components of the second heart sound and the loudest murmurs. The microphone placed over the apex is connected to special filters which allow the recording of low-frequency sounds, as those associated with atrial and ventricular gallops, as well as higher-frequency sounds, as those associated with mitral regurgitation and ventricular septal defect. To assure an accurate recording, the examiner also uses audiophones to monitor the sounds and an oscilloscope to monitor cardiac impulses. — **phonocardiographic,** adj.

-phony, 1. a combining form meaning 'sound': echophony, laryngophony. 2. a combining form meaning a 'speech disorder' of a (specified) type: *autophony, egophony, gutturophony.* Also **-phonia.**

phor-, a combining form meaning 'bearing, carrying': *phoresis, phoroblast, phorology.*

-phore, a combining form meaning a 'bearer or possessor': *gluciphore, physaliphore, trochophore.* Also **-phor.**

-phoresis, a combining form meaning a 'movement in a (specified) manner or medium': *aphoresis, cataphoresis, diaphoresis.*

-phoria, 1. a combining form meaning '(condition of the) visual axes of the eye': *anophoria, esophoria, exophoria.* 2. a combining form meaning an 'emotional state': *adiaphoria, euphoria, ideaphoria.*

phosphatase (fos'fəteis), an enzyme that acts as a catalyst in chemical reactions involving phosphorus. See also **catalyst, enzyme.**

phosphate, a compound of phosphoric acid. Phosphates are extremely important in living cells, particularly in the storage and utilization of energy and the transmission of genetic information within a cell and from one cell to another. See also **adenosine diphosphate, adenosine triphosphate, phosphorus.**

phosphoglycerate kinase (fos'fouglıs'əreit), an enzyme that catalyzes the reversible transfer of a phosphate group from adenosine triphosphate to D-3-phosphoglycerate, forming D-1, 3-diphosphoglycerate. The reaction is one of the steps in glycolysis.

Phospholine Iodide, a trade name for a cholinergic (echothiophate iodide).

phospholipid (fos'foulip'ıd), one of a class of compounds, widely distributed in living cells, containing phosphoric acid, fatty acids, and a nitrogenous base. Two kinds of phospholipids are **lecithin, sphingomyelin.**

phosphomevalonate kinase (fos'fouməvæl'əneit), an enzyme that catalyzes the transfer of a phosphate group from adenosine triphosphate to produce adenosine diphosphate and 5-pyrophosphomevalonate.

phosphoric acid, a clear, colorless, odorless liquid that is irritating to the skin and eyes and moderately toxic if ingested. Phosphoric acid is used in the production of fertilizers, soaps, detergents, animal feeds, and certain drugs.

phosphorus (P), a nonmetallic chemical element occurring extensively in nature as a component of phosphate rock. Its atomic number is 15; its atomic weight is 30.975. Phosphorus forms a series of sulfides used commercially in the manufacture of matches. It can be prepared in yellow or white, red, and black allotropic forms. Phosphorus is essential for the metabolism of protein, calcium, and glucose. The body uses phosphorus in its combined forms, which are obtained from such nutritional sources as milk, cheese, meat, egg yolk, whole grains, legumes, and nuts. A deficiency of phosphorus in the body can cause weight loss, anemia, and abnormal growth. Phosphorus is essential to the body for the production of adenosine triphosphate and for the process of glycolysis. Elemental white or yellow phosphorus is extremely poisonous and produces severe gastrointestinal irritation. If ingested, it can produce hemorrhage, cardiovascular failure, and death. Chronic poisoning from phosphorus is characterized by anemia, cachexia, bronchitis, and necrosis of the mandible.

phosphorus poisoning, a toxic condition caused by the ingestion of white or yellow phosphorus, sometimes found in rat poisons, certain fertilizers, and fireworks. Intoxication is characterized initially by nausea, throat and stomach pain, vomiting, diarrhea, and an odor of garlic on the breath. Following a few days of apparent recovery, nausea, vomiting, and diarrhea recur with renal and hepatic dysfunction. Treatment includes gastric lavage, and administration of mineral oil, vitamin K, intravenous fluids, and medication to counteract shock. Physical contact with the vomitus and feces of the patient are avoided.

Phosphotope, a trade name for an antineoplastic (sodium phosphate P 32).

phot-. See **photo-.**

-photic, a combining form meaning 'pertaining to the ability to see at a (specified) light level': *euryphotic, stenophotic, sthenophotic.*

photo-, phot-, a combining form meaning 'of or pertaining to light': *photoelectric, photoreceptor, phototropism.*

photoallergic, exhibiting a delayed hypersensitivity reaction after exposure to light. Compare **phototoxic.** See also **photoallergic contact dermatitis.**

photoallergic contact dermatitis, a papulovesicular, eczematous, or exudative skin reaction occurring 24 to 48 hours after exposure to light in a previously sensitized person. The sensitizing substance concentrates in the skin and requires chemical alteration by light to become an active antigen. Among common photosensitizers are phenothiazines, hexachlorophene, oral hypoglycemic agents, and sulfanilamide. Prevention requires avoidance of the photosensitizer and sunlight. Treatment is the same as that for any other inflammatory dermatitis.

photochemotherapy, a kind of chemotherapy in which the effect of the administered drug is enhanced by exposing the patient to light, as the treatment of psoriasis with oral methoxsalen followed by exposure to ultraviolet light. See also **chemotherapy.**

photophobia (fou'toufou'biə), **1.** abnormal sensitivity to light, especially by the eyes. The condition is prevalent in albinism and various diseases of the conjunctiva and cornea and may be a symptom of such disorders as measles, psittacosis, encephalitis, Rocky Mountain spotted fever, and Reiter's syndrome. **2.** (in psychiatry) a morbid fear of light with an irrational need to avoid light places. The anxiety disorder is seen more often in women than in men

and is usually caused by a repressed intrapsychic conflict symbolically related to light. Treatment consists of psychotherapy to uncover the cause of the phobic reaction followed by behavior therapy, often using the techniques of systemic desensitization and flooding. — **photophobic,** *adj.*

photosensitive, increased reactivity of skin to sunlight caused by a disorder, as albinism or porphyria, or more frequently resulting from the use of certain drugs. Relatively brief exposure to sunlight or to an ultraviolet lamp may cause edema, papules, urticaria, or acute burns in individuals with endogenous or acquired photosensitivity. Drugs inducing photosensitivity include phenothiazine tranquilizers, antibiotic tetracycline, antimycotic griseofulvin, antibacterial nalidixic acid, oral hypoglycemic agents, the artificial sweetener calcium cyclamate, the oral contraceptive agents mestranol and norethynodrel, and halogenated salicylanides used in antifungal soaps. Treatment involves avoidance of exposure to sunlight or the photosensitizing agent. Methoxsalen and trioxsalen are potent photosensitizers sometimes used to enhance pigmentation or increase tolerance to sunlight, but overexposure or overdosage can cause severe reactions.

photosensitivity, any abnormal response to exposure to light, specifically, a skin reaction requiring the presence of a sensitizing agent and exposure to sunlight or its equivalent. Photosensitivity includes photoallergic and phototoxic reactions.

photosynthesis (fou'tousɪn'fhəsɪs), a process by which green plants containing chlorophyll synthesize chemical substances, chiefly carbohydrates, from atmospheric carbon dioxide and water, using light for energy and liberating oxygen in the process.

phototherapy, the treatment of disorders by the use of light, especially ultraviolet light. Ultraviolet light may be employed in the therapy of acne, decubiti and other indolent ulcers, psoriasis, and hyperbilirubinemia. — **phototherapeutic,** *adj.*

phototherapy in the newborn, a treatment for hyperbilirubinemia and jaundice in the newborn that involves the exposure of an infant's bare skin to intense fluorescent light. The blue range of light accelerates the excretion of bilirubin in the skin, decomposing it by photo-oxidation.

■ METHOD: The infant is placed nude under the fluorescent lights with the eyes and genitalia covered. The baby is turned frequently and the body temperature is monitored, using a skin thermistor. All vital signs are carefully noted, and details regarding position of the bulbs, time and duration of treatment, and the infant's response are charted. Adverse effects of phototherapy include dehydration: an infant may need 25 per cent more fluid during treatment. Loose stools, priapism, and 'bronze-baby' syndrome may occur.

■ NURSING ORDERS: The nurse performs phototherapy and may be responsible for collecting specimens for serial tests for bilirubin in the blood. The lights may scorch the nurse's hair and irritate the eyes; as protection, a cap and sunglasses may be worn. Breast feeding may be discontinued during treatment but often is not; additional water is always given. The family is encouraged to visit and to participate in caring for the infant. They may be told that the eyeshields are necessary but do not seem to bother the infant.

■ OUTCOME CRITERIA: Bilirubin levels usually decrease by 3 to 4 mg/100 ml in the first 8 to 12 hours of therapy; thus, simple jaundice clears rapidly. Excess bilirubin and jaundice that are the result of hemolytic disease or infection may be controlled with phototherapy, but the underlying cause is treated separately. Recovery is usually complete. The long-term safety of phototherapy has not been established; short-term efficacy and practicality of use are certain.

phototoxic, characterized by a rapidly developing, non-immunologic reaction of the skin when it is exposed to a photosensitizing substance and light. Compare **photoallergic.** See also **phototoxic contact dermatitis.**

phototoxic contact dermatitis, a rapidly appearing, sunburnlike response of areas of skin that have been exposed to the sun after contact with a photosensitizing substance. Hyperpigmentation may follow the acute reaction. Among known photosensitizing materials are coaltar derivatives, oil of bergamot (often used in cosmetics), and many plants containing furocoumarin (cowslip, buttercup, carrot, parsnip, mustard, yarrow, etc.). Treatment includes Burow's solution, acid mantle cream, and topical corticosteroids.

-phragma, a combining form meaning a 'septum or musculomembranous barrier between cavities': *inophragma, mesophragma, telophragma.* Also **-phragm.**

-phrasia, a combining form meaning an 'abnormal condition of speech': *aphrasia, echophrasia, embolophrasia.*

phren-, 1. a combining form meaning 'of or related to the mind': *phrenasthenia, phrenoblabia, phrenology.* 2. a combining form meaning 'of or related to the diaphragm': *phrenodynia, phrenogastric, phrenohepatic.*

-phrenia, a combining form meaning a 'disordered condition of mental activity': *hebephrenia, ideophrenia, kolyphrenia.*

phrenic (fren′ĭk), 1. of or pertaining to the diaphragm. 2. of or pertaining to the mind.

-phrenic, 1. a combining form meaning the 'diaphram or adjacent regions of the body': *costophrenic, postphrenic, subphrenic.* 2. a combining form meaning 'characteristic of a disorder of the mind': *hebephrenic, ideophrenic, schizophrenic.*

phrenic nerve, one of a pair of muscular branches of the cervical plexus, arising from the fourth cervical nerve.

It contains about half as many sensory as motor fibers and is generally known as the motor nerve to the diaphragm, although the lower thoracic nerves also help to innervate the diaphragm. The phrenic nerve lies on the ventral surface of the scalenus anterior, crossing from its lateral to its medial border. It continues with the scalenus anterior between the subclavian vein and the subclavian artery, enters the thorax, passes over the cupula of the pleura, along the lateral aspect of the pericardium, and reaches the diaphragm, where it divides into terminal branches. The right phrenic nerve is deeper and shorter than the left. The pleural branches of the phrenic nerve are very fine filaments supplying the mediastinal pleura. The pericardial branches are delicate filaments passing to the upper pericardium. The terminal branches diverge after passing separately through the diaphragm and are distributed on the abdominal surface of the diaphragm. On the right side, a branch near the inferior vena cava communicates with the phrenic plexus in association with a phrenic ganglion. There is no phrenic ganglion on the left side. Also called **internal respiratory nerve of Bell.** Compare **accessory phrenic nerve.**

phthi-, a combining form meaning 'decay, wasting away': *phthisiogenesis, phthisiomania, phthisis.*

Phthirus (thī′rəs), a genus of bloodsucking lice that includes the species *Phthirus pubis,* the pubic louse, or crab.

-phthongia, a combining form meaning a 'condition of speech': *aphthongia, diphthongia, heterophthongia.*

phyco-, a combining form meaning 'of or pertaining to seaweed': *phycochrome, phycocyan, phycology.*

phycomycosis (faɪ′koumaɪkou′sɪs), a fungal infection caused by a species of the order Phycomycetes. These organisms are common in the soil and are not usually pathogenic. Severe nosocomial pulmonary phycomycosis sometimes occurs with advanced diabetes mellitus that is untreated or out of control and complicated by ketoacidosis. See also **mucormycosis, zygomycosis.**

phyl-, a combining form meaning 'guarding or preservation': *phylacagogic, phylactic, phylaxis.*

-phyll, a combining form meaning a 'coloring matter in plants': *chlorophyll, leukophyll.* Also **-phyl.**

phyllo-, a combining form meaning 'of or pertaining to leaves': *phyllochlorin, phyllode, phyllosan.*

phylloquinone (fɪl′əkwɪn′oun). See **vitamin K₁.**

phylo-, a combining form meaning 'type, kind': *phylobiology, phylogenesis, phylogeny.*

phylogenesis. See **phylogeny.**

phylogenetic, phylogenic, 1. of, relating to, or acquired during phylogeny. 2. that which is based on a natural evolutionary relationship, as a system of classification.

phylogeny (fɪloj′ɪni), the development of the structure of a particular race or species as it evolved from simpler forms of life. Compare **ontogeny.**

-phyma, a combining form meaning a 'swelling tumor': *adenophyma, celiophyma, onychophyma.*

physi-. See **physio-.**

-physical, a combining form meaning 'natural': *iatrophysical, medicophysical, psychophysical.*

physical allergy, an allergic response to physical factors, as cold, heat, light, or trauma. Usually, specific antibodies are found in people having physical allergies. Common characteristics include pruritis, urticaria, and angioedema. There may be photosensitivity, owing to the use of certain cosmetics or drugs. Prophylaxis usually includes an attempt to remove the stimulus, and treatment involves the use of antihistamines or steroids. Compare **contact dermatitis.** See also **atopic.**

physical assessment, the part of the health assessment representing a synthesis of the information obtained in a physical examination.

physical chemistry, the natural science dealing with the relationship between chemical and physical properties of matter.

physical diagnosis, the diagnostic process accomplished by the study of the physical manifestations of health and illness revealed in the physical examination, as guided by the patient's complete history and supported by various laboratory tests. Physical diagnosis is to medicine what the health assessment is to nursing.

physical examination, an investigation of the body to determine its state of health, using any or all of the techniques of inspection, palpation, percussion, auscultation, and smell. The physical examination, medical history, and initial laboratory tests constitute the data base on which a diagnosis is made and on which a plan of treatment developed.

physical science, the study of the laws and properties of nonliving matter. Some kinds of physical science are **chemistry, geology,** and **physics.** Compare **life science.**

physical therapist, a person who is licensed to assist in the examination, testing, and treatment of physically disabled or handicapped people through the use of special exercise, application of heat or cold, use of sonar waves, and other techniques. A physical therapist usually becomes qualified by taking a four-year college course leading to a B.S. in physical therapy or a special 12-month certificate course after obtaining a bachelor's degree in a related field.

physical therapy, the treatment of disorders with physical agents and methods, as massage, manipulation, therapeutic exercises, cold, heat (including shortwave, microwave, and ultrasonic diathermy), hydrotherapy, electrical stimulation, and light, to assist in rehabilitating patients and in restoring normal function following an illness or injury. Also called **physiotherapy.**

physician, 1. a health professional who has earned a degree of Doctor of Medicine (M.D.) after completing an approved course of study at an approved medical school. Satisfactory completion of National Board Examinations, usually given during both the second and the final years of medical school and after graduation, is also required. An M.D. usually enters a hospital internship program for one year of postgraduate training before beginning practice or further training in a specialty. In order to practice medicine, an M.D. is required to obtain a license from the state in which professional services will be performed. 2. a health professional who has earned a degree of Doctor of Osteopathy (D.O.) by satisfactorily completing a course of education in an approved college of osteopathy. Osteopathic physicians and medical physicians follow nearly identical courses of training and modes of practice, except that osteopathic medicine places special emphasis on the study of mechanical derangement of tissues as a cause of illness and on treatment that involves manipulation of body structures.

physician's assistant (PA), a person trained in certain aspects of the practice of medicine to provide assistance to a physician. A physician's assistant is trained by physicians and practices under the direction and supervision and within the legal license of a physician. Training programs vary in length from a few months to two years. Health-care experience or academic preparation may be a prerequisite to admission to some programs. Most physician's assistants are prepared for the practice of primary care, but some practice subspecialities, including surgical assisting, dialysis, or radiology. National certification is available to qualified graduates of approved training programs. The national organization is the American Association of Physician's Assistants (AAPA). Also called **physician's associate.**

physician's associate. See **physician's assistant.**

***Physician's Desk Reference* (PDR),** a compendium compiled annually, containing information about drugs, primarily prescription drugs and products used in diagnostic procedures, supplied by their manufacturers.

physics, the study of the laws and properties of matter and energy, particularly as related to motion and force.

-physics, a combining form meaning the 'science of the nature of' something specified: *cytophysics, medicophysics, microphysics.*

physio-, physi-, a combining form meaning 'related to nature or to physiology': *physiochemical, physiognosis, physiotherapy.*

physiological chemistry. See **biochemistry.**

physiological dead space, an area in the respiratory system that includes the anatomical dead space together with the space in the alveoli occupied by air that does not contribute to the oxygen-carbon dioxide exchange. Compare **anatomical dead space.**

physiological motivation, a bodily need, as food or water, that initiates behavior directed toward satisfying the particular need. Also called **organic motivation.** Compare **achievement motivation, social motivation.**

physiologic contracture, a temporary condition in which muscles may contract and shorten for a considerable period of time. Drugs, extremes of temperature, and local accumulation of lactic acid are causes. Compare **functional contracture.**

physiologic dwarf. See **primordial dwarf.**

physiologic psychology, the study of the interrelationship of physiologic and psychologic processes, especially the effects of a change from normal to abnormal.

physiologic retraction ring, a ridge around the inside of the uterus that forms during the second stage of normal labor at the junction of the thinned lower uterine segment and thickened upper segment as a result of progressive lengthening of the muscle fibers of the lower segment and concomitant shortening of the muscle fibers of the upper segment. Compare **constriction ring, pathologic retraction ring.**

physiologic third heart sound, a low-pitched extra heart sound heard early in diastole in a healthy child or young adult. It is of no clinical significance and usually disappears with age. The same sound, heard in an older person who has heart disease is an abnormal finding called a ventricular gallop. See also **gallop.**

physiotherapy. See **physical therapy.** —**physiotherapeutic,** adj. **physiotherapist,** n.

-physis, a combining form meaning a 'growth or growing': *metaphysis, onychophysis, zygapophysis.*

physo-, a combining form meaning 'of or pertaining to air or gas': *physocele, physocephaly, physometra.*

physostigmine (fai'soustɪg'mɪn), a cholinergic.

■ INDICATIONS: It is prescribed in the treatment of some forms of glaucoma.

■ CONTRAINDICATIONS: Narrow-angle glaucoma, iridocyclitis, or known hypersensitivity to this drug prohibits its use.

■ ADVERSE EFFECTS: Among the more serious adverse reactions are bradycardia, dyspnea, bronchospasm, anorexia, and convulsions.

phytanic acid storage disease (faitæn'ık), a rare genetic disorder of lipid metabolism in which there are accumulations of phytanic acid in the plasma and tissues. The condition is characterized by ataxia, peripheral neuropathy, retinitis pigmentosa, and abnormalities of the bone and skin. Also called **Refsum's syndrome.**

-phyte, a combining form meaning a 'plant which grows in or on or produces': *epiphyte, paraphyte, pteridophyte.*

phyto-, a combining form meaning 'of or pertaining to a plant or plants': *phytobezoar, phytochemistry, phytoncide.*

phytonadione (fai'tounədai'oun). See **vitamin K₁.**

P.I., (in the patient record) abbreviation for *present illness.*

pia mater (pi'ə mei'tər), the innermost of the three meninges covering the brain and the spinal cord. It is closely applied to both structures and carries a rich supply of blood vessels, which nourish the nervous tissue. The cranial pia mater covers the surface of the brain and dips deeply into the fissures and the sulci of the cerebral hemispheres. Extending into the transverse cerebral fissure, the cranial pia mater forms the tela choroidea of the third ventricle, combines with the ependyma to form the choroid plexuses of the third and the lateral ventricles, and passes over the roof of the fourth ventricle to form its tela choroidea and its choroid plexus. The spinal pia mater is thicker, firmer, and less vascular than the cranial pia mater and consists of two layers. The outer layer is composed of longitudinal collagenous fibers which are concentrated along the anterior median fissure as the linea splendens. The inner layer closely wraps the entire spinal cord and, at the end of the cord, is prolonged into the filum terminale. The pia mater also forms the denticulate ligament which extends the entire length of the spinal cord on both sides between the dorsal and the ventral spinal nerve roots. Compare **arachnoid, dura mater.**

pian (piæn'). See **yaws.**

pica (pai'kə), a craving to eat substances that are not foods, as dirt, clay, chalk, glue, starch, or hair. The appetite disorder may occur with some nutritional deficiency states, pregnancy, and in some forms of mental illness.

Pick's disease, a form of presenile dementia occurring in middle age. This disorder affects mainly the frontal and temporal lobes of the brain and characteristically produces neurotic behavior, slow disintegration of intellect, personality, and emotions, and degeneration of cognitive abilities. See also **dementia.**

Pickwickian syndrome, an abnormal condition characterized by obesity, decreased pulmonary function, somnolence, and polycythemia.

pico-, a combining form meaning 'one trillionth' (10^{-12}) of the unit designated: *picogram, picoliter, picometer.*

picornavirus (paikɔr'nəvai'rəs), a member of a group of small RNA viruses that includes the enteroviruses, rhinoviruses, and causative organisms of encephalomyocarditis and foot-and-mouth disease.

picro-, a combining form meaning 'bitter': *picroadonidin, picropyrine, picrotoxin.*

picrotoxin (pɪk'routok'sɪn), a central nervous system stimulant obtained from the seeds of *Anamirta cocculus.* It was formerly used as an antidote for acute barbiturate poisoning.

PID, abbreviation for **pelvic inflammatory disease.**

P.I.E., abbreviation for *pulmonary infiltrate with eosinophilia,* a hypersensitivity reaction, characterized by infiltration of alveoli with eosinophils and large mononuclear cells, edema, and inflammation of the lungs. Simple pulmonary eosinophilia, in which patchy, migratory infiltrates cause minimal symptoms, is a self-limited reaction that is elicited by helminthic infections and by certain drugs, as para-aminosalicylic acid, sulfonamides, and chlorpropamide. A more prolonged illness, characterized by fever, night sweats, cough, dyspnea, weight loss, and more severe tissue reaction, occurs in certain drug allergies and bacterial, fungal, and parasitic infections. Tropical eosinophilia with paroxysmal nocturnal asthma, dyspnea, cough, low-grade fever, and malaise is related to filarial infection, and P.I.E. may occur in longstanding asthma and periarteritis nodosa.

piebald (pai'bɔld), having patches of white hair or skin owing to an absence of melanocytes in those nonpigmented areas. It is a hereditary condition. Compare **albinism**. See also **vitiligo**.

Piedmont fracture, an oblique fracture of the distal radius, with fragments of bone pulled into the ulna.

Pierre Robin syndrome, a complex of congenital anomalies including a small mandible, cleft lip, cleft palate, other craniofacial abnormalities, and defects of the eyes and ears. Intelligence is usually normal. Plastic surgery may achieve satisfactory cosmetic repair, but speech therapy, orthodontia, and psychological counseling and support are often necessary.

piez-, a combining form meaning 'of or related to pressure': *piezesthesia, piezallochromy, piezotherapy.*

pigeon breast, a congenital structural defect characterized by a prominent anterior projection of the xiphoid and the lower part of the sternum and by a lengthening of the costal cartilages. It may cause cardiorespiratory complications but rarely warrants surgical correction. —**pigeon-breasted**, *adj.*

pigeon breeder's lung, a respiratory disorder caused by acquired hypersensitivity to antigens in bird droppings. Also called **bird breeder's lung**.

piggyback port, a special coupling for the primary I.V. tubing which allows a supplementary, or piggyback, solution to run into the I.V. system. The piggyback port includes a backcheck valve which automatically prevents the primary I.V. solution from flowing while the piggyback solution is flowing. When the piggyback solution stops flowing, the backcheck valve starts the flow of the primary I.V. solution. Piggyback ports are part of piggyback I.V. sets, which are used solely for intermittent drug administration.

pigment, 1. any organic coloring material produced in the body, as melanin. 2. any colored, paintlike, medicinal preparation applied to the skin surface. —**pigmentary**, **pigmented**, *adj.*, **pigmentation**, *n.*

pigmy. See **pygmy**.

pilar cyst, an epidermoid cyst of the scalp. Its keratinized contents are firmer and less cheesy than the material in epidermoid cysts found elsewhere. The cyst originates from the middle portion of the epithelium of a

hair follicle. Treatment is surgical excision. Also called **sebaceous cyst, wen**. Compare **epidermoid cyst**.

piles. See **hemorrhoids**.

pill. See **tablet**.

pillion fracture (pɪl'yən), a T-shaped fracture of the distal femur with displacement of the condyles posterior to the femoral shaft, caused by a severe blow to the knee.

pilo-, a combining form meaning 'resembling or composed of hair': *pilocystic, pilomotor, pilose.*

Pilocar Ophthalmic, a trade name for a cholinergic (pilocarpine hydrochloride).

pilocarpine (pai'loukar'pin), a topical cholinergic antiglaucoma agent for ophthalmic use.
■ INDICATIONS: It is prescribed to induce miosis and to decrease intraocular pressure in chronic forms of open-angle glaucoma and in angle-closure glaucoma.
■ CONTRAINDICATIONS: It is used with caution in the presence of asthma, keratitis, conjunctivitis, and iritis. Known hypersensitivity to this drug prohibits its use.
■ ADVERSE REACTIONS: Among the more serious adverse reactions are dyspnea, wheezing, muscle tremors, diaphoresis, and hyperptyalism. Blurred vision, eye pain, and headache may occur.

pilocarpine and epinephrine, a fixed-combination drug used in the treatment of glaucoma, containing a cholinergic (pilocarpine hydrochloride) and an adrenergic vasoconstrictor (epinephrine bitartrate). Both ingredients reduce intraocular pressure.

pilocarpine and physostigmine, a fixed-combination drug used in the treatment of glaucoma, containing a cholinergic (pilocarpine hydrochloride) and a short-acting cholinesterase inhibitor (physostigmine salicylate). Both ingredients reduce intraocular pressure.

pilocarpine hydrochloride, an ophthalmic cholinergic.
■ INDICATIONS: It is prescribed as a miotic in treating primary open-angle and acute-angle closure glaucoma.
■ CONTRAINDICATION: Known hypersensitivity to this drug prohibits its use.
■ ADVERSE EFFECTS: Among the most serious adverse reactions are ciliary spasm with pain and allergic reactions.

Pilocel, a trade name for a cholinergic (pilocarpine hydrochloride).

Pilomiotin, a trade name for a cholinergic (pilocarpine hydrochloride).

pilomotor reflex (pai'loumou'tər), erection of the hairs of the skin in response to a chilly environment, emotional stimulus, or irritation of the skin. This normal reaction is abolished below the level of a transverse spinal cord lesion and may be exaggerated on the affected side in a patient with hemiplegia. Also called **gooseflesh, horripilation**.

pilonidal cyst (pai'lonai'dəl), a cyst in the midline of the upper portion of the gluteal fold, formed during embryologic development by the inclusion of a small amount of endothelial tissue in a space beneath the skin. Pilonidal cysts may sometimes be recognized at birth by a depression, sometimes a hairy dimple, in the midline of the back, sacrococcygeal area. Usually these cysts do not cause any problems, but occasionally a sinus or fistula develops in early adulthood that communicates with the skin, resulting in infection. A fistula may also develop to the spinal tract from a pilonidal cyst. If a cyst becomes infected or inflamed it is excised, and the space is surgically closed after the infection or inflammation has been effectively treated.

pilonidal fistula, an abnormal channel containing a tuft of hair, situated most frequently over or close to the tip of the coccyx but also occurring in other regions of the body. Also called **pilonidal sinus.**

pilonidal sinus. See **pilonidal fistula.**

pilosebaceous (pai'lousɪbei'ʃəs), of or pertaining to a hair follicle and its oil gland.

Pima, a trade name for an expectorant (potassium iodide).

pimaricin (pɪmær'ɪsɪn). See **natamycin.**

pimelo-, a combining form meaning 'of or related to fat': *pimeloma, pimelopterygium, pimelorrhea.*

pimozide (pɪm'əzaid), an investigational antipsychotic agent.

pimple, a small papule, pustule, or furuncle.

pin, 1. (in orthopedics) to secure and immobilize fragments of bone with a nail. **2.** See **nail,** def. 2. **3.** (in dentistry) a small metal rod or peg, used as a support in rebuilding a tooth.

pineal body (pɪn'iəl), a small, somewhat flattened, cone-shaped structure about 8 mm long, suspended by a stalk in the epithalamus. It consists of glial cells and pinealocytes and apparently elaborates the hormone melatonin.

pineal gland, a cone-shaped structure in the brain, situated between the superior colliculi, the pulvinar, and the splenium of the corpus callosum. Its precise function has not been established. It may secrete the hormone melatonin which appears to inhibit the secretion of luteinizing hormone. Also called **epiphysis cerebri, pineal body.**

pinealocytoma (pɪn'iəlousaitou'mə). See **pinealoma.**

pinealoma (pɪn'iəlou'mə), *pl.* **pinealomas, pinealomata.** a rare neoplasm of the pineal body in the brain, characterized by hydrocephalus, papillary changes, gait disturbances, headache, nausea, and vomiting. Precocious puberty occurs in some cases, probably owing to extension of the tumor into the hypothalamus. Also called **pinealocytoma.**

pineal tumor, a neoplasm of the pineal body. See also **pinealoma.**

pine tar, a topical antieczematic and a rubefacient. It is a common ingredient in creams, soaps, and lotions used in the treatment of chronic skin conditions, as eczema or psoriasis.

ping-ponging, *Slang.* a fraudulent practice involving passing a patient from one physician to another so that a health program or facility can charge a third party for several cursory examinations.

pinhole test, a test performed in examining a person who has diminished visual acuity to distinguish a refractve error from organic disease. A refractive error may be corrected with glasses and is not medically dangerous. Loss of visual acuity owing to organic disease is serious as it may indicate a systemic, particularly a neurologic, disease and may signal the development of avoidable blindness. The test is simple to perform. Several pinholes are punched in a card; the patient selects one and looks through it with one eye at a time, without wearing glasses. If visual acuity is improved, the defect is refractive; if not, it is organic. The pinhole effect results from blocking peripheral light waves, those most distorted by refractive error.

pinkeye. See **conjunctivitis.**

Pinkus' disease (pɪŋ'kəsəz). See **lichen nitidus.**

pinna (pɪn'ə), *pl.* **pinnas, pinnae.** See **auricula.** – **pinnal,** *adj.*

pinocytosis (pi'nousaitou'sɪs), the process by which extracellular fluid is taken into a cell. The cell membrane develops a saccular indentation filled with extracellular fluid, then closes around it, forming a vesicle or a vaccule of fluid within the cell.

pinta, an infection of the skin caused by *Treponema carateum*, a common organism in South and Central America. The bacterium gains entry into the body through a break in the skin. Prolonged exposure and close contact appear to be necessary for transmission. The primary lesion is a slowly enlarging papule with regional lymph node enlargement, followed in one to twelve months by a generalized red to slate-blue macular rash. Eventually these lesions become depigmented. Diagnosis is based on serologic tests and darkfield microscopic examination of scrapings from skin lesions. Treatment with penicillin G is effective. The major complication of the disease is social ostracism resulting from the permanently disfiguring mottling of the skin. Also called **azul, carate, mal del pinto.** Compare **yaws.**

pin track infection, an abnormal condition associated with skeletal traction and characterized by infection of superficial, deeper, or soft tissues or by osteomyelitis. These infections may develop at skeletal traction pin sites. Some of the signs of pin track infection are erythema at the pin sites, drainage and odor, pin slippage, elevated temperature, and pain. Superficial infection at the pin site is treated with antibiotics administered topically or orally. Deeper infection at the pin sites usually requires removal of the pins and antibiotic therapy.

pinworm. See *Enterobius vermicularis.*

pio-, a combining form meaning 'of or pertaining to fat': *pionemia, piorthopnea, pioscope.*

pion (paiʹon). See **negative pi meson.**

piperacetazine (pai′pərəsetʹəzin), a phenothiazine tranquilizer.

■ INDICATION: It is prescribed in the treatment of psychotic disorders.

■ CONTRAINDICATIONS: Parkinson's disease, concomitant administration of central nervous system depressants, liver or renal dysfunction, severe hypotension, or known hypersensitivity to other phenothiazine medication prohibits its use.

■ ADVERSE EFFECTS: Among the more serious adverse effects are hypotension, liver toxicity, blood dyscrasias, hypersensitivity reactions, and a variety of extrapyramidal reactions, including post-treatment tardive dyskinesia.

piperazine citrate (pi per′əzin), an anthelmintic.

■ INDICATIONS: It is prescribed to treat infestation by pinworms or roundworms.

■ CONTRAINDICATIONS: Impaired liver or kidney function, convulsive disorders, or known hypersensitivity to this drug prohibits its use.

■ ADVERSE EFFECTS: Among the more serious adverse reactions, usually due to overdosage, are abdominal cramps, diarrhea, vertigo, blurring of vision, and fever.

Piper forceps. See **obstetric forceps.**

pipette (paipet′, pipet′), **1.** a calibrated, transparent open-ended tube of glass or plastic used for measuring or transferring small quantities of a liquid or gas. **2.** using a pipette to dispense liquid.

pipobroman (pai′pəbrou′mən), an antineoplastic.

■ INDICATIONS: It is prescribed in the treatment of polycythemia vera and chronic granulocytic leukemia.

■ CONTRAINDICATIONS: Bone marrow depression or known hypersensitivity to this drug prohibits its use.

■ ADVERSE EFFECTS: Among the more serious adverse reactions are nausea, abdominal cramps, and fever.

piriform aperture, the anterior nasal opening in the skull.

piriformis (pir′ifor′mis), a flat, pyramidal muscle lying almost parallel with the posterior margin of the gluteus medius. It is partly within the pelvis and partly at the back of the hip joint. It arises from the sacrum, the greater sciatic foramen, and the sacrotuberous ligament, and it inserts, by a rounded tendon, into the greater trochanter of the femur. The piriformis is innervated by branches of the first and the second sacral nerves and functions to rotate the thigh laterally and to abduct and to help extend it. Compare **obturator externus, obturator internus.**

Pirquet test (pərkəi′), a tuberculin skin test that consists of scratching the tuberculin material onto the skin. Also called **von Pirquet test.** See also **tuberculin test.**

pisiform bone (fis′ifərm), a small, spheroidal carpal bone in the proximal row of carpal bones. It articulates with the triangular bone and is attached to the flexor retinaculum, the flexor carpi ulnaris, and the abductor digiti minimi.

pitch, the quality of a tone or sound dependent on the relative rapidity of the vibrations by which it is produced.

Pitocin, a trade name for an oxytocic (oxytocin).

Pitocin Citrate, a trade name for an oxytocic (oxytocin citrate).

Pitressin, a trade name for an antidiuretic hormone (vasopressin).

pitting, 1. small, punctate indentations in fingernails or toenails, often a result of psoriasis. **2.** an indentation that remains for a short time after pressing edematous skin with a finger. **3.** small, depressed scars in the skin or other organ of the body. **4.** the removal by the spleen of material from within erythrocytes without damage to the cells.

pituit-, a combining form meaning 'of or related to phlegm': *pituita, pituitary, pituitous.*

pituitary adamantinoma. See **craniopharyngioma.**

pituitary cachexia. See **postpubertal panhypopituitarism.**

pituitary dwarf, a dwarf whose retarded development is owing to a deficiency of growth hormone resulting from hypofunction of the anterior lobe of the pituitary. In most cases the cause is unknown, and the defect is limited to a lack of somatotropin, although in some instances gonadotropins, adrenocorticotropic hormone, and thyroid-stimulating hormone may also be deficient. The body is properly proportioned, with no facial or skeletal deformities, and there is normal mental and sexual development. The condition is usually diagnosed in childhood by radiographic examination of the bones and radioimmunoassay of levels of plasma growth hormone. Also called **hypophyseal dwarf, Lévi-Lorain dwarf, Paltauf's dwarf.**

pituitary gland, the small gland attached to the hypothalamus and couched in the sphenoid bone, supplying numerous hormones that govern many vital processes. It is divided into an anterior adenohypophysis and a smaller posterior neurohypophysis. The adenohypophysis secretes growth hormone (somatotrophin), thyrotrophic hormone, adrenocorticotrophic hormone (ACTH), two gonadotrophic hormones, follicle-stimulating hormone (FSH), luteinizing hormone (LH), and prolactin, the hormone that promotes milk secretion. The neurohypophysis stores two hormones, oxytocin and vasopressin. Oxytocin stimulates the contraction of smooth muscle, especially in the uterus. Vasopressin inhibits diuresis and raises blood pressure. The pituitary gland is larger in a woman than in a man and becomes further enlarged during pregnancy. Also called **hypophysis cerebri.** See also **adenohypophysis, neurohypophysis.**

pituitary nanism, a type of dwarfism associated with hypophyseal infantilism. See also **pituitary dwarf.**

pituitary snuff lung, a type of hypersensitivity pneumonitis that sometimes occurs among takers of pituitary snuff. The antigens to which the hypersensitivity reaction occurs are found in serum proteins of cows and pigs and in pituitary tissue. Symptoms of the acute form of the disease include chills, cough, fever, dyspnea, anorexia, nausea, and vomiting. The chronic form of the disease is characterized by fatigue, chronic cough, weight loss, and dyspnea on exercise.

Pituitrin, a trade name for an extract of the antidiuretic and oxytocic hormone of the posterior pituitary gland.

pit viper, any one of a family of venomous snakes found in the Western Hemisphere and Asia, characterized by a heat-sensitive pit between the eye and nostril on each side of the head and hollow, perforated fangs that are usually folded back in the roof of the mouth. With the exception of coral snakes, all indigenous poisonous snakes in the United States are pit vipers. See also **copperhead, cottonmouth, rattlesnake.**

pityriasis alba (pɪtəraɪ'əsɪs), a common idiopathic dermatosis characterized by round or oval, finely scaling patches of hypopigmentation. The lesions are sharply demarcated, occasionally pruritic, and occur primarily in children and adolescents. The condition may recur, but spontaneous clearing is the usual prognosis. Treatment includes lubricating creams, topical corticosteroids, and, less commonly, coal tar creams. Compare **pityriasis rosea.**

pityriasis rosea, a self-limited skin disease in which a slightly scaling, pink, macular rash spreads over the trunk and other unexposed areas of the body. A characteristic feature is the **herald patch,** a larger, more scaly lesion which precedes the diffuse rash by several days. The smaller lesions tend to line up with the long axis parallel to normal lines of cleavage of the skin. Mild itching is the only symptom. The disease lasts four to eight weeks and rarely recurs. It is unusual, apparently not contagious, and its cause is unknown.

pivot joint, a synovial joint in which movement is limited to rotation. The joint is formed by a pivotlike process that may turn within a ring composed partly of bone and partly of ligament. The proximal radioulnar articulation is a pivot joint in which the head of the radius rotates within the ring formed by the radial notch of the ulna and the annular ligament. Also called **trochoid joint.** Compare **gliding joint, hinge joint.** See also **condyloid joint.**

PK, abbreviation for **psychokinesis.**

PKD, abbreviation for **polycystic kidney disease.**

PK test, abbreviation for **Prausnitz-Küstner test.**

PKU, abbreviation for **phenylketonuria.**

placebo (pləsi'bou), an inactive substance, as saline, distilled water, or sugar, or a less than effective dose of a harmless substance, as a water-soluble vitamin prescribed as if it were an effective dose of a needed medication. Placebos are used in experimental drug studies to com-
pare the effects of the placebo with those of the experimental drug. They are also prescribed for patients who cannot be given the medication they request or who, in the judgment of the health care provider, do not need that medication. Placebo therapy is effective in some cases, and side effects often occur as they would from the actual medication. The benefit to the patient of a placebo should clearly outweigh the ethical, moral, and legal problems posed by its administration.

placebo effect, a physical or emotional change occurring after a substance is taken or administered that is not the result of any special property of the substance. The change is usually beneficial and reflects the expectations of the patient and, often, the expectations of the person giving the substance.

placent-, a combining form meaning 'a cakelike mass': *placenta, placentapepton, placentogenesis.*

placenta, a highly vascular fetal organ through which the fetus absorbs oxygen, nutrients, and other substances and excretes carbon dioxide and other wastes. It begins to form on approximately the eighth day of gestation when the blastocyst touches the wall of the uterus and adheres to it. The blastocyst becomes surrounded by an outer layer of syncytiotrophoblast and an inner layer of cytotrophoblast. The trophoblast is able to digest cells of the endometrium, causing a small erosion on the uterine wall in which an embryo nidates. Under the influence of increasing amounts of progesterone, secreted by the corpus luteum of the ovary, the embryo and the placenta continue to develop. A hormone, chorionic gonadotropin, is secreted by the developing placenta and is present in the maternal blood and urine. The trophoblastic layer continues to infiltrate the maternal tissues with fingerlike projections, called chorionic villi. Separating the villi are lakes of blood in the eroded tissue. The maternal blood flows into the lakes surrounding the villi, allowing nutrients, gases, and other substances to pass into the fetal circulation by diffusion, hydrostatic pressure, and osmosis. The placenta is able to secrete large amounts of progesterone by the third month of pregnancy, enough to relieve the corpus luteum of that function. At term the normal placenta weighs one seventh to one fifth of the weight of the infant. The maternal surface is lobulated and divided into cotyledons. It has a dark red, rough, liverlike appearance. The fetal surface is smooth and shiny, covered with the fetal membranes, marked by the large white blood vessels beneath the membranes that fan out from the centrally inserted umbilical cord. The time between the delivery of the infant and the expulsion of the placenta is the third and last stage of labor.

-placenta, a combining form meaning an 'organ shaped lake a flat cake': *ectoplacenta, hemiplacenta, subplacenta.*

placental hormone, one of the several hormones produced by the placenta, including human placental lactogen, chorionic gonadotropin, estrogen, progesterone, and a thyrotropinlike hormone.

placental insufficiency, an abnormal condition of pregnancy, manifested clinically by retardation of the rate of fetal and uterine growth. One or more placental abnormalities cause dysfunction of maternal-placental or fetal-placental circulation sufficient to compromise fetal nutrition and oxygenation. Some of the abnormalities that can result in placental insufficiency are abnormal implantation of the placenta, multiple pregnancy, abnormal attachments of the umbilical cord or anomalies of the cord itself, and abnormalities of the placental membranes. Histopathologic abnormalities that can cause placental insufficiency include intravillous thrombi, placental infarction, and breaks in the placental membrane that result in fetal bleeding into the maternal circulation. Placental insufficiency may also result from placental senescence in postmaturity, from systemic diseases, as erythroblastosis fetalis and diabetes melitus, or from bacterial, viral, parasitic, or fungal infections. See also **intrauterine growth retardation, postmature infant syndrome.**

placenta previa, a condition of pregnancy in which the placenta is implanted abnormally in the uterus so that it impinges upon or covers the internal os of the uterine cervix. It is the most common cause of painless bleeding in the third trimester of pregnancy. Its etiology is unknown. The incidence of the condition increases with increased parity from approximately 1 in 1,500 primiparas to approximately 1 in 20 grand multiparas. Even slight dilatation of the internal os can cause enough local separation of an abnormally implanted placenta to result in bleeding. If severe hemorrhage occurs, immediate Caesarean section is usually required to stop the bleeding and to save the mother's life; it is performed regardless of the stage of fetal maturity. Prior to hemorrhage, placenta previa may be diagnosed by ultrasonography and treated with complete bed rest under close observation. Even at rest, sudden massive hemorrhage can occur without warning. Vaginal examination is usually contraindicated if placenta previa is present or suspected because palpation can cause local placental separation and precipitate hemorrhage. Cautious and very gentle intracervical palpation may be performed to determine the existence and exact extent of previa. Before this examination, an intravenous infusion is begun, the woman's blood is typed and crossmatched, and preparations for immediate Caesarean section are made. If the placenta is next to or near, rather than touching or covering the cervical os, labor and vaginal delivery may be attempted. Also called *Informal. previa.* Kinds of placenta previa are **central placenta previa, marginal placenta previa, partial placenta previa.** Compare **abruptio placenta.**

Placidyl, a trade name for a sedative (ethchlorvynol).

Plafon fracture, a fracture that involves the buttress portion of the malleolus of a bone.

plagiocephaly (plei'jiousef'əli), **plagiocephalism,** a congenital malformation of the skull in which premature or irregular closure of the coronal or lambdoidal sutures results in asymmetrical growth of the head, giving it a twisted, lopsided appearance so that the maximum length is not along the midline but on a diagonal. See also **craniostenosis.** – **plagiocephalic, plagiocephalous,** *adj.*

plague, an infectious disease caused by the bite of a flea infected by a rat infected with the bacillus *Yersinia pestis.* Plague is primarily an infectious disease of rats: the rat fleas feed on humans only when their preferred hosts have been killed by the plague in a rat epizootic; therefore, epidemics occur after rat epizootics. Kinds of plague include **bubonic plague, pneumonic plague, septicemic plague.** See also *Yersinia pestis.*

plague vaccine, an active immunizing agent prepared with killed plague bacilli.

■ INDICATION: It is prescribed for immunization against plague following probable exposure.

■ CONTRAINDICATIONS: Immunosuppression or acute infection prohibits its use.

■ ADVERSE EFFECTS: Among the most serious adverse reactions are allergic reactions, inflammation at the site of injection, headache, and malaise.

plaintiff, (in law) a person who files a lawsuit initiating a legal action. The plaintiff complains or sues for remedial relief and names a complainant in various civil actions. In criminal actions, the prosecution is the plaintiff, acting in behalf of the people of the jurisdiction.

-plakia, a combining form meaning 'patches on mucous membrane': *leukoplakia, malocoplakia, melanoplakia.*

planar xanthoma, a yellow or orange flat macule or slightly raised papule containing foam cells and occurring in clusters in localized areas, as the eyelids, or widely distributed over the body, as in generalized planar xanthoma or xanthelasmatosis. Also called **plane xanthoma, xanthoma planum.** See also **xanthelasma, xanthelasmatosis.**

plane, 1. a flat surface determined by three points in space. 2. an extension of a longitudinal section through an axis, as the coronal, the horizontal, and the sagittal planes used to identify the position of various parts of the body in the study of anatomy. 3. the act of paring or of rubbing away. 4. a superficial incision in the wall of a cavity or between tissue layers, especially in plastic surgery. – **planar,** *adj.*

planes of anesthesia. See **Guedel's signs.**

-plania, a combining form meaning the 'deviation from its normal location': *choloplania, pyoplania, spiloplania.*

planned parenthood, a philosophical framework central to the development of contraceptive methods, contraceptive counseling, and family planning programs and clinics. Advocates hold that as it is the right of each woman to decide when to conceive and bear children, and that contraceptive and gynecologic care and information should be available to her to help her to become or to avoid becoming pregnant.

planning, (in five-step nursing process) a category of nursing behavior in which a strategy is designed for the achievement of the goals of care for an individual client, as established in assessing and analyzing. Planning includes developing and modifying a care plan for the client, cooperating with other personnel, and recording relevant information. To develop the plan the nurse anticipates the client's needs according to established priorities; involves the client and the client's family and significant others in designing the plan; uses all information necessary for managing care of the patient, including recorded information from other health professionals, and the age, sex, culture, ethnicity, and religion; plans for the client's comfort, activity, and function; and chooses nursing measures that are necessary to deliver care as planned. With the cooperation of other health personnel, the nurse coordinates care for the benefit of the client and identifies resources in the hospital or community for social or health assistance as needed by the client or the client's family. All information relevant to the management of the client's care plan is recorded. Planning follows analyzing and precedes implementing in the five-step nursing process. See also **assessing, evaluating.**

plano-, a combining form meaning 'wandering': *planocyte, planotopokinesia.*

plantago seed (plæntei'gou), a bulk forming laxative. Also called **psyllium seed.**

■ INDICATION: It is prescribed in the treatment of constipation.

■ CONTRAINDICATIONS: Symptoms of appendicitis, intestinal obstruction, or gastrointestinal ulceration prohibits its use.

■ ADVERSE EFFECTS: Among the more serious adverse effects are intestinal obstruction and allergic reactions.

plantar (plæn'tər), of or pertaining to the sole of the foot. Also called **volar.**

plantar aponeurosis, the tough fascia surrounding the muscles of the soles of the feet. Also called **plantar fascia.**

plantar fascia. See **plantar aponeurosis.**

plantaris (plænta'rɪs), one of three superficial muscles at the back of the leg, between the soleus and the gastrocnemius. The plantaris is a small muscle that arises from the distal part of the linea aspera of the femur and from the oblique popliteal ligament of the knee joint. It has a small fusiform belly, ending in a long, slender tendon that inserts into the calcaneus. The plantaris is innervated by a branch of the tibial nerve, containing fibers from the fourth and the fifth lumbar and the first sacral nerves. It flexes the foot and the leg. Compare **gastrocnemius, soleus.**

plantar neuroma, a neuroma of the sole of the foot.

plantar reflex, the normal response, elicited by firmly stroking the outer surface of the sole from heel to toes, characterized by flexion of the toes. Compare **Babinski's reflex.**

plantar wart, a painful verrucous lesion on the sole of the foot, primarily at points of pressure, as over the metatarsal heads and the heel. Caused by the common wart virus, it appears as a soft, central core and is surrounded by a firm, hyperkeratotic ring resembling a callus. Multiple, tiny, black spots on the surface represent bits of coagulated blood in the wart. Treatment methods include electrodesiccation, cryotherapy, topical acids, cantharadin, and even mental suggestion. See also **mosaic wart, verruca vulgaris.**

plantigrade (plæn'tɪgreɪd), of, pertaining to, or characterizing the human gait; walking on the sole of the foot with the heel touching the ground.

plaque, 1. a flat, often raised, patch on the skin or any other organ of the body. 2. a patch of atherosclerosis. 3. Also called **dental plaque.** a thin film on the teeth made up of mucin and colloidal material found in saliva and often secondarily invaded by bacteria.

Plaquenil Sulfate, a trade name for an antimalarial, anti-arthritic, and lupus erythematosus suppressant (hydroxychloroquine sulfate).

-plasia, a combining form meaning '(condition of) formation or development': *alloplasia, anosteoplasia, cacoplasia.*

-plasm, a combining form meaning 'cell or tissue substance': *deutoplasm, mitoplasm, phytoplasm.* Also **-plasma.**

plasma, the watery, colorless, fluid portion of the lymph and the blood in which the leukocytes, erythrocytes, and platelets are suspended. It contains no cells and is made up of water, electrolytes, proteins, glucose, fats, bilirubin, and gases. It is essential for carrying the cellular elements of the blood through the circulation, transporting nutrients, maintaining the acid-base balance of the body, and transporting wastes from the tissues. Plasma and interstitial fluid correspond closely in content and concentration of proteins; therefore, plasma is important in maintaining the osmotic pressure and the exchange of fluids and electrolytes between the capillaries and the tissues. Compare **serum.**

plasma-, a combining form meaning 'the liquid portion of the blood': *plasmablast, plasmacyte, plasmapheresis.*

-plasma, a combining form meaning 'fluid part of cytoplasm or protoplasm': *ectoplasma, hydroplasma, ovoplasma.*

plasma cell, a lymphoid or lymphocyte-like cell found in the bone marrow, connective tissue, and, sometimes, in the blood. It contains an eccentric nucleus with deeply staining chromatin material arranged in a pattern like the spokes of a wheel or a clock face. Plasma cells are involved in the immunologic mechanism and are formed in large numbers in multiple myeloma. See also **multiple myeloma.**

plasma cell leukemia, an unusual neoplasm of blood-forming tissues in which the predominant cells in peripheral blood are plasmacytes. The disease may develop in the course of multiple myeloma or arise independently. Bence Jones proteinuria, abnormal serum globulins, hepatomegaly, and splenomegaly are usual in plasma cell leukemia. In most cases plasma cell leukemia is rapidly fatal, but some patients respond to treatment with alkylating agents and glucocorticoids.

plasma cell myeloma. See **multiple myeloma.**

plasma cell tumor. See **plasmacytoma.**

plasmacytoma (plæz′mɔsaitou′mɔ), *pl.* **plasmacytomas, plasmacytomata.** a focal neoplasm containing plasma cells. It may develop in the bone marrow, as in multiple myeloma, or outside the bone marrow, as in certain tumors of the viscera and the mucosa of the nasal, oral, and pharyngeal areas. Also called **peripheral plasma cell myeloma, plasma cell tumor.**

Plasma-Lyte, a trade name for a nutritional supplement containing various electrolytes with or without dextrose.

plasma membrane. See **cell membrane.**

plasmaphoresis (plæz′mɔfɔri′sɪs), a laboratory procedure in which the plasma proteins are separated by electrophoresis for identification and evaluation of the proportion of the various proteins.

plasma protein, any one of the various proteins, including albumin, fibrinogen, prothrombin, and the gamma globulins, which constitute about 6 to 7 per cent of the blood plasma in the body. These substances aid in the maintenance of water balance affecting osmotic pressure, increase blood viscosity, and help maintain blood pressure. Fibrinogen and prothrombin are essential to blood coagulation, and the gamma globulins are important in immunoregulation. All the plasma proteins except the gamma globulins, are synthesized in the liver. See also **serum.**

plasma thromboplastin antecedent (PTA), a blood factor essential in the coagulation process. Thromboplastin cannot be formed in its absence. Also called **antihemophilic C factor, factor IX complex.**

plasma thromboplastin component deficiency. See **hemophilia.**

plasmid, (in bacteriology) any type of intracellular inclusion considered to have a genetic function, especially a molecule of DNA separate from the bacterial chromosome that determines traits not essential for the viability of the organism but that in some way changes the organism's ability to adapt. R (resistance) factor is an example: a bacterium containing the factor is able to resist many antibacterial drugs that act in many different ways. Plasmid may be passed from one bacterium to another, and it

is replicated in later generations of any bacterium carrying it.

plasmidotrophoblast (plæz′mɪdoutrou′fɔblæst). See **syncytiotrophoblast.**

plasmin. See **fibrinolysin.**

plasminogen (plæzmɪn′ɔjɪn). See **fibrinogen.**

plasmo-, a combining form meaning 'of or related to plasma, or to the substance of a cell': *plasmocyte, plasmodium, plasmosome.*

Plasmodium (plæzmou′diɔm), a genus of protozoa several species of which cause malaria, transmitted to man by the bite of an infected Anopheles mosquito. ***Plasmodium falciparum*** causes falciparum malaria, the most severe form of the disease; *P. malariae* causes quartan malaria; *P. ovale* causes mild tertian malaria with oval red blood cells; and *P. vivax* causes common tertian malaria. See also ***Anopheles,*** **blackwater fever, malaria.**

plasmosome, plasmasome (plæz′mɔsoum), the true nucleolus of a cell as distinguished from the karyosomes in the nucleus.

plast-, a combining form meaning 'formed': *plastidogenetic, plastodynamia, plastogamy.*

-plast, a combining form meaning a 'primitive cell': *chondroplast, gymnoplast, osteoplast.*

plaster, 1. any composition of a liquid and a powder that hardens when it dries, used in shaping a cast to support a fractured bone as it heals, as plaster of Paris. **2.** a home remedy consisting of a semisolid mixture applied to a part of the body as a counterirritant or for other therapeutic reasons, as a mustard plaster.

-plastia, a combining form meaning '(condition of) cell or tissue formation or development': *anaplastia, macroplastia, mastplastia.* Also **-plasia.**

-plastic, a combining form meaning 'pertaining to the development of' something specified: *entoplastic, hemoplastic, rhinoplastic.*

plastic surgery, the alteration, replacement, or restoration of visible portions of the body, performed to correct a structural or cosmetic defect. In performing corrective plastic surgery, the surgeon may use tissue from the patient or from another person or an inert material that is nonirritating, has a consistency appropriate to the use, and is able to hold its shape and form indefinitely. Implants are commonly used in mammoplasty for breast augmentation. Skin grafting is the most common procedure in plastic surgery. Z-plasty and Y-plasty are simpler techniques often performed instead of a graft in areas of the body covered by skin that is loose and elastic, as the neck, axilla, throat, and inner aspect of the elbow. Dermabrasion is used to remove pockmarks, scars from acne, or signs of traumatic skin damage. Chemical peeling is another technique in corrective plastic surgery; it is used primarily for removing fine wrinkles on the face. Tattooing, in which a pigment is tattooed into the skin of a graft, is performed to change the color of the graft to resemble more closely the surrounding skin. Reconstructive plastic surgery is performed to correct birth defects, to repair structures destroyed by trauma, and to replace tissue removed in other surgical procedures. Cleft lip and cleft palate repair and other maxillofacial surgical procedures, including rhinoplasty, otoplasty, and rhytidoplasty, are among these reconstructive procedures. Care of the person before and after plastic surgery may require considerable sensitivity and tact. The patient may be exceedingly uncomfortable about the real or perceived appearance of the defect. An accepting, nonjudgmental attitude on the part of all staff members is to the patient's benefit. Optimal nutritional status helps a graft to 'take' and speeds healing. Each procedure and technique involves particular kinds of care in the preoperative and postoperative periods. Instructions and assistance in self-care activities are also specific to the various procedures. Success of most of the procedures depends greatly on the patient's cooperation and fastidious nursing care. The correction of a visible abnormality may be of inestimable benefit to the patient's assurance, self-esteem, and function in society. See also specific procedures.

-plasty, a combining form meaning 'plastic surgery on a (specified) body part or by (specified) means': *bronchoplasty, cervicoplasty, uveoplasty.*

plate, a flat structure or layer, as a thin layer of bone or the frontal plate between the sides of the ethmoid cartilage and the sphenoid bone in the fetus.

platelet, the smallest of the cells in the blood. Platelets are disc-shaped and contain no hemoglobin. They are essential for the coagulation of blood. Normally between 200,000 and 300,000 platelets are found in 1 cu mm of blood. See also **thrombocytopenia, thrombocytosis.**

Platinol, a trade name for an antineoplastic (cisplatin).

platinum (Pt), a silvery-white, soft metallic element. Its atomic number is 78; its atomic weight is 195.09. Platinum is used in jewelry and in the manufacture of chemical apparatus that must withstand high temperatures.

platy-, a combining form meaning 'broad or flat': *platybasia, platycephalous, platyenemic.*

platypelloid pelvis (plæt′əpel′oid), a rare type of pelvis in which the inlet is round like the gynecoid type in the anterior section, but the posterior section is foreshortened by its flat and heavy border. The sacrum is hollow and inclines posteriorly, and the sidewalls are convergent. In the midplane, the transverse diameter is much wider than the narrowed anteroposterior diameter. Vaginal delivery is not usually possible in women who have platypelloid pelves. This type of pelvis is present in 3 per cent of women.

platysma (plətɪz′mə), one of a pair of wide muscles at the side of the neck. It arises from the fascia covering the superior parts of the pectoralis major and the deltoideus, crosses the clavicle, and rises obliquely and medially along the side of the neck. The anterior fibers of the platysma interlace, inferior and posterior to the symphysis menti, with the fibers of the muscle of the opposite side. The posterior fibers of the platysma cross the mandible, some inserting into the bone below the oblique line, others into the skin and the subcutaneous tissue of the lower part of the face. Many of the fibers blend with the muscles at the angle and the lower part of the mouth. The platysma covers the external jugular vein as the vein descends from the angle of the mandible to the clavicle. The platysma is innervated by the cervical branch of the facial nerve and serves to draw down the lower lip and the corner of the mouth. When the platysma fully contracts, the skin over the clavicle is drawn toward the mandible, increasing the diameter of the neck.

play, any spontaneous or organized activity that provides enjoyment, entertainment, amusement, or diversion. It is essential in childhood for the development of a normal personality and as a means for developing physically, intellectually, and socially. Play provides an outlet for releasing tension and stress as well as a means for testing and experimenting with new or fearful roles or situations. It is an indispensable part of the nursing care of children, especially in the hospital. It helps to relieve the tension and anxiety of being in unfamiliar surroundings and separated from parents, and it gives the child a sense of security and a means of expressing fears and fantasies. Play also offers the nurse one of the most effective methods of communicating with and gaining the trust of the child and helping the child to understand treatments and procedures. Kinds of play include **active play, associative play, cooperative play, dramatic play, parallel play, passive play, skill play, solitary play.** See also **play therapy.**

play therapy, a form of psychotherapy in which a child plays in a protected and structured environment with games and toys provided by a therapist, who observes the behavior, affect, and conversation of the child in order to gain insight into his thoughts, feelings, and fantasies. As conflicts are discovered, the therapist often helps the child to understand and work through them.

pleasure principle, (in psychoanalysis) the need for immediate gratification of instinctual drives. Compare **reality principle.**

pledget (plej′it), a small, flat compress made of cotton gauze, or a tuft of cotton wool, lint, or a similar synthetic material, used to wipe the skin, absorb drainage, or clean a small surface.

-plegia, a combining form meaning 'a (specified) paralysis': *colicoplegia, esophagoplegia, proctoplegia.*

-plegic, 1. a combining form meaning 'of or pertaining to a specific paralysis': *cycloplegic, ganglionoplegic, pharyngoplegic.* 2. a combining form meaning a 'sufferer from a specific paralysis': *diplegic, ophthalmoplegic, psychoplegic.*

Plegine, a trade name for an anorexiant (phendimetrazine tartrate).

pleiades (pli′ədiz), *Obsolete.* a mass of enlarged lymph nodes.

pleio-. See **pleo-.**

pleiotropy (plæiot′rəpi), (in genetics) a variable factor that modifies basic patterns of inheritance. It is the multiple, different, and apparently unrelated manifestation of a particular disorder, as the cluster of symptoms in Marfan's syndrome, aortic aneurysm, dislocation of the optic lens, skeletal deformities, and arachnodactyly, any or all of which may be present.

pleo-, pleio-, a combining form meaning 'more': *pleochromatic, pleomastia, pleomorphism.*

plessimeter (plesɪm′ɪtər). See **pleximeter.**

plethysmogram (pləθɪz′məgræm), a tracing produced by a plethysmograph.

plethysmograph (pləθɪz′məgræf), an instrument which measures and records changes in the sizes and volumes of extremities and organs by measuring changes in their blood volumes. — **plethysmographic,** *adj.,* **plethysmography,** *n.*

pleur-. See **pleuro-.**

pleura (plur′ə), *pl.* **pleurae.** a delicate serous membrane enclosing the lung, composed of a single layer of flattened mesothelial cells resting on a delicate membrane of connective tissue. Beneath the membrane is a stroma of collagenous tissue containing yellow elastic fibers. The pleura divides into the visceral pleura, which covers the lung, dipping into the fissures between the lobes, and the parietal pleura, which lines the chest wall, covers the diaphragm, and reflects over the structures in the mediastinum. The parietal and visceral pleurae are separated from each other by a small amount of fluid that acts as a lubricant as the lungs expand and contract during respiration. See also **pleural cavity, pleural space.** — **pleural,** *adj.*

pleural cavity, the cavity within the thorax that contains the lungs. Between the ribs and the lungs are the visceral and parietal pleurae.

pleural effusion, an abnormal accumulation of fluid in the interstitial and air spaces of the lungs, characterized by fever, chest pain, dyspnea, and nonproductive cough. The fluid involved is an exudate or a transudate from inflamed pleural surfaces. A transudate which accumulates in pulmonary edema is commonly aspirated. An exudate may result from pulmonary infarction, trauma, tumor, or infection, as tuberculosis. The specific cause of the exudate is treated and the exudate may be aspirated or surgically drained. Other treatment may include the administration of corticosteroids, diuretics, and vasodilators, oxygen therapy, and intermittent positive pressure breathing.

pleural space, the potential space between the visceral and parietal layers of the pleurae. The space contains a small amount of fluid that acts as a lubricant, allowing the pleurae to slide smoothly over each other as the lungs expand and contract with respiration.

pleurisy, inflammation of the parietal pleura of the lungs, characterized by dyspnea and stabbing pain, leading to restriction of ordinary breathing with spasm of the chest on the affected side. A friction rub may be heard on auscultation. Simple pleurisy with undetectable exudate is called fibrinous or dry; pleural effusion indicates extensive inflammation with considerable amounts of exudate in the pleural spaces. Common causes of pleurisy include bronchial carcinoma, lung or chest wall abscess, pneumonia, pulmonary infarction, and tuberculosis. The condition may result in permanent adhesions between the pleura and adjacent surfaces. Treatment consists of relief of pain and therapy for the primary disease. See also **pleural effusion, pleurodynia, pulmonary edema.**

pleuro-, pleur-, a combining form meaning 'of or pertaining to the pleura, to a side, or to a rib': *pleurocentrum, pleurography, pleuropulmonary.*

pleurodynia, 1. acute inflammation of the intercostal muscles and the muscular attachment of the diaphragm to the chest wall. It is characterized by sudden severe pain and tenderness, fever, headache, and anorexia. These symptoms are aggravated by movement and respiration. The lungs are not affected and characteristically there is no cough or pleural effusion. 2. See **epidemic pleurodynia.**

pleuropericardial rub, an abnormal coarse friction sound heard on auscultation of the lungs during late inspiration and early expiration. It is caused by the visceral and parietal pleural surfaces rubbing against each other. The sound is not affected by coughing. A pleural rub indicates primary inflammatory, neoplastic, or traumatic pleural disease, or inflammation secondary to infection or neoplasm. See also **breath sound, Kussmaul breathing, rales, rhonchi, wheeze.**

pleuroperitoneal cavity. See **splanchnocoele.**

pleuropneumonia (plur′ounumoun′yə), 1. a combination of pleurisy and pneumonia. 2. an infection of cattle resulting in inflammation of both the pleura and lungs, caused by microorganisms of the *Mycoplasma* group. See also **mycoplasma, pleuropneumonialike organism.**

pleuropneumonialike organism (PPLO) (plur′ounumou′myəlaɪk). a group of filterable organisms of the genus *Mycoplasma* similar to *M. mycoides,* the cause of pleuropneumonia in cattle.

pleurothotonos (plur′əθhot′ənəs), an involuntary, severe, prolonged contraction of the muscles of one side of the body, resulting in an acute arch to that side. It is usually associated with tetanus infection or strychnine poisoning. Compare **emprosthotonos, opisthotonos, orthotonos.** — **pleurothotonic,** *adj.*

plex-, a combining form meaning 'a stroke or to strike': *plexalgia, pleximeter, plexor.*

-plex, a combining form meaning a 'network': *brachiplex, cerviplex, veniplex.* Also **-plexus.**

-plexia, a combining form meaning '(condition resulting from a) stroke': *apoplexia, pagoplexia, selenoplexia.* Also **-plexy.**

plexiform neuroma, a neoplasm composed of twisted bundles of nerves. Also called **Verneuil's neuroma.**

pleximeter (pleksɪm'ɪtər), a mediating device, as a percussor or finger, used to receive light taps in percussion. Also called **plessimeter.** See also **percussion.**

Plexonal, a trade name for a central-nervous-system, fixed-combination drug containing a sedative-hypnotic (phenobarbital sodium), a sedative (butalbital sodium), an antiadrenergic (dihydroergotamine mesylate), and an anticholinergic (scopolamine hydrobromide).

plexor. See **percussor.**

plexus, *pl.* **plexuses.** a network of intersecting nerves and blood vessels or of lymphatic vessels. The body contains many plexuses, as the brachial plexus, the cardiac plexus, the cervical plexus, and the solar plexus.

-plexy. See **-plexia.**

plic-, a combining form meaning a 'fold or ridge': *plicadentin, plication, plicotomy.*

plica (plai'kə), *pl.* **plicae** (plai'si). a fold of tissue within the body, as the plicae transversales of the rectum and the plicae circulares of the small intestine. − **plical,** *adj.*

plica circularis, *pl.* **plicae circulares.** See **circular fold.**

plicae transversales recti, semilunar, transverse folds in the rectum that support the weight of feces. Also called **Houston's valves.** See also **rectum.**

plica semilunaris, the semilunar fold of the conjunctiva that extends laterally from the lacrimal caruncle. It has a concave free border directed toward the cornea. In some individuals it contains smooth muscular fibers.

plica umbilicalis lateralis. See **lateral umbilical fold.**

plica umbilicalis mediana. See **middle umbilical fold.**

Plimmer's bodies (plɪm'ərz), small, round, encapsulated bodies found in cancers once thought to be the causative parasites. Also called **Behla's bodies, cancer bodies.**

-ploid, a combining form meaning 'having a (specified) number of chromosome sets': *heptaploid, octaploid, polyploid.*

ploidy (plɔi'di), the status of a cell nucleus in regard to the number of complete chromosome sets it contains.

-ploidy, a combining form meaning the 'condition of having a (specified) number of chromosome sets': *alloploidy, haploidy, heteroploidy.*

plug, a mass of tissue cells, mucus, or other matter that blocks a normal opening or passage of the body.

Plummer's disease, goiter characterized by a hyper-functioning nodule or adenoma and thyrotoxicosis. Also called **toxic nodular goiter.**

Plummer-Vinson syndrome (pləm'ərvɪn'sən), a rare disorder associated with severe and chronic iron-deficiency anemia, characterized by dysphagia owing to esophageal webs at the level of the cricoid cartilage. Also called **sideropenic dysphagia.** Compare **Patterson-Kelly syndrome.**

plunging goiter. See **diving goiter.**

pluri-, a combining form meaning 'more': *pluriceptor, plurimenorrhea, pluritissular.*

pluricentric blastoma (plur'isen'trɪk). See **blastoma.**

pluripolar mitosis (plur'ɪpou'lər). See **multipolar mitosis.**

plutonium (Pu), a man-made, transuranic metallic element. Its atomic number is 94; its atomic weight is 242. A highly toxic waste product of nuclear power plants, plutonium was used in the assembly of early nuclear weapons.

Pm, symbol for **promethium.**

PMB, a trade name for a hormonal, fixed-combination drug containing esterified estrogen and a sedative (meprobamate).

P.M.D., abbreviation for *private medical doctor.* Also called **L.M.D.**

PMI, abbreviation for **point of maximum impulse.**

PMT, abbreviation for **premenstrual tension.**

PND., **1.** abbreviation for **post nasal drip. 2.** abbreviation for **paroxysmal nocturnal dyspnea.**

-pnea, a combining form meaning 'breath or breathing': *brachypnea, bromopnea, dyspnea.* Also **-pnoea.**

pneo-, a combining form meaning 'of or pertaining to the breath, or to breathing': *pneodynamics, pneograph, pneoscope.*

pneuma-. See **pneumato-.**

pneumato-, pneuma-, a combining form meaning 'of or related to air or gas, or to respiration': *pneumatology, pneumatophore, pneumatothorax.*

pneumo-, pneumono-, a combining form meaning 'of or related to the lungs, to air, or to the breath': *pneumobacillin, pneumocele, pneumolith.*

pneumococcal (nu'moukok'əl), of or pertaining to bacteria of the genus *Pneumococcus.*

pneumococcal vaccine, an active immunizing agent containing antigens of the fourteen types of *Pneumococcus* associated with 80 per cent of the cases of pneumococcal pneumonia.

■ INDICATIONS: It is prescribed for people over two years of age who are at high risk of developing severe pneumococcal pneumonia.

■ CONTRAINDICATIONS: Pregnancy, early childhood (under two years of age), or known hypersensitivity to the vaccine prohibits its use.

■ ADVERSE EFFECTS: Among the more serious adverse

reactions are inflammation at the site of injection, fever, and hypersensitivity reactions.

pneumococcus (nu'məkok'əs,) *pl.* **pneumococci** (nu'-məkok'saɪ). a gram-positive diplococcal bacterium of the species *Diplococcus pneumoniae,* the most common cause of bacterial pneumonia. More than 85 subtypes of this organism are known. See also **lobar pneumonia, pneumonia.**

pneumoconiosis (nu'moukou'niou'sɪs), any disease of the lung caused by chronic inhalation of dust, usually mineral dusts of occupational or environmental origin. Some kinds of pneumoconioses are **anthracosis, asbestosis, silicosis.**

pneumocystosis (nu'mousɪstou'sɪs), infection with the parasite *Pneumocystis carinii,* usually seen in infants or debilitated or immunosuppressed people and characterized by fever, cough, tachypnea, and, frequently, cyanosis. The diagnosis is difficult to make and usually requires lung biopsy and special staining techniques. Mortality nears 100 per cent in untreated patients. Treatment with pentamidine isethionate or a combination of trimethoprim and sulfamethoxazole is effective. Also called **interstitial plasma cell pneumonia.**

pneumoencephalogram, a radiograph of the brain made during pneumoencephalography.

pneumoencephalography (nu'mouensef'əlog'rəfi), a procedure for the radiographic visualization of the ventricular space, basal cisterns, and subarachnoid space overlying the cerebral hemispheres of the brain. Air, helium, or oxygen is injected into the lumbar subarachnoid space after the intermittent removal of the cerebrospinal fluid by lumbar puncture. See also **encephalography, ventriculography.** — **pneumoencephalographic,** *adj.*

pneumogastric nerve. See **vagus nerve.**

pneumomediastinum (nu'moumi'diəstaɪ'nəm), the presence of air or gas in the mediastinal tissues, which in infants may lead to pneumothorax or pneumopericardium, especially in those with respiratory distress syndrome or aspiration pneumonitis. In older children the condition may result from bronchitis, acute asthma, pertussis, cystic fibrosis, or bronchial rupture from cough or trauma.

pneumonia, an acute inflammation of the lungs, usually owing to inhaled pneumococci of the species *Diplococcus pneumoniae,* causing the alveoli and bronchioles of the lungs to become plugged with a fibrous exudate. Pneumonia may be caused by other bacteria, as well as by viruses, rickettsiae, and fungi, but in 85 per cent of the cases, pneumococcus infection is the cause.

■ OBSERVATIONS: Characteristic of pneumonia are severe chills, a high fever (which may reach 105°F), headache, cough, and chest pain. Inflammation of the lower lobe of the right lung may produce a pain suggesting appendicitis. An effusion of red blood cells into the alveolar spaces, resulting from histolytic damage by the microorganism, causes a rust-colored sputum that may be a diagnostic sign of pneumococcal infection. As the disease progresses, sputum may become thicker and more purulent, and the person may experience painful attacks of coughing. Respiration usually becomes more difficult, painful, shallow, and rapid. The pulse increases in rapidity, often measuring 120 or more beats a minute. Other signs may include profuse sweating and cyanosis. Gastrointestinal disorders and an outbreak of herpes simplex about the face may also occur. In children, pneumonia may be accompanied by convulsion. As the alveoli become filled with exudate, the affected area of a lobe becomes increasingly firm and consolidated. A distinctive kind of rale is heard on auscultation. X-ray films are taken to evaluate consolidation; laboratory analysis of sputum and cultures of the blood help in identifying the causative organism.

■ INTERVENTION: The treatment of pneumonia includes bed rest, fluids, antibiotics, analgesics, and, if necessary, oxygen. The antibiotic prescribed is specific for the bacterium identified in the laboratory analysis of sputum or blood. Crystalline penicillin G is usually prescribed for pneumococcal pneumonia. The antibiotic is administered intramuscularly until the patient's temperature is normal for two days. Analgesics are given as needed for relief of chest pain. Oxygen is administered by tent, mask, or catheter to patients who are cyanotic, very weak, or delirious; the amount of oxygen to be given is determined through serial laboratory analyses of blood gases. Expectorants, postural drainage, and aspiration of the bronchi are often prescribed. Chest x rays are advised during the acute phase, after therapy has been completed, and on a follow-up examination four to six weeks later. Mild pneumonia is often treated without hospitalization.

■ NURSING CONSIDERATIONS: Fluid and electrolytes are often lost during prolonged high fever; intravenous replacement is often required. Ice packs or cold, wet compresses may be needed to reduce the fever. Fever, loss of fluids, and breathing through the mouth result in a need for care of the mouth and the nares, where herpes lesions frequently develop. The nurse collects samples of sputum for laboratory analysis, administers antibiotics and other medications, and notes the temperature, pulse, and respiration as often as necessary. *(See next page for table)*

-pneumonia, a combining form meaning an 'inflammation of the lungs': *necropneumonia, splenopneumonia, typhopneumonia.*

-pneumonic, 1. a combining form meaning 'related to pneumonia': *bronchopneumonic, peripneumonic, pleuropneumonic.* **2.** a combining form meaning 'related to the lungs': *gastropneumonic, hepatopneumonic.*

pneumonic plague, a highly virulent and rapidly fatal form of plague characterized by bronchopneumonia. There are two forms: **primary pneumonic plague** results from involvement of the lungs in the course of bubonic

Comparison of the three major bacterial pneumonias

	Pneumococcal pneumonia	Staphylococcal pneumonia	Streptococcal pneumonia
Etiology and epidemiology	Most common agent in lobar pneumonia (approximately 90% of all pneumonias) Occurs most often in late winter and early spring Organisms transmitted by droplet infection Highest attack rate during the first 4 years and declines with increasing age Uncommon in infants less than 1 year of age	Most common agent in bronchopneumonia Greatest incidence in first 2 years of life; 30% of all cases occur in children less than 3 months of age; 70% before 1 year of age Occurs most often in winter months Usually contracted as primary infection Cross contamination common in hospitals	Usually lobular Less common than other bacterial pneumonias Usually occurs as complication of influenza or measles
Pathology	Usually lobar but may be lobular Progresses through four stages: (1) engorgement—lobe is congested, heavy, and dark with effusion of blood and serum into alveoli; (2) red heparinization—lobe is solid, dark red, and airless; alveoli contain fibrin, serum red blood cells, neutrophils, and pneumococci; (3) gray heparinization—lobe is larger than normal, firm, gray, and pleural surface appears dull; fibrin present in alveoli but decreased cellular elements and bacteria; (4) resolution	Localized abscesses in older children; more diffuse in infants Exotoxin causes necrosis and sloughing of bronchial mucous membranes Formation of peribronchial abscesses Pneumatocele formation—frequently, abscesses erode bronchial wall, abscess material is discharged into lumen; air enters abscess cavity and becomes trapped to form pneumatoceles visible on radiographs (pathognomonic of staphylococcus pneumonia), which usually develop during the first 10 days of illness; most disappear within a few weeks	Interstitial pneumonia Spreads via lymphatics Although usually lobular, areas of consolidation may coalesce to become lobar
Radiographic findings	Areas of consolidation, usually patchy in children in one or more lobes; may involve entire lung	Patchy clouding in one or more lobes Pneumatoceles of varying sizes appear as thin-walled translucencies	Disseminated infiltration
Laboratory findings	Elevated white blood cell count—15,000-40,000/mm^3 Positive sputum culture Positive blood culture in 30% of cases	Leukocytosis of 20,000/mm^3 or more in older children; may be normal in infants Bacteremia in 10% of cases	Polymorphonuclear leukocytosis Blood cultures positive Elevated antistreptolysin O titer
Complications	Fibrinous pleurisy Pleural effusion Empyema Occasionally postpneumatic pneumatocele formation	Empyema Tension pneumothorax Pyopneumothorax	Pleural effusion Empyema in approximately 20% of cases Streptococcal foci may appear in other areas; for example, bones

Clinical manifestations	Infants:
	  Usually preceded by upper respiratory tract infection
	  Fretfulness and diminished appetite followed by abrupt onset of fever, 39°–40.5°C (102°–105°F)
	  May be accompanied by convulsions
	  Restlessness
	  Apprehension
	  Respiratory distress
	  Appears acutely ill
	  Moderate to severe air hunger
	  Flushed cheeks
	  Circumoral cyanosis
		Usually in infants less than 1 year of age, often with history of staphylococcal skin lesion and preceded by upper respiratory tract manifestations
		Abrupt onset of fever, listlessness and lethargy when undisturbed, irritability on arousal, anorexia, nasal discharge, cough, grunting respirations, progressively severe dyspnea that may include subcostal and sternal retractions and cyanosis
		Shocklike state may be present
		Symptoms of complications; for example, pneumothorax, empyema, and septicemia
			May appear without evidence of illness
			May follow streptococcal infection of upper respiratory tract or as complication of contagious disease
			Symptoms similar to those of pneumococcal pneumonia
			Onset sudden
			High temperature
			Chills
			Signs of respiratory distress
			At times, extreme prostration
			Occasionally, only mild symptoms
			Tachypnea usually mild
			Rales generally unilateral and exaggerated by deep inspiration

Comparison of the three major bacterial pneumonias—cont'd

	Pneumococcal pneumonia	Staphylococcal pneumonia	Streptococcal pneumonia
Clinical manifestations—cont'd	Physical—may be decreased breath sounds and crackling rales; exaggerated breath sounds on opposite side; pleural friction rub may be heard Older children: Usually follows an upper respiratory tract infection Shaking chill followed by high fever, 40°–40.5°C (104°–105°F) Chest pain Drowsiness with intermittent periods of restlessness Tachypnea Hacking, unproductive cough (initially) Anxiety Occasionally, delirium Circumoral cyanosis Splinting of side caused by pleurisy pain Physical—dullness; diminished breath sounds, tactile and vocal fremitus; consolidation on second or third day evidenced by dullness, increased fremitus, tubular breath sounds, and disappearance of rales With resolution—moist rales; productive cough with large amounts of blood-tinged mucus	Some infants have gastrointestinal disturbances; for example, vomiting, diarrhea, and sometimes abdominal distention Rapid progression of symptoms characteristic Physical findings—early, diminished breath sounds, rales, and rhonchi with effusion or pneumothorax; dullness on percussion; breath sounds diminished; respiratory lag on affected side; exaggerated excursion on opposite side; tubular breathing above fluid level and on unaffected side	
Antibiotic therapy	Pneumococcus highly susceptible to penicillin G and therefore the preferred drug Administered IV or IM, 25,000–50,000 U/kg/day or 300,000–400,000 U orally every 6–8 hours Continued 4–5 days after temperature returns to normal Alternate drugs—ampicillin, tetracycline, chloramphenicol, erythromycin, and sulfonamides Resolution begins about 24 hours after initiation of therapy	Methicillin, 250–300 mg/kg/day parenterally Equally effective are oxacillin, cloxacillin, dicloxacillin, or nafcillin For penicillin-sensitive organisms, penicillin G, 100,000–200,000 U/kg/day, may be given Duration of treatment usually 3 weeks If empyema—aspiration of empyema fluid and instillation of penicillin May require closed chest drainage for a while	Penicillin G (IV or IM) is highly effective—30,000–50,000 U/kg/day for infants; 500,000–1 million U/kg/day for children
Prognosis	Good when recognized and treated early Mortality less than 1%; higher in debilitated children Rapid recovery with treatment	Prognosis ranges from 5% to 40% mortality and varies with length of illness before treatment Course is usually prolonged, often 6–10 weeks Early recognition and treatment usually effective	Variable in duration Radiographic findings may be seen for 3 or 4 weeks, with spontaneous resolution

plague; **secondary pneumonic plague** results from the inhalation of infected particles of sputum from a person having pneumonic plague. Compare **bubonic plague, septicemic plague.** See also **plague,** *Yersinia pestis.*

pneumonitis (nu'mǝnai'tɪs), *pl.* **pneumonitides.** inflammation of the lung. Pneumonitis may be caused by a virus or it may be a hypersensitivity reaction owing to allergy to chemicals or organic dusts, as bacteria, bird droppings, or molds. It is usually an interstitial, granulomatous, fibrosing inflammation of the lung, especially of the bronchioles and alveoli. Dry cough is a common symptom. Treatment depends on the cause but includes removal of any offending agents and the administration of corticosteroids to reduce inflammation. Compare **pneumonia.**

pneumono-. See **pneumo-.**

pneumothorax (nu'mouθɔr'æks), a collection of air or gas in the pleural space causing the lung to collapse. Pneumothorax may be the result of an open chest wound that permits the entrance of air, the rupture of an emphysematous vesicle on the surface of the lung, or a severe bout of coughing, or it may occur spontaneously without apparent cause.

■ OBSERVATIONS: The onset of pneumothorax is accompanied by a sudden, sharp chest pain, followed by difficult, rapid breathing, cessation of normal chest movements on the affected side, tachycardia, a weak pulse, hypotension, diaphoresis, an elevated temperature, pallor, dizziness, and anxiety.

■ INTERVENTION: The patient is assured that the condition can be treated, is urged to remain quiet, and is placed in bed in Fowler's position. Oxygen is administered through a nasal cannula, unless contraindicated, and the air is immediately aspirated from the pleural space. A chest tube is inserted and attached to a water seal drainage system; the tube is not removed until air no longer is expelled through the underwater drainage system and an x ray shows that the lung is completely expanded. Pain may be controlled by administering appropriate analgesics, but the use of respiratory depressants is avoided. Intermittent positive pressure breathing may be administered, and the patient is taught how to turn, cough, breathe deeply, and perform passive exercises and is told to avoid stretching, reaching, or making sudden movements.

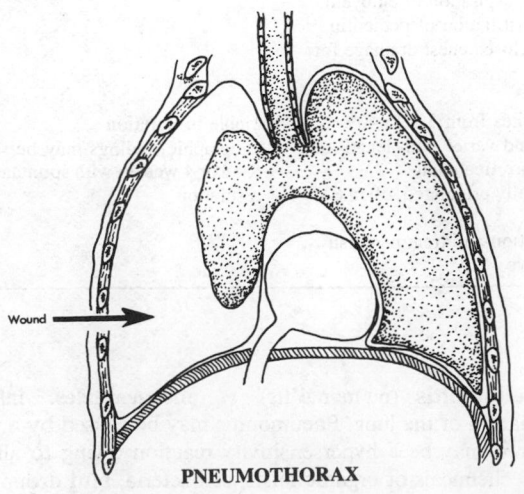

PNEUMOTHORAX

■ NURSING CONSIDERATIONS: The nurse plays an important role in the patient's rehabilitation in the hospital and in preparing the individual for discharge. The patient is advised not to smoke, to drink fluids copiously, to exercise, to avoid fatigue and strenuous activity, and to report any symptoms of recurrence, to the physician, as chest pain, difficult breathing, fever, or respiratory infection.

PNH, abbreviation for **paroxysmal nocturnal hemoglobinuria.**

-pnoea. See **-pnea.**

PNP, abbreviation for **pediatric nurse practitioner.**

Po, symbol for **polonium.**

Po₂, symbol for *partial pressure of oxygen.* See **partial pressure.**

pod-. See **podo-.**

podiatrist. See **chiropodist.**

podiatry (pədai'ətri), the diagnosis and treatment of diseases and other disorders of the feet. See also **chiropody.**

-podium, a combining form meaning 'something footlike': *axiopodium, phyllopodium, pseudopodium.*

podo-, pod-, a combining form meaning 'of or related to the foot': *podogram, podology, podotrochilitis.*

podophyllotoxin, any one of a group of substances derived from the roots of *Podophyllum peltatum,* a common plant species known as May apple, or mandrake. Podyphillin, a resinous preparation of podophyllotoxin is prescribed in the topical treatment of condyloma acuminatum. Several semisynthetic podophyllotoxins are being studied for their antineoplastic effects, including the inhibition of mitosis. Podophyllotoxins are not recommended for use in early pregnancy.

podophyllum (pod'əfɪl'əm), the dried rhizome and roots of *Podophyllum peltatum,* from which a caustic resin is derived for use in removing certain warts.

poecil-. See **poikilo-.**

-poesis. See **-poiesis.**

-poetic, a combining form meaning 'referring to production of something specified': *cholepoetic, oenopoetic, uropoetic.* Also **-poietic.**

-poiesis, a combining form meaning 'production of': *cholanopoiesis, erythropoiesis, hemopoiesis.* Also **-poesis.**

-poietic, a combining form meaning 'producing something specified': *cholepoietic, gonepoietic, hemapoietic.* Also **-poetic.**

poikilo-, a combining form meaning 'varied or irregular': *poikilocarynosis, poikiloderma, poikilothymia.* Also **pecilo-, poecil-.**

poikilocytosis (poi'kɪlousaitou'sis), an abnormal degree of variation in the shape of the erythrocytes in the blood. Compare **macrocytosis, microcytosis.**

poikiloderma atrophicans vasculare, an abnormal skin condition characterized by hyperpigmentation or hypopigmentation, telangiectasia, and atrophy of the epidermis. It may be symmetrical or patchy, localized or widespread. It tends to be permanent.

poikiloderma of Civatte, a common benign, progressive dermatitis characterized by erythmatous patches on the face and neck that become dry and scaly. As the condition progresses, pigment is deposited around the hair follicles extending down the lateral aspects of the neck. Photosensitivity is sometimes associated with this dermatitis.

poikilothermic (poi′kɪlouθər′mɪk). See **cold-blooded.**

point of maximum impulse (PMI), the place in the fifth intercostal space of the thorax, just medial to the left midclavicular line.

poison, any substance that impairs health or destroys life when ingested, inhaled, or absorbed by the body in relatively small amounts. Some toxicologists suggest that, depending on dosages, all substances are poisons. Many experts state that it is impossible to categorize any chemical as either safe or toxic and that the real concern is the risk or hazard associated with the use of any substance, as the high risk that may be associated with a life-saving drug that would not be acceptable as a food additive. Clinically, all poisons are divided into those which respond to specific treatments or antidotes and those for which there is no specific treatment. Research continues to develop effective antitoxins for poisons, but there are relatively few effective antidotes and the treatment of poisoned individuals is based mainly on eliminating the toxic agent from the body before it can be absorbed. Maintaining respiration and circulation is the most important aspect of such treatment. Some substances which may be poisonous are the saps of certain plants, bacterial toxins, animal venoms, corrosives, heavy-metal compounds, certain gases, various volatile and nonvolatile substances, industrial chemicals, and numerous drugs. The toxic effects of poisons may be reversible or irreversible. The capacity of body tissue to recover from poison determines the reversibility of the effect. Poisons that injure the central nervous system (CNS) create irreversible effects because CNS neurons of the brain cannot regenerate. Toxic effects of chemicals may be divided into local effects and systemic effects. Local effects, as those caused by the ingestion of caustic substances and the inhalation of irritants, involve the site of the first contact between the biological system and the toxicant. Systemic effects depend on the absorption and the distribution of the toxicant. Systemic toxicity most often affects the CNS but may also affect the circulatory system, the blood and hematopoietic system, the skin, and the visceral organs, as the liver, kidney, and lung. The muscles and the bones are less often affected by systemic toxicity. The precise incidence of poisoning in the United States is not known, but about 150,000 cases are voluntarily reported to the National Clearinghouse for Poison Control Centers each year. Authorities, however, estimate that the real incidence is at least 10 times the number of reported cases. The total number of poisoning cases increases each year, but the incidence of poisoning in children under five years of age has significantly decreased, probably because of safer packaging of household drugs and products. About 60 per cent of all poisoning involves children 1 to 2 years old and the ingestion of chemicals other than drugs. Approximately 75 per cent of the cases of poisoning in individuals over 15 years of age are drug related. About 4,000 persons die each year in the United States from poisoning by toxic liquid and solid substances. Another 7,000 persons are bitten by poisonous snakes, as the pit viper and coral snake. Such bites may cause severe pain and swelling, numbness, respiratory distress, paralysis, impaired coagulation, coma, and death. Snake bites may be treated with antivenin, tetanus toxoid, and broad spectrum antibiotics. Antihistamines and topical antipyretics are commonly used to treat toxic skin reactions from poisonous plants, as poison ivy, poison sumac, and poison oak. The saps or juices of such plants may cause severe reactions through skin contact or through ingestion. Authorities stress the importance of prompt treatment of acute poisoning from toxic chemicals and liquids. Some common treatments in such cases involve emesis and gastric lavage. Most toxic effects of drugs occur shortly after administration, but carcinogenic effects of chemicals may take 15 to 45 years to develop fully. Chemical carcinogenesis is a complex process involving the conversion of secondary carcinogens into primary carcinogens and the possible development of tumors through reactions of the toxicant with deoxyribonucleic acid. **–poisonous,** *adj.*

poison control center, one of a nearly worldwide network of facilities that provide information regarding all aspects of poisoning or intoxication, maintain records of their occurrence and refer patients to treatment centers.

poisoning, 1. the act of administering a toxic substance. 2. the condition or physical state produced by the ingestion, injection, inhalation, or exposure of a poisonous substance. Identification of the poison and the presentation of a container label are critical to expeditious diagnosis and treatment. Kinds of poisoning include **creosote poisoning, food poisoning, heavy metals poisoning, petroleum distillate poisoning, salicylate poisoning.** See also **alcohol poisoning, carbon monoxide poisoning, nicotine, pesticide poisoning, poison ivy, poison oak, poison sumac.**

poison ivy, any of several species of climbing vine of the genus *Rhus,* characterized by shiny, three-pointed leaves. It is common in North America and causes severe allergic contact dermatitis in many people. Localized vesicular eruption with itching and burning results and may be treated with antipruritic lotions, cold compresses, or topical corticosteroid ointment or cream. Severe cases may require corticosteroids given intramuscularly or orally. In people who are hypersensitive, prophylactic

---

Actions in selected situations with a conscious victim who has ingested poison

Corrosive substances
  Household cleaners: do *not* induce vomiting; give milk
  Paint (liquid); do *not* induce vomiting; give milk
  Ammonia: do *not* induce vomiting; give *citrus juice*

Noncorrosive substances
  Insecticides: induce vomiting; give milk
  Medicines: induce vomiting; give milk
  Cosmetics: induce vomiting; give milk
  Plants: induce vomiting; give milk

Methods of inducing vomiting

1. Give 1 or 2 glasses of warm water followed by tickling the back of the throat.
2. Give 1 tbsp (15 ml) syrup of Ipecac followed by 1 glass of water. (Dose can be repeated once only if vomiting does not occur within 15 to 20 min.)
3. Give 1 tbsp salt *or* 1 to 2 tsp mustard in 1 glass of *warm* water. (Mix dry mustard with water just before drinking.)
4. Physician's order: Apomorphine hydrochloride 0.03 mg/lb subcutaneously. (Contraindicated if respiratory depression present.)

---

treatment with *Rhus* antigen may be given after contact, before symptoms develop. Careful washing of the exposed skin after suspected contact may prevent the reaction. See also **rhus dermatitis, urushiol.**

poison oak, any of several species of shrub of the genus *Rhus,* common in North America. Skin contact results in allergic dermatitis in many people. The characteristics and the treatment of the condition are similar to those of poison ivy. See also **rhus dermatitis, urushiol.**

poison sumac (su′mæk), a shrub of the genus *Rhus,* common in North America. Skin contact results in allergic dermatitis in many people. The characteristics and the treatment of the condition are similar to those of poison ivy. See also **rhus dermatitis, urushiol.**

poker spine. See **bamboo spine.**

Polaramine, a trade name for an antihistaminic (dexchlorpheniramine maleate).

polar body, one of the small cells produced during the two meiotic divisions in the maturation process of female gametes, or ova. It is nonfunctional and incapable of being fertilized. See also **oogenesis.**

polarity (poulær′ɪti), **1.** the existence or manifestation of opposing qualities, tendencies, or emotions, like pleasure and pain, love and hate, strength and weakness, depend-

ence and independence, masculinity and femininity. The concept is central to various psychotherapeutic approaches, as client-centered therapy, in which the key to self-actualization lies in accepting polarity within oneself. **2.** (in physics) the distinction between a negative and a positive electrical charge.

pole, 1. (in biology) an end of an imaginary axis drawn through the symmetrically arranged parts of a cell, organ, ovum, or nucleus. **2.** (in anatomy) the point on a nerve cell at which a dendrite originates. — **polar,** *adj.*

polio, *Informal.* **poliomyelitis.**

polio-, a combining form meaning 'of or related to gray matter in the nervous system': *polioclastic, polioencephalitis, poliomyelitis.*

polioencephalitis (pou′liɔuensef′əlaɪ′tɪs), an inflammation of the gray matter of the brain caused by infection of the brain by a poliovirus.

polioencephalomyelitis (pou′liɔuensef′əloumaɪ′əlaɪ′tɪs), inflammation of the gray matter of the brain and the spinal cord, caused by infection by a poliovirus.

poliomyelitis (pou′liɔumaɪ′əlaɪ′tɪs), an infectious disease caused by one of the three polioviruses. Asymptomatic, mild, and paralytic forms of the disease occur. Several factors influence susceptibility to the virus and the course of the disease: more boys than girls are severely affected, stress increases susceptibility, more pregnant than nonpregnant women acquire the paralytic form of the disease, and the severity of the infection increases with age. It is transmitted from person to person through fecal contamination or oropharyngeal secretions. Also called *Informal.* **polio.** See also **poliovirus.**

■ OBSERVATIONS: Asymptomatic infection has no clinical features, but it confers immunity. Abortive poliomyelitis lasts only a few hours and is characterized by minor illness with fever, malaise, headache, nausea, vomiting, and slight abdominal discomfort. Nonparalytic poliomyelitis is longer lasting and is marked by meningeal irritation with pain and stiffness in the back and by all the signs of abortive poliomyelitis. Paralytic poliomyelitis begins as abortive poliomyelitis. The symptoms abate, and for several days the person seems well. Malaise, headache, and fever recur; pain, weakness, and paralysis develop. The peak of paralysis is reached within the first week. In spinal poliomyelitis viral replication occurs in the anterior horn cells of the spine causing inflammation, swelling, and, if severe, destruction of the neurons. The large proximal muscles of the limbs are most often affected. Bulbar poliomyelitis results from viral multiplication in the brain stem. Bulbar and spinal poliomeylitis often occur together.

■ INTERVENTION: Treatment of the abortive and nonparalytic forms of the disease is symptomatic, consisting of bed rest, good nutrition, and avoidance, for at least two weeks, of overexertion, stress, and fatigue. Treatment

of the paralytic form includes hospitalization with observation for advance of the disease, the application of hot packs and the giving of baths, range-of-motion exercise, and assisted ventilation when necessary. As soon as the acute febrile stage is over, active, comprehensive rehabilitation is promptly begun.
■ NURSING CONSIDERATIONS: The more quickly function returns, the better the outcome. The pain and muscle spasm of the acute period cause the person to want to remain immobile. Such immobility enhances the tendency to deformity, and the nurse may be of great help in encouraging the person to exercise and to participate actively in the rehabilitative program. Poliomyelitis, which has not been eradicated, may be prevented by immunization. Families are encouraged to obtain the complete series for all family members. Formerly, when epidemic, poliomyelitis was seen chiefly in the summer. Now the few cases occurring are sporadic rather than seasonal.

poliomyelitis vaccine. See **poliovirus vaccine.**

poliosis (pou'liou'sɪs), depigmentation of the hair on the scalp, eyebrows, eyelashes, mustache, beard, or body. The condition may be inherited and generalized or acquired and localized in patches. Acquired localized poliosis often occurs in alopecia areata.

poliovirus, the causative organism of poliomyelitis. There are three serologically distinct types of this very small RNA virus. Infection or immunization with one type does not protect against the others.

poliovirus vaccine, a vaccine prepared from poliovirus to confer immunity to it. TOPV, the trivalent live oral form of vaccine, is recommended for all children under eighteen years of age who have no specific contraindications. The inactivated poliovirus vaccine (IPV) is recommended for infants and children who are immunodeficient and for unvaccinated adults. TOPV is called Sabin vaccine; IPV is called Salk vaccine. IPV is given subcutaneously. Rarely, vaccine associated paralysis occurs following administration of TOPV; this reaction has not occurred with IPV.

pollakiuria (pol'əkiyur'iə), an abnormal condition characterized by unduly frequent passage of the urine.

pollen coryza, acute seasonal rhinitis caused by exposure to an allergenic. Also called **hay fever.** See also **coryza.**

pollinosis (pol'ɪnou'sɪs). See **hay fever.**

polonium (Po), a radioactive element which is one of the disintegration products of uranium; its atomic number is 84; its atomic weight is approximately 210.

polus (pou'ləs), *pl.* **poli.** either of the opposite ends of any axis; the official anatomical designation for the extremity of an organ. See also **pole.** – **polar,** *adj.*

poly-, a combining form meaning 'many or much': *poly-acid, polycholia, polydactylia.*

polyarteritis (pol'iar'tərai'tɪs), an abnormal inflammatory condition of several arteries.

polyarteritis nodosa, a severe and poorly understood collagen vascular disease in which there is widespread inflammation and necrosis of small and medium-sized arteries and ischemia of the tissues they serve. Any organ or organ system may be affected. The disease attacks men and women between the ages of 20 and 50. Its cause is unknown, although immunologic factors are suspected. Polyarteritis nodosa may be acute and rapidly fatal, or chronic and wasting. It is characterized by fever, abdominal pain, weight loss, neuropathy, and, if the kidneys are affected, hypertension, edema and uremia. Some symptoms may mimic gastrointestinal or cardiac disorders. Diagnosis is based upon the clinical signs, laboratory tests, and biopsy of sites affected by the disease. Mortality in polyarteritis nodosa is high, especially if there is kidney involvement. Aggressive treatment includes massive doses of corticosteroids. Immunosuppressive drugs have been used experimentally with some success. Physical therapy helps the patient to maintain muscle tone and prevents or slows the development of disability.

polychromasia (pol'ikroumei'ʒə). See **polychromatophilia.**

polychromatophile (pol'ikroumæt'əfail), any cell that may be stained by several different dyes.

polychromatophilia (pol'ikrou'mætəfɪl'iə), an abnormal tendency of a cell, particularly an erythrocyte, to be dyed by a variety of laboratory stains. Also called **polychromasia.**

Polycillin, a trade name for an antibacterial (ampicillin).

Polycillin-N, a trade name for an antibacterial (ampicillin sodium).

polyclonal (pol'iklou'nəl), **1.** of, pertaining to, or designating a group of identical cells or organisms derived from several identical cells. **2.** of, pertaining to, or designating several groups of identical cells or organisms (clones) derived from a single cell.

polyclonal gammopathy. See **gammopathy.**

Polycose, a trade name for a nutritional supplement containing glucose polymers derived from corn starch.

polycystic kidney disease (PKD), an abnormal condition in which the kidneys are enlarged and contain many cysts. There are three forms of the disease. **Childhood polycystic disease (CPD)** is uncommon and may be differentiated from adult or congenital polycystic disease by genetic, morphologic, and clinical facets. Death usually occurs within a few years as the result of portal hypertension and liver and kidney failure. A portocaval shunt may prolong life into the twenties. **Adult polycystic disease (APD)** may be unilateral, bilateral, acquired, or congenital. The condition is characterized by flank pain and high blood pressure. Kidney failure eventually develops, progressing to uremia and death. **Congenital polycystic dis-**

ease **(CPD)** is a rare congenital aplasia of the kidney involving all or only a small segment of one or both kidneys. Severe bilateral aplasia results in death shortly after birth. Minor aplasia may cause no dysfunction and may never be diagnosed.

polycystic ovary, an abnormal condition characterized by anovulation, amenorrhea, hirsutism, and infertility. It is caused by an endocrine imbalance with increased levels of testosterone, estrogen, and luteinizing hormone (LH) and decreased secretion of follicle-stimulating hormone (FSH). The increased level of LH associated with this disorder may be the result of an increased sensitivity of the pituitary to stimulation by releasing hormone or of excessive stimulation by the adrenal gland. Polycystic ovary may also be associated with a variety of problems in the hypothalamic-pituitary-ovarian axis, with extragonadal sources of androgens, or with androgen-producing tumors. This condition is transmitted as an X-linked dominant or autosomal dominant trait. The depressed but continuous production of FSH associated with this disorder causes continuous partial development of ovarian follicles. Numerous follicular cysts, 2 to 6 mm in diameter, may develop. The affected ovary commonly doubles in size and is invested by a smooth, pearly-white capsule. The increased level of estrogen associated with this abnormality raises the risk of cancers of the breast and the endometrium. Depending on the severity of symptoms and whether or not the patient wants to become pregnant, treatment involves suppression of hormonal stimulation of the ovary, usually using female hormones or resection of part of one or both ovaries.

polycythemia (pol′isaithi′miə), an abnormal increase in the number of erythrocytes in the blood. It may be secondary to pulmonary disease or heart disease or to prolonged exposure to high altitudes. In the absence of a demonstrable cause, it is considered idiopathic. Also called **Osler's disease, polycythemia vera.** Compare **leukemia.** See also **erythrocytosis.**

polydactyly, polydactylia, polydactylism, a congenital anomaly characterized by the presence of more than the normal number of fingers or toes. The condition is usually inherited as an autosomal dominant characteristic and can usually be corrected by surgery shortly after birth. Also called **hyperdactyly.**

polydipsia (pol′idip′siə), **1.** excessive thirst characteristic of several different conditions, including diabetes mellitus in which an excessive concentration of glucose in the blood osmotically increases the excretion of fluid via increased urination, which leads to hypovolemia and thirst. In diabetes insipidus, the deficiency of the pituitary antidiuretic hormone results in excretion of copious amounts of dilute urine, reduced fluid volume in the body, and polydipsia. In nephrogenic diabetes insipidus, there is also copious excretion of urine and consequent

polydipsia. Polyuria resulting from other forms of renal dysfunction also leads to polydipsia. The condition may also be psychogenic in origin. **2.** *Informal.* alcoholism.

polyestradiol phosphate, an antineoplastic estrogen compound.

■ INDICATION: It is prescribed for cancer of the prostate.

■ CONTRAINDICATIONS: Male breast cancer, estrogen-dependent neoplasia, thrombophlebitis, or known hypersensitivity to this drug prohibits its use.

■ ADVERSE EFFECTS: Among the more serious adverse reactions are loss of libido, impotence, gynecomastia, fluid retention and edema, and, rarely, cholestatic jaundice.

polygene (pol′ijin′), any of a group of nonallelic genes that individually exert a small effect but together interact in a cumulative manner to produce a particular characteristic within an individual, usually of a quantitative nature, as size, weight, skin pigmentation, or degree of intelligence. Also called **cumulative gene, multiple factor, multiple gene.** See also **multifactorial inheritance.** — **polygenic** (pol′ijen′ik), *adj.*

polygenic inheritance. See **multifactorial inheritance.**

polyhybrid, (in genetics) pertaining to or describing an individual, organism, or strain that is heterozygous for more than three specific traits, that is the offspring of parents differing in more than three specific gene pairs, or that is heterozygous for more than three particular characteristics or gene loci being followed.

polyhybrid cross, (in genetics) the mating of two individuals, organisms, or strains that have different gene pairs that determine more than three specific traits or in which more than three particular characteristics or gene loci are being followed.

polyhydramnios. See **hydramnios.**

polyleptic (pol′ilep′tik), describing a disease or condition marked by numerous remissions and exacerbations.

polyleptic fever, a fever occurring paroxysmally, as smallpox and relapsing fever.

polymicrogyria (pol′imaï′krouJaï′riə). See **microgyria.**

polymorphism (pol′imor′fizəm), **1.** the state or quality of existing or occurring in several different forms. **2.** the state or quality of appearing in different forms at different stages of development. Kinds of polymorphism are **balanced polymorphism, genetic polymorphism.** — **polymorphic,** *adj.*

polymorphocytic leukemia (pol′imor′fəsit′ik), a neoplasm of blood-forming tissues in which mature, segmented granulocytes are predominant. Also called **mature cell leukemia, neutrophilic leukemia.**

polymorphonuclear (pol′imor′founu′kliər), having a nucleus with a number of lobules or segments connected by a fine thread.

polymorphonuclear leukocyte, a white blood cell containing a segmented lobular nucleus; an eosinophil, basophil, or neutrophil. See also **granulocyte.**

polymorphous (pol'imɔr'fəs), occurring in many varying forms, possibly changing in structure or appearance at different stages.

polymorphous light eruption, a common, recurrent, superficial vascular reaction to sunlight or ultraviolet light in susceptible individuals. Within one to four days after exposure to the light, small, erythematous papules and vesicles appear on otherwise normal skin, then disappear within two weeks. A delayed allergic response is a possible cause. Tanning reduces the severity of the reaction.

Polymox, a trade name for an antibacterial (amoxicillin).

polymyalgia arteritica (pol'imaiæl'jə). See **polymyalgia rheumatica.**

polymyalgia rheumatica, a chronic, episodic, inflammatory disease of the large arteries that usually develops in people over the age of 60 years. Polymyalgia rheumatica and cranial arteritis are believed to represent the same disease process with slightly different symptoms. Polymyalgia rheumatica primarily affects the muscles, and it is characterized by pain and stiffness of the back, shoulder, or neck, usually becoming more severe on rising in the morning. There may also be a cranial headache, as in cranial arteritis, which affects the temporal and occipital arteries, causing a severe, throbbing headache. Serious complications include arterial insufficiency, coronary occlusion, stroke, or blindness. Usually, patients with polymyalgia rheumatica or cranial arteritis have marked elevations of the erythrocyte sedimentation rate. Both forms of the disease may follow a self-limited course; however, adrenocorticosteroids have proven highly effective in reducing inflammation and in speeding recovery. Both forms are probably autoimmune conditions. Also called **polymyalgia arteritica, temporal arteritis.**

polymyositis (pol'imai'ousai'tis), inflammation of many muscles, usually accompanied by deformity, edema, insomnia, pain, sweating, and tension. Some forms of polymyositis are associated with malignancy. See also **dermatomyositis.**

polymyxin, an antibiotic.
- INDICATION: It is used topically and systemically in the treatment of gram-negative bacterial infections.
- CONTRAINDICATIONS: Hypersensitivity to this drug prohibits its use. It is used with great caution in patients with impaired renal function.
- ADVERSE EFFECTS: Among the more serious adverse reactions when this drug is used systemically are nephrotoxicity and various neurological alterations, including blockade of neuromuscular junction. Pain or phlebitis at the site of injection also may occur. When applied locally, irritation and allergic reactions of the skin or mucosa are sometimes seen.

polymyxin B sulfate, an antibiotic.
- INDICATION: It is prescribed for infections caused by microorganisms sensitive to this drug.
- CONTRAINDICATIONS: Known hypersensitivity to this drug prohibits its use. Extreme caution is necessary when it is given systemically to people with impaired renal function.
- ADVERSE EFFECTS: Among the more serious adverse reactions when given systemically are nephrotoxicity, neurotoxicity, and drug fever. When given topically allergies are the most common problem.

polyneuritic psychosis. See **Korsakoff's psychosis.**

polypeptide (pol'ipep'taid), a chain of amino acids joined by peptide bonds. A polypeptide has a larger molecular weight than a peptide but a smaller molecular weight than a protein. Polypeptides are formed by parital hydrolysis of proteins or by synthesis of amino acids into chains.

polyphagia (pol'ifei'jiə), eating to the point of gluttony. See also **bulimia.**

polyploid (pol'əploid), **polyploidic. 1.** of or pertaining to an individual, organism, strain, or cell that has more than the two complete sets of chromosomes normal for the somatic cell. The multiple of the haploid number characteristic of the species is denoted by the appropriate prefix, as in triploid, tetraploid, pentaploid, hexaploid, heptaploid, octaploid, and so on. Polyploidy is rare in animals, producing organisms that are abnormal in appearance and usually infertile, but it is common in plants, which are generally larger, have larger cells, and are more hardy than those with the normal diploid number. **2.** such an individual, organism, strain, or cell. Compare **aneuploid.**

polyploidy (pol'iploi'di), the state or condition of having more than two complete sets of chromosomes.

polypoid adenocarcinoma. See **papillary adenocarcinoma.**

polyradiculitis (pol'irədɪk'yulai'tis), inflammation of many nerve roots, as found in the Guillain-Barré syndrome.

polyribosome. See **polysome.**

Polysal, a trade name for an electrolyte solution containing various electrolytes with or without dextrose.

polysome, (in genetics) a group of ribosomes joined together by a molecule of messenger RNA containing the genetic code. The structure is found in the cytoplasm during protein synthesis. Also called **ergosome, polyribosome.** See also **translation.**

polysomy (pol'əsou'mi), the presence of a chromosome in at least triplicate in an otherwise diploid somatic cell as the result of chromosomal nondisjunction during meiotic division in the maturation of gametes. The chromosome may be duplicated three times (trisomy), four times (tetrasomy), or more times. In males with Klinefelter's syn-

A polyp - a tumor ē a pedicle

drome the genotype may be XXXXY or XXXXXY instead of the usual XXY associated with the syndrome and among polysomic females with three, four or five X chromosomes there is a higher frequency of mental retardation.

Polysporin, a trade name for an ophthalmic and topical, anti-infective, fixed-combination drug containing antibacterials (polymyxin B sulfate and bacitracin).

Polytar Bath, a trade name for a fixed-combination drug containing two topical antieczematics (coal tar and pine tar).

polytene chromosome, an excessively large type of chromosome consisting of bundles of unseparated chromonemata filaments. It is found primarily in the saliva of certain insects. See also **giant chromosome.**

polythiazide, a diuretic and antihypertensive.

■ INDICATIONS: It is prescribed in the treatment of hypertension and edema.

■ CONTRAINDICATIONS: Anuria or known hypersensitivity to this drug, other thiazides, or sulfonamide derivatives prohibits its use.

■ ADVERSE EFFECTS: Among the more serious adverse reactions are hypokalemia, hyperglycemia, hyperuricemia, and various hypersensitivity reactions.

polyunsaturated fatty acid. See **unsaturated fatty acid.**

polyuria (pol'iyur'iə), the excretion of an abnormally large quantity of urine. Some causes of polyuria are diabetes insipidus, diabetes mellitus, diuretics, excessive fluid intake, hypercalcemia.

polyvalent antiserum. See **antiserum.**

Poly-Vi-Flor, a trade name for an oral, pediatric, fixed-combination drug containing several vitamins and sodium fluoride.

polyvinyl chloride (PVC), a common synthetic thermoplastic material.

POMP, acronym for a combination drug regimen used in the treatment of cancer, containing three antineoplastics, Purinethol (mercaptopurine), Oncovin (vincristine sulfate), methotrexate, and prednisone (a glucocorticoid).

Pomp's disease, a form of muscle glycogen storage disease in which there is a generalized accumulation of glycogen, resulting from a deficiency of acid maltase (alpha-1, 4-glucosidase). It is usually fatal in infants, owing to cardiac or respiratory failure. Children with Pompe's disease appear imbecilic and hypotonic, seldom living beyond twenty years of age. In adults muscle weakness is progressive, but the disease is not fatal. Also call **glycogen storage disease, type II.** See also **glycogen storage disease.**

pompholyx (pom'fəlɪks). See **dyshidrosis.**

POMR, abbreviation for **problem-oriented medical record.**

Pondimin, a trade name for an anorexiant (fenfluramine hydrochloride).

pono-, a combining form meaning 'of or related to pain': *ponograph, ponopalmosis, ponophobia.*

ponos. See **kala-azar.**

pons (ponz), *pl.* **pontes** (pon'tiz). **1.** any slip of tissue connecting two parts of a structure or an organ of the body. **2.** Also called **bridge of Varolius.** a prominence on the ventral surface of the brain stem, between the medulla oblongata and the cerebral peduncles of the midbrain. The pons consists of white matter and a few nuclei and is divided into a ventral portion and a dorsal portion. The ventral portion consists of transverse fibers separated by longitudinal bundles and small nuclei. The dorsal portion comprises the tegmentum, which is a continuation of the reticular formation of the medulla. The tegmentum contains the nucleus of the abducens nerve, the nucleus of the facial nerve, the motor nucleus of the trigeminal nerve, the sensory nuclei of the trigeminal nerve, the nucleus of the cochlear division of the eighth nerve, the superior olive, and the nuclei of the vestibular division of the eighth nerve.

Ponstel, a trade name for an anti-inflammatory and analgesic (mefenamic acid).

pont-, a combining form meaning 'bridge': *pontic, ponticulus, pontimeter.*

Pontiac fever. See **Legionnaires' disease.**

Pontocaine Hydrochloride, a trade name for a local anesthetic (tetracaine hydrochloride).

pooled plasma, a liquid component of whole blood, collected and pooled to prepare various plasma products or to use directly as a plasma expander when whole blood is unavailable or is contraindicated. It is useful in surgery and in the treatment of hypovolemia because of its stability and availability in freeze-dried form. It is collected from blood banks or prepared directly from donors by plasmapheresis. It is thin and colorless or slightly yellow. Of the total volume of normal blood, 55 to 65 per cent is plasma.

poorly differentiated lymphocytic malignant lymphoma, a lymphoid neoplasm containing many cells resembling lymphoblasts that have a fine nuclear structure and one or more nucleoli. Also called **lymphoblastic lymphoma, lymphoblastic lymphosarcoma, lymphoblastoma.**

popliteal artery (pop lɪt'iəl, pop'lɪti'əl), a continuation of the femoral artery, extending from the opening in the abductor magnus, passing through the popliteal fossa at the knee, dividing into eight branches, and supplying various muscles of the thigh, leg, and foot. Its branches are the superior muscular, sural, cutaneous, medial superior genicular, lateral superior genicular, middle genicular, medial inferior genicular, and lateral inferior genicular.

popliteal node, a node in one of the groups of lymph glands in the leg. Approximately seven small popliteal nodes are imbedded in the fat of the popliteal fossa at the back of the knee. One node is near the terminal section of the saphenous vein and drains the area around the vein. Another node lying between the popliteal artery and the posterior surface of the knee joint drains that region. The other popliteal nodes lie along the popliteal vessels and receive the afferent trunks accompanying the anterior and posterior tibial vessels. Most of the efferents of the popliteal nodes course along the femoral vessels to the deep inguinal nodes. Compare **anterior tibial node, inguinal node.**

popliteal pulse, the pulse of the popliteal artery, palpated behind the knee of a person lying prone with the knee flexed.

population, 1. (in genetics) an interbreeding group of individuals, organisms, or plants characterized by genetic continuity through several generations. 2. a group of individuals collectively occupying a particular geographical locale. 3. any group that is distinguished by a particular trait or situation. 4. any group measured for some variable characteristic from which samples may be taken for statistical purposes.

population at risk, a group of people who share a characteristic that causes each member to be vulnerable to a particular event, as nonimmunized children who are exposed to poliovirus or immunosuppressed people who are exposed to herpesvirus.

population genetics, a branch of genetics that applies Mendelian inheritance to groups and studies the frequency of alleles and genotypes in breeding populations. See also **Hardy-Weinberg equilibrium principle.**

por-, a combining form meaning 'passage or pore': *porencephalia, porion, porotomy.*

-pore, a combining form meaning 'passage-way': *metapore, myelopore, neuropore.*

poriomania (pɔr'ioumei'niə), a tendency to leave home impulsively or to be a vagabond.

pork tapeworm. See *Taenia solium.*

pork tapeworm infection, an infection of the intestine or the tissues, caused by the adult and larval forms of the tapeworm *Taenia solium.* The pork tapeworm is unique in that it can use humans as both intermediate hosts for larvae and definitive hosts for the adult worm. Humans are usually infected with the adult worm after eating contaminated, undercooked pork. The infection is rare in the United States but relatively common in South America, Asia, and Russia. See also **cysticercosis, tapeworm infection.**

poro-, a combining form meaning 'callus': *porokeratosis, poroma, porosis.*

porphobilinogen (pɔr'foubilin'əjən), a substance that appears in the urine of persons with porphyria, representing an error of metabolism. See also **porphyria.**

porphyria (pɔrfir'iə), a group of inherited disorders in which there is abnormally increased production of substances called porphyrins. Two major classifications of porphyria are **erythropoietic porphyria,** characterized by the production of large quantities of porphyrins in the blood-forming tissue of the bone marrow, and **hepatic porphyria,** in which large amounts of porphyrins are produced in the liver. Clinical signs common to both classifications of porphyria are photosensitivity, abdominal pain, and neuropathy.

porphyrin (pɔr'fərin), any iron- or magnesium-free pyrrole derivative occurring in many plant and animal tissues.

portacaval shunt, a shunt created surgically to increase the flow of blood from the portal circulation by carrying it into the vena cava.

Portagen, a trade name for a nutritional supplement containing protein, carbohydrate, and fat.

porta hepatis. See **portal fissure.**

portal fissure, a fissure on the visceral surface of the liver along which the portal vein, the hepatic artery, and the hepatic ducts pass. Also called **porta hepatis.**

portal hypertension, an increased venous pressure in the portal circulation caused by compression or by occlusion in the portal or hepatic vascular system. It results in splenomegaly, large collateral veins, ascites, and, in severe cases, systemic hypertension and esophageal varices. Portal hypertension is frequently associated with alcoholic cirrhosis. Also called **renovascular hypertension.**

portal system, the network of veins that drains the blood from the abdominal portion of the digestive tube, the spleen, the pancreas, and the gallbladder and conveys blood from these viscera to the liver.

portal-systemic encephalopathy. See **hepatic coma.**

portal vein, a vein that ramifies like an artery in the liver and ends in capillary-like sinusoids that convey the blood to the inferior vena cava through the hepatic veins. In the adult, the portal vein has no valves; but in the fetus and during a brief postnatal period the tributaries of the portal vein contain valves that soon atrophy and disappear. In some individuals, the valves persist as degenerate structures. About eight cm long, the portal vein is formed at the level of the second lumbar vertebra by the junction of the superior mesenteric and the splenic veins. The portal vein passes behind the duodenum and ascends through the lesser omentum to the porta hepatis, where it divides into the right and the left branches. The vein is surrounded by the hepatic plexus of nerves and accompanied by numerous lymphatic vessels and some lymph nodes. Accompanied by corresponding branches of the hepatic artery, the right branch of the portal vein enters the right lobe of the liver and the left branch enters the left lobe. The tributaries of the portal vein are the lienal vein, the superior mesenteric vein, the coronary vein, the pyloric vein, the cystic vein, and the parumbilical vein.

Porter-Silber reaction, a reaction, visible as a change in color to yellow, that indicates the amount of adrenal steroids (the 17-hydroxycorticosteroids), excreted per day in the urine. The test is used to evaluate adrenocortical function.

port-wine stain. See **nevus flammeus.**

position, any one of many postures of the body, as the anatomical position, lateral recumbent position, or semi-Fowler's position. See specific positions.

-position, a combining form meaning 'to put, set in place': *electrodeposition, juxtaposition, reposition.*

positive, 1. (of a laboratory test) indicating that a substance or a reaction is present. 2. (of a sign) indicating on physical examination that a finding is present, often meaning that there is pathologic change. 3. (of a substance) tending to carry or carrying a positive chemical charge.

positive end expiratory pressure (PEEP), (in respiratory therapy) ventilation controlled by a flow of air delivered in cycles of constant pressure through the respiratory cycle. The patient is intubated and a respirator cycles the air through an endotracheal tube. PEEP is used for the relief of respiratory distress secondary to prematurity, pancreatitis, shock, pulmonary edema, trauma, surgery, or other conditions in which spontaneous respiratory efforts are inadequate and arterial levels of oxygen are deficient. During PEEP therapy close observation is necessary; the patient often needs to be sedated in order to help stop resistance to the respirator. Blood gases and vital signs are monitored closely. If PEEP does not significantly improve the patient's condition, it is not continued. Compare **continuous positive airway pressure.**

positive euthanasia. See **active euthanasia.**

positive feedback, 1. (in physiology) an increase in function in response to a stimulus, as micturition increases once the flow of urine has started or as the uterus contracts more frequently and with greater strength once it has begun to contract in labor. 2. *Informal.* an encouraging, favorable, or otherwise positive response from one person to what another person has communicated.

positive identification, the unconscious modeling of one's personality on that of another who is admired and esteemed. See also **identification.**

positive pressure, 1. a greater-than-ambient atmospheric pressure. 2. (in respiratory therapy) any technique in which compressed air or gas or air is delivered to the respiratory passages at greater-than-ambient pressure. Positive pressure techniques in respiratory therapy require a flow-regulating device and a delivery system, as a cannula, mouthpiece, endotracheal tube, or tracheostomy tube.

positive-pressure breathing unit. See **IPPB unit.**

positive relationship, (in research) a direct relationship between two variables; as one increases the other can be expected to increase. Also called **direct relationship.** Compare **negative relationship.**

positive signs of pregnancy, three unmistakable signs of pregnancy: fetal heart tones, heard on auscultation; fetal skeleton, seen on x-ray film or ultrasonogram; and fetal parts, felt on palpation.

positron emission tomography (PET), a computerized radiographic technique that employs radioactive substances to examine the metabolic activity of various body structures. In PET studies the patient either inhales or is injected with a biochemical, as glucose, carrying a radioactive substance that emits positively charged particles, or positrons, that combine with negatively charged electrons normally found in the cells of the body. When the positrons combine with these electrons, gamma rays are emitted. The electronic circuitry and computers of the PET device detect the gamma rays and convert them into color-coded images which indicate the intensity of the metabolic activity of the organ involved. The radioactive substances used in the PET technique are very short-lived so that patients undergoing a PET scan are exposed to very small amounts of radiation. Researchers use PET to study blood flow and the metabolism of the heart and the blood vessels. There is also a growing application of the technique in the study and diagnosis of cancer and in studies of the biochemical activity of the brain.

post-, a combining form meaning 'after or behind': *postarbortal, postcerebellar, postdiastolic.*

postcommissurotomy syndrome (poust′kəmĭsh′yŭrot′-əmi), a condition of unknown etiology occurring within the first few weeks following cardiac valvular surgery, characterized by intermittent episodes of pain and fever, which may last weeks or months and then resolve spontaneously.

postconcussional syndrome, a condition following head trauma, characterized by dizziness, poor concentration, headache, hypersensitivity, and anxiety. It usually resolves itself without treatment.

posterior, 1. of or pertaining to or situated in the back part of a structure, as of the dorsal surface of the human body. 2. the back part of something. 3. toward the back.

posterior asynclitism. See **asynclitism.**

posterior atlantoaxial ligament, one of five ligaments connecting the atlas to the axis. It is broad and thin and fixed to the inferior border of the anterior arch of the atlas and to the ventral surface of the body of the axis. Compare **anterior atlantoaxial ligament.**

posterior atlanto-occipital ligament. See **posterior atlanto-occipital membrane.**

posterior atlanto-occipital membrane, one of a pair of thin, broad fibrous sheets that form part of the atlanto-occipital joint between the atlas and the occipital bone and contain an opening for the vertebral artery and the suboccipital nerve. Also called **posterior atlanto-occipital ligament.** Compare **anterior atlanto-occipital membrane.**

posterior auricular artery, one of a pair of small branches from the external carotid arteries, dividing into auricular and occipital branches and supplying parts of the ear, scalp, and other structures in the head.

posterior common ligament. See **posterior longitudinal ligament.**

posterior costotransverse ligament, one of the five ligaments of each costotransverse joint, comprised of a fibrous band passing from the neck of each rib to the base of the vertebra above. Compare **superior costotransverse ligament.**

posterior fontanel. See **fontanel.**

posterior fossa, a depression on the posterior surface of the humerus, above the trochlea, that lodges the olecranon of the ulna when the elbow is extended.

posterior longitudinal ligament, a thick, strong ligament attached to the dorsal surfaces of the vertebral bodies, extending from the occipital bone to the coccyx. Also called **posterior common ligament.**

posterior mediastinal node, a node in one of three groups of thoracic visceral nodes, connected to the part of the lymphatic system that serves the esophagus, pericardium, diaphragm, and convex surface of the liver. Most of the efferents of the posterior mediastinal nodes end in the thoracic duct, but some join the tracheobronchial nodes. Compare **anterior mediastinal node.**

posterior mediastinum, the irregularly shaped caudal portion of the mediastinum, parallel with the vertebral column. It is bounded ventrally by the pericardium, caudally by the diaphragm, dorsally by the vertebral column from the fourth to the twelfth thoracic vertebra, and laterally by the mediastinal pleurae. It contains the bifurcation of the trachea, two primary bronchi, esophagus, thoracic duct, many large lymph nodes, and various vessels, as the thoracic portion of the aortic arch. Compare **anterior mediastinum, middle mediastinum, superior mediastinum.**

posterior nares, a pair of posterior openings in the nasal cavity that connect the nasal cavity with the nasopharynx and allow the inhalation and the exhalation of air. Each is an oval aperture that measures about 2.5 cm vertically and is about 1.5 cm in diameter. Also called **choana.** Compare **anterior nares.**

posterior neuropore, the opening at the caudal end of the embryonic neural tube. It closes at about the 25 somite stage, which indicates the end of horizon XII in the numerical anatomical charting of human embryonic development. Compare **anterior neuropore.** See also **horizon.**

posterior pituitary. See **neurohypophysis.**

posterior pituitary gland. See **neurohypophysis.**

posterior tibial artery, one of the divisions of the popliteal artery, starting at the distal border of the popliteus muscle, passing behind the tibia, dividing into eight branches, and supplying various muscles of the lower leg, foot, and toes. Its eight branches are the peroneal, nutri-

ent (tibial), muscular, posterior medial malleolar, communicating, medial calcaneal, medial plantar, and lateral plantar. Compare **anterior tibial artery.**

posterior tibialis pulse, the pulse of the posterior tibialis artery palpated on the medial aspect of the ankle, just posterior to the prominence of the ankle bone.

posterior vein of left ventricle, one of the five tributaries of the coronary sinus that drains blood from the capillary bed of the myocardium. It courses along the diaphragmatic surface of the left ventricle, accompanying the circumflex branch of the left coronary artery. In some individuals, it ends in the great cardiac vein. Compare **great cardiac vein, middle cardiac vein, small cardiac vein.**

postero-, a combining form meaning 'of or related to the posterior part': *posteroanterior, posteromedian, posterosuperior.*

post gastrectomy care, nursing care following the removal of all or part of the stomach. Drainage of the nasogastric tube normally changes from bright red to dark in the first 24 hours. If the tube becomes blocked, this fact is reported at once, since gastric distension strains the suture lines. Adequate medication for pain allows deeper breathing and coughing, since the incision is close to the diaphragm. When bowel sounds reappear and a small amount of water given by the ounce is retained, the nasogastric tube is removed. Small, bland meals are offered hourly as tolerated. An increase in temperature or dyspnea indicates a leakage of oral fluids around the anastomosis. The diet is changed slowly to a regular diet, with five or six dry small feedings daily. Fluids are given hourly between meals. The most common complication of gastrectomy is the dumping syndrome, with fullness and discomfort, including vertigo, sweating, palpitation, and nausea occuring 5 to 30 minutes after eating, as food enters the small bowel. Small, dry meals, eaten lying down, along with sedatives and antispasmodics, may prevent the symptoms, though they may persist up to a year after surgery. Other possible complications include marginal peptic ulcer, in which gastric acids come into contact with a suture line; afferent loop syndrome, in which the duodenal loop is blocked and pancreatic juices and bile flow back into the stomach; Vitamin B_{12} and folic acid deficiency; reduced absorption of calcium and Vitamin D; and functional hyperinsulinism, in which carbohydrates now passing directly into the small bowel cause an outpouring of insulin into the bloodstream and a resultant hypoglycemia within 2 hours.

posthepatic cirrhosis. See **cirrhosis.**

postictal (poust'ĭktəl), of or pertaining to the period following a convulsion. —**postictus,** *n.*

post-infectious, occurring after an infection.

post-infectious encephalitis. See **encephalitis.**

post-infectious glomerulonephritis, the acute form of glomerulonephritis, which may follow one to six weeks after a streptococcal infection. Characteristic of the disease are hematuria, oliguria, and proteinuria, especially in the form of granular casts. There is slight impairment of renal function, but most patients recover fully in one to three months. There is no specific treatment for this form of glomerulonephritis; the dietary restriction of protein and the prescription of diuretics may be necessary until kidney function returns to normal. See also **glomerulonephritis.**

postmastectomy exercises, exercises essential to the prevention of shortening of the muscles and contracture of the joints following mastectomy.

■ METHOD: The woman is asked to flex and extend the fingers of the affected arm and to pronate and supinate the forearm immediately on return to her room after recovery from anesthesia and surgery. On the first postoperative day she is asked to squeeze a rubber ball in her hand. Brushing her teeth and hair are encouraged as effective exercises. Other exercises are usually taught, including four that are called climbing the wall, arm swinging, rope pulling, and elbow spreading. They are performed as follows:

Climbing the wall: The patient stands facing a wall, toes close to the wall. The elbows are bent and the palms of the hands are placed on the wall at shoulder height. The hands are moved up the wall together until the woman feels pain or pulling on the incision, then returned to the starting position.

Arm swinging: While standing, the patient bends forward from the waist, allowing both arms to relax and hang naturally. The arms are swung together from the shoulders from left to right and then in circles parallel to the floor, clockwise and counterclockwise. She straightens up slowly.

Rope pulling: A rope is attached over a shower rod or a hook. Each end of the rope is grasped and the patient alternately pulls each end, raising one arm after the other to the height at which incisional pain or pulling is felt. The rope is shortened until the affected arm is raised almost directly overhead.

Elbow spreading: The hands are clasped behind the neck and the elbows are slowly raised to chin level while holding the head erect. Gradually, the elbows are spread apart to the point at which incisional pain or pulling is felt.

■ NURSING ORDERS: Specific exercises may be ordered. The patient is shown how to do them and is encouraged to continue them at home.

■ OUTCOME CRITERIA: With proper exercise, full range of motion returns, both arms can be extended fully and equally high over the head. The woman benefits from having something active to do to help herself during the difficult period of adjustment following mastectomy. Many activities of daily life provide good exercise, as reaching high shelves, hanging clothes, and gardening.

postmature, 1. overly developed or matured. 2. of or pertaining to a postmature infant. See also **dysmaturity.** – **postmaturity,** *n.*

postmature infant, an infant, born after the end of the forty-second week of gestation, bearing the physical signs of placental insufficiency. Characteristically, the baby has dry, peeling skin, long fingernails and toenails, and folds of skin on the thighs and, sometimes, on the arms and buttocks. Hypoglycemia and hypokalemia are common. Postmature infants often look as if they have lost weight in utero. The newborn is fed early and the calcium and potassium levels in the blood are monitored and corrected, if necessary, to avoid seizures and neurologic damage. To avoid the syndrome, labor may be induced as gestation approaches forty-two weeks. To anticipate the problems associated with the syndrome, the fetus and the mother may be electronically monitored through labor.

postmenopausal, 1. of or pertaining to the period of life following the menopause. 2. being postmenopausal.

post-mortem, 1. after death. 2. *Informal.* Also called **autopsy, necropsy.** post-mortem examination.

postmyocardial infarction syndrome, a condition that may occur days or weeks after an acute myocardial infarction. It is characterized by fever, pericarditis with a friction rub, pleurisy, pleural effusion, and joint pain. It tends to recur and often provokes severe anxiety, depression, and fear that it is another heart attack. Treatment includes aspirin, reassurance, and a short course of corticosteroids. Nursing care includes close observation and emotional support, especially when debilitating anxiety and depression are present.

postnasal drip (PND), a drop-by-drop discharge of nasal mucus into the posterior pharynx, often accompanied by a feeling of obstruction, an unpleasant taste, and fetid breath, caused by rhinitis, chronic sinusitis, or hypersecretion by the nasopharyngeal mucosa. Methods of treatment include the application of drops or sprays of phenylephrine or ephedrine sulfate to constrict blood vessels and reduce hyperemia, sinus irrigation to improve drainage, and the use of appropriate antibiotics. Therapy for allergies may be indicated in some cases, and surgery may be required if the nasal passages are obstructed by polyps or a deviated septum.

postnecrotic cirrhosis, a nodular form of cirrhosis that may follow hepatitis or other inflammation of the liver. Also called **posthepatic cirrhosis.** See also **cirrhosis.**

postoperative, of or pertaining to the period of time following surgery. It begins with the patient's emergence from anesthesia and continues through the time required for the acute effects of the anesthetic or surgical procedures to abate.

postoperative atelectasis, a form of atelectasis in which collapse of lung tissue is caused by the depressant effects of anesthetic drugs. Deep breathing and coughing are encouraged at frequent intervals postoperatively to prevent this condition.

postoperative bed, a bed prepared for a patient who is weak or unconscious, as when recovering from anesthesia. The bed is in the flat position. The bottom sheet may be covered with a cotton bath blanket that is tucked tightly beneath the mattress. The top linen is fan-folded to the far side of the bed and not tucked in. The bed is made in this way to simplify transferring a patient from a stretcher into the bed.

postoperative care, the management of a patient following surgery. See also **preoperative care.**

■ METHOD: On the patient's discharge from the operating room, the surgical drapes, ground plate, and restraints are removed and a sterile dressing is applied to the incision. The patency and connections of all drainage tubes and the flow rate of parenteral infusions are checked. The patient's cleanliness and dryness is given attention and the gown is changed, avoiding exposing the individual. Four people transfer the patient slowly and cautiously to a recovery room bed, maintaining body alignment and protecting the limbs. When indicated, an oral or nasal airway is inserted or a previously inserted endotracheal tube is suctioned; respiration may be supported with a pulmonator or intermittent positive pressure breathing (IPPB); if respiration remains impaired the anesthesiologist is notified. The blood pressure, pulse, and respirations are initially reported to the anesthesiologist and are then checked every 15 minutes or as ordered. At similar intervals, the level of consciousness, reflexes, and movements of extremities are observed, and the incision, drainage tubes, and intravenous infusion site are inspected. Nothing is given orally; medication, blood or blood components, oxygen, and IPPB are administered as ordered, and fluid intake and output are measured. Pain is controlled by giving narcotics in one fourth, one third, or one half doses until the patient reacts fully. The patient is kept warm, dry, and positioned for optimal ventilation and comfort; if necessary, the arms are restrained. At the first sign of vomiting, the head is turned to one side and suction is applied. Oral hygiene is administered every one to two hours to keep the mouth and tongue moist. The chest is auscultated for breath sounds every 30 minutes and the patient, when reactive, is helped to turn, cough, and deep breathe every one to two hours. The rectal or axillary temperature is taken every one to four hours. When completely awake, able to move the extremities well, and after having exhibited stable vital signs for an hour, the patient may be medicated for pain and transferred to the assigned room, provided the drainage tubes are functioning, the dressings show no bleeding or excessive drainage, and the anesthesiologist approves the move. The family is informed of the patient's progress and expectations in the postoperative period. The airway patency, rate, depth, and character of respirations, pulse, blood pressure, temperature, skin color, level of consciousness, and condition of dressings and drainage tubes are assessed. If respirations are noisy, the patient is assisted in coughing. A rapid, weak, thready pulse may indicate increased bleeding and is reported, especially if other signs of impending shock, as hypotension or decreased consciousness, are evident. The dressing is examined at frequent intervals and excessive drainage is reported immediately. The patient is positioned for comfort and good ventilation with the side rails of the bed raised for safety and the head slightly elevated, except after spinal anesthesia, neurosurgery, and certain kinds of ocular surgery. A cardiac monitor may be connected. Parenteral fluids and medication for pain are administered as ordered; vitamin C may be indicated to promote the healing of a wound. Fluid intake and output are measured; range-of-motion exercises to extremities are performed, and ambulation, when ordered, is assisted.

■ NURSING ORDERS: The recovery room nurse performs the immediate postoperative procedures, and the clinical unit nurse provides ongoing care, emotional support, and instructions for the patient and his family. Special attention is given to preventing trauma postoperatively, as may occur when confused or elderly patients fall getting out of bed. Falls by postoperative patients are second to errors in medication as the most common incidents reported by hospitals.

■ OUTCOME CRITERIA: Meticulous postoperative care prevents falls, infections, and other complications and promotes the healing of the incision and restoration of the patient to health.

postoperative cholangiography, (in diagnostic radiology) a procedure for outlining the major bile ducts. A radio-opaque contrast material is injected into the common bile duct via a T-tube inserted during surgery. It is usually performed after a cholecystectomy to discover any residual calculi. See also **cholangiography.**

postpartal care, care of the mother and her newborn baby during the first few days of the puerperium. See also **newborn intrapartal care.**

■ METHOD: The physical and physiologic changes of involution in the mother are observed for deviation from the normal. The uterus contracts after delivery, causing bleeding from the site of placental implantation to diminish. It is the size of a softball; the fundus is below the umbilicus. The lochia changes color and consistency during the first few days. Red lochia rubra flows for up to a week, followed by straw-colored lochia serosa, and, finally, by clear, sticky lochia alba. The abdominal wall is soft, but muscle tone returns with time and exercise. On the third day the milk usually begins to fill the breasts.

■ NURSING CONSIDERATIONS: Maternal-infant bonding may be augmented by increased contact between the mother and baby. The nurse is the source of most of the teaching that occurs in the postpartum phase. Breastfeeding, bottle feeding, nutrition, care of the umbilical and diaper areas, baby baths, safety practices and accident prevention, and exercises for physical reconditioning are taught during the postpartum phase.

■ OUTCOME CRITERIA: During the first hours and days after delivery the nurse encourages frequent mother-infant contact. The mother's nuturing abilities are fostered and developed; many new mothers need time and contact with the baby to acquire skills of infant care and to develop feelings of love. As the mother gives to the baby she gains satisfaction. If the baby is prevented from taking, or the mother from giving, both become frustrated. Toxemia, hemorrhage, and infection are the chief medical problems of the puerperium, but they are not common and are largely avoidable. Fatigue, breast engorgement, psychological depression, and superficial thrombophlebitis are more common, but not usual.

postpartum (poustpar'təm), after giving birth.

postpartum depression, an abnormal psychiatric condition that occurs following childbirth, typically, from three days to six weeks postpartum. It is characterized by symptoms that range from mild "postpartum blues" to an intense, suicidal, depressive psychosis. Severe postpartum depression occurs approximately once in every two to three thousand pregnancies. The etiology is not proven; neurochemical and psychologic influences have been implicated. Approximately one third of patients are found to have had some degree of psychiatric abnormality predating the pregnancy. The disorder recurs in subsequent pregnancies in 25 per cent of cases. Some women at risk for postpartum depression may be identified during the prenatal period by their having made no preparations for the expected baby, by their expressing unrealistic plans for postpartum work or travel, or by their denying the reality of the responsibilities of parenthood. Depending on the severity of the disorder, psychoactive medication or psychiatric hospitalization may be necessary.

post-perfusion syndrome, a cytomegalovirus (CMV) infection, occurring between 2 and 4 weeks after the transfusion of fresh blood containing CMV. It is characterized by prolonged fever, hepatitis, rash, atypical lymphocytosis, and occasionally, jaundice. No specific treatment is yet available.

postpericardiotomy syndrome (poust'perıkar'diot'əmi), a condition that sometimes occurs days or weeks after pericardiotomy, characterized by symptoms of pericarditis, often without any fever. It appears to be an autoimmune response to damaged muscle cells of the myocardium and pericardium. See also **pericarditis.**

post-pill amenorrhea, failure of normal menstrual cycles to resume within three months following discontinuation of oral contraceptive. The pathophysiology of this uncommon condition is poorly understood. Post-pill amenorrhea is rarely permanent. See also **amenorrhea, oral contraceptive.**

postpolycythemic myeloid metaplasia, a common late development in polycythemia vera, characterized by anemia owing to sclerosis of the bone marrow. The production of red blood cells then occurs only in extramedullary tissue, as the liver and spleen. This condition is frequently complicated by leukemia, especially if the patient has been treated with ionizing radiation. See also **myeloid metaplasia, polycythemia.**

postprandial, after a meal.

postpubertal panhypopituitarism, insufficiency of pituitary hormones, caused by postpartum pituitary necrosis resulting from thrombosis of the circulation of the gland during or after delivery. The disorder, characterized initially by weakness, lethargy, failure to lactate, amenorrhea, loss of libido, and intolerance to cold, leads to loss of axillary and pubic hair, bradycardia, hypotension, premature wrinkling of the skin, and atrophy of the thyroid and adrenal glands. Treatment consists of the administration of ACTH, thyroid-stimulating hormone, or thyroid, adrenal, and sex hormones. Also called **Simmonds' disease, hypophyseal cachexia, pituitary cachexia.**

postpuberty, postpubescence, a period of approximately one to two years following puberty during which skeletal growth slows and the physiologic functions of the reproductive years are established. — **postpuberal, postpubertal, postpubescent,** adj.

postsynaptic, 1. situated after a synapse. 2. occurring after a synapse has been crossed.

postsynaptic element, any neurological structure, as a neuron, situated distal to a synapse.

post-term infant. See **postmature infant.**

post-traumatic stress disorder, an anxiety disorder characterized by an acute emotional response to a traumatic event or situation involving severe environmental stress, like a natural disaster, airplane crash, serious automobile accident, military combat, and physical torture. Symptoms of the condition include recurrent, intrusive recollections or nightmares, diminished responsiveness to the external world, hyperalertness or an exaggerated startle response, sleep disturbances, irritability, memory impairment, difficulty in concentrating, depression, anxiety, headaches, and vertigo. Treatment usually consists of sedation in extreme cases followed by supportive psychotherapy. Also called **stress reaction, stress response syndrome.** See also **combat fatigue, shell shock.**

postural albuminuria. See **orthostatic proteinuria.**

postural drainage, the use of positioning to drain secretions from specific segments of the bronchi and the lungs into the trachea. Coughing normally expels secretions from the trachea.

■ METHOD: Positions are selected that promote drainage

from the affected parts of the lungs. Pillows and raised sections of the hospital bed are used to support or elevate parts of the body. The procedure is begun with the patient level, and the head is gradually lowered to a full Trendelenburg position. Inhalation through the nose and exhalation through the mouth is encouraged. Simultaneously the nurse may use cupping and vibration over the affected area of the lungs to dislodge and mobilize secretions. The person is then helped to a position conducive to coughing and is asked to breathe deeply at least three times and to cough at least twice. See also **cupping and vibrating.**

■ OUTCOME CRITERIA: Effectiveness of the procedure depends on positioning that allows drainage by gravity and

CORRECT POSITIONS FOR POSTURAL DRAINAGE

on liquefaction, ciliary action, and effective breathing. As the secretions are cleared the patient becomes better able to breathe, is more comfortable, and may move about more freely; thus, the respiratory passages may remain freer of obstructing secretions and regain their normal function.

■ NURSING ORDERS: A patient who is dyspneic, or who has hemoptysis or signs of cerebral hemorrhage, increased intracerebral pressure, or lung abscess is not placed in a head-down position without caution and a specific medical order. Suction is kept available in all cases in which the patient might not be able to expel the secretions that have drained into the trachea. The patient's tolerance for the procedure and the position is carefully observed; fatigue is avoided.

postural hypotension. See **orthostatic hypotension.**

postural proteinuria. See **orthostatic proteinuria.**

postural vertigo. See **cupulolithiasis.**

posture, the position of the body with respect to the surrounding space. A posture is determined and maintained by coordination of the various muscles that move the limbs, by proprioception, and by the sense of balance.

pot-, a combining form meaning 'of or related to drinking': *potable, potocytosis, potomania.*

potassium chloride (KCL), an electrolyte replenisher.

■ INDICATIONS: It is prescribed in the treatment of hypokalemia owing to a variety of causes and in treating digitalis intoxication.

■ CONTRAINDICATIONS: Hyperkalemia, concomitant use of spironolactone or triamterene, or known hypersensitivity to this drug prohibits its use.

■ ADVERSE EFFECTS: Among the most serious adverse reactions are hyperkalemia, and, when given orally, ulceration of the small bowel.

potassium hydroxide (KOH), a white, soluble, highly caustic compound. Occasionally used in solution as an escharotic for bites of rabid animals, KOH has many laboratory uses as an alkalinizing agent, including the preparation of clinical specimens for examination for fungi under the microscope.

potassium iodide, a bronchodilator.

■ INDICATIONS: It is prescribed in the treatment of bronchitis, bronchiectasis, and asthma.

■ CONTRAINDICATIONS: Acute bronchitis, known or suspected pregnancy, or known hypersensitivity to this drug or to any iodide prohibits its use.

■ ADVERSE EFFECTS: Among the more serious adverse reactions are hypersensitivity, goiter, myxedema, gastrointestinal disturbance, and skin lesions.

potassium (K), an alkali-metal element, the seventh most abundant element in the earth's crust. Its atomic number is 19; its atomic weight is 39.100. Potassium occurs in a wide variety of silicate rocks; in its elemental form it is easily oxidized and extremely reactive. Potas-

sium salts are necessary to the life of all plants and animals. Potassium in the body constitutes the predominant intracellular cation, helping to regulate neuromuscular excitability and muscle contraction. Sources of potassium in the diet are whole grains, meat, legumes, fruit, and vegetables. The average adequate daily intake for most adults is 2 to 4 gm. Potassium is important in glycogen formation, protein synthesis, and in the correction of imbalances of acid-base metabolism, especially in association with the action of sodium and hydrogen ions. Most of the dietary potassium in the body is absorbed from the gastrointestinal tract and, in homeostasis, the amount of potassium excreted in the urine is essentially equal to the amount of potassium in the diet. Potassium salts are very important as therapeutic agents but are extremely dangerous if used improperly. The kidneys play an important role in controlling its secretion and absorption. Aldosterone stimulates sodium reabsorption and potassium secretion by the kidneys; the major extrarenal adaptation to this process involves the absorption of potassium by the body tissues, especially the tissues of the muscles and the liver. The intracellular concentrations of potassium and hydrogen are higher than those of the extracellular fluid of the body, and when the extracellular hydrogen ion concentration increases, as in acidosis, potassium ions move from the cells into the extracellular fluid. When the extracellular hydrogen ion decreases, as in alkalosis, potassium ions move from the extracellular fluid into the cells. Extracellular acidosis produces hyperkalemia. Extracellular alkalosis produces hypokalemia. Potassium is most commonly depleted in the body by an increased rate of excretion by the kidneys or the gastrointestinal tract, or more rarely, by the skin. Increased renal excretion may be caused by diuretic therapy, large doses of anionic drugs, or by renal disorders. Increased gastrointestinal secretion of potassium may occur with the loss of gastrointestinal fluid through vomiting, diarrhea, surgical drainage, or the chronic use of laxatives. Potassium loss through the skin is rare but can result from perspiring during excessive exercise in a hot environment.

potassium penicillin V. See **penicillin V.**

potassium-sparing diuretic. See **diuretic.**

potassium triplex, a fixed-combination electrolyte replenisher.

■ INDICATION: It is prescribed in the treatment of potassium deficiency.

■ CONTRAINDICATIONS: Severe kidney impairment, untreated Addison's disease, adynamia episodica hereditaria, acute dehydration, heat cramps, or hyperkalemia from any cause prohibits its use.

■ ADVERSE EFFECTS: Among the more serious adverse reactions are flaccid paralysis, heart block, and hyperkalemia.

potency, (in embryology) the range of developmental possibilities of which an embryonic cell or part is capable, regardless of whether the stimulus for growth or differentiation is natural, artificial, or experimental. See also **competence.**

-potent, a combining form meaning 'able to do' something specified: *pluripotent, unipotent, viripotent.*

potential trauma, (in dentistry) a change in tissue that may occur because of existing malocclusion or dental disharmony.

potentiation (pouten'shiei'shan), a synergistic action in which the effect of two drugs given simultaneously is greater than the effect of the drugs given separately.

Pott's disease, tuberculosis of the spine. This form of tuberculosis is rare but results in bone destruction and marked kyphosis if not treated early in the course of infection.

Pott's fracture, a fracture of the fibula near the ankle, often accompanied by a break of the malleolus of the tibia or rupture of the internal lateral ligament. Also called **Dupuytren's fracture.**

potty-chair, a small chair that has an open seat over a removable pot, used for the toilet training of young children.

pouch of Douglas (dəg'ləs). See **cul-de-sac of Douglas.**

poultice (poul'tis), a soft, moist, pulp spread between layers of gauze or cloth and applied hot to an area to provide heat or counterirritation. A kind of poultice is a **mustard poultice.**

Povan, a trade name for an anthelmintic (pyrvinium pamoate).

povidone-iodine (pou'vɪdounai'ədain), an antiseptic microbicide.
■ INDICATIONS: It is prescribed as a topical microbicide for disinfection of wounds, as a preoperative surgical scrub, for vaginal infections, and for antiseptic treatment of burns.
■ CONTRAINDICATIONS: Known hypersensitivity to this drug or to iodine prohibits its use.
■ ADVERSE EFFECTS: Among the more serious adverse reactions are local skin irritation, redness, and swelling.

Powassan virus infection, an uncommon form of encephalitis caused by a tick-borne arbovirus found in eastern Canada and the northern United States.

powder bed, a treatment in which large areas of a patient's body are kept in contact with a powdered medication for a certain length of time. It is usually repeated three times a day, as necessary. An already made bed is prepared by placing a full-sized sheet lengthwise over the linen. The powder is spread on the sheet from a shaker. The patient lies supine on the powdered sheet. Areas of skin that are apposed are separated with gauze, and powder is shaken over the patient's body. The powdered sheet is then wrapped around the limbs and the trunk from the side in order to keep the powder in contact with the body. The patient is virtually helpless during treatment and requires close attention from the nurse.

pox, 1. any of several vesicular or pustular exanthematous diseases. 2. the pitlike scars of smallpox. 3. *Archaic.* syphilis.

poxvirus, a member of a family of viruses that includes the organisms which cause molluscum contagiosum, smallpox, and vaccinia.

PPD, abbreviation for **purified protein derivative,** the material used in testing for tuberculin sensitivity. Also called **PPD of Seibert, PPD-S.** See also **Mantoux test, tine test, tuberculin test, tuberculosis.**

PPLO, abbreviation for **pleuropneumonialike organism.** See **mycoplasma.**

PPO, abbreviation for **diphengloxazole,** a scintillator used in radiology.

PPV, abbreviation for *positive pressure ventilation.* See **positive pressure,** def. 2.

Pr, symbol for **praseodymium.**

practical anatomy. See **applied anatomy.**

practice theory, (in nursing research) a theory that describes, explains, and prescribes nursing practice in general. It serves as the basis for specific items in the curriculum of nursing education and for the development of theories in the administration of nursing and nursing education.

practicing medicine without a license, (in law) practicing activities defined under state law in the medical practice act without physician supervision, direction, or control.

practitioner, a person qualified to practice in a special professional field, as a nurse practitioner.

Prader-Willi syndrome, a metabolic condition characterized by congenital hypotonia, hyperphagia, obesity, mental retardation and the development of diabetes mellitus in later life. The syndrome is associated with a less-than-normal secretion of gonadotropic hormones by the pituitary gland.

prae-. See **pre-.**

-pragia, a combining form meaning 'quality of action': *bradypragia, dyspragia, tachypragia.*

Pragmatar, a trade name for a topical, fixed-combination drug containing an antieczematic (cetyl alcohol-coal tar distillate), a keratolytic (salicylic acid), and a scabicide (precipitated sulfur).

pralidoxime chloride (præl'ədok'sim), a cholinesterase reactivator.
■ INDICATION: It is prescribed as an antidote for organophosphate poisoning or drug overdosage in the treatment of myasthenia gravis.
■ CONTRAINDICATION: Known hypersensitivity to this drug prohibits its use.
■ ADVERSE EFFECTS: Among the most serious adverse re-

actions are dizziness, tachycardia, hyperventilation, and muscle weakness. These reactions are most common when the drug is injected too rapidly.

Pramasone, a trade name for a topical, fixed-combination drug containing a glucocorticoid (hydrocortisone acetate) and a topical anesthetic (pramoxine hydrochloride).

prandial (præn′diəl), pertaining to a meal; it is used in relation to timing, as postprandial or preprandial. –**prandiality,** n.

Prantal, a trade name for an anticholinergic (diphemanil methylsulfate).

praseodymium (Pr), a rare-earth metallic element. Its atomic number is 59; its atomic weight is 140.91.

Prausnitz-Küstner (PK) test (praus′nıtskyst′nər), a skin test in which an allergic response is transferred to a nonallergic person who acts as a surrogate to permit identification of the allergen. After screening the allergic patient for hepatitis and other serum-borne diseases, a small amount of the patient's serum is injected intradermally into several sites on a nonallergic person (usually a relative). After 24 to 48 hours, suspected antigens are applied to these sites on the nonallergic person. A sensitive skin response (wheal and flare reaction), indicates that the suspect antigen is indeed causing hypersensitivity in the allergic patient. The Prausnitz-Küstner test is only performed when skin sensitivity testing cannot be performed directly on the allergic person. Also called **passive transfer test, PK test.** Compare **patch test, radioallergosorbent test.** See also **anaphylaxis.**

-praxia, a combining form meaning a 'condition concerning the performance of movements': *dyspraxia, eupraxia, hypopraxia.*

-praxis, a combining form meaning a 'therapeutic treatment involving a (specified) method': *actinopraxis, echopraxis, parapraxis.*

prazosin hydrochloride (pra′zəsın), an antihypertensive.

■ INDICATION: It is prescribed in the treatment of hypertension.

■ CONTRAINDICATION: Known hypersensitivity to this drug prohibits its use.

■ ADVERSE EFFECTS: Among the more serious adverse reactions are tachycardia, fainting, drowsiness, angina, and a sudden drop in blood pressure following the initial dose.

pre-, a combining form meaning 'before': *preataxic, precritical, pregenital.* Also **prae-.**

preagonal ascites, a rapid accumulation of fluid within the peritoneal cavity, representing the transudation of serum from the circulatory system. Preagonal ascites immediately precedes death in some cases. See also **ascites.**

preanesthetic medication. See **premedication.**

preaortic node (pri′eiɔr′tık), a node in one of the three sets of lumbar lymph nodes that serve various abdominal viscera supplied by the celiac, superior mesenteric, and inferior mesenteric arteries. The preaortic nodes lie ventral to the aorta and are divided into the celiac nodes, superior mesenteric nodes, and inferior mesenteric nodes. Most of the efferents from the preaortic nodes unite to form the lymphatic intestinal trunk which enters the cisterna chyli. Compare **lateral aortic node, retroaortic node.**

precancerous dermatitis. See **intraepidermal carcinoma.**

precipitate (1. prısıp′ıteit, 2, 3. prısıp′ıtıt), **1.** to cause a substance to separate or to settle out of solution. **2.** a substance that has separated from or settled out of a solution. **3.** occurring hastily or unexpectedly.

precipitate delivery (prısıp′ıtıt), childbirth that occurs with such speed or in such a situation that the usual preparations cannot be made. See also **emergency childbirth.**

precipitin (prısıp′ıtın), an antibody that causes formation of an insoluble complex when combined with a specific soluble antigen.

Precision, a trade name for a nutritional supplement free of lactose, cholesterol, and gluten.

precocious, pertaining to the early, often premature, development of physical or mental qualities.

precocious dentition, the abnormal acceleration of the eruption of the deciduous or permanent teeth, usually associated with an endocrine imbalance, as excess pituitary growth hormone or hyperthyroidism. Compare **retarded dentition.**

preconscious, 1. prior to the development of self-consciousness and self-awareness. **2.** (in psychiatry) the mental function in which thoughts, ideas, emotions, or memories not in immediate awareness can be brought into the consciousness, usually through associations, without encountering any intrapsychic resistance or repression. **3.** the mental phenomena capable of being recalled, although not present in the conscious mind.

precordial (prikɔr′diəl), of or pertaining to the precordium, which forms the region over the heart and the lower part of the thorax.

precordial movement, any motion of the anterior wall of the thorax localized in the area over the heart. Kinds of precordial movements include **apical impulse, left ventricular thrust, right ventricular thrust.**

Pred, a trade name for a glucocorticoid (prednisolone acetate).

Predalone, a trade name for a hormonal, fixed-combination drug containing glucocorticoids (prednisolone acetate and prednisolone sodium phosphate).

predeciduous dentition, the epithelial structures found in the mouth of the infant preceding the eruption of the deciduous teeth. See also **deciduous dentition, teething.**

predictive hypothesis, (in research) a hypothesis that predicts the nature of a relationship among the variables to be studied.

predictive validity, validity of a test or a measurement tool that is established by demonstrating its ability to predict the results of an analysis of the same data using another test instrument or measurement tool. See also **validity.**

predictor variable. See **independent variable.**

Prednis, a trade name for a glucocorticoid (prednisolone).

prednisolone (prednɪsʹəloun), a glucocortocoid.
- INDICATION: It is prescribed as an anti-inflammatory agent.
- CONTRAINDICATIONS: Fungal infections or known hypersensitivity to this drug prohibits its systemic use. Viral or fungal infections of the skin, impaired circulation, or known hypersensitivity to this drug prohibits its topical use.
- ADVERSE EFFECTS: Among the more serious adverse reactions to the systemic administration of this drug are gastrointestinal, endocrine, neurologic, fluid, and electrolyte disturbances. A variety of skin reactions may occur from topical administration of this drug.

prednisone (predʹnɪsoun), a glucocorticoid.
- INDICATION: It is prescribed as an anti-inflammatory agent.
- CONTRAINDICATIONS: Fungal infections or known hypersensitivity to this drug prohibits its systemic use. Viral or fungal infections of the skin, impaired circulation, or known hypersensitivity to this drug prohibits its use.
- ADVERSE EFFECTS: Among the more serious adverse reactions to the systemic administration of the drug are gastrointestinal, endocrine, neurologic, and fluid and electrolyte disturbances. A variety of skin reactions may occur from topical administration of this drug.

Predulose, a trade name for an ophthalmic, fixed-combination drug containing a glucocorticoid (prednisolone acetate).

preeclampsia (priʹɪklæmpʹsiə), an abnormal condition of pregnancy characterized by the onset of acute hypertension after the 24th week of gestation. The classic triad of preeclampsia is hypertension, proteinuria, and edema. The etiology of the disease remains unknown despite 100 years of research by thousands of investigators. It occurs in 5 to 7 per cent of pregnancies, most often in primigravidas, and is more common in some areas of the world than others; the incidence is particularly high in the southeastern portion of the United States. The incidence increases with increasing gestational age, and it is more common with multiple gestation, hydatidiform mole, or hydramnios. A typical lesion in the kidneys, glomeruloendotheliosis, is pathognomonic. Termination of the pregnancy results in resolution of the signs and symptoms of the disease and in healing of the renal lesion. Preeclampsia is classified as mild or severe. Mild preeclampsia is diagnosed if one or more of the following signs develop after the 24th week of gestation: systolic blood pressure of 140 mm/Hg or more or a rise of 30 mm or more above the woman's usual systolic blood pressure; diastolic blood pressure of 90 mm/Hg or more or a rise of 15 mm or more above the woman's usual diastolic blood pressure; proteinuria; edema. Severe preeclampsia is diagnosed if one or more of the following is present: systolic blood pressure of 160 mm/Hg or more or a diastolic blood pressure of 110 mm/Hg or more on two occasions 6 hours apart with the woman at bed rest; proteinuria of 5 gm or more in 24 hours; oliguria of less than 400 cc in 24 hours; ocular or cerebral vascular disorders; cyanosis or pulmonary edema. Preeclampsia commonly causes abnormal metabolic function, including negative nitrogen balance, increased central nervous system irritability, hyperactive reflexes, compromised renal function, hemoconcentration and alterations of fluid and electrolyte balance. Complications include premature separation of the placenta, hypofibrinogenemia, hemolysis, cerebral hemorrhage, ophthalmologic damage, pulmonary edema, hepatocellular changes, fetal malnutrition, and lowered birth weight. The most serious complication is eclampsia, which can result in maternal and fetal death. Healthy living conditions, including a diet high in protein, calories and essential nutritional elements, and rest and exercise are associated with a decreased incidence of preeclampsia. Treatment includes rest, sedation, magnesium sulfate and antihypertensives. Ultimately, if eclampsia threatens, delivery by induction of labor or Caesarean section may be necessary. See also **eclampsia, toxemia of pregnancy.**

preferential anosmia, the inability to smell certain odors. The condition is often caused by psychological factors concerning either a particular smell or the situation in which the smell occurs.

prefix, a portion of a word, usually derived from Latin or Greek, occurring at the beginning of a compound word. In this dictionary, prefixes are called "combining forms." In the words *antiseptic, epidermis, hypoglycemia, periosteum,* and *semipermeable, anti-, epi-, hypo-, peri-,* and *semi-* are prefixes. Compare **suffix.**

preformation, an early theory in embryology in which the organism is contained in minute and complete form within the germ cell and after fertilization grows from microscopic to normal size. Compare **epigenesis.**

Pregestimil, a trade name for a hypoallergenic, nutritional supplement for infants.

pregnancy, the gestational process, comprising the growth and development within a woman of a new individual from conception through the embryonic and fetal periods to birth. Pregnancy lasts approximately 266 days (38 weeks) from the day of fertilization, but it is clinically considered to last 280 days (40 weeks; 10 lunar months; 9⅓ calendar months) from the first day of the last menstrual period. The estimated date of confinement (EDC) is calculated on the latter basis even if a woman's periods are irregular. If a woman is certain that coitus occurred only once during the month of conception and if she knows the date on which coitus occured, the EDC may be calculated as 266 days from that date. Pregnancy begins following coitus at or near the time of ovulation (usually about 14 days prior to a woman's next expected menstrual period). Of the millions of ejaculated sperm cells, thousands reach the female ovum in the outer end of the Fallopian tube, but usually only one penetrates the egg for union of the male and female pronuclei and conception. The zygote, genetically a unique entity, begins cell division as it is transported to the uterine cavity where it implants in the uterine wall. Maternal and embryologic elements together form the beginnings of the placenta, which grow into the substance of the uterus. The placenta functions in maternal-fetal exchange of nutrients and waste products, though the maternal and fetal bloods do not normally mix. The conceptus is, in some aspects, like a foreign graft or transplant in the mother. Though the mother does not activate an immune response, all of her tissues and organs undergo change, many of them profound and some of them permanent.

■ PSYCHOLOGICAL CHANGES: The emotional experiences of pregnancy, as reported by pregnant women, are normal and healthy, but extraordinary. A pregnant woman is "herself," but in a very unfamiliar way. She has a sense of heightened function and expectancy. Being keenly aware of the rapid and inevitable changes her body is undergoing, she is more intensely interested in herself. Her concern for the perfection of her baby, her anticipation of the exertion of labor, and her contemplation of the new or expanded responsibilities of motherhood all serve to intensify her emotional tone.

■ CARDIOVASCULAR CHANGES: Cardiac output increases 30 to 50 per cent in pregnancy. The increase begins at about the 6th week, reaches a maximum about the 16th week, declines slightly after the 30th week, and then rapidly falls off following delivery. It returns to pre-pregnancy level about the 6th week post partum. The stroke-volume of the heart increases and the pulse rate becomes more rapid: normal pulse rate in pregnancy is approximately 80 to 90 beats per minute. Blood pressure may drop slightly after the 12th week of gestation and return to its usual level after the 26th week. The circulation of blood to the pregnant uterus near term is about one liter per minute, requiring about 20 per cent of the total cardiac output. Total blood volume also increases in pregnancy; plasma volume increases more than red cell volume, and this results in a drop in the hematocrit, owing to dilution. The white blood cells increase: the normal WBC count in pregnancy is often over 9000/ml.

■ PULMONARY CHANGES: Though vital capacity and Po_2 remain the same in pregnancy, respiratory rate, tidal and minute volumes, and plasma pH increase. Inspiratory and expiratory reserves, residual volume and residual capacity, and plasma Pco_2 diminish.

■ RENAL CHANGES: The glomerular filtration rate (GFR) and the renal plasma flow increase approximately 30 to 50 per cent in pregnancy; the pattern of change closely parallels that of cardiac function. A marked dilatation of the execretory tract often occurs and is called hydronephrosis of pregnancy. It is the result of the pressure exerted on the ureters by the enlarging uterus and by the influence of the hormone, progesterone. Blood urea nitrogen (BUN) normally increases as much as 10 mg/100 ml, and blood creatinine drops to approximately 0.7 mg/100 ml. Positional influences on renal function are more marked in pregnancy because of the pressure of the uterus on the great vessels. Renal function is better in the recumbent position than in the standing position and is better in the left lateral recumbent position than in the supine position.

■ GASTROINTESTINAL CHANGES: Progesterone, which is increased in pregnancy, causes some relaxation of gastrointestinal smooth muscle. Heartburn may result from delayed gastric emptying and relaxation of the sphincter at the gastroesophageal junction. Decreased colonic motility and pressure on the rectum and sigmoid colon from the enlarging uterus may result in constipation. Nausea and vomiting may occur, usually early in pregnancy, probably owing to the effect of human chorionic gonadotropin. The incidence of gall-bladder disease is slightly increased.

■ ENDOCRINE CHANGES: Protein binding is increased in pregnancy. As most hormones are circulated in protein-bound forms, the function of most endocrine glands is altered. Thyroid function changes markedly in a way that mimics hyperthyroidism as indicated by thyroid test. Adrenal hormone levels are increased and are probably responsible for stria gravidarum, which are similar to the stria of hyperadrenalism. Sugar metabolism is altered by estrogen, progesterone, and glucocorticoids; the need for insulin is increased. The placenta produces four hormones: human chorionic gonadotropin (HCG), progesterone, estrogen, and human placental lactogen (HPL). HCG prolongs the life of the corpus leuteum early in pregnancy. Progesterone functions to support the modified endometrium of the uterus, called the decidua, and to stimulate the development of the breast acini. Estrogen stimulates uterine and breast growth. HPL stimulates the growth and development of breast tissue in preparation for lactation; it also has an anti-insulin effect for the sparing of maternal glucose for the benefit of the fetus.

■ BREAST CHANGES: The breasts become firm and tender early in pregnancy. This tenderness constitutes a subjective symptom of pregnancy. As the breasts enlarge and soften, the tenderness disappears. The areola around the nipple becomes more deeply pigmented, and the sebaceous Montgomery glands within the areola become prominent. As the tubules and acini of the mammary glands develop, a clear or whitish watery material, called colostrum, begins to issue from the nipple.

■ SKIN CHANGES: Perspiration increases. Erythema of the thenar and hypothenar eminences of the palms becomes apparent. Hair growth may be stimulated. Telangiectasias are extremely common. Stria over the abdomen, breasts, and buttocks appear in some women. New deposits of the pigment melanin cause freckles to intensify; the linea nigra in the midline of the lower abdomen becomes darker and may extend nearly to the xiphoid process. There may be a darkening of the skin of the face over the nose across the malar eminences and above the eyebrows. This is called chloasma, or the "mask of pregnancy."

■ WEIGHT CHANGES: Normal weight gain may vary within wide limits in pregnancy. Average weight gain is 20 to 25 pounds, but greater increases are common without ill effects.

■ NUTRITIONAL CHANGES: Requirements for dietary iron, protein, and calcium increase out of proportion to the need for an overall increase in intake of calories and other nutrients.

pregnancy luteoma. See **luteoma.**

pregnancy rate, (in statistics) the ratio of pregnancies per 100 woman-years, calculated as the product of the number of pregnancies in the women observed multiplied by 1,200 (months) divided by the product of the number of women observed multiplied by the number of months observed. For example, if 50 women used one contraceptive method for 12 months and 5 of them became pregnant, the pregnancy rate would be 10 per 100 woman-years.

pregnanediol (pregnein'diol), a crystalline, biologically inactive compound found in the urine of women during pregnancy or the secretory phase of the menstrual cycle. A dihydroxy derivative of the saturated steroid pregnane, pregnanediol is formed by the reduction of progesterone.

preinvasive carcinoma. See **carcinoma in situ.**

Preisner model (prais'nər). See **nurse therapist model.**

Preludin, a trade name for an anorexiant (phenmetrazine hydrochloride).

premalignant fibroepithelioma, an elevated flesh-colored sessile neoplasm formed of interlacing ribbons of epithelial cells on a hyperplastic mesodermal stroma. The tumor occurs most often on the lower trunk of older people and may be found in association with a superficial basal cell carcinoma or may develop into a basal cell carcinoma.

Premarin, a trade name for conjugated estrogens.

Premarin with Methyltestosterone, a trade name for a hormonal, fixed-combination drug containing Premarin and an androgen (methyltestosterone).

premature, 1. not fully developed or mature. 2. occurring before the appropriate or usual time. 3. of or pertaining to an infant born before 37 weeks of gestation. – **prematurity,** n.

premature atrial contraction, a cardiac arrhythmia characterized by an atrial beat occurring before the expected excitation, indicated electrocardiographically as an early P wave followed by a normal QRS complex. Premature atrial beats may occur occasionally, in a regular pattern, or several may occur in sequence. The arrhythmia may be the result of atrial enlargement or ischemia, or may be caused by stress, caffeine, or nicotine. Isolated premature atrial beats usually have no significance, but their frequent occurrence may lead to atrial tachycardia or fibrillation, and to decreased cardiac output.

premature ejaculation, uncontrollable, untimely ejaculation of semen often owing to anxiety during sexual intercourse. Behavioral techniques can be learned by the man and his partner to extend the length of time between erection and ejaculation. See also **ejaculation, erection.**

premature infant, any neonate, regardless of birth weight, born prior to 37 weeks of gestation. Since exact gestational age is often difficult to determine, low birth weight is a significant criterion for identifying the high-risk infant with incomplete organ system development. Predisposing factors associated with prematurity include multiple pregnancy, toxemia, chronic disease, acute infection, sensitization to blood incompatibility, and any severe trauma that may interfere with normal fetal development. In most instances the etiology is unknown. The incidence of prematurity is highest among women from low socioeconomic circumstances for whom poor nutrition and lack of prenatal medical care are often precipitating factors. The premature infant usually appears small and scrawny, with a large head in relation to body size, and weighs less than 2,500 gm. The skin is bright pink, smooth, shiny, and translucent with the underlying vessels clearly visible. The arms and legs are extended, not flexed, as in the full-term infant. There is little subcutaneous fat, sparse hair, few creases on the soles and palms, and poorly developed ear cartilage. In boys, the scrotum has few rugae and the testes may be undescended; in girls, the labia gape and the clitoris is prominent. Among the common problems of the premature infant are variations of body temperature, chilling, apnea, respiratory distress, sepsis, poor sucking and swallowing reflexes, small stomach capacity, lowered tolerance of the alimentary tract that may lead to necrotizing enterocolitis, immature renal function, hepatic dysfunction often associated with hyperbilirubinemia, incomplete enzyme systems, and susceptibility to various metabolic upsets, as hypoglycemia, hyperglycemia, and hypocalcemia. The degree of complications and the rate of survival of premature infants are directly related to the state of physiological and anatomical maturity of the various organ systems at the time of birth, the condition of the infant other than prematurity, and the quality of postnatal care. With treatment in a neonatal intensive care unit, survival rates improve yearly. Increasing numbers of very small babies develop normally, and those who do not have seizures or apneic spells in the first few days will not suffer neurologic or physical sequelae of their prematurity. Of primary concern for the nurse caring for the premature infant is the stabilization of body temperature by maintaining a neutral thermal environment, the maintenance of respiration, the prevention of infection, the provision of adequate nutrition and hydration, and the conservation of energy. Important functions of the nurse are to involve the parents in the care of the infant, to explain therapeutic procedures, and to facilitate attachment between the infant and family. Also called **preterm infant.** Compare **postmature infant.**

premature labor, labor that occurs earlier in pregnancy than normal, either before the fetus has reached a weight of 2,000 to 2,500 gm or before the 37th or 38th week of gestation. No single measure of fetal weight or gestational age is used universally to designate premature birth; local or institutional policy dictates which of several standards is applied. Prematurity is a concomitant of 75 per cent of births that eventuate in neonatal mortality. It may occur spontaneously, or it may be brought about iatrogenically. The incidence of premature labor increases in inverse proportion to maternal age, weight, and socioeconomic status. Incidence is higher for black women, for women who have not had adequate prenatal care or whose obstetric history is abnormal, and for women who smoke or whose diets are deficient in protein or calories. Predisposing conditions include maternal infection, low weight gain, uterine bleeding, multiple gestation, polyhydramnios, uterine abnormalities, incompetent cervix, premature rupture of membranes, and intrauterine fetal growth retardation. The etiology of premature labor is poorly understood; in some cases, there may be several contributing causes. In some pregnancies, premature labor may be homeostatic, resulting in the best possible outcome under the particular, abnormal conditions. If premature labor itself constitutes a threat to the fetus, the outcome of pregnancy may be improved if labor can be inhibited. Determining accurately which pregnancies are likely to benefit from the inhibition of labor and which are not is difficult. Medications used to stop labor are not always effective. Misdiagnosis of gestational age and fetal condition may lead to induction of labor that is inadvertently premature; premature babies whose births have been brought about inappropriately early account for 15 per cent of admissions to newborn intensive care nurseries. Also called **preterm labor.** See also **prematurity, small-for-gestational-age, tocolysis.**

premature thelarche. See **thelarche.**

premature ventricular contraction (PVC), a cardiac arrhythmia characterized by a ventricular beat preceding the expected electrical impulse, shown on the electrocardiogram as an early, wide QRS complex without a preceding P wave. Premature ventricular contractions may occur occasionally, in a regular pattern, or as several in sequence. They may be caused by stress, acidosis, electrolyte imbalance, hypoxemia, hypercapnia, ventricular enlargement, or a toxic reaction to drugs, especially to digitalis or quinidine. Isolated PVCs are not clinically significant but they may produce tachycardia, and frequent occurrence of the arrhythmia indicates myocardial irritability and may be a precursor of ventricular tachycardia or fibrillation and lead to inadequate cardiac output. Agents used in treating PVCs include procainamide, lidocaine, oxygen, sodium bicarbonate, and potassium. Also called **premature ventricular beat.**

premedication, 1. any sedative, tranquilizer, hypnotic, or anticholinergic medication administered prior to anesthesia. Pentobarbital, secobarbital, phenobarbital, morphine, scopolamine, and atropine are commonly used. The choice of drug depends on such variables as the patient's age and physical condition and the specific operative procedure. 2. the administration of such medications. —**premedicate,** v.

premenopausal, 1. of or pertaining to the time of life preceding the menopause. 2. being premenopausal.

premenstrual tension (PMT), a syndrome of nervous tension, irritability, weight gain, edema, headache, mastalgia, dysphoria, and lack of coordination occurring during the last few days of the menstrual cycle preceding the onset of menstruation. There are several theories that attempt to explain the etiology of the syndrome, including nutritional deficiency, stress, hormonal imbalance, and various emotional disorders. None has proved valid.

premolar (primou′lər), one of eight teeth, four in each dental arch, located lateral to and posterior to the canine teeth. The premolars appear during childhood and remain until old age. They are smaller and shorter than the canine teeth. The crown of each premolar is compressed anteroposteriorly and surmounted by two cusps. The neck of the premolar is oval; the root is usually single and compressed, with an anterior and a posterior groove. The upper premolars are larger than the lower premolars. Also called **bicuspid.** Compare **canine tooth, incisor, molar.**

premolar tooth. See **bicuspid.**

prenatal, prior to birth; occurring or existing before birth, referring both to the care of the woman during pregnancy and the growth and development of the fetus. Also called **antenatal.** See also **antepartal care.**

prenatal development, the entire process of growth, maturation, differentiation, and development that occurs between conception and birth. On approximately the

fourteenth day before the next expected menstrual period, ovulation usually occurs. If the egg is fertilized it immediately begins the course to fetal maturity and birth. During the first two weeks the fertilized ovum undergoes cell division several times, becoming a morula, and then a blastocyst that is able to implant in the uterine wall. From the beginning of the third to the end of the seventh week of embryonic development, implantation deepens and completes. Primitive uteroplacental circulation originates between the enlarging trophoblast and the maternal endometrial tissue of the uterus. The amniotic cavity appears as an opening between the inner cell mass and the invading trophoblast. A thin lining in the cavity becomes the amnion. At this point the embryo is a two-layered embryonic disc composed of an ectoderm and an endoderm. As the disc thickens in the middle, giving rise to the third cell layer, or mesoderm, the basic structural systems of the body begin to form. The neural tube develops as a precursor of the central nervous system in the midline of the cranial portion of the ectoderm. Primitive blood vessels and blood cells, a heart tube, and umbilical vessels are formed and begin to function. Arm and leg buds may be seen, and rudimentary gut, lungs, and kidneys form. By the fifth week, the brain has begun to grow rapidly, the heart tube is divided into chambers, the palate and the upper lip are forming, and the urogenital system is developing. By the end of the seventh week, all essential systems are present. The period of time from the eighth week to birth is called the fetal stage. From the eighth to the tenth week the fetus continues to grow and develop rapidly. The head is almost one half of its total length, and arms, legs, and face are clearly recognizable. The fetus floats in the amniotic fluid of the amniotic sac within the uterus; the umbilical vessels in the cord extend to a rapidly growing placenta. By the twelfth week the features of the face are formed and the eyelids are present but not yet closed, as they have not divided into upper and lower eyelids. The palate is fusing, there is a neck between the large head and the body, and tooth buds and nail beds have begun to form. Identification of the external genitalia is possible for the first time. From the thirteenth to the sixteenth weeks, the arms, legs, and trunk grow rapidly, and the fetus is active. Scalp hair develops. The skeleton of the fetus is calcified and may be seen on an x-ray film. Respiratory movements may sometimes be detected by a sonogram. Between the seventeenth and the twentieth weeks of pregnancy, the mother usually first feels the baby move. The fetus looks like a very small baby at this time. There are eyebrows and tiny nipples; during fetoscopic examination, the fetus has been seen and photographed sucking its thumb and grasping its own umbilical cord. At the twenty-fourth week the external ears are smooth and soft and the skin is wrinkled and translucent. The body is covered with lanugo and vernix and weighs a little more than a pound. At twenty-eight weeks subcutaneous fat begins to develop, fingernails and toenails are present, the eyelids are separate and the eyes may open, scalp hair is well developed, and, in males, the testes are at the internal inguinal ring or below. In a modern neonatal intensive care unit more than 80 per cent of the babies born at twenty-eight weeks survive. By the thirty-second week, the fetus weighs between three and four pounds. The hair is fine and woolly, the fingernails and toenails have grown to the tips of the fingers and toes and there are one or two creases on the anterior part of the soles of the feet. The areolae of the breasts are visible, but flat. In females, the clitoris is prominent and the labia majora are small and separated. At thirty-six weeks, the body and the limbs are fuller and more rounded, creases involve the anterior two thirds of the soles, and the skin is thicker and less translucent. As the fetus reaches term, between 38 and 42 weeks, the vernix decreases, and the ear cartilage is developed. In males, the testes are in the scrotum; in females, the labia majora meet in the midline and cover the labia minora and the clitoris. At forty weeks, the average fetus weighs 7¼ pounds and is between 19 and 22 inches long. Prenatal development may be adversely affected by several factors. Between two and fourteen weeks of gestation, ionizing radiation and some drugs may have profound effects on morphologic and functional development. During the first ten days of development any damage usually kills the conceptus. Various viruses, malnutrition, trauma, or maternal disease may also affect the morphologic development of a rapidly differentiating structure or organ during the embryologic or early fetal stage. After fourteen weeks when all the organs, systems, and parts of the body have formed, any adverse effects are largely functional; major morphologic damage does not occur.
(See next page for illustration)

prenatal diagnosis, any of various diagnostic techniques to determine if a developing fetus in the uterus is affected with a genetic disorder or other abnormality. Such procedures as x-ray examination and ultrasound scanning can be used to follow fetal growth and detect structural abnormalities; amniocentesis enables fetal cells to be obtained from the amniotic fluid for culture and biochemical assay to detect metabolic disorders and for chromosomal analysis; fetoscopy enables fetal blood to be withdrawn from a blood vessel on the placenta and examined for disorders, as thalassemia, sickle cell anemia, and Duchenne's muscular dystrophy. If any of the tests are positive and the child is likely or certain to be born with a severe defect or disease, the parents need support and advice from genetic counselors on whether to terminate the pregnancy. If the parents decide to have the baby, the nurse can help to educate them about the specific disorder and to prepare them for the special care required of a handicapped or genetically defective child. Also called

PRENATAL DEVELOPMENT

(large numbers, weeks; small numbers, days)

antenatal diagnosis. See also **genetic counseling, genetic screening.**

preoperative, of or pertaining to the period of time preceding a surgical procedure. Commonly, the preoperative period begins with the first preparation of the patient for surgery, as when, 12 hours before scheduled procedure, fluids or food by mouth is forbidden. It ends with the induction of surgical anesthesia in the operating suite.

preoperative care, the preparation and management of a patient prior to surgery.

■ METHOD: The patient's nutritional and hygienic state, medical and surgical history, allergies, current medication, physical handicaps, signs of infection, and elimination habits are noted and recorded. The person's understanding of the operative, preoperative, and postoperative procedures, the person's ability to verbalize anxieties, and the family's knowledge of the planned surgery are ascertained. The signed informed consent statement, the physician's preoperative orders, and the patient's identification bands, willingness to receive blood if necessary, and understanding of the use of the call bell and the purpose of the bed's side rails are checked. Blood pressure, temperature, pulse, and respiration are recorded, and any abnormalities are reported to the physician. The physician is also informed if the electrocardiogram, chest x ray, or laboratory studies show any abnormalities. On completion of the patient's blood typing, the number of matched blood units required to be held for a possible blood transfusion is determined. When ordered, an enema is given, a bowel preparation is completed, a nasogastric tube or indwelling catheter is inserted, and parenteral fluids are administered. Before bedtime, the patient showers, using an antibacterial soap; nothing is given orally after midnight unless ordered. After preoperative medication is administered, the side rails of the bed are raised. Before leaving for the operating room with the completed chart, the patient voids, and any dentures, contact lenses, and valuables are removed for safekeeping.

■ NURSING ORDERS: The nurse performs and explains the preoperative procedures, reinforces the physician's explanation of the operation, provides instruction and emotional support, answers the patient's questions as honestly as possible, avoiding standard clichés in responding to any anxiety, and reassures the patient that medication will be available to relieve postoperative pain. Depending on the surgical procedure, the nurse shows the patient how to turn, cough, deep breathe, and support the incision during coughing. The nurse informs the patient and the patient's family about the postoperative period in the recovery room or the intensive care unit, if indicated.

■ OUTCOME CRITERIA: The patient who is carefully prepared for an operation, psychologically as well as physically, experiences less anxiety and is more likely to make an uneventful recovery.

prepared childbirth. See **natural childbirth.**

prepatellar bursa, a bursa between the tendon of the quadriceps and the lower part of the femur continuous with the cavity of the knee joint.

preprandial, before a meal.

prepubertal panhypopituitarism, insufficiency of pituitary hormones, caused by damage to the gland usually associated with a suprasellar cyst or craniopharyngioma, occurring in childhood. The disorder is characterized by dwarfism with normal body proportions, subnormal sexual development, impaired thyroid and adrenal function, and yellow, wrinkled skin. Diabetes insipidus is frequently present, and there may be bitemporal hemaniopia or complete blindness, but the patient's mentality is usually normal. X rays show delayed fusion of the epiphyses, suprasellar calcification, and the sella turcica is often destroyed. The condition is treated with cortisone, thyroid and gonadotrophic hormones, and, if available, human growth hormone.

prepuberty, the period immediately preceding puberty, lasting approximately two years and characterized by preliminary physical changes, as accelerated growth and appearance of secondary sex characteristics, that lead to sexual maturity. — **prepuberal, prepubertal.** *adj.*

prepubescence (pri′pyubes′əns), the state of being prepubertal. — **prepubescent,** *adj.*

prepuce (pri′pyus), a fold of skin that forms a retractable cover, as the foreskin of the penis or the fold around the clitoris. — **prepucial, preputial,** *adj.*

Presamine, a trade name for an antidepressant (imipramine hydrochloride).

Pre-Sate, a trade name for an anorexiant (chlorphentermine hydrochloride).

presbycardia (prez′bıkar′dıə), an abnormal cardiac condition, especially affecting elderly individuals and associated with heart failure in the presence of other complications, as heart disease, fever, anemia, mild hyperthyroidism, and excess fluid administration. Presbycardia may be associated with decreased elasticity of the musculature of the heart and with mild fibrotic changes of the heart valves, but the basis for these changes and the associated pigmentation of the heart is not known. Some authorities believe that presbycardia only rarely produces heart failure but that the condition does decrease the adaptive capacity of the heart and predisposes elderly patients to heart failure in the presence of other illnesses.

presbyopia (prez′biou′piə), farsightedness resulting from a loss of elasticity of the lens of the eye. The condition commonly develops with advancing age. — **presbyopic,** *adj.*

prescreen, 1. to evaluate a patient or a group of patients to identify those who are at greater risk of developing a particular condition in order to select those who are in particular need of special diagnostic procedures or health care. 2. *Informal.* a rapid, superficial examination of a person who does not appear to be acutely ill. It may include taking a medical history.

prescribe, 1. to write an order for a drug, treatment, or procedure. 2. to recommend or encourage a course of action.

prescription, an order for medication, therapy, or a therapeutic device given by a properly authorized person to a person properly authorized to dispense or perform the order. A prescription is usually in written form and includes the name and address of the patient, the date, the ℞ symbol (superscription), the medication prescribed (inscription), directions to the pharmacist or other dispenser (subscription), directions to the patient that must appear on the label, the prescriber's signature, and, in some instances, an identifying number.

prescription drug, a drug that can be dispensed to the public only with a prescription. The designation of a drug as a prescription drug is made by the Food and Drug Administration. See also **ethical drug.**

prescriptive theory, a theory that is comprised of a description of a specific activity, a statement of the goal of the activity, and an analysis of the elements of the

Vertex   Brow   Face   Shoulder

Breech   Fundus   Fetal back and small parts

Engagement of presenting part   Cephalic prominence

PALPATION OF FETAL PRESENTATION

activity that, together, constitute a prescription for reaching the goal.

presenile dementia. See **Alzheimer's disease.**

presentation, the position of a baby in utero with reference to the part of the baby that is directed toward or into the birth canal. Kinds of presentations are **breech presentation, brow presentation, face presentation, shoulder presentation, transverse presentation, vertex presentation.** Also called **fetal lie.** — **present,** v.

present health, (in a health history) a chronologic, succinct account of any recent changes in the health of the patient and of the circumstances or symptoms that prompted the person to seek health care.

presenting symptom. See **symptom.**

presomite embryo (prisou′mait), an embryo in any stage of development prior to the appearance of the first pair of somites, which, in humans, usually occurs around 19 to 21 days following fertilization of the ovum.

pressor (pres′ər), describing a substance that tends to cause a rise in blood pressure.

pressure, a force, or stress, applied to a surface by a fluid or an object, usually measured in units of mass per unit of area, as pounds per square inch.

pressure acupuncture, a system of acupuncture involving the application of pressure, as by the tip of a finger, to certain specified points of the body. See also **acupuncture.**

pressure bandage, a bandage applied to stop bleeding, prevent edema, or provide support for varicose veins.

pressure dressing, a dressing firmly applied to exert pressure, usually on a wound for hemostasis.

pressure point, **1.** a point over an artery where the pulse may be felt. Pressure on the point may be helpful in stopping the flow of blood from a wound distal to the point. **2.** a site that is extremely sensitive to pressure, as the phrenic pressure point along the phrenic nerve between the sternocleidomastoid and the scalenus anticus on the right side; pressure at this site may be symptomatic of gall bladder dysfunction.

pressure sore. See **decubitus ulcer.**

preswing stance stage, one of the five stages in the stance phase of walking or gait, involving a brief transitional period of double limb support during which one leg of the body is rapidly relieved of body-bearing weight and prepared for the swing forward. The type of preswing used by an individual is a factor in the diagnoses of many abnormal orthopedic conditions. Compare **initial contact stance stage, loading response stance stage, midstance, terminal stance.** See also **swing phase of gait.**

presynaptic, 1. situated near or before a synapse. 2. occurring before a synapse is crossed.

presynaptic element, any neurological structure, as a neuron, situated proximal to a synapse.

presystolic, of or pertaining to the period preceding systole.

preterm infant. See **premature infant.**

preterm labor. See **premature labor.**

pretibial (pritɪb'iəl), of or pertaining to the area of the leg in front of the tibia.

pretibial fever, an acute infection caused by *Leptospira autumnalis,* characterized by headache, chills, fever, enlarged spleen, myalgia, low white blood cell count, and a rash on the anterior surface of the legs. Also called **Fort Bragg fever.**

pretrial discovery. See **discovery.**

prevalence (prev'ələns), (in epidemiology) the number of all new and old cases of a disease or occurrences of an event during a particular period of time. Prevalence is expressed as a ratio in which the number of events is the numerator and the population at risk is the denominator. See also **rate.**

prevention, (in nursing care) any action directed toward preventing illness and promoting health in order to avoid the need for primary, secondary, or tertiary health care. Prevention includes such nursing actions as assessment and promotion of health potential; application of prescribed measures, as immunization; health teaching; early diagnosis and treatment; recognition of disability limitations and rehabilitation potential. In acute care nursing, many interventions are simultaneously therapeutic and preventive.

preventive, tending to slow, stop, or interrupt the course of an illness or to decrease the incidence of a disease.

preventive care, a pattern of nursing and medical care that focuses on the prevention of disease and health maintenance and includes early diagnosis of disease, discovery and identification of people at risk of developing specific problems, counseling, and other intervention to avert a health problem. Screening tests, health education, and immunization programs are common examples of preventive care.

preventive health care. See **preventive care.**

preventive treatment, a procedure, measure, substance, or program designed to prevent a disease from occurring or a mild disorder from becoming more severe. Various diseases are prevented by immunizations with vaccines, antiseptic measures, the avoidance of smoking, regular exercise, a prudent diet, adequate rest, the correction of congenital anomalies, and screening programs for the detection of preclinical signs of disorders. Also called **prophylactic treatment.**

previa, praevia (pri'viə), *Informal.* placenta previa.

previllous embryo (privil'əs), an embryo of a placental mammal at any stage prior to the development of the chorionic villi, which, in humans, begin to form between the first and second months following fertilization of the ovum.

previtamin (privai'təmɪn). See **provitamin.**

priapism (prai'əpɪz'əm), an abnormal condition of prolonged or constant penile erection, often painful and seldom associated with sexual arousal. It may result from a lesion within the penis or the central nervous system. It sometimes occurs in men who have acute leukemia.

priapitis (prai'əpai'tɪs), inflammation of the penis.

priapus (praiei'pəs). See **penis.**

prickle cell layer. See **stratum spinosum.**

prickly heat. See **miliaria.**

prilocaine hydrochloride (prɪl'oukein), a local anesthetic agent of the amide family, used for nerve block, epidural and regional anesthesia. It is not used for spinal or topical anesthesia. Prilocaine hydrochloride is about one half as toxic as lidocaine, but since methemoglobinemia is a possible reaction, prilocaine hydrochloride is not used for patients with hypoxic conditions of any kind.

prim-, a combining form meaning 'first': *primerite, primigravida, primitiae.*

primaquine phosphate (prai'məkwɪn), an antimalarial.
■ INDICATION: It is prescribed in the treatment of malaria.
■ CONTRAINDICATIONS: Lupus erythematosus, rheumatoid arthritis, concomitant use of bone marrow depressants or hemolytic drugs, or known hypersensitivity to this drug prohibits its use.
■ ADVERSE EFFECTS: Among the more serious adverse reactions are hemolytic anemia, agranulocytosis, and abdominal distress.

primary, 1. first in order of time, place, development, or importance. 2. not derived from any other source or cause, specifically the original condition or set of symptoms in disease processes, as a primary infection or a primary tumor. 3. (in chemistry) noting the first and most simple compound in a related series, formed by the substitution of one of two or more atoms or of a group in a molecule, as in amine or carboxyl radicals. Compare **secondary, tertiary.**

primary afferent fiber, a sensory nerve fiber that transmits impulses from the intrafusal fibers of the muscle spindle to the central nervous system during muscle contraction. See also **gamma efferent fiber.**

primary amenorrhea. See **amenorrhea.**

primary amputation, amputation performed after severe trauma, after the patient has recovered from shock, and before infection has set in. Compare **secondary amputation.** See also **amputation.**

primary apnea, a self-limited condition characterized by an absence of respiration. It may follow a blow to the head and is common immediately after birth in the newborn who breathes spontaneously when the carbon dioxide in the circulation reaches a certain level. Reflexes are present and the heart is beating, but the skin color may be pale or blue and muscle tone is diminished. No treatment is necessary, but careful observation, maintenance of body temperature, and oral pharyngeal aspiration are usually performed. Within seconds the baby usually begins breathing, becomes pinker, moves the arms and legs, and cries. Compare **periodic apnea of the newborn, secondary apnea.**

primary atelectasis, failure of the lungs to expand fully at birth, most commonly seen in premature infants or those narcotized by maternal anesthesia. The infant is usually cared for in an incubator in which the temperature and humidity may be closely monitored. Nursing care includes frequent changes of position of the infant to assist respiration, suctioning to remove bronchial secretions, and very slow feedings to avoid abdominal distention.

primary atypical pneumonia. See **mycoplasma pneumonia.**

primary biliary cirrhosis, a chronic inflammatory condition of the liver. It is characterized by generalized pruritus, enlargement and hardening of the liver, weight loss, and diarrhea with pale, bulky stools. Petechiae, epistaxis, or hemorrhage resulting from hypoprothrombinemia may also be evident. Pathological fractures and collapsed vertebrae may develop as the result of the associated malabsorption of vitamin D and calcium. Xanthomas commonly develop when the serum cholesterol level exceeds 450 mg/100 ml. The etiology of primary biliary cirrhosis is unknown; the condition most often affects women aged 40 to 60. The diagnosis is confirmed by liver biopsy and cholangiography. Jaundice, dark urine, pale stools, and cutaneous xanthosis may occur in the later stages of this disease. Treatment commonly includes the administration of fat-soluble vitamins A, D, E, and K to prevent and correct deficiencies caused by malabsorption. Drugs, including methyltestosterone or norethandrolene, may relieve associated pruritus. Some studies indicate that *D*-penicillamine may help correct this disorder over the long term. When treatment is begun in the early, asymptomatic stages of the condition the prognosis is excellent. The life expectancy is about 5 years for symptomatic

patients after the onset of jaundice. Compare **secondary biliary cirrhosis.**

primary bronchus, one of the two main air passages that branch from the trachea and convey air to the lungs as part of the respiratory system. The right primary bronchus is about 2.5 cm long, wider and shorter than the left primary bronchus, and enters the right lung nearly opposite the fifth thoracic vertebra. The left primary bronchus is about 5 cm long, passes under the aortic arch, and courses ventral to the esophagus, the thoracic duct, and the descending aorta before dividing into bronchi for the superior and the anterior lobes of the lung. The bronchi, like the trachea, are composed of rings of hyaline cartilage, fibrous tissue, mucous membrane, and glands. The carina at the bottom of the trachea separates the two primary bronchi and is situated to the left of the middle line so that the right primary bronchus is a more direct extension of the trachea than the left. Hence, foreign objects entering the trachea usually drop into the right bronchus rather than the left.

primary carcinoma, a neoplasm at its site of origin.

primary constriction. See **centromere.**

primary cutaneous melanoma, a primary melanoma on the skin.

primary degenerative dementia. See **senile psychosis.**

primary dental caries, dental caries developing in the enamel of a tooth that was previously unaffected.

primary dentition. See **deciduous dentition.**

primary dysmenorrhea. See **dysmenorrhea.**

primary fissure, a fissure that marks the division of the anterior and posterior lobes of the cerebellum.

primary gain, a benefit, primarily relief from emotional conflict and freedom from anxiety, attained through the use of a defense mechanism or other psychological process. Compare **secondary gain.**

primary health care, a basic level of health care that includes programs directed at the promotion of health, early diagnosis of disease or disability, and prevention of disease. Primary health care is provided in an ambulatory facility to limited numbers of people, often those living in a particular geographic area. In any episode of illness, it is the first patient contact with the health care system. It may be continuing health care, as provided by a family nurse practitioner, or it may be care at the point of entry into the health care system, as offered by an emergency room that provides care and referral.

primary host. See **definitive host.**

primary hypertension. See **hypertension.**

primary nurse, a nurse who is responsible for the planning, implementation, and evaluation of the nursing care of one or more clients twenty-four hours a day for the duration of the hospital stay. In primary nursing, nursing care usually includes the development and implementation of a care plan, participation in conferences on the care of a client, collaboration with the client, the health care team members, and the client's family, referral to community resources, and evaluation of the outcome of care.

primary nursing, a system for the distribution of nursing care in which care of one patient is managed for the entire 24-hour day by one nurse who directs and coordinates nurses and other personnel, schedules all tests, procedures, and daily activities for that patient, and cares for that patient personally when on duty. In an acute-care situation, the primary-care nurse might be responsible for only one patient; in an intermediate-care situation, the primary-care nurse might be responsible for three or more patients. Primary nursing is a new concept. Nurse-midwives and other nurse practitioners practice primary nursing, and many hospital nursing services are replacing team nursing with primary nursing. Some advantages are continuity of care for the patient, accountability of the nurse for that care, patient-centered care that is comprehensive, individualized, and coordinated, and the professional satisfaction of the nurse. Compare **team nursing.**

primary organizer, the part of the dorsal lip of the blastopore that is self-differentiating and induces the formation of the neural plate that gives rise to the main axis of the embryo.

primary physician, 1. the physician who usually takes care of a person; the physician who first sees a patient for the care of a given health problem. **2.** a family practice physician or general practitioner. See also **family medicine.**

primary proximal renal tubular acidosis. See **proximal renal tubular acidosis (proximal RTA).**

primary sequestrum, a piece of dead bone that completely separates from sound bone during the process of necrosis. Compare **secondary sequestrum.**

primary shock, a state of physical collapse comparable to fainting. It may be the result of slight pain, as that produced by venipuncture, or may be caused by fright. Primary shock is usually mild, self-limited, and of short duration. Severe injury may prolong and merge primary shock with secondary shock. Compare **hemorrhagic shock.**

primary tooth. See **deciduous tooth.**

primary tuberculosis, the childhood form of tuberculosis, most commonly occurring in the lungs, the posterior pharynx, or, rarely, the skin. Infants lack resistance to the disease, being easily infected and especially vulnerable to rapid and extensive spread of the infection through their bodies. In childhood, the disease is usually brief and benign, characterized by regional lymphadenopathy, calcification of the tubercles, and residual immunity. The tuberculin test will be positive for life. See also **tuberculosis.**

prime mover, a muscle that acts directly to produce a desired movement amid other muscles acting simultaneously to produce indirectly the same movement. Most movements of the body require the combined action of numerous muscles. Compare **antagonist, fixation muscle, synergist.**

primidone (prai′mədoun), an anticonvulsant.
■ INDICATIONS: It is prescribed in the treatment of seizure disorders.
■ CONTRAINDICATIONS: Porphyria or known hypersensitivity to this drug or to phenobarbital prohibits its use.
■ ADVERSE EFFECTS: The most serious adverse reaction, seen on rare occasions, is megaloblastic anemia. Drowsiness, ataxia, and dizziness are common. Other adverse effects of phenobarbital may be seen.

primigravida (prim′igræv′idə), a woman who is pregnant for the first time. Also called **gravida 1.** — **primigravid,** adj.

primitive, 1. undeveloped; undifferentiated; rudimentary; showing little or no evolution. **2.** embryonic; formed early in the course of development; existing in an early or simple form. Compare **definitive. 3.** first or early in terms of time; original; primary.

primitive fold. See **primitive ridge.**

primitive groove, a furrow in the posterior region of the embryonic disc that indicates the cephalocaudal axis resulting from the active involution of cells forming the primitive streak.

primitive gut. See **archenteron.**

primitive line. See **primitive streak.**

primitive node, a knoblike accumulation of cells at the cephalic end of the primitive streak in the early stages of embryonic development in man and the higher animals. It consists of mesoderm cells that give rise to the notochord, and it corresponds to the dorsal lip of the blastopore in lower animals. Also called **Hensen's node.**

primitive pit, a minute indentation at the anterior end of the primitive groove in the early developing embryo. It lies posterior to the primitive node and probably functions as an opening into the notochordal canal in man and the higher animals and into the neurenteric canal in the lower animals.

primitive reflex, any reflex not normally found in an adult but normal in an infant or fetus. The presence of such a reflex in an adult usually indicates serious neurological disease. Some kinds of primitive reflexes are **grasp reflex, Moro reflex, sucking reflex.**

primitive ridge, a ridge that bounds the primitive groove in the early stages of embryonic development. Also called **primitive fold.** See also **primitive streak.**

primitive streak, a dense area on the central posterior region of the embryonic disc, formed by the morphogenetic movement of a rapidly proliferating mass of cells that spreads between the ectoderm and endoderm, giving rise to the mesoderm layer. This seamlike elongation indicates the cephalocaudal axis along which the embryo develops, and it corresponds to the blastopore of lower animal groups. Also called **primitive line.**

primordial (praɪmɔr′dɪəl), **1.** characteristic of the most undeveloped or primitive state, specifically those cells or tissues that are formed in the early stages of embryonic development. **2.** first or original; primitive.

primordial dwarf, a person of extremely short stature who is otherwise perfectly formed, with the usual proportions of body parts and normal mental and sexual development. The condition may be genetically related, involving some defect in the ability to utilize growth hormone, or it may occur sporadically within a particular population. Also called **hypoplastic dwarf, normal dwarf, physiologic dwarf, pure dwarf, true dwarf.** See also **pituitary dwarf, pygmy.**

primordial germ cell, any of the large spherical diploid cells that are formed in the early stages of embryonic development and are precursors of the oogonia and spermatogonia. They are formed outside of the gonads and migrate to the embryonic ovaries and testes for maturation. See also **oogenesis, spermatogenesis.**

primordial image (praɪmɔr′dɪəl), (in analytic psychology) the archetype or original parent, representing the source of all life. It occurs in the memory as a stage preceding the differentiation of the actual mother and father. See also **collective unconscious.**

primordium (praɪmɔr′dɪəm), *pl.* **primordia.** the first recognizable stage in the embryonic development and differentiation of a particular organ, tissue, or structure; anlage; rudiment.

principal cell. See **chief cell.**

Principen, a trade name for an antibacterial (ampicillin).

PR interval, the component of the cardiac cycle shown on an electrocardiogram as an inverted U-shaped curve from the beginning of the P wave that tails off in an abrupt, flat downward direction (Q wave) until it angles sharply upward to a peak (R wave). It represents the interval of time required for atrial depolarization and for the impulse from the sinoatrial node to reach the ventricles, preparing them for contraction.

Prinzmetal's angina, a form of angina pectoris in which the attacks occur during rest and are associated with an elevation of the ST segment on the electrocardiogram.

Priscoline Hydrochloride, a trade name for a peripheral vasodilator (tolazoline hydrochloride).

-privia, a combining form meaning a '(specified) condition of loss or deprivation': *calciprivia, hormonoprivia, paraprivia.*

Privine Hydrochloride, a trade name for an adrenergic (naphazoline hydrochloride).

PRL, abbreviation for **prolactin.**

p.r.n., (in prescriptions) abbreviation for *pro re nata,* a Latin phrase meaning 'as needed.' The times of administration are determined by the needs of the patient.

pro-, a combining form meaning 'first, or in front of': *procallus, procheilon, progravid.*

proaccelerin. See **factor V.**

Probana, a trade name for a nutritional supplement for infants.

proband (prou′bænd). See **propositus.**

Pro-Banthine, a trade name for an anticholinergic (propantheline bromide).

probenecid (prouben′əsɪd), a uricosuric.
- ■ INDICATIONS: It is prescribed in the treatment of gout and as an adjunct prolonging the activity of penicillin or cephalosporins in some infections.
- ■ CONTRAINDICATIONS: Uric acid kidney stones, blood dyscrasias, or known hypersensitivity to this drug prohibits its use. It is not initiated during acute attack of gout but is continued if an attack intervenes during treatment. It is not given to children under two years of age. Concomitant administration of salicylates decreases the effect of probenecid.
- ■ ADVERSE EFFECTS: Among the most serious adverse reactions are gastrointestinal disturbances, headache, urinary frequency, and minor allergic reactions. It is involved in many drug interactions.

problem-oriented medical record (POMR), a method of recording data about the health status of a client in a problem-solving system. The POMR preserves the data in an easily accessible way that encourages ongoing assessment and revision of the health-care plan by all members of the health-care team. The particular format of the system used varies from setting to setting, but the components of the method are similar. A database is collected prior to beginning the process of identifying the client's problems. The database consists of all information available that contributes to this end, as information collected in an interview with the client and family or others, information from a health assessment or physical examination of the client, and information from various laboratory tests. Weed recommends that the database be as complete as possible, limited only by potential hazard or pain or discomfort to the patient or by excessive expense of the diagnostic procedure. The interview, augmented by prior records, provides the patient's history, including the reason for contact, an identifying statement that is a descriptive profile of the person, a family illness history, a history of the current illness, a history of past illness, an account of the patient's current health practices, and a review of systems. The physical examination or health assessment comprises the second major part of the database. The extent and depth of the examination varies from setting to setting and depends on the services offered and the condition of the client. The next section of the POMR is the master problem list. The formulation of the problems on the list is similar to the assessment phase of the nursing process. Each problem as identified represents a conclusion or a decision resulting from examination, investigation, and analysis of the database. A problem is defined as anything that causes concern to the patient or to the care-giver, including physical abnormalities, psychologic disturbance, and socioeconomic problems. The master problem list usually includes active, inactive, temporary, and potential problems. The list serves as an index to the rest of the record and is arranged in five columns: a chronological list of problems; the date of onset; the action taken; the outcome of the problem (often its resolution); and its date. Problems may be added, and intervention or plans for intervention may be changed; thus, the status of each problem is available for the information of all members of the various professions involved in caring for the client. The third major section of the POMR is the initial plan, in which each separate problem is named and described, usually written on the progress note in a SOAP format: S stands for the subjective data from the patient's point of view; O stands for the objective data acquired by inspection, percussion, auscultation, and palpation and from laboratory tests; A is an assessment of the problem that is an analysis of the subjective and objective data; and P is the plan, including further diagnostic work, therapy, and education or counseling. After an initial plan for each problem is formulated and recorded, the problems are followed in the progress notes by narrative notes in the SOAP format or by flow sheets showing the significant data in a tabular manner. A discharge summary is formulated and written, relating the overall assessment of progress during treatment and the plans for follow-up or referral. The summary allows a review of all the problems initially identified and encourages continuity of care for the patient.

problem solving approach to patient-centered care, (in nursing) a conceptual framework that incorporates the overt physical needs of a patient with covert psychological, emotional, and social needs. It provides a model for caring for the whole person as an individual, not as an example of a disease or a medical diagnosis. Nursing is defined within this model as a problem-solving process. The patient is viewed as a person who is in an impaired state, less than usually able to perform self-care activities. Nursing problems are conditions experienced by the patient or the patient's family in which the nurse may provide professional service. The nurse makes a nursing diagnosis that identifies the impaired state and determines the care needed to augment the patients' ability to perform self-care. The requirements for care are classified in four levels. Care given to sustain life is sustenal care; care given to assist the patient in self-care is remedial care; care that helps the patient to develop new skills and goals in self-care is restorative care; care given to guide the patient to a level of self-help beyond the normal level is preventive care. Twenty-one nursing problems are identified and sorted into four groups: problems relating to comfort, hygiene, and safety; physiological balance; psychological and social factors; and sociologic and community factors.

procainamide hydrochloride (prōukein'əmaid, prōu'-keinæm'aid), an antiarrhythmic agent.
- INDICATIONS: It is prescribed in the treatment of a variety of cardiac arrhythmias.
- CONTRAINDICATIONS: Myasthenia gravis, heart block, or known hypersensitivity to this drug, to procaine, or to related local anesthetics prohibits its use.
- ADVERSE EFFECTS: Among the more serious adverse reactions are gastrointestinal disturbances, hypersensitivity reactions, agranulocytosis, and a syndrome resembling lupus erythematosus.

procaine hydrochloride, a local anesthetic of the ester family.
- INDICATIONS: Procaine is administered for local anesthesia by infiltration and injection and for caudal, epidural, and other regional anesthetic procedures. It is not used for topical anesthesia.
- CONTRAINDICATIONS: Known hypersensitivity to anesthetics of the ester group prohibits its use. It is not injected into inflamed or infected tissue, and large doses are not given to patients with heart block.
- ADVERSE EFFECTS: Among the most serious adverse reactions are potentially serious neurological and cardiovascular reactions that result from inadvertent intravascular administration. Allergic reactions may also occur.

procarbazine hydrochloride, an antineoplastic.
- INDICATIONS: It is prescribed in the treatment of a variety of neoplasms, including Hodgkin's disease.
- CONTRAINDICATIONS: Bone marrow depression or known hypersensitivity to this drug prohibits its use.
- ADVERSE EFFECTS: Among the most serious adverse reactions are bone marrow depression and gastrointestinal disturbances, particularly nausea and vomiting.

procaryon (prōukær'ion). See **prokaryon.**

procaryosis (prōu'kæriou'sıs). See **prokaryosis.**

Procaryotae (prōukær'iou'ti), (in bacteriology) a kingdom of plants that includes all microorganisms in which the nucleoplasm has no basic protein and is not surrounded by a nuclear membrane. The kingdom has two divisions, Cyanobacteria and Bacteria.

procaryote (prōukær'iout). See **prokaryote.** —**procaryotic,** *adj.*

procerus (prōusir'əs), one of three muscles of the nose. Arising from the fascia of the nasal bone and the lateral nasal cartilage and inserting into the skin over the lower part of the forehead between the eyebrows, it is a small pyramidal muscle, innervated by buccal branches of the facial nerve. The procerus functions to draw down the eyebrows and wrinkle the nose. Compare **depressor septi, nasalis.**

process, 1. a series of related events that follow in sequence from a particular state or condition to a conclusion or resolution. 2. a natural growth that projects from a bone or other part. 3. to put through a particular series of interdependent steps.

process recording, (in nursing education) a system used for teaching nursing students to understand and analyze verbal and nonverbal interaction. The conversation between nurse and patient is written on special forms or in a special format. The student nurse is instructed to record observations, perceptions, thoughts, and feelings as well as the words exchanged. The process recording is then studied by the nursing instructor to discover and to help the student nurse identify patterns of difficulty in communicating with the patient.

process schizophrenia, a form of schizophrenia caused by organic changes in the brain rather than by environmental influences. The onset of the disease is usually gradual, but it progresses rapidly or slowly to irreversible psychosis. Compare **reactive schizophrenia.** See also **schizophrenia.**

prochlorperazine, a phenothiazine antipsychotic and anti-emetic.
■ INDICATIONS: It is prescribed in the treatment of psychotic disorders and for the control of nausea and vomiting.
■ CONTRAINDICATIONS: Parkinson's disease, the concurrent administration of central nervous system depressants, liver or renal dysfunction, severe hypotension, or known hypersensitivity to any phenothiazine prohibits its use.
■ ADVERSE EFFECTS: Among the more serious adverse effects are hypotension, liver toxicity, extrapyramidal reactions, blood dyscrasias, and hypersensitivity reactions.

prochlorperazine maleate. See **prochlorperazine.**

prochromosome (prɔukrɔu′məsoum). See **karyosome.**

proconvertin. See **factor VII.**

proct-. See **procto-.**

-proctia, a combining form meaning '(condition of the) anus': *ankyloproctia, cacoproctia, coloproctia.*

proctitis (proktaı′tıs), inflammation of the rectum and anus caused by infection, trauma, drugs, allergy, or radiation injury. Acute or chronic, it is accompanied by rectal discomfort and the repeated urge to pass feces with the inability to do so. Pus, blood, or mucus may be present in the stools, and tenesmus may be present. Also called **rectitis.**

procto-, proct-, a combining form meaning 'of or pertaining to the rectum': *proctocele, proctorrhea, proctoscopy.*

Proctocort, a trade name for a glucocorticoid (hydrocortisone).

proctodeum, proctodaeum, *pl.* **proctodea, proctodaea.** an invagination of the ectoderm, behind the urorectal septum of the developing embryo, that forms the anus and anal canal when the cloacal membrane ruptures. Compare **stomodeum.** – **proctodaeal, proctodeal.** *adj.*

Proctodon, a trade name for a local anesthetic agent (diperodon hydrochloride).

proctologist (proktol′əjıst), a physician who specializes in proctology.

proctology (proktol′əji), the branch of medicine concerned with treating disorders of the colon, rectum, and anus.

proctoscope, an instrument used to examine the rectum and the distal portion of the colon. It consists of a light mounted on a tube or speculum. Compare **sigmoidoscope.**

procyclidine hydrochloride (prɔusaı′klədin), an anticholinergic.
■ INDICATION: It is prescribed in the treatment of parkinsonism.
■ CONTRAINDICATIONS: Narrow angle glaucoma, asthma, obstruction of the genitourinary or gastrointestinal tract, severe ulcerative colitis, or known hypersensitivity to this drug prohibits its use.
■ ADVERSE EFFECTS: Among the more serious adverse effects are blurred vision, central nervous system effects, tachycardia, dry mouth, decreased sweating, and hypersensitivity reactions.

prodromal labor, the early period in parturition before uterine contractions become forceful and frequent enough to result in progressive dilatation of the uterine cervix.

prodrome, 1. an early sign of a developing condition or disease. 2. the earliest phase of a developing condition or disease. – **prodromal,** *adj.*

productive cough, a sudden, noisy expulsion of air from the lungs that effectively removes sputum from the respiratory tract and helps to clear the air passages, permitting oxygen to reach the alveoli. Coughing is stimulated by irritation or by inflammation of the respiratory tract caused most frequently by infection. Deep breathing, with contraction of the diaphragm and intercostal muscles and forceful exhalation, promotes productive coughing in patients with respiratory infections. Mucolytic agents liquefy mucus in the respiratory tract so that it can be raised and expectorated more easily. Anticholinergic drugs, as atropine, decrease respiratory secretions. See also **nonproductive cough.**

professional corporation (PC), a corporation formed according to the law of a particular state for the purpose of delivering a professional service. In some states, corporations may not practice law, medicine, surgery, or dentistry, and in some states nurses may form or be partners in a professional corporation. According to the laws of the various states professional corporations may offer legal and tax benefits to the members of the corporation. ▸

professional liability, a legal concept describing the obligation of a professional person to pay a patient or client for damages caused by the professional's act of omission, commission, or negligence. Professional liability better describes the responsibility of all professionals to their clients than does the concept of malpractice, but the idea of professional liability is central to malpractice.

professional network, (in psychiatric nursing) the network of professional resources available to support the psychiatric outpatient in the community. The network may include a therapist, a hospital day treatment program, social work agency, and other agencies.

professional organization, an organization, whose members share a professional status, created to deal with issues of concern to the professional group or groups involved.

Professional Standards Review Organization (PSRO), an organization formed under Social Security Act Amendments of 1972 to review the services provided under Medicare, Medicaid, and Maternal Child Health programs. Review is conducted by physicians to ascertain the need for the program, to ensure that it is carried out in accord with certain criteria, norms, and standards, and, in institutional situations, in a proper setting. The PSRO requires that regional organizations be formed to conduct these reviews throughout the nation.

profibrinolysin (prou'faibrinol'isin). See **plasminogen.**

progenitive, capable of producing offspring; reproductive.

progenitor, 1. a parent or ancestor. 2. one who or anything that originates or precedes; precursor.

progeny (proj'əni), 1. offspring; an individual or organism resulting from a particular mating. 2. the descendants of a known or common ancestor.

progeria (prouji'riə), an abnormal congenital condition characterized by premature aging and the appearance in childhood of gray hair and wrinkled skin and by small stature, absence of pubic and facial hair, and the posture and habitus of an aged person. Death usually occurs before the age of twenty years. Compare **infantilism.**

progestagen. See **progestogen.**

Progestasert, a trade name for a progestin (progesterone).

progestational (prou'jestei'shənəl), of or pertaining to a drug with effects similar to those of progesterone, the hormone produced by the corpus luteum and adrenal cortex during the luteal phase of the menstrual cycle that prepares the uterus for reception of the fertilized ovum. Natural and synthetic preparations of progesterone and its derivative medroxyprogesterone acetate are used in the treatment of secondary amenorrhea and abnormal uterine bleeding. Progestational compounds, as norethindrone and norgestrel, are constituents of oral contraceptives. The use of progestogens to prevent habitual or threatened abortion is no longer recommended.

progesterone (prəjes'təroun), a natural progestational hormone.

■ INDICATIONS: It is prescribed in the treatment of various menstrual disorders, infertility owing to luteal phase dysfunction, and repeated spontaneous abortion.

■ CONTRAINDICATIONS: Thrombophlebitis, liver dysfunction, breast cancer, missed abortion, or hypersensitivity to this drug prohibits its use.

■ ADVERSE EFFECTS: Among the more serious adverse reactions are pain at the site of injection, catabolic effects, and electrolyte disturbances.

progestogen, progestagen, any natural or synthetic progestational hormone. Also called **progestin.**

proglottid (prouglot'id), an egg-bearing segment of a tapeworm, containing both male and female reproductive organs.

prognosis, a prediction of the probable outcome of a disease based on the condition of the person and the usual course of the disease as observed in similar situations.

progressive, describing the course of a disease or condition in which the characteristic signs and symptoms become more prominent and severe, as progressive muscular atrophy.

progressive myonecrosis. See **myonecrosis.**

progressive patient care, a system of care in which patients are placed in units on the basis of their needs for care as determined by the degree of illness rather than in units based on a medical specialty. The usual levels or stages of progressive patient care are intensive care, intermediate care, and minimal care.

progressive resistance exercise, a method of increasing the strength of a weak or injured muscle by gradually increasing the resistance against which the muscle works, as by using graduated weights over a period of time. Also called **graduated resistance exercise.** See also **active resistance exercise.**

progressive spinal muscular atrophy of infants. See **Werdnig-Hoffmann disease.**

progressive systemic sclerosis (PSS), the most common form of scleroderma.

progress notes, (in the patient record) notes made by a nurse and physician that describe the patient's condition and the treatments given or planned. Progress notes may follow the problem-oriented medical record format. The physician's progress notes usually focus on the medical or therapeutic aspects of the patient's condition and care; the nurse's progress notes, while noting the medical conditions of the patient, usually focus on the objectives stated in the nursing care plan. These objectives might include the person's ability to perform activities of daily living or acceptance or understanding of a particular condition or treatment. Progress notes in an in-hospital setting are recorded daily; progress notes in a clinic or office setting are usually preceded by an episodic or an interval history and are written as an account of each visit.

Progynon, a trade name for an estrogen (estradiol).

projection, 1. a protuberance; anything that thrusts or juts outward. 2. the act of perceiving an idea or thought as an objective reality. 3. (in psychology) an unconscious defense mechanism by which an individual attributes his own unacceptable traits, ideas, or impulses to another.

projective test, a kind of diagnostic, psychological or personality test that uses unstructured or ambiguous stimuli, like inkblots, a series of pictures, abstract patterns, or incomplete sentences, to illicit responses that reflect a projection of various aspects of the subject's personality. See also **Rorschach test.**

prokaryocyte, procaryocyte (proukær'iəsait), a cell without a true nucleus and with nuclear material scattered throughout the cytoplasm. Prokaryocytic organisms include bacteria, viruses, rickettsiae, chlamydiae, mycoplasmas, actinomycetes, and certain algae. Compare **eukaryocyte.**

prokaryon, procaryon (proukær'ion), 1. nuclear elements that are not bound by a membrane but are spread throughout the cytoplasm, as in bacteria, viruses, and other unicellular organisms. 2. an organism containing such unbound nuclear elements. Compare **eukaryon.**

prokaryosis, procaryosis, the condition of not containing a true nucleus surrounded by a nuclear membrane, as in bacteria and viruses. Compare **eukaryosis.**

prokaryote, procaryote (proukær'iout), an organism that does not contain a true nucleus surrounded by a nuclear membrane, characteristic of lower forms, as bacteria, viruses, and blue-green algae. The nuclear elements are spread throughout the cytoplasm and division occurs through simple fission. Compare **eukaryote.** —**prokaryotic,** adj.

Proketazine Maleate, a trade name for a phenothiazine tranquilizer (carphenazine maleate).

prolactin (PRL) (proulæk'tin), a hormone produced and secreted into the blood stream by the anterior pituitary. Prolactin, acting with estrogen, progesterone, thyroxine, insulin, growth hormone, glucocorticoids, and human placental lactogen, stimulates the development and growth of the mammary glands. After parturition, prolactin together with glucocorticoids is essential for the initiation and maintenance of milk production. Prolactin synthesis and release from the pituitary is mediated by the central nervous system in response to suckling by the infant. When suckling or its mechanical equivalent ceases, prolactin secretion slows and milk production ceases. Prolactin is similar to growth hormone in its chemical structure. It is unknown in males. Also called **lactogen, lactogenic hormone, luteotropin.**

prolapse (prou'læps, proulæps'), the falling, sinking, or sliding of an organ from its normal position or location in the body, as a prolapsed uterus.

Proloid, a trade name for a thyroid hormone preparation (thyroglobulin).

prolonged release, designed to deliver a dose of a drug over an extended period of time. The most common device for this purpose is a soft, soluble capsule containing minute pellets of the drug for release at different rates in the gastrointestinal tract, depending on the thickness and nature of the oil, fat, wax, or resin coating on the pellets. Another system consists of a porous plastic carrier impregnated with the drug and a surfactant which facilitates the entry of gastrointestinal fluids that slowly leach out the drug. Ion exchange resins that bind to drugs and liquids containing suspensions of slow release drug granules are also used to provide medication over an extended period. Various mechanisms and vehicles have also been developed to prolong the release of drugs after injection intramuscularly or subcutaneously.

Proloprim, a trade name for an antibacterial (trimethoprim).

Promapar, a trade name for an antiemetic and tranquilizer (chlorpromazine hydrochloride).

promethazine hydrochloride, a phenothiazine antiemetic and antihistamine.

■ INDICATIONS: It is prescribed in the treatment of nausea, rhinitis, itching, and skin rash.

■ CONTRAINDICATIONS: Known hypersensitivity to this drug or to other phenothiazines prohibits its use.

■ ADVERSE EFFECTS: Drowsiness, hypotension, and dry mouth are the most common adverse reactions.

promethium (Pm), a radioactive, rare-earth, metallic element. Its atomic number is 61; its atomic weight is 147.

promoter, (in molecular genetics) a DNA sequence that initiates RNA transcription of the genetic code.

prompt insulin zinc suspension, a fast-acting noncrystalline semilente insulin prescribed in the treatment of diabetes mellitus when a prompt, intense, and short-acting response is desired. This type of insulin is only slightly slower to act than insulin injection. See also **fast acting insulin.**

promyelocyte (proumai'ələsait), a large mononuclear blood cell abnormally present in the circulating blood. It contains a single, regular, symmetric nucleus and a few undifferentiated cytoplasmic granules. It is intermediate in development between a myeloblast and a myelocyte and is indicative of leukemia. See also **leukemia, metamyelocyte, myeloblast.**

pronation (prounei'shən), 1. assumption of a prone position, one in which the ventral surface of the body faces downward. 2. of the arm, the rotation of the forearm so that the palm of the hand faces downward and backward.

3. of the foot, the lowering of the medial edge of the foot while turning it outward. — **pronate,** *v.,* **prone,** *adj.*

pronator reflex (prōunei′tər), a reflex elicited by holding the patient's hand vertically and tapping the distal end of the radius or ulna, resulting in pronation of the forearm. Hyperactivity of the reflex may be seen with lesions of the pyramidal system above the level of the sixth cervical nerve root.

pronator teres, a superficial muscle of the forearm, arising from a humeral and an ulnar head. The humeral head is the larger and more superficial, originating near the medial epicondyle, from the tendon common to the superficial muscles of the forearm, from certain intermuscular septa, and from the antebrachial fascia. The ulnar head originates in the coronoid process of the ulna. Fibers from both portions of the muscle pass obliquely across the forearm, ending in a flat tendon that inserts into the radius. The pronator teres is innervated by a branch of the median nerve, which contains fibers from the sixth and the seventh cervical nerves, and it functions to pronate the hand. Compare **flexor carpi ulnaris, flexor carpi radialis, flexor digitorum superficialis, palmaris longus.**

Pronemia, a trade name for a hematinic, fixed-combination drug containing iron, vitamin B_{12}, intrinsic factor concentrate, vitamin C, and folic acid.

proneness profile, a screening process that evaluates the probability of developmental problems occurring in the early years of a child's life. Screening ideally begins in the course of prenatal care and continues after delivery. Several of the variables in the proneness profile that appear to be significant in selecting the infants who are at risk are the perinatal health status of the mother and infant, especially complications of pregnancy, delivery, the neonatal period and the puerperium; characteristics of the mother, especially her temperament, educational level, perception of the life situation, and perception of the infant; characteristics of the infant, including alertness, activity pattern, and responsiveness; and the behaviors of the infant and care-giver as they interact. The proneness profile is followed by a developmental profile that assesses the current status of the infant and care-giver. Three areas to be considered are: characteristics of the infant, including adaptation and response to the environment, the ability to give interpretable cues, and the developmental progress as compared with established norms; characteristics of the care-giver, including adaptation to the new infant, sensitivity to cues from the infant, and techniques for relieving distress; and the healthful quality of the environment, including health, safety, comfort, and stimulation.

pronephric duct, one of the paired ducts that connects the tubules of each of the pronephros with the cloaca in the early developing vertebrate embryo. They later become the functional mesonephric ducts. Also called **archinephric canal, archinephric duct.**

pronephric tubule, any of the segmentally arranged excretory units of the pronephros in the early developing vertebrate embryo. The tubules open into the pronephric duct and communicate with the coelom through a nephrostoma. In man and the higher vertebrates the tubules are present only in vestigial form; in lower animals, they are functional.

pronephron (prōunef′ron), *pl.* **pronephra.** See **pronephros.**

pronephros, pronephron, *pl.* **pronephroi, pronephra.** the primordial excretory organ in the developing vertebrate embryo. It consists of a series of pronephric tubules that arise along the anterior portion of the nephrotome and empty into the cloaca by way of the pronephric duct. In man and other mammals the structure is nonfunctional, representing the first of three excretory systems that are formed one after the other in an anterior to posterior sequence and that disappear with the formation of the mesonephros. The organ is functional in certain primitive fishes, as lampreys, and serves as a provisional kidney in some fishes and amphibians. Also called **archinephron, head kidney.** See also **mesonephros, metanephros.** — **pronephric,** *adj.*

Pronestyl, a trade name for a cardiac depressant (procainamide hydrochloride).

pronucleus, *pl.* **pronuclei.** the nucleus of the ovum or the spermatozoon after fertilization but prior to the fusion of the chromosomes to form the nucleus of the zygote. Each contains the haploid number of chromosomes, is larger than the normal nucleus, and is diffuse in appearance. The female pronucleus of the mature ovum is formed only after penetration by the sperm and the completion of the second mitotic division and polar body formation. The nucleus then loses its nuclear envelope to release the chromosomes so that synapsis can occur with the chromosomes of the male pronucleus, which is contained in the head of the spermatozoon. Also called **germ nucleus, germinal nucleus.** See also **oogenesis, spermatogenesis.**

Propadrine Hydrochloride, a trade name for an adrenergic (phenylpropanolamine hydrochloride).

propantheline bromide, an anticholinergic.

■ INDICATION: It is prescribed as an adjunct in peptic ulcer therapy.

■ CONTRAINDICATIONS: Narrow angle glaucoma, asthma, obstruction of the genitourinary or gastronintestinal tract, severe ulcerative colitis, or known hypersensitivity to this drug prohibits its use.

■ ADVERSE EFFECTS: Among the more serious adverse reactions are blurred vision, central nervous system effects, tachycardia, dry mouth, decreased sweating, and hypersensitivity reactions.

proparacaine hydrochloride (prōupær′əkein), a rapid-acting, topical anesthetic of the amide family used for ophthalmologic procedures. It is used for tonometry, gonioscopy, removal of foreign objects from the eye, and other minor optical procedures and preoperatively for major eye surgery. One drop gives 15 minutes of optical anesthesia. Prolonged use may injure the eye. Proparacaine hydrochloride is not administered to individuals with cardiac disease, hyperthyroidism, or multiple allergies. People given the drug should be warned not to touch their eyes until the anesthetic has worn off. Adverse optical reactions may occur with proparacaine, but systemic reactions are rare. Also called **proxymetacaine.**

prophase (prou'feiz), the first of four stages of nuclear division in mitosis and in each of the two divisions of meiosis. In mitosis, the chromosomes progressively shorten and thicken to form individually recognizable elongated double structures composed of two chromatids held together by a centromere; the nucleolus and nuclear membrane disappear, the spindle and polar bodies are formed, and the chromosomes begin to migrate toward the midplane of the developing spindle. In the first meiotic division, prophase is complex and subdivided into five stages: leptotene, zygotene, pachytene, diplotene, and diakinesis. In the second meiotic division, the same processes occur as in mitotic prophase. See also **anaphase, interphase, meiosis, metaphase, mitosis, telophase.**

prophylactic (prou'filæk'tik), **1.** preventing the spread of disease. **2.** an agent that prevents the spread of disease. — **prophylactically,** *adv.*

prophylactic forceps. See **low forceps.**

prophylactic treatment. See **preventive treatment.**

prophylaxis (prou'filæk'sis), prevention of or protection against disease, often involving the use of a biological, chemical, or mechanical agent to destroy or prevent the entry of infectious organisms.

Propine, a trade name for an ophthalmic adrenergic (dipivefrin hydrochloride).

propionicacidemia (prou'pion'ikæs'idi'miə), a rare inherited metabolic defect caused by the failure of the body to metabolize the amino acids threonine, isoleucine, and methionone, characterized by lethargy and mental and physical retardation. Acidosis occurs as a result of the accumulation of propionic acid in the body. A diet low in these amino acids is difficult to achieve but is the only treatment. — **propionicacidemic,** *adj.*

propionic fermentation, the production of propionic acid by the action of certain bacteria on sugars or lactic acid.

Proplex, a trade name for human clotting factor IX.

propositus, a person from whom a genealogical lineage is traced, as is done to discover the pattern of inheritance of a familial disease or a physical trait.

propoxyphene (proupok'səfin), a mild centrally acting narcotic analgesic.

■ INDICATION: It is prescribed to relieve mild to moderate pain.

■ CONTRAINDICATIONS: Concurrent administration of tranquilizers or antidepressant drugs, current alcohol or drug abuse, or known hypersensitivity to aspirin, phenacetin, caffeine, or this drug prohibits its use. It is not recommended for use by people who are suicidal or prone to alcohol or drug addiction or by women who are pregnant because neonatal withdrawal symptoms have been observed.

■ ADVERSE EFFECTS: Among the more serious reactions are hepatic dysfunction and severe depression of the central nervous system occurring with overdose or drug interraction. A small number of people may experience nausea, dizziness, sedation, or vomiting when correctly taking a usual, prescribed dosage.

propoxyphene hydrochloride, an analgesic.

■ INDICATION: It is prescribed for the relief of mild to moderate pain.

■ CONTRAINDICATION: Known hypersensitivity to this drug prohibits its use.

■ ADVERSE EFFECTS: Among the more serious adverse reactions are respiratory depression, paradoxical excitement, and convulsions.

propranolol hydrochloride, a beta-adrenergic blocking agent.

■ INDICATIONS: It is prescribed in the treatment of angina pectoris, cardiac arrhythmias, and hypertension.

■ CONTRAINDICATIONS: Asthma, certain arrhythmias, congestive heart failure, concomitant use of monamine oxidase inhibitors, or known hypersensitivity to this drug prohibits its use.

■ ADVERSE EFFECTS: Among the more serious adverse reactions are heart failure, heart block, increased airway resistance, augmentation of hypoglycemic response, gastrointestinal disturbances, and hypersensitivity reactions. Withdrawal syndrome has been observed in some patients.

proprietary, **1.** of or pertaining to an institution or other organization that is operated for profit. **2.** of a product, as a drug or device, made for profit.

proprietary hospital, a hospital operated as a profitmaking organization. Many proprietary hospitals are owned by physicians who operate the hospital primarily for their own patients but also accept patients from other physicians. Some proprietary hospitals are owned by investor groups or large corporations.

proprietary medicine, any pharmaceutical preparation or medicinal substance that is protected from commercial competition because its ingredients or method of manufacture are kept secret or are protected by trademark or copyright.

proprioception (prou'priəsep'ʃhən), sensation pertaining to stimuli originating from within the body regarding spatial position and muscular activity or to the sensory receptors that they activate. Compare **exteroceptive, interoceptive.**

proprioceptive reflex (prou'priǝsep'tɪv), any reflex initiated by stimulation of proprioceptive receptors, as the increase in respiratory rate and volume induced by impulses arising from muscles and joints during exercise.

proprioceptor, any sensory nerve ending, as those located in muscles, tendons, joints and the vestibular apparatus, that responds to stimuli originating from within the body regarding movement and spatial position. Compare **exteroceptor, interoceptor.** See also **mechanoreceptor, proprioceptive nervous system, receptor.**

proptosis (proptou'sɪs), bulging, protrusion, or forward displacement of a body organ or area.

propylformic acid (prou'pɪlfǝr'mɪk). See **butyric acid.**

propylhexedrine, an adrenergic vasoconstrictor.
- INDICATION: It is prescribed to relieve nasal congestion.
- CONTRAINDICATIONS: Concommitant use of monoamine oxidase inhibitors or known hypersensitivity to this or other sympathomimetics prohibits its use.
- ADVERSE EFFECTS: Among the more serious adverse reactions are systemic sympathomimetic effects. Irritation of the nasal mucosa and rebound congestion may occur.

propylthiouracil, an inhibitor of thyroid hormone biosynthesis.
- INDICATION: It is prescribed in the treatment of hyperthyroidism.
- CONTRAINDICATION: Known hypersensitivity to this drug prohibits its use.
- ADVERSE EFFECTS: Among the more serious adverse reactions are gastrointestinal distress, pruritus, and rashes. Rarely, blood dyscrasia occurs.

proscribe, to forbid, as forbidding of certain acts or services by the members of an organization by its bylaws. – **proscriptive,** adj.

prosencephalon (pros'ensef'ǝlon), the portion of the brain that includes the diencephalon and the telencephalon. It develops from the anterior of the three primary vesicles of the embryonic neural tube and contains various structures, as the thalamus and hypothalamus, which control important body functions and affect the consciousness, the appetite, and the emotions. Also called **forebrain.** Compare **mesencephalon.** – **prosencephalic,** adj.

proso-, pros-, a combining form meaning 'forward, or anterior': prosocoele, prosodemic, prosogaster.

Pro Sobee, a trade name for a commercial milk-substitute formula that is prepared from a soy isolate base and is lactose free, prescribed for infants with galactosemia and persons with lactose intolerance. It is supplemented with other nutrients, fortified with vitamins and minerals, and is available in both powder and liquid forms. See also **Neo-Mull-Soy, Nutramigen, Soyalac.**

prosopalgia (prou'soupæl'jiǝ). See **trigeminal neuralgia.**

-prosopia, a combining form meaning '(condition of the) face': ateloprosopia, lipoprosopia, schizoprosopia.

prosopo-, a combining form meaning 'of or related to the face': prosopoanoschisis, prosopodiplegia, prosoponeuralgia.

prosoposternodidymus (pros'ǝpoustǝr'noudɪd'ǝmǝs), a fetal monster consisting of conjoined twins united laterally from the head through the sternum.

prosopothoracopagus (pros'ǝpouθɔr'ǝkop'ǝgǝs), conjoined symmetrical twins who are united laterally in the frontal plane from the thorax through most of the head region.

prospective study, a study designed to determine the relationship between a condition and a characteristic shared by some members of a group. The population selected is healthy at the beginning of the study. Some of the members of the group share a particular characteristic, as cigarette smoking. The researcher follows the population group over a period of time, noting the rate at which a condition, as lung cancer, occurs in the smokers and in the nonsmokers. A prospective study may involve many variables or only two; it may seek to demonstrate a relationship that is an association or one that is causal. The kinds of data collected, the numbers of people studied, and other details of the design of the study affect the kind of analysis and the interpretation of the data.

prostaglandin (PG) (pros'tǝglæn'dɪn), one of several potent hormonelike unsaturated fatty acids that act in exceedingly low concentrations on local target organs. They are produced in small amounts and have a large array of significant effects. Prostaglandins given by nebulizer, in tablets, or in solutions for oral or intravenous use, effect changes in vasomotor tone, capillary permeability, smooth-muscle tone, aggregation of platelets, endocrine and exocrine functions, and in the autonomic and central nervous systems. Some of the pharmacologic uses for the prostaglandins are termination of pregnancy and treatment of asthma and gastric hyperacidity.

Prostaphlin, a trade name for an antibacterial (oxacillin sodium).

prostate (pros'teit), a gland in men that surrounds the neck of the bladder and the urethra and elaborates a secretion that liquefies coagulated semen. It is a firm structure about the size of a chestnut, composed of muscular and glandular tissue. It is located in the pelvic cavity, below the caudal part of the symphysis pubis and ventral to the rectum, through which it can be felt, especially when enlarged. A depression on its cranial border accommodates the entry of the two ejaculatory ducts and divides the posterior surface of the gland into the middle lobe above, and a larger, lower portion below. A sinus about 6 mm long runs upward and backward in the gland behind the middle lobe and is part of the urethra. The prominent lateral surfaces of the prostate are covered by a plexus of veins and by the ventral portions of the levator ani. The portion of the gland in front of the urethra is comprised of dense muscular tissue. In most men the urethra lies along the junction of the anterior portion and the middle third of the prostate. The ejaculatory ducts pass obliquely through the posterior part of the gland. The prostatic secretion consists of alkaline phosphatase, citric acid, and various proteolytic enzymes. – **prostatic,** *adj.*

prostatectomy, surgical removal of a portion of the prostate gland, as performed for benign prostatic hypertrophy, or the total excision of the gland, as performed for malignancy. An indwelling urinary catheter is inserted, and a type and cross-match of blood is done to prepare for possible transfusion. Either a general or a spinal anesthetic is used. Kinds of approaches include transurethral, the most common, in which a resectoscope is inserted and through it shavings of prostatic tissue are cut off at the bladder opening with a loop, suprapubic, and retropubic. The perineal approach is used for biopsy when early cancer is suspected or for the removal of calculi. In a suprapubic approach, the patient returns with a large catheter positioned into the bladder through the abdomen. Wound drains are left in place in both the perineal and the suprapubic types. After surgery, hematuria is expected for several days; on the first day the bleeding is frank, usually venous, and may be controlled by increasing the pressure in the balloon end of the urethral catheter. If arterial in nature, the bleeding will be bright red with numerous clots and increased viscosity and may lead to hemorrhagic shock, requiring transfusion and surgical intervention. The catheters are connected to a closed system of either constant or intermittent drainage. Meticulous aseptic technique is required to prevent infection when tending catheters, tubings, and collection bags, as well as when changing the dressing. Catheter patency is assured, and pain is assessed, as blockage or kinking of the drainage tubes may be the cause. Accidental removal or dislodging of catheters is avoided. Bladder spasm may occur if a catheter becomes blocked or from the irritation of the balloon of the catheter in the bladder. Antispasmodic drugs may prevent spasm but are not given in severe cardiac disease or if glaucoma is present. The nurse also assesses the patient's ability to void in adequate amounts when the urethral catheter is removed. Complications of prostatectomy include urethral stricture (especially with the transurethral approach), urinary incontinence, and impotence.

prostatic (prostæt′ɪk), pertaining to the prostate gland.

prostatic catheter, a catheter that is approximately 16 inches long and has an angled tip. It is used in male catheterization to pass an enlarged prostate gland obstructing the urethra.

prostatic ductule (dək′tyul), any one of 12 to 20 tiny excretory tubes that convey the alkaline secretion of the prostate gland and open into the floor of the prostatic portion of the urethra. The ductules are joined together by areolar tissue, supported by extensions of the fibrous capsule of the prostate and its muscular stroma, and wrapped in a delicate network of capillaries.

prostatic utricle, the portion of the urethra in men that forms a cul-de-sac about six mm long behind the middle lobe of the prostate. It is composed of fibrous tissue, muscular fibers, and mucous membrane; numerous small glands open on its inner surface. It is derived from the atrophied paramesonephric ducts and is homologous with the uterus in women. Also called **uterus masculinis.** See also **prostate.**

prostatitis (pros′tətaɪ′tɪs), acute or chronic inflammation of the prostate gland, usually the result of infection. The patient complains of burning, frequency, and urgency. Treatment consists of administration of antibiotics, sitz baths, bed rest, and fluids. Compare **benign prostatic hypertrophy.**

prosthesis (prosfhi′sɪs), *pl.* **prostheses, 1.** an artificial replacement for a missing part of the body. **2.** a device designed and applied to improve function, as a hearing aid. See also **artificial limb, maxillofacial prosthesis, Starr-Edwards prothesis.**

prosthodontics (pros′fhədon′tɪks), a branch of dentistry devoted to the construction of artificial appliances that replace missing teeth or restore parts of the face.

Prostigmin, a trade name for a neuromuscular blocking agent (neostigmine) used as an adjunct to anesthesia.

Prostin F2 Alpha, a trade name for a prostaglandin abortifacient (dinoprost tromethamine).

prot-. See **proto-.**

protactinium, (Pa), a radioactive element. Its atomic number is 91; its atomic weight is 231. The most long lived isotope of protactinium is p-231 which has a half life of 34,000 years and is produced as an intermediate in the radioactive decay of uranium-235.

protamine sulfate (prou′təmin), a heparin antagonist.

■ INDICATION: It is prescribed to diminish or reverse the anticoagulant effect of heparin.

■ CONTRAINDICATION: Known hypersensitivity to this drug prohibits its use.

■ ADVERSE EFFECTS: Among the more serious adverse reactions are hypotension, dyspnea, and bradycardia. Dosage greater than needed to neutralize heparin causes the toxic and anticoagulant effects of protamine itself.

protamine zinc insulin suspension, a long-acting insulin that is absorbed slowly at a steady rate. Some patients can be treated with only one injection daily, but combination therapy with regular insulin may be necessary for adequate control.

protanopia (prou'tənou'piə). See **daltonism.**

protease (prou'tieis), an enzyme that is a catalyst in the breakdown of protein. See also **proteolytic.**

protein, any of a large group of naturally occurring, complex, organic nitrogenous compounds. Each is composed of large combinations of amino acids containing the elements carbon, hydrogen, nitrogen, oxygen, usually sulfur, and, occasionally, phosphorus, iron, iodine, or other essential constituents of living cells. Twenty-two amino acids have been identified as vital for proper growth, development, and maintenance of health. The body can synthesize fourteen of these amino acids, called nonessential, while the remaining eight must be obtained from dietary sources and are termed essential. Protein is the major source of building material for muscles, blood, skin, hair, nails, and the internal organs. It is necessary for the formation of hormones, enzymes, and antibodies, as a source of heat and energy, and it functions as an essential element in proper elimination of waste materials. Rich dietary sources are meat, poultry, fish, eggs, milk, and cheese, which are classified as complete proteins since they contain the eight essential amino acids. Nuts and legumes, including navy beans, chick peas, soybeans, and split peas, are also good sources but are incomplete proteins, since they do not contain all the essential amino acids. Protein deficiency causes abnormal growth and tissue development in children, leading to kwashiorkor and marasmus, while in adults it results in lack of vigor and stamina, weakness, mental depression, poor resistance to infection, impaired healing of wounds, and slow recovery from disease. Excessive intake of protein may in some conditions result in fluid imbalance.

protein-bound iodine (PBI), iodine that is firmly bound to protein in serum, the measurement of which indirectly indicates the concentration of circulating thyroxine (T_4). PBI less than the normal range of 4 to 8 μ/ml of serum is indicative of hypothyroidism and a PBI of more than the normal values indicates hyperthyroidism. The test is currently used less frequently because of the availability of more sensitive measurements of T_4.

protein hydrolysate injection, a fluid and nutrient replenisher.

■ INDICATIONS: It is prescribed to correct a negative nitrogen balance and in other clinical situations requiring parenteral nutrition.

■ CONTRAINDICATIONS: Renal failure, anuria, severe liver disease, hepatic coma, or known hypersensitivity to one or more of the amino acids prohibits the use of this drug.

■ ADVERSE EFFECTS: Among the more serious adverse reactions are hypotension, abdominal pain, convulsions, phlebitis, thrombosis, and edema.

protein kinase, a protein that catalyzes the transfer of a phosphate group from adenosine triphosphate to produce a phosphoprotein.

protein metabolism, the processes whereby protein foodstuffs are used by the body to make tissue proteins, together with the processes of breakdown of tissue proteins in the production of energy. Food proteins are first broken down into amino acids, then absorbed into the bloodstream, and finally used in body cells to form new proteins. Amino acids in excess of the body's needs may be converted by liver enzymes into keto acids and urea. The keto acids may be used as sources of energy via the Krebs citric acid cycle, or they may be converted into glucose or fat for storage. Urea is excreted in urine and sweat. Growth hormones and androgens stimulate protein formation, and adrenal cortical hormones tend to cause breakdown of body proteins. Diseases affecting protein metabolism include homocystinuria, liver disease, maple sugar urine disease, and phenylketonuria.

proteinuria (prou'tinyur'iə), the presence in the urine of abnormally large quantities of protein, usually albumin. Healthy adults excrete less than 250 mg of protein per day. Persistent proteinuria is usually a sign of renal disease or renal complications of another disease, as hypertension, heart failure. However, proteinuria can result from heavy exercise or fever. Also called **albuminuria, proteinuria.**

proteo-, a combining form meaning 'of or pertaining to protein': *proteocrasis, proteolysis, proteopepsis.*

proteolipid (prou'tioulip'id), a type of lipoprotein in which lipid material forms more than half of the molecule. It is insoluble in water and occurs primarily in the brain.

proteolysis (prou'tiol'əsis), a process in which water added to the peptide ponds of proteins breaks the protein molecule. Numerous enzymes may catalyze this process. The action of mineral acids and heat may also induce proteolysis.

proteolytic (prou'tiəlit'ik), of or pertaining to any substance that promotes the breakdown of protein.

Proteus (prou'tiəs), a genus of motile, gram-negative bacilli often associated with nosocomial infections, normally found in feces, water, and soil. *Proteus* may cause urinary tract infections, pyelonephritis, wound infections, diarrhea, bacteremia, and endotoxic shock. Some species are sensitive to penicillin; most respond to the aminoglycoside antibiotics.

prothrombin (prouthrom'bin), a plasma protein that is the precursor to thrombin. It forms thrombin, the first step in blood clotting, when exposed to thromboplastin and calcium. It is synthesized in the liver if adequate vitamin K is present. Also called **Factor II.** See also **blood coagulation.**

prothrombin time (PT), a one-stage test for detecting certain plasma coagulation defects owing to a deficiency of factors V, VII or X. Thromboplastin and calcium are added to a sample of the patient's plasma and, simultaneously, to a sample from a normal control. The length of time required for clot formation in both samples is observed. Thrombin is formed from prothrombin in the presence of adequate calcium, thromboplastin, and the essential tissue coagulation factors. A prolonged PT therefore indicates deficiency in one of the factors, as in liver disease, vitamin K deficiency, or anticoagulation therapy with the drug coumarin. Compare **partial thromboplastin.** See also **blood clotting.**

protiptyline hydrochloride, a tricyclic antidepressant.
■ INDICATION: It is prescribed in the treatment of mental depression.
■ CONTRAINDICATIONS: Concomitant administration of monoamine oxidase inhibitors, recent myocardial infarction, or known hypersensitivity to any tricyclic medication prohibits its use. It is used with caution where anticholinergics are contraindicated, in seizure disorders, and in patients with cardiovascular disease.
■ ADVERSE EFFECTS: Among the more serious adverse reactions are sedation and anticholinergic side effects. A variety of gastrointestinal, cardiovascular, and neurological reactions may occur. This drug interacts with many other drugs.

proto-, prot-, a combining form meaning 'first': *protoblast, prototoxin, protopathic.*

protocol (prou'təkɔl), a written plan specifying the procedures to be followed in giving a particular examination, in conducting research, or in providing care for a particular condition. See also **standing orders.**

protokylol hydrochloride (prou'təkai'loul), an adrenergic bronchodilator.
■ INDICATIONS: It is prescribed in the treatment of asthma, emphysema, bronchiectasis, and pulmonary fibrosis.
■ CONTRAINDICATIONS: Cardiac arrhythmia, coronary insufficiency, or known hypersensitivity to this drug or to other sympathomimetic medication prohibits its use.
■ ADVERSE EFFECTS: Among the more serious adverse reactions are tachycardia and palpitation, dizziness, tremor, insomnia, and central nervous system disturbances.

proton, a positively charged particle that is a fundamental component of the nucleus of all atoms. The number of protons in the nucleus of an atom equals the atomic number of the element. Compare **electron, neutron.** See also **atomic weight.**

Protopam Chloride, a trade name for a cholinesterase reactivator (pralidoxime chloride).

protoplast (prou'təplæst), **1.** (in biology), the protoplasm of a cell without its containing membrane. **2.** a first entity or an original. — **protoplastic,** *adj.*

protoporphyria (prou'touporfir'iə). increased excretion of protoporphyrin in the feces.

protoporphyrin (prou'touporfirɪn), a kind of porphyrin

that combines with iron and protein to form a variety of important organic molecules including catalase, hemoglobin, and myoglobin.

protostoma. See **blastopore.**

protozoa (prou'təzou'ə), *sing.* **protozoon.** single-celled microorganisms of the class Protozoa, the lowest form of animal life. Protozoa are more complex than bacteria, forming a self-contained unit with organelles that carry on such functions as locomotion, nutrition, excretion, respiration, and attachment to other objects or organisms. Approximately 30 protozoa are pathogenic to man. — **protozoal, protozoan,** *adj.*

protozoal infection, any disease caused by single-celled organisms of the class Protozoa. Some kinds of protozoal infections are **amebic dysentery, kala azar, malaria, trichomonas vaginitis.**

protracted dose, (in radiotherapy) a low amount of radiation delivered continuously over a relatively long period of time.

protrusio bulbi. See **exophthalmia.**

proud flesh, excessive granulation tissue. See also **pyogenic granuloma.**

Provera, a trade name for a progestin (medroxyprogesterone acetate).

Provincial Territorial Nurses' Association (PTNA), an association of nurses organized at the provincial or territorial level. The Canadian Nurses' Association is a federation of the eleven PTNAs.

provitamin (prouvai'təmin), a precursor of a vitamin; a substance found in certain foods that in the body may be converted into a vitamin. Also called **previtamin.**

provocative diagnosis, a diagnosis in which the identity and etiology of an illness are discovered by inducing an episode of the condition, as in immunology an allergen causing an allergic response is shown to be an etiologic factor in the patient's allergic condition.

proximal (prok'siməl), nearer to a point of reference, frequently the trunk of the body, than other parts of the body. Proximal interphalangeal joints are those closest to the hand.

proximal radioulnar articulation, the pivot joint between the circumference of the head of the radius and the ring formed by the radial notch of the ulna and the annular ligament. The joint allows the rotary movements of the head of the radius in pronation and supination. Also called **superior radioulnar joint.** Compare **distal radioulnar articulation.**

proximal renal tubular acidosis (proximal RTA), an abnormal condition characterized by excessive acid accumulation and bicarbonate excretion. It is caused by the defective reabsorption of bicarbonate in the proximal tubules of the kidney and the resulting flow of excessive bicarbonate into the distal tubules which normally secrete hydrogen ions. This disruption impedes the formation of titratable acids and ammonium for excretion and ultimately leads to metabolic acidosis. Treatment is as for renal tubular acidosis. In **primary proximal RTA** the defective reabsorption of bicarbonate is the sole causative factor. In **secondary proximal RTA** the reabsorptive defect is one of several causative factors and may result from tubular cell damage produced by various disorders, as Fanconi's syndrome. Compare **distal renal tubular acidosis.**

proxymetacaine (prok'simet'əkein). See **proparacaine hydrochloride.**

prurigo (prʊraiˈgou), any of a group of chronic inflammatory conditions of the skin characterized by severe itching and multiple, dome-shaped, small papules capped by tiny vesicles. Later, as a result of repeated scratching, crusting and lichenification may occur. Some causes of prurigo are allergies, drugs, endocrine abnormalities, malignancies, and parasites. Specific treatment depends on the cause. Symptomatic therapy is the same as for pruritus. A mild form of the disease is called **prurigo mitis** and a more severe form, **prurigo agria** or **prurigo ferox.** See also **pruritus.** — **pruriginous,** *adj.*

pruritus (prʊraiˈtəs), the symptom of itching, an uncomfortable sensation leading to the urge to scratch. Scratching often results in secondary infection. Some causes of pruritus are allergy, infection, jaundice, lymphoma, and skin irritation. Treatment is best directed at the cause; symptomatic relief may be obtained by antihistamines, starch baths, topical corticosteroids, cool water, or alcohol applications. — **pruritic,** *adj.*

pruritus ani, a common chronic condition of itching of the skin around the anus. Some causes are candida infection, contact dermatitis, external hemorrhoids, pinworms, psoriasis, and psychogenic illness. Treatment is best directed at the specific cause; however, symptomatic relief may be obtained by careful cleansing, soothing creams or lotions, topical corticosteroids, antihistamines, and tranquilizers.

pruritus vulvae, itching of the external genitalia of a female. The condition may become chronic and result in lichenification, atrophy, and occasionally malignancy. Some causes of pruritus vulvae are contact dermatitis, lichen sclerosus et atrophicus, psychogenic pruritus, trichomoniasis, and vaginal candidiasis. Treatment of the condition depends on its cause.

psammo-, a combining form meaning 'of or related to sand or to sandlike material': *psammocarcinoma, psammoma, psammosarcoma.*

psammoma (sæmouˈmə), *pl.* **psammomas, psammomata.** a neoplasm containing small calcified granules (psammoma bodies) that occurs in the meninges, choroid plexus, pineal body, and ovaries. Also called **sand tumor.**

psammoma body, a round, layered mass of calcareous material occurring in benign and malignant epithelial and connective tissue neoplasms and in some chronically inflamed tissue.

-pselaphesia, a combining form meaning '(condition of the) tactile sense': *apselaphesia, hyperpselaphesia, hypopselaphesia.* Also **-pselaphesis.**

pseudesthesia (su'desfhi'ʒhə), a sensation experienced without an external stimulus or a sensation which does not correspond to the causative stimulus, as phantom limb pain.

pseudo-, pseud-, a combining form meaning 'false': *pseudoangina, pseudocyst, pseudorubella.*

pseudoallele (su'douəlil'), (in genetics) one of two or more closely linked genes on a chromosome that appear to function as a single member of an allelic pair but occupy distinct, nearly corresponding loci on homologous chromosomes. Such gene pairs produce a mutant effect in the diploid state when located on homologous chromosomes but are capable of being separated by crossing over during meiosis to produce a wild-type effect when recombined on either of the homologues. — **pseudoallelic,** *adj.,* **pseudoallelism,** *n.*

pseudoanorexia (su'douæn'ourek'siə), a condition in which an individual eats secretly while claiming a lack of appetite and inability to eat. Also called **false anorexia.**

pseudochylous ascites (su'doukai'lɔs), the abnormal accumulation in the peritoneal cavity of a milky fluid that resembles chyle. The turbidity of the fluid is caused by cellular debris in the fluid. Pseudochylous ascites is indicative of an abdominal tumor or infection. Compare **chylous ascites.** See also **ascites.**

pseudocoxalgia (su'doukoksæl'jə). See **Perthes' disease.**

pseudocyst, a space or cavity containing gas or liquid but without a lining membrane. Pseudocysts commonly occur after pancreatitis when digestive juices break through the normal ducts of the pancreas and collect in spaces lined by fibroblasts and surfaces of adjacent organs. Symptoms are owing to displacement of abdominal structures or fluid or to atelectasis at the base of the left lung. Ultrasound and computerized tomography are useful in diagnosis; surgical drainage is the best therapy. See also **pancreatitis.**

pseudoephedrine hydrochloride, an adrenergic that acts as a vasoconstrictor and bronchodilator.

■ INDICATION: It is prescribed for the relief of nasal congestion and eustachian tube congestion.

■ CONTRAINDICATIONS: Known hypersensitivity to sympathomimetic drugs prohibit its use. It is prescribed with caution in patients who have hypertension, glaucoma, heart disease, diabetes, or urinary retention.

■ ADVERSE EFFECTS: Among the more serious adverse reactions are central nervous system stimulation, headache, and tachycardia.

pseudoephedrine sulfate. See **pseudoephedrine hydrochloride.**

pseudogene (su'doujin'), (in molecular genetics) a sequence of nucleotides that resembles a gene and may be derived from one but lacks a genetic function.

pseudogout (su'dougaut'). See **chondrocalcinosis.**

pseudohermaphrodism (su'douhərmæf'rədiz'əm). See **pseudohermaphroditism.**

pseudojaundice, a yellow discoloration of the skin that is not caused by hyperbilirubinemia. The excessive ingestion of carotene results in a form of pseudojaundice.

pseudomembranous enterocolitis. See **necrotizing enterocolitis.**

pseudomembranous stomatitis, a severe inflammation of the mouth that produces a membranelike exudate. The inflammation may be caused by a variety of bacteria or by chemical irritants. It may produce dysphagia, pain, fever, and swelling of the lymph glands, or it may remain localized and mild.

pseudomonad (sudom'ənæd), a bacterium of the genus *Pseudomonas.*

Pseudomonas (sudom'ənæs), a genus of gram-negative bacteria that includes several free-living species of soil and water and some opportunistic pathogens, as *Pseudomonas aeruginosa,* isolated from wounds, burns, and infections of the urinary tract. Pseudomonads are notable for their fluorescent pigments and their resistance to disinfectants and antibiotics.

pseudoneurotic schizophrenia. See **latent schizophrenia.**

pseudopsychopathic schizophrenia. See **latent schizophrenia.**

pseudorubella. See **roseola infantum.**

pseudosclerema (su'douskliri'mə). See **adiponecrosis subcutanea neonatorum.**

pseudotumor (su'doutu'mər), a false tumor. Kinds of pseudotumors are **orbital pseudotumor, pseudotumor cerebri.**

pseudotumor cerebri, a condition characterized by increased intracranial pressure, headache, vomiting, and papilledema without neurological signs, except, occasionally, palsy of the sixth cranial nerve. Also called **benign intracranial hypertension, meningeal hydrops.**

pseudoxanthoma elasticum (su'douzænθou'mə). See **Grönblad-Strandberg syndrome.**

psilocybin (sai'lousai'bin, sai'lousib'in), a psychedelic drug and an active ingredient of various Mexican hallucinogenic mushrooms of the genus *Psilocybe mexicana.* It can produce altered states of mood and consciousness and has no acceptable medical use in the United States. Psilocybin is controlled under Schedule I of the Comprehensive Drug Abuse Prevention and Control Act of 1970, which bans the prescription of psilocybin and numerous other drugs and allows their procurement and use only for special research projects authorized by the Drug Enforcement Administration of the United States Department of Justice.

psittacosis (sit'əkou'sis), an infectious illness caused by the bacterium *Chlamydia psittaci,* characterized by respiratory, pneumonialike symptoms and transmitted to humans by infected birds, especially parrots. The clinical manifestations of the disease are extremely variable and resemble a great number of infectious diseases, but fever, cough, anorexia, and severe headache are almost always present. A history of exposure to birds is highly suggestive, because all chlamydiae are difficult to isolate and culture. A demonstrated rise in antibody titer confirms a diagnosis. Tetracycline is usually used to treat psittacosis and is continued for 10 to 14 days after the fever subsides. Isolation is advised. Also called **ornithosis, parrot fever.** See also *Chlamydia.*

psoas major (sou'əs), a long abdominal muscle originating from the transverse processes of the lumbar vertebrae and the fibrocartilages and sides of the vertebral bodies of the lower thoracic vertebrae and the lumbar vertebrae. It joins the iliacus to form the iliopsoas deep in the pelvis as it passes under the inguinal ligament and inserts in the lesser trochanter. It acts to flex and laterally rotate the thigh and to flex and laterally bend the spine.

psoas minor, a long, slender muscle of the pelvis, ventral to the psoas major. Many individuals do not have this muscle. It arises from the bodies of the twelfth thoracic and the first lumbar vertebrae and from the disc between them and ends in a long, flat tendon that inserts into the pectineal line of the pelvis and into the iliac fascia. The psoas minor is innervated by a branch of the first lumbar nerve and functions to flex the spine. Compare **iliacus, psoas major.**

psor-, a combining form meaning 'of or related to itching': *psora, psorocomium, psorous.*

psoralen-type photosynthesizer, any one of the chemical compounds that contain photosensitizing psoralen and that react on exposure to ultraviolet light to increase the melanin in the skin. Naturally occurring psoralen photosynthesizers, as 5- and 8-methoxypsoralen, are found in buttercups, carrot greens, celery, clover, cockleburs, dill, figs, limes, parsley, and meadow grass. Some psoralen-type photosynthesizers produced as pharmaceuticals are methoxsalen and trioxalen; both are used to enhance skin pigmentation or tanning in the treatment of skin diseases, as psoriasis and vitiligo. Such drugs are carefully administered to avoid over-sensitization of the skin and other complications. Psoralen-type photosynthesizers are also used in the manufacture of some perfumes, colognes, and pomades. Such chemicals cause unique skin reactions, as Berlock dermatitis, in some individuals. Oil of bergamot, extracted from the peels of small oranges grown in southern France and Italy is a photosynthesizing psoralen used by the perfume industry.

psoriasis (sərai′əsıs), a common, chronic, heritable, skin disorder, characterized by circumscribed red patches covered by thick, dry, silvery, adherent scales that are the result of excessive development of epithelial cells. Exacerbations and remissions are typical. Lesions may be anywhere on the body but are more common on extensor surfaces, bony prominences, scalp, ears, genitalia, and the perianal area. An arthritis, particularly of distal small joints, may accompany the skin disease. Treatment includes topical and intralesional corticosteroids, ultraviolet light, tar solution baths, creams and shampoos, methotrexate, and photochemotherapy. Subcategories of psoriasis include **guttate psoriasis** and **pustular psoriasis**. See also **photochemotherapy, psoriatic arthritis**. — **psoriatic,** (sər′iæt′ık) *adj.*

psoriatic arthritis, a form of rheumatoid arthritis associated with psoriatic lesions of the skin and nails, particularly at the distal interphalangeal joints of the fingers and toes.

PSP, a trade name for a glucocorticoid (prednisolone sodium phosphate).

PSRO, abbreviation for **Professional Standards Review Organization.**

PSS, abbreviation for **progressive systemic sclerosis.**

PSSO, abbreviation for **peer specialist second opinion.**

psych-. See **psycho-.**

psychasthenia (sai′kəsthi′niə). See **obsessive-compulsive neurosis.**

psyche (sai′ki), **1.** the aspect of one's mental faculty that encompasses the conscious and unconscious processes. **2.** the vital mental or spiritual entity of the individual as opposed to the body or soma. **3.** (in psychoanalysis) the total components of the id, ego, and superego, including all conscious and unconscious aspects. Compare **soma.**

psychedelic (sai′kıdel′ık), **1.** of or describing a mental state characterized by altered sensory perception and hallucination, accompanied by euphoria or fear, usually caused by the deliberate ingestion of drugs or other substances known to produce this effect. **2.** of or describing any drug or substance that causes this state, as mescaline or psilocybin.

psychiatric disorder. See **mental disorder.**

psychiatric nurse practioner, a nurse practitioner who, by advanced study and clinical practice, as in a master's program in psychiatric nursing, has gained expert knowledge in the care and prevention of mental disorders. See also **psychiatric nursing.**

psychiatric nursing, the branch of nursing concerned with the prevention and cure of mental disorders and their sequelae. It employs theories of human behavior as its scientific framework and requires the use of the self as its art or expression in nursing practice. Some of the activities of the psychiatric nurse include the provision of a safe therapeutic milieu; working with patients, or clients, concerning the real day-to-day problems that they face; identifying and caring for the physical aspects of the patient's problems, including drug reactions; assuming the role of social agent or parent for the patient in various

Professional Standards Review Organization

Local PSRO Structure

recreational, occupational, and social situations; conducting psychotherapy; and providing leadership and clinical assistance for other nurses and health care workers. Psychiatric nurses work in many settings; their responsibilities vary with the setting and with the level of expertise, experience, and training of the individual nurse. Also called **mental health nursing.**

psychiatry, the branch of medical science that deals with the causes, treatment, and prevention of mental, emotional, and behavioral disorders. Some kinds of psychiatry are **community psychiatry, descriptive psychiatry, dynamic psychiatry, existential psychiatry, forensic psychiatry, orthopsychiatry.** – **psychiatric,** *adj.*

-psychic, a combining form meaning 'relating to the relation between mind and body': *allopsychic, biopsychic, physiopsychic.*

psychic contagion. See **psychic infection.**

psychic infection, the spread of neurotic or psychic effects or influences on others, on a small scale, as in folie à deux, or on a large scale, as in the dance and witch manias of the Middle Ages or the spread of hysterical or panic reactions in a crowd. Also called **psychic contagion.** See also **sympathy.**

psychic suicide, the termination of one's own life without the use of physical means or agents, as an older person widowed after many years of marriage becomes sufficiently depressed to lose "the will to live."

psychic trauma, an emotional shock or injury or a distressful situation that produces a lasting impression, especially on the subconscious mind. Common causes of psychic trauma are abuse or neglect in childhood, rape, and loss of a loved one. Psychotherapeutic sessions in which the injured person can ventilate feelings can help to alleviate psychic trauma.

psycho-, psych-, a combining form meaning 'of or related to the mind': *psychoauditory, psychodynamics, psycholepsy.*

psychoanalysis, a branch of psychiatry founded by Sigmund Freud devoted to the study of the psychology of human development and behavior. From its systematized method for investigating the processes of the mind evolved a system of psychotherapy based on the concepts of a dynamic unconscious, utilizing such techniques as free association, dream interpretation, and the analysis of defense mechanisms, especially resistance and transference. Through these devices, emotions and behavior are traced to the influence of repressed instinctual drives in the unconscious. Treatment consists of helping the individual become aware of the existence of repressed emotional conflicts, analyzing their origin, and through the process of insight bringing them into the consciousness so that irrational and maladaptive behavior can be altered. See also **psychosexual development.**

psychoanalyst, a psychotherapist, usually a psychiatrist, who has had special training in psychoanalysis and who applies the techniques of psychoanalytic theory. A primary requisite for training is that the person himself undergo psychoanalysis.

psychoanalytic, 1. of or pertaining to psychoanalysis. 2. using the techniques or principles of psychoanalysis.

psychobiology, 1. the study of personality development and functioning in terms of the interaction of the body and the mind. 2. a school of psychiatric thought introduced by Adolf Meyer that stresses total life experience, including biological, emotional, and sociocultural factors, in assessing the psychological makeup or mental status of an individual. Mental disorders are interpreted as dynamic adaptive reactions of the individual to stress or conflict, with little or no emphasis placed on unconscious factors. Also called **biopsychology.** See also **distributive analysis and synthesis.**

psychocatharsis (saiˈkoukəθharˈsis). See **catharsis.**

psychodrama, a form of group therapy, originated by J. L. Moreno, in which people act out their emotional problems through dramatization and role playing. Also called **role-playing therapy.**

psychogenesis (saiˈkoujenˈəsis), 1. the development of the mind or of a mental function or process. 2. the development or production of a physical symptom or disease from mental or psychic origins rather than organic factors. 3. the development of emotional states, either normal or abnormal, from the interaction of conscious and unconscious psychological forces. Compare **somatogenesis.**

psychogenic (saiˈkəjenˈik), **psychogenetic** (saiˈkəjinetˈik), 1. originating within the mind. 2. any physical symptom, disease process, or emotional state that is of psychological rather than physical origin. Compare **somatogenic.** See also **psychosomatic.**

psychogenic pain disorder, a disorder characterized by persistent and severe pain for which there is no apparent organic cause. The condition is often accompanied by other sensory or motor dysfunction, as paresthesia or muscle spasm. The cause may be one or many unresolved needs or conflicts. Treatment consists of immediate alleviation of the symptoms followed by long-term psychotherapy aimed at uncovering the unconscious emotional conflicts that influenced the development and maintenance of the pain. See also **psychogenesis.**

psychokinesia (saiˈkoukini'ˈʑhə, saiˈkoukaini'ˈʑhə), 1. impulsive, maniacal behavior resulting from deficient or defective inhibitions. 2. (in parapsychology) psychokinesis.

psychokinesis (PK) (saiˈkoukiniˈsis, saiˈkoukainiˈsis), the direct influence of the mind or will upon matter usually resulting in the production of motion in objects without the intervention of the physical senses or a physical force.

psychokinetics (sai′koukɪnet′ɪks, sai′koukainet′ɪks), the study of psychokinesis.

psychological test, any of a group of standardized tests designed to measure or ascertain such characteristics of an individual as intellectual capacity, motivation, perception, role behavior, values, level of anxiety or depression, coping mechanisms, and general personality integration. Compare **achievement test, aptitude test, intelligence test, personality test.**

psychologist, a specialist in the study of psychology.

psychology, 1. the study of behavior and of the functions and processes of the mind, especially as related to environment. 2. a profession that involves the practical applications of knowledge, skills, and techniques in the understanding of, prevention of, or solution to individual or social problems, especially in regard to the interaction between the individual and the physical and social environment. 3. the mental, motivational, and behavioral characteristics and attitudes of an individual or group of individuals. Kinds of psychology include **analytic psychology, animal psychology, behaviorism, clinical psychology, cognitive psychology, experimental psychology, humanistic psychology, social psychology.** – **psychologic, psychological,** *adj.,* **psychologically,** *adv.*

psychometrics (sai′koume′trɪks), **psychometry** (saikom′ɪtri), the development, administration, or interpretation of psychological and intelligence tests.

psychomotor development, the progressive attainment by the child of skills that involve both mental and muscular activity, as the ability of the infant to turn over, sit, or crawl at will and of the toddler to walk, talk, control bladder and bowel functions, and begin solving cognitive problems. The mean chronologic ages at which certain psychomotor skills are attained by most children follow.

12 weeks	looks at own hand.
20 weeks	able to grasp objects voluntarily.
24 weeks	able to roll from back to front at will.
44 weeks	creeps with abdomen off the floor and imitates speech sounds.
15 months	able to walk without help.
24 months	has a vocabulary of 300 or more words and uses pronouns.
30 months	able to jump with both feet.
3 years	able to ride a tricycle and to feed self well.
4 years	able to hop and skip on one foot, catch and throw a ball; is independent, boasts, tattles, and shows off.
5 years	able to tie shoelaces, cut with scissors, tries to please, interested in facts about world, gets along more easily with parents.

psychomotor seizure, a temporary impairment of consciousness, often associated with temporal lobe disease and characterized by psychic symptoms, loss of judgment, automatic behavior, and abnormal acts. No apparent convulsions occur, but there may be loss of consciousness or amnesia for the episode. During the seizure the individual may appear drowsy, intoxicated, or violent; asocial acts or crimes may be committed but normal activities, as driving a car, typing, or eating, may continue at an automatic level. Psychic symptoms, including visual and auditory hallucinations, a sense of unreality, and déjà vu may be present and may be accompanied by visceral symptoms, as chest pain, transient respiratory arrest, tachycardia, and gastrointestinal discomfort and by abnormal sensations of smell and taste.

psychoneurosis. See **neurosis.**

psychoneurotic. See **neurotic.**

psychoneurotic disorder. See **neurotic disorder.**

psychopath, a person who has an antisocial personality disorder. Also called **sociopath.**

psychopathia (sai′koupæth′iə). See **psychopathy.**

psychopathia sexualis (sek′s̸huæl′ɪs), a mental disease characterized by sexual perversion.

psychopathic, of or pertaining to antisocial behavior. Also called **sociopathic.** See also **antisocial personality, antisocial personality disorder.**

psychopathic personality. See **antisocial personality.**

psychopathologist, one who specializes in the study and treatment of mental disorders. – **psychopathology,** *n.*

psychopathology, 1. the study of the causes, processes, and manifestations of mental disorders. 2. the behavioral manifestation of any mental disorder.

psychopathy (saikop′əfhi), any disease of the mind, congenital or acquired, not necessarily associated with subnormal intelligence. Also called **psychopathia.**

psychopharmacology, the scientific study of the effects of drugs in the treatment of mental disorders.

psychophylaxis (sai′koufɪlæk′sɪs). See **mental hygiene.**

psychophysical preparation for childbirth, a program that prepares women for giving birth by teaching them the physiology of the process, by teaching them exercises to improve muscle tone and physical stamina, and by teaching them various techniques of breathing and relaxation to promote control and comfort during labor and delivery. There are several methods of psychophysical preparation for childbirth. Among the goals of all of the methods are a decrease in the mother's fear and pain, a decrease in or elimination of the use of analgesia and anesthesia in childbirth, and an increase in the mother's participation and cooperation, thus requiring less obstetric intervention. Methods of psychophysical preparation for childbirth include **Bradley method, Lamaze method, Read method.**

psychophysics, the branch of psychology concerned with the relationships between physical stimuli and sensory responses.

psychophysiologic, 1. of or pertaining to psychophysiology. 2. having physical symptoms resulting from psychogenic origins; psychosomatic.

psychophysiological disorder, any of a large group of mental disorders characterized by the dysfunction of an organ or organ system controlled by the autonomic nervous system, as a peptic ulcer, which may be caused or aggravated by emotional factors, like stress or anxiety. The disorders are named and classified according to the organ system involved, such as cardiovascular, respiratory, musculoskeletal, and gastrointestinal. Also called **psychosomatic illness, psychosomatic reaction.**

psychophysiology, 1. the study of physiology as it relates to various aspects of psychological or behavioral function. See also **psychophysiological disorder.** 2. the study of mental activity by physical examination and observation.

psychoprophylactic preparation for childbirth, a system of prenatal education for giving birth using the Lamaze method of natural childbirth.

psychosexual, of or pertaining to the psychological and emotional aspects of sex. See also **psychosexual development, psychosexual disorder.** — **psychosexuality,** n.

psychosexual development, (in psychoanalysis) the emergence of the personality through a series of stages from infancy to adulthood, each stage relatively fixed in time and characterized by a dominant mode of achieving libidinal pleasure through the interaction of the person's biological drives and the restraints of the environment. Resolution of the conflicts encountered at each of the stages theoretically leads to a balanced, heterosexual adjustment and normal development, while a lack of resolution results in personality disturbances, fixated at the stage during which the unresolved conflicts occurred. Such disturbances may be latent or may result in various behavioral or personality disorders. The stages of development are the oral stage, anal stage, phallic stage, latency stage, genital stage. Also called **libidinal development.** See also **psychomotor development.**

psychosexual disorder, any condition characterized by abnormal sexual attitudes, desires, or activities resulting from psychological rather than organic causes. See also **gender identity disorder, paraphilia, psychosexual dysfunction.**

psychosexual dysfunction, any of a large group of sexual maladjustments or disorders caused by an emotional or psychological problem.

psychosis, pl. **psychoses.** any major mental disorder of organic or emotional origin characterized by extreme derangement or disorganization of the personality, often accompanied by severe depression, agitation, regressive behavior, illusions, delusions, and hallucinations that so greatly impair perception, thinking, emotional response, and personal orientation that the individual loses touch with reality, is incapable of functioning normally in society, and usually requires hospitalization. Kinds of psychoses include **affective psychosis, alcoholic psychosis, bipolar disorder, Korsakoff's psychosis, paranoia, schizophrenia, senile psychosis.** See also **major affective disorder, organic mental disorder.**

-psychosis, a combining form meaning a 'serious mental disorder': *autopsychosis, encephalopsychosis, pharmacopsychosis.*

psychosocial assessment, an assessment of a person's mental and social status and function. The person's self-image and self-esteem, goals, values, beliefs, and relationships are observed and evaluated in the process of making a psychosocial assessment.

psychosocial development, (in child development) a description devised by Erik Erikson of the normal serial development of trust, autonomy, identity, and intimacy; the development begins in infancy and progresses as the infantile ego interacts with the environment. For the child to reach a new stage, the preceding one must be fully realized. The sequence and chronology of the stages coincide with the psychosexual stages of development as described by Freud.

psychosomatic (sāī'kousəmæt'ɪk), 1. of or pertaining to psychosomatic medicine. 2. relating to, characterized by, or resulting from the interaction of the mind or psyche and the body. 3. the expression of an emotional conflict through physical symptoms. See also **psychogenic, psychophysiological disorder.**

psychosomatic approach, the interdisciplinary or holistic study of physical and mental disease from a biological, psychosocial, and sociocultural point of view.

psychosomatic illness. See **psychophysiological disorder.**

psychosomatic medicine, the branch of medicine concerned with the interrelationships between mental and emotional reactions and somatic processes, in particular the manner in which intrapsychic conflicts influence physical symptoms. It maintains that the body and mind are one inseparable entity and that both physiological and psychological techniques should be applied in the study and treatment of illness. Also called **psychosomatics.**

psychosomatic reaction. See **psychophysiological disorder.**

psychosomatics. See **psychosomatic medicine.**

psychosurgery, surgical interruption of certain nerve pathways in the brain, performed to treat selected cases of chronic, unremitting anxiety, agitation, or obsessional neuroses when the condition is severe and when alternative treatments, as psychotherapy, drugs, and electroshock, have proven ineffective. The procedure may be a limited prefrontal lobotomy (in which connecting fibers in the frontal region are cut) or a modified bifrontal tractotomy (in which nerve tracts of the brain stem are severed). Light general anesthesia is given. Postoperative nursing care includes observation for signs of leakage of cerebrospinal fluid. A marked alteration of personality is unavoidable. Various cognitive and affective functions are also affected, depending on the location of the induced lesion, the extent of destruction of nerve tissue, and the age, sex, and condition of the patient. Modern psychotherapeutic drugs have replaced psychosurgery in most cases.

psychotherapeutics, the treatment of personality disorders by means of psychotherapy.

psychotherapist, one who practices psychotherapy, including psychiatrists, licensed psychologists, psychiatric nurses, psychiatric social workers, and persons trained in counseling. The specific requirements for education and training differ markedly in content, breadth, and duration, depending on the form of psychotherapy practiced. Licensing procedures and definitions of practice vary from state to state. Compare **psychoanalyst.**

psychotherapy, any of a large number of related methods of treating mental and emotional disorders by psychological techniques rather than by physical means. Included among these techniques, which are used either with individuals or with groups, are reinforcement, persuasion, suggestion, reassurance, support, and abreaction. Some of the aims of psychotherapy are to change maladaptive behavioral patterns, improve interpersonal relationships, resolve inner conflicts that cause personal distress, modify inaccurate assumptions about the self and the environment, and foster a definite sense of self-identity in order to promote individual growth leading to a more meaningful and fulfilling existence. Kinds of psychotherapy are **behavior therapy, group therapy, humanistic-existential therapy, interpersonal therapy, psychoanalysis.**

psychotic, 1. of or pertaining to psychosis. 2. a person exhibiting the characteristics of a psychosis.

psychotic disorder. See **psychosis.**

psychotic reaction. See **psychosis.**

psychro-, a combining form meaning 'of or pertaining to cold': *psychrometer, psychrophilic, psychrophore.*

psyllium seed (sɪl′ɪəm). See **plantago seed.**

Pt, symbol for **platinum.**

PT, abbreviation for **prothrombin time.**

PTA, abbreviation for **plasma thromboplastin antecedent.**

PTCA, abbreviation for **percutaneous transluminal coronary angioplasty.**

pteroylglutamic acid. See **folic acid.**

pterygium (tərɪj′ɪəm), a thick, triangular bit of pale tissue that extends medially from the nasal border of the cornea to the inner canthus of the eye.

-pterygium, a combining form meaning a '(specified) ab-

PTERYGIUM

normality of the conjunctiva': *loxopterygium, pimelopterygium, symblepharopterygium.*

pterygoideus lateralis, one of the four muscles of mastication. Extending almost horizontally from the infratemporal fossa and the condyle of the mandible, it is a short, thick, somewhat conical muscle, arising by two heads from the great wing of the sphenoid, the infratemporal crest, and the lateral pterygoid plate. It inserts into the condyle of the mandible and into the articular disc of the temporomandibular articulation. The pterygoideus lateralis is innervated by the lateral pterygoid nerve and functions to open the jaws, protrude the mandible, and move the mandible from side to side. Also called **external pterygoid muscle.** Compare **masseter, pterygoideus medialis, temporalis.**

pterygoideus medialis, one of the four muscles of mastication. Arising from the pyramidal process of the palatine bone and from the tuberosity of the maxilla and inserting into the medial surface of the ramus of the mandible, it is innervated by the medial pterygoid nerve and acts to close the jaws. Also called **internal pterygoid muscle.** Compare **masseter, pterygoideus lateralis, temporalis.**

pterygoid plexus (ter′ɪɡɔɪd), one of a pair of extensive networks of veins between the temporalis and the pterygoideus lateralis, extending between surrounding structures in the infratemporal fossa. The plexus receives deoxygenated blood from various tributaries that correspond with branches of the maxillary artery; it communicates with the cavernous sinus through the foramen of Vesalius and with the facial vein through the deep facial and angular veins. Compare **maxillary vein.**

PTNA, abbreviation for **Provincial Territorial Nurses' Association.**

ptoma-, a combining form meaning 'of or related to a corpse': *ptomaine, ptomatopsia, ptomatopsy.*

ptosis (tou′sɪs), an abnormal condition of one or both upper eyelids in which the eyelid droops owing to a congenital or acquired weakness of the levator muscle or paralysis of the third cranial nerve. Partial ptosis and a small pupil may be caused by an unusual hemologic disorder of the sympathetic portion of the autonomic nervous system. The condition may be treated surgically by shortening the levator muscle.

-ptosis, a combining form meaning a 'prolapse of an organ': *esophagoptosis, hepaptosis, uvulaptosis.*

PTOSIS

ptotic kidney (tou'tik), a kidney that is abnormally situated in the pelvis, usually over the sacral promontory behind the peritoneum. The condition of having a ptotic kidney may be either congenital or secondary to trauma. It is usually asymptomatic, but pregnancy may result in obstruction of the flow of urine from the kidney.

PTT. See **partial thromboplastin time.**

ptyalin (tai'əlɪn), a starch-digesting enzyme present in saliva. Also called **amylase.**

ptyalism (tai'əlɪz'əm), excessive salivation, as sometimes occurs in the early months of pregnancy. Also called **hyperptyalism.**

ptyalo-, a combining form meaning 'of or related to the saliva': *ptyalocele, ptyalogenic, ptyalography.*

-ptysis, a combining form meaning a 'spitting of matter': *albuminoptysis, hemoptysis, plasmoptysis.*

Pu, symbol for **plutonium.**

pub-, a combining form meaning 'adult': *puberal, puberty, pubescence.*

pubarche (pyubar'ki, pyu'barki), the onset of puberty, marked by the beginning of the development of secondary sexual characteristics.

puberulic acid (pyuber'yəlɪk), an antibiotic isolated from the mold *Penicillium puberulum* that prevents the replication of gram-positive bacteria.

-pubic, a combining form meaning 'of, referring, or relating to the frontal part of the pelvis': *iliopubic, retropubic, vesicopubic.*

pubic bone. See **pubis.**

pubic symphysis, the slightly movable interpubic joint of the pelvis, consisting of two pubic bones separated by a disc of fibrocartilage and connected by two ligaments. Also called **symphysis pubis.**

pubis (pyu'bɪs), *pl.* **pubes.** one of a pair of pubic bones that, with the ischium and the ilium, form the hip bone and join the pubic bone from the opposite side at the pubic symphysis. The pubis forms one fifth of the acetabulum and is divisible into the body, the superior ramus, and the inferior ramus. The external surface of the pubis is rough and serves as the origin of the adductor longus, the obturator externus, the adductor brevis, and the proximal part of the gracilis. The internal surface of the pubis is smooth; it forms part of the anterior wall of the pelvis, giving origin to the levator ani and the obturator internus, and attachment to the puboprostatic ligaments and a few muscular fibers from the bladder. The pubic crest affords attachment to the rectus abdominus, the pyramidalis, and the inguinal falx. The lateral portion of the superior ramus of the pubis presents the superior, the inferior, and the dorsal surfaces. The superior surface presents the iliopectineal line, and the inferior ramus gives origin to the gracilis, a portion of the obturator externus, the adductor brevis, the adductor magnus, the obturator internus, and the constrictor urethrae. Compare **ilium, ischium.**

publish or perish, *Informal.* a practice followed in many academic institutions in which a contract for employment is renewed at the same or higher rank only if a candidate has demonstrated scholarship and professional status by having had work published in a book or in a reputable, usually national, professional journal. This work is in addition to whatever obligations for teaching or professional practice are entailed by the position.

pubococcygeus exercises (pyu'boukoksɪj'iəs), a regimen of isometric exercises in which a woman executes a series of voluntary contractions of the muscles of her pelvic diaphragm and perineum in an effort to increase the contractility of her vaginal introitus or to improve her retention of urine. Also called **Kegel exercises.**

■ METHOD: The exercise involves the familiar muscular squeezing action that is required to stop the urinary stream while voiding; that action is performed in an intensive, repetitive, and systematic way throughout each day.

■ NURSING ORDERS: The woman is instructed in how to duplicate the squeezing, pulling-up action. A woman whose muscles are particularly attenuated may have difficulty understanding or feeling the muscular action involved. It is often helpful for her to be told that the action is exactly the same as that which is required to stop the flow of urine. When the woman can effect the contraction required she is asked to hold the contraction for 6 to 10 seconds, allowing the muscles to relax completely between contractions. She is then advised to perform 4 to 6 repetitions of the contraction in a series and to repeat the series 3 to 4 times each day. She is further advised that the physiology of muscular exercise is such that weakened muscles may make gains in strength during the early phases of an exercise program, and that, with diligence, she can expect to notice significant improvement in control that will continue as she maintains the regimen of exercise.

■ OUTCOME CRITERIA: Laxity and weakness of the pubococcygeus muscles, often a result of childbirth, may predispose certain women to looseness of the vaginal introitus and to stress incontinence. These problems may be ameliorated as the strength and tone of the muscles are increased through exercise. The rapidity with which a woman can, during voiding, close off the urinary stream is taken as a measure of the strength and tone of her pubococcygeus muscles. Ideally, she should be able to perform the action completely and almost instantly.

pudendal block, a form of regional anesthetic block administered to relieve the discomfort of the expulsive second stage of labor. The pudendal nerves are anesthetized by the injection of a local anesthetic in the trunk of each nerve as it passes over the sacrospinous ligament, just below the ischial spine. A 10 ml syringe, a long needle, and a guide, usually an Iowa trumpet, are used in the procedure. The injection is most easily performed transvaginally; the transperitoneal approach is technically more difficult and is more uncomfortable for the woman. Pudendal block anesthetizes the perineum, vulva, clitoris, labia majora, and the perirectal area without affecting the muscular contractions of the uterus. When the block is properly administered the risk is minimal.

pudendal canal. See **Alcock's canal.**

pudendal nerve, one of the branches of the pudendal plexus that arises from the second, third, and fourth sacral nerves, passes between the piriformis and coccygeus, and leaves the pelvis through the greater sciatic foramen. It crosses the spine of the ischium and reenters the pelvis through the lesser sciatic foramen. It accompanies the internal pudendal vessels through a fascial tunnel along the lateral wall of the ischiorectal fossa and divides into two terminal branches near the urogenital diaphragm. The branches of the pudendal nerve are the inferior rectal nerve, perineal nerve, and dorsal nerve of the penis or of the clitoris. See also **pudendal plexus.**

pudendal plexus, a network of motor and sensory nerves formed by the anterior branches of the second and the third and all of the fourth sacral nerves. It is often considered part of the sacral plexus. The pudendal plexus lies in the posterior hollow of the pelvis, on the ventral surface of the piriformis. The branches of the plexus are the visceral branches, the muscular branches, and the pudendal nerve. The visceral branches arise from the second, third, and fourth sacral nerves and supply the bladder, prostate, seminal vesicles, uterus, external genitalia, and some of the intestinal tract. The muscular branches arise from the fourth, and, sometimes, the third and fifth sacral nerves and supply the levator ani, sphincter ani, and coccygeus. The pudendal nerve arises from the second, third, and fourth sacral nerves and divides into five branches supplying the genital structures and the pelvic region. Compare **lumbar plexus, sacral plexus.**

pudendum (pyuden'dəm), *pl.* **pudenda.** the external genitalia, especially of women. In a woman it comprises the mons veneris, the labia majora, the labia minora, the vestibule of the vagina, and the vestibular glands. In a man it comprises the penis, scrotum, and testes. —**pudendal,** *adj.*

puer-, a combining form meaning 'child': *puericulture, puerilism, puerperium.*

puericulture (pyu'ərɪkəl'chər), the specialty of rearing and training children. —**puericulturist,** *n.*

puerile (pyu'ərɪl, pyuər'ail), of or pertaining to children or childhood; juvenile. —**puerility,** *n.*

puerperal (pyuər'pərəl), **1.** of or pertaining to the period immediately after childbirth. **2.** of or pertaining to a woman (puerpera) who has just given birth to an infant.

puerperal endometritis. See **puerperal fever.**

puerperal fever, a syndrome associated with systemic bacterial infection and septicemia that occurs following childbirth, usually as a result of unsterile obstetric technique. It is characterized by endometritis, fever, tachycardia, uterine tenderness, and foul lochia; if untreated, prostration, renal failure, bacteremic shock, and death may occur. The causative organism is most often one of the hemolytic streptococci. Puerperal fever was little known before hospital childbirth became common, early in the nineteenth century; but then it became an endemic and frequently epidemic scourge that resulted in the deaths of many thousands of mothers and infants. Maternal mortality rates of twenty per cent and higher were not uncommon in parts of the world where childbirth occurred in hospitals. Ignaz Philipp Semmelweis, in Vienna, noted that women attended by midwives were much less likely to contract the disease than those attended by physicians and medical students. Midwives did not perform frequent vaginal examinations during labor and did not participate in autopsies. Though the germ theory of disease had not yet been elaborated, Semmelweis deduced that the causative agent of the disease was being transmitted by doctors and students from the infected cadavers in the autopsy room to women in labor on the maternity wards. By instituting a policy requiring that the hands and instruments of obstetric attendants be disinfected, maternal mortality in his clinic dropped dramatically. His work was widely ignored or discredited for almost half a century because physicians were unwilling to believe that they were the agents of transmission. Late in the nineteenth century, following Pasteur's discovery of microbes, Semmelweis was posthumously vindicated. Sterile techniques were gradually instituted, but not until the fourth decade of the twentieth century did puerperal fever cease to be the leading cause of maternal death. Postpartum uterine infection is not uncommon but is effectively treated with massive parenteral doses of antibiotics before it becomes a systemic illness. Also called **childbed fever, puerperal sepsis.**

puerperal mania, a rare, acute mood disorder that sometimes occurs in women following childbirth, characterized by a severe manic reaction. See also **mania**.

puerperal metritis. See **puerperal fever**.

puerperium (pyu'ərpir'iəm), the time following childbirth, lasting approximately six weeks, during which the anatomic and physiologic changes brought about by pregnancy resolve, and a woman adjusts to the new or expanded responsibilities of motherhood and nonpregnant life.

Pulex (pyu'leks), a genus of fleas some species of which transmit arthropod-borne infections, as plague and epidemic typhus.

pulmo-, pulmon-, a combining form meaning 'of or pertaining to the lungs': *pulmogram, pulmolith, pulmometer*.

pulmonary, pulmonic, of or pertaining to the lungs or the respiratory system.

pulmonary alveolus, one of the numerous terminal air sacs in the lungs in which oxygen and carbon monoxide are exchanged.

pulmonary anthrax. See **woolsorter's disease**.

pulmonary arteriolar resistance (PAR), pressure loss per unit of blood flow from the pulmonary artery to a pulmonary vein.

pulmonary atrium, any of the spaces at the end of an alveolar duct into which alveoli open.

pulmonary carcinosis. See **alveolar cell carcinoma**.

pulmonary disease, an abnormal condition of the respiratory system, characterized by cough, chest pain, dyspnea, hemoptysis, sputum production, stridor, and wheezing. Less common symptoms may be anxiety, arm and shoulder pain, tenderness in the calf of the leg, erythema nodosum, swelling of the face, headache, hoarseness, polyarthralgia, and somnolence. Diagnostic procedures used for pulmonary diseases include bronchoscopy, cytological, serological and biochemical examination of bronchial secretions, laryngoscopy, pulmonary function tests, and radiography. Pulmonary diseases are either obstructive or restrictive. Obstructive respiratory diseases are the result of an obstacle in the airway that impedes the flow of air, especially during expiration. Such obstructions may be bronchospasm, edema of the bronchial mucosa, loss of lung elasticity, or thick bronchial secretions. Obstructive diseases are characterized by reduced expiratory flow rates and increased total lung capacities. Acute obstructive respiratory diseases include asthma, bronchitis, and bronchiolitis; chronic conditions are combinations of emphysema and bronchitis. Patients with obstructive diseases may have acute failure from any respiratory stress, as infections or general anesthesia. Restrictive respiratory diseases are caused by conditions that limit lung expansion by an actual reduction of the volume of inspired air, as fibrothorax, a neuromuscular disorder, kyphosis, scoliosis, spondylitis, or surgical removal of lung tissue. Characteristic features of restrictive respiratory diseases are decreased forced vital capacity and total lung capacity, with increased work of breathing and inefficient exchange of gases. Acute restrictive conditions are the most common pulmonary cause of acute respiratory failure.

pulmonary edema, the accumulation of extravascular fluid in lung tissues and alveoli, caused most commonly by congestive heart failure and also occurring in barbiturate and opiate poisoning, diffuse infections, hemorrhagic pancreatitis, renal failure, and following a stroke, skull fracture, near-drowning, the inhalation of irritating gases, and the rapid administration of whole blood, plasma, serum albumin, or intravenous fluids. In congestive heart disease serous fluid is pushed back through the pulmonary capillaries into alveoli and quickly enters bronchioles and bronchi.

■ OBSERVATIONS: The patient with pulmonary edema breathes rapidly and shallowly with difficulty, is usually restless, apprehensive, hoarse, pale or cyanotic, and may cough up frothy, pink sputum. The peripheral and neck veins are usually engorged; the blood pressure and heart rate are increased, and the pulse may be full and bounding or weak and thready. There may be edema of the extremities, rales in the lungs, respiratory acidosis, and profuse diaphoresis.

■ INTERVENTION: Acute pulmonary edema is an emergency requiring prompt treatment. The patient is placed in bed in a high Fowler's position and the immediate administration of intravenous morphine sulfate is usually ordered to relieve pain, quiet breathing, and allay apprehension. A cardiotonic, often digitalis, a fast-acting diuretic, often furosemide or ethacrynic acid, and a bronchodilator, often aminophylline, may be given, and intermittent positive pressure breathing (IPPB) of humidified oxygen may be ordered. IPPB decreases the passage of fluid in the alveoli by exerting counterpressure on alveolar capillaries and decreases venous return to the heart by increasing pleural pressure. The use of rotating tourniquets may be ordered to pool blood in the extremities in order to reduce the load on the heart. The tourniquets usually are placed on three extremities at one time and are so rotated that each of the four extremities is occluded for 45 minutes of every hour in which this kind of therapy is given. While the patient is acutely ill the blood pressure, respiration, apical pulse, and breath sounds are checked every hour or continually monitored. Parenteral fluids, if indicated, are infused slowly in limited quantities; a low-sodium diet is served and the patient's intake and output of fluids are measured. The patient is weighed daily and any sudden gain is noted and reported.

■ NURSING CONSIDERATIONS: In addition to providing continued care and emotional support, the nurse teaches the patient to exercise to tolerance, plan frequent rest periods, report any symptoms, avoid smoking, and follow the regimen ordered for medication, diet, and return checkups.

pulmonary embolism (PE), the blockage of a pulmonary artery by foreign matter as fat, air, tumor tissue, or a thrombus that usually arises from a peripheral vein. Predisposing factors include an alteration of blood constituents with increased coagulation, damage to blood vessel walls, and stagnation or immobilization, especially when associated with childbirth, congestive heart failure, polycythemia vera, or surgery. Pulmonary embolism is difficult to distinguish from myocardial infarction and pneumonia. It is characterized by dyspnea, sudden chest pain, shock, and cyanosis. Pulmonary infarction, which often occurs within 6 to 24 hours after the formation of a pulmonary embolus, is further characterized by pleural effusion, hemoptysis, leukocytosis, fever, tachycardia and atrial arrhythmias, and a striking distension of the neck veins. Analysis of blood gases reveals arterial hypoxia and reduced arterial carbon dioxide tension. Pulmonary embolism is detected by chest x rays, pulmonary angiography, and radioscanning of the lung fields. Two thirds of patients with a massive pulmonary embolus die within two hours. Initial resuscitative measures include external cardiac massage, oxygen, vasopressor drugs, embolectomy, and correction of acidosis. The formation of further emboli is prevented by the use of anticoagulants, and, sometimes, streptokinase or urokinase. Ambulation, exercise, and electrical stimulation of the calf muscles are also recommended.

pulmonary function test (PFT), a procedure for determining the capacity of the lungs to exchange oxygen and carbon dioxide efficiently. There are two general kinds of respiratory function tests. One measures ventilation or the ability of the bellows action of the chest and lungs to move gas in and out of alveoli; the other kind measures the diffusion of gas across the alveolar capillary membrane and the perfusion of the lungs by blood. Efficient gas exchange in the lungs requires a balanced ventilation/perfusion ratio, with areas receiving ventilation well perfused and areas receiving blood flow capable of ventilation. Basic ventilation studies are performed with a spirometer and recording device as the patient breathes through a mouthpiece and connecting tube; a nose clip prevents nasal breathing. Measurements or calculations are made of the tidal volume (TV), or gas inspired and expired in a normal breath; the inspiratory reserve volume (IRV), or the maximal volume that can be inspired after a normal respiration; the expiratory reserve volume (ERV), or the maximal volume that can be expired forcefully after a normal expiration; the residual volume (RV), or the gas remaining in the lungs following maximal expiration; and the minute volume, or the gas inspired and expired in a minute of normal breathing. The vital capacity of the lungs is equal to TV + IRV + ERV and the total lung capacity to TV + IRV + ERV + RV. The forced expiratory volume (FEV), or the amount of air forcefully expelled in the first second after a maximal inspiration, and the maximal breathing capacity (MBC), or the amount of gas exchanged per minute with maximal rate and depth of respiration, each have special clinical significance. Bronchospirometric measurements of the ventilation and oxygen consumption of each lung separately are performed using a specially constructed double-lumen catheter with two balloons; one balloon is inflated to seal off the contralateral lung when the other lung is tested. Arterial blood gas studies, including determinations of the acidity, partial pressure of carbon dioxide and of oxygen, and the oxyhemoglobin saturation, provide information on the diffusion of gas across the alveolar capillary membrane and the adequacy of oxygenation of tissues.

pulmonary infiltrate with eosinophilia. See **P.I.E.**

pulmonary sulcus tumor, a destructive, invasive neoplasm that develops at the apex of the lung and infiltrates the ribs, vertebrae, and the brachial plexus. Also called **Pancoast's tumor.**

pulmonary surfactant, a surfactant agent found in the lungs that functions to reduce the surface tension of the fluid on the surface of the cells of the lower respiratory system, enhancing the elasticity of the alveoli and bronchioles and, thus, the exchange of gases in the lungs.

pulmonary trunk, the short, wide vessel that conveys venous blood from the right ventricle of the heart to the lungs. It is approximately 5 cm long and 3 cm in diameter and it ascends obliquely, dividing into right and left branches.

pulmonary tuberculosis. See **tuberculosis.**

pulmonary valve, a cardiac structure composed of three semilunar cusps that close during each heartbeat to prevent blood from flowing back into the right ventricle from the pulmonary artery. The cusps are separated by sinuses which resemble tiny buckets when they are closed and filled with blood. These flaps grow from the lining of the pulmonary artery and, when they collapse from the inflow of ventricular blood, open the valve and allow deoxygenated blood to flow through the pulmonary artery and on to the lungs. Also called **semilunar valve.** Compare **aortic valve, mitral valve, tricuspid valve.**

pulmonary vascular resistance (PVR), pressure loss per unit of blood flow from the pulmonary artery to the left ventricle.

pulmonary vein, one of a pair of large vessels that return oxygenated blood from each lung to the left atrium of the heart. The right pulmonary veins pass dorsal to the right atrium and the superior vena cava. The left pulmonary veins pass ventral to the descending thoracic aorta. Compare **pulmonary trunk.**

pulmonary Wegener's granulomatosis, a rare, fatal disease of young or middle-aged men, characterized by granulomatous lesions of the respiratory tract, focal necrotizing arteritis, and, finally, widespread inflammation of body organs. Pulmonary infarction and glomerulonephritis may occur.

pulmonic, See **pulmonary.**

-pulmonic, a combining form meaning 'relating to the lungs': *apulmonic, gastropulmonic, intrapulmonic.*

pulmonic stenosis, an abnormal cardiac condition, generally characterized by concentric hypertrophy of the right ventricle with relatively little increase in diastolic volume. When the ventricular septum is intact this condition may be caused by valvular stenosis, by infundibular stenosis, or by both; it produces a pressure difference during systole between the right ventricular cavity and the pulmonary artery. Pulmonic stenosis is most often congenital but may also be produced after birth by any of a number of types of lesions. Severe pulmonic stenosis may result in heart failure and death, but mild to moderate forms of this disorder are relatively well tolerated by some individuals. See also **valvular heart disease.**

pulp, any soft, spongy tissue, as that contained within the spleen, the pulp chamber of the tooth, or the distal phalanges of the fingers and the toes. – **pulpy,** *adj.*

pulpitis (pəlpai′tıs), infection or inflammation of the dental pulp. See also **caries.**

pulse, 1. a rhythmical beating or vibrating movement. 2. a brief electromagnetic wave. 3. the regular, recurrent expansion and contraction of an artery produced by waves of pressure caused by the ejection of blood from the left ventricle of the heart as it contracts. The phenomenon is easily detected on superficial arteries, as the radial and carotid arteries, and corresponds to each beat of the heart. The normal number of pulse beats per minute in the average adult varies from 50 to 100, with fluctuations occurring with exercise, injury, illness, and emotional reactions.

pulse deficit, the discrepancy between the ventricular rate auscultated at the apex of the heart and the arterial rate of the radial pulse.

pulseless disease. See **Takayasu's arteritis.**

pulse point, any one of the sites on the surface of the body where arterial pulsations can be easily palpated. The most commonly used pulse point is over the radial artery at the wrist. Other pulse points are over the temporal artery in front of the ear, over the common carotid artery at the lower level of the thyroid cartilage, and over the facial artery at the lower margin of the jaw.

pulse pressure, the difference between the systolic and diastolic pressures, normally 30 to 40 mm Hg.

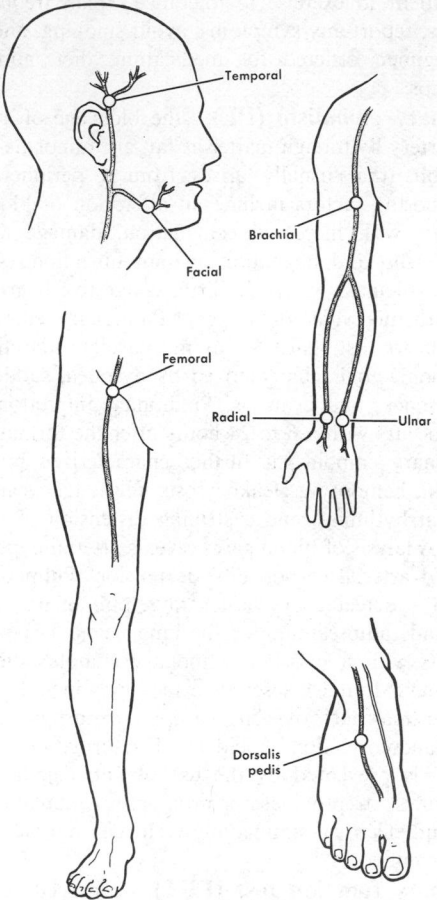

PULSE POINTS

-pulsion, a combining form meaning the 'action or condition of pushing': *compulsion, lateropulsion, retropulsion.*

pulsus alternans (pəl′səs ɔl′tərnænz), a pulse characterized by a regular alternation of weak and strong beats without changes in the length of the cycle.

pulsus paradoxus, an abnormal decrease in systolic pressure and pulse-wave amplitude during inspiration. The normal fall in pressure is less than 10 mm Hg, and an excessive decline may be a sign of cardiac tamponade in acute pericarditis.

pump, 1. an apparatus used to move fluids or gases by suction or by positive pressure, as an infusion pump, or stomach pump. 2. a physiologic mechanism by which a substance is moved, usually by active transport across a cell membrane, as a sodium pump. 3. to move a liquid or gas by suction or positive pressure.

pump lung. See **congestive atelectasis.**

punch biopsy, the removal of living tissue for microscopic examination, usually bone marrow from the sternum, by means of a punch.

punch forceps,   a surgical instrument used to cut out a disc of dense or resistant tissue, as bone and cartilage. The ends of the blades of the punch forceps are perforated to grip the involved tissue. There are several varieties of this instrument, with blades and tips specially designed for different surgical needs.

punct-,   a combining form meaning 'a point, or like a point': *punctate, punctiform, punctograph.*

punctum lacrimale (pəngk′təm), *pl.* **puncta lacrimalia.**   a tiny aperture in the margin of each eyelid that opens into the lacrimal duct. The puncta release the tears that travel from the lacrimal glands through the lacrimal ducts to the conjunctiva. Puncta clogged with mucus or dirt cause irritation and discomfort.

puncture wound,   a traumatic injury caused by the penetration of the skin by a narrow object, as a knife, nail, or slender fragment of metal, wood, glass, or other material. In such an injury to the eye, a lung, or a visceral organ, the object or implement is not removed until the person has been transported to a medical facility. Minor puncture wounds are treated with thorough cleansing. If a puncture wound is allowed to close at the skin before deeper healing has occurred suppuration often results. A tetanus booster inoculation is usually given for such wounds.

punitive damages.   See **damages.**

Punnett square,   a checkerboard, graphlike diagram, used in charting genetic ratios, that shows all of the possible combinations of male and female gametes when one or more pairs of independent alleles are crossed. Letters representing the male gametes are placed along the Y-axis and those of the female along the X-axis, with the results of the various crossings occupying the squares in a geometric pattern. See also **pedigree.**

pupil,   a circular opening in the iris of the eye, located slightly to the nasal side of the center of the iris. The pupil lies behind the anterior chamber of the eye and the cornea and in front of the lens. Its diameter changes with contraction and relaxation of the muscular fibers of the iris as the eye responds to changes in light, emotional states, and other kinds of stimulation. The pupil is the window of the eye through which light passes to the lens and the retina. See also **dilatator pupillae, sphincter pupillae.** – **pupillary,** *adj.*

pupill-.   See **pupillo-.**

pupillary reflex,   1. See **light reflex.** 2. See **accommodation reflex.**

pupillary-skin reflex.   See **ciliospinal reflex.**

pupillo, pupill-,   a combining form meaning 'of or pertaining to the pupil': *pupillometer, pupilloplegia, pupillostatometer.*

pur-,   a combining form meaning 'of or related to pus': *puric, puriform, purohepatitis.*

pure dwarf.   See **primordial dwarf.**

pure science.   See **science.**

pure tone audiometry.   See **audiometry.**

pure vegetarian.   See **strict vegetarian.**

purgation.   See **catharsis.**

purge,   1. to evacuate the bowels, as with a cathartic. 2. a cathartic. – **purgation,** *n.,* **purgative,** *n., adj.*

purified protein derivative (PPD),   a dried form of tuberculin used in testing for past or present infection with tubercle bacilli. This product is usually introduced into the skin during such tests and may produce a tuberculin reaction within 48 to 72 hours.

purine (pyur′in, pyur′ın),   any one of a large group of nitrogenous compounds. Purines are produced as end products in the digestion of certain proteins in the diet, but some are synthesized in the body. Purines are also present in many medications and other substances, including caffeine, theophylline, and various diuretics, muscle relaxants, and myocardial stimulants. Hyperuricemia may develop in some people as a result of an inability to metabolize and excrete purines. A low-purine diet or a purine-free diet may be required. Foods that are high in purines include anchovies and sardines, sweetbreads, liver, kidneys, and other organ meats, legumes, and poultry. The foods lowest in purine content include vegetables other than legumes, eggs, fruit, cheese, nuts, sugar, and gelatin.

Purinethol,   a trade name for an antineoplastic (mercaptopurine).

Purkinje network (pərkın′ji),   a complex network of muscle fibers that spread through the right and the left ventricles of the heart and carry the impulses that contract those chambers almost simultaneously. The Purkinje fibers ramify from cardiac muscle fibers spreading into the right ventricle and are continuous with the muscle of the right ventricle. The fibers that connect with the Purkinje fibers start in the atrioventricular (AV) node in the right atrium of the heart, along the lower part of the interatrial septum. Impulses generated in the sinuatrial (SA) node travel swiftly through the muscle fibers of both atria of the heart, starting atrial contraction. As the impulse enters the AV node from the right atrium it slows and allows both atria to contract completely before traveling into the ventricles. The velocity of the impulse increases after the impulse leaves the AV node and spreads to the Purkinje fibers. The Purkinje fibers, which can be identified only with the aid of a microscope, are larger in diameter than ordinary cardiac muscle and contain relatively few peripheral myofibrillae. They have abundant sarcoplasm and larger central nuclei than ordinary cardiac muscle.

Purodigin,   a trade name for a cardiotonic (digitoxin).

purpur-, a combining form meaning 'purple': *purpuriferous, purpuriparous, purpurogenous.*

purpura (pər'pyurə), any of several bleeding disorders characterized by hemorrhage into the tissues, particularly beneath the skin or mucous membranes, producing ecchymoses or petechiae. The two major kinds of purpura are **thrombocytopenic purpura** and **nonthrombocytopenic purpura.** — **purpuric,** *adj.*

purulent (pyur'ulənt), producing or containing pus.

pus, a creamy, viscous, pale yellow or yellow-green fluid exudate that is the result of liquefaction necrosis. Its main constituent is an abundance of polymorphonuclear leukocytes. Bacterial infection is its most common cause. The character of the pus, including its color, consistency, quantity, or odor may be of diagnostic significance.

pustular psoriasis, a severe form of psoriasis consisting of bright red patches and sterile pustules all over the body. Crops of lesions lasting four to seven days occur every few days in cycles over weeks or months. Recurrences are inevitable. Fever, leukocytosis, and hypoalbuminemia are associated. In rare cases, hypovolemia and kidney failure occur. Hospitalization may be necessary for fluid replacement, steroid therapy, and sedation. Compare **guttate psoriasis.** See also **psoriasis.**

pustule (pəs'chul), a small, circumscribed elevation of the skin containing fluid that is usually purulent. — **pustular,** *adj.*

P value, (in research) the statistical probability attached to the occurrence of a given finding by chance alone in comparison with the known distribution of possible findings, considering the kinds of data, the technique of analysis, and the number of observations. The P value may be noted as a decimal: $p < .01$ means that the likelihood of the phenomena tested occurring by chance alone is less than 1 per cent.

PVC, **1.** abbreviation for **polyvinyl chloride. 2.** abbreviation for **premature ventricular contraction.**

P.V. Carpine, a trade name for a cholinergic (pilocarpine nitrate).

PVR, abbreviation for **pulmonary vascular resistance.**

P wave, the component of the cardiac cycle shown on an electrocardiogram as an inverted U-shaped curve that follows the end of the T wave and precedes the spike of the QRS complex. It represents atrial depolarization, during which the atria contract, pumping blood into the ventricles from the superior vena cava and the pulmonary vein.

PWP, abbreviation for *pulmonary wedge pressure.*

pyel-. See **pyelo-.**

pyelitis (pai'lai'tis), *Obsolete.* an inflammation of the pelvis of the kidney. See **pyelonephritis.**

pyelo-, pyel-, a combining form meaning 'of or pertaining to the pelvis of the kidney': *pyelocaliectasis, pyelocystitis, pyelograph.*

pyelogram (pai'ələgræm'), an x ray of the kidneys and ureters. An intravenous pyelogram (IVP), taken following the injection of a radiopaque dye, shows the size and location of the kidneys, the outline of the ureters and bladder, the filling of the renal pelves, the patency of the urinary tract, and any cysts or tumors within the kidneys. Preparation for an IVP includes bowel cleansing, withholding of fluids for eight hours, and testing for sensitivity to the iodine in the radiopaque dye; persons with known sensitivity are not tested lest anaphylaxis occur. Patients able to tolerate the dye may feel warm and experience a salty taste when the material is injected. Retrograde pyelograms, which demonstrate filling of the renal collecting structures, are taken after the contrast medium is injected into the ureters by means of catheters in a cystoscope introduced through the urethra into the bladder.

pyelography (pai'ilog'rəfi). See **intravenous pyelography.**

pyelonephritis (pai'iloun1frai'tis), a diffuse pyogenic infection of the pelvis and parenchyma of the kidney. **Acute pyelonephritis** is usually the result of an infection that ascends from the lower urinary tract to the kidney. *Escherischia coli* contamination of the urethral meatus is a common cause in females. Infection may spread to the kidney from other locations in the body. The onset of acute pyelonephritis is rapid, characterized by fever, chills, pain in the flank, nausea, and urinary frequency. A urinalysis reveals the presence of bacteria and white blood cells. Antimicrobial treatment is continued for ten days to two weeks. Relapse or reinfection is common. **Chronic pyelonephritis** develops slowly following bacterial infection of the kidney and may progress to renal failure. Most cases are associated with some form of obstruction, as a stone or a stricture of the ureter. Treatment includes removal of the cause of obstruction and long-term antimicrobial therapy.

pygmalianism (pigmei'liəniz'əm), a psychosexual abnormality in which the individual directs erotic fantasies toward an object that he has created.

pygmy, pigmy, an extremely small person whose bodily parts are proportioned accordingly; a primordial dwarf.

pygo-, a combining form meaning 'of or pertaining to the buttocks': *pygoamorphus, pygodidymus, pygopagus.*

pygoamorphus (pai'gouəmor'fəs), asymmetrical, conjoined twins in which the parasitic member is represented by an undifferentiated amorphous mass attached to the autosite in the sacral region.

pygodidymus (pai'goudid'əməs), **1.** a malformed fetus that has a double pelvis and hips. **2.** conjoined twins that are fused in the cephalothoracic region but separated at the pelvis.

pygomelus (paigom'ələs), a malformed fetus that has an extra limb or limbs attached to the buttock. Also called **epipygus.**

pygopagus (pāigop′əgəs), conjoined twins consisting of two fully formed or nearly formed fetuses that are united in the sacral region so that they are back to back.

pyknic (pɪk′nɪk), describing a body structure characterized by short, round limbs, a full face, a short neck, stockiness and a tendency toward obesity. Compare **asthenic habitus, athletic habitus.** See also **endomorph.**

pykno-, a combining form meaning 'thick, compact, or frequent': *pyknocardia, pyknohemia, pyknomorphous.*

pyle-, a combining form meaning 'of or related to the portal vein': *pylemphraxis, pylephlebectasis, pylephlebitis.*

pyloric orifice (pāilər′ɪk), the opening of the stomach into the duodenum lying to the right of the middle line at the level of the cranial border of the first lumbar vertebra. The orifice is usually indicated on the surface of the stomach by the circular, duodenopyloric constriction.

pyloric sphincter, a thickened muscular ring in the stomach, separating the pylorus from the duodenum. Also called **pyloric valve.**

pyloric stenosis, a narrowing of the pyloric sphincter at the outlet of the stomach, causing an obstruction which blocks the flow of food into the small intestine. The condition occurs as a congenital defect in one of 200 newborns and, occasionally, in older adults secondary to an ulcer or fibrosis at the outlet. Diagnosis is made in infants by the presence of forceful projectile vomiting and palpation of a hard, prominent pylorus and in adults by x ray following a barium meal. Surgical correction is done under light general anesthesia, after the stomach is emptied. The muscle fibers of the outlet are cut, without severing the mucosa, and the opening is widened. After surgery, a stomach tube remains in place and observation is maintained for signs of hemorrhage or of blockage of the tube.

pyloric ulcer. See **peptic ulcer.**

pyloro-, a combining form meaning 'of or related to the pylorus': *pylorodilator, pyloroplasty, pyloroptosis.*

pyloroplasty (pāilər′əplæs′ti), a surgical procedure performed to relieve pyloric stenosis resulting from chronic gastric ulcer. Before surgery, any electrolyte imbalances or fluid deficiencies are corrected; sodium chloride and potassium chloride solutions may be given to correct ion losses from vomiting, which is characteristic of the condition. Under light general anesthesia, the passageway is dilated. As treatment for the duodenal ulcer, the operation allows the alkaline secretions of the duodenum to flow back into the stomach. Branches of the vagus nerve that supply the acid-secreting portion of the stomach may be cut, reducing the acidity of the stomach contents. Diarrhea is a common postoperative complication.

pylorospasm (pāilər′əspæz′əm), a spasm of the pyloric sphincter of the stomach, as occurs in pyloric stenosis.

pylorus (pāilər′əs), *pl.* **pylori, pyloruses.** a tubular portion of the stomach that angles to the right from the body of the stomach toward the duodenum. The most common position of the pylorus is about 3 cm to the right of the sagittal axis. It is distinctively marked by the thickening of the pyloric sphincter and its lining is composed of an intestinal kind of epithelium rather than the gastric kind common to the body of the stomach. — **pyloric,** *adj.*

pyo-, a combining form meaning 'of or related to pus': *pyocalyx, pyocele, pyocyte.*

Pyocidin Ophthalmic, a trade name for an ophthalmic, fixed-combination drug containing antibacterials (polymyxin B sulfate, neomycin sulfate, and bacitracin zinc).

Pyocidin-Otic, a trade name for an otic, fixed-combination drug containing a glucocorticoid (hydrocortisone) and an antibacterial (polymyxin B sulfate).

pyoderma (pāi′oudər′mə), any purulent skin disease, as impetigo.

pyogenic (pāi′əjen′ɪk), pus-producing.

pyogenic granuloma, a small, nonmalignant mass of excessive granulation tissue, usually found at the site of an injury. Most often a dull-red color, it contains numerous capillaries, bleeds easily, and is very tender; it may be attached by a narrow stalk. Treatment is with electric cautery or topical silver nitrate. Also called **telangiectatic granuloma.**

Pyopen, a trade name for an antibacterial (carbenicillin disodium).

pyorrhea (pāi′əri′ə), 1. a discharge of pus. 2. a purulent inflammation of the tissues surrounding the teeth. — **pyorrheal,** *adj.*

pyosalpinx (pāi′ousæl′pɪŋks), an accumulation of pus in a Fallopian tube. See also **salpingitis.**

Pyracort-D, a trade name for an adrenergic (phenylephrine hydrochloride).

Pyradyne, a trade name for a respiratory, fixed-combination drug containing an antihistaminic (pyrilamine maleate), analgesics (salicylamide and phenacetin), and a stimulant (caffeine).

pyramidal (pɪræm′ɪdəl), of or pertaining to the shape of a pyramid.

pyramidalis (pɪræm′ɪdei′lɪs), one of a pair of anterolateral muscles of the abdomen, contained in the lower end of the sheath of the rectus abdominis. It is a small, triangular muscle that arises from the pubis and inserts into the linea alba. It is innervated by a branch of the twelfth thoracic nerve and functions to tense the linea alba. Compare **obliquus externus abdominis, obliquus internus abdominis, rectus abdominis, transversus abdominis.**

pyramidal tract, a pathway comprised of groups of nerve fibers in the white matter of the spinal cord through which motor impulses are conducted to the anterior horn cells from the opposite side of the brain. These descending fibers, the nerve cells of which are found in the precentral cortex, regulate the voluntary and reflex activity of the muscles through the anterior horn cells.

pyrantel pamoate, an anthelmintic.

■ INDICATIONS: It is prescribed in the treatment of infestation by roundworms or pinworms.

■ CONTRAINDICATION: Known hypersensitivity to this drug prohibits its use.

■ ADVERSE EFFECTS: Among the more serious adverse reactions are nausea, abdominal cramps, diarrhea, dizziness, and skin rash.

pyrazinamide (pai'rəzın'əmaid), an antimycobacterial.

■ INDICATION: It is prescribed in combination chemotherapy in the treatment of tuberculosis.

■ CONTRAINDICATIONS: Severe liver damage or known hypersensitivity to this drug prohibits its use.

■ ADVERSE EFFECTS: Among the more serious adverse reactions are hepatotoxicity and hyperuricemia.

pyrethrins and piperonyl butoxide, a fixed-combination scabicide and pediculocide.

■ INDICATIONS: It is prescribed in the treatment of infestations of head, body, and pubic lice.

■ CONTRAINDICATIONS: Known hypersensitivity to ragweed or to this drug prohibits its use.

■ ADVERSE EFFECTS: Among the more serious adverse reactions are irritation of the skin and the mucous membranes.

pyreto-, a combining form meaning 'of or pertaining to fever': *pyretogen, pyretography, pyretotherapy.*

pyrexia (pairek'siə). See **fever.**

-pyrexia, a combining form meaning a 'febrile condition': *apyrexia, electropyrexia, physiopyrexia.*

Pyribenzamine Citrate, a trade name for an antihistamine (tripelennamine citrate).

Pyribenzamine Hydrochloride, a trade name for an antihistaminic (tripelennamine hydrochloride).

Pyridium, a trade name for an analgesic (phenazopyridine hydrochloride).

pyridostigmine bromide (pır'ıdoustıg'min), a cholinergic.

■ INDICATIONS: It is prescribed in the treatment of myasthenia gravis and is used as an antagonist to nondepolarizing muscle relaxants.

■ CONTRAINDICATIONS: Intestinal or urinary obstruction or known hypersensitivity to this drug or to other anticholinesterases prohibits its use.

■ ADVERSE EFFECTS: Among the more serious adverse reactions are nausea, diarrhea, abdominal cramps, muscle cramps, and weakness.

pyridoxal phosphate (pır'ədok'səl), an enzyme in the body that acts with pyridoxamine phosphate and transaminase to catalyze the reversible transfer of an amino group from an alpha-amino acid to an alpha-keto acid, especially alpha-ketoglutaric acid. Such processes are essential to metabolism.

pyridoxamine phosphate (pır'ədok'səmin), an enzyme that participates with pyridoxal phosphate and trans-

aminase in the reversible transfer of an amino group from an alpha-amino acid to an alpha-keto acid, especially alpha-ketoglutaric acid. Such transfers are essential in the metabolism of the body.

pyridoxine (pır'ıdok'sin), a water-soluble, white, crystalline vitamin that is part of the B complex group, derived from pyridine, and converted in the body to pyridoxal and pyridamin for synthesis. It functions as a coenzyme essential for the synthesis and breakdown of amino acids, the conversion of tryptophan to niacin, the breakdown of glycogen to glucose-1-phosphate, the production of antibodies, the formation of heme in hemoglobin, the formation of hormones important in brain function, the proper absorption of vitamin B_{12}, the production of hydrochloric acid and magnesium, and the maintenance of the balance of sodium and potassium, which regulates body fluids and the functioning of the nervous and musculoskeletal systems. Rich dietary sources are meats, especially organ meats, whole-grain cereals, soybeans, peanuts, wheat germ, and brewer's yeast; milk and green vegetables supply smaller amounts. The most common symptoms of deficiency are seborrheic dermatitis about the eyes, nose, mouth, and behind the ears, cheilosis, glossitis and stomatitis, nervousness, depression, peripheral neuropathy, and lymphopenia, leading to convulsions in infants and anemia in adults. Treatment and prophylaxis consist of administration of the vitamin and a diet rich in foods containing it. Several drugs interfere with the use of pyridoxine, notably isoniazid and penicillamine, and supplements of the vitamin are recommended with their use. The need for increased amounts of pyridoxine occurs during pregnancy, lactation, exposure to radiation, cardiac failure, aging, and use of oral contraceptives. The vitamin is considered nontoxic. Also called **vitamin B_6.**

pyridoxine hydrochloride. See **vitamin B_6.**

pyrilamine maleate, an antihistamine.

■ INDICATIONS: It is prescribed in the treatment of a variety of hypersensitivity reactions, including rhinitis, skin rash, and pruritus.

■ CONTRAINDICATIONS: Asthma or known hypersensitivity to this drug prohibits its use. It is not given to newborn infants or lactating mothers.

■ ADVERSE EFFECTS: Drowsiness, skin rash, hypersensitivity reactions, dry mouth, and tachycardia commonly occur.

Pyrilgin, a trade name for an analgesic and antipyretic (dipyrone).

pyrimethamine (pır'ımefh'əmin), an antimalarial.

■ INDICATIONS: It is prescribed in the treatment of malaria and toxoplasmosis.

■ CONTRAINDICATIONS: There are no known contraindications.

■ ADVERSE EFFECTS: Among the more serious adverse

reactions, primarily with large doses, are megaloblastic anemia, atrophic glossitis, leukopenia, and convulsions.

pyrimidine (pīrĭm′ədin), an organic compound of heterocyclic nitrogen found in nucleic acids and in many drugs, including the antiviral drugs, acyclovir, ribavirin, and trifluridine.

pyro-, a combining form meaning 'of or related to fire or heat, or produced by heating': *pyrocatechin, pyrodextrin, pyromania.*

pyrogen (pī′rĭjen), any substance or agent that tends to cause a rise in body temperature, as some bacterial toxins. See also **fever.** — **pyrogenic,** *adj.*

pyrolagnia (pī′rōlæg′niə), sexual stimulation or gratification from watching or setting fires.

pyromania (pī′rōmei′niə), an impulse neurosis characterized by an uncontrollable urge to set fires. The condition is found predominantly in men and is usually associated with alcohol intoxication, chronic personal frustrations, resentment of authority figures, or some other psychological disturbance or psychosexual dysfunction. Those with the condition experience an increased sense of tension before setting the fire and intense gratification while watching it burn; they may often display satisfaction from the resulting destruction, although many show signs of depression, anxiety, and guilt over the possibility of being apprehended. Treatment consists of psychotherapy to uncover the causative emotional problems and often institutionalization for the protection of the person and of society.

pyromaniac (pī′rōmei′niæk), **1.** a person with or displaying characteristics of pyromania. **2.** of, pertaining to, or exhibiting pyromania. — **pyromaniacal,** *adj.*

pyrosis (pīrou′sis), a precordial, substernal, or epigastric burning sensation, often associated with the eructation of acid contents of the stomach. It may be a symptom of esophagitis. Also called **heartburn.**

pyrrole (pīroul′, pīr′oul), any of several organic compounds whose derivatives may be added to whole blood or to plasma as a preservative.

Pyrroxate, a trade name for a respiratory, fixed-combination drug containing an adrenergic (methoxyphenamine hydrochloride), an antihistaminic (chlorpheniramine maleate), analgesics (aspirin and phenacetin), and a stimulant (caffeine).

pyruvate kinase, an enzyme in all body tissues that catalyzes the transfer of a phosphate group from adenosine triphosphate to produce adenosine diphosphate and phosphoenolpyruvate.

pyruvate kinase deficiency, a congenital hemolytic disorder transmitted as an autosomal recessive trait. The homozygous condition is characterized by severe chronic hemolysis. The heterozygous form may occur with a mild to severe anemia but is usually asymptomatic and of no clinical significance.

pyruvic acid (pīru′vĭk), a compound formed as an end product of glycolysis, the anaerobic stage of glucose metabolism. Exposed to oxygen and acetylcoenzyme A at the entrance to the Krebs' citric acid cycle, the compound is changed to citric acid.

pyrvinium pamoate (pīrvĭn′iəm pæm′oueit), an anthelmintic.

■ INDICATION: It is prescribed in the treatment of infestation by pinworms.

■ CONTRAINDICATION: Known hypersensitivity to this drug prohibits its use.

■ ADVERSE EFFECTS: Among the more serious adverse effects are nausea, cramping, diarrhea, and hypersensitivity reactions.

pyuria (pāiyur′iə), the presence of white blood cells in the urine, usually a sign of an infection of the urinary tract. See also **bacteriuria.**

Q

Q, symbol for **blood volume.**

Q̇, symbol for **rate of blood flow.**

q.d., (in prescriptions) abbreviation for *quaque die,* a Latin phrase meaning 'everyday.' Also called **quotid.**

Q fever, an acute febrile illness, usually respiratory, caused by the rickettsia, *Coxiella burnetii (Rickettsia burnetii).* The disease is spread through contact with infected domestic animals, either by inhaling the rickettsiae from their hides, drinking their contaminated milk, or being bitten by a tick harboring the organism. Onset is abrupt and high fever may persist for three weeks or more. The illness is especially common among those who work with sheep, goats, and cattle. Treatment with tetracycline is usually effective in 36 to 48 hours. People who are regularly exposed to domestic animals can be vaccinated against Q fever. Also called **Australian Q fever.**

q.h., (in prescriptions) abbreviation for *quaque hora,* a Latin phrase meaning 'every hour'.

q.2h., (in prescriptions) abbreviation for *quaque secunda hora,* a Latin phrase meaning 'every two hours.'

q.3h., (in presescriptions) abbreviation for *quaque tertia hora,* a Latin phrase meaning 'every three hours.'

q.4h., (in prescriptions) abbreviation for *quaque quarta hora,* a Latin phrase meaning 'every four hours.'

q.6h., (in prescriptions) abbreviation for *quaque sex hora,* a Latin phrase meaning 'every six hours.'

q.8h., (in prescriptions) abbreviation for *quaque octa hora,* a Latin phrase meaning 'every eight hours.'

q.i.d., (in prescriptions) abbreviation for *quater in die,* a Latin phrase meaning 'four times a day.'

QRS complex, the component of the cardiac cycle shown on an electrocardiogram as a sharp narrow inverted V following the shorter, less acute curve of the P wave and preceding the ST segment. It represents ventricular depolarization, in which the impulse is conducted over the bundle of His and the Purkinje fibers, causing ventricular contraction.

q.s., (in prescriptions) abbreviation for *quantum sufficiat,* a Latin phrase meaning 'quantity required.'

Q's test. See **Queckenstedt's test.**

Quaalude, a trade name for a sedative-hypnotic (methaqualone).

quack. See **charlatan.**

quadr-, a combining form meaning 'four': *quadrangular, quadribasic, quadrivalent.*

quadratus labii superioris. See **zygomaticus minor.**

quadriceps femoris, the great extensor muscle of the anterior thigh, comprised of the rectus femoris, the vastus lateralis, the vastus medialis, and the vastus intermedius. The quadriceps forms a large dense mass covering the front and sides of the femur. Tendons of the four parts of the muscle unite at the distal part of the thigh, forming a single strong tendon that inserts into the patella. The quadriceps is innervated by branches of the femoral nerve, which contain fibers from the second, third, and fourth lumbar nerves, and it functions to extend the leg.

quadriceps reflex. See **patellar reflex.**

quadrigeminal (kwod′rɪjem′ɪnəl), **1.** in four parts. **2.** a fourfold increase in size or frequency.

quadrigeminal pulse, a pulse in which a pause occurs after every fourth beat.

Quadrinal, a trade name for a respiratory, fixed-combination drug containing a smooth-muscle relaxant (theophylline calcium salicylate), an adrenergic (ephedrine hydrochloride), an expectorant (potassium iodide), and a sedative-hypnotic (phenobarbital).

quadriplegia (kwod′rəpli′jə), an abnormal condition characterized by paralysis of the arms, the legs, and the trunk of the body below the level of an associated injury to the spinal cord. Trauma usually causes this condition, which affects about 150,000 Americans, the majority of whom are men between the ages of 20 and 40. This disorder may be caused by spinal cord injury, especially in the area of the fifth to the seventh vertebrae. Automobile accidents and sporting mishaps are common causes.

■ OBSERVATIONS: The signs and symptoms of quadriplegia commonly include flaccidity of the arms and the legs and the loss of power and sensation below the level of the injury. Cardiovascular complications may also develop from any injury that damages the spinal cord above the fifth cervical vertebra because of an associated block of the sympathetic nervous system. A major cause of death from such injury is respiratory failure. Other symptoms may include low body temperature, bradycardia, impaired peristalsis, and autonomic dysreflexia. Diagnosis is based on a complete physical and neurologic examination with x rays of the head, chest, and abdomen to rule out underlying injuries. Extensive laboratory tests assess other body conditions, as CBC, electrolytes, urine creatinine clearance, and prothrombin time. Spinal x rays and myelography show any fractures and spinal cord blockages.

■ INTERVENTION: Treatment starts at the accident scene, where the neck and the spine of the patient are immobilized. Additional immobilization at the hospital commonly includes the use of halo traction and Stryker frame, the insertion of a Foley catheter, aggressive respiratory therapy, and the administration of diuretics to decrease spinal cord edema. After an appropriate period of therapy, surgery is commonly performed to fuse unstable spinal sections and remove bone fragments.

■ NURSING CONSIDERATIONS: Maintaining adequate respiration and the integrity of the gastrointestinal system is very important in quadriplegia. Complications, as hypothermia, bradycardia, catheter obstruction, and fecal impaction, require immediate nursing attention. A quadriplegic patient who suffers hypothermia is wrapped in blankets instead of being warmed with hotwater bottles or electromechanical devices because such devices can burn the skin of the patient experiencing severe sensory loss. Abdominal binders and antiembolism hose are used when placing the patient in an upright position. Patients who develop bradycardia are commonly connected to a cardiac monitor and intravenously administered an antimuscarinic drug, as atropine. Fecal impaction may cause hypertension and is always a possible complication. Manipulation of the rectum to free such impaction may aggravate the associated hypertension. A common precaution in removing an obstructive fecal mass is first to apply a topical anesthetic ointment, as tetracaine. Throughout the therapy for quadriplegia, constant psychological support from attending nurses benefits the patient and family and encourages healthy communication. Compare **hemiplegia, paraplegia.**

quadruplet (kwad'rʊplɪt, kwadru'plɪt), any one of four offspring born of the same gestation period during a single pregnancy. See also **Hellin's law.**

quale (kwei'li), pl. **qualia** (kwei'liə). **1.** the quality of a particular thing. **2.** a quality considered as an independent entity. **3.** (in psychology) a feeling, sensation, or other conscious process that has its own unique, particular quality regardless of its external meaning or frame of reference.

qualitative, of or pertaining to the quality, value, or nature of something.

quality assurance, (in health care) any evaluation of services provided and the results achieved as compared to accepted standards. In one form of quality assurance various attributes of health care, as cost, place, accessibility, treatment, and benefits, are scored in a two-part process. First, the actual results are compared with standard results; then, any deficiencies noted or identified serve to prompt recommendations for improvement.

quantitative inheritance. See **multifactorial inheritance.**

quantum mechanics. See **quantum theory.**

quantum theory, (in physics) a theory dealing with the interaction of matter and electromagnetic radiation, particularly at the atomic and subatomic levels, according to which radiation consists of small units of energy called quanta. Radiation can be absorbed only in whole quanta and the energy content of a quantum is inversely proportional to its wavelength. Also called **quantum mechanics.**

quarantine, **1.** isolation of people with communicable disease or of those exposed to communicable disease during the contagious period in an attempt to prevent spread of the illness. **2.** the practice of detaining travelers or vessels coming from places of epidemic disease, originally for forty days, for the purpose of inspection or disinfection.

quartan (kwɔr'tən), recurring on the fourth day, or at about 72-hour intervals. See also **quartan malaria.**

quartan malaria, a form of malaria, caused by the protozoan *Plasmodium malariae,* characterized by febrile paroxysms that occur every 72 hours. Compare **falciparum malaria, tertian malaria.** See also **malaria.**

quarti-, a combining form meaning 'fourth': *quartipara, quartisect, quartisternal.*

quartz silicosis. See **silicosis.**

Queckenstedt's test (kwek'ɪnstet'), a test for an obstruction in the spinal canal in which the large veins on each side of the neck are compressed alternately. The pressure of the spinal fluid is measured by a manometer connected to a lumbar puncture needle or catheter. Normally, occlusion of the veins of the neck causes an immediate rise in spinal fluid pressure; if the vertebral canal is blocked no rise occurs. If increased intracranial pressure is suspected, this test should not be performed. See also **spinal canal.**

Queensland tick typhus, an infection caused by *Rickettsia australis,* occurring in Australia, transmitted by ticks, and resembling mild Rocky Mountain spotted fever. Treatment includes the administration of chloramphenicol or tetracycline. Prevention depends on avoiding tick bites and on the prompt removal of attached ticks. Compare **boutonneuse fever, North Asian tick-borne rickettsiosis, Rocky Mountain spotted fever.**

Quelicin, a trade name for a depolarizing agent (succinylcholine chloride), used as an adjunct to anesthesia.

Quelidrine, a trade name for a respiratory, fixed-combination drug containing adrenergics (phenylephrine hydrochloride and ephedrine hydrochloride), an antihistaminic (chlorpheniramine maleate), an antitussive (dextromethorphan hydrobromide), and an expectorant (ammonium chloride).

quellung reaction (kwel'əŋ), the swelling of the capsule of a bacterium, seen in the laboratory when the organism is exposed to specific antisera. This phenomenon is used to identify the genera, species, or subspecies of the

PQ
R

bacteria causing a disease, including *Haemophilus influenzae, Neisseria meningitides,* and many kinds of streptococci. Also called **capsular swelling test.**

Quengle cast (kwen′gəl), a two-section, hinged orthopedic cast for immobilizing the lower extremities from the foot or ankle to below the knee and the upper thigh to a level just above the knee. The two parts of the cast are connected by special hinges at knee level, medially and laterally. The Quengle cast is used for the gradual correction of knee contractures.

quercetin (kwər′sıtın), a yellow, crystalline, flavonoid pigment found in oak bark, the juice of lemons, asparagus, and other plants. It is used to reduce abnormal capillary fragility.

querulous paranoia (kwer′yuləs), a form of paranoia characterized by extreme discontent and habitual complaining, usually about imagined slights by others. Also called **paranoia quaerula.**

Questran, a trade name for an ion-exchange resin (cholestyramine resin).

Quibron, a trade name for a respiratory, fixed-combination drug containing a smooth-muscle relaxant (theophylline) and an expectorant (guaifenesin).

quickening, the first feeling by a pregnant woman of movement of her baby in utero, usually occurring between sixteen and twenty weeks of gestation.

Quide, a trade name for a tranquilizer (piperacetazine).

quin-, a combining form meaning 'of or related to quinine': *quiniretin, quinometry, quinotoxin.*

-quin, a combining form naming antimalarial medicinal compounds from quinine: *aminoquin, diodoquin, floraquin.* Also **-quine.**

quinacrine hydrochloride, an anthelmintic and an antimalarial.
■ INDICATIONS: It is prescribed in the treatment of giardiasis, cestodiasis, and in the treatment and suppression of malaria.
■ CONTRAINDICATIONS: Pregnancy, concomitant administration of primaquine, or known hypersensitivity to this drug prohibits its use. It is used with caution in patients having a history of psychosis and in patients over 60 years of age.
■ ADVERSE EFFECTS: Among the more serious adverse reactions are severe psoriasis, aplastic anemia, acute hepatic necrosis, nausea, vomiting, and jaundice.

Quinaglute, a trade name for a cardiac depressant (quinidine gluconate).

Quincke's pulse (kvırɪ′kız), an abnormal alternate blanching and reddening of the skin that may be observed in several ways, as by pressing the front edge of the fingernail and watching the blood in the nail bed recede and return. This pulsation is characteristic of aortic insufficiency and other abnormal conditions but may also occur in otherwise normal individuals. Formerly, it was thought to be caused by pulsation of the capillaries, but study has shown it is owing to pulsation of subpapillary arteriolar and venous plexuses. Also called **capillary pulse.**

quinethazone (kwəneth′əzoun), a diuretic and antihypertensive.
■ INDICATIONS: It is prescribed in the treatment of hypertension and edema.
■ CONTRAINDICATIONS: Known hypersensitivity to this drug, to other thiazide medication, or to sulfonamide derivatives prohibits its use.
■ ADVERSE EFFECTS: Among the more serious adverse effects are hypokalemia, hyperglycemia, hyperuricemia, and hypersensitivity reactions.

Quinidex, a trade name for a cardiac depressant (quinidine sulfate).

quinidine (kwın′ədin, kwın′ədın), an antiarrhythmic agent. Also called **quinidine gluconate.**
■ INDICATION: It is prescribed in the treatment of certain cardiac arrhythmias.
■ CONTRAINDICATIONS: Known hypersensitivity to this drug prohibits its use. It is contraindicated in some arrhythmias, particularly those associated with heart block.
■ ADVERSE EFFECTS: Among the most serious adverse reactions are cardiac arrhythmia, hypertension, and cinchonism. Rare, but potentially fatal hypersensitivity reactions, as anaphylaxis and thrombocytopenia, may occur. Diarrhea, nausea, and vomiting are common.

quinidine gluconate. See **quinidine.**

quinine (kwai′nain), a white, bitter crystalline alkaloid, made from cinchona bark, used in antimalarial medications.

quinine dihydrochloride, an antimalarial. See **quinine sulfate.**

quinine sulfate, an antimalarial with antipyretic, analgesic, and muscle relaxant activity.
■ INDICATIONS: It is prescribed in the treatment of malaria and nocturnal leg cramps.
■ CONTRAINDICATIONS: Glucose-6-phosphate dehydrogenase deficiency and certain arrhythmias prohibit its use.
■ ADVERSE EFFECTS: Among the more serious adverse reactions are symptoms of cinchonism or known hypersensitivity to this drug, including tinnitus, headache, and visual, hearing, and gastrointestinal disturbances. Hemolysis, blood dyscrasia, and various hypersensitivity reactions also may occur.

Quinora, a trade name for a cardiac depressant (quinidine sulfate).

quinque-, a combining form meaning 'five': *quinquecuspid, quinquetubercular, quinquevalent.*

quinsy (kwın′zi). See **peritonsillar abscess.**

quint-, a combining form meaning 'fifth, or five-fold': *quintessence, quintipara, quintuplet.*

quintan (kwɪnʹtən), recurring on the fifth day, or at about 96-hour intervals. See also **Trench fever**.

quintana fever (kwɪntænʹə). See **trench fever**.

quintuplet (kwɪnʹtʊplɪt, kwɪntuʹplɪt), any one of five offspring born of the same gestation period during a single pregnancy. See also **Hellin's law**.

Quotane Hydrochloride, a trade name for a local anesthetic (dimethysoquin hydrochloride).

quotid. See **q.d.**

Q wave, the component of the cardiac cycle shown on an electrocardiogram as a short abrupt downward line from the end of the tail of the P wave before the sudden sharp ascent of the R wave. It represents the first part of the QRS complex.

R

R, 1. abbreviation for **metabolic respiratory quotient.** 2. abbreviation for **respiratory exchange ratio.**

Ra, symbol for **radium.**

rabbit fever. See **tularemia.**

rabies (rei'biz), an acute usually fatal viral disease of the central nervous system transmitted from animals to people by infected blood, tissue, or, most commonly, saliva. Also called *Obsolete.* **hydrophobia.** —**rabid** (ræb'ıd), *adj.*
■ OBSERVATIONS: The reservoir of the virus is chiefly wild animals, including skunks, bats, foxes, dogs, raccoons, and cats—almost never rodents. After introduction into the human body, often by a bite of an infected animal, the virus travels along nerve pathways to the brain and, later, to other organs. An incubation period ranges from ten days to one year and is followed by a prodromal period characterized by fever, malaise, headache, paresthesia, and myalgia. After several days, severe encephalitis, delirium, agonizingly painful muscular spasms, seizures, paralysis, coma, and death ensue.
■ INTERVENTION: Few nonfatal cases have been documented in humans; survival in those cases has been the result of intensive supportive nursing and medical care. There is no treatment once the virus has reached the tissue of the nervous system. Local treatment of wounds inflicted by rabid animals may prevent the disease. The wound is cleansed with soap, water, and a disinfectant. A deep wound may be cauterized and rabies immune globulin (RIG) injected directly into the base of the wound. A series of subcutaneous injections with a vaccine is begun. As this is painful and prolonged, great effort is made to locate and examine the animal. The animal that is suspected of being rabid is not immediately killed but put in isolation and carefully observed. If the animal is well in ten days there is no danger of rabies developing from the bite. Tissue from the animal's brain may be examined microscopically or by fluorescent antibody screening techniques.
■ NURSING CONSIDERATIONS: Rabies virus infection may be eradicated from most communities by prophylactic immunization of domestic animals, stringent measures for the control of domestic animals, and the elimination of any wild animals acting as reservoirs of infection. The nurse and other health workers may encourage compliance with such efforts and teach the necessity of avoiding wild animals and the importance of immediate first aid for any animal bite.

rabies immune globulin (RIG), a solution of antirabies immune globulin.
■ INDICATIONS: It is used in conjunction with rabies duck embryo vaccine for possible protection against rabies in persons suspected of exposure to rabies.
■ CONTRAINDICATIONS: Previous administration of this preparation or known hypersensitivity to this solution, to gamma globulin, or to thimerosal prohibits its use.
■ ADVERSE EFFECTS: Among the more serious adverse reactions are soreness at the site of injection, fever, and hypersensitivity reactions.

rabies vaccine, a sterile suspension of killed rabies virus prepared from duck embryo. Also called **DEV.**
■ INDICATION: It is prescribed for immunization against rabies.
■ CONTRAINDICATIONS: A history of allergic reaction to chicken or duck eggs or to protein prohibits its use.
■ ADVERSE EFFECTS: Among the most serious adverse reactions are severe hypersensitivity reactions and pain and inflammation at the site of injection.

race, a group of genetically related people who share certain physical characteristics.

racemose (ræs'əmous'), like a bunch of grapes, used in describing a structure in which many branches terminate in nodular, cystlike forms.

racemose aneurysm, a pronounced dilatation of lengthened and tortuous blood vessels, some of which may be distended to 20 times their normal size. Also called **cirsoid aneurysm.**

Racet, a trade name for a topical fixed-combination drug containing a glucocorticoid (hydrocortisone) and a topical anti-infective (iodochlorhydroxyquin).

rachi-. See **rachio-.**

rachio-, a combining form meaning 'of or related to the spine': *rachiocampsis, rachiotome, rachiotomy.* Also **rachi-, rhachi.**

rachiopagus (rei'kiop'əgəs), **rachipagus,** conjoined symmetrical twins that are united back to back along the spinal column.

rachischisis (rəkıs'kəsıs). See **spina bifida.**

rachischisis totalis. See **complete rachischisis.**

rachitic (rəkıt'ık), 1. of or pertaining to rickets. 2. resembling or suggesting the condition of one afflicted with rickets.

rachitic dwarf, a person whose retarded growth is owing to rickets. See also **Fanconi's syndrome.**

rachitis (rəkai′tɪs), **1.** rickets. **2.** an inflammatory disease of the vertebral column.

racial immunity, a form of natural immunity shared by most of the members of a race. Compare **individual immunity, species immunity.**

racial unconscious. See **collective unconscious.**

rad, radiation absorbed dose; the basic unit of absorbed dose of ionizing radiation. One rad is equal to the absorption of 100 ergs of radiation energy per gram of matter. See also **rem.**

radi-, a combining form meaning 'root': *radiciform, radicotomy, radiectomy.*

radial artery, an artery in the forearm, starting at the bifurcation of the brachial artery, passing in 12 branches to the forearm, wrist, and hand. In the forearm, it extends from the neck of the radius to the forepart of the styloid process; in the wrist, from the styloid process to the carpus; in the hand, from the carpus, across the palm, to the little finger. In the forearm, the branches of the radial artery are the radial recurrent, muscular, palmar carpal, and superficial palmar; in the wrist, the branches are the dorsal carpal and the first dorsal metacarpal. In the hand, the branches are the princeps pollicis, radialis indicis, deep palmar arch, palmar metacarpal, perforating, and recurrent.

RADIAL ARTERY

radial keratotomy, a surgical procedure in which a series of tiny shallow incisions are made on the cornea, causing it to bulge slightly. The operation is performed under local anesthesia and requires only 30 minutes. Hospitalization is not necessary. Radial keratotomy corrects myopia.

radial nerve, the largest branch of the brachial plexus, arising on each side as a continuation of the posterior cord. It supplies the skin of the arm and forearm and their extensor muscles. It crosses the tendon of the latissimus dorsi beneath the axillary artery, passes the inferior border of the teres major, and winds around the medial side of the humerus to enter the triceps between the medial and the long heads of that muscle. It spirals down the arm close to the humerus in the groove separating the origins of the medial and the long heads of the triceps, accompanied by the deep brachial artery. On the lateral side of the arm it pierces the lateral intermuscular septum, runs between the brachialis and the brachioradialis, and divides into the superficial and the deep branches. The branches of the radial nerve are the medial muscular branches, the posterior brachial cutaneous nerve, the posterior muscular branches, the posterior antebrachial cutaneous nerve, the lateral muscular branches, the superficial branch, and the deep branch. Also called **musculospiral nerve.** Compare **median nerve, musculocutaneous nerve, ulnar nerve.**

radial notch of ulna, the narrow, lateral depression in the coronoid process of the ulna that receives the head of the radius.

radial pulse, the pulse of the radial artery palpated at the wrist over the radius. The radial pulse is the one most often taken, owing to the ease with which it is palpated.

radial recurrent artery, a branch of the radial artery, arising just distal to the elbow, ascending between the branches of the radial nerve, and supplying several muscles of the arm and the elbow.

radial reflex, a normal reflex elicited by tapping over the distal radius, with the response being flexion of the forearm. Flexion of the fingers may also occur if the reflex is hyperactive.

radiant energy, the energy emitted by electromagnetic radiation, as radio waves, visible light, x rays, and gamma rays.

radiate, to diverge or spread from a common point. —**radiation,** *n.*

radiate ligament, a ligament that connects the head of a rib with a vertebra and an associated intervertebral disc. Each of the 24 radiate ligaments consists of three flat fasciculi attached to the head of a rib. The superior fasciculus connects with the vertebra above, the inferior fasciculus connects with the vertebra below, and the middle fasciculus connects to the disc between the two vertebrae. Radiate ligaments to the tenth, eleventh, and twelfth ribs have only two fasciculi.

radiation, 1. the emission of energy, rays, or waves. **2.** (in medicine) the use of a radioactive substance in the diagnosis or treatment of disease. —**radiate,** *adj., v.*

radiation caries, tooth decay caused by ionizing radiation of the oral and maxillary structure. Radiation caries is often a side effect of treatment for oral malignancies. See also **dental caries.**

radiation detector, a device for converting radiant energy to an observable form, used for detecting the presence and sometimes the amount of radiation. A Geiger-Müller detector counts and registers the number of particles or photons reaching it from a radioactive source and can be designed with sufficient sensitivity to detect cosmic radiation. An ionization chamber detects exposure to radiation by collecting the ion pairs formed by the passage of radiation through the device.

radiation exposure, a measure of the ionization produced in air by x rays or gamma rays. It is the sum of the electrical charges on all ions of one sign that are produced when all electrons liberated by photons in a volume of air are completely stopped, divided by the mass of air in the volume element. The unit of exposure is the roentgen.

radiation sickness, an abnormal condition resulting from exposure to ionizing radiation. The severity of the condition is determined by the volume of radiation, the length of time of exposure, and the area of the body affected. Moderate exposure may cause headache, nausea, vomiting, anorexia, and diarrhea; long-term exposure may result in sterility, damage to the fetus in pregnant women, leukemia or other forms of cancer, alopecia, and cataracts.

radiation syndrome. See **radiation sickness.**

radiation therapy. See **radiotherapy.**

radical, 1. a group of atoms that acts together and forms a component of a compound. The group tends to remain bound together when a chemical reaction removes it from a compound and attaches it to another. A radical does not exist freely in nature. 2. drastic therapy, as the surgical removal of an organ, limb, or other part of the body.

radical dissection, the surgical removal of tissue in an extensive area surrounding the operative site. Most often it is performed to identify and excise all tissue that may possibly be malignant in order to decrease the chance of recurrence.

radical mastectomy, surgical removal of an entire breast, pectoral muscles, axillary lymph nodes and all fat, fascia, and adjacent tissues. It is performed in the treatment of cancer of the breast. Preoperatively, in addition to giving usual preoperative care, the staff encourages verbalization of the patient's fears of the disease, of the surgery, and of the loss of her breast. Her self-image is usually severely threatened, and she characteristically grieves in anticipation of a loss of femininity. The postoperative period is physically and emotionally painful; the woman is best warned by supportive but realistic explanations prior to surgery. Edema of the arm on the affected side is the rule, as the axillary lymphatic structures that drain the lymph from the arm are removed during surgery. Atelectasis may develop if deep breathing and coughing are not regularly performed. The incision is painful but may be expected to become less so during the first few days; it should not become more inflamed or painfully swollen. A pressure dressing is usually applied and left in place until bleeding and drainage have decreased. A drain is usually left in the wound for several days. The woman may be anxious, depressed, angry, with-

Characteristics and uses of some commonly used radioactive agents

Radiation source	Half-life (where applicable)	Rays emitted	Appearance or form	Method of administration
X-ray	—	Gamma	Invisible rays	X-ray machine
Radium	1600 years	Alpha Beta Gamma	In needles, plaques, molds	Interstitial (needles) Intracavitary (plaques, molds)
Radon	4 days	Alpha Beta Gamma (low intensity)	In seeds, needles	Interstitial (seeds, needles)
Cesium (^{137}Cs)	33 years	Beta Gamma	In needles, capsules	Interstitial (needles) Intracavitary (capsules)
Cobalt (^{60}Co)	5 years	Beta Gamma	External (cobalt unit) Internal (needles, seeds, molds)	Machine (teletherapy) Interstitial (needles, seeds)
Iodine (^{131}I)	8 days	Beta Gamma (low intensity)	Clear liquid	By mouth
Phosphorus (^{32}P)	14 days	Beta	Clear liquid	By mouth, intracavitary, intravenous
Gold (^{198}Au)	3 days	Beta Gamma	Purple liquid	Intracavitary
Iridium (^{192}Ir)	74 days	Beta Gamma (low intensity)	In needles, wires, seeds	Interstitial
Yttrium (^{90}Y)	3 days	Beta	Beads, needles	Interstitial

drawn, or reflect hopelessness. In addition to the usual postoperative measures, the nurse elevates the affected arm above the level of the right atrium; checks the color, sensation, and motion of the fingers; checks the graft site if a graft was performed; and applies reinforcement to the pressure dressing as necessary. Later in the postoperative period, the patient is assisted in range of motion exercises for all extremities and is taught, with assistance, to perform gradually increasing arm and shoulder exercises. In discussion and in providing physical care, the loss of the breast is dealt with frankly; to avoid the fact is not helpful to the patient. Slowly the patient is involved in caring for herself more completely, a process that continues as she gradually resumes her normal daily activities. On discharge, she is encouraged to shower daily, to apply an emollient, like cocoa butter, to the incision, and to examine the remaining breast monthly. Reach to Recovery may be involved in counseling and support before and after a mastectomy. Chemotherapy and radiation therapy may continue after surgery. The woman is told never to allow blood to be drawn from the affected arm; intravenous injection is also to be avoided in that arm. Blood pressure measurement, vaccination, and other injections are best performed on the other arm. Compare **modified radical mastectomy, simple mastectomy.**

radical neck dissection, dissection and removal of all lymph nodes and removable tissues under the skin of the neck, performed to prevent the spread of malignant tumors of the head and neck that have a reasonable chance of being controlled. Before surgery, thorough mouth hygiene is given and antibiotics are begun. Under general anesthesia, a tracheostomy is done; the tumor, surrounding tissues, and the lymph nodes on the affected side are then removed in one mass from the angle of the jaw to the clavicle, forward to midline, and back to the angle of the jaw. A total laryngectomy may be done as part of the surgery. After surgery, the nurse suctions the tracheostomy as necessary, and observes vital signs for indications of hemorrhage or difficulty in breathing. A humidifier or vaporizer will ease coughing and production of mucus. I.V. fluids are continued in the arm not used for writing. Extensive work with a speech pathologist may be necessary to learn esophageal speech. Radiation of the tumor site may be begun and chemotherapy may continue. Compare with **neck dissection.**

radical therapy, 1. a treatment intended to cure, not palliate. 2. a definitive, extreme treatment; not conservative, as radical mastectomy rather than simple or partial mastectomy.

radical vulvectomy. See **vulvectomy.**

radio-, a combining form meaning 'of or related to radiation, sometimes specifically to emission of radiant energy, to radium, or to the radius': *radioactive, radiobiology, radiohumeral.*

radioactive, giving off radiation as the result of the disintegration of the nucleus of an atom.

radioactive contamination, the undesirable addition of radioactive material to the skin or part of the environment, as clothing or equipment. Beta radiation contamination of the body of health-care personnel is only possible through the ingestion, inhalation, or absorption of the source, as when the skin is contaminated with a beta emitter contained in an absorbable chemical form. Instruments, drapes, surgical gloves, and clothing that come in contact with serous fluids, blood, and urine of patients containing beta or gamma radiation emitters may be contaminated. The severity of the contamination is directly related to the elapsed time between the administration of the isotope and surgery; on completion of the procedure possibly contaminated material is isolated and checked; if found to be contaminated, it is disposed of according to institutional or federal standards for the disposal of radioactive waste.

radioactive contrast media, a solution or colloid containing materials of high atomic number, used for visualizing soft tissue structures in diagnostic radiology. Diagnostic radiopharmaceuticals indicate their positions in the body by their gamma ray emissions.

radioactive decay, the disintegration of the nucleus of an unstable nuclide by the spontaneous emission of charged particles, or photons, or both.

radioactive element, an element subject to spontaneous degeneration of its nucleus accompanied by the emission of alpha particles, beta particles, or gamma rays. All elements with atomic numbers greater than 83 are radioactive. Several radioactive elements not found in nature have been produced by the bombardment of stable elements with atomic particles in a cyclotron. Some kinds of radioactive elements are radium, thorium, uranium. Compare **stable element.** See also **radioactivity.**

radioactive iodine (RAI), a radioactive isotope of iodine, used as a tracer in biology and medicine.

radioactive iodine excretion, the elimination by the body of radioactive iodine (RAI) administered in a test of thyroid function and in the treatment of hyperthyroidism. Most RAI is excreted in urine, but small amounts may be found in sputum, perspiration, feces, and vomitus.

radioactive iodine excretion test, a method of evaluating thyroid function by measuring the amount of radioactive iodine (RAI) in urine after the patient is given an oral tracer dose of the radioisotope ^{131}I. Normally, 5 to 35 per cent of the dose is absorbed by the thyroid, but absorption is increased in hyperthyroidism and decreased in hypothyroidism, and the amount excreted in urine is inversely proportional to the uptake of RAI. Following administration of the tracer, a scintillation detector is placed over the patient's neck at 2, 6, and 24 hours to measure the RAI accumulated by the thyroid, and the amount excreted is assayed in urine collected for 24 hours after the oral dose. Diarrhea, can result in low values of RAI in urine; renal failure, by decreasing excretion, can cause high readings. See also **radioactive iodine uptake.**

radioactive iodine uptake (RAIU), the absorption and incorporation by the thyroid of radioactive iodine (RAI), administered orally as a tracer dose in a test of thyroid function and as larger doses for the treatment of hyperthyroidism. The radioisotope ^{131}I is rapidly absorbed in the stomach and is concentrated in the thyroid. A normal thyroid absorbs 5 to 35 per cent of a tracer dose, while the uptake is increased in hyperthyroidism, and patients receiving a large therapeutic dose of RAI may require hospitalization for several days. See also **radioactive iodine excretion test.**

radioactivity, the emission of corpuscular or electromagnetic radiations as a consequence of nuclear disintegration. Natural radioactivity is a property exhibited by all chemical elements with an atomic number greater than 83; artificial or induced radioactivity is manmade through the bombardment of naturally occurring isotopes with subatomic particles or high levels of gamma or x radiation.

radioallergosorbent test (RAST) (rei'diouælər'gousɔr'-bənt),   a test in which a technique of radioimmunoassay is used to identify and quantify IgE in serum that has been mixed with any of 45 known allergens. If an atopic allergy to a substance exists, an antigen-antibody reaction occurs with characteristic conjugation and clumping. The test is an in vitro method of demonstrating allergic reactions. Compare **patch test, Prausnitz-Küstner test.**

radiobiology, the branch of the natural sciences dealing with the effects of radiation on biological systems. — **radiobiologic, radiobiological,** *adj.*

radiocarpal articulation, the condyloid joint at the wrist that connects the radius and distal surface of an articular disc with the scaphoid, the lunate, and the triangular bones. The joint involves four ligaments and allows all movements but rotation. Also called **wrist joint.**

radiochemistry, the branch of chemistry that deals with the properties and behavior of radioactive materials and the use of radionuclides in the study of chemical and biological problems.

radiographic magnification, visualization of small areas through magnification achieved with a small x-ray tube having a small focal point, a common diagnostic tool in orthopedics.

radiography (rei'diog'rəfi), the production of shadow images on photographic emulsion through the action of ionizing radiation. The image is the result of the differential attenuation of the radiation in its passage through the object being radiographed. — **radiographic,** *adj.*

radioimmunoassay (RIA) (rei'diouimyu'nouæs'ei), a technique in radiology used to determine the concentra-

tion of an antigen, antibody or other protein in the serum. A radioactively labeled substance known to react in a certain way with the suspected protein is injected and any reaction is monitored.

radioiodine (rei'diouai'ədain), a radioactive isotope of iodine used in radiotherapy. It is used especially in the treatment of some thyroid conditions and in diagnostic radiology by various scanning techniques. A common form of radioiodine is I^{131}.

radioisotope (rei'diouai'sətoup), a radioactive isotope of an element, used for therapeutic and diagnostic purposes.

radioisotope scan, a two-dimensional representation of the gamma rays emitted by a radioisotope, showing its concentration in a body site, as the thyroid gland, brain, or kidney. Radioisotopes used in diagnostic scanning may be administered intravenously or orally.

radiologist, a physician who specializes in radiology.

radiology, the branch of medicine concerned with radioactive substances and, using various techniques of visualization, with the diagnosis and treatment of disease using any of the various sources of radiant energy. — **radiologic, radiological,** *adj.*

radiopaque, not permitting the passage of x rays or other radiant energy. Bones are relatively radiopaque and therefore show as white areas on an exposed x-ray film. Lead is markedly radiopaque and therefore is widely used to shield x-ray equipment and atomic power sources. See also **radioactive element, radioactivity, radiopaque dye.** — **radiopacity,** *n.*

radiopaque dye, a chemical substance that does not permit the passage of x rays. Various radiopaque iodine compounds are used to outline the interior of hollow organs such as heart chambers, blood vessels, respiratory passages, and the biliary tract in x-ray or fluoroscopic pictures.

radiopharmaceutical, a drug that exhibits spontaneous disintegration of unstable nuclei with the emission of nuclear particles or photons. Kinds of radiopharmaceuticals are **diagnostic radiopharmaceutical, research radiopharmaceutical, therapeutic radiopharmaceutical.**

radiopharmacist, a trained professional responsible for the formulation and dispensing of prescribed radioactive tracers and for the clinical aspects of radiopharmacy. Radiopharmacists are required to receive training in radioactive tracer techniques, in the safe handling of radioactive materials, in the preparation and quality control of drugs for administration to humans, and in the basic principles of nuclear medicine. Some states require that radioactive drugs be dispensed by licensed pharmacists, while others recognize radiopharmaceutical specialists who are not necessarily graduates of a school of pharmacy.

radiopharmacy, a facility for the preparation and dispensing of radioactive drugs and for the storage of radioactive materials, inventory records, and prescriptions of radioactive substances. The radiopharmacy is usually the correlation point for radioactive wastes, the unit responsible for waste disposal or storage, and a center for clinical investigations employing radioactive tracers. It may also be a center for research and for the training of students and residents in radiology and nuclear medicine.

radioresistance, the relative resistance of cells, tissues, organs, organisms, chemical compounds, or any substances to the effects of radiation. Compare **radiosensitivity.** —**radioresistant,** *adj.*

radioresistant, unchanged by or protected against damage by radioactive emissions such as x rays, alpha particles, or gamma rays. Compare **radiosensitive.** See also **radioactivity.**

radiosensitive, capable of being changed by or reacting to radioactive emissions such as x rays, alpha particles, or gamma rays. Compare **radioresistant.** See also **radioactivity.**

radiosensitivity, the relative susceptibility of cells, tissues, organs, organisms, or any living substances to the effects of radiation. Cells of self-renewing systems, as those in the crypts of the intestine, are the most radiosensitive. Cells that divide regularly but mature between divisions, as spermatogonia and spermatocytes, are next in radiosusceptibility. Long-lived cells that usually do not undergo mitosis unless there is a suitable stimulus include the less radiosensitive liver, kidney, and thyroid cells. Least sensitive are fixed postmitotic cells that have lost the ability to divide, as neurons. Connective tissue and blood vessels are intermediate in radiosensitivity; parenchymal cells are affected by moderate doses of radiation that do not damage connective tissue.

radiotherapy, the treatment of neoplastic disease by using x rays or gamma rays, usually from a cobalt source, to deter the proliferation of malignant cells by decreasing the rate of mitosis or impairing DNA synthesis.

■ METHOD: Prior to radiotherapy, the procedure, its purpose, duration, painlessness, and the need to remain completely still during irradiation are explained to the patient. Potential sequelae, as erythema, edema, desquamation, hyperpigmentation, atrophy, pruritus, or skin pain, altered taste, anorexia, nausea, vomiting, headache, hair loss, malaise, tachycardia, and increased susceptibility to infection may be discussed in response to specific questions raised by the patient. A preliminary visit to the radiology department may be arranged so that the equipment and the room in which the patient will be positioned on a table can be seen. From this position the patient is able to communicate with the radiotherapist in an adjoining booth. Daily hygiene measures are completed before treatment; on returning from irradiation, the patient is placed in a noninfectious environment or, if necessary, in protective isolation; friends, family, other patients and staff members with infections, especially upper respiratory infections, are not permitted to visit. Skin care is administered following irradiation and every four hours thereafter, but the ink markings placed by the radiologist on the skin to mark the focus of treatment are not removed between treatments, and the treated area is not washed with water; sterile mineral oil, lanolin, or petroleum jelly may be applied if the radiologist approves. The patient wears loose garments, rests on an air mattress, foam or gel pad, or sheepskin, and a footboard or bed cradle is used to elevate the top sheet and blanket. Cosmetics are avoided and underarm deodorants or antiperspirants are contraindicated if the axillary area is irradiated. If hair loss occurs, the patient may wear a wig, scarf, cap, or toupee. High-protein supplements, soothing gelatins and ice cream are provided, and other food is served when desired by the patient; six small, bland feedings may be tolerated more easily than regular meals. Quiet periods are maintained before and after meals. Antiemetics and vitamins are administered as ordered, and tube feedings or total parenteral nutrition may be indicated if the patient's food intake is severely decreased. Oral hygiene, using a soft-bristled brush and dilute mouth wash or, if needed, foam or sponge swabs and a saline rinse, is administered whenever required, and a fluid intake of 2,000 to 3,000 ml daily is maintained, unless contraindicated. In preparation for discharge, the patient is instructed to follow the hospital practices for skin care, oral hygiene, fluid intake and a high protein, nutritious diet, but to avoid eating immediately before and after irradiation. The patient is told to avoid tight clothing, extremes of temperature, exposure to sunlight, tub baths or showers until ordered, and persons with infections and to report to the physician any symptom of infection, inability to eat, severe diarrhea, increasing headache, and fatigue, or increasing redness, swelling, itching, or pain at the site of therapy.

■ NURSING ORDERS: The nurse offers thorough explanation of the radiotherapy, provides care after treatment, and prepares the patient for discharge and, if indicated, continued therapy on an outpatient basis.

■ OUTCOME CRITERIA: Radiotherapy can control or arrest the development of a number of forms of cancer and provide palliation in some inoperable tumors; the maintenance of adequate nutrition and meticulous care of the skin may allow the person to avoid the most serious and unpleasant side effects of radiotherapy.

radioulnar articulation, the articulation of the radius and the ulna, consisting of a proximal articulation, a distal articulation, and three sets of ligaments.

radium (Ra), a radioactive metallic element of the alkaline-earth group. Its atomic number is 88. Four radium isotopes occur naturally and have different atomic weights: 223, 224, 226, and 228. The isotope with atomic weight 226 is the most abundant. It is formed by the disintegration of uranium[238], has a halflife of 1,620 years, and decays by alpha emission to form radon[222]. Radium occurs in the uranium minerals carnotite and pitchblende, which contain about 3×10^{-7} gm of radium per gm of uranium. Radium salts have been used extensively as radiation sources in the treatment of cancer but are gradually being replaced in such therapy by cobalt and cesium.

radius, *pl.* **radii.** one of the bones of the forearm, lying parallel to the ulna. Its proximal end is small and forms a part of the elbow joint. The distal end is large and forms a part of the wrist joint. The radius receives the insertions of various muscles and articulates with the humerus, ulna, scaphoid, and lunate bones.

radix (rei′dıks), *pl.* **radices** (ræd′ısiz). See **root.** — **radical,** *adj.*

radon (Rn), a radioactive, inert, gaseous, nonmetallic element. Its atomic number is 86; its atomic weight is 222. Radon is used in radiation cancer therapy.

RAI, abbreviation for **radioactive iodine.**

RAIU, abbreviation for **radioactive iodine uptake.**

RA latex test, abbreviation for **rheumatoid arthritis latex test.** See **latex fixation test.**

rale, a common abnormal respiratory sound heard on auscultation of the chest during inspiration, characterized by discontinuous bubbling noises. Fine rales have a crackling sound produced by air entering distal bronchioles or alveoli which contain serous secretions, as in congestive heart failure, pneumonia, or early tuberculosis. Coarse rales originates in the larger bronchi or trachea and have a lower pitch. Kinds of rales are **sibilant rale, sonorous rale.** Compare **rhonchus, wheeze.**

rami-, a combining form meaning 'branch': *ramicotomy, ramification, ramisection.*

Ramsay Hunt's syndrome, a neurologic condition resulting from invasion of the seventh nerve ganglia and the geniculate ganglion by varicella zoster virus, characterized by severe ear pain, facial nerve paralysis, vertigo, hearing loss, and, often, mild, generalized encephalitis. The vertigo may last days or weeks, but usually resolves itself. The facial paralysis may be permanent, and the hearing loss, which is rarely permanent, may be partial or total. Treatment usually includes the prescription of corticosteroid drugs. Also called **herpes zoster oticus.**

ramus (rei′məs), *pl.* **rami.** a small, branchlike structure extending from a larger one or dividing into two or more parts, as a branch of a nerve or artery or one of the rami of the pubis. — **ramification,** *n.* **ramify,** *v.*

random genetic drift. See **genetic drift.**

range of motion exercise, any body action involving the muscles, the joints, and natural directional movements, as abduction, extension, flexion, pronation, and rotation. Such exercises are usually applied actively or passively in the treatment of orthopedic deformities, in the assessment of injuries and deformities, and in athletic conditioning.

ranula (ræn′yulə), a cyst beneath the tongue owing to obstruction of a salivary duct or mucous gland.

rape, a sexual assault, homosexual or heterosexual, the legal definitions for which vary from state to state. Rape is a crime of violence or one committed under the threat of violence, and its victims are treated for medical and psychologic trauma. See also **statutory rape.**

Rape preventive measures

Prevention of attack

Set house lights to go on and off by timer
Keep light on at all entrances
Place safety locks on windows and doors
Have key ready before reaching door of house or car
Look in car before entering
Insist on identification before letting a stranger in house; check identification with agency if suspicious
Do not list first name on mailbox or in telephone directory
Make arrangements with neighbor for needed assistance
Be alert when walking in street; walk in lighted areas
Walk down center of street if possible
Avoid lonely or enclosed areas

If attacked

Run toward a lighted house; yell ''Fire''
Spit in rapist's face; act bizarre; vomit
Rip off rapist's glasses
Step hard on his foot (instep)
Aim at eyes—try to gouge eyes, scrape face
Hit throat at Adam's apple (larynx)
Use fighting and screaming with caution; this may scare some rapists, encourage others
Try talking to avoid rape
If powerless, make close observations about rapist, car, location.

■ OBSERVATIONS: Characteristically, the person is frightened, feels vulnerable, humiliated, and personally violated. General physical examination may reveal cuts, bruises, and other injuries. Pelvic or genital examination may show traumatic injury to the internal or external genitalia or anus.

■ INTERVENTION: Careful physical examination is performed and a detailed history obtained. Specimens are obtained as indicated. Ideally, counseling is available and offered immediately to all victims of rape. In the case of a woman who has been raped by a man, a pregnancy test is performed and specific injuries are treated. If the test is positive, prophylaxis against conception may be administered. Usually, antibiotics are given to prevent the development of venereal disease. Arrangements for ongoing emotional support are made.

■ CONSIDERATIONS: A trained, sympathetic nurse of the

same sex is assigned to stay with the person. Privacy for the history, examination, and police interview is assured. The person may or may not choose to talk to the police, but the police must be informed in every case. The victim must sign a special form to allow specimens to be released to a law enforcement agency. In general, it is the role of the nurse and other medical workers to examine, to treat, and to collect specimens as necessary, not to decide that rape has occurred. Before discharge, it should be ascertained that someone can be with the person, as depression, anger, guilt, and fear are common following rape.

rape counseling, counseling by a trained person provided to a victim of rape. Rape counseling ideally begins at the time the crime is first reported, as in an emergency room. Initially, the counselor offers sensitive support for the victim by accepting the person in a nonprejudicial, noncritical way. The person's response to the trauma of the assault is empathetically elicited, and three basic statements are made: the counselor is sorry that the rape happened, is glad that the injuries are not worse, and does not think that the victim was wrong or did anything wrong. Counseling personnel may provide supportive services and advocacy and liaison between the victim and medical, legal, and law-enforcement authorities. This involves staying with the person during medical examination, police or district attorney's questioning, and throughout the criminal justice process.

rape-trauma syndrome, a nursing diagnosis accepted by the Fourth National Conference on the Classification of Nursing Diagnoses. The syndrome results from the experience of being raped and includes an acute phase of disorganization and a longer phase of reorganization in the victim's life. The etiology of the syndrome is the trauma of the rape. The defining characteristics are divided into three subcomponents: rape-trauma, compound reaction, and silent reaction. The defining characteristics of rape-trauma in the acute phase are emotional reactions of anger, guilt, and embarrassment, fear of physical violence and death, humiliation, wish for revenge, and multiple physical complaints, including gastrointestinal distress, genitourinary discomfort, tension, and disturbance of the normal patterns of sleep, activity, and rest. The long-term phase of rape-trauma is characterized by changes in the usual patterns of daily life (even a change in residence), nightmares and phobias, and a need for support from friends and family. The compound reaction is characterized by all of the defining characteristics of rape-trauma, reliance on alcohol or drugs, or the reoccurrence of the symptoms of previous conditions, including psychiatric illness. The silent reaction sometimes occurs in place of the rape-trauma or compound reaction. The defining characteristics of the silent reaction are an abrupt change in the person's usual sexual relationships,

an increase in nightmares, an increasing anxiety during the interview about the rape incident, a marked change in sexual behavior, denial of the rape or refusal to discuss it, and the sudden development of phobic reactions. See also **nursing diagnosis.**

raphe, rhaphe (rei'fi), a line of union of the halves of various symmetrical parts, as the abdominal raphe of the linea alba or the raphe penis, which appears as a narrow, dark streak on the inferior surface of the penis.

rapid-acting insulin. See **short-acting insulin.**

rapid eye movement (REM). See **sleep.**

rapport (rapɔr'), a sense of mutuality and understanding; harmony, accord, confidence, and respect underlying a relationship between two persons, an essential bond between a therapist and patient in psychotherapy.

raptus (rap'tus), 1. a state of intense emotional or mental excitement, often characterized by uncontrollable activity or behavior resulting from an irresistible impulse; ecstasy; rapture. 2. any sudden or violent seizure or attack. Kinds of raptus include **raptus haemorrhagicus, raptus maniacus, raptus melancholicus, raptus nervorum.**

raptus haemorrhagicus (hem'ɔrei'jikəs), a sudden, massive hemorrhage.

raptus maniacus (manai'əkus), a sudden violent attack of mania. See also **mania.**

raptus melancholicus (mel'ənkou'likus), an attack of extreme agitation or frenzy that occurs during the course of depression.

raptus nervorum (nervɔr'um), a sudden, violent attack of nervousness.

rare-earth element, a metallic element having an atomic number between 57 to 71 inclusive. These closely related substances are classified in three groups: the cerium metals are lanthanum, cerium, pracsodynium, neodynium, promethium and samarium; the terbium metals are europium, gadolinium, and terbium; the yttrium metals are dysprosium, holmium, erbium, thulium, yttrium, ytterbium, and lutetium. Also called **rare-earth metal.**

rare-earth metal. See **rare-earth element.**

RAS, abbreviation for **reticular activating system.**

rash, a skin eruption. Kinds of rashes include **butterfly rash, diaper rash, drug rash, heat rash.**

Rashkind procedure (ræsh'kind), the enlargement of an opening in the cardiac septum between the right and left atria, performed to relieve congestive heart failure in newborns with certain congenital heart defects by improving the oxygenation of the blood. The procedure allows more mixing between oxygenated blood from the lungs and systemic blood without the risk of surgery, sustaining life until the infant is 2 to 3 years of age and a shunt can be created to carry systemic blood to the lungs. Preoperatively, a cardiac catheterization is done to pinpoint the defect. Under light general anesthesia, a deflated balloon is passed through the foramen ovale into the left atrium.

The balloon is inflated and pulled across the septum to enlarge the opening. Postoperatively, the infant is observed carefully for respiratory difficulty, signs of hypoxia, or decreasing cardiac output. Humidified oxygen is administered. Fluids and electrolytes are closely monitored. Also called **balloon septostomy.**

Rasmussen's aneurysm (ræs'myusənz), a localized dilatation of a blood vessel in a tuberculous cavity that causes hemorrhage when it ruptures.

RAST. See **radioallergosorbent test.**

ratbite fever, either of two distinct infections transmitted to man by the bite of a rat or mouse, characterized by fever, headache, malaise, nausea, vomiting, and rash. In the United States, the disease is more commonly caused by *Streptobacillus moniliformis,* and its unique features are rash on palms and soles, painful joints, prompt healing of the wound, and a duration of two weeks. In the Far East, ratbite fever is usually caused by *Spirillum minus* and is associated with an asymmetric rash on the extremities, no joint symptoms, a relapsing fever, swelling at the site of the wound, regional lymphadenopathy, and a duration of from four to eight weeks. Relapse is common. Penicillin administered intramuscularly is effective in treating either form of the disease. Ratbite fever resulting from infection caused by *Streptobacillus moniliformis* is also called **Haverhill fever;** infection caused by *Spirillum Minus* is also called **sodoku.**

rate, a numerical ratio, often used in the compilation of data concerning the prevalence and incidence of events, in which the number of actual occurrences appears as the numerator and the number of possible occurrences appears as the denominator, as when one person in fifteen fails an examination the failure rate is said to be 1/15 (or "one in fifteen"). Standard rates are stated in conventional units of population, as neonatal mortality per 1,000 or maternal mortality per 100,000.

Rathke's pouch tumor (rat'kiz). See **craniopharyngioma.**

ratio, the relationship of one quantity to one or more other quantities expressed as a proportion of one to the others, and written either as a fraction (8/3) or linearly (8:3).

rational 1. of or pertaining to a measure, method, or procedure based on reason. 2. of or pertaining to a therapeutic method based on an understanding of the cause and mechanisms of a specific disease and the potential effects of the drugs or procedures used in treating the disorder. 3. sane; capable of normal reasoning or behavior.

rationale (ræsh'ənæl'), a system of reasoning or a statement of the reasons used in explaining data or phenomena.

rational emotive therapy (RET), a form of psychotherapy, originated by Albert Ellis, that emphasizes a reorganization of one's cognitive and emotional functions, a redefinition of one's problems, and a change in one's attitudes in order to develop more effective and suitable patterns of behavior. RET is conducted with individuals or with groups.

rational treatment. See **treatment.**

rattle, an abnormal sound heard by ascultation of the lungs in some forms of pulmonary disease. It consists of a coarse vibration caused by the movement of moisture and the separation of the walls of small air passages during respiration.

rattlesnake, a poisonous pit viper with a series of loosely connected, horny segments at the end of the tail that make a noise like a rattle when shaken. More than 25 species of rattlesnakes are found in the Americas, including many parts of the United States. They have a hematoxin in their venom, and they are responsible for most of the poisonous snake bites in the United States. See **snakebite.**

rat typhus. See **murine typhus.**

Raudixin, a trade name for an antihypertensive (purified *Rauwolfia serpentina*).

Rau-Sed, a trade name for an antihypertensive (reserpine).

Rauwiloid, a trade name for an antihypertensive (alseroxylin).

rauwolfia, the dried roots of *Rauwolfia serpentina* which provide the extracts for hypotensive agents and tranquilizing alkaloid drugs, like reserpine.

rauwolfia alkaloid, any one of more than 20 alkaloids derived from the root of a climbing shrub, *Rauwolfia serpentina,* indigenous to India and the surrounding area. Formerly used as an antipsychotic agent, its use today is confined to the treatment of hypertension. Numerous trade name formulations of the principal alkaloid reserpine are available.

rauwolfia serpentina, the dried root from *Rauwolfia serpentina,* used as an antihypertensive.

■ INDICATION: It is prescribed in the treatment of mild hypertension.

■ CONTRAINDICATIONS: Mental depression, peptic ulcer, ulcerative colitis, electroconvulsive therapy, or known hypersensitivity to this drug prohibits its use.

■ ADVERSE EFFECTS: Among the more serious adverse reactions are symptoms resembling Parkinsonism, glaucoma, cardiac arrhythmias, and gastrointestinal bleeding.

Rauzide, a trade name for a cardiovascular, fixed-combination drug containing a diuretic (bendroflumethiazide) and an antihypertensive (*Rauwolfia serpentina*).

ray, a beam of radiation, as heat or light, moving away from a source.

Raynaud's sign (reinouz'). See **acrocyanosis.**

razoxane (rəzok'sein), an investigational antineoplastic drug being studied for use in the management of certain neoplasms.

Rb, symbol for **rubidium.**

RBC, abbreviation for red blood cell. See **erythrocyte.**

RBE, abbreviation for **relative biological effectiveness.**

R.C.P., abbreviation for **Royal College of Physicians.**

RCPSC, abbreviation for **Royal College of Physicians and Surgeons of Canada.**

R.C.S., abbreviation for **Royal College of Surgeons.**

RDS, abbreviation for *respiratory distress syndrome.* See **respiratory distress syndrome of the newborn.**

re-, a combining form meaning 'back, again, contrary, etc.': *reaction, recombination, recurrent.*

Re, symbol for **rhenium.**

Reach to Recovery, a national volunteer organization that offers counseling and support to women who have breast cancer and to their families. Many of the members have had mastectomies themselves.

reaction, a response in opposition to a substance, treatment, or other stimulus, as an antigen-antibody reaction in immunology, a hypersensitivity reaction in allergy, or an adverse reaction in pharmacology. — **react,** *v.,* **reactive,** *adj.*

reaction formation, a defense mechanism in which a person avoids anxiety through overt behavior and attitudes that are the opposite of his repressed impulses and drives and that serve to conceal those unacceptable feelings.

reactive depression, an emotional disorder characterized by an acute feeling of despondency, sadness, and depressive dysphoria, which varies in intensity and duration. The condition is caused by an unrealistic and inappropriate reaction to some identifiable external situation or intrapsychic conflict and is relieved when the circumstance is altered or the conflict understood and resolved. Also called **exogenous depression, situational depression.** Compare **endogenous depression.** See also **depression.**

reactive schizophrenia, a form of schizophrenia caused by environmental factors rather than by organic changes in the brain. The onset of the disease is usually rapid; symptoms are of brief duration, and the affected individual appears well both immediately before and following the schizophrenic episode. Compare **process schizophrenia.** See also **schizophrenia, schizophreniform disorder.**

reading, (in molecular genetics) the linear process in which the genetic information contained in a nucleotide sequence is decoded, as in the translation of the messenger RNA directives for the sequence of the amino acids in a polypeptide.

Read method (rid), a method of psychophysical preparation for childbirth designed by Dr. Grantly Dick-Read. It was the first "natural childbirth" program, a term coined by Dr. Read. Basically, Read held that childbirth is a normal, physiologic procedure and that the pain of labor and delivery is of psychologic origin—the fear-tension pain syndrome. He countered womens' fears with education about the physiologic process, encouraged a positive, welcoming attitude, corrected false information, and led tours of the hospital before birth. To decrease tension, he developed a series of breathing exercises for use during the various stages of labor. To foster relaxation and optimal physical function in labor and in recovery after delivery, he incorporated a series of physical exercises to be performed regularly in classes and in practice at home during pregnancy. The woman is helped to manage labor and delivery using the Read method in the following way: during the early and mid-first stage of labor, before cervical dilatation has reached 7 cm, contractions are 2 to 5 minutes apart and last for 30 to 40 seconds. The mother lies on her back with her knees bent. Abdominal breathing is used during contractions. Her hands are placed over her lower abdomen, fingers touching. She breathes deeply and slowly—in through her nose and out through her mouth. The abdominal wall rises with each inhalation, which she can feel with her hands. The rate of breathing is no more than 6 breaths in 30 seconds, or 12 to 18 in one contraction. During the late part of the first stage of labor, after 7 cm of cervical dilatation, the contractions are 1½ to 2 minutes apart and last for 40 to 60 seconds. Costal or diaphragmatic breathing is used during contractions. Her hands are placed on her sides, over the ribs. She breathes in more shallowly, feeling her ribs move sideways against her hands. Each breath is drawn in through her nose and exhaled through her mouth. The abdominal wall does not rise and fall with this kind of breathing. The rate of breathing is no more than 6 breaths in 30 seconds, or 12 to 18 in one contraction. At the end of the first stage of labor, near full dilatation, contractions may be very strong, occurring every 1½ to 2 minutes and lasting 60 to 90 seconds. The mother lies on her back with her knees bent. Panting respirations are used during the contractions. The mother holds one of her hands on her sternum, which rises and falls as she pants lightly and rapidly through her mouth. Panting continues through the end of the first stage to full dilatation as the urge to push grows. Panting helps the woman to avoid pushing. During the second, or expulsive, stage of labor after full dilatation of the cervix, the contractions occur every 1½ to 2 minutes, last 60 to 90 seconds, and are accompanied with an urge to bear down and push. The woman lies back, head and shoulders supported in a semi-sitting position. She is helped to draw her legs up, holding them with her hands behind the lower thighs, thighs on her abdomen and spread apart. As each contraction begins, she raises her head, takes a deep breath, tucks her chin on her chest, blocks the escape of air from her lungs, and bears down. During each contraction she may need to blow the air out, refill her lungs and push again 2 or 3 times. Throughout labor she is helped to understand what is occurring and to participate and accept the experience in anticipation of the birth of the baby. Currently, many authorities who advocate use of other aspects of the Read method strongly recommend that a woman in labor not lie on her back. Supine hypotension is frequently the result of this position, as the uterus can fall back, occluding the vena cava and decreasing the volume of blood returned to the heart, thus reducing the volume of the cardiac output. Maternal hypotension follows, resulting in decreased placental perfusion and an inadequate supply of oxygen to the fetus. Today, the woman using the Read method spends most of labor lying on her side or in a semi-sitting position with her knees, back, and head well supported. Compare **Bradley method, Lamaze method.**

readthrough, (in molecular genetics) transcription of RNA beyond the normal termination sequence in the DNA template, caused by the occasional failure of RNA polymerase to respond to the end point signal.

reagent (riei′jɪnt), a chemical substance known to react in a specific way. A reagent is used to detect or synthesize another substance in a chemical reaction.

reagin, 1. an antibody associated with human atopy, as asthma and hay fever. It attaches to mast cells and basophils and sensitizes the skin and other tissues. It is associated with gamma-E-globulin and, when involved in antigen-antibody reactions, triggers the release of histamine and other mediators that cause atopic symptoms. 2. a nonspecific, nontreponemal antibodylike substance found in the serum of individuals with syphilis. It can combine with an antigen prepared as a lipid extract of normal tissue, a phenomenon that constitutes the basis of the serologic tests for syphilis. — **reaginic,** *adj.*

reagin-mediated disorder, a hypersensitivity reaction, as hay fever or an allergic response to an insect sting, produced by reaginic antibodies (IgE immunoglobulins) that bind exogenous antigen to the surface of mast cells and basophils, causing degranulation and the release of histamine, bradykinin, serotonin, and other vasoactive amines. An initial sensitizing dose of the antigen induces the formation of specific IgE antibodies, and their attachment to mast cells and basophils results in hypersensitivity to a subsequent challenging dose of the antigen. Reactions range from a simple wheal and flair on the skin to life-threatening anaphylactic shock, depending on the amount and route of entrance of the sensitizing dose and challenging dose, the amount and distribution of IgE antibodies, the responsiveness of the host, the timing of exposure to the allergen, and the tissues in which the antigen-antibody reaction occurs. The abundance of mast cells in the skin, nose, and lungs makes those areas susceptible to IgE mediated reactions. Allergens that commonly cause these reactions include plant spores, pollens, animal danders, stings, serum proteins, foods, and certain drugs. See also **allergy, generalized anaphylaxis, hay fever.**

reality principle, an awareness of the demands of the environment and the need for an adjustment of behavior to meet those demands, expressed primarily by the renunciation of immediate gratification of instinctual pleasures in order to obtain long-term and future goals. In psychoanalysis, this function is held to be performed by the ego. Compare **pleasure principle.**

reality testing, a process of evaluating the physical and social aspects of one's environment so as to differentiate between external reality and any inner imaginative world and to behave in a manner that exhibits an awareness of accepted norms and customs. Distortion of reality is indicative of a disturbance in ego functioning that may lead to psychosis.

reality therapy, a form of psychotherapy in which the aims are to help define and assess basic values within the framework of a current situation and to evaluate the person's present behavior and future plans in relation to those values. The emphasis in treatment is on the present rather than the past; it focuses on responsible behavior as a means of personal fulfillment.

reapproximate (ri′əprok′sɪmeit), to rejoin tissues separated by surgery or trauma so that their anatomic relationship is restored. — **reapproximation,** *n.*

reasonable person, (in law) a hypothetical person who possesses the qualities that are used as an objective standard upon which to judge a defendant's action in a negligence suit. In such suits, it must be decided whether or not a reasonable person, under the same circumstances, would have acted in the same way as the defendant.

rebound, 1. recovery from illness. 2. a sudden contraction of muscle following a period of relaxation, often seen in conditions in which inhibitory reflexes are lost.

rebound tenderness, a sign of inflammation of the peritoneum in which pain is elicited by the sudden release of a hand pressing on the abdomen. See also **appendicitis, peritonitis.**

rebreathing bag, (in anesthesia) a flexible bag attached to a mask. The rebreathing bag may function as a reservoir for anesthetic gases during surgery or for oxygen during resuscitation. It may be squeezed to pump the gas or air into the lungs.

recapitulation theory, the theory, formulated by German naturalist Ernst Heinrich Haeckel, that an organism during the course of embryonic development passes through stages that resemble the structural form of several ancestral types of the species as it evolved from a lower to a higher form of life. It is summarized by the statement "Ontogeny recapitulates phylogeny." Also called **biogenetic law, Haeckel's law.**

receiver, (in communication theory) the person or persons to whom a message is sent.

recess, a small hollow cavity, as the epitympanic recess in the tympanic cavity of the inner ear or the retrocecal recess extending as a small pocket behind the cecum.

recessive, of, pertaining to, or describing a gene the effect of which is masked or hidden if there is a dominant gene at the same locus. If both genes are recessive and produce the same trait the trait is expressed in the individual. See also **dominance.**

recessive gene, the member of a pair of genes that lacks the ability to express itself in the presence of its more dominant allele; it is expressed only in the homozygous state. Compare **dominant gene.**

reciprocal gene. See **complementary gene.**

reciprocal inhibition, a theory in behavior therapy that if an anxiety-producing stimulus occurs simultaneously with a response that diminishes anxiety, the stimulus may cause less anxiety, as deep chest or abdominal breathing and relaxation of the deep muscles appear to diminish anxiety and pain in childbirth. See also **systemic desensitization.**

reciprocal translocation, the mutual exchange of genetic material between two nonhomologous chromosomes. Also called **interchange.**

Recklinghausen's canal (rek'lɪŋhɑu'zənz), the small lymph space in the connective tissues of the body.

Recklinghausen's disease. See **neurofibromatosis.**

Recklinghausen's tumor, a benign tumor, derived from smooth muscle containing connective tissue and epithelial elements, that occurs in the wall of the oviduct or posterior uterine wall.

reclining, leaning backward. —**recline,** v.

recluse spider (rek'lus). See **brown spider.**

recombinant, 1. the cell or organism that results from the recombination of genes within the DNA molecule, regardless of whether naturally or artificially induced. 2. of or pertaining to such an organism or cell. See also **recombinant DNA.**

recombinant DNA, a DNA molecule in which rearrangement of the genes has been artificially induced. Enzymes are used to break isolated DNA molecules into fragments that are then rearranged in the desired sequence. Portions of DNA material from another organism of the same or a different species may also be introduced into the molecule, which is then replicated, resulting in both genotypic and phenotypic alterations in the organism. See also **genetic engineering.**

recombination, (in genetics) the formation of new combinations and arrangements of genes within the chromosome as a result of independent assortment of unlinked genes, crossing over of linked genes, or intracistronic crossing over of nucleotides. See also **recombinant DNA.**

recon (ri'kon), (in molecular genetics) the smallest genetic unit that is capable of recombination, thought to be a triplet of nucleotides.

recovery room (R.R., RR), an area adjoining the operating room to which surgical patients are taken while still under anesthesia, before being returned to their rooms. Vital signs and adequacy of ventilation are carefully observed as the patient recovers conciousness. The recovery room has equipment and a specially trained nursing staff with a nurse anesthetist or anesthesiologist available. See also **postoperative care.**

recreational therapy, a form of adjunctive psychotherapy in which games or other group activities are used as a means of modifying maladaptive behavior, awakening social interests, or improving the ability to communicate in depressed, withdrawn people.

recrudescent hepatitis, a form of acute viral hepatitis marked by a relapse during the period of recovery. A minority of patients experience it, and the prognosis for ultimate recovery is rarely affected.

recrudescent typhus. See **Brill-Zinsser disease.**

rectal anesthesia, general anesthesia achieved by the insertion, injection, or infusion of an anesthetic agent into the rectum; this procedure is performed rarely because of the unpredictability of absorption of the drug into the blood.

rectal cancer. See **colorectal cancer.**

rectal instillation of medication, the instillation of a medicated suppository, cream, or gel into the rectum. Some conditions treated by this method are constipation, pruritus ani, and hemorrhoids. The patient lies on the side, with the lower leg extended and the upper leg flexed. The nurse or physician unwraps the suppository and, wearing a glove, raises the upper buttock, exposing the anus. The suppository may be self-lubricating, or it may need to be lubricated with a water-soluble lubricant. The suppository is then gently inserted past the anal sphincter. Occasionally, a drug may be given in a medicated enema. See also **enema.**

Rectal Medicone, a trade name for a rectal, fixed-combination drug containing a topical anesthetic (benzocaine), an antiseptic (oxyquinoline sulfate), an astringent (zinc oxide), and a protectant, (Peruvian balsam).

rectal reflex, the normal response (defecation) to the presence of an accumulation of feces in the rectum. Also called **defecation reflex.**

rectitis (rektaɪ'tɪs). See **proctitis.**

rectocele (rek'təsil), a protrusion of the rectum and the posterior wall of the vagina into the vagina. The condition, which occurs after the muscles of the vagina and pelvic floor have been weakened by childbearing, old age, or surgery, may reflect a congenital weakness in the wall and may, if severe, result in dyspareunia and difficulty in evacuating the bowel. Reconstructive surgery is often helpful and is combined with any other necessary perineal, pelvic, or vaginal repair. Also called **proctocele.** Compare **cystocele.**

rectosigmoid, a portion of the anatomy that includes the lower portion of the sigmoid and the upper portion of the rectum.

rectouterine excavation (rek′touyu′tərɪn). See **cul-de-sac of Douglas.**

rectouterine pouch. See **cul-de-sac of Douglas.**

rectum (rek′təm), *pl.* **rectums, recta.** the portion of the large intestine, about 12 cm long, continuous with the descending sigmoid colon, just proximal to the anal canal. It follows the sacrococcygeal curve, ends in the anal canal, and usually contains three transverse semilunar folds: one situated proximally on the right side, a second one extending inward from the left side, and a third and largest fold projecting caudally. Each fold is about 12 mm wide. The folds overlap when the intestine is empty. –**rectal,** *adj.*

rectus abdominis, one of a pair of anterolateral muscles of the abdomen, extending the whole length of the ventral aspect of the abdomen. The pair is separated by the linea alba. Each rectus arises in a lateral tendon from the crest of the pubis and is interlaced by a medial tendon with that of the opposite side. The rectus abdominis inserts into the fifth, the sixth, and the seventh ribs. It is innervated by branches of the seventh through the twelfth intercostal nerves and functions to flex the vertebral column, tense the anterior abdominal wall, and assist in compressing the abdominal contents. Compare **obliquus externus abdominis, obliquus internus abdominis, pyramidalis, transversus abdominis.**

rectus femoris, a fusiform muscle of the anterior thigh, one of the four parts of the quadriceps femoris. It arises in an anterior tendon originating in the iliac spine and in a posterior tendon originating in the brim of the acetabulum. The two tendons unite and spread into a broad, thick aponeurosis, that extends downward over the thigh in the center of the quadriceps femoris. The aponeurosis narrows into a flattened tendon that inserts into the base of the patella. The rectus femoris is innervated by branches of the femoral nerve, which contain fibers from the second, third, and fourth lumbar nerves, and it functions to flex the leg. Compare **vastus intermedius, vastus lateralis, vastus medialis.** See also **quadriceps femoris.**

rectus muscle, a muscle of the body that has a relatively straight form. Some kinds of rectus muscles are **rectus abdominis, rectus capitis anterior, and rectus capitis lateralis.**

recumbent (rɪkəm′bənt), lying down or leaning backward. See also **reclining.** –**recumbency,** *n.*

recurrent bandage, a bandage which is wrapped several times around itself, usually applied to the head or an amputated stump.

recurrent fever. See **relapsing fever.**

recurvatum (ri′kərvei′təm), backward thrust of the knee caused by weakness of the quadriceps.

red blood cell (RBC). See **erythrocyte.**

Red Book of the American Academy of Pediatrics, a book that serves as the standard reference source of immunization procedures for children and adults. It is available from the American Academy of Pediatrics Inc., Evanston, Illinois.

red bug. See **chigger.**

red cell. See **erythrocyte.**

red cell indices, a series of relationships that characterize the red cell population in terms of size, hemoglobin content, and hemoglobin concentration. Derived mathematically from the red cell count and the hemoglobin and hematocrit values, the indices are useful in making differential diagnoses of several kinds of anemia. The values reported are the mean corpuscular hemoglobin (MCH), the mean corpuscular hemoglobin concentration (MCHC), and the mean corpuscular volume (MCV).

red corpuscle. See **erythrocyte.**

Red Cross. 1. See **International Red Cross Society. 2.** See **American Red Cross.**

red fever. See **dengue.**

red hepatization. See **hepatization.**

red marrow, the red vascular substance consisting of connective tissue and blood vessels containing primitive blood cells, macrophages, megakaryocytes, and fat cells. It is found in the cavities of many bones, including the flat and the short bones, the bodies of the vertebrae, the sternum, the ribs, and the articulating ends of the long bones. Red marrow manufactures and releases leukocytes and erythrocytes into the blood stream. Compare **yellow marrow.**

redon, the smallest unit of the DNA molecule capable of recombination; it may be as small as one deoxyribonucleotide pair. Compare **cistron, muton.**

reduce, (in surgery) the restoration of a part to its original position after displacement, as in the reduction of a fractured bone by bringing ends or fragments back into alignment or of a hernia by returning the bowel to its normal position. A fracture may be reduced under local or general anesthesia. If performed by outside manipulation alone, the reduction is said to be closed; if surgery is necessary, it is said to be open. See also **fracture, hernia, invagination, traction.** –**reduce,** *v.*

reduction, 1. Also called **hydrogenation.** the addition of hydrogen to a substance. **2.** the removal of oxygen from a substance. **3.** the decrease in the valence of the electronegative part of a compound. **4.** the addition of one or more electrons to a molecule or atom of a substance. **5.** the correction of a fracture, hernia, or luxation. **6.** the reduction of data, as in converting interval data to an ordinal or nominal scale of measurement.

reduction diet, a diet that is low in calories, used for reduction of body weight. The diet must supply fewer calories than the individual expends each day while supplying all the essential nutrients for maintaining health. A usual diet of this type provides 1,200 calories per day from the basic food groups. Meats are usually broiled, roasted, stewed, or sautéed, vegetables are steamed or eaten raw; starches and fats are limited; and fresh fruits replace desserts. Foods to be avoided are sweetened carbonated beverages, fried foods, pastries, and most snack foods. Vitamin and mineral deficiencies may result if such a diet is not carefully planned. Also called **low-caloric diet, reducing diet.**

reduction division. See **meiosis.**

Reed-Sternberg cell (rid'stərn'bərg), one of a number of large, abnormal, multinucleated reticuloendothelial cells in the lymphatic system in Hodgkin's disease. The number and proportion of Reed-Sternberg cells identified are the basis for the histopathologic classification of Hodgkin's disease.

reefer. *Slang.* See **cannabis.**

refereed journal, a professional or literary journal in which articles or papers are selected for publication by a panel of referees who are experts in the field. They read and evaluate each of the articles submitted for publication. The important national professional journals in medicine and nursing are refereed.

referential idea. See **idea of reference.**

referred pain, pain felt at a site different from that of an injured or diseased organ or part of the body. Angina, the pain of coronary artery insufficiency, may be felt in the left shoulder, arm, or jaw. In disease of the gall bladder, pain may be felt in the right shoulder or scapular region.

refined birth rate, the ratio of total births to the total female population, considered during a period of one year. Compare **birth rate, crude birth rate, true birth rate.**

reflex action, the involuntary functioning or movement of any organ or part of the body in response to a particular stimulus. The function or action occurs immediately, without the involvement of the will or consciousness. See also **reflex arc.**

reflex apnea, involuntary cessation of respiration owing to irritating, noxious vapors or gases.

reflex bladder. See **spastic bladder.**

reflex dyspepsia, an abnormal condition characterized by impaired digestion associated with the disease of an organ not directly involved with digestion. See also **dyspepsia.**

reflux, an abnormal backward or return flow of a fluid. Kinds of reflux include **gastroesophageal reflux, hepatojugular reflux, vesicoureteral reflux.**

refracting medium. See **medium.**

refraction, 1. the change of direction of energy as it passes from one medium to another of different density. 2. an examination to determine and to correct refractive errors of the eye.

refractory period, the interval following the excitation of a neuron or the contraction of a muscle during which repolarization of the cell membrane occurs. The period is divided into two phases: the absolute refractory period and the relative refractory period. During the absolute stage the cell is incapable of responding to any stimulus, regardless of its strength, because of total depolarization. During the relative phase, as repolarization is underway, a stimulus intensity above the threshold may elicit a response even though the normal resting potential of the cell has not been reached.

Refsum's syndrome (ref'sumz), a rare, hereditary disorder of lipid metabolism in which phytanic acid cannot be broken down. The syndrome is characterized by ataxia, abnormalities of the bones and skin, peripheral neuropathy, and retinitis pigmentosa. Foods containing phytanic acid must be avoided to prevent progressive deterioration. Also called **phytanic acid storage disease.**

regional, of or pertaining to a geographical area, as a regional medical facility, or to a part of the body, as regional anesthesia.

regional anatomy, the study of the structural relationships within the organs and the parts of the body. Kinds of regional anatomy are **surface anatomy** and **cross-sectional anatomy.**

regional anesthesia, anesthesia of an area of the body by injecting a local anesthetic to block a group of sensory nerve fibers. Kinds of regional anesthesia include **brachial plexus anesthesia, epidural anesthesia, intercostal anesthesia, paracervical anesthesia, pudendal anesthesia, spinal anesthesia.**

regional enteritis. See **Crohn's disease.**

regionalization, (in health care planning) the organization of a system for the delivery of health care within a region to avoid costly duplication of services and to ensure availability of essential services. Hospitals are classified as primary, secondary, and tertiary health centers, depending on the facilities and personnel available, the population served, the number of beds in the institution, and other criteria.

registered nurse (RN), 1. *U.S.* a professional nurse who has completed a course of study at a school of nursing accredited by the National League for Nursing and who has taken and passed the State Board Test Pool Examination. A registered nurse may use the initials RN following the signature. RNs are licensed to practice by individual states. 2. *Canada.* a professional nurse who has completed a course of study at an approved school of nursing and who has taken and passed an examination administered by the Canadian Nurses Association Testing Service. See also **nurse, nursing.**

Registered Therapist (R.T.), a title awarded by the American Registry of Radiologic Technicians as certification of qualification to act as an x-ray technician.

registrar, an administrative officer whose responsibility is to maintain the records of an institution.

registry, 1. an office or agency in which lists of nurses and records pertaining to nurses seeking employment are maintained. 2. (in epidemiology) a listing service for incidence data pertaining to the occurrence of specific diseases or disorders, as a tumor registry.

Regitine, a trade name for an alpha-adrenergic blocking agent (phentolamine), used as an adjunct to anesthesia.

Regitine Hydrochloride, a trade name for an alpha-adrenergic blocking agent (phentolamine hydrochloride).

Reglan, a trade name for a gastrointestinal stimulant (metoclopramide hydrochloride).

Regonal (reg'ınəl), a trade name for a neuromuscular blocking agent (pyridostigmine), used as an adjunct to anesthesia.

regression, 1. a retreat or backward movement in conditions, signs, or symptoms. 2. a return to an earlier, more primitive form of behavior. 3. a tendency in physical development to become more typical of the population than of the parents, as a child who attains a height closer to the average than that of tall or short parents. —**regress,** v.

Regroton, a trade name for a cardiovascular, fixed-combination drug containing a diuretic (chlorthalidone) and an antihypertensive (reserpine).

regular diet, a full, well-balanced diet containing all of the essential nutrients needed for optimal growth, repair of the tissues, and normal functioning of the organs. Such a diet contains foods rich in proteins, carbohydrates, fats, minerals, and vitamins in proportions that meet the specific caloric requirements of the individual. Also called **full diet, normal diet.**

Regular Iletin, a trade name for insulin injection (crystalline zinc insulin).

Regular Insulin, a trade name for insulin injection (crystalline zinc insulin).

regulative cleavage. See **indeterminate cleavage.**

regulative development, a type of embryonic development in which the fertilized ovum undergoes indeterminate cleavage, producing blastomeres that have similar developmental potencies and are each capable of giving rise to a single embryo. Determination of the particular organs and parts of the embryo occurs during later stages of development and is influenced by inductors and intercellular interaction. Damage or destruction of various cells during the early stages of development results in readjustments and substitutions so that a normal organism is formed. Compare **mosaic development.**

regulatory gene, (in molecular genetics) a genetic unit that regulates or suppresses the activity of one or more structural genes.

regulatory sequence, (in molecular genetics) a series of DNA nucleotides that regulate the expression of a gene.

regurgitation, 1. the return of swallowed food into the mouth. 2. the backward flow of blood through a defective heart valve, named for the affected valve, as in **aortic regurgitation.**

rehabilitation, the restoration of an individual or a part to normal or near normal function following a disabling disease, injury, addiction, or incarceration. —**rehabilitate,** v.

rehabilitation center, a facility providing therapy and training for rehabilitation. The center may offer occupational therapy, physical therapy, vocational training, and special training, like speech therapy. See also **rehabilitation.**

Rehfuss stomach tube (rei'fəs), a specially designed gastric tube with a graduated syringe, used for withdrawing specimens of the contents of the stomach for study following a test meal.

Reifenstein's syndrome (rai'fənstäinz), male hypogonadism of unknown etiology, marked by azoospermia, undescended testes, gynecomastia, testosterone deficiency, and elevated gonadotropin titers. The condition appears to be inherited as an x-linked recessive trait, but no chromosomal abnormality has been identified.

reinforcement, (in psychology) a process in which a response is strengthened by the fear of punishment or the anticipation of reward.

Reiter's syndrome (rai'tərz), an arthritic disorder of adult males, believed to result from a myxovirus or *Mycoplasma* infection. The syndrome most often affects the ankles, feet, and sacroiliac joints and is usually associated with conjunctivitis and urethritis. The onset may be marked by unexplained diarrhea and low-grade fever, followed in 2 to 4 weeks by conjunctivitis. Lesions that become superficial ulcers may form on the palms and the soles. Arthritis usually persists after the conjunctivitis and urethritis subside, but it may become episodic. Treatment includes a short course of tetracycline to treat the infection and phenylbutazone to relieve pain and inflammation in the joint. Recovery is expected, but recurrent arthritic symptoms may continue for several years.

rejection, 1. (in medicine) an immunological response to organisms or substances that the system recognizes as foreign, including grafts or transplants. 2. (in psychiatry) the act of excluding or denying affection to another person.

Rela, a trade name for a skeletal muscle relaxant (carisoprodol).

relapse, 1. to exhibit again the symptoms of a disease from which a patient appears to have recovered. 2. the recurrence of a disease after apparent recovery. —**relapsing,** adj.

relapsing fever, any one of several acute infectious diseases, marked by recurrent febrile episodes, caused by various strains of the spirochete *Borrelia.* The disease is transmitted by both lice and ticks and is often seen during wars and famines. It has occurred in several western states of the United States but is more commonly found in South America, Asia, and Africa. The first episode usually starts with a sudden high fever (104° to 105°F), accompanied by chills, headache, neuromuscular pains, and nausea. A rash may appear over the trunk and extremities, and jaundice is common during the later stages. Each attack lasts two or three days and culminates in a crisis of high fever, profuse sweating, and a rise in heart and respiratory rate. This is followed by an abrupt drop in temperature and a return to normal blood pressure. People typically relapse after seven to ten days of normal temperature and eventually recover completely. In louse-borne disease, there is usually only a single relapse; in tick-borne disease, several successively milder relapses may occur. To make a diagnosis, the spirochete must be seen on a blood smear obtained during an attack. Treatment is with a long-acting penicillin, tetracycline, or chloramphenicol. Antimicrobial therapy may induce a Herxheimer reaction, so treatment is withheld during a febrile crisis. Bed rest, sponge baths, and aspirin alleviate the symptoms. Disinfection of clothing and bedding is necessary to destroy any lice or ticks. Also called **African tick fever, famine fever, recurrent fever, spirillum fever, tick fever.**

relapsing polychondritis, a rare disease of unknown cause resulting in inflammation and destruction of cartilage with replacement by fibrous tissue. Autoimmunity may be involved in this condition. Most commonly the ears and noses of middle-aged people are affected with episodes of tender swelling, often accompanied by fever, arthralgias, and episcleritis. Consequences include floppy ears, collapsed nose, hearing loss, or hoarseness and airway obstruction owing to laryngeal and tracheal cartilage involvement. Corticosteroids suppress the activity of the disease.

relation searching, (in nursing research) a study design used to discover and describe relationships between and among variables. It may be used to describe various nursing situations in order to examine the efficacy of certain aspects of nursing care.

relative biological effectiveness (RBE), (in radiotherapy) the ratio of the effect of an absorbed dose of a form of radiation under study to the effect of a standard, reference form of radiation.

relative cephalopelvic disproportion. See **cephalopelvic disproportion.**

relative growth, the comparison of the various increases in size of similar organisms, tissues, or structures at different time intervals.

relative refractory period. See **refractory period.**

relative risk, an assessment of the degree or incidence of adverse effects that may be expected in the presence of a particular factor or event as compared to the expected adverse effects in the absence of the factor or event.

relaxation, 1. a reducing of tension, as when a muscle relaxes between contractions. 2. a lessening of pain.

relaxation therapy, treatment in which patients are taught to perform breathing and relaxation exercises and to concentrate on a pleasant situation when a noxious stimulus is applied. An integral part of the Lamaze method of childbirth, relaxation therapy is also used to relieve various kinds of pain and physical manifestations of stress. Various yoga exercises and aspects of hypnotherapy may be included in the treatment program, and biofeedback techniques may be used to demonstrate actions that induce relaxation. Some patients learn through relaxation therapy to relax taut muscles at will, to abort migraine attacks, or to reduce their blood pressure. See also **Lamaze method.**

releasing hormone (RH), one of several peptides produced by the hypothalamus and secreted directly to the anterior pituitary via a portal vein. Each of the releasing hormones stimulates the pituitary to secrete a specific trophic hormone; thus, corticotrophic releasing hormone stimulates the pituitary to secrete adrenocorticotrophic hormone, while growth hormone releasing hormone stimulates the secretion of growth hormone.

reliability, (in research) the extent to which a test measurement or a device produces the same results with different investigators, observers, or administration of the test over time. The repeated use of the same measurement tool on the same sample produces the same consistent results if the measurement is reliable.

rem, roentgen equivalent man. A dose of ionizing radiation that produces in man the same effect as one roentgen of x radiation or gamma radiation.

REM, abbreviation for **rapid eye movement.** See **sleep.**

remission, the partial or complete disappearance of the clinical and subjective characteristics of a chronic or malignant disease. Remission may be spontaneous or the result of therapy. In some cases remission is permanent and the disease is cured. Compare **cure.**

remittent fever, diurnal variations of an elevated temperature with exacerbations and remissions but never a return to normal.

remote afterloading, (in radiotherapy) a technique in which an applicator, as an acrylic mold of an area to be irradiated, is placed in or on the patient and then loaded from a safe source with a high-activity radioisotope. The mold or applicator contains grooves for the insertion of nylon tubes into which the radioactive material can be introduced. Remote afterloading is used in the treatment of head, neck, vaginal, and cervical tumors.

Remsed, a trade name for an antiemetic and antihistaminic (promethazine hydrochloride).

ren-, a combining form meaning 'of or pertaining to the kidneys': *renicardiac, reniform, renocortical.*

renal (ri′nəl), of or pertaining to the kidney.

renal adenocarcinoma. See **clear cell carcinoma of the kidney.**

renal artery, one of a pair of large, visceral branches of the abdominal aorta, arising caudal to the superior mesenteric artery at the level of the disc between the first and second lumbar vertebrae. The left renal artery is somewhat more cranial than the right. Before reaching the kidney, each divides into four branches. The renal arteries supply the kidney, suprarenal glands, and the ureters.

renal biopsy, the removal of kidney tissue for microscopic examination, conducted to establish the diagnosis of a renal disorder and to aid in determining the stage of the disease, the appropriate therapy, and the prognosis. An open biopsy involves an incision, permits better visualization of the kidney, and carries a lower risk of hemorrhage; a closed or percutaneous biopsy performed by aspirating a specimen of tissue with a needle requires a shorter period of recovery and is less likely to cause infection.

■ METHOD: Prior to biopsy, the procedure is explained and the patient is medically evaluated and tested for bleeding or coagulation time. The patient's blood is usually typed and cross matched with two units of donor blood that are held for a possible transfusion until there is no threat of bleeding after the procedure. An open biopsy is generally carried out in the operating room, but the percutaneous procedure may be performed in the radiology department or in the patient's room. The location of the kidney, determined by a plain x-ray film, dye contrast study, or fluoroscopic examination, is marked on the patient's skin in ink for a needle biopsy. The patient is then placed prone over a sandbag and soft pillow with the body bent at the level of the diaphragm, the shoulders on the bed, and the spine in straight alignment. A local anesthetic is injected and the physician inserts the biopsy needle in the lower pole of the kidney, since this area contains the smallest number of large renal vessels. The needle is quickly withdrawn and, after pressure is applied to the site for 20 minutes, a pressure bandage is applied; the patient is turned and kept supine and motionless for the next four hours. The dressing, blood pressure, and pulse are checked every 15 to 60 minutes for two hours, the temperature every four hours for 24 hours; excessive drainage, decreased blood pressure, tachycardia, or elevated temperature are reported to the physician. Fluids are forced to the maximum allotted for the patient's condition; the amount and character of urinary output are noted and the physician is informed if hematuria occurs. The patient is kept in bed for at least 24 hours and is cautioned not to lift any heavy objects for ten days.

■ NURSING ORDERS: The nurse offers an explanation of the procedure, prepares and positions the patient for the percutaneous procedure, and, on its completion, provides care and emotional support.

■ OUTCOME CRITERIA: A biopsy is the most accurate measure for determining the nature and stage of a renal pathologic condition.

renal calculus. See **urinary calculus.**

renal calyx, the first unit in the system of ducts in the kidney carrying urine from the renal pyramid of the cortex to the renal pelvis for excretion through the ureters. There are two divisions: the **minor calyx,** with several others, drains into a larger **major calyx,** which in turn joins other major calyces to form the renal pelvis.

renal cell carcinoma, a malignant neoplasm of the kidney, composed predominantly of large cells with clear cytoplasm that originate in tubular epithelium. The tumor may develop in any part of the kidney, becoming a large mass which may grow into the tributaries of the renal vein. Hematuria and pain are usually present. Metastasis, especially to the lungs and bones, may occur early in the course of development. Treatment includes surgery and radiotherapy. Also called **adenocarcinoma of the kidney, clear cell carcinoma of the kidney.** See also **Wilms' tumor.**

renal colic, sharp, severe pain in the lower back over the kidney, radiating forward into the groin. Renal colic usually accompanies forcible dilation of a ureter followed by spasm as a stone is lodged or passed through it. See also **urinary calculus.**

renal corpuscle. See **Malpighian corpuscle.**

renal cortex, the soft, granular, outer layer of the kidney, containing approximately 1.25 million renal tubules which remove body wastes in the form of urine.

renal diet, a diet prescribed in chronic renal failure and designed to control the intake of protein, potassium, sodium, phosphorus, and fluids, depending on individual conditions. Carbohydrates and fats are the principal sources of energy. Protein is limited; the amount is determined by the patient's condition and is usually supplied from milk, eggs, and meat. Cereals, bread, rice, and pasta are the primary sources of calories. Some vegetables and fruits are included, depending on the degree of restriction of potassium and phosphorus. Special commercial flours and breads have been developed that are protein-free and low in potassium and sodium. The low potassium level of the diet also makes it useful in hyperkalemia. The diet is nutritionally inadequate and should be supplemented with vitamins and electrolytes. See also **Giordano-Giovannetti diet.**

renal dwarf, a dwarf whose retarded growth is caused by renal failure.

renal failure, inability of the kidneys to excrete wastes, concentrate urine, and conserve electrolytes. The condition may be acute or chronic. **Acute kidney failure** is characterized by oliguria and by the rapid accumulation of nitrogenous wastes in the blood. It is caused by hemorrhage, trauma, burn, toxic injury to the kidney, acute pyelonephritis or glomerulonephritis, or lower urinary tract obstruction. Many forms of acute renal failure are reversible after the underlying cause has been identified. Treatment includes restricted intake of fluids and of all substances that require excretion by the kidney. Antibiotics and diuretics are also used. **Chronic renal failure** may result from many other diseases. The early signs include sluggishness, fatigue, and mental dullness. Later, anuria, convulsions, gastrointestinal bleeding, malnutrition and various neuropathies may occur. The skin may turn yellow-brown and become covered with uremic frost. Congestive heart failure and hypertension are frequent complications, the results of hypervolemia. Urinalysis reveals greater than normal amounts of urea and creatinine, waxy casts, and a constant volume of urine regardless of variations in water intake. Anemia frequently occurs. The prognosis depends upon the underlying cause. Treatment usually includes restricted water and protein intake and the use of diuretics. When medical measures have been exhausted, long-term hemodialysis is often begun, and kidney transplantation is considered.

renal hypertension, hypertension resulting from kidney disease, including chronic glomerulonephritis, chronic pyelonephritis, renal carcinoma, and renal calculi. Analgesic abuse and certain drug reactions may also result in renal hypertension. Therapy depends on the cause and may include administration of antibiotics or diuretics or surgery. Untreated renal hypertension is likely to result in kidney damage and cardiovascular disease.

renal nanism, dwarfism associated with infantile renal osteodystrophy.

renal papilla. See **papilla.**

renal rickets, a condition characterized by rachitic changes in the skeleton and caused by chronic nephritis.

renal tubular acidosis (RTA), an abnormal condition associated with persistent dehydration, metabolic acidosis, hypokalemia, hyperchloremia, and nephrocalcinosis. It is caused by the inability of the kidneys to conserve bicarbonate and to adequately acidify the urine. Some forms of RTA are more prevalent in females, older children, and young adults. Prolonged RTA can cause hypercalciuria and the formation of kidney stones. Depending on treatment and the extent of renal damage prognosis is usually good. Compare **distal renal tubular acidosis, proximal renal tubular acidosis, metabolic acidosis, respiratory acidosis.**

■ OBSERVATIONS: Some common signs and symptoms of RTA, especially in children, may include anorexia, vomiting, constipation, retarded growth, polyuria, nephrocalcinosis, and rickets. In children and adults RTA can also cause urinary tract infections and pyelonephritis. Confirming diagnosis of distal RTA is based on laboratory tests which show impaired urine acidification in association with systemic metabolic acidosis. Confirming diagnosis of proximal RTA is based on tests that show bicarbonate wasting owing to impaired reabsorption. Other significant laboratory findings may show decreased sodium bicarbonate, pH, potassium, and phosphorus, increased serum chloride, alkaline phosphatase, urinary bicarbonate, and potassium, and urine with low specific gravity.

■ INTERVENTION: Treatment seeks to replace excessively secreted substances, especially bicarbonate, and may include the administration of sodium bicarbonate tablets, potassium to counter low potassium levels, vitamin D to preserve calcium metabolism, and antibiotics to counter pyelonephritis. Surgery may be required to excise renal calculi.

■ NURSING CONSIDERATIONS: The nurse carefully monitors all laboratory tests, especially those involving potassium levels and urine pH. The urine of the patient is strained to capture any kidney stones for analysis and the nurse is alert to any signs of hematuria. Patients with low potassium levels are usually advised to eat potassium-rich foods, as bananas, oranges, and baked potatoes. The patient and family also benefit from advice and encouragement in seeking genetic counseling and RTA screening.

Rendu-Osler-Weber syndrome (rendu′ous′lərweb′ər). See **Osler-Weber-Rendu syndrome.**

Renese, a trade name for a diuretic and antihypertensive (polythiazide).

renin (ri′nin), a proteolytic enzyme, produced by and stored in the juxtaglomerular apparatus that surrounds each arteriole as it enters a glomerulus. The enzyme affects the blood pressure by catalyzing the change of angiotensinogen to angiotensin, a strong pressor. Compare **rennin.**

rennin (ren′in), a milk-curdling enzyme that occurs in the gastric juices of infants and is also contained in the rennet produced in the stomach of calves and other ruminants. It is an endopeptidase that converts casein to paracasein and was formerly used extensively as a curdling agent by the cheese industry. An artifically produced microbial rennet, rather than the enzyme extracted from rennet in calves, is used in half the cheese produced in the United States today. Compare **renin.**

Renoquid, a trade name for an antibacterial (sulfacytine).

renovascular hypertension. See **portal hypertension.**

reovirus (ri′ouvai′rəs), any one of three ubiquitous, double-stranded RNA viruses found in the respiratory and alimentary tracts in healthy and in sick people. Reoviruses have been implicated in some cases of upper respiratory disease and infantile gastroenteritis.

Repen-VK, a trade name for an antibacterial (penicillin V potassium).

repetition compulsion, an unconscious need to revert to and repeat earlier situations, patterns of behavior, and acts in order to experience previously felt emotions or relationships. See also **compulsion.**

replacement, the substitution of a missing part or substance with a similar structure or substance, as the replacement of an amputated limb with a prosthesis or the replacement of lost blood with donor blood.

replication, 1. a process of duplicating, reproducing, or copying; literally, a folding back of a part to form a duplicate. 2. (in research) the exact repetition of an experiment performed to confirm the initial findings. 3. Also called **semiconservative replication.** (in genetics) the duplication of the polynucleotide strands of DNA, or the synthesis of DNA. The process involves the unwinding of the double helix molecule to form two single strands, each of which acts as a template for the synthesis of a complementary strand. The two resulting molecules of DNA each contain one new and one parental strand which coil to form the double helix. —**replicate,** v.

replicator, (in genetics) the segment of the DNA molecule that initiates and controls the replication of the polynucleotide strands.

replicon (rep′lǝkon), (in genetics) a replication unit; the segment of the DNA molecule that is undergoing replication. The unit is regulated by a section of the molecule, called the regulator, which controls replication and coordinates it with cell division.

Repoise Maleate, a trade name for a phenothiazine tranquilizer (butaperazine maleate).

report, (in nursing) the transfer of information from the nurses on one shift to the nurses on the following shift. Report is given systematically at the time of change of shift. The head nurse, team leader, or primary nurse conducts the report, summarizing the progress and status of each patient, for the nurses who will next assume responsibility for the care. The provider of the information is said to 'give report' and the oncoming staff to 'take report.' Report may be given to the assembled oncoming staff, or it may be taperecorded so that staff members can listen to it individually or in a group on their own schedule. The Kardex and medcard of each patient are updated before report, and staff members are informed of the changes during report.

repression, 1. the act of restraining, inhibiting, or suppressing. 2. (in psychoanalysis) an unconscious defense mechanism whereby unacceptable thoughts, feelings, ideas, impulses, or memories, especially those concerning some traumatic past event, are pushed from the consciousness because of their painful guilt association or disagreeable content and are submerged in the unconscious, where they remain dormant but operant and dynamic. Such repressed emotional conflicts are the source of anxiety which may lead to any of the anxiety disorders. Compare **suppression.** —**repress,** v, **repressive,** adj.

repressor, (in molecular genetics) a protein that binds to a sequence of nucleotides regulating an adjacent gene. The repressor, when bound, blocks the transcription of the gene.

repressor gene, (in molecular genetics) a unit of genetic information that represses the activity of another gene.

reproduction, 1. the process by which animals and plants give rise to offspring; procreation; the sum total of the cellular and genetic phenomena involved in the transmission of organic life from one organism to successive generations similar to the parents so that the perpetuation and continuity of the species is maintained. In humans, the germ cells, the spermatozoa in the male and the ova in the female, which are produced by the testes and ovaries, unite during fertilization to form the new individual. 2. the creation of a similar structure, situation, or phenomenon; duplication; replication. 3. (in psychology) the recalling of a former idea, impression, or something previously learned. Kinds of reproduction include **asexual reproduction, cytogenic reproduction, sexual reproduction, somatic reproduction, unisexual reproduction.** See also **fertilization, oogenesis, pregnancy, spermatogenesis.** —**reproductive,** adj.

repulsion, 1. the act of repelling, disjoining; a force that separates two bodies or things. 2. (in genetics) the situation in linked inheritance in which the alleles of two or more mutant genes are located on homologous chromosomes so that each chromosome of the pair carries one or more mutant and wild-type genes, which are located close enough to be inherited together. Compare **coupling.** See also **trans configuration.**

request for proposal (RFP), a solicitation by a funding agency for proposals to accomplish a particular goal. The RFP lists the requirements a project must meet to receive funding.

RES, abbreviation for **reticuloendothelial system.**

rescinnamine (rɪsɪn′ǝmɪn), an alkaloid antihypertensive.
■ INDICATION: It is prescribed in the treatment of mild hypertension.
■ CONTRAINDICATIONS: Mental depression, electroconvulsive therapy, or known hypersensitivity to this drug prohibits its use.
■ ADVERSE EFFECTS: Among the more serious adverse reactions are gastrointestinal, cardiovascular, and central nervous system disturbances.

research instrument, a testing device for measuring a given phenomenon, as a paper-and-pencil test, a questionnaire, an interview, or a set of guidelines for observation.

research measurement, an evaluation of the quantity or incidence of a given variable as obtained by using a research instrument.

research radiopharmaceutical, a drug that is labeled with a small quantity of a radioactive tracer in order to study its biodistribution; it may later be used in a nonradioactive form.

resect, to remove tissue from the body by surgery. Resection of an organ may be partial or complete.

resection, the cutting out of a significant portion of an organ or structure. A kind of resection is a **wedge resection.**

reserpine (res'ərpin), an antihypertensive.

■ INDICATION: It is prescribed in the treatment of high blood pressure.

■ CONTRAINDICATIONS: Mental depression, peptic ulcer, ulcerative colitis, or known hypersensitivity to this drug prohibits its use.

■ ADVERSE EFFECTS: Among the more serious adverse reactions are mental depression, extrapyramidal reactions, impotence, aggravation of peptic ulcer, and paradoxical excitement.

reserve, a potential capacity to maintain the vital functions of the body in homeostasis by adjusting to increased need, as cardiac reserve, pulmonary reserve, and alkali reserve. See also **homeostasis.**

reserve cell carcinoma. See **oat cell carcinoma.**

reservoir bag, a component of an anesthesia machine in which gas accumulates, forming a reserve supply of gas for use when the quantity of flow is inadequate. This component also permits "bagging," or manual control of ventilation, and serves as a visible monitor of machine function.

reservoir host, a nonhuman host that serves as a means of sustaining an infectious organism as a potential source of human infection. Wild monkeys are reservoir hosts for the yellow fever virus, which may at times spread from the jungle to infect humans.

reservoir of infection, a continuous source of infectious disease. People, animals, and plants may be reservoirs of infection.

resident, a physician in one of the postgraduate years of clinical training following the first, or internship year. The length of residency varies according to the specialty. See also **PGY.**

residual volume, the volume of gas in the lungs at the end of a maximum expiration.

residue schizophrenia, a form of schizophrenia in which there is a history of at least one psychotic schizophrenic episode and objective signs of the illness, in which social withdrawal, eccentric behavior, illogical thinking, and inappropriate emotional reactions persist. The symptoms are less severe than those manifested by persons classified as psychotic. See also **schizophrenia.**

res ipsa loquitur (reis' ɪp'sə lok'wɪtʊr), *Latin. literal.* 'the thing speaks for itself.' a legal concept that is important in many malpractice suits. It describes a situation in which an injury occurred when the defendant was solely and exclusively in control and in which the injury would not have occurred had due care been exercised. Classic examples of res ipsa loquitur are a sponge left in the abdomen after abdominal surgery and the amputation of the wrong extremity.

resistance transfer factor. See **R factor.**

resonance, an echo or other sound produced by percussion of an organ or cavity of the body during a physical examination. – **resonant,** *adj.*

resorcinated camphor (rɪzɔr'sɪnei'tɪd), a mixture of camphor and resorcinol, used for the treatment of pediculosis and itching.

resorcinol test. See **Boas' test.**

respiration, the process of the molecular exchange of oxygen and carbon dioxide within the pulmonary system. The rate varies with the age and condition of the person. Some kinds of respiration are **Biot's respiration, Cheyne-Stokes respiration, Kussmaul respiration.**

respirator, an apparatus used to modify air for inspiration or to improve pulmonary ventilation. See also **nebulizer, negative phase ventilator.**

respiratory (res'pərətori, rɪspair'ətɔr'i), of or pertaining to respiration.

respiratory acidosis, an abnormal condition characterized by increased arterial PCO_2, excess carbonic acid, and increased plasma hydrogen-ion concentration. It is caused by reduced alveolar ventilation, which can result from various disorders, as airway obstruction, medullary trauma, neuromuscular disease, chest injuries, pneumonia, pulmonary edema, emphysema, and cardiopulmonary arrest. It may also be caused by the suppression of respiratory reflexes with narcotics, sedatives, hypnotics, or anesthetics. The hypoventilation associated with this condition inhibits the excretion of carbon dioxide, which consequently combines with water in the body to produce excessive carbonic acid and thus reduces blood pH. Compare **metabolic acidosis.** See also **metabolic alkalosis, respiratory alkalosis.**

■ OBSERVATIONS: Some common signs and symptoms of respiratory acidosis are headache, dyspnea, fine tremors, tachycardia, hypertension, and vasodilation. Confirming diagnosis is usually based on arterial blood gas values for PCO_2 over the normal 45 mm/Hg and on pH values below the normal range of 7.35 to 7.45. Ineffective treatment of acute respiratory acidosis can lead to coma and death.

■ INTERVENTION: Treatment of this condition seeks to remove or to inhibit the underlying causes of associated hypoventilation. Any airway obstructions are immediately removed. Treatment may include oxygen therapy and the intravenous administration of bronchodilators and sodium bicarbonate.

■ NURSING CONSIDERATIONS: The patient with respiratory acidosis is carefully monitored for any changes in respiratory, cardiovascular, and CNS functions, arterial blood gas pressures, and electrolyte concentrations. In patients requiring mechanical ventilation, clear airways are maintained and tracheal tubes are regularly suctioned. Adequate hydration is also important.

respiratory alkalosis, an abnormal condition characterized by decreased PCO_2, decreased hydrogen-ion concentration, and increased blood pH. It is caused by pulmonary and nonpulmonary problems. Some pulmonary causes are acute asthma, pulmonary vascular disease, and pneumonia. Some nonpulmonary causes are aspirin toxicity, anxiety, fever, metabolic acidosis, inflammation of the central nervous system, gram-negative septicemia, and hepatic failure. The hyperventilation associated with respiratory alkalosis most commonly stems from extreme anxiety. Compare **metabolic alkalosis.** See also **metabolic acidosis, respiratory acidosis.**

■ OBSERVATIONS: Deep and rapid breathing at rates as high as 40 respirations per minute is a major sign of respiratory alkalosis. Other symptoms are light-headedness, dizziness, peripheral paresthesia, spasms of the hands and the feet, muscle weakness, tetany, and cardiac arrhythmia. Confirming diagnosis is often based on PCO_2 levels below 35 mm Hg, but the measurement of blood pH is critical in differentiating between metabolic acidosis and respiratory alkalosis. In the acute stage, blood pH rises in proportion to the fall in PCO_2, but in the chronic stage remains within the normal range of 7.35 to 7.45. The carbonic acid concentration is normal in the acute stage of this condition but below normal in the chronic stage.

■ INTERVENTION: Treatment of respiratory alkalosis concentrates on removing the underlying causes. Severe cases, especially those caused by extreme anxiety, may be treated by having the patient breathe into a paper bag and inhale exhaled carbon dioxide to compensate for the deficit being created by hyperventilation. Sedatives may also be administered to decrease the respiration rate.

■ NURSING CONSIDERATIONS: The nurse monitors neurologic, neuromuscular, and cardiovascular functions, arterial blood gases, and serum electrolytes. The patient benefits from explanations about laboratory tests and treatment.

respiratory assessment, an evaluation of the condition and function of a person's respiratory system.

■ METHOD: The nurse asks if the person coughs, wheezes, is short of breath, tires easily, or experiences chest or abdominal pain, chills, fever, excessive sweating, dizziness, or swelling of feet and hands. Signs of confusion, anxiety, restlessness, flaring nostrils, cyanotic lips, gums, earlobes, or nails, clubbing of extremities, fever, anorexia, and a tendency to sit upright are noted if present. The person's breathing is closely observed for evidence of slow, rapid, irregular, shallow, or Cheyne-Stokes respiration, hyperventilation, a long expiratory phase or periods of apnea, and for retractions in the suprasternal, supraclavicular, substernal, or intercostal areas during breathing. The presence of tachycardia, bradycardia, or sinus arrhythmia or evidence of congestive heart failure, as rales, rhonchi, edema, hepatosplenomegaly, abdominal distention, and pain, is recorded. The thorax is examined for scoliosis, kyphosis, funnel or barrel chest, or unequal shoulder height and is palpated for indications of thoracic expansion, tracheal deviation, crepitations, and fremitus. Percussion is performed to evaluate resonance, hyperresonance, tympany, dull or flat sounds; rales, rhonchi, wheezing, friction rubs, the transmission of spoken words through the chest wall, and decreased or absent breath sounds are detected by auscultation. Background information pertinent to the evaluation includes allergies, recent exposure to infection, immunizations, exposure to environmental irritants, previous respiratory disorders and operations, preexisting chronic conditions, medication currently taken, the person's smoking habits, and the family history. Valuable diagnostic aids are a chest x ray, complete blood count, electrocardiogram, pulmonary function tests, bronchoscopy, determinations of blood gases and electrolytes, studies of sputum, throat, or nasopharyngeal cultures, and gastric washings, lung scans, and biopsies.

■ NURSING ORDERS: The nurse collects the background information and the results of diagnostic tests and may perform the examination. In a respiratory care unit, a nurse clinician or practitioner may have greatly expanded responsibilities, as interpreting data from electrocardiographic tracings, setting up and adjusting a respirator, titrating medications, and obtaining specimens for blood-gas determination.

■ OUTCOME CRITERIA: An accurate and thorough assessment of respiratory function is an essential component of the physical examination and is vital to the diagnosis or ongoing care of a respiratory illness.

respiratory bronchiole. See **bronchiole.**

respiratory burn, tissue damage to the respiratory system resulting from the inhalation of a hot gas or burning particles, as may occur in a fire or explosion. Immediate hospitalization and oxygen therapy are recommended. Compare **smoke inhalation.**

respiratory center, a group of nerve cells in the pons and medulla of the brain that control the rhythm of breathing in response to changes in levels of oxygen and carbon dioxide in the blood and cerebrospinal fluid. Change in the concentration of oxygen and carbon dioxide or hydrogen ion levels in the arterial circulation and in cerebrospinal fluid activate central and peripheral chemoreceptors; these send impulses to the respiratory center, increasing or decreasing the breathing rate. This response is essential for normal breathing. In patients with retention of carbon dioxide, as in chronic bronchitis or emphysema, the respiratory center becomes insensitive to carbon dioxide, and the main stimulus to ventilation is then hypoxemia. If such patients inhale gases with a high oxygen content, breathing is depressed, leading to a further rise of blood carbon dioxide. The respiratory center is inhibited by barbiturates, anesthetics, tranquilizing agents, and morphine. See also **hyperventilation, hypoventilation.**

respiratory distress syndrome of the newborn (RDS), an acute lung disease of the newborn, characterized by airless alveoli, inelastic lungs, more than 60 respirations a minute, nasal flaring, intercostal and subcostal retractions, grunting on expiration, and peripheral edema. The condition occurs most often in premature babies and in babies of diabetics. It is caused by a deficiency of pulmonary surfactant, resulting in overdistended alveoli and at times, hyaline membrane formation, alveolar hemorrhage, severe right-to-left shunting of blood, increased pulmonary resistance, decreased cardiac output, and severe hypoxemia. The disease is self-limited; the infant dies in 3 to 5 days or completely recovers with no aftereffects. Treatment includes measures to correct shock, acidosis, and hypoxemia and use of continuous positive airway pressure especially developed for infants to prevent alveolar collapse. Also called **hyaline membrane disease.** Compare **adult respiratory distress syndrome.**

respiratory exchange ratio (R), the ratio of the net expiration of carbon dioxide to the concurrent net inspiration of oxygen, expressed by the formula $\dot{V}CO_2/\dot{V}O_2$.

respiratory failure, the inability of the cardiac and pulmonary systems to maintain an adequate exchange of oxygen and carbon dioxide in the lungs. Respiratory failure may be hypoxemic or ventilatory. Hypoxemic failure is characterized by hyperventilation and occurs in diseases which affect the alveoli or interstitial tissues of the lobes of the lungs, as alveolar edema, emphysema, fungal infections, leukemia, lobar pneumonia, lung carcinoma, various pneumoconioses, pulmonary eosinophilia, sarcoidosis, or tuberculosis. Ventilatory failure, characterized by increased arterial tension of carbon dioxide, occurs in acute conditions in which retained pulmonary secretions cause increased airway resistance and decreased lung compliance, as in bronchitis and emphysema. Ventilation may also be reduced by depression of the respiratory center by barbiturates or opiates, hypoxia, hypercarbia, intracranial diseases, trauma, or by lesions of the neuromuscular system or thoracic cage. Respiratory failure in pre-existing chronic lung diseases may be precipitated by added stress, as with cardiac failure, surgery, anesthesia, or upper respiratory tract infections. Treatment of respiratory failure includes clearing the airways by suction,

bronchodilators, or tracheostomy, antibiotics for infections usually present, anticoagulants for pulmonary thromboemboli, and electrolyte replacement in fluid imbalance. Oxygen may be administered in some cases; in others it may further decrease the respiratory reflex by removing the stimulus of an elevated level of carbon dioxide. Respiratory failure may result in cor pulmonale with congestive heart failure and respiratory acidosis. See also **airway obstruction, carbon dioxide, hypercapnia, hyperventilation, hypoxemia, hypoxia, respiratory acidosis.**

respiratory rate, the rate of breathing at rest, about 14 breaths per minute. The hydrogen ion concentration in the cerebrospinal fluid controls the rate of respiration. The rate may be more rapid in fever, acute pulmonary infection, diffuse pulmonary fibrosis, gas gangrene, left ventricular failure, thyrotoxicosis, and in states of tension. Slower breathing rates may result from head injury, coma, or narcotic overdose.

respiratory rhythm, a regular oscillating cycle of inspiration and expiration, controlled by neuronal impulses transmitted between the muscles of inspiration in the chest and the respiratory centers in the brain. The normal breathing pattern may be altered by a prolonged expiratory phase in obstructive diseases of the airway, as asthma, chronic bronchitis, and emphysema, or by Cheyne-Stokes respiration in patients with raised intracranial pressure or heart failure. See also **apnea, Biot's respiration, Hering-Breuer reflex, hyperventilation, hypoventilation, tachypnea.**

respiratory syncytial virus (RS), a member of a subgroup of myxoviruses which in tissue culture causes formation of giant cells or syncytia. It is a common cause of epidemics of acute bronchiolitis, bronchopneumonia, and the common cold in young children and sporadic acute bronchitis and mild upper respiratory infections in adults. Symptoms of infection with this virus include fever, cough, and severe malaise. Occasional fatalities occur in infants. Systemic invasion by the virus does not happen, and secondary bacterial invasion is uncommon. Treatment includes rest and the administration of aspirin and nasal decongestants. No effective vaccine for prevention is available. See also **bronchiolitis, bronchitis, bronchopneumonia, common cold, rhinovirus.**

respiratory system. See **respiratory tract.**

respiratory therapy (RT), 1. any treatment that maintains or improves the ventilatory function of the respiratory tract. 2. *Informal.* the department in a health-care facility that provides respiratory therapy for the clients of the facility.

respiratory tract, the complex of organs and structures that performs the pulmonary ventilation of the body and the exchange of oxygen and carbon dioxide between the ambient air and the blood circulating through the lungs. It also warms the air passing into the body and assists in the speech function by providing air for the larynx and the vocal cords. Every 24 hours about 500 cubic feet of air passes through the respiratory tract of the average adult, who breathes in and out between 12 and 18 times a minute. The respiratory tract is divided into the upper respiratory tract and the lower respiratory tract. Also called **respiratory system.**

respiratory tract infection, any infectious disease of the upper or lower respiratory tract. **Upper respiratory infections** include the common cold, pharyngitis, rhinitis, sinusitis and tonsillitis. **Lower respiratory infections** include bronchitis, bronchiolitis, pneumonia, and tracheitis.

respondeat superior (respon'diæt səpir'iɔr), *Latin.* 'let the master answer.' a doctrine stating that an employer may be held liable for torts committed by employees acting within the scope of their employment.

respondent conditioning. See **classical conditioning.**

resting cell, a cell that is not undergoing division. See also **interphase.**

resting tremor. See **passive tremor.**

restless legs syndrome, a benign condition of unknown etiology characterized by an irritating sensation of uneasiness, tiredness, and itching deep within the muscles of the leg, especially the lower part of the limb, accompanied by twitching and, sometimes, by pain. The only relief is walking or moving the legs. The condition may be associated with various psychiatric disorders, probably as a form of extrapyramidal hyperkinesis. Also called **anxietas tibiarum, Ekbom syndrome, Wittmaack-Ekbom syndrome.**

restraint, any one of numerous devices used in aiding the immobilization of patients, especially children in traction. Some kinds of restraints are specially designed slings, jackets, or diapers. Restraints often involve a certain amount of emotional trauma for the patient involved and are carefully employed. They are most effective when used consistently. Restraints that are too tight may cause skin irritation, while those that fit too loosely do not serve their purpose. During the course of any therapy, restraints are usually removed every four hours to assess skin integrity and provide skin care, often a massage of the area involved and an alcohol rub.

restraint of trade, an illegal act that interferes with free competition in a commercial or business transaction so as to restrict the production of a product or the provision of a service, affect the cost of a product or a service, or control the market in any way to the detriment of the consumers or purchasers of the service or product. The Clayton Act and the Sherman Antitrust Act are federal statutes that embody the basic concepts of the definition and of the illegal nature of restraint of trade.

restriction endonuclease (en'dounu'klieis), (in molecular genetics) an enzyme that cleaves DNA at a specific site. Each of the many different endonucleases isolated from various bacteria acts at a species-specific cleavage site, making it possible for researchers to divide DNA into discrete segments.

resuscitation, the process of sustaining the vital functions of a person in respiratory or cardiac failure while reviving him, using techniques of artificial respiration and cardiac massage, correcting acid-base imbalance and treating the cause of failure. See also **cardiopulmonary resuscitation.** –**resuscitate,** *v.*

resuscitator (risəs'itei'tər), an apparatus for pumping air into the lungs. It consists of a mask snugly applied over the mouth and nose, a reservoir for air, and a manually or electrically powered pump. Often oxygen may be added to the air in the reservoir.

RET, abbreviation for **rational emotive therapy.**

retarded, (of physical, intellectual, social, or emotional development) abnormally slow. –**retard,** *v.,* **retardation,** *n.*

retarded dentition, the abnormal delay of the eruption of the deciduous or permanent teeth resulting from malnutrition, malposition of the teeth, a hereditary factor, or a metabolic imbalance, as hypothyroidism. Also called **delayed dentition.** Compare **precocious dentition.**

retarded depression, the depressive phase of bipolar disorder.

retch, a strong attempt to vomit without bringing up anything. Compare **eructation, vomit.**

rete (ri'ti), a network, especially of arteries or veins. –**retial,** *adj.*

retention, 1. a resistance to movement or displacement. 2. the ability of the digestive system to hold food and fluid. 3. the inability to urinate or defecate. 4. the ability of the mind to remember information acquired from reading, observation, or other processes. –**retain,** *v.*

retention of urine, an abnormal, involuntary accumulation of urine in the bladder as a result of a loss of muscle tone in the bladder, neurologic dysfunction or damage to the bladder, obstruction of the urethra, or the administration of a narcotic analgesic, especially morphine.

Retet, a trade name for an antibiotic (tetracycline).

reticul-, a combining form meaning 'netlike': *reticulation, reticulocyte, reticulopod.*

reticular (ritik'yələr), (of a tissue or surface) having a netlike pattern or structure of veins.

reticular activating system (RAS), a functional (rather than a morphologic) system in the brain essential for wakefulness, attention, concentration, and introspection. A network of nerve fibers in the thalamus, hypothalamus, brain stem, and cerebral cortex contribute to the system.

reticular formation, a small thick cluster of neurons, nestled within the brain stem, that controls breathing, the heart beat, the blood pressure, the level of consciousness, and other vital functions of the body. The reticular formation constantly monitors the state of the body through connections with the sensory and the motor tracts. Certain nerve cells in the formation regulate the flow of hydrochloric acid in the stomach; other cells regulate swallowing, tongue movements, and movements of the face, eyes, and tongue.

reticulocyte (rɪtɪk'yuləsait), an immature erythrocyte characterized by a meshlike pattern of threads and particles at the former site of the nucleus. Reticulocytes normally make up less than 1 per cent of the circulating erythrocytes; a greater proportion reflects an increased rate of erythropoiesis.

reticuloendothelial system (RES) (rɪtɪk'yulouen'douthi'liəl), a functional, rather than anatomical system of the body involved primarily in defense against infection and in disposal of the products of the breakdown of cells. It is made up of macrophages, the Kupffer cells of the liver, and the reticulum cells of the lungs, bone marrow, spleen, and lymph nodes. Disorders of this system include **eosinophilic granuloma, Gaucher's disease, Hand-Schüller-Christian disease, Niemann-Pick disease.**

reticuloendotheliosis (rɪtɪk'yəlouen'douthi'liou'sɪs), an abnormal condition characterized by increased growth and proliferation of the cells of the reticuloendothelial system. See **reticuloendothelial system.**

reticulosarcoma (rɛtɪk'yulousarkou'mə). See **undifferentiated malignant lymphoma.**

reticulum cell sarcoma. See **histiocytic malignant lymphoma.**

retina (ret'ɪnə), a ten-layered, delicate nervous tissue membrane of the eye, continuous with the optic nerve, that receives images of external objects and transmits visual impulses through the optic nerve to the brain. The retina is soft, semitransparent, and contains rhodopsin which gives it a purple tint. The retina becomes clouded and opaque if exposed to direct sunlight. It develops from the embryonic optic cup in the eighth month of pregnancy and consists of the outer pigmented layer and the nine-layered retina proper. These nine layers, starting with the most internal, are the internal limiting membrane, the stratum opticum, the ganglion cell layer, the inner plexiform layer, the inner nuclear layer, the outer plexiform layer, the outer nuclear layer, the external limiting membrane, and the layer of rods and cones. The outer surface of the retina is in contact with the choroid; the inner surface with the vitreous body. The retina is thinner anteriorly where it extends nearly as far as the ciliary body and thicker posteriorly, except for a thin spot in the exact center of the posterior surface where focus is best. The nervous fibers end anteriorly in the jagged ora serrata at the ciliary body, but the membrane of the retina extends over the back of the ciliary processes and the iris. See also **Jacob's membrane, macula, optic disc.**

Retin-A, a trade name for a keratolytic (tretinoin).

retinaculum (ret'ɪnæk'yuləm), *pl.* **retinacula. 1.** a structure that retains an organ or tissue. **2.** an instrument for retracting tissues during surgery.

retinaculum extensorum manus, the thick band of antebrachial fascia that wraps tendons of the extensor muscles of the forearm at the distal ends of the radius and the ulna. Also called **dorsal carpal ligament, extensor retinaculum of the hand.** Compare **retinaculum flexorum manus.**

retinaculum flexorum manus, the thick, fibrous band of antebrachial fascia that wraps the carpal canal surrounding the tendons of flexor muscles of the forearm at the distal ends of the radius and the ulna. Also called **flexor retinaculum of the hand, volar ligament.**

retinal, an aldehyde preform of vitamin A produced by the enzymatic dehydration of retinol. It is the active form of the vitamin necessary for night, day, and color vision. See also **retinene, vitamin A.**

retinal detachment, a separation of the retina from the choroid in the back of the eye, usually resulting from a hole in the retina that allows the vitreous humor to leak between the choroid and the retina. Severe trauma to the eye, as a contusion or penetrating wound, may be the proximate cause, but in the great majority of cases retinal detachment is the result of internal changes in the vitreous chamber associated with aging, or, less frequently, owing to inflammation of the interior of the eye.

■ OBSERVATIONS: In most cases retinal detachment develops slowly. The first symptom is often the sudden appearance of a large number of spots floating loosely suspended in front of the affected eye. The person may not seek help, as the number of spots tends to decrease during days and weeks following the detachment. The person may also notice a curious sensation of flashing lights as the eye is moved. Because the retina does not contain sensory nerves that relay sensations of pain, the condition is painless. Detachment usually begins at the thin peripheral edge of the retina and extends gradually beneath the thicker, more central areas. The person perceives a shadow that begins laterally and grows in size slowly encroaching on central vision. As long as the center of the retina is unaffected, the vision, when looking straight ahead, is normal; when the center becomes affected, the eyesight is distorted, wavy, and indistinct. If the process of detachment is not halted, total blindness of the eye ultimately results. The condition does not spontaneously resolve itself.

■ INTERVENTION: Surgery is usually required to repair the hole and prevent the leakage of vitreous humor that separates the retina from its source of nourishment, the choroid. If the condition is discovered early, when the hole is small and the volume of vitreous humor lost is not large, the retinal hole may be closed by causing a scar to form on the choroid and to adhere to the retina around the hole. The scar may be produced by heat, electrical current, or cold. The scar is held against the retina by local pressure achieved by a variety of surgical techniques.

■ NURSING CONSIDERATIONS: Retinal detachment requires treatment. The degree of restoration of sight depends on the extent and duration of separation; maximum vision is achieved within three months after surgery. A detached retina slowly dies unless replaced after several years of detachment. Blindness resulting from retinal detachment is irreversible.

retinene (ret'ınin), either of the two carotenoid pigments found in the rods of the retina that are preforms of vitamin A and are activated by light. See also **retinal, retinol.**

retinoblastoma (ret'ınoublæstou'mə), *pl.* **retinoblastomas, retinoblastomata.** a congenital, hereditary neoplasm developing from retinal germ cells. It is the most common malignancy of the eye in childhood. Characteristic signs are diminished vision, strabismus, retinal detachment, and an abnormal pupillary reflex. The rapidly growing tumor may invade the brain and matastasize to distant sites. Treatment includes removal of the eye and as much of the optic nerve as possible, followed by radiation and chemotherapy.

retinocerebral angiomatosis (ret'ınousıri'brəl). See **cerebroretinal angiomatosis.**

retinol (ret'ınol), the cis-trans form of vitamin A. It is found in the retinas of mammals. Also called **vitamin A₁.**

retraction of the chest, the visible sinking-in of the soft tissues of the chest between and around the firmer tissue of the cartilagenous and bony ribs, as occurs with increased inspiratory effort. Retraction begins in the intercostal spaces. If increased effort is needed to fill the lungs, supraclavicular and infraclavicular retraction may be seen. In infants, sternal retraction occurs with only slight increase in respiratory effort, owing to the pliability of their chests. Compare **intercostal bulging.**

retractor, an instrument for holding back the edges of tissues and organs in order to maintain exposure of the underlying anatomy, particularly during surgery, as an army retractor, a double-ended Richardson retractor, or a vaginal retractor.

retro-, a combining form meaning 'backward, or located behind': *retronasal, retroperitoneal, retroversion.*

retroaortic node (re'trɔueiɔr'tık), a node in one of three sets of lumbar lymph nodes that serve various structures in the abdomen and the pelvis. They lie below the cisterna chyli on the bodies of the third and the fourth lumbar vertebrae and receive the lymphatic trunks from the lateral aortic nodes and preaortic nodes. The efferents from the retroaortic nodes end in the cisterna chyli. Compare **lateral aortic node, preaortic node.**

retrograde, 1. moving backward; moving in the opposite direction to that which is considered normal. 2. de-

generating; reverting to an earlier state or worse condition. 3. catabolic.

retrograde amnesia, the loss of memory for events occurring before a particular time in a person's life. The condition may result from disease, brain injury or damage, or a traumatic emotional incident. Compare **anterograde amnesia.** See also **amnesia.**

retrograde cystoscopy, a technique in radiology for examining the bladder in which a catheter is inserted through the urethra into the bladder, allowing the urine present in the bladder to pass through the catheter. A radiopaque medium is introduced, filling the bladder, and the contour of the bladder is observed, using serial x rays or fluoroscopy, as the contrast medium is voided. See also **cystogram, retrograde pyelography.**

retrograde infantilism. See **acromegalic eunuchoidism.**

retrograde pyelography, a technique in radiology for examining the structures of the collecting system of the kidneys that is especially useful in locating an obstruction in the urinary tract. A radiopaque contrast medium is injected through a urinary catheter into the ureters and the calyces of the pelves of the kidneys. Rarely, severe anaphylactoid reaction to the medium may occur, owing to a patient's hypersensitivity to the iodine in the medium, and infection or trauma may result from the catheterization.

retrograde pyelography, a technique in radiology for examining the structures of the collecting system in the kidneys that does not depend on kidney function. A catheter is passed through the urethra and bladder, and each ureter and kidney is injected with a contrast medium, then visualized in turn on x-ray films or a fluoroscopy screen. This test is useful in locating an obstruction in the urinary tract. Infection and trauma may result from the manipulation required to insert the catheter.

retrograde urography. See **retrograde pyelography.**

retrogression, a return to a less complex state, condition, or behavioral adaptation; degeneration; deterioration. See also **regression.**

retroperitoneal (re'trouper'ıtəni'əl), of or pertaining to organs closely attached to the abdominal wall and partly covered by peritoneum, rather than suspended by that membrane.

retroperitoneal fibrosis, a chronic inflammatory process, usually of unknown cause, in which fibrous tissue surrounds the large blood vessels in the lower lumbar area. It frequently causes constriction of the midportion of the ureters, which may lead to hydronephrosis and azotemia. Occasionally the fibrosis spreads upward to involve the duodenum, bile ducts, and superior vena cava. Symptoms include low-back and abdominal pain, weakness, weight loss, fever, and, with urinary tract involvement, frequency of urination, hematuria, polyuria, or anuria. Methysergide, taken to prevent migraine headaches, is one known cause of this condition. Treatment includes stopping methysergide and instituting surgical release of the ureters from the fibrosis with transplantation laterally or intraperitoneally.

retroperitoneal lymph node dissection, surgical removal of lymph nodes behind the peritoneum, usually performed in an attempt to eliminate sites of lymphoma or metastases from malignancies originating in pelvic organs or genitalia.

retropharyngeal abscess, a collection of pus in the tissues behind the pharynx accompanied by difficulty in swallowing, fever, and pain. Occasionally, the airway becomes obstructed. Treatment includes appropriate parenteral antibiotics and surgical drainage. Tracheostomy may be necessary. Compare **parapharyngeal abscess, peritonsillar abscess.**

retroplacental (re'trouplǝsen'tǝl), behind the placenta.

retrospective chart audit, a format for an audit developed by the Joint Commission on the Accreditation of Hospitals. The audit involves several steps that outline a procedure for evaluating the effectiveness of the care given at a particular institution and for correcting any deficiencies found by reviewing the patient's records after discharge and comparing the data with standards held to be adequate by the Commission.

retrospective nursing audit. See **nursing audit.**

retrospective study, a study in which a search is made for a relationship between one (usually current) phenomenon or condition and another that occurred in the past, as a study to discover the family histories of young women diagnosed as having clear-cell adenomas of the vagina which yielded a relationship between the administration of diethylstilbestrol to the mothers of the women during pregnancy and the development of the condition.

retrouterine (re'trouyu'tǝrɪn), behind the uterus.

retroversion (ret'rouvǝr'zhǝn), a common condition in which an organ is tipped backward, usually without flexion or other distortion. The uterus may be retroverted in as many as one fourth of normal women. Uterine retroversion is measured as first-, second-, or third-degree, depending upon the angle of tilt with respect to the vagina. No treatment is necessary. Compare **anteversion.** See also **anteflexion, retroflexion.** −**retrovert,** v.

retrovirus (ret'rouvai'rǝs), a member of a family of viruses that includes the oncoviruses.

Reverdin's needle (ʀǝveʀdǣz'), a surgical needle with an eye that can be opened and closed with a slide.

reverse anaphylaxis. See **inverse anaphylaxis.**

reverse Barton's fracture, a fracture of the volar articular surface of the radius with associated displacement of the carpal bones and radius.

reversed bandage, a roller bandage that is reversed on itself with a half twist so that it lies smoothly, conforming to the contour of the extremity. See also **roller bandage.**

reversed coarctation. See **Takayasu's arteritis.**

reverse isolation, isolation procedures designed to protect a patient from infectious organisms that might be carried by the staff, other patients, or visitors or on droplets in the air or on equipment or materials. Absolute reverse isolation is rarely necessary and requires elaborate specialized equipment. Protective modified reverse isolation is less restrictive but is not prolonged needlessly as the patient usually comes to feel lonely and sensorily deprived. Handwashing, gowning, gloving, sterilization or disinfection of materials brought into the area, and other details of housekeeping vary with the reason for the isolation and the usual practices of the hospital.

review of systems (ROS), (in a health history) a system-by-system review of the functions of the body. The ROS is begun during the initial interview with the patient and completed during the physical examination, as physical findings prompt, further questions. One outline of the systems and some of the signs and symptoms that might be noted or reported are as follows:

■ SKIN: bruising, discoloration, pruritus, birthmarks, moles, ulcers, decubiti, changes in the hair or nails.

■ HEMATOPOIETIC: spontaneous or excessive bleeding, fatigue, enlarged or tender lymph nodes, pallor, history of anemia.

■ HEAD AND FACE: pain, traumatic injury, ptosis.

■ EARS: ringing in the ears, change in hearing, running or discharge from the ears, deafness, dizziness.

■ EYES: change in vision, pain, inflammation, infections, double vision, scotomata, blurring, tearing.

■ MOUTH AND THROAT: dental problems, hoarseness, dysphagia, bleeding gums, sore throat, ulcers or sores in the mouth.

■ NOSE AND SINUSES: discharge, epistaxis, sinus pain, obstruction.

■ BREASTS: pain, change in contour or skin color, lumps, discharge from the nipple.

■ RESPIRATORY TRACT: cough, sputum, change in sputum, night sweats, nocturnal dyspnea, wheezing.

■ CARDIOVASCULAR SYSTEM: chest pain, dyspnea, palpitations, weakness, intolerance of exercise, varicosities, swelling of extremities, known murmur, high blood pressure, asystole.

■ GASTROINTESTINAL SYSTEM: nausea, vomiting, diarrhea, constipation, quality of appetite, change in appetite, dysphagia, gas, heartburn, melena, change in bowel habits, use of laxatives or other drugs to alter the function of the GI tract.

■ URINARY TRACT: dysuria, change in color of urine, change in frequency of urination, pain with urgency, incontinence, edema, retention.

■ GENITAL TRACT: (male) penile discharge, pain or discomfort, pruritus, skin lesions, hematuria, history of venereal disease.

■ GENITAL TRACT: (female) menstrual history, obstetric history, contraceptive use, discharge, pain or discomfort, pruritus, history of venereal disease.

■ SKELETAL SYSTEM: heat, redness, swelling, limitation of function, deformity, crepitation, pain in a joint or an extremity, the neck, or back, especially with movement.

■ NERVOUS SYSTEM: dizziness, tremor, ataxia, difficulty in speaking, change in speech, paresthesia, loss of sensation, seizures, syncope.

■ ENDOCRINE SYSTEM: tremor, palpitations, intolerance of heat or cold, polyuria, polydipsia, polyphagia, diaphoresis, exophthalmos, goiter.

■ PSYCHOLOGIC STATUS: nervousness, instability, depression, phobia, sexual disturbances, criminal behavior, insomnia, night terrors, mania, memory loss, perseveration, disorientation.

Reye's syndrome (reiz), a combination of acute encephalopathy and fatty infiltration of the internal organs that may follow acute viral infections. This syndrome has been associated with influenza B, chicken pox (varicella), the enteroviruses, and the Epstein-Barr virus. It usually affects people under 18 years old, characteristically causing an exanthematous rash, vomiting, and confusion about one week after the onset of a viral illness. In the late stage, there may be extreme disorientation followed by coma, seizures, and respiratory arrest. Laboratory tests reveal greater than normal amounts of SGOT and SGPT, bilirubin, and ammonia in the blood. A specimen obtained by liver biopsy shows fatty degeneration and confirms the diagnosis. Mortality varies between 20 and 80 per cent, depending on the severity of symptoms. The cause of Reye's syndrome is unknown and there is no specific treatment available. Insulin, antibiotics, and mannitol may be given. Blood gases, blood pH, and blood pressure are monitored frequently. Intensive, supportive nursing care with meticulous monitoring of all vital functions and prompt correction of any imbalance are of extreme significance in the outcome of this syndrome.

R factor, an episome in bacteria that is responsible for drug resistance and is transmissible to progeny and to other bacterial cells by conjugation. The portion of the episome involved in replication and transmission is called resistance transfer factor.

RFP, abbreviation for **request for proposal.**

RF (rheumatoid factor) test. See **latex fixation test.**

Rh, symbol for **rhodium.**

Rh negative. See **Rh factor.**

-rh-. For combining forms containing -rh-, see -(r)rh ..., as -(r)rhachia, -(r)rhage, etc.

rhabdo-, rhabdi-, a combining form meaning 'rod-shaped, or of or pertaining to a rod': *rhabdocyte, rhabdomyoma, rhabdosarcoma.*

rhabdomyoma (ræb′doumaiou′mə), *pl.* **rhabdomyomas, rhabdomyomata.** a tumor of striated muscle that may

occur in the uterus, vagina, pharynx, and tongue, and in the heart as congenital neoplastic nodules. Also called **myoma striocellulare.**

rhabdomyosarcoma (ræb′doumaï′ousarkou′mə), *pl.* **rhabdomyosarcomas, rhabdomyosarcomata.** a highly malignant tumor, derived from primitive striated muscle cells, that occurs most frequently in the head and neck and is also found in the genitourinary tract, extremities, body wall, and retroperitoneum. In some cases, the onset is associated with trauma. The initial symptoms depend on the site of tumor development and indicate local tissue or organ destruction, as dysphagia, vaginal bleeding, hematuria, or obstruction of the flow of urine. Diagnostic measures may include barium x-ray studies, angiography, or tomography. Embryonal rhabdomyosarcoma occurs in the head, neck, or trunk of young children; alveolar rhabdomyosarcoma is usually seen in the extremities of adolescents, and the pleomorphic form is most common in the legs of adults. Surgical excision is rarely possible, because the tumor is poorly encapsulated and tends to spread. Amputation of an affected limb or extremity may be curative. Radiotherapy and chemotherapy with combinations of actinomycin D, adriamycin, cyclophosphamide, and vincristine may greatly increase the length of survival.

rhabdovirus (ræb′douvaï′rəs), a member of a family of viruses that includes the organism causing rabies.

rhachi-. See **rachio-.**

rhagades (ræg′ədiz), cracks or fissures in skin that has lost its elasticity, especially common around the mouth. See also **cheilosis.**

rhaphe. See **raphe.**

Rh₀(D) immune globulin, a passive immunizing agent.

■ INDICATION: It is prescribed to prevent Rh sensitization.

■ CONTRAINDICATION: It is not given to an Rh₀(D) positive patient or to the infant.

■ ADVERSE EFFECTS: The most serious adverse reaction is anaphylaxis.

rhenium (Re), a hard brittle metallic element. Its atomic number is 75; its atomic weight is 186.2. Rhenium has a high melting point and is used in thermometers for measuring high temperatures.

rheo-, a combining form meaning 'of or pertaining to electric current, or to a flow': *rheobase, rheoscope, rheotaxis.*

Rheomacrodex, a trade name for a plasma expander (dextran 40).

Rhesus factor (ri′səs). See **Rh factor.**

-rheumatic, a combining form meaning 'relating to or exhibiting traits of rheumatism': *postrheumatic, prerheumatic, pseudorheumatic.*

rheumatic, of or pertaining to rheumatism.

rheumatic aortitis, an inflammatory condition of the aorta, occurring in rheumatic fever and characterized by disseminated focal lesions that may progressively form patches of fibrosis.

rheumatic arteritis, a complication of rheumatic fever characterized by generalized inflammation of arteries and arterioles. Fibrin, mixed with cellular debris, may invade, thicken, and stiffen the vessel wall, and the vessel may be surrounded by hemorrhage and exudate.

rheumatic chorea. See **Sydenham's chorea.**

rheumatic fever, an inflammatory disease that may develop as a delayed reaction to inadequately treated Group A beta-hemolytic streptococcal infection of the upper respiratory tract. This disorder usually occurs in young school-age children and may affect the brain, heart, joints, skin, or subcutaneous tissues. See also **rheumatic heart disease.**

■ OBSERVATIONS: The onset of rheumatic fever is usually sudden, often occurring in from one to five symptom-free weeks following recovery from a sore throat or from scarlet fever. Early symptoms usually include fever, joint pains, nose bleeds, abdominal pain, and vomiting. The major manifestations of this disease include migratory polyarthritis affecting numerous joints and carditis, which causes palpitations, chest pain, and, in severe cases, symptoms of cardiac failure. Sydenham's chorea, which may develop, is usually the sole, late sign of rheumatic fever and may initially be manifested as an increased awkwardness and an associated tendency to drop objects. As the chorea progresses irregular body movements may become extensive, occasionally involving the tongue and the facial muscles, resulting in incapacitation of the affected individual. Other developments may include transient erythema marginatum with circular lesions and subcutaneous rheumatic nodules on various joints and tendons, the spine, and the back of the head. There is no specific diagnostic test for rheumatic fever. The development of serum antibodies to streptococcal antigens is a positive diagnostic sign. Affected individuals may also develop leukocytosis, moderate anemia, and proteinuria. C-reactive protein, evaluated in a specimen of blood, is abnormally high. Recurrences of rheumatic fever are common. Except for carditis, all the manifestations of this disease usually subside without any permanent effects. Mild cases may last 3 to 4 weeks. Severe cases with associated arthritis and carditis may last 2 to 3 months.

■ INTERVENTION: Management of this disease includes bed rest and severe restriction of normal activity. Penicillin is often administered, even if throat cultures are negative, and steroids or salicylates may be used, depending on the severity of any associated carditis and arthritis.

■ NURSING CONSIDERATIONS: The nurse is alert to signs of toxicity associated with salicylate and steroid therapies. Symptoms largely determine the type of nursing care.

Large volumes of fluids are usually administered, and the nurse routinely helps minimize joint pains by properly positioning the patient. Throughout the course of the disease the patient benefits from emotional support and appropriate diversions.

rheumatic heart disease, damage to heart muscle and heart valves caused by episodes of rheumatic fever. When a susceptible person acquires a group A beta hemolytic streptococcal infection, an autoimmune reaction may occur in heart tissue, resulting in permanent deformities of heart valves or chordae tendineae. Involvement of the heart may be evident during acute rheumatic fever, or it may be discovered long after the acute disease has subsided. See also **aortic stenosis, mitral stenosis, rheumatic fever.**

■ OBSERVATIONS: Rheumatic heart disease is characterized by heart murmurs owing to stenosis or insufficiency of the valves and by compensatory alterations in the size of the chambers of the heart and the thickness of their walls. Abnormalities of pulse rate and rhythm, heart block, and congestive heart failure are also common. Deaths are usually due to heart failure or bacterial endocarditis.

■ INTERVENTION: Episodes of acute rheumatic fever must be vigorously treated and supportive therapy given for heart failure, if needed. Chronic rheumatic heart disease may require no immediate treatment except for close observation. If signs of inefficient or decompensating heart action occur, digitalis, diuretics, and a low-sodium diet are often prescribed. In some patients, surgical commissurotomy or valve replacement is necessary. Patients with a history of rheumatic fever or evidence of rheumatic heart disease, in order to prevent streptococcal infection, should receive daily prophylactic penicillin by mouth or monthly intramuscular injections of benzathene penicillin, at least during childhood and adolescence. Patients with evidence of deformed heart valves should be given prophylactic antibiotics before surgical and dental procedures to prevent bacterial endocarditis.

■ NURSING CONSIDERATIONS: In addition to the care of patients with acute rheumatic fever, nurses have a responsibility to help educate them about their disease and about how to recognize the early symptoms and signs of its complications. It is especially important to stress the regular use of prophylactic penicillin to prevent streptococcal infections and the need to take special prophylactic antibiotics to be taken before surgery and all dental procedures.

rheumatism, 1. *Nontechnical.* any of a large number of inflammatory conditions of the bursae, joints, ligaments, or muscles characterized by pain, limitation of movement, and structural degeneration of single or multiple parts of the musculoskeletal system. 2. *Nontechnical.* the syndrome of pain, limitation of movement, and structural degeneration of elements in the musculoskeletal system as may occur in gout, rheumatoid arthritis, systemic lupus erythematosus, ankylosing spondylitis, and many other diseases. —**rheumatic,** *adj.,* **rheumatoid,** *adj.*

rheumatoid arthritis, a chronic, destructive, sometimes deforming, collagen disease that has an autoimmune component. Rheumatoid arthritis is characterized by symmetrical inflammation of the synovium and increased synovial exudate, leading to thickening of the synovium and swelling of the joint. Rheumatoid arthritis usually first appears in early middle age, between 36 and 50 years of age, and most commonly in women. The course of the disease is variable but is most frequently marked by remissions and exacerbation. A kind of rheumatoid arthritis that occurs in younger people is **Still's disease.** Also called **arthritis deformans, atrophic arthritis.**

■ OBSERVATIONS: Rheumatoid arthritis may first present itself with constitutional symptoms, including fatigue, weakness, and poor appetite. Other early signs include low-grade fever, anemia, and an increased erythrocyte sedimentation rate. The symptoms listed by the American Rheumatism Association include morning stiffness, joint pain or tenderness, swelling of at least two joints, subcutaneous nodules (called arthritic nodules and usually found at pressure points, as the elbows), structural changes in the joint seen on x-ray film, a positive rheumatoid factor agglutination test, decreased precipitation of mucin from synovial fluid, and characteristic histologic changes on pathologic examination of the fluid. Immune complexes are characteristically present in both the blood serum and the synovial fluid. Rheumatoid factor (RF) is present in serum and joint fluid of most persons with rheumatoid arthritis, and higher titers of rheumatoid factor are correlated with more severe forms of the disease, in particular those forms with extra-articular manifestations. Antinuclear antibodies and special rheumatoid precipitins are also occasionally present. Extra-articular manifestations may include cardiac involvement, vasculitis, pulmonary disease, and proteinuria. There may also be a thickening of the synovium, called pannus formation. In long-term, severe, chronic rheumatoid arthritis, Felty's syndrome may be present.

■ INTERVENTION: The basic principles of treatment include sufficient rest, exercise to maintain joint function, medication for the relief of pain and the reduction of inflammation, orthopedic intervention to prevent or correct deformities, and excellent nutrition—with weight loss, if necessary. Salicylates are usually given. If improvement is not achieved other anti-inflammatories, as indomethacin, phenylbutazone, antimalarials, gold salts, or some antineoplastic drugs may be used. Corticosteroids are prescribed with caution because of side effects, including gastric ulcer, adrenal suppression, and osteoporosis. Other treatments, including diathermy, ultrasound, warm paraffin applications, exercise under water, and applications of heat are occasionally used.

■ NURSING CONSIDERATIONS: As rheumatoid arthritis is not always progressive, deforming, or debilitating and as early treatment may help the person to recover and perhaps to avoid future attacks, the nurse can play an important role by monitoring drug treatment so that adequate medication is taken, by noting side effects, and by adjusting treatment. Most people who have rheumatoid arthritis may continue in their jobs. The nurse encourages the person to get sufficient sleep and to rest the weight-bearing joints. Suggestions about the most effective use of heat, instruction in muscle-strengthening exercise and methods for easing pain and preventing deformities, as the proper use of pillows, splints, or molds, as well as emotional support are often given by the nurse. As stress often precedes exacerbation of the condition, the person is counseled to avoid situations known to cause anxiety, worry, fatigue, infection, and other stressors.

rheumatoid coronary arteritis, an abnormal condition, characterized by a thickening of the tunica intima of the coronary arteries, which may produce coronary insufficiency. Rheumatoid coronary arteritis is collagen disease that affects the connective tissue by inflammation and fibrinoid degeneration. It is commonly treated with glucocorticoids.

rheumatoid factor (RF), antiglobulin antibodies often found in the serum of patients with a clinical diagnosis of rheumatoid arthritis. Rheumatoid factors are present in about 70 per cent of such cases, but they may also be found in such widely divergent diseases as tuberculosis, parasitic infections, leukemia, and connective tissue disorders. See also **latex fixation test.**

rheumatologist, a specialist in rheumatology.

rheumatology, the study of disorders characterized by inflammation, degeneration, or metabolic derangement of connective tissue and related structures of the body. These disorders are sometimes referred to collectively as rheumatism.

Rh factor, an antigenic substance present in the erythrocytes of most people. A person having the factor is Rh+ (Rh positive); a person lacking the factor is Rh− (Rh negative). If an Rh− person receives Rh+ blood, hemolysis and anemia occur. Rh+ infants may be exposed to antibodies to the factor produced in the Rh− mother's blood, resulting in red cell destruction and erythroblastosis fetalis. Transfusion, blood typing, and crossmatching depend on Rh+ and ABO classification. The Rh factor was first isolated and identified in the blood of a species of the rhesus monkey. It is present in the red cells of 85 per cent of people. See also **Rhogam.**

rhigo-, a combining form meaning 'cold': *rhigolene, rhigosis, rhigotic.*

rhin-. See **rhino-.**

Rh incompatibility, (in hematology) a lack of compatibility between two groups of blood cells that are antigenically different owing to the presence of the Rh factor in one group and its absence in the other. See also **Rh factor.**

rhinencephalon (rai'nensef'əlon), *pl.* **rhinencephala.** a portion of each cerebral hemisphere that contains the limbic system, which is associated with the emotions. The rhinencephalon develops in the embryo from a longitudinal ridge at the rostral extremity of the cerebral hemisphere. The rostral part of the ridge becomes the primitive olfactory lobe; the caudal part becomes the piriform lobe. In an adult, the caudal part of the piriform lobe is absorbed into the gyrus hippocampus. See also **limbic system.** — **rhinencephalic,** *adj.*

rhinitis (rainai'tis), inflammation of the mucous membranes of the nose, usually accompanied by swelling of the mucosa and a nasal discharge. It may be complicated by sinusitis. Rhinitis may be acute, allergic, atrophic, or vasomotor. Also called **coryza.**

rhino-, rhin-, a combining form meaning 'of or pertaining to the nose, or to a noselike structure': *rhinocephalia, rhinolalia, rhinoplasty.*

rhinopathy (rainop'əthi), any disease or malformation of the nose.

rhinophyma (rai'noufai'mə), a form of rosacea in which there is sebaceous hyperplasia, redness, prominent vascularity, swelling, and distortion of the skin of the nose. Treatment includes dermabrasion, electrosurgery, and plastic surgery. See also **rosacea.**

rhinoplasty (rai'nəplæs'ti), a procedure in plastic surgery in which the structure of the nose is changed. Bone or cartilage may be removed, tissue grafted from another part of the body, or synthetic material implanted to alter the shape. Under local anesthesia intranasal incisions are made and the nose is reshaped. Postoperatively, any respiratory difficulty is reported immediately and the patient is kept in mid-Fowler's position. Frequent oral care is given and ice compresses are applied to decrease the pain and edema that usually occur. Edema and discoloration around the eyes is expected to last for several days. The procedure is most frequently performed for cosmetic reasons.

rhinoscope (rai'nəskoup), an instrument for examining the nasal passages through the anterior nares or through the nasopharynx.

rhinoscopy (rainos'kəpi), an examination of the nasal passages to inspect the mucosa and detect inflammation, deformities, or asymmetry, as in deviation of the septum. The nasal passages may be examined anteriorly, by introducing a speculum into the anterior nares, or posteriorly, by introducing a rhinoscope through the nasopharynx. — **rhinoscopic,** *adj.*

rhinosporidiosis (rai'nouspərid'iou'sis), an infection caused by the fungus *Rhinosporidium seeberi,* characterized by fleshy red polyps on mucous membranes of nose, conjunctiva, nasopharynx, and soft palate. The disease may be acquired by swimming or bathing in infected water. The most effective treatment is electrocautery.

rhinotomy (rainot'əmi), a surgical procedure in which an incision is made along one side of the nose, performed to drain accumulated pus from an abscess or a sinus infection. Under local anesthesia, the flap of skin and lining of the nose are turned back to provide a full view of the nasal passages for radical sinus surgery.

rhinovirus (rai'nouvai'rəs), any of about 100 serologically distinct, small RNA viruses that cause about 40 per cent of acute respiratory illnesses. Infection is characterized by dry, scratchy throat, nasal congestion, malaise, and headache. Fever is minimal. Nasal discharge lasts two or three days. Children may also develop a cough. Type specific antibodies may last for two to four years, without serious complications. The treatment is nonspecific and may include rest, analgesics, antihistamines, and nasal decongestants. Complete recovery is usual. Compare **adenovirus, parainfluenza virus, respiratory syncytial virus.** See also **common cold.**

rhitid-. See **rhytid-.**

rhitidosis (rit'idou'sis), **rhytidosis,** a wrinkling, especially of the cornea.

rhizo-, a combining form meaning 'of or related to a root': *rhizodontropy, rhizome, rhizotomist.*

Rhodesian trypanosomiasis, an acute form of African trypanosomiasis, caused by the parasite *Trypanosoma brucei rhodesiense.* The disease may progress rapidly, causing encephalitis, coma, and death in only a few weeks. Also called **kaodzera.** Compare **Gambian trypanosomiasis.** See also **African trypanosomiasis.**

rhodium (Rh), a grayish-white metallic element. Its atomic number is 45; its atomic weight is 102.91. Rhodium is used for providing a hard lustrous coating on other metals and in the making of mirrors.

rhodo-, a combining form meaning 'red': *rhodocyte, rhodopsin, rhodotoxin.*

rhodopsin (roudop'sin), the purple pigmented compound in the rods of the retina, formed by a protein, opsin, and a derivative of vitamin A, retinal. Rhodopsin gives the outer segments of the rods a purple color and adapts the eye to low-density light. The compound breaks down when struck by light and this chemical change triggers the conduction of nerve impulses. Brief periods of darkness allow the opsin and the retinal to reconstitute the rhodopsin, which accounts for the short delay a person experiences in adapting to sudden or drastic changes in lighting, as when moving out of bright sunlight into a darkened room or from darkness into bright light. Closing the eyes is a natural reflex that allows reconstitution of rhodopsin. Compare **iodopsin.**

RhoGAM, a trade name for a passive immunizing agent ($R_0(D)$ immune human globulin).

rhomboideus major (rombɔi′diəs), a muscle of the upper back below and parallel to the rhomboideus minor. Arising from the spinous processes of the third, fourth, and fifth thoracic vertebrae and inserting into the lower half of the medial border of the scapula, it is innervated by the dorsal scapular nerve from the brachial plexus and, with the rhomboideus minor, functions to draw the scapula toward the vertebral column while supporting it and drawing it slightly upward. Compare **latissimus dorsi, levator scapulae, rhomboideus minor, trapezius.**

rhomboideus minor, a muscle of the upper back, above and parallel to the rhomboideus major. It arises from the ligamentum nuchae and from the spinous processes of the seventh cervical and first thoracic vertebrae. It inserts into the upper part of the medial border at the root of the spine of the scapula. It is innervated by the dorsal scapular nerve from the brachial plexus, which contains fibers from the fifth cervical nerve, and, with the rhomboideus major, acts to draw the scapula toward the vertebral column while supporting the scapula and drawing it slightly upward. Compare **latissimus dorsi, levator scapulae, rhomboideus major, trapezius.**

rhomboid glossitis. See **median rhomboid glossitis.**

rhonchi (roŋ′kai), *sing.* **rhonchus.** abnormal sounds heard on auscultation of a respiratory airway obstructed by thick secretions, muscular spasm, neoplasm, or external pressure. The continuous rumbling sounds are more pronounced during expiration, and they characteristically clear on coughing, which rales do not. Rhonchi may be sibilant or sonorous. Sibilant rhonchi are high pitched and are heard in the small bronchi, as in asthma. Sonorous rhonchi are lower pitched and are heard in the large bronchi, as in tracheobronchitis. Dry rales are called rhonchi. Compare **rale, wheeze.**

rhotacism (rou′təsiz′əm), a speech disorder characterized by a defective pronunciation of words containing the sound "r," or by the excessive use of the sound "r," or by the substitution of another sound for "r." Compare **lallation, lambdacism.**

Rh positive. See **Rh factor.**

rhus dermatitis, a skin rash resulting from contact with a plant of the genus *Rhus,* as poison ivy, poison oak, or poison sumac. See also **contact dermatitis.**

rhyp-, a combining form meaning 'of or pertaining to filth': *rhyparia, rhypophagy, rhypophobia.*

rhythm method. See **natural-family planning method.**

rhytid-, rhitid-, a combining form meaning 'wrinkle, or wrinkled': *rhytidectomy, rhytidosis.*

rhytidoplasty (ritid′ouplæs′ti), **rhitidoplasty,** a procedure in reconstructive plastic surgery in which the skin of the face is tightened, wrinkles are removed, and the skin is made to appear firm and smooth. An incision is made at the hairline, and excess skin is separated from the supporting tissue and excised. The edges of the remaining skin are pulled up and back and sutured at the hairline. A pressure dressing is applied and left in place for 24 to 48 hours. Postoperative medication for pain is often necessary. The sutures are removed several days after discharge in an outpatient facility or in the surgeon's office.

rhytidosis (rit′idou′sis). See **rhitidosis.**

RIA. See **radioimmunoassay.**

rib, one of the twelve pairs of elastic arches of bone forming a large part of the thoracic skeleton. The first seven ribs on each side are called **true ribs** because they articulate directly with the sternum and the vertebrae. The remaining five ribs are called **false ribs,** the first three attaching ventrally to ribs above; the last two are free at their ventral extremities and are called **floating ribs.**

riboflavin, a yellow crystalline, water-soluble pigment, one of the heat-stable components of the B vitamin complex. It combines with specific flavoproteins and functions as a coenzyme in the oxidative processes of carbohydrates, fats, and proteins. It is also important in the prevention of some visual disorders, especially cataracts. Small amounts of riboflavin are found in the liver and kidneys, but it is not stored to any great degree in the body and must be supplied regularly in the diet. Common sources are organ meats, milk, cheese, eggs, green leafy vegetables, meat, whole grains, and legumes. Deficiency of riboflavin produces cheilosis, local inflammation, desquamation, and encrustation, glossitis, photophobia, corneal opacities, proliferation of corneal vessels, seborrheic dermatitis about the nose, mouth, forehead, ears, and scrotum, trembling, sluggishness, dizziness, edema, inability to urinate, and vaginal itching. There is no known toxicity of riboflavin. Also called **vitamin B_2.** See also **ariboflavinosis.**

ribonucleic acid (RNA) (rai′bounukli′ik), a nucleic acid, found in both the nucleus and cytoplasm of cells, that transmits genetic instructions from the nucleus to the cytoplasm. In the cytoplasm, RNA functions in the assembly of proteins. See also **deoxyribonucleic acid.**

ribosome, a cytoplasmic organelle composed of ribonucleic acid and protein that functions in the synthesis of cellular protein. Ribosomes interact with messenger RNA and transfer RNA to join together amino acid units into a polypeptide chain according to the sequence determined by the genetic code. The structures appear singly or in clusters as polysomes or they may be attached to endoplasmic reticulum. See also **translation.**

rice diet, a diet consisting only of rice, fruit, fruit juices, and sugar, supplemented with vitamins and iron. Salt is strictly forbidden. It is prescribed for the treatment of hypertension, chronic renal disease, and obesity. The diet is somewhat modified after blood pressure is lowered and other symptoms are alleviated. It should not be followed for any length of time, since the severe dietary restrictions may lead to nutritional deficiencies or imbalance. Also called **Duke diet, Kempner rice-fruit diet.**

Richards, Linda (1841–1930), a nurse considered to be the first American-trained nurse, being graduated in the first class of the New England Hospital for Women and Children. She then studied at the Nightingale Training School in London and, in 1873, organized the Massachusetts General Hospital Training School on the same lines. In 1885, she was sent to Japan to develop a training school at the Charity Hospital. In 1891, she took charge of the Philadelphia Visiting Nurse Society. She is credited with being the first to keep written records on patients, a practice she started when she worked as night superintendent at Bellevue Hospital in New York under Sister Helen.

rickets, a condition caused by the deficiency of vitamin D, calcium, and, usually, phosphorus, seen primarily in infancy and childhood, and characterized by abnormal bone formation. Symptoms include soft pliable bones causing such deformities as bowlegs and knock-knees, nodular enlargements on the ends and sides of the bones, muscle pain, enlarged skull, chest deformities, spinal curvature, enlargement of the liver and spleen, profuse sweating, and general tenderness of the body when touched. Prophylaxis and treatment include a diet rich in calcium, phosphorus, and vitamin D and adequate exposure to sunlight. Kinds of rickets include **acute rickets, adult rickets, celiac rickets, renal rickets, vitamin D resistant rickets.** See also **osteodystrophy, osteomalacia, vitamin D.**

rickettsia (rıket′siə), *pl.* **rickettsiae.** any organism of the genus *Rickettsia.* Rickettsiae are small, round, or rod-shaped, specialized bacteria that live as intracellular parasites in lice, fleas, ticks, and mites. They are transmitted to humans by bites from these insects. Rickettsial diseases have been responsible for many of history's worst epidemics. The various species are distinguished on the basis of similarities in the diseases they cause: the spotted fever group includes Rocky mountain spotted fever, rickettsialpox, and others; the typhus group includes endemic and epidemic typhus; the tsutsugamushi group includes scrub typhus; a miscellaneous group includes Q fever and trench fever. Rickettsial diseases are uncommon in parts of the world where insect and rodent populations are well controlled. Tetracycline or chloramphenicol is usually prescribed in the treatment of rickettsial diseases. – **rickettsial,** *adj.*

rickettsialpox (rıket′siəlpoks), a mild, acute infectious disease caused by *Rickettsia akari* and transmitted from mice to humans by mites. It is characterized by an asymptomatic, crusted primary lesion, chills, fever, headache, malaise, myalgia, and a rash resembling chicken pox. About one week after onset of symptoms, small,

discrete, maculopapular lesions appear on any part of the body, but rarely on palms or soles. These lesions become vesicular and dry and form scabs. Eventually the scabs fall off, leaving no scars. Chloramphenicol or tetracycline will hasten recovery. Prevention is the elimination of house mice. Also called **Kew Gardens spotted fever.** Compare **chickenpox, smallpox.** See also *Rickettsia.*

rickettsiosis (rıket′siouˊsıs), *pl.* **rickettsioses.** any of a group of infectious diseases caused by microorganisms of the genus *Rickettsia.* Kinds of rickettsioses include a spotted fever group (**boutonneuse fever, rickettsialpox, Rocky Mountain spotted fever**), a typhus group (**epidemic typhus, murine typhus, scrub typhus**), and a miscellaneous group (**Q-fever, trench fever**). See also *Rickettsia.*

rider's bone, a bony deposit that sometimes develops in horseback riders on the inner side of the lower end of the tendon of the adductor muscle of the thigh. Also called **cavalry bone.**

ridge, a projection or projecting structure, as the gastrocnemial ridge on the posterior surface of the femur, giving attachment to the gastrocnemius muscle.

Riedel's struma (riˊdəlz). See **fibrous thyroiditis.**

Riedel's thyroiditis. See **fibrous thyroiditis.**

Rieder cell leukemia (riˊdər), a malignant neoplasm of blood-forming tissues, characterized by the presence in blood of large numbers of atypical myeloblasts with immature cytoplasm and relatively mature lobulated, indented nuclei.

Rifadin, a trade name for an antibacterial (rifampin).

rifampin, an antibacterial.

■ INDICATION: It is prescribed in the treatment of tuberculosis.

■ CONTRAINDICATIONS: Liver dysfunction or disease or known hypersensitivity to this drug or to rifamycin prohibits its use.

■ ADVERSE EFFECTS: Among the more serious adverse reactions are liver toxicity and a syndrome resembling influenza. Gastrointestinal distress, aches and cramps, discoloration of urine, saliva, and sweat commonly occur. This drug interacts with many other drugs.

Rift Valley fever, an arbovirus infection of east and south Africa spread by mosquitoes or by handling infected sheep and cattle. It is characterized by abrupt fever, chills, headache, and generalized aching, followed by epigastric pain, anorexia, loss of taste, and photophobia. The disease is of short duration, and recovery is usually complete. There is no specific treatment. A killed virus vaccine that provides protection for two years is available for those at risk, as laboratory workers and veterinarians.

RIG, abbreviation for **rabies immune globulin.**

right atrioventricular valve. See **tricuspid valve.**

right brachiocephalic vein, a vessel, about 2.5 cm long, that starts in the root of the neck at the junction of the internal jugular and the subclavian veins on the right side and descends vertically from behind the sternal end of the clavicle to join the left brachiocephalic vein and form the superior vena cava. The right brachiocephalic vein, like the left, receives various tributaries, as the vertebral vein, the internal thoracic vein, and the inferior thyroid vein. Compare **left brachiocephalic vein.**

right bundle branch block, an abnormal cardiac condition, characterized by an impaired electrical signal associated with the bundle of fibers that transmit impulses from the atrioventricular (AV) bundle to the right ventricle. This dysfunction may be a complete or an incomplete block of action impulses for ventricular contraction and may be caused by a small focal lesion in the AV bundle. A right bundle branch block is often associated with right ventricular hyperatrophy, especially in individuals under 40 years of age. In older individuals a right bundle branch block is commonly caused by coronary artery disease. A complete right bundle branch block commonly occurs following surgical closure of a ventricular defect.

right common carotid artery, the shorter of the two common carotid arteries, springing from the brachiocephalic trunk, passing obliquely from the level of the sternoclavicular articulation to the cranial border of the thyroid cartilage, and dividing into the right internal and the right external carotid arteries. Compare **left common carotid artery.**

right coronary artery, one of a pair of branches of the ascending aorta, arising in the right posterior aortic sinus, passing along the right side of the coronary sulcus, dividing into the right interventricular artery and a large marginal branch, supplying both ventricles, the right atrium and the sinuatrial node. Compare **left coronary artery.**

right coronary vein. See **small cardiac vein.**

right-handedness, a natural tendency to favor the use of the right hand. Also called **dextrality.** See also **cerebral dominance, handedness.**

right-heart failure, an abnormal cardiac condition characterized by the impairment of the right side of the heart and congestion and elevated pressure in the systemic veins and capillaries. Right-heart failure is usually related to left-heart failure because both sides of the heart are part of a circuit and what affects one side will eventually affect the other. The most common cause of right-heart failure is left-heart failure. However, research indicates that experimentally induced pure failure of one ventricle may produce hemodynamic and biochemical abnormalities in the opposite ventricle without the usual signs of failure. In failure associated with either side of the heart, cardiac output may be normal, decreased, or increased. Also called **right-sided failure.** Compare **left-heart failure.**

right hepatic duct, the duct that drains bile from the right lobe of the liver into the common bile duct.

righting reflex, any reflex that tends to return an animal to its normal body position in space when it has been moved from the normal position. These reflexes involve a number of sensory receptors including the eyes, labyrinth, and muscles.

right interventricular artery. See **dorsal interventricular artery.**

right lymphatic duct, a vessel that conveys lymph from the right upper quadrant of the body into the blood stream in the neck at the junction of the right internal jugular and the right subclavian veins. About 1.25 cm long, it courses over the medial border of the scalenus anterior. At its orifice are two semilunar valves that prevent venous blood from flowing backward into the duct. Lymph drains into the right lymphatic duct from numerous capillaries and vessels and from three lymphatic trunks in the right quadrant. Compare **thoracic duct.** See also **lymphatic system.**

right pulmonary artery, the longer and slightly larger of the two arteries conveying venous blood from the heart to the lungs, rising from the pulmonary trunk, bending to the right behind the aorta, and dividing into two branches at the root of the right lung. Compare **left pulmonary artery.**

right sided failure. See **right-heart failure.**

right subclavian artery, a large artery that arises from the brachiocephalic artery. It has several important branches: the axillary, vertebral thoracic, and internal thoracic arteries and the cervical and costocervical trunks, perfusing the right side of the upper body.

rigidity, a condition of hardness, stiffness, or inflexibility. —**rigid,** *adj.*

rigidus (rɪj′ɪdəs), a deformity characterized by limited motion, especially dorsiflexion of the great toe. This condition causes pain and may ultimately produce degenerative changes of involved joints.

rigor, **1.** a rigid condition of the tissues of the body, as in rigor mortis. **2.** a violent attack of shivering that may be associated with chills and fever.

rigor mortis, the rigid stiffening of skeletal and cardiac muscle shortly after death.

rim-, a combining form meaning 'crack, fissure': *rimal, rimose, rimula.*

Rimactane, a trade name for an antibacterial (rifampin).

rima glottidis. See **glottis.**

Rimso-50, a trade name for an anti-inflammatory agent (dimethyl sulfoxide), used in the treatment of interstitial cystitis.

ring chromosome, a circular chromosome formed by the fusion of the two ends. It is the primary type of chromosome found in bacteria.

Ringer's lactate, a fluid and electrolyte replenisher.

■ INDICATION: It is prescribed for correction of extracellular volume depletion.

■ CONTRAINDICATIONS: Kidney failure, congestive heart failure, or hypoproteinemia prohibits its use.

■ ADVERSE EFFECTS: Among the more serious adverse reactions are sodium excess and fluid overload, which may lead to pulmonary and peripheral edema.

ringworm. See **tinea.**

Rinne tuning fork test (rin′i), a method of assessing auditory acuity, useful in distinguishing conductive from sensorineural hearing loss. The test is performed with tuning forks of 256, 512, and 1,024 cycles and while each ear is tested the other is masked. The stem of a vibrating fork is alternately placed 0.5 inch from the external auditory meatus of the ear and on the adjacent mastoid bone until the sound is no longer heard at each of these positions. The person with normal hearing perceives the sound for a longer period when conduction is by air than by bone. If the patient has a conductive loss, the sound is heard for a longer period when conducted by bone than by air. In sensorineural loss, the sound is heard longer when conducted by air, but perception by both air and bone conduction is diminished.

Rio Grande fever. See **abortus fever.**

risk factor, a factor that causes a person or a group of people to be particularly vulnerable to an unwanted, unpleasant, or unhealthful event, as immunosuppression, which increases the incidence and severity of infection, or cigarette smoking, which increases the risk of developing a respiratory or cardiovascular disease.

risorius (risor′iəs), one of the 12 muscles of the mouth. Arising in the fascia over the masseter and inserting into the skin at the corner of the mouth, it is innervated by mandibular and buccal branches of the facial nerve and acts to retract the angle of the mouth, as in a smile.

Risser cast (ris′ər), an orthopedic device for encasing the entire trunk of the body, extending over the cervical area to the chin. In rare cases it extends over the hips to the knees. The Risser cast is of plaster of Paris or fiberglass and is used to immobilize the trunk of the body in the treatment of scoliosis and in the preoperative or the postoperative correction or the maintenance of correction of scoliosis. Compare **body jacket, turnbuckle cast.**

risus sardonicus (ri′səs sardon′ikəs), a wry, mask-like grin caused by spasm of the facial muscles, as seen in tetanus.

Ritalin Hydrochloride, a trade name for a central nervous system stimulant (methylphenidate hydrochloride).

ritodrine hydrochloride, a beta sympathomimetic agent.

■ INDICATION: It is prescribed to stop the uterus from contracting in preterm labor.

■ CONTRAINDICATIONS: It is not given before the 20th week of gestation. Known hypersensitivity to this drug prohibits its use.

■ ADVERSE EFFECTS: Among the more serious adverse reactions are tachycardia, palpitations, headache, nausea, and alterations in blood pressure. Pulmonary edema and death have occurred when it has been given concomitantly with corticosteroids to prevent the development of respiratory distress syndrome in the premature neonate.

Ritter's disease, a rare, staphylococcal infection of newborns which begins with red spots about the mouth and chin, gradually spreading over the entire body and followed by generalized exfoliation. Vesicles and yellow crusts may also be present. Ritter's disease is usually fatal unless treated with antibiotics, which should be selected on the basis of bacterial sensitivity tests. Also called **dermatitis exfoliativa neonatorum.** Compare **toxic epidermal necrolysis.**

river blindness. See **onchocerciasis.**

r-loop, (in molecular genetics) a distinctive loop formation seen under an electron microscope. It is composed of a single helical strand of DNA, wound with a hybrid strand containing another single strand of DNA with a strand of RNA.

RMSF, abbreviation for **Rocky Mountain spotted fever.**

Rn, symbol for **radon.**

RN, abbreviation for **registered nurse.**

RNA, abbreviation for **ribonucleic acid.**

RNA nucleotidyltransferase (nu′klioutai′diltræns′-fəreis). See **RNA polymerase.**

RNA polymerase, (in molecular genetics) an enzyme that catalyzes the assembly of ribonucleoside triphosphates into RNA, with single-stranded DNA serving as the template. Also called **RNA nucleotidyltransferase.**

RNA splicing, (in molecular genetics) the process by which base pairs that interrupt the continuity of genetic information in DNA are removed from the precursors of messenger RNA.

Robaxin, a trade name for a skeletal muscle relaxant (methocarbamol).

Robb, Isabel Hampton (1860–1910), a Canadian-born American nursing educator and writer. She was the first to institute a systematic, step-by-step course for nursing students that integrated clinical experience and classwork and the first educator to arrange for the affiliation of her students at other hospitals for specialized training. She also helped to establish university affiliation for nursing education and for postgraduate courses. When the Johns Hopkins School of Nursing was established in Baltimore, in 1889, she became its first director and while there set the high standards for both the practical and theoretical aspects of nursing education that became the base from which she worked to establish national standards. She was one of the founders of *The American Journal of Nursing* and of the forerunner of the American Nurses' Association.

Robertsonian translocation, the exchange of entire chromosome arms, with the break occurring at the centromere, usually between two nonhomologous acrocentric chromosomes, to form one large metacentric chromosome and one extremely small chromosome that carries little genetic material and through successive cell divisions may be lost, leading to a reduction in total chromosome number.

Robicillin VK, a trade name for an antibiotic (penicillin V potassium).

Ro-Bile, a trade name for a gastrointestinal fixed-combination drug containing a variety of digestive enzymes.

Robimycin, a trade name for an antibacterial (erythromycin).

Robinul, a trade name for an anticholinergic (glycopyrrolate).

Robitet, a trade name for an antibiotic (tetracycline or tetracycline hydrochloride).

Robitussin, a trade name for an expectorant (guaifenesin), available plain, in an aromatic syrup, or in various fixed-combination preparations with an antihistamine used as a cough suppressant or a bronchodilator.

Rocaltrol, a trade name for a regulator of calcium (calcitriol).

rock fever. See **brucellosis.**

Rocky Mountain spotted fever (RMSF), a serious tick-borne infectious disease occurring throughout the temperate zones of North and South America, caused by *Rickettsia rickettsii* and characterized by chills, fever, severe headache, myalgia, mental confusion, and rash. Erythematous macules first appear on wrists and ankles, spreading rapidly over the extremities, trunk, face, and, usually, on the palms and soles. Hemorrhagic lesions, constipation, and abdominal distention are also common. The diagnosis is based on clinical examination and is confirmed by laboratory analyses, including immunofluorescent antibody screens, complement fixation test, and Weil-Felix test. Early treatment with chloramphenicol or tetracycline is important, as more than 20 per cent of untreated patients die from shock and renal failure. A diet high in protein is important to avoid hypoproteinemia. Nursing care is especially important to avoid decubitus ulcers and hypostatic or aspiration pneumonia. Immunity follows recovery. Prevention includes the use of insect repellents, the wearing of protective clothing, frequent inspection of the body and careful removal of wood or dog ticks, and immunization with killed vaccine for those frequently exposed to ticks. Care must be taken not to crush ticks, since infection may be acquired through skin abrasions. Also called **mountain fever, mountain tick fever, spotted fever.** Compare **measles, meningococcemia, rickettsialpox, scrub typhus, typhus.**

rod, **1.** a straight cylindrical structure. **2.** one of the tiny cylindrical elements arranged perpendicular to the surface of the retina. Rods contain the chemical rhodopsin which adapts the eye to detect low intensity light and gives the

rods a purple color. Each rod is 40 to 60 μ in length and about 2 μ thick and consists of a slender, reactive outer segment and an inner granular segment. When bright light strikes a rod, rhodopsin rapidly breaks down; it reforms gradually in low intensity light. Compare **cone.** See also **iodopsin, Jacob's membrane.**

rodenticide poisoning, a toxic condition caused by the ingestion of a substance intended for the control of rodent populations. See also **phosphorus poisoning, thallium poisoning, warfarin poisoning.**

rodent ulcer, a slowly developing serpiginous ulceration of a basal cell carcinoma of the skin. See also **basal cell carcinoma.**

roentgen (rent′gən, rent′jən), the quantity of x or gamma radiation that creates one electrostatic unit of ions in one ml of air at 0°C and 760 mm of pressure or 0.001293 gm of air. In radiotherapy or radiodiagnosis, the roentgen is the unit of the emitted dose. See also **rad, rem.**

roentgen fetometry, the use of radiographic techniques to measure the fetus in utero.

roentgenology (rent′gɪnol′əji, rent′jinol′əji), the study of the diagnostic and therapeutic uses of x rays. See also **radiology, roentgen, x ray.**

roentgen ray (rent′gən, rent′jən). See **x ray.**

Rokitansky's disease (rou′kɪtæn′skiz). See **Budd-Chiari syndrome.**

Rolando's fracture (roulæn′douz), a fracture of the base of the first metacarpal.

role playing, a psychotherapeutic technique in which a person acts out a real or simulated situation as a means of understanding intrapsychic conflicts.

role-playing therapy. See **psychodrama.**

Rolfing. See **structural integration.**

roller bandage, a long, tightly wound strip of material which may vary in width. It is generally applied as a circular bandage.

roller clamp, a device, usually made of plastic, equipped with a small roller which may be rolled counterclockwise to close off primary intravenous tubing or clockwise to open it. The roller clamp may also be manipulated to increase and decrease the flow of the intravenous solution and is easily moved with the thumb, thus making it a one-handed convenience in the administration of intravenous therapy. Compare **screw clamp, slide clamp.**

rolling effleurage, a circular rubbing stroke used in massage to promote circulation and muscle relaxation, especially on the shoulder and buttocks. It is performed with the hand flat, the palm and closely held fingers acting as a unit. Compare **effleurage, pétrissage.**

Romberg sign (rom′bərg), an indication of loss of the sense of position in which the patient loses balance when standing erect, feet together, and eyes closed. Also called **Romberg test.**

Romilar, a trade name for an antitussive (dextromethorphan hydrobromide).

Rondec-DM, a trade name for a fixed-combination drug containing an antihistamine (carbinoxamine maleate), an antitussive (dextromethorphan hydrobromide), and an adrenergic decongestant and bronchodilator (pseudoephedrine hydrochloride).

Rondomycin, a trade name for an antibiotic (methacycline hydrochloride).

rongeur forceps (rɒnźhər′), a kind of biting forceps that is strong and heavy, used for cutting bone. Also called **rongeur.**

Roniacol, a trade name for a peripheral vasodilator (nicotinyl alcohol).

room, any area surrounded by four walls within a building, especially one in which a patient is housed, treated, or cared for.

rooming-in, (in a hospital) a recent practice that allows mothers and new babies to share accommodations, remaining together in the hospital as they would at home rather than being separated.

root, the lowest part of an organ or a structure by which something is firmly attached, as the anatomical root of the tooth, which is covered by cementum. Also called **radix.**

rooting reflex, a normal response in newborns when the cheek is touched or stroked along the side of the mouth to turn the head toward the stimulated side and to begin to suck. The reflex disappears by three to four months of age but in some infants may persist until 12 months.

Rorschach test (rɔr′shak), a projective personality assessment test developed by the Swiss psychiatrist Hermann Rorschach. It consists of ten pictures of inkblots, five in black and white, three in black and red, and two multicolored, to which the subject responds by telling in as many interpretations as is desired, what images and emotions each design evokes. Replies are evaluated according to whether the response is to the entire or only part of the image; whether color, shading, shape, or location of individual elements is significant; whether movement is seen; and the degree of complexity to which each interpretation is given. Scoring is primarily subjective and is based on both the subject's responses and the general reaction to the circumstances under which the test is administered. The test is designed to assess the degree to which intellectual and emotional factors are integrated in the subject's perception of the environment. See also **Holtzman inkblot technique.**

ROS, abbreviation for **review of systems.**

rosacea (rɒuzei′shiə), a chronic form of acne seen in adults of all ages and associated with telangiectasia especially of the nose, forehead, and cheeks. Also called **acne rosacea.** See also **rhinophyma.**

rose fever, a common misnomer for seasonal allergic rhinitis caused by pollen, most frequently of grasses, that is airborne at the time roses are in bloom. Roses are not the cause of common spring and summer allergic reactions; their pollen is not dispersed by the wind but is carried from flower to flower by insects.

Rosenmüller's organ (rɒu′zənmyl′ərs). See **epoophoron.**

Rosenthal's syndrome (rɒu′zəntal′). See **hemophilia C.**

roseola (rɒuzi′ələ), 1. any rose-colored rash. 2. See **roseola infantum.**

roseola infantum, a benign, presumably viral, endemic illness of infants and young children, characterized by abrupt, high sustained or spiking fever, mild pharyngitis, and lymph node enlargement. Febrile convulsions may occur. After four or five days the fever suddenly drops to normal and a faint, pink, maculopapular rash appears on the neck, trunk, and thighs. The rash may last a few hours to two days. Diagnosis is based on high fever with rather mild illness and the rash. Sequelae may occur as a result of the convulsions. There is no specific therapy or vaccine. Aspirin or acetaminophen are often used to try to control fever. Anticonvulsive medication may be indicated. Also called **exanthem subitum, sixth disease, Zahorsky's disease.**

rose spots, small erythematous macules occurring on the upper abdomen and anterior thorax and lasting two or three days, characteristic of typhoid and paratyphoid fevers.

rost-, a combining form meaning 'of or pertaining to a beak': *rostellum, rostrad, rostriform.*

rostral (ros′trəl), beak-shaped. — **rostrum,** *n.*

rot-, a combining form meaning 'turned, or to turn': *rotate, rotatory, rotexion.*

rotameter (rɒutæm′ɪtər), a device operated by a needle valve in an anesthetic gas machine that measures gases by speed of flow, according to their viscosity and density. Also called **flowmeter.**

rotating tourniquet, one of four constricting devices used in a rotating order to pool blood in the extremities in order to relieve congestion in the lungs in the treatment of acute pulmonary edema.

■ METHOD: Tourniquets are applied to the upper parts of three extremities at one time. Every 15 minutes, in clockwise order, a tourniquet is placed on the nonconstricted extremity, and one tourniquet is removed; as a result of this rotation, the blood vessels of each of the four extremities are constricted for 45 minutes of each hour of the procedure. If a rotating tourniquet machine is used, blood pressure cuffs placed on all four extremities are automatically inflated and deflated in a rotating sequence. Rotating tourniquets are contraindicated for patients in shock and are not placed on an extremity receiving parenteral fluids. The patient who is to undergo the procedure is placed in a high Fowler's position. Peripheral pulses, as the brachial, radial, popliteal, and pedal, are palpated and are not occluded in applying the tourniquets. During the procedure, blood pressure, respirations, and the apical pulse are checked, and peripheral pulses are palpated every 15 minutes. The chest is auscultated for breath sounds every 30 minutes. Signs of phlebothrombosis and pulmonary embolism are watched for, and if the color of an extremity does not return to normal on release of a tourniquet the physician is informed. At the termination of the procedure, one tourniquet is removed every 15 minutes in the rotation sequence. If pulmonary edema recurs, the tourniquets are reapplied and the physician is notified immediately.

■ NURSING ORDERS: The nurse applies the tourniquets, keeping a time schedule and rotation diagram at bedside. She explains the procedure and remains with the patient as much as possible to provide emotional support.

■ OUTCOME CRITERIA: Rotating tourniquets are beneficial in some cases but are used less frequently than in the past. Some authorities believe the effect of this therapeutic modality on patients whose condition is poor is worse than that of pulmonary edema.

rotation, **1.** a turning around an axis. **2.** one of the four basic kinds of motion allowed by various joints; the rotation of a bone around its central axis which may lie in a separate bone, as in the pivot formed by the dens of the axis around which the atlas turns. A bone, as the humerus, may also rotate around its own longitudinal axis, or the axis of rotation may not be quite parallel to the long axis of the rotating bone, as in movement of the radius on the ulna during pronation and supination of the hand. Compare **circumduction.** See also **angular movement, gliding.**

Rotor syndrome (rou'tər), a rare condition of the liver inherited as an autosomal recessive trait. It is similar to Dubin-Johnson syndrome but can be distinguished by the normal functioning of the gall bladder and normal pigmentation of the liver. See also **Dubin-Johnson syndrome.**

rotula (rot'yulə). See **troche.**

roughage. See **dietary fiber.**

rouleaux (rulou'), *sing.* **rouleau.** an aggregation of red cells in what looks like a stack of coins or checkers. The formation may sometimes be caused by abnormal proteins, as in multiple myeloma or macroglobulinemia, but it is most often a microscopic artifact. Compare **hemagglutination.** See also **erythrocyte sedimentation rate.**

rounds, *Informal.* a teaching conference or a meeting in which the clinical problems encountered in the practice of nursing, medicine, or other service are discussed. Kinds of rounds include **grand rounds, nursing rounds, teaching rounds, walking rounds.**

roundworm, any worm of the class Nematoda, including *Ancylostoma duodenale, Ascaris lumbricoides, Enterobius vermicularis,* and *Strongyloides stercoralis.*

route of administration, (of a drug) any one of the ways in which a drug may be administered, as intramuscularly, intranasally, intravenously, orally, rectally, subcutaneously, sublingually, topically, or vaginally. Some medications can be given only by one route because absorption occurs by that route only or because the specific substance is toxic or damaging when given by another route.

Rovsing's sign (rov'sɪŋz), an indication of acute appendicitis in which pressure on the left lower quadrant of the abdomen causes pain in the right lower quadrant. See also **appendicitis.**

Royal College of Physicians (R.C.P.), a professional organization of physicians in the United Kingdom.

Royal College of Physicians and Surgeons of Canada (RCPSC), a national Canadian organization that recognizes and confers membership on certain qualified physicians and surgeons.

Royal College of Surgeons (R.C.S.), a professional organization of surgeons in the United Kingdom.

RPF, abbreviation for **renal plasma flow.**

RP-Mycin, a trade name for an antibacterial (erythromycin).

R.R., RR, abbreviation for **recovery room.**

-(r)rachia, a combining form meaning a '(specified) foreign chemical substance': *calciorrhachia, glycorrhachia, polypeptidorrhachia.*

-(r)rhage, a combining form meaning a 'rupture, an excessive fluid discharge': *hemorrhage, lymphorrhage, phleborrhage.*

-(r)rhagia, a combining form meaning a 'fluid discharge of excessive quantity': *lymphorrhagia, meningorrhagia, tracheorrhagia.*

-(r)rhagic, a combining form meaning 'of, pertaining, or referring to a kind or condition of excessive fluid discharge': *haemorrhagic, lymphorrhagic, serohemorrhagic.*

-(r)rhaphy, a combining form meaning a 'suturing in place': *cysticorrhaphy, meningeorrhaphy, osteorrhaphy.* Also **-(r)rhaphia.**

-(r)rhea, a combining form meaning: 'fluid discharge, flow': *anarrhea, cystirrhea, laryngorrhea.* Also **-(r)rhoea, -(r)rhoeica.**

-(r)rheal. See **-(r)rheic.**

-(r)rheic, a combining form meaning 'pertaining to a fluid discharge': *cryptorrheic, diarrheic, pyorrheic.* Also **-(r)rheal, -(r)rhetic, -(r)rhoeic.**

-(r)rhetic. See **-(r)rheic.**

-(r)rhexis, a combining form meaning a 'rupture of a (specified) body part': *arteriorrhexis, cardiorrhexis, plasmarrhexis.*

-(r)rhine, a combining form meaning 'having a (specified sort of) nose': *leptorrhine, mesorrhine, platyrrhine.*

-(r)rhinia, a combining form meaning '(condition of the) nose': *arrhinia, birhinia, microrhinia.*

-(r)rhoeica, a combining form meaning 'fluid discharge': *seborrhoeica, dysmenorrhoeica, gonorrhoeica.* Also **-(r)rhea, -(r)rhoea.**

-(r)rhythmia, a combining form meaning '(condition of the) heartbeat or the pulse': *bradyrhythmia, dysrhythmia, tachyrhythmia.*

R-R interval, the interval from the peak of one QRS complex to the peak of the next as shown on an electrocardiogram. See also **cardiac cycle.**

RSV, abbreviation for *respiratory syncytial virus.* See **bronchiolitis.**

RT, abbreviation for **respiratory therapy.**

R.T., abbreviation for **Registered Therapist.**

RTA, abbreviation for **renal tubular acidosis.**

r.t.c., abbreviation for **return to clinic,** noted on the chart, usually followed by a date on which a subsequent appointment has been made for the patient.

Ru, symbol for **ruthenium.**

rub-, a combining form meaning 'red': *rubedo, ruber, rubor.*

rubber, *Informal.* **condom.**

rubbing alcohol, a disinfectant for skin and instruments. It contains 70 per cent ethyl alcohol by volume, the remainder consisting of water and denaturants, with or without color or perfume. It may cause dryness of the skin. Rubbing alcohol is for external use only and is flammable.

rubefacient (ru'bəfei'shənt), **1.** a substance or agent that increases the reddish coloration of the skin. **2.** increasing the reddish coloration of the skin.

rubella, a contagious viral disease characterized by fever, symptoms of a mild upper respiratory infection, lymph node enlargement, arthralgia, and a diffuse, fine, red, maculopapular rash. The virus is spread by droplet infection and the incubation time is from 12 to 23 days. Also called **German measles, three-day measles.** Compare **measles, scarlet fever.**

■ OBSERVATIONS: The symptoms usually last only two or three days except for arthralgia, which may persist longer or recur. One attack confers lifelong immunity. If a woman acquires rubella in the first trimester of pregnancy, fetal anomalies may result, including heart defects, cataracts, deafness, and mental retardation. An infant exposed to the virus in utero at any time during gestation may shed the virus for up to 30 months after birth. Complications of postnatal rubella are rare.

■ INTERVENTION: The illness itself is mild and needs no special treatment. Live attenuated rubella vaccine is advised for all children to reduce chances of an epidemic and thus to protect pregnant women. The vaccine is not given to women already pregnant, and it is recommended that pregnancy be avoided for three months after the administration of rubella vaccine. Spread of the virus from a recently vaccinated individual rarely occurs. Immune serum globulin containing rubella antibodies may help prevent fetal infection in exposed susceptible pregnant women, but ordinary gamma globulin will not protect the fetus.

■ NURSING CONSIDERATIONS: Temporary arthralgia is common after vaccination. Women of childbearing age working with children may be tested for immunity to rubella and vaccinated if not immune. The only proof of immunity is the laboratory demonstration of antibodies to the rubella virus. The rash and malaise of rubella resemble those of scarlet fever, some cases of mononucleosis, and allergic drug reactions, leading some people to think they have had rubella when they have not.

rubella and mumps virus vaccine, a suspension containing live attenuated mumps and rubella viruses.

■ INDICATIONS: It is prescribed for immunization against rubella and mumps.

■ CONTRAINDICATIONS: Acute infection or known hypersensitivity to avian proteins prohibits its use. It is not given to a patient whose immune function is compromised or to a pregnant woman. It is not given for three months following the use of plasma, whole blood, or an immune serum globulin. Pregnancy is avoided for three months following immunization.

■ ADVERSE EFFECTS: Among the more serious adverse effects are mild to severe hypersensitivity reactions.

rubella embryopathy, any congenital abnormality in an infant caused by maternal rubella in the early stages of pregnancy.

rubella panencephalitis. See **panencephalitis.**

rubella virus vaccine, a suspension containing live attenuated rubella virus.

■ INDICATION: It is prescribed for immunization against rubella.

■ CONTRAINDICATIONS: Compromised immune function, fever, acute infection, untreated tuberculosis, or hypersensitivity to proteins of the animal of the vaccine prohibits its use. It is not given to pregnant women, nor is it given for three months following the use of plasma, whole blood, or immune serum globulin. Pregnancy should be avoided for three months following immunization.

■ ADVERSE EFFECTS: Among the most serious adverse reactions are severe hypersensitivity reactions.

rubeola (rubi'ələ). See **measles.**

rubescent (rubes'ənt), reddening.

rubidium (Rb), a soft metallic element of the alkali metals group. Its atomic number is 37; its atomic weight is 85.47. Slightly radioactive, it is used in radioisotope scanning.

Rubin's test, a test performed in the process of evaluating the cause of infertility by assessing the patency of the Fallopian tubes. Carbon dioxide gas (CO_2) is introduced into the tubes under pressure through a cannula inserted into the cervix. The CO_2 is passed through it from a syringe connected to a manometer at pressures of up to 200 mm Hg. If the tubes are open, the gas enters the abdominal cavity and the recorded pressure falls below 180 mm/Hg. A high-pitched bubbling can be heard through the abdominal wall with the stethoscope as the gas escapes from the tubes. The patient may complain of shoulder pain from diaphragmatic irritation; an x ray will show free gas under the diaphragm. If the tubes are blocked, gas cannot escape from the tubes into the abdominal cavity; the pressure recorded on the manometer remains at 200 mm/Hg. A tracing may be made to show tubal peristalsis, any leakage in the system, tubal spasm, or partial obstruction. After the test, the patient rests for a three-hour period. Crampy pain, dizziness, nausea, and vomiting may occur; positioning with the pelvis higher than the head, in knee-chest position, or in Trendelenberg's position, allows the gas to stay in the pelvis and give some relief by avoiding diaphragmatic irritation.

rubivirus (ru'bivai'rəs), a member of the togavirus family, which includes the rubella virus.

rubor (ru'bər), redness, especially when accompanying inflammation.

Rubramin PC, a trade name for vitamin B_{12} (cyanocobalamin).

ructus (rək'təs). See **eructation.**

rudiment, an organ or tissue that is incompletely developed or nonfunctional. —**rudimentary,** *adj.*

Ruffini's corpuscles (rufi'niz), a variety of oval-shaped nerve endings in the subcutaneous tissue of the human finger, located principally at the junction of the corium and the subcutaneous tissue. Ruffini's corpuscles consist of strong connective-tissue sheaths enclosing nerve fibers with many branches that end in small knobs. Compare **Golgi-Mazzoni corpuscles, Pacini's corpuscles.**

ruga (ru'gə), *pl.* **rugae** (ru'ji). a ridge or fold, as the rugae of the stomach, which presents large folds in the mucous membrane of that organ.

rule of nines, a formula for estimating the amount of body surface covered by burns by assigning nine per cent to the head and each arm, twice nine per cent to each leg, and the anterior and posterior trunk, and one per cent to the perineum.

rumination (ru'minei'shən), habitual regurgitation of small amounts of undigested food with little force after every feeding, a condition commonly seen in infants. It may be a symptom of overfeeding, of eating too fast, or

of swallowing air. It has little or no clinical significance. More copious and forceful regurgitation may indicate a more serious condition, as an allergic intestinal reaction, an infectious disease, an obstruction of the intestinal tract, or a metabolic disorder. See also **vomit.**

rupture, 1. a tear or break in the continuity or configuration of an organ or body tissue, including those instances when other tissue protrudes through the opening. See also **hernia.** 2. to cause a break or tear.

ruptured intervertebral disc. See **herniated disc.**

Rural Clinics Assistance Act, an act of Congress that permitted the establishment of clinics in certain areas designated rural and underserved and in some inner cities. The clinics are designed to provide primary care through teams of physicians and nurse practitioners. The act is significant to nursing by being the first federal legislation which allows third-party reimbursement directly to nurses practicing in expanded roles.

Russell's bodies, the mucoprotein inclusions found in globular plasma cells in cancer. The bodies contain surface gamma globulins, probably derived from the condensation of internal cellular secretions. Also called **cancer bodies, fuchsin bodies.**

Russell dwarf, a person affected with Russell's syndrome, a congenital disorder in which short stature is associated with various anomalies of the head, face, and skeleton and with varying degrees of mental retardation.

Russell traction, a unilateral or a bilateral orthopedic mechanism which combines suspension and traction to immobilize, position, and align the lower extremities in the treatment of fractured femurs and hip and knee contractures and in the treatment of disease processes of the hip and the knee. Russell traction is applied as adhesive or nonadhesive skin traction and employs a sling to relieve the weight of the lower extremities subjected to traction pull. A jacket restraint is often incorporated to help immobilize the patient. Compare **split Russell traction.**

Russian bath, a hot steam bath followed by a cold plunge. Also called **Finnish bath.**

ruthenium (Ru), a hard, brittle, metallic element. Its atomic number is 44; its atomic weight is 101.07.

rutin (ru'tin), a bioflavonoid obtained from buckwheat and used in the treatment of capillary fragility.

RV, abbreviation for **residual volume.**

RVC, abbreviation for *responds to verbal commands.*

R wave, the component of the cardiac cycle shown on an electrocardiogram as a steep, straight line to the beginning of the sharp downward slant of the S wave. It represents the middle part of the QRS complex.

S

s, symbol for **steady state.**

S, 1. symbol for **saturation of hemoglobin.** 2. symbol for **sulfur.**

S₁, the first heart sound in the cardiac cycle occurring with ventricular systole. It is associated with closure of the mitral and tricuspid valves and is synchronous with the apical pulse. Auscultated at the apex, it is louder, longer, and lower than the second sound (S₂), which follows it.

S₂, the second heart sound in the cardiac cycle. It is associated with closure of the aortic and pulmonary valves just before ventricular diastole. Auscultated at the base of the heart, the second sound is louder than the first.

S₃, the third heart sound in the cardiac cycle. Normally, it is audible only in children and physically active young adults. It is an abnormal finding in older people and usually indicates myocardial failure. It is heard with the bell of a stethoscope placed lightly over the apex of the heart with the patient lying down, tipped to the left.

S₄, the fourth heart sound in the cardiac cycle. It occurs late in diastole upon contraction of the atria. Rarely heard in normal subjects, it indicates an abnormally increased resistance to ventricular filling, as in hypertensive cardiovascular disease, coronary artery disease, myocardiopathy, and aortic stenosis.

SA, 1. abbreviation for **surgeon's assistant.** 2. abbreviation for **sinoatrial.** 3. abbreviation for **surface area.** 4. abbreviation for **surgeon's assistant.**

Sabin-Feldman dye test (sei'bɪnfeld'mən), a diagnostic test for toxoplasmosis which depends on the presence of specific antibodies that block the uptake of methylene blue dye by the cytoplasm of the *Toxoplasma* organisms.

Sabin Vaccine. See **poliovirus vaccine.**

sac, a pouch or a baglike organ, as the abdominal sac of the embryo that develops into the abdominal cavity.

sacchari-. See **saccharo-.**

saccharide (sæk'əraid'), any of a large group of carbohydrates including all sugars and starches. Almost all carbohydrates are saccharides. See also **carbohydrate, sugar.**

saccharin (sæk'ərɪn), **saccharine** (sæk'ərɪn, sæk'əraɪn'), 1. a white, crystalline substance many times sweeter than table sugar (sucrose). Saccharin is often used as a substitute for sugar. 2. having a sweet taste, especially cloyingly sweet.

saccharo-, sacchari-, a combining form meaning 'of or pertaining to sugar': *saccharobiose, saccharorrhea, saccharosuria.*

Saccharomyces (sæk'əroumai'siz), a genus of yeast fungi, including brewer's and baker's yeast as well as some pathogenic fungi that cause such diseases as bronchitis, moniliasis, and pharyngitis.

saccharomycosis (sæk'əroumaikou'sɪs), 1. infection with yeast fungi, as the genera *Candida,* or *Cryptococcus.* 2. *Obsolete.* cryptococcosis or European blastomycosis.

saccule (sæk'yul), a small bag or sac, as the air saccules of the lungs. See also **sacculus.** —**saccular,** *adj.*

sacculus (sæk'yuləs), *pl.* **sacculi.** a little sac or bag, especially the smaller of the two divisions of the membranous labyrinth of the vestibule, which communicates with the cochlear duct through the ductus reuniens in the inner ear. See also **saccule.**

Sachs' disease. See **Tay-Sachs disease.**

sacral (sei'krəl, sæk'rəl), of or pertaining to the sacrum.

sacral foramen, one of several openings between the fused segments of the sacral vertebrae in the sacrum through which the sacral nerves pass.

sacral node, a node in one of the seven groups of parietal lymph nodes of the abdomen and the pelvis, situated within the sacrum. The sacral nodes are located in relation to the middle and the lateral sacral arteries and receive lymphatics from the rectum and the posterior wall of the pelvis. Compare **lumbar node.** See also **lymph, lymphatic system, lymph node.**

sacral plexus, a network of motor and sensory nerves formed by the lumbosacral trunk from the fourth and fifth lumbar, and by the first, second, and third sacral nerves. They converge toward the caudal portion of the greater sciatic foramen and unite to become a large, flattened band, most of which continues into the thigh as the sciatic nerve. The plexus lies against the posterior, lateral wall of the pelvis between the piriformis and the internal iliac vessels embedded in the pelvic subserous fascia. The nerves of the plexus, except for the third sacral nerve, divide into ventral and dorsal portions. Branches from these divisions are the nerve to the quadratus femoris and the gemellus inferior, the nerve to the obturator internus and the gemellus superior, the nerve to the piriformis, the superior gluteal nerve, the inferior gluteal nerve, the posterior femoral cutaneous nerve, the perforating cutaneous nerve, the sciatic nerve, and the pudendal nerve. Compare **lumbar plexus.**

sacral vertebra, one of the five segments of the vertebral column that fuse in the adult to form the sacrum. The ventral border of the first sacral vertebra projects into the pelvis. The bodies of the other sacral vertebrae are smaller than that of the first and are flattened and curved ventrally, forming the convex, anterior surface of the sacrum. The rudimentary spinous processes of the first several sacral vertebrae surmount the middle sacral crest, and the transverse processes of the sacral vertebrae form the lateral sacral crests. The sacral hiatus at the caudal end of the sacral canal develops from the incomplete growth of the spinous processes of the last two sacral vertebrae. The resultant widened aperture is used by anaesthesiologists for the insertion of a needle to administer caudal analgesia. Compare **cervical vertebra, coccygeal vertebra, lumbar vertebra, thoracic vertebra.** See also **sacrum, vertebra.**

sacro-, a combining form meaning 'of or pertaining to the sacrum': *sacrococcyx, sacroiliac, sacrolumbalis.*

sacroiliac articulation, an immovable joint in the pelvis formed by the articulation of each side of the sacrum with an iliac bone.

sacrospinalis (seik′rouspæinæl′ɪs), a large, fleshy muscle of the back that divides into a lateral iliocostalis column, an intermediate longissimus column, and a medial spinalis column. Each column consists of three parts. The sacrospinalis is sheathed in the fascia thoracolumbalis and arises in a broad, thick tendon from the sacrum, the ilium, and the lumbar vertebrae. It inserts into the ribs and into certain cervical vertebrae and is innervated by the branches of the dorsal primary divisions of the spinal nerves. It extends and flexes the vertebral column and the head, and it draws the ribs downward. Also called **erector spinae.**

sacrum (sei′krəm, sæk′rəm), the large, triangular bone at the dorsal part of the pelvis, inserted like a wedge between the two hip bones. The base of the sacrum articulates with the last lumbar vertebra, and its apex articulates with the coccyx; various muscles attach to its spinal crest. The sacrum is shorter and wider in women than in men. — **sacral,** *adj.*

saddle block anesthesia, a form of regional nerve block in which the parts of the body anesthetized are those that would touch a saddle, were the patient sitting astride one. It is performed by injecting a local anesthetic into the spinal cavity as the patient sits with the head on the chest, back curved, and legs down. As soon as the anesthetic has been injected, the patient is laid flat and the blood pressure and vital signs are noted. Saddle block anesthesia is common in some centers for anesthesia during childbirth. See also **obstetric anesthesia.**

saddle joint, a synovial joint in which surfaces of contiguous bones are reciprocally concavo-convex. A saddle joint permits no axial rotation but allows flexion, extension, adduction, and abduction, as in the carpometacarpal joint of the thumb. Also called **articulatio sellaris.** Compare **condyloid joint, pivot joint.**

sadism, 1. abnormal pleasure derived from inflicting physical or psychological pain or abuse on others; cruelty. 2. (in psychiatry) a psychosexual disorder characterized by the infliction of physical or psychological pain or humiliation on another person, either a consenting or nonconsenting partner, in order to achieve sexual excitement or gratification. The condition is usually chronic in form, is seen predominantly in men, may result from conscious or unconscious motivations or desires, and, in severe cases, can lead to rape, torture, and murder. Kinds of sadism are **anal sadism, oral sadism.** Also called **active algolagnia.** Compare **masochism.** See also **algolagnia, sadomasochism.** — **sadist,** *n.,* **sadistic,** *adj.*

sadist, a person who is afflicted with or practices sadism.

sadomasochism, a personality disorder characterized by traits of sadism and masochism. Also called **algolagnia.**

safe period. See **natural family-planning method.**

sagittal (sæj′ətəl), (in anatomy) of or pertaining to a suture or an imaginary line extending from the front to the back in the midline of the body or a part of the body.

sagittal plane, the anterioposterior plane or the section parallel to the median plane of the body. Compare **coronal plane, median plane, transverse plane.**

sagittal suture, the serrated connection between the two parietal bones of the skull, coursing down the midline from the coronal suture to the upper part of the lambdoidal suture.

SaH, SAH, abbreviation for **subarachnoid hemorrhage.**

SAIN, abbreviation for **Society for Advancement in Nursing.**

Salamide, a trade name for an analgesic (salicylamide).

salicylanilide (sæl′ɪsɪlæn′ɪlæid), a topical antifungal prescribed in the treatment of tinea capitis caused by *Microsporum audouini.* It is applied to the scalp in a 3 to 5 per cent ointment.

salicylate (səlɪs′əleit), any of several widely prescribed drugs derived from salicylic acid. Salicylates exert analgesic, antipyretic, and anti-inflammatory actions. The most important is acetylsalicylic acid, or aspirin. Sodium salicylate has also been used systemically, and it exerts similar effects. Many of the actions of aspirin appear to result from its ability to inhibit cyclo-oxygenase, a rate limiting enzyme in prostaglandin biosynthesis. Aspirin is used in a wide variety of conditions, and, in the usual analgesic dosage, it causes only mild adverse effects. Severe occult gastrointestinal bleeding or gastric ulcers may occur with frequent use. Large doses taken over a long period can cause significant impairment of hemostasts. Occasionally, an asthma-like reaction is produced in hypersensitive individuals. Because of ready availability of aspirin, accidental and intentional overdosage is common. Symptoms of salicylate intoxication include tinnitus, gastrointestinal disturbances, abnormal respiration, acid-base imbalance, and central nervous system disturbances. Fatalities have occurred from ingestion of as little as 10-30 grains of aspirin in adults or as little as 4 ml of methyl salicylate in children. In addition to aspirin and sodium salicylate, which are used systemically, methyl salicylate is used topically as a counterirritant in ointments and liniments. Methyl salicylate can be absorbed through the skin in amounts capable of causing systemic toxicity. Another salicylate, salicylic acid, is too irritating to be used systemically and is used topically as a keratolytic agent, as for removing warts.

salicylate poisoning, a toxic condition caused by the ingestion of salicylate, most often in aspirin or oil of wintergreen. Intoxication is characterized by rapid breathing, vomiting, headache, irritability, ketosis, hypoglycemia, and, in severe cases, by convulsions and respiratory failure. Treatment usually includes prompt induced emesis or gastric lavage with activated charcoal, the administration of a saline cathartic, a parenteral infusion of sodium bicarbonate, injection of vitamin K if bleeding is present, and correction of dehydration, hypoglycemia, and hypokalemia. Sodium bicarbonate by mouth is contraindicated.

salicylazosulfapyridine. See **sulfasalazine.**

salicylic acid (sæl'ɪsɪl'ɪk), a keratolytic agent.
- INDICATIONS: It is prescribed in the treatment of hyperkeratotic skin conditions and as an adjunct in fungal infections.
- CONTRAINDICATIONS: Diabetes, impaired circulation, or known hypersensitivity to this drug prohibits its use.
- ADVERSE EFFECTS: Among the more serious adverse reactions are skin inflammation and salicylism.

saline cathartic, one of a large group of cathartics administered to achieve prompt, complete evacuation of the bowel. A watery semi-fluid evacuation usually occurs within three to four hours. The most common indication for the administration of any of these agents is preparation of the bowel for diagnostic examination. Various preparations, including magnesium sulfate, sodium phosphate, sodium sulfate, and several naturally occurring mineral waters, may be used to achieve catharsis. The palatability, cost, and adverse systemic reactions of the saline cathartics depend on the particular agent used and the dose of the agent given.

saline infusion, the therapeutic introduction of a physiologic salt solution into a vein.

saline irrigation, the washing out of a body cavity or wound with a stream of salt solution, usually an isotonic aqueous solution of sodium chloride.

saline solution, a solution containing sodium chloride.

Depending on the use, it may be hypotonic, isotonic, or hypertonic with body fluids.

saliva, the clear, viscous fluid secreted by the salivary and mucous glands in the mouth. Saliva contains water, mucin, organic salts, and the digestive enzyme ptyalin. It serves to moisten the oral cavity, to initiate the digestion of starches, and to aid in the chewing and swallowing of food.

salivary, of or pertaining to saliva or to the formation of saliva.

salivary duct, any one of the ducts through which saliva passes. Kinds of salivary ducts are **Bartholin's duct, duct of Rivinus, parotid duct, submandibular duct.**

salivary fistula, an abnormal communication from a salivary gland or duct to an opening in the mouth or on the skin of the face or neck.

salivary gland, one of the three pairs of glands that pour their secretions into the mouth, thus aiding the digestive process. The salivary glands are the parotid, the submandibular, and the sublingual glands. They are racemose structures consisting of numerous lobes subdivided into smaller lobules connected by dense areolar tissue, vessels and ducts. The ducts ramify inside each lobule, ending in alveoli. One kind of alveolus secretes a viscid fluid containing mucin. The other kind secretes serous fluid. The sublingual gland secretes mucus; the parotid gland, serous fluid; the submandibular gland, both mucus and serous fluid. The lobules of the salivary glands are richly supplied with blood vessels and fine plexuses of nerves. The hilum of the submandibular gland contains Langley's ganglion of nerve cells.

salivary gland cancer, a malignant neoplastic disease of a salivary gland, occurring most frequently in a parotid gland. About 75 per cent of tumors that develop in the salivary glands are benign, characteristically slow-growing, painless, mobile masses that are cystic or rubbery in consistency. In contrast, malignant tumors are rapid-growing, hard, lumpy, fixed, and frequently tender. Pain, trismus, and facial palsy may occur. Diagnostic measures include x rays, with sialographic studies and mandibular and chest films to detect metastases, and cytologic studies of saliva from Stensen's duct. Direct biopsies are not recommended. The most common malignant neoplasms are mucoepidermoid, adenoid cystic, solid, and squamous cell carcinomas. Treatment usually consists of the surgical removal of the lobe containing a benign tumor and total parotidectomy with a radical neck dissection if the lesion is advanced. Radiotherapy is administered for residual, recurrent, or inoperable cancers, and chemotherapy may be palliative.

Salk Vaccine. See **poliovirus vaccine.**

salmon calcitonin. See **calcitonin.**

Salmonella (sæl'mənel'ə), a genus of motile, gram-negative, rod-shaped bacteria that includes species causing typhoid fever, paratyphoid fever, and some forms of gastroenteritis. See also **salmonellosis.**

salmonellosis (sæl'mənəlou'sıs), a form of gastroenteritis, caused by ingestion of food contaminated with a species of *Salmonella,* characterized by an incubation period of 6 to 48 hours followed by sudden, colicky abdominal pain, fever, and bloody, watery diarrhea. Nausea and vomiting are common and abdominal signs may resemble acute appendicitis or cholecystitis. Symptoms usually last from two to five days, but diarrhea and fever may persist for up to two weeks. Dehydration may occur. There is no specific treatment. Antibiotics may prolong the excretion of *Salmonella* in stools and are usually not indicated. Adequate cooking, good refrigeration, and careful handwashing may reduce the frequency of outbreaks. See also **food poisoning.**

salol camphor (sæl'ɔl), a clear, oily mixture of two parts of camphor and three parts of phenyl salicylate, used as a local antiseptic.

Salonica fever (səlon'ıkə). See **trench fever.**

salpingectomy (sæl'pınjek'təmi), surgical removal of one or both Fallopian tubes, performed to remove a cyst or tumor, excise an abcess, or, if both tubes are removed, as a sterilization procedure. Often the operation is done with a hysterectomy or an oophorectomy. Either spinal block or general anesthesia may be given. Postoperatively, the patient is instructed to avoid sharply flexing the thighs or the knees. Persistent low back pain or the presence of bloody or scanty urine indicates that a ureter may have been nicked during surgery.

salpingitis (sæl'pınjai'tıs), an inflammation or infection of the Fallopian tube. See also **pelvic inflammatory disease.**

salpingo-, a combining form meaning 'of or pertaining to a tube, especially a Fallopian tube': *salpingocele, salpingolysis, salpingoplasty.*

salpingostomy (sæl'pıŋgos'təmi), the formation of an artificial opening in a Fallopian tube, performed to restore patency in a tube whose fimbriated opening has been closed by infection or by chronic inflammation or in order to drain an abcess or an accumulation of fluid. Either regional or general anesthesia is used. A prosthesis may be inserted to maintain the patency of the Fallopian tube and to direct the route of the ova to assist fertilization. Postoperatively, the nurse cautions the patient against sharply flexing the thighs or the knees. Low back pain or scanty or bloody urine may indicate that a ureter has been nicked, requiring surgical intervention.

salpinx (sæl'pıŋks), *pl.* **salpinges** (sælpın'jiz). a tube, as the *salpinx auditiva* and the *salpinx uterina.* — **salpingian,** *adj.*

salt, **1.** a compound formed by the chemical reaction of an acid and a base. Salts are usually composed of a metal and a nonmetal. Some salts contain groups of atoms that behave chemically as metals or nonmetals. **2.** sodium chloride (common table salt). **3.** a substance, as magnesium sulfate (Epsom salt), used as a purgative.

saltation (sæltei'shən), (in genetics) a mutation causing a significant difference in appearance between parent and offspring or an abrupt variation in the characteristics of the species. — **saltatorial, saltatoric, saltatory,** *adj.*

saltatory evolution, the appearance of a sudden, abrupt change within a species, caused by mutation; the progression of a species by sudden major changes rather than by the gradual accumulation of minor changes. The phenomenon occurs predominantly in plants as a result of polyploidy. See also **emergent evolution.**

salt depletion, the loss of salt from the body through excessive elimination of body fluids by perspiration, diarrhea, vomiting, or urination, without corresponding replacement. See also **electrolyte balance, heat exhaustion.**

Salter fracture (sol'tər). See **epiphyseal fracture.**

salt-free diet. See **low-sodium diet.**

Saluron, a trade name for an antihypertensive and diuretic (hydroflumethiazide).

salve (sæv). See **ointment.**

samarium (Sm), a rare-earth, metallic element. Its atomic number is 62; its atomic weight is 150.35.

sand bath, the application of warm, dry sand or of damp sand to the body.

sand flea. See *Tunga penetrans.*

sandfly fever. See **phlebotomus fever.**

Sandhoff's disease, a variant of Tay-Sachs disease that includes defects in both the enzymes hexosaminidase A and B. It is characterized by a progressively more rapid course and is found in the general population, not restricted as is Tay-Sachs disease. Also called **gangliosidosis type II.** See also **Tay-Sachs disease.**

Sandoptal, a trade name for a sedative (butalbital).

Sandril, a trade name for an antihypertensive (reserpine).

sand tumor. See **psammoma.**

sangui-, a combining form meaning 'of or pertaining to blood': *sanguicolous, sanguiferous, sanguinolent.*

sanguineous (sæŋgwın'iəs), pertaining to blood.

sanita-, a combining form meaning 'of or pertaining to health': *sanitarium, sanitas, sanitation.*

San Joaquin fever (sæn'wokin'), the primary stage of coccidioidomycosis.

SA node. See **sinoatrial node.**

Sanorex, a trade name for an anorexiant (mazindol).

Sansert, a trade name for a vasoconstrictor (methysergide maleate).

Santyl, a trade name for an enzyme (collagenase).

saphenous nerve (səfi'nəs), the largest and longest branch of the femoral nerve, supplying the skin of the medial side of the leg. It courses deep to the sartorius, accompanied by the femoral artery posteriorly, and crosses from the lateral to the medial side of the sartorius, within the fascial cover of the adductor canal. At the tendinous arch in the adductor magnus, it leaves the artery, pierces the fascia of the adductor canal, descends along the medial side of the knee, penetrates the fascia lata between the tendons of the sartorius and the gracilis, and becomes subcutaneous. It accompanies the great saphenous vein along the medial side of the leg, and at the medial border of the tibia in the distal third of the leg divides into two terminal branches. One branch joins the medial cutaneous and the obturator nerves to form the subsartorial plexus. A large infrapatellar branch passes to the skin over the patella and on the lateral side of the knee joins with branches of the lateral femoral cutaneous nerve to form the patellar plexus. One branch of the saphenous nerve below the knee supplies the ankle. Another branch below the knee supplies the medial side of the foot. See also **femoral nerve.**

saphenous vein. See **great saphenous vein.**

sapo-, a combining form meaning 'of or pertaining to soap': *sapogenin, saponaceous, sapotoxin.*

saponin (sæp'ənɪn), a soapy material found in some plants, especially soapwort (Bouncing Bet) and certain lilies. It is used in demulcent medications to provide a sudsy quality. Natural saponins have largely been replaced by synthetic preparations.

-sarc, a combining form meaning '(specified type of) flesh': *ectosarc, endosarc, perisarc.*

sarco-, a combining form meaning 'of or related to the flesh': *sarcoadenoma, sarcode, sarcolyte.*

sarcoidosis (sar'kɔɪdou'sɪs), a chronic disorder of unknown etiology characterized by the formation of tubercles of nonnecrotizing epithelioid tissue. Common sites are the lungs, spleen, liver, skin, mucous membranes, and lacrimal and salivary glands, usually with involvement of the lymph glands. Diminished reactivity to tuberculin frequently accompanies the disorder. The lesions usually disappear over a period of months or years but progress to widespread granulomatous inflammation and fibrosis. Also called **Boeck's sarcoid.**

sarcoidosis cordis, a form of sarcoidosis in which granulomatous lesions develop in the myocardium. The number and the size of the growths vary. Mild cases with few infiltrates are asymptomatic. In severe cases the myocardium may be infiltrated with many tumors and cardiac failure may follow. See also **sarcoidosis.**

sarcoma (sarkou'mə), *pl.* **sarcomas, sarcomata.** an uncommon, malignant neoplasm of the soft tissues arising in fibrous, fatty, muscular, synovial, vascular, or neural tissue, usually first presenting as a painless swelling. About 40 per cent of sarcomas occur in the lower extremities, 20 per cent in the upper extremities, 20 per cent in the trunk, and the rest in the head, neck, or retroperineum. The tumor, composed of closely packed cells in a fibrillar or homogeneous matrix, tends to be vascular and is usually highly invasive. Trauma probably does not play a role in the etiology, but sarcomas may arise in burn or radiation scars. Small tumors may be managed by local excision and postoperative radiotherapy, but bulky sarcomas of the extremities may require amputation followed by irradiation for local control and combination chemotherapy to eliminate small foci or neoplastic cells. See specific sarcomas.

-sarcoma, a combining form meaning a 'malignant neoplasm': *angiosarcoma, hemangiosarcoma, myelosarcoma.*

sarcoma botryoides (bo'trioi'diz), a tumor derived from primitive striated muscle cells, occurring most frequently in young children and characterized by a painful, edematous, polypoid grapelike mass in the upper vagina or on the uterine cervix or the neck of the urinary bladder. See also **rhabdomyosarcoma.**

sarcomagenesis (sarkou'məjen'ɪsɪs), the process of initiating and promoting the development of a sarcoma. Compare **carcinogenesis, oncogenesis, tumorigenesis.** — **sarcomagenetic,** *adj.*

sarcoplasmic reticulum, a network of tubules and sacs in skeletal muscles that plays an important role in muscle contraction and relaxation by releasing and storing calcium ions. This network is analogous, but not identical, to the endoplasmic reticulum of other cells.

Sarcoptes scabiei (sarkop'tiz skei'biai), the genus of itch mite that causes scabies.

sartorius (sartɔr'ias), the longest muscle in the body, extending from the pelvis to the calf of the leg. It is a narrow muscle that arises from the anterior superior iliac spine, passes obliquely across the proximal anterior part of the thigh from the lateral to the medial side, and inserts, by a tendon and an aponeurosis, into the tibia. It is innervated by branches of the femoral nerve. It acts to flex the thigh and rotate it laterally and to flex the leg and rotate it medially. Compare **quadriceps femoris.**

S.A.S. 500, a trade name for a sulfonamide (sulfasalazine), used to treat ulcerative colitis.

saturated fatty acid, any of a number of glyceryl esters of certain organic acids in which all the atoms are joined by single valence bonds. These fats are chiefly of animal origin and include beef, lamb, pork, veal, whole milk products, butter, most cheeses, and a few plant fats such as chocolate, coconut oil, and palm oil. Ordinary oleomargarine and hydrogenated shortenings also contain saturated fatty acids. A diet high in saturated fatty acids may contribute to a high serum cholesterol level and, in some studies of some population groups, it is associated with an increased incidence of coronary heart disease. Compare **unsaturated fatty acid.**

saturated solution, a solution in which the solvent contains the maximum amount of solute it can take up. See also **solute, solvent.**

saturn-, a combining form meaning 'lead': *saturnine, saturnism, saturnotherapy.*

satyriasis (sæt′ıraı′əsıs), excessive and uncontrollable sexual desire in the male, of organic or psychological origin. Also called **satyromania.** Compare **nymphomania.**

satyromania (sæt′ıroumeı′nıə). See **satyriasis.**

sauna bath, a bath in which hot vapor is used to induce sweating, followed by rubbing of the body, and ending with a cold shower. Also called **Finnish bath, Russian bath.**

saur-, a combining form meaning 'lizard, or reptile': *sauriasis, sauriderma, sauroid.*

Savacort, a trade name for a glucocorticoid (prednisolone acetate).

Sayre's jacket (seırz), a cast applied for support and immobilization in the treatment of certain abnormalities of the spinal column.

Sb, symbol for **antimony.**

SBE, abbreviation for **self-breast examination.**

S.B.P., a trade name for a central nervous system sedative-hypnotic fixed-combination drug containing three barbiturates (phenobarbital, secobarbital, and butabarbital).

Sc, symbol for **scandium.**

scab. See **eschar.**

scabicide (skæb′ısaıd), any one of a large group of drugs that destroy the itch mite, *Sarcoptes scabiei.* These drugs are applied topically in a lotion or cream-based preparation. All are potentially toxic and irritating to the skin. They are used with caution in treating children. Kinds of scabicides include **benzene benzoate, crotamiton, gamma benzene hexachloride, lindane.**

scabies (skeı′biz), a contagious disease caused by *Sarcoptes scabiei,* the itch mite, characterized by intense itching of the skin and excoriation from scratching. The mite, transmitted by close contact, as in institutions, burrows into outer layers of the skin where the female lays eggs. Two to four months after the first infection, sensitization to the mites and their products begins, resulting in a pruritic papular rash most common on the webs of fingers, flexor surfaces of wrists, and thighs. Secondary bacterial infection may occur. Diagnosis may be made by microscopic identification of adult mites, larvae, or eggs in scrapings of the burrows. All contacts are treated simultaneously with a sulfur ointment, benzyl benzoate, or other scabicide applied locally. Oral antihistamines and salicylates reduce itching.

scag, *Slang.* heroin.

scalded skin syndrome. See **toxic epidermal necrolysis.**

scale, 1. a small, thin flake of keratinized epithelium. 2. to remove incrusted material from the surface of a tooth.

scalp, the skin covering the head, not including the face and ears.

scalp medication, 1. a cream, ointment, lotion, or shampoo used to treat dermatologic conditions of the scalp. 2. the application of a medication to the scalp. If a cream ointment or lotion is to be applied, a shampoo is usually given first. The hair is dried, combed, and parted in the middle and the medication is spread with the fingertips. After treatment, the medication may need to be washed off the scalp and hair with an alkaline shampoo.

scalp-vein needle, a thin-gauge needle designed for use on small veins, as in children.

SCALP-VEIN NEEDLES SECURED

scamping speech, abnormal speech in which consonants or whole syllables are left out of words owing to the person's inability to shape the sounds.

scandium (Sc), a grayish metallic element. Its atomic number is 21; its atomic weight is 44.956.

scanning, carefully studying an area, organ, or system of the body by recording and displaying an image of the concentration of an injected radioactive substance that has an affinity for that specific tissue. The liver, brain, and thyroid can be examined, tumors can be located, and function can be evaluated by various scanning techniques. See **specific scanning techniques.** – **scan,** *n., v.*

scanning electron microscope (SEM), an instrument similar to an electron microscope in that a beam of electrons instead of visible light is used to scan the surface of a specimen. An SEM differs from an electron microscope in that the sample may be of any convenient size or shape, and the image, produced on a television screen, appears three-dimensional. Compare **electron microscope, transmission scanning electron microscope.**

scanning electron microscopy, the technique using a scanning electron microscope in which a beam of electrons is accelerated and focused on an electrically conducting sample. The beam is moved in a point-to-point manner over the surface of the specimen. The number of electrons emerging from the sample is proportionate to the shape, density, and other properties of the sample. These electrons are deflected, collected, accelerated, and directed against a scintillator. The large number of photons thus created are converted into an electrical signal that modulates an electron beam in a cathode-ray tube; that beam, in turn, modulates the beam scanning the surface of the specimen. The image produced is of less magnification than that produced by an electron microscope, but it appears to be three-dimensional and lifelike. Compare **electron microscopy, transmission scanning electron microscope.**

scanning speech, abnormal speech in which the words are clipped and broken because the person pauses between syllables.

Scanzoni rotation (skænzou′ni), an obstetric operation in which forceps having a curved shank are applied to the fetal head while it is still high in the pelvis. The head is displaced upward and rotated to the occiput anterior position. The forceps are removed and repositioned, and the delivery is accomplished by axis traction. The operation is not often performed in modern obstetrics because Caesarean section is usually safer for the mother and the baby. See also **forceps delivery, obstetric forceps.**

scapho-, a combining form meaning 'boat-shaped': *scaphocephaly, scaphohydrocephaly, scaphoid.*

scaphocephaly (skæf′ousef′əli), **scaphocephalis, scaphocephalism,** a congenital malformation of the skull in which premature closure of the sagittal suture results in restricted lateral growth of the head, giving it an abnormally long, narrow appearance with a cephalic index of 75 or less. The condition is often associated with mental retardation. Also called **dolichocephaly, mecocephaly.** See also **craniostenosis.** –**scaphocephalic, scaphocephalous,** *adj.*

scaphoid bone, either of two similar bones of the hand and the foot. The scaphoid bone of the hand is slanted at the radial side of the carpus and articulates with the radius, trapezium, trapezoideum, capitate, and lunate bones. The scaphoid bone of the foot is located at the medial side of the tarsus between the talus and cuneiform bones and articulates with the talus, the three cuneiform bones, and, occasionally, with the cuboid bone. Also called **navicular bone.**

scapula, one of the pair of large, flat, triangular bones that form the dorsal part of the shoulder girdle. It has two surfaces, three borders, three angles, and a prominent dorsal spine. The acromion of the scapula forms the summit of the shoulder. The coracoid process, resembling a raven's beak, accommodates the attachment of various muscles, including the pectoralis minor, and ligaments, including the trapezoid. Also called **shoulder blade.**

-scapula, a combining form meaning a 'shoulderblade or a part of it': *mesoscapula, prescapula, proscapula.*

scapulohumeral, of or pertaining to the structures of muscles and the area around the scapula and humerus that make up the shoulder girdle.

scapulohumeral muscular dystrophy, a form of limb-girdle muscular dystrophy that begins in the shoulder girdle. Also called **Erb's muscular dystrophy.**

scapulohumeral reflex (skæp′yulouhyu′mərəl), a normal response to tapping the vertebral border of the scapula, resulting in adduction of the arm. Absence of the reflex may indicate a lesion in the region of the fifth cervical segment of the spinal cord.

scar. See **cicatrix.**

scarification (skær′ıfıkei′ʃhən), multiple superficial scratches or incisions in the skin, as are made for the introduction of a vaccine. Erroneously used to mean 'producing a scar.'

scarify (skær′əfaı), to make multiple superficial incisions into the skin; to scratch. Vaccination against smallpox is achieved by scarifying the skin under a drop of vaccine. –**scarification,** *n.*

scarlatina (skar′ləti′nə). See **scarlet fever.**

scarlatiniform (skar′ləti′nıfɔrm), resembling the rash of **scarlet fever.**

scarlet fever, an acute contagious disease of childhood caused by an erythrotoxin-producing strain of group A hemolytic *Streptococcus.* The infection is characterized by sore throat, fever, enlarged lymph nodes in the neck, prostration, and a diffuse bright red rash. Also called **scarlatina.**

scarlet red, an azo dye that has been used to impart color to pharmaceutical preparations.

scato-, skato, a combining form meaning 'of or related to dung, or to fecal matter': *scatophagy, scatophilia, scatoscopy.*

scattergram, a graph representing the distribution of two variables in a sample population. One variable is plotted on the vertical axis; the second on the horizontal axis. The scores or values of each sample unit are usually represented by dots. A scattergram demonstrates the degree or tendency to which the variables occur in association with each other.

scattering, (in radiology) a change in direction of the path of subatomic particles caused by collision or interaction with one another.

scavenging system. See **gas scavenging system.**

scel-, a combining form meaning 'leg': *scelalgia, scelotyrbe.*

-scelia, a combining form meaning '(condition of the) legs': *macroscelia, polyscelia, rhaeboscelia.*

Schedule I, a category of drugs not considered legitimate for medical use. Among the substances so classified by the Drug Enforcement Agency are mescaline, LSD, heroin, and marijuana. Special licensing procedures must be followed to use these or other Schedule I substances.

Schedule II, a category of drugs considered to have a strong potential for abuse or addiction, but which have legitimate medical use. Among the substances so classified by the Drug Enforcement Agency are morphine, cocaine, pentobarbital, oxycodone, alphaprodine, and methadone.

Schedule III, a category of drugs that have less potential for abuse or addiction than Schedule II or I drugs. Among the substances so classified by the Drug Enforcement Agency are glutethimide and various analgesic compounds containing codeine.

Schedule IV, a category of drugs that have less potential for abuse or addiction than those of Schedules III to V. Among the substances so classified by the Drug Enforcement Agency are chloral hydrate, chlordiazepoxide, meprobamate, and oxazepam.

Schedule V, a category of drugs that have a small potential for abuse or addiction. Among the substances so classified by the Drug Enforcement Agency are many commonly prescribed medications that contain small amounts of codeine or diphenoxylate. The specific drugs in Schedule V vary greatly from state to state.

Schedule of Drugs, a classification system that categorizes drugs by their potential for abuse. The schedule is divided into five groups: Schedules I to V. The assignment of drugs to the categories varies from state to state. All substances in Schedules II to V require a written prescription signed by a physician. Schedule I substances are not approved for medical use. Specific regulations for dispensing these substances vary from state to state and from institution to institution. See also specific schedules.

Scheuermann's disease (shoi'ərmanz), an abnormal skeletal condition characterized by a fixed kyphosis that develops at puberty and is caused by wedge-shaped deformities of one or several vertebrae. The cause of the disease is unknown, but authorities have speculated that it may result from such pathologies as infection, inflammatory processes, aseptic necrosis, disc deterioration, mechanical influences, inadequate circulation during rapid growth, or disturbances of epiphyseal growth resulting from protrusion of the intervertebral disc through deficient or defective cartilaginous plates. The most striking pathologic feature of Scheuermann's disease is the presence of wedge-shaped vertebral bodies, seen on radiographic examination, that create an excessive curvature. Scheuermann's disease occurs most frequently in children between the ages of 12 and 16, with the onset at puberty, and the incidence is greater in girls than in boys. The onset is insidious and often associated with a history of unusual physical activity or participation in sports. The most frequent symptom is poor posture with accompanying symptoms of fatigue and pain in the involved area. Tenderness and stiffness may also affect the area involved or may affect the entire spinal column. In most affected individuals the kyphosis is within the thoracic vertebrae. If the disease is diagnosed at the onset, the associated posture may be corrected actively and passively. Otherwise, the associated posture becomes fixed within a period

of 6 to 9 months. The most effective treatment of Scheuermann's disease is immobilization with a plaster cast or with a Milwaukee brace. The immobilization is continuous for 10 to 12 months, with additional immobilization at night for about the same length of time. Immobilization is usually supplemented with an exercise program that is continued after the immobilization is terminated. In adults, persistent pain in the thoracic area may indicate a degenerative alteration secondary to this disease process, and spinal arthrodesis may be required to relieve the symptoms. Also called **adolescent vertebral epiphysitis, juvenile kyphosis.**

Schick test, a skin test to determine immunity to diphtheria in which diphtheria toxin is injected intradermally. A positive reaction, indicating susceptibility, is marked by redness and swelling at the site of injection; a negative reaction, indicating immunity, is marked by absence of redness or swelling.

Schilder's disease (shil'dərz), an eponym for a group of progressive, severe, neurologic diseases beginning in childhood. All are characterized by demyelination of the white matter of the brain with muscle spasticity, optic neuritis, aphasia, deafness, adrenal insufficiency, and dementia. Many of the signs resemble those of multiple sclerosis. There is no known treatment. The cause may be viral or genetic.

Schiller's test, a procedure for indicating areas of abnormal epithelium in the vagina or on the cervix of the uterus as a guide in selecting biopsy sites for cancer detection. A potassium iodide or aqueous iodine solution is painted on the vaginal walls and cervix under direct visualization. Normal epithelium contains glycogen and stains a deep brown color; abnormal epithelium, containing no glycogen, will not stain, and nonstaining sites may then be included in tissue biopsies. The test is not specific for malignancy, since inflammation, ulceration, and keratotic lesions also may not accept the iodine stain.

Schilling's leukemia (shil'ingz). See **monocytic leukemia.**

Schilling test, a diagnostic test for pernicious anemia in which vitamin B_{12} tagged with radioactive cobalt is administered orally, and gastrointestinal absorption is measured by determining the radioactivity of urine samples collected over a 24-hour period. In persons with pernicious anemia, the ability to absorb vitamin B_{12} is reduced, so that excretion of radioactive material in the urine is reduced.

Schiötz tonometer, a tonometer used to measure intraocular pressure by observing the depth of indentation of the cornea made by the weighted plunger on the device.

schisto-, a combining form meaning 'split, or cleft': *schistocelia, schistocephalus, schistomelia.*

Schistosoma (shĭs'tə̄sou'mə), a genus of blood flukes that may cause urinary, gastrointestinal, or liver disease in man and that requires fresh water snails as intermediate hosts. *Schistosoma hematobium,* found chiefly in Africa and the Middle East, affects the bladder and pelvic organs, causing painful, frequent urination and hematuria. *S. japonicum,* found in Japan, the Philippines, and Eastern Asia, causes gastrointestinal ulcerations and fibrosis of the liver. *S. mansoni,* found in Africa, the Middle East, the Caribbean, and South America, causes symptoms similar to those caused by *S. japonicum.* See also **schistosomiasis.**

schistosomiasis, a parasitic infection caused by a species of fluke of the genus *Schistosoma,* transmitted to man, the definitive host, by contact with fresh water contaminated by human feces. A single fluke may live in one part of the body, depositing eggs frequently, for up to 20 years. The eggs are irritating to mucous membrane, causing it to thicken and become papillomatous. Symptoms depend on the part of the body infected. *Schistosoma* may be found in the bladder, rectum, liver, lungs, spleen, intestines, and portal venous system. Pain, obstruction, dysfunction of the affected organ, and anemia may result. Diagnosis requires morphologic identification of the ova or the parasite. Treatment is difficult; antimony drugs may be effective but are so toxic they seldom can be given. Inoculation with a small dose of *Klebsiella pneumoniae* has been effective experimentally in killing some species of *Schistosoma.* Prevention is more effective. Proper disposal of human waste, chlorination of water, and eradication of the intermediate host, the fresh water snail *Australorbis glabratus,* are totally effective. Second only to malaria in the number of people affected, schistosomiasis is particularly prevalent in the tropics and in the Orient. Also called **bilharziasis.** See also **blood fluke,** *Schistosoma.*

schistosomicide (shĭs'tə̄sou'mə̄saĭd), a drug destructive to schistosomes, blood flukes transmitted by snails to human hosts in many parts of Africa, Brazil and Asia. Niridazole, metrifonate, oxamniquine hycanthone hydrochloride, and various salts of antimony, including stibophen, are potent antischistosomal agents. — **schistosomicidal,** *adj.*

schizo-, a combining form meaning 'divided, or related to division': *schizocephalia, schizogenesis, schizophrenia.*

schizoaffective disorder, a condition that includes characteristics of schizophrenia and bipolar disorder or of other major affective disorders.

schizogenesis (skĭt'sə̄jen'ĭsĭs), reproduction by fission. — **schizogenetic, schizogenic, schizogenous,** *adj.*

schizogony (skĭtsog'ə̄ni), **1.** reproduction by multiple fission. **2.** the asexual reproductive stage of sporozoans, specifically the portion of the life cycle of the malarial

parasite that occurs in the erythrocytes or liver cells. See also *Plasmodium,* — **schizogonic, schizogonous.** *adj.*

schizoid (skĭt'soĭd, skĭz'oĭd), **1.** characteristic of or resembling schizophrenia; schizophrenic. **2.** a person, not necessarily a schizophrenic, who exhibits the traits of a schizoid personality.

schizoid personality, a functioning but maladjusted person whose behavior is characterized by extreme shyness, oversensitivity, introversion, seclusiveness, and avoidance of close interpersonal relationships. See also **schizoid personality disorder, schizophrenia.**

schizoid personality disorder, a condition characterized by a defect in the ability to form social relationships, as shown by emotional coldness and aloofness, withdrawn and seclusive behavior, and indifference to praise, criticism, and the feelings of others. The person is unable to express hostility and ordinary aggressive feelings and reacts to disturbing experiences with apparent detachment. The condition may precede schizophrenia.

schizont (skĭt'sont), the multinucleated cell stage during the sexual reproductive phase in the life cycle of a sporozoan, specifically the malarial parasite *Plasmodium.* It is produced by the multiple fission of the trophozoite in a cell of the vertebrate host and subsequently segments into merozoites. Also called **agamont.** Compare **sporont.** See also **schizogony.**

schizonticide (skĭtson'tə̄saĭd'), a substance that destroys schizonts. — **schizonticidal,** *adj.*

schizophasia (skĭt'sə̄fei'zhə, skĭz'ə̄fei'zhə), the disordered, incomprehensible speech characteristic of some forms of schizophrenia. See also **word salad.**

schizophrene (skĭt'sə̄frin, skĭz'ə̄frin), a person afflicted with schizophrenia.

schizophrenia (skĭt'sə̄fri'niə, skĭz'ə̄fri'niə), any one of a large group of psychotic disorders characterized by gross distortion of reality, disturbances of language and communication, withdrawal from social interaction, and the disorganization and fragmentation of thought, perception, and emotional reaction. Apathy and confusion; delusions and hallucinations; rambling or stylized patterns of speech, as evasiveness, incoherence, and echolalia; withdrawn, regressive, and bizarre behavior; and emotional lability often occur. The condition may be mild or require prolonged hospitalization. No single cause of the disease is known; genetic, biochemical, psychological, interpersonal, and sociocultural factors are usually involved. Treatment often requires the use of tranquilizers and antidepressant and antianxiety drugs. Milieu therapy and group psychotherapy may be extremely helpful in providing a safe environment in which the person may test reality, develop an increased ability to communicate with other people, and learn better ways to cope with stress. Kinds of schizophrenia include **acute schizophrenia, catatonic schizophrenia, childhood schizophrenia, disorganized**

schizophrenia, latent schizophrenia, paranoid schizophrenia, process schizophrenia, reactive schizophrenia, residual schizophrenia. Also called **schizophrenic disorder, schizophrenic reaction.**

schizophrenic (skɪt'səfren'ɪk, skɪz'əfren'ɪk), **1.** of or pertaining to schizophrenia. **2.** a person afflicted with schizophrenia.

schizophrenic disorder. See **schizophrenia.**

schizophrenic reaction. See **schizophrenia.**

schizophreniform disorder, a condition exhibiting the same symptoms as schizophrenia but characterized by an acute onset with resolution in two weeks to six months.

schizophrenogenic (skɪt'səfren'əjen'ɪk, skɪz'əfren'əjen'ɪk), tending to cause or produce schizophrenia.

Schizotrypanum cruzi (skɪz'outrɪp'ənəm kru'zaɪ). See **Chagas' disease.**

schizotypal personality disorder (skɪt'soutaɪpəl), a condition characterized by oddities of thought, perception, speech, and behavior that are not severe enough to meet the clinical criteria for schizophrenia. Symptoms include magical thinking, as superstitiousness, clairvoyance, telepathy, and bizarre fantasies; ideas of reference; recurrent illusions, as sensing the presence of a force or person not actually present; social isolation; peculiar speech patterns, including ideas expressed unclearly or words used deviantly; and exaggerated anxiety or hypersensitivity to real or imagined criticism. See also **schizoid personality disorder, schizophrenia.**

Schlatter-Osgood disease (shlæt'əroz'gud). See **Osgood-Schlatter disease.**

Schlatter's disease (shlæt'ərz). See **Osgood-Schlatter disease.**

Schlemm's canal (shlemz). See **canal of Schlemm.**

Schneiderian carcinoma (shnaidir'iən), an epithelial malignancy of the nasal mucosa and paranasal sinuses.

School Nurse Practitioner (S.N.P.), a registered nurse who is qualified by a postgraduate course of study to act as a nurse practitioner in a school.

school phobia, an extreme separation anxiety disorder of children, usually in the elementary grades, characterized by a persistent, irrational fear of going to school or being in a schoollike atmosphere. Such children are usually oversensitive, shy, timid, nervous, and emotionally immature and have pervasive feelings of inadequacy. They typically try to cope with their fears by becoming overdependent on others, especially the parents. Often the fear of being separated from the parents in order to go to school or the emotional conflict symbolically manifested by the school atmosphere subsides with age and the development of relationships with school-age peers. In more severe cases, psychotherapy and behavior therapy, especially in structured group environments within an educational setting, may be necessary and effective.

Schultz-Carlton phenomenon, a cutaneous reaction to the intradermal injection of scarlatina antiserum in a person who has a scarletiniform rash. The rash blanches.

Schwann-cell tumor (shwan'sel'). See **schwannoma.**

schwannoma (shwanou'mə), *pl.* **schwannomas, schwannomata.** a benign, solitary, encapsulated tumor arising in the neurilemma (Schwann's sheath) of peripheral, cranial, or autonomic nerves. Also called **Schwann-cell tumor, neurilemoma.**

Schwann's sheath (shwanz). See **neurilemma.**

Schwartz bed. See **hyperextension bed.**

Schwartzman-Sanarelli phenomenon, a phenomenon induced experimentally in the investigation of the role of coagulation in renal disease. Animals injected twice with a bacterial endotoxin develop massive disseminated intravascular coagulation with thrombosis of the blood vessels in the kidneys. Also called **Schwartzman phenomenon.**

scia-. See **skia-.**

sciatic (saiæt'ɪk), near the ischium, as the sciatic nerve or the sciatic vein.

SCID, abbreviation for **severe combined immunodeficiency disease.**

science, a systematic attempt to establish theories to explain observed phenomena and the knowledge obtained through these efforts. **Pure science** is concerned with the gathering of information solely for the sake of obtaining new knowledge. **Applied science** is the practical application of scientific theory and laws. See also **hypothesis, law, scientific method, theory.**

scientific method, a systematic, ordered approach to the gathering of data and the solving of problems. The basic approach is the statement of the problem followed by the statement of a hypothesis. An experimental method is established to help prove or disprove the hypothesis. The results of the experiment are observed, and conclusions are drawn from the observed results. The conclusions may tend to uphold or to refute the hypothesis.

scirrho-, a combining form meaning 'hard, or related to a hard cancer or scirrhus': *scirrhoid, scirrhoma, scirrhosarca.*

scirrhous carcinoma, a hard, fibrous, particularly invasive tumor in which the malignant cells occur singly or in small clusters or strands in dense connective tissue. It is the most common form of breast cancer. Also called **carcinoma fibrosum.** See also **breast cancer.**

scissors, a sharp instrument composed of two opposing cutting blades, held together by a central pin on which the blades pivot. It has circular handles and straight or curved blades. The most common dissecting scissors are the straight **Mayo,** for cutting sutures; the **Snowden-Pencer,** for deep, delicate tissue; the long, curved **Mayo,** for deep, heavy, or tough tissue; the short, curved **Metzenbaum,** for superficial, delicate tissue; and the long, blunt, curved **Metzenbaum,** for deep, delicate tissue.

scler-. See **sclero-.**

sclera (sklir′ə), the tough, inelastic, opaque membrane covering the posterior five sixths of the eye bulb. It maintains the size and form of the bulb and attaches to muscles that move the bulb. Posteriorly, it is pierced by the optic nerve and, with the transparent cornea, comprises the outermost of three tunics covering the eye bulb.

scleredema (sklir′ədi′mə), an idiopathic skin disease characterized by nonpitting induration beginning on the face or neck and spreading downward over the body, sparing the hands and feet. There also may be swelling of the tongue, restriction of the movements of the eyes, and pericardial, pleural, and peritoneal effusions. Resolution occurs after several months, but recurrences are common. The condition often follows a streptococcal infection or an exanthem of childhood. There is no specific treatment. Compare **scleroderma.**

scleredema neonatorum. See **sclerema neonatorum.**

sclerema adiposum. See **sclerema neonatorum.**

sclerema neonatorum, a progressive generalized hardening of the skin and subcutaneous tissue of the newborn. It is usually a fatal condition that occurs as a result of severe cold stress in severely ill premature infants subject to such life-threatening conditions as metabolic acidosis, hypoglycemia, gastrointestinal or respiratory infection, or gross malformation. Also called **scleredema neonatorum, sclerema adiposum.**

sclero-, scler-, a combining form meaning 'hard,' often used to show relationship to the sclera: *scleroadipose, sclerocorneal, sclerodesmia.*

sclerodactyly (skler′oudæk′tıli), a musculoskeletal deformity affecting the hands of patients with scleroderma. The fingers are fixed in a semiflexed position, and the fingertips are pointed and ulcerated.

scleroderma (skler′oudər′mə), a relatively rare autoimmune disease affecting the blood vessels and connective tissue. The disease is characterized by fibrous degeneration of the connective tissue of the skin, lungs, and internal organs, especially the esophagus and kidneys. Scleroderma is most common in middle-aged women.
■ OBSERVATIONS: The most common initial complaints are changes in the skin of the face and fingers. Raynaud's phenomenon occurs with a gradual hardening of the skin and swelling of the distal extremities. In the early stages, the disease may be confused with rheumatoid arthritis or Raynaud's disease. As the disease progresses, there is deformity of the joints and pain on movement. Skin changes include edema, then pallor; then the skin becomes firm; finally, it becomes slightly pigmented and fixed to the underlying tissues. At this stage the skin of the face is taut, shiny, and masklike, and the patient may have difficulty in chewing and swallowing. Scleroderma may occur in a mild form with the person living 30 to 50 years, or there may be early death owing to cardiac, renal, pulmo-

nary, or intestinal involvement. Localized forms of scleroderma may occur; these cases are benign and occur only as small circumscribed patches on the skin. A biopsy of the lesion may be done to diagnose the condition. X-ray examination of the lungs and gastrointestinal tract may be diagnostic in the systemic form of the disease. Blood tests may reveal antinuclear antibodies.
■ INTERVENTION: There is no specific drug prescribed to cure scleroderma; however, corticosteroids may be useful in treating the symptoms of the disease and salicylates and mild analgesics are given to ease pain in the joints. Physical therapy slows the development of muscle contracture and resultant deformity and debility.
■ NURSING CONSIDERATIONS: Severe renal disease is a major cause of death, although death may occur owing to the involvement of other organs. The usual indication that renal disease is present is the abrupt onset of severe arterial hypertension that does not respond to medication. Nephrectomy or renal transplant may be performed. In the advanced stages of scleroderma, patients often require help in order to eat, and mouth and skin care are particularly important. As the patient becomes more helpless there is a need for considerable emotional support.

-scleroma, a combining form meaning an 'induration, a hardening of the tissues': *laryngoscleroma, pharyngoscleroma, rhinoscleroma.*

scleromalacia perforans, a condition of the eyes in which devitilization and sloughing of the sclera occur as a complication of rheumatoid arthritis. The pigmented uvea becomes exposed and glaucoma, cataract formation, and detachment of the retina may result.

sclerose, to harden or to cause hardening. — **sclerotic,** *adj.*

sclerosing hemangioma, a solid, cellular tumorlike nodule of the skin or a mass of histiocytes, thought to arise from a hemangioma by the proliferation of endothelial and connective tissue cells.

sclerosis (sklırou′sıs), a condition characterized by hardening of tissue resulting from any of several causes, including inflammation, the deposit of mineral salts, and infiltration of connective tissue fibers. — **sclerotic,** *adj.*

sclerotome, (in embryology) the part of the segmented mesoderm layer in the early developing embryo that originates from the somites and gives rise to the skeletal tissue of the body, specifically, the paired segmented masses of mesodermal tissue that lie on each side of the notochord and develop into the vertebrae and ribs. See also **somite.**

scoleco-, a combining form meaning 'of or pertaining to a worm': *scolecoid, scolecoidectomy, scolecology.*

scolex (skou′leks), *pl.* **scoleces** (skou′ləsiz). the headlike segment or organ of an adult tapeworm that has hooks, grooves, or suckers by which it attaches itself to the wall of the intestine.

scolio-, a combining form meaning 'twisted or crooked': *scoliodontic, scoliokyphosis, scoliosiometry.*

scoliosis (skou'liou'sɪs), lateral curvature of the spine, a common abnormality of childhood. Causes include congenital malformations of the spine, poliomyelitis, skeletal dysplasias, spastic paralysis, and unequal leg length. Unequal heights of hips or shoulders may be a sign of this condition. Early recognition and orthopedic treatment may prevent progression of the curvature. Treatment includes braces, casts, exercises, and corrective surgery. See also **kyphoscoliosis, kyphosis, lordosis, spinal curvature.**

NORMAL SPINE   SCOLIOSIS

scop-, a combining form meaning 'to examine, observe': *scopograph, scopometer, scopophilia.*

-scope, a combining form meaning an 'instrument for observation': *ciliariscope, episcope, pelviscope.*

-scopia, a combining form meaning 'observation': *aknephascopia, mixoscopia, phantasmoscopia.*

scopolamine hydrobromide, an anticholinergic.
■ INDICATIONS: It is prescribed in the treatment of nausea and vomiting, as a sedative and pre-anesthetic medication, and as a cycloplegic and mydriatic medication in ophthalmic procedures.
■ CONTRAINDICATIONS: Narrow angle glaucoma, asthma, obstruction of the genitourinary or gastrointestinal tracts, severe ulcerative colitis, or known hypersensitivity to this drug prohibits its use.
■ ADVERSE EFFECTS: Among the more serious adverse reactions are blurred vision, central nervous system effects, tachycardia, dry mouth, decreased sweating, and hypersensitivity reaction.

scopophilia (skou'pəfɪl'iə, skou'pəfil'yə), **scoptophilia** (skop'təfɪl'iə, skop'təfil'yə), **1.** sexual pleasure derived from looking at sexually stimulating scenes or at another person's genitals; voyeurism. **2.** a morbid desire to be seen; exhibitionism. —**scopophiliac, scopophilic, scoptophiliac, scoptophic.** *adj., n.*

scopophobia (skou'pəfou'biə), an anxiety disorder characterized by a morbid fear of being seen or stared at by others. The condition is commonly seen in schizophrenia. See also **phobia.**

-scopy, a combining form meaning 'observation': *bioscopy, stomachoscopy, thoracoscopy.*

-scorbic, a combining form meaning 'of or referring to the prevention or treatment of scurvy': *antiscorbic, ascorbic, glucoascorbic.*

-scorbutic, a combining form meaning 'pertaining to scurvy': *antiscorbutic, postscorbutic, scorbutic.* Also **-scorbic, -scorbutical.**

scorbutic pose (skɔrbyu'tɪk), the characteristic posture of a child with scurvy, with thighs and legs semiflexed and hips rotated outward. The child usually lies motionless without voluntary movements of the extremities because of the pain that accompanies any motion. See also **scurvy.**

scorbutus (skɔrbyu'təs). See **scurvy.**

scorpion sting, a painful wound produced by a scorpion, an arachnid with a hollow stinger in its tail. The stings of many species are only slightly toxic, but some, including *Centruroides sculpturatus* of the southwestern United States, may inflict fatal injury, especially in small children. Initial pain is followed within several hours by numbness, nausea, muscle spasm, dyspnea, and convulsion. Treatment includes ice applied to the wound and intravenous calcium gluconate to control muscle spasm, if necessary. Severe cases may require oxygen and respiratory assistance. Narcotic analgesia is contraindicated. An antivenin is available in some areas.

scoto-, a combining form meaning 'of or related to darkness': *scotodinia, scotogram, scotographic.*

scratch test, a skin test for identifying an allergen, performed by placing a small quantity of a solution containing a suspected allergen on a lightly scratched area of the skin. If a wheal forms within 15 minutes, allergy to the substance is indicated.

screamer's nodule. See **vocal cord nodule.**

screening, 1. a preliminary procedure, as a test or examination, to detect the most characteristic sign or signs of a disorder that may require further investigation. **2.** the examination of a large sample of a population to detect a specific disease or disorder, as hypertension.

screen memory, a consciously tolerable memory that replaces one that is emotionally painful to recall.

screw clamp, a device, usually made of plastic, equipped with a screw that can be manipulated to close and open the primary I.V. tubing for regulating the flow of intravenous solution. Turning the screw clockwise closes the tubing; turning it counterclockwise opens the tubing. Different positions of the screw between the open and the closed positions allow the intravenous fluid to flow at different rates. Compare **roller clamp, slide clamp.**

scrib-, script-, a combining form meaning 'write': *scribble, scribomania, prescription.*

Scribner shunt, a type of arteriovenous bypass, used in hemodialysis, consisting of a special tube connection outside the body.

scrofula (skrof′yulə), *Archaic.* primary tuberculosis with abscess formation, usually of the cervical lymph nodes.

scrofulous keratitis. See **phyctenular keratoconjunctivitis.**

scrotal cancer, an epidermoid malignancy of the scrotum, characterized initially by a small sore that may ulcerate. The lesion occurs most frequently in elderly men who have been exposed to soot, pitch, crude oil, mineral oils, polycyclic hydrocarbons, or arsenical fumes from copper smelting. Treatment involves wide surgical excision of the tumor and resection of inguinal nodes. In the 18th century, Sir Percival Pott associated scrotal cancer in chimney-sweeps with exposure to soot. It is the first malignancy shown to be caused by an environmental carcinogen. Also called **chimney-sweeps' cancer, soot wart.**

scrotum (skrou′təm), the pouch of skin containing the testes and parts of the spermatic cords. It is divided on the surface into two lateral portions by a ridge which continues ventrally to the undersurface of the penis and dorsally along the middle line of the perineum to the anus. In young, robust individuals the scrotum is short, corrugated, and closely wraps the testes. In older persons, debilitated individuals and in warm environments, the scrotum becomes elongated and flaccid. The lateral left portion of the scrotum hangs lower than the right, corresponding with the longer length of the left spermatic cord. The two layers of the scrotum are the skin and the dartos tunic. The skin is very thin, has a brownish color and is usually wrinkled. It is supplied with sebaceous follicles which secrete a substance with a characteristic odor and has thinly scattered, kinky hairs with roots that are visible through the skin. The dartos tunic is composed of a thin layer of unstriated muscular fibers around the base of the

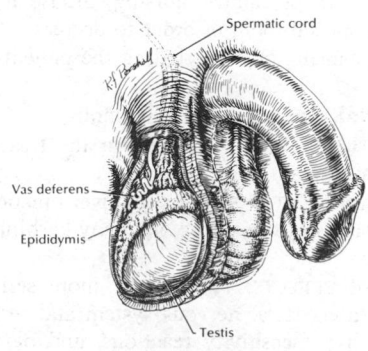

Spermatic cord

Vas deferens

Epididymis

Testis

SCROTUM

scrotum, continuous with the two layers of the superficial fascia of the groin and the perineum. The tunic projects an internal septum which divides the pouch into two cavities for the testes, extending between the scrotal ridge and the root of the penis. The tunic is closely united to the skin but separated from subjacent parts by a distinct fascial cleft on which it glides. The scrotum is highly vascular and contains no fat. See also **testis.** – **scrotal,** *adj.*

scrub. See **surgical scrub.**

scrub room, a special hospital area where surgeons and surgical teams use disposable sterile brushes and bactericidal soaps to wash and scrub their fingernails, hands, and forearms before performing or assisting in surgical operations. Scrub rooms and meticulous washing techniques improve the sterile environment of the operating room and reduce the risk of bacterial infection.

scrub typhus, an acute, febrile disease of Asia, India, northern Australia, and the western Pacific islands, caused by several strains of the genus *Rickettsia tsutsugamushi* and transmitted from infected rodents to man by mites. The clinical course ranges from mild to severe and is characterized by a necrotic papule or black eschar at the site of the esion caused by the bite of the small arachnid. Tender, enlarged regional lymph nodes, fever, severe headache, eye pain, muscle aches, and a generalized rash usually occur. In severe cases, the myocardium and the central nervous system may be involved. The Weil-Felix reaction and indirect fluorescent antibody tests are useful in diagnosis. Treatment with broad-spectrum antibiotics, as chloramphenicol, doxycycline, or tetracycline, has reduced mortality to nearly zero. Person-to-person transmission is not known to occur. No effective vaccine is available, and second attacks are common owing to antigenic differences in various strains of rickettsiae. Prevention includes avoiding mite-infested terrain, reducing the rodent population, destroying scrub vegetation, and using insect repellents. Also called **Japanese river fever, mite typhus, tsutsugamushi disease.** Compare **Q-fever, Rocky Mountain spotted fever, typhus.**

scruple, a measure of weight in the apothecaries' system, equal to 20 grains or 1.296 gm. See also **apothecaries' weight, metric system.**

scultetus bandage (skəlti′təs), a many-tailed bandage with an attached central piece. The tails are overlapped; the last two tied or pinned act to secure the others. A scultetus bandage may be opened or removed without moving the bandaged part of the body.

scurvy, a condition resulting from lack of ascorbic acid in the diet. It is characterized by weakness, anemia, edema, spongy gums, often with ulceration and loosening of the teeth, a tendency to mucocutaneous hemorrhages and induration of the muscles of the legs. Treatment and prophylaxis of the disease consist of administration of ascorbic acid and the inclusion of fresh vegetables and fruits in the diet. Also called **scorbutus.** See also **ascorbic acid, citric acid, infantile scurvy.**

scut work, *Slang, derogatory.* menial tasks, usually of a nontherapeutic nature, that are a necessary part of the work routine performed by the staff of a health-care facility.

scyt-, a combining form meaning 'skin': *scytitis, scytoblastema.*

Se, symbol for **selenium.**

sealed source, (in radiotherapy) a source of radiant energy in which the radioactive material is permanently encased in a container or bonding material in a manner to prevent leakage. Sealed sources, as seeds, needles, and specially designed applicators, are used in the implantation of cesium-137, iodine-125, iridium-192, radium-226, and other radionuclides for the treatment of various malignant tumors.

seal limbs. See **phocomelia.**

seatworm. See *Enterobius vermiculans.*

sea urchin sting, an injury inflicted by any of a variety of sea urchins, in which the skin is punctured and in some species, venom released. A venomous sting is characterized by pain, muscular weakness, numbness around the mouth, and dyspnea. Immediate removal of the spines is necessary and may require the use of a local anesthetic. An antiseptic and a dressing are applied until the wound is healed. In all cases the broken spines cause local pain and irritation. Infection may result. See also **stingray.**

seawater bath, a bath taken in warm seawater or in saline solution.

sebaceous (sɪbeiʹshəs), fatty, oily, or greasy, usually referring to the oil-secreting glands of the skin or to their secretions.

sebaceous cyst, a misnomer for epidermoid cyst or pilar cyst.

sebaceous gland, one of the many small sacculated organs in the dermis. They are located throughout the body in close association with all types of body hair but are especially abundant in the scalp, the face, the anus, the nose, the mouth, and the external ear. They are wanting in the palms of the hands and the soles of the feet. Each gland consists of a single duct which emerges from a cluster of oval alveoli. Each alveolus is composed of a transparent basement membrane enclosing epithelial cells. The outer cells are small and polyhedral and continuous with the cells lining the duct. The remainder of the alveolus is comprised of larger cells containing lipid, except in the center, where disintegrated cells leave a cavity filled with their debris and a mass of sebum cutaneum. The ducts from most sebaceous glands open into the hair follicles but some open on the general surface of the skin, as in the labia minora and the free margin of the lips. The sebum secreted by the glands oils the hair and the surrounding skin, helps to prevent evaporation of sweat, and aids in the retention of body heat. The sebaceous glands in the nose and the face are large, lobulated, and often swell with accumulated secretion. Compare **sweat gland.**

seborrhea (sebʹəriʹə), any of several common skin conditions in which there is an overproduction of sebum resulting in excessive oiliness or dry scales. See also **seborrheic blepharitis, seborrheic dermatitis.** —**seborrheic,** *adj.*

seborrheic blepharitis, a form of seborrheic dermatitis in which the eyelids are erythematous and the margins are covered with a granular crust.

seborrheic dermatitis, a common, chronic, inflammatory skin disease characterized by dry or moist, greasy scales and yellowish crusts. Common sites are the scalp, eyelids, face, external surfaces of the ears, axillae, breasts, groin, and gluteal folds. In acute stages there may be exudate and infection resulting in secondary furunculosis. Occasionally generalized exfoliation results. In some people seborrheic dermatitis is associated with paralysis agitans, diabetes mellitus, malabsorption disorders, epilepsy, or an allergic reaction to gold or arsenic. Treatment includes selenium sulfide shampoos, topical and oral corticosteroids, topical antibiotics, proper therapy for any underlying systemic disorder, and avoidance of sweating and external irritants. Kinds of seborrheic dermatitis include **cradle cap, dandruff, seborrheic blepharitis.**

seborrheic keratosis, a benign, well-circumscribed, slightly raised, tan to black, warty lesion of the skin of the face, neck, chest, or upper back. The macules are loosely covered with a greasy crust that leaves a raw pulpy base when removed. Itching is common. Treatment includes curettage or electrodesiccation or cryotherapy under local anesthesia.

seborrheic wart. See **seborrheic keratosis.**

sebum (siʹbəm), the normal secretion of the sebaceous glands of the skin, composed of keratin, fat, and cellular debris. Combined with sweat, sebum forms a moist, oily, acidic film that is mildly antibacterial and antifungal and protects the skin against drying.

Seckel's syndrome. See **bird-headed dwarf.**

seclusion, (in psychiatric nursing) the isolation of a patient in a special room in order to decrease stimuli which might be causing or exacerbating the patient's emotional distress.

secobarbital, a sedative and hypnotic.

■ INDICATIONS: It is prescribed in the treatment of insomnia and as an anticonvulsant.

■ CONTRAINDICATIONS: Impaired liver function or known hypersensitivity to this drug or to any barbiturate prohibits its use.

■ ADVERSE EFFECTS: Among the more serious adverse reactions are central nervous system and respiratory depression, hypersensitivity reactions, and paradoxical excitement. Kidney damage may result from the polyethylene glycol that is used as a diluent in injectable preparations of the drug.

Seconal, a trade name for a sedative-hypnotic (secobarbital).

secondary, second in importance or in incidence or belonging to the second order of sophistication or development, as a secondary health care facility or secondary education.

secondary amenorrhea. See **amenorrhea.**

secondary amputation, amputation performed after suppuration has begun following severe trauma. An area is left open for drainage, and antibiotics are given. Compare **primary amputation.** See also **amputation.**

secondary apnea, an abnormal condition in which respiration is absent and will not begin again spontaneously. Resuscitation is begun immediately with artificial respiration; oxygen, cardiac massage, analysis of blood gases, and other treatment and medication specific to the underlying cause may be necessary. Secondary apnea may result from any event that severely impedes the absorption of oxygen into the blood stream. Compare **primary apnea.**

secondary areola, a second ring appearing around the areola of the breast during pregnancy that is more pigmented than the areola before pregnancy.

secondary biliary cirrhosis, an abnormal hepatic condition characterized by obstruction of the bile duct with or without infection. It involves periportal inflammation with progressive fibrosis, destruction of parenchymal cells, and nodular degneration. Compare **primary biliary cirrhosis.**

secondary bronchus, a lobar or segmental bronchus. See also **bronchus, primary bronchus.**

secondary dementia, dementia resulting from another, concurrent form of psychosis. See also **dementia.**

secondary dental caries, dental caries developing in a tooth already affected by the condition; often a new cavity forms adjacent to or beneath the restorative filling of an old cavity.

secondary dentition. See **permanent dentition.**

secondary dysmenorrhea. See **dysmenorrhea.**

secondary fissure, a fissure between the uvula and the pyramid of the cerebellum.

secondary fracture. See **pathologic fracture.**

secondary gain, an indirect benefit, usually obtained through an illness or debility. Such gains may include monetary and disability benefits, personal attentions, or escape from unpleasant situations and responsibilities. Compare **primary gain.**

secondary health care, an intermediate level of health care that includes diagnosis and treatment, performed in a hospital having specialized equipment and laboratory facilities. Secondary health care is provided to a larger group of people from a larger geographical area than those served by primary care.

secondary host. See **intermediate host.**

secondary hypertension. See **hypertension.**

secondary hypertrophic osteoarthropathy. See **clubbing.**

secondary nutrient, a substance that acts as a stimulant to activate the flora of the gastrointestinal tract to synthesize other nutrients.

secondary port, a control device for regulating the flow of a primary and a secondary intravenous solution. It consists of a Y-shaped plastic apparatus that attaches to the primary I.V. tubing and allows the primary and secondary I.V. solutions to flow separately or to flow simultaneously. Compare **piggyback port.**

secondary proximal renal tubular acidosis. See **proximal renal tubular acidosis.**

secondary sequestrum, a piece of dead bone that partially separates from sound bone during the process of necrosis but may be pushed back into position. Compare **primary sequestrum.**

secondary sex characteristic, any of the physical characteristics of sexual maturity secondary to hormonal stimulation that develops in the maturing individual. These characteristics include the adult distribution of hair and the development of the penis or breasts and the labia.

secondary shock, a state of physical collapse and prostration caused by numerous traumatic and pathological conditions. It develops over a period of time following severe tissue damage and may merge with primary shock, accompanied by various signs, as weakness, restlessness, low body temperature, low blood pressure, cold sweat, and reduced urinary output. Blood pressure drops progressively in this state, and death may occur within a relatively short time after onset unless appropriate treatment intervenes. Secondary shock is often associated with heat stroke, crushing injuries, myocardial infarction, poisoning, fulminating infections, burns, and other life-threatening conditions. The pathology of this state reflects changes in the capillaries, which become dilated and engorged with blood. Petechial hemorrhages develop in the serous membranes, edema swells the soft tissues, and the vital organs undergo degenerative changes. Compare **hemorrhagic shock, primary shock.**

secondary thrombocytosis. See **thrombocytosis.**

second cuneiform bone. See **intermediate cuneiform bone.**

second filial generation. See F_2.

second intention. See **intention.**

second nerve. See **optic nerve.**

second sight, an improvement in the near vision of the aged owing to the myopia associated with increasing lenticular nuclear sclerosis. This type of sclerosis commonly leads to the development of nuclear cataracts.

secrete, to discharge a substance into a cavity, vessel, or organ or onto the surface of the skin, as a gland. — **secretion,** *n.*

secretin (sıkri′tın),   a digestive hormone produced by certain cells lining the duodenum and jejunum when acidic, partially digested food enters the intestine from the stomach. It stimulates the pancreas to produce a fluid high in salts but low in enzymes. Secretin has a limited stimulating effect on the production of bile. See also **pancreas.**

secretin test,   a test of pancreatic function following stimulation with a hormone, secretin. The test measures the volume and bicarbonate concentration of pancreatic secretions. A lower than normal volume suggests an obstructing malignancy. Reduced bicarbonate and amylase concentration is usually diagnostic of chronic pancreatitis.

secretory duct,   (of a gland) a small duct that has a secretory function and joins with an excretory duct.

secretory phase,   the phase of the menstrual cycle following the release of an ovum from a mature ovarian follicle. The corpus luteum, stimulated by luteinizing hormone (LH), develops from the ruptured follicle. It secretes progesterone, which stimulates the development of the glands and arteries of the endometrium, causing it to become thick and spongy. In a negative-feedback response to the increased level of progesterone in the blood, the secretion of LH from the pituitary decreases. In the absence of an embryo and its secretion of chorionic gonadotropin, the secretory phase ends. The corpus luteum involutes, progesterone levels plummet, and menstruation occurs. Also called **luteal phase.** Compare **proliferative phase.**

sect-,   a combining form meaning 'to cut': *sectio, section, sector.*

-sect,   a combining form meaning 'to cut': *dissect, medisect, quadrisect.*

secund-,   a combining form meaning 'second, or following': *secundigravida, secundina, secundine.*

secundigravida (səkən′dəgræv′ıdə),   a woman who is pregnant for the second time. Also called **gravida 2.** — **secundigravid,** *adj.*

Sedamyl,   a trade name for a sedative-hypnotic (acetylcarbromal).

sedation,   an induced state of quiet, calmness, or sleep, as by means of a sedative or hypnotic medication.

sedative,   **1.** of or pertaining to a substance, procedure, or measure that has a calming effect. **2.** an agent that decreases functional activity, diminishes irritability, and allays excitement. Some sedatives have a general effect on all organs; others affect principally the activities of the heart, stomach, intestines, nerve trunks, respiratory system, or vasomotor system. Barbiturates and nonbarbiturate sedatives, as carbromal, chloral hydrate, ethinamate, furazepam, glutethimide, and various minor tranquilizers, are used to induce sleep, reduce pain, facilitate the induction of anesthesia, and treat convulsive con-

ditions, anxiety states, and irritable bowel syndrome. See also **sedative-hypnotic.**

sedative bath,   the immersion of the body in water for a prolonged period of time, used especially as a calming procedure for agitated patients.

sedative-hypnotic,   a drug that reversibly depresses the activity of the central nervous system, used chiefly to induce sleep and to allay anxiety. Barbiturates and many nonbarbiturate sedative-hypnotics with divers chemical and pharmacologic properties share the ability to depress the activity of all excitable tissue, but the arousal center in the brainstem is especially sensitive to their effects. Various sedative-hypnotics and minor tranquilizers with similar effects are used in the treatment of insomnia, acute convulsive conditions, anxiety states, and to facilitate the induction of anesthesia. Although sedative-hypnotics have a soporific effect, they may interfere with rapid eye movement (REM) sleep associated with dreaming and, when administered to patients with fever, may act paradoxically and cause excitement rather than relaxation. Sedative-hypnotics may interfere with temperature regulation, depress oxygen consumption in various tissues, produce nausea and skin rashes, and, in elderly patients, may cause dizziness, confusion, and ataxia. Drugs in this group have a high potential for abuse that often results in physical and psychological dependence; treatment of dependence involves gradual reduction of the dosage, since abrupt withdrawal frequently causes serious disorders, including convulsions. Acute reactions to an overdose of a sedative-hypnotic may be treated with an emetic, activated charcoal, gastric lavage, and measures to maintain airway patency. Among nonbarbiturate sedative-hypnotics are chloral hydrate, ethchlorvynol, ethinamate, glutethimide, methaqualone, paraldehyde, triclos sodium, minor tranquilizers (chlordiazepoxide, flurazepam, diazepam), diphenhydramine, and meprobamate. See also **barbiturate.**

sedimentation rate.   See **erythrocyte sedimentation rate.**

sed. rate,   *Informal.* erythrocyte sedimentation rate.

segmental bronchus,   a bronchus branching from a lobar bronchus to a bronchiole.

segmental fracture,   a bone break in which several large bone fragments seperate from the main body of a fractured bone. The ends of such fragments may pierce the skin, as in an open fracture, or may be contained within the skin, as in a closed fracture.

segmental resection,   a surgical procedure in which a part of an organ, gland, or other part of the body is excised, as a segmental resection of a part of an ovary performed to diminish the hormonal secretion of the gland by decreasing the amount of secretory tissue in the gland.

segmentation,   **1.** the repetition of structured parts or the process of dividing into segments or similar parts, as the formation of somites or metameres. **2.** the division of the zygote into blastomeres; cleavage.

segmentation cavity. See **blastocoele.**

segmentation cell. See **blastomere.**

segmentation nucleus, the nucleus of the zygote resulting from the fusion of the male and female pronuclei in the fertilized ovum. It is the final stage in fertilization and initiates the first cleavage of the zygote. Also called **cleavage nucleus.**

segmented hyalinizing vasculitis, a chronic, relapsing inflammatory condition of the blood vessels of the lower legs associated with nodular or purpuric skin lesions that may become ulcerated and leave scars. Also called **livedo vasculitis.**

segregation, (in genetics) a principle stating that the pairs of chromosomes bearing genes derived from both parents are separated during meiosis. Chance alone determines which gene, maternal or paternal, will travel to which gamete. See also **dominance, independent assortment.**

seizure. See **convulsion.**

seizure threshold, the amount of stimulus necessary to produce a convulsive seizure. All humans can have seizures if the provocation is sufficient. Those who have spontaneous convulsions are said to have a 'low seizure threshold.'

selection, **1.** the act or product of choosing. **2.** (in genetics) the process by which various factors or mechanisms determine and modify the reproductive ability of a genotype within a specific population, thus influencing evolutionary change. Kinds of selection are **artificial selection, natural selection, sexual selection.**

selective angiography, a graphic procedure that allows selective visualization of the aorta, the major arterial systems, or a particular vessel. It is performed using a percutaneous catheter. A few milliliters of a radiopaque substance are injected when the catheter is in place. As the radiopaque substance is excreted quickly by the kidneys, films are taken of the fluoroscopic image, using a special camera. The patient is observed for signs of sensitivity to the radiopaque medium, including chills, tremor, or shortness of breath. After the procedure, the catheter is withdrawn, and pressure is placed on the puncture site to prevent bleeding. Blood pressure is checked every 15 minutes for 2 hours.

selenium, (Se), a metalloid element of the sulfur group. Its atomic number is 34; its atomic weight is 78.96. Selenium occurs mainly in iron, copper, lead, and nickel ores and in the form of metallic selenides. One of the chief sources commercially is the flue dust produced by the burning of pyrites to make sulfuric acid. Selenium occurs as a trace element in foods, and research continues to determine the most effective daily allowances for different age groups. Dietary experts say that the estimated safe,

adequate intake of selenium for infants six months old is .04 mg, for adults .05 to 0.2 mg. Although selenium deficiency can result in liver problems and degeneration of muscles in some animals, in humans its need has not yet been clearly defined. Authorities stress that all intakes of selenium and other trace elements in foods are considered safe and effective within recommended ranges, but consumption of greater amounts or smaller amounts over extended periods of time will increase the risk of marginal toxicity or marginal deficiency, respectively. The bright orange, insoluble powder selenium sulfide is used externally in the control of seborrheic dermatitis, dandruff, and other forms of dermatosis. Selenium sulfide, employed as a lotion, is used in some therapeutic shampoos containing 2.5 per cent of selenium sulfide in a detergent vehicle; it is sold without prescription as a 1 per cent detergent suspension in a scented detergent vehicle. Adverse effects may include conjunctivitis if the preparation enters the eyes, increased oiliness or dryness of the hair, and orange tinting of gray hair. The antidandruff effectiveness of selenium sulfide is thought to stem from its antimitotic activity and its residual adherence to the hair after shampooing. Normal skin absorbs very little of the drug, but inflamed or damaged skin absorbs it readily. Burns and dermatitis venenata may result from prolonged skin contact.

selenium sulfide, an antifungal and antiseborrheic.

■ INDICATIONS: It is prescribed for dandruff and for seborrheic dermatitis of the scalp.

■ CONTRAINDICATIONS: Acute scalp inflammation or known hypersensitivity to this drug prohibits its use.

■ ADVERSE EFFECTS: Among the more serious adverse reactions are dermatitis after prolonged skin contact or keratitis after accidental conjunctival contact.

self, *pl.* **selves. 1.** the total essence or being of a person; the individual. **2.** those affective, cognitive, and spiritual qualities that distinguish one person from another; individuality. **3.** a person's awareness of his own being or identity; consciousness; ego. See also **personality.**

self-actualization, (in humanistic psychology) the fundamental tendency toward the maximum realization and fulfillment of one's human potential.

self-alien. See **ego-dystonic.**

self-alienation. See **depersonalization.**

self-anesthesia, the self-administered inhalational anesthesia in which whiffs of anesthetic gas are inhaled from a hand-held breathing device controlled by the patient. This form of anesthesia is most common in England; trilene is the usual gas.

self-breast examination (SBE), a procedure in which a woman examines her breasts and their accessory structures for evidence of change that could indicate malignant process. The SBE is usually performed one week to ten days after the first day of the menstrual cycle, when the breasts are smallest and cyclic nodularity is least apparent. Self-examination is encouraged during all phases of a woman's adult life; a woman who regularly and carefully performs the examination is better able to detect small abnormalities than is a woman who is not familiar with her own breasts. The techniques are similar to those of the examination of the breast as performed in the health assessment or physical examination. Also called **breast self-examination.** See also **breast examination.**

self-care, **1.** the personal and medical care performed by the patient, usually in collaboration with and after instruction by a professional medical person. The need of a patient for assistance and the ability to develop a higher level of self-care must be evaluated in forming any nursing care plan. Maximal self-care appropriate to the condition and to the patient is often the ultimate goal of nursing care. **2.** the medical care by laypersons of their families, friends, and themselves, including identification and evaluation of symptoms, medication, and treatment. Self-care is self-limited, voluntary, and wholly outside professional health-care systems but may include consultation with a physician or other health-care professional as a resource. **3.** personal care accomplished without technical assistance, as eating, washing, dressing, using the telephone, attending to one's own elimination, appearance, and hygiene. The goal of rehabilitation medicine is maximal personal self-care.

self-care deficit: feeding, bathing/hygiene, dressing/ grooming, toileting, a nursing diagnosis accepted by the Fourth National Conference on the Classification of Nursing Diagnoses. The etiology of the condition may be an intolerance for activity owing to decreased strength or endurance, pain or discomfort, impairment of cognitive or perceptual function, depression or marked anxiety, or impairment of mobility or of neuromuscular or musculoskeletal function. The kinds of deficit are separated into functional categories and are graded from 0 – functions independently, to 4 – requires total assistance. The defining characteristics of a self-feeding deficit is an inability or a relative lack of ability to bring food to the mouth from a receptacle. The defining characteristics of a self-bathing/hygiene deficit include an inability to get or get to water for bathing and an inability to regulate properly the temperature of the water. The critical characteristic of this deficit is an inability to wash the body or parts of the body. The defining characteristics of a deficit in self-dressing or self-grooming include an impaired ability to fasten clothing, to obtain or replace articles of clothing, and to maintain a satisfactory appearance. The critical defining characteristic is an impaired ability to don or to remove necessary items of clothing. The fourth component of the deficit, self-toileting, carries the following critical defining characteristics: an inability to get to the toilet or to the commode, to sit down on or to arise from the toilet or commode, to get the necessary clothing on or off, and to perform the usual toilet hygiene. In addition, the person may not be able to flush the toilet or to empty the commode. See also **nursing diagnosis.**

self-care theory, a model, used to provide a conceptual framework for nursing care directed toward self-care by the client to the greatest degree possible. The model requires an assessment of the client's capability for self-care and need for care. The need for care includes biophysical and psychosocial needs and the specific needs that are the result of the illness.

self-catheterization, a procedure performed by a patient to empty the bladder and prevent it from becoming overdistended with urine. The patient who cannot empty the bladder completely but can retain urine for two to four hours at a time can be taught self-catheterization if the person is willing to learn and has some manual dexterity and the ability to palpate the bladder.

■ METHOD: Necessary equipment consists of a pan or toilet, two 14 French catheters, a water-soluble lubricant, soap, water, and a clean washcloth and towel; women usually require a magnifying mirror initially to identify the urethral meatus and men may prefer to perform the procedure sitting on a low stool rather than on a toilet. Women are taught to perform self-catheterization initially in a semi-Fowler's position, using a pan, but later they generally can carry out the procedure sitting on or standing over a toilet. The patient is instructed to clean the urinary meatus and labia or glans penis with soap and water, to grasp the catheter three or four inches from the tip, and to lubricate the tip before it is gently inserted in the meatus: women insert 3 to 5 cm of the catheter and men insert 20 cm. Urine is allowed to flow into the pan or toilet until the bladder is empty. The catheter is then removed, washed in soap and water, thoroughly rinsed, dried by rolling it in a clean towel, and placed in a clean plastic or paper bag for the next self-catheterization.

■ NURSING ORDERS: The nurse teaches the procedure, ensures that the patient understands its purpose, the need to perform it at designated times, and the importance of forcing fluids up to 3,000 ml daily, unless contraindicated. The nurse makes certain that the patient is able to identify the urinary meatus.

■ OUTCOME CRITERIA: Regular self-catheterization by the patient who cannot empty the bladder allows the person to work and participate in the normal activities of daily living and to prevent kidney infection and other renal pathology.

self-concept, the composite of ideas, feelings, and attitudes that a person has about his own identity, worth, capabilities, and limitations. Such factors as the values and opinions of others, especially in the formative years of early childhood, play an important part in the development of the self-concept.

self-concept, disturbance in: body image, self-esteem, role performance, personal identity, a nursing diagnosis accepted by the Fourth National Conference on the Classification of Nursing Diagnoses. The disturbance represents a disruption in the way one sees oneself. There are four subcomponents, each with its own etiology and defining characteristics. The etiology of a disturbance in body image may be a biophysical, cognitive, perceptual, psychosocial, cultural, or spiritual factor. The defining characteristics of the deficit include verbal or nonverbal responses to a real or perceived change in structure or function, a missing body part, personalization of the missing part by giving it a name, refusal by the client to look at a part of the body, negative feelings about the body, trauma to a nonfunctioning part, a change in general social involvement or life style, and a fear of rejection by others. The etiology of a disturbance in self-esteem is to be developed at a later conference. The defining characteristics of a disturbance in self-esteem are an inability to accept praise or encouragement, a lack of participation in treatment and therapy, observed self-neglect, self-destructive behavior, or a lack of eye contact with others. The etiology of a disturbance in role performance is to be developed at a later conference. The defining characteristics of a disturbance in role performance include a change in the person's perception of the role or a denial of the role, a change in the physical capacity to perform the actions of the role, and a lack of knowledge of the functions of the role. The etiology and the defining characteristics of a disturbance in personal identity are to be developed at a later conference. See also **nursing diagnosis.**

self-conscious, 1. the state of being aware of oneself as an individual entity that experiences, desires, and acts. 2. a heightened awareness of oneself and one's actions as reflected by the observations and reactions of others; socially ill-at-ease. – **self-consciousness,** *n.*

self-differentiation, specialization and diversification of a tissue or part resulting solely from intrinsic factors.

self-disclosure, the process by which one person lets his inner being, his thoughts and emotions, be known to another. It is important for psychological growth in individual and group psychotherapy.

self-fulfilling prophecy, a principle that states that a belief in or the expectation of a particular resolution is a factor that contributes to its fulfillment.

self-help group, a group of people who meet to improve their health through discussion and special activities. Characteristically, self-help groups are not led by a professional. A women's self-help group may be primarily supportive or it may be concerned with learning to perform basic tests, like a Pap test, or with identification and treatment of common gynecologic problems, as vaginal infections. Compare **group therapy.**

self-image, the total concept, idea, or mental image one has of oneself and of one's role in society; the person one believes oneself to be.

self-limited, (of a disease or condition) tending to end without treatment.

self-radiolysis, a process in which a compound is damaged by radioactive decay products originating in an atom within the compound.

self-retaining catheter, an indwelling urinary catheter that has a double lumen. One channel allows urine to drain from the bladder into a collecting bag; the other channel has a balloon at the bladder end, and a diaphragm at the other end. Several centimeters of air or sterile water are injected through the diaphragm to fill the balloon in the bladder and hold the catheter in place. To remove the catheter, the air or water is withdrawn through the diaphragm or allowed to escape by cutting the diaphragm off the tube.

self-theory, a personality theory that utilizes one's self-concept in integrating the function and organization of the personality. See also **humanistic psychology.**

sella turcica (sel′ə tər′sıkə), a transverse depression crossing the midline on the superior surface of the body of the sphenoid bone and containing the pituitary gland.

Selsun, a trade name for an antifungal and antiseborrheic (selenium sulfide), used as a shampoo.

SEM. See **scanning electron microscope.**

Semap, a trade name for an investigational antipsychotic (penfluridol).

-seme, a combining form meaning '(one) having an orbital index of less than 84, more than 89, or in between' as specified by the prefix: *megaseme, mesoseme, microseme.*

semeio-, a combining form meaning 'sign, or symptom': *semeiography, semeiology, semeiotic.*

semen (si′mən), the thick, whitish secretion of the male reproductive organs discharged from the urethra upon ejaculation. It contains various constituents, including spermatozoa in their nutrient plasma and secretions of the prostate, seminal vesicles, and of various other glands. Also called **seminal fluid, sperm.** – **seminal,** *adj.*

semi-, a combining form meaning 'one-half': *semicoma, semisupination, semivalent.*

semicircular canal, any of three bony, fluid-filled loops in the osseous labyrinth of the internal ear, associated with the sense of balance. The posterior, superior, and lateral canals, each about 0.8 mm in diameter, open into the cochlea. The posterior canal is the longest.

semicircular duct, one of three ducts that make up the membranous labyrinth of the inner ear. See also **membranous labyrinth.**

semicoma (sem′ikou′mə). See **coma.** – **semicomatose,** *adj.*

semiconservative replication. See **replication.**

semi-Fowler's position, placement of the patient in an inclined position, with the upper half of the body raised by elevating the head of the bed.

semilente insulin. See **intermediate-acting insulin.**

semilunar bone. See **lunate bone.**

semilunar valve, 1. a valve with half-moon-shaped cusps, as the aortic valve and the pulmonary valve. **2.** any one of the cusps constituting such a valve. Also called **tricuspid valve.** See also **heart valve.**

semimembranosus (sem'imem'brənou'səs), one of three posterior femoral muscles. Situated at the back and medial side of the thigh, it originates in a thick tendon attached to the tuberosity of the ischium and inserts into the horizontal groove on the medial condyle of the tibia. The tendon of insertion passes some fibers laterally and upward to insert on the lateral condyle of the femur and form part of the oblique popliteal ligament behind the knee. The tendon of insertion forms one of the two medial hamstrings. The muscle is innervated by several branches of the tibial portion of the sciatic nerve, containing fibers from the fifth lumbar and the first two sacral nerves, and functions to flex the leg, to rotate it medially after flexion and to extend the thigh. Compare **biceps femoris, hamstring muscle, semitendinosus.**

seminal duct, any duct through which semen passes, as the deferent duct or the ejaculatory duct.

seminal fluid. See **semen.**

seminal vesiculitis, inflammation of a seminal vesicle.

seminarcosis (sem'inarkou'sis). See **twilight sleep.**

semitendinosus (sem'iten'dinou'səs), one of three posterior femoral muscles of the thigh, remarkable for the great length of its tendon of insertion. It is a fusiform muscle located in the posterior and medial portion of the thigh, arising from the tuberosity of the ischium. It ends just distal to the middle of the thigh in a long, round tendon that curves around the medial condyle of the tibia and inserts into the tibia. The muscle is innervated by branches of the tibial portion of the sciatic nerve, containing fibers from the fifth lumbar and the first two sacral nerves. It functions to flex the leg and rotate it medially after flexion and to extend the thigh. Compare **biceps femoris, hamstring muscle, semimembranosus.**

semustine, an antineoplastic.

■ INDICATIONS: It is prescribed in the treatment of Lewis lung carcinoma and of other carcinomas.

■ CONTRAINDICATIONS: Acute myelosuppression or known hypersensitivity to this drug prohibits its use. It is not given during pregnancy or to lactating mothers.

■ ADVERSE EFFECTS: Among the more serious adverse reactions are delayed bone-marrow depression and thrombocytopenia.

sender, (in communication theory) the person by whom a message is encoded and sent.

senescent (sines'ənt), aging or growing old. See also **senile.** —**senescence,** *n.*

Sengstaken-Blakemore tube, a thick catheter having a triple lumen and two balloons, used to produce pressure by balloon tamponade in order to arrest hemorrhaging from esophageal varices. Attached to a tube, one balloon is blown up in the stomach and exerts pressure against the upper orifice. Similarly attached, another longer and narrower balloon exerts pressure on the walls of the esophagus. The third tube is used for withdrawing gastric contents. See also **tube.**

Traction sponge

Gastric balloon

Gastric suction

Esophageal balloon

Sphygmomanometer for inflating balloons

SENGSTAKEN-BLAKEMORE TUBE

senile, of, pertaining to, or characteristic of old age or the process of aging, especially the physical or mental deterioration accompanying aging. —**senescent,** *adj.,* **senility,** *n.*

senile angioma. See **cherry angioma.**

senile cataract, a kind of cataract, associated with aging, in which a hard opacity forms in the nucleus of the lens of the eye.

senile delirium, disorientation and mental feebleness associated with extreme age and characterized by restlessness, insomnia, aimless wandering, and less commonly, by hallucination. See also **delirium, senile psychosis.**

senile dementia. See **senile psychosis.**

senile dental caries, tooth decay occurring at an advanced age. Senile dental caries is usually characterized by cavity formation in or around the cementum layer of the tooth. See also **dental caries.**

senile endometritis, *Obsolete.* endometritis in a postmenopausal woman.

senile involution, a pattern of retrograde changes occurring with advancing age and resulting in the progressive shrinking and degeneration of tissues and organs.

senile keratosis. See **actinic keratosis.**

senile memory. See **anterograde memory.**

senile nanism, dwarfism associated with progeria.

senile psychosis, an organic mental disorder of the aged, resulting from the generalized atrophy of the brain with no evidence of cerebrovascular disease. Symptoms include loss of memory, impaired judgment, decreased moral and aesthetic values, inability to think abstractly, periods of confusion, confabulation, and irritability, all of which may range from mild to severe. The condition, which is irreversible, is more common in women than in men, runs a gradual and progressive course, and may be a late form of Alzheimer's disease. Although the exact cause of brain deterioration in the aged is not known, there are several theories being studied, including autoimmunity, slow infection, and cholinergic deficiency. Also called **primary degenerative dementia, senile onset.** See also **multi-infarct dementia.**

senile wart. See **actinic keratosis.**

senna, the dried leaflets or pods of *Cassia acutifolia* or *Cassia augustifolia,* used as a cathartic.

sens-, a combining form meaning 'perception, or feeling': *sensation, sensimeter, sensitinogen.*

sensible perspiration, loss of fluid from the body through the secretory activity of the sweat glands in a quantity sufficient to be observed. Compare **insensible perspiration.**

sensitivity, **1.** capacity to feel, transmit, or react to a stimulus. **2.** susceptibility to a substance, as a drug or an antigen. See also **allergy, hypersensitivity.** – **sensitive,** *adj.*

sensitivity-training group, a group that offers members a supportive atmosphere in which to experiment with and alter behavioral patterns and interpersonal reactions. The focus of sensitivity training is on learning what occurs during group interactions, testing and refining new behavioral responses in light of the reactions they evoke, and applying those responses to situations outside the group setting. Also called **T-group.** See also **encounter group, psychotherapy.**

sensitization, **1.** an acquired reaction in which specific antibodies develop in response to an antigen. This is deliberately caused in immunization by injecting a disease-causing organism that has been altered in such a way that it can no longer cause disease yet remains able to cause the production of antibodies to fight the disease. Allergic reactions are hypersensitivity reactions that result from excess sensitization to a foreign protein. **2.** a photodynamic method of destroying microorganisms by inserting into a solution substances, as fluorescing dyes, that absorb visible light and emit energy at wavelengths destruc-

tive to the organism. **3.** *Nontechnical.* anaphylaxis. – **sensitize,** *v.*

sensorineural hearing loss, a form of hearing loss in which sound is conducted through the external and middle ear in a normal way but a defect in the inner ear results in its distortion, making discrimination difficult. Amplification of the sound with a hearing aid will help some people with sensorineural hearing loss, but many have an intolerance to loud noises and will not be helped. Compare **conductive hearing loss.**

sensory apraxia. See **ideational apraxia.**

sensory deprivation, an involuntary loss of physical awareness caused by detachment from external sensory stimuli. Such deprivation often results in psychological disorders, as panic, mental confusion, depression, and hallucinations. Sensory deprivation may be associated with various handicaps and conditions, as blindness, heavy sedation, and prolonged isolation.

sensory nerve, a nerve consisting of afferent fibers that conduct sensory impulses from the periphery of the body to the brain or spinal cord via the dorsal spinal roots. Compare **motor nerve.**

sensory-perceptual alterations: visual, auditory, kinesthetic, gustatory, tactile, olfactory perception, a nursing diagnosis accepted by the Fourth National Conference on the Classification of Nursing Diagnoses. The etiology of the alteration may be excessive or insufficient environmental stimulation, changes in the reception, transmission, or integration of stimuli, endogenous or exogenous chemical alteration in the perception of stimuli, or psychological stress or disturbance. The defining characteristics of the disturbance include disorientation, change in the ability to abstract, conceptualize, or solve problems, change in behavior and in sensory acuity, restlessness, irritability, inappropriate response to stimuli, and hallucination. See also **nursing diagnosis.**

SEP, abbreviation for **somatosensory evoked potential.**

separation anxiety, fear and apprehension caused by separation from familiar surroundings and significant persons. The syndrome occurs commonly in an infant when separated from its mother or from its mothering figure or when it is approached by a stranger. See also **anxiety, anxiety neurosis.**

seps-, a combining form meaning 'of or pertaining to decay': *sepsin, sepsis, sepsometer.*

sepsis (sep'sis), infection, contamination. Compare **asepsis.** – **septic,** *adj.*

-sepsis, a combining form meaning 'decay due to a (specified) cause or of a (specified) sort': *colisepsis, endosepsis, typhosepsis.*

sept-, **1.** a combining form meaning 'of or pertaining to the nasal septum': *septectomy, septometer, septotomy.* **2.** a combining form meaning 'seven': *septigravida, septipara, septivalent.*

septal defect, an abnormal, usually congenital defect in the wall separating two chambers of the heart. Depending on the size and the site of the defect, various amounts of oxygenated and deoxygenated blood mix, causing a decrease in the amount of oxygen carried in the blood to the peripheral tissues. Kinds of septal defects are **atrial septal defect, ventricular septal defect.**

-septic, a combining form meaning 'referring to decay of a sort or due to a (specified) cause': *aseptic, colyseptic, uroseptic.*

septic abortion, spontaneous or induced termination of a pregnancy in which the life of the mother may be threatened because of the invasion of germs into the endometrium, myometrium, and beyond, requiring immediate and intensive care, massive antibiotic therapy, evacuation of the uterus, and, often, emergency hysterectomy to prevent death from overwhelming infection and septic shock. Compare **infected abortion.** See also **criminal abortion, induced abortion.**

septic arthritis, an acute form of arthritis, characterized by bacterial inflammation of a joint caused by the spread of bacteria through the bloodstream from an infection elsewhere in the body or by contamination of a joint during trauma or surgery. The joint is stiff, painful, tender, warm, and swollen. The diagnosis is confirmed by bacteriologic identification of an organism in a specimen obtained by aspiration of the joint. Parenteral antibiotics are given to prevent destruction of the joint and are continued for several weeks after inflammation has resolved. Repeated aspiration of the joint or surgical incision and drainage may be performed to relieve pressure on the joint. Physical therapy as the joint heals is helpful to restore it to full range of motion. Also called **acute bacterial arthritis.**

septicemia (sep'tısi'miə), systemic infection in which pathogens are present in the circulating blood stream, having spread from an infection in any part of the body. It is diagnosed by culture of the blood and is vigorously treated with antibiotics. Characteristically, septicemia causes fever, chill, prostration, pain, headache, nausea, or diarrhea. Also called **blood poisoning.** Compare **bacteremia.** See also **septic shock.** — **septicemic,** *adj.*

-septicemia, a combining form meaning '(condition of the) blood caused by virulent microorganisms': *hemorrhagicsepticemia, pyosepticemia, streptosepticemia.* Also **-septicaemia.**

septicemic plague, a rapidly fatal form of bubonic plague in which septicemia with meningitis occurs before buboes have had time to form. Compare **bubonic plague, pneumonic plague.** See also **plague,** *Yersinia pestis.*

septic fever, an elevation of body temperature associated with infection by pathogenic microorganisms or in response to a toxin secreted by a microorganism.

septic shock, a form of shock that occurs in septicemia when endotoxins are released from certain bacteria in the blood stream. The endotoxins cause decreased vascular resistance, resulting in a drastic fall in the blood pressure. Fever, tachycardia, increased respirations, and confusion or coma may also occur. Septic shock is usually preceded by signs of severe infection, often of the genitourinary or gastrointestinal system. The causative organism is most frequently gram-negative. Antibiotics, vasopressors, and intravenous fluids and volume expanders are usually given. In some cases an antitoxin may be available and effective. Also called **bacteremic shock.** A kind of septic shock is **toxic shock syndrome.**

Septra, a trade name for the antibacterial, co-trimoxazole (a 1:5 mixture of the antibacterials trimethoprim and sulfamethoxazole.)

septum (sep'təm), *pl.* **septa.** a partition, as the interauricular septum that separates the atria of the heart.

sequela (sıkwi'lə), *pl.* **sequelae.** any abnormal condition that follows and is the result of a disease, treatment, or injury, as paralysis following poliomyelitis, deafness following treatment with an ototoxic drug, or a scar following a laceration.

sequential imaging, (in nuclear medicine) a diagnostic procedure in which a series of closely timed images of the rapidly changing distribution of an administered radioactive tracer is used to determine a physiologic process or processes within the body.

sequester, to detach, separate, or isolate, as a patient sequestered to prevent the spread of an infection.

sequestered antigens theory, a theory of autoimmunity, stressing the relationship between antigen exposure, immunogenic cells, and body cells, maintaining that immunologic tolerance depends on a certain degree of contact between immunologic cells and body cells and on a certain degree of antigen exposure. The theory holds that certain sequestered antigens in the brain, the lenses of the eye, and spermatozoa are isolated from the circulations of the blood and the lymph and do not contact the immune system. When body tissues are damaged, the sequestered antigens suddenly are exposed to the immune system but are not recognized as such by the body, and an autoimmune reaction results. Compare **forbidden clone theory.**

sequestered edema, edema localized in the tissues surrounding a newly created surgical wound.

sequestrum (sıkwes'trəm), *pl.* **sequestra.** a fragment of dead bone that is partially or entirely detached from the surrounding or adjacent healthy bone.

sequestrum forceps, a forceps with small, powerful teeth used for extracting necrotic or sharp fragments of bone from surrounding tissue.

sequoiasis (sıkwoi'əsıs), a type of hypersensitivity pneumonitis common among workers in sawmills where redwood is processed. The antigens are the fungus *Pullu-*

laria pullulans and species of the genus *Graphium,* found in moldy redwood sawdust. Characteristics of the acute disease include chills, fever, cough, dyspnea, anorexia, nausea, and vomiting. Symptoms of the chronic disease include productive cough, dyspnea on exertion, fatigue, and weight loss.

Ser-Ap-Es, a trade name for an antihypertensive, fixed-combination drug containing a diuretic (hydrochlorothiazide) and antihypertensives (reserpine and hydralazine hydrochloride).

Serax, a trade name for a tranquilizer (oxazepam).

Serentil, a trade name for a phenothiazine tranquilizer (mesoridazine).

series, a chain of objects or events arranged in a predictable order, as the series of stages through which a mature blood cell develops.

Sernylan, a trade name for a veterinary anesthetic (phencyclidine hydrochloride), used illicitly as a euphoric. Also called **PCP.**

sero-, a combining form meaning 'of or pertaining to blood serum': *seroculture, serogenesis, serolin.*

serological diagnosis, a diagnosis that is made through laboratory examination of antigen-antibody reactions in the serum. Also called **immunodiagnosis, serum diagnosis.**

serology (sɪrol'əji), the branch of laboratory medicine that studies blood serum for evidence of infection by evaluating antigen-antibody reactions *in vitro.* —**serologic, serological,** *adj.*

Seromycin, a trade name for a tuberculostatic (cycloserine).

serosa (sɪrou'sə), any serous membrane, as the tunica serosa which lines the walls of body cavities and secretes a watery exudate.

serosanguinous (sɪ'rousæŋ'gwɪnəs), (of a discharge) thin and red; composed of serum and blood.

serotonin (ser'ətou'nɪn), a naturally occurring derivative of tryptophan found in platelets and in cells of the brain and the intestine. Serotonin is released from platelets upon damage to the blood vessel walls. It acts as a potent vasoconstrictor. Serotonin in intestinal tissue stimulates the smooth muscle to contract. In the central nervous system, it acts as a neurotransmitter. Lysergic acid diethylamide interferes with the action of serotonin in the brain.

serous membrane, one of the many thin sheets of tissue that line closed cavities of the body, as the pleura lining the thoracic cavity, the peritoneum lining the abdominal cavity, and the pericardium lining the sac that encloses the heart. Between the visceral layer of serous membrane covering various organs and the parietal layer lining the cavity containing such organs is a potential space moistened by serous fluid. The fluid reduces the friction of the structures covered by the serous membrane, as the lungs, which move against the thoracic walls in respiration. Compare **mucous membrane, skin, synovial membrane.**

Serpasil, a trade name for an antihypertensive (reserpine).

Serpasil-Apresoline, a trade name for a fixed-combination drug containing two antihypertensives (reserpine and hydralazine hydrochloride).

Serpasil-Esidrix, a trade name for an antihypertensive fixed-combination drug containing a diuretic (hydrochlorothiazide) and an antihypertensive (reserpine).

serpent ulcer, an ulceration of the skin that heals in one area while extending to another. Also called **serpiginous ulcer.**

serpiginous ulcer. See **serpent ulcer.**

Serratia (sɪrei'shə), a genus of motile, gram-negative bacilli capable of causing infection in humans, including bacteremia, pneumonia, and urinary tract infections. *Serratia* organisms are frequently acquired in hospitals. See also **nosocomial infection.**

serratus anterior, a thin muscle of the chest wall extending from the ribs under the arm to the scapula. Arising from the outer surface and upper border of the first eight or nine ribs, it inserts into the medial angle, the vertebral border, and the inferior angle of the scapula. It is innervated by the long thoracic nerve of the brachial plexus which contains fibers of the fifth, the sixth, and the seventh cervical nerves. It acts to rotate the scapula and to raise the shoulder, as in full flexion and abduction of the arm. Compare **pectoralis major, pectoralis minor, subclavius.**

Sertoli-Leydig cell tumor (sər'təlilai'dɪg). See **arrhenoblastoma.**

serum, 1. See also **blood clotting.** the clear, thin, and sticky fluid portion of the blood. Like plasma, it contains no blood cells or platelets; unlike plasma it contains no fibrinogen. The fibrinogen present in whole cells or platelets; unlike plasma it blood is consumed by the clotting process, leaving the serum separate, as can be seen in a standing tube of clotted blood. 2. a vaccine or toxoid prepared from the serum of a hyperimmune donor for prophylaxis against a particular infection or poison.

serum albumin, a major protein in blood plasma that is important in maintaining the oncotic pressure of the blood.

serum C-reactive protein. See **C-reactive protein.**

serum diagnosis. See **serological diagnosis.**

serum glutamic oxaloacetic transaminase (SGOT), a catalytic enzyme found in various parts of the body, especially the heart, liver, and muscle tissue. Increased amounts of the enzyme occur in the serum as a result of myocardial infarction, acute liver disease, the actions of certain drugs, and any disease or condition in which cells are seriously damaged. See also **transaminase.**

serum glutamic pyruvic transaminase (SGPT), a catalytic enzyme normally found in high concentration in the liver. Greater than normal amounts in the serum indicate liver damage. See also **transaminase.**

serum hepatitis. See **hepatitis B.**

serum sickness, an immunologic disorder that may occur 2 to 3 weeks after the administration of an antiserum. It is caused by an antibody reaction to an antigen in the donor serum and is characterized by fever, splenomegaly, swollen lymph glands, skin rash, and joint pain. Treatment is symptomatic and supportive and may include corticosteroids. See also **antigen-antibody reaction, Arthus reaction.**

service of process, (in law) the delivery of a writ, summons, or complaint to a defendant. Once delivered or left with the party for whom it is intended, it is said to have been served. The original of the document is shown; a copy is served. Service of process gives reasonable notice to allow the person to appear, testify, and be heard in court.

sesamoid bone, any one of numerous small, round, bony masses embedded in certain tendons that may be subjected to compression as well as tension. The largest sesamoid bone is the patella, which is embedded in the tendon of the quadriceps femoris at the knee.

sesqui-, a combining form meaning 'one and a half': *sesquibasic, sesquibo, sesquihora.*

sessile (ses'əl), **1.** (in biology) attached by a base rather than by a stalk or a peduncle, as a leaf which is attached directly to its stem. **2.** permanently connected.

set-, a combining form meaning 'of or related to a bristle': *setaceous, setiferous, seton.*

Setamine, a trade name for a gastrointestinal fixed-combination drug containing anticholinergics (atropine sulfate, scopolamine hydrobromide, and hyoscyamine sulfate) and a sedative-hypnotic (phenobarbital).

settlement, (in law) an agreement made between parties to a suit before a judgment is rendered by a court.

seventh nerve. See **facial nerve.**

severe combined immunodeficiency disease (SCID), an abnormal condition characterized by the complete absence or by the marked deficiency of B cells and T cells with the consequent lack of humoral immunity and cell-mediated immunity. This disease occurs as an X-linked recessive disorder only in males and as an autosomal recessive disorder affecting both males and females. It results in a pronounced susceptibility to infection and is usually fatal. The precise cause of SCID is not known, but research indicates it may be caused by a cytogenic dysfunction of the embryonic stem cells in differentiating B cells and T cells. The affected individual consequently has a very small thymus and little or no protection against infection.

■ OBSERVATIONS: Pronounced susceptibility to infection usually becomes obvious in affected individuals 3 to 6 months after birth, when maternal immunoglobulin reserves are diminishing. Diagnosis is difficult because B cell immunity dysfunction is hard to detect in any individual until five months after birth, when immunoglobulin levels should be one per cent of normal. Infants with SCID commonly fail to thrive and develop a variety of complications, as sepsis, watery diarrhea, persistent pulmonary infections, and common viral infections that are often fatal. Some infants with SCID develop mild infections and low-grade fevers that last for several months, while the infant uses maternal immunoglobulin stores, and then flare into serious, fatal conditions when maternal antibodies are totally depleted, usually within one year. Some of the more obvious symptoms after the infant has used most of the maternal immunoglobulin stores are cyanosis, rapid respirations, and normal chest sounds with an abnormal chest x ray. Maternal IgG is persistent and gram-negative infections in the infant usually do not appear until after the sixth month of life. Normal infants less than five months old have very small amounts of IgM and IgA, and normal IgG levels only reflect maternal IgG. The combination of several symptoms may confirm the diagnosis of SCID. Such symptoms include the absence or the severe reduction of T cell and B cell immunity, a lymph node biopsy that shows no lymphocytes, plasma cells, or lymphoid follicles, and no skin reaction to swabbing with dinitrochlorobenzene. Most infants with SCID die from severe infection within one year after birth.

■ INTERVENTION: Treatment of SCID seeks to develop the immune system and to prevent infection. The only satisfactory treatment available to correct immunodeficiency is histocompatible bone marrow transplant, but such a procedure may cause a graft-versus-host reaction, thus increasing the risk of infection and fatal consequences. Placing the infant with SCID in a completely sterile environment for a long time is a method of treatment that has prolonged the lives of some affected individuals, but this option does not prove successful if the infant involved has already had recurring infections.

■ NURSING CONSIDERATIONS: Supportive treatment is the primary approach in caring for the SCID patient. Nurses commonly try to promote an encouraging atmosphere of growth and development while providing the parents of SCID infants with spiritual and psychological support in the face of the nearly inevitable early death of the patient. The infant must remain in strict protective isolation and benefits from frequent parental visits, gifts of toys, and frequent nursing attention. Toys brought to an infant in protective isolation should be the kind that can be easily sterilized.

Sevin, a trade name for carbaryl, a widely used carbamate insecticide that causes reversible inhibition of cholinesterase. Although less toxic than parathion, carbaryl, when concentrated, may produce skin irritation and systemic poisoning characterized by nausea, vomiting, cramps, diarrhea, diaphoresis, excessive salivation, dyspnea, weakness, loss of coordination, and slurred speech; large doses may cause coma and death. Carbaryl on the skin is promptly removed by washing with water. Treatment of systemic poisoning includes the immediate intravenous or intramuscular injection of 1.0 to 4.0 mg of atropine sulfate, the administration of artificial respiration and oxygen, gastric lavage, and intravenous isotonic saline to correct dehydration.

sex, 1. a classification of male or female based on many criteria, among them anatomic and chromosomal characteristics. 2. coitus. Compare **gender**.

sex-, a combining form meaning 'six': *sexdigitate, sexivalent, sextan*.

sex chromatin, a densely staining mass within the nucleus of all nondividing cells of normal mammalian females. It represents the facultative heterochromatin of the inactivated X chromosome. Examination of cells obtained by amniocentesis for the presence or absence of sex chromatin is a technique used for determining the sex of a baby before birth. Sex chromatin is also found as a drumsticklike mass attached to one of the nuclear lobes in polymorphonuclear leukocytes in normal females. Also called **Barr body**. See also **Lyon hypothesis**.

sex chromosome, a chromosome that is responsible for the sex determination of offspring; it carries genes that transmit sex-linked traits and conditions. In man and other mammals there are two distinct sex chromosomes, the X and the Y chromosomes, which are unequally paired and appear in females in the XX combination and in males as XY. Compare **autosome**.

sex chromosome mosaic, an individual or organism whose cells contain variant chromosomal numbers involving the X or Y chromosomes. Such variations are found in most of the syndromes associated with sex chromosome aberrations, primarily Turner's syndrome, and may be caused by nondisjunction of the chromosomes during the second meiotic division of gametogenesis or by some error in chromosome distribution during cell division of the fertilized ovum. Sex chromosome mosaics often have sexual abnormalities, but because of the sex hormones the overall phenotype is uniform and not mosaic in external characteristics, as in certain animals and insects. See also **intersexuality**.

sex-controlled. See **sex-influenced**.

sex factor. See **F factor**.

sex-influenced, of or pertaining to an autosomal genetic trait or condition, as patterned baldness or gout, that in one sex is expressed phenotypically in both homozygotes and heterozygotes, while in the other sex a phenotypic

effect is produced in homozygotes only. Also called **sex-controlled**.

sexism, a belief that one sex is superior to the other and that the superior sex has endowments, rights, prerogatives, and status greater than those of the inferior sex. Sexism results in discrimination in all areas of life and acts as a limiting factor in educational, professional, and psychological development. — **sexist**, *n.*

sex-limited, of or pertaining to an autosomal genetic trait or condition that is expressed phenotypically in only one sex, although the genes for them may be carried by both sexes. Such traits or conditions are typically influenced by hormonal or environmental conditions.

sex-linked, pertaining to genes or to the normal or abnormal characteristics or conditions they transmit. The genes are carried on the sex chromosomes, specifically the X chromosome. See also **sex-linked disorder, X-linked inheritance, Y-linked inheritance**. — **sex linkage**, *n.*

sex-linked disorder, any disease or abnormal condition that is determined by the sex chromosomes. These may involve a deviation in the number of either the X or Y chromosomes, as occurs in Turner's syndrome and Kleinfelter's syndrome, most occurrences of which are caused as a result of nondisjunction during meiosis. Such aberrations in the number of sex chromosomes do not produce the severe clinical effects that are associated with autosomal aberrations, although some degree of mental deficiency is usually apparent. Other sex-linked disorders are transmitted by single gene defects carried on the X chromosome. X-linked dominant mutants, as hypophosphatemic vitamin D resistant rickets, are rare, and males are more seriously affected than females. In inheritance patterns, X-linked dominant conditions are transmitted by affected males to all of their daughters but none of their sons, by affected heterozygous females to one half of their children regardless of sex, and by affected homozygous females to all of their children. X-linked recessive mutants are more common and are responsible for such traits and disorders as colorblindness, ocular albinism, the Xg blood types, hemophilia, the Duchenne type of muscular dystrophy, and inborn errors of metabolism. Such conditions are always transmitted by females so that those predominantly affected are males, since they have only one X chromosome and all genes, whether recessive or dominant, are expressed. Affected males never transmit the condition to their sons, but all of their daughters will be carriers; they, in turn, will transmit the trait to half of their sons. Occasionally, heterozygous females for X-linked recessive disorders show varying degrees of expression but never as severe as those of the affected male. There are no known clinically significant traits or conditions associated with the genes on the Y chromosome; its only known function is triggering the development of male characteristics.

sex-linked ichthyosis, a congenital skin disorder characterized by large, thick, dry scales that are dark in color and that cover the neck, scalp, ears, face, trunk, and flexor surfaces of the body, as the folds of the arms and the backs of the knees. It is transmitted by females as an X-linked recessive trait and appears only in males. The condition is managed by topical applications of emollients and the use of keratolytic agents to facilitate removal of the scales. Also called **X-linked ichthyosis.** See also **ichthyosis.**

sex mosaic. See **sex chromosome mosaic.**

sexual, of or pertaining to sex.

sexual dwarf, an adult dwarf whose genital organs are normally developed.

sexual dysfunction, a nursing diagnosis accepted by the Fourth National Conference on the Classification of Nursing Diagnoses. The etiology of the condition may be a biological, psychological, or social alteration in sexuality caused by an ineffectual or absent role model, physical abuse, psychosocial abuse, as in a harmful relationship, misinformation or lack of information, a conflict in values, a lack of privacy, or an alteration in body structure or function, as may result from surgery, congenital anomalies, or trauma. The defining characteristics of the condition include a statement by the client of the perceived dysfunction, a physical alteration or limitation imposed by disease or treatment, a reported inability to achieve sexual satisfaction, an alteration in the sexual relationship with the partner, and a change in interest in the self or in others. See also **nursing diagnosis.**

sexual generation, reproduction by the union of male and female gametes.

sexual harassment, an aggressive, sexually motivated act of physical or verbal violation of a person over whom the aggressor has some power. Sexual harassment of women in the workplace is against the law, as it represents an abridgment of the victim's right to equal opportunity, privacy, and freedom from assault. Sexual harassment may be heterosexual or, as is common in prison, homosexual.

sexual history, (in a patient record) the portion of the patient's personal history concerned with sexual function and dysfunction. A sexual history is particularly important in gathering data from a patient who has a disease of the reproductive tract, who experiences sexual dysfunction, or who requests contraception, abortion, or sterilization. The extent of the history varies with the patient's age and condition and the reason for securing the history. A short sexual history is recommended as part of every complete physical examination. The therapist needs a detailed sexual history to understand the patient's complaint and to plan treatment. It may include age at onset of sexual intercourse, the kind and frequency of sexual activity, and the satisfaction derived from it.

sexual intercourse. See **coitus.**

sexuality, 1. the sum of the physical, functional, and psychologic attributes that are expressed by one's gender identity and sexual behavior, whether or not related to the sex organs or to procreation. 2. the genital characteristics that distinguish male from female.

sexually transmitted disease. See **venereal disease.**

sexual melancholia, *Obsolete.* a state of depression in a man resulting from the belief that he is impotent. See also **bipolar disorder, depression.**

sexual psychopath, an individual whose sexual behavior is openly perverted, antisocial, and criminal. See also **antisocial personality disorder.**

sexual reassignment, a change in the gender identity of a person by legal, surgical, hormonal, or social means.

sexual reflex, (in males) a reflex in which tactile or cerebral stimulation results in penile erection, in priapism, or in ejaculation. Also called **genital reflex.**

sexual sadism. See **sadism.**

sexual selection, the theory that mates are chosen according to the attraction of or preference for certain characteristics, as coloration or behavior patterns, so that eventually only those particular traits appear in succeeding generations. The theory explains the wide variety of sexual characteristics among the various species.

SFD, abbreviation for **small-for-dates.** See **small-for-gestational-age infant.**

SGA, abbreviation for **small-for-gestational-age.** See **small-for-gestational-age infant.**

SGOT, abbreviation for **serum glutamic oxaloacetic transaminase.**

SGPT, abbreviation for **serum glutamic pyruvic transaminase.**

shadow chart, a copy of the data contained in the permanent patient record, made for use when it is important to have the information at hand and when retrieval of the record from the record room may be difficult or time-consuming.

shaping, a procedure used for conditioning a person undergoing behavior therapy in order to develop new behavioral responses. Initially, any act remotely resembling the desired behavior is reinforced; gradually, the criterion is made more stringent until the desired response is attained.

shared paranoid disorder, a psychopathological condition characterized by identical manifestations of the same mental disorder, usually ideas, in two closely associated or related persons. Also called **folie à deux.**

SHCC, abbreviation for **Statewide Health Coordinating Committee.**

sheath, a tubular structure that surrounds an organ or any other part of the body, as the sheath of the rectus abdominis muscle or the sheath of Schwann, which covers various nerve fibers.

sheep cell test, a method that mixes human blood cells with the red blood cells of sheep to determine the absence or the deficiency of human T-lymphocytes. When mixed with human blood cells the red blood cells of sheep cluster around the human T-lymphocytes and form characteristic rosettes. An electron microscope is used to examine the rosettes. An absence or a decrease in the number of rosettes indicates a deficiency or absence of T cells. The sheep cell test is used to diagnose several diseases, as DiGeorge's syndrome, which decreases or destroys the cellular immunity provided by T cells.

sheet bath, the application of wet sheets to the body, used primarily as an antipyretic procedure.

shellfish poisoning, a toxic, neurologic condition that results from eating clams or mussels that have ingested the poisonous protozoa commonly called the "red tide." The characteristic symptoms appear within a few minutes and include nausea, light-headedness, vomiting, and tingling or numbness around the mouth, followed by paralysis of the extremities and, possibly, respiratory paralysis. Saxitoxin, the causative agent, is not destroyed by cooking; however, the severity of the illness is diminished if the water used in cooking is not consumed. Treatment includes an intravenous injection of a weak solution of prostigmin methylsulfate and the administration of oxygen and artificial respiration.

shell shock, any of a number of mental disorders, ranging from extreme fear to dementia, believed to be caused by the noise and concussion resulting from exploding shells or bombs but actually owing to a traumatic reaction to the stress of combat. See also **combat fatigue, post-traumatic stress disorder.**

shield, (in radiation technology) a material for preventing or reducing the passage of charged particles or radiation. A shield may be designated by the radiation it is intended to absorb, as a gamma-ray shield, or according to the kind of protection it is intended to give, as a background, biological, or thermal shield. Lucite and aluminum can be used for beta-radiation shields, but lead is required for gamma-ray shields. The amount of material needed to provide shielding is expressed as the half-value layer, which is the quantity required to reduce the radiation intensity at a point in space by one half.

shift, (in nursing) the particular hours of the day during which a nurse is scheduled to work. The day shift is usually 7:00 a.m. to 3:00 p.m. or 8:00 a.m. to 4:00 p.m. The evening shift is usually 3:00 p.m. to 11:00 p.m. or 4:00 p.m. to 12:00 midnight, and the night shift the remaining hours. The evening shift is also called 'relief,' presumably because nurses originally worked 12-hour shifts and the evening and night shift was thought to be relief for the day nurse. Nurses are said to 'work shift' when they work assigned hours. Other nurses do not 'work shift' but set their own hours. Many innovations in staffing practice currently allow variations on the traditional five-day, forty-hour week, as a nurse electing to work a shorter week, preferring longer hours for fewer days.

shift to the left, *Informal.* a predominance of immature lymphocytes, noted in a differential white blood cell count. It is usually indicative of an infection or inflammation. The term derives from a graph of blood components in which immature cell frequencies appear on the left side of the graph.

shift to the right, (in hematology) a preponderance of polymorphonuclear neutrophils having three or more lobes, indicating maturity of the cell. The phenomenon is common in severe liver disease and advanced pernicious anemia. It indicates a relative lack of blood-forming activity.

Shigella (shĭgel'ə), a genus of gram-negative pathogenic bacteria that causes gastroenteritis and bacterial dysentery, as *Shigella dysenteriae.* See also **shigellosis.**

shigellosis (shĭg'ĭlou'sĭs), an acute bacterial infection of the bowel, characterized by diarrhea, abdominal pain, and fever, that is transmitted by hand-to-mouth contact with the feces of individuals infected with bacteria of a pathogenic species of the genus *Shigella* species. These organisms may be carried in the stools of asymptomatic people for up to several months and may be spread through contact with contaminated objects, food, or flies, especially in poor, crowded areas. The disease occurs in isolated outbreaks in the United States but is endemic in underdeveloped areas of the world. It is especially common and usually most severe in children. Diagnosis is made by isolating and identifying *Shigella* in a specimen of stool. The likelihood of encountering or engendering antibiotic-resistant organisms is very high, so the preferred treatment for shigellosis is supportive, and the major goal is to prevent dehydration. Antimicrobials are given if the disease is severe or if the likelihood of further transmission is great. Isolation and strict handwashing precautions are instituted. Shigellosis infections must be reported to the public health department. Also called **bacillary dysentery.**

shin bone. See **tibia.**

shindylesis, an articulation of certain bones of the skull in which a thin plate of one bone enters a cleft formed by the separation of two layers of another bone, as the insertion of the vomer bone into the fissure between the maxillae and the palatine bones.

shingles. See **herpes zoster.**

shin splints, a painful condition of the lower leg caused by strain of the long flexor muscle of the toes following strenuous athletic activity, like running. In many instances it is the result of inadequate training. Treatment usually involves rest and exercise therapy. Surgery is sometimes necessary.

Shirodkar's operation (s̆hır'odkarz'), a surgical procedure called a cerclage in which the cervical canal is closed by a purse-string suture embedded in the uterine cervix encircling the canal. It is performed to correct an incompetent cervix that has failed to retain previous pregnancies. Under spinal block or general anesthesia, a 5 mm-wide band of nonabsorbable material is buried beneath the mucosa of the cervix and pulled in a purse-string manner to close the cervix. The band may be left in place permanently, in which case subsequent deliveries are by Caesarean section. Occasionally, a temporary cerclage is done, sewing in the band and leaving the ends exposed in the vagina. The band is then removed prior to labor and vaginal delivery. Postoperatively, infection or vaginal fistula may occur. If labor begins with the suture in place it is removed promptly or the infant is delivered by Caesarean section, before rupture of the uterus occurs.

shock, an abnormal physiological state, the first phase of the body's alarm reaction to trauma. The common clinical signs of shock include reduced cardiac output, circulatory insufficiency, tachycardia, hypotension, restlessness, pallor, and diminished urinary output. Shock often results from severe tissue damage and may be primary, secondary, or hemorrhagic. See also **cardiogenic shock, electric shock, hypovolemic shock.**

(See next column for table)

shock lung, pulmonary damage occurring early in shock and characterized by acute respiratory distress, atelectasis, and pulmonary edema. Pulmonary vessels may become plugged with blood cells and platelets, causing anoxia and damage to epithelial cells of alveoli and capillaries. Fluid often leaks into the alveoli, decreasing surfactant, with the result that they may collapse and general hypoxia of tissues may ensue.

shock trousers, pneumatic trousers designed to counteract hypotension, associated with internal or external bleeding, and hypovolemia. Shock trousers may be contraindicated in patients with pulmonary edema, cardiogenic shock, increased intracranial pressure, or eviscerations.

■ METHOD: The patient for whom shock trousers are required is losing consciousness, has a decreased or falling blood pressure, and shows signs of respiratory distress, as dyspnea, rapid breathing, a cough, and pink, frothy sputum. The leg pulses may be diminished or absent, and the feet may appear pale, mottled, and cold. Before the pressurized trousers are applied, they are checked for tears or leaks and the proper functioning of their valves; any kinks or twists in the tubes connecting the trousers to the pneumatic pump are removed. The patient is placed in a flat, supine position over the open trousers and the leg sections and portion that encircles the abdomen just below the rib cage are firmly secured in place by closing the Velcro straps or zippers. The exact times at which the

---

Parameters for assessing status of the patient in shock

Hemodynamic monitoring
Blood pressure
Pulse
Central venous pressure (CVP)
Pulmonary wedge pressure (PWP)
Cardiac output (CO)
Electrocardiogram

Respiratory monitoring
Respiratory rate, depth
Breath sounds
Blood gases
  pH
  Po_2
  Pco_2
  Percent saturation

Fluid and electrolyte monitoring
Serum electrolytes
Blood lactate and pyruvate levels
Intake
Output
  Urinary
  Gastrointestinal tract
  Sweating
  Dressings
Weight
Creatinine serum level
Blood urea nitrogen level (BUN)
Serum and urinary osmolarity
Urinary specific gravity

Neurological monitoring
Alertness
Orientation

Hematological monitoring
Erythrocytes
Hematocrit and hemoglobin levels
Leukocytes
Platelets
Prothrombin and partial thromboplastin time
Clotting time

Others
Bowel sounds
Skin temperature

---

trousers' sections are inflated are recorded, and the inflated sections are checked every 15 minutes. The patient's blood pressure, respiration, apical and peripheral pulses are also checked every 15 minutes and chest sounds are auscultated hourly. Parenteral fluids, whole blood, plasmanate, and other plasma volume expanders are administered as ordered; the flow rate of expanders is adjusted according to central venous pressure readings.

An indwelling urethral catheter is connected to a closed gravity drainage system, and fluid intake and output are measured hourly; if less than 30 ml of urine per hour are excreted, renal failure may occur. Monitoring of blood gases and intermittent suctioning through a nasogastric tube may be ordered. The trousers are not deflated or removed until the blood volume replacement is stable and the patient's physician is in attendance. As each section of the trousers, starting with the abdominal section, is gradually deflated, the patient's blood pressure, respiration, and apical pulse are checked every 5 to 10 minutes; if the blood pressure drops 4 to 6 mm Hg, deflation is stopped.

■ NURSING ORDERS: The nurse checks, applies, and inflates the shock trousers and remains with the patient during the entire procedure. The vital signs are monitored at frequent intervals, parenteral fluids and plasma volume expanders are given, measures of the intake and output are taken and recorded, and emotional support is provided.

short-acting, 1. pertaining to or characterizing a therapeutic agent, usually a drug, with a brief period of effectiveness, generally beginning soon after the substance or measure is administered. 2. denoting insulin for injection that begins to act within an hour of administration and remains effective for four to six hours, in the case of regular insulin, or five to eight hours, when crystalline zinc insulin is used.

short-acting insulin, an aqueous preparation of the antidiabetic principle of beef pancreas or pork pancreas that begins to act within an hour of injection and reaches a peak of action in two to four hours. The duration of action of regular insulin is four to six hours and of crystalline zinc insulin five to eight hours. Also called **rapid-acting insulin.** See also **insulin.** Compare **intermediate-acting insulin, long-acting insulin.**

shortage area, a geographic area, county as a census tract, or designated by the federal government as being undersupplied with certain kinds of health-care services, hence possibly eligible for aid under certain federal programs, including the National Health Service Corps or the Rural Clinics Assistance Act.

short arm cast, an orthopedic cast applied to immobilize the hand or the wrist. The short arm cast incorporates the hand below the wrist; it is used in treating fractures, for postoperative positioning, and for correction or maintenance of correction of deformities of the hand and the wrist. Compare **long arm cast.**

shorting, the fraudulent practice of dispensing a quantity of drug less than that called for in the prescription and of charging for the quantity specified in the prescription. See also **kiting.**

short leg cast, an orthopedic cast used for immobilizing fractures in the lower extremities from the toes to the knee. The short leg cast is also used in severe sprains and torn soft tissue of the ankle, for postoperative positioning and immobilization of the foot and the ankle, and for correction or maintenance of correction of a deformity of the foot or the ankle. Compare **long leg cast.**

short leg cast with walker, an orthopedic cast applied to immobilize the lower extremities from the toes to the knee while allowing the patient to walk by incorporating a rubber walker on the bottom of the cast. The short leg cast with walker is used when weight-bearing ambulation is desired during the period immobilization is achieved with a short leg cast.

short sight. See **myopia.**

short-term memory, memory of recent events.

shotgun therapy, *Informal.* any treatment that has a wide range of effect and which, therefore, can be expected to correct the abnormal condition even though the particular cause is unknown. Shotgun therapy may cause more than an acceptable rate of side effects and is rarely desirable or necessary.

shoulder blade. See **scapula.**

shoulder joint, the ball-and-socket articulation of the humerus with the scapula. The joint includes eight bursae and five ligaments, including the glenoidal labrum which deepens the articular cavity and protects the edges of articulating bones. Also called **humeral articulation.**

shoulder spica cast, an orthopedic cast applied to immobilize the trunk of the body to the hips, the wrist, and the hand. It incorporates a diagonal shoulder support between the hip and arm portions. The shoulder spica cast is used in the treatment of shoulder dislocations and injuries or in the positioning and immobilization of the shoulder following surgery.

show. See **vaginal bleeding.**

shreds, glossy filaments of mucus in the urine, indicating inflammation in the urinary tract. Also called **mucous shreds.**

shunt, 1. to redirect the flow of a body fluid from one cavity or vessel to another. 2. a tube or device implanted in the body to redirect a body fluid from one cavity or vessel to another.
(See next page for illustration)

Shy-Drager syndrome (shai'drei'gər), a rare, progressive neurologic disorder of young and middle-aged adults. It is characterized by orthostatic hypotension, bladder and bowel incontinence, atrophy of the iris, anhidrosis, tremor, rigidity, incoordination, ataxia, and muscle wasting. Treatment includes drug therapy to control motor symptoms and to maintain an adequate blood pressure. Antigravity stockings may prevent pooling of blood in the lower extremities. See also **orthostatic hypotension.**

Si, symbol for **silicon.**

SIADH, abbreviation for **syndrome of inappropriate antidiuretic hormone secretion.**

SCRIBNER SHUNT

sial-. See **sialo-.**

-sialia, a combining form meaning '(condition of the) saliva': *asialia, oligosialia, polsialia.*

sialo-, a combining form meaning 'of or related to saliva or to the salivary glands': *sialoaerophagy, sialoangitis, sialostenosis.* Also **sial-.**

sialogogue, anything that stimulates the secretion of saliva.

sialography (sai'əlog'rəfi), a technique in radiology in which a salivary gland is filmed after an opaque substance is injected into its duct. — **sialogram** (saiæl'əgræm), *n.*, **sialographic** (sai'ələgræf'ık), *adj.*

sialolith (saiæl'əlıfh), a calculus formed in a salivary gland or duct.

Siamese twins, conjoined, equally developed twin fetuses that were produced from the same ovum. The severity of the condition ranges from superficial fusion, as of the umbilical vessels, to that in which the heads or complete torsos are united and several internal organs are shared. With modern surgical techniques, most Siamese twins can be successfully separated. See also **conjoined twins.**

Siberian tick typhus, a mild, acute febrile illness seen in north, central, and east Asia, caused by *Rickettsia siberica,* transmitted by ticks, and characterized by a diffuse maculopapular rash, headache, conjunctival inflammation, and a small ulcer or eschar at the site of the tick bite. Treatment with chloramphenicol or tetracycline is associated with an excellent prognosis. Also called **North Asian tick typhus.** See also **rickettsia, typhus.**

sibilant rale, an abnormal whistling sound that may emanate from the lungs of an individual with a respiratory disorder or disease. It is caused by the passage of air through a lumen narrowed by the accumulation of mucus or other viscid fluid.

Siblin, a trade name for a bulk laxative containing psyllium seed.

sibling, 1. Also called *Informal.* **sib.** one of two or more children who have both parents in common; a brother or sister. The number, age differences, sex, and birth order of siblings can greatly affect the childhood environment and relationships within a family. Sibling rivalry and jealousy are common in first-born children, especially when there is a two- to four-year difference in age. In general, sibling relationships help to teach the child important social patterns and moral values, as competitiveness, loyalty, and sharing. 2. of or pertaining to a brother or sister.

sibship, 1. the state of being related by blood. 2. a group of people descended from a common ancestor who are used as a basis for genetic studies. 3. brothers and sisters considered as a group.

sicc-, a combining form meaning 'dry': *siccative, siccolabile, siccostabile.*

sickle cell, an abnormal, crescent-shaped red blood cell containing hemoglobin S, an abnormal form of hemoglobin characteristic of sickle cell anemia.

sickle cell anemia, a severe, chronic, incurable, anemic condition that occurs in people homozygous for hemoglobin S (Hb S). The abnormal hemoglobin results in distortion and fragility of the erythrocytes. Sickle cell anemia is characterized by crises of joint pain, thrombosis, and fever and by chronic anemia, with splenomegaly, lethargy, and weakness.

SICKLE CELL INHERITANCE PATTERN

sickle cell crisis, an acute, episodic condition that occurs in children with sickle cell anemia. The crisis may be vaso-occlusive, resulting from the aggregation of misshapen erythrocytes, or anemic, resulting from bone marrow aplasia, increased hemolysis, folate deficiency, or splenic sequestration of erythrocytes. See also **sickle cell anemia.**

■ OBSERVATIONS: Painful vaso-occlusive crisis is the most common of the sickle cell crises. It is usually preceded by an upper respiratory or gastrointestinal infection without an exacerbation of anemia. The clumps of sickled erythrocytes obstruct blood vessels, resulting in occlusion, ischemia, and infarction of adjacent tissue. Characteristic of this kind of crisis are leukocytosis, acute abdominal pain from visceral hypoxia, painful swelling of the soft tissue of the hands and feet (hand-foot syndrome), and migratory, recurrent, or constant joint pain, often so severe that movement of the joint is limited. Persistent headache, dizziness, convulsions, visual or auditory disturbances, facial nerve palsies, coughing, shortness of breath, and tachypnea may occur if the central nervous system or lungs are affected. Other problems associated with vaso-occlusion include priapism, hematuria, and retinopathy. Anemic crisis is characterized by a dramatic, rapid drop in hemoglobin levels resulting from various causes. Aplastic crisis resulting in severe anemia occurs as red blood cell production is diminished by acute viral, bacterial, or fungal infection. Megaloblastic anemia (another form of anemic crisis) results from folic acid deficiency during periods of accelerated erythropoiesis. Severe anemia between crises is not common unless there is a generalized state of malnutrition. Hyperhemolytic crisis, characterized by anemia, jaundice, and reticulocytosis, results from glucose-6-phosphate dehydrogenase deficiency or in reaction to multiple transfusions. Acute sequestration crisis, which occurs in young children aged six months to five years, results when large quantities of blood suddenly accumulate in the spleen, causing massive splenic enlargement, severe anemia, shock, and, ultimately, death. Susceptibility to infection is a common problem of young children with sickle cell anemia and may be greatly increased during periods of crisis. Systemic infection and septicemia from *Pneumococcus* or *Haemophilus influenzae* are not uncommon and may be rapidly fatal. In older children, local infection, especially osteomyelitis, rather than generalized septicemia is frequently a complicating factor.

■ INTERVENTION: Therapy consists of immediate transfusion of packed red cells in the acute anemic crisis and alleviation of severe abdominal and joint pain with analgesics or narcotics as needed in vaso-occlusive crisis. Short-term oxygen therapy, hydration by oral or intravenous means, electrolyte replacement to counteract metabolic acidosis resulting from hypoxia, and antibiotics to treat any existing infection may be necessary. Pneumococcal and meningococcal vaccine is recommended for children between the ages of two and five years because they are highly susceptible to infection. Partial exchange transfusions are often mandatory in life-threatening crises, as when sickling occurs in the vessels of the brain or lungs, and may be used as a preventive technique, although multiple transfusions increase the risk of hepatitis, hemosiderosis, and transfusion reactions. Oral anticoagulants have been used to relieve the pain of vaso-occlusion, but these increase the risk of bleeding. Priapism, a painful condition frequently seen in vaso-occlusive crisis, may be treated by aspirating the corpora cavernosa. In children with recurrent splenic sequestration, splenectomy may be a life-saving procedure. The process is not routinely recommended because surgery increases the risk of acidosis and hypoxia from anesthesia, and, in time, the spleen usually atrophies through progressive fibrotic changes. Infarction of tissue in any organ is a potential hazard in sickle cell crisis, and special management and treatment are warranted by the specific site of damage. Typical complications include uremia (requiring renal transplantation or hemodialysis), chronic functional pulmonary impairment, aseptic necrosis of the hip, and microvascular occlusion that may lead to venous thrombosis.

■ NURSING CONSIDERATIONS: The primary concern of the nurse during a crisis is to initiate procedures that reduce sickling. Foremost is prevention of tissue deoxygenation and resulting hypoxia by maintaining bed rest to minimize energy expenditure and oxygen utilization, although some exercise is necessary to promote circulation. Hydration and electrolyte balance are essential. A complete record of fluid intake and output is maintained, and adequate therapy is calculated accordingly. Serum sodium is monitored closely to avoid hyponatremia. Oxygen is given in severe anoxia, although prolonged administration depresses bone marrow activity and thus aggravates anemia. Management of pain in vaso-occlusion is often difficult and may require experimentation with various drugs and schedules before adequate relief is achieved. The application of warmth is often soothing; cold is contraindicated, as it enhances vasoconstriction and sickling. The nurse constantly monitors the child's condition for splenomegaly, infection, evidence of shock or cerebrovascular accident, hypervolemia, transfusion reaction, or increasing anemia. An important aspect of nursing care is the continued emotional support for parents whose child has a chronic illness that is potentially fatal.

sickle cell thalassemia, a heterozygous blood disorder in which the genes for sickle cell and for thalassemia are both inherited. A mild form and a severe form may be identified, depending on the degree of suppression of beta-chain synthesis by the thalassemia gene. In the mild form synthesis is only partially suppressed, and the red cell may contain from 25 per cent to 35 per cent normal hemoglobin A along with a somewhat greater concentration of hemoglobin S. The clinical course is relatively mild. When beta-chain synthesis is completely suppressed, as in the severe form, only hemoglobin S appears in the red cells, and the clinical course is generally as severe, as in homozygous sickle cell anemia. See also **hemoglobinopathy, hemoglobin variant.**

sickle cell trait, the heterozygous form of sickle cell anemia, characterized by the presence of both hemoglobin S and hemoglobin A in the red blood cells. It is of little clinical significance. Anemia and the other signs of sickle cell anemia do not occur. People who have the trait are informed and counseled regarding the possibility of having an infant with sickle cell disease if both parents have the trait. See **hemoglobin S.**

sick role, a pattern of behavior in which a person adopts the symptoms of a physical or mental disorder in order to be cared for, sympathized with, and protected from the demands and stresses of life.

sidero-, a combining form meaning 'of or pertaining to iron': *siderocyte, siderofibrous, sideropenic.*

sideroblastic anemia (sɪd'əroublæs'tɪk), any one of a heterogenous group of chronic hematologic disorders characterized by normocytic or slightly macrocytic anemia, hypochromic and normochromic red blood cells, and decreased erythropoiesis and hemoglobin synthesis. The red blood cells contain a perinuclear ring of iron-stained granules. The condition may be acquired or hereditary, primary or secondary to another condition or situation. The etiology of the disease is not understood. Treatment may include extract of liver, pyridoxine, folic acid, and blood transfusion. Compare **iron-deficiency anemia, siderosis.**

sideropenic dysphagia (sɪd'əroupi'nɪk). See **Plummer-Vinson syndrome.**

siderosis (sɪd'ərou'sɪs), **1.** a variety of pneumoconiosis caused by the inhalation of iron dust or particles. **2.** the introduction of color in any tissue owing to the presence of excess iron. **3.** an increase in the amounts of iron in the blood. See also **hemochromatosis, hemosiderosis.**

Sidonna, a trade name for a gastrointestinal fixed-combination drug containing anticholinergics (atropine sulfate, scopolamine hydrobromide, and hyoscyamine sulfate) and a sedative (butabarbital sodium).

SIDS, abbreviation for **sudden infant death syndrome.**

sigh. See **periodic deep inspiration.**

sight. See **vision.**

Sigma Theta Tau (sɪg'mə fhei'tə tau'), a national honor society for nurses.

sigmoid (sɪg'mɔid), **1.** of or pertaining to an S shape. **2.** the sigmoid colon.

sigmoid colon, the portion of the colon that extends from the end of the descending colon in the pelvis to the juncture of the rectum.

sigmoidectomy (sɪg'mɔidek'təmi), excision of the sigmoid flexure of the colon, most commonly performed to remove a malignant tumor. A large percentage of cancers of the lower bowel occur in the sigmoid colon.

sigmoid flexure (flek'ʃhər). See **sigmoid colon.**

sigmoid mesocolon (mez'oukou'lən), a fold of peritoneum that connects the sigmoid colon with the pelvic wall, forming a curved line of attachment, the apex of the curve located at the division of the left common iliac artery. The fold is continuous with the iliac mesocolon and ends in the median plane over the rectum at the level of the third sacral vertebra. Between the two layers of the fold are the sigmoid and the superior rectal vessels. Compare **mesentery proper, transverse mesocolon.**

sigmoidoscope (sɪgmɔi'dəskoup'), an instrument used to examine the lumen of the sigmoid colon. It consists of a tube and a light, allowing direct visualization of the mucous membrane lining the colon. Compare **proctoscope.**

sign, an objective finding as perceived by an examiner, as a fever, a rash, the whisper heard over the chest in pleural effusion, or the light band of hair seen in children following recovery from kwashiorkor. Many signs accompany symptoms, as erythema and a maculopapular rash are often seen when a patient complains of pruritus. Compare **symptom.**

signal symptom. See **symptom.**

significance, **1.** (in research) the statistical probability that a given finding is very unlikely to have occurred by chance alone. The conventional standard for attributing significance is a finding that occurs fewer than 5 times in 100 by chance alone ($p < .05$). **2.** the importance of a study in developing a practice or theory, as in nursing practice.

silent mutation, (in molecular genetics) an alteration in a sequence of nucleotides that does not result in an amino acid change.

silicone, any organic silicon polymer compound used in medicine, as an adhesive, a lubricant, or a substitute for rubber, especially in prosthetic devices.

silicon (Si), a nonmetallic element, second to oxygen as the most abundant of the elements. Its atomic number is 14; its atomic weight is 14. It occurs in nature as silicon dioxide and in silicates. The silicates are used as detergents, corrosion inhibitors, adhesives, and sealants. Elemental silicon is used in metallurgy and in transistors and other electronic components. About 60 per cent of the rocks in the earth's crust contain silicon, and silica dusts are associated with many mining operations. Protracted inhalation of silica dusts can cause silicosis, which increases the susceptibility to other pulmonary diseases.

silicosis (sɪl'ɪkou'sɪs), a lung disorder caused by continued, long-term inhalation of the dust of an inorganic compound, silicon dioxide, which is found in sands, quartzes, flints, and in many other stones. Silicosis is characterized by the development of nodular fibrosis in the lungs. In advanced cases, severe dyspnea may develop. The incidence of silicosis is highest among industrial workers exposed to silica powder in manufacturing processes, in those who work with ceramics, sand, or stone, and in those who mine silica. Also called **grinder's disease, quartz silicosis.** See also **chronic obstructive pulmonary disease, inorganic dust.**

silk suture, a braided, fine, black suture material, usually used to close incisions, wounds, and cuts in the skin. It is not absorbed by the body and is removed after approximately seven days. Compare **chromic suture.**

silo filler's disease, a rare, acute, respiratory condition seen in agricultural workers who have inhaled nitrogen oxide as they work with fermented fodder in closed, poorly ventilated spaces like silos. Characteristically, symptoms of respiratory distress and pulmonary edema occur several hours after exposure. Observation in the hospital and respiratory assistance are often required. The condition is rarely fatal.

Silvadene, a trade name for an antibacterial (sulfadiazine silver).

silver (Ag), a whitish, precious metal occurring mainly as a sulfide. Its atomic number is 47; its atomic weight is 107.88. It is quite soft and is usually alloyed with small amounts of copper to increase its durability. Silver dissolves readily in nitric acid and is used extensively to produce silver halides used in photographic emulsions. It is frequently associated in small amounts with the ores of zinc, copper, and lead and is used extensively as a component of amalgams of dental fillings and many medications, especially antiseptics and astringents. Some antiseptics containing silver are mild silver protein and strong silver protein, preparations which render silver colloidal in the presence of protein. Mild silver protein contains not less than 19 and not more than 23 per cent silver. Strong silver protein contains not less than 7.5 and not more than 8.5 per cent silver. Both preparations are used externally as antiseptics but do not have irritating properties. Silver nitrate is also used externally as an antiseptic and astringent, especially in the prevention of ophthalmia neonatorium. Silver picrate, the ionizable salt of silver, is used in the treatment of trichomoniasis and in the treatment of moniliasis of the vagina.

Silver dwarf, a person who has Silver's syndrome, a congenital disorder in which short stature is associated with lateral asymmetry, various anomalies of the head, face, and skeleton, and precocious puberty.

silver-fork fracture. See **Colles' fracture.**

silver nitrate, a topical anti-infective.
■ INDICATIONS: It is prescribed for the prevention of gonococcal ophthalmia in newborns and for use on wet dressings.
■ CONTRAINDICATION: Known sensitivity to this drug prohibits its use.
■ ADVERSE EFFECTS: Among the more serious adverse reactions are severe local inflammation, burns, and argyria.

silver salts poisoning, a toxic condition caused by the ingestion of silver nitrate, characterized by discoloration of the lips, vomiting, abdominal pain, dizziness, and convulsions. Treatment includes gastric lavage with salt water, followed by demulcents and fluid therapy. Anticonvulsant and antihypotensive therapy may be necessary.

silver sulfadiazine, a topical antimicrobial.
■ INDICATIONS: It is prescribed to prevent or treat infection in second- and third-degree burns.
■ CONTRAINDICATIONS: Known hypersensitivity to this drug, to silver, or to sulfonamides prohibits its use. It is not given in the last weeks of pregnancy or to newborn or premature infants.
■ ADVERSE EFFECTS: Among the most serious adverse reactions are rashes.

simethicone, an antiflatulent.
■ INDICATION: It is prescribed to decrease excess gas in the gastrointestinal tract.
■ CONTRAINDICATIONS: There are no known contraindications.
■ ADVERSE EFFECTS: There are no known adverse reactions.

simian crease, a single crease across the palm from the fusion of proximal and distal palmar creases; seen in congenital disorders, as Down's syndrome. Also called **simian line.**

simian line. See **simian crease.**

simian virus 40, a vacuolating virus isolated from the kidney tissue of Rhesus monkeys.

simil-, a combining form meaning 'like': *Similac, similimum.*

Similac preparations, a trade name for a group of commercial modified milk products that are prepared especially for infant feeding. They are made from a nonfat base of cow's milk supplemented with such substances as lactose, coconut and soy oils, mono- and disaccharides, and fortified with vitamins and minerals. The ratio of the various nutrients is altered in the different preparations in order to accommodate infants with particular nutritional requirements, as iron or one of the other minerals, or nutritional problems, as nephrogenic diabetes insipidus. The formulas are packaged in both powder and liquid form.

Simmonds' disease. See **postpubertal panhypopituitarism.**

simple angioma, a tumor consisting of a network of small vessels or distended capillaries surrounded by connective tissue.

simple fission. See **binary fission.**

simple fracture, an uncomplicated, closed fracture in which the bone does not break the skin. Compare **compound fracture.**

simple mastectomy, a surgical procedure in which a breast is completely removed and the underlying muscles and adjacent lymph nodes are left intact. The procedure may be performed to remove small malignant neoplasms of the breast, or it may be done as a palliative measure to remove an ulcerated carcinoma in advanced breast cancer. Postoperatively, the process of recovery from a simple mastectomy is less uncomfortable and faster than from a radical or modified radical mastectomy, but nursing care is similar. Compare **modified radical mastectomy, radical mastectomy.**

simple phobia, an anxiety disorder characterized by a persistent, irrational fear of specific things, such as animals, dirt, light, or darkness. Some kinds of simple phobias are **algophobia, gynephobia, mysophobia, nyctophobia, photophobia, zoophobia.** Compare **social phobia.** See also **phobia.**

simple protein, a protein that yields amino acids as the only or chief product upon hydrolysis. The class includes albumins, globulins, glutelins, alcohol-soluble proteins, albuminoids, histones, and protamines. See **complex protein.**

simple schizophrenia, a slow, insidiously progressive form of schizophrenia characterized by apathy, withdrawal, lack of initiative, gradual depletion of emotional reactions, and an impoverishment in human relationships. See also **schizotypal personality disorder.**

simple tubular gland, one of the many multicellular glands with only one tube-shaped duct, as various glands within the epithelium of the intestine.

simple vulvectomy. See **vulvectomy.**

Simpson forceps. See **obstetric forceps.**

Sims's position, a position in which the patient lies on the left side with the right knee and thigh drawn upward toward the chest.

sin-, a combining form meaning 'hollow, cavity': *sinography, sinus, sinusotomy.*

sinap-, a combining form meaning 'of or related to mustard': *sinapine, sinapiscopy, sinapism.*

Sinemet, a trade name for a central-nervous-system fixed-combination drug containing decarboxylase inhibitor (carbidopa) and an antiparkinsonian (levodopa).

Sinequan, a trade name for a tricyclic antidepressant (doxepin hydrochloride).

sinew (sın′yu), the tendon of a muscle, as the thick, flattened tendon attached to the short head of the biceps brachii. See also **tendon.**

singer's nodule. See **vocal cord nodule.**

single-blind study, an experiment in which either the subject or the person collecting data does not know whether the subject is in the control group or the experimental group. See also **double-blind study.**

single footling breech. See **footling breech.**

single monster, a fetus with a single body and head but severely malformed or duplicated parts or organs.

singultus (sıŋgəl′təs). See **hiccup.**

sinistrality. See **left-handedness.**

sinistro-, a combining form meaning 'left, or related to the left side': *sinistrocardia, sinistrophobia, sinistrotorsion.*

sinoatrial (SA) block (sai′nouei′triəl), a conduction disturbance in the heart during which an impulse formed within the S-A node is blocked from depolarizing the atrial myocardium. The condition is indicated on the electrocardiogram by the absence of some P waves. Causes include excessive vagal stimulation, acute infections, and atherosclerosis. S-A block may also be an adverse reaction to quinidine or digitalis. Treatment for symptomatic S-A block includes the use of atropine, isoproterenol, and, if these are not effective, stimulation and regulation of the heart with an electronic impulse generated by a pacemaker.

sinoatrial (SA) node, a cluster of hundreds of cells located in the right atrial wall of the heart, near the opening of the superior vena cava. It comprises a knot of modified heart muscle that generates impulses which travel swiftly throughout the muscle fibers of both atria, causing them to contract. Specialized pacemaker cells in the node have an intrinsic rhythm that is independent of any stimulation by nerve impulses from the brain and the spinal cord. Slender fusiform cells comprising the sinoatrial node are largely filled with sarcoplasm but contain a few striated fibrillae. The cells are irregularly grouped together and, at the edge of the node, merge with the atrial musculature. The sinoatrial node will normally "fire" at a rhythmic rate of 70 to 75 beats per minute. If the node fails to generate an impulse, pacemaker function will shift to another excitable component of the cardiac conduction system, as the atrioventricular node or the Purkinje fibers. Certain hormones and various autonomic impulses can affect the sinoatrial node and cause it to 'fire' faster, as during strenuous physical activity. During a lifetime of 70 years the node generates about two billion impulses. Surgical implantation of an artificial pacemaker is a common procedure for individuals suffering from a defective sinoatrial node, and more than 150,000 persons are leading active lives with permanently implanted devices. Also called **Keith-Flack node, pacemaker.** Compare **atrioventricular node, Purkinje network.**

sinus bradycardia. See **bradycardia.**

sinusitis (sai′nəsai′tıs), an inflammation of one or more paranasal sinuses. It may be a complication of an upper respiratory infection, dental infection, allergy, a change in atmosphere, as in air travel or underwater swimming, or a structural defect of the nose. With swelling of nasal mucous membranes the openings from sinuses to the nose may be obstructed, resulting in an accumulation of sinus secretions, causing pressure, pain, headache, fever, and local tenderness. Complications include cavernous sinus thrombosis and spread of infection to bone, brain, or meninges. Treatment includes steam inhalations, nasal decongestants, analgesics, and, if infection is present, antibiotics. Surgery to improve drainage may be performed in the treatment of chronic sinusitis.

sinus venosus defect. See **atrial septal defect.**

sippy diet, a severely restricted dietary regimen for peptic ulcer patients. It consists of hourly servings of milk and cream for several days, with the gradual addition of eggs, refined cereals, puréed vegetables, crackers, and other simple foods as tolerated until the regular bland diet is reached. Since the diet restricts all fresh vegetables and fruits, supplementary iron and vitamins are indicated to prevent deficiency states. See also **bland diet.**

sireniform fetus (saɪren'ɪfɔrm). See **sirenomelus.**

sirenomelia (saɪ'rənəmi'liə), a congenital anomaly in which there is complete fusion of the lower extremities and no feet. Also called **apodial symmelia.**

sirenomelus (saɪ'rənom'ɪləs), an infant who has sirenomelia. Also called **sireniform fetus, sympus apus.**

siriasis (sɪraɪ'əsɪs), sunstroke. See also **heat hyperpyrexia.**

-sis, a combining form meaning an 'action, process, or result of': *centesis, genesis, stasis.*

Sister Kenny's treatment, poliomyelitis therapy in which the patient's limbs and back are wrapped in warm, moist woolen cloths and, after the pain subsides, the patient is taught to exercise affected muscles, especially by swimming.

-site, a combining form meaning an 'organism living inside another form from which it derives sustenance': *celiosite, hemosite, histosite.*

site visit, a visit made by designated officials to evaluate or to gather information about a department or institution. A site visit is a step in the accreditation of an institution and in the funding of many major projects.

-sitia, a combining form meaning '(condition of) appetite for food': *apositia, asitia, eusitia.*

sito-, a combining form meaning 'of or pertaining to food': *sitomania, sitophobia, sitotherapy.*

sitosterol (saɪtos'tərɔl), a mixture of sterols derived from plants, used for treating hyperbetalipoproteinemia and hypercholesterolemia, that are unresponsive to dietary measures. Its use is controversial, for a dispersing action in the mixture tends to cause loose bowel movements and may lead to diarrhea or interfere with the absorption of concomitantly administered medications. Use in pregnancy is not recommended.

situational anxiety, a state of apprehension, discomfort, and anxiety precipitated by the experience of new or changed situations or events. Situational anxiety is not abnormal and requires no treatment; it usually disappears as the person adjusts to the new experiences. See also **anxiety, anxiety neurosis.**

situational crisis, (in psychiatry) a crisis that arises suddenly in response to an external event or a conflict concerning a specific circumstance. The symptoms are transient and the episode is usually brief.

situational depression, (in psychiatry) an episode of emotional and psychological depression that occurs in response to a specific set of external conditions or circumstances.

situational psychosis, (in psychiatry) a psychotic episode that results from a specific set of external circumstances.

situational therapy, (in psychiatry) a kind of psychotherapy in which the milieu is part of the treatment program. See also **milieu therapy.**

situation relating, (in nursing research) a study design used to explain or predict phenomena in nursing practice in which a relationship is thought to exist among certain practices or characteristics of the population being studied.

situation therapy. See **milieu therapy.**

situs (saɪ'təs), the normal position or location of an organ or part of the body.

sitz bath (sɪts, zɪts), a bath in which only the hips and buttocks are immersed in water or saline solution. The procedure is used for patients who have had rectal or perineal surgery. Also called **hip bath.**

sixth disease. See **roseola infantum.**

sixth nerve. See **abducent nerve.**

Sjögren-Larsson syndrome (shou'grenlar'sən), a congenital condition, inherited as an autosomal recessive trait, characterized by ichthyosis, mental deficiency, and spastic paralysis.

SK-65 Compound, a trade name for a fixed-combination drug containing analgesics (propoxyphene hydrochloride, aspirin, and phenacetin) and a stimulant (caffeine).

SK-Ampicillin, a trade name for an antibacterial (ampicillin).

skato-. See **scato-.**

SK-Bamate, a trade name for a sedative (meprobamate).

Skelaxin, a trade name for a skeletal muscle relaxant (metaxalone).

skeletal enchondromatosis. See **enchondromatosis.**

skeletal fixation, any method of holding together the fragments of a fractured bone by the attaching of wires, screws, plates, or nails. See also **external pin fixation.**

skeletal muscle. See **striated muscle.**

skeletal traction, one of the two basic kinds of traction used in orthopedics for the treatment of fractured bones and the correction of orthopedic abnormalities. Skeletal traction is applied to the affected structure by a metal pin or wire inserted in the tissue of the structure and attached to traction ropes. Skeletal traction is often used when continuous traction is desired to properly immobilize, position, and align a fractured bone during the healing process. Infection of the pin tract is one of the complications that may develop with skeletal traction, and careful scrutiny of pin sites is an important precaution. Some common signs of infection of the pin tracts are erythema, drainage, noxious odor, pin slippage, temperature elevation, and pain. Superficial infection of pin tracts is often treated with antibiotic therapy. Deeper infections usually require pin removal and antibiotic therapy. Compare **skin traction.**

skeleton, the supporting framework for the body, comprising 206 bones which protect delicate structures, provide attachments for muscles, allow body movement, serve as major reservoirs of blood, and produce red blood cells. The skeleton is divided into the axial skeleton which has 74 bones, the appendicular skeleton with 126 bones, and the six auditory ossicles. The skeleton is derived from the mesoderm which grows from the primitive streak as skeletal cells multiply, change, and migrate into various regions and form the membranous skeleton. Most of the membranous skeleton changes to cartilaginous skeleton in which ossification centers spread to form the bony skeleton. The four types of bones comprising the skeleton are the long bones, including the humerus, the ulna, the femur, the tibia, the fibula, and the phalanges of the fingers and the toes; the short bones, including the carpals and the tarsals; the flat bones, including the frontal bone and the parietal bone of the cranium, the ribs, and the shoulder bones; and the irregular bones, including the vertebrae, the bones of the sacrum, the bones of the coccyx, and certain bones of the skull, as the sphenoid, the ethmoid, and the mandible. The skeleton changes throughout life as bone formation and bone destruction proceed concurrently. During childhood and adolescence, bone formation proceeds faster than bone destruction. Between the ages of 35 and 40 bone destruction proceeds faster than bone formation. In advanced age bone destruction increases, bones become thin and brittle, vertebrae somewhat collapse, and height decreases. See also **bone.** – **skeletal,** *adj.*

Skene's duct (skinz). See **paraurethral duct.**

Skene's glands, the largest of the glands that open into the urethra of women. They contain ducts that open just within the urethral orifice.

SK-Estrogens, a trade name for esterified estrogens.

skew, a deviation from a line or symmetrical pattern, as data in a research study that do not follow the expected statistical curve of distribution owing to the unwitting introduction of another variable.

skia-, scia-, a combining form meaning 'of or related to shadows, especially of internal structures as produced by roentgen rays': *skiabaryt, skiagenol, skiagraph.*

skilled nursing facility (SNF), an institution or part of an institution that meets criteria for accreditation established by the sections of the Social Security Act that determine the basis for Medicaid and Medicare reimbursement for skilled nursing care, including rehabilitation and various medical and nursing procedures. Written policies and protocols are formulated with appropriate professional consultation. It is required by law that these policies include a designation of which level of care-giver is responsible for implementation of each policy, that the care of every patient be under the supervision of a physician, that a physician be available on an emergency basis, that records be maintained regarding the condition and care of every patient, that nursing service be available 24 hours a day, and that at least one full-time registered nurse be employed. Other criteria stipulate that the facility have appropriate facilities for storing and dispensing drugs and biologicals, that it maintain a utilization review plan, that all licensing requirements of the state in which it is located be met, and that an overall budget be maintained.

Skillern's fracture (skɪl'ərnz), an open fracture of the distal radius associated with a greenstick fracture of the distal ulna.

skill play, a form of play in which a child persistently repeats an action or activity until it has been mastered, as throwing or catching a ball.

skimmed milk, milk from which the fat has been removed. Most of the vitamin A is removed with the cream, although all other nutrients remain. It is available as fluid skimmed milk, fortified skimmed milk, nonfat dry milk, and buttermilk. Also called **nonfat milk.**

skimming, a practice, sometimes employed by health programs that receive their income on a prepaid or capitation basis, of seeking to enroll only relatively healthy individuals as a means of increasing profits by decreasing costs. See also **skimping.**

skimping, a practice, sometimes employed by health programs that receive their income on a prepaid or capitation basis, of delaying or denying services to enrolled members of the program as a means of increasing profits by decreasing costs.

skin, the tough, supple cutaneous membrane that covers the entire surface of the body. It is the largest organ of the body and in different people varies in area from 1.6 to 1.9 square meters. It weighs an average of two kilograms and serves as a waterproof covering that also protects the body against parasites, bacteria, and viruses. This versatile membrane also serves as the outer sensory network of the body, lubricates the exterior of the body with secretions, and helps to control body temperature. The main layers of the skin are the epidermis, and the thicker underlying dermis. A tough, scaly layer of dead cells on the surface of the skin constantly flakes away and is replaced by new epidermal cells which fill with keratin as they migrate to the surface. The dermis is elastic and durable and contains a complex network of nerve endings, sweat glands, hair follicles, lymphatic vessels, and blood vessels. Just below the dermis are fat cells that store energy and help provide the substance and the shape of the human form. All the hairs of the body grow from the dermis; the only parts of the body without hair are the palms of the hands and the soles of the feet. The color of the skin varies according to the amount of melanin in the epidermis. Genetic differences determine the amount of melanin in different persons, accounting for different skin colors among different races. The ultraviolet rays of the sun stimulate the production of melanin, which absorbs the rays and simultaneously tans the skin. Modified skin continues into various parts of the body as mucous membrane, as in the lining of the vagina, the bladder, the lungs, the intestines, the nose, and the mouth. Mucous membrane lacks the heavily keratinized layer of the outside skin. It secretes the mucus that lubricates and protects associated structures. The skin helps to cool the body when the temperature rises by radiating the heat of increased blood flow in expanded blood vessels and by providing a surface for the evaporation of sweat. When the temperature drops, the blood vessels constrict and the production of sweat diminishes. Also called **cutaneous membrane, integument.**

skin cancer, a cutaneous neoplasm caused by ionizing radiation, certain genetic defects, or chemical carcinogens, including arsenicals, petroleum, tar products, and fumes from some molten metals, or by overexposure to the sun. Skin cancers, the most common and most curable malignancies, are also the most frequent secondary lesions in patients with cancer in other sites. Risk factors are a fair complexion, xeroderma pigmentosa, vitiligo, senile and seborrheic keratitis, Bowen's disease, radiation dermatitis, and hereditary basal cell nevus syndrome. The most common skin cancers are basal cell carcinomas and squamous cell carcinomas. Tumors of the sebaceous glands or sweat glands occur infrequently and are adenocarcinomas. Basal cell carcinomas, typically raised, hard, reddish lesions with a pearly surface, do not metastasize in contrast to scaly, slightly elevated squamous cell tumors that may become exophytic, friable growths with extensive ulceration and a nonhealing scab. A definitive diagnosis may be established by incisional biopsy or by excisional biposy, which may be the only treatment required for small lesions. Surgery is usually indicated if the lesion is large, if bone or cartilage is invaded, or if lymph nodes are involved. Radiotherapy may be preferable for some smaller facial lesions and is commonly recommended for the treatment of skin tumors without distinct margins, but, because of the possiblity of late carcinogenesis, surgery is favored for the treatment of younger patients. Topical zinc chloride may be used in treating fairly common recurrent skin cancers; topical 5-fluorouracil is recommended for refractory premalignant actinic keratosis and for superficial basal cell carcinomas. An immunotherapeutic method is based on the induction of delayed hypersensitivity and consists of painting the lesions with a cream containing dinitrochlorobenzene (DNCB) and triethylene-immuno-benzoquinone (TEIB). Despite the curability of skin cancer it causes many deaths because people fail to obtain treatment. Lesions caused by actinic rays are easily prevented by applying a sun screen containing para-aminobenzoic acid (PABA).

skinfold calipers, an instrument used to measure the breadth of a fold of skin, usually on the posterior aspect of the upper arm or over the lower ribs of the chest.

skin graft, a portion of skin implanted to cover areas where skin has been lost through burns, injury, or by surgical removal of diseased tissue. To prevent tissue rejection, the graft is taken from the patient's own body or from the body of an identical twin. Skin from another person can be used as a temporary cover for large burned areas to decrease fluid loss. The area from which the graft is taken is called the donor site, that on which it is placed is called the recipient site. Various techniques are used including pinch, split-thickness, full-thickness, pedicle, and mesh grafts. In pinch grafting, one-quarter-inch pieces of skin are placed as small islands on the donor site which they will grow to cover. These will grow even in areas of poor blood supply and are resistant to infection. The split-thickness graft consists of sheets of superficial and some deep layers of skin. Grafts of up to four inches wide and ten to twelve inches long are removed from a flat surface—abdomen, thigh, or back—with an instrument called a dermatone. The grafts are sutured into place; compression dressings may be applied for firm contact, or the area may be left exposed to the air. A split-thickness graft cannot be used for weight-bearing parts of the body or to cover those subject to friction, as the hand or foot. A full-thickness graft contains all of the layers of skin and is more durable and effective for weight-bearing and friction-prone areas. A pedicle graft is one in which a portion remains attached to the donor site while the remainder is transferred to the recipient site. Its own blood supply remains intact, and it is not detached until the new blood supply has fully developed. This type is often used on the face, neck, or hand. A mesh graft is composed of multiple slices of new skin. A successful new graft of any type is well established in about 72 hours and can be expected to survive unless a severe infection or trauma occurs. The procedure may be done under local anesthesia. Preoperatively, both the donor and the recipient site must be free of infection and the recipient site must have a good blood supply. Postoperatively, stretching or motion of the recipient site is prevented. Strict sterile technique is used for handling dressings, and antibiotics may be given prophylactically to prevent infection. Good nutrition with a high protein, high caloric diet is essential. The nurse may roll the surface of the graft regularly with a sterile applicator to express accumulated fluid to the edge of the graft, allowing better adhesion.

skin integrity, impairment of: actual, a nursing diagnosis accepted by the Fourth National Conference on the Classification of Nursing Diagnoses. The etiology of the condition may be environmental (external) or somatic (internal). Environmental factors that may affect the development of impaired skin integrity include heat, cold, or chemical substances; mechanical factors, as a shearing force or pressure, restraint, or laceration; radiation; physical immobilization; and humidity. Somatic factors that may result in impairment of integrity of the skin include drugs, obesity or emaciation, malnutrition, metabolic disturbance, circulatory disturbance, altered sensation or pigmentation, developmental factors, immunologic deficit, or change in the turgor of the skin. The defining characteristics of the problem are disruption of the surface of the skin, destruction of cell layers of the skin, and invasion of structures of the body through the skin. See also **nursing diagnosis.**

skin integrity, impairment of: potential, a nursing diagnosis accepted by the Fourth National Conference on the Classification of Nursing Diagnoses. The defining characteristics of the problem are the environmental (external) or somatic (internal) risk factors that may contribute to the etiology of the breakdown of the integument. Among the environmental factors are hypothermia or hyperthermia; presence of an injurious chemical substance; shearing force or pressure, restraint, or laceration; radiation; physical immobilization; presence on the skin of excretions or secretions; and an abnormally high humidity. Somatic factors include reaction to some medications; obesity or emaciation; an abnormal metabolic state; alteration in circulation, sensory function, or pigmentation; bony prominences; adverse developmental factors; decrease in normal skin turgor; and psychogenic or immunologic abnormalities. See also **nursing diagnosis.**

Skinner box, a boxlike laboratory apparatus used in operant conditioning in animals, usually containing a lever or other device that when pressed produces reinforcement by either giving a reward, as food or an escape outlet, or avoiding a punishment, as an electric shock. Also called **standard environmental chamber.** See also **operant conditioning.**

skin prep, a procedure for cleansing the skin with an antiseptic before surgery or venipuncture. Skin preps are performed to kill bacteria and pathologic organisms and to reduce the risk of infection. Various skin prep devices are available for this procedure. Such devices are commonly constructed of plastic, filled with a specific antiseptic, and equipped with an applicator. The antiseptic is applied by rubbing the device in a circular motion over the skin. Some of the most common antiseptics contained in skin prep devices are iodine, povidone-iodine, and ethyl alcohol. Each antiseptic has associated advantages and disadvantages. The iodine skin prep kills bacteria, fungi, viruses, protozoa, and yeasts and is an inexpensive and reliable device. The disadvantages of iodine, in addition to its discoloring of the skin, are that it may burn or chap the skin and may cause an allergic reaction. Povidone-iodine, which consists of water-soluble complexes of iodine and organic compounds, is less irritating than iodine tinctures or solutions and does not stain the skin as much as iodine. However, povidine-iodine is less effective than regular iodine solutions, may be absorbed through the skin during prolonged use, and may cause an allergic reaction. Ethyl alcohol, which is not effective against spore-forming organisms, viruses, and tubercle bacilli, is composed of alcohol and ethanol; it is effective as a fat solvent and a germicidal when used in concentrations of 70 to 80 per cent and may be used as a substitute skin prep antiseptic when the patient is allergic to iodine. Some disadvantages of ethyl alcohol are that it evaporates quickly, is explosively flammable, and dries the skin excessively. Most skin prep devices are prepackaged and are disposable items for one-time use. To prep the skin with such a device before a venipuncture, the device is moved in a circular motion with the applicator rubbing the skin at the intended venipuncture site. The venipuncture site is swabbed with the antiseptic for about one minute. The antiseptic is spread over an area about two inches in diameter with the venipuncture site at the center.

skin tag. See **cutaneous papilloma.**

skin test, a test to determine the reaction of the body to a substance by observing the results of injecting the substance intradermally or of applying it topically to the skin. Skin tests are used to detect allergens, to determine immunity, and to diagnose disease. Kinds of skin tests include **patch test, Schick test, tuberculin test.**

skin traction, one of the two basic types of traction used in orthopedics for the treatment of fractured bones and the correction of orthopedic abnormalities. Skin traction applies pull to an affected body structure by straps attached to the skin surrounding the structure. Kinds of skin traction are **adhesive skin traction, nonadhesive skin traction.** Compare **skeletal traction.**

sklero-. See **sclero-.**

SK-Penicillin VK, a trade name for an antibacterial (penicillin V potassium).

SK-Pramine, a trade name for a tricyclic antidepressant (imipramine hydrochloride).

SK-Tetracycline, a trade name for an antibiotic (tetracycline).

SK-Tetracycline Hydrochloride, a trade name for an antibiotic (tetracycline hydrochloride).

skull, the bony structure of the head, consisting of the cranium and the skeleton of the face. The cranium, which contains and protects the brain, consists of eight bones. The skeleton of the face is composed of fourteen bones.

SL, abbreviation for **soda lime.**

slander, any words spoken with malice that are untrue and prejudicial to the reputation, professional practice, commercial trade, office, or business of another person. Formerly, slander included published defamation, but at present it is limited to spoken accusation. To bring legal action in slander, the slandered person must be able to demonstrate real temporal damages—except for cases in which the defamation relates to the person's business or profession or in which the malicious words question the person's chastity or accuse the person of being a criminal or of having a loathsome disease. Compare **libel.**

SLE, abbreviation for **systemic lupus erythematosus.**

sleep, a state marked by reduced consciousness, diminished activity of the skeletal muscles, and depressed metabolism. People normally experience sleep in patterns that follow four observable, progressive stages. A device such as an encephalograph is used to record the recurrent pattern of brain waves during the stages: during Stage 1, the brain waves are of the theta type, followed in Stage 2 by the appearance of distinctive sleep spindles; during Stages 3 and 4, the theta waves are replaced by delta waves. These four stages represent three fourths of a period of typical sleep and are called collectively, **nonrapid eye movement (NREM)** sleep. The remaining time is usually occupied with **rapid eye movement (REM)** sleep, which can be detected with electrodes placed on the skin around the eyes so that tiny electrical discharges from contractions of the eye muscles are transmitted to recording equipment. The REM sleep periods, lasting from a few minutes to half an hour, alternate with the NREM periods. Dreaming occurs during REM time. Individual sleep patterns normally change throughout life as daily requirements for sleep gradually diminish from as much as 20 hours a day in infancy to as little as six hours a day in old age. Infants tend to begin a sleep period with REM sleep, whereas REM activity usually follows the four stages of NREM sleep in adults.

sleeping pill, *Informal.* **1.** a sedative taken for insomnia or for postoperative sedation. **2.** an over-the-counter pill, classified pharmaceutically as an aid to sleeping. Antihistamines, as pyrilamine maleate and doxylamine succinate depend for sedative action on side effects, which may disappear with continued use of such agents. The use of all drugs that depress the central nervous system is contraindicated for pregnant and lactating women and for patients with asthma, glaucoma, or prostatic hypertrophy.

sleeping sickness. See **African trypanosomiasis.**

sleep pattern disturbance, a nursing diagnosis accepted by the Fourth National Conference on the Classification of Nursing Diagnoses. The condition is a disruption of the hours of sleep, causing discomfort or interference with normal daily activities. The etiology of the problem may be change in bodily sensation, illness, psychological disturbance, stress, or various environmental changes. Characteristics of a sleep pattern disturbance include changes in behavior and performance, as increased irritability, restlessness, disorientation, lack of energy, and fatigue. The critical defining characteristics, at least one of which must be present in order to make the diagnosis, are difficulty in falling asleep, wakening earlier than usual, interruption of the night's sleep by periods of wakefulness, or not feeling rested after sleep. See also **nursing diagnosis.**

sleep terror disorder, a condition occurring during stages 3 or 4 of nonrapid eye movement sleep that is characterized by repeated episodes of abrupt awakening, usually with a panicky scream, accompanied by intense anxiety, confusion, agitation, disorientation, unresponsiveness, marked motor movements, and total amnesia concerning the event. The disorder is seen usually in children, is more common in boys than in girls, and is extremely variable in frequency but is more likely to occur if the individual is fatigued, under stress, or has been given a tricyclic antidepressant or neuroleptic at bedtime. Compare **nightmare.** See also **pavor nocturnus.**

sleepwalking. See **somnambulism.**

slide clamp, a device, usually constructed of plastic, employed to regulate the flow of intravenous solution. The slide clamp has a graduated opening through which the intravenous tubing passes. Pushing the tube into the narrow end of the opening constricts the tube and reduces the flow rate of the intravenous solution. Sliding the wide end of the opening over the tube increases the flow rate. Compare **roller clamp, screw clamp.**

sling, a bandage or device used to support an injured part of the body.

sling restraint, a therapeutic device, usually constructed of felt, used to assist in the immobilization of patients, especially orthopedic patients in traction. The sling is placed over the pelvis to reduce pelvic motion with lower extremity traction or over the abdominal area as countertraction with Dunlop traction. With lower extremity tractions, the sling restraint is attached to both sides of the bedspring frame. With Dunlop traction the sling restraint is attached to the opposite side of the bedspring frame. If the Dunlop traction is used in association with a Bradford frame, the sling restraint is attached under the frame. The sling restraint is rarely used with balanced suspension and is not usually used with Cotrel traction, halofemoral traction, halo-pelvic traction, or with suspension for elevation. Compare **diaper restraint, jacket restraint.**

slip-on blood pump, a plastic mesh device with an attached squeeze bulb, rubber tubing, and pressure gauge, used to help administer large amounts of blood quickly. The plastic mesh slips over the blood bag and applies pressure to the bag when the bulb is squeezed. The pressure gauge displays a danger zone, usually marked in red, and indicates pressure limits for safe blood administration. Forcing blood into the veins at excessive pressure may damage the red blood cells or may disconnect the primary intravenous line.

slipped disc. *Informal.* See **herniated intervertebral disc.**

slit lamp, an instrument used in ophthalmology for examining the conjunctiva, lens, vitreous humor, iris, and cornea. A high-intensity beam of light is projected through a narrow slit, and a cross section of the illuminated part of the eye is examined through a magnifying lens.

slit lamp microscope, a microscope for ophthalmic examination. It permits the viewer to examine the endothelium of the posterior surface of the cornea in a projected band of light that is shaped like a slit.

Slo-Phyllin, a trade name for a bronchodilator (theophylline).

slough (slǝf), **1.** to shed or cast off dead tissue cells of the endometrium, which are shed during menstruation. **2.** the tissue that has been shed.

slow-acting insulin. See **long-acting insulin.**

Slow-K, a trade name for a slow-release tablet of an electrolyte replacement (potassium chloride).

slow virus, a virus that remains dormant in the body after initial infection. Years may elapse before symptoms occur. Several degenerative diseases of the central nervous system are believed to be caused by slow viruses, including subacute sclerosing panencephalitis and kuru.

Sm, symbol for **samarium.**

SMA, a trade name for a nutritional supplement for infants.

SMA 12, SMA 24, a trade name for a system that uses a small computer to perform 12 or 24 different blood chemistry tests from a single blood sample.

smack, *Slang.* heroin.

small calorie. See **calorie.**

small cardiac vein, one of the five tributaries of the coronary sinus that drains blood from the myocardium. It runs through the coronary sulcus between the right atrium and the right ventricle and opens into the right side of the coronary sinus. It conveys blood from the back of the right atrium and the right ventricle and, in some individuals, is joined by the right marginal vein. Also called **right coronary vein.** Compare **great cardiac vein, middle cardiac vein, oblique vein of left atrium, posterior vein of left ventricle.**

small cell carcinoma. See **oat cell carcinoma.**

smallest cardiac vein, one of the tiny vessels that drain deoxygenated blood from the myocardium into the atria. A few of these vessels end in the ventricles. Also called **vein of Thebesius.** Compare **anterior cardiac vein.** See also **coronary vein.**

small-for-dates (SFD) infant. See **small-for-gestational-age infant.**

small-for-gestational-age (SGA) infant, an infant whose weight and size at birth falls below the tenth percentile of appropriate-for-gestational-age infants, whether delivered at term or earlier or later than term. Factors associated with smallness or retardation of intrauterine growth other than genetic influences include any disorder causing short stature, as dwarfism; malnutrition owing to placental insufficiency; and certain infectious agents, including cytomegalovirus, rubella virus, and *Toxoplasma gondii*. Other factors associated with the smallness of an SGA infant include cigarette smoking by the mother during pregnancy, her addiction to alcohol or heroin, and her having received methadone treatment. Asphyxia may be a significant risk for the SGA infant during labor and delivery if the condition is the result of placental insufficiency. Such an infant has a low Apgar score, becomes acidotic in labor and at birth, and is likely to develop hypoglycemia within the first hours or days of life. Given adequate nutrition and caloric intake, some SGA infants show phenomenal catch-up growth. Also called **small-for-dates infant.** Compare **large-for-gestational-age infant.** See also **dysmaturity.**

small intestine, the longest portion of the digestive tract, extending for about 7 m from the pylorus of the stomach to the iliocecal junction. It is divided into the duodenum, jejunum, and ileum. Decreasing in diameter from beginning to end, it is situated in the central and caudal part of the abdominal cavity, surrounded by large intestine. Compare **large intestine.**

small omentum. See **lesser omentum.**

smallpox, a highly contagious viral disease characterized by fever, prostation, and a vesicular, pustular rash. It is caused by one of two species of poxvirus, variola minor (alastrim) or variola major. As man is the only reservoir for the virus, worldwide vaccination with vaccinia, a related poxvirus, has been effective in eradicating smallpox. For several years no natural case of the disease has been known to occur. Also called **variola.**

smallpox vaccine, a vaccine prepared from dried smallpox virus.

■ INDICATION: It is prescribed for immunization against smallpox.

■ CONTRAINDICATIONS: Immunosuppression, eczema or other dermatologic conditions, pregnancy, or known hypersensitivity to this drug prohibits its use.

■ ADVERSE EFFECTS: Among the more serious adverse effects are secondary infection at the site of injection and hypersensitivity reactions. Encephalitis may occur.

smear, a laboratory specimen for microscopic examination prepared by spreading a thin film of tissue on a glass slide. A dye, stain, reagent, diluent, or lysing agent may be applied to the specimen, depending on the purpose of the examination.

smegma (smeg′mə), a secretion of sebaceous glands, especially the cheesy, foul-smelling secretion found under the foreskin of the penis and at the base of the labia minora near the glans clitoris.

Smith fracture, a reverse Colles' fracture of the wrist, involving volar displacement and angulation of a distal bone fragment.

Smith-Hodge pessary. See **pessary.**

Smith-Petersen nail (smɪth′pi′tərsən), a three-flanged stainless steel nail used in orthopedic surgery to anchor the fractured neck of the femur to its head. It is introduced below the prominence of the greater trochanter and passed through the fractured part into the head of the femur. See also **nail, pin.**

smoke inhalation, the inhalation of noxious fumes or irritating particulate matter that may cause severe pulmonary damage. Respiratory burns are difficult to distinguish from simple smoke inhalation. Chemical pneumonitis, asphyxiation, and physical trauma to the respiratory passages may occur.

■ OBSERVATIONS: Characteristics include irritation of the upper respiratory tract, singed nasal hairs, dyspnea, hypoxia, dusty gray sputum, rhonchi, rales, restlessness, anxiety, cough, and hoarseness. Pulmonary edema may develop up to 48 hours after exposure.

■ INTERVENTION: Respiration is assisted by means of an airway and humidified oxygen, administered as necessary. Intravenous fluids, endotracheal intubation or tracheostomy, nasogastric tube, and bronchodilators may be ordered. Arterial blood gases are monitored, and corticosteroids may be given.

■ CONSIDERATIONS: The characteristics of smoke inhalation and its treatment vary with the nature of the fumes or matter inhaled and the extent of exposure; it is therefore important to know the circumstances, nature, and period of exposure and whether the person has a history of chronic respiratory or cardiac disease. Observation for at least several hours is usual; if pulmonary edema is anticipated, observation may be required for up to 48 hours.

smooth muscle, one of two kinds of muscle, composed of elongated, spindle-shaped cells in muscles not under voluntary control, as the smooth muscle of the intestines, stomach, and other visceral organs. The heart muscle is an exception because it is a striated involuntary muscle. The nucleated cells of smooth muscle are arranged parallel to one another and to the long axis of the muscle they form. Smooth muscle fibers are shorter than striated muscle fibers, have only one nucleus per fiber, and are smooth in appearance. Biofeedback devices may help many people gain partial control of contractions of involuntary

smooth muscles. Also called **involuntary muscle, unstriated muscle.** Compare **striated muscle, cardiac muscle.**

Sn, symbol for **tin.**

S.N., abbreviation for **student nurse,** used in signing nursing notes.

SNA, 1. abbreviation for **State Nurses' Association.** 2. abbreviation for **Student Nurses' Association.**

snail, an invertebrate of the order Gastropoda, several species of which are intermediate hosts of the blood flukes that cause schistosomiasis in humans. See also **bilharziasis,** *Schistosoma.*

snakebite, a wound resulting from penetration of the flesh by the fangs of a snake. Bites by snakes known to be nonvenomous are treated as puncture wounds; those produced by an unidentified or poisonous snake require immediate attention. The person is kept still, and a partially constrictive tourniquet or an ice pack is applied to retard the absorption of the venom. Incision of the skin through the bite marks is made and suction applied to assist bleeding and in removing the toxin. An appropriate antivenin may be given that protects against the venom of most pit vipers, including the rattlesnakes, copperheads, and cottonmouths that are responsible for 98 per cent of the poisonous snakebites in the United States. Bites of pit vipers are characterized by pain, redness, and edema, followed by weakness, dizziness, profuse perspiration, nausea, vomiting, or weak pulse, subcutaneous hemorrhage, and in severe cases, shock. Treatment includes the use of analgesics and sedatives, antibiotics, and antitetanus prophylaxis to prevent infections from pathogens found in the mouths of snakes. Patients sensitive to horse serum in antivenin may require cortisone for the control of hives, urticaria, and other allergic reactions. Coral snakes rarely bite but their venom contains a neurotoxin that can cause respiratory paralysis.

snare, a device designed for holding a wire noose, used in removing small pedunculated growths. The operator tightens the wire around the peduncle, thus removing the growth.

sneeze, a sudden, forceful, involuntary expulsion of air through the nose and mouth occurring as a result of irritation to the mucous membranes of the upper respiratory tract, as by dust, pollen, or viral inflammation. Also called **sternutation.**

Snellen chart, one of several charts used in testing visual acuity. Letters, numbers, or symbols are arranged on the chart in decreasing size from top to bottom. *(See next page for illustration)*

Snellen test, a test of visual acuity using a Snellen chart. The person being tested stands twenty feet from the chart and reads as many of the symbols as possible, reading each line and proceeding downward from the top. A score is assigned in the form of a ratio, comparing the subject's performance to that of a statistically normal

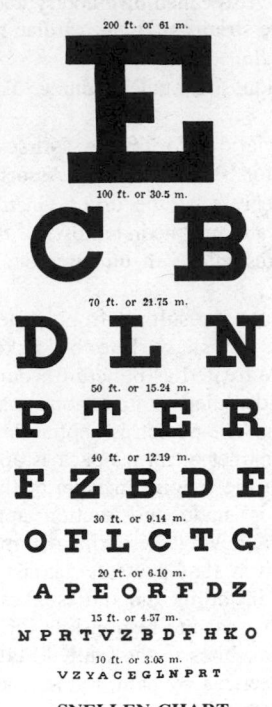

200 ft. or 61 m.

100 ft. or 30.5 m.

70 ft. or 21.75 m.

50 ft. or 15.24 m.

40 ft. or 12.19 m.

30 ft. or 9.14 m.

20 ft. or 6.10 m.

15 ft. or 4.57 m.

10 ft. or 3.05 m.

SNELLEN CHART

subject's performance. A person who can read what the average person can read at twenty feet has 20/20 vision.

SNF, abbreviation for **skilled nursing facility.**

snout reflex, an abnormal sign elicited by tapping the nose, resulting in a marked facial grimace. It usually indicates bilateral corticopontine lesions.

Snowden-Pencer scissors (snou′dınpen′sər). See **scissors.**

SNP, abbreviation for **sodium nitroprusside.**

S.N.P., abbreviation for **School Nurse Practitioner.**

snuffles, a nasal discharge in infancy characteristic of congenital syphilis. See **syphilis.**

soap, 1. a compound of fatty acids and an alkali. Soap cleanses because molecules of fat are attracted to molecules of soap in a water solution and are pulled off the dirty surface into the water. 2. a metallic salt of any salt produced from an acid. Compare **detergent.**

SOAP, (in a problem-oriented medical record) an acronym for subjective, objective, assessment, and plan, the four parts of the written account of the health problem. It is not in general use in Canada but is commonly used in the United States.

SOAP method, a method of taking and charting the patient history and physical examination in which information is classified as subjective (S), objective (O), with assessment (A), and plan (P). This SOAP statement is made for each syndrome, problem, symptom, or diagno-

sis. Charting by this is said to be 'soap-ed' and charts produced using it are called 'soap charts.' See also **problem-oriented medical record (POMR).**

socialization, 1. the process by which an individual learns to live in accordance with the expectations and standards of a group or society, acquiring the beliefs, habits, values, and accepted modes of behavior primarily through imitation, family interaction, and educational systems; the procedure by which society integrates the individual. 2. (in psychoanalysis) the process of adjustment that begins in early childhood by which the individual becomes aware of the need to accommodate inner drives to the demands of external realty. See also **internalization.**

socialized medicine, a system for the delivery of health care in which the expense of care is borne by a governmental agency supported by taxation rather than being paid for directly by the client on a fee-for-service or contract basis.

social medicine, an approach to the prevention and treatment of disease that is based on the study of human heredity, environment, social structures, and cultural values.

social motivation, an incentive or drive resulting from a sociocultural influence that initiates behavior toward a particular goal. Compare **achievement motivation, physiological motivation.**

social phobia, an anxiety disorder characterized by a compelling desire for the avoidance of and a persistent, irrational fear of situations in which the individual may be exposed to scrutiny by others, as speaking, eating, or performing in public, or using public lavatories or transportation. Some kind of social phobias are **erythrophobia, laliophobia, scopophobia, xenophobia.** Compare **simple phobia.** See also **phobia.**

social psychiatry, a branch of psychiatry based on the study of social influences on the development and course of mental diseases. In treatment, social psychiatry favors the use of milieu or other situational approaches to therapy.

social psychology, (in psychology) the study of the effects of group membership on the behavior, attitudes, and beliefs of the individual.

Social Security Act, a federal statute that provides for a national system of old age assistance, survivors' and old age insurance benefits, unemployment insurance and compensation, and other public welfare programs, including Medicare and Medicaid.

Society for Advancement in Nursing (SAIN), a group established for advancment of the profession of nursing through higher education.

sociopath (sou′sioupæfh′). See **psychopath.**

sociopathic (sou′sioupæfh′ık). See **psychopathic.**

sociopathic personality. See **antisocial personality.**

soda, a compound of sodium, particularly sodium bicarbonate, sodium carbonate, or sodium hydroxide.

soda lime (SL), a chemical compound used to absorb exhaled carbon dioxide in an anesthesia rebreathing system.

sodium (Na), a soft, grayish metal of the alkaline metals group. Its atomic number is 11; its atomic weight is 22.99. Sodium is one of the most important elements in the body. Sodium ions are involved in acid-base balance, water balance, the transmission of nerve impulses, and the contraction of muscles. The recommended daily intake of sodium is 250-750 mg for infants six months to one year of age, 900-2,700 mg for children 11 years of age or older and 1,100-3,300 mg for adults. Sodium is an important component of more than 8 liters of secretions produced by the body every day. These secretions include saliva, gastric and intestinal secretions, bile, and pancreatic fluid. The total daily secretion of sodium into these alimentary tract fluids averages between 1,200 and 1,400 mEq. A 154-pound adult has a total body pool of 2,800 to 3,000 mEq. Sodium is also linked to chlorine, which is the most important extracellular anion in the body. Sodium is the chief electrolyte in interstitial fluid, and its interaction with potassium as the main intracellular electrolyte is critical to survival. A decrease in the sodium concentration of the interstitial fluid immediately decreases osmotic pressure, making it hypotonic to intracellular fluid osmotic pressure. The kidney is the chief regulator of sodium levels in body fluids and will excrete sodium-free urine when the body needs to conserve sodium. In high temperatures, as those associated with fever, the body loses sodium through sweat, further diluting sodium reserves with additional water drunk by the affected individual. To avoid serious complications, depleted sodium must be replaced. Sodium salts, as sodium bicarbonate, are widely used in medications. Sodium bicarbonate has an immediate and rapid antacid action on the stomach, but any excess rapidly enters the intestine so that the substance has a shorter action than other antacids. Sodium bicarbonate, which is very effective in rendering the urine alkaline, is an ingredient in many solutions used as douches, mouthwashes, and enemas. Sodium is also important in the transport of sodium and potassium ions through the cytoplasmic membrane.

sodium acid glutamate. See **sodium glutamate.**

sodium arsenite poisoning, a toxic condition caused by the ingestion of sodium arsenite, an insecticide and weed-killer. The characteristic symptoms of arsenite poisoning are similar to those of arsenic poisoning, as is the treatment.

sodium bicarbonate, an antacid, an electroylyte, a urinary alkalinizing agent.

■ INDICATIONS: It is prescribed in the treatment of acidosis, gastric acidity, peptic ulcer, and indigestion.

■ CONTRAINDICATIONS: Pyloric obstruction, renal disease, congestive heart failure, or bleeding ulcer prohibits its use.

■ ADVERSE EFFECTS: Among the more serious adverse reactions are gastric distention, acid rebound, and bicarbonate-induced alkalosis.

sodium chloride, common table salt (NaCl), used as a fluid and electrolyte replenisher, isotonic vehicle, irrigating solution, and enema.

sodium chloride and dextrose. See **dextrose and sodium chloride injection.**

sodium etidronate. See **etidronate disodium.**

sodium glutamate, a salt of glutamic acid used for the treatment of hepatic coma and the enhancement of the flavor of foods. Also called **monosodium glutamate, sodium acid glutamate.**

sodium hypochlorite solution, a 5 per cent aqueous solution of NaOCl used as a disinfectant for utensils not harmed by its bleaching action.

sodium iodide, an iodine supplement.

■ INDICATIONS: It is prescribed in the treatment of thyrotoxic crisis, neonatal thyrotoxicosis, and in the management of hyperthyroidism prior to thyroidectomy.

■ CONTRAINDICATIONS: Hyperkalemia or known hypersensitivity to this drug prohibits its use.

■ ADVERSE EFFECTS: Among the more serious adverse reactions are salivary gland swelling, metallic taste, rashes, and gastrointestinal disturbances. Acute poisoning may result in angioedema and pulmonary edema.

sodium lactate injection, an electrolyte replenisher that has been prescribed for metabolic acidosis.

sodium morrhuate. See **morrhuate sodium injection.**

sodium nitroprusside (SNP), a vasodilator.

■ INDICATIONS: It is prescribed primarily in the emergency treatment of hypertensive crises and in heart failure.

■ CONTRAINDICATIONS: Certain compensatory forms of hypertension or known hypersensitivity to the drug prohibits its use.

■ ADVERSE EFFECTS: Among the most serious adverse reactions are a rapid fall in blood pressure or symptoms of cyanide poisoning (cyanide is produced by the metabolism of nitroprusside). Muscle spasms also may occur.

sodium phosphate, a saline cathartic.

■ INDICATIONS: It is prescribed to achieve prompt, thorough evacuation of the bowel and, in lower dosage, for laxative effect.

■ CONTRAINDICATIONS: Congestive heart failure, hypovolemia, or hypersensitivity to this drug prohibits its use. Frequent administration in any dosage is not recommended.

■ ADVERSE EFFECTS: Among the more severe adverse reactions are dehydration, hypovolemia, and electrolyte imbalance.

sodium phosphate P32, an antineoplastic, antipolycythemic, radioactive agent.

■ INDICATIONS: It is prescribed for polycythemia vera and for neoplasms, including myelocytic leukemia.

■ CONTRAINDICATIONS: Polycythemia vera with leukopenia or decreased platelet count, chronic myelocytic leukemia with leukopenia or erythrocytopenia, concurrent administration of other alkalating agents, or hypersensitivity to this drug prohibits its use.

■ ADVERSE EFFECT: The most serious adverse reaction is radiation sickness.

sodium pump, a theoretical mechanism for transporting sodium ions across cell membranes against an opposing concentration gradient. Sodium is normally moved from a region of low concentration within a cell to the extracellular fluid which contains a much higher concentration. Energy for this transport system is obtained from the hydrolysis of adenosine triphosphate by special enzymes. See also **calcium pump, electrolyte balance.**

sodium-restricted diet. See **low-sodium diet.**

sodium salicylate, an analgesic, antipyretic, and antirheumatic.

■ INDICATIONS: It is prescribed to relieve pain and fever.

■ CONTRAINDICATIONS: Gastrointestinal ulceration or bleeding or known hypersensitivity to this drug or to other salicylates prohibits its use. It is not given to a newborn infant.

■ ADVERSE EFFECTS: Among the most serious adverse reactions are gastrointestinal bleeding and salicylate poisoning owing to overdose. Abdominal pain, nausea, and vomiting also may occur.

sodium stibocaptate, an investigational parasiticide for certain schistosomal infections. It is available from the Center for Disease Control. Also called **stibocaptate.**

sodium sulfate, a saline cathartic.

■ INDICATIONS: It is prescribed to achieve prompt, thorough evacuation of the bowel and, in lower dosage, for laxative effect.

■ CONTRAINDICATIONS: Congestive heart failure, hypovolemia, or hypersensitivity to this drug prohibits its use. Frequent administration, in any dosage, is not recommended.

■ ADVERSE EFFECTS: Among the more severe adverse reactions are dehydration, hypovolemia, and electrolyte imbalance.

Sodium Versenate, a trade name for a metal chelating agent (edetate disodium).

sodoku (sou′dəku). See **ratbite fever.**

sodomy, 1. unnatural sexual intercourse. 2. anal intercourse by a man with another man. 3. intercourse with an animal. 4. oral or anal intercourse or copulation between persons who are not husband and wife or con-senting adult members of the opposite sex. — **sodomite,** n., **sodomize,** v.

soft diet, a diet that is soft in texture, low in residue, easily digested, and well tolerated. It provides the essential nutrients in the form of liquids and semisolid foods, as milk, fruit juices, eggs, cheese, custards, tapioca and puddings, strained soups and vegetables, rice, ground beef and lamb, fowl, fish, mashed, boiled, or baked potatoes, wheat, corn, or rice cereals, and breads. Omitted are raw fruits and vegetables, coarse breads and cereals, rich desserts, strong spices, all fried foods, veal, pork, nuts, and raisins. It is commonly recommended for people who have gastrointestinal disturbances, acute infections, or for anyone unable to tolerate a normal diet.

soft fibroma, a fibroma which contains many cells. Also called **fibroma molle.**

soft money, *Informal.* (in a university, school, or agency) income from unstable sources, as grants or contracts.

soft palate, the structure composed of mucous membrane, muscular fibers, and mucous glands, suspended from the posterior border of the hard palate forming the roof of the mouth. When the soft palate rises, as in swallowing and in sucking, it completely separates the nasal cavity and the nasopharynx from the posterior part of the oral cavity and the oral portion of the pharynx. The posterior border of the soft palate hangs like a curtain between the mouth and the pharynx. Suspended from the posterior border is the conical, pendulous, palatine uvula. Arching laterally from the base of the uvula are the two curved, musculomembranous pillars of the fauces. Compare **hard palate.**

soft radiation, radiation of low energy and low penetrating power.

-sol, a combining form meaning a 'colloidal solution': *electrosol, nitromersol, plastisol.*

solar-, a combining form meaning 'of or pertaining to the sun': *solarium, solarization, solarize.*

solar fever. 1. See **dengue.** 2. See **sunstroke.**

solarium (souleir′iəm), a large, sunny room serving as a lounge for ambulatory patients in a hospital.

solar plexus, a dense network of nerve fibers and ganglia that surrounds the roots of the celiac and the superior mesenteric arteries at the level of the first lumbar vertebra. It is one of the great autonomic plexuses of the body in which the nerve fibers of the sympathetic system and the parasympathetic system combine. The denser part of the solar plexus lies between the suprarenal glands, on the ventral surface of the crura of the diaphragm and on the abdominal aorta. The preganglionic parasympathetic fibers reach the plexus through the anterior and the posterior vagi on the stomach. The preganglionic sympathetic fibers reach the plexus through the greater and the lesser splanchnic nerves. Secondary plexuses emerging from the solar plexus are the abdominal aortic plexus, the hepatic plexus, the inferior mesenteric plexus, the phrenic plexus, the renal plexus, the spermatic plexus, the superior gastric plexus, the splenic plexus, the superior hypogastric plexus, the superior mesenteric plexus, and the suprarenal plexus. Also called **celiac plexus.**

solar radiation, the emission and diffusion of rays from the sun. Overexposure may result in sunburn, keratosis, skin cancer, or lesions associated with photosensitivity.

Solatene, a trade name for an ultraviolet screen (beta-carotene), used in the treatment of erythropoietic protoporphyria.

soleus (sou'liəs), one of three superficial posterior muscles of the leg. It is a broad flat muscle lying just under the gastrocnemius and arising by tendinous fibers from the head of the fibula, from the popliteal line, and from the medial border of the tibia. The fibers of the soleus merge near the middle of the leg with those of the gastrocnemius to form the tendo calcaneus, which inserts into the calcaneus of the foot. The soleus is innervated by a branch of the tibialis nerve, containing fibers from the first and the second sacral nerves. The soleus plantar flexes the foot. Compare **gastrocnemius, plantaris.**

Solfoton, a trade name for an anticonvulsant and sedative-hypnotic (phenobarbital).

Solganal, a trade name for an antirheumatic (aurothioglucose).

solid, 1. a body, figure, structure, or substance that has length, breadth, and thickness; contains no cavity or hollowness; is not a liquid or a gas; and has no breaks or openings on its surface. 2. describing such a body, figure, structure, or substance.

solitary play, a form of play among a group of children within the same room or area in which each child engages in an independent activity using toys that are different from the others', concentrating solely on the particular activity, and showing no interest in joining in or interfering with the play of others. Compare **cooperative play.** See also **associative play, parallel play.**

-soluble, a combining form meaning 'able to be dissolved': *acetosoluble, hydrosoluble, liposoluble.*

Solu-Cortef, a trade name for a glucocorticoid (hydrocortisone sodium succinate).

Solu-Medrol, a trade name for a glucocorticoid (methylprednisolone sodium succinate).

solute (sol'yut, sou'lut), a substance dissolved in a solution.

solution, a mixture of two or more substances dissolved in another substance. The molecules of each of the substances disperse homogenously and do not change chemically. A solution may be a gas, a liquid, or a solid. Compare **colloid, suspension.** See also **solute, solvent.**

-solve, a combining form meaning 'to loosen': *dissolve, resolve.*

solvent, any liquid in which another substance can be dissolved. Informally, the term is used to refer to organic liquids like benzene, carbon tetrachloride, and other volatile petroleum distillates that when inhaled can cause intoxication as well as damage to mucous membranes of the nose and throat and the tissues of the kidney, liver, and brain. Repeated, prolonged exposure can result in addiction, brain damage, blindness, and other serious consequences, some of them fatal. See also **benzene poisoning, carbon tetrachloride, glue sniffing, petroleum distillate poisoning.**

soma (sou'mə), *pl.* **somata, somas.** 1. the body as distinguished from the mind or psyche. 2. the body, excluding germ cells. 3. the body of a cell. — **somatic, somal** *adj.*

Soma, a trade name for a skeletal muscle relaxant (carisoprodol).

soma-. See **somato-.**

-soma, a combining form meaning a 'body or portion of a body': *hystersoma, microsoma, prosoma.*

-somatia, a combining form meaning '(condition of the) body, especially concerning size': *diplosomatia, macrosomatia, microsomatia.*

somatic (soumæt'ık), pertaining to the body. Compare **psychic.** See also **psychosomatic.** — **soma,** *n.*

-somatic, 1. a combining form meaning the 'cause of effects on the body': *exsomatic, neurosomatic, psychosomatic.* 2. a combining form meaning 'concerning a type of human body': *eurysomatic, leptosomatic.*

somatic cavity. See **coelom.**

somatic cell, any of the cells of body tissue that have the diploid number of chromosomes as distinguished from germ cells, which contain the haploid number. Compare **germ cell.**

somatic chromosome, any chromosome in a diploid or somatic cell, as contrasted to those in a haploid or gametic cell; an autosome.

somatic delusion, a false notion or belief concerning body image or body function. See also **delusion.**

somatist (sou'mətıst), a psychotherapist or psychiatrist who believes that every neurosis and psychosis has an organic cause.

somatization disorder, a disorder characterized by recurrent, multiple, physical complaints and symptoms for which there is no organic cause. The condition typically occurs in adolescence or in the early adult years and is rarely seen in men. The symptoms vary according to the individual and the underlying emotional conflict. Some common symptoms are gastrointestinal dysfunction, paralysis, temporary blindness, cardiopulmonary distress, painful or irregular menstruation, sexual indifference, and pain during intercourse. Hypochondriasis may develop if the condition is untreated. Also called **Briquet's syndrome.**

somato-, soma-, a combining form meaning 'of or pertaining to the body': *somatoceptor, somatogenic, somatopleural.*

somatoform disorder, any of a group of neurotic disorders, characterized by symptoms suggesting physical illness or disease, for which there are no demonstrable organic causes or physiological dysfunctions. The symptoms are usually the physical manifestations of some unresolved intrapsychic factor or conflict. Kinds of somatoform disorders are **conversion disorder, hypochondriasis, psychogenic pain disorder, somatization disorder.**

somatogenesis (sou'mætəjen'ɪsɪs), **1.** (in embryology) the development of the body from the germ plasm. **2.** the development of a physical disease or of symptoms from an organic pathophysiologic cause. Compare **psychogenesis.** — **somatogenic, somatogenetic,** *adj.*

somatoliberin. See **growth hormone releasing factor.**

somatomegaly (sou'mætoumeg'əli), a condition in which the body is abnormally large owing to an excessive secretion of somatotropin or an inadequate secretion of somatostatin.

somatoplasm, the nonreproductive protoplasmic material of the body cells as distinguished from the reproductive material of the germ cells. Compare **germ plasm.**

somatopleure (soumæt'əplur), the tissue layer that forms the body wall of the early developing embryo. Consisting of an outer layer of ectoderm lined with somatic mesoderm, it continues as the amnion and chorion external to the embryo. Compare **splanchnopleure.** — **somatopleural,** *adj.*

somatosensory evoked potential (SEP), evoked potential elicited by repeated stimulation of the pain and touch systems. It is the least reliable of the evoked potentials currently being studied as monitors of neurologic function during surgery.

somatosplanchnic (soumæt'ousplæŋk'nɪk), of or pertaining to the trunk of the body and the visceral organs.

somatostatin (sou'mætoustæt'ɪn), a hormone produced in the hypothalamus that inhibits the factor that stimulates release of somatotropin from the anterior pituitary gland. It also inhibits the release of certain hormones, including thyrotropin, adrenocorticotropic hormone, glucagon, insulin, and cholecystokinin, and of some enzymes, including pepsin, renin, secretin, and gastrin. Also called **growth hormone-release-inhibiting hormone.**

somatotropic hormone (sou'mətətrop'ɪk). See **growth hormone.**

somatotropin (sou'mətətrou'pɪn). See **growth hormone.**

-some, a combining form meaning 'a body' of a specified sort: *chromosome, microsome, sarcosome.*

-somia, a combining form meaning '(condition of) possessing body': *agenosomia, diplosomia, microsomia.*

somite, any of the paired, segmented masses of mesodermal tissue that form along the length of the neural tube during the early stage of embryonic development in vertebrates. These structures give rise to the vertebrae and differentiate into various tissues of the body, including the voluntary muscle, bones, connective tissue, and the dermal layers of the skin. The first somite to appear is in the future occipital region and the formation of new somites continues in a caudal direction until 36 to 38 have developed.

somite embryo, an embryo in any stage of development between the formation of the first and the last pairs of somites, which in humans occurs in the third and fourth weeks following fertilization of the ovum.

somn-. See **somni-.**

Somnafac, a trade name for a sedative-hypnotic (methaqualone hydrochloride).

somnambulism (somnæm'byəlɪz'əm), **1.** Also called **noctambulation, sleepwalking.** a condition occurring during stages 3 or 4 of nonrapid eye movement sleep that is characterized by complex motor activity, usually culminating in leaving the bed and walking about, with no recall of the episode on awakening. The episodes, which usually last from several minutes to half an hour or longer, are seen primarily in children, more commonly in boys than in girls, and are more likely to occur if the individual is fatigued, under stress, or has taken a sedative or hypnotic medication at bedtime. Seizure disorders, central nervous system infections, and trauma may be predisposing factors, but the condition is more commonly related to anxiety. In adults, the condition is less common and is classified as a dissociative reaction. **2.** a hypnotic state in which the person has full possession of the senses but no recollection of the episode.

somni-, somn-, a combining form meaning 'of or pertaining to sleep': *somnifacient, somniferous, somnipathy.*

-somnia, a combining form meaning '(condition of or like) sleep': *asomnia, hyposomnia, hypersomnia.*

somnolent, **1.** the condition of being sleepy or drowsy. **2.** tending to cause sleepiness. — **somnolence,** *n.*

Somnos, a trade name for a sedative-hypnotic (chloral hydrate).

Somophyllin, a trade name for a bronchodilator (aminophylline).

-somus, a combining form meaning a 'fetal monster with a body': *disomus, hemisomus, pleurosomus.*

son-, a combining form meaning 'of or pertaining to sound': *sonitus, sonometer, sonotone.*

sonogram (son'əgræm). See **ultrasonography.**

sonography (sənog'rəfi). See **ultrasonography.**

sonorous rale, a snoring sound that may be produced by the vibration of a mass of thick secretion lodged in a bronchus. This sound is associated with various lung or respiratory disorders.

soot wart. See **scrotal cancer.**

Sopor, a trade name for a sedative-hypnotic (methaqualone).

soporific (sop'ərıf'ık), **1.** of or pertaining to a substance, condition, or procedure that causes sleep. **2.** a soporific drug. See also **hypnotic, sedative.**

sorbic acid (sɔr'bık), a compound occurring naturally in berries of the mountain ash. Commercial sorbic acid derived from acetaldehyde is used in fungicides, food preservatives, lubricants, and plasticizers.

Sorbitrate, a trade name for an antianginal (isosorbide dinitrate).

sordes (sɔr'diz), *pl.* **sordes.** dirt or debris, especially the crusts consisting of food, microorganisms, and epithelial cells which accumulate on teeth and lips during a febrile illness or one in which the patient takes nothing by mouth. Sordes gastricae is undigested food and mucus in the stomach.

sore, **1.** a wound, ulcer, or lesion. **2.** tender or painful.

s.o.s., (in prescriptions) abbreviation for *si opus sit,* a Latin phrase meaning 'if necessary.'

souffle (su'fəl), a soft murmur heard through a stethoscope usually over the uterus in a pregnant woman. It is coincident with the maternal pulse and is caused by blood circulating in the large uterine arteries.

sound, an instrument used to locate the opening of a cavity or canal, to test the patency of a canal, to ascertain the depth of a cavity, or to reveal the contents of a canal or cavity. A sound is used to determine the depth of the uterus, to detect stones in the bladder, and, less commonly, to assist in correctly inserting a urinary catheter in the urethra through the urinary meatus.

South African genetic porphyria. See **variegate porphyria.**

South American blastomycosis. See **paracoccidioidomycosis.**

South American trypanosomiasis. See **Chagas' disease.**

Southey's tube (sau'ðiz), *Obsolete.* a small, very thin cannula introduced into edematous tissue to withdraw fluid, especially from the legs or feet, to relieve the edema of congestive heart failure. Also called **Southey-Leech tube.** See also **cannula, tube.**

Soyalac, a trade name for a commercial milk-substitute formula that is prepared from a soy isolate base and is lactose free for infants with galactosemia and persons with lactose intolerance. It is supplemented with other nutrients and fortified with vitamins and minerals. It is packaged in both powder and liquid form. See also **Neo-Mull-Soy, Nutramigen, Pro Sobee.**

sp. *pl.* **sp., spp.** abbreviation for **species.**

space, an actual or a potential cavity of the body, as the complemental spaces in the pleural cavity that are not occupied by lung tissue and the lymph spaces occupied by lymph.

Spalix, a trade name for a gastrointestinal fixed-combination drug containing three anticholinergics (atropine sulfate, scopolamine hydrobromide, and hyoscyamine sulfate) and a sedative-hypnotic (phenobarbital).

Spanish fly. See **cantharis.**

spano-, a combining form meaning 'scanty or scarce': *spanogyny, spanomenorrhea, spanopnea.*

sparganosis (spar'gənou'sıs), an infection with larvae of the fish tapeworm, characterized by painful subcutaneous swellings or swelling and destruction of the eye. It is acquired by ingesting larvae in contaminated water or in inadequately cooked, infected frog flesh. Treatment includes surgery and local injection of ethyl alcohol to kill the larvae.

Sparine, a trade name for a phenothiazine antipsychotic and antiemetic (promazine hydrochloride).

sparteine sulfate, an oxytocic formerly used to reduce uterine bleeding during the third stage of labor.

spasm, **1.** an involuntary muscle contraction of sudden onset, as habit spasms, hiccups, stuttering, or a tic. **2.** a convulsion or seizure. **3.** a sudden, transient constriction of a blood vessel, bronchus, esophagus, pylorus, ureter or other hollow organ. Compare **stricture.** See also **bronchospasm, pylorospasm.**

-spasm, a combining form meaning a 'convulsion' of a specified sort: *gastrospasm, neurospasm, vasospasm.*

spasmo-, a combining form meaning 'of or pertaining to spasm(s)': *spasmodermia, spasmophemia, spasmophilia.*

-spasmodic, a combining form meaning 'of, pertaining, or referring to a convulsion': *angiospasmodic, antispasmodic, postspasmodic.* Also **-spasmodical.**

spasmodic torticollis, a form of torticollis characterized by episodes of spasms of the neck muscles. The condition is often transient in nature, and examination seldom reveals a physical cause. In some cases, severe stress and muscular spasm may be the cause.

spastic, of or pertaining to spasms or other uncontrolled contractions of the skeletal muscles. See also **cerebral palsy.** — **spasticity,** *n.*

spastic aphonia, a condition in which a person is unable to speak because of spasmodic contraction of the abductor muscles of the throat.

spastic bladder, a form of neurogenic bladder caused by a lesion of the spinal cord above the voiding reflex center. It is marked by loss of bladder control and bladder sensation, incontinence, and automatic, interrupted, incomplete voiding. It is most often caused by trauma, but may be a result of tumor or multiple sclerosis. Also called **reflex bladder, automatic bladder.** Compare **flaccid bladder.**

spastic colon. See **irritable bowel syndrome.**

spastic entropion. See **entropion.** See also **ectropion.**

spastic paralysis, an abnormal condition characterized by the involuntary contraction of one or more muscles with associated loss of muscular function. Compare **flaccid paralysis.**

spastic pseudoparalysis. See **Creutzfeldt-Jakob disease.**

spatial summation. See **summation,** def. 2.

SPE, abbreviation for **sucrose polyester.**

Spearman's rho (spir'mənz rou'), (in statistics) a statistical test for correlation between two rank-ordered scales. It yields a statement of the degree of interdependence of the scores of the two scales.

special gene system, a plasmid, transposon, or other genetic fragment that is able to transfer genetic information from one cell to another.

specialing, *Informal.* **1.** (in psychiatric nursing) the constant attendance of a professional staff member upon a disturbed patient to protect the patient from harming himself or others and to observe the patient's behavior. The patient so 'specialed' is accompanied in all activities by the staff member. **2.** (in nursing) the giving of nursing care to only one person, as when acting as a private duty nurse or when caring for a patient whose needs are so great that a nurse is required at all times.

specialist, a health care professional who practices a specialty. A specialist usually has advanced clinical training and may have a postgraduate academic degree.

special sense, the sense of sight, smell, taste, or hearing.

specialty, a branch of medicine or nursing in which the professional is specially qualified to practice by having attended an advanced program of study, by having passed an examination given by an organization of the members of the specialty, or by having gained experience by extensive practice in the specialty.

species, (Sp) (spi'ŝhiz, spi'siz), the category of living things below genus in rank. A species includes individuals of the same genus who are similar in structure and chemical composition and who can interbreed. See also **genus.**

species immunity, a form of natural immunity shared by all members of a species. Compare **individual immunity, racial immunity.**

specific activity, (in nuclear medicine) **1.** the radioactivity of a radioisotope per unit mass of the element or compound, expressed in microcuries per millimol or disintegrations per second per milligram. **2.** the relative activity per unit mass, expressed as counts per minute per milligram. The specific activity of potassium in the human body is the same as that of the environment or diet, and, since potassium is associated chiefly with muscle tissue, a whole body count of ^{40}K, following administration of the radioisotope, can be used to distinguish lean body mass from total body mass.

specific gravity, the ratio of the density of a substance to the density of another substance accepted as a standard. The usual standard for liquids and solids is water. Thus, a liquid or solid with a specific gravity of four is four times as dense as water. Hydrogen is the usual standard for gases. See also **density, mass.**

specific treatment. See **treatment.**

specimen, a small sample of something, intended to show the nature of the whole, as a urine specimen.

spectinomycin hydrochloride, an antibiotic.
■ INDICATION: It is prescribed in the treatment of gonorrhea.
■ CONTRAINDICATION: Known hypersensitivity to this drug prohibits its use.
■ ADVERSE EFFECTS: Among the more serious adverse reactions are oliguria, urticaria, chills, fever, dizziness, and nausea.

spectr-, a combining form meaning 'image': *spectrograph, spectrophobia, spectrum.*

Spectra-Sorb UV 9, a trade name for an ultraviolet screen (oxybenzone).

Spectrocin, a trade name for a topical, fixed-combination drug containing antibacterials (neomycin sulfate and gramicidin).

spectrometer (spektrom'itər), an instrument for measuring wavelengths of rays of the spectrum, the deviation of refracted rays, and the angles between faces of a prism. Kinds of spectrometer are **mass spectrometer, Mössbauer spectrometer.**

spectrometry (spektrom'itri), the procedure of measuring wavelengths of light and other electromagnetic waves. See also **spectrometer.** **– spectrometric,** *adj.*

spectrophotometry (spek'troufətom'itri), the measurement of color in a solution by determining the amount of light absorbed in the ultraviolet, infrared, or visible spectrum, widely used in clinical chemistry to calculate the concentration of substances in solution. **– spectrophotometric,** *adj.*

spectrum, *pl.* **spectra. 1.** a range of phenomena or properties occurring in increasing or decreasing magnitude. Radiant or electromagnetic energy is arranged on the basis of wavelength and frequency. Electromagnetic radiation includes spectra of radio waves, infrared, visible light, ultraviolet, x rays, and gamma rays. **2.** the range of effectiveness of an antibiotic. A broad-spectrum antibiotic is effective against a wide range of microorganisms. See also **antibiotic, electromagnetic radiation, wave.**

speculum (spek'yuləm), a retractor used to separate the walls of a cavity to make examination possible, as an ear speculum, an eye speculum, or a vaginal speculum. *(See next page for illustration)*

speech audiometry. See **audiometry.**

speech dysfunction, any defect or abnormality of speech, including aphasia, alexia, stammering, stuttering, aphonia, and slurring. Speech problems may develop from any of a variety of causes, among them neurologic injury to the cerebral cortex, muscular paralysis owing to trauma, disease, or cerebrovascular accident, structural

Graves   Pederson

SPECULUMS

abnormality of the organs of speech, emotional or psychological tension, strain, or depression, hysteria, and severe mental retardation.

speech pathologist. See **speech therapist.**

speech pathology, 1. the study of abnormalities of speech or of the organs of speech. **2.** the diagnosis and treatment of abnormalities of speech as practiced by a speech pathologist or a speech therapist.

speech therapist, a person trained in speech pathology who treats people with disorders affecting normal oral communication.

speed, 1. Compare **velocity.** the rate of change of position with time. **2.** *Slang.* any stimulating drug, as amphetamine.

speed shock, a sudden adverse physiological reaction of a patient to intravenous medications or drugs that are administered too quickly. Some signs of speed shock are a flushed face, headache, a tight feeling in the chest, irregular pulse, loss of consciousness, and cardiac arrest.

sperm. 1. See **semen. 2.** See **spermatozoon.**

-sperm, a combining form meaning a 'seed': *gymnosperm, oosperm, zygosperm.*

spermatic cord, a structure extending from the deep inguinal ring in the abdomen to the testis, descending nearly vertically into the scrotum. The left spermatic cord is usually longer than the right, consequently the left testis usually hangs lower than the right. Each cord is comprised of arteries, veins, lymphatics, nerves, and the excretory duct of the testis.

spermatic duct. See **deferent duct.**

spermatic fistula, an abnormal passage communicating with a testis or a seminal duct.

spermatid, a male germ cell that arises from a spermatocyte and that becomes a mature spermatozoon in the last phase of the continual process of spermatogenesis.

spermato-, spermo-, a combining form meaning 'of or

pertaining to seed, specifically to the male generative element': *spermatoblast, spermatocyst, spermatogenesis.*

spermatocele (spərmæt'əsil, spər'mətəsil), a cystic swelling, either of the epididymis or of the rete testis, that contains spermatozoa. It lies above, behind, and separate from the testis; it is usually painless and requires no therapy.

spermatocide (spərmæt'əsaid, spər'mətəsaid), a chemical substance that kills spermatozoa by reducing their surface tension, causing the cell wall to break down by a bactericidal effect or by creating a highly acidic environment. Among many spermatocidal agents used in various contraceptive creams are lactic acid, phenylmercuric acetate, chloramine polyethylene glycol, benzethonium chloride, and certain quinine compounds. Also called **spermicide.**

spermatocyte, a male germ cell that arises from a spermatogonium. Each spermatocyte gives rise to two haploid secondary spermatocytes that become spermatids.

spermatocytogenesis (spərmæt'ousai'toujen'ısıs, spər'mətousai'toujen'ısıs). See **spermatogenesis.**

spermatogenesis (spərmæt'əjen'ısıs, spər'mətoujen'ısıs), the process of development of spermatozoa, including the first stage, called spermatogenesis, in which spermatogonia become spermatocytes that develop into spermatids, and the second stage, called spermiogenesis, in which the spermatids become spermatozoa. Also called spermiogenesis.

spermatogonium, *pl.* **spermatogonia.** a male germ cell that gives rise to a spermatocyte early in spermatogenesis.

spermatozoon (spər'mətəzou'ən, spərmæt'əzou'ən), *pl.* **spermatozoa.** a mature male germ cell that develops in the seminiferous tubules of the testes. Resembling a tadpole, it is about 50 micrometers ($\frac{1}{500}$ inch) long, and has a head with a nucleus, a neck, and a tail that provides propulsion. Developed in vast numbers after puberty, it is the generative component of the semen, impregnating the ovum and resulting in fertilization. See **spermatogenesis.**

-spermia, a combining form meaning '(condition of) possessing or producing seed': *aspermia, asthenospermia, necrospermia.* Also **-spermy.**

spermicidal, destructive to spermatozoa.

spermicide (spər'məsaid). See **spermatocide.**

spermiogenesis (spər'mioujen'ısıs). See **spermatogenesis.**

spermo-. See **spermato-.**

-spermy. See **-spermia.**

sphacel-, a combining form meaning 'of or pertaining to gangrene': *sphaceloderma, sphacelotoxin, sphacelus.*

sphaero-. See **sphero-.**

spheno-, a combining form meaning 'of or pertaining to the sphenoid bone, or to a wedge': *sphenocephaly, sphenoidotomy, sphenotemporal.*

sphenoidal fissure, a cleft between the great and small wings of the sphenoid bone.

sphenoidal sinus, one of a pair of cavities in the sphenoid bone of the skull, lined with mucous membrane that is continuous with that of the nasal cavity. Each sinus is approximately spheroidal, with a diameter of about 2 cm but its shape, and size vary from person to person. A large sphenoidal sinus may extend into the roots of the pterygoid processes, into the great wings, or into the occipital bone. The cavities are very small at birth and develop largely after puberty. Compare **ethmoidal air cells, frontal sinus, maxillary sinus.**

sphenoid bone, the bone at the base of the skull, anterior to the temporal bones and the basilar part of the occipital bone. It resembles a bat with its wings extended.

sphenomandibular ligament (sfi′noumændib′yələr), one of a pair of flat, thin ligaments comprising part of the temporomandibular joint between the mandible of the jaw and the temporal bone of the skull. It is attached to the spine of the sphenoid bone and becomes broader as it descends to the lingula of the mandibular foramen.

-sphere, 1. a combining form meaning a 'spherical body': *chondriosphere, onconosphere, somosphere.* **2.** a combining form meaning a 'realm that supports life': *biosphere, vivosphere, zoosphere.* Also **-sphaera, -sphaere.**

sphero-, sphaero-, a combining form meaning 'round, or pertaining to a sphere': *spherocyte, spherolith, spherometer.*

spherocyte (sfir′əsait), an abnormal spherical red cell that contains more than the normal amount of hemoglobin. It can be seen and identified under the microscope on the stained specimen of blood. Its presence in large numbers causes increased osmotic fragility of the red blood cells. — **spherocytic,** *adj.*

spherocytic anemia, a hematologic disorder characterized by hemolytic anemia owing to the presence of red blood cells that are spherical rather than round and biconcave. The cells are fragile and tend to hemolyze in the oxygen-poor peripheral circulatory system. Episodic crises of abdominal pain, fever, jaundice, and splenomegaly occur. As repeated transfusions are often needed to treat the anemia, siderosis may develop. Splenectomy may then be necessary. The condition is inherited as an autosomal dominant trait.

spherocytosis (sfir′ousaitou′sis), the abnormal presence of spherocytes in the blood. Compare **elliptocytosis.**

spheroidea (sfiroi′diə). See **ball-and-socket joint.**

sphincter (sfiŋk′tər), a circular band of muscle fibers that constricts a passage or closes a natural opening in the body, as the hepatic sphincter in the muscular coat of the hepatic veins near their union with the superior vena cava, and the external anal sphincter, which closes the anus.

sphincter pupillae, a muscle that expands the iris, nar-rowing the diameter of the pupil of the eye. It is composed of circular fibers arranged in a narrow band about one mm wide, surrounding the margin of the pupil toward the posterior surface of the iris. The circular fibers near the free margin of the iris are closely packed; those that are near the periphery of the band are more separated and form incomplete circles. The fibers of the sphincter pupillae blend with the fibers of the dilatator pupillae near the margin of the pupil and are innervated by a motor root of the ciliary ganglion from the oculomotor nerve. Compare **dilatator pupillae.**

sphingomyelin lipidosis, (sfiŋ′goumai′əlin), any of a group of diseases characterized by an abnormality in the ability of the body to store sphingolipids. Kinds of sphingomyelin lipidosis include **Gaucher's disease, Niemann-Pick disease, Tay-Sachs disease.** See also **Fabry's disease.**

sphygm-, sphygmo-, a combining form meaning 'pulse': *sphygmodynamometer, sphygmoid, sphygmomanometer.*

-sphygmia, a combining form meaning '(condition of the) pulse': *anisosphygmia, hemisphygmia, sychnosphygmia.*

sphygmo-, a combining form meaning 'of or related to the pulse': *sphygmobologram, sphygmoscope, sphygmosignal.*

sphygmogram (sfig′məgræm), a tracing produced by a sphygmograph. A curve occurs on the tracing with each atrial pulsation. An upward, primary elevation is followed by a sudden drop to a point slightly above the baseline. The curve then gradually descends to the baseline in small decrements of amplitude. Sphygmographic abnormalities of rate, rhythm, and form may be diagnostically useful in an assessment of cardiovascular function.

sphygmograph (sfig′məgræf), an instrument that records the force of the atrial pulse on a tracing called a sphygmogram. — **sphyamographic,** *adj.*

sphygmomanometer (sfig′moumənom′itər), a device for measuring the arterial blood pressure, consisting of a cuff for the arm or leg that has an air bladder connected to a tube with a bulb for pumping air into the bladder, and having a gauge for indicating the amount of air pressure being exerted over the artery. See also **manometer.**

spica bandage (spai′kə), a figure-of-eight bandage in which each turn generally overlaps the next to form a succession of V-like designs. It may be used to give support, to apply pressure, or to hold a dressing in place on the chest, limbs, thighs, or pelvis.

spica cast, an orthopedic cast applied to immobilize part or all of the trunk of the body and part or all of one or more extremities. It is used to treat various fractures, as of the hip and the femur, and in correcting or maintaining the correction of hip deformities. Kinds of spica casts are **bilateral long leg spica cast, one-and-a-half spica cast, shoulder spica cast, unilateral long leg spica cast.**

spicule (spɪk′yul), a sharp body with a needlelike point.

spider angioma, a form of telangiectasis characterized by a central, elevated, red dot the size of a pinhead from which small blood vessels radiate. Spider angiomas are often associated with elevated estrogen levels as occur in pregnancy or when the liver is diseased and unable to detoxify estrogens. Also called **spider nevus.** See also **telangiectasia.**

spider antivenin. See **black widow spider antivenin.**

spider bite, a puncture wound produced by the bite of a spider, an arachnid related to ticks and mites. Fewer than 100 of some 30,000 species of spiders are known to bite. Two of them, the black widow spider and the brown spider, found in the United States, are poisonous.

spider nevus. See **spider angioma.**

spina (spaɪ′nə), *pl.* **spinae.** a spine or a thornlike projection, as the bony projection on the anterior border of the ilium, forming the anterior end of the iliac crest.

spina bifida (spaɪ′nə bɪf′ədə, baɪ′fədə), congenital neural tube defect characterized by a developmental anomaly in the posterior vertebral arch. Spina bifida is relatively common, occurring approximately 10 to 20 times per 1,000 births. It may occur with only a small deformed lamina separated by a midline gap, or it may be associated with the complete absence of laminae surrounding a large area. In cases where the separation is wide enough, contents of the spinal canal protrude posteriorly, and a myelomeningocele is evident. This more serious deformity is associated with gross deficits not normally manifested in spina bifida. Neurologic deficits do not usually accompany the anomalies involving only bony deformity. Direct signs and symptoms are rarely noted in spina bifida, which is frequently diagnosed accidentally during radiographic examinations required for other reasons. Spina bifida that does not involve herniation of the meninges or the contents of the spinal canal rarely requires treatment. Also called **spinal dysrhaphis.**

spina bifida anterior, incomplete closure along the anterior surface of the vertebral column. The defect is often associated with developmental anomalies of the abdominal and thoracic viscera.

spina bifida cystica, a developmental defect of the central nervous system in which a hernial cyst containing meninges (meningocele), spinal cord (myelocele), or both (myelomeningocele) protrudes through a congenital cleft in the vertebral column. The protruding sac is encased in a layer of skin or a fine membrane that can easily rupture, causing the leakage of cerebrospinal fluid and an increased risk of meningeal infection. The severity of neurological dysfunction and associated defects depends directly on the degree of nerve involvement. The most severe type is lumbosacral myelomeningocele, which is frequently associated with hydrocephalus and the Arnold-Chiari malformation. Compare **spina bifida occulta.** See also **myelomeningocele, neural tube defect.**

spina bifida occulta, defective closure of the laminae of the vertebral column in the lumbosacral region without hernial protrusion of the spinal cord or meninges. The defect, which is quite common, occurs in about five per cent of the population and is identified externally by a skin depression or dimple, dark tufts of hair, telangiectasis, or soft, subcutaneous lipomas at the site. Since the neural tube has closed, there are usually no neurological impairments associated with the defect. However, any abnormal adhesion of the spinal cord to the area of the malformation may lead to neuromusucular disturbances, usually problems with gait and foot weakness and with the bowel and bladder sphincters. Compare **spina bifida cystica.**

spinal, **1.** of or pertaining to a spine, especially the spinal column. **2.** *Informal.* spinal anesthesia, as saddle block or caudal anesthesia.

spinal accessory nerve. See **accessory nerve.**

spinal aperture, a large opening formed by the body of a vertebra and its arch.

spinal canal, the cavity within the vertebral column.

spinal caries, decay, cavity and abscess formation in the vertebrae owing to tuberculosis. Characteristic symptoms include stiffness of the back and pain when the spine is moved or touched in the affected area. Less frequently, spinal caries may be marked by abdominal pain, local abscess formation, or paralysis. Children and young adults are more commonly affected by spinal caries than are older people. Treatment includes antituberculosis medication, drainage of pus to relieve pressure on the spinal cord, and removal of the carious portion of the bone. The affected vertebrae may be surgically immobilized to prevent curvature of the spine and to promote healing. Also called **Pott's disease, tuberculous spondylitis.**

spinal column. See **vertebral column.**

spinal cord, a long, nearly cylindrical structure lodged in the vertebral canal and extending from the foramen magnum at the base of the skull to the upper part of the lumbar region. A major component of the central nervous system, the adult cord is approximately 1 cm in diameter with an average length of 42 to 45 cm and a weight of 30 gm. The cord conducts sensory and motor impulses to and from the brain and controls many reflexes. 31 spinal nerves originate from the cord: 8 cervical, 12 thoracic, 5 lumbar, 5 sacral, and 1 coccygeal. It has an inner core of gray material consisting mainly of nerve cells and is enclosed by three protective membranes (meninges): the dura mater, arachnoid, and pia mater. The cord is an extension of the medulla oblongata of the brain and ends caudally between the 12th thoracic and third lumbar vertebrae, often at or adjacent to the disc between the first and second lumbar vertebrae. Until the third month of fetal life, the cord occupies the entire length of the vertebral canal. Thereafter, the canal lengthens faster than the cord. By the sixth fetal month, the caudal end of the cord reaches only as far as the upper sacrum. At birth it is on a level with the third lumbar vertebra. Originating in the ectoderm, like the entire nervous system, the cord develops from the caudal portion of the embryonic neural plate. Also called **chorda spinalis, medulla spinalis.**

spinal cord compression, an abnormal and often serious condition resulting from pressure on the spinal cord. The symptoms range from temporary numbness of an extremity to permanent quadriplegia, depending on the cause, severity, and location of the pressure. Causes include spinal fracture, vertebral dislocation, tumor, hemorrhage, and edema associated with contusion. See also **herniated disc, spondylolisthesis.**

spinal cord injury, any one of the traumatic disruptions of the spinal cord, often associated with extensive musculoskeletal involvement. Common spinal cord injuries are spinal fractures and dislocations, as those commonly suffered by individuals involved in car accidents, airplane crashes, or other violent impacts. Such trauma may cause varying degrees of paraplegia and quadriplegia. Injuries to spinal structures below the first thoracic vertebra may produce paraplegia. Injuries to the spine above the first thoracic vertebra may cause quadriplegia. Injuries that completely transect the spinal cord cause permanent loss of motor and sensory functions activated by neurons below the level of the lesions involved. Spinal cord injuries produce a state of spinal shock, characterized by placid paralysis, and complete loss of skin sensation at the time of the injury. Within a few weeks the muscles affected may become spastic, and the skin sensation may return to a slight degree. The motor and the sensory losses that prevail a few weeks after the injury are usually permanent. Musculoskeletal complications are associated with the neurologic involvement of spinal cord injuries, and prevention of decubitis ulcers and the treatment of any loss of bladder and bowel control are continuing concerns. Treatment of spinal cord injuries varies considerably and involves numerous approaches, as orthopedic exercises, ambulatory techniques, and special physical and psychological therapy.

spinal cord tumor, a neoplasm of the spinal cord of which more than 50 per cent are extramedullary, about 25 per cent are intramedullary, and the rest are extradural. Symptoms usually develop slowly and may progress from unilateral paresthesia and a dull ache to lancinating pain, weakness in one or both legs, abnormal deep tendon reflexes, and, in advanced cases, monoplegia, hemiplegia, or paraplegia. Function of the autonomic nervous system is sometimes disturbed, causing areas of dry, cold, bluish-pink skin or profuse sweating of the lower extremities. The diagnosis is made by x-ray and myelographic examination. About 30 per cent of spinal cord tumors are circumscribed, encapsulated meningiomas, and 25 per cent are schwannomas; these two kinds are found chiefly in the thoracic region. Some 20 per cent are gliomas, and the others consist of congenital lipomas, epidermoids, and metastatic lesions. The dura is resistant to invasion, but many extradural tumors are metastatic lesions from primary cancers in the prostate, lung, breast, thyroid, and gastrointestinal tract. Most extramedullary and nonmetastatic extradural tumors are surgically removed; intermedullary lesions are enucleated, whenever possible; and inoperable tumors are treated with radiotherapy and chemotherapy. Tumors of the spinal cord may arise at any age but appear most frequently in the third decade of life and are one fourth as common as brain neoplasms.

spinal curvature, any persistent, abnormal deviation of the vertebral column from its normal position. Kinds of spinal curvature are **kyphoscoliosis, kyphosis, lordosis, scoliosis.**

spinal dysrhaphis. See **spina bifida.**

spinal fasciculi (fəsɪk′yʊlaɪ). See **spinal tract.**

spinal fluid. See **cerebrospinal fluid.**

spinal fusion, the fixation of an unstable segment of the spine, accomplished by skeletal traction or immobilization of the patient in a body cast but most frequently by a surgical procedure. Operative ankylosis may be performed in the treatment of spinal fractures or following discectomy or laminectomy for the correction of a herniated vertebral disc. Surgical fusion involves the stabilization of a spinal section with a bone graft introduced through a posterior incision in the lumbar region; in the less frequently fused cervical region the incision may be anterior or posterior. Also called **spondylosyndesis.**

spinal headache, a headache occurring after spinal anesthesia or lumbar puncture, caused by a loss of cerebrospinal spinal fluid (CSF) from the subarachnoid space, resulting in traction of the meninges on the pressure-sensitive intracranial structures. Severe spinal headache may be accompanied by diminished aural and visual acuity. Treatment usually includes keeping the patient flat in bed to relieve the meningeal irritation, encouraging an increased fluid intake to increase the intravascular volume to increase the production and volume of cerebrospinal fluid, and administering analgesics to reduce pain. If severe headache persists, an anesthesiologist may perform an autologous blood patch procedure in which a clot of the patient's blood is formed and planted over the leaking puncture site in the dura to prevent further loss of CSF. Meningeal irritation and backache may persist for several days. The incidence of spinal headache is greatest when a large-bore needle is used for the initial anesthetis or diagnostic procedure.

spinal manipulation, the forced passive flexion, extension, and rotation of vertebral segments, carrying the elements of articulation beyond the usual range of movement to the limit of anatomic range. Spinal manipulation may be used effectively in physiotherapy for the treatment of vertebral and sacroiliac dislocations, sprains, and adhesions.

spinal nerves, the 31 pairs of nerves without special names that are connected to the spinal cord and numbered according to the level of the cord at which they emerge. There are eight cervical, twelve thoracic, five lumbar, and five sacral pairs, and one coccygeal pair. The first cervical pair of nerves emerges from the spinal cord in the space between the first cervical vertebra and the occipital bone. The rest of the cervical pairs and all the thoracic pairs emerge horizontally through the intervertebral foramen of their respective vertebrae, as the second cervical pair, which emerges through the foramina above the second cervical vertebra. The lumbar, the sacral, and the coccygeal nerve pairs descend from their points of origin at the lower end of the cord before reaching the intervertebral foramina of their respective vertebrae. Each spinal nerve attaches to the spinal cord by an anterior root and a posterior root. The posterior roots accompany a distended spinal ganglion within the vertebral foramina. Emerging from the cord, each spinal nerve divides into the anterior, the posterior and the white rami, the anterior and the posterior rami serving the voluntary nervous system, the white rami serving the autonomic nervous system. The posterior rami subdivide into lesser nerves that extend into the muscles and the skin of the posterior surface of the head, the neck, and the trunk. The anterior rami, except for those of the thoracic nerves, subdivide and pass fibers to the skeletal muscles and the skin of the extremities. Subdivisions of the anterior rami form complex plexuses, as the brachial plexus, from which smaller nerves emerge to innervate the hand and most of the arm. The brachial plexus in the shoulder region is sometimes damaged during birth and must be treated or the injured baby may develop a withered arm. A broken neck may damage the right and the left phrenic nerves which come from the third, fourth, and fifth cervical nerves. Such damage may prevent nerve impulses from reaching the phrenic nerves, which supply the diaphragm, and thus stop respiration. The sacral plexus in the pelvic cavity is comprised of certain spinal nerve fibers from the lumbar and the sacral regions and gives rise to the great sciatic nerve in the back of the thigh, often the site of painful sciatica. See also **spinal cord.**

spinal puncture. See **lumbar puncture.**

spinal tract, any one of the ascending and descending pathways for motor or sensory nerve impulses that is found in the white matter of the spinal cord. Twenty-one different tracts lie within the dorsal, the ventral, and the lateral funiculi of the white substance. Ascending tracts conduct impulses up the spinal cord to the brain; descending tracts conduct impulses down the cord from the brain. The four major ascending tracts are the lateral spinothalmic, the ventral spinothalmic, the fasciculi gracilis and cuneatus, and the spinocerebellar. The four major descending tracts are the lateral corticospinal, the ventral corticospinal, the lateral reticulospinal, and the medial reticulospinal. Touch, pressure, proprioception, temperature, and pain are sensory stimuli transmitted via the spinal tracts. Reflex and voluntary motor activity are regulated by motor nerve stimulation from the brain and brain stem to the motor neurons of the spinal cord.

spindle, 1. the fusiform figure of achromatin in the cell nucleus during the late prophase and the metaphase of mitosis. It consists of tiny fibers radiating out from the centrosomes and connecting them with one another. 2. a type of brain wave, consisting of a short series of changes in electrical potential with a frequency of 14 per second. 3. any one of the special receptor organs comprising the neurotendinous and the neuromuscular spindles distributed throughout the body. These kinds of spindles serve as special receptor organs which detect the degree of stretch in a muscle or at the junction of a muscle with its tendon and are essential in maintaining muscle tone.

spindle cell carcinoma, a rapidly growing neoplasm composed of fusiform squamous cells. It may be difficult to distinguish from a sarcoma.

spindle cell nevus. See **benign juvenile melanoma.**

spinnbarkheit (spin'barkait), the clear, slippery, elastic consistency characteristic of cervical mucus during ovulation. It has the consistency of an uncooked egg white, and it is a valuable sign of the peak fertile period in a woman's menstrual cycle. Observation of spinnbarkheit is useful in natural methods of family planning, in the clinical evaluation of infertility, and in discovering the optimum time for artificial insemination. Spinnbarkheit may be evaluated by the length to which a string of mucus can be drawn between the fingers before breaking. See also **ovulation method of family planning.**

spino-, a combining form meaning 'of or pertaining to the spine': *spinocain, spinoglenoid, spinotransversarius.*

spinocerebellar (spai'nouser'ibel'ər), of or pertaining to the spinal cord and the cerebellum.

spinocerebellar disorder, an inherited disorder characterized by a progressive degeneration of the spinal cord and cerebellum, often involving other parts of the nervous system as well. These disorders tend to occur within families and can be inherited as dominant or recessive traits. Onset is usually early, during childhood or adolescence. No effective treatment is known. Some kinds of spinocerebellar degeneration are **ataxia telangiectasia, Charcot-Marie-Tooth atrophy, Dejerine-Sottas disease, Friedreich's ataxia, olivopontocerebellar atrophy, Refsum's syndrome.**

spinofallopian tube shunt (spai'noufəlou'piən). See **ventriculofallopian tube shunt.**

spinth-, a combining form meaning 'spark': *spinthariscope, spintherometer, spintheropia.*

spir-, **1.** a combining form meaning 'a coil, or coiled': *spiradenitus, spireme, spirillum.* **2.** a combining form meaning 'of or pertaining to the breath, or to breathing': *spiracle, spirogram, spirophore.*

spiral fracture, a bone break in which the disruption of bone tissue is spiral, oblique, or transverse to the long axis of the fractured bone.

spiral organ of Corti. See **Corti's organ.**

spiral reverse bandage, a spiral bandage that is turned and folded back on itself as necessary to make it fit the contour of the body more securely.

spirillary ratbite fever (spai′rıler′i). See **ratbite fever.**

spirillum fever. See **ratbite fever.**

spirit, **1.** any volatile liquid, particularly one that has been distilled. **2.** a volatile substance dissolved in alcohol. See also **volatile.**

spiritual distress (distress of the human spirit), a nursing diagnosis accepted by the Fourth National Conference on the Classification of Nursing Diagnoses. The etiology of the condition may be separation from religious or cultural ties or a change in beliefs or value system, intense suffering, severe stress, or prolonged treatment. The defining characteristics include stated anger against the deity or questions about the meaning of the suffering being experienced. The client may joke in a macabre fashion, have nightmares, cry, act in a hostile or apathetic manner, express anger or resentment against religious figures, and cease participation in religious practices. See also **nursing diagnosis.**

spirochete (spai′rəkit′), any bacterium that is motile and spiral-shaped. Kinds of spirochetes include the organisms responsible for leptospirosis, relapsing fever, syphilis, yaws. Compare **bacillus, coccus, vibrio.** − **spirochetal,** *adj.*

spirogram (spai′rougræm), a visual record of respiratory movements made by a spirometer, used in the assessment of pulmonary function and capacity.

spirograph (spai′rəgræf), a device for recording respiratory movements. See also **spirometer.** − **spirographic,** *adj.*

spirometer (spairom′ıtər), an instrument that measures and records the volume of inhaled and exhaled air, used to assess pulmonary function. Volumetric information is recorded on a chart, called a spirogram. − **spirometric,** *adj.*

spirometry (spairom′ıtri), laboratory evaluation of the air capacity of the lungs by means of a spirometer. Compare **blood gas determination.** − **spirometric,** *adj.*

Spitz nevus. See **benign juvenile melanoma.**

SPL. See **Staphage Lysate.**

splanchn-. See **splanchno-.**

splanchnic (splæŋk′nık), of or pertaining to the internal organs; visceral.

-splanchnic, a combining form meaning 'viscera, entrails': *somaticosplanchnic, trisplanchnic, vagosplanchnic.*

splanchno-, splanchn-, a combining form meaning 'of or pertaining to a viscus, or to the splanchnic nerve': *splanchnocele, splanchnography, splanchnoptosis.*

splanchnocele, **1.** See **splanchnocoele.** **2.** hernial protrusion of any abdominal viscera.

splanchnocoele, splanchnocele (splæŋk′nousil′), a part of the embryonic body cavity, or coelom, that gives rise to the abdominal, pericardial, and pleural cavities. Also called **pleuroperitoneal cavity.**

splanchnopleure (splæŋk′nouplur′), a layer of tissue in the early developing embryo, formed by the union of endoderm and splanchnic mesoderm. It gives rise to the embryonic gut and the visceral organs and continues external to the embryo as the yolk sac and allantois. Compare **somatopleure.** − **splanchnopleural,** *adj.*

S-plasty, a technique of plastic surgery in which an S-shaped instead of a straight-line incision is made to reduce tension and improve healing in areas where the skin is loose.

spleen, a soft, highly vascular, roughly ovoid organ situated between the stomach and the diaphragm in the left hypochondriac region of the body. It is considered part of the lymphatic system, because it contains lymphatic nodules. It has a dark purple color and varies in shape in different indivuals and within the same individual at different times. The precise function of the spleen has baffled physiologists for more than 100 years, but the most recent research indicates it performs various tasks, as defense, homopoiesis, blood storage, and the destruction of red blood cells and platelets. Macrophages lining the sinuses of the spleen destroy microorganisms by phagocytosis. The spleen also produces leukocytes, monocytes, lymphocytes, and plasma cells. It produces red cells before birth and is believed to produce red cells after birth only in extreme and hemolytic anemia. If the body suffers severe hemorrhage the spleen can increase the blood volume from 350 ml to 550 ml in less than 60 seconds. In the adult the spleen is usually about 12 cm long, 7 cm wide, and 3 cm thick. Its weight increases from 17 gm or less in the first year to about 170 gm at 20 years, then slowly decreases to about 122 gm at 75 to 80 years. The variation in the weight of adult spleens is 100 to 250 gm and, in extreme cases, 50 to 400 gm. The size of the spleen increases during and after digestion and often increases during illness. It can weigh as much as 9 kg in a victim of malarial fever. The splenic nerves are derived from the celiac plexus and are mostly unmyelinated, distributing to the blood vessels of the organ and to the smooth muscle of the splenic capsule and trabeculae. Compare **thymus.** − **splenic,** *adj.*

splen-. See **spleno-.**

splenectomy, the surgical excision of the spleen.

-splenia, a combining form meaning '(condition of the spleen': *asplenia, eusplenia, microsplenia.*

splenic flexure syndrome, a recurrent pain and abdominal distention in the left upper quadrant of the abdomen owing to a pocket of gas trapped in the large intestine below the spleen, at the flexure of the transverse and descending colon. The symptoms are relieved by defecation or passing flatus.

splenic gland. See **pancreaticolienal node.**

splenic vein. See **lienal vein.**

splenius capitis, one of a pair of deep muscles of the back. Arising from the ligamentum nuchae, the seventh cervical vertebra, and the first three or four thoracic vertebrae, it inserts in the occipital bone and the mastoid process of the temporal bone. The muscle is innervated by the lateral branches of the dorsal primary divisions of the middle and the lower cervical nerves and acts to rotate, extend, and bend the head.

splenius cervicis, one of a pair of deep muscles of the back. Arising from a narrow tendinous band from the spinous processes of the third through the sixth thoracic vertebrae, it inserts into the transverse processes of the upper two or three cervical vertebrae. The muscle is innervated by the lateral branches of the dorsal primary divisions of the middle and the lower cervical nerves. The splenius cervicis acts to rotate, bend, and extend the head and neck. Also called **splenius colli.**

spleno-, splen-, a combining form meaning 'of or pertaining to the spleen': *splenocele, splenodiagnosis, splenomalacia.*

splenomedullary leukemia (spli'noumed'ələr'i). See **acute myelocytic leukemia, chronic myelocytic leukemia.**

splenomegaly (spli'noumeg'əli, splen'oumeg'əli), an abnormal enlargement of the spleen, as associated with portal hypertension, hemolytic anemia, Niemann-Pick disease, or malaria.

splenomyclogenous leukemia (spli'noumai'əloj'ənəs). See **acute myelocytic leukemia, chronic myelocytic leukemia.**

splint, 1. an orthopedic device for immobilization, restraint, or support of any part of the body. It may be rigid (of metal, plaster, or wood) or flexible (of felt or leather). 2. (in dentistry) a device for anchoring the teeth or modifying the bite. Compare **brace, cast.**

splinter fracture, a comminuted fracture with thin, sharp bone fragments.

splinter hemorrhage, linear bleeding under a finger- or toenail, resembling a splinter. It is seen after trauma and in patients with bacterial endocarditis.

split gene, (in molecular genetics) a genetic unit whose continuity is interrupted.

split personality. See **multiple personality.**

split Russell traction, an orthopedic mechanism which combines suspension and traction to immobilize, position, and align the lower extremities in the treatment of congenital hip dislocation, hip and knee contractures, and in the correction of orthopedic deformities. Split Russell traction, usually applied as adhesive or nonadhesive skin traction, employs a sling to relieve the weight of the lower extremities. The traction weights are suspended from pulley and rope systems at the foot and the head of the patient's bed; a jacket restraint is often incorporated to help immobilize the patient. Split Russell traction may be applied as a unilateral or as a bilateral mechanism. Compare **Russell traction.**

spodo-, a combining form meaning 'of or pertaining to waste materials': *spodogenous, spodophagous, spodophorous.*

-spondylic, a combining form meaning 'referring to the vertebrae': *cyclospondylic, monospondylic, tectospondylic.*

spondylitis (spon'dəlai'tis), an inflammation of any of the spinal vertebrae, usually characterized by stiffness and pain. The condition may follow traumatic injury to the spine, or it may be the result of infection or rheumatoid disease. See also **ankylosing spondylitis.**

spondylo-, a combining form meaning 'of or pertaining to a vertebra, or to the spinal column': *spondylocace, spondylodidymia, spondylolysis.*

spondylolisthesis (spon'dıloulıs(hi'sıs), the partial forward dislocation of one vertebra over the one below it, most commonly the fifth lumbar vertebra over the first sacral vertebra. See also **spinal cord compression.**

spondylosis (spon'dılou'sıs), a condition of the spine characterized by fixation or stiffness of a vertebral joint. See also **Marie-Strümpell disease, spondylitis.**

spondylosyndesis (spon'dılousın'dısıs). See **spinal fusion.**

sponge, 1. a resilient, absorbent mass used to absorb fluids, to apply medication, or to cleanse. The sponge may be the internal skeleton of a certain marine animal, or it may be manufactured from cellulose, rubber, or synthetic material. 2. *Informal.* a folded gauze square used in surgery.

sponge bath, the procedure of washing the patient with a damp washcloth or sponge, used when a full bath is not necessary or as a method of reducing body temperature.

spongio-, a combining form meaning 'like a sponge, or related to a sponge': *spongioblast, spongiopilin, spongiosis.*

spongioblastoma (spən'jioublæstou'mə), *pl.* **spongioblastomas, spongioblastomata.** a neoplasm composed of spongioblasts, embryonic epithelial cells that develop around the neural tube and transform into cells of the supporting connective tissue of nerve cells or cells of lining membranes of the ventricles and the spinal cord canal. A kind of spongioblastoma is **spongioblastoma unipolare.** Also called **glioblastoma, gliosarcoma, spongiocytoma.**

spongioblastoma multiforme. See **glioblastoma multiforme.**

spongioblastoma unipolare, a rare neoplasm composed of approximately parallel spongioblasts. It may occur near the third ventricle, in the pons and brain stem, in basal ganglia, or in the terminal filament of the spinal cord.

spongiocytoma (spən'jiousaitou'mə). See **spongioblastoma.**

spontaneous, occurring naturally and without apparent cause, as spontaneous remission.

spontaneous abortion, a termination of pregnancy prior to the twentieth week of gestation as a result of abnormalities of the conceptus or maternal environment. More than 10 per cent of pregnancies end as spontaneous abortions, almost all owing to blighted ova that have congenital defects incompatible with life. Compare **induced abortion.**

spontaneous delivery, a vaginal birth occurring without the mechanical assistance of obstetric forceps or vacuum aspirator.

spontaneous evolution, the unassisted delivery of a fetus in the transverse position See also **Denman's spontaneous evolution.**

spontaneous fracture. See **pathologic fracture.**

spontaneous generation, the theoretical origin of living organisms from inanimate matter; abiogenesis.

spontaneous labor, a labor beginning and progressing without mechanical or pharmacologic stimulation.

spor-. See **sporo-.**

sporadic, (of a number of events) occurring at scattered, intermittent, and apparently random intervals.

-sporangium, a combining form meaning an 'encasement of spores': *haplosporangium, oosporangium, sporangium.*

spore, 1. a reproductive unit of some genera of fungi or protozoa. 2. a form assumed by some bacteria that is resistant to heat, drying, and chemicals. Under proper environmental conditions the spore may revert to the actively multiplying form of the bacterium. Diseases caused by spore-forming bacteria include anthrax, botulism, gas gangrene, and tetanus.

-spore, a combining form meaning a 'reproductive element': *archespore, chlamydospore, hemispore.*

sporicide (spɔr'isaid), any agent effective in destroying spores, as compounds of chlorine and formaldehyde, and the gluteraldehydes.

sporiferous (spɔrif'ərəs), producing or bearing spores.

sporo-, spor-, a combining form meaning 'of or pertaining to a spore': *sporocyst, sporogenesis, sporogeny.*

sporoblast, any cell that gives rise to a sporozoite or spore during the sexual reproductive phase of the life cycle of a sporozoan, specifically the cells resulting from

the multiple fission of the encysted zygote of the malarial parasite *Plasmodium* from which the sporozoites develop.

sporocyst, 1. any structure containing spores or reproductive cells. 2. a saclike structure, or oocyst, secreted by the zygote of certain protozoa prior to sporozoite formation. 3. the second larval stage in the life cycle of parasitic flukes. The saclike organism develops from the miracidium, or first larval stage, in the body of a freshwater snail host and contains germinal cells that give rise to either daughter sporocysts that develop into cercariae or to rediae. See also **fluke.**

sporogenesis (spɔr'oujen'əsis), 1. the formation of spores; sporogeny. 2. reproduction by means of spores. – **sporogenic,** *adj.*

sporogenous (spɔroj'ənəs), describing an animal or plant that reproduces by spores.

sporogeny (spɔroj'əni), the formation of spores.

sporogony (spɔrog'əni), reproduction by means of spores, specifically the formation of sporozoites during the sexual stage of the life cycle of a sporozoan, primarily the malarial parasite *Plasmodium.* Fusion of the sex cells occurs in the body of the invertebrate host, the female *Anopheles* mosquito in the case of *Plasmodium,* where the encysted zygote undergoes multiple division, giving rise to the sporozoites. Compare **schizogony.**

sporont (spɔr'ont), a mature protozoan parasite in the sexual reproductive stage of its life cycle. It undergoes conjugation to form a zygote, which produces sporozoites by multiple fission. Compare **schizont.** See also **sporogony.**

sporonticide, any substance that destroys sporonts, as chloroquine and other antimalarial drugs. – **sporonticidal,** *adj.*

sporophore, that part of an organism or plant that produces spores.

sporophyte, the asexual, spore-bearing stage in plants that reproduce by alternation of generations.

sporotrichosis (spɔr'outrikou'sis), a common, chronic fungal infection caused by the species *Sporothrix schenckii,* usually characterized by skin ulcers and subcutaneous nodules along lymphatic channels. It rarely spreads to involve bones, lungs, joints, or muscles. The fungus is found in soil and decaying vegetation and usually enters the skin by accidental injury. Treatment may include amphotericin B.

Sporotrichum (spɔrot'rikəm), a genus of soil-inhabiting fungi formerly thought to cause sporotrichosis.

Sporozoa, a class of parasite in the phylum Protozoa that is characterized by the absence of any external organs of locomotion. Included in this class are the genera *Toxoplasma* and *Plasmodium.*

sporozoite, any of the cells resulting from the sexual union of spores during the life cycle of a sporozoan. It refers specifically to the elongated nucleated cells produced by the multiple fission of the zygote contained in the oocyst in the female *Anopheles* mosquito during the sexual reproductive stage of the life cycle of the malarial parasite *Plasmodium*. Upon release from the oocyst, the sporozoites migrate to the salivary glands of the mosquito where they are transmitted to man and develop within the parenchymal cells of the liver as merozoites. Also called **falciform body**. See also **malaria**, *Plasmodium*.

sport, (in genetics) **1.** an individual or organism that differs drastically from its parents or others of its type because of genetic mutation; a mutant. **2.** a genetic mutation. **3.** See **lusus naturae**.

sporulation (spor'yəlei'shən), **1.** a type of reproduction that occurs in lower plants and animals, as fungi, algae, and protozoa, and involves the formation of spores by the spontaneous division of the cell into four or more daughter cells each of which contains a portion of the original nucleus. **2.** the formation of a refractile body, or resting spore, within certain bacteria that makes the cell resistant to unfavorable environmental conditions. The cell regains its viability when the conditions become favorable. See also **spore**.

spotted fever. See **Rocky Mountain spotted fever**.

sprain, a traumatic injury to the tendons, muscles, or ligaments around a joint, characterized by pain, swelling, and discoloration of the skin over the joint. The duration and severity of the symptoms vary with the extent of damage to the supporting tissues. Treatment requires support, rest, and alternating cold and heat. Ultrasound therapy may speed recovery. X-ray pictures are often indicated to be certain that no fracture has occurred.

sprain fracture, a fracture that results from the separation of a tendon or ligament at the point of insertion, associated with the separation of a bone at the same insertion site.

spring forceps, a kind of forceps that includes a spring mechanism, used for grasping an artery to arrest or prevent hemorrhage. Also called **bulldog forceps**.

spring lancet, a lancet with a spring-triggered blade. It may be used for collecting small specimens of blood for laboratory tests. See also **lancet**.

sprinter's fracture, a fracture of the anterior superior or the anterior inferior spine of the ilium, caused by a fragment of bone being forcibly pulled by a violent muscle spasm.

sprue, a chronic disorder resulting from malabsorption of nutrients from the small intestine and characterized by a broad range of symptoms, including diarrhea, weakness, weight loss, poor appetite, pallor, muscle cramps, bone pain, ulceration of the mucous membrane lining the digestive tract, and a smooth, shiny tongue. It occurs in both tropical and nontropical forms and affects both children and adults. Also called **catarrhal dysentery**. See also **malabsorption syndrome, nontropical sprue, tropical sprue**.

SPRX, a trade name for an anorexiant (phendimetrazine tartrate).

SPSS, (in statistics) abbreviation for **Statistical Package for the Social Sciences,** a computer program often used in research in clinical nursing for the analysis of complex data from large samples.

spurious aperture of facial canal, an opening in the petrous part of the temporal bone for the greater petrosal nerve and a branch of the middle meningeal artery.

sputum (spyu'təm), material coughed up from the lungs and expectorated through the mouth. It contains mucus, cellular debris, microorganisms, and it may also contain blood or pus. The amount, color, and constituents of the sputum are important in the diagnosis of many illnesses, including tuberculosis, pneumonia, cancer of the lung, and the pneumoconiosis.

squam-, a combining form meaning 'of or pertaining to scales': *squamatization, squamocellular, squamopetrosal*.

squamous cell carcinoma, a slow-growing, malignant tumor of squamous epithelium, frequently found in the lungs and skin and occurring also in the anus, cervix, larynx, nose, bladder, and other sites. The typical skin lesion, a firm, red, horny, painless nodule, ranging from less than one to several centimeters in size, is often the result of overexposure to the sun. The neoplastic cells characteristically resemble prickle cells and form keratin pearls on the surface of lesions. Also called **epidermoid carcinoma**.

squeeze dynamometer, a dynamometer for measuring the muscular strength of the grip of the hand.

squint. See **strabismus**.

squinting eye, the abnormal eye in a person with strabismus that cannot be focused with the fixated eye. See also **strabismus**.

Sr, symbol for **strontium**.

ss, abbreviation for **steady state**.

SSKI, a trade name for an expectorant (potassium iodide).

SSSS, abbreviation for **staphylococcal scalded skin syndrome**.

S's test. See **Sulkowitch's test**.

stab form. See **band**.

-stabile, a combining form meaning 'stable, resistant to change': *coctostabile, hydrostabile, tempostabile*.

stable element, a nonradioactive element, one not subject to spontaneous nuclear degeneration. Some kinds of stable elements are calcium, iron, lead, potassium, sodium. Compare **radioactive element**. See also **element**.

staccato speech, abnormal speech in which the person pauses between words, breaking the rhythm of the phrase or sentence. The condition is sometimes observed in association with multiple sclerosis.

stadium, *pl.* **stadia.** a stage in a fever or illness, as the fastigium of a febrile illness or the prodromal stage of a viral infection.

Stadol, a trade name for an opioid analgesic (butorphanol tartrate), used as an adjunct to anesthesia.

staff, 1. the people who work toward a common goal and are employed or supervised by someone of higher rank, as the nurses in a hospital. 2. a designation by which a staff nurse is distinguished from a head nurse or other nurse. 3. (in nursing education) the nonprofessional employees of the institution, as librarians, technicians, secretaries, and clerks. 4. (in nursing service administration) the units of the organization that provide service to the 'line,' or administratively defined hierarchy, as the personnel office is 'staff' to the director of nursing and the nursing service administration.

staff development, (in nursing) a process that assists individual nurses in attaining new skills and knowledge, gaining increasing levels of competence, and growing professionally. Various resources outside the agency employing the nurse may be used. The process may include such programs as orientation, in-service education, and continuing education. Many fields outside of nursing also develop and utilize programs for staff development which are specific to their needs.

staffing pattern, (in hospital or nursing administration) the number and kinds of staff assigned to the particular units and departments of a hospital. Staffing patterns vary with the unit, department, and shift.

staff of Æsculapius, a staff carried by Æsculapius, the Greek god of medicine. It is used as the traditional symbol of the physician. A single serpent entwines the staff of Æsculapius, which is often confused with the caduceus, a staff with two serpents, symbolizing the U.S. Army Medical Corps.

-stage, a combining form meaning a '(specified) phase': *aecidiostage, multistage, uredostage.*

stages of anesthesia. See **Guedel's signs.**

stages of dying, the four emotional and behavioral stages that often occur after a person first learns of approaching death. The stages, identified and described by Elizabeth Kubler-Ross, are denial and shock, anger, bargaining, and acceptance. The stages may occur in sequence or they may recur, as the person moves forward and backward—especially between denial, anger, and bargaining. Caring for a dying person requires sensitivity to the signs of each stage. At first, shock may be accompanied by signs of panic. The person may refuse care and deny the diagnosis and prognosis. Denial serves as a defense against the shock. Anger often follows this stage. It is characterized by abusive language, refusal to perform basic self-care responsibilities, negative criticism of anyone who wants to help, and other kinds of angry behavior. The third stage, bargaining, reflects the need of the person for time to accept the situation. A common obser-

vation of this period is the patient's attempt to make a bargain, "If I could live until Christmas, . . ." Commonly, the person goes back and forth from anger to bargaining: sometimes silent, sometimes grieving, and sometimes apathetic, depressed, insomniac, and distant. Nursing care includes administering adequate pain relief, ensuring privacy and dignity, and giving sensitive, honest emotional support to both patient and family. See also **hospice.**

stain, 1. a pigment, dye, or substance used to impart color to microscopic objects or tissues in order to facilitate their examination and identification. Kinds of stains include **acid-fast stain, Gram's stain, Wright's stain.** 2. to apply pigment to a substance or tissue in order to examine it under a microscope. 3. an area of discoloration.

-stalsis, a combining form meaning a 'contraction in the alimentary canal': *antistalsis, catastalsis, retrostalsis.*

stance phase of gait, the first phase of the normal gait cycle that begins with the strike of the heel on the ground and ends with the lift of the toe at the beginning of the swing phase of gait: the brief period in which both feet are on the ground.

standard, 1. an evaluation that serves as a basis for comparison for evaluating similar phenomena or substances, as a standard for the preparation of a pharmaceutical substance, or a standard for the practice of a profession. 2. a pharmaceutical preparation or a chemical substance of known quantity, ingredients, and strength which is used to determine the constituents or the strength of another preparation. 3. of known value, strength, quality, or ingredients. —**standardize,** v., **standardization,** n.

standard death certificate, a form for a death certificate that is commonly used throughout the United States. It is the preferred form of the United States Census Bureau.

standard deviation, (in statistics) a mathematical statement of the dispersion of a set of values or scores from the mean. Each sample value is subtracted from the sample mean and squared, and the squares are summed. The square root of the summed squares gives a mathematically standardized value so that sample deviations can be compared.

standard environmental chamber. See **Skinner box.**

standard error, (in statistics) the variability in scores that can be expected if measurements are made on random samples of the same size from the same universe of population, phenomena, or observations. The standard error provides a framework within which a determination of the difference between groups may be made. It is an element used in determining statistical significance by means of a wide variety of formulas and methods.

standardized death rate, the number of deaths per 1,000 people of a specified population during one year. This rate is adjusted to avoid distortion by the age composition of the population. A standard population is used for determining this rate. Also called **adjusted death rate.**

standing orders, a written document containing rules, policies, procedures, regulations, and orders for the conduct of patient care in various stipulated clinical situations. The standing orders are usually formulated collectively by the professional members of a department in a hospital or other health care facility. Standing orders usually name the condition and prescribe the action to be taken in caring for the patient, including the dosage and route of administration for a drug or the schedule for the administration of a therapeutic procedure.

stann-, a combining form meaning 'of or pertaining to tin': *stanniferous, stanniform, stannoxyl.*

stanozolol (stɔnou′zɔlol, stənou′zəloul), an androgenic anabolic steroid.

■ INDICATIONS: It is prescribed in the treatment of aplastic anemia and osteoporosis.

■ CONTRAINDICATIONS: Cancer of the breast or prostate, nephrosis, pregnancy or known hypersensitivity to this drug prohibits its use.

■ ADVERSE EFFECTS: Among the most serious adverse reactions are various androgenic effects and allergic reactions. Gastrointestinal disturbances also may occur.

stapedectomy (stei′pıdek′təmi), removal of the stapes of the middle ear and insertion of a graft and prosthesis, performed to restore hearing in the treatment of otosclerosis. The stapes which has become fixed is replaced so that vibrations again transmit sound waves through the oval window to the fluid of the inner ear. Under local anesthesia, the stapes is removed and the opening into the inner ear is covered with a graft of body tissue. One end of a small plastic tube or piece of stainless steel wire is attached to the graft; the other end is attached to the two remaining bones of the middle ear, the malleus and the incus. Headache and dizziness are expected early in the postoperative period. The patient's hearing does not improve until the edema subsides and the packing is removed. Possible complications include infection of the outer, middle, or inner ear, displacement or rejection of the graft or the prosthesis, and leaking of perilymph around the prosthesis into the middle ear, with ringing in the ear and dizziness. Compare **incudectomy.**

stapes (stei′piz), one of the three ossicles in the middle ear, resembling a tiny stirrup. It transmits sound vibrations from the incus to the internal ear. Compare **incus, malleus.** See also **middle ear.**

Staphage Lysate (SPL), a trade name for an active immunizing agent (staphylococcal antigen phage lysed), used in staphylococcal infection.

Staphcillin, a trade name for an antibacterial (methicillin sodium).

staphyl-,-. See **staphylo-.**

staphylo-, staphyl-, a combining form meaning 'resem-

bling a bunch of grapes,' used especially to show relationship to the uvula: *staphyloangina, staphylococcide, staphylolysin.*

staphylococcal antigen phage lysed. See **Staphage Lysate.**

staphylococcal infection, an infection caused by any one of several pathogenic species of *Staphylococcus,* commonly characterized by the formation of abscesses of the skin or other organs. Staphylococcal infections of the skin include carbuncles, folliculitis, furuncles, and hidradenitis suppurativa. Bacteremia is common and may result in endocarditis, meningitis, or osteomyelitis. Staphylococcal pneumonia often follows influenza or other viral disease and may be associated with chronic or debilitating illness. Acute gastroenteritis may result from an enterotoxin produced by certain species of staphylococci in contaminated food. Treatment usually includes bed rest, analgesics, and an antimicrobial drug that is resistant to penicillinase, an enzyme secreted by many species of *Staphylococcus.* Surgical drainage, especially of deep abscesses, is often necessary.

staphylococcal scalded skin syndrome (SSSS), an abnormal skin condition, characterized by epidermal erythema, peeling, and necrosis, that gives the skin a scalded appearance. This disorder primarily affects infants one to three months old and children, but it may also affect adults. It is caused by strains of *Staphylococcus aureus,* especially phage type 71. Individuals contracting the disease may be predisposed to it by deficient immune functions and by renal insufficiency. SSSS is more common in the newborn infant because of undeveloped immunity and renal systems.

■ OBSERVATIONS: A prodromal upper respiratory tract infection with concomitant purulent conjunctivitis is commonly associated with SSSS. Epidermal complications develop in the erythemal stage, the exfoliation stage, and the desquamation stage. Erythema often spreads around the mouth and other orifices and may extend over the entire body in wide circles as the skin becomes tender and the superficial layer of the skin sloughs from friction. The exfoliation stage follows the erythema stage by 24 to 48 hours and is commonly manifested by slight crusting and erosion, which may spread from around the orifices to wider skin areas. More severe forms of SSSS may cause large, soft bullae to erupt and extend over wide skin areas. The eventual rupture of these bullae reveals areas of denuded skin. The desquamation stage of SSSS, following the exfoliation stage, is characterized by the drying up of affected areas and the formation of powdery scales. Normal skin replaces the scales within 5 to 7 days. Diagnosis is based on close observation of the development of SSSS through its three characteristic stages. Erythema multiforme and drug-induced toxic epidermal necrolysis are similar to SSSS but may be ruled out in differential diagnosis by exfoliative cytology and biopsy. Confirming diagnosis is usually made on the basis of isolation of Group 2 *Staphylococcus aureus* in cultures of skin lesions. The mortality in SSSS is 2 to 3 per cent, death usually being caused by complications of fluid and electrolyte loss, sepsis, and involvement of other body systems.

■ INTERVENTION: Treatment of SSSS commonly includes the administration of systemic antibiotics to prevent secondary infections and the replacement of body fluids to maintain fluid and electrolyte balance.

■ NURSING CONSIDERATIONS: The nursing role in the treatment of this disorder focuses on special care for the neonate, as maintenance of body temperature by placing the infant in an incubator, careful monitoring of intake and output, administration of I.V. fluids, maintenance of skin integrity, and careful, regular checks of vital signs. Nurses caring for SSSS patients are especially alert for any sudden rise in temperature, which could be an indication of sepsis and of the immediate need for aggressive treatment. To maintain skin integrity, the nurse uses a strict aseptic technique to prevent any secondary infection. The aseptic technique in skin care is especially important during the SSSS exfoliation stage, when open lesions increase the risk of infection. The patient is loosely clothed and covered to minimize friction, which sloughs off the affected skin. Cotton is inserted between the affected fingers and toes to prevent webbing. During the recovery period, warm baths and soaks aid the healing, and gentle debridement of exfoliated areas hastens the healing process. Helpful to parents is the justifiable assurance from the nurse that complications and residual scars from SSSS rarely occur.

Staphylococcus (stæf'ɪloʊkok'əs), a genus of nonmotile, spherical, gram-positive bacteria. Some species are normally found on the skin and in the throat; certain species cause severe, purulent infections or produce an enterotoxin, which may cause nausea, vomiting, and diarrhea. Life-threatening staphylococcal infections may arise within hospitals. *Staphylococcus aureus* is a species frequently responsible for abscesses, endocarditis, impetigo, osteomyelitis, pneumonia, and septicemia. *S. epidermidis,* formerly called *S. albus,* occasionally causes endocarditis in the presence of intracardiac prostheses. See also **staphylococcal infection.** —**staphylococcal,** *adj.*

staphylokinase (stæf'əloʊkaɪ'neɪs), an enzyme, produced by certain strains of staphylococci, that catalyzes the conversion of plasminogen to plasmin in various animal hosts of the microorganism.

starch, the principal molecule used for the storage of food in plants. Starch is a polysaccharide and is composed of long chains of glucose subunits. In animals, excess glucose is stored as glycogen. The molecular structure of glycogen is similar to that of starch. See also **carbohydrate, glucose, glycogen.**

Starr-Edwards prosthesis (star'ed'wərdz), an artificial cardiac valve. A caged-ball form of device, it obstructs the valve opening and prevents the backward flow of blood. See also **prosthesis.**

start codon (koʊ'don). See **initiation codon.**

startle reflex. See **Moro reflex.**

start point, (in molecular genetics) the initial nucleotide transcribed from the DNA template in the formation of messenger RNA.

starvation, 1. a condition resulting from the lack of essential nutrients over a long period of time and characterized by multiple physiologic and metabolic dysfunctions. 2. the act or state of starving or being starved. See also **malnutrition.**

stas-, a combining form meaning 'stopped, or relation to standing or walking': *stasibasiphobia, stasidynic, stasis.*

-stasia, 1. a combining form meaning a '(specified) condition involving the ability to stand': *astasia, ananastasia, dysstasia.* 2. a combining form meaning '(condition of) stoppage or inhibition': *cholestasia, hemostasia, menostasia.* Also **-stasis.**

stasis (stei'sɪs, stæs'ɪs), 1. a disorder in which the normal flow of a fluid through a vessel of the body is slowed or halted. 2. stillness.

-stasis, a combining form meaning a 'stoppage': *enterostasis, mecystasis, proctostasis.*

stasis dermatitis, a common result of venous insufficiency of the legs beginning with ankle edema and progressing to tan pigmentation, patchy erythema, petechiae, and induration. Ultimately, there may be atrophy and fibrosis of the skin and subcutaneous tissue, with ulcerations that are slow to heal. The tan pigment is hemosiderin from blood leaking through capillary walls under elevated venous pressure. The involved skin is very easily irritated or sensitized to topical medications. The underlying venous insufficiency must be treated. The dermatitis is often treated by bed rest, Burow's solution for oozing lesions, antibiotics for infection, and corticosteroids to reduce inflammation. Also called **venous stasis dermatitis.** See also **stasis ulcer.**

stasis ulcer, a necrotic craterlike lesion of the skin of the lower leg owing to chronic venous congestion. The ulcer is often associated with stasis dermatitis and varicose veins. Healing is slow, and good nursing care to prevent irritation and infection is essential. Potentially sensitizing agents should not be used. Bed rest, elevation, and pressure bandages are usually ordered and appropriate antibiotics, Burow's solution compresses, Unna's paste boot, pinch grafts, and surgery to improve venous flow are useful in treatment. Also called **varicose ulcer.** See also **stasis dermatitis.**

-stat, 1. a combining form meaning a 'device for keeping stationery': *catheterostat, hysterostat, ophthalmostat.* 2. a combining form meaning an 'instrument for the regulation of something specified: *hemostat, rheostat, thermostat*. **3.** a combining form meaning an 'apparatus for the reflection of in one direction of' something specified: *siderostat*. **4.** a combining form meaning a 'device for studying in a state of rest': *hydrostat, orbitostat, microstat*. **5.** a combining form meaning an 'agent for stopping the growth of': *bacteriostat, fungistat, mycostat*.

-state, a combining form meaning the 'result of a (specified) process': *anastate, catastate, mesostate*.

State Board Test Pool Examination, an examination prepared by the National Council of State Boards of Nursing for testing the competency of a person to perform safely as a newly licensed registered nurse. Each jurisdiction within the United States and its territories regulates entry into the practice of nursing; each requires the candidate to pass the examination. The content of the examination is planned to test the candidates' knowledge of the nursing process as applied to the broad areas of nursing practice, including maternal and child health, medical and surgical nursing, and psychiatric nursing. The process includes five steps: assessing, analyzing, planning, implementing, and evaluating. Knowledge, comprehension, application, and analysis of the nursing process are tested as they apply to decision-making situations.

state medicine. *Informal.* See **socialized medicine.**

State Nurses' Association (SNA), an association of nurses at the state level. The various State Nurses' Associations are constituent units of the American Nurses' Association.

Statewide Health Coordinating Committee (SHCC), a component of the national network of Health Systems Agencies.

static, without motion, at rest, in equilibrium. Compare **dynamic.**

static imaging, (in nuclear medicine) a diagnostic procedure in which a radioactive substance is administered to a patient to visualize an internal organ or body compartment. An image or set of images is made of the fixed or slowly changing distribution of the radioactivity.

Statistical Package for the Social Sciences. See **SPSS.**

station, the level of the biparietal plane of the fetal head relative to the level of the ischial spines of the maternal pelvis. An imaginary plane at the level of the spines is designated "zero station." Higher and lower stations are numbered at intervals of one centimeter; minus above, plus below. For example, "station minus three" is 3 cm above the spines, and "station plus two" is 2 cm below the spines. In breech presentation, the bitrochanteric diameter of the breech is used to determine station. See also **dilatation, effacement, labor.**

Statobex, a trade name for an anorexiant (phendimetrazine tartrate).

statotonic reflex (stæt'ɔton'ɪk). See **attitudinal reflex.**

Statrol Ophthalmic, a trade name for an ophthalmic, fixed-combination drug containing antibacterials (polymyxin B sulfate and neomycin sulfate).

status, 1. a specified state or condition, as emotional status. **2.** an unremitting state or condition, as status asthmaticus.

status asthmaticus, an acute, severe, and prolonged asthma attack in which bronchospasm does not respond to oral medication. Hypoxia, cyanosis, and unconsciousness may follow. Treatment includes aminophylline given intravenously, controlled positive pressure ventilation, heavy sedation, frequent bronchial hygiene therapy, and emotional support. A bronchodilator may be given by aerosol inhalation from a ventilator.

status dysraphicus. See **dysraphia.**

status epilepticus, a medical emergency characterized by continual attacks of convulsive seizures occurring without intervals of consciousness. Unless convulsions are arrested, irreversible brain damage results. Status epilepticus can be precipitated by the sudden withdrawal of anticonvulsant drugs, inadequate body levels of glucose, a brain tumor, a head injury, a high fever, or by poisoning. Therapy includes intravenous administration of anticonvulsant drugs, nutrients, and electrolytes, preferably given in an intensive care unit. An adequate airway is usually maintained with an oral pharyngeal or endotracheal tube.

statute of limitations, (in law) a statute that sets a limit of time during which a suit may be brought or criminal charges may be made. In a malpractice suit, dispute may arise as to whether the time set by the particular statute of limitations begins to run at the time of the injury or at the time of the discovery of the injury.

statutory rape, (in law) sexual intercourse with a female below the age of consent, which varies from state to state. See also **rape.**

steady state (ss), a basic physiologic concept implying that the various forces and processes of life are in a state of homeostasis. Living organisms are in constant flux, working to balance the internal and external environments in an effort to avoid a deficiency or an excess that might cause illness. Steady state is a complete state of well-being involving total adaptation.

steap-. See **stearo-.**

stear-. See **stearo-.**

-stearic, a combining form meaning '(specified) fat or fat derivatives': *aleostearic, ketostearic, neurostearic*.

Stearns' alcoholic amentia, a form of insanity brought on by alcohol, characterized by an emotional disturbance of a less severe nature than that of delirium tremens but of longer duration and with greater mental clouding and amnesia.

stearo-, steap-, stear-, steato-, a combining form meaning 'of or pertaining to fat': *stearoconotum, stearodermia, stearopten*.

stearyl alcohol, a solid substance, prepared by the catalytic hydrogenation of stearic acid, used in various ointments.

steato-. See **stearo-.**

steatorrhea (sti'ətəri'ə), greater than normal amounts of fat in the feces, characterized by frothy, foul-smelling fecal matter that floats, as in celiac disease, some malabsorption syndromes, and any condition in which fats are poorly absorbed by the small intestine.

Steele-Richardson-Olszewski syndrome, a rare, progressive, neurologic disorder of unknown etiology, occurring in middle age, more often in men. It is characterized by paralysis of eye muscles, ataxia, neck and trunk rigidity, pseudobulbar palsy, and parkinsonian facies. Dementia and inappropriate emotional responses are also common. Treatment usually includes the antiparkinsonian drug levodopa for control of extrapyramidal symptoms. See also **Parkinson's disease.**

steeple head. See **oxycephaly.**

Stelazine, a trade name for a phenothiazine tranquilizer (trifluoperazine).

stell-, a combining form meaning 'of or pertaining to a star': *stellate, stellectomy, stellula.*

stellate (stel'ıt, stel'eit), star-shaped or arranged in the pattern of a star.

stellate fracture, a fracture that involves the central point of impact or injury and radiates numerous fissures throughout surrounding bone tissue.

stem cell leukemia, a malignant neoplasm of blood-forming organs in which the predominant neoplastic cell is too immature to classify. The disease is extremely acute and has a rapid, relentless course. Also called **embryonal leukemia, hemoblastic leukemia, hemocytoblastic leukemia, lymphoidocytic leukemia, undifferentiated cell leukemia.**

stem cell lymphoma. See **undifferentiated malignant lymphoma.**

Stemex, a trade name for a glucocorticoid (paramethasone acetate).

stem pessary. See **pessary.**

steno-, a combining form meaning 'contracted or narrow': *stenobregmate, stenocephaly, stenothorax.*

stenosis (stınou'sıs), an abnormal condition characterized by the constriction or narrowing of an opening or passageway in a body structure. Kinds of stenosis include **aortic stenosis, pyloric stenosis.** —**stenotic,** *adj.*

Stensen's duct. See **parotid duct.**

stent, 1. a compound used in making dental impressions and medical molds. 2. a mold or device made of stent, used in anchoring skin grafts and for supporting body openings and cavities during grafting or vessels and tubes of the body during surgical anastomosis.

step reflex. See **dance reflex.**

Sterane, a trade name for a glucocorticoid (prednisolone).

Sterapred, a trade name for a glucocorticoid (prednisone).

sterco-, a combining form meaning 'of or pertaining to feces': *stercobilin, stercolith, stercoremia.*

stereo-, a combining form meaning 'solid, three dimensional, or firmly established': *stereoblastula, stereograph, stereopsis.*

stereognostic perception (ster'iognos'tık), the ability to recognize objects by the sense of touch.

stereoscopic microscope, a microscope that produces three-dimensional images through the use of double eye-pieces and double objectives. The three-dimensional image is created because the double optical systems have independent light paths. Also called **Greenough microscope.**

stereoscopic parallax. See **binocular parallax.**

stereotypy (ster'iətai'pi), the persistent, inappropriate, mechanical repetition of actions, body postures, or speech patterns, usually occurring with a lack of variation in thought processes or ideas. It is often seen in patients with schizophrenia. —**stereotypical,** *adj.*

sterile (ster'ıl), 1. barren; unable to produce children owing to a physical abnormality, often the absence of spermatogenesis in a man or blockage of the Fallopian tubes in a woman. Compare **impotence.** 2. aseptic. —**sterility,** *n.*

sterilization, 1. a process or act that renders a person unable to produce children. See also **hysterectomy, tubal ligation, vasectomy.** 2. a technique for destroying microorganisms using heat, water, chemicals, or gases. —**sterilize,** *v.*

-sternal, a combining form meaning 'pertaining to the sternum': *adsternal, presternal, suprasternal.*

sternal node (stər'nəl), a node in one of the three groups of thoracic parietal lymph nodes. They are situated at the anterior ends of the intercostal spaces, adjacent to the internal thoracic artery. The afferent vessels of the sternal nodes drain the lymph from breast, the diaphragmatic surface of the liver, and the deep, ventral thoracic wall. The efferent vessels of the sternal nodes usually form a single lymphatic trunk on each side. The trunk may open directly into the junction of the internal jugular and the subclavian veins; or the trunk on the right side may join the right lymphatic subclavian trunk, and the trunk on the left side may join the thoracic duct. Also called **internal mammary node.** Compare **diaphragmatic node, intercostal node.** See also **lymphatic system, lymph node.**

-sternia, a combining form meaning '(condition of the) sternum': *asternia, koilosternia, schistosternia.*

sterno-, a combining form meaning 'of or pertaining to the sternum': *sternocleidal, sternocostal, sternopagus.*

sternoclavicular articulation, the double gliding joint between the sternum and the clavicle. It involves the sternal end of the clavicle, the superior and lateral part of the manubrium, the cartilage of the first rib, and six ligaments.

sternocostal articulation, the gliding articulation of the cartilage of each true rib and the sternum, except for the articulation of the first rib in which the cartilage is directly united with the sternum to form a synchondrosis. Each sternocostal articulation also involves five ligaments.

sternohyoideus (stər'nouhaioi'diəs), one of the four infrahyoid muscles. Arising from the medial end of the clavicle, the posterior sternoclavicular ligament, and the manubrium sterni and inserting into the inferior border of the hyoid bone, it is a thin, narrow muscle innervated by fibers from the first, second, and third cervical nerves. It acts to depress the hyoid bone. Also called **sternohyoid muscle.** Compare **omohyoideus, sternothyroideus, thyrohyoideus.**

sternothyroideus (stər'noufhairoi'diəs), one of the four infrahyoid muscles. Arising from the dorsal surface of the manubrium sterni and inserting into the thyroid cartilage, it is innervated by fibers from cervical nerves 1, 2, and 3, through the ansa cervicalis. It acts to depress the thyroid cartilage. Also called **sternothyroid muscle.** Compare **omohyoideus, sternohyoideus, thyrohyoideus.**

sternothyroid muscle. See **sternothyroideus.**

sternum, the elongated, flattened bone forming the middle portion of the thorax. It supports the clavicles, articulates with the first seven pairs of ribs, and comprises the manubrium, the gladiolus, and the xiphoid process. It is composed of highly vascular tissue covered by a thin layer of bone and is a site for needle puncture for biopsy of bone marrow specimens. The sternum is longer in men than in women.

sternutation (stər'nyutei'shən). See **sneeze.**

sterognosis, 1. the faculty of perceiving and understanding the form and nature of objects by the sense of touch. 2. perception by the senses of the solidity of objects. — **sterognostic,** *adj.*

sthen-. See **stheno-.**

stertorous (stər'tərəs), having a snoring sound.

steth-. See **stetho-.**

stetho-, steth-, a combining form meaning 'of or pertaining to the chest': *stethometer, stethomyitis, stethospasm.*

stethoscope, an instrument, used in mediate auscultation, consisting of two earpieces connected by means of flexible tubing to a diaphragm, which is placed against the skin of the patient's chest or back.
(See next page for illustration)

Stevens-Johnson syndrome, a serious, sometimes fatal inflammatory disease affecting children and young adults. It is characterized by the acute onset of fever, bullae on the skin, and ulcers on the mucous membranes of the lips, eyes, mouth, nasal passage, and genitalia. Pneumonia, pain in the joints, and prostration are com-

mon. The syndrome may be an allergic reaction to certain drugs, or it may follow pregnancy, herpesvirus I, or other infection. It is seen rarely in association with malignancy or with radiation therapy. Treatment includes bed rest, antibiotics for pneumonia, glucocorticoids, analgesics, mouthwashes, and sedatives.

Stewart, Isabel Maitland (1878–1963), a Canadian-born American nursing educator and writer. The first nurse to receive a master's degree from Columbia University in New York, she succeeded Mary Adelaide Nutting as Professor of Nursing at Teachers College at that university. She was instrumental in upgrading the nursing curriculum and in directing educational policies and became an important figure in international nursing affairs.

-sthenia, a combining form meaning 'power or strength': *angiosthenia, eusthenia, hyposthenia.*

sthenic fever, high body temperature associated with thirst, dry skin, and, often, delirium.

stheno-, sthen-, a combining form meaning 'of or pertaining to strength': *sthenometer, sthenoplastic, sthenopyra.*

-sthenuria, a combining form meaning '(condition of) urination or of the specific gravity of urine': *hyposthenuria, isosthenuria, normosthenuria.*

stib-, a combining form meaning 'of or pertaining to antimony': *stibamine, stibophen, stiburea.*

stibocaptate. See **sodium stibocaptate.**

stibogluconate sodium, an antileishmanial available from the Center for Disease Control. It is a drug of choice for the visceral form of leishmaniasis and has some effect on other forms.

stibophen (stib'əfin), a schistosomicide.

■ INDICATIONS: It is prescribed in the treatment of infestations of *Schistosoma japonicum.* or *S. haematobium.*

■ CONTRAINDICATIONS: Severe hepatic, renal, or cardiac insufficiency or known hypersensitivity to this drug prohibits its use.

■ ADVERSE EFFECTS: Among the more serious adverse reactions are pain at the site of injection, gastrointestinal disturbances, fever, and blood dyscrasias.

-stichia, a combining form meaning a 'condition involving rows of eyelashes': *distichia, tristichia, polystichia.*

sticky ends. See **cohesive termini.**

Stieda's fracture (sti'dəz), a fracture of the internal condyle of the femur.

stiff lung. See **congestive atelectasis.**

stigma, *pl.* **stigmata.** 1. a moral or physical blemish. 2. a physical characteristic that serves to identify a disease or a condition.

stilet (stai'lit), **stilette** (stilet'). See **stylet.**

stilbestrol (stilbes'trol). See **diethylstilbestrol.**

stillbirth, 1. the birth of a fetus that died before or during delivery. 2. a fetus, born dead, that weighs more than 1,000 gm and would usually have been expected to live.

Anterior thorax

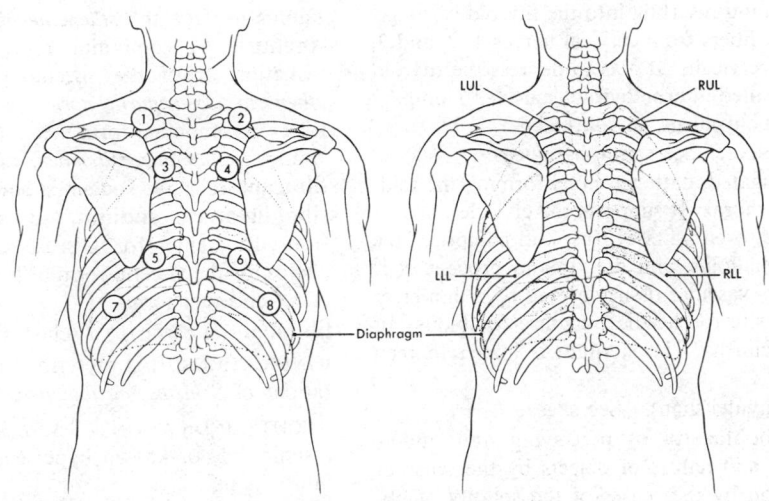

Posterior thorax

STETHOSCOPE PLACEMENT

stillborn, **1.** an infant that was born dead. **2.** of or pertaining to an infant that was born dead.

Still's disease, a form of rheumatoid arthritis, usually affecting the larger joints of children under 16 years of age. As bone growth in children is dependent on the epiphyseal plates of the distal epiphyses, skeletal development may be impaired if these structures are damaged. Treatment includes analgesia, anti-inflammatory medication, and rest. The recovery rate in this juvenile form is better than in the adult forms of rheumatoid arthritis. Also called **juvenile rheumatoid arthritis.**

Stilphostrol, a trade name for an estrogen (diethylstilbestrol diphosphate).

stimulant cathartic, a cathartic that acts by promoting the motility of the bowel, especially the longitudinal peristalsis of the colon. Kinds of stimulant cathartics are **cascara, senna.**

stimulating bath, a bath taken in water that contains an aromatic substance, an astringent, or a tonic.

stimulus, *pl.* **stimuli.** anything that excites or incites an organism or part to function, become active, or respond. —**stimulate,** *v.*

stimulus duration, the length of time a stimulus must be applied in order for the resulting nerve impulse to produce excitation in the receptor tissue. In general, more intense stimuli require shorter excitation times to effect cellular response. Any stimulus that acts for a period of time too brief to overcome the threshold intensity of the receptor cell will not elicit a response.

sting, an injury caused by a sharp, painful penetration of the skin, often accompanied by exposure to an irritating chemical or the venom of an insect or other animal. In cases of hypersensitivity, a highly venomous sting, or multiple stings, anaphylactic shock may occur. Kinds of stings include **bee stings, jellyfish stings, scorpion stings, sea urchin stings, shellfish stings.** See also **stingray, wasp.**

stingray, a flat, long-tailed fish bearing barbed spines on its back that are connected to sacs of venom. Spasm of the skeletal muscles, severe local pain, seizures, and dyspnea may occur if the skin is broken by the spines. The wound is washed with cold salt water, and the injured limb is placed in very hot water for 30 to 60 minutes; an antiseptic is applied and tetanus prophylaxis is administered. See also **sea urchin sting.**

St. Louis encephalitis, an arbovirus infection of the brain transmitted from birds to man by the bite of an infected mosquito. It occurs most commonly in the central and southern portions of the United States and is characterized by headache, malaise, fever, stiff neck, delirium, and convulsions. Sequelae may include visual and speech disturbances, difficulty in walking, and personality changes. Convalescence may be prolonged, and death may result. Compare **California encephalitis, equine encephalitis.** See also **encephalitis.**

stoker's cramp. See **heat cramp.**

Stokes-Adams syndrome. See **Adams-Stokes syndrome.**

-stole, a combining form referring to the contraction, retraction, or dilation of various organs: *anastole, diastole, peristole.*

stoma, *pl.* **stomas, stomata. 1.** a pore, orifice, or opening on a surface. **2.** an artificial opening of an internal organ on the surface of the body, created surgically, as for a colostomy, ileostomy, or tracheostomy. **3.** a new opening created surgically, between two body structures, as for a gastroenterostomy, pancreaticogastrostomy, pancreatoduodenostomy, or pyeloureterostomy.

-stoma, a combining form meaning a 'mouth': *hypostoma, metastoma, tetrastoma.*

stomach, the major organ of digestion, located in the right upper quadrant of the abdomen and divided into a body and a pylorus. It receives and partially processes food and drink funneled from the mouth and esophagus and moves nutritional bulk into the intestines. The stomach lies in the epigastric and left hypogastric regions bounded by the anterior abdominal wall and the diaphragm between the liver and the spleen. The shape of the stomach is modified by the amount of contents, stage of digestion, development of gastric musculature, and condition of the intestines. It is lined with a mucous coat, a submucous coat, a muscular coat, and a serous coat, all

richly supplied with blood vessels and nerves, and contains fundic, cardiac, and pyloric gastric glands. Also called **gaster.**

stomach pump, a pump for withdrawing the contents of the stomach through a tube passed through the mouth or nose into the stomach.

stomadeum. See **stomodeum.**

stomal peptic ulcer, a marginal peptic ulcer. See also **peptic ulcer.**

stomatitis (stou'mətai'tis), any inflammatory condition of the mouth. It may result from infection by bacteria, viruses or fungi, from exposure to certain chemicals or drugs, from vitamin deficiency, or from a systemic inflammatory disease. Kinds of stomatitis include **aphthous stomatitis, pseudomembranous stomatitis, thrush, Vincent's infection.**

stomato-, stomo-, a combining form meaning 'of or pertaining to the mouth': *stomatodysodia, stomatogastric, stomatopathy.*

-stomia, a combining form meaning '(condition of the) mouth': *atelostomia, atretostomia, hygrostomia.*

stomo-. See **stomato-.**

stomodeum, stomodaeum, *pl.* **stomodeums, stomodea, stomodaeums, stomodaea, stomadeums, stomadea.** an invagination in the ectoderm located in the foregut of the developing embryo that forms the mouth. Compare **proctodeum.** — **stomodeal, stomodaeal, stomadeal,** *adj.*

-stomy, a combining form meaning 'surgical opening': *gastrostomy, lobostomy, tracheostomy.*

stone. See **calculus.**

-stone, a combining form meaning a 'calculus in a human organ or duct': *bilestone, gallstone, wombstone.*

stool. See **feces.**

stool softener. See **fecal softener.**

stop needle, a needle with a shoulder flange that stops it from penetrating beyond a certain distance.

storing fermentation, the rapid, gaseous clotting of milk caused by *Clostridium perfringens.*

stork bite. See **telangiectatic nevus.**

Stoxil, a trade name for an antiviral (idoxuridine).

STP, *Slang.* a psychedelic agent [dimethoxy-4 methylampetamine (DOM)]. STP is an abbreviation for serenity, tranquility, and peace.

STPD, abbreviation for *standard temperature, standard pressure, dry.*

strab-, a combining form meaning 'squinting': *strabismometer, strabometry, strabotomy.*

strabismus, an abnormal ocular condition in which the eyes are crossed. There are two kinds of strabismus, paralytic and nonparalytic. Paralytic strabismus results from the inability of the ocular muscles to move the eye owing to neurologic deficit or muscular dysfunction. The muscle that is dysfunctional may be identified by watching as the patient attempts to move the eyes to each of the cardinal positions of gaze. If the affected eye cannot be directed to a position, the examiner infers that the associated ocular muscle is the dysfunctional one. As this kind of strabismus may be caused by tumor, infection, or injury to the brain or the eye, an ophthalmologic examination is recommended. Nonparalytic strabismus is a defect in the position of the two eyes in relation to each other. The condition is inherited. The person cannot use the two eyes together but has to fix with one or the other. The eye that looks straight at a given time is the fixing eye. Some people have alternating strabismus, using one eye and then the other; some have monocular strabismus affecting only one eye. Visual acuity diminishes with diminished use of an eye, and suppression amblyopia may develop. Nonparalytic strabismus and suppression amblyopia are treated most successfully in early childhood. Treatment consists mainly of covering the fixing eye, forcing the child to use the deviating eye. The earlier it is begun the more rapid and effective the treatment. By the age of six years a deviating eye has usually become so suppressed that treatment is not effective and permanent visual loss has occurred. The eyes might be straightened by surgery but suppression amblyopia will not be corrected. Also called **squint**. – **strabismal, strabismic, strabismical,** *adj.*

Convergent

Divergent

STRABISMUS

straight-line blood set, a common device, composed of plastic components, for delivering blood infusions. It includes the plastic tubing, the clamp, the drip chamber, and the filter. Some kinds of straight-line blood sets contain filters within drip chambers; others have separate filters. The latter kind can be filled by squeezing the attached drip chamber but must not be squeezed itself or it may rupture. The former kind can be filled by squeezing the section of the blood set that contains the filter and the drip chamber. Before infusion, the filter of either kind is tapped with the fingers to dislodge any trapped air bubbles. Compare **component drip set, component syringe set, microaggregate recipient set, Y-set.**

straight sinus, one of the six posterior superior venous channels of the dura mater, draining blood from the brain into the internal jugular vein. It has no valves and is located at the junction of the falx cerebri with the tentorium cerebelli. It is triangular in section and increases in size as it runs posteriorly from the end of the inferior sagittal sinus to the transverse sinus of the opposite side. It receives the inferior sagittal sinus, the great cerebral vein, and the superior cerebellar veins. Compare **inferior sagittal sinus, superior sagittal sinus, transverse sagittal sinus.**

strain, 1. to exert excessive physical force in a manner that may result in injury, usually muscular. 2. to separate solids or particles from a liquid with a filter or sieve. 3. the damage, usually muscular, that results from excessive physical effort. 4. a taxon that is a subgroup of a species. 5. an emotional state reflecting mental pressure or fatigue.

strait jacket, a coatlike garment of canvas with long sleeves that can be tied behind the wearer's back to prevent movement of the arms. It is used for restraining violent or uncontrollable people who might be a danger to themselves or to others.

strangulation, the constriction of a tubular structure of the body, as the trachea, a segment of bowel, or the blood vessels of a limb, that impedes circulation or prevents function. See also **intestinal strangulation.** – **strangulate,** *v.,* **strangulated,** *adj.*

strapping, the application of overlapping strips of adhesive tape to an extremity or body area to exert pressure and hold a structure in place, performed in the treatment of strains, sprains, dislocations, and certain fractures.

strati-, a combining form meaning 'layer': *stratification, stratiform, stratigraphy.*

stratiform cartilage (stræt′ɪfɔrm). See **fibrocartilage.**

stratiform fibrocartilage, a structure made of fibrocartilage that forms a thin coating of osseous grooves through which tendons of certain muscles glide. Small masses of stratified fibrocartilage also develop in the tendons of some muscles that glide over bones, as in the tendons of the peroneus longus and the tibialis posterior. Compare **circumferential fibrocartilage, connecting fibrocartilage, interarticular fibrocartilage.**

stratum (strei′təm, stræt′əm), *pl.* **strata.** a uniformly thick sheet or layer, usually associated with other layers, as the stratum basale and the stratum spinosum of the epidermis.

stratum corneum, the horny, outermost layer of the skin, composed of dead cells converted to keratin that continually flakes away. The thickness of the layer is correlated with the normal wear of the area it covers. The stratum corneum is thick on the palms of the hands and the soles of the feet but thin over more protected areas. Also called **horny layer.** Compare **stratum basale, stratum**

granulosum, stratum lucidum, stratum spinosum. See also **skin.**

stratum germinativum. See **stratum basale.**

stratum granulosum, one of the five layers of the epidermis, situated just below the stratum corneum except in the palms of the hands and the soles of the feet, where it lies just under the stratum lucidum. The stratum granulosum contains visible granules in the cytoplasm of its cells, which die, become keratinized, move to the surface, and flake away. Compare **stratum basale, stratum corneum, stratum lucidum, stratum spinosum.** See also **skin.**

stratum lucidum, one of the five layers of the epidermis, situated just beneath the stratum corneum and present only in the thick skin of the palms of the hands and the soles of the feet. It contains translucent eleidin which forms keratin. Compare **stratum basale, stratum corneum, stratum granulosum, stratum spinosum.** See also **skin.**

stratum spinosum, one of the five layers of the epidermis, composed of several layers of polygonal cells. It lies on top of the stratum basale and beneath the stratum granulosum and contains tiny fibrils within its cellular cytoplasm. When the cells of the stratum spinsosum are pulled apart, they present minute spines at their surfaces. Also called **prickle cell layer.** Compare **stratum basale, stratum corneum, stratum granulosum, stratum lucidum.** See also **skin.**

stratum spongiosum, one of the three layers of the endometrium of the uterus, containing tortuous, dilated uterine glands and a small amount of interglandular tissue. With the stratum compactum it forms the functional part of the endometrium during pregnancy. Compare **stratum basale, stratum compactum.** See also **decidua, placenta.**

strawberry gall bladder, a tiny, yellow gall bladder spotted with deposits on the red mucous membrane, characteristic of cholesterolosis.

strawberry hemangioma, a bright red, superficial vascular tumor that is soft and raised and resembles a strawberry. It is fragile, and extensive bleeding may occur if the vessel walls are broken. Strawberry angiomas are present at birth and tend to increase in size for the first few months of life, then to decrease in size and color, and finally to disappear in early childhood. Also called **hemangioma simplex.**

strawberry mark. See **capillary hemangioma.**

streak, a line or a stripe, as the primitive streak at the caudal end of the embryonic disc.

strepho-, streph-, a combining form meaning 'twisted': *strephopodia, strephosymbolia, strephotome.*

strep throat, *Informal.* an infection of the oral pharynx and tonsils caused by a hemolytic species of *Streptococcus,* usually belonging to group A. The infection is characterized by sore throat, chills, fever, swollen lymph nodes in the neck, and, sometimes, by nausea and vomiting. The symptoms usually begin abruptly a few days after exposure to the organism in airborne droplets or after direct contact with an infected person. Also called **streptococcal sore throat.**

■ OBSERVATIONS: The throat is diffusely red and tonsils often are covered with a yellow or white exudate. Diagnosis is confirmed by bacteriologic culture and identification of the streptococcal bacteria in a specimen taken from the throat. Complications of strep throat are otitis media, scarlet fever, and sinusitis; other complications include acute glomerulonephritis and acute rheumatic fever.

■ INTERVENTION: Treatment usually includes intramuscular injection of benzathene penicillin G or the administration of penicillin for ten days. Erythromycin may be given to people allergic to penicillin. For recurrent infections, tonsillectomy may be recommended.

■ NURSING CONSIDERATIONS: Analgesics and throat irrigation with warm saline solution may give relief from pain. Family members and other contacts are observed for signs of infection, and those for whom streptococcal infection presents a special risk are treated prophylactically.

strepto-, a combining form meaning 'twisted': *streptobacilli, streptococcal, streptomicrodactyly.*

streptobacillary rat-bite fever (strep'toubæs'ıler'i). See **Haverhill fever.**

Streptobacillus (strep'toubəsil'əs), a genus of necklace-shaped bacteria that can cause rat-bite fever in humans.

streptococcal infection, an infection caused by pathogenic bacteria of one of several species of the genus *Streptococcus* or their toxins. Almost any organ of the body may be involved. The infections occur in many forms including cellulitis, endocarditis, erysipelas, impetigo, meningitis, pneumonia, scarlet fever, tonsillitis, and urinary tract infection. See also **strep throat.**

streptococcal sore throat. See **strep throat.**

Streptococcus (strep'təkok'əs), a genus of nonmotile, gram-positive, cocci classified by serologic types (Lancefield groups A through T), by hemolytic action (alpha, beta, gamma) when grown on blood agar, and by reaction to bacterial viruses (phage types 1 to 86). Many species cause disease in humans. *Streptococcus fecalis,* a penicillin-resistant, Group D enterococcus and normal inhabitant of the gastrointestinal tract, may cause infection of the urinary tract or endocardium. *S. pneumoniae* (formerly, *Diplococcus pneumoniae*) causes 90 per cent of the cases of bacterial pneumonia in the United States. *S. pyogenes* belongs to group A and may cause tonsillitis, respiratory, urinary, or skin infections. Some beta-hemolytic strains may lead to rheumatic fever or to glomerulonephritis. *S. viridans,* a member of the normal flora of the mouth, is the most common cause of bacterial endocarditis, especially when introduced into the blood stream during dental procedures.

streptokinase (strep'təkai'neis), an enzyme, produced by streptococci, that catalyzes the conversion of plasminogen to plasmin in various animal hosts of the microorganism.

streptokinase-streptodornase (strep'toukai'neis-strep'toudɔr'neis), two enzymes derived from a strain of *Streptococcus hemolyticus.*

■ INDICATIONS: It is prescribed for debridement of purulent exudates, clotted blood, or fibrinous deposits resulting from trauma or infection.

■ CONTRAINDICATIONS: Active hemorrhage, acute cellulitis, or danger of reopening bronchopleural fistulas prohibits its use.

■ ADVERSE EFFECTS: Among the more serious adverse reactions are pyrogenic reactions and irritation.

streptolysin (streptol'əsin), a filterable substance, produced by various streptococci, that liberates hemoglobin from red blood cells.

streptomycin sulfate, an aminoglycoside antibiotic.

■ INDICATIONS: It is prescribed in the treatment of tuberculosis and certain other infections.

■ CONTRAINDICATIONS: Known hypersensitivity to this drug prohibits its use. It must be used with caution in impaired renal function.

■ ADVERSE EFFECTS: Among the most serious adverse reactions are ototoxicity, nephrotoxicity, muscle weakness, and allergic reactions.

streptozocin, an investigational antineoplastic used in the treatment of a variety of neoplasms, including metastatic islet-cell tumors of the pancreas. It is an antibiotic substance from *Streptomyces acromogenes.*

stress, any emotional, physical, social, economic, or other factor that requires a response or change, as dehydration, which can cause an increase in body temperature, or a separation from parents, which can cause a young child to cry. Stress may also be applied therapeutically to promote change, as implosion therapy for phobic patients, in which the patient is given support while being exposed to the situation that produces anxiety and is thereby gradually desensitized. The nature and degree of stress observed in a patient are frequently evaluated by the nurse as part of her ongoing holistic nursing assessment.

stress fracture, a fracture, especially of one or more of the metatarsal bones, caused by repeated, prolonged, or abnormal stress.

stress reaction. **1.** See **general adaptation syndrome.** **2.** See **post-traumatic stress disorder.**

stress response syndrome. See **post-traumatic stress disorder.**

(See next page for illustration)

stress test, a test that measures the function of a system of the body when subjected to carefully controlled amounts of stress. The data produced allow the examiner to evaluate the condition of the system being tested. Cardiopulmonary function, respiratory function, and intrauterine fetal-placental function are tested with stress tests. See also **exercise electrocardiogram, oxytocin challenge test.**

stress ulcer, a gastric or duodenal ulcer that develops in previously unaffected individuals subjected to severe stress, as when severely burned. See also **Curling's ulcer.**

stretch mark. See **stria.**

stri-, a combining form meaning 'line or streak': *striation, striocellular, striomuscular.*

stria (strai'ə), *pl.* **striae.** a streak or a linear scar which often results from rapidly developing tension in the skin, as seen on the abdomen after pregnancy. Purplish striae are one of the classical findings in hyperadrenocorticism. Also called **stretch mark.**

striated muscle, one of two kinds of muscle, including all the skeletal muscles. Striated muscles are composed of bundles of parallel, striated fibers under voluntary control; the heart, a striated involuntary muscle, is an exception. Each striated muscle is covered by a thin connective epimysium and divided into bundles of sheathed fibers containing smaller myofibrils. Each myofibril is comprised of thick filaments that consist of molecules of myosin and of thin filaments that consist of actin and two other protein compounds. Muscle contraction occurs when an electrochemical impulse crosses the myonevral junction, causing the thin filaments to shorten. Also called **skeletal muscle, voluntary muscle.** Compare **cardiac muscle, smooth muscle.**

stricture, an abnormal temporary or permanent narrowing of the lumen of a hollow organ, as the esophagus, pylorus of the stomach, ureter, or urethra, owing to inflammation, external pressure, or scarring. Treatment varies depending on the cause. Compare **spasm.**

strict vegetarian, a vegetarian whose diet excludes the use of all foods of animal origin. Such diets, unless adequately planned, may be deficient in many essential nutrients. Also called **pure vegetarian, vegan.**

stridor (strai'dɔr), an abnormal, high-pitched, musical respiratory sound, caused by an obstruction in the trachea or larynx. It is usually heard during inspiration. Stridor may indicate several neoplastic or inflammatory conditions, including glottic edema, asthma, diphtheria, laryngospasm, or papilloma. Compare **pleuropericardial rub, rales, rhonchi, wheeze.**

strike, an action taken by the employees of a company or institution in which they stop reporting for work in an effort to cause the employer to accede to certain demands. A strike usually follows unsuccessful negotiations between representatives of the union and management.

string carcinoma, a malignancy of the large intestine,

STRESS RESPONSE SYNDROME

usually of the ascending or transverse colon that, on radiologic visualization, causes the intestine to appear to be tied in segments like a string of large beads.

strip membranes, (in obstetrics) a procedure in which an examiner digitally frees the membranes of the amniotic sac from the wall of the lower segment of the uterus in the small area around the cervical os. It is done to stimulate labor, but, as infection or hemorrhage may result, it is not recommended.

stripping, *Nontechnical.* a surgical procedure for the removal of the long and the short saphenous veins of the legs. See also **milking, varicose veins.**

stroke. See **cerebrovascular accident.**

-stroke, a combining form meaning a 'condition caused by or resembling an apoplectic stroke': *bloodstroke, lightstroke.*

stroke prone profile, a predictive index using a complex of risk factors that indicate susceptibility of a person to cerebrovascular accident (CVA). The factors include advanced age, hypertension, a history of transient ischemic attacks, cigarette smoking, heart disorders, associated embolism, family hisory of CVA, use of oral contraceptives, diabetes mellitus, physical inactivity, obesity,

hypercholesteremia, and hyperlipidemia.

stroma-, a combining form meaning 'a covering': *stromatin, stromatogenous, stromatosis.*

stroma (strou'mə), *pl.* **stromata.** the supporting tissue or the matrix of an organ as distinguished from its parenchyma. Some kinds of stromata are the vitreous stroma, which encloses the vitreous humor of the eye, and Rollet's stroma, which contains the hemoglobin of a red blood cell. — **stromatic,** *adj.*

-stroma, a combining form meaning the 'supporting tissue of an organ': *blastostroma, mesostroma, myostroma.*

Strongyloides (stron'jɪlɔɪ'diz), a genus of parasitic intestinal nematode. A species of *Strongyloides, S. stercoralis,* causes strongyloidiasis.

strongyloidiasis (stron'jəlɔɪdaɪ'əsɪs), infection of the small intestine by the roundworm *Strongyloides stercoralis,* acquired when larvae from the soil penetrate intact skin, incidentally causing a pruritic rash. The larvae pass to the lungs via the bloodstream, sometimes causing pneumonia. Larvae then migrate up the air passages to the pharynx, are swallowed, and develop into adult worms in the small intestine. Bloody diarrhea and intestinal malabsorption may result. Rarely, fatal disseminated strongyloidiasis occurs. Diagnosis depends on finding larvae in freshly passed feces. Treatment often includes administration of thiabendazole. Proper sanitary methods for the disposal of excrement could eliminate the disease. Wearing shoes prevents contagion from contaminated soil.

strontium (Sr), a metallic element. Its atomic number is 38; its atomic weight is 87.62. Chemically similar to calcium, it is found in bone tissue. Isotopes of strontium are used in radioisotope scanning procedures of bone. Strontium-85 (^{85}Sr) and strontium-87 (^{87}Sr) mimic calcium metabolism and are used in studies of bone physiology and disorders. These radionuclides can be counted with any standard detector or imaged at a very early stage in bone disease, whereas x rays of bone without the use of a radioactive tracer can show decreased density only after approximately 50 per cent of bone is decalcified. Most ^{85}Sr or ^{87}Sr is deposited in bone within an hour following injection; increased deposition of these radionuclides is strongly linked to osteoblastic activity and new bone formation. In addition to four naturally occurring isotopes (^{88}Sr, ^{87}Sr, ^{86}Sr, and ^{84}Sr), 12 artificial strontium isotopes are produced by nuclear reactions. Strontium-90, the longest lived, is the most dangerous constituent of fallout from atomic bomb tests. It can replace some of the calcium in food, become concentrated in teeth and bones, and continue to emit electrons that can cause death in the host. Cows concentrate strontium-90 in their milk.

-strophe, a combining form meaning 'turning or twisting': *cardianastrophe, enstrophe, phallanastrophe.* Also **-strophy.**

stropho-, a combining form meaning 'twisted': *strophocephalus, strophosomus.*

-strophy, a combining form meaning a 'twisting or turning': *dystrophy, exstrophy, polystrophy.* Also **-strophe.**

structural chemistry, the science dealing with the molecular structure of chemical substances.

structural gene, (in molecular genetics) a unit of genetic information that specifies the amino acid sequence of a polypeptide.

structural integration, a technique of deep massage intended to help in the realignment of the body by altering the length and tone of myofascial tissues. The basis of the practice is the belief that misalignment of myofascial tissues, occurring as a result of improper posture and emotional and physical traumas, may have an overall detrimental effect on a person's energy level, self-image, muscular efficiency, perceptions, and general health. Also called **Rolfing.**

structure, a part of the body, as the heart, a bone, a gland, a cell, or a limb.

strum-, a combining form meaning 'of or pertaining to a goiter, or to scrofula': *strumectomy, strumiform, strumitis.*

struma lymphomatosa (stru'mə). See **Hashimoto's disease.**

Strycin, a trade name for an antibacterial (streptomycin sulfate).

Stryker wedge frame, an orthopedic bed that allows the patient to be rotated as required to either the supine or prone position. Like the Foster bed, the Stryker wedge frame is used in the immobilization of patients with unstable spines, postoperative management of multilevel spinal fusions, and in the management of severe burn patients. Use of the Stryker wedge frame is not recommended if hyperextension of the spine is required or if lower extremity traction is needed. The Stryker wedge frame comes in only one size, the only accommodation to different body builds being an adjustable crossbar on the anterior circle of the frame. If the crossbar is properly adapted, the patient is held firmly between the frames without the addition of pillows or extra padding. The Stryker wedge frame is constructed of lightweight aluminum mounted at the head end to a base by two posts, anterior for the prone frame and posterior for the supine frame. Each frame is fastened to its corresponding post by a knurled nut. The foot ends of the frame are secured by resting on crossbars within a ring, which, when closed, secures the patient between the frames. The ring has two handles to permit turning of the patient by one person, although most hospitals usually require two staff members to turn patients confined to such frames. The ring is released for turning when the red knob or turning lock is pulled. For safety, unintentional rotation of the frames is prevented by a pin at the head end of the frames. The pin is pulled prior to releasing the ring by pulling a red knob. The crossbars of the frame are wedge-shaped, and the patient is always turned toward the apex of the wedge formed by the crossbars. The lower frame always locks when it is horizontal and level. The ring may then be unlocked and opened for removal of the upper frame. Half of the circle may be removed for exercises, but the circle is usually closed for added security. The Stryker wedge frame is usually equipped with armboards which may be turned up as protective siderails at night. The frame is also often equipped with a reading table. To prevent injury to the arms, the armboards and the reading table are lowered when the frame is rotated. The armboards may also be adjusted toward the head end of the frame for support when the patient is prone or toward the foot end when the patient is supine. The bedpan shelf on the frame is adjustable but must be lowered to allow free rotation of the frame. As with all horizontal turning frames, the level of the trochanters must be aligned with the bottom edge of the torso canvas to prevent hyperextension of the lumbosacral spine when the bedpan portion of the frame is open. Loose linen and catheter tubes can become entrapped in the ring during rotation of the frame unless excess top covers are removed and catheter tubing is placed between the patient's legs, with the drainage bag at the foot end of the frame. The elevation lock of the wedge is useful for elevating the head end of the anterior frame when the patient is prone. In the immediate postoperative period it is also useful for increasing pulmonary expansion by decreasing visceral pressure on the diaphragm. When a patient is in halo or tong cervical traction, the elevation lock provides countertraction up to a maximum of seven inches. Most hospitals provide the nursing staff with charts to determine the elevation needed for countertraction according to the weight of the patient and the pull forces of traction weights. Compare **Foster bed, hyperextension bed.**

ST segment, the component of the cardiac cycle shown on an electrocardiogram as a short, gradual upward curve following the spiked QRS complex, preceding the ascent of the T wave. It represents the interval between complete depolarization at the end of ventricular contraction and the beginning of repolarization.

Stuartnatal 1 + 1, a trade name for an oral, prenatal, fixed-combination drug containing vitamins and minerals.

Stuart-Power factor. See **factor X.**

stump, the part of a limb following amputation that is proximal to the portion amputated.

stump hallucination, the sensation of the continued presence of an amputated limb. See also **hallucination, phantom limb syndrome.**

stupor, a state of lethargy and unresponsiveness in which a person seems unaware of his surroundings. The condition occurs in neurologic as well as psychiatric disorders. Kinds of stupor are **anergic stupor, benign stupor, delusion stupor, epileptic stupor.**

Sturge-Weber syndrome (stərj'web'ər), a congenital neurocutaneous disease marked by a port wine-colored capillary hemangioma over a sensory dermatome of a branch of the trigeminal nerve of the face. X-ray examination of the skull reveals intracranial calcification. The cerebral cortex may atrophy, and generalized or focal seizures, angioma of the choroid, secondary glaucoma, optic atrophy, and new cutaneous hemangiomas may develop. There is no known cure. Treatment is supportive and includes anticonvulsive medication.

sty, stye, a purulent infection of a Meibomian or sebaceous gland of the eyelid, often caused by a staphylococcal organism. Also called **hordeolum.**

-style, a combining form meaning a 'bone attached to an internal structure': *cephalostyle, sarcostyle, zygostyle.*

stylet (stai'lɪt, stailet'), **stilet, stilette,** a thin metal probe for inserting into or passing through a needle, tube, or catheter to clean the hollow bore or for inserting in a soft, flexible catheter to make it shift as the catheter is placed in a vein or passed through an orifice of the body.

stylo-, a combining form meaning 'like a stake or pole,'

used especially to show relationship to the styloid process of the temporal bone: *stylomastoid, stylomyloid, stylostixis.*

stylohyoid bone (stai'louhai'oid). See **stylohyoideus.**

stylohyoideus (stai'louhaioi'diəs), one of four suprahyoid muscles, lying anterior and superior to the posterior belly of the digastricus. It is a slender muscle that arises from the styloid process and inserts into the hyoid bone. It is pierced near its insertion by the tendon of the digastricus. It is innervated by fibers of the mandibular branch of the facial nerve, and it serves to draw the hyoid bone up and back. Also called **stylohyoid bone.** Compare **digastricus, geniohyoideus, mylohyoideus.**

stylohyoid ligament, the ligament attached to the tip of the styloid process of the temporal bone and to the lesser cornu of the hyoid bone. It frequently contains a small cartilage in its center and is often partially ossified.

stylomandibular ligament, one of a pair of specialized bands of cervical fascia, forming an accessory part of the temporomandibular joint. It extends from the styloid process of the temporal bone to the ramus of the mandible between the masseter and pterygoideus muscles and separates the parotid gland from the submandibular gland. Compare **sphenomandibular ligament.**

styptic (stɪp'tɪk), **1.** a substance used as an astringent, often to control bleeding. A chemical styptic induces coagulation of blood. A cotton pledget used as a compress to control bleeding is a mechanical styptic. **2.** acting as an astringent or agent to control bleeding.

sub-, a combining form meaning 'under, near, almost, or moderately': *subacid, subcapsular, subdental.* Also **suf-, sup-.**

subacromial bursa, the bursa separating the acromion and deltoid muscle from the insertion of the supraspinatus muscle and the greater tubercle of the humerus.

subacute, **1.** less than acute. **2.** of or pertaining to a disease or other abnormal condition present in a person who appears to be clinically well. The condition may be identified or discovered by means of a laboratory test or by radiologic examination.

subacute bacterial endocarditis (SBE), a chronic bacterial infection of the valves of the heart, characterized by a slow, quiet onset with fever, heart murmur, splenomegaly, and the development of clumps of abnormal tissue, called vegetations, around an intracardiac prosthesis or on the flaps of a valve. Various species of *Streptococcus* or *Staphylococcus* are commonly the cause of SBE. Dental procedures are associated with infection by *Streptococcus viridans,* surgical procedures with *Streptococcus fecalis,* and self-infection (especially by drug abusers) with *Staphylococcus aureus.* See also **endocarditis, Janeway's spots.**

■ OBSERVATIONS: The infected vegetations may separate from the valve or prosthesis and form emboli. Oster's nodes, petechiae, Roth's spots, and splinter hemorrhages under the fingernails are common manifestations of blood-borne metastases of these emboli. Bacteriologic examination of cultures of the blood may allow specific diagnosis and treatment.

■ INTERVENTION: Treatment requires prolonged and regular administration of an antibiotic that is known to be effective against the causative organism. If a prosthesis has become infected, it is usually removed. Before surgery or a dental procedure, prophylactic antibiotics are given. During the acute phase of illness, the fever is treated with antipyretic medication and bed rest; adequate high-protein diet and fluids are encouraged.

■ NURSING CONSIDERATIONS: Sometimes bed rest and hospitalization may be necessary for several weeks. Emotional and psychological support from the nurse may help the patient to adjust to the necessary inactivity and to understand that SBE is a chronic illness.

subacute glomerulonephritis, an uncommon noninfectious disease of the glomerulus of the kidney characterized by proteinuria, hematuria, decreased production of urine, and edema. Of unknown cause, the disease may progress rapidly, and renal failure may occur. Kidney transplantation and dialysis are the only treatments available. See also **acute glomerulonephritis, chronic glomerulonephritis, uremia.**

subacute sclerosing panencephalitis, an uncommon, slow-virus infection caused by the measles virus and characterized by diffuse inflammation of brain tissue, personality change, seizures, blindness, dementia, fever, and death. The condition occurs in children and in adolescents who have had measles at a very early age. No effective therapy is known. See also **slow virus.**

subacute thyroiditis. See de Quervain's thyroiditis.

subarachnoid (səb'əræk'noid), situated under the arachnoid membrane and above the pia mater.

subarachnoid block anesthesia, a form of spinal anesthesia involving the injection of an anesthetic into the space between the arachnoidea and pia mater. This procedure is an especially effective form of rapid spinal anesthesia but one requiring great skill to avoid contamination or neurologic trauma. See also **obstetric anesthesia.**

subarachnoid hemorrhage (SaH, SAH), an intracranial hemorrhage into the cerebrospinal fluid-filled space between the arachnoid and pial membranes on the surface of the brain. The hemorrhage may extend into the brain if the force of the bleeding from the broken vessel is sudden and severe. The cause may be trauma, or rupture of a berry aneurysm or an arteriovenous anomaly.

■ OBSERVATIONS: The first symptom of a subarachnoid hemorrhage is a sudden extremely severe headache that begins in one localized area and then spreads, becoming dull and throbbing. The localized pain results from vascular distortion and injury. The generalized ache is the result of meningeal irritation from blood in the subarachnoid space. Other characteristics of subarachnoid hemorrhage include dizziness, rigidity of the neck, pupillary inequality, vomiting, drowsiness, sweating and chills, stupor, and loss of consciousness. A brief period of unconsciousness immediately following the rupture is common; severe hemorrhage may result in continued unconsciousness, coma, and death. Delirium and confusion often persist through the first weeks of recovery and permanent brain damage is not uncommon.

■ INTERVENTION: Observation of the initial localization of the headache may be diagnosistically important. Treatment has three basic goals: preservation of the person's life, limitation of disability, and prevention of recurrence. Bed rest is recommended for as long as four to six weeks. Care for the person who is unconscious owing to a subarachnoid hemorrhage is the same as for the person who is unconscious from other neurologic causes; an airway is maintained, the bladder is emptied, and fluid and electrolyte balance is maintained. The patient who is conscious needs relief from pain, especially in the first days after hemorrhage. Surgical repair of a vessel or excision of an aneurysm may be performed if the patient is conscious, relatively young, healthy, and normotensive.

■ NURSING CONSIDERATIONS: The person is given nothing by mouth for the first 24 hours. Because delirium and restlessness commonly occur, the staff tries to keep the environment around the patient quiet and nonstimulating. A family member may be encouraged to stay with the patient, and treatments, procedures, and examinations are kept to a minimum. Constipation is to be avoided, as straining to evacuate the bowel may raise intracranial pressure and cause another hemorrhage.

subcapital fracture, a fracture of tissue just distal to the head of a bone that pivots in a ball-and-socket joint, as the head of the femur.

subclavian (səbklei'viən), situated under the clavicle, as the subclavian vein.

subclavian artery, one of a pair of arteries that vary in origin, course, and the height to which they rise in the neck but having six similar main branches supplying the vertebral column, spinal cord, ear, and brain. See also **left subclavian artery, right subclavian artery.**

subclavian steal syndrome, a vascular syndrome caused by an occlusion in the subclavian artery proximal to the origin of the vertebral artery. The block results in a reversal of the normal blood pressure gradient in the vertebral artery and decreased blood flow distal to the occlusion. This condition is characterized by episodes of flaccid paralysis of the arm, pain in the mastoid and occipital areas, and a diminished or absent radial pulse on the involved side. Markedly different blood pressure measurements obtained from the arms are sometimes indicative of the condition.

subclavian vein, the continuation of the axillary vein in the upper body, extending from the lateral border of the first rib to the sternal end of the clavicle, where it joins the internal jugular to form the brachiocephalic vein. It usually contains a pair of valves near its junction with the internal jugular vein. The subclavian vein receives deoxygenated blood from the external jugular vein and, on the left side, at the junction with the internal jugular vein, receives lymph from the thoracic duct. On the right side, at the corresponding junction, it receives lymph from the right lymphatic duct.

subclavius (səbkleɪ′viəs), a short muscle of the chest wall. It is a small, cylindrical muscle between the clavicle and the first rib and arises in a short, thick tendon from the junction of the first rib and its cartilage. It inserts into the groove on the inferior surface of the clavicle between the costoclavicular and the conoid ligaments. The subclavius is innervated by a special nerve from the lateral trunk of the brachial plexus, which contains fibers from the fifth and sixth cervical nerves, and it acts to draw the shoulder down and forward. Compare **pectoralis major, pectoralis minor, serratus anterior.**

subclinical, of or pertaining to a disease or abnormal condition that is so mild it produces no symptoms.

subconscious, 1. imperfectly or partially conscious. 2. *Obsolete.* (in psychiatry) the preconscious and the unconscious. —**subconsciousness,** *n.*

subconscious memory, a thought, sensation, or feeling that is not immediately available for recall to the conscious mind.

subcutaneous (səb′kyuteɪ′niəs), beneath the skin.

subcutaneous fascia, a continuous layer of connective tissue over the entire body between the skin and the deep fascial investment of the specialized structures of the body, as the muscles. It is comprised of an outer, normally fatty layer, and an inner, thin elastic layer. Between the two layers lie superficial blood vessels, nerves, lymphatics, the mammary glands, most of the facial muscles, and the platysma. Compare **deep fascia, subserous fascia.**

subcutaneous fat necrosis. See **adiponecrosis subcutanea neonatorum.**

subcutaneous infusion. See **hypodermoclysis.**

subcutaneous injection, a hypodermic injection into the subcutaneous tissue beneath the skin, usually on the upper arm, thigh, or abdomen. A 24- or 25-gauge needle 2 cm long is used. The drug is prepared and drawn into the syringe. The cleansed area of skin is held flat by the thumb and forefinger to tense and steady the injection site. The needle is inserted at an angle of 45 to 60 degrees, piercing the skin quickly and advancing steadily to minimize the pain. The barrel or plunger is withdrawn slightly to ascertain whether or not the syringe of the needle has inadvertently entered a blood vessel. If no blood is aspirated, the drug is injected slowly, the needle is withdrawn, and the skin is massaged gently with a sterile alcohol sponge. Certain drugs that are extremely irritating to the skin are injected into the deep subcutaneous tissues using a variation of the technique. The skin tissue overlying the injection site is grasped with the thumb and forefinger but elevated in a roll, rather than tensed and flattened. The angle of injection may be as great as 90° to the skin. Heparin, insulin, and emetine are injected in this way. If subcutaneous injections are repeated, each is performed at least 5 cm from the previous site. A diagram of a plan for the rotation of injection sites helps to avoid overuse of one area of skin.

SUBCUTANEOUS INJECTION

subcutaneous mastectomy, a surgical procedure in which all the breast tissue of one or both breasts is removed leaving the skin, areola, and nipple intact. The adjacent lymph nodes and the pectoralis major and pectoralis minor are not removed. It may be performed on women who are at great risk of developing breast cancer. Reconstruction of the breasts is performed, with the assistance of a plastic surgeon, through the insertion of prostheses to return the normal contour to the breasts.

subcutaneous nodule, a small, solid boss, or node, beneath the skin that can be detected by touch. Subcutaneous nodules consisting chiefly of Aschoff bodies are found in patients with rheumatic fever. Minute subcutaneous nodules formed by the perivascular infiltration of mononuclear cells occur in typhus fever.

subcutaneous test. See **intradermal test.**

subdural (səbdur′əl), situated under the dura mater and above the arachnoid membrane.

suberosis (su′bərou′sɪs). See **cork worker's lung.**

subgerminal cavity. See **blastocoele.**

subinvolution, delayed or absent involution of the uterus during the postpartum period. The causes of subinvolution include retained fragments of placenta, uterine fibromyomas, and infection. Regardless of the cause of the condition, it is characterized by longer and heavier bleeding after childbirth and, on pelvic examination, a larger and softer uterus than would be expected at that time. Treatment includes ergonovine given by mouth for two or three days, and, if an infection is present, an antibiotic. The hemoglobin or hematocrit is also evaluated and iron is given if necessary. A follow-up examination is performed two weeks later.

subjective, 1. pertaining to the essential nature of an object as perceived in the mind rather than to a thing in itself. 2. existing only in the mind. 3. that which arises within or is perceived by the individual as contrasted with something that is modified by external circumstances or something that may be evaluated by objective standards. 4. a person who places excessive importance on his own moods, attitudes, or opinions; egocentric.

subjective data collection, the process in which data relating to the client's problem are elicited from the client. The interviewer encourages a full description of the onset, the course, and the character of the problem and any factors that aggravate or ameliorate it. Compare **objective data collection.**

sublethal gene, a gene whose presence causes abnormalities or impairs the functioning of an organism but does not cause its death. Compare **lethal gene.**

subleukemic leukemia, a malignant neoplasm characterized by anemia, thrombocytopenia, and abnormally functioning leukocytes that infiltrate tissues but are not present in circulating blood in abnormal numbers. Also called **aleukemic leukemia, aleukocythemic leukemia, hypocytic leukemia, leukopenic leukemia.**

sublimate, to refine or divert instinctual impulses and energy from their immediate goal to one that can be expressed in a social, moral, or aesthetic manner acceptable to the person and to society.

sublimation, 1. a defense mechanism by which an unacceptable instinctive drive is unconsciously diverted to and expressed through a personally approved, socially accepted means. 2. (in psychoanalysis) the process of diverting certain components of the sex drive to a socially acceptable, nonsexual goal. Compare **displacement.**

Sublimaze, a trade name for a narcotic analgesic (fentanyl), used as an adjunct to anesthesia.

Sublimaze Citrate, a trade name for a narcotic analgesic (fentanyl citrate).

subliminal, taking place below the threshold of sensory perception or outside the range of conscious awareness.

sublingual (səbliŋ'gwəl), beneath the tongue.

sublingual administration of a medication, the administration of a drug, usually in tablet form, by placing it beneath the tongue until the tablet dissolves.

sublingual duct. 1. See **Bartholin's duct.** 2. See **duct of Rivinus.**

sublingual gland, one of a pair of small salivary glands situated under the mucous membrane of the floor of the mouth, beneath the tongue. It is a narrow, almond-shaped structure, and weighs about two gm. It is in relation, inferiorly, with the mylohyoideus; posteriorly, with the submandibular gland; laterally, with the mandible; and medially, with the genioglossus from which it is separated

by the lingual nerve and the submandibular duct. It has from 8 to 20 ducts, some of which join to form the sublingual duct. The sublingual gland secretes mucus produced by its alveoli. Compare **parotid gland, submandibular gland.**

subluxation (səb'ləksei'shən), a partial dislocation.

submandibular duct, a duct through which a submandibular gland secretes saliva. Also called **submaxillary duct.**

submandibular gland, one of a pair of round, walnutsized salivary glands in the submandibular triangle, reaching anteriorly to the anterior belly of the diagastricus and posteriorly to the stylomandibular ligament. The ligament lies between the submandibular gland and the parotid gland. The submandibular gland extends superiorly under the inferior border of the mandible and extends a deep process anteriorly above the mylohyoideus muscle. The upper portion of the superficial surface of the gland lies partly against the submandibular depression on the inner surface of the mandible and partly on the pterygoideus medialis. The lower part is covered by skin, superficial fascia, platysma, and deep cervical fascia. The submandibular duct is about 5 cm long, starts at the deep surface of the gland, runs between the sublingual gland and the genioglossus, and opens on a small papilla at the side of the frenulum linguae. The gland secretes both mucus and a thinner serous fluid, which aid the digestive process. Compare **sublingual gland, parotid gland.** See also **salivary gland.**

submaxillary duct. See **submandibular duct.**

submetacentric (səb'metəsen'trik), pertaining to a chromosome in which the centromere is located approximately equidistant between the center and one end so that the arms of the chromatids are not equal in length. Compare **acrocentric, metacentric, telocentric.**

submucous, beneath a mucous membrane.

subperiosteal fracture (səb'perios'tiəl), a fracture in a bone beneath the periosteum and does not disrupt the periosteal covering.

subpoena, (in law) a document from a court commanding that a person appear at a certain time and place to testify on a specific matter. Subpoenas are governed by federal rules for criminal procedure or for civil procedure.

subpoena duces tecum, (in law) a subpoena commanding a person to bring books, papers, records, or other items to the court.

subserous fascia, one of three kinds of fascia, lying between the internal layer of deep fascia and the serous membranes lining the body cavities in much the same manner as the subcutaneous fascia lies between the skin and the deep fascia. It is thin in some areas, as between the pleura and the chest wall, and thick in other areas, where it forms a pad of adipose tissue. Compare **deep fascia, subcutaneous fascia.**

subspecialty, (in nursing) a nurse's particular professional and highly specialized field of practice, as nursing in dialysis, oncology, neurology, or newborn intensive care. Compare **specialty.**

substance P, a neurotransmitting substance that is synthesized by the body and acts to stimulate vasodilation and contraction of intestinal and other smooth muscles. It also plays a part in salivary secretion, diuresis, and natriuresis, and it affects the function of the peripheral and central nervous systems. It has been isolated from certain cells of the gastrointestinal and biliary tracts.

substernal goiter, an enlargement of the thyroid gland, a portion of which is beneath the sternum.

subthalamus (sǝbſhæl'ǝmǝs), a portion of the diencephalon that serves as a correlations center for optic and vestibular impulses relayed to the globus pallidus. It is a transition zone between the thalamus and the tegmentum mesencephali, squeezed between the cerebral peduncle and the mammillary area. It accommodates prolongations of the red nucleus and the substantia nigra and contains fibrous masses of the fields of Forel. Compare **epithalamus, hypothalamus, metathalamus, thalamus.** — **subthalamic,** *adj.*

subtle, having a low intensity; not severe and having no serious sequelae, as a mild infection or inflammation.

subungual (sǝbʌŋ'gwǝl), under a finger- or toenail.

subungual hematoma, a collection of blood beneath a nail, usually resulting from trauma. The pain accompanying this condition may be quickly alleviated by burning or drilling a small hole through the nail to release the blood.

succ-, a combining form meaning 'of or pertaining to a juice': *succagogue, succorrhea, succus.*

succinic acid (sʌksɪn'ɪk), a compound found in certain hydatid cysts and in lichens, amber, and fossils. Commercial succinic acid, produced by the fermentation of ammonium tartrate, is used in lacquer and dyes. Succinic acid was formerly used in the treatment of diabetic ketoacidosis.

Succinyl-Astra (sǝk'sɪnǝlæs'trǝ), a trade name for a muscle relaxant (succinylcholine chloride), used as an adjunct to anesthesia.

succinylcholine chloride (sǝk'sɪnɪlkoʊ'lin), a skeletal muscle relaxant.

■ INDICATIONS: It is prescribed as an adjunct to anesthesia or to reduce muscle contractions caused by pharmacologically or electrically induced convulsions.

■ CONTRAINDICATIONS: Known hypersensitivity to this drug prohibits its use. Caution is used in administering this drug to patients with low pseudocholinesterase levels and in patients with myasthenia gravis or renal failure.

■ ADVERSE EFFECTS: Among the more serious adverse reactions are cardiac arrhythmia and severe respiratory depression.

succus (sǝk'ǝs), *pl.* **succi** (sǝk'sai). a juice or fluid, usually one secreted by an organ of the digestive tract.

succussion splash (sǝkǝsh'ǝn), the sound elicited by shaking the body of an individual who has free fluid and air or gas in a hollow organ or body cavity. This sound may be present over a normal stomach but may also be heard with hydropneumothorax, large hiatal hernia, or intestinal or pyloric obstruction.

suck, 1. to draw a liquid or semiliquid into the mouth by creating a partial vacuum through motions of the lips and tongue. 2. to hold on the tongue and dissolve by the movements of the mouth and action of the saliva. 3. to draw fluid into the mouth, specifically to draw milk from the breast or nursing bottle.

sucking blisters, the pale, soft pads on the upper and lower lips of a baby that look like blisters but are not. They form as soon as the baby begins to suck well, at the breast or on a bottle. They seem to augment the seal of the lips around the nipple or breast. Some babies are born with them, having sucked on their own fingers, hand, or arm before birth.

sucking reflex, involuntary sucking movements of the circumoral area in newborns in response to stimulation. The reflex continues throughout infancy and often occurs without stimulation, as during sleep. Compare **rooting reflex.**

suckle, 1. to provide nourishment, specifically to breast feed. 2. to take in as nourishment, especially by feeding from the breast.

suckling, an infant that has not been weaned.

Sucostrin, a trade name for a depolarizing agent (succinylcholine), used as an adjunct to anesthesia.

Sucostrin Chloride, a trade name for a skeletal muscle relaxant (succinylcholine chloride).

sucrose, sugar derived from sugar cane, sugar beets, and sorghum.

sucrose polyester (SPE), a synthetic, nonabsorbable fat that, when added to the diet, reduces plasma cholesterol levels by increasing the excretion of cholesterol in the feces. It is formulated to have the characteristic texture, taste, and consistency of regular margarine or vegetable oil and adds no calories to the diet.

suction curettage, a method of curettage in which a specimen of the endometrium or the products of conception are removed by aspiration. Under local or light general anesthesia the cervix is dilated, a catheter is introduced into the uterus, and suction is applied. Postoperative care includes monitoring vital signs for symptoms of blood loss. Also called **vacuum aspiration.** Compare **dilatation and curettage.**

suction drainage. See **drainage.**

Sudafed, a trade name for an adrenergic vasoconstrictor (pseudoephedrine hydrochloride), used as a decongestant and bronchodilator.

sudden infant death syndrome (SIDS), the unexpected and sudden death of an apparently normal and healthy infant that occurs during sleep and with no physical or autopsic evidence of disease. It is the most common cause of death in children between the ages of two weeks and one year, with an incidence rate of one in every 300 to 350 live births. The etiology is unknown but multiple causes have been proposed, including lack of biotin in the diet, abnormality of the endogenous-opioid system, mechanical suffocation, a defect in respiratory mucosal defense, prolonged apnea, an unknown virus, anatomical abnormality of the larynx, and immunoglobulin abnormalities. It is known that the condition occurs more often in infants 10 to 14 weeks old, especially those born prematurely, in males more often than in females, during the winter months, that it is seen more often among babies who have recently had a minor illness such as upper respiratory infection, or in infants born to women less than 20 years of age who have had at least one previous child, who begin prenatal care in the third trimester, or who smoke or are anemic or drug dependent. The syndrome is neither contagious nor hereditary, although there is a greater than average risk of its occurrence within the same family, which may indicate the influence of polygenic factors. Controversy exists as to whether or not home monitoring systems are of value for infants who are at risk or who have had a "near miss" episode. Nursing considerations consist predominantly of support and counseling, as assessing how the parents feel about the death in order to help them through the resolution of grief, learning what they know about the syndrome and supplying them with whatever information and literature they need, finding out how they are coping with any guilt feelings, and how the siblings, if any, are coping with the death. The nurse can also supply information about local groups of parents who have lost a child from SIDS. Also called **cot death, crib death.** See also **parental grief.**

sudo-, a combining form meaning 'of or pertaining to sweat': *sudogram, sudokeratosis, sudorrhea.*

sudoriferous duct, a duct leading from a sweat gland to the surface of the skin. Also called **sweat duct.**

sudoriferous gland, one of about three million tiny structures within the dermis that produce sweat. The average quantity of sweat secreted in 24 hours varies from 700 to 900 gm. Most of these glands are eccrine glands, producing sweat which carries away sodium chloride, the waste products urea and lactic acid, and the breakdown products from garlic, spices, and other substances. Apocrine sweat glands associated with the coarse hair of the armpits and the pubic region are larger and secrete fluid which is much thicker than that secreted by the eccrine glands. Each sudoriferous gland consists of a single tube with a deeply coiled body and a superficial duct. In the superficial layers of the dermis the duct is straight; in the

deeper layers it is convoluted. In the thick dermis of the palms of the hands and the soles of the feet the duct is spirally coiled. The number of glands per square centimeter of skin varies in different parts of the body, the sudoriferous glands being very plentiful on the palms of the hands and on the soles of the feet and least numerous in the neck and the back; they are completely absent in the deeper portions of the external auditory meatus, the prepuce, and the glans penis, and are more numerous in the fingers of Filipinos, Hindus, and American Negroes than in the fingers of American whites. Compare **sebaceous gland.**

sudorific (su'dərıfık), **1.** of or pertaining to a substance or condition, as heat or emotional tension, that promotes sweating. **2.** a sudorific agent. Sweat glands are stimulated by cholinergic drugs. The alkaloid pilocarpine is a potent sudorific drug, but it is rarely used for that purpose in modern medicine. Also called **diaphoretic.**

suf-. See **sub-.**

suffix, a portion of a word occurring at the end of a compound word. In this dictionary, a suffix is called a "combining form." In the words *appendectomy, bronchoscopy, nephrology, pharyngitis,* and *tracheotomy,* the suffixes are *-ectomy, -scopy, -logy, -itis,* and *-tomy.* Compare **prefix.**

suffocative goiter, an enlargement of the thyroid gland causing a sensation of suffocation on pressure.

sugar, any of several water-soluble carbohydrates. The two principal categories of sugars are monosaccharides and disaccharides. A monosaccharide is a single sugar, as glucose, fructose, or galactose. A disaccharide is a double sugar, as sucrose (table sugar) or lactose. See also **carbohydrate, fructose, galactose, glucose, saccharide, sucrose.**

sugar alcohol, an alcohol produced by the reduction of an aldehyde or ketone of a sugar.

suggestion, **1.** the process by which one thought or idea leads to another, as in the association of ideas. **2.** the use of persuasion, exhortation, or other device to implant an idea, thought, attitude, or belief in the mind of another as a means of influencing or altering behavior or states of mind. See also **hypnosis. 3.** an idea, belief, or attitude implanted in the mind of another. Compare **autosuggestion.**

Sugracillin, a trade name for an antibacterial (penicillin G potassium).

suicidal, of, relating to, or tending toward self-destruction.

suicidal melancholia, *Obsolete.* a state of severe depression in which suicidal tendencies are prominent. See also **suicidal.**

suicide, **1.** the intentional taking of one's own life. **2.** *Informal.* the ruin or destruction of one's own interests. **3.** a person who commits or attempts self-destruction. Early signs of suicidal intent include depression; expressions of guilt, tension, and agitation; insomnia; loss of weight and appetite; neglect of personal appearance; and direct or indirect threats to commit suicide.

suicide gesture, (in psychiatric nursing) an apparent attempt by a patient to cause self-injury without lethal consequences and generally without actual intent to commit suicide. A suicide gesture serves to attract attention to the patient's disturbed emotional status but is not as serious as a suicide attempt.

suicidolgy (su'ɪsaɪdol'əji), the study of the prevention and the causes of suicide. – **suicidologist,** *n.*

Suladyne, a trade name for an anti-infective, fixed-combination drug containing antibacterials (sulfamethizole and sulfadiazine) and a urinary antiseptic (phenazopyridine hydrochloride).

Sulamyd Sodium, a trade name for an antibacterial (sulfacetamide sodium).

sulcus (səl'kəs), *pl.* **sulci** (səl'saɪ). a shallow groove, a depression, or a furrow on the surface of an organ, as a sulcus that separates the convolutions of the cerebral hemisphere. A sulcus is usually not as deep as a fissure, but, in the terminology of anatomy, *sulcus* and *fissure* are often used interchangeably. – **sulcate,** *adj.*

sulcus centralis cerebri. See **fissure of Rolando.**

sulcus pulmonalis, a depression on each side of the vertebral bodies that accommodates the posterior portion of the lung.

Sulfacel-15, a trade name for an antibacterial (sulfacetamide sodium).

sulfacetamide (səl'fæset'əmaɪd), a topical antibacterial.
■ INDICATIONS: It is most commonly prescribed for the prophylaxis of infection after injury to the cornea and in the treatment of bacterial conjunctivitis.
■ CONTRAINDICATION: Known hypersensitivity to the drug or to other sulfonamides prohibits its use.
■ ADVERSE EFFECT: The only known adverse effect is hypersensitivity reaction to the drug.

sulfacetamide sodium, a sulfonamide antibacterial agent.
■ INDICATIONS: It is prescribed in the prophylaxis of infection following corneal injury and in the treatment of some forms of acute bacterial conjunctivitis.
■ CONTRAINDICATION: Known hypersensitivity to this drug prohibits its use.
■ ADVERSE EFFECTS: Among the more serious adverse reactions are allergic reactions and local irritation.

Sulfacet-R, a trade name for a topical, fixed-combination drug containing a scabicide (sulfur), an antibacterial (sulfacetamide sodium), and an antiseptic and astringent (zinc oxide).

sulfachlorpyridazine (səl'fəklɔr'oupɪrɪd'əzin), a sulfonamide antibacterial.
■ INDICATIONS: It is prescribed in the treatment of infection, particularly of the urinary tract.
■ CONTRAINDICATIONS: Porphyria, urinary tract obstruc-

tion, or known hypersensitivity to this or to other sulfonamides prohibits its use.
■ ADVERSE EFFECTS: Among the more serious adverse reactions are crystalluria, severe allergic reactions, photosensitivity, and blood dyscrasias.

sulfacytine, a sulfonamide antibacterial.
■ INDICATION: It is prescribed in the treatment of infection, particularly of the urinary tract.
■ CONTRAINDICATIONS: Porphyria, urinary tract obstruction, or known hypersensitivity to sulfonamides prohibits its use.
■ ADVERSE EFFECTS: Among the more serious adverse reactions are crystalluria, photosensitivity, severe allergic reactions, and blood dyscrasias.

sulfadiazine (səl'fədaɪ'əzin), a sulfonamide antibacterial.
■ INDICATION: It is prescribed in the treatment of infection, particularly of the urinary tract.
■ CONTRAINDICATIONS: Porphyria, urinary tract obstruction, or known hypersensitivity to sulfonamides prohibits its use.
■ ADVERSE EFFECTS: Among the more serious adverse effects are crystalluria, photosensitivity, severe allergic reactions, and blood dyscrasias.

sulfameter, a long-acting sulfonamide antibacterial.
■ INDICATIONS: It is prescribed in the treatment of urinary tract infections.
■ CONTRAINDICATIONS: Porphyria, urinary tract obstruction, or known hypersensitivity to this drug or to other sulfonamide medications prohibits its use. It is not given to children under 12 years of age.
■ ADVERSE EFFECTS: Among the more serious adverse reactions are crystalluria, blood dyscrasias, and severe hypersensitivity, reactions, including Stevens-Johnson syndrome.

sulfamethazine, an antibacterial sulfonamide; salicylazosulfapuridine.
■ INDICATION: It is prescribed in the treatment of certain infections, especially of the urinary tract.
■ CONTRAINDICATIONS: Porphyria, urinary tract obstruction, or known hypersensitivity to this drug or to other sulfonamide medication prohibits its use.
■ ADVERSE EFFECTS: Among the more serious adverse reactions are crystalluria, blood dyscrasias, and severe hypersensitivity reactions.

sulfamethizole, a sulfonamide antibacterial.
■ INDICATION: It is prescribed in the treatment of infection, particularly of the urinary tract.
■ CONTRAINDICATIONS: Porphyria, urinary tract obstruction, or known hypersensitivity to sulfonamides prohibits its use.
■ ADVERSE EFFECTS: Among the more serious adverse reactions are crystalluria, photosensitivity, blood dyscrasias, and severe allergic reactions.

sulfamethoxazole, a sulfonamide antibacterial.

■ INDICATIONS: It is prescribed in the treatment of certain infections, especially of the urinary tract.

■ CONTRAINDICATIONS: It is not given during the last trimester of pregnancy, during lactation, or to children under two months of age. Known hypersensitivity to this drug or other sulfonamides prohibits its use.

■ ADVERSE EFFECTS: Among the more serious adverse reactions are crystalluria and rash, fever, and other allergic reactions.

sulfamethoxazole and trimethoprim, a fixed-combination antibacterial.

■ INDICATIONS: It is prescribed in the treatment of urinary tract infections, otitis media, and shigellosis.

■ CONTRAINDICATIONS: It is used with caution in patients with impaired renal or hepatic function, with possible folate deficiency, or in patients with known hypersensitivity to either drug or to sulfonomides. It is not recommended for use in infants under two months of age or in the third trimester of pregnancy.

■ ADVERSE EFFECTS: Among the more serious adverse reactions are crystalluria and rashes, fever, and other allergic reactions.

sulfamethoxypyridazine, a long-acting sulfonamide antibacterial.

■ INDICATION: It is prescribed in the treatment of infections of the urinary tract.

■ CONTRAINDICATIONS: Urinary tract obstruction, porphyria, or known hypersensitivity to this drug or to other sulfonamide medications prohibits its use.

■ ADVERSE EFFECTS: Among the more serious adverse effects are crystalluria, blood dyscrasias, and severe hypersensitivity reactions.

Sulfamylon, a trade name for a topical anti-infective (mafenide acetate).

sulfanilic acid (səl'fənɪl'ɪk), a red-tinged, white crystalline compound used in the synthesis of sulfonamides and as a reagent in tests for phenol, fecal matter in water, albumen, aldehydes, and glucose. Also called **anilinparasulfonic acid.**

Sulfapred, a trade name for a topical fixed-combination drug containing a glucocorticoid (prednisolone acetate), an antibacterial, (sulfacetamide sodium), and an adrenergic (phenylephrine hydrochloride).

sulfapyridine (səl'fəpɪr'ədin), a sulfonamide antibacterial.

■ INDICATION: It is prescribed in the treatment of dermatitis herpetiformis.

■ CONTRAINDICATIONS: Porphyria, urinary tract obstruction, or known hypersensitivity to sulfonamides prohibits its use.

■ ADVERSE EFFECTS: Among the more serious adverse reactions are crystalluria, blood dyscrasias, and severe allergic reactions.

sulfasalazine, a sulfonamide; salicylazosulfapyridine.

■ INDICATION: It is prescribed in the treatment of ulcerative colitis.

■ CONTRAINDICATIONS: Urinary obstruction, porphyria, or known hypersensitivity to this drug, to other sulfonamide medication, or to salicylates prohibits its use. It is not given during the last trimester of pregnancy.

■ ADVERSE EFFECTS: Among the more serious adverse reactions are crystalluria, blood dyscrasias, and severe hypersensitivity reactions. Gastrointestinal symptoms and anorexia commonly occur.

sulfate, a salt of sulfuric acid. A sulfate is usually a combination of a metal with sulfuric acid. Natural sulfates, as sodium sulfate, calcium sulfate, and potassium sulfate, are plentiful in the body.

sulfathiazole (səl'fəfhæi'əzoul), a sulfonamide antibacterial no longer commonly used.

sulfhemoglobin, a form of hemoglobin containing an irreversibly bound sulfur molecule that prevents normal oxygen binding. It is present in the blood in trace amounts.

sulfinpyrazone (səl'fɪnpɪr'əzoun), a uricosuric.

■ INDICATION: It is prescribed in the treatment of chronic gout.

■ CONTRAINDICATIONS: Peptic ulcer, ulcerative colitis, renal dysfunction, or known hypersensitivity to this drug or to phenylbutazone prohibits its use. It is not usually given during an acute attack of gout.

■ ADVERSE EFFECTS: Among the more serious adverse reactions are gastrointestinal ulcers, blood dyscrasias, and dermatitis.

sulfisoxazole, a sulfonamide antibacterial.

■ INDICATION: It is prescribed in the treatment of urinary tract infections.

■ CONTRAINDICATIONS: Porphyria, urinary tract obstruction, or known hypersensitivity to this drug or to sulfonamide medication prohibits its use. It is not given during the last trimester of pregnancy or to children under two months of age.

■ ADVERSE EFFECTS: Among the more serious adverse reactions are crystalluria, blood dyscrasias, and severe hypersensitivity reactions.

sulfo-, a combining form naming chemical compounds, showing presence of divalent sulfur or of the group SO_2OH: *sulfoamide, sulfomethane, sulfophenol.*

sulfobromophthalein (səl'fəbrou'məfhæl'in, səl'fəbrou'-məfhæl'iɪn), a substance used in its disodium salt form for evaluating the function of the liver. See also **Bromsulphalein test.**

sulfonamide, (səlfon'əmaid'), one of a large group of synthetic, bacteriostatic drugs that are effective in treating infections caused by many gram-negative and gram-positive microorganisms. The drugs act by preventing the normal growth, development, and multiplication of the bacteria but do not kill mature organisms. They are bacteriostatic rather than bactericidal. Some sulfonamides are short-acting, some are intermediate-acting, and some are long-acting, depending on the speed with which they are excreted. They are used in treating many urinary tract infections. In the past they have been used to treat gramnegative enteric infections, including those caused by species of Shigella, and as a 'bowel prep' before and after intestinal surgery. Some people are hypersensitive to the drugs. Sulfonamides are given with caution to people who have impaired liver or kidney function, and they are not given in the last trimester of pregnancy or to young infants, as mental retardation sometimes occurs. Hemolytic anemia, agranulocytosis, thrombocytopenia, or aplastic anemia, drug fever, and jaundice may occur, particularly with long-acting sulfonamides given for more than ten days. Dosage varies with the particular drug and with the age, size, and condition of the person. Most sulfonamides are given orally.

sulfonylurea (səl'fənɪlyʊriə), an oral antidiabetic agent that stimulates the pancreatic production of insulin. Hypersensitivity to sulfonamides is a contraindication for using such agents, and ethanol consumption is incompatible with all sulfonylureas. The safety of these drugs for use in pregnant women has not been established, making insulin the preferred drug in treating diabetes in pregnancy. Aspirin or other salicylates taken with any sulfonylurea intensifies the hypoglycemic effect.

sulfosalicylic acid (səl'fousælɪsɪl'ɪk), a white or faintly pink crystalline substance that is highly water-soluble, used as a reagent in tests for albumin and as an intermediate compound in the manufacture of dyes and surfactants.

Sulfose, a trade name for an antibacterial (trisulfapyrimidines).

Sulfoxyl, a trade name for a topical fixed-combination drug containing a disinfectant (benzoyl peroxide) and a scabicide (sulfur).

sulfur, sulphur (S), a nonmetallic, multivalent, tasteless, odorless chemical element that occurs abundantly in yellow crystalline form or in masses, especially in volcanic areas. Its atomic number is 16; its atomic weight is 32.006. It is used to produce sulfuric acid and used commercially in metallurgy, rubber vulcanization, petroleum refining, and many other industrial processes. Sulfur has been used in the treatment of gout, rheumatism, and bronchitis and as a mild laxative. The sulfonamides, or sulfa drugs, are used in the treatment of various bacterial infections.

-sulfuric, a combining form meaning 'compounds containing sulfur, especially in its highest valences': *hydrosulfuric, persulfuric, thiosulfuric.* Also **-sulphuric.**

sulfuric acid, a clear, colorless, oily, highly corrosive liquid that generates great heat when mixed with water.

An extremely toxic substance, sulfuric acid causes severe skin burns, blindness on contact with the eyes, serious lung damage if the vapors are inhaled, and death if it is ingested. In industry, sulfuric acid is used in the manufacture of fertilizers, dyes, glue, and other acids, in the purifying of petroleum, and in the pickling of metals. Weak solutions of sulfuric acid are used in the treatment of gastric hypoacidity and serous diarrhea. It was formerly called **oil of vitriol.**

sulindac, an anti-inflammatory agent.

■ INDICATIONS: It is prescribed in the treatment of arthritis and ankylosing spondylitis.

■ CONTRAINDICATIONS: Pregnancy, lactation, or known hypersensitivity to this drug, to aspirin, or to nonsteroidal anti-inflammatory drugs prohibits its use. It is used with caution in patients who have upper gastrointestinal tract disease or impaired renal function.

■ ADVERSE EFFECTS: Among the more serious adverse reactions are gastrointestinal upset, peptic ulcer, dizziness, tinnitus, and skin rash. This drug interacts with many other drugs.

Sulkowitch's test (səl'kawɪtʃ), an examination of the urine for the presence of calcium. A reagent, containing oxalic acid, ammonium oxalate, and glacial acetic acid, mixed with urine, causes calcium to precipitate out of the urine. Also called **S's test.** See also **hypercalciuria.**

Sulla, a trade name for an antibacterial (sulfameter).

Sultrin, a trade name for a vaginal fixed-combination drug containing antibacterials (sulfathiazole, sulfacetamide, and sulfabenzamide).

summary judgment, (in law) a judgment requested by any party to a civil action to end the action when it is believed that there is no genuine issue or material fact in dispute. Summary judgment may be directed toward part or all of a claim or defense and may be based on the proceedings in court or on affadavits or other outside materials.

summation, 1. an accumulative effect or action; a total aggregate; totality. 2. (in neurology), the accumulation of the concentration of a neurotransmitter at a synapse, either by increasing the frequency of nerve impulses in each fiber (temporal summation) or by increasing the number of fibers stimulated (spatial summation), so that the threshold of the postsynaptic neuron is overcome and an impulse is transmitted. See also **facilitation,** def. 2.

summons, (in law) a document issued by a clerk of the court upon the filing of a complaint. A sheriff, marshall, or other appointed person serves the summons, notifying a person that an action has been begun against him. See also **service of process.**

Sumycin, a trade name for an antibiotic (tetracycline hydrochloride).

sun bath, the exposure of the naked body to the sun.

Sundare, a trade name for an ultraviolet screen (cinoxate).

sundowning, a condition in which elderly institutionalized patients tend to become confused or disoriented at the end of the day. Many of them have diminished visual acuity and varying degrees of sensorineural and conduction hearing loss. With less light, they lose visual cues that help them to compensate for their sensory impairments.

sunstroke, a morbid condition caused by overexposure to the sun and characterized by a high fever, convulsions, and coma. See also **heat hyperpyrexia.**

sup-. See **sub-.**

Supen, a trade name for an antibacterial (ampicillin).

super-, a combining form meaning 'above, or implying excess': *superduct, superfunction, supernumerary.*

superego (su′pəri′gou, su′pəreg′ou), (in psychoanalysis) that part of the psyche, functioning mostly in the unconscious, that develops as the standards of the parents and of society are incorporated into the ego. The superego has two parts, the conscience and the ego ideal. See also **ego, ego ideal, id.**

superfecundation, the fertilization of two or more ova released during one menstrual cycle by spermatozoa from the same or different males during separate acts of sexual intercourse.

superfetation, the fertilization of a second ovum after the onset of pregnancy, resulting in the presence of two fetuses of different degrees of maturity developing within the uterus simultaneously. Also called **superimpregnation.**

superficial, 1. of or pertaining to the skin or another surface. 2. not grave or dangerous.

superficial fading infantile hemangioma, a superficial, transient, salmon-colored patch in the center of the forehead, face, or occiput of many newborns. It fades during the first two years of life, but it may temporarily deepen in color if the child becomes flushed or angry.

superficial implantation, (in embryology) the partial embedding of the blastocyst within the uterine wall so that it and, later, the chorionic sac protrude into the uterine cavity. Also called **central implantation, circumferential implantation.**

superficial inguinal node, a node in one of the two groups of inguinal lymph glands in the upper femoral triangle of the thigh. The nodes form a chain distal to the inguinal ligament and receive afferents from the skin of the penis, scrotum, perineum, buttocks, and abdominal wall below the level of the umbilicus. Compare **anterior tibial node, popliteal node.**

superficial reflex, any neural reflex initiated by stimulation of the skin. Kinds of superficial reflexes are **abdominal reflex, cremasteric reflex.** Compare **deep tendon reflex.**

superficial sensation, the awareness or perception of feelings in the superficial layers of the skin in response to touch, pressure, temperature, and pain. Such sensations are conveyed to the brain via the spinothalamic system. Compare **deep sensation.**

superficial spreading melanoma, a melanoma that grows outward, spreading over the surface of the affected organ or tissue, most commonly on the lower legs of women. Occurring in late middle age, it is raised and palpable, is usually unevenly pigmented, and has an irregular shape and unclear border.

superficial temporal artery, an artery at each side of the head that can be easily felt in front of the ear and is often used for taking the pulse. It is the smaller of the two terminal branches of the external carotid and arises in the substance of the parotid gland. It crosses the zygomatic process of the temporal bone and about 5 cm above the process divides into the frontal branch and the parietal branch. Compare **deep temporal artery, middle temporal artery.**

superficial vein, one of the many veins between the subcutaneous fascia just under the skin. Compare **deep vein.**

superimpregnation. See **superfetation.**

superinfection, an infection occurring during antimicrobial treatment for another infection. It is usually a result of change in the normal tissue flora favoring replication of some organisms by diminishing the vitality and then the number of competing organisms, as yeast microbes flourish during penicillin therapy prescribed to cure a bacterial infection.

Superinone, a trade name for a detergent (tyloxapol.)

superior, situated above or oriented toward a higher place as the head is superior to the torso. Compare **inferior.**

superior aperture of minor pelvis, an opening bounded by the crest and pecten of the pubic bones, the arch-shaped lines of the ilia, and the anterior margin of the base of the sacrum.

superior aperture of thorax, an elliptical opening at the summit of the thorax bounded by the first thoracic vertebra, the first ribs, and the upper margin of the sternum.

superior costotransverse ligament, one of five ligaments associated with each costotransverse joint, except that of the first rib. It passes from the neck of each rib to the transverse process of the vertebra immediately above and is associated with the intercostal vessels and the intercostal nerves. The first rib has no superior costotransverse ligament. Compare **posterior costotransverse ligament.**

superior gastric node, a node in one of two sets of gastric lymph glands, accompanying the left gastric artery, and divided into the upper group of nodes on the stem of the artery, the lower group of nodes accompanying branches of the artery along the cardiac half of the lesser curvature of the stomach, and the paracardial group of nodes around the neck of the stomach. The superior gastric nodes receive their afferents from the stomach and pass their efferents to the celiac group of preaortic nodes. Compare **inferior gastric node.**

superior hemorrhagic polioencephalitis. See **Wernicke's encephalopathy.**

superior mediastinum, the cranial portion of the mediastinum in the middle of the thorax, containing the trachea, the esophagus, the aortic arch, and the origins of the sternohyoidei and the sternothyroidei. The superior mediastinum is bounded by the superior aperture of the thorax, the plane of the superior limit of the pericardium, the manubrium, the upper four thoracic vertebrae, and laterally by the mediastinal aspect of the parietal pleurae of the lungs. Compare **anterior mediastinum, middle mediastinum, posterior mediastinum.**

superior mesenteric artery, a visceral branch of the abdominal aorta, arising caudal to the celiac artery, dividing into five branches, and supplying most of the small intestine and parts of the colon. The branches are the inferior pancreaticoduodenal, intestinal, ileocolic, right colic, and middle colic.

superior mesenteric node, a node in one of the three groups of visceral lymph nodes that serve the viscera of the abdomen and the pelvis. The superior mesenteric nodes are associated with branches of the superior mesenteric artery and are divided into mesenteric nodes, iliocolic nodes, and mesocolic nodes. Compare **gastric node, inferior mesenteric node.**

superior mesenteric vein, a tributary of the portal vein that drains the blood from the small intestine, the cecum, and the ascending and the transverse colons. It begins in the right iliac fossa, ascends between the two mesenteric layers to the right of the superior mesenteric artery, and joins the lienal vein to form the portal vein, dorsal to the neck of the pancreas. The tributaries of the superior mesenteric vein are the intestinal vein, the ileocolic vein, the right colic vein, the middle colic vein, the gastroepiploic vein, and the pancreaticoduodenal vein. See also **portal vein.**

superior profunda artery. See **deep brachial artery.**

superior radioulnar joint. See **proximal radioulnar articulation.**

superior sagittal sinus, one of the six venous channels in the posterior of the dura mater, draining blood from the brain into the internal jugular vein. It has no valves and presents a triangular section as the sinus courses posteriorly through a groove in the frontal bone and passes along the convex margin of the falx cerebri to the occipital protuberance, usually continuing as the right transverse sinus. The superior sagittal sinus receives the superior cerebral veins, veins from the diploe, and, near the posterior extremity of the sagittal suture, the anasto-

mosing emissary veins from the pericranium and the veins from the dura mater. It also anastomoses with veins of the nose, the scalp, and the diploe. Compare **inferior sagittal sinus, straight sinus, transverse sinus.**

superior subscapular nerve (səbskæp′yulər), one of two small nerves on opposite sides of the body that arise from the posterior cord of the brachial plexus. It supplies the superior part of the subscapularis. Compare **inferior subscapular nerve.**

superior thyroid artery, one of a pair of arteries in the neck, usually rising from the external carotid artery, that supplies the thyroid gland and several muscles in the head.

superior ulnar collateral artery, a long, slender division of the brachial artery, arising just distal to the middle of the arm, descending to the elbow, and anastomosing with the posterior ulnar recurrent and inferior ulnar collateral arteries.

superior vena cava, the second largest vein of the body, returning deoxygenated blood from the upper half of the body to the right atrium. It is about two cm in diameter and seven cm long and is formed by the junction of the two brachiocephalic veins at the level of the first intercostal space behind the sternum on the right side. The section of the superior vena cava closest to the heart comprises about half of the vessel's length and is within the pericardial sac, covered by the serous pericardium. It has no valves and just before it enters the pericardium, receives the azygous vein and several small pericardial veins. Compare **inferior vena cava.**

Supertah, a trade name for an antieczematic ointment containing coal tar, zinc oxide, and starch.

supervisor, (in hospital or public health nursing) the midlevel management position between the director of nursing and head nurses of a division or of several units. The title is sometimes considered old-fashioned; in many hospitals 'clinical director' is preferred. The supervisor's responsibilities are primarily administrative, although they may also include clinical leadership for the nurses working in a group of units, wards, or divisions.

supination (su′pɪneɪ′ʃən), **1.** the position of lying on the back, face up. **2.** one of the kinds of rotation allowed by certain skeletal joints, as the elbow and the wrist joints, which allow the palm of the hand to turn up. Compare **pronation.** —**supinate,** v., **supine,** adj.

supinator longus (su′pɪneɪ′tər). See **brachioradialis.**

supine (səpaɪn′, su′paɪn), lying horizontaly on the back. Compare **prone.** See also **body position.**

supplemental inheritance, the acquisition or expression of a genetic trait or condition from the presence of two independent pairs of nonallelic genes that interact in such a way that one gene supplements the action of the other.

supplementary gene, one of two pairs of nonallelic genes that interact in such a way that one pair needs the presence of the other to be expressed, while the other pair can produce an effect independent of the first.

support, 1. to sustain, hold up, or maintain in a desired position or condition, as in physically supporting the abdominal muscles with a scultetis binder or emotionally supporting a client under stress. 2. the assistance given to this end, as physical support, emotional support, or life support.

supportive psychotherapy, a form of psychotherapy that concentrates on creating an effective means of communication with an emotionally disturbed person rather than on trying to produce psychological insight into his underlying conflicts. Through such supportive measures as reassurance, reinforcement of the person's defenses, direction, suggestion, and persuasion, the therapist participates directly in the solution of specific problems. Compare **nondirective therapy.**

supportive treatment. See **treatment.**

suppository, an easily melted medicated mass for insertion in the rectum, urethra, or vagina. Theobroma oil, glycerinated gelatin, and high-molecular-weight polyethylene glycols are common vehicles for drugs in suppositories that are cone- or spindle-shaped for insertion in the rectum, globular or egg-shaped for use in the vagina, and pencil-shaped for insertion in the urethra. Drugs administered by rectal suppository are absorbed systemically, and this route is especially useful in babies, uncooperative patients, and in cases of vomiting.

suppressant (səpres′ənt), an agent that suppresses or diminishes a physical or mental activity, as a medication that reduces hyperkinetic behavior or the excretory or secretory activity of a gland.

suppression, (in psychoanalysis) the conscious inhibition or effort to conceal unacceptable or painful thoughts, desires, impulses, feelings, or acts. Compare **repression.**

suppression amblyopia, a partial loss of vision, usually in one eye, owing to cortical suppression of central vision to avoid diplopia. It occurs commonly in strabismus in the eye that deviates and does not fixate. Early recognition of strabismus and amblyopia is essential, as occlusive therapy that forces use of the bad eye may dramatically improve the child's vision if begun early. It is ineffective after the age of six years, and near blindness in the affected eye may result.

suppressor gene, (in molecular genetics) a genetic unit that is able to reverse the effect of a specific kind of mutation in other genes.

suppressor mutation, (in molecular genetics) a mutation that partially or completely restores a function lost by a primary mutation occurring in a different genetic site.

suppressor T cell. See **T cell.**

suppurate (səp′yureit), to produce purulent matter. – **suppuration,** *n.,* **suppurative,** *adj.,*

supra-, a combining form meaning 'above or over': *suprabuccal, supradural, suprarenalism.*

supraclavicular nerve (su′prəkləvik′yulər), one of a pair of cutaneous branches of the cervical plexus, arising from the third and the fourth cervical nerves, mostly from the fourth nerve. It emerges from the posterior border of the sternocleidomastoideus and crosses the posterior triangle of the neck under the deep fascia. Near the clavicle it pierces the fascia and the platysma in the anterior, the middle, and the posterior groups. The anterior group supplies the skin of the infraclavicular region, the middle group supplies the skin over the pectoralis major and the deltoideus, and the posterior group supplies the skin of the cranial and the dorsal parts of the shoulder.

supracondylar fracture (su′prəkon′dılər), a fracture involving the area between the condyles of humerus or the femur.

suprainfection, a secondary infection usually caused by an opportunistic pathogen, as a fungal infection following the antibiotic treatment of another infection or pneumonia in a patient debilitated by another illness.

suprapubic (su′prəpyu′bık), located above the symphysis pubis.

suprarenal (su′prəri′nəl), situated above the kidney, as the suprarenal gland.

suprascapular nerve (su′prəskæp′yulər), one of a pair of branches from the cords of the brachial plexus. It arises from the superior trunk, passes to the scapular notch, and, in the supraspinatous fossa, branches to the supraspinatus, the shoulder joint, the infraspinatus, and the scapula.

suprasellar cyst. See **craniopharyngioma.**

supraspinal ligament, the ligament that connects the apices of the spinous processes from the seventh cervical vertebra to the sacrum. Between the spinous processes it is continuous with the interspinal ligaments; from the seventh cervical vertebrae it continues upward to the external occipital protuberance and the medial nuchal line as the ligamentum nuchae.

suramin sodium (sur′əmın), an antitrypanosomal and an antifilarial available from the Center for Disease Control. It is used primarily for treatment and prophylaxis of African trypanosomiasis.

Surfacaine, a trade name for a local anesthetic agent (cyclomethycaine sulfate).

surface anatomy, the study of the structural relationships of the external features of the body to the internal organs and parts. Compare **cross sectional anatomy.**

surface anesthesia. See **topical anesthesia.**

surface area (SA), the total area exposed to the outside environment. The surface area of an object increases with the square of the object's linear dimensions;

volume increases as the cube of the object's linear dimensions. Thus, the larger of two objects of the same shape will have less surface area per unit volume than the smaller object. Most loss of body heat takes place from the body surface.

surface biopsy, the removal of living tissue for microscopic examination by scraping the surface of a lesion. The procedure is used primarily to diagnose cancer of the uterine cervix. See also **exfoliative cytology.**

surface tension, the tendency of the surface of a liquid to minimize the area of its surface by contracting. This property causes liquids to rise in a capillary tube, affects the exchange of gases in the pulmonary alveoli, and alters the ability of various liquids to wet another surface.

surface therapy, a form of radiotherapy administered by placing one or more radioactive sources on or near an area of body surface. The resulting array of sources is called a surface mold, surface applicator, or plaque.

surface thermometer, a device that detects and indicates the temperature of the surface of any part of the body.

surfactant (sərfæk′tənt), **1.** an agent, like soap or detergent, dissolved in water to reduce its surface tension or the tension at the interface between the water and another liquid. **2.** certain lipoproteins that reduce the surface tension of pulmonary fluids, allowing the exchange of gases in the alveoli of the lungs and contributing to the elasticity of pulmonary tissue. See also **alveolus, atelectasis, surface tension.**

Surfadil, a trade name for a topical fixed-combination drug containing an antihistaminic (methapyrilene hydrochloride) and a topical anesthetic (cyclomethycaine sulfate).

Surlak, a trade name for a stool softener (docusate calcium).

surfer's nodules, nodules on the skin of the knees, ankles, feet, or toes of a surfer caused by repeated contact of the skin with an abrasive, sandy surfboard. The nodules will slowly diminish in size and disappear if surfing is discontinued. When treatment is necessary, injection of corticosteroids is usually effective.

surgeon's assistant (SA), a medical professional trained to assist in surgery and in the preoperative and postoperative periods under the supervision of a licensed medical doctor. An SA is required to attend two years of college studying anatomy, physiology, pharmacology, and other subjects, followed by two years of special clinical training and clinical experience.

surgery, a branch of medicine concerned with diseases and trauma requiring operative procedures. — **surgical,** *adj.*

-surgery, a combining form meaning the 'treatment of illness or deformity': *cardiosurgery, chemosurgery, radiosurgery.* Also **-chirurgia.**

surgical abdomen. See **acute abdomen.**

surgical anatomy, (in applied anatomy) the study of the structure and morphology of the tissues and organs of the body as they relate to surgery.

surgical anesthesia, the third stage of general anesthesia. See also **general anesthesia, Guedel signs.**

surgical diathermy. See **electrocoagulation.**

surgical induction of labor. See **induction of labor.**

surgical microscope. See **operating microscope.**

surgical pathology, the study of disease by the study of tissue specimens obtained during surgery. The surgical pathologist often examines specimens during surgery to determine how the operation should be modified or completed. Various techniques are used. The appearance of the specimen is first noted; then slices of the tissue are prepared by the paraffin or frozen section method and microscopically examined by a physician trained in pathology.

surgical scrub, 1. a bactericidal soap or solution used by surgeons and surgical nurses before performing or assisting in surgery. **2.** the act of washing the fingernails, hands, and forearms with a bactericidal soap or solution before a surgical procedure.

surgical treatment. See **treatment.**

Surital Sodium, a trade name for a barbiturate (thiamylal sodium), used as a general anesthetic.

Surmontil, a trade name for an antidepressant (trimipramine maleate).

surrogate, 1. a substitute; a person or thing that replaces another. **2.** (in psychoanalysis) a substitute parental figure, a symbolic image or representation of another, as may occur in a dream. The identity of the person represented often remains unconscious.

sursum-, a combining form meaning 'upward': *sursumduction, sursumvergence, sursumversion.*

susceptibility, the condition of being more than normally vulnerable to a disease or disorder. — **susceptible,** *adj.*

suspension, 1. a liquid in which small particles of a solid are dispersed, but not dissolved, and in which the dispersal is maintained by stirring or shaking the mixture. If left standing, the solid particles settle at the bottom of the container. **2.** a treatment, used primarily in spinal disorders, consisting of suspending the patient by the chin and shoulders. **3.** a temporary cessation of pain or of a vital process.

supensory ligament of the lens. See **zonula ciliaris.**

sustained release. See **prolonged release.**

sustenance, 1. the act or process of supporting or maintaining life or health. **2.** the food or nutrients essential for maintaining life.

sutilains (su′tĭleinz), a proteolytic enzyme.
■ INDICATIONS: It is prescribed for debridement of certain wounds and second- and third-degree burns.

■ CONTRAINDICATIONS: Wounds communicating with major body cavities, wounds containing exposed major nerves or nervous tissue, or fungating neoplastic ulcers prohibits its use. It is not given during pregnancy.

■ ADVERSE EFFECTS: Among the more serious adverse reactions are bleeding, paresthesias, and dermatitis.

sutura (sutur′ə), *pl.* **suturae.** an immovable, fibrous joint in which certain bones of the skull are connected by a thin layer of fibrous tissue. Compare **gomphosis, syndesmosis.**

sutura dentata, an immovable fibrous joint that is one kind of true suture in which toothlike processes interlock along the margins of connecting bones of the skull. Compare **sutura limbosa, sutura serrata.**

sutura limbosa, an immovable fibrous joint that is one kind of true suture in which beveled and serrated edges of certain connecting bones of the skull, as the parietal and temporal bones, overlap and interlock. Compare **sutura dentata, sutura serrata.**

sutura plana, a fibrous joint that is one kind of false suture in which rough, contiguous edges of certain bones of the skull, as the maxillae, form a connection. Compare **sutura squamosa.**

sutura serrata, an immovable fibrous joint that is one kind of true suture in which connecting bones interlock along serrated edges that resemble fine-toothed saws. Compare **sutura dentata, sutura limbosa.**

sutura squamosa, an immovable fibrous joint that is one kind of false suture in which overlapping, beveled edges unite certain bones of the skull, as the temporal and the parietal bone. Compare **sutura plana.**

suture (su′chər), **1.** a border or a joint, as between the bones of the cranium. **2.** to stitch together cut or torn edges of tissue with suture material. **3.** a surgical stitch taken to repair an incision, tear, or wound. **4.** material used for surgical stitches, as absorbable or nonabsorbable silk, catgut, wire, or synthetic material.

Sux-Cert, a trade name for a skeletal muscle relaxant (succinylcholine chloride).

SV40, abbreviation for **simian virus 40.**

swab, a stick or clamp for holding absorbent gauze or cotton, used for washing, cleansing, or drying a body surface, for collecting a specimen for laboratory examinations, or for applying a topical medication.

swamp fever. 1. See **leptospirosis. 2.** See **malaria.**

Swan-Ganz catheter, a long, thin cardiac catheter with a tiny balloon at the tip. It is used during anesthesia for open-heart surgery in order to determine left ventricular function by measuring left atrial wedge pressure.
(See next page for illustration)

swan neck deformity, a structural abnormality of the kidney tubules associated with rickets. The kidney tubule connecting the glomerulus with the convoluted portion of the tubule is narrowed into a configuration referred to as 'swan neck.' There is also a thinning and atrophy of the distal tubule and a shortening of the convoluted portion.

S wave, the component of the cardiac cycle shown on an electrocardiogram as a line slanting downward sharply from the peak of the R wave to the beginning of the upward curve of the T wave. It represents the final phase of the QRS complex.

sweat. See **perspiration.**

sweat bath, a bath given to induce sweating.

sweat duct, any one of the tiny tubules conveying sweat to the surface of the skin from about two million sweat glands throughout the body. Each sweat duct is the most superficial part of a coiled tube that forms the body of each sweat gland and opens onto the surface through a funnel-shaped opening. The sweat ducts in the armpits and in the groin are larger than in other parts of the body. Ducts and sweat glands abound on the palms of the hands and the soles of the feet. There are about 370 sweat ducts rising from a corresponding number of sweat glands per square centimeter on each palm. Each duct is composed of a basement membrane with two or three layers of polyhedral cells and is lined with a thin cuticle.

sweat gland. See **sudoriferous gland.**

sweating. See **diaphoresis.**

sweat test, a method for evaluating sodium and chloride excretion from the sweat glands, often the first test performed in the diagnosis of cystic fibrosis. The sweat glands are stimulated with a drug, as pilocarpine, and the perspiration produced is analysed. The exocrine glands of patients with cystic fibrosis produce sodium and chloride concentrations that are three to six times that of the normal. Chloride levels above 60 mEq/liter are considered diagnostic for the disease. The test is very reliable, and while it may be useful at any age, it is usually performed on infants from two weeks to one year old. See also **cystic fibrosis.**

swimmer's ear, *Informal.* otitis externa resulting from infection transmitted in the water of a swimming pool.

swimmer's itch, an allergic dermatitis caused by sensitivity to schistosome cercarias which die under the skin, leading to erythema, urticaria, and a papular rash lasting one or two days. Treatment usually includes oral antihistamines and antipruritic lotions. See also **schistosomiasis.**

swimming pool conjunctivitis. See **pharyngoconjunctival fever.**

swing phase of gait, one of the two phases in the rhythmic process of walking. The swing phase of gait follows the stance phase and is divided into the initial swing stage, the midswing stage, and the terminal swing stage. The analyses of pathological gaits and the diagnoses of many abnormal orthopedic conditions focus on walking as a specilized function of the musculoskeletal system and the swing phase of gait as the kinetic conclusion of one complete gait cycle. By studying the two

Placement of
flow-directed catheter
via superior vena cava

Balloon inflated and
wedged in
pulmonary artery

SWAN-GANZ CATHETER

phases of stance and swing in the gait of any individual, orthopedists can often determine gait deviations associated with many abnormal conditions or deformities of the spine, hip, pelvis, legs, or feet, and weaknesses in associated muscles. Compare **stance phase of gait.**

sy-. See **syn-.**

sycosis barbae, an inflammation of hair follicles of skin that has been shaved. Treatment includes light and infrequent shaving, topical and systemic antibiotics, and daily plucking of infected hairs. Also called **barber's itch, sycosis vulgaris.**

sycosis vulgaris. See **sycosis barbae.**

Sydenham's chorea (sɪd'ənhæmz), a form of chorea associated with rheumatic fever, usually occurring during childhood. The cause is a streptococcal infection of the vascular and perivascular tissues of the brain. The choreic movements increase over the first two weeks, reach a plateau, and then diminish. The child is usually well within ten weeks. With undue exertion or emotional strain, the condition may recur. Also called **chorea minor, rheumatic chorea.**

syl-. See **syn-.**

sylvatic plague, an endemic disease of wild rodents caused by *Yersinia pestis* and transmissable to man by the bite of an infected flea. It is found on every continent except Australia. See also **bubonic plague.**

sym-. See **syn-.**

symbiosis (sɪm'bɪoʊ'sɪs), 1. (in biology) a mode of living characterized by close association between organisms of different species, usually in a mutually beneficial relationship. 2. (in psychiatry) **a.** a state in which two mentally disturbed people are emotionally dependent on each other. **b.** pathologic inability of a child to separate from its mother emotionally and, sometimes, physically. — **symbiotic,** *adj.*

symbol, 1. an image, object, action, or other stimulus that represents something else by reason of conscious association, convention, or other relationship. 2. an object, mode of behavior, or feeling that disguises a repressed emotional conflict through an unconscious association rather than through an objective relationship, as in dreams and neuroses.

-symbolia, a combining form meaning '(condition involving) the ability to interpret symbols': *asymbolia, dyssymbolia, strephosymbolia.*

symbolism, 1. the representation or evocation of one idea, action, or object by the use of another as in systems of writing, poetic language, or dream metaphor. 2. (in psychiatry) an unconscious mental mechanism characteristic of all human thinking in which a mental image stands for but disguises some other object, person, or thought, especially one associated with emotional conflict. The mechanism is a principal factor in the formation of dreams and in various symptoms resulting from such neurotic and psychotic conditions as conversion reactions, obsessions, and compulsions. Also called **symbolization.**

symbolization. See **symbolism.**

symelus (sım'ıləs). See **symmelus.**

symmelia, a fetal anomaly characterized by the fusion of the lower limbs with or without feet. Kinds of symmelia are **apodial symmelia, dipodial symmelia, monopodial symmelia, tripodial symmelia.**

symmelus, symelus (sım'ıləs), a malformed fetus characterized by symmelia.

Symmer's disease (sım'ərz). See **giant follicular lymphoma.**

Symmetrel, a trade name for an antiviral (amantadine hydrochloride).

symmetrical, symmetric, (of the body or parts of the body) equal in size or shape; different in placement or arrangement about an axis. Compare **asymmetrical.** – **symmetry,** *n.*

symmetrical lipomatosis. See **nodular circumscribed lipomatosis.**

symmetric tonic neck reflex, a normal response in infants to assume the crawl position by extending the arms and bending the knees when the head and neck are extended. The reflex disappears when neurological and muscular development enables independent limb movement for actual crawling. Also called **crawling reflex.** See also **tonic neck reflex.**

sympathectomy (sım'pəθek'təmi), a surgical interruption of part of the sympathetic nerve pathways, performed for the relief of chronic pain in vascular diseases, as arteriosclerosis, claudication, Buerger's disease, and Raynaud's phenomenon. The sheath around an artery carries the sympathetic nerve fibers that control constriction of the vessel. Removal of the sheath causes the vessel to relax and expand and allows more blood to pass through it. The operation may also be done with a vascular graft, to increase the blood flow through the graft area. Preoperatively the physician may assess the effect of surgery by injecting sympathetic ganglia with alcohol to interrupt temporarily the sympathetic nerve impulses. The nerves lie along the spinal column and are approached through the back or the neck, under local anesthesia. Postoperatively, the adequacy of circulation in the affected extremity is monitored. An arteriogram shows a widened pathway.

sympathetic nervous system. See **autonomic nervous system.**

sympathetic ophthalmia, a granulomatous inflammation of the uveal tract of both eyes occurring after an injury to the uveal tract of one eye. Corticosteroids may be helpful in treatment, but surgical enucleation of the originally injured eye may be necessary to preserve vision in the uninjured eye. Also called **metastatic ophthalmia, migratory ophthalmia.**

sympathetic trunk, one of a pair of chains of ganglia extending along the side of the vertebral column from the base of the skull to the coccyx. Each trunk is part of the sympathetic nervous system and consists of a series of ganglia connected by cords containing various types of fibers. The cranial end of the trunk is formed by the superior cervical ganglion from the internal carotid nerve of the head. In some individuals the caudal ends of both trunks merge into a single ganglion at the coccyx. Interconnection of the trunks is common but rarely occurs above the fifth lumbar nerve. In addition to the ganglia, the trunks contain the preganglionic fibers, which are small and myelinated, the postganglionic fibers, which are mostly unmyelinated, some myelinated afferent fibers, and some unmyelinated afferent fibers. The central ganglia of each trunk are irregularly shaped structures with diameters ranging from 1 to 10 mm. Each sympathetic trunk distributes branches with postganglionic fibers to the autonomic plexuses, the cranial nerves, the individual organs, the nerves accompanying arteries, and the spinal nerves.

sympathizing eye, (in sympathetic ophthalmia) the uninfected eye that becomes infected by lymphatic or blood-born metastasis of the microorganism.

sympatholytic (sım'pæθhəlıt'ık). See **antiadrenergic.**

sympatholytic agent. See **antiadrenergic.**

sympathomimetic (sım'pəθoumımet'ık), noting a pharmacologic agent that mimics the effects of stimulation of organs and structures by the sympathetic nervous system by occupying adrenergic receptor sites and acting as an agonist or by increasing the release of the neurotransmitter norepinephrine at postganglionic nerve endings. Various sympathomimetic agents are used as decongestants of nasal and ocular mucosa, as bronchodilators in the treatment of asthma, bronchitis, bronchiectasis, and emphysema and as vasopressors and cardiac stimulants in the treatment of acute hypotension and shock; they are also used for maintaining normal blood pressure during operations under spinal anesthesia. Drugs in this group include cyclopentamine, dobutamine, dopamine, ephedrine, isoproterenol, levarterenol, metaraminol, metaproterenol, mephentermine, methoxamine, methoxyphenamine, naphazoline, phenylephrine, phenylpropanolamine, propylhexedrine, protokylol, pseudoephedrine, terbutaline sulfate, tetrahydrozoline, tuaminoheptane, xylmetazoline, and epinephrine, a synthetic isomer of the hormone secreted by the adrenal medulla. Adverse effects of sympathomimetic drugs may be nervousness, severe headache, anxiety, vertigo, nausea, vomiting, dilated pupils, glycosuria, and dysuria. Also called **adrenergic.**

sympathomimetic amine. See **adrenergic.**

sympathy,   **1.** an expressed interest or concern regarding the problems, emotions, or states of mind of another. Compare **empathy. 2.** the relation that exists between the mind and body causing the one to be affected by the other. **3.** mental contagion or the influence exerted by one individual or group on another and the effects produced, as the spread of panic, uncontrollable laughter, or yawning. **4.** the physiologic or pathologic relationship between two organs, systems, or parts of the body. — **sympathetic,** *adj.,* **sympathize,** *v.*

symphalangia (sɪmˈfəlænˈjiə),   **1.** a condition, usually inherited, characterized by ankylosis of the fingers or toes. **2.** a congenital anomaly in which webbing of the fingers or toes occurs in varying degrees, often in conjunction with other defects of the hands or feet. Also called **symphalangism.** See also **syndactyly.**

symphocephalus,   twin fetuses joined at the head. It is often used as a general designation for fetuses with varying degrees of the anomaly. See also **cephalothoracopagus, craniopagus, syncephalus.**

symphysic teratism,   a congenital anomaly in which there is a fusion of normally separated parts or organs, as a horseshoe kidney, or in which parts close prematurely, as the skull bones in craniostenosis.

symphysis (sɪmˈfəsɪs), *pl.* **symphyses** (sɪmˈfəsiz),   **1.** a line of union, especially a cartilaginous joint in which adjacent bony surfaces are firmly united by fibrocartilage. Also called **fibrocartilaginous joint. 2.** *Informal. symphysis pubis.* — **symphysic,** *adj.*

symphysis pubis (sɪmˈfisɪs).   See **pubic symphysis.**

sympodia (sɪmpouˈdiə),   a congenital developmental anomaly characterized by fusion of the lower extremities. See also **sirenomelus, sympus.**

symptom,   a subjective indication of a disease or a change in condition as perceived by the patient. The halo symptom of glaucoma is the seeing by the patient of colored rings around a single light source. Many symptoms are accompanied by objective signs, as pruritus, which is often reported with erythema and a maculopapular eruption on the skin. Some symptoms may be objectively confirmed, as numbness of a body part, which may be confirmed by absence of response to a pin prick. Compare **sign.**

symptomatic nanism,   dwarfism associated with defects in bone growth, tooth formation, and sexual development.

symptomatic treatment. See **treatment.**

symptothermal method of family planning,   a natural method of family planning that incorporates the ovula-tion and basal body temperature methods of family planning. It is more effective than either method used alone and requires fewer days of abstinence, because it enables the fertile period of the menstrual cycle to be more precisely identified.

sympus (sɪmˈpəs),   a malformed fetus in which the lower extremities are completely fused or rotated and the pelvis and genitalia are defective. Kinds of sympuses are **sirenomelus, sympus dipus, sympus monopus.** See also **symmelus.**

sympus apus (eiˈpəs).   See **sirenomelus.**

sympus dipus (diˈpəs),   a malformed fetus in which the lower extremities are fused and both feet are formed.

sympus monopus (monˈəpəs),   a malformed fetus in which the lower extremities are fused and one foot is formed. Also called **monopodial symmelia, uromelus.**

syn-, sy-, syl-, sym-,   a combining form meaning 'union, or association': *synalgia, syncephalus, synchronous.*

synadelphus, syndelphus, *pl.* **synadelphi.**   a conjoined twin fetal monster with a single head and trunk and eight limbs. Also called **cephalothoracoiliopagus.**

Synalar,   a trade name for a glucocorticoid (fluocinolone acetonide).

Synalgos,   a trade name for a fixed-combination drug containing the phenothiazine antiemetic-antihistamine (promethazine hydrochloride) and APC (aspirin, phenacetin, and caffeine), used for the relief of mild to moderate pain.

synapse (sɪnˈæps),   **1.** the region surrounding the point of contact between two neurons or between a neuron and an effector organ, across which nerve impulses are transmitted through the action of a neurotransmitter, as acetylcholine or norepinephrine. When an impulse reaches the terminal point of one neuron, it causes the release of the neurotransmitter, which diffuses across the gap between the two cells to bind with receptors in the other neuron, muscle, or gland, triggering electrical changes that either inhibit or continue the transmission of the impulse. Synapses are polarized so that nerve impulses travel in only one direction; they are also subject to fatigue, oxygen deficiency, anesthetics, and other chemical agents. **2.** to form a synapse or connection between neurons. **3.** (in genetics) to form a synaptic fusion between homologous chromosomes during meiosis. Kinds of synapses include **axoaxonic synapse, axodendritic synapse, axodendrosomatic synapse, axosomatic synapse, dendrodendritic synapse.** Compare **ephapse.** — **synaptic,** *adj.*

(See next page for illustration)

synapsis (sɪnæpˈsɪs), *pl.* **synapses.**   the pairing of homologous chromosomes during the early meiotic prophase stage in gametogenesis to form double or bivalent chromosomes. — **synaptic,** *adj.*

synaptic cleft,   the microscopic, extracellular space at the synapse that separates the membrane of the terminal

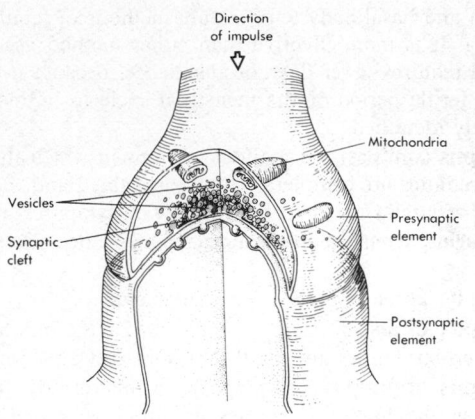

Direction of impulse

Mitochondria

Vesicles

Synaptic cleft

Presynaptic element

Postsynaptic element

SYNAPSE ANATOMY

nerve endings of a presynaptic neuron and the membrane of a postsynaptic cell. Nerve impulses are transmitted across this cleft by means of a neurotransmitter. See also **myoneural junction.** Also called **synaptic gap.**

synaptic junction, the membranes of both the presynaptic neuron and the postsynaptic receptor cell together with the synaptic cleft. See also **synapse.**

synaptic transmission, the passage of a neural impulse across a synapse from one nerve fiber to another by means of a neurotransmitter. Compare **ephaptic transmission.**

synarthrosis (sɪn'arˈθrou'sɪs), pl. **synarthroses.** See **fibrous joint.**

syncephalus, a conjoined twin monster having a single head and two bodies. Also called **monocephalus.**

synchilia, syncheilia (sɪŋki'liə), a congenital anomaly in which there is complete or partial fusion of the lips; atresia of the mouth.

synchondrosis (sɪŋ'kondrou'sɪs), pl. **synchondroses.** a cartilaginous joint between two immovable bones, as the synchondroses of the cranium, the pubic symphysis, the sternum, and the manubrium.

synchorial (sɪŋkor'iəl), pertaining to multiple fetuses that share a common placenta, as in monozygosity.

Syncillin, a trade name for an antibacterial (phenethicillin potassium).

synclitism (sɪŋ'klɪtɪzəm), **1.** (in obstetrics) a condition in which the sagittal suture of the fetal head is in line with the transverse diameter of the inlet, equidistant from the maternal symphysis pubis and sacrum. This position is usually found on examination either late in pregnancy or early in labor, as the fetal head descends into the pelvic inlet. As labor progresses, posterior asynclitism develops and, as the head descends further, anterior asynclitism is evident owing to the shape of the true pelvis below the inlet. **2.** (in hematology) the normal condition

in which the nucleus and the cytoplasm of the blood cells mature simultaneously and at the same rate.

syncopal attack, any episode of unconsciousness or fainting, especially one associated with fear or pain. Many individuals especially men, suffer such attacks during violent coughing spells because of associated rapid changes in arterial blood pressure. Syncopal attacks also occur as the result of any of a number of cardiovascular disorders.

syncope (sɪŋ'kəpi), a brief lapse in consciousness caused by transient cerebral hypoxia. It is usually preceded by a sensation of light-headedness and may often be prevented by lying down or by sitting with the head between the knees. It may be caused by many different factors, including emotional stress, vagal stimulation, vascular pooling in the legs, diaphoresis, or sudden change in environmental temperature or body position.

syncretic thinking, a stage in the development of the cognitive thought processes of the child. During this phase thought is based purely on what is perceived and experienced. The child is incapable of reasoning beyond the observable or of making deductions or generalizations. Through imaginative play, questioning, interaction with others, and the increasing use of language and symbols to represent objects, the child begins to learn to make associations between ideas and to elaborate concepts. In Piaget's classification, this stage occurs between 2 and 7 years of age and is preceded by the sensorimotor stage of development when the child progresses from reflex activity to repetitive and imitative behavior. Compare **abstract thinking, concrete thinking.** — **syncresis,** n.

Syncurine, a trade name for a depolarizing skeletal muscle relaxant (decamethonium bromide).

syncytial trophoblast. See **syncytiotrophoblast.**

syncytiotrophoblast, the outer syncytial layer of the trophoblast of the early mammalian embryo that erodes the uterine wall during implantation and gives rise to the villi of the placenta. Also called **plasmidotrophoblast, syncytial trophoblast, syntrophoblast.** Compare **cytotrophoblast.** — **syncytiotrophoblastic,** adj.

syndactylus, a person with webbed fingers or toes.

syndactyly (sɪndæk'təli), **syndactylia, syndactylism,** a congenital anomaly characterized by the fusion of the fingers or toes. It varies in degree of severity from incomplete webbing of the skin of two digits to complete union of digits and fusion of the bones and nails. — **syndactyl, syndactylous,** adj.

syndelphus, pl. **syndelphi.** See **synadelphus.**

syndesmo-, a combining form meaning 'of or pertaining to the connective tissue or particularly the ligaments': syndesmochorial, syndesmography, syndesmoma.

syndesmosis (sɪn'desmou'sɪs), pl. **syndesmoses.** a fibrous articulation in which two bones are connected by interosseous ligaments, as the anterior and the posterior ligaments in the tibiofibular articulation. Compare **gomphosis, sutura.**

syndrome, a complex of signs and symptoms resulting from a common cause or appearing, in combination, to present a clinical picture of a disease or inherited abnormality. See also specific syndromes.

syndrome of inappropriate antidiuretic hormone secretion (SIADH), an abnormal condition characterized by the excessive release of antidiuretic hormone (ADH) which upsets the fluid and electrolytic balances of the body. It results from various malfunctions, as the inability of the body to produce and secrete dilute urine, water retention, increased extracellular fluid volume, and hyponatremia. SIADH develops in association with diseases that affect the osmoreceptors of the hypothalamus. Oat cell carcinoma of the lung is the most common cause, affecting about 80 per cent of involved patients. Less common causes are disorders that affect the central nervous system, as brain tumors and lupus erythematosis, pulmonary diseases, as pneumonia, cancers of the pancreas and the prostate, and pathological reactions to various drugs, as chlorpropamide, vincristine sulfate, carbamazepine, and clofibrate. Prognosis depends on the underlying disease and the response of the patient to treatment.

■ OBSERVATIONS: Common signs and symptoms of SIADH are weight gain despite anorexia, vomiting, nausea, muscle weakness, and irritability. In some patients SIADH may produce coma and convulsions. Most of the free water associated with this syndrome is intracellular, and associated edema is rare unless excess water volume exceeds 4 milliosmols. Confirming diagnosis is based on urine osmolality that exceeds 150 milliosmols/kg of water and serum osmolality of less than 280 milliosmols/kg of water. Normal urine osmolality is 1.5 times serum osmolality. Other significant results include less than normal concentrations of blood urea nitrogen, serum creatinine, and albumin and a concentration of sodium in the urine higher than normal.

■ INTERVENTION: Treatment of SIADH commonly includes restriction of water intake and may require administration of normal saline to raise the serum sodium level if water intoxication is severe. Furosemide may be administered to block circulatory overload, and drugs, as demeclocycline hydrochloride and lithium, may be administered to block renal response to ADH. Surgery and chemotherapy are other alternatives to remove or destroy neoplasms that may be the underlying causes of this syndrome.

■ NURSING CONSIDERATIONS: Nurses monitor the SIADH patient for any signs of hyponatremia, weight change, and fluid imbalance. The patient is carefully advised on the importance of restricted water intake to prevent water intoxication and is closely observed for any indications of restlessness, congestive heart failure, and convulsions.

synechia (sɪnek'ɪə), *pl.* **synechiae.** an adhesion, especially of the iris to the cornea or lens of the eye. It may develop from glaucoma, cataracts, uveitis, keratitis, or as a complication of surgery or trauma to the eye. Synechiae prevent or impede flow of aqueous fluid between the anterior and posterior chambers of the eye and may lead rapidly to blindness. Immediate treatment consists of dilating the pupils with a mydriatic agent, followed by treatment of the underlying cause.

Synemol, a trade name for a glucocorticoid (fluocinolone acetonide).

synergism. See synergy.

synergist (sɪn'ərjɪst), an organ, agent, or a substance that augments the activity of another organ, agent, or substance. – **synergistic, synergetic,** *adj.*

synergy (sɪn'ərji), the process in which two organs, substances, or agents work simultaneously to enhance the function and effect of one another. Also called **synergism.** – **synergistic,** *adj.*

Synkayvite, a trade name for a synthetic preparation of vitamin K (menadiol sodium diphosphate).

synophthalmia (sɪn'ofthæl'mɪə). See **cyclopia.**

Synophylate, a trade name for a bronchodilator (theophylline sodium glycinate).

synotia (sɑɪnou'shə), a congenital malformation characterized by the union or approximation of the ears in front of the neck, often accompanied by the absence or defective development of the lower jaw. Compare **agnathia.** See also **otocephaly.**

synotus (sɑɪnou'təs), a fetus with synotia.

synovia (sɪnou'vɪə), a transparent, viscous fluid, resembling the white of an egg, secreted by synovial membranes and acting as a lubricant for many joints, bursae, and tendons. Also called **synovial fluid.** – **synovial,** *adj.*

synovial bursa, one of the many closed sacs filled with synovial fluid in the connective tissue between the muscles, the tendons, the ligaments, and the bones. The synovial bursae facilitate the gliding of muscles and tendons over bony and ligamentous prominences. Compare **synovial membrane, synovial tendon sheath.**

synovial chondroma, a rare cartilaginous growth developing in the connective tissue below the synovial membrane of the joints, tendon sheaths, or bursa. Foci on the surface may develop stalks and then detach, resulting in numerous loose bodies within the joint. Also called **synovial chondromatosis.**

synovial chondromatosis, a rare condition in which masses of cartilage develop in the synovial membranes of bursae, joints, and tendon sheaths. Metaplastic foci on the membrane surface may become sessile, pedunculate, and then separate, forming loose masses.

synovial crypt, a pouch in the synovial membrane of a joint.

synovial fluid (sınou′viəl), the clear, viscid fluid secreted in the bursae and tendon sheaths of the joints. It contains mucin, albumin, fat, and mineral salts, and serves to lubricate the joints.

synovial joint, a freely movable joint in which contiguous bony surfaces are covered by articular cartilage and connected by ligaments lined with synovial membrane. Kinds of synovial joints are **ball-and-socket joint, condyloid joint, gliding joint, hinge joint, pivot joint, saddle joint, uniaxial joint.** Compare **cartilaginous joint, fibrous joint.**

synovial membrane, the inner layer of an articular capsule surrounding a freely movable joint. The synovial membrane is loosely attached to the external fibrous capsule. It secretes into the joint a thick fluid that normally lubricates the joint but that may accumulate in painful amounts when the joint is injured. Compare **synovial bursa, synovial tendon sheath.**

synovial sarcoma, a malignant tumor, composed of synovioblasts, that begins as a soft swelling and often metastasizes through the blood stream to the lung before it is discovered.

synovial sheath, any one of the membranous sacs that enclose a tendon of a muscle and facilitate the gliding of a tendon through a fibrous or a bony tunnel, as that under the flexor retinaculum of the wrist.

synovial tendon sheath, one of the many membranous sacs enclosing various tendons that glide through fibrous and bony tunnels in the body, as those under the flexor retinaculum of the wrist. One layer of the synovial sheath lines the tunnel; the other covers the tendon. The sheath secretes synovial fluid, which lubricates the tendon. Compare **synovial bursa, synovial membrane.**

synovitis (sın′əvaɪ′tıs), an inflammatory condition of the synovial membrane of a joint as the result of an aseptic wound or a traumatic injury, as a sprain or severe strain. The knee is most commonly affected. Fluid accumulates around the capsule, the joint is swollen, tender, and painful, and motion is restricted. In most cases, the inflammation subsides, and the fluid is resorbed without medical or surgical intervention.

synteny (sın′təni), (in genetics) the presence on the same chromosome of two or more genes that may or may not be transmitted as a linkage group but that appear to be able to undergo independent assortment during meiosis. The term is used primarily in human genetics where linked inheritance patterns are more difficult to determine. See also **linkage.**

-synthesis, a combining form meaning 'putting together or formation of': *narcosynthesis, psychosynthesis, velosynthesis.*

synthetic, of or pertaining to a substance that is produced by an artificial rather than a natural process or material.

synthetic chemistry, the science dealing with the formation of chemical compounds from simpler substances.

synthetic oleovitamin D. See **viosterol.**

Synthroid, a trade name for a thyroid hormone (levothyroxine sodium).

Syntocinon, a trade name for an oxytocic (oxytocin).

syntrophoblast. See **syncytiotrophoblast.**

syphilis, a venereal infection caused by the spirochete, *Treponema pallidum,* usually transmitted by sexual contact and characterized by distinct stages of effects over a period of years. Any organ system may become involved. The spirochete is able to pass through human placenta, producing congenital syphilis.

■ OBSERVATIONS: The first stage **(primary syphilis)** is marked by the appearance of a small, painless, red pustule on the skin or mucous membrane between 10 and 90 days after exposure. The lesion may appear anywhere on the body where contact with a lesion on an infected person has occurred, but is seen most often in the anogenital region. It quickly erodes, forming a painless, bloodless ulcer, called a chancre, exuding a fluid that swarms with spirochetes. The chancre may not be noticed by the patient, and many people may become infected. It heals spontaneously within 10 to 40 days, often creating the mistaken impression that the sore was not a serious event. The second stage **(secondary syphilis)** occurs about two months later, after the spirochetes have increased in number and spread throughout the body. This stage is characterized by general malaise, anorexia, nausea, fever, headache, alopecia, bone and joint′ pain, or the appearance of a morbiliform rash that does not itch, flat white sores in the mouth and throat, or condylomata lata papules on the moist areas of the skin. The disease remains highly contagious at this stage and can be spread by kissing. The symptoms usually continue for from three weeks to three months but may be recurrent over a period of two years. The third stage **(tertiary syphilis)** may not develop for 3 to 15 or more years. It is characterized by the appearance of soft, rubbery tumors, called gummas, that ulcerate and heal by scarring. Gummas may develop anywhere on the surface of the body and in the eye, liver, lungs, stomach, or reproductive organs. Tertiary syphilis may be painless, unnoticed except for gummas, or it may be accompanied by deep, burrowing pain. The ulceration of the gummas may result in punched-out areas of the palate, nasal septum, or larynx. Various tissues and structures of the body, including the central nervous system, myocardium, and the valves of the heart may be damaged or destroyed, leading to mental or physical disability and premature death. **Congenital syphilis** resulting from prenatal infection may result in the birth of a deformed or blind infant. In some cases, the infant appears to be well until, at several weeks of age, snuffles, sometimes with a blood-stained or mucopurulent discharge, and skin lesions are observed, particularly on the palms and soles or in the genital region. Such children may also have visual or hearing defects and progeria and poor health may develop. Diagnosis of syphilis is made by darkfield microscopy of fluid from primary or secondary stage lesions, by bacteriologic study of blood samples, and by an examination of cerebrospinal fluid. Because of the slow development of the disease during the early stages, the various serological tests, including the Wassermann, may not be accurate until months after exposure. Repeated tests and crosschecking with more than one test may be required in some cases. The report by a person that exposure to syphilis has occurred is often the only evidence available to the clinician.

■ INTERVENTION: Patients with primary or secondary syphilis are usually given benzathine penicillin or an equivalent in a single dose of 2.4 million units or in two doses of 1.2 million units intramuscularly. The objective is to maintain penicillin in the bloodstream for a number of days, because *Treponema pallidum* divides at an average rate of once every 33 hours, and the antibiotic is most effective during the stage of cell division. Larger doses of penicillin, of between 7.2 and 9 million units, are administered over a period of two to three weeks for tertiary syphilis. Infants and small children with congenital syphilis are usually given 50,000 units/kg intramuscularly. Treatment of an infected mother with penicillin during the first four months of pregnancy usually prevents the development of congenital syphilis in the fetus. Treating the mother with antibiotics later in the pregnancy usually eliminates the infection but may not protect the fetus.

■ NURSING CONSIDERATIONS: Special care and aseptic precautions are taken while handling the highly contagious fluid from syphilitic lesions used in diagnostic

Evolution of a typical case of syphilis

Stage	Duration	Clinical disease	Activity of Treponema pallidum	Diagnosis	Tissue change
Incubation	2 to 6 weeks (most often 3 to 4 weeks)	None	Spirochetes actively proliferate at entry site, spread over body	Identification of *Treponema pallidum*: a. Dark-field microscopy b. Fluorescent antibody technique	Chancre appears at inoculation site
Primary	8 to 12 weeks	1. Chancre present at inoculation site 2. Regional lymphadenopathy	Chancre teeming with them	1. Dark-field microscopy of chancre 2. STS* become positive	Chancre present
Primary latent	4 to 8 weeks	None	Inconspicuous	STS positive	None demonstrable; chancre has healed with little scarring
Secondary	Variable over period of 5 years (latent periods with recurrences)	1. Skin and mucosal lesions ("mucous patches") 2. Generalized lymphadenopathy	Skin and mucosal lesions rich in spirochetes (highly infectious)	1. Dark-field microscopy of lesions 2. STS positive	1. Infection active: a. Vascular changes b. Cuffs of inflammatory round cells about small blood vessels 2. Resolution spontaneous—little scarring
Latent	Few months to a lifetime (average 6 to 7 years)	None	Inconspicuous	STS positive (can be negative)	
Tertiary	Variable—rest of patient's life	Related to organ system diseased and the incapacity thereof	Paucity of spirochetes in classic lesions	1. STS positive or negative 2. Special silver stains of tissue lesions may show spirochetes	1. Gumma 2. Definite predilection to heal in lesions 3. Scarring 4. Tissue distortion and abnormal function

*Serological tests for syphilis.

testing, because the infection may be acquired through a cut or break in the skin. The nurse is often the person delegated to discuss the disease and its treatment with the patient. The need for and the nearly total effectiveness of the antibiotic are stressed. The extremely contagious nature of the infection is explained, and the importance of treatment for all who may have been exposed is emphasized. Tact, patience, and understanding are required to reassure the usually upset, frightened patient, to secure the patient's cooperation in accepting treatment and in assisting in the identification and location of others needing treatment. In many states, active, serologically documented cases of syphilis must, by law, be reported to the Department of Health. See also **chancre, Hutchinson's teeth, snuffles.**

syphilitic aortitis, an inflammatory condition of the aorta, occurring in tertiary syphilis and characterized by diffuse dilatation with gray, wheallike plaques containing calcium on the inner coat and scars and wrinkles on the outer coat. The middle layer of the vascular wall is usually infiltrated with plasma cells and contains fragments of damaged elastic tissue and many newly formed blood vessels. There may be damage to the aortic valves, narrowing of the mouths of the coronary arteries, and the formation of thrombi. Cerebral embolism may result. Signs of syphilitic aortitis are substernal pain, dyspnea, bounding pulse, and high systolic blood pressure. Penicillin may slow the course of the disease, but it cannot reverse the structural damage to the vessels and the heart. Also called **luetic aortitis, Döhle-Heller disease.**

syphilitic meningoencephalitis. See **general paresis.**

syphilitic periarteritis, an inflammatory condition of the outer coat of one or more arteries occurring in tertiary syphilis and characterized by soft gummatous perivascular lesions infiltrated with lymphocytes and plasma cells. Also called **periarteritis gummosa.** See also **syphilitic aortitis.**

Syraprim, a trade name for an antibacterial (trimethoprim).

syring-. See **syringo-.**

syringe, a device for withdrawing, injecting, or instilling fluids. A syringe for the injection of medication usually consists of a calibrated glass or plastic cylindrical barrel having a close-fitting plunger at one end and a small opening at the other to which the head of a hollow-bore needle is fitted. Medication of the desired amount may be pulled up into the barrel by suction as the plunger is withdrawn and injected by pushing the plunger back into the barrel, forcing the liquid out through the needle. A syringe for irrigating a wound or body cavity or for extracting mucus or another body fluid from an orifice or body cavity is usually larger than the kind used for injection. It often has a rubber bulb at one end and a blunt, soft-tipped, flexible tube with an opening at the other

end. The bulb is squeezed to eject a fluid and is released to withdraw one. Kinds of syringe include **asepto syringe, bulb syringe, hypodermic syringe, Luer-lock syringe, tuberculin syringe.**

syringo-, syring-, a combining form meaning 'of or pertaining to a tube or a fistula': *syringobulbia, syringocystoma, syringomyelitis.*

syringomyelocele (sĭrĭng'gōmī'əlōsil'), a hernial protrusion of the spinal cord through a congenital defect in the vertebral column in which the cerebrospinal fluid within the central cavities of the cord is greatly increased so that the cord tissue forms a thin-walled sac that lies close to the membrane of the cavity. See also **myelomeningocele, neural tube defect, spina bifida.**

system, a collection or assemblage of parts that, unified, make a whole. Physiologic systems, as the cardiovascular or reproductive systems, are made up of structures specifically able to engage in processes that are essential for a vital function in the body.

systematic tabulation, (in research) mechanical or manual techniques for recording and classifying data for statistical analysis.

systemic (sĭstem'ĭk), of or pertaining to the whole body rather than to a localized area or regional portion of the body.

systemic desensitization, a technique used in behavior therapy for eliminating maladaptive anxiety associated with phobias. The procedure involves the construction by the person of a hierarchy of anxiety-producing stimuli and the general presentation of these stimuli until they no longer elicit the initial response of fear. Also called **desensitization.** Compare **flooding.** See also **reciprocal inhibition.**

systemic lupus erythematosus (SLE), a chronic inflammatory disease affecting many systems of the body. The pathophysiology of the disease includes severe vasculitis, renal involvement, and lesions of the skin and nervous system. The primary cause of the disease has not been determined; viral infection or dysfunction of the immune system has been suggested. Adverse reaction to certain drugs may also cause a lupuslike syndrome. Four times more women than men have SLE.

■ OBSERVATIONS: The initial manifestation is often arthritis. An erythematous rash over the nose and malar eminences, weakness, fatigue, and weight loss are also frequently seen early in the disease. Photosensitivity, fever, skin lesions on the neck, and alopecia where the skin lesions extend beyond the hairline may occur. The skin lesions may spread to the mucous membranes and other tissues of the body. They do not ulcerate but cause degeneration of the tissues affected. Depending on the organs involved, the patient may also have glomerulonephritis, pleuritis, pericarditis, peritonitis, neuritis, or anemia. Renal failure and severe neurologic abnormalities are among the most serious manifestations of the disease. Diagnosis

of SLE is made by subjective and objective findings based on physical examination and laboratory findings, including antinuclear antibody in the cerebrospinal fluid and a positive lupus erythematosus (LE) cell reaction in a lupus erythematosus preparation (LE prep). Other laboratory examinations may be useful, depending on the organs, tissues, and systems affected by the disease.
■ INTERVENTION: In many cases SLE may be controlled with corticosteroid medication administered systemically. Care and treatment vary with the severity and nature of the disease and the body systems that are affected. Topical steroids may be applied to the rash; salicylates may be given to alleviate pain and swelling in the joints. Fatigue and stress are avoided, and all body surfaces are protected from direct sunlight. Antimalarial drugs are sometimes given to treat cutaneous lesions, but retinal damage may occur with prolonged use.
■ OUTCOME CRITERIA: The timing, dosage, side effects, and toxic reactions to the medications are explained before discharge. The steroids must be taken exactly as prescribed and, in the event that the patient cannot take them, the doctor is to be consulted promptly. An identification card is carried bearing the patient's diagnosis, a list of all medications and their dosage, and the doctor's name and telephone number. As in any disease marked by chronic remission and exacerbation of many distressing symptoms, the patient may require extensive emotional and psychological support. Also called **disseminated lupus erythematosus, lupus erythematosus.**

systemic remedy, a medicinal substance that is given orally, parenterally, or rectally to be absorbed into the circulation for treatment of a health problem. Many remedies or medications administered locally or regionally are to some degree absorbed systemically. Medication administered systemically may have various local effects, but the intent is to treat the whole body.

systemic vein, one of a number of veins that drain deoxygenated blood from most of the body. Systemic veins arise in tiny plexuses that receive blood from the billions of capillaries lacing the body tissues and converge into trunks which increase in size as they pass toward the heart. They are larger and more numerous than the arteries, have thinner walls, and collapse when they are empty. Kinds of systemic veins are identified according to location, as deep veins, superficial veins, and venous sinuses. Groups of systemic veins include the coronary veins, the superior vena cava and its tributaries in the upper body, and the inferior vena cava and its tributaries in the lower body.

system of care, a framework within which health care is delivered, comprised of actors or agents; recipients, consumers, or patients; energy resources or dynamics; organizational and political contexts or frameworks; and processes or procedures. Current theory recognizes that an analysis of the delivery of health care requires knowledge of the systems of care.

systole (sıs′təli), the normal contraction of the heart, especially of the ventricles, driving blood into the aorta and pulmonary artery. The occurrence of systole is indicated by the first heart sound heard on auscultation, by the palpable apex beat, and by the peripheral pulse. Systole is sometimes described as occurring in three phases: pre-ejection, ejection, and relaxation periods.

-systole, a combining form referring to 'types and locations of the higher blood pressure measurement': *dyssystole, hysterosystole, tachysystole.*

systolic click (sıstol′ık), an extra heart sound that occurs in midsystole or in late systole. It is usually of no significance but may be associated with abnormal function of the mitral valve. Compare **ejection click.**

systolic gradient, the difference in pressure in the left atrium and left ventricle during systole.

systolic murmur, cardiac murmur occurring during systole. Systolic murmurs are generally less significant than diastolic murmurs and occur in many people with no evidence of heart disease. Systolic murmurs include ejection murmurs often heard in pregnancy or in people with anemia, thyrotoxicosis, or aortic or pulmonary stenosis, pansystolic murmurs heard in people with incompetence of the mitral or tricuspid valve, and late systolic murmurs, also caused by mitral valve incompetence.

T

T, **1.** abbreviation for **tumor** in the TNM system for staging malignant neoplastic disease. See **cancer staging.** **2.** symbol for **temperature.**

T₃, symbol for **triiodothyronine.**

T₄, symbol for **thyroxine.**

Ta, symbol for **tantalum.**

TA, abbreviation for **transactional analysis.**

ta-. See **tono-.**

tabe-, a combining form meaning 'of or pertaining to wasting (away)': *tabefaction, tabescent, tabetiform.*

tabes dorsalis, an abnormal condition characterized by the slow degeneration of all or part of the body and the progressive loss of peripheral reflexes. This disease involves the posterior columns and the posterior roots of the spinal cord and destroys the large joints of affected limbs in some individuals. It is often accompanied by incontinence and impotence and severe flashing pains in the abdomen and the extremities. The cause of tabes dorsalis is unclear and it is believed to be an uncommon disorder. Some surveys have indicated that about 10 per cent of individuals with late syphilis and 40 per cent of those with clinical neurosyphilis have tabes dorsalis.

tablet, a small, solid dosage form of a medication. It may be compressed or molded in its manufacture, and it may be of almost any size, shape, weight, and color. Most tablets are intended to be swallowed whole, but some may be dissolved in the mouth, chewed, or dissolved in liquid before swallowing; some may be placed in a body cavity.

Tacaryl, a trade name for an antihistamine (methdilazine).

TACE, a trade name for an estrogen (chlorotrianisene).

tacho-, a combining form meaning 'of or pertaining to speed': *tachogram, tachography, tachometer.*

tachy-, a combining form meaning 'swift or rapid': *tachycardia, tachyphrenia, tachysystole.*

tachycardia (tæk′ıkar′diə), an abnormal circulatory condition in which the myocardium contracts regularly but at a rate of 100 to 150 beats per minute. The heart rate normally accelerates in response to fever, exercise, or nervous excitement. Pathologic tachycardia accompanies anoxia, as caused by anemia, congestive heart failure, hemorrhage, or shock. Bradycardia develops as the heart muscle becomes anoxic and cannot maintain the acceler-

ated pace. Tachycardia acts to increase the amount of oxygen delivered to the cells of the body by increasing the amount of blood circulated through the vessels.

tachyphylaxis (tæk′əfəlæk′sıs), **1.** (in pharmacology) a phenomenon in which the repeated administration of some drugs results in a marked decrease in effectiveness. **2.** (in immunology) Also called **mithridatism.** rapidly developing immunity to a toxin owing to previous exposure, as from previous injection of small amounts of the toxin.

tachypnea (tæk′ıpni′ə), an abnormally rapid rate of breathing, as seen with hyperpyrexia. See also **respiratory rate.**

tact-, a combining form meaning 'of or pertaining to touch': *tactile, tactilogical, taction.*

-tactic, **1.** a combining form meaning 'exhibiting agent-controlled orientation or movement': *chemotactic, eosinotactic, thermotactic.* **2.** a combining form meaning 'having an arrangement of something': *cytotactic, leukotactic, phyllotactic.* Also **-tactical, -taxic.**

tactile (tæk′təl), of or pertaining to the sense of touch.

tactile anesthesia, the absence or lack of the sense of touch in the fingers, possibly resulting from injury or disease. This condition can be congenital or psychosomatic and may cause the patient to incur severe burns, serious cuts, contusions, or abrasions. See also **traumatic anesthesia.**

tactile corpuscle, any one of many small, oval end organs associated with the sense of touch, widely distributed throughout the body in peripheral areas, as the papillae of the corium of the hand and foot, front of the forehead, skin of the lips, mucous membrane of the tongue, palpebral conjunctivae, and skin of the mammary papillae. Each corpuscle consists of a tiny, round structure surrounded by a capsule penetrated by a nerve fiber which spirals through the interior of the capsule and ends in globular enlargements. Also called **Meissner's corpuscle.**

tactile corpuscle of Meissner. See **Wagner-Meissner corpuscle.**

tactile fremitus, a tremulous vibration of the chest wall during respiration that is palpable on physical examination. It may indicate inflammation, infection, congestion, or, most commonly, consolidation of a lung or a part of a lung.

tactile image, a mental concept of an object as perceived through the sense of touch. See also **image.**

Taenia (ti′niə), a genus of large, parasitic, intestinal flatworm of the family Taeniidae, class Cestoda, having an armed scolex and a series of segments in a chain. Taeniae are among the most common parasites infecting humans and include *Taenia saginata,* the beef tapeworm, and *T. solium,* the pork tapeworm.

taenia-. See **tenia-.**

Taenia saginata, a species of tapeworm that inhabits the tissues of cattle during its larval stage and infects the intestine of humans in its adult form. *Taenia saginata* may grow to a length of between 12 and 25 feet and is the tapeworm species that most often infects humans. Also called **beef tapeworm.** See also **tapeworm, tapeworm infection.**

taeniasis (tinai′əsis), an infection with a tapeworm of the genus *Taenia.* See also **tapeworm infection.**

Taenia solium, a species of tapeworm that most commonly inhabits the tissues of pigs during its larval stage and infects the intestine of humans in its adult form. Infrequently, humans will serve as the intermediate hosts for this tapeworm, and larval infestation of the muscle and brain tissue may occur. Also called **pork tapeworm.** See also **cysticercosis, tapeworm, tapeworm infection.**

Tagamet, a trade name for a histamine H² receptor antagonist (cimetidine).

tail bud. See **end bud.**

tail fold, a curved ridge formed at the caudal end of the early developing embryo. It consists of the tail bud, which in lower animals gives rise to the caudal appendage and in man forms the hindgut.

tailor's bottom. See **weaver's bottom.**

Takayasu's arteritis (ta′kəya′suz), a disorder characterized by progressive occlusion of the brachiocephalic trunk and the left subclavian and left common carotid arteries above their origin in the aortic arch. Signs of the disorder are absence of a pulse in both arms and in the carotid arteries, transient paraplegia, transient blindness, and atrophy of facial muscles. Also called **brachiocephalic arteritis, Martorell's syndrome, pulseless disease, reversed coarctation.**

Takayasu's disease. See **aortic arch syndrome.**

talbutal, a barbiturate sedative hypnotic.

■ INDICATION: It is prescribed as a hypnotic in the treatment of insomnia.

■ CONTRAINDICATIONS: Previous addiction to sedative-hypnotics, porphyria, impaired hepatic function, or known hypersensitivity to this drug or to other barbiturates prohibits its use.

■ ADVERSE EFFECTS: Among the more serious adverse effects are respiratory depression, drug hangover, allergic reactions, porphyria, and physical dependence.

talip-, a combining form meaning 'club-footed': *taliped, talipes, talipomanus.*

talipes (tæl′ıpiz′), a deformity of the foot, usually congenital, in which the foot is twisted and relatively fixed in an abnormal position. Kinds of talipes include **talipes calcaneovarus, talipes equinovarus.** See also **pes cavus, pes planus.**

talipes cavus. See **pes cavus.**

talo-, a combining form meaning 'of or pertaining to the ankle': *talocalcaneal, talocrural, talofibular.*

talus (tei′ləs), *pl.* **tali.** the second largest tarsal bone. It supports the tibia, rests on the calcaneus, and articulates with the malleoli and with the navicular bones. It consists of a body, neck, and head. Also called **ankle bone, astragalus.**

Talwin, a trade name for an analgesic (pentazocine).

tamoxifen (təmok′səfın), a nonsteroidal antiestrogen used in the palliative treatment of advanced breast cancer in postmenopausal women whose tumors are estrogen-dependent.

tampon, a pack of cotton, a sponge, or other material for checking bleeding or absorbing secretions in cavities or canals or for holding displaced organs in position.

tamponade (tæm′pəneid′), stoppage of the flow of blood to an organ or a part of the body by pressure, as by a tampon or a pressure dressing applied to stop a hemorrhage or by the compression of a blood vessel by an accumulation of fluid, as in cardiac tamponade.

Tandearil, a trade name for an anti-inflammatory and antirheumatic (oxyphenbutazone).

Tangier disease (tænjir′), a rare familial deficiency of high-density lipoproteins, characterized by low blood cholesterol and an abnormal orange or yellow discoloration of the tonsils and pharynx. There may also be enlarged lymph nodes, liver, and spleen, muscle atrophy, and peripheral neuropathy. No specific treatment is known.

tannin, any of a group of astringent substances obtained from plants, used for the tanning of leather. Tannic acid, a mixture of tannins, is used in the treatment of burns.

tanning, a process in which the pigmentation of the skin deepens as a result of exposure to ultraviolet light. Skin cells containing melanin darken immediately. New melanin is formed within 2 to 3 days and moves upward rapidly, allowing the darkening process to continue.

tantalum (Ta), a silvery metallic element. Its atomic number is 73; its atomic weight is 180.95. Relatively inert chemically, tantalum is used in prosthetic devices such as skull plates and wire sutures.

tantrum, a sudden outburst or violent display of rage, frustration, and bad temper, usually occurring in a maladjusted child and certain emotionally disturbed persons. The activity is usually not directed at anyone or anything specific but toward the environment in general and is used primarily as a device for attempting to control others and the surroundings. Also called **temper tantrum.**

TAO, a trade name for an antibacterial (troleandomycin).

Tapazole, a trade name for a thyroid inhibitor (methimazole).

tapeworm, a parasitic, intestinal worm belonging to the class Cestoda and having a scolex and a ribbon-shaped body composed of segments in a chain. Humans usually acquire tapeworms by eating the undercooked meat of intermediate hosts contaminated by the larval form of the tapeworm. In the human alimentary canal the worm develops into an adult with an attaching head, or scolex, and numerous hermaphroditic segments, or proglottids, each of which is capable of producing eggs. Kinds of tapeworm include *Diphyllobothrium latum, Taenia saginata, Taenia solium.* Also called **cestode.**

tapeworm infection, an intestinal infection by one of several species of parasitic worms, caused by eating raw or undercooked meat infested with tapeworm or its larvae. Tapeworms live as larvae in one or more vertebrate intermediate hosts and grow to adulthood in the intestine of humans. Symptoms of intestinal infection with adult worms are usually mild or absent, but diarrhea, epigastric pain, and weight loss may occur. Diagnosis is made when eggs or portions of the adult worm are passed in the stool. The drugs niclosamide and quinacrine are used to loosen and dissolve the worm so that it may be excreted. Sanitary disposal of fecal material from affected patients is necessary to prevent the passage of larvae or eggs to humans or other hosts. Certain species of tapeworm can infect humans during the larval stage, causing a serious, often cystic, condition of larval infestation. Also called **cestodiasis.** See also **cysticercosis, tapeworm.**

tapho-, a combining form meaning 'of or pertaining to the grave': *taphophilia, taphophobia.*

tapotement (tʌpɔtmã′), a type of massage in which the body is tapped in a rhythmical manner with the tips of the fingers or the sides of the hands, using short, rapid, repetitive movements. The procedure is often used on the chest wall of patients with bronchitis to help loosen the mucus in the air passages. See also **massage.**

Taractan, a trade name for a tranquilizer (chlorprothixene).

Tarbonis, a trade name for a topical antieczematic containing coal tar.

Tarcortin, a trade name for a topical fixed-combination drug containing a glucocorticoid (hydrocortisone) and an antieczematic (crude coal tar).

tardive dyskinesia (tar′dɪv), an abnormal condition characterized by involuntary, repetitious movements of the muscles of the face, the limbs, and the trunk. This disorder most commonly affects older people who have been treated for extended periods with phenothiazine

drugs to alleviate the symptoms of parkinsonism. The involuntary movements associated with the condition may slacken or disappear after weeks or months and have been significantly reduced in some individuals by the administration of large doses of choline chloride.

tardy peroneal nerve palsy, an abnormal condition and a type of mononeuropathy in which the peroneal nerve is excessively compressed where it crosses the head of the fibula. Such compression may occur when an individual falls asleep with the legs crossed.

tardy ulnar nerve palsy, an abnormal condition characterized by atrophy of the first dorsal interosseous muscle and difficulty in the performance of fine manipulations. It may be caused by injury of the ulnar nerve at the elbow and commonly affects individuals with a shallow ulnar groove or those who persistently rest their weight on their elbows. Signs and symptoms of this disorder may include numbness of the small finger, of the contiguous half of the proximal and the middle phalanges of the ring finger, and of the ulnar border of the hand. Treatment of this condition concentrates on the prevention of further injury of the ulnar nerve. Therapy may include the use of a doughnut cushion for the elbow to relieve the pressure on the ulnar nerve. Severe cases of this disorder may be corrected by surgical procedures that mobilize and transplant the nerve to a site in front of the medial epicondyle.

target cell, 1. Compare **discocyte, spherocyte.** an abnormal red blood cell characterized, when stained and examined under a microscope, by a densely stained center surrounded by a pale unstained ring circled by a dark, irregular band. Target cells occur in the blood after splenectomy, in anemia, in hemoglobin C disease, and in thalassemia. 2. any cell having a specific receptor that reacts with a specific hormone, antigen, antibody, antibiotic, sensitized T cell, or other substance.

target organ, 1. (in radiotherapy) an organ intended to receive a therapeutic dose of irradiation, as the kidney when high-energy x rays or gamma rays are beamed to the renal area for the treatment of a tumor. 2. (in nuclear medicine) an organ intended to receive the greatest concentration of a diagnostic radioactive tracer, as the liver, which accumulates [99]technetium sulfur colloid when it is injected intravenously to detect hepatic lesions. 3. (in endocrinology) an organ most affected by a specific hormone, as the thyroid gland, which is the target organ of thyroid-stimulating hormone secreted by the anterior pituitary gland.

Tarpaste, a trade name for a topical fixed-combination drug containing an antieczematic (tar distillate) in a paste.

tarsal (tar′səl), of or pertaining to the tarsus, or ankle bone.

tarsal bone, any one of seven bones comprising the

tarsus of the foot, consisting of the talus, calcaneus, cuboid, navicular, and the three cuneiforms.

tarsal gland, one of numerous modified sebaceous glands on the inner surfaces of the eyelids. About 30 tarsal glands, resembling tiny, parallel strings of pearls, line each upper eyelid and somewhat fewer tarsal glands line each lower eyelid. They are embedded in grooves in the inner surfaces of the tarsi, their lengths corresponding to the width of the tarsal plates. The ducts of the tarsal glands open by tiny apertures on the free margins of the eyelids. Each gland consists of a single straight follicle with numerous lateral branches. The follicles are supported by a basement membrane and lined at their mouths by stratified epithelium. Polyhedral cells line the deeper parts of the follicles and their lateral diverticula. Acute localized bacterial infection of a tarsal gland causes a sty. Also called **Meibomian gland.** Compare **ciliary gland.**

tarsal tunnel syndrome, an abnormal condition and a kind of mononeuropathy, characterized by pain and numbness in the sole of the foot. This disorder may be caused by fractures of the ankle which compress the posterior tibial nerve and may be corrected by appropriate orthopedic therapy or by surgery.

tarso-, a combining form meaning 'of or pertaining to the edge of the foot, or to the eyelid': *tarsoclasis, tarsomalacia, tarsometatarsal.*

tarsometatarsal, of or pertaining to the metatarsal bones and the tarsus of the foot, especially the articulations of the metatarsal bones with the cuneiform and cuboid bones at the instep of the foot.

Tarsum, a trade name for a shampoo containing coal tar and salicylic acid.

tarsus, *pl* **tarsi. 1.** the area of articulation between the foot and the leg. **2.** Also called **tarsal plate.** any one of the plates of cartilage about 2.5 cm long forming the eyelids. One tarsal plate shapes each eyelid. The superior tarsal plates form the upper eyelids. The inferior tarsal plates the lower eyelids. The superior tarsal plates are semilunar, about 10 mm wide at the center, and attach anteriorly to the levator palpebrae superioris. The inferior tarsal plates are thin, elliptical, and about 5 mm in vertical diameter. The free margins of the plates are thick and straight, the orbital margins attached to the circumference of the orbit by the orbital septum, the lateral angles attached to the zygomatic bones by the lateral palpebral raphes. The medial angles of the two plates on each side end at the lacus lacrimalis and attach to the frontal process of the maxilla by the medial palpebral ligament. —**tarsal,** *adj.*

tartar, 1. a hard, gritty deposit composed of organic matter, phosphates, and carbonates that collects on the teeth and gums. An excessive accumulation of tartar may cause gum disease and other dental problems. See also gingivitis, pyorrhea. **2.** any of several compounds containing tartrate, the salt of tartaric acid. See **tartar emetic.**

tartar emetic. See **antimony potassium tartrate.**

tartaric acid (tärtær'ĭk), a colorless or white powder found in various plants and prepared commercially from maleic anhydride and hydrogen peroxide. It is used in baking powder, certain beverages, and in tartar emetic.

-tas, a noun-forming combining form: *fragilitas, graviditas, infertilitas.*

taste, the sense of perceiving different flavors in soluble substances that contact the tongue and trigger nerve impulses to special taste centers in the cortex and the thalamus of the brain. The four basic traditional tastes are sweet, salty, sour, and bitter. The front of the tongue is most sensitive to salty and sweet substances; the sides of the tongue are most sensitive to sour substances; and the back of the tongue is most sensitive to bitter substances. The middle of the tongue produces virtually no taste sensation. Chemoreceptor cells in the taste buds of the tongue detect different substances. Adults have about 9,000 taste buds, most of them situated on the upper surface of the tongue. The sense of taste is intricately linked with the sense of smell, and taste discrimination is very complex. Many experts believe the capacity to perceive different tastes involves a synthesis of chemoreactive nerve impulses and coordinating brain processes, still not completely understood.

taste bud, any one of many peripheral taste organs distributed over the tongue and the roof of the mouth. The four basic taste sensations registered by chemical stimulation of the taste buds are sweet, sour, bitter, and salty. All other tastes perceived are combinations of these four basic flavors. Each taste bud rests in a spherical pocket, which extends through the epithelium. Gustatory cells and supporting cells form each bud, which has a surface opening and an opening in the basement membrane. Also called **gustatory organ.**

TAT, abbreviation for **tetanus antitoxin.**

tattoo, a permanent coloration of the skin by the introduction of foreign pigment. A tattoo may accidentally occur when a bit of graphite from a broken pencil point is embedded in the skin. Small tattoos can be removed by surgical excision. Dermabrasion is preferred for removal of extensive areas of pigment. —**tattoo,** *v.*

tauto-, a combining form meaning 'same': *tautomenial, tautomeral, tautomerism.*

tax-, a combining form meaning 'order or arrangement': *taxis, taxology, taxonomy.*

-taxia, 1. a combining form meaning '(condition of) impaired mental or physical control': *acroataxia, cardiataxia, hypotaxia.* **2.** a combining form meaning '(condition of) internal ordering or arrangement': *cataxia, heterotaxia, prostaxia.* Also **-taxis, -taxy.**

-taxic. See **-tactic.**

-taxis, 1. a combining form meaning a '(specified) arrangement': *biotaxis, heterotaxis, homotaxis.* **2.** a combining form meaning a 'movement of an organism in response to a stimulus': *aerotaxis, electrotaxis, geotaxis.* Also **-taxia, -taxy.**

taxonomy (tækson'əmi), a system for classifying organisms on the basis of natural relationships and assigning them appropriate names. — **taxonomic,** *adj.*

Taylor brace, a padded steel brace used to support the spine. Also called **Taylor splint.**

Taylor, Effie J. (1874–1970), a Canadian-born American nurse who was graduated from Johns Hopkins School of Nursing. After graduation she continued at Johns Hopkins at the Phipps Psychiatric Institute, served as a nurse in World War I, and went to Yale University School of Nursing in 1923, succeeding Annie Goodrich as Dean in 1934. She served as President of the International Council of Nurses during World War II.

Taylor splint. See **Taylor brace.**

Tay-Sachs disease (tei'sæks'), an inherited, neurodegenerative disorder of lipid metabolism caused by a deficiency of the enzyme hexosaminidase A, which results in the accumulation of sphingolipids in the brain. The condition, which is transmitted as an autosomal recessive trait, occurs predominantly in families of Eastern European Jewish origin, specifically the Ashkenazic Jews, and is characterized by progressive mental and physical retardation and early death. Symptoms first appear by six months of age, after which no new skills are learned and there is progressive loss of those skills already acquired. Convulsions and atrophy of the optic nerve head occur after one year, followed by blindness, with a cherry-red spot on each retina, spasticity, dementia, and paralysis. Most children die between the ages of two and four years. There is no specific therapy for the condition, and intervention is purely symptomatic and supportive. The disease can be diagnosed in utero through amniocentesis. Also called **amaurotic familial idiocy, gangliosidosis type I, infantile cerebral sphingolipidosis, Sachs' disease.** See also **Sandhoff's disease.**

Tay's spot. See **cherry red spot.**

Tb, symbol for **terbium.**

TB, abbreviation for **tuberculosis.**

T bandage, a bandage in the shape of the letter T. It is used for the perineum and sometimes for the head. Also called **crucial bandage, Heliodorus' bandage.**

TBP, 1. abbreviation for **bithionol. 2.** abbreviation for *total bypass.*

TBT, abbreviation for **tracheobronchial tree.**

TBZ, abbreviation for *tetrabenazine,* an anesthetic adjuvant.

t.c., abbreviation for *telephone call.*

Tc, symbol for **technetium.**

TC, abbreviation for **therapeutic community.**

T cell, a small circulating lymphocyte produced in the bone marrow that matures in the thymus or as a result of exposure to thymosin secreted by the thymus. T cells, which live for years, have several functions but primarily mediate cellular immune responses, as graft rejection and delayed hypersensitivity. One kind of T cell, the **helper cell,** affects the production of antibodies by B cells; a **suppressor T cell,** suppresses B cell activity. Compare **B cell.** See also **immune response.**

TD, abbreviation for **toxic dose.**

TD50. See **median toxic dose.**

tDNA, abbreviation for **transfer DNA.**

Te, symbol for **tellurium.**

tea. *Slang.* See **cannabis.**

teacher's nodule. See **vocal cord nodule.**

teaching rounds, the somewhat informal conferences held regularly—often at the beginning of the day. Various members of the department and staff may attend, including nurses, residents, interns, students, attending physicians, and faculty. Specific problems in the care of people who are current patients are discussed. See also **nursing rounds.**

team nursing, a decentralized system in which the care of a patient is distributed among the members of a team. The charge nurse delegates authority to a team leader who must be a professional nurse. This nurse leads the team—usually of four to six members—in the care of between fifteen and twenty-five patients. The team leader assigns tasks, schedules care, and instructs team members in details of care. A conference is held at the beginning and at the end of each shift to allow team members to exchange information, and the team leader to make changes in the nursing care plan for any patient. Compare **primary nursing.**

team practice, professional practice by a group of professionals that may include physicians, nurses, and others, as a social worker, nutritionist, or physical therapist, who manage the care of a specified number of patients as a team, usually in an outpatient setting.

teardrop fracture, an avulsion fracture of one of the short bones, as a vertebra, causing a tear-shaped disruption of bone tissue.

tear duct, any duct that carries tears, including the lacrimal ducts, nasolacrimal ducts, and the excretory ducts of the lacrimal glands.

tearing, watering of the eye usually caused by excessive tear production, as by strong emotion, infection, or mechanical irritation by a cinder or other foreign body. If the normal amount of fluid tears is produced but not drained into the lacrimal punctum at the nasal border of the eye, tearing will occur. If the lacrimal punctum, sac, cuniculi, or nasolacrimal duct becomes blocked, tears will also overflow. Also called **epiphora.**

technetium (Tc), a radioactive, metallic element. Its atomic number is 43; its atomic weight is 99. The first man-made element, technetium also occurs in nature. Isotopes of technetium are used in radioisotope scanning procedures of internal organs, as the liver and spleen. Formerly called **masurium.**

-technics, a combining form meaning 'the art or mechanics of': *balneotechnics, mnemotechnics, psychotechnics.* Also **-technology, -techny.**

technique, technic, the method and details followed in performing a procedure, as those used in conducting a laboratory test, a physical examination, a psychiatric interview, a surgical operation, or any process requiring certain skills or an ordered sequence of actions.

-technique, a combining form meaning 'the skillful way in which something is done': *iatrotechnique, microtechnique, zymotechnique.* Also **-technic.**

techno-, a combining form meaning 'art': *technopsychology, technocausis, technology.*

-techny, a combining form meaning 'the art or mechanics of' a specified area: *odontotechny, zootechny, zymotechny.* Also **-technics, -technology.**

tecto-, a combining form meaning 'rooflike': *tectocephalic, tectorial, tectum.*

Tedral, a trade name for a respiratory fixed-combination drug containing a bronchodilator (theophylline), an adrenergic (ephedrine hydrochloride), and a sedative-hypnotic (phenobarbital).

teenager. See **adolescent.**

teether, an object, as a teething ring, on which an infant can bite or chew during the teething process.

teething, the physiological process of the eruption of the deciduous teeth through the gums. It normally begins between the sixth and eighth months of life and occurs periodically until the complete set of 20 teeth has appeared at about 30 months. Discomfort and inflammation result from the pressure exerted against the periodontal tissue as the crown of the tooth breaks through the membranes. General signs of teething include excessive drooling, biting on hard objects, irritability, difficulty in sleeping, and refusal of food. Fever or diarrhea often occurs during teething but is indicative of illness rather than of teething. The pain and inflammation may usually be soothed by cold, as with a frozen teething ring, cold metal spoon, or ice wrapped in a washcloth. Use of teething powders and procedures, as rubbing or cutting the gums, are discouraged because of the possibility of infection or complications from ingestion of the medication. — **teethe,** *v.*

teething ring, a circular device, usually made of plastic or rubber, on which an infant may chew or bite during the teething process.

Teflon, a trade name for a substance (polytetrafluor-ethylene), used for the construction of surgical implants in restorative surgery.

teg-, a combining form meaning 'of or pertaining to a cover': *tegmen, tegmental, tegument.*

Tegopen, a trade name for an antibacterial (cloxacillin sodium).

Tegretol, a trade name for an analgesic and anticonvulsant (carbamazepine).

TEIB, abbreviation for *triethylene-immuno-benzoquinone.*

tela-, a combining form meaning 'a web or weblike structure': *telalgia, telangiectasia, telangitis.*

-tela, a combining form meaning a 'weblike membrane': *aulatela, epitela, metatela.*

telangiectasia (təlæn′jiektei′zhə), permanent dilatation of groups of superficial capillaries and venules. Common causes are actinic damage, atrophy-producing dermatoses, rosacea, elevated estrogen levels, and collagen-vascular diseases. See also **Rendu-Osler-Weber syndrome, spider angioma.**

telangiectatic epulis, a benign, red tumor of the gingiva, containing prominent blood vessels. Low-grade or chronic irritation is usually associated, and the lesion is easily traumatized.

telangiectatic fibroma. See **angiofibroma.**

telangiectatic glioma, a tumor composed of glial cells and a network of blood vessels, which give the mass a vivid pink appearance.

telangiectatic granuloma. See **pyogenic granuloma.**

telangiectatic lipoma. See **angiolipoma.**

telangiectatic nevus, a common skin condition of neonates, characterized by flat, deep-pink localized areas of capillary dilatation that occur predominantly on the back of the neck, lower occiput, upper eyelids, upper lip, and bridge of the nose. The areas disappear permanently by about two years of age. Also called **capillary flames, stork bite.**

telangiectatic sarcoma, a malignant tumor of mesodermal cells with an unusually rich vascular network.

tele-, 1. a combining form meaning 'of or related to the end': *telencephalon, teleneuron, telesystolic.* 2. a combining form meaning 'operating at a distance, or far away': *telecardiogram, teleceptor, telemetry.*

telepathist (təlep′əthist), 1. a person who believes in telepathy. 2. a person who has or claims to have telepathic powers.

telepathy (təlep′əthi), the communication of thought from one person to another by means other than the physical senses. Also called **thought transference.** See also **extrasensory perception, parapsychology.** — **telepathic,** *adj.,* **telepathize,** *v.*

tellurium (Te), an element exhibiting metallic and nonmetallic chemical properties. Its atomic number is 52; its atomic weight is 127.60. Inhaling vapors of tellurium results in a garlicky breath.

telo-, a combining form meaning 'of or pertaining to the end': *telobiosis, telodendron, telosynapsis.*

telocentric (tel′əsen′trık), pertaining to a chromosome in which the centromere is located at the end, so that the chromatids appear as straight filaments. Compare **acrocentric, metacentric, submetacentric.**

telophase (tel′əfeiz), the final of the four stages of nuclear division in mitosis and in each of the two divisions in meiosis. The newly produced daughter chromosomes from the preceding anaphase stage assemble at the poles of the division spindle and become long and slender, the nuclear membrane forms around them, the nucleolus reappears, and the cytoplasm begins to divide. See also **anaphase, interphase, meiosis, metaphase, mitosis, prophase.**

Temaril, a trade name for an antihistamine (trimeprazine tartrate).

temperate phage, a bacteriophage whose genome is incorporated into the host bacterium. It persists through many cell divisions of the bacterium without destroying the host, in contrast to a virulent phage that lyses and kills its host.

temperature, **1.** a relative measure of sensible heat or cold. **2.** (in physiology) a measure of sensible heat associated with the metabolism of the human body, normally maintained at a constant level of 98.6°F or 37°C by the thermotaxic nerve mechanism which balances heat gains and heat losses. **3.** *Informal.* a fever.

temper tantrum. See **tantrum.**

template (tem′plıt), (in genetics) the strand of DNA that acts as a mold for the synthesis of messenger RNA. This messenger RNA contains the same sequence of nucleic acids as the DNA strand and carries the code to the ribosomes, which are located in the cytoplasm, for the synthesis of proteins.

tempo-, a combining form meaning 'of or pertaining to time': *tempolabile, temporal, tempostabile.*

temporal arteritis, a progressive, inflammatory disorder of cranial blood vessels, principally the temporal artery, occurring most frequently in women over the age of 70. Characteristic changes in the involved vessels include granulomatous disruption of the elastic layer and engulfment of fiber fragments by giant cells in the intimal and medial layers. Symptoms are intractable headache, difficulty in chewing, weakness, rheumatic pains, and loss of vision if the central retinal artery becomes occluded. Also called **cranial arteritis, giant cell arteritis, Horton's arteritis.**

temporal artery, any one of three arteries on each side of the head: the superficial temporal artery, the middle temporal artery, and the deep temporal artery.

temporal bone, one of a pair of large bones forming part of the lower cranium and containing various cavities and recesses associated with the ear, as the tympanic cavity and the auditory tube. Each temporal bone consists of three portions: the squama, the petrous, and the tympanic.

temporal bone fracture, a break of the temporal bone of the skull, sometimes characterized by bleeding from the ear. Diminished hearing, facial paralysis, or infection of the tympanic cavity leading to meningitis may occur.

temporalis (tem′pərael′ıs), one of the four muscles of mastication. It is a broad, radiating muscle that arises from the whole of the temporal fossa and from the surface of the temporal fascia. It inserts into the ramus of the mandible near the last molar tooth, and it is innervated by the anterior and the posterior temporal nerves. The temporalis acts to close the jaws and retract the mandible. Also called **temporal muscle.** Compare **masseter, pterygoideus lateralis, pterygoideus medialis.**

temporal lobe, the lateral region of the cerebrum, below the lateral fissure. Within the temporal lobe of the brain is the center for smell, some association areas for memory and learning, and a region where choice is made of thoughts to express. Compare **frontal lobe, occipital lobe, parietal lobe.**

temporal lobe epilepsy. See **psychomotor seizure.**

temporal muscle. See **temporalis.**

temporal summation. See **summation,** def. 2.

temporary tooth. See **deciduous tooth.**

temporomandibular joint, one of two joints connecting the mandible of the jaw to the temporal bone of the skull. It is a combined hinge and gliding joint, formed by the anterior parts of the mandibular fossae of the temporal bone, the articular tubercles, the condyles of the mandible, and five ligaments.

temporomandibular joint pain-dysfunction syndrome, an abnormal condition characterized by facial pain and by mandibular dysfunction, apparently caused by a defective or dislocated temporomandibular joint. Some common indications of this syndrome are the clicking of the joint when the jaws move, limitation of jaw movement, subluxation, and temporomandibular dislocation. Also called **myofacial pain-dysfunction syndrome.**

temporoparietalis (tem′pəroupərai′ıtæl′ıs), one of a pair of broad, thin muscles of the scalp, divided into three parts, which fan out over the temporal fascia and insert into the galea aponeurotica. The three parts include an anterior temporal portion, a superior parietal portion, and a triangular portion in between. The temporoparietalis was formerly considered part of the superior and the inferior auricularis. On both sides, it acts in combination with the occipitofrontalis to wrinkle the forehead, to widen the eyes, and to raise the ears. It is innervated by branches of the facial nerve. Compare **occipitofrontalis.**

TEN, abbreviation for **toxic epidermal necrolysis.**

tenaculum (tənæk′yuləm), *pl.* **tenacula.** a clip or clamp with long handles used to grasp, immobilize, and hold an organ or a piece of tissue. Kinds of tenacula include the **abdominal tenaculum,** which has long arms and small hooks, the **forceps tenaculum,** which has long hooks and is used in gynecologic surgery, and the **uterine** or **cervical tenaculum,** which has short hooks or open, eye-shaped clamps used to hold the cervix.

tendinitis, tendonitis (ten'danaï'tɪs), an inflammatory condition of a tendon, usually resulting from strain. Treatment may include rest, corticosteroid injections, and support.

tendinous cords (ten'dɪnəs). See **chordae tendineae.**

tendo calcaneus (ten'dou), the common tendon of the soleus and gastrocnemius. It is the thickest and strongest tendon in the body and begins near the middle of the posterior part of the leg. In an adult it is about 15 cm long. The tendon becomes contracted about 4 cm above the heel and flares out again to insert into the calcaneus. Also called **Achilles tendon, tendon of Achilles.**

tendon, one of many white, glistening fibrous bands of tissue that attach muscle to bone. Except at points of attachment, tendons are sheathed in delicate fibroelastic connective tissue. Larger tendons contain a thin internal septum, a few blood vessels, and specialized sterognostic nerves. Tendons are extremely strong and flexible, inelastic, and occur in various lengths and thicknesses. Compare **ligament.** — **tendinous,** *adj.*

tendon of Achilles. See **tendo calcaneus.**

tendon reflex. See **deep tendon reflex.**

tenesmus (tənez'məs), persistent, ineffectual spasms of the rectum or bladder, accompanied by the desire to empty the bowel or bladder. Intestinal tenesmus is a common complaint in inflammatory bowel disease and irritable bowel syndrome.

tenia-, taenia-, a combining form meaning 'ribbon, band': **teniasis, teniafuge, taenidium.**

tennis elbow. See **lateral humeral epicondylitis.**

teno-, a combining form meaning 'of or pertaining to a tendon': *tenodesis, tenodynia, tenomyotomy.* Also **tenonto-.**

Tenon's capsule (ten'ənz). See **fascia bulbi.**

tenonto-. See **teno-.**

tenosynovitis (ten'ousɪn'əvai'tɪs), inflammation of a tendon sheath caused by calcium deposits, repeated strain or trauma, high levels of blood cholesterol, rheumatoid arthritis, gout, or gonorrhea. In some instances, movement yields crackling noise over the tendon. Most cases not associated with systemic disease respond to rest. Local injections of adrenocorticosteroids may provide relief; surgery is indicated if the condition persists.

tenotomy (tɪnot'əmi), the total or partial severing of a tendon, performed to correct a muscle imbalance, as in the correction of strabismus of the eye or in clubfoot.

Tensilon (ten'sɪlon), a trade name for a cholinesterase reactivator (edrophonium), used as an adjunct to anesthesia.

tension, 1. the act of pulling or straining until taut. 2. the condition of being taut, tense, or under pressure. 3. a state or condition resulting from the psychological and physiological reaction to a stressful situation, characterized physically by a general increase in muscle tonus, heart rate, respiration rate, and alertness and psychologically by feelings of strain, uneasiness, irritability, and anxiety. See also **stress.**

-tension. See **-tention².**

tension headache, a pain that affects the occipital region of the body as the result of overwork or emotional strain, tensing the body and inhibiting rest and relaxation.

tensor, any one of the muscles of the body that tenses a structure, as the tensor fasciae latae of the thigh. Compare **abductor, adductor, depressor, sphincter.**

tensor fasciae latae, one of the ten muscles of the gluteal region, arising from the outer lip of the iliac crest, the iliac spine, and the deep fascia lata. It inserts between the two layers of fascia lata in the proximal third of the thigh. The tensor fasciae latae is innervated by a branch of the superior gluteal nerve, which contains fibers from the fourth and fifth lumbar and the first sacral nerves, and it functions to flex the thigh and to rotate it slightly medially. Also called **tensor fasciae femoris.**

tent, 1. a transparent cover, usually of plastic, supported over the upper part of a patient by a frame. Used in the treatment of respiratory conditions, it provides a controlled environment into which steam, oxygen, vaporized medication, or droplets of cool water may be sprayed, as an oxygen tent. 2. a cone made of various materials inserted into a cavity or orifice of the body to dilate its opening, as a laminaria tent. 3. a pack placed in a wound to hold it open in order to ensure that healing progresses from the base of the wound upward to the skin.

tenth nerve. See **vagus nerve.**

-tention¹, a combining form meaning the 'condition of being held': *historetention, retention.*

-tention², a combining form meaning 'condition of being stretched': *attention, distention, intention.* Also **-tension.**

tentorial herniation, the protrusion of brain tissue into the tentorial notch, caused by increased intracranial pressure resulting from edema, hemorrhage, or a tumor. Characteristic signs are severe headache, fever, flushing, sweating, abnormal pupillary reflex, drowsiness, hypotension, and loss of consciousness. Also called **transtentorial herniation.**

tentorium (tentor'iəm), *pl.* **tentoria.** any part of the body that resembles a tent, as the tentorium of the cerebellum which supports the occipital lobes and covers the cerebellum.

tentorium cerebelli, one of the three extensions of the dura mater that separates the cerebellum from the occipital lobe of the cerebrum. Compare **falx cerebelli, falx cerebri.**

Tenuate, a trade name for an anorexiant (diethylpropion hydrochloride).

tenure, (in a university) a faculty appointment without a limit on the number of years it may be held; a permanent appointment usually awarded to a person who has advanced to the rank of professor and who demonstrates scholarship and excellence in a specific field of study.

Tepanil, a trade name for an anorexiant (diethylpropion hydrochloride).

tephr-, a combining form meaning 'ash-colored': *tephromalacia, tephromyelitis, tephrylometer.*

tepid, moderately warm to the touch.

teramorphous, of the nature of or characteristic of a monster.

teras (ter'əs), *pl.* **terata.** a severely deformed fetus; a monster. **– teratic,** *adj.*

teratism, any congenital or developmental anomaly that is produced by inherited or environmental factors, or by a combination of the two; any condition in which a severely malformed fetus is produced. Kinds of teratism include **atresic teratism, ceasmic teratism, ectopic teratism, ectrogenic teratism, hypergenetic teratism, symphysic teratism.** Also called **teratosis.**

terato-, a combining form meaning 'of or related to a monster': *teratoblastoma, teratogenesis, teratoma.*

teratogen, any substance, agent, or process that interferes with normal prenatal development, causing the formation of one or more developmental abnormalities in the fetus. Teratogens act directly on the developing organism or indirectly, affecting such supplemental structures as the placenta or some maternal system. The type and extent of the defect are determined by the specific kind of teratogen and its mode of action, the embryonic process affected, genetic predisposition, and the stage of development at the time the exposure occurred. The period of highest vulnerability in the developing embryo is from about the third through the twelfth week of gestation, when differentiation of the major organs and systems occurs. Susceptibility to teratogenic influence decreases rapidly in the later periods of development, which are characterized by growth and elaboration. Among the known teratogens are chemical agents, including such drugs as thalidomide, alkylating agents, and alcohol; infectious agents, especially the rubella virus and cytomegalovirus; ionizing radiation, particularly x rays; and environmental factors, as the age and general health of the mother or any intrauterine trauma that may affect the fetus, especially during the later stages of pregnancy. Compare **mutagen. – teratogenic,** *adj.*

teratogenesis (ter'ətoujen'əsɪs), the development of physical defects in the embryo. **– teratogenetic,** *adj.*

teratogeny (ter'ətoj'əni). See **teratogenesis. – teratogenic,** *adj.*

teratoid (ter'ətoid), of or pertaining to abnormal physical development; resembling a monster.

teratoid tumor. See **dermoid cyst.**

teratologist, one who specializes in the science of teratology.

teratology, the study of the causes and effects of congenital malformations and developmental abnormalities. **– teratologic, teratological,** *adj.*

teratoma, *pl.* **teratomas, teratomata.** a tumor composed of different kinds of tissue, none of which normally occur together or at the site of the tumor. Teratomas are most common in the ovaries or testes.

teratosis. See **teratism.**

terbium (Tr), a rare-earth metallic element. Its atomic number is 65; its atomic weight is 158.294.

terbutaline sulfate, a beta-adrenergic stimulant.

■ INDICATIONS: It is prescribed as a bronchodilator in the treatment of asthma, bronchitis, and emphysema and as a uterine relaxant to treat premature labor.

■ CONTRAINDICATIONS: Cardiac arrhythmias or known hypersensitivity to this drug prohibits its use.

■ ADVERSE EFFECTS: Among the most serious reactions are dizziness and palpitations. Nervousness and tremor are common reactions.

teres (tɪ'riz, ter'iz), *pl.* **teretes** (ter'ətɪs, tər'ətiz). a long, cylindrical muscle, as the teres minor or the teres major. **– teres,** *adj.*

teres major, a thick, flat muscle of the shoulder. Arising from the dorsal surface of the scapula and from the fibrous septa between the teres major, the teres minor, and the infraspinatus, it is innervated by a branch of the lower subscapular nerve from the brachial plexus, which contains fibers from the fifth and the sixth cervical nerves, and it functions to adduct, extend, and rotate the arm medially. Compare **teres minor.**

teres minor, a cylindrical, elongated muscle of the shoulder. Arising from the dorsal surface of the scapula and from two aponeurotic laminae, one of which separates it from the teres major, the other from the infraspinatus, it is inserted into the humerus and is innervated by a branch of the axillary nerve, which contains fibers from the fifth cervical nerve. The teres minor functions to rotate the arm laterally, weakly adduct the arm, and draw the humerus toward the glenoid fossa of the scapula, strengthening the shoulder joint. Compare **teres major.**

terminal, (of a struture or process) near or approaching its end, as a terminal bronchiole or a terminal disease. **– terminate,** *v.,* **terminus,** *n.*

terminal bronchiole. See **bronchiole.**

terminal nerve, a small nerve originating in the cerebral hemisphere in the region of the olfactory trigone, classified by most anatomists as part of the olfactory, or first cranial, nerve. The terminal nerve courses anteriorly along the olfactory tract and passes through the ethmoid bone. Most filaments of the nerve form a single strand which passes to the membrane near the anterior superior border of the nasal septum and communicates in the nasal cavity with the ophthalmic division of the trigeminal nerve. The central connections of the terminal nerve end in the septal nuclei, the olfactory lobe, and the posterior commissural and supraoptic regions of the brain.

terminal stance, one of the five stages in the stance phase of a walking gait, directly associated with the continuation of single limb support or the period during which the body moves forward on the supporting foot. Double limb support is initiated during the latter part of terminal stance, which is often a factor in the analysis of many abnormal orthopedic conditions and the diagnosis of weaknesses that may develop in certain muscles used in walking, as the quadriceps femoris and the gluteus maximus. Compare **initial contact stance stage, loading response stance stage, midstance, preswing stance stage.** See also **swing phase of gait.**

terminal sulcus of right atrium, a shallow channel on the external surface of the right atrium between the superior and inferior venae cavae.

termination codon, (in molecular genetics) a unit in the genetic code that specifies the end of the sequence of amino acids in a polypeptide.

termination sequence, (in molecular genetics) a DNA segment at the end of a unit that is transcribed to messenger RNA from the DNA template.

term infant, any neonate, regardless of birth weight, born after the end of the thirty-seventh and before the beginning of the forty-third week of gestation. Infants delivered at term usually measure from 48 to 53 cm from head to heel and weigh between 2,700 and 4,000 gm.

terpin hydrate and codeine elixir, a preparation of the expectorant, terpin hydrate, with sweet orange peel tincture, benzaldehyde, glycerin, alcohol, syrup, water, and the antitussive narcotic codeine. Terpin hydrate diminishes secretions and promotes healing of the mucous membrane, while codeine depresses the cough center in the medulla oblongata; prolonged use may lead to addiction.

Terra-Cortril, a trade name for a topical fixed-combination drug containing a glucocorticoid (hydrocortisone) and an antibiotic (oxytetracycline).

Terramycin, a trade name for an antibiotic (oxytetracycline).

Terrastatin, a trade name for a fixed-combination drug containing an antifungal (nystatin) and an antibiotic (oxytetracycline).

terti-, a combining form meaning 'third': *tertiary, tertigravida, tertipara.*

tertian (tər'shən), occurring every three days, including the first day of occurrence, as vivax or tertian malaria, in which fever occurs every third day. Compare **quartan.** See also **malaria.**

tertian malaria, a form of malaria, caused by the protozoan *Plasmodium vivax* or *Plasmodium ovale,* characterized by febrile paroxysms that occur every 48 hours. **Vivax malaria,** caused by *Plasmodium vivax,* is the most common form of malaria, and although it is rarely fatal, it is the most difficult form to cure. Relapses are common. **Ovale malaria,** caused by *Plasmodium ovale,* is usually milder and causes only a few, short attacks. Both types of tertian malaria are treated with chloroquine. Compare **falciparum malaria, quartan malaria.** See also **malaria.**

tertiary (tər'shieri, tərsh'əri), third in frequency or in order of use; belonging to the third level of sophistication of development, as a tertiary health care facility.

tertiary health care, a specialized, highly technical level of health care that includes diagnosis and treatment of disease and disability in sophisticated, large research and teaching hospitals. Specialized intensive-care units, advanced diagnostic support services, and highly specialized personnel are usually characteristic of tertiary health care. It offers a highly centralized care to the population of a large region; in some cases, to the world.

Teslac, a trade name for an antineoplastic (testolactone).

Tessalon, a trade name for a local anesthetic agent (benzonatate).

test, 1. an examination or trial intended to establish a principle or determine a value. 2. a chemical reaction or reagent that has clinical significance. 3. to detect, identify, or conduct a trial. See also **laboratory test.**

test-, a combining form meaning 'of or pertaining to the testicles': *testicond, testitoxicosis, testosterone.*

testcross, 1. (in genetics) the cross of a dominant phenotype with a recessive phenotype to determine either the degree of genetic linkage or whether the dominant phenotype is homozygous or heterozygous. 2. the subject undergoing such a test.

testicle (tes'tikəl). See **testis.**

testicular (testik'yulər), of or pertaining to the testicle.

testicular artery, one of a pair of long, slender branches of the abdominal aorta, arising caudal to the renal arteries and supplying the testis.

testicular cancer, a malignant neoplastic disease of the testis occurring most frequently in men between the ages of 20 and 35. An undescended testicle is often affected. In many cases the tumor is detected following an injury, but trauma is not considered an etiologic factor. Patients with early testicular cancer are often asymptomatic, and metastases may be seeded in lymph nodes, the lungs, and liver before the primary lesion is palpable. In the later stages there may be pulmonary symptoms, ureteral obstruction, gynecomastia, and an abdominal mass. Diagnostic measures include transillumination of the scrotum, excretory urography, lymphangiography, and a urine or serum test to evaluate circulating levels of luteinizing hormone. Tumors develop more often in the right than in the left testis. Seminomas are the most curable lesions and the most common, representing 40 per cent of all testicular tumors. Embryonal carcinomas are more highly malignant and represent 15 to 20 per cent of these tumors. Teratocarcinomas, and choricarcinomas also occur. Radiotherapy and surgical excision are usually recommended to treat seminoma. Chemotherapy using combinations of drugs is recommended for nonseminomatous tumors. Chemotherapeutic agents, used in various combinations, are increasing the survival of patients with testicular cancer. Some of these drugs are actinomycin D, bleomycin, cis-platinum, cyclophosphamide, methotrexate, and vincristine.

testicular duct.   See **deferent duct.**

testicular vein,   one of a pair of veins that emerge from convoluted venous plexuses, forming the greater mass of the spermatic cords. Veins from each plexus start from small veins at the back of the testes, ascend along the spermatic cords, anterior to the ductus deferens, and pass through the deep inguinal ring and unite to form a single vein. The right testicular vein opens into the inferior vena cava; the left testicular vein into the left renal vein. Both testicular veins contain valves. Compare **ovarian vein.**

testis (tes′tıs), *pl.* **testes.**   one of the pair of male gonads that produce semen. The adult testes are suspended in the scrotum by the spermatic cords; in early fetal life they are contained in the abdominal cavity behind the peritoneum. Before birth they descend into the scrotum and during development are covered with layers of tissue derived from the serous, the muscular, and the fibrous layers of the abdominal parietes. The coverings of the testes are the skin and the dartos tunic of the scrotum, the external spermatic fascia, the cremastic layer, the internal spermatic fascia, and the tunica virginalis. Each testis is a laterally compressed oval body about 4 cm long, 2.5 cm wide, and weighs about 12 gm. It is positioned obliquely in the scrotum, with the cranial extremity directed ventrally and slightly laterally, the caudal end directed dorsally and slightly medially. The anterior border, the lateral surfaces, and the extremities of the organ are convex, free, smooth, and covered by the tunica virginalis. The convoluted epididymis lying on the posterior border of the testis is about 20 feet long and connects with the vas deferens through which spermatozoa pass during ejaculation. Each testis consists of several hundred conical lobules containing the tiny coiled seminiferous tubules, each about 75 mm long, in which spermatozoa develop. In early life the tubules are pale in color but in old age become invested with yellow fatty matter. The tubules converge to form the rete testis which is drained by the efferent ducts into the head of the epididymis. The testis,

developed in the lumbar region, may be retained in the abdomen, the deep inguinal ring, or the inguinal canal. A man with both testes undescended is sterile but may not be impotent. The testes are supplied with blood by the two internal spermatic arteries which arise from the aorta, are served by the testicular veins which form the pampiniform plexuses constituting the greater part of the spermatic cords, and are innervated by the spermatic plexuses of nerves from the celiac plexuses of the autonomic nervous system. Compare **ovary.** See also **scrotum.**

testolactone,   an antineoplastic androgen analog.

■ INDICATION: It is prescribed in the treatment of breast cancer.

■ CONTRAINDICATIONS: Pregnancy, lactation, or known hypersensitivity to this drug prohibits its use. It is not given to men.

■ ADVERSE EFFECTS: Among the more serious adverse reactions are hypercalcemia and peripheral neuropathies with numbness or tingling.

testosterone (testos′tərɔun),   a naturally occurring androgenic hormone.

■ INDICATIONS: It is prescribed for androgen deficiency, female breast cancer, and for stimulation of growth, weight gain, and red blood cell production.

■ CONTRAINDICATIONS: Cancer of the male breast or prostate, liver disease, pregnancy or suspected pregnancy, or known hypersensitivity to this drug prohibits its use.

■ ADVERSE EFFECTS: Among the more serious adverse reactions are fluid retention, masculinization, acne, and erythrocytemia.

testosterone cyclopentylpropionate.   See **testosterone cypionate.**

testosterone cypionate,   a long-acting form of testosterone.

testosterone derivative.   See **anabolic steroid.**

testosterone enanthate,   a long-acting form of testosterone.

testosterone propionate,   an androgen given intramuscularly. See also **testosterone.**

test tube,   a tube made of transparent material having one open end. It is used in the growth of bacteriologic specimens, in the analysis of some chemical functions, and in many other common laboratory functions. See also **tube.**

-tetanic,   a combining form meaning 'relating to or producing tetanus or tetany': *antitetanic, posttetanic, subtetanic.*

tetano-,   a combining form meaning 'of or pertaining to tetanus': *tetanolysin, tetanometer, tetanophilic.*

tetanus (tet′ənəs),   an acute, potentially fatal infection of the central nervous system caused by an exotoxin, tetanospasmin, elaborated by an anaerobic bacillus, *Clostridium tetani.* More than 50,000 people a year die of tetanus infection, worldwide. The toxin is a neurotoxin and is one of the most lethal poisons known. *C. tetani* infects only wounds that contain dead tissue. The bacillus is a common resident of the superficial layers of the soil and a normal inhabitant of the intestinal tracts of cows and horses; therefore, barnyards and fields fertilized with manure are heavily contaminated.

■ OBSERVATIONS: The bacillus may enter the body through a puncture wound, laceration, or burn, via the uterus into the blood stream in septic abortion or postpartum sepsis, or through the stump of the umbilical cord of the newborn. The dead tissue of the area is low in oxygen; this is the environment essential for the replication of *C. tetani*. The infection occurs in two clinical forms: one with an abrupt onset, high mortality, and a short incubation period (3 to 21 days); the other with less severe symptoms, a lower mortality, and a longer incubation period (4 to 5 weeks). Wounds of the face, head, and neck are the ones most likely to result in fatal infection, as the bacillus may travel rapidly to the brain. The disease is characterized by irritability, headache, fever, and painful spasms of the muscles resulting in lockjaw, risus sardonicus, opisthotonos, and laryngeal spasm; eventually, every muscle of the body is in tonic spasm. The motor nerves transmit the impulses from the infected central nervous system to the muscles. There is no lesion; even at autopsy no organic lesion is seen and the cerebrospinal fluid is clear and normal.

■ INTERVENTION: Prompt and thorough cleansing and debridement of the wound are essential for prophylaxis. A booster shot of tetanus toxoid is given to previously immunized people; tetanus immune globulin and a series of three injections of tetanus toxoid are given to those not immunized. People who are known to have been adequately immunized within 5 years do not usually require immunization. The treatment of people who have the infection includes maintenance of an airway, giving an antitoxin as soon as possible, sedation, control of the muscle spasms, and assuring a normal fluid balance. The room is kept quiet and benzodiazepines may be given to reduce hypertonicity; penicillin G is administered for infection; and a tracheostomy is performed and oxygen given for ventilation.

■ NURSING CONSIDERATIONS: The nurse may encourage everyone to be actively immunized against the infection. The vaccine is safe and effective. Immunization more often than required is not recommended.

tetanus and diphtheria toxoids, an active immunizing agent containing detoxified tetanus and diphtheria toxoids that slowly produce an antigenic response to the diseases.

■ INDICATIONS: It is prescribed for immunization against tetanus and diphtheria in children under seven years of age when pertussis vaccine present in the usual diphtheria, pertussis, and tetanus tri-valent vaccine is contraindicated.

■ CONTRAINDICATIONS: Immunosuppression, concomitant use of corticosteroids, or acute infection prohibits its use.

■ ADVERSE EFFECTS: Among the most serious adverse reactions are allergic reactions and stinging at the site of injection.

tetanus antitoxin (TAT), a tetanus immune serum that neutralizes exotoxins in tetanus infection.

■ INDICATION: It is prescribed for short-term immunization against tetanus following possible exposure to the organism.

■ CONTRAINDICATIONS: It is not given if the more effective tetanus immune globulin is available or if there is a known sensitivity to equine serum.

■ ADVERSE EFFECTS: Among the most serious adverse reactions are allergic reactions and pain and inflammation at the site of injection.

tetanus immune globulin (TIG), an injectible solution prepared from the globulin of an immune human. It is effective and much safer than tetanus antitoxin.

■ INDICATION: It is prescribed for short-term immunization against tetanus following possible exposure to the organism.

■ CONTRAINDICATION: Known hypersensitivity to this drug prohibits its use.

■ ADVERSE EFFECTS: The most serious adverse reaction is hypersensitivity. Pain and inflammation at the site of injection may occur.

tetanus toxoid, an active immunizing agent prepared from detoxified tetanus toxin that produces an antigenic response in the body, conferring permanent immunity to tetanus infection.

■ INDICATION: It is prescribed for active immunization against tetanus.

■ CONTRAINDICATIONS: Immunosuppression or acute infection prohibits its use.

■ ADVERSE EFFECTS: The most serious adverse reaction is hypersensitivity. Pain and inflammation at the site of injection may occur.

tetany (tet'əni), a condition characterized by cramps, convulsions, twitching of the muscles, and sharp flexion of the wrist and ankle joints. These symptoms are sometimes accompanied by attacks of stridor. Tetany is a manifestation of an abnormality in calcium metabolism, which can occur in association with vitamin D deficiency, hypoparathyroidism, alkalosis, or the ingestion of alkaline salts. Kinds of tetany are **duration tetany, grass tetany, hyperventilation tetany, lactation tetany.** Compare **tetanus.**

tetart-, a combining form meaning 'fourth': *tetartanopia, tetartocone, tetartoconoid.*

tetra-, a combining form meaning 'four': *tetracycline, tetrahydric, tetranopsia.* Also **tetro-.**

Tetrachel, a trade name for an antibiotic (tetracycline hydrochloride).

tetrachlormethane (tet'rəklɔrmeth'ein). See **carbon tetrachloride.**

tetrachloroethylene, an anthelmintic.

- INDICATION: It has been prescribed in the treatment of infestation by hookworm.
- CONTRAINDICATIONS: Liver degeneration or known hypersensitivity to this drug prohibits its use. It is not recommended for use in small, severely ill children.
- ADVERSE EFFECTS: Among the more serious adverse reactions are nausea, vomiting, liver toxicity and abdominal cramps.

tetracycline, a broad spectrum antibiotic.

- INDICATIONS: It is prescribed for the treatment of many bacterial and rickettsial infections.
- CONTRAINDICATIONS: Significantly impaired liver or renal function or known hypersensitivity to this drug prohibits its use. Because it may cause permanent discoloration of the teeth, its use is contraindicated in the last half of pregnancy and during a child's first eight years of life.
- ADVERSE EFFECTS: Among the more serious adverse reactions are renal toxicity, hepatotoxicity, severe gastrointestinal disturbances, enterocolitis, inflammatory lesions with monilial overgrowth in the anogenital area, hemolytic anemia, thrombocytopenia, eosinophilia, and rashes.

tetracycline hydrochloride (tet'rəsāi'klin, tet'rəsāi'klın), a tetracycline antibiotic.

- INDICATIONS: It is prescribed in the treatment of a variety of infections.
- CONTRAINDICATIONS: Known hypersensitivity to this drug or to other tetracyclines prohibits its use. Use during pregnancy or in children under 8 years of age may result in discoloration of the child's teeth. It is to be administered with caution with renal or liver impairment.
- ADVERSE EFFECTS: Among the most serious reactions are potentially serious suprainfections, various allergic reactions, phototoxicity, and gastrointestinal disturbances.

Tetracyn, a trade name for an antibiotic (tetracycline hydrochloride).

tetrad (tet'ræd), (in genetics) a group of four chromatids of a synapsed pair of homologous chromosomes during the first meiotic prophase stage of gametogenesis. The group is formed in preparation for the two meiotic divisions in the maturation process of gametes. —**tetradic,** *adj.*

tetrahydrocannabinol (THC), the active principle, occurring as two psychomimetic isomers, in the hemp plant *Cannabis sativa,* used in the preparation of marijuana, hashish, bhang, and ganja. THC, a rapidly metabolized beta-adrenergic antagonist, increases pulse rate, causes conjunctival reddening, a feeling of euphoria, and has variable effects on blood pressure, respiratory rate, and pupil size. The drug affects memory, cognition, and the sensorium, decreases motor coordination, and increases appetite. Propranolol blocks the peripheral effects of THC but not the psychic effects. Overdoses of THC may be treated by "talking down" the patient and administering sedative barbiturates or diazepam parenterally. Nonintoxicating doses of THC are used experimentally in the treatment of glaucoma and to relieve nausea and increase the appetite in patients receiving cancer chemotherapy. See also **cannabis.**

tetrahydrozoline hydrochloride, an adrenergic vasoconstrictor.

- INDICATIONS: It is prescribed for the treatment of nasal congestion and as an ophthalmic vasoconstrictor.
- CONTRAINDICATIONS: Glaucoma or known hypersensitivity to this drug or to other vasoconstrictors prohibits its use. It is used with caution in patients who have cardiovascular disease.
- ADVERSE EFFECTS: Among the more serious adverse reactions are irritation to mucosa, rebound nasal congestion, and effects associated with systemic absorption, including sedation and alterations in cardiovascular function.

tetraiodothyronine. See **thyroxine.**

tetralogy of Fallot (fælou'), a congenital cardiac anomaly that consists of four defects: pulmonic stenosis, ventricular septal defect, malposition of the aorta so that it arises from the septal defect or the right ventricle, and right ventricular hypertrophy. The primary symptoms in the infant are cyanosis and hypoxia, usually during crying, difficulty in feeding, failure to gain weight, and poor development. In older children a typical squatting position and clubbing of the fingers and toes are evident. A pansystolic murmur is usually heard and the second heart sound is faint or absent. Diagnosis of the condition is primarily based on the history and physical symptoms, although cardiac catheterization is performed to evaluate the severity of the defects. Treatment consists mainly of supportive measures and palliative surgical procedures, primarily systemic-to-pulmonary anastomoses, to decrease tissue hypoxia and prevent complications until the child is old enough to tolerate total corrective surgery. The optimal age for surgical repair is approximately four or five years. Also called **blue baby, Fallot's syndrome.** See also **congenital cardiac anomaly, trilogy of Fallot.**

tetraploid (4n), 1. Also **tetraploidic.** of or pertaining to an individual, organism, strain, or cell that has four complete sets of chromosomes, quadruple the normal haploid number characteristic of the species. In humans, the tetraploid number is 92 and is extremely rare, found only occasionally in abortuses and stillborn fetuses. **2.** such an individual, organism, strain, or cell. Compare **diploid, haploid, triploid.** See also **polyploid.**

tetraploidy (tet'rəploi'di), the state or condition of having four complete sets of chromosomes.

Tetrastatin, a trade name for an anti-infective fixed-combination drug containing an antifungal (nystatin) and an antibiotic (tetracycline hydrochloride).

Tetrex, a trade name for an antibiotic (tetracycline phosphate complex.)

tetro-. See **tetra-.**

Texacort, a trade name for a topical preparation containing a glucocorticoid (hydrocortisone).

T fracture, an intercondylar fracture in which the fracture lines are T-shaped.

TGF, abbreviation for **transforming growth factor.**

T-group. See **sensitivity-training group.**

Th, symbol for **thorium.**

thalamus (thǎl'əməs), *pl.* **thalami.** one of a pair of large, oval organs forming most of the lateral walls of the third ventricle of the brain and part of the diencephalon. It relays sensory impulses to the cerebral cortex, measures about four cm long and 1.5 cm wide and consists of numerous nuclei arranged in anterior, lateral, intralaminar, medial, and posterior groups. On each side the thalamus extends caudally beyond the third ventricle, with its medial and superior surfaces exposed in the ventricle and its inferior and lateral surfaces buried against other structures. It is composed mainly of gray substance and translates impulses from appropriate receptors into crude sensations of pain, temperature, and touch. It also participates in associating sensory impulses with pleasant and unpleasant feelings, in the arousal mechanisms of the body, and in the mechanisms that produce complex reflex movements. Compare **epithalamus, hypothalamus, subthalamus.** – **thalamic,** *adj.*

thalassemia (thǎl'əsi'mǐə), hemolytic anemia characterized by microcytic, hypochromic, and short-lived red blood cells caused by deficient hemoglobin synthesis. People of Mediterranean origin are more often affected than others. It is an autosomal recessive, genetically transmitted disease occurring in two forms. **Thalassemia major** (the homozygous form) evident in infancy, is recognized by anemia, fever, failure to thrive, and splenomegaly and confirmed by characteristic changes in the red blood cells on microscopic examination. Frequent transfusions are necessary to maintain oxygen-carrying capacity of the blood. Red cells are rapidly destroyed, freeing large amounts of iron to be deposited in the skin, which becomes bronzed and freckled. The iron is also deposited in the heart, liver, and pancreas, which become fibrotic and dysfunctional. The spleen may become so enlarged that respiratory excursion is impeded, and the abdominal organs are crowded. Headache, abdominal pain, fatigue, and anorexia often occur. There is no cure. The nurse is aware that the child is uncomfortable and that growth and sexual development are usually retarded. Rarely, a child with thalassemia major is able to function without transfusions, thereby avoiding the massive ill effects of accumulated iron deposits. **Thalassemia minor** (the heterozygous form) is characterized only by a mild anemia and minimal red blood cell changes. Nursing considerations in the care of thalassemia patients and their families should include observation for ill effects of transfusion, education and counseling about the disease, and referral for genetic counseling. Also called **Cooley's anemia.** See also **hemochromatosis, hemosiderosis.**

thalasso-, a combining form meaning 'of or pertaining to the sea': *thalassophobia, thalassotherapy.*

thalidomide, a formerly used sedative-hypnotic, withdrawn because of its potential for teratogenic effects, particularly phocomelia, when taken during pregnancy.

thallium (Tl), a soft, bluish-white metallic element that exhibits some nonmetallic chemical properties. Its atomic number is 81; its atomic weight is 204.37. Many of its compounds are highly toxic. Thallium sulfate is widely used as a rat poison.

thallium poisoning, a toxic condition caused by the ingestion or the absorption through the skin of thallium salts, especially thallium sulfate. Characteristic of the condition are abdominal pain, vomiting, bloody diarrhea, tremor, delirium, and alopecia. Treatment may include gastric lavage, chelation with Prussian blue, and a laxative. Anticonvulsant and antihypotensive medication may be necessary. Thallium has been used in insect and rodent poisons, fireworks, and in some cosmetic hair removers, but this extremely toxic and cumulative poison was banned for use in household products in 1965.

THAM, a trade name for a buffering agent (tromethamine), used in the treatment of acid-base disturbances.

thanato-, a combining form meaning 'of or pertaining to death': *thanatobiologic, thanatognomonic, thanatology.*

thanatology (thǎn'ətol'əji), the study of death and dying. – **thanatologist** (thǎn'ətol'əjist), *n.*

thanatophoric dwarf, an infant with severe micromelia, the limbs usually extending straight out from the trunk, an extremely narrow chest, and flattened vertebral bodies with wide intervertebral spaces. Death usually occurs from respiratory complications shortly after birth.

thanotopsy (thǎn'ətop'si). See **autopsy.**

THC, abbreviation for **tetrahydrocannabinol.**

The Blues, *Informal.* a designation for Blue Cross (an insurance system that pays the costs of treatment by a hospital or clinic) and Blue Shield (an insurance system that pays the costs of treatment by a professional).

thec-, a combining form meaning 'of or pertaining to a sheath, as of a tendon': *thecal, thecitis, thecodont.*

theca (thi'kə), *pl.* **thecae** (thi'si). a sheath or capsule, as the theca cordis or pericardium.

theca cell tumor, an uncommon, benign fibroid tumor of the ovary, composed of theca cells and usually containing granulosa (follicular) cells. These tumors, characteristically solid masses with yellow, fatty streaks, are frequently associated with excessive estrogen production and tend to develop cystic degeneration. Also called **fibroma thecocellulare xanthomatodes, thecoma.**

-thecium, a combining form meaning a 'sack or container': *bdellepithecium, epithecium, perithecium.*

thecocellulare xanthomatodes (fhɪ'kousel'yuleɪr zæn'fhəmæt'ədiz). See **theca cell tumor.**

thecoma (fhɪkou'mə), *pl.* **thecomas, thecomata.** See **theca cell tumor.**

Theden's bandage (tei'dənz), a roller bandage applied below the injury and continued upward over a compress, used to stop bleeding. Also called **Genga's bandage.**

Theelin, a trade name for an estrogen (estrone).

thel-, a combining form meaning 'of or pertaining to the nipple': *thelalgia, theleplasty, thelitis.*

thelarche (fhɪlar'ki), the beginning of female pubertal breast development that normally occurs prior to puberty at the beginning of the phase of rapid growth between 9 and 13 years of age. **Premature thelarche** is precocious breast development in a female without other evidence of sexual maturation. Compare **menarche.**

-thelia, a combining form meaning '(condition of the) nipples': *epithelia, hyperthelia, microthelia.*

-thelioma, a combining form meaning a 'tumor in a cellular tissue': *celiothelioma, hemendothelioma, perithelioma.*

-thelium, a combining form meaning a 'layer of (specified kind of) cellular tissue': *desmepithelium, mesothelium, retothelium.*

thely-, a combining form meaning 'female': *thelyblast, thelygenic, thelyplasty.*

thenar (fhi'nar), **1.** the bulky mass of tissue on the lateral side of the palm of the hand; the ball of the thumb. **2.** of or pertaining to the palm.

theo-, a combining form meaning 'of or pertaining to a god': *theomania, theophobia, theotherapy.*

Theobid, a trade name for a respiratory fixed-combination drug containing a smooth muscle relaxant (theophylline) and a sedative (butabarbital).

Theo-Dur, a trade name for a bronchodilator (theophylline).

Theolair, a trade name for a bronchodilator (theophylline), used for the relief of acute bronchial asthma.

theoretical effectiveness, (of a contraceptive method) the effectiveness of a medication, device, or method in preventing pregnancy if used consistently and exactly as intended, without human error by the user. Compare **use effectiveness.**

theory, an abstract statement formulated to predict, explain, or describe the relationships among concepts, constructs, or events. Theory is developed and tested by observation and research, using factual data.

theotherapy (fhi'oufher'əpi), a therapeutic approach to the prevention, diagnosis, and treatment of disease and

dysfunction based on religious or spiritual practices and beliefs.

therapeutic, 1. beneficial. **2.** of or pertaining to a treatment.

-therapeutic, a combining form meaning 'pertaining to medical treatment by (specified) techniques': *eutherapeutic, kinetotherapeutic, orthotherapeutic.*

therapeutic abortion, 1. a termination of early pregnancy deemed necessary for medical or psychiatric reasons by the physician. **2.** *Informal.* any legal, induced abortion. Compare **elective abortion.** See also **induced abortion.**

therapeutic communication, (in psychiatric nursing) a process in which the nurse consciously influences a client or helps the client to a better understanding through verbal or nonverbal communication.

therapeutic community (TC), (in mental health) a treatment facility in which the entire milieu is part of the treatment. The physical environment, the other clients, the staff, and the policies of the facility influence the function of the individual in the activities of daily living in the community. The concept of a therapeutic community is integral to milieu therapy.

therapeutic equivalent, a drug that has essentially the same effect in the treatment of a disease or condition as one or more other drugs. A drug that is a therapeutic equivalent may or may not be chemically equivalent, bioequivalent, or generically equivalent. See also **bioequivalent, chemical equivalent, generic equivalent.**

therapeutic exercise, any exercise planned and performed to attain a specific physical benefit, as maintenance of the range of motion, strengthening of weakened muscles, increased flexibility of a joint, or improved cardiovascular and respiratory function.

therapeutic radiopharmaceutical, a radioactive drug administered to a patient to deliver radiation to body tissues internally, as iodide-131, which is used to ablate thyroid tissue in hyperthyroid patients, or cesium-137, iridium-192, radium-226, or strontium-90, which is implanted in a sealed source for the treatment of malignant tumors.

-therapeutics, a combining form meaning 'medical treatment by (specified) techniques': *hydrotherapeutics, physicotherapeutics, radiotherapeutics.*

-therapia, a combining form meaning 'medical care': *balneotherapia, odontotherapia.* Also **-therapy.**

therapy, the treatment of any disease or a pathological condition, as inhalation therapy, which administers various medicines for patients suffering from diseases of the respiratory tract. —**therapeutic,** *adj.*

-therapy, 1. a combining form meaning 'medical treatment of disease' by specified means: *chemotherapy, hypnotherapy, kinesitherapy.* **2.** a combining form meaning 'medical treatment of a (specified) disorder or body area': *cardiotherapy, sarcotherapy, urotherapy.* Also **-therapia.**

therio-, a combining form meaning 'of or pertaining to beasts': *theriomimicry, theriotherapy, theriotomy.*

therm-. See **thermo-.**

-therm, a combining form meaning an 'animal with a (specified) body temperature': *allotherm, endotherm, poikilotherm.*

thermal, thermic, of or pertaining to the production, application, or maintenance of heat.

thermal burn, tissue injury, usually of the skin, caused by exposure to extreme heat. See also **burn.**

-thermia, 1. a combining form meaning a 'state of body temperature': *monothermia, normothermia, pantothermia.* 2. a combining form meaning 'generation of body heat': *azothermia, diathermia, transthermia.* Also **-thermy.**

thermic fever. See **heat hyperpyrexia.**

thermistor (thərmɪs′tər), a kind of thermometer for measuring minute changes in temperature. The resistance of a thermistor varies with the ambient temperature, thereby enabling accurate measurements of small temperature changes. See also **temperature, thermometer.**

thermo-, therm-, a combining form meaning 'of or pertaining to heat': *thermochemistry, thermogenesis, thermopalpation.*

thermocautery (thər′moukə′təri), the use of a needle or snare heated by direct flame, a heated hydrocarbon vapor, or an electric current in the destruction of tissue. See also **Paquelin's cautery.**

thermogenesis (thər′moujen′ɪsɪs), production of heat, especially by the cells of the body. — **thermogenetic,** *adj.*

thermography (thərmog′rəfi), a technique for sensing and recording on film hot and cold areas of the body by means of an infrared detector, used to study blood flow to the limbs and to detect breast tumors — **thermographic,** *adj.*

thermolabile (thər′məlei′bəl), easily destroyed or altered by heat. Also called **heat labile.** Compare **thermostable.**

thermometer, an instrument for measuring temperature. It usually consists of a sealed glass tube, marked in degrees of Centigrade or Fahrenheit, containing liquid, as mercury or alcohol. The liquid rises or falls as it expands or contracts according to changes in temperature. Some kinds of thermometers are **clinical thermometer, digital thermometer, electronic thermometer.**

thermopenetration, the use of diathermic techniques to produce warmth within the body tissues for therapeutic purposes. Also called **transthermia.**

thermoradiotherapy, a therapeutic process that applies ionizing radiation to any part of the body in which the temperature has been raised by artificial means. Thermoradiography seeks to increase the radiosensitivity of the body part being treated.

thermostable, unaffected by or resistant to change by an increase in temperature. Compare **thermolabile.**

thermostat, a device for the automatic control of a heating or cooling system. — **thermostatic,** *adj.*

thermotherapy, the treatment of disease by the application of heat. Thermotherapy may be administered as dry heat with heat lamps, diathermy machines, electric pads, or hot water bottles or as moist heat with warm compresses or immersion in warm water. Warm soaks or compresses may be used to treat local infections, to relax muscles and relieve pain in patients with motor problems, and to promote circulation in peripheral vascular disorders, as thrombophlebitis. — **thermotherapeutic,** *adj.*

-thermy. See **-thermia.**

theta rhythm. See **theta wave.**

theta wave, one of the four types of brain waves, characterized by a relatively low frequency of 4 to 7 Hz and a low amplitude of 10 microvolts. Theta waves are the "drowsy waves" of the temporal lobes of the brain and are observed in electroencephalograms when the individual is awake but relaxed and sleepy. Also called **theta rhythm.** Compare **alpha wave, beta wave, delta wave.**

-thetic, a combining form meaning 'to put, place, set': *metathetic, prosthetic, synthetic.* Also **-thetical.**

thiabendazole, an anthelmintic.

■ INDICATION: It is prescribed in the treatment of a variety of worm infestations.

■ CONTRAINDICATION: Known hypersensitivity to this drug prohibits its use.

■ ADVERSE EFFECTS: Among the more serious adverse reactions are anorexia, severe gastrointestinal disturbances, dizziness, and hypotension.

thiamine, thiamin, a water-soluble, crystalline compound of the B complex vitamin group, essential for normal metabolism and for the health of the cardiovascular and nervous systems. Thiamine combines with pyruvic acid to form a coenzyme necessary for the breakdown of carbohydrates into glucose. Rich sources of thiamine are pork, organ meats, green leafy vegetables, legumes, sweet corn, egg yolk, corn meal, brown rice, yeast, the germ and husks of grains, berries, and nuts. It is not stored in the body and must be supplied daily. A deficiency of thiamine affects chiefly the nervous system, the circulation, and the gastrointestinal tract. Symptoms include irritability, emotional disturbances, loss of appetite, multiple neuritis, increased pulse rate, dyspnea, reduced intestinal motility, and heart irregularities. Severe deficiency causes beriberi. Thiamine is not known to cause any toxic effects. Also called **antiberiberi factor, antineuritic vitamin, vitamin B$_1$.**

thiazide diuretic. See **diuretic.**

thiethylperazine maleate, a phenothiazine anti-emetic.

■ INDICATION: It is prescribed to control nausea and vomiting.

■ CONTRAINDICATIONS: Parkinson's disease, central nervous system disorders, liver or renal dysfunction, severe hypotension, or known hypersensitivity to phenothiazine medication prohibits its use.

■ ADVERSE EFFECTS: Among the more serious adverse effects are hypotension, liver toxicity, a variety of extrapyramidal reactions, blood dyscrasias, and hypersensitivity reactions.

thigh, the section of the lower limb between the hip and the knee.

thigh bone. See **femur.**

thigm-, a combining form meaning 'of or pertaining to touch': *thigmesthesia, thigmocyte, thigmotropic.*

thimerosal (thaimer′əsæl), an anti-infective.

■ INDICATIONS: It is prescribed as a topical and ophthalmic antiseptic and as a preoperative and postoperative skin disinfectant.

■ CONTRAINDICATIONS: Concurrent administration of permanganates, strong acids, salts of heavy metals, or known hypersensitivity to this drug or to mercury-containing compounds prohibits its use.

■ ADVERSE EFFECTS: Among the more serious adverse reactions are erythematous, vesicular, and papular eruptions at the site of application. Mercury poisoning has been reported when large doses of this drug are given.

thinking, 1. the cognitive process of forming mental images or concepts. 2. the process of cognitive problem solving through the sorting, organizing, and classification of facts. Kinds of thinking include **abstract thinking, concrete thinking, syncretic thinking.** See also **imagination.**

thio-, a combining form designating the presence of sulfur: *thioarsenite, theocarbamide, thiocyanate.*

thioamide derivative, one of a group of antithyroid drugs prescribed in the treatment of hyperthyroidism. Thioamide drugs act by inhibiting the synthesis of thyroid hormone. The principal thioamides are propylthiouricil, methimazole, methylthiouricil, and carbamizole. Adverse reactions include agranulocytosis, hypersensitivity, and a mild transient pruritus. As agranulocytosis may occur very rapidly, serial white blood and cell counts are not useful in diagnosing that complication of treatment. Instead, the patient is requested to report immediately instances of sore throat and fever, which often herald the onset of agranulocytosis. Prompt discontinuation of the drug, before serious depletion of granulocytic white cells develops, usually results in complete recovery. Use of antithyroid medications in pregnancy may result in fetal hypothyroidism, goiter, and cretinism.

thioctic acid (thaiok′tik), a pyruvate-oxidation factor found in liver and yeast, used in bacterial culture media.

thioguanine (thai′ougwa′nin), an antineoplastic.

■ INDICATIONS: It is prescribed in the treatment of a variety of malignant neoplastic diseases, including the acute leukemias.

■ CONTRAINDICATIONS: Known hypersensitivity or resistance to this drug prohibits its use. It is not given to pregnant women.

■ ADVERSE EFFECTS: Among the most serious adverse reactions are bone marrow depression, gastrointestinal distress, and stomatitis.

Thiomerin, a trade name for a mercurial diuretic (mercaptomerin sodium).

thiopental sodium, a potent, short-acting barbiturate, used as a general anesthetic for surgical procedures that are expected to require 15 minutes or less, as an induction agent for other general anesthetics, as a hypnotic component in balanced anesthesia, and as an adjunct to regional anesthesia. It is administered intravenously in adults; in children it is occasionally given rectally. By depressing the CNS, thiopental sodium induces hypnotic sleep in less than a minute after infusion. It has no analgesic properties and therefore must be supplemented by analgesics. It is a powerful respiratory and myocardial depressant and may be habit-forming. See also **barbiturate.**

thioridazine hydrochloride, a phenothiazine antipsychotic.

■ INDICATIONS: It is prescribed in the treatment of psychotic disorders.

■ CONTRAINDICATIONS: Parkinson's disease, concurrent administration of central nervous system depressants, hepatic or renal dysfunction, severe hypotension, known hypersensitivity to this drug or to other phenothiazine medication prohibits its use.

■ ADVERSE EFFECTS: Among the more serious adverse reactions are hypotension, hepatotoxicity, a variety of extrapyramidal reactions, blood dyscrasias, and hypersensitivity reactions.

Thiosulfil, a trade name for a sulfonamide antibacterial (sulfamethizole).

thiotepa (thai′outep′ə), an antineoplastic alkylating agent.

■ INDICATIONS: It is prescribed in the treatment of a variety of malignant neoplastic diseases, including adenocarcinoma of the breast and ovary.

■ CONTRAINDICATIONS: Bone marrow depression, pregnancy, liver or kidney dysfunction, or known hypersensitivity to this drug prohibits its use.

■ ADVERSE EFFECTS: Among the most serious adverse reactions are bone marrow depression, anorexia, nausea, and headache.

thiothixene, a thioxanthene antipsychotic.

■ INDICATIONS: It is prescribed in the treatment of psychotic disorders.

■ CONTRAINDICATIONS: Parkinson's disease, concurrent administration of central nervous system depressants, hepatic or renal dysfunction, severe hypotension, known hypersensitivity to this drug or to other phenothiazine medication prohibits its use.

■ ADVERSE EFFECTS: Among the more serious adverse reactions are hypotension, hepatotoxicity, a variety of extrapyramidal reactions, blood dyscrasias, and hypersensitivity reactions.

thioxanthine derivative, any one of a group of antipsychotic drugs, each of which is similar to the phenothiazenes in indication, action, and adverse effects.

thiphenamil hydrochloride, an anticholinergic agent.

■ INDICATIONS: It is prescribed in the treatment of gastrointestinal pain owing to hypermotility and spasm.

■ CONTRAINDICATIONS: Narrow angle glaucoma, asthma, obstruction of the genitourinary or gastrointestinal tract, severe ulcerative colitis, or known hypersensitivity to this drug prohibits its use.

■ ADVERSE EFFECTS: Among the more serious adverse reactions are blurred vision, central nervous system effects, tachycardia, dry mouth, decreased sweating, and hypersensitivity reactions.

third cuneiform bone. See **lateral cuneiform bone.**

third nerve. See **oculomotor nerve.**

third-party reimbursement, reimbursement for services rendered to a person in which an entity other than the giver or receiver of the service is responsible for the payment. Third-party reimbursement for the cost of a subscriber's health care is commonly paid by insurance plans, as Blue Shield or Blue Cross.

third ventriculostomy (ventrik'yulos'təmi), a surgical procedure for draining cerebrospinal fluid into the cisterna chiasmatis of the subarachnoid space in hydrocephalus, usually in the newborn. The procedure is not commonly performed and is used chiefly when the cisterna magna is not available for the Torkildsen procedure. The third ventriculostomy makes an opening on the anterior wall of the floor of the third ventricle into the interpeduncular cistern and is performed to correct an obstructive type of hydrocephalus.

thirst, a perceived desire for water. The sensation of thirst is usually referred to the mouth and throat.

Thiry's fistula (thai'riz), an artificial passage from the abdominal surface of an experimental animal to an isolated intestinal segment, created surgically for the study of internal secretions. The continuity of the animal's gut is restored by anastomosis of the severed sections, and the isolated segment's vascular and nervous connections are maintained. One end of the isloated internal segment is closed, and the other is attached to an opening in the skin of the abdomen.

Thiry-Vella fistula (thai'rivel'ə), an artificial passage from the abdominal surface of an experimental animal to an isolated intestinal loop, created surgically for the study of intestinal secretions. The continuity of the animal's gut is restored by anastomosis of the severed sections, and the isolated loop's vascular connections and mesenteric attachment are preserved. The ends of the isolated segment

are attached to two openings in the skin of the abdomen to form a closed internal loop.

Thiuretic, a trade name for a diuretic (hydrochlorothiazide).

thixo-, a combining form meaning 'of or pertaining to touch': *thixolabile, thixotropic, thixotropy.*

Thomas splint, **1.** a rigid splint constructed of steel bars that are curved to fit the involved limb and held in place by a cast or a rigid bandage. It is used in the treatment of chronic joint diseases. **2.** Also called **Thomas ring splint.** A rigid metal splint that extends from a ring at the hip to beyond the foot. It is used in the treatment of a fractured leg and, in conjunction with various traction and suspension devices, to immobilize and position a fractured femur of the preoperative or the postoperative patient.

Thomsen's disease (tom'sənz). See **myotonia congenita.**

thoracentesis (thor'əsenti'sis). See **thoracocentesis.**

thoracic (thoræs'ik), of or pertaining to the thorax.

-thoracic, a combining form meaning 'of, referring, or relating to the chest': *abdominothoracic, extrathoracic, intrathoracic.*

thoracic actinomycocis. See **actinomycosis.**

thoracic aorta, the large, upper portion of the descending aorta, starting at the caudal border of the fourth thoracic vertebra, dividing into seven branches, and supplying many parts of the body, as the heart, ribs, chest muscles, and stomach. Its seven branches are the pericardial, bronchial, esophageal, mediastinal, posterior intercostal, subcostal, and superior phrenic. See also **descending aorta.** Compare **abdominal aorta.**

thoracic duct, the common trunk of all the lymphatic vessels in the body, except those on the right side of the head, the neck, and the thorax, the right upper limb, the right lung, the right side of the heart and the diaphragmatic surface of the liver. In the adult it is 38 to 45 cm long and 3 to 5 mm in diameter. It begins high in the abdomen at the cisterna chyli, ventral to the second lumbar vertebra, enters the thorax through the aortic hiatus of the diaphragm, and ascends into the neck through the posterior mediastinum, between the aorta and the azygous vein. In the neck it arches over the clavicle and opens into the junction of the left internal jugular and the left subclavian veins. The thoracic duct contains various valves, including two at this orifice that prevent venous blood from flowing into the lymphatic system. Compare **right lymphatic duct.** See also **lymphatic system.**

thoracic fistula, an abnormal opening in the chest wall that ends blindly or that communicates with the thoracic cavity.

thoracic medicine, the branch of medicine concerned with the diagnosis and treatment of disorders of the structures and organs of the chest, especially the lungs.

thoracic nerves, the 12 spinal nerves on each side of the thorax, including 11 intercostal nerves and one subcostal nerve. They are distributed mainly to the walls of the thorax and the abdomen. The thoracic nerves do not enter a plexus but follow independent courses, making them different from other spinal nerves. The first two intercostal nerves innervate the upper limb as well as the thorax; the next four supply only the thorax; and the lower five supply the walls of the thorax and the abdomen. Each subcostal thoracic nerve innervates the abdominal wall and the skin of a buttock. The thoracic portion of the sympathetic trunk contains a series of ganglia often coalesced in a single mass that, when independent, corresponds approximately to the thoracic spinal nerves. The roots of the ganglia are supplied by each thoracic nerve. The first thoracic ganglion, larger than the rest, is elongated, lying in the medial end of the first intercostal space, and usually combined with the inferior cervical ganglion into a stellate ganglion. The second to the tenth ganglia lie opposite the intervertebral disc associated with but slightly lower than the corresponding thoracic nerve. In most individuals the last thoracic ganglion lies on the body of the twelfth thoracic vertebra and, by its connection to both the eleventh and the twelfth thoracic nerves, serves a dual role as a single ganglion. See also **sympathetic nervous system.**

thoracic outlet syndrome, an abnormal condition and a type of mononeuropathy characterized by paresthesia of the fingers. It may be caused by a nerve-root compression by a cervical disc or by carpal tunnel syndrome.

thoracic parietal node, one of the lymph glands in the thorax, associated with various lymphatic vessels and divided into sternal nodes, intercostal nodes, and diaphragmatic nodes. See also **lymphatic system, lymph node.**

thoracic vertebra, one of the 12 bony segments of the spinal column of the upper back, designated T1 to T12. T1 is just below the seventh cervical vertebra (C7) and T12 is just above the first lumbar vertebra (L1). The thoracic portion of the spine is flexible and has a concave ventral curvature. Each vertebra has a broad, thick lamina; long, obliquely directed spinous processes; and thick, strong articular facets. The vertebrae are separated from each other by intervertebral discs. The vertebrae become thicker and heavier in descending order from T1 to T12. Compare **cervical vertebra, lumbar vertebra, sacral vertebra.**

thoracic visceral node, a node in the three groups of lymph nodes connected to the part of the lymphatic system that serves certain structures within the thorax, as the thymus, pericardium, esophagus, trachea, lungs, and bronchi. The thoracic visceral nodes include the anterior mediastinal nodes, the posterior mediastinal nodes, and the tracheobronchial nodes. Compare **thoracic parietal node.** See also **lymph, lymphatic system, lymph node.**

thoraco-, a combining form meaning 'of or pertaining to the chest': *thoracobronchotomy, thoracocentesis, thoracomyodynia.*

thoracocentesis (thor'əkōusenti'sis), **thoracentesis** (thor'əsenti'sis), the surgical perforation of the chest wall and pleural space with a needle for the aspiration of fluid for diagnostic or therapeutic purposes or for the removal of a specimen for biopsy. The procedure is usually performed under local anesthesia, with the patient in an upright position. Thoracocentesis may be used in the treatment of pleural effusion, as may occur in bronchogenic carcinoma. Fluid samples may be examined for erythrocyte, leukocyte, and differential white cell counts, protein, glucose, and amylase concentrations and may be cultured for studies of microorganisms that may be present.

thoracodorsal nerve (thor'əkōudor'səl), a branch of the brachial plexus, usually arising between the two subscapular nerves. It courses along the posterior wall of the axilla and terminates in branches that supply the latissimus dorsi.

thorax, the cage of bone and cartilage containing the principal organs of respiration and circulation and covering part of the abdominal organs. It is formed ventrally by the sternum and costal cartilages and dorsally by the twelve thoracic vertebrae and the dorsal parts of the twelve ribs. The thorax of women has less capacity, a shorter sternum, and more movable upper ribs than that of men. Also called **chest.**

Thorazine, a trade name for a phenothiazine (chlorpromazine), used as an antiemetic and tranquilizer.

thorium (Th), a heavy, grayish, radioactive, metallic element. Its atomic number is 90; its atomic weight is 232.04. Thorium is used in radiographic procedures and in radiation therapy.

thought processes, alterations in, a nursing diagnosis accepted by the Fourth National Conference on the Classification of Nursing Diagnoses. The etiology of the condition is to be developed at a later conference. The defining characteristics of the problem include distraction, egocentrism, abnormal cognitive function, abnormal interpretations of the environment, and attention to environmental cues that is more or less acute than might normally be expected. See also **nursing diagnosis.**

thought transference. See **telepathy.**

threadworm. See *Enterobius vermiculans.*

thready pulse, an abnormal pulse that is weak and often fairly rapid; the artery does not feel full, and the rate may be difficult to count. It is characteristic of hypovolemia, as occurs with severe hemorrhage.

threatened abortion, a condition in pregnancy prior to the twentieth week of gestation characterized by uterine bleeding and cramping sufficient to suggest that miscarriage may result. A threatened abortion is generally managed with rest and observation. Compare **incomplete abortion, inevitable abortion, imminent abortion.**

three day fever. See **phlebotomus fever.**

three-day measles. See **rubella.**

threp-, a combining form meaning 'of or pertaining to nutrition': *threpsis, threpology, threptic.*

threshold, the point at which a stimulus is great enough to produce an effect, as a pain threshold is the point at which a person becomes aware of pain.

thrill, a fine vibration, felt by an examiner's hand on the body of a patient over the site of an aneurysm or on the precordium, indicating the presence of an organic murmur of grade four or greater intensity. Compare **bruit, murmur.**

throat. See **pharynx.**

throb, a deep, pulsating kind of discomfort or pain. – **throbbing,** *adj.*

thrombasthenia (throm'bæsthi'niə), a rare hemorrhagic disease characterized by a defect in platelet mediated hemostasis owing to an abnormality in the membrane surface of the platelet. The platelets do not aggregate, a clot does not form, and hemorrhage ensues, often from the mucous membrane. Transfusion with platelets is usually effective in stopping the hemorrhage. The condition is congenital, and is inherited as an autosomal recessive trait.

thrombectomy (thrombek'təmi), the removal of a thrombus from a blood vessel, performed as emergency surgery to restore circulation to the affected part. Before surgery, anticoagulant therapy is begun, and an arteriogram is done to locate the thrombus. Under general anesthesia, a longitudinal incision is made into the blood vessel and the clot is removed. Postoperatively, the blood pressure is maintained close to its preoperative level, as a decrease would predispose to further clotting. Compare **embolectomy.**

thrombin (throm'bɪn), an enzyme formed in plasma during the clotting process from prothrombin, calcium, and thromboplastin. Thrombin causes fibrinogen to change to fibrin, essential in the formation of a clot. See also **blood clot.**

thrombo-, a combining form meaning 'of or pertaining to a clot, or thrombosis': *thromboarteritis, thrombocystis, thrombolysis.*

thromboangiitis obliterans (throm'bouæn'jiai'tɪs), an occlusive vascular condition, usually of a leg or a foot, in which the small and medium-sized arteries become inflamed and thrombotic. Early signs of the condition are burning, numbness, and tingling of the foot or leg distal to the lesion. Phlebitis and gangrene may develop as the disease progresses. Pulsation in the limb below the damaged blood vessels is often absent. The goal of therapy is to avoid all factors that decrease the blood supply to the extremity, as cigarette smoking, and to use all means possible to increase the supply. Amputation may be necessary if the condition progresses to gangrene with chronic infection and extensive tissue destruction. Men are affected 75 times more often than women; most of the affected men smoke and are between the ages of 20 and 40. Also called **Buerger's disease.**

thrombocyte (throm'bəsait). See **platelet.**

thrombocytopathy (throm'bousaitop'əfhi), any disorder of the blood coagulation mechanism owing to an abnormality or dysfunction of platelets. Kinds of thrombocytopathies include **thrombocytopenia, thrombocytosis.** – **thrombocytopathic,** *adj.*

thrombocytopenia (throm'bousai'təpi'niə), an abnormal hematologic condition in which the number of platelets is reduced, usually by destruction of erythroid tissue in bone marrow owing to certain neoplastic diseases or to an immune response to a drug. There may be decreased production of platelets, decreased survival of platelets, increased consumption of platelets, and splenomegaly. Thrombocytopenia is the most common cause of bleeding disorders. Bleeding is usually from many small capillaries. Treatment requires a specific diagnosis of the cause. All drugs are stopped, as any drug may cause the condition. Adrenal corticosteroids may be administered, and transfusion may be necessary.

thrombocytopenic purpura, a bleeding disorder characterized by a marked decrease in the number of platelets, resulting in multiple bruises, petechiae, and hemorrhage into the tissues. It may occur secondary to a number of causes, including infection and drug sensitivity and toxicity. Until recently it was called idiopathic thrombocytopenic purpura (ITP), a diagnosis reached only by the exclusion of other causes. Today it is considered to be a manifestation of an autoimmune response. Two distinct entities, acute and chronic thrombocytopenia can be differentiated from clinical manifestations alone. The acute form usually occurs in children between 2 and 6 years of age and is benign, with complete recovery usually apparent within 6 weeks. The chronic form usually occurs in adults between 20 and 50 years of age. Recovery is rarely spontaneous and often requires adrenocortical steroids, or, possibly, splenectomy. Compare **disseminated intravascular coagulation.** See also **hemophilia, hemorrhagic diathesis, thrombasthenia.**

thrombocytosis (throm'bousaitou'sɪs), an abnormal increase in the number of platelets in the blood. **Benign,** or **secondary thrombocytosis** is asymptomatic and usually occurs following splenectomy, inflammatory disease, hemolytic anemia, hemorrhage, or iron deficiency, as a response to exercise, or following treatment with vincristine. It may also occur in advanced carcinoma or Hodgkin's disease or in other lymphomas. **Essential thrombocythemia** is characterized by episodes of spontaneous bleeding alternating with thrombotic episodes. The platelets may reach levels exceeding 1,000,000/cu mm. Compare **thrombocytopenia.** See also **polycythemia.**

thromboembolism, a condition in which a blood vessel is blocked by an embolus carried in the blood stream from the site of formation of the clot. The area supplied by an obstructed artery may tingle and become cold, numb, and cyanotic. Treatment includes quiet bed rest, warm wet packs, and anticoagulants to prevent the formation of additional thrombi. Embolectomy may be indicated, especially if the aorta or common iliac artery is obstructed. An embolus in the lungs causes a sudden, sharp, thoracic or upper abdominal pain, dyspnea, a violent cough, fever, and hemoptysis. Obstruction of the pulmonary artery or one of its branches may be rapidly fatal. Emboli in smaller pulmonary arteries may be diagnosed by x-ray films and other radiologic techniques, including lung scans and angiography.

thrombophlebitis (fhrom'boufləbai'tıs), inflammation of a vein, often accompanied by formation of a clot. It occurs most commonly as the result of trauma to the vessel wall, hypercoagulability of the blood, infection, chemical irritation, postoperative venous stasis, prolonged sitting, standing, or immobilization, or a long period of intravenous catheterization. Also called **phlebitis.**

■ OBSERVATIONS: Thrombophlebitis of a superficial vein is generally evident; the vessel feels hard and thready or cordlike and is extremely sensitive to pressure; the surrounding area may be erythematous and warm to the touch, and the entire limb may be pale, cold, and swollen. Deep vein thrombophlebitis is characterized by aching or cramping pain, especially in the calf when the patient walks or dorsiflexes the foot (Homan's sign).

■ INTERVENTION: Thrombophlebitis of a vein of the arm or hand caused by the irritation of an intravenous catheter is usually treated by removing the catheter, elevating the arm, and applying moist heat. When the condition occurs in a vein of the leg, the person is maintained on complete bed rest in a comfortable position that does not restrict venous return. The legs are elevated, if ordered, but pillows are not used and the knees are never bent unless the foot of the bed is raised. Anticoagulant therapy and streptokinase may be administered and moist heat is applied to the affected area; intense heat, which may burn edematous skin, is avoided. Every four hours the blood pressure, temperature, pulse, respiration, circulation of the affected extremity, skin condition, and pulses in all the extremities are checked; a Doppler ultrasonic sensing device may be used. The patient is kept warm and dry and is helped to turn, cough, and deep-breathe every two hours; the chest is auscultated for breath sounds every four hours. Observation for signs of pulmonary embolism, myocardial infarction, cardiovascular accident, or decreased renal function is constant. The affected limb is covered with a bed cradle, is not washed or massaged, and is measured daily, with the size recorded. Active and passive range of motion exercises are performed with the unaffected extremities. Constipation is avoided, and during the acute phase the patient is lifted on and off the bedpan. When phlebography is ordered, the patient is told how the contrast medium will be injected prior to an x-ray study of the affected vein. As inflammation subsides, the use of support or antiembolic stockings is demonstrated, and an exercise program is initiated. The patient is instructed to alternate exercise with bed rest, never to dangle the legs, to walk ten minutes every hour, to avoid prolonged standing, to avoid becoming overweight, and, when sitting, to elevate the legs, flex the calf muscles, and contract the quadriceps ten minutes per hour, as well as to avoid constricting circulation in the groin or crossing the legs at the knees.

■ NURSING CONSIDERATIONS: Thrombophlebitis is a common and often avoidable complication of various treatments and conditions in the hospitalized patient. Much routine nursing care is directed toward avoiding thrombophletitis. Early postoperative and postpartum ambulation, range of motion exercises for the immobilized patient, good technique in intravenous catheterization, attention to fluid balance, and proper positioning of the patient are common nursing measures to promote good circulation and reduce venous stasis and the development of thrombophlebitis.

thrombophlebitis migrans. See **migratory thrombophlebitis.**

thrombophlebitis purulenta, an inflammation of a vein associated with the formation of a soft, purulent thrombus that infiltrates the wall of the vessel.

thromboplastin, a complex substance that initiates the clotting process by converting prothrombin to thrombin in the presence of calcium ion. It is found in most tissue cells and, in somewhat different form, in red cells and leukocytes. See also **blood clotting, coagulation.**

thrombosis, *pl.* **thromboses.** an abnormal vascular condition in which thrombus develops within a blood vessel of the body. See also **blood coagulation.**

thrombotic phlegmasia. See **phlegmasia alba dolens.**

thrombotic thrombocytopenic purpura (TTP), a disorder characterized by thrombocytopenia, hemolytic anemia, and neurological abnormalities. It is accompanied by a generalized purpura together with the deposition of microthrombi within the capillaries and smaller arterioles. It is seen in a chronic form and in an acute fulminating form that may be fatal in weeks. Therapy includes corticosteroids and splenectomy. Compare **disseminated intravascular coagulation.** See also **thrombocytopenic purpura.**

thrombus (fhrom'bəs), *pl.* **thrombi.** an aggregation of platelets, fibrin, clotting factors, and the cellular elements of the blood attached to the interior wall of a vein or artery, sometimes occluding the lumen of the vessel. Kinds of thrombi include **agonal thrombus, hyaline thrombus, laminated thrombus, marasmic thrombus, parasitic thrombus, white thrombus.** Also called **blood clot.** Compare **embolus.**

thrush. See also *Candida albicans.*

thulium (Tm), a rare-earth metallic element. Its atomic number is 69; its atomic weight is 168.93. Thulium that has been irradiated in a nuclear reactor gives off x rays and has been used in portable x-ray devices.

thumb, the first and shortest digit of the hand, classified by some anatomists as one of the fingers because its metacarpal bone ossifies in the same manner as those of the phalanges. Other anatomists classify the thumb separately, regarding it as composed of one metacarpal bone and only two phalanges. The metacarpal bone of the thumb articulates with the trapezium of the carpus and is controlled by the thenar muscles, which occupy the radial side of the hand, and by the abductor pollicis longus, the extensor pollicis brevis, and the extensor pollicis longus. The thenar muscles include the abductor pollicis longus, the opponens pollicis, the flexor pollicis brevis, and the adductor pollicis. The nerves that innervate the various muscles controlling the thumb include branches of the radial nerve, the deep palmar branch of the ulnar nerve, and a branch of the median nerve. The metacarpal bone of the thumb, like the metacarpals of the other digits, ossifies from a center in the body of the bone and from a center at the distal end. Ossification begins in the middle of the eighth or ninth week of fetal life. About the third year of life the base extremity of the metacarpal of the thumb starts to ossify, uniting with the body of the metacarpal about the twentieth year of life. The phalanges of the thumb ossify from centers in the bodies of the phalanges and from centers at their proximal extremities. Ossification of the phalangeal body begins about the eighth week of fetal life.

thumb-sucking, the habit of sucking the thumb for oral gratification. It is normal in infants and young children as a pleasure-seeking or comforting device, especially when the child is hungry or tired. The habit reaches its peak when the child is between 18 and 20 months of age, and it normally disappears as the child develops and matures. Thumb-sucking beyond four to six years of age may lead to malocclusion of the teeth and deformation of the bony tissue of the thumb. Excessive thumb-sucking, especially in older children, may be indicative of some emotional problem.

-thymia, a combining form meaning '(condition of the) mind or will': *amphithymia, barythymia, poikilothymia.*

thymic (thaī'mĭk), of or pertaining to the thymus gland.

thymic hypoplasia. See **DiGeorge syndrome.**

thymic parathyroid aplasia. See **DiGeorge syndrome.**

thymo-, 1. a combining form meaning 'of or pertaining to the thymus gland': *thymocyte, thymolysis, thymoma.* 2. a combining form meaning 'of or pertaining to the spirit or mind': *thymogenic, thymopathy, thymopsyche.*

thymol (thaī'mol), a synthetic or natural thyme oil, used as an antibacterial and antifungal, that is an ingredient in some over-the-counter preparations for the treatment of hemorrhoids, acne, and tinea pedis. It is also used as a stabilizer in various pharmaceutical preparations.

thymoma (thaīmou'mə), *pl.* **thymomas, thymomata.** a usually benign tumor of the thymus gland that may be associated with myasthenia gravis or abnormal or excessive erythropoesis.

thymosin (thaī'məsin), 1. a naturally occurring immunologic hormone secreted by the thymus gland. It is present in greatest amounts in young children and decreases in amount throughout life. 2. an investigational drug derived from bovine thymus extracts and prescribed as an immunomodulator in experimental treatments for certain diseases, as systemic lupus erythematosus or rheumatoid arthritis.

thymus (thaī'məs), *pl.* **thymuses, thymi.** a single, unpaired gland that is located in the mediastinum, extending superiorly into the neck to the lower edge of the thyroid gland and inferiorly as far as the fourth costal cartilage. It was once considered a minor vestigial structure, but research has established that the thymus is the primary central gland of the lymphatic system. The endocrine activity of the thymus is believed to depend on the hormone thymosin, which is composed of biologically active peptides critical to the maturation and the development of the immune system. The T cells of the cell-mediated immune response develop in this gland before migrating to the lymph nodes and the spleen. The gland consists of two lateral lobes closely bound by connective tissue, which also encloses the entire organ in a capsule. Superficial to the gland is the sternum. Lying deep to the thymus are the great vessels and the cranial portion of the pericardium. The two lobes of the gland differ in size, and, in many individuals, the right lobe overlaps the left lobe. The thymus is about 5 cm long, 4 cm wide, and 6 mm thick. The lobes are composed of numerous lobules, which vary from 0.5 to 2 mm in diameter. The lobules are separated by delicate connective tissue. Each lobule is composed of a dense cellular cortex and an inner, less dense medulla. The cortices are composed almost entirely of small lymphocytes secured by reticular tissue with relatively few reticular cells. The medullae contain far fewer lymphocytes than the cortices and are composed of reticular tissue that contains more reticular cells. The thymus develops in the embryo from the third branchial pouch and increases in size until attaining a weight of 12 to 14 gm before birth. The size of the organ relative to the rest of the body is largest when the individual is about two years old. The thymus usually attains its greatest absolute size at puberty, when it weighs about 35 gm. After puberty, the organ undergoes involution as the small lymphocytes of the cortices disappear and the reticular tissue is compressed. Adipose tissue often replaces the receding thymic tissue, but the connective tissue capsule of the gland may persist. With aging, the gland may change in color from pinkish gray to yellow, and in the elderly individual may appear as small islands of thymic tissue covered with fat and surrounded by the yellowish capsule. The normal involution of the thymus may be superseded by rapid accidental involution caused by starvation or by acute disease. The gland is supplied by arteries derived from the internal thoracic and from the superior and the inferior thyroids. The veins of the gland end in the left brachiocephalic vein and in the thyroid veins. The lymphatics of the thymus end in the anterior mediastinal, the tracheobronchial, and the sternal nodes. The gland is innervated by tiny nerves derived from the vagi and the sympathetic. Branches from the descendens hypoglossi and the phrenic nerve reach the thymic capsule but do not penetrate the glandular tissue.

Thypinone, a trade name for the synthetic thyrotropin-releasing hormone (protirelin), used as an adjunctive agent in the diagnostic assessment of thyroid function.

Thyrar, a trade name for thyroid hormone.

-thyrea, a combining form meaning a 'condition of the thyroid gland': *athyrea, hypothyrea, hyperthyrea.* Also **-thyreosis, -thyroidism.**

-thyreosis. See **-thyrea.**

thyro-, a combining form meaning 'of or pertaining to the thyroid gland': *thyroactive, thyroidectomy, thyroiditis.*

thyrocalcitonin. See **calcitonin.**

thyrocervical trunk, one of a pair of short, thick, arterial branches, arising from the first portion of the subclavian arteries, close to the medial border of the scalenus anterior, supplying numerous muscles and bones in the head, neck, and back. Each is divided into three branches: the inferior thyroid, suprascapular, and transverse cervical.

thyroglobulin, a purified extract of porcine thyroid. See also **thyroid hormone.**

■ INDICATIONS: It is prescribed in the treatment of cretinism, myxedema, goiter, and other hypothyroid states.

■ CONTRAINDICATIONS: Hypopituatarism or known hypersensitivity to this drug prohibits its use.

■ ADVERSE EFFECTS: Among the more serious adverse reactions are tremors, nervousness, palpitation and tachycardia, and arrythmias when given in excessive doses.

thyroid acropathy, swelling of subcutaneous tissue of the extremities and clubbing of the digits, occurring rarely in patients with thyroid disease and usually associated with pretibial myxedema or exophthalmos.

thyroid cancer, a neoplasm of the thyroid gland, usu-

ally characterized by slow growth and a slower and more prolonged clinical course than that of other malignancies. A significant carcinogenic effect of exposure to ionizing radiation is demonstrated by the high rate of thyroid cancer in survivors of atomic bomb explosions and in individuals who have been treated with radiotherapy for an enlarged thymus in infancy or for acne or other skin disorders in adolescence. Nontoxic colloid goiters and follicular adenomas may be precursors of malignant thyroid tumors. The first sign of cancer may be an increase in size of the thyroid gland, a palpable nodule, hoarseness, dysphagia, dyspnea, or pain on pressure. Diagnostic measures include x-ray examination, transillumination of the gland, radioisotope scanning, needle biopsy, and ultrasonic examination. More than one half of thyroid malignancies are papillary carcinomas, about one third are follicular carcinomas, and the rest consist of rapidly growing invasive anaplastic carcinomas, medullary carcinomas that secrete calcitonin, and metastatic lesions from primary tumors in the breast, kidneys, or lungs. Total or subtotal thyroidectomy with excision of involved lymph nodes is usually recommended. Radioactive iodine may be administered postoperatively, and high doses of exogenous thyroid are often used to suppress thyroid-stimulating hormone (TSH) in an effort to cause the regression of residual tumor dependent on TSH. Various chemotherapeutic agents, especially adriamycin, may be effective in patients with metastatic thyroid cancer that is unresponsive to conventional treatment. Cancer of the thyroid is twice as common in women as in men; although it is diagnosed most frequently in people between the ages of 30 and 50, it may occur in children and elderly individuals.

thyroid cartilage, the largest cartilage of the larynx, consisting of two laminae fused together at an acute angle in the middle line of the neck to form the Adam's apple. Immediately above this prominence the laminae are separated by the superior thyroid notch. An oblique line runs caudally from the outer surface of each lamina and serves for the attachment of the sternothyroideus, the thyrohyoideus, and the constrictor pharyngis inferior. The cranial border of the thyroid cartilage secures the thyrohyoid membrane; the caudal border holds the cricoid cartilage, and the dorsal border receives insertions of the stylopharyngeus and the pharyngopalatinus. Compare **cricoid.**

thyroid dermoid cyst, a tumor derived from embryonal tissues that is believed to have developed in the thyroid gland or in the thyrolingual duct.

thyroidectomy (thaī'roidek'təmi), the surgical removal of the thyroid gland, performed for colloid goiter, removal of tumors, or hyperthyroidism that does not respond to iodine therapy and antithyroid drugs. All but five to ten per cent of the gland is removed; regrowth usually begins shortly after surgery, and thyroid function may return to normal. For cancer of the thyroid, the entire gland is removed, along with surrounding structures from neck to collarbone, in a radical neck dissection. Before surgery, the basal metabolism rate is lowered to normal by giving iodine and antithyroid drugs. If a tumor is present a frozen section of the affected tissue is examined by a pathologist. If malignant cells are found, most or all of the gland is removed. After surgery the patient is most comfortable in semi-Fowler's position with continuous mist inhalation administered to liquefy oral secretions. Oral suctioning may be necessary. A tracheotomy set and oxygen are kept in the room. Postoperatively, the patient is observed for signs of hemorrhage, respiratory difficulty due to edema of the glottis, the muscular twitching of tetany from accidental removal of a parathyroid gland, and thyroid storm.

thyroid function test, any of several laboratory tests performed to evalute the function of the thyroid gland. Often several of the tests are performed simultaneously. Thyroid function tests include protein-bound iodine, butanol-extractable iodine, T-3, T-4, free thyroxine index, thyroxin-binding globulin, thyroid-stimulating hormone, long-acting thyroid stimulator, radioactive iodine uptake, radioactive iodine excretion.

thyroid gland, a highly vascular organ at the front of the neck, usually weighing about 30 gm, consisting of bilateral lobes connected in the middle by a narrow isthmus. It is slightly heavier in women than in men and enlarges during pregnancy. The thyroid gland secretes the hormone thyroxin directly into the blood and is part of the endocrine system of ductless glands. It is essential to normal body growth in infancy and childhood, and its removal greatly reduces the oxidative processes of the body, producing a lower metabolic rate characteristic of hypothyroidism. The apices of the conical lobes of the gland are directed cranially and laterally as far as the lower middle of the thyroid cartilage. The bases of the lobes are on the level with the fifth or the sixth tracheal ring. Each lobe is about 5 cm long, a maximum of 3 cm wide, and usually about 2 cm thick. The lateral surface is convex and covered by the skin, the sternocleidomastoideus, the omohyoideus, the sternohyoideus, and the sternothyroideus. The deep fascia forms a capsule for the gland. The thyroid is activated by the pituitary thyrotrophic hormone and requires iodine to elaborate thyroxine. The arteries of the thyroid are remarkably large and form numerous anastomoses. Compare **parathyroid gland.**

thyroid hormone, an iodine-containing compound secreted by the thyroid gland, predominantly as thyroxine (T_4) and in smaller amounts as four times more potent triiodothyronine (T_3). These hormones increase the rate of metabolism, affect body temperature, regulate protein, fat, and carbohydrate catabolism in all cells, maintain growth hormone secretion, skeletal maturation, the cardiac rate, force, and output, promote central nervous system development, stimulate the synthesis of many enzymes, and are necessary for muscle tone and vigor. Derivatives of thyronine, T_4 and T_3 are synthesized in the thyroid gland by a complex process involving the uptake, oxidation, and incorporation of iodide and the production of thyroglobulin; the form in which the hormones apparently are stored in thyroid follicular colloid. Following the proteolysis of thyroglobulin, T_4 and T_3 are released and transported in the blood in strong, but noncovalent, association with certain plasma proteins; T_4 accounts for approximately 90 per cent of iodine in circulation and T_3 for five per cent. All phases of the production and the release of T_4 and T_3 are regulated by the thyroid stimulating hormone (TSH) secreted by the anterior pituitary gland. The production of thyroid hormones is excessive in Graves' disease and toxic nodular goiter (Plummer's disease), diminished in myxedema, and absent in cretinism. T_4's normal six to seven day half-life in blood is reduced to three or four days in hyperthyroidism and extended to nine or ten days in myxedema. T_3 has a normal half-life of two days or less and, like T_4, is metabolized most actively in the liver. Pharmaceutical preparations of thyroid hormones extracted from animal glands and the synthetic compounds levothyroxine sodium and liothyronine sodium are used as replacement therapy in patients with hypothyroidism. The dosage is initially low and is gradually increased to the optimal level based on the patient's clinical response and tests of the basal metabolic rate, radioactive iodine uptake, protein-bound iodine, and deep tendon reflexes. Overdosage or too rapid increase in the dosage may result in signs of hyperthyroidism, as nervousness, tremor, tachycardia, cardiac arrhythmia, and menstrual irregularity.

-thyroidism. See -thyrea.

thyroiditis (thai'roidai'tis), inflammation of the thyroid gland. Acute thyroiditis, caused by staphylococcal, streptococcal, or other infections, is characterized by suppuration and abscess formation and may progress to subacute, diffuse disease of the gland. Subacute thyroiditis is marked by fever, weakness, sore throat, and a painfully enlarged gland containing granulomas composed of colloid masses surrounded by giant cells and mononuclear cells. Chronic lymphocytic thyroiditis (Hashimoto's disease), characterized by lymphocyte and plasma cell infiltration of the gland and by diffuse enlargement, seems to be transmitted as a dominant trait and may be associated with various autoimmune disorders. Another chronic form of thyroiditis is Riedel's struma, a rare progressive fibrosis, usually of one lobe of the gland but sometimes involving both lobes, the trachea, and surrounding muscles, nerves, and blood vessels. Radiation thyroiditis occasionally occurs seven to ten days following the treatment of hyperthyroidism with radioactive iodine$_{131}$.

thyroid-stimulating hormone (TSH), a chemical substance, secreted by the anterior lobe of the pituitary gland, that controls the release of thyroid hormone and is necessary for the growth and function of the thyroid gland. The secretion of TSH is regulated by thyrotropin releasing factor, elaborated in the median eminence of the hypothalamus. Also called **thyrotropin.** See also **thyroid hormone.**

thyroid storm, a crisis in uncontrolled hyperthyroidism caused by the release into the blood stream of increased amounts of thyroid hormones. The storm may occur spontaneously or be precipitated by infection, stress, or a thyroidectomy performed on a patient who is inadequately prepared with antithyroid drugs. Characteristic signs are fever that may reach 106°F., a rapid pulse, acute respiratory distress, apprehension, restlessness, irritability, and prostration. The patient may become delirious, lapse into a coma, and die of heart failure.

Thyrolar, a trade name for a thyroid hormone (liotrix).

thyronine. See under **thyroid hormone.**

thyrotoxicosis (thaĭ′routok′sĭkou′sĭs). See **Graves' disease.**

thyrotropin. See **thyroid-stimulating hormone.**

thyrotropin (systemic) (thaĭrot′rəpĭn, thaĭ′rətrou′pĭn), a preparation of bovine thyroid-stimulating hormone that increases the uptake of radioactive iodine in the thyroid and the secretion of thyroxine by the thyroid.

■ INDICATIONS: It is prescribed in diagnostic tests and to enhance uptake of ^{131}I in the treatment of thyroid cancer.

■ CONTRAINDICATIONS: Coronary thrombosis or known hypersensitivity to this drug prohibits its use. It is not be given in untreated Addison's disease or following myocardial infarction.

■ ADVERSE EFFECTS: Among the most serious adverse reactions are symptoms of hyperthyroidism, allergic reactions, hypotension, and arrhythmias.

thyrotropin releasing factor (TRF), a chemical substance, secreted by the median eminence of the hypothalamus, that regulates the secretion of thyroid stimulating hormone by the anterior lobe of the pituitary gland.

thyrotropin releasing hormone, a substance elaborated in the median eminence of the hypothalamus that stimulates the release of thyrotropin (thyroid stimulating hormone) from the anterior pituitary gland. Also called **thyrotropin releasing factor, TSH releasing factor.**

thyroxine (T$_4$), a hormone of the thyroid gland, derived from tyrosine, that influences metabolic rate. Also called **tetraiodothyronine.**

thyroxine-binding globulin, a plasma protein that binds with and transports thyroxine in the blood.

Thytropar, a trade name for bovine thyrotropin.

Ti, symbol for **titanium.**

TI, abbreviation for *therapeutic index.*

TIA, abbreviation for **transient ischemic attack.**

tibia, the second longest bone of the skeleton, located at the medial side of the leg. It articulates with the fibula laterally, the talus distally, and the femur proximally, forming part of the knee joint. The tibia attaches to the ligament of the patella and to various muscles, including the popliteus and the flexor digitorum longus. Also called **shin bone.**

tibialis anterior, one of the anterior crural muscles of the leg, situated on the lateral side of the tibia. It is a thick, fleshy muscle proximally and tendinous distally, arising from various origins, as the lateral side of the tibia, and inserting into the first cuneiform bone and the first metatarsal bone. It is innervated by a branch of the deep peroneal nerve, in which there are fibers from the fourth and the fifth lumbar and the first sacral nerves. The tibialis anterior dorsiflexes and supinates the foot. Also called **tibialis anticus.** Compare **extensor digitorum longus.**

tibialis anticus (tĭb′ĭæl′ĭs ænti′kəs). See **tibialis anterior.**

tibial torsion, a lateral or a medial twisting rotation of the tibia on its longitudinal axis, as in the pronation of the hand owing to the contraction of the pronator teres and the pronator quadratus, or the supination of the hand, owing to the contraction of the supinator muscle. Compare **femoral torsion.**

tic. See **mimic spasm.**

tic douloureux (tĭk′ du′luru′). See **trigeminal neuralgia.**

tick bite, a puncture wound produced by the toothed beak of a blood-sucking tick, a small, tough-skinned, arachnid. Ticks transmit several diseases to humans and a few species carry a neurotoxin in their saliva that may cause ascending paralysis beginning in the legs. Nervousness, loss of appetite, tingling and headache, followed by muscle pain, and, in extreme cases, respiratory failure may occur. Symptoms often disappear when the attached tick is carefully removed with forceps. Placing a drop of alcohol or ether on the tick or coating it with petrolatum or nail polish facilitates removal. See also **Lyme arthritis, Q fever, relapsing fever, Rocky Mountain spotted fever, tularemia.**

tick fever. See **relapsing fever.**

tick paralysis, a rare, progressive, reversible disorder caused by several species of ticks that release a neurotoxin that causes weakness, incoordination, and paralysis. The tick must feed on the host for several days before the symptoms appear, and removal of the tick leads to rapid recovery. Since respiratory or bulbar paralysis can cause death, it is important to search for ticks, frequently hidden in scalp hair, on a patient with these symptoms.

t.i.d., (in prescriptions) abbreviation for *ter in die,* a Latin phrase meaning 'three times a day.'

tidal drainage. See **drainage.**

tidal volume (TV), the amount of air inhaled and exhaled during normal ventilation. Inspiratory reserve volume, expiratory reserve volume, and tidal volume make up vital capacity. See also **pulmonary function test.**

tide, a variation, increase or decrease, in the concentration of a particular component of body fluids. — **tidal,** *adj.*

Tietze's syndrome (tit′siz), **1.** a disorder characterized by nonsuppurative swellings of one or more costal cartilages causing pain that may radiate to the neck, shoulder, or arm and mimic the pain of coronary artery disease. The syndrome may accompany chronic respiratory infections, and, if the costal swellings are extremely painful, infiltration with procaine and hydrocortisone may provide relief. **2.** albinism, except for normal eye pigment, accompanied by deaf mutism and hypoplasia of the eyebrows.

TIG, abbreviation for **tetanus immune globulin.**

T-I-Gammagee, a trade name for a passive immunizing agent (tetanus immune globulin).

Tigan, a trade name for an antiemetic (trimethobenzamide hydrochloride).

timed release. See **prolonged release.**

timolol maleate, a beta-adrenergic receptor blocking agent.

■ INDICATION: It is prescribed for reducing intraocular pressure in glaucoma.

■ CONTRAINDICATIONS: Known hypersensitivity to this drug prohibits its use. It is used with caution in patients with contraindications to systemic use of beta-adrenergic receptor blocking agents.

■ ADVERSE EFFECTS: The most serious adverse reaction is blurring of vision. Mild eye irritation also may occur.

Timoptic, a trade name for a beta-adrenergic receptor blocking agent (timolol maleate).

Tinactin, a trade name for an antifungal (tolnaftate).

Tindal Maleate, a trade name for a phenothiazine (acetophenazine maleate), used as a tranquilizer.

tinea (tin′iə), a group of fungal skin diseases caused by dermatophytes of several kinds, characterized by itching, scaling, and, sometimes, painful lesions. Tinea is a general term that refers to infections of various etiologies, which are seen on several sites; the specific type is usually designated by a modifying term. Diagnosis is made by demonstrating fungus on smear or by culture. Also called **ringworm.**

tinea capitis, a contagious fungal disease characterized by circular, bald patches of from one to 6 cm in diameter with slight erythema, scaling, and crusting. Diagnosis is made by bright fluorescence of infected hairs under Wood's light, by microscopic examination of infected hairs, and by culture of the fungus. Treatment consists of three to six weeks of griseofulvin given orally. Also called **ringworm.**

tinea corporis, a superficial fungal infection of the nonhairy skin of the body, most prevalent in hot, humid climates and usually caused by species of *Trichophyton* or *Microsporum.* Topical fungicides, as miconazole, are used for moderate cases; severe infection calls for griseofulvin.

tinea cruris (kru′ris), a superficial fungal infection of the groin, caused by species of *Trichophyton* or *Epidermophyton floccosum.* It is most common in the tropics and among males. Topical antifungals, as miconazole and clotrimazole, are often prescribed. Griseofulvin is used only for severe, resistant cases. Also called **jock itch.**

tinea pedis, a chronic, superficial fungal infection of the foot, especially of the skin between the toes and on the soles. It is common worldwide and is usually caused by *Trichophyton mentagrophytes, T. rubrum,* and *Epidermophyton floccosum.* Adults are most susceptible, and the wearing of constricting footwear, as sneakers, seems to induce the infection. Drying the feet well after bathing and applying powder between the toes help to prevent it. Griseofulvin is the most effective treatment, but miconazole and tolnaftate are also used. Recurrence is common. Also called **athlete's foot.**

tinea unguium, a superficial fungal infection of the nails caused by various species of *Trichophyton* and, occasionally, by *Candida albicans.* It is more common on the toes than the fingers and can cause complete crumbling and destruction of the nails. Griseofulvin is the drug of choice, but it must be continued until the nail has regrown completely.

tinea versicolor, a fungous infection of the skin characterized by finely desquamating, pale tan patches on the upper trunk and upper arms that may itch and do not tan. In dark-skinned persons the lesions may be depigmented. The fungus fluoresces under Wood's light and may be easily identified in scrapings viewed under a microscope. Treatment usually includes a single application of selenium sulfide left on overnight and rinsed off by thorough showering in the morning. The pale patches may persist for up to a year after successful treatment.

Tinel's sign (tinelz′), an indication of irritability of a nerve, resulting in a distal tingling sensation upon percussion of a damaged nerve. The sign is often present in the carpal tunnel syndrome and is produced by tapping over the median nerve on the volar aspect of the wrist.

tine test, a tuberculin skin test in which a small disposable disc with multiple tines bearing tuberculin antigen is used to puncture the skin. The method is widely used to test for sensitivity to the tuberculin antigen. Induration around the puncture site indicates previous exposure or active disease, requiring further testing. See also **tuberculin test.**

tingling, a prickly sensation in the skin or a part of the body, accompanied by diminished sensitivity to stimulation of the sensory nerves, felt by a person as the area is numbed by local anesthetic or by exposure to the cold, or as it "goes to sleep" from pressure on a nerve.

tinnitus (tɪnaɪ'təs), tinkling or ringing heard in one or both ears. It may be a sign of acoustic trauma, Ménière's disease, otosclerosis, or presbycusis or of an accumulation of cerumen impinging on the eardrum or occluding the external auditory canal.

tin (Sn), a whitish metallic element. Its atomic number is 50; its atomic weight is 118.69. Tin oxide is used in dentistry as a polishing agent for teeth and in some restorative procedures.

T-Ionate-P.A., a trade name for an androgen (testosterone cypionate).

tissue activator. See **fibrinokinase.**

tissue committee, a group that evaluates all surgery performed in a hospital or other health-care facility. The evaluation is usually made on the basis of the extent of agreement of the preoperative, postoperative, and pathological diagnoses and on the relevance and acceptability of the diagnostic procedures. See also **tissue review.**

tissue dextrin. See **glycogen.**

tissue dose, (in radiotherapy) the amount of radiation absorbed by tissue in the region of interest, expressed in rads.

tissue fixation, a process in which a tissue specimen is placed in a fluid that preserves the cells as nearly as is possible in their natural state.

tissue fixative, a fluid that preserves cells in their natural state, so that they may be identified and examined.

tissue kinase. See **fibrinokinase.**

tissue perfusion, alteration in: cerebral, cardiopulmonary, renal, gastrointestinal, peripheral, a nursing diagnosis accepted by the Fourth National Conference on the Classification of Nursing Diagnoses. The etiology of the diagnosis may be interruption of the venous or arterial circulation to the affected part of the body, hypovolemia or hypervolemia, or a condition that causes abnormal exchange of fluids and nutrients to or from the cells to the circulation. The defining characteristics of the condition include coldness of the affected extremity, paleness on elevation of the extremity, diminished arterial pulses, and changes in the arterial blood pressure when measured in the affected extremity. Claudication, gangrene, brittle nails, slowly healing ulcers or wounds, shiny skin, and lack of hair are also commonly seen. See also **nursing diagnosis.**

tissue response, any reaction or change in living cellular tissue when it is acted upon by disease, toxin, or other external stimulus. Some kinds of tissue responses are **immune response, inflammation, necrosis.**

tissue review, a review of the surgery performed in a hospital or other health-care facility. The evaluation is usually made on the basis of the extent of agreement of the preoperative, postoperative, and pathological diagnoses and on the relevance and acceptability of the diagnostic procedures. See also **tissue committee.**

tissue typing, a systematized series of tests to evaluate the intraspecies compatibility of tissues of a donor and a recipient prior to transplantation. This is accomplished by identifying and comparing a large series of human leukocyte antigens (HLA) in the cells of the body. See also **HLA, immune system, transplant.**

titanium (Ti), a grayish, brittle metallic element. Its atomic number is 22; its atomic weight is 47.90. An alloy of titanium is used in the manufacture of orthopedic prostheses. Titanium dioxide is the active ingredient in a number of topical ointments and lotions.

title, a section of the Social Security Act that provides for the establishment, funding, and regulation of a service to a specific segment of the population, as Title XIX, which includes medical coverage under Medicaid, and Title X which awards lump-sum grants for family planning programs.

titubation (tɪch'ubei'shən), unsteady posture characterized by a staggering or stumbling gait and a swaying head or trunk while sitting. It may be a manifestation of cerebellar disease. Compare **ataxia.**

Tl, symbol for **thallium.**

TLC, 1. abbreviation for **total lung capacity. 2.** *Informal.* abbreviation for *tender loving care.*

Tm, symbol for **thulium.**

TNM, a system for staging malignant neoplastic disease. See also **cancer staging.**

t.n.t.c., abbreviation for *too-numerous-to-count,* usually applied to organisms or cells viewed on a slide under a microscope.

t.o., abbreviation for *telephone order.*

toadstool poisoning, a toxic condition caused by ingestion of certain varieties of poisonous mushrooms. See **mushroom poisoning.**

tobacco, a plant, the leaves of which are dried and used for smoking and chewing, and in snuff. See also **nicotine.**

tobramycin sulfate, an aminoglycoside antibiotic.

■ INDICATION: It is prescribed in the treatment of serious infection.

■ CONTRAINDICATIONS: Kidney dysfunction, use of potent diuretics, or known hypersensitivity to this or other aminoglycosides prohibits its use.

■ ADVERSE EFFECTS: Among the more serious adverse reactions are ototoxicity and nephrotoxicity.

Tobruk plaster (tou'brʊk), a plaster cast splint with tapes for skin traction coming through openings in the plaster and connected with a Thomas splint. It covers and immobilizes the leg from foot to groin. Also called **Tobruk splint.**

-tocia, 1. a combining form meaning 'conditions of labor': *mogitocia, omotocia, tomotocia.* 2. a combining form meaning the 'product of parturition': *deuterotocia, dystrophiadystocia, odontocia.*

toco-, toko-, a combining form meaning 'pertaining to childbirth or labor': *tocodynamometer, tocography, tocomania.*

tocodynamometer, tokodynamometer (touˈkoudaiˈnəmomˈɪtər), an electronic device for monitoring and recording contractions in labor. It consists of a pressure transducer that is applied to the fundus of the uterus by means of a belt, which is connected to a machine that records the duration of the contractions and the interval between them on graph paper. The relative intensity of the contractions is also indicated but cannot be quantified. The tocodynamometer is a component of external monitoring in childbirth. See also **electronic fetal monitor.**

tocopherol (toukofˈərol), any of a group of pale-yellow, fat-soluble, oily liquid phenolic compounds that possess vitamin E activity in varying degrees. They are stable to heat and acids and unstable to alkalis, ultraviolet light, and oxygen. All are powerful antioxidants and occur naturally in various vegetable oils, oils from seeds (especially wheat germ and cottonseed), and fish-liver oils. Alphatocopherol is the physiologically most active form of the group. See also **vitamin E.**

toddler, a child between the ages of 12 and 36 months. During this period of development the child acquires a sense of autonomy and independence through the mastery of various specialized tasks, as control of bodily functions, refinement of motor and language skills, and acquisition of socially acceptable behavior, especially toleration of delayed gratification and acceptance of separation from the mother or parents. The period is characterized by exploration of the environment and by rapid cognitive development as the child strives for self-assertion and personal interaction with others while struggling with parental discipline and sibling rivalry. Of primary importance for the nurse is the understanding of the dynamics of the growth and development of the toddler in order to help parents deal effectively with appropriate nutrition, toilet training, temper tantrums, prevention of accidental injury– primarily from falls, poisoning, burns, and childhood fears, especially anxiety as a result of separation from the parents.

toddlerhood, the state or condition of being a toddler.

toe, any one of the digits of the feet.

toenail, one of the heavy ungual structures covering the terminal phalanges of the toes. Also called **unguis.**

Tofranil, a trade name for a tricyclic antidepressant (imipramine hydrochloride).

togavirus (touˈgəvaiˈrəs), a family of viruses that includes the organisms causing encephalitis, dengue, yellow fever, and rubella.

toilet training, the process of teaching a child to control the functions of the bladder and bowel. Training programs vary, but all emphasize a positive, consistent, nonpunitive, and nonpressured approach, and each program is individualized, depending on the mental and physical age and state of the child, the parent-child relationship, and readiness of the child to learn. Training often begins between 18 and 24 months of age, when voluntary control of the anal and urethral sphincters is achieved by most children. When the child has mastered some motor skills, is aware of his ability to control the body, and can communicate adequately, training is likely to be easy. Resistance occurs if the parents try to train the child before the child is physiologically and psychologically ready. Bowel training is usually accomplished before bladder training because the urge to evacuate the bowel is stronger than the urge to empty the bladder, and the need is less frequent and more regular. Nighttime bladder control may not be achieved until the child is four or five years of age or older. Behavior modification, using a system of rewards for each of the various phases of the training, has been successful with both normal and mentally retarded children. A major nursing function is to identify the readiness of the child to learn, to work with the parents, advising them in a nonauthoritarian way of the various techniques.

token economy, a technique of reinforcement used in behavior therapy in the management of a group of people, as in hospitals, institutions, or classrooms. Individuals are rewarded for specific activities or behavior with tokens they can exchange for desired objects or privileges.

toko-. See **toco-.**

tokodynamometer (touˈkoudaiˈnəmomˈɪtər). See **tocodynamometer.**

tolazamide, a sulfonylurea and antidiabetic.

■ INDICATION: It is prescribed in the treatment of stable adult onset diabetes mellitus.

■ CONTRAINDICATIONS: Unstable diabetes, serious impairment of renal, hepatic, or thyroid function, pregnancy, or known hypersensitivity to this drug or to other sulfonylurea medication prohibits its use.

■ ADVERSE EFFECTS: Among the more serious adverse effects are hypoglycemia and skin reactions. Blood dyscrasias may occur.

tolazoline hydrochloride, a peripheral vasodilator.

■ INDICATIONS: It is prescribed in the treatment of spastic peripheral vascular disorders.

■ CONTRAINDICATIONS: Coronary artery disease, cerebrovascular accident, or known hypersensitivity to this drug prohibits its use.

■ ADVERSE EFFECTS: Among the more serious adverse reactions are cardiac arrhythmia, hypertension, exacerbation of peptic ulcer, and a paradoxical response in seriously damaged limbs.

tolbutamide, an oral sulfonylurea antidiabetic.

■ INDICATION: It is prescribed in the treatment of stable adult-onset diabetes mellitus.

■ CONTRAINDICATIONS: Unstable diabetes, serious impairment of renal, hepatic, or thyroid function, pregnancy, or known hypersensitivity to this drug or to other sulfonylurea medication prohibits its use.

■ ADVERSE EFFECTS: Among the more serious adverse reactions are hypoglycemia and skin reactions. Blood dyscrasias may occur.

Tolectin, a trade name for nonsteroidal anti-inflammatory (tolmetin sodium).

tolerance, the ability to endure hardship, pain, or ordinarily injurious substances like drugs without apparent physiological or psychological injury. A kind of tolerance is **work tolerance.**

tolerance dose, (in radiotherapy) the amount of radiation that can be delivered to a body structure before irreversible damage occurs.

Toleron, a trade name for a hematinic (ferrous fumarate).

Tolinase, a trade name for an antidiabetic (tolazamide).

tolmetin sodium (tol′mətin), a nonsteroidal anti-inflammatory agent.

■ INDICATION: It is prescribed primarily in the treatment of rheumatoid arthritis.

■ CONTRAINDICATIONS: Impaired renal function, gastrointestinal disease, or known hypersensitivity to this drug, to aspirin, or to nonsteroidal anti-inflammatory medication prohibits its use.

■ ADVERSE EFFECTS: Among the more serious adverse reactions are peptic ulcer and gastrointestinal distress. Dizziness, skin rash, and tinnitus commonly occur. This drug interacts with many other drugs.

tolnaftate (tolnæf′teit), an antifungal.

■ INDICATIONS: It is prescribed in the treatment of superficial fungus infections of the skin.

■ CONTRAINDICATION: Known hypersensitivity to this drug prohibits its use.

■ ADVERSE EFFECTS: Among the more common adverse reactions are hypersensitivity reactions and mild irritation of the skin.

-tome, 1. a combining form meaning a 'cutting instrument': *labiotome, neurotome, thyrotome.* 2. a combining form meaning a '(specified) segment or region': *dermomyotome, pleurotome, viscerotome.*

-tomic, a combining form meaning 'related to incisions or sections of tissue': *dermatomic, phlebotomic, somatomic.* Also **-tomical.**

tomography (təmog′rəfi), an x-ray technique that produces a film representing a detailed cross section of tissue structure at a predetermined depth. It is a valuable diagnostic tool for the discovery and identification of space-occupying lesions, as might be found in the brain, liver, pancreas, and gall bladder.

-tomy, a combining form meaning a 'surgical incision': *cystotomy, oncotomy, phlebotomy.*

tone. See **tonus.**

tongue, the principal organ of the sense of taste that also assists in the mastication and the deglutition of food. It is located in the floor of the mouth within the curve of the mandible. Its root is connected to the hyoid bone posteriorly by the hypoglossi and the genioglossi muscles. It is also connected to the epiglottis by three folds of mucous membrane, to the soft palate by the glossopalatine arches, and to the pharynx by the constrictores pharyngis superiores and by the mucous membrane. The apex of the tongue rests anteriorly against the lingual surfaces of the lower incisors. The mucous membrane connecting the tongue to the mandible reflects over the floor of the mouth to the lingual surface of the gum and, in the midline of the floor is raised into a vertical fold. The dorsum of the tongue is divided into symmetrical halves by a median sulcus, which ends posteriorly in the foramen cecum. A shallow sulcus terminalis runs from this foramen laterally and forward on either side to the margin of the organ. From the sulcus, the anterior two thirds of the tongue is covered with papillae. The posterior third is smoother and contains numerous mucous glands and lymph follicles. The use of the tongue as an organ of speech is not anatomical, but a secondary acquired characteristic. Also called **lingua.**

-tonia, a combining form meaning '(condition or degree of) tonus of a sort or in a region of the body': *angiotonia, hemotonia, vasotonia.* Also **-tony.**

-tonic, 1. a combining form meaning the 'quality of muscle contraction or tonus': *hypertonic, myatonic, normotonic.* 2. a combining form meaning a 'solution with a comparative concentration': *hypertonic, hypotonic, isotonic.*

tonicity (tounis′iti), the quality of possessing tone, or tonus.

tonic labyrinthine reflex, a normal postural reflex in animals, abnormally accentuated in decerebrate humans, characterized by extension of all four limbs when the head is positioned in space at an angle above the horizontal in quadripeds or in the neutral, erect position in humans. Also called **decerebrate rigidity.**

tonic neck reflex, a normal response in newborns to extend the arm and the leg on the side of the body to which the head is quickly turned while the infant is supine and to flex the limbs of the opposite side. The reflex, which prevents the infant from rolling over until adequate neurological and motor development occurs, disappears by three to four months of age to be replaced by symmetric positioning of both sides of the body. Absence or persistence of the reflex may indicate central nervous system damage. Also called **asymmetric tonic neck reflex.** See also **symmetric tonic neck reflex.**

tono-, a combining form meaning 'pertaining to tone or tension': *tonoclonic, tonoscillograph, tonoplast.*

tonometer (tounom′ɪtər), an instrument used in measuring tension or pressure, especially intraocular pressure.

tonometry (tounom′ɪtri), the measuring of intraocular pressure by determining the resistance of the eyeball to indentation by an applied force. Several kinds of tonometers are used. The air-puff tonometer, which does not touch the eye, records deflections of the cornea from a puff of pressurized air. The aplanation tonometer records the pressure needed to flatten the corneal surface.

tonsil, a small, rounded mass of tissue, especially lymphoid tissue, as that comprising the palatine tonsils in the oropharynx. Compare **intestinal tonsil, lingual tonsil, palatine tonsil, pharyngeal tonsil.**

tonsillectomy, the surgical excision of the palatine tonsils, performed to prevent recurrent streptococcal tonsillitis. Before surgery, several laboratory tests, including a bleeding and clotting time, complete blood count, and urinalysis are done. Tonsillar tissue is dissected and removed, usually under general anesthesia, and bleeding areas are sutured or cauterized. An airway remains in place until swallowing returns. An increase in pulse rate, falling blood pressure, restlessness, or frequent swallowing warns of possible hemorrhage. On recovery from anesthesia, ice chips or clear liquids without a drinking straw may be offered. Tonsillectomy is often combined with adenoidectomy.

tonsillitis, an infection or inflammation of a tonsil. Acute tonsillitis, frequently caused by streptococcus infection, is characterized by severe sore throat, fever, headache, malaise, difficulty in swallowing, earache, and enlarged, tender lymph nodes in the neck. Acute tonsillitis may accompany scarlet fever. Treatment includes systemic antibiotics, analgesics, and warm irrigations of the throat. Soft foods and ample fluids are given. Tonsillectomy is sometimes performed for recurrent tonsillitis or tonsillar abscess. See also **peritonsillar abscess, scarlet fever, strep throat.**

tonus (tou′nəs), **tone,** **1.** the normal state of balanced tension in the tissues of the body, especially the muscles. Partial contraction or alternate contraction and relaxation of neighboring fibers of a group of muscles hold the organ or the part of the body in a neutral, functional position without fatigue. Tone is essential for many normal body functions, like holding the spine erect, the eyes open, and the jaw closed. **2.** the state of the tissues of the body being strong and fit.

-tony, a combining form meaning a 'condition of motor control': *arteriotony, neurotony, vagotony.* Also **-tonia.**

tooth, *pl.* **teeth.** one of numerous dental structures that develop in the jaws as part of the digestive system and are used to cut, grind, and process food in the mouth for ingestion. Each tooth consists of a crown, which projects above the gum; two to four roots, embedded in the alveolus; and a neck, which stretches between the crown and the root. Each tooth also contains a cavity filled with pulp, richly supplied with blood vessels and nerves that enter the cavity through a small aperture at the base of each root. The solid portion of the tooth consists of dentin, enamel, and a thin layer of bone on the surface of the root. The dentin comprises the bulk of the tooth. The enamel covers the exposed portion of the crown. Two sets of teeth appear at different periods of life: the 20 deciduous teeth appear during infancy, the 32 permanent teeth during childhood and early adulthood. See also **deciduous teeth, permanent tooth.**

tooth germ, a primitive cell in the embryo that is the precursor of a tooth.

tophus (tou′fəs), *pl.* **tophi.** a calculus, containing sodium urate deposits, that develops in periarticular fibrous tissue, typically in patients with gout.

-topia, a combining form meaning '(condition of) placement of organs in the body': *heterotopia, normotopia, skeletopia.* Also **-topy.**

topical, **1.** of or pertaining to the surface of a part of the body. **2.** of or pertaining to a drug or treatment applied topically.

topical anesthesia, surface analgesia produced by application of a topical anesthetic in the form of a solution, gel, or ointment to the skin, mucous membrane, or cornea. The most common ingredients include benzocaine, butamben, cyclomethycaine, dibucaine, dimethisoquin, diperodon, dyclonine, lidocaine, piperocaine, pramoxine, hexylcaine, and tetracaine. Cocaine may be applied in solution to the mucous membranes of the nasal passages in certain otolaryngeal or maxillofacial procedures. Also called **surface anesthesia.** Compare **local anesthesia.**

Topicort, a trade name for a topical glucocorticoid (desoximethasone).

topo-, a combining form meaning 'place': *topognosis, toponarcosis, topoparesthesia.*

Topsyn, a trade name for a glucocorticoid (fluocinonide).

TORCH, an acronym for toxoplasmosis, other, rubella virus, cytomegalovirus, and herpes simplex viruses, a group of agents that can infect the fetus or the newborn infant causing a constellation of morbid effects called the TORCH syndrome.

TORCH syndrome, infection of the fetus or newborn by one of the TORCH agents. The outcome of a pregnancy complicated by a TORCH agent may be abortion or stillbirth, intrauterine growth retardation, or premature delivery.

■ OBSERVATIONS: At delivery and during the first days after birth an infant infected with any one of the organisms may demonstrate various clinical manifestations, as fever, lethargy, poor feeding, petechiae on the skin, purpura, pneumonia, heptosplenomegaly, jaundice, hemolytic and other anemias, encephalitis, microcephaly, hydrocephalus, intracranial calcifications, hearing deficits, chorioretinitis and micro-ophthalmia. In addition, each of the agents is associated with several other abnormal clinical findings involving abnormal immune response, cataracts, glaucoma, vesicles, ulcers, and congenital cardiac defects.

■ INTERVENTION: Before pregnancy women may be tested for susceptibility to the rubella virus and inoculated against it if not immune. There are currently no vaccines that confer immunity to the other TORCH agents, but the mother may be serologically tested for antibody levels to them. During pregnancy toxoplasmosis is asymptomatic in about 90 per cent of cases, making diagnosis unlikely. If infection is suspected, serial paired serologic tests are performed: a high, rising titre indicates recent infection. Transplacental infection occurs in 35 per cent of mothers infected during pregnancy. If it is contracted in the first trimester, before the placenta is fully developed, the infant may not become infected; if the infection is contracted, severe congenital manifestations of the syndrome usually occur. If the fetus is infected after the first trimester, the baby is usually born with asymptomatic or mild disease; the infection may be spread from the baby during the newborn period. Sulfadiazone, pyrimethamine, and folinic acid are sometimes given to treat the infection.

Primary cytomegalovirus infection during pregnancy is usually asymptomatic. If the infection is suspected serologic testing may be performed to demonstrate primary infection, as infants born to mothers infected for the first time during pregnancy are much more likely to develop severe congenital anomalies than if the infection were a reactivation of previous cytomegalovirus infection. There is no specific treatment. The child is considered to be infectious, but contagion among newborns from a congenitally infected infant has not been proven.

Transplacental rubella virus infection in pregnancy during the first eight weeks is likely to cause infection in 50 per cent of fetuses and to result in demonstrable defects in 85 per cent of those infected. The risk becomes less as gestation increases to 24 weeks, after which time infection has not been known to result in defects. Rubella is the only TORCH virus that is usually symptomatic, and, therefore, it is often recognized. Many mothers infected during the first trimester choose to abort the pregnancy. There is no treatment for the infection, but screening and immunization before pregnancy could prevent virtually all cases of congenital rubella.

Herpesvirus infection (HSV) in pregnancy may rarely be transplacentally transmitted to the fetus. Primary infection during pregnancy may sometimes result in spontaneous abortion or premature delivery. In the newborn the infection is usually systemic and life-threatening. The fetus is most apt to become infected by the virus shed from an active genital lesion during vaginal delivery or as the result of vaginal examination or the placement of an intrauterine catheter or a fetal scalp electrode during labor. There is no treatment: if the mother has active, genital herpesvirus lesions intrapartal internal monitoring is contraindicated, vaginal exams are often omitted, regional anesthetic techniques are avoided, and the infant is delivered by Caesarean section.

The TORCH infections caused by other agents are asymptomatic in pregnancy, revealing themselves by the syndrome after birth. The congenital effects are not amenable to change or to amelioration by any known treatment.

■ NURSING CONSIDERATIONS: Newborn infants who are infected with a TORCH agent or who bear the stigmata of TORCH syndrome are considered to be potential sources of neonatal spread of infection. Rubella screening and vaccination are encouraged. Only 10 per cent of the cases of TORCH syndrome are proven to be associated with a known agent (toxoplasmosis, rubella virus, cytomegalovirus, or herpesvirus); 90 per cent are the result of 'other' infections; therefore, pregnant women are instructed to avoid contact with people ill with infectious diseases to the greatest extent possible.

Torecan Maleate, a trade name for a phenothiazine antiemetic (thiethylperazine maleate).

Torkildsen procedure (tor′kıldsın). See **ventriculocisternostomy.**

torpid idiocy, *Obsolete.* severe mental retardation associated with dullness and inactivity.

torque (tork), a moment of force that tends to produce rotation, or torsion, as the forces produced by contraction of the medial femoral muscles tend to rotate the thigh medially.

torr (tor), a unit of pressure, commonly used to mean 1 mm Hg, the amount of pressure required to raise a column of mercury 1 mm.

tors-, a combining form meaning 'twisted': *torsiometer, torsive, torsiversion.*

torsion, 1. the process of twisting or turning away from the normal position. It may be positive (clockwise) or negative (counterclockwise). 2. the state of being turned.

torsion dystonia. See **dystonia musculorum deformans.**

torsion fracture, a spiral fracture, usually caused by a torsion injury.

torsion of the testis, the axial rotation of the spermatic cord that cuts off the blood supply to the testicle, epididymis, and other structures. Complete ischemia for six hours may result in gangrene of the testis. Partial loss of circulation may result in atrophy. Certain testes are anatomically predisposed to torsion because of inadequate connective tissue, but the condition may be caused by trauma with severe swelling. Torsion of the testis occurs more often on the left than on the right side and is most frequent in the first year of life and during puberty. Surgical correction is required in most cases; if performed within five hours of the onset of symptoms, the testis can usually be saved.

torsion spasm. See **dystonia musculorum deformans.**

tort, (in law) a civil wrong, other than a breach of contract. Torts include negligence, false imprisonment, assault, and battery. The elements of a tort are: a legal duty owed by the defendant to the plaintiff, a breach of duty, and damage from the breach of duty. A tort may be constitutional, in which one person deprives another of a right or immunity guaranteed by the Constitution; personal, in which a person or a person's reputation or feelings are injured; or intentional, in which the wrong is a deliberate act that is unlawful. Many other kinds of tort exist. **tortious,** *adj.*

tort feasor, a person who commits a tort.

torticollis (tor'tıkol'ıs), an abnormal condition in which the head is inclined to one side as a result of the contraction of the muscles on that side of the neck. It may be congenital or acquired. Treatment may include surgery, heat, support, or immobilization depending on the cause and the severity of the condition. Also called **wryneck.** See also **spasmodic torticollis.**

Torula histolytica (tor'yulə hıstəlıt'ıkə). See ***Cryptococcus neoformans.***

torulopsosis (tor'yulop'səsıs), an infection with the yeast *Torulopsis glabrata,* a normal inhabitant of the oropharynx, gastrointestinal tract, and skin, that causes disease in severely debilitated patients, in those with impaired immune function, or, sometimes, in patients having prolonged urinary catheterization. Systemic infection is usually treated with amphotericin B or fluorocytosine.

torulosis (tor'yulou'sıs). See **cryptococcosis.**

torus fracture (tor'əs). See **lead pipe fracture.**

Totacillin, a trade name for an antibacterial (ampicillin).

total anomalous venous return, a rare congenital cardiac anomaly in which the pulmonary veins attach directly to the right atrium or to various veins draining into the right atrium rather than directing flow to the left atrium. Clinical manifestations include cyanosis, pulmonary congestion, and heart failure. Other cardiac defects may also be present, as atrial septal defect, which shunts unoxygenated systemic blood to the left side of the heart and helps to decompress the right atrium. Corrective surgery is indicated, usually after one year of age, but may be necessary at an earlier age if pulmonary venous obstruction or severe congestive heart failure is present. See also **congenital cardiac anomaly.**

total cleavage, mitotic division of the fertilized ovum into blastomeres. Compare **partial cleavage.**

total lung capacity (TLC), the volume of gas in the lungs at the end of a maximum inspiration.

total parenteral nutrition (TPN), the administration of a nutritionally adequate hypertonic solution consisting of glucose, protein hydrolysates, minerals, and vitamins through an indwelling catheter into the superior vena cava. The high rate of blood flow results in rapid dilution of the solution and full nutritional requirements can be met indefinitely. The procedure is used in prolonged coma, severe uncontrolled malabsorption, extensive burns, gastrointestinal fistulas, and other conditions in which feeding by mouth cannot provide adequate amounts of the essential nutrients. Strict asepsis must be maintained as infection is a grave and present danger of this therapy. Other solutions are never instilled through this catheter. Also called **hyperalimentation.**

total renal blood flow (TRBF), the total volume of blood that flows into the renal arteries. The average TRBF in a normal adult is 1200 ml per minute.

touch deprivation, a lack of tactile stimulation, especially in early infancy, which if continued for a sufficient length of time may lead to serious developmental and emotional disturbances, like stunted growth, personality disorders, and social regression. In severe cases, a child who is deprived of adequate physical handling and emotional stimulation may not survive infancy. See also **hospitalism.**

tourniquet (tur'nıkıt, tur'nıkıt), a device used in controlling hemorrhage, consisting of a wide constricting band applied to the limb proximal to the site of bleeding. The use of a tourniquet is a drastic measure and is to be employed only if the hemorrhage is life-threatening and if other, safer measures have proved ineffective. See also **hemorrhage.**

tourniquet test, a test of capillary fragility, in which a blood pressure cuff is applied for five minutes to a person's arm and is inflated to a pressure halfway between his diastolic and systolic blood pressure. The number of petechiae within a circumscribed area of the skin may be counted, or the results may be reported in a range from negative (no petechiae) to +4 positive (confluent petechiae).

tower head, See **oxycephaly.** Also called **tower skull.**

tower skull. See **oxycephaly.**

town-gown, of or pertaining to any aspect of the relationship between an educational institution and the community in which it is situated.

toxemia (toksi'miə), 1. Also called **blood poisoning.** the presence of toxins in the bloodstream 2. See **pre-eclampsia.** —**toxemic,** *adj.*

-toxemia, a combining form meaning a '(specified) toxic substance in the blood': *ectotoxemia, gonotoxemia, ophiotoxemia.* also **-toxaemia.**

toxemia of pregnancy. See **pre-eclampsia.**

-toxia, a combining form meaning 'condition resulting from a poison in a (specified) region of the body': *neurotoxia, thyrotoxia, urotoxia.*

toxic, 1. of or pertaining to a poison. 2. (of a disease or condition) severe and progressive.

-toxic, a combining form meaning 'pertaining to poison': *cardiotoxic, hematoxic, spermatoxic.* Also **-toxical.**

toxic amblyopia, partial loss of vision owing to retro-optic bulbar neuritis, caused by poisoning with quinine, lead, wood alcohol, arsenic, or certain other poisons.

toxic dementia, dementia resulting from excessive use of or exposure to a poisonous substance. See also **dementia.**

toxic dose (TD), (in toxicology) the amount of a substance that may be expected to produce a toxic effect. See also **median toxic dose.**

toxic epidermal necrolysis (TEN), a rare skin disease, characterized by epidermal erythema, superficial necrosis, and skin erosions. This condition, which affects mainly adults, makes the skin appear scalded, often leaving scars. The cause of TEN is unknown, but it may result from toxic or hypersensitive reactions. It is commonly associated with drug reactions, as those associated with butazones, sulfonamides, penicillins, barbiturates, and hydantoins. Other drugs may be involved, and the disease has also been associated with airborne toxins, as carbon monoxide. TEN may also indicate an immune response, or it may be associated with severe physiologic stress.

■ OBSERVATIONS: Early signs of the condition include inflammation of the mucous membranes, fever, malaise, a burning sensation in the conjunctivae, and pervasive tenderness of the skin. The first phase of TEN is manifested by diffuse erythema. The second phase involves vesiculation and blistering. The third phase is marked by extensive epidermal necrolysis and desquamation. As the disease progresses, large, flaccid bullae develop and rupture, exposing wide expanses of denuded skin. Tissue fluids and electrolytes are consequently lost, resulting in extensive systemic complications, as pulmonary edema, bronchopneumonia, gastrointestinal and esophageal hemorrhage, sepsis, shock, renal failure, and disseminated intravascular coagulation. These extreme conditions contribute to the high mortality associated with TEN—about 30 per cent—especially among the infirm and the elderly. Confirming diagnosis is based on symptoms in the third phase of the disease, as skin denuded by even slight friction, affecting the areas of erythema. Diagnosis is commonly supported by bacteriologic culture and Gram's stains of lesions to determine if infection exists. The presence of leukocytosis, fluid and electrolyte imbalances, albuminuria, and elevated transaminase levels are characteristic and help to confirm the diagnosis. Erythema multiforme and exfoliative dermatitis may be ruled out by exfoliative biopsy and cytology.

■ INTERVENTION: Treatment of TEN commonly involves the administration of I.V. fluids to replace body fluids and to maintain electrolyte balance. Frequent laboratory analyses are necessary to monitor hematocrit and hemoglobin, serum proteins, electrolytes, and blood gases.

■ NURSING CONSIDERATIONS: Nursing care of patients with TEN requires meticulous monitoring of vital signs, central venous pressure, and urinary output. Any signs of renal failure, as decreased urinary output, and of bleeding are of immediate concern. It is important to detect and quickly treat any septic infection. Temperature elevations are reported immediately and all laboratory work, as blood cultures and sensitivity tests, are performed promptly. Ocular lesions are common with TEN, and frequent eye care is often needed to remove exudate. Protective isolation and prophylactic antibiotic therapy may be required to prevent secondary infection. Nurses also make sure that the TEN patient does not wear tight clothing and is covered loosely to minimize the friction that causes skin sloughing. A Stryker frame or a CircOlectric bed may be helpful in caring for the patient. Analgesics are administered as needed, and cool, sterile compresses may be applied to relieve discomfort. Psychological and emotional support for the patient and the family is also a key nursing concern.

toxic erythema of the newborn. See **erythema toxicum neonatorum.**

toxic gastritis. See **corrosive gastritis.**

toxic goiter, an enlargement of the thyroid gland associated with exophthalmia and systemic disease. See also **Graves' disease.**

toxic hemoglobinuria. See **hemoglobinuria.**

toxicity, 1. the degree to which something is poisonous. 2. a condition that results from exposure to a toxin or to toxic amounts of a substance that does not cause adverse effects in smaller amounts.

toxic nodular goiter, an enlarged thyroid gland characterized by numerous discrete nodules and hypersecretion of thyroid hormones, occurring most frequently in elderly individuals. Typical signs of thyrotoxicosis, as nervousness, tremor, weakness, fatigue, weight loss, and irritability, are usually present, but exophthalmia is rare; anorexia is more common than hyperphagia, and cardiac arrhythmia or congestive heart failure may be a predominant manifestation. When clinical findings suggest thyrotoxicosis a therapeutic trial of antithyroid drugs, as propylthiouracil or methimazole, is indicated, but once the diagnosis is established, radioactive iodine is considered the treatment of choice and large doses are usually required.

toxico-, toxo-, a combining form meaning 'pertaining

to poison, poisonous': *toxicodendrol, toxicomucin, toxicosozin.* Also **toxo-.**

toxicologist, a specialist in toxicology.

toxicology, the scientific study of poisons, their detection, their effects, and methods of treatment for conditions they produce. – **toxicologic, toxicological,** *adj.,* **toxicologist,** *n.*

toxic shock syndrome (TSS), a severe acute disease caused by infection with strains of *Staphylococcus aureus,* phage group I, that produces a unique toxin, enterotoxin F. It is most common in menstruating women using high absorbency tampons but has been seen in newborn infants, children, and men.

■ OBSERVATIONS: The onset of the syndrome is characterized by sudden high fever, headache, sore throat with swelling of the mucous membranes, diarrhea, nausea, and erythroderma. Acute renal failure, abnormal liver function, confusion, and refractory hypotension usually follow, and death may occur. It is probable that mild forms of the syndrome are not reported and, therefore, are not diagnosed. There does not appear to be any seasonal or geographic factor in the etiology of the disease, and there is no evidence of contagion among household or sexual contacts of people who have TSS. Bacteremia, or discernible local infection, is absent in most cases. *Staphylococcus aureus* may be cultured from many sites, including the pharynx, nares, and cervix, but the drastic effects of infection are the result of the toxin released from the organism rather than from the infection itself.

■ INTERVENTION: Aggressive volume expansion by the administration of large amounts of intravenous fluid, assisted ventilation, and administration of vasopressors may be necessary in treating severe TSS. Early recognition and active supportive treatment greatly improve the survival rates and decrease both prolonged morbidity and recurrence.

■ NURSING CONSIDERATIONS: The use of highly absorbent tampons is associated with a greater incidence of the disease than the use of regular tampons, but a few cases have occurred in women who have never used tampons. The nurse counsels women to avoid the high absorbency tampons and to report any illness occurring during the menses that is accompanied by nausea, diarrhea, and fever. Recurrence is likely; a mild, undiagnosed episode during a preceding menstrual period is often reported when severe TSS is diagnosed. Women who have had TSS are usually advised to avoid using any kind of tampons for at least several months.

toxin, a poison, usually one produced by or occurring in a plant or microorganism. See also **endotoxin, exotoxin.**

-toxin, a combining form meaning 'poison': *cynotoxin, hypnotoxin, zootoxin.*

toxo-. See **toxico-.**

toxocariasis (tok'soukərai'əsis), infection with the larvae of *Toxocara canis,* the common roundworm of dogs and cats. Ingestion of viable eggs, commonly found in soil, leads to the spread of tiny larvae throughout the body, resulting in respiratory symptoms, enlarged liver, skin rashes, eosinophilia, and delayed ocular lesions. Children who eat dirt are particularly subject to this disease. Specific drug therapy is not very useful; the outcome is usually good without therapy. Regular worming of pets helps prevent infection. Also called **visceral larva migrans.**

toxoid, a toxin that has been treated with chemicals or with heat to decrease its toxic effect but that retains its antigenic power. It is given to produce immunity by stimulating the creation of antibodies. See also **toxin, vaccine.**

Toxoplasma (tok'souplæz'mə), a genus of protozoa with only one known species, *Toxoplasma gondii,* an intracellular parasite of cats and other hosts that causes toxoplasmosis in man.

toxoplasmosis (tok'souplæzmou'sis), a common infection with the protozoan intracellular parasite *Toxoplasma gondii,* characterized in the congenital form by liver and brain involvement with cerebral calcification, convulsions, blindness, microcephaly or hydrocephaly, and mental retardation. The acquired form is characterized by rash, lymphadenopathy, fever, malaise, central nervous system disorders, myocarditis, and pneumonitis.

■ OBSERVATIONS: Cats acquire the organism by eating infected birds and mice. Cysts of the organism are transmitted from cat feces to humans or by human ingestion of inadequately cooked meat containing the cysts. Transplacental transmission occurs only during acute infection of the mother, but the disease is very serious in the fetus and in those with an impaired immune system. Diagnosis is made by demonstrating rising antibody titers or by immunofluorescent antibody tests. Infection confers immunity.

■ INTERVENTION: Combinations of sulfonamides with pyrimethamine are recommended as treatment, possibly reducing the severity of the illness in the fetus.

■ NURSING CONSIDERATIONS: All meat should be heated to at least 140°F throughout to kill this parasite. Pregnant women who are not immune are advised not to handle cats, cat feces, or litter boxes.

TPAL. See **parity.**

TPN, abbreviation for **total parenteral nutrition.**

trabecula carnea (trəbek'yulə), *pl.* **trabeculae carneae.** any one of the irregular bands and bundles of muscle which project from the inner surfaces of the ventricles, except in the arterial cone of the right ventricle. Some of these trabeculae are ridges of muscle along the ventricular walls; others are short projections into the ventricular cavities; still others form the ventricular papillary muscles. Compare **chorda tendinea.** See also **heart, left ventricle, right ventricle.**

trabecula septomarginalis. See **moderator band.**

trace element, an element essential to nutrition or physiological processes, found in such minute quantities that analysis yields a presence of virtually zero amounts.

trace gas, a gas or vapor that escapes into the atmosphere during an anesthetic procedure. Because these substances may have adverse effects on the health of personnel exposed to them, scavenging equipment is often installed in operating rooms to clean the air. See also **gas scavenging system.**

tracer, **1.** See also **radioisotope scan.** a radioactive isotope that is used in diagnostic x-ray techniques to allow a biologic process to be seen. The tracer, which is introduced into the body, binds with a specific substance and is followed with a scanner or fluoroscope as it passes through various organs or systems in the body. Kinds of tracers include **radioactive iodine (^{131}I), radioactive carbon(^{14}C). 2.** a mechanical device which graphically records the outline or movements of an object, or part of the body. **3.** a dissecting instrument which is used to isolate vessels and nerves. — **trace,** *v.*

tracer depot method, (in nuclear medicine) a technique used to determine local skin or muscle blood flow, based on the rate at which a radioactive tracer deposited in a tissue is removed by diffusion into the capillaries and washed out by the local blood supply. If blood flow is diminished or absent, as in dead skin, the deposited tracer does not wash out.

trachea (trei′kiə), a nearly cylindrical tube in the neck, composed of cartilage and membrane, that extends from the larynx at the level of the sixth cervical vertebra to the fifth thoracic vertebra, where it divides into two bronchi. The trachea conveys air to the lungs; it is about 11 cm long and 2 cm wide. The ventral surface of the tube is covered in the neck by the isthmus of the thyroid gland and various other structures, as the sternothyroideus and the sternohyoideus. Dorsally, the trachea is in contact with the esophagus. Also called **windpipe.** See also **primary bronchus.** — **tracheal,** *adj.*

tracheal breath sound, a normal breath sound heard in auscultation of the trachea. Inspiration and expiration are equally loud, the expiratory sound being heard during the greater part of expiration, whereas the inspiratory sound stops abruptly at the height of inspiration, with a pause before the sound of expiration is heard. Compare **vesicular breath sound.**

tracheitis (trei′kiai′tɪs), any inflammatory condition of the trachea. It may be acute or chronic, resulting from infection, allergy, or physical irritation.

trachelo-, a combining form meaning 'pertaining to the neck or a necklike structure': *trachelobregmatic, trachelocystitis, tracheloschisis.*

trachelodynia (træk′əloudɪn′iə). See **cervicodynia.**

tracheo-, a combining form meaning 'pertaining to the trachea': *tracheobronchial, tracheomalacia, tracheorrhaphy.*

tracheobronchial tree (TBT), an anatomical complex that includes the trachea, the bronchi, and the bronchial tubes. It conveys air to and from the lungs and is a primary structure in respiration. See also **bronchial tree.**

tracheobronchitis (trei′kioubroŋkai′tɪs), inflammation of the trachea and bronchi, a common form of respiratory infection.

tracheostomy (trei′kios′təmi), an opening through the neck into the trachea with an indwelling tube inserted. The incision and stoma are created surgically to establish an airway when the pharynx is obstructed by a foreign body, tumor, or edema of the glottis. In an emergency, the operation may be rapidly performed at the site of the accident or incident. In the operating room, local or general anesthesia is usually given. The patient's neck is hyperextended, an incision is made below the Adam's apple, a small opening is made in the fibrous tissues of the trachea, and a tube is slipped in while the hole is held open with a small hemostat like a mosquito forceps. Following tracheostomy the patient's chest is auscultated for breath sounds indicative of pulmonary congestion; mucous membranes and fingertips are observed for cyanosis; humidified oxygen is given via tent or directly into the tracheostomy tube. The patient is reassured that the tube is open and that air can pass through it. The tube is

TRACHEOSTOMY TUBE WITH CUFF

suctioned frequently to keep it free from tracheobronchial secretions using a suction catheter attached to a Y-connector. The catheter is inserted 6 to 8 inches into the tube. The catheter is rotated and intermittent suction applied for no longer than 5 seconds. The patient is taught to cough to move secretions up and out of the bronchi. The nurse holds the tube stable during intense coughing to prevent its displacement. Should the outer tube be expelled, the nurse uses a dilator or hemostat to hold the trachea open until another tube can be inserted. A fluid intake of 3,000 ml per day is recommended. The dressing is changed as necessary, the area is kept dry and clean, and frequent oral care is given. Pen and paper or a magic slate is kept available for communication because the patient cannot speak. Complications of tracheostomy include pneumothorax and mediastinal emphysema. If the procedure was done as an emergency, the tracheostomy is closed once normal breathing is restored. If the tracheostomy is permanent, as with a laryngectomy, the patient is taught self-care. Compare **tracheotomy.**

tracheotomy (trei′kiot′əmi),   an incision made into the trachea through the neck below the larynx, performed to gain access to the airway below a blockage with a foreign body, tumor, or edema of the glottis. The opening may be made as an emergency measure at an accident site or at a hospitalized patient's bedside or in the operating room as part of a tracheostomy. Local or general anesthesia may be used, if available. The patient's neck is hyperextended and an incision is made through the skin below the Adam's apple. A small hole is made in the fibrous tissue of the trachea and the opening is then dilated to allow the intake of air. In an emergency any available instrument may be used as a dilator, even the barrel of a ballpoint pen with the inner portion removed, if only that is available. The patient is brought to the hospital for medical care. If the blockage persists a tracheostomy tube is inserted; if not, the incision is closed once normal respirations are established. After surgery the patient is observed for recurrent respiratory difficulty or cyanosis. Compare **tracheostomy.**

trachoma (trəkou′mə),   a chronic, infectious disease of the eye caused by the bacterium *Chlamydia trachomatis,* characterized initially by inflammation, pain, photophobia, and lacrimation. If untreated, follicles form on the upper eyelids and grow larger until the granulations invade the cornea, eventually causing blindness. Tetracycline, erythromycin, and topical sulfonamides usually provide effective treatment. Scarred eyelids may be surgically repaired. Trachoma is a significant cause of blindness and is endemic to hot, dry, poverty-ridden areas. In the United States, it is found on Indian reservations in the Southwest. Teaching an affected population about the spread of trachoma and having an adequate water supply for washing hands, towels, and handkerchiefs are important factors in eliminating the disease. Also called **Egyptian ophthalmia, granular conjunctivitis.**

tract,   an elongate group of tissues and structures that function together as a pathway, like the digestive tract or the respiratory tract.

90-90 traction,   an orthopedic mechanism, used especially in pediatrics, that combines skeletal traction and suspension with a short leg cast or a splint to immobilize and position the lower extremity in the treatment of a displaced fractured femur. This type of traction is usually unilateral with the opposite leg in Buck's traction or in split Russell traction for immobilization. The pin used in this kind of skeletal traction is inserted into bone in the knee area and attached to a riser running through a pulley on an overhead traction frame to a pulley and weight system fitted over the foot of the bed. The pulley and weight system at the foot of the bed also accommodates additional attachments to the short leg cast or splint of the involved lower limb. Application of 90-90 traction may also incorporate a jacket restraint to help immobilize the patient. A variation of this type of traction is often used with adults in the treatment of low back pain.

traction,   **1.** (in orthopedics) the process of putting a limb, bone, or group of muscles under tension by means of weights and pulleys to align or to immobilize the part or to relieve pressure on it. **2.** the process of pulling a part of the body along, through, or out of its socket or cavity, as axis traction with obstetric forceps in delivering an infant.

traction frame,   an orthopedic apparatus that supports the pulleys, the ropes, and the weights by which traction is applied to various parts of the body or by which various parts of the body are suspended. Traction frames are used in the treatment of bone fractures and dislocations, disease processes of the musculoskeletal system, in the correction of various orthopedic deformities, and in the general immobilization of specific areas of the body. The main components of a traction frame are metal uprights which attach to the bed and support an overhead metal bar. In addition to traction equipment, traction frames are often rigged with trapeze bars which the patient can grasp to help in changing positions and to exercise the muscles of the arms and the trunk. The components of a traction frame are securely clamped together when in use but can be easily disassembled and reassembled. Compare **I.V.-type traction frame, claw-type traction frame, Balkan traction frame.**

trade name,   the registered trademark assigned to a product by its manufacturer. See also **generic name.**

tragus (trei′gəs), *pl.* **tragi** (trei′jai).   a projection of the cartilage of the auricle at the opening of the external auditory meatus.

trained reflex.   See **conditioned response.**

traineeship,   a grant of money allocated to an individual for study in a given field. In nursing, many graduate students have been awarded federal traineeships which provide funds for tuition and living expenses.

training grant,   a grant of money or other resources to provide training in a particular field. Many schools of nursing receive federal or state grants to provide specific educational programs. Funds may be allocated for faculty salaries, student aid, or other expenses.

trait,   **1.** a characteristic mode of behavior or any mannerism or physical feature that distinguishes one individual or culture from another. **2.** any characteristic quality or condition that is genetically determined and inherited as a specific genotype. A trait is expressed in the phenotype as dominant or recessive for the particular characteristic; it is inherited in the genotype as either homozygous dominant, homozygous recessive, or heterozygous in the ratio of 1:2:1. In medicine, trait is used specifically to denote the heterozygous state of a recessive disorder, as the sickle cell trait. See also **dominance, gene, Mendel's laws, recessive.**

Tral, a trade name for an anticholinergic (hexocyclium methylsulfate).

trance, 1. a sleeplike state characterized by the complete or partial suspension of consciousness and loss or diminution of motor activity, as seen in hypnosis, the dissociative form of hysterical neurosis, and various cataleptic and ecstatic states. 2. a dazed or bewildered condition; stupor. 3. a state of detachment from one's immediate surroundings, as in deep concentration or daydreaming. Kinds of trances are **alcoholic trance, death trance, hypnotic trance, hysterical trance, induced trance**.

Trancopal, a trade name for an antianxiety agent (chlormezanone).

Tranmep, a trade name for an antianxiety agent (meprobamate).

tranquilizer, a drug prescribed to calm anxious or agitated people, ideally without decreasing their consciousness. Major tranquilizers, as derivatives of phenothiazine, butyrophenone, and thioxanthene, are used in the treatment of psychoses. Minor tranquilizers prescribed for the treatment of anxiety, irritability, tension, or psychoneurosis include chlordiazepoxide, diazepam, and hydroxyzine. Tranquilizers tend to induce drowsiness and have the potential for causing physical and psychological dependence. See also **antipsychotic.**

trans-, a combining form meaning 'across, through, over': *transabdominal, transferase, transplacental.*

transactional analysis (TA), a form of psychotherapy developed by Eric Berne, based on a theory that three different, coherent, organized egos exist throughout life simultaneously in every person, representing the child, the adult, and the parent. Interactions between people are transactions, originating from a person in one of the ego states, received by another person who may be in a complementary or a crossed ego state. Transactions are motivated by a need for recognition and contact called "strokes." Transactions occur in six kinds of "time structure": withdrawal, rituals, pastimes, games, activities, and intimacy. The way in which a person structures time reflects internal conflicts and patterns adopted to cope with those conflicts. The goal of transactional analysis is to give the adult ego state decision-making power over the child and the parent.

transaminase (trænsæm'ɪneɪs), an enzyme which catalyzes the transfer of an amino group from an alpha-amino acid to an alpha-keto acid, with pyridoxal phosphate and pyridoxamine phosphate acting as coenzymes. Glutamic-oxaloacetic transaminase (GOT), normally present in serum and various tissues, especially in the heart and liver, is released by damaged cells, and, as a result, a high serum level of GOT may be diagnostic in myocardial infarction or hepatic disease. Glutamic-pyruvic transaminase (GPT), a normal constituent of serum and various tissues, especially in the liver, is released by injured tissue and may be present in high concentrations in the sera of patients with acute liver disease. Also called **aminotransferase.**

transcondylar fracture (trænzkon'dɪlər), a fracture that occurs transversally and distal to the epicondyles of any one of the long bones.

trans configuration, trans arrangement, trans position, (in genetics) 1. the presence of the dominant allele of one pair of genes and the recessive allele of another pair on the same chromosome. 2. the presence of at least one mutant gene and one wild-type gene of a pair of pseudoalleles on each chromosome of a homologous pair. Compare **cis configuration.**

transcortical apraxia. See **ideomotor apraxia.**

transcription, (in molecular genetics) the process by which RNA is formed from a DNA template in the process of manufacturing a protein.

transcultural nursing, a field of nursing in which the nurse transcends ethnocentricity and practices nursing in other cultural environments. As current nursing process and theory are not culturally bound and the needs of each person are considered individually, transcultural nursing is potentially a part of all nursing practice.

transduction (trænzdək'shən), (in molecular genetics) a method of genetic recombination by which DNA is transferred from one cell to another by a viral vector. Various bacteriophages transduce genetic material from one species of bacteria to another.

transfection, (in molecular genetics) the process by which a cell is infected with DNA or RNA isolated from a virus or a viral vector. Acute transfection is short-term infection.

transfer DNA (tDNA), (in molecular genetics) DNA transferred from its original source and present in transformed cells.

transference, 1. the shifting of symptoms from one part of the body to another, as occurs in conversion disorder. 2. (in psychiatry) an unconscious defense mechanism whereby feelings and attitudes originally associated with important people and events in one's early life are attributed to others in current interpersonal situations. 3. (in psychoanalysis and psychotherapy) the feelings of a patient for the analyst to whom the patient has attributed or assigned the qualities, attitudes, and feelings of a person or persons significant in his emotional development, usually a figure from his childhood. The phenomenon is used as a tool in understanding the emotional problems of the patient and their origins. See also **countertransference, parataxic distortion.**

transfer factor, a leukocyte extract that transfers delayed hypersensitivity from one person to another. Transfer factor is being studied for its possible use in the treatment of chronic mucocutaneous candidiasis and Wiskott-Aldrich syndrome and as a means of transferring antitumor immunity in patients with various types of cancer.

transferrin (trænzfer′ın), a trace protein present in the blood that is essential in the transport of iron. Its major function is to move iron from the intestine into the blood stream, making it available to the normoblasts of the bone marrow. It may also take part in a slower exchange with ferritin, hemosiderin, and other iron forms in the tissues. See also **hemosiderin, iron transport.**

transfer RNA (tRNA), (in molecular genetics) a kind of RNA that transfers the genetic code from messenger RNA for the production of a specific amino acid. There are at least 20 different kinds of tRNA, each of which is able to combine covalently with a specific amino acid and to bond with at least one messenger RNA nucleotide triplet. Also called **adaptor RNA.**

transformation, (in molecular genetics) the process in which exogenous genes are integrated into chromosomes in a form which is recognized by the replicative and transcriptional apparatus of the host cell. Transformation occurs rarely in most cell populations.

transforming growth factor (TGH), a protein or a group of proteins produced by the cells of a tumor that, when inoculated into a normal cell culture, causes a disorderly and abnormal increase in the number of cells in the culture.

transfusion, the introduction into the blood stream of whole blood or blood components, as plasma, platelets, or packed red cells. Whole blood may be infused into the recipient directly from a donor matched for the ABO blood group and antigenic subgroups, but more frequently the donor's blood is collected and stored by a blood bank. See also **blood transfusion.**

transfusion reaction, a systemic response by the body to the administration of blood incompatible with that of the recipient. The causes include red cell incompatibility, allergic sensitivity to the leukocytes, the platelets, or the plasma protein components of the transfused blood or to the potassium or citrate preservative in the banked blood.

■ OBSERVATIONS: Fever is the most common transfusion reaction; urticaria is a relatively common allergic response. Asthma, vascular collapse, and renal failure occur less commonly. A hemolytic reaction from red cell incompatibility is serious and must be diagnosed and treated promptly. Symptoms begin shortly after beginning the transfusion, before 50 ml have been given, and include a throbbing headache, sudden, deep and severe lumbar

pain, precordial pain, dyspnea, and restlessness. Objective signs include ruddy facial flushing followed by cyanosis and distended neck veins, rapid, thready pulse, diaphoresis, and cold, clammy skin. Profound shock may occur within one hour.

■ INTERVENTION: The administration of antihistamines is usually beneficial in urticaria but offers no benefit for febrile reactions. When a hemolytic reaction is suspected, the transfusion is promptly terminated and the infusion line kept open with a normal solution of intravenous fluid for therapeutic purposes. The remaining bank blood is saved for a repeat type and cross-match against a fresh sample of blood from the recipient. Direct and indirect Coomb's tests are usually ordered to detect hemolytic antibodies, and a sample of urine is examined for free hemoglobin. Immediate treatment may include I.V. mannitol and a solution of 5 per cent dextrose in water to maintain urine flow of more than 100 ml/hr. In the presence of oliguria, the possibility of acute renal failure is evaluated and the patient managed accordingly. Hypovolemia is corrected with saline or plasma expanders but the administration of more whole blood is avoided, if possible.

■ NURSING CONSIDERATIONS: The need for exceptional care to assure that typed and cross-matched blood conforms to compatibility standards is emphasized. The identifying information on the container of blood is always checked against the transfusion record. Questioning the patient about previous transfusions may elicit warning indications of possible adverse reactions. Once the transfusion is started, the patient is watched for objective signs of a transfusion reaction and is questioned for subjective symptomatology. Routine temperature checks are done to detect febrile reactions that can be controlled by antipyretic drugs.

transient ischemic attack (TIA), an episode of cerebrovascular insufficiency, usually owing to a partial occlusion of an artery by an atherosclerotic plaque or an embolism. The symptoms vary with the site and the degree of occlusion. Disturbance of normal vision in one or in both eyes, dizziness, weakness, dysphasia, numbness, or unconsciousness may occur. The attack is usually brief, lasting a few minutes; rarely, symptoms may continue for several hours.

transillumination, 1. the passage of light through a solid or liquid substance. 2. the passage of light through body tissues for the purpose of examining a structure interposed between the observer and the light source. A diaphanoscope is an instrument introduced into a body cavity to transilluminate tissues.

transitional cell carcinoma, a malignant, usually papillary tumor derived from transitional stratified epithelium, occurring most frequently in the bladder, ureter, urethra, or renal pelvis. The majority of tumors in the collecting system of the kidney are of this kind. They have a better prognosis than squamous cell carcinomas in the same site.

transitional dentition. See **mixed dentition.**

transitory mania, a mood disorder characterized by the sudden onset of manic reactions that are of short duration, usually lasting from an hour to a few days. See also **mania.**

translation, (in molecular genetics) the process in which the genetic information carried by nucleotides in messenger RNA directs the amino acid sequence in the synthesis of a specific polypeptide.

translocation, (in genetics) the rearrangement of genetic material within the same chromosome or the transfer of a segment of one chromosome to another nonhomologous one. In simple translocations, one end segment of one chromosome is transferred onto the end of another nonhomologous one, involving a single break in only one of the chromosomes. Translocations in which material from the middle of one chromosome is shifted to the middle of another one are more complex and involve at least three breaks in the participating chromosomes. Such shifting of genetic material can result in serious disorders, as Down's syndrome, which is caused by a 14/21 translocation, and chronic granulocytic leukemia, in which part of the long arm of the 22 chromosome is translocated to the short arm of chromosome 9. Kinds of translocations are **balanced translocation, reciprocal translocation, Robertsonian translocation.**

transmission, the transfer or conveyance of a thing or condition, as a neural impulse, infectious or genetic disease, or a hereditary trait, from one person or place to another. — **transmissible,** *adj.*

transmission electron microscopy. See **electron microscopy.**

transmission scanning electron microscope, an instrument that transmits a highly magnified, well-resolved, three-dimensional image on a television screen, thus combining the advantages of the electron and the scanning electron microscopes. Compare **electron microscope, scanning electron microscope.**

transmission scanning electron microscopy (TSEM), a technique using a transmission scanning electron microscope in which the atomic number of the portion of the sample being scanned is determined and used to modulate a beam of electrons in a cathode ray tube and in the beam scanning the sample. The image produced is clear, three-dimensional, and highly magnified. Compare **electron microscopy, scanning electron microscopy.**

transmitter substance. See **neurotransmitter.**

transneuronal degeneration, degeneration of irreparably damaged nerve cells that may progress proximally or distally to involve neurons more than one synapse removed.

transovarial transmission, the transfer of pathogens to succeeding generations through invasion of the ovary and infection of the egg, as occurs in arthropods, primarily ticks and mites.

transplacental (træn'pləsen'təl), across or through the placenta, specifically in reference to the exchange of nutrients, waste products, and other material between the developing fetus and the mother.

transplant, 1. to transfer an organ or tissue from one person to another or from one body part to another in order to replace a diseased structure or to restore function. Skin and kidneys are the most frequently transplanted structures; others include cartilage, bone, corneal tissue, portions of blood vessels and tendons, and recently but infrequently, hearts and livers. Preferred donors are identical twins or persons having the same blood type and immunologic characteristics. Success of the transplant depends upon overcoming the rejection of the donor tissue by the immune system of the recipient. Under local or general anesthesia, the recipient site is prepared and the donor structure grafted in place; its oxygenation and blood supply are preserved during the procedure until the circulation can be restored at the new site. After surgery, circulation in the area is observed for signs of impairment. Antilymphocytic serum may be given, with steroids, to suppress the production of antibodies to the foreign tissue proteins. Signs of rejection reaction include fever, pain, and loss of function, usually occuring in the first 4 to 10 days following transplantation. An abcess may form if the reaction is not subdued promptly. The grafted structure may require several weeks to become established. Late rejection may occur several months or even a year later. 2. any tissue or organ that is transplanted. 3. of or pertaining to a tissue or organ that is transplanted or to a recipient of a donated tissue or organ or to a phenomenon associated with the procedure. Also called **graft.** — **transplantation,** *n.*

transposable element, (in molecular genetics) a DNA fragment or segment that can move or be moved from one site in the genome to another.

transposase (trænz'pəzeis), (in molecular genetics) an enzyme involved in the movement of a DNA fragment or segment from one site in the genome to another.

transposition, 1. an abnormality occuring during embryonic development in which a part of the body normally on the left is found on the right or vice versa. 2. the shifting of genetic material from one chromosome to another at some point in the reproductive process, often resulting in a congenital anomaly. — **transpose,** *v.*

transposition of the great vessels, a congenital cardiac anomaly in which the pulmonary artery arises from the left ventricle and the aorta from the right ventricle so that there is no communication between the systemic and pulmonary circulations. Life is impossible without associated cardiac defects, as septal defects or a patent ductus arteriosus, which enable the mixing of oxygenated and unoxygenated blood. The severity of the condition depends on the type and size of the associated defect. The primary symptoms are cyanosis and hypoxia, especially in infants with small septal defects, although cardiomegaly is usually evident a few weeks after birth. Signs of congestive heart failure develop rapidly, especially in those infants with large ventricular septal defects. Definitive diagnosis is based on cardiac catheterization. Surgical correction of the defect is postponed, if possible, until after six months of age when the infant can better tolerate the procedure. Immediate palliative surgical procedures, as balloon septostomy, may be performed to decrease pulmonary vascular resistance and prevent congestive heart failure. See also **congenital cardiac anomaly.**

transposon, a gene or a group of genes that are mobile and, like plasmids, act to transfer genetic instructions from one place to another. Transposons travel piggyback from virus to virus on bacteriophages. The genetic material is incorporated into the virus when the virus infects a bacterial cell. As the bacteria replicates itself, it also copies the genetic instructions brought by the transposon.

transtentorial herniation (trænz'tentɔr'iəl), a bulge of brain tissue out of the cranium through the tentorial notch, caused by increased intracranial pressure. See also **tentorial herniation.**

transthermia (trænzfhər'miə). See **thermopenetration.**

transudate (træn'sudeit'), a fluid passed through a membrane or squeezed through a tissue or into the space between the cells of a tissue. It is thin and watery and contains few blood cells or other large proteins. See also **edema.**

transudative ascites (trænsyu'dətıv), an abnormal accumulation in the peritoneal cavity of a fluid that characteristically contains scant amounts of protein and cells. Ascitic fluids with protein counts of less than 2.5 gm per ml are considered to be transudates. Transudative ascites is indicative of cirrhosis or congestive heart failure rather than infection, inflammation, or the presence of a tumor.

transurethral (trænz'yuri'fhrəl), through the urethra, as in transurethral prostatectomy. Compare **suprapubic.**

transverse, at right angles to the long axis of any common part, as the planes that cut the long axis of the body into upper and lower portions and are at right angles to the sagittal and frontal planes.

transverse colon, the segment of the colon that extends from the end of the ascending colon at the hepatic flexure on the right side across the midabdomen to the beginning of the descending colon at the splenic flexure on the left side.

transverse fissure, a fissure dividing the dorsal surface of the diencephalon and the ventral surface of the cerebral hemisphere. Also called **fissure of Bichat.**

transverse fracture, a fracture that occurs at right angles to the longitudinal axis of the bone involved.

transverse lie, abnormal presentation of a fetus in which the long axis of the baby's body is horizontal to the long axis of the mother's body; unless the baby turns spontaneously or is turned by means of external or internal version, vaginal delivery is impossible.

transverse ligament of the atlas, a thick, strong ligament stretched across the ring of the atlas, holding the dens against the anterior arch. As it crosses the dens it arches cranially and caudally, forming the cruciate ligament of the atlas. The transverse ligament divides the circular opening of the atlas into posterior and anterior parts. The posterior part transmits the spinal cord and its membranes; the anterior part contains the dens.

transverse mesocolon (mez'ɔukou'lən), a broad fold of the peritoneum connecting the transverse colon to the dorsal wall of the abdomen. It is continuous with the greater omentum along the ventral surface of the transverse colon and contains between its layers the vessels which supply the transverse colon. Its two layers diverge along the anterior border of the pancreas. Compare **mesentery proper, sigmoid mesocolon.**

transverse palatine suture, the line of junction between the processes of the maxilla and the horizontal portions of the palatine bones that form the hard palate.

transverse plane, any one of the planes that cut across the body perpendicular to the sagittal and the frontal planes, dividing the body into caudal and cranial portions. Compare **frontal plane, median plane, sagittal plane.**

transverse sinus, one of a pair of large venous channels in the posterior superior group of sinuses serving the dura mater. Each transverse sinus starts at the internal occipital protuberance and one, usually the right, is a direct continuation of the superior sagittal sinus, the other a continuation of the straight sinus. Each tranverse sinus curves slightly to the base of the petrous portion of the temporal bone and within the margin of the tentorium. It leaves the tentorium and becomes the sigmoid sinus, which curves inferiorly and medially to the jugular foramen and ends in the internal jugular vein. The transverse sinuses are often of different size, the larger one usually formed by the superior sagittal sinus. Each transverse sinus receives the blood from the superior petrosal sinus at the base of the temporal bone; each anastomoses with the veins of the pericranium through the mastoid and the condyloid emissary veins; and each receives some of the inferior cerebral and the inferior cerebellar veins and some of the veins from the diploe. Compare **confluence of the sinuses, inferior sagittal sinus, occipital sinus, straight sinus, superior sagittal sinus.**

transversus abdominis, one of a pair of transverse abdominal muscles that are the anterolateral muscles of the abdomen, lying immediately under the obliquus internus abdominis. Arising from the inguinal ligament, the iliac crest, the thoracolumbar fascia, and the last six ribs, it inserts into the linea alba. It is innervated by branches of the seventh through the twelfth intercostal nerves and by the iliohypogastric and the ilioinguinal nerves. It serves to constrict the abdomen and, by compressing the contents, to assist in micturition, defecation, emesis, parturition, and forced expiration. Compare **obliquus externus abdominis, obliquus internus abdominis, pyramidalis, rectus abdominis.**

Tranxene, a trade name for a tranquilizer (chlorazepate dipotassium).

tranylcypromine sulfate (træn′əlsɪp′rəmin), a monoamine oxidase inhibitor that acts as an antidepressant.

■ INDICATIONS: It is prescribed in the treatment of mental depression.

■ CONTRAINDICATIONS: Heart disease, paranoid schizophrenia, liver dysfunction, alcoholism, pheochromocytoma, or known hypersensitivity to this drug prohibits its use. It is not given to children under 16 years of age.

■ ADVERSE EFFECTS: Among the most serious adverse reactions are severe hypertensive episodes which can be precipitated by ingestion of foods rich in tyramine or by concurrent administration of many sympathomimetic drugs. Common side effects include headache, vertigo, dry mouth, blurred vision, and orthostatic hypertension.

trapezium (trəpi′ziəm), *pl.* **trapeziums, trapezia.** a carpal bone in the distal row of carpal bones. It has a deep groove on the palmar surface between the scaphoid and first metacarpal bones. The lateral surface is broad and rough for the attachment of ligaments. A deep groove in its palmar surface transmits the tendon of the flexor carpi radialis. The opponens pollicis and the abductor brevis originate on the palmar surface. The trapezium articulates with the scaphoid proximally, the first metacarpal distally, and the trapezoideum and the second metacarpal medially. Also called **greater multangular, os trapezium.**

trapezius (trəpi′ziəs), a large flat triangular muscle of the shoulder and upper back. It arises from the occipital bone, the ligamentum nuchae and the spinous processes of the seventh cervical and all the thoracic vertebrae. It is innervated by the third and fourth cervical nerves and by the spinal accessory nerve. It acts to rotate the scapula, raise the shoulder, and abduct and flex the arm.

trapezoid bone, the smallest carpal bone, located in the distal row of carpal bones between the trapezium and the capitate. It resembles a wedge with the broad end at the dorsal surface, the narrow end at the palmar surface. The trapezoid articulates with the scaphoid proximally, the second metacarpal distally, the trapezium laterally, and the capitate medially. Also called **lesser multangular bone, os trapezoideum.**

Trasentine Hydrochloride, a trade name for an anti-

cholinergic and smooth muscle relaxant (adiphenine hydrochloride).

trauma (trau′mə), **1.** physical injury caused by violent or disruptive action, or by the introduction into the body of a toxic substance. **2.** psychic injury resulting from a severe emotional shock. — **traumatic,** *adj.,* **traumatize,** *v.*

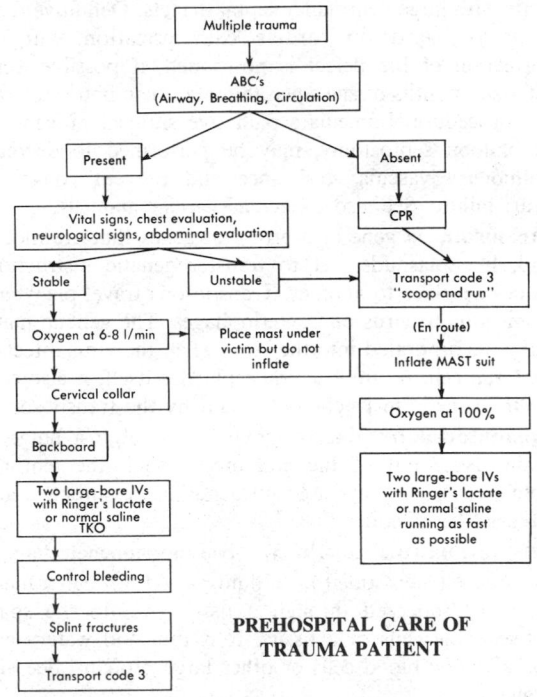

PREHOSPITAL CARE OF TRAUMA PATIENT

-trauma, a combining form meaning a 'wound or injury, psychic or physical': *arthrotrauma, barotrauma, neurotrauma.*

traumatic anesthesia, a total lack of normal sensation in a part of the body, resulting from injury, destruction of nerves, or interruption of nerve pathways. See also **tactile anesthesia.**

traumatic delirium, delirium following severe head injury, characterized by alertness and conciousness with disorientation, confabulation, and amnesia apparent. See also **delirium.**

traumatic fever, an elevation in body temperature secondary to mechanical trauma, particularly a crushing injury. Such fevers may last one or two days. The increased body temperature may help provide resistance to subsequent infection, and increased wound temperature may accelerate local healing.

traumatic idiocy, *Obsolete.* severe mental retardation resulting from injury to the brain received at birth, during infancy, or in early childhood.

traumatic myositis, inflammation of the muscles resulting from a wound or other trauma.

traumatic neuroma, a tangled mass of nerve elements and fibrous tissue produced by the proliferation of Schwann cells and fibroblasts following severe injury to a nerve. A kind of traumatic neuroma is **amputation neuroma.**

traumato-, a combining form meaning 'pertaining to trauma, or to an injury or wound': *traumatogenic, traumatopnea, traumatopyra.*

traumatology (trɔ'mətol'əji), **1.** the study of wounds and injuries. **2.** a surgical specialty dealing with the treatment of wounds, injuries, and resulting disabilities. — **traumatologic, traumatological,** *adj.*

traumatopathy (trɔ'mətop'əthi), a pathologic condition resulting from a wound or injury. — **traumatopathic,** *adj.*

traumatophilia (trɔ'mətoufil'iə, trɔ'mətoufil'yə), a psychological state in which the individual derives unconscious pleasure from injuries and surgical operations. — **traumatophiliac,** *n.,* **traumatophilic,** *adj.*

traumatopnea (trɔ'mətop'niə), partial asphyxia with collapse of the patient, caused by a penetrating thoracic wound permitting air to enter the pleural space and compress the lungs.

traumatopyra (trɔ'mətoupai'rə), an elevated temperature resulting from a wound or injury.

traumatotherapy (trɔ'mətouther'əpi), the medical, surgical, and psychological treatment of wounds, injuries, and disabilities resulting from trauma. — **traumatotherapeutic,** *adj.*

traumatropism (trɔmæt'rəpɪz'əm), the tendency of damaged tissue to attract microorganisms and to promote their growth, frequently causing infections following injuries, especially burns.

travail (trəveil'), **1.** physical or mental exertion, especially when distressful. **2.** (in obstetrics) the effort of labor and childbirth.

Travase, a trade name for a protcolytic enzyme (sutilains).

traveler's diarrhea, any of several diarrheal disorders commonly seen in people visiting regions of the world other than their own. Some strains of *Escherichia coli,* which produce a powerful exotoxin, are the common cause. Other etiologic organisms include *Giardia lamblia* and species of *Salmonella* and *Shigella.* Symptoms last for a few days and include abdominal cramps, nausea, vomiting, slight fever, and watery stools. Relapse is rare. Treatment depends on identification of the cause and includes rehydration with beverages containing electrolytes. Preventive measures include using pure or boiled water for drinking and brushing the teeth and eating only fruits and vegetables that have a skin or peel. Also called **turista.**

TRBF, abbreviation for **total renal blood flow.**

Treacher Collins' syndrome (tri'ĉhərkol'ɪnz), an inherited disorder, characterized by mandibulofacial dysostosis. See also **Pierre Robin syndrome.**

treatment, 1. the care and management of a patient in order to combat, ameliorate, or prevent a disease, disorder, or injury. **2.** a method of combating, ameliorating, or preventing a disease, disorder, or injury. Active or curative treatment is designed to cure; palliative treatment is directed to relieve pain and distress; prophylactic treatment is for the prevention of a disease or disorder; causal treatment focuses on the etiology of a disorder; conservative treatment avoids radical measures and procedures; empiric treatment employs methods shown to be beneficial by experience; rational treatment is based on a knowledge of a disease process and the action of the measures used. Treatment may bc pharmacological, using drugs; surgical, involving operative procedures; or supportive, building the patient's strength. It may be specific for the disorder, or symptomatic to relieve symptoms without effecting a cure.

treatment room, a room in a patient-care unit, usually in a hospital, in which various treatments or procedures requiring special equipment are performed, as removing sutures, draining a hematoma, packing a wound, or performing an examination.

Trecator-SC, a trade name for a tuberculostatic (ethionamide).

Trechona (trɪkon'ə), a genus of spiders, family Dipluridae, the bite of which is toxic and irritating to humans.

tree, (in anatomy) an anatomical structure with branches that spread out like those of a tree, as the bronchial trcc and the tracheobronchial tree.

-trema, 1. a combining form meaning a 'hole, orifice, opening': *gonotrema, helicotrema, peritrema.* **2.** a combining form meaning 'creatures possessing an opening': *Eurytrema, Monotrema, Troglotrema.*

trematode (trem'ətoud), any species of flatworm of the class Trematoda, some of which are parasitic to humans, infecting the liver, the lungs, and the intestines. Kinds of trematodes include the organisms causing **clonorchiasis, fascioliasis, paragonimiasis, schistosomiasis.** Also called **fluke.**

Tremin, a trade name for an anticholinergic (trihexyphenidyl hydrochloride).

tremor, rhythmic, purposeless, quivering movements resulting from the involuntary alternating contraction and relaxation of opposing groups of skeletal muscles, occurring in some elderly individuals, in certain families, and in patients with various neurodegenerative disorders. Senile tremor is characterized by fine, quick movements, especially of the hands, rhythmic head nodding, and increased trembling during purposeful movements. Familial tremor, which may be hereditary, and the tremor occurring in multiple sclerosis also increase during voluntary movement and may be intensified by anxiety, excitement, and self-consciousness. The tremors of Graves' disease, alcoholism, mercury poisoning, and other toxicoses are usually less rhythmic, and the tremor in lead poisoning often affects the lips. The fine, quick, continuous tremor present in Parkinson's disease sometimes disappears during purposeful movements. Kinds of tremors are **continuous tremor, intention tremor.**

trench fever, a self-limited infection, caused by *Rochalimaea quintana,* a rickettsial organism transmitted by body lice, characterized by weakness, fever, rash, and leg pains. It was common during World War I but is now rare. Also called **quintana fever.**

trench mouth, an infection of the mouth and gums characterized by ulcerative, destructive lesions of the mucous membrane. It usually occurs in debilitated, malnourished people. The fusiform bacillus and the spirochete found in the ulcers are not the cause; they represent secondary infection.

Trendelenburg gait (trendel'ənbərg), an abnormal gait associated with a weakness of the gluteus medius. The Trendelenburg gait is characterized by the dropping of the pelvis on the unaffected side of the body at the moment of heelstrike on the affected side. In this deviation, the pelvic drop during the walking cycle lasts until heelstrike on the unaffected side and is accompanied by an apparent lateral protrusion of the affected hip. The patient with a Trendelenburg gait also shortens the step on the unaffected side and displays a lateral deviation of the entire trunk and the affected side during the stance phase of the affected lower limb. The Trandelenburg gait is one of the more common gait deviations. Also called **uncompensated gluteal gait.** Compare **compensated gluteal gait.**

Trendelenburg position, a position in which the head is low and the body and legs are on an inclined plane. It is sometimes used in pelvic surgery to displace the abdominal organs upward, out of the pelvis, or to increase the flow of blood to the brain in hypotension and shock.

Trendelenburg's operation, the ligation of varicose veins whose valves are ineffective, performed to remove weakened portions of veins and pockets in which thrombi might lodge. With the patient under general anesthesia the saphenous vein is ligated at the groin, where it joins the femoral vein. A wire device, called a stripper, is threaded through the lumen of the vein from groin to ankle; the wire and the vein are then pulled from the groin incision. Incisions may be made at several sites along the leg. Bleeding is minimal. After surgery a pressure bandage is applied from foot to thigh and the foot of the bed is elevated 6 to 9 inches raising the legs above the level of the heart. The patient is encouraged to walk, but discouraged from standing or sitting. Cyanosis of the toes indicates possible constriction by the dressings. Elastic bandages remain in place until the seventh day after sur-

gery when the sutures are usually removed. Possible complications include hemorrhage, infection, nerve damage, and thrombosis.

Trendelenburg test, a simple test for incompetent valves in a person who has varicose veins. The person lies down and elevates the leg to empty the vein, then stands, and the vein is observed as it fills. If the valves are incompetent, the vein fills from above; if the valves are normal they do not allow back-flow of blood, and the vein fills from below.

trephine (trɪfāin', trɪfin'), a circular, sawlike instrument used in removing pieces of bone or tissue, usually from the skull. Also called **trepan.**

Treponema (trep'əni'mə), a genus of spirochetes, including some pathogenic to man, as the organisms causing bejel, pinta, syphilis, and yaws.

Treponema pallidum, an actively motile, slender spirochetal organism that causes syphilis.

treponematosis (trep'əni'mətou'sɪs), pl. **treponematoses.** any disease caused by spirochetes of the genus *Treponema.* All of these infections are effectively treated with penicillin; often one dose, given intramuscularly, results in cure. Kinds of treponematoses are **bejel, pinta, syphilis, yaws.**

-tresia, a combining form meaning 'perforation': *atresia, proctotresia, sphenotresia.*

Trest, a trade name for an anticholinergic smooth muscle relaxant (methixene hydrochloride).

tretinoin, a keratolytic.

■ INDICATION: It is prescribed in the treatment of acne vulgaris.

■ CONTRAINDICATION: Known hypersensitivity to this drug prohibits its use.

■ ADVERSE EFFECTS: Among the more serious adverse reactions are red, edematous, blistered, or crusted skin.

TRF, abbreviation for **thyrotropin releasing factor.**

tri-, a combining form meaning 'three or thrice': *triage, tribrachia, tridermoma.*

triacetin (traiæs'ɪtɪn), an antifungal.

■ INDICATIONS: It is prescribed in the treatment of superficial fungus infections of the skin, including athlete's foot.

■ CONTRAINDICATIONS: There are no known contraindications.

■ ADVERSE EFFECTS: There are no known adverse effects.

triacetyloleandomycin. See **troleandomycin.**

triage (triaẑh'), 1. (in military medicine) a classification of casualties of war and other disasters according to the gravity of injuries, urgency of treatment, and place for treatment. 2. a process in which a group of patients is sorted according to their need for care. The kind of illness or injury, the severity of the problem, and the facilities available govern the process. 3. (in disaster medicine) a process in which a large group of patients is sorted in order that care be concentrated on those who are likely to survive.

Triage rating systems

Five-tier system (used in military triage)
  Dead or will die
  Life-threatening—readily correctable
  Urgent—must be treated within 1 to 2 hours
  Delayed—noncritical or ambulatory
  No injury—no treatment necessary
Four-tier system
  Immediate—seriously injured, reasonable chance of survival
  Delayed—can wait or care after simple first aid
  Expectant—extremely critical, moribund
  Minimal—no impairment of function, can either treat self or
    be treated by a nonprofessional
Three-tier system
  Life-threatening—readily correctable
  Urgent—must be treated within 1 to 2 hours
  Delayed—no injury, noncritical, or ambulatory
Two-tier system
  Immediate versus delayed
    Immediate—life-threatening injuries that are readily cor-
      rectable on scene and those that are urgent
    Delayed—no injury, noncritical injuries, ambulatory
      victims, moribund, and dead

---

trial forceps, an obstetric operation consisting of an attempt to deliver an infant with obstetric forceps. The forceps are applied to the baby's head and moderate traction is applied. The delivery is completed only if the trial indicates that delivery can be accomplished safely. The procedure is abandoned if proper application of the forceps or rotation of the baby's head is not possible or if the trial indicates that completion of the delivery with forceps will require inordinately heavy traction likely to be more traumatic to mother or baby than Caesarean section. Trial forceps is usually performed with a double setup so that Caesarean section can be carried out immediately if necessary. Compare **failed forceps.** See also **double setup.**

triamcinolone (trai'æmsɪn'əloun), a glucocorticoid.
■ INDICATIONS: It is prescribed as an anti-inflammatory agent.
■ CONTRAINDICATIONS: Fungal infections or known hypersensitivity to this drug prohibits its systemic use. Viral or fungal infections of the skin, impaired circulation, or known hypersensitivity to this drug prohibits its topical use.
■ ADVERSE EFFECTS: Among the more serious adverse reactions to the systemic administration of the drug are gastrointestinal, endocrine, neurologic, fluid, and electrolyte disturbances. A variety of skin reactions may occur from topical administration of this drug.

triamterene (traiæm'tərin), a potassium-sparing diuretic.
■ INDICATIONS: It is usually prescribed alone or with another diuretic in the treatment of edema, hypertension, and congestive heart failure.
■ CONTRAINDICATIONS: Anuria, severe liver or kidney dysfunction, hyperkalemia, or known hypersensitivity to this drug prohibits its use.
■ ADVERSE EFFECTS: Among the most serious adverse reactions are electrolyte disturbances, particularly hyperkalemia. Gastrointestinal disturbances also may occur.

triangular bandage, a square of cloth folded or cut into the shape of a triangle. It may be used as a sling, a cover, or a thick pad to control bleeding.

triangular bone, the pyramidal carpal bone in the proximal row on the ulnar side of the wrist. It articulates with the lunate bone laterally, the pisiform anteriorly, the hamate distally, and with the triangular articular disc which separates it from the lower end of the ulna. Also called **cuneiform bone, os triquetrum.**

Triavil, a trade name for a central nervous system fixed-combination drug containing a phenothiazine tranquilizer (perphenazine) and a tricyclic antidepressant (amitriptyline hydrochloride).

-tribe, a combining form meaning a 'surgical instrument used to crush a body part': *cephalotribe, sphenotribe, vasotribe.*

tribromoethyl alcohol (traibrou'mouefh'ɪl). See **tribromoethanol.**

TRIC, acronym for trachoma inclusion conjunctivitis agent, which refers to *Chlamydia trachomatis,* the organism that causes both inclusion conjunctivitis and trachoma. See also *Chlamydia.*

tricarboxylic acid cycle (trai'karboksɪl'ɪk). See **Kreb's citric acid cycle.**

triceps. See **triceps brachii.**

triceps brachii, a large muscle that extends the entire length of the dorsal surface of the humerus. Proximally, it has a long head, a lateral head, and a medial head. The long head arises in a flattened tendon originating on the scapula; the lateral head arises from the posterior surface of the humerus, the lateral border of the humerus, and the lateral intermuscular septum; the medial head arises from the posterior body of the humerus, the medial body of the humerus, and the whole length of the medial intermuscular septum. The three portions of the muscle converge in a long tendon and insert in the posterior aspect of the olecranon. The triceps brachii is innervated by branches of the radial nerve, contains fibers from the seventh and the eighth cervical nerves, and functions to extend the forearm and to adduct the arm. Also called **triceps, triceps extensor cubiti.** Compare **biceps brachii.**

triceps extensor cubiti. See **triceps brachii.**

triceps jerk. See **triceps reflex.**

triceps reflex, a deep tendon reflex elicited by tapping sharply the triceps tendon proximal to the elbow with the forearm in a relaxed position. The response is a definite extension movement of the forearm. The reflex is accentuated by lesions of the pyramidal tract above the level of the seventh or eighth vertebra. Also called **triceps jerk.** See also **deep tendon reflex.**

triceps surae limp, an abnormal action in the walking or gait cycle, associated with a deficiency in the elevating and the propulsive factors on the affected side of the body, especially a deficiency of the triceps surae. Such a deficiency prevents the triceps surae from raising the pelvis and carrying it forward during the walking cycle. The pelvis consequently sags below its normal level and lags behind in the walking movement.

-trichia, **1.** a combining form meaning a 'pathological condition of the hair': *leukotrichia, melanotrichia, sclerotrichia.* **2.** a combining form meaning a '(specified) hairiness': *glossotrichia, polytrichia.* Also **-trichosis.**

trichiasis (trɪkaɪ′əsɪs), an abnormal inversion of the eyelashes that irritates the eyeball. It usually follows infection or inflammation. Compare **ectropion.**

trichinosis (trɪk′ɪnou′sɪs), infestation with the parasitic roundworm *Trichinella spiralis,* transmitted by eating raw or undercooked pork or bearmeat. Early symptoms of infection include abdominal pain, nausea, fever, and diarrhea; later, muscle pain, tenderness, fatigue, and eosinophilia are observed. Light infections may be asymptomatic. Also called **trichinellosis, trichiniasis.**

■ OBSERVATIONS: Encysted larvae in improperly cooked pork mature in the intestines of the host, with mature worms depositing their larvae in the intestinal wall. The larvae penetrate the intestinal mucosa and move to other parts of the body through the blood and lymphatic systems, ultimately invading skeletal muscles, especially the diaphragm and the chest muscles, where they encyst. Larval penetration of the brain or the heart may result in death. Serologic tests, skin sensitivity tests, and microscopic examination of specimens of infested muscle obtained by a biopsy often contribute to the diagnosis.

■ INTERVENTION: There is no specific treatment. Analgesics, thiabendazole, and corticosteroids may relieve symptoms. Bed rest is recommended to prevent relapse and possible death. After two or three months, the organisms are completely encysted and cause no further symptoms.

■ NURSING CONSIDERATIONS: Prevention requires cooking pork or wild game at 350° F for 35 minutes a pound. Freezing at 10° F for 20 days also kills the larvae. Pork or pork products should never be eaten raw, and even smoked or salted meat may still harbor viable larvae. Routine inspection of carcasses for trichinella organisms is not performed in the United States, where the disease is on the decline.

trichlormethiazide (traɪ′klɔrməfhaɪ′əzaɪd), a thiazide diuretic and antihypertensive.

■ INDICATIONS: It is prescribed in the treatment of hypertension and edema.

■ CONTRAINDICATIONS: Anuria or known hypersensitivity to this drug, to thiazide medication, or to sulfonamide derivatives prohibits its use.

■ ADVERSE EFFECTS: Among the more serious adverse effects are hypokalemia, hyperglycemia, hyperuricemia, and various hypersensitivity reactions.

trichloroethylene (traɪklɔr′ouefh′ɪlin), a general anesthetic, administered by mask with N_2O, for dentistry, minor surgery, and the first stages of labor. It is too cardiotoxic for deep anesthesia; even in light planes of anesthesia, arrhythmias may occur but may be reversed by administering oxygen and discontinuing the anesthesia. Trichloroethylene must not be given by rebreathing circuits using soda lime, as highly toxic gases may result. Its safety for use in early pregnancy has not been documented. It is contraindicated in severe cardiac disease of any kind, eclampsia or preeclampsia, and should not be combined with epinephrine.

tricho-, a combining form meaning 'pertaining to hair': *trichobezoar, trichomycosis, trichorrhea.*

trichobasalioma hyalinicum (trɪk′oubeisæl′iou′mə). See **cylindroma** def. 2.

trichoepithelioma (trɪk′ouep′ɪthi′liou′mə), *pl.* **trichoepitheliomas, trichoepitheliomata.** a benign cutaneous nodule derived from the basal cells of the follicles of the fine body hair of the fetus. Trichoepithelioma is an inherited condition and usually occurs as multiple growths. Also called **acanthoma adenoides cysticum, epithelioma adenoides cysticum.**

trichoid (trɪk′oid), resembling a hair.

trichologia (trɪk′əlou′jiə), an abnormal condition in which a person pulls out his own hair, usually seen only in delirium.

trichomonacide, an agent destructive to *Trichomonas vaginalis,* a parasitic protozoan flagellate that causes a refractory type of vaginitis, cystitis, and urethritis. Metronidazole is used in the treatment of women with trichomoniasis and their asymptomatic partners. – **trichomonacidal,** *adj.*

Trichomonas vaginalis (trɪk′əmon′əs), a motile protozoan parasite that causes vaginitis with a copious malodorous discharge and pruritus. See also **trichomoniasis.**

trichomoniasis (trɪk′əmənaɪ′əsɪs), a vaginal infection caused by the protozoan *Trichomonas vaginalis,* characterized by itching, burning, and frothy, pale yellow-to-green, malodorous vaginal discharge. With chronic infection all symptoms may disappear, although the organisms are still present. In the male, infection is usually asymptomatic but may be evidenced by a persistent or recurrent urethritis. Infection is transmitted by sexual intercourse, rarely by moist washcloths or, in newborns, by passage through the birth canal. Diagnosis is by microscopic examination of fresh vaginal secretions. Treatment is by oral metronidazole. Reinfection is common if sexual partners are not treated simultaneously.

trichophytic granuloma. See **Majocchi's granuloma.**

Trichophyton (trɪkof′ɪton), a genus of fungi that infects skin, hair, and nails. See also **dermatomycosis, dermatophyte.**

-trichosis. See **-trichia.**

trichostrongyliasis (trɪk′oustron′jəlaɪ′əsɪs), infestation with *Trichostrongylus,* a genus of nematode worm. Also called **trichostrongylosis.** See also **Nematode.**

Trichostrongylus (trɪk′oustron′jɪləs), a genus of roundworm, some species of which are parasitic to man, as *Trichostrongylus orientalis.* See also **trichostrongyliasis.**

trichotillomania (trɪk′outɪl′oumeɪ′niə), **trichomania** (trɪk′əmeɪ′niə), a morbid impulse or desire to pull out one's hair, frequently seen in cases of severe mental retardation and delirium. Also called **hair pulling.** See also **trichologia.** – **trichotillomanic, trichomanic,** *adj.*

trichuriasis (trɪk′yuraɪ′əsɪs), **trichiuriasis** (trɪk′iyuraɪ′əsɪs), infestation with the roundworm *Trichuris trichiura.* The condition is usually asymptomatic but heavy infestation may cause nausea, abdominal pain, diarrhea, and, occasionally, anemia and rectal prolapse. It is common in tropical areas with poor sanitation. Eggs are passed in feces. Contamination of the hands, food, and water results in ingestion of the eggs which hatch in the intestines, where the adult worms embed two thirds of their length in the mucosa. The worms may live 15 to 20 years. Treatment is with mebendazole, prevention includes proper disposal of feces and good personal hygiene.

Trichuris (trɪkyur′ɪs), a genus of parasitic roundworms of which the species *Trichuris trichiura* infects the intestinal tract. Adult worms, which are 30 to 50 mm long, resemble a whip, with a threadlike anterior and a thicker posterior. Also called **whipworm.** See also **trichuriasis.**

triclofos sodium, a sedative-hypnotic.

■ INDICATIONS: It is prescribed to treat insomnia in adults, to calm children, and to induce sleep for electroencephalography.

■ CONTRAINDICATIONS: Marked liver or kidney damage or known hypersensitivity to this drug or to chloral hydrate prohibits its use. It is not given to women in labor or to neonates.

■ ADVERSE EFFECTS: Among the most serious adverse reactions are development of drug dependence, gastrointestinal disturbances, and drug hangover.

Triclos, a trade name for a sedative-hypnotic (triclofos sodium).

Tricofuron, a trade name for a vaginal fixed-combination drug containing the antimicrobials furazolidone and nifuroxime, prescribed topically.

tricrotic pulse (traɪkrot′ɪk), an abnormal pulse that has three peaks of elevation on a sphygmogram, representing the pressure wave from the heart in systole followed by two pressure waves in diastole.

tricuspid (traɪkəs′pɪd), **1.** of or pertaining to three points or cusps. **2.** of or pertaining to the tricuspid valve of the heart.

tricuspid atresia, a congenital cardiac anomaly characterized by the absence of the tricuspid valve so that there is no opening between the right atrium and right ventricle. Other cardiac defects, as atrial and ventricular septal defects, are usually present, allowing some shunting of blood into the lungs. Clinical manifestations include severe cyanosis, dyspnea, anoxia, and signs of right-sided heart failure. Definitive diagnosis is made by cardiac catheterization, although radiographic studies usually reveal a small, underdeveloped right ventricle and large atria, giving the heart a round shape, and decreased pulmonary vascularity. Immediate palliative treatment includes pulmonary-to-artery anastomoses to increase blood flow to the lungs and atrial septostomy if the atrial septal defect is small. Total corrective surgery has been successful in a limited number of older children. See also **congenital cardiac anomaly.**

tricuspid stenosis. See **valvular heart disease.**

tricuspid valve, a valve with three main cusps situated between the right atrium and the right ventricle of the heart. The cusps of the tricuspid valve include the ventral, dorsal, and medial cusps. The ventral cusp is the largest, the posterior cusp the smallest. The cusps are composed of strong fibrous tissue and are anchored to the papillary muscles of the right ventricle by several tendons. As the right and the left ventricles relax during the diastyle phase of the heartbeat, the tricuspid valve opens, allowing blood to flow into the ventricle. In the systole phase of the heartbeat both blood-filled ventricles contract, pumping out their contents, while the tricuspid and mitral valves close to prevent any backflow. Also called **right atrioventricular valve.** Compare **mitral valve, semilunar valve.** See also **cuspid valve, heart valve.**

tricyclic antidepressant. See **antidepressant.**

tricyclic compound, a chemical substance containing three rings in the molecular structure, especially a tricyclic antidepressant drug, as imipramine, amitriptyline, doxepin, and nortriptyline, used in the treatment of reactive or endogenous depression. These drugs also have anticonvulsant, antihistaminic, anticholinergic, hypotensive, and sedative effects. See also **antidepressant.**

Tridesilon, a trade name for a glucocorticoid (desonide).

tridihexethyl chloride, an anticholinergic.

■ INDICATION: It is prescribed in the treatment of gastrointestinal muscle spasm.

■ CONTRAINDICATIONS: Narrow angle glaucoma, asthma, obstruction of the genitourinary or gastrointestinal tract, severe ulcerative colitis, or known hypersensitivity to this drug prohibits its use.

■ ADVERSE EFFECTS: Among the more serious adverse effects are blurred vision, tachycardia, dry mouth, decreased sweating, and hypersensitivity reactions.

Tridione, a trade name for an anticonvulsant (trimethadione).

triethanolamine polypeptide oleate-condensate, a ceruminolytic agent prescribed to reduce excessive earwax, used as a solution in propylene glycol. A possible serious adverse effect is severe contact dermatitis.

trifacial nerve. See **trigeminal nerve.**

trifluoperazine hydrochloride (traɪ'fluɒuper'əzin), a phenothiazine tranquilizer.

■ INDICATIONS: It is prescribed in the treatment of psychotic disorders and as an anti-emetic.

■ CONTRAINDICATIONS: Parkinson's disease, concurrent administration of central nervous system depressants, hepatic or renal dysfunction, severe hypotension, or known hypersensitivity to this drug prohibits its use.

■ ADVERSE EFFECTS: Among the more serious adverse effects are hypotension, hepatotoxicity, a variety of extrapyramidal reactions, blood dyscrasias, and hypersensitivity reactions.

trifluorothymidine (traɪflur'ɒuthaɪ'mədin), an antiviral. Also called **trifluridine.**

■ INDICATIONS: It is prescribed in the treatment of keratoconjunctivitis, herpetic keratitis, and other forms of keratitis caused by herpes simplex virus.

■ CONTRAINDICATION: Known hypersensitivity to this drug prohibits its use.

■ ADVERSE EFFECTS: Among the more serious adverse effects are hypersensitivity reactions, stromal edema, and increased ocular pressure.

triflupromazine hydrochloride, a phenothiazine tranquilizer.

■ INDICATIONS: It is prescribed in the treatment of psychotic disorders and for the control of severe vomiting.

■ CONTRAINDICATIONS: Parkinson's disease, concurrent administration of central nervous system depressants, liver or renal dysfunction, severe hypotension, or known hypersensitivity to this drug or to other phenothiazine medication prohibits its use.

■ ADVERSE EFFECTS: Among the more serious adverse effects are hypotension, liver toxicity, a variety of extrapyramidal reactions, blood dyscrasias, and hypersensitivity reactions.

trifluridine, an experimental ophthalmic antiviral agent.

■ INDICATIONS: It is being tested for the treatment of herpesvirus I keratoconjunctivitis and keratitis.

■ CONTRAINDICATION: Known hypersensitivity to this drug prohibits its use.

■ ADVERSE EFFECTS: Among the more serious adverse effects are epithelial keratopathy and allergic reactions. Burning and stinging and palpebral edema may also occur.

trigeminal nerve, either of the largest pair of cranial nerves, essential for the act of chewing, general sensibility of the face, and muscular sensibility of the obliquus superior. The trigeminal nerves have sensory, motor, and intermediate roots and connect to three areas in the brain. Also called **fifth nerve, nervus trigeminus, trifacial nerve.**

trigeminal neuralgia, a neurologic condition of the trigeminal facial nerve, characterized by paroxysms of flashing, stablike pain radiating along the course of a branch of the nerve from the angle of the jaw. It is caused by degeneration of the nerve or by pressure on it. Any of the three branches of the nerve may be affected. Neuralgia of the first branch results in pain around the eyes and over the forehead; of the second branch, in pain in the upper lip, nose, and cheek; of the third branch, in pain on the side of the tongue and the lower lip. The momentary bursts of pain recur in clusters lasting many seconds; paroxysmal episodes of the pains may last for hours. Also called **prosopalgia, tic douloureux.**

trigeminal pulse, an abnormal pulse in which every third beat is absent. See also **bigeminal pulse, trigeminy.**

trigeminy (traɪjem'ɪni), 1. grouping in threes. 2. a cardiac arrhythmia characterized by the occurrence of three heartbeats in rapid succession. — **trigeminal,** adj.

triglyceride (traɪglɪs'əraɪd), a compound consisting of a fatty acid (oleic, palmitic, or stearic) and glycerol. Triglycerides make up most animal and vegetable fats and are the principal lipids in the blood where they circulate, bound to a protein, forming high- and low-density lipoproteins. The total amount of triglyceride, and the amount and proportion of the kinds of lipoproteins are important in the diagnosis and treatment of many diseases and conditions including diabetes, hypertension, and heart disease. Normally the total amount of triglyceride in the blood does not exceed 200 mg to 300 mg/100 ml.

trigone (traɪ'goun), 1. a triangle. 2. the first three dominant cusps, considered collectively, of an upper molar.

trigonitis (traɪ'gənaɪ'tɪs), inflammation of the trigone of the bladder, which often accompanies urethritis.

trihexyphenidyl hydrochloride, an anticholinergic agent.

■ INDICATIONS: It is prescribed in the treatment of Parkinson's disease and to control drug-induced extrapyramidal reactions.

■ CONTRAINDICATIONS: Narrow angle glaucoma, asthma, obstruction of the genitourinary or gastrointestinal tract, severe ulcerative colitis, or known hypersensitivity to this drug prohibits its use.

■ ADVERSE EFFECTS: Among the more serious adverse effects are blurred vision, central nervous system effects, tachycardia, dry mouth, decreased sweating, and hypersensitivity reactions.

trihybrid, (in genetics) pertaining to or describing an individual, organism, or strain that is heterozygous for three specific traits, that is the offspring of parents differing in three specific gene pairs, or that is heterozygous for three particular characteristics or gene loci being followed.

trihybrid cross, (in genetics) the mating of two individuals, organisms, or strains that have different gene pairs that determine three specific traits or in which three particular characteristics or gene loci are being followed.

trihydric alcohol, an alcohol containing three hydroxyl groups.

triiodothyronine (T₃) (trai'aiou'doufhai'rənin), a hormone which helps to regulate growth and development, helps to control metabolism and body temperature, and, by a negative feedback system, acts to inhibit the secretion of thyrotropin by the pituitary. Triiodothyronine is produced mainly from the metabolism of thyroxine in the peripheral tissues but is also synthesized by and stored in the thyroid gland as an amino acid residue of the protein thyroglobulin. Triiodothyronine circulates in the plasma where it is bound mainly to thyroxine-binding globulin and thyroxine-binding prealbumin, proteins which protect the hormone from metabolism and excretion during its half-life of 2 days or less before it is degraded in the liver. The hormone acts principally by complementing thyroxine in the control of protein synthesis. It is a component of various drugs, as liotrix and liothyronine sodium, used in the treatment of hypothyroidism and simple goiter. See also **thyroid hormone.**

Trilafon, a trade name for a phenothiazine tranquilizer (perphenazine).

trilaminar blastoderm, the stage of embryonic development in which all three of the primary germ layers, the ectoderm, mesoderm, and entoderm, have formed. Compare **bilaminar blastoderm.**

trilogy of Fallot (fælou'), a congenital cardiac anomaly consisting of the combination of pulmonic stenosis, interatrial septal defect, and right ventricular hypertrophy. See also **congenital cardiac anomaly, tetralogy of Fallot.**

trimalleolar fracture (trai'mæliou'lər). See **Cotton's fracture.**

trimeprazine tartrate (traimep'rəzin), an antipruritic.

■ INDICATIONS: It is prescribed in the treatment of hypersensitivity reactions of the skin.

■ CONTRAINDICATIONS: Coma, bone marrow depression, lactation, or known hypersensitivity to this drug prohibits its use. It is not given to children under six months of age

or to patients receiving large amounts of central nervous system depressants.

■ ADVERSE EFFECTS: Among the more serious reactions are paradoxical excitement, parkinsonlike problems, hepatitis, and gastrointestinal disturbance.

trimester (traimes'tər, trai'mes'tər), one of the three periods of approximately three months into which pregnancy is divided. The first trimester includes the time from the first day of the last menstrual period to the end of twelve weeks. The second trimester, closer to four months in length than three, extends from the twelfth to the twenty-eighth week of gestation. The third trimester begins at the twenty-eighth week and extends to the time of delivery.

trimethadione (trai'mefhədai'oun), an anticonvulsant.

■ INDICATION: It is prescribed to prevent seizures in petit mal epilepsy.

■ CONTRAINDICATIONS: Severe renal or hepatic impairment, blood dyscrasias, or known hypersensitivity to this drug prohibits its use.

■ ADVERSE EFFECTS: Among the more serious adverse reactions are exfoliative dermatitis, blood dyscrasias, and aplastic anemia. Sedation and hemeralopia may occur.

trimethaphan camsylate, a ganglionic blocking agent.

■ INDICATIONS: It is prescribed to produce controlled hypotension during surgery and to lower blood pressure in hypertensive emergencies.

■ CONTRAINDICATIONS: It is not used where hypotension places a patient in undue risk or when hypersensitivity to this drug prohibits its use.

■ ADVERSE EFFECTS: The most serious adverse reaction is severe hypotension.

trimethobenzamide hydrochloride, an antiemetic.

■ INDICATIONS: It is prescribed for the relief of nausea and vomiting.

■ CONTRAINDICATIONS: Reye's syndrome or known hypersensitivity to this drug prohibits its use.

■ ADVERSE EFFECTS: Among the most serious adverse reactions with high doses are drowsiness, diarrhea, allergic reactions, and extrapyramidal reactions. Adverse reactions are rare at usual dosages.

trimethoprim (traimefh'əprim), an antibacterial.

■ INDICATIONS: It is prescribed in the treatment of various infections, particularly of the urinary tract, middle ear, and bronchi.

■ CONTRAINDICATION: Known hypersensitivity to this drug prohibits its use.

■ ADVERSE EFFECTS: Among the more serious adverse reactions are blood dyscrasias and allergic, gastrointestinal, and central nervous system disorders.

trimethoprim and sulfalene, a new, experimental fixed-combination drug for the treatment of chloroquine-resistant falciparum malaria. It is not yet approved for use by the FDA.

trimethoprim and sulfamethoxazole. See **sulfameth-oxazole and trimethoprim.**

trimethylene (traɪmeth′ɪlin). See **cyclopropane.**

trimipramine maleate (trɪmɪp′rəmin), an antidepressant.

■ INDICATIONS: It is prescribed in the treatment of anxiety, depression, and insomnia.

■ CONTRAINDICATIONS: Concomitant use of a monoamine oxidase inhibitor within 14 days or known hypersensitivity to this drug prohibits its use. It is not given during recovery from myocardial infarction or to schizophrenic patients. It is not recommended for children.

■ ADVERSE EFFECTS: Among the more serious adverse reactions are tachycardia, seizures, parkinsonism, blurred vision, hypotension, and aggravation of glaucoma.

Trimpex, a trade name for an antibacterial (trimethoprim).

Trinsicon, a trade name for a hematinic fixed-combination drug containing iron, vitamin B_{12}, and intrinsic factor concentrate.

trioxsalen, a melanizing agent.

■ INDICATIONS: It is prescribed for repigmentation of the skin in idiopathic vitiligo and to increase tolerance to sunlight.

■ CONTRAINDICATIONS: Diseases associated with photosensitivity, as porphyria, acute lupus erythematosus, or leukoderma of infectious origin, or the concomitant use of drugs having any photosensitizing activity prohibits its use.

■ ADVERSE EFFECTS: Among the most serious adverse reactions are severe burns from excessive exposure to ultraviolet light. Gastric irritation and nausea also may occur.

tripelennamine citrate. See **tripelennamine hydrochloride.**

tripelennamine hydrochloride, an antihistamine.

■ INDICATIONS: It is prescribed in the treatment of rhinitis and hypersensitivity reactions of the skin.

■ CONTRAINDICATIONS: Asthma, glaucoma, difficulty in emptying the bladder, concomitant administration of a monoamine oxidase inhibitor, or known hypersensitivity to this drug prohibits its use. It is not given to premature or newborn infants or to lactating mothers.

■ ADVERSE EFFECTS: Among the more serious adverse reactions are sedation, tachycardia, and gastrointestinal upset.

triple commitment, a threefold obligation for a faculty member to teach, practice, and perform research. A triple commitment is usual for faculty appointments in schools of medicine and nursing.

triple-dye treatment, the therapy of burns by applying 6.0 per cent gentian violet, 1.0 per cent brilliant green, and 0.1 per cent acriflavin base.

triple response, a triad of phenomena that occur in sequence following the intradermal injection of histamine. First, a red spot develops, spreading outward for a few millimeters, reaching its maximal size within one minute and then turning bluish. Next, a brighter red flush of color spreads slowly in an irregular flare around the original red spot. Finally, a wheal, filled with fluid, forms over the original spot. Also called **triple response of Lewis.**

triple response of Lewis. See **triple response.**

triple sugar iron reaction, any one of several reactions seen in certain bacterial cultures growing on triple sugar iron agar, a culture medium used to aid in the identification of *Escherichia coli, Proteus, Salmonella, Shigella,* and other pathogenic enteric bacteria.

triple sulfonamides. See **trisulfapyrimidines.**

triplet, **1.** any one of three offspring born of the same gestation period during a single pregnancy. See also **Hellin's law.** **2.** (in genetics) the unit of three consecutive bases in one polynucleotide chain of DNA or RNA that codes for a specific amino acid. See also **codon, genetic code.**

triple X syndrome. See **XXX syndrome.**

triploid, (3n), **1.** Also called **triploidic.** of or pertaining to an individual, organism, strain, or cell that has three complete sets of chromosomes, triple the normal haploid number characteristic of the species. In humans, the triploid number is 69, found in rare cases of aborted or stillborn fetuses. Of those triploid fetuses born alive, all are characterized by gross and multiple malformations; they live only for a few hours. **2.** such an individual, organism, strain, or cell. Compare **diploid, haploid, tetraploid.** See also **polyploid.**

triploidy (trɪp′loɪdi), the state or condition of having three complete sets of chromosomes.

tripodial symmelia (traɪpoʊ′diəl), a fetal anomaly characterized by the fusion of the lower extremities and the presence of three feet.

triprolidine hydrochloride, an antihistamine.

■ INDICATIONS: It is prescribed in the treatment of a variety of hypersensitivity reactions, including rhinitis, skin rash, and pruritus.

■ CONTRAINDICATIONS: Asthma or known hypersensitivity to this drug prohibits its use. It is not given to newborn infants or lactating mothers.

■ ADVERSE EFFECTS: Drowsiness, skin rash, hypersensitivity reactions, dry mouth, and tachycardia may occur.

-tripsis, a combining form meaning a 'chafing or wearing away': *anatripsis, entripsis, syntripsis.*

-tripsy, a combining form meaning a 'crushing of a body part by a surgical instrument': *basiotripsy, lithotripsy, sarcotripsy.*

trismus (trɪz′məs), a prolonged tonic spasm of the muscles of the jaw. Also called, *Informal.* **lockjaw.** See also **tetanus.**

trisomy (trai'səmi), **trisomia** (traisou'miə), a chromosomal aberration characterized by the presence of one more than the normal number of chromosomes in a diploid complement; in humans the trisomic cell contains 47 chromosomes and is designated $2n + 1$. The additional member can join any of the normal homologous pairs, although most human trisomies involve the small chromosomes, such as those in the E or G group, or the sex chromosomes. Partial trisomy occurs when only a portion of a chromosome attaches to another. In genetic nomenclature, trisomies are indicated by the exact chromosome or karyotypic group in which the addition is made, as trisomy 13 or trisomy D. Compare **monosomy**. See also **trisomy syndrome**. – **trisomic**, *adj.*

trisomy 8, a congenital condition associated with the presence of an extra chromosome 8 within the C group. Those with the condition are slender, of normal height, have a large, asymmetric head, prominent forehead, deepset eyes, low-set prominent ears, and thick lips. There is mild to severe mental and motor retardation, often with delayed and poorly articulated speech. Skeletal anomalies and joint limitation, especially camptodactyly, may occur, and there are unusually deep palmar and plantar creases, which are diagnostically significant. Most trisomy 8 individuals are mosaic, with no abnormal or only slight clinical manifestations, or they are only partially trisomic, with part of the extra chromosome 8 missing, and show varying degrees of the clinical symptoms. In general, trisomy 8 is a less severe condition than other trisomies, especially trisomy 13 and trisomy 18, so that the mortality rate is low. Also called **trisomy C syndrome**.

trisomy 13, a congenital condition caused by the presence of an extra chromosome in the D group, predominantly chromosome 13, although in rare instances chromosome 14 or 15. It is characterized by multiple midline anomalies and central nervous system defects, including holoprosencephaly, microcephaly, myelomeningocele, microphthalmos, and cleft lip and palate. There are also severe mental retardation, polydactyly, deafness, convulsions, and abnormalities of the heart, viscera, and genitalia. Most infants with the condition are severely affected and do not survive beyond the first six months of life. Also called **Patau's syndrome, trisomy D syndrome, trisomy 13-15**.

trisomy 13-15. See **trisomy 13**.

trisomy 16-18. See **trisomy 18**.

trisomy 18, a congenital condition caused by the presence of an extra chromosome 18, characterized by severe mental retardation and multiple deformities. Among the most common defects are scaphocephaly or other skull abnormalities, micrognathia, abnormal facies with low-set malformed ears and prominent occiput, cleft lip and palate, clenched fists with overlapping fingers, especially the index over the third finger, clubfeet, and syndactyly. Ven-

tricular septal defect, patent ductus arteriosus, atrial septal defect, and renal anomalies are also common. The condition occurs predominantly in females, according to a 3:1 sex ratio, and survival for more than a few months is rare. Also called **Edward's syndrome, trisomy E syndrome, trisomy 16-18**.

trisomy 21. See **Down's syndrome**.

trisomy 22, a congenital condition caused by the presence of an extra chromosome 22 in the G group, characterized by psychomotor retardation and various developmental anomalies. Common defects include microcephaly, micrognathia, hypotonia, hypertelorism, abnormal ears with preauricular tags or fistulas, and congenital heart disease. In partial trisomy 22, the extra chromosome is much smaller than the normal pair and causes coloboma of the iris or anal atresia, or both, as well as various other defects. See also **cat-eye syndrome**.

trisomy C syndrome. See **trisomy 8**.

trisomy D syndrome. See **Patau's syndrome**.

trisomy E syndrome. See **Edward's syndrome**.

trisomy G syndrome. See **Down's syndrome**.

trisomy syndrome, any condition caused by the addition of an extra member to a normal pair of homologous autosomes or to the sex chromosomes or by the translocation of a portion of one chromosome to another. Most trisomies occur as a result of complete or partial nondisjunction of the chromosomes during cell division. The more severe conditions are related to trisomies of the autosomes rather than the sex chromosomes. The most common trisomy syndromes with clearly established clinical manifestations are trisomy 8, trisomy 13, trisomy 18, trisomy 21, trisomy 22.

Trisoralen, a trade name for a pigmentation agent (trioxsalen).

trisulfapyrimidines, three antibacterials in combination (sulfadiazine, sulfamerazine, and sulfamethazine), rarely prescribed today.

Tri-Vi-Flor, a trade name for an oral pediatric fixed-combination drug containing sodium fluoride and vitamins A, C, and D.

tRNA, abbreviation for **transfer RNA**.

Trobicin, a trade name for an antibacterial (spectinomycin hydrochloride).

trocar (trou'kar), a sharp, pointed rod that fits inside a tube. It is used to pierce the skin and the wall of a cavity or canal in the body in order to aspirate fluids, to instill a medication or solution, or to guide the placement of a soft catheter. The trocar is usually removed and the catheter, tube, or instrument is left in place. See also **cannula**.

trochanter (troukæn'tər), one of the two bony projections on the proximal end of the femur that serve for the attachment of various muscles. The two protuberances are the greater trochanter and the lesser trochanter.

troche (trou'ki), a small oval, round, or oblong tablet containing a medicinal agent incorporated in a flavored, sweetened mucilage or fruit base that dissolves in the mouth, releasing the drug. Also called **lozenge, rotula, trochiscus.**

trochiscus (troukıs'kəs). See **troche.**

trochlea (trok'liə), a pulley-shaped part or structure. — **trochlear,** adj.

trochlear nerve, either of the smallest pair of cranial nerves, essential for eye movement and eye muscle sensibility. The trochlear nerves branch to the obliquus superior and communicate with the ophthalmic division of the trigeminal nerve, connecting with two areas in the brain. Also called **fourth nerve, nervus trochlearis.**

trochlear notch of ulna, a large depression in the ulna, formed by the olecranon and coronoid processes, that articulates with the trochlea of the humerus.

trochoid joint. See **pivot joint.**

Trocinate, a trade name for an anticholinergic (thiphenamil hydrochloride).

troleandomycin, a macrolide antibiotic.

■ INDICATIONS: It is prescribed in the treatment of certain infections.

■ CONTRAINDICATION: Known hypersensitivity to this drug prohibits its use.

■ ADVERSE EFFECTS: Among the more serious adverse effects are gastrointestinal disturbances, mild to severe allergic reactions (including anaphylaxis), and hepatotoxicity.

trombiculosis (trombık'yulou'sıs), an infestation with mites of the genus *Trombicula,* some species of which carry scrub typhus.

tromethamine, an alkalizer.

■ INDICATION: It is prescribed to correct acidosis.

■ CONTRAINDICATIONS: Anuria or uremia prohibits its use. It is not given during pregnancy except in acute life-threatening situations.

■ ADVERSE EFFECTS: Among the more serious adverse reactions are hypoglycemia, respiratory depression, and local tissue damage at the site of injection.

-tron, a combining form meaning a '(specified) type of vacuum tube': *dynatron, magnetron, thyratron.*

Tronothane Hydrochloride, a trade name for a local anesthetic (pramoxine hydrochloride).

trop-, tropo-, combining forms meaning 'turn, turning' or 'tendency, affinity': *tropism, tropomyosin.* See also **troph-, tropho-,** with which they are sometimes confused.

-tropal. See **-tropic.**

-trope, a combining form meaning 'influencing or influenced by': *gonadotrope, heliotrope, rheotrope.*

troph-. See **tropho-.**

-troph, **1.** a combining form meaning 'that which nourishes an embryo': *embryotroph, hemotroph, histotroph.* **2.** a combining form meaning an 'organism that gets nourish-

ment from a (specified) source': *autotroph, metatroph, prototroph.*

trophectoderm. See **trophoblast.**

-trophic, a combining form meaning 'referring to a type of nutrition or nutritional requirement': *chondrotrophic, lipotrophic, viscerotrophic.*

trophic fracture, a fracture resulting from the weakening of bone tissue owing to nutritional disturbances.

trophic ulcer, a decubitus ulcer caused by external trauma to a part of the body that is in poor condition owing to disease, vascular insufficiency, or loss of afferent nerve fibers. Trophic ulcers may be painless or associated with severe causalgia. See also **decubitus ulcer.**

tropho-, troph-, a combining form meaning 'pertaining to food or nourishment': *trophoblast, trophoedema, trophoneurosis.*

trophoblast, the layer of tissue that forms the wall of the blastocyst of placental mammals in the early stages of embryonic development. It functions in the implantation of the blastocyst in the uterine wall and in supplying nutrient to the embryo. At implantation the cells differentiate into two layers, the inner cytotrophoblast, which forms the chorion, and the syncytiotrophoblast, which develops into the outer layer of the placenta. Also called **trophectoderm.** — **trophoblastic,** adj.

trophoblastic cancer, a malignant neoplastic disease of the uterus derived from chorionic epithelium, characterized by the production of high levels of human chorionic gonadotropin (HCG). The tumor may be an invasive hydatid mole (chorioadenoma destruens) formed by grossly enlarged, vesicular chorionic villi or a malignant uterine choriocarcinoma that arises from nonvillous chorionic epithelium. Half the cases of choriocarcinoma follow a molar pregnancy, 25 per cent an abortion, 22.5 per cent a normal pregnancy, and 2.5 per cent an ectopic pregnancy. A hydatid mole invades the myometrium and often forms extrauterine nodules that may spread to distant sites. Choriocarcinoma forms a dark red, hemorrhagic, nodular tumor on or in the uterine wall and metastasizes early in its course to the lungs, brain, liver, bones, vagina, or vulva. Initial symptoms are vaginal bleeding and a profuse, foul-smelling discharge; a persistent cough or hemoptysis signals pulmonary involvement. As the disease progresses there may be frequent hemorrhage, weakness, and emaciation. Diagnostic measures include serial assays to determine if the HCG level in the blood is elevated and histologic examination of specimens obtained by curettage. Hysterectomy is indicated in most cases, but surgery does not eliminate the possibility of a recurrence. Chemotherapy is effective in curing a large percentage of patients with trophoblastic tumors. Single-agent chemotherapy with methotrexate or actinomycin D is recommended for low-risk patients, those with disease of less than four months duration, and those with lung or vaginal metastases. Treatment of high-risk patients with more prolonged disease and liver or brain metastases is usually individualized but may include radiotherapy and a combination of methotrexate, actinomycin D, and chlorambucil. See also **choriocarcinoma, hydatid mole.**

trophozoite, a motile protozoon, as an ameba. Diseases in which trophozoites may be isolated by bacteriologic studies include amebic dysentery, malaria, and trichomonas vaginitis.

-trophy, a combining form meaning a 'condition of nutrition or growth': *cyotrophy, embryotrophy, lipotrophy.* Also **-trophia.**

-tropia, a combining form meaning '(condition of) deviation in the visual axis': *cyclotropia, parectropia, talantropia.*

-tropic, 1. a combining form meaning a 'turn or change in the visual axis': *anatropic, hemitropic, stereotropic.* **2.** a combining form meaning a 'tendency to have an influence on, or be influenced by': *corticotropic, pancreatropic, radiotropic.* Also **-tropal, -tropous.**

tropical medicine, the branch of medicine concerned with the diagnosis and treatment of diseases commonly occurring in tropical and subtropical regions of the world, generally between 30 degrees north and south of the equator.

tropical sore. See **oriental sore.**

tropical sprue, a malabsorption syndrome of unknown etiology that is endemic in the tropics and subtropics. It is characterized by abnormalities in the mucosa of the small intestine resulting in protein malnutrition and multiple nutritional deficiencies, often complicated by severe infection. Symptoms include diarrhea, anorexia, and weight loss. Megaloblastic anemia may result from folic acid- and vitamin B_{12} deficiency. Treatment includes administration of antibiotics, particularly tetracycline, folic acid, iron, calcium, and vitamins A, D, K, and the B complex group, as well as a balanced diet high in protein and normal in fat content. See also **nontropical sprue.**

tropical typhus. See **scrub typhus.**

tropicamide, an anticholinergic mydriatic.

■ INDICATIONS: It is prescribed as a cycloplegic and mydriatic medication for diagnostic purposes in ophthalmology.

■ CONTRAINDICATIONS: Glaucoma or known hypersensitivity to this drug prohibits its use.

■ ADVERSE EFFECTS: Among the more serious adverse reactions are photophobia and tachycardia.

-tropism, a combining form meaning a 'condition of having an affinity for something (specified)': *parasitotropism, phototropism, sitotropism.* Also **-tropy.**

-tropo. See **-trop.**

-tropous. See **-tropic.**

-tropy, a combining form meaning 'influenced by or having an affinity for' something specified: *allotropy, ergotropy, syntropy.* Also **-tropism.**

Trousseau's sign (trusouz'), a test for latent tetany in which carpal spasm is induced by inflating a sphygmomanometer cuff on the upper arm to a pressure exceeding systolic blood pressure for three minutes. A positive test may be seen in hypocalcemia and hypomagnesemia.

true birth rate, the ratio of total births to the total female population of child-bearing age, between the ages of 15 and 45. Compare **birth rate, crude birth rate, refined birth rate.**

true chondroma. See **enchondroma.**

true dwarf. See **primordial dwarf.**

true glottis. See **glottis.**

true neuroma, any neoplasm composed of nerve tissue.

true rib. See **rib.**

true suture, an immovable fibrous joint of the skull in which the edges of bones interlock along a series of processes and indentations. The three kinds of true sutures are the sutura dentata, the sutura limbosa, and the sutura serrata. Compare **false suture.**

true twins. See **monozygotic twins.**

true vocal cord. See **vocal cord.**

truncus arteriosus, the embryonic arterial trunk that initially opens from both ventricles of the heart and later divides into the aorta and the pulmonary trunk, the two portions separated by the bulbar septum.

trunk incurvation reflex. See **Galant reflex.**

truss, an apparatus worn to prevent the herniation of the intestines or other organ through an opening in the abdominal wall.

Trypanosoma (trɪp'ənousou'mə), a genus of parasitic organisms, several species of which can cause significant diseases in man. Most *Trypanosoma* organisms live part of their life cycle in insects and are transmitted to man by insect bites. See also **trypanosome, trypanosomiasis.**

Trypanosoma brucei gambiense. See **Gambian trypanosomiasis.**

Trypanosoma brucei rhodesiense. See **Rhodesian trypanosomiasis.**

Trypanosoma cruzi. See **Chagas' disease.**

trypanosomal infection. See **trypanosomiasis.**

trypanosome (trɪp'ənousoum', trɪpæn'əsoum'), any organism of the genus *Trypanosoma.* See also **trypanosomiasis.** — **trypanosomal,** *adj.*

trypanosomiasis (trɪp'ənousoumaɪ'əsɪs, trɪpæn'əsoumaɪ'əsɪs), an infection by an organism of the *Trypanosoma* genus. Kinds of trypanosomiasis are **African trypanosomiasis, Chagas' disease.**

trypanosomicide (trɪp'ənousou'məsaɪd), a drug destructive to trypanosomes, especially the species of the protozoan parasite transmitted to man by various insect vectors common in Africa and Central and South America. Various arsenical preparations are used to treat African sleeping sickness, caused by *Trypanosoma gambiense* and *T. rhodesiense,* and Chagas' disease, caused by *T. cruzi,* in the Americas.   **– trypanosomicidal,** *adj.*

trypsin crystallized, a proteolytic enzyme from the pancreas of the ox, *Bos taurus,* that has been used as a debriding agent for open wounds and ulcers.

Tryptacin, a trade name for an amino acid (L-tryptophan), used as an antidepressant and to induce sleep.

tryptophan (trɪp′təfæn), an amino acid essential for normal growth in infants and for nitrogen balance in adults. Tryptophan is the precursor of several substances, including serotonin and niacin. About 50 per cent of the daily requirement of tryptophan is provided through the metabolism of niacin. The rest is derived from dietary protein, especially legumes, grains, and seeds. See also **amino acid, protein metabolism.**

TSEM, abbreviation for **transmission scanning electron microscopy.**

tsetse fly (tset′si, tsi′tsi), an insect of the genus *Glossina,* found in Africa, which carries the organisms of trypanosomiasis.

TSH, abbreviation for **thyroid-stimulating hormone.**

TSH releasing factor. See **thyrotropin releasing hormone.**

TSS, abbreviation for **toxic shock syndrome.**

tsutsugamushi disease (tsu′tsʊgəmu′ʃhi). See **scrub typhus.**

TTP, abbreviation for **thrombotic thrombocytopenic purpura.**

T-tube, a tubular device in the shape of a T, inserted through the skin into a cavity or a wound, used for drainage.

Tuamine, a trade name for an adrenergic vasoconstrictor (tuaminoheptane).

tuaminoheptane (tu′æminoʊhep′tein), an adrenergic vasoconstrictor.
- INDICATION: It is used to reduce nasal congestion.
- CONTRAINDICATIONS: The concomitant use of a monoamine oxidase inhibitor or tricyclic antidepressant or known hypersensitivity to this drug or to other adrenergic drugs prohibits its use.
- ADVERSE EFFECTS: Among the adverse reactions are reflex swelling of the nasal mucosa, palpitations, nausea, and central nervous system stimulation.

tubal abortion, a condition of pregnancy in which an embryo, ectopically implanted, is expelled from the uterine tube into the peritoneal cavity. Tubal abortion is often accompanied by significant internal bleeding causing acute abdominal and pelvic pain, but may be asymptomatic, the products of conception being resorbed. Rarely, the conceptus reimplants on the peritoneum and continues growing to become an abdominal pregnancy. See also **abdominal pregnancy, ectopic pregnancy.**

tubal dermoid cyst, a tumor derived from embryonal tissues that develops in an oviduct.

tubal ligation, one of several sterilization procedures in which both Fallopian tubes are blocked to prevent conception from occurring. Spinal or local anesthesia is used unless the procedure accompanies major surgery. Through a small abdominal incision, the Fallopian tubes are ligated in two places with suture, and intervening segment is burnt, crushed, or excised. The procedure is less commonly performed vaginally. Complications of the procedure, which are rare but serious, include pulmonary embolism, hemorrhage, infection, and tubal pregnancy. The requirements for informed consent for sterilization procedures vary among states and institutions.

tubal pregnancy, an ectopic pregnancy in which the conceptus implants in the Fallopian tube. Approximately 2 per cent of all pregnancies are ectopic; of these, approximately 90 per cent are tubal. Tubal pregnancy seldom occurs in primigravidas. The most important predisposing factor is prior tubal injury. Pelvic infection, scarring and adhesions from surgery, or IUD complications may result in damage that diminishes the motility of the tube. Transport of the ovum through the tube after fertilization is slowed, and implantation takes place before the conceptus reaches the uterine cavity. Most often the tube, which cannot long contain the growing fetus, ruptures, precipitating an intraperitoneal hemorrhage which, if not stopped, can lead rapidly to shock and, often, death. Occasionally, the conceptus does not firmly implant in the tube and is extruded from the fimbriated end of the tube as a tubal abortion. Some conceptuses apparently die and are resorbed in the tube. Diagnosis of tubal pregnancy is often difficult. With rupture of the Fallopian tube, women commonly experience sudden sharp pain in one side of the lower abdomen, but signs and symptoms of tubal pregnancy are insidiously variable, and the classic triad of amenorrhea, pelvic pain, and a tender adnexal mass are present only 50 per cent of the time. Recovery of blood from the cul-de-sac by means of culdocentesis is highly suggestive of a ruptured Fallopian tube and tubal pregnancy; it requires immediate surgical exploration of the abdomen. Absence of blood on culdocentesis does not rule out the presence of an unruptured tubal pregnancy; laparoscopy or laparotomy may be required, particularly if a woman's pregnancy test is positive, the pelvic findings are suggestive, and sonography of the pelvis cannot demonstrate an intrauterine pregnancy. Because of the lethal potential of an undiagnosed tubal pregnancy, women who report any of the characteristic symptoms early in their pregnancies, particularly during the time before the existence of a normal intrauterine pregnancy can be confirmed, must be considered susceptible. In women who have a history of prior pelvic disease and in those who have symptoms or signs that are of tubal pregnancy, emergency treatment requires an immediate intravenous infusion via a large-bore intravenous catheter, type and cross match of blood for blood replacement, and treatment of shock as necessary. Treatment is surgical and involves laparotomy, removal of the entire products of conception and any intraperitoneal blood present, and the removal or repair of the involved tube. Conditions that predispose to a first tubal pregnancy also predispose to a second; a woman who has had one tubal pregnancy has one chance in five of having another in a subsequent pregnancy. Depending on the location of the developing embryo, the condition is classified as an ampullary, fimbrial, or interstitial tubal pregnancy.

Tubarine, a trade name for a skeletal muscle relaxant (tubocurarine chloride).

tube, a hollow, cylindrical piece of equipment or structure of the body.

tube feeding, the administration of nutritionally balanced liquefied foods through a tube inserted into the stomach or duodenum. The procedure is used following mouth or gastric surgery, in severe burns, in paralysis or obstruction of the esophagus, in severe cases of anorexia nervosa, and for unconscious patients or those unable to chew or swallow. Also called **gavage feeding, nasogastric feeding.** See also **parenteral nutrition.**

tube feeding care, the nursing care and management of a patient receiving nourishment through a nasogastric tube.

■ METHOD: The tip of a nasogastric tube is lubricated with a water-soluble lubricant, inserted into a nostril, and rapidly advanced into the stomach as the patient, if conscious, is asked to swallow hard repeatedly. Correct placement of the tube may be determined by aspirating the gastric contents, which are subsequently returned to prevent loss of electrolytes. Placement may also be checked by listening for a bubbling sound through a stethoscope placed over the stomach, as 5 ml of air is injected into the tube. If a stream of bubbles is observed when the proximal end of the tube is submerged in water or if the patient coughs forcefully when 1 or 2 ml of water are injected into the tube, it is placed in the upper respiratory tract rather than the stomach. The tube, held securely and comfortably by a tape across the nose or upper lip, may be left in place in adults and older children but usually is removed and reinserted for each feeding in infants. Before each feeding the patient is helped up to a semi-Fowler's position or is turned on the right side if unconscious. If a cuffed tracheostomy tube or endotracheal tube is in place the cuff is inflated. The nasogastric tube is checked for proper placement and for the amount of residual formula in the stomach. Any solid medication to be given with the feeding is dissolved in water. The normal liquefied diet formula contains a mixture of milk, eggs, sugar, skim milk powder, and protein hydrolysates. A low-residue formula

consists of amino acids, sugars, vitamins, and minerals. Depending on the patient's preference, the formula is at or below room temperature when administered slowly by gravity at a rate of no more than 300 ml an hour. During feeding the patient is observed for respiratory distress, nausea, vomiting, abdominal cramps, and restlessness. At the completion of the procedure, the tube is flushed with water as ordered and then clamped. The patient receives oral hygiene, lubrication and cleaning of the nares, and is maintained in the same position for 30 minutes after feeding; at that time the cuff on the tracheostomy or endotracheal tube is deflated.

■ NURSING ORDERS: The nurse positions the patient for feeding, checks the tube placement, notes and replaces the amount of residual formula, and reports residual volume in excess of 100 ml. The nurse administers the feeding, ensures that the patient and family members understand the purpose of the procedure, and cautions the patient to report symptoms, as nausea, abdominal cramps, diarrhea, or constipation.

■ OUTCOME CRITERIA: A formula containing the proper proportions of protein, carbohydrate, and fat administered through a nasogastric tube can provide adequate nutrition over a short term. A high content of simple sugars may cause diarrhea. Concentrated mixtures containing too little water or large volumes administered rapidly may dehydrate the patient.

tubercle (tu'bərkəl), **1.** a nodule or a small eminence, as that on a bone. **2.** a nodule, especially an elevation of the skin that is larger than a papule, as Morgagni's tubercles of the areolae of the breasts. **3.** a small rounded nodule produced by infection with mycobacterium tuberculosis, consisting of a gray translucent mass of small spherical cells surrounded by connective cells.

tuberculin purified protein derivative, a solution containing a purified protein fraction derived from isolated culture filtrates of strains of *Mycobacterium tuberculosis.* It is used as an aid in the diagnosis of tuberculosis, in the Mantoux test and, for the same purpose in a dried form, in multiple puncture devices. See also **Mantoux test, Tine test.**

tuberculin test, a test to determine past or present tuberculosis infection based on a positive skin reaction, using one of several methods. A purified protein derivative (PPD) of tubercle bacilli, called tuberculin, is introduced into the skin by scratch, puncture, or intradermal injection. If a raised, red, or hard zone forms surrounding the tuberculin test site, the person is said to be sensitive to tuberculin, and the test is read as positive. However, a negative tuberculin reaction does not rule out a diagnosis of previous or active tuberculosis. Sputum and gastric cultures, acid-fast staining, and x rays are often needed to establish a diagnosis of tuberculosis. Kinds of tuberculin tests include **Heaf test, Mantoux test, Pirquet test, tine test.**

tuberculoid leprosy. See **leprosy.**

tuberculoma (tubər'kyulou'mə), a rare tumorlike growth of tuberculous tissue in the central nervous system, characterized by symptoms of an expanding cerebral, cerebellar, or spinal mass. Treatment consists of the administration of antimicrobial drugs to resolve the primary growth and to prevent meningitis.

tuberculosis (TB), a chronic, granulomatous infection caused by an acid-fast bacillus, *Mycobacterium tuberculosis,* generally transmitted by the inhalation or ingestion of infected droplets and usually affecting the lungs, although infection of other organ systems by other modes of transmission occurs.

■ OBSERVATIONS: Listlessness, vague chest pain, pleurisy, anorexia, fever, and weight loss are early symptoms of pulmonary tuberculosis. Night sweats, pulmonary hemorrhage, expectoration of purulent sputum, and dyspnea develop as the disease progresses. The lung tissues react to the bacillus by producing protective cells that engulf the disease organism, forming tubercles. Untreated, the tubercles enlarge and merge to form larger tubercles that undergo caseation, eventually sloughing off into the cavities of the lungs. Hemoptysis occurs as a result of cavitary spread. Physical examination reveals apical rales, amphoric bronchial sounds, decreased respiratory excursion, and, in advanced cases, cyanosis. Laboratory examination demonstrates leukocytosis and an increased sedimentation rate, and microscopic study of a specimen of sputum stained with carbol-fuchsin may be diagnostic. Culture of the tubercle bacillus is slow and requires darkness, carefully controlled temperature, and inoculation on special media. The infecting organism does not produce endotoxins or hemolysins, but tuberculin, a toxic substance, is released as the bacillus disintegrates. Tuberculin has no effect in people who have never been infected but produces a characteristic skin reaction when injected intradermally in people who have or have had tuberculosis. Purified protein derivative (PPD) is a stable, purified active preparation used to test for current or past infection. X-ray films of the lungs reveal infiltrates, mediastinal lymphadenopathy, caseation, pleural effusion, and calcification. Tuberculosis may spread from the lungs via the lymphatics and blood vessels; such miliary infection is characterized by tiny, seedlike tubercles in the liver, spleen, and other organs.

■ INTERVENTION: The bacillus is generally sensitive to isoniazid (INH), para-aminosalicylic acid, streptomycin, rifampin, dihydrostreptomycin, to ultra-violet radiation, and to heat. A combination of drugs is prescribed, with regular tests of the function of the kidneys, liver, eyes, and ears performed to discover early signs of drug toxicity. This is particularly important because drug therapy

will usually continue for more than a year. The person is usually hospitalized for the first weeks of treatment to limit the possible spread of infection, to encourage rest and excellent nutrition, to insure complete compliance with the prescribed drug regimen, and to observe for adverse drug effects. Samples of sputum are regularly examined. The disease is not infectious once the bacillus is no longer present in the sputum. Care of an outpatient includes continued medication, evaluation for adverse drug effects, sputum analyses, and encouragement to complete the long course of treatment. All contacts are tested periodically with PPD. People who are at increased risk of infection may be treated empirically, without a positive diagnosis having been made.

■ NURSING CONSIDERATIONS: Before discharge, the patient is taught the following: how to prevent the spread of the disease, the elements of good nutrition, the name, dose, action, and side effects of all medications prescribed, the need to take the drugs regularly, and how and where to get the next supply of drugs. Plans for follow-up are discussed; they include date, time, and place of the next laboratory tests, and a reminder that a cough, weight loss, fever, night sweats, and hemoptysis are danger signals that are to be reported immediately. See also **miliary tuberculosis, tuberculin test.**

tuberculosis vaccine. See **BCG vaccine.**

tuberculous spondylitis, a rare, grave form of tuberculosis caused by the invasion of *Mycobacterium tuberculosis* into the spinal vertebrae. The intervertebral discs may be destroyed, resulting in the collapse and wedging of affected vertebrae and the shortening and angulation of the spine. Thoracic vertebrae are more frequently involved than the vertebrae of the lumbar, the cervical, or the sacral segments of the spine. More than one area of the spine may be affected, and normal vertebrae may be evident between affected and unaffected sections. The infection characteristically dissects vertebrae anterolaterally and produces abscesses. The pressure of the abcess may cause ischemic paralysis in the subjacent spinal cord, and abscesses in the cervical area may displace or obstruct the trachea and the esophagus. Also called **Pott's disease, spinal caries.** See also **tuberculosis.**

tuberosity (tu'bəros'ıti), an elevation or protuberance, especially of a bone.

tuberosity of the tibia, a large oblong elevation at the proximal end of the tibia that attaches to the ligament of the patella.

tuberous carcinoma, a scirrhous carcinoma of the skin, characterized by nodular projections. Also called **carcinoma tuberosum.**

tuberous sclerosis, a familial, neurocutaneous disease characterized by epilepsy, mental deterioration, adenoma sebaceum, nodules and sclerotic patches on the cerebral cortex, retinal tumors, depigmented leaf-shaped macules on the skin, tumors of the heart or kidneys, and cerebral calcifications. There is no effective treatment. Also called **epiloia.** See also **adenoma sebaceum.**

tuberous xanthoma. See **xanthoma tuberosum.**

Tubex unit, a trade name for a unit consisting of a cartridge and needle that fits into a holder that has a plunger. The cartridge may be empty or prefilled with a standard dose of a medication. The needle is covered with a rubber protective guard and is permanently attached to the cartridge. The plunger may be unscrewed to allow the cartridge-needle unit to be slipped in place. The cartridge is then twisted clockwise to secure it in the holder. The plunger is replaced and screwed onto a small projection on top of a rubber diaphragm on the cartridge. As the plunger is depressed, forcing the diaphragm into the cartridge, medication is forced out through the needle. The cartridge-needle unit is sterile and disposable. The holder requires no special care and is reuseable.

tubocurarine chloride, a skeletal muscle relaxant.

■ INDICATIONS: It is prescribed as an adjunct to anesthesia and electroshock therapy and in the diagnosis of myasthenia gravis.

■ CONTRAINDICATION: Asthma or known hypersensitivity to this drug prohibits its use.

■ ADVERSE EFFECTS: Among the more serious adverse effects are hypotension, bronchospasm (in asthmatics), and allergic reaction. Many drugs act to increase the activity of tubocurarine.

tubule (tu′byul), a small tube, as one of the collecting tubules in the kidneys, the seminiferous tubules of the testes, or Henle's tubules between the distal and proximal convoluted tubules. — **tubular,** *adj.*

tuft fracture, fracture of any one of the distal phalanges.

Tuinal, a trade name for a central nervous system fixed-combination drug containing two sedative-hypnotics (amobarbital sodium and secobarbital sodium).

tularemia (tu′ləri′miə), an infectious disease of animals caused by the bacillus *Francisella (Pasteurella) tularensis,* which may be transmitted by insect vectors or direct contact. It is characterized in humans by fever, headache, and an ulcerated skin lesion with localized lymph node enlargement or by eye infection, gastrointestinal ulcerations, or pneumonia, depending on the site of entry and the response of the host. Treatment includes streptomycin, chloramphenicol, and tetracycline. Recovery produces lifelong immunity. A vaccine is available. Also called **deerfly fever, rabbit fever.**

-tumescence, a combining form meaning a 'swelling': *detumescence, intumescence, tumescence.*

tumor, **1.** a swelling or enlargement occurring in inflammatory conditions. **2.** Also called **neoplasm.** a new growth of tissue characterized by progressive, uncontrolled proliferation of cells. The tumor may be localized or invasive, benign or malignant. A tumor may be named for its location, for its cellular makeup, or for the person who first identified it.

tumor albus, a white swelling occurring in a tuberculous bone or joint.

tumoricide (tumor′isaid), a substance capable of destroying a tumor. — **tumoricidal,** *adj.*

tumorigenesis (tu′mərɪjen′əsɪs), the process of imitating and promoting the development of a tumor. Compare **carcinogenesis, oncogenesis, sarcomagenesis.** — **tumorigenic,** *adj.*

tungsten (W), a metallic element. Its atomic number is 74; its atomic weight is 183.85. It has the highest melting point of all metals.

tunica vasculosa bulbi. See **uvea.**

tuning fork, a small metal instrument consisting of a stem and two prongs that produces a constant pitch when either prong is struck. It is used in auditory tests of nerve function and of air and bone conduction.

turban tumor, a benign neoplasm consisting of multiple pink or maroon nodules that may cover the entire scalp and may also occur on the trunk and extremities. The growth is apparently familial and often recurs after excision.

turbidimetry (tər′bɪdɪm′ɪtri), measurement of the turbidity (cloudiness) of a solution or suspension in which the amount of transmitted light is quantified with a spectrophotometer or estimated by visual comparison with solutions of known turbidity.

turbinate (tər′bɪnɪt), **1.** of or pertaining to a scroll shape. **2.** the concha nasalis.

turgid (tər′jɪd), swollen, hard, and congested, usually as a result of an accumulation of fluid. — **turgor,** *n.*

turgor (tər′gər), the normal resiliency of the skin caused by the outward pressure of the cells and interstitial fluid. Dehydration results in decreased skin turgor, manifested by lax skin which, when grasped and raised between two fingers, slowly returns to a position level with the adjacent tissue. Marked edema or ascites results in increased turgor manifested by smooth, taut, shiny skin that cannot be grasped and raised. An evaluation of the turgor of the skin is an essential part of physical assessment.

turista (turis′tə). See **traveler's diarrhea.**

turnbuckle cast, an orthopedic device used to encase and immobilize the entire trunk, one arm to the elbow, and the opposite leg to the knee. It is constructed of plaster of Paris or fiberglass and incorporates hinges as part of its design in the treatment of scoliosis. The hinges are placed at the level of the apex of the curvature. Employed for preoperative and postoperative positioning, it is used less frequently than the Risser cast. An adaptation of the turnbuckle cast is used occasionally as a hyperextension cast for the treatment of kyphosis or kyphoscoliosis.

Turner's sign. See **Grey Turner's sign.**

Turner's syndrome, a chromosomal anomaly seen in about one in 3,000 live female births, characterized by the absence of one X chromosome, congenital ovarian failure, genital hypoplasia, cardiovascular anomalies, dwarfism, short metacarpals, "shield chest," extosis of tibia, and underdeveloped breasts, uterus, and vagina. Spatial disorientation and moderate degrees of learning disorders are common. Treatment includes hormone therapy (estrogens, androgens, pituitary growth hormone) and, often, surgical correction of cardiovascular anomalies and the webbing of the neck skin. Also called **Bonnevie-Ullrich syndrome, monosomy X.**

turricephaly (tər'əsef'əli). See **oxycephaly.**

-tuse, 1. a combining form meaning 'dull or blunt': *obtuse.* **2.** a combining form meaning 'to beat or thrust': *contuse.*

Tussionex, a trade name for a fixed-combination drug containing an antitussive (hydrocodone bitartrate) and an antihistamine (phenyltoloxamine citrate).

TV, abbreviation for **tidal volume.**

T wave, the component of the cardiac cycle shown on an electrocardiogram as a short, inverted, U-shaped curve following the ST segment. It represents repolarization, the last phase of the cardiac cycle as the heart recovers from contraction and prepares to begin the cycle again with atrial depolarization during the P wave.

twelfth nerve. See **hypoglossal nerve.**

24-hour-clock system, a method of designating time by using the numerical sequence from 00 to 23 for the hours and the numbers 00 to 59 for the minutes in a daily cycle beginning with 0000 (midnight) and ending with 2359 (one minute before the following midnight). The system provides a clear distinction between prenoon and afternoon time without requiring the designations A.M. and P.M.

twilight sleep, *Obsolete.* light anesthesia obtained by the parenteral administration of a mixture of morphine and scopolamine to reduce pain and obtund recall in childbirth.

twin, either of two offspring born of the same pregnancy and developed from either a single ovum or from two ova that were released from the ovary simultaneously and fertilized at the same time. The incidence of twin births is approximately one in 80 pregnancies. Kinds of twins include **conjoined twins, dizygotic twins, interlocked twins, monozygotic twins, Siamese twins, unequal twins.** See also **Hellin's law.**

twin monster. See **double monster.**

twinning, 1. the development of two or more fetuses during the same pregnancy, either spontaneously or through external intervention for experimental purposes in animals. **2.** the duplication of like structures or parts by division.

two-way catheter, a catheter that has a double lumen, one channel for injection of medication or fluids and the other for removal of fluid or specimens.

tybamate (tai'bəmeit), a minor tranquilizer.
■ INDICATIONS: It is prescribed to reduce anxiety and tension in psychoneurotic disorders.
■ CONTRAINDICATIONS: Acute intermittent porphyria or known hypersensitivity to this drug or related compounds, as carisoprodol, mebutamate, or meprobamate, prohibits its use.
■ ADVERSE EFFECTS: Among the most serious effects are drowsiness or dizziness. Rashes and other reactions also may occur.

Tybatran, a trade name for a tranquilizer (tybamate).

Tylenol, a trade name for an analgesic and antipyretic (acetaminophen).

tyloxapol (tailok'səpol), a respiratory tract detergent prescribed for bronchitis, emphysema, pulmonary abcess, bronchiectasis, or atelectasis.

tympanic (tımpæn'ık), of or pertaining to a structure that resonates when struck; drumlike, as a **tympanic abdomen** that resonates on percussion because the intestines are distended with gas. – **tympanum,** *n., pl.* **tympana;** *genitive* **tympani.**

tympanic antrum, a relatively large, irregular cavity in the superior anterior portion of the mastoid process of the temporal bone, communicating with the mastoid air cells and lined by the extension of the mucous membrane of the tympanic cavity. The bony tegmen tympani separates the tympanic antrum from the middle fossa of the cranial cavity, and the lateral semicircular canal of the internal ear projects into the antrum. See also **mastoid process.**

tympanic cavity. See **middle ear.**

tympanic membrane, a thin, semitransparent membrane in the middle ear that transmits sound vibrations to the internal ear by means of the auditory ossicles. It is nearly oval in form, with a vertical diameter of about 10 mm, and separates the tympanic cavity from the bottom of the external acoustic meatus. Also called **ear drum, membrana tympani.**

tympanic reflex, the reflection of a beam of light shining on the eardrum. In a normal ear a bright, wedge-shaped reflection is seen; its apex is at the end of the malleus, and its base is at the anterior inferior margin of the eardrum. In disorders of the middle ear or eardrum, this shape may be distorted. Also called **light reflex.**

tympanoplasty (tımpæn'əplæs'ti), any of several operative procedures on the eardrum or ossicles of the middle ear, designed to restore or improve hearing in patients with conductive deafness. These operations may be used to repair a perforated eardrum, for otosclerosis, dislocation of the incus, or necrosis of one of the small bones of the middle ear. See also **myringoplasty.**

-type, a combining form meaning a 'representative form or class': *lysotype, serotype, somatotype.*

type I hyperlipidemia, a familial form of primary lipoproteinemia. A rare disease transmitted as a recessive trait, it is characterized by the accumulation of triglycerides in the blood stream, resulting in recurrent bouts of acute pancreatitis. The symptoms begin in childhood. The disease is caused by a deficiency in the activity of an enzyme, lipoprotein lipase, that normally removes triglycerides from the blood. The accumulation of triglycerides is proportional to the amount of dietary fat. Treatment is primarily dietary; both saturated and unsaturated fats are restricted to amounts that produce less than 500 mg/100 ml of blood, evaluated after an overnight fast. Also called **exogenous hyperlipemia.**

type II hyperlipoproteinemia. See **familial hypercholesterolemia.**

type I hypersensitivity. See **anaphylactic hypersensitivity.**

type II hypersensitivity. See **cytotoxic hypersensitivity.**

type III hypersensitivity. See **immune complex hypersensitivity.**

type IV hypersensitivity. See **cell-mediated immune response.**

typhlitis (tɪflaiʹtɪs), *Obsolete.* appendicitis.

typhlo-, **1.** a combining form meaning 'pertaining to the cecum': *typhlocolitis, typhlostenosis, typhlostomy.* **2.** a combining form meaning 'pertaining to blindness': *typhlolexia, typhlology, typhlosis.*

-typhoid, **1.** a combining form meaning a '(specified) form of typus': *bronchotyphoid, meningotyphoid, nephrotyphoid.* **2.** a combining form meaning 'of or resembling typhus': *antityphoid, paratyphoid, posttyphoid.* Also **-typhoidal.**

typhoid fever, a bacterial infection usually caused by *Salmonella typhi,* transmitted by contaminated milk, water, or food and characterized by headache, delirium, cough, watery diarrhea, rash, and a high fever. Compare **cholera, paratyphoid fever, salmonellosis.**

■ OBSERVATIONS: The incubation period may be as long as 60 days. Characteristic maculopapular rosy spots are scattered over the skin of the abdomen. Splenomegaly and leukopenia develop first. The diagnosis is made by bacteriologic culture of blood and stool and by a rising titer of agglutinins in the Widal test. The disease is serious and may be fatal. Complications include intestinal hemorrhage or perforation and thrombophlebitis. The disease is spread by food, milk, or water contaminated by human excreta. Some people who recover from the disease continue to be carriers and excrete the organism, spreading the disease.

■ INTERVENTION: Chloramphenicol, ampicillin, amoxicillin, and trimethoprim-sulfamethoxazole are all useful in treatment. Prolonged administration of antibiotics or cho-

lecystectomy may eliminate the carrier state. Typhoid vaccine gives some protection but requires annual booster doses for best effect.

■ NURSING CONSIDERATIONS: To lower the temperature, sponge baths are preferred to salicylates because salicylates may cause hypothermia or hypotension. Laxatives and enemas are contraindicated because of the danger of bowel perforation. Proper disposal of human wastes is essential to prevent epidemics, and carriers should not be permitted to prepare food.

typhoid pellagra, a form of pellagra in which the symptoms also include continued high temperatures.

typhoid vaccine, a bacterial vaccine prepared from an inactivated, dried strain of *Salmonella typhi.*

■ INDICATION: It is prescribed for immunization against typhoid fever.

■ CONTRAINDICATIONS: Acute infection or concomitant use of corticosteroids prohibits its use.

■ ADVERSE EFFECTS: Among the more serious adverse reactions are anaphylaxis and pain and inflammation at the site of injection.

typhus, any of a group of acute infectious diseases caused by various species of *Rickettsia* and usually transmitted from infected rodents to man by the bites of lice, fleas, mites, or ticks. These diseases are all characterized by headache, chills, fever, malaise, and a maculopapular rash. Kinds of typhus are **epidemic typhus, murine typhus, scrub typhus.** See also **Brill-Zinsser disease.**

typhus vaccine, any one of three vaccines, each of which is prepared for the different rickettsial organisms that cause epidemic typhus, murine typhus, or Brill-Zinsser disease.

■ INDICATION: Each of the vaccines is prescribed for immunization against a form of typhus.

■ CONTRAINDICATIONS: Acute infection, debilitating disease, concomitant use of corticosteroids, or hypersensitivity to eggs prohibits its use.

■ ADVERSE EFFECTS: Among the most serious adverse reactions are anaphylaxis and various allergic reactions. Pain at the site of injection also may occur.

-typia, a combining form meaning '(condition of) conformity to type': *atypia, ectypia, zelotypia.*

typing, the process of ascertaining the classification of a specimen of blood, tissue, or other substance. See also **blood typing, tissue typing.**

tyramine, an amino acid synthesized in the body from the essential acid tyrosine. Tyramine stimulates the release of the catecholamines epinephrine and norepinephrine. It is important that people taking monoamine oxidase inhibitors avoid the ingestion of foods and beverages containing tyramine, including beer, wine, broad beans, some cheeses (brie, cheddar, Camembert, Stilton), Chianti wine, chicken livers, caffeine, chocolate, cola drinks, liver, herring, tea, yogurt, and yeast. See also **adrenergic drug, amine, catecholamine, epinephrine, norepinephrine, vasoconstriction.**

tyro-, a combining form meaning 'pertaining to cheese': *tyrogenous, tyroid, tyrometosis.*

tyroma (taɪrou'mə), *pl.* **tyromas, tyromata.** a new growth or nodule with a cascous or cheesy consistency.

tyromatosis (taɪ'roumətou'sɪs), a process in which necrotic tissue is broken down and degenerates to a granular, amorphous, caseous mass.

tyrosine (taɪ'rəsin'), an amino acid synthesized in the body from the essential amino acid phenylalanine. Tyrosine is found in most proteins and is a precursor of melanin and several hormones, including epinephrine and thyroxin. See also **amino acid, hormone, melanin.**

tyrosinemia (taɪ'rousɪni'miə), **1.** Also called a **neonatal tyrosinemia.** a benign, transient condition of the newborn, especially premature infants, in which an excessive amount of the amino acid tyrosine is found in the blood and urine. The disorder is caused by an anomaly in amino acid metabolism, usually delayed development of the enzymes necessary to metabolize tyrosine, and is controlled by dietary measures and vitamin C therapy. The metabolic defect disappears with treatment, or it may disappear spontaneously. **2.** Also called **hereditary**

tyrosinemia. an hereditary disorder involving an inborn error of metabolism of the amino acid tyrosine. The condition, which is transmitted as an autosomal recessive trait, is caused by an enzyme deficiency and results in liver failure or hepatic cirrhosis, renal tubular defects that can lead to renal rickets and renal glycosuria, generalized aminoaciduria, and mental retardation. Treatment consists of a diet low in tyrosine and phenylalanine and high in doses of vitamin C.

tyrosinosis (taɪ'rousɪnou'sɪs), a condition resulting from a defect in amino acid metabolism and characterized by the excretion of an excessive amount of parahydroxyphenylpyruvic acid, an intermediate product of tyrosine, in the urine. See also **tyrosinemia.**

Tyzine, a trade name for an alpha-adrenergic drug (tetrahydrozoline hydrochloride).

Tzanck test (tsæŋk), a microscopic examination of cellular material from skin lesions in order to help diagnose certain vesicular diseases. The tissue is scraped from the base of a vesicle, placed on a slide, and stained with Wright's or Giemsa's stain. Multinucleated giant cells are diagnostic of herpesvirus or varicella. Typical pemphigus and other cells can also be identified.

U

u, symbol sometimes used to stand for **micron** (properly μ), as in u/ml, representing μ/ml.

U, symbol for **uranium**.

UICC, abbreviation for *International Union Against Cancer, Union internacional contra el cancer, Union internationale contre le cancer, Unio internationalis contra cancrum, Unione internazionale contro il cancro.*

-ular, 1. a combining form meaning 'pertaining to' something specified: *appendicular, molecular, pedicular.* 2. a combining form meaning 'resembling' something specified: *circular, globular, tubular.*

ulcer, a circumscribed, craterlike lesion of the skin or mucous membrane resulting from necrosis that accompanies some inflammatory, infectious, and malignant processes. An ulcer may be shallow, involving only the epidermis, as in phemphigus, or deep, as in a rodent ulcer. Some kinds of ulcer are **decubitus ulcer, peptic ulcer, serpent ulcer.** – ulcerate, *v.,* ulcerative, *adj.*

ulcerative blepharitis, a form of blepharitis in which a staphylococcal infection of the follicles of the eyelashes and glands of the eyelids results in sticky crusts forming on the lid margins. If the crusts are pulled off, the skin beneath bleeds. Tiny pustules develop in the follicles of the eyelashes and break down to form shallow ulcers. Other symptoms include burning, itching, swelling, and redness of the eyelids; a loss of eyelashes; irritation of the conjunctiva with tearing; photophobia; and gluing together of the eyelids during sleep by the dried secretions. Compare **nonulcerative blepharitis.**

ulcerative colitis, a chronic, episodic, inflammatory disease of the large intestine and rectum, characterized by profuse watery diarrhea containing varying amounts of blood, mucus, and pus.
■ OBSERVATIONS: The attacks of diarrhea are accompanied by tenesmus, severe abdominal pain, fever, chills, anemia, and weight loss. Children with the disease may suffer retarded physical growth. The debilitating symptoms often prevent persons with ulcerative colitis from carrying on the normal activities of daily living. Diagnosis of the disease is based upon clinical signs, the results of barium x rays of the colon, and colonoscopy with biopsy. It is often difficult to differentiate between ulcerative colitis and Crohn's disease.
■ INTERVENTION: Medical treatment with corticosteroids or other anti-inflammatory agents may help to control the symptoms in some persons. Those with severe disease or life-threatening complications usually require surgery. Total proctocolectomy with ileostomy is a permanent cure for ulcerative colitis.
■ NURSING CONSIDERATIONS: Some of the many systemic complications of ulcerative colitis include peripheral arthritis, ankylosing spondylitis, kidney and liver disease, and inflammation of the eyes, skin, and mouth. Persons with severe disease may develop toxic megacolon, a dangerous complication which may lead to perforation of the bowel, septicemia, and death. Ulcerative colitis also carries an increased risk of developing cancer of the colon, and periodic colonoscopy is performed to rule out this complication. A person with ulcerative colitis is suffering from a chronic, life-threatening illness, and requires frequent evidence of support and understanding during prolonged hospitalization.

ule-. See ulo-, def.2.

-ule. 1. See -ulum. 2. See -ulus.

-ulent, a combining form meaning 'full of, characterized by': *feculent, pulverulent, succulent.*

ulna, the bone on the medial or little finger side of the forearm, lying parallel with the radius. Its proximal end bulges into the olecranon and the coronoid processes and dips into the trochlear and the radial notches. The ulna articulates with the humerus and the radius. Also called **elbow bone.**

ulnar artery, a large artery branching from the brachial artery, supplying muscles in the forearm, wrist, and hand; arising near the elbow, it passes obliquely in a distal direction to become the superficial palmar arch. It has nine branches: four in the forearm, two in the wrist, and three in the hand. The forearm branches are the anterior ulnar recurrent, posterior ulnar recurrent, common interosseous, and muscular. The two branches in the wrist are the palmar carpal and dorsal carpal. The branches in the hand are the deep palmar, superficial palmar arch, and common palmar digital.

ulnar nerve, one of the terminal branches of the brachial plexus that arises on each side from the medial cord of the plexus and supplies the muscles and the skin on the ulnar side of the forearm and the hand. It can be easily palpated as the 'funny bone' of the elbow as it courses along the groove between the olecranon process and the medial epicondyle of the humerus. It first passes medial to the axillary artery and the brachial artery to the middle of the arm, pierces the medial intermuscular septum, and follows along the medial head of the triceps to the olecranon. It descends into the forearm and in the distal portion on the ulnar side is covered only by the skin and the fascia. Just above the wrist it gives off a large dorsal branch and continues into the hand where it gives off the digital and the muscular branches. The ulnar nerve usually has no branches above the elbow. Below the elbow its branches are the articular branches to the elbow joint, two muscular branches, the palmar cutaneous branch, the dorsal branch, the palmar branch, the superficial branch, and the deep branch. Compare **median nerve, musculocutaneous nerve, radial nerve.**

ulo-, **1.** a combining form meaning 'pertaining to a scar or cicatrix': *ulodermatitis, uloid, ulotomy.* **2.** Also **ule-.** a combining form meaning 'pertaining to the gums or gingivae': *ulocase, ulorrhagia, ulotripsis.*

ulocarcinoma (yu'lɔukar'sɪnɔu'mə), *pl.* **ulocarcinomas, ulocarcinomata.** any malignant neoplastic disease of the gums that is classified as a carcinoma.

ultra-, a combining form meaning 'beyond, farther, beyond a certain limit': *ultragaseous, ultrasound, ultravirus.*

Ultracef, a trade name for the cephalosporin antibiotic (cefadroxil monohydrate).

ultracentrifuge (əl'trəsen'trɪfyuj), a high-speed centrifuge with a rotation rate fast enough to produce sedimentation of viruses, even in blood plasma. It is used in many kinds of biochemical analyses, including the measurement and separation of some proteins and viruses. Use of an attached microscope may make it possible to see the sediment.

Ultralente Iletin, a trade name for insulin zinc suspension.

ultralente insulin. See **long-acting insulin.**

ultramicroscopy (əl'trəmaɪkros'kəpi). See **darkfield microscopy.**

ultrasonic cardiography. See **echocardiography.**

ultrasonography (əl'trəsonog'rəfi), the process of representing deep structures of the body by measuring and recording the reflection of pulsed or continuous high-frequency sound waves. It is valuable in many medical situations, including the diagnosis of fetal abnormalities, length of gestation of a fetus, gallstones, heart defects, and tumors. Also called **sonography.**

ultrasound, sound waves at the very high frequency of over 20,000 vibrations per second. Ultrasound has many medical applications, including fetal monitoring, imaging of internal organs, and, at an extremely high frequency, cleaning dental and surgical instruments.

ultraviolet, light beyond the range of human vision, at the short end of the spectrum. It occurs naturally in sunlight; it burns and tans the skin and converts precursors in the skin to vitamin D. Ultraviolet lamps are used in the control of infectious, airborne bacteria and viruses and in the treatment of psoriasis and other skin conditions. Black light is ultraviolet light used in fluoroscopy. See also **angstrom, light, radiation, spectrum.**

ultraviolet microscopy. See **fluorescent microscopy.**

ultraviolet radiation, a range of electromagnetic waves extending from the violet or short-wavelength end of the spectrum to the beginning of the x-ray spectrum. Near-ultraviolet radiation covers a range of wavelengths from 380 to 320 millimicrons; middle-ultraviolet radiation covers a range from 320 to 280 millimicrons; and far-ultraviolet radiation extends from 280 to about 10 millimicrons. About 5 per cent of the radiation from the sun is in the ultraviolet range, but little of this type of energy reaches the earth because much is absorbed by oxygen and ozone in the atmosphere. Window glass also absorbs this radiation. Artificial sources of ultraviolet radiation include the iron arc, the carbon arc, and the mercury-vapor arc. For maximum transmission, quartz or fluorite envelopes, which are transparent to ultraviolet radiation, must be used instead of glass. Prisms and lenses used for work in the ultraviolet region must also be made of quartz or fluorite or of synthetic halides. In medicine, ultraviolet radiation is used in the treatment of rickets and certain skin conditions. Milk and some other foods become activated with vitamin D when exposed to this type of energy. Ultraviolet radiation also causes fluorescence and phosphorescence, a useful characteristic in such diverse applications as lighting and the identification of minerals.

-ulum, a combining form meaning 'small one': *ovulum, scutulum, speculum.* Also **-ule.**

-ulus, a combining form meaning 'small one': *homunculus, nodulus, ramulus.* Also **-ule.**

-um, a combining form marking singular nouns: *cerebellum, dextrum, quantum.*

umbilical (əmbɪl'ɪkəl), **1.** of or pertaining to the umbilicus. **2.** of or pertaining to the umbilical cord.

umbilical catheterization, a procedure in which a radiopaque catheter is passed through an umbilical artery to provide a newborn infant with parenteral fluid, to obtain blood samples, or both, or through the umbilical vein for an exchange transfusion or the emergency administration of drugs, fluids, or volume expanders.

■ METHOD: Within an hour of the insertion of the catheter the position of the tip is validated by x-ray examination. The infant is maintained in a neutral thermal environment as parenteral fluids are delivered by an infusion pump; the rate of flow is checked hourly, and the intravenous bottle is never allowed to empty. All connections to the umbilical line are checked every 30 to 60 minutes, and only grounded electrical equipment is used on or near the infant. At hourly intervals the young patient is repositioned, and the cardiac and respiratory rates are monitored; the auxiliary temperature is taken every two to three hours, and the pedal pulses are checked every two to four hours. The condition of the cord is observed every two to three hours for signs of infection, as redness, edema, or drainage at the catheter insertion site; the intravenous tubing is retaped when required, the cord dressing is changed, and antibiotic or antiseptic ointment is applied as ordered. If the umbilical line is displaced, pressure is quickly applied to the cord with a sterile four-by-four-inch gauze, and an associate is delegated to notify the physician immediately. Fluid intake and output are measured. The infant is observed for oliguria or anuria, signs of vasospasm, as blanching, mottling, or darkening of the legs and absence of peripheral pulses, and for evidence of sepsis, hemorrhage, or oozing from the catheter insertion site, thromboembolism, and abdominal distention and vomiting, which may indicate necrotizing enterocolitis.

■ NURSING ORDERS: The nurse provides ongoing care, monitoring the catheterized infant for any signs of complications, which are promptly reported. The family is included in the care of the infant as much as possible.

■ OUTCOME CRITERIA: Umbilical catheterization can be an effective method of administering therapeutic fluids and agents or of obtaining diagnostic blood samples from a high-risk newborn, but great care is required in inserting and monitoring the tube.

umbilical cord, a flexible structure connecting the umbilicus with the placenta in the gravid uterus and giving passage to the umbilical arteries and vein. In the newborn it is about 2 feet long and ½ inch in diameter. First formed during the fifth week of pregnancy, it contains the yolk sac and the body stalk with the enclosed allantois. Also called the **chorda umbilicalis, funiculus umbilicalis.** See also **cord.**

umbilical duct. See **vitelline duct.**

umbilical fissure, a groove on the inferior surface of the liver that holds the ligamentum teres and separates the right and left lobes of the liver.

umbilical fistula, an abnormal passage from the umbilicus to the intestine or more frequently to the remnant of the canal in the median umbilical ligament that connects the fetal bladder with the allantois.

umbilical hernia, a soft, skin-covered protrusion of intestine and omentum through a weakness in the abdominal wall around the umbilicus. It usually closes spontaneously within one to two years, although large hernias may require surgical closure.

umbilical vein, one of a pair of embryonic vessels that return the blood from the placenta and fuse to form a single trunk in the body stalk. They remain separate for a short time in the embryo, opening into the sinus venosus. Development of the fetal liver breaks the connection between the umbilical veins and the sinus venosus, whereupon the right umbilical vein shrivels and disappears. The

left umbilical vein remains attached to the placenta, and is contained, with the fetal arteries, in the umbilical cord. After birth, the left umbilical vein and the ductus venosus atrophy and form respectively the ligamentum teres and the ligamentum venosum of the liver.

umbilical vesicle, a pear-shaped structure formed from the yolk sac at about the fourth week of prenatal development that protrudes into the cavity of the chorion and connects to the developing embryo by the yolk stalk at the region of the future midgut.

umbilicus, the point on the abdomen at which the umbilical cord joined the fetal abdomen. In most adults it is marked by a depression; in some it is marked by a small protrusion of skin. Also called **belly button, navel.**

unciform bone. See **hamate bone.**

uncompensated gluteal gait. See **Trendelenburg gait.**

unconditioned response, a normal, instinctive, unlearned reaction to a stimulus; one that occurs naturally and is not acquired by association and training. Also called **inborn reflex, instinctive reflex, unconditioned reflex.** Compare **conditioned response.**

unconscious, 1. unaware of the surrounding environment; insensible; incapable of responding to sensory stimuli. 2. (in psychiatry) the part of the mental function in which thoughts, ideas, emotions, or memories are outside awareness and not subject to ready recall. It contains data that have never been conscious or that were conscious at one time, usually for a brief period, and later repressed. Compare **preconscious.** See also **collective unconscious, personal unconscious.**

unconsciousness, a state of complete or partial unawareness or lack of response to sensory stimuli as a result of injury, shock, illness, or other bodily disorder, as alcoholic excess, narcotic overdose, poisoning, and sunstroke. Various degrees of unconsciousness can occur during stupor, fugue, catalepsy, and dream states. See also **coma.**

(See next page for table)

unction (əŋk′shən). See **ointment.**

undecylenic acid, an antifungal.

■ INDICATIONS: It is prescribed in the treatment of athlete's foot and ringworm.

■ CONTRAINDICATIONS: Known hypersensitivity to this drug prohibits its use. It is not used in the eyes or on mucous membranes.

■ ADVERSE EFFECTS: Among the more serious adverse effects are skin irritation and hypersensitivity reactions.

underwater exercise, any physical activity performed in a pool or large tub, as a Hubbard tank, where the buoyancy of the water facilitates the movement of weak or injured muscles. See also **exercise.**

underweight, less than normal in body weight after adjustment for height, body build, and age.

undescended testis. See **cryptorchidism, monorchidism.**

Possible causes of unconsciousness

Hypoxia (decreased oxygen to brain)

1. Respiratory insufficiency
    Airway obstruction from foreign body, secretions
    Pneumothorax
    Spinal cord injury
2. Shock
    Cardiogenic: cardiac arrest
    Hypovolemic: hemorrhage

Metabolical (chemical brain depressants)

1. Extrinsic
    a. Drugs: alcohol, narcotics, barbiturates, antihistamines, tranquilizers
    b. Poisons: carbon monoxide, carbon tetrachloride, hydrocarbons, methane gas
2. Intrinsic
    a. Ketones: diabetic ketoacidosis, starvation
    b. Glucose: hypoglycemia, hyperglycemia
    c. Ammonia: liver failure
    d. Urea: kidney failure
    e. Hormonal hypofunction: hypothyroidism, Addison's disease
    f. Electrolyte imbalance: sodium, potassium, calcium, hydrogen ions

Brain pathology

1. Trauma: concussion, brainstem contusion, intracranial hematoma
2. Seizures: epilepsy, tumors, idiopathology
3. Cerebral vascular accident: cerebral hemorrhage, thrombosis
4. Tumors: benign, malignant
5. Infections: meningitis, encephalitis

---

undifferentiated cell leukemia. See **stem cell leukemia.**

undifferentiated malignant lymphoma, a lymphoid neoplasm containing many large stem cells that have large nuclei, small amounts of pale cytoplasm, and borders that are not well defined. Also called **reticulosarcoma, stem cell lymphoma.**

undifferentiated schizophrenia. See **acute schizophrenia.**

undisplaced fracture, a bone break in which cracks in the osseous tissue may radiate in several directions without the separation or displacement of fragmented sections.

undulant fever. See **brucellosis.**

unengaged head, a floating fetal head. See **engagement.** See also **ballottement.**

unequal cleavage, mitotic division of the fertilized ovum into blastomeres that are larger near the yolk portion of protoplasm, or vegetal pole, and smaller near the nucleus, or animal pole. Compare **equal cleavage.**

unequal twins, two nonjoined fetuses born of the same pregnancy in which only one of the pair is fully formed, with the other showing various degrees of developmental defects.

ungual phalanx. See **distal phalanx.**

unguent (əng′gwənt). See **ointment.**

unguis (əng′gwis), *pl.* **ungues.** See **nail.** — **ungual,** *adj.*

uni-, a combining form meaning 'one': *unibasal, uniceps, unifocal.*

UNICEF, abbreviation for **United Nations International Children's Emergency Fund.**

unicellular reproduction, the formation of a new organism from a female egg that has not been fertilized; parthenogenesis.

unicentric blastoma. See **blastoma.**

unidose. See **unit dose.**

unification model, a theoretical framework based on the close relationship of nursing education and clinical nursing service at the University of Rochester. The faculty of the school of nursing hold joint appointments to the school and the hospital, teaching nursing students and providing clinical leadership in nursing service in the hospital. See also **joint appointment.**

unilateral long leg spica cast, an orthopedic cast applied to immobilize one leg and the trunk of the body cranially as far as the nipple line. It is used to treat a fractured femur or for the correction or the maintenance of the correction of a hip deformity. Compare **bilateral long leg spica cast, one-and-a-half spica cast.**

unilateral papalysis. See **hemiplegia.**

uniovular, developing from a single ovum as in monozygotic twins as contrasted with dizygotic twins. Also called **monovular.** Compare **binovular.**

uniovular twins. See **monozygotic twins.**

Unipen, a trade name for an antibacterial (nafcillin sodium).

unipolar lead, **1.** an electrocardiographic conductor in which the exploring electrode is placed on the precordium or a limb while the indifferent electrode is in the central terminal. **2.** *Informal.* a tracing produced by such a lead on an electrocardiograph.

unit, **1.** a single item. **2.** a quantity designated as a standard of measurement.

unitary man conceptual framework, a complex theory in nursing that emphasizes the importance of holistic health care and an understanding of "man" in relation to the universal environment.

unit dose, a method of preparing medications in which individual doses of patient medications are prepared by the pharmacy and delivered in individual labeled packets to the patient's unit to be administered by the nurses on the ordered schedule. Also called **unidose.**

United Nations International Children's Emergency Fund (UNICEF), a fund established by the General Assembly of the United Nations in 1946 to aid children in devastated areas of the world. It is funded by contributions from the member nations and acts to prevent disease, including tuberculosis, whooping cough, and diphtheria, and provides food and clothing to needy children in more than 50 countries. In 1953, UNICEF was made a permanent organization of the United Nations.

United States Pharmacopeia (USP), a compendium, recognized officially by the Federal Food, Drug, and Cosmetic Act, that contains descriptions, uses, strengths, and standards of purity for selected drugs and for all of their forms of dosage.

United States Public Health Service (USPHS), an agency of the federal government responsible for the control of the arrival from abroad of any people, goods, or substances that may affect the health of U.S. citizens. The agency sets standards for the domestic handling and processing of food and the manufacture of serums, vaccines, cosmetics, and drugs. It supports and performs research, aids localities in times of disaster and epidemics, and provides medical care for certain groups of Americans. The agency employs physicians, nurses, social workers, laboratory technicians, and many other specified health workers.

univalent (yu'nɪveil'ənt), the capacity of one atom of a chemical element to attract one atom of hydrogen or to displace one atom of hydrogen. See also **valence.**

univalent antiserum. See **antiserum.**

universal antidote, a mixture of 50 per cent activated charcoal, 25 per cent magnesium oxide, and 25 per cent tannic acid, formerly thought to be useful as an antidote for most types of acid, heavy metal, alkaloid, and glycoside poisons. It is now believed that the mixture is no more effective than activated charcoal given with water.

universal donor, a person with blood of type O, Rh factor negative. Such blood may be used for emergency transfusion with minimal risk of incompatibility. See also **blood donor, blood group, transfusion.**

Unna's paste boot (u'nəz), a dressing for varicose ulcers formed by applying a layer of a gelatin-glycerin-zinc oxide paste to the leg and then a spiral bandage which is covered with successive coats of paste to produce a rigid boot.

unsaturated alcohol, an alcohol derived from an unsaturated hydrocarbon, as an alkene or olefin.

unsaturated fatty acid, any of a number of glyceryl esters of certain organic acids in which some of the atoms are joined by double or triple valence bonds. These bonds are easily split in chemical reactions and other substances are joined to them. Monounsaturated fatty acids have only one double or triple bond per molecule and are found in such foods as fowl, almonds, pecans, cashew nuts, peanuts, and olive oil. Polyunsaturated fatty acids have more than one double or triple bond per molecule and are found in fish, corn, walnuts, sunflower seeds, soybeans, cottonseeds, and safflower oil. Diets high in polyunsaturated fatty acids and low in saturated fatty acids have been correlated with low serum cholesterol levels in some study populations. Compare **saturated fatty acid.**

unsocialized aggressive reaction, a behavior disorder of childhood characterized by overt and covert hostility, disobedience, physical and verbal aggression, vengefulness, quarrelsome behavior and destructiveness, often manifested in such acts as lying, stealing, temper tantrums, vandalism, and physical violence against others. The condition, which is more prevalent in boys than in girls, results typically from an unstable home environment that is characterized by harsh and inconsistent application of discipline, general frustration, rejection, marital discord, separation, or divorce. Punitive treatment is ineffective. Recommended psychotherapeutic techniques reinforce desirable behavioral patterns and attempt to modify unfavorable environmental conditions. If untreated, the condition may lead to antisocial personality disorder.

unstriated muscle. See **smooth muscle.**

upper extremity suspension, an orthopedic procedure used in the treatment of bone fractures and the correction of orthopedic abnormalities of the upper limbs. The procedure uses traction equipment, including metal frames, ropes, and pulleys to relieve the weight of the upper limb involved rather than to exert traction. Upper extremity suspension is usually unilateral but may also be used bilaterally in the postoperative, posttraumatic, or postreduction control of edema. Compare **balanced suspension, hyperextension suspension, lower extremity suspension.**

upper motor neuron paralysis, an injury to the lesion in the brain or spinal cord that causes damage to the cell bodies, or axons, or both, of the upper motor neurons, which extend from the cerebral centers to the cells in the spinal column. Clinical manifestations include increased muscle tone and spasticity of the muscles involved with little or no atrophy, hyperactive deep-tendon reflexes, diminished or absent superficial reflexes, the presence of pathological reflexes, as the Babinski and Hoffmann reflexes, and no local twitching of muscle groups. Compare **lower motor neuron paralysis.**

upper respiratory infection (URI). See **respiratory tract infection.**

upper respiratory tract, one of the two divisions of the respiratory system. The upper respiratory tract consists of the nose, the nasal cavity, the ethmoidal air cells, the frontal sinuses, the sphenoidal sinuses, the maxillary sinus, the larynx, and the trachea. The upper respiratory tract conducts air to and from the lungs and filters, moistens, and warms the air during each inspiration. Infection and irritation of the upper respiratory tract are common and often spread to the lower respiratory tract, where they may cause serious complications. See also **larynx, nose, trachea.** Compare **lower respiratory tract.**

ur-. See **uro-.**

uranium (U), a heavy, radioactive metallic element. Its atomic number is 92; its atomic weight is 238.03. Uranium is the heaviest of the natural elements. Isotopes of uranium are used in nuclear power plants to provide neutrons for the nuclear reactions that result in release of energy.

urano-, a combining form meaning 'pertaining to the palate': *uranoplasty, uranoplegia, uranoschism.*

urate (yur′eit), a salt of uric acid, normally present in the urine. See also **gout, uric acid.**

urban typhus. See **murine typhus.**

urea, a systemic osmotic diuretic and topical keratolytic.
■ INDICATIONS: It is prescribed to reduce cerebrospinal and intraocular fluid pressure and is used topically as a keratolytic agent.
■ CONTRAINDICATIONS: Severely impaired kidney function, active intracranial bleeding, marked dehydration, or liver damage prohibits its systemic use.
■ ADVERSE EFFECTS: Among the more serious adverse reactions are pain and necrosis at the site of injection, headache, gastrointestinal disturbances, and dizziness. There are no known severe reactions to topical use.

-urea, a combining form meaning a 'compound containing urea': *glycolylurea, plenylurea, solurea.*

Ureaphil, a trade name for an osmotic diuretic (urea).

Ureaplasma urealyticum, a sexually transmitted microorganism that is a common inhabitant of the urogenital systems of men and women in whom infection is asymptomatic. Neonatal death, prematurity, and perinatal morbidity are statistically associated with colonization of the chorionic surface of the placenta by *Ureaplasma urealyticum.* The mechanisms by which the unfavorable effects on pregnancy occur are not understood. There is no characteristic lesion in the fetus or newborn.

Urechline, a trade name for a cholinergic (bethanechol chloride).

uremia, 1. the presence of excessive amounts of urea and other nitrogenous waste products in the blood. 2. the abnormal condition of having an excessive amount of these substances in the blood, as occurs in renal failure. Also called **azotemia.**

uremic frost, a pale, frostlike deposit of white crystals on the skin owing to kidney failure and uremia. Urea compounds and other waste products of metabolism that cannot be excreted by the kidneys into the urine are excreted through the small superficial capillaries into the skin, where they collect on the surface.

Urestrin, a trade name for natural estrogenic substances.

-uret, a combining form designating a binary compound: *bromuret, phosphuret, sulphuret.*

ureter (yuri′tər), one of a pair of tubes, about 30 cm long, that carry the urine from the kidney into the bladder. They are thick-walled, vary in diameter along their length from 1 mm to 1 cm and are divided into an abdominal portion and a pelvic portion. The abdominal portion lies behind the peritoneum on the medial side of the psoas major and enters the pelvic cavity by crossing either the termination of the common iliac artery or the commencement of the external iliac artery. In men, the pelvic portion of the ureter runs caudal along the lateral wall of the pelvic cavity and reaches the lateral angle of the bladder just ventral to the upper tip of the seminal vesicle. In women, the pelvic portion of the ureter forms the posterior boundary of the ovarian fossa and runs medially and ventrally along the upper part of the vagina. The ureter enters the bladder through an oblique tunnel that functions as a valve to prevent backflow of urine into the ureter when the bladder contracts. Connecting with the kidneys, the ureters expand into funnel-shaped renal pelves which branch into calyces, each calyx containing a renal papilla. Urine draining through renal tubules drops into the papillae, passes through the calyces and the pelvis and down each ureter into the bladder. The openings of the ureters in the bladder lie at the lateral angles of the trigone, spaced about 2 cm apart when the bladder is empty, about 5 cm apart when the bladder is distended. Urine is pumped through the ureters by peristaltic waves that occur an average of three times a minute. Each ureter is composed of a fibrous, a muscular, and a mucous coat and is perfused by arterial branches of the renal, the testicular, the internal iliac, and the inferior vesical arteries. It is innervated by nerves derived from the inferior mesenteric, the testicular, and the pelvic plexi. —**ureteral,** *adj.*

ureteral dysfunction, a disturbance of the normal peristaltic flow of urine through a ureter, resulting from dysfunction of ureteral motor nerves. See also **megaloureter.**

ureteritis (yuri′tərai′tis), an inflammatory condition of a ureter caused by infection or by the mechanical irritation of a stone.

ureterocele (yuri′tərousil), a prolapse of the terminal portion of the ureter into the bladder. The condition may lead to obstruction of the flow of urine, hydronephrosis, and loss of renal function. Cystoscopy and pyelography reveal the prolapsed ureter. Surgical correction is performed to prevent permanent damage to the kidney. Compare **cystocele.**

urethra (yuri′thrə), a small tubular structure that drains urine from the bladder. In women, it is about 3 cm long and lies directly behind the symphysis pubis, anterior to the vagina. In men, it is about 20 cm long and begins at the bladder, passes through the center of the prostate gland, goes between two sheets of tissue connecting the pubic bones, and, finally, passes through the urinary meatus of the penis. In men, the urethra serves as a passageway for semen during ejaculation as well as a canal for urine during voiding. See also **ureter.**

urethral (yʊri′θrəl), of or pertaining to the urethra.

urethral papilla. See **papilla.**

urethritis (yʊr′ɪθraɪ′tɪs), an inflammatory condition of the urethra that is characterized by dysuria, usually the result of an infection in the bladder or kidneys. Medications, as a sulfonamide or other antibacterial, a urinary antiseptic, and an analgesic are usually prescribed once the causative organism is identified by bacteriologic culture of a urine specimen. See also **nongonococcal urethritis.**

urethro-, a combining form meaning 'pertaining to the urethra': *urethrocele, urethrocystitis, urethrophraxis.*

urethrocele (yʊri′θrəsil), (in women) a herniation of the urethra. It is characterized by a protusion of a segment of the urethra and the connective tissue surrounding it into the anterior wall of the vagina. The herniation may be slight and high in the vagina and only palpable on digital examination when the patient strains downward, or it may be large and low in the anterior wall with visible bulging at the vaginal introitus. A large cystocele may result in difficulty in voiding, some degree of incontinence, urinary tract infection, and dyspareunia. The condition may be congenital or acquired, secondary to obesity, parturition, and poor muscle tone. Surgical repair is the usual treatment.

Urex, a trade name for an antibacterial (methenamine hippurate).

-urgy, a combining form meaning the 'art of working with (specified) tools': *chemurgy, micrurgy, zymurgy.*

URI, abbreviation for **upper respiratory infection.** See **respiratory tract infection.**

-uria, 1. a combining form meaning the 'presence of a substance in the urine': *ammoniuria, calciuria, enzymuria.* 2. a combining form meaning '(condition of) possessing urine': *paruria, polyuria, pyuria.*

uric acid, a product of the metabolism of protein present in the blood and excreted in the urine. See also **gout, kidney, liver, purine, urine.**

uricaciduria (yʊr′ɪkæs′ɪdʊr′iə), a greater than normal amount of uric acid in the urine, often associated with urinary calculi or gout.

urico-, a combining form meaning 'pertaining to uric acid': *uricocholia, uricosuria, uricotelic.*

urinalysis, a physical, microscopic, or chemical examination of urine. The specimen is physically examined for color, turbidity, specific gravity and pH. Then it is spun in a centrifuge to allow collection of a small amount of sediment that is examined microscopically for blood cells, casts, crystals, pus, and bacteria. Chemical analysis may be performed for the identification and quantification of any of a large number of substances but most commonly for ketones, sugar, protein, and blood. The nurse collects the urine specimen for chemical analysis in the amount, at the time, and according to the directions of the specific laboratory.

urinary, of or pertaining to urine or to the formation of urine.

urinary bladder, the muscular membranous sac in the pelvis that stores urine for discharge through the urethra. Urine reaches its reservoir from the kidneys via the ureters.

urinary calculus, a calculus formed in any part of the urinary tract. Calculi may be large enough to cause an obstruction in the flow of urine or small enough to be passed with the urine. See also **calculus.**

urinary elimination, alteration in patterns, a nursing diagnosis accepted by the Fourth National Conference on the Classification of Nursing Diagnoses. The etiology of the diagnosis may involve several factors, including anatomical or physical obstruction, impairment of sensory innervation or muscular function of the bladder, or urinary tract infection. Among the characteristics that define the condition are dysuria, urinary frequency, hesitancy, incontinence, nocturia, and urgency of urination. See also **nursing diagnosis.**

urinary frequency, a greater than normal frequency of the urge to void without an increase in the total daily volume of urine. The condition is characteristic of inflammation in the bladder or urethra or of diminished bladder capacity or other structural abnormalities. Burning and urgency with increased frequency herald an infection of the urinary tract. Infection requires precise diagnosis and specific antibacterial medication; structural abnormality may require surgical correction. See also **cystitis, cystocele.**

urinary hesitancy, a decrease in the force of the stream of urine, often with difficulty in beginning the flow. Hesitancy is usually the result of an obstruction or stricture between the bladder and the urethral opening; in men it may indicate an enlargement of the prostate gland, in women, stenosis of the urethral opening. Cold, stress, dehydration, and various neurogenic and psychogenic factors are common causes of this condition.

urinary incontinence, involuntary passage of urine, with the failure of voluntary control over bladder and urethral sphincters. Among the causes are neurogenic bladder dysfunction resulting from lesions of the brain and spinal cord, a neoplasm of calculus in the bladder, multiple sclerosis, obstruction of the lower urinary tract, trauma, aging, and multiparity in women. In children, incontinence may be psychogenic or the result of allergy. Treatment with medication, surgery, or psychotherapy appropriate to the underlying cause is often effective.

urinary infection. See **urinary tract infection.**

urinary output, the total volume of urine excreted daily, normally between 700 and 2,000 ml. Various metabolic and renal diseases may change the normal urinary output, resulting in increased or decreased flow of urine. See also **anuria, oliguria, polyuria.**

urinary system assessment, an evaluation of the condition and functioning of the kidneys, bladder, ureters, and urethra and an investigation of concurrent and previous disorders that may be factors in abnormalities in the urinary system.

■ METHOD: In an interview the patient is asked if dysuria, frequency or burning on urination, dribbling, a decreased urinary stream, nocturia, stress incontinence, headache, back pain, or increased thirst has occurred. The color, odor, and amount of urine voided without a catheter and with one in place are determined. The patient's vital signs, any distention of the bladder, the condition of the skin, neurologic changes, and the location, duration, and character of pain, and the presence of bladder spasms are recorded. It is determined whether or not the patient has hypertension, diabetes, a venereal disease, vaginal or urethral drainage or discharge, or a history that includes cystitis, pyelonephritis, kidney stones, prostatectomy, renal surgery, a kidney transplant, or a venereal infection. The patient's sexual activity, use of coffee, tea, cola beverages, alcohol, perfumed soaps, feminine hygiene sprays, prescribed and over-the-counter medication, and habit of bathing in a tub or shower are ascertained. A family history of polycystic kidney disease, hypertension, diabetes, or cancer is noted in the assessment, together with laboratory studies of the specific gravity, casts, protein, red and white cells in the patient's urine, and the serum creatinine level. Diagnostic procedures may include cystoscopy, excretory and intravenous urography, renal angiography, retrograde studies, and x rays of the kidneys, ureters, and bladder.

■ NURSING ORDERS: The nurse interviews the patient, reports the objective data, and assembles the background information and the results of the diagnostic tests.

■ OUTCOME CRITERIA: A comprehensive assessment of the patient's urinary system aids the urologist in establishing the diagnosis.

urinary tract, all organs and ducts involved in the secretion and elimination of urine from the body.

urinary tract infection (UTI), an infection of one or more structures in the urinary tract. Most of these infections are caused by gram-negative bacteria, most commonly *Escherichia coli* or species of *Klebsiella, Proteus, Pseudomonas,* or *Enterobacter.* The condition is more common in women than in men and may be asymptomatic. Urinary tract infection is usually characterized by urinary frequency, burning, pain with voiding, and, if the infection is severe, visible blood and pus in the urine. Diagnosis of the cause and the location of the infection is made by microscopic examination of the sediment and supernatant portion of a centrifuged urine specimen, by physical examination of the patient, by bacteriologic culture of a specimen of urine, and, if necessary, by various radiologic techniques, as retrograde pyelography, or by cystoscopy. Treatment includes antibacterial, analgesic, and urinary antiseptic medications. Kinds of urinary tract infections include **cystitis, pyelonephritis, urethritis.**

urination, the act of passing urine. See also **micturition.**

urine, the fluid secreted by the kidneys, transported by the ureters, stored in the bladder, and voided through the urethra. Normal urine is clear, straw-colored, slightly acid, and has the characteristic odor of urea. The normal specific gravity of urine is between 1.005 and 1.030. Its normal constituents include water, urea, sodium chloride and potassium chloride, phosphates, uric acid, organic salts, and the pigment urobilin. Abnormal constituents indicative of disease include ketone bodies, protein, bacteria, blood, glucose, pus, and certain crystals. See also **bacteriuria, glycosuria, hematuria, ketonuria, proteinuria.**

urinoma (yur′ɪnou′mə), *pl.* **urinoma, urinomata.** a cyst filled with urine.

urinometer (yur′ɪnom′ɪtər), any device for determining the specific gravity of urine, including gravitometers and hydrometers.

Urised, a trade name for a urinary fixed-combination drug containing an antibacterial (methenamine), an analgesic (phenyl salicylate), anticholinergics (atropine sulfate and hyoscyamine), an antifungal (benzoic acid), and an antiseptic (methylene blue).

Urispas, a trade name for a smooth muscle relaxant (flavoxate hydrochloride).

Uristix, a trade name for paperstrips used in testing urine for sugar and albumin by dipping the stick into a urine sample. Bands containing reagents at the end of the strip change color depending on the amount of sugar or albumin present in the urine. The colors of the bands on the strips are evaluated by comparing them to a chart of normal and abnormal values.

Uritone, a trade name for a urinary antibacterial (methenamine).

uro-, ur-, urono-, a combining form meaning 'pertaining to urine, the urinary tract, or urination': *urocrisia, uromancy, uropterin.*

urobilin (yur′əbai′lɪn), a brown pigment formed by the oxidation of urobilinogen, normally found in feces and, in small amounts, in urine.

urobilinogen (yur′əbailɪn′əjɪn), a colorless compound formed in the intestine after the breakdown of bilirubin by bacteria. Some of this substance is excreted in feces, and some is resorbed and excreted again in bile or urine. See also **urobilin.**

Urobiotic, a trade name for a urinary, fixed-combination drug containing antibacterials (oxytetracycline hydrochloride and sulfamethizole) and an analgesic (phenazopyridine hydrochloride).

urogenital (yʊr'ɔujen'ɪtəl), of or pertaining to the urinary and the reproductive systems. Also called **genitourinary.**

urogenital sinus, one of the elongated cavities, formed by the division of the cloaca in early embryonic development, into which open the ureter, mesonephric and paramesonephric ducts, and bladder. It also gives rise to the vestibule, urethra, and part of the vagina in the female and part of the urethra in the male.

urogenital system, the urinary and genital organs and the associated structures that develop in the fetus to form the kidneys, the ureters, the bladder, the urethra, and the genital structures of the male and female. In women these are the ovaries, the uterine tubes, the uterus, the clitoris, and the vagina. In men these are the testes, the seminal vesicles, the seminal ducts, the prostate, and the penis. Also called **genitourinary system.**

urogram (yʊr'ɔgræm), an x-ray film of the urinary tract, obtained by urography. See also **pyelogram.**

urography (yʊrog'rəfi), any of a group of x-ray techniques used to examine the urinary system. A radiopaque substance is injected, and x rays are taken as the substance is passed through or excreted from the part of the system being studied. Some kinds of urography are **cystoscopic urography, intravenous pyelography, retrograde pyelography.**

urokinase (yʊr'ɔkɑɪ'neɪs), an enzyme, produced in the kidney and found in urine, that is a patent activator of the fibrinolytic system. A pharmaceutical preparation of urokinase is administered intravenously in the treatment of pulmonary embolism.

urolithiasis (yʊr'ɔlɪθɑɪ'ɔsɪs). See **urinary calculus.**

urologist, a licensed physician who has completed an approved residency program and who specializes in the practice of urology.

urology, the branch of medicine concerned with the study of the anatomy and physiology, the disorders, and the care of the urinary tract in men and women and of the male genital tract.

uromelus (yʊrom'ələs). See **sympus monopus.**

urono-. See **uro-.**

uropathy (yʊrop'əθi), any disease or abnormal condition of any structure of the urinary tract. — **uropathic,** *adj.*

uroporphyria (yʊr'ɔupɔrfir'iə), a rare, genetic disease characterized by excessive secretion of uroporphyrin in the urine, blistering dermatitis, photosensitivity, splenomegaly, and hemolytic anemia. Corticosteroid ointments may be helpful for the skin lesions; splenomegaly may be necessary to alleviate the hemolytic anemia. Most patients die from hematologic complications before middle age. See also **porphyria.**

uroporphyrin (yʊr'ɔupɔr'fɪrɪn), a porphyrin normally excreted in the urine in small amounts. See also **uroporphyria.**

urorectal septum, a ridge of mesoderm covered with endoderm that in the early developing embryo divides the endodermal cloaca into the urogenital sinus and the rectum. Also called **cloacal septum.**

urticaria (ər'tɪker'iə), a pruritic skin eruption characterized by transient wheals of varying shapes and sizes with well-defined erythematous margins and pale centers, caused by local release of histamine or other vasoactive substances. Acute urticaria is usually of allergic origin; in chronic cases, causative agents are rarely discovered. Some of the most common causes of urticaria are drugs, foods, insect bites, inhalants, and exposure to the cold or sun. Also called **hives.** — **urticarial,** *adj.*

urticaria pigmentosa, an uncommon form of mastocytosis characterized by pigmented skin lesions that become urticarial upon mechanical or chemical irritation. Although duration of the condition is unpredictable, prognosis is good. Treatment is symptomatic and usually includes antihistamines for relief of itching. See also **mastocytosis.**

urushiol (əru'ʃiol), a toxic resin in the sap of certain plants of the genus *Rhus,* as poison ivy, poison oak, and poison sumac, that produces allergic contact dermatitis in many people.

-us, a combining form signaling singular nouns: *echolalus, thalamus, tonus.*

USAN, an acronym for *United States Adopted Names,* a list of approved drugs compiled and published by U.S. Pharmacopeial Convention, Inc. (USPC).

use effectiveness, (of a contraceptive method) the actual effectiveness of a medication, device, or method in preventing pregnancy. Inconsistent use and human error usually reduce the theoretical effectiveness of any particular method of contraception. Compare **theoretical effectiveness.**

use test, a procedure used to identify offending allergens in foods, cosmetics, or fabrics by the systematic elimination and addition of specific items associated with the lifestyle of the patient involved. Allergic reactions to the use test may be immediate or may be spread over a considerable period of time. Some patients undergoing the test become frustrated and discouraged, requiring regular encouragement to continue the search for the sources of their allergies by this method. See also **allergy testing.**

USP. See *United States Pharmacopeia.*

USPHS, abbreviation for **United States Public Health Service.**

uta (yu'tə), a mild cutaneous form of American leishmaniasis, occurring in the Andes of Peru and Argentina, caused by *Leishmania peruana.* See also **American leishmaniasis, leishmaniasis.**

uterine anteflexion, an abnormal position of the uterus in which the uterine body is bent forward on itself at the juncture of the isthmus of the uterine cervix and the lower uterine segment.

uterine anteversion, a position of the uterus in which the body of the uterus is directed ventrally. Mild degrees of anteversion are of no clinical significance. On speculum examination of the vagina, acute anteversion of the uterus may be deduced from the location of the cervix in the posterior of the vaginal vault. Slight anteversion is the most common position of the uterus; on speculum examination the cervix is in the middle of the top of the vagina vault, and it protrudes directly downward toward the vaginal orifice.

uterine cancer, any malignancy of the uterus. It may be cervical cancer affecting the cervix or endometrial cancer affecting the lining of the body of the uterus. See also **cervical cancer, endometrial cancer.**

uterine retroflexion, a position of the uterus in which the body of the uterus is bent backward on itself at the isthmus of the cervix and the lower uterine segment. It has no clinical significance; it does not prevent conception or adversely affect pregnancy. On speculum examination of the vagina, the condition may be deduced by the location of the cervix in the anterior of the vaginal vault.

uterine retroversion, a position of the uterus in which the body of the uterus is directed away from the midline, toward the back. Mild degrees of retroversion are common and have no clinical significance. Severe retroversion may be accompanied by vague persistent pelvic discomfort and dyspareunia and may prevent the fitting and use of a contraceptive diaphragm. Compare **uterine anteversion.** See also **uterine retroflexion.**

uterine tenaculum. See **tenaculum.**

uterine tube. See **Fallopian tube.**

uteritis (yu'tərai'tɪs). See **metritis.**

uteroglobulin. See **blastokinin.**

utero-ovarian varicocele, a swelling of the veins of the pampiniform plexus of the female pelvis. Compare **varicocele, ovarian varicocele.**

uteroplacental apoplexy. See **Couvelaire uterus.**

uterovesical (yu'tərouves'ɪkəl). See **vesicouterine.**

uterus, the hollow, pear-shaped internal female organ of reproduction in which the fertilized ovum is implanted and the fetus develops, and from which the decidua of menses flows. Its anterior surface lies on the superior surface of the bladder separated by a fold of peritoneum, the vesicouterine pouch. Its posterior surface, also covered with peritoneum, is adjacent to the sigmoid colon and some of the coils of the small intestine. The uterus is comprised of three layers: the endometrium, the myometrium, and the parametrium. The endometrium lines the uterus and becomes thicker and more vascular in pregnancy and during the second half of the menstrual cycle

under the influence of the hormone progesterone. The myometrium is the muscular layer of the organ. Its muscle fibers wrap around the uterus obliquely, laterally, and longitudinally. After childbirth the meshlike network of fibers contracts, creating a mass of natural ligatures that stop the flow of blood from the large blood vessels supplying the placenta. The parametrium is the outermost layer of the uterus. It is composed of serous connective tissue and extends laterally into the broad ligament. In the adult, the organ measures about 7.5 cm long, 5 cm wide at its fundus, and weighs approximately 40 gm. During pregnancy it is able to grow to many times its usual size, almost entirely by cellular hypertrophy. Few new cells develop. The uterus has two parts: a body and a cervix. The body extends from the fundus to the cervix, just above the isthmus. The cavity within the body is only a potential space. The walls of the body touch, unless the woman is pregnant. The cervix has a vaginal portion, protruding into the vagina, and a supravaginal portion at the juncture of the lower uterine segment. The principal ligaments of the uterus are the broad ligaments, which extend laterally from the sides of the isthmus of the cervix between the folds of the broad ligaments; the cardinal ligaments, crossing the pelvic diaphragm from the top of the cervix to the large muscles of the pelvic outlet; and the uterosacral ligaments, curving back from the cervix to the sacrum around the cul-de-sac of Douglas. The body of the uterus is thus free in the abdominal cavity, fixed only at its base by the series of ligaments from the cervix.

uterus masculinis. See **prostatic utricle.**

UTI, abbreviation for **urinary tract infection.**

Uticillin VK, a trade name for an antibacterial (penicillin V potassium).

utilization review, an assessment of the appropriateness and economy of an admission to a health care facility or a continued hospitalization. The length of the hospital stay is also compared to the average length of stay for similar diagnoses.

utricle, the larger of two membranous pouches in the vestibule of the membranous labyrinth of the ear. It is an oblong structure that communicates with the semicircular ducts by five openings and receives utricular filaments of the acoustic nerve. Compare **saccule.**

utriculosaccular duct, a duct connecting the utricle with an endolymphatic duct of the membranous labyrinth.

uvea (yu'viə), the fibrous tunic beneath the sclera that includes the iris, the ciliary body, and the choroid of the eye. Also called **tunica vasculosa bulbi, uveal tract.** —**uveal,** adj.

uveal tract. See **uvea.**

uveitis (yu'viai'tɪs), inflammation of the uveal tract of the eye, including the iris, ciliary body, and choroid. It may be characterized by an irregularly shaped pupil, inflammation around the cornea, pus in the anterior chamber, opaque deposits on the cornea, pain, and lacrimation. Causes include allergy, infection, trauma, diabetes, collagen disease, and skin diseases. A major complication may be glaucoma. See also **chorioretinitis, choroiditis, iritis.**

uvula (yu′vyulə), *pl.* **uvulae.** the small, cone-shaped process, suspended in the mouth from the middle of the posterior border of the soft palate. —**uvular,** *adj.*

uvulitis (yu′vyəlai′tıs), inflammation of the uvula. Common causes are allergy and infection.

V

v, symbol for *venous blood*.

V, symbol for **vanadium**.

V̇, symbol for **rate of gas flow**.

vaccination, any injection of attenuated microorganisms, as bacteria, viruses, or rickettsias, administered to induce immunity or to reduce the effects of associated infectious diseases. Historically, the first vaccinations were administered to immunize against smallpox. Vaccinations are now available to immunize against many diseases, as typhoid, measles, and mumps. — **vaccinate** (væk′səneit), *v.*

vaccine (væksin′, væk′sin, væk′sɪn), a suspension of attenuated or killed microorganisms administered intradermally, intramuscularly, orally, or subcutaneously to induce active immunity to infectious disease. Viruses and rickettsiae used in certain vaccines are grown in avian embryos, rabbit brain tissue, or monkey kidney tissue, and the organisms are usually inactivated by formalin, phenol, or beta-propiolactone. Bacteria for various vaccines may be inactivated by acetone, formalin, heat, or phenol. Vaccines may be used as single agents or in combinations.

-vaccine, a combining form meaning a 'preparation containing microorganisms for producing immunity to disease': *autovaccine, enterovaccine, heterovaccine.*

vaccinia (væksɪn′iə), an infectious disease of cattle caused by a poxvirus which may be transmitted to humans by direct contact or by deliberate inoculation as a protection against smallpox. A pustule develops at the site of infection, usually followed by malaise and fever which last for several days. After two weeks the pustule becomes a crust which eventually drops off, leaving a scar. Satellite lesions may occur, and the virus may be spread to other sites by scratching. Individuals with eczema or other preexisting skin disease may develop generalized vaccinia. Rarely, a severe encephalitis may follow vaccinia. Also called **cowpox**. Compare **smallpox**. See also **vaccination**.

vacuole (væk′yuoul), **1.** a clear space or cavity within a cell. **2.** a small space in the body enclosed by a membrane, usually containing fat, secretions, or cellular debris. — **vacuolar, vacuolated,** *adj.*

vacuum aspiration, a method of abortion in which the fetus and placenta are removed by suction to terminate an early pregnancy, up to the 14th week. Under local or light general anesthesia, the cervix is dilated and the uterus emptied with suction. Postoperative care includes the close observation of vital signs for symptoms of blood loss. Also called **suction curettage**. Compare **dilatation and curettage**. See also **therapeutic abortion**.

vagal (vei′gəl), of or pertaining to the vagus nerve.

vagina, the part of the female genitalia that forms a canal from the orifice through the vestibule to the uterine cervix. It is behind the bladder and in front of the rectum. In the adult woman the anterior wall of the vagina is about 7 cm long and the posterior wall is about 9 cm long. The canal is actually a potential space; the walls usually touch. The vagina widens from the vestibule upward and narrows toward the top, forming a curved vault around the protruding cervix. The vagina is lined with mucosa covering a layer of erectile tissue and muscle. The mucous membrane of the vagina forms two longitudinal columns from which transverse rugae extend around the canal. The muscular coat is composed of a strong, external longitudinal layer and an internal circular layer. The lower end of the vagina is surrounded by the erectile tissue of the bulb of the vestibule and the bulbocavernosus muscle. The muscular layer is highly vascular. The muscles of the vagina are innervated by the pudendal nerve and perfused by the vaginal artery.

vagina bulbi. See **fascia bulbi**.

vaginal bleeding, an abnormal condition in which blood is passed from the vagina, other than during the menses. It may be caused by abnormalities of the uterus or cervix by an abnormal pregnancy; by endocrine abnormalities; by abnormalities of one of both ovaries or one or both Fallopian tubes; or by an abnormality of the vagina. The following terms are commonly used in describing the approximate amount of vaginal bleeding: **heavy vaginal bleeding** is that which is greater than heaviest normal menstrual flow; **moderate vaginal bleeding** is that which is equal to heaviest normal menstrual flow; **light vaginal bleeding** is that which is less than heaviest normal menstrual flow; **vaginal staining** is a very light flow of blood barely requiring the use of a sanitary napkin or tampon; **vaginal spotting** is the passage vaginally of a few drops of blood; **bloody show** is an episode of light vaginal bleeding as often occurs in early labor, during labor, and, particularly, at the time of full dilatation of the cervix at the end of the first stage of labor.

vaginal cancer, a malignancy of the vagina occurring rarely as a primary neoplasm and more often as a secondary lesion or extension of vulvar, cervical, endometrial, or ovarian cancer. Clear cell adenocarcinoma occurs in young women exposed in utero to diethylstilbestrol given the mother to prevent abortion, but most primary vaginal cancers arise in white women over 50 years of age. A predisposing factor is cervical carcinoma. Vaginal leukoplakia, erythematosis, erosion, or granulation of the mucosa may prove to be carcinoma in situ. Symptoms of invasive lesions are postmenopausal bleeding, purulent discharge, pain, and dysuria. Diagnostic measures include cervical, endocervical, and vaginal Pap smears, colposcopy, biopsy, and Schiller's iodine test in which malignant cells do not stain dark brown. Ninety per cent of vaginal cancers are squamous cell carcinomas; others are clear cell or undifferentiated adenocarcinomas, malignant melanomas, and sarcomas. Depending on the patient's age and condition and the site and extent of the lesion, treatment may be by irradiation or vaginectomy and radical hysterectomy with lymph node dissection. Cryosurgery, topical 5-fluorouracil, and dinitrochlorobenzene (DNCB) may be used, but chemotherapy is not usually effective.

vaginal discharge, any discharge from the vagina. A clear or pearly-white discharge occurs normally. Throughout the reproductive years the amount varies greatly from woman to woman, and the amount and character vary in each woman at different times in her menstrual cycle. Before menarche and after menopause, the quantity of discharge is usually less than during the reproductive years. The discharge is largely composed of secretions of the endocervical glands. Inflammatory conditions of the vagina and cervix often cause an increase in the discharge, which may then have a foul odor and cause pruritus of the perineum and external genitalia.

vaginal instillation of medication, the instillation of a medicated cream, a suppository, or a gel into the vagina, usually performed to treat a local infection of the vagina or uterine cervix. The woman voids prior to the treatment. She then lies back, recumbent or semirecumbent. The nurse or physician, wearing gloves, separates the labia majora, exposing the vaginal orifice. The medication is instilled gently. A cream or gel is squeezed into an applicator from a tube and is then placed in the vagina by depressing the plunger of the applicator while withdrawing the device from the vagina. A tablet or suppository is usually placed in the vagina near the cervix with another style of applicator that holds the medication in a slotted receptacle at its tip. The woman remains recumbent after the instillation to prevent escape of the medication from the vagina. Most applicators may be washed after each instillation and reused for the same woman for the next dose. They are discarded after a course of treatment. Vaginal instillation may easily be taught to the woman.

vaginal jelly, a contraceptive product containing a spermicide in a jelly medium. It is usually used in conjunction with a contraceptive diaphragm or cervical cap. Some antimicrobial medications are also supplied in the form of a vaginal jelly.

vaginal spotting. See **vaginal bleeding.**

vaginal staining. See **vaginal bleeding.**

vaginismus (væj′ınız′məs), a psychophysiologic genital reaction of women, characterized by intense contraction of the perineal and paravaginal musculature tightly closing the vaginal introitus. It occurs in response to fear of painful intromission prior to coitus or pelvic examination. Vaginismus is considered abnormal if it occurs in the absence of genital lesions and if it conflicts with a woman's desire to participate in coition or to permit examination, but it may be a normal or physiologic response if painful genital conditions exist or if forcible or premature intromission is anticipated. Abnormal vaginismus is uncommon. Sexual adjustment can often be achieved through educative and supportive measures that lead to improved sexual self-awareness and response. In some cases, the condition is a manifestation of serious mental illness and requires formal psychiatric evaluation and treatment. Gender identity conflict, a history of trauma from rape or incest, or an intense suppression of sexuality in childhood and adolescence are factors that are often seen in association with vaginismus.

vagino-, a combining form meaning 'pertaining to the vagina': *vaginodynia, vaginolabial, vaginopexy.*

Vagisec, a trade name for a vaginal douche containing polyoxyethylene nonyl phenol, edetate sodium, and dioctyl sodium sulfosuccinate, used to treat trichomoniasis.

Vagitrol, a trade name for a vaginal fixed-combination drug containing an antibacterial (sulfanilamide) and a topical anti-infective (aminacrine hydrochloride).

vagotomy (veigot′əmi), the cutting of certain branches of the vagus nerve, performed with gastric surgery, to reduce the amount of gastric acid secreted and lessen the chance of recurrence of a gastric ulcer. With the patient under general anesthesia, a gastrectomy is performed and the appropriate branches of the vagus nerve are excised. Since peristalsis will be diminished, a pyloroplasty or an anastomosis of the stomach to the jejunum is done to assure proper emptying of the stomach. See also **anastomosis, gastrectomy, gastric ulcer, pyloroplasty, vagus nerve.**

vagotonus (vei′gətou′nəs), an abnormal increase in the activity and the effects of the stimulation of the vagus nerve, especially bradycardia with decreased cardiac output, faintness, and syncope. Vagotonus may occur in suctioning the oropharynx of a newborn as the syringe, laryngoscope blade, or catheter is inadvertently pressed on

UVW

the back of the throat, stimulating the nerve. It also occurs in some women following surgical treatment or simple manipulation of the uterine cervix.

vagovagal reflex (vei'gouvei'gəl), a stimulation of the vagus nerve by reflex in which irritation of the larynx or the trachea results in slowing of the pulse rate.

vagus nerve, either of the longest pair of cranial nerves essential for speech, swallowing, and the sensibilities and functions of many parts of the body. The vagus nerves communicate through 13 main branches, connecting to four areas in the brain. Also called **nervus vagus, pneumogastric nerve, tenth nerve.**

valence (veil'əns), **1.** (in chemistry) a numerical expression of the capability of an element to combine chemically with atoms of hydrogen or their equivalent. A negative valence indicates the number of hydrogen atoms to which one atom of a chemical element can bond. A positive valence indicates the number of hydrogen atoms that one atom of a chemical element can displace. An element is considered univalent (or monovalent) if each of its atoms can react with only one hydrogen atom or its equivalent; bivalent (or divalent) if each atom can react with two hydrogen or equivalent atoms; tervalent (or trivalent) if each atom can react with three hydrogen atoms; multivalent (or polyvalent) if each atom can react with many hydrogen atoms. **2.** (in immunology) an expression of the number of antigen-binding sites for one molecule of any given antibody or the number of antibody-binding sites for any given antigen. Most antibody molecules, and those belonging to the IgG, IgA, and IgE immunoglobulin classes have two antigen-binding sites. Most large antigen molecules are multivalent.

-valence, a combining term meaning the 'combining capacity of an atom compared with that of one hydrogen atom': *quantivalence, trivalence, univalence.* Also **-valency.**

-valent, a combining form meaning 'having a valency of a (specified) magnitude': *octavalent, pentavalent, tetravalent.*

valeric acid (vələr'ik), an organic acid with a penetrating odor found in the roots of *Valeriana officinalis.* Commercially prepared, it is used in the production of perfumes, flavors, lubricants, and certain drugs.

valgus (væl'gəs), an abnormal position in which a part of a limb is bent or twisted outward, away from the midline, as the heel of the foot in **talipes valgus.** Compare **varus.** See also **hallux valgus.**

validity, (in research) the extent to which a test measurement or other device measures what it is intended to measure. Kinds of validity include **content validity, current validity, construct validity, face validity, predictive validity.**

valine, an essential amino acid produced in the body by the digestion of proteins. It is needed for optimal growth in infants and for nitrogen equilibrium in adults.

Valisone, a trade name for a glucocorticoid (betamethasone valerate).

Valium, a trade name for an antianxiety agent (diazepam), used as an adjunct to anesthesia.

vallecula (vəlek'yələ), (in anatomy) **1.** any groove or furrow on the surface of an organ or structure. **2.** *Informal.* **vallecula epiglottica.** — **vallecular,** *adj.*

vallecula epiglottica, a furrow between the glossoepiglottic folds of each side of the posterior oropharynx.

vallecular dysphagia, difficulty or pain on swallowing owing to inflammation of the vallecula epiglottica. Compare **contractile ring dysphagia, dysphagia lusoria.**

Vallestril, a trade name for an estrogen (methallenestril).

valley fever. See **coccidioidomycosis.**

Valmid, a trade name for a sedative (ethinamate).

Valpin, a trade name for an anticholinergic (anisotropine methylbromide).

valproic acid, an anticonvulsant.

■ INDICATIONS: It is prescribed to prevent certain types of seizure activity.

■ CONTRAINDICATIONS: It is not recommended for use during pregnancy or lactation. Known hypersensitivity to this drug prohibits its use.

■ ADVERSE EFFECTS: Among the more severe adverse reactions are decreased platelet function and hepatotoxicity. Gastrointestinal disturbances are common, and alopecia, rash, headache, and insomnia may also occur.

Valsalva maneuver, any forced expiratory effort against a closed airway, as when an individual holds his breath and tightens his muscles in a concerted, strenuous effort to move a heavy object or to change position in bed. Most healthy individuals perform Valsalva maneuvers during normal daily activities without any injurious consequences; but such efforts are dangerous for many patients with cardiovascular diseases, especially if they become dehydrated, increasing the viscosity of their blood and the attendant risk of blood clotting. Constipation increases the risk of cardiovascular trauma in such patients, especially if they perform the Valsalva maneuver in trying to move their bowels. On relaxing after each muscular effort with held breath, the blood of such individuals rushes to the heart, often overloading the cardiac system and causing cardiac arrest. Orthopedic patients often use the Valsalva maneuver in changing their position in bed with the aid of an overhead trapeze bar. Patients who may be endangered by performing the Valsalva maneuver are commonly instructed to exhale instead of holding their breath when they move. The exhalation decreases the risk of cardiovascular trauma.

Valsalva's test (vælsæl'vəz), a method for testing the patency of the eustachian tubes. With mouth and nose kept tightly closed, a forced expiratory effort is made; if the eustachian tubes are open, air will enter into the middle ear cavities and the subject will hear a popping sound. See also **Valsalva maneuver.**

value system, the accepted mode of conduct and the set of norms, goals, and values binding any social group. Such guidelines for determining what is right or wrong, good or bad, desirable or undesirable serve as a frame of reference for the individual in reaching decisions and in achieving a meaningful life.

valve, a natural structure or artificial device in a passage or vessel that prevents reflux of the fluid contents passing through it. Valves in veins are membranous folds that prevent backflow of blood. — **valvular,** *adj.*

Tricuspid valve
(closed and seen from above)

Cusps

Cordae
tendineae

Papillary
muscle

Mitral valve
(closed and seen from above)

Mitral valve (open)

VALVES

-valve, a combining form meaning 'a thing that regulates the flow of': *bivalve, pseudovalve, trivalve.*

valve of Kerkring (kǝrk'rıŋ). See **circular fold.**

valve of lymphatics, one of the tiny semilunar structures in the vessels and trunks of the lymphatic system that help to regulate the flow of lymph and prevent venous blood from entering the system. There are no valves in the capillaries of the system but there are many in the collecting vessels. The valves are attached by their convex edges to the walls of the vessels, leaving their concave edges free and directed along the course of the current of lymph. Usually, two valves of equal size are found opposite each other. They are more numerous near the lymph nodes and more prevalent in the lymphatic vessels of the neck and the arms than in the vessels of the legs. The wall of the vessel just above the attachment of each valve bulges with a small sinus that gives the vessel its beaded appearance. See also **lymphatic system.**

valvotomy (vælvot'ǝmi), the incision into a valve, especially one in the heart, to correct a defect and allow proper opening and closure. Before surgery a cardiac catheterization is performed. With the patient under general anesthesia, the damaged valve is repaired, if possible, or removed and a prosthetic valve suture put in its place. Complications peculiar to prosthetic valve surgery are displacement of the valve owing to broken sutures, heart

block, leakage and regurgitation from chamber to chamber, infection, and embolus.

valvular heart disease, an acquired or congenital disorder of a cardiac valve, characterized by stenosis and obstructed blood flow or by valvular degeneration and regurgitation of blood. Diseases of aortic and mitral valves are most common and may be caused by congenital defects, bacterial endocarditis, syphilis, or, most frequently, by rheumatic fever. Episodes of rheumatic fever often affect cardiac valves, causing them to degenerate and remain open or causing the cusps of the valves to become stiff, calcified, and constricted. Valvular dysfunction results in changes in intracardiac pressure and in pulmonary and peripheral circulation. It may lead to cardiac arrhythmia, heart failure, and cardiogenic shock.

■ OBSERVATIONS: Malaise, anorexia, embolism, pulmonary edema, and ventricular failure often accompany valvular heart disease. In moderate or severe **aortic stenosis,** pulse pressure is decreased; the carotid pulse is small and slow with a long upstroke, but the apical pulse may be strong and sustained during systole. There may be a pansystolic thrill or generally harsh heart sounds, or the second systolic sound may be diminished or absent. The patient may experience anginal pain and syncope, and the electrocardiogram may show evidence of left ventricular hypertrophy, conduction defects, or complete heart block. Characteristic signs of aortic regurgitation are dyspnea, profuse sweating, flushed skin, bounding pulsations in neck arteries, and a blowing heart murmur throughout diastole. The electrocardiogram may be normal or reveal left ventricular hypertrophy. The patient with **mitral stenosis** tires easily, is short of breath on exertion, may have paroxysmal nocturnal dyspnea, and may develop hemoptysis and systemic embolism. The first heart sound usually is increased and the second is followed by a decrescendo opening snap. There may be atrial fibrillation, right ventricular hypertrophy, and increased pressure in the left atrium, pulmonary artery, and right ventricle. Mitral regurgitation is typified by dyspnea, fatigue, intolerance of exercise, heart palpitation, and a large, laterally placed apical pulse. There may be an apical systolic murmur; a diminished first heart sound; a third heart sound; atrial arrhythmia; or elevated wedge pressure in the left atrium, pulmonary artery, or pulmonary vein. **Tricuspid stenosis** is relatively uncommon, is usually associated with lesions in other valves resulting from rheumatic fever, and, in rare cases, is caused by carcinoid heart disease or endomyocardial fibrosis. Characteristics of tricuspid stenosis are a diastolic pressure gradient between the right atrium and ventricle, jugular vein distention, pulmonary congestion, and, in severe cases, hepatic congestion and splenomegaly. Tricuspid regurgitation, usually secondary to marked dilatation of the right ventricle and the ring of the valve, commonly occurs in late stages of cardiac failure in rheumatic or congenital heart disease with severe pulmonary hypertension. Typical signs include engorged neck veins, hepatomegaly, systolic pulsations of the liver, edema, and ascites. The pulmonic valve is affected by rheumatic fever much less frequently than other cardiac valves. **Pulmonic stenosis** may cause the intraventricular septum to bulge into the right ventricular chamber and regurgitation is a consequence of severe pulmonary hypertension, but destruction of the valve does not cause heart failure unless pulmonary hypertension is a serious problem.

■ INTERVENTION: Cardiotonics, diuretics, analgesics, sodium restriction, and antibiotics, if indicated, are used in the conservative treatment of valvular heart disease, but surgery is usually performed when the symptoms are incapacitating. A stenosed aortic valve may be repaired by removing the calcium deposits and opening the fused commissures, by removing a cusp and reconstructing the valve, or it may be replaced with a porcine or artificial valve. Defective mitral and tricuspid valves may also be replaced or repaired surgically.

■ NURSING CONSIDERATIONS: The patient undergoing cardiac valve repair or replacement may be hospitalized for from four to six weeks and requires diversional activities as well as the standard pre- and post-operative care provided for open-heart surgery.

valvular stenosis, a narrowing or constricture of any of the valves of the heart. The condition may result from a congenital defect, or it may be caused by some disease process. See also **aortic stenosis, congenital cardiac anomaly, mitral stenosis, pulmonic stenosis.**

valvulitis (væl′vyulɑi′tɪs), an inflammatory condition of a valve, especially a cardiac valve. Inflammatory changes in the aortic, mitral, and tricuspid valves of the heart are caused most commonly by rheumatic fever and less frequently by bacterial endocarditis and syphilis. Infected valves degenerate or their cusps become stiff and calcified, resulting in stenosis and obstructed blood flow.

VAMP, an acronym for a combination drug regimen, used in the treatment of cancer, containing three antineoplastics (vincristine sulfate, methotrexate, and mercaptopurine) and a glucocorticoid (prednisone).

vanadium (V), a grayish metallic element. Its atomic number is 23; its atomic weight is 50.942. Absorption of vanadium compounds results in a condition called vanadiumism, characterized by anemia, conjunctivitis, pneumonitis, and irritation of the respiratory tract.

van Bogaert's disease (vænbou′gɑrts), a rare familial disorder of lipid metabolism in which the substance cholestanol is deposited in the nervous system, blood, and connective tissue. Persons with the disease develop progressive ataxia and dementia, premature atherosclerosis, cataracts, and xanthomas of the tendons. No effective treatment has been found.

Vanceril, a trade name for a glucocorticoid (beclomethasone dipropionate), used for oral inhalation therapy in asthma.

Vancocin Hydrochloride, a trade name for an antibacterial (vancomycin hydrochloride).

vancomycin hydrochloride, an antibiotic.

■ INDICATIONS: It is prescribed in the treatment of infections caused by vancomycin-susceptible microorganisms.

■ CONTRAINDICATIONS: Concomitant administration of neurotoxic, nephrotoxic, or ototoxic drugs, or known hypersensitivity to this drug prohibits its use.

■ ADVERSE EFFECTS: Among the more serious adverse reactions are anaphylaxis, dizziness, and tinnitus.

van den Bergh test (væn′dənbərg′), a test for the presence of bilirubin in the blood serum. Blood is obtained from a patient who has fasted overnight, and the diluted serum is added to diazo reagent. A blue or violet color indicates the presence of bilirubin. The rate and magnitude of the color change are noted. Normal total bilirubin ranges from 0.2 to 1.4 mg. per 100 ml of serum, of which about 15 per cent should be what is called direct, or conjugated bilirubin.

Vandid, a trade name for an analeptic agent (ethamivan).

vanillylmandelic acid (VMA) (væ′nɪlɪlmændel′ɪk), a urinary metabolite of epinephrine and norepinephrine. A greater than normal amount of VMA is characteristic of a pheochromocytoma of the adrenal medulla.

Vanobid, a trade name for an antifungal (candicidin).

Vanoxide, a trade name for a topical fixed-combination drug containing an antibacterial (benzoyl peroxide) and a keratolytic drying agent (chlorhydroxyquinoline).

Van Rensselaer (væn ren′səlir), **Euphenia** (1840–1912), an American socialite who entered the first class of the Bellevue Hospital Training School for Nurses in New York. She designed the first nurses' uniform, a blue and white seersucker dress with collar and cuffs, apron, and cap. She succeeded Sister Helen as superintendent of Bellevue and later joined the Sisters of Charity, for whom she established a mission in Nassau. She organized the Seton Hospital for Tuberculosis in New York.

Vaponefrine, a trade name for an adrenergic agent (epinephrine hydrochloride), used as a bronchodilator.

vapor bath, the exposure of the body to vapor, as steam.

variable behavior, a response, activity, or action that may be modified by individual experience. Compare **invariable behavior.**

variance, **1.** (in statistics) a numerical representation of the dispersion of data around the mean in a given sample. It is represented by the square of the standard deviation and is used principally in performing an analysis of variance. **2.** *Nontechnical.* the general range of a group of findings.

varicella (vær'ısel'ə). See **chickenpox**.

varicella zoster virus (VZV), a member of the herpesvirus family, which causes the diseases varicella (chickenpox) and herpes zoster (shingles). The virus has been isolated from vesicle fluid in chickenpox, is highly contagious, and may be spread by direct contact or droplets. Dried crusts of skin lesions do not contain active virus particles. Herpes zoster is produced by reactivation of latent varicella virus, usually several years after the initial infection. There is no simple test for measuring antibodies to this virus; however, zoster immune globulin (ZIG) obtained from convalescing zoster patients, if injected within three days of exposure, will prevent varicella in susceptible children. The temporary nature of this protection and the relative scarcity of ZIG warrant reservation of its use to children receiving immunosuppressive therapy or suffering from immune deficiency diseases. See also **chickenpox, herpesvirus hominis, herpes zoster.**

varicelliform (vær'ısel'ıfɔrm), resembling the rash of chickenpox.

varicocele (vær'əkousil'), a dilatation of the pampiniform venous complex of the spermatic cord. The varicocele forms a soft, elastic swelling that can cause pain. It is most common in men between the ages of 15 and 25 and affects the left spermatic cord more often than the right. It is usually more pronounced and painful in the standing position. Compare **ovarian varicocele, utero-ovarian varicocele.**

varicose (vær'əkous), 1. (of a vein) exhibiting varicosis, or a varicosity. 2. abnormally and permanently distended, as the bulging veins in some individuals.

varicose ulcer. See **stasis ulcer.**

varicose vein, a tortuous, dilated vein with incompetent valves. Causes include congenitally defective valves, thrombophlebitis, pregnancy, and obesity. Varicose veins are common, especially in women. The saphenous veins of the legs are most often affected. Elevation of the legs and use of elastic stockings are frequently sufficient therapy for uncomplicated cases. Surgery (ligation and stripping) may be required in severe cases. Injection of sclerosing solutions helps to prevent or to treat postphlebitic syndrome.

varicosis, a common condition characterized by one or more tortuous, abnormally dilated, or varicose veins, usually in the legs or the lower trunk, occurring between the ages of 30 and 60. Varicosis may be caused by congenital defects of the valves or walls of the veins or by congestion and increased intraluminal pressure resulting from prolonged standing, poor posture, pregnancy, abdominal tumor, or chronic systemic disease. Symptoms include pain and muscle cramps with a feeling of fullness and heaviness in the legs. Dilation of superficial veins is often evident before the condition produces discomfort. Varicose veins may be treated conservatively by elevating the affected limb periodically or by wearing an elastic bandage or stocking. Ligation of the vein above the varicosity and removal of the distal portion of the vessel may be indicated for more severe cases if deeper vessels can maintain the return of venous blood.

varicosity, 1. an abnormal condition, usually of a vein, characterized by swelling and tortuosity. 2. a vein in this condition.

variegate (ver'iəgeit), having characteristics that vary, especially as to color.

variegate porphyria, an uncommon form of hepatic porphyria, characterized by skin lesions and photosensitivity. The condition may be congenital or acquired. The congenital form is more serious, resulting in crises of acute abdominal pain and in certain neurologic complications. See also **porphyria.**

variola (vərai'ələ). See **smallpox.**

variola major. See **smallpox.**

variola minor. See **alastrim.**

varioloid (veir'iəloid), 1. resembling smallpox. 2. a mild form of smallpox in a vaccinated person or one who has previously had the disease.

varix (vær'ıks), *pl.* **varices** (vær'əsiz). 1. a tortuous, dilated vein. 2. an enlarged, tortuous artery or a distended, twisting lymphatic.

varus (ver'əs), an abnormal position in which a part of a limb is turned inward toward the midline, as the heel and foot in **talipes varus.** Compare **valgus.**

vas (væs), *pl.* **vasa** (vei'sə), any one of the many vessels of the body, especially those that convey blood, lymph, or spermatozoa.

Vasal, a trade name for a smooth-muscle relaxant (papaverine hydrochloride).

vascular (væs'kyulər), of or pertaining to a blood vessel.

vascular hemophilia. See **Von Willebrand's disease.**

vascular insufficiency, inadequate peripheral blood flow caused by occlusion of vessels with atherosclerotic plaques, thrombi, or emboli, by damaged, diseased, or intrinsically weak vascular walls, arteriovenous fistulas, hematologic hypercoagulability, or heavy smoking. Signs of vascular insufficiency include pale, cyanotic, or mottled skin over the affected area, swelling of an extremity, absent or reduced tactile sensation, tingling, diminished sense of temperature, muscle pain, as intermittent claudication in the calf, and, in advanced disease, atrophy of muscles of the involved extremity. Diagnosis may be made by checking and comparing peripheral pulses in contralateral extremities, by angiography, plethysmography, ultrasonography, and skin temperature tests. Treatment of vascular insufficiency may include a diet low in saturated fats, moderate exercise, sleeping on a firm mattress, avoidance of smoking, prolonged standing, or prolonged sitting with the knees bent, the use of vasodilating drug, and, if indicated, surgical repair of an

arteriovenous fistula or aneurysm. See also **arterial insufficiency.**

vascularization,   the process by which body tissue becomes vascular and develops proliferating capillaries. It
may be natural or may be induced by surgical techniques.
–**vascularize,** *v.*

vascular leiomyoma,   a neoplasm composed of a coil of
blood vessels surrounded by a mesh of smooth-muscle
fibers.

vascular spider.   See **spider angioma.**

vasculitis (væs'kyulaɪ'tɪs),   an inflammatory condition of
the blood vessels that is characteristic of certain systemic
diseases or that is caused by an allergic reaction. Kinds of
vasculitis are **allergic vasculitis, necrotizing vasculitis, segmented hyalinizing vasculitis.**

vas deferens (def'ərenz), *pl.* **vasa deferentia** (def'əren'-
s̆hiə).   the extension of the epididymis of the testis that
ascends from the scrotum and joins the seminal vesicle to
form the ejaculatory duct. It is enclosed by fibrous connective tissue with blood vessels, nerves, and lymphatics
and passes through the inguinal canal as part of the spermatic cord. Extending from the scrotum into the abdominal cavity it passes over the top, then down the posterior
surface of the bladder, becomes wider and convoluted,
and joins the ampulla of the seminal vesicle. A vasectomy
severs the vas deferens and makes a man sterile by interrupting the route spermatozoa must take to the exterior
from the epididymis. Compare **testis.**

vasectomy (væsek'təmi),   a procedure for male sterilization involving the bilateral surgical removal of a portion
of the vas deferens. Vasectomy is most commonly performed as an office procedure under local anesthesia. The
procedure is also performed routinely prior to removal of
the prostate gland in order to prevent inflammation of the
testes and epididymides. Potency is not affected. A signed
and witnessed form indicating informed consent is usually
required prior to performance of the procedure.

vaso-,   a combining form meaning 'pertaining to a vessel
or duct': *vasoconstrictor, vasodilation, vasoganglion.*

vasoactive (vei'zoʊæk'tɪv),   (of a drug) tending to cause
vasodilation or vasoconstriction.

Vasocidin,   a trade name for a topical fixed-combination
drug containing a glucocorticoid (prednisolone sodium
phosphate) an antibacterial (sulfacetamide sodium), and
an adrenergic (phenylephrine hydrochloride).

Vasocon,   a trade name for an adrenergic (naphazoline
hydrochloride).

vasoconstriction (væs'oʊkənstrɪk'S̆hən),   a narrowing of
the lumen of any blood vessel, especially the arterioles
and the veins in the blood reservoirs of the skin and the

Bilateral incision to expose sheath

Vas exposed and occluded

Segment excised

Vas replaced and skin sutured

VASECTOMY

abdominal viscera. It is accomplished by various mechanisms that together control blood pressure and the distribution of blood throughout the body. Vasoconstriction depends on the stimulation of the vasomotor constriction center in the medulla. Impulses from this center travel along the sympathetic nerve fibers and contract the smooth muscle layers of the arteries, the arterioles, the venules, and the veins, causing the constriction of these vessels. Vasoconstriction is also induced by vasomotor pressure reflexes, chemical reflexes, the medullary ischemic reflex, and vasomotor impulses from the cerebral cortex and the hypothalamus. Compare **vasodilatation.**

vasoconstrictor (væs'oukənstrɪk'tər), **1.** of or pertaining to a process, condition, or substance that causes the constriction of blood vessels. **2.** an agent that promotes vasoconstriction. Cold, fear, stress, and nicotine are common exogenous vasoconstrictors. Internally secreted epinephrine and norepinephrine cause blood vessels to contract by stimulating adrenergic receptors of peripheral sympathetic nerves. Other endogenous vasoconstrictors are angiotensin, which is formed in the blood through the action of renin, and antidiuretic hormone, which is secreted by the pituitary. Adrenergic sympathomimetic drugs cause some degree of vasoconstriction, and several of these agents are used for this action in maintaining blood pressure during anesthesia and in treating pronounced hypotension resulting from hemorrhage, myocardial infarction, septicemia, sympathectomy, or drug reactions. Among these therapeutic agents are methoxamine hydrochloride, metaraminol litartrate, and levarterenol (norepinephrine). See also **vasopressor.**

Vasodilan, a trade name for a vasodilator (isoxsuprine hydrochloride).

vasodilatation (vei'zoudɪl'ətei'shən, vei'zoudæ'lətei'shən), **vasodilation** (vei'zoudailei'shən), widening or distention of blood vessels, particularly arterioles, usually owing to nerve impulses or to certain drugs that cause relaxation of smooth muscle in the walls of the blood vessels. Compare **vasoconstriction.**

vasodilator (vei'zoudai'leitər), **1.** a nerve or agent that causes dilatation of blood vessels. **2.** pertaining to the relaxation of the smooth muscle of the vascular system. **3.** producing dilatation of blood vessels. Vasodilators are a recent, important addition to the treatment of heart failure. Included are hydralazine, nitroglycerin, nitroprusside, and trimethaphan. They have proven very useful in the treatment of acute heart failure in myocardial infarction, in cases associated with severe mitral insufficiency, and in failure resulting from myocardial disease.

vasomotor (væs'oumou'tər), of or pertaining to the nerves and muscles that control the caliber of the lumen of the blood vessels. Circularly arranged fibers of the muscles of arteries can contract, causing vasoconstriction, or they can relax, causing vasodilation.

vasomotor rhinitis, chronic rhinitis and nasal obstruction, without allergy or infection, characterized by sneezing, rhinorrhea, nasal obstruction, and vascular engorgement of the mucous membranes of the nose. A vaporizer or humidifier and systemic vasoconstrictive agents are used to alleviate discomfort. Nose drops and nasal sprays are avoided, as continued use may cause further vasodilation of the mucous membrane and aggravation of the condition. Vasomotor rhinitis is common in pregnancy.

vasomotor system, that part of the nervous system that controls the constriction and dilatation of the blood vessels. See also **vasoconstriction, vasodilatation.**

vasopressin. See **antidiuretic hormone.**

Vasospan, a trade name for a smooth muscle relaxant (papaverine hydrochloride).

Vasosulf, a trade name for an ophthalmic fixed-combination drug containing an antibacterial (sulfacetamide sodium) and an adrenergic (phenylephrine hydrochloride).

vasovasostomy (væs'ouvəsos'təmi), a surgical procedure in which the function of the vas deferens on each side of the testes is restored, having been cut and ligated in a preceding vasectomy. The procedure is performed if a man wants to regain his fertility. In most cases, the patency of the canals is achieved, but in many cases fertility does not result, probably owing to circulating autoantibodies that disrupt normal sperm activity. The antibodies apparently develop following vasectomy as the developing sperm cannot be excreted through the urogenital tract.

Vasoxyl, a trade name for an alpha-adrenergic (methoxamine hydrochloride).

vastus intermedius, one of the four muscles of the quadriceps femoris, situated in the center of the thigh. It arises from the front and lateral surfaces of the femur and from the lateral intermuscular septum. Its fibers end in a superficial aponeurosis which forms the deep part of the quadriceps femoris tendon inserted into the patella. The vastus intermedius is innervated by branches of the femoral nerve, which contain fibers from the second, third, and fourth lumbar nerves, and it functions with the other three muscles of the quadriceps to extend the leg. Also called **crureus.** Compare **rectus femoris, vastus lateralis, vastus medialis.**

vastus internus. See **vastus medialis.**

vastus lateralis, the largest of the four muscles of the quadriceps femoris, situated on the lateral side of the thigh. It is a large, dense mass originating in a broad aponeurosis that is attached to the intertrochanteric line of the femur, the greater trochanter, the lateral lip of the gluteal tuberosity, and to the lateral lip of the linea aspera. The fibers of the muscle are gathered to form a strong aponeurosis that converges to become a flat tendon before inserting into the patella. The vastus lateralis is innervated by branches of the femoral nerve, which contain fibers from the second, third, and fourth lumbar nerves, and it functions to help extend the leg. Compare **rectus femoris, vastus intermedius, vastus medialis.**

vastus medialis, one of the four muscles of the quadriceps femoris, situated in the medial portion of the thigh. It originates from the intertrochanteric line of the femur, the linea aspera, the medial supracondylar line, the tendons of the adductor longus and the adductor magnus, and the medial intermuscular septum. The vastus medialis extends to the lower anterior aspect of the thigh and inserts by an aponeurosis into the patella and the quadriceps femoris tendon. An expansion of the aponeurosis passes to the capsule of the knee joint. The muscle is innervated by branches of the femoral nerve, which contain fibers from the second, third, and fourth lumbar nerves, and it functions in combination with other parts of the quadriceps femoris to extend the leg. Also called **vastus internus.** Compare **rectus femoris, vastus intermedius, vastus lateralis.**

VC, abbreviation for **vital capacity.**

V-Cillin, a trade name for an antibacterial (penicillin V).

V-Cillin K, a trade name for an antibacterial (penicillin V potassium).

VD, abbreviation for **venereal disease.**

VDRL test, abbreviation for *Venereal Disease Research Laboratory test,* a serological flocculation test for syphilis. It is also positive in other treponemal diseases, as yaws. False positive and false negative results may occur. A positive test must be confirmed by further, more definitive testing.

V̇e, symbol for *expired volume.*

V̇E, symbol for *volume expired in one minute.*

vector, 1. a quantity having direction and magnitude, usually depicted by a straight arrow whose length represents magnitude and whose head represents direction. 2. a carrier, especially one which transmits disease. A **biological vector** is usually an arthropod in which the infecting organism completes part of its life cycle. A **mechanical vector** transmits the infecting organism from one host to another but is not essential to the life cycle of the parasite. Kinds of vectors include dogs, which carry rabies, mosquitoes, which transmit malaria, and ticks, which carry Rocky Mountain spotted fever. —**vector,** *v.,* **vectorial,** *adj.*

Vectrin, a trade name for a tetracycline antibiotic (minocycline hydrochloride).

VEE, abbreviation for **Venezuelan equine encephalitis.** See **equine encephalitis.**

Veetids, a trade name for an antibacterial (penicillin V potassium).

vegan (vej'æn). See **strict vegetarian.**

veganism (vej'əniz'əm), the adherence to a strict vegetable diet, with the exclusion of all protein of animal origin.

vegetable albumin, albumin produced in plants.

vegetal pole, vegetative pole, the relatively inactive part of the ovum protoplasm where the food yolk is situated, usually opposite the animal pole. Also called **antigerminal pole.** Compare **animal pole.**

vegetarian (vej'əteir'iən), a person whose diet is restricted to foods of vegetable origin, including fruits, grains, and nuts. Many vegetarians eat eggs and milk products but avoid all animal flesh. Kinds of vegetarians are **lacto-ovo-vegetarian, lacto-vegetarian, strict vegetarian.**

vegetarianism (vej'əteir'iəniz'əm), the theory or practice of restricting the diet to food substances of vegetable origin, including fruits, grains, and nuts.

vegetation, an abnormal growth of tissue around a valve, composed of fibrin, platelets, and bacteria.

vegetative (vej'ɪtei'tɪv), 1. of or pertaining to nutrition and growth. 2. of or pertaining to the plant kingdom. 3. denoting involuntary function, as produced by the parasympathetic nervous system. 4. resting, not active; denoting the stage of the cell cycle in which the cell is not replicating. 5. leading a secluded, dull existence without social or intellectual activity; sluggish; lacking animation. 6. (in psychiatry) emotionally withdrawn and passive, as may occur in schizophrenia and in the depressive phase of bipolar disorder. —**vegetate,** *v.*

vegetative nervous system. See **autonomic nervous system.**

vehicle, 1. an inert substance with which a medication is mixed to facilitate measurement and administration or application. 2. any fluid or structure in the body that passively conveys a stimulus.

Veillonella (vei'yənel'ə), a genus of gram-negative anaerobic bacteria. The species *Veillonella parvula* is normally present in the alimentary tract, especially in the mouth.

Veillon's tube (veiyounz'), a transparent tube, the ends of which are closed with removable stoppers, one cotton and one rubber. It is used for the laboratory growth of bacteriologic cultures.

vein, one of the many vessels that convey blood from the capillaries to the heart as part of the pulmonary venous system, the systemic venous network, or the portal venous complex. Most of the veins of the body are systemic veins that convey blood from the whole body (except the lungs) to the right atrium of the heart. Each vein is a macroscopic structure enclosed in three layers of different kinds of tissue homologous with the layers of the heart. The outer tunica adventitia of each vein is homologous with the epicardium, the tunica media with the myocardium, and the tunica intima with the endocardium. Deep veins course through the more internal parts of the body and superficial veins lie near the surface, where many of them can be seen through the skin. Veins have thinner coatings and are less elastic than arteries and collapse when cut. They also contain semilunar valves at various intervals.

Compare **artery**. See also **portal vein, pulmonary vein, systemic vein.**

vein ligation and stripping, a surgical procedure consisting of the ligation of the saphenous vein and its removal from groin to ankle, performed for the treatment of recurrent thrombophlebitis or severe varicosities or for obtaining a blood vessel to graft in another site, as in a coronary bypass operation.

vein of Thebesius (thĭbi'siəs). See **smallest cardiac vein.**

veins of the vertebral column, the veins that drain the blood from the vertebral column, the adjacent muscles, and the meninges of the spinal cord. Along the entire vertebral column these veins form plexuses which are divided into internal and external groups, according to their locations inside or outside the vertebral canal. The plexuses and the veins of the vertebral network are the external plexus, the internal plexus, the basivertebral veins, the intervertebral veins, and the spinal cord veins.

Velban, a trade name for an antineoplastic (vinblastine sulfate).

vellus hair. See **lanugo.**

velocity, the rate of change in the position of a body moving in a particular direction. Velocity along a straight line is linear velocity. Angular velocity is that of a body in circular motion. Compare **speed.**

velopharyngeal closure (vi'loufərɪn'jiəl), the blocking of any escape of air by the raising of the soft palate and the contraction of the posterior pharyngeal wall. Compare **closure, flask closure.**

velopharyngeal insufficiency, an abnormal condition resulting from a congenital defect in the structure of the velopharyngeal sphincter; closure of the oral cavity beneath the nasal passages is not complete, as seen in cleft palate. Food may be regurgitated through the nose, and speech is impaired. Surgical correction is usually successful.

Velosef, a trade name for a cephalosporin antibiotic (cephradine).

Velpeau's bandage (velpouz'), a roller bandage that immobilizes the elbow and shoulder by holding the brachium against the side and the flexed forearm on the chest. The palm of the hand rests on the clavicle of the opposite side.

vena cava (vi'nə kei'və), pl. **venae cavae.** one of two large veins returning blood from the peripheral circulation to the right atrium of the heart. See also **inferior vena cava, superior vena cava.** — **vena caval,** adj.

vena comes (vi'nə kou'miz), pl. **venae comites** (vi'ni kom'itiz). one of the deep paired veins that accompany the smaller arteries, one on each side of the artery. The three vessels are wrapped together in one sheath. Some of the arteries accompanied by such venous pairs are the brachial, the ulnar, and the tibial.

venereal (vɪnir'iəl), pertaining to or caused by sexual intercourse or genital contact.

venereal disease (VD), any contagious condition acquired by sexual intercourse or genital contact. Kinds of venereal diseases include **chancroid, gonorrhea, granuloma inguinale, herpes simplex Type II, lymphogranuloma venereum, syphilis.**

venereal sore. See **chancre.**

venereal wart. See **condylomatum acuminatum.**

venereology (vɪnir'iol'əji), the study of venereal diseases. — **venereologic, venereological,** adj., **venereologist,** n.

venesection (ven'əsek'shən). See **phlebotomy.**

Venezuelan equine encephalitis (VEE). See **equine encephalitis.**

venipuncture (ven'ɪpəngk'chər), a technique in which a vein is punctured transcutaneously by a sharp rigid stylet or cannula carrying a flexible plastic catheter or by a steel needle attached to a syringe or catheter. The purpose of the procedure is to withdraw a specimen of blood, to perform a phlebotomy, to instill a medication, to start an intravenous infusion, or to inject a radiopaque substance for radiologic examination of a part or system of the body.

■ METHOD: The specific steps in performing a venipuncture vary with the purpose of the procedure and the equipment to be used, but in most instances it begins as follows: a convenient vein is selected, usually on the outside of the forearm, on the back of the hand, or in the antecubital fossa. The vein is palpated, and to dilate the vein a tourniquet is wrapped around the arm proximal to the intended site of puncture. The site is cleansed, and the vein is immobilized by applying traction on the skin around the puncture site. The stylet or needle is held at an angle of 30° for direct venipuncture. In performing direct venipuncture the tip of the needle is pointed in the direction of the flow of blood and is advanced through the skin directly into the vein. The tip is usually inserted bevelside up, but if a large bore needle must be used in a small vein, it is preferable to insert the needle bevelside down, as it is less likely to perforate the posterior wall of the vein. After the skin is punctured little resistance is felt as the tip passes through the subcutaneous tissue, but a sudden, slight resistance may be felt as the tip hits the wall of the vein. At this point, the tip is cautiously advanced, with the needle or stylet held nearly flush with the skin. Slight upward pressure aids in keeping the tip in the vein as it is advanced into the lumen of the intravenous space. Blood flows back into the hub of the needle or into the catheter attached to the needle or covering the stylet, and the tip of the needle can usually be felt to be in the vein. If these signs are absent, the tip is not in the vein, in which case it is usually best to remove the needle or stylet, apply pressure to the puncture site, and start the procedure again, using new equipment.

■NURSING CONSIDERATIONS: Wing-tipped 'butterfly' needles, various kinds of intracatheters, and single or multiple venipuncture needles require familiarity and practice for correct insertion and stabilization. A sterile dressing and an antimicrobial ointment are applied over the insertion site. The cleansing agent used to prepare the injection site may be iodine, povidone-iodine, or ethyl alcohol. If an iodine preparation or solution is to be used, the patient is first asked about any previous allergic reaction to iodine. To aid insertion of the tip into the vein, the patient may be asked to clench the fist to further dilate the vein. If the patient is unable to do this a second tourniquet may be placed several inches distal to the puncture site. This tourniquet is released when the needle or stylet has been placed in the vein.

■OUTCOME CRITERIA: Aseptic technique is required to avoid infection. A quick, skillful insertion is nearly painless for the patient. Specific sequelae to venipuncture vary with the techniques and equipment used. See also **intravenous infusion, phlebotomy.**

veno-, a combining form meaning 'pertaining to a vein': *venoclysis, venopressor, venovenostomy.*

venogram (vi'nəgræm, ven'əgræm). See **phlebogram.**

venography (vinog'rəfi). See **phlebography.**

venom, a toxic fluid substance secreted by some snakes, arthropods, and other animals and transmitted by their stings or bites.

venom-extract therapy, the administration of antivenin as prophylaxis against the toxic effects of the bite of a specific poisonous snake or spider, or other venomous animal.

venom immunotherapy, the reduction of sensitivity to the bite of a venomous insect or animal by the serial administration of gradually increasing amounts of the specific antigenic substance secreted by the insect or animal.

venous (vi'nəs), of or pertaining to a vein.

-venous, a combining form meaning 'of or referring to veins': *endovenous, lymphovenous, perivenous.*

venous blood gas, the oxygen and carbon dioxide in venous blood measured by various methods to assess the adequacy of oxygenation and ventilation and to determine the acid-base status. The oxygen tension of venous blood normally averages 40 mm Hg; the dissolved oxygen averages 0.1 per cent by volume, the total oxygen content 15.2 per cent, and the oxygen saturation of venous hemoglobin 75 per cent. The carbon dioxide tension normally averages 46 mm Hg, the dissolved carbon dioxide 2.9 per cent by volume, and the total carbon dioxide content 50 per cent. The normal average pH of venous plasma is 7.37. Venous blood in an extremity when analyzed for gas content provides data chiefly pertaining to that limb.

Since a sample from a central venous catheter is usually an incomplete mix of venous blood from various parts of the body, a specimen of completely mixed blood may be obtained from the right ventricle or pulmonary artery for an accurate determination of venous blood gases.

venous insufficiency, an abnormal circulatory condition characterized by decreased return of the venous blood from the legs to the trunk of the body. Edema is usually the first sign of the condition; pain, varicosities, and ulceration may follow. Treatment usually consists of elevation of the legs, use of elastic hose, and correction of the underlying condition.

venous pressure, the stress exerted by circulating blood on the walls of veins, normally 60 to 120 mm of water in peripheral veins but elevated in congestive heart failure, acute or chronic constrictive pericarditis, and in venous obstruction caused by a clot or external pressure against a vein. Indications of increased pressure are continued distention of veins on the back of the hand when it is raised above the sternal notch and distention of the neck veins when the individual is sitting with the head elevated 30 to 45 degrees. Central venous pressure, normally 40 to 100 mm of water, is determined by inserting a catheter into a major vein and threading it through the superior vena cava to the right atrium. The catheter is attached by a three-way stopcock to a water manometer, and a solution, usually five per cent glucose in water, is allowed to drip slowly into the vein. Prior to taking a reading, the stopcock is opened to fill the manometer with the intravenous solution; then the stopcock is turned to the venous opening, and the fluid level in the manometer, which fluctuates with each respiration, is allowed to stabilize. The highest level of the fluid column is used for the reading, and, as soon as it is recorded, the stopcock is turned to the solution position and the infusion is continued.

venous pulse, the pulse of a vein usually palpated over the internal or external jugular veins in the neck. The pulse in the jugular vein is taken to evaluate the pressure of the pulse and the form of the pressure wave, especially in a person with a cardiac conduction defect or cardiac arrhythmia.

venous sinus, one of many sinuses that collect blood from the dura mater and drain it into the internal jugular vein. Each sinus is formed by the separation of the two layers of the dura mater, the outer coat of the sinus consisting of fibrous tissue, the inner coat consisting of endothelium continuous with that of the veins.

venous stasis dermatitis. See **stasis dermatitis.**

venous thrombosis, a condition characterized by the presence of a clot in a vein in which the wall of the vessel is not inflamed. Pain, swelling, and inflammation may follow if the vein is significantly occluded. Also called **phlebothrombosis.** Compare **thrombophlebitis.**

ventilate, 1. to provide with fresh air. 2. to provide the lungs with air from the atmosphere and to aerate or oxygenate blood in the pulmonary capillaries. 3. (in psychiatry) to open discussion, as to ventilate feelings. —**ventilation,** *n.*

ventilation, the process by which gases are moved into and out of the lungs. Compare **respiration.** —**ventilatory,** *adj.*

ventilator, any of several devices used in respiratory therapy to provide assisted respiration and intensive positive-pressure breathing. Kinds of ventilators are **pressure limited ventilator, volume ventilator.** See also **IPPB unit.**

venting, (in intravenous therapy) a method for allowing air to enter the vacuum of the intravenous bottle and displace the intravenous solution as it flows out. Glass intravenous bottles are usually equipped with a venting tube attached to the primary I.V. tubing or to a vent port incorporated with the bottle stopper. Venting is not required with a plastic I.V. bag, because the bag collapses as the fluid runs out. The air vent attached to primary I.V. tubing is removable to allow the injection of medication.

ventral, of or pertaining to a position toward the belly of the body; frontward; anterior. Compare **dorsal.**

-ventral, a combining form meaning 'of the stomach or abdominal region': *biventral, dorsoventral, uteroventral.*

ventral hernia. See **abdominal hernia.**

ventri-. See **ventro-.**

ventricle (ven'trikəl), a small cavity, as one of the cavities filled with cerebrospinal fluid in the brain, or the right and the left ventricles of the heart. —**ventricular,** *adj.*

ventricular (ventrik'yulər), of or pertaining to a ventricle.

ventricular aneurysm, a localized dilatation or saccular protrusion in the wall of the left ventricle, occurring most often following a myocardial infarction. Scar tissue is formed in response to the inflammatory changes of the infarction. This tissue weakens the myocardium, allowing its walls to bulge outward when the ventricle contracts. A typical sign of the lesion is a recurrent ventricular arrhythmia that does not respond to treatment with antiarrhythmic drugs, as procainamide or quinidine. Diagnostic measures are x-ray studies and cardiac catheterization. Treatment may consist of the administration of propranolol, digoxin, or procainamide but usually involves surgical removal of the scar tissue. Also called **cardiac aneurysm.**

ventricular fibrillation, a cardiac arrhythmia marked by rapid, disorganized depolarizations of the ventricular myocardium. The condition is characterized by a complete lack of organized electrical impulse, conduction, and ventricular contraction. Blood pressure falls to zero, resulting in unconsciousness. Death may occur within four minutes. Defibrillation and ventilation must be initiated immediately.

ventricular gallop, an abnormal cardiac rhythm in which a low-pitched extra heart sound is heard early in diastole on auscultation of the heart. When it is heard in an older person with heart disease it indicates myocardial failure. The same sound, heard in a healthy child or young adult is a physiologic finding (called a physiologic third heart sound) that usually disappears with age. See also **gallop.**

ventricular gradient, the algebraic sum of the areas within the QRS complex and within the T wave in the electrocardiogram.

ventricular septal defect (VSD), an abnormal opening in the septum separating the ventricles, permitting blood to flow from the left ventricle to the right ventricle and to recirculate through the pulmonary artery and lungs. It is the most common congenital heart defect, with openings that may be single or multiple and may range in size from 1 to 2 mm to several cm. Children with small defects are usually asymptomatic, while those with large defects may present with congestive heart failure, associated with lower respiratory tract infections, rapid breathing, poor weight gain, restlessness, and irritability. Small defects may close spontaneously; larger ones may lead to bacterial endocarditis, pulmonary vascular obstructive disease, aortic regurgitation, or congestive heart failure. Diagnosis is established by electrocardiography, cardiac catheterization, and angiography. Treatment consists of surgical repair of the defect, preferably in early childhood.

ventriculo-, a combining form meaning 'pertaining to a ventricle of the heart or brain': *ventriculocisternostomy, ventriculopuncture, ventriculostium.*

ventriculoatrial shunt (ventrik'yəlouei'triəl), a surgically created passageway, consisting of plastic tubing and one-way valves, implanted between a cerebral ventricle and the right atrium of the heart in order to drain excess cerebrospinal fluid from the brain in hydrocephalus.

ventriculocisternostomy, a surgical procedure performed to treat hydrocephalus. An opening is created that allows cerebrospinal fluid to drain through a shunt from the ventricles of the brain into the cisterna magna. Also called **Torkildsen's procedure.**

ventriculofallopian tube shunt (ventrik'yuloufəlou'-piən), a surgical procedure with limited effectiveness for diverting cerebrospinal fluid into the peritoneal cavity. The procedure passes a polyethylene tube from the lateral ventricle or from the spinal subarachnoid space into a ligated fallopian tube and finally into the peritoneal cavity, where the shunted cerebrospinal fluid is absorbed. This procedure is used to correct both the obstructive and the communicating types of hydrocephalus. Also called **spinofallopian tube shunt.**

ventriculography (ventrık'yulog'rəfi), **1.** an x-ray examination of the head, following injection of air or another contrast medium into the cerebral ventricles. **2.** an x-ray examination of a ventricle of the heart, following injection of a radiopaque contrast medium.

ventriculoperitoneal shunt, a surgically created passageway, consisting of plastic tubing and one-way valves, between a cerebral ventricle and the peritoneum for the draining of excess cerebrospinal fluid from the brain in hydrocephalus.

ventriculoperitoneostomy (ventrık'yulouper'ıtounios'-təmi), a surgical procedure for temporarily diverting cerebrospinal fluid in hydrocephalus, usually in the newborn. In this procedure, which spares the kidney but is less efficient than a ventriculoureterostomy, a polyethylene tube is passed from the lateral ventricle subcutaneously down the dorsal spine and is reinserted into the peritoneal cavity where the diverted fluid is absorbed. This procedure is used to correct both the communicating and the obstructive types of hydrocephalus.

ventriculopleural shunt (ventrık'yulouplur'əl), a surgical procedure for diverting cerebrospinal fluid from engorged ventricles in hydrocephalus, usually in the newborn. In this procedure, cerebrospinal fluid is diverted from the lateral ventricle into the pleural cavity. It is used to correct both the obstructive and the communicating types of hydrocephalus.

ventriculoureterostomy (ventrık'yulouyuri'təros'təmi), a surgical procedure for directing cerebrospinal fluid into the general circulation performed in the treatment of hydrocephalus, usually in the newborn. In this procedure a polyethylene tube is passed from the lateral ventricle down the dorsal spine subcutaneously to the twelfth rib; the tube is inserted through the paraspinal muscles into a ureter. Rarely used, the method is an alternative to auriculoventriculostomy, especially if the obstruction to cerebrospinal fluid includes the basilar and the cerebral subarachnoid spaces, posterior fossa, and the spinal subarachnoid spaces. The procedure is performed to correct an obstructive type of hydrocephalus.

ventro-, ventri-, a combining form meaning 'pertaining to the belly or to the front of the body': *ventrodorsal, ventrolateral, ventroptosia.*

venule (ven'yul), any one of the small blood vessels that gather blood from the capillary plexuses and anastomose to form the veins. – **venular,** *adj.*

VEP, abbreviation for **visual evoked potential.**

Veracillin, a trade name for an antibiotic (dicloxacillin sodium).

verbal aphasia. See **motor aphasia.**

Vercyte, a trade name for an antineoplastic (pipobroman).

Verequad, a trade name for a respiratory fixed-combination drug containing a bronchodilator (theophylline cal-

cium salicylate), an adrenergic (ephedrine hydrochloride), an expectorant (guaifenesin), and a sedative-hypnotic (phenobarbital).

vermicide, an agent that kills worms, particularly those in the intestine. Compare **anthelmintic, vermifuge.**

vermiform appendix, a wormlike, blunt process extending from the cecum. Its length varies from 3 to 6 inches and its diameter is about 1/3 inch. Also called **appendix vermiformis, cecal appendix.** See also **appendicitis.**

vermifuge, an agent that causes the evacuation of intestinal worms.

vermis (vər'mıs), *pl.* **vermes. 1.** a worm. **2.** a structure resembling a worm, as the median lobe of the cerebellum. – **vermiform,** *adj.*

Vermox, a trade name for an anthelmintic (mebendazole).

vernal conjunctivitis, a chronic, bilateral form of conjunctivitis, thought to be allergic in origin, that occurs most frequently in young men under 20 years during the spring and summer months. Most common symptoms include itense itching and crusting discharge. Topical corticosteroids may be applied and desensitization to pollen may be helpful. Compare **allergic conjunctivitis.**

Verneuil's neuroma (vərnoız'). See **plexiform neuroma.**

vernix caseosa (vər'nıks kæs'iou'sə), a grayish-white, cheeselike substance, consisting of sebaceous gland secretions, lanugo, and desquamated epithelial cells, that covers the skin of the fetus and newborn. It acts as a protective agent during intrauterine life and is thought to have an insulating effect against heat loss.

verruca (veru'kə), a fungating, warty skin lesion with a rough, papillomatous surface. Methods of treatment include salicylic acid, cantharidin, electrodesiccation, solid carbon dioxide, liquid nitrogen, and mental suggestion. Also called **wart.** – **verrucose, verrucous,** *adj.*

verruca plana, a small, slightly elevated, smooth, tan or flesh-colored wart, sometimes occuring in large numbers on the face, neck, back of the hands, wrists, and knees, especially in children. Also called **flat wart.**

verruca senillis. See **basal cell papilloma.**

verruca vulgans. See **wart.** Also called *verruca vulgaris.*

verrucous carcinoma, a well-differentiated squamous cell neoplasm of soft tissue of the oral cavity, larynx, or genitalia. A slow-growing tumor, it tends to displace rather than invade surrounding tissue; it does not usually metastasize.

verrucous dermatitis, any skin rash with wartlike lesions.

verruga peruana (vəru'gə per'ua'nə). See **bartonellosis.**

Versapen, a trade name for an antibacterial (hetacillin).

-verse, 1. a combining form meaning 'to turn': *reverse, sacrotransverse, transverse.* **2.** combining form meaning 'turned, changed': *inverse, reverse.*

Versene Acid, a trade name for a common chelating agent (edetic acid).

version and extraction, an obstetric operation in which a baby presenting head first is turned and delivered feet first. It is performed by reaching deeply into the uterus, grasping the baby's feet and pulling them down, and extracting the infant. The procedure is considered outmoded and hazardous and has been replaced by Caesarean section, although it may still be done to deliver a second twin. Also called **internal podalic version and total breech extraction.** Compare **external version.** See also **breech extraction, breech presentation.**

-vert, a combining form meaning a 'person who has turned (metaphorically)' in a specified direction: *extrovert, introvert, invert.*

vertebra, *pl.* **vertebrae.** any one of the 33 bones of the spinal column, comprising the seven cervical, twelve thoracic, five lumbar, five sacral, and four coccygeal vertebrae. The vertebrae, with the exception of the first and second cervical vertebrae, are much alike and are composed of a body, an arch, a spinous process for muscle attachment, and pairs of pedicles and processes. The first cervical vertebra is called the atlas and has no vertebral body. The second cervical vertebra is called the axis and forms the pivot on which the atlas rotates. The body of the axis also extends into a strong, bony process.

-vertebral, a combining form referring to the spinal column: *paravertebral, pelvivertebral, subvertebral.*

vertebral artery, each of two arteries branching from the subclavian arteries, arising deep in the neck from the cranial and dorsal subclavian surfaces. Each vertebral artery divides into two cervical and five cranial branches, supplying deep neck muscles, the spinal cord and spinal membranes, and the cerebellum. The cervical branches are the spinal and the muscular. The cranial branches are the meningeal, posterior spinal, anterior spinal, posterior inferior cerebellar, and the medullary.

vertebral body, the weight-supporting, solid central portion of a vertebra. The pedicles of the arch project from its dorsolateral surfaces.

vertebral column (vər′təbrəl, vərti′brəl), the flexible structure that forms the longitudinal axis of the skeleton and in the adult includes 26 separate vertebrae arranged in a straight line from the base of the skull to the coccyx. The vertebrae are separated by intervertebral discs. They provide attachment for various muscles, as the iliocostalis thoracis and the longissimus thoracis, which give the column strength and flexibility. The vertebral column includes seven cervical, twelve thoracic, five lumbar, five sacral, and four coccygeal vertebrae. In the adult, the sacral and the coccygeal vertebrae fuse to form the sacrum and the coccyx. The average length of the vertebral column in men is about 71 cm. The cervical part measures about 12.5 cm, the thoracic part about 28 cm, the lumbar part about 18 cm, and the sacrum and the coccyx about 12.5 cm. The vertebral column in women measures approximately 61 cm. Several curves in the column increase its strength, as the cervical, thoracic, lumbar, and pelvic curves. The cervical curve is convex ventrally from the apex of the dens to the middle of the second thoracic vertebra and is the least marked of all the curves. The thoracic curve, concave ventrally, starts at the middle of the second and ends at the middle of the twelfth thoracic vertebra. The lumbar curve, more pronounced in women than in men, begins at the middle of the last thoracic vertebra and ends at the sacrovertebral angle. The pelvic curve starts at the sacrovertebral articulation, and it ends at the point of the coccyx. The thoracic and the sacral curves constitute primary curves, present during fetal life; the cervical and the lumbar curves constitute secondary curves, which develop after birth. The cervical curve develops when the child is able to hold up its head, usually three to four months after birth; the lumbar curve develops 12 to 18 months after birth, when the child starts to walk. The vertebral column also presents a slight lateral curve, which in most individuals presents a convexity toward the right side. The vertebral canal courses through the vertebral column and contains the spinal cord. The canal is formed by the posterior arches of the vertebrae and is large and triangular in the cervical and the lumbar sections of the column, the most flexible portions. The canal is small and rounded in the thoracic region, where motion is more restricted. Also called **spinal column, spine.** See also **vertebra.**

vertebro-, a combining form meaning 'pertaining to the vertebral column or to a vertebra': *vertebrocostal, vertebrodymus, vertebrosternal.*

vertex presentation, (in obstetrics) a fetal presentation in which the vertex of the fetus is the part nearest to the cervical os and can be expected to be born first.

vertical plane. See **cardinal frontal plane.**

vertical transmission, the transfer of a disease, condition, or trait from one generation to the next, either genetically or congenitally, as the spread of an infection through breast milk or through the placenta.

vertigo. See **dizziness.**

very low-density lipoprotein, a plasma protein that is composed chiefly of triglycerides with small amounts of cholesterol, phospholipid, and protein. It transports triglycerides primarily from the liver to peripheral sites in the tissues for utilization or storage. The triglycerides are quickly converted to smaller, more soluble intermediate lipoproteins and eventually to low-density lipoproteins.

vesical fistula, an abnormal passage connecting to the urinary bladder. Vesical fistulae may communicate with the skin, vagina, uterus, or rectum.

vesicle (ves′ıkəl), a tiny blister; a small, thin-walled, raised skin lesion containing clear fluid. Compare **bulla.** – **vesicular,** *adj.*

vesicle reflex, the sensation of a need to urinate when the bladder is moderately distended. See also **micturition reflex.**

vesico-, a combining form meaning 'pertaining to the bladder or to a blister': *vesicocavernous, vesicosigmoid, vesicourethral.*

vesicoureteral reflux, an abnormal backflow of urine from the bladder to the ureter, resulting from a congenital defect, obstruction of the outlet of the bladder, or infection of the lower urinary tract. Reflux increases the hydrostatic pressure in the ureters and kidneys. The condition is characterized by abdominal or flank pain, enuresis, pyuria, hematuria, proteinuria, and bacteriuria accompanied by persistent or recurrent urinary tract infections. Diagnosis is made by cystoscopy and voiding cystourethrogram. Obstruction or defective implantation of the ureter in the bladder may be surgically corrected. Antibacterial medication, urinary tract antiseptics, and analgesia are usually prescribed for any infection that causes or results from this condition.

vesicouterine (ves′ɪkouyu′tərɪn, ves′ɪkouyu′tərain), of or pertaining to the bladder and uterus. Also called **uterovesical.**

vesicular appendix, a cystic structure on the fimbriated end of each of the Fallopian tubes. It represents a remnant of the mesonephric ducts.

vesicular breath sound, a normal sound of rustling or swishing heard with a stethoscope over the lung periphery, characteristically higher pitched during inspiration and fading rapidly during expiration. Compare **tracheal breath sound.**

vesicular mole. See **hydatid mole.**

vesiculitis (vəsɪk′yulai′tɪs), inflammation of any vesicle, particularly the seminal vesicles. Clinical manifestations of this condition are minimal; it is usually associated with prostatitis.

Vesprin, a trade name for a phenothiazine tranquilizer (triflupromazine hydrochloride) for intramuscular injection.

vessel, any one of the many tubules throughout the body that convey fluids, as blood and lymph. The main kinds of vessels are the arteries, the veins, and the lymphatic vessels.

vestibular (vestɪb′yulər), of or pertaining to a vestibule, as the vestibular portion of the mouth, which lies between the cheeks and the teeth.

vestibular gland, any one of four small glands, two on each side of the vaginal orifice. One pair of the small structures constitute the greater vestibular glands; the other pair constitute the lesser vestibular glands. The vestibular glands secrete a lubricating substance. Compare **Cowper's gland.** See also **Bartholin's gland.**

vestibule (ves′tɪbyul), a space or a cavity that serves as the entrance to a passageway, as the vestibule of the vagina or the vestibule of the ear.

vestibulocochlear nerve (vestɪb′yuloukok′liər). See **acoustic nerve.**

vestige, an imperfectly developed, relatively useless organ or other structure of the body that had a vital function at an earlier stage of life or in a more primitive form of life. The vermiform appendix is a vestigial organ. – **vestigial,** *adj.*

viable, capable of developing, growing, and otherwise sustaining life, as a normal human fetus at 28 weeks of gestation. – **viability,** *n.*

viable infant, an infant who at birth weighs 1,000 gm or is 28 weeks or more of gestational age.

Viadril, a trade name for a steroid (hydroxydione) derived from pregnanediol, used as an anesthetic agent.

Vibramycin, a trade name for a tetracycline antibiotic (doxycycline).

Vibramycin Hyclate, a trade name for a tetracycline antibiotic (doxycycline hyclate).

Vibramycin Monohydrate, a trade name for a tetracycline antibiotic (doxycycline monohydrate).

vibrating. See **cupping and vibrating.**

vibration, a type of massage administered by quick tapping with the fingertips, alternating the fingers in a rhythmical manner, or by a mechanical device. See also **massage.**

vibrio (vɪb′riou), any bacterium that is curved and motile, as those belonging to the genus *Vibrio*. Cholera and several other epidemic forms of gastroenteritis are caused by members of the genus.

Vibrio cholerae, the species of comma-shaped, motile bacillus that is the cause of cholera.

vibrio gastroenteritis, an infectious disease acquired from contaminated seafood and characterized by nausea, vomiting, abdominal pain, and diarrhea, caused by *Vibrio parahaemolyticus.* Headache, mild fever, and bloody stools may also be present. Spontaneous recovery usually occurs in two to five days. Compare **salmonellosis, shigellosis.**

Vibrio parahaemolyticus (pær′əhi′moulɪt′ɪkəs), a species of microorganisms of the genus *Vibrio,* the causative agent in food poisoning associated with the ingestion of uncooked or undercooked shellfish, especially crabs and shrimp. This microorganism is a common cause of gastroenteritis in Japan, aboard cruise ships, and in the eastern and southeastern coastal areas of the United States. Thorough cooking of seafood prevents the infection associated with *Vibrio parahaemolyticus,* which causes watery diarrhea, abdominal cramps, vomiting, headache, chills, and fever. This microorganism has an incubation period of 2 to 48 hours, after which the symptoms of infection appear. The food poisoning from this agent usually subsides spontaneously within two days but may be more severe, even fatal, in debilitated and elderly persons. Confirming diagnosis must rule out other causes of food poisoning and acute gastrointestinal disorders and requires bacteriologic examination of the vomitus, stool, and blood. Treatment usually includes bed rest and the oral replacement of fluids. Intravenous replacement of fluids is seldom required.

vidarabine, an antiviral agent.
■ INDICATIONS: It is used systemically to treat herpes simplex encephalitis and locally to treat herpesvirus I keratoconjunctivitis and keratitis.
■ CONTRAINDICATIONS: It is used in pregnancy only when the risk of teratogenicity is outweighed by benefits. Known hypersensitivity to this drug prohibits its use.
■ ADVERSE EFFECTS: Among the more serious adverse reactions to systemic administration are severe nausea and other symptoms of gastrointestinal distress, various central nervous system effects, and bone marrow depression. Local irritation, photophobia and corneal edema may occur in topical ophthalmic applications.

villioma (vil'iou'mǝ). See **villoma.**

villoma (vilou'mǝ), *pl.* **villomas, villomata.** a villous neoplasm or papilloma, occurring chiefly in the rectum. Also called **villioma.**

villous adenoma (vil'ǝs), a slow-growing, soft, spongy, potentially malignant papillary growth of the mucosa of the large intestine.

villous carcinoma, an epithelial tumor with many long, velvety papillary outgrowths. Also called **carcinoma villosum.**

villous papilloma, a benign tumor with long, slender processes, usually occurring in the bladder, breast, or a cerebral ventricle.

villus, *pl.* **villi.** one of the many tiny projections, barely visible to the naked eye, clustered over the entire mucous surface of the small intestine. The villi diffuse and transport fluids and nutrients. They are quite irregular in size and are larger in some parts of the intestine than in others, flattening out when the intestine distends. Each villus has a core of delicate areolar and reticular connective tissue supporting the epithelium, various capillaries, and usually a single lymphatic lacteal which fills with milky white chyle during the digestion of a fatty meal. – **villous,** *adj.*

vinblastine sulfate (vinblæs'tin, vinblæs'tin), an antineoplastic.
■ INDICATIONS: It is prescribed in the treatment of many neoplastic diseases.
■ CONTRAINDICATIONS: Leukopenia, bacterial infection, or known hypersensitivity to this drug prohibits its use. It is not prescribed in pregnancy.
■ ADVERSE EFFECTS: Among the most serious adverse reactions are leukopenia and neurotoxicity. Nausea, diarrhea, stomatitis, and alopecia also may occur.

Vincent's angina. See **acute necrotizing gingivitis.**
Vincent's infection. See **acute necrotizing gingivitis.**

vincristine sulfate (vinkris'tin, vinkris'tin), an antineoplastic.
■ INDICATIONS: It is prescribed in the treatment of many neoplastic diseases.
■ CONTRAINDICATION: Known hypersensitivity to this drug prohibits its use.
■ ADVERSE EFFECTS: Among the most serious adverse reactions are neurotoxicity and leukopenia. Constipation, abdominal pain, alopecia, and inflammation at the site of injection also may occur.

Viocin, a trade name for a tuberculostatic antibiotic (viomycin).

Vioform, a trade name for an antiamebic and topical anti-infective (iodochlorhydroxyquin).

Viokase, a trade name for an enzyme (pancreatin).

violence, potential for: self-directed or directed at others, a nursing diagnosis accepted by the Fourth National Conference on the Classification of Nursing Diagnoses. The etiology of the condition may be complex and may involve an antisocial personality, mania, organic brain syndrome, panic, rage, suicidal behavior, temporal lobe epilepsy, or a toxic reaction to a medication. Characteristics of clients who are potentially violent include anxiety, fear of the self or other people, lack of verbal ability, complaining or demanding vocalization, provocative, argumentative or overreactive behavior, poor self-esteem, or psychological depression. Many other factors may also be present, as a history of self-destructive behavior, pacing, excitement, agitation, or the possession of a weapon. See also **nursing diagnosis.**

viomycin sulfate, a tuberculostatic antibiotic.
■ INDICATION: It is prescribed in the treatment of tuberculosis.
■ CONTRAINDICATION: Known hypersensitivity to this drug prohibits its use.
■ ADVERSE EFFECTS: Among the more serious adverse reactions are nephrotoxicity, ototoxicity, and various allergic reactions.

viosterol (vaios'tǝrol), synthetic vitamin D_2 in an oil base. Also called **synthetic oleovitamin D.** See also **calciferol, ergosterol.**

VIP, abbreviation for a *very important person.* A VIP suite in a hospital is one reserved for such persons.

Vira-A, a trade name for an antiviral (vidarabine).

viral disease. See **viral infection.**

viral hepatitis, a viral, inflammatory disease of the liver, caused by one of the hepatitis viruses, A, B, or non-A, non-B. Transmission, speed of onset, and probable course of the illness vary with the kind and strain of virus, but the characteristics of the disease and its treatment are the same. See also **hepatitis A; hepatitis B; non-A, non-B hepatitis.**

■ OBSERVATIONS: Characteristic of viral hepatitis are anorexia, malaise, headache, pain over the liver, fever, jaundice, clay-colored stools, dark urine, nausea and vomiting, and diarrhea. Laboratory analyses reveal increased amounts of serum glutamic oxalacetic transaminase (SGOT) and bilibrubin and an abnormal coagulation of the blood. Severe infection, especially with hepatitis B virus, may be prolonged and result in tissue destruction, cirrhosis, and chronic hepatitis or in hepatic coma and death.

■ INTERVENTION: Treatment of viral hepatitis is largely supportive. It includes bed rest; isolation, if necessary; fluids; a low-fat, high-protein, high-calorie diet; special skin care if pruritus is present; emotional support; vitamins B_{12}, K, and C; and monitoring of liver and kidney function. Sedatives, analgesics, antiemetics, and steroids may be ordered. However, the patient is carefully observed for adverse reaction to medication, as the liver may not be able to break down and detoxify the drugs. Decrease in the amount or frequency of administration or change of the medication may be necessary.

■ NURSING CONSIDERATIONS: The person is taught the importance of rest and of avoiding fatigue, of washing the hands carefully after urinating or defecating in order to avoid spreading the virus, of eating well, of following written dietary instructions after discharge, and of avoiding alcohol, usually for at least one year. The patient is encouraged to have certain blood tests performed periodically, including SGOT and serum bilirubin, to report any symptoms of recurrence immediately, and to avoid contact with people having infections. The person is told not to donate blood and not to take over-the-counter drugs without medical consultation.

viral infection, any of the diseases caused by one of approximately 200 viruses pathogenic to humans. Some are the most communicable and dangerous diseases known; some are mild and transient conditions that pass virtually unnoticed. If cells are damaged by the viral attack, disease exists. The signs of the infection reflect the anatomic location of the damaged cells. Viruses are introduced into the body through a break in the skin or through a transfusion into blood stream, by droplet infection through the respiratory tract, or by ingestion through the digestive tract into the gastrointestinal system. The pathogenicity of the particular virus depends on the rapidity of action, the enzymes released, the part of the body infected, and the particular action of the virus. The general process of viral infection reflects the life cycle of a virus. The first step in the cycle, after entry into the body, is the attachment of the virus to a susceptible cell and the cell's adsorption of the virus. This is followed by penetration of the viral nucleic acid into the parasitized cell. The dissembled virus at this point causes no symptoms and cannot be recovered from the cells in infectious form. The virus begins to mature within the cell and, carrying its own genetic information, begins to replicate itself, using chemical building blocks and energy available in the parasitized cell. The virus has now taken over the cell. After a variable period of time, masses of fully grown viruses appear, each able to survive outside the cells until susceptible cells are found. In poliovirus infection, one parasitized cell may produce more than 100,000 poliovirus particles in a few hours. Techniques used in viral identification and immunization are based on the essential fact that viruses can multiply only inside living cells. Inoculation of susceptible animals, of tissue culture media, and of chick embryos allows cultivation of viruses for study and identification and for the preparation of vaccine. Diagnosis of the cause of viral infection is also possible using various other techniques, including serologic tests, fluorescent antibody microscopic examination, microscopic examination, and skin tests. In many viral diseases, including mumps, smallpox, and measles, one attack confers permanent immunity. In others, immunity is short-lived. The incubation period for viral infection is short, the viruses do not circulate in the blood stream, antibodies do not form and, most often, immunity does not develop. Exposure to a few viruses results in immunity to that virus and to other closely related viruses. Some vectors are able to spread several viruses, but only one at a time. Other mechanisms of natural resistance to viral infection are poorly understood, but susceptibility to a particular virus is somehow species-specific, as chickenpox, caused by the varicellazoster virus, is seen only in humans. A protective substance, interferon, is elaborated naturally in small amounts in the body. It is cell-specific and species-specific but not virus-specific. Interferon may act as a broad-spectrum antiviral agent, protecting the body from the effects of many viral infections by stopping the synthesis of viral nucleic acid within the parasitized cell. See also specific viral infections.

viral pneumonia, 1. pulmonary infection caused by a virus. 2. *Informal.* mycoplasma pneumonia.

viremia (vairi′miə), the presence of viruses in the blood. Compare **bacteremia, fungemia, parasitemia.**

virile (vɪr′əl), 1. of, pertaining to, or characteristic of an adult male; masculine; manly. 2. possessing or exhibiting masculine strength, vigor, force, or energy. 3. of or pertaining to the male sexual functions; capable of procreation. Compare **virilism,** −**virility,** *n.*

virilism, 1. See virilization. 2. pseudohermaphrodism in a female. 3. premature development of masculine characteristics in the male. Kinds of virilism are **adrenal virilism, prosopopilary virilism.**

virilization, a process in which secondary, male sexual characteristics are acquired by a female, usually as the result of adrenal dysfunction or hormonal medication. Also called **masculinization.** See also **adrenal virilism.**

virion (vai′riən), a rudimentary virus particle with a central nucleoid surrounded by a protein sheath or capsid. The complete nucleocapsid with a nucleic acid core may constitute a complete virus, as the adenoviruses and the picornaviruses, or it may be surrounded by an envelope, as in the herpesviruses and the myxoviruses. Such an envelope is a membrane that contains lipids, proteins, and carbohydrates and projects spikelike structures from its surface. See also **capsid.**

virologist (vairol′əjist, virol′əjist), a specialist who studies viruses and diseases caused by viruses.

virology (vairol′əji, virol′əji), the study of viruses and viral diseases. — **virologic, virological,** adj.

Viroptic, a trade name for an ophthalmic antiviral (trifluridine).

virulence (vir′yələns), the power of a microorganism to produce disease. — **virulent,** adj.

virulent (vir′yulənt), of or pertaining to a very pathogenic or rapidly progressive condition. — **virulence,** n.

virus, a minute microorganism much smaller than a bacterium which, having no independent metabolic activity, may only replicate within a cell of a living plant or animal host. A virus consists of a core of nucleic acid (DNA or RNA) surrounded by a coat of antigenic protein sometimes surrounded by an envelope of lipoprotein. The virus provides the genetic code for replication, and the host cell provides the necessary energy and raw materials. More than 200 viruses have been identified as capable of causing disease in humans. Some kinds of viruses are **adenovirus, arenavirus, enterovirus, herpesvirus, rhinovirus.** See also **viral infection.** — **viral,** adj.

visceral (vis′ərəl), of or pertaining to the viscera, or internal organs in the abdominal cavity. Also called **splanchnic.**

visceral afferent fibers, the nerve fibers of the visceral nervous system that receive stimuli and carry impulses toward the central nervous system and share the sensory ganglia of the cerebrospinal nerves with the somatic sensory fibers. Peripheral distribution of the visceral afferent fibers constitutes the main difference between them and the somatic afferents. The visceral afferents produce sensations different from those of the somatic afferents. The visceral efferent fibers connect with both the somatic and visceral afferents; the number and extent of the visceral afferents is not clearly established. Their peripheral processes reach the ganglia by various routes. Most of the visceral afferents accompany blood vessels for part of their course, and various afferent fibers run in the cerebrospinal nerves. Some of the parts of the body with visceral afferents are the face, scalp, nose, mouth, descending colon, lungs, abdomen, and rectum. See also **autonomic nervous system, parasympathetic nervous system, sympathetic nervous system.**

visceral larva migrans, infestation with parasitic larvae or *Toxocara* or, occasionally, *Ascaris, Strongyloides,* or other nematodes. See **toxocariasis.**

visceral leishmaniasis. See **kala-azar.**

visceral lymph node, a small oval nodular gland that filters lymph circulating in the lymphatic vessels of the thoracic, abdominal, and pelvic viscera. The visceral lymph nodes of the thorax include the anterior mediastinal nodes, posterior mediastinal nodes, and tracheobronchial nodes. The visceral lymph nodes of the abdomen and pelvis include those that follow the course of the celiac artery, superior mesenteric artery, and inferior mesenteric artery. Compare **parietal lymph node.** See also **lymph, lymphatic system, lymph node.**

visceral nervous system, the visceral portion of the peripheral nervous system that comprises the whole complex of nerves, fibers, ganglia, and plexuses by which impulses travel from the central nervous system to the viscera and from the viscera to the central nervous system. It contains the usual afferent fibers that receive stimuli and carry impulses toward the central nervous system and efferent fibers that carry impulses from the appropriate centers to the active effector organs, as the nonstriated muscle, cardiac muscle, and glands of the body. Also called **involuntary nervous system.** Compare **parasympathetic nervous system, sympathetic nervous system.** See also **autonomic nervous system.**

visceral pain, abdominal pain caused by any abnormal condition of the viscera. It is characteristically severe, diffuse, and difficult to localize.

visceral peritoneum, one of two portions of the largest serous membrane in the body, that invests the viscera. The free surface of the visceral peritoneum is a smooth layer of mesothelium exuding a serous fluid which lubricates the viscera and allows them to glide freely against the wall of the abdominal cavity or over each other. The attached surface of the membrane is connected to the viscera and the abdominal wall by subserous fascia. Compare **parietal peritoneum.** See also **peritoneal cavity.**

viscero-, a combining form meaning 'pertaining to the organs of the body': *viscerocranium, visceropleural, viscerosomatic.*

viscid (vis′id), **viscous** (vis′kəs), sticky or glutinous.

viscous fermentation, the formation of viscous material in milk, urine, and wine by the action of various bacilli.

viscus (vis′kəs), *pl.* **viscera** (vis′ərə). any one of the large internal organs contained in the abdominal, the thoracic, or the pelvic cavities of the body. — **visceral,** adj.

vision, the capacity for sight.

visit, 1. a meeting between a practitioner and a client or patient. In the hospital and the home, the practitioner makes a visit to the patient; in the clinic or office the patient makes a visit to the practitioner. 2. (of a patient) to meet a practitioner to obtain professional services or (of a practitioner) to see a patient or client in order to render a professional service.

Vistaril, a trade name for a tranquilizer (hydroxyzine hydrochloride).

Vistaril IM, a trade name for a tranquilizer (hydroxyzine hydrochloride).

Vistaril Pamoate, a trade name for a tranquilizer (hydroxyzine pamoate).

Vistrax, a trade name for a gastrointestinal fixed-combination drug containing an anticholinergic (oxyphencyclimine hydrochloride) and a tranquilizer (hydroxyzine hydrochloride).

visual accommodation, a process by which the eye adjusts and is able to focus, producing a sharp image at various, changing distances from the object seen. The convexity of the anterior surface of the lens may be increased or decreased by contraction or relaxation of the ciliary muscle. With increasing age the lens becomes harder and less flexible, resulting in a loss of accommodation, and, usually, the ability to focus on nearby objects. Compare **presbyopia.**

visual evoked potential (VEP), an evoked potential elicited by a repeatedly flashing light. The waves produced are too variable to be reliable predictors of injury to nerve tissue. High-risk infants are monitored with VEP to evaluate visual function.

visual field defect, one or more spots or defects in the vision that move with the eye, unlike a floater. This fixed defect is usually caused by damage to the retina or visual pathways, as by chorioretinitis, traumatic injury, macular degeneration, glaucoma, or a vascular occlusion of the eye or the brain. Sudden loss of a noticeable portion of the visual field warrants ophthalmologic examination. Defects in the field of vision may be detected using an Amsler grid.

visual memory, the ability to create an eidetic image of visual experiences. Also called **eye memory.**

visual pathway, a pathway over which a visual sensation is transmitted from the retina to the brain. A pathway consists of an optic nerve, the fibers of an optic nerve traveling through or along the sides of the optic chiasm to the lateral geniculate body of the thalamus, and an optic tract terminating in an occipital lobe. Each optic nerve contains fibers from only one retina. The optic chiasm contains fibers from the nasal portions of the retinas of both eyes; these fibers cross to the opposite side of the brain at the optic chiasm. The fibers from the temporal portion of each eye bypass the optic chiasm and pass through the lateral geniculate body on the same side of the brain continuing back to the occipital lobe. Thus the optic tracts, occipital lobe, lateral geniculate bodies of the thalamus, and optic chiasm each contain nerve fibers from both eyes. If the right optic tract were destroyed a person would lose partial vision in both eyes—the right nasal and the left temporal fields of vision.

visual purple. See **rhodopsin.**

vita-, a combining form meaning 'pertaining to life': *vitaglass, vital, vitascope.*

vital capacity (VC), a measurement of the amount of air that can be expelled after a maximum inspiration, representing the greatest possible breathing capacity. The average normal values of 4,000 to 5,000 ml are affected by age, physical dimensions of the chest cage, physical fitness, posture, and sex. The vital capacity may be reduced by a decrease in functioning lung tissue, owing to atelectasis, edema, fibrosis, pneumonia, pulmonary resection, or tumors, by limited chest expansion, resulting from ascites, chest deformity, neuromuscular disease, pneumothorax, or pregnancy, or by airway obstruction. Compare **expiratory reserve volume, residual volume, tidal volume.**

vital signs, the measurements of pulse rate, respiration rate, and body temperature. Although not strictly a vital sign, blood pressure is also customarily included. Abnormalities of vital signs are often clues to diseases, and alterations in vital signs are used to evaluate a patient's progress. See also **blood pressure, pulse, respiration, temperature.**

vital statistics, data relating to births or natality, deaths or mortality, marriages, health, and disease or morbidity.

vitamin, an organic compound essential in small quantities for normal physiologic and metabolic functioning of the body. With few exceptions, vitamins cannot be synthesized by the body and must be obtained from the diet or dietary supplements. No one food contains all the vitamins. Vitamin-deficiency diseases produce specific symptoms usually alleviated by the administration of the appropriate vitamin. Vitamins are classified according to their fat- or water-solubility, their physiologic effects, or their chemical structures, and they are designated by alphabetical letters or specific names. The fat-soluble vitamins are A, D, E, and K; the B complex and C vitamins are water-soluble. See also **avitaminosis, hypervitaminosis, oleovitamin, provitamin,** specific vitamins.

(See page 1142 for table)

vitamin A, a fat-soluble, solid terpene alcohol essential for skeletal growth, maintenance of normal mucosal epithelium, and visual acuity. It is derived from various carotenoids, mainly carotene, and is present in leafy green vegetables, yellow fruits and vegetables, the liver oils of the cod and other fish, liver, milk, cheese, butter, and egg yolk. Deficiency leads to atrophy of epithelial tissue resulting in keratomalacia, xerophthalmia, night blindness, and lessened resistance to infection of mucous membranes. Symptoms of hypervitaminosis A are irritability, fatigue, lethargy, abdominal discomfort, painful joints, severe throbbing headache, insomnia and restlessness, night sweats, loss of body hair, brittle nails, and exophthalmus. Also called **anti-infection vitamin, antixerophthalmic vitamin.** See also **oleovitamin A.**

vitamin B₁. See **thiamine.**

vitamin B₂. See **riboflavin.**

vitamin B₆. See **pyridoxine.**

vitamin B complex, a group of water-soluble vitamins differing from each other structurally and in their biologic effect. All of the B vitamins are found in large quantities in liver and yeast, and they are present separately or in combination in many foods. Heat and prolonged cooking, especially cooking with water, destroys the B vitamins. See also **folic acid,** vitamins B₁ through B₁₂.

vitamin C. See **ascorbic acid.**

vitamin D, a fat-soluble vitamin chemically related to the steroids and essential for the normal formation of bones and teeth and for the absorption of calcium and phosphorus from the gastrointestinal tract. The vitamin is present in natural foods in small amounts, and requirements are usually met by artificial enrichment of various foods, especially milk and dairy products, and exposure to sunlight. Ultraviolet rays activate a form of cholesterol in the oil of the skin and convert it to a form of the vitamin, which is then absorbed. The natural foods containing vitamin D are of animal origin and include saltwater fish, especially salmon, sardines, and herring, organ meats, fish-liver oils, and egg yolk. Deficiency of the vitamin results in rickets in children, osteomalacia, osteoporosis, and osteodystrophy. Hypervitaminosis D produces a toxicity syndrome characterized by anorexia, vomiting, headache, drowsiness, diarrhea, and calcification of the soft tissues of the heart, blood vessels, renal tubules, and lungs. Treatment consists of discontinuing the vitamin dosage and initiating a low-calcium diet until symptoms resolve. See also **calciferol, vitamin D₃.**

vitamin D₃, an antirachitic, white, odorless, crystalline, unsaturated alcohol that is the predominant form of vitamin D of animal origin. It is found in most fish-liver oils, butter, brain, and egg yolk and is formed in the skin, fur, and feathers of animals and birds exposed to sunlight or ultraviolet rays. Also called **activated 7-dehydrocholesterol, cholecalciferol.**

vitamin deficiency, a state or condition resulting from the lack of or inability to utilize one or more vitamins. The symptoms and manifestations of each deficiency vary depending on the specific function of the vitamin in promoting growth and development and maintaining body health.

vitamin D resistant rickets, a disease clinically similar to rickets but resistant to treatment with large doses of vitamin D. It is caused by a congenital defect in renal tubular reabsorption of phosphate and is usually seen in men. See also **rickets.**

vitamin E, any or all of the group of fat-soluble vitamins that consist of the tocopherols and are essential for normal reproduction, muscle development, resistance of erythrocytes to hemolysis, and various other biochemical functions. It is an intracellular antioxidant and acts in maintaining the stability of polyunsaturated fatty acids and other fatlike substances, including vitamin A and hormones of the pituitary, adrenal, and sex glands. Deficiency results in muscle degeneration, abnormalities in the vascular system, megaloblastic anemia, hemolytic anemia, infertility, creatinuria, and liver and kidney damage and is associated with the aging process. The richest dietary sources are wheat-germ, soybean, cottonseed, peanut, and corn oils, margarine, whole raw seeds and nuts, soybeans, eggs, butter, liver, sweet potatoes, and the leaves of many vegetables, as turnip greens. It is stored in the body for long periods of time so that severe deficiency is rare. It is considered nontoxic except in hypertensive patients and those with chronic rheumatic heart disease. See also **tocopherol.**

vitamin H. See **biotin.**

vitamin K, a group of fat-soluble vitamins known as quinones that are essential for the synthesis of prothrombin in the liver and of several related proteins involved in the clotting of blood. It is also involved with the process of phosphorylation and electron transport. The vitamin is widely distributed in foods, especially leafy green vegetables, pork liver, yogurt, egg yolk, kelp, alfalfa, fish-liver oils, and blackstrap molasses and is synthesized by the bacterial flora of the gastrointestinal tract. It is also produced synthetically. Deficiency results in hypoprothrombinemia, characterized by poor coagulation of the blood and hemorrhage, and usually occurs from inadequate absorption of the vitamin from the gastrointestinal tract or the inability to utilize it in the liver. It is used to reduce the clotting time in patients with obstructive jaundice and in hemorrhagic states associated with intestinal diseases and diseases of the liver; it is given prophylactically to infants to prevent hemorrhagic disease of the newborn. A form of the vitamin is used as a preservative to control fermentation in foods. Natural vitamin K is stored in the body and produces no toxicity. Excessive doses of synthetic vitamin K may cause anemia in newborn infants and hemolysis in persons with glucose-6-phosphate deficiency. See also **vitamins K₁, K₂, K₃.**

vitamin K₁, a yellow, viscous, oil-soluble vitamin, occurring naturally, especially in alfalfa, and produced synthetically. It is used as a prothrombinogenic agent. Also called **phylloquinone, phytonadione.**

vitamin K₂, a pale-yellow, fat-soluble crystalline vitamin of the vitamin K₂ group that is more unsaturated than vitamin K₁ and slightly less active biologically. It is isolated from putrefied fish meal and synthesized by various bacteria in the gastrointestinal tract. See also **vitamin K.**

Vitamins and their nutritional significance

Vitamins	Physiological function	RDA*	Sources
A (retinol)	Necessary component in formation of pigment rhodopsin (visual purple) Formation and maintenance of epithelial tissue	Infants—1400-2000 IU†; others‡—2000-5000 IU	Natural form—liver, kidney, fish oils, milk and non-skimmed milk products, egg yolk
Provitamin A (carotene)			Carrots, sweet potatoes, squash, apricots, spinach, collards, broccoli, cabbage, artichokes
B_1 (thiamine)	Coenzyme (with phosphorus) in carbohydrate metabolism	Infants—0.3-0.5 mg; others— 0.7-1.5 mg (usually calculated in relation to caloric intake as 0.5 mg/1000 kcal)	Meats—pork, beef, or liver Legumes, nuts, and whole or enriched grains
B_2 (riboflavin)	Coenzyme (with phosphorus) in protein metabolism	Infants—0.4-0.6 mg; others— 0.8-1.8 mg (usually calculated in relation to caloric intake as 0.6 mg/1000 kcal)	Milk and its products, eggs, organ meats (liver, kidney, and heart), enriched cereals, some green leafy vegetables, and legumes
Niacin (nicotinic acid, nicotinamide)	Coenzyme (with riboflavin) in protein and fat metabolism	Infants—5.0-8.0 mg; others— 9-20 mg (tryptophan is a precursor; 60 g = 1 mg of niacin)	Meat, fish, peanuts, beans, peas, whole or enriched grains except corn and rice
B_6 (pyridoxine)	Coenzyme in protein, carbohydrate, and fat metabolism Possibly involved in metabolism of polyunsaturated fatty acids	Infants—0.3-0.4 mg; others— 0.6-2.0 mg	Meats, especially liver and kidney, cereal grains (wheat and corn), yeast, soybeans, and peanuts
B_9 (folic acid) (reduced form is called folinic acid or citrovorum factor)	Coenzyme for single-carbon transfer (purines, thymine, hemoglobin)	Infants—50 μg; others— 100-400 μg	Green leafy vegetables (spinach), asparagus, liver, kidney, nuts
B_{12} (cobalamin)	Coenzyme in protein synthesis, indirect effect on formation of red blood cells (particularly on formation of nucleic acids and folic acid metabolism)	Infants—0.3 μg; others— 1.0-3.0 μg	Meat, liver, kidney, milk, eggs, and cheese

C (ascorbic acid)	Intercellular cement substance
	General metabolism
	  Increases utilization of iron for hemoglobin formation
	  Enhances conversion of folic to folinic acid
	  Affects cholesterol synthesis and conversion of proline to hydroxyproline
	  Probably a coenzyme in metabolism of tyrosine and phenylalanine
	  May play role in hydroxylation of adrenal steroids
	  May have stimulating effect on phagocytic activity of leukocytes and formation of antibodies
		Infants—35 mg; others— 40-45 mg	Citrus fruits, berries, tomatoes, melon, cabbage, green and yellow vegetables

*RDA—Recommended Dietary Allowances represent the amount of nutrients needed daily by healthy individuals, plus an excess of 30% to 50% to allow for
†One international unit (IU) is approximately equivalent to 1 milligram (mg).
‡Others—1 to 18 years of age

Results of deficiency	Results of overdose
Night blindness Keratinization of the epithelium, xerophthalmia, conjunctivitis, phrynoderma, and drying of the respiratory, gastrointestinal, and genitourinary tracts Defective tooth enamel Retarded growth Impaired bone formation Decreased thyroxine formation	Early signs—irritability, anorexia, pruritus, fissures at the corners of nose and lips Later signs—hepatomegaly, jaundice, retarded growth, poor weight gain, thickening of the cortex of long bones with pain and fragility, hard tender lumps in extremities and occiput of the skull NOTE: Overdose only results from ingestion of large quantities of the vitamin, not the provitamin; large amounts of carotene (carotenemia) cause yellow or orange discoloration of the skin (not the sclera as in jaundice), but none of the above symptoms

Beriberi
  Gastrointestinal—anorexia, constipation, indigestion
  Neurological—apathy, fatigue, emotional instability, polyneuritis, convulsions, and coma (in infants)
  Circulatory—cardiac failure, peripheral vasodilation, edema
	None

Ariboflavinosis
  Lips—cheilosis, perlèche
  Tongue—glossitis
  Nose—irritation and cracks at nasal angle
  Eyes—burning, itching, tearing, photophobia, cornea vascularization, cataracts
  Skin—seborrheic dermatitis, delayed wound healing and tissue repair
	None

Pellagra
  Oral—stomatitis, glossitis
  Cutaneous—scaly dermatitis on exposed areas
  Gastrointestinal—anorexia, weight loss, diarrhea, fatigue
  Neurological—apathy, anxiety, confusion, depression, dementia
	Nicotinic acid—potent vasodilator, circulatory disturbances, skin flushing, itching, and increased peristalsis

Scaly dermatitis, convulsions, peripheral neuritis, anemia, retarded growth	None
Macrocytic anemia, bone marrow depression, glossitis, intestinal malabsorption	None

Pernicious anemia
  General signs of severe anemia
  Lemon yellow tinge to skin
  Spinal cord degeneration
	Unknown

Scurvy
  Skin—dry, rough, petechiae, perifollicular hyperkeratotic papules
  Musculoskeletal—bleeding into muscles and joints, pseudoparalysis from pain, swelling of joints, costochondral beading (scorbic rosary)
  Gums—spongy, friable, swollen, bleed easily, bluish red or black color, teeth loosen and fall out
  General disposition—irritable, anorexic, apprehensive, in pain, refuses to move
  Signs of anemia
  Decreased wound healing
  Increased susceptibility to infection
	None, controversial reports of beneficial effects of megadoses in prevention of infection (common cold)

continued.

individual variations and conditions of stress. RDA set by Food and Nutrition Board of the National Academy of Sciences—National Research Council (1974).

Vitamins and their nutritional significance—cont'd

Vitamins	Physiological function	RDA	Sources
D₂ (ergocalciferol) and D₃ (cholecalciferol)	Absorption of calcium and phosphorus and decreased renal excretion of phosphorus	400 IU	Cod liver oil, herring, mackerel, salmon, tuna, sardines, direct sunlight Enriched food sources—milk, milk products, cereals, margarine, breads, many breakfast drinks
E (tocopherol)	Production of red blood cells Muscle and liver integrity Antioxidant agent Coenzyme factor in tissue respiration Reproduction (demonstrated only in animals) Minimizes oxidation of polyunsaturated fatty acids and vitamin A in intestinal tract and tissues	Infants—4-5 IU; others—10-15 IU	Vegetable oils, wheat germ, milk, eggs, muscle meats, fish, cereal, nuts, legumes, green leafy vegetables
K	Catalyst for production of prothrombin and blood clotting factors II, VII, IX, and X by the liver	Not established	Pork, liver, green leafy vegetables (spinach, kale, cabbage), tomatoes, egg yolk, cheese

vitamin K₃. See **menadione.**

vitaminology (vai'təmɪnol'əji), the study of vitamins, including their structures, modes of action, and function in maintaining the health of the body.

vitamin P. See **bioflavonoid.**

vitamin P₂. See **calciferol.**

vitellin (vɪtel'ɪn), a phosphoprotein containing lecithin, found in the yolk of eggs. Also called **ovovitellin.**

vitelline artery (vɪtel'ɪn), any of the embryonic arteries that circulate blood from the primitive aorta of the early developing embryo to the yolk sac. Also called **omphalomesenteric artery.**

vitelline circulation, the circulation of blood and nutrients between the developing embryo and the yolk sac by way of the vitelline arteries and veins. Also called **omphalomesenteric circulation.** See also **fetal circulation.**

vitelline duct, (in embryology) the narrow channel connecting the yolk sac with the intestine. Also called **umbilical duct.**

vitelline membrane, the delicate cytoplasmic membrane surrounding the ovum. Also called **yolk membrane.** See also **zona pellucida.**

vitelline sac. See **yolk sac.**

vitelline sphere. See **morula.**

vitelline vein, any of the embryonic veins that return blood from the yolk sac to the primitive heart of the early developing embryo. Also called **omphalomesenteric vein.**

vitellogenesis (vɪtel'oujen'ɪsɪs), the formation or production of yolk. — **vitellogenetic,** adj.

vitellus (vɪtel'əs, vaitel'əs), the yolk of an ovum. — **vitelline,** adj.

vitiligo (vɪt'ɪli'gou), a benign, acquired skin disease of unknown cause, consisting of irregular patches of various sizes totally lacking in pigment and often having hyperpigmented borders. Exposed areas of skin are most often affected. Treatment using 8-methoxypsoralen requires extreme care and carefully regulated sun exposure. Waterproof cosmetics are often used to cover the patches. Compare **albinism, piebald.** — **vitiliginous,** adj.

vitriol, oil of. See **sulfuric acid.**

vitreous body. See **vitreous humor.**

vitreous cavity, the cavity posterior to the lens that contains the vitreous body and vitreous membrane and is transected by the vestigial remnants of the hyaloid canal.

vitreous hemorrhage, a hemorrhage into the vitreous humor of the eye.

vitreous humor, a transparent, semigelatinous substance contained in a thin hyoid membrane filling the cavity behind the crystalline lens of the eye. Some indications of the hyaloid canal may persist in the vitreous humor, but it is not penetrated by any blood vessels and is nourished at its periphery by vessels of the retina and the ciliary processes. The vitreous humor is concave anteriorly to accommodate the crystalline lens and is closely applied to the retina around the wall of the eyeball. Also called **corpus vitreum, vitreous body.**

vitreous membrane, a membrane that lines the posterior cavity of the eye and surrounds the vitreous body.

Results of deficiency	Results of overdose
Rickets	Acute—vomiting, dehydration, fever, abdominal cramps, bone pain, convulsions, and coma
Head—craniotabes, bossing of the frontal bones, deformed shape (skull flat and depressed toward middle), delayed closure of fontanels	Chronic—lassitude, mental slowness, anorexia, failure to thrive, thirst, urinary urgency, polyuria, vomiting, diarrhea, abdominal cramps, bone pain, pathological fractures
Chest—rachitic rosary, pigeon chest, Harrison's groove	Calcification of soft tissue—kidneys, lungs, adrenal glands, vessels (hypertension), heart, gastric lining
Spine—kyphosis, scoliosis, lordosis	Osteoporosis of long bones
Abdomen—potbelly, constipation	Elevated serum levels of calcium and phosphorus
Extremities—bowing of arms and legs, knock-knee, saber shins, instability of hip joints, pelvic deformity, enlargement of epiphysis at ends of long bones	
Teeth—delayed calcification, especially of permanent teeth	
Not well established; may involve red blood cell hemolysis, especially in premature infants, and focal necrosis of tissues	Unknown
Causes infertility in rats, but not in humans (does *not* increase human male virility or potency)	
Hemorrhage	Hyperbilirubinemia in infants
	Hemolytic anemia in patients who are deficient in glucose-6-phosphate dehydrogenase

Vivactil, a trade name for a tricyclic antidepressant (protriptyline hydrochloride).

vivax malaria (vai'væks). See **tertian malaria.**

viviparous (vivip'ərəs), bearing living offspring rather than eggs, as most mammals and some fishes and reptiles. Compare **oviparous, ovoviviparous.**

Vivonex, a trade name for a nutritional supplement containing protein, carbohydrate, and fat.

VMA, abbreviation for **vanillylmandelic acid.**

V̇o₂, symbol for *oxygen uptake.*

vocal cord, either of two strong bands of yellow elastic tissue in the larynx enclosed by membranes called vocal folds and attached ventrally to the angle of the thyroid cartilage and dorsally to the vocal process of the arytenoid. Also called **true vocal cord, vocal ligament.** Compare **false vocal cord.**

vocal cord nodule, a small, inflammatory or fibrous growth that develops on the vocal cords of people who constantly strain their voices. Also called **screamer's nodule, singer's nodule, teacher's nodule.** See also **chorditis.**

vocal fremitus, the vibration of the chest wall as a person speaks or sings that allows the person's voice to be heard by the examiner during auscultation of the chest with a stethoscope. Vocal fremitus is decreased in emphysema, pleural effusion, pulmonary edema or bronchial obstruction.

voice-box. See **larynx.**

void, to empty, or evacuate, as urine from the bladder.

volar (vou'lər), of or pertaining to the palm of the hand or the sole of the foot.

volar ligament. See **retinaculum flexorum manus.**

volatile, (of a liquid) having the characteristics of boiling at a low temperature and evaporating at room temperature.

volatile solvent, an easily evaporated liquid capable of dissolving a substance.

-volemia, a combining form meaning '(condition of the) volume of plasma in the body': *hypervolemia, hypovolemia, normovolemia.*

volition (vəlɪ'shən), **1.** the act, power, or state of willing or choosing. **2.** the conscious impulse to perform or to abstain from an act. — **volitional,** *adj.*

Volkmann's canal (foulk'manz), any one of the small canals connecting Haversian canals in bone tissue. Compare **Haversian canaliculus.** See also **Haversian system.**

Volkmann's contracture, a serious, persistent flexion contraction of forearm and hand owing to ischemia. A pressure or crushing injury in the region of the elbow usually precedes this condition, and pressure from a cast or tight bandage about the elbow are common causes. Permanent fibrosis, muscle degeneration, and a clawlike hand may result. Nurses must watch for swelling, pallor, coldness, cyanosis, or pain distal to the injury site so that prompt loosening of constriction can restore circulation. Also called **ischemic contracture.**

Volkmann splint, a splint that supports and immobilizes the lower leg. It has a footpiece attached to two sides that extends from the foot to the knee, allowing ambulation.

volsella forceps (volsel'ə), a kind of forceps having a

small, sharp-pointed hook at the end of each blade. Also called **volsella, volsellum forceps, vulsella forceps.**

volt, the unit of electric potential. In an electrical circuit a volt is the force required to send one ampere of current through one ohm of resistance, or the difference in potential between two points on a conductor carrying a charge of one ampere when there is a dissipation of one watt between them. See also **ampere, circuit, current, ohm, watt.**

volume, the amount of space occupied by a body, expressed in cubic units.

volume-control fluid chamber, any one of several types of transparent, plastic reservoirs with graduated volumetric markings, used to regulate the flow of intravenous solutions. These devices are components of intravenous volume control sets and accommodate the injection and the mixing of medications by means of special built-in ports. The volume-control fluid chamber contains a filter which must be primed to function.

volume dose. See **integral dose.**

voluntary, (of an action, thought, etc.) originated, undertaken, controlled or accomplished as a result of a person's free will or choice.

voluntary agency, a service agency legally controlled by volunteers rather than by owners or a paid staff. Most public health nursing agencies are voluntary; most hospitals, which are legally controlled by hospital boards, are composed of lay and professional members who are not paid for their services.

voluntary muscle. See **striated muscle.**

-volute, a combining form meaning 'to roll, turn around': *cicumvolute, involute, revolute.*

volvulus (vol′vyuləs), a twisting of the bowel on itself, causing intestinal obstruction. The condition is frequently the result of a prolapsed segment of mesentery and occurs most often in the ileum, the secum, or the sigmoid portions of the bowel. If it is not corrected, the obstructed bowel becomes necrotic, peritonitis and rupture of the bowel occur, and death may ensue. Severe, gripping pain, nausea and vomiting, an absence of bowel sounds, and a tense, distended abdomen suggest the diagnosis, which is confirmed by x-ray examination. Compare **intussusception.**

volvulus neonatorum, an intestinal obstruction in a newborn baby resulting from a twisting of the bowel due to malrotation or nonfixation of the colon. Typical symptoms include abdominal distention, persistent regurgitation, often accompanied by fecal vomiting, and nonpassage of stools. Characteristic barium enema x rays confirm the diagnosis. The condition requires immediate surgical correction to prevent necrosis and gangrene of the affected segment of bowel.

vomer (vou′mər), the bone forming the posterior and inferior part of the nasal septum and having two surfaces and four borders.

vomit, **1.** to expel the contents of the stomach through the esophagus and out of the mouth. Also called **emesis, vomitus.** **2.** the material expelled.

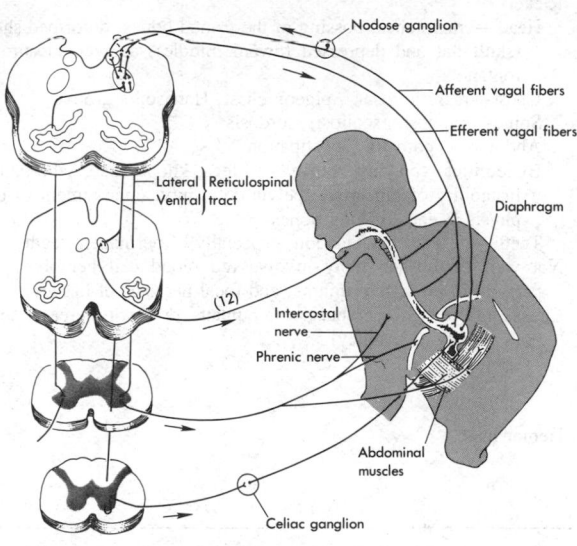

BRAIN CIRCUITS INVOLVED IN INITIATING VOMITING REFLEX

von Economo's encephalitis (von′ɪkon′əmouz). See **epidemic encephalitis.**

von Gierke's disease (vongir′kəz), a form of glycogen storage disease in which abnormally large amounts of glycogen are deposited in the liver and kidneys. The disorder is characterized by hypoglycemia, ketoacidosis, and hyperlipemia. Biopsy of the affected organs reveals the absence of glucose-6-phosphate dehydrogenase (G-6-PD), an enzyme necessary for glycogen metabolism. There is no effective treatment for the disorder. Medical efforts are directed at preventing hypoglycemia and ketoacidosis. Also called **glycogen storage disease, type I.** See also **glycogen storage disease.**

von Hippel-Lindau disease. See **cerebroretinal angiomatosis.**

von Pirquet test (vonpərkei′). See **Pirquet test.**

von Recklinghausen's disease (vanrek′lɪŋhau′zənz). See **neurofibromatosis.**

Vontrol, a trade name for an antiemetic (diphenidol).

von Willebrand's disease, an inherited disorder characterized by abnormally slow coagulation of the blood and spontaneous epistaxis and gingival bleeding owing to a deficiency of Factor VIII. Excessive bleeding is common postpartum, during menstruation, and following injury or surgery. Compare **angiohemophilia.** See also **hemophilia, thrombasthenia.**

Voranil, a trade name for an anorexiant (clortermine hydrochloride).

-vorous, a combining form meaning 'of or referring to feeding on' something specified: *leguminivorous, panivorous, proteinivorous.*

vortex, *pl.* **vortexes, vortices.** a whirlpool effect produced by the whirling of a more or less cylindrical mass of fluid (liquid or gas). The velocity of the motion increases as the radius of the circle described by the motion decreases; the velocity decreases as the radius increases. Tornadoes and whirlpools are examples of free vortexes.

vox (voks), voice, as vox cholerica, the barely audible, hoarse voice of a patient in an advanced and severe case of cholera.

vox cholerica. See **vox.**

voyeur (voiyər′, *French* vwayœr′), one whose sexual desire is gratified by the practice of voyeurism. Also called **Peeping Tom.**

voyeurism (voi′yəriz′əm, voiyər′izəm), a psychosexual disorder in which a person derives sexual excitement and gratification from looking at the naked bodies and genital organs or observing the sexual acts of others, especially from a secret vantage point.

VSD, abbreviation for **ventricular septal defect.**

vulsella forceps (vəlselə). See **volsella forceps.**

vulva (vəl′və). See **pudendum.** — **vulvar,** *adj.*

vulvar (vəl′vər), of or pertaining to the vulva.

vulvectomy (vəlvek′təmi), the surgical removal of part or all of the tissues of the vulva, performed most frequently in the treatment of malignant or premalignant neoplastic disease. **Simple vulvectomy** includes the removal of the skin of the labia minora, the labia majora, and the clitoris. **Radical vulvectomy** involves excision of the labia majora, labia minora, clitoris, the surrounding tissues, and pelvic lymph nodes.

vulvocrural (vəl′voukrur′əl), of or pertaining to the vulva and the thigh.

vulvovaginal (vəl′vouvæj′ɪnəl), of or pertaining to the vulva and the vagina.

VZV, abbreviation for **varicella zoster virus.**

W

W, symbol for **tungsten.**

Wagner-Meissner corpuscle (vag′nərmaɪs′nər), one of a number of small, special sensory end organs with a connective tissue capsule and tiny stacked plates in the corium of the hand and foot, the front of the forearm, the skin of the lips, the mucous membrane of the tongue, the palpebral conjunctiva, and the skin of the mammary papilla. A single nerve fiber penetrates each oval capsule, spirals through the interior, and ends as a globular mass. Also called **tactile corpuscle of Meissner.** Compare **Golgi-Mazzoni corpuscles, Krause's corpuscles.**

Wagstaffe's fracture (wæg′stæfs), a fracture characterized by separation of the internal malleolus.

waking imagined analgesia (WIA), the pain relief experienced by a patient who employs the psychological technique, usually with the help of an attending nurse or a hospital aide, of concentrating on previous pleasant personal experiences that produced tranquility, as lying on a summer beach beside cooling ocean water or drifting down a quiet river in a canoe. The patient employing the WIA technique is encouraged to verbalize such experiences, thereby reinforcing recollection with attendant soothing biological responses. This technique is often effective in reducing mild to moderate pain, especially when used with a mild nonnarcotic analgesic and the compassionate interaction of an attending health care professional. See also **pain evaluation, pain intervention, pain mechanism.**

Waldenström's disease (val′dənstrœmz). See **Perthes' disease.**

Wald (wɔld), **Lillian** (1867–1940), an American public-health nurse, settlement leader, and social reformer. She founded the Henry Street Settlement in New York to bring nursing care into the homes of the poor, which led to the development of the Visiting Nurse Service of New York. She was also instrumental in establishing the school nursing system, the federal government's Children's Bureau, and the Nursing Service Division of the Metropolitan Life Insurance Company. She was the first nurse to be elected into the Hall of Fame for Great Americans.

walker, an extremely light, movable apparatus, about waist high, made of metal tubing, used to aid a patient in walking. It has four widely placed, sturdy legs. The patient holds onto the walker and takes a step, then moves the walker forward and takes another step. Compare **crutch.**

walking pneumonia. See **mycoplasma pneumonia.**

walking rounds, rounds in which the clinician responsible leads a group of junior clinicians on a tour to visit the patients for whom they are collectively responsible. In some hospitals nurses may participate in walking rounds in lieu of or in addition to report.

wall, a limiting structure within the body, as the wall of the abdominal, the thoracic, or the pelvic cavities, or the wall of a cell.

wander, 1. to move about purposelessly. 2. to cause to move back and forth in an exploratory manner, as, in inserting an intrauterine catheter, the tip of the inserter must usually be wandered around the fetal head in the cervix in order to find a space through which the catheter may be passed upward into the uterus.

wandering goiter. See **diving goiter.**

Wangensteen apparatus (wæŋ′ənstin′), a nasogastroduodenal catheter and a suction apparatus used for constant, gentle drainage and decompression of the stomach or duodenum. It may be used to relieve abdominal distention that often occurs postoperatively or that may complicate a gastrointestinal disorder, especially an intestinal obstruction. See also **Wangensteen tube.**

Wangensteen tube, the catheter portion of a Wangensteen apparatus.

Wans, a trade name for an fixed-combination drug containing an antihistamine antiemetic (pyrilamine maleate) and a sedative-hypnotic (pentobarbital sodium).

warfarin poisoning, a toxic condition caused by the ingestion of warfarin, accidentally in the form of a rodenticide or by overdose with the substance in its pharmacologic anticoagulant form. The poison accumulates in the body and results in nosebleed, bruising, hematuria, melena, and internal hemorrhage. Treatment may include gastric lavage, a cathartic, vitamin K, and blood transfusion. The goal of therapy is to eliminate the poison and to reestablish normal coagulation.

warfarin sodium, an anticoagulant.

■ INDICATIONS: It is prescribed for the prophylaxis and treatment of thrombosis and embolism.

■ CONTRAINDICATIONS: Hemorrhage or known hypersensitivity to this drug prohibits its use.

■ ADVERSE EFFECTS: The most serious adverse reaction is

hemorrhage. Many other drugs interact with this drug to increase or decrease its effects.

warm-blooded, having a relatively high and constant body temperature, as the temperatures maintained by humans, other mammals, and birds, despite changes in environmental temperatures. Heat is produced in the warm-blooded human body by the catabolism of foods in proportion to the amount of work performed by the tissues in the body. Heat is lost from the body by evaporation, radiation, conduction, and convection. About 80 per cent of the body heat that is dissipated in humans is lost through the skin; the rest is lost through the mucous membranes of the respiratory, the digestive, and the urinary systems. The temperature of the average healthy human is 98.6°F or 37°C. The human body's tolerance for change in its temperature is very small, and significant changes can have drastic, even fatal consequences. The control mechanism for temperature in the human body consists of thermal receptive neurons in the anterior portion of the hypothalamus, more than two million sweat glands, and the vast network of blood vessels in the skin. Reduced heat loss results from less secretion and slower evaporation of sweat and from vasoconstriction of blood vessels. Increased heat gain results from shivering, which increases the work of body tissues and, hence, increases catabolism. Fever, which raises internal body temperature, temporarily resets the thermostatic control of the hypothalamus by the action of chemical pyrogens from bacteria and viruses and by the function of the prostaglandins that the pyrogens release. The temperature control mechanisms of the body serve to restore normal heat levels during fever. Aspirin and other antipyretic drugs foil the synthesis of prostaglandins. Also called **homoiothermal, homothermal.** Compare **cold-blooded.**

war neurosis. See **combat fatigue, shell shock.**

wart. See **verruca.**

Warthin's tumor. See **papillary adenocystoma lymphomatosum.**

washout, the elimination or expulsion of one gas or volatile anesthetic agent by the administration of another.

wasp, a slender, narrow-waisted insect with two pairs of membranous wings that are folded lengthwise when at rest like parts of a fan. Many species of wasps may give painful stings that may have severe results in hypersensitive persons. Treatment is as for bee stings.

Wassermann test (was′ərmən), a diagnostic blood test for syphilis based on the complement-fixation reaction.

wasting, a process of deterioration marked by weight loss and decreased physical vigor, appetite, and mental activity.

water (H₂O), a chemical compound, one molecule of which contains one atom of oxygen and two atoms of hydrogen. Almost three quarters of the earth's surface is covered by water. Essential to life as it exists on this planet, water comprises more than 70 per cent of living things. Pure water freezes at 0°C (32°F) and boils at 100°C (212°F) at sea level.

waterborne, carried by water, as a waterborne epidemic of typhoid fever.

Waterhouse-Friderichsen syndrome (wɔ′tərhaus′frīd′ərīk′sən), overwhelming bacteremia, characterized by the sudden onset of fever, cyanosis, petechiae, and collapse from massive bilateral adrenal hemorrhage. The syndrome requires immediate emergency treatment, hospitalization, and intensive care. Emergency treatment includes vasopressor drugs, intravenous fluids, plasma, and oxygen. No sedatives or narcotics are given. Specific treatment for bacteremia is intensive antibiotic therapy, given parenterally and continued for several days after symptoms subside. Nursing management includes close observation and the maintenance of adequate provision of fluids and nutrients.

water moccasin. See **cottonmouth.**

waters. *Informal.* See **amniotic fluid.**

watt, the unit of electrical power or work in the meter/kilogram/second system of notation. The watt is the product of the voltage and the amperage. One watt of power is dissipated when a current of one ampere flows across a difference in potential of one volt. See also **ampere, current, ohm, volt.**

wave, a disturbance in which energy moves through a medium without permanently altering the constituents of the medium. Electromagnetic waves, as light, x rays, and radio waves, can travel through a vacuum. Sound waves can be transmitted only through matter. See also **electromagnetic radiation, light, sound, x ray.**

wavelength, the distance between a given point on one wave cycle and the corresponding point on the next successive wave cycle. A pure color is produced by light of a specific wavelength. Electromagnetic waves of different wavelengths account for many of the transmission characteristics of radio and television.

wax. See **cerumen.**

wax bath. See **paraffin bath.**

waxy flexibility. See **cerea flexibilitas.**

WBC, abbreviation for **white blood cell.** See **leukocyte.**

W chromosome, Z chromosome, the sex chromosomes of certain insects, birds, and fishes. Females of such species are heterogametic and have one W and one Z chromosome, whereas males are homogametic and have two Z chromosomes. The ZZ-ZW system of nomenclature was chosen to differentiate the chromosomes from the XX-XY type, which occurs in man and various other animals and in which the female is homogametic and the male is heterogametic.

W/D, symbol for *well-developed,* often used in the initial identifying statement in a patient record. It is used so frequently as to have lost all meaning or use in identifying or describing the patient.

wean, **1.** to induce a child to give up breast feeding and to accept other food in place of breast milk. Many children are ready for weaning during the second half of the first year; some wean themselves. **2.** to detach or withdraw a person from something on which he is dependent. – **weanling,** *n.*

weanling, a child who has recently been weaned.

weaver's bottom, a form of bursitis affecting the ischial bursae of the hips of people whose work requires prolonged sitting in one position. Also called, *Obsolete,* **tailor's bottom.**

web, a network of fibers forming a tissue or a membrane, as the laryngeal web that spreads between the vocal cords.

Weber tuning fork test, a method of assessing auditory acuity, especially useful in determining if defective hearing in an ear is a conductive loss caused by a middle-ear problem or a sensorineural loss, resulting from a disorder in the inner ear or auditory nerve system. The test is performed by placing the stem of a vibrating 256 tuning fork in the center of the person's forehead or on the maxillary incisors. The loudness of the sound is equal in both ears if hearing is normal. If the person has a sensorineural loss in one ear, the unaffected ear perceives the sound as louder. When conductive hearing loss is present, the sound is louder in the affected ear, because it does not hear ordinary background noise conducted through the air and receives only sound vibrations by bone conduction.

wedge fracture, a fracture of vertebral structures with anterior compression.

wedge pressure, the capillary pressure in the left atrium, determined by measuring the pressure in a cardiac catheter wedged in the most distal segment of the pulmonary artery.

wedge resection, the surgical excision of part of an organ, as a part of an ovary containing a cyst. The segment excised may be wedge-shaped.

WEE, abbreviation for **Western equine encephalitis.** See **equine encephalitis.**

weed. *Slang.* See **cannabis.**

weeping, **1.** crying, lacrimating. **2.** oozing or exuding fluid, as a sore or rash.

Wegener's granulomatosis (veiʹgənərz), an uncommon, chronic inflammatory process leading to the formation of nodules or tumorlike masses in the air passages, necrotizing vasculitis, and glomerulonephritis. Symptoms, depending on the organs involved, may include sinus pain, a bloody, purulent nasal discharge, saddle-nose deformity, chest discomfort and cough, weakness, anorexia, weight loss, and skin lesions. Glomerulonephritis, as a complication, was formerly fatal in a few months, but with the use of cytotoxic drugs, especially cyclophosphamide, a high percentage of patients achieve long-term remissions.

weight, the force exerted on a body by the gravity of the earth. On the surface of the earth, mass and weight are the same. As a body moves away from the earth, the weight of the body decreases, but the mass remains constant. In space, a body has mass but no weight. Weight is sometimes measured in units of force, as newtons or poundals, but it is usually expressed in pounds or kilograms, as is mass. See also **mass.**

Weil's disease (vailz). See **leptospirosis.**

Weismannism (vaisʹmənizʹəm), the basic concepts of heredity and development as proposed by German biologist August Weismann. These state that the vehicle of inheritance is the germ plasm, which is distinct from the somatoplasm and is transmitted from one generation to the next; that during embryonic development the hereditary components are dispersed to the somatoplasm to give rise to inherited characteristics; and that changes in somatoplasm do not affect germ plasm, so that acquired characteristics cannot be inherited. Also called **germ plasm theory.** Also called **Weismann's theory.** Compare **pangenesis.** – **Weismannian,** *adj., n.*

Weiss's sign (vaisʹiz). See **Chvostek's sign.**

well-baby care, periodic health supervision for infants and children in order to promote optimal physical, emotional, and intellectual growth and development. Such health-care measures include routine immunizations to prevent disease, screening procedures for early detection and treatment of illness, and parental guidance and instruction in proper nutrition, accident prevention, and specific care and rearing of the child at various stages of development. The recommended preventive health-care schedule for children who are developing normally is monthly for the first six months of life, every two months until one year of age, every three months during the second year, every six months during the third year, followed by annual visits. Well-baby care may be provided in a clinic, a convenient local meeting place, a private doctor's office, the Public Health Nurse's office, or a school. Nurses or nurse practitioners frequently provide the care.

well-differentiated lymphocytic malignant lymphoma, a lymphoid neoplasm characterized by the predominance of mature lymphocytes. Also called **lymphocytic lymphoma, lymphocytic lymphosarcoma, lymphocytoma.**

wellness, a dynamic state of health.

wen (wen). See **pilar cyst.**

Wenckebach heart block. See **Mobitz I heart block.**

Wenckebach periodicity, a form of second-degree atrioventricular block with a progressive beat-to-beat prolongation of the PR interval, finally resulting in a nonconducting P wave. At this point, the PR interval shortens to normal and the sequence recurs. Also called **Wenckebach phenomenon.** See also **atrioventricular block.**

Werdnig-Hoffmann disease (verd′nɪghɔf′man), a genetic disorder beginning in infancy or young childhood, characterized by progressive atrophy of the skeletal muscle resulting from degeneration of the cells in the anterior horn of the spinal cord and the motor nuclei in the brain stem. Onset occurs within the first year of life, with the condition usually apparent at birth. Symptoms include congenital hypotonia, absence of stretch reflexes, flaccid paralysis, especially of the trunk and limbs, lack of sucking ability, fasciculations of the tongue and, sometimes, of other muscles, and, often, dysphagia. Treatment is symptomatic and death generally occurs in early childhood, often from respiratory complications. The condition is transmitted as an autosomal recessive trait and occurs more frequently in siblings than in successive generations. Also called **familial spinal muscular atrophy, Hoffmann's atrophy, infantile spinal muscular atrophy, progressive spinal muscular atrophy of infants, Werdnig-Hoffmann paralysis.** See also **floppy infant syndrome.**

Werlhof's disease (verl′hofs). See **thrombocytopenic purpura.**

Wernicke's encephalopathy (vər′nɪkiz en′sefəlop′əthi), an inflammatory, hemorrhagic, degenerative condition of the brain, characterized by lesions in several parts of the brain including the hypothalamus, mamillary bodies, and tissues surrounding ventricles and aqueducts. The condition is characterized by double vision, involuntary and rapid movements of the eyes, lack of muscular coordination, and decreased mental function, which may be mild or severe. Wernicke's encephalopathy is caused by a thiamine deficiency and is seen in association with chronic alcoholism. It also occurs as a complication of gastrointestinal tract disease and hyperemesis gravidarum owing to malabsorption and malnutrition.

West African sleeping sickness. See **Gambian trypanosomiasis.**

Westcort, a trade name for a glucocorticoid (hydrocortisone valerate).

western equine encephalitis (WEE). See **equine encephalitis.**

West nomogram, a nomogram used in estimating the body surface area of children or adults. See also **nomogram.**

wet cough. *Nontechnical.* See **productive cough.**

wet dream. See **nocturnal emission.**

wet dressing, a moist dressing used to relieve symptoms of some skin diseases. As the moisture evaporates, it cools and dries the skin beneath it, softens dried blood and sera, and stimulates drainage. Medication may be added if necessary.

wet lung, an abnormal condition of the lungs, characterized by a persistent cough and rales at the lung bases. It occurs in workers exposed to pulmonary irritants, as ammonia, chlorine, sulfur dioxide, volatile organic acids, dusts, and vapors of corrosive chemicals. Treatment consists of removing the person from exposure to the irritant and therapy for possible pulmonary edema. Compare **pulmonary edema.** See also **pleural effusion, pleurisy.**

wet nurse, a woman who cares for and breast feeds another's infant.

W/F, symbol for *white female,* often used in the initial identifying statement in a patient record.

Wharton's jelly, a gelatinous tissue that remains when the embryonic body stalk blends with the yolk sac within the umbilical cord.

wheal (hwil), an individual lesion of urticaria.

wheat weevil disease, a hypersensitivity pneumonitis caused by allergy to weevil particles found in wheat flour.

wheelchair, a mobile chair equipped with large wheels and brakes. If longterm use of the chair is expected, a physical therapist may prescribe certain personalized requirements, as size, left- or right-hand propulsion, type of brakes, height of armrests, special seat pads, and various other features.

wheeze, **1.** a form of rhonchus, characterized by a high-pitched musical quality. It is caused by a high velocity flow of air through a narrowed airway and is heard both during inspiration and expiration. Wheezes are associated with asthma and chronic bronchitis. Unilateral wheezes are characteristic of bronchogenic carcinoma, foreign bodies, and inflammatory stenosing lesions. An asthmatoid wheeze is caused by an obstruction in the trachea or bronchus. **2.** to breathe with a wheeze. See also **rales, rhonchi.**

whiplash injury, *Informal.* an injury to the cervical vertebrae or their supporting ligaments and muscles causing pain and stiffness, usually resulting from sudden acceleration or deceleration of the body, as in a rear-end car collision.

Whipple's disease, a rare intestinal disease characterized by severe intestinal malabsorption, steatorrhea, anemia, weight loss, arthritis, and arthralgia. Persons with the disease are severely malnourished and have abdominal pain, chest pain, and a chronic nonproductive cough. The diagnosis is made by jejunal biopsy. Penicillin and tetracycline may alleviate the symptoms. See also **malabsorption syndrome.**

whipworm. See **Trichuris.**

whirlpool bath, the immersion of the body or a part of the body in a tank of hot water agitated by a jet of equally hot water and air.

white blood cell (WBC). See **leukocyte.**

white cell, *Informal.* white blood cell. See **leukocyte.**

white corpuscle. See **leukocyte.**

white damp. See **damp.**

white fibrocartilage, a mixture of tough, white fibrous tissue and flexible cartilaginous tissue. It is one of the three kinds of cartilage in the body and is divided into interarticular fibrocartilage, connecting fibrocartilage, circumferential fibrocartilage, and stratiform fibrocartilage. Compare **hyaline cartilage, yellow cartilage.**

whitehead. See **milia.**

white leg. See **phlegmasia alba dolens.**

white matter. See **white substance.**

white substance, the tissue surrounding the gray substance of the spinal cord, consisting of many myelinated nerve fibers and unmyelinated nerve fibers, embedded in a spongy network of neuroglia. It is subdivided in each half of the spinal cord into three funiculi: the anterior, the posterior, and the lateral white column. Each column subdivides into tracts that are closely associated in function. The anterior column divides into two ascending tracts and five descending tracts. The posterior column divides into two large ascending tracts, one small descending tract, and one intersegmental tract. The lateral column divides into six ascending tracts and four descending tracts. Also called **white matter.** Compare **gray substance.** See also **spinal cord, spinal tract.**

white thrombus, 1. an aggregation of blood platelets, fibrin, clotting factors, and cellular elements containing few or no erythrocytes. 2. a thrombus comprised chiefly of white blood cells. 3. a thrombus composed primarily of blood platelets and fibrin.

whitlow (hwɪt'lou), an inflammation of the end of a finger or toe that results in suppuration. See also **felon.**

WHO, abbreviation for **World Health Organization.**

whole blood, blood that is unmodified except for the presence of an anticoagulant. It is used for transfusion. Various components and factors may be separated from whole blood for infusion to replace or to augment a component or factor that is deficient in amount or function owing to a variety of diseases and conditions.

whooping cough. See **pertussis.**

whorl (hwərl), a spiral turn, as one of the turns of the cochlea or of the dermal ridges that form fingerprints.

WIA, abbreviation for **waking imagined analgesia.**

Widal test (vidal'), an agglutination test used to aid in the diagnosis of salmonella infections, as typhoid fever. A fourfold increase in titer of agglutinins is highly suggestive of active infection. A high titer may persist for years after the disease or after immunization against typhoid fever.

Wiedenbach (wi'dənbæk), **Ernestine** (1900–), a German-born American nursing educator and writer. She taught maternal and newborn health nursing at Yale School of Nursing, was a leader in family-centered maternity nursing, and developed the full range of the art and science of obstetrical nursing.

Wigraine, a trade name for a fixed-combination drug containing anticholinergics (belladonna alkaloids), an analgesic (phenacetin), and a vasoconstrictor (ergotamine tartrate), used to treat migraine.

wild-type gene, a normal or standard form of a gene, as contrasted with a mutant form.

will, 1. the mental faculty that enables one consciously to choose or decide upon a course of action. 2. the act or process of exercising the power of choice. 3. a wish, desire, or deliberate intention. 4. a disposition or attitude toward another or others. 5. determination or purpose; willfulness.

Willis's circle (wɪl'ɪsɪz). See **circle of Willis.**

Willis's disease. See **diabetes mellitus.**

willow fracture. See **greenstick fracture.**

Wilms' tumor (vɪlm'zɪz), a malignant neoplasm of the kidney, occurring in young children, before the fifth year in 75 per cent of the cases. The most frequent early sign of this large malignant tumor of childhood is hypertension, followed by the appearance of a palpable mass, pain, and hematuria. Diagnosis usually can be established by an excretory urogram with tomography. The tumor, an embryonal adenomyosarcoma, is well encapsulated in the early stage, but it may later extend into lymph nodes and the renal vein or vena cava and metastasize to the lungs or other sites. Prompt removal of resectable tumors by transperitoneal nephrectomy is recommended. Radiotherapy is used preoperatively or postoperatively; it may be used palliatively in inoperable cases. Cyclic chemotherapy with actinomycin-D and vincristine combined with surgery and irradiation is proving highly effective.

Wilpo, a trade name for an anorexiant (phentermine hydrochloride).

Wilson's disease, a rare, inherited disorder of copper metabolism, in which copper accumulates slowly in the liver and is then released and taken up in other parts of the body. Hemolysis, then hemolytic anemia occur as the copper accumulates in the red blood cells. Accumulation in the brain destroys certain tissue and may cause tremors, muscle rigidity, dysarthria, and dementia. Kidney function is diminished; the liver becomes cirrhotic. Treatment of Wilson's disease includes a reduction of copper in the diet and the prescription of copper-binding agents and penicillamine. Also called **hepatolenticular degeneration.**

Winckel's disease (wɪŋ'kəlz). See **hemoglobinuria.**

wind chill, the loss of heat from the body when it is exposed to wind of a given speed at a given temperature and humidity. The **wind-chill index** is expressed in kilocalories per hour per square meter of skin surface. The **wind-chill factor** is expressed in degrees Celsius or Fahrenheit as the effective temperature felt by a person exposed to the weather.

winding sheet, a shroud for wrapping a dead body.

window, a surgically created opening in the surface of a structure or an anatomically occurring opening in the surface or between the chambers of a structure.

windowed, (of an orthopedic cast) having an opening, especially to relieve pressure that may irritate and inflame the skin.

Winstrol (wɪn′strɔl), a trade name for an androgen (stanozolol), used as an anabolic agent.

winter cough, *Nontechnical.* a chronic condition characterized by a persistent cough occasioned by cold weather. See also **cough.**

wintergreen oil. See **methyl salicylate.**

winter itch, pruritus occurring in cold weather in people who have dry skin, particularly in those who have atopic dermatitis. Warmer temperature, increased humidity, and topical, antipruritic emollients may offer relief.

wiry pulse, an abnormal pulse that is strong but small.

wisdom tooth, either of the last teeth on each side of the upper and lower jaw. These are third molars and are the last teeth to erupt, usually between the ages of 17 and 21, often causing considerable pain, dental problems, and the need for extraction. Also called **dens serotinus.** See also **molar.**

wish fulfillment, 1. the gratification of a desire. 2. (in psychology) the satisfaction of a desire or the release of emotional tension through such processes as dreams, daydreams, and neurotic symptoms. 3. (in psychoanalysis) one of the primary motivations for dreams in which an unconscious desire or urge, unacceptable to the ego and superego because of sociocultural restrictions or feelings of personal guilt, is given expression.

wishful thinking, the interpretation of facts or situations according to one's desires or wishes rather than as they exist in reality, usually used as an unconscious device to avoid painful or unpleasant feelings.

Wiskott-Aldrich syndrome (wɪs′kotɔl′drɪ̆ch), immunodeficiency inherited as a recessive, X-linked trait, characterized by thrombocytopenia, eczema, inadequate T and B cell function, and an increased susceptibility to viral, bacterial, and fungal infections and to cancer. Treatment includes the prescription of appropriate antibiotics for specific infectious organisms and the administration of transfer factor from activated lymphocytes to increase the resistance to infection and to clear the eczema. See also **transfer factor.**

witch hazel, 1. a shrub, *Hamamelis virginiana,* indigenous to North America, from which an astringent extract is derived. 2. Also called **hamamelis water.** a solution comprised of the extract, alcohol, and water, used as an astringent.

witch's milk, a milklike substance secreted from the breast of the newborn, caused by circulating maternal lactating hormone. Also called **hexenmilch.**

withdrawal, 1. See also **schizophrenia.** a common response to physical danger or severe stress characterized by a state of apathy, lethargy, depression, retreat into oneself, and, in grave cases, catatonia and stupor. It is pathologic if it interferes with a person's perception of reality and the ability to function in society, as in the various forms of schizophrenia. 2. the removal of the penis from the vagina in sexual intercourse prior to ejaculation in an attempt to prevent conception. Withdrawal is not an effective method of contraception. Also called **coitus interruptus.**

withdrawal bleeding, the passage of blood from the uterus, associated with the shedding of endometrium that has been stimulated and maintained by hormonal medication. It occurs when the medication is discontinued. In the endocrine evaluation of a woman with amenorrhea, withdrawal bleeding constitutes evidence that the woman's endometrium is reponsive to hormonal stimulation and that the cause of her amenorrhea is probably not uterine.

withdrawal method, a contraceptive technique in coitus wherein the penis is pulled from the vagina prior to ejaculation. It is not reliable because small amounts of seminal fluid carrying millions of spermatozoa may be emitted without sensation prior to full ejaculation. Also called **coitus interruptus.**

withdrawal symptom. See **symptom.**

withdrawal symptoms, the unpleasant, sometimes life-threatening physiologic changes that occur when some drugs are withdrawn after prolonged, regular use. The effects may occur following use of a narcotic, tranquilizer, stimulant, barbiturate, alcohol, or other substance to which the person has become physiologically or psychologically addicted.

withdrawn behavior, a condition in which there is a blunting of the emotions and a lack of social responsiveness.

Wittmaack-Ekbom syndrome (vɪt′makek′bom). See **restless legs syndrome.**

W/M, symbol for *white male,* often used in the initial identifying statement in a patient record.

W/N, symbol for *well-nourished,* often used in the initial identifying statement in a patient record. It is used so frequently as to have lost all meaning or use in identifying or describing the patient.

Wolffian body (vɔl′fiən). See **mesonephros.**

Wolffian duct (vɔl′fiən). See **mesonephric duct.**

Wolff-Parkinson-White syndrome (wɔlf′par′kɪnsənhwait′), a disorder of atrioventricular conduction, characterized by two AV conduction pathways. This syndrome is often identified by a characteristic deltawave seen on an electrocardiogram. See also **Lown-Ganong-Levine syndrome.**

wolfram (W). See **tungsten.**

woman-year, (in statistics) a year in the reproductive life of a sexually active woman; a unit that represents 12 months of exposure to the risk of pregnancy. Woman-years are used in calculating a pregnancy rate in the assessment of the effectiveness of the various methods of family planning and of the adverse effect on the birth rate of various environmental factors.

womb. See **uterus.**

wood alcohol. See **methanol.**

Wood's glass, a nickel-oxide filter that holds back all light except for a few violet rays of the visible spectrum and ultraviolet wavelengths of about 365 nm. It is used extensively to help diagnose fungus infections of the scalp and erythrasma and to reveal porphyrins and fluorescent materials.

Wood's light, an ultraviolet light used to diagnose certain scalp and skin diseases. The light causes hairs infected with a fungus, as *tinea capitis,* to become brilliantly fluorescent. Also called **Wood's glass, Wood's lamp, Wood's rays.**

woolsorter's disease, the pulmonary form of anthrax, so named because it is an occupational hazard to those who handle sheep's wool. Early symptoms mimic influenza, but the patient soon develops high fever, respiratory distress, and cyanosis. If the disease is not treated at this stage, it is often fatal. Also called **pulmonary anthrax.** See also **anthrax.**

word association. See **controlled association.**

word association test. See **association test.**

word salad, a jumble of words and phrases that lacks logical coherence and meaning, often characteristic of disoriented individuals and schizophrenics.

work therapy, a therapeutic approach in which the client performs a useful activity or learns an occupation, as in occupational therapy.

work tolerance, the kind and amount of work that a physically or mentally ill person can or should perform.

work-up, the process of performing a complete evaluation of a patient, including history, physical examination, laboratory tests, and x-ray or other diagnostic procedures in order to acquire an accurate data base upon which a diagnosis and treatment plan may be based.

World Health Organization (WHO), an agency of the United Nations, affiliated with the Food and Agricultural Organization of the UN, the International Atomic Energy Agency, the International Labor Organization, the Pan American Health Organization, and UNESCO. The WHO is primarily concerned with worldwide or regional health problems, but in emergencies it is authorized to render local assistance on request. Its functions include furnishing technical assistance, stimulating and advancing epidemiologic investigation of diseases, recommending health regulations, promoting cooperation among scientific and professional health groups, and providing information and counsel relating to health matters. Its headquarters are in Geneva, Switzerland. Also called **Organisation Mondiale de la Santé, OMS.**

worm, any of the soft-bodied, elongated invertebrates of the phyla Annelida, Nemathelminthes, or Platyhelminthes. Some kinds of worms parasitic for humans are **hookworm, pinworm, tapeworm.** See also **fluke, roundworm.**

wormian bone (vɔr′miən), any of several tiny, smooth, segmented bones that are soft, moist, and tepid to the touch, usually found as the serrated borders of the sutures between the cranial bones. Wormian bones were named for the Danish anatomist Claus Worm.

wound, **1.** any physical injury involving a break in the skin, usually caused by an act or accident rather than by a disease, as a chest wound, gunshot wound, puncture wound. **2.** to cause an injury, especially one that breaks the skin.

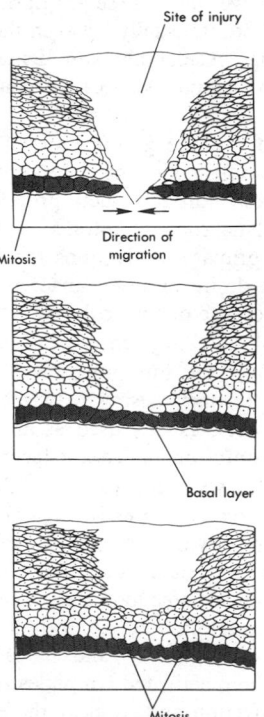

WOUND REPAIR IN SKIN

wound irrigation, rinsing a wound or the cavity formed by a wound using a medicated solution, water, or an antimicrobial liquid preparation.

■ METHOD: The dressing is removed and wrapped for disposal. The patient is assisted to an appropriate position. Using equipment from a sterile irrigation pack or tray, an irrigating solution is then poured into a graduated measure. It is then warmed in a basin of warm water unless the solution's action depends on antibiotic or enzyme activity, which would be inhibited by warming. An emesis or kidney basin is then fitted snugly against the patient's body beneath the wound. It may be held in place by the patient or by an assistant. A catheter is held with sterile gloves or forceps and gently inserted into the wound to a prescribed depth and at a prescribed angle. A syringe filled with irrigating solution is then attached to the catheter and the solution is gently instilled. The catheter is pinched before the empty syringe is removed to prevent aspiration of the return irrigation flow during disconnection. The syringe is filled and attached again and the wound is irrigated until the returning solution runs clear. If a catheter is not used, the solution is sprayed directly on the wound from the syringe until the wound looks clean. After irrigation is completed, the body area is dried with sterile sponges working from the wound out to the area around it, and a dry sterile dressing is applied.

■ OUTCOME CRITERIA: Wounds are irrigated in order to remove secretions and dried blood and to keep the wound surface open in order to encourage healing from the inside out. When the irrigation solution returns clear, the wound is considered clean.

■ NURSING ORDERS: Frequency of irrigation, type of solution, and amount of solution to be used are specifically prescribed. The condition of the wound, amount of irrigating solution used, and the appearance of the returned solution are noted by the nurse.

Wright's stain (rīts), a stain containing methylene blue and eosin, used to color blood specimens for microscopic examination, as for complete blood count and, particularly, for malarial parasites.

wrist. See **carpus.**

wrist joint. See **radiocarpal articulation.**

writer's cramp, a painful involuntary contraction of the muscles of the hand when attempting to write. It often occurs following long periods of writing. Also called **graphospasm.**

wrongful death statute, (in law) a statute existing in all states that provides that the death of a person can give rise to a cause of legal action brought by the person's beneficiaries in a civil suit against the person whose willful or negligent acts caused the death. Prior to the existence of these statutes, a suit could be brought only if the injured person survived the injury.

wrongful life action, (in law) a civil suit usually brought against a physician or health facility on the basis of negligence that resulted in the wrongful birth or life of an infant. The parents of the unwanted child seek to obtain payment from the defendant for the medical expenses of pregnancy and delivery, for pain and suffering, and for the education and upbringing of the child. Wrongful life actions have been brought and won in several situations, including malpracticed tubal ligations, vasectomies, and abortions. Failure to diagnose pregnancy in time for abortion and incorrect medical advice leading to the birth of a defective child have also led to malpractice suits for a wrongful life.

wryneck. See **torticollis.**

Wuchereria (vu'kəri'riə), a genus of filarial worms found in tropical climates. *Wuchereria bancrofti,* transmitted by mosquitoes, is the cause of elephantiasis. See also **filariasis.**

Wyamine Sulfate, a trade name for an alpha-adrenergic agent (mephentermine sulfate).

Wycillin, a trade name for an antibacterial (penicillin G procaine).

Wydase, a trade name for an enzyme (hyaluronidase).

X

xanthelasma palpebrarum (zæn'thɪlæz'mə pæl'pəbrə'-rəm). See **xanthoma palpebrarum.**

xanthelasmatosis (zæn'fhɪlæz'mətou'sɪs), a dissemi-nated, generalized form of planar xanthoma frequently associated with reticuloendothelial disorders, especially multiple myeloma.

xanthemia (zænfhi'miə). See **carotenemia.**

xanthine (zæn'fhin), a nitrogenous by-product of the metabolism of nucleoproteins. It is normally found in the muscles, liver, spleen, pancreas, and urine. – **xanthic,** *adj.*

xanthine derivative, any one of the closely related al-kaloids, caffeine, theobromine, or theophylline. They are found in plants widely distributed geographically and are variously ingested as components in different beverages, as coffee, tea, cocoa, and cola drinks. The xanthine deriv-atives or methylxanthines have pharmacological proper-ties that stimulate the central nervous system, produce diuresis, and relax smooth muscles. Theobromine has low potency and is seldom used as a pharmaceutical. Theo-phylline produces more dangerous central nervous system stimulation than caffeine. Some experiments have shown that caffeine increases the capacity for sustained intellec-tual effort, decreases reaction time, and improves the as-sociation of ideas. Caffeine and theophylline also affect the circulatory system, tending to dilate the systemic blood vessels but increasing cerebrovascular resistance with an associated decrease in cerebral blood flow and the oxygen tension of the brain. Some authorities believe it is this vasoconstriction that accounts for the relief of hyper-tensive headaches in individuals who drink beverages that contain any of the xanthine derivatives. The ability of the xanthine derivatives to relax smooth muscle is especially important in certain treatments of asthma. Theophylline is most effective in such treatment and markedly increases vital capacity. The methylxanthines reinforce the release of certain secretions of various endocrine and exocrine tissues, except for mast cells and, possibly, certain other mediators of inflammation. Caffeine can induce chromo-somal abnormalities in plant cells and in mammalian cells in culture, and it strongly augments mutations of micro-organisms. Such effects are apparently associated with the retardation of DNA-repair mechanisms but only occur at caffeine concentrations much higher than those in xan-thine beverages, as coffee. Several studies offer contradic-

tory conclusions as to whether daily ingestion of more than 5 to 6 cups of coffee increases the susceptibility to myocardial infarction. Research continues in an effort to determine the effect of caffeine on pregnant women who ingest it in large amounts. Various studies indicate that the per capita consumption of caffeine in the United States is 200 mg daily, about 90 per cent of which comes from coffee. One cup of coffee contains approximately 85 mg of caffeine; one cup of tea contains about 50 mg of caffeine and 1 mg of theophylline. One cup of cocoa contains about 250 mg of theobromine and 5 mg of caf-feine. A 350 ml bottle of a cola beverage contains about 50 mg of caffeine. Consumption of xanthine beverages may cause various problems, including restlessness and inability to sleep, gastrointestinal irritation, and excessive myocardial stimulation characterized by premature sys-tole and tachycardia.

xanthinuria (zæn'fhɪnyur'iə), **1.** the presence of exces-sive quantities of xanthine in the urine. **2.** a rare disorder of purine metabolism, resulting in the excretion of large amounts of xanthine in the urine owing to the absence of an enzyme, xanthine oxidase, that is necessary in xanthine metabolism. This inherited deficiency may cause the de-velopment of kidney stones made of xanthine precipitate.

xantho-, a combining form meaning 'yellow': *xan-thochroia, xanthogen, xanthophore.*

xanthochromic (zæn'fhəkrou'mɪk),**xanthochromatic** (zæn'fhəkroumæt'ɪk), having a yellowish color, as cer-ebrospinal fluid that contains blood or bile.

xanthogranuloma (zæn'fhougræn'yulou'mə), *pl.* **xantho-granulomas, xanthogranulomata.** a tumor or nodule of granulation tissue containing lipid deposits. A kind of xanthogranuloma is **juvenile xanthogranuloma.**

xanthoma (zænfhou'mə), *pl.* **xanthomas, xanthomata.** a benign, fatty, fibrous, yellowish plaque, nodule, or tumor that develops in the subcutaneous layer of skin, often around tendons. The lesion is characterized by the intra-cellular accumulation of cholesterol and cholesterol esters.

xanthoma disseminatum, a benign, chronic condition in which small orange or brown papules and nodules develop on many body surfaces, especially on the mucous membrane of the oropharynx, larynx, and bronchi, and in skin folds and fissures. Also called **xanthoma multiplex.**

xanthoma eruptivum. See **eruptive xanthoma.**

xanthoma multiplex. See **xanthoma disseminatum.**

xanthoma palpebrarum, a soft, yellow spot or plaque usually occurring in groups on the eyelids. Also called **xanthelasma, xanthelasma palpebrarum.**

xanthoma planum. See **planar xanthoma.**

xanthomasarcoma (zæn'fhoumǝsarkou'mǝ), a giant cell sarcoma of the tendon sheaths and aponeuroses which contains xanthoma cells.

xanthoma striatum palmare, a yellow or orange flat plaque or slightly raised nodule occurring in groups on the palms of the hands.

xanthoma tendinosum, a yellow or orange elevated or flat round papule or nodule occurring in clusters on tendons, especially the extensor tendons of the hands and feet, of individuals with hereditary lipid storage disease.

xanthomatosis (zæn'fhoumǝtou'sis), an abnormal condition in which there are deposits of yellowish fatty material in the skin, internal organs, and reticuloendothelial system. It may be associated with hyperlipoproteinemia, paraproteinemia, lipoid storage diseases, and other disorders of adipose tissue. Also called **xanthosis.** See also **hyperlipidemia, xanthoma, xanthoma palpebrarum.**

xanthoma tuberosum, a yellow or orange, flat or elevated round papule occurring in clusters on the skin of joints, especially the elbows and knees, usually in people who have a hereditary lipid storage disease, as hyperlipoproteinemia. The xanthomatous papules may also be associated with biliary cirrhosis and myxedema. Also called **tuberous xanthoma, xanthoma tuberosum multiplex.**

xanthopsia (zænfhop'siǝ), an abnormal visual condition in which everything appears to have a yellow hue. It is sometimes associated with jaundice or digitalis toxicity.

xanthosis (zænfhou'sis), 1. a yellowish discoloration sometimes seen in degenerating tissues of malignant diseases. 2. See **xanthomatosis.** 3. a reversible yellow discoloration of the skin most commonly caused by the ingestion of large amounts of yellow vegetables containing carotene pigment. The antimalarial drug quinacrine, if taken over a prolonged period, may produce a similar skin color. Xanthosis may be differentiated clinically from jaundice since the sclerae are colored yellow in jaundice but are not discolored in xanthosis. Also called **carotenosis.** See also **carotenemia.**

xanthureic acid (zænfh'yuri'ik), a metabolite of tryptophan that occurs in normal urine and in elevated levels in patients with vitamin B_6 deficiency.

X chromosome, a sex chromosome that in humans and many other species is present in both sexes, appearing singly in the cells of normal males and in duplicate in the cells of normal females. The chromosome is carried as a sex determinant by all of the female gametes and half of all male gametes, is morphologically much larger than the Y chromosome, and has many sex-linked genes associated with clinically significant disorders, as hemophilia, Duchenne's muscular dystrophy, and Hunter's syndrome. Compare **Y chromosome.**

Xe, symbol for **xenon.**

xeno-, a combining form meaning 'strange or pertaining to foreign matter': *xenodiagnosis, xenogenous, xenology.*

xenogenesis (zen'ǝjen'ǝsis), 1. alternation of generations; heterogenesis. 2. the theoretical production of offspring that are totally different from both of the parents. — **xenogenetic, xenogenic,** *adj.*

xenograft (zen'ǝgræft'). See **heterograft.**

xenon (Xe), an inert, gaseous, nonmetallic element. Its atomic number is 54; its atomic weight is 131.30.

xenophobia (zen'ǝfou'biǝ), an anxiety disorder characterized by a pervasive, irrational fear or uneasiness in the presence of strangers, especially foreigners, or in new surroundings. See also **phobia.**

xero-, a combining form meaning 'pertaining to dryness': *xerocheilia, xeromenia, xerophthalmia.*

xeroderma (zir'ǝdǝr'mǝ), a chronic skin condition characterized by dryness and roughness.

xeroderma pigmentosum, a rare, inherited skin disease characterized by sensitivity to ultraviolet light, exposure to which results in freckles, telangiectases, keratoses, papillomas, carcinoma, and, possibly, melanoma. Keratitis and tumors developing on the eyelids and cornea may result in blindness. Exposure to sunlight must be avoided.

xerogram (zi'rǝgræm), an x-ray image produced by xerography.

xeroradiography (zi'rourei'diog'rǝfi), a diagnostic x-ray technique in which an image is produced electrically rather than chemically, permitting lower exposure times and radiation of lower energy than that of ordinary x rays. It is used most commonly to discover breast tumors.

X-inactivation theory. See **Lyon hypothesis.**

xerosis (zirou'sis). See **dry skin.**

xiphi-. See **xipho.**

xiphisternal articulation, the cartilaginous connection between the xiphoid process and the body of the sternum. This joint usually ossifies at puberty. Compare **manubriosternal articulation.**

xiphisternum (zif'istǝr'nǝm). See **xiphoid process.**

xipho-, xiphi-, a combining form meaning 'pertaining to a sword or to the xiphoid process': *xiphodymus, xiphoiditis, xiphopagus.*

xiphoid appendix. See **xiphoid process.**

xiphoid process, the smallest of three parts of the sternum, articulating caudally with the body of the sternum and laterally with the seventh rib. Several muscles of the abdominal wall are attached to the xiphoid process, including the rectus abdominis and the linea alba. Also called **ensiform process, xiphisternum, xiphoid appendix.** Compare **manubrium.**

X-linked, pertaining to genes or to the characteristics or conditions they transmit that are carried on the X chromosome. Most X-linked traits and conditions, as hemophilia, are recessive and therefore occur predominantly in males, since they have only one X chromosome. Women may inherit the genes but the recessive effects are usually masked by the normal dominant alleles carried on the second X chromosome. Compare **Y-linked.** See also **sex-linked disorder.** $-$ **X linkage,** *n.*

X-linked dominant inheritance, a pattern of inheritance in which the transmission of a dominant gene on the X chromosome causes a characteristic to be manifested. Affected individuals all have an affected parent. All of the daughters of an affected male are affected but none of the sons. Half of the sons and half of the daughters of an affected female are affected. Normal children of an affected parent have normal offspring. The inheritance shows a clear positive family history. Hypophosphatemic vitamin D-resistant rickets is an example of this pattern. X-linked dominant inheritance closely resembles autosomal dominant inheritance. Compare **X-linked recessive inheritance.**

X-linked ichthyosis. See **sex-linked ichthyosis.**

X-linked inheritance, a pattern of inheritance in which the transmission of traits varies according to the sex of the person, because the genes on the X chromosome have no counterparts on the Y chromosome. The inheritance pattern may be recessive or dominant. The characteristic determined by a gene on the X chromosome is always expressed in males. Transmission from father to son does not occur. Compare **autosomal inheritance.** See also **X-linked dominant inheritance, X-linked recessive inheritance.**

X-linked mucopolysaccharidosis. See **Hunter's syndrome.**

X-linked recessive inheritance, a pattern of inheritance in which transmission of an abnormal recessive gene on the X chromosome results in a carrier state in females and characteristics of the condition in males. Affected people have unaffected parents (except for the rare situation in which the father is affected and the mother is a carrier). Half of the female siblings of an affected male carry the trait. Unaffected male siblings do not carry the trait. Sons of affected males are unaffected and daughters of affected males are carriers. Unaffected male children of a carrier female do not carry the trait.

XO, (in genetics) the designation for the presence of only one sex chromosome; either the X or Y chromosome is missing so that each cell is monosomic and contains a total of 45 chromosomes. See also **Turner's syndrome.**

x ray, 1. Also called **roentgen ray.** electromagnetic radiation of shorter wavelength than visible light. X rays are produced when electrons, traveling at high speed, strike certain materials, particularly heavy metals like tungsten. They can penetrate most substances and are used to investigate the integrity of certain structures, to therapeutically destroy diseased tissue, and to make photographic images for diagnostic purposes, as in radiography and fluoroscopy. **2.** a radiograph made by projecting x rays through organs or structures of the body onto a photographic plate. As some tissue, like bone, is more radiopaque (allowing fewer x rays to pass through) than other tissue, like skin or fat, a shadow is created on the plate that is the image of a bone or of a cavity filled with a radiopaque substance. **3.** to make a radiograph. See also **contrast medium, electron, fluoroscopy, radiopaque.** $-$ **x-ray,** *adj.*

x-ray microscope, a microscope that produces images by x-rays and records them on fine-grain film or projects them as enlargements. Film images produced by x-ray microscopes may be examined at quite large magnifications with a light microscope.

x-ray pelvimetry, a radiographic examination used to determine the dimensions of the bony pelvis of a pregnant woman and, if possible, the biparietal diameter of her baby's head. It is performed when there is doubt that the head can pass safely through the pelvis in labor. Images of the pelvis and the baby are projected radiographically onto film. After the film is developed the images are measured. The measurements are corrected for distortion, and the true dimensions of the birth canal and head are calculated. Often the cephalopelvic relationship cannot be accurately evaluated from the films, because the baby's head may be positioned in such a way that the biparietal diameter cannot be visualized. Because minor degrees of cephalopelvic disproportion are often overcome safely in labor by molding of the fetal skull, and because major disproportions may be detected by clinical pelvimetry without x ray, the value of x-ray pelvimetry is frequently judged to be insufficient to warrant the risk of radiation exposure. Other diagnostic tools, among them ultrasonography, often provide the necessary information with less apparent risk. Compare **clinical pelvimetry.** See also **cephalopelvic disporportion, contraction, dystocia.**

XX, (in genetics) the designation for the normal sex chromosome complement in the human female. See also **X chromosome.**

XXX syndrome, a human sex chromosomal aberration characterized by the presence of three X chromosomes and two Barr bodies instead of the normal XX complement, so that somatic cells contain a total of 47 chromosomes. The condition occurs approximately once in every 1,000 live female births and is confirmed diagnostically by the presence of the extra Barr body in the cells. Individuals with the anomaly show no significant clinical manifestations, although there is usually some degree of mental retardation. Since there is selective migration of the X chromosome during meiosis, half of the offspring of a trisomy X female will be both chromosomally and phenotypically normal. Also called **triple X syndrome.**

XXXX, XXXXX, (in genetics) the designation for an abnormal sex chromosome complement in the human female in which there are four or five instead of the normal two X chromosomes so that each somatic cell contains a total of 48 or 49 chromosomes. Although there is no consistent phenotype associated with such aberrations, the risk of congenital anomalies and mental retardation in the affected individual increases significantly with the increase in the number of X chromosomes.

XXXY, XXXXY, XXYY, (in genetics) the designation for an abnormal sex chromosome complement in the human male in which there are more than the normal one X chromosome, resulting in a total of 48, 49, or more chromosomes in each somatic cell. The aberration is a variant of Kleinfelter's syndrome and, in general, the more X chromosomes there are, the greater the number of congenital defects and the severity of mental retardation in the affected individual. See also **Kleinfelter's syndrome.**

XXY syndrome. See **Kleinfelter's syndrome.**

XY, (in genetics) the designation for the normal sex chromosome complement in the human male. See also **X chromosome, Y chromosome.**

xylitol (zaɪ′lɪtɒl), a sweet, crystalline pentahydroxy alcohol obtained by the reduction of xylose and used as an artificial sweetener.

xylo-, a combining form meaning 'pertaining to wood': *xyloketosuria, xylose, xylosuria.*

Xylocaine, a trade name for a local anesthetic (lidocaine).

xylometazoline hydrochloride, an adrenergic vasoconstrictor.

■ INDICATION: It is prescribed in the treatment of nasal congestion.

■ CONTRAINDICATIONS: Glaucoma, known hypersensitivity to this drug or to sympathomimetic medication prohibits its use. It is used with caution in patients having cardiovascular disease.

■ ADVERSE EFFECTS: Among the more serious adverse reactions are irritation to the mucosa, rebound nasal congestion, effects associated with systemic absorption, including sedation and alterations in cardiovascular function.

XYY syndrome, the phenotypic manifestation of an extra Y chromosome, which has a positive effect on height and may have a negative effect on mental and psychological development. See also **trisomy.**

Y

Y, symbol for **yttrium.**

yaws (yoz), a nonvenereal infection caused by the spirochete *Treponema pertenue,* transmitted by direct contact and characterized by chronic, ulcerating sores anywhere on the body with eventual tissue and bone destruction, leading to crippling if untreated. It is a disease of unsanitary tropical living conditions and may be effectively treated with penicillin G. All serologic tests for syphilis may be positive in yaws. The infection may afford protection against syphilis. Also called **bouba, buba, frambesia, parangi, patek, pian.** Compare **bejel, pinta, syphilis.**

Yb, symbol for **ytterbium.**

Y chromosome, a sex chromosome that in humans and many other species is present only in the male, appearing singly in the normal male. It is carried as a sex determinant by half of the male gametes and none of the female gametes, is morphologically much smaller than the X chromosome, and has genes associated with triggering the development and differentiation of male characteristics. There are no known medically significant traits or conditions associated with the genes on the Y chromosome. Compare **X chromosome.**

yeast, any unicellular, usually oval, nucleated fungus that reproduces by budding. *Candida albicans* is a kind of pathogenic yeast.

yellow cartilage, the most elastic of the three kinds of cartilage, consisting of elastic fibers in a flexible fibrous matrix. It is yellow and is located in various parts of the body, as the external ear, the auditory tube, the epiglottis, and the larynx. Also called **elastic cartilage.** Compare **hyaline cartilage, white fibrocartilage.**

yellow fever, an acute arbovirus infection transmitted by mosquitoes, characterized by headache, fever, jaundice, vomiting, and bleeding. There is no specific treatment and mortality is about five per cent. Recovery is followed by lifelong immunity. Immunization for travelers to endemic areas is advised. Nonhuman primates are a reservoir of infection.

yellow fever vaccine, a vaccine produced from live, attenuated yellow fever virus grown in chick embryos.

■ INDICATION: It is prescribed for immunization against yellow fever.

■ CONTRAINDICATIONS: Immunosuppression, pregnancy, or known hypersensitivity to chicken or egg protein prohibits its use.

■ ADVERSE EFFECTS: Among the more serious adverse effects are fever, malaise, and hypersensitivity reactions.

yellow journal, *Informal. The American Journal of Psychiatry,* so named for the color of its cover. Compare **green journal, grey journal.**

yellow marrow. See **bone marrow.**

Yersinia arthritis (yərsın′iə), a polyarticular inflammation occurring a few days to one month after the onset of infection caused by *Yersinia enterocolitica* or *Y. pseudotuberculosis* and usually persisting longer than a month. Knees, ankles, toes, fingers, and wrists are most often affected. Cultures of synovial fluid yield no infectious organism. The clinical presentation may mimic juvenile rheumatoid arthritis, rheumatic fever, or Reiter's syndrome and may be associated with erythema nodosum or erythema multiforme. Treatment is with antibiotics.

Yersinia pestis (yərsın′iə), a small, gram-negative bacillus that causes plague. The primary host is the rat, but other small rodents also harbor the organism. A person without symptoms may be a carrier, but this happens rarely. *Yersinia pestis* is hardy, living for long periods in infected carcasses, the soil of the host's habitat, or in sputum. Also called *Pasteurella pestis.* See also **plague.**

Y fracture, a Y-shaped intercondylar fracture.

-yl, a combining form used in naming radicals: *benzoyl, ethyl, hydroxyl.*

Y-linked, pertaining to genes or to the characteristics or conditions they transmit that are carried on the Y chromosome. Such traits, as hypertrichosis of the pinna of the ear, can be expressed only in males. Compare **X-linked.** See also **sex-linked disorder** — **Y linkage,** *n.*

Yodoxin, a trade name for an antiamebic (diiodohydroxyquin).

yogurt, a slightly acid, semisolid, curdled milk preparation made from either whole or skimmed cow's milk and milk solids by fermentation with organisms from the genus *Lactobacillus.* It is rich in vitamins of the B complex group and a good source of protein. It also provides a medium in the gastrointestinal tract that inhibits the growth of harmful bacteria and aids in the absorption of minerals.

yolk, the nutritive material, rich in fats and proteins, contained in the ovum to supply nourishment to the developing embryo. The amount and distribution of the yolk within the egg depend upon the species of animal and type of reproduction and development of offspring. In humans and most mammals the yolk is absent or greatly diffused through the cell, since embryos absorb nutrients directly from the mother through the placenta. See also **deutoplasm**.

yolk membrane. See **vitelline membrane**.

yolk sac, a structure that develops in the inner cell mass of the embryo and expands into a vesicle with a thick part that becomes the primitive gut and a thin part that grows into the cavity of the chorion. The cells of the extraembryonic mesoderm differentiate to develop endothelium, primitive blood plasma, and hemoglobin. After supplying the nourishment for the embryo, the yolk sac usually disappears during the seventh week of pregnancy. See also **allantois, Meckel's diverticulum**.

yolk sphere. See **morula**.

yolk stalk, the narrow duct connecting the yolk sac with the midgut of the embryo during the early stages of prenatal development. It connects at the region of the future ileum and usually undergoes complete obliteration but occasionally may appear as a diverticulum. Also called **omphalomesenteric duct, umbilical duct, vitelline duct.** See also **Meckel's diverticulum**.

Yomesan, a trade name for an anthelmintic (niclosamide).

Young's rule, a method for the calculation of the appropriate dose of a drug for a child of 2 years or more using the formula (age in years) ÷ (age + 12) × adult dose.

Y-plasty, a method of surgical revision of a scar, using a Y-shaped incision to reduce scar contractures. See also **Z-plasty**.

Y-set, a device composed of plastic components, used for delivering intravenous fluids through a primary intravenous line connected to a combination drip chamber-filter section from which two separate plastic tubes lead to fluid sources. The Y-set also includes three clamps, one for the primary intravenous line and one for each of the two separate tubes. It is often used to transfuse packed blood cells which must be diluted with saline solution to decrease their viscosity. In such a transfusion one of the tubes is connected to the container enclosing the packed cells; the other tube is connected to the receptacle containing the saline solution. During a prolonged transfusion of packed blood cells, the tubing of the Y-set must be changed every four hours. Compare **component drip set, component syringe set, microaggregate recipient set, straight-line blood set**.

ytterbium (Yb), a rare-earth metallic element. Its atomic number is 70; its atomic weight is 173.04.

yttrium (Y), a scaly, grayish metallic element. Its atomic number is 39; its atomic weight is 88.905. Radioactive isotopes of yttrium have been used in cancer therapy.

Yutopar, a trade name for a beta-adrenergic drug (ritodrine hydrochloride), used to stop premature labor.

XY
Z

Z

Zactirin, a trade name for a fixed-combination drug containing analgesics (aspirin and ethoheptazine citrate).

Zahorsky's disease (zəhor'skiz). See **roseola infantum.**

Zakrzewski (zakshef'ski), **Marie** (1829–1902), a Polish-German midwife who studied medicine in Berlin and spent some time in Kaiserswerth, Germany, before emigrating to the United States. In New York she met Elizabeth Blackwell, who encouraged her to continue her medical studies. After receiving her medical degree in Cleveland, she worked at Blackwell's New York Infirmary before going to Boston. In 1872 she organized the first successful American school of nursing at the New England Hospital for Women and Children.

Zanosar, a trade name for an antineoplastic (streptozocin).

Zarontin, a trade name for an anticonvulsant (ethosuximide).

Zaroxolyn, a trade name for a diuretic and antihypertensive (metolazone).

Z chromosome, a sex chromosome of certain insects, birds, and fishes, appearing singly in normal females of the species and doubly in the males. See also **W chromosome.**

Zenker's diverticulum, a circumscribed herniation of the mucous membrane of the pharynx as it joins the esophagus. Food may become trapped in the diverticulum and may be aspirated. Diagnosis is confirmed by x-ray studies. In most cases it is small, causes no dysfunction, is not diagnosed, and requires no treatment.

Zentron, a trade name for a hematinic fixed-combination drug containing iron and vitamins.

Zephiran Chloride, a trade name for a disinfectant (benzalkonium chloride).

Zestē, a trade name for esterified estrogens.

Zetar, a trade name for a topical antieczematic containing coal tar.

Ziehl-Neelson test (zil'nil'sən), one of the most widely used methods of acid-fast staining, commonly used in the microscopic examination of a smear of sputum suspected of containing *Mycobacterium tuberculosis.* See also **acid-fast stain.**

ZIG, abbreviation for **zoster immune globulin.**

zinc (Zn), a bluish white crystalline metal commonly associated with lead ores. Its atomic number is 30; its atomic weight is 65.38. Zinc is ductile in its pure form and occurs abundantly in minerals such as sphalerite, zincite, and franklinite. It has many commercial uses, as a protective coating for steel and in printing plates. Zinc is an essential nutrient in the body and is used in numerous pharmaceuticals, as zinc acetate, zinc oxide, zinc permanganate, and zinc stearate. Zinc acetate is used as an emetic, a styptic, and as an astringent. Zinc oxide is used internally as an antispasmodic and as a protective in ointments. Zinc permanganate is used as an astringent and in the treatment of urethritis by injection or douche in a 1:4000 solution. Zinc stearate is used as a water-repellent protective agent in the treatment of acne, eczema, and other skin diseases.

zinc chill. See **metal fume fever.**

zinc deficiency, a condition resulting from insufficient amounts of zinc in the diet, characterized by abnormal fatigue, decreased alertness, a decrease in taste and odor sensitivity, poor appetite, retarded growth, delayed sexual maturity, prolonged healing of wounds, and susceptibility to infection and injury. Other conditions that may precipitate the deficiency include alcoholic cirrhosis and other liver diseases, ulcers, myocardial infarction, Hodgkin's disease, mongolism, and cystic fibrosis. Prophylaxis and treatment consist of a diet of foods high in protein, which are also rich in zinc, including meats, eggs, liver, seafood, legumes, nuts, peanut butter, milk, and whole-grain cereals.

zinc gelatin, a topical protectant for varicosities and other lesions of the lower limbs. It is available as a smooth jelly containing zinc oxide (10%), gelatin (15%), glycerin (40%), and purified water (35%). It is also available impregnated in gauze.

zinc oxide, a topical protectant prescribed for a wide range of minor skin irritations.

zinc salt poisoning, a toxic condition caused by the ingestion or inhalation of a zinc salt. Symptoms of ingestion include a burning sensation of the mouth and throat, vomiting, diarrhea, abdominal and chest pain, and, in severe cases, shock and coma. Treatment includes gastric lavage, followed by a demulcent and chelation with calcium edetate, and fluid therapy. Inhalation of zinc salts may cause metal fume fever; skin contact may produce blisters.

zinc sulfate, an ophthalmic astringent given in drops for nasal congestion or irritation of the eye, applied topically in deodorants, and given orally in tablets to promote healing and as a dietary supplement.

ZIP, abbreviation for *zoster immune plasma*. See **chicken pox.**

zirconium (Zr), a steel-gray, tetravalent metallic element. Its atomic number is 40; its atomic weight is 91.22. It occurs widely in combined form, especially in zircon and baddeleyite. It is usually extracted from sands containing zircon by heating with carbon and chlorine and passing the resulting volatile zirconium tetracholoride into hot molten magnesium or into sodium to yield a spongy form of the free metal. A component of zirconium dioxide was formerly used in some ointments for the treatment of poison ivy skin rashes, but such ointments caused skin granulomas in some individuals. Similar skin conditions developed in individuals using deodorants containing zirconium sodium lactate, and the use of zirconium compounds, except for zirconyl hydroxychloride, has been discontinued in the manufacture of skin ointments. Zirconyl hydroxychloride is still used in antiperspirants.

Zn, symbol for **zinc.**

zoanthropy (zouæn'ſhrəpi), the delusion that one has assumed the form and characteristics of an animal. —**zoanthropic,** *adj.*

-zoite, a combining form meaning a 'simple organism' of a specified sort: *merozoite, saprozoite, sporozoite.*

Zollinger-Ellison syndrome (zol'ɪnjərel'ɪsən), a condition characterized by severe peptic ulceration, gastric hypersecretion, elevated serum gastrin, and gastrinoma of the pancreas or the duodenum. The syndrome is uncommon but not rare; it may occur in early childhood, but is seen more frequently in persons between 20 and 50 years of age. Two thirds of the tumors are malignant. Total gastrectomy may be necessary, but the administration of cimetidine in large doses may control gastric hypersecretion and allow the ulcers to heal. See also **peptic ulcer.**

Zomax, a trade name for a nonsteroidal analgesic and anti-inflammatory (zomepirac sodium).

zomepirac sodium, an analgesic and anti-inflammatory agent.

■ INDICATION: It is prescribed to reduce mild to moderately severe pain.

■ CONTRAINDICATIONS: Known hypersensitivity to this drug or to any nonsteroidal anti-inflammatory agent prohibits its use. It is used with caution in patients having upper gastrointestinal disease. It is not given to pregnant or lactating women.

■ ADVERSE EFFECT:Among the more serious adverse reactions are gastrointestinal bleeding, palpitations, depression, and skin rash.

zona (zou'nə), *pl.* **zonae.** a girdlelike, usually striated segment of a rounded or spherical structure. Some kinds of zona are **zona arcuata, zona orbicularis, zona pellucida.**

zona ciliaris. See **ciliary zone.**

zona pellucida (pelu'sɪdə), the thick, transparent, noncellular membrane that encloses the mammalian ovum. It is secreted by the ovum during its development in the ovary and is retained until near the time of implantation. Also called **oolemma.** See also **vitelline membrane.**

zona radiata (rei'dia'tə), a zona pellucida that has a striated appearance caused by radiating canals within the membrane. Also called **zona striata.**

zona striata. See **zona radiata.**

Zondek-Ascheim test (tson'dekæſh'haim). See **Ascheim-Zondek test.**

zone, an area with specific boundaries and characteristics, as the epigastric, the mesogastric, or the hypogastric zones of the abdomen.

zone therapy, the treatment of a disorder by mechanical stimulation and counterirritation of a body area in the same longitudinal zone as the affected organ or region.

zonula, *pl.* **zonulae.** a small zone. Also called **zonule.**

zonula ciliaris, a ligament composed of straight fibrils radiating from the ciliary body of the eye to the crystalline lens, holding the lens in place and relaxing by the contraction of the ciliary muscle. Relaxation of the ligament allows the lens to become more convex. Also called **zonule of Zinn.**

zonule of Zinn (zoun'yul). See **zonula ciliaris.**

zoo-, zo-, a combining form meaning 'pertaining to an animal': *zooamylon, zoogony, zoonosis.*

zooerastia (zou'ouеræs'tiə). See **bestiality.**

zoogenous (zouoj'ɪnəs), acquired from or originating in animals. See also **zoonosis.**

zoograft, tissue of an animal transplanted to a person, as the use of a heart valve from a pig to replace a damaged heart valve in a human.

zoology, the study of animal life.

zoomania (zou'əmei'niə), a psychopathological state characterized by an excessive fondness for and preoccupation with animals. —**zoomaniac,** *n.*

-zoon, a combining form meaning a 'living being': *dermatozoon, entozoon, hepatozoon.*

zoonosis (zouon'əsɪs, zou'ənou'sɪs), a disease of animals that is transmissible to humans from its primary animal host. Some kinds of zoonoses are **equine encephalitis, leptospirosis, rabies, yellow fever.**

zooparasite (zou'əpær'əsait), any parasitic animal organism. Kinds of zooparasites are **arthropods, protozoa, worms.** —**zooparasitic,** *adj.*

zoopathology, the study of the diseases of animals.

zoophilia (zou'əfɪl'iə, zou'əfil'yə), **zoophilism** (zouof'ɪlɪz'əm), **1.** an abnormal fondness for animals. **2.** (in psychiatry) a psychosexual disorder in which sexual excitement and gratification are derived from the fondling of animals or from the fantasy or act of engaging in sexual activity with animals. See also **paraphilia.** —**zoophile,** *n.,* **zoophilic, zoophilous,** *adj.*

zoophobia (zou'əfou'biə), an anxiety disorder characterized by a persistent, irrational fear of animals, particularly dogs, snakes, insects, and mice. The condition is seen more often in women than in men, nearly always begins in childhood, and can typically be traced to some frightening or unpleasant experience involving an animal. Treatment consists of psychotherapy to uncover the cause of the phobic reaction followed by behavior therapy, specifically the techniques of systemic desensitization and flooding.

zoopsia (zouop'siǝ), a visual hallucination of animals or insects, often occurring in delirium tremens.

zootoxin (zou'ǝtok'sɪn), a poisonous substance from an animal, as the venom of snakes, spiders, and scorpions. — **zootixic,** *adj.*

Zorane, a trade name for an oral contraceptive containing an estrogen (ethinyl estradiol) and a progestin (norethindrone acetate.)

zoster (zos'tǝr). See **herpes zoster.**

zosteriform (zoster'ɪfɔrm), resembling the pocks seen in herpes zoster infection.

zoster immune globulin (ZIG), a passive immunizing agent currently in limited experimental use for preventing or attenuating herpes zoster virus infection in immunosuppressed individuals who are at great risk of severe herpes zoster virus infection.

Z-plasty, a method of surgical revision of a scar or closure of a wound using a Z-shaped incision to reduce contractures of the adjacent skin. See also **Y-plasty.**

Zr, symbol for **zirconium.**

zwieback, a sweetened bread that is enriched with eggs and baked, then sliced and toasted until dry and crisp. It is used as a snack food for children, especially teething infants.

zyg-, zygo-, a combining form meaning 'union or fusion, yoked or joined, pertaining to a junction, or a pair': *zygomatic, zygogenesis, zygote.*

zygogenesis (zai'goujen'ɪsɪs), 1. the formation of a zygote. 2. reproduction by the union of gametes. — **zygogenetic, zygogenic,** *adj.*

zygoma (zaigou'mǝ, zɪgou'mǝ), 1. a long slender zygomatic process of the temporal bone, arising from the lower part of the squamous portion of the temporal bone, passing forward to join the zygomatic bone, and forming part of the zygomatic arch. 2. the zygomatic bone that forms the prominence of the cheek.

zygomatic bone, one of the pair of bones that forms the prominence of the cheek, the lower part of the orbit of the eye, and parts of the temporal and infratemporal fossae.

zygomatic head. See **zygomaticus minor.**

zygomaticus major (zai'goumæt'ɪkǝs), one of the 12 muscles of the mouth. Arising from the zygomatic bone and inserting into the corner of the mouth, it is innervated by buccal branches of the facial nerve and acts to draw the angle of the mouth up and back to smile or laugh. Also called **zygomaticus.** Compare **zygomaticus minor.**

zygomaticus minor, one of the 12 muscles of the mouth. Arising from the malar surface of the zygomatic bone and inserting into the upper lip, it is innervated by buccal branches of the facial nerve and acts to deepen the nasolabial furrow in a sad facial expression. Also called **quadratus labii superioris, zygomatic head.** Compare **zygomaticus major.**

zygomycosis (zai'goumaikou'sɪs), an acute, often fulminant and sometimes fatal fungous infection caused by a class of water mold, seen primarily in patients with chronic debilitating diseases, especially uncontrolled diabetes mellitus. Characteristically, it begins with fever and with pain and discharge in the nose and paranasal sinuses that progresses to invade the eye and lower respiratory tract. The fungus may enter blood vessels and spread to the brain and other organs. Transmission is usually by inhalation. The diagnosis is confirmed by biopsy and pathologic examination of sputum. Treatment includes improved control of diabetes mellitus, extensive debridement of craniofacial lesions, and amphotericin B administered intravenously. Also called **mucormycosis.** Compare **phycomycosis.**

zygonema (zai'gǝni'mǝ), the synaptic chromosome formation that occurs in the zygotene stage of the first meiotic prophase of gametogenesis. — **zygonematic,** *adj.*

zygosis (zaigou'sɪs), a form of sexual reproduction in unicellular organisms, consisting of the union of the two cells and fusion of the nuclei. — **zygotic,** *adj.*

zygosity (zaigos'ɪti), the characteristics or conditions of a zygote. The form occurs primarily as a suffix-combining form to denote genetic makeup, referring specifically to whether the paired alleles determining a particular trait are identical (homozygosity) or different (heterozygosity) or to the condition in twins of having developed from the fertilization of one ovum (monozygosity) or two (dizygosity).

zygosperm. See **zygospore.**

zygospore, the spore resulting from the conjugation of two isogametes, as in certain fungi and algae.

zygote (zai'gout), (in embryology) the developing ovum from the time it is fertilized until, as a blastocyst, it is implanted in the uterus.

zygotene (zai'gǝtin), the second stage in the first meiotic prophase of gametogenesis in which synapsis of homologous chromosomes occurs. See also **diakinesis, diplotene, leptotene, pachytene.**

Zyloprim, a trade name for a xanthine oxidase inhibitor (allopurinol).

-zyme, a combining form meaning a 'ferment or enzyme': *lysozyme, opzyme, serozyme.*

zymo-, a combining form meaning 'pertaining to an enzyme, or to fermentation': *zymocide, zymohexase, zymophore.*

zymogenic cell. See **chief cell.**

COLOR ATLAS OF HUMAN ANATOMY

SKELETAL SYSTEM

CLINICAL NOTE • The skeletal system

It is impossible to demonstrate all 208 skeletal bones in the space alloted, but the complexity of the bony structures within the locomotor system is well demonstrated by the figures on these pages.

In studying the diseases of bones and joints, whether localized or more widespread disorders, there can be a problem with x-rays. At a certain total dosage (the amount depending on individual patient variation) there is a risk of developing radiation-induced diseases such as leukemia. Although radioisotopes also emit radiation in clinical use, the amounts involved are very small because of their short half-life and the high sensitivity of detectors such as the gamma camera and the crystal scintillator.

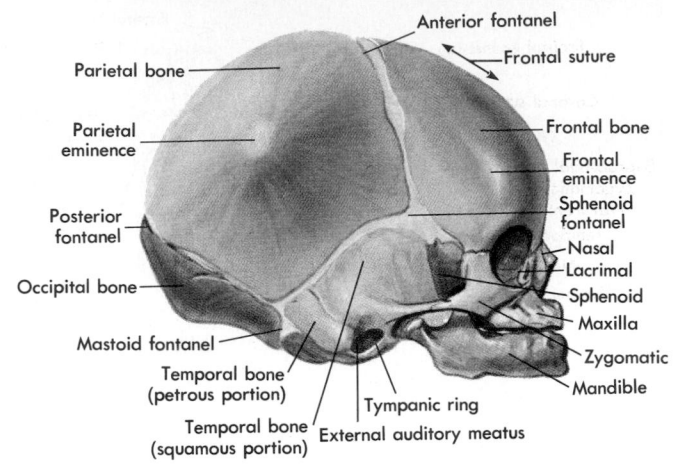

FETAL SKULL

**ANTERIOR AND POSTERIOR
VIEWS OF SKELETAL SYSTEM**

Anterior

Posterior

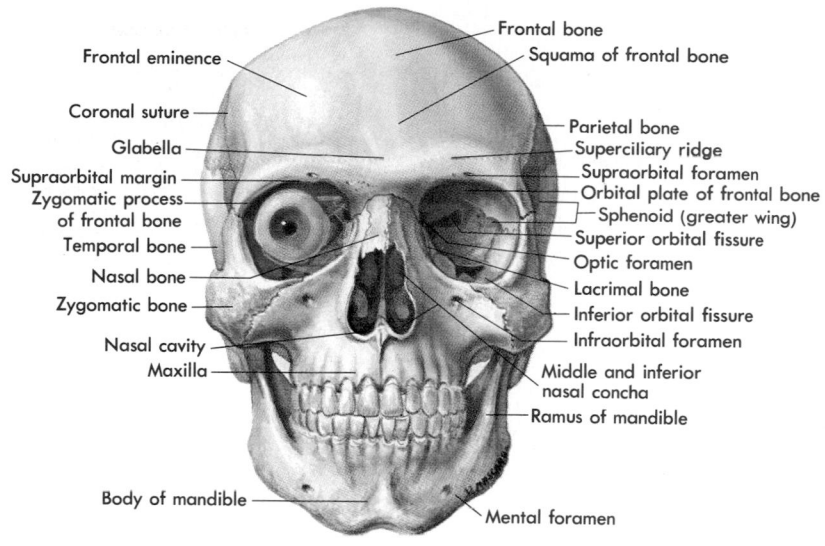

Frontal bone
Squama of frontal bone
Frontal eminence
Coronal suture
Parietal bone
Glabella
Superciliary ridge
Supraorbital margin
Supraorbital foramen
Zygomatic process
of frontal bone
Orbital plate of frontal bone
Sphenoid (greater wing)
Temporal bone
Superior orbital fissure
Nasal bone
Optic foramen
Zygomatic bone
Lacrimal bone
Inferior orbital fissure
Nasal cavity
Infraorbital foramen
Maxilla
Middle and inferior
nasal concha
Ramus of mandible
Body of mandible
Mental foramen

ANTERIOR VIEW OF SKULL

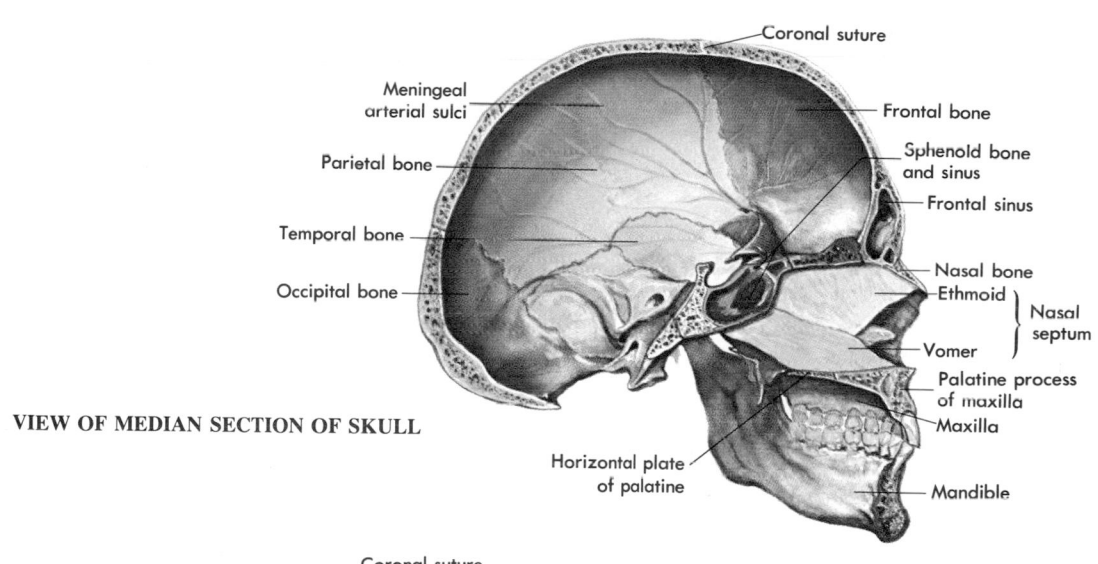

Coronal suture
Meningeal
arterial sulci
Frontal bone
Sphenoid bone
and sinus
Parietal bone
Frontal sinus
Temporal bone
Nasal bone
Ethmoid
Nasal
septum
Occipital bone
Vomer
Palatine process
of maxilla
Maxilla
Horizontal plate
of palatine
Mandible

VIEW OF MEDIAN SECTION OF SKULL

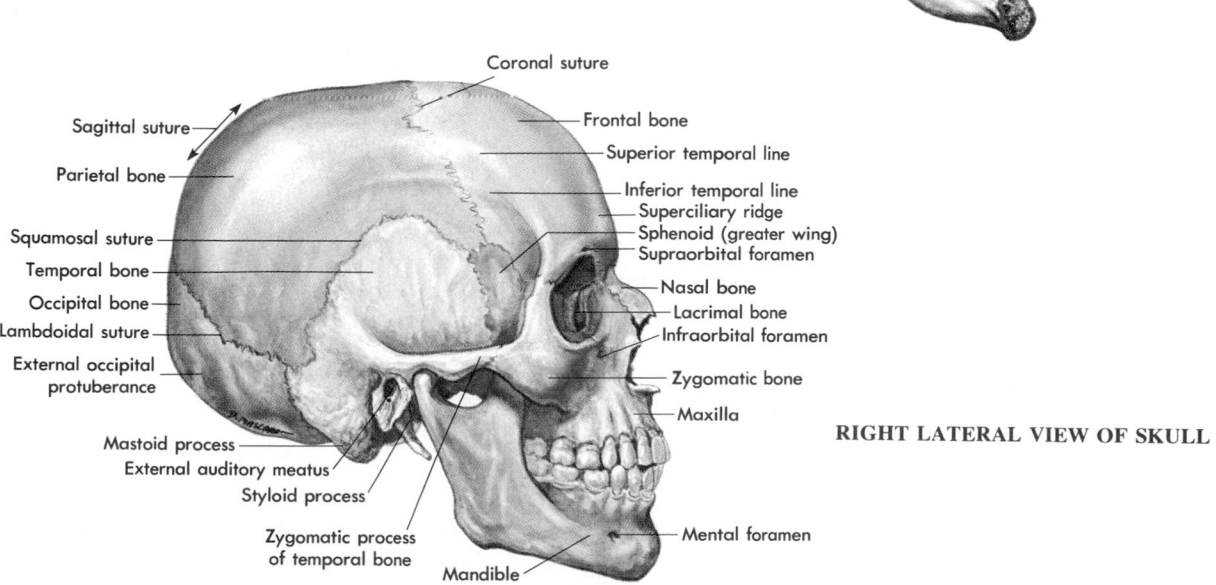

Coronal suture
Sagittal suture
Frontal bone
Superior temporal line
Parietal bone
Inferior temporal line
Superciliary ridge
Squamosal suture
Sphenoid (greater wing)
Supraorbital foramen
Temporal bone
Nasal bone
Occipital bone
Lacrimal bone
Lambdoidal suture
Infraorbital foramen
External occipital
protuberance
Zygomatic bone
Maxilla
Mastoid process
External auditory meatus
Styloid process
Zygomatic process
of temporal bone
Mental foramen
Mandible

RIGHT LATERAL VIEW OF SKULL

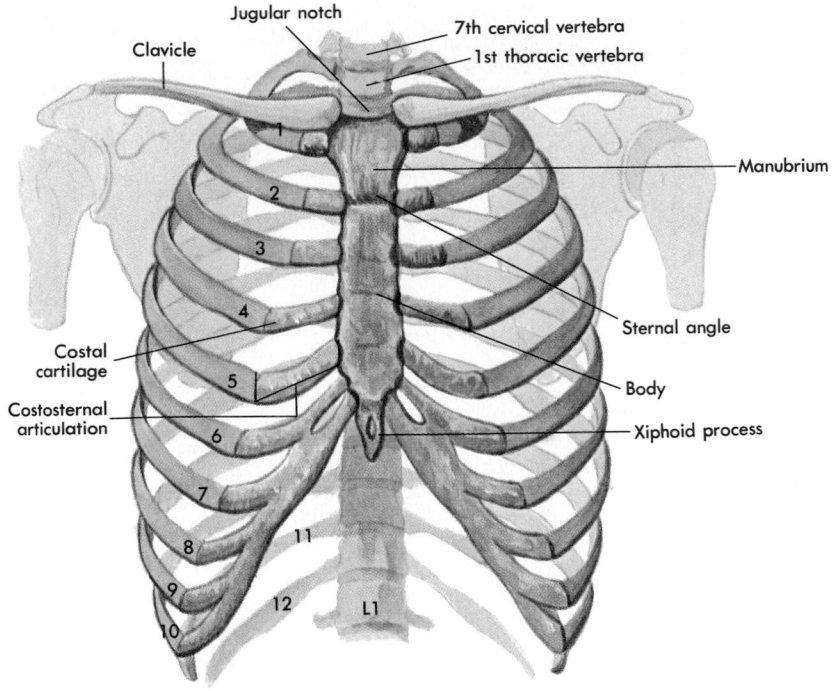

Jugular notch

Clavicle

7th cervical vertebra

1st thoracic vertebra

Manubrium

Sternal angle

Costal cartilage

Body

Costosternal articulation

Xiphoid process

THORAX AND RIBS

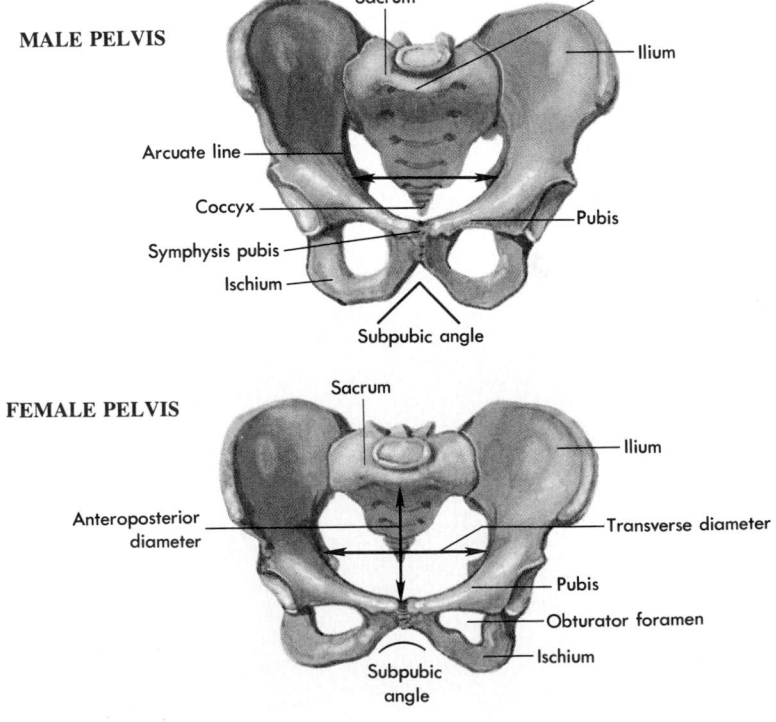

MALE PELVIS

Sacrum

Sacral promentory

Ilium

Arcuate line

Coccyx

Pubis

Symphysis pubis

Ischium

Subpubic angle

FEMALE PELVIS

Sacrum

Ilium

Anteroposterior diameter

Transverse diameter

Pubis

Obturator foramen

Ischium

Subpubic angle

Haversian system

Concentric lamellae

Canaliculi

Lacuna containing osteocyte

Blood vessel

Trabeculae

Compact bone | Spongy bone | Compact bone

DETAIL OF STRUCTURE OF A SEGMENT OF LONG BONE

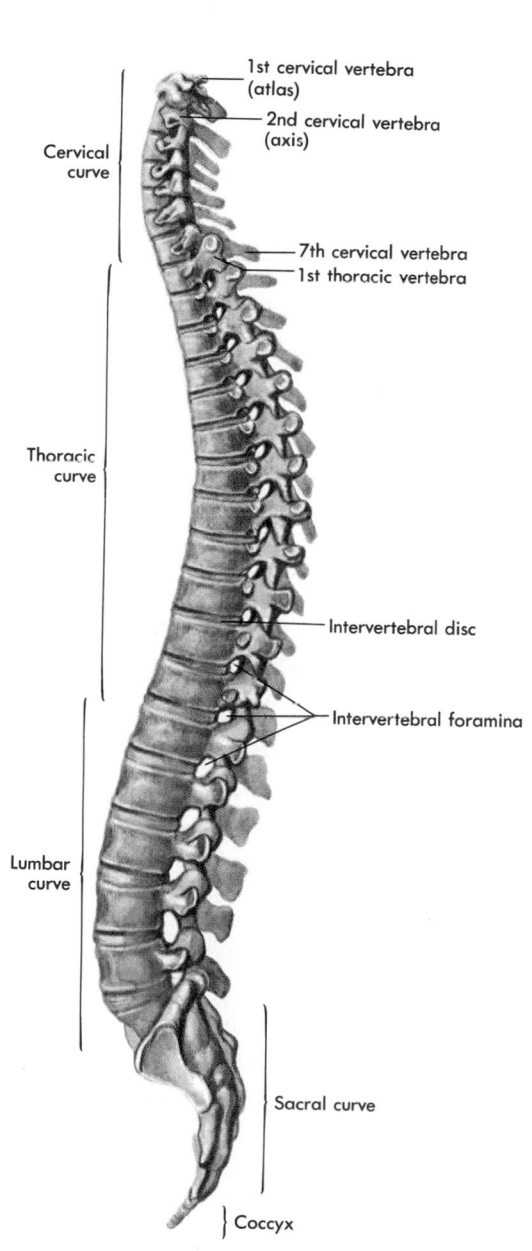

Cervical curve

1st cervical vertebra (atlas)

2nd cervical vertebra (axis)

7th cervical vertebra

1st thoracic vertebra

Thoracic curve

Intervertebral disc

Intervertebral foramina

Lumbar curve

Sacral curve

Coccyx

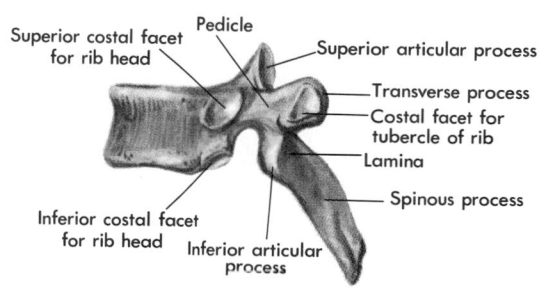

Superior costal facet for rib head

Pedicle

Superior articular process

Transverse process

Costal facet for tubercle of rib

Lamina

Spinous process

Inferior costal facet for rib head

Inferior articular process

INDIVIDUAL VERTEBRA

LATERAL VIEW OF VERTEBRAL COLUMN

MUSCULAR SYSTEM

Cranial muscles

Facial muscles

Sternocleidomastoid

Trapezius

Deltoid

Pectoralis major

Biceps brachii

Serratus anterior

Linea alba

Rectus abdominis

Flexors of
wrist and fingers

Extensors of
wrist and fingers

External
oblique

Adductors
of thigh

Tensor
fascia lata

Flexor retinaculum

Sartorius

Vastus lateralis

Rectus femoris

Vastus medialis

Patella

Patellar tendon

Gastrocnemius

Tibialis anterior

Extensor digitorum longus

Peroneus longus

Peroneus brevis

Soleus

Extensor hallucis
longus tendon

Superior extensor
retinaculum

ANTERIOR VIEW

Sternocleidomastoid

Splenius capitis

7th cervical vertebra

Trapezius

Deltoid

Teres minor

Teres major

Infraspinatus

Portion of rhomboid

Triceps

Latissimus dorsi

External oblique

Extensors of
wrist and fingers

Gluteus maximus

Semitendinosus

Adductor magnus

Gracilis

Biceps femoris

Iliotibial tract

Semimembranosus

Plantaris

Gastrocnemius

Gastrocnemius tendon
(Achilles tendon)

Soleus

Peroneus longus

Peroneus brevis

Superior peroneal
retinaculum

POSTERIOR VIEW

CLINICAL NOTE • Chest wall muscles

The many insertions of dorsal muscles into the ribs and vertebrae allow for precision in control and flexibility in twisting and turning movements of the trunk. The fibers of the intercostal muscles run obliquely, but at right angles to each other; thus they play an important part in increasing thoracic volume during respiration.

Galea aponeurotica

Temporalis

Temporalis fascia

Superior auricular

Anterior auricular

Occipitalis

Posterior auricular

Masseter

Sternocleidomastoid

Trapezius

Frontalis

Corrugator

Orbicularis oculi

Procerus

Levator labii superioris alaeque nasi

Levator labii superioris

Zygomaticus minor

Levator anguli oris

Zygomaticus major

Orbicularis oris

Risorius (cut)

Mentalis

Depressor labii inferioris

Depressor anguli oris

Buccinator

Omohyoid

Sternohyoid

LATERAL AND ANTERIOR VIEWS OF MUSCLES OF FACE AND ANTERIOR CRANIUM AND SEVERAL MUSCLES OF MASTICATION

Galea aponeurotica (frontal portion)

Epicranius (frontal belly)

Orbicularis oculi (orbital portion)

Medial palpebral ligament

Orbicularis oculi (palpebral portion)

Levator labii superioris

Zygomaticus minor

Parotid gland

Zygomaticus major

Risorius

Levator anguli oris

Depressor anguli oris

Depressor labii inferioris

Corrugator

Temporalis

Procerus

Levator labii superioris alaeque nasi

Zygomaticus minor and major (cut)

Nasalis

Levator anguli oris (cut)

Masseter

Buccinator

Orbicularis oris

Mentalis

Platysma (part)

SUPERFICIAL MUSCLES OF UPPER CHEST AND SHOULDERS

Deltoid (cut)

Coracobrachialis

Deltoid

Pectoralis major

Serratus anterior

Biceps brachii

Long head of the triceps

Semispinalis capitis

Splenius capitis

Sternocleidomastoid

Trapezius

Sternocleidomastoid tendon (cut)

Levator scapulae (cut)

Splenius cervicis

7th cervical vertebra

Rhomboid minor

Rhomboid major

SUPERFICIAL MUSCLES OF POSTERIOR NECK AND UPPER BACK

SOME SUPERFICIAL MUSCLES
OF BACK

Levator scapulae

Rhomboid minor
Rhomboid major
Supraspinatus
Infraspinatus
Teres minor
Dotted line indicates
attachment of latissimus
dorsi to humerus

Teres major
Thoracolumbar
fascia
Latissimus dorsi

12th thoracic
vertebra

External oblique

Splenius capitis
Dotted line indicates
outline of trapezius

Serratus posterior
superior
Rhomboids (cut edge)
Dotted line indicates
outline of trapezius
Longissimus thoracis

Iliocostalis thoracis
Spinalis thoracis
Serratus posterior
inferior

Internal oblique

Erector spinae

Muscle

Muscle fascicle

Muscle fiber

Myofibril

Myofilaments

Sarcoplasmic
reticulum
Cisternae   Transverse tubule
Mitochondria
Sarcolemma

I band

A band

Myofibrils   Z line

H band
A band
Z
H band
I band

Sarcomere

STRUCTURE OF
SKELETAL MUSCLE

F-actin filament

G-actin molecules

Myosin filament   Myosin molecule   Light meromyson   Heavy
meromyson

1172

CIRCULATORY SYSTEM

Transverse cervical artery
Suprascapular artery
Descending scapular artery

Acromial branch
Axillary artery (rib 1 to teres tendon)
Posterior humeral circumflex artery
Anterior humeral circumflex artery

Subscapular artery

Brachial artery

Inferior thyroidal artery
Common carotid artery
Thyrocervical trunk
Subclavian artery
Brachiocephalic artery
Highest thoracic artery
Internal thoracic artery
Thoracoacromial artery
Thoracic branch
Lateral thoracic artery

AXILLARY ARTERIES

PRINCIPAL VEINS AND ARTERIES

Principal arteries

1 Angular
2 Anterior tibial
3 Aorta
4 Arcuate
5 Axillary
6 Brachial
7 Celiac
8 Common carotid, left
9 Common carotid, right
10 Common iliac, right
11 Coronary, left
12 Deep femoral
13 Deep medial
   circumflex femoral
14 Digital
15 Dorsal metatarsal
16 Dorsalis pedis
17 External carotid
18 External iliac
19 Femoral
20 Hepatic
21 Metacarpal
22 Inferior mesenteric
23 Internal iliac
   (hypogastric)
24 Palmar arch, deep
25 Palmar arch, superficial
26 Peroneal
27 Popliteal
28 Posterior tibial
29 Pulmonary
30 Radial
31 Renal
32 Splenic
33 Subclavian, left (cut)
34 Subclavian, right
35 Superficial temporal
36 Superior mesenteric
37 Ulnar

Principal veins

1 Anterior tibial
2 Axillary
3 Basilic
4 Brachial
5 Cephalic
6 Cervical plexus
7 Colic
8 Common iliac, left
9 Digital
10 Dorsal venous arch
11 External jugular
12 Femoral
13 Great saphenous
14 Hepatic
15 Inferior mesenteric
16 Inferior sagittal sinus
17 Inferior vena cava
18 Brachiocephalic, left
19 Internal jugular, left
20 Internal jugular, right
21 Lateral thoracic
22 Median cubital
23 Peroneal
24 Popliteal
25 Portal
26 Posterior tibial
27 Pulmonary
28 Subclavian, left
29 Superior mesenteric
30 Superior sagittal sinus
31 Superior vena cava

BECK

Circulatory system

Aorta

Left pulmonary artery

Left pulmonary veins

Left atrium

Circumflex branch of
left coronary artery

Great cardiac vein

Oblique vein

Posterior vein of
left ventricle

Left ventricle

Apex

Azygos vein

Superior vena cava

Right pulmonary artery

Right pulmonary veins

Right atrium

Right auricle

Inferior vena cava

Small cardiac vein

Right coronary artery

Coronary sinus

Right ventricle

Posterior interventricular sulcus

Middle cardiac vein

Right interventricular artery

**CORONARY VESSELS
(POSTERIOR VIEW)**

HUMAN HEART IN FRONTAL SECTION

Brachiocephalic artery

Left common carotid artery

Right common
carotid artery

Right internal
jugular vein

Right subclavian
vein

Superior vena cava

Right pulmonary
arteries

Right pulmonary veins

Right atrium

Aortic valve (dotted lines)

Section of right
ventricle intact

Tricuspid valve

Right ventricle

Inferior vena cava

Papillary muscle

Left subclavian artery

Aortic arch

Ligamentum arteriosus

Pulmonary trunk

Left pulmonary arteries

Left pulmonary veins

Pulmonary valve leaflet

Left atrium and mitral valve

Chordae tendineae

Papillary muscle

Left ventricle

Interventricular septum

Myocardium

Superior vena cava

Right pulmonary
arteries

Right auricle

Right atrium

Coronary sulcus

Right coronary artery

Anterior cardiac veins

Right ventricle

Small cardiac vein

Inferior vena cava

Marginal artery

Aorta

Left pulmonary
arteries

Left auricle

Circumflex artery

Left coronary artery

Anterior longitudinal sulcus

Anterior descending branch of
left coronary artery

Left ventricle

Apex

**CORONARY VESSELS
(ANTERIOR VIEW)**

1174

CLINICAL NOTE • Fetal circulation

In fetal circulation, the lungs are inactive. A flap valve allows mixing of blood in the left ventricular chamber, but this valve closes soon after the first breath is taken. Some cardiac malformations cause cyanosis due to improper oxygenation of arterial blood. Fallot's tetralogy is an example. The stenosed pulmonary artery, ventricular septal defect, poorly positioned aorta, and right ventricular hypertrophy are all characteristic but are usually correctable by surgery.

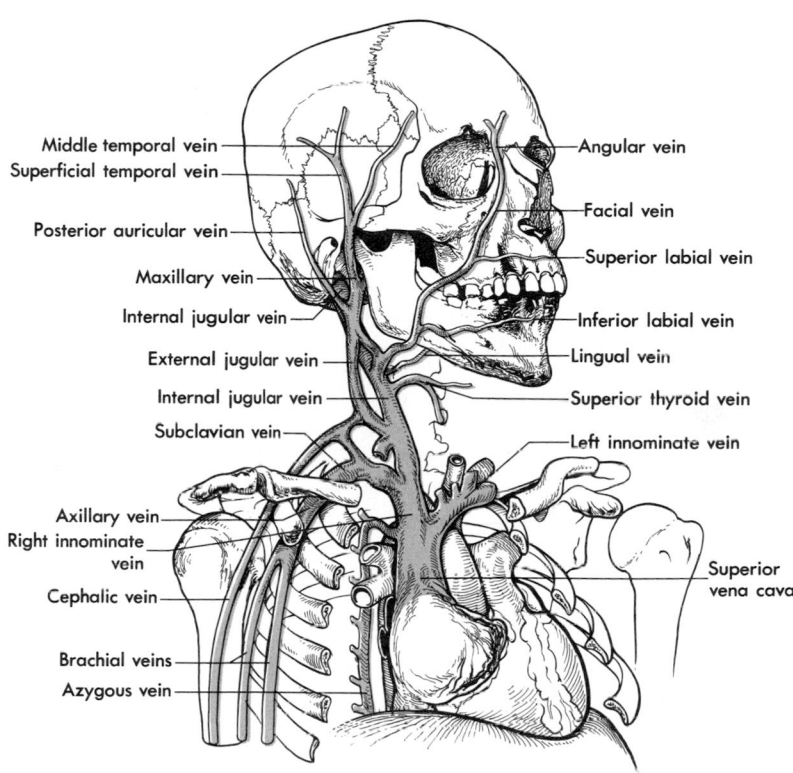

VEINS FORMING SUPERIOR VENA CAVA

TETRALOGY OF FALLOT

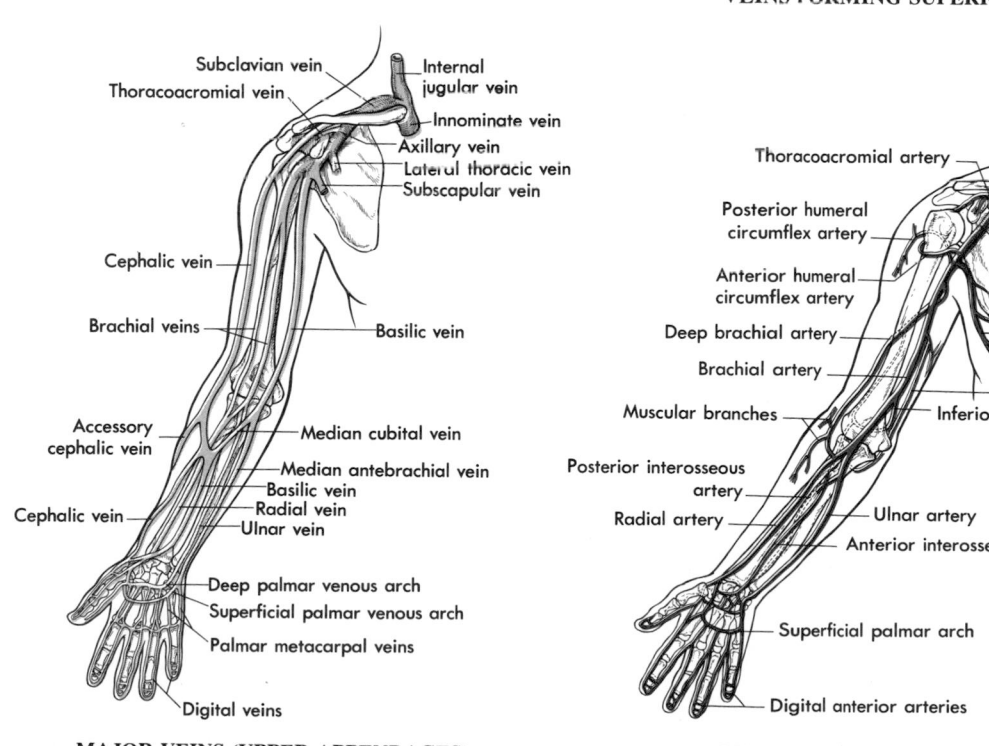

MAJOR VEINS (UPPER APPENDAGES)

MAJOR ARTERIES (UPPER APPENDAGES)

ENDOCRINE SYSTEM

Corpus callosum

Pineal

Area of hypothalamus

Optic chiasm

Anterior pituitary

Posterior pituitary

LOCATION OF PITUITARY AND PINEAL GLANDS

CLINICAL NOTE • Pituitary gland

Near the base of the pituitary gland the optic chiasma has a cross-over point (not shown) for nerve fibers running backward from each retina. Pituitary tumors may cause pressure here and therefore produce disturbances in vision.

DETAIL OF PITUITARY GLAND

Infundibular stalk

Pars tuberalis

Posterior pituitary

Anterior pituitary

Hypophysis (pituitary)

Thyroid gland with parathyroids on posterior surface

Adrenal gland

Adrenal gland

Pancreas

Cortex

Medulla

Ovary in females

Testis in males

Suprarenal artery

Capsule

Cortical capillaries

Medullary capillaries

Central vein

ANATOMY OF ADRENAL GLAND

ENDOCRINE SYSTEM

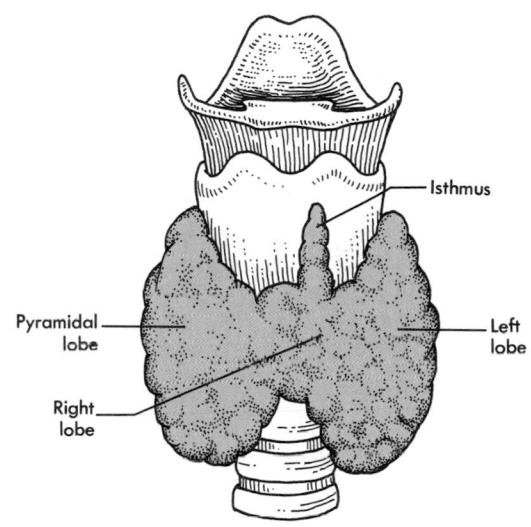

Isthmus

Pyramidal
lobe

Left
lobe

Right
lobe

STRUCTURE OF THYROID GLAND

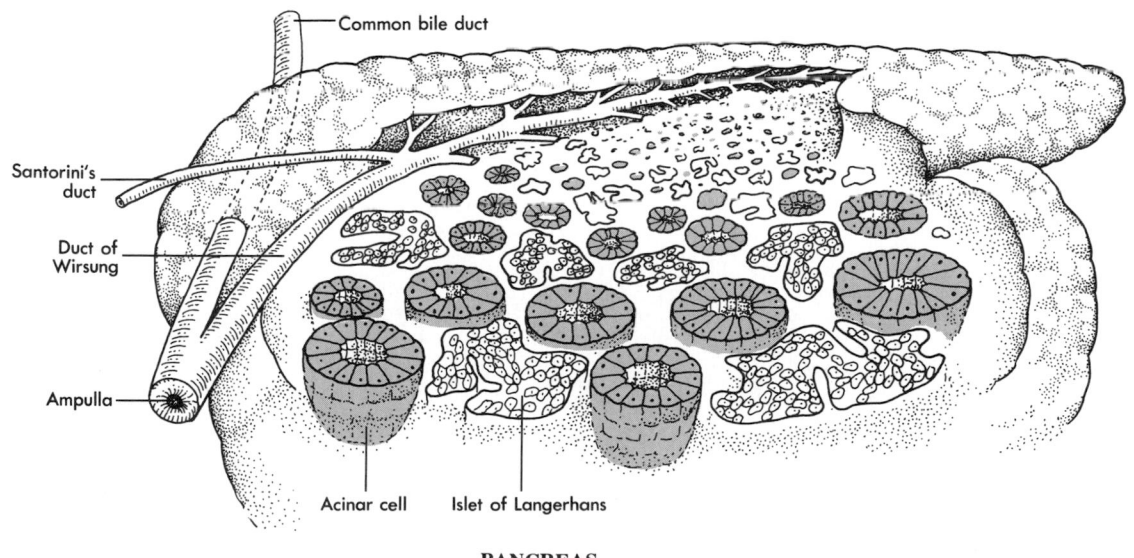

Common bile duct

Santorini's
duct

Duct of
Wirsung

Ampulla

Acinar cell

Islet of Langerhans

PANCREAS

LYMPHATIC SYSTEM

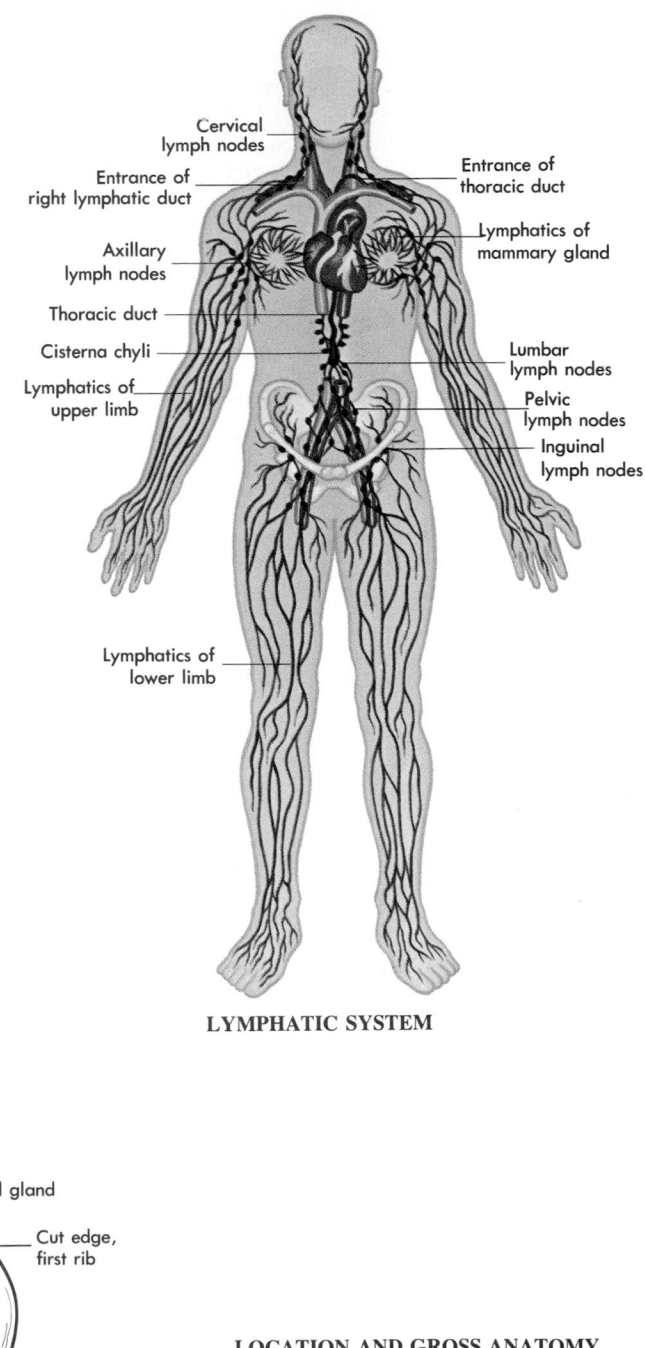

Cervical lymph nodes

Entrance of right lymphatic duct

Axillary lymph nodes

Thoracic duct

Cisterna chyli

Lymphatics of upper limb

Entrance of thoracic duct

Lymphatics of mammary gland

Lumbar lymph nodes

Pelvic lymph nodes

Inguinal lymph nodes

Lymphatics of lower limb

LYMPHATIC SYSTEM

Thyroid gland

Cut edge, first rib

Lobes of the thymus

Heart

Lung

LOCATION AND GROSS ANATOMY OF THYMUS

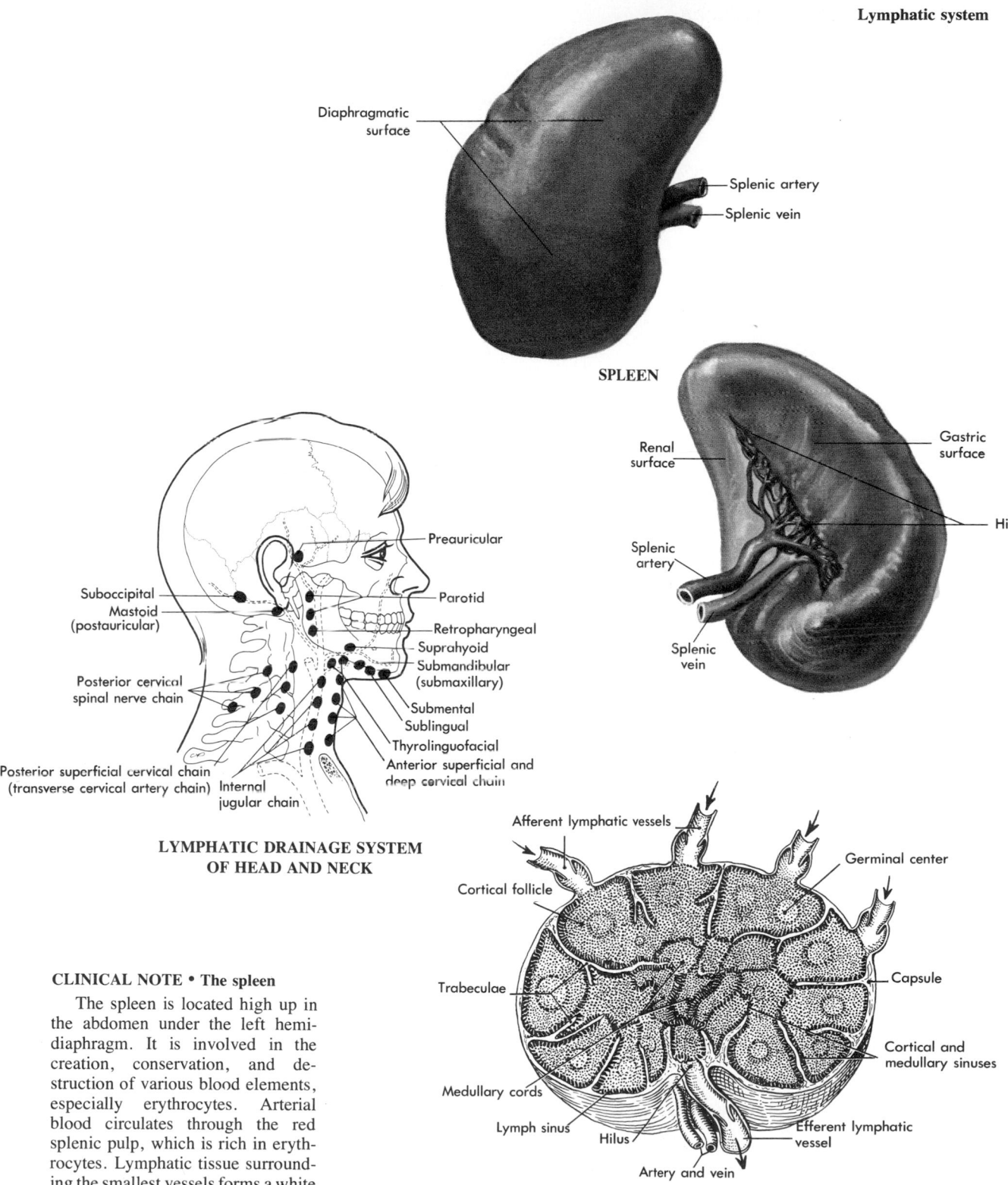

SPLEEN

**LYMPHATIC DRAINAGE SYSTEM
OF HEAD AND NECK**

Diaphragmatic surface

Splenic artery

Splenic vein

Renal surface

Gastric surface

Hilus

Splenic artery

Splenic vein

Preauricular

Suboccipital

Mastoid (postauricular)

Parotid

Retropharyngeal

Suprahyoid

Submandibular (submaxillary)

Posterior cervical spinal nerve chain

Submental

Sublingual

Thyrolinguofacial

Anterior superficial and deep cervical chain

Posterior superficial cervical chain (transverse cervical artery chain)

Internal jugular chain

Afferent lymphatic vessels

Germinal center

Cortical follicle

Trabeculae

Capsule

Cortical and medullary sinuses

Medullary cords

Lymph sinus

Hilus

Efferent lymphatic vessel

Artery and vein

CLINICAL NOTE • The spleen

The spleen is located high up in the abdomen under the left hemidiaphragm. It is involved in the creation, conservation, and destruction of various blood elements, especially erythrocytes. Arterial blood circulates through the red splenic pulp, which is rich in erythrocytes. Lymphatic tissue surrounding the smallest vessels forms a white pulp material.

DIAGRAMMATIC REPRESENTATION OF A LYMPH NODE

NERVOUS SYSTEM

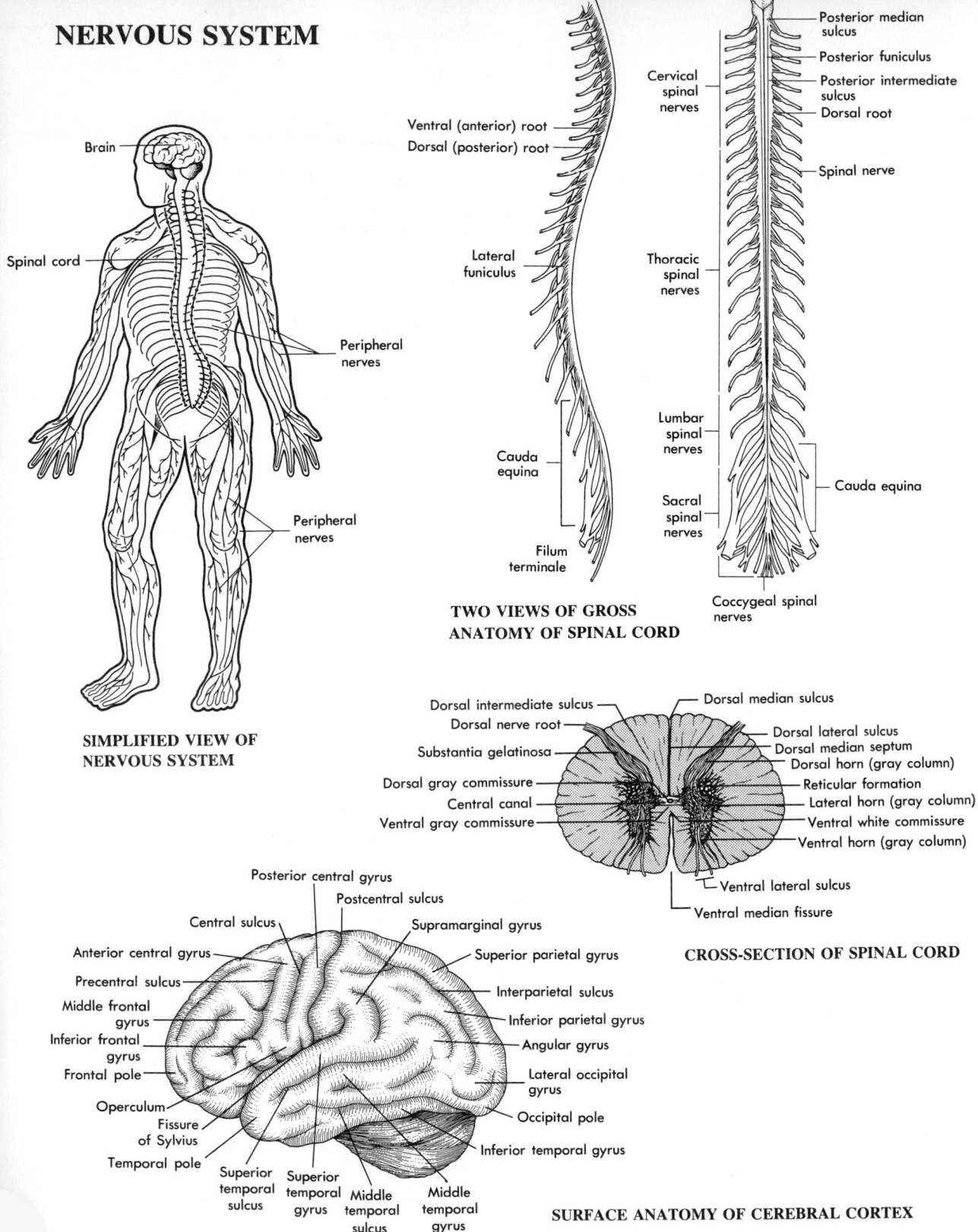

Brain

Spinal cord

Peripheral nerves

Peripheral nerves

SIMPLIFIED VIEW OF NERVOUS SYSTEM

Ventral (anterior) root
Dorsal (posterior) root

Lateral funiculus

Cauda equina

Filum terminale

Cervical spinal nerves

Thoracic spinal nerves

Lumbar spinal nerves

Sacral spinal nerves

Posterior median sulcus
Posterior funiculus
Posterior intermediate sulcus
Dorsal root

Spinal nerve

Cauda equina

Coccygeal spinal nerves

TWO VIEWS OF GROSS ANATOMY OF SPINAL CORD

Dorsal intermediate sulcus
Dorsal nerve root
Substantia gelatinosa
Dorsal gray commissure
Central canal
Ventral gray commissure

Dorsal median sulcus
Dorsal lateral sulcus
Dorsal median septum
Dorsal horn (gray column)
Reticular formation
Lateral horn (gray column)
Ventral white commissure
Ventral horn (gray column)

Ventral lateral sulcus
Ventral median fissure

CROSS-SECTION OF SPINAL CORD

Posterior central gyrus
Postcentral sulcus
Central sulcus
Supramarginal gyrus
Anterior central gyrus
Superior parietal gyrus
Precentral sulcus
Interparietal sulcus
Middle frontal gyrus
Inferior parietal gyrus
Inferior frontal gyrus
Angular gyrus
Frontal pole
Lateral occipital gyrus
Operculum
Occipital pole
Fissure of Sylvius
Inferior temporal gyrus
Temporal pole
Superior temporal sulcus
Superior temporal gyrus
Middle temporal sulcus
Middle temporal gyrus

SURFACE ANATOMY OF CEREBRAL CORTEX

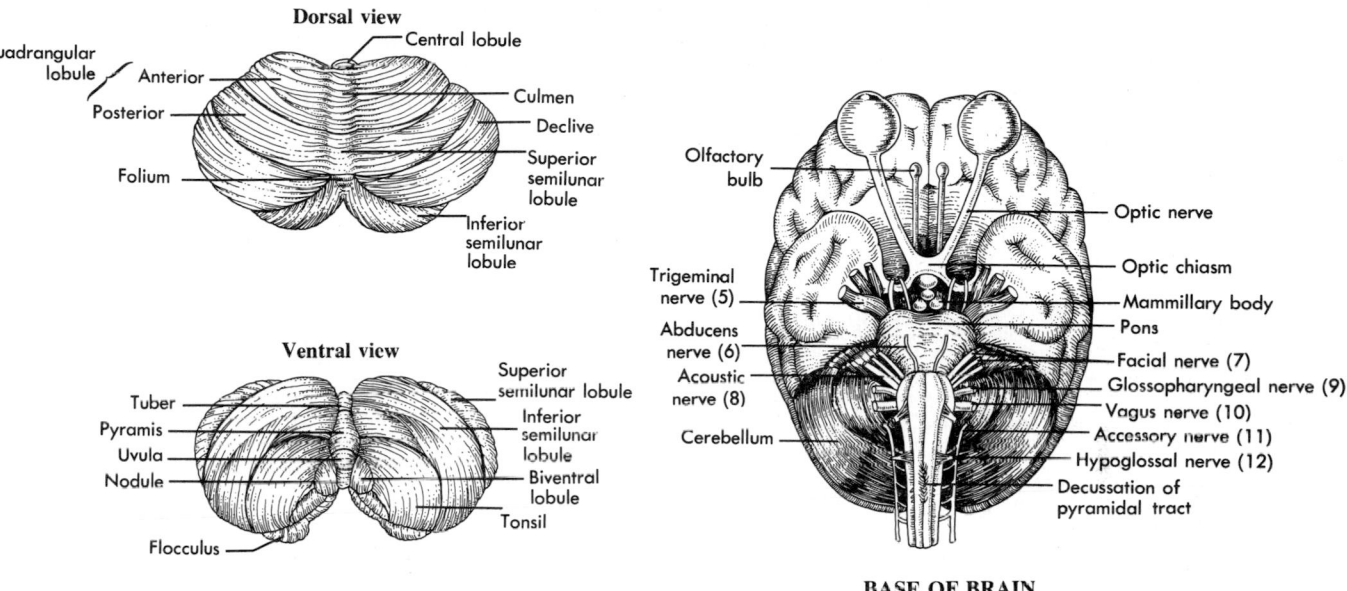

Dorsal view

Quadrangular lobule — Central lobule

Anterior

Posterior

Folium

Culmen

Declive

Superior semilunar lobule

Inferior semilunar lobule

Ventral view

Tuber

Pyramis

Uvula

Nodule

Flocculus

Superior semilunar lobule

Inferior semilunar lobule

Biventral lobule

Tonsil

ANATOMY OF CEREBELLUM

Olfactory bulb

Trigeminal nerve (5)

Abducens nerve (6)

Acoustic nerve (8)

Cerebellum

Optic nerve

Optic chiasm

Mammillary body

Pons

Facial nerve (7)

Glossopharyngeal nerve (9)

Vagus nerve (10)

Accessory nerve (11)

Hypoglossal nerve (12)

Decussation of pyramidal tract

BASE OF BRAIN

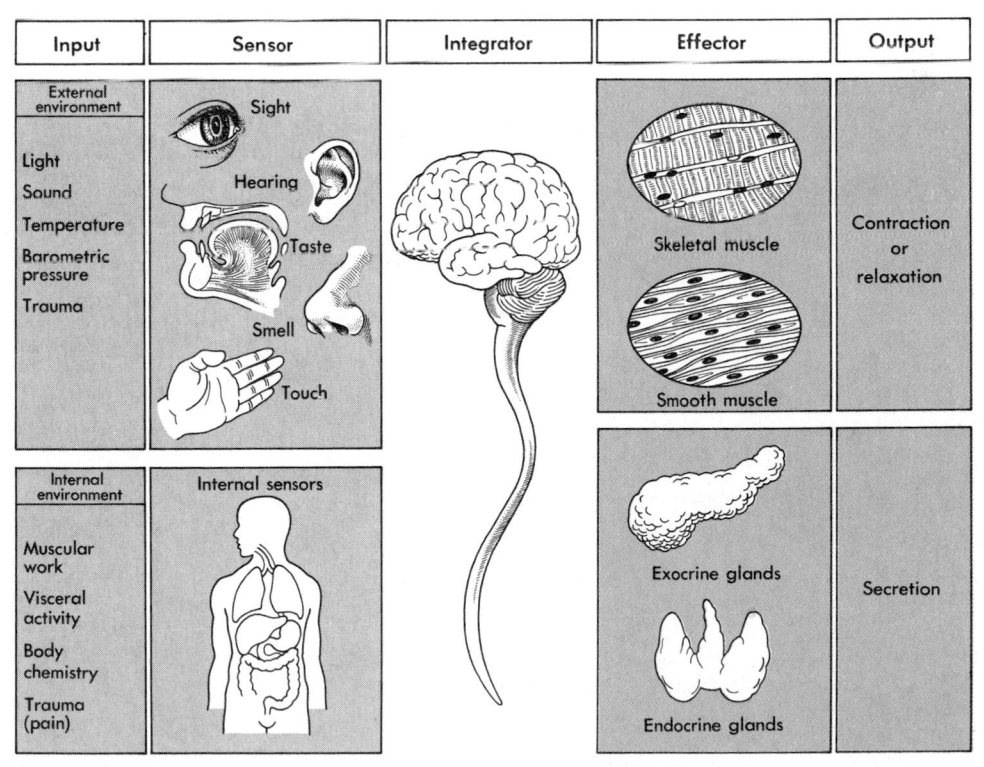

Input	Sensor	Integrator	Effector	Output
External environment Light Sound Temperature Barometric pressure Trauma	Sight Hearing Taste Smell Touch		Skeletal muscle Smooth muscle	Contraction or relaxation
Internal environment Muscular work Visceral activity Body chemistry Trauma (pain)	Internal sensors		Exocrine glands Endocrine glands	Secretion

COMPONENTS OF NERVOUS SYSTEM

1181

CLINICAL NOTE • The neuron

The neuron (see below) is the basic excitable cell unit of the nervous system. Neurons display a variety of shapes and sizes. Usually they have a large number of dendritic processes but a single axonal extension. Axons appear as elongated, and bundles of axons, called tracts, make up the white matter that surrounds the gray matter of spinal nerve cells.

TWO MAJOR TYPES OF NEURONS IN THE BODY (SPINAL NERVES SHOWN)

Nissl body

Dendrite

Neurofibrils

Axon

Axon

Nucleus of Schwann cell

Myelin lamellae

Neurolemma

Node of Ranvier

Neurofibrils

Neuromuscular junction

Axon

Dendrite

Neurolemma
Myelin lamellae
Nucleus of Schwann cell

Nerve ending in skin

Midbrain

Medulla

(3)

(7)

(9)

(10)

C1
C2
C3
C4
C5
C6
C7
C8
T1
T2
T3
T4
T5
T6
T7
T8
T9
T10
T11
T12
L1
L2
L3
L4
L5
S1
S2
S3
S4
S5

Ciliary ganglion

Eye

Submaxillary ganglion

Submaxillary gland

Superior cervical ganglion

Parotid gland

Otic ganglion

Middle cervical ganglion

Stellate ganglion

Greater splanchnic nerve

Heart

Celiac ganglion

Stomach

Lesser splanchnic nerve

Small intestine

Superior mesenteric ganglion

Adrenal medulla

Inferior mesenteric ganglion

Colon

Bladder

Sympathetic trunk

Pelvic nerve

SYMPATHETIC AND PARASYMPATHETIC DIVISIONS OF THE AUTONOMIC NERVOUS SYSTEM AND CONNECTIONS OF EACH

— Sympathetic

— Parasympathetic

=== Postganglionic fibers

RESPIRATORY SYSTEM

STRUCTURE OF THE NOSE

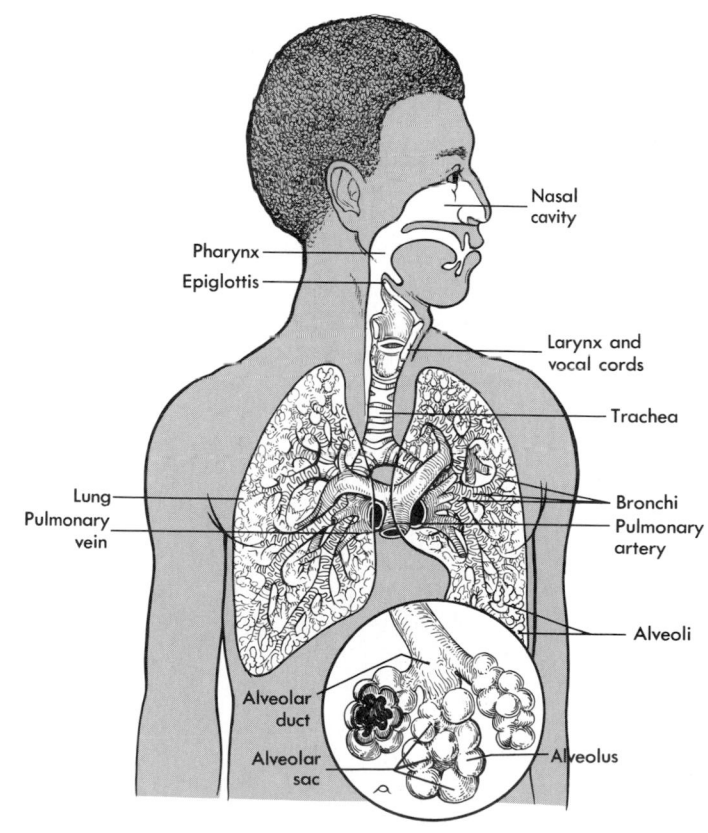

**RESPIRATORY SYSTEM AND DETAILED
ENLARGEMENT OF ALVEOLAR SACS**

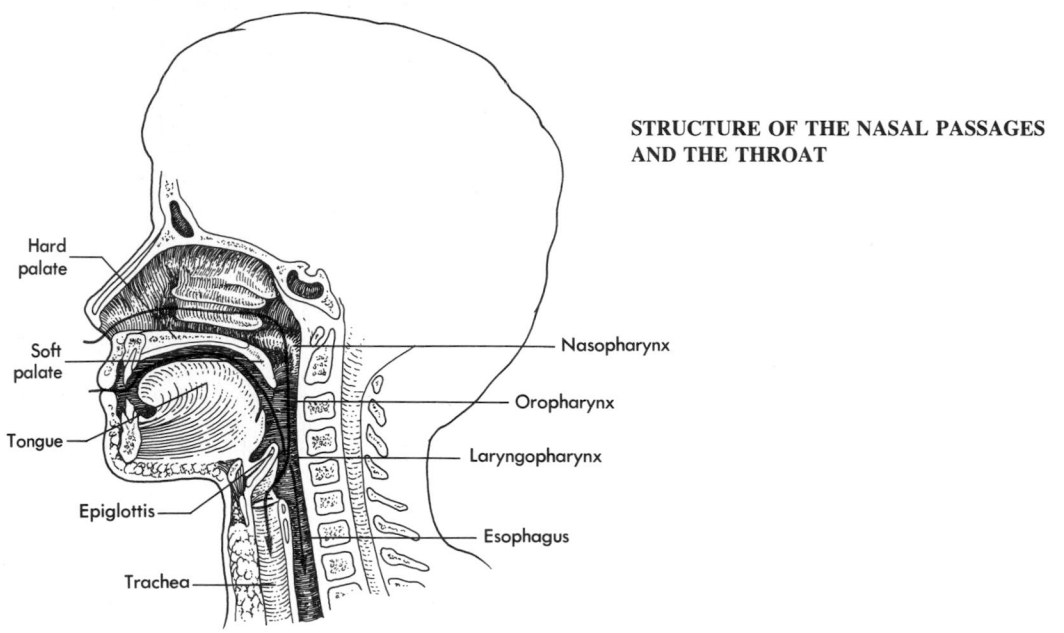

**STRUCTURE OF THE NASAL PASSAGES
AND THE THROAT**

Hard palate

Soft palate

Tongue

Epiglottis

Trachea

Nasopharynx

Oropharynx

Laryngopharynx

Esophagus

**ANATOMY OF AIR-EXCHANGING
SURFACE OF THE LUNGS**

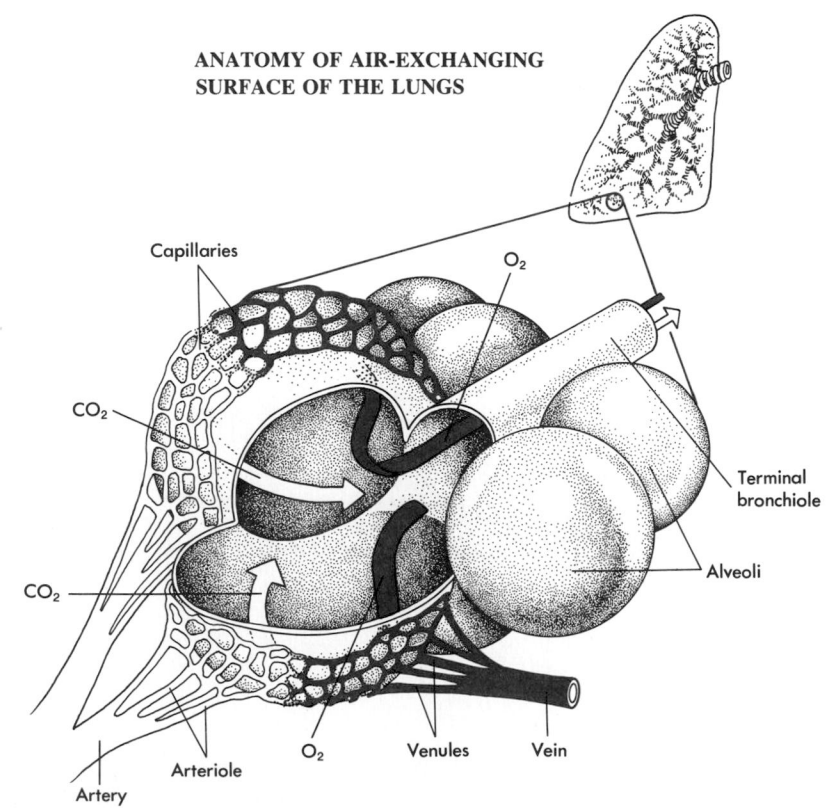

Capillaries

O_2

CO_2

CO_2

Terminal bronchiole

Alveoli

O_2

Venules

Vein

Arteriole

Artery

1184

Muscles of inspiration   Muscles of expiration

External
intercostals
(elevate ribs)

Diaphragm

Internal
intercostals

Rectus
abdominus

External
oblique

Internal
oblique

MECHANICS OF RESPIRATION; MUSCLES REQUIRED FOR INSPIRATION AND EXPIRATION

Right lung   Left lung

Superior
lobe

Superior
lobe

Middle
lobe

Inferior
lobe

Inferior
lobe

LOBES OF THE LUNG

Flexibility of trachea

Membrane

CLINICAL NOTE • Respiratory muscles

Unlike cardiac muscle, respiratory muscles are skeletal and striated and possess no inherent rhythm. The periodic nature of respiratory movements results instead from the activity of certain pontine and medullary cells belonging to the reticular formation. Some stimulate breathing movements, others the opposite (inspiratory and expiratory centers).

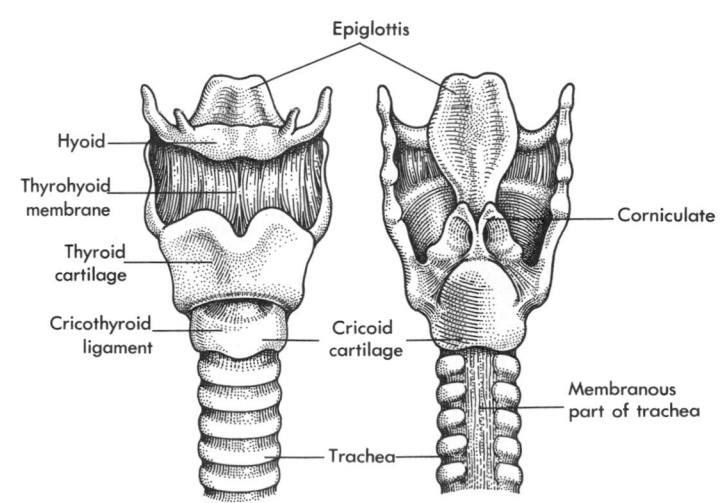

Epiglottis

Hyoid

Thyrohyoid
membrane

Thyroid
cartilage

Cricothyroid
ligament

Corniculate

Cricoid
cartilage

Membranous
part of trachea

Trachea

CARTILAGINOUS STRUCTURE OF THE LARYNX AND UPPER TRACHEA

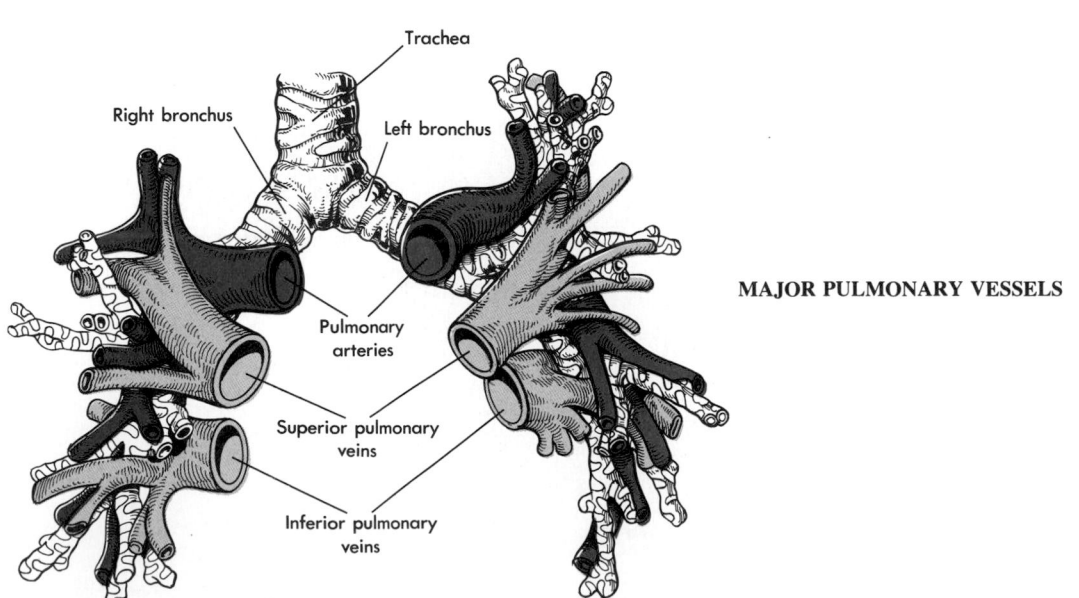

BRONCHOPULMONARY SEGMENTS

Apical

Posterior

Apical

Anterior

Lateral

Lateral basal

Anterior basal

Medial

Right lung—lateral view

Apicoposterior

Anterior

Apical

Superior lingular

Inferior lingular

Anterior basal

Lateral basal

Left lung—lateral view

Posterior

Apical

Anterior

Apical

Posterior basal

Medial

Medial basal

Lateral

Anterior basal

Lateral basal

Right lung—medial view

Apicoposterior

Anterior

Apical

Superior lingular

Inferior lingular

Posterior basal

Medial basal

Lateral basal

Anterior basal

Left lung—medial view

Trachea

Right bronchus

Left bronchus

MAJOR PULMONARY VESSELS

Pulmonary arteries

Superior pulmonary veins

Inferior pulmonary veins

DIGESTIVE SYSTEM

CLINICAL NOTE • Digestive system

A malignant growth of the descending colon can take different forms and has several potential pathways for spreading. The growth may be polypoid, or annular, causing stenosis and obstruction of the large bowel, or plaque-like with a rolled edge and ulcerated center. Distant implantation of cancer cells is called metastasis. How soon this occurs depends on the type of cancer cells and the speed of their growth. Early invasion of pericolic veins may result in clumps of cells passing to the liver where they form metastatic nodules. Lymphatic penetration proceeds to involvement of the regional lymph nodes, and direct seeding can occur to other parts of the large bowel. The aim of surgery is to remove the primary growth and to restore bowel continuity by end-to-end anastomosis or, if necessary to create a colostomy.

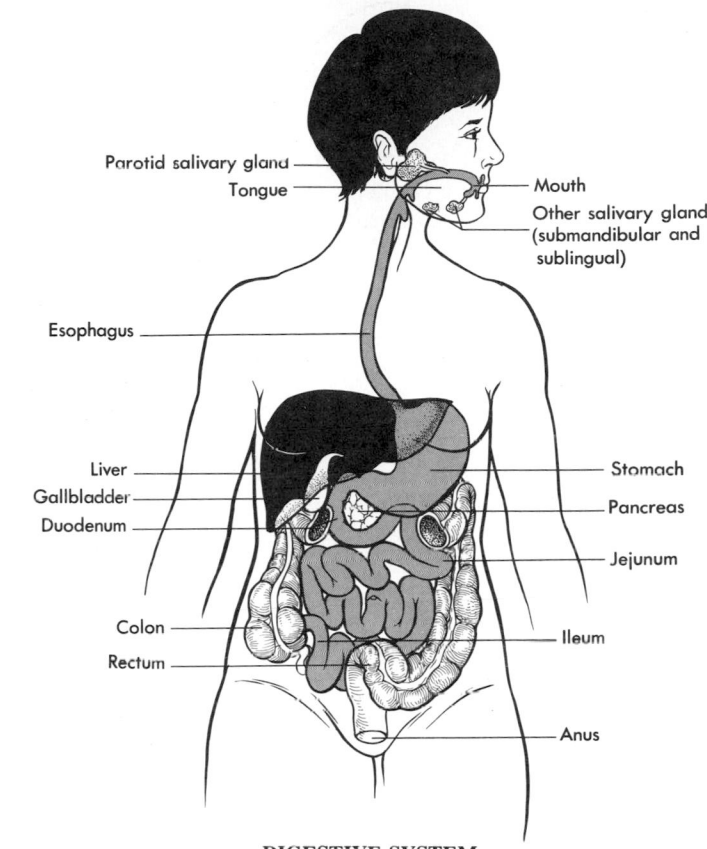

DIGESTIVE SYSTEM

Anatomy of the stomach, the spleen, and the pancreas, illustrating the relationship and distribution of the branches of the celiac artery.

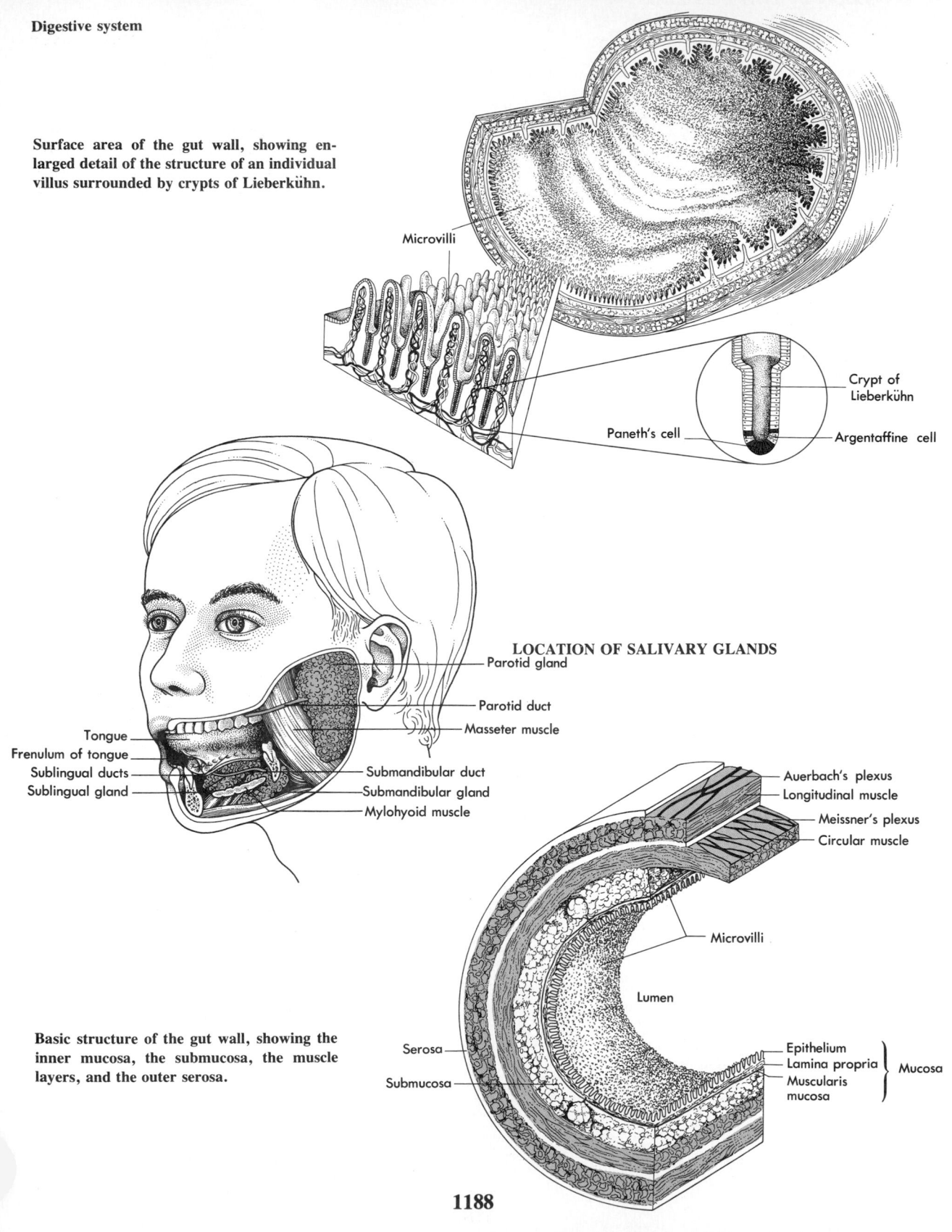

Surface area of the gut wall, showing enlarged detail of the structure of an individual villus surrounded by crypts of Lieberkühn.

Microvilli

Crypt of Lieberkühn

Paneth's cell

Argentaffine cell

LOCATION OF SALIVARY GLANDS

Parotid gland

Parotid duct

Masseter muscle

Tongue

Frenulum of tongue

Sublingual ducts

Sublingual gland

Submandibular duct

Submandibular gland

Mylohyoid muscle

Auerbach's plexus

Longitudinal muscle

Meissner's plexus

Circular muscle

Microvilli

Lumen

Epithelium

Lamina propria

Muscularis mucosa

Mucosa

Serosa

Submucosa

Basic structure of the gut wall, showing the inner mucosa, the submucosa, the muscle layers, and the outer serosa.

1188

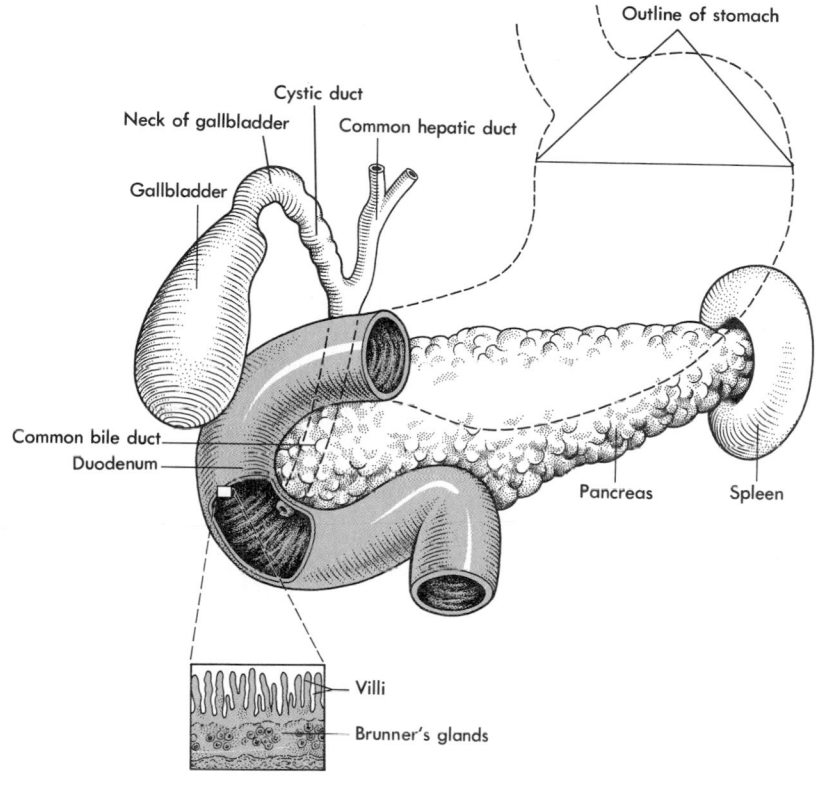

Outline of stomach

Cystic duct

Neck of gallbladder

Common hepatic duct

Gallbladder

Common bile duct

Duodenum

Pancreas

Spleen

Villi

Brunner's glands

Sources of intestinal secretion: bile from the gallbladder, pancreatic juice from the exocrine pancreas, and mucus secretion from Brunner's glands in the duodenal wall.

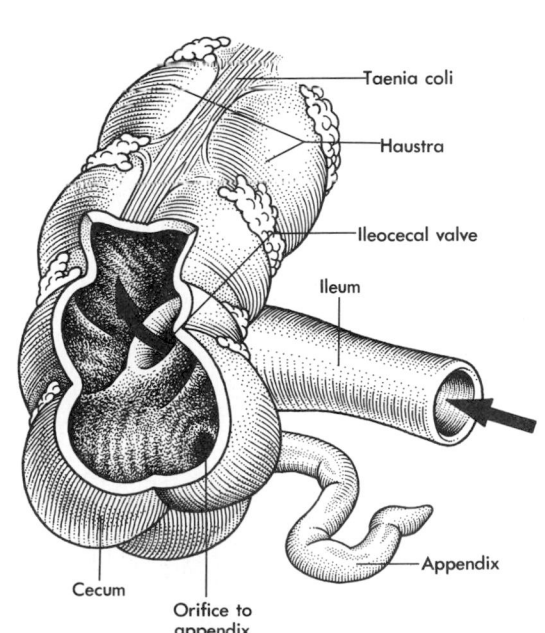

Taenia coli

Haustra

Ileocecal valve

Ileum

Appendix

Cecum

Orifice to appendix

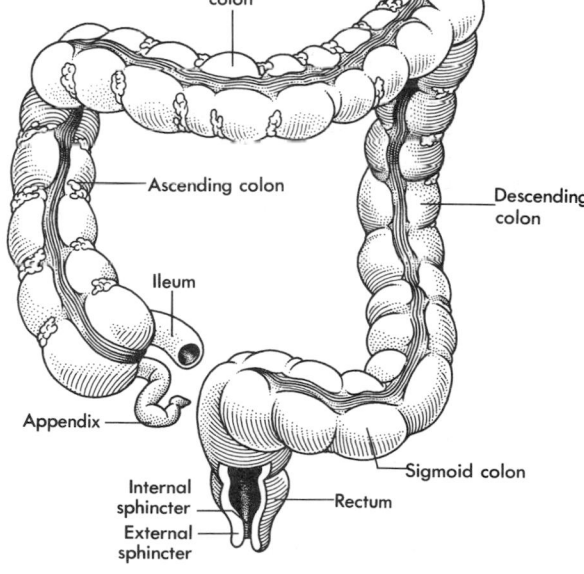

Transverse colon

Ascending colon

Descending colon

Ileum

Appendix

Internal sphincter

External sphincter

Rectum

Sigmoid colon

Anatomy of the large intestine, rectum, and anus. Enlarged detail shows the junction between the large and small intestines and the valve-like entry of the ileum into the cecum.

REPRODUCTIVE SYSTEM

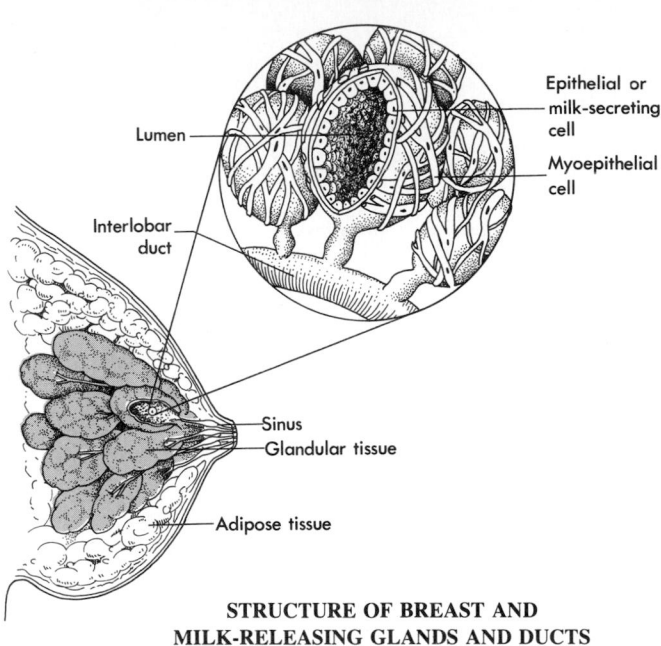

CLINICAL NOTE • Female reproductive system

Immense structural changes occur within the uterus during pregnancy. However, if fertilization does not take place, then the endometrial lining is shed cyclically under hormonal control in the phenomenon of menstruation.

**STRUCTURE OF BREAST AND
MILK-RELEASING GLANDS AND DUCTS**

FEMALE REPRODUCTIVE SYSTEM

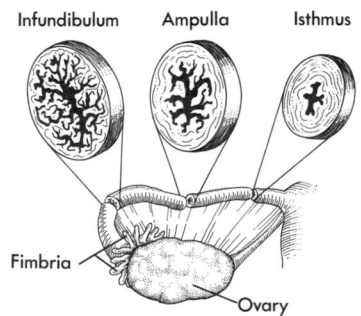

**DETAILED STRUCTURE OF
FALLOPIAN TUBES**

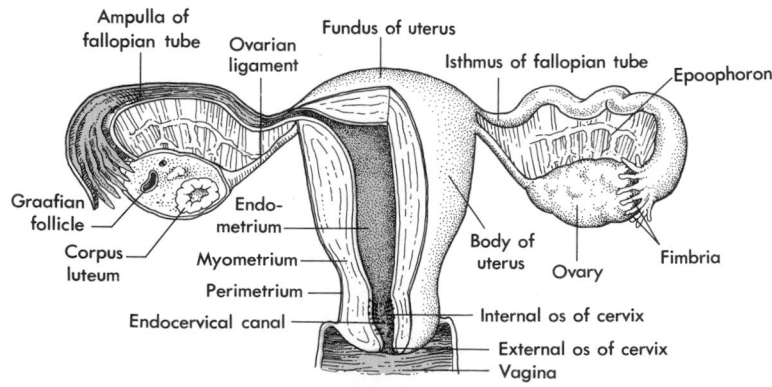

ANATOMY OF FALLOPIAN TUBES AND UTERUS

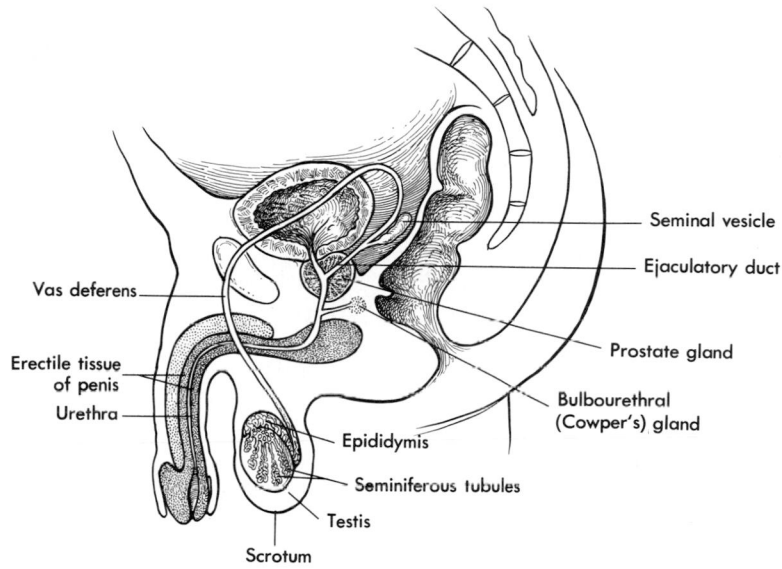

Seminal vesicle

Ejaculatory duct

Vas deferens

Prostate gland

Erectile tissue
of penis

Bulbourethral
(Cowper's) gland

Urethra

Epididymis

Seminiferous tubules

Testis

Scrotum

MALE REPRODUCTIVE SYSTEM

Acrosome

Principal
piece

Head

Nucleus

Front   Side

Middle piece

End
piece

ANATOMY OF A SPERM

1191

URINARY SYSTEM

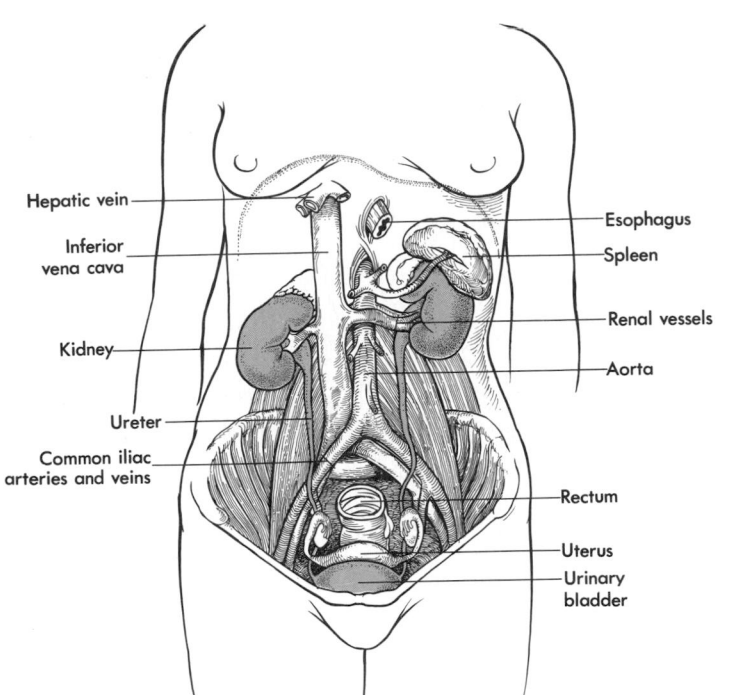

Hepatic vein
Inferior vena cava
Kidney
Ureter
Common iliac arteries and veins

Esophagus
Spleen
Renal vessels
Aorta
Rectum
Uterus
Urinary bladder

**URINARY SYSTEM AND
SOME ASSOCIATED STRUCTURES**

**GROSS ANATOMY OF KIDNEY,
SHOWING ARRANGEMENT OF KIDNEY
TUBULES IN CORTEX AND MEDULLA**

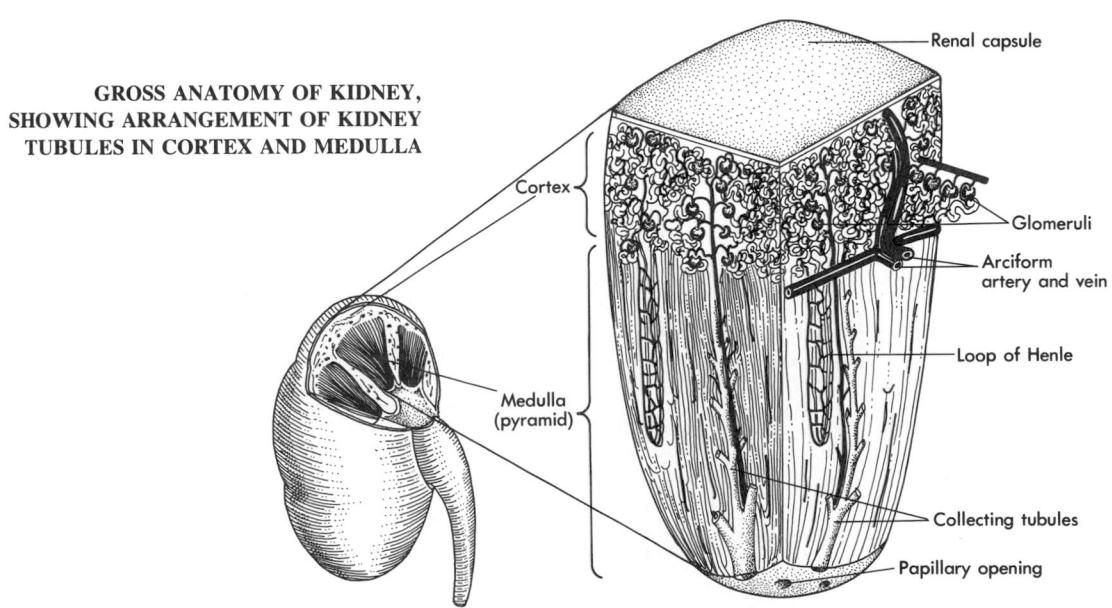

Cortex
Medulla (pyramid)

Renal capsule
Glomeruli
Arciform artery and vein
Loop of Henle
Collecting tubules
Papillary opening

**LOBULAR ARRANGEMENT OF KIDNEY,
SHOWING THE BASIC BLOOD SUPPLY PATTERN**

ANATOMY OF URINARY TRACT

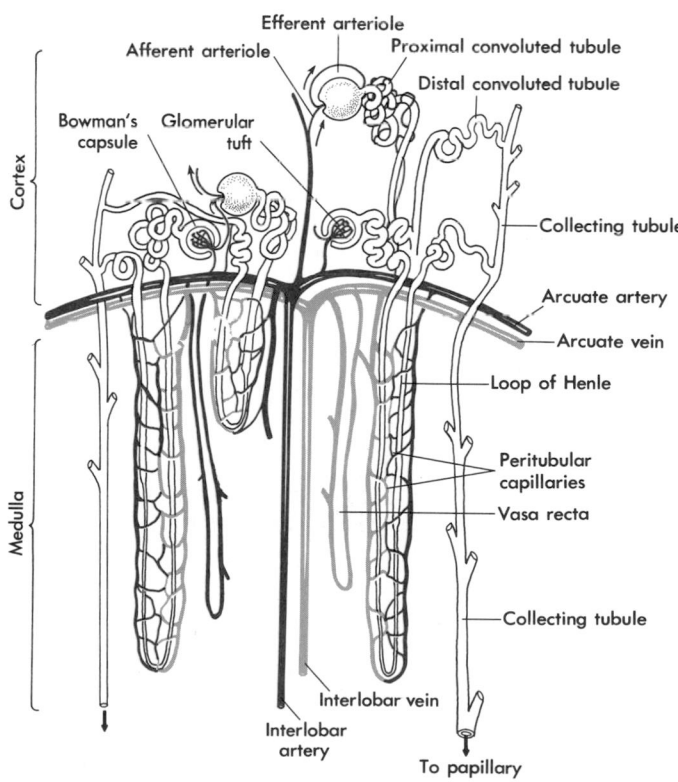

**MICROSCOPIC DETAIL OF THE NEPHRON,
THE STRUCTURAL AND FUNCTIONAL
UNIT OF THE KIDNEY**

1193

SPECIAL SENSES

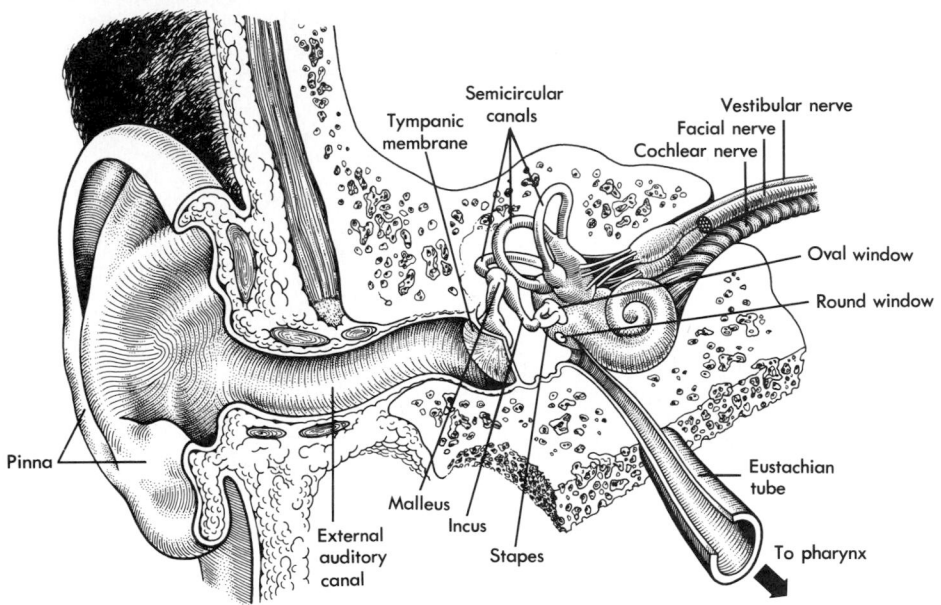

Semicircular canals

Tympanic membrane

Vestibular nerve

Facial nerve

Cochlear nerve

Oval window

Round window

Pinna

Malleus

Incus

Stapes

Eustachian tube

External auditory canal

To pharynx

GROSS ANATOMY OF THE EAR

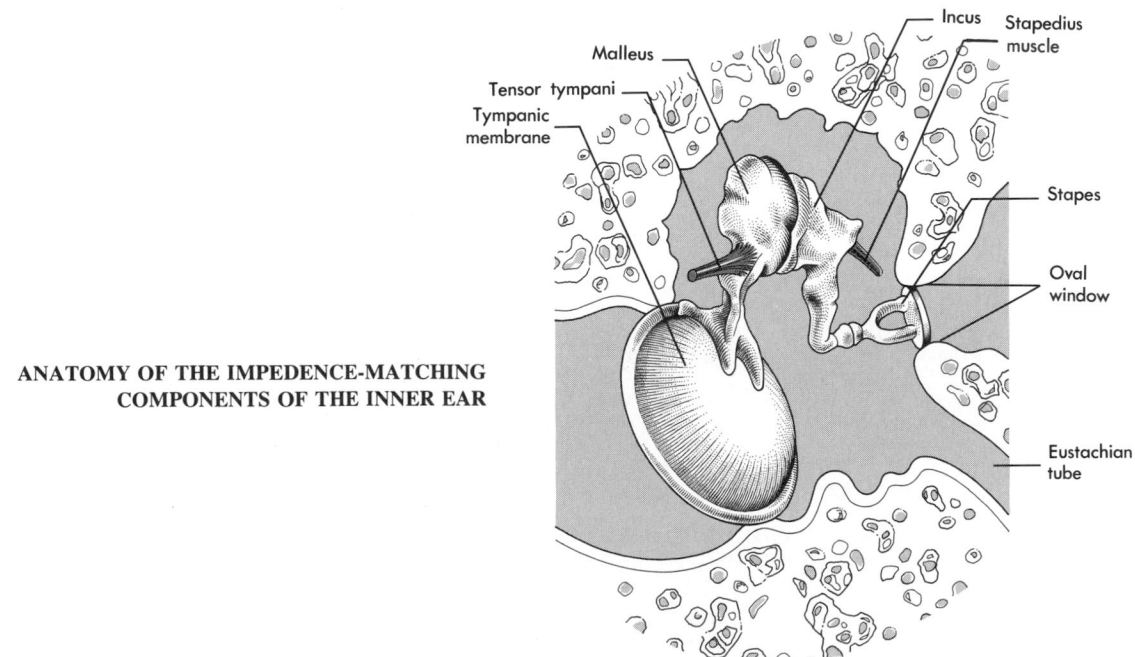

Incus

Stapedius muscle

Malleus

Tensor tympani

Tympanic membrane

Stapes

Oval window

ANATOMY OF THE IMPEDENCE-MATCHING COMPONENTS OF THE INNER EAR

Eustachian tube

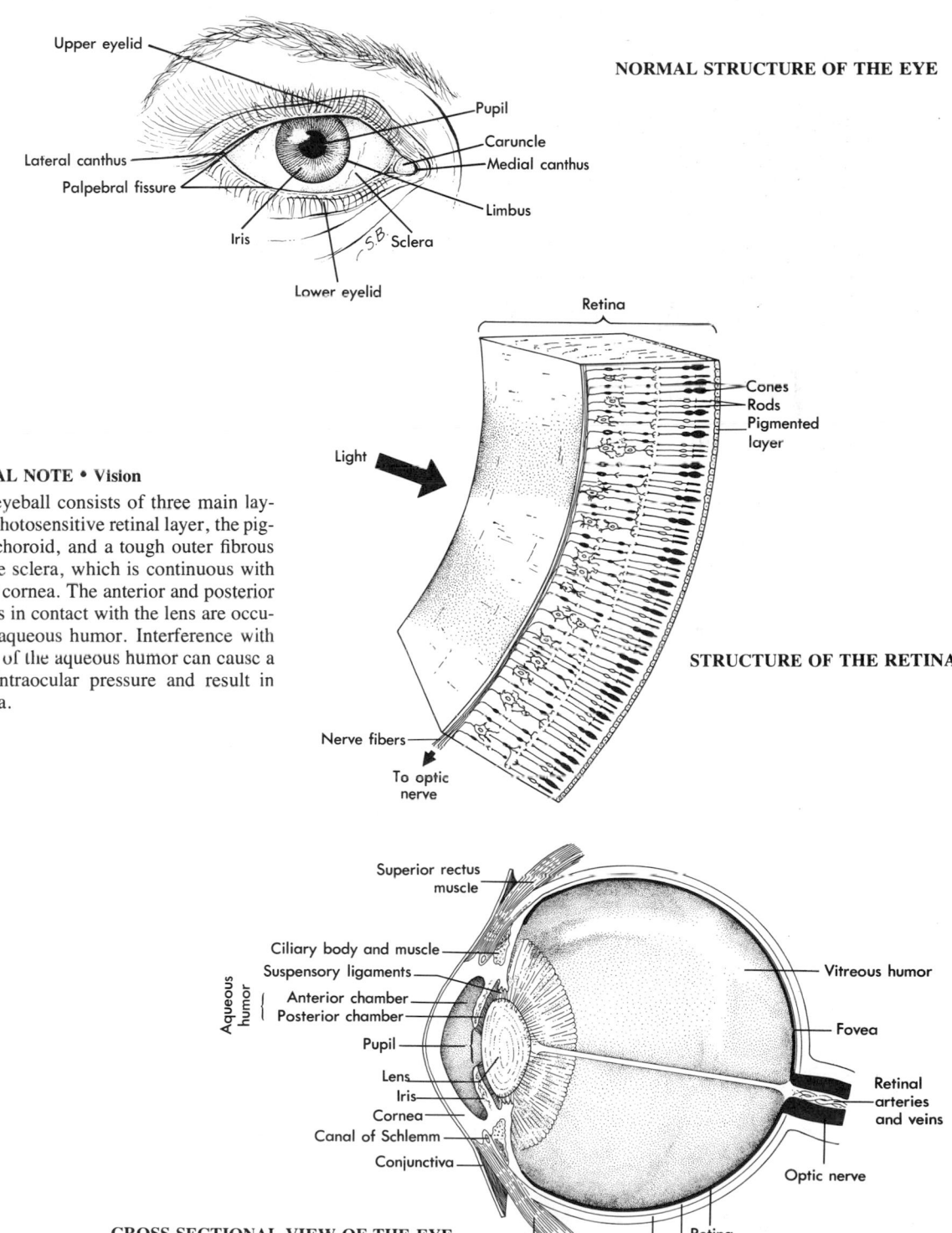

NORMAL STRUCTURE OF THE EYE

Upper eyelid

Pupil

Caruncle

Lateral canthus

Medial canthus

Palpebral fissure

Limbus

Iris

S.B. Sclera

Lower eyelid

Retina

Cones

Rods

Pigmented layer

Light

CLINICAL NOTE • Vision

The eyeball consists of three main layers: the photosensitive retinal layer, the pigmented choroid, and a tough outer fibrous layer, the sclera, which is continuous with the clear cornea. The anterior and posterior chambers in contact with the lens are occupied by aqueous humor. Interference with drainage of the aqueous humor can cause a rise in intraocular pressure and result in glaucoma.

STRUCTURE OF THE RETINA

Nerve fibers

To optic nerve

Superior rectus muscle

Ciliary body and muscle

Suspensory ligaments

Vitreous humor

Aqueous humor

Anterior chamber

Posterior chamber

Pupil

Fovea

Lens

Iris

Retinal arteries and veins

Cornea

Canal of Schlemm

Conjunctiva

Optic nerve

CROSS-SECTIONAL VIEW OF THE EYE

Inferior rectus muscle

Retina

Choroid

Sclera

STRUCTURE OF THE SKIN

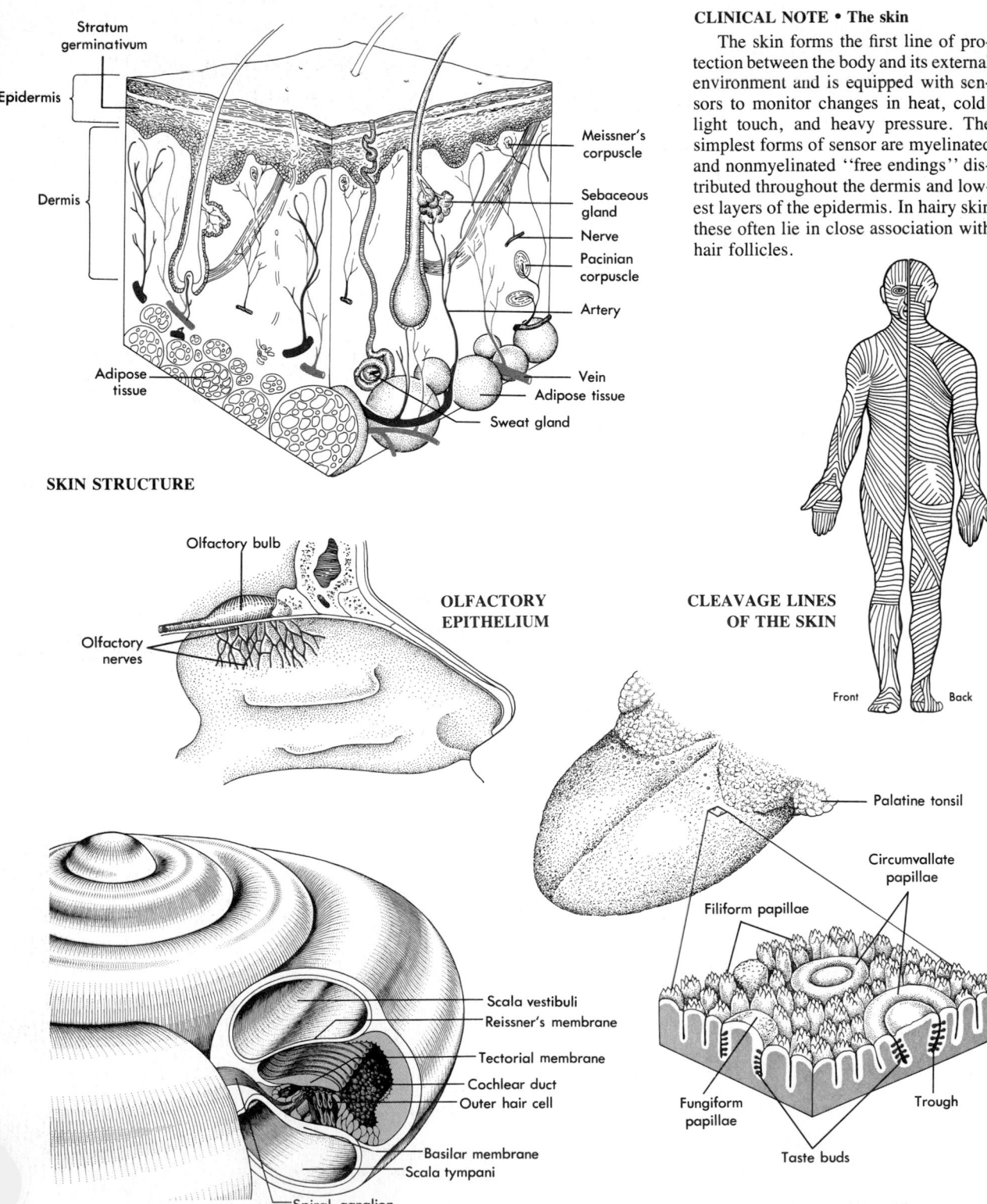

Stratum germinativum

Epidermis

Dermis

Meissner's corpuscle

Sebaceous gland

Nerve

Pacinian corpuscle

Artery

Adipose tissue

Vein

Adipose tissue

Sweat gland

SKIN STRUCTURE

CLINICAL NOTE • The skin

The skin forms the first line of protection between the body and its external environment and is equipped with sensors to monitor changes in heat, cold, light touch, and heavy pressure. The simplest forms of sensor are myelinated and nonmyelinated "free endings" distributed throughout the dermis and lowest layers of the epidermis. In hairy skin these often lie in close association with hair follicles.

Olfactory bulb

Olfactory nerves

OLFACTORY EPITHELIUM

CLEAVAGE LINES OF THE SKIN

Front

Back

Palatine tonsil

Circumvallate papillae

Filiform papillae

Fungiform papillae

Trough

Taste buds

Scala vestibuli

Reissner's membrane

Tectorial membrane

Cochlear duct

Outer hair cell

Basilar membrane

Scala tympani

Spiral ganglion

ANATOMY OF THE COCHLEA

1196

PAPILLAE ON THE TONGUE AND LOCATION OF TASTE BUDS

APPENDICES

APPEN-
DIX

APPENDIX 1 • Units of measurement

1-1. Conversion factors

Conversion rules: To convert units of one system into the other, multiply the number of units in the first column by the equivalent factor in the second column.

WEIGHT

Unit	Equivalent
1 milligram	0.015432 grain
1 gram	15.432 grains
1 gram	0.25720 apothecaries' dram
1 gram	0.03527 avoirdupois ounce
1 gram	0.03215 apothecaries' or troy ounce
1 kilogram	35.274 avoirdupois ounces
1 kilogram	32.151 apothecaries' or troy ounces
1 kilogram	2.2046 avoirdupois pounds
1 grain	64.7989 milligrams
1 grain	0.0648 gram
1 apothecaries' dram	3.8879 grams
1 avoirdupois ounce	28.3495 grams
1 apothecaries' or troy ounce	31.1035 grams
1 avoirdupois pound	453.5924 grams

CAPACITY (FLUID OR LIQUID)

Unit	Equivalent
1 milliliter	16.23 minims
1 milliliter	0.2705 fluid dram
1 milliliter	0.0338 fluid ounce
1 liter	33.8148 fluid ounces
1 liter	2.1134 pints
1 liter	1.0567 quart
1 liter	0.2642 gallon
1 fluid dram	3.697 milliliters
1 fluid ounce	29.573 milliliters
1 pint	473.166 milliliters
1 quart	946.332 milliliters
1 gallon	3.785 liters

VOLUME (AIR OR GAS)

Unit	Equivalent
1 cubic centimeter	0.06102 cubic inch
1 cubic meter	35.314 cubic feet
1 cubic meter	1.3079 cubic yard
1 cubic inch	16.3872 cubic centimeters
1 cubic foot	0.02832 cubic meter

MISCELLANEOUS CONVERSION FACTORS
Pressure

To obtain	Multiply	By
lb/sq in	atmospheres	14.696
lb/sq in	in of water	0.03609
lb/sq in	ft of water	0.4335
lb/sq in	in of mercury	0.4912
lb/sq in	kg/sq meter	0.00142
lb/sq in	kg/sq cm	14.22
lb/sq in	cm of mercury	0.1934
lb/sq ft	atmospheres	2116.2
lb/sq ft	in of water	5.1981
lb/sq ft	ft of water	62.378
lb/sq ft	in of mercury	70.727
lb/sq ft	cm of mercury	27.845
lb/sq ft	kg/sq meter	0.20482
lb/cu in	gm/ml	0.03613
lb/cu ft	lb/cu in	1728.0
lb/cu ft	gm/ml	62.428
lb/US gal	gm/ml	8.345
in of water	in of mercury	13.60
in of water	cm of mercury	5.3524
ft of water	atmospheres	33.93
ft of water	lb/sq in	2.311
ft of water	kg/sq meter	0.00328
ft of water	in of mercury	1.133
ft of water	cm of mercury	0.4460
atmospheres	ft of water	0.02947
atmospheres	in of mercury	0.03342
atmospheres	kg/sq cm	0.9678
bars	atmospheres	1.0133
in of mercury	atmospheres	29.921
in of mercury	lb/sq in	2.036
mm of mercury	atmospheres	760.0
gm/ml	lb/cu in	27.68
gm/sq cm	lb/sq in	70.31
gm/sq cm	kg/sq meter	0.1
kg/sq meter	in of water	25.38
kg/sq meter	in of mercury	345.32
kg/sq meter	cm of mercury	135.95
kg/sq meter	atmospheres	10332.0
kg/sq cm	atmospheres	1.0332

Flow rate

To obtain	Multiply	By
cu ft/hr	cc/min	0.00212
cu ft/hr	L/min	2.12
L/min	cu ft/hr	0.472

Parts per million

Conversion of parts per million (ppm) to percent: 1 ppm = 0.0001%, 10 ppm = 0.001%, 100 ppm = 0.01%, 1000 ppm = 0.1%, and 10,000 ppm = 1%.

1-2. Metric doses and apothecary equivalents

LIQUID MEASURE

Metric	Approximate apothecary equivalents
Milliliters	
1000	1 quart
750	1½ pints
500	1 pint
250	8 fluid ounces
200	7 fluid ounces
100	3½ fluid ounces
50	1¾ fluid ounces
30	1 fluid ounce
15	4 fluid drams
10	2½ fluid drams
8	2 fluid drams
5	1¼ fluid drams
4	1 fluid dram
3	45 minims
2	30 minims
1	15 minims
0.75	12 minims
0.6	10 minims
0.5	8 minims
0.3	5 minims
0.25	4 minims
0.2	3 minims
0.1	1½ minims
0.06	1 minim
0.05	¾ minim
0.03	½ minim

WEIGHT

Metric	Approximate apothecary equivalents
Grams	Grains
.0002	1/300
.0003	1/200
.0004	1/150
.0005	1/120
.0006	1/100
.001	1/60
.002	1/30
.005	1/12
.010	1/6
.015	1/4
.025	3/8
.030	1/2
.050	3/4
.060	1
.100	1½
.120	2
.200	3
.300	5
.500	7½
.600	10
1	15
2	30
4	60

1-3. Units of length, volume, and weight

Arabic numbers are used with weights and measures, as 10 gm or 3 ml. Portions of weights and measures are usually expressed decimally. For practical purposes, 1 cc is equivalent to 1 ml and 1 drop (gtt) of water is equivalent to 1 minim ($\mathfrak{m}$).

UNITS OF LENGTH

	Millimeters	Centimeters	Inches	Feet	Yards	Meters
1 mm =	1.0	0.1	0.03937	0.00328	0.0011	0.001
1 cm =	10.0	1.0	0.3937	0.03281	0.0109	0.01
1 in =	25.4	2.54	1.0	0.0833	0.0278	0.0254
1 ft =	304.8	30.48	12.0	1.0	0.333	0.3048
1 yd =	914.40	91.44	36.0	3.0	1.0	0.9144
1 m =	1000.0	100.0	39.37	3.2808	1.0936	1.0

1 μ = 1 mu = 1 micrometer = 0.001 millimeter. 1 mm = 1000 μ.
1 Km = 1 kilometer = 1000 meters = 0.6215 mile.
1 mile = 5280 feet = 1.609 kilometers.

VOLUME CONVERSIONS (METRIC AND APOTHECARY)

Milliliters	Minims	Fluid drams	Fluid ounces	Pints		Liters	Gallons	Quarts	Fluid ounces	Pints
1	16.2	.27	.0333	.0021		1	.2642	1.057	33.824	2.114
.0616	1	1/60	1/480	1/7680		3.785	1	4	128	8
3.697	60	1	1/8	1/128		.946	1/4	1	32	2
29.58	480	8	1	1/16		.473	1/8	1/2	16	1
473.2	7680	128	16	1		.0296	1/128	1/32	1	1/16

WEIGHT CONVERSIONS (METRIC AND AVOIRDUPOIS)

Grams	Kilograms	Ounces	Pounds
1	.001	.0353	.0022
1000	1	35.3	2.2
28.35	.02835	1	1/16
454.5	.4545	16	1

LINEAR MEASURE

1 inch = 2.54 centimeters
40 rods = 1 furlong
8 furlongs = 1 statute mile

12 inches = 1 foot
3 feet = 1 yard
5.5 yards = 1 rod

1 statute mile = 5280 feet
3 statute miles = 1 statute league

TROY WEIGHT (USED FOR WEIGHING GOLD, SILVER, AND JEWELS)

24 grains = 1 pennyweight
20 pennyweights = 1 ounce
12 ounces = 1 pound

WEIGHT CONVERSIONS (METRIC AND APOTHECARY)

Grams	Milligrams	Grains	Drams	Ounces	Pounds
1	1000	15.4	.2577	.0322	.00268
.001	1	.0154	.00026	.0000322	.00000268
.0648	64.8	1	1/60	1/480	1/5760
3.888	3888	60	1	1/8	1/96
31.1	31104	480	8	1	1/12
373.25	373248	5760	96	12	1

APPROXIMATE* HOUSEHOLD MEASUREMENT EQUIVALENTS (VOLUME)

		1 tsp =		5 ml
		1 tbsp = 3 tsp =		15 ml
		1 fl oz = 2 tbsp = 6 tsp =		30 ml
	1 cup =	8 fl oz	=	240 ml
1 pt =	2 cups =	16 fl oz	=	480 ml
1 qt = 2 pt =	4 cups =	32 fl oz	=	960 ml
1 gal = 4 qt = 8 pt =	16 cups =	128 fl oz	=	3840 ml

*Household measures are not precise. For instance, 1 household tsp will hold from 3 ml to 5 ml of liquid. Therefore do not substitute household equivalents for prescribed medication.

MISCELLANEOUS WEIGHTS AND MEASURES

Apothecaries' weight

20 grains = 1 scruple

3 scruples = 1 dram

Avoirdupois weight

27.343 grains = 1 dram

2000 pounds = 1 short ton

1 oz troy = 480 grains

1 lb troy = 5760 grains

16 drams = 1 ounce

100 pounds = 1 hundredweight

2240 pounds = 1 long ton

1 oz avoirdupois = 437.5 grains

1 lb avoirdupois = 7000 grains

Circular measure

60 seconds = 1 minute

90 degrees = 1 quadrant

60 minutes = 1 degree

4 quadrants = 360 degrees = circle

Cubic measure

1728 cubic inches = 1 cubic foot

2150.42 cubic inches = 1 standard bushel

1 cubic foot = about four-fifths of a bushel

27 cubic feet = 1 cubic yard

268.8 cubic inches = 1 dry gallon (US)

128 cubic feet = 1 cord (wood)

Dry measure

2 pints = 1 quart   8 quarts = 1 peck   4 pecks = 1 bushel

Liquid measure

1000 milliliters = 1 liter

4 gills = 1 pint

31.5 gallons = 1 barrel (US)

2 barrels = 1 hogshead (US)

Barrels and hogsheads vary in size. One US gallon is equal to 0.8327 British gallon; therefore, 1 British gallon is equal to 1.201 US gallons. 1 liter is equal to 1.0567 quarts.

1-4. Temperature

To convert Centigrade or Celsius degrees to Fahrenheit degrees: multiply the number of Centigrade degrees by $9/5$ and add 32 to the result. *To convert Fahrenheit degrees to Centigrade degrees:* Subtract 32 from the number of Fahrenheit degrees and multiply the difference by $5/9$.

Fahrenheit and Celsius equivalents: body temperature range

F°	C°	F°	C°	F°	C°	F°	C°	F°	C°
94.0	34.44	97.0	36.11	100.0	37.78	103.0	39.44	106.0	41.11
94.2	34.56	97.2	36.22	100.2	37.89	103.2	39.56	106.2	41.22
94.4	34.67	97.4	36.33	100.4	38.00	103.4	39.67	106.4	41.33
94.6	34.78	97.6	36.44	100.6	38.11	103.6	39.78	106.6	41.44
94.8	34.89	97.8	36.56	100.8	38.22	103.8	39.89	106.8	41.56
95.0	35.00	98.0	36.67	101.0	38.33	104.0	40.00	107.0	41.67
95.2	35.11	98.2	36.78	101.2	38.44	104.2	40.11	107.2	41.78
95.4	35.22	98.4	36.89	101.4	38.56	104.4	40.22	107.4	41.89
95.6	35.33	98.6	37.00	101.6	38.67	104.6	40.33	107.6	42.00
95.8	35.44	98.8	37.11	101.8	38.78	104.8	40.44	107.8	42.11
96.0	35.56	99.0	37.22	102.0	38.89	105.0	40.56	108.0	42.22
96.2	35.67	99.2	37.33	102.2	39.00	105.2	40.67		
96.4	35.78	99.4	37.44	102.4	39.11	105.4	40.78		
96.6	35.89	99.6	37.56	102.6	39.22	105.6	40.89		
96.8	36.00	99.8	37.67	102.8	39.33	105.8	41.00		

Fahrenheit and Celsius equivalents

F°	C°	F°	C°	F°	C°	F°	C°	F°	C°
−40	−40.0	11	−11.67	62	16.67	113	45.0	164	73.33
−39	−39.44	12	−11.11	63	17.22	114	45.56	165	73.89
−38	−38.89	13	−10.56	64	17.78	115	46.11	166	74.44
−37	−38.33	14	−10.0	65	18.33	116	46.67	167	75.0
−36	−37.78	15	−9.44	66	18.89	117	47.22	168	75.56
−35	−37.22	16	−8.89	67	19.44	118	47.78	169	76.11
−34	−36.67	17	−8.33	68	20.0	119	48.33	170	76.67
−33	−36.11	18	−7.78	69	20.56	120	48.89	171	77.22
−32	−35.56	19	−7.22	70	21.11	121	49.44	172	77.78
−31	−35.0	20	−6.67	71	21.67	122	50.0	173	78.33
−30	−34.44	21	−6.11	72	22.22	123	50.56	174	78.89
−29	−33.89	22	−5.56	73	22.78	124	51.11	175	79.44
−28	−33.33	23	−5.0	74	23.33	125	51.67	176	80.0
−27	−32.78	24	−4.44	75	23.89	126	52.22	177	80.56
−26	−32.22	25	−3.89	76	24.44	127	52.78	178	81.11
−25	−31.67	26	−3.33	77	25.0	128	53.33	179	81.67
−24	−31.11	27	−2.78	78	25.56	129	53.89	180	82.22
−23	−30.56	28	−2.22	79	26.11	130	54.44	181	82.78
−22	−30.0	29	−1.67	80	26.67	131	55.0	182	83.33
−21	−29.44	30	−1.11	81	27.22	132	55.56	183	83.89
−20	−28.89	31	−0.56	82	27.78	133	56.11	184	84.44
−19	−28.33	32	0.0	83	28.33	134	56.67	185	85.0
−18	−27.78	33	0.56	84	28.89	135	57.22	186	85.56
−17	−27.22	34	1.11	85	29.44	136	57.78	187	86.11
−16	−26.67	35	1.67	86	30.0	137	58.33	188	86.67
−15	−26.11	36	2.22	87	30.56	138	58.89	189	87.22
−14	−25.56	37	2.78	88	31.11	139	59.44	190	87.78
−13	−25.0	38	3.33	89	31.67	140	60.0	191	88.33
12	−24.44	39	3.89	90	32.22	141	60.56	192	88.89
−11	23.89	40	4.44	91	32.78	142	61.11	193	89.44
−10	−23.33	41	5.0	92	33.33	143	61.67	194	90.0
−9	−22.78	42	5.56	93	33.89	144	62.22	195	90.56
−8	−22.22	43	6.11	94	34.44	145	62.78	196	91.11
−7	−21.67	44	6.67	95	35.0	146	63.33	197	91.67
−6	−21.11	45	7.22	96	35.56	147	63.89	198	92.22
−5	−20.56	46	7.78	97	36.11	148	64.44	199	92.78
−4	−20.0	47	8.33	98	36.67	149	65.0	200	93.33
−3	−19.44	48	8.89	99	37.22	150	65.56	201	93.89
−2	−18.89	49	9.44	100	37.78	151	66.11	202	94.44
−1	−18.33	50	10.0	101	38.33	152	66.67	203	95.0
0	−17.78	51	10.56	102	38.89	153	67.22	204	95.56
1	−17.22	52	11.11	103	39.44	154	67.78	205	96.11
2	−16.67	53	11.67	104	40.0	155	68.33	206	96.67
3	−16.11	54	12.22	105	40.56	156	68.89	207	97.22
4	−15.56	55	12.78	106	41.11	157	69.44	208	97.78
5	−15.0	56	13.33	107	41.67	158	70.0	209	98.33
6	−14.44	57	13.89	108	42.22	159	70.56	210	98.89
7	−13.89	58	14.44	109	42.78	160	71.11	211	99.44
8	−13.33	59	15.0	110	43.33	161	71.67	212	100.0
9	−12.78	60	15.56	111	43.89	162	72.22		
10	−12.22	61	16.11	112	44.44	163	72.78		

1-5. Physical elements*

Element	Symbol	Valence	Atomic number	Atomic weight†	Element	Symbol	Valence	Atomic number	Atomic weight†
Actinium	Ac	3	89	(227.0278)	Mendelevium	Md		101	(257.0956)
Aluminum	Al	3	13	26.98154	Mercury	Hg	1,2	80	200.59
Americium	Am	3,4,5,6	95	(243.0614)	Molybdenum	Mo	3,4,6	42	95.94
Antimony	Sb	3,5	51	121.75	Neodymium	Nd	3	60	144.24
Argon	Ar	0	18	39.948	Neon	Ne	0	10	20.179
Arsenic	As	3,5	33	74.9216	Neptunium	Np	4,5,6	93	237.0482
Astatine	At	1,3,5,7	85	(209.987)	Nickel	Ni	2,3	28	58.70
Barium	Ba	2	56	137.34	Niobium	Nb	3,5	41	92.9064
Berkelium	Bk	3,4	97	(247.0703)	Nitrogen	N	3,5	7	14.0067
Beryllium	Be	2	4	9.01218	Nobelium	No		102	(255.0933)
Bismuth	Bi	3,5	83	208.9804	Osmium	Os	2,3,4,8	76	190.2
Boron	B	3	5	10.81	Oxygen	O	2	8	15.9994
Bromine	Br	1,3,5,7	35	79.904	Palladium	Pd	2,4,6	46	106.4
Cadmium	Cd	2	48	112.40	Phosphorus	P	3,5	15	30.98376
Calcium	Ca	2	20	40.08	Platinum	Pt	2,4	78	195.09
Californium	Cf	3	98	(251.0796)	Plutonium	Pu	3,4,5,6	94	(244.0642)
Carbon	C	2,4	6	12.011	Polonium	Po	2,4	84	(208.9824)
Cerium	Ce	3,4	58	140.12	Potassium	K	1	19	39.098
Cesium	Cs	1	55	132.9054	Praseodymium	Pr	3	59	140.9077
Chlorine	Cl	1,3,5,7	17	35.453	Promethium	Pm	3	61	(144.9128)
Chromium	Cr	2,3,6	24	51.996	Protactinium	Pa		91	(231.0359)
Cobalt	Co	2,3	27	58.9332	Radium	Ra	2	88	(226.0254)
Columbium	See:	Niobium			Radon	Rn	0	86	(222.0176)
Copper	Cu	1,2	29	63.546	Rhenium	Re		75	186.207
Curium	Cm	3	96	(247.0704)	Rhodium	Rh	3	45	102.9055
Dysprosium	Dy	3	66	162.50	Rubidium	Rb	1	37	85.4678
Einsteinium	Es		99	(254.0881)	Ruthenium	Ru	3,4,6,8	44	101.07
Erbium	Er	3	68	167.26	Samarium	Sm	2,3	62	150.4
Europium	Eu	2,3	63	151.96	Scandium	Sc	3	21	44.9559
Fermium	Fm		100	(257.0951)	Selenium	Se	2,4,6	34	78.96
Fluorine	F	1	9	18.9984	Silicon	Si	4	14	28.086
Francium	Fr	1	87	(223.0198)	Silver	Ag	1	47	107.868
Gadolinium	Gd	3	64	157.25	Sodium	Na	1	11	22.98977
Gallium	Ga	2,3	31	69.72	Strontium	Sr	2	38	87.62
Germanium	Ge	4	32	72.59	Sulfur	S	2,4,6	16	32.06
Glucinum	See:	Beryllium			Tantalum	Ta	5	73	180.9479
Gold	Au	1,3	79	196.9665	Technetium	Tc	6,7	43	96.9062
Hafnium	Hf	4	72	178.49	Tellurium	Te	2,4,6	52	127.60
Helium	He	0	2	4.0026	Terbium	Tb	3	65	158.9254
Holmium	Ho	3	67	164.9304	Thallium	Tl	1,3	81	204.37
Hydrogen	H	1	1	1.0079	Thorium	Th	4	90	232.0381
Indium	In	3	49	114.82	Thulium	Tm	3	69	168.9342
Iodine	I	1,3,5,7	53	126.9045	Tin	Sn	2,4	50	118.69
Iridium	Ir	3,4	77	192.22	Titanium	Ti	3,4	22	47.90
Iron	Fe	2,3	26	55.847	Tungsten	W	6	74	183.85
Krypton	Kr	0	36	83.30	Uranium	U	4,6	92	238.029
Lanthanum	La	3	57	138.9055	Vanadium	V	3,5	23	50.9414
Lawrencium	Lw		103	(256.0986)	Xenon	Xe	0	54	131.30
Lead	Pb	2,4	82	207.2	Ytterbium	Yb	2,3	70	173.04
Lithium	Li	1	3	6.941	Yttrium	Y	3	39	88.9059
Lutetium	Lu	3	71	174.97	Zinc	Zn	2	30	65.38
Magnesium	Mg	2	12	24.305	Zirconium	Zr	4	40	91.22
Manganese	Mn	2,3,4,6,7	25	54.938					

*The 103 chemical elements known at present are included in this table. Some of those recently discovered have been obtained only as unstable isotopes.
†Based on Carbon-12. Figures enclosed in parentheses represent the mass number of the most stable isotope.

1-6. Height and weight table for adults

Desirable weights for persons age 25 and over (weight in pounds according to frame [in indoor clothing])

Men					Women*				
Height (with shoes on) 1-inch heels		Small frame	Medium frame	Large frame	Height (with shoes on) 2-inch heels		Small frame	Medium frame	Large frame
ft	in	lb	lb	lb	ft	in	lb	lb	lb
5	2	112-120	118-129	126-141	4	10	92- 98	96-107	104-119
5	3	115-123	121-133	129-144	4	11	94-101	98-110	106-122
5	4	118-126	124-136	132-148	5	0	96-104	101-113	109-125
5	5	121-129	127-139	135-152	5	1	99-107	104-116	112-128
5	6	124-133	130-143	138-156	5	2	102-110	107-119	115-131
5	7	128-137	134-147	142-161	5	3	105-113	110-122	118-134
5	8	132-141	138-152	147-166	5	4	108-116	113-126	121-138
5	9	136-145	142-156	151-170	5	5	111-119	116-130	125-142
5	10	140-150	146-160	155-174	5	6	114-123	120-135	129-146
5	11	144-154	150-165	159-179	5	7	118-127	124-139	133-150
6	0	148-158	154-170	164-184	5	8	122-131	128-143	137-154
6	1	152-162	158-175	168-189	5	9	126-135	132-147	141-158
6	2	156-167	162-180	173-194	5	10	130-140	136-151	145-163
6	3	160-171	167-185	178-199	5	11	134-144	140-155	149-168
6	4	164-175	172-190	182-204	6	0	138-148	144-159	153-173

*For girls between 18 and 25, subtract 1 pound for each year under 25.

1-7. Height and weight tables for children

Girls (juvenile and adolescent ages)

Height (in)	5 yr	6 yr	7 yr	8 yr	9 yr	10 yr	11 yr	12 yr	13 yr	14 yr	15 yr	16 yr	17 yr	18 yr
38	33	33												
39	34	34												
40	36	36	36											
41	37	37	37											
42	39	39	39											
43	41	41	41	41										
44	42	42	42	42										
45	45	45	45	45	45									
46	47	47	47	48	48									
47	49	50	50	50	50	50								
48		52	52	52	52	53	53							
49			54	55	55	56	56							
50			56	57	58	59	61	62						
51			59	60	61	61	63	65						
52			63	64	64	64	65	67						
53			66	67	67	68	68	69	71					
54				69	70	70	71	71	73					
55				72	74	74	74	75	77	78				
56					76	78	78	79	81	83				
57					80	82	82	82	84	88	92			
58						84	86	86	88	93	96	101		
59						87	90	90	92	96	100	103	104	
60						91	95	95	97	101	105	108	109	111
61							99	100	101	105	108	112	113	116
62							104	105	106	109	113	115	117	118
63								110	110	112	116	117	119	120
64								114	115	117	119	120	122	123
65								118	120	121	122	123	125	126
66									124	124	125	128	129	130
67									128	130	131	133	133	135
68									131	133	135	136	138	138
69										135	137	138	140	142
70										136	138	140	142	144
71										138	140	142	144	145

Boys (juvenile and adolescent ages)

Height (in)	5 yr	6 yr	7 yr	8 yr	9 yr	10 yr	11 yr	12 yr	13 yr	14 yr	15 yr	16 yr	17 yr	18 yr	19 yr
38	34	34													
39	35	35													
40	36	36													
41	38	38	38												
42	39	39	39	39											
43	41	41	41	41											
44	44	44	44	44											
45	46	46	46	46	46										
46	47	48	48	48	48										
47	49	50	50	50	50	50									
48		52	53	53	53	53									
49		55	55	55	55	55	55								
50		57	58	58	58	58	58	58							
51			61	61	61	61	61	61	61						
52			63	64	64	64	64	64	64						
53			66	67	67	67	67	68	68						
54				70	70	70	70	71	71	72					
55				72	72	73	73	74	74	74					
56				75	76	77	77	77	78	78	80				
57					79	80	81	81	82	83	83				
58					83	84	84	85	85	86	87				
59						87	88	89	89	90	90	90			
60						91	92	92	93	94	95	96			
61							95	96	97	99	100	103	106		
62							100	101	102	103	104	107	111	116	
63							105	106	107	108	110	113	118	123	127
64								109	111	113	115	117	121	126	130
65								114	117	118	120	122	127	131	134
66									119	122	125	128	132	136	139
67									124	128	130	134	136	139	142
68										134	134	137	141	143	147
69										137	139	143	146	149	152
70										143	144	145	148	151	155
71										148	150	151	152	154	159
72											153	155	156	158	163
73											157	160	162	164	167
74											160	164	168	170	171

1-8. Pound to kilogram conversion*

Pounds	0	1	2	3	4	5	6	7	8	9
0	0.00	0.45	0.90	1.36	1.81	2.26	2.72	3.17	3.62	4.08
10	4.53	4.98	5.44	5.89	6.35	6.80	7.25	7.71	8.16	8.61
20	9.07	9.52	9.97	10.43	10.88	11.34	11.79	12.24	12.70	13.15
30	13.60	14.06	14.51	14.96	15.42	15.87	16.32	16.78	17.23	17.69
40	18.14	18.59	19.05	19.50	19.95	20.41	20.86	21.31	21.77	22.22
50	22.68	23.13	23.58	24.04	24.49	24.94	25.40	25.85	26.30	26.76
60	27.21	27.66	28.12	28.57	29.03	29.48	29.93	30.39	30.84	31.29
70	31.75	32.20	32.65	33.11	33.56	34.02	34.47	34.92	35.38	35.83
80	36.28	36.74	37.19	37.64	38.10	38.55	39.00	39.46	39.91	40.37
90	40.82	41.27	41.73	42.18	42.63	43.09	43.54	43.99	44.45	44.90
100	45.36	45.81	46.26	46.72	47.17	47.62	48.08	48.53	48.98	49.44
110	49.89	50.34	50.80	51.25	51.71	52.16	52.61	53.07	53.52	53.97
120	54.43	54.88	55.33	55.79	56.24	56.70	57.15	57.60	58.06	58.51
130	58.96	59.42	59.87	60.32	60.78	61.23	61.68	62.14	62.59	63.05
140	63.50	63.95	64.41	64.86	65.31	65.77	66.22	66.67	67.13	67.58
150	68.04	68.49	68.94	69.40	69.85	70.30	70.76	71.21	71.66	72.12
160	72.57	73.02	73.48	73.93	74.39	74.84	75.29	75.75	76.20	76.65
170	77.11	77.56	78.01	78.47	78.92	79.38	79.83	80.28	80.74	81.19
180	81.64	82.10	82.55	83.00	83.46	83.91	84.36	84.82	85.27	85.73
190	86.18	86.68	87.09	87.54	87.99	88.45	88.90	89.35	89.81	90.26
200	90.72	91.17	91.62	92.08	92.53	92.98	93.44	93.89	94.34	94.80

*Numbers in the farthest left column are 10-pound increments; numbers across the top row are 1-pound increments. The kilogram equivalent of weight in pounds is found at the intersection of the appropriate row and column. For example, to convert 34 pounds, read down the left column to 30 and then across that row to 4: 34 pounds = 15.42 kilograms.

1-9. Grams to pounds and ounces conversion for weight of newborns

Pounds / Ounces	0	1	2	3	4	5	6	7	8	9	10	11	12	13	14	15
0	—	28	57	85	113	142	170	198	227	255	283	312	430	369	397	425
1	454	482	510	539	567	595	624	652	680	709	737	765	794	822	850	879
2	907	936	964	992	1021	1049	1077	1106	1134	1162	1191	1219	1247	1276	1304	1332
3	1361	1389	1417	1446	1474	1503	1531	1559	1588	1616	1644	1673	1701	1729	1758	1786
4	1814	1843	1871	1899	1928	1956	1984	2013	2041	2070	2098	2126	2155	2183	2211	2240
5	2268	2296	2325	2353	2381	2410	2438	2466	2495	2523	2551	2580	2608	2637	2665	2693
6	2722	2750	2778	2807	2835	2863	2892	2920	2948	2977	3005	3033	3062	3090	3118	3147
7	3175	3203	3232	3260	3289	3317	3345	3374	3402	3430	3459	3487	3515	3544	3572	3600
8	3629	3657	3685	3714	3742	3770	3799	3827	3856	3884	3912	3941	3969	3997	4026	4054
9	4082	4111	4139	4167	4196	4224	4252	4281	4309	4337	4366	4394	4423	4451	4479	4508
10	4536	4564	4593	4621	4649	4678	4706	4734	4763	4791	4819	4848	4876	4904	4933	4961
11	4990	5018	5046	5075	5103	5131	5160	5188	5216	5245	5273	5301	5330	5358	5386	5415
12	5443	5471	5500	5528	5557	5585	5613	5642	5670	5698	5727	5755	5783	5812	5840	5868
13	5897	5925	5953	5982	6010	6038	6067	6095	6123	6152	6180	6290	6237	6265	6294	6322
14	6350	6379	6407	6435	6464	6492	6520	6549	6577	6605	6634	6662	6690	6719	6747	6776

1 pound = 453.59 grams. 1 ounce = 28.35 grams. Grams can be converted to pounds and tenths of a pound by multiplying the number of grams by .0022.

APPENDIX 2 • Symbols

℥	Dram	+	Plus; excess; acid reaction; positive
f℥	Fluid dram	−	Minus; deficiency; alkaline reaction; negative
℥	Ounce	±	Plus or minus; either positive or negative; indefinite
f℥	Fluid ounce	#	Number; following a number; pounds
O	Pint	÷	Divided by
℔	Pound	×	Multiplied by; magnification
℞	Recipe; take	=	Equals
M	Misce; mix	≅	Approximately equals
A, Å	Angstrom unit	≠	Not equal to
C′	Complement	>	Greater than; from which is derived
E_0	Electroaffinity	<	Less than; derived from
F_1	First filial generation	≮	Not less than
F_2	Second filial generation	≯	Not greater than
$m\mu$	Millimicron, micromillimeter	≦	Equal to or less than
μg	Microgram	≧	Equal to or greater than
mEq	Milliequivalent	√	Root; square root; radical
mg	Milligram	$\sqrt[2]{}$	Square root
m%	Milligrams percent; milligrams per 100 ml	$\sqrt[3]{}$	Cube root
$Q\ O_2$	Oxygen consumption	∞	Infinity
m-	Meta-	:	Ratio; "is to"
o-	Ortho-	°	Degree
p-	Para-	%	Percent
Po_2	Partial pressure of oxygen	π	3.1416—ratio of circumference of a circle to its diameter; pi
Pco_2	Partial pressure of carbon dioxide		
μm	Micrometer	□, ♂	Male
μ	Micron (common term for micrometer)	○, ♀	Female
$\mu\mu$	Micromicron	⇌	A reversible reaction

APPENDIX 3 • A tabular atlas of the anatomy and physiology of the human body

3-1. Basic structures and functions of the body

Cells

Cell structures	Functions
Cytoplasmic membrane	Serves as the boundary of the cell, maintaining its integrity; protein molecules on outer surface of cytoplasmic membrane perform various functions; for example, they serve as markers that identify cells of each individual, receptor molecules for certain hormones and neurotransmitters provide means of communication between cells, receptor molecules for foreign proteins function to produce immunity
Endoplasmic reticulum (ER)	Serves as a cell's own circulatory system
Golgi apparatus	Synthesizes carbohydrate, combines it with protein, and packages the product as globules of glycoprotein
Mitochondria	Catabolism; ATP synthesis; a cell's "powerhouse"
Lysosomes	A cell's "digestive system"
Ribosomes	Synthesize proteins; a cell's "protein factory"
Nucleus	Dictates protein synthesis, thereby playing essential role in other cell activities, namely, active transport, metabolism, growth, and heredity
Nucleoli	Play essential role in the formation of ribosomes

Tissues

Tissue	Location	Function
Epithelial		
Simple squamous	Alveoli of lungs	Absorption by diffusion of respiratory gases between alveolar air and blood
	Lining of blood and lymphatic vessels (called endothelium; classed as connective tissue by some histologists)	Absorption by diffusion; filtration; osmosis
	Surface layer of pleura, pericardium, peritoneum (called mesothelium; classed as connective tissue by some histologists)	Absorption by diffusion; osmosis; also, secretion
Stratified squamous	Surface of lining of mouth and esophagus	Protection
	Surface of skin (epidermis)	Protection
Simple columnar	Surface layer of lining of stomach, intestines, and part of respiratory tract	Protection; secretion; absorption; moving of mucus (by ciliated columnar)

Tissues—cont'd

Tissue	Location	Function
Muscle		
Skeletal (striated voluntary)	Muscles that attach to bones	Movement of bones
	Extrinsic eyeball muscles	Eye movements
	Upper third of esophagus	First part of swallowing
Visceral (nonstriated involuntary or smooth)	In walls of tubular viscera of digestive, respiratory, and genitourinary tracts	Movement of substances along respective tracts
	In walls of blood vessels and large lymphatic vessels	Change diameter of blood vessels, thereby aiding in regulation of blood pressure
	In ducts of glands	Movement of substances along ducts
	Intrinsic eye muscles (iris and ciliary body)	Change diameter of pupils and shape of lens
	Arrector muscles of hairs	Erection of hairs (gooseflesh)
Cardiac (striated involuntary)	Wall of heart	Contraction of heart
Connective (most widely distributed of all tissues)		
Reticular tissue	Spleen, lymph nodes, bone marrow	Defense against microbes and harmful substances by filtration from blood and lymph by reticular network; phagocytosis by reticular cells; synthesis of reticular fibers by reticular cells
Loose, ordinary (areolar)	Between other tissues and organs	Connection
	Superficial fascia	Connection
Adipose (fat)	Under skin	Protection
	Padding at various points	Insulation
		Support
		Reserve food
Dense fibrous	Tendons	Flexible but strong connection
	Ligaments	
	Aponeuroses	
	Deep fascia	
	Dermis	
	Scars	
	Capsule of kidney, etc.	
Bone	Skeleton	Support
		Protection
Cartilage		
Hyaline	Part of nasal septum	Firm but flexible support
	Covering articular surfaces of bones	
	Larynx	
	Rings in trachea and bronchi	
Fibrous	Disks between vertebrae	
	Symphysis pubis	
Elastic	External ear	
	Eustachian tube	
Hemopoietic		
Myeloid (bone marrow)	Marrow spaces of bones	Formation of red blood cells, granular leukocytes, platelets; also reticuloendothelial cells and some other connective tissue cells
Lymphatic	Lymph nodes	Formation of lymphocytes and monocytes; also plasma cells and some other connective tissue cells
	Spleen	
	Tonsils and adenoids	
	Thymus gland	
Blood	In blood vessels	Transportation
		Protection
Nervous		
	Brain	Irritability; conduction
	Spinal cord	
	Nerves	

3-2. The skeletal system

Bones of the skeleton

APPENDICULAR SKELETON (126 bones)			Bones that are appended to axial skeleton; upper and lower extremities, including shoulder and hip girdles
Part of body	**Name of bone**	**Number**	**Identification**
Upper extremities (including shoulder girdle) (64 bones)	Clavicle	2	Collar bones; shoulder girdle joined to axial skeleton by articulation of clavicles with sternum; scapula does not form joint with axial skeleton
	Scapula	2	Shoulder blades; scapulae and clavicles together comprise shoulder girdle
	Humerus	2	Long bone of upper arm
	Radius	2	Bone of thumb side of forearm
	Ulna	2	Bone of little finger side of forearm; longer than radius
	Carpals (scaphoid, lunate, triquetrum, pisiform, trapezium, trapezoid, capitate, and hamate)	16	Arranged in two rows at proximal end of hand
	Metacarpals	10	Long bones forming framework of palm of hand
	Phalanges	28	Miniature long bones of fingers, 3 in each finger, 2 in each thumb
Lower extremities (62 bones)	Ossa coxae or innominate bones	2	Large hip bones; with sacrum and coccyx, these 3 bones form basin-like pelvic cavity; lower extremities attached to axial skeleton by pelvic bones
	Femur	2	Thigh bone; largest, strongest bone of body
	Patella	2	Kneecap; largest sesamoid bone of body*; embedded in tendon of quadriceps femoris muscle
	Tibia	2	Shin bone
	Fibula	2	Long, slender bone of lateral side of lower leg
	Tarsals (calcaneus, talus, navicular, first, second, and third cuneiforms, cuboid)	14	Bones that form heel and proximal or posterior half of foot
	Metatarsals	10	Long bones of feet
	Phalanges	28	Miniature long bones of toes; 2 in each great toe, 3 in other toes
TOTAL		206*	

*An inconstant number of small, flat, round bones known as *sesamoid bones* (because of their resemblance to sesame seeds) is found in various tendons in which considerable pressure develops. Because the number of these bones varies greatly between individuals, only 2 of them, the patellae, have been counted among the 206 bones of the body. Generally, 2 of them can be found in each thumb (in flexor tendon near metacarpophalangeal and interphalangeal joints) and great toe plus several others in the upper and lower extremities. *Wormian bones,* the small islets of bone frequently found in some of the cranial sutures, have not been counted in this list of 206 bones either because of their variable occurrence.

Part of body	Name of bone	Number	Identification
AXIAL SKELETON (80 bones)			Bones that form upright axis on body—skull, hyoid, vertebral column, sternum, and ribs
Skull (28 bones)			
Cranium (8 bones)			Cranium forms floor for brain to rest on and helmetlike covering over it
	Frontal	1	Forehead bone; also forms most of root of orbits (eye sockets) and anterior part of cranial floor
	Parietal	2	Prominent, bulging bones behind frontal bone; form topsides of cranial cavity
	Temporal	2	Form lower sides of cranium and part of cranial floor; contain middle and inner ear structures
	Occipital	1	Forms posterior part of cranial floor and walls
	Sphenoid	1	Keystone of cranial floor; forms its midportion; resembles bat with wings outstretched and legs extended downward posteriorly; lies behind and slightly above nose and throat; forms part of floor and sidewalls of orbit
	Ethmoid	1	Complicated irregular bone that helps make up anterior portion of cranial floor, medial wall of orbits, upper parts of nasal septum, and sidewalls and part of nasal roof; lies anterior to sphenoid and posterior to nasal bones
Face (14 bones)	Nasal	2	Small bones forming upper part of bridge of nose
	Maxillary	2	Upper jaw bones; form part of floor of orbit, anterior part of roof of mouth, and floor of nose and part of sidewalls of nose
	Zygomatic (malar)	2	Cheekbones; form part of floor and sidewall of orbit
	Mandible	1	Lower jawbone; largest, strongest bone of face
	Lacrimal	2	Thin bones about size and shape of fingernail; posterior and lateral to nasal bones in medial wall of orbit, help form sidewall of nasal cavity, often missing in dry skull
	Palatine	2	Form posterior part of hard palate floor, and part of sidewalls of nasal cavity and floor of orbit
	Inferior conchae (turbinates)	2	Thin scroll of bone forming kind of shell along inner surface of sidewall of nasal cavity; lies above roof of mouth
	Vomer	1	Forms lower and posterior part of nasal septum; shaped like ploughshare
Ear bones (6 bones)	Malleus (hammer)	2	Tiny bones referred to as auditory ossicles in middle ear cavity in temporal bones; resemble, respectively, miniature hammer, anvil, and stirrup
	Incus (anvil)	2	
	Stapes (stirrup)	2	
Hyoid bone		1	U-shaped bone in neck between mandible and upper part of larynx; claims distinction as only bone not forming a joint with any other bone; suspended by ligaments from styloid processes of temporal bones
Sternum and ribs (25 bones)			Sternum, ribs, and thoracic vertebrae together form bony cage known as *thorax;* ribs attach posteriorly to vertebrae, slant downward anteriorly to attach to sternum (see description of false ribs below)
	Sternum	1	Breastbone; flat dagger-shaped bone
	True ribs	7 pairs	Upper 7 pairs; fasten to sternum by costal cartilages
	False ribs	5 pairs	False ribs do not attach to sternum directly; upper 3 pairs of false ribs attach by means of costal cartilage of seventh ribs; last 2 pairs do not attach to sternum at all; therefore called *"floating"*
Vertebral column (26 bones)			Not actually a column but a flexible segmented rod shaped like an elongated letter S; forms axis of body; head balanced above, ribs and viscera suspended in front, and lower extremities attached below; encloses spinal cord
	Cervical vertebrae	7	First or upper 7 vertebrae
	Thoracic vertebrae	12	Next 12 vertebrae; 12 pairs of ribs attached to these
	Lumbar vertebrae	5	Next 5 vertebrae
	Sacrum	1	Five separate vertebrae until about 25 years of age; then fused to form 1 wedge-shaped bone
	Coccyx	1	Four or 5 separate vertebrae in child but fused into 1 in adult

Identification of bone markings

SPECIAL FEATURES OF SKULL

Marking	Description
Sutures	Immovable joints between skull bones
1 Sagittal	1 Line of articulation between two parietal bones
2 Coronal	2 Joint between parietal bones and frontal bone
3 Lambdoidal	3 Joint between parietal bones and occipital bone
Fontanels	"Soft spots" where ossification incomplete at birth; allow some compression of skull during birth; also important in determining position of head before delivery; 6 such areas located at angles of parietal bones
1 Anterior (or frontal)	1 At intersection of sagittal and coronal sutures (juncture of parietal bones and frontal bone); diamond shaped; largest of fontanels; usually closed by 1½ years of age
2 Posterior (or occipital)	2 At intersection of sagittal and lambdoidal sutures (juncture of parietal bones and occipital bone); triangular in shape; usually closed by second month
3 Anterolateral (or sphenoid)	3 At juncture of frontal, parietal, temporal, and sphenoid bones
4 Posterolateral (or mastoid)	4 At juncture of parietal, occipital, and temporal bones; usually closed by second year
Sinuses	
1 Air (or bony)	1 Spaces or cavities within bones; those that communicate with nose called *paranasal sinuses* (frontal, sphenoidal, ethmoidal, and maxillary); mastoid cells communicate with middle ear rather than nose, therefore not included among paranasal sinuses
2 Blood	2 Veins within cranial cavity
Orbits formed by	
1 Frontal	1 Roof of orbit
2 Ethmoid	2 Medial wall
3 Lacrimal	3 Medial wall
4 Sphenoid	4 Lateral wall
5 Zygomatic	5 Lateral wall
6 Maxillary	6 Floor
7 Palatine	7 Floor
Nasal septum formed by	Partition in midline of nasal cavity; separates cavity into right and left halves
1 Perpendicular plate of ethmoid bone	1 Forms upper part of septum
2 Vomer bone	2 Forms lower, posterior part
3 Cartilage	3 Forms anterior part
Wormian bones	Small islands of bones within suture

FRONTAL

Marking	Description
Supraorbital margin	Arched ridge just below eyebrow
Frontal sinuses	Cavities inside bone just above supraorbital margin; lined with mucosa; contain air
Frontal tuberosities	Bulge above each orbit; most prominent part of forehead
Superciliary arches	Ridges caused by projection of frontal sinuses; eyebrows lie over these ridges
Supraorbital notch (sometimes foramen)	Notch or foramen in supraorbital margin slightly mesial to its midpoint; transmits supraorbital nerve and blood vessels
Glabella	Smooth area between superciliary ridges and above nose

SPHENOID

Marking	Description
Body	Hollow, cubelike central portion
Greater wings	Lateral projections from body; form part of outer wall of orbit
Lesser wings	Thin, triangular projections from upper part of sphenoid body; form posterior part of roof of orbit
Sella turcica (or *Turk's saddle*)	Saddle-shaped depression on upper surface of sphenoid body; contains pituitary gland
Sphenoid sinuses	Irregular air-filled mucosa-lined spaces within central part of sphenoid
Pterygoid processes	Downward projections on either side where body and greater wing unite; comparable to extended legs of bat if entire bone is likened to this animal; form part of lateral nasal wall
Optic foramen	Opening into orbit at root of lesser wing; transmits second cranial nerve
Superior orbital fissure	Slitlike opening into orbit; lateral to optic foramen; transmits third, fourth, and part of fifth cranial nerves
Foramen rotundum	Opening in greater wing that transmits maxillary division of fifth cranial nerve
Foramen ovale	Opening in a greater wing that transmits mandibular division of fifth cranial nerve

ETHMOID

Marking	Description
Horizontal (cribriform) plate	Olfactory nerves pass through numerous holes in this plate
Crista galli	Meninges attach to this process
Perpendicular plate	Forms upper part of nasal septum
Ethmoid sinuses	Honeycombed, mucosa-lined air spaces within lateral masses of bone
Superior and middle turbinates (conchae)	Help to form lateral walls of nose
Lateral masses	Compose sides of bone; contain many air spaces (ethmoid cells or sinuses); inner surface forms superior and middle conchae

Identification of bone markings—cont'd

TEMPORAL

Marking	Description
Mastoid process	Protuberance just behind ear
Mastoid air cells	Air-filled mucosa-lined spaces within mastoid process
External auditory meatus (or canal)	Opening into ear and tube extending into temporal bone
Zygomatic process	Projection that articulates with malar (or zygomatic) bone
Internal auditory meatus	Fairly large opening on posterior surface of petrous portion of bone; transmits eighth cranial nerve to inner ear and seventh cranial nerve on its way to facial structures
Squamous portion	Thin, flaring upper part of bone
Mastoid portion	Rough-surfaced lower part of bone posterior to external auditory meatus
Petrous portion	Wedge-shaped process that forms part of center section of cranial floor between sphenoid and occipital bones; name derived from Greek word for stone because of extreme hardness of this process; houses middle and inner ear structures
Mandibular fossa	Oval-shaped depression anterior to external auditory meatus; forms socket for condyle of mandible
Styloid process	Slender spike of bone extending downward and forward from undersurface of bone anterior to mastoid process; often broken off in dry skull; several neck muscles and ligaments attach to styloid process
Stylomastoid foramen	Opening between styloid and mastoid processes where facial nerve emerges from cranial cavity
Jugular fossa	Depression on undersurface of petrous portion; dilated beginning of internal jugular vein lodged here
Jugular foramen	Opening in suture between petrous portion and occipital bone; transmits lateral sinus and ninth, tenth, and eleventh cranial nerves
Carotid canal (or foramen)	Channel in petrous portion; best seen from undersurface of skull; transmits internal carotid artery

PALATINE

Marking	Description
Horizontal plate	Joined to palatine processes of maxillae to complete part of hard palate

MANDIBLE

Marking	Description
Body	Main part of bone; forms chin
Ramus	Process, one on either side, that projects upward from posterior part of body
Condyle (or head)	Part of each ramus that articulates with mandibular fossa of temporal bone
Neck	Constricted part just below condyles
Alveolar process	Teeth set into this arch
Mandibular foramen	Opening on inner surface of ramus; transmits nerves and vessels to lower teeth
Mental foramen	Opening on outer surface below space between two bicuspids; transmits terminal branches of nerves and vessels that enter bone through mandibular foramen; dentists inject anesthetics through these foramina
Coronoid process	Projection upward from anterior part of each ramus; temporal muscle inserts here
Angle	Juncture of posterior and inferior margins of ramus

MAXILLA

Marking	Description
Alveolar process	Arch containing teeth
Maxillary sinus or antrum of Highmore	Large air-filled mucosa-lined cavity within body of each maxilla; largest of sinuses
Palatine process	Horizontal inward projection from alveolar process; forms anterior and larger part of hard palate
Infraorbital foramen	Hole on external surface just below orbit; transmits vessels and nerves
Lacrimal groove	Groove on inner surface; joined by similar groove on lacrimal bone to form canal housing nasolacrimal duct

OCCIPITAL

Marking	Description
Foramen magnum	Hole through which spinal cord enters cranial cavity
Condyles	Convex, oval processes on either side of foramen magnum; articulate with depressions on first cervical vertebra
External occipital protuberance	Prominent projection on posterior surface in midline short distance above foramen magnum; can be felt as definite bump
Superior nuchal line	Curved ridge extending laterally from external occipital protuberance
Inferior nuchal line	Less well-defined ridge paralleling superior nuchal line short distance below it
Internal occipital protuberance	Projection in midline on inner surface of bone; grooves for lateral sinuses extend laterally from this process and one for sagittal sinus extends upward from it

Identification of bone markings—cont'd

VERTEBRAL COLUMN

Marking	Description
General features	Anterior part of vertebra (except first two cervical) consists of body; posterior part of neural arch, which, in turn, consists of 2 pedicles, 2 laminae, and 7 processes projecting from laminae
Thoracic vertebrae	
1 Body	1 Main part; flat, round mass located anteriorly; supporting or weight-bearing part of vertebra
2 Pedicles	2 Short projections extending posteriorly from body
3 Laminae	3 Posterior part of vertebra to which pedicles join and from which processes project
4 Neural arch	4 Formed by pedicles and laminae; protects spinal cord posteriorly; congenital absence of one or more neural arches known as *spina bifida* (cord may protrude right through skin)
5 Spinous process	5 Sharp process projecting inferiorly from laminae in midline
6 Transverse processes	6 Right and left lateral projections from laminae
7 Superior articulating processes	7 Project upward from laminae
8 Inferior articulating processes	8 Project downward from laminae; articulate with superior articulating processes of vertebrae below
9 Spinal foramen	9 Hole in center of vertebra formed by union of body, pedicles, and laminae; spinal foramina, when vertebrae superimposed one on other, form spinal cavity that houses spinal cord
Cervical vertebrae	
1 General features	1 Foramen in each transverse process for transmission of vertebral artery, vein, and plexus of nerves; short bifurcated spinous processes except on seventh vertebrae, where it is extra long and may be felt as protrusion when head bent forward; bodies of these vertebrae small, whereas spinal foramina large and triangular
2 Atlas	2 First cervical vertebra; lacks body and spinous processes; superior articulating processes concave ovals that act as rockerlike cradles for condyles of occipital bone; named atlas because supports head as Atlas was thought to have supported world
3 Axis (epistropheus)	3 Second cervical vertebra, so named because atlas rotates about this bone in rotating movements of head; *dens,* or odontoid process, peglike projection upward from body of axis, forming pivot for rotation of atlas

Marking	Description
Lumbar vertebrae	Strong, massive; superior articulating processes directed inward instead of upward; inferior articulating processes, outward instead of downward; short, blunt spinous process
Sacral promontory	Protuberance from anterior, upper border of sacrum into pelvis; of obstetrical importance because its size limits anteroposterior diameter of pelvic inlet
Intervertebral foramina	Opening between vertebrae through which spinal nerves emerge
Curves	Curves have great structural importance because increase carrying strength of vertebral column, make balance possible in upright position (if column were straight, weight of viscera would pull body forward), absorb jars from walking (straight column would transmit jars straight to head), and protect column from fracture
1 Primary	1 Column curves at birth from head to sacrum with convexity posteriorly; after child stands, convexity persists only in *thoracic* and *sacral* regions, which, therefore, are called primary curves
2 Secondary	2 Concavities in *cervical* and *lumbar* regions; cervical concavity results from infant's attempts to hold head erect (3 to 4 months); lumbar concavity, from balancing efforts in learning to walk (10 to 18 months)
3 Abnormal	3 *Kyphosis,* exaggerated convexity in thoracic region (hunchback); *lordosis,* exaggerated concavity in lumbar region, a very common condition; *scoliosis,* lateral curvature in any region

SCAPULA

Marking	Description
Borders	
1 Superior	1 Upper margin
2 Vertebral	2 Margin toward vertebral column
3 Axillary	3 Lateral margin
Spine	Sharp ridge running diagonally across posterior surface of shoulder blade
Acromion process	Slightly flaring projection at lateral end of scapular spine; may be felt as tip of shoulder; articulates with clavicle
Coracoid process	Projection on anterior surface from upper border of bone; may be felt in groove between deltoid and pectoralis major muscles, about 1 inch below clavicle
Glenoid cavity	Arm socket

Identification of bone markings—cont'd

STERNUM

Marking	Description
Body	Main central part of bone
Manubrium	Flaring, upper part
Xiphoid process	Projection of cartilage at lower border of bone

RIBS

Marking	Description
Head	Projection at posterior end of rib; articulates with corresponding thoracic vertebra and one above, except last three pairs, which join corresponding vertebrae only
Neck	Constricted portion just below head
Tubercle	Small knob just below neck; articulates with transverse process of corresponding thoracic vertebra; missing in lowest 3 ribs
Body or shaft	Main part of rib
Costal cartilage	Cartilage at sternal end of true ribs; attaches ribs (except floating ribs) to sternum

HUMERUS

Marking	Description
Head	Smooth, hemispherical enlargement at proximal end of humerus
Anatomical neck	Oblique groove just below head
Greater tubercle	Rounded projection lateral to head on anterior surface
Lesser tubercle	Prominent projection on anterior surface just below anatomical neck
Intertubercular	Deep groove between greater and lesser tubercles; long tendon of biceps muscle lodges here
Surgical neck	Region just below tubercles; so named because of its liability to fracture
Deltoid tuberosity	V-shaped, rough area about midway down shaft where deltoid muscle inserts
Radial groove	Groove running obliquely downward from deltoid tuberosity; lodges radial nerve
Epicondyles (medial and lateral)	Rough projections at both sides of distal end
Capitulum	Rounded knob below lateral epicondyle; articulates with radius; sometimes called radial head of humerus
Trochlea	Projection with deep depression through center similar to shape of pulley; articulates with ulna
Olecranon fossa	Depression on posterior surface just above trochlea; receives olecranon process of ulna when lower arm extends
Coronoid fossa	Depression on anterior surface above trochlea; receives coronoid process of ulna in flexion of lower arm

ULNA

Marking	Description
Olecranon process	Elbow
Coronoid process	Projection on anterior surface of proximal end of ulna; trochlea of humerus fits snugly between olecranon and coronoid processes
Semilunar notch	Curved notch between olecranon and coronoid process, into which trochlea fits
Radial notch	Curved notch lateral and inferior to semilunar notch; head of radius fits into this concavity
Head	Rounded process at distal end; does not articulate with wrist bones but with fibrocartilaginous disk
Styloid process	Sharp protuberance at distal end; can be seen from outside on posterior surface

RADIUS

Marking	Description
Head	Disk-shaped process forming proximal end of radius; articulates with capitulum of humerus and with radial notch of ulna
Radial tuberosity	Roughened projection on ulnar side, short distance below head; biceps muscle inserts here
Styloid process	Protuberance at distal end on lateral surface (with forearm supinated as in anatomical position)

FEMUR

Marking	Description
Head	Rounded, upper end of bone; fits into acetabulum
Neck	Constricted portion just below head
Greater trochanter	Protuberance located inferiorly and laterally to head
Lesser trochanter	Small protuberance located inferiorly and medially to greater trochanter
Linea aspera	Prominent ridge extending lengthwise along concave posterior surface
Gluteal tubercle	Rounded projection just below greater trochanter; rudimentary third trochanter
Supracondylar ridges	Two ridges formed by division of linea aspera at its lower end; medial supracondylar ridge extends inward to inner condyle, lateral ridge to outer condyle
Condyles	Large, rounded bulges at distal end of femur; one on medial and one on lateral surface
Adductor tubercle	Small projection just above inner condyle; marks termination of medial supracondylar ridge
Trochlea	Smooth depression between condyles on anterior surface; articulates with patella
Intercondyloid notch	Deep depression between condyles on posterior surface; cruciate ligaments that help bind femur to tibia lodge in this notch

Identification of bone markings—cont'd

OS COXAE

Marking	Description
Ilium	Upper, flaring portion
Ischium	Lower, posterior portion
Pubic bone or pubis	Medial, anterior section
Acetabulum	Hip socket; formed by union of ilium, ischium, and pubis
Iliac crests	Upper, curving boundary of ilium
Iliac spines	
1 Anterior superior	1 Prominent projection at anterior end of iliac crest; can be felt externally as "point" of hip
2 Anterior inferior	2 Less prominent projection short distance below anterior superior spine
3 Posterior superior	3 At posterior end of iliac crest
4 Posterior inferior	4 Just below posterior superior spine
Greater sciatic notch	Large notch on posterior surface of ilium just below posterior inferior spine
Gluteal lines	Three curved lines across outer surface of ilium—posterior, anterior, inferior, respectively
Iliopectineal line	Rounded ridge extending from pubic tubercle upward and backward toward sacrum
Iliac fossa	Large, smooth, concave inner surface of ilium above iliopectineal line
Ischial tuberosity	Large, rough, quadrilateral process forming inferior part of ischium; in erect sitting position body rests on these tuberosities
Ischial spine	Pointed projection just above tuberosity
Symphysis pubis	Cartilaginous, amphiarthrotic joint between pubic bones
Superior pubic ramus	Part of pubis lying between symphysis and acetabulum; forms upper part of obturator foramen
Inferior pubic ramus	Part extending down from symphysis; unites with ischium
Pubic arch	Angle formed by two inferior rami
Pubic crest	Upper margin of superior ramus
Pubic tubercle	Rounded process at end of crest
Obturator foramen	Large hole in anterior surface of os coxa; formed by pubis and ischium; largest foramen in body
Pelvic brim (or inlet)	Boundary of aperture leading into true pelvis; formed by pubic crests, iliopectineal lines, and sacral promontory; size and shape of this inlet has great obstetrical importance, since if any of its diameters too small, infant skull cannot enter true pelvis for natural birth
True (or lesser) pelvis	Space below pelvic brim; true "basin" with bone and muscle walls and muscle floor; pelvic organs located in this space
False (or greater) pelvis	Broad, shallow space above pelvic brim, or pelvic inlet; name "false pelvis" is misleading, since this space is actually part of abdominal cavity, not pelvic cavity

Marking	Description
Pelvic outlet	Irregular circumference marking lower limits of true pelvis; bounded by tip of coccyx and two ischial tuberosities
Pelvic girdle (or bony pelvis)	Complete bony ring; composed of two hip bones (ossa coxae), sacrum, and coccyx; forms firm base by which trunk rests on thighs and for attachment of lower extremities to axial skeleton

TIBIA

Marking	Description
Condyles	Bulging prominences at proximal end of tibia; upper surfaces concave for articulation with femur
Intercondylar eminence	Upward projection on articular surface between condyles
Crest	Sharp ridge on anterior surface
Tibial tuberosity	Projection in midline on anterior surface
Popliteal line	Ridge that spirals downward and inward on posterior surface of upper third of tibial shaft
Medial malleolus	Rounded downward projection at distal end of tibia; forms prominence on inner surface of ankle

FIBULA

Marking	Description
Lateral malleolus	Rounded prominence at distal end of fibula; forms prominence on outer surface of ankle

TARSALS

Marking	Description
Calcaneus	Heel bone
Talus	Uppermost of tarsals; articulates with tibia and fibula; boxed in by medial and lateral malleoli
Longitudinal arches	Tarsals and metatarsals so arranged as to form arch from front to back of foot
1 Medial	1 Formed by calcaneus, talus, navicular, cuneiforms, and 3 medial metatarsals
2 Lateral	2 Formed by calcaneus, cuboid, and 2 lateral metatarsals
Transverse (or metatarsal) arch	Metatarsals and distal row of tarsals (cuneiforms and cuboid) so articulated as to form arch across foot; bones kept in 2 arched positions by means of powerful ligaments in sole of foot and by muscles and tendons

Classification of joints

Joints	Description	Movement	Example
Fibrous			
Sutures	Thin layer of fibrous tissue (extension of periosteum); grows between articulating surfaces of bones; fibrous connection replaced by bone in older adults	None (synarthroses)	Sutures between certain skull bones
Syndesmoses	Same as sutures, but fibrous tissue not eventually replaced by bone	None (synarthroses)	Distal tibiofibular
Cartilaginous			
Symphyses	Fibrocartilage connects articulating surfaces of bones; joint capsule present, and sometimes a joint cavity	Slight (amphiarthroses)	Symphysis pubis; joints between bodies of vertebrae
Synchondroses	Hyaline cartilage connects epiphyses to diaphysis of growing bones	Ordinarily none	In all growing long bones
Synovial			
Ball and socket (spheroidal, endarthroses)	Ball-shaped head fits into concave socket	Widest range of all joints; triaxial	Shoulder joint and hip joint
Hinge (ginglymus)	Spool-shaped surface, fits into concave surface	In one plane about single axis (uniaxial); like hinged-door movement, namely, flexion and extension	Elbow, knee, ankle, and interphalangeal joints
Pivot (trochoid)	Arch-shaped surface rotates about rounded or peglike pivot	Rotation; uniaxial	Between axis and atlas; between radius and ulna
Ellipsoidal (condyloid, ovoid)	Oval-shaped condyle fits into elliptical cavity	In two planes at right angles to each other—specifically, flexion, extension, abduction, and adduction; biaxial	Wrist joint (between radius and carpals)
Saddle	Saddle-shaped bone fits into socket that is concave-convex in opposite direction; modification of condyloid joint	Same kinds of movement as condyloid joint but freer; like rider in saddle; biaxial	Thumb, between first metacarpal and trapezium, is only saddle joint
Gliding (arthrodia)	Articulating surfaces; usually flat	Gliding—a nonaxial movement	Between carpals and between tarsals

Description of individual joints

Name	Articulating bones	Type	Movements
Atlantoepistropheal	Anterior arch of atlas rotates about dens of axis (epistropheus)	Diarthrotic (pivot type)	Pivoting or partial rotation of head
Vertebral	Between bodies of vertebrae	Amphiarthrotic, cartilaginous	Slight movement between any two vertebrae but considerable motility for column as whole
	Between articular processes	Diarthrotic (gliding)	
Sternoclavicular	Medial end of clavicle with manubrium of sternum; only joint between upper extremity and trunk	Diarthrotic (gliding)	Gliding; weak joint that may be injured comparatively easily
Acromioclavicular	Distal end of clavicle with acromion of scapula	Diarthrotic (gliding)	Gliding; elevation, depression, protraction, and retraction
Thoracic	Heads of ribs with bodies of vertebrae	Diarthrotic (gliding)	Gliding
	Tubercles of ribs with transverse processes of vertebrae	Diarthrotic (gliding)	Gliding
Shoulder	Head of humerus in glenoid cavity of scapula	Diarthrotic (ball and socket type)	Flexion, extension, abduction, adduction, rotation, and circumduction of upper arm; one of most freely movable of joints
Elbow	Trochlea of humerus with semilunar notch of ulna; head of radius with capitulum of humerus	Diarthrotic (hinge type)	Flexion and extension
	Head of radius in radial notch of ulna	Diarthrotic (pivot type)	Supination and pronation of lower arm and hand; rotation of lower arm on upper as in using screwdriver
Wrist	Scaphoid, lunate, and triquetral bones articulate with radius and articular disk	Diarthrotic (condyloid)	Flexion, extension, abduction, and adduction of hand
Carpal	Between various carpals	Diarthrotic (gliding)	Gliding
Hand	Proximal end of first metacarpal with trapezium	Diarthrotic (saddle)	Flexion, extension, abduction, adduction, and circumduction of thumb and opposition to fingers; motility of this joint accounts for dexterity of human hand compared with animal forepaw
	Distal end of metacarpals with proximal end of phalanges	Diarthrotic (hinge)	Flexion, extension, limited abduction, and adduction of fingers
	Between phalanges	Diarthrotic (hinge)	Flexion and extension of finger sections
Sacroiliac	Between sacrum and two ilia	Diarthrotic (gliding); joint cavity mostly obliterated after middle life	None or slight, for example, during late months of pregnancy and during delivery
Symphysis pubis	Between two pubic bones	Synarthrotic (or amphiarthrotic), cartilaginous	Slight, particularly during pregnancy and delivery
Hip	Head of femur in acetabulum of os coxae	Diarthrotic (ball and socket)	Flexion, extension, abduction, adduction, rotation, and circumduction
Knee	Between distal end of femur and proximal end of tibia; largest joint in body	Diarthrotic (hinge type)	Flexion and extension; slight rotation of tibia
Tibiofibular	Head of fibula with lateral condyle of tibia	Diarthrotic (gliding type)	Gliding
Ankle	Distal ends of tibia and fibula with talus	Diarthrotic (hinge type)	Flexion (dorsiflexion) and extension (plantar flexion)
Foot	Between tarsals	Diarthrotic (gliding)	Gliding; inversion and eversion
	Between metatarsals and phalanges	Diarthrotic (hinge type)	Flexion, extension, slight abduction, and adduction
	Between phalanges	Diarthrotic (hinge type)	Flexion and extension

3-3. The muscular system

Muscles grouped according to location

Location	Muscles	Location	Muscles
Neck	Sternocleidomastoid	Thigh	
Back	Trapezius	Anterior surface	Quadriceps femoris group
	Latissimus dorsi		Rectus femoris
Chest	Pectoralis major		Vastus lateralis
	Serratus anterior		Vastus medialis
Abdominal wall	External oblique		Vastus intermedius
Shoulder	Deltoid	Medial surface	Gracilis
Upper arm	Biceps brachii		Adductor group (brevis, longus, magnus)
	Triceps brachii	Posterior surface	Hamstring group
	Brachialis		Biceps femoris
Forearm	Brachioradialis		Semitendinosus
	Pronator teres		Semimembranosus
Buttocks	Gluteus maximus	Leg	
	Gluteus minimus	Anterior surface	Tibialis anterior
	Gluteus medius	Posterior surface	Gastrocnemius
	Tensor fascia latae		Soleus
		Pelvic floor	Levator ani
			Levator coccygeus
			Rectococcygeus

Muscles grouped according to function

Part moved	Example of flexor	Example of extensor	Example of abductor	Example of adductor
Head	Sternocleidomastoid	Semispinalis capitis		
Upper arm	Pectoralis major	Trapezius	Deltoid	Pectoralis major with latissimus dorsi
		Latissimus dorsi		
Forearm	With forearm supinated: biceps brachii	Triceps brachii		
	With forearm pronated: brachialis			
	With semisupination or semipronation: brachioradialis			
Hand	Flexor carpi radialis and ulnaris	Extensor carpi radialis, longus, and brevis	Flexor carpi radialis	Flexor carpi ulnaris
	Palmaris longus	Extensor carpi ulnaris		
Thigh	Iliopsoas	Gluteus maximus	Gluteus medius and gluteus minimus	Adductor group
	Rectus femoris (of quadriceps femoris group)			
Leg	Hamstrings	Quadriceps femoris group		
Foot	Tibialis anterior	Gastrocnemius	Evertors	Invertor
		Soleus	Peroneus longus	Tibialis anterior
			Peroneus brevis	
Trunk	Iliopsoas	Sacrospinalis		
	Rectus abdominis			

Muscles that move the head

Muscle	Origin	Insertion	Function	Innervation
Sternocleidomastoid	Sternum Clavicle	Temporal bone (mastoid process)	Flexes head (prayer muscle) One muscle alone, rotates head toward opposite side; spasm of this muscle alone or associated with trapezius called torticollis or wryneck	Accessory nerve
Semispinalis capitis	Vertebrae (transverse processes of upper six thoracic, articular processes of lower four cervical)	Occipital bone (between superior and inferior nuchal lines)	Extends head; bends it laterally	First five cervical nerves
Splenius capitis	Ligamentum nuchae Vertebrae (spinous processes of upper three or four thoracic)	Temporal bone (mastoid process) Occipital bone	Extends head Bends and rotates head toward same side as contracting muscle	Second, third, and fourth cervical nerves
Longissimus capitis	Vertebrae (transverse processes of upper six thoracic, articular processes of lower four cervical)	Temporal bone (mastoid process)	Extends head Bends and rotates head toward contracting side	

Muscles of facial expression and of mastication

Muscle	Origin	Insertion	Function	Innervation
Muscles of facial expression				
Epicranius (occipitofrontalis)	Occipital bone	Tissues of eyebrows	Raises eyebrows, wrinkles forehead horizontally	Cranial nerve VII
Corrugator supercilii	Frontal bone (superciliary ridge)	Skin of eyebrow	Wrinkles forehead vertically	Cranial nerve VII
Orbicularis oculi	Encircles eyelid		Closes eye	Cranial nerve VII
Orbicularis oris	Encircles mouth		Draws lips together	Cranial nerve VII
Platysma	Fascia of upper part of deltoid and pectoralis major	Mandible (lower border) Skin around corners of mouth	Draws corners of mouth down—pouting	Cranial nerve VII
Buccinator	Maxillae	Skin of sides of mouth	Permits smiling Blowing, as in playing a trumpet	Cranial nerve VII
Muscles of mastication				
Masseter	Zygomatic arch	Mandible (external surface)	Closes jaw	Cranial nerve V
Temporal	Temporal bone	Mandible	Closes jaw	Cranial nerve V
Pterygoids (internal and external	Undersurface of skull	Mandible (mesial surface)	Grate teeth	Cranial nerve V

Muscles that move the shoulder

Muscle	Origin	Insertion	Function	Innervation
Trapezius	Occipital bone (protuberance) Vertebrae (cervical and thoracic)	Clavicle Scapula (spine and acromion)	Raises or lowers shoulders and and shrugs them Extends head when occiput acts as insertion	Spinal accessory, second, third, and fourth cervical nerves
Pectoralis minor	Ribs (second to fifth)	Scapula (coracoid)	Pulls shoulder down and forward	Medial and lateral anterior thoracic nerves
Serratus anterior	Ribs (upper eight or nine)	Scapula (anterior surface, vertebral border)	Pulls shoulder forward; abducts and rotates it upward	Long thoracic nerve

Muscles that move the upper arm

Muscle	Origin	Insertion	Function	Innervation
Pectoralis major	Clavicle (medial half) Sternum Costal cartilages of true ribs	Humerus (greater tubercle)	Flexes upper arm Adducts upper arm anteriorly; draws it across chest	Medial and lateral anterior thoracic nerves
Latissimus dorsi	Vertebrae (spines of lower thoracic, lumbar, and sacral) Ilium (crest) Lumbodorsal fascia*	Humerus (intertubercular groove)	Extends upper arm Adducts upper arm posteriorly	Thoracodorsal nerve
Deltoid	Clavicle Scapula (spine and acromion)	Humerus (lateral side about halfway down—deltoid tubercle)	Abducts upper arm Assists in flexion and extension of upper arm	Axillary nerve
Coracobrachialis	Scapula (coracoid process)	Humerus (middle third, medial surface)	Adduction; assists in flexion and medial rotation of arm	Musculocutaneous nerve
Supraspinatus	Scapula (supraspinous fossa)	Humerus (greater tubercle)	Assists in abducting arm	Suprascapular nerve
Teres major	Scapula (lower part, axillary border)	Humerus (upper part, anterior surface)	Assists in extension, adduction, and medial rotation of arm	Lower subscapular nerve
Teres minor	Scapula (axillary border)	Humerus (greater tubercle)	Rotates arm outward	Axillary nerve
Infraspinatus	Scapula (infraspinatus border)	Humerus (greater tubercle)	Rotates arm outward	Suprascapular nerve

*Lumbodorsal fascia—extension of aponeurosis of latissimus dorsi; fills in space between last rib and iliac crest.

Muscles that move the lower arm

Muscle	Origin	Insertion	Function	Innervation
Biceps brachii	Scapula (supraglenoid tuberosity) Scapula (coracoid)	Radius (tubercle at proximal end)	Flexes supinated forearm Supinates forearm and hand	Musculocutaneous nerve
Brachialis	Humerus (distal half, anterior surface)	Ulna (front of coronoid process)	Flexes pronated forearm	Musculocutaneous nerve
Brachioradialis	Humerus (above lateral epicondyle)	Radius (styloid process)	Flexes semipronated or semisupinated forearm; supinates forearm and hand	Radial nerve
Triceps brachii	Scapula (infraglenoid tuberosity) Humerus (posterior surface—lateral head above radial groove; medial head, below)	Ulna (olecranon process)	Extends lower arm	Radial nerve
Pronator teres	Humerus (medial epicondyle) Ulna (coronoid process)	Radius (middle third of lateral surface)	Pronates and flexes forearm	Median nerve
Pronator quadratus	Ulna (distal fourth, anterior surface)	Radius (distal fourth, anterior surface)	Pronates forearm	Median nerve
Supinator	Humerus (lateral epicondyle) Ulna (proximal fifth)	Radius (proximal third)	Supinates forearm	Radial nerve

Muscles that move the hand

Muscle	Origin	Insertion	Function	Innervation
Flexor carpi radialis	Humerus (medial epicondyle)	Second metacarpal (base of)	Flexes hand Flexes forearm	Median nerve
Palmaris longus	Humerus (medial epicondyle)	Fascia of palm	Flexes hand	Median nerve
Flexor carpi ulnaris	Humerus (medial epicondyle) Ulna (proximal two thirds)	Pisiform bone Third, fourth, and fifth metacarpals	Flexes hand Adducts hand	Ulnar nerve
Extensor carpi radialis longus	Humerus (ridge above lateral epicondyle)	Second metacarpal (base of)	Extends hand Abducts hand (moves toward thumb side when hand supinated)	Radial nerve
Extensor carpi radialis brevis	Humerus (lateral epicondyle)	Second, third metacarpals (bases of)	Extends hand	Radial nerve
Extensor carpi ulnaris	Humerus (lateral epicondyle) Ulna (proximal three fourths)	Fifth metacarpal (base of)	Extends hand Adducts hand (move toward little finger side when hand supinated)	Radial nerve

Muscles that move the trunk

Muscle	Origin	Insertion	Function	Innervation
Sacrospinalis (erector spinae)			Extend spine; maintain erect posture of trunk Acting singly, abduct and rotate trunk	Posterior rami of first cervical to fifth lumbar spinal nerves
Lateral portion Iliocostalis lumborum	Iliac crest, sacrum (posterior surface), and lumbar vertebrae (spinous processes)	Ribs, lower six		
Iliocostalis dorsi	Ribs, lower six	Ribs, upper six		
Iliocostalis cervicis	Ribs, upper six	Vertebrae, fourth to sixth cervical		
Medial portion Longissimus dorsi	Same as iliocostalis lumborum	Vertebrae, thoracic ribs		
Longissimus cervicis	Vertebrae, upper six thoracic	Vertebrae, second to sixth cervical		
Longissimus capitis	Vertebrae, upper six thoracic and last four cervical	Temporal bone, mastoid process		
Quadratus lumborum (forms part of posterior abdominal wall)	Ilium (posterior part of crest) Vertebrae (lower three lumbar)	Ribs (twelfth) Vertebrae (transverse processes of first four lumbar)	Both muscles together extend spine One muscle alone abducts trunk toward side of contracting muscle	First three or four lumbar nerves
Iliopsoas	See muscles that move the thigh		Flexes trunk	

Muscles that move the chest wall

Muscle	Origin	Insertion	Function	Innervation
External intercostals	Rib (lower border; forward fibers)	Rib (upper border of rib below origin)	Elevate ribs	Intercostal nerves
Internal intercostals	Rib (inner surface, lower border; backward fibers)	Rib (upper border of rib below origin)	Probably depress ribs	Intercostal nerves
Diaphragm	Lower circumference of thorax (of rib cage)	Central tendon of diaphragm	Enlarges thorax, causing inspiration	Phrenic nerves

Muscles that move the abdominal wall

Muscle	Origin	Insertion	Function	Innervation
External oblique	Ribs (lower eight)	Ossa coxae (iliac crest and pubis by way of inguinal ligament)* Linea alba† by way of an aponeurosis‡	Compresses abdomen Important postural function of all abdominal muscles is to pull front of pelvis upward, thereby flattening lumbar curve of spine; when these muscles lose their tone, common figure faults of protruding abdomen and lordosis develop	Lower seven intercostal nerves and iliohypogastric nerves
Internal oblique	Ossa coxae (iliac crest and inguinal ligament) Lumbodorsal fascia	Ribs (lower three) Pubic bone Linca alba	Same as external oblique	Last three intercostal nerves; iliohypogastric and ilioinguinal nerves
Transversalis	Ribs (lower six) Ossa coxae (iliac crest, inguinal ligament) Lumbodorsal fascia	Pubic bone Linea alba	Same as external oblique	Last five intercostal nerves; iliohypogastric and ilioinguinal nerves
Rectus abdominis	Ossa coxae (pubic bone and symphysis pubis)	Ribs (costal cartilage of fifth, sixth, and seventh ribs) Sternum (xiphoid process)	Same as external oblique; because abdominal muscles compress abdominal cavity, they aid in straining, defecation, forced expiration, and childbirth; abdominal muscles are antagonists of diaphragm, relaxing as it contracts and vice versa Flexes trunk	Last six intercostal nerves

*Inguinal ligament (or Poupart's)—lower edge of aponeurosis of external oblique muscle, extending between the anterior superior iliac spine and the tubercle of the pubic bone. This edge is doubled under like a hem on material. The inguinal ligament forms the upper boundary of the femoral triangle, a large triangular area in the thigh; its other boundaries are the adductor longus muscle mesially and the sartorius muscle laterally.
†Linea alba—literally, a white line; extends from xiphoid process to symphysis pubis; formed by fibers of aponeuroses of the right abdominal muscles interlacing with fibers of aponeuroses of the left abdominal muscles; comparable to a seam up the midline of the abdominal wall, anchoring its various layers. During pregnancy the linea alba becomes pigmented and is known as the linea niger.
‡Aponeurosis—sheet of white fibrous tissue that attaches one muscle to another or attaches it to bone or other movable structures, for example, the right external oblique muscle attaches to the left external oblique muscle by means of an aponeurosis.

Muscles of the pelvic floor

Muscle	Origin	Insertion	Function	Innervation
Levator ani	Pubis (posterior surface) Ischium (spine)	Coccyx	Together form floor of pelvic cavity; support pelvic organs; if these muscles are badly torn at childbirth or become too relaxed, uterus or bladder may prolapse, that is, drop out	Pudendal nerve
Coccygeus (posterior continuation of levator ani)	Ischium (spine)	Coccyx Sacrum	Same as levator ani	Pudendal nerve

Muscles that move the thigh

Muscle	Origin	Insertion	Function	Innervation
Iliopsoas (iliacus and and psoas major)	Ilium (iliac fossa) Vertebrae (bodies of twelfth thoracic to fifth lumbar)	Femur (small trochanter)	Flexes thigh Flexes trunk (when femur acts as origin)	Femoral and second to fourth lumbar nerves
Rectus femoris	Ilium (anterior, inferior spine)	Tibia (by way of patellar tendon)	Flexes thigh Extends lower leg	Femoral nerve
Gluteal group				
Maximus	Ilium (crest and posterior surface) Sacrum and coccyx (posterior surface) Sacrotuberous ligament	Femur (gluteal tuberosity) Iliotibial tract*	Extends thigh—rotates outward	Inferior gluteal nerve
Medius	Ilium (lateral surface)	Femur (greater trochanter)	Abducts thigh—rotates outward; stabilizes pelvis on femur	Superior gluteal nerve
Minimus	Ilium (lateral surface)	Femur (greater trochanter)	Abducts thigh; stabilizes pelvis on femur Rotates thigh medially	Superior gluteal nerve
Tensor fasciae latae	Ilium (anterior part of crest)	Tibia (by way of iliotibial tract)	Abducts thigh Tightens iliotibial tract*	Superior gluteal nerve
Piriformis	Vertebrae (front of sacrum)	Femur (medial aspect of greater trochanter)	Rotates thigh outward Abducts thigh Extends thigh	First or second sacral nerves
Adductor group				
Brevis	Pubic bone	Femur (linea aspera)	Adducts thigh	Obturator nerve
Longus	Pubic bone	Femur (linea aspera)	Adducts thigh	Obturator nerve
Magnus	Pubic bone	Femur (linea aspera)	Adducts thigh	Obturator nerve
Gracilis	Pubic bone (just below symphysis)	Tibia (medial surface behind sartorius)	Adducts thigh and flexes and adducts leg	Obturator nerve

*The iliotibial tract is part of the fascia enveloping all the thigh muscles. It consists of a wide band of dense fibrous tissue attached to the iliac crest above and the lateral condyle of the tibia below. The upper part of the tract encloses fasciae latae muscle.

Muscles that move the lower leg

Muscle	Origin	Insertion	Function	Innervation
Quadriceps femoris group				
Rectus femoris	Ilium (anterior, inferior spine)	Tibia (by way of patellar tendon)	Flexes thigh Extends leg	Femoral nerve
Vastus lateralis	Femur (linea aspera)	Tibia (by way of patellar tendon)	Extends leg	Femoral nerve
Vastus medialis	Femur	Tibia (by way of patellar tendon)	Extends leg	Femoral nerve
Vastus intermedius	Femur (anterior surface)	Tibia (by way of patellar tendon)	Extends leg	Femoral nerve
Sartorius	Os innominatum (anterior, superior iliac spines)	Tibia (medial surface of upper end of shaft)	Adducts and flexes leg Permits crossing of legs tailor fashion	Femoral nerve
Hamstring group				
Biceps femoris	Ischium (tuberosity)	Fibula (head of)	Flexes leg	Hamstring nerve (branch of sciatic nerve)
	Femur (linea aspera)	Tibia (lateral condyle)	Extends thigh	Hamstring nerve
Semitendinosus	Ischium (tuberosity)	Tibia (proximal end, medial surface)	Extends thigh	Hamstring nerve
Semimembranosus	Ischium (tuberosity)	Tibia (medial condyle)	Extends thigh	Hamstring nerve

Muscles that move the foot

Muscle	Origin	Insertion	Function	Innervation
Tibialis anterior	Tibia (lateral condyle of upper body)	Tarsal (first cuneiform) Metatarsal (base of first)	Flexes foot Inverts foot	Common and deep peroneal nerves
Gastrocnemius	Femur (condyles)	Tarsal (calcaneus by way of Achilles tendon)	Extends foot Flexes lower leg	Tibial nerve (branch of sciatic nerve)
Soleus	Tibia (underneath gastrocnemius) Fibula	Tarsal (calcaneus by way of Achilles tendon)	Extends foot (plantar flexion)	Tibial nerve
Peroneus longus	Tibia (lateral condyle) Fibula (head and shaft)	First cuneiform Base of first metatarsal	Extends foot (plantar flexion) Everts foot	Common peroneal nerve
Peroneus brevis	Fibula (lower two thirds of lateral surface of shaft)	Fifth metatarsal (tubercle, dorsal surface)	Everts foot Flexes foot	Superficial peroneal nerve
Tibialis posterior	Tibia (posterior surface) Fibula (posterior surface)	Navicular bone Cuboid bone All three cuneiforms Second and fourth metatarsals	Extends foot (plantar flexion) Inverts foot	Tibial nerve
Peroneus tertius	Fibula (distal third)	Fourth and fifth metatarsals (bases of)	Flexes foot Everts foot	Deep peroneal nerve

3-4. The endocrine system

Production, control, and effects of pituitary hormones

Pituitary gland (hypophysis cerebri)	Hormone	Source (cell type or location)	Control mechanism	Effect
Anterior pituitary gland (adenohypophysis)	Growth hormone (GH, somatotropin [STH])	Acidophils	GRH (growth hormone–releasing hormone) from hypothalamus	Promotes body growth, protein anabolism, and mobilization and catabolism of fats; decreases glucose catabolism; increases blood glucose levels
Pars anterior	Prolactin (lactogenic or luteotropic hormone [LTH])	Acidophils	Prolactin inhibitory factor (PIF; prolactin-releasing factor (PRF) from hypothalamus and high blood levels of oxytocin	Stimulates milk secretion and development of secretory alveoli; helps maintain corpus luteum
	Thyrotropin (TH); thyroid-stimulating hormone (TSH)	Basophils	Thyrotropin-releasing hormone (TRH) from hypothalamus	Growth and maintenance of thyroid gland and stimulation of thyroid hormone secretion
	Adrenocorticotropin (ACTH)	Basophils	Corticotropin-releasing factor (CRF) from hypothalamus	Growth and maintenance of adrenal cortex and stimulation of cortisol and other glucocorticoid secretions
	Follicle-stimulating hormone (FSH)	Basophils	Follicle-stimulating hormone–releasing hormone (FSH-RH) from hypothalamus	In female—stimulates follicle growth and maturation and estrogen secretion
				In male—stimulates development of seminiferous tubules and maintains spermatogenesis
	Luteinizing hormone (LH in female, ICSH in male)	Basophils	Luteinizing hormone–releasing hormone (LH-RH) from hypothalamus	In female (LH)—induces ovulation and stimulates formation of corpus luteum and progesterone secretion
				In male (ICSH)—stimulates interstitial cell secretion of testosterone
Pars intermedia	Melanocyte-stimulating hormone (MSH); intermedin	Basophils	Unknown in humans	May cause darkening of skin by increasing melanin production
Posterior pituitary gland (neurohypophysis)	ADH (vasopressin)	Hypothalamus, mainly supraoptic nucleus	Osmoreceptors in hypothalamus stimulated by increase in blood osmotic pressure, decrease in extracellular fluid volume, and stress	Decreased urine output
	Oxytocin	Hypothalamus, paraventricular nucleus	Nervous stimulation of hypothalamus caused by stimulation of nipples (nursing)	Contraction of uterine smooth muscle and ejection of milk into lactiferous ducts

Names and locations of endocrine glands

Name	Location	Name	Location
Pituitary gland (hypophysis cerebri) and hypothalamus	Cranial cavity	Adrenal glands	Abdominal cavity (retroperitoneal)
Anterior lobe (adenohypophysis)		Adrenal cortex	
Intermediate lobe (pars intermedia)		Adrenal medulla	
		Islands of Langerhans	Abdominal cavity (pancreas)
Posterior lobe (neurohypophysis)		Gastric and intestinal mucosa	Abdominal cavity
Pineal gland (epiphysis)	Cranial cavity	Ovaries	Pelvic cavity
Thyroid gland	Neck	Graafian follicle	
Parathyroid glands	Neck	Corpus luteum	
Thymus	Mediastinum	Testes (interstitial cells)	Scrotum
		Placenta	Pregnant uterus

3-5. The nervous system

Major ascending tracts of the spinal cord

Name	Function	Location	Origin*	Termination†
Lateral spinothalamic	Pain, temperature, and crude touch opposite side	Lateral white columns	Posterior gray column opposite side	Thalamus
Ventral spinothalamic	Crude touch, pain, and temperature	Anterior white columns	Posterior gray column opposite side	Thalamus
Fasciculi gracilis and cuneatus	Discriminating touch and pressure sensations, including vibration, stereognosis, and two-point discrimination; also conscious kinesthesia	Posterior white columns	Spinal ganglia same side	Medulla
Spinocerebellar	Unconscious kinesthesia	Lateral white columns	Posterior gray column	Cerebellum

*Location of cell bodies of neurons from which axons of tract arise.
†Structure in which axons of tract terminate.

Major descending tracts of the spinal cord

Name	Function	Location	Origin*	Termination†
Lateral corticospinal (or crossed pyramidal)	Voluntary movement, contraction of individual or small groups of muscles, particularly those moving hands, fingers, feet, and toes of opposite side	Lateral white columns	Motor areas cerebral cortex (mainly areas 4 and 6) opposite side from tract location in cord	Intermediate or anterior gray columns
Ventral corticospinal (direct pyramidal)	Same as lateral corticospinal except mainly muscles of same side	Lateral white columns	Motor cortex but on same side as tract location in cord	Intermediate or anterior gray columns
Lateral reticulospinal	Mainly facilitatory influence on motoneurons to skeletal muscles	Lateral white columns	Reticular formation, midbrain, pons, and medulla	Intermediate or anterior gray columns
Medial reticulospinal	Mainly inhibitory influence on motoneurons to skeletal muscles	Anterior white columns	Reticular formation, medulla mainly	Intermediate or anterior gray columns

*Location of cell bodies of neurons from which axons of tract arise.
†Structure in which axons of tract terminate.

Spinal nerves and peripheral branches

Spinal nerves	Plexuses formed from anterior rami	Spinal nerve branches from plexuses	Parts supplied
Cervical 1 2 3 4	Cervical plexus	Lesser occipital Great auricular Cutaneous nerve of neck Anterior supraclavicular Middle supraclavicular Posterior supraclavicular Branches to numerous neck muscles	Sensory to back of head, front of neck, and upper part of shoulder; motor to numerous neck muscles
		Phrenic (branches from cervical nerves before formation of plexus; most of its fibers from fourth cervical nerve)	Diaphragm
		Suprascapular and dorsoscapular	Superficial muscles* of scapula
		Thoracic nerves, medial and lateral branches	Pectoralis major and minor
		Long thoracic nerve	Serratus anterior
Cervical 5 6		Thoracodorsal	Latissimus dorsi
		Subscapular	Subscapular and teres major muscles
7 8	Brachial plexus	Axillary (circumflex)	Deltoid and teres minor muscles and skin over deltoid
Thoracic (or dorsal) 1		Musculocutaneous	Muscles of front of arm (biceps brachii, coracobrachialis, and brachialis) and skin on outer side of forearm
2 3 4 5 6 7	No plexus formed; branches run directly to intercostal muscles and skin of thorax	Ulnar	Flexor carpi ulnaris and part of flexor digitorum profundus; some of muscles of hand; sensory to medial side of hand, little finger, and medial half of fourth finger
8 9 10 11		Median	Rest of muscles of front of forearm and hand; sensory to skin of palmar surface of thumb, index, and middle fingers
12		Radial	Triceps muscle and muscles of back of forearm; sensory to skin of back of forearm and hand
		Medial cutaneous	Sensory to inner surface of arm and forearm

*Although nerves to muscles are considered motor, they do contain some sensory fibers that transmit proprioceptive impulses.

†Sensory fibers from the tibial and peroneal nerves unite to form the *medial cutaneous* (or sural) *nerve* that supplies the calf of the leg and the lateral surface of the foot. In the thigh the tibial and common peroneal nerves are usually enclosed in a single sheath to form the *sciatic nerve,* the largest nerve in the body with its width of approximately ¾ of an inch. About two thirds of the way down the posterior part of the thigh, it divides into its component parts. Branches of the sciatic nerve extend into the hamstring muscles.

Spinal nerves and peripheral branches—cont'd

Spinal nerves	Plexuses formed from anterior rami	Spinal nerve branches from plexuses	Parts supplied
Lumbar 1 2 3 4 5 Sacral 1 2 3 4 5 Coccygeal 1	Lumbosacral plexus	Iliohypogastric } Sometimes fused Ilioinguinal	Sensory to anterior abdominal wall Sensory to anterior abdominal wall and external genitalia; motor to muscles of abdominal wall
		Genitofemoral	Sensory to skin of external genitalia and inguinal region
		Lateral cutaneous of thigh	Sensory to outer side of thigh
		Femoral	Motor to quadriceps, sartorius, and iliacus muscles; sensory to front of thigh and medial side of lower leg (saphenous nerve)
		Obturator	Motor to adductor muscles of thigh
		Tibial† (medial popliteal)	Motor to muscles of calf of leg; sensory to skin of calf of leg and sole of foot
		Common peroneal (lateral popliteal)	Motor to evertors and dorsiflexors of foot; sensory to lateral surface of leg and dorsal surface of foot
		Nerves to hamstring muscles	Motor to muscles of back of thigh
		Gluteal nerves, superior and inferior	Motor to buttock muscles and tensor fasciae latae
		Posterior cutaneous nerve	Sensory to skin of buttocks, posterior surface of thigh, and leg
		Pudendal nerve	Motor to perineal muscles; sensory to skin of perineum

Sympathetic and parasympathetic neurons compared to location

	Sympathetic	Parasympathetic
Preganglionic neurons		
Dendrites and cell bodies	In lateral gray columns of thoracic and first four lumbar segments of spinal cord	In nuclei of brainstem and cord (in lateral gray columns of sacral segments of cord)
Axons	In anterior roots of spinal nerves, to spinal nerves (thoracic and first four lumbar), to white rami, and then in any of three following pathways: (1) ganglia; (2) through white rami to and through sympathetic ganglia, then up or down sympathetic trunk before synapsing in a sympathetic ganglion; (3) through white rami to and through sympathetic ganglia, to and through splanchnic nerves to collateral ganglia (celiac, superior, and inferior mesenteric ganglia)	From brainstem nuclei through cranial nerve III to ciliary ganglion From nuclei in pons: through cranial nerve VII to sphenopalatine or submaxillary ganglion From nuclei in medulla through cranial nerve IX to otic ganglion or through cranial nerves X and XI to cardiac and celiac ganglia, respectively
Postganglionic neurons		
Dendrites and cell bodies	In sympathetic and collateral ganglia	In parasympathetic ganglia (for example, ciliary, sphenopalatine, submaxillary, otic, cardiac, celiac) located in or near visceral effector organs
Axons	In autonomic nerves and plexuses that innervate thoracic and abdominal viscera and blood vessels in these cavities In gray rami to spinal nerves, to smooth muscle of skin blood vessels and hair follicles, and to sweat glands	In short nerves to various visceral effector organs

Cranial nerves

Nerve*	Sensory fibers†			Motor fibers†		Functions‡
	Receptors	Cell bodies	Termination	Cell bodies	Termination	
I Olfactory	Nasal mucosa	Nasal mucosa	Olfactory bulbs (new relay of neurons of olfactory cortex)			Sense of smell
II Optic	Retina	Retina	Nucleus in thalamus (lateral geniculate body); some fibers terminate in superior colliculus of midbrain			Vision
III Oculomotor	External eye muscles except superior oblique and lateral rectus	?	?	Midbrain (oculomotor nucleus and Edinger-Westphal nucleus)	External eye muscles except superior oblique and lateral rectus; fibers from Edinger-Westphal nucleus terminate in ciliary ganglion and then to ciliary and iris muscles	Eye movements, regulation of size of pupil, accommodation, proprioception (muscle sense)
IV Trochlear	Superior oblique	?	?	Midbrain	Superior oblique muscle of eye	Eye movements, proprioception
V Trigeminal	Skin and mucosa of head, teeth	Gasserian ganglion	Pons (sensory nucleus)	Pons (motor nucleus)	Muscles of mastication	Sensations of head and face, chewing movements, muscle sense
VI Abducens	Lateral rectus			Pons	Lateral rectus muscle of eye	Abduction of eye, proprioception
VII Facial	Taste buds of anterior two thirds of tongue	Geniculate ganglion	Medulla (nucleus solitarius)	Pons	Superficial muscles of face and scalp	Facial expressions, secretion of saliva, taste
VIII Acoustic						
1 Vestibular branch	Semicircular canals and vestibule (utricle and saccule)	Vestibular ganglion	Pons and medulla (vestibular nuclei)			Balance or equilibrium sense
2 Cochlear or auditory branch	Organ of Corti in cochlear duct	Spiral ganglion	Pons and medulla (cochlear nuclei)			Hearing

IX Glossopharyngeal	*Pharynx; taste buds and other receptors of posterior one third of tongue*	*Jugular and petrous ganglia*	*Medulla (nucleus solitarius)*		*Taste and other sensations of tongue,* **swallowing movements, secretion of saliva,** *aid in reflex control of blood pressure and respiration*
			Medulla (nucleus ambiguus)	**Muscles of pharynx**	
		Carotid sinus and carotid body	*Medulla (respiratory and vasomotor centers)*		
			Medulla at junction of pons (nucleus salivatorius)	**Otic ganglion and then to parotid gland**	
X Vagus	*Pharynx, larynx, carotid body, and thoracic and abdominal viscera*	*Jugular and nodose ganglia*	*Medulla (nucleus, solitarius), pons (nucleus of fifth cranial nerve)*		*Sensations and movements or organs supplied; for example,* **slows heart, increases peristalsis, and contracts muscles for voice production**
			Medulla (dorsal motor nucleus)	**Ganglia of vagal plexus and then to muscles of pharynx, larynx, and thoracic and abdominal viscera**	
XI Spinal accessory	?	?	?		**Shoulder movements, turning movements of head, movements of viscera, voice productions,** *proprioception?*
			Medulla (dorsal motor nucleus of vagus and nucleus ambiguus)	**Muscles of thoracic and abdominal viscera and pharynx and larynx**	
			Anterior gray column of first five or six cervical segments of spinal cord	**Trapezius and sternocleidomastoid muscle**	
XII Hypoglossal	?	?	**Medulla (hypoglossal nucleus)**	**Muscles of tongue**	**Tongue movements,** *proprioception?*

---

*The first letters of the words in the following sentence are the first letters of the names of the cranial nerves. Many generations of anatomy students have used this sentence as an aid to memorizing these names. It is "On Old Olympus Tiny Tops, A Finn and German Viewed Some Hops." (There are several slightly differing versions of this mnemonic.)

†Italics indicate sensory fibers and functions. Boldface type indicates motor fibers and functions.

‡An aid for remembering the general function of each cranial nerve is the following 12-word saying: "Some say marry money but my brothers say bad business marry money." Words beginning with S indicate sensory function. Words beginning with M indicate motor function. Words beginning with B indicate both sensory and motor functions. For example, the first, second, and eighth words in the saying start with S, which indicates that the first, second, and eighth cranial nerves perform sensory functions.

Cranial nerves contrasted with spinal nerves

	Cranial nerves	Spinal nerves
Origin	Base of brain	Spinal cord
Distribution	Mainly to head and neck	Skin, skeletal muscles, joints, blood vessels, sweat glands, and mucosa except of head and neck
Structure	Some composed of sensory fibers only; some of both motor axons and sensory dendrites; some motor fibers belong to somatic nervous system, some to autonomic	All of them composed of both sensory dendrites and motor axons; some of latter, somatic, some autonomic
Function	Vision, hearing, sense of small, sense of taste, eye movements	Sensations, movements, and sweat secretion

Autonomic functions

Visceral effectors	Sympathetic impulses	Parasympathetic impulses
Cardiac muscle	Stimulate pacemaker, accelerate rate and strength of heartbeat	Inhibit pacemaker; decrease rate and strength of heartbeat
Smooth muscle of blood vessels		
Skin blood vessels	Stimulate; constrict	No parasympathetic fibers
Skeletal muscle blood vessels	Inhibit; dilate	No parasympathetic fibers
Coronary blood vessels	Inhibit; dilate	No parasympathetic fibers
Blood vessels in cerebrum and abdominal viscera	Stimulate; constrict	Inhibit; dilate; no parasympathetic fibers to some viscera
Blood vessels in external genitalia	Inhibit; dilate	Stimulate; constrict
Smooth muscle of hollow organs and sphincters		
Bronchi	Inhibit; dilate	Stimulate; constrict
Digestive tract, except sphincters	Inhibit; decrease peristalsis	Stimulate; increase peristalsis
Sphincters of digestive tract	Stimulate; close	Inhibit; open
Urinary bladder	Inhibit; relax	Stimulate; contract
Urinary sphincters	Stimulate; close	Inhibit; open
Eye		
Iris	Stimulate radial muscle; dilate pupil	Stimulate circular muscle; constrict pupil
Ciliary	Inhibit; accommodate for far vision	Stimulate; accommodate for near vision
Hairs (pilomotor muscles)	Stimulate; produce "goose pimples" (pilo-erection)	No parasympathetic fibers
Glands		
Sweat	Stimulate; increase sweat	No parasympathetic fibers
Digestive (salivary, gastric, etc.)	Inhibit; decrease secretion of saliva; not known for others	Stimulate; increase secretion of saliva
Pancreas, including islets	Inhibit; decrease secretion	Stimulate; increase secretion of pancreatic juice and insulin
Liver	Stimulate glycogenolysis; increase blood sugar level	No parasympathetic fibers
Adrenal medulla	Stimulate; increase epinephrine secretion	No parasympathetic fibers

3-6. The circulatory system

White blood cells (leukocytes)

Class	Differential count*	
	Normal range (%)	Typical normal (%)
Those with granular cytoplasm and irregular nuclei		
Neutrophils (neutral staining)	65 to 75	65
Eosinophils (acid staining)	2 to 5	3
Basophils (basic staining)	½ to 1	1
Those with nongranular cytoplasm and regular nuclei		
Lymphocytes (large and small)	20 to 25	25
Monocytes	3 to 8	6
TOTAL		100

*In any differential count the sum of the percentages of the different kinds of leukocytes must, of course, total 100%

Blood cells

Cells	Number	Function	Formation (hemopoiesis)	Destruction
Red blood cells (erythrocytes)	4.5 to 5.5 million/mm³ (total of approximately 30 trillion in adult body)	Transport oxygen and carbon dioxide	Red marrow of bones (myeloid tissue)	Reticuloendothelial cells in lining of blood vessels in liver, spleen, and bone marrow phagocytose old red blood cells; live about 105 to 120 days in bloodstream
White blood cells (leukocytes)	Usually about 5000 to 9000/mm³	Play important part in producing immunity; for example, phagocytosis by neutrophils and monocytes; antibody formation by lymphocytes and their descendents, plasma cells; production of *heparin* by basophils; detoxification by eosinophils	Granular leukocytes in red marrow; before birth and for a few months after, some lymphocytes are formed in thymus gland; later, most lymphocytes and monocytes formed in lymph nodes and other lymphatic tissues	Not known definitely; probably some destroyed by phagocytosis
Plateletes (thrombocytes)	150,000 to 350,000/mm³	Initiate blood clotting and hemostasis	Red marrow, lungs, and spleen	Unknown

Coronary arteries

Right coronary artery	Left coronary artery
Divides into two main branches:	Divides into two main branches:
1 Posterior descending artery—sends branches to both ventricles	1 Anterior descending artery—sends branches to ventricles
2 Marginal artery—sends branches to right ventricle and right atrium	2 Circumflex artery—sends branches to left ventricle and left atrium

Structure of blood vessels

	Arteries	Veins	Capillaries
Coats	Outer coat (tunica adventitia or externa) of white fibrous tissue; causes artery to stand open instead of collapsing when cut	Same three coats but thinner and fewer elastic fibers; veins collapse when cut; semilunar valves present at intervals	Only lining coat present; therefore walls only one cell thick
	Muscle coat (tunica media) of smooth muscle, elastic, and some white fibrous tissues; this coat permits constriction and dilation		
	Lining (tunica intima) of endothelium		

Blood supply

Endothelial lining cells supplied by blood flowing through vessels; exchange of oxygen, etc., between cells of middle coat and blood by diffusion; outer coat supplied by tiny vessels known as *vasa vasorum* or "vessels of vessels"

Nerve supply

Smooth muscle cells of tunica media innervated by autonomic fibers

Abnormalities

Atherosclerosis—hardening of walls of arteries (arteriosclerosis) characterized by lipid deposits in tunica intima
Aneurysm—saclike dilation of artery wall
Varicose veins—stretching of walls, particularly around semilunar valves
Phlebitis—inflammation of vein; "milk leg," phlebitis of femoral vein of women after childbirth

Main arteries

Artery	Branches (only largest ones named)
Ascending aorta	Coronary arteries (two, to myocardium)
Aortic arch	Innominate (or brachiocephalic) artery
	Left subclavian
	Left common carotid
Innominate	Right subclavian
	Right common carotid
Subclavian (right and left)	Vertebral*
	Axillary (continuation of subclavian)
Axillary	Brachial (continuation of axillary)
Brachial	Radial
	Ulnar
Radial and ulnar	Palmer arches (superficial and deep arterial arches in hand formed by anastomosis of branches of radial and ulnar arteries; numerous branches to hand and fingers)
Common carotid (right and left)	Internal carotid (brain, eye, forehead, and nose)*
	External carotid (thyroid, tongue, tonsils, ear)
Descending thoracic aorta	Visceral branches to pericardium, bronchi, esophagus, mediastinum
	Parietal branches to chest muscles, mammary glands, and diaphragm
Descending abdominal aorta	Visceral branches:
	1 Celiac axis (or artery), which branches into gastric, hepatic, and splenic arteries (stomach, liver, and spleen)
	2 Right and left suprarenal arteries (suprarenal glands)
	3 Superior mesenteric artery (small intestine)
	4 Right and left renal arteries (kidneys)
	5 Right and left spermatic (or ovarian) arteries (testes or ovaries)
	6 Inferior mesenteric artery (large intestine)
	Parietal branches to lower surface of diaphragm, muscles and skin of back, spinal cord, and meninges
	Right and left common iliac arteries—abdominal aorta terminates in these vessels in an inverted Y formation
Right and left common iliac	Internal iliac or hypogastric (pelvic wall and viscera)
	External iliac (to leg)
External iliac (right and left)	Femoral (continuation of external iliac after it leaves abdominal cavity)
Femoral	Popliteal (continuation of femoral)
Popliteal	Anterior tibial
	Posterior tibial
Anterior and posterior tibial	Plantar arch (arterial arch in sole of foot formed by anastomosis of terminal branches of anterior and posterior tibial arteries; small arteries lead from arch to toes)

*The right and left vertebral arteries extend from their origin as branches of the subclavian arteries up the neck, through foramina in the transverse processes of the cervical vertebrae, and through the foramen magnum into the cranial cavity and unite on the undersurface of the brainstem to form the *basilar artery,* which shortly branches into the right and left *posterior cerebral arteries.* The internal carotid arteries enter the cranial cavity in the midpart of the cranial floor, where they become known as the *anterior cerebral arteries.* Small vessels, the *communicating arteries,* join the anterior and posterior cerebral arteries in such a way as to form an arterial circle (the *circle of Willis*) at the base of the brain, a good example of arterial anastomosis.

APPENDIX 4 • Prefixes and Suffixes

The ability to break down medical terms into separate components or to recognize a complete word depends on the mastery of the combining forms (a stem or root with an "o" attached), roots or stems that appear in medical terms, and prefixes and suffixes that alter or modify meaning and usage of a term.

PREFIXES

Prefixes, the most frequently used elements in the formation of Greek and Latin words, consist of one or more syllables (prepositions or adverbs) placed before words or roots to show various kinds of relationships. They are never used independently, but when added before verbs, adjectives, or nouns, they modify the meaning. Most prefixes are a part of words in ordinary speech and do not refer specifically to medical or scientific terminology, but many occur frequently in medical terminology.

Prefix	Translation of Greek or Latin	Examples
a (an before vowel)	Without, lack of	Apathy (lack of feeling), apnea (without breath), aphasia (without speech), anemia (lack of blood)
ab	Away from	Abductor (leading away from), aboral (away from mouth)
ad	To, toward, near to	Adductor (leading toward), adhesion (sticking to), adnexia (structures joined to), adrenal (near the kidney)
ambi	Both	Ambidextrous (ability to use hands equally), ambilaterally (both sides)
amphi	About, on both sides, both	Amphibious (living on both land and in water)
ampho	Both	Amphogenic (producing offspring of both sexes)
ana	Up, back, again, excessive	Anatomy (a cutting up), anagenesis (reproduction of tissue) anasarca (excessive serum in cellular tissues of body)
ante	Before, forward	Antecubital (before elbow), anteflexion (forward bending)
anti	Against, opposed to, reversed	Antiperistalsis (reversed peristalsis), antisepsis (against infection)
apo	From, away from	Apolepsis (stopping a function)
bi	Twice, double	Biarticulate (double joint), bifocal (two foci), bifurcation (two branches)
cata	Down, according to, complete	Catabolism (breaking down), catalepsy (diminished movement)
circum	Around, about	Circumflex (winding about), circumference (surrounding), circumarticular (around joint)
com	With, together	Commissure (sending or coming together)
con	With, together	Conductor (leading together), concrescence (growing together), concentric (having a common center)
contra	Against, opposite	Contralateral (opposite side), contraception (prevention of conception), contraindicated (not indicated)
de	Away from	Dehydrate (remove water), dedentition (removal of teeth), decompensation (failure of compensation)
dia	Through, apart, across, completely	Diaphragm (wall across), diapedesis (ooze through), diagnosis (complete knowledge)
dis	Reversal, apart from, separation	Disinfection (apart from infection), disparity (apart from equality), dissect (cut apart)
e, ex	Out, away from	Enucleate (remove from), eviscerate (take out viscera or bowels), exostosis (outgrowth of bone)
ec	Out from	Ectopic (out of place), eccentric (away from center), ectasia (stretching out or dilation)
ecto	On outer side, situated on	Ectoderm (outer skin), ectoretina (outer layer of retina)
em, en	In	Empyema (pus in), encephalon (in the brain)
endo	Within	Endocardium (within heart), endometrium (within uterus)
epi	Upon, on	Epidural (upon dura), epidermis (on skin)
exo	Outside, on outer side, outer layer	Exogenous (originating outside), exocolitis (inflammation of outer coat of colon)
extra	Outside	Extracellular (outside cell), extrapleural (outside pleura)

Prefix	Translation of Greek or Latin	Examples
hyper (hy′per)	Over, above, excessive	Hyperemia (excessive blood), hypertrophy (overgrowth), hyperplasia (excessive formation)
hypo (hi′po)	Under, below, deficient	Hypotension (low blood pressure), hypothyroidism (deficiency or underfunction of thyroid)
im, in	In, into	Immersion (act of dipping in), infiltration (act of filtering in), injection (act of forcing fluid into)
im, in	Not	Immature (not mature), involuntary (not voluntary), inability (not able)
infra	Below	Infraorbital (below eye), infraclavicular (below clavicle or collar bone)
inter	Between	Intercostal (between ribs), intervene (come between)
intra	Within	Intracerebral (within cerebrum), intraocular (within eye), intraventricular (within ventricles)
intro	Into, within	Introversion (turning inward), introduce (lead into)
meta	Beyond, after, change	Metamorphosis (change of form), metastasis (beyond original position), metacarpal (beyond wrist)
opistho	Behind, backward	Opisthotic (behind ears), opisthognathous (beyond jaws)
para	Beside, beyond, near to	Paracardiac (beside the heart), paraurethral (near the urethra)
per	Through, excessive	Permeate (pass through), perforate (bore through), peracute (excessively acute)
peri	Around	Periosteum (around bone), periatrial (around atrium), peribronchial (around bronchus)
post	After, behind	Postoperative (after operation), postpartum (after childbirth), postocular (behind eye)
pre	Before, in front of	Premaxillary (in front of maxilla), preoral (in front of mouth)
pro	Before, in front of	Prognosis (foreknowledge), projection (throw forward)
re	Back, again, contrary	Reflex (bend back), revert (turn again to), regurgitation (backward flowing, contrary to normal)
retro	Backward, located behind	Retrocervical (located behind cervix), retrograde (going backward), retrolingual (behind tongue)
sub	Under	Subcutaneous (under skin), subarachnoid (under arachnoid), subungual (under nail)
super	Above, upper, excessive	Supercilia (upper brows), supernumerary (excessive number), supermedial (above middle)
supra	Above, upon	Suprarenal (above kidney), suprasternal (above sternum), suprascapular (on upper part of scapula)
sym, syn	Together, with	Symphysis (growing together), synapsis (joining together), synarthrosis (articulation of joints together)
trans	Across, through, beyond	Transection (cut across), transduodenal (through duodenum), transmit (send beyond)
ultra	Beyond, in excess	Ultraviolet (beyond violet end of spectrum), ultraligation (ligation of vessel beyond point of origin), ultrasonic (sound waves beyond the upper frequency of hearing by human ear)

SUFFIXES

Suffixes are the one or more syllables or elements added to the root or stem of a word (the part that indicates the essential meaning) to alter the meaning or indicate the intended part of speech.

To make a word pronounceable, the last letter or letters of the root to which the suffix is attached may be changed. The last vowel may be changed to an "o," or an "o" may be inserted if it is not already present before a suffix beginning with a consonant, as in cardiology. The final vowel in the root may be dropped before a suffix beginning with a vowel, as in neuritis.

Most suffixes are in common use in English, but some are peculiar to medical science. The suffixes most commonly used to indicate disease are *itis,* meaning inflammation; *oma,* meaning tumor; and *osis,* meaning a condition, usually morbid. The suffixes listed occur often in medical terminology, but they are also in use in ordinary language. These suffixes apply to Greek and Latin words.

Suffix	Use	Examples
ize, ate	Add to nouns or adjectives to make verbs expressing to use and to act like, to subject to, make into	Visualize (able to see), impersonate (act like), hypnotize (put into state of hypnosis)
ist, or, er	Add to verbs to make nouns expressing agent or person concerned or instrument	Anesthetist (one who practices the science of anesthesia), dissector (instrument that dissects or person who dissects), donor (one who donates)
ent	Add to verbs to make adjectives or nouns of agency	Recipient (one who receives), concurrent (happening at the same time)
sia, y, tion	Add to verbs to make nouns expressing action, process, or condition	Therapy (treatment), inhalation (act of inhaling), anesthesia (process or condition of not feeling)
ia, ity	Add to adjectives or nouns to make nouns expressing quality or condition	Septicemia (poisoning of blood), disparity (inequality), acidity (condition of excess acid), neuralgia (pain in nerves)
ma, mata, men, mina, ment, ure	Add to verbs to make nouns expressing result of action or object of action	Trauma (injury), foramina (openings), ligament (tough fibrous band holding bone or viscera together), fissure (groove)
ium, olus, olum, culus, culum, cule, cle	Add to nouns to make diminutive nouns	Bacterium, alveolus (air sac), follicle (little bag), cerebellum (little brain), molecule (little mass), ossicle (little bone)
ible, ile	Add to verbs to make adjectives expressing ability or capacity	Contractile (ability to contract), edible (capable of being eaten), flexible (capable of being bent)
al, c, ious, tic	Add to nouns to make adjectives expressing relationship, concern, or pertaining to	Neural (referring to nerve), neoplastic (referring to neoplasm), cardiac (referring to the heart), delirious (suffering from delirium)
id	Add to verbs or nouns to make adjectives expressing state or condition	Flaccid (state of being weak or lax), fluid (state of being liquid)
tic	Add to a verb to make an adjective showing relationship	Caustic (referring to burn), acoustic (referring to sound or hearing)
oid, form	Add to nouns to make adjectives expressing resemblance	Polypoid (resembling polyp), plexiform (resembling a plexus), fusiform (resembling a fusion), epidermoid (resembling epidermis)
ous	Add to nouns to make adjectives expressing material	Ferrous (composed of iron), serous (composed of serum), mucinous (composed of mucin)

APPENDIX 5 • Normal laboratory values

5-1. Tables of normal values

ABBREVIATIONS USED IN TABLES

<	less than
>	greater than
dl	deciliter, 100 ml
g	gram (SI)
gm	gram
IU	International Unit
kg	kilogram
kPa	kilopascal (SI)
kU	kilounit
l	liter
mEq	milliequivalent
mg	milligram
ml	milliliter
mM	millimole
mmol	millimole (SI)
mmHg	millimeters of mercury
mIU	milliInternational Unit
mOsm	milliosmole
mμ	millimicron
MUU	mouse uterine units
ng	nanogram
nmol	nanomole
pg	picogram
pMol	picomole
μEq	microequivalent
μg	microgram
μIU	microInternational Unit
μl	microliter
μM	micromole
μU	microunit
s	second
U	unit

Whole blood, serum, and plasma chemistry

Component	System	Typical reference intervals		
		In conventional units	Factor*	In SI units†
Acetoacetic acid				
Qualitative	Serum	Negative		Negative
Quantitative	Serum	0.2-1.0 mg/dl	98	19.6-98.0 μmol/l
Acetone				
Qualitative	Serum	Negative		Negative
Quantitative	Serum	0.3-2.0 mg/dl	172	51.6-344.0 μmol/l
Albumin, quantitative	Serum	3.2-4.5 gm/dl (salt fractionation)	10	32-45 g/l
		3.2-5.6 gm/dl (electrophoresis)	10	32-56 g/l
		3.8-5.0 gm/dl (dye binding)	10	38-50 g/l
Alcohol, ethyl	Serum or whole blood	Negative—but not presented as mg/dl	0.22	Negative—but presented as mmol/l
Aldolase	Serum: adults	3-8 Sibley-Lehninger U/dl at 37° C	7.4	22-59 mU/l at 37° C
	children	Approximately 2 times adult levels		Approximately 2 times adult levels
	newborn	Approximately 4 times adult levels		Approximately 4 times adult levels
Alpha-amino acid nitrogen	Serum	3.6-7.0 mg/dl	0.714	2.6-5.0 mmol/l
δ-Aminolevulinic acid	Serum	0.01-0.03 mg/dl	76.3	0.76-2.29 μmol/l
Ammonia	Plasma	20-120 μg/dl (diffusion)	0.554	22.2-44.3 μmol/l
		40-80 μg/dl (enzymatic method)	0.554	11.1-67.0 μmol/l
		12-48 μg/dl (resin method)	0.554	6.7-26.6 μmol/l
Amylase	Serum	60-160 Somogyi units/dl	1.85	111-296 IU/l
Argininosuccinate lyase	Serum	0-4 U/dl	10	0-40 IU/l
Arsenic‡	Whole blood	<7 μg/dl	0.13	<0.91 μmol/l
Ascorbic acid (vitamin C)	Plasma	0.6-1.6 mg/dl	56.8	34-91 μmol/l
	Whole blood	0.7-2.0 mg/dl	56.8	40-114 μmol/l
Barbiturates	Serum, plasma, or whole blood	Negative	—	Negative
Base excess	Whole blood			
	male	−3.3 to +1.2 mEq/l	1	−3.3 to +1.2 mmol/l
	female	−2.4 to +2.3 mEq/l	1	−2.4 to +2.3 mmol/l
Base, total	Serum	145-160 mEq/l	1	145-160 mmol/l
Bicarbonate	Plasma	21-28 mM	1	21-28 mmol/l
Bile acids	Serum	0.3-3.0 mg/dl	10	3.0-30.0 mg/l
Bilirubin	Serum			
Direct (conjugated)		Up to 0.3 mg/dl	17.1	Up to 5.1 μmol/l
Indirect (unconjugated)		0.1-1.0 mg/dl	17.1	1.7-17.1 μmol/l
Total		0.1-1.2 mg/dl	17.1	1.7-20.5 μmol/l
Newborn total		1-12 mg/dl	17.1	17.1-205.0 μmol/l
Blood gases				
pH	Whole blood	7.38-7.44 (arterial)	1	7.38-7.44
		7.36-7.41 (venous)	1	7.36-7.41
Pco_2	Whole blood	35-40 mmHg (arterial)	0.133	4.66-5.32 kPa
		40-45 mmHg (venous)	0.133	5.32-5.99 kPa
Po_2	Whole blood	95-100 mmHg (arterial)	0.133	12.64-13.30 kPa
Bromide	Serum	0-5 mg/dl	0.125	0-0.63 mmol/l
BSP (Bromsulphalein) (5 mg/kg)	Serum	Less than 6% retention 45 min after injection	0.01	Less than 0.06 retention 45 min after injection

*Factor—Number factor (note that units are not presented).

†Value in SI units—Value in conventional units × factor.

‡Usually not measured in blood (preferred specimen is urine, hair, or nails except in acute cases when gastric contents are used).

Whole blood, serum, and plasma chemistry—cont'd

Component	System	Typical reference intervals		
		In conventional units	Factor*	In SI units†
Calcium				
Ionized	Serum	4-4.8 mg/dl	0.25	1.0-1.2 mmol/l
		2.0-2.4 mEq/l	0.5	
		30-58% of total	0.01	0.30-0.58 of total
Total		9.2-11.0 mg/dl	0.25	2.3-2.8 mmol/l
		4.6-5.5 mEq/l	0.5	23-28 mmol/l
Carbon dioxide (CO_2 content)	Whole blood (arterial)	19-24 mM	1	19-24 mmol/l
	Plasma or serum (arterial)	21-28 mM	1	21-28 mmol/l
Carbon dioxide	Whole blood (venous)	22-26 mM	1	22-26 mmol/l
	Plasma or serum (venous)	24-30 mM	1	24-30 mmol/l
CO_2 combining power	Plasma or serum (venous)	24-30 mM	1	24-30 mmol/l
CO_2 partial pressure (PCO_2)	Whole blood (arterial)	35-40 mmHg	0.133	4.66-5.32 kPa
	Whole blood (venous)	40-45 mmHg	0.133	5.32-5.99 kPa
Carbonic acid (H_2CO_3)	Whole blood (arterial)	1.05-1.45 mM	1	1.05-1.45 mmol/l
	Whole blood (venous)	1.15-1.50 mM	1	1.15-1.50 mmol/l
	Plasma (venous)	1.02-1.38 mM	1	1.02-1.38 mmol/l
Carboxyhemoglobin (carbon monoxide hemoglobin)	Whole blood Suburban non-smokers	< 1.5% saturation of hemoglobin	0.01	< 0.015 saturation of hemoglobin
	Smokers	1.5-5.0% saturation	0.01	0.015-0.050 saturation
	Heavy smokers	5.0-9.0% saturation	0.01	0.050-0.090 saturation
Carotene, beta	Serum	40-200 µg/dl	0.0186	0.75-3.72 µmol/l
Ceruloplasmin	Serum	23-50 mg/dl	10	230-500 mg/l
Chloride	Serum	95-103 mEq/l	1	95-103 mmol/l
Cholesterol				
Total	Serum	150-250 mg/dl (varies with diet, sex, and age)	0.026	3.90-6.50 mmol/l
Esters	Serum	65-75% of total cholesterol	0.01	0.65-0.75 of total cholesterol
Cholinesterase	Erythrocytes	0.65-1.3 pH units	1	0.65-1.3 units
(Pseudocholinesterase)	Plasma	0.5-1.3 pH units	1	0.5-1.3 units
		8-18 IU/l at 37° C	1	8-18 U/l at 37° C
Citrate	Serum or plasma	1.7-3.0 mg/dl	52	88-156 µmol/l
Copper	Serum, plasma			
Male		70-140 µg/dl	0.157	11.0-22.0 µmol/l
Female		80-155 µg/dl	0.157	12.6-24.3 µmol/l
Cortisol	Plasma			
8 AM-10 PM		5-23 µg/dl	27.6	138-635 nmol/l
4 PM-6PM		3-13 µg/dl	27.6	83-359 nmol/l
Creatine as creatinine	Serum or plasma			
Male		0.1-0.4 mg/dl	76.3	7.6-30.5 µmol/l
Female		0.2-0.7 mg/dl	76.3	15.3-53.4 µmol/l
Creatine kinase (CK)	Serum			
Male		55-170 U/l at 37° C	1	55-170 U/l at 37° C
Female		30-135 U/l at 37° C	1	30-135 U/l at 37° C
Creatinine	Serum or plasma	0.6-1.2 mg/dl (adult)	88.4	53-106 µmol/l
		0.3-0.6 mg/dl (children <2 yr)	88.4	27-54 µmol/l

Whole blood, serum, and plasma chemistry—cont'd

Component	System	Typical reference intervals		
		In conventional units	Factor*	In SI units†
Creatinine clearance (endogenous)	Serum or plasma and urine			
	Male	107-139 ml/min	0.167	1.78-2.32 ml/s
	Female	87-107 ml/min	0.0167	1.45-1.79 ml/s
Cryoglobulins	Serum	Negative	—	Negative
Electrophoresis				
Protein	Serum	Percent	0.01	0.52-0.65 of total protein
Albumin		52-65% of total protein	0.01	0.025-0.05 of total protein
Alpha-1		2.5-5.0% of total protein	0.01	0.07-0.13 of total protein
Alpha-2		7.0-13.0% of total protein	0.01	0.08-0.14 of total protein
Beta		8.0-14.0% of total protein	0.01	0.12-0.22 of total protein
Gamma		12.0-22.0% of total protein		
	Serum	Concentration	10	32-56 g/l
Albumin		3.2-5.6 gm/dl		1-4 g/l
Alpha-1		0.1-0.4 gm/dl		4-12 g/l
Alpha-2		0.4-1.2 gm/dl		5-11 g/l
Beta		0.5-1.1 gm/dl		5-16 g/l
Gamma		0.5-1.6 gm/dl		
Fats, neutral (see Triglycerides)				
Fatty acids				
Total (free and esterified)	Serum	9-15 mM	1	9-15 mmol/l
Free (non-esterified)	Plasma	300-480 μEq/l	1	300-480 μmol/l
Fibrinogen	Plasma	200-400 mg/dl	0.01	2.00-4.00 g/l
Fluoride	Whole blood	< 0.05 mg/dl	0.53	< 0.027 mmol/l
Folate	Serum	5-25 ng/ml (bioassay)	2.27	11-56 nmol/l
		> 2.3 ng/ml (radioassay)	2.27	> 5.2 nmol/l
	Erythrocytes	166-640 ng/ml (bioassay)	2.27	376-1452 nmol/l
		> 140 ng/ml (radioassay)	2.27	> 318 nmol/l
Galactose	Whole blood			
	Adults	None	0.055	None
	Children	< 20 mg/dl	0.055	< 1.1 mmol/l
Gamma globulin	Serum	0.5-1.6 gm/dl	10	5-16 g/l
Globulins, total	Serum	2.3-3.5 gm/dl	10	23-35 g/l
Glucose, fasting	Serum or plasma	70-110 mg/dl	0.055	3.85-6.05 mmol/l
	Whole blood	60-100 mg/dl	0.055	3.30-5.50 mmol/l
Glucose tolerance	Serum or plasma			
Oral	Fasting	70-110 mg/dl	0.055	3.85-6.05 mmol/l
	30 min	30-60 mg/dl above fasting	0.055	1.65-3.30 mmol/l above fasting
	60 min	20-50 mg/dl above fasting	0.055	1.10-2.75 mmol/l above fasting
	120 min	5-15 mg/dl above fasting	0.055	0.28-0.83 mmol/l above fasting
	180 min	Fasting level or below	0.055	Fasting level or below
	Serum or plasma			
Intravenous	Fasting	70-110 mg/dl	0.055	3.85-6.05 mmol/l
	5 min	Max of 250 mg/dl	0.055	Max of 13.75 mmol/l
	60 min	Significant decrease	0.055	Significant decrease
	120 min	Below 120 mg/dl	0.055	Below 6.60 mmol/l
	180 min	Fasting level	0.055	Fasting level

*Factor—Number factor (note that units are not presented).
†Value in SI units—Value in conventional units × factor.
‡Usually not measured in blood (preferred specimen is urine, hair, or nails except in acute cases when gastric contents are used).

Whole blood, serum, and plasma chemistry—cont'd

Component	System	Typical reference intervals		
		In conventional units	Factor*	In SI units†
Glucose 6-phosphate dehydrogenase (G6PD)	Erythrocytes	250-500 units/10^6 cells	1	250-500 units/10^6 cells
		1200-2000 mIU/ml packed erythrocytes	1	1200-2000 U/l packed erythrocytes
γ-Glutamyl transferase	Serum	5-40 IU/l	1	5-40 U/l at 37° C
Glutathione	Whole blood	24-37 mg/dl	0.032	0.77-1.18 mmol/l
Growth hormone	Serum	<10 ng/ml	1	<10 μg/l
Guanase	Serum	<3 nM/ml/min	1	<3 U/l at 37° C
Haptoglobin	Serum	60-270 mg/dl	.01	0.6-2.7 g/l
Hemoglobin	Serum or plasma			
Qualitative		Negative	10	Negative
Quantitative		0.5-5.0 mg/dl	10	5-50 mg/l
	Whole blood			
Female		12.0-16.0 gm/dl	10	1.86-2.48 mmol/l
Male		13.5-18.0 gm/dl	10	2.09-2.79 mmol/l
α-Hydroxybutyric dehydrogenase	Serum	140-350 U/ml	1	140-350 kU/l
17-Hydroxycorticosteroids	Plasma			
Male		7-19 μg/dl	10	70-190 μg/l
Female		9-21 μg/dl	10	9-21 μg/l
After 24 USP units of ACTH IM		35-55 μg/dl	10	350-550 μg/l
Immunoglobulins	Serum			
IgG		800-1801 mg/dl	0.01	8.0-18.0 g/l
IgA		113-563 mg/dl	0.01	1.1-5.6 g/l
IgM		54-222 mg/dl	0.01	0.54-2.2 g/l
IgD		0.5-3.0 mg/dl	10	5.0-30 mg/l
IgE		0.01-0.04 mg/dl	10	0.1-0.4 mg/dl
Insulin	Plasma			
Bioassay		11-240 μIU/ml	0.0417	0.46-10.00 μg/l
Radioimmunoassay		4-24 μIU/ml	0.0417	0.17-1.00 μg/l
Insulin tolerance (0.1 unit/kg)	Serum			
Fasting		Glucose of 70-110 mg/dl	0.055	Glucose of 3.85-6.05 mmol/l
30 min		Fall to 50% of fasting level	0.01^b	Fall to 0.5 of fasting level
90 min		Fasting level		Fasting level
Iodine				
Butanol-extractable (BEI)	Serum	3.5-6.5 μg/dl	0.079	0.28-0.51 μmol/l
Protein-bound (PBI)	Serum	4.0-8.0 μg/dl		0.32-0.63 μmol/l
Iron, total	Serum	60-150 μg/dl	0.179	11-27 μmol/l
Iron binding capacity	Serum	300-360 μg/dl	0.179	54-64 μmol/l
Iron saturation	Serum	20-55%	0.01^b	0.20-0.55 of total iron binding capacity
Isocitric dehydrogenase	Serum	50-240 units/ml at 25° C (Wolfson-Williams Ashman units)	0.0167	0.83-4.18 U/l at 25° C
Ketone bodies	Serum	Negative	—	Negative
17-Ketosteroids	Plasma	25-125 μg/dl	0.01	0.25-1.25 mg/l
Lactic acid (as lactate)	Whole blood			
Venous		5-20 mg/dl	0.111	0.6-2.2 mmol/l
Arterial		3-7 mg/dl		0.3-0.8 mmol/l
Lactate dehydrogenase (LDH)	Serum	80-120 units at 30° C (lactate → pyruvate)	0.48	38-62 U/l at 30° C (lactate → pyruvate)
		185-640 units at 30° C (pyruvate → lactate)	0.48	90-310 U/l at 30° C (pyruvate → lactate)
		100-190 IU/l at 37° C (lactate → pyruvate)	1	100-190 U/l at 37° C (lactate → pyruvate)

Whole blood, serum, and plasma chemistry—cont'd

Component	System	Typical reference intervals		
		In conventional units	Factor*	In SI units†
Lactate dehydrogenase iso-enzymes	Serum			
LDH$_1$ (anode)		17-27%	0.01	0.17-0.27 of total LDH
LDH$_2$		27-37%		0.27-0.37 of total LDH
LDH$_3$		18-25%		0.18-0.25 of total LDH
LDH$_4$		3-8%		0.03-0.08 of total LDH
LDH$_5$ (cathode)		0.5%		0.00-0.05 of total LDH
Lactate dehydrogenase (heat stable)	Serum	30-60%	0.01	0.3-0.6 of total LDH
Lactose tolerance	Serum	Serum glucose changes similar to glucose tolerance test	—	Serum glucose changes similar to glucose tolerance test
Lead	Whole blood	0-50 μg/dl	0.048	0.2-4 μmol/l
Leucine aminopeptidase (LAP)	Serum			
Male		80-200 U/ml (Goldbarg-Rutenberg)	0.24	19.2-48.0 U/l
Female		75-185 U/ml (Goldbarg-Rutenberg)	0.24	18.0-44.4 U/l
Lipase	Serum	0-1.5 U/ml (Cherry-Crandall)	278	0-417 U/l
		14-280 mIU/ml	1	14-280 U/l
Lipids, total	Serum	400-800 mg/dl	0.01	4.00-8.00 g/l
Cholesterol		150-250 mg/dl	0.026	3.9-6.5 mmol/l
Triglycerides		10-190 mg/dl	0.109	1.09-20.71 mmol/l
Phospholipids		150-380 mg/dl	0.01	1.50-380 g/l
Fatty acids (free)		9.0-15.0 mM/l	1	9.0-15.0 mmol/l
		300-480 μEq/l	0.01	300-480 μmol/l
Phospholipid phosphorous		8.0-11.0 mg/dl	0.323	2.58-3.55 mmol/l
Lithium	Serum	Negative	—	Negative
Therapeutic interval		0.5-1.4 mEq/l	1	0.5-1.4 mmol/l
Long-acting thyroid-stimulating hormone (LATS)	Serum	None	—	None
Luteinizing hormone (LH)	Serum			
Male		6-30 mIU/ml	0.23	1.4-6.9 mg/l
Female		Midcycle peak: 3 times baseline value	0.23	Midcycle peak: 3 times baseline value
		Premenopausal <30 mIU/ml	0.23	Premenopausal <5 times baseline value
		Postmenopausal >35 mIU/ml		Postmenopausal >5 times baseline value
Macroglobulins, total	Serum	70-430 mg/dl	0.01	0.7-4.3 g/l
Magnesium	Serum	1.3-2.1 mEq/l	0.5	0.7-1.1 mmol/l
		1.8-3.0 mg/dl	0.41	0.7-1.1 mmol/l
Methemoglobin	Whole blood	0-0.24 gm/dl	10	0.2-2.4 g/l
		<3% of total hemoglobin	0.01	<.03 of total hemoglobin
Mucoprotein	Serum	80-200 mg/dl	0.01	0.8-2.0 g/l
Non-protein nitrogen (NPN)	Serum or plasma	20-35 mg/dl	0.714	14.3-25.0 mmol/l
	Whole blood	25-50 mg/dl	0.714	17.9-35.7 mmol/l
5'Nucleotidase	Serum	0-1.6 units at 37° C	1	0-1.6 units at 37° C
Ornithine carbamyl transferase	Serum	8-20 mIU/ml at 37° C	1	8-20 U/l at 37° C
Osmolality	Serum	280-295 mOsm/kg	1	280-295 mOsm/l

*Factor—Number factor (note that units are not presented).
†Value in SI units—Value in conventional units × factor.
‡Usually not measured in blood (preferred specimen is urine, hair, or nails except in acute cases when gastric contents are used).

Whole blood, serum, and plasma chemistry—cont'd

Component	System	Typical reference intervals		
		In conventional units	Factor*	In SI units†
Oxygen				
Pressure (Po₂)	Whole blood (arterial)	95-100 mmHg	0.133	12.64-13.30 kPa
Content	Whole blood (arterial)	15-23 volume %	0.01	0.15-0.23 of volume
Saturation	Whole blood (arterial)	94-100%	0.01	0.94-1.00 of total
pH	Whole blood (arterial)	7.38-7.44	1	7.38-7.44
	Whole blood (venous)	7.36-7.41	1	7.36-7.41
	Serum or plasma (venous)	7.35-7.45	1	7.35-7.45
Phenylalanine	Serum			
Adults		<3.0 mg/dl	0.061	<0.18 mmol/l
Newborns (term)		1.2-3.5 mg/dl	0.061	0.07-0.21 mmol/l
Phosphatase				
Acid phosphatase	Serum	0.13-0.63 U/l at 37° C (paranitrophenylphosphate)	16.67	2.2-10.5 U/l at 37° C (p-nitrophenylphosphate)
Alkaline phosphatase	Serum	20-90 IU/l at 30° C (paranitro-phenylphosphate in AMP buffer)	1	20-90 U/l at 30° C (p-nitrophenylphosphate) 25-97 U/l at 37° C (p-nitrophenylphosphate)
Phospholipid phosphorus	Serum	8-11 mg/dl	0.323	2.6-3.6 mmol/l
Phospholipids	Serum	150-380 mg/dl	0.01	1.50-3.80 g/l
Phosphorus, inorganic	Serum			
Adults		2.3-4.7 mg/dl	0.323	0.78-1.52 mmol/l
Children		4.0-7.0 mg/dl	0.323	1.29-2.26 mmol/l
Potassium	Plasma	3.8-5.0 mEq/l	1	3.8-5.0 mmol/l
Prolactin	Serum	1-25 ng/ml (females)	1	1-25 μg/l
		1-20 ng/ml (males)	1	1-20 μg/l
Proteins	Serum			
Total		6.0-7.8 g/dl	10	60-78 g/l
Albumin		3.2-4.5 g/dl	10	32-45 g/l
Globulin		2.3-3.5 g/dl	10	23-35 g/l
Protein fractionation		See Electrophoresis		See Electrophoresis
Protoporphyrin	Erythrocytes	15-50 μg/dl	0.018	0.27-0.90 μmol/l
Pyruvate	Whole blood	0.3-0.9 mg/dl	114	34-103 μmol/l
Salicylates	Serum	Negative	—	Negative
Therapeutic interval		15-30 mg/dl	0.072	1.44-1.80 mmol/l
		150-300 μg/ml	0.0072	1.08-2.16 mmol/l
Sodium	Plasma	136-142 mEq/l	1	136-142 mmol/l
Sulfate, inorganic	Serum	0.2-1.3 mEq/l	0.5	0.10-0.65 mmol/l
		0.9-6.0 mg/dl as SO₄⁻⁻	0.104	0.09-0.62 mmol/l as SO₄⁻⁻
Sulfhemoglobin	Whole blood	Negative	—	Negative
Sulfonamides	Serum or whole blood	Negative	—	Negative
Testosterone	Serum or plasma			
Male		300-1200 ng/dl	0.035	10.0-42.0 nmol/l
Female		30-95 ng/dl	0.035	1.1-3.3 nmol/l
Thiocyanate	Serum	Negative	—	Negative
Thymol flocculation	Serum	0-5 units	1	0-5 units

Whole blood, serum, and plasma chemistry—cont'd

Component	System	Typical reference intervals		
		In conventional units	Factor*	In SI units†
Thyroid hormone tests	Serum			
(a) Expressed as thyroxine				
T_4 by column		5.0-11.0 μg/dl	13.0	65-143 nmol/l
T_4 by competitive binding—Murphy-Pattee		6.0-11.8 μg/dl	13.0	78-153 nmol/l
T_4 RIA		5.5-12.5 μg/dl	13.0	72-163 nmol/l
free T_4		0.9-2.3 ng/dl	13.0	12-30 pmol/l
(b) Expressed as iodine				
T_4 by column		3.2-7.2 μg/dl	79.0	253-569 nmol/l
T_4 by competitive binding—Murphy-Pattee		3.9-7.7 μg/dl	79.0	308-608 nmol/l
free T_4		0.6-1.5 ng/dl		47-119 pmol/l
T_3 resin uptake		25-38 relative % uptake	0.01	0.25-0.38 relative uptake
Thyroxine-binding globulin (TBG)	Serum	10-26 μg/dl	10	100-260 μg/l
TSH	Serum	<10 μU/ml	1	<10^{-3} IU/l
Transferases				
Aspartate amino transferase (AST or SGOT)	Serum	10-40 U/ml (Karmen) at 25° C	0.48	8-29 U/l at 30° C
		16-60 U/ml (Karmen) at 30° C		8-33 U/l at 37° C
Alanine amino transferase (ALT or SGPT)	Serum	10-30 U/ml (Karmen) at 25° C		
		8-50 U/ml (Karmen) at 30° C	0.48	4-24 U/l at 30° C
				4-36 U/l at 37° C
Gamma glutamyl transferase (GGT)		5-40 IU/l at 37° C	1	5.40 U/l at 37° C
Triglycerides	Serum	10-190 mg/dl	0.011	0.11-2.09 mmol/l
Urea nitrogen	Serum	8-23 mg/dl	0.357	2.9-8.2 mmol/l
Urea clearance	Serum and urine			
Maximum clearance		64-99 ml/min	0.0167	1.07-1.65 ml/s
Standard clearance		41-65 ml/min, or more than 75% of normal clearance	0.0167	0.68-1.09 ml/s or more than 0.75 of normal clearance
Uric acid	Serum			
Male		4.0-8.5 mg/dl	0.059	0.24-0.5 mmol/l
Female		2.7-7.3 mg/dl	0.059	0.16-0.43 mmol/l
Vitamin A	Serum	15-60 μg/dl	0.035	0.53-2.10 μmol/l
Vitamin A tolerance	Serum			
Fasting 3 hr or 6 hr after 5000 units vitamin		15-60 μg/dl	0.035	0.53-2.10 μmol/l
A/kg 24 hrs		200-600 μg/dl Fasting values or slightly above		7.00-21.00 μmol/l Fasting values or slightly above
Vitamin B_{12}	Serum	160-950 pg/ml	0.74	118-703 pmol/l
Unsaturated vitamin B_{12} binding capacity	Serum	1000-2000 pg/ml	0.74	740-1480 pmol/l
Vitamin C	Plasma	0.6-1.6 mg/dl	56.8	34-91 μmol/l

*Factor—Number factor (note that units are not presented).
†Value in SI units—Value in conventional units × factor.
‡Usually not measured in blood (preferred specimen is urine, hair, or nails except in acute cases when gastric contents are used).

Whole blood, serum, and plasma chemistry—cont'd

Component	System	Typical reference intervals		
		In conventional units	Factor*	In SI units†
Xylose absorption	Serum			
	Normal	25-40 mg/dl between 1 and 2 hr	0.067	1.68-2.68 mmol/l between 1 and 2 hr
	In malabsorption	Maximum approximately 10 mg/dl		Maximum approximately 0.67 mmol/l
Dose				
Adult		25 g D-xylose	0.067	0.167 mol D-xylose
Children		0.5 g/kg D-xylose		3.33 mmol/kg D-xylose
Zinc	Serum	50-150 μg/dl	0.153	7.65-22.95 μmol/l

*Factor—Number factor (note that units are not presented).
†Value in SI units—Value in conventional units × factor.
‡Usually not measured in blood (preferred specimen is urine, hair, or nails except in acute cases when gastric contents are used).

Urine

Component	Type of urine specimen	Typical reference intervals		
		In conventional units	Factor	In SI units
Acetoacetic acid	Random	Negative	—	Negative
Acetone	Random	Negative	—	Negative
Addis count	12-hr collection	WBC and epithelial cells		
		1,800,000/12 hr	1	$1.8 \times 10^6/12$ hr
		RBC 500,000/12 hr	1	$0.5 \times 10^6/12$ hr
		Hyaline casts		
		0-5000/12 hr	1	$5.0 \times 10^3/12$ hr
Albumin				
Qualitative	Random	Negative	—	Negative
Quantitative	24 hr	15-150 mg/24 hr	1	0.015-0.150 g/24 hr
Aldosterone	24 hr	2-26 μg/24 hr	2.77	5.5-72.0 nmol/24 hr
Alkapton bodies	Random	Negative	—	Negative
Alpha-amino acid nitrogen	24 hr	100-290 mg/24 hr	0.0714	7.14-20.71 mmol/24 hr
δ-aminolevulinic acid	Random			
	Adult	0.1-0.6 mg/dl	76.3	7.6-45.8 μmol/l
	Children	<0.5 mg/dl	76.3	<38.1 μmol/l
	24 hr	1.5-7.5 mg/24 hr	7.63	11.15-57.2 μmol/24 hr
Ammonia nitrogen	24 hr	20-7-mEq/24 hr		
		500-1200 mg/24 hr	0.071	35.5-85.2 mmol/24 hr
Amylase	2 hr	35-260 Somogyi units/hr	0.185	6.5-48.1 U/hr
Arsenic	24 hr	<50 μg/l	0.013	<0.65 μM/l
Ascorbic acid	Random	1-7 mg/dl	0.057	0.06-0.40 mmol/l
	24 hr	>50 mg/24 hr	0.0057	>0.29 mmol/24 hr
Bence Jones protein	Random	Negative	—	Negative
Beryllium	24 hr	<0.05 μg/24 hr	111	<5.55 nmol/24 hr
Bilirubin, qualitative	Random	Negative	—	Negative
Blood, occult	Random	Negative	—	Negative
Borate	24 hr	<2 mg/l	16	<32 μmol/l
Calcium				
Qualitative (Sulkowich)	Random	1 + turbidity	1	1 + turbidity
Quantitative	24 hr			
	Average diet	100-240 mg/24 hr	0.025	2.50-6.25 mmol/24 hr
	Low calcium diet	<150 mg/24 hr	0.025	<3.75 mmol/24 hr
	High calcium diet	240-300 mg/24 hr	0.025	6.25-7.50 mmol/24 hr

Urine—cont'd

Component	Type of urine specimen	Typical reference intervals		
		In conventional units	Factor	In SI units
Catecholamines	Random	0-14 µg/dl	0.059	0-0.83 µmol/1
	24 hr	<100 µg/24 hr (varies with activity)	0.0059	<0.59 µmol/24 hr
Epinephrine		<10 ng/24 hr	5.46	<55 nmol/24 hr
Norepinephrine		<100 ng/24 hr	5.91	<590 nmol/24 hr
Total free catecholamines		4-126 µg/24 hr	5.91	24-745 nmol/24 hr
Total metanephrines		0.1-1.6 mg/24 hr	5.07	0.5-8.1 µmol/24 hr
Chloride	24 hr	140-250 mEq/24 hr	1	140-250 mmol/24 hr
Concentration test (Fishberg)	Random—after fluid restriction			
Specific gravity		>1.025	1	>1.025
Osmolality		>850 mOsm/l	1	>850 mOsm/l
Copper	24 hr	0-30 µg/24 hr	0.016	0-0.48 µmol/24 hr
Coproporphyrin	Random			
Adult		3-20 µg/dl	0.015	0.045-0.30 µmol/l
	24 hr			
Adult		50-160 µg/24 hr	0.0015	0.075-0.24 µmol/24 hr
Children		0-80 µg/24 hr	0.0015	0.00-0.12 µmol/24 hr
Creatine	24 hr			
Male		0-40 mg/24 hr	0.0076	0-0.30 mmol/24 hr
Female		0-100 mg/24 hr	0.0076	0-0.76 mmol/24 hr
		Higher in children and during pregnancy		Higher in children and during pregnancy
Creatinine	24 hr			
Male		20-26 mg/kg/24 hr	0.0088	0.18-0.23 mmol/kg/24 hr
		1.0-2.0 g/24 hr	8.8	8.8-17.6 mmol/24 hr
Female		14-22 mg/kg/24 hr	0.0088	0.12-0.19 mmol/kg/24 hr
		0.8-1.8 g/24 hr	8.8	7.0-15.8 mmol/24 hr
Crystine, qualitative	Random	Negative	—	Negative
Crystine and cysteine	24 hr	10-100 mg/24 hr	.0083	0.08-0.83 mmol/24 hr
Diacetic acid	Random	Negative	—	Negative
Epinephrine	24 hr	0-20 µg/24 hr	0.0055	0.00-0.11 µmol/24 hr
Estrogens				
Total	24 hr			
Male		5-18 µg/24 hr	1	5-18 µg/24 hr
Female				
Ovulation		28-100 µg/24 hr	1	28-100 µg/24 hr
Luteal Peak		22-80 µg/24 hr	1	22-80 µg/24 hr
At menses		4-25 µg/24 hr	1	4-25 µg/24 hr
Female				
Pregnancy		Up to 45,000 µg/24 hr	1	Up to 45,000 µg/24 hr
Postmeno-pausal		Up to 10 µg/24 hr	1	Up to 10 µg/24 hr
Fractionated	24 hr nonpreg-nant, midcycle			
Estrone (E[1])	—	2-25 µg/24 hr	3.7	7-93 nmol/24 hr
Estradiol (E[2])	—	0-10 µg/24 hr	3.7	0-37 nmol/24 hr
Estriol (E[3])	—	2-30 µg/24 hr	3.5	7-105 nmol/24 hr
Fat, qualitative	Random	Negative	—	Negative
FIGLU (formiminoglutamic acid)	24 hr	<3 mg/24 hr	5.7	<17.0 µmol/8 hr
	After 15 gm of L-histidine	4 mg/8 hr	5.7	23.0 µmol/8 hr
Fluoride	24 hr	<1 mg/24 hr	0.053	0.053 mmol/24 hr

Urine—cont'd

Component	Type of urine specimen	Typical reference intervals		
		In conventional units	Factor	In SI units
Follicle-stimulating hormone (FSH)	24 hr			
	Adult	6-50 MUU/24 hr	1	4-25 mIU/ml
	Prepubertal	<10 MUU/24 hr	1	4-30 mIU/ml
	Postmeno-pausal	>50 MUU/24 hr	1	40-50 mIU/ml
	Midcycle	2+ baseline		
Fructose	24 hr	30-65 mg/24 hr	0.0056	0.17-0.36 mmol/24 hr
Glucose				
Qualitative	Random	Negative	—	Negative
Quantitative	24 hr			
Copper-reducing substances		0.5-1.5 g/24 hr	1	0.5-1.5 g/24 hr
Total sugars		Average 250 mg/24 hr	1	Average 250 mg/24 hr
Glucose		Average 130 mg/24 hr	0.0056	Average 0.73 mmol/24 hr
Gonadotropins, pituitary (FSH and LH)	24 hr	10-50 MUU/24 hr	1	10-50 MUU/24 hr
Hemoglobin	Random	Negative	—	Negative
Homogentisic acid	Random	Negative	—	Negative
Homovanillic acid (HVA)	24 hr	<15 mg/24 hr	5.5	<83.0 μmol/24 hr
17-Hydroxycorticosteroids	24 hr			
	Male	5.5-14.5 mg/24 hr	1	5.5-145 mg/24 hr
	Female	4.9-12.9 mg/24 hr	1	4.9-12.9 mg/24 hr
5-Hydroxyindoleacetic acid (5-HIAA)				
Qualitative	Random	Negative	—	Negative
Quantitative	24 hr	9 mg/24 hr	5.2	47 μmol/24 hr
Ketone bodies	Random	Negative		Negative
17-Ketosteroids	24 hr			
	Male	8-20 mg/24 hr	1	8.0-20 mg/24 hr
	Female	4-15 mg/24 hr		4.0-15 mg/24 hr
Androsterone	24 hr			
	Male	2.0-5.9 mg/24 hr	3.44	6.9-17.2 μmol/24 hr
	Female	0.8-3.0 mg/24 hr		2.8-10.3 μmol/24 hr
Etiocholanolone	24 hr			
	Male	1.4-5.0 mg/24 hr	3.44	4.8-17.2 μmol/24 hr
	Female	0.8-4.0 mg/24 hr	3.44	2.8-13.8 μmol/24 hr
Dehydroepiandrosterone	24 hr			
	Male	0.2-2.0 mg/24 hr	3.46	0.7-6.9 μmol/24 hr
	Female	0.2-1.8 mg/24 hr	3.46	0.7-6.2 μmol/24 hr
11-Ketoandrosterone	24 hr			
	Male	0.2-1.0 mg/24 hr	3.28	0.7-3.3 μmol/24 hr
	Female	0.2-0.8 mg/24 hr	3.28	0.7-2.6 μmol/24 hr
11-Ketoetiocholanolone	24 hr			
	Male	0.2-1.0 mg/24 hr	3.28	0.7-3.3 μmol/24 hr
	Female	0.2-0.8 mg/24 hr	3.28	0.7-2.6 μmol/24 hr
11-Hydroxyandosterone	24 hr			
	Male	0.1-0.8 mg/24 hr	3.26	0.3-2.6 μmol/24 hr
	Female	0.0-0.5 mg/24 hr	3.26	0.0-1.6 μmol/24 hr
11-Hydroxyetiocholanolone	24 hr			
	Male	0.2-0.6 mg/24 hr	3.26	0.7-2.0 μmol/24 hr
	Female	0.1-1.1 mg/24 hr	3.26	0.3-3.6 μmol/24 hr
Lactose	24 hr	14-40 mg/24 hr	2.9	41-116 μmol/24 hr
Lead	24 hr	<100 μg/24 hr	0.0048	<0.48 μmol/24 hr
Magnesium	24 hr	6.0-8.5 mEq/24 hr	0.5	3.0-4.3 mmol/24 hr
Melanin, qualitative	Random	Negative	—	Negative

Urine—cont'd

Component	Type of urine specimen	Typical reference intervals		
		In conventional units	Factor	In SI units
3-Methoxy-4-hydroxyman-delic acid (VMA)	24 hr			
	Adults	1.5-7.5 mg/24 hr	5.05	7.6-37.9 μmol/24 hr
	Infants	83 μg/kg/24 hr	0.0051	0.4 μmol/kg/24 hr
Mucin	24 hr	100-150 mg/24 hr	1	100-150 mg/24 hr
Myoglobin				
Qualitative	Random	Negative	—	Negative
Quantitative	24 hr	<4 mg/l	1	<4 mg/l
Osmolality	Random	500-800 mOsm/kg water	1	500-800 mOsm/kg water
Pentoses	24 hr	2-5 mg/kg/24 hr	1	2-5 mg/kg/24 hr
pH	Random	4.6-8.0	1	4.6-8.0
Phenolsulfonphthalein (PSP)	Urine timed after 6 mg PSP IV			
	15 min	20-50% dye excreted	0.01	0.2-0.5 dye excreted
	30 min	16-24% dye excreted	0.01	0.16-0.24 dye excreted
	60 min	9-17% dye excreted	0.01	0.09-0.17 dye excreted
	120 min	3-10% dye excreted	0.01	0.03-0.10 dye excreted
Phenylpyruvic acid Qualitative	Random	Negative	—	Negative
Phosphorus	Random	0.9-1.3 g/24 hr	32	29-42 mmol/24 hr
Porphobilinogen				
Qualitative	Random	Negative	—	Negative
Quantitative	24 hr	0-1.0 mg/24 hr	4.42	0-4.4 μmol/24 hr
Potassium	24 hr	40-80 mEq/24 hr	1	40-80 mmol/24 hr
Pregnancy tests	Concentrated morning specimen	Positive in normal pregnancies or with tumors producing chorionic gonadotropin	1	Positive in normal pregnancies or with tumors producing chorionic gonadotropin
Pregnanediol	24 hr			
	Male	0-1.5 mg/24 hr	3.12	0-4.7 μmol/24 hr
	Female	1-8 mg/24 hr	3.12	3-25 μmol/24 hr
	Peak	1 week after ovulation	3.12	1 week after ovulation 156 μmol/24 hr
	Pregnancy	50 mg/24 hr	3.12	
	Children	Negative	—	Negative
Pregnanetriol	24 hr			
	Male	0.4-2.4 mg/24 hr	2.97	1.2-7.1 μmol/24 hr
	Female	0.5-2.0 mg/24 hr	2.97	1.5-5.9 μmol/24 hr
	Children	Up to 1 mg/24 hr	2.97	Up to 3 μmol/24 hr
Protein, qualitative	Random	Negative	—	Negative
	24 hr	40-150 mg/24 hr	1	40-150 mg/24 hr
Reducing substances, total	24 hr	0.5-1.5 mg/24 hr	1	0.5-1.5 mg/24 hr
Sodium	24 hr	75-200 mEq/24 hr	1	75-200 mmol/24 hr
Solids, total	24 hr	55-70 gm/24 hr	1	55-70 g/24 hr
		Decreases with age to 30 gm/24 hr		Decreases with age to 30 g/24 hr
Specific gravity	Random	1.016-1.022 (normal fluid intake)	1	Relative density (urine 20° C/water 20° C)
				1.016-1.022 (normal fluid intake)
		1.001-1.035 (range)		1.001-1.034 (range)
Sugars (excluding glucose)	Random	Negative	—	Negative
Titratable acidity	24 hr	20-50 mEq/24 hr	1	20-50 mmol/24 hr
Urea nitrogen	24 hr	6-17 gm/24 hr	0.0357	0.21-0.60 mol/24 hr
Uric acid	24 hr	250-750 mg/24 hr	0.0059	1.48-4.43 mmol/24 hr

Urine—cont'd

Component	Type of urine specimen	Typical reference intervals		
		In conventional units	Factor	In SI units
Urobilinogen	2 hr	0.3-1.0 Ehrlich units	—	
	24 hr	0.05-2.5 mg/24 hr or 0.5-4.0 Ehrlich units/24 hr	1.69	0.09-4.23 μmol/24 hr
Uropepsin	Random	14-45 units/hr (Anson)	7.37	111-332 U/hr
	24 hr	1500-5000 units/24 hr (Anson)	7.37	11-37 kU/hr
Uroporphyrins				
Qualitative	Random	Negative	—	Negative
Quantitative	24 hr	10-30 μg/24 hr	0.0012	0.012-0.037 μmol/24 hr
Vanillylmandelic acid (VMA)	24 hr	1.5-7.5 mg/24 hr	5.05	7.6-37.9 μmol/24 hr
Volume, total	24 hr	600-1600 ml/24 hr	0.001	0.6-1.61/24 hr
Zinc	24 hr	0.15-1.2 mg/24 hr	15.3	2.3-18.4 μmol/24 hr

Synovial fluid

Component	Typical reference intervals		
	In conventional units	Factor	In SI units
Blood-serum-synovial fluid glucose difference	<10 mg/dl	0.055	<0.55 mmol/l
Differential cell count	Granulocytes 25% of nucleated cells	0.01	Granulocytes 0.25 of nucleated cells
Fibrin clot	Absent	—	Absent
Mucin clot	Abundant	—	Abundant
Nucleated cell count	<200 cells/μl	10^6	<2 × 10^8 cells/1
Viscosity	High	—	High
Volume	<3.5 ml	0.001	<0.00351

Seminal fluid

Component	Typical reference intervals		
	In conventional units	Factor	In SI units
Liquefaction	Within 20 min	1	Within 20 min
Sperm morphology	>70% normal, mature spermatozoa	0.01	>0.7 normal, mature spermatozoa
Sperm motility	>60%	0.01	>0.06
pH	>7.0 (average 7.7)	1	>7.0 (average 7.7)
Sperm count	60-150 million/ml	10^3	60-150 × 10^9/1
Volume	1.5-5.0 ml	0.001	0.0015-0.005/1

Hematology

Component	Typical reference intervals		
	In conventional units	**Factor**	**In SI units**
Red cell volume			
Male	25-35 ml/kg body wt	0.001	0.025-0.035 l/kg body wt
Female	20-30 ml/kg body wt	—	0.020-0.030 l/kg body wt
Plasma volume			
Male	40-50 ml/kg body wt	0.001	0.040-0.050 l/kg body wt
Female	40-50 ml/kg body wt	—	0.040-0.050 l/kg body wt
Coagulation tests			
Bleeding time (Ivy)	1-6 min	1	1-6 min
Bleeding time (Duke)	1-3 min	1	1-3 min
Clot retraction	1/2 in the original mass in 2 hr	1	0.5 the original mass in 2 hr
Dilute blood clot lysis time	Clot lysis between 6 and 10 hr at 37° C	1	Clot lysis between 6 and 10 hr at 37° C
Euglobin clot lysis time	Clot lysis between 2 and 6 hr at 37° C	1	Clot lysis between 2 and 6 hr at 37° C
Partial thromboplastin time	60-70 sec	1	60-70 s
Kaolin activated	35-50 sec	1	35-50 s
Prothrombin time	12-14 sec	1	12-14 s
Venous clotting time			
3 tubes	5-15 min	1	5-15 min
2 tubes	5-18 min	—	5-8 min
Whole blood clot lysis time	None in 24 hr	—	None in 24 hr
Complete blood count (CBC)			
Hematocrit			
Male	40-54%	0.01	0.40-0.54
Female	38-47%	—	0.38-0.47
Hemoglobin			
Male	13.5-18.0 gm/dl	0.155	2.09-2.79 mmol/l
Female	12.0-16.0 gm/dl	—	1.86-2.48 mmol/l
Red cell count			
Male	$4.6\text{-}6.2 \times 10^6/\mu l$	0.155	$4.6\text{-}6.2 \times 10^{12}/l$
Female	$4.2\text{-}5.4 \times 10^6/\mu l$	—	$4.2\text{-}5.4 \times 10^{12}/l$
White cell count	$4.5\text{-}11.0 \times 10^3/\mu l$	10^6	$4.5\text{-}11.0 \times 10^9/l$
Erythrocyte indices			
Mean corpuscular volume (MCV)	80-96 cu microns	1	80-96 fl
Mean corpuscular hemoglobin (MCH)	27-31 pg	1	27-31 pg
Mean corpuscular hemoglobin concentration (MCHC)	32-36%	0.01	0.32-0.36

*All percentages are multiplied by 0.01 to give mean fraction.

Hematology—cont'd

Component	In conventional units		Factor	In SI units	
	Typical reference intervals				
Component	**In conventional units**		**Factor**	**In SI units**	
White blood cell differential (adult)	Mean percent	Range of absolute counts		Mean fraction*	Range of absolute count
Segmented neutrophils	56%	1800-7000/μl	10^6	0.56	1.8-7.0 × 10^9/l
Bands	3%	0-700/μl	10^6	0.03	0-0.70 × 10^9/l
Eosinophils	2.7%	0-450/μl	10^6	0.027	0-0.45 × 10^9/l
Basophils	0.3%	0-200/μl	10^6	0.003	0.020 × 10^9/l
Lymphocytes	34%	1000-4800/μl	10^6	0.34	1.0-4.8 × 10^9/l
Monocytes	4%	0-800/μl	10^6	0.04	0-0.80 × 10^9/l
Hemoglobin A_2	1.5-3.5% of total hemoglobin		0.01	0.015-0.035 of total hemoglobin	
Hemoglobin F	<2%		0.01	<0.02	
Osmotic fragility	% NaCl	% Lysis	% NcCl—171	NaCl	Fractional lysis
		Fresh 24 hr at 37° C	% Lysis—0.01 mmol/l		Fresh 24 hr at 37° C
	0.2	— 95-100		34.2	— 0.95-1.00
	0.3	97-100 85-100		51.3	0.97-1.00 0.85-1.00
	0.35	90-99 75-100		59.8	0.90-0.99 0.75-1.00
	0.4	50-95 65 100		68.4	0.50-0.95 0.65-1.00
	0.45	5-45 55-95		77.0	0.05-0.45 0.55-0.95
	0.5	0-6 40-85		85.5	0-0.06 0.40-0.85
	0.55	0 15-70		94.1	0 0.15-0.70
	0.6	— 0-40		102.6	— 0-0.40
	0.65	— 0-10		111.2	— 0-0.10
	0.7	— 0-5		119.7	— 0-0.05
	0.75	— 0		128.3	— 0
Platelet count	150,000-400,000/μl		10^6	0.15-0.4 × 10^{12}/l	
Reticulocyte count	0.5-1.5%		0.01	0.005-0.015	
	25,000-75,000 cells/μl		10^6	25-75 × 10^9/l	
Sedimentation rate (ESR) (Westergren)					
Men under 50 yrs	<15 mm/hr		1	<15 mm/hr	
Men over 50 yrs	<20 mm/hr		1	<20 mm/hr	
Women under 50 yrs	<20 mm/hr		1	<20 mm/hr	
Women over 50 yrs	<30 mm/hr		1	<30 mm/hr	
Viscosity	1.4-1.8 times water		1	1.4-1.8 times water	
Zega sedimentation ratio	41-54%		0.01	0.41-0.54	

Gastric fluid

Component	Typical reference intervals		
	In conventional units	Factor	In SI units
Fasting residual volume	<50 ml	0.001	<.05/l
pH (stimulated specimen)	<2.0	1	<2.0
Basal acid output (BAO)	0-6 mEq/hr	1	0-6 mmol/hr
Maximum acid output (MAO) (after histamine stimulation)	5-40 mEq/hr	1	5-40 mmol/hr
BAO/MAO ratio	<0.4	1	<0.4

Amniotic fluid

Component	Typical reference intervals		
	In conventional units	Factor	In SI units
Appearance			
Early gestation	Clear	—	Clear
Term	Clear or slightly opalescent	—	Clear or slightly opalescent
Albumin			
Early gestation	0.39 gm/dl	1	3.9 g/l
Term	0.19 gm/dl	1	1.9 g/l
Bilirubin			
Early gestation	<0.075 mg/dl	17.1	<1.28 μmol/l
Term	<0.025 mg/dl	17.1	<0.43 μmol/l
Chloride			
Early gestation	Approx equal to serum chloride	—	Approx equal to serum chloride
Term	Generally 1-3 mEq/l lower than serum chloride	1	Generally 1-3 mmol/l lower than serum chloride
Creatinine			
Early gestation	0.8-1.1 mg/dl	88.4	70.7-97.2 μmol/l
Term	1.8-4.0 mg/dl (generally >2 mg/dl)	88.4	159.1-353.6 μmol/l (generally >176.8 μmol/l)
Estriol			
Early gestation	<10 μg/dl	0.035	<0.35 μmol/l
Term	>60 μg/dl	0.035	>2.1 μmol/l
Lecithin/sphingomyelin			
Early (immature)	<1:1	1	<1:1
Term (mature)	>2:1	1	>2:1

5-2. Selected pediatric reference values*

S + -acid phosphatase
  Newborn   7.4-19.4 U/l
  2-13 yrs   6.4-15.2 U/l
S-aldolase
  Newborn   to 4 × adult value
  Child   to 2 × adult value
S-alkaline phosphatase
  Newborn   40-300 U/l
  Child   60-270 U/l
S-alpha fetoprotein
  Newborn   up to 100 mg/1
  2 weeks   undetectable
S-amylase
  Newborn   little if any amylase activity
  1 year   adult values
S-aspartate aminotransferase
  Newborn   16-74 U/l
  1-3 yrs   6-30 U/l
S-bilirubin
  Newborn

	Pre-term	Full-term
24 hr	17.1-102.8 μmol/l (10-60 mg/l)	34.2-102.8 μmol/l (20-60 mg/l)
48 hr	102.8-137.0 μmol/l (60-80 mg/l)	102.8-119.9 μmol/l (60-70 mg/l)
3-5 day	171.0-266.5 μmol/l (100-150 mg/1)	68.6-205.2 μmol/l (40-120 mg/l)

S-calcium
  Pre-term, first week   1.5-2.5 mmol/l (60-100 mg/l)
  Full-term, first week   1.75-3.00 mmol/l (70-120 mg/l)
  1-2 yr   2.5-3.0 mmol/l (100-120 mg/l)
  2-16 yr   2.25-2.88 mmol/l (90-115 mg/l)
U + -catecholamines

	Norepinephrine	Epinephrine
1 yr	29.5-86.8 nmol/day (5.4-15.9 μg/day)	0.6-25.4 nmol/day (0.1-4.3 μg/day)
1-5 yr	44.2-168.1 nmol/day (8.1-30.8 μg/day)	4.7-53.8 nmol/day (0.8-9.1 μg/day)
6-15 yr	103.7-388.1 nmol/day (19.0-71.1 μg/day)	7.7-62.1 nmol/day (1.3-10.5 μg/day)
>15 yr	188.8-474.8 nmol/day (34.4-87.0 μg/day)	20.7-78.0 nmol/day (3.5-13.2 μg/day)

U-chloride
  Infant   1.7-8.5 mmol/day (1.7-8.5 mEq/24 hr)
  Child   17-34 mmol/day (17-34 mEq/24 hr)
S-cholesterol
  Cord blood   1.2-2.5 mmol/l (460-980 mg/l)
  1-2 yr   1.8-4.9 mmol/l (700-1900 mg/l)
  2-16 yr   3.5-6.5 mmol/l (1350-2500 mg/l)
U-cortisol (free)
  4 mo-10 yr   5.5-74.4 nmol/day (2-27 μg/day)
  11-20 yr   1.9-151.7 nmol/day (0.7-55 μg/day)
S-creatine kinase
  Newborn   3 × adult values
  3 wk-3 mo   1.5 × adult values
  >1 yr   at adult values

*S = serum; U = urine.

S-creatinine
Upper reference value

Up to 5 yr	44 μmol/l (5.0 mg/l)
Up to 6 yr	53 μmol/l (6.0 mg/l)
Up to 7 yr	62 μmol/l (7.0 mg/l)
Up to 8 yr	70 μmol/l (8.0 mg/l)
Up to 9 yr	79 μmol/l (9.0 mg/l)
Up to 10 yr	88 μmol/l (10.0 mg/l)
>10 yr	106 μmol/l (12.0 mg/l)

S-estradiol

0-2 yr	0-26 pmol/l (0-7 pg/ml)
2-4 yr	0.26 pmol/l (0-7 pg/ml)
4-6 yr	0-51 pmol/l (0-14 pg/ml)
6-8 yr	0-37 pmol/l (0-10 pg/ml)
8-10 yr	0-367 pmol/l (0-100 pg/ml)
10-12 yr	0-367 pmol/l (0-100 pg/ml)
12-14 yr	0-367 pmol/l (0-100 pg/ml)
14-16 yr	26-285 pmol/l (7-105 pg/ml)
16-25 yr	26-1175 pmol/l (7-320 pg/ml)

Fecal fat

Pre-term newborn	up to 40% excreted
Full-term newborn	up to 20% excreted
3 mo-1 yr	up to 15% excreted
1 yr	up to 8.5% excreted

P-nonesterified fatty acids

Newborn	0-1845 mmol/l
4 mo-10 yr	300-1100 mmol/l

S-glucose

Pre-term newborn	1.2-3.6 mmol/l (200-656 mg/l)
Full-term newborn	1.1-6.0 mmol/l (200-1100 mg/l)
Child	3.3-5.8 mmol/ (600-1050 mg/l)

S-y-glutamyltransferase

Premature newborn	56-233 U/l
Newborn-3 wk	10-103 U/l
3 wk-3 mo	4-111 U/l
1-5 yr	2-23 U/l
6-15 yr	2-23 U/l
16 yr-adult	2-35 U/l

S-haptoglobin

Newborn	detectable haptoglobin in only 10-20%
1 yr and older	at adult values

S-immunoglobulin IgG

0-5 wk	7500-15,000 mg/l
6 mo	1500-7000 mg/l
1 yr	1400-10,300 mg/l
5 yr	3700-15,000 mg/l
10 yr	4400-15,500 mg/l

S-immunoglobulin IgA

0-5 wk	none
6 mo	200-1300 mg/l
1 yr	200-1300 mg/l
5 yr	300-2000 mg/l
10 yr	500-2300 mg/l

S-immunoglobulin IgM

0-5 wk	less than 200 mg/l
6 mo	300-600 mg/l
1 yr	300-1600 mg/l
5 yr	200-2200 mg/l
10 yr	300-1700 mg/l

Inulin clearance

<1 mo	29-88 ml/min per 1.73 m^2 of body surface
1-6 mo	40-112 ml/min per 1.73 m^2 of body surface
6-12 mo	62-121 ml/min per 1.73 m^2 of body surface
>1 yr	78-164 ml/min per 1.73 m^2 of body surface

U-17 ketosteroids

0-3 day	0-0.5 mg/day	
1-3 yr	<2.0 mg/day	
3-6 yr	0.5-3.0 mg/day	
6-9 yr	0.8-4.0 mg/day	
10-12 yr	male	0.7-6.0 mg/day
	female	0.7-5.0 mg/day
Adolescent	male	3-15 mg/day
	female	3-12 mg/day

S-lactate dehydrogenase

1-3 day	up to 2 × adult values

S-phosphorus (inorganic)

	Pre-term	Full-term
Newborn	1.8-2.6 mmol/l (56.0-80.0 mg/l)	1.6-2.5 mmol/l (50.0-78.0 mg/l)
6-10 day	2.0-3.8 mmol/l (61-117 mg/l)	1.6-2.9 mmol/l (49-89 mg/l)
4 mo	1.6-2.6 mmol/l (48-81 mg/l)	
1 yr	1.25-2.1 mmol/l (39-60 mg/l)	
2-16 yr	0.9-1.5 mmol/l (26-50 mg/l)	

S-potassium

Pre-term newborn	4.5-7.2 mmol/l (4.5-7.2 mEq/l)
Full-term newborn	5.0-7.7 mmol/l (5.0-7.7 mEq/l)
2 day-2 wk	4.0-6.4 mmol/l (4.0-6.4 mEq/l)
2 wk-3 mo	4.0-6.2 mmol/l (4.0-6.2 mEq/l)
3 mo-1 yr	3.7-5.6 mmol/l (3.7-5.6 mEq/l)
1-16 yr	3.6-5.2 mmol/l (3.6-5.2 mEq/l)

S-testosterone

Age	Male	Female
0-2 yr	0.1-1.3 nmol/l (40-370 ng/l)	0.2-0.6 nmol/l (70-180 ng/l)
2-4 yr	0.2-0.6 nmol/l (50-160 ng/l)	0.2-0.7 nmol/l (70-200 ng/l)
4-6 yr	0.3-1.4 nmol/l (80-400 ng/l)	0.3-0.7 nmol/l (100-200 ng/l)
6-8 yr	0.2-1.0 nmol/l (60-280 ng/l)	0.5-1.0 nmol/l (150-300 ng/l)
8-10 yr	0.3-1.7 nmol/l (90-500 ng/l)	0.7-1.4 nmol/l (200-400 ng/l)
10-12 yr	0.3-10.1 nmol/l (80-2900 ng/l)	0.7-1.7 nmol/l (200-500 ng/l)
12-14 yr	0.2-24.6 nmol/l (50-7600 ng/l)	1.0-2.4 nmol/l (300-700 ng/l)
14-16 yr	3.1-19.5 nmol/l (900-5600 ng/l)	1.2-3.3 nmol/l (350-950 ng/l)
16-18 yr	9.0-25.4 nmol/l (2600-7300 ng/l)	1.4-3.3 nmol/l (400-950 ng/l)
18-20 yr	13.9-25.0 nmol/l (4000-7200 ng/l)	1.4-3.3 nmol/l (400-950 ng/l)
20-25 yr	11.8-38.9 nmol/l (3400-11,200 ng/l)	1.4-3.3 nmol/l (400-950 ng/l)

S-thyroxine

1-3 day	142-296 nmol/l (11-23 μg/dl)
1 wk-1 mo	116-232 nmol/l (9-18 μg/dl)
1-4 mo	97-212 nmol/l (7.5-16.5 μg/dl)
4-12 mo	71-187 nmol/l (5.5-14.5 μg/dl)
1-6 yr	71-174 nmol/l (5.5-13.5 μg/dl)
6-10 yr	64-161 nmol/l (5.0-12.5 μg/dl)

6-1. Recommended daily dietary allowances, revised 1980

Recommended daily dietary allowances of some selected nutrients for pregnancy and lactation

Nutrients	Nonpregnant girl 12-14 yr 47 kg (103 lb)	Nonpregnant girl 14-18 yr 55 kg (120 lb)	Nonpregnant woman 25 yr 58 kg (128 lb)	Pregnancy Added need	Pregnancy Girl 12-14 yr	Pregnancy Girl 14-18 yr	Pregnancy Woman 25 yr	Lactation (850 ml daily) Added need	Lactation Girl 12-14 yr	Lactation Girl 14-18 yr	Lactation Woman 25 yr
Calories	2,200	2,100	2,000	300	2,500	2,400	2,300	500	2,700	2,600	2,500
Protein (g)	46	46	44	30	76	76	74	20	66	68	64
Calcium (g)	1.2	1.2	0.8	0.4	1.6	1.6	1.2	0.4	1.6	1.6	1.2
Iron (mg)	18	18	18	‡	18+	18+	18+	‡	18+	18+	18+
Vitamin A (RE)*	800	800	800	200	1,000	1,000	1,000	400	1,200	1,200	1,200
Thiamin (mg)	1.1	1.1	1.0	0.4	1.5	1.5	1.4	0.5	1.6	1.6	1.5
Riboflavin (mg)	1.3	1.3	1.2	0.3	1.6	1.6	1.5	0.5	1.8	1.8	1.7
Niacin equivalent and tryptophan (mg)	15	14	13	2	17	16	15	5	20	19	18
Ascorbic acid (mg)	50	60	60	20	70	80	80	40	90	100	100
Vitamin D (µg)†	10	10	5	5	15	15	10	5	15	15	10

*Retinol equivalents.
†Cholecalciferol; 10 µg equals 400 IU vitamin D.
‡Required iron supplement 30-60 mg.

Recommended daily dietary allowances for growth

	Age (yr)	Weight kg	Weight lb	Height cm	Height in	Energy (kcal)	Protein (g)	Fat-soluble vitamins Vit. A µg RE	Vit. A IU	Vit. D (µg*)	Vit. E (mgαTE)
Infants	Birth-0.5	6	13	60	24	kg × 115	kg × 2.2	420	1,400	10	3
	0.5-1	9	20	71	28	kg × 105	kg × 2.0	400	2,000	10	4
Children	1-3	13	29	90	35	1,300	23	400	2,000	10	5
	4-6	20	44	112	44	1,700	30	500	2,500	10	6
	7-10	28	62	132	52	2,400	34	700	3,300	10	7
Males	11-14	45	99	157	62	2,700	45	1,000	5,000	10	8
	15-18	66	145	176	69	2,800	56	1,000	5,000	10	10
Females	11-14	46	101	157	62	2,200	46	800	4,000	10	8
	15-18	55	120	163	64	2,100	46	800	4,000	10	8

*As cholecalciferol; 10 µg cholecalciferol = 400 IU vitamin D.

Mean heights and weights and recommended energy intake*

Category	Age (years)	Weight kg	Weight lb	Height cm	Height in	Energy needs (with range) kcal		Energy needs (with range) MJ
Infants	0.0-0.5	6	13	60	24	kg × 115	(95-145)	kg × .48
	0.5-1.0	9	20	71	28	kg × 105	(80-135)	kg × .44
Children	1-3	13	29	90	35	1300	(900-1800)	5.5
	4-6	20	44	112	44	1700	(1300-2300)	7.1
	7-10	28	62	132	52	2400	(1650-3300)	10.1
Males	11-14	45	99	157	62	2700	(2000-3700)	11.3
	15-18	66	145	176	69	2800	(2100-3900)	11.8
	19-22	70	154	177	70	2900	(2500-3300)	12.2
	23-50	70	154	178	70	2700	(2300-3100)	11.3
	51-75	70	154	178	70	2400	(2000 2800)	10.1
	76+	70	154	178	70	2050	(1650-2450)	8.6
Females	11-14	46	101	157	62	2200	(1500-3000)	9.2
	15-18	55	120	163	64	2100	(1200-3000)	8.8
	19-22	55	120	163	64	2100	(1700-2500)	8.8
	23-50	55	120	163	64	2000	(1600-2400)	8.4
	51-75	55	120	163	64	1800	(1400-2200)	7.6
	76+	55	120	163	64	1600	(1200-2000)	6.7
Pregnancy						+300		
Lactation						+500		

*From: Recommended Dietary Allowances, Revised 1980. Food and Nutrition Board National Academy of Sciences-National Research Council, Washington, D.C.

The data in this table have been assembled from the observed median heights and weights of children together with desirable weights for adults for the mean heights of men (70 in) and women (64 in) between the ages of 18 and 34 years as surveyed in the U.S. population (HEW/NCHS data).

The energy allowances for the young adults are for men and women doing light work. The allowances for the two older age groups represent mean energy needs over these age spans, allowing for a 2% decrease in basal (resting) metabolic rate per decade and a reduction in activity of 200 kcal per day for men and women between 51 and 75 years, 500 kcal for men over 75 years, and 400 kcal for women over 75. The customary range of daily energy output is shown for adults in parentheses and is based on a variation in energy needs of ±400 kcal at any one age, emphasizing the wide range of energy intakes appropriate for any group of people.

Energy allowances for children through age 18 are based on median energy intakes of children these ages followed in longitudinal growth studies. The values in parentheses are 10th and 90th percentiles of energy intake, to indicate the range of energy consumption among children of these ages.

Water-soluble vitamins							Minerals					
Vit. C (mg)	Folacin (μg)	Niacin (mg)	Riboflavin (mg)	Thiamin (mg)	Vit. B₆ (mg)	Vit. B₁₂ (μg)	Calcium (mg)	Phosphorus (mg)	Iodine (μg)	Iron (mg)	Magnesium (mg)	Zinc (mg)
35	30	6	0.4	0.3	0.3	0.5	360	240	40	10	50	3
35	45	8	0.6	0.5	0.6	1.5	540	360	50	15	70	5
45	100	9	0.8	0.7	0.9	2.0	800	800	70	15	150	10
45	200	11	1.0	0.9	1.3	2.5	800	800	90	10	200	10
45	300	16	1.4	1.2	1.6	3.0	800	800	120	10	250	10
50	400	18	1.6	1.4	1.8	3.0	1,200	1,200	150	18	350	15
60	400	18	1.7	1.4	2.0	3.0	1,200	1,200	150	18	400	15
50	400	15	1.3	1.1	1.8	3.0	1,200	1,200	150	18	300	15
60	400	14	1.3	1.1	2.0	3.0	1,200	1,200	150	18	300	15

6-2. Daily dietary guide—the basic four food groups

Food group	Main nutrients	Daily amounts*
Milk		
Milk, cheese, ice cream, or other products made with whole or skimmed milk	Calcium Protein Riboflavin	Children under 9: 2-3 cups Children 9-12: 3 or more cups Teen-agers: 4 or more cups Adults: 2 or more cups Pregnant women: 3 or more cups Nursing mothers: 4 or more cups (1 cup = 8 oz fluid milk or designated milk equivalent†)
Meats		
Beef, veal, lamb, pork, poultry, fish, eggs	Protein Iron Thiamin	2 or more servings Count as 1 serving 2-3 oz of lean, boneless, cooked meat, poultry, or fish 2 eggs
Alternates: dry beans, dry peas, nuts, peanut butter	Niacin Riboflavin	1 cup cooked dry beans or peas 4 tbsp peanut butter
Vegetables and fruits		4 or more servings Count as 1 serving ½ cup of vegetable or fruit or a portion such as 1 medium apple, banana, orange, potato, or ½ a medium grapefruit, melon Include
	Vitamin A	A dark-green or deep-yellow vegetable or fruit rich in vitamin A at least every other day
	Vitamin C (ascorbic acid)	A citrus fruit or other fruit or vegetable rich in vitamin C daily
	Smaller amounts of other vitamins and minerals	Other vegetables and fruits including potatoes
Bread and cereals		4 or more servings of whole grain, enriched or restored Count as 1 serving
	Thiamin	1 slice of bread
	Niacin	1 oz (1 cup) ready to eat cereal, flake or puff varieties
	Riboflavin	½-¾ cup cooked cereal
	Iron	½-¾ cup cooked pastes (macaroni, spaghetti, noodles)
	Protein	Crackers: 5 saltines, 2 squares graham crackers

*Use additional amounts of these foods or added butter, margarine, oils, sugars, etc., as desired or needed.
†Milk equivalents: 1 oz cheddar cheese, 3 servings cottage cheese, 1 cup fluid skimmed milk, 1 cup buttermilk, ½ cup dry skimmed milk powder, 1 cup ice milk, 1⅔ cups ice cream, ½ cup evaporated milk.

6-3. Vitamins and minerals

Summary of fat-soluble vitamins

Vitamin	Physiological functions	Results of deficiency	Requirement	Food sources
A (retinol) Provitamin A (carotene)	Production of rhodopsin (visual purple) Formation and maintenance of epithelial tissue Toxic in large amounts	Xerophthalmia Night blindness Keratinization of epithelium Follicular hyperkeratosis Skin and mucous membrane infections Faulty tooth formation	Adult male: 1,000 μg RE (5,000 IU) Adult female: 800 μg RE (4,000 IU) Pregnancy: 1,000 μg RE (5,000 IU) Lactation: 1,200 μg RE (6,000 IU) Children: 400 μg RE (2,000 IU) to 800 μg RE (4,000 IU)	Liver Cream, butter, whole milk Egg yolk Green and yellow vegetables Yellow fruits Fortified margarine
D (calciferol)	Absorption of calcium and phosphorus Calcification of bones Renal phosphate clearance Toxic in large amounts	Rickets Faulty bone growth Osteomalacia in adults	Adult: 5-10 μg cholecalciferol (200-400 IU) Pregnancy and lactation: 10-12.5 μg (400-500 IU) depending on age Children: 10 μg (400 IU)	Fish oils Fortified or irradiated milk
E (tocopherol)	Related to action of selenium Antioxidant with vitamin A and unsaturated fatty acids Hemopoiesis Reproduction (in animals)	Hemolysis of red blood cells; anemia Possible protection of unsaturated fatty acids Sterility (in rats)	Adult: 8-10 mg αTE Pregnancy and lactation: 10-11 mg αTE Children: 3-10 mg αTE	Vegetable oils
K (menadione)	Blood clotting, necessary for synthesis of prothrombin Possible coenzyme in oxidation phosphorylation Toxic in large amounts	Hemorrhagic disease of the newborn Bleeding tendencies in biliary disease or surgical procedures Deficiency in intestinal malabsorption (sprue, celiac disease, colitis) Prolonged antibiotic therapy Anticoagulant therapy (dicumarol counteracts)	Unknown	Green leafy vegetables Cheese Egg yolk Liver

Summary of vitamin C (ascorbic acid)

Physiological functions	Clinical applications	Requirement	Food sources

Intercellular cement substance:
  1. Collagen formation
  2. Firm capillary walls
General metabolism:
  1. Makes iron available for hemoglobin and maturation of red blood cells
  2. Influences conversion of folic acid to "citrovorum factor" (folinic acid)
	Scurvy (deficiency)
	Megaloblastic anemia
	Wound healing; tissue formation
	Fevers and infections
	Stress reactions
	Growth periods
		60 mg daily (adults)	Citrus fruits
			Tomatoes
			Cabbage
			Potatoes
			Strawberries
			Melon
			Chili peppers

Summary of B-complex vitamins

Vitamin	Physiological functions	Clinical applications	Requirement	Food sources
Thiamin (B₁)	Coenzyme in carbohydrate metabolism: TPP—decarboxylation TDP—transketolation	Beriberi (deficiency) GI*: anorexia, gastric atony, indigestion, deficient hydrochloric acid CNS*: fatigue, apathy, neuritis, paralysis CV*: cardiac failure, peripheral vasodilation, and edema of extremities	0.5 mg/1000 calories	Pork, beef, liver, whole or enriched grains, legumes
Riboflavin (B₂)	Coenzyme in protein of energy metabolism (flavoproteins) FMN (flavin mononucleotide) FAD (flavin-adenine dinucleotide)	Wound aggravation Cheilosis Glossitis Eye irritation; photophobia Seborrheic dermatitis	0.6 mg/1000 calories	Milk, liver, enriched cereals
Niacin (nicotinic acid) (precursor—tryptophan)	Coenzyme in tissue oxidation to produce energy (ATP) NAD (nicotinamide-adenine dinucleotide) NADP (nicotinamide-adenine dinucletide phosphate)	Pellagra (deficiency) Weakness, lassitude, anorexia Skin: scaly dermatitis CNS: neuritis, confusion	14-20 mg (NE)	Meat, peanuts, enriched grains
Pyridoxine (B₆)	Coenzyme in amino acid metabolism Decarboxylation Deamination Transamination Transsulfuration Niacin formation from tryptophan Heme formation Amino acid absorption	Anemia (hypochromic microcytic) CNS: hyperirritability, convulsions, neuritis Isoniazid is an antagonist for pyridoxine Pregnancy: anemia	2 mg	Wheat, corn, meat, liver
Pantothenic acid	Coenzyme in formation of active acetate (CoA)—acetylation	Contributes to: Lipogenesis Amino acid activation Formation of cholesterol Formation of steroid hormones Formation of heme Excretion of drugs		Liver, egg, skimmed milk
Lipoic acid (sulfur-containing fatty acid)	Coenzyme (with thiamin) in carbohydrate metabolism to reduce pyruvate to active acetate Oxidative decarboxylation	Undetermined (see thiamin)		Liver, yeast
Biotin	Coenzyme in decarboxylation (synthesis of fatty acids, amino acids, purines); deamination	Undetermined		Egg yolk, liver
Folic acid (B₉)	Coenzyme for single carbon transfer—purines, thymine, hemoglobin Transmethylation	Blood cell regeneration in pernicious anemia but not control of its neurological problems Megaloblastic anemia Macrocytic anemia of pregnancy Sprue treatment Aminopterin is antagonist	400 μg Pregnancy: 800 μg Lactation: 800 μg	Liver, green leafy vegetables, asparagus
PABA (part of folic acid)		Treatment of rickettsial diseases Anemias (see folic acid)		Same as folic acid
Cobalamin (B₁₂)	Coenzyme in protein synthesis Formation of nucleic acid and cell proteins—red blood cells Transmethylation	Extrinsic factor in pernicious anemia—combines with intrinsic factor of gastric secretions for absorption; forms red blood cells (with folic acid) Sprue treatment (with folic acid)	3 μg	Liver, meat, milk, egg, cheese
Inositol	Lipotropic agent (?)	Undetermined		Citrus fruit, grains, meat, milk
Choline	Lipotropic agent Forms nerve mediator—acetylcholine	Fatty liver—hepatitis, cirrhosis (undetermined in human nutrition)		Meat, cereals, egg yolk

*GI = Gastrointestinal; CNS = Central nervous system; CV = Cardiovascular.

Summary of major minerals

Mineral	Metabolism	Physiological functions	Clinical application	Requirement	Food sources
Calcium (Ca)	Absorption according to body need, aided by vitamin D, favored by protein, lactose, acidity; hindered by excess fats and binding agents (phosphates, oxalates, phytate) Excretion chiefly in feces, 70% to 90% of amount ingested Deposition-mobilization in bone compartment constant; deposition aided by vitamin D Parathyroid hormone controls absorption and mobilization	Bone formation Teeth Blood clotting Muscle contraction and relaxation Heart action Nerve transmission Cell wall permeability Enzyme activation (ATPase)	Tetany—decrease in ionized serum calcium Rickets Renal calculi Hyperparathyroidism Hypoparathyroidism	Adults: 0.8 gm Pregnancy and lactation: 1.2 gm Infants: 360-540 mg Children: 0.8-1.2 gm	Milk Cheese Green leafy vegetables Whole grains Egg yolk Legumes, nuts
Phosphorus (P)	Absorption with calcium aided by vitamin D, hindered by excess binding agents (calcium, aluminum, iron) Excretion chiefly by kidney according to renal threshold blood level Parathyroid hormone controls renal excretion balance with blood level Deposition-mobilization in bone compartment constant	Bone formation Overall metabolism: Absorption of glucose and glycerol (phosphorylation) Transport of fatty acids Energy metabolism (enzymes, ATP) Buffer system	Growth Hypophosphatemia: Recovery state from diabetic acidosis Sprue, celiac disease (malabsorption) Bone diseases (upset Ca:P balance) Hyperphosphatemia: Renal insufficiency Hypoparathyroidism Tetany	Adults: 1½ times calcium intake Pregnancy and lactation: 1.2 gm Infants: 240-400 mg Children: 0.8-1.2 gm	Milk Cheese Meat Egg yolk Whole grains Legumes, nuts
Magnesium (Mg)	Absorption increased by parathyroid hormone, hindered by excess fat, phosphate, calcium Excretion regulated by kidney	In bones and teeth Activator and coenzyme in carbohydrate and protein metabolism Essential intracellular fluid (ICF) cation Muscle, nerve irritability	Tremor, spasm; low serum level following gastrointestinal losses	300-350 mg Deficiency in humans unlikely	Whole grains Nuts Meat Milk Legumes
Sodium (Na)	Readily absorbed Excretion chiefly by kidney, controlled by aldosterone, acid base balance	Major extracellular fluid (ECF) cation Water balance, osmotic pressure Acid-base balance Cell permeability; absorption of glucose Muscle irritability; transmission of electrochemical impulse and resulting contraction	Fluid shifts and control Buffer system Losses in gastrointestinal disorders	About 0.5 gm Diet usually has more: 2-6 gm	Table salt (NaCl) Milk Meat Egg Baking soda Baking powder Carrots, beets, spinach, celery
Potassium (K)	Secreted and reabsorbed in digestive juices Excretion guarded by kidney according to blood levels; increased by aldosterone	Major ICF cation Acid-base balance Regulates neuromuscular excitability and muscle contraction Glycogen formation Protein synthesis	Fluid shifts Losses in starvation, diabetic acidosis, adrenal tumors Heart action—low serum potassium (tachycardia, cardiac arrest) Treatment of diabetic acidosis (rapid glycogen production reduces serum potassium) Tissue catabolism—potassium loss	About 2-4 gm Diet adequate in protein, calcium, and iron contains adequate potassium	Whole grains Meat Legumes Fruits Vegetables
Chlorine (Cl)	Absorbed readily Excretion controlled by kidney	Major ECF anion Acid-base balance—chloride-bicarbonate shift Water balance Gastric hydrochloric acid—digestion	Hypochloremic alkalosis in prolonged vomiting, diarrhea, tube drainage	About 0.5 gm Diet usually has more: 2-6 gm	Table salt
Sulfur (S)	Absorbed as such and as constituent of sulfur-containing amino acid, methionine Excreted by kidney in relation to protein intake and tissue catabolism	Essential constituent of cell protein Activates enzymes High-energy sulfur bonds in energy metabolism Detoxification reactions	Cystine renal calculi Cystinuria	Diet adequate in protein contains adequate sulfur	Meat Egg Cheese Milk Nuts, legumes

Summary of trace minerals

Mineral	Metabolism	Physiological functions	Clinical application	Requirement	Food source
Iron (Fe)	Absorption according to body need controlled by mucosal block—ferritin mechanism, aided by vitamin C, gastric hydrochloric acid Transport—transferrin Storage—ferritin, hemosiderin Excretion from tissue in minute quantities, body conserves and reuses	Hemoglobin formation Cellular oxidation (cytochrome system producing ATP)	Growth (milk anemia) Pregnancy demands Deficiency—anemia Excess—hemosiderosis; hemochromatosis	Men 10 mg Women 18 mg Pregnancy 18+ mg Lactation; 18 mg Children: 10-18 mg	Liver Meats Egg yolk Whole grains Enriched bread and cereal Dark green vegetables Legumes, nuts
Copper (Cu)	Transported bound to an α-globulin as ceruloplasmin Stored in muscle, bone, liver, heart, kidney, and central nervous system	Associated with iron in Enzyme systems Hemoglobin synthesis Absorption and transport of iron Involved in bone formation and maintenance of brain tissue and myelin sheath in nervous system	Hypocupremia: Nephrosis Malabsorption Wilson's disease—excess copper storage	2-2.5 mg Diet provides 2-5 mg	Liver Meat Seafood Whole grains Legumes, nuts Cocoa Raisins Food cooked in copper utensils
Iodine (I)	Absorbed as iodides, taken up by thyroid gland under control of thyroid-stimulating hormone (TSH) Excretion by kidney	Synthesis of thyroxine, the thyroid hormone, which regulates cell oxidation	Deficiency—endemic colloid goiter; cretinism	Men: 140 μg Women: 100 μg Infants: 35-45 μg Children 60-140 μg	Iodized salt Seafood
Manganese (Mn)	Absorption limited Excretion mainly by intestine	Activates reactions in Urea formation Protein metabolism Glucose oxidation Lipoprotein clearance and synthesis of fatty acids	No clinical deficiency observed in humans Inhalation toxicity in miners	2.5-7 mg (estimated) Diet provides 3-9 μg	Cereals, whole grain Soybeans Legumes, nuts Tea, coffee Vegetables Fruits
Cobalt (Co)	Absorbed chiefly as constituent of vitamin B_{12}	Constituent of vitamin B_{12}; essential factor in red blood cell formation	Deficiency associated with deficiency of vitamin B_{12}—pernicious anemia	Unknown	Supplied by preformed vitamin B_{12}
Zinc (Zn)	Transported with plasma proteins Excretion largely intestinal Stored in liver, muscle, bone, and organs	Essential enzyme constituent: Carbonic anhydrase Carboxypeptidase Lactic dehydrogenase Combined with insulin for storage of the hormone	Possible relation to liver disease Wound healing Taste and smell acuity Retarded sexual and physical development	Adults: 15 mg Children: 10 mg Infants: 3-5 mg	Widely distributed Liver Seafood, especially oysters Eggs Milk Whole grains

Summary of trace minerals—cont'd

Mineral	Metabolism	Physiological functions	Clinical application	Requirement	Food source
Molybdenum (Mo)	Minute traces in the body	Constituent of specific enzymes involved in Purine conversion to uric acid Aldehyde oxidation		450-500 μg (estimated)	Organ meats Milk Whole grains Leafy vegetables Legumes
Fluorine (Fl)	Deposited in bones and teeth Excreted in urine	Associated with dental health	Small amount prevents dental caries Excess causes endemic dental fluorosis	1-3 mg (estimated)	Water (1 ppm Fl)
Selenium (Se)	Active as cofactor in cell oxidation enzyme systems	Associated with fat metabolism	Constituent of "factor 3," which acts with vitamin E to prevent fatty liver	Under 100 μg (estimated)	Seafoods Meats Whole grains
Chromium (Cr)	Improves faulty uptake of glucose by body tissues	Associated with glucose metabolism; raises abnormally low fasting blood sugar levels	Infants unable to metabolize sugar, and adult diabetics show definite improvement when small amounts of chromium added to diet Possible link with cardiovascular disorders and diabetes	20-50 μg (estimated)	Animal proteins, especially meats (except fish) Whole grains
Nickel (Ni)	Binding by phytate reduces intestinal absorption	Constituent of the protein nickeloplasmin Associated with thyroid hormone High in RNA	Plasma levels decreased in cirrhosis and chronic uremia	Under 0.6 μg (estimated)	Whole grains Legumes Vegetables Fruits
Tin (Sn)		Structural element in protein synthesis Associated with cell enzyme systems in energy metabolism	Wound healing Tissue growth	Under 1 mg (estimated)	Meats Whole grains Legumes Vegetables Fruits Acid juices canned in tin
Silicon (Si)		Essential agent in formation of bone, cartilage, connective tissue	Bone calcification and healing	Unknown	All plant foods
Vanadium (V)		High in teeth; may have role in bone and tooth formation	Possible relation to lipid metabolism, blood lipid levels	0.1-0.3 mg (estimated)	Grains, breads Root vegetables Nuts Vegetable oils

6-4. Nutritive values of the edible part of foods[1]

Food, approximate measure, and weight (in grams)		weight (in grams)	Food energy (calories)	Protein (g)	Fat (total lipid) (g)	Saturated (total) (g)	Fatty acids Unsaturated Oleic (g)	Fatty acids Unsaturated Linoleic (g)	Carbohydrate (g)	Calcium (mg)	Iron (mg)	Vitamin A value (IU)	Thiamin (mg)	Riboflavin (mg)	Niacin (mg)	Ascorbic acid (mg)
Milk, cream, cheese (related products)																
Milk, cow's																
Fluid, whole (3.5% fat)	1 cup	244	160	9	9	5	3	Trace	12	288	0.1	350	0.08	0.42	0.1	2
Fluid, nonfat (skim)	1 cup	246	90	9	Trace	—	—	—	13	298	.1	10	.10	.44	.2	2
Buttermilk, cultured, from skim milk	1 cup	246	90	9	Trace	—	—	—	13	298	.1	10	.09	.44	.2	2
Evaporated, unsweetened, undiluted	1 cup	252	345	18	20	11	7	1	24	635	.3	820	.10	.84	.5	3
Condensed, sweetened, undiluted	1 cup	306	980	25	27	15	9	1	166	802	.3	1,090	.23	1.17	.5	3
Dry, whole	1 cup	103	515	27	28	16	9	1	39	936	.5	1,160	.30	1.50	.7	6
Dry, nonfat, instant	1 cup	70	250	25	Trace	—	—	—	36	905	.4	20	.24	1.25	.6	5
Milk, goat's																
Fluid, whole	1 cup	244	165	8	10	6	2	Trace	11	315	.2	390	.10	.27	.7	2
Cream																
Half-and-half (cream and milk)	1 cup	242	325	8	28	16	9	1	11	261	.1	1,160	.08	.38	.1	2
	1 tbsp	15	20	Trace	2	1	1	Trace	1	16	Trace	70	Trace	.02	Trace	Trace
Light, coffee or table	1 cup	240	505	7	49	27	16	1	10	245	.1	2,030	.07	.36	.1	2
	1 tbsp	15	30	Trace	3	2	1	Trace	1	15	Trace	130	Trace	.02	Trace	Trace
Whipping, unwhipped (volume about double when whipped)																
Light	1 cup	239	715	6	75	41	25	2	9	203	.1	3,070	.06	.30	.1	2
	1 tbsp	15	45	Trace	5	3	2	Trace	1	13	Trace	190	Trace	.02	Trace	Trace
Heavy	1 cup	238	840	5	89	49	29	3	7	178	.1	3,670	.05	.26	.1	2
	1 tbsp	15	55	Trace	6	3	2	Trace	Trace	11	Trace	230	Trace	.02	Trace	Trace
Cheese																
Blue or Roquefort type	1 oz	28	105	6	9	5	3	Trace	1	89	.1	350	.01	.17	.1	0
Cheddar or American																
Ungrated	1 inch cube	17	70	4	5	3	2	Trace	Trace	128	.2	220	Trace	.08	Trace	0
Grated	1 cup	112	445	28	36	20	12	1	2	840	1.1	1,470	.03	.51	.1	0
	1 tbsp	7	30	2	2	1	1	Trace	Trace	52	.1	90	Trace	.03	Trace	0
Cheddar, process	1 oz	28	105	7	9	5	3	Trace	1	219	.3	350	Trace	.12	Trace	0
Cheese foods, Cheddar	1 oz	28	90	6	7	4	2	Trace	2	162	.2	280	.01	.16	Trace	0
Cottage cheese, from skim milk																
Creamed	1 cup	225	240	31	9	5	3	Trace	7	212	0.7	380	0.07	.56	0.2	0
	1 oz	28	30	4	1	1	Trace	Trace	1	27	.1	50	.01	.07	Trace	0

Food	Measure	Grams	Food energy	Protein (g)	Fat (g)	Saturated (g)	Oleic (g)	Linoleic (g)	Carbohydrate (g)	Calcium (mg)	Iron (mg)	Vitamin A (IU)	Thiamine (mg)	Riboflavin (mg)	Niacin (mg)	Ascorbic acid (mg)
Uncreamed	1 cup	225	195	38	1	Trace	Trace	Trace	6	202	.9	20	.07	.63	.2	0
	1 oz	28	25	5	Trace	Trace	Trace	Trace	1	26	.1	Trace	.01	.08	Trace	0
Cream cheese	1 oz	28	105	2	11	6	4	Trace	1	18	.1	440	Trace	.07	Trace	0
	1 tbsp	15	55	1	6	3	2	Trace	Trace	9	Trace	230	Trace	.04	Trace	0
Swiss (domestic)	1 oz	28	105	8	8	4	3	Trace	1	262	.3	320	Trace	.11	Trace	0
Milk beverages																
Cocoa	1 cup	242	235	9	11	6	4	Trace	26	285	.9	390	.09	.45	.4	2
Chocolate-flavored milk drink (made with skim milk)	1 cup	250	190	8	6	3	2	Trace	27	270	.4	210	.09	.41	.2	2
Malted milk	1 cup	270	280	13	12	—	—	—	32	364	.8	670	.17	.56	.2	2
Milk desserts																
Cornstarch pudding, plain (blanc mange)	1 cup	248	275	9	10	5	3	Trace	39	290	.1	390	.07	.40	.1	2
Custard, baked	1 cup	248	285	13	14	6	5	1	28	278	1.0	870	.10	.47	.2	1
Ice cream, plain, factory packed																
Slice or cut brick, ⅛ of quart brick	1 slice or cut brick	71	145	3	9	5	3	Trace	15	87	.1	370	.03	.13	.1	1
Container	3½ fld oz	62	130	2	8	4	3	Trace	13	76	.1	320	.03	.12	.1	1
Container	8 fld oz	142	295	6	18	10	6	1	29	175	.1	740	.06	.27	.1	1
Ice milk	1 cup	187	285	9	10	6	3	Trace	42	292	.2	390	.09	.41	.2	2
Yogurt, from partially skimmed milk	1 cup	246	120	8	4	2	1	Trace	13	295	.1	170	.09	.43	.1	2
Eggs																
Eggs, large, 24 ounces per dozen																
Raw																
Whole, without shell	1 egg	50	80	6	6	2	3	Trace	Trace	27	1.1	590	.05	.15	Trace	0
White of egg	1 white	33	15	4	Trace	—	—	—	Trace	3	Trace	0	Trace	.09	Trace	0
Yolk of egg	1 yolk	17	60	3	5	2	2	Trace	Trace	24	.9	580	.04	.07	Trace	0
Cooked																
Boiled, shell removed	2 eggs	100	160	13	12	4	5	1	1	54	2.3	1,180	.09	.28	.1	0
Scrambled, with milk and fat	1 egg	64	110	7	8	3	3	Trace	1	51	1.1	690	.05	.18	Trace	0
Meat, poultry, fish, shellfish (related products)																
Bacon, broiled or fried, crisp	2 slices	16	100	5	8	3	4	1	1	2	.5	0	.08	.05	.8	—
Beef, trimmed to retail basis², cooked																
Cuts braised, simmered, or pot-roasted																
Lean and fat	3 oz	85	245	23	16	8	7	Trace	0	10	2.9	30	.04	.18	3.5	—
Lean only	2.5 oz	72	140	22	5	2	2	Trace	0	10	2.7	10	.04	.16	3.3	—
Hamburger (ground beef), broiled																
Lean	3 oz	85	185	23	10	5	4	Trace	0	10	3.0	20	.08	.20	5.1	—
Regular	3 oz	85	245	21	17	8	8	Trace	0	9	2.7	30	.07	.18	4.6	—

¹Reprinted from Nutritive value of foods, U.S. Department of Agriculture, Home and Garden Bulletin No. 72.
Dashes show that no basis could be found for imputing a value although there was some reason to believe that a measurable amount of the constituent might be present.

Food, approximate measure, and weight (in grams)	(grams)	Food energy (calories)	Protein (g)	Fat (total lipid) (g)	Fatty acids Saturated (total) (g)	Unsaturated Oleic (g)	Unsaturated Linoleic (g)	Carbohydrate (g)	Calcium (mg)	Iron (mg)	Vitamin A value (IU)	Thiamin (mg)	Riboflavin (mg)	Niacin (mg)	Ascorbic acid (mg)
Roast, oven-cooked, no liquid added															
Relatively fat, such as rib															
Lean and fat 3 oz	85	375	17	34	16	15	1	0	8	2.2	70	.05	.13	3.1	—
Lean only 1.8 oz	51	125	14	7	3	3	Trace	0	6	1.8	10	.04	.11	2.6	—
Relatively lean, such as heel of round															
Lean and fat 3 oz	85	165	25	7	3	3	Trace	0	11	3.2	10	.06	.19	4.5	—
Lean only 2.7 oz	78	125	24	3	1	1	Trace	0	10	3.0	Trace	.06	.18	4.3	—
Steak, broiled															
Relatively fat, such as sirloin															
Lean and fat 3 oz	85	330	20	27	13	12	1	0	9	2.5	50	.05	.16	4.0	—
Lean only 2.0 oz	56	115	18	4	2	2	Trace	0	7	2.2	10	.05	.14	3.6	—
Relatively lean, such as round															
Lean and fat 3 oz	85	220	24	13	6	6	Trace	0	10	3.0	20	.07	.19	4.8	—
Lean only 2.4 oz	68	130	21	4	2	2	Trace	0	9	2.5	10	.06	.16	4.1	—
Beef, canned															
Corned beef 3 oz	85	185	22	10	5	4	Trace	0	17	3.7	20	.01	.20	2.9	—
Corned beef hash 3 oz	85	155	7	10	5	4	Trace	9	11	1.7	—	.01	.08	1.8	—
Beef, dried or chipped 2 oz	57	115	19	4	2	2	Trace	0	11	2.9	—	.04	.18	2.2	—
Beef and vegetable stew 1 cup	235	210	15	10	5	4	Trace	15	28	2.8	2,310	.13	.17	4.4	15
Beef potpie, baked: individual pie, 4¼-inch diameter, weight before baking about 8 oz 1 pie	227	560	23	33	9	20	2	43	32	4.1	1,860	.25	.27	4.5	7
Chicken, cooked															
Flesh only, broiled 3 oz	85	115	20	3	1	1	1	0	8	1.4	80	.05	.16	7.4	—
Breast, fried ½ breast															
With bone 3.3 oz	94	155	25	5	1	2	1	1	9	1.3	70	.04	.17	11.2	—
Flesh and skin only 2.7 oz	76	155	25	5	1	2	1	1	9	1.3	70	.04	.17	11.2	—
Drumstick, fried															
With bone 2.1 oz	59	90	12	4	1	2	1	Trace	6	.9	50	.03	.15	2.7	—
Flesh and skin only 1.3 oz	38	90	12	4	1	2	1	Trace	6	.9	50	.03	.15	2.7	—
Chicken, canned, boneless 3 oz	85	170	18	10	3	4	2	0	18	1.3	200	.03	.11	3.7	3
Chicken potpie. See Poultry potpie.															
Chile con carne, canned															
With beans 1 cup	250	335	19	15	7	7	Trace	30	80	4.2	150	.08	.18	3.2	—
Without beans 1 cup	255	510	26	38	18	17	1	15	97	3.6	380	.05	.31	5.6	—
Fish and shellfish															
Bluefish, baked or broiled 3 oz	85	135	22	4	—	—	—	0	25	.6	40	.09	.08	1.6	—
Clams															
Raw, meat only 3 oz	85	65	11	1	—	—	—	2	59	5.2	90	.08	.15	1.1	8

Food	Measure	Grams	Food energy (cal.)	Protein (g)	Fat (g)	Saturated (g)	Oleic (g)	Linoleic (g)	Carbohydrate (g)	Calcium (mg)	Iron (mg)	Vitamin A (I.U.)	Thiamine (mg)	Riboflavin (mg)	Niacin (mg)	Ascorbic acid (mg)
Canned, solids and liquid	3 oz	85	45	7	1	—	—	—	2	47	3.5	—	.01	.09	.9	—
Crabmeat, canned	3 oz	85	85	15	2	—	—	—	1	38	.7	—	.07	.07	1.6	—
Fish sticks, breaded, cooked, frozen; stick 3.8 by 1.0 by 0.5 inch	10 sticks or 8 oz package	227	400	38	20	5	4	10	15	25	.9	—	.09	.16	3.6	—
Haddock, fried	3 oz	85	140	17	5	—	—	—	5	34	1.0	—	0.03	0.06	2.7	2
Mackerel																
Broiled, Atlantic	3 oz	85	200	19	13	—	—	—	0	5	1.0	450	.13	.23	6.5	—
Canned, Pacific, solids and liquid[3]	3 oz	85	155	18	9	—	—	—	0	221	1.9	20	.02	.28	7.4	—
Ocean perch, breaded (egg and breadcrumbs), fried	3 oz	85	195	16	11	—	—	—	6	28	1.1	—	.08	.09	1.5	—
Oysters, meat only. Raw, 13-19 medium selects	1 cup	240	160	20	4	—	—	—	8	226	13.2	740	.33	.43	6.0	—
Oyster stew, 1 part oysters to 3 parts milk by volume, 3-4 oysters	1 cup	230	200	11	12	—	—	—	11	269	3.3	640	.13	.41	1.6	—
Salmon, pink, canned	3 oz	85	120	17	5	1	1	Trace	0	[4]167	.7	60	.03	.16	6.8	—
Sardines, Atlantic, canned in oil, drained solids	3 oz	85	175	20	9	—	—	—	0	372	2.5	190	.02	.17	4.6	—
Shad, baked	3 oz	85	170	20	10	—	—	—	0	20	.5	20	.11	.22	7.3	—
Shrimp, canned, meat only	3 oz	85	100	21	1	—	—	—	1	98	2.6	50	.01	.03	1.5	—
Swordfish, broiled with butter or margarine	3 oz	85	150	24	5	—	—	—	0	23	1.1	1,780	.03	.04	9.3	—
Tuna, canned in oil, drained solids	3 oz	85	170	24	7	—	—	—	0	7	1.6	70	.04	.10	10.1	—
Heart, beef, lean, braised	3 oz	85	160	27	5	—	—	—	1	5	5.0	20	.21	1.04	6.5	1
Lamb, trimmed to retail basis,[2] cooked																
Chop, thick, with bone, broiled	1 chop, 4.8 oz	137	400	25	33	18	12	1	0	10	1.5	—	.14	.25	5.6	—
Lean and fat	4.0 oz	112	400	25	33	18	12	1	0	10	1.5	—	.14	.25	5.6	—
Lean only	2.6 oz	74	140	21	6	3	2	Trace	0	9	1.5	—	.11	.20	4.5	—
Leg, roasted																
Lean and fat	3 oz	85	235	22	16	9	6	Trace	0	9	1.4	—	.13	.23	4.7	—
Lean only	2.5 oz	71	130	20	5	3	2	Trace	0	9	1.4	—	.12	.21	4.4	—
Shoulder, roasted																
Lean and fat	3 oz	85	285	18	23	13	8	1	0	9	1.0	—	.11	.20	4.0	—
Lean only	2.3 oz	64	130	17	6	3	2	Trace	0	8	1.0	—	.10	.18	3.7	—
Liver, beef, fried	2 oz	57	130	15	6	—	—	—	3	6	5.0	30,280	.15	2.37	9.4	15
Pork, cured, cooked																
Ham, light cure, lean and fat, roasted	3 oz	85	245	18	19	7	8	2	0	8	2.2	0	.40	.16	3.1	—

[2] Outer layer of fat on the cut was removed to within approximately ½ inch of the lean. Deposits of fat within the cut were not removed.

[3] Vitamin values based on drained solids.

[4] Based on total contents of can. If bones are discarded, value will be greatly reduced.

Food, approximate measure, and weight (in grams)		Food energy (calories)	Protein (g)	Fat (total lipid) (g)	Fatty acids			Carbohydrate (g)	Calcium (mg)	Iron (mg)	Vitamin A value (IU)	Thiamin (mg)	Riboflavin (mg)	Niacin (mg)	Ascorbic acid (mg)
					Saturated (total) (g)	Unsaturated Oleic (g)	Unsaturated Linoleic (g)								
Luncheon meat															
Boiled ham, sliced	2 oz	57	135	11	10	4	4	1	0	6	1.6	0	.25	.09	1.5	—
Canned, spiced or unspiced	2 oz	57	165	8	14	5	6	1	1	5	1.2	0	.18	.12	1.6	—
Pork, fresh, trimmed to retail basis,[2] cooked															
Chop, thick, with bone	1 chop, 3.5 oz	98	260	16	21	8	9	2	0	8	2.2	0	.63	.18	3.8	—
Lean and fat	2.3 oz	66	260	16	21	8	9	2	0	8	2.2	0	.63	.18	3.8	—
Lean only	1.7 oz	48	130	15	7	2	3	1	0	7	1.9	0	.54	.16	3.3	—
Roast, oven-cooked, no liquid added															
Lean and fat	3 oz	85	310	21	24	9	10	2	0	9	2.7	0	.78	.22	4.7	—
Lean only	2.4 oz	68	175	20	10	3	4	1	0	9	2.6	0	.73	.21	4.4	—
Cuts, simmered															
Lean and fat	3 oz	85	320	20	26	9	11	2	0	8	2.5	0	.46	.21	4.1	—
Lean only	2.2 oz	63	135	18	6	2	3	1	0	8	2.3	0	.42	.19	3.7	—
Poultry potpie (based on chicken potpie). Individual pie, 4¼-inch diameter, weigh before baking	1 pie	227	535	23	31	10	15	3	42	68	3.0	3,020	.25	.26	4.1	5
Sausage															
Bologna, slice, 4.1 by 0.1 inch	8 slices	227	690	27	62	—	—	—	2	16	4.1	—	.36	.49	6.0	—
Frankfurter, cooked	1	51	155	6	14	—	—	—	1	3	.8	—	.08	.10	1.3	—
Pork, links or patty, cooked	4 oz	113	540	21	50	18	21	5	Trace	8	2.7	0	.89	.39	4.2	—
Tongue, beef, braised	3 oz	85	210	18	14	—	—	—	Trace	6	1.9	—	.04	.25	3.0	—
Turkey potpie. *See* Poultry potpie															
Veal, cooked															
Cutlet, without bone, broiled	3 oz	85	185	23	9	5	4	Trace	—	9	2.7	—	.06	.21	4.6	—
Roast, medium fat, medium done; lean and fat	3 oz	85	230	23	14	7	6	Trace	0	10	2.9	—	.11	.26	6.6	—
Mature dry beans and peas, nuts, peanuts (related products)															
Almonds, shelled	1 cup	142	850	26	77	6	52	15	28	332	6.7	0	.34	1.31	5.0	Trace
Beans, dry Common varieties, such as Great Northern, navy, and others, canned:															
Red	1 cup	256	230	15	1	—	—	—	42	74	4.6	Trace	.13	.10	1.5	—
White, with tomato sauce															
With pork	1 cup	261	320	16	7	3	3	1	50	141	4.7	340	.20	.08	1.5	5
Without pork	1 cup	261	310	16	1	—	—	—	60	177	5.2	160	.18	.09	1.5	5
Lima, cooked	1 cup	192	260	16	1	—	—	—	48	56	5.6	Trace	.26	.12	1.3	Trace

Food	Measure	Weight (g)	Calories	Protein (g)	Fat (g)	Saturated	Oleic	Linoleic	Carbohydrate (g)	Calcium (mg)	Iron (mg)	Vitamin A (IU)	Thiamine (mg)	Riboflavin (mg)	Niacin (mg)	Ascorbic acid (mg)
Brazil nuts	1 cup	140	915	20	94	19	45	24	15	260	4.8	Trace	1.34	.17	2.2	—
Cashew nuts, roasted	1 cup	135	760	23	62	10	43	4	40	51	5.1	140	.58	.33	2.4	—
Coconut																
Fresh, shredded	1 cup	97	335	3	34	29	2	Trace	9	13	1.6	0	.05	.02	.5	3
Dried, shredded sweetened	1 cup	62	340	2	24	21	2	Trace	33	10	1.2	0	.02	.02	.2	0
Cowpeas or blackeye peas, dry, cooked	1 cup	248	190	13	1	—	—	—	34	42	3.2	20	.41	.11	1.1	Trace
Peanuts, roasted, salted																
Halves	1 cup	144	840	37	72	16	31	21	27	107	3.0	—	.46	.19	24.7	0
Chopped	1 tbsp	9	55	2	4	1	2	1	2	7	.2	—	.03	.01	1.5	0
Peanut butter	1 tbsp	16	95	4	8	2	4	2	3	9	.3	—	.02	.02	2.4	0
Peas, split, dry, cooked	1 cup	250	290	20	1	—	—	—	52	28	4.2	100	.37	.22	2.2	—
Pecans																
Halves	1 cup	108	740	10	77	5	48	15	16	79	2.6	140	.93	.14	1.0	2
Chopped	1 tbsp	7.5	50	1	5	Trace	3	1	1	5	.2	10	.06	.01	.1	Trace
Walnuts, shelled																
Black or native, chopped	1 cup	126	790	26	75	4	26	36	19	Trace	7.6	380	.28	.14	.9	—
English or Persian																
Halves	1 cup	100	650	15	64	4	10	40	16	99	3.1	30	.33	.13	.9	3
Chopped	1 tbsp	8	50	1	5	Trace	1	3	1	8	.2	Trace	.03	.01	.1	Trace
Vegetables and vegetable products																
Asparagus																
Cooked, cut spears	1 cup	175	35	4	Trace	—	—	—	6	37	1.0	1,580	.27	.32	2.4	46
Canned spears, medium																
Green	6 spears	96	20	2	Trace	—	—	—	3	18	1.8	770	.06	.10	.8	14
Bleached	6 spears	96	20	2	Trace	—	—	—	4	15	1.0	80	.05	.06	.7	14
Beans																
Lima, immature, cooked	1 cup	160	180	12	1	—	—	—	32	75	4.0	450	.29	.16	2.0	28
Snap, green																
Cooked																
In small amount of water, short time	1 cup	125	30	2	Trace	—	—	—	7	62	.8	680	.08	.11	.6	16
In large amount of water, long time	1 cup	125	30	2	Trace	—	—	—	7	62	0.8	680	0.07	0.10	0.4	13
Canned																
Solids and liquid	1 cup	239	45	2	Trace	—	—	—	10	81	2.9	690	.08	.10	.7	9
Strained or chopped (baby food)	1 oz	28	5	Trace	Trace	—	—	—	1	9	.3	110	.01	.02	.1	Trace
Bean sprouts. *See* Sprouts																
Beets, cooked, diced	1 cup	165	50	2	Trace	—	—	—	12	23	.8	40	.04	.07	.5	11
Broccoli spears, cooked	1 cup	150	40	5	Trace	—	—	—	7	132	1.2	3,750	.14	.29	1.2	135
Brussels sprouts, cooked	1 cup	130	45	5	1	—	—	—	8	42	1.4	680	.10	.18	1.1	113
Cabbage																
Raw																
Finely shredded	1 cup	100	25	1	Trace	—	—	—	5	49	.4	130	.05	.05	.3	47
Coleslaw	1 cup	120	120	1	9	2	2	5	9	52	.5	180	.06	.06	.3	35

[2] Outer layer of fat on the cut was removed to within approximately ½ inch of the lean. Deposits of fat within the cut were not removed.

Food, approximate measure, and weight (in grams)		Food energy (calories)	Protein (g)	Fat (total lipid) (g)	Fatty acids			Carbohydrate (g)	Calcium (mg)	Iron (mg)	Vitamin A value (IU)	Thiamin (mg)	Riboflavin (mg)	Niacin (mg)	Ascorbic acid (mg)
					Saturated (total) (g)	Unsaturated Oleic (g)	Linoleic (g)								
Cooked															
In small amount of water, short time	1 cup	170	35	2	Trace	—	—	—	7	75	.5	220	.07	.07	.5	56
In large amount of water, long time	1 cup	170	30	2	Trace	—	—	—	7	71	.5	200	.04	.04	.2	40
Cabbage, celery or Chinese															
Raw, leaves and stalk, 1-inch pieces	1 cup	100	15	1	Trace	—	—	—	3	43	.6	150	.05	.04	.6	25
Cabbage, spoon (or pakchoy), cooked	1 cup	150	20	2	Trace	—	—	—	4	222	.9	4,650	.07	.12	1.1	23
Carrots															
Raw															
Whole, 5½ by 1 inch, (25 thin strips)	1	50	20	1	Trace	—	—	—	5	18	.4	5,500	.03	.03	.3	4
Grated	1 cup	110	45	1	Trace	—	—	—	11	41	.8	12,100	.06	.06	.7	9
Cooked, diced	1 cup	145	45	1	Trace	—	—	—	10	48	.9	15,220	.08	.07	.7	9
Canned, strained or chopped (baby food)	1 oz	28	10	Trace	Trace	—	—	—	2	7	.1	3,690	.01	.01	.1	1
Cauliflower, cooked, flowerbuds	1 cup	120	25	3	Trace	—	—	—	5	25	.8	70	.11	.10	.7	66
Celery, raw															
Stalk, large outer, 8 by about 1½ inches, at root end	1 stalk	40	5	Trace	Trace	—	—	—	2	16	.1	100	.01	.01	.1	4
Pieces, diced	1 cup	100	15	1	Trace	—	—	—	4	39	.3	240	.03	.03	.3	9
Collards, cooked	1 cup	190	55	5	1	—	—	—	9	289	1.1	10,260	.27	.37	2.4	87
Corn, sweet															
Cooked, ear 5 by 1¾ inches[5]	1 ear	140	70	3	1	—	—	—	16	2	.5	[6]310	.09	.08	1.0	7
Canned, solids and liquid	1 cup	256	170	5	2	—	—	—	40	10	1.0	[6]690	.07	.12	2.3	13
Cowpeas, cooked, immature seeds	1 cup	160	175	13	1	—	—	—	29	38	3.4	560	.49	.18	2.3	28
Cucumbers, 10 oz, 7½ by about 2 inches															
Raw, pared	1	207	30	1	Trace	—	—	—	7	35	.6	Trace	.07	.09	.4	23
Raw, pared, center slice ⅛-inch thick	6 slices	50	5	Trace	Trace	—	—	—	2	8	.2	Trace	.02	.02	.1	6
Dandelion greens, cooked	1 cup	180	60	4	1	—	—	—	12	252	3.2	21,060	.24	.29	—	32
Endive, curly (including escarole)	2 oz	57	10	1	Trace	—	—	—	2	46	1.0	1,870	.04	.08	.3	6
Kale, leaves including stems, cooked	1 cup	110	30	4	1	—	—	—	4	147	1.3	8,140	—	—	—	68

Food	Measure	Grams	Calories	Protein	Fat				Carbohydrate	Calcium	Iron	Vitamin A	Thiamine	Riboflavin	Niacin	Ascorbic acid
Lettuce, raw																
Butterhead, as Boston types; head, 4-inch diameter	1 head	220	30	3	Trace	—	—	—	6	77	4.4	2,130	.14	.13	.6	18
Crisphead, as Iceberg; head, 4¾-inch diameter	1 head	454	60	4	Trace	—	—	—	13	91	2.3	1,500	.29	.27	1.3	29
Looseleaf, or bunching varieties, leaves	2 large	50	10	1	Trace	—	—	—	2	34	.7	950	.03	.04	.2	9
Mushrooms, canned, solids and liquid	1 cup	244	40	5	Trace	—	—	—	6	15	1.2	Trace	.04	.60	4.8	4
Mustard greens, cooked	1 cup	140	35	3	1	—	—	—	6	193	2.5	8,120	.11	.19	.9	68
Okra, cooked, pod 3 by ⅜ inch	8 pods	85	25	3	Trace	—	—	—	5	78	.4	420	.11	.15	.8	17
Onions																
Mature																
Raw, onion 2½-inch diameter	1	110	40	2	Trace	—	—	—	10	30	0.6	40	0.04	0.04	0.2	11
Cooked	1 cup	210	60	3	Trace	—	—	—	14	50	.8	80	.06	.06	.4	14
Young green, small, without tops	6	50	20	1	Trace	—	—	—	5	20	.3	Trace	.02	.02	.2	12
Parsley, raw, chopped	1 tbsp	3.5	1	Trace	Trace	—	—	—	Trace	7	.2	300	Trace	.01	Trace	6
Parsnips, cooked	1 cup	155	100	2	1	—	—	—	23	70	.9	50	.11	.13	.2	16
Peas, green																
Cooked	1 cup	160	115	9	1	—	—	—	19	37	2.9	860	.44	.17	3.7	33
Canned, solids and liquid	1 cup	249	165	9	1	—	—	—	31	50	4.2	1,120	.23	.13	2.2	22
Canned, strained (baby food)	1 oz	28	15	1	Trace	—	—	—	3	3	.4	140	.02	.02	.4	3
Peppers, hot, red, without seeds, dried (ground chili powder, added seasonings)	1 tbsp	15	50	2	2	—	—	—	8	40	2.3	9,750	.03	.17	1.3	2
Peppers, sweet																
Raw, medium, about 6 per pound																
Green pod without stem and seeds	1 pod	62	15	1	Trace	—	—	—	3	6	.4	260	.05	.05	.3	79
Red pod without stem and seeds	1 pod	60	20	1	Trace	—	—	—	4	8	.4	2,670	.05	.05	.3	122
Canned, pimentos, medium	1 pod	38	10	Trace	Trace	—	—	—	2	3	.6	870	.01	.02	.1	36
Potatoes, medium (about 3 per pound raw)																
Baked, peeled after baking	1	99	90	3	Trace	—	—	—	21	9	.7	Trace	.10	.04	1.7	20

[5] Measure and weight apply to entire vegetable or fruit including parts not usually eaten.

[6] Based on yellow varieties; white varieties contain only a trace of cryptoxanthin and carotenes, the pigments in corn that have biological activity.

Food, approximate measure, and weight (in grams)		Food energy (calories)	Protein (g)	Fat (total lipid) (g)	Fatty acids Saturated (total) (g)	Unsaturated Oleic (g)	Linoleic (g)	Carbohydrate (g)	Calcium (mg)	Iron (mg)	Vitamin A value (IU)	Thiamin (mg)	Riboflavin (mg)	Niacin (mg)	Ascorbic acid (mg)
Boiled															
Peeled after boiling	1	136	105	3	Trace	—	—	—	23	10	.8	Trace	.13	.05	2.0	22
Peeled before boiling	1	122	80	2	Trace	—	—	—	18	7	.6	Trace	.11	.04	1.4	20
French-fried, piece 2 by ½ by ½ inch															
Cooked in deep fat	10 pieces	57	155	2	7	2	2	4	20	9	.7	Trace	.07	.04	1.8	12
Frozen, heated	10 pieces	57	125	2	5	1	1	2	19	5	1.0	Trace	.08	.01	1.5	12
Mashed															
Milk added	1 cup	195	125	4	1				25	47	.8	50	.16	.10	2.0	19
Milk and butter added	1 cup	195	185	4	8	4	3	Trace	24	47	.8	330	.16	.10	1.9	18
Potato chips, medium, 2-inch diameter	10 chips	20	115	1	8	3	2	4	10	8	.4	Trace	.04	.01	1.0	3
Pumpkin, canned	1 cup	228	75	2	1				18	57	.9	14,590	.07	.12	1.3	12
Radishes, raw, small, without tops	4	40	5	Trace	Trace				1	12	.4	Trace	.01	.01	.1	10
Sauerkraut, canned, solids and liquid	1 cup	235	45	2	Trace				9	85	1.2	120	.07	.09	.4	33
Spinach															
Cooked	1 cup	180	40	5	1				6	167	4.0	14,580	.13	.25	1.0	50
Canned, drained solids	1 cup	180	45	5	1				6	212	4.7	14,400	.03	.21	.6	24
Canned, strained or chopped (baby food)	1 oz	28	10	1	Trace				2	18	.2	1,420	.01	.04	.1	2
Sprouts, raw															
Mung bean	1 cup	90	30	3	Trace				6	17	1.2	20	.12	.12	.7	17
Soybean	1 cup	107	40	6	2				4	46	.7	90	.17	.16	.8	4
Squash															
Cooked															
Summer, diced	1 cup	210	30	2	Trace				7	52	.8	820	.10	.16	1.6	21
Winter, baked, mashed	1 cup	205	130	4	1				32	57	1.6	8,610	.10	.27	1.4	27
Canned, winter, strained and chopped (baby food)	1 oz	28	10	Trace	Trace				2	7	.1	510	.01	.01	.1	1
Sweetpotatoes															
Cooked, medium, 5 by 2 inches, weight raw about 6 oz															
Baked, peeled after baking	1	110	155	2	1	—	—	—	36	44	1.0	8,910	.10	.07	.7	24
Boiled, peeled after boiling	1	147	170	2	1	—	—	—	39	47	1.0	11,610	.13	.09	.9	25
Candied, 3½ by 2¼ inches	1	175	295	2	6	2	3	1	60	65	1.6	11,030	.10	.08	.8	17

Food	Measure	Grams	Food energy (Cal.)	Protein (g)	Fat (g)	Saturated (g)	Oleic (g)	Linoleic (g)	Carbohydrate (g)	Calcium (mg)	Iron (mg)	Vitamin A (IU)	Thiamine (mg)	Riboflavin (mg)	Niacin (mg)	Ascorbic acid (mg)
Canned, vacuum or solid pack	1 cup	218	235	4	Trace	—	—	—	54	54	1.7	17,000	.10	.10	1.4	30
Tomatoes																
Raw, medium, 2 by 2½ inches, about 3 per pound	1	150	35	2	Trace	—	—	—	7	20	.8	1,350	.10	.06	1.0	34[7]
Canned	1 cup	242	50	2	Trace	—	—	—	10	15	1.2	2,180	.13	.07	1.7	40
Tomato juice, canned	1 cup	242	45	2	Trace	—	—	—	10	17	2.2	1,940	.13	.07	1.8	39
Tomato catsup	1 tbsp	17	15	Trace	Trace	—	—	—	4	4	.1	240	.02	.01	.3	3
Turnips, cooked, diced	1 cup	155	35	1	Trace	—	—	—	8	54	.6	Trace	.06	.08	.5	33
Turnip greens																
Cooked																
In small amount of water, short time	1 cup	145	30	3	Trace	—	—	—	5	267	1.6	9,140	.21	.36	.8	100
In large amount of water, long time	1 cup	145	25	3	Trace	—	—	—	5	252	1.4	8,260	.14	.33	.8	68
Canned, solids and liquid	1 cup	232	40	3	1	—	—	—	7	232	3.7	10,900	.04	.21	1.4	44
Fruits and fruit products																
Apples, raw, medium, 2½-inch diameter, about 3 per pound[5]	1	150	70	Trace	Trace	—	—	—	18	8	.4	50	.04	.02	.1	3
Apple brown betty	1 cup	230	345	4	8	3	4	Trace	68	41	1.4	230	.13	.10	.9	3
Apple juice, bottled or canned	1 cup	249	120	Trace	Trace	—	—	—	30	15	1.5	—	.01	.04	.2	2
Applesauce, canned																
Sweetened	1 cup	254	230	1	Trace	—	—	—	60	10	1.3	100	.05	.03	.1	3
Unsweetened or artifically sweetened	1 cup	239	100	Trace	Trace	—	—	—	26	10	1.2	100	.04	.02	.1	2
Applesauce and apricots, canned, strained or junior (baby food)	1 oz	28	25	Trace	Trace	—	—	—	6	1	.1	170	Trace	Trace	Trace	1
Apricots																
Raw, about 12 per pound[5]	3 apricots	114	55	1	Trace	—	—	—	14	18	.5	2,890	.03	.04	.7	10
Canned in heavy syrup																
Halves and syrup	1 cup	259	220	2	Trace	—	—	—	57	28	.8	4,510	.05	.06	.9	10
Halves (medium) and syrup	4 halves; 2 tbsp syrup	122	105	1	Trace	—	—	—	27	13	.4	2,120	.02	.03	.4	5
Dried																
Uncooked, 40 halves, small	1 cup	150	390	8	1	—	—	—	100	100	8.2	16,350	.02	.23	4.9	19
Cooked, unsweetened, fruit and liquid	1 cup	285	240	5	1	—	—	—	62	63	5.1	8,550	.01	.13	2.8	8
Apricot nectar, canned	1 cup	250	140	1	Trace	—	—	—	36	22	.5	2,380	.02	.02	.5	7

[5] Measure and weight apply to entire vegetable or fruit including parts not usually eaten.

[7] Year-round average. Samples marketed from November through May average around 15 milligrams per 150-gram tomato; from June through October, around 39 milligrams.

Food, approximate measure	Weight (in grams)	Food energy (calories)	Protein (g)	Fat (total lipid) (g)	Fatty acids — Saturated (total) (g)	Unsaturated — Oleic (g)	Unsaturated — Linoleic (g)	Carbohydrate (g)	Calcium (mg)	Iron (mg)	Vitamin A value (IU)	Thiamin (mg)	Riboflavin (mg)	Niacin (mg)	Ascorbic acid (mg)
Avocados, raw															
California varieties, mainly Fuerte															
10-ounce avocado, about 3½ by 4¼ inches, peeled, pitted — ½	108	185	2	18	4	8	2	6	11	.6	310	.12	.21	1.7	15
½-inch cubes — 1 cup	152	260	3	26	5	12	3	9	15	.9	440	.16	.30	2.4	21
Florida varieties															
13 oz avocado, about 4 by 3 inches, peeled, pitted — ½	123	160	2	14	3	6	2	11	12	.7	360	.13	.24	2.0	17
½-inch cubes — 1 cup	152	195	2	17	3	8	2	13	15	.9	440	.16	.30	2.4	21
Bananas, raw, 6 by 1½ inches, about 3 per pound[5] — 1	150	85	1	Trace	—	—	—	23	8	.7	190	.05	.06	.7	10
Blackberries, raw — 1 cup	144	85	2	1	—	—	—	19	46	1.3	290	.05	.06	.5	30
Blueberries, raw — 1 cup	140	85	1	1	—	—	—	21	21	1.4	140	.04	.08	.6	20
Cantaloups, raw; medium, 5-inch diameter, about 1⅔ pounds[5] — ½	385	60	1	Trace	—	—	—	14	27	.8	[8]6,540	.08	.06	1.2	63
Cherries															
Raw, sweet, with stems[5] — 1 cup	130	80	2	Trace	—	—	—	20	26	.5	130	.06	.07	.5	12
Canned, red, sour, pitted, heavy syrup — 1 cup	260	230	2	1	—	—	—	59	36	.8	1,680	.07	.06	.4	13
Cranberry juice cocktail, canned — 1 cup	250	160	Trace	Trace	—	—	—	41	12	.8	Trace	.02	.02	.1	(9)
Cranberry sauce, sweetened, canned, strained — 1 cup	277	405	Trace	1	—	—	—	104	17	.6	40	.03	0.3	.1	5
Dates, domestic, natural and dry, pitted, cut — 1 cup	178	490	4	1	—	—	—	130	105	5.3	90	.16	.17	3.9	0
Figs															
Raw, small, 1½-inch diameter, about 12 per pound — 3 figs	114	90	1	Trace	—	—	—	23	40	.7	90	.07	.06	.5	2
Dried, large, 2 by 1 inch — 1 fig	21	60	1	Trace	—	—	—	15	26	.6	20	.02	.02	.1	0
Fruit cocktail, canned in heavy syrup, solids and liquid — 1 cup	256	195	1	1	—	—	—	50	23	1.0	360	.04	.03	1.1	5
Grapefruit															
Raw, medium, 4¼-inch diameter, size 64															
White[5] — ½	285	55	1	Trace	—	—	—	14	22	.6	10	.05	.02	.2	52
Pink or red[5] — ½	285	60	1	Trace	—	—	—	15	23	.6	640	.05	.02	.3	52
Raw sections, white — 1 cup	194	75	1	Trace	—	—	—	20	31	.8	20	.07	.03	.3	72

Canned, white														
Syrup pack, solids and liquid	1 cup	249	175	1	Trace	—	44	32	.7	20	.07	.04	.5	75
Water pack, solids and liquid	1 cup	240	70	1	Trace	—	18	31	.7	20	.07	.04	.5	72
Grapefruit juice														
Fresh	1 cup	246	95	1	Trace	—	23	22	.5	(10)	.09	.04	.4	92
Canned, white														
Unsweetened	1 cup	247	100	1	Trace	—	24	20	1.0	20	.07	.04	.4	84
Sweetened	1 cup	250	130	1	Trace	—	32	20	1.0	20	.07	.04	.4	78
Frozen, concentrate, unsweetened														
Undiluted, can, 6 fluid oz	1 can	207	300	4	1	—	72	70	.8	60	.29	.12	1.4	286
Diluted with 3 parts water, by volume	1 cup	247	100	1	Trace	—	24	25	.2	20	.10	.04	.5	96
Frozen, concentrate, sweetened														
Undiluted, can, 6 fluid oz	1 can	211	350	3	1	—	85	59	.6	50	.24	.11	1.2	245
Diluted with 3 parts water, by volume	1 cup	249	115	1	Trace	—	28	20	.2	20	.08	.03	.4	82
Dehydrated														
Crystals, can, net weight 4 oz	1 can	114	430	5	1	—	103	99	1.1	90	.41	.18	2.0	399
Prepared with water (1 pound yields about 1 gal)	1 cup	247	100	1	Trace	—	24	22	.2	20	.10	.05	.5	92
Grapes, raw														
American type (slip skin), such as Concord, Delaware, Niagara, Catawba, and Scuppernong[5]	1 cup	153	65	1	1	—	15	15	.4	100	.05	.03	.2	3
European type (adherent skin), such as Malaga, Muscat, Thompson Seedless, Emperor, and Flame Tokay[5]	1 cup	160	95	1	Trace	—	25	17	.6	140	.07	.04	.4	6
Grape juice, bottled or canned	1 cup	254	165	1	Trace	—	42	28	.8	—	.10	.05	.6	Trace
Lemons, raw, medium, 2½-inch diameter, size 150[5]	1 lemon	106	20	1	Trace	—	6	18	.4	10	.03	.01	.1	38
Lemon juice														
Fresh	1 cup	246	60	1	Trace	—	20	17	.5	40	.08	.03	.2	113
	1 tbsp	15	5	Trace	Trace	—	1	1	Trace	Trace	Trace	Trace	Trace	7
Canned, unsweetened	1 cup	245	55	1	Trace	—	19	17	.5	40	.07	.03	.2	102

[5] Measure and weight apply to entire vegetable or fruit including parts not usually eaten.

[8] Value based on varieties with orange-colored flesh, for green-fleshed varieties value is about 540 IU per ½ melon.

[9] About 5 milligrams per 8 fluid ounces is from cranberries. Ascorbic acid is usually added to approximately 100 milligrams per 8 fluid ounces.

[10] For white-fleshed varieties value is about 20 IU per cup; for red-fleshed varieties, 1,080 IU per cup.

| Food, approximate measure, and weight (in grams) | | Food energy (calories) | Protein (g) | Fat (total lipid) (g) | Fatty acids | | | Carbo-hydrate (g) | Cal-cium (mg) | Iron (mg) | Vita-min A value (IU) | Thia-min (mg) | Ribo-flavin (mg) | Niacin (mg) | Ascorbic acid (mg) |
| | | | | | Satu-rated (total) (g) | Unsaturated | | | | | | | | | |
						Oleic (g)	Linoleic (g)								
Lemonade concentrate, frozen, sweetened															
Undiluted, can, 6 fluid oz	1 can	220	430	Trace	Trace	—	—	—	112	9	.4	40	.05	.06	.7	66
Diluted with 4½ parts water, by volume	1 cup	248	110	Trace	Trace	—	—	—	28	2	.1	10	.01	.01	.2	17
Lime juice															
Fresh	1 cup	246	65	1	Trace	—	—	—	22	22	.5	30	.05	.03	.03	80
Canned	1 cup	246	65	1	Trace	—	—	—	22	22	.5	30	.05	.03	.3	52
Limeade concentrate, frozen, sweetened															
Undiluted, can, 6 fluid oz	1 can	218	410	Trace	Trace	—	—	—	108	11	.2	Trace	.02	.02	.3	26
Diluted with 4⅓ parts water, by volume	1 cup	248	105	Trace	Trace	—	—	—	27	2	Trace	Trace	Trace	Trace	Trace	6
Oranges, raw															
California, Navel (winter), 2⅘,5-inch diameter, size 88[5]	1 orange	180	60	2	Trace	—	—	—	16	49	.5	240	.12	.05	.5	75
Florida, all varieties, 3-inch diameter[5]	1	210	75	1	Trace	—	—	—	19	67	.3	310	.16	.06	.6	70
Orange juice															
Fresh															
California, Valencia (summer)	1 cup	249	115	2	1	—	—	—	26	27	.7	500	.22	.06	.9	122
Florida varieties															
Early and mid-season	1 cup	247	100	1	Trace	—	—	—	23	25	.5	490	.22	.06	.9	127
Late season, Valencia	1 cup	248	110	1	Trace	—	—	—	26	25	.5	500	.22	.06	.9	92
Canned, unsweetened	1 cup	249	120	2	Trace	—	—	—	28	25	1.0	500	.17	.05	.6	100
Frozen concentrate															
Undiluted, can, 6 fluid oz	1 can	210	330	5	Trace	—	—	—	80	69	.8	1,490	.63	.10	2.4	332
Diluted with 3 parts water, by volume	1 cup	248	110	2	Trace	—	—	—	27	22	.2	500	.21	.03	.8	112
Dehydrated															
Crystals, can, net weight 4 oz	1 can	113	430	6	2	—	—	—	100	95	1.9	1,900	.76	.24	3.3	406
Prepared with water, 1 lb yields about 1 gal	1 cup	248	115	1	Trace	—	—	—	27	25	.5	500	.20	.06	.9	108
Orange and grapefruit juice															
Frozen concentrate															
Undiluted, can, 6 fluid oz	1 can	209	325	4	1	—	—	—	78	61	.8	790	.47	.06	2.3	301

Food	Measure															
Diluted with 3 parts water, by volume	1 cup	248	110	1	Trace	—	—	—	26	20	.3	270	.16	.02	.8	102
Papayas, raw, ½-inch cubes[5]	1 cup	182	70	1	Trace	—	—	—	18	36	.5	3,190	.07	.08	.5	102
Peaches																
Raw																
Whole, medium, 2-inch diameter, about 4 per pound[5]	1	114	35	1	Trace	—	—	—	10	9	.5	[11]1,320	.02	.05	1.0	7
Sliced	1 cup	168	65	1	Trace	—	—	—	16	15	.8	[11]2,230	.03	.08	1.6	12
Canned, yellow-fleshed, solids and liquid																
Syrup pack, heavy																
Halves or slices	1 cup	257	200	1	Trace	—	—	—	52	10	.8	1,100	.02	.06	1.4	7
Halves (medium) and syrup	2 halves and 2 tbsp syrup	117	90	Trace	Trace	—	—	—	24	5	.4	500	.01	.03	.7	3
Water pack	1 cup	245	75	1	Trace	—	—	—	20	10	.7	1,100	.02	.06	1.4	7
Strained or chopped (baby food)	1 oz	28	25	Trace	Trace	—	—	—	6	2	.1	140	Trace	.01	.2	1
Dried																
Uncooked	1 cup	160	420	5	1	—	—	—	109	77	9.6	6,240	.02	.31	8.5	28
Cooked, unsweetened, 10-12 halves and 6 tbsp liquid	1 cup	270	220	3	1	—	—	—	58	41	5.1	3,290	.01	.15	4.2	6
Frozen																
Carton, 12 oz, not thawed	1 carton	340	300	1	Trace	—	—	—	77	14	1.7	2,210	.03	.14	2.4	[12]135
Can, 16 oz, not thawed	1 can	454	400	2	Trace	—	—	—	103	18	2.3	2,950	.05	.18	3.2	[12]181
Peach nectar, canned	1 cup	250	120	Trace	Trace	—	—	—	31	10	.5	1,080	.02	.05	1.0	1
Pears																
Raw, 3 by 2½-inch diameter[5]	1	182	100	1	1	—	—	—	25	13	.5	30	.04	.07	.2	7
Canned, solids and liquid																
Syrup pack, heavy																
Halves or slices	1 cup	255	195	1	1	—	—	—	50	13	.5	Trace	.03	.05	.3	4
Halves (medium) and syrup	2 halves and 2 tbsp syrup	117	90	Trace	Trace	—	—	—	23	6	.2	Trace	.01	.02	.2	2
Water pack	1 cup	243	80	Trace	Trace	—	—	—	20	12	.5	Trace	.02	.05	.3	4
Strained or chopped (baby food)	1 oz	28	20	Trace	Trace	—	—	—	5	2	.1	10	Trace	.01	.1	1
Pear nectar, canned	1 cup	250	130	1	Trace	—	—	—	33	8	.2	Trace	.01	.05	Trace	1
Persimmons, Japanese or kaki, raw, seedless, 2½-inch diameter[5]	1	125	75	1	Trace	—	—	—	20	6	.4	2,740	.01	.02	.1	11

[5] Measure and weight apply to entire vegetable or fruit including parts not usually eaten.

[11] Based on yellow-fleshed varieties; for white-fleshed varieties value is about 50 IU per 114-gram peach and 80 IU per cup of sliced peaches.

[12] Average weighted in accordance with commercial freezing practices. For products without added ascorbic acid, value is about 37 milligrams per 12-ounce carton and 50 milligrams per 16-ounce can; for those with added ascorbic acid, 139 milligrams per 12 ounces and 186 milligrams per 16 ounces.

| Food, approximate measure, and weight (in grams) | | Food energy (calories) | Protein (g) | Fat (total lipid) (g) | Fatty acids | | | Carbohydrate (g) | Calcium (mg) | Iron (mg) | Vitamin A value (IU) | Thiamin (mg) | Riboflavin (mg) | Niacin (mg) | Ascorbic acid (mg) |
					Saturated (total) (g)	Unsaturated Oleic (g)	Linoleic (g)								
Pineapple															
Raw, diced	1 cup	140	75	1	Trace	—	—	—	19	24	.7	100	.12	.04	.3	24
Canned, heavy syrup pack, solids and liquid															
Crushed	1 cup	260	195	1	Trace	—	—	—	50	29	.8	120	.20	.06	.5	17
Sliced, slices and juice	2 small or 1 large and 2 tbsp juice	122	90	Trace	Trace	—	—	—	24	13	.4	50	.09	.03	.2	8
Pineapple juice, canned	1 cup	249	135	1	Trace	—	—	—	34	37	.7	120	.12	.04	.5	22
Plums, all except prunes															
Raw, 2-inch diameter, about 2 ounces[5]	1	60	25	Trace	Trace	—	—	—	7	7	.3	140	.02	.02	.3	3
Canned, syrup pack (Italian prunes)															
Plums (with pits) and juice[5]	1 cup	256	205	1	Trace	—	—	—	53	22	2.2	2,970	.05	.05	.9	4
Plums (without pits) and juice	3 plums and 2 tbsp juice	122	100	Trace	Trace	—	—	—	26	11	1.1	1,470	.03	.02	.5	2
Prunes, dried, "softenized," medium															
Uncooked[5]	4	32	70	1	Trace	—	—	—	18	14	1.1	440	.02	.04	.4	1
Cooked, unsweetened, 17-18 prunes and ⅓ cup liquid[5]	1 cup	270	295	2	1	—	—	—	78	60	4.5	1,860	.08	.18	1.7	2
Prunes with tapioca, canned, strained or junior (baby food)	1 oz	28	25	Trace	Trace	—	—	—	6	2	.3	110	.01	.02	.1	1
Prune juice, canned	1 cup	256	200	1	Trace	—	—	—	49	36	10.5	—	.02	.03	1.1	4
Raisin, dried	1 cup	160	460	4	Trace	—	—	—	124	99	5.6	30	.18	.13	.9	2
Raspberries, red															
Raw	1 cup	123	70	1	1	—	—	—	17	27	1.1	160	.04	.11	1.1	31
Frozen, 10 oz carton, not thawed	1 carton	284	275	2	1	—	—	—	70	37	1.7	200	.06	.17	1.7	59
Rhubarb, cooked, sugar added	1 cup	272	385	1	Trace	—	—	—	98	212	1.6	220	.06	.15	.7	17
Strawberries															
Raw, capped	1 cup	149	55	1	1	—	—	—	13	31	1.5	90	.04	.10	1.0	88
Frozen, 10-oz carton, not thawed	1 carton	284	310	1	1	—	—	—	79	40	2.0	90	.06	.17	1.5	150
Frozen, 16-ounce can, not thawed	1 can	454	495	2	1	—	—	—	126	64	3.2	150	.09	.27	2.4	240
Tangerines, raw, medium, 2½-inch diameter, about 4 per pound[5]	1	114	40	1	Trace	—	—	—	10	34	.3	350	.05	.02	.1	26

Food	Measure	g	cal	Protein	Fat	Sat.	Oleic	Lino.	Carb.	Ca	Fe	Vit. A	Thiamine	Riboflavin	Niacin	Ascorbic
Tangerine juice, Canned, unsweetened	1 cup	248	105	1	Trace	—	—	—	25	45	.5	1,040	.14	.04	.3	56
Frozen concentrate, Undiluted, can, 6 fluid oz	1 can	210	340	4	1	—	—	—	80	130	1.5	3,070	.43	.12	.9	202
Diluted with 3 parts water, by volume	1 cup	248	115	1	Trace	—	—	—	27	45	.5	1,020	.14	.04	.3	67
Watermelon, raw, wedge, 4 by 8 inches (1/16 of 10 by 16-inch melon, about 2 pounds with rind)[5]	1 wedge	925	115	2	1	—	—	—	27	30	2.1	2,510	.13	.13	.7	30
Breads and cereals																
Barley, pearled, light, uncooked	1 cup	203	710	17	2	—	—	—	160	32	4.1	0	.25	.17	6.3	0
Biscuits, baking powder with enriched flour, 2½-inch diameter	1	38	140	3	6	2	3	1	17	46	.6	Trace	.08	.08	.7	Trace
Bran flakes (40 percent bran) added thiamine	1 oz	28	85	3	1	—	—	—	23	20	1.2	0	.11	.05	1.7	0
Bread																
Boston brown bread, slice, 3 by ¾ inch	1 slice	48	100	3	1	—	—	—	22	43	.9	0	.05	.03	.6	0
Cracked-wheat bread																
Loaf, 1-pound, 20 slices	1 loaf	454	1,190	39	10	2	5	2	236	399	5.0	Trace	.53	.42	5.8	Trace
Slice	1	23	60	2	1	—	—	—	12	20	.3	Trace	.03	.02	.3	Trace
French or Vienna bread																
Enriched, 1-pound loaf	1 loaf	454	1,315	41	14	3	8	2	251	195	10.0	Trace	1.26	.98	11.3	Trace
Unenriched, 1-pound loaf	1 loaf	454	1,315	41	14	3	8	2	251	195	3.2	Trace	.39	.39	3.6	Trace
Italian bread																
Enriched, 1-pound loaf	1 loaf	454	1,250	41	4	Trace	1	—	256	77	10.0	0	1.31	.93	11.7	0
Unenriched, 1-pound loaf	1 loaf	454	1,250	41	4	Trace	1	—	256	77	3.2	0	.39	.27	3.6	0
Raisin bread																
Loaf, 1-pound, 20 slices	1 loaf	454	1,190	30	13	3	8	2	243	322	5.9	Trace	.24	.42	3.0	Trace
Slice	1	23	60	2	1	—	—	—	12	16	.3	Trace	.01	.02	.2	Trace
Rye bread																
American, light (⅓ rye, ⅔ wheat)																
Loaf, 1-pound, 20 slices	1 loaf	454	1,100	41	5	—	—	—	236	340	7.3	0	.81	.33	6.4	0
Slice	1	23	55	2	Trace	—	—	—	12	17	.4	0	.04	.02	.3	0
Pumpernickel, loaf, 1 pound	1 loaf	454	1,115	41	5	—	—	—	241	381	10.9	0	1.05	.63	5.4	0

Measure and weight apply to entire vegetable or fruit including parts not usually eaten.

Food, approximate measure, and weight (in grams)		weight (g)	Food energy (calories)	Protein (g)	Fat (total lipid) (g)	Fatty acids Saturated (total) (g)	Unsaturated Oleic (g)	Unsaturated Linoleic (g)	Carbohydrate (g)	Calcium (mg)	Iron (mg)	Vitamin A value (IU)	Thiamin (mg)	Riboflavin (mg)	Niacin (mg)	Ascorbic acid (mg)
White bread, enriched																
1 to 2 percent nonfat dry milk																
Loaf, 1-pound, 20 slices	1 loaf	454	1,225	39	15	3	8	2	229	318	10.9	Trace	1.13	.77	10.4	Trace
Slice	1 slice[13]	23	60	2	1	Trace	Trace	Trace	12	16	.6	Trace	.06	.04	.5	Trace
3 to 4 percent nonfat dry milk[13]																
Loaf, 1-pound	1	454	1,225	39	15	3	8	2	229	381	11.3	Trace	1.13	.95	10.8	Trace
Slice, 20 per loaf	1	23	60	2	1	Trace	Trace	Trace	12	19	.6	Trace	.06	.05	.6	Trace
Slice, toasted	1	20	60	2	1	Trace	Trace	Trace	12	19	.6	Trace	.05	.05	.6	Trace
Slice, 26 per loaf	1	17	45	1	1	Trace	Trace	Trace	9	14	.4	Trace	.04	.04	.4	Trace
5 to 6 percent nonfat dry milk																
Loaf, 1-pound, 20 slices	1 loaf	454	1,245	41	17	4	10	2	228	435	11.3	Trace	1.22	.91	11.0	Trace
Slice	1	23	65	2	1	Trace	Trace	Trace	12	22	.6	Trace	.06	.05	.6	Trace
White bread, unenriched																
1 to 2 percent nonfat dry milk																
Loaf, 1-pound, 20 slices	1 loaf	454	1,225	39	15	3	8	2	229	318	3.2	Trace	.40	.36	5.6	Trace
Slice	1	23	60	2	1	Trace	Trace	Trace	12	16	.2	Trace	.02	.02	.3	Trace
3 to 4 percent nonfat dry milk[13]																
Loaf, 1-pound	1 loaf	454	1,225	39	15	3	8	—	228	381	3.2	Trace	.31	.39	5.0	Trace
Slice, 20 per loaf	1 slice	23	60	2	1	Trace	Trace	Trace	12	19	.2	Trace	.02	.02	.3	Trace
Slice, toasted	1	20	60	2	1	Trace	Trace	Trace	12	19	.2	Trace	.01	.02	.3	Trace
Slice	1 slice	17	45	1	1	Trace	Trace	Trace	9	14	.1	Trace	.01	.01	.2	Trace
5 to 6 percent nonfat dry milk																
Loaf, 1-pound, 20 slices	1 loaf	454	1,245	41	17	4	10	2	228	435	3.2	Trace	.32	.39	4.1	Trace
Slice	1	23	65	2	1	Trace	Trace	Trace	12	22	.2	Trace	.02	.03	.2	Trace
Whole-wheat bread, made with 2 percent nonfat dry milk																
Loaf, 1-pound, 20 slices	1 loaf	454	1,105	48	14	3	6	3	216	449	10.4	Trace	1.17	.56	12.9	Trace
Slice	1	23	55	2	1	Trace	Trace	Trace	11	23	.5	Trace	.06	.03	.7	Trace
Slice, toasted	1	19	55	2	1	Trace	Trace	Trace	11	22	.5	Trace	.05	.03	.6	Trace
Breadcrumbs, dry, grated	1 cup	88	345	11	4	1	2	1	65	107	3.2	Trace	.19	.26	3.1	Trace
Cakes[14]																
Angelfood cake; sector, 2-inch (1/12 of 8-inch-diameter cake)	1 sector	40	110	3	Trace	—	—	—	24	4	.1	0	Trace	.06	.1	0
Chocolate cake, chocolate icing; sector, 2-inch (1/16 of 10-inch-diameter layer cake)	1 sector	120	445	5	20	8	10	1	67	84	1.2	[15]190	.03	.12	.3	Trace

Food	Measure	Weight (g)	Food energy (cal)	Protein (g)	Fat (g)	Saturated (g)	Unsaturated Oleic (g)	Unsaturated Linoleic (g)	Carbohydrate (g)	Calcium (mg)	Iron (mg)	Vitamin A (IU)	Thiamine (mg)	Riboflavin (mg)	Niacin (mg)	Ascorbic acid (mg)
Fruitcake, dark (made with enriched flour); piece, 2 by 2 by ½ inch	1 piece	30	115	1	5	1	3	1	18	22	.8	[15]540	.04	.04	.2	Trace
Gingerbread (made with enriched flour); piece, 2 by 2 by 2 inches	1 piece	55	175	2	6	1	4	Trace	29	37	1.3	50	.06	.06	.5	0
Plain cake and cupcakes, without icing																
Piece, 3 by 2 by 1½ inches	1	55	200	2	8	2	5	1	31	35	.2	[15]590	.01	.05	.1	Trace
Cupcake, 2¾-inch diameter	1	40	145	2	6	1	3	1	22	26	.2	[15]570	.01	.03	.1	Trace
Plain cake and cupcakes, with chocolate icing																
Sector, 2-inch (1/16 of 10-inch-layer cake)	1	100	370	4	14	5	7	1	59	63	.6	[15]180	.02	.09	.2	Trace
Cupcake, 2¾-inch diameter	1	50	185	2	7	2	4	Trace	30	32	.3	[15]590	.01	.04	.1	Trace
Poundcake, old-fashioned (equal weights flour, sugar, fat, eggs); slice, 2¾ by 3 by ⅝ inch	1 slice	30	140	2	9	5	5	1	14	6	.2	[15]580	.01	.03	.1	0
Sponge cake; sector, 2-inch (1/12 of 8-inch-diameter cake)	1	40	120	3	2	1	1	Trace	22	12	.5	180	.02	.06	.1	Trace
Cookies																
Plain and assorted, 3-inch diameter	1 cooky	25	120	1	5	1	2	1	18	9	.2	20	.01	.01	.1	Trace
Fig bars, small	1	16	55	1	1	—	—	—	12	12	.2	20	.01	.01	.1	Trace
Corn, rice and wheat flakes, mixed, added nutrients	1 oz	28	110	2	Trace	—	—	—	24	11	.5	0	.11	—	.9	0
Corn flakes, added nutrients																
Plain	1 oz	28	110	2	Trace	—	—	—	24	5	.4	0	.12	.02	.6	0
Sugar-covered	1 oz	28	110	1	Trace	—	—	—	26	3	.3	0	.12	.01	.5	0
Corn grits, degermed, cooked																
Enriched	1 cup	242	120	3	Trace	—	—	—	27	2	[16].7	[17]150	[16].10	[16].07	[16]1.0	0
Unenriched	1 cup	242	120	3	Trace	—	—	—	27	2	.2	[17]150	.05	.02	.5	0
Cornmeal, white or yellow, dry																
Whole ground, unbolted	1 cup	118	420	11	5	1	2	1	87	24	2.8	[17]600	.45	.13	2.4	0
Degermed, enriched	1 cup	145	525	11	2	Trace	1	Trace	114	9	[16]4.2	[17]640	[16].64	[16].38	[16]5.1	0
Corn muffins, made with enriched degermed cornmeal and enriched flour; muffin, 2¾-inch diameter	1 muffin	48	150	3	5	1	2	Trace	23	50	.8	[18]80	.09	.11	.8	Trace

[13]When the amount of nonfat dry milk in commercial white bread is unknown, values for bread with 3 to 4% nonfat dry milk are suggested.

[14]Unenriched cake flour and vegetable cooking fat used unless otherwise specified.

[15]If the fat used in the recipe is butter or fortified margarine, the vitamin A value for chocolate cake with chocolate icing will be 490 IU per 2-inch sector; 100 IU for fruitcake; for plain cake without icing, 300 IU per piece; 220 IU per cupcake; for plain cake with icing, 440 IU per 2-inch sector; 220 IU per cupcake; and 300 IU for poundcake.

[16]Iron, thiamine, riboflavin, and niacin are based on the minimum levels of enrichment specified in standards of identity promulgated under the Federal Food, Drug, and Cosmetic Act.

[17]Vitamin A value based on yellow product. White product contains only a trace.

[18]Based on recipe using white cornmeal; if yellow cornmeal is used, the vitamin A value is 140 IU per muffin.

Food, approximate measure, and weight (in grams)		Food energy (calories)	Protein (g)	Fat (total lipid) (g)	Saturated (total) (g)	Unsaturated Oleic (g)	Unsaturated Linoleic (g)	Carbohydrate (g)	Calcium (mg)	Iron (mg)	Vitamin A value (IU)	Thiamin (mg)	Riboflavin (mg)	Niacin (mg)	Ascorbic acid (mg)
Corn, puffed, pre-sweetened, added nutrients	1 oz — 28	110	1	Trace	—	—	—	26	3	.5	0	.12	.05	.6	0
Corn, shredded, added nutrients	1 oz — 28	110	2	Trace	—	—	—	25	1	.7	0	.12	.05	.6	0
Crackers															
Graham, plain	4 small or 2 medium — 14	55	1	1	—	—	—	10	6	.2	0	.01	.03	.2	0
Saltines, 2 inches squares	2 crackers — 8	35	1	1	—	—	—	6	2	.1	0	Trace	Trace	.1	0
Soda															
Cracker, 2½ inches square	2 crackers — 11	50	1	1	Trace	1	Trace	8	2	.2	0	Trace	Trace	.1	0
Oyster crackers	10 crackers — 10	45	1	1	Trace	1	Trace	7	2	.2	0	Trace	Trace	.1	0
Cracker meal	1 tbsp — 10	45	1	1	Trace	1	Trace	7	2	.1	0	.01	Trace	.1	0
Doughnuts, cake type	1 doughnut — 32	125	1	6	1	4	Trace	16	13	[19]4	30	[19].05	[19].05	[19]4	Trace
Farina, regular, enriched, cooked	1 cup — 238	100	3	Trace	—	—	—	21	10	[16].7	0	[16].11	[16].07	[16]1.0	0
Macaroni, cooked															
Enriched															
Cooked, firm stage (8 to 10 minutes; undergoes additional cooking in a food mixture)	1 cup — 130	190	6	1	—	—	—	39	14	[16]1.4	0	[16].23	[16].14	[16]1.9	0
Cooked until tender	1 cup — 140	155	5	1	—	—	—	32	11	[16]1.3	0	[16].19	[16].11	[16]1.5	0
Unenriched															
Cooked, firm stage (8 to 10 minutes; undergoes additional cooking in a food mixture)	1 cup — 130	190	6	1	—	—	—	39	14	.6	0	.02	.02	.5	0
Cooked until tender	1 cup — 140	155	5	1	—	—	—	32	11	.6	0	.02	.02	.4	0
Macaroni (enriched) and cheese, baked	1 cup — 220	470	18	24	11	10	1	44	398	2.0	950	.22	.44	2.0	Trace
Muffins, with enriched white flour; muffin, 2¾-inch diameter	1 — 48	140	4	5	1	3	Trace	20	50	.8	50	.08	.11	.7	Trace
Noodles (egg noodles), cooked															
Enriched	1 cup — 160	200	7	2	1	1	Trace	37	16	[16]1.4	110	[16].23	[14].14	[16]1.8	0
Unenriched	1 cup — 160	200	7	2	1	1	Trace	37	16	1.0	110	.04	.03	.7	0
Oats (with or without corn) puffed, added nutrients	1 oz — 28	115	3	2	Trace	1	1	21	50	1.3	0	.28	.05	.5	0

Food	Measure															
Oatmeal or rolled oats, regular or quick-cooking, cooked	1 cup	236	130	5	2	Trace	1	1	23	21	1.4	0	.19	.05	.3	0
Pancakes (griddlecakes), 4-inch diameter																
Wheat, enriched flour (home recipe)	1 cake	27	60	2	2	Trace	1	Trace	9	27	.4	30	.05	.06	.3	Trace
Buckwheat (buckwheat pancake mix, made with egg and milk)	1 cake	27	55	2	1	1	1	Trace	6	59	.4	60	.03	.04	.2	Trace
Piecrust, plain, baked																
Enriched flour																	
Lower crust, 9-inch shell	1	135	675	8	45	10	29	3	59	19	2.3	0	.27	.19	2.4	0
Double crust, 9-inch pie	1	270	1,350	16	90	21	58	7	118	38	4.6	0	.55	.39	4.9	0
Unenriched flour																	
Lower crust, 9-inch shell	1	135	675	8	45	10	29	3	59	19	.7	0	.04	.04	.6	0
Double crust, 9-inch pie	1	270	1,350	16	90	21	58	7	118	38	1.4	0	.08	.07	1.3	0
Pies (piecrust made with unenriched flour); sector, 4-inch, 1/7 of 9-inch-diameter pie																
Apple	1 sector	135	345	3	15	4	9	1	51	11	.4	40	.03	.02	.5	1
Cherry	1 sector	135	355	4	15	4	10	1	52	19	.4	590	.03	.03	.6	1
Custard	1 sector	130	280	8	14	5	8	1	30	125	.8	300	.07	.21	.4	0
Lemon meringue	1 sector	120	305	4	12	4	7	1	45	17	.6	200	.04	.10	.2	4
Mince	1 sector	135	365	3	16	4	10	1	56	38	1.4	Trace	.09	.05	.5	1
Pumpkin	1 sector	130	275	5	15	5	7	Trace	32	66	.6	3,210	.04	.13	.6	Trace
Pizza (cheese); 5½-inch sector; ⅛ of 14-inch diameter pie	1 sector	75	185	7	6	2	3	Trace	27	107	.7	290	.04	.12	.7	4
Popcorn, popped, with added oil and salt	1 cup	14	65	1	3	2	Trace	Trace	8	1	.3	—	.01	—	.2	0
Pretzels, small stick	5 sticks	5	20	Trace	Trace	—	—	—	4	1	0	0	Trace	Trace	Trace	0
Rice, white (fully milled or polished), enriched, cooked																
Common commercial varieties, all types	1 cup	168	185	3	Trace	—	—	—	41	17	[20]1.5	0	[20].19	[20].01	[20]1.6	0
Long grain, parboiled	1 cup	176	185	4	Trace	—	—	—	41	33	[20]1.4	0	[20].19	[20].02	[20]2.0	0
Rice, puffed, added nutrients (without salt)	1 cup	14	55	1	Trace	—	—	—	13	3	.3	0	.06	.01	.6	0
Rice flakes, added nutrients	1 cup	30	115	2	Trace	—	—	—	26	9	.5	0	.10	.02	1.6	0

[14] Unenriched cake flour and vegetable cooking fat used unless otherwise specified.

[16] Iron, thiamine, riboflavin, and niacin are based on the minimum levels of enrichment specified in standards of identity promulgated under the Federal Food, Drug, and Cosmetic Act.

[19] Based on product made with enriched flour. With unenriched flour, approximate values per doughnut are: Iron, 0.2 milligram; thiamine, 0.01 milligram; riboflavin, 0.03 milligram; niacin, 0.2 milligram.

[20] Iron, thiamine, and niacin are based on the minimum levels of enrichment specified in standards of identity promulgated under the Federal Food, Drug, and Cosmetic Act. Riboflavin is based on unenriched rice. When the minimum level of enrichment for riboflavin specified in the standards of identity becomes effective the value will be 0.12 milligram per cup of parboiled rice and of white rice.

Food, approximate measure, and weight (in grams)	weight (g)	Food energy (calories)	Protein (g)	Fat (total lipid) (g)	Fatty acids Saturated (total) (g)	Unsaturated Oleic (g)	Unsaturated Linoleic (g)	Carbohydrate (g)	Calcium (mg)	Iron (mg)	Vitamin A value (IU)	Thiamin (mg)	Riboflavin (mg)	Niacin (mg)	Ascorbic acid (mg)
Rolls															
Plain, pan; 12 per 16 ounces															
Enriched, 1 roll	38	115	3	2	Trace	1	Trace	20	28	.7	Trace	.11	.07	.8	Trace
Unenriched, 1 roll	38	115	3	2	Trace	1	Trace	20	28	.3	Trace	.02	.03	.3	Trace
Hard, round; 12 per 22 oz, 1 roll	52	160	5	2	Trace	1	Trace	31	24	.4	Trace	.03	.05	.4	Trace
Sweet, pan; 12 per 18 oz, 1 roll	43	135	4	4	1	2	Trace	21	37	.3	30	.03	.06	.4	Trace
Rye wafers, whole-grain, 1⅞ by 3½ inches, 2 wafers	13	45	2	Trace	—	—	—	10	7	.5	0	.04	.03	.2	0
Spaghetti															
Cooked, tender stage (14 to 20 minutes)															
Enriched, 1 cup	140	155	5	1	—	—	—	32	11	[16]1.3	0	[16].19	[16].11	[16]1.5	0
Unenriched, 1 cup	140	155	5	1	—	—	—	32	11	.6	0	.02	.02	.4	0
Spaghetti with meat balls in tomato sauce (home recipe), 1 cup	250	335	19	12	4	6	1	39	125	3.8	1,600	.26	.30	4.0	22
Spaghetti in tomato sauce with cheese (home recipe), 1 cup	250	260	9	9	2	5	1	37	80	2.2	1,080	.24	.18	2.4	14
Waffles, with enriched flour, ½ by 4½ by 5½ inches, 1	75	210	7	7	2	4	1	28	85	1.3	250	.13	.19	1.0	Trace
Wheat, puffed															
With added nutrients (without salt), 1 oz	28	105	4	Trace	—	—	—	22	8	1.2	0	.15	.07	2.2	0
With added nutrients, with sugar and honey, 1 oz	28	105	2	1	—	—	—	25	7	.9	0	.14	.05	1.8	0
Wheat, rolled; cooked, 1 cup	236	175	5	1	—	—	—	40	19	1.7	0	.17	.06	2.1	0
Wheat, shredded, plain (long, round, or bite-size), 1 oz	28	100	3	1	—	—	—	23	12	1.0	0	.06	.03	1.2	0
Wheat and malted barley flakes, with added nutrients, 1 oz	28	110	2	Trace	—	—	—	24	14	.7	0	.13	.03	1.1	0
Wheat flakes, with added nutrients, 1 oz	28	100	3	Trace	—	—	—	23	12	1.2	0	.18	.04	1.4	0
Wheat flours															
Whole-wheat, from hard wheats, stirred, 1 cup	120	400	16	2	Trace	1	1	85	49	4.0	0	.66	.14	5.2	0
All-purpose or family flour															
Enriched, sifted, 1 cup	110	400	12	1	Trace	Trace	Trace	84	18	[16]3.2	0	[16].48	[16].29	[16]3.8	0
Unenriched, sifted, 1 cup	110	400	12	1	Trace	Trace	Trace	84	18	.9	0	.07	.05	1.0	0
Self-rising, enriched, 1 cup	110	385	10	1	Trace	Trace	Trace	82	292	[16]3.2	0	[16].49	[16].29	[16]3.9	0
Cake or pastry flour, sifted, 1 cup	100	365	8	1	Trace	Trace	Trace	79	17	.5	0	.03	.03	.7	0

Food	Measure	Weight (g)	Food energy	Protein	Fat	Saturated	Oleic	Linoleic	Carbohydrate	Calcium	Iron	Vitamin A	Thiamine	Riboflavin	Niacin	Ascorbic acid
Wheat germ, crude, commercially milled	1 cup	68	245	18	7	1	2	4	32	49	6.4	0	1.36	.46	2.9	0
Fats, oils																
Butter, 4 sticks per pound																
Sticks, 2	1 cup	227	1,625	1	184	101	61	6	1	45	0	[21]7,500	—	—	—	0
Stick, ⅛	1 tbsp	14	100	Trace	11	6	4	Trace	Trace	3	0	[21]460	—	—	—	0
Pat or square (64 per pound)	1	7	50	Trace	6	3	2	Trace	Trace	1	0	[21]230	—	—	—	0
Fats, cooking																
Lard	1 cup	220	1,985	0	220	84	101	22	0	0	0	0	0	0	0	0
Lard	1 tbsp	14	125	0	14	5	6	6	0	0	0	0	0	0	0	0
Vegetable fats	1 cup	200	1,770	0	200	46	130	14	0	0	0	—	0	0	0	0
Vegetable fats	1 tbsp	12.5	110	0	12	3	8	1	0	0	0	—	0	0	0	0
Margarine, 4 sticks per pound																
Sticks, 2	1 cup	227	1,635	1	184	37	105	33	1	45	0	[22]7,500	—	—	—	0
Stick, ⅛	1 tbsp	14	100	Trace	11	2	6	2	Trace	3	0	[22]460	—	—	—	0
Pat or square (64 per pound)	1 pat	7	50	Trace	6	1	3	1	Trace	1	0	[22]230	—	—	—	0
Oils, salad or cooking																
Corn	1 tbsp	14	125	0	14	1	4	7	0	0	0	—	0	0	0	0
Cottonseed	1 tbsp	14	125	0	14	4	3	7	0	0	0	—	0	0	0	0
Olive	1 tbsp	14	125	0	14	2	11	1	0	0	0	—	0	0	0	0
Soybean	1 tbsp	14	125	0	14	2	3	7	0	0	0	—	0	0	0	0
Salad dressings																
Blue cheese	1 tbsp	16	80	1	8	2	2	4	1	13	Trace	30	Trace	.02	Trace	Trace
Commercial, mayonnaise type	1 tbsp	15	65	Trace	6	1	1	3	2	2	Trace	30	Trace	Trace	Trace	—
French	1 tbsp	15	60	Trace	6	1	1	3	3	2	.1	—	—	—	—	Trace
Home cooked, boiled	1 tbsp	17	30	1	2	1	1	Trace	3	15	.1	80	.01	.03	Trace	—
Mayonnaise	1 tbsp	15	110	Trace	12	2	3	6	Trace	3	.1	40	Trace	.01	Trace	Trace
Thousand Island	1 tbsp	15	75	Trace	8	1	2	4	2	2	.1	50	Trace	Trace	Trace	Trace
Sugars, sweets																
Candy																
Caramels	1 oz	28	115	1	3	2	1	Trace	22	42	.4	Trace	.01	.05	Trace	Trace
Chocolate, milk, plain	1 oz	28	150	2	9	5	3	Trace	16	65	.3	80	.02	.09	.1	Trace
Fudge, plain	1 oz	28	115	1	3	2	1	Trace	21	22	.3	Trace	.01	.03	.1	Trace
Hard candy	1 oz	28	110	0	Trace	—	—	—	28	6	.5	0	0	0	0	0
Marshmallows	1 oz	28	90	1	Trace	—	—	—	23	5	.5	0	0	Trace	0	0
Chocolate syrup, thin type	1 tbsp	20	50	Trace	Trace	Trace	Trace	Trace	13	3	.3	—	Trace	.01	Trace	Trace
Honey, strained or extracted	1 tbsp	21	65	Trace	0	—	—	—	17	1	.1	0	Trace	.01	.1	0
Jams and preserves	1 tbsp	20	55	Trace	Trace	—	—	—	14	4	.2	Trace	Trace	.01	Trace	Trace
Jellies	1 tbsp	20	55	Trace	Trace	—	—	—	14	4	.3	Trace	Trace	.01	Trace	1

[16]Iron, thiamine, riboflavin, and niacin are based on the minimum levels of enrichment specified in standards of identity promulgated under the Federal Food, Drug, and Cosmetic Act.

[21]Year-round average.

[22]Based on the average vitamin A content of fortified margarine. Federal specifications for fortified margarine require a minimum of 15,000 IU of vitamin A per pound.

Food, approximate measure, and weight (in grams)		Food energy (calories)	Protein (g)	Fat (total lipid) (g)	Fatty acids			Carbohydrate (g)	Calcium (mg)	Iron (mg)	Vitamin A value (IU)	Thiamin (mg)	Riboflavin (mg)	Niacin (mg)	Ascorbic acid (mg)
					Saturated (total) (g)	Unsaturated Oleic (g)	Unsaturated Linoleic (g)								
Molasses, cane															
Light (first extraction)	1 tbsp	20	50	—	—	—	—	13	33	.9	—	.01	.01	Trace	—
Blackstrap (third extraction)	1 tbsp	20	45	—	—	—	—	11	137	3.2	—	.02	.04	.4	—
Sirup, table blends (chiefly corn, light and dark)	1 tbsp	20	60	0	—	—	—	15	9	.8	0	0	0	0	0
Sugars (cane or beet)															
Granulated	1 cup	200	770	0	0	—	—	199	0	0	0	0	0	0	0
	1 tbsp	12	45	0	0	—	—	12	0	Trace	0	0	0	0	0
Lump, 1⅛ by ¾ by ⅜	1 lump	6	25	0	0	—	—	6	0	Trace	0	0	0	0	0
Powdered, stirred before measuring	1 cup	128	495	0	0	—	—	127	0	.1	0	0	0	0	0
	1 tbsp	8	30	0	0	—	—	8	0	Trace	0	0	0	0	0
Brown, firm-packed	1 cup	220	820	0	0	—	—	212	187	7.5	0	.02	.07	.4	0
	1 tbsp	14	50	0	0	—	—	13	12	.5	0	Trace	Trace	Trace	0
Miscellaneous items															
Beer (average 3.6 percent alcohol by weight)	1 cup	240	100	1	0	—	—	9	12	Trace	—	.01	.07	1.6	—
Beverages, carbonated															
Cola type	1 cup	240	95	0	0	—	—	24	—	—	0	0	0	0	0
Ginger ale	1 cup	230	70	0	0	—	—	18	—	—	0	0	0	0	0
Bouillon cube, ⅝ inch	1 cube	4	5	1	Trace	—	—	Trace	—	—	—	—	—	Trace	—
Chili powder. *See* Vegetables, peppers															
Chili sauce (mainly tomatoes)	1 tbsp	17	20	Trace	Trace	—	—	4	3	.1	240	.02	.01	.3	3
Chocolate															
Bitter or baking	1 oz	28	145	3	15	8	6	Trace	8	22	1.9	20	.01	.07	.4	0
Sweet	1 oz	28	150	1	10	6	4	Trace	16	27	.4	Trace	.01	.04	.1	Trace
Cider. *See* Fruits, apple juice															
Gelatin, dry															
Plain	1 tbsp	10	35	9	Trace	—	—	—	—	—	—	—	—	—	—
Dessert powder, 3 oz package	½ cup	85	315	8	0	—	—	75	—	—	—	—	—	—	—
Gelatin dessert, ready-to-eat															
Plain	1 cup	239	140	4	0	—	—	34	—	—	—	—	—	—	—
With fruit	1 cup	241	160	3	Trace	—	—	40	—	—	—	—	—	—	—
Olives, pickled															
Green	4 medium or 3 extra large or 2 giant	16	15	Trace	2	Trace	2	Trace	Trace	8	.2	40	—	—	—	—

Food	Amount	Weight (g)	Food energy (Cal)	Protein (g)	Fat (g)	Saturated (g)	Oleic (g)	Linoleic (g)	Carbohydrate (g)	Calcium (mg)	Iron (mg)	Vitamin A (IU)	Thiamin (mg)	Riboflavin (mg)	Niacin (mg)	Ascorbic acid (mg)
Ripe: Mission	3 small or 2 large	10	15	Trace	2	Trace	2	Trace	Trace	9	.1	10	Trace	Trace	—	—
Pickles, cucumber																
Dill, large, 4 by 1¾ inches	1	135	15	1	Trace	—	—	—	3	35	1.4	140	Trace	.03	—	8
Sweet, 2¾ by ¾ inches	1	20	30	Trace	Trace	—	—	—	7	2	.2	20	Trace	Trace	—	1
Popcorn. *See* Grain products																
Sherbet, orange	1 cup	193	260	2	2	—	—	—	59	31	Trace	110	.02	.06	Trace	4
Soups, canned; ready-to-serve (prepared with equal volume of water)																
Bean with pork	1 cup	250	170	8	6	1	2	2	22	62	2.2	650	.14	.07	1.0	2
Beef noodle	1 cup	250	70	4	3	1	1	1	7	8	1.0	50	.05	.06	1.0	Trace
Beef bouillon, broth, consomme	1 cup	240	30	5	0	0	0	0	3	Trace	.5	Trace	Trace	.02	1.2	—
Chicken noodle	1 cup	250	65	4	2	Trace	1	1	8	10	.5	50	.02	.02	.8	Trace
Clam chowder	1 cup	255	85	2	3	—	—	—	13	36	1.0	920	.03	.03	1.0	—
Cream soup (mushroom)	1 cup	240	135	2	10	1	3	5	10	41	.5	70	.02	.12	.7	Trace
Minestrone	1 cup	245	105	5	3	—	1	1	14	37	1.0	2,350	.07	.05	1.0	—
Pea, green	1 cup	245	130	6	2	1	1	Trace	23	44	1.0	340	.05	.05	1.0	7
Tomato	1 cup	245	90	2	2	Trace	—	1	16	15	.7	1,000	.05	.05	1.1	12
Vegetable with beef broth	1 cup	250	80	3	2	—	—	—	14	20	.8	3,250	.05	.02	1.2	—
Starch (cornstarch)	1 cup	128	465	Trace	Trace	—	—	—	112	0	0	0	0	0	0	0
	1 tbsp	8	30	Trace	Trace	—	—	—	7	0	0	0	0	0	0	0
Tapioca, quick-cooking granulated, dry, stirred before measuring	1 cup	152	535	1	Trace	—	—	—	131	15	.6	0	0	0	Trace	0
	1 tbsp	10	35	Trace	Trace	—	—	—	9	1	Trace	0	0	0	0	0
Vinegar	1 tbsp	15	2	0	—	—	—	—	1	1	.1	—	—	—	—	—
White sauce, medium	1 cup	265	430	10	33	18	11	1	23	305	.5	1,220	.12	.44	.5	Trace
Yeast																
Baker's																
Compressed	1 oz	28	25	3	Trace	—	—	—	3	4	1.4	Trace	.20	.47	3.2	Trace
Dry active	1 oz	28	80	10	Trace	—	—	—	11	12	4.6	Trace	.66	1.53	10.4	Trace
Brewer's, dry, debittered	1 tbsp	8	25	3	Trace	—	—	—	3	17	1.4	Trace	1.25	.34	3.0	Trace
Yogurt. *See* Milk, cream, cheese, related products																

6-5. Sodium and potassium content of foods, 100 gm, edible portion[1]

Food and description	Sodium (mg)	Potassium (mg)	Food and description	Sodium (mg)	Potassium (mg)
Almonds			Beans, lima—cont'd		
dried	4	773	canned		
roasted and salted	198	773	regular pack, solids and liquid	236[2]	222
Apples			special dietary pack (low-sodium), solids and liquid	4	222
raw, pared	1	110			
frozen, sliced, sweetened	14	68	frozen, thin-seeded types, commonly called baby limas, cooked, boiled, drained	129	394
Apple brown betty	153	100			
Apple butter	2	252			
Apple juice, canned or bottled	1	101	mature seeds, dry, cooked	2	612
Applesauce, canned, sweetened	2	65	Beans, mung, sprouted seeds, cooked, boiled, drained	4	156
Apricots					
raw	1	281	Beans, snap		
canned, syrup pack, light	1	239	green		
dried, sulfured, cooked, fruit, and liquid	8	318	cooked, boiled, drained	4	151
			canned		
Apricot nectar, canned (approx. 40% fruit)	Trace	151	regular pack, solids and liquid	236[2]	95
			special dietary pack (low sodium), solids and liquid	2	95
Asparagus					
cooked spears, boiled, drained	1	183	frozen, cut, cooked, boiled, drained	1	152
canned spears, green			yellow or wax		
regular pack, solids and liquid	236[2]	166	cooked, boiled, drained	3	151
special dietary pack (low-sodium), solids and liquids	3	166	canned		
			regular pack, solids and liquid	236[2]	95
frozen			special dietary pack (low-sodium), solids and liquid	2	95
cuts and tips, cooked, boiled, drained	1	220			
spears, cooked, boiled, drained	1	238	frozen, cut, cooked, boiled, drained	1	164
Avocados, raw, all commercial varieties	4	604	Beans and frankfurters, canned	539	262
			Beef		
Bacon, cured, cooked, broiled or fried, drained	1021	236	retail cuts, trimmed to retail level		
			round	60	370
Bacon, Canadian, cooked, broiled or fried, drained	2555	432	rump	60	370
			hamburger, regular ground, cooked	47	450
Baking powders					
home use			Beef and vegetable stew, canned	411	174
straight phosphate	8220	170	Beef, corned, boneless		
special low-sodium preparations	6	10,948	cooked, medium-fat	1740	150
Bananas, raw, common	1	370	canned corned-beef hash (with potato)	540	200
Barbecue sauce	815	174			
Bass, black sea, raw	68	256	Beef, dried, cooked, creamed	716	153
Beans, common, mature seeds, dry			Beef potpie, commercial, frozen, unheated	366	93
white					
cooked	7	416	Beets, common, red		
canned, solids and liquid, with pork and tomato sauce	463	210	canned		
			regular pack, solids and liquid	236[2]	167
red, cooked	3	340	special dietary pack (low-sodium), solids and liquid	46	167
Beans, lima					
immature seeds					
cooked, boiled, drained	1	422			

[1]Numbers in parentheses denote values imputed—usually from another form of the food or from a similar food. Dashes denote lack of reliable data for a constituent believed to be present in measurable amount.

[2]Estimated average based on addition of salt in the amount of 0.6% of the finished product.

Food and description	Sodium (mg)	Potassium (mg)	Food and description	Sodium (mg)	Potassium (mg)
Beet greens, common, cooked, boiled, drained	76	332	Brazil nuts	1	715
Beverages, alcoholic			Breads		
beer, alcohol 4.5% by volume	7	25	cracked-wheat	529	134
(3.6% by weight)	7	25	French or vienna, enriched	580	90
gin, rum, vodka, whisky			Italian, enriched	585	74
80-proof (33.4% alcohol by weight)	1	2	raisin	365	233
86-proof (36.0% alcohol by weight)	1	2	rye, American ($^1/_3$ rye, $^2/_3$ clear flour)	557	145
90-proof (37.9% alcohol by weight)	1	2	white, enriched, made with 3%-4% non-fat dry milk	507	105
94-proof (39.7% alcohol by weight)	1	2	whole-wheat, made with 2% non-fat dry milk	527	273
100-proof (42.5% alcohol by weight)	1	2	Bread crumbs, dry, grated	736	152
wines			Bread stuffing mix and stuffings prepared from mix		
dessert, alcohol 18.8% by volume (15.3% by weight)	4	75	mix, dry form	1331	172
table, alcohol 12.2% by volume (9.9% by weight)	5	92	Broccoli		
Biscuits, baking powder, made with enriched flour	626	117	cooked spears, boiled, drained	10	267
Biscuit dough, commercial, frozen	910	86	frozen, spears, cooked, boiled, drained	12	220
Biscuit mix, with enriched flour, and biscuits baked from mix			Brussels sprouts, frozen, cooked, boiled, drained	14	295
mix, dry form	1300	80	Buffalo fish, raw	52	293
biscuits, made with milk	973	116	Bulgur (parboiled wheat)		
Blackberries, including dewberries, boysenberries, and youngberries, raw	1	170	canned, made from hard red winter wheat		
Blackberries, canned, solids and liquid			unseasoned[3]	599	87
water pack, with or without artificial sweetener	1	115	seasoned[4]	460	112
syrup pack, heavy	1	109	Butter[5]	987	23
Blueberries			Buttermilk, fluid, cultured (made from skim milk)	130	140
raw	1	81	Cabbage		
frozen, not thawed, sweetened	1	66	common varieties (Danish, domestic, and pointed types)		
Bluefish, cooked			raw	20	233
baked or boiled	104	—	cooked, boiled until tender, drained, shredded, cooked in small amount of water	14	163
fried	146	—	red, raw	26	268
Boston brown bread	251	292	Cabbage, Chinese (also called celery cabbage or petsai)	23	253
Bouillon cubes or powder	24,000	100	Cakes		
Boysenberries, frozen, not thawed, sweetened	1	105	baked from home recipes		
Bran, added sugar and malt extract	1060	1070	angelfood	283	88
Bran flakes (40% bran), added thiamine	925	—	fruitcake, made with enriched flour, dark	158	496
Bran flakes with raisins, added thiamine	800	—	gingerbread, made with enriched flour	237	454
			plain cake or cupcake, without icing	300	79
			pound, modified	178	78

[3]Processed, partially debranned, whole-kernel wheat with salt added.
[4]Processed, partially debranned, whole-kernel wheat with chicken fat, chicken stock base, dehydrated onion flakes, salt, monosodium glutamate, and herbs.
[5]Values apply to salted butter. Unsalted butter contains less than 10 mg of either sodium or potassium per 100 gm. Value for vitamin A is the year-round average.

Food and description	Sodium (mg)	Potassium (mg)
Cakes—cont'd		
frozen, commercial, devil's food, with chocolate icing	420	119
Candy		
caramels, plain or chocolate	226	192
chocolate, sweet	33	296
chocolate-coated, chocolate fudge	228	193
gum drops, starch jelly pieces	35	5
hard	32	4
marshmallows	39	6
peanut bars	10	448
Carp, raw	50	286
Carrots		
raw	47	341
canned		
regular pack, solids and liquid	236[2]	120
special dietary pack (low-sodium), solids and liquid	39	120
Cashew nuts	15[6]	464
Catfish, freshwater, raw	60	330
Cauliflower		
cooked, boiled, drained	9	206
frozen, cooked, boiled, drained	10	207
Caviar, sturgeon, granular	2200	180
Celery, all, including green and yellow varieties		
raw	126	341
cooked, boiled, drained	88	239
Chard, Swiss, cooked, boiled, drained	86	321
Cheese straws	721	63
Cheeses		
natural cheeses		
cheddar (domestic type, commonly called American)	700	82
cottage (large or small curd)		
creamed	229	85
uncreamed	290	72
cream	250	74
parmesan	734	149
Swiss (domestic)	710	104
pasteurized process cheese, American	1136[7]	80
pasteurized process cheese spread, American	1625[7]	240
Cherries		
raw, sweet	2	191
canned		
sour, red, solids and liquid, water pack	2	130

Food and description	Sodium (mg)	Potassium (mg)
Cherries—cont'd		
sweet, solids and liquid, syrup pack, light	1	128
frozen, not thawed, sweetened	2	130
Chicken		
all classes		
light meat without skin, cooked, roasted	64	411
dark meat without skin, cooked, roasted	86	321
Chicken potpie, commercial, frozen, unheated	411	153
Chicory, Witloof (also called French or Belgian endive), bleached head (forced), raw	7	182
Chili con carne, canned, with beans	531	233
Chocolate, bitter or baking	4	830
Chocolate syrup, fudge type	89	284
Chop suey, with meat, canned	551	138
Chow mein, chicken (without noodles), canned	290	167
Citron, candied	290	120
Clams, raw		
soft, meat only	36	235
hard or round, meat only	205	311
Clams, canned, including hard, soft, razor, and unspecified solids and liquids	—	140
Cocoa and chocolate-flavored beverage powders		
cocoa powder with non-fat dry milk	525	800
mix for hot chocolate	382	605
Cocoa, dry powder		
high-fat or breakfast		
plain	6	1,522
processed with alkali	717	651
Coconut cream (liquid expressed from grated coconut meat)	4	324
Coconut meat, fresh	23	256
Cod		
cooked, broiled	110	407
dehydrated, lightly salted	8100	160
Coffee, instant, water-soluble solids		
dry powder	72	3,256
beverage	1	36
Coleslaw, made with French dressing (commercial)	268	205
Collards, cooked, boiled, drained, leaves, including stems, cooked in small amount of water	25	234

[2] Estimated average based on addition of salt in the amount of 0.6% of the finished product.

[6] Applies to unsalted nuts. For salted nuts, value is approximately 200 mg per 100 gm.

[7] Values for phosphorus and sodium are based on use of 1.5% anhydrous disodium phosphate as the emulsifying agent. If emulsifying agent does not contain either phosphorus or sodium, the content of these two nutrients in milligrams per 100 gm is as follows:

	P	Na
American process cheese	444	650
Swiss process cheese	540	681
American cheese food	427	—
American cheese spread	548	1139

Food and description	Sodium (mg)	Potassium (mg)	Food and description	Sodium (mg)	Potassium (mg)
Cookies			Cream, fluid, light, coffee, or table, 20% fat	43	122
assorted, packaged, commercial	365	67	Cream substitutes, dried, containing cream, skim milk (calcium re-duced), and lactose	575	—
butter, thin, rich	418	60			
gingersnaps	571	462			
molasses	162	138	Cream puffs with custard filling	83	121
oatmeal with raisins	162	370	Cress, garden, raw	14	606
sandwich type	483	38	Croaker, Atlantic, cooked, baked	120	323
vanilla wafer	252	72	Cucumbers, raw, pared	6	160
Cookie dough, plain, chilled in roll, baked	548	48	Custard, baked	79	146
			Dates, domestic, natural and dry	1	648
Corn, sweet			Doughnuts, cake type	501	90
Cooked, boiled, drained, white and yellow, kernels, cut off cob before cooking	Trace	165	Duck, domesticated, raw, flesh only	74	285
			Eggs, chicken		
			raw		
canned			whole, fresh and frozen	122	129
regular pack, cream style, white and yellow, solids and liquid	236[2]	(97)	whites, fresh and frozen	146	139
			yolks, fresh	52	98
special dietary pack (low-so-dium), cream style, white and yellow, solids and liquid	2	(97)	Eggplant, cooked, boiled, drained	1	150
			Endive (curly endive and escarole), raw	14	294
frozen, kernels cut off cob, cooked, boiled, drained	1	184	Farina		
			enriched		
Corn fritters	477	133	regular		
Corn grits, degermed, enriched, dry form	1	80	dry form	2	83
			cooked	144	9
Corn products used mainly as ready-to-eat breakfast cereals			quick-cooking, cooked	165	10
			instant-cooking, cooked	188	13
corn flakes, added nutrients	1005	120	enriched, regular, dry form	2	83
corn, puffed, added nutrients	1060	—	Figs, canned, solids and liquid, syrup pack, light	2	152
corn, rice, and wheat flakes, mixed, added nutrients	950	—			
			Flatfishes (flounders, soles, and sand dabs), raw	78	342
Cornbread, baked from home recipes, southern style, made with degermed cornmeal, enriched	591	157			
			Fruit cocktail, canned, solids and liquid, water pack, with or without artificial sweetener	5	168
Cornbread mix and cornbread baked from mix, cornbread, made with egg, milk	744	127			
			Garlic, cloves, raw	19	529
Cornmeal, white or yellow, de-germed, enriched, dry form	1	120	Ginger root, fresh	6	264
			Gizzard, chicken, all classes, cooked, simmered	57	211
Cornstarch	Trace	Trace			
Cowpeas, including blackeye peas			Goose, domesticated, flesh only, cooked, roasted	124	605
immature seeds, canned, solids and liquid	236[2]	352			
			Gooseberries, canned, solids and liquid, syrup pack, heavy	1	98
young pods, with seeds, cooked, boiled, drained	3	196			
			Grapefruit		
Crab, canned	1000	110	raw, pulp, pink, red, white, all varieties	1	135
Crackers					
butter	1092	113	canned, juice, sweetened	1	162
graham, plain	670	384	Grapefruit juice and orange juice blended, canned, sweetened	1	184
saltines	(1100)	(120)			
sandwich type, peanut-cheese	992	226	Grapes, raw, American type (slip skin) such as Concord, Delaware, Niagara, Catawba, and Scup-pernong	3	158
soda	1100	120			
Cranberries, raw	2	82			
Cranberry juice cocktail, bottled (approx. 33% cranberry juice)	1	10			
	1	10	Grapejuice, canned or bottled	2	116
Cranberry sauce, sweetened, canned, strained	1	30	Guavas, whole, raw, common	4	289
			Haddock, cooked, fried	177	348

[2]Estimated average based on addition of salt in the amount of 0.6% of the finished product.

Food and description	Sodium (mg)	Potassium (mg)	Food and description	Sodium (mg)	Potassium (mg)
Hake, including Pacific hake, squirrel hake, and silver hake or whiting; raw	74	363	Muffin mixes, corn, and muffins baked from mixes		
Halibut, Atlantic and Pacific, cooked, broiled	134	525	muffins, made with egg, milk	479	110
Ham croquette	342	83	muffins, made with egg, water	346	104
Heart, beef, lean, cooked, braised	104	232	Mushrooms		
Herring			raw	15	414
raw, Pacific	74	420	canned, solids and liquid	400	197
smoked, hard	6231	157	Muskmelons, raw, cantaloupes, other netted varieties	12	251
Honey, strained or extracted	5	51	Mussels, Atlantic and Pacific, raw, meat only	289	315
Horse-radish, prepared	96	290	Mustard greens, cooked, boiled, drained	18	220
Ice cream and frozen custard			Mustard, prepared		
regular, approximately 10% fat	63[8]	181	brown	1307	130
Ice cream cones	232	244	yellow	1252	130
Ice milk	68[8]	195	Nectarines, raw	6	294
Jams and preserves	12	88	New Zealand spinach, cooked, boiled, drained	92	463
Kale, cooked, boiled, drained, leaves including stems	43	221	Noodles, egg noodles, enriched, cooked	2	44
Kingfish; southern, gulf, and northern (whiting); raw	83	250	Oat products used mainly as hot breakfast cereals oatmeal or rolled oats		
Lake herring (cisco), raw	47	319	dry form	2	352
Lamb, retail cuts	70	290	cooked	218	61
Lemon juice, canned or bottled, unsweetened	1	141	Oat products used mainly as ready-to-eat breakfast cereals		
Lettuce, raw crisphead varieties such as Iceberg, New York, and Great Lakes strains	9	175	oats (with or without corn), puffed, added nutrients	1267	—
Lime juice, canned or bottled, unsweetened	1	104	Ocean perch, Atlantic (redfish)		
Liver, beef, cooked, fried	184	380	raw	79	269
Lobster, northern, canned or cooked	210	180	cooked, fried	153	284
Loganberries, canned, solids and liquid, syrup pack, light	1	111	Ocean perch, Pacific, raw	63	390
Macadamia nuts	—	164	Oils, salad or cooking	0	0
Macaroni, unenriched, dry form	2	197	Okra		
Macaroni and cheese, canned	304	58	raw	3	249
Margarine[9]	987	23	cooked, boiled, drained	2	174
Marmalade, citrus	14	33	Olives, pickled; canned or bottled		
Milk, cow			green	2400	55
fluid (pasteurized and raw)			ripe, Ascolano (extra large, mammoth, giant jumbo)	813	34
whole, 3.7% fat	50	144	ripe, salt-cured, oil-coated, Greek style	3288	—
skim	52	145			
canned, evaporated (unsweetened)	118	303	Onions, mature (dry), raw	10	157
dry, skim (non-fat solids), regular	532	1745	Onions, young green (bunching varieties), raw bulb and entire top	5	231
malted					
dry powder	440	720	Oranges, raw, peeled fruit, all commercial varieties	1	200
beverage	91	200	Orange juice		
chocolate drink, fluid, commercial			raw, all commercial varieties	1	200
made with skim milk	46	142	canned, unsweetened	1	199
made with whole (3.5% fat) milk	47	146	frozen concentrate, unsweetened, diluted with 3 parts water, by volume	1	186
Molasses, cane					
first extraction or light	15	917			
third extraction or blackstrap	96	2927			

[8]Value for product without added salt.

[9]Values apply to salted margarine. Unsalted margarine contains less than 10 mg per 100 gm of either sodium or potassium. Vitamin A value based on the minimum required to meet federal specifications for margarine with vitamin A added, namely 15,000 IU of vitamin A per pound.

Food and description	Sodium (mg)	Potassium (mg)	Food and description	Sodium (mg)	Potassium (mg)
Oysters			Pineapple		
raw, meat only, Eastern	73	121	raw	1	146
cooked, fried	206	203	frozen chunks, sweetened, not thawed	2	100
frozen, solids and liquid	380	210	Pizza, with cheese, from home recipe, baked		
Oyster stew, commercial frozen, prepared with equal volume of milk	366	176	with cheese topping	702	130
Pancake and waffle mixes and pancakes baked from mixes plain and buttermilk, made with egg, milk	564	154	with sausage topping	729	168
Parsnips, cooked, boiled, drained	8	379	Plate dinners, frozen, commercial, unheated		
Peaches			beef pot roast, whole oven-browned potatoes, peas, and corn	259	244
raw	1	202	chicken, fried; mashed potatoes; mixed vegetables (carrots, peas, corn, beans)	344	112
canned, solids and liquid, water pack, with or without artificial sweetener	2	137	meat loaf with tomato sauce, mashed potatoes, and peas	393	115
frozen, sliced, sweetened, not thawed	2	124	turkey, sliced; mashed potatoes; peas	400	176
Peanuts			Plums		
roasted with skins	5	701	raw, Damson	2	299
roasted and salted	418	674	canned, solids and liquid, purple (Italian prunes), syrup pack, light	1	145
Peanut butters made with small amounts of added fat, salt	607	670	Popcorn, popped		
Pears			plain	(3)	—
raw, including skin	2	130	oil and salt added	1940	—
canned, solids and liquid, syrup pack, light	1	85	Pork, fresh		
Peas, green, immature			retail cuts, trimmed to retail level loin	65	390
cooked, boiled, drained	1	196	Pork, cured, light-cure, commercial, ham, medium-fat class, separable lean, cooked, roasted	930	326
canned, Alaska (Early or June peas)			Pork, cured, canned		
regular pack, solids and liquid	236[2]	96	ham, contents of can	(1100)	(340)
special dietary pack (low-sodium), solids and liquid	3	96	Potatoes		
frozen, cooked, boiled, and drained	115	135	cooked, boiled in skin	3[10]	407
Peas, mature seeds, dry, whole, raw	35	1005	dehydrated mashed		
Peas and carrots, frozen, cooked, boiled, drained	84	157	flakes without milk		
Pecans	Trace	603	dry form	89	1600
Peppers, hot, chili, mature, red, raw, pods excluding seeds	25	564	prepared, water, milk, table fat added	231	286
Peppers, sweet, garden varieties, immature, green, raw	13	213	Pretzels	1680[11]	130
Perch, yellow, raw	68	230	Prunes		
Pickles, cucumber, dill	1428	200	dried, "softenized," cooked (fruit and liquid), with added sugar	3	262
Pies			Pudding mixes and puddings made from mixes with starch base		
baked, piecrust made with unenriched flour			pudding made with milk, cooked	129	136
apple	301	80	pudding made with milk, without cooking	124	129
cherry	304	105	Pumpkin, canned	2	240
mince	448	178	Radishes, raw, common	18	322
pumpkin	214	160			
Piecrust or plain pastry, made with enriched flour, baked	611	50			
Pike, walleye, raw	51	319			

[2]Estimated average based on addition of salt in the amount of 0.6% of the finished product.
[10]Applies to product without added salt. If salt is added, an estimated average value for sodium is 236 mg per 100 gm.
[11]Sodium content is variable. For example, very thin pretzel sticks contain about twice the average amount listed.

Food and description	Sodium (mg)	Potassium (mg)	Food and description	Sodium (mg)	Potassium (mg)
Raisins, natural (unbleached)			Rusk	246	161
cooked, fruit and liquid, added sugar	13	355	Rutabagas, cooked, boiled, drained	4	167
Raspberries			Rye, flour, medium	(1)	203
canned, solids and liquid, water pack, with or without artificial sweetener, red	1	114	Rye wafers, whole-grain	882	600
			Salad dressings, commercial[13]		
			Blue and Roquefort cheese		
			regular	1094	37
frozen, red, sweetened, not thawed	1	100	special dietary (low-calorie)		
			low-fat (approx. 5 cal per tsp)	1108	34
Rennin products			French		
tablet (salts, starch, renin enzyme)	22,300	—	regular	1370	79
tablet (salts, starch, rennin enzyme)			special dietary (low-calorie)		
			low-fat (approx. 5 cal per tsp)	787	79
dessert mixes and desserts prepared from mixes			mayonnaise	597	34
chocolate, dessert made with milk	52	125	Thousand island		
			regular	700	113
other flavors (vanilla, caramel, fruit flavorings)			special dietary (low-calorie, approx. 10 cal per tsp)	700	113
mix, dry form	6	—	Salmon		
dessert, made with milk	46	128	Coho (silver)		
Rhubarb, cooked, added sugar	2	203	raw	48[15]	421
Rice			canned, solids and liquid	351[14]	339
brown			Salt pork, raw	1212	42
raw	9	214	Salt sticks, regular type	1674	92
cooked	282	70	Sandwich spread (with chopped pickle)		
white (fully milled or polished) enriched			regular	626	92
common commercial varieties, all types			special dietary (low-calorie, approx. 5 cal per tsp)	626	92
raw	5	92	Sardines, Atlantic, canned in oil, drained solids	823	590
cooked	374	28	Sardines, Pacific, in tomato sauce, solids and liquid	400	320
Rice products used mainly as ready-to-eat breakfast cereals			Sauerkraut, canned, solids and liquid	747[16]	140
rice flakes, added nutrients	987	180	Sausage, cold cuts, and luncheon meats		
rice, puffed; added nutrients, without salt	2	100	bologna, all samples	1300	230
rice, puffed or open-popped, pre-sweetened, honey and added nutrients	706	—	frankfurters, raw, all samples	1100	220
			luncheon meat, pork, cured ham or shoulder, chopped, spiced or unspiced, canned	1234	222
Rockfish, including black, canary, yellowtail, rasphead, and bocaccio, cooked, oven-steamed	68	446	pork sausage, links or bulk, cooked	958	269
Roe, cooked, baked or broiled, cod and shad[12]	73	132	Scallops, bay and sea, cooked, steamed	265	476
Rolls and buns			Soups, commercial, canned		
commercial			beef broth, bouillon, and con-somme, prepared with equal volume of water	326	54
ready-to-serve					
Danish pastry	366	112	chicken noodle, prepared with equal volume of water	408	23
hard rolls, enriched	625	97			
plain (pan rolls), enriched	506	95			
sweet rolls	389	124			

[12]Prepared with butter or margarine, lemon juice or vinegar.

[13]Values apply to products containing salt. For those without salt, sodium content is low, ranging from less than 10 mg to 50 mg per 100 gm; the amount usually is indicated on the label.

[14]For product canned without added salt, value is approximately the same as for raw salmon.

[15]Sample dipped in brine contained 215 mg sodium per 100 gm.

[16]Values for sauerkraut and sauerkraut juice are based on salt content of 1.9% and 2.0%, respectively, in the finished products. The amounts in some samples may vary significantly from this estimate.

Food and description	Sodium (mg)	Potassium (mg)	Food and description	Sodium (mg)	Potassium (mg)
Soups, commercial, canned—cont'd			Tomato catsup, bottled	1042[17]	363
tomato			Tomato juice		
prepared with equal volume of water	396	94	canned or bottled		
			regular pack	200	227
prepared with equal volume of milk	422	167	special dietary pack (low-sodium)	3	227
vegetable beef, prepared with equal volume of water	427	66	Tomato juice cocktail, canned or bottled	200	221
Soy sauce	7325	366	Tomato puree, canned		
Spaghetti, enriched, cooked, tender stage	1	61	regular pack	399	426
			special dietary pack (low-sodium)	6	426
Spaghetti, in tomato sauce with cheese, canned	382	121	Tongue, beef, medium-fat, cooked, braised	61	164
Spinach			Tuna, canned		
cooked, boiled, drained	50	324	in oil, solids and liquid	800	301
canned			in water, solids and liquid	41[18]	279[18]
regular pack, drained solids	236[2]	250	Turkey, all classes		
special dietary pack (low-sodium), solids and liquid	34	250	light meat, cooked, roasted	82	411
	34	250	dark meat, cooked, roasted	99	398
frozen, chopped, cooked, boiled, drained	52	333	Turkey potpie, commercial, frozen, unheated	369	114
Squash, summer, all varieties, cooked, boiled, drained	1	141	Turnips, cooked, boiled, drained	34	188
Squash, frozen			Turnip greens, leaves, including stems		
summer, yellow crookneck, cooked, boiled, drained	3	167	canned, solids and liquid	236[2]	243
			frozen, cooked, boiled, drained	17	149
winter, heated	1	207	Veal, retail cuts, untrimmed	80	500
Strawberries			Vinegar, cider	1	100
raw	1	164	Waffles, frozen, made with enriched flour	644	158
frozen, sweetened, not thawed, sliced	1	112	Walnuts		
Sturgeon, cooked, steamed	108	235	black	3	460
Succotash (corn and lima beans), frozen, cooked, boiled, drained	38	246	Persian or English	2	450
Sugars, beet or cane, brown	30	344	Watercress leaves including stems, raw	52	282
Sweet potatoes			Watermelon, raw	1	100
cooked, all, baked in skin	12	300	Wheat flours		
canned, liquid pack, solids and liquid, regular pack in syrup	48	(120)	whole (from hard wheats)	3	370
			patent		
dehydrated flakes, prepared with water	45	140	all-purpose or family flour, enriched	2	95
Tangerines, raw (Dancy variety)	2	126	self-rising flour, enriched (anhydrous monocalcium phosphate used as a baking aid)[19]	1079	—[20]
Tapioca, dry	3	18			
Tapioca desserts, tapioca cream pudding	156	135	Wild rice, raw	7	220
Tartar sauce, regular	707	78	Yeast		
Tea, instant (water-soluble solids),	—	4530	baker's, compressed	16	610
carbohydrate added dry powder beverage	—	25	brewer's, debittered	121	1894
Tomatoes, ripe			Yogurt, made from whole milk	47	132
raw	3	244	Zwieback	250	150
canned, solids and liquid, regular pack	130	217			

[2]Estimated average based on addition of salt in the amount of 0.6% of the finished product.

[17]Applies to regular pack. For special dietary pack (low sodium), values range from 5 to 35 mg per 100 gm.

[18]One sample with salt added contained 875 mg of sodium per 100 gm and 275 mg of potassium.

[19]The acid ingredient most commonly used in self-rising flour. When sodium acid pyrophosphate in combination with either anhydrous monocalcium phosphate or calcium carbonate is used, the value for calcium is approximately 120 mg per 100 gm; for phosphorus, 540 mg; for sodium 1360 mg.

[20]90 mg of potassium per 100 gm contributed by flour. Small quantities of additional potassium may be provided by other ingredients.

6-6. Cholesterol content of foods

Item	Amount of cholesterol in		Refuse from item as purchased (%)	Item	Amount of cholesterol in		Refuse from item as purchased (%)
	100 gm edible por-tion[1] (mg)	Edible por-tion of 450 gm (1 lb) as purchased (mg)			100 gm edible por-tion[1] (mg)	Edible por-tion of 450 gm (1 lb) as purchased (mg)	
Beef, raw				Liver, raw	300	1360	0
with bone[2]	70	270	15	Lobster			
without bone[2]	70	320	0	whole[2]	200	235	74
Brains, raw	>2000	>9000	0	meat only[2]	200	900	0
Butter	250	1135	0	Margarine			
Cavier or fish roe	> 300	>1300	0	all vegetable fat	0	0	0
Cheese				two-thirds animal fat,	65	295	0
cheddar	100	455	0	one-third vege-			
cottage, creamed	15	70	0	table fat			
cream	120	545	0	Milk			
other (25% to 30% fat)	85	385	0	fluid, whole	11	50	0
Cheese spread	65	295	0	dried, whole	85	385	0
Chicken, flesh only, raw	60	—	0	fluid, skim	3	15	0
Crab				Mutton			
in shell[2]	125	270	52	with bone[2]	65	250	16
meat only[2]	125	565	0	without bone[2]	65	295	0
Egg, whole	550	2200	12	Oysters			
Egg white	0	0	0	in shell[2]	> 200	> 90	90
Egg yolk				meat only[2]	> 200	> 900	0
fresh	1500	6800	0	Pork			
frozen	1280	5800	0	with bone[2]	70	260	18
dried	2950	13,380	0	without bone[2]	70	320	0
Fish				Shrimp			
steak[2]	70	265	16	in shell[2]	125	390	31
fillet[2]	70	320	0	flesh only[2]	125	565	0
Heart, raw	150	680	0	Sweetbreads (thymus)	250	1135	0
Ice cream	45	205	0	Veal			
Kidney, raw	375	1700	0	with bone[2]	90	320	21
Lamb, raw				without bone[2]	90	410	0
with bone[2]	70	265	16				
without bone[2]	70	320	0				
lard and other animal fat	95	430	0				

[1]Data apply to 100 gm of edible portion of the item, although it may be purchased with the refuse indicated and described or implied in the first column.
[2]Designate items that have the same chemical composition for the edible portion but differ in the amount of refuse.

6-7. Examples of intentional food additives

Function	Chemical compound	Common food uses
Acids, alkalis, buffers	Sodium bicarbonate	Baking powder
	Tartaric acid	Fruit sherbets
		Cheese spreads
Antibiotics	Chlortetracycline	Dip for dressed poultry
Anticaking agents	Aluminum calcium silicate	Table salt
Antimycotics	Calcium propionate	Bread
	Sodium propionate	Bread
	Sorbic acid	Cheese
Antioxidants	Butylated hydroxyanisole (BHA)	Fats
	Butylated hydroxytoluene (BHT)	Fats
Bleaching agents	Benzoyl peroxide	Wheat flour
	Chlorine dioxide	
	Oxides of nitrogen	
Color preservative	Sodium benzoate	Green peas
		Maraschino cherries
Coloring agents	Annotto	Butter, margarine
	Carotene	
Emulsifiers	Lecithin	Bakery goods
	Monoglycerides and diglycerides	Dairy products
	Propylene glycol alginate	Confections
Flavoring agents	Amyl acetate	Soft drinks
	Benzaldehyde	Bakery goods
	Methyl salicylate	Candy; ice cream
	Essential oils; natural extractives	
	Monosodium glutamate	Canned meats
Nonnutritive sweeteners	Saccharin, calcium, and sodium cyclamates	Diet packed canned fruit Low-calorie soft drinks
Nutrient supplements	Potassium iodide	Iodized salt
	Vitamin C	Fruit juices
	Vitamin D	Milk
	Vitamin A	Margarine
	B vitamins, iron	Bread and cereal
Sequestrants	Sodium citrate	Dairy products
	Calcium pyrophosphoric acid	
Stabilizers and thickeners	Pectin	Jellies
	Vegetable gums (carob bean, carrageenan, guar)	Dairy desserts and chocolate milk Confections
	Gelatin	"Low-calorie" salad dressings
	Agar-agar	
Yeast foods and dough conditioners	Ammonium chloride	Bread, rolls
	Calcium sulfate	
	Calcium phosphate	

I. Chief complaint of client
   A. Location
   B. Character
   C. Chronology
   D. Situational determinants
   E. Aggravating or alleviating factors
   F. Previous attempts at therapy and their effectiveness
   G. Disability resulting from this complaint
II. Social systems
   A. Social development
      *1. Age
      *2. Sex
      *3. Developmental tasks
      *4. Psychosocial personality development (Erickson's Eight Stages of Man)
      *5. Diversional, recreational interests (what to do to pass time while ill)
      *6. Roles in family, community, work, and perceived performance of them
      *7. Degree of independence-dependence
      *8. Child's favorite play activity
      *9. Socially oriented habits (include alcohol, drugs), frequency of use, and response to use
   B. Family or significant others
      *1. Others in living group
      *2. Significant others outside living group
      *3. Visiting preferences and who is able to visit
      *4. Marital status
      *5. Alterations for family's life because of ill member
      *6. Interaction patterns (observe this also)
      *7. Presence of disease in other family members
   C. Work
      *1. Occupation
      *2. Source of income
      *3. Insurance (hospitalization)
      *4. Changes in work pattern because of illness
      *5. Feelings about work and being away from productivity and routine
   D. Religion
      *1. Religious affiliation
      *2. Desire for chaplain visit
      *3. Practices or beliefs that might affect reaction to health care (proscriptions against immunization or blood transfusion, dietary laws, beliefs about disease causation, death)

E. Education
   *1. Formal education
   *2. Satisfaction and progress with school
F. Community
   *1. Type of housing
   *2. Contacts or previous referrals to social agencies
   *3. Availability and pattern of utilization of health care facilities (physician, dentist), frequency and reason for visits
   *4. Immunizations (type, date)
G. Ethnic-cultural system
   *1. Factors that may influence reaction to hospitalization, therapy, illness
   *2. Food preferences
   *3. Response to stress (e.g., pain)
H. Environment
   *1. Effect of present environment on health status and developmental level (e.g., lighting, noise, activity, color—variation, consistency excessive or absent)
   *2. Arrangement of environmental in relation to functional abilities or disabilities
   *3. Safety factors
      a. Mobility (arrangement of objects in physical environment)
      b. Use of prosthetic or supportive devices (e.g., crutches, wheelchair)
   *4. Infection control
      a. Ready sources of infection
      b. Barriers to infection (isolation technique, hand-washing facility)
III. Psychological systems
   A. Cognition
      *1. Level of consciousness (response to sensory stimuli)
      *2. Orientation to time, place, person
      *3. Mental skills
         a. Ability to read and write
         b. Vocabulary
         c. Ability to comprehend and follow directions
         d. Attention and memory span
      *4. Intellectual development relative to chronological age (e.g., Piaget's formulation)
      *5. Understanding of and reaction to health concern and goals of medical-nursing therapy
      *6. Desired information about present tests and treatment
      *7. Previous experience with and reaction to illness and hospitalization
      *8. Name child or adolescent prefers
   B. Emotion
      *1. Quality of mood, expression, intensity of reaction
      *2. Activity level (active, sluggish, hyperactive)
      *3. Effect of illness on life and expectation of future effects

---

*Key data to collect for all clients. Data not marked are collected if dysfunction is found in system.

     *4. Feelings about hospitalization
     *5. Coping patterns in stressful situations (describe stressful situations); availability, need for, and effectiveness of internal-external support systems
     *6. Special concerns or fears
     *7. Patterns of relating to others (e.g., verbal, congenial)
     *8. Self-concept (body image before and in relation to current health problem)
     *9. Comfort, rest and sleep patterns (hours, time, nap periods, feeling of being rested) before and since illness
    *10. Aids used to sleep
    *11. Presence of pain or discomfort (location, duration, degree, character, precipitating factors, change in pattern)
    *12. Use of aids to relieve pain

IV. Biological systems
  A. Gas transport and exchange
    1. Cardiovascular
      *a. Past or present disease of cardiovascular system
      *b. Syncope
      *c. Dizziness
      *d. Fatigue, activity tolerance
      *e. Chest pain
        (1) Type
        (2) Pattern
        (3) Precipitating factors
        (4) Relief measures
      *f. Subjective feeling of warmth or coldness of body parts
      *g. Medications taken to affect CV system
      *h. Edematous body parts
    2. Respiratory
      *a. Past or present diseases of respiratory system
      *b. Cough
        (1) Frequency
        (2) Duration
      *c. Sputum
        (1) Color
        (2) Odor
        (3) Amount
      *d. Shortness of breath
        (1) Precipitating factors
        (2) Frequency
        (3) Effect on activity
      *e. Allergies
      *f. Smoking
        (1) Amount
        (2) Duration
        (3) Attempts and success at stopping
      *g. Medications taken to affect respiratory system
      h. Orthopnea
      i. Hemoptysis
      j. Fever
      k. Frequency of colds and sore throat
      l. Activity tolerance
      m. Factors affecting breathing
        (1) Emotion
        (2) Pollution
        (3) Position

  B. Nutrition and elimination
    1. Gastrointestinal
      *a. Past or present disease of GI system
      *b. Dietary habits
        (1) Amount of basic four food groups
        (2) Amount of fluid intake daily
        (3) Likes
        (4) Dislikes
        (5) Number of meals and snacks
        (6) Time of meals
        (7) Assistance needed with eating
        (8) Alcohol intake
      *c. Appetite, thirst, stability of weight
      *d. Factors related to ingestion
        (1) Nonoral intake
        (2) Chewing
        (3) Swallowing
        (4) Oral hygiene habits
      *e. Factors related to digestion
        (1) Ease
        (2) Nausea
        (3) Vomiting
        (4) Belching
        (5) Pain in abdomen
      *f. Bowel elimination pattern
        (1) Time and frequency of bowel movements
        (2) Degree of child's independence in toileting
        (3) Words used by child regarding elimination
        (4) Character of stools
        (5) Ease (constipation, diarrhea)
        (6) Hemorrhoids
        (7) Passage of flatus, blood
      *g. Abdominal pain and character
      *h. Medicines taken to alter digestion and metabolism of foods
    2. Urinary
      *a. Past or present diseases of urinary system
      *b. Fluid intake
      *c. Urination pattern
        (1) Amount
        (2) Color
        (3) Odor
        (4) Frequency, night or day urgency
        (5) Dysuria
      *d. Vaginal or urethral discharge
      *e. Degree of independence in toileting
      *f. Edema
  C. Sensorimotor
    1. Musculoskeletal
      *a. Past or present diseases of musculoskeletal system
      *b. Abnormal innervation to muscles (paralysis, weakness, spasticity)
      *c. Activity endurance
      *d. Method of ambulation
        (1) Assistance needed with dressing, hygiene
        (2) Safety measures needed
      *e. Range of motion limitation
      *f. Muscle weakness
      *g. Medicines taken to affect musculoskeletal subsystem

2. Nervous
   *a. Past or present diseases of nervous system
   *b. Visual status
      (1) Acuity
      (2) Deficits and corrective devices
   *c. Auditory status
      (1) Deficits and corrective devices
      (2) Unusual sensations (ringing, buzzing, vertigo, pain)
   *d. Olfactory status
   *e. Gustatory status
   *f. Tactile status (ability to discriminate sharp-dull, light-firm, heat-cold sensations)
   *g. Mobility (coordination, balance)
   *h. Medicines taken to affect nervous system
D. Protective mechanisms
   1. Integument
      *a. Past or present diseases of integumentary system
      *b. Factors predisposing to skin breakdown
      *c. Personal hygiene
         (1) Bathing (kind, type, frequency)
         (2) Frequency, time of shaving
         (3) After bath skin care
      *d. Medicines taken to affect integumentary system

   2. Immune mechanism
      *a. Past or present allergy
      *b. Past or present sensitivities to drugs or other agents (pollens, insect bites)
      *c. Past or present high susceptibility to infection
E. Endocrine mechanisms
   *1. Abnormal function of endocrine gland(s) and effect; past or present diseases
   *2. Growth patterns
   *3. Medicines taken to affect endocrine system
F. Sexuality and reproduction
   *1. Past or present alterations of reproduction system
   *2. Reproductive data
      a. Number of pregnancies
      b. Live births
      c. Living children
      d. Family planning (methods used)
      e. Menstrual pattern
      f. Menopause (age of onset and associated factors)
   *3. Breast self-examination routine
   *4. Frequency of Pap smears
   *5. Sexual libido and performance
   *6. Level of sexual development
   *7. Attitudes toward own sexuality
   *8. Medicines taken to affect reproductive system

APPENDIX 8 · Maternity and obstetrics

8-1. Standard laboratory values in the neonatal period

Hematological values

	Neonatal	
Clotting factors	2 min	
Activated clotting time (ACT)	2 min	
Bleeding time (Ivy)	1-8 min	
Clot retraction	Complete 1-4 hr	
Clotting time		
2 tubes	5-8 min	
3 tubes	5-15 min	
Fibrinogen	150-300 mg/dl	
Fibrinolysin (plasminogen)	Lysis of clot	
Partial thromboplastin time (PTT)	<90-120 sec	
Prothrombin time, one-stage (PT)	12-21 sec	
Thromboplastin generation test (TGT)	8-24 sec in 6 min tube	

	Term	Preterm
Hemoglobin (gm/dl)	17-19	15-17
Hematocrit (%)	57-58	45-55
Sedimentation rate, erythrocytes (ESR) mm/hr	0-2	1-5
Reticulocytes (%)	3-7	Up to 10
Fetal hemoglobin (% of total)	40-70	80-90
Nucleated RBC/cu mm (per 100 RBC)	200 (0.05)	(0.2)
Platelet count/cu mm	100-300,000	120-180,000
WBC/cu mm	15,000	10,000-20,000
Neutrophils (%)	45	47
Eosinophils and basophils (%)	3	
Lymphocytes (%)	30	33
Monocytes (%)	5	4
Immature WBC (%)	10	16

Biochemical values

		Neonatal
Ammonia		100-150 μg/dl
Amylase		0-1000 IU/lu
Antistreptolysin 0 titer, group B		
Normal		12-100 Todd units
Recent streptococcal infection		200-2500 Todd units
Bilirubin, direct		0-1 mg/dl
Bilirubin, total	Cord:	<2 mg/dl
	Peripheral blood: 0-1 day	6 mg/dl
	1-2 day	8 mg/dl
	3-5 day	12 mg/dl
Blood gases	Arterial:	pH 7.31-7.45
		P_{CO_2} 33-48 mmHg
		P_{O_2} 50-70 mmHg
	Venous:	pH 7.28-7.42
		P_{CO_2} 38-52 mmHg
		P_{O_2} 20-49 mmHg
Calcium, ionized		2.1-2.6 mEq/L
Calcium, total		4-7.0 mEq/L
Catecholamines (μg/24 hr)		
Neonatal: norepinephrine, 2-12; epinephrine, 1-2		
Newborn: norepinephrine, 2-4; epinephrine, 0-1		
Ceruloplasmin (p-phenylenediamine dihydrochloride, 37 C)		1-30 mg/dl
Chloride		95-110 mEq/L
Cholesterol, esters		42% to 71% of total
Cholesterol, total		45-170 mg/dl

Biochemical values—cont'd　　　　　　　　　　　　　　　　　　*Neonatal*

Copper	20-70 μg/dl
Cortisol	
AM specimen	15-25 μg/dl
PM specimen	5-10 μg/dl
C-reactive protein (CRP)	0
Creatine	0.2-1 mg/dl (higher in females)
Creatine phosphokinase (CPK) (creatine phosphate, 30 C)	10-300 IU/L
Creatinine	0.3-1 mg/dl
Electrophoresis, total protein	Preterm: 4.3-7.6 gm/dl
	Newborn: 4.6-7.4 gm/dl

    Preterm: albumin, 3.1-4.2; α_1-globulin, 0.1-0.5; α_2-globulin,
      0.3-0.7; β-globulin, 0.3-1.2; γ-globulin, 0.3-1.4
    Newborn: albumin, 3.6-5.4; α_1-globulin, 0.1-0.3; α_2-globulin,
      0.2-0.5; β-globulin, 0.2-0.6; γ-globulin, 0.2-1.2.

Fatty acids, free	0.4-1 mg/L
α_1-fetoprotein	0
Fibrinogen	150-300 mg/dl
Glucose, fasting (FBS)	
Hepatitis-associated (Australia) antigen	0
Immunoglobulin levels, serum, newborn	660-1.439 mg/dl
IgG 645-1.244	
IgM 5-30	
IgA 0-11	
Iodine, butanol extractable (BEI)	3-13 μg/dl
Iodine, T_4-by-column (thyroxine)	3-12 μg/dl
Iodine, T_4 (competitive protein-binding thyroxine)	3-12 μg/dl
Iodine, total serum organic (PBI)	4-14 μg/dl
Iron	100-200 μg/dl
Iron-binding capacity (IBC)	60-175 μg/dl
17-Ketogenic steroids (17-KGS)	2.4 mg/24 hr
17-Ketosteroids (17-KS)	0.5-2.5 mg/24 hr
Lactic dehydrogenase (LDH) (pyruvate, 30 C)	300-1500 IU/L
Lipids, total	170-450 mg/dl
Lipoproteins, newborn (mg/dl)	
Alpha 70-180	
Beta 50-160	
Chylo 50-110	
Magnesium	1.4-2.9 mEq/L
Malate dehydrogenase (MDH) (oxaloacetic acid, 37 C)	41-68 IU/L
Phosphatase, acid	10.4-16.4 IU/L
Phosphatase, alkaline	50-275 IU/L
Phospholipids	75-170 mg/dl
Phosphorus	3.5-8.6 mg/dl
Potassium	4-7 mg/L
Pregnanetriol	0 mg/24 hr
Protein, total	4.3-7.6 gm/dl
Sodium	140-160 mEq/L
Transaminases, serum	
Glutamic-oxaloacetic (SGOT) (aspartate, 30 C)	5-70 IU/L
Glutamic-pyruvic (SGPT)	5-50 IU/L
Triglycerides	5-40 mg/dl
Urea nitrogen (BUN)	5-15 mg/dl
Vanillylmandelic acid (VMA)	0-1 mg/24 hr

Urinalysis

Volume: 20-40 ml excreted daily in the first few days; by 1 wk, 24 hr urine volume close to 200 ml
Protein: may be present in first 2-4 days
Casts and WBCs: may be present in first 2-4 days
Osmolarity (mOsm/L): 100-600
pH: 5-7
Specific gravity: 1.001-1.020

Cerebrospinal fluid

Calcium	2-3 mg/L
Cell count	WBCs/cu mm 0-15
	RBCs/cu mm 0-500
Chloride	110-120 mg/L
Color	May be xanthochromic
Glucose	24-40 mg/dl
Lactate dehydrogenase (LDH)	5-80 IU/L
Magnesium	3-3.3 mg/dl
Pándy's test (for excess globulins)	Negative
pH (at 37 C)	7.33-7.42
Pressure	50-80 mmHg
Protein, total	20-120 mg/dl
Sodium	130-165 mg/L
Specific gravity	1.007-1.009
Transaminase, glutamic-oxaloacetic (GOT)	2-10 IU/L
Volume	5 ml

Cardiorespiratory determinations

Blood pressure at birth
  Term: systolic, 78 mm Hg; diastolic, 42 mm Hg
  Preterm: systolic, 50-60 mm Hg; diastolic, 30 mm Hg
Respiratory rate: 30-60/min
Heart rate, fetus
  Baseline: 120-160/min
    Tachycardia: >160 beats/min (with maternal complication)
    Bradycardia: <120 beats/min (with maternal hypotension and hypoxia)
    Acceleration: tachycardia >160 beats/min with uterine contraction—normal (usually)
  Beat-to-beat variability: disappears with fetal distress
  With uterine contraction
    Early deceleration: bradycardia with onset of contraction—benign
    Variable deceleration: bradycardia due to cord compression—usually benign
    Late deceleration: bradycardia after lag period caused by fetal hypoxia—ominous sign
Heart rate, term infant: 140 ± 20 beats/min

Urine screening tests for inborn errors of metabolism

Benedict's test: for reducing substances in the urine—glucose, galactose, fructose, lactose; phenylketonuria, alkaptonuria, tyrosyluria, and tyrosinosis *may* give positive Benedict's test.

Ferric chloride test: an immediate, green color for phenylketonuria, histidinemia, and tyrosinuria; a gray to green color for presence of phenothiazines, isoniazid; red to purple color for presence of salicylates or ketone bodies.

Dinitrophenylhydrazine test: for phenylketonuria, maple syrup urine disease, Lowe's syndrome.

Cetyltrimethyl ammonium bromide test: for mucopolysaccharides; immediate positive reaction in gargoylism (Hurler's syndrome); delayed, moderately positive reaction for Marfan's, Morquio-Ullrich, and Murdoch syndromes.

Metachromatic stain (of urine sediment): Granules (free or as inclusion bodies in cells) are seen in metachromatic leukodystrophy; may also be seen rarely in Tay-Sachs and other lipid diseases of the central nervous system.

Amino acid chromatography: Aminoaciduria may be normal in newborns; chromatography may be helpful to detect hypophosphatasia and argininosuccinicaciduria.

Diagnostic tests for phenylketonuria

Test	Method	Use
Urine tests		
Diaper test	10% ferric chloride dropped on freshly wet diaper; green spot (positive): probable PKU	Inexpensive; useful in screening large groups of infants but not of value until infant is at least 6 wk of age
Phenistix test	Prepared test stick pressed against wet diaper or dipped in urine; green color reaction: probable PKU	Simple; more accurate than diaper test; useful in screening large groups of infants but not of value until after infant is 6 wk of age
Dinitrophenyl-hydrazine (DNPH) test	0.5-1 ml of urine placed in test tube, equal amount of DNPH solution added; immediate pale yellow-orange color reaction: negative; gradual change to opaque bright yellow: positive, indicates probable PKU	Inexpensive; accurate but more complicated than diaper test or Phenistix; most useful in clinical setting to confirm these tests

Test	Method	Use
Blood serum phenylalanine tests		
Guthrie inhibition assay methods	Drops of blood placed on filter paper; laboratory uses bacterial growth inhibition test; phenylalanine level above 8 mg/dl blood: diagnostic of PKU	Effective in newborn period; used also to monitor PKU diet; blood easily obtained by heel or finger puncture; inexpensive; used for wide-scale screening
LaDu-Michael method	5 ml of blood; serum separated and tested for phenyl-alanine; level above 8 mg/dl blood: PKU; in persons with PKU, phenylalanine level above 8-12 mg/dl blood: loss of dietary control	Useful diagnostic tool and to monitor PKU diet; requires blood drawn from person; laboratory method difficult (test not available in many laboratories)
McCaman and Robins fluorometric method	5 ml of blood; serum separated and tested for phenyl-alanine; level above 8 mg: PKU or loss of dietary control	Diagnostic and diet monitoring tool; laboratory procedure more simple than LaDu-Michael method; test not available in many laboratories

8-2. Relationship of drugs to breast milk and effect on infant

Drug	Excreted in milk	Amount in milk after therapeutic dose	Effect on infant
Analgesics and anti-inflammatory drugs (nonnarcotic)			
Acetaminopen (Datril, Tylenol)	Yes		Detoxified in liver. Avoid in immediate postdelivery period, otherwise no problems with therapeutic dose.
Aspirin	Yes	1-3 mg/dl	Long history of experience shows complications rare. Can cause interference with platelet aggregation and diminished factor XII (Hageman factor) at birth. When mother requires high, continuing level of medication for arthritis, aspirin is drug of choice. Observe infant for bruisability. Platelet aggregation can be evaluated. Salicylism only seen in maternal overdosing. Mother should increase vitamin C and vitamin K intake.
Donnatal (phenobarbital, hyoscy-amine sulfate, atropine sulfate, hyoscine hydrobromide)	Yes		Consider for its component parts. Can be given to children but can accumulate in neonate.
Flufenamic acid (Arlef)	Yes	0.50 μg/ml (mean)	No apparent effect on infant when maternal dosage was 200 mg, three times a day. Infant able to excrete via urine.
Indomethacin (Indocin)	Yes		Convulsions in breast-fed neonate (case report). Used to close patent ductus arteriosus. Insufficient data as to effect on other vessels. May be nephrotoxic.
Mefenamic acid (Ponstel)	Yes	Trace amounts	No apparent effect on infant at therapeutic doses; infant able to excrete via urine.
Naproxen (Naprosyn, synaxsyn, naprosine, naxen, proxen)	Yes	1% of maternal plasma; binds to plasma protein	Less toxic in adults than some other organic derivatives.
Oxyphenbutazone (Tandearil)	Yes	In milk of 2 of 55 mothers, 10% to 80% of maternal plasma level	No known effect.
Pentazocine (Talwin)	No		Withdrawal in neonatal period from ingestion during pregnancy.
Percodan (oxycodone [derived from opiate thebaine] aspirin, phenace-tin, caffeine)	Yes		Consider for its component parts. In neonatal period sleepiness and failure to feed, which increase maternal engorgement and neonatal weight loss, have been observed, probably caused by oxycodone.
Phenylbutazone (Butazolidin)	Yes	0.63 mg ml 90 min after 750 mg given IM	Very potent drug; risk to infant not well defined but considerable. Not given directly to children; may accumulate in infant.

Drug	Excreted in milk	Amount in milk after therapeutic dose	Effect on infant
Propoxyphene (Darvon)	Yes	0.4% of maternal* dose	Only symptoms detectable would be failure to feed and drowsiness. On daily, around-the-clock dosage infant could consume 1 mg/day.

Antibiotics

Drug	Excreted in milk	Amount in milk after therapeutic dose	Effect on infant
Amantadine (Symmetrel)	Yes	Not defined	Vomiting, urinary retention, rash. Contraindicated.
Ampicillin (Polycillin, Amcill, Omnipen, Penbritin)	Yes	0.07 μg/ml	Sensitivity due to repeated exposure; diarrhea or secondary candidiasis.
Carbenicillin (Pyopen, Geopen)	Yes	0.265 μg/ml 1 hr after 1 g given	Levels not significant. Drug is given to neonate.
Cefazolin (Ancef, Kefzol)	Yes	1.5 μg/ml (0.075% of dose)	Probably not significant.
Cephalexin (Keflex)	No		
Cephalothin (Keflin)	No		
Chloramphenicol (Chloromycetin)	Yes	Half blood level; 2.5 mg/dl	Gray syndrome. Infant does not excrete drug well, and small amounts may accumulate. Contraindicated. May be tolerated in older infant with mature glycuronide system.
Chloroquine (Aralen)	Yes	2.7 mg in 2 days†	Can be use to *treat* child under 6 mo of age who is wholly breast-fed.
Colistin (Colymycin)	Yes	0.05-0.09 mg/dl	Not absorbed orally.
Demeclocycline (Declomycin)	Yes	0.2-0.3 mg/dl	Not significant in therapeutic doses. Can be given to infants.
Erythromycin (Ilosone, E-Mycin, Erythrocin)	Yes	0.05-0.1 mg/dl; 3.6-6.2 μg/ml	Higher concentrations have been reported in milk than in plasma. Should not be given under 1 mo of age because of risk of jaundice. Dose in milk higher when given IV to mother.
Gentamicin	Unknown		Not absorbed from gastrointestinal tract, may change gut flora. Drug is given to newborns directly.
Isoniazid (Nydrazid)	Yes	0.6-1.2 mg/dl‡	Infant at risk for toxicity, but need for breast milk may outweigh risk.
Kanamycin (Kantrex)	Yes	18.4 μg/ml after 1 gm given IM	Infant absorbs little from gastrointestinal tract. Infants can be given drug.
Lincomycin (Lincocin)	Yes	0.5-2.4 mg/dl	Not significant in therapeutic doses to affect child.
Mandelic acid	Yes	0.3 gm/24 hr after dose of 12 gm/day	Not significant in therapeutic doses to affect child.
Methacycline (Rondomycin)	Yes	½ plasma level; 50-260 μg/dl	Same precautions as with tetracycline.
Methenamine (Hexamine)	Yes		Not significant in therapeutic doses to affect child.
Metronidazole (Flagyl)	Yes	Level comparable to serum§	Caution should be exercised because of its high milk concentrations. Contraindicated when infant under 6 mo, may cause neurologic disorders and blood dyscrasia.
Nalidixic acid (Neggram)	Yes	0.4 mg/dl	Not significant in therapeutic doses beyond neonatal period. Hemolytic anemia in an infant attributed to nalidixic acid in G6PD deficiency or when mother has renal failure.
Nitrofurantoin (Furadantin)	Yes	Trace to 0.5 μg/ml	Not significant in therapeutic doses to affect child except in G6PD deficiency.
Novobiocin (Albamycin, cathomycin)	Yes	0.36-0.54 mg/dl	Infant can be given drug directly.
Nystatin (Mycostatin)	No	Not absorbed orally	Can be given to infant directly.
Oxacillin (Prostaphlin)	No		
Para-aminosalicylic acid	No		
Penethamate (Leocillin)	No	24-74 μg/dl	Animal study suggests it be avoided.

*Shown by animal experiments. Milk plasma ratio (M/P) = ½.
†Peaks in 6 hr.
‡Same concentration in milk as in maternal serum.
§Gives serum levels in infants of 0.05 to 0.4 μg/ml.

Drug	Excreted in milk	Amount in milk after therapeutic dose	Effect on infant
Antibiotics—cont'd			
Penicillin G, benzathine (Bicillin)	Yes	10-12 units/dl	Clinical need should supersede possible allergic responses.
Penicillin G, potassium	Yes	Up to 6 units/dl; 1.2-3.6 μg/dl	Infant can be given penicillin directly. Parents should be told to inform physician that infant has been exposed to penicillin because of potential sensitivity.
Pyrimethamine (Daraprim)	Yes	0.3 mg/dl (3% of dose)	Significant in therapeutic doses when infant under 6 mo and entirely breast-fed.
Quinine sulfate	Yes	0-0.1 mg/dl after maternal dose of 300-600 mg	In therapeutic doses, no effect on child except rare thrombocytopenia.
Sodium fusidate	Yes	0.02 μg/ml	Not significant in therapeutic doses to affect child.
Streptomycin	Yes	Present for long periods in slight amounts when given as dihydrostreptomycin	Not to be given more than 2 wk. Ototoxic and nephrotoxic with long use. Is given to infants directly.
Sulfanilamide	Yes	9 mg/dl after dose of 2-4 gm/24 hr	Not significant in therapeutic doses; may cause a rash or hemolytic anemia. Should be avoided for first month after delivery.
Sulfapyridine	Yes	3-13 mg/dl after dose of 3 gm/24 hr	To be avoided; has caused skin rash.
Sulfathiazole	Yes	0.5 mg/dl after dose of 3 gm/24 hr	Not significant in therapeutic doses to affect child after 1 mo of age.
Sulfisoxazole (Gantrisin)	Yes	Concentration similar to plasma level.	To be avoided during first month after delivery; may cause kernicterus.
Tetracycline HCl (Achromycin, Panmycin, Sumycin)	Yes	0.5-2.6 μg/ml after dose of 500 mg four times a day	Not enough to treat an infection in an infant. May cause discoloration of the teeth in the infant; the antibiotic, however, may be largely bound to the milk calcium. Do not give over 10 days or repeatedly.
Anticoagulants			
Coumarin derivatives Dicumarol (bishydroxycoumarin) Warfarin (Panwarfin)	Yes	Probably little but may be cumulative*	Monitor prothrombin time. Give vitamin K to infant. Discontinue if surgery or trauma occurs. Drug of choice if mother to continue nursing.
Ethyl biscoumacetate (Tromexan)	Yes	0-0.17 mg/dl†	Hemorrhage around umbilical stump and cephalhematoma reported. Prothrombin normal in infants with hemorrhage. Vitamin K has no effect. Contraindicated while nursing.
Heparin	No		Heparin ineffective orally.
Phenindione (Hedulin) (Dindevan)	Yes		Breast milk a major route of excretion. Reports of serious hemorrhage in infant. Prothrombin times prolonged in infant. Contraindicated while nursing.
Anticonvulsants and sedatives‡			
Barbital (Veronal)	Yes	8-10 mg/L after 500 mg dose	May produce sedation in infant. In general, barbiturates pass into milk but do not sedate infant. Watch for symptoms.
Carbamazepine (Tegretol)	Yes	60% of plasma levels§	Animal studies show lack of weight gain, unkempt appearance.
Chloral hydrate (Noctec, Somnos)	Yes	Up to 1.5 mg/dl	No significant symptoms, can be given to infants directly.
Phenytoin (Dilantin)	Yes	1.5 to 2.6 μg/ml after 300 mg/24 hr dose	One case of hemolytic reaction reported. Other infants appear to tolerate the small doses. Therapeutic plasma level 10-20 μg/ml.
Mephenytoin (Mesantoin) (hydantoin homologue of mephobarbital)	Unknown		Detoxified in liver. No information.

*Reports conflict.
†No correlation with dosage, continues in milk after plasma clear.
‡All barbitals appear in breast milk.
§When plasma 13.0 μmoles/L, 7.5 μmoles/L in milk.

Drug	Excreted in milk	Amount in milk after therapeutic dose	Effect on infant
Pentobarbital (Nembutal)	Yes		Depends on liver for detoxification so may accumulate in first week of life until infant able to detoxify. No problem for older infant in usual doses.
Phenobarbital (Luminal)	Yes	0.1-0.5 mg when plasma level 0.6-1.8 mg	Sleepiness and decreased sucking possible. On usual analeptic doses infants alert and feed well. On hypnotic doses infant depressed and difficult to rouse.
Phensuximide (Milontin)			No specific data.
Primidone (Mysoline)	Yes		Causes drowsiness and decreased feeds. May cause bleeding due to hypoprothrombinemia. Infant needs vitamin K. Avoid drug during lactation.
Sodium bromide (Bromo-Seltzer and over-the-counter sleeping aids)	Yes	Up to 6.6 mg/dl	Drowsy, decreased crying, rash, decreased feeding.
Trimethadione (Tridione)			No specific data.
Antihistaminics			
Brompheniramine (Dimetane) Diphenhydramine (Benadryl) Methdilazine (Tacaryl) Tripelennamine (Pyribenzamine)	Yes	No specific data available. All pass into milk.	Drug is used in neonates. May cause sedation, decreased feeding, or may produce stimulation and tachycardia. Should avoid long-acting preparations, which may accumulate in infant. When combined with decongestants, may cause decrease in milk.
Autonomic drugs			
Atropine sulfate*	Yes	0.1 mg/dl	Hyperthermia, atropine toxicity, infants especially sensitive; also inhibits lactation. Infant dose 0.01 mg/kg.
Carisoprodol (Soma, Rela)	Yes	Two to four times maternal plasma	Blocks interneuronal activity in descending reticular formation and spinal cord; drowsiness, hypotonia, poor feed.
Ergot (Cafergot)	Yes	Unknown	90% of infants had symptoms of ergotism: vomiting and diarrhea to weak pulse and unstable blood pressure. Short-term therapy for migraine should not exceed 6 mg. Cafergot also contains 100 mg caffeine.
Mepenzolate bromide (Cantil)	No		Postganglionic parasympathetic inhibitor used to diminish gastric acidity and decrease spasm of colon. Oral absorption low.
Methocarbamol (Robaxin)	Yes	Minimum	Too little in milk to produce effect.
Neostigmine	No		No known harm to infant.
Propantheline bromide (Pro-Banthine)	No	Uncontrolled data indicate no measurable levels	Drug rapidly metabolized in maternal system to inactive metabolite. Moher should avoid long-acting preparations, however.
Scopolamine (hyoscine)	Yes		Usually given as single dose and of no problem to neonate. No data on repeated doses.
Cardiovascular drugs			
Diazoxide (Hyperstat)			Arteriolar dilators and antihypertensive, only given IV, not active orally.
Dibenzyline†			No data available.
Digoxin	Yes	0.96-0.61 ng/ml‡	Digoxin 20% bound to protein; infant receives <1/100 of dose. If mother at toxic level of 5 ng/ml, milk would have 4.4 ng/ml and infant would receive only $\frac{1}{20}$ daily dose.
Guanethidine (Ismelin)§	Yes		Not significant in therapeutic doses to affect child.
Hydralazine (Apresoline)	Yes		Jaundice, thrombocytopenia, electrolyte disturbances possible.
Methyldopa (Aldomet)§	Yes		Galactorrhea. No specific data except as affects mother's milk production.

*Ingredient in many prescription and nonprescription drugs.
†α blocking agent.
‡Peak level occurs 4-6 hr after dose given. Maternal plasma level was higher, M/P = 0.9 and 0.8; infant's plasma level was 0.
§Adrenergic blocking agent.

Drug	Excreted in milk	Amount in milk after therapeutic dose	Effect on infant
Cardiovascular drugs—cont'd			
Propranolol (Inderal)*	Yes	40 ng/ml of maternal plasma†	Insignificant amount. Infants reported had no symptoms noted. Should watch for hypoglycemia and/or "β-blocking" effects.
Quinidine	Yes		Arrhythmia may occur.
Reserpine (Serpasil)‡	Yes		May produce galactorrhea, lethargy, diarrhea, or nasal stuffiness.
Cathartics			
Aloin	Yes	Low	Occasionally gave symptoms, caused colic and diarrhea in infant.
Anthraquinone laxatives such as di-hydroxyanthraquinone (Dorbane and Dorbantyl)	Yes	High	Caused colic and diarrhea in infant.
Calomel	No	None	None.
Cascara	Yes	Low	Caused colic and diarrhea in infant.
Milk of magnesia	No	None	No effect.
Mineral oil	No	None	No effect.
Phenolphthalein	Unknown	Unknown§	Reported to cause symptoms in some.
Rhubarb	Unknown	None	None in syrup form. Fresh rhubarb may give symptoms of colic and diarrhea.
Saline cathartics	No	None	No effect.
Senna	No	None	None.
Stool softeners and bulk-forming laxatives	No	None	No effect.
Suppositories (for constipation)	No	None	Not absorbed.
Diagnostic materials and proceures			
Barium	No		Not absorbed.
Iopanoic acid (Telepaque)	Yes		Not sufficient to produce problem in infant on single dose. Does contain iodine radical.
Radioactive compounds			
Radioactive sodium	Yes	0.5% to 1.3% of dose/L‖	Diminished after 24 hr; discontinue nursing 24 hr.
[^{67}Ga] citrate	Yes		Discontinue nursing until ^{67}Ga has cleared, usually 24 hr.
^{125}I, ^{131}I	Yes	M/P = 0.13 μCi/0.002 μCi¶	^{131}I content in milk proportional to amount of milk. Most excreted in 24 hr. Discontinue nursing for 48 hr or check milk before resuming feeding if under 48 hr.
^{90}Sr	Yes	M/P = $^1/_{10}$	Less than in cow's milk. Bottle infant doubles stores in 1 mo.
^{99m}Tc	Yes		Reported to clear in 6-22 hr. Discontinue breast feeding 24 hr. ^{99m}Tc preferentially picked up by breast tissue.
Tuberculin test	No		Tuberculin-sensitive mothers can adoptively immunize their infants through breast milk, and that immunity may last several years.
X-ray films	No		No effect.
Diuretics			
Acetazolamide (Diamox)	Probable	No specific data available but probably similar to sulfonamide	Acts as enzyme inhibitor on carbonic anhydrase non-bacteriostatic sulfonamide. Observe only for dehydration and electrolyte loss by monitoring urine and turgor.

*β blocking agent.
†Total daily dose to infant via milk is 15-20 μg.
‡Adrenergic blocking agent.
§Reports differ.
‖Peak in 2 hr; detectable for 96 hr.
¶27% of dose in 48 hr.

Drug	Excreted in milk	Amount in milk after therapeutic dose	Effect on infant
Furosemide (sulfamoylanthranilic acid) (Lasix)	No		Drug is given to children under medical management.
Mercurial diuretics (Dicurin, Thiomerin)	Yes		In addition to diuretic effect, there is risk of mercury deposition. However, drug not absorbed orally.
Spironolactone (Aldactone)	Yes	Canrenone, a metabolite, appears	Acts as antagonist of aldosterone; causes sodium excretion and potassium retention. The metabolite apparently has some activity.
Thiazides (Diuril, Enduron, Esidrix, Hydrodiuril, Oretic, Thiuretic tablets)	Yes	>0.1 mg/dl*	Risk of dehydration and electrolyte imbalance, especially sodium loss, which would require monitoring. Watching weight and wet diapers and taking an occasional specific gravity reading of the urine and serum sodium would indicate status of infant. Risk, however, is extremely low. May suppress lactation due to dehydration in mother.

Environmental agents

Aldrin	Yes	Varies by location	Not a reason to wean from breast. No need to test milk unless inordinate exposure.
Benzene hexachloride (BHC)	Yes	Varies by location	Not a reason to wean from breast. No need to test milk unless inordinate exposure.
Dichlorodiphenyltrichloroethane (DDT or DDE)	Yes	Varies by location	Not a reason to wean from breast. No need to test milk unless inordinate exposure.
Dieldrin	Yes	Varies by location	Also found in permanently mothproofed garments. Avoid these. Not a reason to wean.
Hexachlorobenzene (HCB)	Yes	Varies by location	Not a reason to wean from breast. No need to test milk unless inordinate exposure.
Heptachlorepoxide	Yes	Varies by location	Not a reason to wean from breast. No need to test milk unless inordinate exposure.
Methyl mercury	Yes	500-1000 ng/ml†	Infant blood level 600 ng/ml in heavy exposure. Only in excessive exposure is testing and/or weaning necessary.
Polybrominated biphenyl (PBB)	Yes	Varies by location	If mother at high risk from the environment or the diet, milk sample should be measured. If level in milk is high, then breast feeding should be discontinued. Those at risk are (1) workers who handle PBB/PCB and (2) individuals who eat game fish from contaminated waters. Crash diets mobilize fats and should be avoided especially if PBB or PCB present.
Polychlorinated biphenyl (PCB)	Yes	Varies by location	
^{90}Sr, ^{89}Sr (strontium)	Yes	$^1/_{10}$ of that in maternal diet	Cow's milk has six times as much as human milk. Cow's milk-fed infant doubles amount in body in 1 mo.

Heavy metals

Arsenic	Yes	Can be measured for given woman	Can accumulate. Check infant's blood level if there is reason to suspect exposure.
Copper	Yes		
Fluorine	Yes		Monitor for excessive dose.
Gold thiomalate (Myocrisin)	Yes	0.022 μg/ml when mother given 50 mg/wk	No proteinuria or aminoaciduria observed.
Halothane	Yes	2 ppm	Nursing mothers who work in environment with halothane should be checked.
Iron	Yes		
Lead	Unknown		Nursing contraindicated if maternal serum 40 μg; conflicting reports, breast milk not always cause of lead poisoning in breast-fed infant.
Magnesium	Yes		Not sufficient to be toxic.
Mercury	Yes		Hazardous to infant.

*Linear relationship between plasma and milk. In 1 L of milk at 0.1 mg/dl there would be 1 mg/24 hr. Infant dose is 20 mg/kg/24 hr.
†M/P = 8.6% in heavy exposure.

Drug	Excreted in milk	Amount in milk after therapeutic dose	Effect on infant
Hormones and contraceptives			
Carbimazole (neo-mercazole)	Yes		Antithyroid effect may cause goiter.
Chlorotrianisene (Tace)	Yes		Has estrogenic effect although does not change consistency of milk. May have feminizing effect on infant.
Contraceptives (oral) Ethinyl estradiol Mestranol 19-Nortestosterone Norethindrone (Norlutin) Norethynodrel (Enovid)	Yes		May diminish milk supply. May decrease vitamins, protein, and fat in milk. One author showed no difference when mothers took norethindrone. Most significant concern is long-range impact of hormone on young infant, which is not certain. Reports of feminization of infant.
Corticotropin	Yes		Destroyed in gastrointestinal tract of infant. No effect.
Cortisone	Yes		Animal studies show 50% lower weight than controls and retarded sexual development and exophthalmos.
Dihydrotachysterol (Hytakerol)	Yes		May cause hypercalcemia; need monitoring of infant serum and urine calcium.
Epinephrine (adrenalin)	Yes		Destroyed in GI tract of infant.
Estrogen	Yes	0.17 µg/dl after 1 gm	Risks as with oral contraceptives.
Fluoxymesterone (Halotestin, Ora-Testryl, Ultandren)	Yes		Suppress lactation; masculinizing.
Insulin	Unknown		Destroyed in gastrointestinal tract.
Liothyronine (Cytomel)	No		Synthetic form of natural thyroid.
Medroxyprogesterone acetate (Provera)	No		
Phenformin HCl	Yes	Minimum	Not sufficient to cause symptoms in infant. Does not cause hypoglycemia in normal infants. No case reports available.
Prednisone	Yes	0.07-0.23% dose/L after 5 mg dose*	Minimum amount not likely to cause effect on infant in short course.
Pregnanediol	Yes		Unknown risk as with other female hormones over a long period of time.
Tolbutamide (Orinase)	Yes		Not recommended in the childbearing years.
Narcotics			
Codeine		0 to trace after 32 mg every 4 hr (6 doses)	No effect in therapeutic level and transient usage. Can accumulate. Individual variation. Watch for neonatal depression.
Heroin	Yes		13 of 22 infants had withdrawal. Historically breast feeding had been used to wean addict's infant. This is no longer recommended.
Marijuana (Cannabis)	Yes		Shown in laboratory animals to produce structural changes in nursling's brain cell; impairs DNA and RNA formation. Infant at risk of inhaling smoke during feeding or when held while smoking.
Meperidine (Demerol)	Yes	>0.1 mg/dl†	Trace amounts may accumulate if drug taken around the clock when infant is neonate. Watch for drowsiness and poor feeding.
Methadone	Yes	0.03 µg/ml or 0.023-0.028 mg/24 hr‡	When dosage not excessive, infant can be breast-fed if monitored for evidence of depression and failure to thrive.
Morphine	Yes	Trace amount	Single doses have minimum effect. Potential for accumulation. May be addicting to neonate. Breast feeding no longer considered appropriate means of weaning infant of an addict.

*0.16 µg/ml after 10 mg dose; 2.67 µg/ml after 2 hr.
†Plasma 0.07-0.1 mg/dl.
‡Mother received 50 mg/24 hr; M/P = 0.83. Peak level 4 hr after oral dose. Results obscured if addict also taking the herbal root golden seal.

Drug	Excreted in milk	Amount in milk after therapeutic dose	Effect on infant
Psychotropic and mood-changing drugs			
Alcohol	Yes	Similar to plasma level	Ordinarily no problem and can be therapeutic in moderation. Infants are more susceptible to effects. Chronic drinking reported to cause obesity in one infant. Ethanol in doses of 1-2 gm/kg to mother causes depression of milk-ejection reflex (dose dependent). No acetaldehyde found in infants.
Amphetamine	Yes		Has caused stimulation in infants with jitteriness, irritability, sleeplessness. Long-acting preparations cumulative.
Benzodiazepines*			
Chlordiazepoxide HCl (Librium)	Yes		Not sufficient to affect infant first week when glucuronyl system needed for detoxification. May accumulate. Older infant, no apparent problem.
Diazepam (Valium)	Yes	90 µg/L†	Detoxified in glucuronyl system. In first weeks of life may contribute to jaundice. Metabolite active. Effect on infant: hypoventilation, drowsiness, lethargy, and weight loss. Single doses over 10 mg contraindicated during nursing. Accumulation in infant possible.
Pineazepam	Yes	Metabolite, 5-11.2 ng/ml; pineazepam, >1.0 ng/ml‡	No data, probably similar to diazepam.
Haloperidol (Haldol)	Yes	Unknown	A butyrophenone antidepressant; animal studies in nurslings show behavior abnormalities.
Lithium carbonate (Eskalith, Lithane, Lithonate)	Yes	$^1/_3$-½ maternal plasma level§	Measurable lithium in infant's serum. Infant kidney can clear lithium; however, lithium inhibits adenosine 3':5'-cyclic monophosphate, significant for brain growth. Also affects amine metabolism. Real effects not measurable immediately. Report of cyanosis and poor muscle tone and ECG changes in nursing infant.
Monoamine oxidase (MAO) inhibitors (Eutonyl, Nardil)			Inhibits lactation.
Meprobamate (Miltown, Equanil)	Yes	2-4 times maternal plasma level	If therapy continued, infant should be followed closely.
Penfluridol‖	Yes	Unknown	Animal studies show learning abnormalities in sucklings. This is a potent long-acting oral neuroleptic drug.
Phenothiazines			
Chlorpromazine (Thorazine)	Yes	$^1/_3$ plasma level¶	Can be safely nursed; minimum in milk. Increases maternal prolactin. No symptoms in infants reported; 5 yr follow-up showed infants normal.
Mesoridazine (Serentil)	Yes	Minimum	
Piperacetazine (Quide)	Yes	Minimum	Probably no effect.
Thioridazine (Mellaril)	Yes	No information	Thioridazine is less potent in general than other phenothiazines. Probably quite safe.
Trifluoperazine (Stelazine)	Yes	Minimum	
Tricyclic antidepressants			Apparently no accumulation. No infants that have been observed showed symptoms. Watch for depression or failure to feed. Increases maternal prolactin secretion.
Amitriptyline HCl (Elavil)	Yes	Minimum amounts	
Desipramine HCl (Norpramin, Pertofrane)	Yes	Minimum amounts	
Imipramine HCl (Tofranil)	Yes	0.1 mg/dl#	

*Alcohol enhances effect of this group.
†10 mg or less yields 45 ng of diazepam/ml and 85 ng of metabolite/ml. P/M ratio is variable. Mean P/M ratio of diazepam is 6.14; of metabolite is 3.64. Effect lasts about 4 days.
‡Both drug and active metabolite appear for about 4 days after dose.
§0.030 mmol/L in infant's serum, 0.57 mmole/L in infant's urine. Milk level was half of maternal serum level in one case report.
‖Neuroleptic drug.
¶If dose <200 mg, milk contains bare trace. Dose of 1200 mg showed trace.
#Plasma level 0.2-1.3 mg/dl.

Drug	Excreted in milk	Amount in milk after therapeutic dose	Effect on infant
Stimulants			
Caffeine	Yes	1% of dose	Accumulates when intake moderate and continual. Causes jitteriness, wakefulness, and irritability. Caffeine present in many hot and cold drinks. Consider if infant very wakeful.
Theobromine	Yes	3.7-8.2 mg/L after 240 mg dose*	No adverse symptoms observed in the infants. Chocolate most common cause of exposure.
Theophylline	Yes	10% of maternal dose†	Irritability, fretfulness.
Thyroid and antithyroid medications			
Carbimazole (neo-mercazole)	Yes		May cause goiter.
Methimazole (Tapazole)	Yes	M/P > 1	Inhibits synthesis of thyroid hormone but does not inactivate existing thyroid. Can inhibit infant thyroid. ⅛ grain/day of thyroid can be given to infant simultaneously.
Potassium iodide	Yes	3 mg/dl‡	May alter thyroid function of infant; may cause goiter in infant.
Propylthiouracil	Yes	M/P > 1;4.5-6% of dose	Risk of goiter and agranulocytosis. With present microtechniques for T_3, T_4, and TSH, close monitoring of infant is possible, as with methimazole.
Radioactive iodine ^{125}I, ^{131}I (as a treatment)	Yes	M/P > 1	*Treatment* doses are excreted via the breast for 1-3 wk. Milk can be checked by Geiger counter if there is a question. Breast feeding should be discontinued until milk is clear.
Thiouracil	Yes	9-12 mg/dl§	Same as for propylthiouracil.
Thyroid and thyroxine	Yes		Does not produce adverse symptoms on long-range follow-up. Noted to improve milk supply of hypothyroid mothers. No contraindication.
Miscellaneous			
Cyclophosphamide	Yes	Present‖	Antineoplastic agent. Any amounts contraindicated.
DPT	Yes	Minimum	Does not interfere with immunization schedule.
Methotrexate	Yes	Minor route of excretion: M/P = 0.08/1.0	Antimetabolite. Infant would receive 0.26 µg/dl, which researchers consider nontoxic for infant.
Nicotine	Yes	Mean 91 ppb (20-512 ppb)¶	Decreases milk production. No apparent effect on infant —perhaps a tolerance is developed in utero. Smoking may interfere with let-down reflex if smoking started before onset of a feeding.
Poliovirus vaccine	No		Live vaccine taken orally. Not necessary to withhod nursing 30 min before and after dose. Provide booster after infant no longer nursing.
Rb antibodies	Yes		Destroyed in gastrointestinal tract; not effective orally.
Rubella virus vaccine	Yes	Minimum	Will not confer passive immunity. Mother should not be given vaccine when at risk for pregnancy.
Smallpox vaccine	No		Exposure is by direct contact. Live virus. No longer given.

*113 gm chocolate bar.
†M/P = 0.7.
‡Dose was 325-650 mg three times a day.
§Maternal plasma level was 3.4 mg/dl after a 1.0 g dose; M/P = 3.
‖Single 500 mg IV dose in milk at 1, 3, 5, and 6 hr after injection.
¶At ½-1½ packs/day. Large variation from single donor.

8-3. Human fetotoxic chemical agents

Maternal medication	Reported effect on fetus or neonate
Analgesics	
Indomethacin	Prolongs gestation (monkey)
Narcotics	70% of maternal level; death, apnea, depression, bradycardia, hypothermia
Salicylates	Death in utero; hemorrhage, methemoglobinemia, ↓ albumin-binding capacity, salicylate intoxication, difficult delivery, ? prolonged gestation
Anesthesia	
Conduction	Indirect effect of maternal hypotension; direct effect—convulsions, death, acidosis, bradycardia, myocardial depression, fetal hypotension, methemoglobinemia
General	Apnea, depression (prolonged inhalation by gravid female), ? congenital malformations, chromosome abnormality; ether has direct narcotic effect on infant
Ether	
Halothane (Fluothane)	
Trichloroethylene (Trilene)	
Hypnosis	Indirect effect of maternal hyperventilation and excessive bearing down
Local	
Paracervical	Methemoglobinemia, fetal acidosis, bradycardia, neurologic depression, myocardial depression
Anticoagulants	
Coumarins	Fetal death, hemorrhage, calcifications
Anticonvulsant agents	
Barbiturates	Irritability and tremulousness 4 to 5 months postdelivery; hemorrhage, enzyme inducer
Diphenylhydantoin and barbiturate	Congenital malformations, cleft lip and palate, congenital heart disease (CHD), CNS and skeletal anomalies, failure to thrive, enzyme inducer, hemorrhage
Paradione	CHD, microophthalmia, mental retardation, abortion
Tridione	
Antidiabetics	See hypoglycemic agents
Antimalarial	
Quinine	? Congenital anomalies of CNS and extremities, thrombocytopenia, hypoplastic optic nerve, congenital deafness
Antimicrobials	All antimicrobials cross placenta
Ampicillin	↓ Maternal urinary and plasma estriol levels
Cephaloridine	Blood levels maintained for hours after delivery; ? false positive direct Coombs' test
Chloramphenicol	Crosses placenta with no reported effect; interferes with biotransformation of tolbutamide, diphenylhydantoin, biohydroxycoumarin (i.e., hypoglycemia may occur if used in combination)
Chloroquine	Death, deafness, retinal hemorrhage
Erythromycin	Possible hepatic injury
Nitrofurantoin	Megaloblastic anemia, G6PD deficiency
Novobiocin	Hyperbilirubinemia
Quinine, quinidine	Possible ototoxicity, thrombocytopenia
Streptomycin	Therapeutic levels reached, nerve deafness
Sulfonamides	
Long and short acting	Icterus, hemolytic anemia, kernicterus, ? growth retardation, thrombocytopenia
Tetracycline	Placental transfer after 4 months' gestation; enamel hypoplasia, delay in bone growth, ? congenital cataract
Antituberculous	
Isoniazid	Toxic blood level in fetus; no reported effect; mother should be on pyridoxine supplement
Pyridoxine	See vitamins
Belladonna derivatives	
Atropine	Intrauterine tachycardia; dilated, nonreacting pupils
Scopolamine	? Delays labor, ? delays respiration, deleterious to premature infant

Maternal medication	Reported effect on fetus or neonate
Cancer chemotherapeutic agents	
Aminopterin	Abortion, congenital anomalies (first trimester); combination of drugs detrimental to fetus; skeletal and cranial malformations, hydrocephalus; questionable long-term effects = slow somatic growth; ovarian agenesis; ↓ immune mechanisms
Busulfan	
Cyclophosphamide	
6-Mercaptopurine	
Methotrexate	
Cardiovascular agents	
Digitoxin	Placental transfer, no reported effect
Propranolol	Indirect effect of delay in cervical dilatation
Cholinesterase inhibitors	Myasthenia-like symptoms for 1 week; muscle weakness in 10% to 20% of infants
Cigarette smoking	Effect equal to number of cigarettes smoked; ↑ incidence of stillbirth; low birth weight; ? effect on later somatic growth and mental development; reduction in O_2 transport to fetus
Diuretics	
Ammonium chloride	Maternal and fetal acidosis; thrombocytopenia, hemorrhage, hypoelectrolytemia, convulsions, respiratory distress, death, hemolysis
Benzothiazides	
Chlorothiazide	
Thiazide	
Diazoxide	Hypertrichosis lanuginosa, alopecia, ? hypoglycemia
Drugs of abuse (usually multiple drugs consumed)	
Alcohol	Blood level equal to mother's; convulsions, withdrawal syndrome, hyperactivity, crying, irritability, poor sucking reflex, low birth weight; cleft palate, ophthalmic malformation, malformation of extremities and heart; poor mental performance; microencephaly, small-for-dates, growth deficiency
Barbiturates	Withdrawal symptoms, convulsions, onset immediately after birth or at 2 weeks of age
Glutethimide	Small-for-dates, irritability
LSD (lysergic acid)	Chromosome breakage, limb and skeletal anomalies
Narcotics	Small-for-dates, 4% to 10% mortality, habituation, withdrawal symptoms, convulsions, sudden death, indirect effect on maternal complications (i.e., infection, hepatitis, venereal disease), ? permanent effect on somatic growth
Heroin	
Methadone	
Fluorine	Placental transfer—utilized for growth and development of bones and teeth of fetus
Hormones	
Androgens	Labioscrotal fusion prior to twelfth week, after 12 weeks' phallic enlargement; ? anomalies; ? ↑ bilirubin, vaginal cancer; cleft lip and palate, CHD, TE fistula, anal atresia, cancer of prostate, testes, and bladder
Estrogens	
Progestins	
Corticosteroids	Adrenal insufficiency, cleft palate, small-for-dates infant
Ovulatory agents	? Anencephaly, ? chromosome abnormalities in abortus, multiple pregnancy
Hypoglycemic agents	
Chlorpropamide	Higher fetal mortality, prolonged hypoglycemia, competes for albumin-binding sites
Insulin	Insulin coma, ? increased fetal damage
Tolbutamide	? Potentiates hypoglycemia in newborn, thrombocytopenia
Hypotensive agents	
Hexamethonium	Paralytic ileus, perforation, death
Reserpine	1% to 15% of infants have symptoms; nasal stuffiness, bradycardia, respiratory distress, hypothermia, abnormal muscle tone (in mice, hyperactivity and increased emotionalism)
Insecticide and pesticides	
Organochlorine	Present in fetus, ? enzyme induction, ? premature labor
Intravenous alcohol	Hypoglycemia; abnormal bone marrow morphology in premature infant
Intravenous fluids	Excessive fluids—hyponatremia, seizures
Muscle relaxants	
Curare	Paralysis in utero (prolonged use), position deformities

Maternal medication	Reported effect on fetus or neonate
Narcotic antagonist	
Nalorphine (Nalline)	Not effective unless large doses of narcotics administered to mother; act as respiratory depressant if cause of depression is other than narcotic
Levallorphan (Lorfan)	
Oxytocin	Thrombocytopenia, fetal bradycardia, water intoxication, ? ↑ bilirubin level; abortions (ergot)
Psychotropic drugs	
Antidepressants	
Aventyl	Withdrawal, coliclike syndrome, cyanosis, irritability, weight loss, hyperhydrosis, respiratory distress, craniofacial anomalies, CNS and skeletal anomalies; urinary retention
Chloropyramine	
Imipramine	
Nortriptyline	
Diazepam (Valium)	High fetal levels; hypotonia, poor sucking reflex, hypothermia; ↑ low Apgar score infants; ↑ resuscitation, ↑ assisted deliveries; dose related
Lithium	Neonatal serum levels reach adult toxic range; lethargy, cyanosis for 10 days; teratogenic—dose related
Phenothiazine	? Effect on eyes; withdrawal; extrapyramidal dysfunction; delay in onset of respiration; maternal hypotension, ? prolongs labor, effective uterine contraction; ? chromosomal breakage; hypotonia, hyperactivity
Radiation	Microencephaly, mental retardation, many unknown effects; nondisjunction of chromosomes
Radiopaque media	Elevated PHI, depressed ^{131}I uptake
Sedatives	
Barbiturate	Apnea, depression, depressed EEG, poor sucking reflex, slow weight gain; concentration of drug in brain; enzyme inducer = lower bilirubin level
Bromides	Growth failure, lethargy, dilated pupils, dermatitis, hypotonia, ? effect on mental development
Magnesium sulfate	Neonatal blood level does not correlate with clinical condition; respiratory depression, hypotonia, convulsions, death; exchange transfusion may be required
Paraldehyde	Apnea, depression
Thalidomide	Administered between thirty-fourth and fiftieth day of gestation causes phocomelia, malformation of cord, angiomas of face, CHD, intestinal stenosis, eye defects, absence of appendix
Thyroid medications	
Iodine	Normal or goitrous infants; euthyroid, hyperthyroid or hypothyroid; respiratory distress due to tracheal compression; thrombocytopenia
Thioureas	
^{131}I	Uptake by fetal thyroid after 12 weeks' gestation; exophthalmus, arrest of brain development
Toxins	
Carbon monoxide	Stillbirth, brain damage equal to anoxia
Heavy metals	
Arsenic	Concentrated in brain
Lead	Abortions, growth retardation, congenital anomalies, sterility
Mercury	Cerebral palsy, mental retardation, convulsions, involuntary movements, defective vision; mother asymptomatic
Naphthalene	Hemolysis
Vitamins	
A and D	Congenital anomalies
K (water-soluble analogues)	Icterus, anemia, kernicterus
Pyridoxine	Withdrawal seizures

8-4. Pregnancy table for expected date of delivery

Find the date of the last menstrual period in the top line (light-face type) of the pair of lines. The dark number (bold-face type) in the line below will be the expected day of delivery.

Month	1	2	3	4	5	6	7	8	9	10	11	12	13	14	15	16	17	18	19	20	21	22	23	24	25	26	27	28	29	30	31	
Jan.	1	2	3	4	5	6	7	8	9	10	11	12	13	14	15	16	17	18	19	20	21	22	23	24	25	26	27	28	29	30	31	
Oct.	**8**	**9**	**10**	**11**	**12**	**13**	**14**	**15**	**16**	**17**	**18**	**19**	**20**	**21**	**22**	**23**	**24**	**25**	**26**	**27**	**28**	**29**	**30**	**31**	**(1**	**2**	**3**	**4**	**5**	**6**	**7**	**Nov.**
Feb.	1	2	3	4	5	6	7	8	9	10	11	12	13	14	15	16	17	18	19	20	21	22	23	24	25	26	27	28				
Nov.	**8**	**9**	**10**	**11**	**12**	**13**	**14**	**15**	**16**	**17**	**18**	**19**	**20**	**21**	**22**	**23**	**24**	**25**	**26**	**27**	**28**	**29**	**30**	**(1**	**2**	**3**	**4**	**5**				**Dec.**
Mar.	1	2	3	4	5	6	7	8	9	10	11	12	13	14	15	16	17	18	19	20	21	22	23	24	25	26	27	28	29	30	31	
Dec.	**6**	**7**	**8**	**9**	**10**	**11**	**12**	**13**	**14**	**15**	**16**	**17**	**18**	**19**	**20**	**21**	**22**	**23**	**24**	**25**	**26**	**27**	**28**	**29**	**30**	**31**	**(1**	**2**	**3**	**4**	**5**	**Jan.**
April	1	2	3	4	5	6	7	8	9	10	11	12	13	14	15	16	17	18	19	20	21	22	23	24	25	26	27	28	29	30		
Jan.	**6**	**7**	**8**	**9**	**10**	**11**	**12**	**13**	**14**	**15**	**16**	**17**	**18**	**19**	**20**	**21**	**22**	**23**	**24**	**25**	**26**	**27**	**28**	**29**	**30**	**31**	**(1**	**2**	**3**	**4**		**Feb.**
May	1	2	3	4	5	6	7	8	9	10	11	12	13	14	15	16	17	18	19	20	21	22	23	24	25	26	27	28	29	30	31	
Feb.	**5**	**6**	**7**	**8**	**9**	**10**	**11**	**12**	**13**	**14**	**15**	**16**	**17**	**18**	**19**	**20**	**21**	**22**	**23**	**24**	**25**	**26**	**27**	**28**	**(1**	**2**	**3**	**4**	**5**	**6**	**7**	**Mar.**
June	1	2	3	4	5	6	7	8	9	10	11	12	13	14	15	16	17	18	19	20	21	22	23	24	25	26	27	28	29	30		
Mar.	**8**	**9**	**10**	**11**	**12**	**13**	**14**	**15**	**16**	**17**	**18**	**19**	**20**	**21**	**22**	**23**	**24**	**25**	**26**	**27**	**28**	**29**	**30**	**31**	**(1**	**2**	**3**	**4**	**5**	**6**		**April**
July	1	2	3	4	5	6	7	8	9	10	11	12	13	14	15	16	17	18	19	20	21	22	23	24	25	26	27	28	29	30	31	
April	**7**	**8**	**9**	**10**	**11**	**12**	**13**	**14**	**15**	**16**	**17**	**18**	**19**	**20**	**21**	**22**	**23**	**24**	**25**	**26**	**27**	**28**	**29**	**30**	**(1**	**2**	**3**	**4**	**5**	**6**	**7**	**May**
Aug.	1	2	3	4	5	6	7	8	9	10	11	12	13	14	15	16	17	18	19	20	21	22	23	24	25	26	27	28	29	30	31	
May	**8**	**9**	**10**	**11**	**12**	**13**	**14**	**15**	**16**	**17**	**18**	**19**	**20**	**21**	**22**	**23**	**24**	**25**	**26**	**27**	**28**	**29**	**30**	**31**	**(1**	**2**	**3**	**4**	**5**	**6**	**7**	**June**
Sept.	1	2	3	4	5	6	7	8	9	10	11	12	13	14	15	16	17	18	19	20	21	22	23	24	25	26	27	28	29	30		
June	**8**	**9**	**10**	**11**	**12**	**13**	**14**	**15**	**16**	**17**	**18**	**19**	**20**	**21**	**22**	**23**	**24**	**25**	**26**	**27**	**28**	**29**	**30**	**(1**	**2**	**3**	**4**	**5**	**6**	**7**		**July**
Oct.	1	2	3	4	5	6	7	8	9	10	11	12	13	14	15	16	17	18	19	20	21	22	23	24	25	26	27	28	29	30	31	
July	**8**	**9**	**10**	**11**	**12**	**13**	**14**	**15**	**16**	**17**	**18**	**19**	**20**	**21**	**22**	**23**	**24**	**25**	**26**	**27**	**28**	**29**	**30**	**31**	**(1**	**2**	**3**	**4**	**5**	**6**	**7**	**Aug.**
Nov.	1	2	3	4	5	6	7	8	9	10	11	12	13	14	15	16	17	18	19	20	21	22	23	24	25	26	27	28	29	30		
Aug.	**8**	**9**	**10**	**11**	**12**	**13**	**14**	**15**	**16**	**17**	**18**	**19**	**20**	**21**	**22**	**23**	**24**	**25**	**26**	**27**	**28**	**29**	**30**	**31**	**(1**	**2**	**3**	**4**	**5**	**6**		**Sept.**
Dec.	1	2	3	4	5	6	7	8	9	10	11	12	13	14	15	16	17	18	19	20	21	22	23	24	25	26	27	28	29	30	31	
Sept.	**7**	**8**	**9**	**10**	**11**	**12**	**13**	**14**	**15**	**16**	**17**	**18**	**19**	**20**	**21**	**22**	**23**	**24**	**25**	**26**	**27**	**28**	**29**	**30**	**(1**	**2**	**3**	**4**	**5**	**6**	**7**	**Oct.**

APPENDIX 9 · Pediatrics

9-1. The Washington guide to promoting development in the young child

Motor skills

Expected tasks	Suggested activities
1 to 3 months	
1. Holds head up briefly when prone	1. Place infant in prone position
2. Head erect and bobbing when supported in sitting position	2. Support in sitting position with his head erect
3. Head erect and steady in sitting position	3. Pull infant to sitting position
4. Follows object through all planes	4. Provide with opportunity to observe people or activity
5. Palmar grasp	5. Hang bright-colored objects and mobiles within reach across crib
6. Moro reflex	6. Provide with opportunity to observe objects or people while in sitting position
	7. Use infant seat
	8. Alternate bright shiny objects with dark and light visual patterns
4 to 8 months	
1. Sits with minimal support, with stable head and back	1. Pull up to sitting position
2. Sits alone steadily	2. Provide opportunity to sit supported or alone when head and trunk control are stabilized
3. Plays with hands, which are open most of time	3. Put bright-colored objects within reach
4. Grasps rattle or bottle with both hands	4. Give toys or household objects: rattles, teething ring, cloth animals or dolls, 1-inch cubes, plastic objects such as cups, rings, and balls
5. Picks up small objects, for example, cube	5. Offer small objects such as cereal to improve grasp
6. Transfers toys from one hand to other	6. Offer a variety of patterns or textures to play with
7. Neck-righting reflex	7. Use squeak toys
9 to 12 months	
1. Rises to sitting position	1. Provide playpen, allow child to pull himself to standing
2. Creeps or crawls, maybe backward at first	2. Give opportunity and space to practice creeping and crawling
3. Pulls to standing position	3. Have child practice moving on knees to improve balance prior to walking
4. Stands alone	4. Have child use walker or straddle toys
5. Cruises	5. Play airplane with child; have child practice catching himself while rolling on large ball
6. Uses index finger to poke	6. Provide with objects such as spoons, plastic bottles, cups, ball, cubes, finger foods, saucepans, and lids
7. Finger-thumb grasp	
8. Parachute reflex	
9. Landau reflex	
13 to 18 months	
1. Walks a few steps without support	1. Provide opportunity to practice walking, climbing stairs with help
2. Balanced when walking	2. Give toys that can be pushed around
3. Walks upstairs with help, creeps downstairs	3. Supervise activity with paper and large crayons
4. Turns pages of book	4. Provide toys such as cubes, cups, saucepans, lids, rag dolls, and other soft, cuddly toys
	5. Begin introducing child to swing
19 to 30 months	
1. Runs	1. Provide opportunity to practice and develop activities
2. Walks up and down stairs, one at a time (not alternating feet)	2. Provide pattern for child while he watches and then encourage him to try
3. Imitates vertical strokes	3. Provide tricycle or similar pedal toys; secure foot on pedal if necessary
4. Imitates building tower of four or more blocks	
5. Throws ball overhand	
6. Jumps in place	
7. Rides tricycle	

Motor skills—cont'd

Expected tasks	Suggested activities
31 to 48 months	
1. Walks downstairs (alternating feet)	1. Continue with blocks, combining materials, toy cars, and trains
2. Hops on one foot	2. Provide clay and other manipulating materials
3. Swings and climbs	3. Give opportunities to swing and climb
4. Balances on one foot for 10 seconds	4. Provide with activities such as finger painting, chalk, and blackboard
5. Copies circle	
6. Copies cross	
7. Draws person with three parts	
49 to 52 months	
1. Balances well	1. Provide with music and games to synchronize hand and foot, tapping with music, skipping, hopping, and dancing rhythmically to improve coordination
2. Skips and jumps	
3. Can heel-toe walk	
4. Copies square	
5. Catches bounced ball	

Feeding skills

Expected tasks	Suggested activities
1 to 3 months	
1. Sucking reflex present	1. Consider a change in nipple or posturing if there is difficulty in swallowing
2. Rooting reflex present	2. Introduce solids, one kind at a time (use small spoon, place food well back on infant's tongue)
3. Ability to swallow pureed foods	3. Hold in comfortable relaxed position while feeding
4. Coordinates sucking, swallowing, and breathing	4. Pace feeding tempo to infant's needs
4 to 8 months	
1. Tongue used in moving food in mouth	1. Give finger foods to develop chewing, stimulate gums, and encourage hand-to-mouth motion (cubes of cheese, bananas, dry toast, bread crust, cookies)
2. Hand-to-mouth motions	2. Encourage upright supported position for feeding
3. Recognizes bottle on sight	3. Promote bottle holding
4. Gums or mouths solid foods	4. Introduce junior foods
5. Feeds self cracker	
9 to 12 months	
1. Holds own bottle	1. Bring child in highchair to table and include in part of or entire meal with family
2. Drinks from cup or glass with assistance	2. Have child in dry comfortable position with trunk and feet supported
3. Finger feeds	3. Encourage self-help in feeding; use of table foods
4. Beginning to hold spoon	4. Offer spoon when interest is indicated
	5. Introduce cup or glass with small amount of fluid
13 to 18 months	
1. Holds cup and handle with digital grasp	1. Continue offering finger foods (wieners, sandwiches)
2. Lifts cup and drinks well	2. Use nontip dishes and cups; dishes should have sides to make filling of spoon easy
3. Beginning to use spoon, may turn bowl down before reaching mouth	3. Give opportunity for self-feeding
4. Difficulty in inserting spoon into mouth	4. Provide fluids between meals rather than having child fill up on fluids at mealtime
5. May refuse food	

Feeding skills—cont'd

Expected tasks	Suggested activities
19 to 30 months 1. Drinks without spilling 2. Holds small glass in one hand 3. Inserts spoon in mouth correctly 4. Distinguishes between food and inedible material 5. Plays with food	1. Encourage self-feeding with spoon 2. Do not rush child 3. Serve foods plainly but in attractive servings 4. Small servings of food will encourage eating more than large servings
31 to 48 months 1. Pours well from pitcher 2. Serves self at table with little spilling 3. Rarely needs assistance 4. Interest in setting table	1. Encourage self-help 2. Give opportunity for pouring (give rice and pitcher to promote pouring skills) 3. Encourage child to help set table 4. Have well-defined rules about table manners
49 to 52 months 1. Feeds self well 2. Social and talkative during meal	1. Socialize with child at mealtime 2. Have child help with preparation, table setting, and serving 3. Include child in conversations at mealtimes by planning special times for him to tell about events, situations, or what he did during the day

Sleep

Expected tasks	Suggested activities
1 to 3 months 1. Night: 4- to 10-hour intervals 2. Naps: frequent 3. Longer periods of wakefulness without crying	1. Provide separate sleeping arrangements away from parents' room 2. Reduce noise and light stimulation when placing in bed 3. Have room at comfortable temperature with no drafts or extremes in heat 4. Reverse position of crib occasionally 5. Place child in different positions from time to time for sleep 6. Alternate from back to side to stomach 7. Keep crib sides up
4 to 8 months 1. Night: 10 to 12 hours 2. Naps: 2 to 3 (1 to 4 hours in duration) 3. Night awakenings	1. Keep crib sides up 2. Refrain from taking child into parents' room if he awakens 3. Check to determine if there is cause for awakenings: hunger, teething, pain, cold, wet, noise, or illness 4. If a baby-sitter is used, attempt to find some person with whom infant is familiar. Explain bedtime and naptime arrangements
9 to 12 months 1. Night: 12 to 14 hours 2. Naps: one to two (1 to 4 hours in duration) 3. May begin refusing morning nap	1. Short crying periods may be source of tension release for child 2. Observe for signs of fatigue, irritability, or restlessness if naps are shorter 3. Provide familiar person to baby-sit who knows sleep routines
13 to 18 months 1. Night: 10 to 12 hours 2. Naps: one in afternoon (1 to 3 hours in duration) 3. May awaken during night crying (associated with wetting bed) 4. As he becomes more able to move about, he may uncover himself, become cold, and awaken	1. Night terrors may be terminated by awakening infant and offering reassurance 2. Check to see that child is covered 3. Avoid hazardous devices to keep child covered, including blanket clips, pins, and garments that enclose child to neck

Sleep—cont'd

Expected tasks	Suggested activities
19 to 30 months 1. Night: 10 to 12 hours 2. Naps: one (1 to 3 hours in duration) 3. Doesn't go to sleep at once—keeps demanding things 4. May awaken crying if wet or soiled 5. May awaken because of environmental change of temperature, change of bed, change of sleeping room, addition of sibling to room, absence of parent from home, hospitalization, trip with family, or relatives visiting	1. Quiet period of socialization prior to bedtime—reading child book or telling story 2. Holding child—talking quietly with him 3. Ritualistic behavior may be present; allow child to carry out routine; helps him overcome fear of unexpected or fear of dark; for example, child may wish to arrange toys in certain way 4. Explain bedtime ritual to baby-sitter 5. Give more reassurance, spend more time before bedtime preparation 6. Provide familiar bedtime toys or items 7. Allow crying-out period if he is safe, comfortable, and tucked in 8. Place in bed before he reaches excessive state of fatigue, excitement, or tiredness 9. Eliminate sources of stimulation or fear 10. Maintain consistent hour of bedtime
31 to 48 months 1. Daily range: 10 to 15 hours 2. Naps: beginning to disappear 3. Prolongs process of going to bed 4. Less dependent on taking toys to bed 5. May awaken crying from dreams 6. May awaken if wet	1. Television programs may affect ability to go to sleep; avoid violent television programs 2. Anxiety about going to bed and desire to stay up with parents—requires limits 3. Regularity and consistency important to promote good sleeping habits 4. Reassurance—night light or leaving door ajar 5. Do not use bedtime or naptime as punishment 6. Encourage naps if signs of fatigue or irritability are evidenced
49 to 52 months 1. Daily range: 9 to 13 hours 2. Naps: rare 3. Quieter during sleep	1. Encourage napping if excessive or strenuous activity occurs and child is overly tired 2. Explain to child if baby-sitter will be there after child is asleep

Play

Expected tasks	Suggested activities
1 to 3 months 1. Quieted when picked up 2. Regards face of others	1. Encourage holding and touching of child by mother 2. Provide with cradle gyms and mobiles, brightly colored, visually interesting objects within arm's distance
4 to 8 months 1. Plays with own body 2. Differentiates strangers from family 3. Seeks out objects 4. Grasps, holds, and manipulates objects 5. Repeats activities he enjoys 6. Bangs toys or objects together	1. Begin patty-cake and peekaboo 2. Provide for periods of solitary play (playpen) 3. Encourage holding and touching of child by mother 4. Provide variety of multicolored and multitextured objects that child can hold 5. Encourage exploration of body parts 6. Provide floating toys for bath
9 to 12 months 1. Puts objects in and out of containers 2. Examines objects held in hand 3. Plays interactive games (peekaboo) 4. Extends toy to other person without releasing 5. Works to get toy out of reach	1. Continue mother-infant games 2. Give opportunity to place objects in containers and pour out 3. Provide large and small objects with which to play 4. Encourage interactive play

Play—cont'd

Expected tasks	Suggested activities
13 to 18 months	
1. Plays by himself—may play near others	1. Introduce to other children even though child may not play with them
2. Has preferred toys	2. Provide music, books, and magazines
3. Enjoys walking activities, pulling toys	3. Encourage imitative activities—helping with dusting, sweeping, stirring
4. Throws and picks up objects, throws again	
5. Imitates, for example, reading newspaper, sweeping	
19 to 30 months	
1. Parallel play—not interactive but plays alongside another child	1. Provide with new materials for manipulating and feeling—finger paints, clay, sand, stones, water, and soap
2. Uses both large and small toys	Wooden toys—cars and animals
3. Rough-and-tumble play	Building blocks of various sizes, crayons, and paper
4. Play periods longer than before—interested in manipulative and constructive toys	Rhythmical tunes and equipment—swing, rocking chair, rocking horse
5. Enjoys rhymes and singing (television programs)	Children's books—short, simple stories with repetition and familiar objects; enjoys simple pictures, brightly colored
	2. Guide child's hand to actively participate with specific activities, for example, using crayons, hammering
31 to 48 months	
1. In playing with others, beginning to interact, sharing toys, taking turns	1. Encourage play with small groups of children
2. Dramatizes, expresses imagination in play	2. Encourage imaginative and dramatic play activities
3. Combining playthings; more use of constructive materials	3. Music: singing and experimenting with musical instruments
4. Prefers two or three children to play with; may have special friend	4. Group participation in rhymes, dancing by hopping or jumping
	5. Drawing and painting (seldom recognizable)
49 to 52 months	
1. Dramatic play and interest in going on excursions	1. Painting and drawing (objects will be out of proportion; details that are most important to child are drawn largest)
2. Fond of cutting and pasting, creative materials	2. Encourage printing of numbers and letters
3. Completes most activities	3. Clay: making recognizable objects
	4. Cutting and pasting
	5. Provide with materials, for example, boxes, chairs, barrels, for building sturdy structures

Language

Expected tasks	Suggested activities
1 to 3 months	
Receptive abilities	
1. Movement of eyes, respiration rate, or body activity changes when bell is rung close to child's head	1. Observe facial expressions, gestures, bodily postures, and movements when vocalizations are being produced
2. Smiles when socially stimulated	2. Smile and talk softly in pleasant tone while holding, touching, and handling infant
3. Has facial, vocal, and generalized bodily responses to faces	3. Hold, touch, and interact frequently with infant for pleasure
4. Reacts differently to adult voices	4. Refrain from letting infant engage in prolonged and incessant crying
Expressive abilities	
1. Makes prelanguage vocalizations that consist of cooing, throaty sounds, for example, gu	
2. Makes "pleasure" sounds that consist of soft vowels	
3. Makes "sucking" sounds	
4. Crying can be differentiated for discomfort, pain, and hunger as reported by mother	
5. An "A" sound as in cat is commonly heard in distress crying	

Language—cont'd

Expected tasks	Suggested activities
4 to 8 months	
Receptive abilities	
1. Eyes locate source of sound	1. Engage in smiling eye-to-eye contact while talking to infant
2. Responds to "hi, there" by looking up at face that is across and in front of him	2. Vocalize in response to inflectional patterns and when infant is producing babbling sounds; echo the sounds he makes
3. Head turns to sound of cellophane held and crunched 2 feet away and at a 135-degree angle on either side of head	3. Observe for subtle communication clues such as eye aversion, struggling to move away, flushing of skin, tension of body, or movement of arms
4. Will turn head to locate sound of "look here" when spoken at a 90-degree angle from head 2 feet away*	4. Vocalize with infant during handling, while feeding, bathing, dressing, diapering, bedtime preparation, and holding
5. Turns head to sound of rattle	5. Stimulate laughing by light tickling
6. Responds differently to vacuum cleaner, phone, doorbell, or sound of dog barking: may cry, whimper, look toward sound, or mother may report change in body tension	6. Observe child's reactions to bells, whistles, horns, phones, laughing, singing, talking, music box, noisemaking toys, and common household noises
7. Responds by raising arms when mother reaches toward child and says "come up"	7. While talking to infant, hold in position so that he can see your face
	8. Have infant placed at position of eye level while talking to him throughout the day
Expressive abilities	9. If crying or laughing sounds are not discerned at this stage, report to family physician, pediatrician, public health nurse, or well-child clinic
1. Uses different inflectional patterns: ah ah uh	
2. Laughs aloud when stimulated	
3. Has differential patterns of crying when hungry, in pain, or angry	
4. Produces vowel sounds and chained syllables (baba, gugu, didi)	
5. Makes "talking sounds" in response to others talking to him	
6. Babbles to produce consonant sounds: ba, da, m-m	
7. Vocalizes to toys	
8. Says "da-da" or "ma-ma" but not specific to presence of parents	
9 to 12 months	
Receptive abilities	
1. Ceases activity when name is pronounced or "no-no" is said	1. Gain child's attention when giving simple commands
2. Gives toys on request when accompanied by facial and bodily gestures	2. Accompany oral directions with gestures
3. Attends to simple commands	3. Vocalize with child during feeding, bathing, and playtimes
	4. Provide sounds that child can reproduce such as lip smacking and tongue clicking
Expressive abilities	5. Repeat direction frequently and have child participate in action: open and close the drawer; move arms and legs up and down
1. Imitates definite speech sounds such as tongue clicking, lip smacking, or coughing	6. Have child respond to verbal directions: stand up, sit down, close door, open door, turn around, come here
2. Should have two words that are *specific* for parents: "mama," "dada," or equivalents	
13 to 18 months	
Receptive abilities	
1. Attends to person speaking to child	1. Incorporate repetition into daily routine of home
2. Finds "the baby" in picture when requested, for example, on baby food jar, in magazine, or in storybooks	a. Feeding: name baby's food and eating utensils; ask if he is enjoying his dessert; concentrate on reviewing a day's events in simple manner
3. Indicates wants by gestures	b. Household duties: mother names each item as she dusts; pronounces word while cooking and preparing foods
4. Looks toward family members or pets when named	c. Playing: identify toys when using them; explain their function
Expressive abilities	2. Let child see mouthing of words
1. Uses three words other than mama and dada to denote *specific* objects, persons, or actions	3. Encourage verbalization and expression of wants
2. Indicates wants by naming object such as cookie	

*Do not test for localization of sound by producing sound directly behind infant's head.

Language—cont'd

Expected tasks	Suggested activities

19 to 30 months

Receptive abilities

1. Points to one named body part
2. Follows two or three verbal directions that are not accompanied by facial or body gestures, for example, put ball on table, give it to mommy, or put toy in box

Expressive abilities

1. Combines two different words, for example, "play ball," "want cookie"
2. Names object in picture, for example, cat, bird, dog, horse, man
3. Refers to self by pronoun rather than by name

Suggested activities

1. Continue to present concrete objects with words; talk about activities child is involved with
2. Include child in conversations during mealtimes
3. Encourage speech by having child express wants
4. Incorporate games into bathing routine by having child name and point to body parts
5. As child gains confidence in remembering and using words appropriately, encourage less use of gestures
6. Count and name articles of clothing as they are placed on child
7. Count and name silverware as it is placed on table
8. Sort, match, and name glassware, laundry, cans, vegetables, and fruit with child
9. Have child keep scrapbook and add new picture every day to increase recognition of vocabulary words
10. Spend 15 to 20 minutes per day going through booklets and naming pictures; have child point to pictures as objects are named
11. Help child develop functional core vocabulary to express safety needs and information about neighborhood
12. Whenever possible, use word (for example, paper), show object, have child handle and use it, encourage him to watch your face while you say the words, and suggest that he repeat it; refrain from undue pressure

31 to 36 months

Receptive abilities

1. Takes turns when asked while playing, eating
2. Attends longer to stories and television programs
3. Demonstrates understanding of two prepositions by carrying out two commands one at a time, for example, "put the block under the chair"
4. Can follow commands asking for two objects or two actions
5. Demonstrates understanding of concepts of big and little, for example, selects larger of two balls when asked for big one
6. Points to additional body parts

Expressive abilities

1. Uses regular plurals, for example, adds "s" to apple, box, orange (does not use irregular plurals, for example, mouse to mice)
2. Gives first and last name
3. Names what he has drawn after scribbling
4. On request, tells you his sex, for example, are you a little boy or a little girl?
5. Can repeat a few rhymes or songs
6. On request, tells what action is going on in picture, for example, the kitten is eating

Suggested activities

1. Read stories with familiar content but with more detail; nonsense rhymes, humorous stories
2. Expect child to follow simple commands
3. Give child opportunity to hear and repeat his full name
4. Listen to child's explanation about pictures he draws
5. Encourage child to repeat nursery rhymes by himself and with others
6. Address child by his first name

37 to 48 months

1. Expresses appropriate responses when asked what child does when tired, cold, or hungry
2. Tells stories
3. Common expression: I don't know
4. Repeats sentence composed of twelve to thirteen syllables, for example, "I am going when daddy and I are finished playing"
5. Has mastered phonetic sounds of p, k, g, v, tf, d, z, lr, hw, j, kw, l, e, w, qe, and o

Suggested activities

1. Provide visual stimuli while reading stories
2. Have child repeat story
3. Arrange trips to zoo, farms, seashore, stores, and movies and discuss with child
4. Give simple explanations in answering questions

Language—cont'd

Expected tasks	Suggested activities
49 to 52 months *Receptive abilities* 1. Points to penny, nickel, or dime on request 2. Carries out in order command containing three parts, for example, "pick up the block, put it on the table, and bring the book to me" *Expressive abilities* 1. Names penny, nickel, or dime on request 2. Replies appropriately to questions such as, "What do you do when you are asleep?" 3. Counts three objects, pointing to each in turn 4. Defines simple words, for example, hat, ball 5. Asks questions 6. Can identify or name four colors	1. Play games in which child names colors 2. Encourage use of please and thank you 3. Encourage social-verbal interactions with other children 4. Encourage correct usage of words 5. Provide puppets or toys with movable parts that child can converse about 6. Provide group activity for child; children may stimulate each other by taking turns naming pictures 7. Allow child to make choices about games, stories, and activities 8. Have child dramatize simple stories 9. Provide child with piggy bank and encourage naming coins as they are handled or dropped into bank

Discipline

Expected tasks	Suggested activities

1 to 3 months
1. Draws attention by crying
 	
2. Infant desires whatever is pleasant and wishes to avoid unpleasant situations
3. Beginning to "wiggle" around
	1. a. Needs should be identified and met as promptly as possible
	   b. Every bit of fussing should not be interpreted as emergency requiring immediate attention
	   c. Infant should not be ignored and permitted to cry for exhaustive periods
	2. Begin to present limit of having to wait so that infant can learn that tension and discomfort are bearable for short periods
	3. Place infant on surfaces that have sides to protect him from falling off

4 to 8 months
1. Begins to respond to "no-no"
 	
2. Infant who is left alone for long periods of time may become bored or fretful; learns that crying and whining result in attention
3. Beginning to show signs of timidity and fretfulness and may whimper and cry when mother separates from him or when strangers pick him up
 	
4. Beginning to grasp objects and bring to mouth, but unable to differentiate safe from hazardous items
	1. a. Reserve "no-no" for times when it is really needed
	   b. Be consistent with word "no-no" for same activity and event that requires it; be friendly and firm with verbal control of limit setting
	2. Make special efforts to attend to infant when he is quiet and amusing himself
	3. a. Gradually introduce strangers into infant's environment
	   b. Refrain from promoting frightening situations with strangers during this stage
	   c. Play hiding games like peekaboo in which mother disappears and reappears
	   d. Allow infant to cling to mother and get used to persons a little at a time
	   e. If baby-sitter is used, find person familiar to infant or introduce for brief periods before mother leaves infant in her care
	   f. Encourage gentle handling by mother, father, and siblings. Discourage rough handling, particularly by strangers
	4. a. Provide toys that do not have small detachable parts
	   b. Check frequently for small objects in his line of reach
	5. When traveling in car, place in crib or seat with safety belts securely fastened

Discipline—cont'd

Expected tasks	Suggested activities
9 to 12 months	
1. Beginning to respond to simple commands, for example, "pick up the ball, put the toy in the box"	1. a. Avoid setting unreasonable number of limits b. Give simple commands one at a time c. Once limit is set, adhere to it firmly each time and connect it immediately with misbehavior d. Respond with consistency in enforcing rule e. Allow time to conform to request f. Gain child's attention
2. Ready to go places on his own and is trying out newly developing motor capacities (not to be confused with naughtiness, "spoiled," or stubbornness)	2. a. Begin setting and enforcing limits on where child is allowed to travel and explore b. Remove tempting objects c. Remove sources of danger such as light sockets, protruding pot handles, hanging table covers, sharp objects, and hanging cords d. Keep child away from fans, heaters, and certain drawers and do not place vaporizer close to infant's crib e. Keep high chair at least 2 feet away from working and cooking surfaces in kitchen f. Use gate to keep child out of kitchen when it is being used g. Be certain that pans, basins, and tubs of hot water are never left unattended h. Remove all possible poisons or substances that are not food that can be eaten or drunk off floor, low-level cabinets, and under sink i. Keep child from objects or surfaces that he may chew, for example, porch rails, windowsills, *repainted* toys or cribs that may contain lead j. Instruct baby-sitter on all safety items
3. Has emerging desires to look at, handle, and touch objects	3. a. Experiment with diversionary measures b. Provide child with own play objects
4. Explores objects by sucking, chewing, and biting	4. a. Remove household poisons, cosmetics, pins, and buttons that he could put in his mouth b. Be certain that objects that go into mouth are hygienic c. Check toys for detachable small parts
5. Beginning to test reactions to certain parental responses during feeding and may become choosy about food	5. a. Once problem behaviors are defined, plan to work on changing only one behavior at a time until child behaves or conforms to expectations b. Be certain that child understands old rules before adding new ones c. Respond with consistency in enforcing old rules: enforce each time, do not ignore next time d. Provide regular pattern of mealtimes e. Refrain from feeding throughout day f. Allow child to decide what he will eat and how much g. Introduce new foods gradually over period of time h. Continue to offer foods that may have been rejected first time i. Do not force food j. Refrain from physically punishing child for changes in eating habits
6. Beginning to test reactions to parental responses at bedtime preparation	6. a. Provide regular time for naps and bedtime b. Avoid excessive stimulation at bedtime or naptime c. Ignore fussing and crying once safety and physical needs are satisfied and usual ritual is carried out d. Keep child in own room e. Refrain from picking up and rocking and holding if needs seem satisfied

Discipline—cont'd

Expected tasks	Suggested activities

13 to 18 months

1. Understands simple commands and requests

  1. a. Begin with one rule; add new ones as appropriate
    b. In selecting new rules, choose on the basis of being able to clearly define it to self and child, having it reasonable and enforceable at all times; demand no more than fulfillment of defined expectations
    c. Plan decisive limits and plan to give consistent attention to them

2. In learning mastery over impulses and self-control, child begins testing out limit setting

  2. a. Immediately correct errors in behavior as they occur
    b. Use consistent enforcement of short-term rules (which are given as verbal commands) and long-term rules (which pertain to chores and family routines)
    c. Ignore temper tantrums
    d. Show child when you approve of his behavior and praise for obedience throughout day

3. With increasing fine motor control, child can manipulate objects that may be hazardous

  3. a. Set limits regarding play with doorknobs and car door handles
    b. Keep away from open windows; latch screens
    c. Supervise around pools and ponds or drain or fence them
    d. Lock cabinets
    e. Keep open jars and bottles out of reach
    f. Use gate to protect child from falling down stairs

19 to 30 months

1. Attention span increasing

  1. a. Gain attention before giving simple commands, one at a time; praise for success
    b. Add new rules as child conforms to old ones
    c. Refrain from expecting *immediate* obedience

2. Begins simple reasoning—asks question why; may be repetitive

  2. Make special efforts to answer questions: give simple explanations; gauge need for simplicity by number of times act is repeated or question asked

3. Interested in further exploration of environment; may lack physical control

  3. a. Supervise on stair rails and waxed floors
    b. Set rules about crossing streets and carrying knives, sharp objects, or glass objects
    c. Have outdoor play area securely fenced or supervised
    d. When riding in car, secure child safely by seat belt or insist on his sitting in back seat; do not permit standing on car seats
    e. Keep matches out of reach
    f. Shield adult tools such as knives, lawnmowers, sharp tools

4. Negativistic behavior is expected; responds more frequently with word ''no''; may show more resistance at bedtime preparation and during mealtime

  4. a. Practice consistency in responding to behavior
    b. Allow more time to conform to expectation

5. Behavior may change if new sibling is introduced into family unit

  5. a. Explain verbally or through play that new child is expected
    b. Exercise more patience with child
    c. Set special times aside for parental attention to child
    d. Allow child to help with special care tasks of new sibling

31 to 48 months

1. Displays more interest in conforming

  1. a. Exercise consistency in parental demands; enforce each time and avoid ignoring behavior next time
    b. Show concrete approval and give immediate recognition for acceptable behavior
    c. Refrain from use of threats that produce fearfulness

2. Shows greater understanding when simple reasoning is communicated

  2. a. Give simple explanations; allow child chance to demonstrate understanding by talking about event, situation, or rule
    b. Eliminate unnecessary and impractical rules
    c. Refrain from constant verbal reprimands
    d. Denial of privileges should not be excessive or prolonged

Discipline—cont'd

Expected tasks	Suggested activities

3. Will respond to simple commands such as putting toys away	3. a. Assign simple household tasks that child can carry out each day; show approval for performance and success
	   b. Decide if child is capable of doing what is asked by observing him
	   c. Determine how much time is necessary to complete a chore or activity before expecting maximum performance

4. Displays a greater independence in general activities	4. a. Be extra cautious about supervising riding tricycles in streets and watching for cars in driveways
	   b. Do not permit dashing into street while playing
	   c. Do not allow child to follow ball into street
	   d. Areas under swings and slides should not be paved
	   e. Provide an imitative model that child can copy, for example, do not jaywalk
	   f. Provide scissors that are blunt tipped

49 to 52 months	
1. Can be given two or three assignments at one time; will carry out in order 2. Complies readily with reasonable, well-defined, and consistent requirements 3. Understands reasoning	1. Give more opportunities to be independent 2. Use simple explanations and reasoning 3. Ask child to define role if he disobeys 4. Have child correct mistakes as they occur 5. Do not use punishment without warnings 6. Praise for successful performance 7. Use gold stars on chart for rewards 8. If leaving for social obligation, vacation, or visiting away from home, let child know 9. Avoid making promises that cannot be kept 10. Avoid bribing, ridicule, shaming, teasing, inflicting pain, using unfavorable comparison with other children, and exhibition of behavior by parents they are trying to stop in child 11. Remember that child may be imitating models of behavior set up by parents, brothers, sisters, a neighborhood child, or maybe a television hero 12. Recognize that there are stress periods in family or child's life that may result in changes in child's behavior including accidents, illness, moving into new neighborhood, separation from friends, death, divorce, and hospitalization of child or parents (be more patient with child's behavior, give more time to conform, show more approval for mastery of tasks, and exercise consistency in handling problems as they occur)

Dressing

Expected tasks	Suggested activities
13 to 18 months	
1. Cooperates in dressing by extending arm or leg 2. Removes socks, hat, mittens, shoes 3. Can unzip zippers 4. Tries to put shoes on	1. Encourage child to remove socks, etc. after task is initiated for him 2. Do not rush child 3. Have him practice with large buttons and with zippers
19 to 30 months	
1. Can undress 2. Can remove shoes if laces are untied 3. Helps dress 4. Tries to unbutton 5. Pulls on simple clothes	1. Provide opportunities to button with extra-large–sized buttons 2. Encourage and allow opportunity for self-help in getting drink, removing clothes with help, hand washing, unbuttoning, etc. 3. Simple clothing 4. Provide mirror at height child can observe himself for brushing teeth, etc.

Dressing—cont'd

Expected tasks	Suggested activities
31 to 48 months	
1. Greater interest and ability in dressing	1. Provide with own dresser drawer
2. Intent on lacing shoes (usually does incorrectly)	2. Simple garments encourage self-help; do not rush child
3. Does not know back from front	3. Provide large buttons, zippers, slipover clothing
4. Washes and dries hands, brushes teeth	4. Self hand washing but help with brushing teeth
5. Can button	5. Provide regular routine for dressing, either in bathroom or bedroom
49 to 52 months	
1. Dresses and undresses with care except for tying shoes and buckling belts	1. Assign regular task of placing clothes in hamper or basket
2. May learn to tie shoes	2. Continue to use simple clothing
3. Combs hair with assistance	3. Encourage self-help in dressing and undressing
	4. Allow child to select clothes he will wear

Toilet training

Expected tasks	Suggested activities
9 to 12 months	
1. Beginning to show regular patterns in bladder and bowel elimination	1. Watch for clues that indicate child is wet or soiled
2. Has one to two stools daily	2. Be sure to change diapers when wet or soiled so that child begins to experience contrast between wetness and dryness
3. Interval of dryness does not exceed 1 to 2 hours	
13 to 18 months	
1. Will have bowel movement if put on toilet at approximate time	1. Sit child on toilet or potty chair at regular intervals for short periods of time throughout day
2. Indicates wet pants	2. Praise child for success
	3. If potty chair is used, it should be located in bathroom
	4. Training should be started when social disruptions are at minimum
	5. Respond promptly to signals and clues of child by taking him to bathroom or changing pants
	6. Use training pants, once toilet training is commenced
	7. Plan to begin training when disruptions in regular routine are minimized, that is, do not begin on vacation
19 to 30 months	
1. Anticipates need to eliminate	1. Continue regular intervals of toileting
2. Same word for both functions	2. Reward success
3. Daytime control (occasional accident)	3. Dress in simple clothing that child can manage
4. Requires assistance (reminding, dressing, wiping)	4. Remind occasionally, particularly after mealtime, juicetime, naptime, and playtime
	5. Take to bathroom before bedtime
	6. Bathroom should be convenient to use, easy to open door
31 to 48 months	
1. Takes responsibility for toilet if clothes are simple	1. May still need reminding
2. Continues to verbalize need to go; apt to hold out too long	2. Dress in simple clothing that child can manage
3. May have occasional accident	3. Ignore accidents; refrain from shame or ridicule
4. Needs help with wiping	
49 to 52 months	
1. General independence (anticipates needs, undresses, goes, wipes, washes hands)	1. Praise child for his accomplishment

9-2. Immunization schedules

Recommended schedule for active immunization of normal infants and children

Age	Immunization recommended
2 months	DTP,* TOPV†
4 months	DTP, TOPV
6 months	DTP‡
1 year	Tuberculin test§
15 months	Measles, rubella, mumps‖
18 months	DTP, TOPV
4-6 years	DTP, TOPV
14-16 years	Td¶—repeat every 10 years

*DTP—diphtheria and tetanus toxoids combined with pertussis vaccine.
†TOPV—trivalent oral poliovirus vaccine. This recommendation is suitable for breast-fed as well as bottle-fed infants.
‡A third dose of TOPV is optional but may be given in areas of high endemicity of poliomyelitis.
§Frequency of tuberculin testing depends on risk of exposure of the child and on the prevalence of tuberculosis in the population group. The initial test should be at or preceding the measles vaccine.
‖May be given at 15 months as measles-rubella or measles-mumps-rubella combined vaccines.
¶Td—combined tetanus and diphtheria toxoids (adult type) for those more than 6 years of age, in contrast to diphtheria and tetanus (DT) toxoids which contain a larger amount of diphtheria antigen.

Primary immunization for children not immunized in early infancy*

| Time interval | Age (years) | |
	Under 6	6 and older
First visit	DTP, TOPV, tuberculin test	Td, TOPV, tuberculin test
1 month later	Measles,† mumps, rubella	Measles, mumps, rubella
2 months later	DTP, TOPV	Td, TOPV
4 months later	DTP, TOPV‡	
8 to 14 months later		Td, TOPV
10 to 16 months later or pre-school	DTP, TOPV	
At age 14-16 years	Td—repeat every 10 years	Td—repeat every 10 years

*The sequence of these schedules may be altered if specific infections are prevalent. For example, measles vaccine might be given on the first visit if an epidemic is occurring.
†Measles vaccine is not routinely given before 15 months of age.
‡Optional.

9-3. Possible side effects and nursing responsibilities of recommended childhood immunizations*

Immunization	Reaction	Nursing responsibilities
Diphtheria	Fever usually within 24-48 hours Soreness, redness, and swelling at site of injection	Instructions for DTP: Advise parents of possible side effects; may recommend prophylactic use of aspirin or acetaminophen if fever occurred following previous DTP immunization; recommend its use if fever occurs following present immunization; advise parents to notify physician immediately of any unusual side effects, such as those listed under pertussis
Tetanus	Same as for diphtheria but may include urticaria and malaise All may have delayed onset and last several days Lump at injection site may last for weeks, even months, but gradually disappears	
Pertussis	Same as for tetanus but may include loss of consciousness, convulsions, and thrombocytopenia	
Poliovirus (TOPV)	Essentially no side effects Vaccine-associated paralysis usually occurs within 2 months of immunization	See general comment to parents*
Measles	Anorexia, malaise, rash, and fever may occur 7 to 10 days after immunization Rarely (estimated risk 1 in 1 million doses) encephalitis may occur	Advise parents of more common side effects and use of antipyretics for fever; if a persistent high fever with other obvious signs of illness occurs, have them notify physician immediately
Mumps	Essentially no side effects other than a brief, mild fever	See general comment to parents*
Rubella	Mild rash that lasts 1 or 2 days within a few days after immunization Arthralgia, arthritis, and/or paresthesia of the hands and fingers may occur about 2 weeks after vaccination and is more frequent in older children and adults	Advise parents of side effects, especially of time delay before joint swelling and pain; assure them that these symptoms will disappear; may recommend use of mild analgesics for pain

*General comment to parents regarding each immunization: The benefit of being protected by the immunization is believed to greatly outweigh the risk from the disease.

9-4. Infectious diseases that occur during early childhood

Diseases	Infectious agent	Source	Transmission	Incubation period	Period of communicability	Clinical manifestations
Chickenpox	Varicella-zoster	Primarily secretions of respiratory tract of infected person; to a lesser degree skin lesions (scabs not infectious)	Direct contact, droplet spread, and objects contaminated by contact with skin lesions and mucous membranes of infectious persons	2-3 weeks; commonly 13-17 days	Probably 1 day before eruption of lesions (prodromal period) to 6 days after first crop of vesicles when crusts have formed; most communicable in early stages of dermal eruptions	Prodromal stage: slight fever, malaise, and anorexia for first 24 hours: rash highly pruritic; begins as macule, rapidly progresses to papule and then vesicle (surrounded by erythematous base, becomes umbilicated and cloudy, breaks easily, and forms crusts); all three stages present in varying degrees at one time. Distribution: centripetal, spreading to face and proximal extremities, but sparse on distal limbs. Constitutional signs and symptoms: lymphadenopathy, temperature, irritability from pruritus
Diphtheria	*Corynebacterium diphtheriae*	Discharges from mucous membranes of nose and nasopharynx, from skin, and from other lesions of infected person	Direct contact with infected person, a carrier, or contaminated articles from discharge of infected person	Usually 2-5 days, possibly longer	Variable; until virulent bacilli are no longer present (identified by three negative cultures); usually 2 weeks or less, but sometimes as long as 4 weeks	Varies according to anatomic location of pseudomembrane. Nasal: resembles common cold, serosanguineous mucopurulent nasal discharge without constitutional symptoms; may be frank epistaxis. Tonsillar/pharyngeal: malaise; anorexia; sore throat; low-grade fever; pulse increased above expected for temperature within 24 hours; smooth, adherent, white or gray membrane; lymphadenitis possibly pronounced (bull's neck); in severe cases, toxemia, septic shock, and death within 6-10 days. Laryngeal: fever, hoarseness, cough, with or without signs of above; potential airway obstruction, apprehensive, dyspneic retractions, cyanosis
Erythema infectiosum (fifth disease)	Probably virus	Infected persons	Presumably direct contact by droplet infection	6-14 days	Uncertain; most outbreaks subside in 1-2 months	Rash appears in three stages: I—erythema on face, chiefly on cheeks, "slapped face" appearance; disappears by 1-4 days. II—about 1 day after rash appears on face, maculopapular red spots appear, symmetrically distributed on upper and lower extremities; rash progresses from proximal and distal surfaces and may last a week or more. III—rash subsides but reappears if skin is irritated or traumatized (sun, hot, cold, friction)

Treatment	Nursing considerations	Control measures	Complications
Specific: none Supportive: benadryl or antihistamines to relieve itching; skin care to prevent secondary bacterial infection	Administer skin care: give daily bath; change clothes and linens daily; administer topical application of calamine lotion or paste of baking soda and water; keep child's fingernails short and clean; apply mittens if child must scratch Lessen pruritus; keep child occupied Remove loose crusts that rub and irritate skin Teach child to apply pressure to pruritic area rather than scratch it If older child, reason with him regarding danger of scar formation from scratching	Immunization not available Isolation of child in home until vesicles have dried (usually 1 week after onset of disease) Isolation of high-risk children (including neonates born of mothers who contract the disease 5 days or less before delivery and infants less than 1 month of age); treatment of exposed high-risk children includes administration of immune serum globulin (ISG) or zoster-immune-globulin (ZIG); one attack confers permanent immunity, although second attack of herpes zoster (shingles) can occur in susceptible children or adults	Secondary bacterial infections (abscesses, cellulitis, pneumonia, sepsis) Encephalitis Varicella pneumonia Hemorrhagic varicella (tiny hemorrhages in the vesicles and numerous petechiae in the skin)
Antitoxin (usually intravenously); preceded by skin or conjunctival test to rule out sensitivity to horse serum Antibiotics (penicillin or erythromycin) Complete bed rest (prevention of myocarditis) Tracheostomy for airway obstruction	Maintain *strict* isolation Participate in sensitivity testing; have epinephrine available Administer antibiotics; observe for signs of sensitivity to penicillin Administer *complete* care to maintain bed rest Use suctioning as needed Regulate humidity for optimal liquefaction of secretions Observe respirations for signs of obstruction	Immunization during infancy and boosters every 10 years after initial series Strict isolation of all symptomatic persons Treatment of infected contacts (positive throat cultures and Schick test) and carriers (positive throat cultures but negative Schick test)	Myocarditis (second week) Neuritis
None necessary	Support parents regarding benign nature of condition	None specific, except isolation of child from other siblings	Self-limited arthritis and arthralgia

Diseases	Infectious agent	Source	Transmission	Incubation period	Period of communicability	Clinical manifestations
Exanthem subitum (roseola)	Probably virus	Unknown	Unknown (limited virtually to children between 6 months and 2 years of age)	Unknown	Unknown	Persistent high fever for 3-4 days in child who appears well Precipitous drop in fever to normal with appearance of rash Rash: discrete rose-pink macules or maculopapules, appearing first on trunk, then spreading to neck, face, and extremities; nonpruritic, fades on pressure, lasts 1-2 days Associated signs and symptoms: cervical/postauricular lymphadenopathy, injected pharynx, occasionally catarrhal otitis media
Measles (rubeola)	Virus	Respiratory tract secretions, blood, and urine of infected person	Usually by direct contact with droplets of infected person; less commonly by airborne or indirect contact with articles freshly contaminated by respiratory tract secretions	10-20 days	From 4 days before to 5 days after rash appears, mostly during catarrhal phase	Prodromal stage: fever and malaise, followed in 24 hours by coryza, cough, conjunctivitis, Koplik spots (small irregular red spots with a minute bluish white center first seen on the buccal mucosa opposite the molars) 2 days prior to rash; symptoms gradually increase in severity until second day after rash appears, when they begin to subside Rash: appears 3-4 days after onset of prodromal stage; begins as erythematous maculopapular eruption on face and gradually spreads downward; more severe in earlier sites (appears confluent) and less intense in later sites (appears discrete); after 3-4 days, assumes brownish appearance and fine desquamation occurs over areas of extensive involvement Constitutional signs and symptoms: anorexia, malaise, generalized lymphadenopathy
Mumps	Virus	Saliva of infected persons	Direct contact with or droplet spread from an infected person	14-21 days	Most communicable immediately before and after swelling begins; virus present in saliva up to 7 days before and 9 days after parotid swelling	Prodromal stage: fever, headache, malaise, and anorexia for 24 hours, followed by "earache" that is aggravated by chewing Parotitis: by third day, parotid gland(s) (either unilateral or bilateral) enlarges and reaches maximal size in 1-3 days; accompanied by pain and tenderness Other manifestations: submaxillary and sublingual infection, orchitis, and meningoencephalitis

Treatment	Nursing considerations	Control measures	Complications
None specific Antipyretics to control fever Anticonvulsives for child with history of febrile seizures	Teach parents measures for lowering temperature (antipyretic drugs and tepid sponge baths) If child is prone to seizures, discuss appropriate precautions Reassure parents regarding benign nature of illness	None	Febrile seizures
Supportive: bed rest during febrile period Antipyretics Antibiotics to prevent secondary bacterial infection in high-risk children	Maintain bed rest during prodromal stage; provide quiet activity Fever: instruct parents to administer antipyretics and cool sponge bath; avoid chilling; if child is prone to seizures, institute appropriate precautions (fever spikes to 40° C [104° F] between fourth and fifth days) Eye care: dim lights if photophobia present; cleanse eyelids with warm saline solution to remove secretions or crusts; keep child from rubbing his eyes; examine cornea for signs of ulceration Coryza/cough: use cool mist vaporizer; protect skin around nares with layer of petrolatum; encourage fluids and soft bland foods Skin care: keep skin clean; use tepid baths as necessary	Immunization with measles virus vaccine at 15 months of age (if given earlier to provide protection during an epidemic, vaccine needs to be repeated at this age because of suppression of immunity by maternal antibodies) Gamma globulin may prevent or modify the illness and prevent complications in unimmunized and high-risk children One attack of measles confers lifelong immunity Isolation only necessary until fifth day of rash; if hospitalized, respiratory precautions are instituted	Otitis media Pneumonia Bronchiolitis Obstructive laryngitis and laryngotracheitis Encephalitis
Symptomatic and supportive: analgesics for pain and antipyretics for fever Intravenous fluid may be necessary for child who refuses to drink or vomits because of meningoencephalitis	Maintain bed rest during prodromal phase until swelling subsides Give analgesics for pain; if child is unwilling to chew medication, use elixir form Encourage fluids and soft bland foods; avoid foods requiring chewing Apply hot or cold compresses to neck, whichever is more comforting To relieve orchitis, provide warmth and local support by means of a nest of absorbent cotton in the diaper or tight-fitting underpants (stretch bathing suit works well)	Immunization of all infants at 15 months of age Passive protection with gamma globulin ineffective Confinement to the home recommended during period of communicability; respiratory isolation is required during hospitalization One attack of bilateral, unilateral, or inapparent infection usually confers permanent immunity	Sensorineural deafness Postinfectious encephalitis Myocarditis Arthritis Hepatitis Sterility (in adult males)

Diseases	Infectious agent	Source	Transmission	Incubation period	Period of communicability	Clinical manifestations
Poliomyelitis	Enteroviruses: type 1—most frequent cause of paralysis, both epidemic and endemic; type 2—least frequently associated with paralysis; type 3—second most frequent	Feces and oropharyngeal secretions of infected persons, especially young children	Direct contact with persons with apparent or inapparent active infection; spread is via fecal-oral and pharyngeal-oropharyngeal routes	Usually 7-14 days, with range of 5-35 days	Not exactly known; virus is present in throat and feces shortly after infection and persists for about 1 week in throat and 4-6 weeks in feces	May be manifest in three different forms: Abortive or inapparent—fever, uneasiness, sore throat, headache, anorexia, vomiting, abdominal pain; lasts a few hours to a few days Nonparalytic—same manifestations as abortive but more severe, with pain and stiffness in neck, back, and legs Paralytic—initial course similar to nonparalytic type, followed by recovery and then signs of central nervous system paralysis; acute stage (about 5-7 days) characterized by headache, vomiting, fever, stiffness of back and neck (tripod sign—unable to sit up straight unless hands are used to brace self), pain in back, limbs, and neck, and finally paralysis; any muscle groups may be involved, but demonstrates predilection for large muscles; respiratory paralysis may occur from damage to nerve cells in cervicothoracic segments of spinal cord or damage to vital centers in medulla (bulbar poliomyelitis); recovery may be complete over several months or associated with residual paralysis
Pertussis (whooping cough)	*Bordetella pertussis*	Discharge from respiratory tract of infected persons	Direct contact or droplet spread from infected person; indirect contact with freshly contaminated articles	5-21 days, usually 10	Greatest during catarrhal stage before onset of paroxysms and may extend to fourth week after onset of paroxysms	Catarrhal stage: begins with symptoms of upper respiratory infection, such as coryza, sneezing, lacrimation, cough, and low-grade fever; symptoms continue for 1-2 weeks, when dry hacking cough becomes more severe Paroxysmal stage: cough that most commonly occurs at night consists of a series of short rapid coughs, followed by a sudden inspiration that is associated with a high-pitched crowing sound or "whoop"; during paroxysms, cheek becomes flushed or cyanotic, eyes bulge, and tongue protrudes; paroxysm may continue until a thick mucus plug is dislodged; vomiting frequently follows an attack; stage generally lasts 4-6 weeks, followed by convalescent stage

Treatment	Nursing considerations	Control measures	Complications
No specific treatment, including antimicrobials or gamma globulin Supportive treatment; complete bed rest during acute phase Assisted respiratory ventilation in case of respiratory paralysis Physical therapy for muscles following acute stage	Maintain complete bed rest Administer mild sedatives as necessary to relieve anxiety and promote rest Participate in physiotherapy procedures (use of moist hot packs and range-of-motion exercise) Position child to maintain body alignment and prevent contractures or decubiti; use footboard Encourage child to move; administer analgesics for maximum comfort during physical activity Observe for respiratory paralysis (difficulty in talking, ineffective cough, inability to hold the breath, shallow and rapid respirations); report such signs and symptoms to physician; have tracheostomy tray at bedside	Immunization of all children with complete series of trivalent oral poliovirus vaccine Vaccination of close contacts who have not been adequately immunized During an epidemic, avoid visiting families with known cases, overexertion or chilling, eating unwashed fresh fruits or vegetables, surgical procedures in nose and oropharynx, and unnecessary injections, including vaccination other than for poliomyelitis	Permanent paralysis Respiratory arrest Hypertension Kidney stones from demineralization of bone during prolonged immobility
Antimicrobial therapy (such as erythromycin) Administration of pertussis-immune globulin Supportive treatment: hospitalization required for infants, children who are dehydrated, or those who have complications Bed rest Increased oxygen intake and humidity Adequate fluids Intubation possibly necessary	Maintain bed rest as long as fever is present Keep child occupied during the day (interest in play is associated with fewer paroxysms) Reassure parents during frightening episodes of whooping cough Provide restful environment and reduce factors that promote paroxysms (dust, smoke, sudden change in temperature, chilling, activity, excitement); keep room well-ventilated Encourage fluids; offer small frequent fluids; refeed child after vomiting Keep child in Croupette with high humidity; suction gently but often to *prevent* choking on secretion Observe for signs of airway obstruction (increased restlessness, apprehension, retractions, cyanosis) Involve public health nurse if child is cared for at home	Immunization during early infancy (2 months of age); no passive immunity from mother and absence of IgM antibodies Value of pertussis-immune globulin in preventing illness is questionable If child is hospitalized, respiratory isolation required One attack usually confers permanent immunity	Pneumonia (usual cause of death) Atelectasis Otitis media Convulsions Hemorrhage (subarachnoid, subconjunctival, epistaxis) Weight loss and dehydration Hernia Prolapsed rectum

Diseases	Infectious agent	Source	Transmission	Incubation period	Period of communicability	Clinical manifestations
Rubella (German measles)	Virus	Primarily nasopharyngeal secretions of persons with apparent or inapparent infection; virus also present in blood, stool, and urine	Direct contact and spread via infected person; indirectly via articles freshly contaminated with nasopharyngeal secretions, feces, or urine	14-21 days	7 days before to about 5 days after appearance of rash	Prodromal phase: absent in children, present in adults and adolescents; consists of low-grade fever, headache, malaise, anorexia, mild conjunctivitis, coryza, sore throat, cough, and lymphadenopathy; lasts for 1-5 days, subsides 1 day after appearance of rash Rash: first appears in face and rapidly spreads downward to neck, arms, trunk, and legs; by end of first day, body is covered with a discrete pinkish-red maculopapular exanthema; disappears in same order as it began and is usually gone by third day Constitutional signs and symptoms: occasionally low-grade fever, headaches, malaise, and lymphadenopathy
Congenital rubella		Primarily nasopharyngeal secretions of persons with apparent or inapparent infection; virus also present in blood, stool, and urine	Direct contact and spread via infected person; indirectly via articles freshly contaminated with nasopharyngeal secretions, feces, or urine	Transplacental	Not applicable; virus is only dangerous to fetus during first trimester	Infants may be infectious for months; virus shedding from throat disappears by 6 months of age in 80% to 90% of cases	Virtually any organ can be affected; classic rubella syndrome characterized by growth retardation, cerebral defects (mental retardation, microcephaly), deafness, eye defects (cataracts, strabismus, retinopathy), congenital heart disease (patent ductus arteriosus [PDA], ventricular septal defect; coarctation of the aorta, pulmonary stenosis), thrombocytopenic purpura, behavioral abnormalities—unusual pleasure in rocking, obsession with lights, lack of recognition of human relationships, little interest in food, difficulties with toilet training
Scarlet fever	Group A beta hemolytic streptococcus	Usually from nasopharyngeal secretions of infected persons and carriers	Direct contact with infected person or droplet spread; indirectly by contact with contaminated articles, ingestion of contaminated milk or other food	2-4 days with range of 1-7 days	During incubation period and clinical illness, approximately 10 days; during first 2 weeks of carrier phase, although may persist for months	Prodromal stage: abrupt high fever, pulse increased out of proportion to fever, vomiting, headache, chills, malaise, abdominal pain

Note: In the "Congenital rubella" row, the columns shift — "Transplacental" belongs under Transmission, "Not applicable; virus is only dangerous to fetus during first trimester" belongs under Incubation period, and "Infants may be infectious for months..." belongs under Period of communicability.

Treatment	Nursing considerations	Control measures	Complications
No treatment necessary other than antipyretics for low-grade fever and analgesics for discomfort Antibiotics not indicated because secondary bacterial infection does not occur	Reassure parents of benign nature of illness Employ comfort measures as necessary Isolate child from pregnant women	Routine immunization of all children (usually at 15 months of age) and of all females before childbearing age See also measures included under congenital rubella	Complications rare (arthritis, encephalitis, or purpura); most benign of all childhood communicable diseases; greatest danger is teratogenic effect on fetus
Strict isolation of neonates with rubella until throat culture is free of virus Medical treatment as indicated by various anomalies (chief causes of death are sepsis, congestive heart failure, and general debility) Rehabilitation of children who survive infancy	Identify neonates with congenital rubella and institute *strict* isolation *immediately* Select nursing personnel to care for infant who are not at high risk for rubella infection	See also preceding discussion of rubella Do not administer rubella vaccine to pregnant women (threat of contracting disease from newly vaccinated children negligible) Immunization of women of childbearing age with low hemagglutination-inhibition (HI) titer who agree to use contraception for 2 months after receiving immunization Use of immune serum globulin in pregnant women exposed to rubella who have low HI antibodies Elective therapeutic abortion for pregnant women with known (or suspected) infection during first trimester Isolate women at risk of contracting rubella from contact with infant	Same as outlined under clinical manifestations
Treatment of choice is a full course of penicillin (or erythromycin in penicillin-sensitive children); fever should subside 24 hours after beginning therapy Supportive measures: bed rest during febrile phase, analgesics for sore throat	Ensure compliance with oral antibiotic therapy (intramuscular benzathine penicillin G [Bicillin] may be given if parents' reliability in giving oral drugs is questionable) Maintain bed rest during febrile phase; provide quiet activity during convalescent period	Respiratory isolation of children with scarlet fever until 24 hours after initiation of treatment Throat cultures of children with sore throat and penicillin therapy for those with positive group A streptococci test Antibiotic therapy for newly diagnosed carriers (nose or throat cultures positive for streptococcus)	Otitis media Peritonsillar abscess Sinusitis Rheumatic fever Glomerulonephritis

Diseases	Infectious agent	Source	Transmission	Incubation period	Period of communicability	Clinical manifestations
						Enanthema: tonsils enlarged, edematous, reddened, and covered with patches of exudate; in severe cases appearance resembles membrane seen in diphtheria; pharynx is edematous and briefly red; during first 1 or 2 days tongue is coated and papillae (become red and swollen (white strawberry tongue); by the fourth or fifth day white coat sloughs off, leaving prominent papillae (red strawberry tongue); palate is covered with erythematous punctate lesions
						Exanthema: rash appears within 12 hours after prodromal signs: red pinhead-sized punctate lesions rapidly become generalized but are absent on the face, which becomes flushed; rash is more intense in folds of joints; by end of the first week, desquamation begins which may be complete by 3 weeks or longer
Smallpox (variola)	Poxvirus (variola)	Respiratory secretions and lesions of skin and mucous membranes of infected person	Prolonged direct contact with infected person; indirectly by articles freshly contaminated with crusts or secretions	12 days, with range of 7-17 days	Onset of first symptom to disappearance of all scabs, usually about 2-3 weeks	Prodromal stage: abrupt onset with chills, fever (reaches peak by end of second day), headache, backaches, and prostration; lasts 2-4 days, and symptoms begin to improve as rash develops
						Eruption period: painful lesions appear on mucous membranes of mouth, throat, and respiratory tract, causing symptoms of sore throat, hoarseness, and cough; macules first appear on face, forearm, trunk, (especially back), and finally lower extremities; intensity of rash is centrifugal—denser on preipheral than on central regions; within a few hours, macules become papules; by sixth day from onset of illness they become vesicles, then pustules, and finally form crusts by end of 14 days; during pustular stage constitutional signs worsen and lesions are painful; dessication of lesions is accompanied by intense pruritis and is followed by 1- to 2-week period of desquamation

Treatment	Nursing considerations	Control measures	Complications
	Relieve discomfort of sore throat with analgesics, gargles, lozenges, antiseptic throat sprays (Chloraseptic), and inhalation of cool mist Encourage fluids during febrile phase; avoid irritating liquids (citrus juices) or rough foods; when child is able to eat, begin with soft diet Advise parents to consult physician if fever persists after beginning therapy Discuss procedures for preventing spread of infection	Prophylactic antibiotic therapy of household contacts, ideally those with cultures positive for streptococcus, regardless of associated symptoms, or an upper respiratory infection Proper food handling (use of pasteurized milk and exclusion of infected persons from handling food)	
No specific treatment available; patients are placed under strict isolation; antibiotics are used if bacterial infection is present Supportive therapy: adequate fluids, calories, and electrolytes (may require gavage feeding because oral and intravenous routes are incapacitated by presence of lesions), analgesics, antipruritics	Ensure strict isolation procedures; maintain complete bed rest; schedule analgesics to ensure optimum comfort Cleanse eyes with sterile saline solution to remove crusts, inspect cornea for evidence of infection Observe patterns of fever (peaks on second to third day and during pustular stage but is only low grade at other times; normal by tenth to twelfth day); unusual spikes may indicate bacterial infection Although no special skin care indicated, change bedclothes and linens at least daily, especially during desquamation phase Prevent child from scratching: use mittens, keep fingernails short and clean, use elbow restraints Participate in immunization procedures of close contacts or general population if epidemic is anticipated	Routine immunization no longer recommended except for groups at risk (military, health personnel, and travelers to areas where disease is endemic) Strict isolation of infected person Vaccination or revaccination of persons presumably exposed to smallpox Use of vaccines of variola-immune globulin (VIG) may prevent or modify disease in exposed individuals	Secondary bacterial infection: impetigo, furuncles, cellulitis, pneumonia, septicemia, osteomyelitis, keratitis, scarring, laryngeal edema, encephalitis, psychoses, abortion in pregnant women

9-5. Contraindications to routine immunizations

Contraindication	Immunization	Rationale	Nursing considerations
Acute febrile illness or chronic debilitating diseases	All	Masks febrile reactions from the immunization, decreases body's natural defense mechanisms	Explain reason for postponing immunization to parent and reschedule it at earliest return visit For chronic diseases, check with physician before administering any immunization
Gastroenteritis	Live poliovirus vaccine	May interfere with colonization of the viruses in the intestines, which is essential for the immune response to occur	Explain reason for postponing immunization and reschedule it as soon as possible
Altered immune system Immunologic disease Generalized malignancy (leukemia, lymphoma) Immunosuppressive therapy (steroids, antimetabolites, radiation)	All live viral vaccines (measles, mumps, rubella, and polio)	Depressed immune defenses may result in extreme reactions to the immunizations	Emphasize to parents the need to prevent their children from exposure to any of these childhood diseases, because they cannot be artificially protected from them
Recently acquired passive immunity Blood transfusion or immune serum globulin within last 6 weeks Maternal antibodies during first year	Measles, mumps, and rubella vaccines	Presence of passive immunity prevents formation of antibodies to the vaccine	Inquire during the history concerning recent blood transfusions or injections of immune serum globulin; wait recommended 6 weeks before administering the immunization; follow suggested schedule for measles, mumps, and rubella (15 months)
Allergy to substances in vaccine, for example, egg protein, neomycin	Live virus vaccines grown on chick embryos, treated with neomycin	Known hypersensitivity to substance will also result in reaction to substance in vaccine	Check manufacturer's product information for specific contraindications and screen child for known allergies to potential foreign substances
History of nervous system disorders Reaction of high fever, somnolence, or convulsions following a DTP immunization	Pertussis vaccine	Danger of serious reaction to pertussis vaccination is greatly increased	Take a detailed neurological history, including past convulsions, fainting spells, tremors, or twitching and specific reactions to DTP; report any such findings to a physician before administering the pertussis vaccine
Pregnancy	All live virus vaccines except for poliovirus	Potential risk to fetus, especially from rubella	Take a careful history of all women of childbearing age regarding the possibility of pregnancy or conception within the next 2 months

10-1. Psychiatric assessment guides

The following assessment guides have been developed to:
1. Identify high-risk factors that may contribute to and/or precipitate the development of mental illness
2. Determine the need for intervention when high-risk factors are present to prevent the development or recurrence of mental illness
3. Understand the interrelationship of biological, psychological, and social factors in the maintenance of mental health and the prevention of mental illness
4. Assess mental health status
5. Assess clients' strengths and weaknesses
6. Develop nursing strategies designed to utilize strengths
7. Develop nursing strategies designed to minimize weaknesses
8. Assess psychocultural perceptions and orientations concerning health and illness
9. Establish mental health goals consistent with clients' perceptions and orientations about health and illness
10. Assess the dynamics of group and family systems
11. View individuals, families, and groups as integral subsystems of a large social system

GUIDE FOR ASSESSMENT OF MENTAL HEALTH

I. Demographic data
  A. Name
  B. Address
  C. Age
  D. Sex
  E. Education
  F. Ethnicity (optional)*
  G. Religion (optional)*
  H. Living arrangements
  I. Marital status
II. Admission data
  A. Date and time of admission
  B. Manner of admission
    1. Self
    2. Relatives
    3. Police
    4. Other (describe)
  C. Form of retention (if hospitalized)
    1. Informal retention
    2. Voluntary retention
    3. Involuntary retention
    4. Emergency
    5. Comments
  D. Reason for admission
  E. Client's primary complaint
  F. Client's premorbid personality
III. History of psychiatric problems
  A. Previous condition: date; problem

B. Assistance sought: native healer; therapist; agency; clergyman; other (describe)
C. Current levels of functioning and coping
IV. Behavioral observations
  A. Thought patterns
    1. Delusion: grandeur; persecution; somatic; self-accusatory
    2. Obsession
    3. Ideas of reference
    4. Phobia
    5. Looseness of association
    6. Flight of ideas
    7. Fugue
    8. Impaired judgment
    9. Impaired insight
    10. Impaired orientation to time, place, or person
    11. Impaired memory
    12. No observable thought disturbance
    13. Comments
  B. Sensory processes
    1. Hallucination: olfactory; auditory; tactile; gustatory; visual
    2. No observable sensory disturbance
    3. Comments
  C. Speech patterns
    1. Blocking
    2. Word salad
    3. Echolalia
    4. Circumstantiality
    5. Irrelevancy
    6. Confabulation
    7. Mutism
    8. Neologism
    9. Perseveration
    10. Stuttering
    11. No observable speech disturbance
    12. Comments
  D. Affect
    1. Elation
    2. Depression
    3. Ambivalence
    4. Apathy
    5. Anger
    6. No observable disturbance of affect
    7. Comments
  E. Motor activity
    1. Hyperactive
    2. Hypoactive
    3. Stereotypical: persistent; aimless; repetitive
    4. Perseveration
    5. Catalepsy: stupor; waxy flexibility
    6. Compulsion
    7. No observable disturbance in motor activity
    8. Comments

*Legislation protects people from being required to reveal ethnicity and religion.

   F. Level of consciousness
     1. Confusion
     2. Stupor
     3. Delirium
     4. Alert
     5. Comments
V. Physical appearance
   A. Posture
     1. Sagging
     2. Rigid
     3. Curled into fetal position
     4. Bent
     5. No observable disturbance in posture
     6. Comments
   B. Facies
     1. Drooping or sagging: deflected eyes; lusterless eyes; drooping eyelids; deep nasolabial folds
     2. Uplifted or retracted: smiling; retracted brow; wide open eyes; darting eyes
     3. Blank: staring into space; distant expression in eyes
     4. Mask-like or ironed-out
     5. Facial tic
     6. No observable disturbance in facies
     7. Comments
   C. Mode of dress
     1. Overly neat
     2. Disheveled
     3. Bizarre
     4. Appropriate
     5. Comments
VI. Physical status
   A. Vital signs: pulse; temperature; respirations; blood pressure
   B. Physical condition
     1. Medical problems: acute; chronic
     2. Physical aids (describe)
     3. Medications: date and time of last dose
     4. Allergies (describe)
     5. Comments
   C. Patterns of daily living
     1. Sleep patterns: restlessness; insomnia; narcoplexy; average number of hours of sleep
     2. Eating patterns: number of meals a day; compulsive eating; anorexia
     3. Drinking patterns: beverage; quantity consumed; frequency of consumption
     4. Sexual patterns: sexual orientation or preference; attitudes about sexuality; sexual activity
     5. Elimination patterns: constipation; diarrhea; urinary frequency; urinary retention
     6. Social patterns: recreation; work; intimacy; community involvement
     7. Comments
   D. Level of self-care
     1. Personal hygiene
     2. Activities of daily living
     3. Comments
VII. Cultural orientation
   A. Place of residence: interethnic neighborhood; ethnic enclave
   B. Family organization: nuclear; extended; members composing family unit; members vested with authority; members involved in child rearing; sense of obligation of family members to one another

   C. Sex-defined roles: stereotyped male and female roles; amount of independence permitted men and women; degree of intimacy permitted between married men and women, unmarried men and women
   D. Communication patterns: language spoken at home; language spoken outside home; use of touching and/or gesturing; interpersonal spacing
   E. Type of dress: traditional ethnic dress; Western-style dress
   F. Type of food: ethnic food; American food
   G. Relationship to people: individualistic; group-oriented; egalitarian; authoritative
   H. Relationship to time: past-oriented; present-oriented; future-oriented
   I. Relationship to the world: personal control; goal directed; fatalistic
   J. Health care patterns: ideas concerning causes of mental illness; ideas concerning treatment of mental illness; people consulted for treatment of mental illness (e.g., family member, native healer, mental health therapist, other [describe])
   K. Comments
VIII. Effective social network
   A. Family
   B. Household members (if different from family)
   C. Friends
   D. Associates: employer; coworkers; neighbors; others
   E. Religious affiliates: clergyman; church elders; congregants
   F. Comments
IX. Stressors
   A. Culture shock
     1. Communication (foreign verbal, kinesic, and proxemic systems)
     2. Mechanical environment (i.e., different types of food, housing, clothing, utilities)
     3. Social isolation from family and friends
     4. Foreign customs, standards, and/or values
     5. Different or new role relationships
   B. Life changes
     1. Affectional: marriage; birth; death; divorce; abandonment
     2. Socioeconomic: promotion; demotion; unemployment; change of employment; change of residence; increased responsibilities
     3. Biophysical: serious illness (acute or chronic); surgery; accident; loss of body part; sexual trauma (e.g., rape, incest)
   C. Other (describe)
   D. No significant stress
   E. Comments
X. Coping mechanisms
   A. Coping mechanisms used (describe)
   B. Effectiveness of coping mechanisms
   C. Client's perception of mechanisms that are effective in reducing stress
   D. Comments
XI. Resources
   A. Personal: interests; leisure time activities; physical and mental abilities; educational achievement; other
   B. Social: interpersonal networks; economic support systems (e.g., health insurance, sick leave, union benefits); food, shelter, clothing; other
   C. Comments

XII. Candidacy for active involvement in treatment program
   A. Developmental level
   B. Interactional ability
   C. Willingness to participate in treatment program
   D. Areas of anticipated need for assistance from nursing staff
   E. Comments

GUIDE FOR ASSESSMENT OF FAMILY PROCESS

I. Demographic data
   A. Names of members
   B. Age of members
   C. Sex of members
   D. Relationship between members: affinal; consanguineous
   E. Educational levels of members
   F. Occupations of members
   G. Ethnicity (optional)*
   H. Religion (optional)*
   I. Family members living in another household (describe relationship)
   J. Nonfamily members living in the household (describe living arrangement)
   K. Other (describe)
II. Family organization
   A. Type of family: nuclear; extended
   B. Type of system: open; closed; boundary maintaining mechanisms (describe); norms; rules
   C. Members involved in child rearing
   D. Members vested with authority
   E. Sense of obligation of family members—roles: peacemaker; protector; attacker; provider; interpreter; rescuer; other
   F. Sex-defined roles: stereotyped male-female relationships; amount of independence permitted men and women
   G. Other (describe)
III. Family world view
   A. Relationship to people: individualistic; group-oriented; egalitarian; authoritarian
   B. Relationship to time: past-oriented; present-oriented; future-oriented
   C. Relationship to the world: personal control; goal-directed; fatalistic
   D. Comments
IV. Family perceptions and definitions
   A. Family
   B. Privacy
   C. Intimacy
   D. Health (mental and physical)
   E. Illness (mental and physical)
   F. Other (describe)
V. Family health care patterns
   A. Ideas concerning causes of illness (mental and physical)
   B. Ideas concerning treatment of illness (mental and physical)
   C. People consulted in times of crisis or for treatment of mental and physical illnesses (e.g., family member; native healer; mental health therapist; pharmacist; physician; other)
   D. Comments
VI. Family living arrangements
   A. Type of residence: multi-familiy dwelling; single-family dwelling; one-room dwelling; other
   B. Environment of residence: urban; surban; rural; interethnic neighborhood; ethnic enclave

   C. Time in residence: length of time in present residence; length of time in previous residences
   D. Sleeping arrangements: number of rooms serving as bedrooms (differentiate between rooms functioning solely as bedrooms and those that have other functions)
   E. Eating arrangements: family members eat together; eat alone; eat in shifts
   F. Privacy arrangements: Rooms or sections of rooms reserved for specific family members; furniture (e.g., chairs) reserved for specific family members
   G. Other (describe)
VII. Family interaction patterns
   A. Communication patterns
      1. Verbal
         a. Language spoken at home
         b. Language spoken outside home
      2. Kinesic
         a. Touching
         b. Gesturing
      3. Proxemic
         a. Interpersonal spacing
         b. Fixed and/or built space
      4. Themes
         a. Double-bind messages
         b. Manipulation
         c. Scapegoating
         d. Intellectualization
         e. Blame placing
         f. Validation
         g. Other (describe)
   B. Behavioral patterns
      1. Physical acting out
      2. Isolation
      3. Detachment
      4. Cooperation
      5. Competition
      6. Overdependency
      7. Other (describe)
   C. Social patterns
      1. Alliances
         a. Among family members
         b. Between family members and members of social network
         c. Conflict between alliances
         d. Resolution of conflict between alliances
      2. Authority
         a. Nominal authority figure(s)
         b. Actual authority figure(s)
         c. Patterns of authority
         d. Implementation of authority: direct; delegated
      3. Decision making
         a. Nominal decision-making figure(s)
         b. Actual decision-making figure(s)
         c. Patterns of decision making
         d. Implementation of decisions
      4. Dissemination of information
         a. Sources of information
         b. Pattern of communicating information
      5. Social interaction
         a. Social network: relatives; friends; employers; co-workers; neighbors; clergy; other (describe)
         b. Community involvement: school; church; union; neighborhood; other (describe)

*Legislation protects people from being required to reveal ethnicity and religion.

c. Patterns of recreation

d. Patterns of intimacy

6. Other (describe)

VIII. Family stressors

A. Culture shock

1. Communication: foreign verbal, kinesic, and proxemic systems

2. Mechanical environment (i.e., different types of food, housing, clothing, utilities)

3. Social isolation from family and friends

4. Foreign customs, standards, and/or values

5. Different or new role relationships

B. Life changes

1. Affectional: marriage; birth; death; divorce; abandonment

2. Socioeconomic: promotion; demotion; unemployment; change of employment; change of residence

3. Biophysical: Accident or serious illness involving a family member (acute or chronic)

C. Other (describe)

D. No significant stress

IX. Family coping mechanisms

A. Coping mechanisms used (indicate whether mechanisms are used only by specific family members)

B. Effectiveness of coping mechanisms

C. Family's perception of mechanisms that are effective in reducing stress

D. Comments

X. Family resources

A. Familial: interests; leisure time activities; physical and mental abilities; other

B. Social: interpersonal networks; economic support systems (e.g., health insurance, sick leave, union benefits); food, shelter, clothing; other

GUIDE FOR ASSESSMENT OF GROUP PROCESS

I. Description of group

A. Type of group (e.g., activity, encounter, remotivation, psychodrama)

B. Goals of group

C. Size of group

D. Composition of group

1. Age of members

2. Sex of members

3. Ethnic background of members (optional)*

4. Behavior exhibited by members

5. Educational levels of members

6. Communicational levels of members (e.g., verbal; mute; speak a foreign language)

7. Reality testing levels of members

8. Other (describe)

---

*Legislation protects people from being required to reveal ethnic background.

II. Characteristics of group

A. Group phase or stage (orientation, working, termination)

B. Level of cohesiveness

C. Level of anxiety

D. Level of conflict

E. Level of resistance

F. Other (describe)

III. Patterns of group interaction

A. Communication patterns

1. Silence

2. Semantic argument

3. Intellectualization

4. Monopolization

5. Scapegoating

6. Other (describe)

B. Behavior patterns

1. Physical activity

2. Withdrawal

3. Detachment

4. Cooperation

5. Competition

6. Other (describe)

C. Social patterns

1. Group norms

2. Group rules

3. Roles (e.g., peacemaker, leader, protector, attacker, interpreter)

4. Alliances among members (subgroups)

5. Conflict between alliances

6. Other (describe)

IV. Patterns of leadership

A. Approach of leader(s)

1. Laissez-faire

2. Democratic

3. Power struggle

4. Authoritarian

5. Other (describe)

B. Competence of leader(s)

1. Provides relaxed, nonjudgmental atmosphere

2. Protects group members from disruptive communication patterns (scapegoating)

3. Accepts all feelings, attitudes, and ideas as valid themes for group discussion

4. Responds to verbal and nonverbal communication

5. Facilitates communication and problem solving by

a. encouraging group members to clarify and describe feelings, attitudes, and ideas

b. summarizing as needed

6. Facilitates group cohesiveness by

a. asking for feedback and validation

b. giving responsibility to the group

c. encouraging the group to make decisions

d. permitting the group to review and revise goals as indicated

e. developing leadership among group members

7. Other (describe)

10-2. DSM-III classification: axes I and II categories and codes

The *Diagnostic and Statistical Manual of Mental Disorders* is published by the American Psychiatric Association and is periodically revised. The third edition (DSM-III) appeared in 1980.

The *Manual* categorizes and codifies psychiatric diagnoses. A description of diagnostic criteria accompanies each diagnosis. Categories and codes are used by physicians when they make diagnoses and by institutional personnel when they compile statistics and complete insurance forms.

All official DSM-III codes and terms are included in ICD-9-CM. However, in order to differentiate those DSM-III categories that use the same ICD-9-CM codes, unofficial non-ICD-9-CM codes are provided in parentheses for use when greater specificity is necessary.

The long dashes indicate the need for a fifth-digit subtype or other qualifying term.

DISORDERS USUALLY FIRST EVIDENT IN INFANCY, CHILDHOOD OR ADOLESCENCE
Mental retardation

Code in fifth digit: 1 = with other behavioral symptoms (requiring attention or treatment and that are not part of another disorder), 0 = without other behavioral symptoms.
317.0(x) Mild mental retardation, _____
318.0(x) Moderate mental retardation, _____
318.1(x) Severe mental retardation, _____
318.2(x) Profound mental retardation, _____
319.0(x) Unspecified mental retardation, _____

Attention deficit disorder

314.01 with hyperactivity
314.00 without hyperactivity
314.80 residual type

Conduct disorder

312.00 undersocialized, aggressive
312.10 undersocialized, nonaggressive
312.23 socialized, aggressive
312.21 socialized, nonaggressive
312.90 atypical

Anxiety disorders of childhood or adolescence

309.21 Separation anxiety disorder
313.21 Avoidant disorder of childhood or adolescence
313.00 Overanxious disorder

Other disorders of infancy, childhood or adolescence

313.89 Reactive attachment disorder of infancy
313.22 Schizoid disorder of childhood or adolescence
313.23 Elective mutism
313.81 Oppositional disorder
313.82 Identity disorder

Eating disorders

307.10 Anorexia nervosa
307.51 Bulimia
307.52 Pica
307.53 Rumination disorder of infancy
307.50 Atypical eating disorder

Stereotyped movement disorders

307.21 Transient tic disorder
307.22 Chronic motor tic disorder
307.23 Tourette's disorder
307.20 Atypical tic disorder
307.30 Atypical stereotyped movement disorder

Other disorders with physical manifestations

307.00 Stuttering
307.60 Functional enuresis
307.70 Functional encopresis
307.46 Sleepwalking disorder
307.46 Sleep terror disorder (307.49)

Pervasive developmental disorders

Code in fifth digit: 0 = full syndrome present. 1 = residual state.
299.0x Infantile autism, _____
299.9x Childhood onset pervasive developmental disorder, _____
299.8x Atypical, _____

Specific developmental disorders

NOTE: These are coded on Axis II.
315.00 Developmental reading disorder
315.10 Developmental arithmetic disorder
315.31 Developmental langauge disorder
315.39 Developmental articulation disorder
315.50 Mixed specific developmental disorder
315.90 Atypical specific developmental disorder

ORGANIC MENTAL DISORDERS

Section 1. Organic mental disorders whose etiology or pathophysiological process is listed below (taken from the mental disorders section of ICD-9-CM).

Dementias arising in the senium and presenium

Primary degenerative dementia, senile onset
290.30 with delirium
290.20 with delusions
290.21 with depression
290.00 uncomplicated
Code in fifth digit: 1 = with delirium, 2 = with delusions, 3 = with depression, 0 = uncomplicated.
290.1x Primary degenerative dementia, presenile onset, _____
290.4x Multi-infarct dementia, _____

Substance-induced

Alcohol
303.00 intoxication
291.40 idiosyncratic intoxication
291.80 withdrawal
291.00 withdrawal delirium
291.30 hallucinosis
291.10 amnestic disorder
Code severity of dementia in fifth digit: 1 = mild, 2 = moderate, 3 = severe, 0 = unspecified.
291.2x Dementia associated with alcoholism, _____

Barbiturate or similarly acting sedative or hypnotic
305.40 intoxication (327.00)
292.90 withdrawal (327.01)
292.00 withdrawal delirium (327.02)
292.83 amnestic disorder (327.04)

Opioid
305.50 intoxication (327.10)
292.00 withdrawal (327.11)

Cocaine
305.60 intoxication (327.20)

Amphetamine or similarly acting sympathomimetic
305.70 intoxication (327.30)
292.80 delirium (327.32)
292.11 delusional disorder (327.35)
292.00 withdrawal (327.31)

Phencyclidine (PCP) or similarly acting arylcyclohexylamine
305.90 intoxication (327.40)
292.81 delirium (327.42)
292.90 mixed organic mental disorder (327.49)

Hallucinogen
305.30 hallucinosis (327.56)
292.11 delusional disorder (327.55)
292.84 affective disorder (327.57)

Cannabis
305.20 intoxication (327.60)
292.11 delusional disorder (327.65)

Tobacco
292.00 withdrawal (327.71)

Caffeine
305.90 intoxication (327.80)

Other or unspecified substance
305.90 intoxication (327.90)
292.00 withdrawal (327.91)
292.81 delirium (327.92)
292.82 dementia (327.93)
292.83 amnestic disorder (327.94)
292.11 delusional disorder (327.95)
292.12 hallucinosis (327.96)
292.84 affective disorder (327.97)
292.89 personality disorder (327.98)
292.90 atypical or mixed organic mental disorder (327.99)

Section 2. Organic brain syndromes whose etiology or pathophysiological process is either noted as an additional diagnosis from outside the mental disorders section of ICD-9-CM or is unknown.

293.00 Delirium
294.10 Dementia
294.00 Amnestic syndrome
293.81 Organic delusional syndrome
293.82 Organic hallucinosis
293.83 Organic affective syndrome
210.10 Organic personality syndrome
294.80 Atypical or mixed organic brain syndrome

SUBSTANCE USE DISORDERS

Code in fifth digit: 1 = continuous, 2 = episodic, 3 = in remission, 0 = unspecified.
305.0x Alcohol abuse, _____
303.9x Alcohol dependence (Alcoholism), _____
305.4x Barbiturate or similarly acting sedative or hypnotic abuse
304.1x Barbiturate or similarly acting sedative or hypnotic dependence, _____
305.5x Opioid abuse, _____
304.0x Opioid dependence, _____
305.6x Cocaine abuse, _____
305.7x Amphetamine or similarly acting sympathomimetic abuse, _____
304.4x Amphetamine or similarly acting sympathomimetic dependence, _____
305.9x Phencyclidine (PCP) or similarly acting arylcyclohexylamine abuse, _____ (328.4x)
305.3x Hallucinogen abuse, _____
305.2x Cannabis abuse, _____
304.3x Cannabis dependence, _____
305.1x Tobacco dependence, _____
305.9x Other, mixed or unspecified substance abuse, _____
304.6x Other specified substance dependence, _____
304.9x Unspecified substance dependence, _____
304.7x Dependence on combination of opioid and other nonalcoholic substance, _____
304.8x Dependence on combination of substances, excluding opioids and alcohol, _____

SCHIZOPHRENIC DISORDERS

Code in fifth digit: 1 = subchronic, 2 = chronic, 3 = subchronic with acute exacerbation, 4 = chronic with acute exacerbation, 5 = in remission, 0 = unspecified.

Schizophrenia
295.1x disorganized, _____
295.2x catatonic, _____
295.3x paranoid, _____
295.9x undifferentiated, _____
295.6x residual, _____

PARANOID DISORDERS

297.10 Paranoia
297.30 Shared paranoid disorder
298.30 Acute paranoid disorder
297.90 Atypical paranoid disorder

PSYCHOTIC DISORDERS NOT ELSEWHERE CLASSIFIED

295.40 Schizophreniform disorder
298.80 Brief reactive psychosis
295.70 Schizoaffective disorder
298.90 Atypical psychosis

NEUROTIC DISORDERS

These are included in Affective, Anxiety, Somatoform, Dissociative, and Psychosexual Disorders. In order to facilitate the identification of the categories that in DSM-II were grouped together in the class of Neuroses, the DSM-II terms are included separately in parentheses after the corresponding categories. These DSM-II terms are included in ICD-9-CM and therefore are acceptable as alternatives to the recommended DSM-III terms that precede them.

AFFECTIVE DISORDERS
Major affective disorders

Code major depressive episode in fifth digit: 6 = in remission, 4 = with psychotic features (the unofficial non-ICD-9-CM fifth digit 7 may be used instead to indicate that the psychotic features are mood-incongruent), 3 = with melancholia, 2 = without melancholia, 0 = unspecified.

Code manic episode in fifth digit: 6 = in remission, 4 = with psychotic features (the unofficial non-ICD-9-CM fifth digit 7 may be used instead to indicate that the psychotic features are mood-incongruent), 2 = without psychotic features, 0 = unspecified.

Bipolar disorder

296.6x mixed, _____
296.4x manic, _____
296.5x depressed, _____

Major depression

296.2x single episode, _____
296.3x recurrent, _____

Other specific affective disorders

301.13 Cyclothymic disorder
300.40 Dysthymic disorder (or Depressive neurosis)

Atypical affective disorders

296.70 Atypical bipolar disorder
296.82 Atypical depression

ANXIETY DISORDERS

Phobic disorders (or phobic neuroses)

300.21 Agoraphobia with panic attacks
300.22 Agoraphobia without panic attacks
300.23 Social phobia
300.29 Simple phobia

Anxiety states (or anxiety neuroses)

300.01 Panic disorder
300.02 Generalized anxiety disorder
300.30 Obsessive compulsive disorder (or Obsessive compulsive neurosis)

Post-traumatic stress disorder

308.30 acute
309.81 chronic or delayed
300.00 Atypical anxiety disorder

SOMATOFORM DISORDERS

300.81 Somatization disorder
300.11 Conversion disorder (or Hysterical neurosis, conversion type).
307.80 Psychogenic pain disorder
300.70 Hypochondriasis (or Hypochondriacal neurosis)
300.70 Atypical somatoform disorder (300.71)

DISSOCIATIVE DISORDERS (OR HYSTERICAL NEUROSES, DISSOCIATIVE TYPE)

300.12 Psychogenic amnesia
300.13 Psychogenic fugue
300.14 Multiple personality
300.60 Depersonalization disorder (or Depersonalization neurosis)
300.15 Atypical dissociative disorder

PSYCHOSEXUAL DISORDERS
Gender identity disorders

Indicate sexual history in the fifth digit of Transsexualism code: 1 = asexual, 2 = homosexual, 3 = heterosexual, 0 = unspecified.
302.5x Transsexualism, _____
302.60 Gender identity disorder of childhood
302.85 Atypical gender identity disorder

Paraphilias

302.81 Fetishism
302.30 Transvestism
302.10 Zoophilia
302.20 Pedophilia
302.40 Exhibitionism
302.82 Voyeurism
302.83 Sexual masochism
302.84 Sexual sadism
302.90 Atypical paraphilia

Psychosexual dysfunctions

302.71 Inhibited sexual desire
302.72 Inhibited sexual excitement
302.73 Inhibited female orgasm
302.74 Inhibited male orgasm
302.75 Premature ejaculation
302.76 Functional dyspareunia
306.51 Functional vaginismus
302.70 Atypical psychosexual dysfunction

Other psychosexual disorders

302.00 Ego-dystonic homosexuality
302.89 Psychosexual disorder not elsewhere classified

FACTITIOUS DISORDERS

300.16 Factitious disorder with psychological symptoms
301.51 Chronic factitious disorder with physical symptoms
300.19 Atypical factitious disorder with physical symptoms

DISORDERS OF IMPULSE CONTROL NOT ELSEWHERE CLASSIFIED

312.31 Pathological gambling
312.32 Kleptomania
312.33 Pyromania
312.34 Intermittent explosive disorder
312.35 Isolated explosive disorder
312.39 Atypical impulse control disorder

ADJUSTMENT DISORDER

309.00 with depressed mood
309.24 with anxious mood
309.28 with mixed emotional features
309.30 with disturbance of conduct
309.40 with mixed disturbance of emotions and conduct
309.23 with work (or academic) inhibitioin
309.83 with withdrawal
309.90 with atypical features

PSYCHOLOGICAL FACTORS AFFECTING PHYSICAL CONDITION

Specify physical condition on Axis III.
316.00 Psychological factors affecting physical condition

PERSONALITY DISORDERS

NOTE: These are coded on Axis II.

301.00 Paranoid
301.20 Schizoid
301.22 Schizotypal
301.50 Histrionic
301.81 Narcissistic
301.70 Antisocial
301.83 Borderline
301.82 Avoidant
301.60 Dependent
301.40 Compulsive
301.84 Passive-Aggressive
301.89 Atypical, mixed or other personality disorder

V CODES FOR CONDITIONS NOT ATTRIBUTABLE TO A MENTAL DISORDER THAT ARE A FOCUS OF ATTENTION OR TREATMENT

V65.20 Malingering
V62.89 Borderline intellectual functioning (V62.88)
V71.01 Adult antisocial behavior
V71.02 Childhood or adolescent antisocial behavior
V62.30 Academic problem
V62.20 Occupational problem
V62.82 Uncomplicated bereavement
V15.81 Noncompliance with medical treatment
V62.89 Phase of life problem or other life circumstance problem
V61.10 Marital problem
V61.20 Parent-child problem
V61.80 Other specified family circumstances
V62.81 Other interpersonal problem

ADDITIONAL CODES

300.90 Unspecified mental disorder (nonpsychotic)
V71.09 No diagnosis or condition on Axis I
799.90 Diagnosis or condition deferred on Axis I

V71.09 No diagnosis on Axis II
799.90 Diagnosis deferred on Axis II

APPENDIX 11 · Dimensions of pharmacology

11-1. Drug interaction guide

HOW TO USE THE APPENDIX

When the interaction of two or more prescription or over-the-counter (OTC) products is in question, look up each individual product in the index following Chart 18. All prescription drugs are listed by both trade name and corresponding generic name. The trade name refers the reader to the generic name and indicates the charts containing the interaction in question.

Column 4 of each chart lists OTC/food items that may interact with the prescription drugs listed in column 1 to produce side effects noted in the introduction to that chart. Most OTC and household remedies are listed in the charts and may not be listed individually in the index. Chart 1 deals primarily with OTC drugs, household remedies, and their interactions.

Prescription medications primarily used in the injectable form and some anesthetics are listed in Chart 18 and may not be listed individually in the index.

Chart 1 Over-the-counter drug interactions

	Any of these OTC drugs may interact with	➡	any of these OTC/food items as described in introductory material.	
This chart deals strictly with products that can be bought over the counter and points out the potentially hazardous reactions that may occur.	Alcoholic beverages		A.P.C. and A.P.C. Compound	PAC
	Beer		A.S.A., A.S.A. Compound	Pamprin
	Cheracol, Cheracol D		Alka-Seltzer	Phensal
As described in the chart, the combination of alcohol-containing products can increase the damage to the stomach lining and possibly cause blood loss.	Cosanyl-DM		Alka-2	Pyrilamine
	Creo-Terpin, Creo-Terpin Plus		Allerest	Robitussin-AC
	Demazin Syrup		Anacin products	Sinutab
	Dristan Cough Formula		Arthritis Strength Bufferin	Sleep-Eze
Also described in this chart is the combination of alcohol-containing OTC products that, when combined with other OTC antihistamine-containing products, may cause drowsiness. Although some cough and cold remedies cause drowsiness when taken alone, combination compounds the decrease in alertness.	Histadyl E.C.		Ascriptin	Sodium salicylate
	Neo Synephrine Tablets		Aspergum	Sominex
	Novahistine-DH and Novahistine Expectorant		Aspirin	Sudafed Plus
	Nyquil		Bayer products	Triaminic liquids
	Pertussin		Bufferin	Triaminicin
	Robitussin, Robitussin-AC, Robitussin DM		Cama	Triaminicol
	Triaminic Expectorant		Chlorpheniramine products	Vanquish
When selecting a product in the OTC category it is always advisable to evaluate the ingredients to avoid any further complications with other OTC products or prescription medications, as pointed out in this and following charts.	Valadol Liquid		Chlor-Trimeton	Vicks Formula 44 Cough Mixture
	Vicks Formula 44 Cough Mixture		Compoz	
			Conar	
			Contac	
			Coricidin products	
The OTC products that interact with other prescription medications are described in the following charts.			Coryban-D Capsules	
			Demazin	
			Dormin	
			Ecotrin	
			Empirin compound	
			Excedrin	
			4-Way Cold Tablets	
			Histadyl E.C.	
			Measurin	
			Midol	
			Neo-Synephrine Tablets	
			Novahistine products	
			Nyquil	
			Nytol	

Chart 2 Antihistamine interactions

	Any of these prescription drugs may interact with	➡ any of these prescription drug groups	➡ and result in this interaction.	OTC/food items
The drugs listed in Chart 2, column 1, are antihistamines, and antihistamine combinations. The combinations listed usually contain a decongestant such as pseudoephedrine or phenylpropanolamine. Indications, depending on the type of antihistamine, include allergies, nasal congestion and drainage, and watery eyes. Antihistamines are commonly employed to aid in the treatment of nausea, vomiting, dizziness, vertigo, and insomnia. Hydroxyzine (Atarax, Vistaril) is an antihistamine but is also indicated to be useful in the management of pruritus resulting from allergic conditions and contact dermatoses. Antihistamines can potentiate other central nervous system–acting drugs, so special precautions should be exercised when these are used in conjunction, especially with narcotics, barbiturates, and alcohol. Antihistamines may cause anticholinergic effects, such as dry mouth, which could be relieved by chewing gum. Smoking tends to cause further irritation and should be avoided. If nausea or upset stomach is a problem, the medication should be taken with food or milk. The interactions denoted here between antihistamines and OTC drugs should be avoided since an increased potential for severe drowsiness or decrease in mental alertness may occur.	Azatadine (Optimine) Brompheniramine (Dimetane) Chlorpheniramine (Chlor-Trimeton, Teldrin) Clemastine (Tavist) Cyproheptadine (Periactin) Dexchlorpheniramine (Polaramine) Dimetapp Diphenhydramine (Benadryl) Disophrol Drixoral Naldecon Nolamine Novafed-A Ornade Promethazine (Phenergan) Pyribenzamine Tripelennamine (PBZ) Triprolidine (Actidil)	Acenocoumarol (Sintrom) Anisindione (Miradon) Bishydroxycoumarin (Dicumarol) Griseofulvin (Fulvicin, Grifulvin) Oral contraceptives Oxyphenbutazone (Tandearil) Phenindione (Hedulin) Phenprocoumon (Liquamar) Phenylbutazone (Azolid, Butazolidin) Phenytoin (Dilantin) Warfarin (Coumadin) ──────────── Atropine products Belladonna products (Donnatal) Dicyclomine (Bentyl) Furazolidone (Furoxone) Glycopyrrolate (Robinul) Isocarboxazid (Marplan) Pargyline (Eutonyl) Phenelzine (Nardil) Procarbazine (Matulane) Propantheline (Pro-Banthine) Tranylcypromine (Parnate) Trihexphenidyl (Artane)	This interaction can cause a decrease in the effectiveness of the prescription drugs listed in column 2. ──────────── The combination of these medications may cause constipation, dry mouth, blurred vision, urine retention, and possible increased heart rate. Also a possibility of decreased mental alertness may occur. See below for additional prescription drug–prescription drug interactions involving antihistamines listed in column 1.	A.R.M. Alcoholic products Allerest Bayer Decongestant Cold Tablets Beer Cheracol, Cheracol D Coldene Compoz Conar Contac Coricidin Coryban-D Cosanyl-DM Creo-Terpin Demazin Dormin Dristan Dristan Cough Formula Histadyl E.C. Neo-Synephrine Novahistine Nyquil Nytol Pertussin Pyrilamine Robitussin-AC & Robitussin DM Sinutab Sleep-Eze Sominex Super Anahist Tea Plus Triaminicin Triaminicol Vicks Formula 44 products Vicks Sinex products

Chart 2 Antihistamine interactions—cont'd

Any of these prescription drugs may interact with	any of these prescription drug groups ▶	and result in this interaction. ▶	OTC/food items

Azatadine (Optimine) Brompheniramine (Dimetane) Chlorpheniramine (Chlor-Trimeton, Teldrin) Clemastine (Tavist) Cyproheptadine (Periactin) Dexchlorpheniramine (Polaramine) Dimetapp Diphenhydramine (Benadryl) Disophrol Drixoral Naldecon Nolamine Novafed-A Ornade Promethazine (Phenergan) Pyribenzamine Tripelennamine (PBZ) Triprolidine (Actidil)	Amobarbital (Amytal) Chloral hydrate (Noctec) Chlordiazepoxide (Librium) Chlorpromazine (Thorazine) Clonazepam (Clonopin) Clorazepate (Tranxene, Azene) Codeine-containing products Cyclobenzaprine (Flexeril) Diazepam (Valium) Esgic Ethchlorvynol (Placidyl) Fiorinal Fluphenazine (Prolixin) Flurazepam (Dalmane) Glutethimide (Doriden) Hydroxyzine (Atarax, Vistaril) Librax Limbitrol Lorazepam (Ativan) Meprobamate (Equanil, Miltown) Oxazepam (Serax) Oxybutynin (Ditropan) Pentobarbital (Nembutal) Perphenazine (Trilafon) Phenobarbital (Luminal) Prazepam (Centrax) Prochlorperazine (Compazine) Promazine (Sparine) Propoxyphene (Darvon, Darvocet) Secobarbital (Seconal) Thioridazine (Mellaril) Thiothixene (Navane) Triclofos (Triclos) Trifluoperazine (Stelazine) Tuinal	The combination of the medications listed in column 2 with the drugs in column 1 could cause an increase in the likelihood of central nervous system depression.
		
		   Such a combination could result in drowsiness, dizziness, blurred vision, loss of appetite, and a decrease in mental alertness.
		
		   Caution must be exercised if operating any type of machinery or driving. It is not advisable to drink alcoholic beverages while taking any of these medications as this may compound the problem of adverse side effects.	

Chart 3 Antidiabetic drug interactions

	Any of these prescription drugs may interact with	any of these prescription drug groups ▶	and result in this interaction. ▶	OTC/ food items
The hypoglycemic agents listed in Chart 3, column 1, aside from insulin, are sulfonamide derivatives devoid of antibacterial effects. These oral agents aid in the stimulation of synthesis of endogenous insulin in the patient with functional pancreatic beta cells.	Acetohexamide (Dymelor) Chlorpropamide (Diabinese) Insulin Tolazamide (Tolinase) Tolbutamide (Orinase)	Acetazolamide (Diamox) Bendroflumethiazide (Naturetin) Benzthiazide (Exna) Chlorothiazide (Diuril) Chlorthalidone (Hygroton) Dichlorphenamide (Daranide) Ethacrynic acid (Edecrin) Ethoxyzolamide (Cardrase, Ethamide) Furosemide (Lasix) Hydrochlorothiazide (Esidrix, HydroDiuril) Methazolamide (Neptazane) Methyclothiazide (Enduron) Metolazone (Diulo, Zaroxolyn) Polythiazide (Renese) Quinethazone (Hydromox) Steroids (Prednisone) Trichlormethiazide (Metahydrin, Naqua)	Reaction may cause an increase in blood glucose level, which could result in excessive thirst and urination (hyperglycemic effect). Drugs in column 2 may work against diabetic medication in column 1. Notify physician if loss of appetite, nausea, or vomiting is noticed. See Chart 7 for additional listing of steroids that can cause this same effect.	Alcoholic beverages Beer Cheracol and Cheracol D Coldene Coryban-D Cosanyl-DM Creo-Terpin Demazin Syrup Dristan Cough Formula Histadyl E.C. Neo-Synephrine Elixir Novahistine-DH and Novahistine Expectorant Nyquil Pertussin Robitussin, Robitussin-AC, and Robitussin DM Triaminic Expectorant Valadol Liquid Vicks Formula 44 Cough Mixture
Contraindications include fever, infections, surgery for severe trauma, ketosis, acidosis, coma, and pregnancy. Transient side effects may include loss of appetite, nausea, and stomach upset. Prolonged discomfort, sore throat, low fever, diarrhea, or dark urine may warrant a change in dosage or discontinuation of the medication. The OTC interactions denoted here involve the cough and cold preparations that could alter the dosage or increase the potential for nausea or stomach upset. Alcoholic beverages should always be avoided, and aspirin or salicylate products could also lower one's blood glucose level when used in combination with these medications.		Alcoholic products Clofibrate (Atromids) Furazolidone (Furoxone) Guanethidine (Ismelin Sulfate) Isocarboxazid (Marplan) Metoprolol (Lopressor) Nadolol (Corgard) Oxyphenbutazone (Tandearil) Pargyline (Eutonyl) Phenelzine (Nardil) Phenylbutazone (Azolid, Butazolidin) Procarbazine (Matulane) Propranolol (Inderal) Tranylcypromine (Parnate)	Reaction may cause a decrease in blood glucose level leading to hunger (excessive), numbness, fatigue, headache, drowsiness, or sweating (hypoglycemic effect). If this occurs use candy or lump sugar to offset this adverse reaction.	

Chart 4 Anticoagulant interactions

The medications listed in Chart 4	Any of these prescription drugs may interact with	any of these prescription drug groups	and result in this interaction.	OTC/ food items

The medications listed in Chart 4, column 1, are probably the most critical group to monitor in terms of interactions. Since these agents are highly but weakly bound to plasma protein (albumin), a significant potential for displacing these drugs by other drugs exists. Even though a particular drug is known to interact with an anticoagulant, it is often difficult to predict a certain patient's response, and thus close monitoring of the patient is mandatory.

The in vivo effect of depressing factors VII, IX, X, and II (prothrombin) depends on the dosage of the drug administered. Oral anticoagulants have no effect on established thrombosis and do not reverse any tissue damage. The aim of treatment is to prevent further complications.

Adverse reactions range from prolonged or excessive bleeding from nose, gums, and cuts to black stools, vomiting, unusual menstrual flow, prolonged diarrhea, headaches, fever, and loss of appetite.

The description of the OTC interactions listed here are described in column 3.

Column 2 — Any of these prescription drugs may interact with:
Acenocoumarol (Sintrom)
Anisindione (Miradon)
Bishydroxy-coumarin (Dicumarol)
Phenindione (Hedulin)
Phenprocoumon (Liquamar)
Warfarin (Coumadin)

Column 3 — any of these prescription drug groups:
Acetohexamide (Dymelor)
Allopurinol (Zyloprim)
Chloral hydrate (Noctec)
Chlorpropamide (Diabinese)
Cimetidine (Tagamet)
Clofibrate (Atromid-S)
Methandrostenolone (Dianabol)
Naldixic acid (NegGram)
Oxymetholone (Anadrol)
Oxyphenbutazone (Oxalid, Tandearil)
Phenylbutazone (Azolid, Butazolidin)
Sulfinpyrazone (Anturane)
Thyroid preparations
Tolazamide (Tolinase)
Tolbutamide (Orinase)

Column 4 — and result in this interaction:
Drug interaction may result in an increased likelihood of increasing the activity of the anticoagulant drugs listed in column 1. See Chart 16 for analgesics that may cause this same effect.

Amobarbital (Amytal)
Butabarbital (Butisol)
Carbamazepine (Tegretol)
Ethchlorvynol (Placidyl)
Glutethimide (Doriden)
Pentobarbital (Nembutal)
Phenobarbital (Luminal)
Rifampin (Rifadin, Rimactane)
Secobarbital (Seconal)
Tuinal
Vitamin K (Synkayvite)

Other prescription drugs including antihistamines (Chart 2), steroids (Chart 7), and alcoholic beverages could produce unpredictable responses to medication, and a physician should be consulted before using these drugs.

Drug interaction may result in an increased likelihood of decreasing the activity of the anticoagulant drugs listed in column 1. See the diuretics (Chart 10) and oral contraceptives (Chart 6), which may cause this same result.

Column 5 — OTC/ food items:
The OTC drugs listed could increase the activity of therapeutic medication and lead to excessive bleeding. The foods listed are high in vitamin K and could reduce the effectiveness of an anticoagulant drug.
A.S.A. and A.S.A. Compound
Aspirin
Alka-Seltzer and Alka-Seltzer Plus.
Alka-2
A.P.C.
Arthritis Strength Bufferin
Ascriptin & Ascriptin A/D
Aspergum
Bayer products
Bufferin
Cama
Coricidin products
Dristan Tablets
Ecotrin
Empirin compound
Excedrin and Excedrin PM
4-Way Cold Tablets
Measurin
Midol
PAC
Pamprin
Phensal
Sodium salicylate
Sominex
Super Anahist
Triaminicin Tablets
Vanquish
Leafy green vegetables, for example, cabbage, spinach, kale, cauliflower, alfalfa

Chart 5 Antiparkinsonism drug interactions

	Any of these prescription drugs may interact with	any of these prescription drug groups ▶	and result in this ▶ interaction.	OTC/ food items
The medications listed in Chart 5, column 1, are referred to as "antiparkinsonism agents." Since the depletion of dopamine in the brain can cause the involuntary movements, levodopa products are used to cross the blood-brain barrier and then are converted to dopamine. Dopamine itself does not cross the barrier.	Levodopa products Bendopa Bio/DOPA Dopar Larodopa L-Dopa Parda Sinemet	Furazolidone (Furoxone) Isocarboxazid (Marplan) Pargyline (Eutonyl) Phenelzine (Nardil) Procarbazine (Matulane) Tranylcypromine (Parnate)	The mixing of antidepressant or antianxiety agents with the medications listed in column 1 may cause a severe increase in blood pressure, flushing, and palpitations.	Allbee-T Beminal-500 Corn Cynal Hexa-Betalin Liver Orexin Pyridoxine tablets Stresstabs 600 Trophite Vio-Bec Vitamin B complex Vitamin B_6 tablets Yeast
In the combination product (Sinemet), carbidopa aids in preventing the systemic decomposition of levodopa, thus allowing more medication to reach the brain. These medications should be used with caution or not at all in patients with a history of peptic ulcers or those who are pregnant or nursing. The OTC interactions here involve reducing or reversing the beneficial effects of levodopa products when combined with foods or drugs containing pyridoxine (vitamin B_6). If a vitamin supplement is necessary, Larobec is one product formulated not to contain any pyridoxine.		Chlorpromazine (Thorazine) Fluphenazine (Prolixin) Haloperidol (Haldol) Mesoridazine (Serentil) Perphenazine (Trilafon) Piperacetazine (Quide) Prochlorperazine (Compazine) Promazine (Sparine) Thioridazine (Mellaril) Trifluoperazine (Stelazine) Triflupromazine (Vesprin)	Various phenothiazine tranquilizers may block or diminish the effectiveness of the prescription medications in column 1. Other tranquilizers should be used with caution. Methyldopa (Aldomet) may increase dopa products' effect, while phenytoin (Dilantin) and papaverine (Pavabid) may diminish the effects. See Chart 13 for additional antianxiety agents that could also cause decreased effects of prescription drugs in column 1.	

Chart 6 Oral contraceptive interactions

	Any of these prescription drugs may interact with	any of these prescription drug groups	and result in this interaction.	OTC/ food items
The oral contraceptives suppress ovulation by increasing the level of estrogen and progestin, which inhibit the follicle-stimulating hormone and luteinizing hormone. Oral contraceptives are also employed for their supplemental effect in other conditions. These medications should not be used if any of the following conditions are present or suspected: breast cancer, history of cerebrovascular accidents, neoplasms, pregnancy, nursing, or abnormal vaginal bleeding. The individual package insert should be consulted for additional warnings and precautions. Cigarette smoking increases the risk of serious cardiovascular side effects with estrogens and should be avoided. These risks also increase with age and amount of smoking. The first group of OTC interactions denoted here involves those vitamins that may be depleted when taking contraceptives and should be corrected by supplementing diet with an OTC product containing these vitamins. The second group, vitamin A products, if taken in excess, could lead to an accumulation of vitamin A within the system.	Brevicon Demulen Enovid Locstrin ModiCon Norinyl Norlestrin Ortho-Novum Ovcon Ovral Ovulen	Ampicillin (Polycillin, Principen) Antihistamines (see Chapter 2) Oxyphenbutazone (Tandearil) Phenylbutazone (Azolid, Butazolidin) Phenytoin (Dilantin) Rifampin (Rifadin, Rimactane)	An increased possibility of breakthrough bleeding or spotting and decrease in the effectiveness of the pill may occur. Another form of contraception may be advisable in these instances. When combining these interacting drugs see Chart 2, column 1, for detailed list of antihistamines that may cause the same effect.	Cyanocobalamin (vitamin B_{12}) Folic acid Pyridoxine (vitamin B_6) Vitamin E Vitamin A products: Adabee Cod liver oil concentrate Dayalets Mi-Cebrin Myadec Optilets-500 Super-D products Theragran Vitamin A
		Acenocoumarol (Sintrom) Anisindione (Miradon) Bishydroxycoumarin (Dicumarol) Phenindione (Hedulin) Phenprocoumon (Liquamar) Warfarin (Coumadin)	The blood-thinning drugs listed in column 2 may be decreased in their effectiveness. Onset and cessation of bleeding should be closely monitored.	

Chart 7 Steroid interactions

	Any of these prescription drugs may interact with	any of these prescription drug groups	and result in this interaction.	OTC/food items

The medications listed in Chart 7, column 1, are referred to as "steroids," or more specifically, adrenocortical steroids. With the exception of fludrocortisone they are all glucocorticoids.

Indications include endocrine, rheumatic, allergic, dermatologic, ophthalmic, respiratory, hematologic, and neoplastic conditions. Individual drug monographs should be consulted.

Stressful situations, vaccinations, and surgery should be avoided while receiving steroid therapy. Patients predisposed to ulcers or who are pregnant or nursing require special monitoring or discontinuance of steroid medication, which is primarily completed by a gradual decrease in the dosage.

Adverse reactions that may require immediate medical attention involve, but are not limited to, sodium and fluid retention, muscle weakness, nausea, persistent thirst, frequent urination, increased intraocular pressure, and blurred vision.

The salicylate- or alcohol-containing OTCs listed here can complicate and increase the potential for nausea, ulceration, or decrease in the steroid effectiveness.

Betamethasone (Celestone)
Cortisone (Cortone)
Dexamethasone (Decadron, Hexadrol)
Fludrocortisone (Florinef)
Hydrocortisone (Cortef, Hydrocortone)
Methylprednisolone (Medrol)
Prednisolone (Delta-Cortef)
Prednisone (Deltasone, Meticorten)
Triamcinolone (Aristocort, Kenacort)

Acetazolamide (Diamox)
Bendroflumethiazide (Naturetin)
Benzthiazide (Exna)
Chlorothiazide (Diuril)
Chlorthalidone (Hygroton)
Dichlorphenamide (Daranide)
Digifortis (Pil-Digis)
Digitoxin (Crystodigin, Purodigin)
Digoxin (Lanoxin)
Ethacrynic acid (Edecrin)
Ethoxzolamide (Cardrase, Ethamide)
Furosemide (Lasix)
Gitalin (Gitaligin)
Hydrochlorothiazide (Esidrix, HydroDiuril)
Methazolamide (Neptazane)
Methyclothiazide (Enduron)
Metolazone (Diulo, Zaroxolyn)
Polythiazide (Renese)
Quinethazone (Hydromox)
Trichlormethiazide (Metahydrin, Naqua)

This combination may cause an increase in the effect of the heart medications in column 2. Too much potassium may be lost, and a physician should be notified if shortness of breath, fatigue, prolonged nausea, abdominal pain, cramps, and blurred vision are noticed. The diuretics listed in column 2 may also increase loss of potassium, so it is imperative to have frequent checkups. See Charts 3 and 9 for additional steroid reactions.

Amobarbital (Amytal)
Chloral hydrate (Noctec, Somnos)
Flurazepam (Dalmane)
Glutethimide (Doriden)
Pentobarbital (Nembutal)
Secobarbital (Seconal)
Tuinal

The sedatives or hypnotics (sleeping medications) listed in column 2 may reduce a steroid's effectiveness.

OTC/food items:

A.P.C. and A.P.C. Compound
A.S.A. and A.S.A. Compound
Alcoholic products
Alka-Seltzer
Alka-2
Allerest
Anacin products
Arthritis Strength Bufferin
Ascriptin
Aspergum
Aspirin
Bayer products
Bufferin
Cama
Chlorpheniramine products
Chlor-Trimeton
Compoz
Conar
Contac
Coricidin products
Coryban-D Capsules
Demazin
Dormin
Ecotrin
Empirin compound
Excedrin
4-Way Cold Tablets
Histadyl E.C.
Measurin
Midol
Neo-Synephrine Tablets
Novahistine products
Nyquil
Nytol
PAC
Pamprin
Phensal
Pyrilamine
Robitussin-AC
Sinutab
Sleep-Eze
Sodium salicylate
Sominex
Sudafed Plus
Triaminic liquids
Triaminicin
Triaminicol
Vanquish
Vicks Formula 44 Cough Mixture

Chart 8 Antispasmodic interactions

	Any of these prescription drugs may interact with	any of these prescription drug ➤ groups	and result in this ➤ interaction.	OTC/food items
The prescription drugs listed in Chart 8, column 1, are referred to as "antispasmodics." Most of these products are used in gastrointestinal disorders, yet some are used primarily in urinary, kidney, and allergic disorders. Since these products may cause some drowsiness, dizziness, or blurred vision, the CNS depressants should be avoided. If dryness of the mouth occurs, relief could be accomplished by chewing gum. If this persists or if a skin rash, flushing, or eye pain develops, further medical attention is necessary. Some of these drugs can decrease perspiration, which could lead to fever or heat stroke, so it is advisable to remain, when possible, in a cool environment. Antacids, if used along with any of these products, should not be taken at the same time. An hour or two should be allowed between them. The OTC interactions noted here can compound the problem of dry mouth, blurred vision, or drowsiness, and these product combinations should be avoided if possible.	Atropine products Belladonna products Benztropin mesylate (Cogentin) Dicyclomine (Bentyl) Glycopyrrolate (Robinul) Librax Propantheline (Pro-Banthine) Trihexyphenidyl (Artane)	Amitriptyline (Elavil, Endep) Chlorpromazine (Thorazine) Cyclobenzaprine (Flexeril) Desipramine (Norpramin, Pertofrane) Disopyramide (Norpace) Haloperidol (Haldol) Imipramine (Tofranil) Meperidine (Demerol) Nortriptyline (Aventyl) Oxybutynin (Ditropan) Prochlorperazine (Compazine) Quinidine (Cin-Quin)	The combination of these medications may cause constipation, dryness of mouth, blurred vision, urine retention, and possible increased heart rate. If to combine the drugs must be used in combination, physician may need to reduce the dose of one or both drugs. Refer to Chart 2 for additional interactions of antispasmodics and antihistamines.	Allerest A.R.M. Bayer Decongestant Cold Tablets Chlorpheniramine Chlor-Trimeton Compoz Conar Contac Coricidin Coryban-D Capsules Demazin Dormin Dristan Histadyl E.C. Neo-Synephrine Tablets Novahistine products Nyquil Nytol Pyrilamine Robitussin-AC Sinutab Sleep-Eze Sominex Super Anahist Tea Plus Triaminic liquids Triaminicin Triaminicol Vicks Formula 44 Cough Mixture Vicks Sinex products

Chart 9 Heart medication interactions

	Any of these prescription drugs may interact with	➡ any of these prescription drug groups	➡ and result in this interaction.	OTC/food items
The medications listed in Chart 9, column 1, are referred to as "cardiac glycosides." They increase the force of myocardial contraction and the refractory period of the atrioventricular (A-V) node. Indications include congestive heart failure, atrial fibrillation, flutter, and tachycardia, but these medications are contraindicated in ventricular fibrillation. Lowered potassium levels sensitize the myocardium to the glycosides, and toxic levels may be reached even with usual dosages. Many arrhythmias for which digitalis is advised closely resemble those reflecting toxic digitalis levels. Nausea and vomiting may also be associated with toxic levels, along with a loss of appetite, weakness, diarrhea, blurred vision, and yellow or green halos around objects. The first group of OTC interactions involves antacids, which, if taken *at the same time,* could decrease the effectiveness of the glycoside. The second group of antiasthmatic products could cause or complicate arrhythmias while a patient is undergoing digitalis therapy.	Digifortis (Pil-Digis) Digitoxin (Crystodigin, Purodigin) Digoxin (Lanoxin) Gitalin (Gitaligin)	Acetazolamide (Diamox) Bendroflu-methiazide (Naturetin) Benthiazide (Exna) Chlorothiazide (Diuril) Chlorthalidone (Hygroton) Dichlorphenamide (Daranide) Ethacrynic acid (Edecrin) Ethoxzolamide (Cardrase, Ethamide) Furosemide (Lasix) Hydrochlorthiazide (Esidrix, HydroDiuril) Methazolamide (Neptazane) Methyclothiazide (Enduron) Metolazone (Diulo, Zaroxolyn) Polythiazide (Renese) Quinethazone (Hydromox) Trichlormethiazide (Metahydrin, Naqua)	Although these drugs are sometimes used together, there is a possibility of a decreasing potassium level, which could lead to toxic levels of a heart pill. A physician should be notified if any of the signs explained in the introduction to Chart 9 or leg cramps are noticed. Steroids (Chart 7) and licorice may also cause a loss in potassium. See Chart 10 for more information on the diuretics listed in column 2. If any potassium supplements (KCl, Kato, K-Lyte, Kaon, Kaochlor, and so on) must be taken, checkups should be frequent to ensure that levels are not too high.	Aludrox Aluminum hydroxide Amphojel Anacin Arthritis Formula Antacids Ascriptin Camalox Dristan Gelusil Kaolin/pectin (Kaopectate) Maalox Magnesium hydroxide Magnesium trisilicate Milk of Magnesia Mylanta Adrenalin Asthmanefrin Breatheasy Bronkaid Mist Epinephrine Histadyl E.C. Medihaler-EPI Primatene Mist Solution A Vaponefrin Va-Tro-Nol
		Metoprolol (Lopressor) Nadolol (Corgard) Propranolol (Inderal) Phenytoin (Dilantin) Reserpine (Serpasil) Reserpine combination (see Chart 11)	The drugs in column 2 are sometimes used together with heart medications, yet could result in irregular heartbeat. Pulse should be taken regularly and any changes in pulse or persistent dizziness should be reported to a physician. See Chart 3 for additional reactions on some of the prescription drugs in column 2.	

Chart 10 Diuretic interactions

	Any of these prescription drugs may interact with	➤ any of these prescription drug groups	➤ and result in this interaction.	OTC/food items
The medications listed in Chart 10, column 1, are referred to as "diuretics." The range of indication includes, but is not limited to, hypertension, edema, cardiac conditions, and renal dysfunction. The carbonic anhydrase inhibitors listed are also sometimes employed in the treatment of glaucoma. The thiazide diuretics tend to cause a depletion of potassium and sodium; thus, close monitoring of potassium levels is necessary, especially in cardiac conditions requiring digitalis therapy. Lowered potassium levels may be indicated by weakness, leg cramping, and joint or foot pain. Spironolactone (Aldactone Aldactazide) and triamterene (Dyazide, Dyrenium) are used to help conserve the loss of potassium, and additional potassium ion supplements may not be necessary or even harmful. The OTC alcoholic interactions denoted here involve products that could increase the potential for severe hypotension and drowsiness. The decongestant products listed could negate the antihypertensive effect or cause an increase in blood pressure.	Acetazolamide (Diamox) Bendroflumethiazide (Naturetin) Benthiazide (Exna) Chlorothiazide (Diuril) Chlorthalidone (Hygroton) Dichlorphenamide (Daranide) Ethacrynic acid (Edecrin) Ethoxzolamide (Cardrase, Ethamide) Furosemide (Lasix) Hydrochlorthiazide (Esidrix, HydroDiuril) Methazolamide (Neptazane) Methyclothiazide (Enduraon) Metolazone (Diulo, Zaroxolyn) Polythiazide (Renese) Quinethazone (Hydromox) Trichlormethiazide (Metahydrin, Naqua)	Digifortis (Pil-Digis) Digitoxin (Crystodigin, Purodigin) Digoxin (Lanoxin) Gitalin (Gitaligin) Acenocoumarol (Sintrom) Anisindione (Miradon) Bishydroxycoumarin (Dicumarol) Phenindione (Hedulin) Phenprocoumon (Liquamar) Warfarin (Coumadin) See Chart 11 for additional prescription drugs used for high blood pressure (antihypertensives).	Although this combination of a heart tablet (column 2 drugs) with a diuretic is often used to treat various illnesses, the diuretic could decrease the potassium level, which could lead to toxic levels of the heart pill. Frequent checkups are recommended, and a physician should be notified if any weakness, leg cramps, shortness of breath, abdominal pain, or blurred or yellow vision is noticed. See Chart 9 for other heart medication interactions. See Charts 3, 4, and 7 for diuretic interactions. Drug interactions could result in an increased likelihood of decreasing the activity of the anticoagulant drugs in column 2. See Chart 4 for more anticoagulant interactions. Lithium (Eskalith) should be used with caution when combined with diuretics.	Adrenalin Alcoholic products Alconefrin Allerest capsules and spray A.R.M. Asthmanefrin Bayer Decongestant Breatheasy Bromo-Quinine Bronkaid Caffeine Coffee Coldene Contac Coricidin Cough Syrup and Nasal Mist Coricidin-D Coryban-D Cosanyl-DM Demazine Repetabs & Syrup Dimacol Dristan tablets, capsules, and liquid Epinephrine Fedrazil 4-Way Cold Tablets and Nasal Spray Histadyl E.C. Medihaler-EPI Neo-Synephrine products No Doz Novahistine products Nyquil Ornacol Ornex Orthoxicol Phenylephrine Phenylpropanolamine Primatene Privine Romilar Cough Syrup Sinutab Cold Tablets and Sinutab II Solution A Sudafed Super Anahist Tea Tea Plus Triaminic products Triaminicol Trind Ursinus Va-Tro-Nol Vicks Inhaler

Chart 11 Antihypertensive interactions

	Any of these prescription drugs may interact with ➤	any of these prescription drug groups ➤	and result in this interaction. ➤	OTC/ food items
The medications listed in Chart 11, column 1, are referred to as "antihypertensives." The diuretic antihypertensives are discussed in Chart 10. When initiating therapy, transient drowsiness or dizziness may occur, and thus the patient should avoid sudden changes in posture and balance. If medications are changed or discontinued, it is advisable to gradually reduce the dosage over a period of days. Adverse reactions that may require further medical attention might include persistent hypotension, fever, fatigue, chills, sore throat, diarrhea, or swelling. The following antihypertensives are listed in other charts: clonidine (Catapres, Combipres) (see Chart 14), metoprolol (Lopressor), nadolol (Corgard), and propranolol (Inderal) (see Charts 3 and 9). The OTC interactions denoted here involve products that could cause or complicate severe drowsiness and dizziness. OTC cold remedies that contain a decongestant should be avoided since an unpredictable response may occur. This should be explained to any patient taking reserpine products, since these naturally tend to cause nasal congestion. A saline nasal spray may be the only product necessary to control this problem without further complications.	Guanethidine (Esimil, Ismelin) Hydralazine (Apresazide, Apresoline) Methyldopa (Aldomet, Aldoril) Reserpine (Serpasil, Reserpoid) Reserpine combinations: Demi-Regroton Diupres Diutensin-R Exna-R Hydropres Hydroserpine Metatensin Naquival Regroton Salutensin Ser-Ap-Es	Furazolidone (Furoxone) Isocarboxazid (Marplan) Pargyline (Eutonyl) Phenelzine (Nardil) Procarbazine (Matulane) Tranylcypromine (Parnate)	This combination may result in a severe increase in blood pressure, fever, convulsion, or dizziness. A physician should be notified if persistent headache, sore throat, diarrhea, or any irregular heartbeat is noticed. See also Chart 15 for other antidepressants that could cause a change in blood pressure when used in combination. Although combinations of different antihypertensive drugs are used together to aid in the control of blood pressure, certain combinations should be avoided or monitored very closely. Propranolol, metoprolol, and nadolol may interact with prazosin (Minipress) or reserpine and reserpine combinations. Hydralazine may interact with minoxidil (Loniten). These reactions could produce severe low blood pressure with resultant dizziness or produce irregular heartbeat.	Alcoholic beverages Beer Cheracol Coryban-D Cosanyl-DM Creo-Terpin Demazin Dristan Cough Formula Histadyl E.C. Neo-Synephrine tablets Novahistine products Nyquil Pertussin Robitussin Triaminic Expectorant Vicks Formula 44 Cough Mixture

Chart 12 Antibiotic interactions

	Any of these prescription drugs may interact with	▶ any of these prescription drug groups	▶ and result in this interaction.	OTC/ food items
The medications listed in Chart 12, column 1, are referred to as "tetracycline" or "tetracycline-combination antibiotics." The combination products contain an antifungal agent to help decrease or eliminate the severity of a diarrhea side effect in those susceptible.	Achromycin V Achrostatin V Bristacycline Cyclopar Kesso-Tetra Mysteclin-F Panmycin QID Tet Robitet SK-Tetracycline Sumycin Tetrachel Tetracycline Tetracyn Tetrex V-Tet	Ampicillin (Polycillin, Principen) Bactocill Cloxacillin (Tegopen) Dicloxacillin (Dycill, Dynapen) Oxacillin (Prostaphlin) Penicillin Penicillin G potassium (Pentids) Penicillin V potassium (Ledercillin, Pen·Vee K, V-Cillin K, Veetids)	A decrease in the effectiveness of the drugs in either column 1 or 2 may occur. The mixing of these drugs should be avoided unless otherwise directed.	Iron preparations Fer-In-Sol Ferrous sulfate Milk & dairy products Antacids & products containing calcium, aluminum, or magnesium Alka-Seltzer Plus Alka-2 Aludrox Aluminum hydroxide Amphojel Anacin Arthritis Formula
Skin sensitivity to the burning rays of the sun is a common occurrence when taking these medications; it is therefore advisable to use a sunscreen agent for protection. Avoidance of these medications is advisable if one is pregnant or nursing. They should also be avoided in infants and young children to prevent any damage to tooth enamel or discoloration of the teeth. Dosage should be taken on an empty stomach, 1 hour before a meal or 2 hours after, unless otherwise directed. A change in medication or dosage may be indicated if severe diarrhea or skin rash occurs. The OTC interactions denoted here involve products that may comply with the tetracycline product and thus result in a decrease in absorption with resultant lower therapeutic levels of the antibiotic.		Acenocoumarol (Sintrom) Anisindione (Miradon) Bishydroxycoumarin (Dicumarol) Phenindione (Hedulin) Phenprocoumon (Liquamar) Warfarin (Coumadin)	An increase in the effect of the blood-thinning drugs in column 2 may occur, which could result in hemorrhage or unusual bleeding.	Ascriptin Bufferin Calcium Calcium carbonate Cama Camalox Creamalin Dicarbosil Antacid Tablets Di-Gel Dristan Tablets Gelusil Maalox & Maalox Plus Magnesium hydroxide Magnesium trisilicate Milk of Magnesia Mylanta and Mylanta III Rolax Titralac Triaminicin Tums Vanquish

Chart 13 Antianxiety medication and sedative interactions

	Any of these prescription drugs may interact with	any of these prescription drug groups	and result in this interaction.	OTC/ food items

Although the medications listed in Chart 13, column 1, include antianxiety drugs, sedatives, hypnotics, antipsychotics, and tranquilizers, they are grouped this way since they have similar or common interactions.

The therapeutic indications of these groups involve, but are not limited to, allergic disorders, nausea, tension, insomnia, muscular disorders, and epilepsy. Other anticonvulsants may also interact in a similar manner as these agents; therefore a full package insert should be consulted.

An adjustment in dosage or medication may be warranted if excessive drowsiness, fatigue, difficulty in concentrating, dizziness, nightmares, irritability, muscle spasm, or dependence develops or if the patient becomes pregnant.

Combination of any of the column 1 drugs may increase central nervous system depression and should be avoided if possible.

The OTC interactions involved here increase the potential for severe central nervous system depression and may still cause this effect a day or two after the prescription medication has been discontinued. Caution should be exercised when in any activity requiring mental alertness.

Any of these prescription drugs may interact with

Amobarbital (Amytal)
Chloral hydrate (Noctec)
Chlordiazepoxide (Limbitrol, Librium)
Chlorpromazine (Thorazine)
Clonazepam (Clonopin)
Clorazepate (Azene, Tranzene)
Diazepam (Valium)
Ethchlorvynol (Placidyl)
Fluphenazine (Prolixin)
Flurazepam (Dalmane)
Glutethimide (Doriden)
Hydroxyzine (Atarax, Vistaril)
Lorazepam (Ativan)
Meprobamate (Equanil, Miltown)
Oxazepam (Serax)
Pentobarbital (Nembutal)
Perphenazine (Trilafon)
Phenobarbital (Luminal)
Prazepam (Centrax)
Prochlorperazine (Compazine)
Promazine (Sparine)
Secobarbital (Seconal, Tuinal)
Triclofos (Triclos)
Trifluoperazine (Stelazine)
Thioridazine (Mellaril)
Thiothixene (Navane)

any of these prescription drug groups

Amitriptyline (Elavil, Endep)
Amoxapine (Asendin)
Cyclobenzaprine (Flexeril)
Desipramine (Norpramin, Pertofrane)
Doxepin (Adapin, Sinequan)
Etrafon
Imipramine (Tofranil)
Limbitrol
Maprotiline (Ludiomil)
Nortriptyline (Aventyl, Pamelor)
Triavil
Trimipramine (Surmontil)

and result in this interaction.

The combination of the drugs in column 1 with any of the medications in column 2 may increase the likelihood of central nervous system depression. This may cause confusion, depression, drowsiness, unusual weakness, slurred speech, headache, or lack of mental alertness. A person taking these medications, whether a drug in column 1, a drug in column 2, or a combination of drugs in both columns, should be familiar with his or her reaction to the medication before driving or undertaking a job requiring mental alertness.

See Chart 2, column 1, drugs, the antihistamines, which could also cause severe nervous system depression and drowsiness if combined with the medications in column 1.

OTC/ food items

Alcoholic products
Allerest
A.R.M.
Bayer Decongestant Cold Tablets
Beer
Cheracol & Cheracol D
Coldene
Compoz
Conar
Contac
Coridin
Coryban-D
Cosanyl-DM
Creo-Terpin
Demazin
Dormin
Dristan & Dristan Cough Formula
Histadyl E.C.
Neo-Synephrine
Novahistine
Nyquil
Nytol
Pertussin
Pyrilamine
Robitussin-AC & Robitussin-DM
Sinutab
Sleep-Eze
Sominex
Super Anahist
Synephricol
Tea Plus
Triaminicin
Triaminicol
Vicks Formula 44 Cough Mixture
Vicks Sinex

Chart 14 Antidepressants-I interactions

	Any of these prescription drugs may interact with	any of these prescription drug groups ➤	and result in this interaction. ➤	OTC/food items
The medications listed in Chart 14, column 1, are referred to as "antidepressants." Some of these medications also have antianxiety effects. Others may be used in enuresis, and one is primarily a muscle relaxant but interacts like a tricyclic. Often these medications may require up to 4 weeks of therapy before noticeable improvement may be seen. Discontinuance of therapy should be gradual to avoid headache or nausea. Transient drowsiness or dryness of the mouth may be experienced when first beginning these medications. If a sore throat develops, further medical attention may be required to adjust or discontinue medication. Drowsiness or blurred vision may occur, which may be transient. Persons predisposed to glaucoma should be monitored closely. The OTC interactions involving alcohol-containing products may result in an increased potential for severe drowsiness and decreased mental alertness. An unpredictable response to the sympathomimetics may occur when combined with the prescription drugs in column 1.	Amitriptyline (Elavil, Endep) Amoxapine (Asendin) Cyclobenzaprine (Flexeril) Desipramine (Norpramin, Pertofrane) Doxepin (Adapin, Sinequan) Etrafon Imipramine (Tofranil) Limbitrol Maprotiline (Ludiomil) Nortriptyline (Aventyl, Pamelor) Triavil Trimipramine (Surmontil)	Clonidine (Catapres, Combipres) Guanethidine (Esimil, Ismelin) <hr>Furazolidone (Furoxone) Isocarboxazid (Marplan) Pargyline (Eutonyl) Phenelzine (Nardil) Procarbazine (Matulane) Tranylcypromine (Parnate) <hr>Amphetamine (Benzedrine) Benzphetamine (Didrex) Chlorphentermine (Pre-Sate) Dextroamphetamine (Dexedrine) Diethylpropion (Tenuate, Tepanil) Ephedrine products Epinephrine products Methamphetamine (Desoxyn) Phendimetrazine (Bontril, Plegine) Phenmetrazine (Preludin) Phenteramine (Fastin, Ionamin)	The drug reaction here can block the blood-pressure-lowering effect of the drugs listed in column 2. A physician may need to adjust the dosage required. <hr>This reaction could cause a severe increase in blood pressure and lead to fever, excitement, convulsions, coma, and possible circulatory collapse. This combination of drugs should be avoided. <hr>This combination may increase or decrease the effects of the drugs in column 2. This could lead to such varied side effects as increased blood pressure and severe headache. Caution should be exercised if these groups are combined. See Charts 13 and 15 for additional antidepressant interactions.	Alcoholic products Allerest A.R.M. Bayer Decongestant Cold Tablets Beer Cheracol and Cheracol D Coldene Compoz Conar Contac Coricidin Coryban-D Cosadein Cosanyl-DM Creo-Terpin Demazin Dormin Dristan & Dristan Cough Formula Histadyl E.C. Neo-Synephrine Novahistine Nyquil Nytol Penetro Pertussin Pyrilamine Robitussin-AC & Robitussin-DM Sinutab Sleep-Eze Sominex Super Anahist Synephricol Tea Plus Triaminicin Triaminicol 2/G DM Vicks Formula 44 Cough Mixture Vicks Sinex products

Chart 15 Antidepressants-II interactions

	Any of these prescription drugs may interact with	→ any of these prescription drug groups	→ and result in this interaction.	OTC/food items

The drugs listed in Chart 15, column 1, are referred to as "monoamine oxidase (MAO) inhibitors." Although the major effects are antidepressant, some are used for anxiety or in chemotherapy procedures.
 	
Because of the potency of these drugs they require special precautions and considerations when used. Transient drowsiness, dizziness, weakness, or blurred vision may occur. If these symptoms persist or severe headaches, rash, dark urine, jaundice, sore throat, or diarrhea occurs, the dosage or drug may need to be changed.
 	
Since the effects of MAO inhibitors may last for up to 2 weeks after discontinuing use, no interacting drug should be started within this period of time.
 	
The interacting OTC and food products listed here could cause severe hypertension, fever, excitement, and convulsions if combined. Therefore it is of the utmost importance to avoid these products high in tyramine and sympathomimetics. Alcohol-containing products should also be avoided if possible.
	Furazolidone (Furoxone)
	Isocarboxazid (Marplan)
	Pargyline (Eutonyl)
	Phenelzine (Nardil)
	Procarbazine (Matulane)
	Tranylcypromine (Parnate)
		Antidepressants (see Chart 14)
		Ephedrine products
		Guanethidine (Esimil, Ismelin)
		Levodopa (Dopar, Larodopa)
		Meperidine (Demerol)
		Methyldopa (Aldomet, Aldoril)
		Methylphenidate (Ritalin)
		OTC diet aids (see Chart 14)
		Phenylephrine (Neo-Synephrine)
		Phenylpropanol-amine (Propadrine)
		Pseudoephedrine (Sudafed)
		Reserpine (Serpasil)
		Reserpine-containing drugs (see Chart 11)
		Tyramine
			A combination of this type could result in a lethal reaction. Concurrent use of any of the drugs in column 2 with any of the medication in column 1 may cause sudden and severe high blood pressure, fever, excitement, and convulsions.
			
			The MAO inhibitors in column 1 should not be combined with any of these drugs, nor should they be used for 14 days after discontinuing an MAO inhibitor.
			
			See Charts 2, 3, 4, 11, and 14 for additional MAO inhibitor interactions.
				Cheeses:
				  Cheddar
				  Emmenthaler
				  Gruyere
				  Stilton
				  Brie
				  Camembert
				Coffee
				Chocolate
				Cola (excessive)
				Fermented sausages, for example, fermented bolognas, salamis, summer sausage, pepperoni
				A.R.M.
				Adrenalin
				Alconefrin
				Allerest capsules and spray
				Asthmanefrin
				Bayer Decongestant Cold Tablets
				Breatheasy
				Bromoquinine
				Bronkaid
				Cheracol Cold Capsules
				Coldene
				Contac
				Coricidin-D
				Cosanyl-DM
				Demazin
				Dimacol
				Dristan
				Epinephrine

Chart 15 Antidepressants-II interactions—cont'd

Any of these prescription drugs may interact with	➡ any of these prescription drug groups	➡ and result in this interaction.	OTC/food items
Furazolidone (Furoxone) Isocarboxazid (Marplan) Pargyline (Eutonyl) Phenelzine (Nardil) Procarbazine (Matulane) Tranylcypromine (Parnate)			Fedrazil Histadyl E.C. Medihaler-EPI Beer Red wines, for example, Chianti, Sherry Bananas Figs (canned) Avocados Fava or yeast extract Chicken liver Beef liver Neo-Synephrine No-Doz Nyquil Ornacol Ornex Orthoxicol OTC diet aids Phenylephrine Phenylpropanol- amine Primatene Privine Romilar Cough Syrup Sinutab Solution A Sudafed Super Anahist Tea Tea Plus Triaminic products Triaminicol Trind Ursinus Va-Tro-Nol Vicks Sinex 4-Way cold products

Chart 16 Analgesic interactions

	Any of these prescription drugs may interact with	any of these prescription drug groups	and result in this interaction.	OTC/food items

The medications listed in Chart 16, column 1, are referred to as "analgesics." The majority are more specifically referred to as "nonsteroidal antiinflammatory agents"; these help control pain and inflammation by a reduction in prostaglandin synthesis.

These medications should be taken with food or milk to minimize the potential for stomach distress or bleeding of the intestinal mucosa.

Patients with a history of allergies to aspirin, bleeding problems, or ulcers may not tolerate these medications. Skin rash, tinnitus, blurred vision, swelling, or unusual weight gian may require a change in dosage or drug. Dizziness may be transient with these medications.

The OTC interactions denoted here involve products containing aspirin, salicylates, or alcohol, which in combination can increase the severity of stomach distress and/or bleeding. Propoxyphene (Darvon, Darvocet) and products containing codeine may react similarly with these OTC products.

Aspirin and salicylate products can decrease the effectiveness of the other prescription analgesics.

Column 1 — prescription drugs:
Aspirin/salicylate products
Fenoprofen (Nalfon
Ibuprofen (Motrin)
Indomethacin (Indocin)
Meclofenamate (Meclomin)
Naproxen (Anaprox, Naprosyn)
Oxyphenbutazone (Oxalid, Tandearil)
Phenylbutazone (Azolid, Butazolidin)
Sulindac (Clinoril)
Zomepirac (Zomax)

Column 2 — prescription drug groups:
Acenocoumarol (Sintrom)
Anisindione (Miradon)
Bishydroxycoumarin (Dicumarol)
Phenindione (Hedulin)
Phenprocoumon (Liquamar)
Warfarin (Coumadin)

Interaction:
When used in combination there is an increase in the likelihood and severity of increasing the effectiveness of the prescription drugs in column 2. This could result in bruising, increased bleeding, or hemorrhage. Some of the prescription drugs in column 1 may not have as much of an effect (for example, Zomax) but still could affect bleeding time.

Probenecid (Benemid) and sulfinpyrazone (Anturane) should normally not be combined with the column 1 drugs (especially with Indocin).

OTC/food items:
Alcoholic beverages
Alka-Seltzer
Alka-2
Anacin
A.P.C.
Bufferin
A.S.A. and A.S.A. compound
Ascriptin
Aspergum
Aspirin
Bayer products
Beer
Cama
Cheracol
Coricidin
Coryban-D
Cosanyl-DM
Creo-Terpin
Demazin Syrup
Dristan Cough Formula and Dristan Decongestant Tablets
Ecotrin
Empirin
Excedrin
4-Way Cold Tablets
Histadyl E.C.
Measurin
Midol
Neo-Synephrine
Novahistine
Nyquil
PAC and PAC Compound
Pamprin
Pepto-Bismol
Pertussin
Phensal
Robitussin
Sodium salicylate
Sominex
Super Anahist
Triaminic Expectorant
Triaminicin
Vanquish
Vicks Formula 44 Cough Mixture

Chart 17 Chemotherapeutic drug interactions

	Any of these prescription drugs may interact with ➡	any of these OTC/food items as described in column 1.	Any of these prescription drugs may interact with ➡	any of these prescription drug groups ➡	and result in this interaction. ➡
The antineoplastic drugs listed in Chart 17 are primarily used in various neoplastic disorders, although methotrexate is sometimes used in psoriatic conditions. The full product description should be consulted when questioning these medications. Persistent diarrhea, fever, chills, sore throat, unusual bleeding, bruising, or jaundice may warrant a change in dosage or drug. Nursing or pregnancy should be avoided for at least 8 weeks following therapy. The patient should avoid stressful situations and maintain a well-balanced diet. The OTC reactions noted here show that if fluorouracil is used orally, acidic foods taken at the same time could significantly decrease the effectiveness of fluorouracil. The OTC interactions regarding methotrexate point out that salicylates can increase the toxic side effects of methotrexate if the two are combined. Methotrexate can also decrease the effects of fluorouracil.	Fluorouracil (5-Fu) Methotrexate	Acidic foods, for example, orange juice Alka-2 Alka-Seltzer Anacin Products A.P.C. Arthritis Strength Bufferin A.S.A. and A.S.A. Compound Ascriptin Aspergum Aspirin Bayer products Bufferin Cama Coricidin products Dristan Ecotrin Empirin Excedrin 4-Way Cold Tablets Measurin Midol PAC and PAC Compound Pamprin Pepto-Bismol Phensal Sodium salicylate Sominex Super Anahist Triaminicin Vanquish	Azathioprine (Imuran) Cyclophosphamide (Cytoxan) Mercaptopurine (Purinethol) Procarbazine (Matulane; see Chart 15)	Allopurinol (Zyloprim)	Even though this combination of two interacting drugs may often be prescribed by the physician, it is usually with a decrease in the dosage or strength of the drugs in column 1. This is done to avoid any toxic or adverse side effects.

Chart 18 Injectable drug and anesthetic interactions

Any of these prescription drugs may interact with	▶ any of these prescription drug groups	▶ and result in this interaction.
Heparin sodium	A.S.A. and salicylates Anticoagulants (oral) (Chart 4)	An increase in the anticoagulant effect may occur; patients should be monitored pro-time. Guaifenesin (Robitussin) and dipyridamole (Persantine) may react with heparin and lead to increased chance of bleeding.
Methotrimeprazine (Levoprome)	Antihypertensives (Chart 11)	An increase in antihypertensive effect resulting in severe hypotension may occur.
	CNS depressants MAO inhibitors (Chart 15)	There is an increase in central nervous system depression and severe and toxic reactions. Avoid MAO inhibitor combination.
	Anticholinergics Succinylcholine chloride (Anectine)	This combination results in decreased blood pressure and effects on the central nervous system from stimulation to delirium. Extrapyramidal symptoms or tachycardia may occur.

Muscle relaxants
  Depolarizing:
    Decamethonium (Syncurine)
    Succinylcholine (Anectine)
  Nondepolarizing:
    Gallamine (Flaxadil)
    Pancuronium (Pavulon)
    (Metubine)
    Tubocurarine
	Anesthetics
	Lithium (Lithane, Eskalith)
	Lidocaine (Mylocaine)
	Clindamycin (Cleocin)
	Lincomycin (Lincocin)
	Quinidine (CinQuin)
	Procainamide (Pronestyl, Procan)
	colymycin-M
	Polymixin B (Aerosporin)
		These combinations result in prolongation in neuromuscular blockade. Respiratory depression or apnea may occur.
		
		Amphotericin B (Fungizone) and aminoglycosides react with muscle relaxants (see below).

Diazoxide (Hyperstat I.V.)	Thiazide diuretics Antidiabetic agents (Chart 3)	Enhanced hyperglycemic effect and hypertension occur. Hyperglycemic effects occur.
	Anticoagulants (Chart 4)	These combinations cause increased anticoagulant effect and possible hemorrhage.
Amphotericin B (Fungizone)	Muscle relaxants (see above) Aminoglycoside (see below) Digitalis (Chart 9)	Increased skeletal muscle effect due to potassium loss occurs. There is an increased possibility of nephrotoxicity. Hypokalemia and increased digitalis toxicity are possible.
	Steroids (Chart 7)	These combinations result in increased potassium loss and possible decrease in infectious resistance, sometimes used together to control drug reaction.

Chart 18 Injectable drug and anesthetic interactions—cont'd

Any of these prescription drugs may interact with	▶ any of these prescription drug groups	▶ and result in this interaction.
Methoxyflurane (Penthrane)	Tetracyclines (Chart 12)	These combinations may cause nephrotoxicity and should be avoided.
Mercaptomerin (Thiomerin)	Digitalis (Chart 9)	These may result in hypokalemia with resultant digitalis toxicity.
Doxorubicin (Adriamycin) Dannorubiecin (Cerubidine)	Cyclophosphamide (Cytoxan)	An increase in cardiotoxicity may occur.
Aminoglycosides Amikacin (Amikin) Gentamicin (Garamycin) Neomycin Kanamycin (Kantrex) Streptomycin Tobramycin (Nebcin)	Anesthetics (see below) Muscle relaxants (see above) Ether Sodium citrate	These combinations result in a possible increase in skeletal muscle response and severe possibility of respiratory paralysis.
	Diuretics Ethacrynic acid (Edecrin) Furosemide (Lasix)	These result in ototoxicity and should be avoided if possible.
	Colistimethate (Coly-Mycin M) Polymixin B (Aerosporin) Viomycin (Viocin) Cephaloridine (Loridine)	There is an increased potential of nephroxicity/neurotoxicity and neuromuscular block with polypeptides. Concurrent use should be avoided if possible. Cephaloridine could increase toxicity when used with diuretics above.
Anesthetics	Metaraminol (Aramine) Epinephrine preparations Dopamine (Intropin)	Ventricular arrhythmias may occur.
	Antihistamines (Chart 2) MAO inhibitors (Chart 15) Methyldopa (Aldomet, Aldoril) *Rauwolfia* alkaloids and reserpine combinations (Chart 11)	Severe increase in hypotension/hypertension and/or central nervous system depression could occur. Physicians should allow 10 to 14 days after discontinuing MAO inhibitors and *Rauwolfia* products before administering anesthetics.
Anesthetics with vasoconstrictor, for example, lidocaine (Xylocaine) with epinephrine	MAO inhibitors (Chart 15) Tricyclic antidepressants (Chart 14) Phenothiazines	Severe hypotension and/or hypertension may occur. Sufficient time should be allowed after discontinuing drugs in column 2 before administering.

11-2. Comparison of selected effects of commonly abused drugs

Some selected effects of commonly abused drugs are summarized in the following table. This table is intended for quick reference only.

Drug category	Physical dependence	Characteristics of intoxication
Opiates	Marked	Analgesia with or without depressed sensorium; pinpoint pupils (tolerance does not develop to this action); patient may be alert and appear normal; respiratory depression with overdose
Barbiturates	Marked	Patient may appear normal with usual dose, but narrow margin between doses needed to prevent withdrawal symptoms and toxic dose is often exceeded and patient appears "drunk," with drowsiness, ataxia, slurred speech, and nystagmus on lateral gaze; pupil size and reaction normal; respiratory depression with overdose
Nonbarbiturate sedatives Glutethimide (Doriden)	Marked	Pupils dilated and reactive to light; coma and respiratory depression prolonged; sudden apnea and laryngeal spasm common
Antianxiety agents ("minor tranquilizers")	Marked	Progressive depression of sensorium as with barbiturates; pupil size and reaction normal; respiratory depression with overdose
Ethanol	Marked	Depressed sensorium, acute or chronic brain syndrome, odor on breath, pupil size and reaction normal
Amphetamines	Mild to absent	Agitation, with paranoid thought disturbance in high doses; acute organic brain syndrome after prolonged use; pupils dilated and reactive; tachycardia, elevated blood pressure, with possibility of hypertensive crisis and CVA; possibility of convulsive seizures
Cocaine	Absent	Paranoid thought disturbance in high doses, with dangerous delusions of persecution and omnipotence; tachycardia; respiratory depression with overdose
Marihuana	Absent	Milder preparations: drowsy, euphoric state with frequent inappropriate laughter and disturbance in perception of time or space (occasional acute psychotic reaction reported); stronger preparations such as hashish: frequent hallucinations or psychotic reaction; pupils normal, conjunctivas injected (marihuana preparations frequently adulterated with LSD, tryptamines, or heroin)
Psychotomimetics LSD, STP, tryptamines, mescaline, morning glory seeds	Absent	Unpredictable disturbance in ego function, manifest by extreme lability of affect and chaotic disruption of thought, with danger of uncontrolled behavioral disturbance; pupils dilated and reactive to light
Phencyclidine	Unknown	Disinhibition, agitation, confusion, chaotic thought disturbance, unpredictable behavior, hypertension, meiosis, respiratory collapse, cardiovascular collapse, death
Anticholinergic agents	Absent	Nonpsychotropic effects such as tachycardia, decreased salivary secretion, urinary retention, and dilated, nonreactive pupils plus depressed sensorium, confusion, disorientation, hallucinations, and delusional thinking
Inhalants*	Unknown	Depressed sensorium, hallucinations, acute brain syndrome; odor on breath; patient often with glassy-eyed appearance

*The term "inhalant" is used to designate a variety of gases and highly volatile organic liquids, including the aromatic glues, paint thinners, gasoline, some anes administration (such as marihuana).

Characteristics of withdrawal	"Flashback" symptoms	Masking of symptoms of illness or injury during intoxication
Rhinorrhea, lacrimation, and dilated, reactive pupils, followed by gastrointestinal disturbances, low back pain, and waves of gooseflesh; convulsions not a feature unless heroin samples were adulterated with barbiturates	Not reported	An important feature of opiate intoxication, due to analgesic action, with or without depressed sensorium
Agitation, tremulousness, insomnia, gastrointestinal disturbances, hyperpyrexia, blepharoclonus (clonic blink reflex), acute brain syndrome, major convulsive seizures	Not reported	Only in presence of depressed sensorium or after onset of acute brain syndrome
Similar to barbiturate withdrawal syndrome, with agitation, gastrointestinal disturbances, hyperpyrexia, and major convulsive seizures	Not reported	Same as in barbiturate intoxication
Similar to barbiturate withdrawal syndrome, with danger of major convulsive seizures	Not reported	Same as in barbiturate intoxication
Similar to barbiturate withdrawal syndrome, but with less likelihood of convulsive seizures	Not reported	Same as in barbiturate intoxication
Lethargy, somnolence, dysphoria, and possibility of suicidal depression; brain syndrome may persist for many weeks	Infrequently reported	Drug-induced euphoria or acute brain syndrome may interfere with awareness of symptoms of illness or may remove incentive to report symptoms of illness
Similar to amphetamine withdrawal	Not reported	Same as in amphetamine intoxication
No specific withdrawal symptoms	Infrequently reported	Uncommon with milder preparations; stronger preparations may interfere in same manner as psychotomimetic agents
No specific withdrawal symptoms; symptomatology may persist for indefinite period after discontinuation of drug	Commonly reported as late as 1 year after last dose	Affective response or psychotic thought disturbance may remove awareness of, or incentive to report, symptoms of illness
No specific withdrawal symptoms	Occasionally reported	Same as in LSD intoxication
No specific withdrawal symptoms; mydriasis may persist for several days	Not reported	Pain may not be reported as a result of depression of sensorium, acute brain syndrome, or acute psychotic reaction
No specific withdrawal symptoms	Infrequently reported	Same as in anticholinergic intoxication

thetic agents, and amylnitrite. The term excludes liquids sprayed into the nasopharynx (droplet transport required) and substances that must be ignited before

11-3. Cross-reference guide to drugs (generic and brand names)

Drugs or drug type	Brand names	Generic name	Drugs or drug type	Brand names	Generic name
Acetaminophen (systemic)	Algophen* Atasol* Atasol Forte* Campain* Datril Empracet* Exdol* Liquiprin Phenaphen Robigesic* Rounox* SK-APAP Tempra Tivrin* Tylenol Tylenol Extra Strength Valadol	Acetaminophen		Hydeltrasol Inflamase Metreton Pred Forte Pred Mild Predulose	Prednisolone
			Adrenocorticoids (otic)	Decadron Maxidex	Dexamethasone
				Hydeltrasol Metreton	Prednisolone
Acetaminophen and codeine (systemic)	Aceta with Codeine Capital with Codeine Empracet with Codeine Papa-Deine Pavadon Phenaphen with Codeine Proval SK-APAP with Codeine Tylenol with Codeine		Adrenocorticoids (topical)	Cyclocort	Amcinonide
				Benisone Betacort* Betaderm* Betnovate* Celestoderm* Celestone Valisone	Betamethasone
				Tridesilon	Desonide
				Topicort	Desoximetasone
Acrisorcin (topical)	Akrinol	Acrisorcin		Aeroseb-Dex Decaderm Decadron Decaspray Hexadrol	Dexamethasone
Adrenocorticoids (dental)	Orabase HCA	Hydrocortisone		Florone	Diflorasone
	Kenalog in Orabase	Triamcinolone		Locacorten* Locorten	Flumethasone
Adrenocorticoids (ophthalmic)	Decadron Maxidex Novadex*	Dexamethasone		Dermalar* Fluoderm* Fluonid Flurosyn Synalar	Fluocinolone
	FML Liquifilm	Fluorometholone		Lidemol* Lidex Topsyn	Fluocinonide
	Cortamed* Cortisol Hydrocortone Optef	Hydrocortisone		Oxylone	Fluorometholone
	HMS Liquifilm	Medrysone		Cordran Drenison*	Flurandrenolide
	AK-Pred AK-Tate Econopred			Halciderm Halog	Halcinonide
				Cortaid Cort-Dome Cortef Corticreme*	

*Not available in the United States.

Drugs or drug type	Brand names	Generic name	Drugs or drug type	Brand names	Generic name
	Cortisol Cortril Dermacort Hyderm* Hydrocortone Hytone Texacort	Hydrocortisone		Aristospan Cinonide Kenacort Kenalog Tramacort	Triamcinolone
	Medrol	Methylprednisolone		Doca Percorten	Desoxycorticoster-one
	Meti-Derm	Prednisolone		Florinef	Fludrocortisone
	Aristocort Aristogel Kenalog Kenalog-E* Spencort Triacet Triaderm* Triamalone* Trimacort*	Triamcinolone	Alcohol and acetone (topical)	Seba-Nil Sebasum Tyrosum	
			Alcohol and sulfur (topical)	Acne Aid Acnomead Epi-Clear Liquimat Postacne Transact Xerac	
Adrenocorticoids (systemic)	Betnelan* Betnesol* Celestone	Betamethasone	Allopurinol (systemic)	Lopurin Purinol* Zyloprim	Allopurinol
	Cortone	Cortisone	Amantadine (systemic)	Symmetrel	Amantadine
	Decadron Dexasone Hexadrol	Dexamethasone	Aminocaproic acid (systemic)	Amicar	Aminocaproic acid
	Alphadrol	Fluprednisolone	Aminoglycosides (systemic)	Amikin	Amikacin
	A-Hydrocort Cortef Cortenema Hydrocortone Solu-Cortef	Hydrocortisone		Apogen Bristagen Cidomycin* Garamycin U-Gencin	Gentamicin
	Betapar	Meprednisone		Kantrex Klebcil	Kanamycin
	A-MethaPred Duralone Medralone Medrol Methylone	Methylprednisolone		Mycifradin	Neomycin
	Haldrone	Paramethasone			Streptomycin
	Delta-Cortef Hydeltrasol Meticortelone Sterone	Prednisolone		Nebcin	Tobramycin
			4-Aminoquinolones (systemic)	Camoquin	Amodiaquine
	Predoxine	Prednisolone, Buf-fered		Aralen	Chloroquine
				Plaquenil	Hydroxychloroquine
	Colisone* Deltasone Meticorten Orasone Sterapred Winpred*	Prednisone	Aminosalicylates (systemic)	Nemasol* P.A.S. Parasal Teebacin	Aminosalicylic acid
	Aristocort		Amphetamines (systemic)	Benzedrine	Amphetamine
				Dexampex Dexedrine	

Drugs or drug type	Brand names	Generic name	Drugs or drug type	Brand names	Generic name
	Diphylets Ferndex Obotan Oxydess Spancap	Dextroamphetamine		Aparkane* Artane Tremin	Trihexyphenidyl
	Desoxyn Methampex	Methamphetamine	Antiglaucoma agents, choliner- gic—long-acting cholinesterase in- hibitors (ophthalmic)	Humorsol	Demecarium
				Echodide Phospholine Iodide	Echothiophate
Amphotericin B (systemic)	Fungizone	Amphotericin B		Floropryl	Isoflurophate
Amphotericin B (topical)	Fungizone	Amphotericin B	Antihistamines (systemic)	Idulian* Optimine	Azatadine
Anthralin (topical)	Anthra-Derm Lasan	Anthralin		Ambodryl Deserol*	Bromodiphenhy- dramine
Anticoagulants (systemic)	Miradon	Anisindione		Bromphen Dimetane Ilvin* Puretane Symptom 3	Brompheniramine
	Dufalone*	Dicumarol			
	Danilone* Hedulin	Phenindione		Allergefon* Clistin	Carbinoxamine
	Liquamar Marcumar*	Phenprocoumon		Chloramate Chlor-Trimeton Histalon* Histaspan Ibioton* Novopheniram* Phenetron Piriton* Teldrin	Chlorpheniramine
	Athrombin-K	Warfarin Potassium			
	Coumadin Panwarfin Warfilone* Warnerin*	Warfarin Sodium			
Antidiabetics, oral (systemic)	Dimelor* Dymelor	Acetohexamide		Tavegil* Tavist	Clemastine
	Chloromide* Chloronase* Diabinese	Chlorpropamide		Cyprodine Nuran* Periactin Vimicon*	Cyproheptadine
	Tolinase	Tolazamide		Polaramine	Dexchlorphenira- mine
	Mobenol* Neo-Dibetic* Novobutamide* Oramide* Orinase Tolbutone*	Tolbutamide		Dramamine Eldodram Gravol* Novodimenate* Travamine*	Dimenhydrinate
Antidyskinetics— anticholinergic agents used to treat Parkinson's dis- ease (systemic)	Bensylate* Cogentin	Benztropine		Dimethpyrindene Forhistal Triten	Dimethindene
	Akineton	Biperiden		Benadryl Bendylate Eldadryl Insomnal* Nautamine* Valdrene	Diphenhydramine
	Pagitane	Cycrimine			
	Parsidol Parsitan*	Ethopropazine			
	Kemadrin	Procyclidine			

*Not available in the United States.

Drugs or drug type	Brand names	Generic name	Drugs or drug type	Brand names	Generic name
	Diafen Hispril	Diphenylpyraline		Bontril PDM Phendiet Plegine	Phendimetrazine
	Decapryn	Doxylamine		Preludin	Phenmetrazine
	Allertoc Mepyramine Neo-Antergan* Thylogen	Pyrilamine		Fastin Ionamin	Phentermine
	Benzoxal* PBZ Pyribenzamine Pyrizil*	Tripelennamine	Asparaginase (systemic)	Elspar	
			Atropine (anticholin- ergics) (ophthalmic)	Atropisol BufOpto Atropine Isopto Atropine	Atropine
	Actidil Actidilon* Pro-Actidil*	Triprolidine		Homatrocel Isopto Homatropine	Homatropine
				Isopto Hyoscine	Scopolamine
Antipyrine, benzo caine, and glycerin (otic)	Auralgan Aurasol		Azathioprine (systemic)	Imuran	Azathioprine
Antithyroid agents (systemic)	Tapazole Thiamazole	Methimazole	Baclofen (systemic)	Lioresal	Baclofen
	Propacil Propyl-Thyracil	Propylthiouracil	Barbiturates (systemic)	Amytal Isobec*	Amobarbital
APC (Aspirin, phen- acetin, and caf- feine) (systemic)	Acetophen Aidant APAC A.S.A. Compound Asalco No. 1 Asphac-G P-A-C Compound Phencaset Sal-Fayne Salphenine Tabloid APC			Buticaps Butisol	Butabarbital
				Sombulex	Hexobarbital
				Mebaral	Mephobarbital
				Gemonil	Metharbital
				Nembutal Nova-Rectal* Pentogen*	Pentobarbital

APC and codeine
(systemic)
	Empirin Compound
	  with Codeine
	A.S.A. and Codeine
	  Compound
	P-A-C Compound
	  with Codeine
	Salatin with Codeine
	Tabloid APC with
	  Codeine
				Eskabarb*
				Gardenal*
				Nova-Pheno*
				Sedadrops
				SK-Phenobarbital
				Solfoton
					Phenobarbital

				Secogen* Seconal Seral*	Secobarbital
				Tuinal	Secobarbital and Amobarbital
Appetite suppres- sants (systemic)	Didrex	Benzphetamine		Lotusate	Talbutal
	Pre-Sate	Chlorphentermine	Beclomethasone (inhalation)	Beclovent Vanceril	Beclomethasone
	Voranil	Clortermine	Belladonna alkaloids and barbiturates (systemic)	Minabel Omnibel Palbar	Atropine, Hyoscya- mine, Scopola- mine, and Buta- barbital
	Dietec* Regibon* Tenuate Tepanil	Diethylpropion			
	Sanorex	Mazindol			

*Not available in the United States.

Drugs or drug type	Brand names	Generic name
	Cyclo-Bell	Atropine, Hyoscyamine, Scopolamine, Butabarbital, Pentobarbital, and Phenobarbital
	Barbidonna Donna-Sed Donnatal Donphen Hasp Hybephen Hyosophen Kinesed Sedralex Setamine Spalix Spasmolin Spasmophen Spasmorel Tri-Spas	Atropine, Hyoscyamine, Scopolamine, and Phenobarbital
	Alised Antrocol Atrobarb	Atropine and Phenobarbital
	Amobell	Belladonna and Amobarbital
	Butibel	Belladonna and Butabarbital
	Belap Bellophen Bello-Phen Chardonna Donabarb Donnabarb Oxoids Phenobel Phenobella Sedajen Valaspas	Belladonna and Phenobarbital
	Hybar	Hyoscyamine, Scopolamine, and Phenobarbital
	Cystospaz-SR	Hyoscyamine and Butabarbital
	Anaspaz PB Levsin-PB Levsin w/Phenobarbital Levsinex w/Phenobarbital	Hyoscyamine and Phenobarbital
Benzodiazepines (systemic)	A-poxide C-Tran* Librium Nack* Novopoxide*	Chlordiazepoxide

Drugs or drug type	Brand names	Generic name
	Relaxil* SK-Lygen	
	Tranxene	Clorazepate
	D-Tran* E-Pam* Novodipam* Valium Vivol*	Diazepam
	Dalmane	Flurazepam
	Ativan	Lorazepam
	Serax	Oxazepam
	Verstran	Prazepam
Benzoyl peroxide (topical)	Benoxyl Benzac Benzagel Clear By Design Dermodex Desquam-X Epi-Clear Fostex BPO Panoxyl Persadox Persa-Gel Porox 7 Teen Topex Xerac BP	Benzoyl peroxide
Beta-adrenergic blocking agents (systemic)	Lopressor	Metoprolol
	Corgard	Nadolol
	Inderal	Propranolol
Bethanechol (systemic)	Duvoid Myotonachol Urecholine	
Bleomycin (systemic)	Blenoxane	Bleomycin
Bromocriptine (systemic)	Parlodel	Bromocriptine
Brompheniramine, giuaifenesin, phenylephrine, and phenylpropanolamine (systemic)	Dimetane expectorant Midatane expectorant Normatene expectorant Puretane expectorant Spentane expectorant	

*Not available in the United States.

Drugs or drug type	Brand names	Generic name	Drugs or drug type	Brand names	Generic name
Brompheniramine, guaifenesin, phenylephrine, phenylpropanolamine, and codeine (systemic)	Dimetane expectorant-DC Midatane DC expectorant Normatane DC expectorant Puretane Expectorant DC Spentane DC expectorant			Mefoxin	Cefoxitin
				Ceporex* Keflex	Cephalexin
				Kafocin	Cephaloglycin
				Ceporan* Loridine	Cephaloridine
				Ceporacin* Keflin Neutral	Cephalothin
				Cefadyl	Cephapirin
Brompheniramine, phenylephrine, and phenylpropanolamine (systemic)	Brompheniramine Compound Bromatapp Dimetapp Eldatapp Puretapp			Anspor Velosef	Cephradine
			Charcoal, activated (oral)	Charcocaps Charcodote Charcotabs	
Busulfan (systemic)	Myleran	Busulfan	Chloral hydrate (systemic)	Aquachloral Chloralex* Chloralvan* Cohidrate Noctec Novochlorhydrate* Oradrate	
Butalbital and APC (systemic)	Fiorinal				
Butalbital, APC, and codeine (systemic)	Fiorinal with codeine				
			Chlorambucil (systemic)	Leukeran	Chlorambucil
Butorphanol (systemic)	Stadol	Butorphanol	Chloramphenicol (ophthalmic)	Chloromycetin Chloroptic Econochlor Fenicol* Ophthochlor Pentamycetin* Sopamycetin*	Chloramphenicol
Calcitonin (systemic)	Calcimar	Calcitonin			
Capreomycin (systemic)	Capastat	Capreomycin			
Carbachol (ophthalmic)	Carbacel Isopto Carbachol Miostat Murocarb	Carbachol	Chloramphenicol (otic)	Chloromycetin	Chloramphenicol
			Chloramphenicol (systemic)	Amphicol Chloromycetin Novochlorocap* Pentamycetin*	Chloramphenicol
Carboprost (systemic)	Prostin/15 M	Carboprost			
Carisoprodol (systemic)	Rela Soma Soprodol	Carisoprodol	Chloramphenicol (topical)	Chloromycetin	Chloramphenicol
Carmustine (systemic)	BiCNU	Carmustine	Chlordiazepoxide and amitriptyline (systemic)	Limbitrol	
Cephalosporins (systemic)	Ceclor	Cefaclor	Chlordiazepoxide and clidinium (systemic)	Librax	
	Duricef Ultracef	Cefadroxil			
	Mandol	Cefamandole	Chloroxine (topical)	Capitrol	Chloroxine
	Ancef Kefzol	Cefazolin			

*Not available in the United States.

Drugs or drug type	Brand names	Generic name	Drugs or drug type	Brand names	Generic name
Chlorpheniramine, phenylpropanolamine, and isopropamide (systemic)	Allernade Capade Ornade		Colchicine (systemic)	Colsalide Improved	Colchicine
			Colestipol (systemic)	Colestid	Colestipol
Chlorzoxazone (systemic)	Paraflex	Chlorzoxazone	Colistin, neomycin, and hydrocortisone (otic)	Coly-Mycin S	
Chlorzoxazone and acetaminophen (systemic)	Chlorofon-F Chlorzone Forte Lobac Miflex Parachlor Parafon Forte Tuzon		Cromolyn (inhalation)	Intal	Cromolyn
			Cyclandelate (systemic)	Cyclospasmol	Cyclandelate
Cholestyramine (oral)	Questran	Cholestyramine	Cyclobenzaprine (systemic)	Flexeril	Cyclobenzaprine
Cimetidine (systemic)	Tagamet	Cimetidine	Cyclopentolate (ophthalmic)	Cyclogyl Mydplegic*	Cyclopentolate
Cisplatin (systemic)	Platinol	Cisplatin	Cyclophosphamide (systemic)	Cytoxan Procytox*	Cyclophosphamide
Clindamycin (topical)	Cleocin T	Clindamycin	Cycloserine (systemic)	Seromycin	Cycloserine
Clofibrate (systemic)	Atromid-S	Clofibrate	Cytarabine (systemic)	Cytosar-U	Cytarabine
Clomiphene (systemic)	Clomid	Clomiphene	Dacarbazine (systemic)	DTIC-Dome	Dacarbazine
Clonidine (systemic)	Catapres	Clonidine	Dactinomycin (systemic)	Cosmegen	Dactinomycin
Clonidine and chlorthalidone (systemic)	Combipres		Danazol (systemic)	Cyclomen* Danocrine	Danazol
			Dantrolene (systemic)	Dantrium	Dantrolene
Clotrimazole (topical)	Lotrimin Mycelex	Clotrimazole	Dapsone (systemic)	Avlosulfon	Dapsone
Clotrimazole (vaginal)	Gyne-Lotrimin	Clotrimazole	Desonide and acetic acid (otic)	Tridesilon	
Coal tar (topical)	DHS tar Estar Medotar Pentrax Tar Pso-Rite Supertah Tar Dak Tarbonis Tarpaste Tersa-Tar Ul-Tar Zetar		Dexamethasone (nasal)	Decadron	Dexamethasone
			Dexbrompheniramine and pseudoephedrine (systemic)	Disophrol Drixoral	
			Diazoxide (oral)	Proglycem	Diazoxide

*Not available in the United States.

Drugs or drug type	Brand names	Generic name	Drugs or drug type	Brand names	Generic name
Dicyclomine (systemic)	Bentyl Bentylol* Cyclobec* Dyspas	Dicyclomine	Epinephrine (ophthalmic)	Epifrin Epitrate Glaucon Murocoll Mytrate	Epinephrine
Digitalis medicines (systemic)	Cedilanid-D	Deslanoside		Epinal Eppy/N	Epinephryl Borate
	Digifortis Pil-Digis	Digitalis	Epinephrine (systemic)	Adrenalin AsthmaHaler Bronitin Bronkaid Medihaler-Epi Primatene	Epinephrine
	Crystodigin Purodigin	Digitoxin		AsthmaNefrin microNEFRIN Vaponefrin	Racepinephrine
	Lanoxin	Digoxin			
	Gitaligin	Gitalin			
	Cedilanid	Lanatoside C			
	Strophanthin-G	Ouabain			
Dimethyl sulfoxide (topical)	Rimso-50	Dimethyl sulfoxide	Ergoloid mesylates (systemic)	Hydergine	
Dinoprost (intra-amniotic)	Prostin F₂ Alpha	Dinoprost	Ergonovine (systemic)	Ergotrate	Ergonovine
Dinoprostone (vaginal)	Prostin E₂	Dinoprostone		Methergine	Methylergonovine
Dione-type anti-convulsants (systemic)	Paradione Tridione	Paramethadione Trimethadione	Ergotamine (systemic)	Ergomar Ergostat Gynergen Medihaler Ergota-mine	Ergotamine tartrate
Diphenoxylate and atropine (systemic)	Colonil Lomotil SK-Diphenoxylate		Ergotamine, bella-donna alkaloids, and phenobarbital (systemic)	Bellergal Bellergal-S	
Dipivefrin (ophthalmic)	Propine	Dipivefrin	Ergotamine and caf-feine (systemic)	Cafergot Cafermine Cafetrate Ergocaf Ergocaffeine Lanatrate Migrastat	
Dipyridamole (systemic)	Persantine	Dipyridamole			
Disopyramide (systemic)	Norpace Rythmodan*	Disopyramide	Ergotamine, caf-feine, belladonna alkaloids, and phenobarbital (systemic)	Cafergot-PB	
Disulfiram (systemic)	Antabuse	Disulfiram			
Doxapram (systemic)	Dopram	Doxapram			
Doxylamine and pyridoxine (systemic)	Bendectin		Erythromycin (ophthalmic)	Ilotycin	Erythromycin
Drocode, prometha-zine, and APC (systemic)	Synalgos-DC		Erythromycin (topical)	Ilotycin	Erythromycin
Ephedrine (systemic)	Ectasule Minus Ephedsol		Erythromycins (systemic)	E-Mycin Erythromid*	

*Not available in the United States.

Drugs or drug type	Brand names	Generic name	Drugs or drug type	Brand names	Generic name
	Ilotycin Novorythro* Robimycin RP-Mycin	Erythromycin		Ovulen	Ethynodiol Diacetate and Mestranol
	Ilosone	Erythromycin Estolate		Ovcon Brevicon Modicon	Norethindrone and Ethinyl Estradiol
	E.E.S. E-Mycin E Pediamycin Wyamycin E	Erythromycin Ethylsuccinate		Norinyl Ortho-Novum	Norethindrone and Mestranol
	Ilotycin	Erythromycin Gluceptate		Norlestrin Loestrin	Norethindrone Acetate and Ethinyl Estradiol
	Erythrocin	Erythromycin Lactobionate		Enovid	Norethynodrel and Mestranol
	Bristamycin Erypar Erythrocin Ethril Pfizer-E SK-Erythromycin Wyamycin S	Erythromycin Stearate		Ovral Lo-Ovral	Norgestrel and Ethinyl Estradiol
			Ethacrynic acid (systemic)	Edecrin	Ethacrynic acid
Estrogens (systemic)	TACE	Chlorotrianisene	Ethambutol (systemic)	Etibi* Myambutol	Ethambutol
	DES Stilphostrol	Diethylstilbestrol	Ethchlorvynol (systemic)	Placidyl	Ethchlorvynol
	Delestrogen Estrace Progynon	Estradiol	Ethinamate (systemic)	Valmid	Ethinamate
	Premarin	Conjugated Estrogens	Ethionamide (systemic)	Trecator-SC	Ethionamide
	Amnestrogen	Esterified Estrogens	Ethylnorepinephrine (systemic)	Bronkephrine	Ethylnorepinephrine
	Theelin	Estrone	Fenfluramine (systemic)	Pondimin	Fenfluramine
	Ogen Piperazine Estrone Sulfate	Estropipate	Fenoprofen (systemic)	Nalfon	Fenoprofen
	Estinyl Feminone	Ethinyl Estradiol	Flucytosine (systemic)	Ancobon Ancotil*	Flucytosine
	Estrovis	Quinestrol	Fluorouracil (systemic)	Adrucil	Fluorouracil
Estrogens (vaginal)	DV Cream	Dienestrol	Fluorouracil (topical)	Efudex Fluoroplex	Fluorouracil
	DES	Diethylstilbestrol	Furosemide (systemic)	Furoside* Lasix Neo-renal Novosemide* Uritol*	Furosemide
	Premarin	Conjugated Estrogens			
	Ogen Piperazine Estrone Sulfate	Estropipate			
Estrogens and progestins—oral contraceptives (systemic)	Demulen	Ethynodiol Diacetate and Ethinyl Estradiol	Gentamicin (ophthalmic-otic)	Garamycin Genoptic	Gentamicin

*Not available in the United States.

Drugs or drug type	Brand names	Generic name	Drugs or drug type	Brand names	Generic name
Gentamicin (topical)	Garamycin	Gentamicin	Guanethidine and hydrochlorothiazide (systemic)	Esimil	
Gentian violet (vaginal)	Genapax Hyva	Gentian violet	Haloperidol (systemic)	Haldol	Haloperidol
Glutethimide (systemic)	Doriden Dormtabs	Glutethimide	Haloprogin (topical)	Halotex	Haloprogin
Glycerin (systemic)	Glyrol Osmoglyn		Heparin (systemic)	Hepalean* Heprinar Lipo-Hepin Liquaemin Panheprin	Heparin
Gold compounds (systemic)	Solganal Myochrysine	Aurothioglucose Gold Sodium Thiomalate			
Griseofulvin (systemic)	Fulvicin P/G Fulvicin-U/F Grifulvin V Grisactin Grisovin-FP* grisOwen Gris-PEG	Griseofulvin	Hydantoin-type anticonvulsants (systemic)	Peganone	Ethotoin
				Mesantoin Methoin*	Mephenytoin
				Dantoin* Dilantin Di-Phen Diphenylan Diphenylhydantoin	Phenytoin
Guaifenesin (systemic)	2/G Anti-Tuss Breonesin Genetuss Glycotuss Glytuss Hytuss Malotuss Nortussin Proco Robitussin	Guaifenesin	Hydralazine (systemic)	Apresoline Rolazine*	Hydralazine
			Hydrocodone (systemic)	Codone Corutol DH* Dicodid Robidone*	Hydrocodone
Guaifenesin and codeine (systemic)	Cheracol Nortussin w/ Codeine Robitussin A-C Tolu-Sed		Hydrocodone and hematropine (systemic)	Hycodan	
Guaifenesin and dextromethorpan (systemic)	Anti-Tuss DM Cheracol D Dextro-Tuss GG 2 G-DM G-Tuss DM Guaiadex Neo-Vadrin Queltuss Robitussin-DM Silexin Tolu-Sed DM Trocal Unproco		Hydrocodone and phenyltoloxamine resin complexes (systemic)	Tussionex	
			Hydrocodone and pseudoephedrine (systemic)	Tussend	
			Hydrocodone, pseudoephedrine, and guaifenesin (systemic)	Tussend expectorant	
			Hydrocortisone (rectal)	Cortifoam Cort-Dome Proctocort	Hydrocortisone
Guanethidine (systemic)	Ismelin	Guanethidine	Hydrocortisone and acetic acid (otic)	VōSol HC	

*Not available in the United States.

Drugs or drug type	Brand names	Generic name	Drugs or drug type	Brand names	Generic name
Hydrocortisone, belladonna, ephedrine, zinc oxide, boric acid, bismuth, and peruvian balsam (rectal)	Wyanoids HC		Iodochlorhydroxyquin (topical)	Vioform	Iodochlorhydroxyquin
Hydrocortisone, bismuth, benzyl benzoate, peruvian balsam, and zinc oxide (rectal)	Anusol-HC		Iodochlorhydroxyquin and hydrocortisone (topical)	Dek-Quin Domeform-HC HCV Mity-Quin Racet Vioform-HC	
Hydroxyurea (systemic)	Hydrea	Hydroxyurea	Iodoquinol (systemic)	Moebiquin Yodoxin	Iodoquinol
Hydroxyzine (systemic)	Atarax Vistaril	Hydroxyzine	Isoetharine (systemic)	Bronkometer Bronkosol	Isoetharine
Ibuprofen (systemic)	Motrin	Ibuprofen	Isometheptene, dichloralphenazone, and acetaminophen (systemic)	Midrin	
Idoxuridine (ophthalmic)	Dendrid Herplex Stoxil	Idoxuridine	Isoniazid (systemic)	INH Isotamine* Nydrazid Rimifon*	Isoniazid
Indomethacin (systemic)	Indocid* Indocin	Indomethacin	Isoproterenol (systemic)	Aerolone Iprenol Isuprel Medihaler-Iso Norisodrine Aerotrol Proternol Vapo-Iso	Isoproterenol
Insulin (systemic)	Actrapid Regular Insulin Regular Iletin II (new) Velosulin	Insulin Injection	Isoproterenol and phenylephrine (systemic)	Duo-Medihaler	
	Globin Insulin	Globin Zinc Insulin Injection			
	Insulatard NPH NPH Iletin II	Isophane Insulin Suspension	Isoxsuprine (systemic)	Vasodilan Vasoprine	Isoxsuprine
	Mixtard	Isophane Insulin Suspension and Insulin Injection	Kanamycin (oral)	Kantrex	Kanamycin
	Lentard Lente Insulin Lente Iletin II Monotard	Insulin Zinc Suspension	Kaolin and pectin (oral)	Kaomead Kaopectate Pargel	
	Ultralente Ultralente Iletin Ultratard	Extended Insulin Zinc Suspension	Kaolin, pectin, belladonna alkaloids, and opium (systemic)	Donnagel-PG	
	Semilente Semilente Iletin Semitard	Prompt Insulin Zinc Suspension	Kaolin, pectin, and paregoric (systemic)	Parepectolin	
	Protamine Zinc & Iletin II PZI	Protamine Zinc Insulin Suspension			

*Not available in the United States.

Drugs or drug type	Brand names	Generic name	Drugs or drug type	Brand names	Generic name
Laxatives, bulk-forming (oral)	Maltsupex	Malt Soup Extract		Cholan-DH Decholin Neocholan	Dehydrocholic Acid
	Cellothyl Cologel Hydrolose	Methylcellulose		Alophen Espotabs Evac-U-Gen Evac-U-Lax Ex-Lax Feen-A-Mint Phenolax Prulet	Phenolphthalein
		Polycarbophil			
	Mitrolan	Polycarbophil Calcium			
	Effersyllium Konsyl L.A. Formula Metamucil Modane Bulk Mucilose Plova Serutan Siblin	Psyllium Mucilloid Psyllium Seed Psyllium		Black Draught Casa Fru Dr. Caldwell's Senna Laxative Fletcher's Castoria Senokot Swiss Kriss X-Prep	Senna
Laxatives, emollient (oral)	Surfak	Docusate Calcium		Glysennid Senokot X-Prep	Sennosides A and B
	Kasof	Docusate Potassium	Levodopa (systemic)	Sinemet	Carbidopa and Levodopa
	Afko-Lube Colace Colax Comfolax Dioctyl Sodium Sulfosuccinate	Docusate Sodium		Bendopa Dopar Larodopa Levopa*	Levodopa
	Alaxin Magcyl	Poloxamer 188	Lime, sulfurated (topical)	Vlem-Dome Vleminckx's solution	
Laxatives, hyperosmotic-lactulose and saline (oral)	Chronulac	Lactulose	Lincomycins (systemic)	Cleocin Dalacin C*	Clindamycin
	Citrate of Magnesia	Magnesium Citrate		Lincocin	Lincomycin
	Adlerika Epsom Salts	Magnesium Sulfate	Lindane (topical)	GBH* Kwell Kwellada*	Lindane
	Phospho-Soda	Sodium Phosphate (or phosphates)	Lithium (systemic)	Eskalith Lithonate Lithobid Lithonate-S Lithane	Lithium Carbonate
	Sal Hepatica	Effervescent Sodium Phosphate			
Laxatives, lubricant (oral)	Liquid petrolatum Nujol	Mineral Oil	Lomustine (systemic)	Cee Nu	Lomustine
	Neo-Cultol	Mineral Oil (Jellied)	Loperamide (systemic)	Imodium	Loperamide
Laxatives, stimulant (oral)	Cenalax Codylax Dulcolax Theralax	Bisacodyl	Loxapine (systemic)	Daxolin Loxitane	Loxapine
	Cascara Sagrada Cas-Evac	Cascara			
	Alphamul Neoloid	Castor Oil			
	Dorbane Modane	Danthron			

*Not available in the United States.

Drugs or drug type	Brand names	Generic name	Drugs or drug type	Brand names	Generic name
Magnesia, milk of (oral)	Magnesia Magnesium hydroxide			Sopor Triador* Tualone*	
Mannitol (systemic)	Osmitrol	Mannitol	Methenamine (systemic)	Hiprex Urex	Methenamine Hippurate
Mecamylamine (systemic)	Inversine	Mecamylamine		Mandelamine Methandine* Prov-U-Sep Sterine*	Methenamine Mandelate
Mechlorethamine (systemic)	Mustargen	Mechlorethamine	Methocarbamol (systemic)	Delaxin Forbaxin Marbaxin-750 Metho-500 Robamol Robaxin Spinaxin Tumol	Methocarbamol
Meclizine (systemic)	Bucladin-S Marezine Antivert Bonine	Buclizine Cyclizine Meclizine			
Meclofenamate (systemic)	Meclomen	Meclofenamate	Methotrexate (systemic)	Mexate	Methotrexate
Melphalan (systemic)	Alkeran	Melphalan	Methoxsalen (systemic)	Oxsoralen	Methoxsalen
Meperidine (systemic)	Demerol Demer-Idine* Pethadol	Meperidine	Methyldopa (systemic)	Aldomet Dopamet* Medimet-250* Novomedopa*	Methyldopa
Meprobamate (systemic)	Equanil Lan-Dol* Medi-Tran* Mep-E* Meprospan Miltown Neo-Tran* Novo-Mepro* Quietal* SK-Bamate Tranmap	Meprobamate	Methyldopa and thiazide diuretics (systemic)	Aldoclor Aldoril	Methyldopa and Chlorothiazide Methyldopa and Hydrochlorothiazide
			Methylphenidate (systemic)	Methidate* Ritalin	Methylpenidate
Meprobamate, ethoheptazine, and aspirin (systemic)	Equagesic Heptogesic Mepro Compound Meprogesic		Methyprylon (systemic)	Noludar	Methyprylon
Mercaptopurine (systemic)	Purinethol	Mercaptopurine	Methysergide (systemic)	Sansert	Methysergide
Metaproterenol (systemic)	Alupent Metaprel	Metaproterenol	Metronidazole (systemic)	Flagyl Neo-Tric* Novonidazole* Trikacide*	Metronidazole
Methadone (systemic)	Dolophine Westadone	Methadone	Metyrosine (systemic)	Demser	Metyrosine
Methaqualone (systemic)	Mequelon* Mequin Parest Quaalude Sedalone*	Methaqualone	Miconazole (systemic)	Monistat	Miconazole
			Miconazole (topical)	Micatin	Miconazole

*Not available in the United States.

Drugs or drug type	Brand names	Generic name	Drugs or drug type	Brand names	Generic name
Miconazole (vaginal)	Monistat	Miconazole	Neomycin, poly-myxin B, and hydrocortisone (otic)	Cortisporin Otobione	
Minoxidil (systemic)	Loniten	Minoxidil	Nicotinyl alcohol (systemic)	Roniacol	Nicotinyl alcohol
Mithramycin (systemic)	Mithracin	Mithramycin	Organic nitrates (other than nitro-glycerin) (systemic)	Cardilate	Erythrityl Tetranitrate
Mitomycin (systemic)	Mutamycin	Mitomycin		Coronex* Dilatrate-SR Iso-Bid Isordil Isotrate Sorate Sorbide Sorbitrate	Isosorbide Dinitrate
Mitotane (systemic)	Lysodren	Mitotane			
Monoamine oxidase (MAO) inhibitors (systemic)	Marplan	Isocarboxazid		Duotrate Kaytrate Pentraspan Pentritol Peritrate	Pentaerythritol Tetranitrate
	Nardil	Phenelzine			
	Parnate	Tranylcypromine			
Nalbuphine (systemic)	Nubain	Nalbuphine			
Nalidixic acid (systemic)	Neg Gram	Nalidixic acid	Nitrofurantoin (systemic)	Cyantin Furadantin Furatine* Macrodantin Nephronex* Nifuran* Novofuran*	
Naproxen (systemic)	Anaprox Naprosyn	Naproxen			
Natamycin (ophthalmic)	Natacyn	Natamycin			
Neomycin (ophthalmic)	Myciguent	Neomycin	Nitroglycerin (systemic)	Glyceryl trinitrate Nitro-Bid Nitroglyn Nitrol Nitrong Nitrospan Nitrostat	Nitroglycerin
Neomycin (oral)	Mycifradin Neobiotic	Neomycin			
Neomycin (topical)	Herisan Antibiotic* Myciguent		Nylidrin (systemic)	Arlidin	Nylidrin
Neomycin, poly-myxin B, and bacitracin (ophthalmic)	Mycitracin Neo-Polycin Neosporin Polyspectrin Pyocidin		Nystatin (oral)	Mycostatin Nadostine* Nilstat	Nystatin
Neomycin, poly-myxin B, and bacitracin (topical)	Mycitracin Neo-Polycin Neosporin		Nystatin (topical)	Candex Mycostatin Nadostine* Nilstat Nyaderm*	Nystatin
Neomycin, poly-myxin B, and gramicidin (ophthalmic)	Neo-Polycin Neosporin		Nystatin (vaginal)	Korostatin Mycostatin Nadostine* Nilstat	Nystatin
Neomycin, poly-myxin B, and hydrocortisone (ophthalmic)	Cortisporin				

*Not available in the United States.

Drugs or drug type	Brand names	Generic name
Nystatin, neomycin, gramicidin, and triamcinolone (topical)	Mycolog Myco Triacet Mytrex Triamcinolone NNG	
Orphenadrine (systemic)	Flexojet Flexon Marflex Myolin Neocyten Norflex Ro-Orphena Tega-Flex X-Otag	
Orphenadrine and APC (systemic)	Norgesic Norgesic Forte	
Oxolinic acid (systemic)	Utibid	Oxolinic acid
Oxtriphylline and guaifenesin (systemic)	Brondecon Brondelate	
Oxycodone and acetaminophen (systemic)	Percocet-5 Tylox	
Oxycodone and aspirin (systemic)	Percodan Percodan-Demi	

Oxymetazoline (nasal)	Afrin
	Duration
	Nafrine*
	St. Joseph
	  Decongestant for
	  Children
		Oxymetazoline

Papaverine (systemic)	Cerebid Cerespan Dipav Dylate Hyobid Kavrin Myobid Orapav P-A-V Pavabid Pavacap Pavacon Pavadur Pavakey Pavased Pavasule Pavatest Pavatran	Papaverine

Drugs or drug type	Brand names	Generic name
	Paverolan Ro-Papav Sustaverine Vasal Vasospan	
Paraldehyde (systemic)	Paral	
Pargyline (systemic)	Eutonyl	
Pemoline (systemic)	Cylert	
Penicillamine (systemic)	Cuprimine Depen	
Penicillins (systemic)	Amoxil Larotid Novamoxin* Penamox* Polymox Robamox Sumox Trimox Utimox Wymox	Amoxicillin
	Amcill Ampicin* Omnipen Penbritin Pensyn Polycillin Principen Supen Totacillin	Ampicillin
	Geocillin Geopen Pyopen	Carbenicillin
	Bactopen* Cloxapen Novocloxin* Tegopen	Cloxacillin
	Cyclapen-W	Cyclacillin
	Dycill Dynapen Pathocil Veracillin	Dicloxacillin
	Versapen Versapen-K	Hetacillin
	Azapen Celbenin Staphcillin	Methicillin
	Nafcil Unipen	Nafcillin

*Not available in the United States.

Drugs or drug type	Brand names	Generic name
	Bactocill Prostaphlin	Oxacillin
	Bicillin Crystapen* Crysticillin Duracillin Megacillin* Penioral* Pentids Permapen Wycillin	Penicillin G
	Betapen-VK Novopen-V* Penapar VK Pen-Vee K Uticillin VK V-Cillin Veetids	Penicillin V
	Ticar	Ticarcillin
Pentazocine (systemic)	Talwin	Pentazocine
Pentazocine and aspirin (systemic)	Talwin Compound	
Pentobarbital and carbromal (systemic)	Carbrital	
Perphenazine and amitriptyline (systemic)	Etrafon Triavil	
Phenazopyridine (systemic)	Azo-100 Azodine Azo-Standard Di-Azo Phen-Azo Phenazodine Pyridiate Pyridium Pyrodine	Phenazopyridine
Phenothiazines (systemic)	Tindal	Acetophenazine
	Repoise	Butaperizine
	Proketazine	Carphenazine
	Chloramead Chlor-Promanyl* Chlorprom* Promapar Promosol* Largactil* Thorazine	Chlorpromazine

Drugs or drug type	Brand names	Generic name
	Modecate* Moditen* Permitil Prolixin	Fluphenazine
	Serentil	Mesoridazine
	Phenazine* Trilafon	Perphenazine
	Quide	Piperacetazine
	Compazine Stemetil	Prochlorperazine
	Norzine* Promanyl* Sparine	Promazine
	Mellaril Novoridazine* Thioril*	Thioridazine
	Clinazine* Novoflurazine* Pentazine* Solazine* Stelazine Terfluzine* Triflurin* Tripazine*	Trifluoperazine
	Psyquil* Vesprin	Triflupromazine
Phenoxybenzamine	Dibenzyline	
Phenylbutazone (systemic)	Oxalid Tandearil	Oxyphenbutazone
	Algoverine* Azolid Butagesic* Butazolidin Intrabutazone* Malgesic* Nadozone* Neo-Zoline* Novobutazone* Phenbutazone*	Phenylbutazone
	Azolid-A Butazolidin Alka Phenylzone-A	Buffered Phenylbutazone
Phenylephrine (nasal)	Alcon-Efrin Allerest Contac Coricidin Isophrin Neo-Mist Neo-Synephrine Pyracort-D	

*Not available in the United States.

Drugs or drug type	Brand names	Generic name	Drugs or drug type	Brand names	Generic name
	Rhinall Sinarest Super Anahist Synasal Vacon			K-Phos M. F. K-Phos Neutral K-Phos No. 2	Monobasic Potassium and Sodium Phosphates
Phenylephrine (ophthalmic)	Efricel Isopto Frin Mydfrin Neo-Synephrine Ocusol Phenoptic Prefrin Soothe Eye Tear-Efrin			Neutra-Phos	Potassium and Sodium Phosphates
			Potassium supplements (systemic)	Potassium Triplex Tri-K Trikates	Potassium Acetate, Potassium Bicarbonate, and Potassium Citrate
				K-Lyte	Potassium Bicarbonate and Citric acid
Phenylpropanolamine (systemic)	Coffee-Break Control Delcopro Diadax Dietac Obestat Pro-Dax 21 Propadrine Rhindecon			KEFF	Potassium Bicarbonate, Potassium Carbonate, and Potassium Chloride
				Klorvess	Potassium Bicarbonate and Potassium Chloride
Phenylpropanolamine, phenylephrine, phenyltoloxamine, and chlorpheniramine (systemic)	Naldecon			K-Lyte/Cl	Potassium Bicarbonate, Potassium Chloride, and Citric Acid
				Kaochlor-Eff	Potassium Bicarbonate, Potassium Chloride, and Potassium Citrate
Physostigmine (ophthalmic)	Eserine Isopto Eserine	Physostigmine		Kaochlor Kaon-Cl Kato Kay-Ciel K-Lor KLOR-10% KLOR-CON Klorvess Klotrix K-Lyte/Cl Slow-K	Potassium Chloride
Pilocarpine (ophthalmic)	Adsorbocarpine Almocarpine Isopto Carpine Miocarpine* Ocusert Pilo Pilocar Pilomiotin P. V. Carpine	Pilocarpine			
Potassium iodide (systemic)	KI-N Pima	Potassium iodide		Kolyum	Potassium Chloride and Potassium Gluconate
Potassium phosphates (systemic)	K-Phos Original	Monobasic Potassium Phosphates		Twin-K	Potassium Citrate and Potassium Gluconate
	Neutra-Phos-K	Potassium Phosphates		Kaon	Potassium Gluconate
Potassium and sodium phosphates (systemic)	Uro-KP-Neutral	Dibasic Potassium and Sodium Phosphates	Prazosin (systemic)	Minipress	Prazosin
			Primidone (systemic)	Mysoline	Primidone

*Not available in the United States.

Drugs or drug type	Brand names	Generic name	Drugs or drug type	Brand names	Generic name
Probenecid (systemic)	Benemid Benuryl* Probalan	Probenecid	Propoxyphene and acetaminophen (systemic)	Darvocet-N Dolacet Dolene AP-65 SK-65-APAP Wygesic	
Probucol (systemic)	Lorelco	Probucol	Propoxyphene and APC (systemic)	Darvon Compound Dolene Compound-65 SK-65 Compound	
Procainamide (systemic)	Procamide Procan Procan SR Procopan Pronestyl Sub-Quin	Procainamide	Propoxyphene and aspirin (systemic)	Darvon with A.S.A. Darvon-N with A.S.A.	
Procarbazine (systemic)	Matulane Natulan*	Procarbazine	Pseudoephedrine (systemic)	Afrinol D-Feda Eltor* Neobid Novafed Pseudofrin* Robindrine* Ro-Fedrin Sudafed Sudrin	Pseudoephedrine
Prochlorperazine and isopropamide (systemic)	Combid				
Progestins (systemic)	Duphaston	Dydrogesterone			
	Delalutin	Hydroxyprogesterone			
	Provera	Medroxyprogesterone	Pyrilamine and pentobarbital (systemic)	Eme-Nil Wans	
	Megace	Megestrol	Pyrithione zinc (topical)	Danex Head and Shoulders Zincon	
	Micronor Nor-Q.D. Norlutin	Norethindrone			
	Norlutate	Norethindrone Acetate	Pyrvinium (systemic)	Pamovin* Povan Pyr-Pam* Vanquin*	Pyrvinium
	Ovrette	Norgestrel			
	Proluton Lipo-Lutin	Progesterone	Quinidine (systemic)	Cardioquin Cin-Quin Duraquin Quinaglute Dura-Tabs Quinate* Quinidex Extentabs Quinora	
Promethazine (systemic)	Historest Phenergan Remsed	Promethazine			
Propantheline (systemic)	Pro-Banthine	Propantheline	Quinine (systemic)	Coco-Quinine Kinine* Quine	Quinine
Propoxyphene (systemic)	Algodex* Darvon Depronal-SA* Dolene Novopropoxyn* Pargesic 65 Pro-65* Proxagesic Proxene SK-65 642*	Propoxyphene	Quinine and aminophylline (systemic)	Quinamm Quinite Strema	
			Rauwolfia alkaloids (systemic)	Harmonyl Raunormine* Raudixin	Deserpidine

*Not available in the United States.

Drugs or drug type	Brand names	Generic name	Drugs or drug type	Brand names	Generic name
	Raulfia Raupoid Rauserpa	Rauwolfia Serpentina	Rifampin and iso- niazid (systemic)	Rifamate	
	Rau-Sed Reserpoid Sandril Serpasil	Reserpine	Salicyclates (systemic)	Bayer Aspirin Ecotrin Empirin Analgesic Measurin St. Joseph Aspirin	Aspirin
Rauwolfia alkaloids and thiazide di- uretics (systemic)	Oreticyl Oreticyl Forte	Deserpidine and Hy- drochlorothiazide		Ascriptin Bufferin CAMA Inlay-Tabs	Buffered Aspirin
	Enduronyl	Deserpidine and Methyclothiazide		Calurin	Carbaspirin
	Rauzide	Rauwolfia Serpen- tina and Bendro- flumethiazide		Arthropan	Choline Salicylate
	Exna-R	Reserpine and Benzthiazide		Parbocyl Uracel	Sodium Salicylate
	Diupres	Reserpine and Chlorothiazide	Salicylic acid (topical)	Calicylic Domerine Fomac	
	Demi-Regroton Regroton	Reserpine and Chlorthalidone		Hydrisalic Ionil Keralyt	
	Hydropres Reserpazide Serpasil-Esidrix	Reserpine and Hy- drochlorothiazide		Mediplast Saligel Sebisol	
	Salutensin Salutensin-Demi	Reserpine and Hy- droflumethiazide		Xseb	
	Diutensen-R	Reserpine and Methyclothiazide	Salicylic acid and sulfur (topical)	Acne-Dome Acno Antiseb	
	Renese-R	Reserpine and Polythiazide		BUF Exzit Fostex	
	Hydromox-R	Reserpine and Quinethazone		Klaron Meted Pernox	
	Metatensin Naquival	Reserpine and Tri- chlormethiazide		Rezamid SAStid Sebex	
Reserpine and hydralazine (systemic)	Serpasil-Apresoline			Sebulex Therac Vanseb	
Reserpine, hydrala- zine, and hydro- chlorothiazide (systemic)	Ser-Ap-Es Tri-Hydroserpine		Salicylic acid, sulfur, and coal tar (topical)	Antiseb-T Sebex-T Sebutone Vanseb-T	
Resorcinol and sulfur (topical)	Acne-Dome Acnomel Cenac Exzit pHisoAc Sulforcin		Selenium sulfide (topical)	Exsel Iosel Selsun Selsun Blue Sul-Blue	
Rifampin (systemic)	Rifadin Rimactane Rofact*	Rifampin	Sodium fluoride (systemic)	Denta-Fl Flo-Tab	

*Not available in the United States.

Drugs or drug type	Brand names	Generic name	Drugs or drug type	Brand names	Generic name
	Fluorident Fluoritab Fluorodex Flura Karidium Luride Luride-SF Nafeen Pedi-Dent Pediaflor Stay-Flo Studaflor		Sulfonamides (vaginal)	AVC Femguard Nil Tricholan Vagidine Vagimine Vagitrol	Sulfanilamide, Aminacrine, and Allantoin
				Sultrin Trysul	Sulfathiazole, Sulfacetamide, and Sulfabenzamide
				Koro-Sulf	Sulfisoxazole
Spironolactone (systemic)	Aldactone	Spironolactone		Vagilia	Sulfisoxazole, Aminacrine, and Allantoin
Spironolactone and hydrochlorothiazide (systemic)	Aldactazide		Sulfonamides and phenazopyridine (systemic)	Azo Gantanol	Sulfamethoxazole and Phenazopyridine
Succinimide-type anticonvulsants (systemic)	Zarontin Celontin Milontin Ethosuximide Methsuximide Phensuximide			Azo Gantrisin Azo-Soxazole Azosul Azo-Sulfizin Suldiazo	Sulfisoxazole and Phenazopyridine
Sulfasalazine (systemic)	Azulfidine S.A.S.-500 Salazopyrin*	Sulfasalazine	Sulindac (systemic)	Clinoril	Sulindac
			Tamoxifen (systemic)	Nolvadex	Tamoxifen
Sulfinpyrazone (systemic)	Anturan* Anturane Zynol	Sulfinpyrazone	Terbutaline (systemic)	Brethine Bricanyl	Terbutaline
Sulfonamides (ophthalmic)	Bleph Cetamide Isopto Cetamide Optosulfex* Sulamyd Sulf-10	Sulfacetamide	Terpin hydrate and codeine (systemic)	Cortussis	
			Testolactone (systemic)	Teslac	Testolactone
	Gantrisin	Sulfisoxazole	Tetracyclines (ophthamic)	Aureomycin	Chlortetracycline
				Achromycin	Tetracycline
Sulfonamides (systemic)	Renoquid	Sulfacytine	Tetracyclines (systemic)	Declomycin	Demeclocycline
	Gantanol Methoxal Methoxanol	Sulfamethoxazole		Doxychel Doxy-Tabs Vibramycin Vibra-Tabs	Doxycycline
	Bactrim Septra	Sulfamethoxazole and Trimethoprim		Rondomycin	Methacycline
	Gantrisin Lipo Gantrisin Novosoxazole* Sosol Sulfalar Sulfizin Sulfizole*	Sulfisoxazole		Minocin Ultramycin*	Minocycline
				Oxlopar Oxy-Kesso-Tetra Terramycin Tetramine	Oxytetracycline

*Not available in the United States.

Drug or drug type	Brand names	Generic name
	Achromycin Bio-Tetra* Bristacycline Cyclopar Medicycline* Neo-Tetrine* Novotetra* Panmycin Retet Robitet Sumycin Tetracrine* Tetracyn	Tetracycline
Tetracyclines (topical)	Aureomycin	Chlortetracycline
	Achromycin Topicycline	Tetracycline
Theophylline, ephed- rine, and barbi- turates (systemic)	Asminyl Asma-lief Phedral Tedfern Tedral Thalfed Thedrizem Theodrine Theofed Theofenal Theoral Theotabs	
Theophylline, ephed- rine, guaifenesin, and barbiturates (systemic)	Broncholate Bronkolixir Bronkotabs Duovent Luftodil Mudrane GG Quibron Plus Verequad	
Theophylline, ephed- rine, and hy- droxyzine (systemic)	Asminorel E.T.H. Compound Hydrophed Marax Theophozine Theozine	
Theophylline and guaifenesin (systemic)	Asbron G Asma Cerylin Dialixir Glybron Glyceryl T Hylate Lanophyllin-GG Quibron Slo-Phyllin GG Synophylate-GG Theo-Col Theo-Guaia	

Drug or drug type	Brand names	Generic name
Thiazide diuretics (systemic)	Naturetin	Bendroflumethiazide
	Aquastat Aquatag Exna Hydrex	Benzthiazide
	Diuril SK-Chlorothiazide	Chlorothiazide
	Hygroton Novothalidone* Uridon	Chlorthalidone
	Anhydron	Cyclothiazide
	Esidrix Hydro-Aquil HydroDIURIL Novohydrazide* Oretic	Hydrochlorothiazide
	Diucardin Saluron	Hydroflumethiazide
	Aquatensen Duretic Enduron	Methyclothiazide
	Diulo Zaroxolyn	Metolazone
	Renese	Polythiazide
	Hydromox	Quinethazone
	Metahydrin Naqua	Trichlormethiazide
Thioxanthenes (systemic)	Taractan Tarasan*	Chlorprothixene
	Navane	Thiothixene
Thyroid hormones (systemic)	Levothroid L-T-S Ro-Thyroxine Synthroid	Levothyroxine
	Cytomel Ro-Thyronine Tertroxin	Liothyronine
	Euthroid	Liotrix
	Proloid	Thyroglobulin
	S-P-T Thyrar Thyrocrine	Thyroid
Thyrotropin (systemic)	Thyrotron Thytropar	Thyrotropin
Timolol (ophthalmic)	Timoptic	Timolol
Tolmetin (systemic)	Tolectin	Tolmetin

*Not available in the United States.

Drug or drug type	Brand names	Generic name
Tolnaftate (topical)	Aftate Tinactin	Tolnaftate
Tretinoin (topical)	Retin-A	Tretinoin
Triamterene (systemic)	Dyrenium	Triamterene
Triamterene and hydrochlorothiazide (systemic)	Dyazide	
Tricyclic antidepressants (systemic)	Amitid Amitil Elavil Endep	Amitriptyline
	Norpramin Pertofrane	Desipramine
	Adapin Sinequan	Doxepin
	Imavate Janimine SK-Pramine Tofranil	Imipramine
	Aventyl Pamelor	Nortriptyline
	Vivactil	Protiptyline
	Surmontil	Trimipramine
Trifluridine (ophthalmic)	Viroptic	Trifluridine
Trimethobenzamide (systemic)	Tigan	Trimethobenzamide
Triprolidine and pseudoephedrine (systemic)	Actifed Allerphed Tagafed	
Tropicamide (ophthalmic)	Mydriacyl	Tropicamide
Undecylenic acid$_1$ compound (topical)	Decylenes Desenex Medaped Quinsana Plus	
Urea (systemic)	Ureaphil	
Valproic acid (systemic)	Depakene	Valproic acid
Vidarabine (ophthalmic)	Vira-A	Vidarabine
Vinblastine (systemic)	Velban Velbe*	Vinblastine

Drugs or drug type	Brand names	Generic name
Vincristine (systemic)	Oncovin	Vincristine
Vitamins and fluoride (systemic)	Vita-Flor Adeflor Mulvidren-F Novacebrin with Fluoride Vi-Penta F Poly-Vi-Flor V-Daylin with Fluoride	Multiple Vitamins and Fluoride
	Cari-Tab Tri-Vi-Flor	Vitamins A, D, and C, and Fluoride
(methyl)-Xanthines (systemic)	Aminodur Aminophyl* Amphylline* Corophyllin* Lixaminol Mini-Lix Somophyllin	Aminophylline
	Aerophylline* Airet Dilin Dilor Lufyllin Neothylline Protophylline*	Dyphylline
	Choledyl	Oxtriphylline
	Accurbron Aerolate Asthmophylline* Bronkodyl Elixicon Elixophyllin Physpan Slophyllin Somophyllin-T Theobid Theoclear Theodur Theolair Theolixir Theophyl Theospan	Theophylline
Xylometazoline (nasal)	4-Way Long Acting Neo-synephrine II Otrivin Rhinall Long Acting Sine-Off Once-A-Day Sinex Long-Acting Sinutab Long Acting Sinus Spray	

*Not available in the United States.

APPENDIX 12 • The nursing profession: associations in the United States and Canada and a directory of health care workers

12-1. Professional nursing associations in the United States

National Organizations

Alpha Tau Delta National Fraternity for Professional Nurses
489 Serento Circle
Thousand Oaks, Calif. 91360

American Association of Colleges of Nursing
Suite 430, 11 DuPont Circle
Washington, D.C. 20036

American Hospital Association
Division of Nursing
840 N. Lake Shore Drive
Chicago, Illinois 60611

American Indian/Alaska Native Nurses Association, Inc.
P.O. Box 1588
Norman, Oklahoma 73070

American Nurses' Association
2420 Pershing Road
Kansas City, Missouri 64108

Committee on Nursing of the Catholic Hospital Association
1438 S. Grand Boulevard
St. Louis, Missouri 63104

Gay Nurses' Alliance
P.O. Box 1015
Brownsville, Texas 78520

Lutheran Hospital Association of America
840 N. Lake Shore Drive
Room 607 W.
Chicago, Illinois 60611

National Black Nurses Association, Inc.
425 Ohio Building
175 S. Main Street
Akron, Ohio 44308

National Center for Nursing Ethics
P.O. Box 2237
Cincinnati, Ohio 45201

National League for Nursing
10 Columbus Circle
New York, New York 10019

National Male Nurse Association
2308 State Street
Saginaw, Michigan 48602

National Nurses for Life
1998 Menold
Allison Park, Pa. 15101

National Student Nurses' Association, Inc.
10 Columbus Circle
New York, New York 10019

Nurses Christian Fellowship
233 Langdon Street
Madison, Wisconsin 53703

Nurses Educational Funds
10 Columbus Circle
New York, New York 10019

Sigma Theta Tau
National Honor Society of Nursing
1100 West Michigan Street
Indianapolis, Indiana 46202

Specialty Associations

American Association for Respiratory Therapy
1720 Regal Row
Dallas, Texas 75235

American Association of Blood Banks
1828 L Street N.W.
Washington, D.C. 20036

American Association of Critical Care Nurses
P.O. Box C-19528
Irvine, California 92664

American Association of Nephrology Nurses and Technicians
Suite 219
505 N. Tustin
Santa Ana, California 92705

American Association of Neurosurgical Nurses
625 North Michigan Avenue
Suite 1519
Chicago, Illinois 60611

American Association of Nurse Anesthetists
111 East Wacker Drive
Suite 929
Chicago, Illinois 60601

American Association of Occupational Health Nurses, Inc.
575 Lexington Avenue
New York, New York 10022

American Board of Urologic Allied Health Professionals
2222 N.W. Lovejoy, Suite 256
Portland, Oregon 97210

American Burn Association
c/o Dr. Charles E. Hartford
Burn Treatment Center
Crozier-Chester Medical Center
15th and Upland Avenue
Chester, Pennsylvania 19013

American College of Nurse-Mid-Wives
Suite 1120
1522 K St., N.W.
Washington, D.C. 20005

American Geriatrics Society
Room 1470
10 Columbus Circle
New York, New York 10019

American Society for Hospital Nursing Service Administrators
840 N. Lake Shore Drive
Chicago, Illinois 60611

American Society of Radiologic Technologists
55 E. Jackson Boulevard
Suite 1820
Chicago, Illinois 60604

American Urological Association Allied
21510 S. Main Street
Carson, California 90745

Association for Practitioners in Infection Control
c/o Katherine R. Holl
557 N. Pinecrest
Wichita, Kansas 67208

Association for the Care of Children in Hospitals
3615 Wisconsin Ave., N.W.
Washington, D.C. 20016

Association of Operating Room Nurses
10170 E. Mississippi Avenue
Denver, Colorado 80231

Association of Pediatric Oncology Nurses
c/o Lorraine Bivalec
Pacific Medical Center
P.O. Box 7999
San Francisco, Calif. 94120

Association of Rehabilitation Nurses
2506 Gross Point Road
Evanston, Illinois 60201

Emergency Department Nurses' Association
666 N. Lake Shore Drive
Suite 1729
Chicago, Illinois 60611

International Association for Enterostomal Therapy
1701 Lake Avenue
Glenview, Illinois 60025

National Association of Orthopaedic Nurses
Scottish Rite Hospital
1001 Johnson Ferry Road, N.E.
Atlanta, Georgia 30342

National Association of Pediatric Nurse Associates and Practitioners
North Woodbury Road, Box 56
Pitman, New Jersey 08071

National Joint Practice Commission
Suite 1990
35 East Wacker Drive
Chicago, Illinois 60601

National Intravenous Therapy Association
Suite Four
93 Concord Ave.
Belmont, Massachusetts 02178

Nurses Association of the American College of Obstetricians & Gynecologists
Suite 2700
1 East Wacker Drive
Chicago, Illinois 60601

Oncology Nursing Society
c/o Donna Liberto
P.O. Box 33
Oakmont, Pennsylvania 15139

State Nurses' Associations

Alabama State Nurses Association
360 N. Hall Street
Montgomery, Alabama 36104

Alaska Nurses Association
1172 Gambell Street
Anchorage, Alaska 99501

Arizona Nurses Association
4525 N. 12th Street
Phoenix, Arizona 85014

Arkansas State Nurses Association
117 S. Cedar
Little Rock, Arkansas 72205

California Nurses Association
790 Market Street
San Francisco, Calif. 94102

Colorado Nurses Association
5453 E. Evans Place
Denver, Colorado 80222

Connecticut Nurses Association
1 Prestige Drive
Meriden, Connecticut 06450

Delaware Nurses Association
Room 201
1003 Delaware Avenue
Wilmington, Delaware 19806

District of Columbia Nurses Association
3000 Connecticut Ave. N.W.
Washington, D.C. 20008

Florida Nurses Association
Box 6985
Orlando, Florida 32853

Georgia Nurses Association
269 10th Street NE
Atlanta, Georgia 30309

Hawaii Nurses Association
677 Ala Moana #1014
Honolulu, Hawaii 96813

Idaho Nurses Association
1134 North Orchard #8
Boise, Idaho 83704

Illinois Nurses Association
6 North Michigan Avenue
Chicago, Illinois 60602

Indiana State Nurses Association
Suite 53
3231 N. Meridian Street
Indianapolis, Indiana 46208

Iowa Nurses Association
810 Walnut
Des Moines, Iowa 50309

Kansas State Nurses Association
Room 520
820 Quincy Street
Topeka, Kansas 66612

Kentucky Nurses Association
P.O. Box 8342, Station E
1400 South First Street
Louisville, Kentucky 40208

Louisiana State Nurses Association
P.O. Box 837
Metairie, Louisiana 70004

Maine State Nurses Association
83 Western Avenue
Augusta, Maine 04330

Maryland Nurses Association
2315-17 St. Paul Street
Baltimore, Maryland 21218

Massachusetts Nurses Association
141 Tremont Street
Boston, Massachusetts 02111

Michigan Nurses Association
120 Spartan Avenue
East Lansing, Michigan 48823

Minnesota Nurses Association
Room N-377
1821 University Avenue
St. Paul, Minnesota 55104

Mississippi Nurses Association
135 Bounds Street
Suite 100
Jackson, Mississippi 39206

Missouri Nurses Association
Box 325
206 East Dunklin Street
Jefferson City, Missouri 65101

Montana Nurses Association
P.O. Box 5718
1716 Ninth Avenue
Helena, Montana 59601

Nebraska Nurses Association
Suite 26
10730 Pacific Street
Omaha, Nebraska 68114

Nevada Nurses Association
3660 Baker Lane
Reno, Nevada 89509

New Hampshire Nurses Association
48 West Street
Concord, New Hampshire 03301

New Jersey State Nurses Association
Room 201
60 S. Fullerton Avenue
Montclair, New Jersey 07042

New Mexico Nurses Association
303 Washington S.E.
Albuquerque, New Mexico 87108

New York State Nurses Association
2113 Western Avenue
Guilderland, New York 12084

North Carolina Nurses Association
Box 12025
Raleigh, North Carolina 27605

North Dakota State Nurses Association
219 N. 7th Street
Bismarck, North Dakota 58501

Ohio Nurses Association
4000 East Main Street
Columbus, Ohio 43213

Oklahoma State Nurses Association
2912 Paseo
Oklahoma City, Oklahoma 73103

Oregon Nurses Association
Room 804
620 S.W. 5th Avenue
Portland, Oregon 97204

Pennsylvania Nurses Association
2515 N. Front Street
Harrisburg, Pa. 17110

Rhode Island State Nurses Association
134 Francis Street
Providence, Rhode Island 02903

South Carolina Nurses Association
1821 Gadsden Street
Columbia, S. Carolina 29201

South Dakota Nurses Association
Suite 6
1505 S. Minnesota
Sioux Falls, S. Dakota 57105

Tennessee Nurses Association
Suite 400
1720 West End Building
Nashville, Tennessee 37203

Texas Nurses Association
Suite 504, 1 Highland Center
314 Highland Mall Boulevard
Austin, Texas 78752

Utah Nurses Association
1058 East 9th South
Salt Lake City, Utah 84105

Vermont State Nurses Association
72 Hungerford Terrace
Burlington, Vermont 05401

Virginia Nurses Association
1311 High Point Avenue
Richmond, Virginia 23230

Washington State Nurses Association
1109 Second Avenue
Seattle, Washington 98101

West Virginia Nurses Association
47 Capital City Building
Charleston, W. Virginia 25301

Wisconsin Nurses Association
206 East Olin Avenue
Madison, Wisconsin 53713

Wyoming Nurses Association
Majestic Building, Room 305
1603 Capitol Avenue
Cheyenne, Wyoming 82001

Guam Nurses Association
Box 3134
Agana, Guam 96910

Virgin Island Nurses Association
P.O. Box 2866
Charlotte Amalie, St. Thomas,
Virgin Islands 00801

12-2. Licensure to practice nursing and directory of state boards of nursing

PURPOSE OF LICENSURE

Protection of the public is the basic purpose of all licensing legislation. Because of its concern for the health and welfare of the public, the American Nurses' Association supports the principle that any person who practices nursing should be licensed. ANA and state nurses' associations, since their establishment, have promoted state laws to regulate the practice of nursing, and they continue to work for the improvement of the existing laws.

Nursing is one of the health professions and occupations regulated by law in every state, the District of Columbia, and U.S. territories—American Samoa, Guam, Puerto Rico, and the Virgin Islands. Individuals desiring to practice nursing must meet the qualifications and standards established by the law of the jurisdiction.

ADMINISTRATION OF THE LAW

Laws regulating the practice of nursing vary from state to state. Generally, the state board of nursing is responsible for:

- Evaluating the personal and educational qualifications of applicants for licensure,
- Determining by examination applicants' competence to practice nursing,
- Issuing licenses to qualified applicants,
- Establishing minimum standards for and approving educational programs preparing persons for licensure, and
- Investigating and taking disciplinary action against violators, imposters, and those who are found unfit to practice nursing.

PROCEDURE FOR OBTAINING A LICENSE

Application forms are obtained directly from the board of nursing in the state in which the nurse wishes to be licensed.

Requirements for licensure include the successful completion of an approved program of study in nursing and an examination as determined by the state board of nursing. State laws may also include other requirements. Specific information regarding requirements is provided by the board of nursing from which the application form is obtained.

Application for initial licensure may be made in the state in which the program of study in nursing was completed or in the state where the individual intends to practice nursing.

A nurse licensed by examination in one state who wishes to practice in another state must submit an application to the board of nursing in that state. The state board of nursing reviews the information submitted and determines if a license may be granted without examination, if examination is indicated, or if supplementary education must be obtained. An examination is usually not required unless the nurse's scores on the initial licensure examination fail to meet the second state's standards.

The procedure for obtaining a license in another state should be completed prior to moving to that state.

THE LICENSING EXAMINATION

Nursing is one of the health professions that utilizes a nationwide standardized examination for licensure. The examinations for registered nurse licensure and practical nurse licensure have been one of the most effective means of facilitating the interstate licensing process for nurses.

The State Board Test Pool Examinations (SBTPE) were administered for the first time in 1944 and were developed through the cooperative efforts of state boards of nursing, the American Nurses' Association, and the National League of Nursing Education. The examinations continue to be developed and their use regulated by the National Council of State Boards of Nursing, Inc., in cooperation with the state boards of nursing. The Division of Measurement of the National League for Nursing is the test service agency for the SBTPE. The examinations are administered by the individual state boards of nursing.

The SBTPE for registered nurse licensure consists of tests in the areas of medical nursing, surgical nursing, obstetric nursing, nursing of children, and psychiatric nursing. Each of these tests includes questions from the biological, physical, and social sciences, nutrition and diet therapy, and pharmacology as they relate to the particular clinical nursing subject. Each test includes 90-125 multiple choice questions. A sixth test of 60 questions in one of the clinical subjects is also administered for statistical analyses of new questions. This sixth test is written only by graduates of U.S. schools of nursing who were graduated within the past 2 years and who are writing the examination for the first time. Two days are required for writing the entire examination.

The SBTPE for practical nurse licensure is an integrated examination with content appropriate to the beginning practice of practical/vocational nursing. For purposes of administration it is divided into two parts. Each part contains 118-125 multiple choice questions. A third test of 60 questions is administered for statistical analyses of new questions. This third test is written only by graduates of U.S. practical/vocational nursing programs who were graduated within the past 2 years and who are writing the licensing examination for the first time. One day is required for writing the entire examination.

Passing scores for the examinations for licensure are determined by the individual state boards of nursing.

Applicants should contact the board of nursing in the state in which they are seeking licensure for information about fees, testing dates, and examination centers. The examinations are administered on uniform dates specified by the National Council of State Boards of Nursing, Inc.

NURSES EDUCATED IN OTHER COUNTRIES

Nurses from other countries are expected to meet the same qualifications for licensure and to follow the same procedure for obtaining a license as graduates of U.S. schools of nursing.

Before leaving their own country, graduates of foreign nursing schools should take the Commission on Graduates of Foreign Nursing Schools (CGFNS) Qualifying Examination, which tests nursing and English language competency. The CGFNS examination is offered in April and October of each year. The CGFNS examination, while similar to the state licensing examination, is not a substitute for the SBTPE. In many states, passing the CGFNS examination is required before a graduate of a foreign nursing school is permitted to take the SBTPE.

A certificate issued by the Commission on Foreign Nurse Graduates is required by the U.S. government in order to secure a nonimmigrant occupational preference visa (H-1) and will soon be a requirement for the immigrant visa (third preference).

Application forms and information about the CGFNS Qualifying Examination may be obtained by writing to the Commission on Graduates of Foreign Nursing Schools, 3624 Market Street, Philadelphia, Pennsylvania 19104.

Once they are in the United States, nurses educated in other countries must successfully complete the licensure examination required by the respective state board of nursing. This examination is offered in February and July of each year. Specific information about the requirements for licensure should be requested directly from the board of nursing in the state where the nurse wishes to practice.

RENEWAL OF LICENSES

Each state law regulating the practice of nursing specifies when the license to practice nursing shall be renewed. The procedure for renewal includes the completion of an application for renewal and the submission of a renewal fee. Some states have additional requirements for renewal such as continuing education.

Nurses who allow their licenses to lapse by failing to renew may be reinstated upon completion of the requirements specified in the law. Nurses who choose to become inactive should inquire whether the state law permits an inactive status, and the requirements for reinstatement to active status. Information about these requirements is obtained from the state board of nursing.

STATE AND TERRITORIAL BOARDS OF NURSING

Alabama
Board of Nursing
One/East Bldg., Suite 203
500 Eastern Blvd.
Montgomery, Alabama 36109
Tel: (205) 832-5747

Alaska
Board of Nursing
142 East 3rd Avenue
Anchorage, Alaska 99501
Tel: (907) 276-7969

Arizona
Board of Nursing
State Occupational and Licensing Bldg.
1645 W. Jefferson, Suite 254
Phoenix, Arizona 85007
Tel: (602) 255-5092

Arkansas
Board of Nursing
Westmark Bldg., Suite 308
4120 West Markham Street
Little Rock, Arkansas 72205
Tel: (501) 371-2751

California
Board of Registered Nursing
1020 N. Street
Sacramento, California 95814
Tel: (916) 322-3350

Colorado
Board of Nursing
115 State Services Bldg.
1525 Sherman Street
Denver, Colorado 80203
Tel: (303) 839-2871

Connecticut
Board of Examiners for Nursing
79 Elm Street, Room 101
Hartford, Connecticut 06115
Tel: (203) 566-3716 or 566-4979

Delaware
Board of Nursing
Cooper Building, Room 234
Dover, Delaware 19901
Tel: (302) 678-4752

District of Columbia
Nurses' Examining Board
614 H. Street N.W., Rm. 112
Washington, D.C. 20001
Tel: (202) 629-4543

Florida
Board of Nursing
111 Coast Line Drive East, Suite 540
Jacksonville, Florida 32202
Tel: (904) 359-6331

Georgia
Board of Nursing
166 Pryor Street S.W.
Atlanta, Georgia 30303
Tel: (404) 656-3944
For Licensing Information
State Examining Boards
166 Pryor Street S.W.
Atlanta, Georgia 30303
Tel: (404) 656-3900

Guam
Administrative Secretary
Board of Nurse Examiners
P.O. Box 20518
Guam Main Facility, 96921

Hawaii
Board of Nursing
P.O. Box 3469
Honolulu, Hawaii 96801
Tel: (808) 548-7471

Idaho
Board of Nursing
413 W. Idaho Street, Rm. 203
Boise, Idaho 83702
Tel: (208) 384-3110

Illinois
Nursing Committee
Department of Registration & Education
Third Floor
628 East Adams Street
Springfield, Illinois 62786
Tel: (217) 785-0800

For Licensing Information
Department of Registration & Education
17th Floor
55 E. Jackson Blvd.
Chicago, Illinois 60604
Tel: (312) 341-9810

Indiana
Board of Nurses' Registration and Nursing
  Education
700 North High School Road
Indianapolis, Indiana 46224
Tel: (317) 633-5787/5705

Iowa
Board of Nursing
State Office Building
300-4th Street
Des Moines, Iowa 50319
Tel: (515) 281-3255

Kansas
Board of Nursing
Box 19235
Topeka, Kansas 66619
Tel: (913) 296-4929

Kentucky
Board of Nursing
4010 Dupont Circle, #430
Louisville, Kentucky 40207
Tel: (502) 897-5143

Louisiana
Board of Nursing
150 Baronne Street, Rm. 907
New Orleans, Louisiana 70112
Tel: (504) 568-5464

Maine
Board of Nursing
295 Water Street
Augusta, Maine 04330
Tel: (207) 289-2921

Maryland
Board of Examiners of Nurses
201 West Preston Street
Baltimore, Maryland 21201
Tel: (301) 383-2084/2085

Massachusetts
Board of Registration in Nursing
1509 Leverett Saltonstall Bldg.
100 Cambridge Street
Boston, Massachusetts 02202
Tel: (617) 727-3060

Michigan
Board of Nursing
P.O. Box 30018
Lansing, Michigan 48909
Tel: (517) 373-1600

Minnesota
Board of Nursing
717 Delaware Street S.E.
Minneapolis, Minnesota 55414
Tel: (612) 296-5493

Mississippi
Board of Nursing
135 Bounds Street, Suite 101
Jackson, Mississippi 39206
Tel: (601) 354-7349

Missouri
Board of Nursing
P.O. Box 656
Jefferson City, Missouri 65101
Tel: (314) 751-2334

Montana
Board of Nurses
Lalonde Bldg.
Helena, Montana 59601
Tel: (406) 449-3737

Nebraska
Board of Nursing
State House Station, P.O. Box 95065
Lincoln, Nebraska 68509
Tel: (402) 471-2001

Nevada
Board of Nursing
1201 Terminal Way, Suite 203
Reno, Nevada 89502
Tel: (702) 786-2778

New Hampshire
Board of Nursing Education & Nurse
   Registration
105 Loudon Road
Concord, New Hampshire 03301
Tel: (603) 271-2323

New Jersey
Board of Nursing
1100 Raymond Boulevard, Rm. 319
Newark, New Jersey 07102
Tel: (201) 648-2691

New Mexico
Board of Nursing
2340 Menaul N.E., Suite 112
Albuquerque, New Mexico 87107
Tel: (505) 842-3026

New York
Board for Nursing
State Education Department
Cultural Education Center
Albany, New York 12230
Tel: (518) 474-3843/3844
For Licensing Information
Division of Professional Licensing Ser.
State Education Department
Cultural Education Center
Albany, New York 12230
Tel: (518) 474-3817

North Carolina
Board of Nursing
P.O. Box 2129
Raleigh, North Carolina 27602
Tel: (919) 828-0740

North Dakota
Board of Nursing
418 East Rosser
Bismarck, North Dakota 58505
Tel: (701) 224-2974

Ohio
Board of Nursing Education & Nurse
   Registration
65 South Front Street, Suite 509
Columbus, Ohio 43215
Tel: (614) 466-3947

Oklahoma
Board of Nurse Registration & Nsg. Ed.
4001 North Lincoln Blvd., Suite 400
Oklahoma City, Oklahoma 73105
Tel: (405) 521-2363

Oregon
Board of Nursing
574 State Office Bldg.
1400 S.W. Fifth Avenue
Portland, Oregon 97201
Tel: (503) 229-5653/5654

Pennsylvania
Board of Nurse Examiners
P.O. Box 2649
Harrisburg, Pennsylvania 17120
Tel: (717) 783-3628

Rhode Island
Board of Nurse Registration and Nursing
   Education
104 Health Dept. Bldg.
75 Davis Street
Providence, Rhode Island 02908
Tel: (401) 277-2827

South Carolina
Board of Nursing
1777 St. Julian Place, Suite 102
Columbia, South Carolina 29204
Tel: (803) 758-2611

South Dakota
Board of Nursing
304 S. Phillips Ave., Suite 205

Sioux Falls, South Dakota 57102
Tel: (605) 334-1243

Tennessee
Board of Nursing
R.S. Gass State Office Bldg.
Ben Allen Road
Nashville, Tennessee 37216
Tel: (615) 741-7256

Texas
Board of Nurse Examiners
510 South Congress, Suite 216
Austin, Texas 78704
Tel: (512) 478-9602

Utah
Board of Nursing
330 East Fourth South Street
Salt Lake City, Utah 84111
Tel: (801) 533-5718

Vermont
Board of Nursing
Division of Registration & Licensing
10 Baldwin Street
Montpelier, Vermont 05602
Tel: (802) 828-2384

Virginia
Board of Nursing
Seaboard Bldg., Suite 453
3600 West Broad Street
Richmond, Virginia 23230
Tel: (804) 257-0350

Virgin Islands
Board of Nurse Examiners
P.O. Box 1442
Charlotte Amalie
St. Thomas, Virgin Islands 00801
Tel: (809) 774-1321, Ext. 254

Washington
Board of Nursing
Division of Professional Licensing
P.O. Box 9649
Olympia, Washington 98504
Tel: (206) 753-3726

West Virginia
Board of Examiners for Registered Nurses
Embleton Bldg., Suite 309
922 Quarrier Street
Charleston, West Virginia 25301
Tel: (304) 348-3596

Wisconsin
Dept. of Regulation & Licensing Division
   of Nurses
1400 E. Washington Avenue
Madison, Wisconsin 53702
Tel: (608) 266-3735

Wyoming
Board of Nursing
Hathaway Building
2300 Capitol Avenue
Cheyenne, Wyoming 82002
Tel: (307) 777-7601

SEPARATE STATE BOARDS OF PRACTICAL NURSING

California
Board of Vocational Nurse & Psychiatric Technician Examiners
1020 N. Street
Sacramento, California 95814
Tel: (916) 445-0739

District of Columbia
Practical Nurses' Examining Board
614 H. Street N.W.
Washington, D.C. 20001
Tel: (202) 629-4543

Georgia
Board of Examiners of Licensed Practical Nurses
166 Pryor Street S.W.
Atlanta, Georgia 30303
Tel: (404) 656-3900
For Licensing Information
State Examining Boards
166 Pryor Street S.W.
Atlanta, Georgia 30303
Tel: (404) 656-3900

Louisiana
Board of Practical Nurse Examiners
150 Baronne Street, Rm. 1408
New Orleans, Louisiana 70112
Tel: (504) 568-5825

Texas
Board of Vocational Nurse Examiners
Commerce Park, Bldg. H, Suite 131
5555 N. Lamar
Austin, Texas 78751
Tel: (512) 458-1203

Washington
Board of Practical Nursing
Division of Professional Licensing
P.O. Box 9649
Olympia, Washington 98504
Tel: (206) 753-3726

West Virginia
Board of Examiners for Licensed Practical Nursing
Embleton Bldg. Suite 506
922 Quarrier Street
Charleston, West Virginia 25301
Tel: (304) 348-3572

12-3. Registered nurses associations in Canada

CANADIAN ASSOCIATIONS

Canadian Association of Enterostomal Therapy

Of the approximately 110 enterostomal therapists in Canada, more than 90 are active members of the Canadian Association of Enterostomal Therapists. Most are registered nurses working in hospitals or home care agencies; all are working to effect the rehabilitation of those persons who undergo 'ostomy surgery'. But they also care for individuals with any kind of draining wound and many are involved in the treatment of pressure sores and the teaching of self-catheterization.

The CAET, a member of the International Association of Enterostomal Therapists, meets annually at a spring conference and a teaching seminar is usually held in the fall. Provincial interest groups are active.

Enterostomal Therapy Centre
Royal Jubilee Hospital
Victoria, B.C.
V8R 1J8

Canadian Association of Neurological and Neurosurgical Nurses

This group was founded in Toronto in 1969 by Miss Jessie Young and was the first group of specialized nurses to form on a national basis. Its objectives are:

- to promote the highest standards of practice in the field of neurological and neurosurgical nursing,
- to foster continuing professional education of the members,
- to provide methods of sharing this knowledge, and
- to establish and maintain lines of communication between nursing and other disciplines practising in the field of neurological sciences.

An affiliate of the Canadian Nurses Association, the association meets annually to present papers of interest to membership and to elect a board of directors and councillors to represent each province. Both active and associate memberships in the association are available. Membership now stands at 341.

296 Palace Road
Kingston, Ontario
K7L 4T3

Canadian Association of Practical and Nursing Assistants

CAPNA, founded in 1971, is the national organization and official spokesman for approximately 80,000 Licensed Practical Nurses, Certified, Licensed and Registered Nursing Assistants. One of the main objectives of CAPNA is to promote the uniformity of curriculum content, standardization of training and registration in all of Canada, to establish a minimum proficiency level of care across the country. The association also strives to promote improved health care and to interpret the role of the practical nurse and nursing assistant on the health care team.

R.R. No. 4
St. Stephen, N.B.
E3L 2Y2

Canadian Association of University Schools of Nursing

In 1942, eight university schools of nursing met and agreed to organize a "provisional council of university schools and departments of nursing" in order to determine desirable standards for existing schools and to support the development of future university schools of nursing. Now the voluntary association represents all 23 university schools of nursing in Canada and membership, which is by institution only, is supported by membership fees from the constituent universities. An associate member of the Association of Universities and College of Canada, CAUSN meets on a national basis to discuss issues in higher education. At present, its objectives include:

- to develop criteria for university education in nursing,
- to promote research in nursing,
- to promote the interchange of nursing knowledge among members,
- to represent the views of the association to educational, professional and other appropriate bodies, and
- to promote understanding by the public that university education in nursing contributes to the development of health services in Canada.

To ensure continuity of thought and activities between council meetings and to consolidate the structure of the association, four regions of the association have been formed: Atlantic, Quebec, Ontario and the Western regions.

CAUSN is the official accreditation agency for university nursing programs in Canada.

1200-151 Slater
Ottawa, Ont.
K1P 5N1

Canadian Council of Cardiovascular Nurses

The C.C.C.N. was founded in 1973 as a scientific council of the Canadian Heart Foundation. With membership open to all registered nurses interested in cardiovascular diseases (membership now stands at approximately 1600) the council works to promote the quality of health care as it relates to cardiovascular functioning.

The C.C.C.N., which has a board of management responsible to the board of directors of the Canadian Heart Foundation, has two main standing committees: the continuing education committee, responsible for educational events, such as traveling lectureship programs on the national level and a variety of workshops and seminars on a provincial level; and the research committee which stimulates and coordinates nursing research as well as encourages publication and dissemination of information on current trends and results of research in the cardiovascular field.

An annual membershp fee of $15 includes many benefits:

- the opportunity to attend an annual meeting and scientific sessions of the Canadian Heart Foundation, the Canadian Cardiovascular Society and of the Council,
- a Quarterly Bulletin, written and published by C.C.C.N., continuing education articles, news happenings, and educational courses being offered,
- seminars and workshops at the provincial level,
- a voice in public education through representation on the Heart Foundation committees,
- entitlement of free subscription to three official journals of the American Heart Association, *(Modern Concepts of Cardiovascular Disease, Cardiovascular Nursing,* and *Current Concepts of Cerebrovascular Disease),*
- access to a central pool of audio-visual aids and bibliographies,
- a nursing research fellowship for nurses seeking advanced preparation at the Masters or doctoral level, and
- reduced fees for council-sponsored programs.

Canadian Council of Cardiovascular Nurses
1200-1 Nicholas St.
Ottawa, Ont.
K1N 7B7

Canadian Hospital Infection Control Association

CHICA was founded in June 1971 to improve and support methods and facilities needed by those engaged in the prevention and control of infections in health care institutions in Canada. The association's objectives include:

- to initiate and develop effective communications,
- to support the development of effective and rational infection control programs in health care agencies,
- to encourage standardization and critical evaluation of infection control practices,
- to promote quality research in practices and procedures related to infection control,
- to initiate the creation of educational programs in infection control, and
- to create regional organizations in order to improve the exchange of scientific knowledge.

Membership in CHICA is extended to all individuals occupationally or professionally involved in the practice of infection control. The CHICA newsletter, the official newsletter of the association, is the primary means of communication among membership which meets annually for a national conference.

McMaster University
Medical Centre
1200 Main St. W.
Hamilton, Ontario
L8S 4J9

Canadian Intravenous Nurses Association

Founded in 1975 with the aim of promoting higher standards in intravenous therapy for better and safer care through communication, education and participation, CINA has been active in meeting this goal and boasts a membership of over 150.

At the request of CINA, a working group was established by Health and Welfare Canada to develop guidelines for the administration of I.V. therapy. Two CINA members represented the association on this project. Currently, representatives of CINA are meeting with community colleges to discuss the possibility of offering courses in intravenous therapy to all personnel interested in this field. In preparation for this, a questionnaire was sent to all hospitals in Ontario asking if such a course was wanted and very favorable replies were received.

Active, inactive and associate memberships are available in the association. An active membership fee is currently $30 and includes a subscription of ten issues of the *American Journal of I.V. Therapy* and a quarterly CINA newsletter. An annual convention attracts a variety of speakers and exhibitors.

CINA
200-4433 Sheppard Ave. E.
Agincourt, Ontario
M1S 1V3

Canadian Nurses Foundation

The Canadian Nurses Foundation (CNF) is the only Canadian foundation that deals exclusively in supporting nursing scholars. Launched in 1962 with a donation from the W.K. Kellogg Foundation, the Foundation's entire source of revenue since 1967 has been from nurses, either by individual memberships, personal donations, or donations from provincial nurses associations.

CNF solicits and holds funds to provide scholarships for nurses undertaking graduate studies in nursing and to provide grants in aid of nursing research; more than 200 nurses have benefited from CNF scholarships. The Foundation has an elected voluntary board of directors chosen every two years from among its membership and has a nurse representative in each province.

Membershp now stands at well over 500. Fees: regular membership, $10; sustaining, $50 and patron $500 (initial fee).

Applicants for an award must be a member of their provincial nurses association and have gained acceptance into graduate school. They must identify the practice area in which they wish to study and have definite career goals.

Canadian Nurses Foundation
50 The Driveway
Ottawa, Ontario
K2P 1E2

Canadian Nurses Respiratory Society

An affiliate of the Canadian Nurses Association, membership in this society is open to all registered nurses working with or interested in alleviating the problems associated with respiratory disease. As a section of the Canadian Lung Association, all members of the society receive the two official publications of the association: the quarterly Bulletin and the bimonthly Canadian Lung Association Newsletter, and, as well, take part in the association's annual meeting. The objectives of the society include:
- to contribute to the promotion of health of Canadians,
- to further objectives of the Canadian Lung Association within the scope of the nursing profession and in conjunction with other related professional organizations,
- to encourage members of the nursing profession to keep up with advances in the prevention, treatment and rehabilitation of respiratory diseases,
- to act in an advisory capacity to nursing and allied professional groups on matters pertinent to respiratory care, and
- to encourage nurses to engage in research related to respiratory health and disease (research grants and funding available).

Currently, the society is compiling a resource index of nurses involved in respiratory care across Canada.

Nurses Section
Canadian Lung Association
908-75 Albert St.
Ottawa, Ont.
K1P 5E7

Canadian Orthopedic Nurses Association

One of the largest and most active national associations in Canada today, CONA boasts over 700 members and nine chapters. Promotion of the highest standards in the practice of orthopedic nursing through continuing education has been the prime objective of this group. To meet this objective CONA publishes a professional quarterly journal and has a very active continuing education committee dedicated to providing nurses with a library of clinical resource material to help solve orthopedic problems. At their annual meeting, which features a wide variety of speakers and exhibitors, two nurses are recognized; one as Orthopedic Nurse of the Year and the second for her contributions to continuing education in the orthopedic nursing field.

Membership is open to all nursing personnel and other health professionals interested in the field of orthopedics for a fee of $15.

The Canadian Orthopedic
Nurses Association
43 Wellesley Street E.
Toronto, Ont.
M4Y 1H1

Canadian University Nursing Students

Promoting professionalism among university nursing students, that is the purpose of CUNSA, a national association which held its first conference in 1968 with representatives from five universities. In 1972, CUNSA became an official association made up of 22 university schools of nursing. Affiliated with CAUSN, the association's objectives include:
- to provide a communication link between university nursing students across Canada,
- to act as the official voice of university nursing students,
- to provide a medium through which students can express their opinions on issues in nursing,
- to provide liaison with other organizations concerned with nursing, and
- to assist and/or initiate nursing research.

CUNSA is divided into four regions: Atlantic, Quebec, Ontario and Western; each with a regional chairperson and representative to the national executive committee. Membership fees are paid by member universities, which pay according to student enrollment. An annual conference and a quarterly newsletter facilitate communications between membership.

This year, CUNSA has compiled a booklet on post RN nursing in Canada and completed a survey of future educational needs cited by current students.

1468 Summer St.
Halifax, N.S.
B3H 3A3

National Conference of Operating Room Nurses

An affiliate of the Canadian Nurses Association, this group is primarily concerned with continuing education for O.R. nurses, in upgrading standards of O.R. care and in increasing communication between O.R. nurses. The most major change for the group has been the appointment of a "National Liaison Officer" to increase communication between each provicincial group. This individual will compile the national newsletter bi-annually, establish a file of each province's constitution, executive and total membership figures, and collect information on upcoming conferences, etc. National conferences are presented every two years.

National Chairperson:	*National Liaison Officer:*
c/o Operating Room	Box 535
St. Boniface General Hospital	Brooks, Alberta
Winnipeg, Manitoba	T0J 0J0
R2H 2A6	

Nursing Sisters Association of Canada

In the 1920's, after World War I, nursing sisters across Canada began to form groups to keep up the friendships which they had developed overseas and to extend assistance to those in need. In 1920, the first group was officially formed in Edmonton and was closely followed by the formation of similar groups across Canada. In July, 1929, at the International Congress of Nurses in Montreal, the National Association of Overseas Nursing Sisters was formed, later, the name was changed to the Nursing Sisters Association of Canada. Currently, membership in the association includes nurses, Home Sisters, dieticians and physiotherapists who have been honorably discharged or are now serving with her Majesty's forces. With a current membership of 891, units still exist in all provinces and a national executive is elected. Their objectives include:
- to stimulate friendship among members,
- to work for national unity and international peace, and
- to give aid and comfort to nurses in need.

Affiliated with the National Council of Veteran Associations of Canada, the association holds biennial meetings during the biennial convention of the Canadian Nurses Association. The Agnes Campbell Neill Memorial Award, presented every two years through the Canadian Nurses Foundation, is sponsored by the Nursing Sisters Association of Canada.

8500 Francis Rd.
Richmond, B.C.
V6Y 1A6

Psychiatric Nurses Association of Canada

This national association had its beginnings in 1950 when representatives of the British Columbia and Saskatchewan associations met and made plans to form the Canadian Council of Psychiatric Nurses. After the 1951 founding conference, attended by delegates from B.C., Saskatchewan and Alberta, Manitoba joined in 1960, Ontario in 1971 and Nova Scotia in 1974. The Northwest Territories was admitted as an associate member in 1977.

The association, whose name was changed in 1965, has a national office, a bi-monthly publication—*The Canadian Journal of Psychiatric Nursing*—and sponsors research and meetings aimed at improved national standards of psychiatric care.

Psychiatric Nurses
Association of Canada
1854 Portage Ave.
Winnipeg, Man.
R3J 0G9

Registered Nurses of Canadian Indian Ancestry

The Registered Nurses of Canadian Indian Ancestry is a group of Indian nurses who are interested in striving for and promoting better health for Canadian Indian people. The idea for the association was conceived in 1974 by a few nurses who were concerned with the poor health of their people as a group. In 1975, during International Women's Year, 43 nurses of Canadian Indian ancestry from across Canada met, the first assembly of Indian professionals in the history of Canada. The following objectives have been adopted:

- to act as an agent in promoting and striving for better health for the Indian people,
- to conduct studies and maintain reporting, compiling information and publishing of material on Indian health, medicine and culture,
- to offer assistance to government and private agencies in developing programs designed to improve health in Indian communities,
- to maintain a consultative mechanism which the association, bands, government and other agencies concerned with Indian health may utilize,
- to develop and encourage courses in the educational system of nursing and health professions on Indian health and cross-cultural nursing.
- to generally encourage and facilitate Indian control of Indian health involvement and decision-making in Indian health care,
- to research cross-cultural nursing and cross-cultural medicine and develop and assemble material on Indian health, and
- to actively develop a means of recruiting more people of Indian ancestry into the medical field and health professions.

500-275 Portage Ave.
Winnipeg, Man.
R3B 2B3

INTERNATIONAL ASSOCIATIONS-CANADIAN DIVISIONS
American Association of Critical Care Nurses, Toronto Chapter

Initially, the American Association of Cardiovascular Nurses, the organization was reincorporated in 1972 to become the American Association of Critical Care Nurses. Today, AACN is the world's largest specialty nursing organization, with an international membership of over 36,000 nurses working in critical care.

The first Canadian chapter, the Toronto chapter was officially sanctioned in 1976. Membership in the association, which costs $42.50, includes: a subscription to *Heart & Lung—The Journal of Critical Care* and *Focus on AACN*, the bi-monthly newsletter, a self-assessment guide published in *Focus* to allow testing of comprehension of editorial content of the journal, a core curriculum for critical care nursing, a compilation of core knowledge for these nurses at reduced cost, a national teaching institute, an annual four-day learning seminar, continuing education opportunities and the Toronto Chapter newsletter.

Toronto Chapter—AACN
P.O. Box 37, Postal Station Z
Toronto, Ontario
M5N 2Z3

Association for the Care of Children's Health

ACCH is an international interdisciplinary organization focusing on the psychosocial needs of children and their families in health care settings. Founded in 1965, the association has more than 200 members, who include individuals in the fields of administration, architecture, child life activities, dietetic, education, medicine, nursing, occupational therapy, psychiatry, psychology, recreation, rehabilitation, social work, as well as concerned consumers. Full individual membership is $30. Members receive a quarterly journal containing research articles, a bi-monthly newsletter, an opportunity for multidisciplinary interaction and legislative input, current publications available at minimum fees and eligibility to attend study sessions that focus on specific issues. There is also an annual four-day conference. Several local affiliates exist across Canada.

ACCH
3615 Wisconsin Ave. N.W.
Washington, D.C.
U.S.A. 20016

Nurses Association of the American College of Obstetricians and Gynecologists

More than 19,000 registered nurses and allied health care personnel make up NAACOG which endorses the philosophy that it must foster and promote the highest standards of practice in obstetrics, gynecologic and neonatal nursing. The association hopes to promote this philosophy through encouraging professional growth, teamwork through their affiliation with the American College of Obstetricians and Gynecologists and liaison with other allied professional associations and continuing education. The Association is divided geographically into eight sections which extend north/south. As a result Canadian provinces are members of four different districts: Atlantic provinces and Quebec, District I; Ontario, District V; Manitoba, Saskatchewan, District VI; and Alberta and British Columbia, District VIII. Membership fees of $50 include a subscription to the *Journal of Obstetric, Gynecologic and Neonatal Nursing*, a Manual of Standards for OGN Nursing with Technical and Practice Resource Bulletins and local newsletters as well as annual conferences and seminars.

N.A.A.C.O.G. Membership Department
One East Wacker Drive, Suite 2700
Chicago, Illinois
U.S.A. 60601

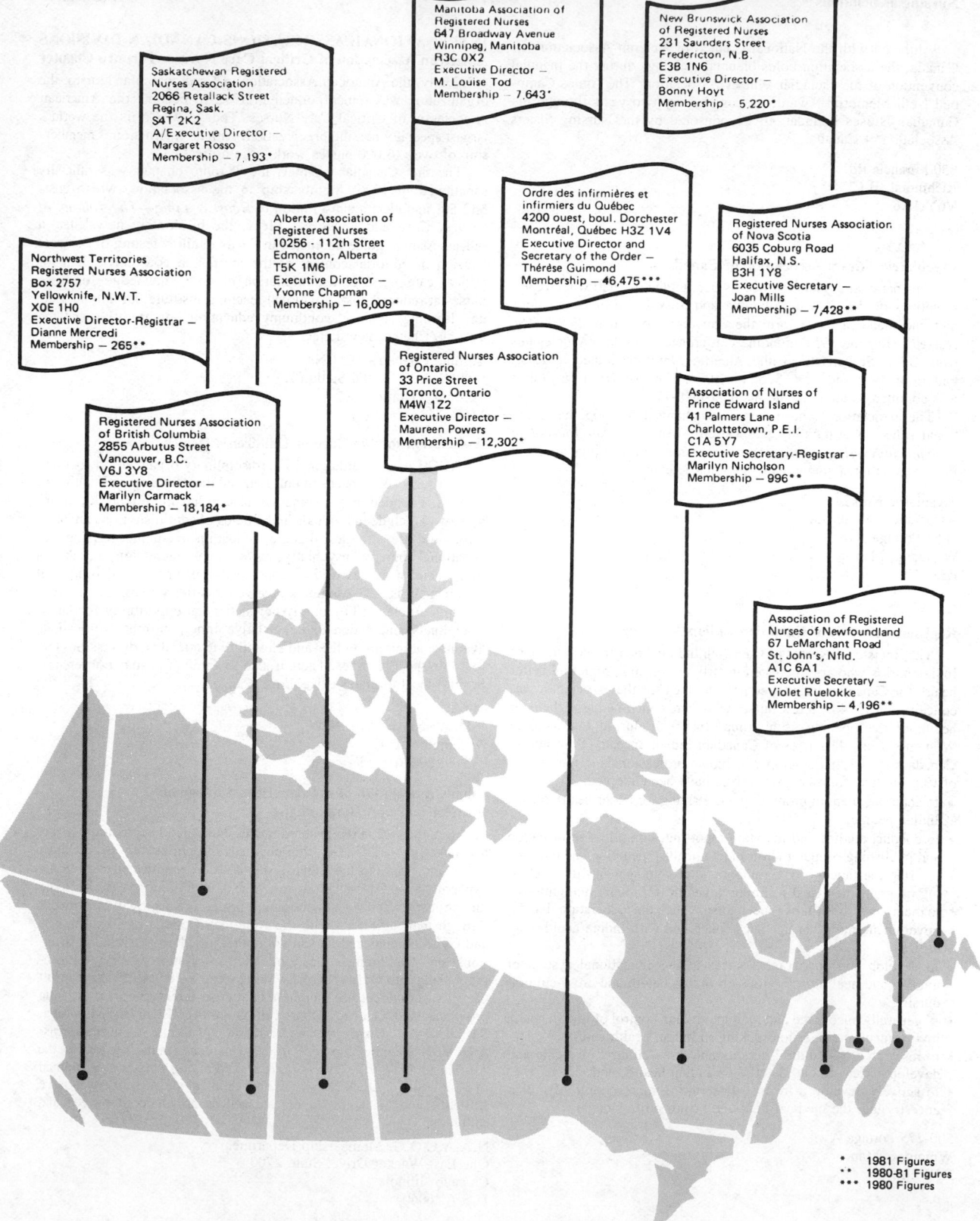

Saskatchewan Registered
Nurses Association
2066 Retallack Street
Regina, Sask.
S4T 2K2
A/Executive Director —
Margaret Rosso
Membership — 7,193*

Manitoba Association of
Registered Nurses
647 Broadway Avenue
Winnipeg, Manitoba
R3C 0X2
Executive Director —
M. Louise Tod
Membership — 7,643*

New Brunswick Association
of Registered Nurses
231 Saunders Street
Fredericton, N.B.
E3B 1N6
Executive Director —
Bonny Hoyt
Membership — 5,220*

Alberta Association of
Registered Nurses
10256 - 112th Street
Edmonton, Alberta
T5K 1M6
Executive Director —
Yvonne Chapman
Membership — 16,009*

Ordre des infirmières et
infirmiers du Québec
4200 ouest, boul. Dorchester
Montréal, Québec H3Z 1V4
Executive Director and
Secretary of the Order —
Thérèse Guimond
Membership — 46,475***

Registered Nurses Association
of Nova Scotia
6035 Coburg Road
Halifax, N.S.
B3H 1Y8
Executive Secretary —
Joan Mills
Membership — 7,428**

Northwest Territories
Registered Nurses Association
Box 2757
Yellowknife, N.W.T.
X0E 1H0
Executive Director-Registrar —
Dianne Mercredi
Membership — 265**

Registered Nurses Association
of Ontario
33 Price Street
Toronto, Ontario
M4W 1Z2
Executive Director —
Maureen Powers
Membership — 12,302*

Association of Nurses of
Prince Edward Island
41 Palmers Lane
Charlottetown, P.E.I.
C1A 5Y7
Executive Secretary-Registrar —
Marilyn Nicholson
Membership — 996**

Registered Nurses Association
of British Columbia
2855 Arbutus Street
Vancouver, B.C.
V6J 3Y8
Executive Director —
Marilyn Carmack
Membership — 18,184*

Association of Registered
Nurses of Newfoundland
67 LeMarchant Road
St. John's, Nfld.
A1C 6A1
Executive Secretary —
Violet Ruelokke
Membership — 4,196**

*   1981 Figures
**   1980-81 Figures
***   1980 Figures

PROVINCIAL TERRITORIAL AND LOCAL ASSOCIATIONS

British Columbia

British Columbia Nursing
Supervisors Group
(RNABC Affiliate)
3318 Napier St.
Vancouver, B.C.
V5K 2X3

British Columbia Occupational
Health Nurses Interest Group
(RNABC Affiliate)
1801 Dublin St.
New Westminster, B.C.
V3M 3A2

British Columbia Operating
Room Nurses Group
(RNABC Affiliate)
4313 Alderwood Crescent
Burnaby, B.C.
V5G 2G7

Community Health Nurses
Interest Group of
British Columbia
(RNABC Affiliate)
P.O. Box 451
Abbotsford, B.C.
V2S 5Z5

Emergency Nurses Group
of British Columbia
(RNABC Affiliate)
P.O. Box 86824
North Vancouver, B.C.
V7L 4L3

Home Care Nurses Group
of British Columbia
(RNABC Affiliate)
5621 Forglen Dr.
Burnaby, B.C.
V5H 3K9

The Licensed Practical Nurses
Association of British Columbia
695 Montague Rd.
Nanaimo, B.C.
V9R 3G4

Nursing Administrators'
Association of British Columbia
Vernon Jubilee Hospital
Vernon, B.C.
V1T 5L2

Registered Psychiatric Nurses
Association of British Columbia
7790 Edmonds Street
Burnaby, B.C.
V3N 1B8

Alberta

Alberta Association of
Registered Nursing Assistants
11435-107th Avenue
Edmonton, Alberta
T5H 0Y6

Alberta Community Health Nurses
811-71 Avenue, N.W.
Calgary, Alberta
T2K 0N6

Alberta Health Care Educators
Interest Group
1212-2010 Ulster Road, N.W.
Calgary, Alberta
T2N 4C2

Alberta Occupational Health
Nurses Association
231 Lake Placid Green, S.E.
Calgary, Alberta
T2J 5G6

Alberta Respiratory Nursing
Association
2-10625-85 Avenue
Edmonton, Alberta
T6E 2K6

Calgary Infection Control Group
Colonel Belcher Hospital
1213-4th Street, S.W.
Calgary, Alberta
T2R 0X7

Canadian Orthopedic Nurses
Association, Alberta Chapter
1315-63 Street
Edmonton, Alberta
T5A 0W9

Consortium of Senior Nurse
Educators, Alberta
University of Lethbridge
Lethbridge, Alberta
T1K 3M4

Emergency Nurse Interest Group
115 Brander Villager
Edmonton, Alberta
T6H 5C9

OCEAN, Oncology Club
Edmonton Alberta Nurses
10930-65 Avenue
Edmonton, Alberta
T6H 4R6

Operating Room Nurses of Alberta
2502-8210-11 St.
Edmonton, Alberta
T6G 2C7

Psychiatric Nurses Association
of Alberta
16314-88 Street
Edmonton, Alberta
T5R 4M7

Western Nurse Midwives
Association
Box 4268
Edmonton, Alberta
T6E 4T3

Saskatchewan

Administrative Nurses Section
(SRNA Interest Group)
SRNA
2066 Retallack St.
Regina, Sask.
S4T 2K2

Saskatchewan Nursing
Assistants' Association
2066 Retallack St.
Regina, Sask.
S4T 2K2

Saskatchewan Psychiatric
Nurses Association
Suite D
2835-13th Avenue
Regina, Sask.
S4T 1N6

Manitoba

Association for the Care
of Children's Health
(Manitoba Affiliate)
Winnipeg Health Sciences Centre
685 Bannatyne Avenue
Winnipeg, Manitoba
R3E 0W1

CAN_3 (Canadian Association
of Neurological and
Neurosurgical Nurses)
1202-411 Cumberland Ave.
Winnipeg, Manitoba
R3B 1T7

Cardiovascular Nurses
Interest Group
630 Cordova St.
Winnipeg, Manitoba
R3N 1B1

Dialysis Interest Group
73 Lennox Ave.
Winnipeg, Manitoba
R2M 1A8

Directors of Nursing Education
Misericordia General Hospital
99 Cornish Avenue
Winnipeg, Manitoba
R3C 1A2

Manitoba Health Care Inservice
Education Interest Group
Deer Lodge Hospital
2109 Portage Ave.
Winnipeg, Manitoba
R3J 0L3

Manitoba Indian
Nurses' Association
2nd Floor
550 Main St.
Winnipeg, Manitoba
R3B 1C4

Manitoba Infection Control Group
Infection Control Nurse
Brandon General Hospital
150 McTavish Ave. E.
Brandon, Manitoba
R7A 2B3

Manitoba Nursing Research Group
St. Boniface General Hospital
School of Nursing
431 Tache Ave.
Winnipeg, Manitoba
R2H 2A7

Manitoba Operating Room
Study Group
MARN building
647 Broadway Ave.
Winnipeg, Manitoba
R3C 0X2

Maternal Child Interest Group
(NAACOG)
477 Boyd Ave.
Winnipeg, Manitoba
R2W 1P7

Nurse Practitioners Interest Group
Klinic Inc.
545 Broadway Ave.
Winnipeg, Mannitoba
R3C 0W3

Nurses Christian Movement of
Manitoba Interest Group
220 Oak St.
Winnipeg, Manitoba
R3M 3R4

Nursing Administration
Interest Group
Box 9600
Selkirk Mental Health Centre
Selkirk, Manitoba
R1A 2B5

Occupational Health Nurses
Interest Group
44 Pleasant Bay
Winnipeg, Manitoba
R2K 0E3

Personal Care Homes
Interest Group
107-35 Valhalla Drive
Winnipeg, Manitoba
R2G 0G5

Phillipine Nurses Association
of Manitoba
824 Cloutier Dr.
Winnipeg, Manitoba
R3V 1L2

Respiratory Interest Group
Canada Arthritis Society
825 Sherbrook St.
Winnipeg, Manitoba
R3G 2L3

Winnipeg Association of
Critical Care Nurses
336 Overdale St.
Winnipeg, Manitoba
R3J 2G4

Ontario

American Association of
Critical Care Nurses
(Toronto Chapter)
P.O. Box 37
Postal Station Z
Toronto, Ontario
M5N 1A0

Association of Nursing Directors
& Supervisors of Ontario Official
Health Agencies
Borough of East York Health Unit
550 Mortimer Avenue
Toronto, Ontario
M4J 2H2

Association of Nursing Executives,
Metro Toronto
Director of Inpatient Services
Etobicoke General Hospital
101 Humber College Blvd.
Rexdale, Ontario
M9V 1R8

Canadian Association of
Quality Care Coordinators
St. Joseph's General Hospital
720 McLaren St.
North Bay, Ontario
P1B 3L9

Canadian Association of
University School of Nursing,
Ontario Region
Laurentian University
Ramsay Lake Rd.
Sudbury, Ontario
P3E 2C6

Emergency Nurses Association
of Ontario
McMaster University
Medical Centre
1200 Main St. W.
Hamilton, Ontario
L8S 4J9

Gerontological Nursing
Association of Ontario
(RNAO Affiliate)
14 Bruce Park Ave.
Toronto, Ontario
M4P 2S3

Lakehead Operating Room
Nurses Association
McKellar General Hospital O.R.
Thunder Bay, Ontario
P7E 1G6

Metro Toronto In-Service
Educators Association
St. Michael's Hospital
30 Bond St.
Toronto, Ontario
M5B 1W8

Niagara Association of
Critical Care Nurses
NACCN
P.O. Box 61
Welland, Ontario
L3B 5N9

Northern Ontario Operating
Room Nurses Interest Group
Kirkland and District Hospital
145 Government Rd. E.
Kirkland Lake, Ontario
P2N 1R2

Northwestern Ontario
Occupational Health Nurses
Association
Health Services
Confederation College
P.O. Box 398
Station F
Thunder Bay, Ontario
P7C 4W1

Nurse Childbirth
Educators' Group
326 Morrison Rd.
Oakville, Ontario
L6J 4J9

Nurse Practitioners
Association of Ontario
(RNAO Affiliate)
50 Verne Crescent
Agincourt, Ontario
M1B 2X1

Nurses' Association of
American College of
Obstetricians & Gynecologists
(Ontario Section)
808-31 Alexander St.
Toronto, Ontario
M4Y 1B2

Ontario Community Mental
Health Nurses Association
Queen St. Mental Health Centre
Southwestern Service
1001 Queen St. W.
Toronto, Ontario
M6J 1H3

Ontario Lung Association
Nurses Section
157 Willowdale Ave.
Willowdale, Ontario
M2N 4Y7

Ontario Association of
Registered Nursing Assistants
112 Merton St.
3rd Floor
Toronto, Ontario
M4S 1A1

Ontario Nurse
Midwives' Association
(RNAO Affiliate)
51 Harvard Ave.
Toronto, Ontario
M6R 1C7

Ontario Occupational Health
Nurses' Association
3209 Rymal Rd.
Mississauga, Ontario
L4Y 3B8

Operating Room Nurses
of Greater Toronto
100-100 Burrows Hall Blvd.
Agincourt, Ontario
M1B 1M7

Psychiatric Nurses' Association
of Ontario
52 Forest St.
Guelph, Ontario
N1G 1H9

Toronto Practitioners in
Infection Control
Mount Sinai Hospital
600 University Ave.
Toronto, Ontario
M5G 1X5

**Registered Nurses Association of
Ontario Interest Groups**

Clinical Nurse Specialist
Interest Group
602-155 Balliol St.
Toronto, Ontario
M4S 1C4

Nursing Administrators
Interest Group
Salvation Army Grace
General Hospital
1156 Wellington St.
Ottawa, Ontario
K1Y 2Z4

Provincial Nurse Educators
Interest Group
3032 Britannia Rd.
RR No. 2
Milton, Ontario
L9T 2X6

Psychiatric Nursing Interest Group
50 Cartier Cres.
Richmond Hill, Ontario
L4C 2N2

Public Health Nurses
109 Queen St.
Guelph, Ontario
N1E 4S1

Registered Nurses in
Private Practice
509-810 Edgeworth
Ottawa, Ontario
K2B 5L5

Quebec

Association des infirmières et
infirmiers en santé du travail
du Québec, Inc.
Northern Telecom Canada Ltée
150, bul. Montréal-Toronto
Lachine, Québec
H8S 1B6

Association des Infirmiéres
Licenciées pour service
privé en nursing
Le Registre Ville-Marie Inc.
1818 est, rue Sherbrooke
Montréal, Québec
H2K 1B3

Association des infirmiéres-sages-
femmes du Québec
C.P. 121
Succursale St. Martin
Montréal, Québec
H7V 3P4

Association of Practitioners for
the Prevention of Infection
1839 Trepanier St.
Ville Brossard, Québec
J4W 2K4

Association Pulmonaire du Québec
La section des Infirmiéres
4200 ouest, boulevard Dorchester
Montréal, Québec
H3Z 1V4

Canadian Orthopedic Nurses
Association, Montreal Chapter
16-4780 Côte des Neiges
Montréal Québec
H3V 1G2

Corporation professionelle des
infirmiéres et infirmicrs
auxiliaries due Québec
1980 ouest, rue Sherbrooke
Suite 920
Montréal, Québec
H3H 1E8

Operating Room Nurses
Group of Quebec
3755 Cote Ste-Catherine Rd.
Montréal, Québec
H3T 1E2

Regroupement des Infirmiéres et
Infirmiers Diplomés des 2e et 3^e
Cycles du Québec
C.P. 1578, Succursale B
Hull, Québec
J8X 3Y5

Societé du Timbre de Noël
du Québec, Inc.,
La section des Infirmiéres
264 rue Chenier
Québec, Québec
G1K 1R2

New Brunswick

Association of New Brunswick
Registered Nursing Assistants
Executive Director
39 Coventry Crescent
Fredericton, New Brunswick
E3B 4P4

New Brunswick Infection Control
Practitioners' Group
(NBARN Interest Group)
310 Gilmour St.
Oromocto, N.B.
E2V 1E5

New Brunswick Mental
Health Nursing Group
10-25 Ocean Court
Churchill Heights
Saint John, N.B.
E2M 4B1

New Brunswick Occupational
Health Nursing Group
(NBARN Interest Group)
MacMillan-Rothesay
P.O. Box 1900
Saint John, N.B.
E2L 4K9

New Brunswick Operating Room
& Recovery Room Nurses Group
(NBARN Interest Group)
285 Southampton Drive
Fredericton, N.B.
E3B 4T5

Nursing Home Nurses Association
(NBARN Interest Group)
Loch Lomond Villa Inc.
185 Loch Lomond Rd.
Saint John, N.B.
E2J 3S3

Nova Scotia

Canadian Association of
Neurological and
Neurosurgical Nurses
Nova Scotia Chapter
1203-1333 South Park St.
Halifax, N.S.
B3J 2K9

Canadian Council of
Cardiovascular Nurses
Nova Scotia Branch
202-58 Manor Lane
Halifax, N.S
B3M 3M7

Canadian Society of
Dialysis Perfusionists
Nova Scotia Chapter
Dialysis Unit
Victoria General Hospital
Tower Road
Halifax, N.S.
B3H 2Y9

Central Service Association
Province of Nova Scotia
Chief Supervisor
Victoria General Hospital
Tower Road
Halifax, N.S.
B3H 2Y9

Evening and Night Supervisory
Interest Group
Harbour View Hospital
Sydney Mines, N.S.
B1V 2Y4

Gerontology Association of
Nova Scotia
Box 103
Falmouth, N.S.
B0P 1L0

Hospital Continuing Education
Association of Nova Scotia
Director, In-service Education
Glace Bay Hospital
197 Main St.
Glace Bay, N.S.
B1A 4Z8

Nova Scotia Operating
Room Nurses
11th Floor, O.R.
Victoria General Hospital
Halifax, N.S.
B3H 2Y9

Nurses Association of the
American College of
Obstetricians and Gynecologists
Reproductive Care Program
Grace Maternity Hospital
5821 University Ave.
Halifax, N.S.
B3H 1W3

Occupational Health Nurses
Association of Nova Scotia
Employee Health Services
Gulf Canada Ltd.
P.O. Box 2006
Port Hawkesbury, N.S.
B0E 2V0

Office Nurses (Ambulatory Care)
Dalhousie Family Medicine Centre
5599 Fenwick St.
Halifax, N.S.
B3H 1R2

Provincial Directors of Nursing
Service of Nova Scotia
Director of Nursing
Colchester General Hospital
Truro, N.S.
B2N 5A1

Psychiatric Nurses Association
of Nova Scotia
P.O. Box 40
Waterville, N.S.
B0P 1V0

Prince Edward Island

Prince Edward Island Licensed
Nursing Assistants Association
Nursing Assistants Programme
Department of Health
P.O. Box 1253
Charlottetown, P.E.I.
C1A 7M8

Newfoundland

Atlantic Maternal and Newborn
Nursing Association/Atlantic
Nurse-Midwives Association
School of Nursing
Memorial University
St. John's, Nfld.
A1C 5S7

Canadian Council of
Cardiovascular Nurses,
Newfoundland Division
14 St. Andrew's Ave.
Glendale-Mount Pearl, Nfld.
A1N 1C7

Council for Nursing Assistant
Department of Health
Confederation Building,
P.O. Box 4750
St. John's, Nfld.
A1C 5T7

Newfoundland Infection
Control Association
4 Glasgow Place
St. John's, Nfld.
A1B 2B4

Newfoundland Tuberculosis and
Respiratory Disease Association,
Nurses' Section
161 Logy Bay Road
St. John's, Nfld.
A1A 1J7

Northwest Territories

The Registered Psychiatric
Nurses' Association of the
Northwest Territories
c/o Yellowknife Correctional
Institute
Yellowknife, N.W.T.

12-4. Health care workers

Primary title	Alternate title	Primary title	Alternate title
Administration		Dental hygienist	
Health administrator	Health officer or commissioner	Dental assistant	
	Environmental control administrator	Dental laboratory technician	Dental laboratory assistant
	Health agency executive director	**Dietetic and nutritional services**	
	Health care administrator	Dietitian	Administrative dietitian
	Hospital administrator		Consultant (public health) dietitian
	Medical care administrator		Research dietitian
	Nursing home administrator		Teaching dietitian
	Public health administrator		Therapeutic dietitian
Health program analyst	Public health analyst	Nutritionist	Public health nutritionist
	Public health specialist	Dietary technician	Dietary (food service) assistant
Health program representative	Public health advisor		Food service manager
			Food service technician
Health systems analyst	Public health representative	Dietary aide	
		Food service supervisor	Dietary (food service) worker
Biomedical engineering		**Environmental health services**	
Biomedical engineer	Bioengineer	Environmental scientist	Sanitary sciences specialist
	Medical engineer		Air pollution meteorologist
Biomedical engineering technician	Medical engineering technician		Environmental control chemist
			Estuarine oceanographer
Biomedical engineering aide			Groundwater hydrologist
			Health physicist
Chiropractic and naturopathy			Limnologist
Chiropractor	Doctor of Chiropractic	Environmental engineer	Sanitary engineer
Naturopath	Naturopathic physician		Air pollution engineer
			Hospital engineer
Clinical laboratory services			Industrial hygiene engineer
Clinical laboratory scientist	Clinical chemist		Public health engineer
			Radiologic health engineer
	Microbiologist	Environmental technologist	Sanitarian
Clinical laboratory technologist	Medical laboratory technologist		Air pollution specialist
	Medical technologist		Industrial hygienist
	Blood banking technologist		Radiologic health specialist
	Chemistry technologist	Environmental technician	Sanitarian technician
	Hematology technologist		Environmental engineering technician
	Microbiology technologist		Radiologic health technician (monitor)
Clinical laboratory technician	Medical laboratory technician		
	Medical technician		
	Cytotechnician	Environmental aide	Sanitarian aide
	Cytotechnologist		Environmental engineering aide
Clinical laboratory aide	Laboratory assistant		Sewage plant assistant
	Certified laboratory assistant		Waterworks assistant
	Histologic aide		
	Histologic technician	**Food and drug protective services**	
	Pathology laboratory aide	Food technologist	
		Food and drug inspector	
Dentistry and allied services		Food and drug analyst	
Dentist	Endodontist	**Health education**	
	Oral pathologist	Health educator	Community health educator
	Oral surgeon		Public health educator
	Orthodontist		School health educator
	Pedodontist		School health coordinator
	Periodontist		
	Prosthodontist	Health education aide	
	Public health dentist		

Primary title	Alternate title	Primary title	Alternate title
Information and communication			Radiologist
Health information specialist	Biomedical communication specialist		Surgeon
Health science writer	Medical writer	M.D.	Thoracic surgeon
Health technical writer	Medical technical writer	or	Urologist
	Medical editor	D.O.	Intern
Medical illustrator	Medical photographer		Resident
			Fellow
Library services		**Midwifery**	
Medical librarian		Midwife	Lay midwife
Medical library assistant			Nurse midwife
Hospital librarian	Patients' librarian	**Natural sciences**	
Mathematical sciences		Anatomist	Cytologist
Mathematician	Biomathematician		Embryologist
	Demographer		Histologist
Statistician	Biostatistician	Botanist	
	Health statistician	Chemist	Bioanalyst
	Vital record registrar		Biochemist
			Clinical chemist
			Environmental control chemist
Medical record services		Ecologist	
Medical record librarian	Medical record specialist	Entomologist	
	Medical record technologist	Epidemiologist	
Medical record technician	Medical record assistant	Geneticist	
Medical record clerk	Medical record aide	Hydrologist	Groundwater hydrologist
		Immunologist	
Medicine and osteopathy		Meteorologist	Air pollution meteorologist
Physician	Doctor of Medicine—M.D.	Microbiologist	Bacteriologist
Osteopathic physician	Doctor of Osteopathy—D.O.		Mycologist
	Allergist		Parasitologist
	Anesthesiologist		Virologist
	Aviation medicine specialist	Nutritionist	
	Cardiovascular disease specialist	Oceanographer	Estuarine oceanographer
	Colon and rectal surgeon (proctologist)	Pathologist	
	Dermatologist	Pharmacologist	Toxicologist
	Forensic pathologist	Physicist	Health physicist
	Gastroenterologist		Biophysicist
	General practitioner	Physiologist	
	Gynecologist	Sanitary sciences specialist	
	Internist	Zoologist	Limnologist
	Manipulative therapy specialist		
	Neurologic surgeon	**Nursing and related services**	
M.D.	Neurologist	Nurse	Registered nurse—R.N.
or	Occupational medicine specialist		Graduate nurse
D.O.	Obstetrician		Professional nurse
	Ophthalmologist		Hospital nurse
	Orthopedic surgeon		Occupational health (industrial) nurse
	Otolaryngologist (otorhinolaryngologist)		Office nurse
	Pathologist		Private duty nurse
	Pediatrician		Public health nurse
	Physiatrist (physical medicine and rehabilitation specialist)		School nurse
	Plastic surgeon		Nurse anesthetist
	Preventive medicine specialist		Nurse midwife
	Psychiatrist		Obstetrical nurse
	Public health physician		Psychiatric nurse
	Pulmonary disease specialist		Pediatric nurse
			Surgical (operating room) nurse

Primary title	Alternate title	Primary title	Alternate title
Practical nurse	Licensed practical nurse Vocational nurse Licensed vocational nurse	Psychologist	Clinical psychologist Counseling psychologist Measurement psychologist (psychometrist) Social psychologist
Nursing aide Orderly Attendant	Nursing assistant Psychiatric (mental health) aide	Sociologist	Medical sociologist
Home health aide	Home aide—homemaker Visiting health aide	**Social work**	
Ward clerk	Floor clerk	Clinical social worker	Medical social worker Psychiatric social worker
Occupational therapy		Clinical social work assistant	
Occupational therapist		Clinical social work aide	Clinical casework aide
Occupational therapy assistant	Occupational therapy technician	**Specialized rehabilitation services**	
Occupational therapy aide		Corrective therapist	
Orthotic and prosthetic technology		Corrective therapy aide	
Orthotist	Orthopedic brace maker	Educational therapist	
Orthotic aide		Manual arts therapist	
Prosthetist	Artificial limb maker	Music therapist	
Prosthetic aide		Recreation therapist	Therapeutic recreation specialist
Restoration technician		Recreation therapy aide	
Pharmacy		Homemaking rehabil- itation consultant	
Pharmacist	Community pharmacist Hospital pharmacist Industrial pharmacist Pharmacy helper	**Speech pathology and audiology**	
		Audiologist	Hearing therapist
Physical therapy		Speech pathologist	Speech therapist
Physical therapist		**Veterinary medicine**	

Physical therapy as-
  sistant
	Physical therapy technician	Veterinarian	Laboratory (animal medicine)
			  veterinarian
			Public health veterinarian

Physical therapy aide			Veterinary laboratory diagnostician
Podiatry			Veterinary pathologist
Podiatrist	Chiropodist Foot orthopedist Foot roentgenologist Podiatric surgeon Pododermatologist		Veterinary microbiologist Veterinary radiologist Veterinary surgeon Veterinary toxicologist
		Veterinary technician	Animal technician
Radiologic technology		**Vision care**	
Radiologic technolo- gist		Ophthalmologist	
Radiologic technician	X-ray technician Radiation therapy technician	Optometrist	
		Vision care technol- ogist	Ocular care technologist Ophthalmic technologist Optometric technologist
Secretarial and office services		Technician	
Secretary	Dental secretary Medical secretary	Vision care techni- cian	Ocular care technician Ophthalmic technician (assistant)
Office assistant	Dentist's office assistant Medical assistant Optometrist's office assistant Physician's office assistant	Orthoptic techni- cian	Optometric technician (assistant) Orthoptist
Social sciences		Optician	Dispensing optician Ophthalmic dispenser (optical fitter)
Anthropologist	Cultural (social) anthropologist Physical anthropologist		Contact lens technician Lens grinder-polisher
Economist	Health economist		Optical (laboratory) mechanic

Primary title	Alternate title	Primary title	Alternate title

Visual care aide	Ocular care aide
	Ophthalmic aide
	Optometric aide
	Visual training aide
		Inhalation therapy:
		  Inhalation therapist
		  Inhalation therapy
		   aide
			Inhalation therapy technician

Vocational rehabilitation counseling		Medical machine technology:	
Vocational rehabilitation counselor	Rehabilitation counselor	Cardiopulmonary technician	
Miscellaneous health services		Electrocardiograph technician	
Assistance for physicians:		Electroencephalo- graph technician	
Physician's associates	Child health associate Pediatric associate	Other	Biomedical instrument technician

Physician's assistant	Anesthesiology assistant
	Orthopedic assistant
		Nuclear medicine:
		  Nuclear medical
		   technologist	

Physician's aide	Obstetrical aide Pediatric aide Surgical aide	Nuclear medical technician	
		Other health services:	
Emergency health service:		Community health aide	Dental health aide Mental health aide (worker) School health aide
Medical emergency technician		Extracorporeal circulation specialist	
Ambulance attendant (aide)		Other	

APPENDIX 13 • Directory of addresses

13-1. Burn centers in the United States

The following list includes Burn centers in the United States. The inclusion of a center on this list should not be interpreted as an endorsement of the institution or the quality of care available at these facilities. For additional information regarding these centers, direct inquiries to the American Burn Association (ABA).

Burn care services in the United States

State	City	Hospital	Telephone number for patient referral	Special burn beds	Burn service medical director or M.D.s most active in burn treatment
Alabama	Birmingham	University of Alabama Hospitals	205/934-3411	13	Alan R. Dimick
		Children's Hospital	205/933-4000	8	Marshall Pitts
	Mobile	University of South Alabama Medical Center Hospital	205/473-0311	5	Byron E. Green Arnold Luterman
Alaska	Anchorage	Providence Hospital	907/276-4511	10	Robert E. Mallin W.J. Mills (hypothermia)
	Fairbanks	Fairbanks Memorial Hospital	907/452-8181	4	William Wennen Richard Parry
Arizona	Phoenix	Maricopa County General Hospital	602/267-5700	20	John M. Stein
		PHS Indian Medical Center	602/263-1200	5	Robert E.G. Norton Frank Zwemer
	Tucson	St. Mary's Hospital	602/795-8700	9	Philip Fleishman
Arkansas	Little Rock	Arkansas Child's Hospital	501/376-4621	12	Fred T. Caldwell
California	Berkeley	Alta Bates Hospital	415/845-7110	6	Jerold Z. Kaplan
	Castro Valley	Eden Hospital	415/537-1234	6	Ronald Iverson Eleanor Kohn
	Chico	Chico Community Memorial Hospital	916/345-2411 or 916/342-7513	6	Donald J. Mangus
	Culver City	Brotman Medical Center	213/652-6630	23	Arthur M. Kahn
	Downey	Rancho Los Amigos Hospital	213/922-7454		G. Brody et al. (Reconstructive only)
	Eureka	St. Joseph's Hospital	707/443-8051		Terry Knapp Russell Pardoe
	Fresno	Valley Medical Center	209/453-4161	6	Steven N. Parks
	Los Angeles	LAC/USC Medical Center	213/226-7991	38	Bruce E. Zawacki William T. Choctaw
	Orange	University of California, Irvine Medical Center	714/634-5304	13	Bruce M. Achauer
	Sacramento	Sacramento Medical Center	916/453-3636	8	Robert Demling
	San Bernardino	San Bernardino Community	714/887-6333 or 714/884-3612	5	David Hess
		San Bernardino County Medical Center	714/383-3131	6	Donald Dressler David Sizemore
	San Diego	University Hospital, University of California Medical Center	714/294-6502	14	Thomas Wachtel Hugh Frank
	San Francisco	St. Francis Memorial Hospital	415/775-4321	10	Edward Falces
		San Francisco General Hospital	415/821-8197	6	Donald D. Trunkey

Burn care services in the United States—cont'd

State	City	Hospital	Telephone number for patient referral	Special burn beds	Burn service medical director or M.D.s most active in burn treatment
	San Jose	Santa Clara Valley Medical Center	408/279-5452	12	R.L. Berkowitz
	San Luis Obispo	San Luis Obispo General Hospital	805/543-1500	5	Jerren Jorgensen et al.
	San Pablo	Brookside Hospital	415/235-7000	6	Robert L. Shapiro
	Sherman Oaks	Sherman Oaks Community Hospital	213/981-7111	30	A. Richard Grossman
	Stockton	Dameron Hospital	209/944-5550	12	Genest de L'Arbre
	Torrance	Torrance Memorial Hospital	213/325-9110	10	Leslie Lee
Colorado (organized as the Colorado burn injury network)	**Burn units**				
	Denver	Children's Hospital	303/861-6906	8	William Carl Bailey
		University Hospital	303/394-8400	5	John Hansbrough
	Burn facilities				
	Colorado Springs	Penrose Hospital	303/630-5770	8	Alfred J. Martin, Jr.
	Denver	St. Anthony's Hospital	303/629-4355		Ian Winspur
	Grand Junction	St. Mary's Hospital	303/242-9127		William Merkel
	Greeley	Weld County Gen. Hospital	303/352-4121		James R. Wheeler
	Pueblo	St. Mary-Corwin Hospital	303/561-5000		Clifford Hoyle
Connecticut	Bridgeport	Bridgeport Hospital	203/384-3000	9	Michael L. D'Aiuto
	Hartford	Hartford Hospital	203/524-2515		Philip E. Trowbridge et al.
	New Haven	Yale-New Haven Hospital	203/436-4404		William Frazier
					Charles Cuono
District of Columbia	Washington	Children's Hospital, National Medical Center	202/745-5016	12	Judson G. Randolph
		Washington Hospital Center	202/541-7241 or 202/541-6662	27	Marion Jordan
Florida	Gainesville	Shands Teaching Hospital	904/392-3055	6	Hal G. Bingham
	Miami	Jackson Memorial Hospital	305/325-7085	8	C. Gillon Ward
	Orlando	Orlando Regional Medical Center	305/841-5176	7	Patricio Quijada
	Tampa	Tampa General Hospital	813/253-0711 or 813/251-7617	18	C. Wayne Cruse
Georgia	Atlanta	Grady Memorial Hospital	404/588-4307	30	H. Harlan Stone (Fulton & DeKalb Co. only)
		St. Joseph's Hospital	404/256-7165		Patrick Shea, Jr.
	Augusta	Doctor's Hospital	404/863-3232	10	Alton Garrison
					Joseph Still
		Eugene Talmadge Memorial Hospital, Medical College of Georgia	404/722-0070	6	Richard C. Treat
	Columbus	Medical Center	404/324-4711	6	Robert K. Worman (Acting)
Illinois	Chicago	Children's Memorial Hospital	312/649-4094		Desmond Kernahan
					Victor Lewis
		Cook County Hospital	312/633-6564 312/633-6570	30	Takayoshi Matsuda
					Marella Hanumadass
		Edgewater Hospital	312/878-6000	4	Ramesh Kharwadkar
		University of Chicago Hospital	312/947-6965	20	Martin Robson
	Evanston	Evanston Hospital	312/492-7720	8	Charles Drueck
	Maywood	Foster G. McGaw Hospital, Loyola University of Chicago	312/531-3988	14	Raymond Warpeha

State	City	Hospital	Telephone number for patient referral	Special burn beds	Burn service medical director or M.D.s most active in burn treatment
	Rock Island	Rock Island Franciscan Hospital	309/793-3173	10	Frank E. Miller
	Rockford	St. Anthony's Hospital	815/226-2000	8	Edward H. Sharp
	Springfield	Memorial Medical Center	217/788-3325	10	Jack Baldwin
Indiana	Fort Wayne	St. Joseph's Hospital	219/422-9387	7	Jack Patterson
	Indianapolis	J.W. Riley Hospital	317/264-3927	8	Bernard L. Swartz (children)
		W.N. Wishard Memorial Hospital	317/630-6471	8	David J. Smith (adults)
Iowa	Iowa City	University of Iowa Hospital & Clinics	319/356-2496	13	Albert E. Cram
	Sioux City	St. Luke's Medical Center	712/279-3440	8	Larry D. Foster
Kansas	Kansas City	University of Kansas Medical Center	913/588-6540	10	Mani M. Mani David W. Robinson
	Wichita	St. Francis Hospital	316/262-3495		Tommy E. Kendall et al.
		Wesley Medical Center	316/688-2688		Richard C. Shaw et al.
Kentucky	Lexington	University Hospital	606/233-5260	4	Edward Luce
	Louisville	Norton-Child's Hospital (admits adult burns)	502/589-8000	8	Harry D. Stambaugh et al.
Louisiana	Baton Rouge	Baton Rouge General Hospital	504/387-7716	14	D.V. Cacioppo
	Marrero	West Jefferson Hospital	504/347-5511	14	Frank C. DiVincenti
	New Orleans	Charity Hospital of Louisiana	504/568-2311	4	Frank C. DiVincenti
	Shreveport	L.S.U. Medical Center Hospital	318/674-6133	12	Edwin Deitch
Maine	Bangor	Eastern Maine Medical Center	207/947-3711		Charles Dixon
	Lewiston	Central Maine Medical Center	207/795-0111		Alan Ingraham
	Portland	Maine Medical Center	207/871-2991	6	Richard Britton
	Presque Isle	Arthur Gould Memorial Hospital	207/769-2511		Raymond Giberson
Maryland	Baltimore	Baltimore City Hospital	301/396-8765	21	Andrew Munster
Massachusetts	Boston	Beth Israel Hospital	617/735-2000	3	Joel Noe Mark Weinstein
		Boston City Hospital	617/424-5204		Erwin Hirsch
		Brigham & Women's Hospital	617/732-7712	10	Douglas W. Wilmore
		Massachusetts General Hospital	617/726-3354	10	John F. Burke
		Shriners Burns Institute	617/722-3000	30	John P. Remensnyder
	Springfield	Baystate Medical Center	413/787-4380		Manu H. Desai
Michigan	Ann Arbor	Michigan Burn Center University Hospital St. Joseph Mercy Hospital Chelsea Community Hospital	313/995-BURN	29	Irving Feller Jai K. Prasad
	Detroit	Children's Hospital of Michigan	313/494-5678	12	James Lloyd
		Detroit Receiving Hospital	313/494-3374	18	Eti Gursel
	Flint	Hurley Medical Center	313/766-0188 or 313/238-3626	13	Musa Haffajee et al.
	Grand Rapids	Blodgett Memorial Medical Center	616/774-7670	8	William Simpson Richard A. Wehrenberg
	Kalamazoo	Bronson Methodist Hospital	616/383-6485 or 1-800/632-3403	14	Frank J. Newman Paul Fierke
	Lansing	Edward R. Sparrow Hospital	517/487-2774	4	Errikos Constant Jorge Gomez
	Marquette	Marquette General Hospital	906/228-9440		James Keplinger Constance N. Arnold

Burn care services in the United States—cont'd

State	City	Hospital	Telephone number for patient referral	Special burn beds	Burn service medical director or M.D.s most active in burn treatment
	Saginaw	St. Mary's Hospital	517/790-5055	6	Syed Akhtar
Minnesota	Duluth	Miller-Dwan Hospital & Medical Center	218/727-8762	12	John W. Wolf
	Minneapolis	Minneapolis Children's Health Center & Hospital	612/871-4551		F.A. McParland
		Hennepin County Medical Center	612/347-2915	11	John Twomey
		North Memorial Medical Center	612/588-0616	6	Fereydoon Mahjouri
	Rochester	St. Mary's Hospital	507/285-5123 or 507/285-5591	6	George B. Irons (adults) Robert Telander (children)
	St. Paul	St. Paul-Ramsey Medical Center	612/221-3351	24	Lynn D. Solem
Mississippi	Greenville	Delta Medical Center	601/378-3783	10	Robert Love
	Jackson	University Hospital	601/987-3916 or 601/987-5566	4	Frederick R. Heckler
Missouri	Columbia	University of Missouri Health Sciences Center	314/882-7994	7	Boyd E. Terry
	Kansas City	Children's Mercy Hospital	816/234-3520	6	Raymond Amoury
	St. Louis	Barnes Hospital	314/454-3244	6	William H. Monafo
		Cardinal Glennon Memorial Hospital	314/865-4000		F.X. Paletta
		St. John's Mercy Medical Center	314/569-6055	17	Vatche H. Ayvazian Dan F. Kopen
	Springfield	St. John's Regional Health Center	417/885-2876	9	Mark Wittmer
Montana	Billings	Saint Vincent Hospital	406/657-7067		David F. Sloan
Nebraska	Lincoln	St. Elizabeth Community Health Center	402/489-7181 or 402/483-9206	10	Robert W. Gillespie
Nevada	Las Vegas	Southern Nevada Memorial Hospital	702/384-7979	9	John Batdord
New Jersey	Hackensack	Hackensack Hospital	201/487-4000		Anthony Barbara
	Livingston	St. Barnabas Medical Center	201/533-5920	12	Frederick Fuller
New Mexico	Albuquerque	University of New Mexico Hospital	505/843-2111	12	William R. Schiller
New York	Albany	Albany Medical Center	518/445-3010	9	Richard M. McShane Dhiraj M. Shah
	Buffalo	Children's Hospital	716/878-7301, 7435		Theodore Jewett Donald R. Cooney
		Millard Fillmore Hospital	716/887-4776	4	Evan J. Evans
		Sheehan Memorial Emergency Hospital	716/842-2200	10	Louis C. Cloutier
	East Meadow	Nassau County Medical Center	516/542-3207	10	Leonard Rubin Roger L. Simpson
	Elmira	St. Joseph's Hospital	607/733-6541	4	James Marshall James Sonsire
	New York City Bronx	Bronx Municipal Hospital Center	212/430-8065	12	Jane Petro
	Brooklyn	Kings County Hospital	212/630-3131	5	Winston Mitchell
	Manhattan	Harlem Hospital Center	212/694-1335	7	Vincent Porter
		NY Hospital-Cornell Medical Center	212/472-5132	24	David N. Herndon (acting)
		St. Vincent's Hospital	212/790-8940	6	Ronald N. Ollstein
	Rochester	Strong Memorial Hospital	716/275-5475	9	Robert M. McCormack

State	City	Hospital	Telephone number for patient referral	Special burn beds	Burn service medical director or M.D.s most active in burn treatment
	Syracuse	Upstate Medical Center	315/473-6083	6	William Clark
	Valhalla	Westchester County Medical Center	914/347-4909	10	Roger E. Salisbury
	West Islip	Good Samaritan Hospital	516/321-2000		Richard A. Giery
North Carolina	Chapel Hill	North Carolina Memorial Hospital	919/966-4131	23	G. Peter Dingeldein (acting)
	Durham	Duke University Hospital	919/681-2404	9	Gregory Georgiade Joseph Moylan
	Winston-Salem	North Carolina Baptist Hospital	919/748-2011	6	Jesse H. Meredith Connell Shearin
North Dakota	Fargo	St. Luke's General Hospital	701/280-5504	4	David W. Todd
Ohio	Akron	Children's Hospital Medical Center (admits adult burns)	216/379-8224	12	C.R. Boeckmann R.L. Klein
	Cincinnati	University of Cincinnati Hospital	513/872-3100	10	Robert P. Hummel
		Shriners Burns Institute	513/751-3900	30	Bruce G. MacMillan
	Cleveland	Cleveland Metropolitan General Hospital	216/459-5627	16	Richard Fratianne
	Columbus	Children's Hospital	614/461-2000	14	E. Thomas Boles
		Ohio State University Hospital	614/422-4516	3	Robert Ruberg
	Dayton	Children's Medical Center	513/226-8300	4	Charles D. Goodwin
		Miami Valley Hospital	513/223-6192	4	R.K. Finley Sidney Miller
	Toledo	St. Vincent's Hospital	419/259-4098	8	George Baibak
Oklahoma	Oklahoma City	Baptist Medical Center	405/949-3345	15	Paul Silverstein
		Oklahoma Children's Memorial Hospital	405/271-4733	12	E. Ide Smith
	Tulsa	Hillcrest Medical Center	918/584-1351	28	Harold F. Dunlap
Oregon	Portland	Oregon Burn Center (at Emanuel Hospital)	503/280-4233	12	Philip Parshley
Pennsylvania	Allentown	Allentown & Sacred Heart Hospital Center	215/821-2058	6	Walter J. Okunski
	Chester	Crozer-Chester Medical Center	215/876-0356	19	Charles E. Hartford
	Danville	Geisinger Medical Center	717/271-6353 or 717/271-6591	4	Philip C. Breen
	Erie	Hamot Medical Center	814/455-0066	8	Charles R. Bales Forrest C. Mischler
	Hershey	Hershey Medical Center	717/534-8521		William P. Graham
	Philadelphia	Saint Agnes Medical Center	215/339-4339	11	Frederick A. DeClement
		St. Christopher's Hospital For Children	215/427-5000	4	Stuart J. Hulnick
	Pittsburgh	Mercy Hospital	412/232-8225	7	Thomas Layton
		Western Pennsylvania Hospital	412/682-4200	18	John Gaisford
	York	York Hospital	717/771-2345	6	Robert Davis Richard W. Dabb
South Carolina	Charleston	Medical University Hospital	803/792-3681 803/792-3851	9	Dabney R. Yarbrough (adult) H. Biemann Othersen Jr. (children)
Tennessee	Chattanooga	Baroness Erlanger Hospital	615/755-7881	6	John R. Reynolds
	Memphis	City of Memphis Hospital	901/528-7100		J. Garnett Murphy Charles White

Burn care services in the United States—cont'd

State	City	Hospital	Telephone number for patient referral	Special burn beds	Burn service medical director or M.D.s most active in burn treatment
	Nashville	Vanderbilt University Hospital	615/322-7311	20	John B. Lynch/J. O'Neill
Texas	Austin	Brackenridge Hospital	512/476-6461		Robert A. Ersek et al.
	Beaumont	Baptist Hospital	713/835-3781	10	Duane Larson Wesley Washburn
	Corpus Christi	Memorial Medical Center	512/844-4511	9	Robert H. Balme
	Dallas	Parkland Memorial Hospital	214/638-1800 or 214/688-3754	30	John Hunt
	El Paso	Sun Towers Hospital	915/532-6281	12	Charles Lyon et al.
	Fort Sam Houston	Brooke Army Medical Center	512/221-4604	40	Basil A. Pruitt, Jr.
	Fort Worth	John Peter Smith Hospital	817/921-3431		Charles Crenshaw et al.
	Galveston	John Sealy Hospital	713/765-1255 (days) 713/765-2023 (nights)	15	Steven J. Blackwell
		Shriners Burns Institute	713/765-2516	30	Donald H. Parks
	Houston	Ben Taub General Hospital	713/791-7000	8	Frank Gerow
	Houston	Hermann Hospital	713/792-5406	13	David E. Beesinger
	San Antonio	Bexar County Hospital	512/696-3030 or 512/691-6151		A.B. Cruz, Jr.
Utah	Salt Lake City	University of Utah Hospital	801/581-2700	12	Glenn Warden Scott Petersen
Vermont	Burlington	Medical Center Hospital of Vermont	802/656-4545		John Davis Richard Gamelli
Virginia	Charlottesville	University of Virginia Medical Center	804/924-5520	6	Richard Edlich
	Norfolk	Norfolk General Hospital	804/628-3117	8	Willcox Ruffin et al.
	Richmond	Medical College of Virginia Hospital	804/786-9240	12	Boyd W. Haynes
Washington	Seattle	Harborview Medical Center	206/223-3127	40	David Heimbach
	Spokane	Sacred Heart Medical Center	509/455-3344		James Brinkman et al.
	Tacoma	St. Joseph's Hospital	206/627-4101 or 206/596-6677	10	Thomas J. Irish
West Virginia	Huntington	Cabell-Huntington Hospital	304/696-6110	4	James A. Coil, Jr.
Wisconsin	Madison	University of Wisconsin Hospitals	608/263-1490 or 608/263-1387	7	Richard Helgerson
	Milwaukee	St. Mary's Hospital	414/289-7000	20	George Collentine

13-2. Burn centers and facilities in Canada

British Columbia
Vancouver General Hospital (23 Beds)
855 West 12th Avenue
(604/875-4000)

Victoria General Hospital (4 beds)
841 Fairfield Road
(604/388-9121)

Alberta
Foothills Provincial General Hospital (8 beds)
1403 29th Street N.W.
(403/270-1110)

University of Alberta Hospital (5 beds)
8505 112th Street
(403/432-8822)

Saskatchewan
Regina General Hospital (5 beds)
1440 14th Avenue
(306/359-4444)

University Hospital (5 beds)
University of Saskatchewan
(306/343-2112)

Ontario
Hamilton General Hospital (8 beds)
237 Baron Street
(416/527-0271)

Hotel Dicu Hospital (Kingston) (2 beds)
Syndeham Street
(613/544-3310)

Ottawa General Hospital (5 beds)
501 Smyth Road
(613/737-7777)

Hospital for Sick Children (21 beds)
555 University, Toronto
(416/597-1500)

Wellesley Hospital (10-12 beds)
160 Wellesley Street
(416/966-6600)

Quebec
Montreal Children's Hospital (4 beds)
2300 Tupper Street
(514/937-8511)

Montreal General Hospital (22 beds)
1650 Cedar Avenue
(514/937-6011)

New Brunswick
Dr. Everett Chalmers Hospital (5 beds)
Box 9000 Fredrickton
(506/452-5400)

Moncton Hospital (3 beds)
135 Mac Beth Avenue
(506/855-1600)

Nova Scotia
Izaak Walton Killam Hospital for Children (3 beds)
5850 University Avenue
(902/424-6111)

Victoria General Hospital (4 beds)
1278 Tower Road, Halifax
(902/428-2110)

13-3. Poison control centers in the United States and Canada

Poison control centers in United States and possessions

City and phone	Location	City and phone	Location
Alabama		Pine Bluff	Jefferson Hospital
State coordinator	EMS Division	501/541-7100 ext. 5350	Emergency Room
205/832-3935	State Office Building	501/541-7111	1515 W. 42nd Avenue
	Room 644		71601
	Montgomery 36130	Harrison	Boone County Hospital
Birmingham	The Children's Hospital	501/741-6141	Emergency Room
205/933-4050	1601 6th Avenue S.	ext. 275, 276, or 277	620 N. Willow Street
800/292-6678	35233		72601
Tuscaloosa	The West Alabama Poison Center	El Dorado	Warner Brown Hospital
205/345-0600	Druid City Hospital	501/863-2266	Emergency Room
	809 University Blvd., East		460 W. Oak Street
	34501		71730
		Osceola	Osceola Memorial Hospital
Alaska		501/563-7000 ext.	Emergency Room
State coordinator	Department of Health & Social Services	7180, 7181, or 7182	611 Lee Avenue, W.
907/465-3100	Juneau 99811	563-3174	72370
Anchorage	Anchorage Poison Center		
907/274-6535	Providence Hospital	Helena	Helena Hospital
	3200 Providence Dr.	501/338-6411 ext. 340	Emergency Room
	99504		Hospital Drive
			72342
Arizona		Fort Smith	St. Edward Mercy Medical Center
State coordinator	Arizona Poison Control System	501/452-5100 ext. 2043	Emergency Room
602/626-6016	College of Pharmacy		7301 Rogers Avenue
800/362-0101	Tucson 85724		72903
Flagstaff	Flagstaff Hospital and Medical Center of	Fort Smith	Sparks Regional Medical Center
602/774-5233	N. Arizona	501/441-5011	Emergency Room
	1215 N. Beaver St.		1311 S. "I" Street
	86001		72901
Phoenix	St. Lukes Hospital and Medical Center		
602/253-3334	525 N. 18th St.	**California**	
	85006	State coordinator	Department of Health and Welfare
Tucson	Arizona Regional Poison Center	916/322-4336	Emergency Medical Services
602/626-6016	Arizona Health Sciences Center		Sacramento
800/362-0101	University of Arizona		95814
(Arizona)	85724	Fresno	Central Valley Regional Poison Control
Yuma	Yuma Regional Medical Center	209/445-1222	Center
602/344-2000	Avenue A and 24th St.		Fresno Community Hospital and Medical
	85364		Center
			P.O. Box 1232
Arkansas			Fresno & R Sts.
State coordinator	Division of Environmental Health		93715
501/661-2301	Protection	Los Angeles	Thomas J. Fleming Memorial Center
	Department of Health	213/664-2121	Children's Hospital of Los Angeles
Little Rock	University of Arkansas Medical Center		P.O. Box 54700
501/661-6161	Emergency Room		4650 Sunset Blvd.
	4301 W. Markham Street		90054
	72201		

City and phone	Location	City and phone	Location
Oakland 415/428-3000	Children's Hospital Medical Center of Northern California 51st & Grove Sts. 94609	203/436-1960	Yale–New Haven Hospital Department of Pediatrics 789 Howard Ave. 06504
Orange 714/634-5988 634-6011	University of California Irvine Medical Center 101 City Drive S. 92688	Norwalk 203/852-2160	Norwalk Hospital 24 Stevens St. 06852
Sacramento 916/453-3692 800/852-7221	Sacramento Medical Center 2315 Stockton Blvd. 95817	Waterbury 203/574-6011	St. Mary's Hospital 56 Franklin St. 06702
San Diego 714/294-6000	San Diego Poison Information Center University Hospital 225 Dickinson St. 92103	**Delaware** State coordinator 302/655-3389	Wilmington Medical Center Delaware Division Wilmington 19801
San Francisco 415/666-2845 800/792-0720	San Francisco Bay Area Regional Poison Control Center 1001 Potrerro Ave. 94102	Wilmington 302/655-3389	Wilmington Medical Center Delaware Division 501 W. 14th St. 19899
San Jose 408/279-5112	Santa Clara Valley Medical Center 751 S. Bascom Ave. 95128	**District of Columbia** State coordinator 202/673-6741 202/673-6736	Department of Human Services Washington, D.C. 20009
Colorado State coordinator 303/320-8476	Department of Health Emergency Medical Services Denver 80220	Washington 202/625-3333	National Capitol Poison Center Georgetown University Hospital 3800 Reservoir Rd. 20007
Denver 303/629-1123 800/332-3073	Rocky Mountain Poison Center Denver General Hospital W. 8th Ave. and Cherokee Sts. 80204	**Florida** State coordinator 904/487-1566	Department of Health and Emergency Medical Services Tallahassee 32301
Connecticut State coordinator 203/674-3456	University of Connecticut Health Center Farmington 06032	Apalachicola 904/653-8853	George E. Weems Memorial Hospital P.O. Box 610 Franklin Sq. 32320
Bridgeport 203/384-3566	Bridgeport Hospital 267 Grant St. 06602	Bradenton 813/746-5111 ext. 466	Manatee Memorial Hospital 206 Second St. E. 33505
203/576-5178	St. Vincent's Hospital 2820 Main St. 06602	Daytona Beach 904/258-2002	Halifax Hospital Emergency Department P.O. Box 1990 32014
Danbury 203/797-7300	Danbury Hospital 95 Locust Ave. 06810	Fort Lauderdale 305/463-3131 ext. 1511	Broward General Medical Center Emergency Department 1600 S. Andrews Ave. 33316
Farmington 203/674-3456	Connecticut Poison Control Center University of Connecticut Health Center 06032	Fort Myers 813/332-1111 ext. 285	Lee Memorial Hospital 2776 Cleveland Ave. P.O. Drawer 2218 33902
Middletown 203/347-9471	Middlesex Memorial Hospital 28 Crescent St. 06457	Fort Walton Beach 904/392-1111 ext. 106	General Hospital of Ft. Walton Beach 1000 Mar-Walt Dr. 32548
New Haven 203/789-3469	The Hospital of St. Raphael 1450 Chapel St. 06511		

Poison control centers in United States and possessions—cont'd

City and phone	Location	City and phone	Location
Gainesville 904/392-3740	Shands Teaching Hospital and Clinics University of Florida 32610	St. Petersburg 813/821-5858	Bay Front Medical Center, Inc. 701 6th St., S. 33701
Inverness 904/726-2800	Citrus Memorial Hospital 502 Highland Blvd. 32650	Sarasota 813/953-1332	Memorial Hospital 1901 Arlington St. 33579
Jacksonville 904/389-7751 ext. 8315	St. Vincent's Medical Center Barrs St. & Johns Ave. 32204	Tallahassee 904/599-5411	Tallahassee Regional Medical Center 1300 Miccosukee Rd. 32304
Lakeland 813/686-4913	Lakeland General Hospital Lakeland Hills Blvd. P.O. Box 480 33802	Tampa 813/251-6995	Tampa General Hospital Davis Island 33606
Leesburg 904/787-7222 ext. 381	Leesburg General Hospital 600 E. Dixie 32748	Titusville 305/268-6111	Jess Parrish Memorial Hospital 951 N. Washington Ave. P.O. Drawer W 32780
Melbourne 305/727-7000 ext. 675	James E. Holmes Regional Medical Center 1350 S. Hickory St. 32901	West Palm Beach 305/655-5511 ext. 4250	Good Samaritan Hospital Palm Beach Lakes Blvd. 33402
Miami 305/325-6799	Jackson Memorial Hospital Attn: Pharmacy 1611 N.W. 12th Ave. 33136	Winter Haven 813/299-9701	Winter Haven Hospital, Inc. 200 Avenue F., N.E. 33880
Naples 813/262-7838	Naples Community Hospital 350 7th St. N. 33940	**Georgia** State coordinator 404/894-5170	Department of Human Resources Emergency Health Section
North Miami Beach 305/653-3333	Parkway General Hospital, Inc. 160 N.W. 170th St. 33169	Albany 912/883-1800 ext. 4152	Phoebe Putney Memorial Hospital 417 Third Ave. 31705
Ocala 904/732-1111 ext. 187	Munroe Memorial Hospital 140 S.E. Orange St. P.O. Box 6000 32670	Athens 405/543-5215	Athens General Hospital 797 Cobb St. 30601
Orlando 305/841-5222	Orlando Regional Medical Center Orange Memorial Division 1414 S. Kuhl Ave. 32806	Atlanta 404/588-4400 800/282-5846 404/525-3323 (Deaf)	Georgia Poison Control Center Grady Memorial Hospital 80 Butler St., S.E. 30303
Panama City 904/769-1511 ext. 415 or 416	Bay Memorial Medical Center 600 N. MacArthur Ave. 32401	Augusta 404/722-9011 ext. 2440	University Hospital 1350 Walton Way 30902
Pensacola 904/434-4611 800/874-1555 800/342-3222	Baptist Hospital 1000 W. Moreno St. (In Florida Only) 32501	Columbus 404/324-4711 ext. 6431	The Medical Center 710 Center St. 31902
Punta Gorda 813/637-2529	Medical Center Hospital 809 E. Marion Ave. 33950	Macon 912/742-1122 ext. 1146	Medical Center of Central Georgia 777 Hemlock St. 31201
Rockledge 305/636-2211 ext. 168	Wuesthoff Memorial Hospital 110 Longwood Ave. 32955	Rome 404/291-2196	Floyd Hospital P.O. Box 233 31061
		Savannah 912/355-5228	Savannah Regional Poison Center Department of Emergency Medicine Memorial Medical Center P.O. Box 23089 31403

City and phone	Location	City and phone	Location
Thomasville 912/226-4121 ext. 169	John D. Archbold Memorial Hospital 900 Gordon Ave. 31792	Springfield 217/753-3330 800/252-2022	St. John's Hospital Regional Poison Resource Center 800 E. Carpenter 62702
Valdosta 912/333-1110	South Georgia Medical Center P.O. Box 1727 31601	**Indiana**	
Waycross 912/283-3030	Memorial Hospital 410 Darling Ave. 31501	State coordinator 317/633-0332	Indiana State Board of Health Hazardous Products Section and Division of Drug Control Indianapolis 46206
Guam		Anderson 317/646-5198	Community Hospital 1515 N. Madison Ave. 46012
State coordinator 646-5801	Guam Memorial Hospital P.O. Box AX Agana 96910	317/646-8251	St. John's Hickey Memorial Hospital 2015 Jackson St. 46014
Agana 344-9265 344-9354	Pharmacy Service, Box 7696 U.S. Naval Regional Medical Center (GUAM) FPO San Francisco, CA 96630	Angola 219/665-2141 ext. 146	Cameron Memorial Hospital, Inc. 416 East Maumee St. 46703
Hawaii		Columbus 812/376-5277	Bartholomew County Hospital 2400 East 17th St. 47201
State coordinator 808/531-7776	Department of Health Honolulu 96801	Crown Point 219/738-2100	St. Anthony Medical Center Main at Franciscan Rd. 46307
Honolulu 800/941-4411 800/362-3585	Kapiolani-Children's Medical Center 1319 Punahou St. 96826	East Chicago 219/392-1700 392-7203	St. Catherine's Hospital 4321 Fir St. 46312
Idaho		Elkhart 219/294-2621 800/382-9697	Elkhart General Hospital 600 East Blvd. 46514
State coordinator 208/334-2241 800/632-8000 (Idaho)	Department of Health and Welfare Boise 83701	Evansville 812/426-3405	Deaconess Hospital 600 Mary St. 47710
Boise 208/376-1211 ext. 707 800/632-8000 (Idaho)	Idaho Poison Center St. Alphonsus Hospital 1055 N. Curtis Rd. 83704	812/426-8000	Welborn Memorial Baptist Hospital 401 S.E. 6th St. 47713
Idaho Falls 208/522-3600	Consolidated Hospitals Emergency Department 900 Memorial Dr. 83401	Fort Wayne 219/458-2211	Lutheran Hospital 3024 Fairfield Ave. 46807
Pocatello 208/232-2733 ext. 244 800/632-9490 (Idaho)	St. Anthony's Hospital 650 North 7th St. 83201	219/484-6636 ext. 6000	Parkview Memorial Hospital 220 Randalia Dr. 46805
Illinois		219/423-2614	St. Joseph's Hospital 700 Broadway 46802
State coordinator 217/785-2080	Division of Emergency Medical Services and Highway Safety Springfield 62761	Frankfort 317/659-4731	Clinton County Hospital 1300 S. Jackson St. 46041
Chicago 312/942-5969 800/942-5969	Rush Presbyterian- St. Luke's Medical Center 1753 W. Congress Pkwy. 60612	Gary 219/886-4710	Methodist Hospital of Gary, Inc. 600 Grant St. 46402
Peoria 309/672-2334 800/322-5330	St. Francis Hospital and Medical Center 530 N.E. Glen Oak Ave. 61637		

Poison control centers in United States and possessions—cont'd

City and phone	Location	City and phone	Location
Goshen 219/533-2141	Goshen General Hospital 200 High Park Ave. 46526	South Bend 219/237-7264	St. Joseph's Hospital 811 E. Madison St. 46622
Hammond 219/932-2300 931-4477	St. Margaret's Hospital 25 Douglas St. 46320	Terre Haute 812/238-7000 ext. 7523	Union Hospital, Inc. 1606 N. Seventh St. 47804
Indianapolis 317/924-3521	Methodist Hospital of Indiana, Inc. 1604 N. Capitol Ave. 46202	Valparaiso 219/464-8611 ext. 232 312 or 334	Porter Memorial Hospital 814 LaPorte Ave. 46383
317/630-7351 800/382-9097	Indiana Poison Center 1001 W. Tenth St. 46202	Vincennes 812/885-3348	The Good Samaritan Hospital 520 S. 7th St. 47591
Kendallville 219/347-1100	McCray Memorial Hospital Hospital Dr. 46755	**Iowa** State coordinator 515/281-4964	Department of Health Des Moines 50319
Kokomo 317/453-8444	Howard Community Hospital 3500 S. LaFountain St. 46901	Des Moines 515/283-6254 800/362-2327	Blank Memorial Hospital 1200 Pleasant St. 50308
Lafayette 317/447-6811	Lafayette Home Hospital 2400 South St. 47902	Dubuque 319/588-8050	Mercy Medical Center Mercy Dr. 52001
317/423-6699	St. Elizabeth's Hospital 1501 Hartford St. 47904	Fort Dodge 515/573-7211 573/3101 (night)	Trinity Regional Hospital Kenyon Rd. 50501
LaGrange 219/463-2144	LaGrange County Hospital Route #1 46761	Iowa City 319/356-2922 800/272-6477 (IA)	University of Iowa Hospital Poison Information Center 52240
LaPorte 219/326-1234	LaPorte Hospital, Inc. 1007 Lincolnway 46350	Waterloo 319/235-3893	Allen Memorial Hospital Emergency Room 1825 Logan Ave. 50703
Lebanon 317/482-2700 ext. 241	Witham Memorial Hospital 1124 N. Lebanon St. 46052	**Kansas**	
Madison 812/265-5211 ext. 109	King's Daughter's Hospital 112 Presbyterian Ave. P.O. Box 447 47250	State coordinator 913/862-9360 ext. 451	Kansas Department of Health and Environment Bureau of Food and Drug Forbes Field Topeka 66620
Marion 317/662-4693	Marion General Hospital Wabash and Euclid Aves. 46952	Atchison 913/367-2131	Atchison Hospital 1301 N. 2nd St. 66002
Muncie 317/747-3241	Ball Memorial Hospital 2401 University Ave. 47303	Dodge City 316/225-9050 ext. 381	Dodge City Regional Hospital Ross & Avenue "A" P.O. Box 1478 67801
Portland 219/726-7131	Jay County Hospital 505 W. Arch St. 47371	Emporia 316/343-6800 ext. 545	Newman Memorial Hospital 12th and Chestnut Sts. 66801
Richmond 317/962-7010	Reid Memorial Hospital 1401 Chester Blvd. 47374	Fort Riley 913/239-7777 239-7778	Irwin Army Hospital Emergency Room 66442
Shelbyville 317/392-3211 ext. 52	William S. Major Hospital 150 W. Washington St. 46176		

City and phone	Location	City and phone	Location
Fort Scott 316/223-2200 223-0476 (night)	Mercy Hospital 821 Burke St. 66701	Owensboro 502/926-3030 ext. 180 or 186	Owensboro-Daviess County Hospital 811 Hospital Ct. 42301
Great Bend 316/792-2511 ext. 115	Central Kansas Medical Center 3515 Broadway 67530	Paducah 502/444-5100 ext. 105 or 180	Western Baptist Hospital 2501 Kentucky Ave. 42001
Hays 913/628-8251	Hadley Regional Medical Center 201 E. 7th St. 67601	Prestonburg 606/886-8511 ext. 132 or 160	Poison Control Center Highlands Regional Medical Center 41653
Kansas City 913/588-6633	University of Kansas Medical Center 39th and Rainbow Blvd. 66103	South Williamson 606/237-1010	Appalachian Regional Hospitals Central Pharmaceutical Service 2000 Central Ave. 25661
Lawrence 913/843-3680 ext. 162 or 163	Lawrence Memorial Hospital 325 Maine St. 66044	**Louisiana** State coordinator 504/342-2600	Bureau of Emergency Medical Services Baton Rouge 70801
Parsons 316/421-4880 ext. 320	Labette County Medical Center S. 21st St. 67357	Alexandria 318/487-8111 ext. 231	Rapides General Hospital Emergency Department P.O. Box 7146 71301
Salina 913/827-5591 ext. 112	St. John's Hospital 139 N. Penn St. 67401	Baton Rouge 504/928-6558	Doctors Hospital 2414 Bunker Hill Dr. 70808
Topeka 913/354-6100	Stormont-Vail Regional Medical Center 10th & Washburn Sts. 66606	Lafayette 318/234-7381	Our Lady of Lourdes Hospital P.O. Box 3827 611 St. Landry St. 70501
Wichita 316/688-2222	Wesley Medical Center 550 N. Hillside Ave. 67214	Lake Charles 318/478-6800	Lake Charles Memorial Hospital P.O. Drawer M 70601
Kentucky State coordinator 502/564-3970	Department for Human Resources Frankfort 40601	Monroe 318/342-3008	School of Pharmacy Northeast Louisiana University 700 University Ave. 71209
Ashland 606/324-2222	King's Daughter's Hospital 2201 Lexington Ave. 41101	318/325-6454	St. Francis Hospital P.O. Box 1901 71301
Fort Thomas 606/292-3216 800/352-9900	St. Lukes Hospital 85 N. Grand Ave. 41075	New Orleans 504/568-5222	Charity Hospital 1532 Tulane Ave. 70140
Lexington 606/278-3411 ext. 363	Central Baptist Hospital 1740 S. Limestone St. 40503	Shreveport 318/425-1524	LSU Medical Center P.O. Box 33932 71130
606/233-5320	Drug Information Center University of Kentucky Medical Center 40536	**Maine** State coordinator 207/871-2950	Maine Poison Control Center Portland 04102
Louisville 502/589-8222 800/722-5725 (KY)	Poison Control Center NKC, Inc. P.O. Box 35070 40232	Portland 207/871-2950 800/442-6305	Maine Medical Center Emergency Division 22 Bramhall St. 04102
Murray 502/753-7588	Murray-Calloway County Hospital 803 Popular 42071		

Poison control centers in United States and possessions—cont'd

City and phone	Location	City and phone	Location
Maryland		Eloise	Wayne County General Hospital
State coordinator	Maryland Poison Center	313/722-3748	30712 Michigan Ave.
301/528-7604 (MD)	University of Maryland School of Pharmacy	313/724-3000 (night)	48132
	Baltimore 21201	Flint	Poison Information Center
		313/766-0111	Hurley Medical Center
Baltimore	Maryland Poison Center	800/572-5396	One Hurley Plaza
301/528-7701	University of Maryland School of		48502
800/492-2414 (MD)	Pharmacy	Grand Rapids	St. Mary's Hospital
	636 W. Lombard St.	616/774-6794	201 Lafayette, S.E.
	21201		49503
Cumberland	Tri-State Poison Center	800/442-4571	Western Michigan Regional Poison
301/722-6677	Sacred Heart Hospital	800/632-2727	Center
	900 Seton Dr.		1840 Wealthy, S.E.
	21502		49506
Massachusetts		Jackson	W. A. Foote Memorial Hospital
State coordinator	Department of Public Health	517/788-4816	205 N. East St.
617/727-2700	Boston 02111		49201
Boston	Massachusetts Poison Control System	Kalamazoo	Midwest Poison Center
617/232-2120	300 Longwood Ave.	616/383-7070	Borgess Medical Center
800/682-9211 (MA)	02115	800/632-4177	1521 Gull Rd.
Michigan		(Michigan)	49001
State coordinator	Department of Public Health	616/383-6409	Bronson Methodist Hospital
517/373-1406	Emergency Medical Services	800/442-4112	252 E. Lovell St.
	Lansing 48909		49006
Adrian	Emma L. Bixby Hospital	Lansing	St. Lawrence Hospital
517/263-2412	818 Riverside Ave.	517/372-5112	1210 W. Saginaw St.
	49221	517/372-5113	48914
Ann Arbor	University Hospital	Marquette	Marquette General Hospital
313/764-5102	1405 E. Ann St.	906/228-9440	420 W. Magnetic Dr.
	48104	800/562-9781	49855
Battle Creek	Community Hospital	(N. Michigan)	
616/963-5521	Pharmacy Dept.	Midland	Midland Hospital
	183 West St.	517/631-8100	4005 Orchard Dr.
	49016		48640
Bay City	Bay Medical Center	Petoskey	Northern Michigan Hospitals, Inc.
517/894-3131	100 15th St.	616/347-0555	416 Connable
	48706		49770
Berrien Center	Berrien General Hospital	Pontiac	Poison Information Center
616/471-7761	Dean's Hill Rd.	313/858-7373	St. Joseph Mercy Hospital
	49102	313/858-7374	900 S. Woodward Ave.
Coldwater	Community Health Center of Branch		48053
517/279-7935	County	Port Huron	Port Huron Hospital
	274 E. Chicago St.	313/987-5555	1001 Kearney St.
	49036	313/987-5000	48060
Detroit	Poison Control Center	Saginaw	Saginaw General Hospital
313/494-5711	Children's Hospital of Michigan	517/755-1111	1447 N. Harrison
800/572-1655	3901 Beaubien		48602
800/462-6642	48201	Traverse City	Poison Information Center
313/927-7000	Mount Carmel Mercy Hospital	616/947-6140	Munson Medical Center
	Pharmacy Dept.		Sixth St.
	6071 W. Outer Dr.		49684
	48235		

City and phone	Location	City and phone	Location
Minnesota		Willmar	Rice Memorial Hospital
State coordinator	State Department of Health	612/235-4543	402 W. 3rd St.
612/296-5281	Minneapolis 55404		56201
Duluth	St. Luke's Hospital Emergency Dept.	Worthington	Worthington Reg. Hospital
218/727-6636	915 E. First St.	507/372-2941	1016 6th Ave.
	55805		56187
218/726-4500	St. Mary's Hospital		
	407 E. 3rd St.	**Mississippi**	
	55805	State coordinator	State Board of Health
Edina	Fairview-Southdale Hospital	601/354-6660	Jackson 39205
612/920-4400	6401 France Ave., So.	Biloxi	Gulf Coast Community Hospital
	55435	601/388-1919	4642 West Beach Blvd.
Fergus Falls	Lake Region Hospital		39531
218/736-5475	56537	601/377-6555	USAF Hospital Keesler
Fridley	Unity Hospital	601/377-6556	Keesler Air Force Base
612/786-2200	550 Osborne Rd.		39534
	55432	Brandon	Rankin General Hospital Pharmacy
Mankato	Immanuel-St. Joseph's Hospital	601/825-2811	Department
507/625-4031	325 Garden Blvd.	ext. 487 or 463	350 Crossgates Blvd.
	56001		39042
Minneapolis	Fairview Hospital	Columbia	Marion County General Hospital
612/371-6402	Outpatient Dept.	601/736-6303	Sumrall Rd.
	2312 S. 6th St.	ext. 217	39429
	55406	Greenwood	Greenwood-Leflore Hospital
612/347-3141	Hennepin Poison Center	601/453-9751	River Rd.
	Hennepin County Medical Center	ext. 2633	38930
	701 Park Ave.	Hattiesburg	Forrest County General Hospital
	55415	601/264-4235	400 S. 28th Ave.
Morris	Stevens County Memorial Hospital		39401
612/589-1313	56267	Jackson	St. Dominic-Jackson Memorial Hospital
Rochester	Southeastern Minnesota	601/982-0121	969 Lakeland Dr.
507/285-5123	Poison Control Center	ext. 2345	39216
ext. 517	St. Mary's Hospital	601/354-6650	State Board of Health
	1216 Second St., S.W.		Bureau of Disease Control
	55901		39205
St. Cloud	St. Cloud Hospital	601/354-7660	University Medical Center
612/251-2700	1406 6th Ave., No.		2500 N. State St.
ext. 221	56301		39216
St. Paul	Bethesda Lutheran Hospital	Laurel	Jones County Community Hospital
612/221-2301	559 Capitol Blvd.	601/649-4000	Jefferson St. at 13th Ave.
	55103	ext. 207, 218, 220, or	39440
612/228-3132	St. John's Hospital	248	
	403 Maria Ave.	Meridian	Meridian Regional Hospital
	55106	601/433-6211	Highway 39, N.
612/298-8402	United Hospitals, Inc.		39301
	300 Pleasant Ave.	Pascagoula	Singing River Hospital Emergency Room
	55102	601/938-5162	2609 Denny Ave.
612/221-2113	St. Paul-Ramsey Hospital		39567
	640 Jackson St.	University	University of Mississippi School of
	55101	601/234-1522	Pharmacy
			38677

Poison control centers in United States and possessions—cont'd

City and phone	Location	City and phone	Location
Missouri		**Montana**	
State coordinator 314/751-2713	Missouri Division of Health Jefferson City 65102	State coordinator 406/449-3895	Department of Health and Environmental Sciences Helena 59620
Cape Girardeau 314/651-6235	St. Francis Medical Center St. Francis Drive 63701	Helena 800/525-5042	Montana Poison Control System Cogswell Bldg. 59620
Columbia 314/882-8091	University of Missouri Medical Center 807 Stadium Rd. 65201	**Nebraska**	
Hannibal 314/221-0414 ext. 101	St. Elizabeth's Hospital c/o Pharmacy Department 109 Virginia St. 63401	State coordinator 402/471-2122	Department of Health Lincoln 68502
Jefferson City 314/635-7141 ext. 215	Charles E. Still Osteopathic Hospital 1125 Madison 65101	Omaha 402/390-5400 800/642-9999 (NE) 800/228-9515 (surrounding states)	Nebraska Reg. Poison Center Children's Memorial Hospital 8301 Dodge 68114
Joplin 417/781-2727 ext. 2305	St. John's Medical Center 2727 McClelland Blvd. 64801	**Nevada**	
Kansas City 816/234-3000	Children's Mercy Hospital 24th at Gillham Rd. 46108	State coordinator 702/885-4750	Department of Human Resources Carson City 89710
Kirksville 816/626-2121	Kirksville Osteopathic Health Center Box 949 #1 Osteopathy Ave. 63501	Las Vegas 702/385-1277	Southern Nevada Memorial Hospital 1800 W. Charleston Blvd. 89102
		702/732-4989	Sunrise Hospital Medical Center 3186 S. Maryland Pkwy. 89109
Poplar Bluff 314/785-7721	Lucy Lee Hospital 2620 N. Westwood Blvd. 63901	Reno 702/789-3013	St. Mary's Hospital 235 W. 6th 89503
Rolla 314/364-1322	Phelps County Memorial Hospital 1000 W. 10th St. 65401	702/785-4129	Washoe Medical Center 77 Pringle Way 89502
St. Joseph 816/271-7580 232-8481	Methodist Medical Center Seventh to Ninth on Faraon St. 64501	**New Hampshire**	
St. Louis 314/772-5200 800/392-9111 (MO)	Cardinal Glennon Memorial Hospital for Children 1465 S. Grand Ave. 63104	State coordinator Hanover 603/643-4000	New Hampshire Poison Center May Hitchcock Hospital Hanover 03755
314/367-2034	St. Louis Children's Hospital 500 S. Kingshighway 63110	**New Jersey**	
		State coordinator 609/292-5666	Department of Health Accident Prevention and Poison Control Program Trenton 08625
Springfield 417/831-9746 800/492-4824	Ozark Poison Center Lester E. Cox Medical Center 1423 N. Jefferson St. 65802	Atlantic City 609/344-4081 ext. 2359	Atlantic City Medical Center 1925 Pacific Ave. 08401
417/885-2115	St. John's Regional Health Center 1235 E. Cherokee 65802	Belleville 201/751-1000 ext. 781, 782, or 783	Clara Maass Memorial Hospital 1A Franklin Ave. 07109
		Boonton 201/334-5000 ext. 186 or 187	Riverside Hospital Powerville Rd. 07055
West Plains 417/256-9111 ext. 258 or 259	West Plains Memorial Hospital 1103 Alaska Ave. 65775	Bridgeton 609/451-6600	Bridgeton Hospital Irving Ave. 08302

City and phone	Location	City and phone	Location
Camden 609/795-5554	West Jersey Hospital Evesham Ave. and Voorhees Turnpike 08104	Orange 201/266-2120	Hospital Center at Orange Emergency Department 188 S. Essex Ave. 07051
Denville 201/627-3000 ext. 6063	St. Clare's Hospital Pocono Rd. 07834	Passaic 201/473-1000 ext. 441	St. Mary's Hospital 211 Pennington Ave. 07055
East Orange 201/672-8400 ext. 223	East Orange General Hospital 300 Central Ave. 07019	Perth Amboy 201/442-3700 ext. 2501	Perth Amboy General Hospital 530 New Brunswick Ave. 08861
Elizabeth 201/527-5059	St. Elizabeth's Hospital 225 Williamson St. 07207	Phillipsburg 201/859-1500 ext. 280	Warren Hospital 185 Roseberry St. 08865
Englewood 201/894-3440	Englewood Hospital 350 Engle St. 07631	Point Pleasant 201/892-1100 ext. 385	Point Pleasant Hospital Osborn Ave. and River Front 08742
Flemington 201/782-2121 ext. 369	Hunterdon Medical Center Route #31 08822	Princeton 609/734-4554	The Medical Center at Princeton 253 Witherspoon St. 08540
Livingston 201/992-5161	St. Barnabas Medical Center Old Short Hills Rd. 07039	Saddle Brook 201/368-6025	Saddle Brook General Hospital 300 Market St. 07662
Long Branch 201/222-2210	Monmouth Medical Center Emergency Department Dunbar and 2nd Ave. 07740	Somers Point 609/653-3515	Shore Memorial Hospital Brighton & Sunny Aves. 08244
Montclair 201/746-6000 ext. 234	Mountainside Hospital Bay and Highland Aves. 07042	Somerville 201/725-4000 ext. 431, 432, or 433	Somerset Medical Center Rehill Ave. 08876
Mount Holly 609/267-7877	Burlington County Memorial Hospital 175 Madison Ave. 08060	Summit 201/522-2232	Overlook Hospital 193 Morris Ave. 07901
Neptune 201/775-5500 800/822-9761 (NJ)	Jersey Shore Medical Center Fitkin Hospital 1945 Corlies Ave. 07753	Teaneck 201/833-3000	Holy Name Hospital 718 Teaneck Rd. 07666
Newark 201/926-7240 926-7241 926-7242 926-7243	Newark Beth Israel Medical Center 201 Lyons Ave. 07112	Trenton 609/396-1077	Helene Fuld Medical Center 750 Brunswick Ave. 08638
New Brunswick 201/828-3000 ext. 425 or 308	Middlesex General Hospital 180 Somerset St. 08903	Union 201/687-1900 ext. 237	Memorial General Hospital 1000 Galloping Hill Rd. 07083
201/745-8527	St. Peter's Medical Center 245 Easton Ave. 08903	Wayne 201/942-6900 ext. 224, 225, or 226	Greater Paterson General Hospital 224 Hamburg Turnpike 07470
Newton 201/383-2121 ext. 270, 271, or 273	Newton Memorial Hospital St. 175 High St. 07860	**New Mexico** State coordinator Albuquerque 505/843-2551 800/432-6866 (NM)	New Mexico Poison, Drug Information and Medical Crisis Center, University of New Mexico Albuquerque 87131
		New York State coordinator 518/474-3785	Department of Health Albany 12237

Poison control centers in United States and possessions—cont'd

City and phone	Location	City and phone	Location
Binghamton 607/723-8929	Southern Tier Poison Center Binghamton General Hospital 13903	Syracuse 315/476-7529 473-5831	Syracuse Poison Information Center 750 E. Adams St. 13210
607/798-5231	Our Lady of Lourdes Memorial Hospital 169 Riverside Dr. 13905	Troy 518/272-5792	St. Mary's Hospital 1300 Massachusetts Ave. 12180
Buffalo 716/878-7000 878-7654 878-7655	Western New York Poison Center Children's Hospital of Buffalo 219 Bryant St. 14222	Utica 315/798-6200 798-6223	St. Luke's Hospital Center P.O. Box 479 13502
Dunkirk 716/366-1111 ext. 414 or 415	Brooks Memorial Hospital 10 W. 6th St. 14048	Watertown 315/788-8700	House of the Good Samaritan Hospital Washington & Pratt Sts. 13602
East Meadow 516/542-2323 542-2324 542-2325	Long Island Poison Center Nassau County Medical Center 2201 Hempstead Turnpike 11554	**North Carolina** State coordinator 919/684-8111	Duke University Medical Center Durham 27710
Elmira 607/737-4100	Arnot Ogden Memorial Hospital Roe Ave. & Grove St. 14901	Asheville 704/255-4490	Western North Carolina Poison Control Center 509 Baltimore Ave. 28801
607/734-2662	St. Joseph's Hospital Health Center 555 E. Market St. 14901	Charlotte 704/379-5827	Mercy Hospital 2001 Vail Ave. 28207
Endicott 607/754-7171	Ideal Hospital 600 High St. 13760	Greensboro 919/379-4105	Moses Cone Hospital 1200 N. Elm St. 27420
Glens Falls 518/792-3151 ext. 456	Glens Falls Hospital 100 Park St. 12801	Hendersonville 704/693-6522 ext. 555 or 556	Margaret R. Pardee Memorial Hospital Fleming St. 28739
Jamestown 716/487-0141 484-8648	W. C. A. Hospital 207 Foote Ave. 14701	Hickory 704/322-6649	Catawba Memorial Hospital Fairgrove-Church Rd. 28601
Johnson City 607/773-6611	Wilson Memorial Hospital 14707	Jacksonville 919/353-7610	Onslow Memorial Hospital Western Blvd. 28540
Kingston 914/331-3131	Kingston Hospital 396 Broadway 12401	Wilmington 919/343-7046	New Hanover Memorial Hospital 2131 S. 17th St. 28401
New York City 212/340-4494 764-7667	NY City Poison Center Dept. of Health Bureau of Laboratories 455 First Ave. 10016	**North Dakota** State coordinator 701/224-2388	Department of Health Bismarck 58505
		Bismarck 701/223-4357	Bismarck Hospital Emergency Dept. 300 N. 7th St. 58501
Nyack 914/353-1000 ext. 451 or 452	Hudson Valley Poison Center Nyack Hospital N. Midland Ave. 10960	Fargo 701/280-5575	St. Luke's Hospital Fifth St. at Mills Ave. 58122
Rochester 716/275-5151	Finger Lakes Poison Center LIFE LINE University of Rochester Medical Center 14620	Grand Forks 701/780-5000	United Hospital 1200 S. Columbia Rd. 58201
Schenectady 518/382-4039 382-4121	Ellis Hospital 1101 Nott St. 12308	Minot 701/857-2553	St. Joseph's Hospital Third St. and Fourth Ave., S.E. 58701

City and phone	Location	City and phone	Location
Williston 701/572-7661	Mercy Hospital 1301 15th Ave., W. 58801	**Oklahoma** State coordinator 405/271-5454 800/522-4611	Oklahoma Poison Control Center Oklahoma Children's Memorial Hospital P.O. Box 26307 Oklahoma City 73126
Ohio State coordinator 614/466-5190	Department of Health Columbus 43216	Ada 405/322-2323 ext. 200	Valley View Hospital 1300 E. 6th St. 74820
Akron 216/379-8562 800/362-9922 (Ohio)	Children's Hospital Medical Center of Akron 281 Locust St. 44308	Ardmore 405/223-5400	Memorial Hospital of Southern Oklahoma 1011-14th Ave. 73401
Canton 216/452-9911 ext. 203	Aultman Hospital Emergency Room 2600 Sixth St., S.W. 44710	Lawton 405/355-8620	Comanche County Memorial Hospital 3401 Gore Blvd. 73501
Cincinnati 513/872-5111	Drug and Poison Information Center Bridge Med. Science Bldg. Room 7701 231 Bethesda Ave. 45267	McAlester 918/426-1800 ext. 240	McAlester General Hospital Inc., W. P.O. Box 669 74501
Cleveland 216/231-4455	Academy of Medicine 11001 Cedar Ave. 44106	Oklahoma City 405/271-5454 800/522-4611 (OK)	Oklahoma Poison Control Center Oklahoma Children's Memorial Hospital P.O. Box 26307 73126
Columbus 614/228-1323	Ohio Poison Center Children's Hospital 700 Children's Dr. 43205	Ponca City 405/765-3321	St. Joseph Medical Center 14th and Hartford 74601
Dayton 513/222-2227	Children's Medical Center One Children's Plaza 45404	Tulsa 918/584-1351 ext. 6165	Hillcrest Medical Center 1653 East 12th 74104
Lorain 216/282-2220	Lorain Community Hospital 3700 Kolbe Rd 44053	**Oregon** State coordinator Portland 503/225-8968 800/452-7165	Oregon Poison Control and Drug Information Center University of Oregon Health Sciences Center Portland 97201
Mansfield 419/522-3411 ext. 545	Mansfield General Hospital 335 Glessner Ave. 44903		
Springfield 513/325-1255	Community Hospital 2615 E. High St. 44505	**Panama** Panama City 52-7105	U.S.A. MEDDAC PANAMA Gorgas U.S. Army Hospital APO Miami 34004
Toledo 419/381-3897	Poison Information Center Medical College Hospital P.O. Box 6190 43679	**Pennsylvania** State coordinator 717/787-2307	Director, Division of Epidemiology Department of Health P.O. Box 90 Harrisburg 17108
Youngstown 216/746-2222	Mahoning Valley Poison Center 1044 Belmont Ave. 44501	Allentown 215/433-2311	Lehigh Valley Poison Center 17th & Chew Sts. 18102
Zanesville 614/454-4221	Poison Information Center Bethesda Hospital 2951 Maple Ave. 43701	Altoona 814/946-3711	Altoona Region Poison Center 2500 Seventh Ave. 16603
		Bloomsburg 717/784-7121	The Bloomsburg Hospital 549 E. Fair St. 17815

Poison control centers in United States and possessions—cont'd

City and phone	Location	City and phone	Location
Bradford 814/368-4143	Bradford Hospital Interstate Pkwy. 16701	Harrisburg 717/782-3639	Harrisburg Hospital S. Front & Mulberry St. 17101
Bryn Mawr 215/896-3577	The Bryn Mawr Hospital 19010	717/782-4141 ext. 4132	Polyclinic Hospital 3rd & Polyclinic Ave. 17105
Chester 215/494-0721 ext. 232	Sacred Heart General Hospital 9th and Wilson St. 19013	Hershey 717/634-6111 534-8955	Capital Area Poison Center The Milton S. Hershey Medical Center University Dr. 17033
Clearfield 814/765-5341	Clearfield Hospital 809 Turnpike Ave. 16830	Jeannete 412/527-3551	Jeannete District Memorial Hospital 600 Jefferson Ave. 15644
Coaldale 717/645-2131	Coaldale State General Hospital 8218	Jersey Shore 717/398-0100	Jersey Shore Hospital Thompson St. 17740
Coudersport 814/274-9300	Charles Cole Memorial Hospital RD #3 Route 6 16915	Johnstown 814/535-5351	Conemaugh Valley Memorial Hospital 1086 Franklin St. 15905
Danville 717/275-6116	Susquehanna Poison Center Geisinger Medical Center North Academy Ave. 17821	814/535-5352	Cambria-Somerset Poison Center Lee Hospital 320 Main St. 15901
Doylestown 215/345-2283	Doylestown Hospital 595 W. State St. 18901	814/535-5353	Mercy Hospital 1020 Franklin St. 15905
East Stroudsburg 717/421-4000	Pocono Hospital 206 E. Brown St. 18301	Lancaster 717/299-5511	Lancaster General Hospital 555 N. Duke St. 17604
Easton 215/258-6221	Easton Hospital 21st & Lehigh St. 18042	717/299-4546	St. Joseph's Hospital 250 College Ave. 17604
Erie 814/454-2120	Doctors Osteopathic Hospital 252 W. 11th St. 16501	Lansdale 215/368-2100	North Penn Hospital 7th and Broad St. 19446
814/864-4031	Erie Osteopathic Hospital 5515 Peach St. 16509	Lebanon 717/272-7611	Good Samaritan Hospital 4th and Walnut Sts. 17042
814/452-4242	Hamot Medical Center 201 State St. 16512	Lehighton 215/377-1300	Gnaden-Huetten Memorial Hospital 11th and Hamilton St. 18235
814/452-3232	Northwest Poison Center St. Vincent's Health Center P.O. Box 740 16512	Lewiston 717/248-5411	Lewistown Hospital Highland Ave. 17044
Gettysburg 717/334-2121	Annie M. Warner Hospital S. Washington St. 17325	Muncy 717/546-8282	Muncy Valley Hospital P.O. Box 340 17756
Greensburg 412/832-4000	Westmoreland Hospital Association 532 W. Pittsburgh St. 15601	Nanticoke 717/735-5000	Nanticoke State Hospital N. Washington St. 18634
Hanover 717/637-3711	Hanover General Hospital 300 Highland Ave. 17331	Paoli 215/648-1043	Paoli Memorial Hospital 19301

City and phone	Location	City and phone	Location
Philadelphia 215/922-5523 922-5524	Philadelphia Poison Information 321 University Ave. 19104	Mayaguez 809/832-8686 ext. 1224	Mayaguez Medical Center Department of Health P.O. Box 1868 00709
Philipsburg 814/342-3320	Philipsburg State General Hospital 16866	Ponce 809/842-8364	District Hospital of Ponce 00731
Pittsburgh 412/681-6669	Children's Hospital 125 Desoto St. 15213	Rio Piedras 809/754-8535 ext. 8535, 8536, 8537, or 8538	Childrens Hospital Center of Puerto Rico 00936
Pittston 717/654-3341	Pittston Hospital Oregon Heights 18640	San Juan 809/753-4849 (information only)	Pharmacy School Medical Sciences Campus 00936
Pottstown 215/327-7000	Pottstown Memorial Medical Center High St. and Firestone Blvd. 19464	**Rhode Island** State coordinator Providence 401/277-5727	Rhode Island Poison Center 593 Eddy Street Rhode Island Hospital Providence 02902
Pottsville 717/622-3400 ext. 270	Good Samaritan Hospital E. Norwegian and Tremont St. 17901		
Reading 215/376-4881 ext. 267	Community General Hospital 145 N. 6th St. 19601	**South Carolina** State coordinator 803/758-5654	Department of Health and Environmental Control Columbia 29201
Sayre 717/888-6666	The Robert Packer Hospital Guthrie Sq. 18840	Charleston 803/792-4201 800/845-7633 800/922-0193	National Pesticides Telecommunications Network Medical University of South Carolina 171 Ashley Ave. 29403
Sellersville 215/257-3611	Grandview Hospital 18960		
Somerset 814/443-2626	Somerset Community Hospital 225 S. Center Ave. 15501	Columbia 803/765-7359 800/922-1117	Palmetto Poison Center University of South Carolina College of Pharmacy 29208
State College 814/238-4351	Centre Community Hospital 16801		
Titusville 814/827-1851	Titusville Hospital 406 W. Oak St. 16354	**South Dakota** State coordinator 605/773-3361	Department of Health Pierre 57501
Tunkhannock 717/836-2161	Tyler Memorial Hospital RD #1 18657	Aberdeen 605/225-1880 800/592-1889	The Dakota Midland Poison Control Center 57401
York 717/843-8623	Memorial Osteopathic Hospital 325 S. Belmont St. 17403	Rapid City 605/341-8222 800/742-8925	Rapid City Regional Hospital Main 353 Fairmont Blvd. 57701
717/771-2311	York Hospital 1001 S. George St. 17405	Sioux Falls 605/336-3894 800/952-0123	McKennan Hospital Poison Center 800 East 21st St. 57101
Puerto Rico State coordinator 809/765-4880 809/765-0615	University of Puerto Rico Rio Piedras	**Tennessee** State coordinator 615/741-2407	Department of Public Health Div. of Emergency Services Nashville 37216
Arecibo 809/878-6467 (information only)	District Hospital of Arecibo 00613	Chattanooga 615/755-6100	T. C. Thompson Children's Hospital 910 Blackford St. 37403
Fajardo 809/863-0939 ext. 202 or 203	District Hospital of Fajardo 00649		

Poison control centers in United States and possessions—cont'd

City and phone	Location	City and phone	Location
Columbia 615/381-4500	Maury County Hospital 1224 Trotwood Ave. 38401	Galveston 713/765-1420	Southeast Texas Poison Center 8th & Mechanic Sts. 77550
Cookeville 615/526-4818	Cookeville General Hospital 142 W. 5th St. 38501	Harlingen 512/421-1860 421-1859	Valley Baptist Hospital P.O. Box 2588 2101 S. Commerce St. 78550
Jackson 901/424-0424	Madison General Hospital 708 W. Forest 38301	Houston 713/654-1701	Southeast Texas Poison Control Center 8th & Mechanic Sts. 77550
Johnson City 615/461-6111	Memorial Hospital Boone & Fairview Ave. 37601	Laredo 512/724-6247	Mercy Hospital 1515 Logan St. 78040
Knoxville 615/971-3261	Memorial Research Center and Hospital 1924 Alcoa Hgwy. 37920	Lubbock 806/792-1011	Methodist Hospital Pharmacy 3615 19th St. 79410
Memphis 901/528-6048	Southern Poison Center University of Tennessee College of Pharmacy 26 Dunlap St. 38163	Midland 915/685-1111	Midland Memorial Hospital 1908 W. Wall 79701
Nashville 615/322-3391	Vanderbilt University Hospital 21st & Garland 37232	Odessa 915/333-7111	Medical Center Hospital P.O. Box 633 79760
Texas		Plainview 806/296-9601	Central Plains Regional Hospital 2601 Dimmitt Rd. 79072
State coordinator 512/458-7254	Texas Department of Health Div. of Occupational Health Austin 78756	San Angelo 915/653-6741 ext. 210	Shannon West Texas Memorial Hospital P.O. Box 1879 9 S. Magdalen St. 76901
Abilene 915/677-7762	Hendrick Hospital 19th & Hickory Sts. 79601	San Antonio 512/223-6361 ext. 295	Dept. of Pediatrics University of Texas Health Sciences Center at San Antonio 7703 Floyd Curl Dr. 78284
Amarillo 806/376-4292	Amarillo Emergency Receiving Center Amarillo Hospital Dist. P.O. Box 1110 2103 W. 6th St. 79106	Tyler 214/597-0351	Medical Center Hospital 1000 S. Beckham St. 75701
Austin 512/478-4490 476-6461	Brackenridge Hospital 14th & Sabine Sts. 78701	Waco 817/756-8611	Hillcrest Baptist Hospital 3000 Herring Ave. 76708
Beaumont 713/833-7409	Baptist Hospital of Southeast Texas P.O. Box 1591 College & 11th St. 77701	Wichita Falls 817/322-6771	Wichita General Hospital 1600 8th St. 76301
Corpus Christi 512/881-4559	Memorial Medical Center P.O. Box 5280 2606 Hospital Blvd. 78405	**Utah**	
El Paso 915/533-1244	R.E. Thomason General Hospital P.O. Box 20009 4815 Alameda Ave. 79905	State coordinator 801/533-6161	Utah Department of Health Division Family Health Services Salt Lake City 84113
Fort Worth 817/927-2007	W. I. Cook Children's Hospital 1212 Lancaster 76102	Salt Lake City 801/581-2151	Intermountain Regional Poison Control Center 50 N. Medical Dr. 84132

City and phone	Location	City and phone	Location
Vermont		Petersburg	Petersburg General Hospital
State coordinator	Department of Health	804/732-7220	Mt. Erin & Adams Sts.
802/862-5701	Burlington 05401		23803
		Portsmouth	U.S. Naval Hospital
Burlington	Vermont Poison Center	804/398-5898	23708
802/658-3456	Medical Center Hospital		
	05401	Richmond	Central Virginia Poison Center
		804/786-9123	Medical College of Virginia
Virginia			Box 763 MCV Station
State coordinator	Bureau of Emergency Medical Services		23298
804/786-5188	Richmond 23219		
		Roanoke	Roanoke Memorial Hospital
Alexandria	Alexandria Hospital	703/981-7336	Belleview at Jefferson St.
703/379-3070	4320 Seminary Rd.		P.O. Box 13367
	22314		24033
Arlington	Arlington Hospital	Staunton	King's Daughter's Hospital
703/558-6161	5129 N. 16th St.	703/885-6848	P.O. Box 2007
	22205		24401
Blacksburg	Montgomery County Community	Waynesboro	Waynesboro Community Hospital
703/951-1111	Hospital	703/942-4096	501 Oak Ave.
	Rt. 460, S.		22980
	24060		
Charlottesville	Blue Ridge Poison Center	Williamsburg	Williamsburg Community Hospital
804/924-5543	University of Virginia Hospital	804/253-6005	1238 Mt. Vernon Ave.
800/446-9876	22903		Drawer H
(deaf out-of-state)			23185
800/552-3723			
(deaf VA only)		**Virgin Islands**	
Danville	Danville Memorial Hospital	State coordinator	Department of Health
804/799-2100	142 S. Main St.	809/774-1321	St. Thomas 00801
ext. 3869	22201	ext. 275	
Falls Church	Fairfax Hospital	St. Croix	Charles Harwood Memorial Hospital
703/698-3600	3300 Gallows Rd.	809/773-1212	Christiansted
698-3111	22046	773-1311	00820
		ext. 221	
Hampton	Hampton General Hospital		
804/727-1131	3120 Victoria Blvd.	809/772-0260	Ingeborg Nesbitt Clinic
	23661	772-0212	Fredericksted
			00840
Harrisonburg	Rockingham Memorial Hospital		
703/433 9706	738 S. Mason St.	St. John	Morris F. DeCastro Clinic
	22801	809/776-1469	Cruz Bay
			00830
Lexington	Stonewall Jackson Hospital		
703/463-9141	22043	St. Thomas	Knud-Hansen Memorial Hospital
		809/774-1321	00801
Lynchburg	Lynchburg Gen. Marshall Lodge	ext. 224 or 225	
804/528-2066	Hospital, Inc.		
	Tate Springs Rd.	**Washington**	
	24504	State coordinator	Department of Social & Health Sciences
		206/522-7478	Seattle 98115
Nassawadox	Northampton-Accomack Memorial		
804/442-8700	Hospital	Seattle	Children's Orthopedic-Hospital and
	23413	206/634-5252	Medical Center
			4800 Sandpoint Way, NE
Newport News	Riverside Hospital		98105
804/599-2050	500 J. Clyde Morris Blvd.		
	23601	Spokane	Deaconess Hospital
		509/747-1077	W. 800 5th Ave.
Norfolk	DePaul Hospital	800/572-5842	99210
804/489-5288	Granby St. at Kingsley La.		
	23505	Tacoma	Mary Bridge Children's Hospital
		206/272-1281	South L Street
		ext. 259	98405

Poison control centers in United States and possessions—cont'd

City and phone	Location
Yakima 509/248-4400 800/572-9176	Central Washington Poison Center Yakima Valley Memorial Hospital 2811 Tieton Dr. 98902
West Virginia State coordinator 304/348-2971	Department of Health Charleston 25305
Charleston 800/642-3625 304/348-4211	West Virginia Poison System 3110 MacCorkle Ave., S.E. 29208
Wisconsin State coordinator 608/267-7174	Department of Health & Social Services Division of Health Madison 53701
Eau Claire 715/835-1515	Luther Hospital 1225 Whipple 54701
Green Bay 414/433-8100	Green Bay Poison Control Center St. Vincent's Hospital 835 S. Van Buren St. 54305
LaCrosse 608/784-3971	St. Francis Hospital 700 West Ave. N. 54601
Madison 608/262-3702	Madison Area Poison Center University Hospital and Clinic 600 Highland Ave. 53792
Milwaukee 414/931-4114	Milwaukee Children's Hospital 1700 W. Wisconsin 53233
Wyoming State coordinator 307/777-7955	Office of Emergency Medical Services Department of Health & Social Services Cheyenne 82001
Cheyenne 307/635-9256	Wyoming Poison Center DePaul Hospital 2600 E. 18th St. 82001

Poison control centers in Canada

City	Location
Newfoundland and Labrador	
Labrador City	Capt. Wm. Jackman Memorial Hospital Dr. I. Arnold 944-2632
Corner Brook	Western Memorial Hospital Mr. S. Gibbons, Director 634-7121
Gander	James Paton Memorial Hospital Mr. J. Hoddinott, Director 651-2500
Grand Falls	Central Newfoundland Hospital Mr. T. Maher, Director 489-6661
St. Anthony	Charles S. Curtis Memorial Hospital (The International Grenfell Association) Dr. J.H. Williams 454-8881
St. John's	The Dr. Charles A. Janeway Child Health Centre Dr. J. Muzychka 722-1110
Prince Edward Island	
Charlottetown	Prince Edward Island Hospital 894-8532
Summerside	Prince County Hospital 436-9131
Nova Scotia	
Halifax	The Izaak Walton Killam Hospital for Children Dr. J.P. Anderson 424-6161
New Brunswick	There is a Poison Treatment Center in the Emergency Service of most of the active treatment hospitals in New Brunswick.
Bathurst	Chaleur General Hospital 546-4666
Campbellton	Hôtel-Dieu St. Joseph 753-5212
Edmundston	Hôtel-Dieu St. Joseph 735-7384
Fredericton	Dr. Everett Chalmers Hospital 452-5400
Moncton	Moncton City Hospital 855-1600
Saint John	Saint John General Hospital Dr. R. Scharf 658-2222

City	Location	City	Location
Quebec	There is a Poison Treatment Center in the Emergency Service of every active treatment hospital in Quebec.	Kirkland Lake	Kirkland and District Hospital Dr. R. Denton 567-5251
		Kitchener	Kitchener-Waterloo Hospital Dr. J.W. Swann 742-3611
Main Centres			St. Mary's General Hospital Dr. J.W. Swann 744-3311
Montréal	Hôpital Sainte-Justine Dr. Luc Chicoine 731-4931	London	Victoria Hospital Dr. K.G. Ferguson 432-2352
	Montreal Children's Hospital Dr. Normal Eade 937-8511	St. Catharines	St. Catharines General Hospital Dr. P. O'Malloran 684-7271
Québec City	Centre Hospitalier de l'Université Laval Centre Régional de Toxicologie Dr. Albert Nantel 656-8090	Sarnia	Sarnia General Hospital Dr. K.R. Singh 344-3661
	Centre anti-poison, Dr. Benoit Dumais 656-8380		St. Joseph's Hospital Dr. K. Threndyle 336-3111
Ontario		Sault Ste. Marie	Plummer Memorial Public Hospital Dr. J.C. Paterson 254-5161
Main Poison Control Information Centers			
Toronto	Hospital for Sick Children Dr. M. McGuigan 979-1900 1-800-268-9017	Simcoe	Norfolk General Hospital Dr. K.R. McGavin 426-0750
Ottawa	Children's Hospital of Eastern Ontario Dr. J.M. Park 521-4040 1-800-267-1373	Sudbury	Sudbury General Hospital 674-3181
		Thunder Bay	McKellar General Hospital Dr. M.W.H. Adams 623-5561
Other Centers:			Port Arthur General Hospital Dr. Arnot R. Hawkins 344-6621
Barrie	Royal Victoria Hospital Dr. Raymond Asquith 728-9802	Toronto	East General and Orthopaedic Hospital Dr. A. Kaminker 461-8272
Belleville	Belleville General Hospital Dr. James E. Nelles 968-5511		
Brantford	Brantford General Hospital Dr. I. Kents 752-7871	Windsor	Hôtel-Dieu de St. Joseph Dr. P. Deturnets 252-3631
Burlington	Joseph Brant Memorial Hospital Dr. P. Korhonen 632-3730 or Zenith 46250	**Manitoba**	Poison Treatment is available in every active hospital emergency department in Manitoba.
Guelph	St. Joseph's Hospital Dr. D. Maharaj 824-2620 Ext: 208		
Kingston	Kingston General Hospital Dr. Murray Taylor 547-2001		Provincial Poison Information Centre Telephone: 787-2591

Poison control centers in Canada—cont'd

City	Location	City	Location
	Health Sciences Children's Centre 685 Bannatyne Avenue Winnipeg, Manitoba R3E0W1 Director: Dr. Tenenbein Telephone: 787-2444	Victoria	Emergency Department Royal Jubilee Hospital 595-9212
Saskatchewan		**Northwest Territories** Fort Smith	Fort Smith Health Centre Box 450 X0E0P0 872-2713
	There is a Poison Treatment Center in the Emergency Service of most of the active treatment hospitals in Saskatchewan.	Hay River	H.H. Williams Memorial Hospital P.O. Box 1280, X0E 0R0 874-6512
Main centers	Regina General Hospital Poison Control Centre Dr. B. Kitchen, Director 352-9227	Yellowknife	Stanton Yellowknife Hospital Pharmacist Yellowknife, N.W.T. X0E1H0 873-3444
	Saskatoon University Hospital Poison Control Centre Dr. W.A. Baker, Director 343-3323	**Yukon Territory** Whitehorse	Emergency Department Whitehorse General Hospital 667-7831
Alberta *Poison Information Centers* Calgary	Calgary General Hospital 841 Centre Ave. E. Calgary, Alberta, T2E0A1 262-5982		
	Emergency Department Foothills General Hospital 1403-29th Street N.W. Calgary, Alberta T2N2T9 270-1315		
Edmonton	Royal Alexandra Hospital 10240 Kingsway Ave. Edmonton, Alberta T5H3V9 474-3431		

Poison control centers for the deaf

City	Location
	University of Alberta Hospital 112 Street and 84 Avenue Edmonton, Alberta T6G2B7 432-8410
Blue Ridge Poison Center	University of Virginia Hospital Charlottesville, VA 22903 800/446-9876 (out-of-state) 800/552-3723 (Virginia only)
Finger Lakes Regional Poison Control Center	LIFE LINE Rochester, New York 716/244-1690
Georgia Poison Control Center	Grady Memorial Hospital 80 Butler St., S.E. Atlanta, GA 30303 404/525-3323
Long Island Regional Poison Control Center	Nassau County Medical Center 2201 Hempstead Turnpike East Meadow, NY 11554 516/542-2323
Massachusetts Poison Control System	300 Longwood Ave. Boston, MA 02115 617/277-3323

Treatment Centers
All active treatment hospitals in Alberta

British Columbia
Poison treatment is available in every active hospital emergency department in British Columbia.

Vancouver — Provincial Reference Centre: Provincial Drug and Poison Information Centre St. Paul's Hospital 1081 Burrard St. 682-2344 Local 2126

APPENDIX 14 • Leading health problems and communicable diseases

Two leading health problems in the United States are cardio-vascular disease and cancer. Nurses and other health care professionals encounter some form of these diseases daily. The following statistics are offered in an effort to increase understanding of the magnitude of the problem and to provide a basis for developing patient teaching strategies. In this way, the health care professional becomes a tool for preventive health care, an increasingly important role in today's health conscious society.

Leading Causes of Death
United States: 1979 Estimate

Cause	Number of Deaths (in thousands)
Disease of Heart and Blood Vessels	975,550
Cancer	403,780
Accidents	105,420
Chronic Obstructive Pulmonary Disease	49,980
Pneumonia and Influenza	44,110
All Other Causes	327,160

Source: National Center for Health Statistics, U.S. Public Health Service, DHHS

14-1. Cardiovascular disease

VITAL STATISICS

- 41,290,000 Americans have one or more forms of heart or blood vessel disease.
- Stroke afflicts 1,780,000 Americans.
- As many as 1.5 million Americans may have a heart attack this year and about 550,000 of them will die.
- High blood pressure afflicts an estimated 35,520,000 American adults.
- 1,820,000 adults and 100,000 children in America have rheumatic heart disease.
- The economic cost of cardiovascular disease will amount to an estimated $50.7 billion in 1982.

Estimated Deaths Due to Cardiovascular Diseases by Major Type of Disorder
United States: 1979 Estimate

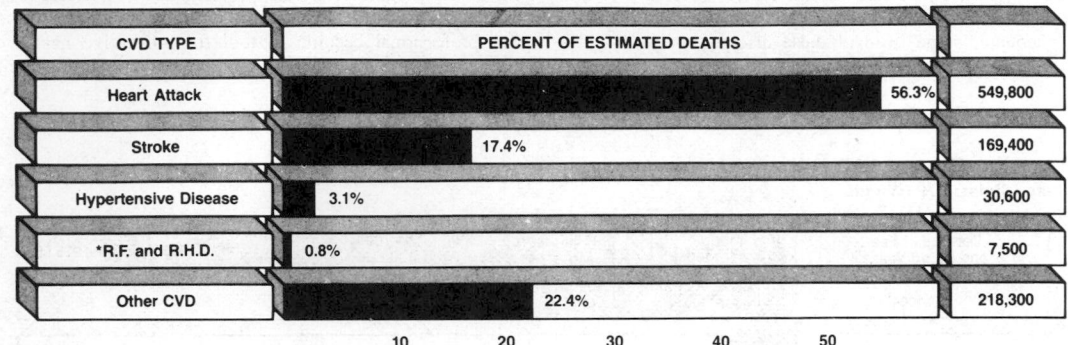

CVD TYPE	PERCENT OF ESTIMATED DEATHS	
Heart Attack	56.3%	549,800
Stroke	17.4%	169,400
Hypertensive Disease	3.1%	30,600
*R.F. and R.H.D.	0.8%	7,500
Other CVD	22.4%	218,300

               10   20   30   40   50

*Rheumatic Fever and Rheumatic Heart Disease

Source: National Center for Health Statistics, U.S. Public Health Service, DHHS

Estimated Economic Costs in Billions of Dollars of Cardiovascular Diseases by Type of Expenditure
United States: 1982 Estimate

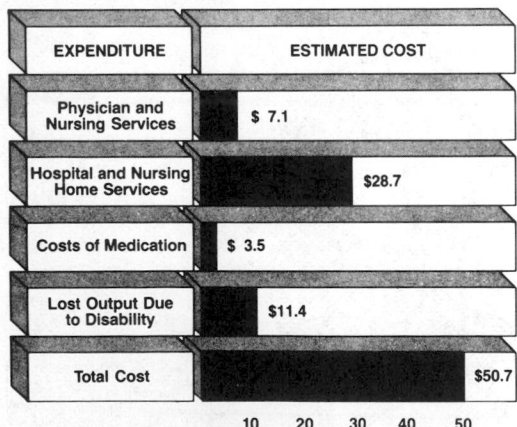

EXPENDITURE	ESTIMATED COST
Physician and Nursing Services	$ 7.1
Hospital and Nursing Home Services	$28.7
Costs of Medication	$ 3.5
Lost Output Due to Disability	$11.4
Total Cost	$50.7

          10   20   30   40   50

Source: American Heart Association

The cost in lives of heart disease and stroke is enormous—nearly one million Americans a year. But the cost in dollars to treat diseases we do not fully understand is enormous as well. The economic costs illustrated in this chart are for physician and nursing services, hospital and nursing home facilities and medications, as well as the lost occupational output as a result of disability. These high costs underline the need to invest in research as a way of understanding cardiovascular disease and reducing the death and disabilty it causes.

Estimated Prevalence of the Major Cardiovascular Disease
United States: 1979 Estimate

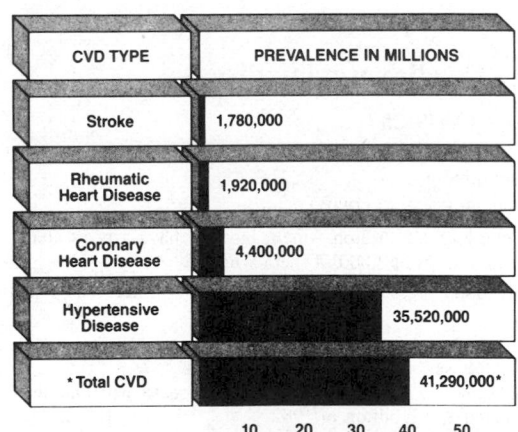

CVD TYPE	PREVALENCE IN MILLIONS
Stroke	1,780,000
Rheumatic Heart Disease	1,920,000
Coronary Heart Disease	4,400,000
Hypertensive Disease	35,520,000
* Total CVD	41,290,000*

          10   20   30   40   50

Source: American Heart Association

*The sum of the individual estimates exceeds 41,290,000 since many persons have more than one cardiovascular disorder.

HEART ATTACK—SIGNALS

Know the warning signals of a heart attack.

- Uncomfortable pressure, fullness, squeezing or pain in the center of your chest, lasting two minutes or more.
- Pain may spread to shoulders, neck or arms.
- Severe pain, dizziness, fainting, sweating, nausea or shortness of breath may also occur.

Not all these signals, however, are always present.

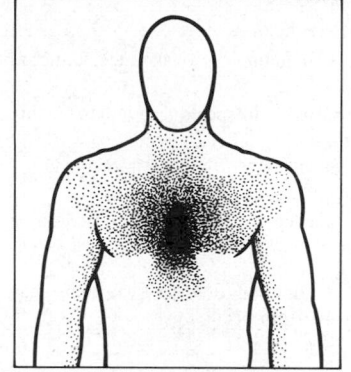

Intensity and Location of Pain

RISK FACTORS OF HEART DISEASE

Major risk factors that cannot be changed.

Heredity—It appears that a tendency toward heart disease or atherosclerosis is hereditary.

Sex—Men have a greater risk of heart attack than women. Even after menopause when women's death rate increases, it never reaches that of men.

Race—Black Americans have a 50% greater chance of having high blood pressure (a contributor to heart attack and stroke) than whites.

Age—Nearly one in four heart attack deaths occurs before 65 years of age.

Major risk factors that can be changed.

Cigarette smoking—The heart attack death rate among people who do not smoke cigarettes is considerably lower than for people who do smoke. For those who have given up the habit, the death rate eventually declines almost to that of people who have never smoked. Do not smoke cigarettes.

High blood pressure—A major risk factor of stroke and heart attack, high blood pressure usually has no specific symptoms but can be detected by a simple, painless test. A person with mild elevations of blood pressure often begins treatment with a program of weight reduction, if overweight, and salt (sodium) restriction before drugs are recommended.

Blood cholesterol levels—Too much cholesterol can cause buildups on the walls of arteries, narrowing the passageway through which blood flows, and leading to heart attack and stroke. A doctor can measure the amount of cholesterol in the blood by a simple test. Since the body gets cholesterol both through diet and by manufacturing it, a diet low in saturated fat and cholesterol will help lower the level of blood cholesterol if it is too high. Medications also are available to maintain cholesterol levels within the normal range.

Diabetes—Diabetes appears most frequently during middle age, more often in people who are overweight. In its mild form, diabetes can escape detection for many years, but it can sharply increase a person's risk of heart attack, making control of other risk factors even more important. A doctor can detect diabetes and prescribe changes in eating habits, weight-control and exercise programs and drugs, if necessary, to keep it in check.

Contributing factors

Obesity—In most cases, obesity simply results from eating too much and exercising too little. It places a heavy burden on your heart. In addition, obesity is associated with coronary heart disease primarily because of its influence on blood pressure, blood cholesterol and precipitating diabetes. To reduce weight, doctors usually recommend a program that combines exercise with a low-calorie diet.

Lack of exercise—Lack of exercise has not been clearly established as a risk factor for heart attack. But when combined with overeating, lack of exercise may lead to excess weight, which is clearly a contributing factor. A doctor should be consulted for the physical activities that best suit the age and physical condition of the individual.

Stress—It's practically impossible to define and measure a person's emotional stress level. Moreover, each of us reacts differently to it. All human beings feel stress—life without it would be dull, indeed. But excessive stress over a long period may create health problems in some people. Most doctors agree that reduction of emotional stress will benefit the health of the average individual.

MAJOR RISK FACTORS THAT CANNOT BE CHANGED	MAJOR RISK FACTORS THAT CAN BE CHANGED	CONTRIBUTING FACTORS
Heredity	Cigarette Smoking	Obesity
Sex	High Blood Pressure	Lack Of Exercise
Race	Blood Cholesterol Levels	Stress
Age	Diabetes	

WARNING SIGNALS OF STROKE

Know the warning signals of stroke.

- Sudden, temporary weakness or numbness of the face, arm and leg on one side of the body.
- Temporary loss of speech, or trouble in speaking or understanding speech.
- Temporary dimness or loss of vision, particularly in one eye.
- Unexplained dizziness, unsteadiness or sudden falls.

Many major strokes are preceded by "little strokes," warning signals like the above, experienced days, weeks, or months before the more severe event.

Prompt medical or surgical attention to these symptoms may prevent a fatal or disabling stroke from occurring.

Brain Damage Affects Opposite Side of Body

RISK FACTORS OF STROKE

Some of the factors that increase the risk of stroke are congenital, while others result from the hazards of life. Some of these factors can be minimized by the individual and with professional help. Other factors cannot be changed.

| RISK FACTORS THAT CANNOT BE CHANGED | Sex |
| Race |
| RISK FACTORS THAT CAN BE CHANGED | High Blood Pressure |
| High Red Blood Cell Count |
| Heart Disease |
| Diabetes Mellitus |

THE AMERICAN HEART ASSOCIATION REGIONS AND AFFILIATES

NORTHWEST-ROCKY MOUNTAIN REGION

Alaska Heart Association
2330 East 42nd Street
Anchorage, AK 99504

Colorado Heart Association
4521 East Virginia Avenue
Denver, CO 80222

Idaho Heart Association
5777 Overland Road
Boise, Idaho 83705

Montana Heart Association
Prof. Bldg., 510 1st Ave., N.
Great Falls, MT 59401

Oregon Heart Association
1500 S.W. 12th Avenue
Portland, OR 97201

Utah Heart Association
250 East 1st South
Salt Lake City, UT 84111

American Heart Association
of Washington
4414 Woodland Park Avenue, N.
Seattle, WA 98103

American Heart Association
of Wyoming
217 West 18th Street
Cheyenne, Wyoming 82001

NORTH CENTRAL REGION

Chicago Heart Association
20 North Wacker
Chicago, IL 60606

Illinois Heart Association
1181 North Dirksen Parkway
Springfield, IL 62708

American Heart Association
Indiana Affiliate
222 South Downey, Suite 222
Indianapolis, IN 46219

Kentucky Heart Association
207 Speed Bldg., 333 Guthrie
Louisville, KY 40202

Michigan Heart Association
Box LV160
16310 W. Twelve Mile Rd.
Southfield, MI 48076

American Heart Association
Northeast Ohio Affiliate
1689 East 115th Street
Cleveland, OH 44106

American Heart Association
Ohio Affiliate
6161 Busch Blvd., Suite 327
Columbus, OH 43229

American Heart Association
Wisconsin Affiliate
795 North Van Buren Street
Milwaukee, WI 53202

SOUTHWEST REGION

American Heart Association
Arizona Affiliate
1445 East Thomas
Phoenix, AZ 85014

American Heart Association
California Affiliate
805 Burlway Road
Burlingame, CA 94010

American Heart Association
of Hawaii
245 North Kukui Street
Honolulu, HI 96817

American Heart Association
Greater Los Angeles Affiliate
2405 West 8th Street
Los Angeles, CA 90057

American Heart Association
Nevada Affiliate
P.O. Box 1218
Chico, CA 95926

American Heart Association
New Mexico Affiliate
Home Office Plaza
Suite W-14
2403 San Mateo Blvd., N.E.
Albuquerque, NM 87110

American Heart Association
Texas Affiliate
860 North Highway 183
Austin, TX 78757

GREAT PLAINS REGION

American Heart Association
Dakota Affiliate
1005 Twelfth Avenue, S.E.
Jamestown, ND 58401

American Heart Association
Iowa Affiliate
3810 Ingersoll Avenue
Des Moines, IA 50312

American Heart Association
Kansas Affiliate
5229 West 7th Street
Topeka, KS 66606

American Heart Association
Minnesota Affiliate
4701 West 77th Street
Minneapolis, MN 55435

American Heart Association
Missouri Affiliate
105 East Ash, Suite 2
Columbia, MO 65201

American Heart Association
Nebraska Affiliate
3624 Farnam
Omaha, NE 68131

UPPER ATLANTIC REGION

American Heart Association
of Delaware
4 Trolley Square
Delaware Ave. & Dupont St.
Wilmington, DE 19806

American Heart Association
New Jersey Affiliate
1525 Morris Avenue
Union, NJ 07083

New York Heart Association
205 East 42nd Street
New York NY 10017

American Heart Association
New York State Affiliate
214 S. Warren St. 8th Floor
Syracuse, NY 13202

American Heart Association
Pennsylvania Affiliate
2743 North Front Street
Harrisburg, PA 17110

Puerto Rico Heart Association
Apartado Postal #1752
554 Cabo Alverio Street
Hato Rey Station
San Juan, PR 00919

MIDDLE ATLANTIC REGION

American Heart Association
Maryland Affiliate
415 North Charles Street
Baltimore, MD 21203

American Heart Association
North Carolina Affiliate
1 Heart Circle, Box 2636
Chapel Hill, NC 27514

American Heart Association
South Carolina Heart
Association Affiliate
5868 Percival Road
Columbia, SC 29260

American Heart Association
Virginia Affiliate
316 East Clay Street
Richmond, VA 23219

American Heart Association
Nation's Capital Affiliate
2233 Wisconsin Avenue, N.W.
Washington, DC 20007

American Heart Association
West Virginia Affiliate
211 35th Street, S.E.
Charleston WV 25304

NEW ENGLAND REGION

American Heart Association
Connecticut Affiliate
71 Parker Avenue
Meriden, CT 06450

American Heart Association
Maine Affiliate
20 Winter Street
Augusta, ME 04330

American Heart Association
Massachusetts Affiliate
33 Broad Street
Boston, MA 02109

New Hampshire Heart
Association
54 South State Street
Concord, NH 03301

American Heart Association
Rhode Island Affiliate
40 Broad Street
Pawtucket, RI 02860

Vermont Heart Association
56 Church Street
Rutland, VT 05701

SOUTHERN REGION

American Heart Association
Alabama Affiliate
1449 Medical Park Drive
Birmingham, AL 35213

American Heart Association
Arkansas Affiliate
909 West 2nd Street
Little Rock, AR 72201

American Heart Association
Florida Affiliate
810 63rd Avenue North
St. Petersburg, FL 33702

American Heart Association
Georgia Affiliate
Broadview Plaza, Level C
2581 Piedmont Rd., N.E.
Atlanta, GA 30324

American Heart Association,
Louisiana
3303 Tulane Avenue
New Orleans, LA 70119

American Heart Association
Mississippi Affiliate
4830 East McWillie Circle
Jackson, MS 39206

American Heart Association
Oklahoma Affiliate
800 Northeast 15th Street
Oklahoma City, OK 73104

American Heart Association
Tennessee Affiliate
Suite 308, 1720 West End Bldg.
Nashville, TN 37203

14-2. Cancer

Cancer around the world—1976-77

Age-adjusted death rates per 100,000 population for selected sites for 42 countries

Country	All sites		Oral		Colon & rectum	
	Male	Female	Male	Female	Male	Female
United States	213.6(17)	136.3(19)	5.8(8)	2.0(7)	26.2(16)	20.2(15)
Argentina	212.5(19)	137.2(18)	4.4(17)	1.0(30)	19.8(22)	17.3(21)
Australia	210.5(22)	129.2(25)	5.3(11)	1.5(16)	28.1(12)	22.7(11)
Austria	248.7(8)	156.3(7)	5.2(14)	0.9(32)	33.4(3)	22.5(13)
Belgium	266.7(3)	147.7(12)	3.5(27)	0.9(32)	29.0(9)	24.6(7)
Bulgaria	158.8(35)	97.7(37)	2.4(37)	0.8(37)	13.5(29)	9.4(32)
Canada	211.2(21)	135.3(20)	5.3(11)	1.6(14)	28.6(10)	23.0(9)
Chile	197.7(23)	153.8(9)	3.3(30)	0.9(32)	9.9(32)	10.0(30)
Costa Rica	163.8(33)	139.5(16)	3.9(23)	1.7(11)	8.2(36)	8.4(34)
Denmark	232.1(12)	170.9(2)	3.1(33)	1.5(16)	32.4(6)	25.9(4)
England & Wales	251.5(7)	156.0(6)	3.7(24)	1.7(11)	29.6(8)	22.8(10)
France	255.7(6)	125.2(29)	18.5(3)	1.5(16)	28.0(13)	18.8(18)
Germany, D.R.	211.8(20)	133.8(22)	3.0(34)	0.9(32)	23.3(19)	19.6(16)
Germany, F.R.	244.8(9)	154.8(8)	3.5(27)	0.9(32)	32.4(6)	24.8(6)
Greece	185.8(28)	103.6(35)	2.2(39)	3.0(5)	8.8(35)	9.2(33)
Honduras	24.5(42)	37.8(40)	0.6(41)	0.4(41)	0.2(41)	0.7(41)
Hong Kong	229.1(14)	125.3(28)	21.2(1)	7.1(1)	16.9(24)	11.9(27)
Hungary	256.9(5)	163.6(4)	7.6(7)	1.4(20)	28.5(11)	22.6(12)
Iceland	170.1(31)	138.7(17)	3.7(24)	1.8(10)	18.4(23)	16.0(24)
Ireland	225.2(15)	161.0(5)	5.3(11)	2.7(6)	36.0(1)	27.2(2)
Israel	170.5(30)	141.3(14)	2.3(38)	1.5(16)	21.4(20)	16.6(23)
Japan	186.7(27)	108.7(33)	2.2(39)	0.8(37)	15.0(26)	11.1(28)
Malta & Gozo	185.1(29)	114.7(31)	9.5(4)	2.0(7)	15.3(25)	13.3(25)
Maritius	100.5(37)	66.9(38)	3.7(24)	1.2(25)	9.9(32)	5.8(37)
Netherlands	261.6(4)	142.6(13)	2.5(36)	0.8(37)	26.9(14)	21.1(14)
New Zealand	221.0(16)	150.7(10)	4.3(20)	1.7(11)	33.0(4)	30.0(1)
Nicaragua	30.6(41)	30.9(41)	0.0(42)	0.0(42)	0.0(42)	0.0(42)
Northern Ireland	229.6(13)	150.4(11)	3.3(30)	1.6(14)	33.5(2)	25.5(5)
Norway	188.0(26)	131.2(23)	4.3(20)	1.1(27)	23.4(18)	19.4(17)
Paraguay	104.1(36)	120.2(30)	4.0(22)	1.1(27)	8.1(37)	5.0(38)
Philippines	62.2(39)	55.1(39)	5.7(10)	4.5(3)	12.8(30)	3.6(39)
Poland	213.4(18)	126.4(27)	5.8(8)	1.3(22)	14.5(28)	11.1(28)
Romania	161.3(34)	105.7(34)	4.4(17)	1.1(27)	9.6(34)	8.0(35)
Scotland	269.8(2)	165.8(3)	4.4(17)	1.9(9)	32.7(5)	26.5(3)
Singapore	242.1(10)	127.7(26)	18.9(2)	6.3(2)	21.2(21)	16.7(22)
Spain	192.5(25)	109.9(32)	4.8(15)	0.8(37)	7.4(38)	12.8(26)
Sweden	197.5(24)	140.9(15)	3.4(29)	1.4(20)	25.0(17)	18.6(19)
Switzerland	236.8(11)	134.2(21)	8.0(6)	1.3(22)	26.6(15)	17.6(20)
Thailand	37.1(40)	24.8(42)	2.6(35)	1.3(22)	3.8(40)	1.2(40)
Uruguay	294.6(1)	180.3(1)	8.3(5)	1.2(25)	14.6(27)	24.5(8)
Venezuela	65.4(38)	130.3(24)	3.3(30)	3.1(4)	7.1(39)	8.0(35)
Yugoslavia	166.5(32)	101.9(36)	4.5(16)	1.0(30)	12.3(31)	10.0(30)

Lung		Breast	Uterus	Skin		Stomach		Prostate	Leukemia	
Male	Female	Female	Female	Male	Female	Male	Female	Male	Male	Female
68.1(6)	17.2(5)	27.3(14)	8.9(30)	3.4(6)	1.9(12)	9.2(37)	4.4(39)	22.3(12)	5.6(23)	5.2(5)
53.9(21)	7.3(22)	24.2(18)	14.0(12)	2.0(22)	1.1(30)	24.0(19)	12.2(22)	17.4(19)	6.7(19)	4.1(25)
61.6(18)	10.3(14)	24.8(16)	7.9(34)	6.6(1)	3.6(2)	15.7(34)	8.4(36)	22.9(11)	8.0(9)	5.0(11)
67.6(7)	8.7(15)	24.7(17)	16.3(8)	2.5(11)	1.9(12)	38.5(7)	20.6(7)	21.9(13)	7.1(16)	4.9(13)
91.5(4)	7.2(23)	27.7(13)	10.1(25)	1.7(26)	1.5(24)	23.4(20)	13.6(19)	25.1(4)	8.0(9)	4.8(17)
44.1(24)	7.7(18)	14.6(29)	9.2(29)	1.4(29)	1.6(18)	36.6(9)	20.3(8)	8.9(33)	5.5(24)	4.1(25)
62.7(14)	12.5(11)	28.4(12)	8.3(33)	2.0(22)	1.8(15)	15.8(33)	7.2(37)	21.0(15)	8.8(2)	5.0(11)
25.3(32)	6.9(25)	14.1(30)	22.3(4)	1.7(26)	1.6(18)	64.9(2)	30.4(3)	17.0(21)	4.6(32)	3.7(30)
14.8(37)	6.1(28)	11.4(34)	24.4(3)	1.9(24)	0.8(32)	61.1(3)	38.8(1)	15.3(23)	4.4(33)	4.9(13)
62.0(15)	15.2(8)	33.8(1)	15.2(11)	3.1(7)	2.7(4)	19.0(29)	9.7(31)	21.1(14)	8.9(1)	5.7(3)
96.5(3)	19.4(4)	33.6(2)	10.4(22)	2.2(18)	1.9(12)	25.1(17)	11.8(24)	18.2(18)	6.6(20)	4.4(20)
48.6(23)	4.6(36)	22.7(21)	11.3(18)	2.2(18)	1.8(15)	20.4(27)	9.4(32)	23.1(9)	8.7(3)	5.2(5)
67.0(8)	6.0(29)	18.8(24)	15.9(9)	2.3(14)	1.5(24)	34.4(12)	16.4(15)	14.2(24)	7.3(14)	4.2(22)
64.0(12)	6.8(26)	25.1(15)	12.1(15)	2.4(13)	1.6(18)	34.4(12)	18.3(10)	24.1(5)	8.2(7)	5.2(5)
55.3(20)	8.2(16)	15.1(28)	7.4(35)	1.4(29)	1.5(24)	17.6(31)	10.6(28)	9.7(31)	8.4(6)	5.2(5)
0.6(41)	0.4(42)	0.1(41)	2.7(41)	0.0(41)	0.1(39)	5.5(40)	3.7(40)	0.2(40)	2.1(40)	1.3(41)
65.6(9)	30.4(1)	10.7(36)	12.1(15)	1.1(33)	0.6(36)	5.8(39)	9.2(33)	2.9(37)	3.8(35)	3.1(36)
65.0(11)	11.2(12)	23.8(19)	19.6(5)	3.6(5)	2.9(3)	47.4(4)	22.6(4)	23.9(6)	7.6(13)	5.1(10)
24.7(33)	14.8(9)	22.2(23)	6.5(38)	1.0(35)	0.0(41)	37.7(8)	21.5(6)	19.2(17)	5.0(27)	3.3(34)
61.8(16)	16.9(6)	32.0(6)	7.2(36)	2.1(20)	2.0(10)	25.1(17)	14.2(17)	23.0(10)	6.2(22)	3.6(31)
32.9(28)	10.5(13)	29.2(10)	5.8(39)	2.5(11)	1.6(18)	18.4(39)	9.2(33)	11.1(29)	8.7(3)	5.9(1)
28.3(31)	8.2(16)	5.7(39)	11.8(17)	1.0(35)	0.7(34)	70.2(1)	34.9(2)	3.6(35)	4.8(31)	3.3(34)
50.3(22)	5.1(34)	33.4(3)	8.7(31)	1.8(25)	1.4(28)	30.1(14)	10.5(29)	11.2(28)	5.0(27)	4.8(17)
15.9(36)	3.7(37)	7.9(37)	11.3(18)	0.5(38)	0.5(37)	22.0(24)	10.5(29)	4.4(34)	2.9(38)	2.4(40)
97.7(2)	6.2(27)	31.5(7)	9.3(28)	2.3(14)	1.6(18)	28.2(15)	13.0(21)	23.8(7)	8.0(9)	5.2(5)
65.6(9)	13.5(10)	30.0(9)	10.2(24)	6.4(2)	3.8(1)	19.1(28)	8.5(35)	23.8(7)	8.5(5)	4.9(13)
0.4(42)	0.5(41)	0.0(42)	1.4(42)	0.0(41)	0.0(41)	2.8(41)	0.6(42)	0.0(42)	3.2(37)	3.0(38)
71.7(5)	16.0(7)	33.0(5)	8.4(32)	2.1(20)	2.1(7)	23.4(10)	14.3(16)	19.9(16)	7.3(14)	3.5(32)
30.5(30)	5.9(31)	22.6(22)	9.9(26)	4.6(3)	2.6(5)	23.8(27)	11.8(24)	29.8(2)	6.6(20)	4.9(13)
9.6(38)	2.7(39)	17.0(25)	36.3(1)	1.5(28)	0.5(37)	23.9(22)	12.1(23)	12.9(26)	5.2(26)	4.4(20)
8.7(39)	3.6(38)	6.7(38)	7.1(37)	1.1(33)	0.7(34)	7.0(38)	5.5(38)	1.9(38)	3.5(36)	2.8(39)
60.2(19)	7.5(20)	16.3(26)	15.7(10)	0.5(38)	2.1(7)	44.6(5)	17.5(12)	10.2(30)	6.8(18)	4.2(22)
37.7(26)	7.2(23)	13.3(32)	18.9(6)	2.3(14)	1.6(18)	36.5(10)	16.7(14)	12.5(27)	4.9(29)	3.5(32)
108.5(1)	23.1(2)	31.3(8)	10.5(21)	2.8(9)	2.0(10)	25.4(16)	13.4(20)	17.2(20)	6.9(17)	4.2(22)
64.0(12)	20.3(3)	11.4(34)	12.7(14)	0.5(38)	0.8(32)	42.2(6)	18.2(11)	3.0(36)	4.9(29)	3.1(36)
18.7(35)	4.8(36)	15.8(27)	10.3(23)	1.0(35)	1.3(29)	15.9(32)	16.8(13)	9.7(31)	2.8(39)	4.1(25)
33.4(27)	7.7(18)	23.5(20)	9.6(27)	3.1(7)	1.7(17)	20.9(25)	10.8(27)	32.3(1)	7.9(12)	5.6(4)
61.7(17)	5.9(31)	28.6(11)	11.2(20)	3.8(4)	2.4(6)	12.0(36)	11.6(25)	28.5(3)	8.1(8)	4.7(19)
4.9(40)	1.9(40)	0.9(40)	3.3(40)	1.3(32)	0.1(39)	1.8(42)	0.8(41)	0.2(40)	0.6(41)	0.4(42)
32.5(29)	6.0(29)	33.3(4)	17.3(7)	1.4(29)	0.9(31)	20.8(26)	18.4(9)	1.6(39)	0.4(42)	5.8(2)
21.3(34)	5.2(33)	12.1(33)	27.5(2)	2.7(10)	2.1(7)	35.0(11)	22.5(5)	16.3(22)	4.0(34)	3.6(31)
43.3(25)	7.4(21)	13.9(31)	12.8(13)	2.3(14)	1.5(24)	15.3(35)	14.0(18)	13.5(25)	5.5(24)	3.8(29)

Cancer deaths—1982 estimated cancer deaths for all sites plus major sites, by state

	All sites		Major sites								
State	Number of deaths	Death rate per 100,000 population	Female breast	Colon-rectum	Lung	Oral	Uterus	Prostate	Stomach	Pancreas	Leukemia
Alabama	7200	170	500	750	2100	125	200	375	200	375	250
Alaska	300	63	20	30	75	5	10	10	10	10	10
Arizona	4700	136	325	550	1200	100	50	225	125	225	150
Arkansas	4600	179	325	500	1400	100	100	275	150	250	200
California	43,000	162	3700	5300	11,000	850	900	2200	1500	2200	1500
Colorado	3800	111	325	500	850	70	70	225	125	200	175
Connecticut	6600	209	650	900	1500	175	125	325	250	350	250
Delaware	1200	190	80	150	300	25	20	50	30	60	30
Dist. of Columbia	1600	293	175	200	375	75	60	100	60	90	40
Florida	25,200	210	1900	3200	7100	450	400	1500	800	1200	750
Georgia	8800	143	650	850	2500	200	250	450	225	425	300
Hawaii	1200	108	75	150	300	30	20	40	90	60	50
Idaho	1300	116	100	150	300	25	25	90	40	70	70
Illinois	22,300	191	2000	3100	5700	500	600	1200	750	1200	900
Indiana	10,100	177	900	1500	2700	200	300	500	250	500	400
Iowa	5700	191	500	950	1300	100	125	350	150	325	275
Kansas	4500	184	425	600	1300	100	100	300	125	250	200
Kentucky	6800	170	475	850	2200	175	175	400	150	350	275
Louisiana	7400	160	550	750	2100	175	175	400	250	375	250
Maine	2400	196	200	350	600	50	60	125	90	100	80
Maryland	8300	187	700	1100	2300	200	175	425	225	375	250
Massachusetts	12,400	215	1200	1900	2900	325	275	600	500	600	425
Michigan	16,300	171	1400	2100	4200	325	400	850	475	800	600
Minnesota	7200	168	650	1000	1600	150	125	475	250	400	325
Mississippi	4500	163	300	450	1200	90	100	325	125	275	200
Missouri	10,100	198	800	1400	2600	200	250	600	275	475	400
Montana	1300	151	100	175	325	30	30	100	50	80	60
Nebraska	3100	189	275	475	700	60	70	200	125	175	150
Nevada	1300	125	80	150	400	25	20	50	10	60	30
New Hampshire	1800	169	150	275	425	40	40	90	40	80	70
New Jersey	16,200	216	1600	2400	4000	350	375	750	650	800	500
New Mexico	1700	112	125	200	350	25	40	80	50	80	50
New York	37,400	220	4000	5800	8800	850	950	1800	1600	2100	1400
North Carolina	10,100	156	750	1100	2600	225	275	550	250	450	375
North Dakota	1200	176	90	175	200	20	20	90	60	80	50
Ohio	21,200	194	1900	3000	5600	425	600	1100	650	1000	800
Oklahoma	5800	171	400	750	1700	100	100	325	150	300	225
Oregon	4800	157	375	550	1300	100	75	300	125	250	200
Pennsylvania	26,000	218	2400	4100	6200	500	700	1300	850	1300	950
Rhode Island	2400	254	250	400	550	60	40	125	100	100	60
South Carolina	4800	136	375	500	1300	100	125	300	125	275	175
South Dakota	1300	183	100	200	300	20	30	100	50	90	80
Tennessee	8500	166	600	900	2400	200	200	450	225	425	300
Texas	22,000	133	1700	2400	6000	425	500	1100	700	1200	1000
Utah	1500	85	150	175	225	20	30	100	50	75	60
Vermont	950	169	80	150	250	20	30	60	30	50	40
Virginia	8700	148	750	1100	2500	175	225	450	250	425	300
Washington	7100	152	600	900	2000	150	150	425	200	375	275
West Virginia	3900	185	275	475	1100	75	100	200	100	200	125
Wisconsin	8800	179	900	1300	1900	175	175	500	325	450	350
Wyoming	650	112	50	70	175	10	10	40	15	40	20
United States	430,000	176	37,000	57,000	111,000	9000	10,000	23,000	14,000	22,000	16,000
Puerto Rico	3000	84	125	225	300	175	150	225	400	100	150

New cancer cases—1982 estimated new cancer cases for all sites plus major sites, by state

State	All sites* Number of cases	Female breast	Colon-rectum	Lung	Oral	Uterus (invasive)	Prostate	Stomach	Pancreas	Leukemia
Alabama	14,000	1600	1600	2300	350	1100	1200	325	425	425
Alaska	600	50	50	100	15	30	20	15	10	20
Arizona	8600	1100	1300	1400	275	550	750	175	250	225
Arkansas	8800	1000	1100	1500	300	650	850	200	300	300
California	82,000	11,300	10,700	13,000	2600	4800	7000	2500	2600	2400
Colorado	7300	1000	1100	1000	175	400	550	175	250	250
Connecticut	13,000	2100	2000	1800	450	800	1100	400	400	400
Delaware	2300	300	350	400	70	150	150	50	50	40
Dist. of Columbia	3200	450	400	450	200	300	325	90	100	60
Florida	49,000	5800	6900	8200	1600	2800	4500	1200	1400	1300
Georgia	17,000	1900	1900	2900	600	1200	1600	400	450	500
Hawaii	2400	300	300	350	100	125	125	175	60	70
Idaho	2700	450	300	350	75	200	275	70	80	100
Illinois	43,000	5900	6600	6600	1500	2700	3500	1400	1300	1200
Indiana	20,000	2700	3000	3100	500	1800	1500	450	550	550
Iowa	11,000	1500	2200	1600	300	800	1200	300	350	400
Kansas	8600	1200	1300	1400	275	700	800	175	300	300
Kentucky	13,000	1400	1800	2500	425	950	1200	275	375	400
Louisiana	14,000	1600	1800	2300	550	950	1300	400	400	400
Maine	4700	600	800	700	150	350	400	150	150	100
Maryland	16,000	2400	2300	2500	650	1100	1400	375	400	400
Massachusetts	24,000	3500	4100	3300	900	1500	2000	850	650	650
Michigan	31,000	4300	4500	4900	950	2200	2900	850	850	900
Minnesota	14,000	2000	2200	1800	375	800	1500	500	450	475
Mississippi	8700	850	1100	1500	250	600	1100	250	300	300
Missouri	20,000	2400	3100	3100	550	1400	1900	500	550	600
Montana	2600	300	400	350	80	150	325	80	80	80
Nebraska	5800	750	1100	850	150	350	500	175	225	225
Nevada	2500	300	300	450	60	150	150	15	60	40
New Hampshire	3600	450	650	500	100	225	275	70	90	125
New Jersey	31,000	4700	5000	4700	1100	2100	2500	1100	900	800
New Mexico	3400	400	450	450	60	250	325	80	90	70
New York	73,000	11,300	12,500	10,300	2600	4800	5800	2800	2400	2000
North Carolina	20,000	2600	2500	3000	650	1400	2000	400	600	500
North Dakota	2500	350	400	250	50	125	300	100	80	70
Ohio	41,000	5900	6300	6600	1300	3000	3300	1200	1300	1300
Oklahoma	11,000	1300	1600	2000	375	650	1000	275	325	325
Oregon	9500	1200	1200	1500	250	600	850	200	300	300
Pennsylvania	52,000	7100	9300	7300	1500	3300	4000	1600	1500	1300
Rhode Island	4700	650	850	700	200	300	400	175	150	80
South Carolina	9400	1200	1100	1500	350	800	900	175	300	250
South Dakota	2500	400	450	350	50	150	300	80	90	100
Tennessee	17,000	1900	2100	2900	550	1100	1500	325	500	475
Texas	43,000	5100	5200	7000	1500	2700	3700	1200	1200	1400
Utah	2900	450	400	250	60	225	300	80	80	80
Vermont	1900	250	300	300	60	150	200	50	50	60
Virginia	17,000	2300	2200	2900	550	1100	1500	400	475	425
Washington	14,000	2000	2000	2200	450	800	1300	350	425	450
West Virginia	7600	850	1000	1200	200	600	650	200	250	200
Wisconsin	17,000	2400	2700	2200	550	950	1700	600	500	550
Wyoming	1200	150	200	200	20	70	80	20	30	30
United States	835,000	112,000	123,000	129,000	27,000	55,000	73,000	24,000	25,000	24,000
Puerto Rico	6000	450	450	350	425	750	400	500	100	175

*Does not include carcinoma in situ or non-melanoma skin cancer.

These estimates are offered as a rough guide and should not be regarded as definitive. They are calculated according to the distribution of estimated 1982 cancer deaths by state. Especially note that year-to-year changes may only represent improvements in the basic data.

Estimated new cancer cases and deaths by sex for all sites—1982*

Site	Estimated new cases			Estimated deaths		
	Both sexes	Male	Female	Both sexes	Male	Female
All sites	**835,000***	**413,000***	**422,000***	**430,000**	**233,000**	**197,000**
Buccal cavity & pharynx (Oral)	26,800	18,600	8200	9150	6300	2850
Lip	4600	4100	500	175	150	25
Tongue	4800	3200	1600	2000	1400	600
Salivary gland				700	450	250
Floor of mouth	9700	5800	3900	525	400	125
Other & unspecified mouth				1550	1000	550
Pharynx	7700	5500	2200	4200	2900	1300
Digestive organs	198,600	102,100	96,500	113,500	59,250	54,250
Esophagus	8900	6300	2600	8300	6000	2300
Stomach	24,200	14,600	9600	13,800	8200	5600
Small intestine	2100	1100	1000	700	350	350
Large intestine } (Colon-	85,000	39,000	46,000	48,600	23,000	25,600
Rectum } rectum)	38,000	21,000	17,000	8500	4600	3900
Liver & Biliary passages	13,100	6100	7000	9900	4800	5100
Pancreas	24,800	12,800	12,000	22,300	11,600	10,700
Other & unspecified digestive	2500	1200	1300	1400	700	700
Respiratory system	143,000	102,100	40,900	116,100	84,000	32,100
Larynx	10,900	9100	1800	3700	3100	600
Lung	129,000	91,000	38,000	111,000	80,000	31,000
Other & unspecified respiratory	3100	2000	1100	1400	900	500
Bone, tissue, and skin	21,500	11,000	10,500	10,300	5900	4400
Bone	1900	1100	800	1750	1000	750
Connective tissue	4800	2600	2200	1650†	800	850
Skin	14,800**	7300**	7500**	6900†	4100	2800
Breast	112,900**	900	112,000	37,300	300	37,000
Genital organs	155,700	78,300	77,400	46,750	24,250	22,500
Cervix, Invasive } Uterus	16,000***	. . .	16,000***	7100	. . .	7100
Corpus, endometrium }	39,000	. . .	39,000	3000	. . .	3000
Ovary	18,000	. . .	18,000	11,400	. . .	11,400
Prostate	73,000	73,000	. . .	23,300	23,300	. . .
Testis, other male genital	5300	5300	. . .	950	950	. . .
Other & unspecified genital, female	4400	. . .	4400	1000	. . .	1000
Urinary organs	55,200	38,300	16,900	18,900	12,300	6600
Bladder	37,100	27,000	10,100	10,600	7300	3300
Kidney & other urinary	18,100	11,300	6800	8300	5000	3300
Eye	1800	900	900	400	200	200
Brain & central nervous system	12,400	6900	5500	10,400	5700	4700
Endocrine glands	11,100	3500	7600	1500	600	900
Thyroid	10,100	2900	7200	1050	350	700
Other endocrine	1000	600	400	450	250	200
Leukemia	23,500	13,000	10,500	15,900	8900	7000
Other blood & lymph tissues	39,600	20,900	18,700	21,100	11,000	10,100
Hodgkin's disease	7000	4000	3000	1600	900	700
Multiple myeloma	9600	4900	4700	6900	3500	3400
Other lymphomas	23,000	12,000	11,000	12,600	6600	6000
All other & unspecified sites	32,900	16,500	16,400	28,700	14,300	14,400

Note: The estimates of new cancer cases are offered as a rough guide and should not be regarded as definitive. Especially note that year-to-year changes may only represent improvements in the basic data. ACS six major sites in boldface.

*Carcinoma in situ and non-melanoma skin cancers not included in totals. Carcinoma in situ of the uterine cervix accounts for over 45,000 new cases annually. Non-melanoma skin cancer accounts for about 400,000 new cases annually.

**Melanoma only

***Invasive cancer only

†Melanoma 5100; other skin 1800

Trends in survival by site of cancer, by race (cases diagnosed in 1960-63 compared to those diagnosed in 1970-73)

Site	White			Black		
	1960-63 Relative 5-year survival (%)	1970-73 Relative 5-year survival (%)	Increase	1960-63 Relative 5-year survival (%)	1970-73 Relative 5-year survival (%)	Increase
Prostate	50	63	13	35	55	20
Kidney	37	46	9	38	44	6
Uterine corpus	73	81	8	31	44	13
Bladder	53	61	8	24	34	10
Colon and rectum	41	48	7	31	35	4
Uterine cervix	58	64	6	47	61	14
Breast	63	68	5	46	51	5
Ovary	32	36	4	32	32	0
Brain and central nervous	18	20	2	19	19	0
Lung and bronchus	8	10	2	5	7	2
Stomach	11	13	2	8	13	5
Esophagus	4	4	0	1	4	3
Hodgkin's disease	40	67	27			
Lymphocytic leukemia-acute	4	28	24			
Lymphocytic leukemia-chronic	35	51	16			
Non-Hodgkin's lymphoma	31	41	10			
Larynx	53	62	9			
Tongue	28	37	9			
Melanoma of skin	60	68	8			
Pharynx	24	28	4			
Thyroid	83	86	3			
Mouth	44	44	0			

FIVE-YEAR CANCER SURVIVAL RATES* FOR SELECTED SITES BY RACE

*Adjusted for normal life expectancy

Source: Biometry Branch, National Cancer Institute

CHARTERED DIVISIONS OF AMERICAN CANCER SOCIETY, INC.

Alabama Division, Inc.
2926 Central Avenue
Birmingham, Alabama 35209
(205) 879-2242

Alaska Division, Inc.
1343 G Street
Anchorage, Alaska 99501
(907) 277-8696

Arizona Division, Inc.
P.O. Box 33187
Phoenix, Arizona 85067
(602) 264-5861

Arkansas Division, Inc.
5520 West Markham Street
P.O. Box 3822
Little Rock, Arkansas 72203
(501) 664-3480-1-2

California Division, Inc.
1710 Webster Street
Oakland, California 94612
(415) 893-7900

Colorado Division, Inc.
1809 East 18th Avenue
P.O. Box 18268
Denver, Colorado 80218
(303) 321-2464

Connecticut Division, Inc.
Barnes Park South
14 Village Lane
P.O. Box 410
Wellingford, Connecticut 06492
(203) 265-7161

Delaware Division, Inc.
Academy of Medicine Bldg.
1925 Lovering Avenue
Wilmington, Delaware 19806
(302) 654-6267

District of Columbia Division, Inc.
Universal Building, South
1825 Connecticut Avenue, N.W.
Washington, D.C. 20009
(202) 483-2600

Florida Division, Inc.
1001 South MacDill Avenue
Tampa, Florida 33609
(813) 253-0541

Georgia Division, Inc.
1422 W. Peachtree Street, N.W.
Atlanta, Georgia 30309
(404) 892-0026

Hawaii Division, Inc.
Community Services Center Bldg.
200 North Vineyard Boulevard
Honolulu, Hawaii 96817
(808) 531-1662-3-4-5

Idaho Division, Inc.
1609 Abbs Street
P.O. Box 5386
Boise, Idaho 83705
(208) 343-4609

Illinois Division, Inc.
37 South Wabash Avenue
Chicago, Illinois 60603
(312) 372-0472

Indiana Division, Inc.
4755 Kingsway Drive, Suite 100
Indianapolis, Indiana 46205
(317) 257-5326

Iowa Division, Inc.
Highway #18 West
P.O. Box 980
Mason City, Iowa 50401
(515) 423-0712

Kansas Division, Inc.
3003 Van Buren Street
Topeka, Kansas 66611
(913) 267-0131

Kentucky Division, Inc.
Medical Arts Bldg.
1169 Eastern Parkway
Louisville, Kentucky 40217
(502) 459-1867

Louisiana Division, Inc.
Masonic Temple Bldg., Room 810
333 St. Charles Avenue
New Orleans, Louisiana 70130
(504) 523-2029

Maine Division, Inc.
Federal and Green Streets
Brunswick, Maine 04011
(207) 729-3339

Maryland Division, Inc.
200 East Joppa Road
Towson, Maryland 21204
(301) 828-8890

Massachusetts Division, Inc.
247 Commonwealth Avenue
Boston, Massachusetts 02116
(617) 267-2650

Michigan Division, Inc.
1205 East Saginaw Street
Lansing, Michigan 48906
(517) 371-2920

Minnesota Division, Inc.
2750 Park Avenue
Minneapolis, Minnesota 55407
(612) 871-2111

Mississippi Division, Inc.
345 North Mart Plaza
Jackson, Mississippi 39206
(601) 362-8874

Missouri Division, Inc.
3322 James Houchin Drive
P.O. Box 1066
Jefferson City, Missouri 65102
(314) 893-4800

Montana Division, Inc.
2820 First Avenue South
Billings, Montana 59101
(406) 252-7111

Nebraska Division, Inc.
8502 West Center Road
Omaha, Nebraska 68124
(402) 393-5800

Nevada Division, Inc.
4100 Boulder Highway
Suite A
Las Vegas, Nevada 89121
(702) 454-4242

New Hampshire Division, Inc.
686 Mast Road
Manchester, New Hampshire 03102
(603) 669-3270

New Jersey Division, Inc.
2600 Route 1
CN2201
North Brunswick, New Jersey 08902
(201) 297-8000

New Mexico Division, Inc.
5800 Lomas Blvd., N.E.
Albuquerque, New Mexico 87110
(505) 262-2333

New York State Division, Inc.
6725 Lyons Street
P.O. Box 7
East Syracuse, New York 13057
(315) 437-7025

Long Island Division, Inc.
535 Broad Hollow Road
(Route 110)
Melville, New York 11747
(516) 420-1111

New York City Division, Inc.
19 West 56th Street
New York, New York 10019
(212) 586-8700

Queens Division, Inc.
111-15 Queens Boulevard
Forest Hills, New York 11375
(212) 263-2224

Westchester Division, Inc.
246 North Central Avenue
Hartsdale, New York 10530
(914) 949-4800

North Carolina Division, Inc.
222 North Person Street
P.O. Box 27624
Raleigh, North Carolina 27611
(919) 834-8463

North Dakota Division, Inc.
Hotel Graver Annex Bldg.
115 Roberts Street
P.O. Box 426
Fargo, North Dakota 58102
(701) 232-1385

Ohio Division, Inc.
453 Lincoln Bldg.
1367 East Sixth Street
Cleveland, Ohio 44114
(216) 771-6700

Oklahoma Division, Inc.
1312 N.W. 24th Street
Oklahoma City, Oklahoma 73106
(405) 525-3515

Oregon Division, Inc.
0330 S.W. Curry
Portland, Oregon 97201
(503) 295-6422

Pennsylvania Division, Inc.
Route 422 & Sipe Avenue
P.O. Box 416
Hershey, Pennsylvania 17033
(717) 533-6144

   Philadelphia Division, Inc.
   21 South 12th Street
   Philadelphia, Pennsylvania 19107
   (215) 665-2900

Puerto Rico Division, Inc.
(Avenue Domenech 273
   Hato Rey, P.R.)
GPO Box 6004
San Juan, Puerto Rico 00936
(809) 764-2295

Rhode Island Division, Inc.
345 Blackstone Blvd.
Providence, Rhode Island 02906
(401) 831-6970

South Carolina Division, Inc.
2442 Devine Street
Columbia, South Carolina 29205
(803) 256-0245

South Dakota Division, Inc.
1025 North Minnesota Avenue
Hillcrest Plaza
Sioux Falls, South Dakota 57104
(605) 336-0897

Tennessee Division, Inc.
2519 White Avenue
Nashville, Tennessee 37204
(615) 383-1710

Texas Division, Inc.
3834 Spicewood Springs Road
P.O. Box 9863
Austin, Texas 78766
(512) 345-4560

Utah Division, Inc.
610 East South Temple
Salt Lake City, Utah 84102
(801) 322-0431

Vermont Division, Inc.
13 Loomis Street, Drawer C
Montpelier, Vermont 05602
(802) 223-2348

Virginia Division, Inc.
3218 West Cary Street
P.O. Box 7288
Richmond, Virginia 23221
(804) 359-0208

Washington Division, Inc.
2120 First Avenue North
Seattle, Washington 98109
(206) 283-1152

West Virginia Division, Inc.
Suite 100
240 Capital Street
Charleston, West Virginia 25301
(304) 344-3611

Wisconsin Division, Inc.
P.O. Box 8370
615 North Sherman Avenue
Madison, Wisconsin 53708
(608) 249-0487

   Milwaukee Division, Inc.
   6401 West Capitol Drive
   Milwaukee, Wisconsin 53216
   (414) 461-1100

Wyoming Division, Inc.
Indian Hills Center
506 Shoshoni
Cheyenne, Wyoming 82001
(307) 638-3331

Affiliate of the
American Cancer Society
Canal Zone Cancer Committee
Drawer A
Balboa Heights, Canal Zone 00101

14-3. Communicable and infectious diseases

Name	Synopsis of symptoms	Incubation period	Mode of transmission	Period of communicability
Actinomycosis	Chronic disease most frequently localized in jaw, thorax, or abdomen; septicemic spread with generalized disease may occur. Lesions are firmly indurated areas of purulence and fibrosis.	Irregular; probably years after colonization in oral tissues, plus days or months after precipitating trauma and actual penetration of tissues.	Contact from person to person as part of normal oral flora.	Time and manner in which *A. israelii* becomes part of normal flora is unknown.
Amebiasis	Infection with a protozoan parasite that exists in two forms: the hardy, infective cyst and the more fragile, potentially invasive trophozoite. Parasite may act as a commensal or invade tissues, giving rise to intestinal or extra-intestinal disease.	Variation—from a few days to several months or years. Commonly 2 to 4 weeks.	Contaminated water or food containing cysts from feces of infected persons, often as complication of another infection such as shigellosis.	During period of cyst passing, which may continue for years.
Ancylostomiasis (hookworm disease, uncinariasis, necatoriasis)	Chronic, debilitating disease with a variety of vague symptoms varying greatly, usually in proportion to degree of anemia and hypoproteinemia.	Symptoms may develop after a few weeks to many months.	Eggs in feces are deposited on ground, and under favorable environmental conditions, hatch; larvae develop in 7 to 10 days. Human infection occurs when infected larvae penetrate skin, usually foot.	Not transmitted from person to person, but infected persons can contaminate soil for several years in absence of treatment.
Arenaviral hemorrhagic fever	Acute febrile illnesses, duration 7 to 15 days. Onset is gradual with malaise, headache, retroorbital pain, conjunctival injection, sustained fever, and sweats, followed by prostration. An exanthem appears on thorax and flanks 3 to 5 days after onset.	Commonly 7 to 16 days.	Saliva and excreta of infected rodents contain virus. May be air-borne transmission by dust contaminated by infected rodent excreta.	Probably not often directly transmitted from person to person (although this has occurred in the Bolivia disease).
A. Arthropod-borne viral diseases (arboviral diseases)				
1. Arthropod-borne viral arthritis and rash	Acute self-limited disease characterized by arthritis, primarily in small joints of extremities that lasts from 2 days to 8 months.	10 to 11 days.	Culicine mosquitoes.	No evidence of transmission from person to person.
2. Arthropod-borne viral encephalitides	Group of acute inflammatory diseases of short duration. Mild cases often occur as	Usually 5 to 15 days.	Infective mosquitoes.	Not directly transmitted from person to person. Virus is not usually demonstrable in blood

Disease	Clinical features	Incubation period	Mode of transmission	Period of communicability
a. Mosquito-borne	aseptic meningitis. Severe infections are usually marked by acute onset, headache, high fever, meningeal signs, stupor, disorientation, coma, tremors, occasionally convulsions, and spastic paralysis.			of humans after onset of disease. Mosquitoes remain infective for life.
b. Tick-borne	Group of diseases resembling mosquito-borne encephalitides, except Russian Spring-Summer type often is associated with flaccid paralysis, particularly of the shoulder girdle.	Usually 7 to 14 days.	By infective ticks or by consuming milk from certain infected animals.	Not directly transmitted from person to person. Tick infected at any stage remains infective for life.
Angiostrongyliasis (eosinophilic meningoencephalitis, eosinophilic meningitis)	Disease of central nervous system caused by a nematode. Invasion may be asymptomatic or mildly symptomatic; more commonly characterized by severe headache, stiffness of neck and back, and various paresthesias. Temporary facial paralysis and low-grade fever may be present.	Usually 1 to 3 weeks.	Ingestion of raw or insufficiently cooked snails, slugs, or land planarians, which are intermediate or transport hosts harboring infective larvae.	Not transmitted from person to person.
Anisakiasis	Disease of human gastrointestinal tract manifested by intestinal colic, fever, and eosinophilic abscesses resulting from ingesting uncooked fish containing larval nematodes of the family Anisakidae.	Stomach involvement may develop within a few hours of ingestion.	Infective larvae live in organs of fish until its death when they invade somatic muscles. When ingested by humans and liberated by digestion in stomach they penetrate gastric or intestinal mucosa.	No direct transmission from person to person.
Anthrax	Acute bacterial disease usually affecting skin but may rarely involve mediastinum or intestinal tract.	Within 7 days, usually 2 to 5 days.	Infection of skin is by contact with tissues of animals dying of the disease or with contaminated animal byproducts (e.g., wool or hides).	No evidence of transmission from person to person. Articles and soil contaminated with spores may remain infective for years.
B. Arthropod-borne viral fevers 1. Mosquito-borne a. Yellow fever	Acute infectious disease of short duration and varying severity. Mildest cases are clinically indeterminate; typical attacks are characterized by dengue-like illness, i.e., sudden onset, fever, headache, backache, prostration, nausea, and vomiting.	3 to 6 days.	In urban and certain rural areas transmitted by infective *Aedes aegypti* mosquitoes.	Blood is infective for mosquitoes shortly before onset of fever and for first 3 to 5 days of illness. Highly communicable where many susceptible persons and abundant vector mosquitoes coexist.
b. Dengue (breakbone fever)	Characterized by sudden onset, fever for about 5 days and intense headache, retro-orbital pains, joint and muscle pains, and rash.	3 to 15 days, commonly 5 to 6 days.	Infective mosquitoes.	Not directly transmitted from person to person.

Name	Synopsis of symptoms	Incubation period	Mode of transmission	Period of communicability
c. Venezuelan equine fever	Clinical manifestations of infection are influenza-like, with abrupt onset of severe headache, chills, fever, myalgia, retro-orbital pain, nausea, and vomiting.	Usually 2 to 6 days, can be as short as 1 day.	Infected mosquitoes.	Person-to-person transmission may occur but has not been demonstrated.
2. Tick-borne a. Colorado tick fever and other tick-borne fevers	Acute febrile, diphasic, dengue-like disease with infrequent rash. Brief remission is usual, followed by second bout of fever lasting 2 or 3 days; neutropenia almost always occurs on fourth or fifth day of fever.	Usually 4 to 5 days.	Infective vector ticks.	Not directly transmitted from person to person except by transfusion. Virus is present during course of fever and, in Colorado tick fever, from 2 to 16 weeks or more after onset.
Ascariasis (roundworm infection)	Helminthic infection of small intestine. Symptoms are variable, often vague or absent, and ordinarily mild; live worms, passed in stools or regurgitated, are frequently first recognized sign of infection.	Worms reach maturity about 2 months after ingestion of embryonated eggs.	By ingestion of infective eggs from soil contaminated with human feces containing eggs, but not directly from person to person.	As long as mature female worms live in intestine. Maximum lifespan of adult worms is under 18 months; however, female produces up to 200,000 eggs a day that can remain viable in soil for months or years.
Aspergillosis	Variety of clinical syndromes can be produced by several *Aspergillus* species.	Probably a few days.	Inhalation of air-borne spores.	Not directly transmitted from person to person.
Babesiosis	Fever, fatigue, and hemolytic anemia lasting several days to a few months.	1 to 12 months.	During the summer months by bite of nymphal *Ixodes* ticks carried by voles or deer mice. Adult tick is normally found on deer.	Transmission from person to person is unlikely except by blood transfusion.
Balantidiasis	Disease of colon characteristically producing diarrhea or dysentery accompanied by abdominal colic, tenesmus, nausea, and vomiting.	Unknown; may be only a few days.	By ingestion of cysts from feces of infected hosts; in epidemics, mainly by fecally contaminated water.	As long as infection persists.
Blastomycosis	Chronic granulomatous mycosis primarily of lungs or skin. *Acute pulmonary blastomycosis* begins with fever and symptoms of respiratory infection and can progress gradually with fever, weight loss, cachexia, cough, and purulent sputum.	Indefinite; probably a few weeks or less to months.	Conidia, typical of the mold or saprophytic growth form, probably are inhaled in spore-laden dust.	Not transmitted directly from humans or from animals to humans.

Disease	Clinical characteristics	Incubation period	Mode of transmission	Period of communicability
Botulism, infant	Illness typically begins with constipation followed by lethargy, listlessness, poor feeding, difficulty in swallowing, loss of head control, hypotonia, generalized weakness, and in some cases, respiratory insufficiency and arrest. Wide spectrum of clinical severity ranging from mild illness to sudden infant death.	Usually unknown, because it cannot be determined precisely when the infant ingested the botulinal spores.	By ingestion of botulinal spores. Sources of spores for infants probably are multiple.	Excretion of *c. botulinum* toxin and organisms. Continues at high levels in patient's feces for weeks to months. No instances of secondary person-to-person transmission have been documented.
Brucellosis (undulant fever)	Systemic disease with acute or insidious onset characterized by continued, intermittent, or irregular fever of variable duration, headache, weakness, profuse sweating, chills, arthralgia, depression, and generalized aching.	Highly variable—usually 5 to 30 days; sometimes several months.	By contact with tissues, blood, urine, vaginal discharges, aborted fetuses and especially placentas, and by ingestion of raw milk or dairy products from infected animals. Airborne infection occurs in humans in laboratories and slaughterhouses	No evidence of communicability from person to person.
Candidiasis (moniliasis, thrush, candidosis)	Mycosis usually confined to superficial layers of skin or mucous membranes with patient having oral thrush, intertrigo, vulvovaginitis, paronychia, or onychomycosis.	Variable, 2 to 5 days in thrush of infants.	Through contact with excretions of mouth, skin, vagina, and especially feces from patients or carriers from patients or carriers from mother to infant during childbirth; and by indogenous spread.	Presumably for duration of lesions.
Capillariasis A. Intestinal capillariasis	Enteropathy with massive protein loss and a malabsorption syndrome that lead to progressive weight loss and extreme emaciation.	Unknown in humans.	Uncertain. Often obtain history of ingesting raw or inadequately cooked fish.	Not transmitted directly from person to person.
B. Hepatic capillariasis (also a pulmonary capillariasis—but only 10 documented cases of human infection recorded).	Uncommon and occasionally fatal disease in humans caused by presence of adult *capillaria hepatica* in liver. Acute or subacute hepatitis with marked eosinophilia resembling visceral larva migrans.	3 to 4 weeks.	Ingesting liver of infected animal.	Not transmitted directly from person to person.
Carditis, Coxsackie (viral carditis, enteroviral carditis)	Acute or subacute myocarditis or pericarditis, which occurs as the only manifestation, or may occasionally be associated with other manifestations.	Usually 3 to 5 days.	Fecal-oral or respiratory droplet contact with infected person.	Apparently during acute stage of disease.
Cat-scratch disease	Subacute, self-limited infectious disease characterized by malaise, granulomatous lymphadenitis, and variable patterns of fever.	Variable; usually 3 to 14 days from innoculation to primary lesions.	90% of patients report history of scratch, bite, lick, or other exposure to healthy cat or kitten.	Unknown. Not directly transmitted from person to person.

Name	Synopsis of symptoms	Incubation period	Mode of transmission	Period of communicability
Chancroid (ulcus molle, soft chancre)	Acute, localized, genital infection characterized by single or multiple painful necrotizing ulcers at site of innoculation, frequently accompanied by painful inflammatory swelling and suppuration of regional lymph nodes. Extragenital lesions have been reported.	From 3 to 5 days, up to 14 days.	By direct sexual contact with discharges from open lesions and pus from buboes; suggestive evidence of asymptomatic infections in women. Sexual promiscuity and uncleanliness favor transmission.	As long as infectious agent persists in original lesion or discharging regional lymph nodes; usually until healed—a matter of weeks.
Chickenpox, herpes zoster (varicella shingles)	Acute generalized viral disease with sudden onset of slight fever, mild constitutional symptoms, and a skin eruption that is maculopapular for a few hours, vesicular for 3 to 4 days, and leaves a granular scab.	From 2 to 3 weeks; commonly 13 to 17 days.	From person to person by direct contact, droplet, or airborne spread of secretion of respiratory tract of chickenpox cases or of vesicle fluid of patients with herpes zoster.	As long as 5 days but usually 1 to 2 days before onset of rash, and not more than 6 days after appearance of first crop of vesicles.
Cholera	Acute intestinal disease with sudden onset, profuse watery stools, occasional vomiting, rapid dehydration, acidosis, and circulatory collapse. Death may occur within a few hours.	From a few hours to 5 days, usually 2 to 3 days.	Through ingestion of food or water contaminated with feces or vomitus of infected persons or with feces of carriers.	Thought to be for duration of stool-positive stage, usually only a few days after recovery. Carrier stage may last for several months.
Chromoblastomycosis (chromomycosis, dermatitis verrucosa)	Chronic spreading mycosis of skin and subcutaneous tissues, usually of a lower extremity. Hematogenous spread to brain has been reported.	Unknown; probably months.	Traumatic contact with contaminated wood or other materials.	Not directly transmitted from person to person.
Clonorchiasis (Chinese or oriental liver fluke disease)	Symptoms result from local irritation of bile ducts by flukes, from toxemia and possibly from secondary bacterial invaders. Loss of appetite, diarrhea, and sensation of abdominal pressure are early common symptoms.	Unpredictable, varies with the number of worms present; flukes reach maturity within 1 month after encysted larvae are ingested.	Humans infected by eating freshwater fish containing encysted larvae (*clonorchis sinensis*).	Not directly transmitted from person to person, but infected individual may pass viable eggs for as long as 30 years.
Coccidioidomycosis (valley fever, desert fever, desert rheumatism, coccidiodal granuloma).	Internal mycosis that begins as respiratory infection. *Primary infection* may be entirely asymptomatic or resemble acute influenza illness with fever, chills, cough, and pleural pain.	1 to 4 weeks in primary infection.	Inhalation of spores from soil and in laboratory accidents from cultures.	Not directly transmitted from humans or animals to humans.
Conjunctivitis, acute bacterial	Clinical syndrome beginning with lacrimation, irritation, and hyperemia of the palpebral and bulbar conjunctivae of one	Usually 24 to 72 hours.	Contact with discharges from conjunctivae or upper respiratory tract of infected persons through contaminated	During course of active infection.

Disease	Description	Incubation period	Mode of transmission	Period of communicability
Conjunctivitis, epidemic hemorrhagic (Apollo 11 disease)	or both eyes, followed by edema of lids, photophobia, and mucopurulent discharge. Virus infection with sudden onset of pain or sensation of a foreign body in eye. Disease rapidly progresses (1 to 2 days) to full case of swollen eyelids, hyperemia of the conjunctivae, often with a cirumcorneal distribution, seromucous discharge, and frequent subconjunctival hemorrhages.	1 to 2 days or even shorter.	fingers, clothing, or other articles. Through direct or indirect contact with discharge from infected eyes and possibly by droplet infection from those with virus in throat.	Unknown, but assumed to be for period of active disease, usually 1 to 2 weeks.
Conjunctivitis, inclusion (swimming pool conjunctivitis, paratrachoma)	In the newborn, acute papillary conjunctivitis with abundant mucopurulent discharge. In children and adults, acute follicular conjunctivitis with pre-auricular lymphadenopathy, often with superficial corneal involvement.	5 to 12 days.	During sexual intercourse; genital discharges of infected persons are infectious.	While genital infection persists; can be longer than 1 year in female.
Contagious pustular dermatitis	Primarily a proliferative cutaneous disease of sheep and goats transmissible to humans and usually a solitary lesion located on hands, arms, or face that is maculopapular or pustular.	Generally 3 to 6 days.	By direct contact with mucous membranes of infected animals.	Unknown. Human lesions show a decrease in number of virus particles as disease progresses.
Herpangina; hand-foot-and-mouth disease, acute lymphonodular pharyngitis	*Herpangina*—grayish papulovesicular pharyngeal lesions on an erythematous base. *Hand-foot-and-mouth disease*—more diffuse oral lesions on buccal surfaces of cheeks, gums, and tongue. *Acute lymphonodular pharyngitis*—lesions are firm, raised, discrete, whitish to yellowish nodules.	3 to 5 days for herpangina and hand-foot-and-mouth disease. 5 days for acute lymphonodular pharyngitis.	Direct contact with nose and throat discharges and feces of infected (possibly asymptomatic) persons and by droplet spread.	During acute stage of illness and longer because virus persists in stools for as long as several weeks.
Cryptococcosis (torulosis, European blastomycosis)	Mycosis, usually subacute or chronic meningoencephalitis. Infection of lung, kidney, prostate, bone, or liver.	Unknown. Pulmonary disease may precede brain infection by months or years.	Presumably by inhalation.	Not directly transmitted from humans or animals to humans.
Cytomegalovirus infections Congenital cytomegalovirus infection Cytomegalic inclusion disease	Most severe form of disease occurs in perinatal period, following congenital infection, with signs and symptoms of severe generalized infection especially involving central nervous system and liver.	Information inexact. 3 to 8 weeks following transfusion with infected blood. 3 to 12 weeks after birth delivery.	Intimate exposure to infectious secretions or excretions. Virus is excreted in urine, saliva, cervical secretions, breast milk, and semen.	Virus is excreted in urine or saliva for months and may persist for several years following primary infection.

Name	Synopsis of symptoms	Incubation period	Mode of transmission	Period of communicability
Dermatophytosis A. Ringworm of scalp and beard (tinea capitis, tinea kerion, favus)	Begins as small papule and spreads peripherally, leaving scaly patches of temporary baldness. Infected hairs become brittle and break off easily. Kerions sometimes develop.	10 to 14 days.	Direct or indirect contact with articles infected with hair from humans or infected animals.	As long as lesions are present and viable fungus persists on contaminated materials.
B. Ringworm of nails (tinea unguium, onychomycosis)	Chronic infectious disease involving one or more nails of hands or feet. Nail thickens, becoming discolored and brittle with an accumulation of caseous-appearing material beneath nail.	Unknown.	Presumably by direct extension from skin or nail lesions of infected persons. Low rate of transmission.	Possibly as long as infected lesion is present.
C. Ringworm of groin and perianal region (dhobie itch, tinea cruris) D. Ringworm of the body (tinea corporis)	Characteristically appears as flat, spreading, ring-shaped lesions. Periphery is usually reddish, vesicular, or pustular and may be dry and scaly or moist and crusted.	4 to 10 days.	Direct or indirect contact with skin and scalp lesions of infected persons or animals.	As long as lesions are present and viable fungus persists on contaminated materials.
E. Ringworm of the foot (tinea pedis, athlete's foot)	Scaling or cracking of skin, especially between toes, or blisters containing thin watery fluid are characteristic. In severe cases vesicular lesions appear on various parts of body.	Unknown.	Direct or indirect contact with skin lesions of infected persons or contaminated floors or shower stalls.	As long as lesions are present and viable spores persist on contaminated materials.
Diarrhea, acute A. Diarrhea caused by *Escherichia Coli*	May be invasive, enterotoxigenic, and enteropathogenic. *Invasive*—fever and mucoid and occasionally bloody diarrhea occur. *Enterotoxigenic*—profuse watery diarrhea without blood or mucous. *Enteropathogenic*—associated with outbreaks of acute diarrhea disease in newborn nurseries.	12 to 72 hours.	Fecal contamination of food, water, or fomites. Persons with diarrhea excrete large numbers of organisms and constitute greatest hazard.	Not known; presumably for duration of fecal excretion, which may be several weeks or longer.
B. Diarrhea caused by *Campylobacter* (vibriosis, vibrionic enteritis)	Acute enteric disease characterized by diarrhea, abdominal pain, malaise, fever, nausea, vomiting, and constitutional complaints.	Range is 1 to 10 days with a usual period of 3 to 5 days.	By ingestion of organisms in food or contaminated water; contact with contaminated animals; drinking unpasteurized milk.	Throughout course of infection from several days to several weeks.

Disease	Clinical characteristics	Incubation period	Mode of transmission	Period of communicability
Diphtheria	Characteristic lesion marked by patch or patches of grayish membrane with surrounding dull red inflammatory zone. Throat is moderately sore in faucial diphtheria, with cervical lymph nodes enlarged and tender; occasionally swelling and edema of neck.	2 to 5 days, sometimes longer.	Contact with patient or carrier; more rarely with articles soiled with discharges from lesions of infected persons. Raw milk has been a vehicle.	Variable, until virulent bacilli have disappeared from discharge and lesions. Usual period is 2 to 4 weeks but chronic carriers may shed organisms for 6 months or more.
Diphyllobothriasis	Symptoms commonly are trivial or absent; depending on severity, vitamin B_{12} deficiency anemia, diarrhea, and toxic symptoms may be present.	From 3 to 6 weeks from ingestion to passage of eggs in stool.	From eating raw or inadequately cooked fish.	Not directly transmitted from person to person.
Dracontiasis	Infection of subcutaneous and deeper tissues by large nematode. Blister appears, usually on a lower extremity, as gravid, meter-long adult female prepares to discharge her larvae.	About 12 months.	Humans swallow infected copepods by drinking water from contaminated step-wells and ponds.	Not directly transmitted from person to person.
Echinococcosis multilocularis infection (alveolar hydatid disease)	Disease primarily of liver caused by poorly circumscribed microvesicular larval masses of *Echinococcus multilocularis*; may be found also in lungs and other organs.	Variable from months to years, depending on number and location of cysts and how rapidly they grow.	By ingestion of infective eggs or by fecally soiled dog fur, harnesses, and environmental fomites.	Not directly transmitted from person to person or from one intermediate host to another.
Enterobiasis (pinworm disease, oxyuriasis)	Intestinal infection with mild or nonspecific symptoms, if any. May be anal itching, disturbed sleep, irritability, and local irritation with secondary infection of scratched skin.	Lifecycle of *Enterobius vermicularis* is 4 to 6 weeks.	Direct transfer of infective eggs by hand from anus to mouth of the same or new host, or indirectly through materials contaminated with eggs of parasite. Dust-borne infection by inhalation is possible.	As long as gravid females are discharging eggs on perianal skin. Continuous reinfection occurs by ano-oral transfer of eggs from self or infected others.
Food poisoning A. Staphylococcal food poisoning	Intoxication (not infection) of abrupt and sometimes violent onset, with severe nausea, cramps, vomiting, usually diarrhea, and prostration; sometimes with subnormal temperature and lowered blood pressure.	Interval between eating food and onset of symptoms is 1 to 6 hours, but usually 2 to 4 hours.	By ingesting of food contacted by food-handler's hands without subsequent cooking or inadequately heated, such as pastries, custards, salads, and meat products.	Not applicable.
B. Botulism	Severe intoxication (not infection as in infant botulism) characterized by clinical manifestations relating primarily to the nervous system. Ptosis, visual difficulty, dry mouth, and sore throat are often first complaints.	Symptoms usually appear within 12 to 36 hours, sometimes several days, after eating contaminated food.	By ingestion of food in which toxin had been formed, primarily from jars or cans inadequately heated during canning, and eaten without subsequent adequate cooking.	Not applicable.

Name	Synopsis of symptoms	Incubation period	Mode of transmission	Period of communicability
C. Clostridial food poisoning (*C. welchii*)	Intestinal disorder characterized by sudden onset of abdominal colic followed by diarrhea. Nausea is common but vomiting and fever are usually absent.	From 6 to 24 hours, usually 10 to 12 hours.	Ingestion of food contaminated by soil or feces in which conditions have permitted multiplication of organism.	Not applicable.
D. *Vibrio parahaemolyticus* food poisoning	Intestinal disorder characterized by watery diarrhea and abdominal cramps; nausea, vomiting, fever, and headache are variably present.	Usually 12 to 24 hours, but can range from 4 to 96 hours.	Ingestion of raw or inadequately cooked seafood.	Not communicable from person to person.
E. *Bacillus cereus* food poisoning	Gastrointestinal disorder characterized in some cases by sudden onset of nausea and vomiting and in others by intense abdominal colic and diarrhea.	From 1 to 5 hours in cases when vomiting is predominant symptom; from 6 to 16 hours when diarrhea is predominant.	Ingestion of food that has been kept at ambient temperatures after cooking, permitting multiplication of organisms.	Not communicable from person to person.
Gastroenteritis, viral A. Epidemic viral gastroenteritis	Usually self-limited mild disease that often occurs in outbreaks with clinical symptoms of nausea, vomiting, diarrhea, abdominal pain, myalgia, headache, malaise, low grade fever, or a combination thereof.	24 to 48 hours; in volunteer studies with Norwalk agent range was 10 to 51 hours.	Unknown; probably by fecal-oral route. Several recent outbreaks strongly suggest food-borne and water-borne transmission.	During acute stage of disease and shortly thereafter.
B. Rotavirus gastroenteritis (sporadic viral gastroenteritis of infants and children)	Sporadic severe gastroenteritis of infants and young children characterized by diarrhea and vomiting, often with severe dehydration and occasional deaths.	Approximately 48 hours.	Probably fecal-oral and possibly respiratory routes.	During acute stage of disease and later while virus shedding continues. Virus is not usually detectable after eighth day of illness.
Giardiasis (giardia enteritis, lambliasis)	Protozoan infection principally of upper small bowel; often asymptomatic, it may also be associated with a variety of intestinal symptoms such as chronic diarrhea, steatorrhea, abdominal cramps, bloating, frequent loose and pale, greasy, malodorus stools, fatigue, and weight loss.	In a water-borne epidemic in United States, clinical illnesses occurred 1 to 4 weeks after exposure; average 2 weeks.	Localized outbreaks occur from contaminated water supplies. By ingestion of cysts in fecally contaminated water and occasionally by fecally contaminated food.	Entire period of infection.
Gonococcal infections A. Gonococcal infection of genitourinary tract (gonorrhea, gonococcal urethritis)	*Males*—purulent discharge from anterior urethra with dysuria appears 2 to 7 days after infecting exposure. *Females*—few days after exposure initial urethritis or cervicitis occurs, frequently so	Usually 2 to 7 days, sometimes longer.	By contact with exudates from mucous membranes of infected persons, almost always result of sexual activity.	May extend for months if untreated, especially in females who frequently are asymptomatic. Specific therapy usually ends communicability within hours except

Disease	Description	Incubation period	Mode of transmission	Period of communicability
	mild as to pass unnoticed. About 20% of patients have uterine invasion at the first, second, or later menstrual period with symptoms of endometritis, salpingitis, or pelvic peritonitis.			with penicillin-resistant strains.
B. Gonococcal conjunctivitis (neonatorum) (gonorrheal ophthalmia neonatorum)	Acute redness and swelling of conjunctiva of one or both eyes, with mucopurulent or purulent discharge in which gonococci are identifiable by microscopic and cultural methods.	Usually 1 to 5 days.	Contact with infected birth canal during childbirth.	While discharge persists if untreated; for 24 hours following initiation of specific treatment.
Granuloma inguinale (donovanosis)	Mildly communicable, nonfatal, chronic and progressive, autoinoculable bacterial disease of skin and mucous membranes of external genitalia, inguinal, and anal region. Small nodule, vesicle, or papule is present.	Unknown; probably 8 to 80 days.	Presumably by direct contact with lesions during sexual activity.	Unknown and probably for duration of open lesions on skin or mucous membranes.
Hemorrhagic nephrosonephritis	Acute infectious disease characterized by abrupt onset of fever of 3 to 8 day duration, conjunctival injection, prostration, anorexia, and vomiting.	Usually 12 to 16 days, but varying from 9 to 35 days.	Unknown; transmission from rodent excreta is presumed.	Apparently not directly transmitted from person to person.
Hepatitis, viral A. Viral hepatitis A (infectious hepatitis, epidemic hepatitis, epidemic jaundice, catarrhal jaundice, Type A hepatitis)	Onset is usually abrupt with fever, malaise, anorexia, nausea, and abdominal discomfort, followed within a few days by jaundice.	From 15 to 50 days, depending on dose; average 28-30 days.	Person to person by fecal-oral route. Common-vehicle outbreaks have been related to contaminated water and food.	Studies indicate maximum infectivity during latter half of incubation period, continuing for a few days, after onset of jaundice.
B. Viral hepatitis B (Type B hepatitis, serum hepatitis)	Onset is usually insidious with anorexia, vague abdominal discomfort, nausea, and vomiting, sometimes arthralgias and rash, often progressing to jaundice. Fever may be absent or mild.	Usually 45 to 160 days, average 60 to 90 days. Variation is related in part to amount of virus in inoculum, mode of transmission, and host factors.	HB_sAG, the infectious agent, has been found in virtually all body secretions, but only blood, saliva, and semen have been shown to be infectious. Transmission usually by percutaneous inoculation of infected blood and blood products; contaminated needles, syringes, and IV equipment.	From several weeks before onset of symptoms through clinical course of disease; carrier state can last for years.

Name	Synopsis of symptoms	Incubation period	Mode of transmission	Period of communicability
C. Hepatitis, non-A, non-B (non-B transfusion–associated hepatitis, hepatitis C)	Chronic infection may be symptomatic or asymptomatic. Differential diagnosis depends on exclusion of hepatitis types A and B.	2 weeks to 6 months, model 6 to 8 weeks.	Most common posttransfusion hepatitis in United States and is more common when paid donors are used. Percutaneous transmission documented and other modes similar to those of Hepatitis B virus are suspected.	Degree of immunity following infection is not known.
Herpes simplex	Viral infection characterized by localized primary lesion, latency, and a tendency to localized recurrence. In perhaps 10% of primary infections overt disease may appear as illness of varying severity marked by fever and malaise lasting 1 week or more.	2 to 12 days.	HSV Type 1: Direct contact with virus in saliva of carriers. HSV Type 2: Sexual contact.	Secretion of virus in saliva has been reported for as long as 7 weeks after recovery from stomatitis. Patients with primary lesions are infective for about 7 to 12 days, with recurrent disease for 4 days to 1 week.
Histoplasmosis, histoplasma capsulatum (Darlings disease, American histoplasmosis)	Systemic mycosis of varying severity with primary lesion, usually in lung. Whereas infection is common, overt clinical disease is not. Five clinical forms are recognized.	Symptoms appear within 5 to 18 days after exposure, commonly 10 days.	Inhalation of air-borne spores.	Not transmitted from person to person.
Influenza	Acute viral disease of respiratory tract characterized by fever, chilliness, headache, myalgia, prostration, coryza, and mild sore throat. Cough is often severe and protracted.	Usually 24 to 72 hours.	By direct contact through droplet infection; probably air-borne among crowded populations in enclosed spaces.	Probably limited to 3 days from clinical onset.
Keratoconjunctivitis, epidemic	Acute viral disease of eye. Onset is sudden with pain, photophobia, blurred vision, occasionally low grade fever, headache, malaise, and tender preauricular lymphadenopathy.	Probably 5 to 12 days.	Direct contact with eye secretions of infected person or indirectly through contaminated instruments or solutions.	From late in incubation period to 14 days after onset.
Lhassa fever	Acute viral illness with duration of 7 to 31 days. Onset is gradual with malaise, fever, headache, sore throat, cough, nausea, vomiting, diarrhea, myalgia, and chest and abdominal pain; fever is persistent or intermittent-spiking.	Commonly 7 to 21 days.	Primarily through direct or indirect contact with urine of infected rodents in dust or on food.	Person-to-person infections occur during acute febrile phase when virus is present in throat. Virus may be excreted in urine of patients for 3 weeks or as long as 60 days.
Legionellosis (legionnaires disease, legionnaires pneumonia, Pontiac fever)	Characterized initially by anorexia, malaise, myalgia, and headache. Within 1 day is usually rapidly rising fever associated with chills. Non-pro-	Legionnaires disease: 2 to 10 days; most often 5 to 6 days. Pontiac fever: 5 to 66 hours; most often 24 to 48 hours.	Evidence supports air-borne transmission.	Person-to-person transmission has not been documented.

Disease	Identification	Incubation period	Mode of transmission	Period of communicability
Leishmaniasis, cutaneous	ductive cough, abdominal pain, and diarrhea often occur. Polymorphic disease of skin and mucous membranes characterized by ulcerating lesions that may be single or multiple and self-limited or indolent, or multiple nodular lesions.	From a few days to many months.	Bite of infective sandfly.	As long as parasites remain in lesions; in untreated cases, 1 year or more.
Leishmaniasis, visceral	Chronic systemic infectious disease characterized by fever, hepatosplenomegaly, lymphadenopathy, anemia with leucopenia, and progressive emaciation and weakness.	Generally 2 to 4 months; range is 10 days to 2 years.	Bite of infective sandfly.	As long as parasites persist in circulating blood or skin. Transmission from person to person, and by blood transfusion, sexual contact, and bites of infected laboratory animals have been reported.
Leprosy (Hansen's disease)	Chronic bacterial disease characterized by lesions of skin and mucous membranes, by involvement and often palpable enlargement of peripheral nerves with consequent anesthesia, muscle weakness, paralysis, and trophic changes in skin, muscle, and bone.	Shortest known is 7 months. Average is probably 3 to 6 years.	Not clearly established, but household and prolonged intimate contact are important. Organisms may gain entrance through broken skin and respiratory tract.	As long as morphologically normal bacilli are demonstrable, infectiousness should be considered possible.
Listeriosis	Bacterial disease usually manifested as acute meningoencephalitis with or without associated septicemia, less frequently septicemia only; very often neonatal. Onset of meningoencephalitis is usually sudden with fever intense headache, nausea, vomiting, and signs of meningeal irritation.	Unknown; probably 4 days to 3 weeks. Fetus is usually infected within several days after maternal disease.	Largely neonatal; infection is transmitted from mother to unborn infant in utero during its passage through infected birth canal.	Mothers of infected newborn infants may shed infectious agent in vaginal discharges or urine for 7 to 10 days after delivery. Period of person-to-person communicability unknown.
Lyme disease	Characterized by distinctive skin lesion (ECM), systemic symptoms, polyarthritis, and neurological and cardiac involvement in varying combination.	From 3 to 21 days after tick exposure.	Presumably tick-borne.	No evidence of transmission from person to person.
Lymphocytic choriomeningitis (LCM, benign (or serous) lymphocytic meningitis)	Viral disease of animals, especially mice, transmissible to man with marked diversity of clinical manifestations. At times it begins with influenza-like attack followed by complete recovery; or after 1 to 2 weeks or remission, meningeal symptoms suddenly appear.	Probably 8 to 13 days; 15 to 20 days to meningeal symptoms.	Virus is excreted in urine, saliva, and feces of infected animals, usually mice transmission to humans, usually through contaminated food or dust.	Not known to be directly transmitted from person to person.

Name	Synopsis of symptoms	Incubation period	Mode of transmission	Period of communicability
Lymphogranuloma venereum (lymphogranuloma inguinale, esthiomene, climatic bubo, tropical bubo)	Venerally acquired infection, beginning with painless evanescent erosion, papule, nodule, or herpetiform lesion on penis or vulva, frequently unnoticed. Regional lymph nodes undergo suppuration followed by extension of inflammatory process to adjacent tissues.	Usually 7 to 12 days, with a range of 4 to 21 days to primary lesion. If bubo is first manifestation, 10 to 30 days, sometimes several months.	Direct contact with open lesions of infected persons usually during sexual intercourse.	Variable, from weeks to years, during presence of active lesions.
Malaria	Fever, chills, sweats, and headache that may progress to icterus coagulation defects, shock, renal and liver failure, acute encephalitis, and coma are symptoms of most serious form (falciparum malaria). Symptoms difficult to differentiate in the four human malarias so laboratory confirmation is needed by demonstration of malaria parasites in blood films.	Average 12 days for *P. falciparum*, 12 days for *P. vivax* and *P. ovale*, and 30 days for *P. malariae*.	By infective female anopheline mosquito.	For infection of mosquitoes, as long as infective gametocytes are present in blood of patients; varies with species and strain of parasite and with response to therapy.
Measles (Rubeola, hard measles, red measles, morbilli)	Acute, highly communicable viral disease with prodromal fever, conjunctivitis, coryza, bronchitis, and Koplik's spots on the buccal mucosa. A characteristic red blotchy rash appears on third to seventh day, beginning on face, becoming generalized, lasting 4 to 7 days and sometimes ending in branny desquamation. Leucopenia is common.	About 10 days varying from 8 to 13 days from exposure to onset of fever; about 14 days until rash appears; uncommonly longer or shorter human normal immune globulin (IG), given later than third day of incubation period for passive protection, may extend the incubation period to 21 days instead of preventing disease.	By droplet spread or direct contact with nasal or throat secretions of infected persons. Measles is one of most readily transmitted communicable diseases.	From slightly before beginning of prodromal period of 4 days after appearance of rash; communicability is minimal after second day of rash.
Melioidosis	Range of clinical manifestations from apparent infection or asymptomatic pulmonary consolidation to rapidly fatal septicemia. May simulate typhoid fever or even tuberculosis.	As short as 2 days; however, several months or years may elapse between presumed exposure and appearance of clinical disease.	Usually by contact with contaminated soil or water through overt or inapparent skin wounds, by aspiration or ingestion of contaminated water or by inhalation of dust from soil.	Person-to-person transmission and laboratory acquired infections are uncommon.
Meningitis, aseptic (viral meningitis, serous meningitis, nonbacterial or abacterial meningitis)	Common, rarely fatal, clinical syndrome with multiple causes, most commonly viral, characterized by sudden onset of febrile illness with signs and symptoms of meningeal involvement. Spinal fluid find-	Varies with specific infectious agent (refer to specific diseases).	Varies with specific infectious agent (refer to specific diseases).	

Disease	Description	Incubation period	Mode of transmission	Period of communicability
Meningitis, bacterial	ings of pleocytosis (usually mononuclear but may be polymorphonuclear in early stages), increased protein, normal sugar, and absence of bacteria. Active illness seldom exceeds 10 days. Clinical signs and symptoms may be indistinguishable from those caused by meningococci including rash. Differentiation is based on smears and bacteriological studies.			
Meningitis, meningococcal (cerebrospinal fever, meningococcemia)	Characterized by sudden onset of fever, intense headache, nausea and often vomiting, stiff neck, and frequently a petechial rash with pink macules or, very rarely, vesicles. Delirium and coma often appear; occasional fulminating cases exhibit sudden prostration, ecchymoses, and shock at onset.	Varies from 2 to 10 days, commonly 3 to 4 days.	By direct contact, including droplets and discharges from nose and throat of infected persons, more often carriers than cases.	Until meningococci are no longer present in discharges from nose and throat. If organisms are sensitive to sulfonamides, meningococci usually disappear from nasopharynx within 24 hours after institution of treatment. They are not fully eradicated from oronasopharynx by penicillin.
Meningitis, hemophilus (meningitis caused by *Hemophilus Influenzae*)	Most common bacterial meningitis in children 2 months to 3 years old in U.S. Otitis media or sinusitis may be precursor. Almost always associated with bacteremia. Onset is sudden with symptoms of fever, vomiting, lethargy, and meningeal irritation.	Probably short—within 2 to 4 days.	By droplet infection and discharges from nose and throat during infectious period. May be purulent rhinitis. Portal of entry is most commonly nasopharyngeal.	As long as organisms are present, which may be for prolonged period even without nasal discharge.
Meningitis, pneumococcal	High fatality rate is associated with this disease. Usually fulminant and occurs with bacteremia but not necessarily with another focus; although there may be otitis media or mastoiditis. Symptoms of high fever, lethargy or coma, and signs of meningeal irritation usually signal onset.			
Meningitis, neonatal	Patients exhibit symptoms of lethargy, seizures, apneic episodes, poor feeding, hypothermia or hyperthermia, and sometimes respiratory distress in first week of life.		Acquired from birth canal. For prevention of early onset form, ampicillin treatment at onset of labor has been recommended for mothers known to be infected with Group B streptococcus.	

Name	Synopsis of symptoms	Incubation period	Mode of transmission	Period of communicability
Meningoencephalitis caused by *Naegleria* and *Acanthamoeba*	*Naegleria:* Disease organisms cause a typical syndrome of fulminating pyogenic meningoencephalitis with severe frontal headache, occasional olfactory hallucinations, nausea, vomiting, high fever, nuchal rigidity and somnolence. *Acanthamoeba:* Disease organisms invade the brain and meninges, usually without involvement of nasal and olfactory tissues, causing disease characterized by insidious onset and prolonged course.	*Naegleria:* 3 to 7 days in documented cases. *Acanthamoeba* Much longer than in *Naegleria.*	*Naegleria:* Infection acquired by forcing infected water into nasal passages. *Naegleria* trophozoites colonize nasal tissues, then invade brain and meninges by extension along olfactory nerves. *Acanthamoeba* trophozoites reach central nervous system by metastasis from skin lesion or other site of primary colonization.	No person-to-person transmission has been observed.
Acanthamebiasis of eye, skin, and vagina	Lesions of conjunctiva, cornea, and inner structures of eye. Granulomatous lesions of the skin have been recorded. Also secondary invasion of central nervous system and occasionally of vagina.			
Molluscum contagiosum	Viral disease of skin that results in pearly pink to white papules with prominent central pore. Papules vary in size from less than 1 mm to 10 mm. Usually multiple lesions, most frequently in the genital area in adults; may occur anywhere in children. Eruption usually clears spontaneously in 6 to 9 months.	2 to 7 weeks.	Usually by direct contact, but transmission by fomites is possible. Sexual transmission occurs.	Unknown, but probably as long as lesions persist.
Mononucleosis, infectious (glandular fever, EBV mononucleosis)	Characterized by fever, sore throat (often with exudative pharyngotonsillitus) and lymphadenopathy (especially posterior cervical). Jaundice occurs in about 4% of infected young adults and splenomegaly in 50%. Duration is from 1 to several weeks.	From 4 to 6 weeks.	Person-to-person spread by oropharyngeal route via saliva. Spread may also occur via blood transfusion to susceptible recipients.	Prolonged; pharyngeal excretion may persist for 1 year after infection; 15% to 20% of healthy adults are oropharyngeal carriers.
Mumps (infectious parotitis)	Acute viral disease characterized by fever, swelling, and tenderness of one or more salivary glands, usually parotid and	About 2 to 3 weeks, commonly 18 days.	By droplet spread and by direct contact with saliva of an infected person.	Virus has been isolated from saliva from 6 days before salivary gland involvement to as long as 9 days thereafter; but

Disease	Clinical characteristics	Incubation period	Mode of transmission	Period of communicability
	sometimes sublingual or submaxillary glands.			height of infectiousness occurs about 48 hours before swelling begins. Urine may be positive for as long as 14 days after onset of illness. Not transmitted from person to person.
Mycetoma, actinomycotic (mycetoma, mycotic)	Characterized by swelling and suppuration of subcutaneous tissues, and formation of sinus tracts with visible granules in pus draining from sinus tracts. Lesions usually are on foot or lower leg.	Usually months.	Subcutaneous implantation of spores or hyphal elements from a saprophytic source by penetrating wounds (thorns, splinters).	
Nocardiosis	Chronic disease often originating in lungs, with hematogenous spread to produce abscesses of brain, subcutaneous tissue and other organs; high fatality rate.	Unknown; probably weeks.	*Nocardia* are presumed to enter by body principally by inhalation of contaminated dust into lung.	Not directly transmitted from humans or animals to humans.
Onchocerciasis	Chronic, nonfatal filarial disease with fibrous nodules in subcutaneous tissues, particularly head and shoulders.	Microfilariae are found in skin usually about 1 year or more after infection.	By infected female blackflies.	Not directly transmitted from person to person; however, humans infect flies as long as living microfilariae occur in skin; i.e., for 10 to 15 years if untreated.
Ornithosis (psittacosis, parrot fever)	Acute generalized infectious disease with variable clinical presentations; fever, headache, myalgia, chills, and upper or lower respiratory tract disease are commonly present.	From 4 to 15 days, commonly 10 days.	Infection is usually acquired by inhaling agent from desiccated droppings of infected birds. Turkeys are usually involved but ducks and pigeons are occasionally responsible for human disease. Household birds are frequent source.	Person-to-person transmission is rare but can occur, especially with paroxysmal coughing.
Paracoccidioidomycosis	Chronic mycosis characterized by patchy pulmonary infiltrates or ulcerative lesions of mucosa (oral, nasal, gastrointestinal) and of skin. Lymphadenopathy is frequent. In disseminated cases all viscera may be affected; adrenal gland is especially susceptible.	Highly variable, from 1 month to many years.	Presumably acquired through inhalation of contaminated soil and dust.	Not known to be transmitted directly from person to person.
Paragonimiasis (pulmonary distomiasis, lung fluke disease)	Clinical signs depend on path of migration and organs parasitized. Lungs are most frequently involved; symptoms are cough and hemoptysis.	Flukes mature and begin to lay eggs approximately 6 weeks after humans ingest infective larvae. Interval until symptoms appear is long and variable depending on organ invaded and number of worms involved.	Infection occurs when raw or partially cooked flesh of freshwater crabs or crayfish containing infective larvae (metacercariae) are eaten.	Not directly transmitted from person to person, but eggs may be discharged by the human host for 20 years or more.

Name	Synopsis of symptoms	Incubation period	Mode of transmission	Period of communicability
Paratyphoid fever	Frequently generalized bacterial enteric infection, often with abrupt onset, continued fever, sometimes rose spots on trunk, usually diarrhea, and involvement of lymphoid tissues of mesentery and intestines.	1 to 3 weeks for enteric fever; 1 to 10 days for gastroenteritis.	Direct or indirect contact with feces or urine of patient or carrier. Spread is by food, especially milk, milk products, and shellfish. Flies may be vectors.	As long as infectious agent persists in excreta, which is from appearance of prodromal symptoms, throughout illness, and for periods up to several weeks or months. Commonly 1 to 2 weeks after recovery.
Pediculosis (lousiness)	Infestation of head, hairy parts of body, or clothing with adult lice, larvae, or nits (eggs), which results in severe itching and excoriation of scalp or scratch marks of body.	Under optimum conditions, eggs of lice hatch in 1 week, reach sexual maturity in approximately 2 weeks.	Direct contact with infected person and indirectly by contact with personal belongings, especially clothing and headgear. Crab lice are usually transmitted through sexual contact.	Communicable as long as lice remain alive on infested person or in clothing, and until eggs in hair and clothing have been destroyed.
Pinta (carate)	Scaling papule with satellite lymphadenopathy appears within 1 to 8 weeks after infection, usually on hands, legs, or dorsum of feet. In 3 to 12 months, a maculopapular, erythematous secondary rash appears and may evolve into tertiary dyschromic macules of variable size. Organ systems are not involved.	3 to 60 days	Presumably person-to-person transmission by direct and prolonged contact with initial and early dyschromic skin lesions; location of primary lesions suggests that trauma provides portal of entry.	Unknown; potentially communicable while dyschromic skin lesions are active, sometimes for many years.
Plague (pest)	Specific zoonosis involving rodents and their fleas that transfer infection to various animals including humans. Initial response is commonly lymphadenitis in node receiving drainage from site of fleabite. Nodes become swollen and tender and fever is often present. Secondary involvement of lungs may result in severe pneumonia with mediastinitis and pleural effusion.	From 2 to 6 days; may be longer in vaccinated individuals.	Plague in humans occurs as result of intrusion into zoonotic transmission cycle or by entry of sylvatic infected animals and their infected fleas into human's habitat.	Fleas may remain infected for days, weeks, or months under suitable conditions of temperature and humidity.
Pleurodynia, epidemic	Acute viral disease characterized by sudden onset of severe pain localized in chest or abdomen that may be intensified by movement, usually accompanied by fever and frequently by headache.	Usually 3 to 5 days.	Probably fecal-oral or respiratory droplet contact with infected person or with articles freshly soiled with feces or throat discharges of infected person who may or may not have symptoms.	Apparently during acute stage of disease.
The pneumonias A. Pneumococcal pneumonia	Acute bacterial infection characterized by sudden onset with single shaking chill, fever,	Not well determined; believed to be 1 to 3 days.	By droplet spread; by direct oral contact or indirectly, through articles freshly soiled with	Presumably until discharges of mouth and nose no longer contain virulent pneumococci in

	pleural pain, dyspnea, cough productive of "rusty" sputum and leukocytosis.		respiratory anisms is common.	significant numbers. Penicillin will render patient noninfectious within 24 to 48 hours.
B. Mycoplasmal pneumonia (primary atypical pneumonia)	Predominantly afebrile lower respiratory infection. Onset is gradual with headache, malaise, cough often paroxysmal, and usually substernal pain (not pleuritic). Sputum, scant at first, may increase later.	14 to 21 days.	Probably by droplet inhalation, direct contact with infected person or with articles freshly soiled with discharges of nose and throat from acutely ill and coughing patient.	Probably less than 10 days; occasionally longer with persisting febrile illness or persistence of the organisms in convalescence (as long as 13 weeks is known).
C. Pneumocystis pneumonia (interstitial plasma-cell pneumonia)	Acute pulmonary disease occurring early in life, especially in malnourished, chronically ill, or premature infants. Characterized by progressive dyspnea, tachypnea, and cyanosis; fever may not be present.	Analysis of data from institutional outbreaks among infants indicates 1 to 2 months.	Unknown.	Unknown.
D. Chlamydial pneumonia (pertussoid eosinophilic pneumonia)	Subacute pulmonary disease occurring in early infancy, primarily in infants of mothers with infection of uterine cervix with causative organism. Characterized by insidious onset, cough, lack of fever, patchy infiltrates on chest x-ray with hyperinflation; eosinophilia, elevated IgM and IgG.	Not known, but pneumonia may occur in infants from 1 to 18 weeks of age (more commonly between 4 and 12 weeks). Nasopharyngeal infection is usually not present before 2 weeks of age.	Presumed to be vertically transmitted from infected cervix to infant during birth, with resultant nasopharyngeal infection (and occasionally conjunctival infection as inclusion conjunctivitis). Direct contact or respiratory transmission has not been established.	Unknown, but length of nasopharyngeal excretion can be at least 2 months.
Poliomyelitis (infantile paralysis)	Acute viral infection whose symptoms include fever, malaise, headache, nausea, vomiting, and stiffness of neck and back with or without paralysis.	Commonly 7 to 14 days for paralytic cases, with a range from 3 to possibly 35 days.	Direct contact through close association. In rare instances milk, foodstuffs, and other fecally-contaminated materials have been incriminated as vehicles. Fecal-oral is major route when sanitation is poor, but during epidemics and when sanitation is good, pharyngeal spread becomes relatively more important.	Not accurately known. Cases are probably most infectious during first few days after onset of symptoms.
Q fever (query fever)	Acute febrile rickettsial disease; onset may be sudden with chills, retrobulbar headache, weakness, malaise, and severe sweats. Pneumonitis occurs in many cases with cough, scanty expectoration, chest pain, and minimal physical findings. Chronic endocarditis, pericarditis, hepatitis, and generalized infections have been reported.	Depends on size of the infecting dose; usually 2 to 3 weeks.	Commonly by air-borne dissemination of rickettsiae in dust from premises contaminated by placental tissues, birth fluids, and excreta of infected animals.	Direct transmission from person to person is very rare, but may occur in cases of pneumonia.

Name	Synopsis of symptoms	Incubation period	Mode of transmission	Period of communicability
Rabies (hydrophobia, lyssa)	Almost invariably fatal acute encephalomyelitis; onset is with sense of apprehension, headache, fever, malaise, and indefinite sensory changes often referred to site of preceding animal bite wound. Disease progresses to paresis or paralysis; spasm of deglutition muscles on attempts to swallow, fear of water, and convulsions.	Usually 2 to 8 weeks, occasionally as short as 10 days or as long as 1 year or more depending on severity and site of wound.	Virus-laden saliva of a rabid animal is introduced by bite or, very rarely, through intact mucous membranes.	In dogs and most other biting animals, for 3 to 5 days before onset of clinical signs and during course of disease.
Rat-bite fever A. Streptobacillary fever	Abrupt onset with chills and fever, headache, and muscle pain is shortly followed by maculopapular or sometimes petechial rash. One or more joints may be swollen, red, and painful. Bacterial endocarditis and focal abscesses may occur late in untreated cases.	3 to 10 days, rarely longer.	Infection is transmitted by secretions of mouth, nose or conjunctival sac of infected animal, most frequently introduced by biting.	Not directly transmitted from person to person.
B. Spirillum fever	Symptoms rarely include arthritic symptoms, but distinctive rash of reddish or purplish plaques is evident.	1 to 3 weeks.		
Relapsing fever	Systemic spirochetal disease in which periods of fever lasting 2 to 9 days alternate with afebrile periods of 2 to 4 days; number of relapses varies from 1 to 10 or more.	5 to 15 days; usually 8 days.	Not directly transmitted from person to person.	Louse becomes infective 4 to 5 days after ingestion of blood from infected person and remains so for life (20 to 40 days).
Respiratory disease (excluding influenza) A. Acute febrile respiratory disease	Viral diseases of respiratory tract are characterized by fever and one or more constitutional reactions such as chills or chilliness, headache, general aching, malaise, and anorexia; in infants by occasional gastrointestinal disturbances.	From a few days to 1 week or more.	Directly by oral contact or by droplet spread, indirectly by hands or other materials soiled by respiratory discharges of infected person.	For duration of active disease; little is known about subclinical or latent infections.
B. Common cold (acute coryza)	Acute catarrhal infections of upper respiratory tract characterized by coryza, sneezing, lacrimation, irritated nasopharynx, chilliness, and malaise lasting 2 to 7 days.		Presumably by direct oral contact or by droplet spread; indirectly by hands and articles freshly soiled by discharges of nose and throat of infected person.	

Disease	Occurrence	Clinical characteristics	Incubation period	Mode of transmission	Period of communicability
Rickettsioses, tick-borne (spotted fever group)					
A. Rocky Mountain spotted fever	Fever is uncommon in children and rare in adults.	Characterized by sudden onset with moderate to high fever that ordinarily persists for 2 to 3 weeks; significant malaise, deep muscle pain, severe headache, chills, and conjunctival injection. A maculopapular rash appears about the third day. Petechiae and hemorrhages are common.	From 3 to about 14 days.	Ordinarily by infected tick.	Not directly transmitted from person to person. Tick remains infective for life; commonly as long as 18 months.
B. Boutonneuse fever		Mild to moderately severe febrile illness of a few days to 2 weeks; characterized by primary lesion at site of tick bite. Lesion (tache noire), usually present at onset of fever, is small ulcer 2 mm to 5 mm in diameter with black center and red areola; regional lymph nodes are enlarged.	Usually 5 to 7 days.	By infected ticks.	Same as in Rocky Mountain spotted fever.
Also: (1) Queensland tick typhus, (2) North Asian tick fever, (3) Rickettsial pox					
Rubella (German measles)					
A. Congenital rubella		Mild febrile infectious disease with diffuse punctate and macular rash. Sometimes resembling that of measles, scarlet fever, or both. May be few or no constitutional symptoms in children but adults may experience 1 to 5 day prodrome characterized by low-grade fever, headache, malaise, mild coryza, and conjunctivitis. As many as 20% to 50% of infections may occur without evident rash; overall 50% are not recognized.	From 16 to 18 days with a range of 14 to 21 days.	Contact with nasopharyngeal secretions of infected person. Infection is by droplet spread or direct contact with patients and indirect contact.	For about 1 week before and at least 4 days after onset of rash. Highly communicable. Infants with congenital rubella syndrome may shed virus for months after birth.
B. Erythema infectiosum (fifth disease)		Mild nonfebrile erythematous eruption occuring as epidemics among children. Characterized by striking erythema of cheeks, reddening of skin, and lace-like serpiginous rash of body.			

Name	Synopsis of symptoms	Incubation period	Mode of transmission	Period of communicability
C. Exanthema subitum (roseola infantum)	Acute illness of probable viral cause characterized by high fever that suddenly appears and lasts 3 to 5 days. A maculopapular rash on trunk and later on rest of body ordinarily follows lysis of fever.			
Salmonellosis	Commonly manifested by acute gastroenteritis. Acute infectious disease with sudden onset of abdominal pain, diarrhea, nausea, and sometimes vomiting. Dehydration may be severe. Fever is nearly always present.	6 to 72 hours, usually about 12 to 36 hours.	By ingestion of organisms in food contaminated by feces of infected person or animal.	Throughout course of infection—extremely variable.
Scabies (sarcoptic acariasis)	Infectious disease of skin caused by mite whose penetration is visible as papules or vesicles, or as tiny linear burrows containing mites and their eggs.	2 to 6 weeks before onset of itching in persons without previous exposure. Persons who have been previously infested develop symptoms 1 to 4 days after reexposure.	Transfer of parasites is by direct skin-to-skin contact and to limited extent from undergarments or soiled bedclothes freshly contaminated by infected persons; frequently acquired during sexual contact.	Until mites and eggs are destroyed by treatment, ordinarily after one or occasionally two courses of treatment 1 week apart.
Shigellosis (bacillary dysentery)	Acute bacterial disease primarily involving large intestine, characterized by diarrhea, accompanied by fever, nausea, sometimes vomiting, cramps, and tenesmus. In severe cases stools contain blood, mucous, and pus.	1 to 7 days, usually 1 to 3 days.	By direct or indirect fecal-oral transmission from patient or carrier. Infection may occur after ingestion of very few organisms.	During acute infection and until infectious agent is no longer present in feces, usually within 4 weeks of illness.
Slow virus infections of central nervous system				
A. Kuru	Signs include cerebellar ataxia, temors, rigidity, progressive wasting, and variable cranial nerve signs in patients 4 years of age or older.	8 to 9 years in childhood cases; range is 4 to more than 30 years.	Exact route of transmission not firmly established. Principally by traditional mortuary practices with intimate contact with infected tissues.	CNS tissues are infectious throughout symptomatic illness.
B. Jakob-Creutzfeldt disease	Insidious onset of confusion, progressive dementia, and variable ataxia in patients 25 years of age or older.	Unknown in most cases.	Unknown.	Same.
Smallpox	Systemic disease with usually characteristic exanthem. Onset is sudden, with fever, malaise, headache, severe backache, prostration, and occasionally abdominal pain. Rash appears after 2 to 4 days and goes	From 7 to 17 days; commonly 10 to 12 days to onset of illness and 2 to 4 days more to onset of rash.	Transmission normally through close contact with respiratory discharges and skin lesions of patients, and material they had recently contaminated. Airborne spread occurred infrequently.	From a few days before development of earliest lesions to disappearance of all scabs; about 3 weeks. Most communicable during first week.

Disease	Identification	Incubation period	Mode of transmission	Period of communicability
Sporotrichosis	Fungal disease, usually of skin, which begins as nodule. As nodule grows, lymphatics draining area become firm and cordlike and form series of nodules, which in turn may soften and ulcerate.	Lymphatic form may develop 1 week to 3 months after injury.	Introduction of fungus through skin following pricks by thorns or barbs, handling of spagnum moss or by slivers from wood or lumber.	Not transmitted from person to person. Environment presumably may be contaminated for duration of active lesion.
Staphylococcal disease A. Staphylococcal disease in community Boils, carbuncles, furuncles Impetigo Cellutitis, abscesses Staphylococcal septicemia Staphylococcal pneumonia Osteomyelitis ondocarditis	Staphylococci produce variety of syndromes with clinical manifestations that range from single lesion to impetigo to septicemia to death. Lesion or lesions containing pus is primary clinical finding, abscess formation is typical.	Variable and indefinite. Commonly 4 to 10 days.	Major site of colonization is anterior nares. Autoinfection is responsible for at least one third of infections. Person with draining lesion or any purulent lesion or who is asymptomatic (usually nasal) carrier of pathogenical strain. Air-borne spread is rare.	As long as purulent lesions continue to drain or carrier state persists.
B. Staphylococcal disease in hospital nurseries Impetigo Abscess of breast	Characteristic lesions develop secondary to colonization of nose or umbilicus, conjunction, circumcision site, or rectum of infants with pathogenical strain.	Commonly 4 to 10 days but may occur several months after colonization.	Spread by hands of hospital personnel is primary mode of transmission within hospitals; to a lesser extent, air-borne.	Same.
C. Staphylococcal disease in medical and surgical wards of hospitals	Lesions vary from simple furuncles or stitch abscesses to extensively infected bedsores or surgical wounds, septic phlebitis, chronic osteomyelitis, fulminating pneumonia, endocarditis, or septicemia.	Variable and indefinite. Commonly 4 to 10 days.	Major site of colonization is anterior nares. Autoinfection is responsible for at least one third of infections. Person with a draining lesion or any purulent lesion or who is an asymptomatic (usually nasal) carrier of a pathogenic strain. Air-borne spread is rare.	As long as purulent lesions continue to drain or carrier state persists.
D. Toxic shock syndrome	Characterized by sudden onset of fever, vomiting, profuse watery diarrhea, and myalgia, followed by hypotension, and in severe cases, shock. An erythematous "sunburnlike" rash is present during acute phase.	Thought to be related to use of tampons; however, mode of transmission is still under investigation.		

(continued from preceding entry) through stages of macules, papules, vesicles, pustules, and finally scabs.

Name	Synopsis of symptoms	Incubation period	Mode of transmission	Period of communicability
Streptococcal diseases caused by group A (beta hemolytic) streptococcal				
A. Streptococcal sore throat	Fever, sore throat, exudative tonsillitis or pharyngitis, and tender anterior cervical lymph nodes	Short, usually 1 to 3 days, rarely longer.	Transmission results from direct or intimate contact with patient or carrier, rarely by indirect contact through objects or hands. Nasal carriers are particularly likely to transmit diseases.	In untreated uncomplicated cases 10 to 21 days; in untreated conditions with purulent discharges, weeks or months.
B. Streptococcal skin infections	Usually superficial, may proceed through vesicular, pustular, and encrusted stages			
C. Scarlet fever	Skin rash and symptoms similar to streptococcal sore throat, enanthem, strawberry tongue, and exanthem. Rash is usually fine erythema.			
D. Erysipelas	Acute cellulitis characterized by fever, constitutional symptoms, leucocytosis, and red, tender, edematous, spreading lesion of skin with definite raised border.			
E. Streptococcal puerperal fever	Acute disease, usually febrile accompanied by local and general symptoms and signs of bacterial invasion of genital tract and sometimes bloodstream in postpartum or postabortion patient.			
Streptococcal (group B) disease of the newborn	Produces diseases of newborn infants including cases of septicemia, evidence of pulmonary involvement, and meningeal involvement.		Acquired during passage through birth canal. Some cases are acquired through environment.	
Stronglyoidiasis	Helminthic infection of duodenum and upper jejunum, asymptomatic in majority of cases. Clinical manifestations include dermatitis, cough, rales, and abdominal symptoms.	From penetration of skin by filariform larvae until rhabitiform larvae appear in feces is about 2 to 3 weeks; period until symptoms appear is variable.	Infective larvae that develop in moist soil contaminated with feces penetrate skin, enter venous circulation, and are carried to lungs.	As long as living worms remain in intestine; up to 35 years.
Syphilis, venereal (Lues)	Acute and chronic treponematosis characterized clinically by primary lesion, secondary	10 days to 10 weeks, usually 3 weeks.	By direct contact with infectious exudates from obvions or concealed moist early lesions of	Variable and indefinite during primary and secondary stages and also in mucocutaneous

(continued from previous page)	eruption involving skin and mucous membranes, long periods of latency, and late lesions of skin, bone, viscerae, and central nervous and cardiovascular systems. Papule appears 3 weeks after exposure at site of initial invasion; after erosion, most common form is indurated chancre.		skin and mucous membrane, body fluids, and secretions of infected persons during sexual contact.	recurrences; some cases may be intermittently communicable for 2 to 4 years.
Syphilis, nonvenereal endemic	Acute disease of limited geographical distribution, characterized clinically by eruption of skin and mucous membrane, usually without evident primary sore.	2 weeks to 3 months.	Direct or indirect contact with infectious early lesions of skin and mucous membranes. Congenital transmission does not occur.	Until moist eruptions of skin and mucous patches disappear—sometimes several weeks or months.
Taeniasis and cysticercosis *Taenia Solium* infection, intestinal form (pork tapeworm) Cysticercosis (cysticerciasis, infection by *Cysticerus cellulosae*) *Taenia Saginata* infection (beef tapeworm)	Taeniasis is intestinal infection with adult stage of large tapeworms. Cysticosis is somatic infection with larvae stage of one species, *Taenia Solium.* Clinical manifestations of infection with adult worm are variable and may include nervousness, insomnia, anorexia, weight loss, abdominal pain, and digestive disturbance. Cysticercosis is serious somatic disease that may involve many different organs. Eggs of tapeworm, when swallowed, hatch in small intestines and larvae migrate throughout body.	For adult tapeworm, from 8 to 14 weeks.	Ova of *Taenia Saginata* passed in stool of infected person are infectious only to cattle. Infection of man follows ingestion of raw or inadequately cooked beef containing cysticerci. Ova of *Taenia Solium* are infectious to both man and pigs. Human infection occurs by direct transfer of eggs in feces of person harboring adult worm to own or another's mouth, or indirectly through ingestion of food or water contaminated with eggs, resulting in somatic cysticercosis. Intestinal infection of humans (taeniasis) follows ingestion of raw or inadequately cooked infected pork.	*Taenia Saginata* is not directly transmitted from person to person but *Taenia Solium* may be; eggs of both species are disseminated into environment as long as worm remains in intestines, sometimes more than 30 years; eggs may remain viable for months.
Tetanus tetanus neonatorum (lockjaw)	Acute disease induced by tetanus bacillus that grows anaerobically at site of injury and produces neurotoxin. Characterized by painful muscular contractions, abdominal rigidity, and generalized spasms. Symptoms usually appear between fifth and twelfth day, most frequently about seventh day.	4 to 21 days, dependent on character, extent, and location of wound; average 10 days. Most cases occur within 14 days.	Tetanus spores introduced into body during injury, usually puncture wound contaminated with soil, street dust, or animal or human feces, but also through lacerations, burns, and trivial or unnoticed wounds.	Not directly transmitted from person to person.

Name	Synopsis of symptoms	Incubation period	Mode of transmission	Period of communicability
Toxocariasis (larva migrans viscervalis, *Toxocara* [Canis] *Toxocara* [Cati] infection, visceral larva migrans syndrome)	Chronic and usually mild disease of young children caused by migration of certain nematode larvae in organs and tissues. Characterized by eosinophilia of variable duration, hepatomegaly, hyperglobulinemia, pulmonary symptoms, and fever.	Probably weeks or months, depending on intensity of infection and sensitivity of patient.	By direct or indirect transmission of infectious *Toxocara* eggs from contamiated soil to mouth; directly related to eating of dirt by young children. Eggs reach soil in feces from infected cats and dogs.	Not directly transmitted from person to person.
Cutaneous larva migrans caused by *Ancylostoma* braziliense resulting from *ancylostoma caninum*	Infective larvae of dog and cat hookworm that causes dermatitis in humans.	Each larva causes serpiginous track, advancing several mm to a few cm a day.	Larva, which enter skin from contact with contaminated soil, migrate intracutaneously for long periods, but eventually penetrate to deeper tissues.	Disease is self-limited, with spontaneous cure after several weeks or months.
Toxoplasmosis (congenital toxoplasmosis)	Systemic protozoal disease. Primary infection is frequently asymptomatic; acute disease may occur with fever, lymphadenopathy, and lymphocytosis persisting for days or weeks. Rare severe manifestations include cerebral signs, pneumonitis, generalized muscle involvement, and death.	Unknown; 10 to 23 days in one outbreak larva vehicle was undercooked meat, and 5 to 20 days in an outbreak associated with infected cats.	Transplacental infection may occur in women with primary infection. Postnatal infections might be acquired by eating raw or undercooked infected meat or more often by ingesting infective oocysts. Drinking water contaminated with feces of *Felidue* has been incriminated.	Not directly transmitted from person to person except in utero.
Trachoma	Communicable keratoconjunctivitis characterized by conjunctival inflammation with papillary hyperplasia, associated with vascular invasion of cornea, and in later stages by conjunctival scarring that may eventually lead to blindness.	5 to 12 days (based on volunteer studies).	By direct contact with ocular discharges and possibly mucoid or purulent discharges of nasal mucous membranes of infected persons or materials. Flies (*Musca sorbens*) may contribute to spread of disease.	As long as active lesions are present in the conjunctivae and adnexal mucous membranes.
Trench fever (Wolhynian fever, quintan fever)	Nonfatal, febrile disease of protean manifestations characterized by headache, malaise, pain, and tenderness especially in shins; onset either sudden or slow with fever, which may be relapsing, typhoid-like, or limited to single short febrile episode lasting several days.	Generally 7 to 30 days.	Not directly transmitted from person to person. Humans infected by inoculation of organism in louse feces through a skin break from either bite of louse or other means.	Organisms may circulate in blood (by which lice can be infected) for weeks, months, or years and may recur with or without symptoms. History of trench fever is permanent contraindication to blood donation.
Trichinosis (trichiniasis, trichinellosis)	Disease caused by larvae of *Trichinella spiralis* that migrate to and become encapsulated in muscles. Clinical manifestations usually include mild febrile disease, but can range	Usually about 10 to 14 days after ingestion by humans of infective meat; varies between 1 and 45 days.	Eating raw or insufficiently cooked flesh of animals containing viable encysted trichinae, chiefly pork and pork products.	Not transmitted directly from person to person. Animal hosts remain infective for months as does meat from such animals for appreciable periods unless processed to kill larvae.

Disease	Clinical characteristics	Incubation period	Mode of transmission	Period of communicability
Trichomoniasis	from inapparent infection to fulminating, fatal disease. Common disease of genitourinary tract, characterized in women by vaginitis, with small petechial or sometimes punctate hemorrhagic lesions and profuse, thin, foamy, yellowish discharge with foul odor; frequently asymptomatic. In men, infectious agent invades and persists in prostate, urethra, or seminal vesicles, but rarely produces symptoms or demonstrable lesions.	4 to 20 days, average 7 days.	By contact with vaginal and urethral discharges of infected persons during sexual intercourse and possibly by contact with contaminated articles.	For duration of infection.
Trichuriasis (trichocephaliasis)	Nematode infection of large intestine, often asymptomatic. Heavy infections result in bloody stools and diarrhea. Rectal prolapse may occur in very heavily infected children.			
Trypanosomiasis, African (African sleeping sickness)	In early stages chancre usually appears at primary tsetse fly bite site with fever, intense headache, insomnia, lymph node enlargement, anemia, local edema, and rash. In late stage is body wasting, somnolence, and signs referable to central nervous system.	In *T. rhodesiense* infection usually 2 to 3 weeks; in *T. gambiense* infection, usually longer and extremely variable—months or even years.	By bite of infective *Glossina*, the tsetse fly. Congenital transmission can occur in humans, as well as direct mechanical transmission by blood on proboscis of *Glossina* and other human-biting flies, or in laboratory accidents.	To tsetse fly, as long as parasite is present in blood of infected person or animal. Parasitemia is extremely variable in untreated cases and occurs in late and early stages of disease.
Trypanosomiasis, American (Chagas' disease)	Acute disease usually occurs in children; chronic manifestations generally appear later in life. Acute disease is characterized by variable fever, malaise, lymphadenopathy and hepatosplenomegaly. Inflammatory response at site of infection (chagoma) may last up to 8 weeks. Unilateral bipalpebral edema occurs in significant percentage of acute cases. Life-threatening or fatal manifestations include myocarditis and meningoencephalitis.	About 5 to 14 days after bite of insect vector; 30 to 40 days if infected by blood transfusion.	By fecal material passed while biting by infected vectors. Infection is through contamination of conjunctiva, mucous membranes, abrasions, or skin wounds by fresh infected bug feces. Transmission also may occur by blood transfusion and organisms may pass through placenta to cause congenital infection.	Organisms are present regularly in blood during acute period and may persist in very small numbers throughout life in symptomatic and asymptomatic persons. Vector becomes infective 10 to 30 days after biting an infective host and remains so for life (as long as 2 years).

Name	Synopsis of symptoms	Incubation period	Mode of transmission	Period of communicability
Tuberculosis	Mycobacterial disease. Initial infection usually goes unnoticed; tuberculin sensitivity appears within a few weeks; lesions commonly heal, leaving no residual changes except pulmonary or tracheobronchial lymph node calcification. May progress to pulmonary tuberculosis or, by lymphohematogenous dissemination of bacilli, to produce miliary, meningeal, or other extrapulmonary involvement.	From infection to demonstrable primary lesion, about 4 to 12 weeks. Whereas subsequent risk of progressive pulmonary or extrapulmonary tuberculosis is greatest within 1 or 2 years after infection, it may persist for a lifetime as latent infection.	Exposure to bacilli in air-borne droplet nuclei from sputum of persons with infectious tuberculosis. Bovine tuberculosis results from exposure to tubercular cattle and ingestion of unpasteurized dairy products.	As long as infectious tubercle bacilli are being discharged.
Tularemia (rabbit fever, deerfly fever, Ohara's disease)	Clinical manifestations related to route of introduction and virulence of strain. Most often ulcer, often on hand, accompanied by swelling of regional lymph nodes. May be no apparent primary ulcer but only enlarged and painful lymph nodes that may suppurate.	Related to virulence of infecting strain and to size of inoculum; 2 to 10 days, usually 3 days.	Inoculation of skin, conjunctival sac, or oropharyngeal mucosa with blood or tissue while handling infected animals; or by fluids from infected flies, ticks, or other animals; or through bite of arthropods.	Not directly transmitted from person to person. Unless treated, infectious agent may be found in blood during first 2 weeks of disease, and in lesions for 1 month from onset—sometimes longer.
Typhoid fever (enteric fever, typhus abdominalis)	Systemic infectious disease characterized by sustained fever, headache, malaise, anorexia, relative bradycardia, enlargement of spleen, rose spots on trunk, nonproductive cough, constipation more commonly than diarrhea, and involvement of lymphoid tissues.	Depends on size of infecting dose; usual range 1 to 3 weeks.	By food or water contaminated by feces or urine of patient or carrier.	As long as typhoid bacilli appear in excreta; usually first week throughout convalescence; variable thereafter. About 10% of untreated patients will discharge bacilli for 3 months after onset of symptoms; 2 to 5% become permanent carriers.
Typhus fever, epidemic louseborne (exanthematic typhus, classical typhus fever)	Onset is variable, often sudden and marked by headache, chills, prostration, fever, and general pains. Macular eruption appears on fifth or sixth day, initially on upper trunk followed by spread to entire body but usually not to face, palms, or soles. Toxemia is usually pronounced and disease terminates by rapid lysis after about 2 weeks of fever.	From 1 to 2 weeks, commonly 12 days.	The body louse, *Pediculus humanis corporis*, is infected by feeding on blood of patient with acute typhus fever. Humans are infected by rubbing feces or crushed lice into bites of louse or other superficial abrasions. Inhalation of infective louse feces as dust may account for some infections.	Disease is not directly transmitted from person to person. Patients are infective for lice during febrile illness and possibly for 2 or 3 days after temperature returns to normal.
Typhus fever, fleaborne (murine typhus, endemic ty-	Course of flea-borne typhus fever resembles that of epidemic louse-borne typhus, but is	From 1 to 2 weeks, commonly 12 days.	Infective rat fleas (usually *Xenopsylla cheopis*) defecate rickettsiae while sucking	Not directly transmitted from person to person. Once infected, fleas remain so for life.

Disease	Description	Incubation	Mode of transmission	Period of communicability
phus fever, shop typhus)	milder. Fatality rate for all ages is about 2%; it increases with age.		blood and contaminate bite site and other fresh skin wounds. Occasional case may follow inhalation of dried infective flea feces.	Not directly transmitted from person to person.
Typhus, scrub (tsutsugamushi disease, mite-borne typhus fever)	Often characterized by primary skin ulcer (eschar) corresponding to site of attachment of infected mite. Acute febrile onset follows within several days, along with headache, profuse sweating, conjunctival injection, and lymphadenopathy.	Usually 10 to 12 days; varies from 6 to 21 days.	By infected larval mites; nymphs and adults do not feed on vertebrate hosts.	
Urethritis, chlamydial Urethritis, nongonorrheal and nonspecific	Sexually transmitted urethritis of males caused by chlamydial agent. Clinical manifestations are usually indistinguishable from gonorrhea but are often milder and include opaque discharge of moderate or scanty quantity, urethral itching, and burning on urination. Infection of women results in cervicitis and salpingitis; infections are often asymptomatic.	5 to 7 days or longer.	Sexual contact.	Unknown.
Verruca vulgaris (warts)	Viral disease manifested by variety of skin and mucous membrane lesions. Include the common wart, a circumscribed, hyperkeratotic, rough textured, painless papule varying in size from pinhead to large masses; also filiform warts, venereal warts, and plantar warts.	About 4 months; range is 1 to 20 months.	Usually by direct contact, but contaminated floors and fomites are frequently implicated. Warts may be autoinoculated. *Condyloma acuminatum* is usually sexually transmitted.	Unknown, but probably as long as visible lesions persist.
Whooping cough (Pertussis)	Acute bacterial disease involving tracheobronchial tree. Initial catarrhal stage has insidious onset with irritating cough that gradually becomes paroxysmal, usually within 1 to 2 weeks, and lasts for 1 to 2 months.	Commonly 7 days; almost uniformly within 10 days, and not exceeding 21 days.	Primarily by direct contact with discharges from respiratory mucous membranes of infected persons by air-borne route, probably by droplets. Frequently brought into home by older sibling.	Highly communicable in early catarrhal stage before paroxysmal cough stage. For control purposes, communicable stage extends from 7 days after exposure to 3 weeks after onset of typical paroxysms in patients not treated with antibiotics; in patients treated with erythromycin, period of infectiousness extends only 5 to 7 days after onset of therapy.

Name	Synopsis of symptoms	Incubation period	Mode of transmission	Period of communicability
Yaws (frambesia, pian, bouba, parang)	Chronic relapsing nonvenereal treponematosis characterized by early cutaneous lesions and noncontagious late, destructive lesions. Typical initial lesion (mother yaw) is papilloma on face or extremities that persists for several weeks or months.	From 2 weeks to 3 months.	Principally by direct contact with exudates of early skin lesions of infected persons. Indirect transmission by contamination from scratching, skin piercing articles, and by flies on open wounds is probable but of undetermined importance.	Variable; may extend intermittently over several years while moist lesions are present. Infectious agent is not usually found in late ulcerative lesions.
Yersinia (pseudotuberculosis)	Acute enteric disease manifested by diarrhea, enterocolitis, acute mesenteric lymphadenitis mimicking appendicitis, low-grade fever, headache, pharyngitis, anorexia, vomiting, erythema nodosum, arthritis, cutaneous ulceration, abscesses, and septicemia.	Probably 3 to 7 days, generally less than 10 days.	Fecal-oral transmission takes place by contact with infected persons or animals (hand-to-mouth), or by eating and drinking contaminated food and water.	Fecal shedding as long as symptoms exist. Chronic carrier state probably exists.
Zygomycosis (mucormycosis, phycomycosis)	Group of mycoses usually caused by fungi of the family *Mucoraceae* of the class *Zygomycetes*. These fungi have affinity for blood vessels, causing thrombosis and infarction. In its craniofacial form is usually nasal or paranasal sinus infections, most often during ketoacidotic episodes of diabetes mellitus.	Unknown. Fungus spreads rapidly in susceptible tissues.	By inhalation or ingestion of fungus by susceptible individuals. Direct inoculation by minor trauma, intravenous catheters, and cutaneous burns are occasionally implicated.	Not directly transmitted from human or animal to human.